Manual of
CLINICAL
MICROBIOLOGY

8TH EDITION

VOLUME 1

Manual of
CLINICAL MICROBIOLOGY

8TH EDITION

EDITOR IN CHIEF

PATRICK R. MURRAY
Clinical Center, National Institutes of Health, Bethesda, Maryland

EDITORS

ELLEN JO BARON
Department of Pathology,
Stanford University Medical School,
Stanford, California

JAMES H. JORGENSEN
Department of Pathology,
University of Texas Health Science Center,
San Antonio, Texas

MICHAEL A. PFALLER
Departments of Pathology and Epidemiology,
University of Iowa College of Medicine
and College of Public Health, Iowa City, Iowa

ROBERT H. YOLKEN
Department of Pediatrics, Stanley Division
of Developmental Neurovirology,
Johns Hopkins Hospital, Baltimore, Maryland

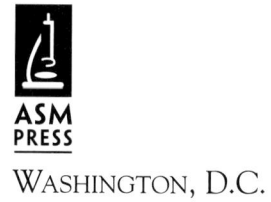

ASM
PRESS

WASHINGTON, D.C.

LIVERPOOL
JOHN MOORES UNIVERSITY
AVRIL ROBARTS LRC
TEL. 0151 231 4022

Address editorial correspondence to ASM Press, 1752 N St. NW,
Washington, DC 20036-2904, USA

Send orders to ASM Press, P.O. Box 605, Herndon, VA 20172, USA
Phone: 800-546-2416; 703-661-1593
Fax: 703-661-1501
E-mail: books@asmusa.org
Online: www.asmpress.org

Library of Congress Cataloging-in-Publication Data

Manual of clinical microbiology/editor in chief, Patrick R. Murray; editors, Ellen Jo Baron . . . [et al.].—8th ed.
  p.; cm.
  Includes bibliographical references and index.
  ISBN 1-55581-255-4 (hardcover set)
  1. Medical microbiology—Handbooks, manuals, etc.   2. Diagnostic microbiology—Handbooks, manu-als, etc.   I. Title: Clinical microbiology.   II. Murray, Patrick R.   III. Baron, Ellen Jo.   IV. American Society for Microbiology.
  [DNLM: 1. Microbiology.   2. Microbiological Techniques.   QW 4 M294 2003]
QR46 .M425 2003
616'.01—dc21

2002074595

Patrick R. Murray's role as editor in chief of this book was carried out in his private capacity and his contribution as an editor does not reflect official support or endorsement by the National Institutes of Health.

Contents

Editorial Board

Contributors

SHARON L. ABBOTT
Microbial Diseases Laboratory, California State Department
of Health Services, 2151 Berkeley Way, Berkeley, CA 94704

MARIA E. AGUERO-ROSENFELD
Clinical Laboratories, Westchester Medical Center, Valhalla,
NY 10595

ANNIKA ALLARD
Department of Virology, Umeå University, S-901 85 Umeå,
Sweden

STEPHEN D. ALLEN
Department of Pathology and Laboratory Medicine, Indiana
University School of Medicine, and Clarian Health Partners,
Methodist-Indiana University-Riley Hospitals, Indianapolis,
IN 46228

MAX Q. ARENS
Department of Pediatrics, Washington University School of
Medicine, St. Louis, MO 63110

SEVTAP ARIKAN
Department of Microbiology and Clinical Microbiology,
Hacettepe University Medical School, 06100 Ankara,
Turkey

MICHAEL ARROWOOD
Division of Parasitic Diseases, National Center for Infectious
Diseases, Centers for Disease Control and Prevention, 4770
Buford Highway NE, Atlanta, GA 30341-3724

LAWRENCE R. ASH
Department of Epidemiology, School of Public Health,
University of California, Los Angeles, CA 90095-1772

DAVID M. ASHER
Laboratory of Bacterial, Parasitic and Unconventional
Agents, Division of Emerging and Transfusion-Transmitted
Diseases, Center for Biologics Evaluation and Research, U.S.
Food and Drug Administration, Rockville, MD 20852-1448

RHODA L. ASHLEY
Department of Laboratory Medicine, University of
Washington at Children's Hospital and Regional Medical
Center, Seattle, WA 98105

TAMMY L. BANNERMAN
Medical Technology Division, The Ohio State University,
Columbus, OH 43210-1234

JAMES BEEBE
Laboratory and Radiation Services Division, Colorado
Department of Public Health and Environment, Denver,
CO 80246-1530

D. BEIGHTON
Department of Oral Microbiology, GKT Dental Institute,
Caldecot Road, Denmark Hill, London SE 9RW, United
Kingdom

WILLIAM J. BELLINI
Measles Virus Section, Respiratory and Enterovirus Branch,
Division of Viral and Rickettsial Diseases, National Center
for Infectious Diseases, Centers for Disease Control and
Prevention, Atlanta, GA 30333

KATHRYN A. BERNARD
Special Bacteriology Section, Health Canada, National
Microbiology Laboratory, Winnipeg, Manitoba R3E 3R2,
Canada

JOHN BESSER
Public Health Laboratory Division, Minnesota Department
of Health, Minneapolis, MN 55414

JACQUES BILLE
Centre National de Référence Listeria, Institut de
Microbiologie, Rue du Bugnon 44, CH-1011 Lausanne,
Switzerland

KAREN BIRKHEAD
Foodborne and Diarrheal Diseases Laboratory Section,
Foodborne and Diarrheal Diseases Branch, Division of
Bacterial and Mycotic Diseases, National Center for
Infectious Diseases, Centers for Disease Control and
Prevention, Atlanta, GA 30333

JOCHEN BOCKEMÜHL
Division of Bacteriology and Virology, Institute of Hygiene,
Marckmannstrasse 129a, D-20539 Hamburg, Germany

ROBERT A. BONOMO
Medical Service, Louis Stokes Cleveland VA Medical
Center, and Department of Medicine, Case Western Reserve
University, Cleveland, OH 44106

CHERYL A. BOPP
Foodborne and Diarrheal Diseases Laboratory Section,
Foodborne and Diarrheal Diseases Branch, Division of
Bacterial and Mycotic Diseases, National Center for
Infectious Diseases, Centers for Disease Control and
Prevention, Atlanta, GA 30333

DONALD H. BOUYER
Department of Pathology, WHO Collaborating Center for
Tropical Diseases, University of Texas Medical Branch,
Galveston, TX 77555-0609

FRANCES W. BRENNER
Foodborne and Diarrheal Diseases Laboratory Section,
Foodborne and Diarrheal Diseases Branch, Division of
Bacterial and Mycotic Diseases, National Center for
Infectious Diseases, Centers for Disease Control and
Prevention, Atlanta, GA 30333

PHILIPPE BROUQUI
Faculté de Médecine, Unité des Rickettsies, CNRS UMR
6020, Marseille Cedex 5, France

EDWIN A. BROWN
Division of Infectious Diseases, Department of Internal
Medicine, Medical University of South Carolina,
Charleston, SC 29425

JUNE M. BROWN
Meningitis and Special Pathogens Branch, Division of
Bacterial and Mycotic Diseases, National Center for
Infectious Diseases, Centers for Disease Control and
Prevention, Atlanta, GA 30333

BARBARA A. BROWN-ELLIOTT
Department of Microbiology, University of Texas Health
Center, Tyler, TX 75799

DAVID A. BRUCKNER
Division of Laboratory Medicine, Department of Pathology
and Laboratory Medicine, UCLA Medical Center, Los
Angeles, CA 90095-1713

CORNELIA BÜCHEN-OSMOND
Columbia Earth Institute, Columbia University, 32540
South Biosphere Road, Oracle, AZ 85623

ANGELA M. CALIENDO
Emory University Hospital and Department of Pathology
and Laboratory Medicine, Emory University School of
Medicine, Atlanta, GA 30322

JOSEPH M. CAMPOS
Department of Laboratory Medicine, Children's National
Medical Center, Washington, DC 20010, and Departments
of Pediatrics, Pathology, and Microbiology/Tropical
Medicine, George Washington University Medical Center,
Washington, DC 20037

ELIZABETH U. CANNING
Department of Biological Sciences, Imperial College of
Science, Technology and Medicine, London SW7 2AZ,
United Kingdom

KAREN C. CARROLL
Department of Pathology, Johns Hopkins University School
of Medicine, Baltimore, MD 21287

LAURA J. CHANDLER
Drexel University College of Medicine, Philadelphia,
PA 19104

KIMBERLE C. CHAPIN
Department of Laboratory Medicine and Department of
Medicine, Division of Infectious Disease, Lahey Clinic
Medical Center, Burlington, MA 01805

MAX A. CHERNESKY
McMaster University, Department of Pathology and
Molecular Medicine, Hamilton Regional Laboratory
Medicine Program, St. Joseph's Healthcare, Hamilton,
Ontario L8N 4A6, Canada

SUNWEN CHOU
Division of Infectious Diseases, Oregon Health and Science
University, Portland, OR 97239

MAY C. CHU
Division of Vector-Borne Infectious Diseases, National
Center for Infectious Diseases, Centers for Disease Control
and Prevention, Fort Collins, CO 80521

DIANE M. CITRON
R. M. Alden Research Laboratory, 1250 16th Street, Santa
Monica, CA 90404, and Microbial Research Laboratory, Los
Angeles County-University of Southern California Medical
Center, 1801 E. Marengo Street, Los Angeles, CA 90033

NIEL T. CONSTANTINE
Department of Pathology, University of Maryland School of
Medicine, Baltimore, MD 21201

BRIAN K. COOMBES
McMaster University, Department of Pathology and
Molecular Medicine, Hamilton Regional Laboratory
Medicine Program, St. Joseph's Healthcare, Hamilton,
Ontario L8N 4A6, Canada

ELLIOT P. COWAN
Center for Biologics Evaluation and Research, U.S. Food
and Drug Administration, Rockville, MD 20852

FRANCIS E. G. COX
Department of Infectious and Tropical Diseases, London
School of Hygiene and Tropical Medicine, London
WC1E 7HT, United Kingdom

NANCY J. COX
Influenza Branch, Division of Viral and Rickettsial Diseases,
National Center for Infectious Diseases, Centers for Disease
Control and Prevention, Atlanta, GA 30333

MELANIE T. CUSHION
Department of Internal Medicine, Division of Infectious
Diseases, University of Cincinnati College of Medicine,
Cincinnati, OH 45267-0560

INGER K. DAMON
Poxvirus Section, Division of Viral and Rickettsial Diseases,
Centers for Disease Control and Prevention, Atlanta,
GA 30333

MARYAM I. DANESHVAR
Meningitis and Special Pathogens Branch, Division of
Bacterial and Mycotic Diseases, National Center for
Infectious Diseases, Centers for Disease Control and
Prevention, Atlanta, GA 30333

GEORGE J. DAWSON
Virus Discovery Group, Abbott Laboratories, 1401 Sheridan
Road, North Chicago, IL 60064

PETER DEPLAZES
Institute of Parasitology, University of Zurich,
Winterthurerstrasse 266a, CH-8057 Zurich, Switzerland

CHARLENE S. DEZZUTTI
HIV and Retrovirology Branch, Division of AIDS, STD, and
TB Laboratory Research, Centers for Disease Control and
Prevention, Atlanta, GA 30333

DANIEL J. DIEKEMA
Medical Microbiology Division, Department of Pathology,
University of Iowa College of Medicine, Iowa City,
IA 52242

DENNIS M. DIXON
Bacteriology and Mycology Branch, Division of Microbiology
and Infectious Diseases, National Institute of Allergy and
Infectious Diseases, National Institutes of Health, Bethesda,
MD 20892

J. STEPHEN DUMLER
Division of Medical Microbiology, Department of Pathology,
The Johns Hopkins Medical Institutions, Baltimore,
MD 21287

CHRISTOPHER L. EMERY
Department of Pathology and Laboratory Medicine, MCP-
Hahnemann University School of Medicine and Medical
College of Pennyslvania-Hahnemann Hospitals,
Philadelphia, PA 19102

ANA V. ESPINEL-INGROFF
Medical Mycology Research Laboratory, Division of
Infectious Diseases, Medical College of Virginia, Virginia
Commonwealth University, Richmond, VA 23298-0049

JOSEPH J. ESPOSITO
National Center for Infectious Diseases, Centers for Disease
Control and Prevention, Atlanta, GA 30333

RICHARD R. FACKLAM
Streptococcus Laboratory, Respiratory Diseases Branch,
Division of Bacterial and Mycotic Diseases, Centers for
Disease Control and Prevention, Atlanta, GA 30333

J. J. FARMER III
Foodborne and Diarrheal Diseases Laboratory Section,
Foodborne and Diarrheal Diseases Branch, Division of
Bacterial and Mycotic Diseases, National Center for
Infectious Diseases, Centers for Disease Control and
Prevention, Atlanta, GA 30333 (retired)

QINGHUA FENG
Department of Pathology, University of Washington,
Seattle, WA 98104

MARY JANE FERRARO
Clinical Microbiology Laboratory, Massachusetts General
Hospital, and Harvard Medical School, Boston, MA 02114

PATRICIA I. FIELDS
Foodborne and Diarrheal Diseases Laboratory Section,
Foodborne and Diarrheal Diseases Branch, Division of
Bacterial and Mycotic Diseases, National Center for
Infectious Diseases, Centers for Disease Control and
Prevention, Atlanta, GA 30333

SYDNEY M. FINEGOLD
Medical Service, VA Medical Center West Los Angeles,
UCLA School of Medicine, Los Angeles, CA 90073

MICHAEL S. FORMAN
Department of Pathology, Division of Microbiology, The
Johns Hopkins Medical Institutions, Baltimore, MD 21287

JAMES G. FOX
Division of Comparative Medicine, Massachusetts Institute
of Technology, Cambridge, MA 02139

RENO FREI
Bacteriology Laboratory, University Hospitals, Basel 6031,
Switzerland

THOMAS R. FRITSCHE
Clinical Microbiology Division, Department of Laboratory
Medicine, University of Washington, Seattle,
WA 98195-7110

ROBERT A. FROMTLING
Regulatory Affairs, International Merck Research
Laboratories, Rahway, NJ 07065-0900

GUIDO FUNKE
Department of Medical Microbiology and Hygiene, Gärtner
& Colleagues Laboratories, D-88250 Weingarten, Germany

LYNNE S. GARCIA
LSG & Associates, 512-12th Street, Santa Monica,
CA 90402-2908

ANNE A. GERSHON
Department of Pediatrics, Columbia University College of
Physicians & Surgeons, New York, NY 10032

SAHEER E. GHARBIA
Genomics, Proteomics, and Bioinformatics Unit, PHLS
Central Public Health Laboratory, London NW9 5HT,
United Kingdom

PETER H. GILLIGAN
Clinical Microbiology-Immunology Laboratories, University
of North Carolina Hospitals, and Department of
Microbiology-Immunology and Pathology-Laboratory
Medicine, University of North Carolina School of Medicine,
Chapel Hill, NC 27514

PAUL A. GRANATO
Department of Microbiology and Immunology, SUNY
Upstate Medical University, Syracuse, NY 13210

MANETH GRAVELL
Laboratory of Molecular Medicine and Neuroscience,
National Institute of Neurological Disorders and Stroke,
Bethesda, MD 20892-4164

DAVID R. GRETCH
Viral Hepatitis Laboratory, University of Washington
Harborview Medical Center, 325 Ninth Avenue, Seattle,
WA 98104

KEVIN C. HAZEN
Division of Clinical Microbiology, Department of Pathology,
University of Virginia Health System, Charlottesville,
VA 22908-0904

DAVID W. HECHT
Department of Microbiology and Immunology and Division
of Infectious Diseases, Loyola University Medical Center,
Maywood, IL 60153, and Hines Veterans Administration
Hospital, Hines, IL 60141

JOHN C. HIERHOLZER
Respiratory and Enteric Viruses Branch, Division of Viral and Rickettsial Diseases, National Center for Infectious Diseases, Centers for Disease Control and Prevention, Atlanta, GA 30333

SHARON L. HILLIER
Magee-Womens Research Institute and Departments of Oral Biology and Obstetrics, Gynecology and Reproductive Sciences, University of Pittsburgh, Pittsburgh, PA 15213

JANET FICK HINDLER
Department of Pathology and Laboratory Medicine, UCLA Medical Center, Los Angeles, CA 90095-1713

RICHARD L. HODINKA
Departments of Pediatrics and Pathology, Clinical Virology Laboratory, Children's Hospital of Philadelphia and University of Pennsylvania School of Medicine, Philadelphia, PA 19104

DANNIE G. HOLLIS
Meningitis and Special Pathogens Branch, Division of Bacterial and Mycotic Diseases, National Center for Infectious Diseases, Centers for Disease Control and Prevention, Atlanta, GA 30333

HARVEY T. HOLMES
Diagnostic Microbiology Section, Epidemiology and Laboratory Branch, Division of Healthcare Quality Promotion, Centers for Disease Control and Prevention, Atlanta, GA 30333

REBECCA T. HORVAT
Department of Pathology and Laboratory Medicine, University of Kansas School of Medicine, Kansas City, KS 66160

JEAN HOU
Laboratory of Molecular Medicine and Neuroscience, National Institute of Neurological Disorders and Stroke, Bethesda, MD 20892-4164

SUSAN A. HOWELL
Department of Medical Mycology, St. Johns Institute of Dermatology, Kings College London, London SE1 7EH, Great Britain

JOSEPH P. ICENOGLE
Measles Virus Section, Respiratory and Enterovirus Branch, Division of Viral and Rickettsial Diseases, National Center for Infectious Diseases, Centers for Disease Control and Prevention, Atlanta, GA 30333

CLARK B. INDERLIED
Department of Pathology and Laboratory Medicine, University of Southern California Keck School of Medicine, and Childrens Hospital of Los Angeles, Los Angeles, CA 90027

PETER B. JAHRLING
Virology Division, USAMRIID, Fort Detrick, Frederick, MD 21702

J. MICHAEL JANDA
Microbial Diseases Laboratory, Division of Communicable Disease Control, California Department of Health Services, Berkeley, CA 94704-1011

WILLIAM M. JANDA
Department of Pathology, University of Illinois Medical Center at Chicago, Chicago, IL 60612

KEITH R. JEROME
Department of Laboratory Medicine, University of Washington Program in Infectious Diseases, Fred Hutchinson Cancer Research Center, Seattle, WA 98109

ROBERT E. JOHNSON
Division of STD Prevention, National Center for HIV, STD, and TB Prevention, Centers for Disease Control and Prevention, Atlanta, GA 30333

JEFFERY L. JONES
Parasitic Epidemiology Branch, Division of Parasitic Diseases, National Center for Infectious Diseases, Centers for Disease Control and Prevention, Atlanta, GA 30341

JAMES H. JORGENSEN
Department of Pathology, The University of Texas Health Science Center, San Antonio, TX 78229-3700

KENNETH C. JOST, JR.
Mycobacteriology Branch, Texas Department of Health, 1100 West 49th Street, Austin, TX 78756

HANNELE R. JOUSIMIES-SOMER
Anaerobe Reference Laboratory, National Public Health Institute, 00300 Helsinki, Finland (deceased)

MOGENS KILIAN
Department of Medical Microbiology and Immunology, University of Aarhus, DK-8000 Aarhus C, Denmark

DEANNA L. KISKA
Microbiology Laboratory, Department of Clinical Pathology, SUNY Upstate Medical University, Syracuse, NY 13210

NANCY B. KIVIAT
Department of Pathology, University of Washington, Seattle, WA 98104

JOAN S. KNAPP
Gonorrhea Research Branch, Division of AIDS, STD, and TB Laboratory Research, Centers for Disease Control and Prevention, Atlanta, GA 30333

PIRKKO KOUKILA-KÄHKÖLÄ
HUS Diagnostics, Mycology Laboratory, Helsinki University Central Hospital, Helsinki, Finland

KAREN KRISHER
Department of Pathology, University of Texas Southwestern Medical Center, Dallas, TX 75230

THOMAS G. KSIAZEK
Special Pathogens Branch, Division of Viral and Rickettsial Diseases, National Center for Infectious Diseases, Centers for Disease Control and Prevention, Atlanta, GA 30333

JAIME A. LABARCA
Internal Medicine Department, Facultad de Medicina, Pontifica Universidad Catolica, Santiago, Chile

RENU B. LAL
HIV Immunology and Diagnostics Branch, Division of AIDS, STD, and TB Laboratory Research, Centers for Disease Control and Prevention, Atlanta, GA 30333

DOLORES P. LANA
Department of Biological Sciences, Villa Julie College, Stevenson, MD 21153

MARIE LOUISE LANDRY
Department of Laboratory Medicine, Yale University School of Medicine, New Haven, CT 06520, and Clinical Virology Laboratory, Yale New Haven Hospital, New Haven, CT 06504

MARK T. LaROCCO
Department of Pathology, St. Luke's Episcopal Health System, and Texas Medical Center, Houston, TX 77030

DAVISE H. LARONE
Department of Pathology and Microbiology, Weill Cornell Medical Center, New York, NY 10021

SANDRA A. LARSEN
Division of AIDS, STD, and TB Laboratory Research, Centers for Disease Control and Prevention, Atlanta, GA 30333 (retired)

PHILIP LaRUSSA
Department of Pediatrics, Columbia University College of Physicians & Surgeons, New York, NY 10032

TSAI-LING LAUDERDALE
Division of Clinical Research, National Health Research Institutes, Taipei 11529, Taiwan, Republic of China

AMY L. LEBER
Quest Diagnostics, Nichols Institute, 33608 Ortega Highway, San Juan Capistrano, CA 92690

KARIN LEDER
Infectious Disease Epidemiology Unit, Department of Epidemiology and Preventive Medicine, Monash University, Victoria 3181, Australia

PAUL N. LEVETT
WHO Collaborating Center on Leptospirosis, Meningitis and Special Pathogens Branch, Division of Bacterial and Mycotic Diseases, National Center for Infectious Diseases, Centers for Disease Control and Prevention, Atlanta, GA 30333

ANNIKA LINDE
Department of Virology, Swedish Institute for Infectious Disease Control, SE-171 82 Solna, Sweden

SHAWN R. LOCKHART
Department of Biological Sciences, University of Iowa, Iowa City, IA 52242

MIKE J. LOEFFELHOLZ
Compunet Clinical Laboratories, 2308 Sandridge Drive, Moraine, OH 45439

NIALL A. LOGAN
School of Biological and Biomedical Sciences, Glasgow Caledonian University, Cowcaddens Road, Glasgow G4 0BA, United Kingdom

GARY LUM
Northern Territory Department of Health and Community Services, Rocklands Drive, Tiwi NT, Australia 0810

DAVID M. LYERLY
TechLab, Inc., 1861 Pratt Drive, Blacksburg, VA 24060-6364

JAMES D. MacLOWRY
Department of Pathology, Oregon Health and Science University, Portland, OR 97201

JAMES B. MAHONY
McMaster University, Department of Pathology and Molecular Medicine, Hamilton Regional Laboratory Medicine Program, St. Joseph's Healthcare, Hamilton, Ontario L8N 4A6, Canada

EUGENE O. MAJOR
Laboratory of Molecular Medicine and Neuroscience, National Institute of Neurological Disorders and Stroke, Bethesda, MD 20892-4164

THOMAS J. MARRIE
Department of Medicine, University of Alberta, Edmonton, Alberta T6H 2B7, Canada

JAMES B. McAULEY
Cermak Health Services, 2800 South California Avenue, Chicago, IL 60608

MICHAEL R. McGINNIS
WHO Collaborating Center for Tropical Diseases, Department of Pathology, University of Texas Medical Branch at Galveston, Galveston, TX 77555-0609

MICHAEL M. McNEIL
Epidemiology and Surveillance Division, National Immunization Program, Centers for Disease Control and Prevention, Atlanta, GA 30333

WILLIAM G. MERZ
Department of Laboratory Medicine, Johns Hopkins Hospital, Baltimore, MD 21287-7093

J. MICHAEL MILLER
Laboratory Response Branch, Bioterrorism Preparedness and Response Program, Centers for Disease Control and Prevention, Atlanta, GA 30333

THOMAS G. MITCHELL
Department of Microbiology and Immunology, Duke University Medical Center, Durham, NC 27710

ROBERT C. MOELLERING, JR.
Department of Medicine, Beth Israel Deaconess Medical Center, and Harvard Medical School, Boston, MA 02215

BERNARD J. MONCLA
Magee-Womens Research Institute and the Schools of Dental Medicine and Medicine, University of Pittsburgh, Pittsburgh, PA 15213

PATRICK R. MURRAY
Department of Laboratory Medicine, National Institutes of Health Clinical Center, Bethesda, MD 20892

MONICA MUSIANI
Department of Clinical Experimental Medicine, Division of Microbiology, University of Bologna, 40138 Bologna, Italy

REINIER MUTTERS
Institute of Medical Microbiology and Hospital Hygiene, Philipps University, D-35037 Marburg, Germany

IRVING NACHAMKIN
Department of Pathology and Laboratory Medicine, University of Pennsylvania School of Medicine, Philadelphia, PA 19104-4283

PHUC NGUYEN-DINH
Division of Parasitic Diseases, Centers for Disease Control and Prevention, Chamblee, GA 30341

STUART T. NICHOL
Special Pathogens Branch, Division of Viral and Rickettsial Diseases, National Center for Infectious Diseases, Centers for Disease Control and Prevention, Atlanta, GA 30333

FREDERICK S. NOLTE
Emory University Hospital and Department of Pathology and Laboratory Medicine, Emory University School of Medicine, Atlanta, GA 30322

STEVEN J. NORRIS
Department of Pathology and Laboratory Medicine, University of Texas Medical School at Houston, Houston, TX 77225

SUSAN M. NOVAK
Microbiology Department, Kaiser Permanente, 11668 Sherman Way, North Hollywood, CA 91605

ERIC NULENS
Department of Medical Microbiology, University Medical Center St. Radboud, 6500 HB Nijmegen, The Netherlands

CAROLINE MOHR O'HARA
Diagnostic Microbiology Section, Epidemiology and Laboratory Branch, Division of Healthcare Quality Promotion, Centers for Disease Control and Prevention, Atlanta, GA 30333

THOMAS C. ORIHEL
Department of Tropical Medicine, School of Public Health and Tropical Medicine, Tulane University, New Orleans, LA 70112

YNES R. ORTEGA
Center for Food Safety and Quality Enhancement, University of Georgia, Griffin, GA 30223

ARVIND A. PADHYE
Mycotic Disease Branch, Division of Bacterial and Mycotic Diseases, National Center for Infectious Diseases, Centers for Disease Control and Prevention, Atlanta, GA 30333

GRAEME P. PALTRIDGE
Bacteriology and Parasitology Laboratory, Canterbury Health Laboratories, Christchurch, New Zealand

PHILIP E. PELLETT
Centers for Disease Control and Prevention, Atlanta, GA 30333

MARTIN PETRIC
Laboratory Services, BC Centre for Disease Control, 655 West 12th Avenue, Vancouver, British Columbia V5Z 4R4, Canada

MICHAEL A. PFALLER
Department of Pathology, University of Iowa College of Medicine, and Department of Epidemiology, University of Iowa College of Public Health, Iowa City, IA 52242

GABY E. PFYFFER
Department of Medical Microbiology, University of Zurich, Swiss National Center for Mycobacteria, Gloriastrasse 30, CH-8028 Zurich, Switzerland

VICTORIA POPE
Division of AIDS, STD and TB Laboratory Research, Centers for Disease Control and Prevention, Atlanta, GA 30333

CLAUDE PUJOL
Department of Biological Sciences, University of Iowa, Iowa City, IA 52242

DIDIER RAOULT
Faculté de Médecine, Unité des Rickettsies, CNRS UMR 6020, Marseille Cedex 5, France

J. KAMILE RASHEED
Division of Healthcare Quality Promotion, National Center for Infectious Diseases, Centers for Disease Control and Prevention, Atlanta, GA 30333

LARRY G. REIMER
Department of Pathology, University of Utah School of Medicine, and Associated Regional and University Pathologists, Salt Lake City, UT 84132

L. BARTH RELLER
Clinical Microbiology Laboratory, Duke University Medical Center, and Departments of Medicine and Pathology, Duke University School of Medicine, Durham, NC 27710

JOHN H. REX
Division of Infectious Diseases, Department of Internal Medicine, Center for the Study of Emerging and Remerging Pathogens, University of Texas Medical School-Houston, and Hermann Hospital, Houston, TX 77030

JUDITH C. RHODES
Department of Pathology and Laboratory Medicine, University of Cincinnati, Cincinnati, OH 45221

LOUIS B. RICE
Medical Service, Louis Stokes Cleveland VA Medical Center, and Department of Medicine, Case Western Reserve University, Cleveland, OH 44106

MALCOLM D. RICHARDSON
Mycology Unit, Department of Bacteriology and Immunology, University of Helsinki, Haartman Institute, 00014 Helsinki, Finland

JOHN D. RIHS
Department of Medicine, University of Pittsburgh, and Infectious Disease Section and Laboratory Medicine and Pathology, VA Medical Center, Pittsburgh, PA 15240

YASUKO RIKIHISA
Department of Veterinary Biosciences, College of Veterinary Medicine, The Ohio State University, Columbus, OH 43210

GLENN D. ROBERTS
Section of Clinical Microbiology, Mayo Clinic and Mayo Foundation, Rochester, MN 55905

JOCELYNE ROCOURT
Food Safety Programme, World Health Organization, Avenue Apia, 1211 Geneva, Switzerland

WILLIAM O. ROGERS
Malaria Program, Naval Medical Research Unit 3, and Noguchi Memorial Institute for Medical Research, Accra, Ghana

PIERRE E. ROLLIN
Special Pathogens Branch, Division of Viral and Rickettsial Diseases, National Center for Infectious Diseases, Centers for Disease Control and Prevention, Atlanta, GA 30333

JOSÉ R. ROMERO
Combined Division of Pediatric Infectious Diseases,
University of Nebraska Medical Center, and Creighton
University, Omaha, NE 68198-2165

HARLEY A. ROTBART
Pediatric Infectious Diseases, University of Colorado Health
Sciences Center, Denver, CO 80262

KATHRYN L. RUOFF
Microbiology Laboratories, Massachusetts General Hospital,
and Department of Pathology, Harvard Medical School,
Boston, MA 02114

DANIEL SAHM
Focus Technologies, 13665 Dulles Technology Drive,
Herndon, VA 20171

IRA F. SALKIN
Department of Biomedical Sciences, School of Public
Health, State University of New York, Albany, NY 12246

WILEY A. SCHELL
Medical Mycology Research Center, Department of
Medicine, Division of Infectious Diseases and International
Health, Duke University Medical Center, and Pathology and
Laboratory Medicine, Veterans Affairs Medical Center,
Durham, NC 27710

GEORGE G. SCHLAUDER
Virus Discovery Group, Abbott Laboratories, 1401 Sheridan
Road, North Chicago, IL 60064

PAUL C. SCHRECKENBERGER
Division of Clinical Pathology, University of Illinois College
of Medicine at Chicago, Chicago, IL 60612

MARTIN E. SCHRIEFER
Centers for Disease Control and Prevention, Rampart Road,
Foothills Campus, Fort Collins, CO 80522

JÖRG SCHÜPBACH
Swiss National Center for Retroviruses, University of Zurich,
CH-8028 Zurich, Switzerland

W. EVAN SECOR
Division of Parasitic Diseases, Centers for Disease Control
and Prevention, Atlanta, GA 30341

DAVID L. SEWELL
Pathology and Laboratory Medicine Service, Veterans
Affairs Medical Center, and Department of Pathology,
Oregon Health and Science University, Portland, OR 97201

ROBERT W. SHAFER
Division of Infectious Diseases, Stanford University,
Stanford, CA 94305

HAROUN N. SHAH
Molecular Identification Services, NCTC, PHLS Central
Public Health Laboratory, London NW9 5HT, United
Kingdom

GILLIAN S. SHANKLAND
Mycology Laboratory, Department of Dermatology,
University of Glasgow, and West Glasgow Hospitals,
University NHS Trust, Glasgow, United Kingdom

SUSAN E. SHARP
University of Missouri Kansas City, and Diagnostic
Microbiology Laboratories, Health Midwest, 2316 East
Meyer Boulevard, Kansas City, MO 64132

ROBYN Y. SHIMIZU
Department of Pathology and Laboratory Medicine, UCLA
Medical Center, Los Angeles, CA 90095-1713

MARGARET C. SHUHART
University of Washington Harborview Medical Center, 325
Ninth Avenue, Seattle, WA 98104

LYNNE SIGLER
Microfungus Collection and Herbarium, Devonian Botanic
Garden, and Medical Microbiology and Immunology,
University of Alberta, Edmonton, Alberta, Canada T6G 2E1

LEONARD N. SLATER
Department of Medicine, University of Oklahoma Health
Sciences Center and Veterans Affairs Medical Center,
Oklahoma City, OK 73104

JEAN S. SMITH
Rabies Laboratory, Viral and Rickettsial Zoonoses Branch,
Division of Viral and Rickettsial Diseases, National Center
for Infectious Diseases, Centers for Disease Control and
Prevention, Atlanta, GA 30333

THOMAS F. SMITH
Division of Clinical Microbiology, Mayo Clinic, Rochester,
MN 55905

JAMES W. SNYDER
Department of Pathology, Division of Laboratory Medicine,
University of Louisville School of Medicine and Hospital,
Louisville, KY 40202

DAVID R. SOLL
Department of Biological Sciences, University of Iowa, Iowa
City, IA 52242

JACK T. STAPLETON
Department of Internal Medicine, University of Iowa
College of Medicine, and The Iowa City Veterans
Administration Medical Center, Iowa City, IA 52242

SHARON P. STEINBERG
Department of Pediatrics, Columbia University College of
Physicians & Surgeons, New York, NY 10032

JANET E. STOUT
Department of Medicine, University of Pittsburgh, and
Infectious Disease Section and Laboratory Medicine and
Pathology, VA Medical Center, Pittsburgh, PA 15240

NANCY A. STROCKBINE
Foodborne and Diarrheal Diseases Laboratory Section,
Foodborne and Diarrheal Diseases Branch, Division of
Bacterial and Mycotic Diseases, National Center for
Infectious Diseases, Centers for Disease Control and
Prevention, Atlanta, GA 30333

PAULA H. SUMMANEN
Research Service, VA Medical Center West Los Angeles,
Los Angeles, CA 90073

RICHARD C. SUMMERBELL
CBS Fungal Biodiversity Center, Uppsalalaan 8, 3584 CT
Utrecht, The Netherlands

DEANNA A. SUTTON
Fungus Testing Laboratory, Department of Pathology,
University of Texas Health Science Center at San Antonio,
San Antonio, TX 78229

BALA SWAMINATHAN
Foodborne and Diarrheal Disease Branch, Division of
Bacterial and Mycotic Diseases, National Center for
Infectious Diseases, Centers for Disease Control and
Prevention, Atlanta, GA 30333

JANA M. SWENSON
Epidemiology and Laboratory Branch, Division of Healthcare
Quality Promotion, Centers for Disease Control and
Prevention, Atlanta, GA 30333

PAUL D. SWENSON
Public Health—Seattle and King County Laboratory,
Seattle, WA 98104

ELLA M. SWIERKOSZ
Departments of Pathology and Pediatrics, Saint Louis
University School of Medicine, St. Louis, MO 63104

DAVID TAYLOR-ROBINSON
Imperial College School of Medicine at St. Mary's Hospital,
Winston Churchill Wing, Paddington, London W2 NY,
United Kingdom

GARY E. TEGTMEIER
Viral Testing Laboratories, Community Blood Center of
Greater Kansas City, Kansas City, MO 64111

LÚCIA MARTINS TEIXEIRA
Instituto de Microbiologia, Universidade Federal do Rio de
Janeiro, Rio de Janeiro, RJ 21941, Brazil

RAYMOND TELLIER
Division of Microbiology, The Hospital for Sick Children,
Toronto, Ontario M5G 1X8, Canada

FRED C. TENOVER
Division of Healthcare Quality Promotion, National Center
for Infectious Diseases, Centers for Disease Control and
Prevention, Atlanta, GA 30333

RICHARD B. THOMSON, JR.
Evanston Northwestern Healthcare and Northwestern
University Medical School, Evanston, IL 60201

GRAHAM TIPPLES
National Microbiology Laboratory, Health Canada, 1015
Arlington Street, Winnipeg, Manitoba R3E 3R2, Canada

DEBRA A. TRISTRAM
Department of Pediatrics, East Carolina School of Medicine,
Greenville, NC 27858

THEODORE F. TSAI
Global Medical Affairs, Wyeth Ayerst Pharmaceuticals, 150
North Radnor-Chester Road, St. Davids, PA 19087

PETER C. B. TURNBULL
Arjemptur Technology Ltd., Porton Down Science Park,
Salisbury SP4 0JQ, United Kingdom

JOHN D. TURNIDGE
Microbiology and Infectious Diseases, Women's and
Children's Hospital, North Adelaide 5006, Australia

ALEXANDRA VALSAMAKIS
Department of Pathology, Division of Microbiology, The
Johns Hopkins Medical Institutions, Baltimore, MD 21287

PETER A. R. VANDAMME
Laboratorium voor Microbiologie, Faculteit Wetenschappen,
Universiteit Gent, K. L. Ledeganckstraat 35, B-9000 Gent,
Belgium

JAMES VERSALOVIC
Departments of Pathology and Molecular Virology and
Microbiology, Baylor College of Medicine, and Department
of Pathology, Texas Children's Hospital, Houston, TX 77030

PAUL E. VERWEIJ
Department of Medical Microbiology, University Medical
Center Nijmegen, Nijmegen, The Netherlands

VÉRONIQUE VINCENT
Reference Laboratory for Mycobacteria, Institut Pasteur,
Paris, France

GOVINDA S. VISVESVARA
Division of Parasitic Diseases, National Center for Infectious
Diseases, Centers for Disease Control and Prevention, 4770
Buford Highway NE, Atlanta, GA 30341-3724

ALEXANDER von GRAEVENITZ
Department of Medical Microbiology, University of Zurich,
Gloriastrasse 32, CH-8028 Zurich, Switzerland

ANDREAS VOSS
Department of Medical Microbiology, University Medical
Center St. Radboud, 6500 HB Nijmegen, The Netherlands

GÖRAN WADELL
Department of Virology, Umeå University, S-901 85 Umeå,
Sweden

KEN B. WAITES
Departments of Pathology and Microbiology, University of
Alabama at Birmingham Schools of Medicine and Dentistry,
University of Alabama Hospital, Birmingham,
AL 35249-7331

DAVID H. WALKER
Department of Pathology, WHO Collaborating Center for
Tropical Diseases, University of Texas Medical Branch,
Galveston, TX 77555-0609

RICHARD J. WALLACE, JR.
Department of Microbiology, University of Texas Health
Center, Tyler, TX 75799

THOMAS J. WALSH
Immunocompromised Host Section, National Cancer
Institute, Bethesda, MD 20892

JOSEPH L. WANER
Department of Pediatrics, Section of Infectious Diseases,
Children's Hospital of Oklahoma, Oklahoma City,
OK 73104-5066

RAINER WEBER
Division of Infectious Diseases and Hospital Epidemiology,
Department of Internal Medicine, University Hospital,
CH-8091 Zurich, Switzerland

MELVIN P. WEINSTEIN
Microbiology Laboratory, Robert Wood Johnson University
Hospital, New Brunswick, NJ 08903

ALICE S. WEISSFELD
Microbiology Specialists, Inc., and Department of Molecular
Virology and Microbiology, Baylor College of Medicine,
Houston, TX 77054

DAVID F. WELCH
Laboratory Corporation of America, and Department of
Pathology, University of Texas Southwestern Medical
Center, Dallas, TX 75230

PETER F. WELLER
Harvard Medical School and Division of Infectious Diseases
and Allergy and Inflammation Division, Beth Israel
Deaconess Medical Center, Boston, MA 02215

JOY G. WELLS
Foodborne and Diarrheal Diseases Laboratory Section,
Foodborne and Diarrheal Diseases Branch, Division of
Bacterial and Mycotic Diseases, National Center for
Infectious Diseases, Centers for Disease Control and
Prevention, Atlanta, GA 30333

FRED W. WESTENFELD
Department of Pathology and Laboratory Medicine, Fletcher
Allen Health Care, Burlington, VT 05401

HANNAH WEXLER
Department of Medicine, UCLA School of Medicine, VA
Medical Center West Los Angeles, Los Angeles, CA 90073

ROBBIN S. WEYANT
Laboratory Safety Branch, Office of Health and Safety,
Centers for Disease Control and Prevention, Atlanta,
GA 30333

R. A. WHILEY
Department of Oral Microbiology, Bart's and the London
Queen Mary School of Medicine and Dentistry, Turner
Street, London E1 2AD, United Kingdom

THEODORE C. WHITE
Department of Pathobiology, School of Public Health and
Community Medicine, University of Washington, and
Seattle Biomedical Research Institute, Seattle, WA 98109

SUSAN WHITTIER
Clinical Microbiology, Meridian Health System, 1945 Route
33, Neptune, NJ 07754

ANDREAS F. WIDMER
Division of Hospital Epidemiology, University Hospitals,
Basel 6031, Switzerland

BETTINA WILSKE
Max von Pettenkofer-Institute, University of Munich,
National Reference Center for Borreliae, D-80336 Munich,
Germany

MARIANNA WILSON
Biology and Diagnostic Branch, Division of Parasitic
Diseases, National Center for Infectious Diseases, Centers for
Disease Control and Prevention, Atlanta, GA 30341

MICHAEL L. WILSON
Department of Pathology and Laboratory Services, Denver
Health Medical Center, Denver, CO 80204, and
Department of Pathology, University of Colorado School of
Medicine, Denver, CO 80262

JANE D. WONG
Microbial Diseases Laboratory, California Department of
Health Services, 2151 Berkeley Way, Berkeley, CA 94704

JOSEPH D. C. YAO
Division of Clinical Microbiology, Mayo Clinic, Rochester,
MN 55902-0002

ROBERT H. YOLKEN
Department of Pediatrics, Stanley Division of
Developmental Neurovirology, Johns Hopkins University
School of Medicine, Baltimore, MD 21287

VICTOR L. YU
Infectious Disease Section and Laboratory Medicine and
Pathology, VA Medical Center, Pittsburgh, PA 15240

REINIIARD ZBINDEN
Department of Medical Microbiology, University of Zurich,
Gloriastrasse 32, CH-8028 Zurich, Switzerland

MARIALUISA ZERBINI
Department of Clinical Experimental Medicine, Division of
Microbiology, University of Bologna, 40138 Bologna, Italy

THEDI ZIEGLER
National Public Health Institute, Mannerheimintie 166,
FIN-00300 Helsinki, Finland

Acknowledgment of Previous Contributors

The *Manual of Clinical Microbiology* is by its nature a continuously revised work which
refines and extends the contributions of authors of previous editions. Since its first edition
in 1970, many eminent scientists have contributed to this important reference work. The
American Society for Microbiology and its Publications Board gratefully acknowledge the
contributions of all of these generous authors over the life of this Manual.

Preface

As we completed the eighth edition of the *Manual of Clinical Microbiology*, we exhaled a breath of relief bordering on exhaustion and then swelled with a feeling of pride. Any book of this magnitude is a labor of love because the number of days spent planning, coordinating, writing, and editing are too numerous to count. However, for every frustrating moment we were blessed with the contributions of talented authors that left us with the satisfied knowledge that we were doing the right thing. Yes, we had our few authors who failed to meet the deadlines, and yes, we had e-mail messages and telephone calls disappear into the black hole of a recalcitrant author's or editor's office. But we did it—141 chapters in two volumes written by more than 230 authors. This is not simply a completed project, but a well-done project—one that each of us is proud to claim. But we cannot take credit for this accomplishment. More important, we want to thank the authors who devoted their time (such a scarce commodity today) and knowledge to produce their chapters and then exercised patience and understanding as the editorial board dissected their chapters and insisted on revisions. It must be noted that this was truly an extraordinary effort because the attention and activities of many authors were preoccupied by the deeds of terrorists. We also thank our section editors—those individuals who worked directly with the authors throughout the entire process of preparing and editing the chapters. Without their efforts this Manual would never have come to fruition. Finally, a special thanks is extended to the staff at ASM Press, whose job it is to handle the myriad of details that most would never see or imagine. It is the policy of ASM to not dedicate the Manual to any one individual, but if we could, this Manual would be dedicated to Susan Birch, the ASM Press Production Manager who simply makes this Manual happen.

PATRICK R. MURRAY
ELLEN JO BARON
JAMES H. JORGENSEN
MICHAEL A. PFALLER
ROBERT H. YOLKEN

GENERAL ISSUES IN CLINICAL MICROBIOLOGY

I

VOLUME EDITOR
JAMES H. JORGENSEN

SECTION EDITOR
MELVIN P. WEINSTEIN

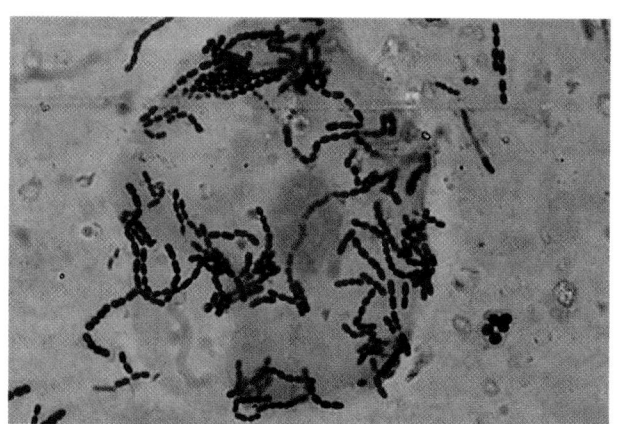

Squamous epithelial cell with mixed bacterial flora.

Introduction to the Eighth Edition of the *Manual of Clinical Microbiology*

PATRICK R. MURRAY

1

This is the third edition of the *Manual of Clinical Microbiology* that I have coordinated. This edition, the eighth in the history of the Manual, represents a major departure from the previous editions. The obvious changes are expansion into two volumes, more than 2,100 pages of text and 141 chapters. However, the substantive changes are those that may be less apparent. I have continued to search for an infusion of new ideas and information. So Jim Jorgensen and five section editors joined the editorial board, and more than 35% of the authors are new. The international character of the Manual has been expanded, with 25% of the authors representing 20 non-U.S. countries.

With the growth of the Manual into two volumes, the constraint of page limits has been less acute, although the editors have done an excellent job of purging the needless phrase, esoteric thesis, or compulsive collection of references. The 141 chapters are organized into 11 sections. Volume 1 contains General Issues; Infection Detection, Prevention, and Control; Diagnostic Technologies; Bacteriology; and Antibacterial Agents and Susceptibility Test Methods. Volume 2 contains Virology; Mycology; and Parasitology; as well as 3 sections covering Antiviral, Antifungal, and Antiparasitic Agents and Susceptibility Test Methods.

Growth presents an opportunity to add and reorganize chapters. The new chapters include ones covering laboratory information systems, bioterrorism, and storage of microorganisms; the coverage of *Mycobacterium* has been expanded into 2 chapters; specimen collection, transport, and processing has expanded from 2 to 5 chapters; reagents, stains, and media has expanded from 3 to 5 chapters; and the chapters discussing antimicrobial agents and susceptibility testing have expanded from 13 to 19. The organized structure of the chapters has been maintained, but the editorial board insisted on the most current taxonomic, diagnostic, and therapeutic information. To underscore this, 25% of the more than 14,000 reference citations in this edition of the Manual were published after the last edition went to press.

With any endeavor of this magnitude, errors of omission and commission are inevitable, and as always, we welcome your suggestions for changes and corrections. However, every chapter was reviewed by three editors, and many hours of editing and revisions were performed by the authors, Manual editors, and ASM Press editorial staff. We believe that the final product is the most current, factual, and comprehensive manual in this discipline, and we hope that the readers agree.

3

Laboratory Management

DAVID L. SEWELL AND JAMES D. MacLOWRY

2

The rapidity and extent of change that has occurred in the health care delivery system in the United States and elsewhere in the last decade have been nothing short of remarkable. For better or worse, microbiology laboratories are part of this change and the directors must obtain the management skills necessary to participate and survive in this new and changing environment.

This chapter is an attempt to expose the reader to the various management concepts and techniques being used today and, more importantly, to stimulate the reader to pursue additional information in this area. The chapter is presented in six parts: (i) basic management concepts, (ii) determination and management of laboratory costs, (iii) analysis of laboratory activities, (iv) quality assessment and control, (v) issues affecting laboratory management, and (vi) regulatory issues affecting the microbiology laboratory. In general, the first three parts of this chapter apply to laboratories worldwide, while the final three sections apply almost exclusively to laboratories in the United States.

The section on management concepts provides an overview of the elements of management such as human resources, the planning and implementation of goals, and the control and improvement of the laboratory process. Facets of managing laboratory costs are reviewed in the second section through a discussion of budgeting, cost accounting, determination of direct and indirect costs, and pricing strategies. The third section outlines approaches to cost containment in the microbiology laboratory. These approaches vary from changing the operation of the laboratory to managing test utilization, and specific suggestions for reducing test costs are included. The final three sections deal with laboratory regulatory issues, basic quality assessment and control concepts, and other issues such as health care practices and workforce changes that affect microbiology laboratories.

Our intent is not to provide an exhaustive and detailed review of all aspects of laboratory management but rather to provoke a discussion of the issues and problems facing the microbiology laboratory today. The laboratory cannot stand alone but must be an active, integrated participant in today's health care delivery system. The key terms and acronyms used in this chapter are presented in Table 1.

BASIC MANAGEMENT CONCEPTS

Management Functions

In the 1800s, creative artisans and apprentices produced unique goods and services in relatively small shops. In 1911, a new theory called "scientific management" was introduced that described the manufacturing process as a set of recognizable and predefined steps that could be standardized (58). This process theory is the basis for the current assembly line concept in which goods and services are produced by using standardized parts and procedures. Communication was in a hierarchical form of directives from top to bottom. Management believed that quality control inspectors ensured quality, that the management process could be optimized by experts, that employees are a commodity which is motivated by fear and reward, and that profits were made by keeping revenues high and costs low (59).

In the 1940s and 1950s a new management concept based on quality was introduced, and this concept has had a major impact on the health care system. Juran, Deming, and Crosby have been the most ardent promoters of the system of management based on the quality of the product. Juran (32, 33) developed a three-part system based on quality planning (determining the needs of the customer), quality control (evaluating actual product performance), and quality improvement (identifying problems and the solutions). Deming, as described by DeAguayo (19), believed that quality is determined and controlled by the employees, that the manufacturing process can always be improved, that employees are not motivated by fear and rewards (such motivation actually destroys teamwork and cooperation), and that profits are generated by loyal customers (19, 68). His strategy is summarized in 14 points (Table 2). Crosby (17) proposed that quality is achieved through compliance with defined specifications and standards and also outlined a 14-step process to achieve this goal (Table 2). These management concepts form the basic quality systems philosophy found in many organizations today.

Associated with this emphasis on the production of a quality product is the recognition that the organization or producer must meet the customer's expectations with regard to the product as well as other service needs. The

TABLE 1 Key terms and acronyms

ABN: Advanced beneficiary notice
    A 1998 initiative of the Centers for Medicare and Medicaid
    Services (CMS) which requires that patients be notified in
    writing that a test will not be reimbursed by CMS and that
    the patient agrees to be billed directly for the test.
CAP: College of American Pathologists
CLIA 88: Clinical Laboratory Improvement Amendments 1988
    Applies to all laboratories that perform testing of human
    specimens for the diagnosis, monitoring, or prevention of
    disease.
CMS: Centers for Medicare and Medicaid Services (previously
    the Health Care Financing Administration)
CPT: Current Procedural Terminology—2001
    Most recent CPT code book
CQI: Continuous quality improvement
    A proactive managerial concept that promotes ongoing QI
    and customer satisfaction. Resolves identified problems and
    seeks improvement where no problems exist.
DHHS: U.S. Department of Health and Human Services
DOT: U.S. Department of Transportation
DRG: Diagnosis-related groups
    System of reimbursement for health care costs.
FDA: Food and Drug Administration
FTE: Full-time equivalent
    Employee who works at least 40 hours per week.
Gatekeeper:
    A health care provider who assesses the need for complex
    testing and provides the least expensive method to
    diagnose a patient's condition.
HCFA: Health Care Finance Administration
    Name has been changed to Centers for Medicare and
    Medicaid Services (CMS)
JCAHO: Joint Commission on Accreditation of Healthcare
    Organizations
LIS: Laboratory information system
OIG: Office of the Inspector General
OSHA: Occupational Safety and Health Administration
POCT: Point-of-care testing
    Testing conducted in the presence of the patient. Also referred
    to as bedside, near-patient, and alternative-site testing.
PPM: Provider-performed microscopy
    Microscopic tests (e.g., wet mounts and KOH) defined by
    CMS that can be performed by physician and nonphysician
    health care personnel and are not subject to routine
    biennial inspection.
QA: Quality assurance
    A planned and systematic process for evaluating and
    monitoring the quality and appropriateness of patient care,
    focusing on problem finding.
QC: Quality control
    A system for detecting and correcting analytical errors by
    establishing performance limits.
QI: Quality improvement
    A system for identifying processes that can be used to
    improve performance and customer satisfaction.
TQM: Total quality management
    A system of managerial programs (team, plans, and
    improvement management) that provide the processes by
    which CQI can be implemented and maintained.
Waived tests:
    Tests that use simple and accurate methodologies, that pose
    no reasonable risk of harm if performed incorrectly, or that
    are approved for home use. Laboratories performing waived
    tests are not inspected routinely, nor are they required to
    meet certain other CLIA 88 requirements.

customer's needs are or should be the driving force in this arrangement. Management attempts to coordinate the actions of the employees to accomplish these goals. Whether the organization is a for-profit or a not-for-profit medical center or a clinical microbiology laboratory, the management team is responsible for the operation of units that include human resources management; directing, planning, and implementation of goals; and control and improvement of the overall process. The essential elements of a quality system are organization, personnel, equipment, purchasing and inventory, process control, documents and records, occurrence management (dealing with errors and problems), internal assessment, process improvement, and service and satisfaction (49). Hardwick and Morrison (27) described the basic elements of management as ideas, things, and people. The tasks associated with these elements are listed in Table 3. To accomplish these tasks, the laboratory manager must be (i) a visionary and strategist, recognizing opportunities for growth and progress; (ii) a teacher, guiding others to identify and solve problems; (iii) a leader, providing a clear course of action and inspiring the employees' commitment to the objectives of the laboratory and the larger organization; and (iv) a problem solver (1).

Although the attempt is often made to manage laboratories by business techniques used in non-health-care environments, the management of laboratories is more complicated due to the complexity of health care delivery and the highly trained personnel who view their profession as a craft, much like the craftsmen of the 1800s. For example, the laboratory produces, interprets, and reports test results to its customers and in many situations also provides research and teaching services. In addition, the laboratory must meet the needs of the patients and the medical staff, as well as the goals, objectives, and missions of the hospital or medical center and the corporate organization. In this complex process, the needs of one group may conflict with other demands placed on the laboratory.

Human Resources Management

Today, most laboratory managers recognize that employees are the key element in the success or failure of an organization. To effectively understand human behavior and manage people, managers need to understand and incorporate the following elements into their managerial skills: (i) motivation, (ii) perception (how a person reacts to a stimulus), (iii) communication, (iv) leadership versus managership, (v) group dynamics, and (vi) morale (60).

The management of people relies on motivation and listening, delegation, and supervision. Appropriate motivation encourages employees to work at a high level of performance and stimulates creativity. Systems that judge, punish, or reward above- or below-average performance do not motivate over the long term, especially in laboratories staffed with highly trained personnel. Persuasion and the use of professional guidelines achieve far better results in this environment. Generally, people are motivated by leaders who understand and appreciate the diversity of people's talents and skills and who allow people to do what is required of them (20).

The good manager is also able to delegate tasks and responsibilities at the level where they can best be accomplished. Supervision ensures that the organizational goals are met and that the policies are followed. Leadership in the health care arena is often more difficult than leadership in other businesses because managers must interact with in-

TABLE 2 Management strategies[a]

Deming's 14 points	Crosby's 14 steps
1. Create constancy of purpose for service improvement	1. Management of commitment
2. Adopt the new philosophy	2. The quality improvement team
3. Cease dependence on inspection to achieve quality	3. Quality measurement
4. End practice of awarding business on the basis of price alone; make partners out of vendors	4. The cost of quality
5. Constantly improve every process for planning, production, and service	5. Quality awareness
6. Institute training and retraining on the job	6. Corrective action
7. Institute leadership for system improvement	7. Zero-defect planning
8. Drive out fear	8. Supervisor training
9. Break down barriers between staff areas	9. Zero-defects day
10. Eliminate slogans, exhortations, and targets for the workforce	10. Goal setting
11. Eliminate numerical quotas for the workforce and numerical goals for the management	11. Error-cause removal
12. Remove barriers to pride of workmanship	12. Recognition
13. Institute a vigorous program of education and self-improvement for everyone	13. Quality councils
14. Put everyone to work on the transformation	14. Do it all over again

[a] Adapted from reference 33a. Deming's 14 points originally appeared in *The Deming Management Method* by Mary Walton, copyright 1986, and is used with permission of G. P. Putnam's Sons, a division of Penguin Putnam, Inc.

dependent, autonomous, and highly skilled health care practitioners.

Planning and Implementation

All change is inherently local, which suggests that the only people who truly understand a process are those individuals who perform it (31). Change is an integral part of today's health care environment of limited resources, and management must plan for change. These plans may include (i) the business plan (which details the laboratory's mission, goals, and objectives); (ii) the marketing plan (which describes customers, test products, and services); (iii) the operation plan (which describes facilities, equipment, capacity, etc.); (iv) the staffing plan (which describes workload and staffing requirements); and (v) the financial plan (which describes needs for capital, financial resources, budget, and reimbursement structure) (61). The best plans are derived from health care professionals working together to optimize and continually improve the processes of providing care.

Juran (32) described the planning process as follows:

Identify the customers (patients, physician, third-party payer) and their needs.

Develop a product that meets the needs of the customer and the laboratory.

Develop and optimize the process to produce the product (procedures and work flow).

Transfer the process to the operating personnel (training and implementation).

Establish a measurement system (evaluate the process).

Cost is a critical element of the laboratory's planning process. Laboratory managers must provide the data to substantiate the fiscal soundness of the laboratory's plan and negotiate an adequate budget to secure the necessary personnel, equipment, and supplies to meet its goals and the needs of its customers.

Control

After the plan is implemented, management must monitor or evaluate the overall process and product quality, compare the results to the initial goals and expectations, and explore possible alternatives. This generally means monitoring the preanalytic phase (prior to the testing of a specimen), the analytic phase (when the test procedure is

TABLE 3 Tasks associated with management[a]

	Management		
Elements	Ideas	Things	People
Tasks	Conceptual thinking	Administration	Leadership
Functions	Analyze problems	Make decisions	Communicate
	Gather facts, ascertain causes, develop alternatives	Establish conclusions	Ensure understanding
Activities	Set objectives	Study work flow and tasks	Monitor performance against standards
	Define performance standards	Establish organizational structure	
	Develop strategies	Select and schedule staff	
	Prepare budgets		
Action items	Plan	Organize and staff	Direct; control

[a] Adapted from Fig. 1.1 of Hardwick and Morrison (27).

performed in the laboratory), and the postanalytic phase (after the test results leave the laboratory) of the test for problems. For the preanalytic phase, the laboratory provides the customer (e.g., the health care provider) with information about specimen collection and transportation, interpretation of results, and test utilization. Producing quality test results during the analytic phase is dependent upon employment of qualified staff, use of written procedures, and availability of adequate resources such as space, supplies, and equipment. During the postanalytic phase, management reviews the accuracy of the released result and its interpretation, its integration into the patient's record, and, if appropriate, the clinical relevance of the test. If the review of these processes reveals problems affecting patient care or inefficiencies, a quality assurance (QA) plan can be instituted. The QA plan should define the problem, propose changes to correct the problem, and monitor the correction process.

Improvement

Quality improvement (QI) is a management tool used to define the customer's expectations, to describe and evaluate the processes used to provide service, and to continuously improve these processes and outcomes (34). QI should focus on the customer's needs rather than process problems and should rely on training and prevention to improve service (65). After identifying the customer's needs and expectations, management describes the process that serves the customer, gathers data on how the process works, identifies areas for improvement based upon the customer's expectations, and implements solutions. Because the customer's and the organization's needs change, the laboratory must continuously monitor and improve this process.

DETERMINATION AND MANAGEMENT OF LABORATORY COSTS

Budget

The budget statement for the laboratory or a section of the laboratory can be viewed as the primary document that summarizes the fiscal management of the laboratory. The budget can be a very deceptive document in that it can create rigid guidelines for the activities of the laboratory or can be used in a more general way with the expectation that only certain predetermined goals will be reached each fiscal year. Aspects of the budget which may be critical to the laboratory have to do with who creates the document, who controls the elements therein, how the ongoing process is monitored, who is actually responsible for meeting the goals of the document, how the budget is integrated into the whole organization's budget, if at all, and how the budget is viewed by the organization as a whole. A few features of the budgetary process and the integration of cost accounting and pricing strategies for the department will be discussed in more detail. This will not be an exhaustive discussion on cost-accounting methods but rather an attempt to point out certain pitfalls in the budget process.

For many laboratories the budgeting process and final document may be imposed by individuals who are outside of the activities of the laboratory but who may have organizational responsibility to "administer the lab." One previously acceptable but now counterproductive consequence of this administrative budgetary oversight rewarded the administrator by increasing the gross revenues assigned to a particular activity. This philosophy rewarded unnecessary

utilization of laboratory activities in the past but now may produce unrealistic pricing strategies that must be corrected by the offering of deep discounts if the laboratory is to be competitive in the market. Another frequently used strategy is "reduction of costs" by making across-the-board decreases in the fiscal resources available to the laboratory. Under these circumstances it is not uncommon that each year a laboratory will be given another cost reduction "goal" that must be reached. Because the major laboratory cost is for labor, it becomes obvious that personnel must be reduced, and this often can be done only by reducing the services provided. Another less obvious consequence of budgeting from "on high" is the difficulty in justifying expenditures in the laboratory, which in the long run may be detrimental, from both quality and fiscal standpoints, to the organization as a whole. Many institutions do not recognize the interconnections of activities in different parts of the system. Such recognition is necessary so that costs can be viewed more globally rather than as being related to just one department. For example, it is possible that rearranging scheduling in the laboratory, and perhaps increasing some cost in doing so, provides laboratory results for inpatients earlier in the day and encourages earlier discharges or that, in the outpatient setting, performing more testing on-site at a greater cost permits clinicians to run their practices more efficiently. Point-of-care testing (POCT), which is more expensive than centralized testing, may be more efficient in the long run if it is used judiciously and creatively. Although these practices are most costly for the laboratory, they may provide overall savings to the institution.

Control of the budget is critical to efficient laboratory activity because repeated personnel reductions made to meet decreased budgeting goals make it virtually impossible for the laboratory to develop a strategy to integrate its activities with organizational needs and goals. For some organizations, the direct labor costs, the direct reagent costs, and the depreciation or reagent rental expenses associated with the test may be the only concerns in deriving the total direct cost of the test, but this omits significant indirect costs, which are often more difficult to identify. These indirect costs, such as space rental, utilities, insurance, and administrative salaries, occur at many organizational levels, including the specific laboratory section, the laboratory, and the institution as a whole. The laboratory rarely has an opportunity to help determine or have input into the institutional indirect costs that may be allocated directly to each test. Many budgets do not include these indirect costs, and they may not need to be included in the budgets, but they are critical when pricing strategies are used to determine competitive fees.

Superficially, it would appear that revenues could be easily defined, but in fact, for many institutions they are not. Depending on the part of the country being considered and the number of Medicare and Medicaid patients being treated, many inpatients are covered under a diagnosis-related group (DRG) global payment for their hospitalization. These payments are not broken down into each of the services provided, and it is difficult to be certain of the revenue generated by the laboratory unless the institution arbitrarily allocates some percentage of the total DRG payments as revenue to the laboratory. Other managed care payers may have more complex allocation of money for laboratory activities for inpatients, and the institution may or may not make the effort to allocate those revenues back to the laboratories. It is often easier for the institution to first determine globally the history of payment for certain health care providers. This percentage of the gross revenues collected is assigned back to the laboratory, and that constitutes the net revenue from that payer. This reimbursed revenue is then compared with the laboratory cost to determine whether or not there is a profit, if it is a for-profit institution, or a revenue margin, if it is a not-for-profit institution. These allocations back to the laboratory may have little to do with the revenues designated for laboratory activities by a particular payer. One consequence of this inadequacy of fiscal management is that the laboratory never really knows whether it is doing well or poorly in terms of reimbursement. If the institution has an expected target for a revenue margin, the laboratory may be viewed negatively when, in fact, the revenues may have been much greater than allocated, or vice versa.

Continued efforts at decreasing costs usually mean decreasing labor costs. Generally, most laboratory directors object to decreasing their labor costs because they feel that the productivity of their personnel is appropriate or the most that can be obtained from the system and that the quality of the work is satisfactory. However, each organization can benefit considerably from looking critically at those things that it does and the ways in which they are done. In the fee-for-service arena, microbiology was rewarded for doing more rather than less work. Readjusting the workload, such that clinically relevant testing is encouraged and nonrelevant testing is either discouraged or not done, can reduce labor costs with no sacrifice of quality. The quality of patient care may improve as the clinicians are presented with fewer data and more clinically appropriate information.

It is difficult to document whether test quality is affected by altering the skill mix of the laboratory personnel. The interest in developing more appropriate skill mixes has to do with trying to match individuals' experiences and educational backgrounds with the tasks that they are performing. Evaluation of the accuracy of test results produced in this environment is extremely difficult and relies very heavily on proficiency testing, which may not be the most reliable way of gauging accuracy.

Another area which may suffer from reductions in the numbers of personnel and which may be more quantitative than qualitative has to do with the availability of services. This includes both the menu of tests offered by a given laboratory and the turnaround times which can be provided by a laboratory. The need to reduce labor costs often translates quickly into reducing hours of service. When that happens, the unavailability of service to the clinicians can have patient care consequences, although they are usually difficult to document. Another area germane to cutting of labor costs is deciding whether or not one should perform a test in-house or send it out. These so-called make-buy decisions are actually very critical to most laboratory functions and are probably underused. As will be discussed shortly, many of these decisions are predicated on the test volume coming to the laboratory, an important consideration with regard to laboratory consolidation, particularly in microbiology.

Cost Accounting

Cost-accounting systems make it possible to respond to budgetary needs, and there are a variety of options available to a laboratory director. There are the more traditional cost-accounting systems, which look globally at the costs incurred for a whole section and determine the cost per test by averaging the cost versus the reported or billable results in determining a unit cost. In these systems, it is difficult to account for a number of nontesting activities such as continuing education, proficiency testing, teaching, and administrative activities. Other more focused cost-accounting methods, such as activity-based cost accounting, can help one determine the cost involved with each activity of the laboratory, but this system comes at a high price in terms of the amount of data which must be collected, stored, and manipulated in order to produce good decisions. Each institution needs to determine its specific needs, how they can best be served, and whether complex cost-accounting methods are worth it either fiscally or intellectually. A concise, laboratory-oriented guideline for cost accounting is available and should be part of each laboratory's library (46).

Laboratory Costs

The definition of direct costs attributed to laboratory tests is sometimes arbitrary, but it is essential that certain components be included. Generally, the costs of labor including benefits, supplies, and reagents, as well as some allocation for instrument depreciation, maintenance, rental, or lease costs, would be considered part of the direct cost because they can be referred back directly to testing activity. If one is involved in a reagent rental or a lease program, a specific termination clause should be included in the contract so that the contract can be canceled on short notice either to upgrade to another instrument or to change the configuration of testing to prevent monies from being committed unnecessarily to a specific instrument.

The indirect costs generally will include all other expenses necessary to do business and are not directly related to a specific instrument or test. The sources of indirect costs may come from the section where the test is being done, from the laboratory itself, or from the institution as a whole or from a network if the hospital is part of a larger group. Usually, these indirect costs are difficult to obtain and document or are part of an institutional formula that assigns some fraction of the direct cost as an indirect cost. These assignments may or may not be based on reality that is appropriate for the laboratory.

Across-the-board cutting of labor costs is not useful for cost control. The analysis of these different components requires a certain amount of experience and creative thoughtfulness as to how specific costs can be controlled or decreased. For example, significant reductions in labor costs can be achieved by readjusting the skill levels required for different processes. In this way, personnel can be used more effectively rather than insisting that all testing in all parts of the laboratory be performed by a microbiologist or medical technologist. On the other hand, labor expense such as overtime is sometimes ignored because it is considered part of the incentive for working in a particular area. Under such circumstances, it is absolutely essential that one look at the possibility of revising schedules creatively, having staff arrive earlier or later, or including as part of a 5-day work week either Saturdays or Sundays in order to decrease overtime. Some administrators are concerned about adding more personnel and would rather pay much more expensive overtime than add another full-time equivalent (FTE) or part of an FTE. Other institutions use compensatory time as a way to reduce overtime costs, but unless it is used sparingly, this can be a self-defeating maneuver. Positions must be covered, and there will have to be an expense for covering that compensatory time. Some institutions may use part-time personnel below the level at which the institution would be required to pay for benefits or at a level at which it pays for reduced levels of benefits. It is hard to know whether or not this is an appropriate solution. It should be noted that the more part-time people used, the more potential there is for increased training. Also, the use of temporary personnel gives the laboratory administration flexibility if there is the potential for future laboratory consolidation. If bargaining units are involved, there would be an opportunity for less severance pay. These attempts at reducing labor costs are often associated with increasing turnover of personnel and cause problems in some of the areas that are more difficult to staff, such as mycology, mycobacteriology, and virology.

Pricing Strategies

A brief comment about pricing strategies is relevant. In the present environment with inpatient DRG-related compensation and the possibility of outpatient prospective payment, some laboratories feel that there is less of a need to be concerned with the fee schedules that they develop. The fee schedules for laboratory testing must accomplish at least two things. First, they must be well based in the cost reality of the laboratory, and second, they must be competitive in the marketplace. Some laboratories have felt that because they have done some client's business for a long time they are immune to the possibility of losing that business. This assumption has repeatedly been proven wrong. Each laboratory needs to be cognizant of its place in the competitive market. Others have suggested that searching for the lowest cost would mean that quality would be sacrificed, but painfully little information is available to document this. The large reference laboratories have resources that permit development of sophisticated quality control systems. Even though many reference laboratories have gone through episodes of embarrassment related to inappropriate billing resulting in staggering fines, it does not follow that the quality of their work is less than that of the local community hospital. One general observation which would seem to be obvious is that it does not make sense to price laboratory tests below the prices on established fee schedules. Laboratories are not philanthropies. Also, laboratory personnel should be cognizant of the way in which the fiscal services department in their organization is applying fees to their tests. Specific formulae sometimes have been used to establish fees that have priced the laboratory out of the marketplace, yet the laboratory was unaware that this particular practice had occurred. It is therefore necessary to work with the fiscal services department to ensure good communication. It must be realized that fiscal services departments are often under great pressure to at least try to increase the gross revenues for an organization, and this is sometimes done in counterproductive ways.

Microbiology CPT Coding Changes

The latest edition of the Current Procedural Terminology (CPT) code book, *CPT 2001* (3a), has extensive changes in the coding of microbiology tests. Although the changes attempted to simplify the coding, they in fact decreased the reimbursement for some microbiology tests. In addition, they created much confusion in laboratories because of the need to change billing activities. These changes were implemented as of April 2001, and there are still interpretive issues regarding the codes.

Professional Reimbursement Issues

A topic that was raised when the Clinical Laboratory Improvement Amendments of 1988 (CLIA 88) were implemented relates to the possibility of reimbursement of Ph.D. microbiologists for consultative activity originating in the diagnostic microbiology laboratory. The Medicare and Medicaid regulations are clear that consultative activity is very restricted, must be requested by the ordering provider, and in order to be billed, must be performed by or signed by an appropriately designated physician. This has caused considerable, often understandable, angst about the recognition of the Ph.D. clinical microbiologist, who may be much better able to make the consultative statement. However, despite efforts to alter this reality, there have thus far been no changes in the regulations. This topic bears close scrutiny to see whether changes can be made in the future.

ANALYSIS OF LABORATORY ACTIVITIES

Management Techniques

The primary goal of the clinical microbiology laboratory is to provide accurate diagnostic testing and high-quality service at the lowest cost for its customers. Achieving this goal requires a detailed analysis of the laboratory's processes and products. Management must, as a first step, clearly and concisely define the laboratory's goals. These goals may include reduction of reagent and labor costs, reduction of lengths of stay for patients, improvement of productivity, improvement of turnaround times (TATs) for tests, improvement of the quality of specimens submitted, and improvement of the clinical relevance of test results.

After the laboratory's goals have been defined, the method or approach to changing the laboratory's operations must be decided. There are four broad approaches to change: (i) reengineering, (ii) downsizing or reorganizing, (iii) process improvement, and (iv) systems analysis (11, 62). The method or methods used are dictated, to some extent, by the degree and rapidity of change deemed necessary by the organization.

Reengineering is a concept that promotes a radical rethinking and redesign of the systems and processes used to produce, deliver, and support patient care. In other words, reengineering means "starting over" and developing an entirely new system, not incrementally changing the current organization. The employees must be involved in the process, and results are expected within 1 to 4 years. Generally, reengineering involves the entire laboratory (optimally, the entire organization) and critically rethinks how health care is produced and delivered. Automation, POCT, computerization, and elimination of traditional laboratory sections are all part of the process.

Downsizing or reorganizing is often considered a part of reengineering, but the approaches to achieving each one are quite different. While reengineering seeks to improve the overall quality of services, downsizing and reorganizing are usually focused on reducing costs, primarily by laying off employees. The goal of management is a quick reduction of costs, and at times this is done without a critical evaluation of the impact on the quality of services produced. It is hoped that this approach is reserved only for the management of crisis situations.

Process improvement (total quality management [TQM] or continuous quality improvement [CQI]) is now a regulatory and accreditation mandate by the Joint Commission on Accreditation of Healthcare Organizations (JCAHO) and the College of American Pathologists (CAP). The implementation of CQI can improve laboratory efficiency, effectiveness, and adaptability when the focus is on results and not on the process of CQI (47). CQI is a systematic, objective approach to improving patient care and uses a bottom-up or team approach to achieve improvements in services. It emphasizes the importance of customer-oriented planning that includes all affected parties and the continuous need to monitor and improve outcomes. The approach focuses on resource use, employee education to reduce errors and minimize delays, adaptation to customers' needs, and efficient use of employees to improve customer satisfaction and reduce costs. Because process improvement examines the performance of processes (not the performance of people) to increase customer satisfaction, it often involves multidisciplinary teams and is a continuous, ongoing exercise. CQI focuses on outcome measurements that affect patient care and seeks to change the process in order to improve outcomes and reduce costs. A number of approaches may be used to improve the processes used in the laboratory (47). The critical goal of CQI is to document that the laboratory test or procedure is clinically relevant and contributes to better patient care and better utilization of the health care resources. The analysis phase identifies the customers, the resources, and the inputs and the outputs of each laboratory activity; how activities are interrelated; and whether the activity improves customer satisfaction and outcome. The process improvement change is introduced, and the process is monitored to determine whether the change produced the desired result. Thus, CQI involves continuous cycles of improvement, which are built into the daily activities of the laboratory and organization.

The systems analysis approach focuses on improving the productivity and efficiency of the organization and reducing costs by analyzing the four basic elements of a laboratory's operation: (i) equipment and technology, (ii) human resources, (iii) reagents and supplies, and (iv) space (62). Laboratory work flow is composed to these four interrelated elements and can be analyzed by breaking the process into three components: (i) the preanalytic (prelaboratory) phase, (ii) the analytic (laboratory) phase, and (iii) the postanalytic (postlaboratory) phase (62).

The focus in the prelaboratory or preanalytic phase includes all processes that occur prior to testing of the specimen in the laboratory. The productivity and efficiency of laboratory operations during this phase can be improved by developing criteria for test selection and utilization through consultation with the health care providers involved (critical pathways); optimization of the collection, transport, and storage of specimens; definition of specimen acceptability; and definition of the tests that are offered. Strategies for controlling test utilization are the most effective means of controlling inappropriate test requests.

The focus in the laboratory or analytic phase is generally on reducing TATs and test costs. Batch processing may negatively affect patient care by causing delays, and better service is obtained with continuous processing. However, this may not be cost-effective. Newer state-of-the-art equipment and technology must be evaluated as to whether it will reduce laboratory reagent and labor costs, reduce TATs, and significantly improve patient care (i.e., whether it will reduce the length of stay and improve test sensitivity and specificity and whether it is clinically relevant). Some questions that must be addressed prior to purchase or implementation include the cost per test, space and staffing

requirements, maintenance, and customer needs. Also, the microbiology tests to be performed (i.e., organism workup, identification, and antimicrobial susceptibility testing) need to be defined for the specimen type and body site to improve the medical relevance of the information produced (71).

The focus in the postlaboratory or postanalytic phase involves the review and reporting of test results. Efficiencies in TAT and ease of access are accomplished with computerized reporting, in which abnormal results are highlighted and an interpretation of the results may be provided. Feedback to the ordering providers on the cost of their overall laboratory utilization may help reduce excessive or inappropriate test requests.

Because labor accounts for 60 to 80% of all direct laboratory costs, increased attention is being focused on improving employee productivity. In general, productivity is most influenced by the work methods and processes, the position description, the facilities layout, personnel scheduling, and material flow (63). Productivity can be improved by increasing the number of tests performed per individual, decreasing the effort necessary to produce the test, and increasing the quality of the test or service with the same effort. Often, productivity improvement is achieved by simply reducing the number of staff. However, other methods, such as changing the staffing mix, consolidating supervisory positions, scheduling more efficiently, eliminating unnecessary and labor-intensive tests, prioritizing or consolidating testing, removing overlapping functions, and providing employee incentives, are available to increase productivity.

Test Utilization Management

In this era of reduced reimbursement for health care services, the laboratory should attempt to manage test utilization to improve patient care practices and laboratory efficiency and to reduce both laboratory and other patient care costs (51, 64, 66). Reductions in the numbers of low-cost tests performed do not significantly lower laboratory or overall costs. Efforts to decrease test utilization should target high-cost and outsourced tests and repetitive testing for inpatients. Repetitive testing may be decreased by the use of an immediate, computer-based intervention informing the health care provider that the test order is redundant (10). Also, tests that produce predictable or questionable results are not an effective use of resources. One means of controlling test utilization is the establishment of a "gatekeeper," who in the larger organization is usually the patient's primary care physician. However, as part of its function the gatekeeper must ensure participation of the laboratory to ensure the use of the least expensive and most clinically relevant test necessary to appropriately manage the patient. If this strategy is to be successful, a consensus must be developed between the medical staff and the laboratory as to the appropriate clinical practice guidelines that should commonly be followed on the basis of the severity and acuteness of the disease process. A well-constructed clinical practice guideline is one that (i) specifies the types of professionals involved in development of the guideline, (ii) defines the strategy and grades the evidence used to produce the guideline, and (iii) provides clear grading of the recommendations (26). Factors that promote acceptance of clinical practice guidelines include regular updating of the guideline, support of the system's opinion leaders, and one-on-one interaction with the users. It is important to remember that the education involved in this process must be bidirectional. The laboratory must comprehend the needs of the medical staff, and the medical staff in turn must understand the laboratory's need to reduce costs without decreasing the quality of testing. This process requires commitment by both groups and must involve the senior staff, long-term rather than short-term interventions, and a mix of strategies (38).

A method of cost reduction that is often tried but that is difficult to achieve is modification of the test-ordering patterns of health care providers (18). The most effective approaches to modifying test utilization are (i) clinical and financial feedback, (ii) education by local experts, and (iii) rationing of care and testing (66). The clinical and financial feedback method informs the physician of his or her test utilization pattern compared to those of his or her peers, the cost of that testing, and the reimbursement received by the hospital. The education approach involves lectures, discussions, written material (e.g., clinical pathways and guidelines or standard protocols), and interpretive laboratory reporting that provides clinically useful information and that addresses the clinical relevance of a particular test. To be effective, the education must be continuous and originate from clinical opinion leaders in the organization or community. Lastly, for the rationing of patient care or testing to be successful, it must be physician directed and consensus among the members of this group must be achieved.

Approaches to Cost Containment in the Clinical Microbiology Laboratory

The following discussion of cost reduction in the clinical microbiology laboratory is not meant to be all inclusive or a mandate for all laboratories. Rather, it is meant to stimulate discussion between clinicians and the clinical microbiologist for implementation of cost-effective, clinically relevant policies. Cost-contaminant policies will not be identical for all laboratories because policies are affected by the patient mix, the needs of the customers, and the form of reimbursement. McLaughlin (37) has published a 10-point plan for the "implementation of cost-effective, clinically relevant diagnostic microbiology policies" that clearly identifies the process that should be followed. A modified version follows:

1. Base changes on published data and opinions of respected experts.
2. Supplement the changes with in-house data when possible.
3. Secure support for the changes from the infectious diseases service.
4. Discuss in advance the changes with the affected groups or the most influential users in the groups.
5. Educate potential users who will be affected by the change.
6. Announce the proposed changes by a means that will reach most users.
7. Educate the technologists who will implement the change.
8. Revise laboratory procedure manuals.
9. Provide users with a mechanism to override the changes in special situations.
10. Provide explanations to users who are uninformed or opposed to the changes.

All major changes are difficult, require a collaborative effort between the laboratory and medical staff, and must have the overall support of the organization's administration (7, 66). It is important for the customer to recognize that the change will improve the overall quality of patient care and is not only a cost reduction for the laboratory. Areas of operations in the clinical microbiology laboratory that may provide opportunities for some cost containment or reduction include (i) automation, (ii) alternative technology or methods, (iii) specimen acceptability, and (iv) extent of specimen workup and organism identification. Cost reduction from volume aggregation through consolidation or merger of laboratories is discussed elsewhere in this chapter.

Automation

Automation is generally thought to be the process that reduces the laboratory's labor costs. In fact, automation tends to redistribute the workload and minimize future staff increases but may not result in an absolute reduction of staffing (62). In some situations, automation may allow the use of lower-salaried employees. The most efficient use of automation occurs when it is interfaced with the laboratory or hospital computer. For automation to be effective, there must be sufficient volume to support its use, the automation must support the pattern of demand and laboratory practice, and, in most cases, the automation must replace a traditional test method, not add to the test menu. Although the clinical microbiology laboratory remains highly labor intensive, automated or semiautomated instruments are available for blood cultures, mycobacterial cultures and susceptibility testing, bacterial susceptibility testing and identification, specimen plating, molecular diagnostics, and immunological or serological testing. Overall cost economies for the health care system may be realized when the test results are rapidly available to the health care provider such that the length of stay is shortened or appropriate therapy is instituted (6, 21).

Alternative Technology or Methods

Traditional multistep methods, procedures, and approaches used for the laboratory diagnosis of infectious diseases need to be replaced by more rapid and accurate tests that reduce overall costs. For example, laboratories might initially test stool specimens submitted for ovum and parasite (O&P) examinations only for *Giardia* and *Cryptosporidium* by an immunoassay. The need for additional testing would be based on the results of the initial test. In addition, the use of rapid, single-substrate, or analyte tests and skilled microbiologists can result in the provision of clinically relevant results in a cost-effective and timely manner (8, 50).

Molecular diagnostics (including DNA chips and microarrays) and other nonculture methods will significantly alter the practice of clinical microbiology over the next decade. However, management must assess the costs of these new test methods in light of the impact on patient care. For example, the use of nucleic acid amplification techniques for the diagnosis of tuberculosis may decrease the time required to detect a positive specimen (with potential savings from exposure costs and additional testing) but significantly increase the cost for the detection of each new case (22). For laboratories that serve a population with a low prevalence of disease, the increased cost may not be justified. However, the increased costs of these tests may be minimized by use of algorithms to identify the specimens that should be tested by the costly tests (14).

Specimen Acceptability

The laboratory can improve the quality of test results and reduce costs by accepting only specimens that are properly collected, transported, and labeled and that are appropriate for the laboratory diagnosis of an infectious disease. The following discussion identifies some general areas of specimen processing where modification of traditional procedures can improve the clinical relevance of microbiological test results, reduce costs, and reduce unnecessary work. Specific information is found in references 24, 55, and 70 (see also chapter 6).

Blood Cultures

Significant data exist regarding the appropriate number of blood samples for culture collected per septic episode, the volume of blood cultured, and the necessity for including an anaerobic blood bottle in the set. As a general rule, no more than two or three blood samples should be submitted per septic episode, with each sample for culture consisting of 20 to 30 ml of blood. Additional samples may need to be cultured for a patient with culture-negative endocarditis or to recover a fastidious microorganism. An anaerobic blood bottle may not be routinely required for each set of cultures, but this should be assessed by each laboratory. Most bacterial pathogens are recovered from blood cultures within 4 or 5 days (71). Bacteremia caused by *Mycobacterium avium* complex can be detected in 85 to 90% of patients with one blood culture, and *M. avium* complex organisms are recovered from nearly 100% of patients with two blood cultures (57, 72). Aerobic blood cultures are adequate for the recovery of most common *Candida* species, but other methods are necessary for recovery of the filamentous fungi (71). One approach to reducing patient care costs is to decrease the number of contaminated blood cultures by use of a dedicated team for blood collections, to use tincture of iodine disinfectant, and to track the contamination rate for each team member.

CSF Specimens

Many bacterial antigen tests are marketed because a rapid and accurate diagnosis of bacterial meningitis is essential for the patient's survival. In general, these tests have not proven to be cost-effective and should not be performed routinely. Bacterial antigen testing may be helpful when the cell count in cerebrospinal fluid (CSF) is abnormal, the Gram stain is negative, and the patient has been treated with antimicrobial agents.

Because tuberculous meningitis is rare is the United States, cultures of CSF for *Mycobacterium tuberculosis* should be performed only when the cell count and the protein and glucose levels in the CSF are consistent with meningitis (2). The laboratory should recommend the collection of ≥5 ml (and, optimally, 10 to 20 ml) of CSF for recovery of *M. tuberculosis* (2, 35).

Neurosyphilis is also infrequently diagnosed in the United States. Therefore, the Venereal Disease Research Laboratory tests should be performed with CSF specimens only when the patient has documented *Treponema pallidum* infection (e.g., a positive serum rapid plasma reagin or fluorescent treponemal antibody absorption test result or a positive result by dark-field examination of an appropriate lesion) and the patient's CSF has abnormalities consistent with neurosyphilis (3). These screening approaches can significantly decrease the number of inappropriate tests performed for the diagnosis of neurosyphilis and tuberculous meningitis.

Stool Cultures and O&P Examinations

It is now accepted laboratory practice to reject for culture and O&P examination stool specimens collected after the patient has been hospitalized for 3 or 4 days (30). The appropriate number of specimens required to detect pathogens in stool specimens is somewhat more controversial. Valenstein et al. (67) currently recommend the use of one or two specimens for the detection of bacterial pathogens and two or three specimens for the detection of stool parasites in a routine workup. Other recommendations include the use of immunological methods that detect specific parasites such as *Giardia, Cryptosporidium,* and *Entamoeba histolytica* in place of the traditional method of concentration and microscopy (25). If the results of these initial tests are negative, a decision for ordering a complete workup for O&P would be determined (30).

For the detection of *Clostridium difficile* disease by a toxin assay, Hines and Nachamkin (30) suggest that testing of two or three specimens obtained over several days is adequate. The second or third specimen is tested only after the prior specimens are determined to be negative. Almost by definition, testing of formed stool specimens is unacceptable in the management of diarrhea, regardless of whether the etiologic agent sought is a parasite or bacterium (including *C. difficile*). However, formed stools may be cultured in order to identify individuals who may be carriers.

Respiratory Cultures

The approach of screening sputum specimens by Gram staining and rejecting specimens on the basis of the relative proportion of leukocytes and squamous epithelial cells is a routine and accepted practice (9, 42). A similar approach is used to screen respiratory secretions collected by endotracheal suction. Morris et al. (40) recommended that specimens collected by endotracheal suction be rejected if more than 10 epithelial cells per low-power field are observed or if no bacteria are seen on the Gram-stained smear. Generally, no more than one sputum specimen should be cultured every 24 to 48 h (71).

Wound, Tissue, and Body Fluid Cultures

The medium inoculated and the length of incubation should be based on the type of specimen submitted and the pathogen(s) sought. Most fungal isolates, with the exception of the dimorphic fungi, are recovered from routine fungal cultures within 14 days (41). The routine use of broth medium for cultures of wound specimens primarily recovers contaminants and does not generally produce clinically useful information (41, 56). However, a broth medium should be inoculated for tissue specimens, CSF specimens from patients with a CSF shunt, and continuous ambulatory peritoneal dialysis fluid specimens (39, 41).

Extent of Workup

Clinical microbiologists have struggled when attempting to define the extent of the workup that should be performed with a specimen. In the past a more complete workup of specimens has contributed to our understanding of the disease process, provided the evidence for the nosocomial spread of organisms within the hospital, and led to the recovery of "new" pathogens and emerging antimicrobial resistance. However, given the current limited resources and cost-containment dictates, the clinician and clinical microbiologist must now determine the clinical importance of the test results produced. Although there are few published data on this topic, a great need exists to achieve a consensus between the laboratory and health care providers.

In determining the extent of the workup, the following factors should be considered: (i) the immune status of the patient, (ii) the severity of the disease, (iii) the type of specimen submitted, (iv) the etiologic agents sought, and (v) the clinical management of the patient. For example, tissue obtained from organ transplantation patients should be more thoroughly evaluated than a clean-catch urine sample submitted from an outpatient with uncomplicated cystitis. The laboratory's goal is to minimize the expenditure of resources producing results of questionable or easily predictable medical value in order to maximize the effort expended on more clinically relevant specimens.

Factors that need to be defined for the different specimen types include (i) the number of different organisms worked up per specimen, (ii) the organisms that require a susceptibility test, (iii) the method of identification, (iv) the testing of replicate specimens from the same patient, and (v) the frequency of repeat susceptibility tests with organisms recovered in subsequent specimens. In general, there is little need to identify or perform susceptibility tests on greater than two gram-negative rods recovered from sputum, two predominant bacteria recovered from a clean-catch urine specimen, or multiple isolates recovered from superficial wounds. Duplicate specimens such as urine, sputum, or stool specimens for detection of C. difficile probably should not be cultured or tested if they are received within 72 h of the time that the initial specimen was positive. Identification and susceptibility tests are generally not performed more frequently than every 3 to 5 days with isolates recovered from the same anatomical site. Spot tests (e.g., indole, oxidase, and catalase tests), pigment, colony morphology, and odor can be used to identify isolates recovered from nonsterile sites such as sputum, urine, or superficial wounds (5, 29, 50). Organisms of little clinical relevance in the disease process should not be worked up without consultation with the laboratory director (13). For example, Haemophilus spp., Corynebacterium spp., and gram-negative rods recovered from cultures of throat swab specimens are not usually associated with pharyngitis and should not be identified. Other considerations include limiting the identification of yeasts and anaerobes from most body sources, eliminating the serotyping of Salmonella isolates (these should be submitted to the state health laboratory), and reporting of coagulase-negative staphylococci from urine or a single blood bottle without further identification. Because outpatients are generally treated empirically, the susceptibilities of urine isolates of Escherichia coli, Proteus spp., Klebsiella spp., and Enterococcus spp.; respiratory isolates of Haemophilus spp. and Moraxella catarrhalis; and genital isolates of Neisseria gonorrhoeae are not usually determined. Laboratories may save these isolates for up to 7 days in the event that a workup is required.

Waived Tests, Provider-Performed Microscopy, and POCT

The waiver of a laboratory test permits the test to be performed without having to meet national personnel, QA, and proficiency testing standards and requires only minimal regulatory oversight. The availability of waived testing and provider-performed microscopy has created an upsurge in POCT in hospitals, clinics, and work sites. POCT is a major

force today in the decentralization of the laboratory. At present, one of four laboratory tests is done by POCT, and the use of POCT is increasing at a rate of 12 to 16% per year (16). The use of POCT for microbiology procedures has and will continue to increase as more procedures are created in formats that can yield high-quality results with a minimum of technical expertise and at a reasonable cost. In addition to moving tests from the laboratory to the bedside, waived tests are moving to the work site (e.g., screening for drugs of abuse) and locations of convenience (e.g., non-hospital-based pharmacies). The potential size of this market guarantees continuous investment in new device concepts and technologies. A list of tests with waived status from the Food and Drug Administration can be found at http://www.accessdata.fda.gov/scripts/cdrh/cfdocs/cfClia/testswaived.cfm or http://www.cap.org/html/lip/waived.html.

The trend toward more home testing, outpatient and home care treatment, and shorter hospitalizations promotes POCT. The ability to provide a sensitive and specific test result, particularly in the outpatient environment, where the patient is available for immediate therapy, is an anticipated goal. At present, only a few microbial antigen or antibody tests are available for use in the setting where waived tests are exclusively performed. Many of the microbiology kits that have been granted waived status are, in fact, less sensitive than the tests routinely performed in the microbiology laboratory. This raises some serious questions regarding the diagnostic accuracies of these tests, the competency of the user, reimbursement for the test, and oversight for performing adequate quality control (QC) and entering the test result into the patient's medical file. The use of these tests may promote cost savings as a result of decreased hospital stays, elimination of additional testing, use of appropriate drugs, and lower labor costs. Often, however, POCT increases overall costs because it becomes an additional service and not a replacement for other laboratory testing.

QUALITY ASSESSMENT AND CONTROL

Basic Quality Assessment Concepts

In general, QA attempts to identify, monitor, evaluate, and improve practices related to patient care. In the past, QA focused on problem finding. Now the focus of quality care has shifted to quality assessment and QI, which, in addition to problem identification, emphasize methods that improve practices. As these quality management concepts matured, the emphasis in the 1990s shifted toward satisfying the needs of the customers through CQI.

CQI is both an organizational philosophy and a systematic process that promotes the enhancement of patient outcomes by measuring customer satisfaction (47). CQI identifies problems that need immediate resolution and seeks to improve processes that are not current problems but that may improve customer satisfaction. Overall, CQI is one approach to managing resources in the constantly changing health care environment.

TQM is a system of managerial programs that includes (i) team management, (ii) plans management, and (iii) improvement management (47). These programs provide the processes by which CQI can be implemented and maintained. All three TQM programs are interrelated, and the success of this approach depends upon the sharing of information by the three programs.

The team management program emphasizes team decision making through leadership skills, education, and delegation of responsibility. This program assesses morale, work attitude, and decision-making skills; provides the support needed to improve these attitudes and skills; and monitors the team's success in these areas. The goal of the team management program is the continuous improvement of employee decision making, which enhances external customer satisfaction. The team management program, if successful, must provide employees with team skills training that may include conflict resolution, motivation, empowerment, opportunity identification, customer-oriented planning, and decision making.

The plans management program strives to improve the organizational process through anticipatory planning consisting of four phases:

Phase 1: Organizational direction
Based on current and future customer needs identified through analysis of data.

Phase 2: Strategic prioritization
Prioritize goals on the basis of the available resources, analysis of the organization's strengths and weaknesses, and external market opportunities. May prioritize by short-, medium-, or long-range goals.

Phase 3: Action planning
Implement the priorities by identifying the goal objectives and tasks and assigning these items to an individual(s).

Phase 4: Action follow-up
Evaluate the actions in improving customer satisfaction and correct the actions when necessary.

The improvement management program achieves CQI through ongoing quality surveillance and identification of current problems as well as processes that will improve customer satisfaction. The program identifies quality indicators or monitors (e.g., specimen acceptability, appropriateness of test utilization, accuracy and timeliness of reports, and customer perceptions); collects and evaluates the data; takes appropriate action to improve the process; and lastly, assesses the effectiveness of the action (52). The first critical step of the improvement management program is to reach a consensus among the customers as to the importance of the monitors or indicators selected. The success of a CQI program rests upon the commitment of the organization's leadership to the concept and to providing the necessary resources to implement the program.

Basic QC Concepts and Guidelines

QC is a concept that includes evaluating product performance, comparing this performance to stated goals, and taking action when the product fails. In the microbiology laboratory, the accuracy of the test information is dependent upon the specimen quality; the correlation of the test method with clinical data; the performance of test procedures, personnel, media, reagents, and instruments; and the method for the reporting of results. The QC program is designed to continuously monitor these elements, identify problems in test performance or process, and correct the problems. Documentation is the cornerstone of a QC program; and all methods, policies, test results, and corrective actions must be recorded. As a minimum, microbiology QC programs should address the following elements: (i) test methods and procedures, (ii) verification and validation of

tests, (iii) content of procedure manuals, (iv) content and storage of records and reports, (v) competency of personnel, (vi) proficiency testing, and (vii) laboratory error.

Test Methods and Procedures

A QC program monitors, evaluates, and documents the performance of all aspects of a test procedure. This includes the quality of the specimen; the performance of reagents, media, and instruments; and the review of test results for errors. Appropriately collected and transported specimens are essential for quality microbiology results. Processing of unsuitable specimens may produce misleading results. The laboratory must specify for the customer (i.e., the health care provider) the appropriate techniques for the collection and transportation of specimens as well as the volume and number of specimens necessary to ensure the reliability of the test result (55) (see chapter 6). Elements of the collection process that can be monitored include volume (e.g., the volume of CSF submitted for multiple cultures and the volume of blood submitted for cultures); the number of specimens (e.g., the number of stool specimens for the detection of diarrheal pathogens); the quality of the specimens (e.g., sputum); and rates of contamination of blood, body fluids, and urine specimens (53). The laboratory should monitor the quality of specimens received and be proactive in improving performance.

Reagents, supplies, and stains are labeled to indicate identity, concentration, storage requirements, preparation and expiration dates, and, if applicable, the type of safety hazard associated with their use. In general, negative and positive controls are required for qualitative tests (e.g., catalase and oxidase tests), and two controls with different titers or concentrations are necessary for quantitative tests (e.g., serology). The QC strains, frequency of testing, and expected results can be found elsewhere (53, 54).

Commercially prepared media that are quality controlled by the manufacturer and listed in the NCCLS publication M22-A2 (44) are exempt from QC by the user except to verify that the media are not dehydrated, hemolyzed, cracked, contaminated, or filled improperly. The manufacturers' quality assurance procedures are listed in publication M22-A2 (44).

Equipment maintenance and function checks are performed and documented as specified by the manufacturer or as established by the user to guarantee accurate test results. These records are retained for the life of the equipment.

The quality and medical relevance of the microbial test information are dependent upon the timeliness and accuracy of the reports. The laboratory should establish clinically useful TATs for critical tests such as body fluid smears, acid-fast bacillus smears, and cultures (53) through consensus of those involved in patient management. When possible, TAT begins with the collection of the specimen and ends when the result is used for patient care. The final report is checked for clerical and computer errors by comparison to the laboratory work card and instrument logs. When an error is detected after the final report is released, the revised report should provide the correct information but must not delete the original error. Clinically significant changes of the test result in the report should be conveyed immediately to the physician. When an error is found, policies and procedures should be modified, if warranted, to prevent recurrences.

Verification and Validation of Tests

New test methods of high complexity must be verified for accuracy and precision before they are used for patient testing, and the laboratory must validate existing methods (23). Verification demonstrates that the laboratory can reproduce the manufacturer's claims or that the new method compares favorably with an accepted reference method. Validation of an existing verified test documents that the test continues to perform satisfactorily on the basis of QC data, proficiency testing, and correlation with clinical data.

Content of Procedure Manuals

The laboratory's policy and procedure manual must contain all material relevant to the operation of the laboratory and production of patients' test results. The procedure's format, where appropriate, should generally adhere to the recommendations specified in NCCLS publication GP2-A3 (45). All original procedures and revisions must be dated, approved, and signed by the current laboratory director. The manual should be readily available to the staff and reviewed annually. Procedures that are no longer in use must be retained for at least 2 years.

Content and Storage of Records and Reports

The laboratory must maintain sufficient records to document all aspects of testing performed on a patient's specimen. The test requisition should contain the patient's name or identifier, the date of collection of the specimen, the date that the specimen was received in the laboratory, the name of the test requester, and the test requested. The procedures performed on the specimen, the personnel performing the test, communication with the requester, and the results obtained should be documented. The final test report also contains the name and address of the laboratory performing the test, appropriate reference ranges, and test interpretation. All records and reports are retained for at least 2 years.

Competency of Personnel

CLIA 88 define the personnel requirements for microbiology laboratories on the basis of a complexity test model (28). Because CLIA 88 reduced the educational requirements for laboratory personnel, annual documentation of the competency of personnel to perform microbiology tests is required, regardless of the individual's experience and education. Written training methods are advised for new employees and for the retraining of other employees (23, 43). The competency of experienced microbiologists may be verified by review of work cards, interpretation of unknowns, the use of proficiency samples, direct observation, or a written examination. The competency information, the annual performance appraisal, past training and certification, and continuing education experiences should be retained in the individual's personnel folder.

Proficiency Testing

All microbiology laboratories must participate in an external proficiency program approved by the U.S. Department of Health and Human Services that reflects the laboratory's specialty and level of expertise (28). Proficiency testing (PT) is a tool that can be used to assess a laboratory's performance compared to the performance of its peers and should be part of the laboratory's CQI program. Limitations of PT are that it addresses only the analytic phase of patient testing and that it may be affected by variables not related to routine testing of patient specimens (48). Some of the approved PT programs are listed elsewhere (53). Sanctions may be imposed on laboratories that fail to submit correct responses for at least 80% of the test samples for two of three testing events.

A voluntary program that may be used in the laboratory's CQI program is Q-Probes, a national interlaboratory program developed by CAP (4). Participants conduct QA studies and receive a critique of the results and recommendations for improving patient testing.

Laboratory Errors

The Institute of Medicine has issued two reports that promise to have an effect on the health care system as we know it. The first report, *To Err Is Human: Building a Safer Health System* (30a), details the frequency of errors associated with the provision of medical care. It has been suggested that this is somewhat of a self-serving, alarmist report, but there is no question that errors do occur, and most laboratories have little or no knowledge of the frequency of errors. Most errors detected relate to preanalytical mix-ups and, occasionally, postanalytical reporting errors that are brought to the laboratory's attention by a puzzled provider. In general, analytical errors are unusual. All laboratories must be diligent in studying the reasons for any inappropriate, unexpected, or questioned result. It is hoped that more sophisticated software programs will help identify unusual results, but most importantly, we must rely on the training, expertise, and professionalism of dedicated laboratory personnel to keep the error rate as close to zero as possible.

The second report, *Crossing the Quality Chasm: A New Health System for the 21st Century* (30b), proposes an overhaul of the entire health care system during the next decade. The emphasis will be on QI of the system through a set of performance expectations, the establishment of new rules to guide patient-clinician relationships, reduction of medical errors and waste, promotion of evidence-based practice, and development of transparent clinical information systems. To gauge improvement in the system, it will be necessary to establish programs to monitor and track performance. In many ways, laboratories have begun this process with the establishment of occurrence logs (for the recording of errors and problems) and determination of solutions through the use of approaches such as root-cause analysis and the use of outcome measurements. More information on the Institute of Medicine's reports can be found at http://www.iom.edu.

ISSUES AFFECTING LABORATORY MANAGEMENT

Health Care Practices

The remarkable changes that have occurred in our health care delivery system in the last decade and particularly in the last 5 years need no specific documentation. It is necessary to reduce the increasing cost of health care, which presently uses approximately one-seventh of the gross national product. The attempts to alter the delivery, reimbursement, extent, and quality of health care have created many varied initiatives that would have been thought impossible not long ago. For example, serious controversy exists regarding the utilization of limited health care resources, and in some states, such as Oregon, there have been legislative initiatives to expand health care to more state citizens. With fixed fiscal resources, legislative solutions have mandated rationing of clinical and laboratory services (12). There exists the conundrum that with decreasing resources, it is hoped that there can be increasing productivity without any compromise in quality. Little information is available on exactly how successful the resolutions of these competing forces are. Health care systems are merging and consolidating, and the numbers of laboratories in physicians' offices and hospitals are decreasing. In the laboratory community, there is considerable concern that patient care will be compromised as specimens are transported to centralized laboratories, but often, these concerns are mainly focused on the loss of jobs and changes from traditional patterns of behavior.

In the area of clinical microbiology there have been attempts to reduce costs by providing more clinically relevant activities. Doing fewer cultures may reduce costs, but as the volume decreases the unit cost increases. Whereas it is obvious in clinical chemistry and hematology that increased volume is associated with decreased costs because automated instrumentation can be used more efficiently, similar changes are not so obvious in clinical microbiology. A few general statements about changing patterns of practice are necessary. First, there will be continuing pressure to reduce laboratory services, which will decrease the test volume for any given laboratory discipline. Second, the reduction in testing is not necessarily a malevolent product of this process, since it must be remembered that we are leaving an era where excessive and often unnecessary testing was fiscally rewarded. Third, there is a great interest in using new technological methods to solve old problems. The mere fact that testing can be done by new methods does not mean that it should be done that way or that it is more cost-effective. Some molecular techniques have extraordinary sensitivities and specificities. However, their costs may well preclude their routine use. Finally, patients are viewed as customers or covered lives, and the laboratory must understand the marketing initiatives that go along with that philosophy.

Consolidation of clinical microbiological laboratories will be discussed from the standpoint of a general conceptual framework as well as personal experience. Consolidation has obvious advantages and a number of potential disadvantages. First, in terms of the advantages of consolidation, the aggregation of volume must be of paramount consideration. Aggregation of volume allows the laboratory to consider the use of multiple diagnostic approaches including potential instrumentation that would otherwise be too costly. More important is the opportunity to decrease reagent costs, increase the skills of personnel, and enhance the efficiency of personnel by working with a larger volume of material. Although the technologist or microbiologist who works with a wide variety of culture specimens as a daily occurrence may find it somewhat more interesting, the ability to concentrate on different specimen types for blocks of time can create a more efficient work flow. Second, consolidation allows a focusing and concentration of intellectual resources in one area. We are fast approaching the time when every laboratory will not have internal to its workforce the expertise needed to provide a high quality of work in all the diverse areas of clinical microbiology. The attempts to maintain this type of a workforce, particularly one that works with small volumes of specimens, as in mycology, mycobacteriology, or virology, often result in the establishment of very inefficient work patterns and encourage the evolution of inefficient performance by these expert

individuals. This focusing of expert resources occurs both at the bench level and at the management level. It is becoming much more difficult to argue that a medium-sized city can justify having more than one centralized community clinical microbiology laboratory. It makes little sense to have these highly trained expert individuals processing specimens when they could be spending their time in the actual evaluation of problem organisms or helping the providers understand the meaning of test results. A third advantage of a consolidated laboratory is that it helps the member organizations develop similar practice patterns for use of the laboratory. These practice patterns should extend to the use of pharmaceutical agents as well, and the more rational interaction between institutions as they use some of these expensive agents not only will decrease operation costs but, more importantly, can also increase the quality of care at each of the institutions. A fourth advantage is that laboratory services performed by more qualified individuals can be made available over longer time frames. With the consolidated laboratory, particularly with creative scheduling, considerable expertise can be made available at all times or at least can quickly be obtained at unusual times. A final general advantage to the consolidation of laboratories is the ability to more constructively interact with the providers in terms of helping both in the definition of appropriate specimens and in the interpretation of the results for those specimens. There is great pressure for health care delivery systems to use individuals, both physicians and nonphysicians, who are much more generalist in their training and experience and who are therefore realistically less able to keep up with all of the nuances and changes which keep occurring in terms of both the diagnostic statements and the therapeutic consequences which are inherent in the clinical microbiology results. Although physician and nonphysician practitioners are trained with the goal of creating a better clinical environment for the patient at lower cost, the training cannot realistically be expected to necessarily increase the quality of care for the patient. It would seem that the laboratory has an opportunity to play a critical role in helping these providers by pooling laboratory expertise and providing higher-quality laboratory services. Some have suggested that specialists, such as infectious disease specialists, will suffer as the laboratory assumes a more proactive role in this interaction with the providers. It is not at all obvious that this will be the case. Infectious disease specialists are under great pressure to decrease their training programs, just as is the case with most specialists. As a consequence, it would seem to be necessary to use those expert individuals in complex clinical situations rather than assume that each unusual organism or strange antibiogram necessarily demands their attention.

Consolidation of laboratories, particularly the clinical microbiology laboratory, is occurring in some geographic areas and may well become more common. The cost of individual microbiology laboratories will stress the health care delivery system, but it is also important that some of the problems associated with consolidation be identified. In our experience, the first and most important problem to be overcome is that of trust between different institutions. Each institution has its own tradition, and usually associated with that tradition is a certain understanding, rightly or wrongly, of how other institutions have acted. The tendency to be competitive rather than cooperative is powerful, and the ability to remember anecdotes that place potential partners in a negative light occurs frequently.

Laboratory directors must interact with each other in a way that creates and fosters professionalism and educational opportunities rather than in a way that detracts from these necessary ventures. The consolidation can occur as a consequence of the coming together of parties with a strong will and cooperative vision, or it can occur when a large group comes in and imposes the consolidation on laboratories. When consolidation happens, there usually is great dislocation, but it is our observation that the ensuing consolidation does not create the clinical havoc that most of the participants predict. Second, a very important aspect of consolidation is the infrastructure that allows the movement of specimens from one point to another. The cost of creating this infrastructure can be considerable. In any evaluation of a merger or consolidation, this issue must be considered very seriously. The more institutions that participate in the courier or transfer service, the greater the ability to distribute transportation costs over a wider base and the smaller the added cost per test. There needs to be retention of some of the "stat" functions at each institution, such as Gram staining of smears and rapid antigen testing, but these should be kept to a minimum, with the majority of testing being done at the centralized laboratory. Third, a considerable problem of consolidation has to do with information exchange. Most institutions are not apt to have the same laboratory information system (LIS), and even if they do have similar systems, they may have different file structures that make the interface between them cumbersome. The goal is an integrated LIS for the network. The considerable cost needs to be clearly identified and then appropriately amortized over the time necessary to get a more cost-effective interaction. Fourth, during consolidation there will of necessity be a reduction in personnel. It makes no sense to consolidate and keep all existing positions. If a consolidation is structured such that there is no reduction of personnel, then one needs to look very seriously at what is being accomplished or who is designing the system. Another cost of consolidation relates to the severance packages that may be necessary, particularly if bargaining units are involved, and this expense needs to be calculated as well.

Technology

In microbiology laboratories that have semiautomated or automated blood culture systems and/or identification and antibiotic susceptibility testing instruments, the instruments may have excess capacity. Consolidation of this excess capacity at a central facility can be a real efficiency, and the ability to decrease the cost of the reagents represents further savings. It is difficult to know exactly where diagnostic microbiology will be moving in the next few years, although many soothsayers predict that molecular diagnostics will replace more traditional methods. It is obvious that in the area of molecular diagnostics there will be opportunities for more sophisticated diagnoses; but with the very considerable pressure on cost containment, it is not clear that these methodologies will be as useful as most proponents would suggest. Unless the costs of molecular diagnostic procedures fall considerably and approach the costs of current procedures, they will continue to be used only very selectively and be confined to a few reference laboratories. The use of robot-based techniques in microbiology will be limited to a relatively few very large volume laboratories.

Workforce Issues

The final concern described in this section has to do with workforce issues. The greatest cost for all laboratories is labor, and therefore, the desire to decrease labor requirements receives much attention. Often, this attention is misdirected in terms of global reductions in labor costs with perhaps some kind of hoped-for increased efficiency. It is our observation that productivity is a considerable variable in individual laboratories; each laboratory defends its traditional productivity. There are few published productivity benchmarks that a manager can use to counsel employees. The attempt to document expectations should be considered more than just an inconvenience but as an adjunct to work guidelines. Most laboratory managers have not been effective in clearly defining expectations for both their supervisory and technical personnel.

A corollary to decreasing FTEs is the popular concept of defining skill mix needs. This is intended to have individuals with various levels of training doing activities that are commensurate with that training. The smaller the laboratory, the more difficult it is to realize efficiencies in this realm, since the use of individuals with less training decreases considerably the flexibility within the whole laboratory environment. The consequence is that highly trained medical technologists and microbiologists may perform tasks, particularly in the processing arena, which do not require their level of skill. The laboratory may struggle with this concept, as it is sometimes difficult to clearly define expectations based on educational background. For example, some individuals with a very modest educational background who are well motivated and have had good on-the-job training are able to easily perform many tasks otherwise assigned to a medical technologist or a microbiology specialist.

Another area of considerable interest is that of cross training of personnel to do a variety of functions either within the laboratory or between the laboratory and other departments such as radiology and perhaps electrocardiography. The advantages of cross training usually are more obvious in smaller hospitals, where a case can be made for the necessity of training individuals in this way. In larger laboratories there is resistance on the part of the medical technologists to perform tasks in areas other than those for which they have had most of their training. The reading of a Gram-stained smear by anyone other than a microbiology technologist may be met with resistance, and the microbiologist may not be able to function adequately in other areas of the laboratory. This is not to say that in appropriate circumstances both cross training and evaluation of skill mix needs are not appropriate goals for the manager. However, the situations for which these techniques are used need to be very carefully defined, and appropriate training programs must be implemented.

Each laboratory must establish its own policies regarding optimal use of its facilities. This is sometimes done in concert with the infectious disease specialist or the physician leadership of the hospital in order to try to decrease repetitive cultures, overculturing, inappropriate culturing, and inpatient parasitological tests and to address the myriad of other suggestions which have been made regarding decreases in the numbers of nonrelevant diagnostic procedures.

There is much anguish over the decrease in fiscal resources, with the assumption generally being made that the previous professional economic milieu was necessary for quality patient care. There is no information that this was in fact the case; and constructive review of procedures, processes, and employee utilization may contribute significantly to more relevant, high-quality, and less costly care. However, there is the hazard that as economic resources are further diminished there will come a point that it is not possible to sustain quality. It is incumbent on the laboratory director to make a documentable case, as the patient advocate, against decreases in quality. It has been suggested that many of the initial savings have been wrung out of the health care system by the managed care initiative.

REGULATORY ISSUES AFFECTING THE MICROBIOLOGY LABORATORY

The continued proliferation of government regulations related to the laboratory is an ongoing concern to all laboratory managers. The general structure of regulatory oversight for the clinical laboratory was described in detail in the sixth edition of the *Manual of Clinical Microbiology* (36). Specific reiteration of the role of the federal government is redundant, and only updates of relevant regulations will be included here. Regular and timely updates are available in the *National Intelligence Report* (69), and laboratory managers are encouraged to monitor these brief synopses, which are published twice monthly. This source has proven to be a very reliable, concise, annotated resource of existing and impending regulatory changes.

With regard to CLIA 88, changes for the clinical microbiology laboratory have been relatively minimal and controlled. The name of the category of microscopy testing which had been called "physician-performed microscopy" has been changed to "provider-performed microscopy" in order to more accurately define some of the individuals who perform this testing. In discussing Gram stains, it should be noted that for those with the moderate-complexity license, only Gram stains related to male and female genital specimens are considered appropriate; Gram staining of all other clinical specimens is considered to be of high complexity.

It should be noted that screening tests are not reimbursed by the Centers for Medicare and Medicaid Services (CMS; previously the Health Care Financing Administration); but there are no definitive guidelines as to when a test moves from a test for diagnosis, to one for monitoring for a recurrence, to one for screening for infections in the future. Also, this requirement applies only to outpatient billing, since the inpatient is covered under a lump-sum payment determined by the DRG code assigned for the hospitalization. If outpatient DRG payments are developed, then much of this extraordinary problem will disappear. Although only CMS is using this payment mechanism for Medicare and Medicaid recipients, it is anticipated that many other third-party payers will follow.

One question which is raised with some frequency by conscientious laboratorians is, "How will anyone find out if we are not adhering strictly to the rules and the letter of the law and all of these multiple layers of CMS and OSHA [Occupational Safety and Health Administration] regulations?" There are probably two answers to this plaintive question. First, most of the violations or the inadvertent failure to adhere to the regulations will, in fact, go unnoticed during the various inspection processes. The second answer is that most violations come to light as a consequence of disgruntled employees making a complaint to the appropriate government agency. In areas where there is

fraud in billing, the employee has an opportunity to recover extraordinary amounts of money as a certain percentage of whatever settlement is levied against the offender. Under the qui tam provisions of the Federal False Claims Act, individuals who not only point out but also are able to document fraudulent claims are able to share in a significant percentage of the judgment.

Accreditation and Licensure of Laboratories

The main changes in the area of accreditation and licensure of laboratories relate to some additional states being given inspection and licensure authority from CMS, with this authority being dependent upon the state adopting regulations which are at least as stringent as the federal regulations. What this means from a practical standpoint is that the state instead of CMS can serve as the inspection authority and that different states may pursue this inspection activity depending on the financial resources available to them or what they feel to be the adequacy of the inspection by agencies such as JCAHO or CAP.

It should also be noted that each state has its own requirements for notification of infectious diseases, and although this list does not change frequently, it is incumbent upon the laboratory director to make sure that the laboratory is in compliance with these state regulations. It might be mentioned that on occasion the state department of health will make certain demands on a laboratory in terms of reporting organisms or providing material to the state department of health in order to satisfy certain requirements of the federal government or because of collaborative investigative work. The laboratory is not necessarily obligated to respond to these demands, although the state may sometimes make it appear as if it is a mandated function. It is appropriate for the laboratory director to press the state for specific documentation of why additional reporting, evaluation of laboratory records, provision of selected organisms, or other general intrusions into laboratory activity are in fact necessary. Also, it should be noted that these invitations to participation usually are done without the provision of funding by the state, and unless the laboratory wishes to participate as a general response of collegiality, participation need not be viewed as a necessary response unless there is a sufficient legal mandate.

It was noted (36) that there is a continued expansion of guidelines that was referred to as "guideline creep." This has not abated. Federal, state, and accrediting agencies have been guilty of encouraging the proliferation of guidelines or documentation requirements which are often couched in terms having to do with the improvement of clinical outcomes, the protection of workers, or the protection of the public at large; but often, little documentation is available to support those claims. Some of these can be resisted or, more importantly, can be evaluated in terms of satisfying the spirit of the law or recommendation in the context of a particular laboratory situation. At times there is a slavish adherence to regulations when, in fact, a well-documented common-sense approach would benefit both the laboratory and the patients much more adequately, and usually, the accrediting agencies are quite willing to accept a well-thought-out, reasonable response to these increasing guidelines. It must be remembered that most of these guidelines are attempts to improve quality but often are then promulgated by individuals who are unfamiliar with their implementation and necessity and proceed from the need for information which may serve their own political territorial needs.

In conclusion, the regulatory initiatives can be viewed as burdensome, frequently misdirected, inadequately documented as to their utility, and generally causing a high level of frustration. However, it needs to be emphasized that these regulatory initiatives are created in the context of the legislative process and that all of us as laboratory directors have an opportunity to provide input into that process. Frequently, there is concern that individual voices will not be heard, but in fact, the government takes very seriously the responses to the proposed regulations. The advantage of being current by using references such as the *National Intelligence Report* (69) or the *Statline* from CAP (15) allows one to know when to look at the *Federal Register* to make comments. There is a tendency for laboratory directors to allow their professional societies such as the American Society for Microbiology, CAP, the American Society for Clinical Pathologists, and the Clinical Laboratory Management Association to make the specific statements of objection or a suggestion for rule making. This is useful, but each laboratory director should try to take time to look at the proposed regulations and, if he or she feels that these regulations are inadequate or inappropriate, should respond directly to whatever agency is identified in the *Federal Register* within the appropriate time frame. A lack of response to these regulations will permit their imposition, and there then should be no complaint if an attempt has not been made to temper the rule making. These rule makings are frequently very complex, and many individuals are quick to comment that the devil is in the details, but in this situation, the devil is probably inappropriately maligned. What is in the details are the desires of special-interest groups, very vocal individuals, or just plain incompetence or ignorance. Much of the rule making is done in a very carefully reasoned and competent fashion and in an attempt to follow the spirit of the usually very vague legislation that prompts the rule making. It is our task and necessary responsibility to help the rule makers promulgate initiatives that will be to the benefit of the patient, that are consonant with patient advocacy, and that can be documented to have relevance to clinical laboratory activities.

Compliance Issues

In the past, compliance referred to whether or not a patient was taking prescribed medications or following a specific plan. Now the concept refers to whether we as health care professionals are following the plans which regulations have defined for our activities. Many aspects of compliance plans relate to trying to root out fraud and abuse. However, there is a component of compliance plans which most of us are expected to endorse that requires us not only to comply ourselves but also to report to appropriate authorities when we detect problems in our own laboratories. This represents a considerable change from previous expectations and one which some take very seriously and others wish to ignore. Suffice it to say, each laboratory must have a coherent compliance policy which follows the federal recommendations and which has been implemented, not just printed, and each laboratory should be able to document that all personnel are involved as part of their initial training and ongoing educational process.

Confidentiality Issues

With the passage of the Health Information Portability and Accountability Act in 1996, issues related to confidentiality have been elevated to a new level of concern. The privacy of patient laboratory information has been of concern to all of us, but that usually referred to privacy within a local medical record. Now that there is recognition of the need for distributing medical information, as our mobile population moves from place to place, there is even greater concern about how privacy can be maintained on the electronic pathways over which it will travel. The level of threat posed by dedicated or thrill-seeking computer hackers who gain access to the data streams that pass between institutions or providers' offices and the potential economic value of the information in those data streams are poorly understood. The implementation of federal regulations will impose a challenge which most of us dimly perceive now and will also probably create many avenues of potential liability that we would prefer to ignore.

Specimen Transport Issues

The federal government, particularly the U.S. Department of Transportation (DOT) and the international agencies with which DOT interacts, has changed the requirement for packaging and labeling of specimens sent by mail, air, train, or bus. It is necessary that the laboratory be aware of these changes as they occur so that specimens will not be rejected for lack of proper labeling or packaging.

REFERENCES

1. **Albrecht, K.** 1988. *Successful Management by Objectives*, p. 1–40. Prentice-Hall, New York, N.Y.
2. **Albright, R. E., C. B. Graham III, R. H. Christianson, W. A. Schell, M. C. Bledsoe, J. L. Emlet, T. P. Mears, L. B. Reller, and K. A. Schneider.** 1991. Issues in cerebrospinal fluid management: acid-fast bacillus smear and culture. *Am. J. Clin. Pathol.* **95:**418–423.
3. **Albright, R. E., Jr., R. H. Christianson, J. L. Emlet, C. B. Graham III, E. G. Estevez, M. L. Wilson, L. B. Reller, and K. A. Schneider.** 1991. Issues in cerebrospinal fluid management: CSF venereal disease research laboratory testing. *Am. J. Clin. Pathol.* **95:**397–401.
3a.**American Medical Association.** 2001. *Current Procedural Terminology 2001.* American Medical Association, Chicago, Ill.
4. **Bachner, P., and P. J. Howanitz.** 1991. Q-Probes: a tool for enhancing your lab's QA. *Med. Lab. Observer* **23**(Nov.):37–46.
5. **Bale, M. J., S. M. McLaws, and J. M. Matsen.** 1985. The spot indole test for identification of swarming *Proteus*. *Am. J. Clin. Pathol.* **83:**87–90.
6. **Barenfanger, J., C. Drake, and G. Kacich.** 1999. Clinical and financial benefits of rapid bacterial identification and antimicrobial susceptibility testing. *J. Clin. Microbiol.* **37:**1415–1418.
7. **Baron, E. J., D. Francis, and K. M. Peddecord.** 1996. Infectious disease physicians rate microbiology services and practices. *J. Clin. Microbiol.* **34:**496–500.
8. **Baron, E. J.** 2001. Rapid identification of bacteria and yeast: summary of a National Committee for Clinical Laboratory Standards proposed guideline. *Clin. Infect. Dis.* **33:**220–225.
9. **Bartlett, R. C.** 1974. *Medical Microbiology: Quality, Cost and Clinical Relevance.* John Wiley & Sons, Inc., New York, N.Y.
10. **Bates, D. W., G. J. Kuperman, E. Ritteberg, J. M. Teich, J. Fiskio, N. Ma'luf, A. Onderdonk, D. Wybenga, J. Winkelman, T. A. Brennan, A. L. Komaroff, and M. Tanasijevic.** 1999. A randomized trial of a computer-based intervention to reduce utilization of redundant laboratory tests. *Am. J. Med.* **106:**144–150.

11. **Bergman, R.** 1994. Reengineering health care. *Hosp. Health Net.* **68:**28–36.

12. **Bodenheimer, T.** 1997. The Oregon health plan—lessons for the nation. *N. Engl. J. Med.* **337:**651–655, 720–723.

13. **Carroll, K., and L. Reimer.** 1996. Microbiology and laboratory diagnosis of upper respiratory tract infections. *Clin. Infect. Dis.* **23:**442–448.

14. **Centers for Disease Control and Prevention.** 2000. Notice to readers: update: nucleic acid amplification tests for tuberculosis. *Morb. Mortal. Wkly. Rep.* **49:**593–594.

15. **College of American Pathologists.** *Statline.* College of American Pathologists, Washington, D.C.

16. **College of American Pathologists.** 2001. *CAP Today*, vol. 15, March. College of American Pathologists, Washington, D.C.

17. **Crosby, P. B.** 1979. *Quality Is Free.* New American Library, New York, N.Y.

18. **Daniels, M., and S. A. Schroeder.** 1977. Variation among physicians in use of laboratory tests: relation to clinical productivity and outcomes of care. *Med. Care* **15:**482–487.

19. **DeAguayo, R.** 1990. *Deming: the American Who Taught the Japanese about Quality*, p. 1–60. Simon and Schuster, New York, N.Y.

20. **DePree, M.** 1989. *Leadership Is an Art.* Bantam/Doubleday/Dell Publishing Group, New York, N.Y.

21. **Doern, G. V., R. Vautour, M. Gaudet, and B. Levy.** 1994. Clinical impact of rapid in vitro susceptibility testing and bacterial identification. *J. Clin. Microbiol.* **32:**1757–1762.

22. **Doern, G. V.** 1996. Diagnostic mycobacteriology: where are we today? *J. Clin. Microbiol.* **34:**1873–1876.

23. **Elder, B. L., S. A. Hanson, J. A. Kellogg, F. J. Marsk, and R. J. Zabransky.** 1997. *Cumitech 31: Verification and Validation of Procedures in the Clinical Microbiology Laboratory.* Coordinating ed., B. W. McCurdy. American Society for Microbiology, Washington, D.C.

24. **Forbes, B. A., and P. A. Granato.** 1995. Processing specimens for bacteria, p. 265–281. *In* P. R. Murray, E. J. Barron, M. A. Pfaller, F. C. Tenover, and R. H. Yolken (ed.), *Manual of Clinical Microbiology*, 6th ed. American Society for Microbiology, Washington, D.C.

25. **Garcia, L. S.** 2000. Current issues related to stool collection, processing, and testing of stool specimens for diagnostic parasitology. *Clin. Microbiol. Newsl.* **22:**140–144.

26. **Gundersen, L.** 2000. The effect of clinical practice guidelines on variations in care. *Ann. Intern. Med.* **133:**317–318.

27. **Hardwick, D. F., and J. I. Morrison.** 1990. *Directing the Clinical Laboratory.* Field and Wood, Inc., New York, N.Y.

28. **Health Care Financing Administration.** 1992. Clinical Laboratory Improvement Amendments of 1988; final rule. *Fed. Regist.* **57:**7137–7186.

29. **Hicks, M. J., and K. J. Ryan.** 1976. Simplified scheme for identification of prompt lactose-fermenting members of the *Enterobacteriaceae. J. Clin. Microbiol.* **4:**511–514.

30. **Hines, J., and I. Nachamkin.** 1996. Effective use of the clinical microbiology laboratory for diagnosing diarrheal diseases. *Clin. Infect. Dis.* **23:**1292–1301.

30a.**Institute of Medicine.** 2000. *To Err Is Human: Building a Safer Health System.* National Academy Press, Washington, D.C.

30b.**Institute of Medicine.** 2001. *Crossing the Quality Chasm: A New Health System for the 21st Century.* National Academy Press, Washington, D.C.

31. **James, B. C.** 1998. Foreword, p. xi–xii. *In* P. Bozzo (ed.), *Cost-Effective Laboratory Management.* Lippincott-Raven Publishers, Philadelphia, Pa.

32. **Juran, J. M.** 1988. Company wide planning for quality, p. 1–51. *In* J. M. Juran and F. M. Gryna (ed.), *Juran's Quality Control Handbook*, 4th ed. McGraw-Hill Book Company, New York, N.Y.

33. **Juran, J. M.** 1989. *Juran on Leadership for Quality: An Executive Handbook*, p. 1–80. Collier MacMillan, New York, N.Y.

33a.**Katz, J. M., and E. Green.** 1997. *Managing Quality.* Mosby-Year Book, Inc., St. Louis, Mo.

34. **Lepoff, R., and P. Romfh.** 1997. Quality management as the basis for cost management, p. 57–75. *In* E. M. Travers (ed.), *Clinical Laboratory Management.* The Williams & Wilkins Co., Baltimore, Md.

35. **Marton, K. I., and A. D. Gean.** 1985. The spinal tap: a new look at an old test. *Ann. Intern. Med.* **104:**840–848.

36. **McGowan, J. E., and J. D. MacLowry.** 1995. Addressing regulatory issues in the clinical microbiology laboratory, p. 67–74. *In* P. R. Murray, E. J. Barron, M. A. Pfaller, F. C. Tenover, and R. H. Yolken (ed.), *Manual of Clinical Microbiology*, 6th ed. American Society for Microbiology, Washington, D.C.

37. **McLaughlin, J.** 1995. The implementation of cost-effective, clinically relevant diagnostic microbiology policies: the approach. *Clin. Microbiol. Newsl.* **17:**70–71.

38. **McQueen, M. J.** 2000. Evidence-based medicine: its application to laboratory medicine. *Ther. Drug Monit.* **22:**1–9.

39. **Meredith, F. T., H. K. Phillips, and L. B. Reller.** 1997. Clinical utility of broth cultures of cerebrospinal fluid from patients at risk for shunt infections. *J. Clin. Microbiol.* **35:**3109–3111.

40. **Morris, A. J., D. C. Tanner, and L. B. Reller.** 1993. Rejection criteria for endotracheal aspirates from adults. *J. Clin. Microbiol.* **31:**1027–1029.

41. **Morris, A. J., S. J. Wilson, C. E. Marx, M. L. Wilson, S. Mirrett, and L. B. Reller.** 1995. Clinical impact of bacteria and fungi recovered only from broth culture. *J. Clin. Microbiol.* **33:**161–165.

42. **Murray, P. R., and J. A. Washington II.** 1975. Microscopic and bacteriologic analysis of expectorated sputum. *Mayo Clin. Proc.* **50:**339–334.

43. **National Committee for Clinical Laboratory Standards.** 1995. *Training Verification for Laboratory Personnel, GP21-A.* National Committee for Clinical Laboratory Standards, Wayne, Pa.

44. **National Committee for Clinical Laboratory Standards.** 1996. *Quality Assurance for Commercially Prepared Microbiological Culture Media, M22-A2.* National Committee for Clinical Laboratory Standards, Wayne, Pa.

45. **National Committee for Clinical Laboratory Standards.** 1996. *Clinical Laboratory Procedure Manuals, GP2-A3.* National Committee for Clinical Laboratory Standards, Wayne, Pa.

46. **National Committee for Clinical Laboratory Standards.** 1998. *Cost Accounting in the Clinical Laboratory, GP11-A.* National Committee for Clinical Laboratory Standards, Wayne, Pa.

47. **National Committee for Clinical Laboratory Standards.** 1999. *Continuous Quality Improvement: Essential Management Approaches and Their Use in Proficiency Testing, GP22-A.* NCCLS, Wayne, Pa.

48. **National Committee for Clinical Laboratory Standards.** 1999. *Using Proficiency Testing (PT) to Improve the Clinical Laboratory, GP-27-A.* NCCLS, Wayne, Pa.

49. **National Committee for Clinical Laboratory Standards.** 1999. *A Quality System Model for Health Care, GP26-A.* NCCLS, Wayne, Pa.

50. **National Committee for Clinical Laboratory Standards.** 2000. *Abbreviated Identification of Bacteria and Yeast; Proposed Guideline, M35-P.* NCCLS, Wayne, Pa.

51. **Robinson, A.** 1994. Rationale for cost-effective laboratory medicine. *Clin. Microbiol. Rev.* **7:**185–199.

52. **Schifman, R. B.** 1994. Quality control and quality assurance, p. 1313–1334. *In* K. D. McClatchey (ed.), *Clinical Laboratory Medicine.* The Williams & Wilkins Co., Baltimore, Md.

53. **Sewell, D. L.** 1998. Quality assessment and control, p. 731–743. *In* H. D. Isenberg (ed.), *Essential Procedures in Clinical Microbiology.* American Society for Microbiology, Washington, D.C.

54. **Sewell, D. L.** 1992. Quality control, p. 13.2.1–13.2.35. *In* H. D. Isenberg (ed.), *Clinical Microbiology Procedures Handbook,* vol. 2. American Society for Microbiology, Washington, D.C.

55. **Shea, Y. R.** 1992. Specimen collection and transport, p. 1.1.1–1.1.30. *In* H. D. Isenberg (ed.), *Clinical Microbiology Procedures Handbook,* vol. 1. American Society for Microbiology, Washington, D.C.

56. **Silletti, R. P., E. Ailey, S. Sun, and D. Tang.** 1997. Microbiologic and clinical value of primary broth cultures of wound specimens collected with swabs. *J. Clin. Microbiol.* **35:**2003–2006.

57. **Stone, B. L., D. L. Cohn, M. S. Kane, M. V. Hildred, M. L. Wilson, and R. R. Reves.** 1994. Utility of paired blood cultures and smears in the diagnosis of disseminated *Mycobacterium avium* complex infection in AIDS patients. *J. Clin. Microbiol.* **32:**841–842.

58. **Taylor, F. W.** 1967. *The Principles of Scientific Management.* W. W. Norton and Company, Inc., New York, N.Y. (Original edition published by Harper & Row, 1911.)

59. **Travers, E. M., and K. D. McClatchey.** 1994. Laboratory management, p. 3–33. *In* K. D. McClatchey (ed.), *Clinical Laboratory Medicine.* The Williams & Wilkins Co., Baltimore, Md.

60. **Travers, E. M.** 1997. Human resource management, p. 121–139. *In* E. M. Travers (ed.), *Clinical Laboratory Management.* The Williams & Wilkins Co., Baltimore, Md.

61. **Travers, E. M.** 1997. The business plan and strategic planning process, p. 101–119. *In* E. M. Travers (ed.), *Clinical Laboratory Management.* The Williams & Wilkins Co., Baltimore, Md.

62. **Travers, E. M.** 1997. Changing operations to improve productivity and reduce costs, p. 435–486. *In* E. M. Travers (ed.), *Clinical Laboratory Management.* The Williams & Wilkins Co., Baltimore, Md.

63. **Travers, E. M.** 1997. Improving productivity and efficiency in laboratories, p. 397–410. *In* E. M. Travers (ed.), *Clinical Laboratory Management.* The Williams & Wilkins Co., Baltimore, Md.

64. **Travers, E. M.** 1997. Methods to manage test utilization and ensure good medical practice, p. 689–714. *In* E. M. Travers (ed.), *Clinical Laboratory Management.* The Williams & Wilkins Co., Baltimore, Md.

65. **Umiker, W.** 1991. *The Customer Orientated Laboratory.* American Society of Clinical Pathologists, Chicago, Ill.

66. **Valenstein, P.** 1996. Managing physician use of laboratory tests. *Clin. Lab. Med.* **16:**749–771.

67. **Valenstein, P., M. Pfaller, and M. Yungbluth.** 1996. The use and abuse of routine stool microbiology: a College of American Pathologists Q-probe study of 601 institutions. *Arch. Pathol. Lab. Med.* **120:**206–211.

68. **Walton, M.** 1986. *The Deming Management Method.* Putnam Publishers, New York, N.Y.

69. **Washington G2 Reports.** *National Intelligence Report.* Washington G2 Reports, Washington, D.C.

70. **Wilson, M. L.** 1996. General principles of specimen collection and transport. *Clin. Infect. Dis.* **22:**766–777.

71. **Wilson, M. L.** 1997. Clinically relevant, cost-effective clinical microbiology. *Am. J. Clin. Pathol.* **107:**154–167.

72. **Yagupsky, P., and M. Menegus.** 1990. Cumulative positivity rates of multiple blood cultures for *Mycobacterium avium-intracellular* and *Cryptococcus neoformans* in patients with the acquired immunodeficiency syndrome. *Arch. Pathol. Lab. Med.* **114:**923–925.

Laboratory Design

MICHAEL L. WILSON AND L. BARTH RELLER

3

A well-designed laboratory is a safe, pleasant, and efficient place in which to work, as well as an enjoyable place to visit. When a new laboratory is being designed or renovation of an existing one is being planned, the design must meet the needs of laboratory staff who spend all or most of their working time there, the needs of workers who spend part of their time there, and the needs of visitors who have to interact with the staff. Above all other considerations, a clinical laboratory must be a safe place. No other aspect of laboratory design carries a higher priority, both for the staff and for visitors. A pleasant environment improves staff morale and productivity, minimizes unnecessary distractions (thereby reducing laboratory errors), and enhances employee recruitment and retention. An efficient clinical laboratory helps to improve productivity, to reduce errors, and to improve patient care by shortening laboratory test turnaround time (TAT). An efficient laboratory also helps to improve staff morale and contributes significantly to a pleasant work environment.

Good laboratory design is based on the concept that form follows function, so the unique functions of a clinical microbiology laboratory (CML) should be reflected in the laboratory design. When designing a CML, it should be remembered that there are three key differences between a CML and other types of clinical laboratories. First, clinical microbiology involves the isolation, propagation, and handling of pathogenic microorganisms that pose a risk to laboratory personnel. To minimize this risk, the entire CML must have the facilities and processes necessary to meet biosafety level 2 criteria and, depending upon the extent and scope of services provided, all or part of the laboratory must also meet the requirements necessary to meet biosafety level 3 criteria (4, 15). Second, the interpretation of cultures, and other microbiologic test results, is based on the ability of the laboratory to isolate pathogenic microorganisms while minimizing microbial contaminants. Again, the laboratory design must be such that the necessary precautions can be taken to minimize contaminants. Third, laboratory design must accommodate specialized equipment used only in microbiology laboratories.

This chapter is intended to be an introduction to the processes of laboratory design, construction, and renovation. Reading this chapter should enable the microbiologist who is beginning a construction or renovation project to communicate with all of the parties who are involved. The informed microbiologist not only will understand the terminology of design and construction, but also will be able to make better decisions as the processes unfold. Being well informed also reduces the likelihood of costly mistakes. Not everything can or should be learned by experience.

GENERAL DESIGN PRINCIPLES

The needs of each laboratory will change over time, often many times between the initial construction of the laboratory and any subsequent renovations. Thus, the best approach to designing is to use the most generic design possible, minimizing features that are unique to circumstances present. Not only does a more generic design facilitate the changing needs of the laboratory, it also reduces the costs of construction, renovations, and ongoing maintenance. Moreover, a generic design is the most flexible one. As stated by Crane and Richmond (5), "the biggest challenge to the laboratory design team is to keep the design simple, not to overdesign the laboratory...." Meeting this challenge requires strong leadership by the laboratory administration and the architect. In particular, leading a design project for either new construction or renovation requires the ability to say "no" to requests for special design features.

Laboratory Location

CMLs providing services for a hospital must be fully integrated with the main hospital laboratory (7, 11, 12). This is a critical factor in providing adequate staffing, ensuring proper specimen processing and handling, reducing errors, and increasing efficiency and productivity. While it is true that off-site reference laboratories serve a useful role in providing esoteric testing and/or routine microbiology services for outpatient clinics and physician offices, we believe that there are important reasons why off-site laboratories do not serve hospitals well. First, use of off-site laboratories may result in delayed specimen processing, which can adversely affect microbial recovery and timely result reporting. Second, use of off-site laboratories decreases interaction between microbiologists and clinicians. This is of particular concern when there is a lack of clinician input into specimen processing, which directly affects the clinical interpretation of microbiological tests. Third, as previously mentioned, loss of integration with the rest of the clinical laboratory, particularly specimen receipt and processing areas, increases the risk of incorrect specimen processing and medical errors. Fourth, laboratory staff members in different laboratory sections are unable to interact on a frequent basis, provide coverage for one another, and act as a cohesive unit. Fifth, added complexity and cost are associated with off-site laboratories (e.g., reliable, timely transport of specimens). Sixth, location of the CML close to the main laboratory facilitates access during off-hours. A laboratory that is remote to the main laboratory is unlikely to be visited by clinicians during off-hours, if ever. Last, location of a CML distant to the site of patient care precludes meaningful training of clinical microbiologists, infectious disease physicians, and other health care professionals (7, 12).

Laboratory Size

Only broad generalizations can be made regarding laboratory size. As a general rule, each bench technologist needs a minimum of 50 ft^2 in which to work, excluding space for large pieces of equipment, walls, corridors, storage, lockers, and offices. Areas such as that used for specimen processing require ample space to accommodate the necessary equipment, the specimen receiving bench itself, and foot traffic. Laboratory sections such as mycobacteriology, mycology, and virology require a larger amount of space relative to the number of technologists who work there. Areas such as a dedicated autoclave room or medium preparation room require additional space. If the number of technologists and supervisors is proportional to the test volume and the laboratory is well-designed with little wasted space, the space allocated for the laboratory should be between 150 and 200 ft^2 per staff member.

Laboratories should be designed with more space than is needed for current workloads and types of services provided. This serves three purposes. First, an efficient laboratory always has the space needed to accommodate short-term expansion of the types and volumes of services provided by that laboratory. Second, extra space (often referred to as swing space) can be used when part of the laboratory is being renovated or repaired. Third, extra space can be used for future expansion of services. It is unwise to design and build a laboratory to meet current needs only.

Transportation

As with other laboratory sections, an effective transportation system is crucial for providing clinical microbiology services. A variety of transportation systems are in use in hospitals today, including manual transportation, robotic systems, and pneumatic tube systems. Manual systems are notoriously unreliable, particularly in large medical centers, and the associated personnel costs make this approach one of the most expensive. While the capital costs of robotic and pneumatic tube systems are high, over time these costs may be less than those associated with a manual transportation system. Robotic systems are not as widely used as pneumatic tube systems for transportation throughout hospitals. Pneumatic tube systems are widely used in hospitals and have been proven to be an effective method for transporting some types of specimens to clinical laboratories. If they are well-designed and maintained, they can play an important role in reducing the costs of transportation, decreasing the number of lost or delayed specimens, and reducing test TAT. In general, however, dedicated pneumatic tube systems are not as useful for CMLs as they are for chemistry and hematology laboratories. This is because most microbiologic tests do not have the same expectation for test TAT, many pneumatic tube systems cannot transport specimens as heavy as full blood culture bottles, and containers used to collect specimens such as urine are prone to leakage when shipped through pneumatic tube systems. Other automated transportation systems are available, but, as with pneumatic tube systems, any benefit to a CML is not as great as it is for other clinical laboratory sections.

Building Codes and Architectural Standards

Laboratorians who have never been involved in the construction or renovation of a laboratory are often unaware of building codes and architectural standards (1). Although it is the responsibility of the architects and engineers to ensure that the plan meets the appropriate codes and standards, laboratory staff members who are involved in a project should understand these issues sufficiently to avoid making requests that are not in compliance with codes and standards. There are definite and specific limits to the way a laboratory can be built.

Interior Design

The design of laboratories that are part of health care systems will often involve meeting organization design standards. In some organizations, the types of materials that are used for construction, color schemes, and many other architectural details are specified from the outset. For some organizations this makes a great deal of sense, as a standard interior design lends a sense of continuity throughout the organization. In many instances it also reduces construction and renovation costs, as the organization can purchase materials in large quantities. For other organizations, however, it makes little sense to adopt interior design schemes developed for one part of the organization for a laboratory. Moreover, not all design schemes are successful, so an organization should not be reluctant to abandon one scheme in favor of a better one. At all costs, one should avoid trendy interior design schemes, as they are less likely to please a large number of employees, become dated more quickly than do more traditional design schemes, and tend to be more expensive. It should always be remembered that one might have to live with a laboratory or office for many years.

Technology

Much of the same logic that applies to interior design also applies to the use of advanced technology in a laboratory. Laboratorians, architects, engineers, and designers are all enamored with technology, and there is a strong temptation to use the most advanced technology in a new laboratory or when renovating an existing one (5). Nonetheless, one should assess carefully the cost of advanced technology versus less advanced but proven technology, evidence that advanced technology has been used successfully in comparable laboratories, and any evidence of long-term durability. Advanced technological products may or may not be better than traditional ones, but the newer they are, the less experience there is with them. Moreover, some advanced technology products are trendy and should therefore be avoided for the same reasons that trendy interior design schemes should be avoided. There are reasons why traditional built-in laboratory casework continues to be used widely and why certain commercial products and vendors have been around for decades.

SPECIFIC DESIGN ISSUES

Laboratory Layout

The laboratory layout is crucial for achieving the goals set forth in the introduction to this chapter. The overall layout of a clinical laboratory is determined by the types of services provided, the numbers and types of specimens that are processed, the physical constraints of the building, and the resources that are available for the construction or renovation project. A laboratory that provides only patient care services has needs that are different from those of one engaged in teaching and/or research. Busy clinical laboratories must be efficient to maximize specimen throughput and to minimize test TAT. Laboratories that support teaching and research missions also need to be efficient but must have the space and facilities to support the broader missions. Decisions regarding the overall layout of the laboratory should be made first and should be immutable during the design process.

Most CMLs are divided into sections according to the way that specimens are handled in those laboratories (e.g., a bench devoted to urine cultures, another to blood cultures, and so on) and/or by discipline (e.g., a mycology section). There are obviously many different ways to organize a laboratory. As noted above, the best approach is to use a generic design so that equipment, staff, and processes can be moved as necessary. Areas that require biosafety level 3 conditions cannot be easily moved, so the laboratory staff should take extra care in choosing a location for these areas.

Specimen Preparation Area

All CMLs need an area to receive and process specimens. This area should be located near the laboratory entrance so that other laboratory staff and couriers do not need to enter the rest of the laboratory to drop off specimens. The area should have ample benchtop space for receiving specimens, for any necessary equipment, and for the handling of specimen requisitions. This area should have a class II biological safety cabinet (BSC) in which all initial specimen processing should be done. All necessary information technology (IT) infrastructure and telecommunications equipment should be provided. This area should have a sink for handwashing and for performing Gram's stain and other direct examinations. Some laboratories place a microscope in this area for reading stains, whereas others place microscopes in a separate area of the laboratory. A refrigerator should be located in the specimen preparation area to hold specimens and media. Some laboratories do not have separate incubators for the specimen processing area, opting to place inoculated media directly in the main laboratory incubators, but unless specimens can be placed in these incubators quickly, a holding incubator should be located in the processing area.

The specific design of a specimen preparation area needs to be tailored to the number of specimens that are received, as well as to the types of microbiologic tests that are performed. There is no single design that is optimal for all laboratories. For this reason, and because this is often one of the busiest areas of any microbiology laboratory, the specimen preparation area should receive emphasis during the design phase of the project. The perspective and wishes of experienced technologists are especially important here. Function should drive design.

General Laboratory Bench Space

Work Areas

Many laboratories are constructed on the basis of U-shaped modules or linear benches. Modules typically measure 10 by 10 ft and can accommodate two or three persons. Advantages to the modular approach include minimized foot traffic in work areas, generous countertop and storage space, corner space that is available for computer workstations (corners otherwise are wasted space), an increased sense of privacy for workers, and use of less floor space for aisles and corridors. Advantages to the linear bench approach include ease of cleaning, ease of moving about the laboratory, a subjective sense of less clutter, easier location of large pieces of equipment such as incubators and refrigerators, ease of moving modular casework, and lower design, construction, and renovation costs. Some laboratories use a combination of modules and linear benches. In many cases, the physical layout and constraints of the building will determine which approach is best for a given laboratory.

The space surrounding workbenches should be sufficient to accommodate ample waste containers, both for paper and for biohazardous waste. It is inefficient for laboratory staff and housekeepers to empty trash containers more often than is necessary. Ample space should be provided so that aisles are unobstructed and free of clutter, yet aisles that are too wide merely waste space.

The laboratory should contain space for storing completed cultures, stock cultures, reference books, and teaching materials (e.g., parasitology slides). It is most efficient for completed cultures and reference materials to be located close to workbenches. Stock cultures should be in a secure location, particularly if the laboratory maintains reference stocks of potential biothreat agents such as *Brucella* spp., *Bacillus anthracis*, *Francisella tularensis*, or *Yersinia pestis*. The principle applies to frozen, lyophilized, or viable cultures.

Casework

Laboratory casework can be built-in (custom) or modular. The type of casework selected for a laboratory is, to a large degree, determined by the size of the laboratory. It is expensive to install custom built-in casework in a large laboratory; vendors are able to give better pricing for installing modular furniture in larger facilities. Thus, larger laboratories almost always find it to be more economical to buy commercial modular furniture. Smaller laboratories, on the other hand, may find the opposite to be true. Before making a decision as to the type of casework, one needs to be familiar with the advantages and disadvantages of each type of casework.

Built-in casework typically is less expensive to install, can be made from a wider variety of building materials to suit individual tastes, can be very strong, and is durable. It is not unusual to see built-in laboratory casework that is decades old but is still functional and aesthetically pleasing. The disadvantages to built-in casework are that it cannot be moved easily, repairs tend to be more difficult and expensive, modifications (e.g., adding additional power and communication lines) also are more difficult and expensive, and, for the most part, it cannot be reused once it is disassembled. From an interior design standpoint, it has the disadvantage of requiring users to live with the aesthetic choices of predecessors and those characteristic of previous eras.

Modular furniture has been, in part, designed to overcome the disadvantages associated with built-in casework.

Specifically, some parts of it can be moved easily, repairs and replacements are easy, modifications are easy and less expensive, and entire units can be disassembled and moved to another location. The converse, however, is equally true: many of the advantages associated with built-in casework are not found in modular furniture. Specifically, modular furniture tends to be more expensive (unless one is buying large quantities, decreasing the unit cost), there is a smaller selection of building materials and colors to suit individual aesthetic tastes, and it tends to be less strong and durable. It should be noted that one of the main advantages to modular furniture, the ability to move it around, tends to be overstated. This is because the stanchions that support the casework are bolted to the floor, plumbing and drains for sinks are not easily moved, and there are practical limits to moving the electrical power supply and IT and telecommunication cables. In fact, with some commercial modular casework systems, only the cabinets, shelves, and countertops can be moved, and even they can be moved only within the confines of the supporting stanchions.

Air, Gas, and Vacuum Supplies

Most modern laboratories have little need for compressed air, gas, and vacuum supplies, except as needed for specific purposes. Use of open flames should be prohibited, so there is no need for a flammable gas supply. Most health care facilities do not have central systems to supply the types of gases used in microbiological incubators. These should be included within the laboratory facility.

A generous amount of space should be allocated for incubators, refrigerators, freezers, floor-model centrifuges, and floor-model diagnostic equipment (e.g., continuous-monitoring blood culture systems). Electrical power, water supply, telecommunications ports, and other features necessary to support such equipment should be part of the design. The load capacity of the facility should be such that it can support the weight of this equipment, particularly if most of it will be located in one part of the laboratory.

Special Laboratory Bench Space

Anaerobic Bacteriology

The anaerobic bacteriology capacities needed by most hospital-based CMLs can be accommodated by countertop jars. For larger laboratories, or those with a special interest in anaerobic bacteriology, sufficient space should be allocated to accommodate an anaerobic chamber and gas supply. Countertop models have replaced most of the floor-model anaerobic tents that once were common in laboratories. Some gas-liquid chromatographs require a dedicated exhaust system for discharged gases. Most of the other equipment needed for anaerobic bacteriology does not require special design features.

Mycobacteriology, Mycology, and Virology

The primary design requirement for mycobacteriology, mycology, and virology laboratories is that they meet biosafety level 3 criteria, as described in the following section. In addition to biosafety issues, these laboratories require special equipment not used elsewhere in the CML, such as refrigerated centrifuges, special diagnostic equipment, and the incubators required to hold specimens at various temperatures. Equipment for performing tissue cultures may also be needed. Mycology and mycobacteriology laboratories must have a certified class II BSC.

Biosafety Level 2 and 3 Conditions

Most routine clinical microbiology procedures can be performed safely under biosafety level 2 conditions (15). Even though biosafety level 2 conditions can be met without use of a BSC, use of a BSC protects laboratory workers from laboratory-acquired infections and protects specimens from contamination (8, 16). Moreover, laboratory staff do not always receive sufficient information with specimen requisition forms to know which specimens are likely to contain pathogens that are risky to process (3). Therefore, it is strongly recommended that all specimen processing be done in a class II BSC. Isolates or cultures that are known or likely to contain high-risk microorganisms should be processed only in a class II BSC, particularly fungal and mycobacterial cultures (3, 15). If possible, positive blood and cerebrospinal fluid cultures should also be processed in a class II BSC. Adequate space, power, and ventilation should be provided for each BSC.

Biosafety level 2 conditions are met largely via use of standard microbiological practices (15). In addition to these practices, biosafety level 2 conditions require that (i) laboratory personnel have specific training in handling pathogenic agents, (ii) personnel be directed by competent scientists, (iii) laboratory access is limited when work is being conducted, (iv) extreme precautions be taken in handling contaminated sharp items, and (v) procedures likely to generate infectious aerosols or splashes are conducted in either a class II BSC or other physical containment equipment (15).

Biosafety level 3 conditions include all of the requirements for biosafety level 2 conditions plus special facilities, equipment, and procedures for handling "pathogenic and potentially lethal agents" (15). For those CMLs that do not have the facilities specified for biosafety level 3 conditions, routine microbiologic procedures should be done using biosafety level 2 conditions. Biosafety level 3 practices and protective equipment should be used when handling agents that pose a risk of serious or lethal infection. The specific requirements needed to meet biosafety level 3 conditions are given in reference 15. In brief, these include (i) limited laboratory access, (ii) written policies and procedures for handling agents, (iii) adequate training, proficiency, and competency for handling agents, (iv) use of a class II BSC for handling highly infectious agents, (v) use of adequate face and respiratory protection for procedures done outside a BSC, and (vi) written policies and procedures for handling spills. The facility requirements are given in reference 15. In brief, these include (i) a separate area with access through two sets of self-closing doors; (ii) sealed floors, walls, and ceilings to facilitate decontamination; (iii) a waste disposal system that is available within the area; (iv) a ducted air system that draws clean air from outside the area, with all of the exhaust air (i.e., none of the air is recirculated) discharged to the outside; and (v) the use of HEPA filters in the exhaust of BSCs, in vacuum lines, and in equipment or devices that may produce aerosols or splashes (e.g., centrifuges).

Molecular Microbiology

As for the general microbiology laboratory, planning for a molecular diagnostics laboratory should optimize workspace flexibility, since this technology is rapidly changing and new equipment, methods, and applications will be available in the next few years (6, 13, 14; K. L. Kaul, personal communication). Prior to establishment of molecular testing, thought must be given to the type of services planned. For example, if the laboratory staff plans to perform only Food and Drug Administration-approved and commercially available kit-based assays, then minimal space and equipment may be all that is needed. Alternatively, if the laboratory staff plans to develop and perform in-house assays, then a significantly greater investment in space, equipment, and technical expertise will be required. In addition, consideration must be given to the specific assays that will be performed, as space and equipment needs vary considerably for different types of assays.

If the laboratory staff plans to perform only commercial amplification kit-based assays, bench space will be needed to accommodate a hood-type work enclosure with a UV light source, an amplification and detection apparatus(es), and a few other pieces of equipment, such as a water bath and microcentrifuge. As little as 15 linear feet of bench space is needed. To reduce the risk of contamination, two geographically separated work areas are needed. Most commercial kit-based assays include methods to prevent carryover amplification, and automated equipment also may reduce the possibility of carryover, both of which minimize the amount of space that is needed. According to the manufacturers of some commercial diagnostic molecular assays, certain assays can now be performed in a single area and with only minimal need for special handling. Experience will show whether this is an acceptable approach, but it is likely that as the technology of molecular diagnosis changes, there will be a decreasing need for separate areas. If this occurs, then laboratories will be able to fully integrate diagnostic molecular assays with the rest of the CML.

Development and performance of in-house methods that involve amplifying nucleic acids require a more elaborate laboratory. A minimum of 500 ft^2 is required for a small molecular diagnostics laboratory, with three separate workspaces. The three work areas include one for reagent preparation, one for specimen preparation, and a third for amplification. General analysis of DNA or RNA requires an assortment of basic laboratory equipment, as well as specialized equipment. Sources of high-grade deionized water, wet ice, and dry ice are needed, as is an autoclave. A fume hood and storage cabinet for solvents and flammables are also needed. Access to a darkroom is advantageous.

The reagent preparation area is the cleanest of the three work areas and can be located in a separate room, in a hood with the fan turned off to minimize aerosolization, or in an enclosed countertop hood or box. This area is used for the preparation of the master mix and other necessary reagents. To minimize contamination, patient samples, prepared DNA, and amplified products must never be brought into this area. Since equipment can become contaminated with DNA, it is imperative that dedicated equipment be used and stored within this area. Reagents should be stored in a refrigerator free of DNA (and especially amplicons), and disposable items such as tubes, tips, and gloves should also be stored in a manner to prevent their contamination. Staff should wear a designated clean laboratory coat along with clean gloves; staff should leave transportable items (e.g., pens, tape, and scissors) in this area.

The second area is the specimen preparation area. In this area, tubes containing the aliquoted master mix should be brought for the addition of nucleic acid; these tubes should not be returned to the reagent preparation area. Specimen preparation activities can be performed in the open laboratory on a bench but might also be performed in an enclosed space such as a benchtop hood or containment box. After nucleic acid is added to the reaction tubes in this area, the tubes are sealed and placed in the thermocycler for amplification. When removed, the tubes should be taken unopened to the third area for product detection.

The third area is the most contaminated of the three work areas. Laboratory staff should take extreme caution to ensure that laboratory coats, gloves, tube racks, and other equipment are never moved back into the reagent or specimen preparation areas. Some laboratories have opted for separate areas for a darkroom/gel electrophoresis room, a room for processing of radioactive samples, and a room for other functions.

Work Flow

Efficient laboratories are designed so that specimens flow in one direction. Traditional microbiologic testing follows a pathway of specimen receipt and plating, incubation, isolate identification, antimicrobial susceptibility testing, and result reporting. Because this sequence is by its nature linear, CMLs benefit from unidirectional work flow. Unidirectional work flow is also important in molecular microbiology laboratories. In this case, the issue is not so much one of efficiency but rather one of minimizing the risk of amplicon carryover and specimen contamination. While much of this can be accomplished by designing unidirectional work processes, the laboratory facility must accommodate the needs of those processes.

Laboratory Storage

Storage space should be adequate but not excessive. Insufficient storage space makes for a cluttered laboratory; unused storage space makes for a dusty one. Short-term storage capacity should meet the daily needs of the staff and no more. Long-term storage of supplies should be in the main laboratory storage room; there is no reason for long-term storage in the CML itself. Storage space, whether on shelves, in overhead cabinets, or in drawers, should be designed so that workers have most of what they need during the day within arm's reach. Storage space should be designed so that it can be cleaned easily.

Incubators, Refrigerators, and Centrifuges

CMLs should have ample space for large floor-model incubators, refrigerators, and centrifuges. Sufficient aisle space should be allocated next to large units so that the aisle remains unobstructed when a door is opened. Adequate electrical power should be incorporated into the area housing these units, as well as any necessary gas or water supplies. The location of these units should help maximize laboratory efficiency and ensure unidirectional work flow. As a general rule, a refrigerator and centrifuge should be located in the specimen processing area. Although some CMLs have adopted the principle of scattering incubators and refrigerators throughout the laboratory, with the rationale of minimizing the distance from workbenches, a more efficient use of space is to have a separate area in the laboratory for these large pieces of equipment. This is because these units almost always are wider than countertops are deep, so locating them throughout a laboratory requires the aisles to be wider than would otherwise be necessary. Because the additional space in the other parts of the aisle is not needed, a significant amount of floor space will be wasted.

Handwashing, Water Supply, and Plumbing

The CML should have sufficient sinks to accommodate staining, waste disposal, and handwashing. To prevent laboratory-acquired infections (3, 15), handwashing sinks should be designed so that they can be operated with knee or foot controls. One sink should be located near the laboratory entrance to facilitate handwashing by staff and visitors as they leave the laboratory. Drainpipes should be able to handle the types and volumes of liquid waste generated within the laboratory.

Plumbing is expensive to install at any time but especially so once laboratory construction is completed. In addition, the plumbing and water supply cannot be moved easily in modern buildings, as one must drill through a concrete floor and then work in the ceiling space of the floor below. This space typically is filled with heating, ventilating, and air-conditioning (HVAC) systems, lighting, IT and telecommunications cables, and electrical power lines, making it difficult and expensive to work there. Such a project is also disruptive to the occupants of the floor below. Therefore, the water supply and plumbing needs should be assessed carefully during the design phase of the project.

Countertops

Countertops at workbenches should be 24 in. deep, with work areas no more than 4 to 5 ft wide. A working space of these dimensions is the most efficient because the entire space is within arm's length for most workers. There should be additional space to each side for storage and equipment. Some countertops will need to be deeper to accommodate countertop-model equipment. Heavy pieces of equipment should be on freestanding tables designed to accommodate the necessary weight. Centrifuges should also be on freestanding tables to minimize the transfer of vibrational forces to adjacent countertops. Sensitive analytical balances should be on freestanding tables. Most modular casework systems include tables that are of the same length and width as the individual countertop pieces and which can be integrated into the overall laboratory layout.

The height of workbenches can be that of a desk (29 to 30 in.) or a counter (36 in.). While there are advantages to both heights, use of one or the other is largely a matter of personal preference. Modular furniture can be adjusted to either height, whereas built-in casework obviously is fixed at one height.

Countertops should be made of materials that can be cleaned and disinfected easily, are durable, and can be replaced or repaired as needed. Most countertops in CMLs do not need to be acid resistant. Countertops that are stain resistant are desirable. Countertops adjacent to sinks should be constructed of water-resistant materials so that constant exposure to water does not damage them. Lighter colors tend to show stains more but have the benefit of making the laboratory brighter. Practical issues aside, colors generally are selected on the basis of interior design needs and personal preference.

Electrical Power Supply

Electrical outlets should be liberal in number and in excess of the current need. These are easily installed during construction, but upgrading the electrical power supply can be expensive and difficult once construction is completed. One important task during the design phase of the project is to perform a comprehensive audit of the electrical needs of the laboratory, particularly as related to 110- versus 220-V power supplies. The need for emergency power supplies should also be assessed, as this requires a separate electrical power supply. Only critical pieces of equipment should be on the emergency power supply. Critical equipment should be wired into a central alarm system so that the appropriate persons can be notified of any power failures.

HVAC

The HVAC system in a clinical laboratory must be designed so that the laboratory meets the necessary biosafety level while maintaining a constant ambient temperature within a narrow range. Thus, the design of an HVAC system is a challenging task for architects and mechanical engineers. Moreover, once installed, an HVAC system cannot be easily modified: it is one of the most expensive parts of construction, it resides in a relatively inaccessible space, and changing the HVAC in one area of a building may have effects in other areas of the building.

Installing an HVAC system is often the most expensive part of the construction project, and revising an HVAC system in a clinical laboratory is expensive or impractical, so it is imperative that the design and installation be done correctly. Balancing the airflow in a CML is challenging, as (i) the laboratory must have a lower air pressure than the adjacent hallway, (ii) the temperature of the laboratory must be maintained within a narrow range, (iii) exhaust air from the CML cannot recirculate into the building, and (iv) the HVAC system must accommodate special needs for odor control. Special plenums that will draw off odors from workbenches can be installed, which is of particular concern in the specimen processing area, parasitology section, anaerobic bacteriology section, and autoclave room, but these can pull large amounts of air out of the laboratory. As a result, balancing the airflow within a CML often requires adjustments to the system after the laboratory has been occupied. Further adjustments may be necessary, as during seasonal changes when the requirements for warm and cool air differ.

IT and Telecommunications

The modern clinical laboratory is highly dependent upon IT and telecommunications systems. IT systems within a laboratory should meet both current and anticipated needs. The IT infrastructure should accommodate the larger institution's (e.g., hospital's) health care information system, the laboratory information system, the facility intranet, and the Internet. Ideally, the IT infrastructure will be designed for high-speed access and will have redundant data storage and processing capacity and sufficient types and numbers of workstations to accommodate changing IT needs. The most efficient laboratories are paperless; the IT infrastructure should support this. Modern telecommunications systems are complex, with a need for support of telefax units, increasingly sophisticated telephone systems, videoconferencing, and other types of telecommunications.

For many laboratory staff members, and certainly for clerical and administrative staff, most of the day is spent using a computer. The computer workstation has become the focus of most offices and many laboratories. A robust IT system supports a variety of applications that are of immediate benefit to the laboratory staff. Any modern laboratory should have the infrastructure needed to support a modern IT system. In particular, the cable plant should be generic in design and have a fiber-optic backbone with a fiber-optic cable to each outlet in the laboratory. This cable architecture will accommodate current IT needs but will also facilitate future transition to voice and video capability. There should be redundancy in the network infrastructure. IT and telecommunications systems should be designed so that information retrieval is limited to those who are authorized to access patient records. The design and installation of the IT and telecommunications systems in a laboratory should be done in close collaboration with the information services within the institution. Once systems have been installed, it is expensive or impractical to make changes to the IT and telecommunications infrastructure.

Offices and Administrative Support

Office space should be located close to but not within the laboratory. Offices should be sufficient to support the managerial, administrative, research, and teaching functions of the laboratory. Just as it makes little sense for a clinical laboratory to be located off-site, it makes equally little sense for the office space that ostensibly supports a laboratory to be in a remote location. Successful clinical and faculty recruitment and retention often hinge on adequate office space. Compared with other parts of a health care facility, office space is inexpensive to build, maintain, and renovate. It is in the long-term interests of the institution to make the modest investment needed for this part of the laboratory.

The process of designing offices should follow the same principles as those that guide the design of a clinical laboratory: offices should be private, quite, efficient, and pleasant places to work or to visit. Although some institutions have opted for an open office plan where low modular barriers separate offices, open offices do not provide the privacy necessary for counseling employees or for discussing confidential matters, nor are they quiet. Offices should be equipped with the office equipment, IT and telecommunications infrastructure, and other features that are necessary to make them efficient. Many offices that are associated with clinical laboratories are too small to be pleasant places to work or to visit. Although offices should be sufficiently large, offices that are too large waste space, which never is in excess. As a general rule, individual offices should be no smaller than 100 ft^2. Traditional furniture is less efficient than modular furniture; office size should be adjusted according to the type of furniture that is used. Laboratory directors and supervisors should have offices that are large enough to accommodate several persons during meetings. Offices of up to 200 ft^2 are not unreasonable for directors.

Work Environment

Ergonomic considerations should receive emphasis in laboratory design. Casework, drawers, shelves, keyboard trays, lighting, and space should all be designed according to ergonomic standards. Both ceiling and task lighting should be abundant and well placed. Signs, bulletin boards, and other means of communication should be placed where laboratory staff and visitors can easily see them. A modest investment in the ergonomic and aesthetic properties in the laboratory will go a long way toward making it a pleasant and efficient workplace.

Safety and Security

As stated in the introduction, above all other considerations, a laboratory should be a safe place. For general safety considerations, this can be achieved by ensuring that the laboratory meets all building codes and architectural standards related to safety. For safety considerations related to the practice of clinical microbiology, this can be achieved by designing the laboratory to meet biosafety level 2 criteria and, where necessary, biosafety level 3 criteria.

Clinical laboratories must meet the safety and security requirements of accrediting and regulatory bodies. Eyewash stations, safety showers, sprinkler systems, fire extinguishers and blankets, fire alarms, spill control kits, and emergency power and lighting should be included as specified by building codes. Water supplies should have either backflow preventers or vacuum breaker devices to prevent the inadvertent contamination of potable water supplies.

The laboratory should be designed so that it can be secured during off-hours, or when staffing is minimal. Institution-specific security concerns will guide the need for more comprehensive security assets such as security cameras, restricted access, or electronic monitoring of access.

Cleaning and Waste Handling

A clinical laboratory should be designed so that it can be cleaned easily. All surfaces should be made of materials that are easily cleaned and disinfected. Carpet should never be used as a floor material in a clinical laboratory. To facilitate cleaning, floors should be kept free of clutter; there is no excuse for using floors in a clinical laboratory for storage space.

The laboratory design should accommodate the handling of the large amounts of biohazardous waste that are generated each day. There should be adequate space for waste containers within the laboratory, for biohazardous waste as well as standard waste. Large bins for both types of waste should be located outside the laboratory but nearby. Large pieces of floor-model equipment should be permanently housed on wheels so that they can be moved easily for cleaning. A housekeeping closet should be located close to the laboratory to facilitate daily cleaning.

Some laboratories maintain an on-site autoclave for medium preparation or decontamination of wastes. Some smaller autoclaves are self-contained, but larger autoclaves require steam lines that must be taken into account early in the design process.

THE DESIGN AND CONSTRUCTION PROCESS

Predesign Phase

Beginning the Process

Architecture, engineering, and construction are complex disciplines. Just as one cannot expect a clinical microbiologist to be familiar with the terminology, processes, and regulations of those disciplines, one should not expect an architect, engineer, or contractor to be familiar with the terminology, processes, and regulations that guide the day-to-day operations of a clinical laboratory. Thus, perhaps the most important skill needed to initiate and complete a design or renovation project is communication. Successful design, construction, and renovation projects are characterized by a commitment to education and communication. This is of particular importance when any of the parties who are involved in the project have little or no prior experience in designing or renovating a laboratory. It is not unusual to meet architects, engineers, or contractors who have no experience with clinical laboratories, just as it is not unusual to meet laboratorians who have never been involved with a laboratory construction or renovation project. It is also not unusual to meet architects, engineers, or contractors who have experience with research or industrial laboratories but not clinical laboratories. Experience with the former does not necessarily translate into expertise in the latter. To facilitate communication and education, it is important to have a clear understanding of the experience and expertise of all the parties who will be involved with the project.

Laboratory Representative

The first step in designing a laboratory is for the laboratory administration to appoint a person who will be the spokesperson throughout the design and construction process. Such an appointment should not be made or taken lightly; this is a significant commitment of time and energy that will extend over 1 or more years. The laboratory administration must give this person the time needed to meet the commitment, as well as the responsibility and authority to make many decisions, often on short notice. Because so many persons are involved in construction and renovation projects, because projects take so long to complete, and because the staff must live with the outcome for many years, the laboratory representative must have a clear understanding of budget constraints, space allocations, laboratory operations, and hospital and clinic operations. There must be clear lines of communication and authority. The laboratory representative should be selected carefully on the basis of communication skills, experience in laboratory administration, and decision-making ability. This person need not be the laboratory director, although the director generally is in a better position to negotiate for necessary resources than is a senior technologist.

Budget and Space Allocations

The next step in designing a laboratory is to assess, realistically and accurately, the current and future needs of the laboratory, as well as the resources required to meet those needs. Both new and renovated laboratories should be designed to accommodate future expansion of test volume and type. This includes planning for office space, specimen receiving and processing, benches, informatics, communications, and the introduction of automation and future test technologies.

The next step is to obtain realistic design and construction budgets. Hospital laboratory construction is expensive. Nonetheless, fiscal constraints should not interfere with designing and building a safe and efficient laboratory. Along the same lines, realistic allocations of space must be done prior to the design phase. It is expensive and wasteful to design a laboratory and then to be faced with redesigning all or part of it to accommodate changes in the budget or space allocations. An adequate investment to do the project right in the first place is the most economical approach to providing a functional laboratory.

Part of developing a realistic and accurate budget is to decide whether to build a new laboratory or to renovate an older one. This obviously involves decisions about the health care facility as a whole. Estimating the costs of new construction (whether for a new building or expansion of an existing one) is generally straightforward. In contrast, estimating the costs of renovations is challenging. First, original construction drawings may not be available or may no longer be accurate due to changes made after the original construction was completed. Thus, the architect and engineer may have limited knowledge of how the laboratory was constructed or modified. Second, laboratories built according to past architectural standards and building codes may not meet current standards and codes. Third, older facilities are likely to contain asbestos in insulating material

and/or floor tiles, as well as lead-based paint. Abating either material is a complex and expensive process. Fourth, older buildings were often built with fixed ceilings and walls, complicating changes in lighting, the HVAC system, IT and telecommunications cabling, plumbing, and the electrical power supply. Fifth, some older buildings do not have the load capacity to support heavy pieces of equipment. Last, construction in older buildings often reveals unexpected issues that must be addressed, adding to the cost and complexity of the project. It is for these and other reasons that it may cost more to renovate an existing building than it would to build a new one.

Design Phase

Several general principles should guide the design phase (10). First, the greater the investment in planning, the more likely a project will be completed on time and under budget. Second, users will be happy with the results of a project only if they believe that they have been able to make significant contributions to it. Third, there need to be clear lines of accountability and communication. Fourth, user expectations should be expressed clearly and unequivocally at the outset; no architect or engineer should be expected to make major changes midway in a project. Last, logic and common sense should guide decisions throughout the process (5).

The first task for the architect, designer, and engineer (the design team) is to understand who the laboratory representative will be, who will have authority to make decisions, and the limits of the budget and space allocations. The next task is for them to learn the needs of the laboratory. These tasks should be undertaken in this order; it is important for the design team to know the constraints of the project before the design phase begins. Once the design team has completed these tasks, the knowledge gained can be used to develop realistic and workable design plans. As the design phase continues, it is for the most part largely one in which the design team works with the laboratory staff to accommodate the needs of the laboratory within the constraints of the project. In many cases, there will be insufficient space or funds to accommodate the needs of the laboratory; in cases such as this, either the laboratory administration must acquire the necessary space or funds or the project will need to be scaled back.

Once preliminary design plans have been drafted and agreed upon, the laboratory staff must address the myriad of details necessary to design a functional laboratory. Every conceivable detail should be thought of and addressed. Nothing should be taken for granted. It is far less expensive and easier to remove features from a design plan than it is to add them at a later point, particularly during the construction phase. The latter process, known as change orders, is one of the most common reasons for construction projects to go over budget. An even thornier problem is the feature that should have been included but cannot be added at any cost once construction has begun.

After final construction documents have been drafted and approved, bids will be requested from general contractors. Any necessary specifications should be included in the request-for-bids document. Once a general contractor has been selected, that contractor will recruit subcontractors to provide services that the general contractor does not provide. The last step prior to construction is for the institution and general contractor to obtain all necessary building permits and other legal documents needed for the project.

Construction Phase

For new laboratory construction, the construction phase generally proceeds for some time before the laboratory representative needs to be involved. The point at which the laboratory representative needs to work closely with the contractor is when the contractor begins to install walls, electrical power, IT and telecommunications cables, plumbing, and casework. From this point on, the laboratory representative will be called upon to make many unexpected decisions, often on short notice, and to clarify ambiguities in construction documents. It is expensive to make changes at this point in the process, but necessary changes should be made at this time rather than years later, when costs are even higher and the disruption in the laboratory makes the changes impractical.

Renovation projects vary in the amount and types of construction that are needed. Many projects require minimal demolition and few changes to the HVAC, plumbing, electrical power supply, and telecommunications and IT systems. In projects such as this, many of the changes are in casework only, or are more cosmetic in nature, and can be accomplished while the laboratory continues to operate. For more extensive renovations, the required demolition makes it necessary to gut the laboratory, in which case the project more closely resembles that of constructing a new laboratory.

Postconstruction Phase

The postconstruction phase is one of the most important, yet often neglected, phases in the process. Almost all construction projects have a warranty, usually for a short period, and the postconstruction phase provides the opportunity to use the warranty to correct things that were not completed or were done incorrectly. The laboratory staff should monitor carefully everything associated with the project, record their findings, and communicate them to the general contractor at the earliest possible time. The longer one waits, the more difficult it becomes for the contractor to return to the site to correct problems. Once the warranty has expired, then it becomes expensive to fix something that could have been done earlier at no cost.

SUMMARY

The construction of a new clinical laboratory, or the renovation of an existing one, is an excellent opportunity to improve the operations and efficiency of a clinical laboratory. It also offers the laboratory staff an opportunity to assess existing laboratory processes and to modify them. A successful construction or renovation project is characterized by the investment of large amounts of time in planning and designing the new facility, good communication between all of the parties involved in the project, a logical and common-sense approach to the project, and realistic expectations. Done well, a new or renovated laboratory facility will accommodate the needs of the laboratory staff for many years.

RESOURCES

Some general resources are listed in the references (1, 2, 5, 9, 10). The reader who needs additional information should consult The American Institute of Architects (http://www.aia.org/). The Institute can provide additional information, including a list of architects in a given area who have experience in designing laboratories and other health care facilities.

REFERENCES

1. **The American Institute of Architects Academy of Architecture for Health and The Facilities Guidelines Institute.** 2001. *Guidelines for Design and Construction of Hospital and Health Care Facilities.* American Institute of Architects, Washington, D.C.
2. **College of American Pathologists.** 1985. *Medical Laboratory Planning and Design.* College of American Pathologists, Skokie, Ill.
3. **Collins, C. H.** 1993. *Laboratory-Acquired Infections,* 3rd ed. Butterworth-Heinemann, Oxford, United Kingdom.
4. **Crane, J. T., and J. F. Riley.** 1997. Design issues in the comprehensive BSL2 and BSL3 laboratory, p. 63–114. *In* J. Y. Richmond (ed.), *Designing a Modern Microbiological/Biomedical Laboratory.* American Public Health Association, Washington, D.C.
5. **Crane, J. T., and J. Y. Richmond.** 2000. Design of biomedical laboratory facilities, p. 283–311. *In* D. O. Fleming and D. L. Hunt (ed.), *Biological Safety: Principles and Practices,* 3rd ed. American Society for Microbiology, Washington, D.C.
6. **Furrows, S. J., and G. L. Ridgway.** 2001. 'Good laboratory practice' in diagnostic laboratories using nucleic acid amplification methods. *Clin. Microbiol. Infect.* **7:**227–229.
7. **Infectious Diseases Society of America.** 2001. Policy statement on consolidation of clinical microbiology laboratories. *Clin. Infect. Dis.* **32:**604.
8. **Kruse, R. H., W. H. Puckett, and J. H. Richardson.** 1991. Biological safety cabinetry. *Clin. Microbiol. Rev.* **4:**207–241.
9. **National Committee for Clinical Laboratory Standards.** 1998. *Laboratory Design. Approved Guideline.* Document GP 18-A. National Committee for Clinical Laboratory Standards, Wayne, Pa.
10. **National Research Council.** 2000. *Laboratory Design, Construction, and Renovation.* National Academy Press, Washington, D.C.
11. **Paxton, A.** 2000. All the oars to the core. *CAP Today* **14:**22–32.
12. **Peterson, L. R., J. D. Hamilton, E. J. Baron, L. S. Tompkins, J. M. Miller, C. M. Wilfert, F. C. Tenover, and R. B. Thomson.** 2001. Role of clinical microbiology laboratories in the management and control of infectious diseases and the delivery of health care. *Clin. Infect. Dis.* **32:**605–610.
13. **Pfaller, M. A., and L. A. Herwaldt.** 1997. The clinical microbiology laboratory and infection control: emerging pathogens, antimicrobial resistance, and new technology. *Clin. Infect. Dis.* **25:**858–870.
14. **Scheckler, W. E., D. Brimhall, A. S. Buck, B. M. Farr, C. Friedman, R. A. Garibaldi, P. A. Gross, J. A. Harris, W. J. Hierholzer, W. J. Martone, L. L. McDonald, and S. L. Solomon.** 1998. Requirements for infrastructure and essential activities of infection control and epidemiology in hospitals: a consensus panel report. *Am. J. Infect. Control* **26:**47–60.
15. **U.S. Department of Health and Human Services, Centers for Disease Control and Prevention, and National Institutes of Health.** 1999. *Biosafety in Microbiological and Biomedical Laboratories,* 4th ed. J. Y. Richmond and R. W. McKinney (ed.). U.S. Government Printing Office, Washington, D.C.
16. **Wilson, M. L., and L. B. Reller.** 1998. Clinical laboratory-acquired infections, p. 343–355. *In* P. Brachman and J. Bennett (ed.), *Hospital Infections,* 4th ed. Lippincott-Raven, Philadelphia, Pa.

Laboratory Consultation, Communication, and Information Systems

JOSEPH M. CAMPOS

4

The flow of information to and from clinical laboratories was revolutionized 30 years ago by the appearance of the first computerized laboratory information system (LIS) (1, 3). The initial major advantage was financial, namely, more efficient billing for laboratory services. Shortly thereafter, the reporting of textual and numerical test results was improved upon by the evolving feature set. Clinical microbiology laboratories began realizing important benefits when it became possible to issue complex culture and antimicrobial susceptibility reports via the LIS.

LISs continue to thrive in the clinical microbiology laboratory environment today. These laboratories furnish vital information to health care providers, especially those who deal frequently with infectious diseases. Laboratory test results essential for diagnosis and treatment of infections are reported. Information that promotes optimum patient management, such as advice on test selection, guidance for specimen collection, interpretation of test results, and suggestions for additional testing, can also be added (5). Clinical microbiologists today are brokers of a wide variety of information that advances patient care (8). The goal of this chapter is to review the state of information management in clinical microbiology laboratories today, emphasizing the central role of LISs.

HEALTH INSURANCE PORTABILITY AND ACCOUNTABILITY ACT OF 1996

A significant event that occurred recently in the United States globally affects the management of health care information. The Health Insurance Portability and Accountability Act of 1996 (HIPAA) has an impact that is so enormous that it is appropriate to begin with a description of its effects. One of its primary purposes is to maintain the security and privacy of information found in patient medical records. The standards also address the mechanisms by which information can be coded and exchanged electronically. This applies directly to the distribution of laboratory test data to clinicians, insurers, and patients.

HIPAA governs the manner in which patient-specific health information can be generated, disseminated, and stored in the United States (17). A related regulation intended to assist in the implementation of HIPAA was also promulgated and is entitled Standards for Privacy of Individually Identifiable Health Information (the Privacy Rule). It was crafted by the Department of Health and Human Services and became effective on 14 April 2001. Most health care institutions and health care plans are obligated to comply with the Privacy Rule by 14 April 2003. Small health care plans may delay compliance until 14 April 2004. Although the provisions of HIPAA and the Privacy Rule do not apply to health care organizations outside of the United States, they establish standards for handling patient information that are relevant to and worthy of consideration by governments in all countries.

The Privacy Rule characterizes the safeguards that health care providers must take to protect the privacy of health information. It establishes standards that protect the medical records and other personal health information of patients. It provides patients more control over their own health data and defines limits on the use and distribution of health records by other entities. It declares that patients are entitled to examine and obtain copies of their own health records and to request that mistaken information be corrected. Patients are also at liberty to find out what disclosures of their health information have been made and to whom. The Privacy Rule holds violators of the standards accountable for their actions by the imposition of civil and criminal penalties. It does, however, permit disclosure of patient-specific health information to public health authorities in order to protect the general public health.

Patient-specific data produced by clinical microbiology laboratories in the United States fall under the jurisdiction of HIPAA. It does not matter whether the information is verbal, written, or electronic. The information may be distributed during the preanalytical, analytical, or postanalytical phases of testing and may be advisory, instructional, results oriented, or interpretive. Clinical microbiologists are expected to deliver this information to health care providers in a timely and comprehensible fashion without violating the tenets of HIPAA.

BUILDING THE MICROBIOLOGY COMPONENTS OF LISs

The modern LIS offers many tools that support communication between the clinical microbiology laboratory and health care providers. In order to take full advantage of these tools, the individuals responsible for building the microbiology component of the LIS must thoroughly understand microbiology testing. These individuals ideally should be clinical microbiologists with a strong interest and commitment to building their module of the LIS. Absent this, the builders of the microbiology module should request and receive guidance from clinical microbiologists during system configuration and validation testing.

In many health care facilities, laboratory tests are not ordered in the LIS but are ordered via a hospital information system (HIS) or a third-party order-entry system that operates as a clinician-friendly front end to the LIS. Under this circumstance, clinical microbiologists must have major input during the selection and formatting of information that will be seen by those ordering microbiology tests in any of these other systems. This may require laboratorians to aggressively seek roles in the external information system building process. Too often, laboratory personnel are overlooked when teams charged with building information systems are assembled.

LISs must handle microbiology testing very differently from the way in which they handle testing in other laboratory disciplines. One reason is that microbiology test results are mostly nonnumerical. Instead, many results are complex composites of text and tables of antimicrobial susceptibility data. In some instances, preliminary findings must be able to initiate orders for "reflex" tests (e.g., ordering antimicrobial susceptibility tests when culture results are positive).

Test Codes

All laboratory tests have codes (mnemonics) and code translations assigned to them as they are built in the LIS. It is advantageous if a rigorously applied convention is used during the code selection process. Logically devised coding conventions encourage the remembrance of codes by LIS users. Most systems permit codes up to six characters in length and allow codes to contain both alphabetical and numerical characters. While most laboratories depend on alphabetical codes abstracted from actual test names (e.g., URICUL for urine culture and BLOCUL for blood culture), some laboratories have chosen predominantly numerical coding schemes to match codes in other institutional information systems and to eliminate code conflicts between test names with similar wording.

A laboratory test may have more than one name in general use (e.g., the serum bactericidal titer and the Schlichter test). It is advisable that cross-references to all synonyms for a test be identified during test building so that user-initiated searches for any of the common names for a test lead to the same test code. Otherwise, LIS users will become frustrated when they are unable to find a test they wish to order and will order it inappropriately as a miscellaneous test.

Entering Results While Ordering Tests

Some LISs allow or even require that one or more components of a test or battery be resulted during the ordering process. This is often true for microbiology cultures in which the specimen description is one of the test or battery components. It may be mandatory to answer the specimen description during the ordering process because the individuals placing orders have the specimens in front of them. When specimen descriptions are predictable for tests (e.g., a pharyngeal swab for a pharyngeal culture) it saves time if the LIS can automatically answer the specimen description with a default code. This streamlines the ordering process

and eliminates ordering errors. Of course, the default specimen description code can be overridden when necessary.

Pending Text

Some LISs can be configured to display informative text automatically while test results are pending (Table 1). Examples of "pending text" that might be used with microbiology tests include the expected turnaround time for test results, a telephone number to call if there are questions regarding the test, or a notice that a reflex test will be ordered if the result is positive. The pending text no longer displays once test results have been entered into the LIS.

Text Code Dictionaries

A major effort during the building of the microbiology section of an LIS is the preparation of text code dictionaries. Several dictionaries must be built, including those for microbiology text codes, microbiology method codes, growth media codes, workload codes, antimicrobial susceptibility codes, specimen description codes, and microorganism name codes.

During the creation of microbiology dictionaries, an important decision must be made regarding the scheme for assigning microorganism name codes. The use of a consistently applied approach that is understood by laboratory personnel simplifies the entry of culture results, since the codes for most microorganisms can be figured out "on the fly." One coding convention in common use is the first letter of the microorganism's genus name and the first several letters of the species name (Table 2). A limitation to this system occurs when codes for different microorganisms turn out to be identical (e.g., ECOLI for both *Escherichia coli* and *Entamoeba coli*). Another system in use is the first three letters of the genus name and the first three letters of the species name (assuming the LIS permits six-letter codes). In this case the mnemonic for *E. coli* the bacterium would be ESCCOL and that for *E. coli* the protozoan would be ENTCOL. However, problems still occur when assigning codes for microorganisms like *Oligella ureolytica* and *Oligella urethralis* (OLIURE in both instances). Any convention selected likely will encounter its own set of problems; thus, a secondary convention should be applied when codes specified by the primary convention are ambiguous (e.g., use ECOLI for the bacterium and ENCOLI for the protozoan).

Some LISs permit the creation of group codes for microorganisms that enable users to refer to a group of

TABLE 1 Sample LIS test and battery names and their pending text[a]

Name	Pending text
Aerobic blood culture	Results in <5 days
CSF culture and Gram stain	Results in <72 hours
Fungal culture	Results in <21 days
GC culture	Results in <72 hours
Bordetella pertussis culture	Results in <7 days
Urine culture	Results in <24 hours
CMV shell vial culture	Results in <48 hours
Res Vir antigen panel	Results in <24 hours
Group A *Streptococcus* detection	Results in <2 hours
RPR	Results in <24 hours

[a] Abbreviations: GC, *Neisseria gonorrhoeae*; CMV, cytomegalovirus; Res Vir, respiratory virus.

TABLE 2 Sample microorganism name codes and their translations

Microorganism code	Translation
AACTI	*Actinobacillus actinomycetemcomitans*
ABAUM	*Acinetobacter baumannii*
ABIOSP	*Abiotrophia* sp. (nutritionally variant *Streptococcus*)
ABOVI	*Actinomyces bovis*
ABSISP	*Absidia* sp.
ACANSP	*Acanthamoeba* sp.
ACAVI	*Aeromonas caviae*
ACHRSP	*Achromobacter* sp.
ACIDSP	*Acidaminococcus* sp.
ACINSP	*Acinetobacter* sp.
ACLAV	*Aspergillus clavatus*

related microorganisms simultaneously. Generally, group members share a property in common (e.g., ANA for anaerobes, GNB for gram-negative bacilli, MOLD for filamentous fungi, and VIRUS for viruses). Assigning microorganisms to group codes should be done by individuals with an understanding of both the microbiology laboratory and the potential uses for microorganism group codes in the LIS.

Antimicrobial Susceptibility Batteries

The creation of antimicrobial susceptibility batteries is an essential phase during the building of the microbiology section of an LIS. This undertaking is preceded by defining antimicrobial agent "tests" that can be answered with numerical or text codes indicating whether isolates are susceptible, intermediately susceptible, or resistant. Groups of these "tests" are then assembled into batteries of antimicrobial agents reflective of the reporting wishes of the laboratory. Separate batteries are usually defined for different categories of isolates like gram-negative bacilli, gram-positive cocci, anaerobes, gram-negative urinary tract isolates, streptococci, and enterococci, among others. In some cases, a separate battery should be created for a single microorganism species (e.g., *Streptococcus pneumoniae*) if that is consistent with National Committee for Clinical Laboratory Standards (NCCLS) guidelines (14). When an isolate belongs to more than one isolate category (e.g., a urine culture isolate of *E. coli* belongs to both the gram-negative bacilli and the gram-negative urinary tract isolate categories), the category that describes the isolate more specifically takes precedence (gram-negative urinary tract isolate battery in this example).

The group of antimicrobial agents assigned to each battery should be based on input from clinicians (particularly infectious diseases physicians), from the microbiology laboratory, and from the recommendations published by the NCCLS (14). Many LISs permit the recording and storage of results for a large group of antimicrobial agents but selective reporting of only a limited group of results (e.g., for those agents present in the hospital formulary). As a cost-containment initiative, some LISs enable the cascading of results so that a result for an expensive agent is displayed only if the result for a less expensive alternative is resistant (e.g., a ceftriaxone result for *E. coli* is reported only if the cefazolin result is resistant). The decisions of which

results to report and when they should be reported should be based on consensus of the groups mentioned above.

Before antimicrobial susceptibility results can be reported, specific text codes (antimicrobial susceptibility codes) must be defined for the standard designations of susceptible, intermediately susceptible, and resistant (e.g., S for susceptible, I for intermediate, and R for resistant). In addition, some LISs offer opportunities for defining extra antimicrobial susceptibility codes that can be used creatively for crafting more functional antimicrobial susceptibility reports (e.g., NREACT for nonreactive and HIDE for ⟨⟨DO NOT REPORT⟩⟩). For example, codes can be in place to serve as reminders to technologists to take specific actions. A code like NOINTP can be used to indicate that testing of a particular antimicrobial agent against a specific microorganism has not been standardized by the NCCLS. A code like DOESBL can be available for reporting cefpodoxime results against *E. coli*, *Klebsiella pneumoniae*, and *Klebsiella oxytoca* when the MIC is > 8 μg/ml. This code would remind technologists to check isolates for extended-spectrum beta-lactamase production before final reports are issued.

Sophisticated antimicrobial susceptibility reports that include cost information and recommended dosages for antimicrobial agents can be created by some LISs. Reports containing relative or actual cost information reduce pharmacy expenditures by encouraging clinicians to select less expensive antimicrobial agents that still show excellent in vitro activity. Reports with dosage recommendations are particularly helpful in hospitals where medical student, intern, and resident training is taking place.

Billing for Laboratory Tests

The driving force that led to the development of the first LIS was a desire to capture laboratory test billing more efficiently than could be accomplished manually. Because billing transactions are initiated automatically by the LIS upon test ordering or specimen receipt, it was no longer necessary to complete paper charge tickets that were manually transcribed into ledgers or stand-alone electronic billing systems.

Billing can be more complicated in the microbiology laboratory than in other laboratory sections due to the automatic ordering of follow-up tests (e.g., a laboratory-initiated order for an antimicrobial susceptibility test when a clinically significant microorganism is detected by culture). Such "reflex" orders may trail initial culture orders by several days, raising the possibility of difficult-to-reimburse late charges if the billing transactions are handled improperly. Fortunately, most LISs are prepared to handle billing for laboratory-initiated orders in a manner satisfactory to payers for laboratory services.

Current procedural terminology (CPT) codes were first devised by the American Medical Association (AMA) in 1966. Among the 8,107 codes in the current 2002 listing is a small group applicable to microbiology testing. Fee-for-service reimbursement for laboratory testing is dependent upon inclusion of the appropriate CPT code(s) in bills for laboratory services rendered. The construction of test or battery billing maintenance in LISs includes an indicator of the applicable CPT code(s) so that these critical bits of information can be forwarded electronically to the hospital billing information system. Although significant improvement in microbiology CPT coding was attained by the AMA in 2001, enough ambiguity yet remains that individuals with microbiology expertise should participate in CPT code selection.

Most LIS vendors have fashioned their microbiology modules so that billing for the most frequent reflex test, antimicrobial susceptibility testing, occurs automatically without user intervention. The billing transaction includes the appropriate CPT code to be sent to the hospital billing information system. It is also feasible with some LISs to use the same automatic billing feature to charge for other reflex tests, such as Western blotting for human immunodeficiency virus type 1 (HIV-1) antibody-positive specimens or confirmatory fluorescent treponemal antibody-absorption testing for rapid plasma reagin (RPR)-positive specimens. In these situations, the reflex test can be built in the same manner as an antimicrobial agent battery. For example, each band on a Western blot strip could be defined as an "antimicrobial agent" test and unique susceptibility result codes could be defined to indicate the presence or absence of each antibody band. Apart from automatic billing, this approach offers the benefit of recalling results from these other reflex tests with "canned" microbiology reports.

Microbiology laboratories are allowed to bill additionally for specific activities performed during specimen processing or while identifying isolates (Table 3). Examples include grinding of tissue prior to culture inoculation and the performance of three or more identification tests on culture isolates. Since these activities apply only to certain specimens or cultures, they need to be billed on an ad hoc basis. This is accomplished via technologist entry of charges into the LIS as the charges are incurred. Alternatively, charges can be entered as a group when final culture results are issued.

TABLE 3 Examples of manually billed microbiology tests[a]

Bill code	Name	CPT code(s)
M8011H	Bacterial ID (aerobic) × 1	87077
M8012H	Bacterial ID (aerobic) × 2	87077×2
M8013H	Bacterial ID (aerobic) × 3	87077×3
M8014H	Bacterial ID (aerobic) × 4	87077×4
M8015H	Bacterial ID (aerobic) × 5	87077×5
M8016H	Bacterial ID (anaerobic) × 1	87076
M8017H	Bacterial ID (anaerobic) × 2	87076×2
M8018H	Bacterial ID (anaerobic) × 3	87076×3
M8025H	ID by nucleic acid probe	87149
M8031H	Yeast ID × 1	87106
M8032H	Yeast ID × 2	87106×2
M8033H	Yeast ID × 3	87106×3
M8035H	Mold ID × 1	87107
M8036H	Mold ID × 2	87107×2
M8037H	Mold ID × 3	87107×3
M8041H	Viral ID	87253
M8051H	Serogrouping by agglutination × 1	87147
M8052H	Serogrouping by agglutination × 2	87147×2
M8053H	Serogrouping by agglutination × 3	87147×3
M8061H	Concentration for infectious agent	87015
M8071H	AFB ID	87118
M8076H	Macroscopic ID (helminth)	87169
M8077H	Macroscopic ID (arthropod)	87168
M8081H	Tissue homogenization	87176

[a] Abbreviations: ID, identification; AFB, acid-fast bacillus.

TABLE 4 Sample group worksheet codes and names

Worksheet code	Worksheet name
BLOOD	Blood cultures
CSF	CSF cultures
MISCEL	Miscellaneous cultures
RESPIR	Respiratory cultures
URINE	Urine cultures
ANA	Anaerobic cultures
MYCOB	Mycobacterial cultures
MYCOL	Mycology cultures
SEROL	Serologic tests
PARA	Parasitology exams
MICRO	Microbiology group
VIROL	Virology group
MICVIR	Microbiology-virology group

LIS Work Sheets

Individual work sheets (or work lists) are used to group similar laboratory tests within the LIS, providing a convenient way to divide work assignments among technologists. Individual work sheets frequently are printed by technologists at the beginning of a work shift to obtain lists of specimens or cultures that require attention that day. They also can be printed at the end of a work shift to double-check that specimens or cultures were not overlooked. The status of tests assigned to individual worksheets can be monitored by calling standard LIS reports. Examples of these reports are those that provide lists of pending tests and overdue test results.

Microbiology tests are usually assigned to work sheets that correspond to laboratory workbenches, such as the blood culture bench, the respiratory culture bench, and the urine culture bench. For this reason, individuals who understand how the microbiology laboratory is organized should have a voice in assignment of tests to work sheets.

Some LISs permit the definition of group work sheets, which are groups of individual work sheets that have characteristics in common (Table 4). Group work sheets are of utility to microbiologists with managerial responsibilities that span more than one workbench. If the microbiology laboratory staff includes separate section supervisors responsible for all bacterial testing, all fungal testing, and all virologic testing, group work sheets can be defined that enable each section supervisor to monitor the status of tests in his or her domain. Similarly, an all-encompassing group work sheet can be defined that includes all of the microbiology individual work sheets. By calling this work sheet, the laboratory supervisor or director can monitor all tests being worked on in the laboratory.

Work sheet maintenance may include the option of defining the number of days following specimen receipt at which tests assigned to individual work sheets are overdue. For the overdue log to be functional, the tests assigned to the same individual work sheets must have the same threshold of days before they become overdue. It would be inadvisable to place routine blood cultures (incubated for 5 days) and fungal blood cultures (incubated for 21 days) on the same work sheet if the overdue log is going to be used.

LIS Rules

LIS rules enable laboratories to automate certain tasks and minimize manual data entry (21). Rules can apply preanalytically to guide the ordering of tests based on the patient's age, the ordering clinician, or earlier results in the patient's laboratory file. They also can flag duplicate test orders to eliminate wastage of reagents and technologist time. Rules can be used analytically to flag questionable antimicrobial susceptibility results or as a reminder to report critical test results by telephone. Rules can be triggered postanalytically that provide clinicians with predefined interpretive comments that clarify the clinical significance of test results. The creation of LIS rules suitable for microbiology testing requires individuals who understand both the laboratory and the capability of the rules engine.

LIS rules usually are defined as "if-then" statements. "If" statements specify the conditions that trigger rules. "Then" statements describe the actions to be taken when "if" conditions are met. An example of a commonly used microbiology rule is: if a *Staphylococcus aureus* isolate is resistant to oxacillin (if statement), then the susceptibility results for all beta-lactam antimicrobial agents should be reported as resistant (then statement). Sophisticated rules engines can process complex if-then statements that include multiple conditions linked by operators such as "and," "or," "greater than," "less than," and "equal to."

Rules should be organized into one or more hierarchies. One hierarchy should define the points at which rules can be executed. This is important because when two or more rules apply during test performance, the corresponding actions should be taken in a logical sequence. For example, separate rules that call for (i) ordering a culture of a "clean-catch" urine specimen for patients older than 18 years and then (ii) reporting the ciprofloxacin susceptibility result if the culture is positive need to be evaluated in the correct order. The execution point for the rule concerning patient age is at the ordering stage, and that for the rule regarding susceptibility testing is at the results stage. The logical order for execution of these rules is (i) order rule and (ii) results rule.

A second necessary hierarchy decides the action sequence when two or more applicable rules have the same execution point. An example here is (i) a rule that prevents ordering of duplicate rotavirus antigen tests for the same patient within 24 h and (ii) a rule that adds rotavirus antigen test orders for stool specimens collected in the emergency department for patients less than 12 months of age between 1 January and 30 April. Many rules engines in this situation would execute the rules in the order in which they were created. Logically, the laboratory's intent is for the rule that prevents the ordering of a second rotavirus assay to take precedence over the rule that automatically orders a rotavirus test.

INFORMATION SHARING DURING THE PREANALYTICAL PHASE OF TESTING

During the preanalytical phase of testing, clinicians wish to select tests that are likely to provide diagnostically useful or therapeutically important information. Clinical microbiologists can be extremely helpful during this phase by supplying information that assists in test selection that leads to quality patient management.

Laboratory Test Menu

The laboratory test menu should be dynamic. When new diagnostic tests become available, whether they are performed in-house or not, the list of tests available to clinicians should be updated. The list should be easily modified so that practitioners have a current group of tests from which to choose. Strong consideration should be given to supplying more than just the names of tests. Test codes, test charges, and expected turnaround times for results are all relevant bits of information.

Another important way in which clinical microbiologists benefit patient care is by assisting clinicians in selecting tests rationally and helping them to collect appropriate specimens. This can be accomplished by fielding telephone queries. However, a more effective method available at all times is developing a catalog of tests that is comprehensive, information rich, and easily accessed.

Many commercial laboratories publish catalogs in book form that are distributed to ordering sites throughout their service areas. Some laboratories prepare them in loose-leaf format that enables easy updating as new tests are added and old tests are deleted. Useful information in these catalogs includes test names and synonyms, required specimens and quantities, specimen transport conditions, turnaround times for test results, the relevant CPT code(s), and prices (Table 5). Interactive electronic catalogs offer the same advantages and more. Catalog contents can be quickly searched by key words or phrases to locate the desired information. They can be modified easily and as often as necessary. They can include links to electronic journal articles and textbooks found on the Internet that contain more information about the tests.

Laboratory Requisitions

Paper requisitions are inflexible when it comes to the addition or removal of tests from the menu. However, they can be used effectively with a little foresight. They should be prepared in small batches that last only a few months. When new batches are ordered, requisition contents should be reviewed and modified where necessary. There should also be a location on the requisition where missing test names can be written in by hand.

Electronic requisitions found in computerized order-entry systems are much more flexible than paper requisitions. These requisitions can be accessed through the LIS, the HIS, an ordering module interfaced to the LIS, or an Internet-based ordering module. The list of tests can be modified quickly whenever there is a change and there is no worry of exhausting the supply of requisitions. As with paper requisitions, there must be a capability for ordering tests that are missing from the electronic list. That is generally accomplished through the use of a "miscellaneous test" in which test specifics (e.g., test name and specimen description) are entered during ordering. When miscellaneous test requests are received by the laboratory, there should be a policy of incorporating them on the electronic requisition for future use.

The Internet is gaining in popularity for ordering of laboratory tests because it is possible to do so from computers anywhere in the world (18). All that is needed on the ordering computer is Internet browsing software and authorized access to the ordering system. A major concern over this mode of order communication is the possibility of unauthorized electronic eavesdroppers acquiring sensitive patient information. Sophisticated means of encrypting the information stream are being used to protect patient confidentiality and achieve HIPAA compliance.

TABLE 5 Sample catalog information about CSF culture and Gram stain[a]

Category	Information
1. Name of test	CSF culture and Gram stain
2. Synonyms or alternate names	Cerebrospinal fluid C/S; culture, CSF
3. Specimen type(s)	CSF, ventricular fluid, or subdural fluid
4. Minimum specimen volume	1 ml
5. Specimen container	Sterile, leak-proof container
6. Transport instructions	Bring to laboratory immediately
7. Information needed	None
8. Special requirements	Send tube no. 2 of 4
9. Test schedule, approximate TAT	Daily, 72 h
10. Laboratory section	Microbiology
11. Prior approval or notice	Not needed
12. Requisition	Microbiology
13. Storage instructions	Refrigeration (4°C)
14. Reflexive order conditions	Antimicrobial susceptibility test if pathogen recovered
15. CPT codes	87070, 87205
16. Comments	Gram stain automatically performed
17. Price	$x.xx

[a] Abbreviations: C/S, culture and sensitivity; TAT, turnaround time.

INFORMATION MANAGEMENT DURING THE ANALYTICAL PHASE OF TESTING

Instead of information flowing predominantly from the laboratory to clinicians, as in the preanalytical and postanalytical phases of testing, the analytical phase finds the laboratory seeking information from internal and external sources. The clinical microbiology laboratory depends heavily on access to repositories of information during the analytical phase of testing. That is because much of the work is visual or decision table oriented. The information received is then acted upon by individuals in the laboratory.

Procedure Manuals

The regulatory agencies overseeing laboratories require up-to-date procedure manuals that are accessible to laboratory workers at all times that testing is in progress. Most laboratories rely on traditional procedure manuals comprised of pages stored in loose-leaf binders. The loose-leaf format lends itself well to preparing photocopies for simultaneous use at multiple workbenches and to replacing outdated procedures with newer versions. A better approach gaining in popularity is conversion of paper procedure manuals into a series of on-line documents that are stored in word-processing format (e.g., x.doc), portable document format (e.g., x.pdf), or Internet browser format (e.g., x.htm) (16). Such documents are easily modified and can be printed to paper, if desired. Documentation of annual review can be accomplished efficiently and unequivocally via electronic signature. Color photographs to illustrate procedural steps can be embedded in the documents. Perhaps their greatest advantage is that the entire procedure manual can be searched rapidly by use of key words or phrases to quickly locate a particular procedure or group of procedures. The NCCLS recently released a revised guideline for the preparation of paper or electronic laboratory procedure manuals (approved guideline GP2-A3) that most laboratories follow (10). In addition, it has made available a computer template that facilitates the preparation of procedures in NCCLS format (approved guideline GP2-A2-C).

Image Libraries

Photographs are indispensable to the accurate identification of many microorganisms. Photographs of gross colonies and microscopic morphologies of a variety of microorganisms can be maintained in image repositories that are useful in differentiating similar microorganisms from one another. Every clinical microbiology laboratory should have a collection of photographs to which technologists can refer during their work. The repository may consist of photographs in a textbook, images in a text atlas, or 35-mm slides maintained in the laboratory.

One of the spin-offs of current technology has been a growing reliance in the laboratory on digital images instead of images recorded on film (20). The reasons are the ability to store high-resolution images on inexpensive magnetic and optical media, the ease with which these images can be manipulated and enhanced with computer software, and the dramatic reductions seen recently in the cost of image capturing hardware (e.g., scanners and cameras). The most significant factor may be the ease of access that laboratories now have to externally stored digital images. Images can be placed on servers located anywhere in the world and yet be viewed and/or downloaded nearly instantaneously over the Internet.

Tables of Microbiological Data

Laboratory identification of many microorganisms is based on a comparison of their physiologic and metabolic properties with those found in reference databases. This can be accomplished manually with a side-by-side assessment, via flowchart analysis, or with the aid of a computer. Many microbiology laboratories still identify microorganisms through analysis of information found in tables and flowcharts in textbooks, journal articles, and government documents. This approach is laborious and time-consuming but has the advantage of including human judgment in the decision-making process.

The use of tables to identify microorganisms determines the best fit between an unknown microorganism and the properties of a group of microorganisms belonging to the same species. These tables usually indicate the percentage of species members that exhibit positive results for particular tests. While this approach is effective when test results for an unknown microorganism closely match those for an established species, it may yield inaccurate identifications when test results are not very similar to those for known species.

The same data found in the identification tables described above can be converted into computerized databases and then quickly and accurately compared with the properties of an unknown microorganism. This has been done for many years in a proprietary fashion by the manufacturers of some automated systems for microbial identification. The sophisticated analysis includes weighting of key properties and pattern recognition to derive best-fit identifications. The likelihood of an identification and the degree of separation from similar microorganisms can also be calculated.

It is also possible for individual clinical microbiologists to convert their own identification tables and those present in the public domain into queriable databases. This can be accomplished by using off-the-shelf database software programs to prepare such databases manually. The same software can then be used to define queries that identify the microorganisms included in the database whose biochemical test results best match those of an unknown microorganism.

Flowchart Algorithms

Flowchart algorithms are another approach to microorganism identification that have been used for many years. This approach differs from the use of tables in that identification test results with the greatest discriminating power are placed at the top of the flowchart and assigned greater weight than results farther down. While the early decisions in the flowchart algorithm are often correct, the accuracy of the later decisions may be compromised by the tests at the bottom of the flowchart that have lower discriminating ability.

Laboratory Work Cards

More than any other area of laboratory medicine, microbiology testing depends on a dependable flow of information between technologists assigned to different work shifts or workdays. That is because very little microbiology testing can be completed in a single work shift and more than one technologist may participate in the testing. Laboratories must have a system for passing information between technologists that accurately conveys the status of testing. Some form of microbiology work card is the choice of most laboratories. Many laboratories, even those with an LIS, still use paper work cards that are maintained at each workstation. Technologists record the work performed daily on individual work cards. Information is documented in the form of handwritten codes, short phrases, or checkoff boxes. Work cards for completed tests are stored for at least 2 years per regulatory requirement.

Almost all LISs can be configured to record microbiology workup information on electronic templates that are accessed by individuals working on the same cultures at later times (Table 6). Information is entered onto the LIS "work card" in the form of text codes or short strings of free text. Entries on the work card are generally organized by isolate or culture medium and then chronologically within each of these categories. The benefits of paperless entry include guaranteed legibility, easy supervisory review of work, and automatic indexing of workup data to simplify

TABLE 6 Sample work card entries for *S. pneumoniae* blood culture isolate

Work card prompt	Response
GRST (Gram stain)	GPCPSM (gram-positive cocci in pairs)
CAT (catalase)	NEG (negative)
PHON (telephone report)	DONE (completed)
OPT (optochin)	POS (positive)
BESC (bile esculin)	NEG (negative)
NACL (6.5% NaCl tolerance)	NEG (negative)
BDIL (broth dilution MIC)	DONE (completed)
PURPLT (purity plate)	AOK (pure culture)
SAVE (save isolate on slant)	DONE (completed)

electronic searches later. The electronic work card also can be used to standardize microorganism workups and accrue the workload for productivity analyses.

Instrument Interfaces

The proliferation of semiautomated and automated instruments in clinical laboratories has dramatically increased the volume of data transfer between instruments and LISs. Information transfer can be accomplished via manual transcription or automatic communication of data via electronic interfaces. Transfer of information to and from instruments that are not electronically interfaced to an LIS is accomplished by manual entry. The number of keystrokes required for this activity can be limited on the LIS side through the use of text codes or keyboard mapping to insert commonly used words, phrases, or even blocks of text. Because of the human component to information entry, transcription errors are an ever-present possibility and the fidelity of data entry should be subjected to supervisory review.

Far easier and much more accurate than manual transcription is the automatic transfer of information between instruments and LISs (12, 13). This can be accomplished through the use of scripted or electronic interfaces. A scripted interface is essentially a very fast electronic typist. It transcribes information from an instrument to the LIS in the same manner that a technologist would—just a lot faster and more accurately. The electronic interface is more complicated in that it converts a stream of data from one system into a format understandable by the other system. Batch interfaces send data on demand, while dynamic interfaces send data as soon as they become available. Unidirectional interfaces transfer information in a single direction—either from the LIS to an instrument (download) or from an instrument to the LIS (upload). Bidirectional interfaces are more costly and complicated to set up since data must be able to flow in either direction.

The decision as to which type of interface is more suitable for a microbiology instrument depends on the timeliness with which the data are needed, the traffic capacity (bandwidth) of the interface, and the cost-benefit ratio of having data flow in one or both directions. Interfaces which download specimen demographic information from an LIS to an instrument are almost always desirable because they eliminate the need for transcribing required information from one system to another. Interfaces which upload data from an instrument to an LIS are valuable when the data sets are large and contain information that will be reported directly to clinicians (e.g., microbial identification and antimicrobial susceptibility data). When the instrument data are only preliminary in nature and require follow-up work at the laboratory workbench (e.g., positive blood culture results from an automated blood culture instrument), justifying the expense of a bidirectional interface is more difficult.

Inventory Management

Inventory management modules are available for some LISs and are intended to help organize and watch over the utilization of laboratory supplies (11). Some modules also assist in the monitoring of equipment maintenance. The modules generate reports regarding ordering patterns for supplies and printing out equipment maintenance logs. They also assist in the performance of cost analysis studies based on supply utilization data. These modules provide a real-time indication of supply levels if the usage of supplies can be entered into the LIS. Some inventory modules also track supply expiration dates by lot number. They alert laboratory personnel when additional supplies should be ordered and may even print order requisitions to be submitted to the purchasing department. When ordered supplies are received, inventory levels can be updated in the LIS. If ordered supplies have not arrived when expected, they remind laboratory personnel to contact the vendor.

Quality Control

The quality control modules found in many LISs aid clinical microbiology laboratory managers by simplifying the entry and review of quality control data. They provide data entry screens and reports that are customized to the requirements of the laboratory. They offer reminders to the laboratory when scheduled quality control data have not been entered. They also send warnings to the laboratory when quality control results are out of range and insist upon the entry of the remedial action taken. When out-of-range quality control results are entered, the LIS immediately alerts the individual entering the results. The LIS then awaits either an acknowledgment that the results are correct or a change to new results that are in range. Acknowledgment of out-of-range results qualifies the entered data for an exception report that should be reviewed daily by supervisory personnel.

Most LISs are able to plot numerical quality control data on an LIS-constructed Levey-Jennings control chart, evaluate the data, and notify users when results are "out of control." A Levey-Jennings control chart is a graphical display of quality control data that indicates the expected mean, the ±2 standard deviation boundary around the mean, and the ±3 standard deviation boundary around the mean. The principle is that current quality control results should exhibit the same distribution as past quality control results, if the test method is stable and being performed correctly. Results beyond the ±2 standard deviation boundary should be encountered no more than 5% of the time, and results beyond the ±3 standard deviation boundary should be seen no more than 1% of the time. When quality control results fall within the specified boundaries, the test is "in control," the results are acceptable, and patient results can be reported. When quality control results are beyond the specified boundaries, the test is "out of control," the results are unacceptable, and patient results cannot be reported. The NCCLS criteria for evaluating antimicrobial susceptibility quality control data are based on principles similar to those used by Levey-Jennings charts.

Many LISs are also able to evaluate numerical quality control according to rules developed by James O. Westgard (22) many years ago (Table 7). The data examined may be limited to a single control or may extend over results from several controls. An example of a Westgard rule violation that applies to a single control is as follows: a single quality control result falls outside the acceptable range, defined as ±2 standard deviations from the mean. An example of a rule infraction that extends over results from several controls is as follows: four consecutive quality control results are more than 1 standard deviation away from the mean in the same direction. The quality control module in most LISs can be set to apply any of the Westgard rules that have been defined within the system. The rules that will be applied usually can be individualized according to the quality control tests being performed.

Quality Assurance

Generic quality assurance rules can be applied automatically to test results to boost the recognition of potential problems. The rules listed below frequently are "hard coded" in the LIS software found in laboratories. Additional site-specific quality assurance rules can be defined by using the rules engine described earlier in this chapter.

1. Normal-Value Checking. Most regulatory agencies mandate that test results be accompanied by the expected values for the test ("normal range"). Expected values for these tests may be a numerical threshold or range for quantitative tests (e.g., expected antistreptolysin O titer, <200 IU/ml) or a text code for qualitative tests (e.g., expected HIV-1 antibody result, negative). Inclusion of the expected value aids clinicians in interpreting the clinical significance of test results. Most LISs provide a mechanism for defining age-specific, gender-specific, and more recently, species-specific expected values for test results. The expected values are incorporated automatically by the LISs into the test report. Results that are outside the normal-value range qualify for a daily quality assurance report. In the microbiology laboratory, normal-value checking generally is limited to nonculture testing.

2. Comparison of Current Results with Past Results. Virtually all LISs have the capability of comparing current test results for a patient to those for the same test last performed within a specified period of time. Sequential

TABLE 7 Examples of Westgard rules

A single quality control result is outside the range of ±2 standard deviations from the mean.

A single quality control result is outside the range of ±3 standard deviations from the mean.

Two consecutive quality control results are on the same side of the mean, more than 2 standard deviations from the mean.

Two of three consecutive quality control results are on the same side of the mean, more than 2 standard deviations from the mean.

Two consecutive quality control results differ by more than 4 standard deviations.

Four consecutive quality control results are more than 1 standard deviation from the mean in the same direction.

Four consecutive quality control results are more than 1 standard deviation from the mean in either direction.

Ten consecutive quality control results are on the same side of the mean.

results that exhibit a user-defined significant difference trigger a "delta check" flag. It is the laboratory's responsibility to investigate flagged results to confirm that the sequential specimens were collected from the same patient. Once confirmation is achieved, the flagged results can be released for viewing by clinicians. Results that elicit a "delta check" flag qualify for a daily quality assurance report. In the microbiology laboratory, "delta checking" is limited typically to nonculture testing.

3. Critical-Value Checking. An avoidable medical error originating from the clinical laboratory is failure to notify clinicians of critical test results as mandated by hospital policy. Almost as important as reporting is documenting that appropriate action was taken by laboratory personnel in response to critical values. Critical test results are typically defined as those that demand immediate interventions of a life-saving nature. Examples in the microbiology laboratory include positive Gram stains of cerebrospinal fluid (CSF) and positive blood cultures. Through the use of LIS-based automatic flagging of critical test results or the use of a rules engine to analyze laboratory data to identify critical results, the LIS can be an important safeguard against these types of medical errors (4, 6). The LIS can also be used to document in the patient's medical record that appropriate action was taken. Results that are deemed critical qualify for a daily quality assurance report. In the microbiology laboratory, automatic critical-value checking is limited to nonculture testing.

4. Comparison of Smear and Culture Results. Some LISs are configured to perform quality assurance checks that are unique to the clinical microbiology laboratory. One of them is comparison of Gram stain and culture results. When Gram stain findings suggest that microorganisms of a particular morphology are present, the LIS alerts users if the culture results do not include a microorganism with that morphology. Deviations between Gram stain and culture results qualify for a daily quality assurance report.

5. Detection of "Bug-Drug" Antimicrobial Susceptibility Result Inconsistencies. Some LISs allow users to define anticipated antimicrobial susceptibility results for specific antimicrobial agents and particular microorganisms. When the results differ from the expected results, a message is displayed requesting that the technologist review the result and either change it or file it manually. Acceptance of an unexpected result qualifies the result for a daily quality assurance report.

INFORMATION SHARING DURING THE POSTANALYTICAL PHASE OF TESTING

Communication of information from the clinical microbiology laboratory is especially vital during the postanalytical phase of testing, for it is this information that is the basis for patient management decisions. The mode of communication may be verbal, written, or electronic and often consists of more than test results.

Test Results Reporting

The information passed on to clinicians most frequently during the postanalytical phase is the test results themselves. With microbiology testing, some results are released in their entirety all at once, and others are issued sequentially as data become available. Examples of the former situation include results from antigen detection tests, nucleic acid probe tests, negative cultures, and certain microscopic assays. Instances of the latter sort include positive

cultures accompanied by a Gram stain report and antimicrobial susceptibility data. All LISs can report Gram stain and initial culture results in clinician-accessible preliminary reports and then release the final reports once antimicrobial susceptibility testing is completed.

Most LISs provide for calculation of the specimen transport time, which is then displayed in the final report. The specimen transport time is the elapsed time between specimen collection by the clinician and specimen receipt by the laboratory, although in some HIS-based ordering systems the specimen collection time may actually be the time that the test was ordered rather than the time that the specimen was collected. Clinical microbiologists should ascertain the meaning of "transport time" as calculated by their LISs before relying upon these data during investigation of delayed specimen transport problems.

Another important time point in the processing of specimens for culture is the plating time—especially when the laboratory inoculating culture media is distant from the specimen collection site. Some LISs now display the plating time in culture reports to identify specimens that may have experienced processing delays. The plating time is also used by LISs in calculating the elapsed time for "no-growth update" reports (e.g., a preliminary blood culture report might read "No growth after 18 hours of incubation").

Microscopic examination and culture results are usually displayed in separate sections of the LIS report. Stained smear results typically are found near the top of the report, since they are available first and acted upon more immediately than culture results. Culture findings frequently evolve with time as one or more isolates are detected and then identified in a stepwise process. For example, a culture that is positive for *Haemophilus influenzae* may be reported initially as "pleomorphic gram-negative coccobacilli consistent with *Haemophilus* sp.," then as "presumptive *Haemophilus* sp.," and finally as "*Haemophilus influenzae* type b" as more information is learned about the isolate.

Advances in taxonomic techniques during the past 25 years have led to the reclassification of some microorganisms into different or newly created genera and species. While microorganism name changes are a nuisance for laboratory personnel as they are forced to adjust to new nomenclature, they can create serious confusion among clinicians trying to interpret the significance of culture results. The LIS can be an effective tool in the ongoing challenge of keeping clinicians up to date with microorganism name changes. By way of illustration, it is no more difficult for an LIS to issue a culture report as "3+ growth of *Moraxella* (*Branhamella*) *catarrhalis*" versus "3+ growth of *Moraxella catarrhalis*." The former report is helpful to clinicians more familiar with the older taxonomic designation.

Interpretive Reports

One of the more effective ways that clinical microbiology laboratories can benefit patients is through provision of interpretive reports that accompany test results. This is especially true for tests that yield complex results like HIV-1 genotyping. Virtually all LISs enable clinical microbiologists to supplement test results with comments that were created and stored previously or with free text comments created in real time when test results are being reported. Libraries of canned comments can be maintained in the LIS and incorporated into reports individually or strung together as a group of comments when the situation warrants.

Supplementation of Microbiology Test Data with Digital Images

While not in common use yet, the potential for enhancement of microbiology reports with digital images is very real. Inclusion of digital photographs of Gram stains, acid-fast stains, ova and parasite preparations, or any other microscopic finding is technologically possible. Similarly, photographs of subjectively read tests such as those for group A streptococcal antigen, *Cryptococcus neoformans* antigen, RPR, and many others could also be stored in the LIS for quality assurance purposes. Data from objectively read tests, such as optical density readings from enzyme immunoassays, are commonly stored in the LIS already. It would seem that a more compelling argument could be made for recording visual evidence of subjectively read tests. The precedent for this has already been set by several currently available pathology and diagnostic imaging information systems. Many offer optional image storage repositories maintained on separate servers. Pathology and radiology reports can include hypertext links that lead users to photographs stored on the image server. In this way, clinicians have the opportunity to view for themselves the images that led to the pathologist's or radiologist's findings. The same could be true for clinical microbiology results.

Antimicrobial Susceptibility Reports

Antimicrobial susceptibility results, in many circumstances, are more valuable to clinicians postanalytically than are culture results. Hence, these data must be displayed in a fashion that advances unequivocal understanding of the results so that correct therapeutic decisions can be made. Most LISs enable laboratories to display antimicrobial susceptibility data in a variety of formats, including linear, columnar, or tabular. Most enable easy addition or deletion of antimicrobial agents to test batteries and also allow the addition of practical information to reports, such as comments pertaining to individual or groups of susceptibility results. In some instances the report can be customized to show antimicrobial agent dosage information, route of administration, achievable levels of antimicrobial agents in the blood and urine, and antimicrobial agent cost indexing.

Virtually all LISs are compatible with the entry of either qualitative (S, I, R) or quantitative (MIC or inhibitory zone diameter) susceptibility data. If quantitative data are entered, the LIS can refer to tables of user-entered interpretive criteria (obtained from the NCCLS or other official agencies) to convert the data to clinician-friendly qualitative results. The accuracy of the interpretive criteria must be updated frequently by laboratory personnel, as important changes are usually made on an annual basis.

The authors of the NCCLS *Performance Standards for Antimicrobial Susceptibility Testing* for many years have recommended carefully worded statements that can be added to susceptibility reports to aid clinicians in the correct interpretation of susceptibility results. Such comments can be added via manual insertion of free text, manual insertion of blocks of stored text, or automatic insertion of blocks of stored text after recognition of an appropriate situation by the LIS rules engine. Whatever the mechanism for their addition, the comments and the situations in which they will be added must be approved by the head of the clinical microbiology laboratory.

Nonculture Test Results Reporting

The development of more rapid technologies for diagnosis of infectious diseases has led to increased numbers of non-culture tests being performed by clinical microbiology laboratories. Most of these tests are quite dissimilar from the traditional microbiology battery of microscopic examination, culture findings, and antimicrobial susceptibility results. They are more similar to tests performed in other sections of the clinical laboratory and thus need to be defined in the LIS very differently from the way in which cultures are defined. Apart from the test results themselves, it is essential that the report include a description of the specimen.

Delivery of Test Results to Clinicians

There are many mechanisms by which microbiology test results can be delivered to clinicians. The requirements that they all have in common are that the results must reach clinicians

1. In a Timely Manner. Results must be available to clinicians within a time frame that enables appropriate interventions to be made.

2. In a Legible and Understandable Format. Results must be easily read and presented in unambiguous language so that suitable action can be taken.

3. In a Form That Is Free of Typographical or Transcriptional Errors. Systems must be in place that reduce the release of misleading or erroneous laboratory data.

The most frequently used means for distributing laboratory test results are still paper reports. Many LISs are configured to print reports daily that are then distributed by couriers to clinicians and patient medical records. Some LISs print the patient's entire laboratory file each day with the expectation that reports from previous days will be discarded. Other LISs print only the patient's "new laboratory activity" so that new reports are added to previously printed reports already in place in the clinician's office or the patient's medical record.

Interim reports show the current laboratory activity for each patient selected. Reports can be limited to new activity since the last interim or cumulative report was printed, or they may be printed for all activity that took place over a specified date range. The test results in interim reports are usually displayed in reverse chronological order, with no further sorting available. Some LISs permit interim reports to be called for groups of patients according to the ordering physician or the patient's location.

Cumulative reports contain results of patient tests grouped by the type of test or the specimen collection site. Examples of cumulative report headers include "bacterial cultures," "fungal cultures," and "nucleic acid probes" for type of test categorization; and "blood cultures," "urine cultures," and "genital nucleic acid probes" for specimen collection site categorization. It should be the province of the clinical microbiology laboratory leadership, with input from clinicians, to decide the style of cumulative report that is most suitable for a particular hospital. Within each group of tests under a cumulative report header, test results usually are sorted in reverse chronological order. Most LISs can call cumulative reports by selected patients, ordering physician, or patient location. Most hospitals depend on postdischarge cumulative reports to serve as the official records of laboratory test results that are appended to patient medical records.

Generation of Ad Hoc (User-Defined) Reports

There are frequent occasions in which none of the "canned" LIS reports available to the laboratory contain the information needed for a specific purpose. Most LISs offer optional modules that permit users to perform ad hoc queries of the LIS database. The queries may be made with proprietary vendor-specific software, or if LIS data are stored in ODBC (open database connectivity)-compliant relational tables, queries may be made with ODBC-compliant software (e.g., Microsoft Access or Crystal Decisions Crystal Report Writer). Such queries are usually intended to gather data for a retrospective review of a particular data set. For example, if one wished to obtain a list of all patients during the past 5 years who had positive blood cultures with simultaneous white blood cell counts greater than 18,000 per mm^3, an ad hoc query would be the easiest manner in which to assemble the data.

Once the ad hoc query is defined and run, the output report is stored in the LIS, usually as a delimited text file. From here the report can be printed to paper or downloaded to a personal computer via a serial port connection to the LIS or via file transfer protocol across the hospital computer network. The ad hoc report file can then be opened on the personal computer by using standard spreadsheet or database software. Spreadsheet tools (e.g., sorting, filtering, and pivot tables from Microsoft Excel) can be used to analyze the data (15). Database tools (e.g., Microsoft Access or Crystal Decisions Crystal Report Writer) can be used to perform further queries or configure attractive displays of the data.

Paperless Reports

The trend toward operating clinical laboratories as essentially paperless activities is gathering momentum. Under this paradigm, LIS reports are not printed on paper but, instead, are placed in files stored on magnetic or optical disk media. Such reports are easily stored in accessible formats, readily distributed to authorized individuals, and quickly retrievable for review at any time. If it is necessary to obtain a paper report, the report file can be sent electronically to a printer for preparation of a conventional hard-copy report.

All LISs provide clinicians on-demand viewing of laboratory test results online. LIS inquiry functions enable clinicians to review patient results for tests of specimens collected on a particular date or range of dates or for a single test or group of tests performed in a particular section of the laboratory. Some LISs enable viewing of serial quantitative data in graphical format, so that numerical trends are more easily spotted.

Many hospitals expect clinicians to order laboratory tests and view laboratory results in an HIS-based information system instead of the LIS. This is accomplished by building an order-entry and results viewing interface between the HIS and the LIS. The advantage to this approach is that clinicians can be trained to perform a wide variety of functions (e.g., ordering and viewing laboratory results, ordering and viewing diagnostic imaging results, ordering pharmaceuticals, and viewing patient vital signs and progress notes) on a single information system. This strategy fits in nicely with the tendency in U.S. hospitals toward greater provider interaction with information systems. The major disadvantage is that the format for displaying laboratory test results may not be as functional in an HIS-based system as it would be in an LIS.

Electronic Delivery of Reports

When the LIS is a node on the hospital local-area or wide-area computer network, it becomes feasible to transmit report files electronically to workstation nodes on the network. Some LISs are equipped with report scheduling capability in which "canned" or ad hoc reports can be run at designated daily, weekly, monthly, quarterly, or annual intervals, "printed" automatically to files, and then sent to workstations or groups of workstations along the network. In fact, a growing number of laboratories no longer print patient discharge cumulative reports to paper. Alternatively, they "print" the reports to a file and send the file via the hospital local-area network to the Health Information Management Department (Medical Records) for inclusion in the patient's electronic medical record.

Another emerging trend among laboratories is granting access to laboratory test results via the Internet (2). Authorized individuals are able to log in to an Internet information server where an up-to-the-minute copy of the laboratory test result database resides. Users then can view results over a secure, encrypted channel from anywhere in the world.

Another very recent technological development is the ability to transmit laboratory test results via a wireless connection to handheld devices such as alphanumeric pagers, digital telephones, or personal data assistants. While still in its infancy, this methodology has the potential to replace the telephoning of critical laboratory values to clinicians. One can also envisage daily downloading of interim reports for a clinician's patient list to a handheld device. It remains to be seen whether the more complex laboratory data found in microbiology reports can be transmitted and viewed effectively on these handheld devices.

Verbal Delivery of Reports

Verbal delivery of laboratory results, in almost every instance, complements results conveyed by other means. Very often verbal reporting is the method of choice for initial issuance of critical values. In the microbiology arena these may be preliminary results, such as the Gram stain morphology of microorganisms growing in blood cultures, or they may be final results such as positive results for a CSF cryptococcal antigen detection test. When noncritical laboratory results are delivered verbally, it is often in situations in which clinicians telephone the laboratory because they do not have access to the standard means of results distribution. Provision of microbiology results in this way must be carried out with caution since it is very easy for complicated results to be confused or misunderstood. The other common context for verbal discussion of test results is during the course of a consultation over results released previously in another manner.

Consultations Concerning Laboratory Reports

Passive consultations from the laboratory perspective are those in which clinicians contact the laboratory for advice in interpreting test results. Such consultations concerning microbiology results should be handled by the laboratory director or supervisor, one of whom should be reachable for this purpose at all times. Active consultations are those in which laboratory directors or supervisors seek out clinicians to discuss the clinical significance of test results and suggest additional tests that should be considered. Although active consultations require commitment and effort on the part of the laboratory staff, the return on investment is easily appreciated in terms of improved patient care.

An underused method of communication between the microbiology laboratory and clinicians is the addition of signed information by the laboratory director to patient medical records. This information can be of great assistance to clinicians in the understanding of test results and can offer valuable suggestions for follow-up testing. The advantages of this route of information sharing are that the clinical microbiologist's observations can be read at the convenience of clinicians and that the information is located in the same place in the medical record location as key information from other clinical services.

Most hospitals and regulatory agencies require that the medical staff bylaws define the individuals who are authorized to place information in patient medical records. It is the responsibility of the microbiology laboratory director and his or her colleagues in laboratory medicine to ensure that they have the necessary authorization.

Preparation of Periodic Antibiogram Reports

A much appreciated service provided by many clinical microbiology laboratories is the distribution of cumulative institutional antimicrobial susceptibility data reports to clinicians (19). These reports generally are prepared on an annual basis, but may be offered more frequently if warranted. In an attempt to standardize the content of antibiogram reports, the NCCLS recently issued document M39-P, entitled *Analysis and Presentation of Cumulative Antimicrobial Susceptibility Test Data* (9). This document recommends methods for recording and analyzing antimicrobial susceptibility data for epidemiologically significant microorganisms. To avoid biasing the data toward more resistant results, the standard recommends including only the first isolate from a patient of a particular species per analysis period and excluding isolates derived from surveillance cultures. To improve the statistical validity of the data, the standard urges limiting the report to organisms tested 10 or more times during the analysis period.

At the time of this writing, LIS vendors are still determining how they will help laboratories comply with the recommendations in the NCCLS document. In the meantime, clinical microbiologists should consider downloading their antimicrobial susceptibility data to a personal computer and then prepare their cumulative antimicrobial susceptibility reports with the aid of spreadsheet or database software (Table 8).

Submission of Laboratory Results to External Repositories

Jurisdictional regulations (e.g., those issued by local, county, state, or national agencies) mandate that hospitals and/or laboratories report positive test results for diagnosis of certain infectious diseases to public health authorities. Traditionally, this has been accomplished via written notification that is either mailed or faxed to the responsible authority. Some LISs are beginning to include in their systems software tools that make it easier for clinical microbiology laboratories to comply with reporting regulations. Autofaxing of reports to designated telephone numbers is now a feature of selected LISs. This capability is being extended by some LISs to submission of HIPAA-compliant encrypted reports via e-mail and the Internet.

SUMMARY

LISs have enabled tremendous progress to be made in the movement of information from the clinical microbiology laboratory to providers of health care (7). Laboratory test data are delivered more efficiently and accurately than ever

TABLE 8 Sample pivot table from Microsoft Excel showing antimicrobial susceptibility data for *S. pneumoniae* tested during calendar year 2001

Culture battery	(All)
Collection month	(All)
Collection year	2001
Order location	(All)
Order physician	(All)
Specimen description	(All)
Gender	(All)

Drug	Result (%)		
	S	I	R
Cefotaxime	80	1	19
Ceftriaxone	80	8	12
Chloramphenicol	95	0	5
Clindamycin	96	0	4
Erythromycin	81	0	19
Penicillin	61	18	21
Tetracycline	90	0	10
Trimeth/sulfa[a]	70	2	27
Vancomycin	100	0	0

[a] Trimeth/sulfa, trimethoprim-sulfamethoxazole.

before. Other information that is imperative to the ordering of correct tests, collection of appropriate specimens, and interpretation of test results can be communicated effectively. The role of these systems in the daily practice of clinical microbiology will only continue to increase in importance. It behooves all clinical microbiologists to become more knowledgeable and comfortable with information systems, for they are perhaps the most powerful tool available to us in our new role as information brokers.

REFERENCES

1. **Becich, M. J.** 2000. Information management: moving from test results to clinical information. *Clin. Leadersh. Manag. Rev.* **14:**296–300.
2. **Friedman, B. A.** 1998. Integrating laboratory processes into clinical processes, Web-based laboratory reporting, and the emergence of the virtual clinical laboratory. *Clin. Lab. Manage. Rev.* **12:**333–338.
3. **Hunter, R. L., Jr.** 1999. The past and future of laboratory information systems. *Ann. Clin. Lab. Sci.* **29:**176–184.
4. **Iordache, S. D., D. Orso, and J. Zelingher.** 2001. A comprehensive computerized critical laboratory results alerting system for ambulatory and hospitalized patients. *Medinfo* **10:**469–473.
5. **Kay, J. D.** 2001. Communicating with clinicians. *Ann. Clin. Biochem.* **38:**103–110.
6. **Kuperman, G. J., J. M. Teich, M. J. Tanasijevic, N. Ma'Luf, E. Rittenberg, A. Jha, J. Fiskio, J. Winkelman, and D. W. Bates.** 1999. Improving response to critical laboratory results with automation: results of a randomized controlled trial. *J. Am. Med. Inform. Assoc.* **6:**512–522.
7. **McPherson, R. A.** 1999. Perspective on the clinical laboratory: new uses for informatics. *J. Clin. Lab. Anal.* **13:**53–58.
8. **Miller, W. G.** 2000. The changing role of the medical technologist from technologist to information specialist. *Clin. Leadersh. Manag. Rev.* **14:**285–288.
9. **NCCLS.** 2001. *Analysis and Presentation of Cumulative Antimicrobial Susceptibility Test Data; Proposed Guideline.* NCCLS document M39-P. NCCLS, Wayne, Pa.

10. **NCCLS.** 1996. *Clinical Laboratory Technical Procedure Manuals,* 3rd ed.; *Approved Guideline.* NCCLS document GP2-A3. NCCLS, Wayne, Pa.

11. **NCCLS.** 1994. *Inventory Control Systems for Laboratory Supplies; Approved Guideline.* NCCLS document GP6-A. NCCLS, Villanova, Pa.

12. **NCCLS.** 2000. *Laboratory Automation: Communications with Automated Clinical Laboratory Systems, Instruments, Devices, and Information Systems; Approved Standard.* NCCLS document AUTO3-A. NCCLS, Wayne, Pa.

13. **NCCLS.** 1995. *Laboratory Instruments and Data Management Systems: Design of Software User Interfaces and End-User Software Systems Validation, Operation, and Monitoring; Approved Guideline.* NCCLS document GP19-A. NCCLS, Wayne, Pa.

14. **NCCLS.** 2002. *Performance Standards for Antimicrobial Susceptibility Testing: 12th Informational Supplement.* NCCLS document M100-S12. NCCLS, Wayne, Pa.

15. **Oakley, S.** 1999. Data mining, distributed networks, and the laboratory. *Health Manage. Technol.* **20:**26–31.

16. **Ruby, S. G., and G. Krempel.** 1998. Intranets: virtual procedure manuals for the pathology lab. *MLO Med. Lab. Obs.* **30:**65–75.

17. **Szabo, J.** 2000. HIPAA compliance could cost dearly. *MLO Med. Lab. Obs.* **32:**8–9.

18. **Todebush, C.** 1999. The Internet-linked laboratory: fundamentally changing the delivery of laboratory information and results. *Am. Clin. Lab.* **18:**10.

19. **Trevino, S.** 2000. Antibiotic resistance monitoring: a laboratory perspective. *Mil. Med.* **165:**40–42.

20. **Uehling, M.** 2000. Digital imaging not picture perfect—yet. *CAP Today* **14:**1, 34–38.

21. **Watine, J.** 1999. Are expert systems "more intelligent" than laboratory doctors? *Clin. Biochem.* **32:**485–486.

22. **Westgard, J. O.** 1994. Selecting appropriate quality-control rules. *Clin. Chem.* **40:**499–501.

Pathogenic and Indigenous Microorganisms of Humans*

PAUL A. GRANATO

5

"The 1990s have been marked by a renewed recognition that our human species is still locked in a Darwinian struggle with our microbial and viral predators." Although this unreferenced quotation was made by Nobel laureate Joshua Lederberg as he was discussing the AIDS and multidrug-resistant *Mycobacterium tuberculosis* epidemics that emerged in the early 1990s, his comment could also apply to most any infectious disease process that has occurred since the recognition of the Germ Theory of Disease in the late 1880s. For as we enter into the 21st century and despite the advances of modern medicine and the continual development of new vaccines and anti-infective therapeutic agents, our human species continues to battle our microbial predators in this Darwinian struggle for survival.

The dynamics of this host-parasite relationship for survival is in a continual state of change. In health, a balance exists between the host and the microbe that allows for the mutual survival and coexistence of both. This balance is best maintained when humans have operative host defense mechanisms (i.e., intact skin and mucous membranes, a functional group of phagocytic cells consisting principally of the reticuloendothelial system, and the ability to produce a humoral immune response). Defects in any one, combination, or all of these host defense mechanisms may shift the balance in favor of the microbe and predispose the host to the risk of developing an infectious disease process. These infections may be acquired from exposure to other infected humans or environmental reservoirs (exogenous source) or from one's own normal microbial flora (endogenous source).

Infectious disease may also occur in individuals with normal operative and functional host defense mechanisms when they are exposed to a particularly pathogenic and virulent microorganism. *Pathogenicity* refers to the ability of a microorganism to cause disease, whereas *virulence* provides a quantitative measure of this property. Virulence factors refer to the properties that enable a microorganism to establish itself on or within a host and enhance the organism's ability to produce disease. Virulence is not generally attributable to a single discrete factor but depends on several parameters related to the organism, the host, and their interaction. Virulence encompasses two general features of pathogenic microorganisms: (i) invasiveness, or the ability to attach, multiply, and spread in tissues, and (ii) toxigenicity, or the ability to produce substances that are injurious to human cells. Highly virulent, moderately virulent, or avirulent strains may occur within a single species of organisms.

NORMAL MICROBIAL FLORA

The terms *normal microbial flora*, *normal commensal flora*, and *indigenous flora* are synonymous in meaning and are used to describe microorganisms that are frequently found in particular anatomic sites in healthy individuals. This microbial flora is associated with the skin and mucous membranes of every human from shortly after birth until death and represents an extremely large and diverse population of microorganisms. The healthy adult consists of about 10 trillion cells and routinely harbors at least 100 trillion microbes (10). The constituents and numbers of the flora vary in different anatomic sites and sometimes at different ages of life. They comprise microorganisms whose morphologic, physiologic, and genetic properties allow them to colonize and multiply under the conditions that exist in a particular body site, to coexist with other colonizing organisms, and to inhibit competing intruders. Thus, each anatomic site that harbors normal microbial flora presents a particular environmental niche for the development of a unique microbial ecosystem.

Local physiologic and environmental conditions at various body sites determine the nature and composition of the normal flora that exists there. These conditions are sometimes highly complex, differing from site to site, and sometimes vary with age. Some of these local, anatomic conditions include the amounts and types of nutrients available for microbial growth, pH, oxidation-reduction potentials, and resistance to local antibacterial substances, such as bile, lysozyme, or short-chain fatty acids. In addition, many bacteria have a remarkable affinity for specific types of epithelial cells to which they adhere and on which they multiply. This adherence, which is mediated by the presence of bacterial pili or fimbriae or other microbial surface components, allows the microbe to attach to specific receptor sites found on the surfaces of certain epithelial cells.

---

* This chapter contains information presented in chapter 3 by Susan E. Sharp in the seventh edition of this Manual.

44

Through this mechanism of adherence, microorganisms are permitted to grow and multiply while avoiding removal by the flushing effects of surface fluids and peristalsis. Various microbial interactions also determine their relative prevalence in the flora. Some of these interactions include competition for nutrients and inhibition by the metabolic products produced by other organisms in the ecosystem (for example, the production of hydrogen peroxide, antibiotics, and/or bacteriocins).

The normal microbial flora plays an important role in health and disease. In health, for example, the normal microbial flora of the intestine plays an important role in human nutrition and metabolism. Certain intestinal bacteria synthesize and secrete vitamin K, which can then be absorbed by the bowel for use in the human. In addition, the enterohepatic circulatory loop is particularly important for the metabolism of steroids and bile salts. These substances are excreted through the bile in conjugated form as glucuronides or sulfates but cannot be reabsorbed in this form. Certain members of the bacterial intestinal flora make glucuronidases and sulfatases that can deconjugate these compounds, thereby allowing their reabsorption and use by the human host (4, 65). Another beneficial role of the normal microbial flora is the antigenic stimulation of the host's immune system. Although the various classes of the immunoglobulins produced from this antigenic exposure are usually present in low concentrations, their presence plays an important role in host defense. In particular, various classes of the immunoglobulin A group of antibodies produced in response to this antigenic stimulation are secreted through mucous membranes. While the role of these immunoglobulins is not well understood, they may play an important role in host defense by interfering with the colonization of deeper tissues by certain normal-flora organisms.

Perhaps one of the most important roles of the normal microbial flora is to help prevent infectious disease following exposure to potential microbial pathogens. The normal commensal flora has the physical advantage of previous occupancy, especially on skin and mucous membranes. Many of these commensal microorganisms adhere to epithelial binding sites, thereby preventing attachment to that receptor site by a potential microbial pathogen. In addition, some commensal microorganisms are capable of producing antibiotics, bacteriocins, or other products that may be inhibitory or lethal to pathogenic microorganisms.

The normal microbial flora, although important for the maintenance of human health, plays a critically important role in infectious disease. In fact, physicians see more patients with infectious diseases acquired from endogenous microbial flora than from exogenous sources (14). Therefore, clinicians and clinical microbiologists must be knowledgeable as to the various microbes that reside as normal flora in different anatomic sites.

Skin

The healthy fetus is sterile in utero until the birth membranes rupture. During and after birth, the infant's skin is exposed to the mother's genital tract flora, skin flora from the mother and other individuals who handle the baby, and a variety of microorganisms acquired by direct contact of the baby with the environment. During the infant's first few days of life, the nature of its microbial skin flora often reflects chance exposure to microorganisms that can grow on particular sites in the absence of microbial competitors. Subsequently, as the infant is exposed to a full range of

human environmental organisms, those best adapted to survive on particular skin sites predominate and establish themselves as part of the resident skin flora. Thereafter, the normal microbial flora resembles that of adult individuals.

The pH of the skin is usually about 5.6. This factor alone may be responsible for inhibiting the establishment of many microbial species. Despite this, skin provides excellent examples of various microenvironments. For instance, quantitative differences in microbial flora characterize each of the three major regions of skin: (i) axilla, perineum, and toe webs; (ii) hands, face, and trunk; and (iii) arms and legs (48). These quantitative differences may relate to differences in skin surface temperature and moisture content as well as the presence of different concentrations in skin surface lipids that may be inhibitory or lethal to various groups of microorganisms at each of these skin sites.

The major groups of microorganisms that are normal residents of skin, even though their numbers may vary as influenced by the microenvironment, include various genera of bacteria and the lipophilic yeasts of the genus *Malassezia*. Nonlipophilic yeasts, such as *Candida* species, are also inhabitants of skin (48). Other bacterial species may be found less commonly on the skin, and some of these include hemolytic streptococci (especially in children), atypical mycobacteria, and *Bacillus* species.

The predominant bacterial flora of the skin are the coagulase-negative staphylococci, micrococci, saprophytic *Corynebacterium* species (diphtheroids), and *Propionibacterium* species. Among this group, *Propionibacterium acnes* is the best studied because of its association with acne vulgaris. *P. acnes* is found briefly on the skin of neonates, but true colonization begins during the 1 to 3 years prior to sexual maturity, when numbers rise from less than 10 to about 10^6 CFU/cm^2, chiefly on the face and upper thorax (43). Various species of coagulase-negative staphylococci are found as normal inhabitants of skin; and some of these include *Staphylococcus epidermidis*, *S. capitis*, *S. warneri*, *S. hominis*, *S. haemolyticus*, *S. lugdunensis*, and *S. auricularis* (31–34). Some of these staphylococci demonstrate ecological niche preferences at certain anatomic sites. For example, *S. capitis* and *S. auricularis* show an anatomic preference for the head and the external auditory meatus, respectively, whereas *S. hominis* and *S. haemolyticus* are found principally in areas where there are numerous aprocrine glands, such as the axillae and pubic areas (31). *Staphylococcus aureus* regularly inhabits the external nares of about 30% of healthy individuals and the perineum, axillae, and toe webs of about 15, 5, and 2% of healthy people, respectively (48). *Micrococcus* spp., particularly *Micrococcus luteus*, are also found on the skin, especially in women and children, where they may be present in large numbers. *Acinetobacter* spp. are found on the skin of about 25% of the population in the axillae, toe webs, groin, and antecubital fossae. Other gram-negative bacilli are found more rarely on the skin, and these include *Proteus* and *Pseudomonas* in the toe webs and *Enterobacter* and *Klebsiella* on the hands. Saprophytic mycobacteria may occasionally be found on the skin of the external auditory canal and of the genital and axillary regions, whereas hemolytic streptococci tend to colonize the skin of children but not adults (48).

The principal fungal flora is the yeast *Malassezia*. Dermatophytic fungi may also be recovered from the skin in the absence of disease, but it is unclear whether they represent normal flora or transient colonizers. The rate of carriage of *Malassezia* spp. probably reaches 100% in adults, but proper determination of carriage rates is obscured by the

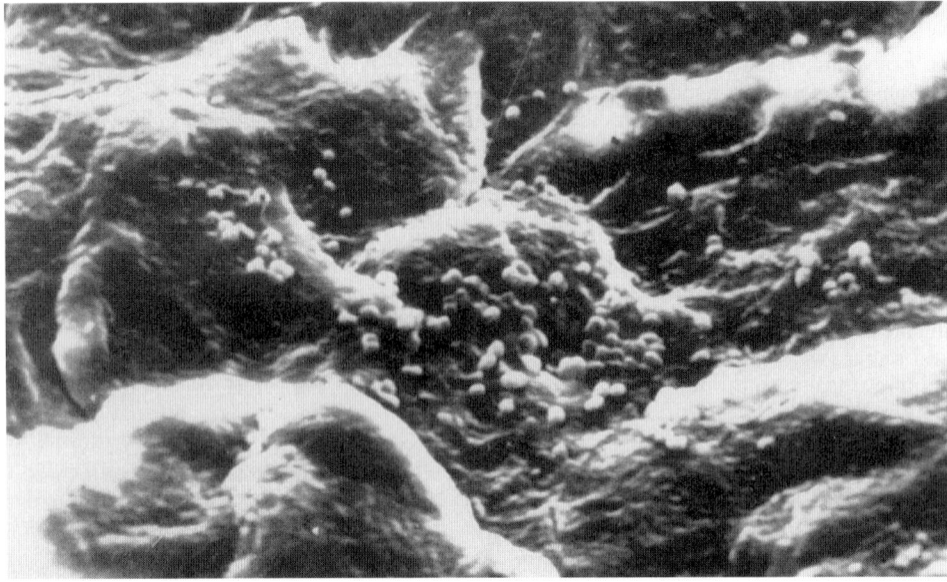

FIGURE 1 Microcolony of cocci on human skin. Reprinted from reference 48 with permission from CRC Press, Boca Raton, Fla.

difficulty of growing some species of these lipophilic yeast in the laboratory (48).

The skin microflora lives both on the skin surface in the form of microcolonies (Fig. 1 and 2) and also in the ducts of hair follicles and sebaceous glands (48). Wolff and Plewig (67) had proposed that *Malassezia* species live near the opening of the duct, the staphylococci live farther down, and the propionibacteria live near the sebaceous glands. A more recent study (38), however, suggests that all three microbial groups are more evenly distributed throughout the follicles. In any event, organisms in the follicles are secreted onto the skin surface along with the sebum, but staphylococci, at least, also exist in microcolonies on the surface. These microcolonies may be of various sizes and are larger (10^3 to 10^4 cells per microcolony) on areas such as the face than on the arms (10^1 to 10^2 cells per microcolony) (48).

Washing may decrease microbial skin counts by 90%, but normal numbers are reestablished within 8 h (15). Abstinence from washing does not lead to an increase in numbers of bacteria on the skin. Normally, 10^3 to 10^4 organisms are found per cm^2. However, counts may increase to $10^6/cm^2$ in more humid areas, such as the groin and axilla. Small numbers of bacteria are dispersed from the skin

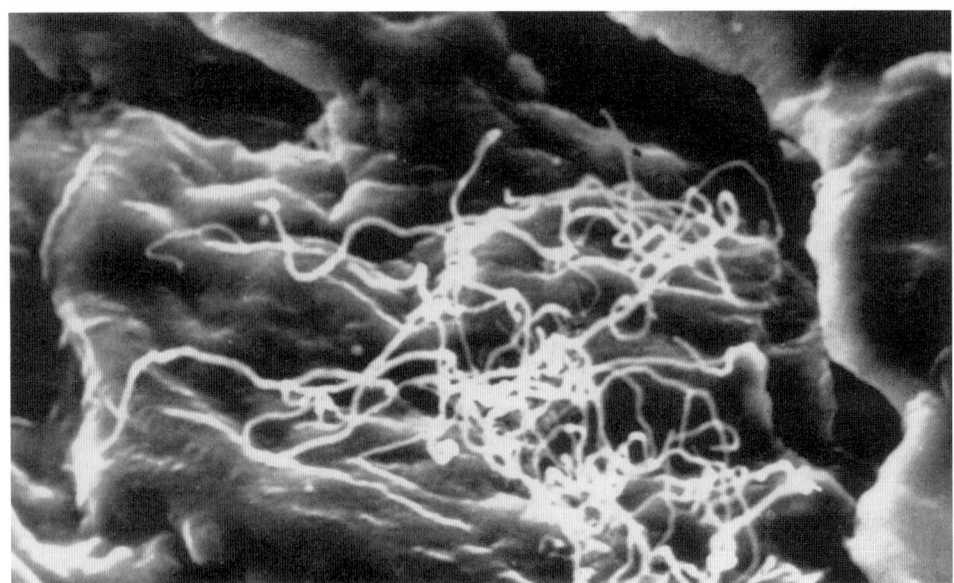

FIGURE 2 Microcolony of coryneforms on human skin. Note the filamentous appearance. Reprinted from reference 48 with permission from CRC Press, Boca Raton, Fla.

to the environment, but certain individuals may shed up to 10^6 organisms in 30 min of exercise. Many of the fatty acids found on the skin may be bacterial products that inhibit colonization by other species. The flora of hair is similar to that of the skin (19).

Eye

The normal microbial flora of the eye contains many of the bacteria found on the skin. However, the mechanical action of eyelids and the washing effect of the eye secretions that contain the bacteriolytic enzyme lysozyme serve to limit the populations of microorganisms normally found on the eye. The predominant normal microbial flora of the eye consists of coagulase-negative staphylococci, diphtheroids, and, less commonly, saprophytic *Neisseria* species and viridans group streptococci.

Ear

The microbiota of the external ear is similar to that of skin, with coagulase-negative staphylococci and *Corynebacterium* species predominating. Less frequently found are *Bacillus*, *Micrococcus*, and saprophytic species of *Neisseria* and mycobacteria. Normal-flora fungi include *Aspergillus*, *Alternaria*, *Penicillium*, and *Candida*.

Respiratory Tract

Nares

In the course of normal breathing, many kinds of microbes are inhaled into the nares to reach the upper respiratory tract. Among these are aerosolized, normal soil inhabitants as well as pathogenic and potentially pathogenic bacteria, fungi, and viruses. Some of these microorganisms are filtered out by the hairs in the nose, while others may land on moist surfaces of the nasal passages, where they may be subsequently expelled by sneezing or blowing one's nose. Generally, in health these airborne microorganisms are transient colonizers of the nose and do not establish themselves as part of the resident commensal flora.

The external 1 cm of the external nares is lined with squamous epithelium and has a flora similar to that found on the skin, except that *S. aureus* is commonly carried as the principal part of the normal flora in some individuals. Approximately 25 to 30% of healthy adults in the community harbor this organism in their anterior nares at any given time, 15% permanently and the remaining 15% transiently (58).

Nasopharynx

Colonization of the nasopharynx occurs soon after birth following aerosal exposure of microorganisms from the respiratory tract from those individuals who are in close contact with the infant (i.e., mother, other family members, etc.). The normal microbial flora of the infant establishes itself within several months and generally remains unchanged throughout life. The nasopharynx has a flora similar to that of the mouth (see below) and is the site of carriage of potentially pathogenic bacteria such as *Neisseria meningitidis*, *Streptococcus pneumoniae*, and *Haemophilus influenzae* (58).

The respiratory tract below the level of the larynx is protected in health by the actions of the epiglottis and the peristaltic movement of the ciliary blanket of the columnar epithelium. Thus, only transiently inhaled organisms are encountered in the trachea and larger bronchi. The accessory sinuses are normally sterile and are protected in a similar fashion, as is the middle ear by the epithelium of the eustachian tubes.

Gastrointestinal Tract

Mouth

Colonization of the mouth begins immediately following birth when the infant is exposed to the microorganisms in the environment, and the numbers present increase rapidly in the first 6 to 10 h after birth (61). During the first few days, several species appear sporadically as transients, many of them not being suitable for the oral environment. During this period, the oral mucosa becomes colonized by its first permanent residents; these are derived mainly from the mouth of the mother and other persons in contact with the infant (63). The child is continuously exposed to transmission of oral bacteria from family members by direct and indirect contact (the latter, for example, via spoons and feeding bottles), as well as by airborne transmission. The various members of the resident microflora become established gradually during the first years of life as growth conditions become suitable for them. This microbial succession is caused by environmental changes related to the host, such as tooth eruption or dietary changes, as well as to microbial interrelations due to, for example, the initial colonizers reducing tissue redox potentials or supplying growth factors.

During the first months of life, the oral microflora mainly inhabits the tongue and is dominated by streptococci, with small numbers of other genera such as *Neisseria*, *Veillonella*, *Lactobacillus*, and *Candida*. *Streptococcus salivarius* is regularly isolated from the baby's first day of life, and often the bacteriocin types are identical to those of the mother (62). *Streptococcus sanguis* colonizes the teeth soon after eruption (6), whereas *Streptococcus mutans* colonizes much more slowly over several years, starting in pits and fissures and spreading to proximal and other surfaces of the teeth (26). Colonization with *S. mutans* and lactobacilli is correlated with dental caries (6, 27), and in fact, their establishment can be inhibited or delayed by use of caries-preventive measures in the infants' mothers (35).

As dental plaque forms on the erupting teeth, the oral microflora becomes more complex and predominately anaerobic. Studies of 4- to 7-year-olds have shown the plaque microflora in the gingival area to be similar to that in adults, with motile rods and spirochetes observed by direct microscopy and the same species of *Actinomyces*, *Bacteroides*, *Capnocytophaga*, *Eikenella*, etc., recovered by cultural techniques (11, 18, 46, 66). In studies of 7- to 19-year-olds, the prevalence of some organisms and the proportions of the flora that they constitute seem, however, to differ with age and hormonal status. Thus, *Prevotella* species and spirochetes increase around puberty, while *Actinomyces naeslundii* and *Capnocytophaga* spp. tend to decrease with increasing age of the children.

In healthy adults, the resident oral microflora consists of more than 200 gram-positive and gram-negative bacterial species as well as several different species of mycoplasmas, yeasts, and protozoa. Only about 100 oral species of bacteria have known genus and species names based upon biochemical and physiologic characteristics (64). With the eruption of teeth and the development of gingival crevices, anaerobic bacteria emerge as the principal flora of the mouth. Concentrations of bacteria vary from approximately 10^8 CFU/ml in the saliva to 10^{12} CFU/ml in the gingival crevices around teeth, with the anaerobic bacteria outnumbering the aerobic bacteria by a ratio of at least 100:1.

The mouth has several different habitats where microorganisms can grow. Each habitat has its own unique environment and is populated by a characteristic community of microorganisms consisting of different populations of various species in each ecosystem. Each species performs a certain functional role as part of the microbial community. Some of the major ecosystems may be found on mucosal surfaces of the palate, gingiva, lips, and cheeks and on the floor of the mouth, on the papillary surface of the tongue, on tooth surfaces with their associated dental plaque, in gingival pockets, etc. In order to remain in the mouth, the microorganisms must adhere to the oral surfaces, resist being eliminated with the stream of saliva swallowed, and grow under the different conditions prevailing at each site. Such sites can harbor extremely numerous and complex microbial communities. For detailed and comprehensive information, the reader is referred to the review in reference 64.

In general, streptococcal species constitute 30 to 60% of the bacterial flora of the surfaces within the mouth. These are primarily viridans group streptococci: *S. salivarius*, *S. mutans*, *S. sanguis*, and *S. mitis* found on the teeth and in dental plaque. Specific binding to mucosal cells or to tooth enamel has been demonstrated with these organisms. Bacterial plaque developing on the teeth may contain as many as 10^{11} streptococci per g, in addition to actinomycetes, *Veillonella*, and *Bacteriodes* species. Anaerobic flora, such as *Prevotella melaninogenica*, treponemes, fusobacteria, clostridia, propionibacteria, and peptostreptococci, are present in gingival crevices, where the oxygen concentration is less than 0.5%. Many of these organisms are obligate anaerobes and do not survive in higher oxygen concentrations. The natural habitat of the pathogenic species *Actinomyces israelii* is the gingival crevice. Among the fungi, species of *Candida* and *Geotrichum* are found in 10 to 15% of individuals (64).

Esophagus

Little attention has been given to characterizing the normal microflora of the esophagus. Essentially, the esophagus is a transit route for food passing from the mouth to the stomach, with approximately 1.5 liters of saliva swallowed per day (2, 49). Although much of this stimulated saliva is swallowed with food, there is a resting rate of saliva secretion estimated to be about 20 ml/h (2) which is swallowed as fluid. In addition, nasal secretions containing the microbial flora of that site may also be swallowed, introducing salt-tolerant organisms, such as staphylococci, from the anterior and posterior nares. As such, normal-flora mouth and nasal microorganisms will be recovered from the esophagus, but it is uncertain whether these organisms represent transient colonization or an established microflora.

Stomach

As for the esophagus, oral and nasal normal-flora microorganisms are swallowed into the stomach, as are microorganisms ingested in food and drink. However, the vast majority are destroyed following exposure to the gastric acid (pH 1.8 to 2.5) (13). The concentrations of bacteria in the healthy stomach are generally low, less than 10^3 CFU/ml, and are composed primarily of relatively acid-resistant species, such as gastric helicobacter, streptococci, staphylococci, lactobacilli, and fungi and even smaller numbers of peptostreptococci, fusobacteria, and *Bacteroides* species (12, 21, 23). Gram-positive organisms predominate in the stomach, with a striking absence of members of the family *Enterobacteriaceae* as well as *Bacteroides* and *Clostridium* species.

The gastric flora can become more complex when the ability to achieve an acid pH is altered by the buffering action of food, by hypochlorhydria due to an intrinsic pathogenic process or surgery (13), or by medications that reduce HCl secretion. In the newborn, the stomach secretes very little gastric acid and does not achieve optimal acid secretion rates until 15 to 20 days after birth (21). As such, during the first few days of life, the stomach does not constitute a microbicidal barrier to gut colonization.

Intestine

A fecal flora is acquired soon after birth (51). The composition of the early flora depends on a number of factors including the method of delivery, the gestational age of the newborn infant, and whether the infant is breast or bottle fed.

After vaginal delivery, the newborn gut is first colonized by facultative organisms acquired from the mother's vaginal flora, mainly *Escherichia coli* and streptococci (51). The guts of infants delivered by cesarean section are usually colonized by *Enterobacteriaceae* other than *E. coli*, with a composition resembling that of the environmental flora of the delivery room (47). Anaerobes appear within the first week or two of life and are acquired more uniformly and more rapidly in bottle-fed rather than breast-fed babies. Virtually 100% of full-term, bottle-fed, and vaginally delivered infants have an anaerobic flora within the first week of life, with *Bacteroides fragilis* predominating, whereas only 59% of similarly delivered but breast-fed infants have anaerobes at this time, and less than 10% harbor *B. fragilis* (30). Breast-fed infants have a marked predominance of *Bifidobacterium* spp. in their colon which exceed the number of *Enterobacteriaceae* by 100- to 1,000-fold (3).

The nature of the gut flora may be influenced by the nutrient content of breast or cow's milk compared to those of infant formulas that are fortified with nutrients such as iron. The presence of iron seems to stimulate a complex flora composed of *Enterobacteriaceae*, *Clostridium* species, and *Bacteroides* species. The low-iron breast or cow's milk diet selects for a simple flora composed predominately of *Bifidobacterium* species and *Lactobacillus* species (24, 60). In breast-fed infants, the *Bifidobacterium* population increases in the first few weeks of life to become the stable and dominant component of the fecal flora until the weaning period (42, 45). The properties of breast milk that promote the dominance of gram-positive bacilli in the feces are not known with certainty but, no doubt, involve both nutritional and immunologic factors.

Weaning results in significant changes in the composition of the gut flora, with increased numbers of *E. coli*, *Streptococcus*, *Clostridium*, *Bacteroides*, and *Peptostreptococcus* species. After weaning, a more stable adult-type flora occurs, in which the number of *Bacteroides* organisms equals or exceeds the number of *Bifidobacterium* organisms, with *E. coli* and *Clostridium* counts decreasing (44).

In adults, the composition of the fecal flora appears to vary more from individual to individual than it does in particular subjects studied over time (12, 21, 23). The numbers and types of bacteria found in the small intestines depend on the flow rate of intestinal contents. When stasis occurs, the small intestine may contain an extensive, complex microbial flora. Normally, flow is brisk enough to wash the microbial flora through to the distal ileum and colon before the microorganisms multiply. As such, the types and numbers of microflora encountered in the duodenum, the jejunum, and the initial portions of ileum are similar to those found in the stomach and on average contain 10^3 CFU/ml (8, 16, 29, 50). Anaerobes only slightly outnumber facultative organisms, with streptococci, lactobacilli, yeasts, and staphylococci also found.

As the ileocecal valve is approached, the number and variety of gram-negative bacteria begin to increase (18, 22, 59). Coliforms are found consistently, and the number of both gram-positive and gram-negative anaerobic organisms (such as *Bifidobacterium*, *Clostridium*, *Bacteroides*, and *Fusobacterium*) rise sharply to 10^5 to 10^6 CFU/ml, on average. In the adult colon, another dramatic increase in the microbial flora occurs as soon as the ileocecal valve is crossed. Here, the number of microorganisms present approaches the theoretical limits of packing cells in space. Nearly one-third of the dry weight of feces consists of bacteria, with each gram of stool containing up to 10^{11} to 10^{12} organisms (41).

Over 98% of the organisms found in the colon are strict anaerobes, with the anaerobes outnumbering aerobes 1,000- to 10,000-fold. The distribution of the major genera of organisms found in the colon per gram of feces is as follows: *Bacteroides*, 10^{10} to 10^{11}; *Bifidobacterium*, 10^{10} to 10^{11}; *Eubacterium*, 10^{10}; *Lactobacillus*, 10^7 to 10^8; coliforms, 10^6 to 10^8; aerobic and anaerobic streptococci, 10^7 to 10^8; *Clostridium*, 10^6; and yeasts, variable numbers (19). Thus, more than 90% of the fecal flora consists of *Bacteroides* and *Bifidobacterium*. Intensive studies of the colonic microbial flora have shown that the average healthy adult harbors well over 200 given species of bacteria alone.

Genitourinary Tract

Urethra

The only portion of the urinary tract in both males and females that harbors a normal microbial flora is the distal 1 to 2 cm of the urethra. The remainder of the urinary tract is sterile in health. The microbial flora of the distal portion of the urethra consists of various members of the family *Enterobacteriaceae*, with *E. coli* predominating. Lactobacilli, diphtheroids, alpha- and nonhemolytic streptococci, enterococci, coagulase-negative staphylococci, *Peptostreptococcus* species, and *Bacteroides* species are also found. In addition, *Mycoplasma hominis*, *Ureaplasma urealyticum*, *Mycobacterium smegmatis*, and *Candida* species may be recovered from this anatomic site in health (58).

Vagina

The normal microbial flora of the vagina varies according to hormonal influences at different ages (28). At birth, the vulva of the newborn child is sterile, but after the first 24 h of life, it gradually acquires a rich and varied flora of saprophytic organisms such as diphtheroids, micrococci, and nonhemolytic streptococci. After 2 to 3 days, estrogen from the maternal circulation induces the deposition of glycogen in the vaginal epithelium, which favors the growth of lactobacilli. The lactobacilli produce acid from glycogen, which lowers the pH of the vagina, and the resultant microbial flora that develops resembles that of a pubertous female. After the passively transferred estrogen is excreted, the glycogen disappears along with the resultant loss of lactobacilli as the predominant vaginal flora and the increase of pH to a physiologic or slightly alkaline level. At this time, the normal microbial flora is mixed, nonspecific, and relatively scanty and contains organisms derived from the flora of the skin and colon. At puberty, the glycogen

reappears in the vaginal epithelium and the adult microbial flora is established. The predominant flora of the vagina in puberty are anaerobic bacteria in concentrations of 10^7 to 10^9 CFU/ml of vaginal secretion, with the anaerobic bacteria outnumbering the aerobic bacteria 100-fold. The major groups of microorganisms represented include lactobacilli, diphtheroids, micrococci, coagulase-negative staphylococci, *Enterococcus faecalis*, microaerophilic and anaerobic streptococci, mycoplasmas, ureaplasmas, and yeasts. During pregnancy, the anaerobic microflora decreases significantly, whereas the numbers of aerobic lactobacilli increase 10-fold (20, 39).

The vaginal flora in postmenopausal women is poorly studied. Specimens are often difficult to obtain from healthy women in this category because they seldom present to a physician unless they have some gynecologic problem, and the amount of vaginal secretion produced and available for sampling is greatly reduced. However, at least one report (9) documents a significant decrease in lactobacilli in the vaginal flora in postmenopausal women due to the lack of circulating estrogen and the resultant decrease in glycogen in the vaginal mucosa.

VIRULENCE FACTORS AND MECHANISMS

The factors that determine the initiation, development, and outcome of an infection involve a series of complex and shifting interactions between the host and the parasite, which can vary with different infecting microorganisms. The microbial factors that contribute to the virulence of a microorganism can be divided into three major categories: (i) those that promote colonization of host surfaces, (ii) those that evade the host's immune system and promote tissue invasion, and (iii) those that produce toxins that result in tissue damage in the human host. Pathogenic microorganisms may have any or all of these factors.

Colonization Factors

Adherence

Most infections are initiated by the attachment or adherence of the microbe to host tissue, followed by microbial replication in order to establish colonization. This attachment can be relatively nonspecific or can require the interaction between structures on the microbial surfaces and specific receptors on host cells. This adherence phenomenon is particularly important in the mouth, small intestine, and urinary bladder, where mucosal surfaces are washed continually by fluids. In these areas, only microorganisms that can adhere to the mucosal surface can colonize that site.

Bacteria adhere to tissues by having pili and/or adhesins. Pili or fimbriae are rod-shaped structures that consist primarily of an ordered array of a single protein subunit called pilin. The tip of the pilus mediates adherence of bacteria by attaching to a receptor molecule on the host cell surface that is composed of carbohydrate residues of either glycoproteins or glycolipids. The binding of the pilus to its host target cell can be quite specific and accounts for the tissue tropism associated with certain bacterial infections. Bacterial pili are easily broken and lost and must be continually reproduced by the bacterium. An important function of pilus replacement, at least for some bacteria, is that it provides a way for the bacterium to evade the host's immune response. Host antibodies that bind to the tips of pili physically block the pili from binding to their host cell targets. Some bacteria can evade this immune defense by growing pili of different antigenic types, thereby rendering the host's immune response ineffective. For example, *Neisseria gonorrhoeae* can produce over 50 pilin types that make it virtually impossible for the host to mount an antibody response that prevents colonization (53).

Bacterial adherence can also be accomplished by a process involving bacterial cell surface structures known as adhesins and complementary receptors on the surfaces of host cells. These adhesins, also known as afimbrial adhesins, are proteins that promote the tighter binding of bacteria to host cells following initial binding by pili. The mechanisms used by a microorganism to adhere to a host cell dictate its ability to enter the cell and set into motion a number of physiologic events. An elegant example of microbial attachment followed by a sequence of pathologic effects is that of enteropathogenic *E. coli* (EPEC). Following initial adhesion, intracellular calcium levels increase, activating actin-severing enzymes and protein kinases, which then lead to vesiculation and disruption of the microvilli. The bacteria are then able to attach to the epithelium in a more intimate fashion, allowing maximal activation of protein kinases. This results in major changes to the cytoskeleton and alterations in the permeability of the membrane to ions. Changes in ion permeation result in ion secretion and reductions in levels of absorption, resulting in the secretory diarrhea that is the hallmark of this disease. It has been found that a majority of EPEC isolates contain a large plasmid that codes for its adhesive properties (1).

In addition to binding to receptors on the host cell surface, some bacteria also form dense, multiorganism layers, called biofilms, in which the first layer of bacteria attaches directly to the surface of the host cells and other layers of bacteria are attached to the basal layer by a polysaccharide matrix. Biofilms have been detected in the vagina, mouth, and intestine, and in fact, the resident microflora of these sites may largely be organized into biofilms. These dense mats of organisms may help explain the barrier function of these sites in protection of the host. However, the formation of biofilms may also be the prelude to disease. For example, dental plaque is a biofilm that is known to cause disease, and *Pseudomonas aeruginosa* has been shown to establish pathogenic biofilms in the lungs of cystic fibrosis patients. Indeed, hospital-acquired infections in patients with indwelling urinary or venous catheters are generally preceded by the formation of a biofilm on the interior wall of the catheter. Organisms within biofilms are more resistant to antibiotics than individual bacteria and are partially protected from phagocytes as well. Biofilm formation on embedded plastic devices provides yet another example of the iatrogenic activities that continue to create new niches that microorganisms can exploit.

Iron Acquisition Mechanisms

Once a microorganism adheres to a body site, it has an obligate requirement for iron for its subsequent growth and multiplication. Although the human body contains a plentiful supply of iron, the majority is not easily accessible to microorganisms. The concentration of useable iron is particularly low because lactoferrin, transferrin, ferritin, and hemin bind most of the available iron, and the amount of free iron remaining is far below the level required to support microbial growth (53). Thus, microorganisms have evolved a number of mechanisms for the acquisition of iron from their environments (40). Microorganisms produce siderophores which chelate iron with a very high affinity and

which compete effectively with transferrin and lactoferrin to mobilize iron for microbial use. In addition, some microbial species can utilize host iron complexes directly without the production of siderophores. For example, *Neisseria* species possess specific receptors for transferrin and can remove iron from transferrin at the cell surface; *Yersinia pestis* can use heme as a sole source of iron; *Vibrio vulnificus* can utilize iron from the hemoglobin-haptoglobin complex; and *H. influenzae* can use hemoglobin, hemoglobin-haptoglobin, heme-hemopexin, and heme-albumin complexes as iron sources. Another mechanism for iron acquisition is the production of hemolysins, which act to release iron complexed to intracellular heme and hemoglobin.

Motility

Some mucosal surfaces, such as the mouth and small intestine, are protected from microbial colonization because they are constantly being washed with fluids. Other mucosal surfaces, such as the colon or vagina, are relatively stagnant areas. In either case, microorganisms that can move directionally toward a mucosal surface will have a better chance of contacting host surfaces than nonmotile organisms. Although motility due to flagella and chemotaxis are appealing candidates as virulence factors, in only a few cases has motility been proven to be essential for virulence (53).

Evading the Host's Immune System

Capsules

A capsule is a loose, relatively unstructured network of polymers that covers the surface of an organism. Most of the well-studied capsules are composed of polysaccharides, but capsules can also be made of proteins or protein-carbohydrate mixtures. The role of capsules in microbial virulence is to protect the organism from complement activation and phagocyte-mediated destruction. Although the host will normally make antibodies directed against the bacterial capsule, some bacteria are able to subvert this response by having capsules that resemble host polysaccharides.

IgA Proteases

Microorganisms that reach mucosal surfaces may often encounter secretory immunoglobulin A (IgA) antibody, which can inhibit their adherence and growth on the epithelium. Certain bacteria that reside and/or cause disease on these mucosal surfaces are able to evade the action of secretory antibody by producing IgA proteases that inactivate IgA antibody. The actual role of IgA proteases in virulence is not well understood, and there is some controversy about their importance; however, the unusual specificities of these enzymes suggest that they must play some role in colonization of mucosal surfaces (53). Examples of bacteria capable of producing IgA proteases include *H. influenzae*, *S. pneumoniae*, *N. meningitidis*, and *N. gonorrhoeae*.

Intracellular Residence

Invasive organisms penetrate anatomic barriers and either enter cells or pass through them to disseminate within the body. To survive under these conditions, organisms have developed special virulence factors that enable them to avoid or disarm host phagocytes. One such antiphagocytic strategy prevents the migration of phagocytes to the site where organisms are growing or limits their effectiveness once the phagocytes are there. Some microbes are capable of producing toxic proteins that kill phagocytes once the phagocytes have arrived, whereas others have developed the ability to survive after phagocytosis by polymorphonuclear cells, monocytes, or macrophages. Strategies for surviving phagocytosis include escaping from the phagosome before it merges with the lysosome, preventing phagosome-lysosome fusion from occurring, or after fusion, enzymatically dissolving the phagolysosome membrane and escaping. *Toxoplasma gondii* is a classic example of an organism that is a successful intracellular parasite. After entry, *T. gondii* resides within a phagosome vacuole that is permanently made incapable of infusion with other intracellular organelles, including lysosomes. The parasite's survival within this vacuole depends on maintaining the appropriate pH, excluding lysosomal contents, and activating specific mechanisms necessary for nutrient acquisition while it is contained inside the vacuole (56).

Serum Resistance

Resistance to the lytic effects of complement is almost a universal requirement for pathogens that traverse mucosal or skin barriers but remain in the extracellular environment. The lytic effect of serum on gram-negative organisms is complement mediated and can be initiated by the classical or alternative pathway. One of the principal targets of complement is the lipopolysaccharide (LPS) layer of gram-negative bacteria. Some pathogens are called "serum resistant" and have evolved defense mechanisms that include (i) failure to bind and activate complement, (ii) shedding of surface molecules that activate the complement system, (iii) interruption of the complement cascade before the formation of C5b-C9, and (iv) enhancement of the formation of nonlytic complexes. Many of the microbes that are able to cause systemic infections are serum resistant, indicating the importance of this trait.

Toxins

Toxins produced by certain microorganisms during growth may alter the normal metabolism of human cells, with damaging and sometimes deleterious effects on the host. Toxins are traditionally associated with bacterial diseases but may play important roles in diseases caused by fungi, protozoa, and helminths. Two major types of bacterial toxins exist: exotoxins and endotoxins. Exotoxins are proteins that are usually heat labile and are generally secreted into the surrounding medium or tissue. However, some exotoxins are bound to the bacterial surface and are released upon cell death and lysis. In contrast, endotoxins are LPSs of the outer membrane of gram-negative bacteria.

Exotoxins

Exotoxins are produced by a variety of organisms, including gram-positive and gram-negative bacteria, and can cause disease through several mechanisms. First, exotoxins may be produced in and consumed along with food. Disease produced by these exotoxins is generally self-limiting because the bacteria do not remain in the body, thus eliminating the toxin source. Second, bacteria growing in a wound or tissue may produce exotoxins that cause damage to the surrounding tissues of the host, contributing to the spread of infection. Third, bacteria may colonize a wound or mucosal surface and produce exotoxins that enter the bloodstream and affect distant organs and tissues. Toxins that attack a variety of different cell types are called cytotoxins, whereas those that attack specific cell types are designated by the cell type or organ affected, such as a neurotoxin, leukotoxin, or hepatotoxin. Exotoxins can also

be named for the species of bacteria that produce them or for the disease with which they are associated, such as cholera toxin, Shiga toxin, diphtheria toxin, and tetanus toxin. Toxins are also named on the basis of their activities, for example, adenylate cyclase and lecithinase, while others are simply given letter designations, such as *P. aeruginosa* exotoxin A.

Five major groups of bacterial exotoxins are known, and they are reviewed in detail elsewhere (54, 57). These exotoxins are typically categorized based upon their mechanisms of action: damage cell membranes, inhibit protein synthesis, activate second messenger pathways, inhibit the release of neurotransmitters, or activate the host immune response. Some of the exotoxins are also known as A-B toxins because the portion of the toxin that binds to a host cell receptor (portion B or binding portion) is separate from the portion that mediates the enzyme activity responsible for its toxicity (portion A or active portion). Two structural types of A-B toxins exist. The simplest kind is synthesized as a single protein with a disulfide bond. A more complex type of A-B toxin has a binding portion that is composed of multiple subunits but that is still attached to the A portion by the disulfide bond. The disulfide bonds are broken when the B portion binds to a specific host cell surface molecule and the A portion is transported into the host cell. Thus, the B portion of the molecule determines the host cell specificity of the toxin. For example, if the B portion binds specifically to the cell receptors found only on the surface of neurons, the toxin will be a specific neurotoxin. Generally speaking, without cell receptor specificity, the A portions of these toxins could kill many cell types if they were to gain entry into the cells. Once having entered the host cell, the A portion becomes enzymatically active and exerts its toxic effect. The A portions of most exotoxins affect the cyclic AMP (cAMP) levels in the host cell by ribosylating the protein that controls cAMP. This causes the loss of control of ion flow, which results in the loss of water from the host tissue into the lumen of the intestine, causing diarrhea. Other toxins have A portions that cleave host cell rRNA, thereby shutting down protein synthesis, as occurs with diphtheria toxin (54, 57).

Another type of exotoxin, membrane-disrupting toxin, lyses host cells by disrupting the integrity of their plasma membranes. There are two types of membrane-disrupting toxins. One is a protein that inserts itself into the host cell membrane by using cholesterol as a receptor and forms channels or pores, allowing cytoplasmic contents to leak out and water to enter. The second type of membrane-disrupting exotoxin consists of phospholipases. These enzymes remove the charged head group from the phospholipids of the cell membrane, which destabilizes the membrane and causes cell lysis. These enzymes are appropriately referred to as cytotoxins.

Some bacterial exotoxins serve as superantigens by acting directly on T cells and antigen-presenting cells of the immune system. Impairment of the immunologic functions of these cells by toxin can lead to serious human disease. One large family of toxins in this category is the pyrogenic toxin superantigens, whose important biologic activities include potent stimulation of the immune cell system, pyrogenicity, and enhancement of endotoxin shock. Examples of bacterial exotoxins that function as superantigens include the staphylococcal and streptococcal exotoxins that are discussed in detail elsewhere (36, 54, 57).

Much more is known about the biology and pathophysiology of exotoxins. Readers who wish additional and more detailed information are referred to the excellent articles and books cited in references 5, 7, 55, and 57.

Endotoxins

Endotoxins are the LPS components of the outer membranes of gram-negative bacteria. The toxic lipid portion (lipid A) is embedded in the outer membrane, with its core antigen extending outward from the bacterial surface. Endotoxins are heat stable, destroyed by formaldehyde, and relatively less toxic than many exotoxins. Lipid A exerts its effects when bacteria lyse by binding to plasma proteins and then interacting with receptors on monocytes, macrophages, and other host cells, thereby forcing the production of cytokines and the activation of the complement and coagulation cascades. The result of these events is an increase in host body temperature, a decrease in blood pressure, damage to vessel walls, disseminated intravascular coagulation, and a decrease in blood flow to essential organs such as the lung, kidney, and brain, leading to organ failure. Activation of the coagulation cascade leads to insufficiency of clotting components, resulting in hemorrhage and further organ damage. Superantigens can also greatly enhance the host's susceptibility to endotoxic shock by acting synergistically with endotoxin to further augment the release of inflammatory cytokines that are lethal to cells of the immune system (36).

Hydrolytic Enzymes

Many pathogenic organisms produce extracellular enzymes such as hyaluronidase, proteases, DNases, collagenase, elastinase, and phospholipases which are capable of hydrolyzing host tissues and disrupting cellular structure. Although not normally considered classic exotoxins, these enzymes can destroy host cells as effectively as exotoxins and are frequently sufficient to initiate clinical disease. For example, *Aspergillus* species secrete a variety of proteases which function as virulence factors by degrading the structural barriers of the host, thereby facilitating the invasion of tissues (37). Other examples are the hyaluronidase and gelatinase enzymes that have long been associated with virulent enterococci. Hyaluronidase-producing enterococci have been implicated as the cause of periodontal disease due to their disruption of the intercellular cementing substances of the epithelium (52). Studies of hyaluronidase in other microorganisms describe it as a spreading factor in *Ancylostoma duodenale* cutaneous larva migrans (25) and as an important factor in the dissemination of *Treponema pallidum* (17).

CONCLUSION

The dynamics of the host-parasite relationship is in a constant state of change throughout life as the balance continues to shift between states of health and disease. As such, the words of Dr. Lederberg continue to have relevance into the 21st century as our human species is still locked in this Darwinian struggle for survival with our microbial and viral predators.

REFERENCES

1. **Baldini, M. M., J. B. Kaper, M. M. Levine, D. C. A. Candy, and H. W. Moon.** 1983. Plasmid-mediated adhesion of enteropathogenic *Escherichia coli. J. Pediatr. Gastroenterol. Nutr.* **2:**534–538.

2. **Bartholomew, B., and M. J. Hill.** 1984. The pharmacology of dietary nitrate and the origin of urinary nitrate. *Food Chem. Toxicol.* **22:**789–791.

3. **Benno, Y., K. Sawada, and T. Mitsuoka.** 1984. The intestinal flora of infants: composition of fecal flora in breast-fed and bottle-fed infants. *Microbiol. Immunol.* **28:** 975–986.

4. **Bokkenheuser, V. D., and J. Winter.** 1983. Biotransformation of steroids, p. 215. *In* D. J. Hentges (ed.), *Human Intestinal Microflora in Health and Disease.* Academic Press, Inc., New York, N.Y.

5. **Brogden, K. A., J. A. Roth, T. B. Stanton, C. A. Bolin, F. C. Minion, and M. J. Wannemuehler (ed.).** 2000. *Virulence Mechanisms of Bacterial Pathogens.* ASM Press, Washington, D.C.

6. **Carlsson, J., H. Grahnen, and G. Jonsson.** 1975. Lactobacilli and streptococci in the mouth of children. *Caries Res.* **9:**333–339.

7. **Cossart, P., P. Boquet, S. Normark, and R. Rappuoli (ed.).** 2000. *Cellular Microbiology.* ASM Press, Washington, D.C.

8. **Cregan, J., and N. J. Hayward.** 1953. The bacterial content of the healthy small intestine. *Br. Med. J.* **i:**1356–1359.

9. **Cruikshank, R., and A. Sharman.** 1936. The biology of the vagina in the human subject. II. The bacterial flora and secretion of the vagina at various age periods and their relation to glycogen in the vaginal epithelium. *J. Obstet. Gynaecol. Br. Emp.* **32:**208–211.

10. **Davis, C. P.** 1996. Normal flora, p. 113–119. *In* S. Baron (ed.), *Medical Microbiology,* 4th ed. The University of Texas Medical Branch at Galveston, Galveston.

11. **Delaney, J. E., S. K. Ratzan, and K. S. Kornman.** 1986. Subgingival microbiota associated with puberty: studies of pre-, circum- and postpubertal human females. *Pediatr. Dent.* **8:**286–291.

12. **Donaldson, R. M., Jr.** 1964. Normal bacterial populations of the intestine and their relationship to intestinal function. *N. Engl J. Med.* **270:**938–945, 994–1001, 1050–1056.

13. **Drasar, B. S., M. Shiner, and G. M. McLeod.** 1969. Studies on the intestinal flora. I. The bacterial flora of the gastrointestinal tract in healthy and achlorhydric persons. *Gastroenterology* **56:**71–79.

14. **Eisenstein, B. I., and M. Schaechter.** 1993. Normal microbial flora, p. 212. *In* M. Schaechter, G. Medoff, and B. I. Eisenstein (ed.), *Mechanisms of Microbial Disease,* 2nd ed. The Williams & Wilkins Co., Baltimore, Md.

15. **Evans, C. A.** 1976. The microbial ecology of human skin. *In* H. M. Stills, W. J. Loesche, and T. C. O'Brien (ed.), *Microbial Aspects of Dental Caries,* vol. 1 (special supplement to *Microbiology Abstracts—Bacteriology*). Information Retrievable, Inc., New York, N.Y.

16. **Finegold, S. M., V. L. Sutter, and G. E. Mathison.** 1983. Normal indigenous intestinal flora, p. 3–31. *In* D. J. Hentges (ed.), *Human Intestinal Microflora in Health and Diseases.* Academic Press, Inc., New York, N.Y.

17. **Fitzgerald, T. J., and L. A. Repesh.** 1987. The hyaluronidase associated with *Treponema pallidum* facilitates treponemal dissemination. *Infect. Immun.* **55:**1023–1028.

18. **Frisken, K. W., J. R. Tagg, A. J. Laws, and M. B. Orr.** 1987. Suspected periodontopathic microorganisms and their oral habitats in young children. *Oral Microbiol. Immunol.* **2:**60–65.

19. **Gallis, H. A.** 1988. Normal flora and opportunistic infections, p. 339. *In* W. K. Joklik, H. P. Willett, D. B. Amos, and C. M. Wilfert (ed.), *Zinsser Microbiology,* 19th ed. Appleton & Lange, Norwalk, Conn.

20. Goperlud, C. P., M. J. Ohm, and R. P. Galask. 1976. Aerobic and anaerobic flora of the cervix during pregnancy and the puerperium. *Am. J. Obstet. Gynecol.* **126:**858–865.

21. Gorbach, S. L. 1971. Intestinal microflora. *Gastroenterology* **60:**1110–1129.

22. Gorbach, S. L., L. Nahas, P. I. Lerver, and L. Weinstein. 1967. Studies of intestinal microflora. I. Effects of diet, age and periodic sampling on numbers of fecal microorganisms in man. *Gastroenterology* **53:**845–855.

23. Gorbach, S. L., A. G. Plant, L. Nahas, L. Weinstein, G. Spanknebel, and R. Levitan. 1967. Studies of intestinal microflora. II. Microorganisms of the small intestine and their relations to oral and fecal flora. *Gastroenterology* **53:**856–867.

24. Hall, M. A., C. B. Cole, and S. L. Smith. 1990. Factors influencing the presence of fecal lactobacilli in early infancy. *Arch. Dis. Child.* **65:**185–189.

25. Hortez, P. J., S. Narasimhan, J. Haggerty, L. Milstone, V. Bhopale, G. A. Schad, and F. F. Richards. 1992. Hyaluronidase from infective *Ancylostoma* hookworm larvae and its possible function as a virulence factor in tissue invasion and in cutaneous larva migrans. *Infect. Immun.* **60:**1018–1023.

26. Ikeda, T., and H. J. Sandham. 1971. Prevalence of *Streptococcus mutans* on various tooth surfaces in Negro children. *Arch. Oral Biol.* **16:**1237–1240.

27. Ikeda, T., H. J. Sandham, and E. L. Bradley, Jr. 1973. Changes in *Streptococcus mutans* and lactobacilli in plaque in relation to the initiation of dental caries in Negro children. *Arch. Oral Biol.* **18:**555–566.

28. Ison, C. A. 1990. Factors affecting the microflora of the lower genital tract of healthy women, p. 111–130. *In* M. J. Hill and P. D. Marsh (ed.), *Human Microbial Ecology.* CRC Press, Inc., Boca Raton, Fla.

29. Justesen, T., O. H. Nielsen, I. E. Jacobsen, J. Lave, and S. N. Rasmussen. 1984. The normal cultivable microflora in upper jejunal fluid in healthy adults. *Scand. J. Gastroenterol.* **19:**279–282.

30. Keusch, G. T., and S. L. Gorbach. 1995. Enteric microbial ecology and infection, p. 1115–1130. *In* W. S. Haubrich, F. Schaffner, and J. E. Berk (ed.), *Gastroenterology,* 5th ed. The W. B. Saunders Co., Philadelphia, Pa.

31. Kloos, W. E. 1986. Ecology of human skin, p. 37–50. *In* P. A. Maardh and K. H. Schleifer (ed.), *Coagulase-Negative Staphylococci.* Almyqvist & Wiksell International, Stockholm, Sweden.

32. Kloos, W. E. 1997. Taxonomy and systematics of staphylococci indigenous to humans, p. 113–137. *In* K. B. Crossley and G. L. Archer (ed.), *The Staphylococci in Human Disease.* Churchill Livingstone, New York, N.Y.

33. Kloos, W. E. 1998. Staphylococcus, p. 577–632. *In* L. Collier, A. Balows, and M. Sussman (ed.), *Topley & Wilson's Microbiology and Microbial Infections,* vol. 2, 9th ed. Edward Arnold, London, United Kingdom.

34. Kloos, W. E., K. H. Schleifer, and F. Gotz. 1991. The genus Staphylococcus, p. 1369–1420. *In* A. Balows, H. G. Truper, M. Dworkin, W. Harder, and K. H. Schleifer (ed.), *The Prokaryotes,* 2nd ed. Springer-Verlag, New York, N.Y.

35. Kohler, B., I. Andreen, and B. Jonsson. 1984. The effect of caries-preventive measures in mothers on dental caries and the oral presence of the bacteria *Streptococcus mutans* and lactobacilli in their children. *Arch. Oral Biol.* **29:**879–883.

36. Kotb, M. 1995. Bacterial pyrogenic exotoxins as superantigens. *Clin. Microbiol. Rev.* **8:**411–426.

37. Kothary, M. H., T. Chase, Jr., and J. D. Macmillan. 1984. Correlation of elastase production by some strains of *Aspergillus fumigatus* with ability to cause pulmonary invasive aspergillosis in mice. *Infect. Immun.* **43:**320–325.

38. Leeming, J. P., K. T. Holland, and W. J. Cunliffe. 1984. The microbial ecology of pilosebaceous units isolated from human skin. *J. Gen. Microbiol.* **130:**803–807.

39. Lindner, J. G. E. M., F. H. F. Plantema, and J. A. A. Hoogkamp-Korstanje. 1978. Quantitative studies of the vaginal flora of healthy women and of obstetric and gynaecological patients. *J. Med. Microbiol.* **11:**233–241.

40. Litwin, C. M., and S. B. Calderwood. 1993. Role of iron in regulation of virulence genes. *Clin. Microbiol. Rev.* **6:**137–149.

41. MacNeal, W. J., L. L. Latzer, and J. E. Kerr. 1909. The fecal bacteria of healthy men. I. Introduction and direct quantitative observations. *J. Infect. Dis.* **6:**123–169.

42. Mata, L. J., and J. J. Urrutia. 1971. Intestinal colonization of breast-fed children in a rural area of low socioeconomic level. *Ann. N. Y. Acad. Sci.* **176:**93–108.

43. McGinley, K. J., G. F. Webster, M. R. Ruggieri, and J. J. Leyden. 1980. Regional variations in density of cutaneous propionibacteria: correlation with *Propionibacterium acnes* populations with sebaceous secretions. *J. Clin. Microbiol.* **12:**672–675.

44. Mevissen-Verhage, E. A., J. H. Marcelis, M. N. deVos, W. C. M. Harmsen-van Amerongen, and J. Verhoef. 1987. *Bifidobacterium, Bacteroides,* and *Clostridium* spp. in fecal samples from breast-fed and bottle-fed infants with and without iron supplement. *J. Clin. Microbiol.* **25:**285–289.

45. Mitsuoka, T., and C. Kaneuchi. 1977. Ecology of the bifidobacteria. *Am. J. Clin. Nutr.* **30:**1799–1810.

46. Moore, L. V. H., W. E. C. Moore, E. P. Cato, R. M. Smibert, J. A. Burmeister, A. M. Best, and R. R. Ranney. 1987. Bacteriology of human gingivitis. *J. Dent. Res.* **66:**989–995.

47. Neut, C., E. Bezirtzoglou, and C. Romand. 1987. Bacterial colonization of the large intestine in newborns delivered by caesarian section. *Zentbl. Bakteriol. Parasitenkd. Infektkrankh. Hyg. Ab to 1 orig. Reihe A* **266:**330–337.

48. Noble, W. C. 1990. Factors controlling the microflora of the skin, p. 131–153. *In* M. J. Hill and P. D. Marsh (ed.), *Human Microbial Ecology.* CRC Press, Inc., Boca Raton, Fla.

49. Parsons, D. S. 1971. Salt transport. *J. Clin. Pathol.* **24**(Suppl. 5):90–98.

50. Plant, A. G., S. L. Gorbach, L. Nahas, L. Weinstein, G. Spanknebe, and R. Levitan. 1967. Studies of intestinal microflora. III. The microbial flora of human small intestinal mucosa and fluids. *Gastroenterology* **53:**868–873.

51. Roberts, A. K. 1988. The development of the infant faecal flora. Ph.D. thesis. Council for National Academic Awards.

52. Rosan, B., and N. B. Williams. 1964. Hyaluronidase production by oral enterococci. *Arch. Oral Biol.* **9:**291–298.

53. Salyers, A. A., and D. D. Whitt. 1994. Virulence factors that promote colonization, p. 30–46. *In* A. A. Salyers and D. D. Whitt (ed.), *Bacterial Pathogenesis: A Molecular Approach.* ASM Press, Washington, D.C.

54. Salyers, A. A., and D. D. Whitt. 1994. Virulence factors that damage the host, p. 47–60. *In* A. A. Salyers and D. D. Whitt (ed.), *Bacterial Pathogenesis: A Molecular Approach.* ASM Press, Washington, D.C.

55. Salyers, A. A., and D. D. Whitt (ed.). 1994. *Bacterial Pathogenesis: A Molecular Approach.* ASM Press, Washington, D.C.

56. Schaechter, M., and B. I. Eisenstein. 1993. Genetics of bacteria, p. 57–76. *In* M. Schaechter, G. Medoff, and B. I.

Eisenstein (ed.), *Mechanisms of Microbial Disease*. The Williams & Wilkins Co., Baltimore, Md.

57. **Schmitt, C. K., K. C. Meysick, and A. D. O'Brien.** 1999. Bacterial toxins: friends or foes? *Emerg. Infect. Dis.* **5:**224–240.

58. **Sherris, J. C.** 1984. Normal microbial flora, p. 50–58. *In* J. C. Sherris, K. J. Ryan, C. G. Ray, J. J. Plorde, L. Corey, and J. Spizizen (ed.), *Medical Microbiology: an Introduction to Infectious Diseases.* Elsevier Science Publishing, New York, N.Y.

59. **Simon, G. L., and S. L. Gorbach.** 1984. The intestinal flora in health and disease: a review. *Gastroenterology* **84:**174–193.

60. **Smith, H. W., and W. E. Crabb.** 1961. The faecal bacterial flora of animals and man: its development in the young. *J. Pathol. Bacteriol.* **82:**53–66.

61. **Socransky, S. S., and S. D. Manganiello.** 1971. The oral microbiota of man from birth to senility. *J. Periodontol.* **42:**485–494.

62. **Tagg, J. R., V. Pybus, and L. V. Phillips.** 1983. Application of inhibitor typing in a study of the transmission and retention in the human mouth of the bacterium *Streptococcus salivarius*. *Arch. Oral. Biol.* **28:**911–915.

63. **Tannock, G. W., R. Fuller, S. L. Smith, and M. A. Hall.** 1990. Plasmid profiling of members of the family *Enterobacteriaceae*, lactobacilli, and bifidobacteria to study the transmission of bacteria from mother to infant. *J. Clin. Microbiol.* **28:**1225–1228.

64. **Theilade, E.** 1990. Factors controlling the microflora of the healthy mouth, p. 1–54. *In* M. J. Hill and P. D. Marsh (ed.), *Human Microbial Ecology.* CRC Press, Inc., Boca Raton, Fla.

65. **Wilson, K. H.** 1999. The gastrointestinal biota, p. 629. *In* T. Yamada, D. H. Alpers, L. Laine, C. Owyang, and D. W. Powell (ed.), *Textbook of Gastroenterology*, 3rd ed. Lippincott Williams & Wilkins, Baltimore, Md.

66. **Wojcicki, C. J., D. S. Harper and P. J. Robinson.** 1987. Differences in periodontal disease-associated microorganisms of subgingival plaque in prepubertal, pubertal and postpubertal children. *J. Periodontol.* **58:**219–223.

67. **Wolff, H. H., and G. Plewig.** 1976. Ultrastruktur der Mikroflora in Follikeln and Komedonen. *Hautarzt* **27:**432–438.

General Principles of Specimen Collection and Handling

J. MICHAEL MILLER, HARVEY T. HOLMES,
AND KAREN KRISHER

6

In terms of the effectiveness of the laboratory, nothing is more important than the appropriate selection, collection, and handling of a specimen for microbiologic diagnosis. When specimen collection and management are not priorities, the laboratory can contribute little to patient care. Consequently, all members of the medical staff involved in this process must understand the critical nature of ensuring specimen quality. It is the responsibility of the laboratory to provide complete and accurate specimen management information in a form that can be easily incorporated into the procedure manuals of those health care workers (i.e., nurses) who have primary responsibility for the collection of specimens. The information provided should address safety, selection, collection, transportation, acceptability, and labeling. This chapter provides an approach for developing a policy for proper collection and handling of specimens destined for analysis in the clinical microbiology laboratory for adult and pediatric patients. Special emphasis and more details are provided for pediatric specimens in this chapter because of the unique character of this patient population and the special procedures often required for obtaining appropriate specimens. Details of specimen management can be found in the relevant chapters for each major group of microorganisms covered in this Manual (bacteriology, chapter 20; virology, chapter 77; mycology, chapter 111; parasitology, chapter 126).

Appropriate specimen management, or the lack of it, affects patient care in several very important ways. It is the key to accurate laboratory diagnosis that directly affects patient care and patient outcome; it influences therapeutic decisions; it affects hospital infection control, patient length of stay, and overall hospital costs; it plays a major role in laboratory costs; and it clearly influences laboratory efficiency. For these reasons, every laboratory should develop a rational, sound, and relevant specimen management policy and enforce it as strictly as possible.

SAFETY

Biosafety at the laboratory bench is of primary concern to laboratorians. Health care workers may be unaware of the potential etiologic agent(s) residing in the specimen being transported to the laboratory. Policies designed to protect laboratory and other personnel from accidental exposure to these agents must be in place. Most microbiology laboratory texts, including chapter 9 of this Manual, have sections on laboratory procedures that should contain safety information related to specimen management. Specific reference material on biosafety should be available in every microbiology laboratory. The reference materials available in the laboratory could include *Biosafety in Microbiological and Biomedical Laboratories*, 4th ed. (68) and *Biosafety in the Laboratory: Prudent Practices for the Handling and Disposal of Infectious Materials* (51).

In general, laboratorians should comply with the following policies for safety in specimen management:

1. Wear gloves, gowns, and, where appropriate, masks and/or goggles when collecting specimens (49).
2. Use leak-proof specimen containers and transport the containers within a sealable, leak-proof plastic bag with a separate compartment for paperwork (50).
3. Never transport syringes with needles to the laboratory. Instead, transfer the contents to a sterile tube or remove the needle with a protective device, recap the syringe, and place it in a sealable, leak-proof plastic bag (59).
4. Do not transport leaking specimen containers to the laboratory or process them. Notify the physician or the responsible nurse of the leaking container and explain the potential compromised nature of the results if processing is continued; ask for a repeat specimen. If a new specimen is submitted, autoclave and discard the leaking one (47). If another specimen cannot be obtained, work with the existing specimen container within a biological safety cabinet.

SELECTION AND COLLECTION OF THE SPECIMEN

Before a specimen is collected for analysis, the specimen or the collection site must be selected and must represent a location of active disease. Even careful collection methods will produce a specimen of little clinical value if it is not obtained from a site where the infection is active. Some of the common sites of infection where ready sources of contamination reside include the bladder, where urethral organisms and those from the perineum may easily contaminate the urine specimen; blood, which is often contaminated by commensal flora from the venipuncture site; the endometrium, which may contain commensal vaginal flora;

fistulas, which may contain organisms from the gastrointestinal tract; the middle ear, a specimen from which will be contaminated with the flora of the external auditory canal if a swab is used to collect the specimen; the nasal sinus, which may contain nasopharyngeal flora; and sites of subcutaneous infections and superficial wounds, which are commonly contaminated by skin and mucous membrane flora.

General specimen selection and collection guidelines should include the following:

1. Avoid contamination from indigenous flora, whenever possible, to ensure a sample representative of the infectious process (9, 47, 59). Specimens from many sites of infection may contain an etiologic agent that would be considered part of the normal flora in a healthy host. This "background noise" of normal flora (i.e., from skin, membranes, and the respiratory tract) could interfere with the interpretation of culture results as well as overgrow and obscure the true agent of disease.

2. Select the correct anatomic site from which to obtain the specimen, and collect the specimen by the proper technique and with the proper supplies, as described in the tables of this and subsequent chapters of this Manual.

3. Optimize the capture of anaerobes from specimens by using the proper precautions, procedures, and supplies; biopsy or needle aspirates are the specimens of choice, while anaerobic swabs are the least desirable (32, 47). Never refrigerate specimens submitted for anaerobic culture but, rather, maintain them at room temperature (29).

4. Collect adequate volumes; insufficient material may yield false-negative results.

5. Place the specimen in a container designed to promote the survival of suspected agents and to eliminate leakage and potential safety hazards.

6. Label each specimen container with the patient's name and identification number, source, specific site, date, time of collection, and initials of the collector (18).

The collection of specimens with swabs may or may not be the method of choice for the collection of a particular specimen for microbiologic analysis (34, 47). It is critical that specimen collectors know the appropriate device and method for the collection of samples. Swab tips for specimen collection are usually made of cotton, Dacron (a polyester), or calcium alginate. Most come with a plastic shaft, although swabs with wooden shafts are available. The swabs with wooden shafts are generally not recommended for routine specimen collection because they may contain toxic products and could inactivate herpes simplex virus and interfere with some *Ureaplasma* identification methods. Cotton-tipped swabs are less popular today because they may contain fatty acids that could interfere with the survival of some bacteria and *Chlamydia* spp. However, most nonfastidious bacteria are not affected if cotton-tipped swabs are used. Cotton-tipped swabs are also suitable for the collection of specimens from the vagina, cervix, or urethra for the detection of *Mycoplasma*. Dacron- and rayon-tipped swabs have a wide range of uses including the collection of specimens for the detection of viruses and can facilitate the survival of *Streptococcus pyogenes*. Calcium alginate-tipped swabs can be toxic for lipid-enveloped viruses and some cell cultures as well as for some strains of *Neisseria gonorrhoeae* and *Ureaplasma urealyticum*. These are useful for the collection of specimens for *Chlamydia* spp. (34). Newer tips of polyurethane foam are finding wide acceptance.

Swabs with flexible wire shafts and small tips are recommended for use for the collection of nasopharyngeal specimens, including sampling for *Bordetella pertussis* and male urethral specimens for diagnosis of gonorrhea. Specimens on plastic-shafted swabs that are labeled by the specimen collector as "nasopharyngeal" are not likely to contain true representatives of the nasopharyngeal flora and may actually contain representatives of the nasal or throat flora (47).

TRANSPORTATION

1. All specimens must be promptly transported to the laboratory, preferably within 2 h (32). If processing is delayed, specimens collected for the detection of bacterial agents may be stored under specified conditions (see chapter 20).

2. In general, do not store specimens for bacterial culture for more than 24 h. Viruses, however, usually remain stable for 2 to 3 days at 4°C (34, 35).

3. Optimal transport of clinical specimens, including specimens for anaerobic culture, depends primarily on the volume of material obtained. Submit small amounts within 15 to 30 min of collection; biopsy tissue may be maintained for up to 20 to 24 h if it is stored at 25°C in an anaerobic transport system (32).

4. Environmentally sensitive organisms include *Shigella* spp. (which should be processed immediately), *Neisseria gonorrhoeae*, *Neisseria meningitidis*, and *Haemophilus influenzae* (which is sensitive to cold temperatures). Never refrigerate spinal fluid, genital, eye, or internal ear specimens (47). Storage conditions for some specimens and agents are summarized in Table 1.

5. Transportation of clinical specimens and transportation of infectious substances from one health care facility or laboratory to another, regardless of the distance, requires strict attention to specimen packaging and labeling instructions (34, 49, 50). Materials for transport must be labeled properly and packaged and protected during transport. The courier vehicles must also be marked and designated as carrying biologic agents. Any clinical specimen, including swabs, scrapings, body fluids, or tissues, that is known or reasonably expected to contain a pathogen is classified as an *infectious substance*.

For specific packaging and shipping instructions, one can refer to a number of sources; the most comprehensive instructions are described by the U.S. Department of Transportation in 49 *Code of Federal Regulations* (http://hazmat. dot.gov/ or http://www.iata.org). Several areas of packaging and shipping are of extreme importance, and one must ensure that everyone involved in packaging and shipping (including courier activities) is current on the specific regulations, including the legal responsibilities of the laboratory as a "shipper," the proper use of certified packaging (only packaging that has been certified by the United Nations for infectious substances can be used), the proper use of necessary package labeling and markings, and proper completion of the required documentation. Frequent referral to the appropriate websites is recommended in order to ensure that compliance with the latest recommendations is accomplished.

Bacterial and Fungal Specimen Transport

Containers for specimen transport and directions on how to use them are often available from the laboratory. The

TABLE 1 Storage conditions for various transport systems and suspected etiologic agents[a]

Preservative or medium type	Specimens held at 4°C	Specimens held at 25°C
No preservative	Autopsy tissue, bronchial wash, intravenous catheter, CSF (viral agent), lung biopsy, pericardial fluid, sputum, urine (all)	CSF (bacterial agents), synovial fluid
Anaerobic transport media		Abdominal fluid, amniotic fluid, anaerobic cultures, aspirates, bile, cul-de-sac material, deep lesion material, IUD for *Actinomyces* spp., lung aspirate, placenta (delivery by cesarean section), sinus aspirate, tissue (surgery), transtracheal aspirate, urine (suprapubic aspirate)
Direct inoculation of media		Corneal scraping, blood cultures, RL or BG plates for *Bordetella* spp., JEMBEC plates for *Neisseria gonorrhoeae*, vitreous humor
Aerobic transport media[b]	Burn wound biopsy, *Campylobacter* spp., ear (external), *Shigella* spp., *Vibrio* spp., *Yersinia* spp.	Bone marrow, *Bordetella* spp., cervix, conjunctiva, *Corynebacterium* spp., ear (internal), genital specimens, nasopharynx, *Neisseria* spp., *Salmonella* spp., upper respiratory tract specimens

[a] Abbreviations: BG, Bordet-Gengou; IUD, intrauterine device; JEMBEC, John E. Martin biological environmental chamber; RL, Regan-Lowe medium.

[b] Stuart's medium, charcoal-impregnated swabs originally formulated for *Neisseria gonorrhoeae* transport; Amies medium, modified Stuart's medium that incorporates charcoal into the medium instead of in the swab; Cary and Blair medium, similar to Stuart's medium but modified for fecal specimens, with the pH increased from 7.4 to 8.4.

potential etiologic agent suspected in the patient dictates the specific collection method and transport system that will support the viability of the agent. Specimens for fungal cultures should not be collected with a swab because of the potential interference of the swab fibers with direct microscopic examination of the specimen. Swabs are acceptable for use for the collection of specimens for the detection of suspected yeast infections, however. Most specimen containers must be sterile since the presence of contaminating flora from nonsterile containers may lead to errors in culture interpretation. Containers for feces need not be sterile but should be clean and should have tight-fitting lids. If there is a question as to whether a specimen container should be sterile for a specific specimen, assume that it should be sterile.

Other useful products and devices include sterile, screw-capped containers for the collection of urine or sputum specimens. The containers should be prepared and packaged for patient use, with directions, including illustrations, that can be understood by patients. Biopsy and tissue specimens may also be placed into these sterile cups, although "biopsy" samples may tend to be smaller than "tissue" samples. To keep these tissues moist, one may add a small amount of nonbacteriostatic saline to the cup rather than wrap the tiny tissue specimen in gauze. Sterile petri dishes or special envelopes can be used to transport hair, skin, or nail scrapings to the mycology laboratory. Commercial transport devices for *Neisseria gonorrhoeae* such as the JEMBEC (John E. Martin biological environmental chamber) system with CO_2 tablets may provide better results than CO_2-containing bottles, especially for transport by courier. The bottles may not have consistent amounts of CO_2, and improper manipulation during inoculation will cause a loss of the atmosphere.

As with bacterial specimens, fungal specimens for culture should be placed into sterile containers and transported to the laboratory promptly. For skin and nail scrapings, cleansing of the site with 70% alcohol is required prior to specimen collection. Nail scrapings for submission to the laboratory must be collected from the deeper, infected portion of the nail, and the initial superficial scrapings should be discarded because they will likely be contaminated. The use of a UV lamp (Wood's lamp) is helpful when selecting infected hair since some dermatophytes will fluoresce. Most other specimens including blood, other sterile body fluids, and urine, respiratory, fecal, and tissue specimens are collected and submitted as described elsewhere for bacterial or mycobacterial specimens. Details can be found in chapter 111.

Virus, Rickettsia, Chlamydia, and Mycoplasma Transport

The methods and media used for the transport of bacteria are inappropriate for the transport of viruses and chlamydiae. Viral transport media (VTM) prevent drying, maintain viral viability during transport, and prevent the overgrowth of contaminating bacteria. Many of the formulations contain either Eagle's minimum essential medium or Hanks' balanced salt solution along with fetal bovine serum (FBS) or bovine serum albumin (BSA). VTM may be prepared in-house or purchased commercially. There is little evidence in the literature that one VTM is better than another. However, in virtually all cases in which a specimen is submitted for viral analysis, the specimen should be selected and collected in a manner appropriate for the target organ (34).

Liquid-based transport systems contain a protein (BSA, gelatin, or FBS) and a combination of antimicrobial agents in a buffered solution. Tissue for viral analysis may also be placed into this type of medium. A phosphate-buffered sucrose-containing transport system (2SP) may be used for virus and chlamydia transport. The antimicrobial agents present in 2SP are not inhibitory to *Chlamydia* spp.

A transport system containing human newborn foreskin fibroblasts is commercially available and useful for recovery and early detection of cytomegalovirus and herpes simplex virus. This cell system has a limited shelf life and is useful only for viruses that grow in fibroblasts.

If specimens arrive in the laboratory after having been inappropriately placed into Stuart's or Amies bacterial transport systems, the swabs may be transferred into one of the systems of liquid VTM.

Recovery of rickettsia seems to be enhanced if glutamate is present in a sodium-free, buffered salt solution. A sucrose-phosphate-glutamate transport medium containing BSA is often used to transport rickettsiae, mycoplasmas, and chlamydiae (34). Manufacturers of nucleic acid probes, amplification systems, or enzyme immunoassay (EIA) antigen detection systems often recommend or supply specific transport media and swabs for the collection and transport of specimens to be tested with their systems.

SPECIMEN ACCEPTABILITY OR REJECTION CRITERIA

At times, specimens arriving in the laboratory may have been improperly selected, collected, or transported. This is essentially the equivalent of a specimen being out of control. This out-of-control process must receive the same attention as an out-of-control identification method or susceptibility test; there must be a corrective action. Processing and reporting of results for these specimens to the physicians may provide misleading information that can lead to misdiagnosis and inappropriate therapy. Consequently, the laboratory must adhere to a strict policy of specimen acceptance and rejection.

Listed below are several examples of situations in which specific laboratory policies must be formulated and enforced to ensure specimen quality:

1. No label. Do not process. Contact the submitting physician or nurse. For specimens obtained by noninvasive means (urine, sputum, or throat swab specimens), have a new specimen submitted. For specimens obtained by invasive procedures (needle aspirates, body fluids, or tissues), process the specimen only after consulting with the physician who obtained the specimen. Note the problem on the report, and document the corrective action taken.

2. Prolonged transport. Do not process. Alert the submitter and request a repeat specimen. Note the problem on the patient's report as "Received after prolonged delay."

3. Improper or leaking container. Do not process. Call the submitter and request a repeat specimen. Note the problem on the patient's report and the corrective action taken.

4. Specimen unsuitable for request (e.g., request for anaerobic culture for a specimen transported aerobically). Do not process. Contact the submitter, clarify the test request, and indicate the discrepancy. Request a proper specimen for the test requested.

5. Duplicate specimens on the same day for the same test request (except blood and tissue). Do not process. Place the specimen in the proper preservative at the correct storage temperature. Call the submitter and indicate the duplication. Note the problem on the report.

There may be instances in which a given specimen must be processed even though its quality is compromised, e.g., a difficult or unusual case, and then only after a consult between the patient's physician and the laboratory director. Table 2 lists specimens that provide little, if any, clinical information; processing of these specimens should be discouraged.

TABLE 2 Specimens to be discouraged due to questionable microbial information

Specimen type	Alternative or comment
Burns, wounds (swabs)	Submit tissue or aspirate
Colostomy discharge	Do not process
Decubiti (swabs)	Submit tissue or aspirate
Foley catheter tip	Do not process
Gangrenous lesion (swab)	Submit tissue or aspirate
Gastric aspirates of newborns	Do not process
Lochia	Do not process
Periodontal lesion (swab)	Submit tissue or aspirate
Perirectal abscess (swab)	Submit tissue or aspirate
Varicose ulcer (swab)	Submit tissue or aspirate
Vomitus	Do not process

Sterile body fluids may be submitted from patients with serious or life-threatening illnesses and must be handled quickly and appropriately. The decision of whether to centrifuge the fluid and culture the specimen on agar media or in blood culture bottles must be incorporated into the laboratory protocol. Table 3 lists some management suggestions for the handling of sterile body fluids (8).

While the above discussion has focused more on general policy issues surrounding specimen management, the details of specimen management for adults will be covered in subsequent and appropriate sections of this Manual. Infants and children represent an important patient population that is often overlooked in specimen management discussions, and there are many instances in which specimens from this patient group require special methods for selection, collection, and transport. The section that follows provides perspective and guidance on these issues.

SPECIMEN MANAGEMENT ISSUES FOR PEDIATRIC PATIENTS

Collection of specimens from pediatric populations may be influenced by factors not encountered when dealing with adults. The types of disease as well as the anatomic areas primarily affected by the infectious agent may differ. Recognition of the critical differences inherent in the collection of specimens for microbiologic assays from infants and children will aid in optimizing the detection of pathogens from this patient population. Table 4 summarizes the salient features of specimen management for this special population.

The volumes of specimen available for testing will vary according to the age and size of the child. Limited volumes are especially pertinent to the collection of blood, urine, cerebrospinal fluid (CSF), other sterile fluids, and tissue samples submitted for culture. Multiple phlebotomies performed for a variety of diagnostic tests can affect the volume of blood collected for culture due to the concern of critical volume depletion in infants and smaller children. The diagnosis of certain types of bacterial meningitis may be hindered by the smaller volumes of CSF available, coupled with the problems inherent in performing lumbar puncture in this age group. The average total volume of CSF in children and infants is approximately 40 to 90 ml, while the volume range for adults is 90 to 150 ml. Lastly, infants and children not only excrete smaller volumes of urine but are also often unable to void on command. In some cases, <1.0 ml of urine may be available for testing.

TABLE 3 Specimen management of sterile body fluids other than blood and CSF[a]

Fluid	Collection container	Concentration	Stain	Comment
Amniotic	Anaerobic tube	No	Gram stain	
Culdocentesis	Anaerobic tube	No	Gram stain	
Dialysis effluent	Isolator tube, urine cup, or Bx2	Centrifuge or filter	Gram stain or AO (low detection rate)	<100 leukocytes/ml is normal; use one-third of filter for one of three media
Pericardial	B and/or anaerobic tube	Cytospin preparation from tube	Gram stain from cytospin sediment	Few leukocytes in normal fluid
Peritoneal (ascites)	Bx2 (10 ml) + anaerobic tube	Cytospin preparation from tube	Gram stain from cytospin sediment	<300 leukocytes/ml is normal
Pleural (effusion, transudate, thoracentesis, empyema)	Anaerobic tube	Cytospin preparation from tube	Gram stain from cytospin sediment	>5 ml needed for fungi; none to a few leukocytes is normal; many leukocytes are found with empyema
Synovial	B + anaerobic tube	Cytospin preparation from tube	Gram stain from cytospin sediment	A few leukocytes is normal

[a] The information in this table is from reference 8. Abbreviations: B, blood culture bottle; Bx2, aerobic and anaerobic blood bottles; AO, acridine orange stain. Cultures and stains can be done from any cytospin sediment.

The greatest challenge, therefore, for laboratories processing specimens from pediatric patients is making the most of the limited amounts of specimens received for culture. Although the procedures for the collection of many specimen types will mirror the protocols used for adult patients, some important differences exist.

Blood Samples for Cultures

Use of proper skin disinfection techniques is even more important in children prior to collection of blood for culture since only one bottle collected during a 24-h period may be available for culture, making the categorization of contaminant versus pathogen difficult to access. Due to the low incidence of anaerobic bacteremia, routine inoculation of an anaerobic blood culture bottle is not warranted. Although the collection of blood from infants and children by venipuncture is achievable by skilled phlebotomists, venous access in pediatric inpatients is often through peripheral or central venous catheters, which eliminates the need for repeated attempts to gain peripheral venous access. Such lines are used primarily for administration of fluids and therapeutic drugs and are infused with heparin to inhibit clotting when not in use. When the catheter is used to obtain blood for culture, the line must be adequately disinfected and flushed of all inhibitory substances before the specimen is obtained. Since volume depletion in the patient is a concern, the amount of fluid to be discarded, as well as the amount of blood available for testing, will be limited. The procedure used most often, the discard method, based the amount of fluid flushed from the line on the weight and size of the child (36). Minimal discard volumes for infants, for example, are in the range of 0.3 to 1.0 ml (58). In response to the decreased volumes of blood that can be obtained from pediatric patients for culture, blood culture bottles that contain approximately 20 ml of broth and that accommodate an inoculation volume of up to 4 ml are available. The smaller volume of broth allows a close approximation of the recommended blood-to-broth ratio necessary to diminish the effect of growth inhibitors and also minimizes the time to detection of a positive culture.

Cerebrospinal Fluid

The primary reason for collection of CSF is for the diagnosis of acute bacterial or viral meningitis or CSF shunt infections. Lumbar puncture is sometimes difficult in an infant or child. A specimen obtained by lumbar puncture that yields only blood is indicative of a failure to access the lumen of the spinal cord (20). If the CSF initially contains a small amount of blood but clears as additional fluid is collected, a repeat lumbar puncture is not required. If only a small amount of fluid is retrieved from the patient due to the patient's age and size, CSF containing clotted blood is sometimes sent for culture pending a repeat lumbar puncture. The clot is homogenized prior to plating, and an acridine orange fluorescent stain of a direct smear of a cytospin preparation is recommended to facilitate the rapid detection of potential pathogens. Gross blood in the specimen may obscure the visualization of organisms when the specimen is stained by Gram's method.

Ventricular shunts are used for drainage in patients who overproduce CSF. Ventricular shunt malfunctions in both children and adults are associated with infection and/or disconnection or obstruction of the catheter (23, 53). The majority of shunt infections are acquired at the time of shunt placement and are associated with organisms usually considered skin flora, such as *Staphylococcus epidermidis* or *Propionibacterium acnes* (12, 66).

Specimens for Detection of Otitis and Sinusitis

Acute otitis media is also a common pediatric disease (11, 52). Uncomplicated otitis media does not require confirmation by culture; however, a persistent infection may require retrieval of fluid from the inner chamber via tympanocentesis for identification of the specific pathogen causing the infection. A swab specimen of the ear canal is unsuitable for diagnosis of acute otitis media or otitis media with effusion. Potential contamination of purulent drainage with resident flora may interfere with accurate analysis of the culture.

Uncomplicated sinusitis is often treated empirically on the basis of the patient's clinical presentation (70). Specimens for culture may be obtained from patients with chronic sinusitis refractory to therapy. Bilateral cultures are

TABLE 4 Requirements for pediatric specimen collection

Specimen type and source	Collection	Comments
Blood for culture		
Peripheral	As for adults. Withdraw a volume of ≥0.5 ml and inoculate the sample into the blood culture bottle.	Collection of larger volumes will aid in retrieval of low concentrations of circulating organisms. Inoculation of one aerobic bottle is usually sufficient.
Peripheral catheter (see comment)	Disinfect the venipuncture site. Insert the catheter and attach a T connector with a syringe to the catheter and withdraw the blood for culture.	A blood sample for culture may be obtained when a peripheral catheter is inserted.
Indwelling central venous catheter	After disinfection, disconnect the extension tubing or cap from the catheter hub. Disinfect the hub. Withdraw a minimum volume of blood and discard. Attach a second sterile syringe and withdraw an additional ≥0.5 ml for culture.	Accidental aspiration of heparin may inhibit the growth of blood-borne pathogens; therefore, flush the catheter with heparin or saline.
Implantable device (for therapy administration)	Disinfect the skin site. Insert a Huber needle through the skin into the apparatus; follow the procedure for collection of blood from a central venous catheter described above.	These devices may rarely be used for vascular access for the retrieval of blood for culture.
CSF		
Lumbar puncture	As for adults.	Difficulties are often encountered in patient positioning and restraint; in addition, there are limitations to the volume of fluid retrievable.
Ventricular shunts	As for adults.	Correct labeling of shunt fluid is important because organisms considered "contaminants" from lumbar punctures may be significant pathogens in ventricular shunt infections.
Dermatologic specimens		
Bacterial and viral cultures		
Pustule or vesicular lesions	Disinfect surface and allow to dry. Unroof the pustule. Aspirate fluid for culture and then insert swab and rotate vigorously to collect fluid and cells from the advancing margin.	Specimens that contain no inflammatory cells are from the superficial areas of the lesion and new specimens must be collected. Viral pathogens are best retrieved from the base of a lesion.
Petechiae, purpura, ecthyma gangrenosa	With a scalpel blade, vigorously scrape the outer margin of the lesion.	A Gram stain of petechial material may give an indication of meningococcal infection.
Fungi	For a dry lesion, scrape the lesion with a scalpel, glass slide, or toothbrush. For moist lesions, use a Dacron swab. For hair, use scissors and forceps. For nails, scrape with a scalpel. Place the scraping directly onto fungal medium or place in a sterile container and send for culture.	A small soft toothbrush is useful for collection of scrapings.
Specimens for detection of scabies	Disinfect the area and allow it to dry. Apply a single drop of mineral oil to the papule and abrade the infested area with a sterile scalpel. Transfer skin scrapings to a sterile container or microscope slide with a coverslip for transport to the lab.	Place the microscope slide with a coverslip in a secure holder so that the coverslip is not dislodged during transit.
Feces		
Bacterial and viral cultures	As for adults. A rectal swab showing feces is suitable for bacterial or viral culture.	Devices that fit into the toilet bowl or techniques such as lining a diaper with plastic wrap facilitate retrieval of feces for testing.

(Continued on next page)

TABLE 4 (*Continued*)

Specimen type and source	Collection	Comments
Clostridium difficile toxin	As for adults.	Toxin-producing strains of *Clostridium difficile* may be normal in some infants <2 years of age. Interpret a positive toxin result for individuals in this age group with caution.
Ovum and parasite examination	As for adults. Submit feces-coated rectal swabs only for antigen detection EIAs, not routine ovum and parasite examinations.	See bacterial and viral cultures. The volume of preservatives present in commercial ovum and parasite collection and transport tubes should be adjusted to retain the recommended stool-to-fixative ratio of 3:1.
Pinworms	Use a commercial paddle sampling device or place the adhesive side of a cellophane tape strip onto a microscope slide. Peel back the tape to expose the adhesive side of the tape. While holding the slide against an applicator, press the tape firmly against the perianal skin. Replace the tape back over the slide and press the adhesive side onto the slide.	The applicator stick provides a safe backing for the glass slide while gentle pressure is applied to the skin for collection of the specimen with the adhesive. Do not use "invisible" or "magic" tape.
Gastric aspirates (may not provide clinically relevant data)	A premeasured length of lubricated catheter is passed gently into the mouth or nasopharynx and is continued through the esophagus into the stomach. The contents are aspirated and placed in a sterile container for immediate transport to the lab. If no gastric secretions are obtained, a lavage of sterile distilled water is collected for specimen processing.	Three consecutive early-morning, fasting specimens are preferred for mycobacterial culture, but infants may not be able to provide such a sample. Collect the aspirate as long after the last feeding as possible. Environmental mycobacterial species may appear in aspirated formula. Neutralization of the specimen must occur upon arrival in the lab.
Genital specimens	Use a small-tipped Dacron swab with a flexible smooth wire. The specimen of choice for a prepubertal female is a vaginal swab or washing. Collect a urethral swab from prepubertal males.	STDs in prepubertal girls involve the vagina as opposed to the cervix. Specimens from adolescents are the same as those collected from adults.
Ear specimens		
Otitis	Cleanse the external auditory canal with an antiseptic.	Needle aspiration of fluid (tympanocentesis) is the recommended method for obtaining a specimen.
Otitis media	Using an otoscope, insert a 1-ml tuberculin syringe with a 3.5-in. 22-gauge spinal needle bent at a 30° angle through the tympanic membrane and aspirate the fluid in the chamber into a sterile vial or syringe.	A purulent discharge from a ruptured membrane can be collected for culture by using a sterile swab
Respiratory specimens		
Bronchoalveolar lavage specimens	As for adults.	Specimens from unsheathed catheters may contain contaminating oropharyngeal flora. For infants and younger children, <10 ml is often retrieved. If >10 ml is collected, centrifuge the sample prior to plating.
Protected brush specimens Nasal specimens	As for adults. Insert a sterile swab at least 1 cm into the opening of the anterior nares.	Used primarily for surveillance for methicillin-resistant *Staphylococcus aureus* or to assess upper respiratory tract colonization in children with immunologic defects.

(*Continued on next page*)

TABLE 4 Requirements for pediatric specimen collection (*Continued*)

Specimen type and source	Collection	Comments
Nasal washes	Aspirate approximately 4 ml of sterile saline into a 1-oz tapered rubber bulb. Tip the patient's head back approximately 70 degrees and insert the bulb into the nostril until it is occluded. Squeeze the bulb to dispense the saline, hold for a few seconds, and then release to collect the secretions. Dispense the specimen into a sterile container and transport to the lab as soon as possible.	A nasal wash or nasal aspirate (see below) is often cited as the preferred specimen type for collection of respiratory secretions for culture for either viruses or *Bordetella pertussis* and direct smear examination for pediatric patients. Transport specimens for viral cultures on ice.
Nasopharyngeal aspirates	Attach a sterile suction catheter to a (mucous) trap and introduce the end of the catheter into the nasopharynx until resistance is encountered. Withdraw the catheter 1–2 cm and apply suction to aspirate the sample. Dispense the specimen into a sterile container and immediately transport it to the lab.	See nasal wash. Transport specimens for viral cultures on ice.
Nasopharyngeal swab specimens	Insert the swab into the nasopharyngeal cavity to the point of resistance and then gently rotate it. Place the swab into an appropriate transport medium and send to the lab immediately.	For young children and infants, use of a swab with a small tip circumference such as a calcium alginate or small-tip Dacron swab. Transport specimens for viral cultures on ice.
Throat swab specimens	Tilt the child's head back and ask the child to open his or her mouth as wide as possible. Carefully insert the sterile swab(s) into the oral cavity and sample the surfaces of the back of the throat and tonsils.	In children, the major pathogen of bacterial pharyngitis is group A streptococcus (GAS). If a rapid screen of a throat swab specimen for GAS is performed, collect two swab specimens to do a culture to confirm negative screening findings or to rule out a possible false-positive result caused by a member of the *Streptococcus anginosus* group. Avoid touching other areas of the oral cavity to prevent contamination of the specimen with oropharyngeal flora.
Tracheal aspirates	After oxygenation of the patient, attach a sterile suction catheter to a (mucous) trap and introduce the end of the catheter into the trachea until resistance is encountered. Withdraw the catheter 1–2 cm and apply suction to aspirate the sample.	Although grading systems for assessment of the quality of pediatric tracheal aspirates have been proposed, careful evaluation is required prior to their implementation.
Transtracheal aspirate	As for adults.	
Sputum specimens	As for adults.	Since children are often unable to produce sputum, tracheal aspirates are more often collected in pediatric populations.
Specimens for detection of viruses	Specimens of choice are similar to others mentioned in this table (45).	Rectal swabs are acceptable for detection of rotavirus antigen.
Specimens for detection of chlamydia	Conjunctival and/or nasopharyngeal swabs are appropriate for screening of neonates.	See genital specimens above. Vaginal (females) or urethral (males) swabs are required for chlamydial culture for the determination of sexual abuse.

recommended (70). Secretions from the region of the maxillary ostium are sampled with a swab under direct vision; however, unless the specimen is obtained very carefully, interpretation of culture results may be hindered by the presence of contaminating flora. Needle aspiration of the sinus is recommended for definitive diagnosis of the etiologic agent of infection (46).

Respiratory Specimens

For the diagnosis of group A streptococcal pharyngitis (10, 14), collection of two pharyngeal swabs is optimal for performance of both a rapid antigen detection assay and culture (one swab for each assay). A single swab shared for both methods may reduce the sensitivity of the antigen detection assay due to a reduction in the concentration of organisms available after culture inoculation (10). Although the reported sensitivities of some rapid assays may suggest that a confirmatory culture may be eliminated in the event that the screen is negative, careful consideration must be given to the possible implications of an undetected infection in some children (10). The collection of nasopharyngeal swab specimens, washes, or aspirates for culture and/or detection of antigens of respiratory viruses and *Bordetella pertussis* is satisfactory (4, 44, 45). Again, collection of more than one swab specimen will increase the chance of isolate detection. Transport of swabs in a suitable holding medium is necessary to ensure organism viability if delays are anticipated between the time of collection and specimen receipt by the laboratory. Due to the small diameter of the nasal passages in some infants and children, coupled with inflammation of the nasal mucosa during the infection, specimen collection with a swab is sometimes more difficult and thus provides an inadequate sample.

A sputum specimen for diagnosis of pneumonia is difficult to obtain from children. More commonly, a tracheal or endotracheal tube aspirate is sent for microbiologic culture. The utility of endotracheal tube aspirates as predictors of pediatric lower respiratory tract infection is influenced by the role that accumulated secretions within the tube play in the promotion of bacterial colonization (27, 61, 74). A bronchoalveolar lavage or the use of a protected brush will provide a superior specimen for intubated children with symptoms of pneumonia (41, 43, 73). Although pediatric bronchoscopes are available, the tubing diameter is sometimes too large for certain pediatric patients. In these situations, a small-diameter catheter is useful for performance of the lavage (2, 40). If an unprotected catheter is used, however, the commensal oral flora will reduce the chances for recognition of the true etiologic agent. Aspiration of gastric secretions is performed for infants and children with presumed pneumonia caused by *Mycobacterium tuberculosis* (1, 60). After the patient has fasted overnight, the swallowed respiratory secretions are aspirated from the stomach by using gastric intubation and sent for diagnostic testing (1, 63). Problems with this method include the inability of infants on a feeding schedule to maintain a fasting state prior to specimen collection. Lastly, many pediatric centers provide care for children with cystic fibrosis. Specimens from these patients are periodically sent to the laboratory for surveillance of lower respiratory tract colonization by various potentially pathogenic microorganisms. Recommended specimens for culture for these types of organisms include sputum, tracheal aspirates, or throat swabs (6, 26, 55).

Genital Specimens

Genital specimens are usually collected from pediatric patients for (i) investigation of possible sexual abuse or rape or (ii) diagnosis of premenarchal vulvovaginitis and/or urethritis. Since these specimens are often irretrievable, every effort must be made to process pediatric urogenital specimens for culture. Although the cervix is the specimen source for diagnosis of gonorrhea and chlamydia in adolescent and adult females, detection of these sexually transmitted diseases (STDs) in prepubertal females requires sampling of the vaginal vault (5). A urethral swab sample is collected from prepubescent males. Culture is required for confirmation of both types of infections (5). Antigen detection assays are not acceptable due to the high reported rates of false positivity (30, 71). Likewise, the performance of molecular methods has not been adequately assessed for detection of STDs in children and is not considered admissible in the event of legal proceedings (31).

Urine Specimens

Collection of uncontaminated urine specimens from pediatric patients is a challenge. The acquisition of a clean-catch specimen from older children is hindered by the same problems experienced with adult patients. A urine specimen collected by catheterization is used for all pediatric age groups and, if performed properly, can yield a specimen free of urethral contaminants (4). Although suprapubic aspiration is considered the optimum method for collection of urine from infants, the technique is frequently unsuccessful in dehydrated patients (4). Specimens must be transported to the lab within 30 min of collection or stored under refrigeration for no longer than 24 h (47). Urine transport systems containing preservatives are available for adult patients, who characteristically excrete larger volumes of urine. For optimum performance, the urine and preservative must be present at the ratio recommended by the manufacturer. At present, no transport system is available to accommodate the lower-volume pediatric urine specimens.

Fecal Specimens

The best clinical predictors of a positive stool culture in children are a combination of persistent diarrhea of >24 h in duration, fever, and either blood in the stool or abdominal pain with nausea and vomiting (17, 42, 56, 60, 65). Many cases of diarrhea occur in children <5 years of age and are caused by pathogens that are endemic to an area, such as rotavirus, shigellae, *Giardia lamblia*, and cryptosporidia (17). Since most diarrheal disease is community acquired, a single stool specimen for culture obtained during the first 72 h after admission to the hospital can be used for diagnosis for almost 98% of children with bacterial gastroenteritis (15, 16, 54). Depending on the age of the child, nosocomially acquired diarrheal disease is most often attributed to rotavirus or *Clostridium difficile* (13, 25). Interpretation of positive *Clostridium difficile* toxin assay results for children <2 years of age may be difficult due to intestinal colonization of this age group with toxin-producing strains (19, 39, 67). A freshly obtained stool sample is preferable for all fecal assays. A rectal swab is less optimal but is acceptable for recovery of bacterial enteric pathogens, surveillance for multidrug-resistant organisms, and performance of certain antigen detection assays. A rectal swab is not recommended for some assays for detection of *Clostridium difficile* toxin. If a delay in transport is anticipated, fecal specimens for either bacterial culture or parasite detection should be placed in an appropriate transport medium or preservative, respectively. In order to maintain the recommended 3:1 ratio of stool to preservative for parasite transport vials, the volume of preservative in the vial may require adjustment prior to inoculation of a small pediatric sample.

Pinworm (*Enterobius vermicularis*) infection is a common ailment of children. After establishment of infection in the colon, the female adult pinworm periodically migrates to the perianal area and deposits her eggs on the skin. Commercial sampling paddles are available for sampling, but cellophane or cellulose tape applied to the perianal skin in the morning, before the patient washes or defecates, will enable collection of the eggs for identification.

Specimens from Neonates

The neonatal nursery and intensive care unit pose unique challenges for the microbiology laboratory. The problems inherent in the decreased sample amounts available from these tiny patients may be compounded by the unpredictable response to infection displayed by neonates (28, 48). For example, isolates retrieved from the mucous membranes, skin, ear canal, nasopharynx, gastric aspirate, or rectum usually do not match the results of blood, CSF, or tissue cultures (28, 48). Differentiation of colonization versus true infection, therefore, may be very difficult. Microorganisms are acquired either through transmission in utero, during delivery, or from nosocomial spread via hospital personnel, various medical devices, or environmental sources (33, 62). Infections reported to occur in neonates include sepsis, meningitis, otitis media, diarrhea, osteomyelitis or septic arthritis, conjunctivitis or orbital cellulitis, pneumonia, and various skin infections (7, 21, 24, 28, 48, 69, 72). Congenital infection is most often caused by agents such as *Toxoplasma gondii* or viruses such as herpes simplex virus, cytomegalovirus, varicella-zoster virus, parvovirus, enterovirus, rubella virus, or hepatitis B virus (22, 28, 38, 48, 64). The collection methods and appropriate specimen types for neonates are similar to those recommended for older infants and children with the exception of blood for culture. Depending on the age of the newborn, recommended sampling sites include the peripheral vein, umbilical artery, and capillary blood (28). Although a minimum volume of 0.5 to 1.0 ml is most often cited as the recommended amount of specimen to be collected, larger volumes are recommended for the optimal recovery of organisms (37, 57).

Viral Specimens

Since smaller specimen volumes are often received from pediatric patients, newer molecular methods may aid in the detection of pediatric systemic or central nervous system viral infections. The antigenemia assay for detection of cytomegalovirus in blood may be impeded by both the smaller specimen volumes and the smaller polymorphonuclear leukocyte concentrations in neutropenic children undergoing transplantation or therapy for oncological problems. Details regarding diagnosis of viral infections can be found in chapter 77 of this Manual.

Dermatologic Specimens

Rashes are a common manifestation of many childhood illnesses. The same techniques are used to sample skin lesions from children and adults. A small, disposable toothbrush is valuable for recovery of scrapings of certain types of dermatophytic fungal lesions and will produce fewer traumas than the use of a scalpel (3). Retrieval of skin samples for detection of scabies often yields no visible organism; however, the distribution of lesions will differ between infants and young children and their older counterparts (3).

REFERENCES

1. **Abadco, D. L., and P. Steiner.** 1992. Gastric lavage is better than bronchoalveolar lavage for isolation of *Mycobacterium tuberculosis* in childhood pulmonary tuberculosis. *Pediatr. Infect. Dis. J.* **11:**735–738.
2. **Alpert, B. E., B. P. O'Sullivan, and H. B. Panitch.** 1992. Nonbronchoscopic approach to bronchoalveolar lavage in children with artificial airways. *Pediatr. Pulmonol.* **13:**38–41.
3. **American Academy of Pediatrics.** 2000. *Red Book.* American Academy of Pediatrics, Elk Grove Village, Ill.
4. **American Academy of Pediatrics.** 1999. Practice parameter: the diagnosis, treatment, and evaluation of the initial urinary tract infection in febrile infants and young children. *Pediatrics* **103:**843–852.
5. **American Academy of Pediatrics.** 1999. Guidelines for the evaluation of sexual abuse of children: subject review. *Pediatrics* **103:**186–191.
6. **Armstrong, D. S., K. Grimwood, J. B. Carlin, R. Carzino, A. Olinsky, and P. D. Phelan.** 1996. Bronchoalveolar lavage or oropharyngeal cultures to identify lower respiratory pathogens in infants with cystic fibrosis. *Pediatr. Pulmonol.* **21:**267–275.
7. **Bale, J. F., and J. R. Murphy.** 1997. Infections of the central nervous system in the newborn. *Clin. Perinatol.* **24:**787–806.
8. **Baron, E. J.** 1994. *Bailey and Scott's Diagnostic Microbiology*, 9th ed. The C.V. Mosby Co., St. Louis, Mo.
9. **Bartlett, R. C.** 1985. Quality control, p. 14–23. *In* E. H. Lennette, A. Balows, W. J. Hausler, Jr., and H. J. Shadomy (ed.), *Manual of Clinical Microbiology*, 4th ed. American Society for Microbiology, Washington, D.C.
10. **Bisno, A.** 2001. Primary care: acute pharyngitis. *N. Engl. J. Med.* **344:**205–211.
11. **Bluestone, C. D., and J. O. Klein (ed.).** 1995. *Otitis Media in Infants and Children*, 2nd ed. The W. B. Saunders Co., Philadelphia, Pa.
12. **Bordes, A., R. Elcuaz, F. J. Noguera, C. Otemin, and G. Egas.** 1997. *Proprionibacterium acnes* infections in patients with CSF shunts. *Enterm. Infecc. Microbiol. Clin.* **15:**24–27.
13. **Brady, M. T., D. L. Pacini, C. T. Budde, and M. J. Connell.** 1989. Diagnostic studies of nosocomial diarrhea in children: assessing their use and value. *Am. J. Infect. Control* **17:**77082.
14. **Carroll, K., and L. Reimer.** 1996. Microbiology and laboratory diagnosis of upper respiratory tract infections. *Clin. Infect. Dis.* **23:**442–448.
15. **Chitkara, Y. K., K. A. McCasland, and L. Kenefic.** 1996. Development and implementation of cost-effective guidelines in the laboratory investigation of diarrhea in a community hospital. *Arch. Intern. Med.* **156:**1445–1448.
16. **Church, D. L., G. Cadrain, A. Kabani, T. Jadavji, and C. Trevenen.** 1994. Practice guidelines for ordering stool cultures in a pediatric population. *Am. J. Clin. Pathol.* **103:**149–153.
17. **Cohen, M. B.** 1991. Etiology and mechanisms of acute infectious diarrhea in infants in the United States. *J. Pediatr.* **118:**S34–S39.
18. **Cook, J. H., and M. Pezzlo.** 1992. Specimen receipt and accessioning. Section 1. Aerobic bacteriology, p. 1.2.1–1.2.4. *In* H. D. Isenberg (ed. in chief), *Clinical Microbiology*

Procedures Handbook. American Society for Microbiology, Washington, D.C.

19. **Craven, D., D. Brick, A. Morrisey, M. A. O'Riordan, V. Petran, and J. R. Schreiber.** 1998. Low yield of bacterial stool culture in children with nosocomial diarrhea. *Pediatr. Infect. Dis. J.* **17:**1040–1044.
20. **Cronan, K. M., and J. F. Wiley.** 1997. Lumbar puncture, p. 541–553. *In* F. M. Henretig and C. King (ed.), *Textbook of Pediatric Emergency Procedures.* The Williams & Wilkins Co., Baltimore, Md.
21. **Dennehy, P. H.** 1987. Respiratory infections in the newborn. *Clin. Perinatol.* **14:**667–682.
22. **Donley, D. K.** 1993. TORCH infections in the newborn. *Semin. Neurol.* **13:**106–115.
23. **Duhaime, A. C., and J. F. Wiley.** 1997. Ventricular shunt and burr hole puncture, p. 553–558. *In* F. M. Henretig and C. King (ed.), *Textbook of Pediatric Emergency Procedures.* The Williams & Wilkins Co., Baltimore, Md.
24. **Eichenwald, E. C.** 1997. Perinatally transmitted neonatal bacterial infections. *Infect. Dis. Clin. N. Am.* **11:**223–239.
25. **Ford-Jones, E. L., C. M. Mindorff, R. Gold, and M. Petric.** 1990. The incidence of viral-associated diarrhea after admission to a pediatric hospital. *Am. J. Epidemiol.* **131:**711–718.
26. **Gilligan, P. H.** 1991. Microbiology of airway disease in patients with cystic fibrosis. *Clin. Microbiol Rev.* **4:**35–51.
27. **Golden, S. E., Z. M. Shehab, J. C. Bjelland, J. R. Kenneth, and C. G. Ray.** 1987. Microbiology of endotracheal aspirates in intubated pediatric intensive care unit patients: correlations with radiographic findings. *Pediatr. Infect. Dis. J.* **6:**665–669.
28. **Gotoff, S. P.** 2000. Infections of the neonatal infant, p. 538–551. *In* R. E. Behrman, R. M. Kleigman, and H. B. Jensen (ed.), *Nelson's Textbook of Pediatrics,* 16th ed. The W. B. Saunders Co., Philadelphia, Pa.
29. **Hagen, J. C., W. S. Wood, and T. Hashimoto.** 1977. Effect of temperature on survival of *Bacteroides fragilis* subsp. *fragilis* and *Escherichia coli* in pus. *J. Clin. Microbiol.* **6:**567–570.
30. **Hammerschlag, M. R.** 1998. Sexually transmitted diseases in sexually abused children: medical and legal implications. *Sex. Transm. Infect.* **74:**167–174.
31. **Hammerschlag, M. R., S. Ajl, and D. Laraque.** 1999. Inappropriate use of nonchlamydia tests for the detection of chlamydia in suspected victims of child sexual abuse: a continuing problem. *Pediatrics* **104:**1137–1139.
32. **Holden, J.** 1992. Collection and transport of clinical specimens for anaerobic culture, 2.2.1–2.2.6. *In* H. D. Isenberg (ed. in chief), *Clinical Microbiology Procedures Handbook.* American Society for Microbiology, Washington, D.C.
33. **Hoogkamp-Korstanje, J. A., B. Cats, R. C. Senders, and I. van Ertgruggen.** 1982. Analysis of bacterial infections in a neonatal intensive care unit. *J. Hosp. Infect.* **393:**275–284.
34. **Isenberg, H. D. (ed. in chief).** 1994. *Clinical Microbiology Procedures Handbook,* vol. 1 and 2. American Society for Microbiology, Washington, D.C.
35. **Johnson, F. B.** 1990. Transport of viral specimens. *Clin. Microbiol. Rev.* **3:**120–131.
36. **Keller, C.** 1994. Methods of drawing blood samples through central venous catheters in pediatric patients undergoing bone marrow transplant: results of a national survey. *Oncol. Nurs. Forum* **21:**879–884.
37. **Kellogg, J. A., F. L. Ferrentino, M. H. Goodstein, S. L. Shapiro, and D. A. Bankert.** 1997. Frequency of low level bacteremia in infants from birth to two months of age. *Pediatr. Infect. Dis. J.* **16:**381–385.
38. **Kinney, J. S., and M. L. Kumar.** 1988. Should we expand the TORCH Complex? A description of clinical and di-

agnostic aspects of selected old and new agents. *Clin. Perinatol.* **15:**727–744.
39. **Knoop, F. C., M. Owens, and I. C. Crocker.** 1993. *Clostridium difficile:* clinical disease and diagnosis. *Clin. Microbiol. Rev.* **6:**251–265.
40. **Koumbourlis, A. C., and G. Kurland.** 1993. Nonbronchoscopic bronchoalveolar lavage in mechanically ventilated infants: technique, efficacy, and applications. *Pediatr. Pulmonol.* **15:**257–262.
41. **Labeene, M., C. Poyart, C. Ranbaud, B. Goldfarb, B. Pron, P. Jouvet, C. Delamare, G. Sebag, and P. Hubert.** 1999. Blind protected specimen brush and bronchoalveolar lavage in ventilated children. *Crit. Care Med.* **27:**2537–2543.
42. **Laney, E. W., and M. B. Cohen.** 1993. Approach to the pediatric patient with diarrhea. *Gastroenterol. Clin. N. Am.* **22:**499–516.
43. **Linder, J., and S. I. Rennard.** 1988. Development and application of bronchoalveolar lavage, p. 1–16. *In Bronchoalveolar Lavage.* ASCP Press, Chicago, Ill.
44. **Marcon, J. J., A. C. Hamoudi, H. J. Cannon, and M. M. Hribar.** 1987. Comparison of throat and nasopharyngeal swab specimens for culture diagnosis of *Bordetella pertussis* infections. *J. Clin. Microbiol.* **25:**1109–1110.
45. **Masters, H. B., K. O. Weber, J. R. Groothuis, C. G. Wren, and B. A. Lauer.** 1987. Comparisons of nasopharyngeal washings and swab specimens for diagnosis of respiratory syncytial virus by EIA, FAT, and cell culture. *Diagn. Microbiol. Infect. Dis.* **8:**101–105.
46. **McBride, T. P., H. W. Davis, and J. S. Reilly.** 1997. Otolaryngology. *In* B. J. Zitelli and H. W. Davis (ed.), *Atlas of Pediatric Physical Diagnosis.* Mosby-Wolfe, St. Louis, Mo.
47. **Miller, J. M. (ed.).** 1999. *A Guide to Specimen Management in Clinical Microbiology,* 2nd ed. ASM Press, Washington, D.C.
48. **Mustafa, M. M., and G. H. McCracken.** 1992. Perinatal infections. *In* R. D. Feigin and J. D. Cherry (ed.), *Textbook of Pediatric Infectious Diseases,* 3rd ed. The W. B. Saunders Co., Philadelphia, Pa.
49. **National Committee for Clinical Laboratory Standards.** 1989. *Guidelines for Laboratory Safety,* p. 11–16. CAP Environment, Safety, and Health Committee, National Committee for Clinical Laboratory Standards, Villanova, Pa.
50. **National Committee for Clinical Laboratory Standards.** 1991. Tentative standard M29-T2. *Protection of Laboratory Workers from Infectious Disease Transmitted by Blood, Body Fluid, and Tissue,* vol. 11, no. 14, p. 28–29. National Committee for Clinical Laboratory Standards, Villanova, Pa.
51. **National Research Council.** 1989. *Biosafety in the Laboratory: Prudent Practices for the Handling and Disposal of Infectious Materials.* National Academy Press, Washington, D.C.
52. **Pichichero, M. E.** 2000. Acute otitis media. Part I. Improving diagnostic accuracy. *Am. Family Physician* **61:**2051–2056.
53. **Renier, D., J. Lacombe, A. Pierre-Kahn, C. Sainte-Rose, and J. F. Hirsch.** 1984. Factors causing acute shunt infection: computer analysis of 1174 operations. *J. Neurosurg.* **61:**1072–1078.
54. **Rohner, P., D. Pittet, B. Pepey, T. Nije-Kinge, and R. Auckenthaler.** 1997. Etiological agents of infectious diarrhea: implications for requests for microbial culture. *J. Clin. Microbiol.* **35:**1427–1432.
55. **Rosenfeld, M., J. Emerson, F. Accurso, D. Armstrong, R. Castile, K. Grimwood, P. Hiatt, K. McCoy, S. McNamara, B. Ramsey, and J. Wagener.** 1999. Diagnostic

accuracy of oropharyngeal cultures in infants and young children with cystic fibrosis. *Pediatr. Pulmonol.* **28:**321–328.

56. **Rudolph, J. A., and M. B. Cohen.** 1999. New causes and treatments for infectious diarrhea in children. *Curr. Gastroenterol. Rep.* **1:**238–244.
57. **Schelonka, R. L., M. K. Chai, B. A. Yoder, D. Hensley, R. M. Brockett, and D. P Ascher.** 1996. Volume of blood required to detect common neonatal pathogens. *J. Pediatr.* **129:**275–279.
58. **Schulman, R. J., S. Phillips, L. Laine, P. Gardner, V. Nichols, T. Reed, and E. Hawkins.** 1993. Volume of blood required to obtain central venous catheter blood cultures in infants and children. *J. Parenteral Enteral Nutr.* **17:**177–179.
59. **Shea, Y. R.** 1992. Specimen collection and transport. Section 1. Aerobic bacteriology, p. 1.1.1–1.1.30. *In* H. D. Isenberg (ed. in chief), *Clinical Microbiology Procedures Handbook.* American Society for Microbiology, Washington, D.C.
60. **Sherman, P. M., M. Petric, and M. B. Cohen.** 1996. Infectious gastroenterocolitides in children: an update on emerging pathogens. *Pediatr. Clin. N. Am.* **43:**391–407.
61. **Slagle, T. A., E. M. Bifano, J. W. Wolf, and S. J. Gross.** 1989. Routine endotracheal cultures for the prediction of sepsis in ventilated babies. *Arch. Dis. Child.* **64:**34–38.
62. **Smith, D. H.** 1979. Epidemics of infectious diseases in newborn nurseries. *Clin. Obstet. Gynecol.* **22:**409–423.
63. **Somu, N., S. Swaminathan, C. N. Paramasivan, D. Vijayasekaran, A. Chandrabhooshanam, V. K. Vijayan, and R. Prabhakar.** 1995. Value of bronchoalveolar lavage and gastric lavage in the diagnosis of pulmonary tuberculosis in children. *Tuber. Lung Dis.* **76:**295–299.
64. **Strodtbeck, R.** 1995. Viral infections of the newborn. *J. Obstet. Gynecol. Neonatal Nurs.* **24:**659–667.
65. **Stutman, H. R.** 1994. Salmonella, Shigella, and Campylobacter: common bacterial causes of infectious diarrhea. *Pediatr. Ann.* **23:**538–543.
66. **Thompson, T. P., and A. L. Albright.** 1998. *Propionibacterium acnes* infections of cerebrospinal fluid shunts. *Childs Nervous System* **14:**378–380.
67. **Tullus, K., B. Aronsson, S. Marcus, and R. Mollby.** 1989. Intestinal colonization with *Clostridium difficile* in infants up to 18 months of age. *Eur. J. Clin. Microbiol. Infect. Dis.* **8:**390–393.
68. **U.S. Department of Health and Human Services.** 1999. *Biosafety in Microbiological and Biomedical Laboratories,* 4th ed. HHS publication no. (CDC) 93-8395. U.S. Department of Health and Human Services, Washington, D.C.
69. **Verbov, J.** 2000. Common skin conditions in the newborn. *Semin. Neonatol.* **5:**303–310.
70. **Wald, E. R.** 1995. Chronic sinusitis in children. *J. Pediatr.* **127:**339–347.
71. **Whittington, W. L., R. J. Rice, J. W. Biddle, and J. S. Knapp.** 1988. Incorrect identification of *Neisseria gonorrhoeae* from infants and children. *Pediatr. Infect. Dis. J.* **7:**3–10.
72. **Wright, P. F.** 1998. Infectious diseases in early life in industrialized countries. *Vaccine* **16:**1355–1359.
73. **Yagoda, M. R., J. Stavola, R. Ward, C. Steinberg, and J. Jones.** 1996. Role of bronchoalveolar lavage in hospitalized pediatric patients. *Ann. Otol. Rhinol. Laryngol.* **105:**863–867.
74. **Zaidi, A. K. M., and L. B. Reller.** 1996. Rejection criteria for endotracheal aspirates from pediatric patients. *J. Clin. Microbiol.* **34:**352–354.

Procedures for the Storage of Microorganisms

LARRY G. REIMER AND KAREN C. CARROLL

7

The maintenance of microorganisms over long periods for future study has long been part of microbiology. Organisms need to be preserved to allow future study for research, clinical, epidemiological, educational, microbiological, and commercial reasons. Individual strains of organisms that have been preserved provide the characteristics that are a permanent record of that organism. Such organisms may narrowly catalog a unique infectious agent in an individual or broadly define the phenotypic and genetic characteristics of a species.

Effective storage means that the organism is being maintained in a viable state free of contamination and without changes in genotypic or phenotypic characteristics. The organism must be easily restored to the same condition it was in prior to preservation.

There are multiple methods for microbial preservation. These have generally been studied by looking at only a single species or small group of microorganisms. Review articles, monographs, and books have been published that provide detailed information about organism storage (1, 10, 13, 14, 22). For clinical microbiology laboratories, simple and broadly applied methods are necessary to maintain organisms for short- and long-term recovery. This chapter presents methods that can be used for storage of bacteria, protozoa, fungi, and viruses.

SHORT-TERM PRESERVATION METHODS

Direct Transfer to Subculture

The simplest method for maintaining short-term viability of organisms, most often used for bacteria, is periodic subculture to fresh medium. Each transfer to a new subculture increases the likelihood of mutation, with undesirable changes in organism characteristics. The space required for organisms kept in this manner can also become an issue depending on the number of specimens and the duration for which they are saved.

The interval between transfers varies among organisms. Additionally, the rate of mutation is quite variable. Some organisms appear stable indefinitely with repeated transfer, while others may change phenotypic traits after as few as two or three passages. The actual rate of mutation, however, has not been studied using sequencing technology.

Issues that must be addressed with direct transfer include the medium to be used, the storage conditions, and the frequency of transfer.

Maintenance Medium

The medium used should support survival of the organism but minimize metabolic processes and slow the rate of growth. The organism should not be placed in too harsh an environment since this may force it to mutate to become more compatible with its surroundings. A medium with too high a nutrient content will induce rapid replication that requires more frequent transfers. Only limited research has been done on ideal maintenance media, and studies that have been published suggest considerable variation from one species to another. Media that have been used include distilled water, tryptic soy broth, and nutrient broths (Becton Dickinson & Co.; Oxoid Ltd.), all of which may be used with or without cryopreservatives.

Storage Conditions

Many laboratories store organisms, most often bacteria, for short periods on routine agar media at the workbench. Cultures kept in this fashion are subject to drying. A better method is to transfer organisms into screw-top test tubes and to store them in an organized location away from light and significant temperature changes. To prevent drying, caps can include rubber liners or film can be wrapped over the top of the tube before or after the cap is screwed on. Storage at lower temperatures (5 to 8°C) slows metabolic processes and maintains viability for longer periods.

Frequency of Transfer

There is no set protocol for the frequency of transfer since the storage conditions, media used, and organisms being kept vary from one laboratory to another. Each laboratory should conduct studies for each organism category to determine acceptable intervals between transfers under the conditions used for storage. Such studies involve performing subcultures at scheduled times until an acceptable interval with complete recovery of the organism is identified.

When transfers are performed, 5 to 10 representative colonies should be used to avoid the possibility of introducing an altered genotypic or phenotypic characteristic.

Quality Control Procedures

Although it is not necessary with each transfer, periodic assessment should be made of the status of specimens. Ongoing viability, stability of phenotype, organism identity, and the rate of contamination of specimens should be determined and noted in a log.

Immersion in Oil

An alternative to simply capping tubes is to add a layer of mineral oil to the top of the specimen. Many bacteria and fungi can be stored for up to 2 to 3 years by this method, and transfers are not needed as frequently. Organisms are still metabolically active in this environment, and mutations can still occur. Contamination of the specimen can occur if the mineral oil is not adequately sterilized.

Mineral oil should be medicinal-grade oil with specific gravity 0.865 to 0.890 (Roxane Laboratories; Becton Dickinson and Co.). For sterilization, it should be heated to 170°C for 1 to 2 h in an oven (10). Autoclaving is not considered acceptable.

To prepare the specimen, an inoculum of 5 to 10 colonies of the organism should be placed on an agar slant or in tubed broth media. Once growth is identified, a layer of mineral oil at least 1 to 2 cm deep is added, and the agar must not be exposed to air. Tests for viability are performed as with simple transfers to establish a transfer schedule. Whereas these transfers are less frequent than when organisms are stored without oil, oil is more difficult to add to vials and to clean up in the event of spills.

Freezing at −20°C

Refrigeration or freezing in ordinary freezers at −20°C is sometimes used to preserve organisms for longer than can be accomplished by repeated transfers. Whereas viability may be maintained for as long as 1 to 2 years for a few organisms, most have poorer survival than at higher or lower temperatures because of damage caused by ice crystal formation (14) and electrolyte fluctuations (10) at this temperature. The media used for storage appear important, since preservation times vary from a few months to 2 years depending on which medium is used (12, 14, 15). Modern self-defrosting freezers with freeze-thaw cycles cannot be used because the repeated temperature fluctuation will destroy the organism.

Drying

Whereas most organisms do not survive drying, some, especially bacteria that form spores and many molds, can be dried and stored for prolonged periods. Soil can be used as a storage medium if it is autoclaved and air dried. Soil should be autoclaved for several hours on two successive days. It is then transferred into sterile glass tubes. A 1-ml suspension of the organism is inoculated into the tube, and the tube is left open to air dry before closing with a sterile stopper. The sample is stored in a refrigerator (10). While potentially effective, soil is not a standardized, defined, and consistent product for use over long periods. Instead, commercial silica gel can be used in small cotton-plugged tubes after heating in an oven to 175°C for 1.5 to 2 h (14), with moderately successful recovery of fungi. Alternatively, a suspension of 10^8 organisms can be inoculated onto sterile filter paper strips or disks. The paper is dried in air or under vacuum and is placed in sterile vials. These vials can be stored in the refrigerator for up to 4 years, and then single strips or disks can be removed as needed (10). This method is commonly used for quality control organisms.

Distilled Water

Most organisms do poorly in distilled water, but some survive for prolonged periods. Many fungi and *Pseudomonas* spp. survive for several years in distilled water at room temperature (14, 18). McGinnis found that, with the exception of fungi that do not easily sporulate, 93% of yeasts, fungi, and aerobic actinomycetes can be easily and inexpensively preserved in this way (18).

LONG-TERM PRESERVATION METHODS

Whereas the methods described above may be used to store organisms for periods up to a few years, ultra-low-temperature freezing and freeze-drying (lyophilization) are the methods now recommended for long-term storage. There are several steps involved in these processes.

Ultra-Low-Temperature Freezing

Microorganisms can be maintained at temperatures of −70°C or lower for prolonged periods. Systems for achieving these temperatures include ultra-low-temperature electric freezers and liquid nitrogen storage units. With either system, unwanted heating can occur due to loss of electrical power or liquid nitrogen. Close observation of the system and an adequate alarm mechanism are essential since any increase in temperature will reduce viability. In the event that the temperature does rise, restoring power and returning to the target storage temperature as quickly as possible seem appropriate, although Pell and Sneath found that the presence of glycerol as a cryopreservant was associated with organism survival for up to several weeks (19). If thawing does occur, there are no guidelines for rapid restoration of the storage condition. Refreezing the sealed vials as described below would seem most appropriate. There are several important components in the process of ultra-low-temperature freezing, and these are described below.

Storage Vials

Storage vials must be able to withstand very low temperatures and maintain a seal for their contents. Plastic (polypropylene) or glass (borosilicate) tubes may be used. Plastic vials with screw tops and silicone washers are much easier to use than glass vials that must be sealed with a flame and then scored and broken to open. Several commercial suppliers stock acceptable vials (Fisher Scientific Products; VWR Scientific; Wheaton Science Products; Becton Dickinson & Co.). Vials come in a variety of sizes. Half-dram vials are available from several suppliers and can be conveniently packaged in a 12-by-12 grid so that 144 vials are stored in one box or layer.

Cryoprotective Agents

To protect microorganisms from damage during the freezing process, during storage, and during thawing, cryoprotective agents are often added to the culture suspension. Whereas most bacteria, fungi, and viruses survive better with such additives, studies have shown that cryoprotective agents significantly damage others. The reader is referred to detailed references for specifics (Table 1) (1, 14). Rapid freezing without additives may still be acceptable for long-term survival of protozoa, although freeze-drying more appropriately preserves some of these.

TABLE 1 Common procedures for preservation of microorganisms

Organism group	Storage methods	Cryopreservative	Storage temp (°C)	Storage duration (yr)
Gram-positive bacteria	Transfer	None	Room temp	0.2–0.3
	Mineral oil	None	4	0.6–2
	Freezing	Sucrose, glycerol	−20	1–3
	Ultra-low-temp freezing	Skim milk, sucrose, glycerol	−70 to −196	1–30
	Lyophilization	Skim milk, sucrose	4	30
Streptococci	Freezing	Skim milk	−20	0.2
	Ultra-low-temp freezing	Skim milk	−70 to −196	0.2–1
	Lyophilization	Skim milk	4	0.5–30
Mycobacteria	Freezing	Skim milk	−20	3–5
	Ultra-low-temp freezing	Skim milk	−70 to −196	3–5
	Lyophilization	Skim milk	4	16–30
Gram-negative bacteria	Transfer	None	Room temp	0.1–0.3
	Mineral oil	None	4	1–2
	Freezing	Sucrose, lactose	−20	1–2
	Ultra-low-temp freezing	Sucrose, lactose, glycerol	−70 to −196	2–30
	Lyophilization	Skim milk + sucrose + lactose	4	30
Spore-forming bacteria	Transfer	None	Room temp	0.2–1
	Mineral oil	None	4	1
	Drying	None	Room temp	1–2
	Freezing	Glucose	−20	1–2
	Ultra-low-temp freezing	Skim milk, glucose	−70 to −196	2–30
	Lyophilization	Skim milk + lactose	4	30
Filamentous fungi	Transfer	None	4 to 25	2–10
	Mineral oil	None	Room temp	1–40
	Distilled water	None	Room temp	1–10
	Drying	Soil, silica gel	Room temp	1–4
	Ultra-low-temp freezing	Glycerol, DMSO	−70 to −196	2–30
	Lyophilization (spore formers)	Glycerol, sucrose, DMSO, skim milk	4	2–30
Yeasts	Distilled water	None	Room temp	1–2
	Drying	Nutrient medium	Room temp	1–2
Protozoa	Freezing	Blood, nutrient broth + DMSO + sucrose	−20 to −40	
	Ultra-low-temp freezing	DMSO or glycerol or blood + nutrient media	−70 to −196	
Viruses	Transfer	Nutrient medium	4	0.5
	Ultra-low-temp freezing	SPGA	−70 to −196	1–30
	Lyophilization	SPGA	4	6–10

There are two types of cryoprotective agents: ones that enter the cell and protect the intracellular environment and others that protect the external milieu of the organism. Glycerol and dimethyl sulfoxide (DMSO) are most often used for the former; sucrose, lactose, glucose, mannitol, sorbitol, dextran, polyvinylpyrrolidone, and polyglycol are used for the latter. Combinations of agents are sometimes used. Other products that have also been studied as cryoprotectants include detergents like Tween 80 and Triton WR 1339, other carbohydrates such as honey, and calcium lactobionate. Cryoprotectants that enter the cell usually provide better protection for bacteria, although individual agents affect unique species differently. Of the internally

incorporated agents, glycerol usually provides better organism survival than DMSO.

Glycerol is added at a concentration of 10% (vol/vol), and DMSO is added at 5% (vol/vol). Prior to use, glycerol is sterilized by autoclaving. Once prepared, it can be stocked at room temperature for months. DMSO must be filter sterilized and can be stored in open containers for only 1 month prior to use.

Of the external products, skim milk is most often used. Dehydrated skim milk is purchased from medical product suppliers (Becton Dickinson and Co.; Oxoid). It is autoclaved and used at a final concentration of 20% (wt/vol) in distilled water (1). This is double the concentration suggested by the manufacturers if the intent is to make a reconstituted equivalent of regular milk.

Preparation of Organisms for Freezing

Organisms are inoculated in a medium that adequately supports maximal growth. Cultures are allowed to mature to late growth or stationary phase before being harvested. Once at this point, broth specimens are centrifuged to create a pellet of organisms. The pellet is withdrawn and resuspended in 2 to 5 ml of broth with the appropriate concentration of cryoprotectant added. For agar specimens, broth containing the cryoprotectant is placed on the surface of the agar. The surface is scraped with a pipette or sterile loop to suspend organisms, and then the broth mixture is pipetted directly into freezer vials. Alternatively, the agar surface can be scraped with a sterile loop. The organisms can then be transferred directly into the vial of cryoprotectant and emulsified into a final dense suspension. The volume of the aliquots to be frozen is typically 0.2 to 0.5 ml.

Freezing Method

The American Type Culture Collection (ATCC) recommends slow, controlled-rate freezing at a rate of 1°C per min until the vials cool to a temperature of at least −30°C, followed by more rapid cooling until the final storage temperature is achieved (1). Controlled-rate freezers are required for the initial phase of cooling. Studies in the 1970s showed that uncontrolled-rate freezing may be just as acceptable for most organisms and is much less expensive and labor-intensive (14). When organisms are to be stored in liquid nitrogen, however, it is still recommended that vials be placed initially in a −60°C freezer for 1 h and then transferred to the liquid nitrogen. When organisms are to be stored permanently at −60 to −70°C, the vials can be placed directly into this freezer.

Small glass beads or plastic beads (Fisher Scientific Products; Wheaton Science Products) can also be added to storage vials before freezing. The culture suspension will coat the beads, and then individual beads can be removed from storage for reconstitution, avoiding the need to thaw the entire sample (8).

Thawing

Damage to microorganisms occurs as they are warmed from the frozen state. The critical temperatures appear to be between −40 and −5°C. Studies suggest that rapid warming through these temperatures improves recovery rates. Hence, recommendations are to rapidly warm stored culture vials by placing them in a 35°C water bath until all ice has disappeared (1, 14). Once a vial is thawed, it should be opened and the organism should be transferred to an appropriate growth medium immediately. Great care must be exercised during the thawing phase since rapid temperature changes and resulting air pressure changes inside vials can cause the vials to explode. Protective clothing and eyewear must be worn during this process.

Freeze-Drying (Lyophilization)

Freeze-drying is considered the most effective way to achieve long-term storage of most bacteria. Better preservation occurs because intracellular ice crystallization contributes greatly to organism loss in the frozen state. Removal of water from the specimen effectively prevents this damage. On the other hand, the process of drying causes extensive damage to molds, protozoa, and most viruses. Hence, these organisms cannot be stored in this way.

Among bacteria, the relative viability with lyophilization decreases from sporeformers to gram-positive bacteria to gram-negative bacteria (14), but overall viability can be maintained for as long as 30 years for bacteria. In addition, dried organisms take up little space, large numbers of vials of organisms can be stored, and organisms preserved in this way can be easily transported long distances at room temperature.

The process combines freezing and dehydration. Organisms are initially frozen and then dried by lowering the atmospheric pressure with a vacuum apparatus. Freeze-drying has been extensively reviewed in the past (13).

Equipment

Equipment includes a vacuum pump connected in-line to a condenser and to the specimens. Specimens can be connected individually to the condenser (manifold method) or can be placed in a chamber where they are dehydrated in one larger air space (chamber or batch method). Alexander et al. (ATCC) and Heckly both have detailed descriptions of equipment options (1, 13).

Storage Vials

Glass vials are used for all freeze-dried specimens. When freeze-drying is performed in a chamber, double glass vials are used. An outer soft glass vial is added for protection, cushioning, and preservation of the dehydrated specimen. Silica gel granules are placed in the bottom of the outer vial before the inner vial is inserted and cushioned with cotton. With the manifold method, a single glass vial is used. For either, the vial containing the actual specimen is lightly plugged with absorbent cotton. The storage vial in the manifold method or the outer vial in the chamber method must be sealed to maintain the vacuum and the dry atmospheric condition. All vials are sterilized prior to use by heating in a hot air oven.

Cryoprotective Agents

Research concerning cryoprotective agents has been extensively reviewed (13). In general, the two most commonly used agents are skim milk and sucrose. Skim milk is used most often for chamber lyophilization and sucrose is used most often for manifold lyophilization. Skim milk is prepared by making a 20% (vol/vol) solution of skim milk in distilled water. It is divided into 5-ml aliquots and autoclaved at 116°C with care taken to prevent overheating and caramelizaton of the solution. The preparation is then used in smaller volumes as described above for freezing. Sucrose is made in an initial mixture of 24% (vol/vol) sucrose in water and added in equal volumes to the organism suspension in growth medium to make a final concentration of 12% (vol/vol).

Preparation of Organisms for Freezing

As with simple freezing, maximum recovery of organisms is achieved by using organisms in the late growth or stationary phase from growth of an inoculum in an appropriate growth medium. High concentrations of organisms are considered important. ATCC recommended a concentration of at least 10^8 CFU/ml (1), while Heckly suggested a concentration of 10^{10} CFU/ml or higher (14).

Freeze-Drying Methods

In the chamber method, inner vials with the organism suspension are placed in a single layer inside a stainless steel container. This container is placed in a low-temperature freezer at −60°C for 1 h. It is then transferred to a chamber containing dry ice and ethyl Cellosolve (Becton Dickinson and Co.) and covered with a sealable vacuum top, which is connected in sequence to a condenser reservoir also filled with dry ice and ethyl Cellosolve and to a vacuum pump. The vacuum is maintained at a minimum of 30 μm of mercury for 18 h. At the same time, the outer vials are prepared by being heated in an oven overnight, filled with silica gel granules and cotton, and placed in a dry cabinet with <10% relative humidity. The freeze-dried inner vials are inserted into the outer vials, and the outer vials are heat sealed. Multiple different strains or species should probably not be processed in the same batch. Cross-contamination rates vary from 0.8 to 3.3% when two different organisms are placed on opposite sides of the same container and are as high as 8.3 to 13.3% when they are intermingled (3).

In the manifold method, a rack of individual vials is used rather than a single container. The rack is placed in a dry ice-ethyl Cellosolve bath. After the freezing process, the vials are connected by individual rubber tubes in sequence to the condenser container filled with dry ice and ethyl Cellosolve and to the vacuum pump. As above, the vacuum is maintained at 30 μm of mercury for 18 h and then the individual vials are sealed.

Storage
Individual vials need to be appropriately labeled and sorted. Storage at room temperature does not maintain viability and is not recommended. Whereas storage at 4°C in an ordinary refrigerator is acceptable, survival may be improved at temperatures of −30 to −60°C (1, 13).

Reconstitution
Care must be taken when opening vials for reconstitution because of the vacuum inside the vial. Safety glasses should always be worn, and vials should be covered with gauze to avoid injury if the vial explodes when air rushes in. Reconstitution should also be conducted in a closed hood to avoid dispersal of organisms. The surface of the vial should be wiped with 70% alcohol, and then the top of the glass vial can be scored and broken off or punctured with a hot needle. A small amount (0.1 to 0.4 ml) of growth medium is injected into the vial with a needle and syringe or Pasteur pipette, the contents are stirred until the specimen is dissolved, and then the entire contents are transferred with the same syringe or pipette to appropriate broth or agar media. A purity check must be done on each specimen because of the possibility of either cross-contamination or mutation during the preservation process.

Procedures for Specific Organisms
Procedures for specific organisms are described below and summarized in Table 1.

Bacteria
All of the material presented in this chapter applies primarily to the preservation of bacteria. Simple transfer, storage under mineral oil, drying, or freezing at −20°C can maintain bacteria for short periods; freezing in ultra-low-temperature electric freezers at −70°C or in liquid nitrogen at −196°C or freeze-drying can provide long-term preservation. A summary of the studies of bacterial preservation has been published (14). In general, serial transfer will preserve bacteria for up to a few months, storage under mineral oil or with drying will last 1 to 2 years, freezing at −20°C will last 1 to 3 years, freezing at −70°C will last 1

to 10 years, and freezing in liquid nitrogen and freeze-drying will last up to 30 years (10).

Protozoa
Information concerning the preservation of protozoa is limited, in keeping with the infrequent need for doing so in clinical microbiology laboratories. Variable methods for individual genera are described. In general, freezing appears to be more appropriate than freeze-drying. All of the following procedures are as described by the ATCC (1).

Acanthamoeba, Leishmania, Naegleria, Trichomonas, and *Trypansoma* can be handled as described above for ultra-low-temperature freezing with 5% (vol/vol) DMSO as the cryoprotecting agent. These organisms should be stored in liquid nitrogen. *Acanthamoeba* and *Naegleria* can also be dried at room temperature onto filter paper. Aliquots of an organism suspension (0.3 ml) are pipetted onto the paper in a shell vial and dried in air for 14 days at room temperature and then in a vacuum desiccator for an additional 1 week. The vials are sealed and stored in liquid nitrogen.

Entamoeba is stored frozen at −40°C. Specimens should be suspended in a mixture of growth medium containing 12% (vol/vol) DMSO and 6% (vol/vol) sucrose.

Leishmania may also be prepared by inoculation of the organism into an animal host. At the peak of infection, the spleen is harvested and homogenized in half the final volume of ATCC medium 811 salt solution. Freezing is completed with 10% glycerol as the cryoprotectant.

Plasmodium spp. can be stored from infected blood samples. At the height of parasitemia, blood is obtained and anticoagulated with the following preparation: 1.33 g of sodium citrate, 0.47 g of citric acid, 3.00 g of dextrose, 200.00 mg of heparin (sodium), and 100 ml of distilled water. The final concentration of anticoagulant added to blood is 10%. To this anticoagulated blood, 30% glycerol in 0.0667 M phosphate buffer is added to a final concentration of 10% (vol/vol) glycerol. Freezing should be carried out in liquid nitrogen.

Trypanosoma spp. must be harvested from an animal host. At the peak of parasitemia, blood is withdrawn into heparinized tubes and diluted 1:1 in Tyrode's solution (8.0 g of NaCl per liter, 0.02 g of KCl per liter, 0.2 g of $CaCl_2$ per liter, 0.1 g of $MgCl_2$ per liter, 0.05 g of NaH_2PO_4 per liter, 1.0 g of $NaHCO_3$ per liter, 1.0 g of glucose per liter) with 1 to 5% phenol red added. Then 5% DMSO is added as the cryoprotectant, and the specimen is stored in liquid nitrogen.

Yeasts and Filamentous Fungi
All of the techniques described above have been applied to the storage of yeasts and fungi (5, 10, 14, 22). The individual method used depends on the species to be preserved and whether or not it sporulates.

Subculturing
Subculturing is the simplest method of maintaining living fungi and involves serial transfer to fresh solid or liquid media. Specimens are stored usually at room or refrigerator temperatures. Fungi may be maintained in this way for a number of years. Care must be taken to avoid aerosolization and contamination of the laboratory or other specimens.

Storage under Oil
Whereas species of *Aspergillus* and *Penicillium* have remained viable under oil for 40 years (22), many species have shown deterioration after 1 to 2 years and must be

transferred periodically. Taddei et. al. also reported the successful storage and recovery of *Actinomyces* spp. stored under paraffin oil for 10 to 30 years (23).

Water Storage

Many fungi can be stored successfully for prolonged periods in distilled water (18, 20). A simple method is to pipette 6 to 7 ml of sterile distilled water onto 2-week-old culture slants in screw-cap tubes. The spores and fragments of hyphae are dislodged by scraping with the pipette, and the suspension is transferred to a sterile 1-g vial, which is tightly capped and stored at 25°C. Organisms are revived by subculturing 0.2 to 0.3 ml of the suspension to appropriate media (4).

An alternative method is to cut agar blocks from the growing edge of a fungal colony and place them in sterile distilled water in bottles with screw cap lids (6). The cultures are stored at 20 to 25°C. The organisms are retrieved by removing a block and placing it mycelium side down on growth media appropriate for that species (22). Contamination (which occurs with 22.8% of samples) is a significant problem with this method (6).

Drying

Drying as described above has been used for fungi. Only 6 of 16 genera of fungi stored in this fashion survived for 4 years (2). The greatest success has been reported for sporulating fungi stored in silica gel or in soil (22).

Freezing

Fungi have been successfully preserved by storage in liquid nitrogen using glycerol or DMSO as cryopreservatives. Broth cultures containing nonpathogenic fungi are disrupted in a Waring blender and suspended in equal parts of DMSO or glycerol to achieve final concentrations of 5 or 10%, respectively. Pathogens should not be disrupted in a mechanical blender because of the potential biohazard associated with aerosolization. *Histoplasma, Paracoccidioides,* and *Blastomyces* should be frozen in the yeast phase and *Coccidioides* should be frozen in the early mycelial phase to minimize exposure of laboratory personnel. Otherwise, procedures for freezing are as described above.

Freeze-Drying

Most spore-forming fungi can be preserved by freeze-drying. Cultures to be stored by freeze-drying should be grown on agar or broth media to the point of maximum sporulation (1) and processed as described above. Survival in storage for many years has been demonstrated (7, 21), but this is true only for sporulating organisms. Young vegetative hyphae of fungi do not survive freeze-drying (22).

Viruses

Viruses tend to be more stable than other microorganisms because of their small size, simple structure, and absence of free water. Many viruses can be stored for months at refrigerator temperatures or for years by ultra-low-temperature freezing or freeze-drying. Storage at −20°C is not recommended (14, 16). Larger viruses tend to be less stable than smaller ones (11).

Ultra-low-temperature freezing is effective in a number of situations. In addition to the cryoprotectants described above, sucrose-phosphate-glutamate containing 1% bovine albumin (SPGA) (14, 16) and hypertonic sucrose are particularly effective, the latter for storing labile viruses such as respiratory syncytial virus (17). If ultra-low-temperature

freezing is employed, the rate of freezing should be as high as possible, using small-volume suspensions (0.1 to 0.5 ml). In addition to freezing pure isolates, stool specimens known to contain viral enteric pathogens have been maintained at −70 to −85°C for 6 to 10 years with reasonable recovery and no change in the morphological characteristics of astroviruses, small round structured viruses, enteric adenoviruses, rotaviruses, or caliciviruses (25).

Gallo and others evaluated five types of media for storage of human immunodeficiency virus-infected peripheral blood lymphocytes and concluded that freezing peripheral blood lymphocytes in RPMI 1640 containing 10% fetal bovine serum and 10% DMSO and storing at −60°C is acceptable for human immunodeficiency virus isolation (9).

Freeze-drying is probably the optimum method for preserving viruses for extended periods. A detailed review of acceptable procedures has been published (11). Virus suspensions freeze-dried in medium supported with SPGA appear to survive better (14, 24). Lyophilization of polioviruses and other enteroviruses works best when electrolytes are removed by dialysis or ultrafiltration (14).

REFERENCES

1. **Alexander, M., P. M. Daggett, R. Gherna, J. Jong, and F. Simione.** 1980. *American Type Culture Collection Methods. I. Laboratory Manual on Preservation, Freezing, and Freeze-Drying as Applied to Algae, Bacteria, Fungi and Protozoa,* p. 1–46. American Type Culture Collection, Rockville, Md.
2. **Antheunisse, J., J. W. DeBruin-Tol, and M. E. Van Der Pol-Van Soest.** 1981. Survival of microorganisms after drying and storage. *Antonie Leeuwenhoek* **47:**539–545.
3. **Barbaree, J. M., and A. Sanchez.** 1982. Cross-contamination during lyophilization. *Cryobiology* **19:**443–447.
4. **Castellani, A.** 1939. Viability of some pathogenic fungi in distilled water. *J. Trop. Med. Hyg.* **42:**225–226.
5. **Crespo, M. J., M. L. Abarca, and F. J. Cabanes.** 2000. Evaluation of different preservation and storage methods for *Malassezia* spp. *J. Clin. Microbiol.* **38:**3872–3875.
6. **De Capriles, C., S. Mata, and M. Middelveen.** 1989. Preservation of fungi in water. *Mycopathologia* **106:**73–79.
7. **Ellis, J. J., and J. A. Roberson.** 1968. Viability of fungus cultures preserved by lyophilization. *Mycologia* **60:**399–404.
8. **Feltham, R. K. A., A. K. Power, P. A. Pell, and P. H. A. Sneath.** 1978. A simple method for storage of bacteria at −76°C. *J. Appl. Bacteriol.* **44:**313–316.
9. **Gallo, D., J. S. Kimpton, and P. J. Johnson.** 1989. Isolation of human immunodeficiency virus from peripheral blood lymphocytes in various transport media and frozen at −60°C. *J. Clin. Microbiol.* **27:**88–90.
10. **Gherna, R. L.** 1981. Preservation, p. 208–217. *In* P. Gerhardt, R. G. E. Murray, R. N. Costilow, E. W. Nester, W. A. Wood, N. R. Krieg, and G. B. Phillips (ed.), *Manual of Methods for General Bacteriology.* ASM Press, Washington, D.C.
11. **Gould, E. A.** 1999. Methods for long-term virus preservation. *Mol. Biotechnol.* **13:**57–66.
12. **Harbec, P. S., and P. Turcotte.** 1996. Preservation of *Neisseria gonorrhoeae* at −20°C. *J. Clin. Microbiol.* **34:** 1143–1146.
13. **Heckly, R. J.** 1961. Preservation of bacteria by lyophilization. *Adv. Appl. Microbiol.* **3:**1–76.
14. **Heckly, R. J.** 1978. Preservation of microorganisms. *Adv. Appl. Microbiol.* **24:**1–53.

15. **Jackson, H.** 1974. Loss of viability and metabolic injury of *Staphylococcus aureus* resulting from storage at 5°C. *J. Appl. Bacteriol.* **37:**59–64.

16. **Johnson, F. B.** 1990. Transport of viral specimens. *Clin. Microbiol. Rev.* **3:**120–131.

17. **Law, T. J., and R. N. Hull.** 1968. The stabilizing effect of sucrose upon respiratory syncytial virus infectivity. *Proc. Soc. Exp. Biol. Med.* **128:**515–518.

18. **McGinnis, M. R., A. A. Padhye, and L. Ajello.** 1974. Storage of stock cultures of filamentous fungi, yeasts, and some aerobic actinomycetes in sterile distilled water. *Appl. Microbiol.* **28:**218–222.

19. **Pell, P. A., and H. A. Sneath.** 1984. A note on survival of bacteria in cryoprotectant medium at temperatures above 0°C. *J. Appl. Bacteriol.* **57:**165–167.

20. **Qiangqiang, Z., W. Jiajun, and L. Li.** 1998. Storage of fungi using sterile distilled water or lyophilization: comparison after 12 years. *Mycoses* **41:**255–257.

21. **Rybnikar, A.** 1995. Long-term maintenance of lyophilized fungal cultures of the genera *Epidermophyton, Microsporum, Paecilomyces* and *Trichophyton. Mycoses* **39:** 145–147.

22. **Smith, D., and A. H. S. Onions.** 1994. *The Preservation and Maintenance of Living Fungi,* 2nd ed. CAB International, Wallingford, United Kingdom.

23. **Taddei, A., M. M. Tremarias, and C. H. deCapriles.** 1999. Viability studies on actinomycetes. *Mycopathologica* **143:**161–164.

24. **Tannock, G. A., J. C. Hierholzer, D. A. Bryce, C. F. Chee, and J. A. Paul.** 1987. Freeze-drying of respiratory syncytial viruses for transportation and storage. *J. Clin. Microbiol.* **25:**1769–1771.

25. **Williams, F. P.** 1989. Electron microscopy of stool-shed viruses: retention of characteristic morphologies after long-term storage at ultraslow temperatures. *J. Med. Virol.* **29:**192–195.

THE CLINICAL MICROBIOLOGY LABORATORY IN INFECTION DETECTION, PREVENTION, AND CONTROL

II

VOLUME EDITOR
MICHAEL A. PFALLER

SECTION EDITOR
JOHN E. McGOWAN, JR.

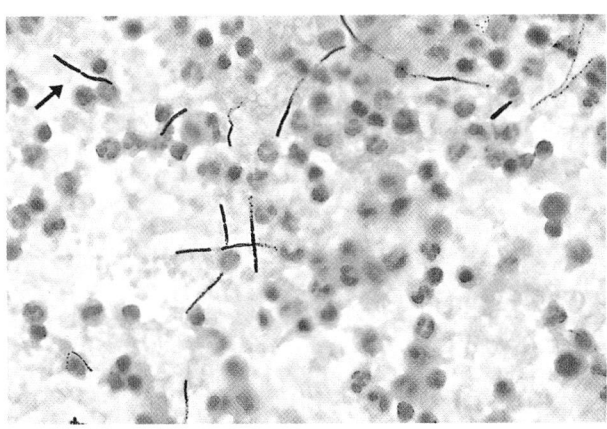

Bacillus anthracis in peripheral blood.

Decontamination, Disinfection, and Sterilization

ANDREAS F. WIDMER AND RENO FREI

8

Decontamination, disinfection, and sterilization are basic components of any infection control program. Patients expect that any reusable instrument or device used for diagnosis or treatment has undergone a process to eliminate any risks for cross-infection. However, many failures of adequate reprocessing have been reported in the literature (11, 88, 150). The basics of the technologies—chemicals for disinfection, heat for sterilization—go well back to the 19th century with Koch, Pasteur, and Lister. However, the principles had already been referenced in the Bible, as the following example shows: "Or if a person touches anything ceremonially unclean—whether the carcasses of unclean wild animals or of unclean livestock or of unclean creatures that move along the ground—even though he is unaware of it, he has become unclean and is guilty" (Lev. 5:2). The burning of victims of the plague in Venice in the 16th century is among the many reports of the use of heat to kill microorganisms to limit the spread of infectious diseases. In addition, much information on disinfection came from the preservation technology used to retard the decay of food.

Long before the introduction of routine antimicrobial prophylaxis, the incidence of postoperative site infection could be limited to <5% if the surgical site was adequately disinfected, strict asepsis was used throughout the procedure, and sterile items were used (37). In the past, surgeons relied predominantly on the knowledge of the operating-room (OR) nurses, who were responsible for adequate reprocessing of surgical instruments and reusable items. The availability and widespread use of disposable or single-use items transferred part of the responsibility of reprocessing from nursing to industry and managers, since the tasks of the central sterilization staff now were refocused primarily on purchasing, storage, and rapid turnaround. Detailed know-how regarding disinfection and sterilization procedures was no longer necessary in hospitals. Expensive electronic items for computer-assisted surgery, the cost of single-use items, environmental concerns, and new low-temperature sterilization technology (e.g., plasma sterilization) were examples of reasons for the return of reprocessing of multiple-use items. In addition, expensive devices for minimally invasive surgery (e.g., video-assisted surgery) and the use of endoscopes challenged reprocessing technologies because most items used for these purposes are heat labile, have narrow lumens, and are difficult to disassemble and clean of proteins and debris. Not surprisingly, there are

dozens of reports of transmission of nosocomial pathogens from contaminated endoscopes (28, 180, 217). Before 1990, it was very difficult to prove a causal relationship between a contaminated device and a subsequent nosocomial infection. Today, state-of-the-art clinical epidemiology supported by molecular typing tools such as pulsed-field gel electrophoresis, PCR amplification, and genome sequencing are available. The tools enable the hospital epidemiologist to ultimately prove a causal relationship between the use of a contaminated device on a patient and a consequent infection. Molecular biology provided the required scientific background to identify the limitations of the available methods and to improve the reprocessing technologies.

Reprocessing starts with the purchase of items and devices based on ample information about their disassembly, cleaning, and disinfection or sterilization. Items and devices that do not meet the basic requirements should not be purchased. Today, the Food and Drug Administration (FDA) has in place a set of requirements demanding the inclusion of detailed information on reprocessing and a telephone number (hotline) of the manufacturer. However, before purchasing it is prudent to ask for specific information about the reprocessing methods for reusable devices. Most of the available disinfectants were introduced to the market more than 20 years ago, and only one new technology for sterilization has been developed during this time. The limited resources available for research into reprocessing explain in part the lack of sound scientific data. Therefore, it is unlikely that major breakthroughs will occur within the next several years, and the standardization and optimized application of the current knowledge rather than the development of newer technologies will be key issues in the near future. Results from clinical or in vitro studies are used throughout the chapter: However, even basic procedures in decontamination, disinfection, and sterilization lack the support of randomized clinical trials. Consequently, results of animal studies, in vitro tests, and expert opinion are used.

PRINCIPLES OF TERMINOLOGY, DEFINITIONS, AND CLASSIFICATION OF MEDICAL DEVICES

Background

There is no uniform terminology for disinfection and sterilization, and many problems arise as a result. Most terms are ill defined even within the United States or Europe. In addition, the testing procedures for disinfectants are not as far advanced and well defined as MIC testing based on the recommendations of the National Committee for Clinical Laboratory Standards (NCCLS). Furthermore, considerable differences exist between the European Union and the United States. For example, liquid sterilization is not considered an appropriate method for sterilization because the process cannot be adequately monitored and validated at this time, whereas monitoring and validation are standardized for autoclaving. Similar to the case when choosing antimicrobial agents for the treatment of infectious diseases, the choice of the optimal liquid chemical germicide or sterilization process depends on a variety of factors, and no single germicide or process is adequate in all circumstances. The principal goal is to reduce the numbers of microorganisms on the device to a level that is insufficient to transmit infection, with a considerable safety margin. The most conservative approach would be to reprocess all items and devices with overkill sterilization. Obviously, not all items must undergo the most vigorous process to eliminate any microorganisms because some items are intended to be used at a nonsterile body site that does not require an overkill sterilization process. For example, a blood pressure cuff that comes into contact with intact skin only does not require sterilization before use between patients. In contrast, only sterilization will provide adequate safety to eliminate any risk of infection if the device comes into contact with a normally sterile body site. The minimum infectious dose required to trigger an infection, the severity of the disease if infection occurs, the feasibility, and, last but not least, human and financial resources are among the factors that ultimately determine the optimum reprocessing method. The optimum choice can also be the use of disposable or single-use items instead of reusable devices, because reprocessing may be more expensive or does not provide the desired level of safety. This may specifically apply to the reprocessing of items that may have been in contact with neural tissue of a patient suffering from any form of Creutzfeldt-Jakob disease (CJD) (224). The most recent research has led to isolation of the infecting agent not only from neural tissue and cerebrospinal fluid but also from tonsils and other lymphatic tissues. The agent of bovine spongiform encephalopathy (BSE) can be transmitted from animals to humans, causing vCJD (58, 109). In addition, current knowledge about prions indicates that the sterilization procedures used to eliminate microorganisms do not provide the desired level of safety for the elimination of prions (http://www.who.int/emc/diseases/bse/).

Therefore, a classification of devices is needed to better define the appropriate method for disinfection and/or sterilization. This classification should balance the potential risks for transmission of infection and the resources available to achieve the necessary or desired level of antimicrobial killing. The most commonly used classification was proposed by Earle H. Spaulding in 1968 (218). He proposed three categories: critical, semicritical, and noncritical (Table 1). This classification has been used by the Centers for Disease Control and Prevention (CDC) in *Guidelines for Handwashing and Hospital Environment Control* and by FDA for approval of sterilants and high-level disinfectants (see http://www.fda.gov/cdrh/index.html) and is used by most infection control professionals worldwide. The use of three classes of devices will guide infection control professionals in selecting the appropriate method for reprocessing. However, this simple classification does not work perfectly for all devices. Even the definition of sterilization as the absence of any viable microorganisms must be revised with the novel concept of a proteinaceous infectious agent as the cause of the vCJD promulgated by the 1997 Nobel Prize winner Stanley Prusiner. Surprisingly little is known about the target of action of disinfectants. Most modes of action

TABLE 1 Spaulding classification of devices

Clinical device	Definition	Example	Infectious risk	Reprocessing procedure	
				FDA classification	EPA classification
Critical device	A medical device that is intended to enter a normally sterile environment, sterile tissue, or the vasculature	Surgical instruments	High	Sterilization by steam, plasma, or ethylene oxide; liquid sterilization acceptable if no other methods feasible	Sterilant or disinfectant
Semicritical device	A medical device that is intended to come in contact with mucous membranes or minor skin breaches	Flexible endoscope	High, intermediate	Sterilization desirable; high-level disinfection acceptable	Sterilant or disinfectant
Noncritical device	A medical device that comes in contact with intact skin	Blood pressure cuff, electrocardiogram electrodes	Low	Intermediate or low level	Hospital disinfectant with label claim for tuberculocidal activity
Medical equipment	A device or a component of a device that does not typically come in direct contact with the patient	Examination table	Low	Low-level disinfection, sanitizer	Hospital disinfectant without label claim for tuberculocidal activity but with claim for virucidal activity against HIV

are ill defined. Generally, disinfectants kill as a result of effects on multiple targets, but the mechanisms, including the problem of the emergence of resistance, remain to be elucidated. Discussion of the presumed or established modes of antimicrobial action of disinfectants is beyond the scope of this chapter, but they are reviewed in detail by Block (31) and Russell and coworkers (154, 188). Basic information is provided below in the sections dealing with the various disinfectants.

Definition and Classification of Devices

FDA has defined medical devices as follows (as defined by the Food, Drug, and Cosmetic Act [FD&C Act]): an instrument, apparatus, implement, machine, contrivance, implant, in vitro reagent, or other similar or related article, including any component, part, or accessory, which is

1. recognized in the official National Formulary, the U.S. Pharmacopeia, or any supplement to them;
2. intended for use in the diagnosis of disease or other conditions or in the cure, mitigation, treatment, or prevention of disease, in humans or animals; or
3. intended to affect the structure or any function of the body of humans or other animals and which does not achieve its primary intended purposes through chemical action within or on the body of humans or other animals and which is not dependent upon being metabolized for the achievement of any of its principal intended purposes.

FDA uses three different levels to classify devices on the basis of a risk analysis (Table 2). These levels regulate the requirements that apply to the device and that the company must adhere to before it is able to legally market a device (Tables 1 and 2). The premarket notification [510 (k)] review determines whether a device is substantially equivalent to an earlier, legally marketed device. A manufacturer must submit a 510 (k) application and receive clearance before it can legally market the device.

The Spaulding classification has been retained because it is simple and easy to understand and applies to the majority of devices. However, this clear-cut classification has limitations with newer technologies such as minimal invasive surgery, computer-assisted surgery, and endoscopy-guided surgery. Therefore, these special cases require more sophisticated approaches, as discussed below.

Classification of Devices for Reprocessing

Critical Items

Items are classified as "critical items" if they enter normally sterile parts of the human body, such as surgical instruments used during an operation, implants, or monitoring devices used during an operation (Table 1). Items classified as critical carry the highest risk for the patient. Therefore, sterilization is the preferred method for reprocessing, and autoclaving is the method of choice if it is feasible. However, some items and devices are heat labile and do not tolerate heat. Alternative methods such as ethylene oxide sterilization and sterilization with plasma require prolonged times, and these methods do not have FDA clearance for use with small dead-end lumens, which are difficult to sterilize. Liquid sterilization with, e.g., a glutaraldehyde-based formulation or peracetic acid is acceptable if sterilization by one of the methods mentioned above is not feasible and the formulation and/or automated device has been cleared by FDA.

Semicritical Items

Semicritical objects come into contact with mucous membranes or skin that is not intact and should be free of microorganisms except spores. Intact mucous membranes generally resist bacterial spores but are susceptible to other microorganisms such as vegetative bacteria (e.g., *Mycobacterium tuberculosis*) or viruses (e.g., human immunodeficiency virus [HIV] and cytomegalovirus). Typical examples are anesthesia equipment, respiratory equipment, and endoscopes. The appropriate process is the use of a high-level disinfectant such as glutaraldehyde, stabilized hydrogen peroxide, peracetic acid, and chlorine compounds. Chlorine compounds, however, corrode items and therefore are rarely used to disinfect devices.

Noncritical Items

Noncritical items come into contact with intact skin only. Intact skin is a very effective barrier against microorganisms, and therefore there is no need for sterilization of such items and devices. Examples are bedside tables, crutches, stethoscopes, furniture, and floors. They pose a very low risk for direct transmission of pathogens and can usually be cleaned at the bedside or where they have been used. Noncritical devices can contribute to the transmission of

TABLE 2 FDA classification of devices

Classification	FDA regulation	Premarket requirements by the FDA	Proposed classification by Global Harmonization Task Force[a]	Examples
Class I	Least regulated, requires fewest regulations	None	A	Band-Aid, tongue depressor
Class II	Must meet federal performance standards	Premarket notification [510 (k)]	B	Surgical gowns, drapes, scrub sponges
			C	Orthopedic implants
Class III	Implanted and life-supporting or life-sustaining devices are required to have FDA approval for safety and effectiveness	Premarket approval	D	Artificial hearts

[a] Details in http://www.fda.gov/cdrh/ocd/sg1-n15r14.html.

pathogens by the indirect route. Contamination of the environment near patients colonized or infected with vancomycin-resistant enterococci is observed in up to 60% of samples. The hands of health care workers (HCWs) may subsequently be contaminated by touching these surfaces and may thereby spread the pathogens to devices or patients. Therefore, it is very important to disinfect noncritical items if contamination by a pathogen is likely. An example is the stethoscope, which can be disinfected by wiping the surface of the membrane with alcohol. Low-level disinfectants may be used to process noncritical items.

DECONTAMINATION AND CLEANING
In Europe, the cleaning process to remove organic material, protein, and fat is called "decontamination." In the United States, this term applies to a process that ensures an item to be "safe to handle" by an HCW without protective attire. This may be simple, manual cleaning but may also include a disinfection and even a sterilization process. In Europe, decontamination basically means cleaning. In the United States, the term describes a cleaning step and any addi-

tional step required to eliminate any risk of infection to HCW during handling. However, cleaning is always part of the decontamination process on both continents. In this chapter, the term is used to describe the removal of debris, blood, and proteins and the bulk of microorganisms which usually, but not necessarily, renders the device "safe to handle" by the HCW without protective attire. Basic definitions are outlined in Table 3. Physical or chemical cleaning, manually or by sonication or with washers, is always the primary step in any reprocessing cycle. It is intended to remove debris, blood, and proteins. All sterilization techniques other than steaming have been shown to fail in 1 to 40% of sterilization cycles if residual proteins and/or salts are not removed by a proper cleaning process (9). Other processes such as high-level disinfection and/or sterilization may follow this cleaning process. The U.S. term "decontamination" applies to the safety of handling of the device by HCWs and not necessarily to the device itself. In Europe, the term most frequently applies only to the device and is used as a synonym for the U.S. term "cleaning." Cleaning is extremely effective in removing microorganisms. Studies with endoscopes have shown reductions of

TABLE 3 Definitions and terms

Term	Standard	Technical-microbiological log CFU reduction	Comment
Sterilization	A (closely monitored) validated process used to render a product free of all forms of viable microorganisms, including all bacterial endospores	$\geq 10^6$ log CFU reduction of the most resistant spores for the sterilization process studied, achieved at the half-time of the regular cycle (ISO 14937)	Prions require an adapted definition because of their high resistance to any form of sterilization
Disinfection	Elimination of most if not all pathogenic microorganisms excluding spores	There is not a clear-cut defined reduction level; a minimum estimate is $\geq 10^3$ log CFU reduction of microorganisms excluding spores, common are 4–5 log units for devices; these are estimates, because there is no international standardization	Some high-level disinfectants achieve microbial reduction, including spores similar to sterilization, if long incubation times and/or temperatures of >25°C are applied; this is called liquid sterilization by sterilants
Decontamination	Reduction of pathogenic microorganisms to a level where items are "safe to handle" without protective attire	Elimination of debris and proteins by cleaning and/or disinfection/sterilization process; in Europe, it is restricted to cleaning only, which achieves a minimum of ≥ 1 log CFU; most cleaning processes achieve 3–5 log CFU reduction; these are estimates, because there is no international standardization	Manual and/or mechanical cleaning with water and detergents or enzymes, a prerequisite before disinfection or sterilization; in Europe, this term is used for cleaning the items; in the United States, it defines an item to be "safe to handle"; it may include a cleaning process but also a disinfection or even a sterilization process; the U.S. term "decontamination" refers to the HCW's safety; in Europe, the term is used for the item only
Antisepsis	Patient related: disinfection of living tissue or skin HCW related: reduction or removal of transient microbiological flora	Preoperative skin preparation with an alcohol-based iodine compound Hand washing: (scrub) Reduction of ≥ 1 log CFU Hand disinfection (rub-in): Reduction of ≥ 2.5 log CFU	Antiseptic agents are handled as drugs by the FDA

>99.99% or 4 log units for viruses (103) and vegetative bacteria. In addition, the activities of disinfectants can be reduced if proteins and debris limit the activity and/or access of the compound to the microorganisms on the surface of the device. In the United States, cleaning is frequently performed manually with water and a detergent. In Europe, many countries rely on washers-disinfectors. They rinse items with cold water and then with warm water plus a detergent. The cycle is completed with hot water at ≥90°C. Items such as bedpans and urinals can be cleaned and disinfected by putting the items into a machine, pushing a button, and removing them after a 2- to 5-min procedure. For noncritical devices such as floors, manual cleaning with a mop and a bucket containing water plus a detergent is almost as effective as cleaning with disinfecting agents. Therefore, a large biological burden should always be reduced before any attempt is made to disinfect and/or sterilize a device. An infectious-disease analogy is the drainage or physical of an abscess by surgery before optimal antimicrobial therapy becomes effective. As in the case of a process involving antibiotics, killing of microorganisms by disinfection or sterilization is a kinetic process, requiring prolonged exposure times if large inocula are present. The presence of protein, blood, and debris after cleaning renders any following disinfection or sterilization process futile.

DISINFECTION

Principles and Antimicrobial Activities of Compounds

Comprehensive, scientifically sound criteria for the evaluation of chemical germicides help to ensure that these agents are safe and effective for their intended use. Therefore, data on antimicrobial activity should ensure that the compounds adequately kill the expected microorganisms on a device or on the skin. MIC data are of little help since the goal of disinfection is to kill rather than inhibit the growth of microorganisms. One important factor in the testing of disinfectants is that almost all compounds need to be inactivated before they are incubated in media or plated, a problem similar to the carryover effect found in studies of MBC and killing curves. For example, bacteria do not grow in the presence of very low concentrations of a disinfectant (inhibitory effect). However, if the compound is inactivated, bacterial growth can be demonstrated. The effect is inhibition only, not killing. The patient may be exposed to a large inoculum because body fluids might dilute and inactivate the compound, releasing vital vegetative bacteria. Therefore, a laboratory testing disinfectants should be familiar with these special methods. It should always present data from dilution experiments to demonstrate the optimal dilutions and concentrations of the inactivating compounds.

In contrast to sterilization, killing curves for disinfectants are not linear, and the rate of log killing decreases at lower inoculum concentrations (as numbers of CFU per milliliter). Therefore, a 3-log-unit killing is more easily achieved with disinfectants if the inoculum is large, e.g., 10^8 CFU, but is rather difficult with an inoculum of 10^4 CFU. As with antibiotics, there is also a lag of regrowth (postantibiotic effect) after bacteria are exposed to a disinfectant. This postexposure effect has recently been quantified for a variety of disinfectants. Alcohols in general have little, if any, postexposure effect, but chlorhexidine delays regrowth after exposure for more than 2 h and chloramine

delays regrowth for even more than 4 h. Disinfectants differ in their spectra of antimicrobial activity, and their use relates to the Spaulding classification (Table 1; Fig. 1): Table 4 summarizes the antimicrobial activities of different compounds. In the last decade, blood-borne viruses have received considerable attention, and disinfection of virus-contaminated devices and spills is critical to protect HCWs. Initially, hepatitis B virus (HBV) was considered to be difficult to eradicate with disinfectants, but several studies showed that even low-level disinfectants are able to kill HBV, hepatitis C virus (HCV), and HIV (32).

Before a disinfectant for critical or semicritical devices can be legally marketed, FDA must grant marketing clearance by

1. issuance of an order in response to a section 510 (k) submission which exempts the device from the FD&C Act's premarket approval requirements, or
2. approval of a premarket approval application; in granting marketing clearance by issuance of a section 510 (k) order exempting a liquid chemical germicide from premarket approval, FDA must find the device to be "substantially equivalent," as the term is defined in section 21 of the U.S. code.

The microbiocidal efficacy testing of liquid chemical sterilants and high-level disinfectants is based on a three-tier approach that includes the following:

1. potency testing, which incorporates Environmental Protection Agency (EPA) test requirements for the registration of germicides, such as the Association of Official Analytical Chemists (AOAC) sporocidal test, tuberculocidal test, etc., and FDA-recommended tests, such as total killing or end-point analysis and comparison of the survivor curve to the predicted curve;
2. simulated use testing with medical devices contaminated with an organic load and the appropriate test microorganisms for the level of disinfection being claimed; the conditions of the artificially contaminated devices represent worst-case postcleaning conditions prior to exposure to the germicide; and
3. "in-use" testing with clinically used medical devices; in-use testing incorporates cleaning of the devices according to the operating procedures of the facility prior to exposure to the germicide.

There is still controversy about the optimal testing procedure to be used to ensure that the germicide achieves the desired log killing. Lipid-enveloped viruses such as HIV and most vegetative bacteria are destroyed even by a low-level disinfectant (Fig. 1). Nonlipid or small viruses such as poliovirus can challenge many disinfectants, including alcohol. For example, isopropyl alcohol has little activity against poliovirus. In contrast, >90% ethanol is very active against these viruses (219). Of the vegetative bacteria, mycobacteria are most resistant to disinfectants. Therefore, FDA includes a tuberculocidal test in its test procedures. This test does not allow for cleaning, uses 2% horse serum as the proteinaceous load, and is performed with a large number of microorganisms (10^5 to 10^6 CFU). Therefore, devices must be exposed to disinfectants for extended immersion times (>45 min) and at elevated temperatures (≥25°C). In the absence of cleaning and the presence of proteinaceous materials with large microbial loads, immersion in 2.4% alkaline glutaraldehyde for 45 min at 25°C is frequently required for complete tuberculocidal killing.

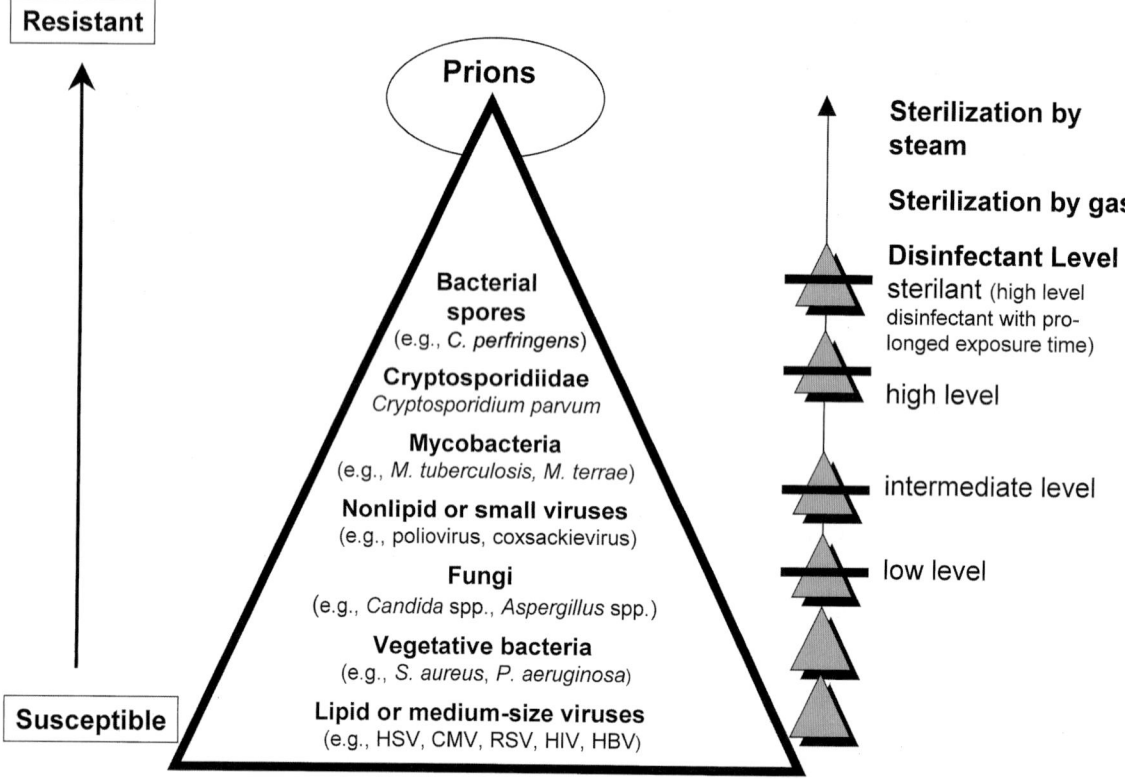

FIGURE 1 Increasing order of resistance of microorganisms to disinfectants.

However, Rutala and Weber conclusively demonstrated that proper cleaning eradicates at least 4 log units of microorganisms (198). In another study, the cleaning of bronchoscopes before disinfection removed all detectable contaminants, with up to an 8-log-unit reduction of viral load (102). Therefore, Rutala and Weber recommended that FDA reconsider its procedures regarding testing for activity against mycobacteria (198). They propose the following: a standardized cleaning protocol and then a 20-min immersion at 20°C with an FDA-cleared disinfectant will be sufficient to achieve a high-level disinfection. However, it must be reiterated that disinfection or sterilization without an antecedent proper cleaning and removal of any debris is a major failure in the decontamination process, and even the use of disinfectants with the highest level of safety is no substitute for appropriate training of HCWs to avoid human errors. An outbreak with *Klebsiella oxytoca* occurred after the concentration of a glutaraldehyde-based surface disinfectant was lowered by 50%. Staff members complained about the strong odor of the disinfectant, and the local infection control committee allowed a reduction in the concentration. The outbreak stopped after reverting to the recommended concentration (178). Use of tap water to rinse disinfected instruments should be discontinued: it harbors many germs including mycobacteria, fungi, and, frequently, mesophilic bacteria. For example, 58 cases were recently reported from an outbreak with *Mycobacterium xenopi* (19). Discovertebral surgery was performed with disinfected instruments that were rinsed with tap water before use (19). The concentration of the disinfectant should be checked regularly if it is diluted at the place of use, even if it is diluted with an electronically monitored dilution device. Failures of the valve or other critical parts of the device can result in an insufficient final concentration, which usually cannot be detected by visual inspection or the odor of the disinfectant.

Definition and Terms (Adapted from FDA and EPA Definitions)

Since FDA regulates the most critical part of disinfection and sterilization, the FDA definitions are used throughout the chapter unless stated otherwise. The most important definitions are given below.

Germicide: an agent that destroys microorganisms. Other terms with the suffix "-cide" (e.g., virucide, fungicide, bactericide, sporicide, and tuberculocide) relate to the killing of the microorganisms identified by the prefix.

Sterilant (chemical): a chemical germicide which achieves sterilization. Only limited data are available to validate the fact that liquid chemical germicides can achieve a defined sterility assurance level (SAL). Liquid chemical germicide sterilization is acceptable only for critical devices that are heat labile or that are otherwise unable to be sterilized by all other sterilization methods that can be biologically monitored.

High-level disinfectant: a germicide that kills all microbial pathogens except large numbers of bacterial endospores when used according to the labeling.

Intermediate-level disinfectant: a germicide that kills all microbial pathogens except bacterial endospores when used according to the labeling.

Low-level disinfectant: a germicide that kills most vegetative bacteria and lipid-enveloped or medium-size viruses when used according to the labeling.

Minimum effective concentration: the minimum effective concentration of a liquid chemical germicide which still

TABLE 4 Overview of common disinfectants[a]

Germicide	Use dilution	Level of disinfection	Active against:						Important characteristics									Typical application in hospitals
			Bacteria	Lipophilic viruses	Fungi	Small or hydrophilic viruses	M. tuberculosis	Bacterial spores	Shelf life of >1 wk	Corrosive/ deleterious effect	Residue	Inactivated by organic matter	Skin irritant	Eye irritant	Respiratory irritant	Toxic	Environmental concerns	
Glutaraldehyde	2–3.2%	High/CS	+	+	+	+	+	+	+	−	+	−	+	+	+	+	−	Endoscopes
Hydrogen peroxide	3–25%	High/CS	+	+	+	+	+	±	+	±	−	±	+	+	−	+	−	Contact lenses
Chlorine	100–1,000 ppm free chlorine	High	+	+	+	+	+	±	−	+	+	+	+	+	+	+	±	Selected semicritical devices
Isopropyl alcohol	60–95%	Int	+	+	+	±	+	−	+	±	−	±	±	+	−	+	−	Small-area surfaces
Glucoprotamine	1.5–4%	Int	+	+	+	+	+	−	+	−	−	−	+	+	−	−	−	Diagnostic instruments
Phenolic compounds	0.4–5% aqueous	Int	+	+	+	±	+	−	+	−	+	−	+	+	−	+	+	Surgical instruments
Iodophors	30–50 ppm free iodine	Int	+	+	+	+	±	−	+	±	+	+	±	+	−	+	−	Medical equipment
Quaternary ammonium compounds	0.4–1.6% aqueous	Low	±	+	±	−	−	−	+	−	+	+	+	+	−	+	−	Disinfection in food preparation areas and floors

[a] Data from references 31, 188, 189, and 227 and from *Laboratory Biosafety Manual*, World Health Organization, Geneva, Switzerland, 1983. Abbreviations: Int, intermediate; CS, chemical sterilant; +, yes; −, no; ±, variable results. Efficacy of the disinfectants is based on an exposure time of less than 30 min at room temperature. Spores require prolonged exposure times (up to 10 h) unless used with a machine at higher temperatures.

achieves the claimed microbicidal activity. Reporting of MICs of disinfectants is not useful, but these reports continue to be published.

Cleaning (or precleaning): the removal of foreign material, e.g., organic or inorganic contaminants, from medical devices as part of a decontamination process.

Guidelines for Choosing a Disinfectant

Several factors should be included in an evaluation of a disinfectant. A prerequisite for a disinfectant is its effectiveness against the expected spectrum of pathogens (Tables 4 and 5). Data on disinfectants should be reviewed, although this process has been performed by EPA or FDA, before registering or clearing the disinfectant. The data required to pass the tests by these agencies include the AOAC tuberculocidal test for a claim of tuberculosis; the AOAC fungicidal test, the AOAC use-dilution tests for *Staphylococcus aureus* ATCC 6538, *Salmonella enterica serovar* Choleraesuis ATCC 10708, and *Pseudomonas aeruginosa*; and EPA virucidal tests for viruses including poliovirus type 2 and herpes simplex virus. In Europe, disinfectants should have been tested by the methods defined by established or proposed European Norms (EN) such as EN 1040 (bactericidal activity) and EN 1275 (fungicidal activity). In addition to the activity of the disinfectant, its compatibility with devices should be reviewed in detail; this should include a review of data on devices that have been immersed for longer than recommended times. Instruments may be forgotten after immersion, and this mistake should not necessarily result in irreparable damage to the device. Other issues are toxicity, odor, and residual activity. In addition to scientific data, knowledge of the hands-on experience of other health care professionals at different institutions helps to avoid simple but sometimes cumbersome problems such as interactions with detergents, unexpected coloring, or odors. At the authors' institution, a change of color of a disinfectant made the otherwise identical disinfectant "not acceptable" to HCWs. Therefore, it is prudent not to switch frequently to other disinfectants with similar or identical active compounds unless there is scientific evidence for improved activity or faster action.

An updated list of low-level and intermediate-level disinfectants registered by EPA or high-level disinfectants and sterilants cleared by FDA is provided on their homepages: http://www.fda.gov/cdrh/ode/germlab.html and http://www.epa.gov/oppad001/chemregindex.htm.

Disinfection by Heat versus Immersion in Germicides

Disinfection by heat—sometimes called pasteurization—is an important tool in Europe and has replaced disinfection with germicides for many applications. The advantages are obvious: automation of the process, monitoring and documentation of the process similar to that for sterilization, lack of emergence of resistance, and, probably, a lower cost per load compared to the cost of germicides. However, there are some obstacles to thermal disinfection: the cost of the purchase and installation of the equipment is much higher than when a germicide is used, and considerable power is needed to heat the water. Vegetative bacteria are killed within seconds at temperatures of >80 to 85°C. The current German recommendation (Bundesseuchengesetz) for manufacturers of washers-disinfectors for thermal disinfection of devices is 10 min at 92°C, a process that kills all vegetative bacteria and viruses including HBV. In the

TABLE 5 ■ Overview of common antiseptic compounds[a]

Compound	Antiseptic effect on:[b]					Rapidity of action	Residual activity[b]	Typical concn (%)	Affected by organic matter	Safety for humans
	Gram-positive bacteria	Gram-negative bacteria	Viruses	Fungi	M. tuberculosis					
Alcohols	+++	+++	++[c]	+++	+++	15–30 s	None	70–95	[e]	Drying, flammable
Chlorhexidine	+++	++	++	+	++	Minutes	+++	4, 2, 0.5 in alcohol	Minimally	Ototoxicity, keratitis
Iodophors	+++	+++	++	++	++	Minutes	+	10, 7.5, 2, 0.5	Yes	Skin irritation
Octenidine[d]	+++	++	++	++	++	Minutes	+++	0.1	Minimally	Limited data
PCMX	++	+	+	+	+	Minutes	+++	0.5–3.75	Minimally	Appears to be safe
Triclosan	++	++	++	±	+	Minutes	+++	0.3–1.0	Minimally	Appears to be safe

[a] Data from references 133, 176, and 241.
[b] ±, poor; +, fair; ++, good; +++, excellent.
[c] Ethanol at >95% is highly effective against small viruses; isopropanol has limited effectiveness against small or nonlipid viruses.
[d] Not available in the United States.
[e] Conflicting data.

United Kingdom, the Department of Health requires 65°C for 10 min, 71°C for 3 min, or 80°C for 1 min (36). Non-spore-forming microorganisms such as enterococci resist temperatures of up to 71°C for 10 min, challenging these recommendations (36). In the United States, this hot-water pasteurization is generally performed at 77°C for 30 min (99), but few scientific data support a certain temperature. Studies by Gurevich et al. (99) indicate that pasteurization with a germicide is more effective than pasteurization without a germicide. However, the washer includes a cleaning process with an average reduction of 4 log units, coupled with heat disinfection (5-log-unit killing), resulting in a total reduction of 8 to 9 log units. This surpasses any international requirements for high-level disinfection. Data on the effectiveness of these machines have been summarized in local reports, but most have not been published in peer-reviewed journals. Washer-disinfectors such as the AMSCO Reliance 430 achieved an inactivation factor of >5 log units (93, 118). At the authors' institution, thermal disinfection has almost completely replaced germicide-based disinfection because it is safer and less expensive once the equipment has been purchased (214). In conclusion, thermal disinfection of devices with a washer-disinfector is an excellent alternative to germicide-based immersion. The decision regarding the basic concept of disinfection should balance the availability and the expense of the equipment, the savings achieved in terms of working hours, and the storage and distribution of disinfectants, HCW safety, and the greater risks for human errors.

Overview of Commonly Used Disinfectants for Devices

Glutaraldehyde

Glutaraldehyde and formaldehyde are the most extensively studied aldehydes among several others that exhibit biocidal activity, including glyoxal, ortho-phthalaldehyde (OPA), succinaldehyde, and benzaldehydes. Extensive reviews may be found elsewhere (17, 187, 189). In commercially available products, glutaraldehyde is the predominant aldehyde. Because of its potent and broad-spectrum microbiocidal activities as well as its noncorrosive properties, glutaraldehyde is often regarded as the high-level disinfectant and chemical sterilant of choice and is widespread in health care facilities. The mechanism of action is complex and is linked to the alkylation of sulfhydryl, hydroxyl, carboxy, and amino groups of microorganisms. Several target sites for the action are known, such as cell wall and membrane components, nucleic acids, enzymes, and other proteins. The biocidal activities of glutaraldehyde solutions are dependent on a variety of variables, such as pH, temperature, concentration at the time of use, the presence of inorganic ions, and the age of the solution (17). Aqueous solutions of glutaraldehyde are usually acidic and are not sporicidal in this form. Therefore, they need to be activated by the addition of an alkalinazing agent. These activated solutions, however, rapidly lose their activity due to polymerization of the glutaraldehyde molecules at an alkaline pH. Therefore, the shelf life of such solutions is limited to 14 days unless other recommendations of the manufacturer are listed. To overcome this problem, novel formulations with longer shelf lives have been developed (e.g., activated dialdehyde solutions containing 2.4 to 3.4% glutaraldehyde with a maximum reuse life of 28 days). The activities of disinfectants increase as the temperature rises. Among eight disinfectants tested, glutaraldehyde was found to be the

chemical most strongly affected by temperature (86). There are stable acid glutaraldehydes that may be used at temperatures of 35 to 55°C at concentrations below 2%. A standard 2% aqueous solution of glutaraldehyde buffered to pH 7.5 to 8.5 is bactericidal, tuberculocidal, sporicidal, fungicidal, and virucidal. It rapidly kills both gram-negative and gram-positive vegetative bacteria. To inactivate spores and mycobacteria, longer exposure times are required. Spores of Bacillus and Clostridium spp. are generally destroyed by 2% glutaraldehyde in 3 h, whereas spores of Clostridium difficile are more rapidly eliminated (195). In contrast, Cryptosporidium parvum oocysts remained viable and infectious after a 10-h treatment in a 2.5% glutaraldehyde product (245). The mycobactericidal activity has been questioned by several investigators. Rubbo et al. (186) demonstrated that glutaraldehyde has a slow action in comparison with alcohols, formaldehyde, iodine, and phenol against Mycobacterium tuberculosis. Ascenzi et al. (18) found in the quantitative suspension test that 2% glutaraldehyde killed only 2 to 3 log units of M. tuberculosis in 20 min at 20°C. Similarly, Collins (60) reported that a standardized suspension of M. tuberculosis could not be completely inactivated within 10 min. Nontuberculous mycobacteria such as M. avium, M. intracellulare, and M. gordonae were more resistant to inactivation than M. tuberculosis (59). These and other data suggest that 20 min (at 20°C) is the minimum exposure time needed to reliably inactivate tuberculous and nontuberculous mycobacteria by 2% glutaraldehyde, provided that the contaminated item has been thoroughly cleaned prior to disinfection (117, 189). Glutaraldehyde-resistant mycobacteria have been isolated from endoscope washers-disinfectors (95, 229) (see "Endoscopes" below). The virucidal activity of glutaraldehyde also extends to the nonenveloped (hydrophilic) viruses, which are generally more resistant to disinfectants than are the enveloped (lipophilic) viruses. Numerous viruses were documented to be inactivated, including HIV, hepatitis A virus (HAV), HBV, poliovirus type 1, coxsackievirus type B, yellow fever virus, and rotavirus (17, 126). Glutaraldehyde is noncorrosive to metal and does not damage rubber and plastic equipment. It retains activity in the presence of organic matter. Glutaraldehyde-based formulations are most commonly used for high-level disinfection of medical equipment such as endoscopes, transducers, dialysis systems, and anesthesia and respiratory therapy equipment (189). Due to dilution, glutaraldehyde concentrations commonly decline during use in manual and automatic baths used for endoscopes (153). Test strips should be used to ensure that the glutaraldehyde concentration has not fallen below 1 to 1.5%. Glutaraldehyde vapor at the level of 0.2 ppm is irritating to the eyes, throat, and nose. In HCWs exposed to glutaraldehyde, allergic contact dermatitis, asthma, rhinitis, and epistaxis have been observed. Measures that may minimize employee exposure include the use of tight-fitting lids on immersion baths, improved ventilation, ducted exhaust hoods or ductless fume hoods with absorbents for the vapor, personal protective equipment, and appropriate automated machines for endoscope disinfection (10, 189). Inadequate rinsing of colonoscopes after immersion in glutaraldehyde may result in proctocolitis (69, 238). In addition, keratopathy caused by ophthalmic instruments that were not properly rinsed after soaking has been reported. Since treatment with formaldehyde prior to autoclaving has stabilized the infectivity of prions (41), aldehydes currently are no longer recommended for disinfecting surgical instruments in Europe (see "Bovine Spongiform Encephalopathy and variant Creutzfeldt-Jacob Disease" below).

ortho-Phthalaldehyde

The 0.55% OPA solution has been recently cleared by the FDA and European countries as a high-level disinfectant. Compared with glutaraldehyde, OPA has demonstrated several advantages. It does not require activation, has increased stability during storage and reuse as well as over a wide range of pH, is not irritating to the eyes and the respiratory tract, has low vapor properties, and produces a barely perceptible odor. In vitro, OPA was more rapidly mycobactericidal than glutaraldehyde and also demonstrated good activity against glutaraldehyde-resistant strains (81). However, 0.5% OPA was found not to be sporicidal within 270 min of exposure (233). OPA stains proteins gray and is a skin irritant. Therefore, it must be handled with appropriate safety precautions (i.e., gloves, fluid-resistant gowns, and eye protection). The material compatibility of OPA is excellent and similar to that of glutaraldehyde. The exposure time for a 0.55% solution at 20°C required for high-level disinfection was set differently: at 12 min in the United States, at 10 min in Canada, and at 5 min in Europe, Asia, and Latin America. Provided that additional and clinical studies corroborate the promising properties, OPA may replace glutaraldehyde in many uses, especially in endoscope disinfection. The new agent appears to be particularly useful in washer-disinfectors, where glutaraldehyde-resistant mycobacteria have emerged (229, 233).

Formaldehyde

Formaldehyde and its condensates are reviewed in depth elsewhere (181). Formaldehyde in aqueous solutions or as a gas has been used as a disinfectant and sterilant for many decades. Its use in the health care setting, however, has sharply decreased for several reasons. The irritating vapors and pungent odor produced by formaldehyde are apparent at very low levels (<1 ppm). In addition, allergy to formaldehyde is not uncommon. The strongest impact on banning formaldehyde for sterilization and disinfection processes was the action of agencies of the U.S. federal government, such as the Occupational Safety and Health Administration, and the Health and Safety Executive of the United Kingdom. They indicated that the inhalation of formaldehyde vapors may pose a carcinogenic risk. The Occupational Safety and Health Administration limits an 8-h time-weighted average exposure in the workplace to a concentration of 0.75 ppm. Elevated levels of occupational exposures have been found among workers in dialysis units and gross anatomy laboratories (6). For these reasons, the use of formaldehyde and formaldehyde-releasing agents in health care institutions is very limited, despite its broad-spectrum microbiocidal activity. The 37% (by weight) water-based solution, called formalin, is still the standard for preserving anatomical, surgical, and biopsy specimens as well as for embalming purposes. Formaldehyde was formerly used for the disinfection of hemodialysis equipment and water dialysate distribution systems but has been largely replaced by peracetic acid. Paraformaldehyde vaporized by heat is still used for the gaseous decontamination of biological safety cabinets.

Chlorine and Chlorine-Releasing Compounds

Among the large number of chlorine compounds commercially available, hypochlorites are the most widely used disinfectants. Hypochlorite has been used for more than a century and remains an important disinfectant. An extensive review of the use of inorganic hypochlorite in health care facilities has been published by Rutala and Weber (199). Aqueous solutions of sodium hypochlorite are usually called household bleach. Bleach commonly contains 5.25% sodium hypochlorite or 52,500 ppm available chlorine; a 1:10 dilution of bleach provides about 300 to 600 mg of free chlorine per liter. Alternative chlorine-releasing compounds frequently used in health care facilities include chloramine-T, sodium dichloroisocyanurate tablets, and demand-release chlorine dioxide. Demand-release chlorine dioxide is an extremely reactive compound and consequently is prepared at the point of use. It is largely used in the chlorination of potable water, swimming pools, and wastewater. Due to its hazardous nature, chlorine gas is rarely used as a disinfectant. In aqueous solution, all chlorine compounds release hypochlorous acid, the most likely active compound. The mechanism of microbiocidal action of hypochlorous acid has not been fully elucidated. Inhibition of some key enzymatic reactions within the cell and denaturation of proteins play major roles in killing. Lowering the pH or raising the temperature or concentration increases its antimicrobial efficacy. Chlorine compounds have broad antimicrobial spectra that include bacterial spores and M. tuberculosis at higher concentrations. Therefore, hypochlorite can be used as a high-level disinfectant for semicritical items. Hypochlorite is fast acting, nonstaining, nonflammable, and inexpensive. However, its use is limited by its corrosive effects, inactivation by organic matter, and relative instability. Although exposure to sodium hypochlorite through direct contact may result in tissue injury, the incidence of injury due to hypochlorite use in health care facilities is extremely low (199). Inhalation of chlorine gas may cause irritation of the respiratory tract, resulting in cough, dyspnea, and pulmonary edema or chemical pneumonitis. Since the potential carcinogens trihalomethanes have been detected in chlorine-treated water, potential health concerns regarding chlorination of water supplies have been raised. High levels of trihalomethanes were found during continuous hyperchlorination of hospital water when the levels of chlorine in hot water exceeded 4 mg/liter (105). The potential hazards and significant benefits of chlorine use are discussed elsewhere (123). Available chlorine concentrations of 100 ppm for contact times of 10 min very effectively inactivate vegetative bacteria and viruses. In suspension tests, significant inactivation of both enveloped and nonenveloped viruses, including HIV, HAV, HBV, herpes simplex virus types 1 and 2, poliovirus, coxsackievirus, and rotavirus has been established (199). In general, endospore-forming bacteria, mycobacteria, fungi, and protozoa are less susceptible, and higher concentrations of chlorine (1,000 ppm) are required to completely destroy these germs. A concentration of 100 ppm eliminated 99.9% of Bacillus subtilis endospores in 5 min (244). In a C. difficile outbreak, the use of sodium hypochlorite solutions (500 ppm and 1,600 ppm) to decontaminate environmental surfaces was associated with both reductions in the levels of surface contamination (79 and 98%, respectively) and control of the outbreak (121). Chloramine-T and sodium dichloroisocyanurate seem to have less sporocidal action than does sodium hypochlorite. Cryptosporidium oocysts remain infective for several days in swimming pool water containing recommended chlorine concentrations. Additionally, because of their small size, these oocysts may not be removed efficiently by conventional pool filters, explaining outbreaks associated with drinking water and swimming pools (50).

Hypochlorites and other chlorine compounds are substantially inactivated in the presence of blood or other organic matter. Consequently, items used for patient care and environmental surfaces must be cleaned before the disinfectant is used. The presence of a biofilm (e.g., in the pipes of a water distribution system) significantly reduces the efficacy of chlorines as well. In addition, the free available chlorine levels in solutions of opened containers can decay to 40 to 50% of the original concentration in 1 month. Therefore, concentrations higher than those established in laboratory experiments should be used in practice. The following conditions of chlorine use favor the stability of available chlorine: use at room temperature, use of diluted solutions, use of solutions in an alkaline pH range, and storage in closed opaque containers. Depending on the concentrations employed, sodium hypochlorite is used in hospitals as a high-level disinfectant for selected semicritical devices (e.g., dental equipment, and mannequins used for cardiopulmonary resuscitation training), as an intermediate-level disinfectant (e.g., hemodialysis equipment), and as a low-level disinfectant for environmental surfaces and hydrotherapy tanks. CDC recommends use of a 1:100 dilution (5,000 ppm) to decontaminate environmental spills of blood and certain other body fluids (46). Because chlorine can be inactivated by blood and other organic material, the use of a full-strength solution or a 1:10 dilution is safer unless the surface is cleaned prior to disinfection (78, 236). Household bleach is also an appropriate laboratory disinfectant for tabletops, incubators, and laboratory spills. For drug addicts, CDC recommends the use of bleach to disinfect syringes before reuse, if no sterile disposable syringes are available (47). Chlorines at low concentrations (usually approximately 0.5 ppm free chlorine) are used in the chlorination of drinking water. Hyperchlorination of institutional water systems contaminated with *Legionella pneumophila* has been successfully used to control epidemic nosocomial legionellosis (105). However, corrosion damage to the water distribution system occurs and represents a long-term problem (105). Stabilized solutions of chlorine dioxide appear to be more efficacious than chlorine for the control of legionellae (100). This compound also has a reputed lower toxicity. A growing number of municipal water treatment plants in the United States are using monochloramine as a residual disinfectant. Chloramination of drinking water has several advantages compared to the use of free chlorine, including better control of Legionnaires' disease at the municipal level or in individual hospitals (130). A list of clinically relevant websites has recently been published (e.g., www.legionella.org) (22).

Hydrogen Peroxide

Hydrogen peroxide is a strong oxidizer used for high-level disinfection and sterilization. It produces destructive hydroxyl free radicals which can attack membrane lipids, DNA, and other essential cell components. Although the catalase produced by anaerobic and some aerobic bacteria may protect cells from hydrogen peroxide, this defense is overwhelmed by the concentrations used for disinfection (141). Generally, a 3% hydrogen peroxide solution is rapidly bactericidal. It is less rapid in its action against organisms with high cellular catalase activity (e.g., *S. aureus* and *Serratia marcescens*) and especially against bacterial spores. Surprisingly, 3% hydrogen peroxide was ineffective against vancomycin-resistant enterococci (212). The use of a 3%

solution for 150 min was shown to destroy 10^6 spores in six of seven exposure trials, whereas use of a 10% concentration for 60 min was always successful (235). *Bacillus subtilis* spores were killed by concentrations of 17.7 and 35.4% in 9.4 and 2.3 min, respectively (139). In a recent investigation, 10% hydrogen peroxide was the most active chemical disinfectant against *B. subtilis* spores among seven liquid agents tested (206). In contrast, other investigators found that the sporicidal activity of hydrogen peroxide was lower than those of peracetic acid and chlorine (8). Killing of spores is greatly enhanced by increased concentration or temperature. Hydrogen peroxide also acts against spores synergistically with ultrasonic energy, UV radiation, and some chemical agents such as peracetic acid. Martin et al. have demonstrated that 0.3% hydrogen peroxide is able to inactivate HIV in 10 min (149). A 3% concentration inactivated rhinovirus in 6 to 8 min at 37°C (155), whereas up to 6% was ineffective against poliovirus in 1 min (227). Hydrogen peroxide has low toxicity to humans and the environment. It is neither carcinogenic nor mutagenic. Concentrated solutions may irritate the eyes, skin, and mucous membranes. Hydrogen peroxide can easily be destroyed by heat or enzymes (catalase and peroxidases). It decomposes to the innocuous end products oxygen and water. Therefore, it is environmentally safe. Stabilized 6% solutions can be used for high-level disinfection of semicritical items, considering the corrosive effects of hydrogen peroxide on copper, zinc, and brass (189). A commercially available product containing 7.5% hydrogen peroxide and 0.85% phosphoric acid (Sporox) for disinfection of flexible endoscopes needs a soaking time of 30 min at 20°C for high-level disinfection. It may be used for reprocessing of flexible endoscopes if compatible with the materials (211). Cases of pseudomembrane-like enterocolitis (pseudolipomatosis) have been associated with exposure to residual hydrogen peroxide in endoscopes (204). Concentrations of 3 to 6% are used for the disinfection of ventilators, soft contact lenses (3% for 2 to 4 h) (112), and tonometer biprisms (141, 189). Corneal damage after the use of hydrogen peroxide-disinfected tonometer tips that were improperly rinsed has been reported (140). For wound cleansing and dental regimens, controversy exists about both the beneficial and the harmful effects of the use of hydrogen peroxide (141). Vaporized hydrogen peroxide is also used for plasma sterilization (see below).

Peracetic Acid

Peracetic acid (or peroxyacetic acid) is an even more potent germicidal agent than hydrogen peroxide. In comparison to other disinfectants, it was the most active agent in several in vitro studies (7, 207). Concentrations of ≤1% are sporicidal even at low temperatures. Accordingly, it is listed as a high-level disinfectant and chemical sterilant by FDA. The mechanism of action of peracetic acid has not been clearly elucidated, but it is likely to function much as hydrogen peroxide and other oxidizing agents. Synergistic sporicidal effects of peracetic acid with alcohols have been observed. Peracetic acid remains effective in the presence of organic matter. At low concentrations it is considerably less stable than hydrogen peroxide; preparations with appropriate stability have been developed and are commercially available. Peracetic acid is corrosive to plain steel, galvanized iron, copper, brass, and bronze. It also attacks natural and synthetic rubbers. Nevertheless, its powerful germicidal activity and its lack of environmentally problematic or toxic residues make peracetic acid very attractive for use in health care settings, most frequently in combination with hydrogen peroxide to disinfect hemodialyzers. However, concerns about the potential toxicity of the combination of peracetic and acetic acids have been raised (104). Feldman et al. reported that dialysis in freestanding facilities that reprocess dialyzers with peracetic and acetic acid was associated with higher mortality rates than was treatment in facilities that discard dialysis filters or use formaldehyde for reprocessing (77). It is not known if the higher death rate arose from the direct toxicity of these disinfectants or other factors related to the patients or facilities. Two commercial products containing a combination of peracetic acid and hydrogen peroxide have been cleared by FDA as liquid sterilant and high-level disinfectant. The use of peracetic acid for chemical sterilization of instruments and endoscopes (STERIS SYSTEM 1) is discussed below.

Alcohols

For centuries, the alcohols have been appreciated for their antimicrobial properties. Ethyl alcohol (ethanol) and isopropyl alcohol (isopropanol) are the alcoholic solutions most often used as surface disinfectants and antiseptic agents in health care institutions. Their antimicrobial efficacies are enhanced in the presence of water, with optimal concentrations being 60 to 90% by volume. The exact mechanism by which alcohols destroy microorganisms is not fully understood. The most plausible explanation for the antimicrobial action is coagulation (denaturation) of proteins, e.g., of enzymatic proteins, leading to the loss of specific cellular functions (136). Ethyl and isopropyl alcohols at appropriate concentrations have broad spectra of antimicrobial activity that include vegetative bacteria, fungi, and viruses. However, they generally do not destroy bacterial spores. Fatal infections due to *Clostridium* spp. were observed when alcohol was used for sterilization of surgical instruments. Against vegetative bacteria, such as *S. aureus*, *Streptococcus pyogenes*, members of the family *Enterobacteriaceae*, and *P. aeruginosa*, alcohols are rapidly bactericidal. These germs were killed by 70 to 80% ethyl alcohol in 10 to 90 s in suspension tests (182). Isopropyl alcohol was found to be slightly more bactericidal than ethyl alcohol (136). It was highly effective against vancomycin-resistant enterococci, in contrast to hydrogen peroxide, which was ineffective in all eight strains tested (212). Isopropyl alcohol has also been demonstrated to have excellent activity against mycobacteria, including M. tuberculosis, and fungi, such as *Candida* spp., *Cryptococcus neoformans*, *Blastomyces dermatitidis*, *Coccidioides immitis*, *Histoplasma capsulatum*, *Aspergillus niger*, and dermatophytes.

Controversial data on the antiviral activity of alcohols have been reported. While both ethyl and isopropyl alcohols are able to inactivate most viruses with a lipid envelope (e.g., influenza virus, herpes simplex virus, and adenovirus), several investigators found that isopropyl alcohol had less virucidal activity against naked, nonenveloped viruses (24, 126). In the experiments by Klein and DeForest, propan-2-ol, even at 95%, could not inactivate the nonenveloped poliovirus type 1 and coxsackievirus type B in 10 min (126). In contrast, these enteroviruses were inactivated by 70% ethanol (126). Against HAV, however, 70% ethanol and 45% propan-2-ol were not effective when their activities were assessed on stainless steel disks contaminated with fecally suspended virus. Among 20 disinfectants tested, only 3 were able to reduce the titer of HAV by greater than 99.9% in 1 min (2% glutaraldehyde, sodium hypochlorite with >5,000 ppm free chlorine, and a quater-

nary ammonium formulation containing 23% HCl) (152). Experiments by Bond et al. (32) and Kobayashi et al. (129) demonstrated that treatment of human plasma containing high-titer HBV with propan-2-ol (70% for 10 min) or ethanol (80% for 2 min) was effective when the treatment was tested by inoculation of the treated plasma into susceptible chimpanzees. In a suspension test, 40% propanol reduced the rotavirus titer by at least 4 logs in 1 min (132). HIV is readily inactivated by both ethyl and isopropyl alcohols. Martin et al. found that 15% ethyl alcohol and 35% isopropyl alcohol were effective in a suspension test (149). More recently, high titers of HIV in suspension have been shown to be rapidly inactivated by 70% ethanol, independent of the protein load. However, the rate of inactivation decreased when virus was dried onto a glass surface and high levels of protein were present (228). Alcohols cannot penetrate protein-rich materials. Therefore, a spray or a wipe with alcohol cannot be guaranteed to disinfect a surface contaminated with blood or other body fluids without preliminary cleaning. The antiviral activities of alcoholic agents found in vitro were confirmed by studies with artificially contaminated hands or fingertips. As an example, both 70% propanol and 70% ethanol reduced the release of rotavirus from the contaminated fingertips by 2.7 log units. In comparison, the mean reductions obtained with liquid soap and an aqueous solution of chlorhexidine gluconate were 0.9 and 0.7 log unit, respectively, which are 100 times lower than the reduction achieved with the alcohols (14).

Alcohols possess many qualities that make them suitable both for disinfection of equipment and for antisepsis of skin. They are fast acting, minimally toxic with topical application, nonstaining, and nonallergenic, and they readily evaporate. The rapid evaporation is advantageous for most disinfection and antisepsis procedures. The uptake of alcohol by intact skin and the lungs when alcohol is used on the skin surface is negligible. Alcohols have better wetting properties than water due to their lower surface tensions. This represents an important feature for skin antisepsis, along with their cleansing and degreasing actions. Repeated application of alcoholic antiseptics, however, may cause drying and irritation of the skin. Therefore, preparations for hand disinfection should contain refatting agents and emollients (see the discussion on hand antisepsis below). Alcohols are also excellent for intermediate-level and low-level disinfection of small and clean surfaces of objects, equipment, and environment (e.g., rubber stoppers of medication vials, stethoscopes, and medication preparation areas). After prolonged and repeated use, alcohols may damage rubber and certain plastic items as well as the shellac mountings of lensed instruments (189). Alcoholic formulations used prior to invasive procedures should be free of spores, a process that is achieved in commercial products by filtration. Since alcohols are flammable, one should consider the flash point. They must not be used on large surfaces, particularly in closed, poorly ventilated areas.

Phenolics

Since the pioneering use of phenol (carbolic acid) as an antiseptic by Lister, a large number of phenol derivatives (or phenolics) have been developed and marketed. Phenol derivatives originate when a functional group (e.g., alkyl, benzyl, phenyl, amyl, or chloro) replaces one of the hydrogen atoms on the aromatic ring. The three phenolics most commonly found as constituents of disinfectants are o-phenylphenol, o-benzyl-p-chlorophenol, and p-tert-amylphenol. The addition of detergents to the basic formulation results in products with excellent detergent properties that clean, dissolve proteins, and disinfect in one step. Phenolics at higher concentrations act as a gross protoplasmic poison, penetrating and disrupting the bacterial cell wall and precipitating the cell proteins (165). Lower concentrations of these compounds inactivate cellular enzyme systems and cause leakage of essential metabolites from the cell. Phenol compounds at concentrations of 2 to 5% are generally considered bactericidal, tuberculocidal, fungicidal, and virucidal against lipophilic viruses (165). However, the manufacturers' efficacy claims against microorganisms have generally not been verified by independent laboratories or EPA (189). A collaborative study by Rutala and Cole documented the fact that randomly selected EPA-registered phenolic detergents and quaternary ammonium compounds do not consistently meet the manufacturers' bactericidal label claims (192). By the AOAC use-dilution method, the phenolics tested at the recommended use dilution failed against *P. aeruginosa* in 33 to 78% of the laboratories. However, extreme variability of test results has been observed among laboratories testing identical products (192). Phenolics at in-use dilutions are not lethal to bacterial spores. A 2% phenolic was shown to kill a wide spectrum of clinically important fungi except *Aspergillus fumigatus* (226). Klein and DeForest found that 12% o-phenylphenol was effective only against lipophilic viruses, although 5% phenol inactivated both lipophilic and hydrophilic viruses (126). Similarly, other investigators demonstrated little or no virucidal effect of a phenolic against coxsackievirus type B4, echovirus type 11, or poliovirus type 1 (163). Martin et al. showed that a 0.5% commercial phenolic formulation (2.8% o-phenylphenol and 2.7% o-benzyl-p-chlorophenol) inactivated HIV (149). In contrast, another commercial product containing phenolics at a final concentration of 1% failed to completely inactivate cell-associated HIV suspended in blood (71). A phenol-based preparation (14.7% phenol diluted 1:256 in tap water) produced a reduction in rotavirus numbers similar to that achieved with a bleach dilution (800 ppm available chlorine) (210). In a further experiment, both the phenolic compound and bleach were able to interrupt the transfer of virus from disks to fingerpads (210). Phenolic compounds are relatively tolerant of anionic and organic matter. They are absorbed by rubber and plastics and leave a residual film. The residual films may cause irritation to the skin and tissues. Depigmentation of the skin caused by preparations containing p-tert-butylphenol and p-tert-amylphenol has been reported. Although differences between the various compounds exist, phenolics are degraded in wastewater at a lower rate than other germicides. Therefore, environmental concerns limit their use in Europe. Phenolic germicidal detergent solutions may be used for intermediate-level and low-level disinfection of surgical instruments and noncritical patient care items. These compounds are also appropriate for the decontamination of the hospital environment, including laboratory surfaces. Their use in nurseries is problematic since hyperbilirubinemia has occurred in phenol-exposed infants. Infant bassinets and incubators should not be disinfected with phenols (189).

Quaternary Ammonium Compounds

A wide variety of quaternary ammonium compounds (quats) exhibiting antimicrobial activity has been introduced in the past decade. Some of the compounds used in health care settings are benzalkonium chloride, alkyldimethylbenzyl ammonium chloride, and didecyldimethyl ammonium chloride. Quats are cationic surface-active detergents. Their biocidal actions appear to result from the disruption of the cell membrane, inactivation of enzymes, and denaturation of cell proteins (156). Quats are nonstaining, odorless, noncorrosive, and relatively nontoxic. However, they have a limited antimicrobial spectrum. Products sold as hospital disinfectants are not sporicidal and are generally not tuberculocidal or virucidal against hydrophilic viruses. Scientific investigations by the AOAC use-dilution method have failed to reproduce the bactericidal and tuberculocidal claims made by manufacturers of quats (193). Manufacturers' label claims and results from in-house evaluations not verified by an independent laboratory should be considered questionable. The overestimation of the germicidal activity may be related to incomplete inactivation of the compounds tested. In this case, the bacteriostatic (inhibitory) activity rather than the bactericidal activity is measured (156). Several outbreaks of infections associated with in-use contamination of quat solutions have been reported. In those solutions, gram-negative bacteria such as *Pseudomonas* spp. and *S. marcescens* were found to survive or grow (79, 162). The contaminated solutions were used for antisepsis on skin and tissue as well as for disinfection of patient care supplies or equipment (i.e., cardiac catheters and cystoscopes). In fact, the quat cetrimide is used in selective media to isolate *P. aeruginosa* in microbiology laboratories. Genes conferring resistance to quats have been detected in 6 to 42% of *S. aureus* isolates collected in Japan and Europe (151). Organic matter, anionic detergents (soaps), and materials such as cotton and gauze pads can reduce the microbiocidal activities of quats. However, quats are excellent cleaning agents. On the basis of their limited antimicrobial spectra, their use in hospitals should be restricted to ordinary environmental sanitation of noncritical surfaces such as floors, furniture, and walls (189) if disinfection of the innate environment is deemed necessary.

Other Germicides of Interest

Glucoprotamine is the conversion product of L-glutamic acid and cocopropylene-1,3-diamine. It possesses a broad antimicrobial spectrum that includes vegetative bacteria, mycobacteria, fungi, and enveloped viruses (67, 158). A clinical study examining used specula from a gynecologic clinic demonstrated the product's >6-log-unit killing of vegetative bacteria excluding spores (A. F. Widmer and R. Frei, *Prog. Abstr. 40th Intersci. Conf. Antimicrob. Agents Chemother.*, abstr. 2329, 2000). Results from the manufacturer's data sheets indicate good compatibility of the compound with humans and the environment as well as various materials. A commercial product is available in Europe for disinfection of instruments and endoscopes.

Peroxygen compounds have been claimed to be effective against a wide variety of microorganisms including bacterial spores. A 1% concentration of a new commercial formulation containing peroxygen achieved a 10^5-fold killing of *B. subtilis* in 2 to 3 h in the absence of blood, but killing was poor in the presence of blood (57). Griffiths et al. have found that peroxygen has poor mycobactericidal activity (95). Likewise, concentrations of 2.3 and 4% and exposure times ranging between 30 and 120 min were not able to inactivate mycobacteria in another study (38).

Superoxidized water is prepared at the point of use by the electrolysis of NaCl solution. The major products generated are hypochlorous acid and a mixture of radicals with strong oxidizing properties. A commercial adaption of this process, i.e., Sterilox, has been recently introduced in the United Kingdom (see "Endoscopes" below) (160). Freshly generated solutions were found to be highly effective and rapidly destroy bacteria including spores and mycobacteria, fungi, and viruses in the absence of organic loading (216). Since Sterilox solutions are unstable, they should be used only once for high-level disinfection. Superoxidized water is claimed to be nondamaging to the environment, nonirritating to the respiratory tract and skin, noncorrosive, and instrument compatible. However, damage to flexible endoscopes has been observed. Further studies are needed to explore the use of this new disinfectant in clinical settings.

Metals such as copper and silver ions inactivate a wide variety of microorganisms (205). Although further work is required, they are used for disinfection of water or medical devices (e.g., intravascular catheters impregnated with silver sulfadiazine). Surfacine is a new silver-based surface germicide that may be applied to inanimate or animate surfaces. Treatment of surfaces resulted not only in immediate elimination of microorganisms but also in long-term residual activity (201). The biocidal activity was retained even when the surface was subjected to repeated dry or wet wiping. In contrast to other topically applied silver compounds, Surfacine transfers the active biocide directly to the microorganism without elution of silver ions into solution. This novel antimicrobial coating might be suitable for a wide range of applications including the prevention of microbial contamination of medical devices if further studies confirm the promising preliminary data.

A more comprehensive review of disinfectants may be found in two renowned references (31, 188). The mode of action and mechanisms of microbial resistance to disinfectants and antiseptics have been recently reviewed by McDonnell and Russell (154). Rutala and Weber have published guidelines for the selection and use of disinfectants and recommendations on the preferred method for disinfection and sterilization of patient care items (189, 190, 237).

Specific Issues

Decontamination in the Event of Biological Terrorism

Intentional release of a harmful biological agent represents one of the most serious terrorist threats. Among numerous biological agents with potential to be used as weapons, the highest priority agents include organisms that pose a risk to national security, i.e., variola major virus (smallpox), *Bacillus anthracis* (anthrax), *Yersinia pestis* (plague), *Clostridium botulinum* toxin (botulism), *Francisella tularensis* (tularemia), and certain filoviruses and arenaviruses (viral hemorrhagic fever). Consensus-based recommendations on medical and public health management following the release of these agents have been recently published (16, 65, 106, 114, 115). Additional and updated information about responding to bioterrorism is available in chapter 10 of this Manual. After the release of a biological agent, environmental decontamination measures may be necessary to decrease the risk of secondary transmission or spreading of the disease. A decontamination agent should be microbiologically effective and readily available at reasonable cost. Therefore, sodium hypochlorite (household bleach) is usually recommended, especially when bacterial spores are involved. It is well suited for various decontamination procedures in the laboratory and health care setting. In

addition, it may be used for decontamination of protective equipment and clothing which should be worn by emergency first responders and decontamination workers.

Smallpox virus does not survive long in the environment but may remain viable for extended periods under favorable conditions. CDC guidelines recommend the following decontamination procedures: sterilization by autoclaving or by ethylene oxide, incineration, vaporization of paraformaldehyde (or use of an Amphyl fogger) to decontaminate spaces and rooms, and use of a 5% aqueous solution of a phenolic germicidal detergent to soak equipment or wipe down surfaces (http://www.bt.cdc.gov/DocumentsApp/Smallpox/RPG/GuideF/Guide-F.pdf). Other disinfectants that are used for standard hospital infection control, such as sodium hypochlorite and quaternary ammonium compounds, are also effective for surface decontamination (106). Since contaminated clothing and bed linen will have spread the virus to personnel who handled laundry, all bedding and clothing of patients must be autoclaved (106). If this is not feasible, they should be laundered in hot water to which bleach has been added. Only vaccinated personnel should perform the decontamination procedures. *B. anthracis* spores have been shown to be extremely stable. Following an intentional release in connection with military tests, they persisted and remained viable for decades in the environment (115). Spores require sterilization procedures, incineration, or sporicidal disinfectants to ensure killing. CDC recommends a 1:10-diluted hypochlorite solution for routine decontamination of spills, items, and surfaces when working with *B. anthracis* in the laboratory (http://www.bt.cdc.gov/Agent/Anthrax/LevelAProtocol/Anthracis20010417.pdf). Decontamination of a building or of large areas contaminated with anthrax spores is extremely difficult. For cleaning environmental surfaces contaminated with infected bodily fluids, however, the standard disinfectants registered for surface disinfection in hospitals are effective (115). *C. botulinum* and its spores are killed by a 1:10 dilution of sodium hypochlorite. Heat (≥85°C for 5 min) or 0.1 M sodium hydroxide (contact time, 20 min) inactivates the toxin (16). Persons with direct exposure to powder or liquid aerosols containing *F. tularensis* should wash body surfaces and clothing with soapy water (65). In the circumstances of a laboratory spill or intentional release, environmental surfaces can be decontaminated with a 1:10-diluted hypochlorite solution. After 10 min, a 70% alcohol solution can be used to further clean the area and reduce the corrosive action of the bleach (65). *Y. pestis* does not survive long outside the host. In a World Health Organization worst-case scenario, a plague aerosol was estimated to be effective and infectious for as long as 1 h. Thus, there is no evidence that environmental decontamination of an area exposed to an aerosol of *Y. pestis* is indicated (114). The list of potential bioterrorism agents also includes the causative agents of Ebola hemorrhagic fever and Marburg hemorrhagic fever (filoviruses), as well as Lassa fever and related diseases (arenaviruses and *Bunyaviridae*). CDC has published guidelines for the management of patients with suspected viral hemorrhagic fever (45). Contaminated equipment or environmental surfaces should be disinfected using a suitable registered hospital disinfectant or a 1:100 dilution of a hypochlorite solution. Serum used in laboratory tests should be pretreated with polyethylene glycol *p-tert*-octylphenyl ether (Triton X-100). Treatment with 10 μl of 10% Triton X-100 per ml of serum for 1 h reduces the titer of hemorrhagic fever viruses in serum. Special precautions are required to avoid contamination of specimen containers (45).

Endoscopes

The shortcomings encountered with the reprocessing of endoscopes are well known, but outbreaks and even outbreaks with deaths continue to be reported. It is probably the most challenging issue in reprocessing for infection control professionals. Flexible endoscopes have an intricate design and have sophisticated small parts that are difficult to clean, but cleaning is a prerequisite for any disinfection process. A large study in several U.S. centers found that 78% of the facilities failed to sterilize all biopsy forceps. In addition, a total of 23.9% of the cultures of specimens from the internal channels of 71 gastrointestinal endoscopes grew $\geq 10^6$ CFU of bacteria (122). These specimens were obtained after the completion of all disinfection and sterilization procedures, and the device had been deemed ready for use on the next patient. Up to 40% of the institutions do not follow published guidelines for endoscope disinfection, thus explaining the frequency of outbreaks (Table 6) (10, 75, 91, 191). In addition, reuse of disposable endoscopic accessories is common in the United States. Items are frequently not sterilized, protocols are not standardized, and therefore reuse of disposable items might become a source of cross-transmission (55). Rigorous mechanical cleaning of the outside of the insertion tube and of all accessible channels is imperative before disinfection. Organic material such as blood, feces, and respiratory secretions may contribute to disinfection failures. Several authors raised concerns about the transmission of C. *difficile* by contaminated endoscopes that may not be fully inactivated by standard reprocessing procedures. However, no cases have been published so far. Likewise, cryptosporidia withstand several hours of exposure to glutaraldehyde (245) but do not survive on dry surfaces (179). Therefore, endoscopes should be stored in a vertical position to facilitate drying. Furthermore, endoscopes should be preferably kept in a cabinet to protect them from dust and accumulation of residual moisture and secondary contamination. More than 20% of all damage to endoscopes is associated with disinfecting agents. Therefore, compatibility of the instrument with the disinfectant is crucial to avoid damage to this expensive equipment (55).

Ample data indicate that a sufficient level of safety can be achieved even with manual disinfection of endoscopes if the guidelines are strictly followed (150). A minimum requirement for an institution is to provide sufficient training for the HCW responsible for endoscope reprocessing. It should include written instructions concerning cleaning, use of disinfectants, immersion times with special attention to all channels, and a system for basic quality assurance. Details are summarized by FDA (http://www.fda.gov/cdrh/safety/endoreprocess.html). Immersion for ≥ 20 min in $\geq 2\%$ glutaraldehyde is required to disinfect endoscopes belonging to the semicritical items. This exposure time and the concentration of glutaraldehyde are sufficient to kill ≥ 3 log units of mycobacteria, the most resistant vegetative bacteria. However, there are reports of glutaraldehyde-resistant mycobacteria, requiring that more stringent guidelines be used to monitor the effectiveness of the disinfection process (95). The glutaraldehyde concentration decreased by more than 50% after 2 weeks in a commercial cleaner-disinfector, promoting the emergence of resistant bacteria (229). Higher concentrations of glutaraldehyde (3.2% instead of 2%) appear to be safe for endoscopes and achieve the required ≥ 3-log-unit killing with a higher margin of safety than achieved with the standard concentration (5). OPA containing 0.55% 1,2-benzenedicarboxaldehyde has several advantages compared to glutaraldehyde (see above): it is stable over a wide pH range of 3 to 9, does not require activation, and is nonirritating to the eyes and nasal passages. Another newer formulation cleared by FDA is peracetic acid plus hydrogen peroxide. Such disinfectants might be corrosive to some endoscopes, and therefore the manufacturer of the endoscope should approve this disinfectant for reprocessing. Endoscopes should be thoroughly rinsed after manual disinfection to remove

TABLE 6 Outbreaks and pseudo-outbreaks associated with contaminated endoscopes or instruments for minimally invasive procedures

Microorganisms	No. of cases	No. of deaths	Yr of publication	Problem identified	Type of outbreak	Reference(s)
M. *xenopi*	58	0	2001	Inappropriate disinfection, use of tap water to rinse before and after disinfection of primarily microsurgical instruments	Disease	19
P. *aeruginosa*	11	2	2000	Failure of washer/disinfector, purchasing without expert advice, poor maintenance	Disease	200, 213
P. *aeruginosa*/mycobacteria	29	0	1999	Problems related to the use of STERIS System 1 processor	Mixed	49
HCV	2	0	1997	Cleaning, immersion	Disease	39
M. *tuberculosis*	2	0	1997	Cleaning, immersion	Disease	159
M. *tuberculosis* (multidrug resistant)	5	1	1997	Cleaning, immersion	Disease	3
P. *aeruginosa*	23	0	1996	Failure of washer-disinfector	Pseudo-outbreak	29
Nontuberculous mycobacteria	4	0	1992	Failure of washer-disinfector	Pseudo-outbreak	
Multiple microorganisms	377	7	1993	Cleaning, immersion, use of tap water, design errors of washer-disinfector	Disease	217 (review)

any residual disinfectant, specifically glutaraldehyde. Otherwise, patients may be exposed to potentially harmful concentrations of glutaraldehyde, resulting in sporadic cases and even outbreaks of colitis (69, 238). Manual reprocessing is more prone to leave residual glutaraldehyde on endoscopes than is the use of automated washer-disinfectors (74). The use of nonimmersable endoscopes is discouraged by FDA (10).

The inherent problem of human errors in manual reprocessing promoted the use of automated washers-disinfectors specifically for endoscopes. They rinse the instruments, clean them in several steps, and run a full-cycle disinfection process. In addition, the time of exposure to disinfectants is given by the machine and cannot be shortened, as it can with manual reprocessing in a busy endoscopy unit. However, none of the current machines fulfill all the demands of infection control professionals. In a study of endoscope washers, microbiological cultures demonstrated growth of gram-negative bacteria and/or mycobacteria in 27% of cultures of specimens obtained before the final alcohol rinse and in 10% of cultures of specimens obtained thereafter. In the same study with specimens obtained at the same times as described above, 37 and 27% of the manually disinfected endoscopes remained contaminated, respectively (80). In 1992, 835 Olympus endoscope washers were recalled: the design of the device allowed colonization by waterborne organisms such as *Pseudomonas* spp. in the internal tanks and tubing (recall no. Z-039/040-2 by FDA). In 1999, CDC reported three outbreaks related to the STERIS SYSTEM 1 (49). This device is supposed to sterilize the endoscopes. However, this machine requires sufficient manual cleaning before using, which introduces the risks for human error (35). Noncompliance with the manufacturer's directions, design flaws, and, most likely, insufficient training of HCWs explain why even today contaminated endoscopes are used on patients after reprocessing in a washer-disinfector. Therefore, extensive review of the current marketed products is crucial before buying a new product (20).

Newer washers-disinfectors should at least continuously monitor the pressure in all channels to detect debris blocking the channels, provide adapters for all kind of endoscopes, use an appropriate disinfection process with an FDA-cleared disinfectant, use filtered water or sterile water for rinsing, and have a built-in automatic disinfection process. FDA recommends the following. The manufacturer should provide a list of all brands and models of endoscopes that are compatible with the washer-disinfector and highlight limitations associated with processing of certain brands and models of endoscopes and accessories. Preferably, they should identify endoscopes and accessories that cannot be reliably reprocessed in the device (negative list). In addition, HCWs should be trained and monitored in the appropriate technique. Although not mandatory, it is prudent to regularly culture the rinsing water of washer-disinfectors for pathogens such as *Pseudomonas* spp. and *Mycobacterium* spp. to identify problems before clinical cases occur. Residual glutaraldehyde may also result in outbreaks after sigmoidoscopy, if water is recycled (101). The latest generation of washers-disinfectors facilitates traceability by monitoring and documenting the disinfecting process similar to autoclaves. Superoxidized water (Sterilox) has similar microbiocidal activity compared to glutaraldehyde and is nontoxic, and nonsensitizing (160). The main products are hypochlorous acid at a concentration of approximately 144 mg/liter and free chlorine radicals. This disinfectant has a pH of 5.0 to 6.5 and is generated at the point of use by passing a saline solution over titanium-coated electrodes with an oxidation-reduction potential of >950 mV. The device is used in the United Kingdom. FDA clearance was pending in 2002. Guidelines for infection prevention and control in flexible endoscopies have recently been updated (10) and should be consulted before choosing a method and/or disinfectant for reprocessing. A checklist adapted from the FDA recommendations may help to avoid errors (http://www.fda.gov/cdrh/safety/endoreprocess.html):

1. All staff must comply with the manufacturer's instructions for cleaning endoscopes.

2. Check if your endoscope is suitable for reprocessing in an automatic washer-disinfector. This is the preferred method.

3. Compare the reprocessing instructions provided by the endoscope and washer-disinfector manufacturers, and resolve any conflicting recommendations.

4. Follow the manufacturer's manual reprocessing instructions for endoscopes as well as the recommendations of the manufacturer of the chemical germicides.

5. Consider incorporating a final drying step in your reprocessing protocol with alcohol.

6. Monitor adherence to the protocols for reprocessing endoscopes.

7. Provide comprehensive and intensive training for all staff assigned to reprocessing endoscopes. Keep records of training.

8. Implement a comprehensive quality control program.

An updated list of sterilants and high-level disinfectants cleared by FDA in a 510 (k) with general claims for processing reusable medical and dental devices can be found on the FDA homepage (http://www.fda.gov/cdrh/ode/germlab.html). Rutala and Weber have added important comments to these FDA cleared substances (200, 201). Endoscopes sent for repairs should be labeled as "contaminated equipment for repair."

Dental Equipment

Dental patients and HCWs may be exposed to a variety of microorganisms by contact with dental instruments or by direct contact with blood or respiratory secretions. Therefore, blood-borne and airborne pathogens are of concern. The most likely mode of transmission is via droplets from infected patients. Typical microorganisms include cytomegalovirus, HBV, HCV, herpes simplex virus types 1 and 2, HIV, and M. *tuberculosis*. Staphylococci and streptococci are commonly isolated but are rarely involved in infections. Pathogens may be transmitted by direct contact with blood, oral fluids, or other secretions; indirect contact with contaminated instruments, operatory equipment, or environmental surfaces; or contact with airborne contaminants present in droplets. Current recommendations are summarized in a report published by CDC in 1993 (48) and a publication of the American Dental Association (ADA) (1). Several issues are outlined: wearing of gloves during procedures, hand disinfection or hand washing between patients, use of a surgical mask and protective eyewear when splashing is likely, and wearing of laboratory coats. The water delivered to patients during nonsurgical dental procedures should consistently contain no more than 200 CFU of aerobic mesophilic heterotrophic bacteria per ml. Critical and semicritical instruments should be sterilized and packaged prior to sterilization if they are not used immediately. The adequacy of sterilization cycles should be verified by the periodic use (e.g., at least weekly) of biological indicators. This recommendation is rarely followed in Europe (97). In fact, 33% of British dentist practices have no policy on general disinfection and sterilization procedures and only 3% own a vacuum autoclave (21).

Routine between-patient sterilization is recommended for all high-speed dental handheld pieces. Handheld pieces that cannot be heat sterilized should be retrofitted to attain heat tolerance; if this is not feasible, they should not be used. Alcohol (70 to 80%) is preferred in Europe for uncovered operating surfaces because of its rapid action (within seconds) and evaporation, but other EPA-registered disinfectants can be used as well. Legionella spp. can contaminate the air-water syringes and high-speed outlets: In one study, 25% of the water samples were contaminated (51). In addition, more than 6% of samples from workbenches, air turbine handheld pieces, holders, suction units, forceps, and dental mirrors were found by PCR to be positive for HCV, indicating extensive HCV contamination of dental surgeries after treatment of HCV-positive patients (169). Therefore, infection control issues, particularly in regard to HCV and HBV, may be more important in dentistry than has been appreciated previously.

ADA recommends immersion or exposure of metal/porcelain in glutaraldehyde and of removable dentures and acrylic/porcelain in iodophors or chlorine compounds. Wax rims or bite plates can be disinfected by a spray containing iodophors. HCWs should have been vaccinated against HBV. Additional information can be found on the homepage of the ADA (http://www.ada.org/prof/prac/issues/topics/icontrol/ic-recs/index.html).

Disinfectants for Living Tissue
Compounds that disinfect living tissue are frequently called antiseptic agents. They must meet many more requirements than compounds used for disinfection of inanimate surfaces, e.g., floors. In addition, some of the agents are considered drugs and thus are regulated by FDA. The antimicrobial spectra of commercially available agents are summarized in Table 5. The choice of the agent should not only be based on their desired effect but should also include consideration of side effects, similar to the case of antibiotics. An example is the observation of anaphylactic shock after the application of chlorhexidine to patients (72, 167). However, side effects are rare, and most agents on the market have excellent safety profiles. Nevertheless, the potential for side effects should be kept in mind when antiseptic agents are used.

Hygienic Hand Washing and Hand Disinfection
The most important issue is not the mechanism of hand washing or hand disinfection or the choice of the disinfectant but the need to motivate the HCW to perform this simple procedure when necessary. Indications for hand washing or disinfection were classified in a hierarchical order by CDC in 1985 and by professional organizations (137). Microorganisms on the hands can be classified into three groups (172): (i) transient flora, which are contaminants taken up from the environment; (ii) resident flora, which are permanent microorganisms on the skin (241); and (iii) the infectious flora. The goal of hand washing or hand disinfection outside the OR is to eliminate the transient flora. Long-term reduction is not desirable, because it may alter the resident flora. The surgical hand scrub or hand disinfection aims to eliminate both transient and resident flora. Hand washing or hand disinfection repre-

sents the single most important procedure for infection control (137). The density of resident bacteria on the skin ranges between 10^2 and 10^3 CFU/cm^2. These resident bacteria limit colonization with more pathogenic microorganisms. The pathogenicity is low, and infections with these bacteria usually require some physical alteration of the host immunity such as placement of an implant or any foreign body. This function is called colonization resistance. HCWs can acquire pathogens from patients during their daily work and can transmit them to susceptible patients. Multiple epidemics have been traced to contaminated hands of HCWs (34, 203, 209, 243, 248). Most of the resident flora is found on the uppermost level of the stratum corneum. The hands of HCWs are frequently contaminated by direct contact while caring for a patient or indirect contact while touching a contaminated surface or device. Several studies indicated that pathogens can be found on the hands of HCWs, such as S. aureus in ≥18% of HCWs (177) and Klebsiella pneumoniae (2), Acinetobacter spp., Enterobacter spp., or Candida spp. in more than 20% of HCWs. Therefore, CDC has set a high priority for hand washing and has issued specific recommendations. Most research was guided by problems concerning effectiveness and compliance with hand washing (68). Studies have proved that a rub-in with a "waterless" alcoholic compound is much more effective at killing bacteria and most viruses than hand washing with a medicated soap (25, 183). However, no sound epidemiological data have demonstrated that a certain level of killing is needed to have an impact on the incidence of nosocomial infection. The level of compliance with hand-washing procedures does not exceed 40% even under controlled study conditions (94, 134). Recent studies prove that compliance with the alcoholic rub-in exceeds that of hand washing (171). Interventions against the bacterial load of the skin should balance two goals: protection of the skin with its resident flora and killing of the transient flora. Intact skin on the hands of HCWs helps to protect both patients and HCWs from contracting or transmitting nosocomial infections. Therefore, any recommendation for hand washing or a hand rub with alcohol should include some advice for skin care, for example, by making a skin care product available free of charge for HCWs. Compliance with hand-washing procedures also depends on the time necessary to adequately perform hand washing and the time available. Hand washing for 15 and 30 s achieves levels of microbial killing of 0.6 to 1.1 and 1.8 to 2.8 log units, respectively (185). However, hand washing for less than 10 s is common in clinical practice, resulting in potentially insufficient killing of the transient flora (135). In fact, a mathematical model estimated that the time required to perform a rub-in with alcohol is only 26% of that required to perform regular hand washing (240). This model was subsequently tested in a tertiary-care center, and similar time savings were observed (231). In addition, a rub-in with alcohol achieves a much higher microbial killing than hand washing does (239). These in vitro and experimental data have also been supported in a crossover clinical trial with surgeons (A. F. Widmer, M. Perschmann, T. C. Gasser, and R. Frei, Program Abstr. 34th Intersci. Conf. Antimicrob. Agents Chemother., abstr. J180, 1994). In addition, sinks are expensive and cannot be installed at locations that are as convenient for HCWs as disinfectant dispensers. HCWs can even contaminate the faucets, as was observed during a Shigella outbreak (157). Therefore, health care institutions in northern Europe have replaced hand washing with alcohol rub-in for many indications for which hand washing was previously the standard of care. At the authors' institution, a rub-in with alcohol replaced hand washing in 85% of opportunities for hand washing, provided that the hands were not visibly soiled (A. Trampuz, N. Lederray, and A. F. Widmer, *Program Abstr. 41st Intersci. Conf. Antimicrob. Agents Chemother.*, abstr. K1335, 2001). An alcohol dispenser is available between all beds at each nurse's desk, and two are available at each bed in intensive care units. A database of the 4,500 HCWs did not identify a single case of documented allergy to the commercial alcohol compound in use, resulting in an incidence density of <1:45,000 person-years. Additional background information has been recently published (241), and a guideline by the CDC is available on the internet (www.cdc.gov).

Surgical Hand Washing (Scrub) or Surgical Hand Disinfection (Rub-in)

The objective of the surgical scrub is to eliminate the transient flora and most of the resident flora. The rationale is to limit bacterial exposure of the surgeon's skin in case the surgical glove is punctured or torn. Tiny holes are observed in ≥ 30% of surgeons' gloves after an operation, even when high-quality gloves are used. In a large study, the incidence of surgical site infection (SSI) after clean surgery was related to punctures in the surgeon's gloves: the incidence of SSI was three times higher if a puncture of the surgeon's gloves was observed than if intact gloves were noted after the procedure (1.7 and 5.7%, respectively) (63). An experimental study demonstrated that the level of bacterial leakage through pinholes ranged between 10^3 and 10^4 CFU (82). In contrast to the hygienic hand wash, a persistent antimicrobial effect is required after washing or disinfection to limit bacterial regrowth underneath the gloves (84). Therefore, agents with a prolonged postexposure effect are preferred. Chlorhexidine is one of the most frequently used agents. However, no controlled clinical trials have demonstrated that it has an impact on the incidence of SSIs. Ethical reasons prohibit such a study (39). In addition, multiple risk factors trigger an SSI, and therefore an extremely large study population would be necessary to quantify the effect. The water supply in the OR may harbor *Pseudomonas* spp. at the sink or the faucet aerator that might contaminate surgical hands after the surgical scrub. Alcoholic preparations are also more effective than any medicated soap for the surgical scrub (185). In addition, they do not alter the skin as much as chlorhexidine washes do (Widmer et al., *34th ICAAC*). Therefore, the presurgical scrub has been replaced in many European countries by the alcoholic rub. The antimicrobial efficacy was also much better in a clinical trial in the OR. The alcoholic compound killed bacteria significantly better than the standard scrub with a chlorhexidine soap did (Widmer et al., *34th ICAAC*). Brushes may harm more than they contribute to cleaning: their use should be restricted to cleaning the fingernails. Alcoholic gels are frequently promoted but are significantly less effective than liquids (170).

Presurgical Skin Disinfection

The aim of skin disinfection is the rapid removal and killing of the skin flora at the site of a planned surgical incision. However, currently available antiseptics do not succeed in sterilizing the operation field. In fact, coagulase-negative staphylococci can be frequently isolated even after three applications of, e.g., iodine-alcohol to the operation field (85), Therefore, routine antimicrobial prophylaxis is recommended for, e.g., orthopedic implant surgery. FDA de-

fines a skin disinfectant as a "fast acting, broad-spectrum and persistent antiseptic-containing preparation that significantly reduces the number of microorganisms on intact skin" (13). Alcohols are well suited for this purpose, but they lack long-term effects. Therefore, iodine is frequently added for this purpose (87). However, for a short-term procedure, alcoholic preparations frequently suffice for skin preparation. Alcohols used for presurgical skin preparation must be free of spores, which is usually achieved by filtration or, in some countries, by adding 0.5% hydrogen peroxide to ethanol (182). Antiseptics should be applied with pressure since friction increases the antibacterial effect: alcohol applied without friction reduces bacterial counts by 1.0 to 1.2 log CFU compared to 1.9 to 3.0 log CFU with friction. In comparison, alcoholic sprays have little antimicrobial effect and produce potentially explosive vapors (143). An extensive review was published by FDA in 1994 (13). The antiseptic should be applied using sterile supplies and gloves or by a no-touch technique, moving from the incision area to the periphery (147). Before the skin preparation of a patient is initiated, the skin should be free of gross contamination (i.e., dirt, soil, or any other debris) (147). Preoperative showering may decrease bacterial counts; it did not reduce the incidence of surgical site infections in a large study, but may help for preparation of clean skin before surgery (184).

Common Antiseptic Compounds

Alcoholic Compounds

The reader is referred to the earlier section on alcohols. As outlined above, alcohol is the most important skin disinfectant. Alcohols used for skin disinfection prior to invasive procedures should generally be free of spores to avoid any contamination. Although the risk of infection is minimal, the low additional cost for a spore-free product is justified.

Chlorhexidine

Chlorhexidine gluconate, a cationic bisbiguanide, has been widely recognized as an effective and safe antiseptic for more than 30 years (66, 176). Its most common formulation is a 4% aqueous solution in a detergent base. The antimicrobial spectrum includes vegetative bacteria, fungi, and viruses. Bactericidal concentrations cause destruction of the bacterial cell membrane, leading to leakage of cellular constituents and coagulation of cell contents (66). Chlorhexidine has been demonstrated to be bactericidal against both gram-positive and gram-negative bacteria. However, Stickler and Thomas found chlorhexidine-resistant bacteria after extensive and long-term use of chlorhexidine prior to bladder catheterization (220). Moreover, microbial contamination of 0.02 and 0.05% chlorhexidine gluconate solutions manufactured in a hospital has been documented (166). The chlorhexidine resistance of vegetative bacteria was thought to be limited to certain gram-negative bacilli (such as *P. aeruginosa*, *Burkholderia* [*Pseudomonas*] *cepacia*, *Proteus mirabilis*, and *S. marcescens*) (220). However, genes conferring resistance to various organic cations, including chlorhexidine, have been recently identified in *S. aureus* clinical isolates (151, 161). Chlorhexidine gluconate shows intermediate rapidity of bactericidal action. In addition, it provides a persistent antimicrobial action that prevents the regrowth of microorganisms for as long as 6 h. This effect is desirable when a sustained reduction in microbial flora reduces infection risk (e.g., during surgical procedures). Chlorhexidine has little activity against bacterial and fungal spores except at high temperatures. Mycobacteria are inhibited but are not killed by aqueous solutions. Yeasts and dermatophytes are usually sensitive, although the fungicidal action varies with the species (66). Chlorhexidine was effective against lipophilic viruses (e.g., HIV, influenza virus, and herpes simplex virus types 1 and 2). Other viruses, such as poliovirus, coxsackievirus, and rotavirus, were not inactivated (66). The antimicrobial activity of chlorhexidine is little affected by blood and other organic material, in contrast to povidone-iodine (142). However, inorganic anions and organic anions such as soaps are incompatible with chlorhexidine. Its activity is also reduced at an extreme acidic or alkaline pH and in the presence of anionic- and nonionic-based moisturizers and detergents. Chlorhexidine absorbed onto the fibers of cotton and certain other fabrics usually resists removal by washing. If a hypochlorite (bleach) is used during the washing procedure, a brown stain may develop (66). Long-term experience with the use of chlorhexidine has demonstrated that the incidence of hypersensitivity and skin irritation is low. However, severe allergic reactions including anaphylaxis have been reported (72, 246). Although cytotoxicity has been observed in exposed fibroblasts, no deleterious effects on wound healing were found in vivo. There is no evidence that chlorhexidine gluconate is toxic if it is absorbed through the skin. However, ototoxicity can occur when chlorhexidine is instilled into the middle ear during surgery. High concentrations and preparations containing other compounds (e.g., alcohols and surfactants) may cause eye damage (222). Chlorhexidine formulations are extensively used for surgical hand disinfection and hygienic hand disinfection. This topic is discussed above. Other applications include preoperative whole-body disinfection, antisepsis in obstetrics and gynecology, management of burns, wound antisepsis, and prevention and treatment of oral disease (plaque control, pre- and postoperative mouthwash, oral hygiene) (66, 176). It is also applied to coat intravenous catheters to prevent catheter-associated infections (145). When chlorhexidine is used orally, its bitter taste must be masked, and tooth staining usually occurs. Chlorhexidine alcoholic preparations have been demonstrated in numerous studies to have superior antimicrobial activity compared with those of detergent-based formulations (138). While they have been used in Europe and Canada for some time, chlorhexidine alcoholic products have been only recently approved by the FDA (http://www.fda.gov/cder/approva/index.htm).

Iodophors

The previously used aqueous iodine and tincture have largely been replaced by the iodophors. The risk of side effects from the use of these compounds, such as staining, irritation of tissue, and resorption, is lower than that from the use of aqueous iodine. Iodophors are chemical complexes with iodine bound to a carrier such as polyvinylpyrrolidone (povidone) or ethoxylated nonionic detergents (poloxamers). These complexes gradually release small amounts of free microbicidal iodine. The most commonly used iodophor is povidone-iodine. Its preparations generally contain 1 to 10% povidone-iodine, which is equivalent to 0.1 to 1.0% available iodine. The active component appears to be free molecular iodine (I_2). A paradoxical effect of dilution on the activity of povidone-iodine has been observed. As the dilution increases, bactericidal activity increases up to a maximum and then falls (92). Commercial povidone-iodine solutions at dilutions of 1:2 to 1:100 killed S. aureus and Mycobacterium chelonae more rapidly than the

stock solutions did (26). S. aureus survived a 2-min exposure to full-strength povidone-iodine solution but did not survive a 15-s exposure to a 1:100 dilution of the iodophor (26). Thus, iodophors must be used at the dilution stated by the manufacturer. The exact mechanism by which iodine destroys microorganisms is not known. It has been postulated that iodine reacts with amino acids and fatty acids of microorganisms, resulting in the destruction of cell structures and enzymes (92). Depending on the concentration of free iodine and other factors, iodophors exhibit a broad range of microbiocidal activity. Commercial preparations are bactericidal, mycobactericidal, fungicidal, virucidal, but not sporicidal at their dilution recommended for use. Prolonged contact times are required to inactivate certain fungi and bacterial spores (189). However, reports on intrinsic contamination of povidone-iodine and poloxamer-iodine solutions with B. (P.) cepacia or P. aeruginosa, which caused pseudobacteremia and peritonitis, have questioned the killing actions of iodophors (27, 61). B. cepacia was found to survive for up to 68 weeks in a contaminated povidone-iodine antiseptic solution (12). The most likely explanation for the prolonged survival of microorganisms in iodophor solutions is mechanical protection of microorganisms by organic and inorganic material and possibly by biofilm formation. Unlike iodine, iodophors are relatively free of toxicity effects. They do not cause irritability and do not corrode metal surfaces (92). They have little if any residual effect. However, for a limited time they may have a residual bactericidal activity on the skin surface, because free iodine diffuses not only into deep regions but also back to the skin surface (92). The antimicrobial efficacy of iodophors is reduced in the presence of organic material such as blood. A body surface treated with an iodine or iodophor solution may absorb free iodine. Consequently, increased serum iodine levels (and serum iodide levels) have been found, especially when large areas were treated for a long period (92). For this reason, hyperthyroidism and other disorders of thyroid functions are contraindications for the use of iodine-containing preparations. Likewise, iodophors should be applied neither to pregnant and nursing women nor to newborns and infants (43). Because severe local and systemic allergic reactions have been observed, iodophors and iodine should not be used in patients with allergies to these preparations (234). Iodophors are widely used for antisepsis of skin, mucous membranes, and wounds. A 2.5% ophthalmic solution of povidone-iodine was shown to be more effective and less toxic than silver nitrate or erythromycin ointment used as prophylaxis against neonatal conjunctivitis (ophthalmia neonatorum) (116). In some countries, povidone-iodine alcoholic solutions are successfully used for skin antisepsis prior to invasive procedures (15). Iodophors containing higher concentrations of free iodine may be used for disinfection of medical equipment (189). Disinfectants for antisepsis are not suitable as hard-surface disinfectants since the concentrations of these disinfectants are usually lower (189).

Triclosan and PCMX

Triclosan (irgasan DP-300, irgacare MP) has been used for more than 30 years in a wide array of skin care products, including handwashes, surgical scrubs, and consumer products. A review of its effectiveness and safety in health care settings has been recently published (119). A concentration of 1% has demonstrated good activity against gram-positive bacteria, including antibiotic-resistant strains, but a lower level of activity against gram-negative organisms, mycobacteria, and fungi. Limited data suggest that triclosan has a relatively broad antiviral spectrum, with high-level activity against enveloped viruses, such as HIV-1, influenza A virus, and herpes simplex virus type 1. However, the nonenveloped viruses proved more difficult to inactivate. Although clinical strains with low-level resistance to triclosan have emerged, the clinical significance of this remains unknown (221). Consequently, concerns have been raised that widespread use of triclosan formulations in non-health care settings and products may select for biocide resistance and even cross-resistance to antibiotics. Triclosan is increasingly being added to soaps, lotions, deodorants, toothpastes, mouthrinses, commonly used household fabrics and plastics, and medical devices. There is evidence that the triclosan resistance mechanisms are similar to those involved in antibiotic resistance. Some of them may account for the observed cross-resistance of laboratory isolates to antibiotics (56). Triclosan solutions produce a sustained residual effect against resident and transient microbial flora that is minimally affected by organic matter. Numerous studies did not show any toxic, allergenic, mutagenic, or carcinogenic potential. According to recent reports, 1% triclosan formulations might be useful in controlling methicillin-resistant S. aureus (MRSA) outbreaks when applied as a personnel handwash or as a bathing cleanser for patients (119). However, a 1% triclosan hand wash failed to eradicate MRSA on the hands of HCWs in a clinical study (73). Although triclosan formulations were shown to be less effective than 2 to 4% chlorhexidine gluconate surgical scrub solutions, properly formulated triclosan solutions may be used for hygienic hand washing.

PCMX (chloroxylenol) is also a common antimicrobial ingredient of hand-washing products. It is available at concentrations of 0.5 to 3.75%. Its properties are similar to those of triclosan. Nonionic surfactants may neutralize PCMX.

Octenidine

Octenidine dihydrochloride is a novel bispyridine compound, which is an effective and safe antiseptic agent. The 0.1% commercial formulation favorably compared with other antiseptics with respect to antimicrobial activity and toxicologic properties. It rapidly killed both gram-positive and gram-negative bacteria as well as fungi in vitro and in vivo (89, 215). Octenidine is virucidal against HIV, HBV, and herpes simplex virus. Similar to chlorhexidine, it has a marked residual effect. No toxicologic problems were found when the 0.1% formulation was applied according to the manufacturer's recommendations. The colorless solution has proved to be useful as an antiseptic for mucous membranes of the female and male genitals and the oral cavity (23). However, its bad taste severely limits its oral application. Octenidine is not registered for use in the United States.

STERILIZATION

Principles, Definitions, and Terms

As outlined in Table 3, sterilization is not a relative term but defines the complete absence of any viable microorganisms including spores. However, this absence cannot be proved by current microbiologic techniques (120). Therefore, sterilization can be defined as a closely monitored, validated process used to render a product free of all forms of viable microorganisms, including all bacterial endo-

spores. To do this, manufacturers of sterilization systems developed a worst-case scenario that allows quantification of the process (log killing) and estimates the probability of process failure. A high degree of conservatism and safety margins have been included for testing purposes. It assumes that items are heavily contaminated with large numbers of spores, soil, and proteins, a scenario that is considered a critical failure of the reprocessing cycle in clinical practice.

The following definitions are based on those of FDA and are required to understand, review, and evaluate data on sterilization. More data on and recommendations for sterilization are provided in reference books (93, 120). The basic prerequisite for any disinfection or sterilization process is reiterated because of its critical importance for adequate reprocessing: Any device undergoing sterilization *must undergo an appropriate cleaning process.* A manufacturer must demonstrate that the sterilizer is effective against a wide range of clinically important microorganisms before being cleared by FDA. In addition, proof of efficacy must be performed with organisms (usually bacterial spores) that have been shown to be the most resistant to the new technology. A validated and reliable biological indicator must be developed, and studies must establish that sterility will be consistently achieved when critical process parameters operate within a defined range. This assures the operator that as long as there is no operational error or equipment failure, sterility is achieved. The most important terms for sterilization are listed to better understand the literature (these definitions are adapted from those of FDA).

Validation: a documented program which provides a high degree of assurance that a specific process will consistently meet its predetermined specifications and quality attributes.

D value (decimal reduction value): the time required to kill 90% (one logarithmic cycle) of a specified population of microorganisms. For calculation purposes, it is assumed that the killing rate follows first-order kinetics.

F value: the time (in minutes) required to kill all the spores in suspension at a temperature of 121°C (250°F) or 132°C (270°F) in the United States (134°C in Europe). The different temperatures used in the United States and Europe are probably guided by temperatures of 121°C (250°F) and 132°C (270°F) (in the United States) or 3 atm of pressure resulting in 134°C (in Europe).

Sterility assurance level (SAL): the expected probability that a microorganism is surviving on each individual product after exposure to a validated sterilization process. SAL is expressed as 10^{-n}, where n is the probability that survivors exist. The Norm ISO 14937 requires a reduction of 10^{-6} CFU of spores at half of the normal cycle to meet the standard. This value is part of the European sterilization definition according to EN 556.

Bioburden: the number and types of viable microorganisms on a medical device prior to exposure to a cleaning and/or microbicidal process.

Kill curves of sterilization processes show a linear decrease in the numbers of CFU on a semilogarithmic scale. Therefore, the required killing is easily computed by drawing a line between measurements of microbial killing. Commercially available spores provide evidence of killing of $\geq 10^6$ CFU if no growth can be detected after an appropriate incubation. The purchases of a sterilizer can expect this level of performance if the device has been cleared by FDA and is operated according to the manufacturer's instructions. Several sources of data have been reviewed in detail and should be read before evaluating a large sterilizer (75, 120, 144, 190, 247). The ISO 11134 (moist heat) and the ISO 11135 (ethylene oxide) documents describe the standards for industrial facility use in the United States. Adaptations for health care facilities have been published by ANSI/AAMI as Standard 46 (moist heat) and Standard 41 (ethylene oxide). These standards are voluntary, but FDA expects that processing will meet the same levels of scientific soundness as these standards. In Europe, EN 550, EN 554, and EN 285 define the standards for steam and ethylene oxide sterilization.

Monitoring

Any sterilization process must be monitored by mechanical, physical, chemical, and facultatively biological methods. Monitoring includes temperature, pressure, and other methods depending on the sterilization method. Before routine use, the performance of the machine should be validated with the most difficult load used at the institution to ensure safety of the process. In addition, a printout of the physical parameters during sterilization should be kept for documentation purposes. Temperature and pressure are routinely recorded in today's sterilizers and are printed out at the end of the sterilization process. In addition, chemical indicators stacked on the tested items change their color if they were exposed to the adequate temperatures and exposure times. Their use is inexpensive and convenient, and they immediately indicate that the item has been exposed to the sterilization process. However, there is no perfect chemical indicator for inadequate sterilization. Some are too sensitive, resulting in false-positive results (194, 197); they may cause an unnecessary recall of adequately sterilized items. Less sensitive chemical indicators do not indicate small deviations in the process. However, good clinical indicators are able to identify a failure of the sterilizer.

The Bowie-Dick test originated in 1963, when Bowie and Dick determined that if residual air remained in a sterilizer after the vacuum phase and there was only one package in the chamber, the air would concentrate in that package (33). A satisfactory test indicates that steam penetration and air removal had occurred. It does not provide information about the sterilization process.

Biological indicators are recognized as being the best monitors of the sterilization process. Most organizations such as CDC and the Joint Commission on Accreditation of Healthcare Organizations (JCAHO) recommend the use of biologic indicators at least weekly. For flash sterilization, the Attest Rapid Readout biological indicator detects the presence of a spore-associated enzyme, α-D-glucosidase, and permits an assessment of sterilization effectiveness within 60 min (230). An important question is whether a load can be distributed before a biological indicator proves adequate sterilization. This is also called parametric release. The JCAHO standard allows the use of appropriate chemical indicators without routine use of a biological indicator. A common approach is to use the sterilized items on the basis of physical and chemical documentation of an adequate sterilization process and not to await the culture results of the biological indicators. A study showed the usefulness of routine biological indicators for monitoring: the biological indicators detected a failure of steam sterilization before nosocomial infections were recorded, supporting the current practice (44). In Europe, routine use of biological indicators is not required if the sterilizer has undergone testing by a validation procedure used for industrial steam sterilization (EN 285, EN 550, EN 554, EN 556). Most

sterilizers in European hospitals probably do not meet these very strict requirements, and consequently, biological indicators are regularly used. These new standards will be implemented for steam sterilization validation in health care organizations because they are already mandated for industrial steam sterilization validation, but the associated expenses are part of an ongoing dispute. The future is likely to involve parametric release with regular validation and/or commissions of the equipment. Legal aspects will probably determine the outcome of this discussion, and lawyers are likely to accept nothing but a zero risk. However, the goal of a zero risk for contamination in central sterilization services will probably contribute to excessive health care costs. Therefore, standards for sterilization should exclude a risk for contamination after the reprocessing cycle but should avoid steps that are performed only for legal reasons.

Packaging, Loading, and Storage

Once items are clean, dry, and inspected, instruments and devices must be wrapped and packaged before sterilization. Wrappers should allow penetration of steam or gas but should serve as a barrier against recontamination after sterilization. For steam, only muslin has limitations, and handling of items made of muslin leads to contamination (242). For gas sterilization, only wrappers approved for use in the sterilization process should be used. Items should be labeled with information, including details of the reprocessing cycle and an expiration date.

Steam Sterilization

The most reliable method of sterilization is one that uses saturated steam under pressure. It is inexpensive, nontoxic, and very reliable; penetrates fabrics; and has an inherent safety margin much higher than that of any other sterilization technique. Therefore, it should be used whenever possible. Pressurized steam destroys microorganisms by irreversible coagulation and denaturation of enzymes and proteins. The pressure allows one to achieve dry 100% saturated steam, without water in the form of a fine mist. Dry air does not provide steam for condensation, and the heat transfer to objects is slowed down. Obviously, this technique cannot be used for plastic, rubber, or objects that are sensitive to heat or moisture, limiting the use of the method for many devices and instruments. The process of sterilization has several cycles: conditioning, exposure, and drying cycle. Common cycles for prevacuum or flash-pressure pulsing steam sterilizers are 121°C for 15 min (121°C for 30 min in a gravity displacement sterilizer) or 132°C for 4 min (FDA addendum to the Sterilizer Guidance, 19 September 1995). The machine should provide this temperature anywhere in the chamber within a narrow margin (0 to +3°C on the basis of EN 554). Several types of autoclaves are available: gravity displacement steam sterilization, prevacuum steam sterilization, and steam flash-pressure pulsing steam sterilization autoclaves. The problem with gravity displacement steam sterilization is the unpredictable performance of the sterilization process (62). Insufficient air removal before the addition of steam at the correct temperature is much more likely with gravity displacement autoclaves than with the more sophisticated systems. The introduction of the prevacuum sterilizer resolved part of the problem and cut the cycle time in half. However, the effectiveness of sterilization can be compromised by small leaks (1 to 10 mm Hg/min) in the sterilizer (120). The most current technology is the steam flash pressure pulsing steam sterilization technique because air leaks do not decrease the effectiveness of the process. It almost eliminates the most important remaining risk in steam sterilization: air in the chamber (62). The steam flash pressure pulsing steam sterilization technique is most useful for general use, since it reduces the thermal lag upon heating of the load to the desired exposure temperature. Detailed reviews including all details on requirements, monitoring, and maintenance of large steam sterilizers have been published (120, 125, 247) and are included in EN 285.

A hot topic is flash sterilization, an emergency process used, for example, after a surgical instrument is dropped but needs to be immediately available during a procedure (144). It exposes unwrapped devices to pressurized steam for 3 min, usually in the OR area, sometimes without a biological indicator. The autoclaves employed are gravity displacement sterilizers that have the problems mentioned above. Flash sterilization is sometimes performed by HCWs without appropriate training. Therefore, several investigators have suggested that this method be strictly limited to emergency situations when no other device from the institution's central sterilization service is available. It is not intended to replace routine regular sterilization because of ease of use and speed (76). As outlined above, the cleaning process may not be observed, which is a prerequisite for an appropriate reprocessing cycle with steam sterilization, and lack of protective packaging can render the device unsterile even after a successful sterilization. In addition, even properly wrapped sterile items can become contaminated if they are transported several times (242) and patient injuries as a result of flash sterilization have been reported (202). Flash sterilization should not be used for reasons of convenience such as avoiding the purchase of extra instrument sets or time saving (147).

Three parameters are critical to ensuring steam sterilization: time of exposure to steam, temperature, and moisture. The D value determines the time frame required to achieve killing of 10^6 CFU of spores most resistant to the sterilization process under study. The temperature is critical for the process. The temperature of any device or instrument must reach the desired temperature, which is not necessarily identical to the gauge display of the autoclave. A drop of only 1.7°C (3°F) results in a 48% increase in the time required to sterilize an item. Pressurized steam allows quick energy transfer to the sterilizer load and, probably, the more rapid denaturation and coagulation of proteins. Without moisture, a temperature of 160°C is required for dry heat sterilization. Therefore, residual air interferes with the sterilization process. Unlike time and temperature, the moisture condition in the autoclave cannot be directly determined. The amount of air within the sterilizer can be estimated by comparing the chamber pressure with the saturated steam pressure calculated from the average chamber temperature. A measured pressure greater than the calculated saturated pressure indicates the presence of residual air in the chamber. Such monitoring devices are common in the United Kingdom.

Ethylene Oxide Gas

Temperature- and/or pressure-sensitive items were traditionally sterilized with ethylene oxide in a standard gas sterilizer that used Freon as a carrier gas. As of 1 January 1996, however, the Clean Air Act banned the use of chlorofluorocarbons as sterilant gases, calling for the use of alternatives for heat-sensitive items and devices. Alternatives include ethylene oxide sterilizers that use 100% ethylene oxide or sterilizers that use other technologies. Ethylene oxide is flammable, explosive, and carcinogenic to laboratory animals, and it requires the use of additional safety precautions. Nitrogen gas is added to remove air from the chamber, or the chamber is evacuated. Items to be sterilized are usually exposed to ethylene oxide at 55°C (130°F). They are then aerated for approximately 12 h to remove any traces of the gas. The total process takes >16 h. Ethylene oxide inactivates all microorganisms including spores, probably by an alkylation process. B. subtilis bacterial spores are among the most resistant, and therefore these are used as a biological monitor. Ethylene oxide is useful only as a surface sterilizer; it is unable to reach blocked-off surfaces. The use of ethylene oxide requires the careful and simultaneous control of six variable but interdependent parameters: gas concentration, vacuum, pressure, temperature, relative humidity, and time of exposure. The gas concentration cannot be measured on-line, limiting the extent of monitoring. Therefore, validation of the concentration is recommended. Another issue is the toxic residues trapped in the wrapper or the items. Polyvinyl chloride and polyurethane are examples of very high absorbers of ethylene oxide. They require long periods to dissipate the oxide. The wrapper itself should be a barrier against recontamination after sterilization, but it also serves as a potential barrier to the access of ethylene oxide to the item. Therefore, only materials with documented ethylene oxide penetration and dissipation properties should be used. The future of ethylene oxide in sterilization is limited, mainly due to environmental concerns surrounding its toxicity. However, plasma sterilization (see below) can only partially replace sterilization with ethylene oxide. No currently available technology could completely replace ethylene oxide. In addition, sterilization with ethylene oxide does not fail as frequently as sterilization with plasma in the presence of residual proteins and/or salts (9). A new rapid-readout ethylene oxide biological indicator will indicate an ethylene oxide sterilization process failure by producing a fluorescence change, which is detected in an autoreader within 4 h of incubation at 37°C, and a visual pH color change of the growth media within 96 h of continued incubation (201).

Plasma Sterilization

Plasma describes any gas that consists of electrons, ions, or neutral particles. The formation of a low-temperature plasma requires a closed chamber, a deep vacuum, and a chemical precursor from which to derive the plasma. In addition, a source of electromagnetic energy, such as radiofrequency energy, creates an electromagnetic field that generates the plasma. The electromagnetic field interacts with the chemical (hydrogen peroxide or a mixture with peracetic acid) and induces the plasma. The resulting free radicals, the chemical precursors, and the UV radiation are among the postulated reactions that rapidly destroy vegetative microorganisms including spores.

Sterrad

The Sterrad 100 sterilizer was the first machine available for health care facilities and has been on the market in Europe since 1990 and in the United States since 1993. Several steps run automatically during a sterilization cycle: medical instruments are placed in the sterilization chamber under a strong vacuum. A solution of 59% hydrogen peroxide and water from a cassette is automatically injected into the sterilization chamber. The solution vaporizes and diffuses throughout the chamber, surrounding the items to be sterilized. Radiofrequency energy is applied to create an electric field, which in turn initiates the generation of the low-temperature plasma, inducing free radicals. The combination of the diffusion pretreatment and plasma phases acts to sterilize the item while eliminating harmful residuals. The radiofrequency energy is turned off, the vacuum is released, and the chamber is filled with filtered air, returning it to normal atmospheric pressure. In August 1997, the Sterrad 100 System was cleared for use in the sterilization of certain surgical instruments with longer and narrower lumens, such as those used in urologic, laparoscopic, and arthroscopic procedures, including single stainless steel lumens of ≥3 and <400 mm in length. Important restrictions are (i) materials that absorb too much hydrogen peroxide such as cellulosics and some nylons, e.g., from connectors, cables, and insulators; (ii) materials that catalytically decompose hydrogen peroxide such as copper and nickel alloys from electrical wire, solder, and surgical instruments; and (iii) materials that react with hydrogen peroxide such as organic dyes (colored anodized aluminum) and organic sulfides (M_2oS of solid lubricant in endoscopic devices). The Sterrad 100S adds one sterilization cycle compared to the Sterrad 100: therefore, the Sterrad 100S fulfills the requirement to kill 10^6 spores at half of the cycle. A smaller device, the Sterrad 50, has been independently tested for efficacy (196). The largest model—the Sterrad 200—is not yet cleared by FDA but is as effective as the smaller models. In addition, it has been independently tested in a university hospital (A. F. Widmer, J. Okpara, R. Frei, B. Jaussi, and M. Borneff-Lipp, *Program Abstr. 41st Intersci. Conf. Antimicrob. Agents Chemother.*, abstr. K1208, 2001). The Sterrad 200 is in use in Europe.

Liquid Sterilization

The STERIS SYSTEM 1 was cleared by FDA for marketing in the United States in 1988. The machine is designed for liquid sterilization with peracetic acid for immersible devices including flexible endoscopes. The machine does not clean the device. The process takes approximately 30 min at ca. 50°C. The items can be used immediately upon completion without aeration. The sterilant concentrate contains 35% liquid peracetic acid and buffering, anticorrosion, wetting, and surface-active agents. Peracetic acid is automatically diluted within the processor with sterile filtered water, and the items are exposed for 12 min. Clinical studies have been performed with bronchoscopes, hysteroscopes, colonoscopes, and rigid endoscopes (35, 232). Independent efficacy tests demonstrated some failures (35, 49). Peracetic acid is an FDA-cleared sterilant and is sporicidal (110, 113). It was the only available cleared sterilizer system for endoscopes with a short turnaround time before the Sterrad 100 plasma sterilizer was cleared for this application by FDA. The STERIS SYSTEM 1 is not considered a sterilizer in Europe (64) since it lacks an appropriate physical and biological monitoring system as required by EN. However, a study demonstrated that commercially available spores can be used for monitoring (131). False-positive test strips were identified from improper clip use (98). Exposure time and temperature are monitored electronically, and conductivity is used as a surrogate marker for peracetic acid concentration. On occasion, the machine has been known to complete its cycle normally and print a concentration of peracetic acid in the normal range even when it is run intentionally without peracetic acid (148). The cost of purchasing and using the equipment is consid-

erably greater than the cost of purchasing and using high-level disinfection with glutaraldehyde (83). It must be reiterated that none of the nonsteam sterilizers is able to meet sterilization requirements if residual debris and/or proteins are present on the items.

Other Sterilization Techniques

Cobalt 60 sterilization is the most common technique used for the commercial sterilization of single-use items. In this process, ionic energy is converted to thermal energy, killing microorganisms and their spores in the process. Design, quality control, and experience rely on experts from industry since this technology is rarely used in hospitals.

REUSE OF SINGLE-USE DEVICES

The legal problems on reprocessing of single-use devices are beyond the scope of this chapter. Current FDA policy states that the responsibility for the safety and performance of reprocessed single-use devices lies in the hands of the reprocessor, not the original manufacturer. FDA considers the hospital to be the manufacturer of a single-use device, if it has been resterilized. Therefore, the reprocessor is responsible not only for the sterility and the absence of toxic substances such as endotoxins or residual ethylene oxide but also for the product's integrity and for ensuring that the material's composition is almost identical to that of a new product. Most hospitals cannot afford to generate appropriate data on the quality and performance of reprocessed single-use items. In addition, a manufacturer can change, for example, an additive to a single-use catheter that would require a reprocessor of single-use devices to redo all analyses for the composition of the catheter before it could legally be marketed after reprocessing. FDA has published a final guidance (see homepage for details: http://www.fda.gov/cdrh/ohip/guidance/1333.html) and keeps track of items that are reused in hospitals. However, the reprocessing of single-use items is performed (sometimes illegally) in many countries throughout the world and may be an important component in the provision of access to state-of-the-art health care in times of limited resources. In the authors' personal opinion, the new reprocessing technologies that use a washer-disinfector coupled with a highly effective low-temperature sterilizer (e.g., the Sterrad 100S plasma sterilizer) are able to provide sufficient levels of safety to ensure the absence of viable microorganisms even in narrow lumens such as cardiac catheters. Infection control professionals will be able to provide the desired level of safety in terms of microbiological and toxicological safety. Some institutions resterilize items that have not been used on patients but that, for instance, have been dropped and/or whose package has been damaged. Even this simple approach, however, creates some risks for the device as a result of the reprocessing. FDA published an alert regarding an ethylene oxide-sterilized implant that had been resterilized with steam. The quality of the implant has been impaired by this reprocessing method (see http://www.fda.gov/cdrh/steamst.html for details). However, unresolved issues are quality, product integrity, and the performance of the frequently plastic or rubber products after reprocessing. An alert has been issued by FDA because outsourcing of reprocessing does not transfer full responsibility to the reprocessor (see full text at http://www.fda.gov/medwatch/safety/1997/device.htm). If a hospital reprocesses a single-use device, the hospital is responsible for ensuring that the device complies with all applicable FDA labeling requirements, even if the device is exempt from the premarket requirements. If the hospital does not ensure that the device complies with FDA labeling requirements, the device is misbranded, and the hospital may be considered responsible for causing the misbranding of the device in violation of section 301(k) of the Act. Class II devices are moderate-risk devices such as a cardiac mapping catheter used to map electrical activity of the heart. FDA enforces premarket filing requirements for reprocessed class II devices as of 14 August 2001 (http://www.fda.gov/cdrh/comp/guidance/1168.pdf) and marketing clearance requirements on 14 February 2002. Reuse of single-use devices may not turn cost-effective with such quality assurance programs. In addition, selling used single-use devices to patients and/or insurance companies as new devices may encounter a legal problem. Many issues are not yet resolved, and, consequently, FDA has set a prioritization scheme (http://www.fda.gov/cdrh/reuse/1156.pdf).

BOVINE SPONGIFORM ENCEPHALOPATHY AND VARIANT CREUTZFELDT-JACOB DISEASE

CJD has been identified on all continents and is thought to occur worldwide. The incidence of CJD is estimated to be about 1 case per 10^6 persons per year, similar to rates in European countries. Most cases of CJD are sporadic: <10% of CJD cases may be related to a genetic autosomal dominant predisposition, and few nosocomial cases are related to contact with contaminated tissue or application of contaminated human growth hormone. The new variant CJD (vCJD) has brought about a major medical and economic crisis in Europe (42, 124, 175). vCJD has a different clinical presentation and occurs at a much younger age (54, 124). The new disease is most probably transmitted by eating BSE agent-contaminated meat (108, 175). As of 2002, more than 105 cases have been reported from the United Kingdom, but cases are also reported from France (3 cases), Ireland (1 case), and Italy (1 case) that fulfill the new WHO case definition of 21 May 2001 (http://www.who.int/emc/diseases/bse/newvCJDdefinition.pdf). Several research groups have tried to estimate the size of the epidemic (174). Latest data indicate that the extent of the epidemic will be lower than predicted (174); however, the 95% confidence limits are still very large.

One striking epidemiological characteristic of vCJD is the young age distribution of the cases. The mean age at death is 28 years; only 6 of 90 patients died at the age of 50 years or older (174). Among several hypotheses that may explain why this age group is most affected are that the incubation period is shorter in the young than in the elderly or they are more susceptible to infection. In the United Kingdom, the number of people exposed to potentially infective doses through food may be extremely high. In the United Kingdom, vigorous actions have been taken at an early stage of evidence, such as requirements for performing tonsillectomies only with disposable instruments. This practice had to be discontinued in 2002 due to serious side effects of the use of disposable instruments.

The origin of this agent remains obscure, but the BSE agent from cattle is most probably responsible for the vCJD in humans. A high incidence of scrapie in sheep and a large proportion of sheep in the mix of carcasses that was rendered for animal feed for livestock may explain why the incidence of BSE in British cattle was more than 10 times

higher than in cattle in any other European country. The problem in Britain began in the mid-1980s because of the elimination several years earlier of a step in tallow extraction from rendered carcasses that allowed some tissue infected with scrapie to survive the process and hence allowed the infectious agent to be recycled as cattle-adapted scrapie or BSE. The animal food was no longer sterilized at 134°C for 20 to 30 min but, rather, was pasteurized before being fed to animals. These carcasses, with encased spinal cords and paraspinal ganglia, were legally processed as hot dogs, sausages, and precooked meat patties (40).

The new agent is not a classic microorganism but an altered prion protein (4, 30, 174, 208). Previously, problems with reprocessing were limited to invasive instruments that came into contact with neural tissue, predominantly instruments used in neurosurgery. However, the detection of the prion agent in lymphoid tissue and tonsils now challenges the idea that it is restricted to neural tissue (124). Studies of naturally infected sheep demonstrated that the infectious agent first appears in tonsil and gut lymphatic tissue, suggesting the oral route as the principal mode of transmission. In fact, multiple studies underline the importance of the B cell in the transmission of the BSE agent (127). Lymphatic organs typically show early accumulation of prions, and B cells and follicular dendritic cells are required for efficient neuroinvasion. The ablation of B lymphocytes prevents neuropathogenesis of prion disease after intraperitoneal inoculation in mice (128). This is probably due to impaired lymphotoxin-dependent maturation of follicular dendritic cells, which are a major extracerebral prion reservoir. The actual entry into the central nervous system probably occurs via peripheral nerves (90). vCJD is highly lymphotropic, so that any instruments used on lymphoid tissues are at risk for contamination with prions (127). Neither classic CJD nor its new variant counterpart vCJD has been shown to be transmissible via blood inoculation. Experimental evidence from animal models indicates that blood can contain prion infectivity, which suggests a potential risk for TSE transmission via proteins isolated from human plasma (111). In the United States, beginning in August 1999, persons who resided in or traveled to the United Kingdom for a total of 6 months from 1980 through 1996 have been deferred from blood donation, as have persons who received bovine insulin derived from cattle in the United Kingdom. Recently, both the American Red Cross and the FDA announced new, expanded geographic deferrals for travel and residence in the United Kingdom and other European countries (52). The United Kingdom no longer collects plasma from its inhabitants and, as a further precautionary measure, has instituted leukocyte reduction (removal of white blood cells) from blood transfusions. As of 2002, no curative therapy is available, but scientists speculate that lymphotoxin beta or antibodies may slow the degenerative process and might even cure it (168). In addition, the antimalarial drug quinacrine and the antipsychotic chlorpromazine prevented the conversion of normal (PrPC) to abnormal (PrPSc) prion protein in vitro and has been used in two patients (130a).

As outlined above, appropriate reprocessing of surgical items includes cleaning, disinfection, and sterilization. Aldehydes enhance the resistance of prions and abolish the inactivating effect of autoclaving (41). Therefore, aldehydes are no longer recommended for disinfecting surgical instruments in most of Europe and are prohibited in Switzerland after 2002. Infectivity of prions may survive autoclaving at 132 to 138°C. These small resistant subpopulations that survive autoclaving are not inactivated by simply reautoclaving and acquire biological characteristics that differentiate them from the main population (223). Therefore, prions challenge reprocessing techniques like never before.

The scientific uncertainties and lack of data do not allow the formulation of scientifically sound guidelines, and this explains the different approaches taken by various European countries. However, vCJD might become self-replicating as a result of contamination of surgical instruments under worst-case assumptions. In January 2001, the British government spent the equivalent of $300 million to improve reprocessing techniques in Central Sterilization Services, and required the use of disposable instruments for tonsillectomies. The French Public Health Office published their recommendations on 14 March 2001. They require sodium hypochlorite for 1 h or NaOH for 1 h and sterilization at 134°C for 18 min on all instruments with potential exposure to lymphatic tissue, central nervous system, or the eyes. If instruments do not tolerate this aggressive approach, double cleaning is followed by the use of various chemicals such as peracetic acid, iodophores, 3% sodium dodecyl sulfate, or 6 M urea and autoclaving at 121°C for 30 min. In Switzerland, all surgical instruments are to be sterilized at 134°C for 18 min after 2002. The background of the Swiss recommendation is that the usual rendering process for carcasses, which was discontinued, resulted in only a 1-log-unit reduction of the infectious particles (225). Therefore, a reduction in the number of infectious particles may suffice to stop transmission. Several methods have been shown to be insufficient for sterilization of prion-contaminated items, including dry heat (160°C for 24 h), formaldehyde sterilization, and standard steam sterilization (70). The minimum requirements for decontamination procedures and precautions for materials potentially contaminated with the agent that causes CJD remain unknown. Limited scientific information provides the basis for recommendations by the CDC (http://www.cdc.gov/ncidod/hip/INFECT/Cjd.htm) or the WHO (http://www.who.int/emc-documents/tse/docs/whocdscsraph2003.pdf):

- Steam autoclave for 1 to 1.5 h at 132 to 134°C.
- Immerse in 1 N sodium hydroxide for 1 h at room temperature.
- Immerse in sodium hypochlorite 0.5% (at least 2% free chlorine) for 2 h at room temperature.

No cases of BSE in cattle or vCJD have yet been identified in the United States despite active surveillance in 1995. Hence, disinfection and sterilization techniques are not required to be adopted in the United States. However, 37 tons of "meals of meat or offal" that were "unfit for human consumption" was sent from the United Kingdom to the United States in 1997, well after the government banned imports of such risky meat (53). In addition, the FDA has raised several concerns about how BSE may have been introduced to the cattle or might be transmitted by imported blood products from Europe. High-risk patients are CJD patients and their family members, patients with a medical history of treatment with pituitary extracts, and cornea transplant patients. In addition, items should be considered prion contaminated if a brain biopsy for the diagnosis of CJD is requested. Instruments used in such procedures should be discarded or placed under quarantine until the histopathological diagnosis is known. However, even given the latest data, the appropriate reprocessing

approach remains unknown (4). The level of knowledge about this situation is similar to that about the HIV epidemic from 1982 to 1984, when the extent of the epidemic was unclear. It is hoped that the vCJD will never become even remotely as epidemic as HIV. However, the long incubation period of the disease and the lack of a therapy may not allow us to wait until scientific knowledge accumulates before adopting guidelines. Therefore, reprocessing techniques in Europe have to be changed now, even at the risk that unnecessary steps are taken at a very high price. The use of disposable instruments in the United Kingdom had to be discontinued because serious side effects, including deaths, occurred as a result of using instruments that apparently were of lower quality than the previous nondisposable instruments. In the United States, scientists believe that the evidence for vCJD is very low, and therefore current recommendations should be followed; the additional steps taken in Europe do not yet appear to be warranted (164). Many approaches have been recommended, but none of them can fulfill the SAL as required for microorganisms. In March 2002, prions were found in skeletal muscle, tissue previously considered as safe (32a). Therefore, the reader is referred to the home pages of CDC, FDA, and WHO to obtain the most recent update on this topic.

REFERENCES

1. **ADA Council on Scientific Affairs and ADA Council on Dental Practice.** 1996. Infection control recommendations for the dental office and the dental laboratory. *J. Am. Dent. Assoc.* **127:**672–680.
2. **Adams, B. G., and T. J. Marrie.** 1982. Hand carriage of aerobic gram-negative rods may not be transient. *J. Hyg.* **89:**33–46.
3. **Agerton, T., S. Valway, B. Gore, C. Pozsik, B. Plikaytis, C. Woodley, and I. Onorato.** 1997. Transmission of a highly drug-resistant strain (strain W1) of *Mycobacterium tuberculosis.* Community outbreak and nosocomial transmission via a contaminated bronchoscope. *JAMA* **278:** 1073–1077.
4. **Aguzzi, A., and C. Weissmann.** 1998. Spongiform encephalopathies. The prion's perplexing persistence. *Nature* **392:**763–764.
5. **Akamatsu, T., K. Tabata, M. Hironaga, and M. Uyeda.** 1997. Evaluation of the efficacy of a 3.2% glutaraldehyde product for disinfection of fibreoptic endoscopes with an automatic machine. *J. Hosp. Infect.* **35:**47–57.
6. **Akbar-Khanzadeh, F., M. U. Vaquerano, M. Akbar-Khanzadeh, and M. S. Bisesi.** 1994. Formaldehyde exposure, acute pulmonary response, and exposure control options in a gross anatomy laboratory. *Am. J. Ind. Med.* **26:**61–75.
7. **Alasri, A., C. Roques, G. Michel, C. Cabassud, and P. Aptel.** 1992. Bactericidal properties of peracetic acid and hydrogen peroxide, alone and in combination, and chlorine and formaldehyde against bacterial water strains. *Can. J. Microbiol.* **38:**635–642.
8. **Alasri, A., M. Valverde, C. Roques, G. Michel, C. Cabassud, and P. Aptel.** 1993. Sporocidal properties of peracetic acid and hydrogen peroxide, alone and in combination, in comparison with chlorine and formaldehyde for ultrafiltration membrane disinfection. *Can. J. Microbiol.* **39:**52–60.
9. **Alfa, M. J., P. DeGagne, and N. Olson.** 1997. Bacterial killing ability of 10% ethylene oxide plus 90% hydrochlorofluorocarbon sterilizing gas. *Infect. Control Hosp. Epidemiol.* **18:**641–645.

10. **Alvarado, C. J., and M. Reichelderfer.** 2000. APIC guideline for infection prevention and control in flexible endoscopy. Association for Professionals in Infection Control. *Am. J. Infect. Control* **28:**138–155.

11. **Alvarado, C. J., S. M. Stolz, and D. G. Maki.** 1991. Nosocomial infections from contaminated endoscope washer. An investigation using molecular epidemiology. *Am. J. Med.* **91:**272S–280S.

12. **Anderson, R. L., R. W. Vess, A. L. Panlilio, and M. S. Favero.** 1990. Prolonged survival of *Pseudomonas cepacia* in commercially manufactured povidone-iodine. *Appl. Environ. Microbiol.* **56:**3598–3600.

13. **Anonymous.** 1994. Tentative final monograph for healthcare antiseptic drug products. *Fed. Regist.* **59:**31401–31452.

14. **Ansari, S. A., S. A. Sattar, V. S. Springthorpe, G. A. Wells, and W. Tostowaryk.** 1989. In vivo protocol for testing efficacy of hand-washing agents against viruses and bacteria: experiments with rotavirus and *Escherichia coli*. *Appl. Environ. Microbiol.* **55:**3113–3118.

15. **Arata, T., T. Murakami, and Y. Hirai.** 1993. Evaluation of povidone-iodine alcoholic solution for operative site disinfection. *Postgrad. Med. J.* **69**(Suppl. 3)**:**S93–S96.

16. **Arnon, S. S., R. Schechter, T. V. Inglesby, D. A. Henderson, J. G. Bartlett, M. S. Ascher, E. Eitzen, A. D. Fine, J. Hauer, M. Layton, S. Lillibridge, M. T. Osterholm, T. O'Toole, G. Parker, T. M. Perl, P. K. Russell, D. L. Swerdlow, and K. Tonat.** 2001. Botulinum toxin as a biological weapon: medical and public health management. *JAMA* **285:**1059–1070.

17. **Ascenzi, J. M.** 1996. Glutaraldehyde-based disinfectants, p. 111–132. *In* J. P. Ascenzi (ed.), *Handbook of Disinfectants and Antiseptics*. Marcel Dekker, Inc., New York, N.Y.

18. **Ascenzi, J. M., R. J. Ezzell, and T. M. Wendt.** 1987. A more accurate method for measurement of tuberculocidal activity of disinfectants. *Appl. Environ. Microbiol.* **53:**2189–2192.

19. **Astagneau, P., N. Desplaces, V. Vincent, V. Chicheportiche, A. Botherel, S. Maugat, K. Lebascle, P. Leonard, J. Desenclos, J. Grosset, J. Ziza, and G. Brucker.** 2001. *Mycobacterium xenopi* spinal infections after discovertebral surgery: investigation and screening of a large outbreak. *Lancet* **358:**747–751.

20. **Axon, A., M. Jung, A. Kruse, T. Ponchon, J. F. Rey, U. Beilenhoff, D. Duforest-Rey, C. Neumann, M. Pietsch, K. Roth, A. Papoz, D. Wilson, I. Kircher-Felgenstreff, M. Stief, R. Blum, K. B. Spencer, J. Mills, E. P. Mart, B. Slowey, H. Biering, and U. Lorenz.** 2000. The European Society of Gastrointestinal Endoscopy (ESGE): check list for the purchase of washer-disinfectors for flexible endoscopes. ESGE Guideline Committee. *Endoscopy* **32:**914–919.

21. **Bagg, J., C. P. Sweeney, K. M. Roy, T. Sharp, and A. Smith.** 2001. Cross infection control measures and the treatment of patients at risk of Creutzfeldt Jakob disease in UK general dental practice. *Br. Dent. J.* **191:**87–90.

22. **Bassetti, S., and A. F. Widmer.** 2002. Internet sources for legionella. *Clin. Infect. Dis.* **34:**1633–1640.

23. **Beiswanger, B. B., M. E. Mallatt, M. S. Mau, R. D. Jackson, and D. K. Hennon.** 1990. The clinical effects of a mouthrinse containing 0.1% octenidine. *J. Dent. Res.* **69:**454–457.

24. **Bellamy, K.** 1995. A review of the test methods used to establish virucidal activity. *J. Hosp. Infect.* **30**(Suppl.)**:** 389–396.

25. **Bellamy, K., R. Alcock, J. R. Babb, J. G. Davies, and G. A. Ayliffe.** 1993. A test for the assessment of 'hygienic' hand disinfection using rotavirus. *J. Hosp. Infect.* **24:**201–210.

26. **Berkelman, R. L., B. W. Holland, and R. L. Anderson.** 1982. Increased bactericidal activity of dilute preparations of povidone-iodine solutions. *J. Clin. Microbiol.* **15:**635–639.

27. **Berkelman, R. L., S. Lewin, J. R. Allen, R. L. Anderson, L. D. Budnick, S. Shapiro, S. M. Friedman, P. Nicholas, R. S. Holzman, and R. W. Haley.** 1981. Pseudobacteremia attributed to contamination of povidone-iodine with *Pseudomonas cepacia*. *Ann. Intern. Med.* **95:**32–36.

28. **Biron, F., B. Verrier, and D. Peyramond.** 1997. Transmission of the human immunodeficiency virus and the hepatitis C virus. *N. Engl. J. Med.* **337:**348–349.

29. **Blanc, D. S., T. Parret, B. Janin, P. Raselli, and P. Francioli.** 1997. Nosocomial infections and pseudoinfections from contaminated bronchoscopes: two-year follow up using molecular markers. *Infect. Control Hosp. Epidemiol.* **18:**134–136.

30. **Blattler, T., S. Brandner, A. J. Raeber, M. A. Klein, T. Voigtlander, C. Weissmann, and A. Aguzzi.** 1997. PrP-expressing tissue required for transfer of scrapie infectivity from spleen to brain. *Nature* **389:**69–73.

31. **Block, S. S.** 2001. *Disinfection, Sterilization, and Preservation*. Lippincott Williams & Wilkins, Philadelphia, Pa.

32. **Bond, W. W., M. S. Favero, N. J. Petersen, and J. W. Ebert.** 1983. Inactivation of hepatitis B virus by intermediate-to-high-level disinfectant chemicals. *J. Clin. Microbiol.* **18:**535–538.

32a.**Bosque, P. J., C. Ryou, G. Telling, D. Peretz, G. Legname, S. J. DeArmond, and S. B. Prusiner.** 2002. Prions in skeletal muscle. *Proc. Natl. Acad. Sci. USA* **99:**3812–3817.

33. **Bowie, J. H., M. H. Kennedy, and I. Robertson.** 1975. Improved Bowie and Dick test. *Lancet* **i:**1135.

34. **Boyce, J. M., G. Potter-Bynoe, S. M. Opal, L. Dziobek, and A. A. Medeiros.** 1990. A common-source outbreak of *Staphylococcus epidermidis* infections among patients undergoing cardiac surgery. *J. Infect. Dis.* **161:**493–499.

35. **Bradley, C. R., J. R. Babb, and G. A. Ayliffe.** 1995. Evaluation of the Steris System 1™ Peracetic Acid Endoscope Processor. *J. Hosp. Infect.* **29:**143–151.

36. **Bradley, C. R., and A. P. Fraise.** 1996. Heat and chemical resistance of enterococci. *J. Hosp. Infect.* **34:**191–196.

37. **Brewer, G. E.** 1915. Studies in aseptic technique. *JAMA* **64:**1369–1372.

38. **Broadley, S. J., J. R. Furr, P. A. Jenkins, and A. D. Russell.** 1993. Antimycobacterial activity of 'Virkon'. *J. Hosp. Infect.* **23:**189–197.

39. **Bronowicki, J. P., V. Venard, C. Botte, N. Monhoven, I. Gastin, L. Chone, H. Hudziak, B. Rhin, C. Delanoe, A. LeFaou, M. A. Bigard, and P. Gaucher.** 1997. Patient-to-patient transmission of hepatitis C virus during colonoscopy. *N. Engl. J. Med.* **337:**237–240.

40. **Brown, P.** 2001. Bovine spongiform encephalopathy and variant Creutzfeldt-Jakob disease. *Br. Med. J.* **322:**841–844.

41. **Brown, P., P. P. Liberski, A. Wolff, and D. C. Gajdusek.** 1990. Resistance of scrapie infectivity to steam autoclaving after formaldehyde fixation and limited survival after ashing at 360 degrees C: practical and theoretical implications. *J. Infect. Dis.* **161:**467–472.

42. **Bruce, M. E., R. G. Will, J. W. Ironside, I. McConnell, D. Drummond, A. Suttie, L. McCardle, A. Chree, J. Hope, C. Birkett, S. Cousens, H. Fraser, and C. J. Bostock.** 1997. Transmissions to mice indicate that 'new variant' CJD is caused by the BSE agent. *Nature* **389:**498–501.

43. **Bryant, W. P., and D. Zimmerman.** 1995. Iodine-induced hyperthyroidism in a newborn. *Pediatrics* **95:**434–436.

44. Bryce, E. A., F. J. Roberts, B. Clements, and S. Mac-Lean. 1997. When the biological indicator is positive: investigating autoclave failures. *Infect. Control Hosp. Epidemiol.* **18:**654–656.

45. Centers for Disease Control. 1995. Management of patients with suspected viral hemorrhagic fever—United States. *Morb. Mortal. Wkly. Rep.* **44:**475–479.

46. Centers for Disease Control and Prevention. 1989. Guidelines for prevention of transmission of human immunodeficiency virus and hepatitis B virus to health-care and public-safety workers. *Morb. Mortal. Wkly. Rep.* **38**(Suppl. 6)**:**1–37.

47. Centers for Disease Control and Prevention. 1996. Community-level prevention of human immunodeficiency virus infection among high-risk populations: the AIDS community demonstration projects. *Morb. Mortal. Wkly. Rep.* **45**(RR6)**:**1–31.

48. Centers for Disease Control and Prevention. 1993. Recommended infection-control practices for dentistry. *Morb. Mortal. Wkly. Rep.* **42:**1–12.

49. Centers for Disease Control and Prevention. 1999. Bronchoscopy-related infections and pseudoinfections—New York, 1996 and 1998. *Morb. Mortal. Wkly. Rep.* **48:**557–560.

50. Centers for Disease Control and Prevention. 2001. Protracted outbreaks of cryptosporidiosis associated with swimming pool use—Ohio and Nebraska, 2000. *Morb. Mortal. Wkly. Rep.* **50:**406–410.

51. Challacombe, S. J., and L. L. Fernandes. 1995. Detecting *Legionella pneumophila* in water systems: a comparison of various dental units. *J. Am. Dent. Assoc.* **126:**603–608.

52. Chamberland, M. E. 2002. Emerging infectious agents: do they pose a risk to the safety of transfused blood and blood products? *Clin. Infect. Dis.* **34:**797–805.

53. Charatan, F. 2001. United States takes precautions against BSE. *West. J. Med.* **174:**235.

54. Chazot, G., E. Broussolle, C. Lapras, T. Blattler, A. Aguzzi, and N. Kopp. 1996. New variant of Creutzfeldt-Jakob disease in a 26-year-old French man. *Lancet* **347:**1181.

55. Cheung, R. J., D. Ortiz, and A. J. DiMarino, Jr. 1999. GI endoscopic reprocessing practices in the United States. *Gastrointest. Endosc.* **50:**362–368.

56. Chuanchuen, R., K. Beinlich, T. T. Hoang, A. Becher, R. R. Karkhoff-Schweizer, and H. P. Schweizer. 2001. Cross-resistance between triclosan and antibiotics in *Pseudomonas aeruginosa* is mediated by multidrug efflux pumps: exposure of a susceptible mutant strain to triclosan selects nfxB mutants overexpressing MexCD-OprJ. *Antimicrob. Agents Chemother.* **45:**428–432.

57. Coates, D. 1996. Sporicidal activity of sodium dichloroisocyanurate, peroxygen and glutaraldehyde disinfectants against *Bacillus subtilis.* *J. Hosp. Infect.* **32:**283–294.

58. Collinge, J. 2001. Prion diseases of humans and animals: their causes and molecular basis. *Annu. Rev. Neurosci.* **24:**519–550.

59. Collins, F. M. 1986. Bactericidal activity of alkaline glutaraldehyde solution against a number of atypical mycobacterial species. *J. Appl. Bacteriol.* **61:**247–251.

60. Collins, F. M. 1986. Kinetics of the tuberculocidal response by alkaline glutaraldehyde in solution and on an inert surface. *J. Appl. Bacteriol.* **61:**87–93.

61. Craven, D. E., B. Moody, M. G. Connolly, N. R. Kollisch, K. D. Stottmeier, and W. R. McCabe. 1981. Pseudobacteremia caused by povidone-iodine solution contaminated with *Pseudomonas cepacia.* *N. Engl. J. Med.* **305:**621–623.

62. Crow, S. 1993. Steam sterilizers: an evolution in design. *Infect. Control Hosp. Epidemiol.* **14:**488–490.

63. Cruse, P. J., and R. Foord. 1973. A five-year prospective study of 23,649 surgical wounds. *Arch. Surg.* **107:**206–210.

64. Daschner, F. 1994. STERIS SYSTEM 1™ in Germany. *Infect. Control Hosp. Epidemiol.* **15:**294, 296.

65. Dennis, D. T., T. V. Inglesby, D. A. Henderson, J. G. Bartlett, M. S. Ascher, E. Eitzen, A. D. Fine, A. M. Friedlander, J. Hauer, M. Layton, S. R. Lillibridge, J. E. McDade, M. T. Osterholm, T. O'Toole, G. Parker, T. M. Perl, P. K. Russell, and K. Tonat. 2001. Tularemia as a biological weapon: medical and public health management. *JAMA* **285:**2763–2773.

66. Denton, G. E. 2001. Chlorhexidine, p. 321–336. *In* S. S. Block (ed.), *Disinfection, Sterilization, and Preservation.* Lippincott Williams & Wilkins, Philadelphia, Pa.

67. Disch, K. 1994. Glucoprotamine—a new antimicrobial substance. *Zentbl. Hyg. Umweltmed.* **195:**357–365.

68. Doebbeling, B. N., G. L. Stanley, C. T. Sheetz, M. A. Pfaller, A. K. Houston, L. Annis, N. Li, and R. P. Wenzel. 1992. Comparative efficacy of alternative handwashing agents in reducing nosocomial infections in intensive care units. *N. Engl. J. Med.* **327:**88–93.

69. Dolce, P., M. Gourdeau, N. April, and P. M. Bernard. 1995. Outbreak of glutaraldehyde-induced proctocolitis. *Am. J. Infect. Control* **23:**34–39.

70. Dormont, D. 1996. How to limit the spread of Creutzfeldt-Jakob disease. *Infect. Control Hosp. Epidemiol.* **17:**521–528.

71. Druce, J. D., D. Jardine, S. A. Locarnini, and C. J. Birch. 1995. Susceptibility of HIV to inactivation by disinfectants and ultraviolet light. *J. Hosp. Infect.* **30:**167–180.

72. Evans, R. J. 1992. Acute anaphylaxis due to topical chlorhexidine acetate. *Br. Med. J.* **304:**686.

73. Faoagali, J. L., N. George, J. Fong, J. Davy, and M. Dowser. 1999. Comparison of the antibacterial efficacy of 4% chlorhexidine gluconate and 1% triclosan handwash products in an acute clinical ward. *Am. J. Infect. Control* **27:**320–326.

74. Farina, A., M. H. Fievet, F. Plassart, M. C. Menet, and A. Thuillier. 1999. Residual glutaraldehyde levels in fiberoptic endoscopes: measurement and implications for patient toxicity. *J. Hosp. Infect.* **43:**293–297.

75. Favero, M. S. 1991. Strategies for disinfection and sterilization of endoscopes: the gap between basic principles and actual practice. *Infect. Control Hosp. Epidemiol.* **12:**279–281.

76. Favero, M. S., and F. A. Manian. 1993. Is eliminating flash sterilization practical? *Infect. Control Hosp. Epidemiol.* **14:**479–480.

77. Feldman, H. I., M. Kinosian, W. B. Bilker, C. Simmons, J. H. Holmes, M. V. Pauly, and J. J. Escarce. 1996. Effect of dialyzer reuse on survival of patients treated with hemodialysis. *JAMA* **276:**1724.

78. Flynn, N., S. Jain, E. M. Keddie, J. R. Carlson, M. B. Jennings, H. W. Haverkos, N. Nassar, R. Anderson, S. Cohen, and D. Goldberg. 1994. In vitro activity of readily available household materials against HIV-1: is bleach enough? *J. Acquir. Immune Defic. Syndr.* **7:**747–753.

79. Frank, M. J., and W. Schaffner. 1976. Contaminated aqueous benzalkonium chloride. An unnecessary hospital infection hazard. *JAMA* **236:**2418–2419.

80. Fraser, V. J., G. Zuckerman, R. E. Clouse, S. O'Rourke, M. Jones, J. Klasner, and P. Murray. 1993. A prospective randomized trial comparing manual and automated endoscope disinfection methods. *Infect. Control Hosp. Epidemiol.* **14:**383–389.

81. **Fraud, S., J. Y. Maillard, and A. D. Russell.** 2001. Comparison of the mycobactericidal activity of ortho-phthalaldehyde, glutaraldehyde and other dialdehydes by a quantitative suspension test. *J. Hosp. Infect.* **48:**214–221.

82. **Furuhashi, M., and T. Miyamae.** 1979. Effect of preoperative hand scrubbing and influence of pinholes appearing in surgical rubber gloves during operation. *Bull. Tokyo Med. Dent. Univ.* **26:**73–80.

83. **Fuselier, H. A. J., and C. Mason.** 1997. Liquid sterilization versus high level disinfection in the urologic office. *Urology* **50:**337–340.

84. **Fuursted, K., A. Hjort, and L. Knudsen.** 1997. Evaluation of bactericidal activity and lag of regrowth (postantibiotic effect) of five antiseptics on nine bacterial pathogens. *J. Antimicrob. Chemother.* **40:**221–226.

85. **Garibaldi, R. A., D. Skolnick, T. Lerer, A. Poirot, J. Graham, E. Krisuinas, and R. Lyons.** 1988. The impact of preoperative skin disinfection on preventing intraoperative wound contamination. *Infect. Control Hosp. Epidemiol.* **9:**109–113.

86. **Gelinas, P., J. Goulet, G. M. Tastayre, and G. A. Picard.** 1991. Effect of temperature and contact time on the activity of eight disinfectants—a classification. *J. Food Prot.* **47:**841–847.

87. **Georgiade, G., R. Riefkohl, N. Georgiade, R. Georgiade, and M. F. Wildman.** 1985. Efficacy of povidone-iodine in pre-operative skin preparation. *J. Hosp. Infect.* **6**(Suppl. A):67–71.

88. **Gerding, D. N., S. Johnson, L. R. Peterson, M. E. Mulligan, and J. Silva, Jr.** 1995. *Clostridium difficile*-associated diarrhea and colitis. *Infect. Control Hosp. Epidemiol.* **16:**459–477.

89. **Ghannoum, M. A., K. A. Elteen, M. Ellabib, and P. A. Whittaker.** 1990. Antimycotic effects of octenidine and pirtenidine. *J. Antimicrob. Chemother.* **25:**237–245.

90. **Glatzel, M., and A. Aguzzi.** 2000. PrP(C) expression in the peripheral nervous system is a determinant of prion neuroinvasion. *J. Gen. Virol.* **81:**2813–2821.

91. **Gorse, G. J., and R. L. Messner.** 1991. Infection control practices in gastrointestinal endoscopy in the United States: a national survey. *Infect. Control Hosp. Epidemiol.* **12:**289–296.

92. **Gottardi, W.** 2001. Iodine and iodine compounds, p. 159–183. *In* S. S. Block (ed.), *Disinfection, Sterilization, and Preservation.* Lippincott Williams & Wilkins, Philadelphia, Pa.

93. **Graham, G. S.** 1997. Decontamination: scientific principles, p. 1–9. *In* M. Reichert and J. H. Young (ed.), *Sterilization Technology.* Aspen Publications, Gaithersburg, Md.

94. **Graham, M.** 1990. Frequency and duration of handwashing in an intensive care unit. *Am. J. Infect. Control.* **18:**77–81.

95. **Griffiths, P. A., J. R. Babb, C. R. Bradley, and A. P. Fraise.** 1997. Glutaraldehyde-resistant *Mycobacterium chelonae* from endoscope washer disinfectors. *J. Appl. Microbiol.* **82:**519–526.

96. **Gubler, J. G., M. Salfinger, and A. von Graevenitz.** 1992. Pseudoepidemic of nontuberculous mycobacteria due to a contaminated bronchoscope cleaning machine. Report of an outbreak and review of the literature. *Chest* **101:**1245–1249.

97. **Gurevich, I., R. Dubin, and B. A. Cunha.** 1996. Dental instrument and device sterilization and disinfection practices. *J. Hosp. Infect.* **32:**295–304.

98. **Gurevich, I., S. M. Qadri, and B. A. Cunha.** 1993. False-positive results of spore tests from improper clip use with the STERIS chemical sterilant system. *Am. J. Infect. Control* **21:**42–43.

99. **Gurevich, I., P. Tafuro, P. Ristuccia, J. Herrmann, A. R. Young, and B. A. Cunha.** 1983. Disinfection of respirator tubing: a comparison of chemical versus hot water machine-assisted processing. *J. Hosp. Infect.* **4:**199–208.

100. **Hamilton, E., D. V. Seal, and J. Hay.** 1996. Comparison of chlorine and chlorine dioxide disinfection for control of Legionella in a hospital potable water supply. *J. Hosp. Infect.* **32:**156–160.

101. **Hanson, J. M., S. M. Plusa, M. K. Bennett, D. A. Browell, and W. J. Cunliffe.** 1998. Glutaraldehyde as a possible cause of diarrhoea after sigmoidoscopy. *Br. J. Surg.* **85:**1385–1387.

102. **Hanson, P. J., D. Gor, J. R. Clarke, M. V. Chadwick, B. Gazzard, D. J. Jeffries, H. Gaya, and J. V. Collins.** 1991. Recovery of the human immunodeficiency virus from fibreoptic bronchoscopes. *Thorax* **46:**410–412.

103. **Hanson, P. J., D. J. Jeffries, and J. V. Collins.** 1991. Viral transmission and fibreoptic endoscopy. *J. Hosp. Infect.* **18**(Suppl. A):136–140.

104. **Held, P. J., R. A. Wolfe, D. S. Gaylin, F. K. Port, N. W. Levin, and M. N. Turenne.** 1994. Analysis of the association of dialyzer reuse practices and patient outcomes. *Am. J. Kidney Dis.* **23:**692–708.

105. **Helms, C. M., R. M. Massanari, R. P. Wenzel, M. A. Pfaller, N. P. Moyer, and N. Hall.** 1988. Legionnaires' disease associated with a hospital water system. A five-year progress report on continuous hyperchlorination. *JAMA* **259:**2423–2427.

106. **Henderson, D. A., T. V. Inglesby, J. G. Bartlett, M. S. Ascher, E. Eitzen, P. B. Jahrling, J. Hauer, M. Layton, J. McDade, M. T. Osterholm, T. O'Toole, G. Parker, T. Perl, P. K. Russell, K. Tonat, and Working Group on Civilian Biodefense.** 1999. Smallpox as a biological weapon: medical and public health management. *JAMA* **281:**2127–2137.

107. **Heppner, F. L., C. Musahl, I. Arrighi, M. A. Klein, T. Rulicke, B. Oesch, R. M. Zinkernagel, U. Kalinke, and A. Aguzzi.** 2001. Prevention of scrapie pathogenesis by transgenic expression of anti-prion protein antibodies. *Science* **294:**178–182.

108. **Hill, A. F., M. Desbruslais, S. Joiner, K. C. Sidle, I. Gowland, J. Collinge, L. J. Doey, and P. Lantos.** 1997. The same prion strain causes vCJD and BSE. *Nature* **389:**448–450.

109. **Hill, A. F., M. Zeidler, J. Ironside, and J. Collinge.** 1997. Diagnosis of new variant Creutzfeldt-Jakob disease by tonsil biopsy. *Lancet* **349:**99–100.

110. **Holton, J., and N. Shetty.** 1997. In-use stability of Nu-Cidex. *J. Hosp. Infect.* **35:**245–248.

111. **Houston, F., J. D. Foster, A. Chong, N. Hunter, and C. J. Bostock.** 2000. Transmission of BSE by blood transfusion in sheep. *Lancet* **356:**999–1000.

112. **Hughes, R., and S. Kilvington.** 2001. Comparison of hydrogen peroxide contact lens disinfection systems and solutions against *Acanthamoeba polyphaga. Antimicrob. Agents Chemother.* **45:**2038–2043.

113. **Hussaini, S. N., and K. R. Ruby.** 1976. Sporicidal activity of peracetic acid against *B. anthracis* spores. *Vet. Rec.* **98:**257–259.

114. **Inglesby, T. V., D. T. Dennis, D. A. Henderson, J. G. Bartlett, M. S. Ascher, E. Eitzen, A. D. Fine, A. M. Friedlander, J. Hauer, J. F. Koerner, M. Layton, J. McDade, M. T. Osterholm, T. O'Toole, G. Parker, T. M. Perl, P. K. Russell, M. Schoch-Spana, K. Tonat, and Working Group on Civilian Biodefense.** 2000. Plague as a biological weapon: medical and public health management. *JAMA* **283:**2281–2290.

115. Inglesby, T. V., D. A. Henderson, J. G. Bartlett, M. S. Ascher, E. Eitzen, A. M. Friedlander, J. Hauer, J. McDade, M. T. Osterholm, T. O'Toole, G. Parker, T. M. Perl, P. K. Russell, K. Tonat, and Working Group on Civilian Biodefense. 1999. Anthrax as a biological weapon: medical and public health management. JAMA 281:1735–1745.

116. Isenberg, S. J., L. Apt, and M. Wood. 1995. A controlled trial of povidone-iodine as prophylaxis against ophthalmia neonatorum. N. Engl. J. Med. 332:562–566.

117. Jackson, J., J. E. Leggett, D. A. Wilson, and D. N. Gilbert. 1996. Mycobacterium gordonae in fiberoptic bronchoscopes. Am. J. Infect. Control 24:19–23.

118. Jette, L. P., and N. G. Lambert. 1988. Evaluation of two hot water washer disinfectors for medical instruments. Infect. Control Hosp. Epidemiol. 9:194–199.

119. Jones, R. D., H. B. Jampani, J. L. Newman, and A. S. Lee. 2000. Triclosan: a review of effectiveness and safety in health care settings. Am. J. Infect. Control 28:184–196.

120. Joslyn, L. J. 2001. Sterilization by heat, p. 695–728. In S. S. Block (ed.), Disinfection, Sterilization, and Preservation. Lippincott Williams & Wilkins, Philadelphia, Pa.

121. Kaatz, G. W., S. D. Gitlin, D. R. Schaberg, K. H. Wilson, C. A. Kauffman, S. M. Seo, and R. Fekety. 1988. Acquisition of Clostridium difficile from the hospital environment. Am. J. Epidemiol. 127:1289–1293.

122. Kaczmarek, R. G., R. M. J. Moore, J. McCrohan, D. A. Goldmann, C. Reynolds, C. Caquelin, and E. Israel. 1992. Multi-state investigation of the actual disinfection/sterilization of endoscopes in health care facilities. Am. J. Med. 92:257–261.

123. Karol, M. H. 1995. Toxicologic principles do not support the banning of chlorine. A Society of Toxicology position paper. Fundam. Appl. Toxicol. 24:1–2.

124. Kawashima, T., H. Furukawa, K. Doh-ura, and T. Iwaki. 1997. Diagnosis of new variant Creutzfeldt-Jakob disease by tonsil biopsy. Lancet 350:68–69.

125. Keene, J. H. 1996. Sterilization and pasteurization, p. 937–946. In C. G. Mayhall (ed.), Hospital Epidemiology and Infection Control. The Williams & Wilkins Co., Baltimore, Md.

126. Klein, M., and A. DeForest. 1963. The inactivation of viruses by germicides. Chem. Spec. Manuf. Assoc. Proc. 49:116–118.

127. Klein, M. A., R. Frigg, E. Flechsig, A. J. Raeber, U. Kalinke, H. Bluethman, F. Bootz, J. Suter, R. M. Zinkernagel, and A. Aguzzi. 1997. A crucial role for B cells in neuroinvasive scrapie. Nature 390:687.

128. Klein, M. A., R. Frigg, A. J. Raeber, E. Flechsig, I. Hegyi, R. M. Zinkernagel, C. Weissmann, and A. Aguzzi. 1998. PrP expression in B lymphocytes is not required for prion neuroinvasion. Nat. Med. 4:1429–1433.

129. Kobayashi, H., M. Tsuzuki, K. Koshimizu, H. Toyama, N. Yoshihara, T. Shikata, K. Abe, K. Mizuno, N. Otomo, and T. Oda. 1984. Susceptibility of hepatitis B virus to disinfectants or heat. J. Clin. Microbiol. 20:214–216.

130. Kool, J. L., J. C. Carpenter, and B. S. Fields. 1999. Effect of monochloramine disinfection of municipal drinking water on risk of nosocomial Legionnaires' disease. Lancet 353:272–277.

130a. Korth, C., B. C. May, F. E. Cohen, and S. B. Prusiner. 2001. Acridine and phenothiazine derivatives as pharmacotherapeutics for prion disease. Proc. Natl. Acad. Sci. USA 98:9836–9841.

131. Kralovic, R. C. 1993. Use of biological indicators designed for steam or ethylene oxide to monitor a liquid

chemical sterilization process. Infect. Control Hosp. Epidemiol. 14:313–319.

132. Kurtz, J. B., T. W. Lee, and A. J. Parsons. 1980. The action of alcohols on rotavirus, astrovirus and enterovirus. J. Hosp. Infect. 1:321–325.

133. Larson, E. 1988. Guideline for use of topical antimicrobial agents. Am. J. Infect. Control 16:253–266.

134. Larson, E., K. Mayur, and B. A. Laughon. 1989. Influence of two handwashing frequencies on reduction in colonizing flora with three handwashing products used by health care personnel. Am. J. Infect. Control 17:83–88.

135. Larson, E., A. McGeer, Z. A. Quraishi, D. Krenzischek, B. J. Parsons, J. Holdford, and W. J. Hierholzer. 1991. Effect of an automated sink on handwashing practices and attitudes in high-risk units. Infect. Control Hosp. Epidemiol. 12:422–428.

136. Larson, E. L. 1991. Alcohols, p. 191–203. In S. S. Block (ed.), Disinfection, Sterilization and Preservation. Lea & Febiger, Philadelphia, Pa.

137. Larson, E. L. 1995. APIC guideline for handwashing and hand antisepsis in health care settings. Am. J. Infect. Control 23:251–269.

138. Larson, E. L., A. M. Butz, D. L. Gullette, and B. A. Laughon. 1990. Alcohol for surgical scrubbing? Infect. Control Hosp. Epidemiol. 11:139–143.

139. Leaper, S. 1984. Influence of temperature on the synergistic sporicidal effect of peracetic acid plus hydrogen peroxide in Bacillus subtilis SA22 (NCA 72-52). Food Microbiol. 1:199–203.

140. Levenson, J. E. 1989. Corneal damage from improperly cleaned tonometer tips. Arch. Ophthalmol. 107:1117.

141. Lever, A. M., and S. V. W. Sutton. 1996. Antimicrobial effects of hydrogen peroxide as an antiseptic and disinfectant, p. 159–176. In J. P. Ascenzi (ed.), Handbook of Disinfectants and Antiseptics. Marcel Dekker, Inc., New York, N.Y.

142. Lowbury, E. J., and H. A. Lilly. 1974. The effect of blood on disinfection of surgeons' hands. Br. J. Surg. 61:19–21.

143. Lowbury, E. J., H. A. Lilly, and J. P. Bull. 1964. Methods for disinfection of operation sites. Br. Med. J. 2:531–533.

144. Maki, D. G., and C. A. Hassemer. 1987. Flash sterilization: carefully measured haste. Infect. Control 8:307–310.

145. Maki, D. G., S. M. Stolz, S. Wheeler, and L. A. Mermel. 1997. Prevention of central venous catheter-related bloodstream infection by use of an antiseptic-impregnated catheter. A randomized, controlled trial. Ann. Intern. Med. 127:257–266.

146. Malakoff, G., and G. Simon. 1991. The matching game. N. Engl. J. Med. 324:778–778.

147. Mangram, A. J., T. C. Horan, M. L. Pearson, L. C. Silver, W. R. Jarvis, and Hospital Infection Control Practices Advisory Committee. 1999. Guideline for prevention of surgical site infection, 1999. Infect. Control Hosp. Epidemiol. 20:250–278.

148. Mannion, P. T. 1995. The use of peracetic acid for the reprocessing of flexible endoscopes and rigid cystoscopes and laparoscopes. J. Hosp. Infect. 29:313–315.

149. Martin, L. S., J. S. McDougal, and S. L. Loskoski. 1985. Disinfection and inactivation of the human T lymphotropic virus type III/lymphadenopathy-associated virus. J. Infect. Dis. 152:400–403.

150. Martin, M. A., M. Reichelderfer, and Association for Professionals in Infection Control and Epidemiology, Inc., 1991, 1992, and 1993 APIC Guidelines Committee. 1994. APIC guidelines for infection prevention and control in flexible endoscopy. Am. J. Infect. Control 22:19–38.

151. **Mayer, S., M. Boos, A. Beyer, A. C. Fluit, and F. J. Schmitz.** 2001. Distribution of the antiseptic resistance genes *qacA*, *qacB* and *qacC* in 497 methicillin-resistant and -susceptible European isolates of *Staphylococcus aureus*. *J. Antimicrob. Chemother.* **47:**896–897.

152. **Mbithi, J. N., V. S. Springthorpe, and S. A. Sattar.** 1990. Chemical disinfection of hepatitis A virus on environmental surfaces. *Appl. Environ. Microbiol.* **56:**3601–3604.

153. **Mbithi, J. N., V. S. Springthorpe, S. A. Sattar, and M. Pacquette.** 1993. Bactericidal, virucidal, and mycobactericidal activities of reused alkaline glutaraldehyde in an endoscopy unit. *J. Clin. Microbiol.* **31:**2988–2995.

154. **McDonnell, G., and A. D. Russell.** 1999. Antiseptics and disinfectants: activity, action, and resistance. *Clin. Microbiol. Rev.* **12:**147–179.

155. **Mentel, R., and J. Schmidt.** 1973. Investigations on rhinovirus inactivation by hydrogen peroxide. *Acta Virol.* **17:**351–354.

156. **Merianos, J. J.** 2001. Surface-active agents, p. 283–320. *In* S. S. Block (ed.), *Disinfection, Sterilization, and Preservation.* Lippincott Williams & Wilkins, Philadelphia, Pa.

157. **Mermel, L. A., S. L. Josephson, J. Dempsey, S. Parenteau, C. Perry, and N. Magill.** 1997. Outbreak of *Shigella sonnei* in a clinical microbiology laboratory. *J. Clin. Microbiol.* **35:**3163–3165.

158. **Meyer, B., and C. Kluin.** 1999. Efficacy of glucoprotamine containing disinfectants against different species of atypical mycobacteria. *J. Hosp. Infect.* **42:**151–154.

159. **Michele, T. M., W. A. Cronin, N. M. Graham, D. M. Dwyer, D. S. Pope, S. Harrington, R. E. Chaisson, and W. R. Bishai.** 1997. Transmission of *Mycobacterium tuberculosis* by a fiberoptic bronchoscope. Identification by DNA fingerprinting. *JAMA* **278:**1093–1095.

160. **Middleton, A. M., M. V. Chadwick, J. L. Sanderson, and H. Gaya.** 2000. Comparison of a solution of superoxidized water (Sterilox) with glutaraldehyde for the disinfection of bronchoscopes, contaminated. *J. Hosp. Infect.* **45:**278–282.

161. **Mitchell, B. A., M. H. Brown, and R. A. Skurray.** 1998. QacA multidrug efflux pump from *Staphylococcus aureus:* comparative analysis of resistance to diamidines, biguanidines, and guanylhydrazones. *Antimicrob. Agents Chemother.* **42:**475–477.

162. **Nakashima, A. K., A. K. Highsmith, and W. J. Martone.** 1987. Survival of *Serratia marcescens* in benzalkonium chloride and in multiple-dose medication vials: relationship to epidemic septic arthritis. *J. Clin. Microbiol.* **25:**1019–1021.

163. **Narang, H. K., and A. A. Codd.** 1983. Action of commonly used disinfectants against enteroviruses. *J. Hosp. Infect.* **4:**209–212.

164. **Newman, L.** 2001. Risk of BSE in USA is low, say US investigators. *Lancet* **358:**2053.

165. **O'Connor, D. O., and J. R. Rubino.** 1991. Phenolic compounds, p. 204–224. *In* S. S. Block (ed.), *Disinfection, Sterilization and Preservation.* Lea & Febiger, Philadelphia, Pa.

166. **Oie, S., and A. Kamiya.** 1996. Microbial contamination of antiseptics and disinfectants. *Am. J. Infect. Control* **24:**389–395.

167. **Parker, F., and S. Foran.** 1995. Chlorhexidine catheter lubricant anaphylaxis. *Anaesth. Intensive. Care* **23:**126.

168. **Peretz, D., R. A. Williamson, K. Kaneko, J. Vergara, E. Leclerc, G. Schmitt-Ulms, I. R. Mehlhorn, G. Legname, M. R. Wormald, P. M. Rudd, R. A. Dwek, D. R. Burton, and S. B. Prusiner.** 2001. Antibodies inhibit prion propagation and clear cell cultures of prion infectivity. *Nature* **412:**739–743.

169. **Piazza, M., G. Borgia, L. Picciotto, S. Nappa, S. Cicciarello, and R. Orlando.** 1995. Detection of hepatitis C virus-RNA by polymerase chain reaction in dental surgeries. *J. Med. Virol.* **45:**40–42.

170. **Pietsch, H.** 2001. Hand antiseptics: rubs versus scrubs, alcoholic solutions versus alcoholic gels. *J. Hosp. Infect.* **48:**S33–S36.

171. **Pittet, D., S. Hugonnet, S. Harbarth, P. Mourouga, V. Sauvan, S. Touveneau, T. V. Perneger, and Infection Control Programme.** 2000. Effectiveness of a hospital-wide programme to improve compliance with hand hygiene. *Lancet* **356:**1307–1312.

172. **Price, P. B.** 1938. The bacteriology of normal skin; a new quantitative test applied to a study of the bacterial flora and the disinfectant action of mechanical cleansing. *J. Infect. Dis.* **63:**301–318.

173. **Proctor, M. E., M. Hamacher, M. L. Tortorello, J. R. Archer, and J. P. Davis.** 2001. Multistate outbreak of *Salmonella* serovar Muenchen infections associated with alfalfa sprouts grown from seeds pretreated with calcium hypochlorite. *J. Clin. Microbiol.* **39:**3461–3465.

174. **Prusiner, S. B.** 1982. Novel proteinaceous infectious particles cause scrapie. *Science* **216:**136–144.

175. **Prusiner, S. B.** 1997. Prion diseases and the BSE crisis. *Science* **278:**245–251.

176. **Ranganathan, N. S.** 1996. Chlorhexidine, p. 235–264. *In* J. P. Ascenzi (ed.), *Handbook of Disinfectants and Antiseptics.* Marcel Dekker, Inc., New York, N.Y.

177. **Reagan, D. R., B. N. Doebbeling, M. A. Pfaller, C. T. Sheetz, A. K. Houston, R. J. Hollis, and R. P. Wenzel.** 1991. Elimination of coincident *Staphylococcus aureus* nasal and hand carriage with intranasal application of mupirocin calcium ointment. *Ann. Intern. Med.* **114:**101–106.

178. **Reiss, I., A. Borkhardt, A. Fussle, A. Sziegoleit, and L. Gortner.** 2000. Disinfectant contaminated with *Klebsiella oxytoca* as a source of sepsis in babies. *Lancet* **356:**310.

179. **Robertson, L. J., A. T. Campbell, and H. V. Smith.** 1992. Survival of *Cryptosporidium parvum* oocysts under various environmental pressures. *Appl. Environ. Microbiol.* **58:**3494–3500.

180. **Roosendaal, R., E. J. Kuipers, A. J. van den Brule, A. S. Pena, A. M. Uyterlinde, J. M. Walboomers, S. G. Meuwissen, and J. de Graaff.** 1994. Importance of the fiberoptic endoscope cleaning procedure for detection of *Helicobacter pylori* in gastric biopsy specimens by PCR. *J. Clin. Microbiol.* **32:**1123–1126.

181. **Rossmoore, H. W., and M. Sondossi.** 1988. Applications and mode of action of formaldehyde condensate biocides. *Adv. Appl. Microbiol.* **33:**223–277.

182. **Rotter, M. A.** 1996. Alcohols for antisepsis of hands and skin, p. 177–234. *In* J. P. Ascenzi (ed.), *Handbook of Disinfectants and Antiseptics.* Marcel Dekker, Inc., New York, N.Y.

183. **Rotter, M. L., W. Koller, G. Wewalka, H. P. Werner, G. A. Ayliffe, and J. R. Babb.** 1986. Evaluation of procedures for hygienic hand-disinfection: controlled parallel experiments on the Vienna test model. *J. Hyg.* **96:**27–37.

184. **Rotter, M. L., S. O. Larsen, E. M. Cooke, J. Dankert, F. Daschner, D. Greco, P. Gronross, O. B. Jepsen, A. Lystad, B. Nystrom, and The European Working Party on Control of Hospital Infections.** 1988. A comparison of the effects of preoperative whole-body bathing with detergent alone and with detergent containing chlorhexidine gluconate on the frequency of wound infections after clean surgery. *J. Hosp. Infect.* **11:**310–320.

185. **Rotter, M. L., R. A. Simpson, and W. Koller.** 1998. Surgical hand disinfection with alcohols at various con-

centrations: parallel experiments using the new proposed European standards method. *Infect. Control Hosp. Epidemiol.* **19:**778–781.

186. **Rubbo, S. D., J. F. Gardner, and R. L. Webb.** 1967. Biocidal activities of glutaraldehyde and related compounds. *J. Appl. Bacteriol.* **30:**78–87.

187. **Russell, A. D.** 1994. Glutaraldehyde: current status and uses. *Infect. Control Hosp. Epidemiol.* **15:**724–733.

188. **Russell, A. D., W. B. Hugo, and G. A. J. Ayliffe.** 1999. *Principles and Practice of Disinfection, Preservation and Sterilization.* Blackwell Science, Oxford, United Kingdom.

189. **Rutala, W. A., and 1994, 1995, and 1996 APIC Guidelines Committee, Association for Professionals in Infection Control and Epidemiology, Inc.** 1996. APIC guideline for selection and use of disinfectants. *Am. J. Infect. Control.* **24:**313–342.

190. **Rutala, W. A.** 1996. Disinfection and sterilization of patient-care items. *Infect. Control Hosp. Epidemiol.* **17:**377–384.

191. **Rutala, W. A., E. P. Clontz, D. J. Weber, and K. K. Hoffmann.** 1991. Disinfection practices for endoscopes and other semicritical items. *Infect. Control Hosp. Epidemiol.* **12:**282–288.

192. **Rutala, W. A., and E. C. Cole.** 1987. Ineffectiveness of hospital disinfectants against bacteria: a collaborative study. *Infect. Control* **8:**501–506.

193. **Rutala, W. A., E. C. Cole, N. S. Wannamaker, and D. J. Weber.** 1991. Inactivation of *Mycobacterium tuberculosis* and *Mycobacterium bovis* by 14 hospital disinfectants. *Am. J. Med.* **91:**267S–271S.

194. **Rutala, W. A., M. F. Gergen, and D. J. Weber.** 1993. Evaluation of a rapid readout biological indicator for flash sterilization with three biological indicators and three chemical indicators. *Infect. Control Hosp. Epidemiol.* **14:**390–394.

195. **Rutala, W. A., M. F. Gergen, and D. J. Weber.** 1993. Inactivation of *Clostridium difficile* spores by disinfectants. *Infect. Control Hosp. Epidemiol.* **14:**36–39.

196. **Rutala, W. A., M. F. Gergen, and D. J. Weber.** 1999. Sporicidal activity of a new low-temperature sterilization technology: the Sterrad® 50 sterilizer. *Infect. Control Hosp. Epidemiol.* **20:**514–516.

197. **Rutala, W. A., S. M. Jones, and D. J. Weber.** 1996. Comparison of a rapid readout biological indicator for steam sterilization with four conventional biological indicators and five chemical indicators. *Infect. Control Hosp. Epidemiol.* **17:**423–428.

198. **Rutala, W. A., and D. J. Weber.** 1995. FDA labeling requirements for disinfection of endoscopes: a counterpoint. *Infect. Control Hosp. Epidemiol.* **16:**231–235.

199. **Rutala, W. A., and D. J. Weber.** 1997. Uses of inorganic hypochlorite (bleach) in health-care facilities. *Clin. Microbiol. Rev.* **10:**597–610.

200. **Rutala, W. A., and D. J. Weber.** 1999. Disinfection of endoscopes: review of new chemical sterilants used for high-level disinfection. *Infect. Control Hosp. Epidemiol.* **20:**69–76.

201. **Rutala, W. A., and D. J. Weber.** 2001. New disinfection and sterilization methods. *Emerg. Infect. Dis.* **7:**348–353.

202. **Rutala, W. A., D. J. Weber, and K. J. Chappell.** 1999. Patient injury from flash-sterilized instruments. *Infect. Control Hosp. Epidemiol.* **20:**458.

203. **Rutala, W. A., D. J. Weber, C. A. Thomann, J. F. John, S. M. Saviteer, and F. A. Sarubbi.** 1988. An outbreak of *Pseudomonas cepacia* bacteremia associated with a contaminated intra-aortic balloon pump. *J. Thorac. Cardiovasc. Surg.* **96:**157–161.

204. **Ryan, C. K., and G. D. Potter.** 1995. Disinfectant colitis. Rinse as well as you wash. *J. Clin. Gastroenterol.* **21:**6–9.

205. **Sagripanti, J. L.** 1992. Metal-based formulations with high microbicidal activity. *Appl. Environ. Microbiol.* **58:**3157–3162.

206. **Sagripanti, J. L., and A. Bonifacino.** 1996. Comparative sporicidal effect of liquid chemical germicides on three medical devices contaminated with spores of *Bacillus subtilis. Am. J. Infect. Control* **24:**364–371.

207. **Sagripanti, J. L., C. A. Eklund, P. A. Trost, K. C. Jinneman, C. J. Abeyta, C. A. Kaysner, and W. E. Hill.** 1997. Comparative sensitivity of 13 species of pathogenic bacteria to seven chemical germicides. *Am. J. Infect. Control* **25:**335–339.

208. **Sailer, A., H. Bueler, M. Fischer, A. Aguzzi, and C. Weissmann.** 1994. No propagation of prions in mice devoid of PrP. *Cell* **77:**967–968.

209. **Samore, M. H., L. Venkataraman, P. C. DeGirolami, R. D. Arbeit, and A. W. Karchmer.** 1996. Clinical and molecular epidemiology of sporadic and clustered cases of nosocomial *Clostridium difficile* diarrhea. *Am. J. Med.* **100:**32–40.

210. **Sattar, S. A., H. Jacobsen, H. Rahman, T. M. Cusack, and J. R. Rubino.** 1994. Interruption of rotavirus spread through chemical disinfection. *Infect. Control Hosp. Epidemiol.* **15:**751–756.

211. **Sattar, S. A., Y. E. Taylor, M. Paquette, and J. Rubino.** 1996. In-hospital evaluation of 7.5% hydrogen peroxide as a disinfectant for flexible endoscopes. *Can. J. Infect. Control* **11:**51–54.

212. **Saurina, G., D. Landman, and J. M. Quale.** 1997. Activity of disinfectants against vancomycin-resistant *Enterococcus faecium. Infect. Control Hosp. Epidemiol.* **18:**345–347.

213. **Schelenz, S., and G. French.** 2000. An outbreak of multidrug-resistant *Pseudomonas aeruginosa* infection associated with contamination of bronchoscopes and an endoscope washer-disinfector. *J. Hosp. Infect.* **46:**23–30.

214. **Scherrer, M., and K. Kümmerer.** 1997. Manual and automated processing of medical instruments—environmental and economic aspects. *Central Serv.* **5:**183–194.

215. **Sedlock, D. M., and D. M. Bailey.** 1985. Microbicidal activity of octenidine hydrochloride, a new alkanediyl-bis[pyridine] germicidal agent. *Antimicrob. Agents Chemother.* **28:**786–790.

216. **Shetty, N., S. Srinivasan, J. Holton, and G. L. Ridgway.** 1999. Evaluation of microbicidal activity of a new disinfectant: Sterilox 2500 against *Clostridium difficile* spores, *Helicobacter pylori,* vancomycin resistant *Enterococcus* species, *Candida albicans* and several *Mycobacterium* species. *J. Hosp. Infect.* **41:**101–105.

217. **Spach, D. H., F. E. Silverstein, and W. E. Stamm.** 1993. Transmission of infection by gastrointestinal endoscopy and bronchoscopy. *Ann. Intern. Med.* **118:**117–128.

218. **Spaulding, E. H.** 1968. Chemical disinfection of medical and surgical materials, p. 517–531. *In* S. Block (ed.), *Disinfection, Sterilization and Preservation.* Lea & Febiger, Philadelphia, Pa.

219. **Steinmann, J., R. Nehrkorn, A. Meyer, and K. Becker.** 1995. Two in-vivo protocols for testing virucidal efficacy of handwashing and hand disinfection. *Zentbl. Hyg. Umweltmed.* **196:**425–436.

220. **Stickler, D. J., and B. Thomas.** 1980. Antiseptic and antibiotic resistance in Gram-negative bacteria causing urinary tract infection. *J. Clin. Pathol.* **33:**288–296.

221. **Suller, M. T., and A. D. Russell.** 2000. Triclosan and antibiotic resistance in *Staphylococcus aureus. J. Antimicrob. Chemother.* **46:**11–18.

222. **Tabor, E., D. C. Bostwick, and C. C. Evans.** 1989. Corneal damage due to eye contact with chlorhexidine gluconate. *JAMA* **261:**557–558.

223. **Taylor, D. M.** 1999. Inactivation of prions by physical and chemical means. *J. Hosp. Infect.* **43**(Suppl.)**:**S69–S76.

224. **Taylor, D. M., H. Fraser, I. McConnell, D. A. Brown, K. L. Brown, K. A. Lamza, and G. R. Smith.** 1994. Decontamination studies with the agents of bovine spongiform encephalopathy and scrapie. *Arch. Virol.* **139:** 313–326.

225. **Taylor, D. M., S. L. Woodgate, A. J. Fleetwood, and R. J. Cawthorne.** 1997. Effect of rendering procedures on the scrapie agent. *Vet. Rec.* **141:**643–649.

226. **Terleckyj, B., and D. A. Axler.** 1987. Quantitative neutralization assay of fungicidal activity of disinfectants. *Antimicrob. Agents Chemother.* **31:**794–798.

227. **Tyler, R., G. A. Ayliffe, and C. Bradley.** 1990. Virucidal activity of disinfectants: studies with the poliovirus. *J. Hosp. Infect.* **15:**339–345.

228. **van Bueren, J., D. P. Larkin, and R. A. Simpson.** 1994. Inactivation of human immunodeficiency virus type 1 by alcohols. *J. Hosp. Infect.* **28:**137–148.

229. **Van Klingeren, B., and W. Pullen.** 1993. Glutaraldehyde resistant mycobacteria from endoscope washers. *J. Hosp. Infect.* **25:**147–149.

230. **Vesley, D., M. A. Nellis, and P. B. Allwood.** 1995. Evaluation of a rapid readout biological indicator for 121 degrees C gravity and 132 degrees C vacuum-assisted steam sterilization cycles. *Infect. Control Hosp. Epidemiol.* **16:**281–286.

231. **Voss, A., and A. F. Widmer.** 1997. No time for handwashing!? Handwashing versus alcoholic rub: can we afford 100% compliance? *Infect. Control Hosp. Epidemiol.* **18:**205–208.

232. **Wallace, J., P. M. Agee, and D. M. Demicco.** 1995. Liquid chemical sterilization using peracetic acid. An alternative approach to endoscope processing. *ASAIO J.* **41:**151–154.

233. **Walsh, S. E., J. Y. Maillard, and A. D. Russell.** 1999. Ortho-phthalaldehyde: a possible alternative to glutaraldehyde for high level disinfection. *J. Appl. Microbiol.* **86:**1039–1046.

234. **Waran, K. D., and R. A. Munsick.** 1995. Anaphylaxis from povidone-iodine. *Lancet* **345:**1506.

235. **Wardle, M. D., and G. M. Renninger.** 1975. Bactericidal effect of hydrogen peroxide on spacecraft isolates. *Appl. Microbiol.* **30:**710–711.

236. **Weber, D. J., S. L. Barbee, M. D. Sobsey, and W. A. Rutala.** 1999. The effect of blood on the antiviral activity of sodium hypochlorite, a phenolic, and a quaternary ammonium compound. *Infect. Control Hosp. Epidemiol.* **20:**821–827.

237. **Weber, D. J., and W. A. Rutala.** 2001. The emerging nosocomial pathogens *Cryptosporidium, Escherichia coli* O157:H7, *Helicobacter pylori,* and hepatitis C: epidemiology, environmental survival, efficacy of disinfection, and control measures. *Infect. Control Hosp. Epidemiol.* **22:**306–315.

238. **West, A. B., S. F. Kuan, M. Bennick, and S. Lagarde.** 1995. Glutaraldehyde colitis following endoscopy: clinical and pathological features and investigation of an outbreak. *Gastroenterology* **108:**1250–1255.

239. **Wewalka, G., M. Rotter, W. Koller, and G. Stanek.** 1977. Comparison of efficacy of 14 procedures for the hygienic disinfection of hands. *Zentbl. Bakteriol.* **165:** 242–249.

240. **Widmer, A. F.** 1994. Infection control and prevention strategies in the ICU. *Intensive Care Med.* **20**(Suppl. 4)**:**S7–S11.

241. **Widmer, A. F.** 2000. Replace hand washing with use of a waterless alcohol hand rub? *Clin. Infect. Dis.* **31:**136–143.

242. **Widmer, A. F., A. Houston, E. Bollinger, and R. P. Wenzel.** 1992. A new standard for sterility testing for autoclaved surgical trays. *J. Hosp. Infect.* **21:**253–260.

243. **Widmer, A. F., R. P. Wenzel, A. Trilla, M. J. Bale, R. N. Jones, and B. N. Doebbeling.** 1993. Outbreak of *Pseudomonas aeruginosa* infections in a surgical intensive care unit: probable transmission via hands of a health care worker. *Clin. Infect. Dis.* **16:**372–376.

244. **Williams, N. D., and A. D. Russell.** 1991. The effects of some halogen-containing compounds on *Bacillus subtilis* endospores. *J. Appl. Bacteriol.* **70:**427–436.

245. **Wilson, J. A., and A. B. Margolin.** 1999. The efficacy of three common hospital liquid germicides to inactivate *Cryptosporidium parvum* oocysts. *J. Hosp. Infect.* **42:**231–237.

246. **Yong, D., F. C. Parker, and S. M. Foran.** 1995. Severe allergic reactions and intra-urethral chlorhexidine gluconate. *Med. J. Aust.* **162:**257–258.

247. **Young, J. H.** 1997. Steam sterilization: scientific principles, p. 124–133. *In* M. Reichert and J. H. Young (ed.), *Sterilization Technology.* Aspen Publications, Gaithersburg, Md.

248. **Zaidi, M., J. Sifuentes, M. Bobadilla, D. Moncada, and S. Ponce de León.** 1989. Epidemic of *Serratia marcescens* bacteremia and meningitis in a neonatal unit in Mexico City. *Infect. Control Hosp. Epidemiol.* **10:**14–20.

Prevention and Control of Laboratory-Acquired Infections

ANDREAS VOSS AND ERIC NULENS

9

Health care workers are known to be at risk for contracting infection from a patient, or in cases of laboratory workers (LWs), from a patient's specimen (3). Laboratories in the United States employ approximately 500,000 LWs who are at occupational risk of exposure to microbiological pathogens that may cause inapparent to life-threatening infections (79). Laboratory-acquired infections (LAIs) are defined as all infections acquired through laboratory activities, regardless of their clinical or subclinical manifestation (83). The actual current risk of contracting LAIs is difficult to estimate, since no regional or national reporting systems are in place and most surveys were conducted years ago. Furthermore, LAIs may be underreported even on a local level due to atypical or subclinical manifestations of infections or the LW's fear of embarrassment. Data on LAIs were collected and published as early as 1949, and reviews of the incidence, consequences, and control of LAIs, such as those by Pike (76) in 1979, stimulated the development of laboratory safety programs. Despite these early guidelines, LAIs still occurred, probably due to a lack of adequate safety instructions and guidelines and/or poor compliance with safe laboratory practices, as examples in this chapter will prove. Stratton (82) assumed that health care workers, perhaps through long exposure to such risks, have become immune to concern about the problem, albeit not to occurrence of infection. Consequently, he advised that a timely reminder of these risks is useful in making sure LWs do not become complacent (82).

The emergence (or reemergence) of human immunodeficiency virus (HIV), hantavirus, hepatitis C virus, and multidrug-resistant *Mycobacterium tuberculosis* has not only renewed interest in biosafety measures but also probably enhanced compliance with these measures. Strategies for the prevention and management of LAIs should be aimed at containing the biohazardous agents and educating LWs about the occupational risks. In general, biosafety programs include recommendations on work practices, laboratory design, personal protective equipment, and safety devices. Adherence to these biosafety guidelines can reduce the risk of exposure and consequent LAIs.

The body of literature on "biosafety" is enormous and includes multiple reviews (78–80), as well as excellent publications from the Centers for Disease Control and Prevention (CDC) (33) and the Occupational Safety and Health Administration (OSHA), which can be found on the respective web sites (http://www.cdc.gov/od/ohs and http://www.osha.gov). In addition to CDC and OSHA, other U.S. agencies issuing guidelines or rules regarding laboratory safety are the National Institute of Occupational Safety and Health, the National Institutes of Health (NIH), the National Committee for Clinical Laboratory Standards (NCCLS), the College of American Pathologists, and the Joint Commission on Accreditation of Healthcare Organizations. In this chapter the basic principles of laboratory safety are described, and examples of specific LAIs and their prevention are given.

LABORATORY-ACQUIRED INFECTION SURVEYS

Sulkin and Pike (83) were the first to study LAIs systematically. By 1976, Pike (76) had published the results of a comprehensive review of the incidence, outcome, and prevention of LAIs after analyzing close to 4,000 cases of LAIs gathered through literature reviews, mail surveys, and personal communications. Despite identifying the major pathogens of LAIs and recognizing that aerosols are the primary route of transmission, Pike's data could not provide information about the denominators to be used to estimate actual risks (79).

Most LAIs (43%) were caused by bacteria, followed by viruses (27%) and rickettsiae (15%) (75). Brucellosis, typhoid fever, and Q fever were the most frequently reported infections (Table 1). The overall mortality rate among more than 3,900 reported cases of LAIs was 4.2%, with the highest mortality rate (7.8%) occurring among LWs with chlamydial infections. These fatalities originated from cases of psittacosis that occurred prior to 1955, at a time when LWs had just begun to implement the use of safe work practices and equipment. Furthermore, Pike (75) pointed out that 97% of the brucellosis and typhoid fever cases were reported before 1955 and that 10 of the 159 agents identified as pathogens responsible for LAIs caused more than 50% of the cases of LAIs. Of all viral LAIs, 36% were caused by a hepatitis virus and Venezuelan equine encephalitis virus, with half of the cases due to the latter agent being reported in only four laboratories. More than 50% of the fungal infections were caused by two pathogens: *Histoplasma capsulatum* and *Coccidioides immitis*. Among cases of LAIs due to rickettsial and parasitic agents, 50 and 24%

TABLE 1 Most frequently reported laboratory-acquired infections in the world and the United States[a]

Infection	Total no. (%) of cases reported for[b]:	
	United States and world (1976)	United States (1969)
Brucellosis	423 (10.8)	274 (9.4)
Q fever	278 (7.1)	184 (6.3)
Typhoid fever	256 (6.5)	292 (10.0)
Hepatitis	234 (6.0)	126 (4.3)
Tularemia	225 (5.7)	129 (4.4)
Tuberculosis	176 (4.5)	174 (6.0)
Dermatomycosis	161 (4.1)	84 (2.9)
Venezuelan equine encephalitis	141 (3.6)	118 (4.1)
Typhus	124 (3.2)	82 (2.8)
Psittacosis	116 (3.0)	70 (2.4)
Coccidioidomycosis	93 (2.4)	108 (3.7)
Leptospirosis	87 (2.2)	43 (1.5)
Streptococcal infection	78 (2.0)	67 (2.3)
Histoplasmosis	71 (1.8)	81 (2.8)
Shigellosis	58 (1.5)	54 (1.9)
Salmonellosis	48 (1.2)	54 (1.9)

[a] Adapted from reference 79.

[b] Entries in the column of data for the United States in 1969 may be larger than the corresponding entries in the column of data for the world and the United States in 1976 due to shifts in the numbers of various LAIs over time.

of the infections were caused by *Coxiella burnetii* and *Toxoplasma gondii*, respectively. After 1955, the relative frequency of fungal and especially viral LAIs increased whereas that of bacterial, chlamydial, and rickettsial infections notably decreased (60, 76).

During the 1980s, the most frequently found pathogens in a series of surveys (40–42, 51, 76, 85) were M. *tuberculosis*, *Salmonella* species, *Shigella* species, hepatitis B virus, and hepatitis non-A, non-B virus. Jacobson et al. (51) described an annual incidence of LAIs of approximately 3 per 1,000 employees in hospital laboratories. The risk of acquiring specific infections seems to differ among the

different types of laboratories. LWs in pathology laboratories had a greater risk of contracting tuberculosis, whereas the microbiology laboratory staff had a greater risk of contracting gastrointestinal infections such as salmonellosis and shigellosis (40, 41, 47, 76, 85). Furthermore, a threefold greater number of LAIs occurred in laboratories with fewer than 25 employees, possibly reflecting the fact that these LWs have less experience in the handling of hazardous agents. In a review of 58 publications between 1980 and 1991, Harding and Lieberman (46) reported 375 infections or seroconversions, resulting in 23 fatalities. A total of 43% (n = 162) of all LAIs were due to rickettsia, with C. *burnetii* accounting for 95% of these infections. Three-fourths of the viral infections (n = 119) were caused by arboviruses and hantaviruses. *Salmonella enterica* serovar Typhi, *Brucella melitensis*, and chlamydial species were the most frequent causes of bacterial LAIs. In general, the relative risk of acquiring an infection with a specific agent is a function of the virulence of the organism, infectious dose, and opportunity for exposure. Therefore, even organisms that are relatively virulent, e.g., *Brucella* or *S. enterica* serovar Typhi, do not cause large numbers of LAIs when the prevalence of the organism is low, which may explain why LAIs with the above-mentioned pathogens are uncommon in the United States today.

EXPOSURE RESULTING IN LABORATORY-ACQUIRED INFECTIONS

The most common types of exposure resulting in LAIs are inhalation, ingestion, inoculation, and contamination of skin and mucous membranes (Table 2). About two-thirds of all LAIs result from direct work with the infectious agent (75). Laboratory accidents were the second greatest source of LAIs, with approximately 70% of the accidents being caused by splashes or sprays, needlesticks, and cuts.

Inhalation

Various procedures in the laboratory, such as mixing, vortexing, grinding, blending, and flaming of a loop, may generate aerosols. After being discharged into the air, droplets may fall onto surfaces or evaporate, leaving droplet

TABLE 2 Routes of exposure associated with LAIs[a]

Route	Laboratory practices and/or accidents
Inhalation	Procedures that produce aerosols:
	Centrifugation
	Spillage and splashes
	Mixing, vortexing, grinding, blending, sonicating
	Separation of two surfaces enclosing a fluid (opening)
Ingestion	Mouth pipetting
	Splashes into mouth
	Eating, drinking, smoking, placing fingers in mouth (e.g., nail biting)
	Leaking contaminated items (labels, pens)
Inoculation	Needlesticks
	Cuts from sharp objects (e.g., blades or broken glassware)
	Animal and insect bites and scratches
Percutaneous or mucosal penetration	Spills and splashes
	Contact with contaminated surfaces and items
	Transfer by hand-to-face actions

[a] Data from references 12 and 79.

nuclei (≤5 μm) that remain suspended in the air and are able to reach the alveoli of the lungs when inhaled (37). Aside from typically airborne pathogens, such as M. tuberculosis, airborne transmission of organisms that do not naturally follow this route may take place in the laboratory. Manipulations of severely contaminated or large volumes of fluids may lead to inhalation of an increased inoculum and an increased probability of infection.

Ingestion

Ingestion may occur through subconscious hand-to-mouth actions, by placing contaminated articles (e.g., pencils) or fingers (e.g., by biting the fingernails) in the mouth. Food consumption in the workplace or lack of hand disinfection before eating and smoking may be other causes. Furthermore, 13% of all accidental LAIs in Pike's study were associated with mouth pipetting, indicating that LWs still neglect basic safety techniques (75).

Inoculation

Parenteral inoculation of infectious materials through accidents with needles, blades, and broken glassware is one of the leading causes of LAIs, with needlesticks and cuts alone accounting for 25.2 and 15.9% of all types of accidents resulting in infections, respectively (32, 75). Needles and sharp objects used by LWs need to be disposed of in appropriate containers in order to reduce the risk of injury of the LWs as well as that of personnel who handle waste.

Contamination of Skin and Mucous Membranes

Splashes onto the mucous membranes of the eyes, nasal cavity, and mouth and hand-to-face actions may lead to the transmission of pathogenic microorganisms. Hand washing and disinfection remain the major means of preventing LAIs.

Intact skin is an efficient barrier against most infectious agents; however, small lesions are frequent and may serve as points of entry. This route of exposure should not be underestimated, especially since Levy et al. (59) found that accidental blood-skin contact may occur between 2 and 10 times a day in LWs. Since Levy's observation originates from the pre-HIV/AIDS period, today's chance for accidental blood-skin contact may be significantly lower, due to the increased precautions we now take in working with blood and blood products.

SPECIFIC LABORATORY-ACQUIRED INFECTIONS AND THEIR AGENTS

Bacterial Infections

Brucella

The genus Brucella consists of six species: B. abortus, B. melitensis, B. suis, B. canis, B. ovis, and B. neotomae, each including different biotypes (48). Of these species, the first four are associated with human disease, with B. melitensis being considered the most virulent (86). Reports have been published of Brucella as an occupational hazard to LWs (86, 89).

As shown in Table 1, brucellosis is the most frequently reported bacterial LAI. All Brucella species are highly contagious when handled in the laboratory, frequently causing small epidemics among laboratory technicians (30, 43, 62, 81) or their families (25). Martin-Mazuelos et al. (62) and Gruner et al. (43) reported on four and five microbiology

technicians with laboratory-acquired B. melitensis infections, respectively (Table 3). Infections may occur when LWs do not expect to encounter this pathogen and neglect to take appropriate safety measures. In the report by Fiori et al. (30), 12 laboratory workers were infected (attack rate, 31%) after an accidental breakage of a centrifuge tube. Furthermore, biochemical misidentification of a Brucella species as a Moraxella species, with consequent mishandling, was shown to be another cause of laboratory-acquired brucellosis (8). Therefore, it seems prudent that clinicians should alert the laboratory when brucellosis is suspected. In addition, clinical specimens should be handled according to the most stringent safety measures (biosafety level 3 [BSL-3]) since the infection can be transmitted by aerosols (70). Still, some investigators from high-endemicity areas report laboratory-acquired infections despite enforcement of stringent safety measures (64, 88). In areas where brucellosis represents 25% of the communicable disease (64) or 10% of the positive aerobic blood culture bottles (88), the problem of LAI with Brucella probably persists, due to the large number of infected specimens handled.

Burkholderia pseudomallei/B. mallei

Burkholderia pseudomallei is the causative agent of melioidosis. In humans, the infection typically produces subclinical disease and an asymptomatic carrier state. Even though clinical illness rarely occurs, it may be associated with a lethal outcome (6). Consequently, LWs need to be trained to handle this bacterium by using safe work procedures and with adequate laboratory facilities. To prevent LAIs, special precautions (BSL-2) should be used, including prohibition of the "sniff" test and the use of centrifugation cups and biological safety cabinets (BSCs) for the processing of sputum, subculturing of stock strains, preparation of antigen, and research studies (6).

In 2000, the first human case of B. mallei in the United States since 1945 was reported in a researcher at the U.S. Army Medical Research Institute (1).

F. tularensis

In the survey published by Pike in 1976 (75), infections due to Francisella tularensis were the third most common bacterial LAIs. Most of the cases occurred in LWs in tularemia research laboratories, probably due to the transmission of infectious aerosols produced during the processing of cultures. Furthermore, infections via damaged skin have been reported in laboratory workers not strictly adhering to safety protocols (54; Basic laboratory protocols for the presumptive identification of Francisella tularensis. [http://www.bt.cdc.gov/Agent/Tularemia/ftu_la_cp_121301.pdf]).

Leptospira

LAIs associated with Leptospira species are mainly due to accidental parenteral exposure (38, 86). Since animals are the natural host of Leptospira, LWs involved in animal care or research are at higher risk of infection (34, 65).

Mycobacterium tuberculosis

The M. tuberculosis complex includes five human pathogens: M. tuberculosis, M. bovis, M. africanum, M. microti, and M. canettii. In the hospital, administrative controls, such as patient screening and risk assessment, followed by prompt isolation and appropriate therapy are the most important components of tuberculosis prevention (14, 15). Among LWs, the risk of exposure to species of the M. tuberculosis complex is especially high in anatomic pathol-

TABLE 3 Examples of bacterial, fungal, parasitic, chlamydial, rickettsial, and viral LAIs reported between 1990 and 2001

Pathogen (infection)	Reference	Comment
Bacteria		
B. melitensis (brucellosis)	Martin-Mazuelos et al. (62)	Outbreak involving four technicians
	Gruner et al. (43)	Outbreak involving five technicians
	Batchelor et al. (8)	Infection due to misidentification
	Memish and Mah (64) and Yagupsky et al. (88)	Cases despite safety procedures, due to high workload in endemic area
	Fiori et al. (30)	Outbreak due to broken centrifuge tube
B. mallei (glanders)	Anonymous (2)	Transmission unknown
Leptospira species (leptospirosis)	Waitkins (86)	Accidental parenteral exposure
	Gilks et al. (38)	Accidental parenteral exposure
M. tuberculosis (tuberculosis)	Mazurek et al. (63)	LAI proven by DNA fingerprinting
	Muller (66)	Higher risk in laboratories
	Shireman (80)	Endometrial tuberculosis
N. meningitidis (meningitis)	Guibourdenche et al. (44)	Transmission confirmed by typing
	Paradis and Grimard (72)	Invasive infection in LW
	Boutet et al. (17)	5 cases in 15 yrs, working outside BSC
Salmonella or *Shigella*	Beers et al. (10)	Nail biters were found to be at higher risk
	Holmes et al. (50)	Handling of strains for proficiency testing
S. enterica serovar Typhi (typhoid fever)	Ashdown and Cassidy (6)	No obvious breakdown in safety techniques
E. coli O157	Burnens et al. (19)	Proven by toxin type and plasmid profile analyses
	Bolten and Aird (16)	LAI, person-to-person
C. jejuni	Penner et al. (73)	Transmission confirmed by typing
Fungi		
Penicillium marneffei	Hilmarsdottir et al.[a]	In an HCW[c] with AIDS
S. schenckii (sporotrichosis)	Cooper et al. (27)	In the absence of apparent trauma
B. dermatitidis, H. capsulatum, and *C. immitis*	Baum and Lerner (9) and Collins (26)	Transmission by inhalation
Protozoa		
Trypanosoma brucei gambiense	Receveur et al.[d]	Trypanosomiasis
T. gondii	Herwaldt and Juranek (49)	Most common protozoal LAI
Leishmania mexicana	Knobloch and Demar (55)	Accidental percutaneous inoculation
Chlamydia		
C. trachomatis	Bernstein et al. (11)	Pneumonitis, lymphadenitis
Rickettsiae		
C. burnetii	Hamadeh et al. (45)	Q-fever epidemics by aerosol transmission
R. rickettsii	Oster et al. (71)	Rocky Mountain spotted fever due to aerosols
Viruses		
Blood-borne pathogens	Jacobson et al. (51)	Despite considerable risk, no attention
	Levy et al. (59)	Due to exposure to HBV-contaminated blood
	Favero and Bond (29)	No evidence of aerosol transmission
Hemorrhagic fever (e.g., Sabia virus)	Gonzales et al. (39) and Barry et al. (7)	Two LAIs caused by strain that caused fatal cases in Sao Paulo, Brazil, 1990
	Gandsman et al. (36) and Ryder and Gandsman[b]	Scientist exposure while purifying the virus from tissue culture
Arenavirus	Vasconcelos et al. (84)	Transmission through aerosols

[a] Hilmarsdottir et al., Letter, *Clin. Infect. Dis.* **19:**357–358, 1994.
[b] R. W. Ryder and E. J. Gandsman, Letter, *N. Engl. J. Med.* **333:**1716, 1995.
[c] HCW, health care worker.
[d] M. C. Receveur, M. LeBras, and P. Vincendeau, Letter, *N. Engl. J. Med.* **329:**209–210, 1993.

ogy laboratories (morgue, frozen-section suite) and is increased in general clinical laboratories and mycobacteriological laboratories (85). In a survey of state and territorial public health laboratories, about 25% of the responding laboratories (13 of 49) reported a total of 21 employees with tuberculin skin test conversion, including 7 with documented LAI (53). Infections were probably due to inadequate isolation procedures, the high volume of specimen handling, and faulty ventilation.

Since the source of laboratory-acquired tuberculosis is often unclear, occupational transmission is difficult to prove. Due to the known characteristics of the strain, Mazurek et al. (63) genotypically proved the transmission of the reference strain M. *tuberculosis* Erdman by using DNA fingerprinting (Table 3). Generally, LAIs with M. *tuberculosis* cause pulmonary infections, but other body sites may be involved. Shireman et al. (80) described a case of granulomatous endometrial tuberculosis that was probably due to respiratory tract exposure as a result of a faulty exhaust hood.

CDC (22) has published regulatory guidelines entitled *Goals for Working Safely with Mycobacterium tuberculosis*. A copy of these draft guidelines may be obtained from the American Society for Microbiology (ASM) at http://www.asmusa.org/pasrc/regulat.htm. ASM specifically questions CDC's advice to apply BSL-3 and respirators in all tuberculosis laboratory operations, providing virtually no stratification of safety standards for different risks and/or settings. At least among health care workers the tuberculin skin test conversion rates did not differ between hospitals in which surgical masks or disposable particulate respirators were used (35), suggesting that respirators certainly are not indicated for all laboratory activities. Still, since the infectious dose of M. tuberculosis is very low (37), all activities that may produce aerosols (e.g., opening of test tubes containing cultures) should be done in BSC. OSHA issued mandatory guidelines regarding tuberculosis exposure in 1993 (69); in March 2002, OSHA reopened discussion of updated regulations—see the OSHA website http://www.osha.gov/SLTC/tuberculosis/index.html (accessed 8 March 2002) for further regulatory developments.

Neisseria meningitidis

Despite regular isolation of *Neisseria meningitidis* in clinical laboratories, it has only infrequently been reported as a cause of LAIs. Guibourdenche et al. (44) proved laboratory transmission of N. meningitidis by using serotyping, outer membrane protein characterization, and enzyme electrophoresis to confirm the identities of the clinical isolates from two laboratory technicians infected with laboratory strains (Table 3). The occupational risk for LWs in particular seems high enough to the Norwegian National Institute of Public Health to justify the development and testing of an N. meningitidis serogroup B vaccine (31). During a 15-year period, five cases of meningococcal disease were identified in LWs in England and Wales (17). All cases actually occurred between 1992 and 1995, and all of the LWs prepared suspensions of the consequently infecting strain on open benches. Recently, the CDC described 2 cases of laboratory-acquired meningococcal diseases and identified an additional 14 cases that were previously unreported (24). This may indicate underreporting of cases or an actual increase of the disease incidence. For the United States (1996 to 2000) an attack rate of 13 per 100,000 was calculated, with a case-fatality rate of 50%. All manipulations of samples that have a risk for droplet or aerosol formation should be performed in a BSC. Further measurements are described in an editorial note on the report of the most recent U.S. cases (24).

Salmonella, Shigella, and Other Stool Pathogens

Salmonellosis and shigellosis are the most commonly reported gastrointestinal LAIs (26, 42, 51, 75, 76). Infections occur from ingestion or, on rare occasions, from inoculation of the stool pathogens from clinical specimens, as well as from the handling of proficiency test strains (50). Chronic nail biters may be at risk, as shown among HCWs in a nursery for newborns (10). The incidences of salmonellosis and shigellosis in Great Britain are reported to be 0.137 and 0.322 infection per 1,000 LWs, respectively (79), but these infections are probably vastly underreported. In a comparison of LWs from clinical laboratories with those from microbiological laboratories, the latter group had an approximately eightfold-higher incidence of laboratory-acquired shigellosis (51). The most serious gastrointestinal infections acquired in the laboratory are probably due to S. enterica serovar Typhi. Genetic and epidemiological evidence for the transmission of LAI with S. enterica serovar Typhi has been obtained by pulsed-field gel electrophoresis (56). A case of laboratory-acquired typhoid fever has been described in a situation in which no obvious breakdown of laboratory safety techniques could be detected (5). In addition to the transmission to or among LWs, cases of typhoid fever may occur among people outside the laboratory (13). Since the infectious dose of S. enterica serovar Typhi and Shigella spp. is smaller than that of most enteric pathogens, handling of specimens containing this pathogens might bear a higher risk of an LAI.

As with S. enterica serovar Typhi, Burnens et al. (19) suggested that the infecting dose of Escherichia coli O157:H7 is low since they found no break in preventive measures preceding a case of LAI caused by this microorganism. Some authorities in the United Kingdom advise that evaluations of the immunization histories of staff working in the microbiological laboratory with regard to their immunity to S. enterica serovar Typhi be performed and recommend a course of typhoid vaccine (74).

Despite causing frequent problems in the hospital, *Clostridium difficile* has not been reported to be a cause of LAIs. Penner et al. (73) used different typing techniques to confirm a laboratory-acquired case of *Campylobacter jejuni* enteritis caused by a frequently passaged laboratory strain.

Chlamydial Infections

To date, only sporadic laboratory cases of chlamydial infections due to *Chlamydophila psittaci* and *Chlamydia trachomatis* have been reported (11, 26). Prior to the 1960s, LWIs with these organisms used to be common and were associated with a high mortality rate (75).

Fungal Infections

Laboratory-acquired fungal infections most commonly originate from inhalation of spores or conidia of *Blastomyces dermatitidis* (9, 26), *Histoplasma capsulatum* (26, 67), and *Coccidioides immitis* (26). These fungal pathogens, as well as *Sporothrix schenckii*, may furthermore lead to cutaneous LAIs after accidental inoculation (26, 27, 58, 75). Cooper et al. (27) reported a case of laboratory-acquired sporotrichosis associated with research activities (Table 3). Since no apparent trauma or other predisposing factors were known, the investigators suggested the possibility that S. schenckii (at least under laboratory conditions) can invade intact, healthy skin.

Despite ranking high on the list of LAI-associated fungal pathogens (Table 1), dermatophytes are not usually seen among LWs in clinical laboratories but are seen among those in animal facilities.

Parasitic Infections

Only a small percentage (~3%) of all LAIs are caused by protozoal agents. *Toxoplasma gondii* is the most frequently observed agent of parasitic LAIs. Other common parasitic LAIs are malaria, leishmaniasis, and trypanosomiasis (49; M. C. Receveur, M. LeBras, and P. Vincendeau, Letter, N. Engl. J. Med. **329**:209–210, 1993). The majority of these cases occur among LWs in animal research facilities. Needlestick injuries were the major source in cases in which an accident could be recalled. Usually, accidents or breaks in laboratory safety measures were not recalled, due to the long incubation period, such as in a patient with

Leishmania mexicana LAI that occurred 8 months after accidental inoculation (55).

Rickettsial Infections

In 1969, Q fever was the second most commonly reported LAI in the world and in the United States (Table 1). More than 30 years later, the question is whether these numbers still reflect the current U.S. experience. LWs in animal research facilities are particularly at risk, since research animals such as sheep may be asymptomatic carriers of *Coxiella burnetii*. As shown with *Brucella* species, aerosol transmission of *C. burnetii* may cause small Q fever epidemics among LWs in the same facility (45). Furthermore, multiple cases of laboratory-acquired Rocky Mountain spotted fever due to aerosol transmission of *Rickettsia rickettsii* have been reported (71).

Viral Infections Caused by Blood-Borne Pathogens

Despite the considerable risk of contraction of hepatitis B virus (HBV) by LWs (29, 51, 59) and the consequential morbidity and mortality from HBV infections among health care workers, it required the advent of the HIV and AIDS epidemic to increase the general level of attention of HCWs to the risk of blood-borne transmission of viral pathogens. In 1994, a total of 32 laboratory technicians were reported by CDC to have documented ($n = 17$) and possible ($n = 15$) cases of HIV infection as a result of occupational transmission (20). Percutaneous exposure was the leading cause in these cases, but, nevertheless, transmissions after mucocutaneous contact were reported.

Parenteral inoculation, percutaneous contact in the presence of skin lesions, and exposure of mucous membranes present a high risk of HIV transmission. So far, no evidence of aerosol HIV transmission exists (29). Evans et al. (28) assessed the risk for occupational exposures to biohazardous agents found in blood by taking environmental samples from a total of 10 clinical and research laboratories. HBV surface antigen was found in 31 of the 800 environmental samples from 11 workstations in three laboratories.

Environmental contamination arises as a result of several factors, such as high workloads, inappropriate behavior, and flawed laboratory techniques. Therefore, a multifactorial approach is necessary to prevent or minimize viral and blood-borne LAIs. Guidelines for prevention of blood-borne infections are in general alike for most of the so-called blood-borne pathogens, such as HBV, HCV, HDV, and HIV. Avoidance of unprotected contact with infectious materials (blood, semen, saliva, tears, urine, cerebrospinal fluid, breast milk, and other excretions or secretions) by the use of BSL-2 practices and containment equipment is the most important means of prevention. For further regulations regarding occupational exposure to blood-borne pathogens, OSHA's rules should be consulted (1, 68). A high educational level and vaccination against hepatitis B are major factors in the prevention of LAIs caused by blood-borne pathogens.

Viral Hemorrhagic Fever

The viral hemorrhagic fever syndrome may be caused by several RNA viruses from the *Filoviridae, Arenaviridae, Bunyaviridae*, and *Flaviviridae* families (18, 61). These viruses are highly infectious by aerosol, and adequate precautions need to be taken when contacting patients and handling their laboratory specimens (4). Filoviruses may infect monkeys and thereby may contaminate cell cultures prepared from monkeys in experimental laboratories (61).

Arenavirus was isolated from a single patient with fatal hemorrhagic fever in the state of Sao Paulo, Brazil, in 1990. A serologically proven LAI transmitted by aerosols was described by Vasconcelos et al. (84) in an LW with symptoms of hemorrhagic fever (Table 3). Attempts to isolate the virus from the LW did not succeed. Several other cases of laboratory-acquired hemorrhagic fever due to Sabia virus have been reported (36, 39; R. W. Ryder and E. J. Gandsman, Letter, *N. Engl. J. Med.* **333:**1716, 1995), including a case of a senior-level visiting research scientist at Yale University, who was exposed to the virus while purifying it from tissue culture fluid (36).

In general, arboviruses are assigned to BSL-1 to BSL-4, depending on their mode of transmission and the consequent severity and/or frequency of LAIs. The most virulent agents, such as Ebola, Lassa, and Marburg viruses, as well as the viruses associated with tick-borne encephalitis, should be handled only in BSL-4 facilities. In 1993, the Subcommittee on Arbovirus Laboratory Safety of the American Society of Tropical Medicine and Hygiene developed and published further recommendations (21).

LWs are exposed to a wide variety of other viral agents, which are described in further detail in a review by Sewell (79).

BIOSAFETY AND INFECTION CONTROL IN THE MICROBIOLOGY LABORATORY

Containment of hazardous agents describes the use of safe methods for managing infectious materials in the laboratory environment. Its purpose is to reduce or eliminate exposure of LWs and the environment to potentially hazardous agents (23). Primary containment involves the protection of personnel and the immediate laboratory environment; secondary containment involves the protection of the environment external to the laboratory (23). Hence, the three most important topics in laboratory safety are: (i) laboratory practice and techniques, (ii) safety equipment, and (iii) facility design.

Laboratory personnel must always be aware of the potential hazards when working with clinical specimens. As a result, strict adherence to standard microbiological practices and techniques is the most important factor in containment. Each laboratory should produce a biosafety manual. To minimize and/or eliminate exposures to certain agents, laboratory personnel must be continually trained to ensure awareness of diagnostic and preventive measures.

Primary barriers (safety equipment) against biological agents include BSC, enclosed containers, and other engineering controls. Safety equipment may also include items for personal protection, such as gloves, face shields, and safety glasses, which are often used in combination with a BSC.

Secondary barriers depend on the risk of transmission of specific agents. The design and construction of the laboratory facility are part of these secondary considerations. These barriers should contribute to the protection of laboratory workers and in addition protect the living environment in the community from infectious agents that may be accidentally released from the laboratory.

Biological Safety Cabinets and Other Primary Barriers

BSCs provide protection for personnel and the environment by minimizing exposures to hazardous biological materials. Class I and II BSCs offer significant levels of protection to laboratory personnel and the environment. The class I BSC has a negative pressure, is ventilated, and is usually operated with an open front. It is designed for general microbiological research with agents of low to moderate risk. Class II cabinets include HEPA-filtered vertical laminar airflow and protect against external contamination with the materials handled inside the BSC. Depending on their inlet flow velocity and the percentage of air that is HEPA filtered and recirculated, class II BSCs are also differentiated into type A and type B class II BSCs. Generally, class IIA BSCs are used for microbiological procedures requiring BSL-2 or BSL-3 containment. Class III BSCs are totally enclosed cabinets with a gas-tight construction and provide the highest possible level of protection to personnel and the environment, thereby being suitable for work requiring BSL-3 or BSL-4 containment (33).

Additional detailed information on BSC construction, certification procedures, instructions for decontamination, and levels of containment for microorganisms can be found in the literature (23, 33, 57) or on the websites of OSHA, NIH, and CDC. Personal protection items such as goggles, respirators, face shields, gloves, and gowns are frequently used in combination with BSCs. Additional equipment used to contain infectious splashes or aerosols includes safety centrifuge cups, which prevent the release of infectious agents that can be transmitted during centrifugation.

Biosafety Levels

In an effort to diminish the risk of LAIs, a system for categorizing infectious agents into groups on the basis of the mode of transmission, availability of preventive measures and antimicrobial treatment, and the type and seriousness of a possible infection was formulated. In regard to the different groups and categories, guidelines that describe appropriate containment equipment, facilities, and procedures to be used by LWs were developed. These guidelines are referred to as biosafety levels (BSLs). In general, four BSLs are described; they consist of the use of combinations of primary and secondary barriers for particular microbiological practices. Each BSL is designed to ensure the safety of personnel and the environment during work with specific infectious agents. With class 1 agents, hazards are minimal; class 4 agents require maximum containment. Detailed information on BSLs recommended for specific bacterial, fungal, parasitic, and viral agents can be found in the Agent Summary Statements in *Laboratory Safety: Principles and Practices* (33) or at the CDC website on Biosafety in Microbiological and Biomedical Laboratories at http://www.cdc.gov/od/ohs/biosfty/biosfty.htm. Categorization of the various organisms is based in particular on the likelihood of their transmission. When working with known organisms, such as in the research setting, the implementation of the appropriate practices for each BSL may be simple. Application of the correct BSL in the clinical laboratory remains difficult, since the infectious nature of the clinical material is typically unknown.

BSL-1 describes the lowest level of containment or microbiological safety and is entirely based on standard laboratory practices. It is recommended for work on an open bench with microorganisms that are not known to cause infections in healthy adults, such as *Bacillus subtilis*, but may behave as opportunistic pathogens in very young or older patients and immunocompromised individuals.

BSL-2 practices are generally applied in bacteriology laboratories during work with moderate-risk agents (e.g., *Salmonella* species and hepatitis B virus) associated with human diseases of various severities. The pathogens may be transmitted by accidental ingestion, percutaneous exposure, or mucous membrane exposure. When standard microbiological practices are applied, the agents may be handled on open benches, especially if primary barriers such as face protection, gowns, and gloves are used when appropriate. BSCs and safety centrifuge cups should be used when exposure to infectious splashes and aerosols is expected.

BSL-3 recommendations are aimed at the containment of hazardous microorganisms transmitted primarily by aerosols, such as *M. tuberculosis* or *C. burnetii*. BSL-3 makes use of stringent practices as well as primary and secondary safety equipment, including specific requirements for the facility, such as a suitable ventilation system. All BSL-3 microorganisms need to be processed in a BSC.

BSL-4 applies to microbiological agents that pose the risk of life-threatening disease which may be transmitted via aerosol or for which there is no available vaccine or therapy (e.g., hemorrhagic fever viruses). Manipulations are generally performed in a class III BSC or by personnel wearing full-body, air-supplied, positive-pressure suits. The facility itself is totally isolated from other laboratories and includes a specialized ventilation and waste management system. A summary of the recommended BSLs for infectious agents is given in Table 4.

Biosafety and Bioterrorism

Until recently, bioterrorism and the agents involved in it were hardly ever encountered in (clinical) laboratories; hence, laboratory personnel were not familiar with the appearance and characteristics of these agents or with the reception, handling, and laboratory treatment of clinical specimens. Due to recent events, clinical laboratories may be requested to process clinical or environmental specimens from real or hoax attacks. Therefore, all microbiological laboratories should be familiar with the methods and precautionary measures involved in handling these agents (Table 5; see chapter 10). Furthermore, special precautions are needed for LWs, since potential bioterrorism agents such as *Brucella* species and *Francisella tularensis* already belong to the group of most commonly reported bacterial LAIs.

CDC has created the Laboratory Response Network to provide an organized response system for the detection and diagnosis of biological warfare agents based on laboratory testing abilities and facilities (52, 54). Laboratories are assigned to four capacity levels (A to D), with each level having designated core-testing competence. Level A laboratories have the minimum core capacity. They rule out suspected isolates by simple tests and refer them to a higher-level laboratory. Level D laboratories, such as CDC, are BSL-4 facilities, having the highest capacity and most advanced techniques. Most clinical, hospital, and private laboratories are classified as a level A, operating at BSL-2. Level A laboratories are most likely to be the first that are contacted or questioned with regard to specimen collection and shipment, culture, and treatment. Despite the fact that these laboratories are not intended to actually handle critical biological agents, they might receive clinical samples

TABLE 4 Summary of recommended BSLs for infectious agents[a]

BSL	Agents	Practices and techniques	Safety equipment	Facilities
1	No disease in healthy adults (e.g., *B. subtilis*)	Standard microbiological practices	None required; laboratory clothing recommended; protection of skin lesions and eyes if indicated	Open bench top resistant and impervious to water; sink required
2	Associated with human disease; transmission generally not via aerosols (e.g., *Salmonella* spp.)	BSL-1 plus limited access, biohazard label; "sharp"-object precautions; biosafety manual (including waste decontamination, immunization policies, training)	Class I or II BSC or other containment devices if infectious aerosols or splashes may occur; appropriate PPE[b]	BSL-1 plus autoclave and eyewash facility
3	Serious or lethal consequences; potential for aerosol transmission (e.g., *M. tuberculosis*)	BSL-2 plus controlled access, decontamination of all waste and clothing, baseline serum sample	Class I or II BSC or other containment devices for all procedures; appropriate PPE	BSL-2 plus negative airflow, air exhaust to outside, self-closing double doors
4	Life-threatening; transmission by aerosol or unknown risk of transmission (e.g., Ebola virus)	BSL-3 plus facility-specific clothing, shower on exit, decontamination of all materials on exit	Class III or class II BSC in combination with full-body air-supplied, positive-pressure suit for all procedures	BSL-3 plus separate building and special engineering and design features

[a] Data from references 12, 33, and 79.
[b] PPE, personal protective equipment (e.g., lab clothing, gloves, and face or respiratory protection).

that are initially not suspected for these agents. Consequently, even level A laboratories should have the necessary facilities, equipment, and competence to process critical biological agents (52).

Therefore, all laboratories handling clinical and environmental specimens should attain a basic standard:

1. Knowledge of the current biosafety level within the laboratory
2. Development and availability of protocols related to the chain of guardianship
3. Collection, preservation, and shipment of specimens as well as culture and identification of targeted agents
4. Location of the nearest higher-level reference laboratory; knowledge of current guidelines to ensure the safe handling and shipment of biological agents
5. Knowledge of the basic characteristics of the current targeted agents (52, 54)

For bacterial warfare agents, activities concerning specimen handling and diagnosis of suspected cultures should be performed at least at a BSL-2 facility. This implies that all specimens after reception and labeling are further handled in a class I or II BSC. Manipulation and production of large quantities of bacterial cultures and other activities which might cause aerosol formation should be avoided and should be referred to a BSL-3 laboratory.

In general, *Bacillus anthracis*, *Yersinia pestis*, and specimens containing botulism toxins can be safely handled using BSL-2 practices, but BSL-3 is recommended for *F. tularensis*, *Brucella* spp., and "modified" *B. anthracis* strains. Smallpox virus and the hemorrhagic fever viruses are extremely infectious, and specimen collection, handling, and further treatment should be referred to a BSL-4 facility (54).

Biosafety Practices

In the United States, biosafety-related issues in microbiology laboratories are regulated by federal agencies, the states, and local jurisdictions. Some of the guidelines published by OSHA; CDC; the National Institute for Occupational Safety and Health (NIOSH), a branch of CDC; the Environmental Protection Agency; NIH; and the Joint Commission on Accreditation of Healthcare Organizations are mandated by law. Others must be seen as "standards of practice."

To ensure biosafety in the individual laboratory, programs should be implemented and documented in writing and LWs should be trained in order to perceive and follow up on these guidelines. The safety program should include LAI surveillance (including surveillance for HBV, HIV, and *M. tuberculosis* infections), vaccination plans, and guidelines that restrict the duties of highly susceptible LWs (e.g., during pregnancy).

The standard laboratory practices that are of utmost importance for the prevention of LAIs are listed in Table 6. Application of CDC's universal precautions to the laboratory area would require that all blood and blood-contaminated specimens be considered "infected." Sharp objects and needles should be used and deposited according to the guidelines, and hands should be disinfected whenever necessary.

Decontamination and Waste Disposal

Decontamination procedures and waste disposal management are described in detail in chapter 8. Nevertheless, a few infection control and biosafety guidelines are mentioned here, since improper waste disposal can be a major source of laboratory accidents.

As a general rule, laboratories should have in writing procedures for waste management, accidents, and spills

TABLE 5 Microbiology biosafety for biological warfare agents

Agent	BSL Specimen handling	BSL Culture handling	Recommended precautions for level A laboratories
Bacillus anthracis	2	2	BSL2: activities involving clinical material collection and diagnostic quantities of infectious cultures BSL3: activities with high potential for aerosol or droplet production
Brucella spp.[a]	2	3	BSL2: activities limited to collection, transport, and plating of clinical material BSL3: all activities involving manipulations of cultures
Clostridium botulinum[b]	2	2	BSL2: activities with materials known or potentially containing toxin must be handled in a BSC (class II) by personnel with a lab coat, disposable surgical gloves, and a faceshield (as needed) BLS3: activities with high potential for aerosol or droplet production
Francisella tularensis[c]	2	3	BLS2: activities limited to collection, transport, and plating of clinical material BLS3: all activities involving manipulations of cultures
Yersinia pestis[d]	2	2	BSL2: activities involving clinical material collection and diagnostic quantities of infectious cultures BSL3: activities with high potential for aerosol or droplet production
Smallpox virus[e]	4	4	BSL4: specimen collection/transport
Hemorrhagic fever viruses[f]	4	4	BSL4: specimen collection/transport

[a] Laboratory acquired brucellosis has occurred by "sniffing" cultures; via aerosols generated by centrifugation; mouth pipetting; accidental parenteral inoculations; sprays into eyes, nose, and mouth; and finally by direct contact with clinical specimens.

[b] Exposure to toxin is the primary laboratory hazard since absorption can occur via direct contact with skin, eyes, or mucous membranes, including the respiratory tract. The toxin can be neutralized by 0.1 M sodium hydroxide. C. botulinum is inactivated by a 1:10 dilution of household bleach. Contact time is 20 min. If material contains both toxin and organisms, the spill must be sequentially treated with bleach and sodium hydroxide for a total contact time of 40 min.

[c] Laboratory-acquired tularemia infection has been more commonly associated with cultures than with clinical materials or animals. Direct skin or mucous membrane contact with cultures, parenteral inoculation, ingestion, and aerosol exposure have resulted in infection.

[d] Special care should be taken to avoid the generation of aerosols.

[e] Ingestion, parenteral inoculation, and droplet or aerosol exposure of mucous membranes or broken skin with infectious fluids or tissues are the primary hazards to LWs.

[f] Respiratory exposure to infectious aerosols, mucous membrane exposure to infectious droplets, and accidental parenteral inoculation are the primary hazards to LWs.

with infectious agents and, moreover, should ensure that LWs are familiar with these guidelines. Potentially infectious waste should be separated immediately at the time of production and should be disposed of in sturdy bags marked with biohazard logos. Puncture-resistant, leakproof containers should be used when disposing of any kind of sharp

TABLE 6 Standard microbiological biosafety practices

Employ constant precautions in handling blood and body fluid (universal precautions).
Deposit sharp objects in special puncture-resistant containers.
Comply with hand disinfection procedures by using alcoholic hand rubs or medicated soaps.
Do not eat, drink, or smoke in the laboratory. Do not store food in refrigerators used for clinical specimens.
Use disposable plastic pipettes, and avoid mouth pipetting by using proper mechanical pipetting devices.
Decontaminate work surfaces daily and after spills.
Wear appropriate personal protective equipment during laboratory work, and remove it before leaving the laboratory area.
Provide well-fitting (latex) gloves in order to increase compliance with glove use.
Wear face shields or masks and eye protection when splashes of blood or body fluids are possible.
Use containment equipment for all laboratory procedures that generate large amounts of aerosols or splashes.

object. Furthermore, tuberculocidal disinfectants should be used for regular decontamination of work surfaces and equipment, and antibacterial soaps or alcoholic hand rubs should be used for hand disinfection.

REFERENCES

1. **Anonymous.** 1993. OSHA's bloodborne pathogens standard: analysis and recommendations. *Health Devices* **22:** 35–92.
2. **Anonymous.** Laboratory-acquired human glanders. 2000. *Morb. Mortal. Wkly. Rep.* **49:**532–535.
3. **Antony, S. J., C. W. Stratton, and M. Decker.** 1999. Prevention of occupational acquired infections in posthospital healthcare workers, p. 1141–1158. *In* C. G. Mayhall (ed.), *Hospital Epidemiology and Infection Control*, 2nd ed. The Williams & Wilkins Co., Baltimore, Md.
4. **Armstrong, L. R., L. M. Dembry, P. M. Rainey, M. B. Russi, A. S. Kahn, S. H. Fischer, S. C. Edberg, T. G. Ksiazek, P. E. Rollin, and C. J. Peters.** Management of a Sabia virus-infected patients in a US hospital. 1999. *Infect. Control Hosp. Epidemiol.* **20:**176–182.
5. **Ashdown, L. R.** 1992. Melioidosis and safety in the clinical laboratory. *J. Hosp. Infect.* **21:**301–306.
6. **Ashdown, L., and J. Cassidy.** 1991. Successive *Salmonella give* and *Salmonella typhi* infections, laboratory-acquired. *Pathology* **23:**233–234.
7. **Barry, M., M. Russi, L. Armstrong, D. Geller, R. Tesh, L. Dembry, J. P. Gonzalez, A. S. Khan, and C. J. Peters.** 1995. Brief report: treatment of a laboratory-acquired Sabia virus infection. *N. Engl. J. Med.* **333:**294–296.

8. **Batchelor, B. I., R. J. Brindle, G. F. Gilks, and J. B. Selkon.** 1992. Biochemical mis-identification of Brucella melitensis and subsequent laboratory-acquired infections. *J. Hosp. Infect.* **22:**159–162.

9. **Baum, G. L., and P. I. Lerner.** 1971. Primary pulmonary blastomycosis: a laboratory-acquired infection. *Ann. Intern. Med.* **73:**263–265.

10. **Beers, L. M., T. L. Burke, and D. B. Martin.** 1989. Shigellosis occurring in newborn nursery staff. *Infect. Control* **10:**147–149.

11. **Bernstein, D. L., T. Hubbard, W. M. Wenman, B. L. Johnson, K. K. Holmes, H. Liebhaber, J. Schachter, R. Barnes, and M. A. Lovett.** 1984. Mediastinal and supraclavicular lymphadenitis and pneumonitis due to Chlamydia trachomatis serovars L1 and L2. *N. Engl. J. Med.* **311:**1543–1546.

12. **Berrouane, Y.** 1997. Laboratory-acquired infections, p. 607–618. *In* R. P. Wenzel (ed.), *Prevention and Control of Nosocomial Infections.* The Williams & Wilkins Co., Baltimore, Md.

13. **Blaser, M. J., and R. A. Feldman.** 1981. Acquisition of typhoid fever from proficiency-testing specimens. *N. Engl. J. Med.* **303:**1481.

14. **Blumberg, H. M.** 1997. Tuberculosis and infection control. *Infect. Control Hosp. Epidemiol.* **18:**538–541.

15. **Blumberg, H. M., D. L. Watkins, J. D. Berschling, A. Antle, P. Moore, N. White, M. Hunter, B. Green, S. M. Ray, and J. E. McGowan, Jr.** 1995. Preventing the nosocomial transmission of tuberculosis. *Ann. Intern. Med.* **122:**658–663.

16. **Bolton, F. J., and H. Aird.** 1998. Verocytotoxin-producing *Escherichia coli* O 157: public health and microbiological significance. *Br. J. Biomed. Sci.* **55:**127–135.

17. **Boutet, R., J. M. Stuart, E. B. Kaczmarski, S. J. Gray, D. M. Jones, and N. Andrews.** 2001. Risk of laboratory-acquired meningococcal disease. *J. Hosp. Infect.* **49:**282–284.

18. **Broussard, L. A.** 2001. Biological agents: weapons of warfare and bioterrorism. *Mol. Diagn.* **6:**323–333.

19. **Burnens, A. P., R. Zbinden, L. Kaempf, I. Heinzer, and J. Nicolet.** 1993. A case of laboratory acquired infection with *Escherichia coli* O157:H7. *Int. J. Med. Microbiol. Virol. Parasitol. Infect. Dis.* **279:**512–517.

20. **Centers for Disease Control and Prevention.** 1994. *HIV/AIDS Surveillance Report.* Report 5. Centers for Disease Control and Prevention, Atlanta, Ga.

21. **Centers for Disease Control and Prevention.** 1994. Laboratory management of agents associated with hantavirus pulmonary syndrome: interim biosafety guidelines. *Morb. Mortal. Wkly. Rep.* **43:**1–7.

22. **Centers for Disease Control and Prevention.** 1997. Goals for working safely with *Mycobacterium tuberculosis. Fed. Regist.,* vol. 62.

23. **Centers for Disease Control and Prevention and National Institutes of Health.** 1999. *Biosafety in Microbiological and Biomedical Laboratories,* 4th ed. U.S. Department of Health and Human Services, Public Health Service, Washington, D.C.

24. **Centers for Disease Control and Prevention.** 2002. Laboratory-acquired meningococcal disease—United States, 2000. *Morb. Mortal. Wkly. Rep.* **51:**141–144.

25. **Chusid, M. J., S. K. Russler, B. A. Mohr, D. A. Margolis, C. A. Hillery, and K. C. Kehl.** 1993. Unsuspected brucellosis diagnosed in a child as a result of an outbreak of laboratory-acquired brucellosis. *Pediatr. Infect. Dis. J.* **12:**1031–1033.

26. **Collins, C. H.** 1993. *Laboratory-Acquired Infections: History, Incidence, Causes, and Prevention.* Butterworth-Heinemann Ltd., Oxford, United Kingdom.

27. **Cooper, C. R., D. M. Dixon, and I. F. Salkin.** 1992. Laboratory-acquired sporotrichosis. *J. Med. Vet. Mycol.* **30:**169–171.

28. **Evans, M. R., D. K. Henderson, and J. E. Bennett.** 1990. Potential for laboratory exposures to biohazardous agents found in blood. *Am. J. Public Health* **80:**423–427. (Erratum, **80:**658.)

29. **Favero, M., and W. W. Bond.** 1995. Transmission and control of laboratory-acquired hepatitis infection, p. 19–32. *In* D. O. Fleming, J. H. Richardson, J. J. Tulis, and D. Vesley (ed.), *Laboratory Safety: Principles and Practices.* American Society for Microbiology, Washington, D.C.

30. **Fiori, P. L., S. Mastrandrea, P. Rappelli, and P. Cappuccinelli.** 2000. *Brucella abortus* infection acquired in microbiology laboratories. *J. Clin. Microbiol.* **38:**2005–2006.

31. **Fischer, M., G. M. Carlone, J. Holst, D. Williams, D. S. Stephens, and B. A. Perkins.** 1999. *Neisseria meningitides* serogroup B outer membrane vesicle vaccine in adults with occupational risk for meningococcal disease. *Vaccine* **14:**2377–2388.

32. **Fleming, D. O.** 1995. Laboratory biosafety practices, p. 203–218. *In* D. O. Fleming, J. H. Richardson, J. J. Tulis, and D. Vesley (ed.), *Laboratory Safety: Principles and Practices.* American Society for Microbiology, Washington, D.C.

33. **Fleming, D. O., J. H. Richardson, J. J. Tulis, and D. Vesley (ed.).** 1995. *Laboratory Safety: Principles and Practices,* 2nd ed. American Society for Microbiology, Washington, D.C.

34. **Fox, J. G., and N. S. Lipman.** 1991. Infections transmitted by large and small laboratory animals. *Infect. Dis. Clin. North Am.* **5:**131–163.

35. **Fridkin, S. K., L. Manangan, E. Boylard, The Society for Healthcare Epidemiology of America, and W. R. Jarvis.** 1995. SHEA-CDC TB survey. II. Efficacy of TB infection control programs at member hospitals 1992. *Infect. Control Hosp. Epidemiol.* **16:**135–146.

36. **Gandsman, E. J., H. G. Aaslestad, T. C. Ouimet, and W. D. Rupp.** 1997. Sabia virus incident at Yale University. *Am. Ind. Hyg. Assoc. J.* **58:**51–53.

37. **Gilchrist, M. J. R.** 1995. Biosafety precautions for airborne pathogens, p. 67–76. *In* D. O. Fleming. J. H. Richardson, J. J. Tulis, and D. Vesley (ed.), *Laboratory Safety: Principles and Practices.* American Society for Microbiology, Washington, D.C.

38. **Gilks, G. F., H. P. Lambert, E. S. Broughton, and C. C. Baker.** 1988. Failure of penicillin prophylaxis in laboratory acquired leptospirosis. *Postgrad. Med. J.* **64:**236–238.

39. **Gonzalez, J. P., M. D. Bowen, S. T. Nichol, and H. R. Rico.** 1996. Genetic characterization and phylogeny of Sabia virus, an emergent pathogen in Brazil. *Virology* **221:**318–324.

40. **Grist, N. R., and J. A. N. Emslie.** 1987. Infections in British clinical laboratories, 1984–85. *J. Clin. Pathol.* **40:**826–829.

41. **Grist, N. R., and J. A. N. Emslie.** 1989. Infections in British clinical laboratories, 1986–87. *J. Clin. Pathol.* **42:**677–681.

42. **Grist, N. R., and J. A. N. Emslie.** 1991. Infections in British clinical laboratories, 1988–89. *J. Clin. Pathol.* **44:**667–669.

43. **Gruner, E., E. Bernasconi, R. L. Galeazzi, D. Buhl, R. Heinzle, and D. Nadal.** 1994. Brucellosis: an occupational hazard for medical laboratory personnel. Report of five cases. *Infection* **22:**33–36.

44. **Guibourdenche, M., J. P. Darchis, A. Boisivon, E. Collatz, and J. Y. Riou.** 1994. Enzyme electrophoresis,

sero- and subtyping, and outer membrane protein characterization of two *Neisseria meningitidis* strains involved in laboratory-acquired infections. *J. Clin. Microbiol.* **32:** 701–704.

45. **Hamadeh, G. N., B. W. Turner, W. Trible, B. J. Hoffmann, and R. M. Anderson.** 1992. Laboratory outbreak of Q-fever. *J. Fam. Pract.* **35:**683–685.
46. **Harding, L., and D. F. Lieberman.** 1995. Epidemiology of laboratory-associated infections, p. 7–15. *In* D. O. Fleming, J. H. Richardson, J. J. Tulis, and D. Vesley (ed.), *Laboratory Safety: Principles and Practices.* American Society for Microbiology, Washington, D.C.
47. **Harrington, J. M., and H. S. Shannon.** 1976. Incidence of tuberculosis, hepatitis, brucellosis and shigellosis in British medical laboratory workers. *Br. Med. J.* **1:**759–762.
48. **Hausler, W. J., N. P. Moyer, and L. A. Holcomb.** 1985. Brucella, p. 382–386. *In* E. H. Lennette, A. Balows, W. J. Hausler, Jr., and H. J. Shadomy (ed.), *Manual of Clinical Microbiology*, 4th ed. American Society for Microbiology, Washington, D.C.
49. **Herwaldt, B. L., and D. D. Juranek.** 1993. Laboratory-acquired malaria, leishmaniasis, trypanosomiasis, and toxoplasmosis. *Am. J. Trop. Med. Hyg.* **48:**313–323.
50. **Holmes, M. B., D. L. Johnson, N. J. Fiumara, and W. M. McCormack.** 1980. Acquisition of typhoid fever from proficiency-testing specimens. *N. Engl. J. Med.* **303:**519–521.
51. **Jacobson, J. T., R. B. Orlob, and J. L. Clayton.** 1985. Infections acquired in clinical laboratories in Utah. *J. Clin. Microbiol.* **21:**486–489.
52. **Jortani, S. A., J. W. Snyder, and R. Valdes, Jr.** 2000. The role of the clinical laboratory in managing chemical or biological terrorism. *Clin. Chem.* **46:**1883–1893.
53. **Kao, A. S., D. A. Ashford, M. M. McNeil, N. G. Warren, and R. C. Good.** 1997. Descriptive profile of tuberculin skin testing programs and laboratory-acquired tuberculosis infections in public health laboratories. *J. Clin. Microbiol.* **35:**1847–1851.
54. **Klietmann, W. F., and K. L. Ruoff.** 2001. Bioterrorism: implications for the clinical microbiologist. *Clin. Microbiol. Rev.* **14:**364–381.
55. **Knobioch, J., and M. Demar.** 1997. Accidental *Leishmania mexicana* infection in an immunosuppressed laboratory technician. *Trop. Med. Int. Health* **12:**1152–1155.
56. **Koay, M. J., D. K. Wong, D. Dudley, M. Houghton, and B. D. Walker.** 1997. Pulsed-field gel electrophoresis as an epidemiological tool in the investigation of laboratory acquired *Salmonella typhi* infection. *Southeast Asian J Trop. Med. Pub. Health* **28:**82–84.
57. **Kruse, R. H., W. H. Puckett, and J. H. Richardson.** 1991. Biological safety cabinetry. *Clin. Microbiol. Rev.* **4:**207–241.
58. **Larson, D. M., M. R. Eckman, C. L. Alber, and V. G. Goldschmidt.** 1983. Primary cutaneous (inoculation) blastomycosis: an occupational hazard to pathologists. *Am. J. Clin. Pathol.* **79:**253–255.
59. **Levy, B. S., J. C. Harris, J. L. Smith, J. W. Washburn, J. Mature, A. Davis, J. T. Crosson, H. Polskey, and M. Hanson.** 1977. Hepatitis B in ward and clinical laboratory employees of a general hospital. *Am. J. Epidemiol.* **106:** 330–335.
60. **Mackel, D. C., and J. E. Forney.** 1986. Overview of the epidemiology of laboratory-acquired infections, p. 37–42. *In* B. M. Miller, J. H. Groschel, J. H. Richardson, D. Vesley, J. R. Songer, R. D. Housewright, and W. E. Barkley (ed.), *Laboratory Safety: Principles and Practices.* American Society for Microbiology, Washington, D.C.

61. **Mahy, B. W.** 1998. Zoonoses and haemorrhagic fever. *Dev. Biol. Stand.* **93:**31–36.
62. **Martin-Mazuelos, E., M. C. Nogales, C. Florez, M. J. Gomez, F. Lozano, and A. Sanchez.** 1994. Outbreak of *Brucella melitensis* among microbiology laboratory workers. *J. Clin. Microbiol.* **32:**2035–2036.
63. **Mazurek, G. H., M. D. Cave, K. D. Eisenach, R. J. Wallace, Jr., J. H. Bates, and J. T. Crawford.** 1991. Chromosomal DNA fingerprint patterns produced with IS6110 as strain-specific markers for epidemiologic study of tuberculosis. *J. Clin. Microbiol.* **29:**2030–2033.
64. **Memish, Z. A., and M. W. Mah.** 2001. Brucellosis in laboratory workers at a Saudi Arabian hospital. *Am. J. Infect. Control* **29:**48–52.
65. **Miller, C. D., J. R. Songer, and J. F. Sullivan.** 1987. A twenty-five year review of laboratory-acquired human infections at the National Animal Disease Center. *Am. Ind. Hyg. Assoc. J.* **48:**271–275.
66. **Muller, H. E.** 1988. Laboratory-acquired mycobacterial infection. *Lancet* **ii:**331.
67. **Murray, J. F., and D. H. Howard.** 1964. Laboratory-acquired histoplasmosis. *Am. Rev. Respir. Dis.* **89:**631–640.
68. **Occupational Safety and Health Administration.** 1991. Occupational exposure to bloodborne pathogens: final rule. *Fed. Regist.* **56:**64003–64182.
69. **Occupational Safety and Health Administration.** 1993. Draft guidelines for preventing the transmission of tuberculosis in healthcare facilities. *Fed. Regist.* **58:**52810–52854.
70. **Olle-Goig, J., and J. C. Canela-Soler.** 1987. An outbreak of *Brucella melitensis* infection by airborne transmission among laboratory workers. *Am. J. Public Health* **77:**335–338.
71. **Oster, C. N., D. S. Burke, R. H. Kenyon, M. S. Ascher, P. Harber, and C. E. Pedersen.** 1977. Laboratory-acquired Rocky Mountain spotted fever. The hazard of aerosol transmission. *N. Engl. J. Med.* **297:**859–863.
72. **Paradis, J. F., and D. Grimard.** 1994. Laboratory-acquired invasive meningococcus—Quebec. *Can. Commun. Dis. Rep.* **20:**12–14.
73. **Penner, J. L., J. N. Hennessy, S. D. Mills, and W. C. Bradbury.** 1983. Application of serotyping and chromosomal restriction endonuclease digest analysis in investigating a laboratory-acquired case of *Campylobacter jejuni*. *J. Clin. Microbiol.* **18:**1427–1428.
74. **Philipott, J., and J. Casewell.** 1994. *Hospital Infection Control.* Saunders, London, United Kingdom.
75. **Pike, R. M.** 1976. Laboratory-associated infections. Summary and analysis of 3921 cases. *Health Lab. Sci.* **13:**105–114.
76. **Pike, R. M.** 1979. Laboratory-associated infections: incidence, fatalities, causes and prevention. *Annu. Rev. Microbiol.* **33:**41–66.
77. **Sepkowitz, K. A.** 1996. Occupational acquired infections in health care workers. 1. *Ann. Intern. Med.* **125:**826–834.
78. **Sepkowitz, K. A.** 1996. Occupationally acquired infections in health care workers. II. *Ann. Intern. Med.* **125:** 917–928.
79. **Sewell, D. L.** 1995. Laboratory-associated infections and biosafety. *Clin. Microbiol. Rev.* **8:**389–405.
80. **Shireman, P. K.** 1992. Endometrial tuberculosis acquired by a health care worker in a clinical laboratory. *Arch. Pathol. Lab. Med.* **116:**521–523.
81. **Staszkiewicz, J., C. M. Lewis, J. Colville, M. Zervos, and J. Band.** 1997. Outbreak of *Brucella melitensis* among microbiology laboratory workers in a community hospital. *J. Clin. Microbiol.* **29:**287–290.

82. **Stratton, C. W.** 2001. Occupationally acquired infections: A timely reminder. *Infect. Control Hosp. Epidemiol.* **22:** 8–9.

83. **Sulkin, S. E., and R. M. Pike.** 1951. Laboratory-acquired infections. *JAMA* **147:**1740–1745.

84. **Vasconcelos, P. F., A. P. Travassos da Rosa, S. G. Rodrigues, R. Tesh, J. F. Travassos da Rosa, and E. S. Travassos da Rosa.** 1993. Laboratory-acquired human infection with SP H 114202 virus (Arenavirus: Arenaviridae family): clinical and laboratory aspects. *Rev. Inst. Med. Trop. Sao Paulo* **35:**521–525.

85. **Vesley, D., and H. M. Hartman.** 1988. Laboratory-acquired infections and injuries in clinical laboratories: a 1986 survey. *Am. J. Public Health* **78:**1213–1215.

86. **Waitkins, R. A.** 1985. Update on leptospirosis. *Br. Med. J.* **290:**1502–1503.

87. **Weaver, R. E., D. G. Hollis, and E. J. Bottone.** 1985. Gram-negative fermentative bacteria and *Francisella tularensis*, p. 309–329. *In* E. H. Lennette, A. Balows, W. J. Hausler, Jr., and H. J. Shadomy (ed.), *Manual of Clinical Microbiology*, 4th ed. American Society for Microbiology, Washington, D.C.

88. **Yagupsky, P., N. Peled, K. Riesenberg, and M. Banai.** 2000. Exposure of hospital personnel to *Brucella melitensis* and occurrence of laboratory-acquired diseases in an endemic area. *Scand. J. Infect. Dis.* **32:**31–35.

89. **Young, E. J.** 1983. Human brucellosis. *Rev. Infect. Dis.* **5:**821–842.

Laboratory Detection of Potential Agents of Bioterrorism

JAMES W. SNYDER AND ALICE S. WEISSFELD

10

Although this is the eighth edition of this text, this is the first time that a chapter on bioterrorism has been added to this Manual. Its inclusion represents the growing recognition, especially after the events of 11 September 2001, by public health officials that clinical microbiology laboratories serve as sentinels for the recognition or raising of suspicion of a possible bioterrorism event and the need to educate clinical microbiologists regarding appropriate laboratory procedures. This chapter is an overview of the most important issues. For other American Society for Microbiology (ASM) publications on this subject, please refer to references (11 and 16) and the second edition of the *Clinical Microbiology Procedures Handbook* (14a).

HISTORY

There is evidence that germ warfare was used by the ancient Greeks, Romans, and Persians, who attempted to pollute their enemies' drinking water supplies by contaminating them with foul-smelling dead animals (6, 23). Of note, this technique was also used during the American Civil War. In the 14th century, Tatar forces catapulted deceased plague victims into the besieged city of Kaffa. The plague epidemic that followed forced the defenders to surrender; it is postulated that some infected people who subsequently left the city may have started the Black Death pandemic in Western Europe. During the French and Indian War (1754 to 1767), the British soldier Sir Jeffrey Amherst provided smallpox-laden blankets and handkerchiefs used by British smallpox victims to Native Americans loyal to the French. These early incidences occurred before individuals understood the germ theory of disease or deliberately set out to produce biological weapons of mass destruction.

The modern age of biowarfare commenced during World War I. Germany was believed to have used *Vibrio cholerae* and *Yersinia pestis* against humans and *Bacillus anthracis* and *Burkholderia mallei* against animals, although their use of mustard gas was more widespread and garnered more attention. In 1925, the Geneva Protocol for the Prohibition of the Use in War of Asphyxiating, Poisonous, or Other Gases, and of Bacteriological Methods of Warfare was signed by a group of nations. Unfortunately, this treaty did not limit or regulate production of such weapons, and a number of countries, including the USSR, Japan, and the United Kingdom, established biological warfare research programs. The Japanese are believed to have conducted tests in Manchuria and China on prisoners; these human subjects were fed contaminated water and food and exposed to aerial spraying of biological agents or small bombs containing plague-infected fleas (12). Outbreaks of plague, cholera, and typhus were attributed to these activities. The Germans used concentration camp victims in a defensive program designed to develop vaccines and effective chemotherapy.

The U.S. Army and Air Force began an offensive biological weapons program in 1942 at Fort Detrick, Md. Research was conducted until 1969, when President Nixon promulgated a biological weapons disarmament declaration. Subsequently, the Biological and Toxic Weapon Convention in 1972 resulted in an agreement that biological weapons development should be stopped worldwide. While most Western governments ceased their offensive program, the former Soviet Union started a clandestine program that was called Biopreparat (7). Monies earmarked for biotechnology were diverted into the development of a variety of different agents, including microorganisms resistant to degradation by heat, light, cold, and UV and ionizing radiation. Strains were also adapted to specific dissemination systems such as cruise missiles. Soviet defector Ken Alibeck, who was Deputy Director of Biopreparat, related valuable insight into this program.

Following the breakup of the former Soviet Union, scientists from Biopreparat are thought to have taken positions in third world countries such as North Korea, Libya, Syria, and Iraq, which are all believed to have active bioweapons programs. In fact, inspectors with the United Nations Special Commission who visited Iraq after the Gulf War believe that it has not abandoned its bioweapons programs.

Fortunately, documented outbreaks of the use of biological agents as weapons of mass destruction are rare. In April 1979, residents living downwind from compound 19, a military microbiology facility in the city of Sverdlovsk in the former Soviet Union, developed anthrax following the accidental release of *B. anthracis* spores (20). The Soviet Ministry of Health initially blamed the outbreak on consumption of contaminated meat; Boris Yeltsin finally revealed the truth in 1992.

In 1984, an outbreak of *Salmonella enterica* serovar Typhimurium in The Dalles, Oreg., caused 750 people to become ill (24). Salad bars at two local restaurants were sprayed with the microorganisms by followers of a religious leader (Bhagwan Shree Rajneesh) to prevent local citizens from voting in an upcoming election. Larry Wayne Harris, a microbiologist linked to white supremacist groups, was apprehended by Federal Bureau of Investigation agents in Las Vegas, Nev., and found to have an avirulent strain of anthrax in the trunk of his car. In the late 1990s, numerous letters allegedly containing anthrax spores were mailed to a variety of agencies, including family planning clinics, and were eventually classified as hoaxes (8, 14, 21). Shortly after the terrorist attacks on the World Trade Center Towers and the Pentagon on 11 September 2001, a case of inhalational anthrax was identified in a journalist in Florida on 4 October 2001 (3). This marked the beginning of the first confirmed outbreak associated with the intentional release of anthrax in the United States. As of 5 December 2001, the Centers for Disease Control and Prevention (CDC) and state and local public health officials had identified a total of 22 cases of anthrax; 11 were confirmed as inhalational anthrax, and 11 (7 confirmed, 4 suspected) were cutaneous (15, 18, 19, 21). These confirmed or suspected cases were concentrated in individuals who worked in the District of Columbia, Florida, New Jersey, and New York (1, 2, 4). One case of inhalational anthrax was discovered in mid-November 2001 in an elderly resident of Connecticut (1). It was determined that the outbreak had resulted from the intentional delivery of *B. anthracis* spores through mailed letters or packages, although the source of the anthrax involved in the Connecticut case was unknown (1, 4).

GENERAL FEATURES OF BIOTERRORISM

Biological terrorism (bioterrorism) is defined as "the intentional use of microorganisms or toxins derived from living organisms to produce death or disease in humans, animals, or plants." From the public and private health perspective, bioterrorism can be defined as the deliberate release of pathogens or their toxins into a civilian population with the intent to cause illness or death (13, 25, 26). In addition to humans, agricultural animals and plants must also be considered as potential targets of bioterrorism (13, 26). The threat posed by bioterrorism was clearly demonstrated during the anthrax outbreak during October and November 2001. Public health officials, along with community health care providers, including clinical laboratories, were inundated with citizens seeking medical treatment and testing for perceived exposure to anthrax spores as a result of encountering powdery substances and a general fear or panic that occurred nationwide following the discovery of additional cases of anthrax. It was no longer a matter of when or if a bioterrorism act would occur, but instead this outbreak was a "wake-up call" to develop or revise and update the respective federal, state, community, and institutional bioterrorism readiness plans. Awareness of and preparation for responding to such an event are essential for clinical microbiologists, who will play a direct role as sentinels in the detection, characterization, and identification of the etiologic agent(s) in addition to alerting the proper authorities. To be effective in preparing for and responding to a suspected or confirmed bioterrorist event, clinical microbiologists should have a general understanding of biological terrorism, including the administrative and technical principles that are necessary for the recognition and management of an event.

Since the threat of bioterrorism has become the focus of attention worldwide, most clinical microbiologists have no or limited experience with bioterrorism, nor have they ever encountered those biological agents that have been targeted as most likely to be used in the commission of an act of bioterrorism. As is common with any discipline, bioterrorism utilizes specific terms, many of which are used interchangeably. As defined above, bioterrorism (biological warfare) refers to the indiscriminate targeting of the masses (e.g., battlefield or civilian population), whereas the term biocrime or biothreat is used when a bioterrorist, which may be one individual who acts alone or a state- or non-state-sponsored group, targets a specific group or individual. The bioterrorism-associated cases of anthrax that occurred in the United States in October and November 2001 represent a biocrime because the primary targets were U.S. politicians and the media rather than the U.S. civilian population. Thus, a biocrime is a criminal act involving the use of biological agents as weapons, and a biothreat is characterized as a suspected but unconfirmed release of a biological agent(s), i.e., microbial pathogens and/or toxins which have been previously considered or used in biological warfare and recent terrorist events (11).

Bioterrorism events are categorized as either overt or covert (Table 1). Of these, the covert pose the greatest challenge to the clinical microbiologist who, along with infectious disease practitioners, in the role as sentinels, will most likely be the first to raise suspicion of a possible event involving a biological agent. The case of inhalational anthrax in the journalist from Florida reported on 4 October 2001 represented a covert event due to the unknown etiology and the associated delay in the eventual diagnosis that was made by a clinician who discovered the presence of gram-positive bacilli in the patient's cerebrospinal fluid. The anthrax cases that followed represented overt events because the letters that were mailed to the targeted politicians and media personnel contained a written message announcing the presence and pending exposure of *B. anthracis* spores. A covert type of event or attack will not have an immediate impact because of the delay between exposure and onset of illness (i.e., incubation period). Consequently, emergency medicine physicians and other primary health care providers, as exemplified in the Florida case, including clinical microbiologists, will most likely identify the first cases (5). Detection and recognition of a possible event will be dependent upon several factors, including an active microbial surveillance and monitoring program, vigilant laboratory staff who are capable of recognizing the unusual or who develop a high index of suspicion, and communication with clinicians (especially emergency medicine personnel), infection control personnel, infectious

TABLE 1 Differentiation of types of bioterrorism

Type of bioterrorism	Recognition	Response	Treatment	Responders
Overt	Early	Early	Early	Front line[a]
Covert	Delayed	Delayed	Delayed	Health care workers[b]

[a] Firefighters, police, hazardous material personnel, and emergency medical services.
[b] Emergency room personnel, primary care physicians, clinical microbiologists, and infection control personnel.

disease specialists, and other local or regional laboratories. The lack of commercially available diagnostic tests and reagents for use in the specific identification of the targeted agents presents a major obstacle to the clinical microbiologist. As a result, confirmation of these agents will require that the specimen or isolate in question be referred to designated laboratories within the Laboratory Response Network that are equipped with the latest diagnostic technologies (state health departments, the CDC, and the U.S. Army Medical Research Institute of Infectious Diseases [USAMRIID]).

Key indicators of a possible act of bioterrorism or biocrime (16; USAMRIID: Biological Warfare and Terrorism Medical Issues and Response Satellite Broadcast, 26 to 28 September 2000) are:

- A disease entity that is unusual or that does not occur naturally in a given geographic area, or combinations of unusual disease entities in the same patient populations
- Multiple disease entities in the same patients, indicating that mixed agents may have been used in the event
- Above-normal rates of morbidity and mortality relative to the number of personnel at risk or within a population that inhabits the same area
- Data suggesting a massive point source outbreak
- Apparent aerosol route of infection
- Illness limited to localized or circumscribed geographical areas
- Low attack rates in personnel who work in areas with filtered air supplies or closed ventilation systems
- Sentinel dead animals of multiple species
- Absence of a competent natural vector in the area of the outbreak (for a biological agent that is vector-borne in nature)

Epidemiologic and microbiologic clues that may signal a biological act of terrorism (16; USAMRIID Satellite Broadcast, 26 to 28 September 2000) include but are not necessarily limited to the following:

- Large numbers of ill persons with a similar disease or syndrome
- Large numbers of cases of unexplained diseases or deaths
- Unusual illness in a population (e.g., unexplained respiratory infection)
- Single case of disease caused by an uncommon agent (e.g., pulmonary anthrax, illness caused by *Burkholderia mallei* or *Burkholderia pseudomallei,* tularemia, viral hemorrhagic fever)
- Several unusual or unexplained diseases coexisting in the same patient without any other explanation
- Higher morbidity and mortality in association with a common disease or syndrome or failure of such patients to respond to usual therapy
- Disease with an unusual geographic or seasonal distribution (e.g., tularemia in an area of nonendemicity, influenza in the summer)
- Illness that is unusual (or atypical) for a given population or age group (e.g., outbreak of measles-like rash in adults)
- Unusual disease presentation (e.g., pulmonary instead of cutaneous anthrax)
- Similar genetic type among agents isolated from distinct sources at different times or locations

TABLE 2 Critical biological agents for bioterrorism and civilian preparedness[a]

Organism	Disease, common name, or toxin	Biothreat level[b]
Bacteria		
Bacillus anthracis[c]	Anthrax	A
Yersinia pestis[c]	Plague	A
Francisella tularensis[c]	Tularemia	A
Coxiella burnetii[c]	Q fever	B
Brucella species[c]	Brucellosis	B
Burkholderia mallei	Glanders	B
Salmonella species	Salmonellosis	B
Shigella dysenteriae	Shigellosis	B
Escherichia coli O157:H7	Hemorrhagic colitis	B
Vibrio cholerae	Cholera	B
Mycobacterium tuberculosis[d]	Tuberculosis	C
Viruses		
Variola major[c]	Smallpox	A
Ebola[c]	Hemorrhagic fever	A
Marburg[c]	Hemorrhagic fever	A
Lassa[c]	Lassa fever	A
Junin[c]	Argentine hemorrhagic fever	A
VEE,[c] WEE, EEE[e]	Encephalomyelitis	B
Nipah	Encephalomyelitis	C
Hantavirus	Hemorrhagic fever, hantavirus pulmonary syndrome	C
Tick-borne viruses	Hemorrhagic fever and/or encephalitis	C
Yellow fever virus	Yellow fever	C
Protozoa		
Cryptosporidium parvum	Cryptosporidiosis	C
Toxin sources		
Clostridium botulinum[c]	Botulinum toxin	A
Staphylococcus aureus[c]	Enterotoxin B	B
Clostridium perfringens	Epsilon toxin	B
Ricinus communis[c] (from castor beans)	Ricin	B
Some marine dinoflagellates	Saxitoxin	
Various species of fungi	Trichothecene mycotoxins	

[a] Adapted with permission from Morse (22).
[b] Biothreat level A, agents that pose the greatest threat due to their infectiousness, relative ease of transmission, or high rate of mortality; biothreat level B, agents having a moderate ease of transmission and morbidity with a low rate of mortality; biothreat level C, emerging pathogens and potential risks for the future.
[c] Organisms categorized as "critical" agents for bioterrorism or biocrime.
[d] Multidrug-resistant strains.
[e] EEE, eastern equine encephalomyelitis; VEE, Venezuelan equine encephalomyelitis; WEE, western equine encephalomyelitis.

- Unusual, atypical, genetically engineered, or antiquated strain of an agent (or antibiotic resistance pattern)
- Stable endemic disease with an unexplained increase in incidence (e.g., tularemia, plague)

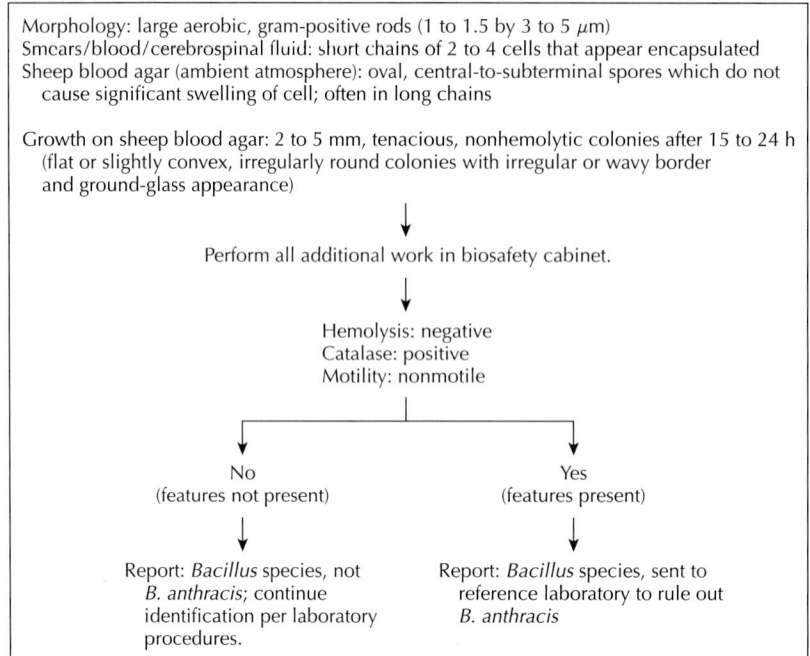

Morphology: large aerobic, gram-positive rods (1 to 1.5 by 3 to 5 μm)
Smears/blood/cerebrospinal fluid: short chains of 2 to 4 cells that appear encapsulated
Sheep blood agar (ambient atmosphere): oval, central-to-subterminal spores which do not
    cause significant swelling of cell; often in long chains

Growth on sheep blood agar: 2 to 5 mm, tenacious, nonhemolytic colonies after 15 to 24 h
    (flat or slightly convex, irregularly round colonies with irregular or wavy border
    and ground-glass appearance)

Perform all additional work in biosafety cabinet.

Hemolysis: negative
Catalase: positive
Motility: nonmotile

No
(features not present)

Yes
(features present)

Report: *Bacillus* species, not
B. anthracis; continue
identification per laboratory
procedures.

Report: *Bacillus* species, sent to
reference laboratory to rule out
B. anthracis

FIGURE 1 *B. anthracis* level A testing.

- Simultaneous clusters of similar illness in noncontiguous areas, domestic or foreign
- Atypical disease transmission through aerosols, food, or water, which suggests deliberate sabotage
- Ill persons who seek treatment at about the same time (point source with compressed epidemic curve)
- No illness in persons who are not exposed to common ventilation systems (i.e., who have separate closed ventilation systems) when illness is seen in persons in proximity who have a common ventilation system
- Unusual pattern of death or illness among animals (which may be unexplained or attributed to an agent of bioterrorism) which precedes or accompanies illness or death in humans

CLASSIFICATION, CHARACTERISTICS, AND CATEGORIZATION OF BIOLOGICAL AGENTS

Biological agents are classified as pathogens, toxins, or biomodulators. Pathogens are used for antipersonnel purposes due to their lethality. Animals serve as the primary target for the utilization of toxins that act primarily as incapacitating agents. Biomodulators are transmissible and are used primarily as antiplant and antimaterial (equipment, apparatus, supplies) agents.

Although it is questionable whether biological agents represent the ultimate weapon, they do possess some unique characteristics not found in chemical or nuclear agents. Although few individuals or terrorist groups possess the scientific and technical resources needed to weaponize and successfully disperse an agent via aerosolization, the most likely mode of dispersal, the targeted agents possess unique advantages that make them suitable for use in the commission of an act of bioterrorism or a biocrime (22):

- Ease of procurement
- Ease of production

- Low cost of production
- Ability to be disseminated at a great distance
- Invisibility of agent cloud
- Difficulty of detection
- Fact that illness is first sign of agent
- Ability to overwhelm medical capacity and capabilities
- Capacity of simple threat to create panic
- Ability of perpetrators to escape before effects felt
- Idealness as a terrorist weapon
- Stability during storage
- Appropriate particle size in aerosol

A targeted (critical) agent list (Table 2) has been developed by the CDC and its affiliated partners based on (i) the public health impact of the agent's ability to cause mass casualties, (ii) the ability of the agent to be widely disseminated, (iii) the ability of the agent to be transmitted from person to person, and (iv) public perception associated with the agent's intentional release. Biothreat levels (A to C) have been established to categorize potential agents on the basis of the threat to national security, morbidity and mortality, and adaptability to being genetically engineered. Category A organisms are considered to pose the greatest threat to national security because they can be easily disseminated or transmitted from person to person; cause high mortality, with potential for major public health impact; may cause public panic and social disruption; and require special action for public health preparedness. Category B agents consist of agents that are moderately easy to disseminate, cause moderate morbidity and low mortality, and challenge the CDC's diagnostic and disease surveillance capacity. This category also includes pathogens that are food borne or waterborne (e.g., *Salmonella* species, *Shigella dysenteriae*, *Escherichia coli* O157:H7, *V. cholerae*, and *Cryptosporidium parvum*). The third highest priority agents are included in category C. These consist primarily of emerging

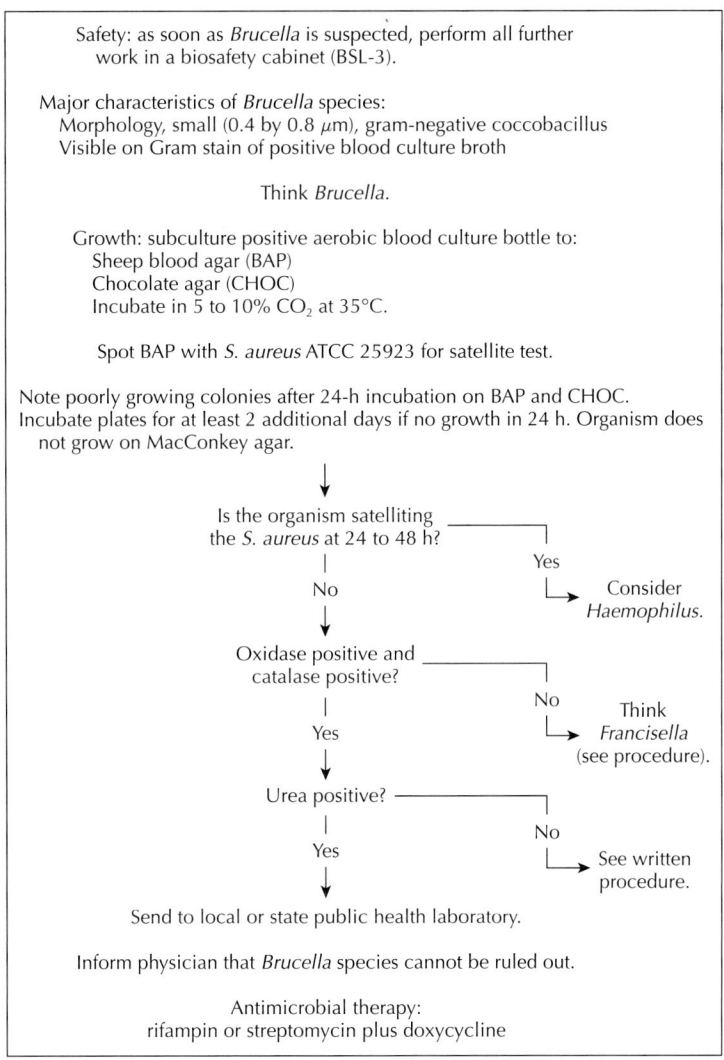

FIGURE 2 *Brucella* sp. level A testing.

pathogens that could be engineered for mass dissemination in the future because of availability, ease of production and dissemination, and their potential for high morbidity, mortality, and major health impact (5, 22). Human, plant, and animal infections caused by these agents are uncommon, especially in the United States, or are limited to certain geographical regions. By virtue of the low incidence or rare occurrence of infections caused by these organisms, the clinical microbiology laboratory must rely on conventional diagnostic technologies for agent identification, especially for category A and B agents. Although some advances have been made in diagnostic techniques (i.e., molecular tests, enzyme immunoassays, and direct and indirect fluorescent-antibody assays), the availability of such tests is limited to specialized research laboratories, federal laboratories (CDC, USAMRIID), and selected state health laboratories. Therefore, public health and private sector laboratory preparedness is dependent upon improvements being made in clinical and laboratory surveillance systems, development and production of commercially available diagnostic reagents and assays, and training of physicians and laboratory personnel (5, 22).

THE UNITED STATES' RESPONSE TO BIOTERRORISM

In response to the risks, vulnerability, and possibility, which eventually became a reality following the events of 11 September 2001, that bioterrorists, either domestic or foreign, could attack the United States, former President Clinton issued Presidential Decision Directive 39 (PPD-39) in 1995 outlining U.S. policy on counterterrorism. The directive designates the Federal Bureau of Investigation as the lead federal agency in charge of immediate crisis management and criminal investigation. The Federal Emergency Management Agency is given the lead role in consequence management and would be assisted by the Departments of Defense, Energy, Agriculture, Transportation, and Health and Human Services and the Environmental Protection Agency.

The Association of Professionals in Infection Control and the CDC have developed a Bioterrorism Preparedness and Response Program to assure a rapid turnaround in the laboratory recognition of a biocrime and its consequences (9, 17). The program includes the following elements:

- Disease surveillance
- Rapid laboratory diagnosis of biological agents
- Epidemiologic investigation
- Open lines of communication between local, state, and federal public health authorities
- Preparedness planning
- Readiness assessment
- Development and maintenance of the National Pharmaceutical Stockpile Program in cooperation with the Department of Health and Human Services Office of Emergency Preparedness

Laboratory Response Network

In order to facilitate rapid laboratory diagnosis of a biocrime, the CDC has established a model in which clinical and public health laboratories are linked in a seamless laboratory network on the basis of the role they will play in the ultimate diagnosis of a biological agent used in a terrorist event (5, 10). The majority of hospital and commercial reference laboratories have been classified as level A. These laboratories act as sentinels for raising suspicion of a bioterrorist event and rule out or refer suspicious isolates only. Furthermore, level A laboratories are restricted to testing human specimens only and forward environmental and animal specimens to a level B or higher laboratory. For example, the isolate that was recovered from the journalist in Florida was suspicious for, but could not be ruled out as the etiological agent of, anthrax. It was referred to the Florida State Department of Health Laboratory (level B), which confirmed the isolate as being *B. anthracis*. Level B laboratories are local or state public health laboratories with biosafety level 2 (BSL-2) facilities that are also equipped to perform animal studies. They perform rapid presumptive microorganism identification using fluorescent-antibody reagents provided by the CDC and/or confirmatory biochemical identification and susceptibility testing. Level B laboratories refer isolates to Level C laboratories (BSL-3), which are larger state public health laboratories that have the capability to perform nucleic acid amplification tests, molecular typing of strains, and toxin or animal testing, where applicable. Level D laboratories are BSL-4 "hot labs" located at the CDC and USAMRIID. These labs are capable of archiving isolates and performing specialized tests.

Since level A laboratories are charged with ruling out, not identifying, suspicious isolates, they must immediately recognize when to refer a specimen to the laboratory at the next higher level. Thus, the proper packaging and shipping of infectious agents is one of their most important functions (refer to chapter 6, "General Principles of Specimen Collection and Handling"). Cultures and clinical specimens known or suspected to contain infectious substances must be packaged according to certain specifications (Infectious Substance Regulations), for example, in a rigid, leakproof secondary container. All laboratories that handle infectious substances (dangerous goods), defined as articles or substances which are capable of posing a significant risk to health, safety, or property when transported by air, must comply with the respective International Air Transport Association (IATA) regulations, 49 Code of Federal Regulations (49 CFR), and Canadian Transportation of Dangerous Goods Regulations (TDGR). These regulations apply worldwide, with some countries, such as Canada and the United States, having specific regulations (TDGR and

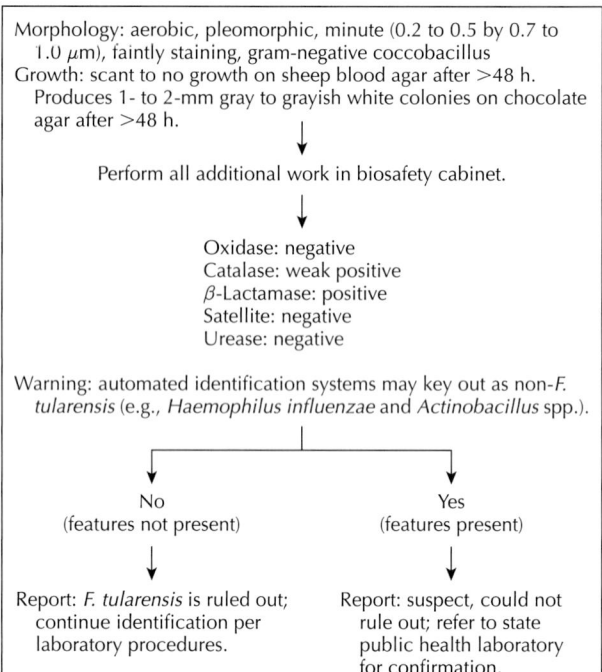

FIGURE 3 *Francisella tularensis* level A testing.

49 CFR, respectively). Formal training in the IATA regulations is recommended, since these regulations are the most restrictive, apply worldwide, and comply with the respective U.S. and Canadian requirements. Anyone, including microbiologists, who ships infectious substances (dangerous goods) is required to complete formal training and become certified in the application of these regulations. Formal training is available through the U.S. Department of Transportation and most commercial suppliers of approved packaging containers (see the websites of Department of Transportation and commercial suppliers).

Organism Identification

Level A laboratories must have a class II certified biological safety cabinet and copies of the level A protocols, laboratory algorithms for ruling out suspicious microorganisms. The protocols are published on the CDC and ASM websites and cover the five most likely bacterial and viral agents. These protocols are a result of a partnership consisting of subject matter experts representing the CDC, ASM, and the Association of Public Health Laboratories. To simplify matters for hospital laboratories, identification of the five most likely microorganisms is based on eight simple conventional tests. The flowcharts from these protocols are reproduced here (Fig. 1 to 4) and are accessible on the ASM and CDC websites (www.asmusa.org/pasrc/biodetection.htm and www.bt.cdc.gov). The agents of smallpox and botulism are not included, since level A laboratories are not to process specimens for these organisms and are required to send representative specimens to the CDC for suspicion of smallpox or to the state public health laboratory for suspicion of botulism (note: not all state health laboratories are equipped to test for botulism toxin). Each level A laboratory should contact its state public health laboratory for information regarding the nearest level B laboratory that tests for botulinum toxin. Hos-

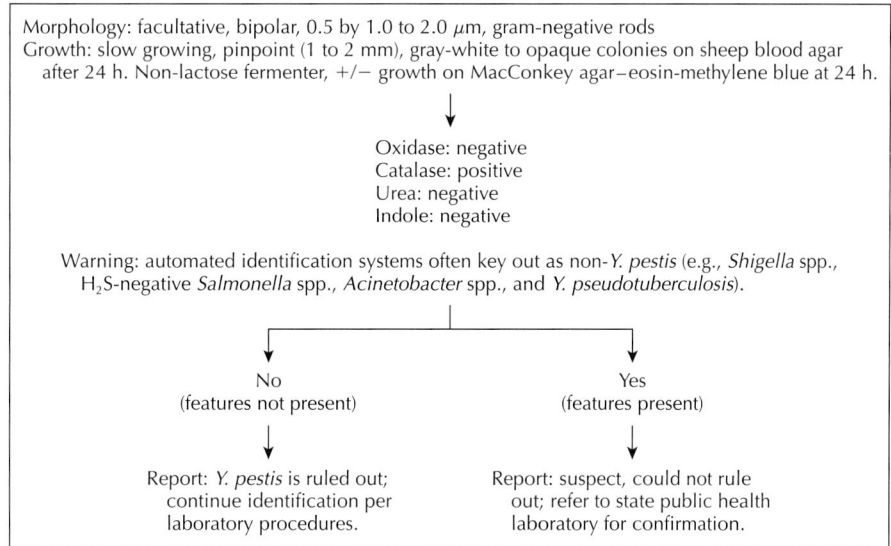

FIGURE 4 *Y. pestis* level A testing.

pital laboratories should maintain a subculture of all suspicious isolates that were referred to the next level of testing pending further investigation. Level A laboratories are not currently required to follow chain-of-custody guidelines. Level A laboratories are not to accept or process nonhuman specimens (animal or environmental). Such specimens are to be forwarded directly to the state public health laboratory under the direction of law enforcement.

All communications with law enforcement individuals should be handled through the facility infection control practitioner. The laboratory director should be notified immediately of suspicious isolates and who is responsible for notifying the attending clinician and infection control practitioner. This chain of command should be outlined in each institution's bioterrorism preparedness program (9). Each state should provide its hospital and commercial laboratories with a list of phone contacts and emergency phone numbers.

Sources for Additional and Updated Information

Information and guidelines on this topic are rapidly changing. The microbiologist is encouraged to remain current with local, state, and federal guidelines. In addition, consultation from the CDC is available at all hours (see their website), and current information can be obtained from a variety of Internet sites, including the following:

1. General information
ASM—www.asmusa.org
CDC Bioterrorism Preparedness and Response Program—www.bt.cd.gov
Johns Hopkins University, Schools of Public Health and Medicine, Center for Civilian Biodefense Studies—www.hopkins-biodefense.org
2. Level A laboratory testing protocols
ASM—www.asmusa.org/pcsrc/biodetection.htm
CDC—www.bt.cdc.gov
3. Bioterrorism readiness plans and templates for health care facilities
Association of Professionals in Infection Control—www.APIC.org

National Center of Infectious Diseases—www.cdc.gov/ncidod/hip
Office of Emergency Preparedness: Counter Bioterrorism Program—www.oep-ndms.dhhs.gov
4. Packaging and shipping regulations
Hazardous Materials Regulations (49 CFR parts 171 to 178, shipment of biological and clinical specimens)—www.dot.gov.rules.html
IATA—www.iata.org
World Health Organization—www.who.org
International Civil Aviation Organization—www.icao.org
U.S. Government Printing Office—www.acess.gpo.gov/nara/cfr
TDGR: Ministry of Supply and Services, Transport Canada, Place de Ville, Tower C, 330 Sparks St., Ottawa, Ontario I1A 0N5, Canada
5. Emergency CDC phone number
The CDC is available for questions and consultation 24/7 at (770) 488-7100 (visit the CDC website for changes in contact telephone numbers). The CDC telephone number for assistance in cases of an unusual nature or occurrence is (770) 488-4819. The local health department should also be contacted regarding emergencies and to report suspected or confirmed exposures to biological agents.

REFERENCES

1. **Centers for Disease Control and Prevention.** 2001. Update: investigation of bioterrorism-related anthrax—Connecticut. *Morb. Mortal. Wkly. Rep.* **50:**1077–1079.
2. **Centers for Disease Control and Prevention.** 2001. Notice to readers: considerations for distinguishing influenza-like illness from inhalational anthrax. *Morb. Mortal. Wkly. Rep.* **50:**984–986.
3. **Centers for Disease Control and Prevention.** 2001. Notice to readers: ongoing investigation of anthrax—Florida. *Morb. Mortal. Wkly. Rep.* **50:**877.
4. **Centers for Disease Control and Prevention.** 2001. Update: investigation of bioterrorism-related anthrax and interim guidelines for clinical evaluation of persons with possible anthrax. *Morb. Mortal. Wkly. Rep.* **50:**941–948.

5. **Centers for Disease Control and Prevention.** 2000. Biological and chemical terrorism: strategic plan for preparedness and response. *Morb. Mortal. Wkly. Rep.* **49:**1–14.

6. **Christopher, G. W., T. J. Cieslak, J. A. Pavlin, and E. M. Eitzen, Jr.** 1997. Biological warfare: a historical perspective. *JAMA* **278:**412–417.

7. **Davis, C. J.** 1999. Nuclear blindness: an overview of the biological weapons programs of the former Soviet Union and Iraq. *Emerg. Infect. Dis.* **5:**509–512.

8. **Dixon, T. C., M. Meselson, J. Guillemin, and P. C. Hanna.** 1999. Anthrax. *N. Engl. J. Med.* **341:**815–826.

9. **English, J. F.** 1999. Overview of bioterrorism readiness plan: a template for health care facilities. *Am. J. Infect. Control* **27:**468–469.

10. **Gilchrist, M. J. R.** 2000. A national laboratory network for bioterrorism: evolution from a prototype network of laboratories performing routine surveillance. *Mil. Med.* **156**(Suppl.):28–34.

11. **Gilchrist, M. J. R., W. P. McKinney, J. M. Miller, and A. S. Weissfeld.** 2000. *Cumitech 33, Laboratory Safety, Management and Diagnosis of Biological Agents Associated with Bioterrorism.* Coordinating ed., J. W. Snyder. ASM Press, Washington, D.C.

12. **Harris, A.** 1992. Japanese biological warfare research on humans: a case study on microbiology and ethics. *Ann. N. Y. Acad. Sci.* **666:**21–52.

13. **Horn, F.** 2000. Agricultural bioterrorism, p. 109–115. *In* B. Roberts (ed.), *Hype or Reality? The "New Terrorism" and Mass Casualty Attacks.* The Chemical and Biological Arms Control Institute, Alexandria, Va.

14. **Inglesby, T. V., D. A. Henderson, J. G. Bartlett, M. S. Ascher, E. Eitzen, A. M. Friedlander, J. Hauer, J. McDade, M. T. Osterholm, T. O'Toole, G. Parker, T. M. Perl, P. K. Russell, and K. Tonat for the Working Group on Civilian Biodefense.** 1999. Anthrax as a biological weapon: medical and public health management. *JAMA* **281:**1735–1745.

14a.**Isenberg, H. D. (ed.).** *Clinical Microbiology Procedures Handbook,* 2nd ed., in press. ASM Press, Washington, D.C.

15. **Jernigan, J. A., D. S. Stephens, D. A. Ashford, C. Omenaca, M. S. Topiel, M. Galbraith, M. Tapper, T. L. Fisk, S. Zaki, T. Popovic, R. F. Meyer, C. P. Quinn, S. A. Harper, S. K. Fridkin, J. J. Sejvar, C. W. Shepard, M. McConnell, J. Guarner, W. J. Shieh, J. M. Malecki, J. L. Gerberding, J. M. Hughes, B. A. Perkins, and members of the Anthrax Bioterrorism Investigation Team.** 2001. Bioterrorism-related inhalational anthrax: the first 10 cases reported in the United States. *Emerg. Infect. Dis.* **7:**933–944.

16. **Klietmann, W. F., and K. L. Ruoff.** 2001. Bioterrorism: implications for the clinical microbiologist. *Clin. Microbiol. Rev.* **14:**364–381.

17. **Lillibridge, S. R., A. J. Bell, and R. S. Roman.** 1999. Centers for Disease Control and Prevention bioterrorism preparedness and response. *Am. J. Infect. Control* **27:**463–464.

18. **Luciana, B., D. Frank, M. Venkat, V. Mani, C. Chirboga, M. Pollanen, M. Ripple, S. Ali, C. DiAngelo, J. Lee, J. Arden, J. Titus, D. Fowler, T. O'Toole, H. Masur, J. Bartlett, and T. Inglesby.** 2001. Death due to bioterrorism-related inhalational anthrax: report of 2 patients. *JAMA* **286:**2554–2559.

19. **Mayer, T. A., S. Bersoof-Matcha, C. Murphy, J. Earls, S. Harper, D. Pauze, M. Nguyen, J. Rosenthall, D. Cerva, Jr., G. Druckenbrod, D. Hanfling, N. Fatteh, A. Napoli, A. Nayyar, and E. L. Berman.** 2001. Clinical presentation of inhalational anthrax following bioterrorism exposure: report of 2 surviving patients. *JAMA* **286:**2549–2553.

20. **Meselson, M., J. Guillemin, M. Hugh-Jones, A. Langmuir, I. Popova, A. Shelokov, and O. Yampolskaya.** 1994. The Sverdlovsk anthrax outbreak of 1979. *Science* **266:**1202–1208.

21. **Moran, G. J.** 1999. Update on emerging infections from the Centers for Disease Control and Prevention: bioterrorism alleging use of anthrax and interim guidelines for management—United States, 1998. *Ann. Emerg. Med.* **34:**229–232.

22. **Morse, S. A.** 2001. Bioterrorism: laboratory security. *Lab. Med.* **32:**303–306.

23. **Poupard, J. A., and L. A. Miller.** 1992. History of biological warfare: catapults to capsomeres. *Ann. N. Y. Acad. Sci.* **666:**9–20.

24. **Torok, T. J., R. V. Tauxe, R. P. Wise, J. R. Livengood, R. Sokolow, S. Mauvais, K. A. Birkness, M. R. Skeels, J. M. Horan, and L. R. Foster.** 1997. A large community outbreak of salmonellosis caused by intentional contamination of restaurant salad bars. *JAMA* **278:**389–395.

25. **Wiener, S. L., and J. Barrett.** 1986. Biological warfare defense, p. 508–509. *In Trauma Management for Civilian and Military Physicians.* W. B. Saunders, Philadelphia, Pa.

26. **Wilkening, D. A.** 1999. BCW attack scenarios, p. 76–114. *In* S. D. Drell, A. D. Sofaer, and G. D. Wilson (ed.), *The New Terror: Facing the Threat of Biological and Chemical Weapons.* Hoover Institution Press, Stanford, Calif.

Infection Control Epidemiology and Clinical Microbiology*

DANIEL J. DIEKEMA AND MICHAEL A. PFALLER

11

In 2000, the Institute of Medicine issued a landmark report on medical errors, estimating that between 44,000 and 98,000 deaths per year in U.S. hospitals are a result of injuries or complications sustained during the delivery of health care (32). Health care-associated (or nosocomial) infections represent one of the most common complications of care, affecting approximately 2 million persons admitted to acute-care hospitals each year (8). For this reason, every health care facility should have an infection control program charged with monitoring, preventing, and controlling the spread of infections in the health care environment. Since infection control requires the ability to detect infections when they occur, the clinical microbiology laboratory is inextricably linked to any comprehensive infection control program. In this chapter we will discuss the impact of nosocomial infections, outline the organization of the hospital infection control program, and describe the important role of the clinical microbiology laboratory in the prevention and control of health care-associated infections.

NOSOCOMIAL INFECTION

Definition

A nosocomial infection is one that is acquired in a hospital or health care facility (i.e., the infection was not present or incubating at the time of admission). For most bacterial infections, an onset of symptoms more than 48 h after admission is evidence for nosocomial acquisition. Other infections (e.g., legionellosis) must be considered in light of their usual incubation periods. Because hospital stays are getting shorter and more patients are treated in the outpatient setting, many health care-associated infections are not recognized during hospitalization. Infection control programs must therefore devise strategies for effective outpatient surveillance to accurately monitor nosocomial infection rates (27).

Infection Rates and Predominant Pathogens

At least 5% of patients may acquire an infection during hospitalization (24). The urinary tract is the most commonly involved site, with 30 to 40% of all nosocomial infections occurring at this site. Surgical wound and lower respiratory tract infections are the next most frequent (15 to 20%), followed by bloodstream infections (5 to 15%). The vast majority of nosocomial infections are related to devices (e.g., urinary tract catheters, endotracheal tubes in ventilated patients, and central venous catheters). For this reason and as a way to adjust for risk when comparing rates over time or between similar units in different facilities, the Centers for Disease Control and Prevention (CDC) recommends calculating nosocomial infection rates in the intensive care unit (ICU) by using device days as the denominator (Table 1).

Table 2 lists the five most common bacterial pathogens isolated from various nosocomial infection sites in U.S. hospital ICUs surveyed in the CDC's National Nosocomial Infections Surveillance System (NNIS) (6). The past 2 decades have seen a gradual shift in the spectrum of nosocomial pathogens from gram-negative to gram-positive organisms and have also seen the emergence of *Candida* spp. as a major problem (42). An important factor associated with the emergence of the staphylococci and enterococci as nosocomial pathogens has been their increasing resistance to antimicrobial agents (10).

Morbidity, Mortality, and Cost

Nosocomial infections cause or contribute to thousands of deaths annually (22, 51). Since patients with the most severe underlying illness are also those most vulnerable to nosocomial infection, it is very difficult to estimate the proportion of crude or overall mortality that is directly attributable to a nosocomial infection. Studies that attempt to address this by carefully controlling for many potentially confounding variables are called attributable-mortality studies. Estimates of the attributable mortality of nosocomial bloodstream infection range from 14% for infections due to coagulase-negative staphylococci (37) to 31 and 37% for infections due to vancomycin-susceptible and -resistant enterococci (14, 34), respectively, to 38% for infections due to *Candida* spp. (58) (Table 3).

---

* This chapter contains information presented in chapter 6 by John E. McGowan, Jr., and Beverly G. Metchock in the seventh edition of this Manual.

TABLE 1 Commonly used terms in health care epidemiology[a]

Term	Definition or summary
Epidemiology	Study of the occurrence, distribution, and determinants of health and disease in a population. Hospital or health care epidemiology is the study of disease occurrence and distribution in the hospital or health care system.
Nosocomial infection	An infection acquired in a hospital or other health care facility.
Endemic infections	Infections occurring as part of the background or usual rate of infection in a specified population.
Epidemic infections	Infections occurring as part of an outbreak (or epidemic) of infection—defined as a significant increase in the usual rate of that infection in the specified population.
Incidence rate	Ratio of the number of new cases of infection in a specified population at risk during a defined period to the overall number of people in the population at risk (the denominator).
Device-associated incidence rate	Ratio of the number of new cases of device-related infection in a specified population at risk during a defined period to the number of days of device utilization in the population at risk.
Prevalence rate	Total number of cases of infection in the defined population at risk at one point in time (point prevalence) or in a given period (period prevalence).
Observational or descriptive study	Study of the natural course of events, without an intervention in the process.
Case control study	Study frequently done as part of an outbreak investigation: a group of patients with the outcome of interest (e.g., cases of nosocomial infection) is compared to a control group of patients without the outcome. A comparison of specific factors between groups (e.g., exposures of interest) may suggest why infection occurred.
Crude or overall mortality rate	Ratio of the number of patients who die to the overall number of patients in a specified population.
Attributable mortality	Ratio of the number of patients who die as a direct result of the disease of interest to the overall population with the disease.

[a] Adapted from reference 38.

Nosocomial infections also increase hospital costs and length of stay (LOS), costing the health care system billions of dollars annually. At the University of Iowa, we have demonstrated a median excess LOS of 8 and 30 days for nosocomial bloodstream infections due to coagulase-negative staphylococci and *Candida* spp., respectively (37, 58).

TABLE 2 Distribution of the five most common nosocomial pathogens isolated from major infection sites in the ICU, January 1992 to May 1999[a]

Pathogen	% of total at each infection site
Bloodstream infection	
CoNS[b]	37.3
Enterococcus spp.	13.5
S. aureus	12.6
C. albicans	5.0
Enterobacter spp.	4.9
Pneumonia	
S. aureus	18.1
P. aeruginosa	17.0
Enterobacter spp.	11.2
K. pneumoniae	7.2
H. influenzae	4.3
Urinary tract infection	
E. coli	17.5
C. albicans	15.8
Enterococcus spp.	13.8
P. aeruginosa	11.0
K. pneumoniae	6.2

[a] Data from NNIS (6).
[b] CoNS, coagulase-negative *Staphylococcus* spp.

Nosocomial bloodstream infections in the ICU are associated with an excess LOS of 24 days and excess hospital costs of $40,000 per survivor (44). Surgical wound infections result in an excess LOS of over 6 days and an increase in hospital costs of over $3,000 per infection (15, 30).

The premise on which infection control programs is based is that many of these life-threatening and costly nosocomial infections are preventable. The Study of the Efficacy of Nosocomial Infection Control indicated that the presence of an active surveillance and infection control program was associated with a 32% decrease in nosocomial infection rates while the absence of such a program was associated with an 18% increase in nosocomial infection rates (25). More recently, the CDC NNIS system of hospitals reported a reduction in risk-adjusted infection rates in ICUs for all monitored infection sites (urinary tract, bloodstream, and lung) during the 1990s. The elements in place in these hospitals that were noted to be critical for rate

TABLE 3 Attributable mortality of nosocomial bloodstream infection due to selected pathogens[a]

Organism	Mortality among cases (%)	Mortality among matched controls (%)	Attributable mortality (%)	Reference
CoNS[b]	31	17	14	37
Enterococcus spp.	43	12	31	34
VRE	67	30	37	14
Candida spp.	57	19	38	58

[a] Adapted from reference 13 with permission of the publisher.
[b] CoNS, coagulase-negative *Staphylococcus* spp.

reduction included targeted surveillance in high-risk populations (using standard definitions), adequate numbers of trained infection control practitioners, data dissemination to health care providers, and links between monitoring of infection rates and prevention efforts (7). Clearly, an effective infection control program improves patient care, saves lives, and decreases health care costs.

THE HOSPITAL INFECTION CONTROL PROGRAM

The hospital infection control program should include surveillance of nosocomial infections, continuing education of medical staff, control of infectious diseases outbreaks, protection of employees from infection, and advice on new products and procedures. The program is generally directed by a physician-epidemiologist and enforced by the infection control committee. Every hospital must also have a working infection control staff, made up of one or more infection control practitioners (ICPs). These professionals are responsible for collecting nosocomial infection-related data and providing the data to the infection control committee.

Infection Control Committee

The infection control committee is responsible for reporting and evaluating nosocomial-infection data and for drafting and implementing policies, procedures, and guidelines pertinent to the practice of infection control. The committee should be multidisciplinary, with representatives from all departments, including clinical microbiology, and should meet every 1 to 3 months to review hospital-specific nosocomial-infection data and to formulate policy. Other responsibilities of the committee include review of technical information about new products, devices, or procedures pertinent to infection control and institution of all necessary control measures in the event of an outbreak or other infection control emergency.

A clinical microbiologist must be on the infection control committee to provide expertise in the interpretation of culture results, advice about the appropriateness and feasibility of microbiological approaches to an infection control problem, and input regarding the laboratory resources necessary to accomplish the goals of the committee. One of the most important contributions of the clinical microbiologist is to inform the infection control committee of the strengths and limitations of methods employed to detect and characterize nosocomial pathogens. He or she should describe the potential impact on infection control of any change in methods for detection, identification, and susceptibility testing of nosocomial pathogens. As just one example, if the laboratory introduces a urinary antigen detection test for diagnosis of legionellosis, the clinical microbiologist is responsible for informing the committee that the test is sensitive and specific only for detection of *Legionella pneumophila* serogroup 1 and that culture is required to test for nosocomial legionellosis due to other species or serogroups. The committee should also be made aware of the budgetary and personnel constraints under which the laboratory operates, to ensure that they do not expend valuable laboratory resources unless there is a clear epidemiologic indication to do so.

Nosocomial Infection Surveillance

Perhaps the most costly and time-consuming activity performed by infection control personnel, systematic surveillance of nosocomial infections is important for many reasons. By monitoring the frequency and types of nosocomial infection, the infection control program may detect outbreaks, evaluate compliance with infection control guidelines, provide data for policy development, and monitor the impact of any infection control interventions on nosocomial-infection rates. Additionally, surveillance is a requirement of national and state accrediting agencies. The most important aspect of surveillance is timely feedback of infection rates to health care providers, along with suggestions for improvement and reemphasis of existing infection control practices. In any case, the existence of an active nosocomial-infection surveillance program is associated with a reduction in infection rates (and their consequent morbidity and mortality) (11, 25).

As outlined above, the association of nosocomial infections with medical devices has led to the recommendation for risk adjustment of nosocomial-infection rates in ICUs by using device days rather than patient days as the denominator for rate calculation. This approach also allows for comparison to national benchmarks for infection rates in selected ICUs (coronary, medical, neurosurgical, etc.) compiled and reported by the CDC NNIS (6). Figure 1 is a sample chart format for reporting changing infection rates in a single tertiary-care center ICU in comparison with national benchmarks. This information should be provided to unit personnel (medical director, nursing manager, and clinicians) and should be accompanied by recommendations for and assistance in improving infection rates. Of course, reporting infection rates using device days as a denominator requires developing a system for counting or accurately estimating device utilization in the ICU.

Since surveillance consumes more resources than any other single infection control activity (16), it is essential that the most efficient surveillance system be employed. The most complete and accurate surveillance program might employ daily chart reviews of all hospitalized patients by an ICP, an approach that is obviously not practical in any but the smallest of hospitals. Limited resources should be focused in the highest-risk areas (ICUs, hematology-oncology units, burn units, and organ transplantation wards), and various screens can be used to increase efficiency. Microbiology reports, nursing-care plans, antibiotic orders, radiology reports, temperature charts, and discharge diagnoses can all be used to determine which charts should be further reviewed.

Review of microbiology reports is probably the most common method for case finding used routinely in nosocomial-infection surveillance. Review of microbiology reports alone compares favorably in some studies to more comprehensive ward-based surveillance (21, 57). For example, Yakoe et al. reported that review of microbiology data alone was both more resource efficient and as effective as applying the CDC NNIS definition for detecting nosocomial bloodstream infection (62). Laboratory-based surveillance allows for the efficient review of large amounts of data, and medical information systems can enhance surveillance further by linking data from many sources, including pharmacy (antimicrobial use), laboratory, radiology, billing (diagnostic codes), and nursing notes (vital signs and care plans).

Although review of microbiology reports is an essential part of surveillance, these data alone may not detect all outbreaks or infections. The sensitivity and specificity of laboratory-based surveillance depend on both the frequency of culturing and the quality of the culture specimens received by the laboratory. Optimal surveillance will include a combination of the above data screens (for example, nursing-care plan and microbiology reports) to help deter-

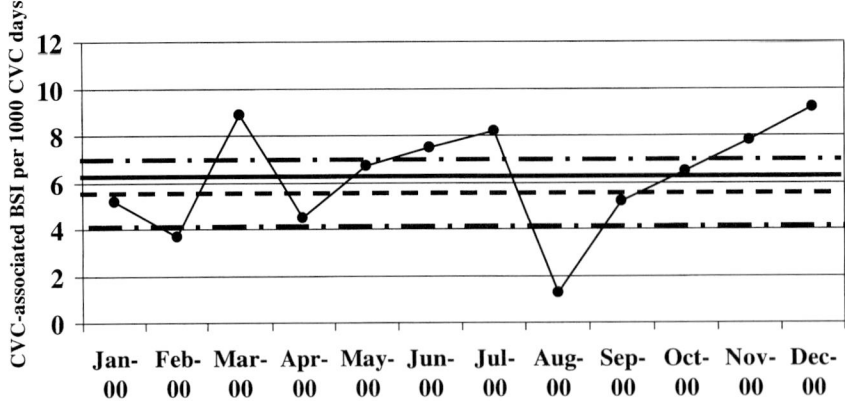

FIGURE 1 Medical ICU catheter-associated bloodstream infection rate. ●———●, central venous catheter (CVC)-associated bloodstream infection rate per 1,000 catheter-days; ———, mean CVC-associated bloodstream infection rate in Hospital A medical ICU; – – – –, pooled mean CVC-associated bloodstream infection rate for the CDC NNIS hospital medical ICUs ($n = 131$); — ▪ —, 25th and 75th percentile for CVC-associated bloodstream infection rate in NNIS hospitals.

mine which charts deserve further review. The frequency of surveillance of specific hospital units should be determined in each hospital by the infection control committee on the basis of available resources, prevailing infection rates, and other factors. In addition, the mechanism by which the laboratory provides specific surveillance information (all positive results, selected or sorted reports, etc.) should be decided by the infection control committee, in consultation with clinical microbiology personnel. The University of Iowa has validated a surveillance strategy using primarily microbiology reports and nursing-care plans and has found the sensitivity and specificity to be 81 and 98%, respectively (4).

ROLE OF THE MICROBIOLOGY LABORATORY IN INFECTION CONTROL

With this overview of the structure and activities of the hospital infection control program in mind, we will now focus on the most important specific roles played by the microbiology laboratory in the day-to-day practice of infection control.

Specimen Collection

Since many nosocomial pathogens are also common colonizing organisms and culture contaminants (e.g., coagulase-negative staphylococci), specimen collection and handling can have an impact on nosocomial infection rates (L. C. McDonald, R. Carrico, B. Simmons, C. Richards, B. Braun, L. Steele, S. Solomon, E. Wong, and S. Kritchevsky, *Abstr. 11th Annu. Meet. Soc. Health Care Epidemiol. Am.*, abstr. 105, 2001). Careful monitoring of specimen quality and enforcement of strict criteria for acceptance of clinical specimens ensure that the most accurate, least misleading microbiological data are reported to both the clinician and the ICP (see chapter 6).

Accurate Identification and Susceptibility Testing of Nosocomial Pathogens

With increasing use of commercial identification and susceptibility testing systems, most laboratories now have the capability to identify microorganisms to species level and

perform antimicrobial susceptibility testing (AST). However, the expanding spectrum of organisms that colonize and infect seriously ill patients continues to challenge the ability of the clinical microbiology laboratory to accurately identify and characterize nosocomial pathogens (41). For example, while many nosocomial pathogens (e.g., *Staphylococcus* spp. and the *Enterobacteriaceae*) are easily detected and identified by commonly used automated systems, many nonfermentative gram-negative organisms also cause nosocomial infection and can be much more difficult to identify. Species level identification of nosocomial pathogens may be the first clue to an outbreak, and so laboratories should establish a system for sending unusual nosocomial pathogens to a reference laboratory for identification. In addition, viral, fungal, and mycobacterial pathogens may cause nosocomial infection and also can be challenging to identify to a level appropriate to infection control needs.

As new antimicrobial resistances emerge and existing resistances increase in frequency, it has become necessary to supplement automated systems with additional methods to guard against significant AST errors for some organism-antimicrobial combinations. Errors are most likely for organisms that display heteroresistance or inducible resistance mechanisms. For example, in the past some systems have underestimated oxacillin resistance among *Staphylococcus* species (60) and have not adequately detected extended-spectrum β-lactamase (ESBL) production among certain members of the *Enterobacteriaceae* (18, 54). Some automated systems have also performed poorly in the detection of certain vancomycin resistance phenotypes in enterococci (53). Conversely, some systems have reported false resistance among gram-negative rods and *S. aureus* (3, 17).

As such problems are brought to the attention of the manufacturers of these systems, improvements can be made in the instrumentation, panels, or software programs to improve accuracy. This process of ongoing independent evaluation of automated systems and feedback to responsive industry representatives is extremely important. Unfortunately, in the era of managed care and shrinking laboratory resources, fewer laboratories have the ability to perform rigorous internal evaluations of new technology. Unrecognized problems in identification or susceptibility testing have obvious, major ramifications for infection control; namely, serious problems and even outbreaks can go unrecognized or, conversely, infection control resources can be diverted toward spurious resistance problems.

Three of the most important resistances emerging as causes of nosocomial infection include ESBL-producing organisms among the *Enterobacteriaceae* (43, 47), glycopeptide resistance among enterococci (10) and staphylococci (9, 48), and methicillin resistance among *S. aureus* strains (MRSA) (12). Effective infection control efforts obviously depend on the ability of the laboratory to detect these epidemiologically important resistant pathogens. The laboratory director must keep up with current literature regarding the ability of automated systems to detect emerging resistances and the need for additional methods to detect or confirm resistance patterns. The CDC maintains fact sheets summarizing current recommendations for laboratory detection of these resistances; laboratories can access them easily on the Internet (http://www.cdc.gov/ncidod/hip/lab/lab.htm). They are also reviewed in chapters 74 and 75.

Rapid Diagnostic Testing

The past decade has seen the increasing development of rapid diagnostic testing using molecular or immunologic methods. The speed with which these methods can produce accurate results can have important implications for infection control. For example, a variety of methods are now available for rapid detection of respiratory syncytial virus (29), *Clostridium difficile* (20), *Mycobacterium tuberculosis* (28), and *Legionella pneumophila* serogroup 1 (45). Rapid methods for detection of important antimicrobial resistances are also under development. Latex agglutination testing for the altered penicillin binding protein 2a (MRSA Screen; Denka Seiken) (63)—or molecular detection of the *mecA* gene responsible for it (5, 64)—may soon provide for more rapid detection of MRSA. A positive result from any of these tests may allow more rapid institution of appropriate isolation precautions and/or early investigation of potential outbreaks. Of course, indiscriminate use or poor quality control of a rapid diagnostic test can lead to errors, including false-positive tests that result in a pseudo-outbreak (36). The clinical microbiologist must provide the ICP with information about the negative predictive value of any rapid tests, which may not be sufficiently high to allow for discontinuation of previously instituted isolation precautions.

Reporting of Laboratory Data

Culture and AST results are an important data source for infection control and are usually reviewed daily by ICPs. However, additional important information should be obtained via direct communication between laboratory and infection control personnel during regular laboratory rounds (e.g., issues of infection versus colonization or the extent to which specimens should be worked up for epidemiologically important organisms). In addition to informal work rounds in the laboratory, we recommend that ICPs and a microbiology laboratory designee attend a weekly "work rounds" to discuss areas of mutual concern (potential clusters of infection, any ongoing outbreaks) and to arrange for the laboratory to proceed with supplementary studies (molecular typing, environmental cultures, etc.).

Some culture results warrant an early phone call from the laboratory to the ICP to ensure that appropriate control measures are implemented. Examples include positive ster-

ile site cultures for *Neisseria meningitidis*, smears or cultures positive for acid-fast bacilli, isolation of the enteric pathogen *Salmonella* or *Shigella*, and the isolation of certain antimicrobial-resistant pathogens such as MRSA and vancomycin-resistant enterococci (VRE). In addition, the detection of new or unusual pathogens (e.g., vancomycin-resistant staphylococci) should also be reported promptly to the ICP.

Routine microbiology laboratory results should be readily accessible to ICPs. In most cases, results are stored in a computer database, facilitating retrieval and analysis. Information stored should include specimen type, date of collection, patient identification, hospital number, hospital service, ward location, organisms identified, AST results, and the results of any specialized testing performed (e.g., typing). Both clinicians and ICPs may benefit from periodic summaries of selected microbiology results: an antibiogram specifically for nosocomial pathogens. These results should be organized into frequency of isolation of various nosocomial pathogens by anatomical site and hospital service. The tables generated should summarize AST results, thereby assisting clinicians in their choice of empiric antimicrobial therapy for patients with nosocomial infection. Inclusion of cost information for the most commonly used antimicrobials may also be appropriate.

Outbreak Recognition and Investigation: Epidemic versus Endemic Infections

The majority of nosocomial infections are not associated with outbreaks; they are endemic rather than epidemic infections. If rates of nosocomial infection are consistently defined by prospective surveillance, outbreaks of nosocomial infection will occasionally be identified by review of these rates—an outbreak being defined as an increase in infection rate beyond the expected during a defined period. However, more often infection control personnel are made aware of potential outbreaks during their interaction with ward, clinic, or laboratory personnel.

When the infection control team detects a cluster or outbreak of nosocomial infection, they must act promptly to define the extent of the outbreak, learn the mode of transmission of the pathogen, and institute appropriate control measures. The clinical microbiology laboratory must provide appropriate laboratory support during this time. Table 4 outlines all the recommended steps of an outbreak investigation and points out the important role of the clinical microbiology laboratory at each step.

Because the demands on the laboratory may be great during outbreak settings, advance preparation should be performed. Laboratory personnel should periodically ask ICPs what types of outbreaks have occurred in the past or could be anticipated in the future and what laboratory resources would be required should such outbreaks occur. The extra costs associated with outbreak investigations should also be anticipated by hospital administration and calculated into annual budgets if possible. Costs should not be borne by the laboratory or charged to individual patients involved in the outbreak.

Some problems and potential pitfalls of outbreak investigation are pertinent to the clinical microbiology laboratory and bear specific mention. Foremost among these is the problem of determining when to proceed with an outbreak investigation in the first place. The number of cases necessary to constitute an outbreak depends on the organism, the patient population, and the institution involved. For example, while numerous cases of *Escherichia coli* urinary

TABLE 4 Steps in nosocomial outbreak investigation, and the role of the laboratory at each step[a]

Investigative step	Role of the clinical microbiology laboratory
Recognize problem	Surveillance and early warning system; notify infection control practitioners of clusters of infections, unusual resistance patterns, and possible patient-to-patient transmission
Establish case definition	Assist and advise regarding inclusion of laboratory diagnosis in case definition
Confirm cases	Perform laboratory confirmation of diagnosis
Complete case finding	Characterize isolates with accuracy; store all sterile site isolates and epidemiologically important isolates; search laboratory database for new cases
Establish background rate of disease, compare to attack rate during suspected outbreak	Provide data for use in ongoing surveillance, which provide baseline rates for selected units and infection sites; search laboratory database for all prior cases of the entity if baseline rate is not prospectively monitored
Characterize outbreak (descriptive epidemiology)	Perform typing of involved strains, compare to previously isolated endemic strains to determine if the outbreak involves a single strain (see chapter 12); this can be done only if selected pathogens are routinely stored (see above).
Generate hypotheses about causation. Reservoir Mode of spread Vector Perform case control study or cohort study	Perform supplementary studies or cultures as needed, but only if justified by epidemiologic link to transmission: personnel, patients, environment
Institute control measures	Adjust laboratory procedures as necessary
Perform ongoing surveillance to document efficacy of control measures	Maintain surveillance and early-warning function of the laboratory

[a] Adapted from reference 38.

tract infection in a long-term care facility may not constitute an outbreak, even a single nosocomial case of group A streptococcal surgical wound infection or vancomycin-intermediate *S. aureus* infection merits an outbreak investigation. We recommend that every clinical laboratory, in consultation with the infection control program, generate a list of epidemiologically important organisms that merit immediate notification of infection control personnel. In addition, laboratories should strongly consider instituting a program for computer-driven recognition of clustering of pathogens within the hospital, followed by typing to evaluate for evidence of outbreaks or patient-to-patient spread. Investigators at Northwestern University Hospital have demonstrated a reduction in nosocomial infection rates temporally associated with implementing such an approach (23).

A second important problem is that of a pseudo-outbreak. A pseudo-outbreak has occurred when an apparent outbreak turns out not to be an outbreak after all. The usual cause of a pseudo-outbreak is either misdiagnosis (e.g., infection has not actually occurred) or misinterpretation of epidemiologic data (e.g., infections have occurred, but clustering or epidemic transmission has not). The microbiology laboratory can be the source of pseudo-outbreaks (2, 17, 26, 33, 35, 49, 55). Quality control problems in the laboratory that often lead to pseudo-outbreaks include contamination of stain preparation reagents (26), false antimicrobial susceptibility test results (17), and culture specimen contam-

ination (often from ongoing construction [35] or cross-contamination during specimen processing [61]). Careful attention to quality control, sterile technique in specimen processing, and construction controls can decrease the likelihood of a laboratory-generated pseudo-outbreak.

Molecular Typing To Support Infection Control Activities

Outbreaks of nosocomial infection often result from exposure of a number of hospitalized patients to a common source or reservoir of a pathogenic agent (e.g., water from a hot-water tank colonized with *Legionella* spp.). The organisms causing the outbreak in these cases are all derived from a single strain (i.e., they can be said to be clonally related). The infection control program may therefore request that the microbiology laboratory characterize potential outbreak strains to determine their genetic relatedness. In the appropriate clinical setting, species level identification and AST results (antibiogram) may provide strong evidence for an epidemiologic link. However, more sensitive methods of strain delineation are often necessary. In this setting, phenotypic typing methods (e.g., AST, biochemical profiles, bacteriophage susceptibility patterns), which discriminate poorly among strains, have been replaced almost completely by genotypic or DNA-based typing methods (1, 46, 56).

The cost-effective application of genotypic typing methods requires that they be used only for well-defined epidemiologic objectives. These objectives include (i) determination of the source and extent of an outbreak, (ii) determination of the mode of transmission of nosocomial pathogens, (iii) evaluation of the efficacy of preventative measures, and (iv) monitoring of infection in high-risk areas (e.g., ICUs), where cross-infection is a recognized hazard.

The ideal genotypic typing system should be standardized, reproducible, stable, sensitive, broadly applicable, readily available, inexpensive, and of proven value in epidemiologic investigation. Further discussion of the relative advantages and disadvantages of the many available typing systems is beyond the scope of this chapter and has been summarized in several recent reviews (1, 39, 46, 52, 56) and in chapter 12 of this Manual.

Organism Storage

Of course, it is impossible to provide the infection control program with supplemental testing like molecular typing if the appropriate isolates have not been saved. The laboratory should plan ahead and be sure to save all epidemiologically important isolates (see chapter 7). Decisions about the number and type of isolates to be banked and the duration of storage will differ from hospital to hospital depending on available resources. We recommend that all isolates from normally sterile sites (e.g., blood and cerebrospinal fluid), important antibiotic-resistant organisms (MRSA, VRE, ESBL-producing Enterobacteriaceae) from any site, and other epidemiologically important pathogens (e.g., M. tuberculosis) be saved for 3 to 5 years.

Cultures of Specimens from Hospital Personnel and the Environment

Cultures of specimens from hospital personnel and the environment (surfaces, air, and water) should be performed rarely and only when the epidemiologic evidence suggests personnel or environmental involvement in the transmission of a nosocomial pathogen. Various potential sources and their appropriate culture methods are outlined in Table 5. Although the use of such cultures is frequently entertained, it should be emphasized that the cultures are often labor-intensive, nonstandardized, and difficult to interpret and rarely provide useful information.

Because the hands of health care workers can act as a vehicle for transmission of nosocomial pathogens from patient to patient, hand cultures are sometimes useful in confirming the mechanism of cross-infection during an outbreak investigation (59). Similarly, because the anterior nares represent the usual reservoir for S. aureus (including MRSA) colonization in humans (31), nares cultures of patients and health care personnel are sometimes appropriate during an S. aureus outbreak.

Any decision to culture hospital personnel during an outbreak investigation should weigh two important factors: (i) finding the outbreak strain on the hands or in the nares of a health care worker does not establish the direction of transmission or definitively implicate the health care worker as the source or reservoir for the outbreak, and (ii) indiscriminate culturing of hospital personnel can lead to confusing results and can generate ill will toward the infection control program. We recommend cultures of spec-

TABLE 5 Cultures of personnel or environmental sources of infection in the hospital[a]

Source	Culture method	Comment
Blood products	Broth culture incubated aerobically and anaerobically at 30–32°C for 10 days	Following transfusion reaction; obtain simultaneous blood cultures by venipuncture
Environmental surfaces	Swab-rinse or impression plate	No evidence that any particular level of contamination correlates with nosocomial infection
Disinfectants and antiseptics	Plating of serial dilutions of the product with and without specific neutralizers	Organisms usually nonfermenting gram-negative aerobic bacilli
Air	Mechanical air sampler (preferred); settling plates (poor)	No uniform agreement on acceptable levels of contamination; lack of correlation with infection
Water (for Legionella spp.)	Membrane filter for water samples, swab of faucets and showerheads	Number of peripheral sites positive for Legionella spp. may correlate with risk of nosocomial cases; culture after confirmed case of nosocomial legionellosis; no data to support routine water cultures
Hands of personnel	Broth-bag: 10–20-ml nutrient broth in sterile plastic bag; wash hands in broth, and plate semiquantitatively	May confirm the mechanism of cross-infection; impress the importance of hand washing
Anterior nares of personnel	Swab culture	Carriage of outbreak strain may be eradicated by application of topical agent (e.g., mupirocin for S. aureus); recolonization with the same strain is frequent

[a] Cultures to be performed only if clearly indicated by epidemiologic data.

imens from hospital personnel only after consultation with a hospital epidemiologist experienced in outbreak investigation. Only health care workers epidemiologically linked to cases should be cultured.

As a general rule, routine cultures of specimens from hospital personnel and the environment should not be performed. Exceptions include routine monitoring of sterilization, infant formula, and other hospital-prepared products; blood components prepared in an "open" system; hemodialysis fluid; and disinfected equipment. Sampling activities that have been specifically identified as unnecessary because of high cost and lack of clinical or epidemiologic benefit include routine culturing of patients or hospital personnel, routine sampling of commercial patient care items, in-use testing of antiseptics and disinfectants, random culturing of blood units, routine culturing of respiratory therapy equipment, routine culturing of peritoneal dialysate, and routine culture of air. These routine cultures are a burden to the laboratory and seldom, if ever, provide useful information or lead to specific interventions (19, 50).

CONCLUSION

The clinical microbiology laboratory is an essential component of any effective infection control program. The development and application of new technologies in the clinical laboratory have the potential to greatly enhance infection control efforts. A good working relationship between clinical laboratory and infection control personnel will greatly facilitate the investigation and control of health care-associated infections.

REFERENCES

1. **Arbeit, R. D.** 1999. Laboratory procedures for the epidemiologic analysis of microorganisms, p. 107–115. *In* P. R. Murray, E. J. Baron, M. A. Pfaller, F. C. Tenover, and R. H. Yolken (ed.), *Manual of Clinical Microbiology*, 7th ed. American Society for Microbiology, Washington, D.C.
2. **Ashford, D. A., S. Kellerman, M. Yakrus, S. Brim, R. C. Good, L. Finelli, W. R. Jarvis, and M. M. McNeil.** 1997. Pseudo-outbreak of septicemia due to rapidly growing mycobacteria associated with extrinsic contamination of culture supplement. *J. Clin. Microbiol.* **35:**2040–2042.
3. **Beidenbach, D. J., and R. N. Jones.** 1995. Interpretive errors using an automated system for the susceptibility testing of imipenem and aztreonam. *Diagn. Microbiol. Infect. Dis.* **21:**57–60.
4. **Broderick, A., M. Mori, M. D. Nettleman, S. A. Streed, and R. P. Wenzel.** 1990. Nosocomial infections: validation of surveillance and computer modeling to identify patients at risk. *Am. J. Epidemiol.* **131:**734–742.
5. **Carroll, K. C., R. B. Leonard, P. L. Newdomb-Gayman, and D. R. Hillyard.** 1996. Rapid detection of the staphylococcal *mecA* gene from BACTEC blood culture bottles by PCR. *Am. J. Clin. Pathol.* **106:**600–605.
6. **Centers for Disease Control and Prevention.** 1999. National Nosocomial Infections Surveillance (NNIS) report, data summary from January 1990–May 1999, issued June 1999. *Am. J. Infect. Control* **27:**520–532.
7. **Centers for Disease Control and Prevention.** 2000. Monitoring hospital-acquired infections to promote patient safety—United States, 1990–1999. *Morb. Mortal. Wkly. Rep.* **49:**149–153.
8. **Centers for Disease Control and Prevention.** 1992. Public health focus: surveillance, prevention and control of nosocomial infections. *Morb. Mortal. Wkly. Rep.* **41:**783–787.
9. **Centers for Disease Control and Prevention.** 1997. Update: *Staphylococcus aureus* with reduced susceptibility to vancomycin—United States, 1997. *Morb. Mortal. Wkly. Rep.* **46:**813–815.
10. **Cormican, M. G., and R. N. Jones.** 1996. Emerging resistance to antimicrobial agents in gram-positive bacteria: enterococci, staphylococci, and non-pneumococcal streptococci. *Drugs* **51**(Suppl. 1):6–12.
11. **Cruse, P. J. E.** 1970. Surgical wound sepsis. *Can. Med. Assoc. J.* **102:**251–258.
12. **Diekema, D. J., M. A. Pfaller, F. J. Schmitz, J. Smayevsky, J. Bell, R. N. Jones, M. L. Beach, and the SENTRY Participants Group.** 2001. Survey of infections due to *Staphylococcus* species: frequency of occurrence and antimicrobial susceptibility of isolated collected in the US, Canada and Latin America for the SENTRY program, 1997–1999. *Clin. Infect. Dis.* **32**(Suppl. 2):S114–S132.
13. **Diekema, D. J., and M. A. Pfaller.** 2001. Role of the clinical microbiology laboratory in hospital epidemiology and infection control, p. 1247–1255. *In* K. McClatchey (ed.), *Clinical Laboratory Medicine*, 2nd ed. Lippincott Williams & Wilkins, New York, N.Y.
14. **Edmond, M. B., J. F. Ober, J. D. Dawson, D. L. Weinbaum, and R. P. Wenzel.** 1996. Vancomycin-resistant enterococcal bacteremia: natural history and attributable mortality. *Clin. Infect. Dis.* **23:**1234–1239.
15. **Emori, T. G., and R. P. Gaynes.** 1993. An overview of nosocomial infections, including the role of the microbiology laboratory. *Clin. Microbiol. Rev.* **6:**428–442.
16. **Emori, T. G., R. W. Haley, and J. S. Garner.** 1981. Technique and use of nosocomial infection surveillance in U.S. hospitals. *Am. J. Med.* **70:**933–940.
17. **Ender, P. T., S. J. Durning, W. K. Woelk, R. M. Brockett, A. Astorga, R. Reddy, and P. A. Meier.** 1999. Pseudo-outbreak of methicillin-resistant *Staphylococcus aureus*. *Mayo Clin. Proc.* **74:**885–889.
18. **Ferraro, M. J., and J. H. Jorgensen.** 1999. Susceptibility testing instrumentation and computerized expert systems for data analysis and interpretation, p. 1593–1600. *In* P. R. Murray, E. J. Baron, M. A. Pfaller, F. C. Tenover, and R. H. Yolken (ed.), *Manual of Clinical Microbiology*, 7th ed. American Society for Microbiology, Washington, D.C.
19. **Garner, J. S., and M. S. Favero.** 1986. Centers for Disease Control guideline for handwashing and hospital environmental control, 1985. *Infect. Control* **7:**231–243.
20. **Gerding, D. N., and J. S. Brazier.** 1993. Optimal methods for identifying *Clostridium difficile* infections. *Clin. Infect. Dis.* **16**(Suppl. 4):S439–S442.
21. **Gross, P. A., A. Beaugard, and C. Van Antwerpen.** 1980. Surveillance for nosocomial infections: can the sources of data be reduced? *Infect. Control* **1:**233–236.
22. **Gross, P. A., H. C. Neu, P. Aswapokee, C. Van Antwerpen, and N. Aswapokee.** 1980. Deaths from nosocomial infections: experience in a university hospital and a community hospital. *Am. J. Med.* **68:**219–223.
23. **Hacek, D. M., T. Suriano, G. A. Noskin, J. Kruszynsky, B. Reisberg, and L. R. Peterson.** 1999. Medical and economic benefit of a comprehensive infection control program that includes routine determination of microbial clonality. *Am. J. Clin. Pathol.* **111:**647–654.
24. **Haley, R. W., D. H. Culver, J. W. White, W. M. Morgan, and T. G. Emori.** 1985. The nationwide nosocomial infection rate. A new need for vital statistics. *Am. J. Epidemiol.* **121:**159–167.
25. **Haley, R. W., D. H. Culver, J. W. White, W. M. Morgan, T. G. Emori, V. P. Munn, and T. M. Hooten.** 1985. The efficacy of infection control surveillance and control programs in preventing nosocomial infections in U.S. hospitals. *Am. J. Epidemiol.* **121:**182–205.

26. **Hopfer, R. L., R. L. Katz, and V. Fainstein.** 1982. Pseudooutbreak of cryptococcal meningitis. *J. Clin. Microbiol.* **15:**1141–1143.

27. **Jarvis, W. R.** 2001. Infection control and changing health-care delivery systems. *Emerg. Infect. Dis.* **7:**170–173.

28. **Kearns, A. M., R. Freeman, M. Steward, and J. G. Magee.** 1998. A rapid PCR technique for detecting M. tuberculosis in a variety of clinical specimens. *J. Clin. Pathol.* **51:**922–924.

29. **Kellogg, J. A.** 1991. Culture versus direct antigen assays for detection of microbial pathogens from lower respiratory tract specimens suspected of containing the respiratory syncytial virus. *Arch. Pathol. Lab. Med.* **115:**451–458.

30. **Kirkland, K. B., J. P. Briggs, S. L. Trivette, W. E. Wilkinson, and D. J. Sexton.** 1999. The impact of surgical-site infections in the 1990's: attributable mortality, excess length of hospitalization, and extra costs. *Infect. Control Hosp. Epidemiol.* **20:**725–730.

31. **Kluytmans, J., A. van Belkum, and H. Verbrugh.** 1997. Nasal carriage of *Staphylococcus aureus*: epidemiology, underlying mechanisms, and associated risks. *Clin. Microbiol. Rev.* **10:**505–520.

32. **Kohn, L. T., J. M. Corrigan, and M. S. Donaldson (ed.).** 2000. *To Err Is Human: Building a Safer Health System.* National Academy Press, Washington, D.C.

33. **Lai, K. K., B. A. Brown, J. A. Westerling, S. A. Fontecchio, Y. Zhang, and R. J. Wallace.** 1998. Long-term laboratory contamination by *Mycobacterium abscessus* resulting in two pseudo-outbreaks: recognition with use of RAPD PCR. *Clin. Infect. Dis.* **27:**169–175.

34. **Landry, S. L., D. L. Kaiser, and R. P. Wenzel.** 1989. Hospital stay and mortality attributed to nosocomial enterococcal bacteremia: a controlled study. *Am. J. Infect. Control* **17:**323–329.

35. **Laurel, V. L., P. A. Meier, A. Astorga, D. Dolan, R. Brockett, and M. G. Rinaldi.** 1999. Pseudoepidemic of *Aspergillus niger* infections traced to specimen contamination in the microbiology laboratory. *J. Clin. Microbiol.* **37:**1612–1615.

36. **Laussucq, S., D. Schuster, W. J. Alexander, W. L. Thacker, H. W. Wilkinson, and J. S. Spika.** 1988. False-positive DNA probe test for *Legionella* species associated with a cluster of respiratory illnesses. *J. Clin. Microbiol.* **26:**1442–1444.

37. **Martin, M. A., M. A. Pfaller, and R. P. Wenzel.** 1989. Mortality and hospital stay attributable to coagulase-negative staphylococcal bacteremia. *Ann. Intern. Med.* **110:**9–16.

38. **McGowan, J. E., and B. G. Metchock.** 1999. Infection control epidemiology and clinical microbiology, p. 107–115. *In* P. R. Murray, E. J. Baron, M. A. Pfaller, F. C. Tenover, and R. H. Yolken (ed.), *Manual of Clinical Microbiology*, 7th ed. ASM Press, Washington, D.C.

39. **Olive, D. M., and P. Bean.** 1999. Principles and applications of methods for DNA-based typing of microbial organisms. *J. Clin. Microbiol.* **37:**1661–1669.

40. **Pfaller, M. A., and M. G. Cormican.** 1997. Microbiology: the role of the clinical laboratory, p. 95–118. *In* R. P. Wenzel (ed.), *Prevention and Control of Nosocomial Infections.* The Williams & Wilkins Co., Baltimore, Md.

41. **Pfaller, M. A., and L. A. Herwaldt.** 1997. The clinical microbiology laboratory and infection control: emerging pathogens, antimicrobial resistance, and new technology. *Clin. Infect. Dis.* **25:**858–870.

42. **Pfaller, M. A.** 1989. Opportunistic fungal infections: the increasing importance of *Candida* species. *Infect. Control Hosp. Epidemiol.* **10:**270–273.

43. **Philippon, A., G. Arlet, and P. H. Lagrange.** 1994. Origin and impact of plasmid-mediated extended spectrum beta-lactamases. *Eur. J. Clin. Microbiol. Infect. Dis.* **13**(Suppl. 1):17–29.

44. **Pittet, D., D. Tarara, and R. P. Wenzel.** 1994. Nosocomial bloodstream infection in critically ill patients: excess length of stay, extra costs, and attributable mortality. *JAMA* **271:**1598–1601.

45. **Plouffe, J. F., T. M. File Jr., R. F. Breiman, B. A. Hackman, S. J. Salstrom, B. J. Marston, B. S. Fields, and the Community Based Pneumonia Incidence Study Group.** 1995. Reevaluation of the definition of Legionnaires' disease: use of the urinary antigen assay. *Clin. Infect. Dis.* **20:**1286–1291.

46. **Sader, H. S., R. J. Hollis, and M. A. Pfaller.** 1995. The use of molecular techniques in the epidemiology and control of infectious diseases. *Clin. Lab. Med.* **15:**407–431.

47. **Sanders, W. E., and C. S. Sanders.** 1988. Inducible beta-lactamases: clinical and epidemiologic implications for use of newer cephalosporins. *Rev. Infect. Dis.* **10:**830–838.

48. **Schwalbe, R. S., J. T. Stapleton, and P. H. Gilligan.** 1987. Emergence of vancomycin resistance in coagulase-negative staphylococci. *N. Engl. J. Med.* **316:**927–931.

49. **Segal-Maurer, S., B. N. Kreiswirth, J. M. Burns, S. Lavie, M. Lim, C. Urban, and J. J. Rahal.** 1998. *Mycobacterium tuberculosis* specimen contamination revisited: the role of laboratory environmental control in a pseudo-outbreak. *Infect. Control Hosp. Epidemiol.* **19:**101–105.

50. **Simmons, B. P.** 1981. Centers for Disease Control guidelines for hospital environmental control/microbiologic surveillance of the environment and of personnel in the hospital. *Infect. Control* **2:**145–146.

51. **Spengler, R. F., and W. E. Greenough III.** 1987. Hospital costs and mortality attributed to nosocomial bacteremias. *JAMA* **240:**2455–2458.

52. **Tenover, F. C., R. D. Arbeit, R. V. Goering, and the Molecular Working Group of the Society for Healthcare Epidemiology of America.** 1997. How to select and interpret molecular strain typing methods for epidemiological studies of bacterial infections: a review for healthcare epidemiologists. *Infect. Control Hosp. Epidemiol.* **18:**426–439.

53. **Tenover, F. C., J. M. Swenson, C. M. O'Hara, and S. A. Stocker.** 1995. Ability of commercial and reference antimicrobial susceptibility testing methods to detect vancomycin resistance in enterococci. *J. Clin. Microbiol.* **33:**1524–1527.

54. **Thompson, K. S., and C. C. Sanders.** 1992. Detection of extended-spectrum beta-lactamases in members of the family *Enterobacteriaceae:* comparison of the double disk and three dimensional test. *Antimicrob. Agents Chemother.* **36:**1877–1882.

55. **Tsakris, A., A. Pantazi, S. Pournaras, A. Maniatis, A. Polyzou, and D. Sofianou.** 2000. Pseudo-outbreak of imipenem-resistant *Acinetobacter baumanii* resulting from false susceptibility testing by a rapid automated system. *J. Clin. Microbiol.* **38:**3505–3507.

56. **Weber, S., M. A. Pfaller, and L. A. Herwaldt.** 1997. Role of molecular epidemiology in infection control. *Infect. Dis. Clin. North Am.* **11:**257–278.

57. **Wenzel, R. P., C. A. Osterman, K. J. Hunting, and J. M. Gwaltney, Jr.** 1976. Hospital-acquired infections. I. Surveillance in a university hospital. *Am. J. Epidemiol.* **103:**251–260.

58. **Wey, S. B., M. Mori, M. A. Pfaller, R. F. Woolson, and R. P. Wenzel.** 1988. Hospital acquired candidemia: attributable mortality and excess length of stay. *Arch. Intern. Med.* **148:**2642–2645.

59. **Widmer, A. F., R. P. Wenzel, A. Trilla, M. J. Bale, R. N. Jones, and B. N. Doebbeling.** 1993. Outbreak of *Pseudomonas aeruginosa* infections in a surgical intensive care unit: probable transmission via hands of a healthcare worker. *Clin. Infect. Dis.* **16:**372–376.

60. **Woods, G. L., D. LaTemple, and C. Cruz.** 1994. Evaluation of Microscan rapid gram-positive panels for detection of oxacillin-resistant staphylococci. *J. Clin. Microbiol.* **32:**1058–1059.

61. **Wurtz, R., P. Demarais, W. Trainor, J. McAuley, F. Kocka, L. Mosher, and S. Dietrich.** 1996. Specimen contamination in mycobacteriology laboratory detected by pseudo-outbreak of multidrug-resistant tuberculosis: analysis by routine epidemiology and confirmation by molecular technique. *J. Clin. Microbiol.* **34:**1017–1019.

62. **Yakoe, D. S., J. Anderson, R. Chambers, M. Connor, R. Finberg, C. Hopkins, D. Lichtenberg, S. Marino,** D. McGlaughlin, E. O'Rourke, M. Samore, K. Sands, J. Strymish, E. Yamplin, N. Vallonde, and R. Platt. 1998. Simplified surveillance for nosocomial bloodstream infections. *Infect. Control. Hosp. Epidemiol.* **19:** 657–660.

63. **Yamazumi, T., S. A. Marshall, W. W. Wilke, D. J. Diekema, M. A. Pfaller, and R. N. Jones.** 2001. Comparison of the Vitek Gram-Positive Susceptibility 106 card and the MRSA-Screen latex agglutination test for determining oxacillin resistance in clinical bloodstream isolates of *Staphylococcus aureus*. *J. Clin. Microbiol.* **39:** 53–56.

64. **Zheng, X., C. P. Kolbert, P. Varga-Delmore, J. Arruda, M. Lewis, J. Kolberg, F. R. Cockerill, and D. H. Persing.** 1999. Direct *mecA* detection from blood culture bottles by branched-DNA signal amplification. *J. Clin. Microbiol.* **37:**4192–4193.

Laboratory Procedures for the Epidemiological Analysis of Microorganisms*

DAVID R. SOLL, SHAWN R. LOCKHART, AND CLAUDE PUJOL

12

In dealing with an infection, one often is immediately faced with species identification in order to prescribe effective treatment. In some clinical cases, however, one must pursue the identity of the infecting organism to the subspecies level. The typing techniques that have evolved for such discrimination at both of these levels of relatedness must be as rapid and accurate as possible. These techniques, therefore, usually focus on phenotypic characteristics and rarely provide the resolution necessary to obtain measurements of genetic relatedness between isolates of the same species or the same subspecies. Such resolution is essential for a number of epidemiological questions now being posed. To accurately identify the origin of a nosocomial infection, transmission of a disease between individuals, the emergence of a new hypervirulent or drug-resistant strain, the microevolution of a commensal or infecting strain, and the general population structure of a pathogen, one must move from species typing to strain and substrain typing. Methods must be selected that provide information on the level of genetic relatedness that is necessary to answer the question posed. In many cases, this requires accurate measures of genetic relatedness in order to group isolates through cluster analyses. Methods have evolved that indeed provide such information, but researchers rarely validate the method they select for characterizing relatedness (130). They rarely ask if the method they have selected has the resolving power to address the question posed. For instance, researchers may select a method with very little resolving power to answer a question that requires distinction between similar but nonidentical isolates. They may ask a question about the stability of an infecting organism but apply a method that cannot discriminate microevolutionary change. Their results may therefore suggest stability when in fact the infecting organism is undergoing rapid microevolution. Alternatively, they may ask a question related to strain grouping that requires the genesis of deep-rooted dendrograms and then apply a method that relies mainly on hypervariable changes. Again, their results may not provide them with a valid answer, in this case because hypervariable changes will affect clustering due to homoplasy, which is the pres-

ence of identical characteristics in distinct phylogenetic lineages that are not acquired by descent but rather through convergence, parallelism, or reversion. It is therefore imperative that one clearly and accurately formulates the question to be answered, defines the level of genetic relatedness that must be attained, selects a genetic fingerprinting method with the resolution necessary to answer that question, and verifies the efficacy of the selected method.

BIOTYPING AND GENETIC FINGERPRINTING TECHNIQUES

Prior to the development of DNA-based techniques for assessing genetic relatedness, scientists relied on biotyping techniques, which measure phenotypic rather than genetic differences. The logic behind this approach was that phenotype reflected genotype, so that if one employed a number of phenotypic parameters, one could obtain a measure of genetic relatedness. In discriminating between genera and species in both bacteria and fungi, biotyping still provides us with fast and reliable diagnostic methods. Kits measuring assimilation patterns (biochemical profiles) are still the mainstay for discriminating among a variety of bacterial and fungal species (21, 25, 74, 76, 95, 100, 150), antibody-based tests continue to be used to discriminate among groups within bacterial species and fungi like *Cryptococcus neoformans* (6, 13, 97, 127), and phage typing continues to be used to discriminate among groups within bacterial species (9, 67). However, these types of methods in general do not provide the kind of genetic discrimination usually necessary for addressing epidemiological questions. First, most of these tests do not provide enough unrelated parameters to obtain a good reflection of genotype. Usually they discriminate among only a limited number of groups, as in the case of serotyping. Second, and more importantly, the expression of many genes is affected by environmental changes and by developmental programs or reversible phenotypic changes, such as high-frequency phenotypic switching in the fungi (11, 129, 136), and phage and plasmids can be transmitted horizontally (19, 23). Most biotyping methods therefore fall short as genetic fingerprinting techniques. There is, however, one major exception, multilocus enzyme electrophoresis (MLEE) (99, 111). MLEE represents a robust fingerprinting method that ex-

---

* This chapter contains information presented in chapter 7 by Robert D. Arbeit in the seventh edition of this Manual.

hibits performance parity with many of the most effective DNA fingerprinting methods (104, 144).

DNA fingerprinting techniques, by virtue of the fact that they assess differences in genetic material, have been assumed to be the most accurate methods for genetic fingerprinting. This is not necessarily the case (130). As noted, some are as effective as MLEE while others fall short. Some are poor indicators of microevolution, while others are good indicators of microevolution, but measure DNA sequences too hypervariable for deep-rooted cluster analyses (104). Some techniques are effective for analyzing bacteria but less effective for analyzing eukaryotes, and vice versa, because of the inherent difference in the prokaryotic and eukaryotic genomes. Finally, while some DNA fingerprinting techniques are excellent for cluster analyses of large collections of isolates, they are not favored by evolutionary biologists because they do not provide codominant markers (138), although this requirement has been challenged quite effectively (142, 143).

What, then, are the general methods of DNA fingerprinting? The methods that will be reviewed in this chapter have, for the most part, been used for bacteria, fungi, and parasites. One of the earliest methods applied to bacteria and fungi took advantage of the fact that in the divergence of strains within a species, restriction sites identified by restriction enzymes, or endonucleases, change, leading to changes in the length of DNA sequences between sites and therefore to differences between strains. These changes accumulate as strains diverge during evolution, and the sum of the changes provides an indicator of evolutionary distance. The pattern of restriction fragments is referred to as the restriction fragment length polymorphism (RFLP) pattern. Differences in the lengths of fragments between genomes represent the polymorphism, and the comparison of the RFLP patterns between different isolates is referred to as RFLP analysis. This method has proven to be very effective in DNA fingerprinting of bacteria, especially with the use of infrequent cutters in combination with pulsed-field gel electrophoresis (PFGE) (139), but less effective, although still popular, in fingerprinting eukaryotic pathogens like the infectious fungi (10, 118). To obtain a more limited or more specific pattern, Southern blots can be hybridized with a DNA probe. Although this method is also referred to as RFLP analysis in the literature, we will distinguish it by calling it RFLP with probe. The probes in this case must distinguish more than one fragment; therefore, they usually contain a repetitive sequence (119, 134, 137), or a combination of unique and repetitive sequences (39, 65, 81). The former are referred to as repetitive element probes, and the latter are called complex probes (130). A second approach to DNA fingerprinting takes advantage of PCR to amplify a variety of sequence fragments from the genome by utilizing sequences identified by the primers used in the PCR. The use of arbitrary primers for amplification has been referred to as random amplification of polymorphic DNA (RAPD) analysis (153, 155). This method has been used to DNA fingerprint a number of prokaryotic and eukaryotic pathogens (79, 91, 96, 144, 153) and can be very effective. In recent years, PCR-based methods have been developed with primers that recognize identified sequences, and in some cases they have been used in combination with RFLP. Some of these methods are preferred by evolutionary biologists since the data they generate represent identified alleles (138). The selection of sequences for amplification differs between bacteria and eukaryotic microbes, and the differences in some cases reflect characteristics unique to

prokaryotic versus eukaryotic genome organization. A third DNA fingerprinting method that has evolved in the last decade is based on PFGE methods for separating chromosome-sized DNA fragments (26, 122). This method has been successfully used to karyotype many fungi (15, 35, 72) and other eukaryotic microorganisms (64, 71) and, in the case of prokaryotes, to separate large fragments generated by infrequent cutters, i.e., endonucleases that identify infrequent restriction sites in the genome under analysis (2, 16, 113). Finally, sequencing of portions of one or several genes represents a basic tool for answering evolutionary questions and a rapidly emerging tool for assessing epidemiological questions (42, 70, 87). Since MLEE and the variety of DNA fingerprinting methods outlined above all represent tools for epidemiological studies of the genetic relatedness of isolates, we will refer to them as genetic fingerprinting methods.

GENERAL REQUIREMENTS OF AN EFFECTIVE GENETIC FINGERPRINTING METHOD

Before considering in detail each DNA fingerprinting method, a consideration of the general requirements of fingerprinting methods is in order. Although a list of requirements will be formulated, it should be immediately realized that different epidemiological questions will require different levels of resolution or stringency.

A Method Should Provide Data That Reflect Genetic Distance at the Level Necessary To Answer the Question Posed

An effective genetic fingerprinting system should do more than demonstrate that two isolates are nonidentical or that a collection of isolates all differ. In many cases, a researcher must know how unrelated (or related) two or more isolates are. If one does not know the resolving power of the genetic fingerprinting method applied, one may conclude that because there are differences in the fingerprinting data, two isolates are unrelated, or because the fingerprinting patterns are identical, the isolates represent the same strain. However, if in the former case the method identifies hypervariable changes in the genome that can occur as frequently as 1 in every 200 cell divisions, the isolates may in fact be highly related, while in the latter case, if the method measures only rare changes, the isolates may in fact be completely unrelated. With this in mind, what are the levels of relatedness we must consider? Because few methods provide a true measure of genetic relatedness, with some functioning better at discriminating one level than another, and because evolutionary time can only be estimated, we will categorize the levels rather than consider them as a continuum. The categories, diagrammed in Fig. 1, are "identical," "highly related but nonidentical," "moderately related," and "unrelated." The utility of using these categories will become evident in the discussion on considering the effectiveness of the separate methods.

A Genetic Fingerprinting Method Should Be Resistant to Environmental Perturbations and High-Frequency Genomic Reorganization

As in MLEE, the targeted sequences of a DNA fingerprinting method must be carefully selected. For instance, plasmid DNA and minichromosomal DNA may in some cases be bad choices since growth rate and cellular phenotype

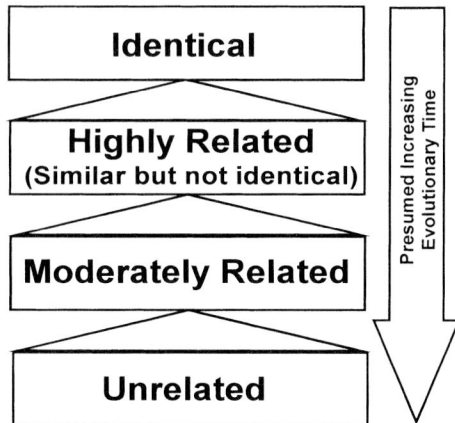

FIGURE 1 Categories of genetic relatedness for isolates within a species.

may affect maintenance of the genetic markers and rate of reorganization (22, 27). Sequences involved in phase transitions in such bacteria as *Salmonella enterica* serovar Typhimurium and *Escherichia coli* undergo reversible transitions (52), as is also the case for the expressed mating type locus in *Saccharomyces cerevisiae* (57). In addition, some genomic reorganization events are repressed by silencing genes (50) and derepressed in mutants (55), while the frequency of other reorganizational events is affected by the expressed phase in phenotypic switching systems (108).

In Most Cases, a Genetic Fingerprinting Method Should Be Fast, Feasible, Affordable, and Amenable to Computer-Assisted Analysis

In many instances, a genetic fingerprinting experiment involves few isolates with limited goals. However, if a study involves large numbers of isolates and requires complex measurements of relatedness and if retrospective use of the data in the future is entertained, one must select a method amenable to automatic computer-assisted analysis and storage. One must also select a method that is within one's technical abilities, that is affordable, that can be accomplished in a reasonable amount of time, and that will answer the question posed.

COMMON GENETIC FINGERPRINTING METHODS

There are several basic genetic fingerprinting methods that have been used repeatedly with prokaryotic and eukaryotic pathogens to answer a variety of epidemiological questions. In the sections that follow, the most commonly used methods are described and evaluated.

Multilocus Enzyme Electrophoresis

It is immediately obvious that a method based on enzyme electrophoresis is not DNA based. However, MLEE fulfills the requirements set forth for DNA-based fingerprinting systems (130) and has been demonstrated to attain resolution at all of the levels categorized in Fig. 1 (99, 104, 111, 144). The MLEE method does rely on phenotypic polymorphisms, but these polymorphisms are rooted in protein structures that usually are reflections of the sequences of the structural genes that encode them. The MLEE method

resolves polymorphisms through differences in the electrophoretic mobilities of the gene products of different alleles of the same gene. Electrophoretic mobility depends primarily on the net charge of the protein, which is a consequence of the primary protein structure but which is also influenced by secondary, tertiary, and quaternary structure. These latter levels of structure can conceal or reveal charged amino acid residues that contribute to the total charge of a protein and therefore to its exact electrophoretic mobility. In addition, MLEE detects polymorphisms only within the coding region of a gene. Mutations affecting the evolution of a gene that occur in promoter regions and introns are not represented in most proteins. Even in coding regions, many mutations do not cause a polymorphism. For instance, because of redundancy in the genetic code, changes in the third base of many codons may not lead to an amino acid change, and the net charge of the protein will therefore not be affected. If an amino acid is replaced by one with equal charge, there may again be no change in the net charge of the protein. Alternatively, an amino acid replacement resulting in a change in net charge may be masked by protein conformation. Conversely, mutations that do not affect the charge of an amino acid may affect conformation, revealing or concealing a charged amino acid and thus affecting electrophoretic mobility. For these reasons, it is difficult to estimate what proportion of base changes leading to amino acid substitutions or other mutations in a protein is detected by the MLEE method. Even so, it is generally accepted that only approximately 15% of the amino acid changes in an average protein can be resolved by the MLEE method (111). This level of sensitivity is sufficient to assess the various levels of genetic relationships outlined in Fig. 1.

In Fig. 2A, a generic version of the MLEE method is presented. The major components of the experimental scheme are (i) preparation of cells, which includes cloning of isolates and growing cells; (ii) preparation of protein extracts, which includes breaking cells, centrifugation, and

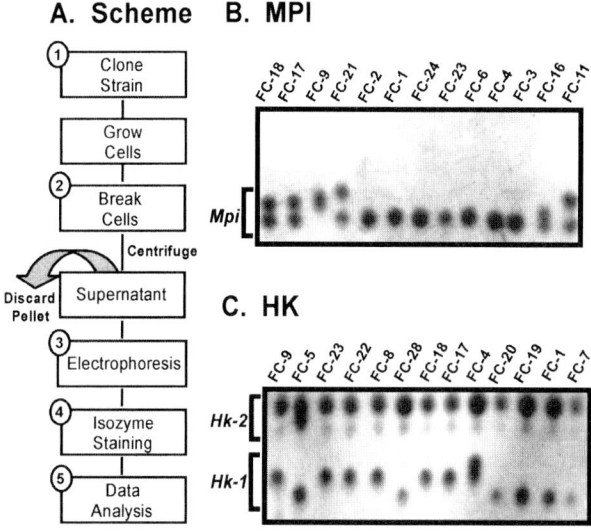

FIGURE 2 MLEE. (A) Generic version of the steps in the MLEE method. (B and C) Examples of enzyme phenotypes using starch gel electrophoresis for mannose-6-phosphate isomerase (MPI) (B) and hexokinase (HK) (C) in 13 *C. albicans* isolates (104). Note that there are two different HK genes, *Hk-1* and *Hk-2*.

collection of the supernatants; (iii) electrophoresis; (iv) isozyme staining; and (v) data analysis. These steps are dealt with individually below.

Preparation of Cells

One must begin with a clone. Therefore, any primary isolate must be diluted and clones must be isolated. Each clone must then be individually grown for protein extraction. For most infectious microorganisms, homogeneous cell populations can be grown in culture to the levels necessary for standard assays. Precaution must be taken, however, in the growth of the different isolates in a test set. Since the expression of genes at the level of protein synthesis represents phenotype, not genotype, it can be affected by environmental conditions. Therefore, growth conditions for isolates must be uniform. If some isolates grow at different rates, reach stationary phase at different times, or express different general phenotypes in the same culture conditions, there may be effects on the isozyme patterns that do not represent changes in DNA sequence. The researcher must be aware of such possibilities.

Preparation of Protein Extracts

One way to describe a general method is to present an example that includes all general aspects of the method. Here, a protocol is described for a generic pathogen. Cells from cultures of cloned isolates are grown in liquid culture to mid-log phase or to stationary phase. Whatever the medium and whatever the growth phase used, they must be uniform for all isolates. Cells are harvested (e.g., pelleted by centrifugation) and washed (e.g., with distilled water). The cell sample (e.g., 200 μl of wet cells) in this example is mixed with glass beads (e.g., 200 μl) and distilled water (e.g., 200 μl) in a 1.5-ml microcentrifuge tube and vortexed. A few important points should be considered at this time. First, the extraction solution must be appropriate for the maintenance of enzyme activity. Although many very specific homogenization solutions have been developed for different organisms and different enzyme activities, distilled water is in many cases appropriate for large, concentrated biological samples. In some cases, proteinase inhibitors must be employed. Second, bead friction during vortexing will produce heat that can denature proteins. To avoid high levels of heat, cooling intervals (e.g., placing the tube in ice water) are interspersed with vortexing pulses. A number of different lysis methods are available, each with different attributes. The method and conditions of disruption or homogenization must be empirically worked out for each organism. Immediately after disruption, samples are centrifuged to remove insoluble materials. For example, if a bead-beating method has been applied, unbroken cells and cellular debris must be removed. The supernatant containing the soluble enzymes of interest can then be divided into small aliquots (e.g., 50-μl aliquots) and immediately used or stored at $\leq 20°C$. It is self evident that enzymes are selected that retain activity through the extraction procedure.

Electrophoresis

Several electrophoretic methods that differ primarily by the supporting medium have been used in MLEE. These include cellulose acetate, agarose, starch, and polyacrylamide. With cellulose acetate, migration of proteins occurs on the surface of gels, in the film created by the buffer. In this case, proteins will migrate as a function of their electrophoretic mobility alone. With both starch and agarose, the supporting gels are made up of a network of constant-size pores,

large enough for the migration of most proteins without retardation due to friction. Therefore, for both starch and agarose gels the majority of proteins will migrate as a function of their electrophoretic mobility alone. With polyacrylamide gels, it is possible to regulate pore size by changing the acrylamide/bisacrylamide ratio. Therefore polyacrylamide gels can be used to separate proteins based on both electrophoretic mobility and size or conformation. All four methods have been successfully used in MLEE. In specific cases, one method may be more effective in separating a particular set of isozymes than another. Regardless of the method, several aspects of electrophoresis must be considered in the context of the MLEE method. First, the enzyme activities must be preserved during electrophoresis. Therefore, electrophoresis must be performed under conditions that support the native conformation of the protein under study. Urea and sodium dodecyl sulfate (SDS), which are used in denaturation gels, can never be included in the electrophoresis procedure. Second, the electrophoretic temperature must usually be maintained close to 4°C to avoid thermal denaturation of the protein. Third, the composition of the electrophoresis buffer must be optimized empirically for the enzymes selected for analysis. Optimization must be worked out for both activity and separation. Buffer characteristics that affect both activity and separation include pH, ionic strength, and the specific concentrations of cations and anions.

Staining of Specific Enzyme Activities

At the completion of electrophoresis, native isozymes have been separated according to electrophoretic mobility or to electrophoretic mobility and size. Once separated, the enzyme positions must be visualized; this is done by using the specific enzyme activity of the isozymes. This basic approach requires that the mutations that affect mobility do not affect enzyme activity. In visualizing enzyme activity, one of the enzyme products is usually stained by a second reaction. Examples of stained isozymes are presented in Fig. 2B and C.

Application and Analysis

As will become clear below, complex data must be collected to assess the many levels of genetic relatedness. If the patterns of a single set of isozymes for a particular gene are used to assess genetic relatedness, the information level is too meager. For a haploid organism, one band is obtained per sample, and for diploids, one or two bands are usually obtained for each isolate. In some cases, for diploids, electrophoretic patterns may be more complex if the enzyme is active in multimeric forms, but this does not increase the information that can be used to assess genetic relatedness. In the patterns generated by MLEE (Fig. 2B and C), the alleles are codominant, which means that for heterozygous loci in diploid organisms, both alleles are expressed. Electrophoretic conditions should therefore be developed that provide the best separation of the different isozymes of each gene. For monomeric enzymes (composed of a single polypeptide), a homozygote exhibits one band and a heterozygote exhibits two bands. For a dimeric enzyme (composed of two polypeptides) in diploid organisms, heterozygotes could show three bands reflecting the three associations of two electromorphs A and B: A can combine with A, B can combine with B, and A can combine with B, at frequencies of 0.25, 0.25, and 0.50, respectively. Similarly, a heterozygote for a tetrameric enzyme should show up to five bands. Such patterns are sometimes difficult to resolve. On rare occasions, enzymes are composed of two or more polypeptides encoded by independent genes, and even greater complications then arise in resolution and interpretation. To generate complex enough data to assess relatedness at all levels (Fig. 1), several genes must be analyzed. On average, 10 to 20 genes should make up the data set for each microorganism (see, e.g., Table 1). The selected genes must exhibit variability among independent isolates. Therefore, for each organism, a set of enzymes must be established empirically. For well-studied organisms, this job usually has already been performed, and so scrutiny of the literature should provide one with a list of enzymes and references to the chemical reactions for visualization. The general approach to selecting enzymes was described by Pujol et al. (104, 105) in developing an MLEE method for the fungal pathogen *Candida albicans*. In two independent studies, 21 enzyme loci were tested in collections of 55 and 29 isolates of *C. albicans*, respectively. In both studies, 13 loci (62%) exhibited variability among the test strains and were selected as the set of analytical enzymes. In recent MLEE studies of bacterial collections, 11 polymorphic enzymes were used to analyze *Streptococcus agalactiae* isolates (106) and 16 polymorphic enzyme loci were used to analyze the genetic diversity of *Helicobacter pylori* (59). In recent MLEE studies of fungal collections, 7 polymorphic enzymes were used to analyze invasive *Aspergillus fumigatus* isolates (17) and 12 polymorphic enzymes were used to analyze strains of *Cryptococcus neoformans* (18). In recent MLEE studies of parasite collections, 22 polymorphic enzyme loci were used to analyze *Trypanosoma cruzi* isolates (12) and 16 polymorphic enzyme loci were used to analyze genetic variability among *Leishmania* isolates (8). Examples of sets of enzymes used effectively in an MLEE study of a bacterium (14), a fungus (104), and a parasite (1) are presented in Table 1.

The result of an MLEE analysis involving, for example, 10 analyzed genes is a phenotype composed of 10 sets of values for each isolate. Each analyzed test isolate must then be compared with every other isolate at every locus to obtain a summed similarity coefficient. The method for doing this will be dealt with later in this chapter.

Restriction Fragment Length Polymorphism without Hybridization

As noted above, one of the earliest methods for DNA fingerprinting infectious microorganisms is restriction enzyme analysis, more commonly referred to as restriction fragment length polymorphism (RFLP) analysis, without probe hybridization. We will refer to this method simply as RFLP. RFLP has been useful in answering limited epidemiological questions posed for a number of lower eukaryotic pathogens, but because of the composition of eukaryotic genomes, RFLP as presently applied has a few severe limitations as a DNA fingerprinting method. For this reason, the application of RFLP to eukaryotic microorganisms will first be described and discussed, and its application to bacteria, which has been far more effective, will follow separately. The basic method of RFLP has also been incor-

TABLE 1 Examples of enzyme sets used to perform MLEE analyses of an infectious bacterium, an infectious fungus, and a protozoan parasite

Enzyme sets used for analysis of:		
Neisseria meningitidis[a,d]	*Candida albicans*[b,d]	*Plasmodium falciparum*[c,d]
ADH (EC 1.1.1.1)	ADH (EC 1.1.1.1)	LDH (EC 1.1.1.27)
ME (EC 1.1.1.40)	SDH (EC 1.1.1.14)	IDH (EC 1.1.1.42)
IDH (EC 1.1.1.42)	MDH (EC 1.1.1.37)	6PGD (EC 1.1.1.44)
G6PD (EC 1.1.1.49)	IDH (EC 1.1.1.42)	NAD-GDH (EC 1.4.1.2)
UDH (EC 1.1.1)	G6PD (EC 1.1.1.49)	GSR (EC 1.6.4.2)
NAD-GDH (EC 1.4.1.2)	SOD (EC 1.15.1.1)	HK (EC 2.7.1.1)
NADP-GDH (EC 1.4.1.4)	AAT (EC 2.6.1.1)	NH-i (EC 3.2.2)
IPO (EC 1.9.3.1)	HK (EC 2.7.1.1)	LAP (EC 3.4.11.1)
AK (EC 2.7.4.3)	PK (EC 2.7.1.40)	PEP1 (EC 3.4.11; Leu-Leu-Leu)
AKP (EC 3.1.3.1)	EST (EC 3.1.1.1)	PEP2 (EC 3.4.11; Leu-Ala)
PEP (EC 3.4)	LAP (EC 3.4.11.1)	ADA (EC 3.5.4.4)
ACO (EC 4.2.1.3)	PEP1 (EC 3.4.13.18; Val-Leu)	GPI (5.3.19)
FUM (EC 4.2.1.2)	PEP2 (EC 3.4.11.4; Leu-Gly-Gly)	
	PEP3 (EC 3.4.13.9; Phe-Pro)	
	MPI (EC 3.5.1.8)	
	ALD (EC 4.1.2.13)	
	FUM (4.2.1.2)	
	GPI (EC 5.3.1.9)	
	PGM (EC 5.4.2.2)	

[a] Data from reference 14.
[b] Data from reference 104.
[c] Data from reference 1.
[d] Enzyme activities are indicated (with Enzyme Commission numbers). ADH, alcohol dehydrogenase; ME, malic enzyme; IDH, isocitrate dehydrogenase; G6PD, glucose-6-phosphate dehydrogenase; UDH, unidentified dehydrogenase; NAD-GDH, glutamate dehydrogenase; NAD$^+$, dependent; NADP-GDH, glutamate dehydrogenase NADP$^+$ dependent; IPO, indophenol oxydase; AK, adenylate kinase; AKP, alkaline phosphatase; PEP, peptidase (the substrates are indicated for the different peptidases used with *C. albicans* and *P. falciparum*); ACO, aconitase; FUM, fumarase; SDH, sorbitol dehydrogenase; MDH, malate dehydrogenase; SOD, superoxide dismutase; AAT, aspartate aminotransferase. HK, hexokinase; PK, pyruvate kinase; EST, esterase; LAP, leucine aminopeptidase; MPI, mannose-6-phosphate isomerase; ALD, aldolase; GPI, glucose-6-phosphate isomerase; PGM, phosphoglucomutase; LDH, lactate dehydrogenase; 6PGD, 6-phosphogluconate dehydrogenase; GSR, glutathione reductase; NH-i, nucleoside hydrolase (substrate inosine); ADA, adenosine deaminase.

porated into a number of additional, more complex finger-printing methods.

Use of RFLP To Analyze Lower Eukaryotic Pathogens

The general RFLP method is relatively straightforward (Fig. 3A). Total cellular DNA is extracted from cells, digested usually with one endonuclease, separated by agarose gel electrophoresis, and stained usually with ethidium bromide. The final banding pattern represents differences in the sizes of the digestion fragments. Differences between patterns are assumed to represent differences in genetic relatedness. Fragment polymorphisms are determined by the positions of restriction sites identified by the particular endonuclease(s) employed. Differences in the banding patterns of two iso-lates of the same species are due to differences in fragment size that can occur as a result of changes in restriction site sequences, secondary modifications of restriction sites, de-letion or insertion of restriction sites, or deletion or inser-tions of sequences between restriction sites. Therefore, se-lecting the most effective endonuclease for generating a pattern must be empirical. A good example of an RFLP pattern of isolates of the yeast pathogen C. albicans is presented in Fig. 3B. One should immediately recognize that not all bands are easily resolvable and that the resolv-able bands represent the most intensely staining ones. Two characteristics of eukaryotic genomes add to the problems encountered when using RFLP without a hybridization probe as a DNA fingerprinting method. First, because of genome complexity, the number of digestion fragments is greater than that for prokaryotes. This reduces the resolu-tion between bands in an agarose gel and leads to the normally smeared appearance of an average RFLP profile. The dominant bands are resolvable, but, unfortunately, these bands represent primarily the repetitive ribosomal cistrons and to a lesser extent the multicopy mitochondrial DNA sequences. Unlike prokaryotes, the multiple ribo-somal cistrons of eukaryotes are clustered on one or two chromosomes (53, 58, 123, 151). The cistrons are in tan-dem with interspersed spacer regions, and structurally quite homogeneous. Therefore, endonuclease digestion that re-sults in a complex RFLP pattern results in a relatively simple ribosomal DNA (rDNA) pattern. To demonstrate this point, the ethidium bromide-stained gel of C. albicans whole-cell DNA in Fig. 3B was destained, Southern blot-ted, and hybridized with an rDNA probe containing the high-molecular-mass (28S), low-molecular-mass (17S), and 5S rDNA sequences (Fig. 3C). Only three intense bands and a few minor bands were resolved with a reasonable degree of resolution in each pattern. The number and variability of the major RFLP bands between independent C. albicans isolates, therefore, do not provide enough com-plexity for resolving differences between moderately or highly related isolates and in some cases may not even be able to distinguish between unrelated isolates. In contrast, the complexity of the pattern of unique-sequence DNA, which should be great enough for assessing genetic distance, is often blurred by the congestion of bands in a normal gel. These general characteristics of RFLPs hold for all eukary-otic pathogens. Even so, RFLP patterns are still used to distinguish between unrelated isolates or identify the same strain in different isolates of eukaryotic pathogens and can sometimes be reasonably effective, if one does not demand resolution at the levels of moderate relatedness (Fig. 1).

In Fig. 3A, a generic version of the RFLP method (116) as applied to eukaryotic pathogens is presented. The major components of the experimental scheme are (i) preparation of cells, which includes cloning strains and growing cells; (ii) preparation of genomic DNA; (iii) endonuclease diges-tion of DNA; (iv) electrophoresis; (v) staining for pattern detection with ethidium bromide; and (vi) analysis of data. These steps are dealt with individually below.

Preparation of Cells

As in the MLEE method, one must begin with a clone. Therefore, any primary isolate must be diluted and clones must be isolated. Each clone must then be individually grown for DNA extraction. In contrast to MLEE, however, one need not worry about uniform growth conditions for different isolates since the genotype is far more stable than the phenotype, by definition.

Preparation of DNA

Many lower eukaryotic pathogens are encased in a cell wall, and in these cases the wall must be removed prior to cell lysis, adding initial steps to the DNA fingerprinting method. Here, a general protocol is described for infectious yeast. Cells from agar cultures are grown to stationary phase in a rich liquid growth medium. Cells are pelleted, washed, and resuspended in medium that removes the cell wall and osmotically maintains the integrity of the resulting sphero-plasts (cells that have had their walls removed). To gener-ate spheroplasts, cells are first suspended in the medium SPP, containing 1 M sorbitol and 50 mM potassium phos-phate (pH 7.4). To remove the cell wall, a variety of enzymes are used, depending on the nature of the wall. To remove yeast cell walls, the snail enzyme Zymolyase can be used. For C. albicans, which has a very tough wall, 15 μl of a solution containing 100 mg of Zymolyase 20 T (Seikagaku America, Ijamsville, Md.) in 800 μl of 50 mM sodium phosphate (pH 6.5)–50% glycerol is added to 0.7 ml of SPP containing 10^{10} cells. The cells are then incubated in suspension for 30 to 90 min at 37°C. The time varies for wall removal, even among strains of the same species. A preparation is assessed microscopically for spheroplast for-

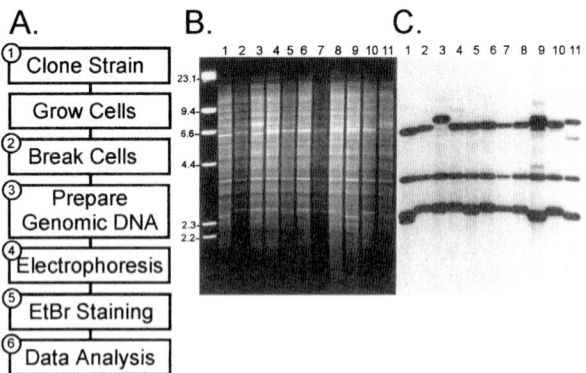

FIGURE 3 RFLP. (A) Generic version of the steps in the RFLP method as it is commonly applied to lower eukaryotic pathogens. EtBr, ethidium bromide. (B) Example of an ethidium bromide-stained gel of EcoRI-digested DNA from 10 test isolates of C. albicans (lanes 2 to 11) and a control isolate (lane 1). The first lane, not numbered, contains molecular mass standards. Molecular sizes (in kilobases) are indicated to the left. (C) The gel in panel B Southern blotted and hybrid-ized with a ribosomal probe that identifies 28, 17, and 5S rDNA.

mation, and the incubation is terminated when the proportion of spheroplasts in the population is >80%. The percentage of spheroplasts can be assessed by adding 1 μl of 10% KOH to a droplet of spheroplasts on a microscope slide and counting the proportion of lysed cells. At the time of 80% lysis, the spheroplasts are pelleted at 2,500 × g for 10 min at room temperature, washed in SPP, and finally resuspended in 500 μl of a lysis buffer containing 50 mM Tris-HCl (pH 7.4) and 20 mM EDTA. Then, 50 μl of 10% SDS is added to the preparation, which is incubated for 30 min at 65°C. A 200-μl volume of 5 M potassium acetate is then added, and the preparation is incubated in an ice bath for 1 h. The lysate is centrifuged at 10,000 × g for 10 min at 4°C, and the supernatant, containing DNA, is extracted with an equal volume of a 1:1 solution of phenol-chloroform. The DNA in the supernatant is then precipitated with an equal volume of cold isopropanol. The DNA is washed twice with 750 μl of 75% ethanol, dried, and resuspended in 100 μl of a solution containing 10 mM Tris-HCl (pH 7.5) and 1 mM EDTA. Contaminating RNA can be removed by adding 2 μl of a 10-mg/ml solution of RNase A and incubating the mixture for 1 h at 37°C. This solution is again extracted with phenol-chloroform and precipitated, as in earlier steps. The final precipitate is then resuspended in 100 μl of the Tris-HCl–EDTA solution and may be stored at 4°C. This solution cannot be frozen.

Endonuclease Digestion

A 3-μg portion of extracted DNA of each test isolate is incubated in 25 μl of reaction buffer containing one or more selected endonucleases as specified by the manufacturer. The units of endonuclease activity should be threefold over the recommended value to ensure complete digestion, a prerequisite for obtaining reproducible, well-separated RFLP patterns. Endonucleases, or restriction enzymes, identify precise sequences throughout the genome. For example, EcoRI identifies and cleaves (cuts) at sites with the sequence 5'GAATTC3', BamHI cleaves at sites with 5'GGATCC3', and HinfI cleaves at sites with 5'GANTC3', where N is any nucleotide. Restriction sites vary in abundance. An infrequent cutter refers to an enzyme that identifies infrequent sites in a particular genome; this is the basis for the RFLP method combined with PFGE frequently applied to prokaryotes. Two examples of infrequent cutters used in fungal studies are NotI, which cleaves sites with the sequence 5'GCGGCCGC3', and SfiI, which cleaves sites with the sequence 5'GGCCNNNNNGG-CC3', where N is again any nucleotide. In bacteria, SmaI represents an infrequent cutter which cleaves sites with the sequence 5'CCCGGG3'. An infrequent cutter will generate a limited number of genomic fragments. These fragments may be too large to be separated by standard gel electrophoresis. On the other hand, some restriction sites are too common, resulting in patterns containing too many bands for good pattern resolution. It should be clear from this brief discussion that one must carefully choose the endonuclease or combination of endonucleases to be used in an RFLP analysis. For an organism not previously analyzed by the RFLP method, selection of the correct endonuclease(s) must be based on empirical data.

Electrophoresis

After digestion is complete and prior to electrophoresis, 3 μl of DNA loading dye (e.g., 40% Ficoll and 0.01% bromophenol blue) is added to each sample. The low-molecular-weight dye will migrate close to the front of the sample and therefore will provide a measure of migration progress. Electrophoresis, in this case, is usually performed in agarose gels cast in and run with 1× TBE buffer, containing 89 mM Tris-HCl (pH 8.1), 89 mM H₃BO₃, and 2 mM EDTA. In a standard experiment, 3 μg of digested DNA is loaded in a well of a 13- by 24-cm gel containing 12 to 15 wells. A set of standards, DNA fragments of known size, should also be loaded on each gel. The percent agarose used will depend on the range of fragment sizes, which will in turn be a function of genome size and the selected restriction enzyme(s). For example, for the gel in Fig. 3B, digestion of C. albicans DNA with the restriction enzyme EcoRI generated a complex pattern separated in a 0.8% agarose gel. For these gel specifications, the dye front should migrate 16 cm from the loading well.

Staining

To visualize the banding patterns of RFLPs, the gel is soaked for 1 h in a solution of 0.2 μg of ethidium bromide per ml. The pattern is then viewed and photographed under a UV light source. It is suggested that a ruler be placed next to the gel when it is photographed, so that values can be assigned to migration distances.

Analysis

The standard RFLP method for eukaryotic pathogens generates patterns that are sometimes difficult to compare. Because of band crowding, automatic computer-assisted analyses are difficult and too much information is lost due to the lack of discrimination. The positions of the major bands in RFLP patterns can be manually digitized into a database, but as noted above, the major bands represent primarily rDNA fragments, and the complexity of the information obtained may not be great enough to obtain meaningful measurements for moderately related isolates. However, when RFLP analyses of lower eukaryotic pathogens involve small numbers of isolates and when all that is demanded from the data is an assessment of identity and nonidentity, qualitative interpretations are sufficient. The problems of RFLP analyses of eukaryotic pathogens are resolved to some extent by applying hybridization probes, the subject of a later section of this chapter.

Use of RFLP To Analyze Prokaryotes

One major approach to fingerprinting bacteria involves the generation of RFLP patterns with restriction enzymes that cut a limited number of times per genome, combined with PFGE. The former generates larger DNA fragments, and the latter separates these fragments in an agarose gel despite their large size. The bacterial genome is usually composed of a single DNA molecule (i.e., a single chromosome). These genomes can vary significantly in size and complexity, but in almost all cases, bacterial genomes are far less complex than lower eukaryotic genomes. One may therefore expect greater resolution in an RFLP pattern generated with a prokaryotic genome, but that is really not the case. When a frequent cutter is used, the ethidium bromide-stained pattern is still crowded. Standard RFLP analysis without probes has therefore not been a popular epidemiological tool for bacteria. Instead, bacterial epidemiologists have used infrequent cutters to generate a limited number of DNA fragments, which are then separated by an electrophoretic method customized for large fragments. In Fig. 4A, a generic version of this method is presented. The components of the experimental scheme are (i) preparation of cells, which includes cloning and growth of cells; (ii) break-

A.

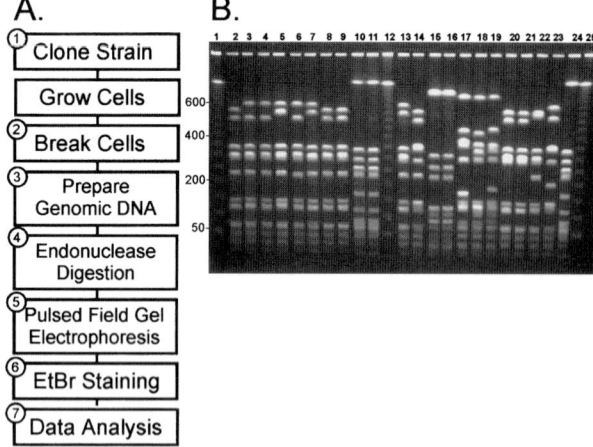

FIGURE 4 RFLP as it is commonly applied to prokaryotic pathogens, using PFGE to separate large DNA fragments. (A) Generic version of the steps in the RFLP-PFGE method. EtBr, ethidium bromide. (B) Example of RFLP-PFGE as it was applied to 22 *Staphylococcus aureus* isolates (provided by M. Pfaller, University of Iowa). Standards were run in lanes 1, 12, and 25. Molecular sizes are given in kilobases.

ing of cells and preparation of DNA; (iii) digestion of DNA; (iv) PFGE; (v) ethidium bromide staining; and (vi) data analysis. A clone is grown to stationary phase in medium recommended for the particular species. In many cases, this represents an overnight growth culture. Cells are usually pelleted by centrifugation and resuspended in a medium customized for the species under analysis. For instance, in a procedure applied to *Staphylococcus aureus* (63), cells are washed in a solution containing 0.15 M NaCl and 10 mM EDTA (pH 8.0) and resuspended in a solution containing 1 M NaCl and 10 mM EDTA (pH 8.0). This cell suspension is then mixed with an equal volume of 1.2% low-temperature-melting agarose, and the mixture is allowed to solidify in a 100-μl mold. The block is then incubated in lysis solution containing 1 M NaCl, 10 mM EDTA, 10 mM Tris-HCl (pH 8.0), and a lysis cocktail that includes 0.5% (wt/vol) Brij 58, 0.2% (wt/vol) deoxycholate, 0.5% (wt/vol) Sarkosyl, 1 mg of lysozyme per ml, and 4 mg of acromopeptidase per ml. The blocks are then incubated at 50°C in a solution containing 0.25 M EDTA, 1% (wt/vol) Sarkosyl, and 0.1 mg of proteinase K per ml and then in a solution containing 10 mM Tris-HCl (pH 8.0), 1 mM EDTA, and 1 mM phenylmethylsulfonyl fluoride. Sections of blocks are then incubated with restriction enzyme and electrophoresed in a 0.9% agarose gel using contour-clamped homogeneous electric field (CHEF) electrophoresis (29), the PFGE system of choice for this form of fingerprinting. Staining and data analysis are as described for RFLP analysis of lower eukaryotes. An example of the application of RFLP-PFGE to *S. aureus* is presented in Fig. 4B. A standardized protocol for the refined preparation of DNA for PFGE analysis has been described by Chang and Chui (28) and should serve as a good starting point for individuals interested in an RFLP method for fingerprinting bacteria. Chung et al. (30) give a protocol for PFGE of *S. aureus* with specific details on troubleshooting problems.

Restriction Fragment End Labeling

Restriction fragment end labeling (RFEL) was developed as a fingerprinting method for bacteria because of the compact size of the bacterial genome. In this method, total genomic DNA is digested with a restriction endonuclease and all the fragments are end labeled using the Klenow fragment of DNA polymerase I. Following labeling, the fragments are separated by electrophoresis through a polyacrylamide-urea gel, such as would be used for DNA sequencing. The number of bands produced and the number of bands that are identifiable will depend on the species and isolate of the bacteria to be analyzed and on the percentage of polyacrylamide and the length of the polyacrylamide gel. In the original analysis of the method, van Steenbergen et al. (148) found that for the 11 species of bacteria they analyzed, they could distinguish between 30 and 50 bands per isolate in the 100- to 400-bp size range. This method has been very successfully applied to the molecular epidemiology of several other bacterial species, including *Streptococcus pneumoniae* (20) and *H. pylori* (146).

Application of Hybridization Probes to RFLPs

In a standard eukaryotic RFLP pattern, ethidium bromide stains all DNA fragments. This is the reason why there are so many bands (Fig. 3B) and why it is difficult, if not impossible, to distinguish between bands in the complex patterns that are generated. Hybridization probes are selective, and because they allow a subset of fragments in an RFLP pattern to be visualized, the resolution of the pattern increases. The increase in resolution is evident in a comparison between the RFLP in Fig. 3B and the Southern blot pattern of the same gel blotted and hybridized with an rDNA probe in Fig. 3C.

Southern blot hybridization of endonuclease-digested DNA with a fingerprinting probe has been used to analyze both prokaryotic and eukaryotic pathogens. The success of this fingerprinting strategy has been mixed, and detailed analysis of this strategy (see, e.g., reference 130) has revealed that the power and efficacy of the method depend on the selected hybridization probe. Therefore, after describing the general method, the caveats of the method and the problems related to the variety of possible probes that have been used will be reviewed. In Fig. 5A, the generic version of the RFLP method with hybridization probe is presented. The major components of the experimental scheme are (i) preparation of cells, which includes cloning isolates and growing cells; (ii) breaking of cells; (iii) preparation of DNA; (iv) endonuclease digestion of DNA; (v) electrophoresis; (vi) staining for the ethidium bromide pattern; (vii) transfer of DNA to a membrane; (viii) hybridization with probe; (ix) visualization of the pattern; and (x) data analysis.

Steps i to vi

Steps i through vi are identical to those already described for the RFLP method without probe and will not be repeated.

Steps vii and viii

To hybridize with a probe, the ethidium bromide-stained DNA must be transferred to a nitrocellulose or nylon membrane, a process referred to as Southern blotting. The method for this process can be found in *Current Protocols in Molecular Biology*, volume 1 (5), or in *Molecular Cloning: a Laboratory Manual* (116). In brief, the gel is first treated

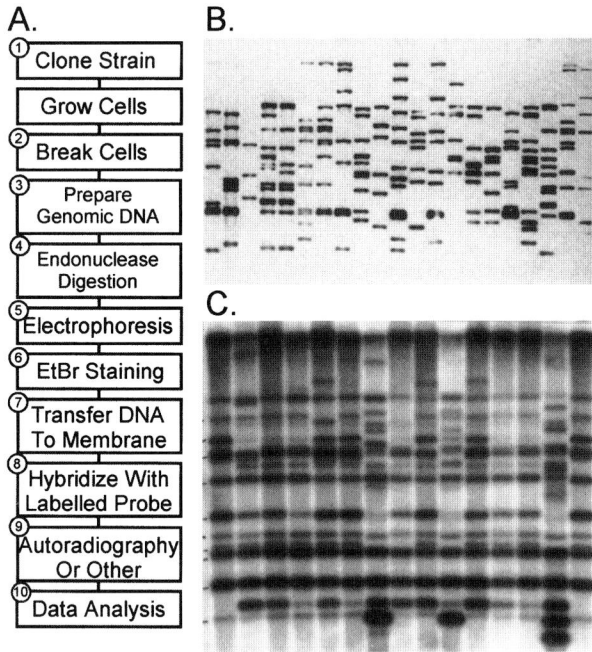

FIGURE 5 RFLP with probe. (A) Generic version of the steps in the RFLP-with-probe method. EtBr, ethidium bromide. (B) Example of RFLP with probe applied to a bacterium, in this case an IS probe applied to *Pvu*II-digested *Mycobacterium tuberculosis* DNA (147). (C) Example of RFLP with probe applied to a yeast, in this case the complex probe Ca3 applied to *Eco*RI-digested *C. albicans* DNA (S. Joly and D. R. Soll, unpublished data).

with 0.25 M HCl. This step results in partial depurination and strand cleavage of DNA. The gel is rinsed in water and soaked in a solution containing 0.5 M NaOH and 1.5 M NaCl. This treatment denatures the DNA, a necessary step prior to hybridization. If a nitrocellulose membrane is used, the gel must then be neutralized to a pH below 9.0. The transfer to the membrane can then be achieved by a number of protocols, the most common ones based on upward or downward capillary transfer (51, 116). The Southern blot is then ready for the hybridization step. The probe must be labeled. The most common method is random priming with $[\alpha\text{-}^{32}P]dCTP$ or $[\alpha\text{-}^{32}P]dATP$. An alternative method, use of a digoxigenin label (62), is a nonradioactive solution, which can generate sharper banding patterns than radioactive probes but is usually less sensitive. For both forms of hybridization, the gel must first be treated with hybridization buffer containing 150 μg of sheared denatured salmon sperm, calf thymus, or other DNA per ml for approximately 4 h at 65°C to block nonspecific binding of the probe. Hybridization is then performed with the same prehybridization buffer containing the labeled probe. One standard hybridization buffer contains 50 mM NaH_2PO_4 (pH 7.5), 50 mM EDTA, 0.9 M NaCl, 5% dextran sulfate, and 0.3% SDS. The hybridization reaction is performed for 16 to 24 h at 65°C. Hybridization is terminated by washing the membrane at 45°C with a solution containing 0.3 M NaCl, 0.03 M sodium citrate (pH 7.0), and 2% SDS.

Step ix

The hybridization pattern generated by a radioactive probe is visualized by exposing the blot to X-ray film with the aid of intensifying screens. Examples of Southern blot hybridization patterns of bacteria and yeast are presented in Fig. 5B and C, respectively. To visualize digoxigenin-labeled patterns, one can treat the gel with antidigoxigenin antibody conjugated to horseradish peroxidase (37). The antibody binds to digoxigenin. Then one adds the substrate luminol under alkaline conditions. Horseradish peroxidase and hydrogen peroxide catalyze luminol oxidation. Oxidized luminol decays, releasing light, which can be visualized again with X-ray film.

Step x

Because hybridization is a result of ionic rather than covalent bonding, one can strip a Southern blot of a probe and rehybridize with additional probes. Different stripping protocols are recommended by different manufacturers. All involve the use of either high temperature or high concentrations of NaOH to separate hybridized DNA strands. The blot can then be rehybridized with subsequent labeled probes, and the patterns can be visualized by the procedure described above.

Selection of a Hybridization Probe

Selecting a probe for fingerprinting a particular organism represents the most crucial step in this process. Since so much time will be invested in collecting specimens, fingerprinting them, and analyzing the data, this decision should be based on a firm understanding of the exact information a particular probe will provide and the level of genetic relatedness it identifies. Some of the first probes used to DNA fingerprint the infectious fungi included single gene sequences, rDNA, or mitochrondrial DNA. It should be evident that a single gene probe will usually hybridize to only one band in a haploid organism and to one or two bands in a diploid organism. Although differences in the size of the fragment carrying the gene may exist between isolates, the data are never sufficient for epidemiological studies that require measurements of moderate relatedness.

The use of rDNA as a fingerprinting probe for both prokaryotic and eukaryotic pathogens was predicated on the idea that single-copy DNA probes would not provide adequate data complexity for deep-rooted relationships in phylogenetic trees. In bacteria, rDNA probes have been quite effective in generating complex patterns and are the basis of the most popular automatic typing systems, such as the Riboprinter Microbial Characterization System (Qualicon, Wilmington, Del.). The reason for the usefulness of rDNA probes in bacteria is that the rRNA cistrons are dispersed throughout the single chromosome (98). Variability in banding sequences leads to multiple rDNA-containing fragments of different size within a single strain, and changes in bordering sequences will lead to pattern variability between strains. Therefore, the RFLP method with ribosomal probes has been used extensively in fingerprinting bacteria (33, 34, 43, 61, 89, 102, 103, 156).

In contrast, the rDNA cistrons of eukaryotes are clustered usually in one of several chromosomes (53, 58, 123, 151). These cistrons are separated by spacers. Endonuclease digestion usually results in a very limited number of bands, generating unexpectedly simple patterns (Fig. 3C), which are not much more complex than those generated by single-copy probes. Therefore, other repetitive sequences were sought that provide more complex patterns. In particular, repetitive sequences were sought that were dispersed throughout the genome. The expectation was that changes in the flanking sequences would generate differences in the patterns of different isolates that could be interpreted in terms of genetic distance. In some bacteria, transposable elements have been used as DNA fingerprinting probes. For instance, in *Mycobacterium tuberculosis*, insertion sequences such as IS6110 (also known as IS986) have been used as probes (60). The copy number of IS6110 per strain varies between 1 and 19, but the majority of strains carry between 8 and 15 copies dispersed throughout the chromosome (109). Therefore, patterns generated with the IS6110 probe and *Pvu*II-digested M. *tuberculosis* DNA are relatively complex and vary among unrelated isolates (Fig. 5B).

In fungal eukaryotes, a variety of moderately repetitive sequences have been used as DNA fingerprinting probes. For instance, poly(GT) and several oligonucleotides, such as (GGAT)$_4$, (GTG)$_5$, (GATA)$_4$, and (GACA)$_4$, have been used to fingerprint *Candida* species (135). These sequences, which identify microsatellite regions, generate complex patterns that may prove to be effective fingerprinting probes, but none have been fully characterized for effectiveness or resolution. In C. *albicans*, the repeat sequence CARE2 (77), which is represented 10 to 14 times in the genome, generates a relatively complex Southern blot hybridization pattern. However, CARE2 and other repetitive sequences that reorganize at a rapid evolutionary rate are sometimes ineffective in identifying clusters of moderately related isolates in a species, a problem we will return to when we consider how to verify the effectiveness of a fingerprinting method later in this chapter.

In the lower fungi, complex probes have been cloned that have proven effective at all levels of relatedness. Complex probes are genomic fragments of 10 to 20 kb that contain and therefore identify highly variable repetitive sequences, moderately variable sequences, and monomorphic sequences. These probes hybridize in a species-specific fashion, and generate patterns that are complex but distinct enough for automatic computer-assisted methods of analysis. They have been cloned from every fungal species so far tested, including C. *albicans* (3, 80, 114), C. *tropicalis* (66), C. *glabrata* (82), C. *dubliniensis* (65), C. *parapsilosis* (39), C. *lusitaniae* (S. Lockhart and D. R. Soll, unpublished results), and *Aspergillus fumigatus* (51). The methods for cloning and characterizing complex probes have been recently reviewed by Lockhart et al. (81). An example of patterns obtained with the Ca3 probe for C. *albicans* is presented in Fig. 5C.

Random Amplification of Polymorphic DNA

RAPD represents one of the most frequently used methods for DNA fingerprinting of eukaryotic organisms (24, 153, 155). As discussed in a following section dealing with verification, this method, when developed correctly, is highly effective in assessing relatedness at all levels of resolution. However, in contrast to RFLP, RFLP-PFGE, and RFLP with hybridization probe, the RAPD method is compromised by problems of reproducibility among laboratories. The method, illustrated in a generic form in Fig. 6, is straightforward. Using random primers of approximately 10 bases, amplicons throughout the genome are amplified by PCR (Fig. 6A). The amplification products are separated on an agarose gel and visualized by ethidium bromide staining. Polymorphisms arise when the distances between primer hybridization sites change or when primer sites appear, disappear, or change location due to insertion, deletion, or recombination. If a primer hybridizes to a large number of sites on opposing Crick-Watson strands (i.e., identifies a significant number of amplicons), that primer will generate a complex pattern. Usually, however, each 10-bp primer

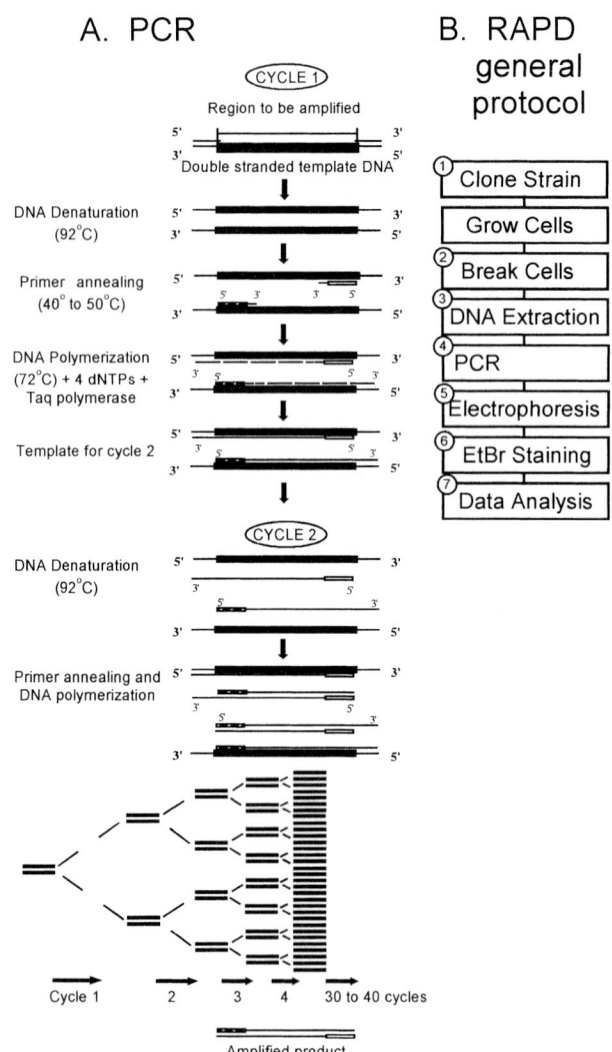

FIGURE 6 RAPD. (A) Description of the PCR amplification. (B) Generic version of the steps in the RAPD method. EtBr, ethidium bromide.

will generate one or a few major bands and a few minor bands (Fig. 7). Because some minor bands may not be highly reproducible in repeat experiments in the same laboratory, only the major bands are usually used for analysis. This irreproducibility is probably the result of low annealing temperature and the short primer sequence, which results in mispairing between primer and template. This produces a pattern with too low a complexity for many of the demands made in epidemiological studies. For that reason, several primers must often be used and the data are pooled to obtain the necessary level of complexity for assessing genetic relatedness. As a general guideline, it is recommended that one use approximately eight primers, each generating at least two reproducible, strong bands, resulting in at least 16 polymorphic bands. As with other genetic fingerprinting methods, the degree of polymorphism should be great enough to resolve genetic variability between isolates. Too low a degree of polymorphism will bias a study. Based on our experience with the RAPD method, we recommend the selection of polymorphic bands

A. OPE-03

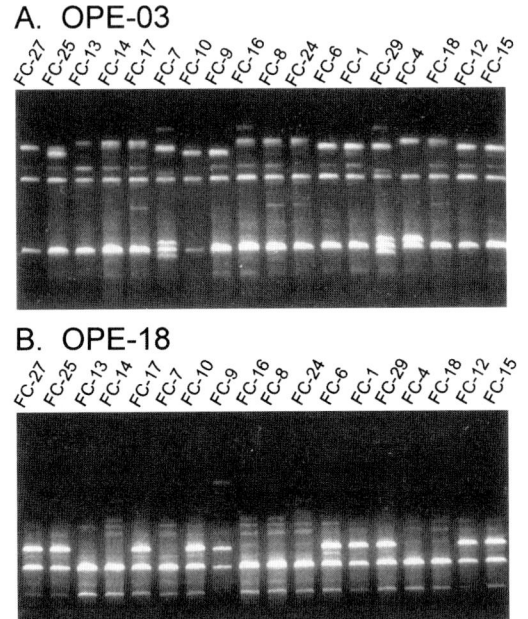

B. OPE-18

FIGURE 7 Examples of RAPD patterns with the primers OPE-03 and OPE-18 applied to 18 isolates of the yeast *C. albicans*. Reprinted from reference 104 with permission.

present in 10 to 90% of isolates (39, 81, 104). To obtain an effective collection of primers, one will have to begin with 30 or 40 primers and test each with a representative collection of isolates if one is setting up one's own RAPD protocol. Primer collections can be readily obtained commercially. The test sequences can usually be obtained from collections used for studies of related organisms. In an analysis of *C. glabrata*, Lockhart et al. (82) selected the following nine primers: GGACTGCAGA, GTGACATGCC, CAGGCCCTTA, TGCCGAGCTG, AATCGGGCTG, GTGATCGCAG, TCGGCGATAG, AGCCAGCGAA, and AGGTGACCGT. In an analysis of *C. albicans*, Pujol et al. (104) selected the following eight primers: CCAGATGCAC, GTGACATGCC, TTATCGCCCC, GGACTGCAGA, ACGGCGTATG, AACGGTGACC, GGAAGCTTGG, and ACGGTACCAG. In an analysis of *Salmonella enterica* serovar Typhimurium isolates, Malorny et al. (88) selected 13 primers, and in an analysis of *Burkholderia pseudomallei* (78), 30 primers were tested for their efficacy in RAPD analysis. In contrast, in several studies, isolates have been grouped using a single primer (31). In some cases, a single primer can give enough data to generate a dendrogram (see, e.g., reference 107).

Once a primer or primers are selected, the method of RAPD analysis is relatively straightforward. In Fig. 6B, a generic version of the RAPD method is presented. The method is described below.

Preparation of Cells
As with the MLEE, RFLP, and RFLP-and-probe methods, one must begin with a clone. Therefore, test isolates are diluted, clones are isolated, and each clone is individually grown for DNA extraction. In contrast to the MLEE method but similar to the RFLP and RFLP-with-probe methods, one need not be as concerned about uniform growth conditions.

Preparation of DNA
The preparation of DNA is similar to that for RFLP, with some modifications. First, since the DNA has to be very pure to facilitate the PCR amplification, several chloroform extractions are necessary to remove phenol and lipid contamination. To prevent DNA degradation during extraction, EDTA can be added during extractions, but EDTA should be absent from the final DNA suspension solutions that will be used as templates since 0.1 μM EDTA can affect the efficiency of *Taq* polymerase in the PCR amplification. The following protocol has been successfully used for RAPD analysis of several fungal species and can be adapted to other organisms. It has proven simpler than many other published methods. A 500-μl suspension of cells (5 × 10^9 cells per ml) in a solution of 10 mM Tris-HCl (pH 8.0)–1 mM EDTA is mixed with an equal volume of glass beads (0.45 mm in diameter) in a 1.5-ml microcentrifuge tube and disrupted in a bead beater. SDS is then added to a final concentration of 2% (wt/vol), and the suspension is mixed by repeatedly inverting the tube. DNA is then purified by two rounds of phenol extraction followed by three rounds of chloroform extraction. DNA is precipitated in 0.3 M sodium acetate (pH 4.5) with 2 volumes of 100% ethanol. The final DNA precipitate is resuspended in distilled water.

PCR Amplification
Unfortunately, PCR is highly sensitive to virtually every aspect of the protocol, and protocols are by no means uniform among laboratories. The following represents a simple version. To a 0.5-ml microcentrifuge tube is added 25 μl of a reaction mixture containing 5 ng of genomic DNA; 2.5 μl of 10× buffer, provided by the manufacturer with purchased *Taq* DNA polymerase; 1.5 mM MgCl$_2$; 0.5 to 1.5 U of *Taq* DNA polymerase; 250 μM each dATP, dCTP, dGTP, and dTTP; and 0.2 mM selected 10-bp primers. Amplification is performed in a thermal cycler programmed for 45 cycles of 1 min at 94°C, 2 min at 36°C, and 2 min at 73°C. Amplification products are separated by electrophoresis in a 1.5% agarose gel run for 4 h at 110 V, so that the bromophenol blue marker dye migrates approximately 10 cm. For the separation of low-molecular-mass (<500 bp) amplification products, acrylamide gels can be used.

Visualization of Bands
The gel is stained with ethidium bromide as described for RFLP gels and viewed under a UV light box.

Problems Inherent in the RAPD Method and Controls That Must Be Applied
Because there is a problem of reproducibility not only among laboratories but also within the same laboratory over time, one must be cognizant of the pitfalls in the procedure. Most aspects of the PCR procedure affect reproducibility (38, 85, 86, 92). First, small differences in the primer-to-template ratio, the concentration of magnesium, and the temperature will produce variation not only in low-intensity bands but also in some high-intensity bands. Second, variation can occur as a result of the source of the *Taq* enzyme. There have been repeated reports that different batches of *Taq* polymerase from different manufacturers and even from the same manufacturer have resulted in quite different RAPD patterns (85, 92). The artifacts were usually in low-intensity bands.

The following steps should therefore be taken to obtain reproducible banding patterns. First, DNA from different strains should be tested at a variety of dilutions to assess the impact of dilution on pattern stability. Second, the DNA of a single strain should be extracted several times to test whether minor variations in the preparation of DNA affect the pattern. Finally, the amplification reaction should be performed in parallel and in sequence for a single DNA preparation that will be used as a control to test intralaboratory reproducibility.

Other PCR-Based Methods for DNA Fingerprinting

Varieties of additional DNA fingerprinting methods continue to be developed that are primarily PCR based and provide advantages. One modification to RAPD is the amplified fragment length polymorphism (AFLP) method, in which restriction fragments are selected for amplification (124, 145, 152). In this method DNA is first digested with a restriction enzyme and random restriction fragments are singled out by using a specific base sequence at the 3' end of the primers. Then, by using PCR conditions more stringent than those used for RAPD amplification, one boosts the reliability of the method. This method can provide a complex fingerprint pattern. While AFLP has been developed to target restriction sites, PCR methods have also been developed to target other known sequences distributed throughout the genome, such as microsatellite sequences and spacer regions between tRNAs or rRNAs. In interrepeat PCR, the variable-length segments found between consecutive repeat elements, rather than the repeat elements themselves, are amplified. Oligonucleotide primers are designed such that they hybridize to the 5' and/or 3' end of repetitive elements, but instead of amplifying the element, they face outward from the element and amplify the internal spacer sequences that are found between copies of the repetitive element. PCR fragments are separated by agarose gel electrophoresis following amplification and are viewed by staining with ethidium bromide. The number of bands produced is dependent on the number of repetitive elements within the genome as well as the number that are adjacent and close enough for *Taq* DNA polymerase to amplify the sequence between them (usually around 5,000 bp). This method has been applied successfully to a number of organisms, and there are a number of variations depending on the organism. Single-primer interrepeat PCR using the M13 core sequence or the microsatellite primers $(GTG)_5$ and $(GACA)_4$ has been successfully used for a number of fungal species including *Candida* spp. (93) and *Cryptococcus neoformans* (94) and the parasite *Leishmania* (120). In bacteria there are at least two commonly used inverted-repeat elements, BOX and ERIC. These elements have been successfully used for typing *Streptococcus pneumoniae* using the single BOXA primer (73) and *Haemophilus influenzae* using primers ERIC1 and ERIC2 (54). A specific protocol for fingerprinting *Mycobacterium tuberculosis* strains, called double-repetitive-element PCR, utilizes two sets of primers, two of which amplify out from the repetitive element IS6110 and two of which amplify out from the polymorphic GC-rich repetitive sequence element PGRS, in order to generate patterns in isolates with a small number of IS6110 repetitive elements (48). Another typing method that is, so far, specific to *Mycobacterium* is spoligotyping. This method uses interrepeat PCR to amplify the regions between a repetitive element known as DR. Rather than separating the interrepeat regions on a gel, one of the primers is end labeled and the products are hybridized to an array of oligonucleotides corresponding to 43 known inter-DR regions (68, 75, 128).

Variable-number-of-tandem-repeat elements (VNTRs) or microsatellites are very short tandem repetitive elements found within the genomes of both prokaryotes and eukaryotes. The VNTR fingerprinting method is PCR based and relies on the amplification of specific VNTRs using primers specific to the outside flanking regions of elements. The bands that are generated are distinguished by size following gel electrophoresis. In a recent article by Lott et al. (84), VNTR profiles were generated for one dimorphic and three polymorphic loci from 114 isolates of *C. albicans*, and the method was verified by comparing the deduced phylogeny to that which was found using some of the same strains in a previously verified fingerprinting system (104). Mazars et al. (90) recently identified 12 VNTR regions within the *M. tuberculosis* genome that had two to eight alleles each in the 72 isolates that were tested. This corresponds to a potential of over 16 million combinations of alleles. VNTR typing has also been successfully applied to the parasite *Plasmodium falciparum*. Anderson et al. (4) described 12 variable-length microsatellite loci and were able to do a population structure analysis of isolates from 465 infections.

Because some evolutionary biologists believe that patterns must account for identified alleles (i.e., a change in a band size in a pattern must be attributed to a change in the size or change of a known sequence), PCR-based methods have been developed that employ genetic markers, either identified or anonymous. Karl and Avise (69) have derived a method that has been applied to a number of lower eukaryotic pathogens, in which arbitrary primers are used to identify monomorphic amplicons, which are then partially sequenced. Customized pairs of primers are then developed for specific bands. Changes in these identifiable bands are then assessed either through RFLP or by single-strand conformational polymorphisms (SSCP) analysis, which involves the isolation of single-base-pair changes in a sequence through nonhomologous renaturation of DNA and separation on a sequencing gel. For the use of these markers in fungi, see the review by Taylor et al. (138). In *C. albicans*, both PCR-SSCP (47, 56) and PCR-RFLP (158, 159) have been used with equally good results. PCR and the use of specific allelic probes have also been applied to this organism (32). Similar approaches have also been developed that target noncoding regions of protein-coding loci. Development of the primer pairs is based on published sequences, and polymorphisms can again be identified by SSCP or RFLP. In these types of PCR-based methods, several pairs of primers must be employed and the pairs must be selected not only because they identify a known sequence but also because they produce the necessary levels of variation among strains. Although these methods have been argued to be superior to standard RFLP because one knows the identity of bands in different strains, analyses of the efficacy of RAPDs in band identification have demonstrated levels of identity between patterns that far exceed those required for effective analysis. Reiseberg (110) tested the homology of 220 pairs of comigrating RAPD fragments from three closely related species (not strains!) of sunflower and found that 91% exhibited homology. Thormann et al. (140) demonstrated an extremely high degree of similarity of hybridization patterns of RAPD bands within several plant species. Both these interspecies and intraspecies analyses support the conclusion that RAPD fragment size within a plant species is a strong indicator of homology, and by inference, this should also be true for microbial pathogens. More importantly, verification of the RAPD method through comparison of its clustering abilities with those of unrelated methods has demonstrated its efficacy, as will be discussed in a later section of this chapter. The bottom line is, it is not necessary to identify the RAPD bands you are analyzing in order to use the RAPD method in genetic fingerprinting, as has been amply argued by Tibayrenc (142–144).

Electrophoretic Karyotyping

Since lower eukaryotes possess multiple chromosomes within the size separation range of PFGE technology, electrophoretic karyotyping (26, 122) has been used as a way of fingerprinting eukaryotic pathogens. A generic scheme for PFGE is outlined in Fig. 8A. If the cell possesses a wall, the wall must be removed. A detailed protocol for the genesis of spheroplasts for infectious yeast was presented in the preceding section on RFLP. Briefly, cells are mixed with enzymes to remove the cell wall, and the resulting spheroplasts are embedded in an agarose plug. Detergent and proteinase are added to remove the membrane, digest the protein, and release the nucleic acid. The agarose matrix reduces shear forces and thus protects the large chromosomal DNAs from fragmenting. The agarose plug is then placed in a well of an agarose slab gel, and electrophoresis is carried out by following the protocol for the specific system used (e.g., orthogonal field-alternating gel electrophoresis [OFAGE] [121], CHEF [29], or transverse alternating-field electrophoresis [TAFE] [49]) and the molecular size range of chromosomal DNAs for the analyzed organism. After electrophoresis, chromosomal DNAs are visualized with ethidium bromide. Chromosomes can then be identified by Southern blot hybridization with chromosome-specific probes. In Fig. 8B, examples are presented of CHEF-separated chromosomes of a number of *C. dubliniensis* isolates demonstrating extreme karyotypic variability. For the infectious yeast, Sangeorzan et al. (117)

demonstrated that patterns were reproducible among experiments and relatively insensitive to the method of preparation. However, other studies have demonstrated pattern variability due to reagents, sample preparation, and eletrophoretic conditions. Thrash-Bingham and Gorman (141) demonstrated that in spite of karyotypic variability among strains, the general organization of the genome was maintained, although some chromosomal translocations contributed to karyotypic variability among strains of *C. albicans*. In addition, it has been demonstrated that the frequency of changes in electrophoretic karyotypes can be dramatically influenced by high-frequency phenotypic switching. In *C. albicans*, cells can be in low- or high-frequency modes of switching (125, 129, 131, 132). In the low-frequency mode, the frequency of karyotypic change is minimal (108). In the high-frequency mode, the frequency of karyotypic change is extremely high, primarily in the chromosomes harboring rDNA cistrons (108). In fact, in a sequence of high-frequency switching, the electrophoretic karyotype of a strain diverged from and then reverted to the original pattern, a process that would invalidate the use of this method for assessing moderate levels of relatedness. There are reasons to believe that the majority of changes in the chromosome harboring rDNA cistrons in *C. albicans* were due to a release from silencing (108), a process involving SIR genes in *Saccharomyces cerevisiae* (50, 55). Whatever the mechanism proves to be, the problem that arises from these observations is that the rate of change identified by PFGE methods may not always reflect genetic distance.

Sequencing

Although sequencing provides the most exact data for assessing divergence and therefore relatedness within a species, its major impact has been in the genesis of phylogenetic trees at the interspecies level. The reason for this is twofold. At the interspecies level, changes in a single sequence prove profound enough for interpreting the phylogeny and evolutionary history of species. However, at the subspecies level, sequence changes at a single locus do not occur fast enough in most cases to discriminate between highly related but nonidentical isolates and do not usually provide enough information for cluster analyses. To obtain such information, multiple loci must be sequenced and the data must be pooled, thus increasing the time necessary to collect the data. Until recently, sequencing was a slow, technically demanding, and expensive procedure. However, in recent years, automatic sequencing has become far more rapid and less expensive. Therefore, sequencing methods have the potential to be highly effective if the hurdles of time and cost can be overcome. These methods should emerge, based on carefully selected sets of primers targeting genes that provide the necessary levels of change for discrimination at the different levels of genetic relatedness (Fig. 1). Such a method, called multilocus sequence typing (MLST), has emerged for bacteria. It was first applied to *Neisseria meningitidis* (87) and has since been applied to a variety of bacteria (36, 40–42).

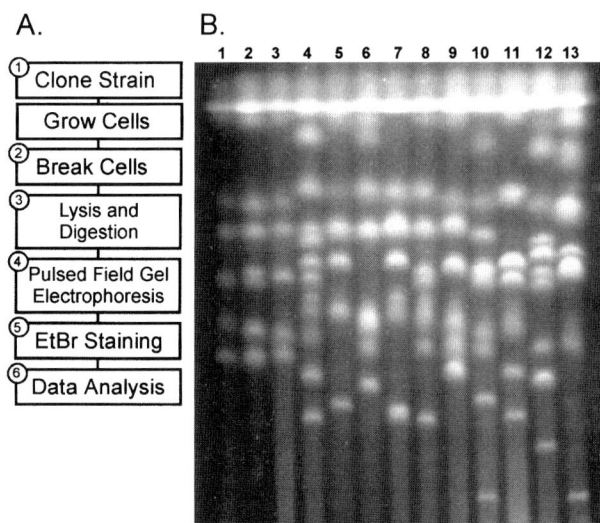

FIGURE 8 PFGE. (A) Generic version of the steps in the PFGE method. EtBr, ethidium bromide. (B) Example of ethidium bromide-stained chromosomes of isolates of the yeasts *C. albicans* (lanes 1 to 3) and *C. dubliniensis* (lanes 4 to 13).

VERIFYING THE EFFICACY OF A GENETIC FINGERPRINTING METHOD

As noted above, one must be sure that a fingerprinting method provides the correct level of genetic resolution for the question posed. Therefore, one must select a method that has already been tested or must perform the tests to verify the method. Perhaps the most straightforward test is through comparison with an unrelated method, using a set of test isolates with known or implied relatedness. The levels to be tested are (i) identical, (ii) highly similar but nonidentical, (iii) moderately related, and (iv) unrelated (Fig. 1). For these respective levels of relatedness, the test collection should include (i) isolates that should be identical (e.g., multiple clones derived immediately from a freshly plated isolate), (ii) isolates that should be highly similar but perhaps nonidentical (e.g., isolates recovered over short intervals in different individuals, body locations, etc., with presumed common origin), (iii) isolates that should be moderately related (e.g., included in a collection of independent isolates from the same geographical locale), and (iv) isolates that are unrelated (e.g., from different, geographically separated locales). The test collection is fingerprinted by the individual methods, and similarity coefficients are computed by the same analytical method for every pair of isolates. Dendrograms based on the independent sets of data are then generated and compared. If the genetically unrelated methods both identify identical isolates as identical, highly related isolates as similar but nonidentical, and unrelated isolates as dissimilar, and if the unrelated methods group isolates into the same clusters, they in essence cross-verify each other's efficacy at every level of relatedness. If they identify as identical presumably identical isolates, identify as similar but nonidentical highly related isolates, but do not cluster in a similar fashion moderately related to unrelated isolates, then one or both methods may be ineffective in assessing lower levels of relatedness. If the two methods cluster isolates into the same general groups but only one discriminates among highly related but nonidentical isolates, then the methods cross-verify each other for general clustering but only one of the two will be effective in discriminating microevolution in a clonal colonizing population. This general method of cross-verification has been used to assess the efficiency of a variety of fingerprinting methods for bacterial, fungal, and parasitic pathogens (see e.g., references 75, 104, and 144). It should be emphasized that without cross-verification, a genetic fingerprinting method is always suspect for the different levels of relatedness (Fig. 1), no matter how valid the system seems to be. One must realize, however, that such cross-verification is possible only for microorganisms with a clonal population structure (104, 142–144).

DATA ANALYSIS

Computing Similarity Coefficients

Genetic fingerprinting data come in different forms. MLEE provides multiple-spot patterns, RAPD provides single- or multiple-band patterns, and RFLP, RFLP with probe, and PFGE provide single- or multiple-band patterns. Regardless of the data form, the goal of a genetic fingerprinting method is to compute similarity coefficients (S_{AB}s) between every pair of isolates in order to generate a dendrogram, or tree. The formula for computing S_{AB} and the formula for generating a tree from the S_{AB}s must be carefully selected, and excellent reviews of these computations are available (44, 126, 154). Here, we will review only the most common of these methods. For a detailed description of the methods, the reader is referred specifically to *Numerical Taxonomy: the Principles and Practice of Numerical Classification* (126).

Band Positions Alone

For methods that produce patterns of bands, the presence or absence of a band is described by the binary values 1 and 0, respectively, n_{AB} is the number of common bands in the two patterns A and B (coded 1,1), a is the number of bands in A with no counterpart in B (coded 1,0), b is the number of bands in B with no counterpart in A (coded 0,1), and c is the number of bands absent in A and B (coded 0,0). The sample size, x, represents the total number of bands, described by the formula $x = n_{AB} + a + b + c$. The number of matches, m, is therefore $m = n_{AB} + c$, and the number of mismatches, u, is $u = a + b$. Using this basic logic, a number of formulas of S_{AB}s based on band position alone have been developed, most notably the coefficient of Jaccard (S_j):

$$S_j = \frac{n_{AB}}{n_{AB} + a + b}$$

the coefficient of Dice (S_D):

$$S_D = \frac{2n_{AB}}{2n_{AB} + a + b}$$

the sample-matching coefficient (S_m):

$$S_m = \frac{n_{AB} + c}{n_{AB} + a + b + c}$$

the Pearson coefficient (S_Ψ):

$$S_\Psi = \frac{(n_{AB}c - ab)}{\sqrt{[(n_{AB} + a)(n_{AB} + b)(b + c)(a + c)]}}$$

and others such as mean square difference/total bands. It should also be noted that data such as that obtained by MLEE or RAPD, in which a series of primers provide binomial data, can be converted to binary values to generate a matrix similar to that obtained with banding data that can then be used to compute S_{AB}s between every pair of isolates. The same formulas for S_{AB}s can then be considered.

Band Position and Intensity

In many cases, the information garnered from band intensity is added to that of band position. In these formulas, X_{iA} and X_{iB} represent the intensities of bands in patterns A and B, respectively, $\bar{X}_{iA}$ and $\bar{X}_{iB}$ represent the respective means of all intensities, and n represents the total number of bands. A number of formulas of S_{AB}s based on band position and intensity have been formulated, most notably Pearson's product-moment correlation coefficient (S_r):

$$S_r = \frac{\sum_{i=1}^{n}[(X_{iA} - \bar{X}_{iA})(X_{iB} - \bar{X}_{iB})]}{\sum_{i=1}^{n}(X_{iA} - \bar{X}_{iA})^2 \sum_{i=1}^{n}(X_{iB} - \bar{X}_{iB})^2}$$

absolute difference/total area (S_{AB}):

$$S_{AB} = 1.0 - \frac{\sum_{i=1}^{n}|X_{iA} - X_{iB}|}{\sum_{i=1}^{n}|X_{iA} + X_{iB}|}$$

and others such as absolute difference/maximum intensity similarity coefficient, mean square difference/intensity similarity coefficient, and mean square difference/maximum intensity similarity coefficient.

In selecting a method for computing S_{AB} values, several points should be kept in mind. First, if the reproducibility of band intensities is not good, an S_{AB} based on band positions alone is obviously more accurate. Second, if a method involves the presence or absence of bands as if they were alleles, $S_{AB}s$ based on band position alone are used. One must realize, however, that in most of the DNA fingerprinting methods employed, allelism is not always verified. Third, it must be realized that in methods based on repeat sequences, band intensities may provide at least as much information on relatedness as does position, and a method based on both may therefore be preferable.

The different similarity coefficients described above do not require the identification of alleles at given loci. For this reason they are favored when cross-verifying methods are applied, since one or more of the methods may rely on dominant markers. Genetic similarity can also be assessed from genetic distances based on the frequencies of codominant markers (44, 126, 154).

Generating Dendrograms

The computation of $S_{AB}s$ leads to a matrix of values generated between every pair of isolates in an epidemiological study. These values are the basis for generating a dendrogram. The most commonly used method for connecting isolates into a tree is the unweighted pair group method using arithmetic averages (UPGMA) first employed by Rohlf (112). This method generates a "rooted" tree. The Fitch-Margoliash method with evolutionary clock (46) also generates a rooted dendrogram, with the additional feature that it tests alternative topologies for the tree by rearranging nodes to minimize the sum of squares computed between genetic distances and branch lengths, making it more time-consuming to perform. There are also methods that do not assume a common molecular clock for all strains and therefore generate unrooted trees. These methods, which include the neighbor-joining method (115) and the Fitch-Margoliash method without evolutionary clock (46), generate unrooted trees that in fact should have more exact topographies. Because the neighbor-joining method and, more particularly, the UPGMA are faster than the other methods, they may be preferable for large experimental samples. There are therefore trade-offs between methods. It should be realized that these methods were developed for generating trees at the species rather than subspecies levels of relatedness, but they still result in interpretable trees at the subspecies and strain levels. If the data are robust, similar dendrograms should be generated no matter which method is applied. Dendrograms generated for intraspecies analysis should not be considered a purely phylogenetic representation of lineages but, rather, a practical tool that provides a visual description of genetic similarities and divergence between strains and that may be useful in identifying groups, or clades. The derived dendrograms represent true phylogenies only when each strain is derived through a purely clonal lineage (i.e., with no genetic exchange) and homoplasy is negligible. These conditions are rarely verified for the markers used in epidemiological studies.

Let us consider how the UPGMA is performed. The S_{AB} matrix is scanned for the most similar isolates. If more than one group (two or more) are identified, the first is arbitrarily taken as group 1. The isolates are joined at the appropriate position along the S_{AB} axis. The matrix is scanned once again for the next most similar isolate or group of isolates, which is then connected along the S_{AB} matrix to the first group, and this function is repeated over and over again until all isolates are incorporated into the tree. A sample dendrogram that includes 67 *C. albicans* isolates is presented in Fig. 9. In this dendrogram, thresholds and landmarks are noted, one (A) which represents identity, at an S_{AB} of 1.00, one (B) which demarcates highly related isolates, at an S_{AB} of 0.90, one (C) which demarcates moderately related groups, in this example at an S_{AB} of 0.70, and one (D) which denotes the average S_{AB} for all strains in the dendrogram, in this example at an S_{AB} of 0.63. The C threshold is the one which best demarcates clades. The selection of thresholds and landmarks in a dendrogram is sometimes somewhat arbitrary (130) but is extremely important in interpreting a tree. Confidence in these values comes with increased familiarity with the origins of isolates and assumptions of relatedness based on those origins.

Testing the Integrity of Clusters and Statistical Analyses

Although the selection of a threshold for defining clusters may be somewhat arbitrary, one can demonstrate that the content of a cluster is stable and that the identity of the cluster is in fact valid. First, the order in which isolates are chosen in the generation of a dendrogram can be randomized (7), an important control when using the UPGMA, since this method is prone to mistakes in higher-order clusters. For instance, one can apply 10 random starts to assess whether a cluster remains intact. Second, "noise" can be introduced by adding or subtracting a set percentage of the S_{AB} values to every pairwise comparison (101). Noise can affect and therefore can be used to assess the stability of second-tier groupings. Third, one can use the comparison of clustering by two independent genetic fingerprinting methods to assess the stability of a cluster (75, 104, 144).

The most common method used by evolutionary biologists to analyze the integrity of clusters is bootstrapping (45). In this process, one generates deletions and duplications by random sampling. This process is normally performed 1,000 times. A consensus tree of all dendrograms is then generated, and a "majority rule consensus" algorithm is used to compute the percentage of occurrence of each node. A percentage above 80% suggests a stable node. In a second common method called jackknifing (157), subsets of the collection are randomly selected approximately 100 times, a consensus dendrogram is generated, and the percentage of occurrence at each node is computed. These methods, however, were developed for DNA fingerprinting methods in which the data represent alleles of identified loci, not for patterns like those generated by RFLP or RAPD. They are therefore not commonly used in general epidemiological studies. They can, however, be used for RAPD data if each primer is considered an independent gene.

For comparing the relatedness of different populations of isolates, it is often the case that the mean S_{AB} of an entire collection is not informative, although comparisons of mean $S_{AB}s$ of different collections may be informative. The Student t test can assess whether mean $S_{AB}s$ are significantly different. In applying the Student t test, a probability value of 0.05 (i.e., less than 5%) usually represents significance.

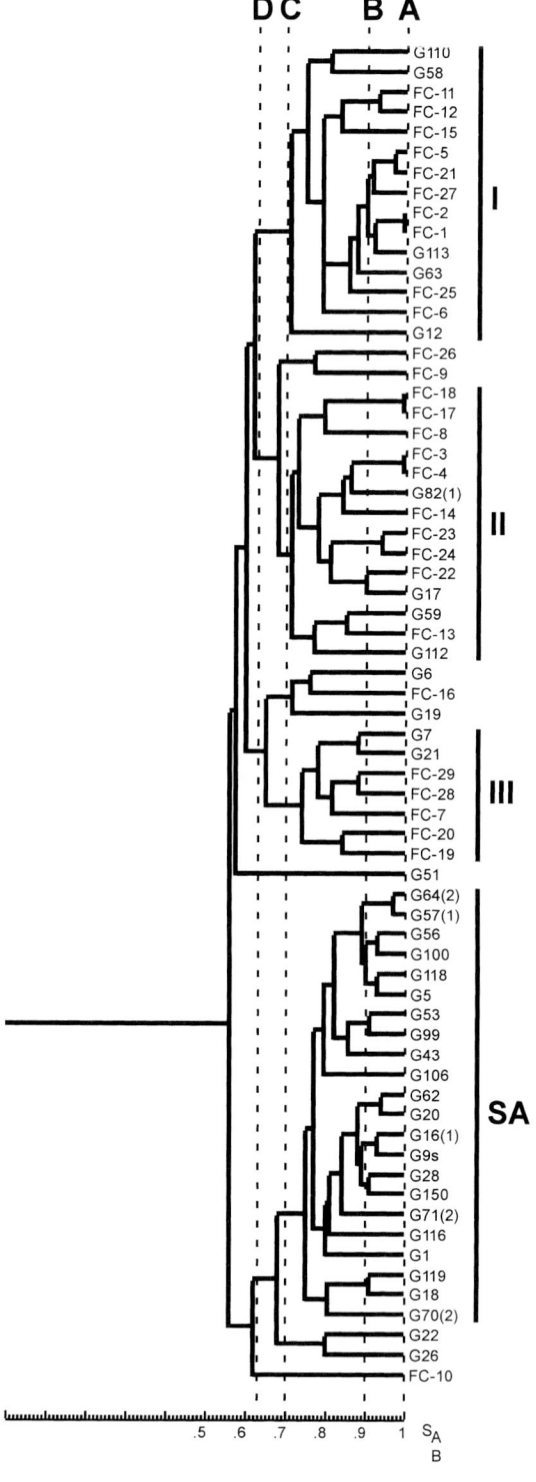

FIGURE 9 Example of a dendrogram. The similarity coefficients (S_{AB}s) were generated from the patterns of 67 isolates of *C. albicans* fingerprinted with the complex Ca3 probe. The value A represents identicalness, at an S_{AB} of 1.00; threshold B demarcates highly related isolates at an S_{AB} of 0.90; threshold C demarcates clades at an S_{AB} of 0.70; and the value D represents the average S_{AB} at 0.63. In this example, a South African-specific clade of *C. albicans* (SA) was identified in addition to the three clades (I, II, and III) present in U.S. collections (E. Blignant, C. Pujol, S. Lockhart, S. Joly, and D. R. Soll, submitted).

ROLE OF COMPUTERS IN GENETIC FINGERPRINTING

For epidemiological studies in which only a few isolates are compared or in which qualitative comparisons are sufficient to obtain an answer, it is simple enough to interpret results, including the computation of similarity coefficients, without the use of computers. However, when dealing with bigger collections, one must recruit a customized computer program. Computer programs are available that can assist in virtually every step in a cluster analysis. For fingerprinting methods that create complex patterns, the systems will automatically acquire the original image and, with the assistance of the user, remove distortion, identify lanes, normalize to a universal standard, identify bands, measure the intensity of bands, compute similarity coefficients, generate dendrograms, identify clusters, and perform statistical tests (130). Computer systems will also store data at any or all levels of analysis for retrospective studies and future comparisons with new collections. An automatic genetic fingerprint analysis system can perform searches based on any aspect of the fingerprinting data (e.g., a particular band length), any characteristic of a patient (e.g., human immunodeficiency virus positive), or any characteristic of the infecting organism (e.g., drug susceptibility). An outline of the steps for computer-assisted analysis of generic complex RFLP, RFLP-with-probe, and select PCR-based patterns follows. The generic software will be referred to simply as the Program.

Digitizing the Pattern

The pattern of an autoradiogram or its equivalent is digitized into the computer's hard drive (Fig. 10A) using a

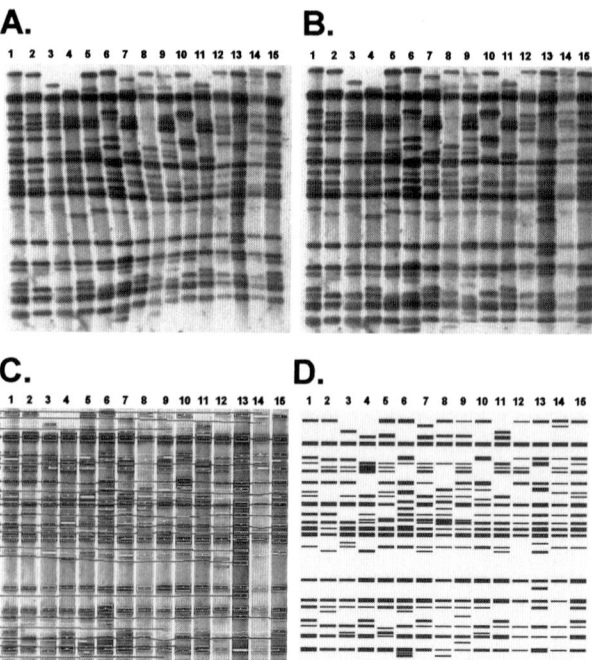

FIGURE 10 Computer-assisted processing and analysis of DNA fingerprint patterns generated with the complex Ca3 probe of 15 isolates of *C. albicans*. (A) Original digitized image with inherent distortions; (B) straightened patterns; (C) correlations of bands with universal standards; (D) model generated from data.

scanner with software that supports grayscale scanning that saves the image in the correct format (e.g., bitmap or tiff). The scanner should be sensitive to a reasonable range of grayscales (e.g., 256 grayscales).

Local Standard

To straighten a pattern for automatic analysis and compare patterns obtained on different gels, landmark bands must exist, either in a set of standards run in lanes alongside test samples, added to the test samples, or as components of the pattern (e.g., monomorphic bands). In all three cases, standards must include bands that span the entire molecular weight range of bands in test patterns.

Global Standard

For studies in which the patterns of multiple gels are compared, each test pattern must be normalized to a global standard in the database. The global standard must share bands in the local standard.

Initial Image Processing

The need for processing stems from artifacts that distort the pattern. First, because of uneven polymerization or electrophoresis, the entire gel pattern may contain "smiles," "frowns," skews, and other linear or nonlinear distortions (Fig. 10A). "Unwarping" is the process of pattern straightening. Local standards are essential for unwarping. Horizontal lines are drawn between common bands for horizontal distortions, and vertical lines are drawn through spaces for vertical distortions. Once drawn and edited, the Program reconstructs the processed pattern (Fig. 10B). Second, because of unequal loading, the pattern in a single lane can be intensified or deintensified.

Automatic Lane and Band Detection

The Program scans and automatically detects lanes and separates them with spaces to facilitate band identification. At this point, the Program should allow editing for final band alignment, which includes lane sliding, stretching, and compressing. This may be necessary if lanes were loaded unequally, which can result in slightly different migration rates for bands with the same molecular weight. Then the Program should perform a densitometric analysis of grayscales along the lane, subtracting background intensity. Integration at peaks or an intensity threshold can be used for band identification, and band intensity can be categorized (e.g., 0 to 5), directly measured, or converted according to a normalization curve. Models of the gel can then be generated from band position and intensity (Fig. 10D).

Calibrating to the Global Standard and Linking

The local standard is calibrated to the global standard (Fig. 10C), providing molecular weights of the standard bands. The Program then automatically links bands in test lanes to bands in the local standard. The user must specify a degree of tolerance for considering bands of the same size. Bands with no correlate in the standard can be linked, and the option should exist for adding new bands to the global standard, if desired.

Creating the Basic Data File

The preceding data provide a text map in which band number, molecular weight, or pixel distance of each band is listed in descending order along the vertical axis of each labeled isolate. At each position, either the binary datum 0 or 1 for position alone, or band intensity is listed. If one has collected binary data using MLEE, RAPD, or other multilocus methods, one can manually generate the data file at this point in the computer program, or the software can combine the data automatically.

Computing Similarity Coefficients and Generating Dendrograms

The Program must provide the user with a choice of formulas for computing S_{AB}s. Once a particular formula is selected, the Program generates a matrix of S_{AB}s between all pairs of isolates. The Program must then provide the user with a choice of algorithms for generating a dendrogram from the S_{AB} matrix and software for separating groups by thresholding, testing the stability of clusters, and statistical analyses (Fig. 9) (7).

Other Useful Functions

The Program should provide accessible storage and comparative capabilities, so that every new set of genetically fingerprinted isolates can be compared with previously fingerprinted isolates in the database. It must also allow searches based on other data elements, such as patient and isolate characteristics. The former includes disease state, treatment, geographical location, anatomical origin of the isolate, age, sex, weight, and predisposing conditions. The latter includes growth characteristics, sugar assimilation patterns, antigenicity, drug susceptibility, switching repertoire, and other phenotypic traits, most notably those involved in virulence and pathogenicity. One must also be able to mine the genetic fingerprint database for particular data characteristics such as the presence of a particular MLEE allele or RFLP fragment.

THE COLLECTION

Because genetic fingerprinting is time-consuming, one must carefully consider the original collection. However, this first step in epidemiological studies is often the most poorly conceived. This problem no doubt stems in part from the assumption that colonizing populations of pathogens are genetically homogenous. It has become increasingly apparent that in many cases, infecting populations, especially in immunocompromised patients, may consist of multiple species, multiple strains of the same species, or diverging substrains. Species heterogeneity has been demonstrated in recurrent infections and commensals (83, 149). In each case in which heterogeneity was demonstrated, care was taken in obtaining the original collection.

In most standard methods of collection, the primary samples are aspirates, tissue, blood, other fluids, or swabs. These materials may be transported to a microbiology laboratory for anaerobic or aerobic culturing. In some cases, the microorganism must be released from the material. Blood cells may be lysed, tissue may be minced, and fluids may be filtered or centrifuged. The problem is clonality. If the sampled colonizing population is homogeneous (i.e., consists of one genetically homogenous strain), there is no problem. However, if the population is heterogeneous (consists of multiple species, strains, or substrains), several problematic scenarios can arise. First, if the culture is genetically heterogeneous at the time of genetic fingerprinting, a mixed fingerprint will arise. Second, if the primary culture contains mixed strains or substrains and is mass cultured, the strain or substrain that grows fastest under the culture conditions employed will be enriched. One therefore runs the risk of beginning with an infecting population that is 98% species or strain A at the site of colonization and

TABLE 2 Rough estimates of the use of the most common genetic fingerprinting methods[a]

Pathogen category	Genus or species	Most common genetic fingerprinting methods
Bacteria	*Streptococcus pneumoniae*	42% RFLP-PFGE; 17% RepE1 PCR; 10% RFEL
	Mycobacterium tuberculosis	54% RFLP + probe; 23% spoligotyping
	Staphylococcus aureus	56% RFLP-PFGE; 13% PCR-RFLP; 11% RAPD
Fungi	*Candida*	30% RAPD; 29% karyotype; 22% RFLP + probe; 12% RFLP
	Aspergillus	71% RAPD; 18% MLEE; 11% RFLP + probe
	Cryptococcus	53% RAPD; 21% karyotype; 18% RFLP + probe
Parasites	*Trypanosoma*	47% MLEE; 30% RAPD
	Leishmania	69% MLEE; 16% RAPD
	Plasmodium	81% PCR-RFLP; 11% RAPD

[a] Estimates were made from a literature search beginning in 1996.

ending with a culture that is 98% species or strain B. Finally, a problem arises when a primary culture containing mixed strains or substrains is cultured and only one clone is picked for analysis. The single clone may not represent the infecting population. The solutions to these problems are straightforward. First, the primary sample can be clonally plated, which may entail assessing the concentration, performing serial dilution, or knowing the approximate density. Second, indicator agars can be used for initial screening of species. Third, more than one colony can be picked for genetic fingerprinting. The number picked and analyzed will depend on the size of the collection and the objectives of the study. These latter considerations apply mainly to bacteria and fungi, but they may be harder to resolve in many parasites that cannot be grown as isolated colonies on agar media.

In addition to sample homogeneity, a second problem arises in some cases that is related to space and time. There is growing evidence of body location specificity in commensalism, geographical specificity of strains, and rapid microevolution (80, 82, 101, 130). It is prudent to consider which body location is sampled, since a pathogen such as *C. albicans* can colonize multiple sites (133). It is also important to realize that if one is testing strain specificity for a particular disease, geographical differences may outweigh disease specialization. For instance, one might find that within a geographical region, isolates from a particular disease state are genetically similar, but when isolates from that disease state are collected from different geographical regions and compared, they may prove genetically dissimilar (101). One must therefore consider restricting the geographical boundaries of the collection or choosing distinct multiple populations. Finally, one must consider the speed of microevolution and timing of the sampling. If one is analyzing substrain specialization, the linear rate of microevolution may outweigh substrain differences related to different disease states or antibiotic resistance. One must therefore consider restricting the time window of collection.

CONCLUDING REMARKS

The preceding survey of methods used to fingerprint microbial pathogens should demonstrate that no dominant method has emerged for all of the pathogen categories (bacteria, fungi, and parasites) or even for all species within a category. For instance, in bacteria, while RFLP-PFGE is the most commonly used method for *Streptococcus pneu-*

moniae and *Staphylococcus aureus*, RFLP with probe is the most commonly used method for *Mycobacterium tuberculosis* (Table 2). The same variability holds true for fungal and parasite species (Table 2). The reason for this variability is twofold. First, differences between the genomes of different species warrant different methods in some cases. Second, different methods are effective for measuring different levels of relatedness. Third, and maybe not as scientific, a particular method may take hold for a particular species due to a consensus of the scientists in that area and the history of the methods first applied. Fourth, selections may be based on expediency in some cases. Whatever the reason, the message of this chapter should be clear. Select a fingerprinting method that will answer the question posed. Make sure the method has been verified for efficacy at the level of genetic relatedness necessary. Use computer-assisted systems, and save data in a format accessible for retrospective analyses and comparisons with new data. Finally, carefully consider the methods used for obtaining the collection.

REFERENCES

1. **Abderrazak, S. B., B. Oury, A. A. Lal, M. F. Bosseno, P. Force-Barge, J. P. Dujardin, T. Fandeur, J. F. Molez, F. Kjellberg, F. J. Ayala, and M. Tibayrenc.** 1999. *Plasmodium falciparum*: population genetic analysis by multilocus enzyme electrophoresis and other molecular markers. *Exp. Parasitol.* **92:**232–238.
2. **Agodi, A., F. Campanile, G. Basile, F. Viglianisi, and S. Stefani.** 1999. Phylogenetic analysis of macrorestriction fragments as a measure of genetic relatedness in *Staphylococcus aureus*: the epidemiological impact of methicillin resistance. *Eur. J. Epidemiol.* **15:**637–642.
3. **Anderson, J. M., T. Srikantha, B. Morrow, S. H. Miyasaki, T. C. White, N. Agabian, J. Schmid, and D. R. Soll.** 1993. Characterization and partial nucleotide sequence of the DNA fingerprinting probe Ca3 of *Candida albicans*. *J. Clin. Microbiol.* **31:**1472–1480.
4. **Anderson, T. J., B. Haubold, J. T. Williams, J. G. Estrada-Franco, L. Richardson, R. Mollinedo, M. Bockarie, J. Molkili, S. Mharakurwa, N. French, J. Whitworth, I. D. Velez, A. H. Brockman, F. Nosten, M. U. Ferreira, and K. P. Day.** 2000. Microsatellite markers reveal a spectrum of population structures in the malaria parasite *Plasmodium falciparum*. *Mol. Biol. Evol.* **17:**1467–1482.
5. **Ausubel, F. M., R. Brent, R. E. Kingston, D. D. Moore, J. G. Seidman, J. A. Smith, and K. Struhl (ed.).** 1994. *Current Protocols in Molecular Biology.* John Wiley & Sons, Inc., New York, N.Y.

6. **Babl, F. E., S. I. Pelton, S. Theodore, and J. O. Klein.** 2001. Constancy of distribution of serogroups of invasive pneumococcal isolates among children: experience during 4 decades. *Clin. Infect. Dis.* **32:**1155–1161.

7. **Backeljau, T., L. De Bruyn, H. De Wolf, K. Jordaens, S. Van Dongen, and B. Winnepenninckx.** 1996. Multiple UPGMA and neighbor-joining trees and the performance of some computer packages. *Mol. Biol. Evol.* **13:**309–313.

8. **Banuls, A. L., J. C. Dujardin, F. Guerrini, S. de Doncker, D. Jacquet, J. Arevalo, S. Noel, D. Le Ray, and M. Tibayrenc.** 2000. Is *Leishmania (Viannia) peruviana* a distinct species? A MLEE/RAPD evolutionary genetics answer. *J. Eukaryot. Microbiol.* **47:**197–207.

9. **Barakate, M. S., Y. X. Yang, S. H. Foo, A. M. Vickery, C. A. Sharp, L. D. Fowler, J. P. Harris, R. H. West, C. Mcleod, and R. A. Benn.** 2000. An epidemiological survey of methicillin-resistant *Staphylococcus aureus* in a tertiary referral hospital. *J. Hosp. Infect.* **44:**19–26.

10. **Barberio, C., R. Fani, A. Raso, A. Carli, and M. Polsinelli.** 1994. DNA fingerprinting of yeast strains by restriction enzyme analysis. *Res. Microbiol.* **145:**659–666.

11. **Barbour, A.** 1989. Antigenic variation in relapsing fever *Borrelia* species: genetic aspects, p. 783–790. *In* D. E. Berg and M. M. Howe (ed.), *Mobile DNA.* American Society for Microbiology, Washington, D.C.

12. **Barnabe, C., K. Neubauer, A. Solari, and M. Tibayrenc.** 2001. *Trypanosoma cruzi*: presence of the two major phylogenetic lineages and of several lesser discrete typing units (DTUs) in Chile and Paraguay. *Acta Trop.* **78:**127–137.

13. **Baro, T., J. M. Torres-Rodriguez, Y. Morera, C. Alia, O. Lopez, and R. Mendez.** 1999. Serotyping of *Cryptococcus neoformans* isolates from clinical and environmental sources in Spain. *J. Clin. Microbiol.* **37:**1170–1172.

14. **Bart, A., I. G. Schuurman, M. Achtman, D. A. Caugant, J. Dankert, and A. van der Ende.** 1998. Randomly amplified polymorphic DNA genotyping of serogroup A meningococci yields results similar to those obtained by multilocus enzyme electrophoresis and reveals new genotypes. *J. Clin. Microbiol.* **36:**1746–1749.

15. **Bart-Delabesse, E., H. van Deventer, W. Goessens, J. L. Poirot, N. Lioret, A. van Belkum, and F. Dromer.** 1995. Contribution of molecular typing methods and antifungal susceptibility testing to the study of a candidemia cluster in a burn care unit. *J. Clin. Microbiol.* **33:**3278–3283.

16. **Bartie, K. L., M. J. Wilson, D. W. Williams, and M. A. Lewis.** 2000. Macrorestriction fingerprinting of "*Streptococcus milleri*" group bacteria by pulsed-field gel electrophoresis. *J. Clin. Microbiol.* **38:**2141–2149.

17. **Bertout, S., F. Renaud, T. De Meeus, M. A. Piens, B. Lebeau, M. A. Viviani, M. Mallie, and J. M. Bastide.** 2000. Multilocus enzyme electrophoresis analysis of *Aspergillus fumigatus* strains isolated from the first clinical sample from patients with invasive aspergillosis. *J. Med. Microbiol.* **49:**375–381.

18. **Bertout, S., F. Renaud, D. Swinne, M. Mallie, and J. M. Bastide.** 1999. Genetic multilocus studies of different strains of *Cryptococcus neoformans*: taxonomy and genetic structure. *J. Clin. Microbiol.* **37:**715–720.

19. **Boerlin, P.** 1999. Evolution of virulence factors in Shiga-toxin-producing *Escherichia coli*. *Cell. Mol. Life Sci.* **56:**735–741.

20. **Bogaert, D., G. A. Syrogiannopoulos, I. N. Grivea, R. de Groot, N. G. Beratis, and P. W. Hermans.** 2000. Molecular epidemiology of penicillin-nonsusceptible *Streptococcus pneumoniae* among children in Greece. *J. Clin. Microbiol.* **38:**4361–4366.

21. **Bourbeau, P. P., and B. J. Heiter.** 1998. Comparison of Vitek GNI and GNI+ cards for identification of gram-negative bacteria. *J. Clin. Microbiol.* **36:**2775–2777.

22. **Brownlie, L., J. R. Stephenson, and J. A. Cole.** 1990. Effect of growth rate on plasmid maintenance by *Escherichia coli* HB101(pAT153). *J. Gen. Microbiol.* **136:**2471–2480.

23. **Brunder, W., and H. Karch.** 2000. Genome plasticity in Enterobacteriaceae. *Int. J. Med. Microbiol.* **290:**153–165.

24. **Caetano-Anolles, G.** 1993. Amplifying DNA with arbitrary oligonucleotide primers. *Genome Res.* **3:**85–94.

25. **Canton, R., M. Perez-Vazquez, A. Oliver, B. Sanchez Del Saz, M. O. Gutierrez, M. Martinez-Ferrer, and F. Baquero.** 2000. Evaluation of the Wider system, a new computer-assisted image-processing device for bacterial identification and susceptibility testing. *J. Clin. Microbiol.* **38:**1339–1346.

26. **Carle, G. F., and M. V. Olson.** 1985. An electrophoretic karyotype for yeast. *Proc. Natl. Acad. Sci. USA* **82:**3756–3760.

27. **Caulcott, C. A., A. Dunn, H. A. Robertson, N. S. Cooper, M. E. Brown, and P. M. Rhodes.** 1987. Investigation of the effect of growth environment on the stability of low-copy-number plasmids in *Escherichia coli*. *J. Gen. Microbiol.* **133:**1881–1889.

28. **Chang, N., and L. Chui.** 1998. A standardized protocol for the rapid preparation of bacterial DNA for pulsed-field gel electrophoresis. *Diagn. Microbiol. Infect. Dis.* **31:**275–279.

29. **Chu, G., D. Vollrath, and R. W. Davis.** 1986. Separation of large DNA molecules by contour-clamped homogeneous electric fields. *Science* **234:**1582–1585.

30. **Chung, M., H. de Lencastre, P. Matthews, A. Tomasz, I. Adamsson, M. Aries de Sousa, T. Camou, C. Cocuzza, A. Corso, I. Couto, A. Dominguez, M. Gniadkowski, R. Goering, A. Gomes, K. Kikuchi, A. Marchese, R. Mato, O. Melter, D. Oliveira, R. Palacio, R. Sa-Leao, I. Santos Sanches, J. H. Song, P. T. Tassios, P. Villari, and Multilaboratory Project Collaborators.** 2000. Molecular typing of methicillin-resistant *Staphylococcus aureus* by pulsed-field gel electrophoresis: comparison of results obtained in a multilaboratory effort using identical protocols and MRSA strains. *Microb. Drug Resist.* **6:**189–198.

31. **Clode, F. E., M. E. Kaufmann, H. Malnick, and T. L. Pitt.** 2000. Distribution of genes encoding putative transmissibility factors among epidemic and nonepidemic strains of *Burkholderia cepacia* from cystic fibrosis patients in the United Kingdom. *J. Clin. Microbiol.* **38:**1763–1766.

32. **Cowen, L. E., C. Sirjusingh, R. C. Summerbell, S. Walmsley, S. Richardson, L. M. Kohn, and J. B. Anderson.** 1999. Multilocus genotypes and DNA fingerprinting do not predict variation in azole resistance among clinical isolates of *Candida albicans*. *Antimicrob. Agents Chemother.* **43:**2930–2938.

33. **Demarta, A., M. Tonolla, A. Caminada, M. Beretta, and R. Peduzzi.** 2000. Epidemiological relationships between *Aeromonas* strains isolated from symptomatic children and household environments as determined by ribotyping. *Eur. J. Epidemiol.* **16:**447–453.

34. **Desjardins, P., B. Picard, B. Kaltenbock, J. Elion, and E. Denamur.** 1995. Sex in *Escherichia coli* does not disrupt the clonal structure of the population evidence from random amplified polymorphic DNA and restriction-fragment-length polymorphism. *J. Mol. Evol.* **41:**440–448.

35. **Dib, J. C., M. Dube, C. Kelly, M. G. Rinaldi, and J. E. Patterson.** 1996. Evaluation of pulsed-field gel electrophoresis as a typing system for *Candida rugosa*: comparison of karyotype and restriction fragment length polymorphisms. *J. Clin. Microbiol.* **34:**1494–1496.

36. **Dingle, K. E., F. M. Colles, D. R. Wareing, R. Ure, A. J. Fox, F. E. Bolton, H. J. Bootsma, R. J. Willems, R. Urwin, and M. C. Maiden.** 2001. Multilocus sequence

typing system for *Campylobacter jejuni. J. Clin. Microbiol.* **39:**14–23.

37. **During, K.** 1993. Non-radioactive detection methods for nucleic acids separated by electrophoresis. *J. Chromatogr.* **618:**105–131.

38. **Ellsworth, D. L., K. D. Rittenhouse, and R. L. Honeycutt.** 1993. Artifactual variation in randomly amplified polymorphic DNA banding patterns. *BioTechniques* **14:**214–217.

39. **Enger, L., S. Joly, C. Pujol, P. Simonson, M. A. Pfaller, and D. R. Soll.** 2001. Cloning and characterization of a complex DNA fingerprinting probe for *Candida parapsilosis. J. Clin. Microbiol.* **39:**658–669.

40. **Enright, M. C., N. P. Day, C. E. Davies, S. J. Peacock, and B. G. Spratt.** 2000. Multilocus sequence typing for characterization of methicillin-resistant and methicillin-susceptible clones of *Staphylococcus aureus. J. Clin. Microbiol.* **38:**1008–1015.

41. **Enright, M. C., and B. G. Spratt.** 1998. A multilocus sequence typing scheme for *Streptococcus pneumoniae:* identification of clones associated with serious invasive disease. *Microbiology* **144:**3049–3060.

42. **Enright, M. C., and B. G. Spratt.** 1999. Multilocus sequence typing. *Trends Microbiol.* **7:**482–487.

43. **Eribe, E. R., and I. Olsen.** 2000. Strain differentiation in *Bacteroides fragilis* by ribotyping and computer-assisted gel analysis. *APMIS* **108:**429–438.

44. **Felsenstein, J.** 1984. Distance methods for inferring phylogenies: a justification. *Evolution* **38:**16–24.

45. **Felsenstein, J.** 1985. Confidence limits on phylogenies: an approach using the bootstrap. *Evolution* **39:**783–791.

46. **Fitch, W. M., and E. Margoliash.** 1967. Construction of phylogenetic trees. *Science* **155:**279–284.

47. **Forche, A., G. Schönian, Y. Gräser, R. Vilgalys, and T. G. Mitchell.** 1999. Genetic structure of typical and atypical populations of *Candida albicans* from Africa. *Fungal Genet. Biol.* **28:**107–125.

48. **Friedman, C. R., M. Y. Stoeckle, W. D. Johnson, Jr., and L. W. Riley.** 1995. Double-repetitive-element PCR method for subtyping *Mycobacterium tuberculosis* clinical isolates. *J. Clin. Microbiol.* **33:**1383–1384.

49. **Gardiner, K., and D. Patterson.** 1989. Transverse alternating field electrophoresis and applications to mammalian genome mapping. *Electrophoresis* **10:**296–302.

50. **Gartenberg, M. R.** 2000. The Sir proteins of *Saccharomyces cerevisiae:* mediators of transcriptional silencing and much more. *Curr. Opin. Microbiol.* **3:**132–137.

51. **Girardin, H., J. P. Latge, T. Srikantha, B. Morrow, and D. R. Soll.** 1993. Development of DNA probes for fingerprinting *Aspergillus fumigatus. J. Clin. Microbiol.* **31:**1547–1554.

52. **Glasgow, A. C., K. T. Hughes, and M. I. Simon.** 1989. Bacterial DNA inversion systems, p. 637–660. *In* D. E. Berg and M. M. Howe (ed.), *Mobile DNA.* American Society for Microbiology, Washington, D.C.

53. **Glover, D. M.** 1983. Genes for ribosomal DNA, p. 207–224. *In* M. Maclean, S. P. Gregory, and R. A. Flavell (ed.), *Eukaryotic Genes: Their Structure and Regulation.* Butterworth & Co., Cambridge, United Kingdom.

54. **Gomez-De-Leon, P., J. I. Santos, J. Caballero, D. Gomez, L. E. Espinosa, I. Moreno, D. Pinero, and A. Cravioto.** 2000. Genomic variability of *Haemophilus influenzae* isolated from Mexican children determined by using enterobacterial repetitive intergenic consensus sequences and PCR. *J. Clin. Microbiol.* **38:**2504–2511.

55. **Gottlieb, S., and R. E. Esposito.** 1989. A new role for a yeast transcriptional silencer gene, *SIR2,* in regulation of recombination in ribosomal DNA. *Cell* **56:**771–776.

56. **Gräser, Y., M. Volovsek, J. Arrington, G. Schönian, W. Presber, T. G. Mitchell, and R. Vilgalys.** 1996. Molecular markers reveal that population structure of the human pathogen *Candida albicans* exhibits both clonality and recombination. *Proc. Natl. Acad. Sci. USA* **93:**12473–12477.

57. **Haber, J. E.** 1998. A locus control region regulates yeast recombination. *Trends Genet.* **14:**317–321.

58. **Hatlan, L. E., and G. Attardi.** 1971. Preparation of the HeLa cell genome complementary to tRNA and 5SRNA. *J. Mol. Biol.* **56:**535–554.

59. **Hazell, S. L., R. H. Andrews, H. M. Mitchell, and G. Daskalopoulous.** 1997. Genetic relationship among isolates of *Helicobacter pylori:* evidence for the existence of a *Helicobacter pylori* species-complex. *FEMS Microbiol. Lett.* **150:**27–32.

60. **Hermans, P. W., D. van Soolingen, J. W. Dale, A. R. Schuitema, R. A. McAdam, D. Catty, and J. D. van Embden.** 1990. Insertion element IS986 from *Mycobacterium tuberculosis:* a useful tool for diagnosis and epidemiology of tuberculosis. *J. Clin. Microbiol.* **28:**2051–2058.

61. **Hesselbarth, J., and S. Schwarz.** 1995. Comparative ribotyping of *Staphylococcus intermedius* from dogs, pigeons, horses, and mink. *Vet. Microbiol.* **45:**11–17.

62. **Holtke, H. J., W. Ankebauer, K. Muhlegger, R. Rein, G. Sagner, R. Seibl, and T. Walter.** 1995. The digoxigenin (DIG) system for non-radioactive labeling and detection of nucleic acids—an overview. *Cell Mol. Biol.* **41:**883–905.

63. **Ichiyama, S. M., M. Ohta, K. Shimokata, N. Kato, and J. Takeuchi.** 1991. Genomic DNA fingerprinting by pulsed-field gel electrophoresis as an epidemiological marker for study of nosocomial infections caused by methicillin-resistant *Staphylococcus aureus. J. Clin. Microbiol.* **29:**2690–2695.

64. **Isaac-Renton, J. L., C. Cordeiro, K. Sarafis, and H. Shahriari.** 1993. Characterization of *Giardia duodenalis* isolates from a waterborne outbreak. *J. Infect. Dis.* **167:**431–440.

65. **Joly, S., C. Pujol, M. Rysz, K. Vargas, and D. R. Soll.** 1999. Development and characterization of complex DNA fingerprinting probes for the infectious yeast *Candida dubliniensis. J. Clin. Microbiol.* **37:**1035–1044.

66. **Joly, S., C. Pujol, K. Schroppel, and D. R. Soll.** 1996. Development of two species specific fingerprinting probes for broad computer-assisted epidemiological studies of *Candida tropicalis. J. Clin. Microbiol.* **34:**3063–3071.

67. **Jorgensen, M., R. Givney, M. Pegler, A. Vickery, and G. Funnell.** 1996. Typing multidrug-resistant *Staphylococcus aureus:* conflicting epidemiological data produced by genotypic and phenotypic methods clarified by phylogenetic analysis. *J. Clin. Microbiol.* **34:**398–403.

68. **Kamerbeek, J., L. Schouls, A. Kolk, M. van Agterveld, D. van Soolingen, S. Kuigper, A. Bunschoten, H. Molhuizen, R. Shaw, M. Goyal, and J. van Embden.** 1997. Simultaneous detection and strain differentiation of *Mycobacterium tuberculosis* for diagnosis and epidemiology. *J. Clin. Microbiol.* **35:**907–914.

69. **Karl, S. A., and J. C. Avise.** 1993. PCR-based assays of mendelian polymorphisms from anonymous single-copy nuclear DNA: techniques and applications for population genetics. *Mol. Biol. Evol.* **10:**342–361.

70. **Kasuga, T., J. W. Taylor, and T. J. White.** 1999. Phylogenetic relationships of varieties and geographical groups of the human pathogenic fungus *Histoplasma capsulatum* Darling. *J. Clin. Microbiol.* **37:**653–663.

71. **Katakura, K., Y. Matsumoto, E. A. Gomez, M. Furuya, and Y. Hashiguchi.** 1993. Molecular karyotype characterization of *Leishmania panamensis, Leishmania mexicana,* and

Leishmania major-like parasites: agents of cutaneous leishmaniasis in Ecuador. *Am. J. Trop. Med. Hyg.* **48:**707–715.

72. **Klepser, M. E., and M. A. Pfaller.** 1998. Variation in electrophoretic karyotype and antifungal susceptibility of clinical isolates of *Cryptococcus neoformans* at a university-affiliated teaching hospital from 1987 to 1994. *J. Clin. Microbiol.* **36:**3653–3656.

73. **Ko, A. I., J. N. Reis, S. J. Coppola, E. L. Gouveia, S. M. Cordeiro, R. S. Lobo, R. M. Pinheiro, K. Salgado, C. M. Ribeiro Dourado, J. Tavares-Neto, H. Rocha, M. Galvao Reis, W. D. Johnson, Jr., and L. W. Riley.** 2000. Clonally related penicillin-nonsusceptible *Streptococcus pneumoniae* serotype 14 from cases of meningitis in Salvador, Brazil. *Clin. Infect. Dis.* **30:**78–86.

74. **Kreger-van Rij, N. J. W. (ed.).** 1984. *The Yeasts: a Taxonomic Study*, 3rd ed. Elsevier Science Publishers B.V., Amsterdam, The Netherlands.

75. **Kremer, K., D. van Soolingen, R. Frothingham, W. H. Hass, P. W. M. Hermans, C. Martin, P. Palittapongarnpim, B. B. Plikaytis, L. W. Riley, M. A. Yakrus, J. M. Musser, and J. D. A. van Embden.** 1999. Comparison of methods based on different molecular epidemiological markers for typing of *Mycobacterium tuberculosis* complex strains: interlaboratory study of discriminatory power and reproducibility. *J. Clin. Microbiol.* **37:**2607–2618.

76. **Krieg, N. R. (ed.).** 1984. *Bergey's Manual of Systematic Bacteriology.* The Williams & Wilkins Co., Baltimore, Md.

77. **Lasker, B. A., L. S. Page, T. J. Lott, and G. S. Kobayashi.** 1992. Isolation, characterization, and sequencing of *Candida albicans* repetitive element 2. *Gene* **116:**51–57.

78. **Leelayuwat, C., A. Romphruk, A. Lulitanond, S. Trakulsomboon, and V. Thamlikitkul.** 2000. Genotype analysis of *Burkholderia pseudomallei* using randomly amplified polymorphic DNA (RAPD): indicative of genetic differences amongst environmental and clinical isolates. *Acta Trop.* **77:**229–237.

79. **Lehmann, P. F., D. Lin, and B. A. Lasker.** 1992. Genotypic identification and characterization of species and strains within the genus *Candida* by using random amplified polymorphic DNA. *J. Clin. Microbiol.* **30:**3249–3254.

80. **Lockhart, S., J. J. Fritch, S. Meier, K. Schroppel, R. Srikantha, R. Galask, and D. R. Soll.** 1995. Colonizing populations of *Candida albicans* are clonal in origin but undergo microevolution through C1 fragment reorganization as demonstrated by DNA fingerprinting and C1 sequencing. *J. Clin. Microbiol.* **33:**1501–1509.

81. **Lockhart, S., C. Pujol, S. Joly, and D. R. Soll.** 2001. Development and use of complex probes for DNA fingerprinting the infectious fungi. *J. Med. Mycol.* **39:**1–8.

82. **Lockhart, S. R., S. Joly, C. Pujol, J. D. Sobel, M. A. Pfaller, and D. R. Soll.** 1997. Development and verification of fingerprinting probes for *Candida glabrata*. *Microbiology* **143:**3733–3746.

83. **Lockhart, S. R., S. Joly, K. Vargas, J. Swails-Wenger, L. Enger, and D. R. Soll.** 1999. Natural defenses against *Candida* colonization breakdown in the oral cavities of the elderly. *J. Dent. Res.* **78:**857–868.

84. **Lott, T. J., B. P. Holloway, D. A. Logan, R. Fundyga, and J. Arnold.** 1999. Towards understanding the evolution of the human commensal yeast *Candida albicans*. *Microbiology* **145:**1137–1143.

85. **Loudon, K. W., A. P. Coke, and J. P. Burnie.** 1995. "Pseudoclusters" and typing by random amplification of polymorphic DNA of *Aspergillus fumigatus*. *J. Clin. Pathol.* **48:**183–184.

86. **Loudon, K. W., A. P. Coke, J. P. Burnie, G. S. Lucas, and J. A. Liu Yin.** 1994. Invasive aspergillosis: clusters and sources? *J. Med. Vet. Mycol.* **32:**217–224.

87. **Maiden, M. C., J. A. Bygraves, E. Feil, G. Morelli, J. E. Russell, R. Urwin, Q. Zhang, J. Zhou, K. Zurth, D. A. Caugant, I. M. Feavers, M. Achtman, and B. G. Spratt.** 1998. Multilocus sequence typing: a portable approach to the identification of clones within populations of pathogenic microorganisms. *Proc. Natl. Acad. Sci. USA* **95:**3140–3145.

88. **Malorny, B., A. Schroeter, C. Bunge, B. Hoog, A. Steinbeck, and R. Helmuth.** 2001. Evaluation of molecular typing methods for *Salmonella enterica* serovar Typhimurium DT104 isolated in Germany from healthy pigs. *Vet. Res.* **32:**119–129.

89. **Masseret, E., J. Boudeau, J. F. Colombel, C. Neut, P. Desreumaux, B. Joly, A. Cortot, and A. Darfeuille-Michaud.** 2001. Genetically related *Escherichia coli* strains associated with Crohn's disease. *Gut* **48:**320–325.

90. **Mazars, E., S. Lesjean, A. Banuls, M. Gilbert, V. Vincent, B. Gicquel, C. Tibayrenc, C. Locht, and P. Supply.** 2001. High-resolution minisatellite-based typing as a portable approach to global analysis of *Mycobacterium tuberculosis* molecular epidemiology. *Proc. Natl. Acad. Sci. USA* **98:**1901–1906.

91. **Mazurier, S. I., A. Audurier, N. Marquet-Van der Mee, S. Notermans, and K. Wernars.** 1992. A comparative study of randomly amplified polymorphic DNA analysis and conventional phage typing for epidemiological studies of *Listeria monocytogenes* isolates. *Res. Microbiol.* **143:**507–512.

92. **Meunier, J. R., and P. A. Grimont.** 1993. Factors affecting reproducibility of random amplified polymorphic DNA fingerprinting. *Res. Microbiol.* **144:**373–379.

93. **Meyer, W., G. N. Latouche, H. M. Daniel, M. Thanos, T. G. Mitchell, D. Yarrow, G. Schonian, and T. C. Sorrell.** 1997. Identification of pathogenic yeasts of the imperfect genus *Candida* by polymerase chain reaction fingerprinting. *Electrophoresis* **18:**1548–1559.

94. **Meyer, W., and T. G. Mitchell.** 1995. Polymerase chain reaction fingerprinting in fungi using single primers specific to minisatellites and simple repetitive DNA sequences strain variation in *Cryptococcus neoformans*. *Electrophoresis* **16:**1648–1656.

95. **Moll, W. M., J. Ungerechts, G. Marklein, and K. P. Schaal.** 1996. Comparison of BBL Crystal ANR ID Kit and API rapid ID 32 A for identification of anaerobic bacteria. *Zentralbl. Bakteriol.* **284:**329–347.

96. **Morgan, U. M., C. C. Constantine, W. K. Greene, and R. C. Thompson.** 1993. RAPD (random amplified polymorphic DNA) analysis of *Giardia* DNA and correlation with isoenzyme data. *Trans. R. Soc. Trop. Med. Hyg.* **87:**702–705.

97. **Nigatu, A.** 2000. Evaluation of numerical analyses of RAPD and API 50 CH patterns to differentiate *Lactobacillus plantarum*, *Lact. fermentum*, *Lact. rhamnosus*, *Lact. sake*, *Lact. parabuchneri*, *Lact. gallinarum*, *Lact. casei*, *Weissella minor* and related taxa isolated from kocho and tef. *J. Appl. Microbiol.* **89:**969–978.

98. **Nomura, M., and E. A. Morgan.** 1977. Genetics of bacterial ribosomes. *Annu. Rev. Genet.* **11:**297–347.

99. **Pasteur, N., G. Pasteur, F. Bonhomme, J. Catalan, and J. Britton-Davidian.** 1988. *Practical Isozyme Genetics.* Halsted Press, New York, N.Y.

100. **Paugam, A., M. Benchetrit, A. Fiacre, C. Tourte-Schaefer, and J. Dupouy-Camet.** 1999. Comparison of four commercialized biochemical systems for clinical yeast identification by colour-producing reactions. *Med. Mycol.* **37:**11–17.

101. **Pfaller, M. A., S. R. Lockhart, C. Pujol, J. A. Swails-Wenger, S. A. Messer, M. B. Edmund, R. N. Jones, R. P. Wenzel, and D. R. Soll.** 1998. Hospital specificity,

region specificity, and fluconazole-resistance of *Candida albicans* bloodstream isolates. *J. Clin. Microbiol.* **36:**1518–1529.

102. **Pfaller, M. A., I. Mujeeb, R. J. Hollis, R. N. Jones, and G. V. Doern.** 2000. Evaluation of the discriminatory powers of the Dienes test and ribotyping as typing methods for *Proteus mirabilis. J. Clin. Microbiol.* **38:**1077–1080.

103. **Priest, F. G., D. A. Kaji, Y. B. Rosato, and V. P. Canhos.** 1994. Characterization of *Bacillus thuringiensis* and related bacteria by ribosomal RNA gene restriction fragment length polymorphism. *Microbiology* **140:**1015–1022.

104. **Pujol, C., S. Joly, S. R. Lockhart, S. Noel, M. Tibayrenc, and D. R. Soll.** 1997. Parity among the randomly amplified polymorphic DNA method, multilocus enzyme electrophoresis, and Southern blot hybridization with the moderately repetitive DNA probe Ca3 for fingerprinting *Candida albicans. J. Clin. Microbiol.* **35:**2348–2358.

105. **Pujol, C., J. Reynes, F. Renaud, M. Raymond, M. Tibayrenc, F. J. Ayala, F. Janbon, M. Mallie, and J. M. Bastide.** 1993. The yeast *Candida albicans* has a clonal mode of reproduction in a population of infected human immunodeficiency virus-positive patients. *Proc. Natl. Acad. Sci. USA* **90:**9456–9459.

106. **Quentin, R., H. Huet, F. S. Wang, P. Geslin, A. Goudeau, and R. K. Selander.** 1995. Characterization of *Streptococcus agalactiae* strains by multilocus enzyme genotype and serotype: identification of multiple virulent clone families that cause invasive neonatal disease. *J. Clin. Microbiol.* **33:**2576–2581.

107. **Radua, S., O. W. Ling, S. Srimontree, A. Lulitanond, W. F. Hin, Yuherman, S. Lihan, G. Rusul, and A. R. Mutalib.** 2000. Characterization of *Burkholderia pseudomallei* isolated in Thailand and Malaysia. *Diagn. Microbiol. Infect. Dis.* **38:**141–145.

108. **Ramsey, H., B. Morrow, and D. R. Soll.** 1994. An increase in switching frequency correlates with an increase in recombination of the ribosomal chromosomes of *Candida albicans* strain 3153A. *Microbiology* **140:**1525–1531.

109. **Ravins, M., H. Bercovier, D. Chemtob, Y. Fishman, and G. Rahav.** 2001. Molecular epidemiology of *Mycobacterium tuberculosis* infection in Israel. *J. Clin. Microbiol.* **39:**1175–1177.

110. **Rieseberg, L. H.** 1996. Homology among RAPD fragments in interspecific comparisons. *Mol. Ecol.* **5:**99–105.

111. **Richardson, B. J., P. R. Baverstock, and M. Adams.** 1986. *Allozyme Electrophoresis, a Handbook for Animal Systematics and Population Studies.* Academic Press Inc., Orlando, Fla.

112. **Rohlf, F. J.** 1963. Classification of *Aedes* by numerical taxonomic methods (Diptera: Culcidae). *Ann. Entomol. Soc. Am.* **56:**798–804.

113. **Rudolph, K. M., A. J. Parkinson, and M. C. Roberts.** 1998. Molecular analysis by pulsed-field gel electrophoresis and antibiogram of *Streptococcus pneumoniae* serotype 6B isolates from selected areas within the United States. *J. Clin. Microbiol.* **36:**2703–2707.

114. **Sadhu, C., M. J. McEachern, E. P. Rustchenko-Bulgac, J. Schmid, D. R. Soll, and J. B. Hicks.** 1991. Telomeric and dispersed repeat sequences in *Candida* yeasts and their use in strain identification. *J. Bacteriol.* **173:**842–850.

115. **Saitou, N., and M. Nei.** 1987. The neighbor-joining method: a new method for reconstructing phylogenetic trees. *Mol. Biol. Evol.* **4:**406–425.

116. **Sambrook, J., E. F. Fritsch, and T. Maniatis.** 1989. *Molecular Cloning: a Laboratory Manual.* Cold Spring Harbor Laboratory Press, Cold Spring Harbor, N.Y.

117. **Sangeorzan, J. A., M. J. Zervos, S. Donabedian, and C. A. Kauffman.** 1995. Validity of contour-clamped homogeneous electric field electrophoresis as a typing system for *Candida albicans. Mycoses* **38:**29–36.

118. **Scherer, S., and D. A. Stevens.** 1987. Application of DNA typing methods to epidemiology and taxonomy of *Candida* species. *J. Clin. Microbiol.* **25:**675–679.

119. **Scherer, S., and D. A. Stevens.** 1988. A *Candida albicans* dispersed, repeated gene family and its epidemiological applications. *Proc. Natl. Acad. Sci. USA* **85:**1452–1456.

120. **Schonian, G., C. Schweynoch, K. Zlateva, L. Oskam, N. Kroon, Y. Graser, and W. Presber.** 1996. Identification and determination of the relationships of species and strains within the genus *Leishmania* using single primers in the polymerase chain reaction. *Mol. Biochem. Parasitol.* **77:**19–29.

121. **Schwartz, D. C., and C. R. Cantor.** 1984. Separation of yeast chromosome-sized DNAs by pulsed field gradient gel electrophoresis. *Cell* **37:**67–75.

122. **Schwartz, D. C., W. Saffran, J. Welsh, R. Haas, M. Goldenberg, and C. R. Cantor.** 1983. New techniques for purifying large DNAs and studying their properties and packaging. *Cold Spring Harbor Symp. Quant. Biol.* **47:**189–195.

123. **Schweizer, E., C. MacKechnie, and H. D. Halvorson.** 1969. The redundancy of ribosomal and transfer DNA genes in *Saccharomyces cerevisiae. J. Mol. Biol.* **40:**261–278.

124. **Singh, D. V., M. H. Matte, G. R. Matte, S. Jiang, F. Sabeena, B. N. Shukla, S. C. Sanyal, A. Huq, and R. R. Colwell.** 2001. Molecular analysis of *Vibrio cholerae* O1, O139, non-O1, and non-O139 strains: clonal relationships between clinical and environmental isolates. *Appl. Environ. Microbiol.* **67:**910–921.

125. **Slutsky, B., J. Buffo, and D. R. Soll.** 1985. High frequency switching of colony morphology in *Candida albicans. Science* **230:**666–669.

126. **Sneath, P. H., and R. R. Sokal.** 1973. *Numerical Taxonomy: the Principles and Practice of Numerical Classification.* W. H. Freeman & Co., San Francisco, Calif.

127. **Soewignjo, S., B. D. Gessner, A. Sutanto, M. Steinhoff, M. Prijanto, C. Nelson, A. Widjaya, and S. Arjoso.** 2001. *Streptococcus pneumoniae* nasopharyngeal carriage prevalence, serotype distribution, and resistance patterns among children on Lombok Island, Indonesia. *Clin. Infect. Dis.* **32:**1039–1043.

128. **Sola, C., S. Ferdinand, C. Mammina, A. Nastasi, and N. Rastogi.** 2001. Genetic diversity of *Mycobacterium tuberculosis* in Sicily based on spoligotyping and variable number of tandem DNA repeats and comparison with a spoligotyping database for population-based analysis. *J. Clin. Microbiol.* **39:**1559–1565.

129. **Soll, D. R.** 1992. High frequency switching in *Candida albicans. Clin. Microbiol. Rev.* **5:**183–203.

130. **Soll, D. R.** 2000. The ins and outs of DNA fingerprinting the infectious fungi. *Clin. Microbiol. Rev.* **13:**332–370.

131. **Soll, D. R.** 2002. The molecular biology of switching in *Candida*, p. 161–182. *In* R. Cihlar and R. Calderone (ed.), *Fungal Pathogenesis: Principles and Clinical Application.* Marcel Dekker, Inc., New York, N.Y.

132. **Soll, D. R.** 2002. Phenotypic switching, p. 123–142. *In* R. A. Calderone (ed.), *Candida and Candidiasis.* ASM Press, Washington, D.C.

133. **Soll, D. R., R. Galask, J. Schmid, C. Hanna, K. Mac, and B. Morrow.** 1991. Genetic dissimilarity of commensal strains of *Candida* spp. carried in different anatomical

locations of the same healthy women. *J. Clin. Microbiol.* **29:**1702–1710.

134. **Suffys, P. N., M. E. Ivens de Araujo, M. L. Rossetti, A. Zahab, E. W. Barroso, A. M. Barreto, E. Campos, D. van Soolingen, K. Kremer, H. Heersma, and W. M. Degrave.** 2000. Usefulness of IS6110-restriction fragment length polymorphism typing of Brazilian strains of *Mycobacterium tuberculosis* and comparison with an international fingerprint database. *Res. Microbiol.* **151:**343–351.

135. **Sullivan, D., D. Bennett, M. Henman, P. Harwood, S. Flint, F. Mulcahy, D. Shanley, and D. Coleman.** 1993. Oligonucleotide fingerprinting of isolates of *Candida* species other than *C. albicans* and of atypical *Candida* species from human immunodeficiency virus-positive and AIDS patients. *J. Clin. Microbiol.* **31:**2124–2133.

136. **Swanson, J., and J. M. Koomey.** 1989. Mechanisms for variation of pili and outer membrane protein II in *Neisseria gonorrhoeae*, p. 743–762. *In* D. E. Berg and M. M. Howe (ed.), *Mobile DNA.* American Society for Microbiology, Washington, D.C.

137. **Symms, C., B. Cookson, J. Stanley, and J. V. Hookey.** 1998. Analysis of methicillin-resistant *Staphylococcus aureus* by IS1181 profiling. *Epidemiol. Infect.* **120:**271–279.

138. **Taylor, J. W., D. M. Geiser, A. Burt, and V. Koufopanou.** 1999. The evolutionary biology and population genetics underlying fungal strain typing. *Clin. Microbiol. Rev.* **12:**126–146.

139. **Tenover, F. C., R. D. Arbeit, R. V. Goering, P. A. Mickelsen, B. E. Murray, D. H. Persing, and B. Swaminathan.** 1995. Interpreting chromosomal DNA restriction patterns produced by pulsed-field gel electrophoresis: criteria for bacterial strain typing. *J. Clin. Microbiol.* **33:**2233–2239.

140. **Thormann, C. E., M. E. Ferreira, L. E. Camargo, J. G. Tivang, and T. C. Osborn.** 1994. Comparison of RFLP and RAPD markers to estimate the genetic relationships within and among cruciferous species. *Theor. Appl. Genet.* **88:**973–980.

141. **Thrash-Bingham, C., and J. A. Gorman.** 1992. DNA translocations contribute to chromosome length polymorphisms in *Candida albicans. Curr. Genet.* **22:**93–100.

142. **Tibayrenc, M.** 1995. Population genetics and strain typing of microorganisms: how to detect departures from panmixia without individualizing alleles and loci. *C. R. Acad. Sci. Ser. III* **318:**135–139.

143. **Tibayrenc, M.** 1996. Towards a unified evolutionary genetics of microorganisms. *Annu. Rev. Microbiol.* **50:**401–429.

144. **Tibayrenc, M., K. Neubauer, C. Barnabe, F. Guerrini, D. Skarecky, and F. J. Ayala.** 1993. Genetic characterization of six parasitic protozoa: parity between randomprimer DNA typing and multilocus enzyme electrophoresis. *Proc. Natl. Acad. Sci. USA* **90:**1335–1339.

145. **Van Der Zwet, W. C., G. A. Parlevliet, P. H. Savelkoul, J. Stoof, A. M. Kaiser, A. M. Van Furth, and C. M. Vandenbroucke-Grauls.** 2000. Outbreak of *Bacillus cereus* infections in a neonatal intensive care unit traced to balloons used in manual ventilation. *J. Clin. Microbiol.* **38:**4131–4136.

146. **van Doorn, N. E., F. Namavar, J. G. Kusters, E. P. van Rees, E. J. Kulipers, and J. de Graaff.** 1998. Genomic DNA fingerprinting of clinical isolates of *Helicobacter pylori* by REP-PCR and restriction fragment end-labeling. *FEMS Microbiol. Lett.* **160:**145–150.

147. **van Soolingen, D., P. W. M. Hermans, P. E. W. de Hans, D. R. Soll, and J. D. A. van Enbden.** 1991. Occurrence and stability of insertion sequences in *Mycobacterium tuberculosis* complex strains: Evaluation of an insertion sequence-dependent DNA polymorphism as a tool in the epidemiology of tuberculosis. *J. Clin. Microbiol.* **29:**2578–2586.

148. **van Steenbergen, T. J., S. D. Colloms, P. W. Hermans, J. de Graaff, and R. H. Plasterk.** 1995. Genomic DNA fingerprinting by restriction fragment end-labeling. *Proc. Natl. Acad. Sci. USA* **92:**5572–5576.

149. **Vargas, K., S. A. Messer, M. Pfaller, S. R. Lockhart, J. Stapleton, J. Hellstein, and D. R. Soll.** 2000. Elevated switching and drug resistance of *Candida* from HIV-positive individuals prior to thrush. *J. Clin. Microbiol.* **38:**3595–3607.

150. **Verweij, P. E., I. M. Breuker, A. J. Rijs, and J. F. Meis.** 1999. Comparative study of seven commercial yeast identification systems. *J. Clin. Pathol.* **52:**271–273.

151. **Vlad, M.** 1977. Quantitative studies of rDNA in amphibians. *J. Cell Sci.* **24:**109–118.

152. **Vos, P., R. Hogers, M. Bleeker, M. Reijans, T. van de Lee, M. Hornes, A. Frijters, J. Pot, J. Peleman, and M. Kuiper.** 1995. AFLP: a new technique for DNA fingerprinting. *Nucleic Acids Res.* **23:**4407–4414.

153. **Welsch, J., and M. McClelland.** 1990. Fingerprinting genomes using PCR with arbitrary primers. *Nucleic Acids Res.* **18:**7213–7224.

154. **Wiley, E. O.** 1981. *Phylogenetics: the Theory and Practice of Phylogenetic Systematics.* John Wiley & Sons, Inc., New York, N.Y.

155. **Williams, J. G., A. R. Kubelik, K. J. Livak, and S. V. Tingey.** 1990. DNA polymorphisms amplified by arbitrary primers are useful as genetic markers. *Nucleic Acids Res.* **18:**6531–6535.

156. **Wolf, B., L. C. Rey, S. Brisse, L. B. Moreira, D. Milatovic, A. Fleer, J. J. Roord, and J. Verhoef.** 2000. Molecular epidemiology of penicillin-resistant *Streptococcus pneumoniae* colonizing children with community-acquired pneumonia and children attending day-care centres in Fortaleza, Brazil. *J. Antimicrob. Chemother.* **46:**757–765.

157. **Wu, C. F. J.** 1986. Jacknife, bootstrap and other resampling plans in regression analysis. *Ann. Stat.* **14:**1261–1295.

158. **Xu, J., T. G. Mitchell, and R. Vilgalys.** 1999. PCR-restriction fragment length polymorphism (RFLP) analyses reveal both extensive clonality and local genetic differences in *Candida albicans. Mol. Ecol.* **8:**59–73.

159. **Xu, J., R. Vilgalys, and T. G. Mitchell.** 1999. Lack of genetic differentiation between two geographically diverse samples of *Candida albicans* isolated from patients infected with human immunodeficiency virus. *J. Bacteriol.* **181:**1369–1373.

Investigation of Foodborne and Waterborne Disease Outbreaks

JOHN BESSER, JAMES BEEBE, AND BALA SWAMINATHAN

13

Foodborne and waterborne illnesses are leading global health problems, accounting for more morbidity and mortality than tuberculosis or malaria. Each year, there are an estimated 4 billion episodes of diarrheal disease, largely foodborne and waterborne, resulting in over 2.2 million deaths (91, 123). An additional 1.5 million individuals contract hepatitis A each year (122). In the United States alone there are an estimated 76 million cases of foodborne disease annually, resulting in approximately 325,000 hospitalizations and 5,000 deaths (87). Between 1993 and 1997, 2,751 foodborne disease outbreaks, affecting a reported 86,058 persons, were reported to the U.S. Centers for Disease Control and Prevention (CDC) (92).

Reported outbreaks are thought to represent only a small proportion of the total number of outbreaks occurring at any time. Most foodborne infections resolve after a few days with or without medical intervention. However, some infections progress to more severe sequelae, such as septicemia, meningitis, meningoencephalitis, hemolytic-uremic syndrome, reactive arthritis, and Guillain-Barré syndrome. Even uncomplicated illness is important from a society-wide point of view because of the large numbers involved. The U.S. Department of Agriculture has estimated that medical costs and productivity losses due to seven specific foodborne pathogens range between 6.5 billion and 34.9 billion dollars annually (4). The total economic burden of foodborne disease in the United States is likely to be much higher.

Water-related infections result in an estimated 3.4 million deaths per year, mostly of children in developing countries (91). Much of the illness is due to endemic disease caused by chronic problems with water supplies, sanitation, and hygiene. Recognized and unrecognized outbreaks, however, probably increase this burden on a continual basis throughout the world and often reach epidemic proportions during natural or anthropogenic disasters. Outbreaks also occur with some regularity in developed nations. In the United States, 689 outbreaks related to drinking water were reported to the CDC from 1971 through 1998 (8, 67, 72, 89). Recreational water was implicated in 83 outbreaks of gastrointestinal disease from 1989 through 1998. Recreational water was also a vehicle for 88 reported outbreaks of meningoencephalitis, dermatitis, and other illnesses. Waterborne disease outbreaks resulting from water microorganisms generally regarded as having low pathogenic potential, such as *Mycobacterium terrae* or *M. fortuitum*, can be a significant problem among hospitalized patients with compromised immune systems (60, 74).

Although only a small proportion of reported cases occur as part of recognized outbreaks, investigation of foodborne and waterborne disease outbreaks provides unique opportunities for prevention. Not only can investigations limit the size and impact of outbreaks, they also can frequently uncover problems in our food and water production and delivery systems that might not otherwise have been discovered. This chapter provides a framework for the investigation of outbreaks due to food or water with a focus on microbiological decisions and procedures. The spectrum of microbial agents known to cause foodborne and waterborne disease outbreaks and methods used to detect outbreaks are discussed. Outbreak detection strategies, general principles of investigation, design of the investigation team, sample selection criteria, and the role of rapid diagnostic methods and molecular subtyping methods are reviewed. Details of clinical specimen collection, transportation to the laboratory, and analytical methodology can be found in other chapters. Sources of standard methods for collection and analysis of clinical, food, water, and environmental samples are described. Although this chapter focuses on investigations of outbreaks in the community, the same general principles apply to hospital or institutional outbreaks. Management of waterborne disease among hospitalized patients is covered in other texts (11, 85).

RATIONALE FOR INVESTIGATING FOODBORNE AND WATERBORNE DISEASE OUTBREAKS

The human and economic costs of foodborne and waterborne disease are high in developed countries and even higher in developing countries. Investigation of foodborne and waterborne disease outbreaks helps reduce those costs by (i) limiting ongoing transmission, (ii) identifying and controlling the underlying problems causing disease, and (iii) identifying trends. A good example of limiting transmission is the 1997 U.S. national outbreak traced to frozen hamburger patties, where 25 million pounds of potentially contaminated meat was recalled (17). Although limiting ongoing transmission is important once an outbreak has occurred, discovery of unforeseen problems in our food and water delivery systems is an even more compelling reason to conduct outbreak investigations. The general requirements of food and water safety are well known, but there is in practice no simple way to achieve universal protection from foodborne or waterborne illness. Food and water safety are complex issues that depend on a combination of environmental, cultural, and socioeconomic factors. For most foodborne and waterborne pathogens, vaccines are not available. Education of consumers and food handlers about basic principles of safe food handling is an important aspect of prevention but is insufficient by itself. Irradiation is very effective at inactivating microorganisms in a number of food matrices but does not prevent contamination during preparation and storage and is not universally accepted by the public. Drinking water delivery systems can be designed to protect consumers, but systems fail, contamination occurs at the point of use, and new pathogens emerge. Direct microbial monitoring of food and water has the potential for detecting problems before consumption but cannot completely ensure safety because of inherent sensitivity, specificity, and economic limitations. In short, problems in our food and water supplies will probably continue into the foreseeable future.

The general strategy for the prevention of foodborne and waterborne diseases is to understand the mechanisms by which contamination and disease transmission occur and to institute appropriate prevention measures. Investigation of outbreaks offers an excellent opportunity to accomplish this objective. Investigations may uncover specific occurrences of contamination or may reveal intrinsic problems in food or water production, processing, storage, distribution, or preparation. Specific control strategies developed as a result of these investigations may be as simple as removing products from distribution, increasing public awareness of safe food-handling practices, or temporary "boil water" orders. Problems uncovered in food or water delivery systems may result in more extensive control measures, such as processing or regulatory changes. Because food production and distribution practices are continually changing and new, unforeseen problems are emerging, the need for continuous monitoring and control efforts is unlikely to diminish. Ultimately, control practices instituted as a result of outbreak investigations help to reduce foodborne and waterborne diseases and improve the overall quality of life of communities and nations.

DEFINITION OF FOODBORNE AND WATERBORNE DISEASE OUTBREAKS

The term "cluster" is often used to describe potential outbreaks before a clear association with a common source has been established. Disease clustering is defined as a closely grouped series of cases of a disease with well-defined distribution patterns in relation to time or place or both (70). The term "outbreak" has been described as follows: "When the observed rate of disease is higher than expected and cases are unusually close together in time and/or space or within the same demographic group, that group of cases is considered an outbreak" (94). A foodborne disease outbreak is generally defined as an incident in which two or more persons experience a similar illness from a common exposure, such as consumption of the same food (92). A similar definition can be used for waterborne disease outbreaks. A single case of certain severe foodborne or waterborne diseases elicits an outbreak-like response because of their unusual nature or potential danger to the community.

This includes such conditions as botulism, gastrointestinal anthrax, primary amebic meningoencephalitis, cholera in an area where disease is not endemic, or variant Creutzfeldt-Jakob disease. The term "waterborne disease outbreaks" includes outbreaks associated with drinking-water supplies and those involving the recreational use of water. Outbreaks caused by contamination of water at point of use, such as outbreaks from vaporizer and whirlpool use, are excluded from the CDC definition of waterborne disease outbreaks (8). This distinction is not made in this chapter, since the source of contamination may not be known at the beginning of an investigation. The complexities of disease transmission sometimes thwart our attempts at precise definition. Since water is used in food processing and preparation, water contamination problems can become food contamination problems. Furthermore, outbreaks initially caused by contaminated food or water may propagate by person-to-person transmission. Both of these situations probably occurred in the 1998 international parsley-associated shigellosis outbreak (23).

GENERAL FEATURES OF FOODBORNE AND WATERBORNE DISEASE OUTBREAKS

The magnitude of foodborne disease outbreaks may range from a small outbreak of only two cases to one that is multinational in scope and involves thousands of cases. Among the largest foodborne disease outbreaks ever recorded are the 1988 outbreak of hepatitis A in Shanghai, China, which was associated with the consumption of raw clams (>300,000 cases) (28); the 1994 nationwide ice cream-associated outbreak of salmonellosis in the United States (>240,000 cases) (50); the outbreak of salmonellosis caused by contaminated pasteurized milk in the midwestern United States (>168,000 cases) (99); and the *Escherichia coli* O157:H7 outbreak among schoolchildren in Japan in 1996 (>6,000 cases) (119). The centralization of food production and globalization of food distribution have greatly increased the chances for large outbreaks of foodborne disease. Waterborne disease outbreaks can also be large, such as the 1993 outbreak of cryptosporidiosis in Milwaukee, Wis. (>400,000 cases) (77), and the *E. coli* O157:H7 outbreak in Walkerton, Ontario, Canada, in 2000 (1,346 cases, 27 cases of hemolytic-uremic syndrome, and 6 deaths) (5). Waterborne disease outbreaks are a frequent consequence of natural disasters. Two examples are leptospirosis in Nicaragua in 1999, due to Hurricane Mitch (16), and widespread diarrheal disease from disruption of water systems due to the 1999 earthquake in Kocaeli, Turkey (112).

The scope of investigations may be narrowly focused on specific disease clusters or may involve broader investigations into the causes of sporadic disease in the population. For example, analyses stimulated by an outbreak investigation identified eggs as the most important source of *Salmonella enterica* serovar Enteritidis infections (106). Other investigations revealed that most sporadic cases of *Campylobacter jejuni* and *C. coli* infections during the summer months appear to be associated with handling and eating undercooked poultry, while the relatively infrequent outbreaks due to *C. jejuni* and *C. coli* occurring during spring and fall are caused by the consumption of unpasteurized milk or untreated surface water (94).

Outbreaks are frequently high-profile events that can have important political, social, and economic consequences. As such, a coherent public message is a hallmark of the well-managed investigation. Successful investigations normally require a high level of coordination between epidemiology and laboratory teams. Often, coordination between public health and food or water regulatory agencies is also necessary, at multiple jurisdictional levels.

Foodborne disease outbreaks occur in communities and, less frequently, in hospitals, nursing homes, and other institutions. Although relatively rare, the cost of foodborne outbreaks in hospitals can be high, estimated in one outbreak to be as high as $400,000 in 1988 dollars (125). Institutional outbreaks are of especial concern when pregnant women or elderly or immunocompromised individuals are involved, since these populations are at risk for increased morbidity and mortality (101, 102). Waterborne gastrointestinal disease outbreaks occur primarily in communities and rarely in hospitals and nursing homes. The source of most drinking-water outbreaks in the United States is contaminated wells, but surface water, springs, and combined sources also have been implicated (8). Waterborne respiratory disease outbreaks are occasionally documented in the community (63, 90), in the workplace (1), and in whirlpool baths (44, 76). These types of outbreaks are frequently reported in hospitals (13, 24, 65, 124).

Agents Responsible for Gastrointestinal Disease Outbreaks

Of the 2,751 foodborne disease outbreaks reported to CDC from 1993 through 1997, 655 (23.8%) were caused by bacteria, 148 (5.4%) were caused by chemicals, 19 (0.7%) were caused by parasites, 56 (4.2%) were caused by viruses, and 1,873 (68.1%) were of unknown etiology. The most commonly reported bacterial agents were *Salmonella*, *E. coli* O157:H7, and *Clostridium perfringens* (92). Outbreaks caused by viruses are probably greatly underestimated due to the lack of widespread testing capability. Human caliciviruses, also known as Norwalk-like agents, alone are thought to be responsible for 9,200,000 (12.1%) of the 76,000,000 cases of foodborne disease in the United States (87) and probably cause a large proportion of unexplained outbreaks.

Of the 691 outbreaks associated with drinking water that were reported to the CDC between 1971 and 1998, 89 (12.9%) were caused by bacteria, 79 (11.4%) were caused by chemicals, 32 (4.6%) were caused by parasites, 53 (7.7%) were caused by viruses, and 336 (48.6%) were of unknown etiology (8). Toxigenic *Vibrio cholerae* O1 and rarely *V. cholerae* O139 are the cause of life-threatening outbreaks in a number of developing countries and may be transmitted by either food or water. The most common agents of foodborne and waterborne disease outbreaks are summarized in Table 1; their incubation period, clinical syndrome, and confirmation criteria are also included.

Agents Responsible for Extraintestinal Disease Outbreaks

Most recognized foodborne outbreaks result in primary gastrointestinal presentation, but some outbreak agents present primarily in other sites. Examples include *Toxoplasma gondii*, *Listeria monocytogenes*, hepatitis A virus, and *Trichinella spiralis*. Foodborne outbreaks of group A streptococcus occasionally occur, although that is not the primary mode of transmission (27). Outbreaks of extraintestinal waterborne disease occur primarily through (i) inhalation of aerosolized water; (ii) ingestion of contaminated tap water or recreational water; (iii) direct contact with contaminated water, as during recreational activity or

hydrotherapy; or (iv) contact with contaminated water on improperly reprocessed medical devices. *Legionella* is responsible for both community and nosocomial outbreaks of Legionnaires' disease and Pontiac fever. Legionnaires' disease occurs after inhalation of large numbers of viable cells in aerosolized water by susceptible hosts, giving rise to primary pneumonia. Pontiac fever occurs after inhalation of dead cells, causing an acute flu-like illness without pneumonia. Although *Legionella pneumophila* is the most commonly implicated agent of Pontiac fever, aerosolized endotoxin from other gram-negative bacteria has been implicated in outbreaks of similar acute febrile illness (1, 90). Nosocomial outbreaks are often caused by the concentration in water-using devices of opportunistic pathogens normally present in potable water, such as *Pseudomonas aeruginosa*, other *Pseudomonas* spp., *Burkholderia cepacia*, *Ralstonia pickettii*, and *Stenotrophomonas maltophilia*. Other water-inhabiting bacteria, such as *Chryseobacterium meningosepticum*, have been implicated in community and nosocomial outbreaks of meningitis. Cases of encephalitis or meningoencephalitis may be caused by parasites such as *Naegleria*, *Acanthamoeba*, or *Balamuthia*. Outbreaks of dermatitis occur due to bacteria such as *P. aeruginosa* or other *Pseudomonas* spp. in improperly treated swimming or spa water or as "swimmer's itch," caused by cercariae of bird schistosomes acquired during recreational water use (71). Rare outbreaks of keratitis due to *Acanthamoeba* spp. have been reported (84). Acute, generalized disease due to *Leptospira interrogans* occurs in an epidemic fashion among swimmers in natural waters or as an aftermath of floods (16, 21, 22). In developed countries, outbreaks of acute schistosomiasis occur among travelers to areas of endemic infection (36).

DETECTION OF OUTBREAKS

Community foodborne and waterborne disease outbreaks are detected either by pathogen-specific surveillance programs for such conditions as salmonellosis, campylobacteriosis, or listeriosis or as a result of self-reporting by consumers or clinicians. Outbreak detection by pathogen-specific surveillance is typically a passive process. For passive surveillance to work, physicians must order bacterial cultures from ill patients and clinical laboratories must recover the pathogens under surveillance. Then, reports and isolates must be forwarded to Public Health Departments. These agencies then must interview patients, further characterize the pathogens, and investigate clusters. The effectiveness of these programs is dependent on routine species identification by diagnostic laboratories. Systematic subspecies identification at public health laboratories is an integral part of a number of surveillance activities, such as serotyping in the U.S. National Salmonella Surveillance System. A good example of outbreak detection by serotype surveillance is the 1995 national ice cream-associated outbreak, which resulted in over 250,000 cases (50). The CDC Salmonella Outbreak Detection Algorithm (SODA) is an automated system which utilizes national serotype data to monitor trends and detect potential outbreaks, including those that are multistate or national in scope (55). Recently, foodborne and waterborne disease surveillance has been yet further enhanced by molecular subtype surveillance utilizing pulsed-field gel electrophoresis (PFGE), allowing the detection of outbreaks that would have previously been unrecognized (9, 10, 35). National networks such as PulseNet in North America (107) and Salm-Net in Europe

TABLE 1 Guidelines for confirmation of foodborne and waterborne disease outbreaks[a]

Etiologic agent	Incubation period	Clinical syndrome	Confirmation
Bacterial			
Bacillus cereus			
Vomiting toxin	1–6 h	Vomiting, occasional diarrhea; fever uncommon	Isolation of organism from stool of two or more ill persons and not from stool of controls OR Isolation of $\geq 10^5$ organisms/g from epidemiologically implicated food, provided the specimen is properly handled
Diarrheal toxin	6–24 h	Diarrhea, abdominal cramps, and vomiting in some patients; fever uncommon	Isolation of organism from stool of two or more ill persons and not from stool of controls OR Isolation of $\geq 10^5$ organisms/g from epidemiologically implicated food, provided the specimen is properly handled
Brucella	Several days to several months, usually >30 days	Weakness, fever, headache, sweats, chills, arthralgia, weight loss, splenomegaly	Two or more ill persons and isolation of organism in culture of blood or bone marrow, greater than fourfold increase in standard agglutination titer (SAT) over several weeks, or single SAT titer of >1:160 in a person with compatible clinical symptoms and history of exposure
Campylobacter	2–10 days, usually 2–5 days	Diarrhea (often bloody), abdominal pain, fever	Isolation of organism from clinical specimens from two or more ill persons OR Isolation of organism from epidemiologically implicated food or water
Clostridium botulinum	2 h–8 days, usually 2–5 days	Illness of variable severity; common symptoms are diplopia, blurred vision, and bulbar weakness; paralysis, which is usually descending and bilateral, may progress rapidly	Detection of botulinal toxin in serum, stool, gastric contents, or implicated food OR Isolation of organism from stool or intestine
Clostridium perfringens	6–24 h	Diarrhea, abdominal cramps; vomiting and fever uncommon	Isolation of $\geq 10^6$ organisms/g in stool of two or more ill persons, provided the specimen is properly handled OR Demonstration of enterotoxin in the stool of two or more ill persons OR Isolation of $\geq 10^5$ organisms/g from epidemiologically implicated food, provided the specimen is properly handled

(Continued on next page)

TABLE 1 Guidelines for confirmation of foodborne and waterborne disease outbreaks[a] (*Continued*)

Etiologic agent	Incubation period	Clinical syndrome	Confirmation
Escherichia coli			
Enterohemorrhagic (*E. coli* O157:H7 and other serotypes that produce Shiga toxins) (EHEC)	1–10 days, usually 4–5 days; approximately 6% go on to develop hemolytic-uremic syndrome (HUS) (children) or thrombotic thrombocytopenic purpura (TTP) (adults)	Diarrhea (often bloody), abdominal cramps (often severe), little or no fever; acute renal failure in HUS or TTP	Isolation of *E. coli* O157:H7 or other Shiga toxin-producing *E. coli* strain from clinical specimen of two or more ill persons OR Isolation of *E. coli* O157:H7 or other Shiga toxin-producing *E. coli* strain from epidemiologically implicated food
Enterotoxigenic *E. coli* (ETEC)	6–48 h	Diarrhea, abdominal cramps, nausea; vomiting and fever less common	Isolation of organisms of the same serotype, which are demonstrated to produce heat-stable (ST) and/or heat-labile (LT) enterotoxin, from stool of two or more ill persons
Enteropathogenic *E. coli* (EPEC)	Variable	Diarrhea, fever, abdominal cramps	Isolation of the same enteropathogenic serotype from stool of two or more ill persons
Enteroinvasive *E. coli* (EIEC)	Variable	Diarrhea (may be bloody), fever, abdominal cramps	Isolation of the same enteroinvasive serotype from stool of two or more ill persons
Legionella spp.	2–10 days (Legionnaires' disease) 5–66 h (Pontiac fever)	Anorexia, malaise, myalgia, headache, fever, cough, pneumonia (Legionnaires' disease)	Evidence of exposure or disease in two or more epidemiologically linked individuals (culture, urine antigen, or fourfold rise in antibody titer); identification of same species epidemiologically in a plausible water source is useful only when isolate matches patient isolates by appropriate molecular subtyping method
Leptospira interrogans	4–19 days (usually 10 days)	Fever, headache, chills, severe myalgia, conjunctival suffusion; occasionally other systemic manifestations including meningitis, myocarditis, or hepatorenal failure	Evidence of disease in two or more epidemiologically linked patients; diagnosis is by culture (cerebrospinal fluid, blood, or urine) using special media, serology (fourfold rise in titers), immunofluorescence, and enzyme immunoassay
Listeria monocytogenes			
Invasive disease	2–6 wk	Meningitis, meningoencephalitis, neonatal sepsis, abortions, stillbirths	Isolation of organism from blood or cerebrospinal fluid of two or more patients and the same serotype and subtype of organism from implicated food(s)
Diarrheal disease	9–32 h	Diarrhea, abdominal cramps, fever	Isolation of organism of same serotype from stool of two or more ill persons exposed to food that is epidemiologically implicated or from which an organism of the same serotype has been isolated
Nontyphoidal *Salmonella*	6 h–10 days, usually 6–48 h	Diarrhea, often with fever and abdominal cramps	Isolation of organism of same serotype and subtype from clinical specimens from two or more ill persons OR Isolation of organism from epidemiologically implicated food

(*Continued on next page*)

TABLE 1 *(Continued)*

Etiologic agent	Incubation period	Clinical syndrome	Confirmation
Salmonella serotype Typhi	3–60 days, usually 7–14 days	Fever, anorexia, malaise, headache, and myalgia; sometimes diarrhea and constipation	Isolation of organism of same serotype from clinical specimens from two or more ill persons OR Isolation of organism from epidemiologically implicated food
Shigella	12 h–6 days, usually 2–4 days	Diarrhea (often bloody), frequently accompanied by fever and abdominal cramps	Isolation of organism of same serotype from clinical specimens from two or more ill persons OR Isolation of organism from epidemiologically implicated food or water
Staphylococcus aureus	30 min–8 h, usually 2–4 h	Vomiting, diarrhea	Isolation of organism of same phage type/molecular subtype from stool or vomitus of two or more ill persons OR Detection of same serotype of enterotoxin in epidemiologically implicated food
Streptococcus group A	1–4 days	Fever, pharyngitis, scarlet fever, upper respiratory infection	Isolation of organism of same M or T type from throats of two or more ill persons OR Isolation of organism of same M or T type from epidemiologically implicated food
Vibrio cholerae O1 or O139	1–5 days	Watery diarrhea, often accompanied by vomiting	Isolation of toxigenic organism from stool or vomitus of two or more ill persons OR Significant rise in vibriocidal, bacterial agglutination, or antitoxin antibodies in acute- and early convalescent-phase sera among persons not recently immunized OR Isolation of toxigenic organism from epidemiologically implicated food or water
Vibrio parahaemolyticus	4–30 h	Diarrhea	Isolation of Kanagawa-positive organism from stool of two or more ill persons OR Isolation of $\geq 10^5$ Kanagawa-positive organisms/g from epidemiologically implicated food or water, provided the specimen is properly handled
Yersinia enterocolitica	1–10 days, usually 4–6 days	Diarrhea, abdominal pain (often severe)	Isolation of organism from clinical specimens of two or more ill persons OR Isolation of pathogenic strain or organism from epidemiologically implicated food

(Continued on next page)

TABLE 1   Guidelines for confirmation of foodborne and waterborne disease outbreaks[a] *(Continued)*

Etiologic agent	Incubation period	Clinical syndrome	Confirmation
Chemical			
Marine toxins			
Ciguatoxin	1–48 h, usually 2–8 h	Usually gastrointestinal symptoms followed by neurologic symptoms (including paresthesia of lips, tongue, throat, or extremities) and reversal of hot and cold sensation	Demonstration of ciguatoxin in epidemiologically implicated fish OR Clinical syndrome among persons who have eaten a type of fish previously associated with ciguatera fish poisoning (e.g., snapper, grouper, or barracuda)
Scombroid toxin (histamine)	1 min–3 h, usually less than 1 h	Flushing, dizziness, burning of mouth and throat, headache, gastrointestinal symptoms, urticaria, and generalized pruritus	Demonstration of histamine in epidemiologically implicated food OR Clinical syndrome among persons who have eaten a type of fish previously associated with histamine fish poisoning (e.g., mahimahi or fish of order Scombroidei)
Paralytic or neurotoxic shellfish poison	30 min–3 h	Paresthesia of lips, mouth, or face, and extremities; intestinal symptoms or weakness, including respiratory difficulty	Detection of toxin in epidemiologically implicated food OR Detection of large numbers of shellfish poisoning-associated species of dinoflagellates in water from which epidemiologically implicated mollusks were gathered OR Demonstration of tetrodotoxin in epidemiologically implicated fish
Puffer fish, tetrodotoxin	10 min–3 h, usually 10–45 min	Paresthesia of lips, tongue, face, or extremities, often following numbness; loss of proprioception or "floating" sensations	Demonstration of tetrodotoxin in epidemiologically implicated fish OR Clinical syndrome among persons who ate puffer fish
Heavy metals (antimony, cadmium, copper, iron, tin, zinc)	5 min–8 h, usually less than 1 h	Vomiting, often a metallic taste	Demonstration of high concentration of metal in epidemiologically implicated food or water
Monosodium glutamate (MSG)	3 min–2 h, usually less than 1 h	Burning sensation in chest, neck, abdomen, or extremities; sensation of lightness and pressure over face or heavy feeling in chest	Clinical syndrome among persons who have eaten food containing MSG (usually ≥1.5 g of MSG)
Mushroom toxins			
Shorter-acting toxins (muscimol, muscarine, psilocybin, coprine [produced by *Coprinus atramentarius*], ibotenic acid)	2 h	Usually vomiting and diarrhea; other symptoms (confusion and visual disturbance [muscimol, ibotenic acid], salivation and diaphoresis [muscarine], hallucinations [psilocybin], disulfiram-like reaction [*C. artementaris* toxin]) differ with toxin	Clinical syndrome among persons who have eaten mushroom identified as toxic type OR Demonstration of toxin in epidemiologically implicated mushroom or mushroom-containing food

(Continued on next page)

TABLE 1 *(Continued)*

Etiologic agent	Incubation period	Clinical syndrome	Confirmation
Longer-acting toxin (e.g., produced by *Amanita* spp.)	6–24 h	Diarrhea and abdominal cramps for 24 h followed by hepatic and renal failure	Clinical syndrome among persons who have eaten mushroom identified as toxic type OR Demonstration of toxin in epidemiologically implicated mushroom or mushroom-containing food
Parasitic			
Cryptosporidium parvum	2–28 days, median 7 days	Diarrhea, nausea, vomiting, fever	Demonstration of organism or antigen in stool or in small-bowel biopsy specimens from two or more ill persons OR Demonstration of organism in epidemiologically implicated food or water
Cyclospora cayetanensis	1–11 days, median 7 days	Fatigue, protracted diarrhea, often relapsing	Demonstration of organism in stool of two or more ill persons
Giardia lamblia	3–25 days, median 7 days	Diarrhea, gas, cramps, nausea, fatigue	Two or more ill persons and detection of antigen in stool or demonstration of organism in stool, duodenal contents, or small-bowel biopsy specimen
Trichinella spp.	1–2 days for intestinal phase; 2–4 wk for systemic phase	Fever, myalgia, periorbital edema, high eosinophil count	Two or more ill persons and positive serologic test or demonstration of larvae in muscle biopsy specimen OR Demonstration of larvae in epidemiologically implicated meat
Viral			
Hepatitis A virus	15–50 days, median 28 days	Jaundice, dark urine, fatigue, anorexia, nausea	Detection of immunoglobulin M anti-hepatitis A virus in serum from two or more persons who consumed epidemiologically implicated food or water
Norwalk family of viruses, small round-structured viruses (NLV)	15–77 h, usually 24–48 h	Vomiting, cramps, diarrhea, headache	Detection of viral RNA in stool or vomitus by RT-PCR OR More than fourfold rise in antibody titer to Norwalk virus or Norwalk-like virus in acute- and convalescent-phase sera in most serum pairs OR Visualization of small, round-structured viruses that react with patient's convalescent-phase sera but not acute-phase sera by immunoelectron microscopy
Astrovirus	15–77 h, usually 24–48 h	Vomiting, cramps, diarrhea, headache	Detection of virus antigen by EIA OR Detection of viral RNA in stool or vomitus by RT-PCR OR Visualization of viruses with characteristic surface morphology by electron microscopy

[a] Modified from reference 18.

(47) have brought molecular subtype surveillance to a national and international scale, allowing the detection of multistate and multinational outbreaks that would otherwise have been considered local problems or would not have been detected at all. An example of enhanced national outbreak detection by molecular subtyping is the multistate outbreak of *Listeria monocytogenes* in 2000, which was traced to contaminated delicatessen meats (20). Both serotyping and subtyping improve the likelihood of identifying potential outbreaks of relatively common pathogens such as *Salmonella* and *E. coli* O157:H7. By classifying the pathogens to the strain level, emerging disease clusters can be differentiated from background sporadic and unrelated cases. Subtype-specific disease surveillance programs are most efficient when (i) standardized protocols are used, (ii) laboratories perform serotyping or subtyping and report results in real time, and (iii) patients are interviewed quickly. Routine examination of data by time, place, person, and agent factors increases the likelihood of recognizing outbreaks as they occur.

Whereas the etiologic agent is usually known in outbreaks detected by pathogen-specific surveillance, the agent must often be determined in outbreaks detected by self-reporting. Under these circumstances, investigators rely on a combination of clinical features of the illness, available laboratory data, and other epidemiological findings to establish presumptive causation. This is the outbreak detection mechanism by which most outbreaks caused by unusual or viral agents are identified. Examples of this include outbreaks of enterotoxigenic *E. coli* (38, 52, 69), hepatitis A virus (54), or Norwalk-like virus (25, 68, 98) infections. This activity also results in the discovery of new or unrecognized agents, such as *Legionella* spp., *Cyclospora cayetanensis* (51, 95), and the enteropathogenic *E. coli*-like *E. coli* O39:NM (49).

THE INVESTIGATION TEAM

Outbreak investigations can be logistically complicated, involving multiple professions, institutions, government agencies, and the public. The successful investigation utilizes a team approach, with clear responsibilities and lines of communication. In general, the team approach involves the following steps: (i) a team of qualified individuals is recruited to conduct the investigation; (ii) a team leader is appointed; (iii) lines of communications are established between team members and important collaborators such as the health care community, public, or media; (iv) team members are assigned responsibilities; and (v) a system is established for data collection, retrieval, and analysis (15). This process generally needs to occur expeditiously to prevent loss of potential information. Rapid formation of the team is critical when ongoing transmission is possible.

The core team generally includes epidemiologists and laboratorians but may also include sanitarians, health care physicians, infection control practitioners, engineers, administrators, statisticians, and media liaisons. Depending on the scope of the outbreak and the jurisdictions involved, the team may include representatives from multiple organizational levels, from individual institutions up to national or international governments. It may also include representatives from multiple government agencies, each handling a different aspect of the problem. When resources are low or for small outbreaks, some individuals may assume multiple roles.

The team leader is often an experienced epidemiologist with primary investigative authority. This individual directs team members to collect, codify, and analyze incoming outbreak information; forms a hypothesis; dispatches sample collectors and oversees their activities; oversees information given to the health care community, the public, and the media regarding the outbreak investigation; and devises immediate intervention strategies.

Epidemiologists are responsible for the collection and analysis of information to determine the cause of the outbreak. They analyze disease case reports, laboratory reports, medical information, patient interviews, and other information under the direction of the team leader. Once an outbreak source has been determined, they are usually involved in various aspects of coordinating and documenting intervention activities.

Sanitarians are charged with examination and analysis of the food preparation and processing methods to search for deviations from standard operating procedures that may have resulted in the foodborne illness. Sanitarians are trained in Good Manufacturing Practice inspections and Hazard Analysis Critical Control Points investigative techniques which are used to identify such food processing and preparation problems as cross-contamination of raw foods with cooked foods and improper cooking and/or holding temperatures (15, 86, 103). Sanitarians receive consumer complaints regarding restaurants, other food service establishments, and food products provided by retail vendors. After review and analysis of complaint information, they decide whether sufficient information has accumulated to warrant the initiation of a formal investigation. More detailed description of the typical procedures used by both epidemiologists and sanitarians during investigations of foodborne illness outbreaks can be found elsewhere (15, 120).

Microbiologists are often the first individuals to notice suspicious clusters and thus can be pivotal in outbreak discovery. They are responsible for analyzing human specimens, food, water, or environmental samples to detect agents of illness or their toxins. Their presence on the team enhances the quality of outbreak management by providing information on the selection, collection, transport, and analysis of samples and the interpretation of results. The laboratory team member is sometimes given responsibility for organizing sample collection, transport, and testing schedules. By communicating with other laboratories, the microbiologist can identify additional cases that are "in the pipeline," i.e., identified by local laboratories but not yet reported to local authorities. The microbiologist is also invaluable in detecting potential or actual pseudo-outbreaks caused by laboratory errors or test malfunctions.

Media professionals often participate in outbreaks that attract attention from electronic and print media. Inconsistent messages can lead to fear and confusion among the public, inappropriate political pressure, and a damaged investigation. The presence of an experienced and knowledgeable information officer who can respond to inquiries from the media and the public can be invaluable (46).

Other types of professionals may be included in the team, depending on circumstances. For instance, outbreaks involving drinking water frequently require experts in plumbing, heating, or cooling systems. Outbreaks involving recreational water may require the experience of civil engineers or park officials. Representatives of emergency response teams or local government officials are necessary in some situations.

STEPS IN AN OUTBREAK INVESTIGATION

The following steps typically occur in an outbreak investigation. These steps do not always happen in the same order, and many activities may occur simultaneously. (i) Establish case definitions(s). (ii) Confirm that cases are "real." (iii) Confirm the outbreak and determine its scope. (iv) Examine the descriptive epidemiological features of the cases. (v) Generate hypotheses. (vi) Test hypotheses. (vii) Collect and test environmental samples (including food and water). (viii) Implement control measures. (ix) Interact with the press and inform the public (96).

A case definition focuses the investigation on ill individuals likely to be related to the outbreak and improves the specificity of the ensuing analyses. This is especially important for gastrointestinal disease outbreaks, since sporadic diarrheal illnesses are likely to be present in any population whether or not an outbreak is occurring. If the outbreak was identified by pathogen-specific surveillance, an individual may be classified as a case simply by being infected by the agent in question during a particular time interval or in a certain location. If the agent is unknown, which is often the circumstance for self-reported outbreaks, the case definition is often based on symptom, time, and place criteria. As new information becomes available, the case definition may be narrowed or broadened, depending on the situation. The case definition can be disseminated to health care providers or the public to detect additional cases.

In some outbreaks, it may be necessary to reconcile case reports with medical and laboratory records to determine if the cases are "real." This is necessary to rule out pseudo-outbreaks, such as those caused by a malfunctioning or misused laboratory test kit. Determining which cases are real can be especially challenging in waterborne outbreaks of Legionnaires' disease, whose symptoms can be nonspecific.

The background rate of disease is examined to determine if the number of observed cases is greater than what can be expected in the population. This determination is relatively straightforward if the outbreak agent is known and if tests for the agent are routinely performed in the community. For example, the background rate of *Listeria* sepsis can generally be determined, since blood cultures and identification are normally performed on patients with sepsis. Background rates can be difficult to determine if the case definition is broad or if the agent is known but testing does not routinely occur in the community. Under these circumstances, it may be necessary to collect and test samples from the community. For example, a team investigating a possible outbreak of Legionnaires' disease in a hospital collected sera not only from hospital staff but also from members of the community. They discovered background rates in the community similar to the rate in the hospital, suggesting that the outbreak was community based rather than hospital based (31). The scope of the outbreak is determined by seeking additional cases, often by publicizing the case definition among health care professionals or the public.

Preliminary outbreak information is summarized in the descriptive epidemiology phase of the investigation. A common way of viewing the data is by time, place, person, and agent factors. Time generally refers to the temporal distribution of disease after exposure to an etiological agent, using such terms as "onset time" and "incubation period." Place refers to common physical locations at which an exposure may have occurred, such as a particular community or restaurant patronized by patients. Person factors include demographic characteristics such as age, gender, race, and ethnicity or other determinants such as health status, belonging to the same organization, or eating the same foods as other patients. Agent factors include species, strain, host range, transmissibility, natural reservoir, antibiotic susceptibility, expected spectrum of illness, and other characteristics. Case information can be displayed using epidemiological curves (time), maps (place), demographic and medical description of cases (person), and compiled laboratory data (agent). These different representations help investigators more easily recognize patterns, often suggest causation, and help with the hypothesis generation.

Hypothesis generation utilizes all existing microbiological and epidemiological data coupled with information about the agent, open-ended interviews of patients, or a wide variety of other possible information sources. The case-control study is a common way of testing the hypothesis in foodborne and waterborne outbreaks. The type of control group varies with the nature of the investigation, but often controls are randomly chosen, non-ill individuals of similar age and gender to the patients and residing in the same community. Patients and controls are interviewed about their exposure histories by using a standard series of questions, which allows a consistent and detailed description of the illness and its relationship to exposures. The case-control study makes it possible to tease out common exposures that are not related to the illness. For instance, in the 1996 outbreak of *Cyclospora cayetansis* in Florida, 87.2% of patients ate bananas and only 65.1% ate raspberries. However, 77.9% of controls also ate bananas but only 6.8% ate raspberries, giving a low degree of association with bananas, and a high association with raspberries (59). Statistical significance itself is not sufficient to identify outbreak causation. It is also necessary to consider confounding factors, effect modifiers, biological plausibility, and secondary person-to-person spread. A dose-response relationship between agent and illness adds strength to the proof of hypothesis. For instance, in the 1999 outbreak of Legionnaires' disease at a Netherlands floral show, exhibitors nearer to a particular whirlpool spa were found to have higher average antibody levels (14). If a common exposure is not identified, additional hypotheses are needed. It is possible that the actual exposure was not considered, patient recall was faulty, or the number of cases was too small (96). The common exposure may be specific, such as a particular product, or may be less specific, such as eating at a particular restaurant or consuming products from one processor. If a product is implicated, a trace-back can be initiated, and the investigation can branch into an examination of the chain of transmission leading to the event. If only a general location is associated with illness, on-site investigation is particularly important. Sanitarians or water system experts are critical at this stage. Specific knowledge about the agent is also invaluable for further identifying problem behaviors, systems, or individual products. For instance, Norwalk virus gastroenteritis is often associated with food handlers who have a recent history of diarrheal illness and inadequate hand hygiene. *S. enterica* serovar Enteritidis is often associated with contaminated eggs or products made with eggs. Cross-contamination with poultry products is suspected in outbreaks of *Campylobacter jejuni*.

Food, water, or environmental samples should be collected and stored as soon as suspicious sources are identified, but testing of food, water, or the environment should ideally be deferred until there is specific epidemiological evidence linking the sample to the illness. A more detailed strategy for testing is provided later in this chapter. Although microbiological confirmation is comforting, it is not always necessary before implementing interventions. If the epidemiological association is sufficiently strong, actions can be taken in the absence of microbiological confirmation, and hence additional cases may be prevented. The intervention could be as simple as recommending procedural changes at a restaurant or as significant as product recalls, "boil-water" orders, or public notices. Concurrently, implicated clinical, food, or environmental samples are tested for the suspect etiologic agent. If the epidemiological association is inconclusive, microbiological confirmation may be essential before interventions are undertaken. Microbial isolates identified in the laboratory may be further analyzed for other markers, such as antibiotic susceptibility, molecular subtype, or specific virulence factors. When all investigations are complete, final analyses are conducted and a long-range prevention strategy is formulated.

Once the cause of the outbreak has been determined, the final job of the team is to explain its findings to those affected by the outbreak. A clear message not only addresses fears and misconceptions of the public but also can be a valuable education tool.

MICROBIOLOGICAL METHODS FOR OUTBREAK DETECTION AND INVESTIGATION

General Strategies for Specimen Selection and Testing

Standardized, validated procedures such as those in the *Clinical Microbiology Procedures Handbook* (56) or the *Bacteriological Analytical Manual* (57) should be used. Improvised culture techniques and attempts to adapt clinical microbiology culture methods to food, water, or environmental analysis are rarely successful and can result in the loss of critical samples to the investigative process. Standard procedures are not available for detection of some types of outbreak-causing agents, such as Norwalk-like virus, or for some types of foods. Under these circumstances, it is sometimes necessary to develop, verify, and validate procedures in-house prior to use or to forward samples to a laboratory with validated procedures. Guidelines are available for verification and validation of clinical microbiology procedures (37). Although there are currently no standard criteria for in-house validation of food testing procedures, discussions to create such a document are under way. Peer review of validation data is available through AOAC International (Gaithersburg, Md.). The principle used in the test should be firmly grounded in the peer-review literature. Any report generated using such a test should reflect its nonstandard status and should clearly state the limitations to be applied to interpretation.

- Isolates or samples known to be unrelated to the outbreak may be needed for control purposes. For example, when performing PFGE on a serotype of *Salmonella* that has not been previously tested, it is important to obtain unrelated isolates of the same serotype to determine that there is sufficient heterogeneity with the conditions used to make a meaningful comparison.

- In certain outbreak situations where the outbreak etiological agent is known, it may be advisable to streamline

the culture protocol. For instance, in a food handler-associated restaurant outbreak of *S. enterica* serovar Typhimurium, employee stool samples may be screened using an abbreviated procedure that does not include protocols specific for *E. coli* O157:H7 or *Campylobacter* spp., which are normally part of the standard test battery.

- Outbreaks of unknown etiology present special challenges for the investigating laboratory. Until the etiology of an outbreak has been determined, it is important to save patient specimens, culture plates, DNA extracts, or other biological material relevant to the investigation for possible further action. If the epidemiological findings suggest an agent that the investigating laboratory does not test for, or if the disease presentation is in any way unusual, assistance from local or regional sources should be sought at the beginning of the investigation. If testing is not performed locally, advice about specimen collection, transport, and testing should be sought. In the United States, state and local public health laboratories should be contacted, which may in turn contact the CDC. Occasionally, outbreaks occur with unusual symptoms that suggest a new or unrecognized agent, such as the Brainerd diarrhea outbreak of 1983 to 1984 (12, 118). In these situations, early consultation with state or national experts is essential for acquiring appropriate patient material.

Criteria for Collection of Fecal Specimens

Fecal specimens collected from ill persons may not yield a pathogen if they were collected at an inappropriate time (for example, after initiation of treatment with antimicrobial agents) or were collected or handled inappropriately. CDC has published detailed recommendations for collection of laboratory specimens associated with gastroenteritis outbreaks (73). Instructions for collection of stool specimens from ill persons for investigations of foodborne disease outbreaks are given in Table 2, which is adapted from the CDC recommendations. Collecting timely specimens in an outbreak setting may require specific effort, such as courier transport of samples from the patient's home.

Criteria for Collection of Food, Water, and Environmental Samples

In general, the decision to test food, water, or the environment should be driven by epidemiological analysis, not vice versa. Mass testing of food, water, or environmental samples is rarely productive, gives erroneous or hard-to-interpret data, and is a poor use of resources. The investigative team may get sidetracked with difficult management decisions that are tangential to the investigation but that cannot be ignored. For instance, if hospital water supplies are tested for *L. pneumophila* after a case has been identified but before an epidemiological investigation, a positive result might be obtained. Since *L. pneumophila* is common in aqueous environments, the significance of this result would be unclear. However, in this scenario even if investigators learn that the infection could not have been acquired in the hospital, the earlier positive water test will force them to consider difficult and expensive remediation decisions. Similarly, screening of all food items in a restaurant outbreak is labor-intensive, only rarely identifies a common vehicle, but similarly often leads to hard-to-interpret findings.

Although mass screening of samples is not recommended, any potentially implicated food, water, or environmental samples should be collected and properly stored

TABLE 2 General instructions for collecting, storing, and transporting stool specimens

Procedure	Instructions regarding specimens to be tested for:		
	Viruses	Bacteria	Parasites
Collection			
When to collect	Within 48 h after onset of illness.	During period of active diarrhea (preferably as soon as possible).	Any time after onset of illness (preferably as soon as possible).
How much to collect	As much stool sample as possible from each of 10 ill persons (a minimum of 10 ml of stool from each); samples may also be obtained from 10 controls.	Two rectal swabs or swabs of each stool from each of 10 ill persons; samples may also be obtained from 10 controls. Also, whole stools may be collected. When testing food handlers or other individuals in a potential chain of transmission, stool cultures should be taken and tested until there are a minimum of two consecutive negative stools collected not less than 24 h apart.	A fresh stool sample from each of 10 ill persons; samples may also be obtained from 10 controls. At least three specimens collected 48 h or more apart should be obtained from each patient.
Method of collection	Place fresh specimens (liquid preferable), unmixed with urine, in clean, dry containers.	For rectal swabs, moisten each of two swabs in an appropriate transport medium (Cary-Blair, Stuart, Amies, etc.; buffered glycerol-saline is suitable for *E. coli*, *Salmonella*, *Shigella*, and *Y. enterocolitica* but not for *Campylobacter* and *Vibrio*) and then insert sequentially into the rectum and gently rotate. Place both swabs into the same Cary-Blair medium tube. Break off top portion of swab sticks and discard.	Collect a bulk stool specimen, unmixed with urine, in a clean container. Place a portion of each stool sample into 10% formalin and polyvinyl alcohol preservatives (or other commercial preservative) at a ratio of 1 part stool to 3 parts preservative. Mix well. A portion of the unpreserved stool may be saved for antigen testing or PCR testing.
Storage	Immediately refrigerate at 4°C. Specimens for electron microscopic examination should not be frozen. A portion of each stool specimen may be stored frozen at −15°C or lower for antigen or PCR testing.	Immediately refrigerate at 4°C if testing is to be done within 48 h after collection. If testing is to be done after 48 h, store samples frozen at −70°C. (Same recommendations apply for whole stools.) A portion of each stool specimen may be stored frozen at −15°C or lower for antigen or PCR testing.	Store at room temperature or refrigerate at 4°C. DO NOT FREEZE. Store unpreserved stool specimen frozen at −15°C or lower for antigen or PCR testing.
Transportation to testing laboratory[a]	Keep refrigerated. Place bagged and sealed specimens on ice or frozen refrigerant packs in an insulated box. Send by overnight mail. DO NOT FREEZE. Send frozen specimens on dry ice for antigen or PCR testing.	Refrigerate as instructed for viral specimens. Place bagged and sealed frozen specimens on dry ice in an insulated box, and send by overnight mail.	Refrigerate preserved stool as instructed for viral specimens. For room temperature specimens, mail in waterproof containers. For antigen and/or PCR testing, place bagged and sealed frozen specimens on dry ice in an insulated box and send by overnight mail.

[a] Label each specimen with a waterproof marker. Pack samples in sealed, waterproof containers. Batch the collection and send by overnight mail to arrive in the testing laboratory on a weekday during business hours, unless other arrangements have been made with the testing laboratory in advance. Give the testing laboratory as much advance notice as possible so that testing can begin as soon as samples arrive.

as soon as possible. In response to outbreaks, food is often discarded, water systems are drained and disinfected, and the environment is cleaned and sanitized. Therefore, it is prudent to collect samples while they are available. For example, with family permission, the entire contents of a refrigerator of a patient with a probable case of botulism can be secured while medical examination and clinical laboratory tests are pending.

Recommendations for collection of food, water, and environmental samples are found in other sources (32, 42, 53). The indications for collection of environmental samples for possible *Legionella* outbreaks have not been clarified, but general strategies have been described (19). The value of water testing for *Legionella* spp. is reduced if human isolates are not available for strain comparison.

Standard Culture Identification and Susceptibility Methods

Standard methods for identification of fecal pathogens in clinical samples can be found in the *Clinical Microbiology Procedures Handbook* (56). Standard measures of water quality, such as total coliform count, fecal coliform count, biochemical oxygen demand (BOD), and *E. coli* count, can provide useful information in waterborne outbreaks. Standard methods for these measures, as well as specific methods for detection and identification of common gastrointestinal pathogens such as *Salmonella*, *C. jejuni*, *Leptospira* spp., or *V. cholerae*, can be found in *Standard Methods for the Examination of Water and Wastewater*, 20th edition (42). Standard procedures for microbial analysis of food and the environment are included in the *Bacteriological Analytical Manual*, 8th ed. (57), *Compendium of Methods for the Microbiological Examination of Foods*, 4th ed. (32), *Official Methods of Analysis of the AOAC International*, 16th ed. (29), and *Standard Methods for the Examination of Dairy Products*, 16th edition (81).

Challenges of Food, Water, and Environmental Culture

The isolation of diarrheal pathogens from food, water, and the environment presents different challenges from their isolation from ill patients. Diarrheal pathogens are usually present in large numbers in acutely ill patients, and the stool environment is relatively predictable. As a result, tests such as *Salmonella* culture are sensitive and relatively easy to perform. By contrast, pathogens are often present sporadically or in small numbers in food, water, or the environment. Even at low levels, pathogens can still cause considerable illness if enough individuals are exposed. For instance, in the 1995 U.S. nationwide ice cream-associated salmonellosis outbreak, samples tested had fewer than six organisms per half cup of product and yet an estimated 224,000 individuals became ill from approximately 1 million implicated gallons (50). In addition to sampling problems, there are a wide variety of possible physical and chemical environments and matrices in food, water, and environmental samples, to which the bacteria are more or less well adapted. Organisms may be trapped in an insoluble matrix, in the presence of inhibitors, or sublethally stressed or injured. As a result, these cultures are subject to results that are false positive (organisms isolated that are not responsible for the observed illness) and false negative (organisms not found that are responsible for the observed illness). Several strategies are used to address these issues. Samples are concentrated, detoxified, diluted, or put into nonselective enrichment media prior to selective culture.

Sublethally injured bacteria are usually sensitive to the selective agents (such as bile salts, dyes, antimicrobials, potassium tellurite, and sodium selenite) that are commonly used in selective enrichment media. These bacteria still may be viable in vivo but are nonviable in culture if placed directly in selective enrichment media. As a result, culture protocols often include a preenrichment in a nonselective nutritionally complete medium to allow the injured cells to repair their damage before being exposed to the selective enrichment medium (29, 32). This is particularly important for isolating pathogenic bacteria from foods which have been preserved by heating, freezing, drying, or addition of acids and other chemicals. Because preenrichment media do not contain selective chemicals, nonpathogenic contaminants may overgrow the pathogen if preenrichment is allowed to proceed for extended periods. Often, nonspecific enrichment broths are used in combination with selective enrichment broth and plating on selective solid media. Although this process overall increases the sensitivity of culture, it is too time-consuming for some outbreak settings. The use of direct plating of sample homogenates or suspension onto solid media in addition to enrichment broths offers the possibility of rapid pathogen recovery when bacterial numbers are large and organisms are not unduly stressed. Selective enrichment methods used by the food regulatory agencies are generally capable of yielding a positive result if the target pathogen is present at a level of at least 1 cell per 25 g of food. The sensitivity of the selective enrichment method can be increased beyond this level by culturing a larger sample of food (450 g of food in 50 ml of enrichment medium). The use of multiple methods can also increase the overall sensitivity of food, water, and environmental testing.

Rapid Methods for Detection of Bacteria and Bacterial Toxins

Rapid methods have been gaining popularity in clinical and food testing laboratories and can play an important role in outbreak investigations. Rapid assays, such as assays for *E. coli* O157:H7 and other Shiga toxin-producing *E. coli* strains (61, 105), are being used to streamline patient diagnosis and in some instances to facilitate outbreak management. These tests do not result in production of a bacterial isolate, which does not allow for further characterization of the agent. Isolates are necessary for antimicrobial resistance testing, which not only helps in patient therapy decisions but also may help guide outbreak management strategies. Isolates may be needed to reveal the presence or absence of virulence factors, such as the *E. coli* attaching and effacing factor (*eae*) in outbreaks of non-O157:H7 Shiga toxin-producing *E. coli* infection (7). Most significantly, isolates are critical for subspecies identification, such as serotyping or subtyping. Serotyping and isolate-dependent molecular subtyping methods, such as PFGE, are pivotal for detecting and managing outbreaks of infection due to *Salmonella*, *Shigella*, *E. coli* O157:H7, and other pathogens. With current technology, the use of isolates is the only way to conduct all of these activities. Therefore, rapid tests should be backed up by culture for pathogens for which culture is the standard method, such as *Salmonella* or *Shigella* spp. At a minimum, culture should be performed on positive samples or arrangements should be made to forward suitable biological material to a Public Health Laboratory for culture. An added benefit of routinely backing up rapid tests with culture is that the rapid test can be maximized for sensitivity, since the culture provides a second level of specificity. Commercial methods for rapid detection of fecal pathogens are described in *Manual of Commercial Methods in Clinical Microbiology* (111) and *Food Microbiology: Fundamentals and Frontiers*, 2nd ed. (40), and on the CDC website (http://www.dpd.cdc.gov).

Rapid tests often expedite the investigation of *L. pneumophila* outbreaks. Assays based on the urinary antigen are noninvasive and are therefore attractive for diagnosis confirmation and detection of new cases. Since the currently available assays detect only serogroup 1, which accounts for 70 to 85% of cases, these tests do not rule out disease caused by other serogroups or species of *Legionella*. Culture should be performed along with rapid tests, since further characterization of the isolate may be critical for determining a linkage between patients and a linkage to an environmental source. Serological testing may play an important role in characterizing the scope of the outbreak, the dose-response effect relative to the common source, etc. However, titers of antibody to *L. pneumophila* have been reported to rise slowly, often reaching maximal levels only after 6 weeks, and often are absent altogether (79, 108). Therefore, the use of serological testing during an outbreak may be limited. Direct fluorescent-antibody staining of sputum specimens can be performed rapidly, but its sensitivity is low and a number of cross-reactions with other genera have been reported (26, 41, 45, 58, 80).

MOLECULAR EPIDEMIOLOGICAL METHODS

Molecular methods, i.e., methods involving analysis of microbial nucleic acids, have become a critical component of disease surveillance and outbreak investigation. Molecular methods have become the mainstay for (i) subspecies identification and (ii) detection of emerging, new, or newly recognized pathogens.

As described above, molecular biology-based subtyping improves the likelihood of identifying outbreaks and focuses investigations, thereby increasing the likelihood of finding a common exposure in a point-source outbreak. The utility of subtyping methods such as PFGE for detecting outbreaks when used on a surveillance basis has been well established for *E. coli* O157:H7 (9) and *S. enterica* serovar Typhimurium (10). PFGE is also invaluable for the management of outbreaks caused by a wide variety of bacterial pathogens (75, 82, 88, 97, 110). Subtyping is effective because it (i) permits the differentiation of emerging disease clusters from unrelated background cases, (ii) reduces the statistical influence of sporadic cases and cases that occur by chance in an outbreak setting, and (iii) allows the resolution of simultaneously occurring outbreaks. By differentiating related and unrelated cases, subtyping increases the statistical association between the illness under investigation and the common exposure. Once a food, water, or environmental source has been implicated by the investigation, molecular subtyping of cultures from those sources can be a valuable confirmation tool, especially when the source is naturally contaminated with similar organisms. The interpretation of PFGE or other subtyping methods for investigation of *Legionella* outbreaks is currently under discussion (33, 66). Although PFGE is the current method of choice for bacterial pathogens in the PulseNet system (107), a wide variety of alternative molecular subtyping methods are under investigation, including amplified fragment length polymorphism analysis (100), multilocus sequence typing (78), and multilocus variable number tandem repeat analysis (62, 113, 115). Table 3 provides information on phenotypic and molecular subtyping methods that are useful for characterizing foodborne pathogens to aid in outbreak investigations. Other chapters in this Manual provide detailed descriptions of molecular subtyping protocols and suggest approaches for interpretation of results. The following points are specifically germane to outbreak investigations.

- Tenover et al. (109) have published guidelines for interpretation of PFGE results, including interpretation of genetic relatedness among patterns that are not exact matches. The inclusion of "closely related" (two or three fragment differences) or "possibly related" (four to six fragment differences) cases in the case-control study using these guidelines has the effect of increasing the study sensitivity at the expense of specificity. This is most appropriate when the number of cases is very small or when the outbreak agent is likely to be polyclonal. However, if the number of cases is large, specificity becomes the more important parameter during the hypothesis generation and testing phase of the investigation. Under these circumstances, use of a strict case definition, such as one which limits inclusion to exact pattern matches, strengthens the statistical association between common-source exposures. Once a significant common source has been identified, interpretative criteria are useful for determining the scope of the outbreak and characterizing the contamination events leading to the outbreak.

- Molecular subtyping tests, such as PFGE, are population-based tests, not diagnostic tests. Therefore, the results are meaningful only in the context of a population. Although valid conclusions can be reached about a population by using these methods, these conclusions cannot be extrapolated back to the individual. For example, a particular subtype may be significantly associated with illness in an outbreak. However, that does not prove that an individual with that subtype was exposed or that a person not having that subtype was not exposed. Having or not having the outbreak subtype only suggests the likelihood of exposure.

Molecular methods are also playing an increasingly important role in the identification and characterization of pathogens that are not easily tested by standard culture or antigenic methods. One important example is human calicivirus, which is thought to be one of the most common diarrheal pathogens and a frequent cause of outbreaks (87, 92). Reverse transcriptase polymerase chain reaction (RT-PCR) is the most sensitive detection method currently available. The methods used to diagnose calicivirus infection, including strategies and targets for RT-PCR in a variety of samples, are the subjects of a recent review (6). Genotyping of calicivirus for the purpose of enhancing epidemiological investigations of calicivirus infection has been accomplished by either hybridization to specific probes (2, 117) or DNA sequencing (3, 39, 116). Use of these molecular methods of detection and subtyping of calicivirus has led to a greater understanding of the epidemiology and prevalence of calicivirus infection in humans, revealing it to be the leading cause of acute gastroenteritis in the United States (39, 43). A second important example of pathogen detection enhanced by molecular methods is enterotoxigenic *E. coli*. Detection of enterotoxigenic *E. coli* typically relies on assaying for the presence of the heat-stable (ST) and heat-labile (LT) enterotoxins or the genes

TABLE 3 Subtyping methods for foodborne and waterborne pathogens

Pathogen	Phenotypic subtyping method(s)	Molecular subtyping methods[a]	Restriction enzyme for RFLP	Comments
Bacillus cereus	Serotyping	RFLP/PFGE	SmaI	
Campylobacter jejuni	Serotyping	*flaA* RFLP	DdeI	
C. coli		RFLP/PFGE	SmaI	
Clostridium botulinum	Toxin typing	RFLP/PFGE	MluI, SmaI, XhoI	Nuclease activity of isolates may present problems
Clostridium perfringens	Serotyping	RFLP/PFGE	SmaI	
E. coli O157	Serotyping, phage typing	RFLP/PFGE	XbaI, AvrII, SpeI	
Listeria monocytogenes	Serotyping, phage typing	REA RFLP/PFGE RAPD	HhaI AscI, ApaI, SmaI	Methods are being standardized by World Health Organization-sponsored international group
Legionella pneumophila	Serotyping	PFGE, RAPD		
Legionella spp.		PFGE, RAPD		
S. enterica serovar Typhimurium	Phage typing, antimicrobial susceptibility	RFLP/PFGE	XbaI, AvrII	
S. enterica serovar Enteritidis	Phage typing	Plasmid profiles, ribotyping, RAPD, PFGE	XbaI, AvrII	No single molecular method has adequate discriminating ability
Other nontyphoidal salmonellae	Phage typing, if available	RFLP/PFGE	XbaI, AvrII	Some strains may not be typeable by PFGE
Shigella spp.		RFLP/PFGE	XbaI, AvrII	
Yersinia enterocolitica	Serotyping	RFLP/PFGE	XbaI, SmaI	
Cryptosporidium parvum		MEE, RAPD, RFLP/repeat DNA, RFLP/18S rRNA + ITS, RFLP/DHFR-TS, PCR/DNA sequence analysis (TRAP-C2)		
Caliciviruses		RT-PCR/sequence analysis		

[a] MEE, multilocus enzyme electrophoresis; RAPD, random amplified polymorphic DNA analysis; RFLP, restriction fragment length polymorphism; ITS, internal transcribed spacer; DHFR-TS, dihydrofolate reductase-thymidylate synthase; TRAP-C2, thrombospondin-related adhesion protein.

encoding these toxins. Kits are commercially available for the detection of ST and LT in culture filtrates and perform well in comparison to classical toxin detection tests (30). In these rapid tests, LT is detected by reverse passive latex agglutination while ST is identified by competitive enzyme immunoassay (EIA). Molecular detection of the toxin genes by PCR is useful for epidemiological studies (64, 114). Multiplex assays have been developed for the simultaneous detection of the genes for ST and LT (93).

Real-time PCR *Legionella* detection assays are very rapid and have shown a high degree of sensitivity and specificity in bronchoalveolar lavage specimens (48) and hospital water systems (121). PCR-based assays have the potential to detect dead cells, making them potentially useful for investigating outbreaks of Pontiac fever. However, due to the near ubiquity of *Legionella* spp. in water, the ability to detect nonviable cells can create difficult interpretation issues.

Although the genetic basis for many types of antimicrobial resistance in a variety of pathogens has been determined and molecular detection assays have been developed, phenotypic antimicrobial susceptibility assays are still the testing standard. Phenotypic assays such as microwell dilution or E test (AB Biodisk, Solna, Sweden) can detect resistance due to a variety of known or unknown resistance mechanisms. Specific molecular biology-based assays, such as those for AmpC-mediated β-lactamase in *Salmonella* (34), may prove important in some outbreak settings.

DEALING WITH INTENTIONAL CONTAMINATION OF FOOD OR WATER

The possibility of intentional contamination of our food and water supply by bioterrorists must be taken seriously (104). Unlike other highly controlled biological agents that have been considered possible threat agents (e.g., smallpox virus), many foodborne disease agents such as *Salmonella*, *V. cholerae*, botulinal toxins, and staphylococcal enterotoxin B are relatively easy to obtain or produce. Many of these agents are stable in the environment and thus can be effectively used to contaminate food and water supplies (83). Some unintentionally contaminated foods that were nationally distributed have caused illness in hundreds of thousands of people within a very short time. Similarly, intentional contamination of the water supply of a town or city can rapidly expose large numbers of people to a pathogen or toxin. These features may make foodborne and waterborne disease agents particularly appealing for the bioterrorist. Unfortunately, it may not be known in the early phases of investigation of a foodborne or waterborne disease cluster that it has been caused by a deliberate act of bioterrorism. Therefore, it is prudent to treat unintentional and intentional contamination of foods in exactly the same way from the surveillance and investigation standpoints. This requires enhanced surveillance for early detection of disease clusters followed by rapid coordinated action to identify the source of illness.

COMMUNICATION AND DOCUMENTATION

Communication is a key ingredient in a well-management outbreak investigation, as it is for any public emergency response. Proper documentation not only serves to clarify communication but also permits organized analysis during an outbreak and is essential for retrospective analysis of issues that invariably come up as a result of outbreak investigations. A detailed resource outlining the sequence of communication activities needed in an infectious-disease outbreak or bioterrorism attack has been published and can be found at the website of Model Emergency Response Communications Plan for Infectious Disease Outbreaks and Bioterrorist Events, Association of State and Territorial Directors of Health Promotion and Public Health Education (www.astdhpphe.org/bioterr/bioterror.pdf). The formation of core information working groups, command centers, local communication and response networks, and players in outbreak communication management is described in this document. Communication is a special problem during community outbreaks, since considerable distances often separate epidemiology and laboratory groups during the entire course of an investigation. The following strategies can facilitate communication and documentation during an investigation.

- An outbreak investigation procedure, written collaboratively by the various investigative units, facilitates a rapid and effective response. This document should include (i) the procedure for collection of complaint data and a standardized format for recording food-related complaints; (ii) a set of guidelines for the initiation of an investigation based on evaluation of epidemiological data; (iii) a set of instructions for the collection, storage, and transport of samples, as well as a list of laboratory tests available; and (iv) an up-to-date list of the principal public health contacts, including phone and fax numbers and e-mail addresses. Examples of standardized forms and procedures are available from the International Association of Milk, Food and Environmental Sanitarians (15).

- The laboratory should be provided with information about the signs and symptoms shown by the patients as well as the suspect agent as soon as that information is available, so that bacteriological media can be prepared, staffing needs can be met, etc. In addition, it should be clarified who is authorized to order tests and to whom the results should be directed. If a specimen or isolate is particularly crucial to the investigation, communication to that effect should occur both at the collection point and at the laboratory so that proper routing is ensured and expedited.

- A requisition should accompany each specimen or set of specimens. For food samples, this document should provide a description of each sample, including quantity, method of collection, time and date of collection, name of the collector, analyses requested, and the agency or individual to whom the report should be sent. Human specimens should be marked with the patient's name and the date and time of collection and should be individually packaged or attached to a test request form, which clearly records the patient's name; the name, address, and phone number of the health care provider; and the tests requested.

- Investigations are often aided by the use of a name or code for the site being investigated (example: "Joe's Restaurant"), especially when team members are dealing with more than one outbreak. The recording of the code on both the food and human test request forms facilitates the laboratory's effort to compile outbreak information in a useful format.

- The investigation team typically establishes a computerized database for the retrieval and analysis of data. EPI-INFO 2000, a database software package made available by CDC, is frequently used for this function.

- Daily updates to all team members by the team leader ensure consistency of action, especially during the earliest phase of investigations when reported cases are fewest and information is fragmentary and sometimes contradictory.

- A telephone bridge conference is often the most effective means of acting interactively when an investigation is occurring in multiple locations.

- Laboratories should begin a file when notified of a possible outbreak; this file may include a basic description of the situation and investigative team makeup, raw and compiled laboratory data, and communication notes.

- To ensure a clear and consistent message throughout the investigation, all requests for information from the public or media should be routed through a central individual, either the team leader or media liaison.

Use of trade names is for identification only and does not imply endorsement by the Public Health Service or by the U.S. Department of Health and Human Services.

REFERENCES

1. **Anderson, K., C. P. McSharry, C. Clark, C. J. Clark, G. R. Barclay, and G. P. Morris.** 1996. Sump bay fever: inhalational fever associated with a biologically contaminated water aerosol. *Occup. Environ. Med.* **53:**106–111.
2. **Ando, T., S. S. Monroe, J. R. Gentsch, Q. Jin, D. C. Lewis, and R. I. Glass.** 1995. Detection and differentiation of antigenically distinct small round-structured viruses ("Norwalk-like viruses") by reverse transcription-PCR and southern hybridization. *J. Clin. Microbiol.* **33:** 64–71.
3. **Ando, T., J. S. Noel, and R. L. Fankhauser.** 2000. Genetic classification of "Norwalk-like viruses." *J. Infect. Dis.* **181**(Suppl. 2)**:**S336–S348.
4. **Anonymous.** 2001. *Food Safety from Farm to Table: a National Food-Safety Initiative. A Report to the President.* Department of Health and Human Services, U.S. Environmental Protection Agency, Washington, D.C.
5. **Anonymous.** 2000. Waterborne outbreak of gastroenteritis associated with a contaminated municipal water supply, Walkerton, Ontario, May–June 2000. *Can. Commun. Dis. Rep.* **26:**170–173.
6. **Atmar, R. L., and M. K. Estes.** 2001. Diagnosis of non-cultivatable gastroenteritis viruses, the human caliciviruses. *Clin. Microbiol. Rev.* **14:**15–37.
7. **Banatvala, N., M. M. Debeukelaer, P. M. Griffin, T. J. Barrett, K. D. Greene, J. H. Green, and J. G. Wells.**

1996. Shiga-like toxin-producing *Escherichia coli* O111 and associated hemolytic-uremic syndrome: a family outbreak. *Pediatr. Infect. Dis. J.* **15:**1008–1011.

8. **Barwick, R. S., D. A. Levy, G. F. Craun, M. J. Beach, and R. L. Calderon.** 2000. Surveillance for waterborne-disease outbreaks—United States, 1997–1998. CDC Surveillance Summaries. *Morb. Mortal. Wkly. Rep.* **49:**1–21.

9. **Bender, J. B., C. W. Hedberg, J. M. Besser, D. J. Boxrud, K. L. MacDonald, and M. T. Osterholm.** 1997. Surveillance by molecular subtype for *Escherichia coli* O157:H7 infections in Minnesota by molecular subtyping. *N. Engl. J. Med.* **337:**388–394.

10. **Bender, J. B., C. W. Hedberg, D. J. Boxrud, J. M. Besser, J. H. Wicklund, K. E. Smith, and M. T. Osterholm.** 2001. Use of molecular subtyping in surveillance for *Salmonella enterica* serotype *typhimurium*. *N. Engl. J. Med.* **344:**189–195.

11. **Bennett, J. V., and P. S. Brachman (ed.).** 1998. *Hospital Infections.* Lippincott-Raven, Philadelphia, Pa.

12. **Blaser, M. J.** 1986. Brainerd diarrhea: a newly recognized raw milk-associated enteropathy. *JAMA* **256:**510–511.

13. **Borella, P., A. Bargellini, S. Pergolizzi, G. Aggazzotti, C. Curti, P. Nizzero, G. Stancanelli, R. Vaiani, G. Gesu, and R. Mazzuconi.** 2000. Prevention and control of *Legionella* infection in the hospital environment. *Ann. Ig* **12:**287–296. (In Italian.)

14. **Boshuizen, H. C., S. E. Neppelenbroek, H. van Vliet, J. F. Schellekens, J. W. Boer, M. F. Peeters, and M. A. Spaendonck.** 2001. Subclinical legionella infection in workers near the source of a large outbreak of Legionnaires' disease. *J. Infect. Dis.* **184:**515–518.

15. **Bryan, F. L., H. W. Anderson, O. D. Cook, K. H. Guzewich, K. H. Lewis, R. C. Swanson, and E. C. D. Todd.** 1989. *Procedures To Investigate Foodborne Illness.* International Association of Milk, Food, and Environmental Sanitarians, Ames, Iowa.

16. **Campanella, N.** 1999. Infectious diseases and natural disasters: the effects of Hurricane Mitch over Villanueva municipal area, Nicaragua. *Public Health Rev.* **27:**311–319.

17. **Centers for Disease Control and Prevention.** 1997. *Escherichia coli* O157:H7 infections associated with eating a nationally distributed commercial brand of frozen ground beef patties and burgers—Colorado. *Morb. Mortal. Wkly. Rep.* **46:**777–778.

18. **Centers for Disease Control and Prevention.** 2000. Guidelines for confirmation of foodborne-disease outbreaks. CDC Sureveillance Summaries, March 17, 2000. *Morb. Mortal. Wkly. Rep.* **49:**52–64.

19. **Centers for Disease Control and Prevention.** 1997. Guidelines for prevention of nosocomial pneumonia. *Morb. Mortal. Wkly. Rep.* **46:**1–79.

20. **Centers for Disease Control and Prevention.** 2000. Multistate outbreak of listeriosis—United States, 2000. *Morb. Mortal. Wkly. Rep.* **49:**1129–1130.

21. **Centers for Disease Control and Prevention.** 1997. Outbreak of leptospirosis among white-water rafters—Costa Rica, 1996. *Morb. Mortal. Wkly. Rep.* **46:**577–579.

22. **Centers for Disease Control and Prevention.** 1998. Update: leptospirosis and unexplained acute febrile illness among athletes participating in triathlons—Illinois and Wisconsin, 1998. *Morb. Mortal. Wkly. Rep.* **47:**673–676.

23. **Centers for Disease Control and Prevention.** 1999. Outbreaks of *Shigella sonnei* infection associated with eating fresh parsley—United States and Canada, July–August 1998. *Morb. Mortal. Wkly. Rep.* **48:**285–289.

24. **Chaudhry, R., B. Dhawan, and A. B. Dey.** 2000. The incidence of *Legionella pneumophila*: a prospective study in a tertiary care hospital in India. *Trop. Doct.* **30:**197–200.

25. **Cheesbrough, J. S., J. Green, C. I. Gallimore, P. A. Wright, and D. W. Brown.** 2000. Widespread environmental contamination with Norwalk-like viruses (NLV) detected in a prolonged hotel outbreak of gastroenteritis. *Epidemiol. Infect.* **125:**93–98.

26. **Chen, S., L. Hicks, M. Yuen, D. Mitchell, and G. L. Gilbert.** 1994. Serological cross-reaction between *Legionella* spp. and *Capnocytophaga ochracea* by using latex agglutination test. *J. Clin. Microbiol.* **32:**3054–3055.

27. **Claesson, B. E., N. G. Svensson, L. Gotthardsson, L. Gotthardsson, and B. Garden.** 1992. A foodborne outbreak of group A streptococcal disease at a birthday party. *Scand. J. Infect. Dis.* **24:**577–586.

28. **Cooksley, W. G.** 2000. What did we learn from the Shanghai hepatitis A epidemic? *J. Viral Hepat.* **7**(Suppl. 1):1–3.

29. **Cunniff, P. (ed.).** 1998. *Official Methods of Analysis of the AOAC International,* 16th ed. AOAC International, Gaithersburg, Md.

30. **Czirok, E., G. Semjen, H. Steinruck, M. Herpay, H. Milch, I. Nyomarkay, Z. Stverteczky, and A. Szeness.** 1992. Comparison of rapid methods for detection of heat-labile (LT) and heat-stable (ST) enterotoxin in *Escherichia coli. J. Med. Microbiol.* **36:**398–402.

31. **Darelid, J., H. Hallander, S. Lofgren, B. E. Malmvall, and A. M. Olinder-Nielsen.** 2001. Community spread of *Legionella pneumophila* serogroup 1 in temporal relation to a nosocomial outbreak. *Scand. J. Infect. Dis.* **33:**194–199.

32. **Downes, F. P., and K. Ito (ed.).** 2001. *Compendium of Methods for the Microbiological Examination of Foods,* 4th ed. American Public Health Association, Washington, D.C.

33. **Drenning, S. D., J. E. Stout, J. R. Joly, and V. L. Yu.** 2001. Unexpected similarity of pulsed-field gel electrophoresis patterns of unrelated clinical isolates of *Legionella pneumophila,* serogroup 1. *J. Infect. Dis.* **183:**628–632.

34. **Dunne, E. F., P. D. Fey, P. Kludt, R. Reporter, F. Mostashari, P. Shillam, J. Wicklund, C. Miller, B. Holland, K. Stamey, T. J. Barrett, J. K. Rasheed, F. C. Tenover, E. M. Ribot, and F. J. Angulo.** 2000. Emergence of domestically acquired ceftriaxone-resistant *Salmonella* infections associated with AmpC beta-lactamase. *JAMA* **284:**3151–3156.

35. **Elbasha, E. H., T. D. Fitzsimmons, and M. I. Meltzer.** 2000. Costs and benefits of a subtype-specific surveillance system for identifying *Escherichia coli* O157:H7 outbreaks. *Emerg. Infect. Dis.* **6:**293–297.

36. **Elcuaz, R., M. Armas, M. Ramirez, F. J. Noguera, M. Bolanos, I. Quinones, and B. Lafarga.** 1998. Outbreak of schistosomiasis in a group of travellers returning from Burkina Faso. *Enferm. Infecc. Microbiol. Clin.* **16:**367–369.

37. **Elder, B. L., S. A. Hansen, J. A. Kellogg, F. J. Marsik, and R. J. Zabransky.** 1997. *Cumitech 31, Verification and Validation of Procedures in the Clinical Microbiology Laboratory.* Coordinating ed., B. W. McCurdy. American Society for Microbiology, Washington, D.C.

38. **Escribano, A., I. Orskov, F. Orskov, and R. Borras.** 1987. Enterotoxigenic *Escherichia coli* O153:H45 from an outbreak of diarrhea in Spain. *Med. Microbiol. Immunol.* (Berlin) **176:**241–244.

39. **Fankhauser, R. L., J. S. Noel, S. S. Monroe, T. Ando, and R. I. Glass.** 1998. Molecular epidemiology of "Norwalk-like viruses" in outbreaks of gastroenteritis in the United States. *J. Infect. Dis.* **178:**1571–1578.

40. **Feng, P.** 2001. Development and impact of rapid methods for detection of foodborne pathogens, p. 775–796. *In* M. P. Doyle, L. R. Beuchat, and T. J. Montville (ed.), *Food Microbiology: Fundamentals and Frontiers,* 2nd ed. ASM Press, Washington, D.C.

41. **Finidori, J. P., D. Raoult, N. Bornstein, and J. Fleurette.** 1992. Study of cross-reaction between *Coxiella burnetii* and *Legionella pneumophila* using indirect immunofluorescence assay and immunoblotting. *Acta Virol.* **36:**459–465.

42. **Franson, M. A. (ed.).** 1998. *Standard Methods for the Examination of Water and Wastewater,* 20th ed. American Public Health Association, American Water Works Association, Water Environment Federation, Washington, D.C.

43. **Glass, R. I., J. Noel, T. Ando, R. Fankhauser, G. Belliot, A. Mounts, U. D. Parashar, J. S. Bresee, and S. S. Monroe.** 2000. The epidemiology of enteric caliciviruses from humans: a reassessment using new diagnostics. *J. Infect. Dis.* **181**(Suppl. 2)**:**S254–S261.

44. **Gotz, H. M., A. Tegnell, B. de Jong, K. A. Broholm, M. Kuusi, I. Kallings, and K. Ekdahl.** 2001. A whirlpool associated outbreak of Pontiac fever at a hotel in Northern Sweden. *Epidemiol. Infect.* **126:**241–247.

45. **Gray, J. J., K. N. Ward, R. E. Warren, and M. Farrington.** 1991. Serological cross-reaction between *Legionella pneumophila* and *Citrobacter freundii* in indirect immunofluorescence and rapid microagglutination tests. *J. Clin. Microbiol.* **29:**200–201.

46. **Gregg, M. B., and J. Parsonnet.** 1997. The principles of an epidemiologic field investigation, p. 537–546. *In* R. Detels, W. W. Holland, J. McEwen, and G. S. Omenn (ed.), *Oxford Textbook of Public Health.* Oxford University Press, London, United Kingdom.

47. **Hastings, L., A. Burnens, B. de Jong, L. Ward, I. Fisher, J. Stuart, C. Bartlett, and B. Rowe.** 1996. Salm-Net facilitates collaborative investigation of an outbreak of *Salmonella tosamanga* infection in Europe. *Commun. Dis. Rep. CDR Rev.* **6:**R100–R102.

48. **Hayden, R. T., J. R. Uhl, X. Qian, M. K. Hopkins, M. C. Aubry, A. H. Limper, R. V. Lloyd, and F. R. Cockerill.** 2001. Direct detection of *Legionella* species from bronchoalveolar lavage and open lung biopsy specimens: comparison of LightCycler PCR, in situ hybridization, direct fluorescence antigen detection, and culture. *J. Clin. Microbiol.* **39:**2618–2626.

49. **Hedberg, C. W., S. J. Savarino, J. M. Besser, C. J. Paulus, V. M. Thelen, L. J. Myers, D. N. Cameron, T. J. Barrett, J. B. Kaper, and M. T. Osterholm.** 1997. An outbreak of foodborne illness caused by *Escherichia coli* O39:NM, an agent not fitting into the existing scheme for classifying diarrheogenic *E. coli. J. Infect. Dis.* **176:**1625–1628.

50. **Hennessy, T. W., C. W. Hedberg, L. Slutsker, K. E. White, J. M. Besser-Wiek, M. E. Moen, J. Feldman, W. W. Coleman, L. M. Edmonson, K. L. MacDonald, M. T. Osterholm, and The Investigation Team.** 1996. A national outbreak of *Salmonella enteritidis* infections from ice cream. *N. Engl. J. Med.* **334:**1281–1286.

51. **Herwaldt, B. L., M. J. Beach, and the Cyclospora Working Group.** 1999. The return of *Cyclospora* in 1997: another outbreak of cyclosporiasis in North America associated with imported raspberries. *Ann. Intern. Med.* **130:**210–220.

52. **Huerta, M., I. Grotto, M. Gdalevich, D. Mimouni, B. Gavrieli, M. Yavzori, D. Cohen, and O. Shpilberg.** 2000. A waterborne outbreak of gastroenteritis in the Golan Heights due to enterotoxigenic *Escherichia coli. Infection* **28:**267–271.

53. **Hurst, C. J., G. R. Knudsen, M. J. McInerney, L. D. Stetzenbach, and M. V. Walter (ed.).** 1997. *Manual of Environmental Microbiology.* ASM Press, Washington, D.C.

54. **Hutin, Y. J., V. Pool, E. H. Cramer, O. V. Nainan, J. Weth, I. T. Williams, S. T. Goldstein, K. F. Gensheimer, B. P. Bell, C. N. Shapiro, M. J. Alter, H. S. Margolis, and the National Hepatitis A Investigation Team.** 1999. A multistate, foodborne outbreak of hepatitis A. *N. Engl. J. Med.* **340:**595–602.

55. **Hutwagner, L. C., E. K. Maloney, N. H. Bean, L. Slutsker, and S. M. Martin.** 1997. Using laboratory-based surveillance data for prevention: an algorithm for detecting *Salmonella* outbreaks. *Emerg. Infect. Dis.* **3:**395–400.

56. **Isenberg, H. D. (ed.)** 2001. *Clinical Microbiology Procedures Handbook.* ASM Press, Washington, D.C.

57. **Jackson, G. J. (ed.)** 1988. *Bacteriological Analytical Manual,* 8th ed. AOAC International, Gaithersburg, Md.

58. **Jimenez-Lucho, V., M. Shulman, and J. Johnson.** 1994. *Bordetella bronchiseptica* in an AIDS patient cross-reacts with *Legionella* antisera. *J. Clin. Microbiol.* **32:**3095–3096.

59. **Katz, D., S. Kumar, J. Malecki, M. Lowdermilk, E. H. Koumans, and R. Hopkins.** 1999. Cyclosporiasis associated with imported raspberries, Florida, 1996. *Public Health Rep.* **114:**427–438.

60. **Kauppinen, J., T. Nousiainen, E. Jantunen, R. Mattila, and M. L. Katila.** 1999. Hospital water supply as a source of disseminated *Mycobacterium fortuitum* infection in a leukemia patient. *Infect. Control Hosp. Epidemiol.* **20:**343–345.

61. **Kehl, K. S., P. Havens, C. E. Behnke, and D. W. Acheson.** 1997. Evaluation of the premier EHEC assay for detection of Shiga toxin-producing *Escherichia coli. J. Clin. Microbiol.* **35:**2051–2054.

62. **Keim, P., L. B. Price, A. M. Klevytska, K. L. Smith, J. M. Schupp, R. Okinaka, P. J. Jackson, and M. E. Hugh-Jones.** 2000. Multiple-locus variable-number tandem repeat analysis reveals genetic relationships within *Bacillus anthracis. J. Bacteriol.* **182:**2928–2936.

63. **Keller, D. W., R. Hajjeh, A. DeMaria, B. S. Fields, J. M. Pruckler, R. S. Benson, S. M. Kludt, P. E. Lett, L. A. Mermel, C. Giorgio, and R. F. Breiman.** 1996. Community outbreak of Legionnaires' disease: an investigation confirming the potential for cooling towers to transmit *Legionella* species. *Clin. Infect. Dis.* **22:**257–261.

64. **Keskimaki, M., L. Mattila, H. Peltola, and A. Siitonen.** 2000. Prevalence of diarrheagenic *Escherichia coli* in Finns with or without diarrhea during a round-the-world trip. *J. Clin. Microbiol.* **38:**4425–4429.

65. **Kool, J. L., D. Bergmire-Sweat, J. C. Butler, E. W. Brown, D. J. Peabody, D. S. Massi, J. C. Carpenter, J. M. Pruckler, R. F. Benson, and B. S. Fields.** 1999. Hospital characteristics associated with colonization of water systems by *Legionella* and risk of nosocomial Legionnaires' disease: a cohort study of 15 hospitals. *Infect. Control Hosp. Epidemiol.* **20:**798–805.

66. **Kool, J. L., U. Buchholz, C. Peterson, E. W. Brown, R. F. Benson, J. M. Pruckler, B. S. Fields, J. Sturgeon, E. Lehnkering, R. Cordova, L. M. Mascola, and J. C. Butler.** 2000. Strengths and limitations of molecular subtyping in a community outbreak of Legionnaires' disease. *Epidemiol. Infect.* **125:**599–608.

67. **Kramer, M. H., B. L. Herwaldt, G. F. Craun, R. L. Calderon, and D. D. Juranek.** 1996. Surveillance for waterborne-disease outbreaks—United States, 1993–1994. CDC Surveillance Summaries. *Morb. Mortal. Wkly. Rep.* **45:**1–33.

68. **Kukkula, M., L. Maunula, E. Silvennoinen, and C. H. von Bonsdorff.** 1999. Outbreak of viral gastroenteritis due to drinking water contaminated by Norwalk-like viruses. *J. Infect. Dis.* **180:**1771–1776.

69. **Kulshrestha, S. B., K. N. Kapoor, S. V. Malik, and P. N. Khanna.** 1989. Enterotoxigenic *Escherichia coli* from an outbreak with cholerigenic syndromes of gastroenteritis. *J. Commun. Dis.* **21:**313–317.

70. **Last, J. M.** 1983. *A Dictionary of Epidemiology.* Oxford University Press, Oxford, United Kingdom.

71. **Leighton, B. J., S. Zervos, and J. M. Webster.** 2000. Ecological factors in schistosome transmission, and an environmentally benign method for controlling snails in a recreational lake with a record of schistosome dermatitis. *Parasitol. Int.* **49:**9–17.

72. **Levy, D. A., M. S. Bens, G. F. Craun, R. L. Calderon, and B. L. Herwaldt.** 1998. Surveillance for waterborne-disease outbreaks—United States, 1995–1996. CDC Surveillance Summaries. *Morb. Mortal. Wkly. Rep.* **47:**1–34.

73. **Lew, J. F., C. W. LeBaron, R. I. Glass, T. Torok, P. M. Griffin, J. G. Wells, D. D. Juranek, and S. P. Wahlquist.** 1990. Recommendations for collection of laboratory specimens associated with outbreaks of gastroenteritis. *Morb. Mortal. Wkly. Rep.* **39:**1–13.

74. **Lockwood, W. W., C. Friedman, N. Bus, C. Pierson, and R. Gaynes.** 1989. An outbreak of *Mycobacterium terrae* in clinical specimens associated with a hospital potable water supply. *Am. Rev. Respir. Dis.* **140:**1614–1617.

75. **Lu, P. L., S. C. Chang, H. J. Pan, M. L. Chen, and K. T. Luh.** 2000. Application of pulsed-field gel electrophoresis to the investigation of a nosocomial outbreak of *Vibrio parahaemolyticus. J. Microbiol. Immunol. Infect.* **33:**29–33.

76. **Luttichau, H. R., C. Vinther, S. A. Uldum, J. Moller, M. Faber, and J. S. Jensen.** 1998. An outbreak of Pontiac fever among children following use of a whirlpool. *Clin. Infect. Dis.* **26:**1374–1378.

77. **MacKenzie, W. R., N. J. Hoxie, M. E. Proctor, M. S. Gradus, K. A. Blair, D. E. Peterson, J. J. Kazmierczak, D. G. Addiss, K. R. Fox, J. B. Rose, et al.** 1994. A massive outbreak in Milwaukee of cryptosporidium infection transmitted through the public water supply. *N. Engl. J. Med.* **331:**161–167.

78. **Maiden, M. C., J. A. Bygraves, E. Feil, G. Morelli, J. E. Russell, R. Urwin, Q. Zhang, J. Zhou, K. Zurth, D. A. Caugant, I. M. Feavers, M. Achtman, and B. G. Spratt.** 1998. Multilocus sequence typing: a portable approach to the identification of clones within populations of pathogenic microorganisms. *Proc. Natl. Acad. Sci. USA* **95:**3140–3145.

79. **Marrie, T. J., S. MacDonald, K. Clarke, and D. Haldane.** 1991. Nosocomial Legionnaires' disease: lessons from a four-year prospective study. *Am. J. Infect. Control* **19:**79–85.

80. **Marshall, L. E., T. C. Boswell, and G. Kudesia.** 1994. False positive *Legionella* serology in *Campylobacter* infection: *Campylobacter* serotypes, duration of antibody response and elimination of cross-reactions in the indirect fluorescent antibody test. *Epidemiol. Infect.* **112:**347–357.

81. **Marshall, R. T. (ed.).** 2001. *Standard Methods for the Examination of Dairy Products,* 16th ed. American Public Health Association, Washington, D.C.

82. **Maslanka, S. E., J. G. Kerr, G. Williams, J. M. Barbaree, L. A. Carson, J. M. Miller, and B. Swaminathan.** 1999. Molecular subtyping of *Clostridium perfringens* by pulsed-field gel electrophoresis to facilitate food-borne-disease outbreak investigations. *J. Clin. Microbiol.* **37:**2209–2214.

83. **Maslanka, S. E., J. Zirnstein, J. Sobel, and B. Swaminathan.** 2001. Foodborne pathogen and toxin diagnostics: current methods and needs assessment from a surveillance, outbreak response, and bioterrorism preparedness perspective, p. 143–163. *In* S. P. Layne, T. J. Beugelsdijk, and C. K. N. Patel (ed.), *FirePower in the Lab: Automation in the Fight against Infectious Disease and Bioterrorism.* Joseph Henry Press, Washington, D.C.

84. **Mathers, W. D., J. E. Sutphin, R. Folberg, P. A. Meier, R. P. Wenzel, and R. G. Elgin.** 1996. Outbreak of keratitis presumed to be caused by *Acanthamoeba. Am. J. Ophthalmol.* **121:**129–142.

85. **Mayhall, C. G. (ed.).** 1999. *Hospital Epidemiology and Infection Control.* Lippincott Williams & Wilkins, Philadelphia, Pa.

86. **McIntyre, C. R.** 1991. Hazard analysis critical control point (HACCP) identification. *Dairy Food Environ. Sanit.* **11:**73–81.

87. **Mead, P. S., L. Slutsker, V. Dietz, L. F. McCaig, J. S. Bresee, C. Shapiro, P. M. Griffin, and R. V. Tauxe.** 1999. Food-related illness and death in the United States. *Emerg. Infect. Dis.* **5:**607–625.

88. **Mitsuda, T., T. Muto, M. Yamada, N. Kobayashi, M. Toba, Y. Aihara, A. Ito, and S. Yokota.** 1998. Epidemiological study of a food-borne outbreak of enterotoxigenic *Escherichia coli* O25:NM by pulsed-field gel electrophoresis and randomly amplified polymorphic DNA analysis. *J. Clin. Microbiol.* **36:**652–656.

89. **Moore, A. C., B. L. Herwaldt, G. F. Craun, R. L. Calderon, A. K. Highsmith, and D. D. Juranek.** 1993. Surveillance for waterborne disease outbreaks—United States, 1991–1992. CDC Surveillance Summaries. *Morb. Mortal. Wkly. Rep.* **42:**1–22.

90. **Muittari, A., P. Kuusisto, and A. Sovijarvi.** 1982. An epidemic of bath water fever—endotoxin alveolitis? *Eur. J. Respir. Dis. Suppl.* **123:**108–116.

91. **Murray, J., and A. Lopez.** 1996. *The Global Burden of Disease.* Harvard School of Public Health, World Health Organization, World Bank.

92. **Olsen, S. J., L. C. MacKinnon, J. S. Goulding, N. H. Bean, and L. Slutsker.** 2000. Surveillance for foodborne-disease outbreaks—United States, 1993–1997. CDC Surveillance Summaries. *Morb. Mortal. Wkly. Rep.* **49:**1–62.

93. **Olsvik, O., and N. A. Strockbine.** 1993. PCR detection of heat-stable, heat-labile, and Shiga-like toxin genes in *Escherichia coli,* p. 271–276. *In* D. H. Persing, T. F. Smith, F. C. Tenover, and T. J. White (ed.), *Diagnostic Molecular Microbiology: Principles and Applications.* American Society for Microbiology, Washington, D.C.

94. **Potter, M. E., and R. V. Tauxe.** 1997. Epidemiology of foodborne diseases: tools and applications. *World Health Stat. Q.* **50:**24–29.

95. **Rabold, J. G., C. W. Hoge, D. R. Shlim, C. Kefford, R. Rajah, and P. Echeverria.** 1994. *Cyclospora* outbreak associated with chlorinated drinking water. *Lancet* **344:**1360–1361.

96. **Reingold, A. L.** 1998. Outbreak investigations—a perspective. *Emerg. Infect. Dis.* **4:**21–27.

97. **Ribot, E. M., C. Fitzgerald, K. Kubota, B. Swaminathan, and T. J. Barrett.** 2001. Rapid pulsed-field gel electrophoresis protocol for subtyping of *Campylobacter jejuni. J. Clin. Microbiol.* **39:**1889–1894.

98. **Russo, P. L., D. W. Spelman, G. A. Harrington, A. W. Jenney, I. C. Gunesekere, P. J. Wright, J. C. Doultree, and J. A. Marshall.** 1997. Hospital outbreak of "Norwalk-like virus." *Infect. Control Hosp. Epidemiol.* **18:**576–579.

99. **Ryan, C. A., M. K. Nickels, N. T. Hargrett-Bean, M. E. Potter, T. Endo, L. Mayer, C. W. Langkop, C. Gibson, R. C. McDonald, R. T. Kenney, et al.** 1987. Massive outbreak of antimicrobial-resistant salmonellosis traced to pasteurized milk. *JAMA* **258:**3269–3274.

100. **Savelkoul, P. H., H. J. Aarts, J. de Haas, L. Dijkshoorn, B. Duim, M. Otsen, J. L. Rademaker, L. Schouls, and J. A. Lenstra.** 1999. Amplified-fragment length polymorphism analysis: the state of an art. *J. Clin. Microbiol.* **37:**3083–3091.

101. **Smith, J. L.** 1998. Foodborne illness in the elderly. *J. Food Prot.* **61:**1229–1239.

102. **Smith, J. L.** 1999. Foodborne infections during pregnancy. *J. Food Prot.* **62:**818–829.

103. Snyder, O. P. 2001. HACCP in the retail food industry. *Dairy Food Environ. Sanit.* **11**:73–81.

104. Sobel, J., A. S. Khan, and D. L. Swendlow. 2002. Threat of a biological terrorist attack on the US food supply: the CDC perspective. *Lancet* **359**:874–880.

105. Stapp, J. R., S. Jelacic, Y. L. Yea, E. J. Klein, M. Fischer, C. R. Clausen, X. Qin, D. L. Swerdlow, and P. I. Tarr. 2000. Comparison of *Escherichia coli* O157:H7 antigen detection in stool and broth cultures to that in sorbitol-MacConkey agar stool cultures. *J. Clin. Microbiol.* **38**:3404–3406.

106. St. Louis, M. E., D. L. Morse, M. E. Potter, T. M. DeMelfi, J. J. Guzewich, R. V. Tauxe, and P. A. Blake. 1988. The emergence of grade A eggs as a major source of *Salmonella enteritidis* infections. New implications for the control of salmonellosis. *JAMA* **259**:2103–2107.

107. Swaminathan, B., T. J. Barrett, S. B. Hunter, and R. V. Tauxe. 2001. PulseNet: the molecular subtyping network for foodborne bacterial disease surveillance, United States. *Emerg. Infect. Dis.* **7**:382–389.

108. Tateda, K., H. Murakami, Y. Ishii, N. Furuya, T. Matsumoto, and K. Yamaguchi. 1998. Evaluation of clinical usefulness of the microplate agglutination test for serological diagnosis of *Legionella pneumonia*. *J. Med. Microbiol.* **47**:325–328.

109. Tenover, F. C., R. D. Arbeit, R. V. Goering, P. A. Mickelsen, B. E. Murray, D. H. Persing, and B. Swaminathan. 1995. Interpreting chromosomal DNA restriction patterns produced by pulsed-field gel electrophoresis: criteria for bacterial strain typing. *J. Clin. Microbiol.* **33**:2233–2239.

110. Threlfall, E. J., M. D. Hampton, L. R. Ward, I. R. Richardson, S. Lanser, and T. Greener. 1999. Pulsed field gel electrophoresis identifies an outbreak of *Salmonella enterica* serotype Montevideo infection associated with a supermarket hot food outlet. *Commun. Dis. Public Health* **2**:207–209.

111. Truant, A. L. (ed.). 2001. *Manual of Commercial Methods in Clinical Microbiology.* ASM Press, Washington, D.C.

112. Vahaboglu, H., S. Gundes, A. Karadenizli, B. Mutlu, S. Cetin, F. Kolayli, F. Coskunkan, and V. Dundar. 2000. Transient increase in diarrheal diseases after the devastating earthquake in Kocaeli, Turkey: results of an infectious disease surveillance study. *Clin. Infect. Dis.* **31**:1386–1389.

113. van Belkum, A., S. Scherer, L. van Alphen, and H. Verbrugh. 1998. Short-sequence DNA repeats in prokaryotic genomes. *Microbiol. Mol. Biol. Rev.* **62**:275–293.

114. van den Schultsz, C. E. J., F. Cobelens, T. Vervoort, A. van Gompel, J. C. Wetsteyn, and J. Dankert. 2000. Diarrheagenic *Escherichia coli* and acute and persistent diarrhea in returned travelers. *J. Clin. Microbiol.* **38**:3550–3554.

115. Viana-Niero, C., C. Gutierrez, C. Sola, I. Filliol, F. Boulahbal, V. Vincent, and N. Rastogi. 2001. Genetic diversity of *Mycobacterium africanum* clinical isolates based on IS6110-restriction fragment length polymorphism analysis, spoligotyping, and variable number of tandem DNA repeats. *J. Clin. Microbiol.* **39**:57–65.

116. Vinje, J., and M. P. Koopmans. 1996. Molecular detection and epidemiology of small round-structured viruses in outbreaks of gastroenteritis in the Netherlands. *J. Infect. Dis.* **174**:610–615.

117. Vinje, J., and M. P. Koopmans. 2000. Simultaneous detection and genotyping of "Norwalk-like viruses" by oligonucleotide array in a reverse line blot hybridization format. *J. Clin. Microbiol.* **38**:2595–2601.

118. Walter, C. W. 1986. The investigation of Brainerd diarrhea. *JAMA* **256**:2963.

119. Watanabe, H., A. Wada, Y. Inagaki, K. Itoh, and K. Tamura. 1996. Outbreaks of enterohaemorrhagic *Escherichia coli* O157:H7 infection by two different genotype strains in Japan, 1996. *Lancet* **348**:831–832.

120. Weitzmen, I., O. D. Cook, and J. P. Massey. 2001. Investigation of foodborne illness outbreaks, p. 257–266. *In* F. P. Downes and K. Ito (ed.), *Compendium of Methods for the Microbiological Examination of Foods.* American Public Health Association, Washington, D.C.

121. Wellinghausen, N., C. Frost, and R. Marre. 2001. Detection of legionellae in hospital water samples by quantitative real-time LightCycler PCR. *Appl. Environ. Microbiol.* **67**:3985–3993.

122. World Health Organization. 2000. Hepatitis A vaccines. *Wkly. Epidemiol. Rec.* **75**:37–44.

123. World Health Organization. 2000. *Health Systems: Improving Performance. World Health Report.* World Health Organization, Geneva, Switzerland.

124. Yu, V. L., and J. E. Stout. 2000. Hospital characteristics associated with colonization of water systems by *Legionella* and risk of nosocomial Legionnaires' disease: a cohort study of 15 hospitals. *Infect. Control Hosp. Epidemiol.* **21**:434–435.

125. Yule, B. F., A. F. Macleod, J. C. Sharp, and G. I. Forbes. 1988. Costing of a hospital-based outbreak of poultry-borne salmonellosis. *Epidemiol. Infect.* **100**:35–42.

DIAGNOSTIC TECHNOLOGIES IN CLINICAL MICROBIOLOGY

III

VOLUME EDITOR
JAMES H. JORGENSEN

SECTION EDITOR
MELVIN P. WEINSTEIN

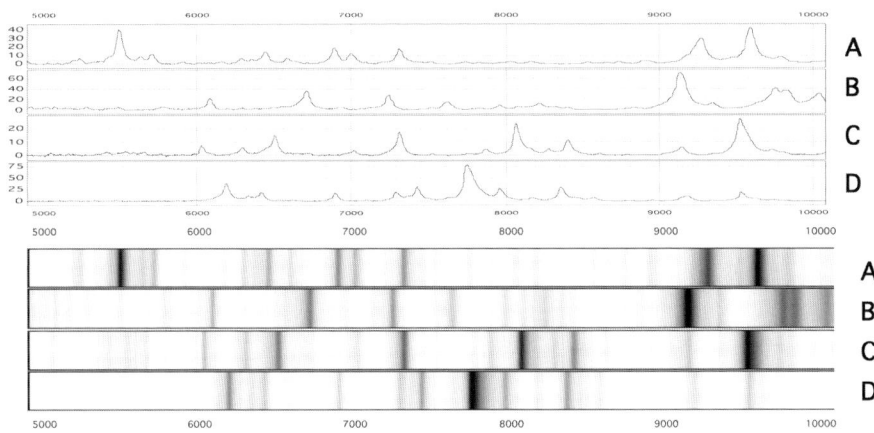

Protein profiles of four bacterial species.

Manual and Automated Systems for Detection and Identification of Microorganisms

CAROLINE MOHR O'HARA, MELVIN P. WEINSTEIN, AND J. MICHAEL MILLER

14

During recent years there has been a trend away from the use of conventional methods for the detection and identification of microorganisms and toward the use of instrument-based methods. In this regard, clinical microbiology laboratories have lagged considerably in comparison with their counterparts in chemistry and hematology. Automation in microbiology first occurred in the early 1970s with the introduction of the first semiautomated blood culture instruments, followed by the early instrumented systems for identification and susceptibility testing of bacteria. In the 1980s, an instrumented screening device for the detection of bacteriuria was introduced. Especially during the past decade, with the development and introduction of automated continuous-monitoring blood culture systems (CMBCSs), this trend toward automation has accelerated. Nevertheless, the fundamental principles that provide the scientific bases for both detection and identification of microorganisms remain important, regardless of whether a laboratory is using manual or automated methods. This chapter reviews the systems used for the detection of microorganisms in clinical specimens, with primary emphasis on the underlying principles and systems for blood cultures, systems for microorganism identification, and criteria for assessing and selecting a system. For an expanded review and discussion of the blood culture issues, the reader is referred to more detailed reviews (13, 46, 62). Discussions relevant to systems for antimicrobial susceptibility testing (chapter 15), immunoassays (chapter 16), molecular diagnostics (chapter 17), and rapid detection of mycobacteria (chapter 36) will be found elsewhere in this Manual.

DETECTION OF MICROORGANISMS

Technical Variables That Affect Blood Cultures

Volume of Blood Cultured

The volume of blood obtained for culture is one of the most important variables in the detection of bloodstream infections (BSIs) (47, 75). It has been well documented that BSIs in adults may be characterized by fewer than a single microorganism per 10 ml of blood. It follows that the sensitivity of detection will be enhanced if a sufficient volume of blood is obtained. Studies have shown a direct relationship between the diagnostic yield of blood cultures and the volume of blood obtained for culture (19, 26, 43, 56). Consensus guidelines recommend obtaining 10 to 30 ml per culture from adults (13), but the optimal volume for maximizing the recovery of microorganisms is 20 to 30 ml per culture (60). The importance of volume for the detection of BSIs in infants and small children has become evident in recent years as well. Isaacman et al. (27) showed that the detection rate from 6 ml of blood was double that from 2 ml of blood from the same blood sample. Kellogg et al. (28) have documented that low-level bacteremia occurs in children and recommends that 4 to 4.5% of a child's blood volume be obtained for optimal detection of BSIs in this patient population.

Culture Medium

A number of different broth formulations have been used to detect microorganisms growing in blood; these include soybean casein digest broth, brain heart infusion broth, Columbia broth, peptone broth, and various anaerobic broths (Table 1). Manufacturers have supplemented the various media with proprietary additives designed to enhance microbial growth, so equivalence among similar basal generic media from different commercial sources cannot be assumed. No one medium or commercial product is capable of optimally detecting all microorganisms. Decisions by microbiologists as to the choice of medium formulations should be based on the needs of the local population and on data from well-controlled field trials in which large numbers of cultures were assessed. The most widely used medium for blood cultures is soybean casein digest broth; brain heart infusion broth may be equivalent or even superior for the recovery of yeasts and some bacteria (76).

Ratio of Blood to Broth

A number of substances in human blood are capable of inhibiting microbial growth, including leukocytes, complement, and lysozyme. Moreover, nearly one-third of patients from whom blood samples for culture were obtained in a recent study (72) were already receiving antimicrobials at the time that the blood samples were obtained. Dilution of blood in broth by at least a ratio of 1:5 has been shown to enhance detection (2, 48), probably by reducing the concentrations of the natural inhibitory substances and antimicrobial agents to subinhibitory levels. Some commercial media, notably, those containing resins, may have blood-

TABLE 1 Blood culture bottles for use with automated blood culture systems

Name	Description	Formulation	Specimen type	Specimen vol	Storage temp (°C)
BacT/ALERT FA	FAN, aerobic	Peptone-enriched tryptic soy broth supplemented with BHI[a] solids and activated charcoal	Blood or SBF[b]	Up to 10 ml	15–30
BacT/ALERT FN	FAN, anaerobic	Peptone-enriched tryptic soy broth supplemented with BHI solids and activated charcoal	Blood or SBF	Up to 10 ml	15–30
BacT/ALERT MB	Mycobacteria, blood	Middlebrook 7H9 broth supplemented with saponin and SPS	Whole blood	3–5 ml	15–30
BacT/ALERT MP	Mycobacteria, process	Supplemented Middlebrook 7H9 broth	Processed sample or SBF other than blood	0.5 ml	4–8
BacT/ALERT PF	Pediatric, FAN	Peptone-enriched tryptic soy broth, supplemented with BHI solids and activated charcoal	Blood	Up to 4 ml	15–30
BacT/ALERT SA	Standard, aerobic	Tryptic soy broth	Blood or SBF	Up to 10 ml	15–30
BacT/ALERT SN	Standard, anaerobic	Tryptic soy broth	Blood or SBF	Up to 10 ml	15–30
BACTEC Lytic/10 Anaerobic F	Anaerobic	Soybean casein digest broth plus a lysing agent	Blood	3–10 ml	2–25
BACTEC Myco/F-Lytic	Mycobacteria, yeasts and fungi from SBF	Modified 7H9 broth	Blood	1–5 ml	2–25
BACTEC PEDS PLUS/F	Pediatric, aerobic	Enriched soybean casein digest broth plus antibiotic-binding resins	Blood	1–3 ml	2–25
BACTEC Plus Aerobic/F	Resin, aerobic	Soybean casein digest broth plus antibiotic-binding resins	Blood	3–10 ml	2–25
BACTEC Plus Anaerobic/F	Resin, anaerobic	Prereduced soybean casein digest broth plus antibiotic-binding resins	Blood	3–10 ml	2–25
BACTEC Standard/10 Aerobic F	Standard, aerobic	Soybean casein digest broth	Blood	3–10 ml	2–25
BACTEC Anaerobic F	Standard, anaerobic	Prereduced soybean casein digest broth	Blood	3–7 ml	2–25
ESP 80A Aerobic broth[c]	Standard, aerobic	Soy casein peptone broth	Blood or SBF	Up to 10 ml	15–30
ESP 80N Anaerobic broth[c]	Standard, anaerobic	Proteose peptone broth	Blood or SBF	Up to 10 ml	15–30
ESP Myco Reagent media	Standard, mycobacteria	Modified 7H9 Middlebrook broth	Blood, SBF, or digested decontaminated specimen	Up to 1 ml	2–8

[a] BHI, brain heart infusion.
[b] SBF, normally sterile body fluid.
[c] Also available as ESP 40A Aerobic broth and ESP 40N Anaerobic broth that are inoculated with only 5 ml of blood or sterile body fluids.

to-broth ratios less than 1:5 (e.g., 1:3); however, these media have sufficiently improved recoveries that the suboptimal blood-to-broth ratios are overcome.

Some manufacturers have marketed "pediatric" blood culture bottles with decreased volumes of broth medium designed to maintain a blood-to-broth ratio of 1:5 to 1:10 when only small volumes of blood can be obtained from young children. The broth media in these bottles are supplemented with X and V factors to enhance the yield of *Haemophilus influenzae* and have reduced concentrations of sodium polyanetholesulfonate (SPS) for improved detection of *Neisseria* species. Although these bottles have become popular, there are few objective data to indicate that they provide higher yields or detect microorganisms earlier than conventional blood culture bottles. Moreover, with the availability of the *H. influenzae* type b vaccine, *H. influenzae* bacteremia in children is now rare. Thus, whether use of pediatric blood culture bottles is truly necessary remains an unanswered question for clinical microbiology laboratories.

Anticoagulants

The yield from blood cultures may be reduced if the blood clots. Therefore, all broth-based blood culture medium formulations contain anticoagulants, the most common being SPS at concentrations of 0.025 to 0.050%. In addition to inhibiting clotting, SPS inhibits lysozyme, inactivates aminoglycoside antibiotics, and inhibits parts of the complement cascade and phagocytosis. However, SPS has some negative attributes, albeit fewer than some other anticoagulants that have been used in blood culture media over the years. SPS has been shown to inhibit the growth of *Neisseria gonorrhoeae*, *Neisseria meningitidis*, *Gardnerella vaginalis*, *Streptobacillus moniliformis*, *Peptostreptococcus anaerobius*, and *Moraxella catarrhalis* (15, 45, 46, 54). In general, higher concentrations of SPS have enhanced the growth of gram-positive cocci but have inhibited the growth of gram-negative bacteria. Although SPS has its limitations, no other anticoagulant has been shown to be superior.

Sodium amylsulfate, an agent without the inhibitory effects of SPS on microbial growth, was evaluated in the 1970s; and its use was shown to result in lower rates of recovery of staphylococci, the *Bacteroides* group, and *Eubacterium* spp. (57). One commercially available medium (ESP; Trek Diagnostic Systems, Inc., Westlake, Ohio) uses proprietary chelators that prevent coagulation by binding to calcium (N. Sullivan, personal communication). Anticoagulants such as heparin and EDTA are toxic to microbes and should not be used (46).

Neutralization and Inactivation of Antimicrobials

Some medium formulations include additives designed to bind to or absorb antimicrobial agents, thereby enhancing the yield of microorganisms. The BACTEC blood culture system (Becton Dickinson Biosciences, Sparks, Md.) uses antibiotic-binding resins on tiny glass beads, whereas the BacT/ALERT blood culture system (bioMérieux Inc., Durham, N.C.) uses activated charcoal and Fuller's earth in a proprietary formulation (Ecosorb). In both systems, culture media containing these additives have been shown to have improved abilities to detect microorganisms overall, especially staphylococci and yeasts, compared to those of medium formulations without the additives (11, 52, 65, 76). More coagulase-negative staphylococcal contaminants may be detected in media containing resins and activated charcoal than in media without these additives (65, 76).

Atmosphere of Incubation

Traditional blood cultures have consisted of two blood culture bottles, one designed to support the growth of aerobes and facultatively anaerobic bacteria and the other designed to support the growth of obligate anaerobes as well as facultatively anaerobic microorganisms. Aerobic blood culture bottles usually contain the ambient atmosphere in the bottle headspace, to which various amounts of carbon dioxide have been added to support the growth of certain microorganisms. Anaerobic blood culture bottles usually contain carbon dioxide and nitrogen but no oxygen in the bottle headspace. With the decrease in the proportion of bacteremias caused by obligate anaerobes in recent decades (13, 32, 41), some investigators have concluded that the routine use of anaerobic blood culture bottles in a culture set is not necessary (39, 41, 50, 79). Rather, use of a second aerobic bottle is recommended to enhance the detection of the more common aerobic and facultative organisms and yeasts and to ensure that 20 ml of blood from adults will be cultured. An anaerobic bottle would be used only selectively for patients deemed at high risk for bacteremia caused by anaerobic microorganisms. Whether only aerobic bottles or a more traditional aerobic and anaerobic pair of bottles should be used remains controversial (13, 62). That said, one should conclude from the foregoing discussion that no one bottle or medium can optimally support the growth and detection of both obligate aerobic and obligate anaerobic microorganisms.

Bottle Agitation

Several studies have assessed the value of bottle agitation during incubation and have documented enhanced yields and improved speeds of detection of microorganisms in positive blood cultures from aerobic bottles (23, 44, 63). All of the commercially available CMBCSs agitate aerobic bottles and, in most instruments, anaerobic bottles as well.

Subcultures

The processing of conventional manual blood cultures includes Gram stains and blind subcultures of the aerobic culture bottles, usually after the first overnight incubation and, if the cultures remain negative, at the end of the incubation period. Blind subcultures of the anaerobic culture bottles in manual systems and of all bottles in instrumented systems are unnecessary (13).

Length of Incubation

In routine situations, manual blood cultures need not be incubated for more than 7 days. Studies of the automated blood culture systems have shown that 5 days of incubation is sufficient for the detection of most pathogens (16, 21, 33, 74). Some investigators have suggested that incubation periods of 4 days (12) or even 3 days (5, 20) may be sufficient for certain systems and media. However, the current standard remains a 5-day duration of incubation. Although it is common to extend the incubation period when infective endocarditis is suspected, Washington (59) has noted that this practice rarely increases the ability to detect the etiologic agent. Similarly, in the best medium formulations of the modern CMBCSs, extended incubation periods appear not to be necessary for the detection of the most common *Candida* species. However, published data for *Candida glabrata* and *Cryptococcus neoformans* are lacking.

Clinical Practices That Affect Blood Cultures

Skin Antisepsis and Prevention of Contamination

The probability that a positive blood culture represents infection rather than contamination is a function of the effectiveness of skin antisepsis at the time of the venipuncture. Growth of blood culture contaminants, especially coagulase-negative staphylococci, which are the most common etiologic agents of catheter-associated bacteremia as well as the most common blood culture contaminants, not only may be confusing to clinicians but also is associated with substantial expense (3). Thus, reducing contamination is a key issue for both the microbiology laboratory and the health care system in general. For many years, contamination rates (number of contaminated blood culture sets/ total number of blood culture sets obtained) of <3% were considered the benchmark for good blood culture practices. A recent 640-institution study done under the auspices of the College of American Pathologists determined the median contamination rate to be 2.5% (49). In that study, the contamination rate for laboratories in the 10th percentile was 5.4%, and that for laboratories in the 90th percentile was 0.9%.

The traditional recommendation for skin preparation has been the application of 70% alcohol followed by the application of either povidone-iodine or 2% iodine tincture. Povidone-iodine preparations require 1.5 to 2 min of contact time for maximum antiseptic effect (62), whereas iodine tincture requires 0.5 min (30). Recently, chlorhexidine has been recommended for use prior to venipuncture; limited published data are available regarding the effectiveness of this preparation for use for skin preparation before the collection of blood for culture (36).

Regardless of the type of skin preparation used, meticulous care and aseptic technique are required to reduce contamination. Studies have demonstrated that a dedicated blood culture team and/or phlebotomists are less likely than other health care workers to contaminate blood samples for culture (61; R. B. Sivadas, B. Vazirani, S. Mirrett, and M. P. Weinstein, *Abstr. 101st Gen. Meet. Am. Soc. Microbiol.*, abstr. C10, 2001). Lastly, blood samples for culture obtained by peripheral venipuncture are less likely than those obtained from indwelling catheters to grow contaminating microorganisms (8, 78; Sivadas et al., *Abstr. 101st Gen. Meet. Am. Soc. Microbiol.*).

Number of Blood Samples Cultured

There is good evidence that the culture of two or three blood samples collected over a 24-h period will detect virtually all BSIs in adults (58, 71). Conversely, the culture of only a single blood sample should be discouraged, if not forbidden altogether (1). The collection of only a single sample for culture will provide insufficient blood volume for the detection of some infections. Moreover, growth of a coagulase-negative staphylococcus, a viridans group streptococcus, or a diphtheroid most often represents contamination from a single blood sample but may represent a clinically important infection (72). Interpretation of the positive result under these circumstances is very difficult.

Timing of Blood Cultures

Few studies have systematically addressed the timing of collection of blood for culture. Although bacteremia is associated with rigors (4), this physiologic event usually precedes fever, and it is the latter that most often triggers the request for a blood culture. Some authorities have recommended that blood samples for culture be drawn at arbitrary intervals (55). However, in a retrospective study, Li et al. (31) showed no difference in yield whether blood samples obtained during a 24-h period were drawn simultaneously or at spaced intervals. The clinician and microbiologist should be guided by the patient's clinical status and suspected diagnosis. In a septic, unstable patient, two to three blood samples should be cultured promptly so that therapy can be instituted. Conversely, if subacute infective endocarditis is suspected in an otherwise stable patient, several blood samples can be obtained at spaced intervals.

BLOOD CULTURE SYSTEMS

Manual Systems

Only three manual blood culture systems are marketed in the United States: Septi-Chek (Becton Dickinson Biosciences), Signal (Oxoid Inc., Ogdensburg, N.Y.), and Isolator (Wampole Laboratories, Cranbury, N.J.).

The Septi-Chek system originally was developed as a labor-saving alternative to conventional blood cultures, which had to be subcultured manually. The system consists of a conventional aerobic broth blood culture bottle to which is attached an agar-coated paddle in a clear plastic cylinder, creating a biphasic system similar to that of the classic Castaneda bottle. After blood is inoculated into the bottle, the paddle is attached and the blood-broth mixture is inverted to flood the agar, inoculating on the agar any microorganisms that may be present. A companion anaerobic bottle that does not use the paddle attachment, which allows oxygen to permeate the system, can be used as well. The bottles are incubated with or without agitation and are inspected macroscopically for evidence of microbial growth once or twice daily. The agar paddle can be removed from its cylinder for better inspection. Following each examination of the agar paddle, the bottle is inverted, in effect repeating the subculture. There are several Septi-Chek medium formulations: casein soybean digest broth with or without 10% sucrose, brain heart infusion broth, Columbia broth, thioglycolate broth, and Schaedler broth. The paddles contain three agars: chocolate, MacConkey, and malt. The Septi-Chek system performed well in published clinical trials (7, 42, 68–70).

The Oxoid Signal system is a one-bottle manual blood culture system that also was developed as a labor-saving alternative to conventional manual blood cultures. After blood is inoculated into the bottle in a conventional fashion, a clear plastic signal device is attached to the top of the bottle; the signal device is anchored by an outer plastic sleeve that slides over the neck of the bottle. Within the device is a long needle that extends beneath the level of the blood-broth mixture. If microbial growth occurs in the bottle, gases are produced in the bottle headspace. This creates increased atmospheric pressure, which forces some of the blood-broth mixture through the needle and into the clear plastic signal cylinder, where it can be detected visually by the microbiologist, who inspects the bottles daily. Only one medium formulation has been marketed. In published controlled clinical trials done in the United States, the Signal system performed less well than its competitors (40, 63, 64, 66).

The Isolator blood culture system is unique in that it is the only commercial system that does not use a broth culture medium. Rather, it is based on the principle of lysis-centrifugation. Blood is inoculated into an Isolator tube that contains a lysing solution consisting of saponin, the anticoagulant EDTA, and a fluorocarbon that acts as a cushion during the centrifugation step of blood processing. After the blood is lysed and centrifuged, the tube's rubber stopper is removed and the supernatant is removed by using a disposable pipette. The pellet is resuspended and inoculated directly to culture media that will support growth of the pathogens for which detection is desired. The Isolator system can be used for detection of routine bacterial pathogens; however, it has been reported to have a reduced ability to detect anaerobes, *Haemophilus* species, and *Streptococcus pneumoniae* if specimens are not processed within 8 h (24, 25, 29, 60). The Isolator system is an excellent system for detecting yeasts and dimorphic fungi, mycobacteria, and *Bartonella* species (6). The system is labor-intensive compared to the newer automated CMBCSs, especially during the initial processing of specimens in the laboratory.

Instrumented Systems

Instrumented blood culture systems were introduced in the United States three decades ago. The detection principle of the first successful instrument, the BACTEC 460 system (Becton Dickinson Biosciences), remains relevant. In the BACTEC 460 system, the blood culture medium contained carbohydrate substrates that incorporated radiolabeled ^{14}C. When growth of microorganisms occurred, the carbohydrate substrates were utilized, with the ^{14}C released as CO_2 in the bottle headspace. As bottles were moved through the instrument's detection unit, needles perforated the rubber diaphragm to sample the headspace. If the amount of ^{14}C was above an arbitrary threshold, the bottle was flagged by the instrument, prompting the technologist to remove it and perform a Gram stain and subculture. ^{14}C is no longer used in these systems because of the problems associated with its disposal. Two of the three commercially available CMBCSs available in the United States still flag bottles as positive, based in part on the pH change associated with CO_2 production in the culture medium.

The introduction of CMBCSs in the early 1990s was associated with a major shift in clinical microbiology laboratories toward the use of instrument-based systems. All of the commercially available systems have a number of characteristics in common. They are modular, a single computer can control as many as 50 incubator units, culture vials are placed in individual cells within an incubating unit, and testing is performed without further manipulation by the technologist (until the instrument flags a bottle as positive), reducing technologist time and effort. In each system, culture vials are monitored individually at intervals of 10 to 15 min for evidence of microbial growth. The instrument's reading of each bottle is transmitted from the incubator unit to its computer for analysis and storage, and growth curves are generated by sophisticated instrument algorithms. Given that culture vials are tested around the clock, it is possible to detect microbial growth approximately 1 to 1.5 days sooner than was the case for the first instrument-based blood culture systems (38, 46, 77). The CMBCSs, perhaps by virtue of the fact that they take more frequent measurements and therefore obtain a greater number of datum points, appear to have fewer false-positive signals than the early systems. Some of the relevant information pertaining to these systems is shown in Table 2.

The CMBCSs have been adapted or modified so that they can be used to detect the growth of mycobacteria; additional information is provided in chapter 36 of this Manual. The CMBCSs have also been used, as have manual and earlier automated systems, to detect the growth of microorganisms from other normally sterile body fluids, for example, peritoneal fluid (18, 51).

The BacT/ALERT system (bioMérieux, Inc.) was the first CMBCS and was marketed in 1990; the system was updated in 1999 as the BacT/ALERT 3D, which has a smaller instrument footprint than the original and a computer touch screen to ease technologist manipulations. Each incubator module has a capacity of 240 culture bottles. At the base of each bottle is a colorimetric CO_2 sensor that is separated from the blood-broth mixture by a CO_2-semipermeable membrane that monitors the amount of CO_2 in the bottle. At the base of each bottle's holding cell in the incubator unit are light-emitting and light-sensing diodes. With microbial growth and production of CO_2, the bottle's sensor changes color, altering the amount of light reflected. The change in reflectance is measured by the instrument, and the information is transmitted to the instrument's computer. The computer has several algorithms that it uses to detect a positive culture, which is noted when (i) the reflectance exceeds an arbitrary threshold, (ii) the instrument recognizes a linear increase in the CO_2 level, or (iii) there is a change in the rate of CO_2 production. Several medium formulations are available: (i) standard aerobic (SA) and anaerobic (SN) media that contain 40 ml of tryptic soy broth and that accept up to 10 ml of blood; (ii) aerobic (FA) and anaerobic (FN) media that contain 30 and 40 ml, respectively, of peptone-enriched tryptic soy broth with brain heart infusion solids, activated charcoal, and Fuller's earth (Ecosorb), which are designed to inactivate or bind to antimicrobial agents in the blood; and (iii) a medium with a lower volume (20 ml) of peptone-enriched tryptic soy broth, brain heart infusion solids, and activated charcoal marketed for use with blood from pediatric patients and those elderly patients from whom it is difficult to obtain larger volumes of blood. A detailed review of published comparative clinical trials is beyond the scope of this chapter, and more comprehensive reviews can be found elsewhere (46, 67). Overall, the system is equivalent to the other commercially available CMBCSs in terms of yield and the speed of detection of microorganisms (67).

There are three instrument formats for the BACTEC 9000 system (Becton Dickinson Biosciences) CMBCS series: the 9240 system, which holds 240 bottles; the 9120 system, which holds 120 bottles; and, for small laboratories, the bench-top 9050 system, which holds 50 bottles. Similar to the BacT/ALERT system, there is a CO_2 sensor at the base of each culture bottle, but unlike the BacT/ALERT system, the BACTEC instrument uses a fluorescence sensing mechanism to detect the growth of microorganisms. When the amount of CO_2 increases, the concomitant increase in fluorescence is detected by the instrument; the principal detection criteria are a linear increase in fluorescence and an increase in the rate of fluorescence. The BACTEC system has multiple medium formulations: (i) standard aerobic and anaerobic media that contain 40 ml of soybean casein digest broth; (ii) aerobic and anaerobic Plus media that contain 25 ml of soybean casein digest broth plus antibiotic-binding resins on glass beads; (iii) an anaerobic lytic medium that contains 40 ml of soybean casein digest broth plus a lysing agent; (iv) a resin medium formulated for pediatric patients; and (v) a medium, designated Myco/F-Lytic, which is designed for improved detection of fungi and mycobacteria but which also supports the growth of bacterial pathogens. Published comparative clin-

TABLE 2 Comparison of features of automated blood culture systems[a]

System	Method for detecting growth	Capacity per module (no. of bottles)	Maximum capacity of system (no. of modules)	Test cycle (min)	Agitation type/speed (no. of back-and-forth strokes/min)	Dimensions (cm)
BacT/ALERT 240	CO_2, colorimetric	240	6	10	Rocking/34	175 by 87 by 66
BacT/ALERT 120	CO_2, colorimetric	120	6	10	Rocking/34	87 by 87 by 55
BacT/ALERT 3D	CO_2, colorimetric	240	12	10	Rocking/34	90 by 49 by 61
BACTEC 9240	CO_2, O_2,[b] fluorescence	240	5/20/50[c]	10	Rocking/30	93 by 128 by 55
BACTEC 9120	CO_2, O_2,[b] fluorescence	120	5/20/50[c]	10	Rocking/30	61 by 129 by 56
BACTEC 9050	CO_2, O_2,[b] fluorescence	50	1	10	Continuous rotation	61 by 72 by 65
ESP 128	Manometric	128	5	12 (aerobic), 24 (anaerobic)	Rotary/160 rpm (aerobic only)	90 by 86 by 65
ESP 256	Manometric	256	5	12 (aerobic), 24 (anaerobic)	Rotary/160 rpm (aerobic only)	199 by 86 by 65
ESP 384	Manometric	384	5	12 (aerobic), 24 (anaerobic)	Rotary/160 rpm (aerobic only)	199 by 86 by 65
VITAL[d]	CO_2, fluorescence	400	3	15	Sinusoidal/150 rpm	108 by 78 by 114
Mini-VITAL[d]	CO_2 fluorescence			15	Sinusoidal/150 rpm	

[a] Adapted from Reimer et al. (46) and Wilson and Weinstein (75) and modified by Weinstein and Reller (67).
[b] O_2 detection is for Myco/F-Lytic medium only.
[c] Maximum number of modules depends on the data management system selected (core, Vision, or Epicenter).
[d] Not available for purchase in the United States.

ical evaluations of the performance of the BACTEC 9000 system versus those of other CMBCSs have demonstrated that the BACTEC 9000 system performs in a relatively equivalent fashion to its competitors in terms of both sensitivity and speed of detection of positive cultures (67).

The ESP blood culture system (Trek Diagnostic Systems, Inc.) differs from the BacT/ALERT and BACTEC 9000 systems in several ways. In this system, bottles are fitted with an adapter and are loaded into the instrument and then monitored for pressure changes within the bottle headspace as gases (oxygen, hydrogen, nitrogen, and carbon dioxide) are either produced or consumed by metabolizing microorganisms. Aerobic bottles are monitored every 12 min, and anaerobic bottles are monitored every 24 min. Pressure changes are plotted against time to yield growth curves, and positive cultures are signaled according to the instrument's proprietary algorithms. Aerobic bottles are agitated orbitally at 160 rpm, whereas agitation is accomplished by gentle rocking in the other two systems. Anaerobic bottles are not agitated in the ESP system, whereas in the other two systems anaerobic bottles are agitated in the same manner as their aerobic companions. In the ESP system, the basal culture media are soy casein peptone broth in the aerobic bottle and proteose peptone broth in the anaerobic bottle. The ESP system was comparable to the BacT/ALERT and BACTEC 9000 systems in studies that used the standard medium formulations of the last two

systems (67). However, the ESP system detected fewer staphylococci and enteric gram-negative rods when it was compared with the BacT/ALERT system by using brain heart infusion broth with activated charcoal (11).

Interpretation of Positive Blood Cultures

In most general hospitals, 8 to 14% of blood samples obtained will be positive by culture. Of the isolates in these positive blood cultures, half to two-thirds will be isolates that are the causes of bacteremia or fungemia, and the remainder will be contaminants or isolates of unknown clinical significance. Thus, interpretation of the clinical significance of positive blood cultures is sometimes a vexing clinical problem. Misinterpretation of positive results can be expensive for both the patient and the institution (3). Several useful criteria may assist in interpretation. These include the identity of the microorganism, the presence of more than a single blood culture positive for the same microorganism, and growth of the same microorganism as that found in the blood from another normally sterile site.

Microorganisms that almost always represent the sources of true infection when isolated from blood include *Staphylococcus aureus*, *Escherichia coli* and other members of the family *Enterobacteriaceae*, *Pseudomonas aeruginosa*, *Streptococcus pneumoniae*, and *Candida albicans* (72). Isolates from blood that rarely represent the causes of true bacteremia include *Corynebacterium* species, *Bacillus* species, and *Pro-*

pionibacterium species (72). Coagulase-negative staphylococci are perhaps the most problematic group with regard to interpreting clinical significance, in part because of their ubiquity and also because 12 to 15% of blood isolates are pathogens rather than contaminants (72). The number of culture bottles positive in a blood culture set is not a reliable criterion for decisions regarding the clinical significance of coagulase-negative staphylococci (37; S. J. Peacock, I. C. J. W. Bowler, and D. W. M. Crook, Letter, *Lancet* **346:**191–192, 1995).

A useful interpretive concept is the number of culture sets that are positive relative to the number of sets obtained. If most or all sets are positive for the same microorganism(s), clinical significance is virtually assured (71). Although ultimately the physician must make the final judgment, the microbiologist may provide important guidance regarding the clinical significance of blood isolates.

Evaluation and Selection of Blood Culture Systems for Laboratories

The process of evaluating, selecting, and validating blood culture systems and media in an individual clinical microbiology laboratory is not an easy task, especially with instrumented systems. These systems tend to take up substantial space, which is at a premium in most labs. Furthermore, even if the manufacturers were willing to provide instruments and media for comparative evaluations on-site, it would not be possible for most laboratories to evaluate and analyze a sample large enough for the investigators to be able to draw valid conclusions. Therefore, most laboratory directors must rely on well-designed, controlled comparative clinical evaluations with large numbers of observations (e.g., more than 5,000 comparisons and more than 500 positive cultures).

Many of the general principles with regard to selection of systems discussed further in this chapter remain applicable, as it is also important to take into consideration the costs of the instrument and the reagents, the space requirements, the ease of use of the system and software, the reliability of the manufacturer's technical support and maintenance personnel, and the cost of service contracts.

IDENTIFICATION OF MICROORGANISMS

Overview of Methods and Mechanisms of Identification

From the early years of diagnostic methods in microbiology until the 1960s, when advances in microbial identification began to emerge, skill in interpretive judgment and the use of tubed and plated media were the bases of microbial identification. Organisms were identified by what we now refer to as "conventional procedures," which include reactions in tubed media and observation of physical characteristics, such as colony morphology and odor, coupled with the results of the Gram stain, agglutination tests, and antimicrobial susceptibility profiles. These conventional procedures eventually defined the genera and species of bacteria and yeasts and became the reference methods by which we confirm the identities of isolates.

The next step in the evolution of identification methods simply miniaturized commonly used biochemical reactions into a more convenient format (22). A system-dependent approach became the industry standard, and it remains the approach upon which most currently used substrate profile systems rely. In a system-dependent methodology, a set of substrates that will allow positive and negative reaction patterns to emerge is carefully selected. These patterns create a metabolic profile that can be compared with an established database profile. In many systems, it is necessary to use different sets of substrates to identify rapidly growing members of the family *Enterobacteriaceae*, slower-growing gram-negative non-*Enterobacteriaceae*, gram-positive cocci, gram-negative cocci, and anaerobes. Yeasts require yet another profile set.

Biochemical profiles are determined by the reactions of individual organisms with each of the substrates in the system. The accuracy of the reactions is dependent upon the users' following the directions of the manufacturer regarding inoculum preparation, inoculum density, incubation conditions, and test interpretation. Most systems rely upon pH changes resulting from utilization of substrate, enzymatic reactions that allow the release of a chromogenic or fluorogenic compound, tetrazolium-based indicators of metabolic activity in the presence of a variety of carbon sources, detection of volatile or nonvolatile acids, or recognition of visible growth (Table 3). Additional tests for microbial identification that use other means of detecting a positive response for a given substrate may also be included.

Although no formal definition of "rapid" exists for describing the time required for results to be generated, most microbiologists expect rapid systems to provide usable results within 2 to 4 h of incubation. Clearly, the generation times of microbes (usually 30 min or longer) will not allow growth-dependent methods to generate detectable biochemical responses within this time. To overcome the problem of generation times, manufacturers of rapid systems use novel substrates with which preformed enzymes, produced by the organisms to be tested, may react to elicit responses detectable within 2 to 4 h.

System Construction

Microbial identification systems are either manual or automated. Manual methods offer the advantage of using the analytical skills of the technologists for reading and interpreting the tests, whereas automated systems offer a hands-off approach, allowing more technologist time for other duties. For all systems, the backbone of accuracy is the strength and utility of the database. Databases are constructed by using known, clinically relevant strains and include the type strains of most taxa. In some cases, before an organism is added to the database, it is evaluated to confirm its relationship to other strains in the same taxon by using the "likelihood fraction." This compares the biochemical characteristics of the new strain to those of a typical culture of the same species.

The number of species included in a database may vary from 200 to as many as 1,200 if the system is to be used not only in clinical laboratory settings but also in environmental and research settings. For most commercial systems, database maintenance is a continuous process, and software upgrades incorporating major taxonomic changes are provided by the manufacturer at intervals of up to every 4 years. Some systems may allow users to make minor changes at the local workstation.

System identifications are supported by algorithm-based decision making that is generally available through a computer. Occasionally, these identifications are compiled into a preprinted index, which is used to manually convert the organism's biochemical profile number into an identification. Bayes's theorem, or modifications of it, is often the basis of algorithm construction from data matrices.

TABLE 3 Basis of identification system reactivity

System reactivity	Need for growth	Analyte	Indicator of positive result	Examples of system
pH-based reactions (mostly 15–24 h)	Yes	Carbohydrate utilization	Color change due to pH indicator; carbohydrate utilization = acid pH; protein utilization or release of nitrogen-containing products = alkaline pH	API, Crystal, Vitek cards, MicroScan conventional panels
Enzyme profile (mostly 2–4 h)	No	Preformed enzymes	Color change due to chromogen or fluorogen release when colorless complex is hydrolyzed by an appropriate enzyme	MicroScan rapid panels; IDS panels, Vitek cards
Carbon source utilization	Yes	Organic products	Color change as a result of metabolic activity transferring electrons to colorless tetrazolium: labeled carbon sources and converting the dye to purple	Biolog
Volatile or nonvolatile acid detection	Yes	Cellular fatty acids	Chromatographic tracing based on detection of end products, which are then compared to a library of known patterns	MIDI
Visual detection of growth	Yes	Various substrates	Turbidity due to growth of organism in presence of a substrate	API 20C AUX

Bayes's theorem is one of the statistical methods that manufacturers use to arrive at an identification of a certain taxon based on the reaction profile produced by the unknown clinical isolate (73). Bayes's theorem considers two important issues in order to arrive at an accurate conclusion: (i) $P(t_i/R)$ is the probability that an organism exhibiting test pattern R belongs to taxon t_i, and (ii) $P(R/t_i)$ is the probability that members of taxon t_i will exhibit test pattern R. Before testing, we make the assumption that an unknown isolate has an equal chance of being any taxon and that each test used to identify the isolate is independent of all other tests. In this case, Bayes's theorem can be written as

$$P(t_i/R) = \frac{P(R/t_i)}{\sum_i P(R/t_i)}$$

By observing reference identification charts derived by conventional biochemical tests, we know the expected pattern of the population of taxon t_i (e.g., *Escherichia coli* is indole positive and citrate negative). R in the formula is the test pattern composed of $R_1, R_2, \ldots R_n$, where R_1 is the result for test 1, R_2 is the result for test 2, etc., for a given taxon. We can then incorporate the percentages (likelihoods that t_i will exhibit R_1, etc.) into Bayes's theorem to arrive at an accurate taxon.

Clinical microbiologists must not, however, become dependent upon these likelihoods and percentages when interpretive judgment would suggest an alternative taxonomic conclusion. Bacteria often tend to stretch the rules of nomenclature when isolated from clinical specimens, and they may not react as expected in a commercial system, even though a legitimate result is produced (e.g., lactose-positive *Salmonella* spp. or H_2S-positive *Escherichia coli*). The result from the most reliable system can be misleading. In these cases, an alternative method of identification must be used. D'Amato et al. (9) have described how the systems use the database profiles and probability matrices to arrive at an identification of an unknown taxon.

The manufacturers of commercial identification systems rely heavily on input from their customers. Laboratories are encouraged to communicate with the product manufacturer about problems such as unusual organism identifications that develop when a method or system is being used. Manufacturers depend on customer satisfaction, and most are willing to assist in problem solving or in projects that could add strength to their systems. These companies, like their users, are clearly interested in the highest quality of cost-effective patient care. Tables 4 to 8 provide a summary of the available identification systems and compare the salient features offered by the automated and nonautomated organism identification methods.

CRITERIA FOR SELECTING A SYSTEM

The laboratorian must consider several issues when selecting an identification system to be used in the laboratory, especially when the equipment will probably provide both organism identification and antimicrobial susceptibility test results. Because the cost of some instrument-based systems may exceed $100,000, purchase of these systems represents a significant capital expenditure and a long-term commitment to that technology. Supervisors and managers in the laboratory should make such major decisions carefully and with expert consultation. Before the first technical representative is seen in the laboratory, several important questions must be answered:

1. Why do I need a new system? Can I justify it as a benefit to the laboratory or the hospital?

2. Will management support the need for a new system? Is funding available?

3. Do I truly need a "rapid" system? Will earlier results actually get to physicians or patient records and affect patient care?

4. On what will I base my final decision? What questions do I need to have answered about the system?

5. Should I buy the system outright or negotiate for a reagent rental contract?

TABLE 4 Summary of identification systems available in 2001

System	Manufacturer	Organisms targeted	Storage temp (°C)	No. of tests	Incubation	Automated
AN Microplate	Biolog	Anaerobes	2–8	95	20–24 h	Reader only[a]
ANI	bioMérieux	Anaerobes	2–8	28	4 h; aerobic	Fill only[b]
API An-IDENT	bioMérieux	Anaerobes	2–8	28	4 h; aerobic	No
API 20A	bioMérieux	Anaerobes	2–8	21	24 h; anaerobic	No
API 20C AUX	bioMérieux	Yeasts	2–8	20	48–72 h	No
API 20E	bioMérieux	Members of the family *Enterobacteriaceae* and nonfermenting gram-negative bacteria	2–8	21	24–48 h	No
API 20 Strep	bioMérieux	Streptococci and enterococci	2–8	20	4–24 h	No
API Coryne	bioMérieux	Corynebacteria and corynebacteria-like organisms	2–8	20	24 h	No
API 20 NE	bioMérieux	Gram-negative non-*Enterobacteriaceae*	2–8	20	24–48 h	No
API NH	bioMérieux	*Neisseria*, *Haemophilus*, and *Moraxella catarrhalis*	2–8	12	2 h	No
API Rapid 20E	bioMérieux	*Enterobacteriaceae*	2–8	21	4 h	No
API Staph	bioMérieux	Staphylococci and micrococci	2–8	20	24 h	No
Crystal Anaerobe	BD[c]	Anaerobes	2–8	29	4 h	No
Crystal E/NF	BD	*Enterobacteriaceae*, some gram-negative nonfermenters	2–8	30	18–20 h	No
Crystal Gram-Positive	BD	Gram-positive cocci and bacilli	2–8	29	18–24 h	No
Crystal MRSA ID	BD	Methicillin-resistant *Staphylococcus aureus*	2–25	1	4 h	No
Crystal *Neisseria/Haemophilus*	BD	*Neisseria*, *Haemophilus*, *Moraxella*, *Gardnerella*, other fastidious pathogens	2–8	29	4 h	No
Crystal Rapid Gram-Positive	BD	Gram-positive cocci and bacilli	2–8	29	4 h	No
Crystal Rapid Stool/Enteric	BD	Gram-negative stool pathogens	2–8	30	3 h	No
Enterotube II	BD	*Enterobacteriaceae*	2–8	15	18–24 h	No
EPS (Enteric Pathogen Screen)	bioMérieux	*Edwardsiella*, *Salmonella*, *Shigella*, *Yersinia*	2–8	10	4–8 h	Fill only
FF Microplate	Biolog	Filamentous fungi and selected yeasts	2–8	95	1–4 h, 7 days	Reader only
Fox Extra Gram Negative MIC/ID	MicroMedia Systems	Enteric and nonenteric gram-negative bacteria	−20–−40	33	18–24 h	No
Fox Extra Gram Positive MIC/ID	MicroMedia Systems	Common staphylococci, micrococci, and streptococci	−20–−40	10	18–24 h	No
GN Microplate	Biolog	Aerobic gram-negative bacteria	2–8	95	4–24 h	Reader only
GNI	bioMérieux	*Enterobacteriaceae* and other nonfermenting bacteria	2–8	29	2–18 h	Yes
GNI+	bioMérieux	*Enterobacteriaceae* and other nonfermenting bacteria	2–8	28	2–12 h	Yes
GP Microplate	Biolog	Aerobic gram-positive bacteria	2–8	95	4–24 h	Reader only
GPI	bioMérieux	Gram-positive cocci and bacilli	2–8	29	2–15 h	Yes
HNID	Dade MicroScan	*Neisseria*, *Haemophilus*, *Moraxella catarrhalis*, and *Gardnerella vaginalis*	2–8	18	4 h	Yes
ID 32 Staph	bioMérieux	Staphylococci	2–8	26	24 h	No
ID-GNB	bioMérieux	Gram-negative fermenting and nonfermenting bacilli	2–8	43	3 h	Yes
ID-GPC	bioMérieux	Gram-positive cocci	2–8	49	2–6 h	Yes
ID-YST	bioMérieux	Yeast	2–8	46	15 h	Yes
ID Tri-Panel	BD	Gram-negative and gram-positive bacteria	−70–−20	30	16–20 h; 40–44 h	Reader only
Micro-ID	Remel	*Enterobacteriaceae*	2–8	15	4 h	No
Micro-ID Listeria	Remel	*Listeria*	2–8			
NEG ID Type 2	Dade MicroScan	*Enterobacteriaceae*, other fermenting and nonfermenting bacteria	2–8	33	15–42 h	Yes
Neisseria Enzyme Test	Remel	*Neisseria* and *Moraxella*	2–8	3	30 min	No
NHI	bioMérieux	*Neisseria* and *Haemophilus*	2–8	15	4 h	No
Oxi/Ferm II	BD	Gram-negative, oxidase-positive glucose fermenters and nonfermenters	2–8	9	24–48 h	No

(Continued on next page)

TABLE 4 Summary of identification systems available in 2001 (*Continued*)

System	Manufacturer	Organisms targeted	Storage temp (°C)	No. of tests	Incubation	Automated
Pos ID 2	Dade MicroScan	Gram-positive cocci and *Listeria*	2–30	27	18–48 h	Yes
RapID ANA II	Remel	Anaerobes	2–8	18	4–6 h; aerobic	No
Rapid Anaerobe	Dade MicroScan	Anaerobes	2–8	24	4 h; aerobic	Yes
RapID CB Plus	Remel	Coryneform bacilli	2–8	18	4 h	No
RAPIDEC STAPH	bioMérieux	Staphylococci	2–8	4	2 h	No
Rapid NEG ID Type 3	Dade MicroScan	*Enterobacteriaceae* and other fermenting and nonfermenting bacteria	2–8	36	2.5 h	Yes
RapID NF Plus	Remel	Nonfermenting gram-negative bacteria	2–8	17	4 h	No
RapID NH	Remel	Members of the family *Neisseriaceae*, *Haemophilus*, and other gram-negative bacteria	2–8	13	4 h; 1 h for gonococci	No
RapID ONE	Remel	*Enterobacteriaceae* and other oxidase-negative bacteria	2–8	19	4 h	No
Rapid POS ID	Dade MicroScan	Gram-positive cocci and *Listeria*	2–8	34	2 h	Yes
RapID SS/u	Remel	Common urinary tract pathogens	2–8	11	2 h	No
RapID STR	Remel	Streptococci	2–8	14	4 h	No
Rapid Yeast ID	Dade MicroScan	Yeast	2–8	27	4 h	Yes
RapID Yeast Plus	Remel	Yeast and yeast-like organisms	2–8	18	4 h	No
r/b Enteric Differential System	Remel	*Enterobacteriaceae*	2–8	15	18–24 h	No
Sensititre AP 80	Trek Diagnostic Systems, Inc.	*Enterobacteriaceae* and nonfermenting gram-negative bacteria	RT[d]	32	5–18 h	Yes
Sensititre AP 90	Trek Diagnostic Systems, Inc.	Gram-positive bacteria	RT	32	24 h	Yes
UID/UID-3	bioMérieux	Urinary tract pathogens directly from urine	2–8	9	1–13 h	Yes
Uni-N/F-Tek	Remel	Gram-negative, fermenting and nonfermenting bacteria	2–8	18	24–48 h	No
Uni-Yeast Tek	Remel	Yeast	2–8	13	24 h–6 days	No
YBC	bioMérieux	Yeast	2–8	26	24–48 h	Yes
YT Microplate	Biolog	Yeast	2–8	94	24–72 h	Reader only

[a] Plates are filled manually, but the system has an automated reading device.
[b] Cards are filled automatically, but read visually.
[c] BD, Becton Dickinson Biosciences.
[d] RT, room temperature.

Once these questions are answered, the next step is to begin the search for the right instrument or system to meet the needs of the laboratory and the medical staff. As a general rule, it is best not to be the first to purchase a new system without having seen in the peer-reviewed literature the results of evaluations performed by reputable clinical laboratories. If microbiology journals are unavailable, the representative can be asked to supply peer-reviewed articles about the ability of the system to correctly identify the range of isolates usually seen in your laboratory. During conversations and demonstrations, the following questions should be answered:

1. Technical applications
   a. Do I like the overall quality of the system? How accurate is it?
   b. How accurate are the identification and antimicrobial susceptibility test results? (Get documentation to prove it.)
   c. What is the turnaround time for a completed test?
   d. What is the cost per test including the costs for the instrument, consumables, and technologist time? What is the cost of quality control testing?
   e. What is the shelf life of the test kits? What are their storage requirements, and do I have adequate space for storage?
   f. Are epidemiology programs available with the software? Can the pharmacy be linked to the system?
   g. Are the printed reports usable?
   h. Who else in this geographic area uses this system?
   i. Do I trust this system to give me accurate results?

TABLE 5 Comparison of features of automated identification systems[a]

Feature	Values for automated identification systems						
	Vitek[b]	Vitek 2[b]	autoSCAN-4[c]	WalkAway SI[c]	Sensititre Aris[d]	Biolog[e]	MIDI[f]
Capacity of system	32/60/120/240/480	60	Unlimited	40/96	192	Unlimited	60
No. of species in database[g] (no. of substrates)							
Gram-negative organisms	116 (30)	108 (43)	142 (24)	142 (24),[h] 149 (44)[i]	140 (32)	501 (95)	480 (NA[i])
Gram-positive organisms	52 (30)	54 (49)	49 (27)	49 (27),[h] (42)[i]	39 (32)	318 (95)	240 (NA)
Anaerobes	85 (29)[k]	No	54 (24)	54 (24)	No	359 (95)	815 (NA)
Fastidious organisms	9 (30)[k]	No	21 (18)	20 (18)	No	Included in tests for gram-negative and gram-positive organisms	50 (NA)
Environmental organisms	No	No	No	No	No	Included in tests for gram-negative and gram-positive organisms	300 (NA)
Yeasts	33 (30)[k]	54 (46)	44 (27)	44 (27)	No	267 (95)	194 (NA)
Mycobacteria	No	No	No	No	No	No	28 (NA)
Inoculation	Automated	Automated	Manual	Manual	Automated	Manual	Automated
Type of incubation, incubation time	On-line	On-line	Off-line	On-line	On-line	Off-line	On-line
Gram-negative organisms	2–18 h	3 h	24 or 48 h	2 or 15–42 h	5–18 h	4–6 or 16–24 h	30 min
Gram-positive organisms	2–15 h	2–6 h	24 or 48 h	2 or 15–42 h	24 h	4–6 or 16–24 h	30 min
Anaerobes	4 h	NA	4 h	4 h	NA	20–24 h	30 min
Fastidious	4 h	NA	4 h	4 h	NA	4–6 or 16–24 h	30 min
Environmental organisms	NA	NA	NA	NA	NA	NA	30 min
Yeasts	24–48 h	15 h	4 h	4 h	NA	24, 48, 72 h	30 min
Mycobacteria	NA	NA	NA	NA	NA	NA	30 min
Manual reagent addition	No	No	Yes	No	No	No	No
Additional tests required before incubation	Yes	No	Yes	Yes	No	Yes	No
Storage temp	2–8°C	2–8°C	RT[l]	RT, 4°C[m]	RT	4°C	RT

(Continued on next page)

TABLE 5 Comparison of features of automated identification systems[a] (Continued)

Feature	Values for automated identification systems						
	Vitek[b]	Vitek 2[b]	autoSCAN-4[c]	WalkAway SI[c]	Sensititre Aris[d]	Biolog[e]	MIDI[f]
Other features							
Susceptibility testing	Yes	Yes	Yes	Yes	Yes	No	No
Urine screen or identification	Yes	No	No	No	No	No	No
DMS[n]	Yes	Yes	Yes	Yes	Yes	Yes	Yes
Computer interface	Yes	Yes	Yes	No	No	Yes	Yes

[a] Modified from Stager and Davis (53) and updated in 2002.
[b] Manufacturer: bioMérieux Inc., 100 Rodolphe St., Durham, NC 27712. Phone: (919) 620-2000, (800) 682-2666.
[c] Manufacturer: Dade Behring Inc., MicroScan Inc., 1584 Enterprise Blvd., West Sacramento, CA 95691. Phone: (916) 372-1900, (800) 677-7226.
[d] Manufacturer: Trek Diagnostic Systems, Inc., 25760 First St., Westlake, OH 44145. Phone: (440) 808-0000, (800) 871-8909.
[e] Manufacturer: Biolog, Inc., 3938 Trust Way, Hayward, CA 94545. Phone: (510) 785-2564.
[f] Manufacturer: Midi, Inc., 125 Sandy Dr., Newark, DE 19713. Phone: (302) 737-4297, (800) 276-8068.
[g] Species in database indicates the groups, genera, or species identified.
[h] Conventional identification panel.
[i] Fluorogenic identification panel.
[j] NA, not applicable.
[k] Although these panels have off-line incubation, they use the Vitek filling module for inoculation and the data management system for generation of identifications.
[l] RT, room temperature.
[m] All rapid identification panels.
[n] DMS, data management system.

2. Manufacturer issues
   a. Can the system be interfaced with our current laboratory computer system? Does it have a one-way or two-way interface?
   b. Is technical and mechanical service available from the company on weekends and holidays?
   c. Is the system expandable?
   d. How much training time is required or suggested by the manufacturer?
   e. What service contracts are recommended? What are their costs?
   f. How much bench space is required? How much does the system weigh, and will this pose an engineering or structural problem in my lab? Are special electrical outlets or communication lines required?
   g. Is the instrument protected from brownouts?
   h. How are software updates handled? Are they free?
   i. Can I trade in my current system?
3. Personnel issues
   a. How much technologist time is required for test setup? For test completion? For quality control?
   b. Is the system usable by all shifts?

It is often helpful to visit other laboratories similar to yours that are using the system under consideration to ask if they like the system, whether they would buy it again, how much downtime they have experienced, whether the service from the manufacturer has been acceptable, and whether the system has been mechanically reliable.

You should select a system that has been fully evaluated and whose accuracy exceeds 90% in its overall ability to identify common and uncommon bacteria normally seen in your hospital or laboratory. The system should be able to identify commonly isolated organisms with at least 95% accuracy compared with those of conventional methods. However, unwarranted expectations should not be placed on the system being considered. Some systems may be unable to identify the more fastidious species accurately, even though these taxa may be listed in the manufacturer's database.

The accuracy of antimicrobial susceptibility testing for combination panels is as important as the accuracy of identification, perhaps more so. Because of the complexities of drug-microbe interactions and the novel resistance mechanisms that are emerging, consultation may be necessary to be assured of the accuracies of the susceptibility test results of a commercial system. Chapter 15 of this Manual discusses the issues involved in instrument susceptibility test methods.

EVALUATING AN INSTRUMENT OR SYSTEM

Anytime an identification system is added to the laboratory, it is necessary to document that the system performs as described by the manufacturer. The first evidence of acceptable performance should be found in published reports by other laboratories that have evaluated the system in a sound, scientific manner (53). These reports should be read carefully, with particular attention given to data that support the conclusions of the paper. Simply reading and accepting the abstract from these published studies may be misleading, especially if the study protocol was poorly conceived (35). The protocols that microbiologists use to evaluate instruments against a "gold standard" or compare one system's performance against another's must be precise in

TABLE 6 Database entries of the *Enterobacteriaceae* (human isolates)[f]

Organism	API 20E, version 4.0	BBL Crystal, version 4.0	IDS RapID onE, version 1.93	Vitek — GNI, version R8.03	Vitek — GNI+, version R8.03	Vitek — ID-GNB, version R02.03	Vitek — ID 32E, version 1.0	MicroScan — Conventional, version 22.28	MicroScan — Rapid, version 22.28	Biolog,[a] version 6.01	MIDI, version 4.0
Budvicia aquatica	X				X		X			X	
Buttiauxella agrestis	X					X	X			X	
Cedecea davisae	X	X	X	X	X	X	X	X	X	X	X
Cedecea lapagei		X	X	X	X	X	X	X	X	X	X
Cedecea neteri		X	X				X	X	X	X	X
Cedecea sp. 3			X					X	"3/5"		
Cedecea sp. 5			X					X	"3/5"		
Citrobacter amalonaticus	X	X	X	X	X	X	X	X	X	X	
Citrobacter braakii	X				X	X			*C. braakii/ C. freundii/ C. sedlakii*	X	X
Citrobacter farmeri	X (*C. koseri*)				X	X				X	
Citrobacter freundii	X	X	X	X	(complex)	X	X	X	X *C. braakii/ C. freundii/ C. sedlakii*	X	X
Citrobacter koseri	X (*C. amalonaticus*)	X	X	X	X	X	X	X	X	X	X
Citrobacter sedlakii					(complex)					X	
Citrobacter murliniae					X (complex)					X	
Citrobacter gillenii					X (complex)					X	
Citrobacter werkmanii					X (complex)				*C. werkmanii / C. youngae*	X	
Citrobacter youngae	X				X (*C. freundii*)	X			*C. werkmanii / C. youngae*	X	
Edwardsiella hoshinae	X	X	X		X	X	X	X		X	X
Edwardsiella tarda	X	X	X	X	X	X	X	X	X	X	X
Enterobacter aerogenes	X	X	X	X	X	X	X		X	X	X

(Continued on next page)

TABLE 6 Database entries of the Enterobacteriaceae (human isolates)[f] (Continued)

Organism	API 20E, version 4.0	BBL Crystal, version 4.0	IDS RapID onE, version 1.93	Vitek — GNI, version R8.03	Vitek — GNI+, version R8.03	Vitek — ID-GNB, version R02.03	Vitek — ID 32E, version 1.0	MicroScan — Conventional, version 22.28	MicroScan — Rapid, version 22.28	Biolog,[a] version 6.01	MIDI, version 4.0
Enterobacter agglomerans group	X		X				X	X	X	X (six spp.)	X
Enterobacter amnigenus group 1	X		X	X	X	X	X (groups 1 and 2)	X	X	X (1 and 2)	X
Enterobacter amnigenus group 2	X		X	X	X	X	X (groups 1 and 2)	X	X	X (1 and 2)	X
Enterobacter asburiae	X	X	X	X	X (*E. cloacae*)	X	X	X	X	X	X
Enterobacter cancerogenus	X	X[b]	X[b]	X[b]	X	X	X	X[b]	X[b]	X[b]	X
Enterobacter cloacae	X	X	X	X	X	X	X	X	X	X	X
Enterobacter gergoviae	X	X	X	X	X	X	X	X	X	X	X
Enterobacter hormaechei	X		X	X	X	X	X	X	X	X	X
Enterobacter intermedius	X		X	X	X	X	X	X	X	X	X
Enterobacter sakazakii	X	X[c]	X	X	X	X	X	X	X	X	X
Escherichia coli	X	X	X	X	X	X	X	X	X	X	X
Escherichia fergusonii	X	X	X	X	X	X	X	X	X	X	X
Escherichia hermannii	X	X	X	X	X	X	X	X	X	X	X
Escherichia vulneris	X	X	X	X	X	X	X	X	X	X	X
Ewingella americana	X	X	X	X	X	X	X	X	X	X	X
Hafnia alvei	X	X	X	X	X	X	X	X	X	X	X
Klebsiella ornithinolytica[d]	X	X	X		X	X	X	X	X	X	X
Klebsiella oxytoca	X	X	X	X (*K. pneumoniae*)	X (*K. pneumoniae*)	X (*K. planticola*, *K. terrigena*)	X	X	X	X	X
Klebsiella ozaenae	X	X	X	X	X	X	X	X	X	X	X
Klebsiella planticola[d]			X	X (*K. oxytoca*)	X		X	X	X	X	X
Klebsiella pneumoniae	X	X	X	X	X (*K. oxytoca*)	X	X	X	X	X	X
Klebsiella rhinoscleromatis	X	X	X	X	X	X	X	X	X	X	X
Klebsiella terrigena[d]	X		X		X		X	X	X	X	X
Kluyvera ascorbata	#[e]	X	X	#	#	#		X	#	X	X
Kluyvera cryocrescens	#	X	X	#	#	#		X	#	X	X
Leclercia adecarboxylata	X	X	X	X	X	X	X	X	X	X	X
Leminorella grimontii			X					#	#	X	X
Leminorella richardii			X					#	#	X	X
Moellerella wisconsensis	X	X	X		X	X	X	X	X	X	X
Morganella morganii	X	X	X	X	X	X	X	X	X	X	X
Pantoea dispersa	X		X			X	X	X	X	X	X

										× (E. agglomerans)
Pantoea agglomerans	× (four spp.)	×		×		×		×	×	×
Pragia fontium								×		
Proteus mirabilis	×	×	×	×	×	×	×	×	×	×
Proteus penneri	×	×	×	×	×	×	×	×	×	×
Proteus vulgaris	×	× (two groups)	×	×	×	×	×	×		×
Providencia alcalifaciens	× (P. rustigianii)	×	×	×	×	×	×	×	×	×
Providencia heimbachae	× (P. alcalifaciens)	×						×	×	×
Providencia rettgeri	×	×	×	×	×	×	×	×	×	×
Providencia rustigianii	×	×	×	×	×	×	×	×	×	×
Providencia stuartii	×	×	×	×	×	×	×	×	×	×
Rahnella aquatilis	×	×	×	×	×	×	×	×	×	×
Salmonella	× (seven groups)	× (three groups)	× (three groups)	× (three groups)	× (five groups)	× (five groups)	× (three groups)	× (four groups)	× (twelve groups)	×
Serratia ficaria	×	×	×	×	×	×	×	×	×	
Serratia fonticola	×	×	×	×	×	×	×	×	×	×
Serratia liquefaciens	×	×	×	×	×	×	×	×	× (S. grimesii)	×
Serratia marcescens	×	×	×	×	×	×	×	×	×	×
Serratia odorifera group 1	×	×	× (groups 1 and 2)	× (groups 1 and 2)	× (groups 1 and 2)	×	×	× (groups 1 and 2)	× (groups 1 and 2)	×
Serratia odorifera group 2	×	×	× (groups 1 and 2)	× (groups 1 and 2)	× (groups 1 and 2)	×	×	× (groups 1 and 2)	× (groups 1 and 2)	×
Serratia plymuthica	×	×	×	×	×	×	×	×	×	×
Serratia rubidaea	×	×	×	×	×	×	×	×	×	×
Shigella spp.	× (two spp.)	× (two groups)	× (three groups)	× (four spp.)	× (three groups)	× (two groups)	× (four groups)	× (two groups)	× (four spp.)	
Tatumella ptyseos	×	×	×	×	×	×	×	×	×	×
Trabulsiella guamensis										
Yersinia enterocolitica	× (group)[g]	×	×	× (group)	× (group)	× (group)	× (group)	× (group)	×	
Yersinia pseudotuberculosis	×		×	×	×				×	
Yersinia frederiksenii	× (Y. intermedia)	× (group)	×	×	×		× (group)		×	
Yersinia intermedia	× (Y. frederiksenii)	× (group)	×	×	×		× (group)		×	
Yersinia kristensenii	×	× (group)	×	×	×		× (group)		×	
Yersinia pestis						×		×	×	
Yersinia ruckeri	×		×	×	×				×	
Yokenella regensburgei	×	× (Koserella)		×		×	×	×	×	

[a]Database also includes 19 additional organisms not listed here.
[b]Reported as *Enterobacter taylorae*.
[c]Includes the ability to differentiate between serogroups O111 and O157.
[d]Recently assigned to the genus *Raoultella*.
[e]#, genus-only designation.
[f]Some products give a choice between two species; the alternate species is indicated in parentheses.
[g]"Group" indicates *Yersinia* group.

TABLE 7 Database entries of the gram-positive organisms (human isolates) for bioMérieux and Dade MicroScan products

Organism	API			Vitek			MicroScan	
	Staph, version 4.0	Rapidec Staph, version 4/99	20 Strep, version 6.0	GPI, version R7.01	ID-GPC, version R02.03	ID32 Staph, version 2.0	Conventional Pos ID 2, version 22.28	Rapid Pos ID, version 22.28
Listeria monocytogenes			×	*Listeria species*			×	×
Micrococcaceae								
Micrococcus (Kocuria) kristinae	×					×	*Micrococcus species*	×
Micrococcus luteus	*Micrococcus species*				×	×		
Micrococcus lylae						×		
Micrococcus (Kocuria) roseus	× (*M. varians*)				×	×	*Micrococcus species*	×
Kocuria varians	× (*M. rosea*)				×	×		
Micrococcus sedentarius								
Staphylococcus arlettae						×		×
Staphylococcus aureus	×	×		×	×	×	×	×
Staphylococcus auricularis	×			×	×	×	×	×
Staphylococcus capitis subsp. *capitis*	×	×		×	×	×	×	×
Staphylococcus capitis subsp. *ureolyticus*							×	
Staphylococcus caprae	×					×		×
Staphylococcus carnosus	×					×		×
Staphylococcus caseolyticus								×
Staphylococcus chromogenes	×					×		
Staphylococcus cohnii subsp. *cohnii*	×			×	×	×	×	×
Staphylococcus cohnii subsp. *urealyticum*	×				×	×	×	
Staphylococcus epidermidis	×	×		×	×	×	×	×
Staphylococcus equorum						×		×
Staphylococcus felis								
Staphylococcus gallinarum						×		×
Staphylococcus haemolyticus	×	×		×	×	×	×	×
Staphylococcus hominis subsp. *hominis*	×			×	×	×	×	×
Staphylococcus hominis subsp. *novobiosepticus*							×	
Staphylococcus hyicus	×			×	×	×	×	× (*S. chromogenes*)
Staphylococcus intermedius				×	×	×	×	×
Staphylococcus kloosii					×	×		×
Staphylococcus lentus	×			×	×	×		×
Staphylococcus lugdenensis	×				×	×	×	×
Staphylococcus pasteuri								
Staphylococcus saccharolyticus								
Staphylococcus saprophyticus	×	×		×	×	×	×	×
Staphylococcus schleiferi	×				×	×	×	×
Staphylococcus sciuri	×			×	×	×	×	×
Staphylococcus simulans	×			×	×	×	×	×
Staphylococcus vitulinus								
Staphylococcus warneri	×			×	×	×	×	×
Staphylococcus xylosus	×	×		×	×	×	×	×
Stomatococcus mucilaginosus						×		
Streptococcaceae								
Aerococcus viridans			×	*Aerococcus species*	×	×	×	×
Alloiococcus otitidis								

(Continued on next page)

TABLE 7 (Continued)

Organism	API			Vitek			MicroScan	
	Staph, version 4.0	Rapidec Staph, version 4/99	20 Strep, version 6.0	GPI, version R7.01	ID-GPC, version R02.03	ID32 Staph, version 2.0	Conventional Pos ID 2, version 22.28	Rapid Pos ID, version 22.28
Dermacoccus nishinomiyaensis						×		
Enterococcus avium			×	×	×		×	×
Enterococcus casseliflavus				×	×		×	
Enterococcus durans			×	×	×		×	×
Enterococcus faecalis			×	×	×		×	×
Enterococcus faecium			×	×	×		×	×
Enterococcus gallinarum			×	×	×		×	
Enterococcus hirae								
Enterococcus malodoratus								
Enterococcus raffinosus							×	
Enterococcus solitarius								
Gemella haemolysans			×					
Gemella morbillorum			×	×	×			×
Globicatella sanguinis								
Helcococcus kunzii								
Lactococcus species								
Leuconostoc species							×	
Pediococcus species							×	
Streptococcus acidominimus			×	×	×			
Streptococcus agalactiae			×	×	×		×	×
Streptococcus anginosus				×	×			
Streptococcus bovis			×	×	×		×	×
Streptococcus constellatus				×	×			
Streptococcus criceti								
Streptococcus cremoris/ thermophilus			×					
Streptococcus crista								
Streptococcus dysgalactiae/ equisimilis			×	×	×			
Streptococcus equi			×	×	×			×
Streptococcus equinus			×	×	×			×
Streptococcis equisimilis			×				×	×
Streptococcus gordonii				× (S. sanguis)	×			
Streptococcus groups E, G, L, P, and U			×					
Streptococcus intermedius				×	×			
Streptococcus lactis/ diacetylactis			×					
Streptococcus milleri group			×	×			×	×
Streptococcus mitis group			×	×	×		×	×
Streptococcus mutans			×	×	×		×	×
Streptococcus oralis				×				
Streptococcus parasanguis								
Streptococcus pneumoniae			×	×	×		×	×
Streptococcus porcinus								
Streptococcus pyogenes			×	×	×		×	×
Streptococcus salivarius				×	×		×	×
Streptococcus sanguinis				×				
Streptococcus sanguis			×	× (S. gordonii)	×		×	×
Streptococcus sobrinus								
Streptococcus uberis			×	×	×			
Streptococcus vestibularis					×			
Streptococcus zooepidemicus			×	×				×
Weisella confusus								

TABLE 8 Database entries of the gram-positive organisms (human isolates) for BD, IDS, Sensititre, Biolog, and MIDI products[d]

Organism	BBL Crystal		IDS RapID STR,[a] version 1.3.97	Pasco Gram-Positive ID,[b] version 4.6	Sensititre AP90, version 2.2	Biolog,[c] version 6.01	MIDI, version 4.0
	Gram-Pos, version 4.0	Rapid Gram-Pos, version 4.0					
Listeria species	× (four species)	× (two species)	*L. monocytogenes*	*L. monocytogenes*	× (two species)	× (seven species)	× (six species)
Micrococcaceae							
Micrococcus (*Kocuria*) *kristinae*	×	×				×	×
Micrococcus luteus	×	×		species	×	×	×
Micrococcus lylae	×					×	×
Micrococcus (*Kocuria*) *roseus*	×	×			×	×	×
Kokuria varians						×	×
Micrococcus (*Kytococcus*) *sedentarius*	×					×	×
Staphylococcus arlettae							
Staphylococcus aureus	×	×		×	×	× (two subspecies)	×
Staphylococcus auricularis	×			×	×	×	×
Staphylococcus capitis subsp. *capitis*	×						×
Staphylococcus capitis subsp. *ureolyticus*	×						
Staphylococcus caprae	×					×	×
Staphylococcus carnosus	×					×	
Staphylococcus caseolyticus							
Staphylococcus chromogenes						×	×
Staphylococcus cohnii subsp. *cohnii*	×			×		×	×
Staphylococcus cohnii subsp. *urealyticum*	×			×			×
Staphylococcus epidermidis	×	×		×	×	×	×
Staphylococcus equorum	×					×	
Staphylococcus felis	×					×	
Staphylococcus gallinarum	×	×				×	×
Staphylococcus haemolyticus	×	×		×	×	×	×
Staphylococcus hominis subsp. *hominis*	×	×		×	×	×	×
Staphylococcus hominis subsp. *novobiosepticus*						×	
Staphylococcus hyicus	×	×				×	×
Staphylococcus intermedius	×	×				×	×
Staphylococcus kloosii	×	×				×	×
Staphylococcus lentus	×	×				×	×
Staphylococcus lugdunensis		×				×	×
Staphylococcus muscae						×	
Staphylococcus pasteuri	×						×
Staphylococcus saccharolyticus	×	×				×	
Staphylococcus saprophyticus	×	×		×	×	×	×
Staphylococcus schleiferi	× (two subspecies)					×	× (two subspecies)
Staphylococcus sciuri	×	×		×		× (two subspecies)	×
Staphylococcus simulans	×	×				×	×
Staphylococcus vitulinus	×			×			×
Staphylococcus warneri		×		×	×	×	×

Organism	1	2	3	4	5	6	7
Staphylococcus xylosus						X	X
Stomatococcus mucilaginosus	X					X	X
Streptococcaceae							
Aerococcus viridans	X (two species)	X	X (*Aerococcus* species)	X (*Aerococcus* species)	X	X (three species)	X (three species)
Alloiococcus otitidis			X			X	
Dermacoccus nishinomiyaensis						X	
Enterococcus avium	X	X	X		X	X	X
Enterococcus casseliflavus	X (*E. gallinarum*)	X (*E. gallinarum*)	X		X	X	X
Enterococcus cecorum	X		X			X	
Enterococcus columbae						X	X
Enterococcus durans	X	X	X		X	X	X
Enterococcus faecalis	X	X	X	X	X	X	X
Enterococcus faecium	X	X	X	X	X	X	X
Enterococcus gallinarum	X (*E. mundtii*)	X			X	X	X
Enterococcus hirae	X		X			X	
Enterococcus malodoratus			X (*E. casseliflavus*)				X
Enterococcus mundtii		X				X	X
Enterococcus raffinosus	X					X	X
Enterococcus solitarius	X						X
Gemella haemolysans	X	X	X		X	X (*G. morbillorum*)	X
Gemella morbillorum	X	X				X (*G. haemolysans*)	X
Globicatella sanguinis	X	X					
Helcococcus kunzii	X	X				X	
Lactococcus species	X (five species)	X (four species)				X (seven species)	X (six species)
Leuconostoc species	X (four species)	X (three species)				X (eight species)	X (five species)
Pediococcus species	X (three species)		X (two species)		X (five species)		X (five species)
Streptococcus acidominimus	X	X	X	X			
Streptococcus agalactiae	X	X	X	X	X	X	X
Streptococcus anginosus	X	X	X	X	X	X	X
Streptococcus bovis	X	X	X	X	X	X	X
Streptococcus constellatus	X	X	X	X	X	X	
Streptococcus criceti	X	X				X	
Streptococcus crista	X	X				X	
Streptococcus dysgalactiae/*Streptococcus equisimilis*	X	X	X	X	X	X	X
Streptococcus equi	X	X			X	X	
Streptococcus equinus	X	X			X	X	
Streptococcis equisimilis	X	X	X (three species)		X		
Streptococcus gordonii	X	X	X	X	X (*S. sanguis*)	X	X
Streptococcus intermedius	X	X	X	X	X	X	X
Streptococcus milleri group	X	X				X	
Streptococcus mitis group	X	X	X	X	X	X	X
Streptococcus mutans	X	X	X		X	X	X
Streptococcus oralis	X	X	X		X	X	X

(Continued on next page)

TABLE 8 Database entries of the gram-positive organisms (human isolates) for BD, IDS, Sensititre, Biolog, and MIDI products (Continued)

Organism	BBL Crystal		IDS RapID STR,[a] version 1.3.97	Pasco Gram-Positive ID,[b] version 4.6	Sensititre AP90, version 2.2	Biolog,[c] version 6.01	MIDI, version 4.0
	Gram-Pos, version 4.0	Rapid Gram-Pos, version 4.0					
Streptococcus parasanguis	×					×	×
Streptococcus pneumoniae	×	×	×	×	×	×	×
Streptococcus porcinus	×					×	×
Streptococcus pyogenes	×	×	×	×	×	×	×
Streptococcus salivarius	×	×	×		×	×	
Streptococcus sanguinis			× (S. gordonii)		×		
Streptococcus sanguis	×	×				×	×
Streptococcus sobrinus	×	×				×	×
Streptococcus uberis	×	×			×	×	×
Streptococcus vestibularis	×	×					×
Streptococcus viridans group		×		×		×	
Streptococcus zooepidemicus	×	×	×				×
Weisella confusus							× (five species)

[a] Manufactured by Remel.
[b] Manufactured by Becton Dickinson Biosciences.
[c] Database also includes 36 additional organisms not listed here.
[d] Some products give a choice between two species; the alternate species is indicated in parentheses.

their experimental design, or the resulting data interpretation could be misleading (14, 35). Because taxonomic definitions are linked to conventional biochemical testing, the results of such testing are usually considered the gold standard against which a system should be measured for determination of its overall accuracy. The use of results from another commercial product as a gold standard may be acceptable when a new product is being introduced into a local laboratory, but such a comparison will not reveal the true accuracy of the system since all commercial products have some drawbacks or weaknesses.

The next evidence of acceptable performance by a new identification instrument should be in-laboratory verification of performance by the purchasing laboratory. Verification is the documentation of test accuracy in the laboratory where the instrument will be used (34). The Clinical Laboratory Improvement Amendments of 1988 (CLIA) (17) specify the following conditions for systems placed into service after 1 September 1992:

> Prior to reporting patient test results, the laboratory must verify or establish, for each method, the performance specifications for the following performance characteristics: accuracy; precision; analytical sensitivity and specificity, if applicable.

Because identification systems provide qualitative information, only accuracy should be addressed. CLIA does not specify how the accuracy verification process is to be done. Each laboratory is responsible for devising its own verification protocol, and verification must be done whether the laboratory is introducing a new system or replacing an old system with a new one.

Smaller laboratories will have fewer resources than larger laboratories for verification of the accuracy of an identification system. Laboratory size, however, has no bearing on the need to ensure the accuracies of laboratory identification methods and of the work performed by a laboratory in support of patient care. It is unreasonable to require that every laboratory reverify what has already been done by the manufacturer and by other laboratories that have published data on the accuracy of a system. A true establishment or verification of accuracy requires exhaustive testing of hundreds of strains. The role of verification by the purchasing laboratory should be to ensure that the personnel using the system can make it perform at the levels of accuracy already documented by the manufacturer and published in the literature. The laboratorian should expect a level of 95% agreement with the existing system or reference method and accept, in the final analysis, no less than 90% agreement. This takes into account the fact that the new system may be more accurate than the old one. If possible, the total cost of verification should be kept within a range of $250 to $1,000, depending upon the size of the laboratory. Toward this end, the laboratory may negotiate with the manufacturer that the purchase be dependent upon successful verification of the system's accuracy and that the manufacturer assist in the process by providing stock strains for that purpose. Verification protocols for identification systems will vary but may be structured around one of the following suggestions:

1. Test the quality control organisms *plus* achieve >90.0% agreement for 1 week of consecutive parallel testing (a minimum of 50 strains) by the existing method. Discrepancies must be arbitrated by a reference laboratory.

2. Test the quality control organisms *plus* two or three known reference strains (stock cultures) of each commonly isolated organism in up to 50 tests (small laboratories) or 100 tests (large laboratories).

3. Test the quality control organisms *plus* ensure that 20 to 50 organism identifications (12 to 15 different species) agree in concurrent testing by the current method or with the results of reference laboratory testing of split samples.

As of early 1998, the Food and Drug Administration (FDA) no longer does premarket [510(K)] evaluations to "clear" automated or manual phenotypic identification systems, nor does it receive or approve quality control protocols from these devices to meet CLIA requirements. Laboratorians must be aware that the identification component of the new or modified system that they are using is not cleared by FDA because this approval is no longer required. This makes it even more important for laboratorians to search the literature for valid evaluations of their chosen instrument and to conduct their own in-house validation to make sure that the instrument meets the claims of the manufacturer regarding identification. Devices and methods incorporating probes, nucleic acid amplification, and other genetic methods, as well as the susceptibility test component of commercial instruments, will continue to be reviewed by FDA for clearance.

LIMITATIONS OF THE SYSTEMS

The databases of microbial identification systems must be revised frequently to accommodate newly named species. For example, had *Enterobacter sakazakii* (the yellow-pigmented variant of *Enterobacter cloacae*) not been added to the databases of these instruments, the clinical correlation of *E. sakazakii* with neonatal meningitis would likely be obscured if only *E. cloacae* was reported. If a physician should ask if an isolate is *Enterococcus faecalis, Enterococcus faecium*, or *Enterococcus gallinarum* and the instrument is unable to distinguish these species because the database has not been updated, clear guidance for empiric therapy against the more drug-resistant organism, *E. faecium*, would take more time or be more difficult. In addition, it would potentially negate the alert to infection control because *E. gallinarum* is likely not a nosocomial pathogen but either of the other two enterococci could be. Laboratorians must be aware that the accuracy of a system is limited to the claims of the manufacturer for the version of the database currently in the instrument and that the database may be outdated.

The laboratory procedure manual must stipulate the action to be taken when a result is questionable either because of the unusual biochemical profile of the organism or because an unexpected susceptibility profile appeared. A backup method must be used to achieve an accurate identification profile. Otherwise the isolate should be sent to a reference laboratory for analysis.

The biochemical properties of closely related species may make it difficult or impossible for the algorithms of the identification process to separate these organisms accurately; however, the inability to distinguish all species within a genus does not always have a negative effect on patient outcome. For example, accurate identification of all of the newly recognized *Citrobacter* species may not be possible for some of the systems. In this case, the effect on patient outcome because of the inability of a system to recognize *Citrobacter werkmanii* may be negligible, and a simple report of "*Citrobacter* species" may provide adequate data for patient management.

Consequently, laboratorians must pay attention to the manufacturer's communications about products, such as letters, notices, or test exclusions regarding the accuracy of their methods, as well as the published literature describing the potential problems encountered by others using these identification systems.

REFERENCES

1. **Aronson, M. D., and D. F. Bor.** 1987. Blood cultures. *Ann. Intern. Med.* **106:**246–253.
2. **Auckenthaler, R., D. M. Ilstrup, and J. A. Washington II.** 1982. Comparison of recovery of organisms from blood cultures diluted 10% (volume/volume) and 20% (volume/volume). *J. Clin. Microbiol.* **15:**860–864.
3. **Bates, D. W., L. Goldman, and T. H. Lee.** 1991. Contaminant blood cultures and resources utilization: the true consequences of false-positive results. *JAMA* **265:**365–369.
4. **Bennett, I. L., Jr., and P. B. Beeson.** 1954. Bacteremia: a consideration of some experimental and clinical aspects. *Yale J. Biol. Med.* **26:**241–262.
5. **Bourbeau, P. P., and J. K. Pohlman.** 2001. Three days of incubation may be sufficient for routine blood cultures with BacT/ALERT FAN blood culture bottles. *J. Clin. Microbiol.* **39:**2079–2082.
6. **Brenner, S. A., J. A. Rooney, P. Manzewitsch, and R. L. Regnery.** 1997. Isolation of *Bartonella* (*Rochalimaea*) *henselae*: effects of methods of blood collection and handling. *J. Clin. Microbiol.* **35:**544–547.
7. **Bryan, L. E.** 1981. Comparison of a slide blood culture system with a supplemented peptone broth culture method. *J. Clin. Microbiol.* **14:**389–392.
8. **Bryant, J. K., and C. L. Strand.** 1987. Reliability of blood cultures collected from intravascular catheter versus venipuncture. *Am. J. Clin. Pathol.* **88:**113–116.
9. **D'Amato, R. F., B. Holmes, and E. J. Bottone.** 1981. The systems approach to diagnostic microbiology. *Crit. Rev. Microbiol.* **9:**1–44.
10. **Doern, G. V., A. Barton, and S. Rao.** 1998. Controlled comparative evaluation of BacT/ALERT FAN and ESP 80A aerobic media as means for detecting bacteremia and fungemia. *J. Clin. Microbiol.* **36:**2686–2689.
11. **Doern, G. V., A. B. Brueggemann, W. M. Dunne, S. G. Jenkins, D. C. Halstead, and J. C. McLaughlin.** 1997. Four-day incubation period for blood culture bottles processed with the Difco ESP blood culture system. *J. Clin. Microbiol.* **35:**1290–1292.
12. **Dorsher, C. W., J. E. Rosenblatt, W. R. Wilson, and D. M. Ilstrup.** 1991. Anaerobic bacteremia: decreasing rate over a 15 year period. *Rev. Infect. Dis.* **13:**633–636.
13. **Dunne, W. M., Jr., F. S. Nolte, and M. L. Wilson.** 1997. *Cumitech 1B, Blood Cultures III.* Coordinating ed., J. A. Hindler. American Society for Microbiology, Washington, D.C.
14. **Edberg, S. C., and L. S. Konowe.** 1982. A systematic means to conduct a microbiology evaluation, p. 268–299. *In* V. Lorian (ed.), *Significance of Medical Microbiology in the Care of Patients,* 2nd ed. The Williams & Wilkins Co., Baltimore, Md.
15. **Eng, J.** 1975. Effect of sodium polyanethol sulfonate in blood cultures. *J. Clin. Microbiol.* **1:**119–123.
16. **Evans, M. R., A. L. Truant, J. Kostman, and L. Locke.** 1991. The detection of positive blood cultures by the BACTEC NR660: the clinical importance of four-day versus seven-day testing. *Diagn. Microbiol. Infect. Dis.* **14:**107–110.

17. *Federal Register.* 1992. Clinical Laboratory Improvement Amendments of 1988; final rule. *Fed. Regist.* **57:**7164.

18. **Fuller, D. D., and T. E. Davis.** 1997. Comparison of BACTEC Plus Aerobic/F, Anaerobic/F, Peds Plus/F, and Lytic/F media with and without fastidious organism supplement to conventional methods for culture of sterile body fluids. *Diagn. Microbiol. Infect. Dis.* **29:**219–225.

19. **Hall, M. M., D. M. Ilstrup, and J. A. Washington II.** 1976. Effect of volume of blood cultured on detection of bacteremia. *J. Clin. Microbiol.* **3:**643–645.

20. **Han, X. Y., and A. L. Truant.** 1999. The detection of positive blood cultures by the AccuMed ESP-384 system: the clinical significance of three-day testing. *Diagn. Microbiol. Infect. Dis.* **33:**1–6.

21. **Hardy, D. J., B. B. Hulbert, and P. C. Migneault.** 1992. Time to detection of positive BacT/ALERT blood cultures and lack of need for routine subculture of 5- to 7-day negative cultures. *J. Clin. Microbiol.* **30:**2743–2745.

22. **Hartman, P. A.** 1968. *Miniaturized Microbiological Methods.* Academic Press, Inc., New York, N.Y.

23. **Hawkins, B. L., E. M. Peterson, and L. M. de la Maza.** 1986. Improvement of positive blood culture detection by agitation. *Diagn. Microbiol. Infect. Dis.* **5:**207–213.

24. **Henry, N. K., C. M. Grewell, P. E. Van Grevenhof, D. M. Ilstrup, and J. A. Washington II.** 1984. Comparison of lysis-centrifugation with a biphasic blood culture medium for the recovery of aerobic and facultatively anaerobic bacteria. *J. Clin. Microbiol.* **20:**413–416.

25. **Henry, N. K., C. A. McLimans, A. J. Wright, R. L. Thompson, W. R. Wilson, and J. A. Washington II.** 1983. Microbiological and clinical evaluation of the Isolator lysis-centrifugation blood culture tube. *J. Clin. Microbiol.* **17:**864–869.

26. **Ilstrup, D. M., and J. A. Washington II.** 1983. The importance of volume of blood cultures in the detection of bacteremia and fungemia. *Diagn. Microbiol. Infect. Dis.* **1:**107–110.

27. **Isaacman, D. J., R. B. Karasic, E. A. Reynolds, and S. I. Kost.** 1996. Effect of number of blood cultures and volume of blood on detection of bacteremia in children. *J. Pediatr.* **128:**190–195.

28. **Kellogg, J. A., J. P. Manzella, and D. A. Bankert.** 2000. Frequency of low-level bacteremia in children from birth to fifteen years of age. *J. Clin. Microbiol.* **38:**2181–2185.

29. **Kiehn, T. E., B. Wong, F. F. Edwards, and D. Armstrong.** 1983. Comparative recovery of bacteria and yeasts from lysis-centrifugation and a conventional blood culture system. *J. Clin. Microbiol.* **18:**300–304.

30. **King, T. C., and P. B. Price.** 1963. An evaluation of iodophors as skin antiseptics. *Surg. Gynecol. Obstet.* **116:**361–365.

31. **Li, J., J. J. Plorde, and L. G. Carlson.** 1994. Effects of volume and periodicity on blood cultures. *J. Clin. Microbiol.* **32:**2829–2831.

32. **Lombardi, D. P., and N. C. Engleberg.** 1992. Anaerobic bacteremia: incidence, patient characteristics, and clinical significance. *Am. J. Med.* **92:**53–60.

33. **Masterson, K. C., and J. E. McGowan, Jr.** 1988. Detection of positive blood cultures by the BACTEC NR660: the clinical importance of five versus seven days of testing. *Am. J. Clin. Pathol.* **90:**91–94.

34. **McCurdy, B. W., B. L. Elder, S. A. Hansen, J. A. Kellogg, F. J. Marsik, and R. J. Zabransky.** 1997. *Cumitech 31, Verification and Validation of Procedures in the Clinical Microbiology Laboratory.* Coordinating ed., B. W. McCurdy. American Society for Microbiology, Washington, D.C.

35. **Miller, J. M.** 1991. Evaluating biochemical identification systems. *J. Clin. Microbiol.* **29:**1559–1561.

36. **Mimoz, O., A. Karim, A. Mercat, M. Cosseron, B. Falissard, F. Parker, C. Richard, K. Samii, and P. Nordmann.** 1999. Chlorhexidine compared with povidone-iodine as skin preparation before blood culture: a randomized, controlled trial. *Ann. Intern. Med.* **131:**834–837.

37. **Mirrett, S., M. P. Weinstein, L. G. Reimer, M. L. Wilson, and L. B. Reller.** 2001. Relevance of the number of positive bottles in determining clinical significance of coagulase-negative staphylococci in blood cultures. *J. Clin. Microbiol.* **39:**3279–3281.

38. **Morello, J. A., C. Leitsh, S. Nitz, J. W. Dyke, M. Andruszewski, G. Maier, W. Landau, and M. A. Beard.** 1994. Detection of bacteremia by Difco ESP blood culture system. *J. Clin. Microbiol.* **32:**811–818.

39. **Morris, A. J., M. L. Wilson, S. Mirrett, and L. B. Reller.** 1993. Rationale for selective use of anaerobic blood cultures. *J. Clin. Microbiol.* **31:**2110–2113.

40. **Murray, P. R., A. C. Niles, R. L. Heeren, M. M. Curren, L. E. James, and J. E. Hoppe-Bauer.** 1988. Comparative evaluation of the Oxoid Signal and Roche Septi-Chek blood culture systems. *J. Clin. Microbiol.* **26:**2526–2530.

41. **Murray, P. R., P. Traynor, and D. Hopson.** 1992. Critical assessment of blood culture techniques: analysis of recovery of obligate and facultative anaerobes, strict aerobic bacteria, and fungi in aerobic and anaerobic blood culture bottles. *J. Clin. Microbiol.* **30:**1462–1468.

42. **Pfaller, M. A., T. K. Sibley, L. M. Westfall, J. E. Hoppe-Bauer, M. A. Keating, and P. R. Murray.** 1982. Clinical laboratory comparison of a slide blood culture system with a conventional broth system. *J. Clin. Microbiol.* **16:**525–530.

43. **Plorde, J. J., F. C. Tenover, and L. G. Carlson.** 1985. Specimen volume versus yield in the BACTEC blood culture system. *J. Clin. Microbiol.* **22:**292–295.

44. **Prag, J., M. Nir, J. Jensen, and M. Arpi.** 1991. Should aerobic blood cultures be shaken intermittently or continuously? *APMIS* **99:**1078–1082.

45. **Reimer, L. G., and L. B. Reller.** 1985. Effect of sodium polyanetholesulfate on the recovery of *Gardnerella vaginalis* from blood culture media. *J. Clin. Microbiol.* **21:**686–688.

46. **Reimer, L. G., M. L. Wilson, and M. P. Weinstein.** 1997. Update on detection of bacteremia and fungemia. *Clin. Microbiol. Rev.* **10:**444–465.

47. **Reller, L. B., P. R. Murray, and J. D. MacLowry.** 1982. *Cumitech 1A, Blood Cultures II.* Coordinating ed., J. A. Washington II. American Society for Microbiology, Washington, D.C.

48. **Salventi, J. F., T. A. Davies, E. L. Randall, S. Whitaker, and J. R. Waters.** 1979. Effect of blood dilution on recovery of organisms from clinical blood cultures in medium containing sodium polyanethol sulfonate. *J. Clin. Microbiol.* **9:**248–252.

49. **Schiffman, R. B., C. L. Strand, F. A. Meier, and P. J. Howantz.** 1998. Blood culture contamination: a College of American Pathologists Q-Probes study involving 640 institutions and 497,134 specimens from adults. *Arch. Pathol. Lab. Med.* **122:**216–221.

50. **Sharp, S. E., J. C. McLaughlin, J. M. Goodman, J. Moore, S. M. Spanes, D. W. Keller III, and R. J. Poppiti, Jr.** 1993. Clinical assessment of anaerobic isolates from blood cultures. *Diagn. Microbiol. Infect. Dis.* **17:**19–22.

51. **Simor, A. E., K. Scythes, H. Meaney, and M. Louie.** 2000. Evaluation of the Bac-T/ALERT microbial detection system with FAN aerobic and FAN anaerobic bottles for culturing normally sterile body fluids other than blood. *Diagn. Microbiol. Infect. Dis.* **37:**5–9.

52. **Smith, J. A., E. A. Bryce, J. H. Ngui-Yen, and F. J. Roberts.** 1995. Comparison of BACTEC 9240 and BacT/

ALERT blood culture systems in an adult hospital. *J. Clin. Microbiol.* **33**:1905–1908.

53. **Stager, C. E., and J. R. Davis.** 1992. Automated systems for identification of microorganisms. *Clin. Microbiol. Rev.* **5**:302–327.

54. **Staneck, J. L., and S. Vincent.** 1981. Inhibition of *Neisseria gonorrhoeae* by sodium polyanetholesulfonate. *J. Clin. Microbiol.* **13**:463–467.

55. **Strand, C. L.** 1988. *Blood Cultures: Consensus Recommendations in 1988.* Microbiology no. MB 88-1 (MB-172). American Society for Clinical Pathologists Check Sample Continuing Education Program. American Society for Clinical Pathologists, Chicago, Ill.

56. **Tenney, J. H., L. B. Reller, S. Mirrett, and W.-L. L. Wang.** 1982. Controlled evaluation of the volume of blood cultured in detection of bacteremia and fungemia. *J. Clin. Microbiol.* **15**:558–561.

57. **Tenney, J. H., L. B. Reller, W.-L. L. Wang, R. L. Cox, and S. Mirrett.** 1982. Comparative evaluation of supplemented peptone broth with sodium polyanetholefulfonate and Trypticase soy broth with sodium amylosulfate for detection of septicemia. *J. Clin. Microbiol.* **16**:107–110.

58. **Washington, J. A., II.** 1975. Blood cultures: principles and techniques. *Mayo Clin. Proc.* **50**:91–98.

59. **Washington, J. A., II.** 1994. Collection, transport, and processing of blood cultures. *Clin. Lab. Med.* **14**:59–68.

60. **Washington, J. A., II, and D. M. Ilstrup.** 1986. Blood cultures: issues and controversies. *Rev. Infect. Dis.* **8**:792–802.

61. **Weinbaum, F. I., S. Lavie, M. Danek, D. Sixsmith, G. F. Heinrich, and S. S. Mills.** 1997. Doing it right the first time: quality improvement and the contaminant blood culture. *J. Clin. Microbiol.* **35**:53–55.

62. **Weinstein, M. P.** 1996. Current blood culture methods and systems: clinical concepts, technology, and interpretation of results. *Clin. Infect. Dis.* **23**:40–46.

63. **Weinstein, M. P., S. Mirrett, L. G. Reimer, and L. B. Reller.** 1989. Effect of agitation and terminal subcultures on yield and speed of detection of the Oxoid Signal blood culture system versus the BACTEC radiometric system. *J. Clin. Microbiol.* **27**:427–430.

64. **Weinstein, M. P., S. Mirrett, L. G. Reimer, and L. B. Reller.** 1990. Effect of altered headspace atmosphere on yield and speed of detection of the Oxoid Signal blood culture system versus the BACTEC radiometric system. *J. Clin. Microbiol.* **28**:795–797.

65. **Weinstein, M. P., S. Mirrett, L. G. Reimer, M. L. Wilson, S. Smith-Elekes, C. R. Chuard, K. L. Joho, and L. B. Reller.** 1995. Controlled evaluation of BacT/ALERT standard aerobic and FAN aerobic blood culture bottles for detection of bacteremia and fungemia. *J. Clin. Microbiol.* **33**:978–981.

66. **Weinstein, M. P., S. Mirrett, and L. B. Reller.** 1988. Comparative evaluation of the Oxoid Signal and BACTEC radiometric blood culture systems for the detection of bacteremia and fungemia. *J. Clin. Microbiol.* **26**:962–964.

67. **Weinstein, M. P., and L. B. Reller.** 2001. Commercial blood culture systems and methods, p. 12–21. *In* A. Truant (ed.), *Manual of Commercial Methods in Clinical Microbiology.* American Society for Microbiology, Washington, D.C.

68. **Weinstein, M. P., L. B. Reller, S. Mirrett, C. W. Stratton, L. G. Reimer, and W.-L. L. Wang.** 1986. Controlled evaluation of the agar slide and radiometric blood culture systems for the detection of bacteremia and fungemia. *J. Clin. Microbiol.* **23**:221–225.

69. **Weinstein, M. P., L. B. Reller, S. Mirrett, W.-L. L. Wang, and D. V. Alcid.** 1985. Controlled evaluation of Trypticase soy broth in agar slide and conventional blood culture systems. *J. Clin. Microbiol.* **21**:626–629.

70. **Weinstein, M. P., L. B. Reller, S. Mirrett, W.-L. L. Wang, and D. V. Alcid.** 1985. Clinical comparison of an agar slide blood culture system with Trypticase soy broth and a conventional blood culture bottle with supplemented peptone broth. *J. Clin. Microbiol.* **21**:815–818.

71. **Weinstein, M. P., L. B. Reller, J. R. Murphy, and K. A. Lichtenstein.** 1983. The clinical significance of positive blood cultures: a comprehensive analysis of 500 episodes of bacteremia and fungemia in adults. I. Laboratory and epidemiologic observations. *Rev. Infect. Dis.* **5**:35–53.

72. **Weinstein, M. P., M. L. Towns, S. M. Quartey, S. Mirrett, L. G. Reimer, G. Parmagiani, and L. B. Reller.** 1997. The clinical significance of positive blood cultures in the 1990s: a prospective comprehensive evaluation of the microbiology, epidemiology, and outcome of bacteremia and fungemia in adults. *Clin. Infect. Dis.* **24**:584–602.

73. **Willcox, W. R., S. P. Lapage, S. Bascomb, and M. A. Curtis.** 1973. Identification of bacteria by computer: theory and programming. *J. Gen. Microbiol.* **77**:317–330.

74. **Wilson, M. L., S. Mirrett, L. B. Reller, M. P. Weinstein, and L. G. Reimer.** 1993. Recovery of clinically important microorganisms from the BacT/ALERT blood culture system does not require testing for 7 days. *Diagn. Microbiol. Infect. Dis.* **16**:31–34.

75. **Wilson, M. L., and M. P. Weinstein.** 1994. General principles in the laboratory detection of bacteremia and fungemia. *Clin. Lab. Med.* **14**:69–82.

76. **Wilson M. L., M. P. Weinstein, S. Mirrett, L. G. Reimer, S. Smith-Elekes, C. R. Chuard, and L. B. Reller.** 1995. Controlled evaluation of BacT/ALERT standard anaerobic and FAN anaerobic blood culture bottles for the detection of bacteremia and fungemia. *J. Clin. Microbiol.* **33**:2265–2270.

77. **Wilson M. L., M. P. Weinstein, L. G. Reimer, S. Mirrett, and L. B. Reller.** 1992. Controlled comparison of the BacT/ALERT and BACTEC 660/730 nonradiometric blood culture systems. *J. Clin. Microbiol.* **30**:323–329.

78. **Wormser G., I. M. Onorato, T. J. Preminger, D. Culver, and W. J. Martone.** 1990. Sensitivity and specificity of blood cultures obtained through intravascular catheters. *Crit. Care Med.* **18**:152–156.

79. **Zaidi, A. K. M., A. L. Knaut, S. Mirrett, and L. B. Reller.** 1995. Value of routine anaerobic blood cultures for pediatric patients. *J. Pediatr.* **127**:263–268.

Susceptibility Testing Instrumentation and Computerized Expert Systems for Data Analysis and Interpretation

MARY JANE FERRARO AND JAMES H. JORGENSEN

15

Clinical microbiology laboratories can choose from among several different manual or instrument-assisted methods for performance of routine antibacterial susceptibility tests. The most popular methods include disk diffusion, broth microdilution, antibiotic gradient, and overnight or short-incubation automated instrument methods (21). This chapter focuses primarily on the instrument systems that are available in the United States that can provide overnight or short-incubation antimicrobial susceptibility testing of common bacterial isolates. Systems are available that provide only computer-assisted data entry and interpretation of visually determined MIC results, while others automate some or most of the individual steps involved in performing an antibacterial susceptibility test. Some instrument systems incorporate "expert" software that can provide automated review of test results for errors or inconsistencies or can analyze susceptibility test results to determine likely mechanisms of resistance.

Among the instrument systems that read and determine test results, some interpret growth end points only when microdilution trays or strips are inserted into a reader device, while other instruments incubate microdilution trays or special test cards to perform serial interpretations of growth patterns in the presence of antimicrobial agents. The instruments that offer the highest degree of automation do so by incorporating some internal robotics to manipulate the test devices during the incubation and reading sequences. Current instruments either use turbidimetric detection of bacterial growth in a liquid medium or detect the hydrolysis of fluorogenic substrates incorporated in a special medium. The suppression of turbidity as evidence of the inhibitory effect of an antimicrobial agent or, conversely, the increase in turbidity in the presence of a drug as an indication of microbial resistance has been firmly established using manual broth dilution susceptibility test methods (59). Determination of susceptibility or resistance on the basis of fluorogenic substrate hydrolysis is a more recent attempt to speed up the measurement of growth during a susceptibility test (3, 53). All of the instruments rely heavily on microprocessor-controlled functions and on the use of dedicated personal computers (PCs) to provide final printed reports and to enable data storage and retrieval. Most of the instruments can also be used to perform additional functions, usually to identify gram-negative or gram-positive bacteria, and to generate combined identification and antimicrobial susceptibility reports (52).

COMPUTER-ASSISTED, SEMIAUTOMATED INSTRUMENTS FOR ANTIMICROBIAL DISK SUSCEPTIBILITY TEST METHODS

Semiautomated devices are available to assist in reading and interpretation of inhibition zones developed on agar plates used for standard disk diffusion susceptibility testing. BIOMIC (Giles Scientific, Inc., Santa Barbara, Calif.), Aura Image (Oxoid, Basingstoke, United Kingdom), Mastascan Elite (Mast, Bootle, United Kingdom), OSIRIS (Bio-Rad, Marnes la Coquette, France), and SIRSCAN (SIRSCAN, Montpellier, France) are plate readers available in the United States or other countries. Depending on the system, disk diffusion plates of various sizes and types of media are inserted manually into the instrument, which determines zone diameters by image analysis in no more than 5 s per plate and interprets the results as susceptibility categories based on appropriate breakpoints. Automated plate readers offer the potential to reduce zone measurement and transcription errors in laboratories that routinely use the disk diffusion susceptibility test method. In addition, the BIOMIC system calculates MICs of individual drugs by computer algorithms from the zone diameter measurements. In limited evaluations (4, 27, 31, 46; T. Kelley, S. B. Killian, C. C. Knapp, P. Anderson, and A. Pereira. Abstr. 98th Gen. Meet. Am. Soc. Microbiol. 1998, abstr. C-475, 1998), these instruments have proven to provide reproducible, generally accurate results compared to those obtained by taking manual measurements. It is recommended, however, that the technologist examine each plate for subtle degrees of growth (e.g., haze or pinpoint colonies within an inhibition zone) that might change the interpretation of the susceptibility report. In such cases, the technologist can adjust the video-assisted readings prior to the release of patient results.

COMPUTER-ASSISTED, MANUAL, OVERNIGHT BROTH MICRODILUTION SUSCEPTIBILITY TEST SYSTEMS

Most manufacturers of broth microdilution panels for antimicrobial susceptibility testing offer a mechanized device for hydration of dried trays and offer reader devices to facilitate manual visualization of results after incubation. Several manufacturers also offer some type of reader device that allows simple recording of the results of manual interpretation of the growth patterns by the use of a light pen, a video display screen resembling the configuration of the tray, or a touch-sensitive template that overlies the microdilution tray. MicroScan touchSCAN-SR (Dade Behring, Inc., West Sacramento, Calif.), Sceptor (Becton Dickinson Diagnostic Instrument Systems, Sparks, Md.), PASCO Data Management System (Becton Dickinson), and Sensititre SensiTouch (Trek Diagnostic Systems, Inc., West Lake, Ohio) are examples of such systems. In addition to recording the manual readings, these devices assist with data recording, application of interpretive breakpoints, and generation of a computer-printed report. The PCs included with these systems enable storage and later retrieval of data for generation of periodic reports, e.g., cumulative susceptibility profiles of various organisms during a defined period.

SEMIAUTOMATED, OVERNIGHT, AND SHORT-INCUBATION BROTH MICRODILUTION TEST SYSTEMS

Automated reading devices that interpret growth patterns in trays or strips represent the next level of instrumentation available from several manufacturers. MicroScan auto-SCAN-4, Becton Dickinson AutoSceptor, and Sensititre AutoReader are examples of instruments for automated interpretation of the results from microdilution panels following overnight incubation in a standard incubator. The mini API (bioMérieux, Marcy l'Etoile, France) can interpret susceptibility test results for members of the family *Enterobacteriaceae* and *Staphylococcus aureus* after strips are incubated off-line for 4 to 5 h, while other organism groups including fastidious bacteria, anaerobes, and yeast require a full 24 h of incubation. These instruments have readers that determine growth either turbidimetrically or fluorometrically and are configured with microcomputers for report preparation, data analysis, and data storage. Although AutoReader, AutoSceptor, and mini API come with an autoinoculator or electronic pipette, these instruments automate only the final, reading step involved in the performance of MIC or breakpoint microdilution tests. Evaluation of one instrument has shown that MIC end points can be interpreted by such instruments with reasonable accuracy (1). However, instances of haze or small pellets of growth that may be important in the determination of resistance can be missed by automated readers (30, 56, 67).

AUTOMATED OVERNIGHT AND SHORT-INCUBATION SUSCEPTIBILITY TEST SYSTEMS

During the past three decades, there have been several attempts at development of automated short-incubation susceptibility test systems. The first of these was the TAAS system, developed in the early 1970s by Technicon Instruments Corp. (Tarrytown, N.Y.) but never marketed (16). The principle of turbidimetric or nephelometric detection of growth was also used in subsequent instruments such as the Autobac System developed and marketed by Pfizer Diagnostics in the early 1970s (later called Autobac Series II; Organon Teknika, Durham, N.C.), the Abbott MS-2 system (later called the Avantage MICROBIOLOGY

CENTER; Abbott Laboratories Diagnostic Division, Irving, Tex.), and, later, COBAS-BACT (Roche Diagnostics, Basel, Switzerland). Although these three systems were commercially available for several years, they are no longer manufactured and are virtually extinct in laboratories today. The VITEK System, formerly called the Auto-Microbic System or AMS (bioMérieux Vitek), and the MicroScan WalkAway (3, 13), formerly called the Auto-Scan W/A (Dade Behring, Inc.), are the only two short-incubation systems currently available for use in clinical laboratories in the United States. Other systems such as the Phoenix (Becton Dickinson), the Sensititre ARIS (Trek, Inc.), and the mini API (bioMérieux) (43) are available in other countries.

To perform a susceptibility test in as little as 4 h, some modifications of conventional susceptibility test methods are required. For example, the density of bacteria in the test inoculum is generally adjusted upward from that used in standard procedures. The actual concentration of the antimicrobial agents in the test wells may be manipulated to provide results comparable to those provided by reference microdilution tests. The MICs determined by the short-incubation instruments may be derived by analysis of growth rates at various drug concentrations. The computer software used with the instruments may allow editing and adjustment of results for certain problematic drug-bacterium combinations. The growth media used in these test systems may include constituents to promote more rapid growth or better detection of resistance for certain bacteria. The specific characteristics of the bioMérieux VITEK, the short-incubation MicroScan WalkAway, and the Becton Dickinson Phoenix systems are described below, in addition to MicroScan and Sensititre systems that employ traditional overnight incubation.

VITEK and VITEK 2 Systems

The VITEK System was a by-product of U.S. space exploration efforts of the 1960s. It was designed and manufactured originally by the McDonnell-Douglas Corp. for the National Aeronautics and Space Administration as an onboard test system for spacecraft to detect and identify common urinary tract pathogens in specimens from astronauts. Because of its intended use aboard a spacecraft, it was highly automated and relatively compact from its inception. Very small plastic reagent cards were designed to contain microliter quantities of biochemical test and selective growth media for the detection and identification of organisms. The VITEK System was modified in the 1970s for clinical laboratory use, principally for the screening and identification of urinary organisms and for qualitative antimicrobial susceptibility testing with susceptible (S), intermediate (I), or resistant (R) results only with *Escherichia coli* or *Proteus mirabilis*. In the 1980s, MIC cards that allowed semiquantitative results for most rapidly growing gram-positive and gram-negative aerobic bacteria in a period of 4 to 10 h were developed.

The conventional VITEK System (now called VITEK Legacy) includes a filler-sealer module for inoculation of the cards; an incubator-reader module that incorporates a carousel-like device to hold the test cards, a robotic system to manipulate the cards, a photometer for measurement of optical density and biochemical reaction color changes in the cards; and a computer module, including a video display monitor and printer (52). The VITEK System also offers an information management system for the storage and retrieval of test data and for the generation of a variety of statistical reports. It uses turbidimetrically determined kinetic measurements of growth in the presence of antimicrobial agents to perform linear regression analysis and, ultimately, to determine algorithm-derived MICs.

Recently, a more automated version of the VITEK System, the VITEK 2, has been developed and marketed in the United States, Europe, and the Asia-Pacific rim. The VITEK 2 automates the initial sample processing, including initial inoculum dilution, density verification, and card-filling and card-sealing steps. This eliminates the need for a separate filler-sealer module and the associated hand labeling and manipulation of cards. The VITEK 2 cards contain 64 wells and are slightly thicker than the 30- or 45-well cards of the original VITEK. In addition, the VITEK 2 cards are labeled by bar coding and the use of a computer chip-containing "smart carrier" that holds and identifies the cards prior to insertion in the instrument. The instrument automatically moves cards through the filling station to the reader-incubator and finally ejects them into a disposal bin at the completion of testing. The VITEK 2 will accommodate a total of 60 simultaneous susceptibility or identification cards, while a larger unit (VITEK 2 XL) will allow twice as many simultaneous tests. The additional automated functions of the VITEK 2 reduce the technical time required to perform each test compared to the VITEK Legacy. Another enhancement provided by the VITEK 2 is the ability to test *Streptococcus pneumoniae* in addition to the gram-positive and gram-negative nonfastidious organisms tested by the VITEK Legacy (14, 20).

MicroScan WalkAway System

The MicroScan WalkAway System was developed in the late 1980s to automate either overnight or, when used in conjunction with MicroScan Rapid Panels, short-incubation susceptibility tests. Recently, an updated version of the same instrument has been renamed the MicroScan rapID/S *plus* system. The instrument consists of a large self-contained incubator-reader unit and a PC and printer (52). Two instrument sizes are available, one that will accommodate 40 tests and a larger version that holds 96 panels. The instrument uses standard-size microdilution trays that are read either photometrically (overnight testing, and now short-incubation with the rapID/S *plus* software) or fluorometrically (short-incubation testing). Once the microdilution trays have been manually inoculated with a multiprong device, they are placed in one of the incubator positions in the instrument. The instrument then incubates the panels for the appropriate period and robotically positions and aligns the trays under the central photometer or fluorometer to perform the readings of growth end points when the value of a growth index exceeds a predetermined level (13). The WalkAway System has offered a choice of MIC or breakpoint testing of gram-positive and gram-negative bacteria after overnight or rapid (3.5- to 15-h) incubation. Special "combo" trays that allow susceptibility testing and organism identification in the same tray are available.

In theory, the detection of fluorescence from a fluorogenic substrate as a marker of growth is more sensitive than detection with turbidimetric readings and would thus allow the more rapid assessment of bacterial growth. However, fluorometric detection of growth is indirect and assumes that all bacteria are capable of metabolizing the fluorogenic substrates, that the enzymatic activity of nonmultiplying cells is insignificant in comparison to that of multiplying cells, and that the fluorogenic substrates do not interfere with the activities of any of the antimicrobial agents tested

(3, 13). Indeed, the early promise of fluorogenic technology has not proven to be superior in practice to that of the turbidimetric approach. For that reason, MicroScan has recently adopted rapid, turbidimetric reading of their standard, dried panels intended for overnight testing, with the rapID/S *plus* version in lieu of further development of the fluorogenic system for susceptibility testing. For organisms that appear to be unequivocally susceptible or highly resistant, results can be available in 4.5 to 5.5 h; for other organisms, results are provided after overnight incubation. The initial reports of the performance of the MicroScan turbidimetric approach appear quite promising (D. Balou, S. Mirrett, J. Hindler, S. Conner, J. O'Connor, G. Williams, and B. L. Zimmer, *Abstr. 101st Gen. Meet. Am. Soc. Microbiol. 2001*, abstr. C229, 2001; J. Hindler, S. Mirrett, D. Balou, S. Connell, J. O'Conner, G. Williams, and B. L. Zimmer, *Abstr. 101st Gen. Meet. Am. Soc. Microbiol. 2001*, abstr. C231, 2001). A side benefit of this approach is the ability to manually read the standard panels after overnight incubation in the case of an instrument failure.

Sensititre ARIS

The Sensititre ARIS was developed in the 1980s and is marketed in the United States only for overnight susceptibility testing, although it has been available in a few other countries for short-incubation testing. The instrument includes an incubator-reader unit that will accommodate 64 panels with an associated PC and printer. Similar to the WalkAway System, the ARIS incorporates the use of standard-size microdilution trays; once the trays are individually inoculated with an autoinoculator module, the instrument incubates the panels, positions them by robotics under the AutoReader for fluorescence measurement, and automatically interprets the growth patterns at the conclusion of the tests. As with the original short-incubation WalkAway System, growth is determined in the ARIS by the Auto-Reader following fluorogenic substrate hydrolysis. The ARIS is capable of performing MIC, breakpoint, or combination susceptibility and identification tests with gram-positive and gram-negative bacteria (37, 53). The ARIS Autoreader has recently been adapted for reading of pneumococcal susceptibility tests using lysed horse blood-containing panels (N. Scalera, T. Kelley, J. Dipersio, M. Kory, S. Killian, and C. Knapp., *Abstr. 101st Gen. Meet. Am. Soc. Microbiol. 2001*, abstr. C97, 2001).

Becton Dickinson Phoenix System

The newest automated susceptibility testing instrument to be developed is the Becton Dickinson Phoenix system. It has recently been marketed in Europe but awaits final approval by the U.S. Food and Drug Administration (FDA) for marketing in the United States. The Phoenix consists of a large, upright instrument that can accommodate 100 simultaneous tests, along with a separate printer. The specially designed test cartridges contain 136 small wells to test up to 16 to 25 different antimicrobial agents, either alone or in combination with wells containing biochemical substrates for simultaneous identification of common gram-positive or gram-negative bacteria. The test panels are inoculated manually by a simple gravity-fed transfer of inoculated medium throughout the disposable cartridge after pouring inoculated broth through an opening in the test device. The Phoenix employs a different approach to growth monitoring by use of a redox indicator system to measure bacterial growth. The indicator (similar to resazurin) is added to the broth at the time of organism inoculation. This approach appears to allow reliable suscepti- bility determinations following approximately 6 to 8 h of incubation (D. Turner, M. Gosnell, J. Sinha, V. Kennedy, T. Wiles, and J. Reuben, *Abstr. 101st Gen. Meet. Am. Soc. Microbiol. 2001*, abstr. C226, 2001; W. Brasso, B. Turng, S. Petti, M. Votta, H. Lilli, M. Deal, and T. Wiles, *Abstr. 101st Gen. Meet. Am. Soc. Microbiol. 2001*, abstr. C228, 2001). The Phoenix instrument will include a rules-based expert system and can be bought with a data management PC and software package called EpiCenter, which will allow networking with other Becton Dickinson microbiol- ogy instruments and a bidirectional interface for a labora- tory information system.

REGULATORY OVERSIGHT OF SUSCEPTIBILITY TEST INSTRUMENTS AND CRITERIA FOR ACCEPTABLE PERFORMANCE

Over the years a variety of criteria for statistically defining the acceptable accuracy of a new susceptibility test system (19, 34, 51, 58) have been proposed. At present none of the professional consensus organizations (e.g., the National Committee for Clinical Laboratory Standards [NCCLS]) promulgates guidelines regarding the specific quality con- trol or performance of short-term incubation susceptibility test methods. Following the enactment of the Federal Food, Drug and Cosmetic Act as amended in May 1976 with the Medical Devices Act, the short-term incubation instru- ments and their drug panels required premarket approval by FDA for clearance to be marketed in the United States. Later, the FDA reclassified short-term incubation systems from the premarket approval review process to the premar- ket notification [510(k)] review process with the use of special controls. When the device is a system employing less than a 16-h (short-term) incubation, the FDA guidance document, *Class II Special Controls Guidance Document: Antimicrobial Susceptibility Test (AST) Systems* serves as that special control (10). Designation of this guidance docu- ment as a special control means that manufacturers must demonstrate that the proposed device complies with either the specific recommendations of this guidance or some alternative control that provides equivalent assurances of safety and effectiveness. These special controls include (i) the use of updated and appropriate "challenge strains," (ii) recommendation of the use of a spectrophotometric device for standardizing the inoculum, and (iii) an "accept- able discrepancy" rate as a range with confidence intervals. This document is intended to ensure well-standardized, reliable, and reproducible performance evaluation for in vitro antibacterial susceptibility testing devices.

Agreement with the NCCLS reference method is used to establish equivalency for all commercial devices for determining the in vitro susceptibility results with organ- isms for each antimicrobial agent. A statistically significant number of organisms including quality control organisms, a challenge set of organisms with known mechanisms of resistance, and fresh or stock clinical isolates representing the spectrum of activity of each antimicrobial agent must be tested. The following would be considered acceptable performance for this type of device: (i) an essential and/or category agreement rate of >89.9%; (ii) a major discrep- ancy rate of ≤3% based on the number of susceptible organisms tested; (iii) a very major discrepancy rate as a function of the total number of resistant organisms tested, with proposed statistical criteria for acceptance that include

an upper 95% confidence limit for the true very major discrepancy rate of ≤7.5% and the lower 95% confidence limit for the true very major discrepancy rate of ≤1.5%; and (iv) growth failure rates in the system of less than 10% for any genus or species tested. For any microorganism, anti- microbial agent, or combination thereof not meeting these specifications, the labeling (package insert) of the device should include this contraindication and should recom- mend the use of an alternative method for testing. In the event that sufficient resistant organisms with an approved indication for use with the antimicrobial agent were not tested, a statement should be included in the labeling stating that the ability to detect resistance to an antimi- crobial agent among these species is unknown because sufficient resistant strains were not available at the time of comparative testing.

The 510(k) review process has been the regulatory mechanism since 1984 for clearance by the FDA for all susceptibility devices that require more than 16 h of in- cubation. The FDA also recommends that this special- controls guidance document be used by manufacturers of overnight incubation systems. The inclusion of the short- term incubation systems in this review category was meant to lessen the burden on antimicrobial susceptibility testing device manufacturers without diminishing the FDA scien- tific review of the performance of these devices.

ADVANTAGES OF CURRENT INSTRUMENTS

The antimicrobial susceptibility testing instruments dis- cussed above are among the most automated instruments applicable to clinical microbiology. However, automation in clinical microbiology has not progressed as rapidly as the level of automation that has been achieved in clinical chemistry, hematology, immunology, or molecular biology. All of the current microbiology instruments offer the po- tential to improve intra- and interlaboratory reproducibil- ities of antimicrobial susceptibility tests, and in some cases they reduce the time required to provide results (e.g., 4 to 8 h versus overnight incubation). Most evaluations have reported that the instruments are mechanically reliable and that well-trained microbiologists readily master their oper- ation. These instruments can offer some degree of labor savings compared to manually performed tests. Because the instruments perform some of the most common tasks in the microbiology laboratory, i.e., organism identification and antimicrobial susceptibility testing, the potential exists to automate a sizable portion of a laboratory's workload with only one instrument. The potential to establish a link between the microcomputer that controls the function of the instrument or its data management system and the laboratory information system affords both potential sav- ings in labor and the elimination of transcription errors associated with manual entry of results. When instruments are interfaced, however, verification of susceptibility data by supervisory personnel is advisable before the automated transfer of data to a patient's file. In addition, the data management systems available with these instruments can archive and periodically provide the cumulative antimicro- bial susceptibilities of the microorganisms encountered in a given medical institution.

Several of the systems allow linkage of the microbiology results with the patient's pharmacy record, thus enabling a review of the antimicrobial therapy regimen. In some in- stitutions, such linkages can ultimately notify the prescrib- ing physician or pharmacist when the isolated organism is resistant to the antimicrobial therapy, when therapy for a clinical isolate for which susceptibility results have been obtained has not been started, or when an antimicrobial agent has been administered for which the algorithm cannot find a clinical isolate or susceptibility test results for the patient (40).

Limited data suggest that rapid susceptibility test results can have a major positive impact on patient care and help to reduce the cost of hospitalization. Some earlier studies (60, 63) showed that providing rapid susceptibility test reports could result in a more timely change to appropriate antimicrobial therapy than if conventional reporting times were used. However, a later study (9) documented a lower mortality rate, as well as direct cost savings attributable to ordering of fewer diagnostic studies and reducing the number of days in an intensive care unit based on rapid susceptibility test reporting. A more recent study also demonstrated cost savings when rapid susceptibility reports were routinely issued (2). This was said to be due to initiating appropriate antibacterial therapy sooner, which led to decreased lengths of hospital stays. Both of these studies claimed very significant potential cost savings that could be achieved through the rapid provision of antimicrobial susceptibility data. However, it is important to note that the rapid generation of any test results in the laboratory can have a clinical impact only when the reports are quickly and efficiently transmitted to physicians (23, 33, 40).

Another advantage of instrument-based susceptibility test systems is the potential to utilize an "expert" software system (7, 15, 40, 48, 49) for automated review and verification of the data generated. Appropriately programmed software can contain algorithms or rules similar to those used by knowledgeable microbiologists to detect impossible or unusual phenotypes or to allow recognition of technical errors that may have occurred in the testing. For example, unusual phenotypes such as ampicillin-susceptible *Klebsiella pneumoniae* or cefazolin-susceptible *Enterobacter cloacae* would be flagged by the system for further testing. Other rules designed to recognize unlikely resistance patterns or rare phenotypes such as imipenem-resistant *E. coli* can also be designed. Following detection, the possibility of potential errors or the detection of unusual phenotypes can be displayed on the data terminal or laboratory report for supervisory review. Expert systems can use an organism's antibiogram to predict resistance mechanisms that can enable laboratories to modify the susceptibility test report to reflect the implications of the mechanism (e.g., resistance to all cephalosporins conferred by an extended-spectrum β-lactamase or the resistance to all penicillins and cephalosporins of a methicillin-resistant *Staphylococcus* spp.). For the mini API, VITEK, VITEK 2, MicroScan, and Phoenix systems, expert software currently exists. The rules and use of computerized expert systems for data analysis and interpretation are further discussed in the last section of this chapter.

DISADVANTAGES OF CURRENT INSTRUMENTS

The instruments discussed in this chapter offer automation of several of the steps involved in the performance of an antimicrobial susceptibility test, but only recently has an instrument (VITEK 2) been able to automate almost the entire process, i.e., to standardize an inoculum and continue through to the final interpretation of results without operator intervention. In all cases, microbiologists must still isolate bacteria by using conventional culture methods and prepare a bacterial suspension of defined density for testing by the instrument. Thus, the automated aspects of the test do not begin until after the manual inoculum preparation. Indeed, inadequacy of the inoculum is a major variable affecting the performance of all of the instruments.

When one of these instruments is purchased, a large capital investment for hardware is required. The disposables used with the rapid systems may be more expensive than the components needed for manual test methods (e.g., disk diffusion testing). In addition to space and electrical requirements, fees for service contracts add to operational costs. Laboratories may wish to gain access to an instrument system by using a reagent rental or lease agreement to avoid a large, initial capital outlay for hardware and to incorporate the costs of maintenance.

A limitation of current instruments is the relative inflexibility of the antimicrobial test batteries available for routine use. Laboratories must select the test panels that most closely conform to their institution's formulary. This may mean that compromises must be made because standard test panels may not exactly match the list of formulary drugs. This also affects the ability of a laboratory to change the test battery or to quickly begin testing when a newly marketed antimicrobial agent is introduced. The NCCLS provides some assistance in selection of agents that are very similar and may serve as surrogates for other closely related drugs when compromises in testing batteries must be made (35, 36). Manufacturers may offer preparation of custom test panels that coincide exactly with a laboratory's needs, although such panels usually are appreciably more expensive than standard panels and may require the purchase of a specified quantify of the panels.

A disadvantage of most of the current instrument-based systems is their inability to test all clinically relevant groups of bacteria. For example, the testing of nutritionally fastidious bacteria, anaerobes, and certain nonfermentative gram-negative bacilli is not possible with some of the current instruments (22). Therefore, alternative susceptibility test methods must be available in the laboratory. Recent notable exceptions include the ability to test *S. pneumoniae* using the VITEK 2 (14, 20) and Sensititre Autoreader (N. Scalera, T. Kelley, J. Dipersio, M. Kory, S. Killian, and C. Knapp. *Abstr. 101st Gen. Meet. Am. Soc. Microbiol. 2001*, abstr. C97, 2001) systems.

In terms of the accuracy of susceptibility test results generated by instrument systems, there are more published evaluations available regarding the VITEK and VITEK 2 than with the other systems (8, 29, 42). At times, reports have pointed out problems with various instruments, which are in turn addressed by the manufacturers through revised reagents or software. For that reason, it is difficult to know the exact level of performance of a system at a given moment. Historically, an incubation period of only 4 to 6 h has not been adequate for expression of all bacterial resistance mechanisms, e.g., inducible β-lactamase-mediated resistance to some enzyme-labile β-lactam antimicrobial agents among gram-negative bacilli (28, 50, 64). This has been particularly true with *Citrobacter freundii*, *Enterobacter* spp., *Serratia* spp., *Morganella morganii*, *Providencia* spp., and *Pseudomonas aeruginosa* (5, 58). Although detection of plasmid-mediated extended-spectrum β-lactamases that confer resistance to all of the cephalosporins and aztreonam is a problem for reference susceptibility test methods, it may be even more so for short-incubation systems (24). Recent inclusion of test wells with low concentrations of broad-spectrum cephalosporins with and without a β-lactamase inhibitor such as clavulanate should help to detect strains with these enzymes (43, 47; J. Spargo, M. J. Ferraro, S. Fitzsimmons, R. Knefel, and G. Jacoby. *Program Abstr. 38th Intersci. Conf. Antimicrob. Agents Chemother.*, abstr. D-44, 1998), which appear to be most common in *Klebsiella* spp. and *E. coli*.

The ability of a susceptibility testing instrument system to detect emerging resistance in key organisms is an important criterion in selecting a system. Low-level vancomycin resistance in *Enterococcus* spp., especially that of the VanB type, may not be detected by some short-incubation susceptibility test systems (12, 17, 39, 44, 56, 57, 62). Since some vancomycin-resistant strains exhibit inducible resistance, failure to detect such strains may be due in part to the short incubation period. Likewise, intrinsic, low-level resistance of the VanC type in *Enterococcus gallinarum* may not always be detected accurately (44, 56). Short-incubation susceptibility testing systems may also not reliably detect the increased, intermediate-level vancomycin MICs that have been reported with rare *S. aureus* strains and certain coagulase-negative staphylococci (55). Recent studies that have focused on fluoroquinolone-resistant gramnegative bacteria have found relatively few very major or major errors with the VITEK and MicroScan systems, although a number of minor interpretive category errors were noted with both systems (54; Hindler et al., *Abstr. 101st Gen. Meet. Am. Soc. Microbiol. 2001*).

Problems with the detection of high-level gentamicin resistance or high-level streptomycin resistance in *Enterococcus* spp. have also been reported for overnight and short-incubation susceptibility test systems (45, 65). For the short-incubation systems, a decrease in the concentration of aminoglycosides in the test medium appeared to correct the problems (38, 68). Failure of an optical reading device to detect subtle amounts of growth in wells with high levels of an aminoglycoside following overnight incubation has been reported (30). Changes in the growth medium used in these wells for overnight systems (65), as recommended by NCCLS (35), or extended incubation (68) seem to have corrected these problems.

Errors in the detection of oxacillin resistance in staphylococci continue to be reported with various testing systems. These include both failure to detect some resistant strains (11) and reporting of false resistance by certain VITEK cards for *S. aureus* (41). Later studies, using newer or different VITEK cards, have reported acceptable accuracy in the detection of methicillin resistance in both *S. aureus* and coagulase-negative staphylococci (32, 69).

False-resistance to aztreonam, especially with *Proteus* and *Morganella* spp., can occur in the systems that detect growth photometrically (D. J. Biedenbach and R. N. Jones, Editorial, *Diagn. Microbiol. Infect. Dis.* **21:**57–60, 1995). This phenomenon may result because elongation of the cells, which occurs just prior to lysis, is interpreted as growth. Additionally, false resistance of various species to imipenem and aztreonam has been reported for both overnight-incubation and short-incubation systems (8, 18, 66; Biedenbach and Jones, Editorial). Overinoculation of VITEK cards results in false resistance for several agents (8, 18). False resistance to imipenem occurs sporadically and may be due to degradation of the antimicrobial agent in the specific test system (66) or to the zinc concentration in the medium (6). However, one report noted false resistance to that agent specifically in *Acinetobacter baumannii* that was not readily explained by technical deviations (61). Mucoid

strains of some species may also confound attempts to accurately interpret the growth in an instrument system (5). Because some of these problems may not be solved easily, manufacturer package inserts may include disclaimers or limitations for certain organism-drug combinations that cannot be tested with their system. If the disclaimed antimicrobial agent is critical to patient care, an alternate procedure is recommended in lieu of reporting the results for that agent.

Quality control is dependent on the use of American Type Culture Collection organisms specified by the manufacturer, since NCCLS does not provide standards for test procedures or quality control of short-incubation susceptibility test systems. Some of the quality control organisms suggested by manufacturers do not produce on-scale quality control values (25, 26). Thus, the routine quality control testing suggested by the manufacturer may not detect subtle deteriorations in instrument or reagent performance.

COMPUTERIZED EXPERT SYSTEMS

Laboratories may purchase a susceptibility test system that has preprogrammed, rule-based expert systems (e.g., VITEK, Phoenix, and MicroScan). Alternatively, the microbiology laboratory information system may allow the custom programming of similar computer algorithms. In either case, the success of the rule-based expert system relies squarely on the expertise of the creators and, potentially, on the customized rules for a specific institution. The medical and laboratory decision support afforded by these programs has several advantages. The algorithms allow continuous monitoring of inconsistent laboratory test results without human intervention, such that there should be more rapid recognition of incorrect or aberrant identification or susceptibility test results. Their use should lead to more uniform reporting both within and among laboratories.

Tables 1, 2, and 3 provide information on resistant and susceptible phenotypes for organisms and their commonly tested antimicrobial agents (35, 36). Table 4 lists expected common phenotypes for organisms that indicate cross-resistance to antimicrobial agents within a similar drug classification. The information in these tables could be used to program a laboratory information system or could be compared to preprogrammed rules available with susceptibility test instrument software. In general, such inconsistencies should lead to verification of the isolate's identity and to a repeat of the susceptibility test by the same or a different method. However, rules more elaborate (7) than those given in this chapter, especially if they are programmed solely on the basis of genetic mechanisms, risk overprediction of clinical resistance.

The full benefit of an expert system generally requires the testing of an array of predictor antimicrobial agents, some of which may not be clinically useful. The VITEK, Phoenix, and MicroScan systems all use a rules-based approach. BioMérieux has taken a different approach with the Advanced Expert System (AES) for the VITEK 2. Instead of a rules-based approach, the new VITEK has used a type of "artificial intelligence" established by testing a large number of isolates that have normal levels of susceptibility for their species, and strains with various acquired resistance mechanisms. In addition, MICs have been entered into the AES database from a large number of published articles to further increase the number of observations for each species and antimicrobial agent. In practice, the AES

TABLE 1 Resistance phenotypes that are rare or that have not been detected

Organism(s)	Antimicrobial agent(s) to which resistance is uncommon
Members of the family *Enterobacteriaceae*	Imipenem, meropenem
Staphylococcus aureus	Vancomycin, linezolid, quinupristin-dalfopristin, teicoplanin
Coagulase-negative staphylococci	Vancomycin, linezolid, quinupristin-dalfopristin
Enterococcus faecalis	Ampicillin, linezolid
Enterococcus faecium	Linezolid, quinupristin-dalfopristin
Beta-hemolytic streptococci groups A, B, C, and G	Penicillin, ampicillin, extended-spectrum cephalosporins
Streptococcus spp. (all)	Vancomycin, linezolid
Haemophilus influenzae	Extended-spectrum cephalosporins, fluoroquinolones
Neisseria gonorrhoeae, Neisseria meningitidis	Extended-spectrum cephalosporins

TABLE 2 Members of the family *Enterobacteriaceae* with expected resistance to commonly tested antimicrobial agents

Organism(s)	Antimicrobial agent(s) to which resistance is expected
Citrobacter, Enterobacter, Klebsiella, Morganella, Providencia, Proteus vulgaris, Proteus penneri, Serratia, Yersinia	Ampicillin
Citrobacter freundii, Enterobacter, Morganella, P. vulgaris, P. penneri, Providencia, Serratia, Yersinia	Cefazolin, cephalothin
Klebsiella	Ticarcillin
C. freundii, Enterobacter, Serratia	Cefoxitin, cefotetan
C. freundii, Enterobacter, P. vulgaris, Serratia	Cefuroxime
Citrobacter, Enterobacter, Serratia	Amoxicillin-clavulanic acid, ampicillin-sulbactam

TABLE 3 *Pseudomonas aeruginosa* and other nonmembers of the family *Enterobacteriaceae* with expected resistance to commonly tested antimicrobial agents

Organism(s)	Antimicrobial agent(s) to which resistance is expected
Acinetobacter baumannii, Aeromonas, Burkholderia cepacia, Pseudomonas aeruginosa, Stenotrophomonas maltophilia	Ampicillin, cefazolin, cephalothin, cefoxitin, cefotetan, cefmetazole
Acinetobacter baumannii	Ticarcillin, mezlocillin, piperacillin
B. cepacia, S. maltophilia	Gentamicin
S. maltophilia	Imipenem, meropenem
P. aeruginosa	Trimethoprim-sulfamethoxazole

TABLE 4 Susceptibility test results that may indicate cross-resistance to other antimicrobial agents

Organism	Antimicrobial agents	
	Primary resistance	Associated resistance
Staphylococcus	Oxacillin	Methicillin, cloxacillin, dicloxacillin, nafcillin, other penicillins, β-lactam–β-lactamase inhibitor combinations, cephems and carbapenems
	Gentamicin	Other aminoglycosides
	Penicillin (β-lactamase positive)	Ampicillin, amoxicillin, azlocillin, carbenicillin, mezlocillin, piperacillin, ticarcillin
	Erythromycin	Azithromycin, clarithromycin
	Ciprofloxacin	Ofloxacin, levofloxacin
Members of the family *Enterobacteriaceae, Pseudomonas aeruginosa*	Gentamicin	Tobramycin
	Amikacin	Gentamicin, tobramycin
	Ciprofloxacin	Ofloxacin, levofloxacin
Klebsiella spp., *Escherichia coli*	Ceftazidime	Cefotaxime, ceftriaxone, ceftizoxime, aztreonam
	Cefotaxime	Ceftazidime, ceftriaxone, ceftizoxime, aztreonam
Enterococcus spp.	High levels of gentamicin	High levels of tobramycin, high levels of amikacin

compares MICs obtained during an individual test with the expected results for that species. If resistance is detected, the phenotypic pattern of resistance is compared with profiles obtained with strains that harbor known resistance mechanisms. This provides an opportunity to describe the most likely mechanisms of resistance encountered in a clinical isolate and the opportunity to correct any inconsistencies in the susceptibility report. Finally, the success of antimicrobial algorithms or expert system approaches is dependent on the correct identification of the organism. Inconsistent phenotypes generally require verification of both organism identification and susceptibility results. Often unusual results are due to transcription errors, contamination, or the use of defective materials. In some cases, use of an alternative identification or susceptibility test method may help to resolve the discrepancy.

SUMMARY

Instruments for the performance of antimicrobial susceptibility testing should be viewed as some of the best examples of automation in clinical microbiology. The performance of susceptibility tests seems well suited to instrumentation, since an objective measurement of microbial growth is the basis for the test. Some instruments provide more rapid results than can be generated by using manual systems, and all have the potential to improve intra- and interlaboratory standardization. Efforts to develop test methods with even shorter analysis times must continue so that rapid reporting can occur in a more compressed and thus more clinically relevant period. Moreover, efforts toward the development of an instrument capable of testing a wide variety of bacteria and accurately detecting clinically relevant resistance mechanisms should continue. Further advances may occur as a result of exploring more innovative means of detecting the inhibitory effects of antimicrobial agents on microorganisms or perhaps the use of large nucleic acid arrays to determine the presence of the genetic determinants of the most common causes of resistance.

REFERENCES

1. **Baker, C. N., S. A. Stocker, D. L. Rhoden, and C. Thornsberry.** 1986. Evaluation of the MicroScan antimicrobial susceptibility system with the AutoScan-4 automated reader. *J. Clin. Microbiol.* **19:**744–747.
2. **Barenfanger, J., C. Drake, and G. Kacich.** 1999. Clinical and financial benefits of rapid identification and antimicrobial susceptibility testing. *J. Clin. Microbiol.* **37:**1415–1418.
3. **Bascomb, S., J. H. Godsey, M. Kangas, L. Nea, and K. M. Tomfohrde.** 1991. Rapid antimicrobial susceptibility testing of gram-positive cocci using Baxter Microscan Rapid Fluorogenic Panels and autoSCAN-W/A. *Pathol. Biol.* **39:**466–470.
4. **Berke, I., and P. M. Tierno.** 1996. Comparison of efficacy and cost-effectiveness of BIOMIC VIDEO and vitek antimicrobial susceptibility test systems for use in the clinical microbiology laboratory. *J. Clin. Microbiol.* **34:**1980–1984.
5. **Burns, J. L., L. Saiman, S. Whittier, J. Krzewinski, Z. Liu, D. Larone, S. A. Marshall, and R. N. Jones.** 2001. Comparison of two commercial systems (Vitek and MicroScan WalkAway) for antimicrobial susceptibility testing of *Pseudomonas aeruginosa* isolates from cystic fibrosis patients. *Diagn. Microbiol. Infect. Dis.* **39:**257–260.
6. **Cooper, G. L., A. Louie, A. L. Baltch, R. C. Chu, R. P. Smith, W. J. Ritz, and P. Michelsen.** 1993. Influence of zinc on *Pseudomonas aeruginosa* susceptibilities to imipenem. *J. Clin. Microbiol.* **31:**2366–2370.
7. **Courvalin, P.** 1996. Interpretive reading of in vitro antibiotic susceptibility tests (the antibiogramme). *Clin. Microbiol. Infect.* **2:**S26–S34.
8. **Doern, G. V., A. B. Brueggemann, R. Perla, J. Daly, D. Halkias, R. N. Jones, and M. A. Saubolle.** 1997. Multicenter laboratory evaluation of the bioMerieux Vitek antimicrobial susceptibility testing system with 11 antimicrobial agents versus members of the family *Enterbacteriaceae* and *Pseudomonas aeruginosa*. *J. Clin. Microbiol.* **35:**2115–2119.
9. **Doern, G. V., R. Vautour, M. Gaudet, and B. Levy.** 1994. Clinical impact of rapid in vitro susceptibility testing and bacterial identification. *J. Clin. Microbiol.* **32:**1757–1762.
10. **Food and Drug Administration.** *Class II Special Controls Guidance Document. Antimicrobial Susceptibility Test (AST) Systems: Final Guidance for Industry and FDA,* in press. Food and Drug Administration, Rockville, Md.
11. **Frebourg, N. B., D. Nouet, L. Lemee, E. Martin, and J. F. Lemeland.** 1998. Comparison of ATB Staph, Rapid ATB Staph, Vitek, and E-test methods for detection of oxacillin heteroresistance in staphylococci possessing mecA. *J. Clin. Microbiol.* **36:**52–57.
12. **Garcia-Garrote, F., E. Cercenado, and E. Bouza.** 2000. Evaluation of a new system, VITEK 2, for identification and antimicrobial susceptibility testing of enterococci. *J. Clin. Microbiol.* **38:**2108–2111.
13. **Godsey, J. H., S. Bascomb, T. Bonnette, M. Kangas, K. Link, K. Richards, and K. M. Tomfohrde.** 1991. Rapid antimicrobial susceptibility testing of gram-negative bacilli using Baxter MicroScan Rapid Fluorogenic Panels and autoSCAN-W/A. *Pathol. Biol.* **39:**461–465.
14. **Goessens, W. H. F., N. Lemmens-den Toom, J. Hageman, P. W. M. Hermans, M. Sluijter, R. de Groot, and H. A. Verbrugh.** 2000. Evaluation of the Vitek 2 system for susceptibility testing of *Streptococcus pneumoniae* isolates. *Eur. J. Clin. Microbiol. Infect. Dis.* **19:**618–622.
15. **Hirtz, P., C. Recule, P. Le Noc, D. Sirot, and J. Croize.** 1992. Detection des beta lactamases e spectre elargi par technique Rapid ATB E. Interet du systeme expert API V2.1.1. *Pathol. Biol.* **40:**551–555.
16. **Isenberg, H. D., A. Reichler, and D. Wiseman.** 1971. Prototype of a fully automated device for determination of bacterial antibiotic susceptibility in the clinical laboratory. *Appl. Microbiol.* **22:**980–986.
17. **Jett, B., L. Free, and D. F. Sahm.** 1996. Factors influencing the Vitek gram-positive susceptibility system's detection of vanB-encoded vancomycin resistance among enterococci. *J. Clin. Microbiol.* **34:**701–706.
18. **Jones, R. N., S. A. Marshall, and L. Zerva.** 1997. Critical evaluation of the Vitek GNS F6 card results compared to standardized, reference susceptibility test methods. *Diagn. Microbiol. Infect. Dis.* **28:**35–40.
19. **Jorgensen, J. H.** 1993. Selection criteria for an antimicrobial susceptibility testing system. *J. Clin. Microbiol.* **31:**2841–2844.
20. **Jorgensen, J. H., A. L. Barry, M. M. Traczewski, D. F. Sahm, M. L. McElmeel, and S. A. Crawford.** 2000. Rapid automated antimicrobial susceptibility testing of *Streptococcus pneumoniae* by use of the bioMerieux VITEK 2. *J. Clin. Microbiol.* **38:**2814–2818.
21. **Jorgensen, J. H., and M. J. Ferraro.** 1998. Antimicrobial susceptibility testing: general principles and contemporary practices. *Clin. Infect. Dis.* **26:**973–980.
22. **Jorgensen, J. H., and M. J. Ferraro.** 2000. Antimicrobial susceptibility testing: special needs for fastidious organisms

and difficult-to-detect resistance mechanisms. *Clin. Infect. Dis.* **30:**799–808.

23. **Jorgensen, J. H., and J. M. Matsen.** 1987. Physician acceptance and application of rapid microbiology instrument test results, p. 209–212. *In* J. H. Jorgensen (ed.), *Automation in Clinical Microbiology.* CRC Press, Inc., Boca Raton, Fla.

24. **Katsanis, G. P., J. Spargo, M. J. Ferraro, L. Sutton, and G. A. Jacoby.** 1994. Detection of *Klebsiella pneumoniae* and *Escherichia coli* strains producing extended-spectrum β-lactamases. *J. Clin. Microbiol.* **32:**691–696.

25. **Kellogg, J. A.** 1984. Inability to control selected drugs on commercially-obtained microdilution MIC panels. *Am. J. Clin. Pathol.* **82:**455–458.

26. **Kellogg, J. A.** 1985. Inability to adequately control antimicrobial agents on AutoMicrobic System gram-positive and gram-negative cards. *J. Clin. Microbiol.* **21:**454–456.

27. **Korgenski, E. K., and J. A. Daly.** 1998. Evaluation of the BIOMIC video reader system for determining interpretive categories of isolates on the basis of disk diffusion susceptibility results. *J. Clin Microbiol.* **36:**302–304.

28. **Lampe, M. F., C. L. Aitken, P. G. Dennis, P. S. Forsythe, K. E. Patrick, F. D. Schoenknecht, and J. C. Sherris.** 1975. Relationship of early readings of minimal inhibitory concentrations to the results of overnight tests. *Antimicrob. Agents Chemother.* **8:**429–433.

29. **Ling, T. K. W., P. C. Tam, Z. K. Liu, and A. F. B. Cheng.** 2001. Evaluation of VITEK 2 rapid identification and susceptibility testing system against gram-negative clinical isolates. *J. Clin. Microbiol.* **39:**2964–2966.

30. **Louie, M., A. E. Simor, S. Szeto, M. Patel, B. Kreiswirth, and D. E. Low.** 1992. Susceptibility testing of clinical isolates of *Enterococcus faecium* and *Enterococcus faecalis.* *J. Clin. Microbiol.* **30:**41–45.

31. **Madeiros, A., and J. Crellin.** 2000. Evluation of the Sirscan automated zone reader in a clinical microbiology laboratory. *J. Clin. Microbiol.* **38:**1688–1693.

32. **Marshall, S. A., M. A. Pfaller, and R. N. Jones.** 1999. Ability of modified Vitek card to detect coagulase-negative staphylococci with *mecA* and oxacillin-resistant phenotypes. *J. Clin. Microbiol.* **37:**2122–2123.

33. **Matsen, J. M.** 1985. Means to facilitate physician acceptance and use of rapid test results. *Diagn. Microbiol. Infect. Dis.* **3:**35S–78S.

34. **Metzler, C. M., and R. M. Dehaan.** 1974. Susceptibility tests of anaerobic bacteria: statistical and clinical considerations. *J. Infect. Dis.* **130:**588–594.

35. **NCCLS.** 2000. *Methods for Dilution Antimicrobial Susceptibility Tests for Bacteria That Grow Aerobically,* 5th ed. *Approved Standard M7-A5.* NCCLS, Wayne, Pa.

36. **NCCLS.** 2002. *Performance Standards for Antimicrobial Susceptibility Testing. Supplement M100-S12.* NCCLS, Wayne, Pa.

37. **Nolte, F. S., K. K. Krisher, L. A. Beltran, N. P. Christianson, and G. E. Sheridan.** 1988. Rapid and overnight microdilution antibiotic susceptibility testing with the Sensititre AutoReader System. *J. Clin. Microbiol.* **261:**1079–1084.

38. **Nolte, F. S., J. M. Williams, K. L. Maher, and B. Metchock.** 1993. Evaluation of modified MicroScan screening tests for high-level aminoglycoside resistance in *Enterococcus faecalis.* *Am. J. Clin. Pathol.* **99:**286–288.

39. **Okabe, T., K. Oana, Y. Kawakami, M. Yamaguchi, Y. Takahashi, Y. Okimura, and T. Katsuyama.** 2000. Limitations of Vitek GPS-418 cards in exact detection of vancomycin-resistant enterococci with the vanB genotype. *J. Clin. Microbiol.* **38:**2409–2411.

40. **Pestotnik, S. L., R. S. Evans, J. P. Burke, P. M. Gardner, and D. C. Classen.** 1990. Therapeutic antibiotic monitor-ing: surveillance using computerized expert system. *Am. J. Med.* **88:**43–49.

41. **Ribeiro, J., F. D. Viera, T. King, J. B. D'Arezzo, and J. M. Boyce.** 1999. Misclassification of susceptible strains of *Staphylococcus aureus* as methicillin-resistant *S. aureus* by a rapid automated susceptibility testing system. *J. Clin. Microbiol.* **37:**1619–1620.

42. **Rittenhouse, S. F., L. A. Miller, L. J. Utrup, and J. A. Poupard.** 1996. Evaluation of 500 gram negative isolates to determine the number of major susceptibility interpretation discrepancies between the Vitek and MicroScan Walkaway for 9 antimicrobial agents. *Diagn. Microbiol. Infect. Dis.* **26:**1–6.

43. **Ronco, E., M. L. Migueres, M. Guenounou, and A. Philippon.** 1991. Detection des beta lactamases a spectre elargi avec le systeme ATB CMI. *Pathol. Biol.* **39:**480–485.

44. **Rosenberg, J., F. C. Tenover, J. Wong, W. Jarvis, and D. J. Vugia.** 1997. Are clinical laboratories in California accurately reporting vancomycin-resistant enterococci. *J. Clin. Microbiol.* **35:**2526–2530.

45. **Sahm, D. F., S. Boonlayangoor, P. C. Iwen, J. L. Baade, and G. L. Woods.** 1991. Factors influencing determination of high-level aminoglycoside resistance in *Enterococcus faecalis.* *J. Clin. Microbiol.* **29:**1934–1939.

46. **Sanchez, M. A., B. Sanchez del Saz, E. Loza, F. Baquero, and R. Canton.** 2001. Evaluation of the OSIRIS Video Reader System for disk susceptibility test reading. *Clin. Microbiol. Infect.* **7:**352–357.

47. **Sanders, C. C., A. L. Barry, J. A. Washington, C. Shubert, E. S. Moland, M. M. Traczewski, C. Knapp, and R. Mulder.** 1996. Detection of extended-spectrum-beta-lactamase-producing members of the family *Enterobacteriaeae* with Vitek ESBL test. *J. Clin. Microbiol.* **34:**2997–3001.

48. **Sanders, C. C., M. Peyret, E. S. Moland, S. J. Cavalieri, C. Shubert, K. S. Thomson, J.-M. Boeufgras, and W. E. Sanders, Jr.** 2001. Potential impact of the VITEK 2 System and the Advanced Expert System on the clinical laboratory of a university-based hospital. *J. Clin. Microbiol.* **39:**2379–2385.

49. **Sanders, C. C., M. Peyret, E. S. Moland, C. Shubert, K. S. Thomson, J.-M. Boeufgras, and W. E. Sanders, Jr.** 2000. Ability of the Vitek 2 Advanced Expert System to identify β-lactam phenotypes in isolates of *Enterobacteriaceae* and *Pseudomonas aeruginosa.* *J. Clin. Microbiol.* **38:**570–574.

50. **Schadow, K. H., D. K. Giger, and C. C. Sanders.** 1993. Failure of the Vitek AutoMicrobic System to detect beta-lactam resistance in *Aeromonas* species. *Am. J. Clin. Pathol.* **100:**308–310.

51. **Sherris, J. C., and K. J. Ryan.** 1982. Evaluation of automated and rapid methods, p. 105. *In* R. C. Tilton (ed.), *Rapid Methods and Automation in Microbiology.* American Society for Microbiology, Washington, D.C.

52. **Stager, C. E., and J. R. Davis.** 1992. Automated systems for identification of microorganisms. *Clin. Microbiol. Rev.* **5:**302–327.

53. **Staneck, J. L., S. D. Allen, E. E. Harris, and R. C. Tilton.** 1985. Automated reading of MIC microdilution trays containing fluorogenic enzyme substrates with the Sensititre Autoreader. *J. Clin. Microbiol.* **22:**187–191.

54. **Steward, C. D., S. A. Stocker, J. M. Swenson, C. M. O'Hara, J. R. Edwards, R. P. Gaynes, J. E. McGowan, Jr., and F. C. Tenover.** 1999. Comparison of agar dilution, disk diffusion, MicroScan and Vitek antimicrobial susceptibility testing methods to broth microdilution for detection of fluoroquinolone-resistant isolates of the family *Enterobacteraceae.* *J. Clin. Microbiol.* **37:**544–547.

55. Tenover, F. C., M. V. Lancaster, B. C. Hill, C. D., Steward, S. A. Stocker, G. A. Hancock, C. M. O'Hara, N. C. Clark, and K. Hiramatsu. 1998. Characterization of staphylococci with reduced susceptibilities to vancomycin and other glycopeptides. *J. Clin. Microbiol.* **36:**1020–1027.

56. Tenover, F. C., J. M. Swenson, C. O'Hara, and S. A. Stocker. 1995. Ability of commercial and reference antimicrobial susceptibility testing methods to detect vancomycin resistance in enterococci. *J. Clin. Microbiol.* **33:** 1524–1527.

57. Tenover, F. C., J. Tokars, J. Swenson, S. Paul, K. Spitalny, and W. J. Jarvis. 1993. Ability of clinical laboratories to detect antimicrobial agent-resistant enterococci. *J. Clin. Microbiol.* **31:**1695–1699.

58. Thornsberry, C., J. P. Anhalt, J. A. Washington II, L. R. McCarthy, F. D. Schoenknecht, J. C. Sherris, and H. J. Spencer. 1980. Clinical laboratory evaluation of the Abbott MS-2 automated antimicrobial susceptibility testing system: report of a collaborative study. *J. Clin. Microbiol.* **12:**375–390.

59. Thrupp, L. D. 1986. Susceptibility testing of antibiotics in liquid media, p. 93–150. *In* V. Lorian (ed.), *Antibiotics in Laboratory Medicine*, 2nd ed. The Williams & Wilkins Co., Baltimore, Md.

60. Trenholme, G. M., R. L. Kaplan, P. H. Karakusis, T. Stine, J. Fuhrer, W. Landau, and S. Levin. 1989. Clinical impact of rapid identification and susceptibility testing of bacterial blood culture isolates. *J. Clin. Microbiol.* **27:** 1342–1345.

61. Tsakris, A., A. Pantazi, S. Pournaras, A. Maniatis, A. Polyzou, and D. Sofianou. 2000. Pseudo-outbreak of imipenem-resistant *Acinetobacter baumannii* resulting from false susceptibility testing by a rapid automated system. *J. Clin. Microbiol.* **38:**3505–3507.

62. van den Braak, N., W. Goessens, A. van Belkum, H. Verbrugh, and H. P. Endtz. 2001. Accuracy of the Vitek 2 system to detect glycopeptide resistance in enterococci. *J. Clin. Microbiol.* **39:**351–353.

63. Vincent, P., D. Izard, T. Lebrun, J. C. Sailly, G. Arbon, A. Hassoun, and H. Leclerc. 1985. Interet cliniques des resultats rapides de bacteriologie au de l'infection nosocomiales: comparaison avec les methods traditionelles. *Presse Med.* **14:**1697–1700.

64. Visser, M. R., L. Bogaards, M. Rozenberg-Arska, and J. Verhoef. 1992. Comparison of the autoSCAN W/A and Vitek Automicrobic Systems for identification and susceptibility testing of bacteria. *Eur. J. Clin. Microbiol. Infect. Dis.* **11:**979–984.

65. Weissmann, D., J. Spargo, C. Wennersten, and M. J. Ferraro. 1991. Detection of enterococcal high-level aminoglycoside resistance with MicroScan freeze-dried panels containing newly modified medium and Vitek gram-positive susceptibility cards. *J. Clin. Microbiol.* **29:**1232–1235.

66. White, R. L., M. B. Kays, L. V. Friedrich, E. W. Brown, and J. R. Koonce. 1991. Pseudoresistance of *Pseudomonas aeruginosa* resulting from degradation of imipenem in an automated susceptibility testing system with predried panels. *J. Clin. Microbiol.* **29:**398–400.

67. Willey, B. M., B. N. Kreiswiri, A. E. Simor, G. Williams, S. R. Scriver, A. Phillips, and D. E. Low. 1992. Detection of vancomycin-resistance in *Enterococcus* spp. *J. Clin. Microbiol.* **30:**1621–1624.

68. Woods, G. L., B. DiGiovanni, M. Levison, P. Pitsakis, and D. LaTemple. 1993. Evaluation of MicroScan rapid panels for detection of high-level aminoglycoside resistance in enterococci. *J. Clin. Microbiol.* **31:**2786–2787.

69. Yamazumi, T., S. A. Marshal, W. W. Wilke, D. J. Diekema, M. A. Pfaller, and R. N. Jones. 2001. Comparison of the Vitek gram-positive susceptibility 106 card and the MRSA-screen latex agglutination test for determining oxacillin resistance in clinical bloodstream isolates of *Staphylococcus aureus*. *J. Clin. Microbiol.* **39:**53–56.

Immunoassays for the Diagnosis of Infectious Diseases*

NIEL T. CONSTANTINE AND DOLORES P. LANA

16

INTRODUCTION

Immunoassays can be considered as analytical methods that incorporate antigens or antibodies as reagents to determine the presence of their corresponding antigens or antibodies in a variety of media (e.g., body fluids, tissues, and environmental substances). Since the first description of the use of antigen-antibody reactions for identification of infectious agents, immunoassays have evolved to offer attractive analytical and performance features that place them among the most widely used methods in clinical and research laboratories (18). Their use crosses all disciplines of clinical pathology, including microbiology, virology, immunology, chemistry, hematology, blood banking, and coagulation. Immunoassays are used not only for diagnosis of infectious diseases, but also for diagnosis of cancer, immunodeficiency diseases, and autoimmune diseases; receptor identification; and the detection and quantification of a wide variety of human and animal proteins. Thus, immunoassays play a critical role in health care, research, and clinical laboratory medicine.

A large variety of immunoassays are used in clinical medicine and research, and each offers important contributions. It is beyond the scope of this chapter to describe all immunoassays; hence, our discussion will focus on those methods that are currently applied or that are being adapted for use in the identification of infectious diseases. The purpose of this chapter is to provide a solid foundation for the types of immunoassays that are available and used in microbiology, the principles upon which their methodologies are based, an understanding of their usage and applications, a basis for how test results are interpreted, and the limitations of the methods.

Terms and Definitions

Immunoassays incorporate antigens or specific antibodies in their procedures and are configured (i) to investigate the presence of specific antibodies (immunoglobulins) that are produced in response to a nonself protein or (ii) to detect any constituents, particularly those of microorganisms, that have antigenic properties. The terms "serology," "serol-ogic," and "serodiagnosis" refer to the study of or the description of the detection of antigen or antibody in serum. However, the term serologic is also used when the medium to be tested is not serum (e.g., saliva or urine), as long as antigens or antibodies are detected. Hence, the term serologic assay can be considered essentially synonymous with the term "immunoassay."

As discussed below, immunoassays that incorporate enzyme-substrate systems as indicator systems are called enzyme immunoassays (EIAs). Because there are a number of configurations of these EIA systems, more specific names may be used, such as the enzyme-linked immunosorbent assay (ELISA), in which an antibody or antigen reagent is adsorbed (sorbent) onto a solid-phase support, or the particle enzyme immunoassay, which incorporates microparticles, for example. Thus, all ELISAs are EIAs, but not all EIAs are ELISAs. If the indicator system uses fluorochromes (fluorescence compounds) or radioactive isotopes, the assays are classified as fluorescence immunoassays or radioactive immunoassays (RIAs), respectively. Additionally, assays may be named according to the format of the assay, such as indirect immunofluorescence assays (IFAs) or direct immunofluorescence assays (DFAs), whereas other assays may be named according to the results that are produced, such as the ones that produce lines (line immunoassays [LIAs]) or dots (dot blot assays). There are many other examples, and the most common will be presented.

Results of immunoassays are expressed in several ways. Most commonly, a result is reported as positive or negative (or reactive versus nonreactive), indicating the presence or absence of detectable antigen or antibody to a particular agent as determined against a cutoff value established within the assay. In other instances, a titer is reported, indicating the amount or concentration of specific antibody or, in the case of antigen detection, a concentration (e.g., picograms per milliliter). The titers of antibodies are determined on the basis of dilutions of sample at particular intervals and reassaying of the sample to determine at which interval final reactivity occurs, i.e., the endpoint. The endpoint titer is defined as the reciprocal of the highest dilution that still produces a positive result; i.e., if the last dilution that yields a positive result was a 1:640 dilution, then the titer is 640. Unfortunately, it is a common error to report titers as the dilution (e.g., 1:640), and this should be avoided. Titers are usually based on serial twofold dilutions

---

* This chapter contains information presented in chapter 12 by James B. Mahony and Max A. Chernesky in the seventh edition of this Manual.

of the sample to yield values such as 8, 16, 32, 64, 128, etc. In other instances, including the determination of bacterial toxins, international units may be used. These are based on international standards so that the resultant values will represent equivalent interpretations regardless of which type of immunoassay is used (ELISA values may represent different concentrations compared to those of agglutination assays). In still other instances, optical density (OD) readings or OD-to-cutoff values may be given (e.g., an OD of <1.5 represents a poor antibody responder).

History and Evolution of Immunoassays

The observation of an antibody binding to an antigen with specificity provided the basis for the initial development of diagnostic immunoassays. The phenomenon of precipitation and agglutination became the basis for development of research tools that would later be adapted for clinical laboratory tests to identify antibodies to infectious bacterial agents such as *Treponema pallidum* and *Salmonella* species. The principle of hemagglutination (HA) was exploited to develop the HA inhibition (HAI) assays that were used widely and effectively for the detection of antibodies to viruses. As the complement system became better understood, it was exploited in immunoassays such as complement fixation (CF) assays to offer a method which, although rigorous, was applicable for the detection of antibodies to a number of infectious agents. Subsequently, immunologic precipitation techniques became popular and offered a means to assess specific immunologic reactions, with the added feature of yielding semiquantitative information. Many of these early assays that were the building blocks for development of newer generations of immunoassays, such as Western blots, are still being used today because of their usefulness and efficiency. Much of the continual development and refinement of immune system-based diagnostic assays can be credited to an increased knowledge of antibodies and antigens and their interactions at the molecular and biochemical levels, to newer methods that offer attractive features, to innovative systems that can significantly increase the sensitivity of assays, and to the advancement in computer technology and instrumentation.

Further advances in immunoassays, such as the incorporation of solid-phase technology during the 1970s (5, 17), were instrumental in improving the simplicity, turnaround times, cost, and throughput of assays for many infectious agents. Immobilization of antigens or antibodies on solid matrices coupled with detection via enzyme-labeled secondary antibodies allowed detection of a wide variety of analytes, including infectious agent antigens or antibodies to these components. Modifications such as the addition of a secondary-antibody amplification step or avidin-biotin systems allowed for an increase in sensitivity (30).

More recent technologies, such as the rapid one-step lateral flow immunoassays, have produced rapid, sensitive, and cost-effective assays that are applicable for a large variety of laboratories with various capabilities (11, 24). They are applicable for use under field conditions, in physicians' offices, and in the homes of consumers. Advances in sample handling have led to the development of fully automated assays that can be applied for the large-scale testing of thousands of samples per day (20, 43). Recent modifications of immunoassays and newer technologies have also allowed for applications that can evaluate epidemiological trends (e.g., detuning assays) and mutational analysis (serotyping). In summary, immunoassays have

evolved because of technologic advances and novel ideas for improvement that have addressed issues of simplicity, turnaround times for results, cost-effectiveness, sensitivity, specificity, safety, standardization, and high throughput using automated platforms.

INTRODUCTION TO IMMUNOASSAYS

Purposes and Uses of Tests

Immunoassays are particularly valuable for diagnosing infection when an infectious agent is difficult to culture or is dangerous to handle. However, the most common uses are for identifying infection and differentiating acute from past infection. A positive result by an antigen assay signals acute infection, as does an immunoglobulin M (IgM) isotype determination and a fourfold or greater rise in titer of IgG antibody to a specific agent. Single point-specific IgG assessments are effective only in verifying past infection, although single IgG avidity determinations and specific IgG antibody titers can sometimes provide information as to the time of infection (see below). The presence of specific IgG to some infectious agents may provide enough information along with clinical data to make a determination about patient management, the need for immunization, and the degree of protection of health care workers in various risk settings. Also, the investigation of titers of antibody to an agent (e.g., hepatitis B virus [HBV] surface antibody) is valuable to determine if sufficient antibody levels are present to protect against infection or if booster injections are required (i.e., poor versus good vaccine responders).

Serologic assays can be used for screening of populations to identify individuals who can benefit from treatment, for protection of the blood supply, for epidemiologic purposes to track infection prevalence (and incidence), for identification of acute infection so that treatment can be instituted in a clinically relevant time frame, for diagnosis of chronic infection, for monitoring of infection or disease progression, and for further understanding of the kinetics of immune responses. The testing of individuals for diagnostic purposes has two major applications: (i) to verify that a patient who presents with symptoms compatible with an infection (or a person at high risk of infection) is truly infected and (ii) to monitor for evidence of infection in an apparently healthy person who is believed to have been exposed to an agent. An important specific application of monitoring for exposure is the unique ability to intervene in infection transmission by using a rapid test for detection of antibodies to the human immunodeficiency virus (HIV). When a health care worker is exposed to blood, the source patient can be tested immediately to determine his or her HIV status. Should the result be positive, the employee has been occupationally exposed and should be considered for immediate antiretroviral treatment to decrease the chance of transmission (7). Similar testing should be performed for women in labor whose HIV status is unknown; here again, a positive result mandates the use of antiretroviral treatment to decrease transmission to the newborn (46).

Requirements of Immunoassays for Screening, Confirming, and Monitoring of Infection

Screening Tests

Screening tests for the serologic identification of infectious agents and infection are designed with the potential to detect all infected individuals. To accomplish this, they must possess exquisite sensitivity, both epidemiologic and analytical (see below). In most infections, IgG antibody responses to microorganisms are substantial and long-lived, and therefore most immunoassays detect established infection quite well. However, early in infection, prior to seroconversion, antibody tests may be ineffective due to an absence of antibody or to the assay's inability to detect low levels of antibody (10). The period after infection but prior to antibody production is referred to as the window period and may last from about 10 days to greater than 6 months (e.g., for hepatitis C virus [HCV]) (2). Newer-generation assays, including the third-generation antigen sandwich assays, can detect antibody earlier due to their ability to detect IgM antibody simultaneously with IgG (52). Alternatively, specific IgM assays are used for many infectious agents and offer effective identification of early infection, reactivation, or reinfection. Therefore, tests to screen for antibody are effective in identifying infection during most periods after infection.

Antigen detection methods can be used as screening methods. They are aimed at detecting organisms or their antigens (e.g., proteins or glycoproteins) directly by using specific antibodies as reagents. Although these methods are usually fast, they require the presence of adequate quantities of antigens for detection; hence, they may lack sensitivity, not because of the tests, but because of the low levels of organisms or their products. However, for most antigen detection methods, clinically significant amounts of infectious agents can be detected. Most notable of the antigen detection methods are the rapid tests based on agglutination or EIA technology that detect bacterial antigens, such as streptococcal antigens (30), or the viral antigens of rotavirus (31, 49), respiratory syncytial virus (RSV) (27), and, more recently, herpes simplex virus type 2 (HSV-2) (POCKIT HSV-2 rapid test; www.Diagnology.com/pockit_test.htm). Antigen detection methods for malaria have now been reported to be effective; in fact, there is much excitement over the use of the new antigen-detecting methods for malaria, since rapid technologies can be instrumental for applications in developing countries (40). For other infections (e.g., HBV and HIV), antigen-detection ELISAs are used because of their enhanced sensitivity compared with rapid assays. As technology improves, the sensitivity of screening methods increases, and newer tests are replacing current ones.

Confirmatory Tests

Confirmatory (supplemental) immunoassays, performed on samples that are found reactive by screening tests, are designed to verify truly infected individuals by increasing the predictive value of a positive result. Accordingly, confirmatory assays have a high specificity and therefore rarely exhibit false-positive results. However, negative results do not always rule out infection, since these assays lack the sensitivity of screening tests, and indeterminate reactions usually require follow-up testing of a subsequent sample for resolution. In such cases, additional tests may help, such as antigen assays, culture, and, more recently, nucleic acid amplification tests.

Monitoring Tests

Immunoassays to monitor infection are few, but those that are available have made important contributions. Most notable are antigen tests for HBV surface antigen (HBsAg) and HIV (p24 antigen). Infectious-agent antigens are produced when the organism replicates, and the antigens spill into blood (antigenemia) at certain intervals during infection. However, antigens may be present but undetectable by current methods; an example is HCV antigen, which until recently was thought not to be present in blood (4). These viral antigens can often be detected prior to seroconversion, thereby indicating acute infection. In addition to their detection during acute infection, some antigens (e.g., HBsAg), if detected for prolonged periods in blood, signal chronic infection and yield some insight into prognosis. HIV p24 antigen detection has also been used with some success to monitor HIV infection in newborns, since interference from maternal antibody is omnipresent.

Testing Algorithms

A test algorithm refers to the selection and sequence of performing two or more tests in tandem to arrive at a conclusion concerning the status of the person being tested. Sometimes, the term "testing strategy" is used synonymously. An algorithm implies that the sequence of additional testing is dependent on a positive result by a previous test in the algorithm, although some facilities may require that a second screening test be used for all samples regardless of the outcome of the first to ensure the accuracy of negative results (e.g., blood screening in some European countries). If any one test were perfect, test algorithms would be unnecessary; indeed, when used alone, antibody tests, antigen tests, nucleic acid tests, and others are usually imperfect for identifying all noninfected and infected individuals. Even two or more tests used in tandem are usually not perfect, and a definitive conclusion sometimes cannot be made. A noninfected individual with a reactive result determined by an antibody test (false-positive screening test result) may never revert to nonreactive and never produce a positive result by confirmatory antibody tests or nucleic acid tests; i.e., it is difficult to rule out infection conclusively until substantial follow-up testing over a long time is conducted. Consequently, strategies to increase the likelihood of correctly classifying individuals, thereby maximizing the negative and positive predictive values, have been derived. Test algorithms can be devised in any way that is effective for a particular testing situation and are often determined on the basis of the availability of different tests. However, in many testing situations, the selection of an algorithm is not a choice but is dictated by regulatory agencies (e.g., blood donor screening in the United States). Some algorithms require the retesting of initially reactive samples (e.g., HCV, human T-cell leukemia virus [HTLV], or HIV), whereas others require titering (rapid plasma reagin [RPR] test, Venereal Disease Research Laboratory [VDRL] test), and others suggest the use of more specific tests (Lyme disease Western blots) to minimize the chance that the reactive screening result was not a biologic false positive.

Immunologic Reactions and Their Characteristics

Immunoassays can be considered to be constructed in two stages. The first is the interaction between antigen and antibody in solution, in a gel, or on a solid-phase support. This reaction is dependent on the specific binding between epitopes on the pathogen or its antigen and the idiotype (antigen binding site) on the antibody. The second is detection of the interaction directly or by incorporation of an indicator system such as a fluorescent dye, a particle that agglutinates, or an enzyme reagent that can catalyze a substrate to produce a color reaction. Each of these stages is discussed below ("Specific Immunoassays for the Detection and Diagnosis of Infectious Diseases").

The ability of a particular antibody to combine with one epitope or antigen defines its specificity; i.e., specific antibodies react with only one epitope of an antigen, whereas nonspecific antibodies can cross-react with similar antigens. For example, when some antigenic determinants are shared by different organisms, a proportion of the antibodies directed against one antigen will also react with another, such as may occur between bacteria that possess cell wall polysaccharides in common with mammalian erythrocytes (heterophile antibodies). The specificity resides in the antibody combining site (Fab or variable portion) or the idiotype of the antibody. Within the variable portion, antigens may combine with several portions, and the closer the fit, the better the specificity. This relationship is referred to as the antibody affinity, where a tightly fitting antibody through noncovalent forces such as hydrophobic or electrostatic bonds has high affinity and affects the utility of the reaction (both in vivo and in immunoassays) (16). In addition, the relationship between antibodies and antigens can be defined in terms of avidity. In contrast to affinity, which describes the interaction of a single antigenic determinant, avidity refers to the interaction between a multivalent antibody and a multivalent antigen. When this involves more than one combining site, the strength of the bonding is significantly increased, resulting in a lesser ability for the antibody and antigen to dissociate (and hence a more pronounced reaction). It is well known that antibody avidity increases as infection progresses due to better tailoring of the immune response. In fact, avidity assays (see below) have been used to determine the relative time of infection.

Determining the Value of Tests: Sensitivity, Specificity, and Predictive Values

Parameters that can be used to determine the relative usefulness or efficiency of a particular test are sensitivity, specificity, and predictive values. Importantly, a valid evaluation must use a large enough sample size to minimize the chance of finding differences between the tests solely due to random error. The parameters used to describe a test's usefulness and accuracy are commonly known as test indices, and the most important ones are discussed below.

Sensitivity

The sensitivity of a diagnostic assay can be analytical or epidemiologic. While the analytical sensitivity of a test is its ability to detect small quantities of antibody and is useful in high-incidence populations, where it could be expected to find individuals who are seroconverting, the epidemiologic sensitivity of a test describes its ability to detect most persons who have established infection (13).

Analytical Sensitivity

Analytical sensitivity refers to the ability of a test to detect very small quantities of antibodies, as occur during seroconversion. Analytical sensitivity is usually dependent on the format of the test, the quantity of antigens incorporated, and the effectiveness of the conjugate (detector) system. To assess the analytical sensitivity, the best means is to test seroconversion panels, i.e., serial samples taken from a person who has recently become infected. These serial samples should have bleed intervals of 1 to 2 weeks so that an assessment can be made at close intervals during the time that antibody levels are rising. Such panels are available commercially (Boston Biomedical, Inc., West Bridge-

water, Mass.) or from investigators who monitor negative persons prospectively and find those who seroconvert (F. Cleghorn, personal communication [Trinidad cohort]).

Epidemiologic Sensitivity

In contrast to analytical sensitivity, epidemiologic sensitivity, sometimes called clinical sensitivity, refers to the ability of a test to detect persons with established infection, i.e., persons who have been infected for some time and have relatively high levels of antibodies. Although it would be expected that all useful tests could detect all persons with high levels of antibodies, this is not always true because the tests may not incorporate the necessary antigens to detect all genotypes or groups of an organism. Thus, the epidemiologic and analytical sensitivities of a test are mutually exclusive. The epidemiologic sensitivity of an assay is assessed by using samples from persons with infection but not those in the seroconversion phase.

Sensitivity can be calculated by the following formula:

$$\text{Sensitivity} = \frac{\text{true positives}}{\text{true positives} + \text{false negatives}} \times 100$$

where true positives are the number of infected persons detected by the test, and false negatives are the number of infected persons who are classified by the test as negative.

Specificity

The specificity of an assay is the ability of the test to identify all noninfected individuals correctly (i.e., produces no false-positive results). The specificity of an assay can be calculated by the following formula:

$$\text{Specificity} = \frac{\text{true negatives}}{\text{true negatives} + \text{false positives}} \times 100$$

where true negatives are the number of noninfected persons classified as negative by the test, and false positives are the number of noninfected persons who are classified by the test as positive.

Predictive Values

Predictive values differ from the above parameters in that they describe the value of tests when the actual prevalence of infection in the population being tested is taken into account. The positive predictive value is the number of correctly classified positive results compared to the total number of positive results; the negative predictive value is calculated similarly, as illustrated below:

% Positive predictive value

$$= \frac{\text{true positives}}{\text{true positives} + \text{false positives}} \times 100$$

% Negative predictive value

$$= \frac{\text{true negatives}}{\text{true negatives} + \text{false negatives}} \times 100$$

An example will illustrate how the positive predictive value changes depending on the prevalence of infection in a population. A test that has a specificity of 99% (1 false positive per 100 tested) will have a positive predictive value of 50% if there is one false positive and one true positive (1/2, i.e., a low-prevalence population). In contrast, in a high-prevalence population where there are 50 true positives (and the 1 false positive), the positive predictive value will be 98% (50/51). Therefore, the chance of a positive result indicating a truly infected person varies dramatically when a single test is used in each population. As is evident, a test with an excellent specificity must be used in a low-risk population to have a result that is meaningful.

SPECIFIC IMMUNOASSAYS FOR THE DETECTION AND DIAGNOSIS OF INFECTIOUS DISEASES

Targets for Detection by Immunoassays

Targets for detection by immunoassays can be antigenic components of infectious agents or antibodies produced in response to infection. Although these targets are similar for a variety of microorganisms (viruses, parasites, fungi), immune responses may vary. For example, viruses are usually detected by identifying structural components (envelope glycoproteins), whereas bacteria can be effectively detected by identifying extracellular products. Two examples will be presented. Humoral immune responses to bacteria vary and are responses to a variety of antigens, including cell surface antigens, intracellular structural components, and enzymes. The specificity of antibodies produced is exemplified in infection by group A streptococci, in which antibodies to a variety of intracellular and extracellular antigens can be identified by serological assays. Judicious selection of the correct commercial antigens is imperative in assays to detect specific antibodies. A common screening test for detection of infection is the Streptozyme agglutination test, which incorporates several different antigens such as streptolysin O, DNase B, streptokinase, and hyaluronidase in an attempt to detect antibodies of diagnostic significance. This test will detect any of these, but if positive, it should be followed by a more specific test for confirmation. Another example of the targets of immunoassays for detection of infection by bacteria is in the serodiagnosis of syphilis. Antibodies to specific *Treponema* structural antigens can be detected, but the tests are expensive and laborious and may require expensive equipment (fluorescent microscope). Alternatively, nonspecific antibodies (Wasserman antibodies) that are present during infection and detected by the RPR or VDRL test can be detected. These antibodies are produced against components of self that occur during the destruction of host tissue by the organism and are detected by flocculation reactions (see below). The tests use cardiolipin-lecithin-cholesterol-derived antigens that aggregate when brought into contact with sera from infected persons that contain antibodies to these proteins (cardiolipin). However, although effective as a screening tool, a positive test must be confirmed with a more specific test such as the fluorescent treponemal antibody absorption test or an HA test using *T. pallidum* antigens.

Detection of viral infections may also involve the identification of multiple antibodies that arise during infection. One example is Epstein-Barr virus (EBV), the causative agent of infectious mononucleosis. Antibody assays for EBV are based upon the detection of several EBV antigen targets, including viral capsid antigens, membrane antigens, and/or EBV nuclear antigen (EBNA) by immunofluorescence or ELISA with anti-IgG or -IgM specific antibodies. The less specific but more appropriate test for screening is detection of heterophile antibodies that result from elevated levels of total serum antibodies secreted from virus-infected B lymphocytes. Heterophile antibodies (IgM) react with red blood cells (RBCs) of certain species, and their detection is exploited by their ability to agglutinate horse or sheep RBCs. In viral hepatitis, the detection of antibodies (and antigens) can provide information about the relative time of infection and the occurrence of chronicity. Examples include identification of the presence of IgM-specific anti-hepatitis A virus antibodies (IgM anti-HAV), antibodies to HBV surface antigen (anti-HBsAg), and antibodies to HBV core antigen (total IgM and IgG anti-HBc and IgM anti-HBc).

Parasitic and fungal infections may be difficult to detect by antibody assays, probably due to the different stages of the organisms and to premunition (long survival of worms through a protective mechanism to decrease antigen expression or enclosure by glycoprotein coats). However, in many parasitic infections, elevated levels of IgE are present in the sera. Serological tests such as agglutination, CF, ELISA, and indirect immunofluorescence have been effective in the diagnosis of some parasitic diseases; immunodiffusion and immunoelectrophoresis are also employed. Serological tests may also be effective in the diagnosis of some fungal infections because isolation and cultivation of fungi are not always successful. Again, a variety of serological assays are used, and the choice of methods is dependent upon the specific fungal organism. Agglutination, immunodiffusion in gels (Ouchterlony technique), immunofluorescence, counterelectrophoresis, and CF assays have proven to be useful for detection of fungal antibodies.

Techniques To Detect Antibody

Classical Immunoassays

Agglutination and Flocculation

Agglutination is a clumping of particles that results in a microscopically or macroscopically visible conglomerate. During the agglutination reaction, a lattice network is formed between the antigen-coated particles and the antibody (or vice versa). This reaction brings about the clumping (agglutination) of particles due to a bivalent antibody attaching to two antigen molecules. Both IgG and IgM antibodies cause agglutination, but IgM antibodies are believed to be several hundred times more efficient (16). The agglutination reaction is read macroscopically (in tubes or in microtiter plates) or with the aid of a microscope. Flocculation assays are similar to agglutination assays except that the agglutinates float rather than sediment. In the most popular flocculation tests (RPR and VDRL), the cardiolipin-charcoal particles are easily viewed as they float in a serum or plasma medium on a paper card or glass microscope well, with visualization enhanced by the presence of colored carbon particles (RPR).

One important limitation of agglutination assays is the potential for false-negative results with high antibody concentrations. This phenomenon, known as a prozone reaction (6), refers to the inhibition of agglutination when excess antibody is present, thereby preventing the visualization of the reaction. In this case, the lattice network does not form optimally; i.e., the high concentration of antibody binds to antigenic sites in such a manner that cross-linking of the complexes cannot occur. Although these false-negative reactions (no agglutination) are not common, they do occur and may be difficult to detect. In this case, antibody in the sample can be detected if the sample is diluted to decrease the antibody concentration and retested.

Tests employing agglutination as the indicator system have been used for diagnosis of infectious diseases for many years and incorporate RBCs, latex particles, gelatin particles, or microbeads as carrier materials. For antibody tests, antigens (e.g., lysates or specific recombinant or synthetic peptide antigens) are adsorbed onto the carrier materials, and these antigen-coated supports become the indicator system for reactions. When antigens are bound without specific attachment (i.e., they are passively adsorbed onto the carriers), the technique is referred to as passive agglutination. If antigens are passively adsorbed onto RBCs, the assay is called a passive HA assay (PHA). If particles other than RBCs are used, such as gelatin particles, the assay may be called a particle agglutination test. Agglutination assays are easy to perform, requiring an initial dilution of serum, addition of coated particles, mixing, and incubation (usually at room temperature); no wash steps are necessary. A control (noncoated or unsensitized particles) should be used to detect nonspecific agglutination due to reactions against the particles themselves. A typical example of a classical agglutination test for bacteria is the Widal test for *Salmonella* O (somatic) and H (flagellar) antigens; because of the poor sensitivity and specificity of this test, it has largely been abandoned. Similarly, for rickettsiae, the Weil-Felix reaction was a classical method but was prone to produce false-positive results (lacked specificity). HA assays are now widely used throughout the world for the detection of antibodies to a variety of infectious agents, including HBV, HCV, HIV, rubella virus, influenza virus, and *T. pallidum* (Fujirebio, Tokyo, Japan) (28, 44, 47). The PHA for *T. pallidum* was developed in the 1980s and uses chicken or sheep RBCs that are sensitized with antigen extracted from the Nichols strain; the test has a high sensitivity and specificity and is recommended for use by the World Health Organization.

Precipitation

Precipitation reactions are perhaps the simplest of serologic techniques by which an insoluble complex is formed between antigen and antibody, simply by mixing the two solutions (e.g., an antigen reagent with patient's serum). These techniques can be done in tubes (solutions), in the more classical procedures, or in gels. When soluble antigens are in contact with antibodies in a zone of equivalence, they form aggregates. Large amounts of these reactants are necessary to form large insoluble lattices that precipitate and are grossly visible. When the antigen concentration is very low with an excess of antibody or vice versa, precipitation does not occur due to the prozone phenomenon. Gel precipitation methods are still used, having evolved from the more basic Ouchterlony method (double diffusion in gels) to radial immunodiffusion and diffusion methods that are enhanced by electrical pulses (e.g., countercurrent electrophoresis for pyogenic meningitis and fungal infections).

CF and HAI

CF is a classical technique developed in the early 1900s that is still used in some laboratories, although its rigorous procedure and standardization are time-consuming. In this technique, antigen is added to a patient's serum (heat inactivated) and supplemented with guinea pig complement. If specific antibody to the antigen is present, the immune complex activates complement where it is "fixed" to the complex. Upon subsequent addition of sheep RBCs, which have been sensitized with rabbit anti-RBCs (hemolysin), the complement is not available to lyse the RBCs

(lysis which would have occurred is prevented); therefore, no lysis represents a positive test (i.e., presence of antibody). The test requires careful standardization of the amounts of antigen, complement, and sensitized RBCs. Nevertheless, it was a powerful technique used for a large number of viruses.

The HAI assay is another classical technique that exploits the phenomenon that certain viruses can agglutinate RBCs; e.g., influenza virus agglutinates human RBCs of blood group O, and rubella virus agglutinates baby chicken cells. In this technique, a known amount of viral antigen (rubella) is mixed with serial dilutions of a patient's serum and the indicator system (baby chicken cells) is added (usually in a microtiter plate). Antibody to rubella will bind to the antigen and prevent the antigen reagent from agglutinating the indicator cells. The dilutions of serum allow for an endpoint titer which is defined as the reciprocal of the highest dilution of serum that prevents HA. As with CF tests, all components of the system must be carefully standardized to prevent false positives and false negatives due to procedural errors; a number of appropriate controls must be included. These assays have mostly been replaced by ELISA methods since they are less technically demanding and have a higher throughput.

Neutralization Assays

In the context of immunoassays, neutralization assays are used not for culture verification, but for confirmation of specific reactivity by ELISA. In the most common examples, neutralization assays are used to verify the presence of HBsAg and HIV p24 antigen. Once the presence of these antigens produces a repeatedly reactive result, a neutralization step follows. The principle is based on the use of very specific antibody reagents that are incubated with the serum to allow true antigen to react, followed by a retesting in the original antigen ELISA. If true antigen is present in the serum, it will be neutralized by the antibody reagent, thereby causing a reduction in the OD reading (compared to that of the original nontreated serum). A reduction of 40 to 50% in reactivity after neutralization signals verification.

RIAs

Sensitivity requirements for immunoassays dictated the need for better methods (51). The sensitivity and specificity afforded by radioactively labeled peptides and other molecules led to the identification and quantification of hormones, drugs, enzymes, sterols, serum proteins, and other molecules. Detection of the HBV antigen in blood and detection of allergen-specific IgE antibodies were two of the earliest applications of RIA in the field of immunology (50). However, RIAs have shortcomings in that radioactive isotopes do decay. For example, ^{131}I has a half-life of only 8 days, and the more commonly used isotope ^{125}I has a half-life of 60 days. Despite the longer half-life of ^{125}I, not all radiolabeled molecules are stable, and problems such as absorption, loss of activity, and structural changes can occur during storage. Safety issues such as exposure to radioactivity, handling, and storage are also of concern and are becoming more so recently due to biowarfare threats. Thus, because of the multiple undesirable traits of radioactive probes, alternative, nonisotopic detection methods with similar sensitivities are actively being applied, e.g., chemiluminescence (3, 25).

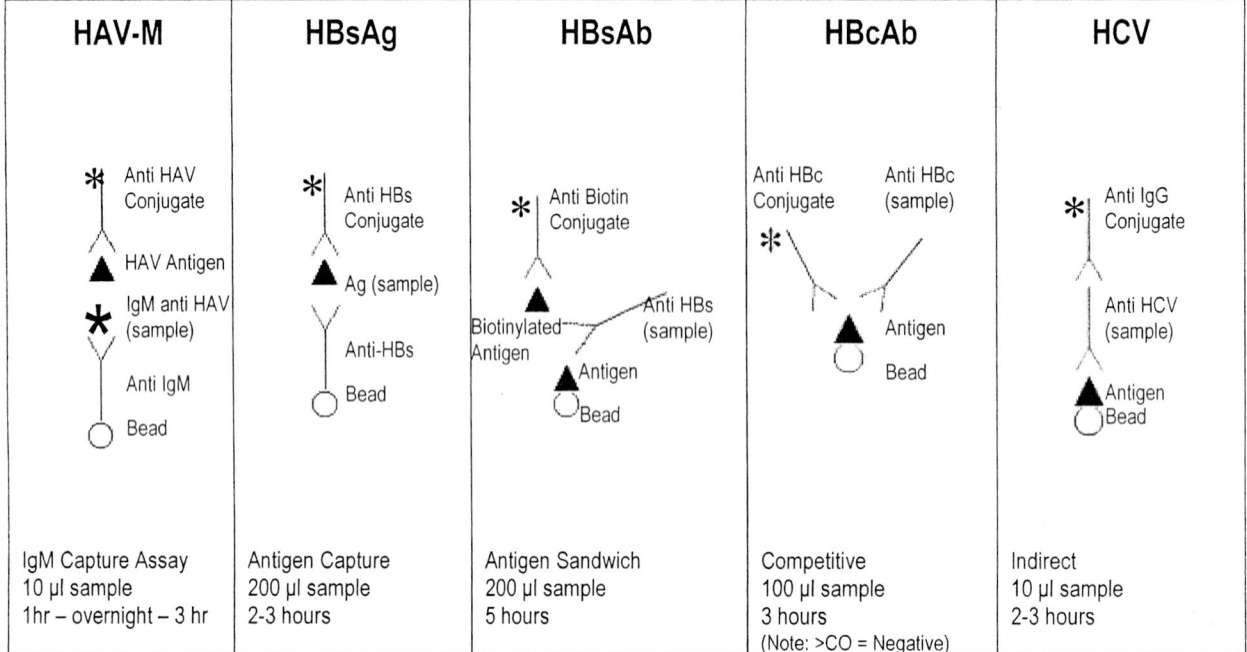

FIGURE 1 Typical ELISA formats. HAV-M, HAV IgM; HBsAg, HBV surface antigen; HBsAb, HBV surface antibody; HBcAb, HBV core antibody; HCV, HCV antibody; *, enzyme or conjugate.

Contemporary Immunoassays

ELISAs

EIAs, of which the ELISA is the most popular, have revolutionized immunoassays. Not only are they used as effective screening tests for a variety of infectious agents, but also they are configured and modified to act as confirmatory assays in some situations. ELISAs are easy to perform, are adaptable for testing of large numbers of samples, do not require the use of radioactive substances, and are sensitive and specific (6). Because they are designed to be very sensitive, a small number of false positives do occur, depending on the specific antibodies used. ELISAs can generally be completed within 2 to 3 h, although some varieties (e.g., competitive) can be completed in half the time. They all offer high throughput and simplicity and are easily adapted to automation. The assays (for antibody) use antigen-coated wells in 96-well microtiter plate formats to capture specific antibody in the sample. Following wash steps to remove unbound material, a conjugate is added, usually consisting of another antibody directed toward human immunoglobulin (anti-IgG or anti-IgG/IgM) which is labeled with an enzyme. Alternative methods include the use of labeled antigen (antigen sandwich method or third-generation assays) that can detect all isotopes of antibody, thereby increasing analytical sensitivity by detecting IgM isotypes, or newer methods such as the fourth-generation assays that increase sensitivity by detecting antigen and antibody simultaneously (37). Subsequently, after another wash, a substrate which has the potential to produce color if the antibody-enzyme or antigen conjugate has been bound in the reaction is added. Indirect ELISAs are the most popular due to their high sensitivity, whereas competitive methods are more specific and faster. Details of the different formats of ELISAs have been published elsewhere (6, 10, 16). Figure 1 shows the principles of different ELISA

formats, indicating the volume of sample required and the approximate assay time.

One potential problem with most immunoassays, particularly sandwich techniques, is the high-dose hook effect (16). This refers to an unexpected fall in signal when the antibody (or antigen) to be assessed is present in very large amounts. The hook effect is similar to the prozone effect of agglutination assays, in which large amounts of the analyte produce a weak or negative result. Although not completely understood, it probably results from a hindrance in the combining of antigen and antibody because of the proximity of multiple molecules, preventing a secondary molecule (detector antibody or conjugate) from binding effectively.

RIPA

The radioimmunoprecipitation assay (RIPA) is extremely sensitive and can be used in conjunction with, or as an alternative to, the Western blot to confirm several infectious diseases, such as HIV and HTLV (10). It has also been used for identification of antibodies to *Trypanosoma cruzi* (28) and HCV (30). Since it is essentially a research technique and requires the use of radioactive substances, it is not used in many clinical laboratories and has largely been replaced with nucleic acid amplification tests.

Western Blots, LIAs, and Recombinant Immunoblots

The Western blot. The Western blot is probably the most widely accepted confirmatory assay (along with the IFA) for the detection of antibodies to a number of infectious agents, most notably HIV, HTLV, HCV, and *Borrelia burgdorferi*. The Western blot technique is considered by many authorities the "gold standard" for validation of results. The Western blot is less sensitive than screening assays but is more specific, and once a positive result is produced, it is rare that it is incorrect. The Western blot is relatively expensive and more labor-intensive to perform than ELISAs.

The Western blot technique owes its exquisite specificity to two factors: component separation and component concentration. As the mixture of viral components is separated by electrophoresis into specific bands, each component becomes relatively pure. In addition, the separation of antigens allows for the identification of specific antibodies to each of the microorganism's antigens. In principle, it is conducted in three parts: (i) separation of antigens from lysates in relation to their molecular weights, (ii) transfer (blotting) of the separated antigens onto nitrocellulose or other absorbent paper, and (iii) testing of the unknown sample directly on the blotted membrane by an EIA method (enzyme-substrate reaction). Most Western blots in use are supplied by commercial companies in kit form with the antigens already electrophoresed and blotted (i.e., only step 3 above needs to be performed). In order to produce a Western blot, large quantities of the infectious agent must be grown in culture and then chemically treated for disruption and inactivation. Antigens are separated through a gel in an electric field in the presence of sodium dodecyl sulfate (SDS) (an anionic detergent that denatures the viral components and yields proteins with net negative charges), and then the proteins are blotted electrophoretically onto nitrocellulose. In the presence of SDS, the negatively charged proteins migrate in polyacrylamide gel according to their molecular weights. Bands of proteins corresponding to certain molecular weights are thus produced. Note that nonagent proteins derived from the host cells in which the agent was grown are also present on the nitrocellulose and can make interpretation difficult. The principles of preparing and performing a Western blot test are depicted in Fig. 2. Some laboratories develop in-house Western blots to save money, but this requires facilities that are capable of propagating the agent and have equipment for electrophoresis and blotting, and the laboratory workers must contend with the hazards associated with handling pathogenic organisms. In addition, the use of preblotted strips from the manufacturers has greatly reduced the variability associated with reagent preparations and therefore helps to standardize the technique.

To perform the Western blot using a manufacturer's product, nitrocellulose strips which already contain the separated antigens are reacted sequentially with sample, conjugate, and substrate, similarly to an ELISA method; a wash step is included after each step to remove nonspecific reactants. The final substrate is precipitable, resulting in the formation of a colored end product (usually purple). The precipitate forms on the nitrocellulose strip at the particular sites where specific antibodies have bound. Depending on the particular antibodies in the sample, Western blot (band) profiles are produced. The type of profile (the combination and intensity of bands that are present) determines whether the individual is considered to be positive, negative, or indeterminate for antibodies to the agent. Figure 3 is a schematic representation showing the virus-specific reactions in a typical HIV Western blot.

LIA and recombinant immunoblot assay. The principle of the LIA is similar to that of the Western blot in that there are separate antigens of the organisms on nitrocellulose strips so that each reaction can be visualized (10); the procedure is also similar to that of the Western blot. The difference is that in LIAs, artificial antigens (synthetic

peptide and/or recombinant) are "painted" on the strips rather than being electrophoresed from lysates of the organisms (35). The advantages of the LIA over Western blots are as follows: (i) the background due to host cell proteins that are often present in lysate preparations if a cell culture system is used is eliminated; (ii) the antigens can be better standardized to minimize lot-to-lot variations; (iii) the antigens can be applied in their optimal concentrations, unlike in Western blots, in which poor recovery of antigens is always a problem (especially glycoprotein antigens); (iv) whole blood can be used; and (v) controls are included on the strips to aid in the scoring of reactions for quality control purposes. Some companies offer an automatic reader for objective and quantitative readings. The use of these artificial antigens helps to eliminate the problems of indeterminate and atypical results that may occur due to antibodies to cellular components of culture systems (10).

The recombinant immunoblot assay (RIBA) is not to be confused with the RIPA technique. The RIBA is identical to the LIA in principle but is given a different name by a different manufacturer and uses only recombinant antigens. RIBAs are used most frequently for HIV, HTLV, HCV, HSV, and *B. burgdorferi*. Figure 4 illustrates a LIA for confirmation and differentiation of HTLV infections. Tests that combine Western blots with RIBAs or LIAs are also available. An example is the augmented blot for HTLV, in which a highly specific recombinant antigen (p21e) and peptides to specific components of HTLV-1 and HTLV-2 on a background of electrophoresed viral lysate antigens are used.

Fluorescence Antibody Assays

Fluorescence assays can be used for the detection of antibodies to organisms or used directly to visualize the agents. Methods include microparticle EIAs for antibody, IFAs for antibody, and DFAs for antigen detection. Those for antigen detection are discussed under "Antigen Detection Technologies" below.

The IFA is a valuable and commonly used immunoassay for detecting antibodies to infectious agents (33). The method is widely used and effective due to its high sensitivity and specificity and its ease of use. However, it requires an expensive fluorescence microscope, results must be read subjectively, and interpretations are sometimes difficult due to nonspecific reactions. Both localization and quantification of antibody reactivity can be accomplished, thereby sometimes yielding information about specific reactions. Also, because of the unique characteristic of fluorochromes, simultaneous detection of multiple antigens by use of different labeled antibodies is possible. The IFA is available for use in the identification of antibodies to a large number of microorganisms, including *T. pallidum*, *Legionella pneumophila*, *B. burgdorferi*, cytomegalovirus, EBV, HSV, HIV, HTLV, varicella-zoster virus, rubella and mumps viruses, and agents of parasitic diseases such as malaria, leishmaniasis, trypanosomiasis, toxoplasmosis, and schistosomiasis (30, 33).

Fluorochromes are excited from a ground state to a higher energy state with UV light by the absorption of photons at one specific wavelength. As the molecules return to a resting state, photons are emitted at a different wavelength (26). Visualization of fluorescence is accomplished with a microscope that employs a dark-field condenser and filters to block out illuminating light of the microscope to create a dark background in which only the emitted fluorescent light is seen. While fluorescently la-

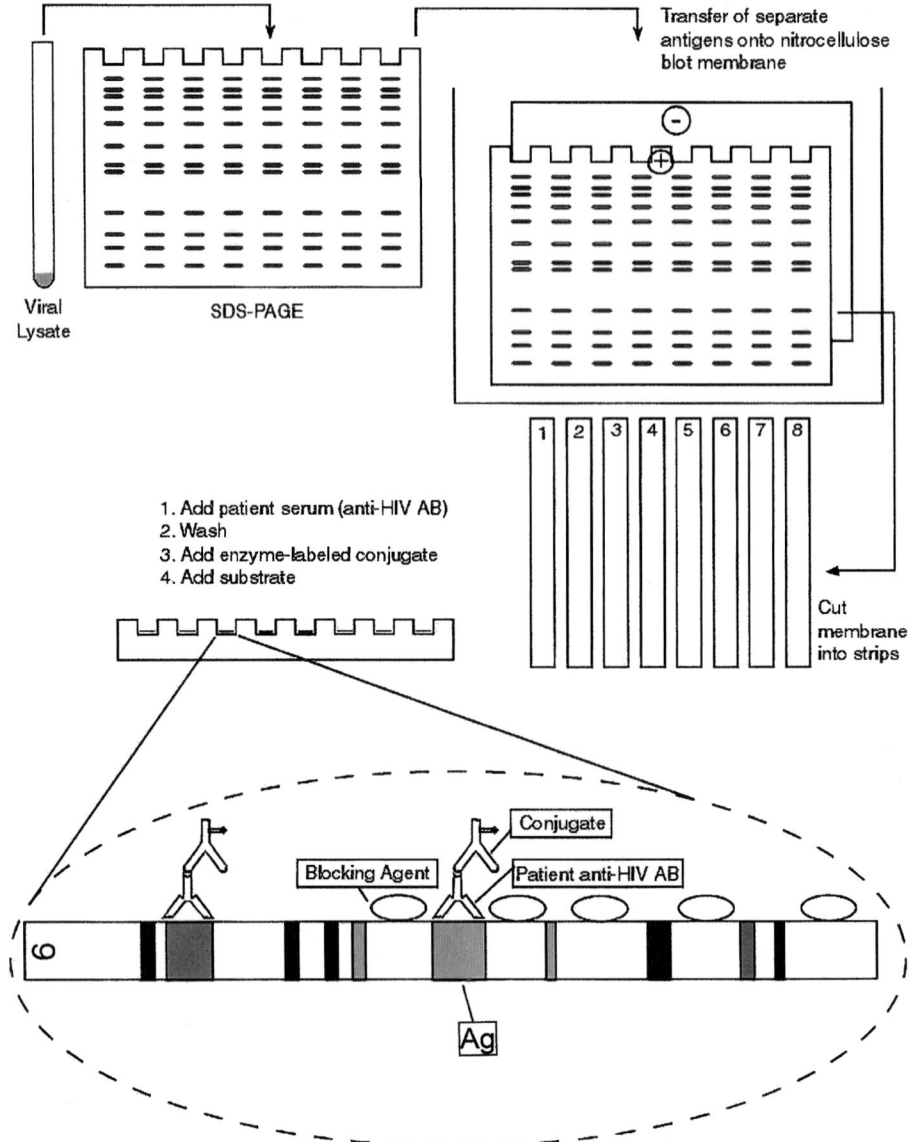

FIGURE 2 Principle of the preparation of a Western blot and the ELISA-type reaction that occurs on the strip. SDS-PAGE, SDS-polyacrylamide gel electrophoresis; AB, antibody; Ag, antigen.

beled probes are extremely stable, fluorescence by organic fluorophores is sometimes emitted from tissue, thereby increasing background noise.

Rapid Tests

One of the most valuable contributions in the field of immunoassays is the development and application of rapid assays that can be completed in less than 30 min and usually without the need for instrumentation. Although some rapid tests have been available for decades (e.g., mononucleosis spot tests and streptococcal tests), the field of rapid diagnostics has been expanded greatly during the last decade. Rapid tests are available for dengue virus (45), chlamydia (9), influenza virus (47), RSV (27), HIV (14), HSV-2 (www.Diagnology.com/pockit_test.htm), and HCV (12, 32).

The earliest of the new generation of rapid tests and the largest variety of different formats for infectious agents are for HIV antibody detection, hence, HIV rapid tests will be used here to exemplify their principles and utility. These tests gained popularity in the early 1990s and, as the technology became refined, proved to be as accurate as other screening tests, including the ELISAs. Applications include use in emergency rooms, physicians' offices, point-of-care testing units, autopsy rooms, funeral homes, and small blood banks and for stat HIV testing (where immediate treatment is recommended for exposures). Importantly, rapid assays are easy to perform and have utility in developing countries where facilities may not be optimal, stable electricity may be unavailable, and formal education programs for laboratory personnel are absent (10).

One class of rapid tests are the dot blot or immunoblot assays, so named because they produce a well-circumscribed colored dot on the solid-phase surface if the test is positive. The procedures for the dot blot assays are similar regardless of the exact format of the test. Most require dropwise

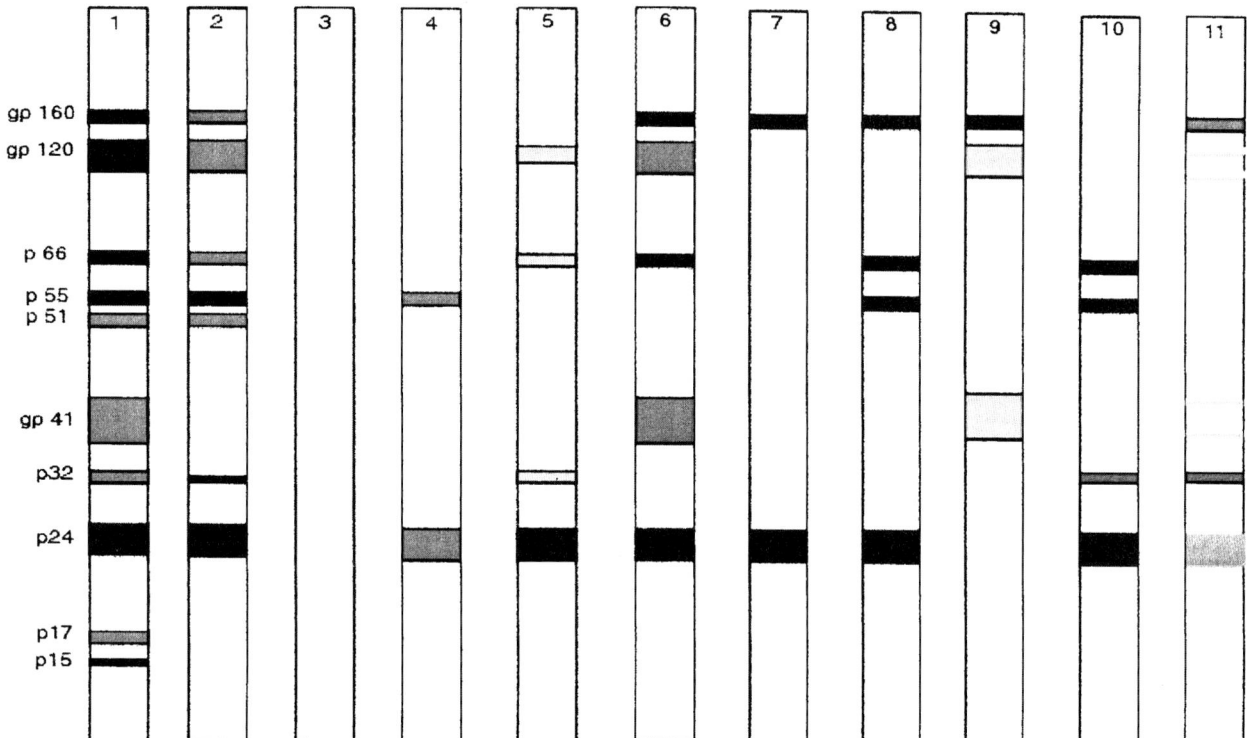

FIGURE 3 Western blot profiles. Lanes: 1, strong positive control; 2, weak positive control; 3, negative control; 4, indeterminate result, possible early infection; 5, minimally positive, possible HIV-2 or HIV-1 group O infections; 6, positive, but rarely may be a false positive (no p32); 7, minimally positive by some criteria, possible infection by a viral variant, or rarely can be a false positive; 8, positive in evolution, or rarely may be a false positive; 9, minimally positive by some criteria, reactivity to only envelope antigens, rarely can be a false positive; 10, minimally positive, suggestive of HIV-2 or HIV-1 group O infections; 11, minimally positive by most criteria, maybe indicating infection by a viral variant.

additions of reagents in the following sequence: buffer, sample, wash buffer, conjugate, wash buffer, substrate, and stop solution. Some assays substitute an IgG binding dye (protein A-gold reagent) for the anti-immunoglobulin conjugate, thereby decreasing the procedure by one step. Most assays now incorporate a built-in control that indicates that the test was performed correctly; this control is an anti-human immunoglobulin that binds any immunoglobulin in the sample and produces a separate indicator when all reagents are added appropriately. There are several varieties of dot blot assays available that include two "dots" which allow the differentiation of types of agents such as HIV type 1 (HIV-1) and HIV-2, and at least one that has three dots to include detection of a particular agent group (HIV-1 group O) has been introduced (14). Other rapid test formats include dipsticks, in which antigen is attached to the "teeth" of comb-like devices; several of these rapid tests have the ability to differentiate HIV-1 and HIV-2. The most recent addition to rapid assays are called lateral flow devices or one-step assays. These offer extreme simplicity and the addition of only one (or no) reagent. They all take advantage of antigens spotted on nitrocellulose membranes with lateral or vertical flow of sample or reagents to interact with immobilized antigen (in-solution kinetics) (24). One variety takes advantage of third-generation kinetics (antigen sandwich) to increase sensitivity. Other major advances in rapid test technology include the use of oral fluid (saliva) and fingerstick whole-blood sample media. One

particular device, the OraQuick HIV-1 (OraSure Technologies), allows the use of fingerstick blood, oral fluid, serum, or plasma for testing in a format that requires no addition of reagents (D. F. York, P. Kiepiela, and A. N. Smith, *Abstr. XIVth Int. AIDS Conf.*, abstr. TuPeC4892, 2002).

Disadvantages of rapid tests include subjective interpretation, difficulty in test interpretation if the laboratorian is color-blind, cost, and lack of automation. Technical errors can be common with these assays if users become careless with the simple procedures. For example, pipettes are not always held in a vertical position as recommended, resulting in an incorrect delivery of reagent volumes. Further, laboratory workers attempt to test multiple samples simultaneously, resulting in inaccuracies due to timing of the steps. Recently, rapid tests have been developed to offer confirmation of HIV infection. These dot blot tests incorporate several antigens of diagnostic significance spotted separately (similar to the LIAs) so that reactivity to different antigens can be visualized (15). Several varieties of rapid tests are shown in Fig. 5.

Antigen Detection Technologies

Antigen detection or direct detection of microorganisms can be accomplished by (i) rapid antigen serologic methods, (ii) ELISA antigen tests (and other antigen detection technologies), (iii) direct and indirect immunofluorescence assays, (iv) culture with staining or the use of probes, and (v) molecular amplification tests to detect nucleic acids. Cul-

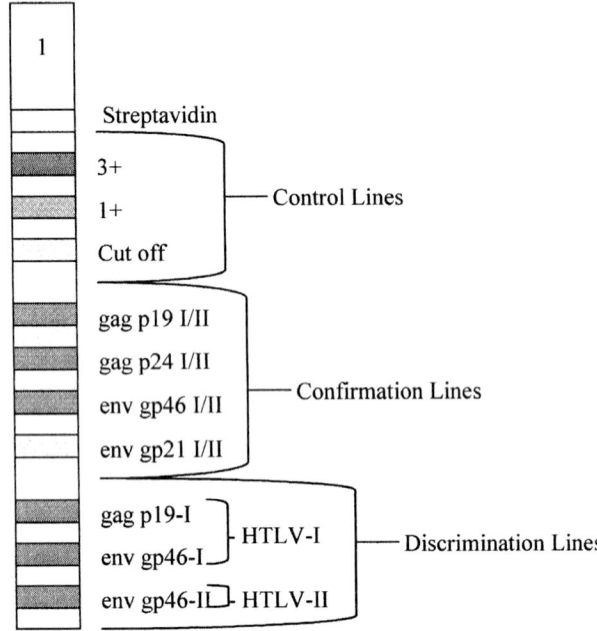

FIGURE 4 A LIA (INNO-LIA, Innogenetics, Belgium) for detection of antibodies to HTLV. Shown are specific antigens that are used to confirm infection and those that can differentiate HTLV-1 from HTLV-2.

ture and molecular methods will not be discussed in this chapter.

Rapid Antigen Serologic Methods

The most popular rapid antigen detection methods are agglutination assays for *Streptococcus pneumoniae*, group A and B streptococci, *Haemophilus influenzae* type B, RSV, *Neisseria meningitidis*, and *Cryptococcus neoformans* (30) and a dot blot antigen assay for rotavirus antigen detection in stool specimens. The agglutination assays usually use latex particles coated with specific antibodies to structural antigens and can detect soluble antigens in urine, cerebrospinal fluid, and serum. In the dot blot type rapid antigen assay, the specimen is spotted on a nitrocellulose membrane and detection is done via a specific antibody in a direct or indirect format. A modification to this method is called the immune complex dot assay, in which preincubation of specimen with antibody results in a complex which is spotted and detected by collodial gold-labeled antibody (48); it has been claimed to be more sensitive than the dot blot test for rotavirus (49). The sensitivity of rapid antigen assays may be less than that of EIA methods (30).

Antigen ELISAs and Immuno-PCR for Antigen Detection

As stated previously, the most common antigen ELISAs are for HIV p24 antigen and HBsAg, although others are available, including ones for HCV antigen, RSV, and rotavirus. In general, these are more sensitive than the rapid membrane or agglutination assays. Their format is a typical antigen capture method in which immobilized specific antibody captures antigen in the specimen and is detected by a detector antibody to a different epitope from that of the capture antibody. Subsequently, a third anti-species immunoglobulin conjugate is used to produce color.

Other antigen detection methods have recently become available, but they are not simple. One such method is immuno-PCR, in which a typical antigen ELISA is coupled with the molecular technique of PCR. In this method, the detector antibody conjugate (which is usually coupled to an enzyme) is coupled instead to a piece of amplifiable DNA. Once attached, PCR is performed to amplify the signal. This method has been shown to detect antigen in the subfemtogram range (8) and is capable of detecting HBV antigen at levels unattainable by ELISA methods (34). It is also being applied for the enhanced sensitivity of detecting HIV p24 antigen (N. Constantine, J. Barletta, E. Feng, D. C. Edelman, and W. E. Highsmith, *Abstr. XIVth Int. AIDS Conf.*, abstr. TuPeC4881, 2002). Figure 6 depicts the principle of the method.

DFAs and IFAs

DFAs are commonly used in immunology, microbiology, and virology laboratories to directly detect the presence of microorganisms. They are fast, easy to perform, and very specific. In this procedure, clinical specimens such as culture material, nasal washes, sputum, cerebrospinal fluid, etc., are centrifuged and washed to remove material that may fluoresce and are fixed on glass slides (usually by heat or cold acetone fixation). The slides are then reacted directly with a specific antibody probe that is labeled with a fluorochrome (fluorescein isothiocyanate), mounting oil and a coverslip are added, and the slides are examined under a fluorescence microscope. Thus, this is essentially a one-step procedure that can be performed (after fixation) within less than 1 h. However, similar to the IFA, it does require an expensive microscope and well-trained personnel. Furthermore, each purified antibody must be individually labeled with a fluorescent molecule and is capable of binding to only a single antigenic site or epitope. Thus, direct assays are limited by the impracticality of preparing hundreds of fluorochrome-labeled antibodies with specificity to a wide variety of microorganisms or other types of peptides or molecules. To increase sensitivity, indirect fluorescent methods to detect antigens can be used to offer a more versatile application, but these assays require about 2 h. This indirect fluorescence assay for direct assessment of antigen should not be confused with the IFA for antibody detection. In the indirect method for antigen detection, a primary IgG antibody (unlabeled) is selected, and its binding to the specific antigen is detected by a secondary fluorescent-labeled antibody having specificity to the primary immunoglobulin molecule. For example, detection of a microorganism by a specific but unlabeled primary antibody made in sheep is done by a secondary fluorescent anti-sheep IgG antibody produced in a goat. Commercially prepared fluorescently labeled secondary antibodies are readily available and can be used in a variety of other immunofluorescent assays employing any primary antibody produced in the same species. The use of this double-antibody system (use of primary and secondary antibodies to detect an antigen versus the use of a single antibody to detect an antigen) increases the sensitivity of the assay. These methods are used widely for *T. pallidum* (21, 33), *Chlamydia trachomatis* (42), and HSV and varicella-zoster virus (particularly in dermal lesion specimens) and are very effective for RSV (19, 29). Further, several fluorochromes can be used simultaneously to detect more than one organism in a given specimen by visualizing different colors under the microscope, particularly for respiratory viruses in nasopharyngeal specimens (19). Figure 7 depicts the methods of

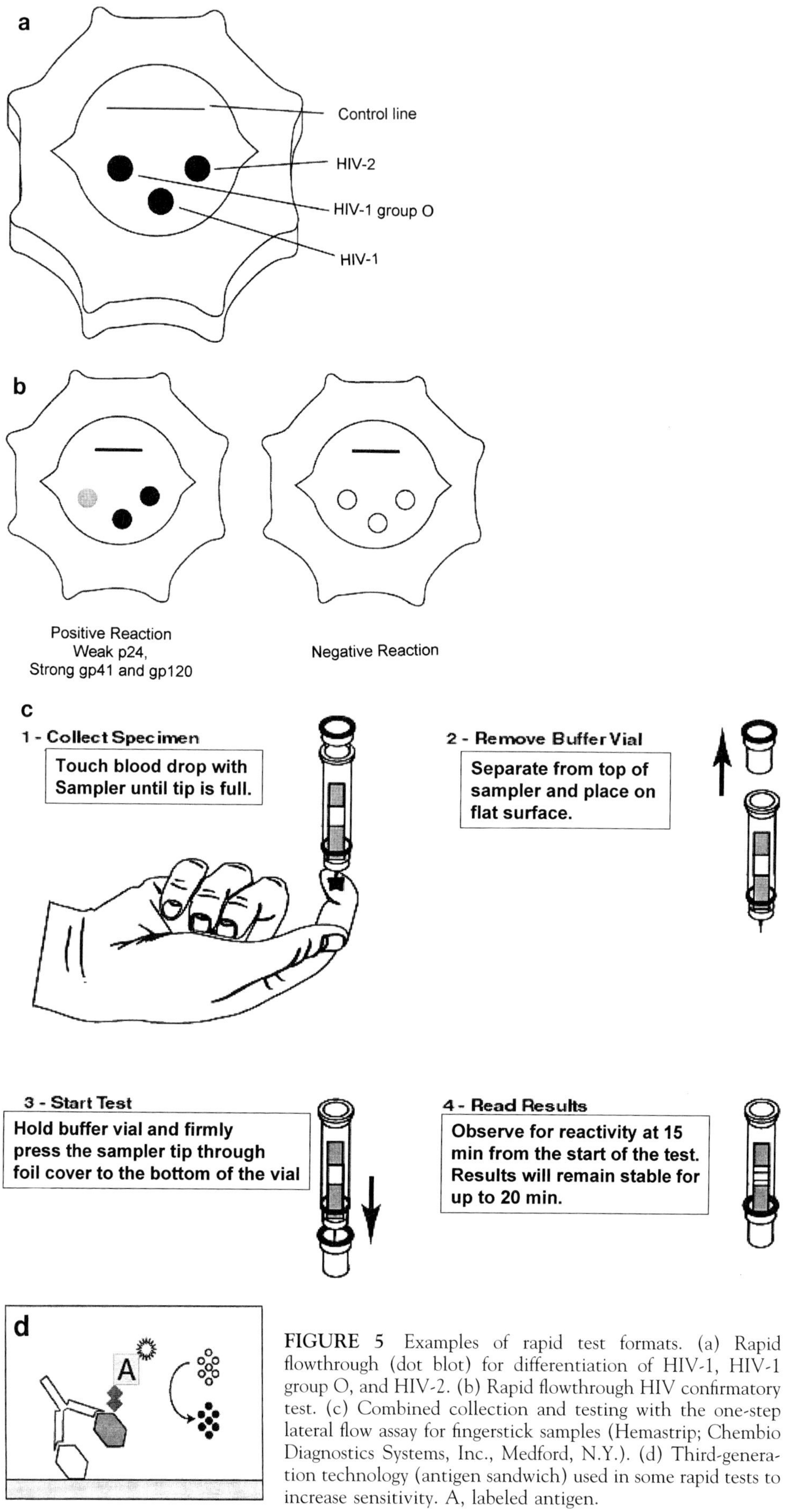

a

Control line

HIV-2

HIV-1 group O

HIV-1

b

Positive Reaction
Weak p24,
Strong gp41 and gp120

Negative Reaction

c

1 - Collect Specimen

Touch blood drop with
Sampler until tip is full.

2 - Remove Buffer Vial

Separate from top of
sampler and place on
flat surface.

3 - Start Test

Hold buffer vial and firmly
press the sampler tip through
foil cover to the bottom of the vial

4 - Read Results

Observe for reactivity at 15
min from the start of the test.
Results will remain stable for
up to 20 min.

d

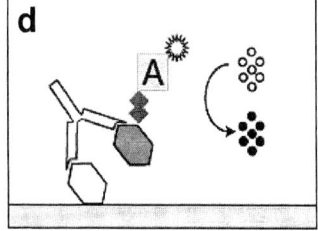

FIGURE 5 Examples of rapid test formats. (a) Rapid
flowthrough (dot blot) for differentiation of HIV-1, HIV-1
group O, and HIV-2. (b) Rapid flowthrough HIV confirmatory
test. (c) Combined collection and testing with the one-step
lateral flow assay for fingerstick samples (Hemastrip; Chembio
Diagnostics Systems, Inc., Medford, N.Y.). (d) Third-generation technology (antigen sandwich) used in some rapid tests to
increase sensitivity. A, labeled antigen.

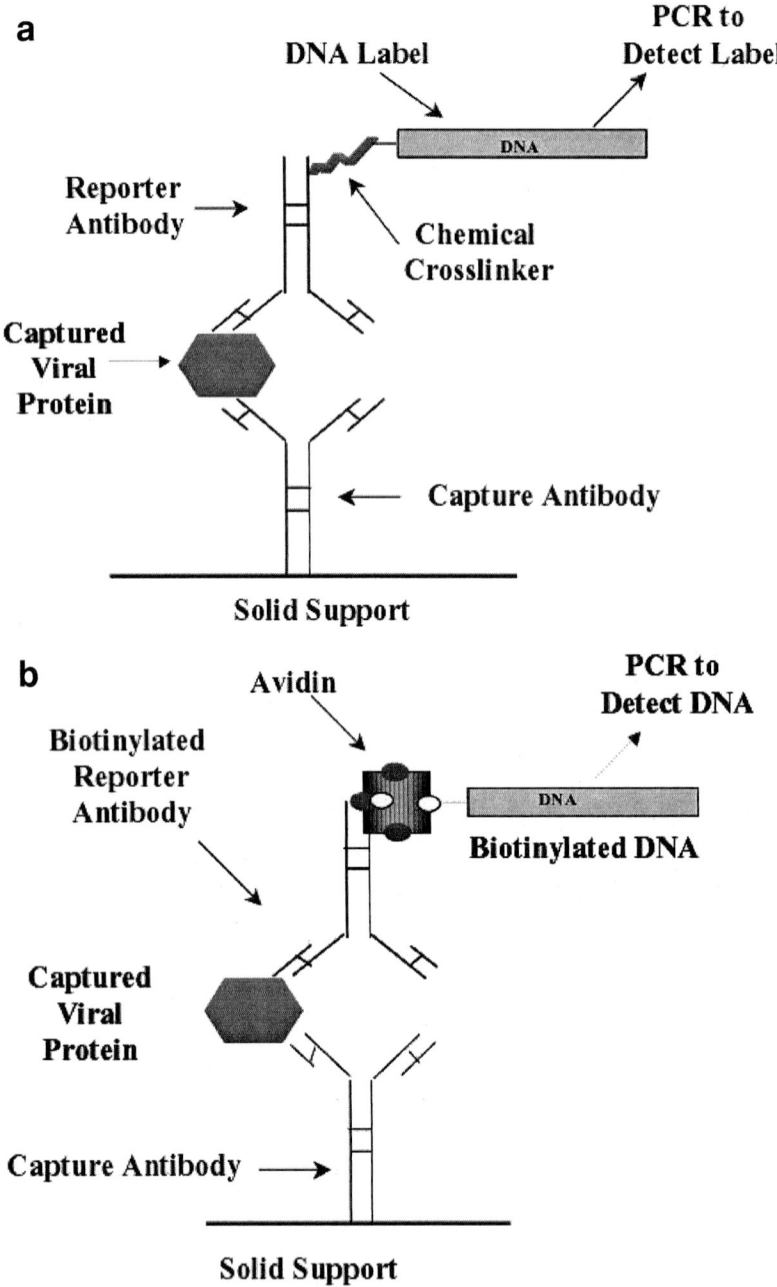

FIGURE 6 Principle of immuno-PCR. (a) DNA directly conjugated to reporter antibody; (b) DNA conjugated via an avidin-biotin reaction.

the DFA and IFA. The most commonly used tests for the detection of infectious agents are listed in Table 1.

Epidemiologic Tools: S/LS (Detuning) Tests

Tests that can be used as epidemiologic tools to estimate incidence in populations have become available. Such estimates are important to identify populations in which high numbers of new infections are occurring and which can benefit from intervention strategies such as vaccination. Sensitive/less sensitive (S/LS) serologic testing strategies, sometimes referred to as detuned assays and more recently as STARHS (serologic testing algorithm for recent HIV

seroconversion), have been developed (22), evaluated (N. Constantine, A. Sill, F. R. Cleghorn, K. Kreisel, J. Edwards, T. Cafarella, N. Jack, C. Bartholomew, and W. A. Blattner, unpublished data), and implemented (38), offering single-point testing in cross-sectional surveys to differentiate individuals with recent HIV infection (e.g., <129 days) from those with established infection. S/LS tests to categorize infected persons are based on the concepts that specific HIV antibody titers rise and plateau over time and that changes (increases) in antibody avidity occur as infection progresses. Therefore, modifications to the procedures of conventional EIA methods have allowed the development

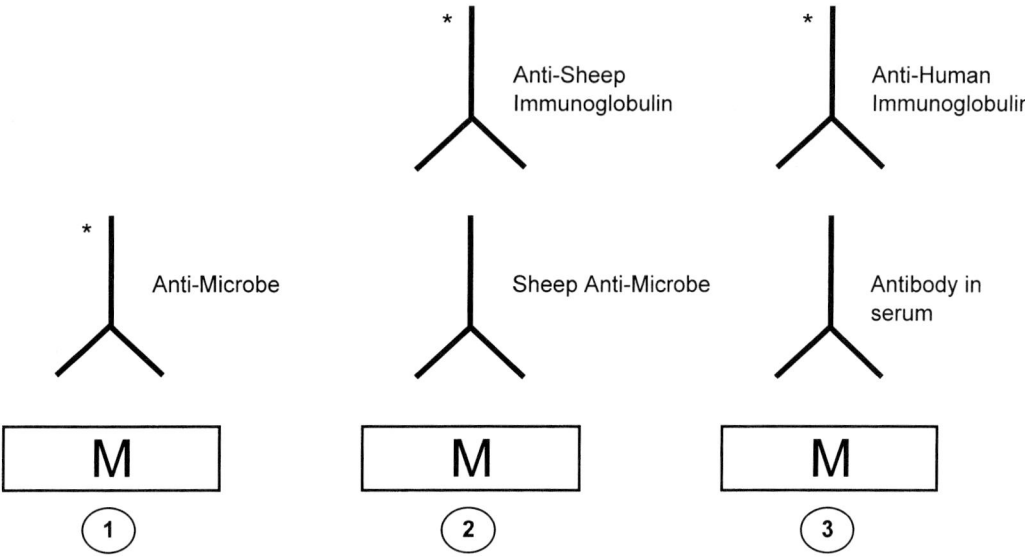

FIGURE 7 Principles of the (1) DFA and (2) IFA for detection of antigen in body fluids or tissues and (3) of the IFA for the detection of antibody in serum. M, organism from body fluids or tissues fixed on a slide (1 and 2) or from commercially supplied sources (3); *, fluorescence signal.

TABLE 1 Partial list of commonly used immunoassays for the detection of antibodies and antigens to some infectious agents[a]

Infectious agent(s)	Screening test(s)	Supplemental test(s)
Viruses		
EBV	ELISA	IFA
HSV	ELISA, rapid	RIBA, IFA
Cytomegalovirus	ELISA, rapid	IFA
HIV	ELISA, rapid, IFA, PHA	WB, RIBA, IFA, LIA
HTLV	ELISA, PHA	RIBA, LIA
Hepatitis (A, B, C, D, E, G) virus	ELISA (IgG, IgM), rapid (Ag), rapid (HCV), MEIA	Neutralization (Ag), WB (HEV), RIBA, (HCV), RIPA
Rubella, mumps, measles virus	ELISA, PHA, HAI, agglutination	IFA
Varicella-zoster virus	ELISA, rapid	IFA
RSV	ELISA (Ag), ELISA (Ab), rapid (Ag), HAI	IFA, DFA, neutralization
Influenza virus	ELISA, HAI	IFA, DFA
Rotavirus	ELISA (Ag), rapid (Ag), HAI	DFA
Bacteria		
Streptococcus spp.	Agglutination	ASO, AHT, DNase B
Treponema spp.	RPR, VDRL	PHA, IFA (FTA)
B. burgdorferi	ELISA	WB, RIBA, IFA
Chlamydia spp.	ELISA, rapid (Ag)	DFA
Fungi	DD, ELISA	IFA
Rickettsiae	CF, agglutination	IFA
Parasites		
Toxoplasma	PHA, ELISA	IFA
T. cruzi	Rapid, ELISA	RIPA, IFA
Others	IgE, DFA, rapid	IFA

[a] Abbreviations: MEIA, microparticle EIA; DD, double diffusion (Ouchterlony); WB, Western blot; Ag, antigen; Ab, antibody; ASO, anti-streptolysin O assay; AHT, anti-hyaluronidase test; rapid, a simple assay that can be performed in less than 30 min.

of a less sensitive test mode that can be used to estimate antibody titer or avidity. Accordingly, modifications of the assay procedure, such as use of higher dilutions of sample and changes in incubation times or the addition of chaotropic reagents, have been shown to be effective in discriminating the time of infection based on antibody titer or antibody avidity, respectively (M. K. Shriver, *Abstr. Assoc. Public Health Lab. Dir.*, abstr. 22, 1999). Recently, a rapid test in conjunction with an EIA has been proposed as a means to increase the accuracy of S/LS methods (F. R. Cleghorn, A. Sill, N. E. Jack, H. Smith, V. Forsythe-Duke, K. Kreisel, D. Banfield-Roche, C. Bartholomew, N. Constantine, and W. A. Blattner, *Abstr. XIVth Int. AIDS Conf.*, abstr. MoOrC1039, 2002).

Flow Cytometric Assays

Flow cytometry, used extensively for quantifying and identifying cell populations, is gaining popularity for infectious diseases in microbiology and virology laboratories. The basic principle of flow cytometry involves illumination with laser light of a continuous stream of suspended cells in a fluid medium. As the individual cells pass through the laser, scattering of the beam in different directions (e.g., forward angle, side scatter) is measured with a set of detectors, and the results are stored and analyzed with computers. The type of diffracted light can yield information such as cell size, cell density, and cell granularity, which can aid in the identification of particular cell types. In addition to assessment by light scatter, cells can be labeled with specific antibodies conjugated to fluorochromes. These allow direct staining of a particular antigen(s), and the laser-induced fluorescence is then measured and analyzed.

Flow cytometry has several advantages over other immunoassays. Analysis is easy and rapid, with greater sensitivity, and is cost-effective when large numbers of samples are tested (1). Its use negates the waiting period for the propagation of microorganisms, it is not labor-intensive, and the results are reproducible (36). From a single sample, simultaneous detection of multiple pathogens is possible. Coupled with monoclonal antibodies, flow cytometry can detect antigenic differences among different strains of the same microorganisms or different microorganisms in the same sample (41). An assessment of the viability of microorganisms, the effectiveness of antimicrobial therapies, detection of bacterial spores, and even determination of whether a bacterium is gram positive or gram negative are just some of the applications of flow cytometry reported in the literature (23). Flow cytometry is also used as an adjunct to the identification of microorganisms, such as in the management and immunological assessment of HIV infection, in which flow cytometry has been used to determine the number of $CD4^+$ lymphocytes in the blood and the level of multiple viral proteases from leukocytes of HIV-positive individuals. The presence of variant HIV strains within an individual or the mutation of an HIV strain over time can also be detected by flow cytometry. As the number of flow cytometers in hospital or clinical diagnostic settings and the knowledge of potential applications continue to increase, a rise in the use of this technique in the diagnosis of microorganisms is imminent. Recently, the use of flow cytometry has been reported for antimicrobial susceptibility testing, offering results after only 1 h for rapidly growing organisms (39).

REFERENCES

1. Álvarez-Barrietnos, A., J. Arroyo, R. Cantón, C. Nombela, and M. Sánchez-Pérez. 2000. Applications of flow cytometry to clinical microbiology. *Clin. Microbiol. Rev.* **13:**167–195.
2. Bansal, J., N. T. Constantine, X. Zhang, J. D. Callahan, V. C. Marsiglia, and K. C. Hyams. 1993. Evaluation of five hepatitis C virus screening tests and two supplemental assays: performance when testing a high risk population in the U.S.A. *Clin. Diagn. Virol.* **1:**113–121.
3. Boeckx, R. L. 1984. Chemiluminescence: applications for the clinical laboratory. *Hum. Pathol.* **15:**104–111.
4. Brojer, E., G. Liszewski, A. Niznik, A. Roseik, M. Letowska, J. E. Petersen, M. Calmann, P. L. Kerrison, and S. R. Lee. 2001. Detection of HCV core antigen in HCV RNA positive, anti-HCV negative blood donations from Polish blood donors. *Transfusion* **41:**304.
5. Butler, J. E. 2000. Enzyme-linked immunosorbent assay. *J. Immunoassay* **21:**165–209.
6. Carpenter, A. B. 1997. Enzyme-linked immunoassays, p. 20–29. *In* N. R. Rose, E. C. de Macario, J. D. Folds, H. C. Lane, and R. M. Nakamura (ed.), *Manual of Clinical Laboratory Immunology*, 5th ed. ASM Press, Washington, D.C.
7. Centers for Disease Control and Prevention. 1998. Guidelines for the management of health care worker exposures to HIV and recommendations for postexposure prophylaxis. *Morb. Mortal. Wkly. Rep.* **47:**3.
8. Chang, T. C., and S. H. Huang. 1997. A modified immuno polymerase chain reaction for the detection of beta glucuronidase from Escherichia coli. *Immunol. Methods* **208:**35–42.
9. Chernesky, M., D. Jang, J. Sellors, P. Coleman, J. Bodner, I. Hrusovsky, S. Chong, and J. Mahony. 1995. Detection of *Chlamydia trachomatis* antigens in male urethral swabs and urines with a microparticle enzyme immunoassay. *Sex. Transm. Dis.* **22:**55–59.
10. Constantine, N. T., J. D. Callahan, and D. M. Watts. 1992. *Retroviral Testing: Essentials for Quality Control and Laboratory Diagnosis.* CRC Press, Boca Raton, Fla.
11. Constantine, N. T. 1993. Serologic tests for the retroviruses: approaching a decade of evolution. *AIDS* **7:**1–13.
12. Constantine, N. T., C. Holm-Hansen, N. Skaug, and F. Vasilescu. 1994. Successful use of two rapid HCV assays in a high prevalence Romanian population. *J. Clin. Lab. Anal.* **8:**332–334.
13. Constantine, N. T., G. van der Groen, E. Belsey, D. Heymann, and H. Tamashiro. 1994. Sensitivity of HIV antibody assays as determined by seroconversion panels. *AIDS* **8:**1715–1720.
14. Constantine, N. T., L. Zekeng, A. Sangare, L. Gutler, R. Saville, H. Anhary, and C. Wild. 1997. Diagnostic challenges for rapid HIV assays: performance using HIV-1 group O, group M, and HIV-2 samples. *J. Hum. Virol.* **1:**46–52.
15. Constantine, N. T., and F. Ketema. 2001. Rapid confirmation of HIV infection. *Int. J. Infect. Dis.* **6:**170–177.
16. Cummings, P. J. 2001. Immunoassay, p. 303–322. *In* R. H. Christenson, J. E. Hutton, G. Shugar, and L. J. Johnson (ed.), *Appleton and Lange's Outline Review Clinical Chemistry.* McGraw-Hill Professional Publishing, New York, N.Y.
17. Engvall, E., and P. Perlman. 1971. Enzyme-linked immunosorbent assay (ELISA). Quantitative assay of immunoglobulin G. *Immunochemistry* **8:**871–874.
18. Gosling, J. P. 1990. A decade of development in immunoassay methodology. *Clin. Chem.* **36:**1408–1427.
19. Grandien, M., C. A. Pettersson, P. S. Gardner, A. Linde, and A. Stanton. 1985. Rapid viral diagnosis of acute respiratory infections: comparison of enzyme-linked im-

munosorbent assay and the immunofluorescence technique for detection of viral antigens in nasopharyngeal secretions. *J. Clin. Microbiol.* **22:**757–760.

20. **Hanson, K. L., and C. P. Cartwright.** 2001. Evaluation of an automated liquid handling system (Tecan Genesis RSP 100) in the AbbottLCx assay for Chlamydia trachomatis. *J. Clin. Microbiol.* **39:**1975–1977.

21. **Hook, E. W., R. E. Roddy, S. A. Lukehart, J. Hom, K. K. Holmes, and M. R. Tam.** 1985. Detection of *Treponema pallidum* in lesion exudates with a pathogen-specific monoclonal antibody. *J. Clin. Microbiol.* **22:**241–244.

22. **Janssen, R. S., G. A. Satten, S. L. Stramer, B. Rawal, T. R. O'Brien, B. J. Weiblen, F. M. Hecht, N. Jack, F. R. Cleghorn, J. O. Kahn, M. A. Chesney, and M. P. Busch.** 1998. New testing strategy to detect early HIV-1 infection for use in incidence estimates and for clinical and prevention purposes. *JAMA* **280:**42–48.

23. **Kaprelyants, A., and D. G. Kell.** 1992. Rapid assessment of bacterial viability and vitality using rhodamine 123 and flow cytometry. *J. Appl. Bacteriol.* **72:**410–422.

24. **Ketema, F., C. Zeh, D. C. Edelman, R. Saville, and N. T. Constantine.** 2001. Assessment of the performance of a rapid, lateral flow assay for the detection of antibodies to HIV. *J. AIDS* **27:**63–70.

25. **Kricka, L. J.** 1997. Chemiluminescence immunoassays, p. 49–53. *In* N. R. Rose, E. C. de Macario, J. D. Folds, H. C. Lane, and R. M. Nakamura (ed.), *Manual of Clinical Laboratory Immunology,* 5th ed. ASM Press, Washington, D.C.

26. **Kumar, V.** 2000. Immunofluorescence and enzyme immunomicroscopy methods. *J. Immunoassay* **21:**235–253.

27. **Lauer, B. A., H. A. Masters, C. G. Wren, and M. J. Levin.** 1985. Rapid detection of respiratory syncytial virus in nasopharyngeal secretions by enzyme-linked immunosorbent assay. *J. Clin. Microbiol.* **22:**782–785.

28. **Leiby, D. A., S. Wendel, E. T. Takaoka, R. M. Fachini, L. C. Oliveira, and M. A. Tibbals.** 2000. Serological testing for *Trypanosoma cruzi*: comparison of radioimmunoprecipitation assay with commercially available indirect immunofluorescence assay, indirect hemagglutination assay, and enzyme-linked immunosorbent assay kits. *J. Clin. Microbiol.* **38:**639–642.

29. **Loeffelholz, M. J.** 2002. Rapid diagnosis of viral infections. *Lab. Med.* **33:**283–286.

30. **Mahony, J. B., and M. A. Chernesky.** 1999. Immunoassays for the diagnosis of infectious diseases, p. 202–214. *In* P. R. Murray, E. J. Baron, M. A. Pfaller, F. C. Tenover, and R. H. Yolken (ed.), *Manual of Clinical Microbiology,* 7th ed. ASM Press, Washington, D.C.

31. **Morinet, F., F. Ferchal, R. Colimon, and Y. Perol.** 1984. Comparison of six methods for detecting human rotavirus in stools. *Eur. J. Clin. Microbiol.* **3:**136.

32. **Mvere, D., N. T. Constantine, E. Katsawde, O. Tobaiwa, S. Dambire, and P. Corcoran.** 1996. Rapid and simple hepatitis assays: encouraging results from a blood donor population in Zimbabwe. *Bull. W. H. O.* **74:**19–24.

33. **Nakamura, R. M., and D. J. Bylund.** 1997. Fluorescence immunoassays, p. 39–48. *In* N. R. Rose, E. C. de Macario, J. D. Folds, H. C. Lane, and R. M. Nakamura (ed.), *Manual of Clinical Laboratory Immunology,* 5th ed. ASM Press, Washington, D.C.

34. **Niemeyer, D. M., M. Adler, and D. Blohm.** 1997. Fluorometric polymerase chain reaction (PCR) enzyme-linked immunosorbent assay for quantification of immuno-PCR products in microplates. *Anal. Biochem.* **246:**140–145.

35. **Pollet, D. E., E. L. Saman, D. C. Peeters, H. M. Warmenbol, L. M. Heyndrickx, C. J. Wouters, G. Beelaert, G. van der Groen, and H. Van Heuverswyn.** 1991. Confirmation and differentiation of antibodies to human

immunodeficiency virus 1 and 2 with a strip-based assay including recombinant antigens and synthetic peptides. *Clin. Chem.* **37:**1700–1707.

36. **Rieseberg, M., C. Kasper, K. F. Reardon, and T. Schepter.** 2001. Flow cytometry in biotechnology. *Appl. Microbiol. Biotech.* **56:**350–360.

37. **Saville, R., N. T. Constantine, F. R. Cleghorn, N. Jack, C. Bartholomew, J. Edwards, and W. A. Blattner.** 2001. Fourth-generation immunoassay for the simultaneous detection of HIV antigen and antibody utilizing an automated platform. *J. Clin. Microbiol.* **39:**2518–2524.

38. **Schwarcz, S., T. Kellog, W. McFarland, B. Louie, R. Kohn, M. Katz, G. Bolan, J. Klausner, and H. Weinstock.** 2001. Differences in temporal trends of HIV seroincidence and seroprevalence among sexually transmitted disease clinic patients, 1989–1998: application of the serologic testing algorithm for recent HIV seroconversion. *Am. J. Epidemiol.* **153:**925–934.

39. **Shapiro, H. M.** 2002. Microbiology applications of flow cytometry. *Adv. Admin. Lab.* **11(4):**61–64.

40. **Singh, N., and M. Shukla.** 2001. An assessment of the usefulness of a rapid immunochromatographic test, "Determine Malaria pf" in evaluating intervention measures in forest villages of central India. *BMC Infect. Dis.* **1:**10–15.

41. **Steen, H. B., E. Boye, K. Skarstad, B. Bloom, T. Goday, and S. Mustafa.** 1982. Applications of flow cytometry on bacteria: cell cycle kinetics, drug effects, and quantitation of antibody binding. *Cytometry* **2:**249–257.

42. **Tam, M. R., W. E. Stamm, H. H. Handsfield, R. Stephens, C. C. Kuo, K. Holmes, K. Ditzenberg, M. Krieger, and R. C. Nowinski.** 1984. Culture-independent diagnosis of Chlamydia trachomatis using monoclonal antibodies. *N. Engl. J. Med.* **310:**1146–1150.

43. **Tomar, R.** 1999. Total laboratory automatic and diagnostic immunology. *Clin. Diagn. Lab. Immunol.* **6:**293–294.

44. **Vaananen, P., V. M. Haiva, P. Koskela, and O. Meurman.** 1985. Comparison of a simple latex agglutination test with hemolysis-in-gel, hemagglutination inhibition, and radioimmunoassay for detection of rubella virus antibodies. *J. Clin. Microbiol.* **21:**793–795.

45. **Vaughn, D. W., A. Nisalak, S. Kalayanarooj, T. Solomon, N. M. Dung, A. Cuzzubbo, and P. L. Devine.** 1998. Evaluation of a rapid immunochromatographic test for diagnosis of dengue virus infection. *J. Clin. Microbiol.* **36:**234–238.

46. **Wade, N. A., G. S. Birkhead, and B. L. Warren.** 1998. Abbreviated regimens of zidovudine prophylaxis and prenatal transmission of the human immunodeficiency virus. *N. Engl. J. Med.* **339:**1409–1414.

47. **Waner, J. L., S. J. Todd, J. Shalaby, P. Murphy, and L. V. Wall.** 1991. Comparison of Directigen FLU-A with viral isolation and direct immunofluorescence for the rapid detection and identification of influenza A virus. *J. Clin. Microbiol.* **29:**470–482.

48. **Wu, B., J. B. Mahony, G. Simon, and M. A. Chernesky.** 1990. Sensitive solid-phase immune electron microscopy double-antibody technique with gold-immunoglobulin G complexes for detecting rotavirus in cell culture and feces. *J. Clin. Microbiol.* **28:**864–868.

49. **Wu, B., J. B. Mahony, and M. A. Chernesky.** 1990. A new immune complex dot assay for detection of rotavirus antigen in feces. *J. Virol. Methods* **29:**157–166.

50. **Yalow, R. S.** 1986. Radioactivity in the service of humanity. *Ala. J. Med. Sci.* **23:**447–453.

51. **Yalow, R. S.** 1991. Remembrance Project: origins of RIA. *Endocrinology* **129:**1694–1695.

52. **Zaaijer, H. L., P. V. Exel-Oehlers, T. Kraaijeveld, E. Altena, and P. N. Lelie.** 1992. Early detection of antibodies to HIV-1 by third-generation assays. *Lancet* **340:**770–772.

Molecular Detection and Identification of Microorganisms*

FREDERICK S. NOLTE AND ANGELA M. CALIENDO

17

Since the publication of the seventh edition of this Manual, significant changes have occurred in the practice of diagnostic molecular microbiology. Nucleic acid amplification techniques are now commonly used to diagnose infectious diseases and manage patients with some infectious diseases. The growth in the number of commercially available test kits has facilitated the use of this technology in the clinical laboratory. Technological advances in real-time PCR techniques, nucleic acid sequencing, and DNA microarrays have invigorated the field and created new opportunities for growth.

Molecular microbiology has emerged as the leading area in molecular pathology in terms of both the numbers of tests performed and clinical relevance. This technology has reduced the dependency of the clinical microbiology laboratory on culture-based methods and created new opportunities for the clinical laboratory to affect patient care. This chapter covers amplified and nonamplified probe techniques, postamplification detection and analysis, clinical applications of these techniques, and the special challenges and opportunities that these techniques provide for the clinical laboratory. Molecular methods used in epidemiological investigations are covered in chapter 12.

NONAMPLIFIED NUCLEIC ACID PROBES

Nucleic acid probes are segments of DNA or RNA labeled with radioisotopes, enzymes, or chemiluminescent reporter molecules that can bind to complementary nucleic acid sequences with high degrees of specificity. Although probes can range from 15 to thousands of nucleotides in size, synthetic oligonucleotides of <50 nucleotides are most commonly incorporated into commercial kits. The probes can be designed to identify microorganisms at any taxonomic level. A number of commercially available DNA probes have been developed for direct detection of pathogens in clinical specimens and identification of pathogens after isolation by culture.

The commonly used formats for probe hybridization include liquid-phase, solid-phase, and in situ hybridization.

The leading method used in clinical microbiology laboratories is a liquid-phase hybridization protection assay (Gen-Probe). In this method a single-stranded DNA probe labeled with an acridinium ester is incubated with the target nucleic acid. Alkaline hydrolysis follows the hybridization step and probe binding is measured in a luminometer after addition of peroxides. For a positive sample, the acridinium ester on the bound probe is protected from hydrolysis and upon addition of peroxides emits light. The hybridization protection assay can be completed in several hours and does not require removal of unbound single-stranded probe or isolation of probe-bound double-stranded sequences (3).

In solid-phase hybridization, target nucleic acids are bound to nylon or nitrocellulose and are hybridized with a probe in solution (112). The unbound probe is washed away and the bound probe is detected by means of fluorescence, luminescence, radioactivity, or color development. Although solid-phase hybridization is a powerful research tool, the length of time required and the complexity of the procedure limit its application in clinical practice.

In situ hybridization is another type of solid-phase hybridization in which the nucleic acid is contained in tissues or cells which are affixed to microscope slides and is governed by the same basic principles described previously (36). In most clinical applications, formalin-fixed, paraffin-embedded tissue sections are used. The sensitivity of in situ hybridization is often limited by the accessibility of the target nucleic acid in the cells.

In general, the application of nonamplified probe techniques to direct detection of pathogens in clinical specimens is limited to those situations in which the number of organisms is large due to the poor analytical sensitivities of these techniques. These include group A streptococcal pharyngitis and genital tract infections with *Neisseria gonorrhoeae* and *Chlamydia trachomatis*. These techniques are used most effectively in culture confirmation assays for mycobacteria and systemic dimorphic fungi. These culture confirmation tests have a positive effect on patient management by providing rapid and accurate diagnoses for these slowly growing, often difficult to identify pathogens.

Nucleic acid probes for direct detection of group A streptococci, *C. trachomatis*, and *N. gonorrhoeae* are available from Gen-Probe. Probes for identification of *Blastomyces dermatitidis*, *Coccidioides immitis*, *Histoplasma capsulatum*, *Campylobacter* spp., enterococci, group A streptococci,

---

* This chapter contains information presented in chapter 13 by Yi-Wei Tang and David H. Persing in the seventh edition of this Manual.

TABLE 1 Nucleic acid amplification methods

Method	Category	Manufacturer (trademark name)	Amplification system	Temp requirement	Nucleic acid target	Reference
bDNA	Signal	Bayer Diagnostics, Emeryville, Calif. (Versant)	Branched DNA probes	Isothermal	DNA, RNA	117
Hybrid capture	Signal	Digene, Gaithersburg, Md. (Hybrid Capture)	Anti-DNA-RNA hybrid antibody	Isothermal	DNA, RNA	66
PCR	Target	Roche Diagnostics, Indianapolis, Ind. (AMPLICOR)	DNA polymerase	Thermal cycle	DNA, RNA	101
NASBA	Target	bioMérieux, Durham, N.C. (NucliSens)	RT, RNA polymerase, RNase H	Isothermal	RNA (DNA)	20
TMA	Target	Gen-Probe, San Diego, Calif. (APTIMA)	RT and RNase H, RNA polymerase	Isothermal	RNA (DNA)	54
SDA	Target	Becton-Dickinson, Sparks, Md. (ProbeTec)	Restriction endonuclease, DNA polymerase	Isothermal	DNA, RNA	120
LCR	Probe	Abbott, Chicago, Ill. (LCx)	DNA ligase	Thermal cycle	DNA, RNA	123
Cleavase-invader	Probe	Third Wave, Madison, Wis.	FEN-1 DNA polymerase (cleavase)	Isothermal	DNA, RNA	96
Cycling Probe	Probe	ID Biomedical Corp, Bothell, Wash.	Chimeric Probe, RNase H	Isothermal	DNA	29

group B streptococci, *Haemophilus influenzae*, *Listeria monocytogenes*, mycobacteria, *N. gonorrhoeae*, *Staphylococcus aureus*, and *Streptococcus pneumoniae* isolated in culture are also available from Gen-Probe.

AMPLIFIED NUCLEIC ACID TECHNIQUES

The development of the PCR by Mullis and colleagues (101) was a milestone in biotechnology and heralded the beginning of molecular diagnostics. Although PCR is the best-developed and most widely used nucleic acid amplification strategy, other strategies have been developed, and several have clinical utility. These strategies are based on signal, target, or probe amplification. Examples of each category will be discussed in the sections that follow. These techniques have sensitivity unparalleled in laboratory medicine, have created new opportunities for the clinical laboratory to have an effect on patient care, and have become the new "gold standards" for laboratory diagnosis of several infectious diseases. Table 1 compares the major features of the different nucleic acid amplification methods.

SIGNAL AMPLIFICATION TECHNIQUES

In signal amplification methods the concentration of probe or target does not increase. The increased analytical sensitivity comes from increasing the concentration of labeled molecules attached to the target nucleic acid. Multiple enzymes, multiple probes, multiple layers of probes, and reduction of background noise have all been used to enhance target detection (53). Target amplification systems generally have greater analytical sensitivity than signal amplification methods, but technological developments, particularly in branched DNA (bDNA) assays, have low-

ered the limits of detection to levels that may rival target amplification assays in some applications (51).

Signal amplification assays have several advantages over target amplification assays. In signal amplification systems, the number of target molecules is not altered, and as a result, the signal is directly proportional to the amount of target sequence present in the clinical specimen. This reduces concerns about false-positive results due to cross-contamination and simplifies the development of quantitative assays. Since signal amplification systems are not dependent on enzymatic processes to amplify target sequence, they are not affected by the presence of enzyme inhibitors in clinical specimens. Consequently, less cumbersome nucleic acid extraction methods may be used. Typically, signal amplification systems use either larger probes or more probes than target amplification systems and, consequently, are less susceptible to errors resulting from target sequence heterogeneity. Finally, RNA levels can be measured directly without the synthesis of a cDNA intermediate.

bDNA Assays

The bDNA signal amplification system is a solid-phase, sandwich hybridization assay incorporating multiple sets of synthetic oligonucleotide probes (77). The key to this technology is the amplifier molecule, a bDNA molecule with 15 identical branches, each of which can bind to three labeled probes.

The bDNA signal amplification system is illustrated in Fig. 1. Multiple target-specific probes are used to capture the target nucleic acid onto the surface of a microtiter well. A second set of target-specific probes also binds to the target. Preamplifier molecules bind to the second set of target probes and up to eight bDNA amplifiers. Three alkaline phosphatase-labeled probes hybridize to each

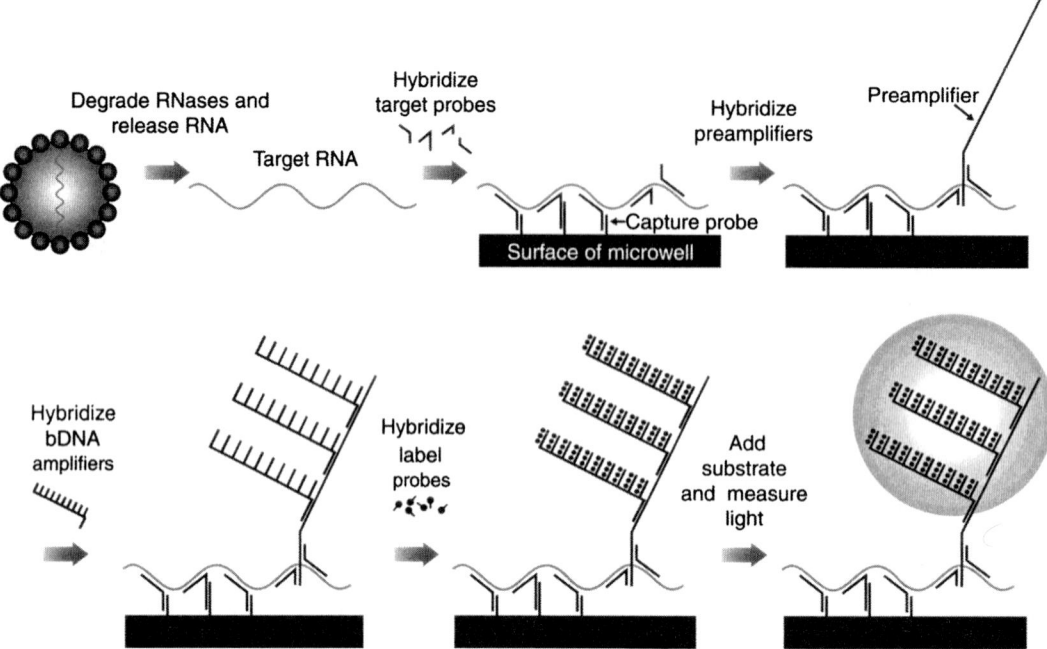

FIGURE 1 bDNA signal amplification.

branch of the amplifier. Detection of bound labeled probes is achieved by incubating the complex with dioxetane, an enzyme-triggerable substrate, and measuring the light emission in a luminometer. The resulting signal is directly proportional to the quantity of target in the sample. The quantity of target in the sample is determined from an external standard curve.

Nonspecific hybridization of any of the amplification probes and nontarget nucleic acids leads to amplification of the background signal. In order to reduce potential hybridization to nontarget nucleic acids, isocytidine (isoC) and isoguanosine (isoG) were incorporated into the preamplifier and labeled probes used in the third-generation bDNA assays (19). IsoC and isoG form base pairs with each other but not with any of the four naturally occurring bases (86). The use of isoC- and isoG-containing probes in bDNA assays increases target-specific signal amplification without a concomitant increase in the background signal, thereby greatly enhancing the detection limits. The detection limit of the third-generation bDNA assay for human immunodeficiency virus (HIV) type 1 (HIV-1) RNA is 50 copies/ml. bDNA assays for the quantitation of hepatitis B virus (HBV) DNA, hepatitis C virus (HCV) RNA, and HIV-1 RNA are commercially available (Bayer). The System 340 platform for bDNA assays automates the incubation, washing, reading, and data-processing steps.

Hybrid Capture Assays

The hybrid capture system is a solution hybridization, antibody capture assay that uses chemiluminescence detection of the hybrid molecules. The target DNA in the specimen is denatured and then hybridized with a specific RNA probe. The DNA-RNA hybrids are captured by antihybrid antibodies that are coated onto the surface of a tube. Alkaline phosphatase-conjugated antihybrid antibodies bind to the immobilized hybrids. The bound antibody conjugate is detected with a chemiluminescent substrate, and

the light emitted is measured in a luminometer. Multiple alkaline phosphatase conjugates bind to each hybrid molecule amplifying the signal. The intensity of the emitted light is proportional to the amount of target DNA in the specimen. Hybrid capture assays for detection of HBV, human papillomavirus (HPV) (21), and cytomegalovirus (CMV) (66) in clinical specimens are commercially available (Digene).

TARGET AMPLIFICATION TECHNIQUES

All of the target amplification systems share certain fundamental characteristics. They use enzyme-mediated processes, in which a single enzyme or multiple enzymes synthesize copies of target nucleic acid. By all of these techniques the amplification products are detected by two oligonucleotide primers that bind to complementary sequences on opposite strands of double-stranded targets. All techniques result in the production of millions to billions of copies of the targeted sequence in a matter of hours, and in each case, the amplification products can serve as templates for subsequent rounds of amplification. Because of this, all of the techniques are sensitive to contamination with product molecules that can lead to false-positive reactions. The potential for cross-contamination is real and should be adequately addressed before any of these techniques are used in the clinical laboratory. However, false-positive reactions can be reduced through special laboratory design, practices, and work flow.

PCR

PCR is a simple, in vitro, chemical reaction that permits the synthesis of essentially limitless quantities of a targeted nucleic acid sequence. This is accomplished through the action of a DNA polymerase that, under the proper conditions, can copy a DNA strand. At its simplest, a PCR consists of target DNA, a molar excess of two oligonucleotide primers, a heat-stable DNA polymerase, an equimolar mixture of deoxyribonucleotide triphosphates (dNTPs; dATP, dCTP, dGTP, and dTTP), $MgCl_2$, KCl, and a Tris-HCl buffer. The two primers flank the double-stranded DNA sequence to be amplified, typically <100 to several hundred bases, and are complementary to opposite strands of the target.

To initiate a PCR, the reaction mixture is heated to separate the two strands of target DNA and is then cooled to permit the primers to anneal to the target DNA in a sequence-specific manner. The DNA polymerase then initiates extension of the primers at their 3′ ends toward one another. The primer extension products are dissociated from the target DNA by heating. Each extension product, as well as the original target, can serve as a template for subsequent rounds of primer annealing and extension.

At the end of each cycle, the PCR products are theoretically doubled. Thus, after n PCR cycles the target sequence can be amplified 2^n-fold. The whole procedure is carried out in a programmable thermal cycler that precisely controls the temperature at which the steps occur, the length of time that the reaction mixture is held at the different temperatures, and the number of cycles. Ideally, after 20 cycles of PCR a 10^6-fold amplification is achieved and after 30 cycles a 10^9-fold amplification occurs. In practice, the amplification may not be completely efficient due to failure to optimize the reaction conditions or the presence of inhibitors of the DNA polymerase. In such cases, the total amplification is best described by the expression $(1 + e)^n$, where e is the amplification efficiency ($0 \leq e \leq 1$) and n is the total number of cycles.

RT-PCR

As it was originally described, PCR was a technique for DNA amplification. Reverse transcriptase (RT) PCR (RT-PCR) was developed to amplify RNA targets. In this process cDNA is first produced from RNA targets by reverse transcription, and then the cDNA is amplified by PCR. As it was originally described, RT-PCR used two enzymes, a heat-labile RT such as avian myeloblastosis virus (AMV) RT and a thermostable DNA polymerase. Because of the temperature requirements of the heat-labile enzyme, cDNA synthesis had to occur at lower temperatures. This presented problems in terms of both nonspecific primer annealing and inefficient primer extension due to the formation of RNA secondary structures. These problems have largely been overcome by the development of a thermostable DNA polymerase derived from *Thermus thermophilus* that under the proper conditions can function efficiently as both an RT and a DNA polymerase (73). RT-PCRs with this enzyme are more specific and efficient than previous protocols with conventional, heat-labile RT enzymes. Commercially available kits (Roche) that use this single-enzyme technology are available for detection of HCV RNA and for quantitation of HIV-1 and HCV RNA in clinical specimens.

Nested PCR

Nested PCR was developed to increase both the sensitivity and the specificity of PCR (37). It uses two pairs of amplification primers and two rounds of PCR. Typically, one primer pair is used in the first round of PCR for 15 to 30 cycles. The products of the first round of amplification are then subjected to a second round of amplification with the second set of primers that anneal to a sequence internal to the sequence amplified by the first primer set. The increased

sensitivity arises from the high total cycle number, and the increased specificity arises from the annealing of the second primer set to sequences found only in the first-round products, thus verifying the identity of the first-round product. The major disadvantage of nested PCR is the high rates of contamination that can occur during the transfer of first-round products to the second tube for the second round of amplification. This can be avoided either by physically separating the first- and second-round amplification mixtures with a layer of wax or oil or by designing single-tube amplification protocols. In practice, the enhanced sensitivity afforded by nested PCR protocols is rarely required in diagnostic applications, and the identity of an amplification product is usually confirmed by hybridization with a nucleic acid probe.

Multiplex PCR

In multiplex PCR, two or more primer sets designed for amplification of different targets are included in the same reaction mixture (11). By this technique more than one target sequence in a clinical specimen can be coamplified in a single tube. The primers used in multiplexed reactions must be carefully selected so that they have similar annealing temperatures and lack complementarity. Multiplex PCRs have proved to be more complicated to develop and are usually less sensitive than PCRs with single primer sets.

Quantitative PCR and RT-PCR

A linear relationship exists between the quantity of input template and the amount of amplification product. However, since the final amount of PCR product depends on exponential amplification of the initial quantity of template, minor differences in amplification efficiency may lead to very large and unpredictable differences in the final product yield (17). The sample-to-sample differences may depend on the sample preparation procedure, nucleic acid purification procedures, the presence of inhibitors, and thermal cycler performance. For these reasons, simple quantitation of the amplified product and the use of external standard reference curves do not provide reliable means of quantitation of the template initially present in the sample.

A variety of PCR-based strategies have been developed to accurately quantitate DNA and RNA targets in clinical specimens. It is generally accepted that a competitive PCR (cPCR) approach is the most reliable and robust. The basic concept behind cPCR is the coamplification in the same reaction tube of two different templates of equal or similar lengths and with the same primer binding sequences. Since both templates are amplified with the same primer pair, identical thermodynamics and amplification efficiencies are ensured. The amount of one of the templates must be known, and after amplification, the products from both templates must be distinguishable from each other. Different types of competitors have been used in cPCR, but in general, those competitors similar in size and base composition to the target work most effectively. RNA competitors should be used in quantitative RT-PCRs to address the problem of variable RT efficiency.

The yield of PCR product is described by the equation $Y = I(1 + e)^n$, where Y is the quantity of PCR product, I is the quantity of template at the beginning of the reaction, e is the efficiency of the reaction, and n is the number of cycles. In cPCR this equation is written for both templates as follows: for the competitor, $Y_c = I_c(1 + e)^n$; for the target, $Y_t = I_t(1 + e)^n$. Since e and n are the same for both the competitor and the target, the relative product ratio

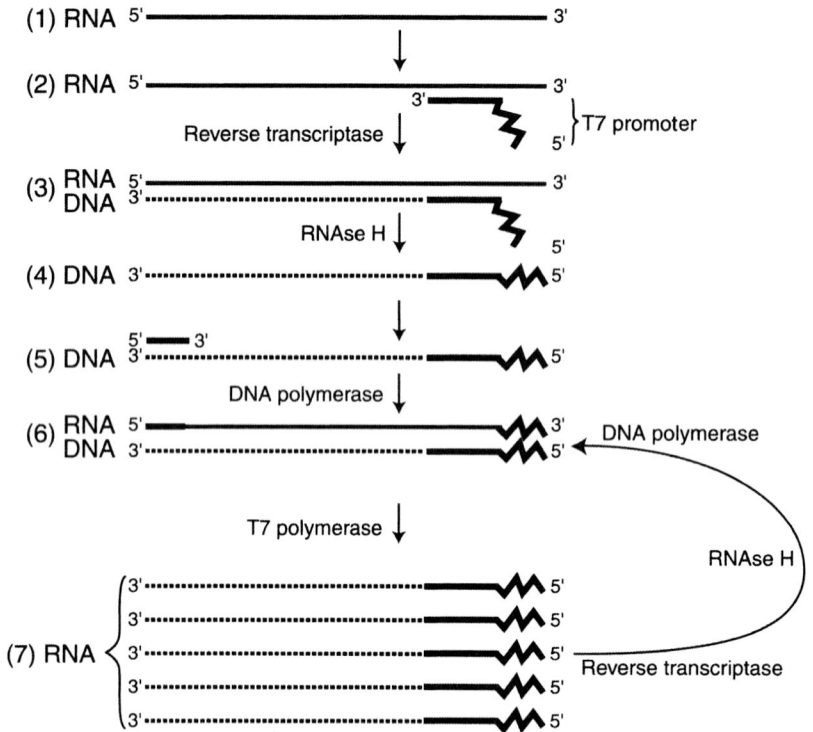

FIGURE 2 Transcription-based amplification.

Y_c/Y_t directly depends on their initial concentration ratio, I_c/I_t, and the function $Y_c/Y_t = I_c/I_t$ is linear.

A single concentration of competitor is sufficient, in theory, to quantitate an unknown amount of target without the use of a standard curve. However, because analysis of two template species present in a sample in widely different amounts may be difficult and imprecise in practice, cPCRs with several concentrations of the competitor within the expected concentration range of the target were generally performed. However, this approach provided no more accurate results than the use of a single concentration of competitor in a study of different approaches to standardization of cPCR (35). The commercially available quantitative PCR and RT-PCR assays for CMV, HIV-1, and HCV (Roche) all use a single concentration of a competitor to determine the initial concentration of the target. The NCCLS (75) has published guidelines for quantitative molecular methods for the detection of infectious diseases that address the development and application of quantitative PCR and other nucleic acid amplification methods.

Transcription Amplification Methods

Nucleic acid sequence-based amplification (NASBA) and transcription-mediated amplification (TMA) are both isothermal RNA amplification methods modeled after retroviral replication (20, 34, 54). The methods are similar in that the RNA target is reversed transcribed into cDNA and then RNA copies are synthesized with an RNA polymerase. NASBA uses AMV RT, RNase H, and T7 bacteriophage RNA polymerase, whereas TMA uses an RT enzyme with endogenous RNase H activity and T7 RNA polymerase.

Amplification involves the synthesis of cDNA from the RNA target with a primer containing the T7 RNA polymerase promoter sequence (Fig. 2). The RNase H then degrades the initial strand of target RNA in the RNA-cDNA hybrid. The second primer then binds to the cDNA and is extended by the DNA polymerase activity of the RT, resulting in the formation of double-stranded DNA containing the T7 RNA polymerase promoter. The RNA polymerase then generates multiple copies of single-stranded, antisense RNA. These RNA product molecules reenter the cycle with subsequent formation of more double-stranded cDNAs that can serve as templates for more RNA synthesis. A 10^9-fold amplification of the target RNA can be achieved in less than 2 h by this method.

The single-stranded RNA products of TMA in the Gen-Probe tests are detected by modification of the hybridization protection assay. Oligonucleotide probes are labeled with modified acridinium esters with either fast or slow chemiluminescent kinetics so that signals from two hybridization reactions can be analyzed simultaneously in the same tube. The NASBA products in the bioMérieux tests are detected by hybridization with probes labeled with tris(2,2' bispyridine)ruthenium and electrochemiluminescence. NASBA has also been used with molecular beacons to create a homogeneous, kinetic amplification system similar to real-time PCR (58).

Transcription-based amplification systems have several strengths, including no requirement for a thermal cycler, rapid kinetics, and a single-stranded RNA product that does not require denaturation prior to detection. Also, single-tube clinical assays and a labile RNA product may help minimize contamination risks. Limitations include the poor performance with DNA targets and concerns about the stability of complex, multienzyme systems. Gen-Probe has developed TMA-based assays for detection of *Mycobacterium tuberculosis*, *C. trachomatis*, *N. gonorrhoeae*, HCV, and HIV-1. NASBA-based kits (bioMérieux) for the de-

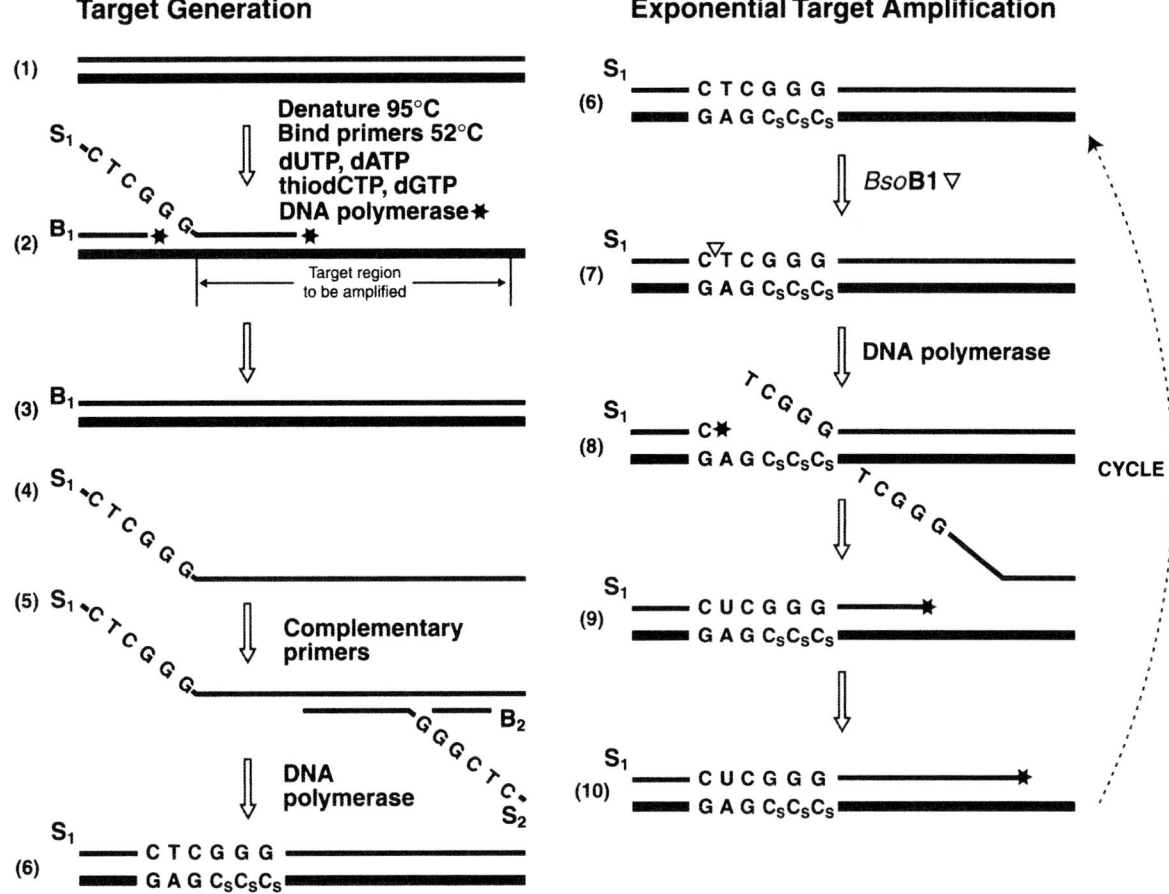

FIGURE 3 SDA. This process is shown for only one strand of a double-stranded DNA target, but amplification occurs on both strands simultaneously.

tection and quantitation of HIV-1 RNA and CMV RNA transcripts are commercially available. A basic NASBA kit is also available for the development of other applications defined by the user.

The commercially available NASBA kit for HIV-1 RNA quantitation uses three synthetic RNA molecules of known low, medium, and high concentrations. These RNA molecules are added to the lysis buffer containing the released nucleic acid and serve as internal calibrators for the assay. Each calibrator has a unique internal sequence that allows discrimination of the calibrator and the target amplicons. Each sample has its own three-point calibration curve, which increases the accuracy and precision of the assay, since small changes in amplification efficiency are internally corrected and do not result in large variations in the results.

Strand Displacement Amplification

Strand displacement amplification (SDA) is an isothermal template amplification technique that can be used to detect trace amounts of DNA or RNA of a particular sequence. SDA as it was first described was a conceptually straightforward amplification process with some technical limitations (119, 120). Since its initial description, however, it has evolved into a highly versatile tool that is technically simple to perform but conceptually complex. Clinical applications of SDA developed by Becton Dickinson include

assays for detection of *M. tuberculosis, C. trachomatis,* and *N. gonorrhoeae* and quantitation of HIV-1 RNA. The Becton Dickinson ProbeTec ET system is based on the simultaneous amplification of nucleic acids by SDA and real-time detection by using fluorescence resonance energy transfer (FRET) (60).

SDA occurs in two discrete phases, target generation and exponential target amplification, as illustrated in Fig. 3. For simplicity, the process is shown for only one strand of a double-stranded DNA target, but the process occurs on both strands simultaneously and yields exponential amplification. In the target generation phase, a double-stranded DNA target (step 1 in Fig. 3) is denatured and allowed to hybridize to two primers, primers B_1 and S_1 (step 2). B_1 is a bumper primer, and S_1 is a primer that contains the single-stranded restriction enzyme sequence for *Bso*B1 located at the 5′ end of the target binding sequence. In the presence of *Bso*B1, an exonuclease-free DNA polymerase, and a dNTP mixture consisting of dUTP, dATP, dGTP, and thioated dCTP (C_s), simultaneous extension products of B_1 (step 3) and S_1 (step 4) are generated. This process displaces the S_1 products, which are available for hybridization with the opposite-strand primers, primers B_2 and S_2 (step 5).

The simultaneous extension of primers B_2 and S_2 produces strands complementary to the S_1 products with C_s incorporated into the *Bso*B1 cleavage site (step 6). This product enters the exponential target amplification phase of the reaction. The BsoB1 enzyme recognizes the double-stranded site, but because one strand contains C_s, it is nicked rather than cleaved by the enzyme (step 7). The DNA polymerase next binds to the nick and begins synthesis of a new strand while simultaneously displacing the downstream strand (steps 8 to 10). This step re-creates the double-stranded species shown in step 7, and the iterative nicking and displacement process repeats. The displaced strands are capable of binding to opposite-strand primers, which produces an exponential amplification at 52.5°C.

These single-stranded products also bind to detector probes for real-time detection. The detection probes are single-stranded DNA molecules containing fluorescein and rhodamine labels. The region between the two labels forms a stem-loop structure. The loop contains the recognition sequence for the BsoB1 enzyme. The target-specific sequence of the probe is located 3' to the rhodamine label. Before specific target amplification the proximal location of rhodamine and fluorescein quenches the fluorescence of fluorescein. The first step in the conversion of the detector probe involves hybridization of an amplification primer and detector probe to a displaced target sequence. The simultaneous extension of the amplification primer and the probe leads to displacement of an extended probe. Next, the extended probe binds to the opposite-strand primer and is extended. This extension step linearizes the stem-loop structure and creates a BsoB1 site that lacks C_s. BsoB1 cleaves rather than nicks because there is no C_s at the recognition site. The cleavage results in physical separation of the quencher and fluorophore such that emission from the excited fluorescein label can be detected. This detection process differs from the 5' nuclease chemistry in several ways, including the use of restriction endonuclease digestion rather than the exonuclease activity of a DNA polymerase to separate the fluorophore and quencher and the lack of a need for thermocycling.

SDA has a reported sensitivity high enough to detect as few as 10 to 50 copies of a target molecule (119). By using a primer set designed to amplify a 10-copy repetitive sequence in the M. tuberculosis genome, the assay is sensitive enough to detect 1 to 5 genome copies of the bacterium. Recently, SDA has been adapted to quantitate RNA by adding an RT step (RT-SDA). In this case, a primer hybridizes to the target RNA and an RT synthesizes a cDNA. This cDNA can then serve as a template for primer incorporation and strand displacement. The products of this strand displacement then feed into the amplification scenario described above. RT-SDA has been used for the determination of HIV-1 viral loads (79).

The main advantage of SDA over PCR is that it can be performed at a single temperature after initial target denaturation. This eliminates the need for expensive thermocyclers. Furthermore, samples can be subjected to SDA in a single tube, with amplification times varying from 30 min to 2 h. The main disadvantage of SDA lies in the fact that, unlike PCR, the relatively low temperature at which SDA is carried out can result in nonspecific primer hybridization to sequences found in complex DNA mixtures. Hence, when the abundance of the target is low compared to the amount of background DNA, nonspecific amplification products can swamp the system, decreasing the sensitivity of the technique. However, the use of organic solvents to increase the stringency of primer binding at low temperatures and the recent introduction of more thermostable polymerases capable of strand displacement have alleviated much of this problem.

PROBE AMPLIFICATION TECHNIQUES

Probe amplification methods differ from target amplification methods in that the amplification products contain only a sequence present in the initial probes. Ligase chain reaction (LCR) (123), cycling probe technology (29), and cleavase-invader technology (63) are all examples of probe amplification methods with commercial potential. To date, only LCR has had a significant impact on the clinical microbiology laboratory.

Ligase Chain Reaction

In a standard LCR two oligonucleotide probes hybridize adjacent to one another on each of the denatured target DNA strands such that a "nick" is formed. A thermostable DNA ligase then seals the nick by joining the 3' end of one probe and the 5' end of the other. Each ligated product, as well as the original target, can serve as a template in subsequent rounds of denaturation, annealing, and ligation, resulting in an exponential accumulation of ligation products (4, 123).

A modification of this technique called gapped LCR (G-LCR) differs from standard LCR in that a short gap of a few nucleotides is formed after annealing of the probes to the template. The gap is filled by a thermostable DNA polymerase, and the resulting nick is then ligated by the DNA ligase (6). Kits based on G-LCR for detection of C. trachomatis and N. gonorrhoeae are commercially available (Abbott). The amplification products are detected by a microparticle enzyme immunoassay in an LCx analyzer. Each individual probe is labeled with either a capture hapten or a detection hapten. The capture hapten is recognized by an antibody attached to microparticles, and the detection hapten is recognized by an antibody conjugated to alkaline phosphatase. The probes are labeled such that the amplification products have a capture hapten at one end and a detection hapten at the other.

In the LCx analyzer, the amplification product is automatically transferred to an incubation well where microparticles coated with antihapten antibody bind to the amplification product as well as to any unligated probes with the capture hapten. The microparticles are washed to remove unligated probes having only the detection hapten. The bound microparticle complexes are then incubated with anti-detection hapten: alkaline phosphatase conjugate. This antibody conjugate binds only to the amplification product. The bound product is detected by the addition of a substrate, which is dephosphorylated to produce a fluorescent molecule.

The LCx analyzer automatically delivers a chelated metal complex and an oxidizing agent after the amplification product has been detected to chemically inactivate it. This helps to reduce the risk of false-positive reactions due to amplification product cross-contamination.

Cleavase-Invader Technology

Invader assays (Third Wave Technologies) are based on a probe amplification method that relies upon the specific recognition and cleavage of particular DNA structures by cleavase, a member of the FEN-1 family of DNA polymerases. These polymerases will cleave the 5' single-stranded flap of a branched base-paired duplex. This enzymatic activity likely plays an essential role in the

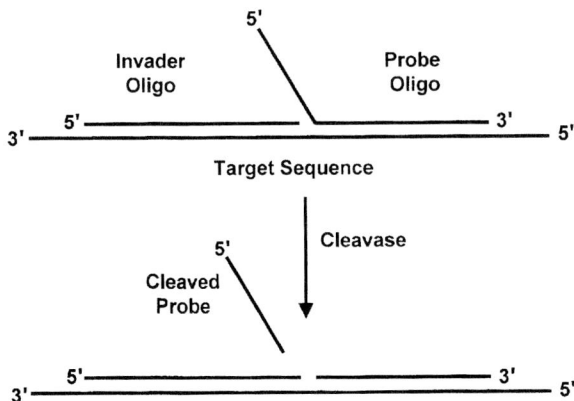

FIGURE 4 Cleavase-invader probe amplification. Oligo, oligonucleotide.

elimination of the complex nucleic acid structures that arise during DNA replication and repair. Since these structures may occur anywhere in a replicating genome, the enzyme recognizes the molecular structure of the substrate without regard to the sequence of the nucleic acids making up the DNA complex (59).

In the invader assays, two primers are designed which hybridize to the target sequence in an overlapping fashion (Fig. 4). Under the proper annealing conditions, the probe oligonucleotide binds to the target sequence. The invader oligonucleotide is designed such that it hybridizes upstream of the probe with a region of overlap between the 3' end of the invader and the 5' end of the probe. Cleavase cleaves the 5' end of the probe and releases it. It is in this way that the target sequence acts as a scaffold upon which the proper DNA structure can form. Since the DNA structure necessary to serve as a cleavase substrate will occur only in the presence of the target sequence, the generation of cleavage products indicates the presence of the target. Use of a thermostable cleavase enzyme allows reactions to be run at temperatures high enough for a primer exchange equilibrium to exist. This allows multiple cleavase products to form off of a single target molecule.

Various methods can be used to detect the cleavage products. Third Wave Technologies uses FRET probes and a second invasive cleavage reaction to detect the target-specific products. Invader technology can be used for genotyping, detection of mutations, and viral load testing.

The invader assay has several inherent advantages. Because the overlap in the invader probe need be only 1 bp, this technology can easily be adapted to detect point mutations of interest by designing the overlap region to encompass the mutation to be detected. The detection of these point mutations would not require postreaction restriction digestion, since the primers would be differentially cleaved on the basis of the presence or the absence of the mutation in question. This feature could be exploited to track mutations in pathogens associated with drug resistance or virulence. In addition, unlike amplification techniques such as PCR, SDA, or TMA, in which the target sequence itself is amplified, the invader assay does not increase the amount of target sequence. As a consequence, invader assays are less prone to problems of false-positive results due to amplicon cross-contamination.

In addition to the invader assay, cleavase can also be used to generate cleavase fragment length polymorphisms

(CFLPs), analogous to restriction fragment length polymorphisms (RFLPs). Heating and rapid cooling of the DNA forms highly reproducible hairpin loop secondary structures which can serve as substrates for cleavase. Since the secondary structures are determined by the nucleotide sequence, sequence polymorphisms are reflected in unique patterns of cleavase products. CFLP analysis has successfully been used to genotype HCV (107). Since hairpin loops occur with a greater diversity than most restriction enzyme recognition sites, CFLP analysis may provide better discrimination among different genotypes than RFLP analysis.

In summary, structure-specific endonucleases can be used to detect nucleic acid targets of a particular sequence, can be used to detect point mutants, and can be applied to generate diverse fragmentation patterns capable of distinguishing complex genotypes. Taken together, these enzymes are powerful tools for nucleic acid analysis.

Cycling Probe Technology

Cycling probe technology (CPT; ID Biomedical Corp., Bothell, Wash.) uses a chimeric DNA-RNA-DNA probe labeled with fluorescein at the 5' end and biotin at the 3' end. The CPT reaction occurs at a constant temperature, which allows the probe to anneal to the target DNA. RNase H cuts the RNA portion of the probe, allowing the cleaved fragments to dissociate from the target DNA, making the target available for further probe cycling. The strip detection system uses a nitrocellulose membrane with streptavidin and anti-mouse immunoglobulin G (IgG) antibody impregnated on the test line and the control line, respectively. In the absence of the target gene, the uncut probe is bound to a mouse antifluorescein antibody-gold conjugate and is then captured by the streptavidin to form a test line. In the presence of the target gene, no test line is formed on the strip. A second line is used as a control for proper sample flow in the strip and develops as a result of the binding of excess antifluorescein antibody to the anti-mouse IgG antibody line.

CPT assays have been developed for detection of the *mecA* gene in isolates of *S. aureus* (29) and for detection of *vanA* and *vanB* genes in isolates of enterococci (71). The *mecA* test (Velogene) is cleared for in vitro diagnostic use by the Food and Drug Administration (FDA).

AUTOMATION

Target and probe amplification assays consist of three major steps: specimen processing, nucleic acid amplification, and product detection. The amplification and detection steps have proved the easiest to automate. Unfortunately, sample processing is usually the most labor-intensive step and represents the biggest challenge for manufacturers of automated test systems. Several stand-alone robotic stations for nucleic acid purification are available for use in clinical laboratories that process large numbers of specimens.

The COBAS system (Roche) automates the amplification and detection steps for PCR. The Abbott LCx system automates the detection of G-LCR products. The System 340 platform for bDNA assays (Bayer) automates the incubation, washing, reading, and data-processing steps. bioMérieux manufactures separate automated sample preparation and detection systems for NASBA assays.

All of the major manufacturers are developing high-throughput, fully automated nucleic acid analyzers. The TIGRIS system (Gen-Probe) is an example of a fully automated and integrated system designed to perform sample processing, nucleic acid amplification, and product detection (67). It was developed to screen the blood supply for HCV and HIV-1 RNA and can process up to 500 nucleic acid detection tests in 8 h.

POSTAMPLIFICATION DETECTION AND ANALYSIS

Gel Analysis

Visualization of amplification products in agarose gels after electrophoresis and ethidium bromide staining was the earliest detection method. After gel electrophoresis DNA is often transferred to a nitrocellulose or nylon membrane and hybridized to a specific probe to increase both the sensitivity and the specificity of detection. Membranes with bound radiolabeled probes are placed in proximity to X-ray film, and the hybrids are visualized as dark bands. Enzyme-labeled probes can be visualized through either light or color production after the addition of the appropriate chemiluminescent or chromogenic substrates. Many of these nonisotopic approaches are at least as sensitive as isotopic methods and are faster. In addition, the enzyme-labeled probes are more stable. Although gel electrophoresis and blotting remain important research tools, these techniques are being replaced by faster and simpler methods in the clinical laboratory.

Single-strand conformation polymorphism (SSCP) analysis and RFLP analysis have been used to ascertain information about the base compositions of the amplification products visualized in a gel. In SSCP analysis the PCR product is denatured and then subject to electrophoresis in a nondenaturing gel (81). Variations in the physical conformations of the PCR products are related to the base composition and are detected by differential gel migration. This technique has successfully been used to detect mutations causing rifampin resistance in M. tuberculosis (111).

RFLP analysis uses restriction endonucleases to cleave amplification products at specific recognition sites. The fragments are separated by electrophoresis, and the resulting banding pattern provides information about the nucleic acid sequence. When coupled with a hybridization reaction, RFLP analysis can also provide information about the location and number of loci homologous to the probe. Both SSCP analysis and RFLP analysis of short products may soon be replaced by direct DNA sequencing as this technology improves and the costs decrease.

Colorimetric Microtiter Plate Systems

Colorimetric microtiter plate (CMP) systems are convenient alternatives to traditional gel and blotting techniques for detection of amplified products. In these systems amplified product is captured in microtiter plate wells by specific oligonucleotide probes coating the plastic surface. Bound product is detected by a color change that takes place after addition of an enzyme conjugate and the appropriate substrate. These systems resemble enzyme immunoassays and use microtiter plate washers and readers commonly found in clinical laboratories. CMP systems are more practical and faster than the traditional membrane hybridization techniques described above.

Several variations of CMP systems are commercially available. In one popular approach, biotinylated primers are used to amplify the target, and the biotin-containing PCR product is denatured and added to the microtiter well. After hybridization with a capture probe, the bound product is detected with a streptavidin-enzyme conjugate and a chromogenic substrate (61). Enzyme-conjugated antibodies directed against double-stranded DNA have also been used to detect PCR product in CMP systems (65). Another approach uses digoxigenin-dUTP to label the PCR product and enzyme-conjugated antidigoxigenin antibodies to detect the captured product (87).

Real-Time (Homogeneous, Kinetic) PCR

Real-time PCR describes methods by which the target amplification and detection steps occur simultaneously in the same tube (homogeneous). These methods require special thermal cyclers with precision optics that can monitor the fluorescence emission from the sample wells. The computer software supporting the thermal cycler monitors the data throughout the PCR at every cycle and generates an amplification plot for each reaction (kinetic).

In its simplest format, the PCR product is detected as it is produced by using fluorescent dyes that preferentially bind to double-stranded DNA. SYBR Green I is one such dye that has been used in this application (72). In the unbound state, the fluorescence is relatively low, but when the dye is bound to double-stranded DNA the fluorescence is greatly enhanced. The dye will bind to both specific and nonspecific PCR products. The specificity of the detection can be improved through melting curve analysis. The specific amplified product will have a characteristic melting peak at its predicted melting temperature (T_m), whereas the primer dimers and other nonspecific products should have different T_ms or give broader peaks (95).

The specificity of real-time PCR can also be increased by including hybridization probes in the reaction mixture. These probes are labeled with fluorescent dyes or with combinations of fluorescent and quencher dyes. In the 5' nuclease PCR assay (Taqman), the 5'-to-3' exonuclease activity of Taq DNA polymerase is used to cleave a nonextendable hybridization probe during the primer extension phase of PCR (45). This approach uses dual-labeled fluorogenic hybridization probes and is illustrated in Fig. 5. One fluorescent dye serves as a reporter, and its emission spectrum is quenched by the second fluorescent dye. The nuclease degradation of the hybridization probe releases the reporter dye, resulting in an increase in its peak fluorescent emission. The increase in fluorescent emission indicates that specific PCR product has been made, and the intensity of fluorescence is related to the amount of product (38).

FRET is the basis of another approach to real-time PCR (56). This method requires two specially designed sequence-specific oligonucleotide probes. These hybridization probes are designed to hybridize next to each other on the product molecule. The 3' end of one probe is labeled with a donor dye, and the 5' end of the other probe is labeled with an acceptor dye. The donor dye is excited by an external light source and instead of emitting light transfers its energy to the acceptor dye by a process called FRET. The excited acceptor dye emits light at a longer wavelength than the unbound donor dye, and the intensity of the acceptor dye light emission is proportional to the amount of PCR product.

Real-time detection and quantitation of PCR product can also be accomplished with molecular beacons (116). Molecular beacons are hairpin-shaped oligonucleotide probes with an internally quenched fluorophore whose fluorescence is restored when they bind to a target nucleic acid (Fig. 6). They are designed in such a way that the loop portion of the probe molecule is complementary to the

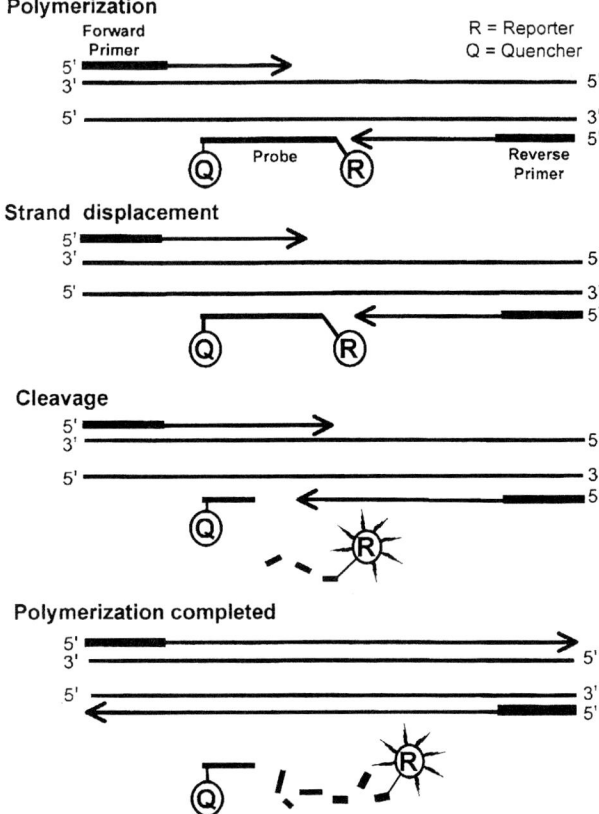

Polymerization

Strand displacement

Cleavage

Polymerization completed

FIGURE 5 Detection of specific PCR product by using the 5' to 3' exonuclease activity of DNA polymerase. The polymerase displaces and then cleaves the dual-labeled hybridization probe during the primer extension phase of PCR. The degradation of the probe separates the fluorescent reporter from the quencher molecule, resulting in an increase in the peak fluorescence of the reporter.

target sequence. The stem is formed by the annealing of complementary arm sequences on the ends of the probe. A fluorescent dye is attached to one end of one arm, and a quenching molecule is attached to the end of the other arm. The stem keeps the fluorophore and quencher in close proximity such that no light emission occurs. When the probe encounters a target molecule, it forms a hybrid that is longer and more stable than the stem and undergoes a conformational change that forces the stem apart, causing the fluorophore and the quencher to move away from each other, restoring the fluorescence.

Figure 7 shows a representative amplification plot and defines the terms used in real-time PCR quantitation. The amplification plot shows the normalized fluorescence signal from the reporter (R_n) at each cycle number. In the initial cycles of PCR there is little change in the fluorescent signal. This defines the baseline for the plot. An increase above the baseline indicates the detection of accumulated PCR product. A fixed fluorescence threshold can be set above the baseline. The cycle threshold (C_T) is defined as the cycle number at which the fluorescence passes the fixed threshold. A plot of the log of the initial target concentration versus C_T for a set of standards is a straight line (41). The amount of target in an unknown sample is determined

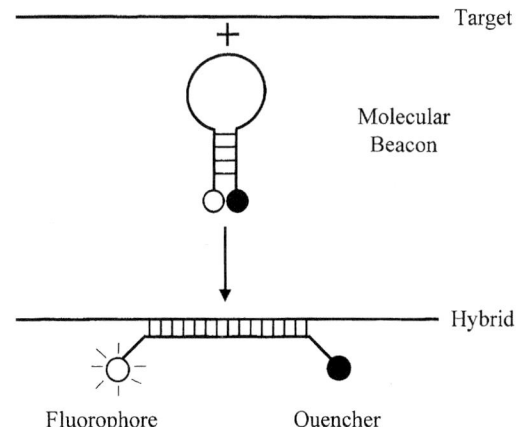

FIGURE 6 Principle of operation of molecular beacon probes.

by measuring the sample C_T and using a standard curve to determine the starting copy number.

Real-time PCR methods decrease the time required to perform nucleic acid assays because there are no post-PCR processing steps. Also, since amplification and detection occur in the same closed tube, these methods eliminate the postamplification manipulations that can lead to laboratory contamination with the amplicon. In addition, real-time PCR methods lend themselves well to quantitative applications because analysis is performed early in the log phase of product accumulation and, as a result, are less prone to error resulting from differences in sample-to-sample amplification efficiency.

Allele-Specific Hybridization

Line probe assays (LiPAs) are manufactured by Innogenetics (Ghent, Belgium) for the genotyping of HCV and HBV, identification of mycobacteria, and analysis for drug resistance mutations in HIV-1, HBV, *M. tuberculosis*, and *Helicobacter pylori* (97, 108, 109). The HCV LiPA is marketed by Bayer Diagnostics. In these assays a series of probes with poly(T) tails are attached to nitrocellulose strips. Biotin-labeled PCR product is then hybridized to the immobilized probes on the strip. The labeled PCR product hybridizes only to the probes that give a perfect sequence match under the stringent hybridization conditions used. After hybrid-

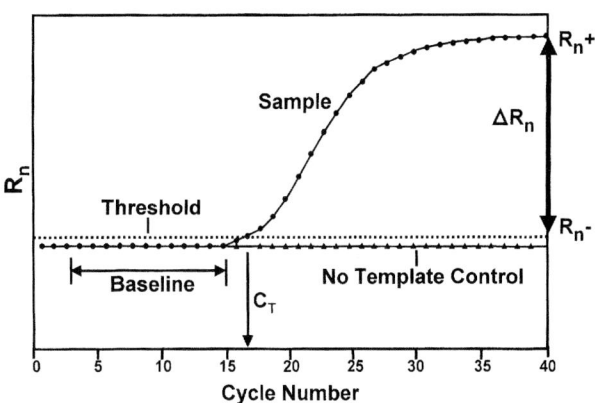

FIGURE 7 Real-time PCR amplification plot showing commonly used terms and abbreviations.

ization, streptavidin labeled with alkaline phosphatase is added and binds to the biotinylated hybrids. Incubation with a chromogen results in a purple precipitate. The pattern of hybridization provides information about the nucleic acid sequence of the amplicon. This method is capable of detecting single nucleotide polymorphisms.

Direct Sequencing

The combination of PCR and dideoxynucleotide chain termination methods can be used to determine DNA sequences in clinical samples (48). The use of fluorescent dye terminator chemistry and laser scanning in a polyacrylamide gel electrophoresis (PAGE) format has been the standard in electrophoretic separation technology. However, the recent application of capillary electrophoresis techniques to the separation of PCR and dideoxy chain termination products has streamlined the sequencing process by eliminating some of the labor-intensive steps (28).

CLIP sequencing (Visible Genetics, Suwanee, Ga.) uses oligonucleotide primers labeled with different fluorescent dyes, standard dideoxynucleotide termination reagents, and PCR to produce extension products that end with a chain-terminating nucleotide. The nucleic acid sequence is deduced from the electrophoretic mobilities of the different extension products from a set of four reactions, each containing a different chain-terminating nucleotide. A unique feature of CLIP sequencing is that one reaction produces sequence information for both nucleic acid strands. CLIP sequencing serves as the basis for commercially available assays for HIV-1 drug resistance and HCV genotyping.

The Viroseq HIV-1 genotyping assays (Applied Biosystems, Foster City, Calif.) also uses dideoxy chain-terminating sequencing, but each dideoxynucleotide is labeled with a different fluorescent dye. Each reaction mixture contains one primer but all four uniquely labeled dideoxynucleotides. Separation of the terminated PCR products can be done by PAGE or capillary electrophoresis.

Although direct sequencing of PCR products by electrophoresis is a powerful research tool, its routine use in the clinical laboratory depends upon the development of high-throughput systems with integrated databases and data analysis software. Such systems are available for HIV-1 and HCV genotyping and for identification of bacteria and fungi by ribosomal DNA sequence analysis.

DNA Microarrays

DNA microarrays are produced by attaching or synthesizing hundreds or thousands of oligonucleotides on a solid support in precise patterns. A labeled amplification product is hybridized to the probes, and hybridization signals are mapped to various positions within the array. If the number of probes is sufficiently large, the sequence of the PCR product can be deduced from the pattern of hybridization. A number of manufacturers are developing DNA microarrays and the instrumentation required to acquire and analyze the data.

One of the most developed approaches brings together advances in synthetic nucleic acid chemistry with photolithography, a process used in the manufacture of semiconductors for the computer industry. This approach uses light to direct the synthesis of short oligonucleotides on a silica wafer (83). On a 15-mm-square chip, thousands of individual sites or features can be established. At each feature specific oligonucleotides are assembled, one nucleotide at a time, by light-activated chemistry.

The DNA chip is incubated in a flow cell with DNA product that has been fragmented and labeled with a fluorophore. After hybridization, a scanning laser confocal microscope evaluates the surface fluorescence intensity of the chip. Automated scanning by the microscope takes only a few minutes to acquire an image of the entire surface of the chip, and computer software analyzes the fluorescent image and determines the nucleic acid sequence of the PCR product. A DNA chip based on this technology for the detection of HIV-1 drug resistance mutations is commercially available (Affymetrix, Santa Clara, Calif.).

Another method of producing DNA microarrays involves the precise micropipetting of premade double-stranded DNA probes (typically 200 to 2,000 bp in length) onto glass slides with a robotic device (103). These microarrays are not suitable for mutation detection due to the size and density of the arrayed DNA probes but have facilitated gene expression profiling. DNA microarrays of this type can be used to determine the activation states (mRNA levels) of thousands of genes simultaneously. Gene expression profiling of pathogens by use of microarrays may provide new insights into pathogenic mechanisms and help identify new therapeutic targets.

The newest developments in DNA chip technology are bioelectronic chips. Nanogen (San Diego, Calif.) has developed a bioelectronic chip with 100 individually addressable electrodes. The silicon chip is manufactured by using the same type of photolithographic and deposition techniques used in the microelectronics industry. The technology uses electrical fields to move biological samples through the chip and direct the samples to the electrodes. Cheng and colleagues (13) used a microelectrode array to separate *Escherichia coli* cells from a whole-blood sample and then to lyse the isolated *E. coli* cells on the chip. The lysate was then transferred to another bioelectronic chip for an electronically enhanced hybridization assay developed previously by this group (106). The development of fully integrated analytical systems that function as a laboratory, the so-called lab on a chip, is the ultimate goal of microchip designers.

A bioelectronic means of detection of nucleic acid sequences is also being developed by Clinical Micro Sensors (Pasadena, Calif.). This technology is based on the electron transfer that occurs when one strand of a nucleic acid hybrid is labeled with an electron donor. The target nucleic acid is captured on the chip surface microelectrode with specific probes attached to a microelectrode through a phenylacetylene "molecular wire." The captured target nucleic acid is hybridized to a signaling probe labeled with an organometallic electron donor, ferrocene. When a voltage is applied to the chip, each ferrocene molecule loses an electron, which is transferred through the molecular wire to the electrode surface. The current generated is proportional to the number of target nucleic acid molecules captured at the electrode surface.

DNA microarrays and bioelectronics hold much promise for molecular diagnostics. However, the current technology has several limitations including the complexity of fabricating the microarrays, limited availability, and high test cost.

CURRENT APPLICATIONS

Molecular methods have created new opportunities for the clinical microbiology laboratory to affect patient care in the areas of initial diagnosis, disease prognosis, and monitoring

TABLE 2 Examples of human pathogens first identified from clinical specimens using molecular approaches[a]

Disease	Pathogen	Reference
Non-A, non-B hepatitis	Hepatitis C virus	15
Bacillary angiomatosis	*Bartonella henselae*	93
Whipple's disease	*Tropheryma whipplei*	94
Disseminated infections in AIDS	*Mycobacterium genavense*	44
Hantavirus pulmonary syndrome	Sin nombre virus	76
Kaposi's sarcoma	Human herpesvirus 8	12

[a] Data from reference 92.

of the response to therapy. However, in most cases the new molecular tests supplement rather than replace the conventional diagnostic tests and add significant expense to the laboratory budget. As a consequence, only those clinical applications that add true value to the overall diagnostic strategy will stand the test of time.

Detection of Slowly Growing and Uncultivable Pathogens

With the development of molecular methods, the clinical microbiology laboratory is no longer solely reliant on the traditional culture methods for detection of pathogens in clinical specimens. Culture-based methods have long been the gold standard for infectious disease diagnosis, but for several diseases nucleic acid-based tests have replaced culture as the gold standard. Hepatitis C, enteroviral meningitis, pertussis, herpes simplex virus (HSV) encephalitis, and genital infections with C. trachomatis are some examples of infectious diseases for which nucleic acid-based tests are the new gold standards for diagnosis. This technology has been used to best advantage in situations in which traditional methods are slow, insensitive, expensive, or not available. These techniques work particularly well with fragile or fastidious microorganisms that may die in transit or that may be overgrown by contaminating flora when cultured. N. gonorrhoeae is an example of an organism whose nucleic acid can be detected under circumstances in which the organism cannot be cultured. The use of improper collection media, inappropriate transport conditions, or delays in transport can reduce the viability of the pathogen but may leave the nucleic acid detectable. It is beyond the scope of this chapter to review all of the possible applications or to provide a compendium of methods for detection of various pathogens. The reader is directed to other excellent resources for this information (84, 85).

Opportunities to actually replace culture for detection of bacterial pathogens in routine practice are limited by the need to isolate the organisms for antibiotic susceptibility testing. In those applications in which culture has actually been replaced by nucleic acid testing, the pathogens are of predictable susceptibility, and consequently, routine susceptibility testing is not performed.

Molecular methods have had the biggest impact in clinical virology, in which the molecular approaches are often faster, more sensitive, and more cost-effective than the traditional approaches. Enteroviral meningitis, HSV encephalitis, and CMV infections in immunocompromised patients are examples of infectious diseases for which nucleic acid-based tests are clinically relevant and cost-effective for diagnosis. The opportunities to replace the conventional methods are greater in virology than in bac-

teriology because the culture-based methods are costly and antiviral susceptibility testing is not routinely performed. In those situations in which antiviral susceptibility testing is required, it is also more amenable to molecular approaches.

Perhaps the greatest impact of molecular methods has been in the discovery of previously unrecognized or uncultivable pathogens. During the past 15 years, a number of infectious agents have been first identified directly from clinical material by molecular methods (Table 2). HCV, the principal etiologic agent of what was once known as non-A, non-B hepatitis, was discovered in 1989 through the application of molecular cloning techniques by investigators from the Centers for Disease Control and the Chiron Corporation (15). Cloning and analysis of the HCV genome led to the production of viral antigens that now serve as the basis of the specific serologic tests used to screen the blood supply and to diagnose hepatitis C. To date, HCV has resisted all attempts at sustained in vitro propagation. As a result, RT-PCR is used to detect, quantitate, and genotype HCV in infected individuals.

Tropheryma whippelii, the causative agent of Whipple's disease, is another example of an uncultivable microorganism which was initially identified by molecular methods (94). It was discovered by the use of broad-range PCR, in which primers are directed against conserved sequences in the bacterial 16S rRNA gene. Sequence analysis of the PCR product and comparison with known 16S rRNA gene sequences were used to characterize the organism and establish its disease association. This approach provides a new paradigm for the discovery of unrecognized pathogens and will be of value for other diseases with features that suggest an infectious etiology (92).

The discoveries of HCV and T. whippelii demonstrate an important new principle in medical microbiology. An etiologic agent can be detected and characterized by molecular methods and its disease association can be established long before its existence can be substantiated by traditional culture and serologic methods.

Identification of Bacteria and Fungi by Nucleic Acid Sequencing

Nucleotide sequence analysis of the bacterial 16S rRNA gene has expanded our knowledge of the phylogenetic relationships among bacteria and is the new standard for bacterial identification. rRNA contains several functionally different regions, with some regions having highly conserved nucleic acid sequences and other regions having highly varied nucleic acid sequences (122). The DNA sequence of the 16S rRNA gene is a stable genotypic signature that can be used to identify an organism at the genus or the species level. The 16S gene sequence can be determined rapidly and provides objective results independent of phenotypic characteristics. As discussed in the preceding section, it can also be used to characterize previously unrecognized species. A similar approach that targets the nuclear large subunit (LSU) of the rRNA gene can be used for the identification of fungi. This gene is universally found in all fungi and contains sufficient variation to identify most fungi accurately to the species level.

The DNA sequencing approach to microbial identification involves extraction of the nucleic acids, amplification of the target sequence by PCR, sequence determination, and a computer software-aided search of an appropriate sequence database. The major limitations to this approach to microbial identification include the high cost of automated nucleic acid sequencers, the lack of appropriate analysis software, and limited databases.

Applied Biosystems has developed ribosomal gene sequencing kits for bacteria and fungi. A sequence from an unknown bacterium is compared with either full or partial 16S rRNA sequences from over 1,000 type strains by using MicroSeq analysis software (110). The software analysis provides percent base pair differences between the unknown bacterium and the 20 most closely related bacteria, alignment tools to show differences between the related sequences, and phylogenetic tree tools to verify that the unknown bacterium actually clusters with the 20 closest bacteria in the database. The MicroSeq fungal identification system is similar to the bacterial identification system but targets the D2 LSU of the rRNA gene. Continued improvements in automation, refinements of analysis software, and decreases in cost should lead to the more widespread use of nucleic acid sequence-based approaches to microbial identification.

Disease Prognosis

Molecular techniques have created opportunities for the laboratory to provide important information that may predict disease progression. Probably the best example is the HIV-1 viral load as a predictor of progression to AIDS and death in HIV-1-infected individuals. This was first demonstrated in 1996 as part of a multicenter AIDS cohort study (69). The investigators showed that the risk of progression to AIDS and death was directly related to the magnitude of the plasma viral load at study entry. The plasma viral load was a better predictor of disease progression than the number of CD4$^+$ lymphocytes. Subsequent studies have confirmed that the baseline viral load critically influences disease progression.

Subtyping of certain viruses by molecular methods may also have prognostic value. Subtyping of respiratory syncytial viruses may provide information about the severity of infection in hospitalized infants, with those infected with group A viruses having poorer outcomes (121). HPV causes dysplasia, intraepithelial neoplasia, and carcinoma of the cervix in women. HPV types 16 and 18 are associated with a high risk of progression to neoplasia, while HPV types 6 and 11 are associated with a low risk of progression (91). A recent study has established the clinical utility of molecular testing for high-risk HPV DNA in the management of women with the cervical cytologic diagnosis of atypical squamous cells of undetermined significance (ASCUS). Women with ASCUS can be triaged to colposcopy on the basis of the detection of high-risk HPV DNA (105).

CMV viral load testing has recently been shown to be useful for decision making regarding when to initiate preemptive therapy in organ transplant recipients and in distinguishing active disease from latent infection. Qualitative PCR assays for CMV DNA have been unable to distinguish patients with latent CMV infection from those with active CMV disease (31, 78). Recently, studies have shown that the level of CMV DNA can predict the development of active CMV disease. With the availability of standardized commercial assays, it is possible to establish the viral load cutoffs that predict the development of CMV disease and that indicate the need for the initiation of preemptive therapy (1, 47). It is likely that quantitative assays will be useful in distinguishing disease from infection with other herpesviruses such as Epstein-Barr virus and human herpesvirus 6.

Response to Therapy

Molecular methods have been developed to detect the genes responsible for resistance to single antibiotics or classes of antibiotics in bacteria and in many cases are superior to the phenotypic, growth-based methods. For example, molecular methods have been used to supplement the growth-based methods for the detection of methicillin resistance in staphylococci, vancomycin resistance in enterococci, and rifampin resistance in M. tuberculosis (113). However, it is difficult to imagine, given our current state of knowledge of the molecular genetics of antimicrobial resistance and the technological limitations of molecular methods, that a genotypic approach to routine antimicrobial susceptibility testing of bacteria could rival the phenotypic methods in terms of information content and cost.

Molecular techniques are playing increasing roles in predicting and monitoring patient responses to antiviral therapy. The laboratory may have a role in predicting the response to therapy by detecting specific drug resistance mutations, determining viral load, and genotyping. Both viral load and genotype are independent predictors of the response to combination therapy with interferon and ribavirin in patients with chronic HCV infections (68). Those patients with high pretreatment viral loads of >2 million copies/ml or with HCV genotype 1 infections have poor sustained response rates. Both of these virological parameters are used in conjunction with other factors to determine the duration of therapy (89).

Quantitative tests for HIV-1 RNA are the standard of practice for guiding clinicians in initiating, monitoring, and changing antiretroviral therapy. Several commercially available HIV-1 viral load assays have been developed, and guidelines for their use in clinical practice have been published (100). Viral load assays have also been used to monitor the response to therapy in patients chronically infected with HBV and HCV (39, 104). In organ transplant recipients, the persistence of CMV after several weeks of antiviral therapy is associated with the development of resistant virus (9).

Drug resistance mutations in HIV-1 RT and protease genes lead to lower levels of sensitivity to antiretroviral agents and are important causes of treatment failure (42). In randomized clinical trials, testing for genotypic resistance was found to have a significant benefit on the virological response because it allowed appropriate therapeutic alternatives to be chosen (23). Prospective randomized trials evaluating the clinical utility of phenotypic resistance testing have shown mixed results (18; D. Melnick, J. Rosenthal, M. Cameron, M. Snyder, S. Griffith-Howard, K. Hertogs, W. Verbiest, N. Graham, and S. Pham, Abstr. 7th Conf. Retrovir. Opportunistic Infect., abstr. 786, 2000). Although more data are needed to document the clinical benefits of assays for the detection of drug resistance mutations, clinical guidelines for their use have been established (43). Testing for resistance is also used to determine an appropriate treatment regimen in patients failing therapy and in pregnant women to optimize treatment and minimize transmission of HIV-1 to the neonate (43).

SPECIAL CONCERNS

The unparalleled analytical sensitivities of nucleic acid amplification techniques coupled with their susceptibilities to cross-contamination present unique challenges to the routine application of these techniques in the clinical laboratory. There are special concerns in the areas of specimen processing, work flow, quality assurance, and interpretation of test results. Additional information can be found in the NCCLS MM3-A document *Molecular Diagnostic Methods for Infectious Diseases: Approved Guideline* (74).

Specimen Collection, Transport, and Processing

Proper collection, transport, and processing of clinical specimens are essential to ensure reliable results from molecular assays. Nucleic acid integrity must be maintained throughout these processes. Important issues to be considered in specimen collection are the timing of specimen collection in relationship to disease state and the proper specimen type. Reliable test results are not possible unless an adequate specimen is obtained. Other factors that come into play include use of the proper anticoagulant, use of the proper transport and storage temperatures, and timely processing of the specimen. For example, the proper conditions for specimen collection, transport, and processing have been well described for HIV-1 viral load testing, and the description of these conditions has provided insight into the importance of these factors. For HIV-1 viral load testing, the plasma needs to be separated from the cells within 6 h of collection to minimize degradation of RNA. Once the plasma has been separated, it can be stored at 4°C for several days, but −70°C is recommended for long-term storage (100). For CMV viral load testing, the viral DNA is stable in whole blood for up to 5 days when it is stored at 4°C (9). This improved stability in whole blood is likely due to the fact that DNA is more stable than RNA. Most types of specimens are best stored at −20 to −70°C prior to processing.

Molecular methods have several advantages over conventional culture with regard to specimen collection. It may be easier to maintain the integrity of nucleic acid than the viability of an organism. Nucleic acid persists in specimens after initiation of treatment (30, 55), thus allowing detection of a pathogen even though the organism can no longer be cultured. Also, due to the increased sensitivity of molecular assays it may be possible to test a smaller volume of specimen or use a specimen that can be obtained by less invasive means.

The major goals of specimen processing are to release nucleic acid from the organism, maintain the integrity of the nucleic acid, render the sample noninfectious, remove inhibiting substances, and, in some instances, concentrate the specimen. These processes need to be balanced with minimization of the manipulation of the specimen. Complex specimen processing methods are time-consuming, may lead to the loss of target nucleic acid, or may result in contamination between specimens. Care must be taken to avoid carryover of inhibitory substances, such as phenol or alcohol, from the nucleic acid isolation step to the amplification reaction mixture.

There are several general methods for nucleic acid extraction. Different methods may be used depending on whether the desire is to purify RNA or DNA, or both. Isolation of RNA can be challenging because RNases can be very difficult to inactivate. RNases are endogenous to the organism from which RNA is to be extracted and can also be introduced through laboratory materials and human hands (24). The use of disposable plastic ware, designated reagents, and work areas only for RNA extraction can be helpful. Another factor to consider when deciding on a nucleic acid extraction method is the type of pathogen sought. Some pathogens, such as viruses, can be very easy to lyse, while mycobacteria, staphylococci, and fungi can be very difficult to lyse. Enzyme digestion or harsh lysis conditions may be required to disrupt the cell walls of these organisms.

DNA isolation methods often use detergents to solubilize the cell wall or membranes, a proteolytic enzyme such as proteinase K to digest proteins, and EDTA to chelate the divalent cations needed for nuclease activity (7, 33). This lysate can be used directly in amplification assays or used after extraction with phenol and chloroform-isoamyl alcohol (24:1) and precipitation of nucleic acids by ethanol. These additional steps remove proteins and traces of organic solvents and concentrate the specimen. In order to successfully use a crude lysate, the target DNA must be present at a relatively high concentration, and the level of inhibitors of amplification present in the sample must be minimal. If these criteria are not met, the additional steps of extraction and precipitation should be used.

Another commonly used method of nucleic acid isolation involves disruption of cells or organisms with the chaotropic agent guanidinium thiocyanate and a detergent (14). After a short incubation the nucleic acid can be precipitated with isopropanol. Guanidinium thiocyanate denatures proteins and is also a strong inhibitor of RNases, making it a very useful method for RNA isolation, although it is also used for purification of DNA. The extraction method of Boom et al. (8) is also based on the lysing and nuclease-inactivating properties of guanidinium thiocyanate, but it uses the acid-binding properties of silica or glass particles to purify the nucleic acid. Clinical specimens are placed in a lysis buffer containing guanidinium thiocyanate, and after a brief incubation silica, which binds to RNA and DNA, is added. After several washing steps to remove proteins and other cellular debris, the nucleic acid is eluted in a low-salt buffer. Over the past several years, various manufacturers have developed commercially available reagents using one of these basic methods or a modification of these methods. These products are easy to use and provide a rapid, reproducible method for purification of nucleic acid from a wide variety of clinical specimens. These reagents tend to be expensive, but the additional cost can be offset by savings in time and the cost of labor.

Tissue samples need to be disrupted prior to the nucleic acid extraction process. This can be accomplished by cutting the tissue specimen into small pieces or mechanically homogenizing the tissue specimen prior to proceeding with one of the extraction methods described above. For preserved tissue specimens, removal of the paraffin with solvents and slicing of the specimen into fine sections are required prior to processing.

Removal of inhibitors of amplification is a key function of the nucleic acid extraction process. Simple methods of nucleic acid extraction that involve boiling of the specimen have been used for relatively acellular specimens such as cerebrospinal fluid (CSF). Although this method is fast and easy, there are problems with inhibitors of amplification that are present in CSF and that are not inactivated by boiling (70). The inhibition rate can be reduced to <1% when a silica-based extraction method is used. Urine specimens are now commonly used for the detection of *C. trachomatis* and *N. gonorrhoeae*. Several of the commercial methods use a crude detergent lysis step to release nucleic acid from cells and organisms. By these methods, between 3 and 7% of urine specimens contain substances that are inhibitory to amplification. Common inhibitory substances include hemoglobin, crystals, β-human chorionic gonadotropin, and nitrates (64). Blood samples are commonly used for detection and/or quantification of a variety of viral pathogens including HIV-1, HCV, and CMV. For example, the effects of different anticoagulants in tests for the determination of HIV-1 viral loads have been well studied. HIV-1 RNA is most stable when it is collected in tubes containing EDTA. Acid citrate dextrose may be used, but the viral load will be decreased by 15% due to the volume of anticoagulant (46, 52). Heparin has been shown to be inhibitory to amplification and should be avoided (5, 50). In addition, very small volumes of whole blood (1%) can be inhibitory to *Taq* DNA polymerase (40). For assays that use whole blood or specimens contaminated with blood, the nucleic acid must be adequately purified.

Contamination Control

Several types of contamination can occur with molecular testing: contamination of specimens during the nucleic acid extraction step, contamination of specimens with positive control material, and carryover contamination of amplified products. Carryover contamination with amplified products can occur with DNA or RNA target amplification and with probe amplification methods. It does not occur with signal amplification assays since no nucleic acid molecules are synthesized by these methods. Contamination that occurs during specimen processing or when handling positive control material can occur with all amplification methods.

Establishing a unidirectional work flow from a DNA-free area for reagent preparation, to a specimen processing area, and, finally, to the area where amplification and detection occur can minimize contamination. When using signal amplification methods it is not necessary to separate the specimen processing area from the amplification and detection area. Each area should have designated pipettors, equipment, and supplies. Other general practices that can minimize the risk of contamination include preparation of reagents in an area that is free of DNA and storing of reagents in single-use aliquots. The application of 2 to 10% solution of sodium hypochlorite is an effective method for the elimination of nucleic acid from work surfaces and equipment (74, 90). Following the application of the sodium hypochlorite, work surfaces and equipment should be wiped down with ethanol (70%) to minimize the corrosive effects of the bleach. UV light exposure of work surfaces can destroy DNA, but the efficiency and the time required vary with the size of the DNA fragment, with the maximum effect achieved after 8 h of exposure (26).

Clinical microbiologists have long been concerned about minimizing contamination between samples with microorganisms during specimen processing. Molecular methods have raised the level of concern considerably, and for good reason, as current methods can detect a few molecules. The previously undetected low levels of contamination that occurred while specimens were processed for routine culture can lead to false-positive results by molecular assays. Prevention of contamination due to target DNA is best done by carefully handling the specimens to avoid splashing, opening only one specimen tube at a time, pulse-spinning tubes prior to opening, using screw-top tubes rather than flip-top tubes to minimize aerosolization, bleaching work surfaces, and using plugged pipette tips. Some of these approaches can be difficult for high-volume laboratories. Prevention of contamination of the laboratory with DNA from a clinical specimen or positive control material is very important, because elimination of contamination with target DNA once it occurs can be very difficult. This is why care should be taken to use a positive control at the lowest concentration that is consistently amplified. The enzymatic and photochemical inactivation methods used to control carryover contamination of amplified products are not effective in preventing contamination with target DNA.

Uracil-N-glycosylase (UNG) is a DNA repair enzyme found in a variety of bacterial species. The normal function of the enzyme is to remove uracil residues from double-stranded DNA molecules. During the PCR dTTP is replaced with dUTP, so that dUTP is incorporated into the newly synthesized DNA products. This allows a distinction between starting template DNA and amplified products; only newly synthesized PCR products will contain deoxyuracil. If UTP-containing amplification products are present as contaminants, the addition of UNG to the reaction mixture will result in the cleavage of deoxyuracil residues, thus destroying the contaminating DNA (62). UNG will not degrade TTP-containing template DNA. UNG is added to the PCR master mixture. After a short incubation period at 50°C, the enzyme is activated, contaminated products are eliminated, and then thermal cycling proceeds. The use of UNG increases the amount of carryover DNA needed to contaminate the reaction mixture by several $\log_{10}$ (82). When using UNG it is important to keep the annealing temperature above 55°C so that the UNG remains inactive, thus avoiding degradation of the newly synthesized product. For the same reason, after completion of amplification, the reaction mixture should be held at 72°C (114). UNG can be inactivated at 94°C, but prolonged inactivation at 94°C may also affect the activity of the polymerase enzyme. UNG will not remove uracil from RNA molecules and is therefore ineffective in controlling contamination with RNA amplification assays, such as TMA and NASBA.

Several issues need to be considered when replacing dTTP with dUTP in the PCR master mixture. The PCR conditions should be reoptimized, as the magnesium requirement may increase. The efficiency of amplification may be reduced when dUTP is substituted for dTTP. This can be overcome by adding a mixture of dUTP and dTTP in the master mixture. dUTP substitution in amplified products may reduce the binding affinities of the oligonucleotide probes used in the detection reaction (10). This can usually be overcome by reducing the stringency of the probe hybridization or washing or using a mixture of dTTP and dUTP in the PCR mixture. Also, the efficiency of inactivation with UNG depends on the size of the amplified product and its G+C content. Inactivation may not be effective with amplified products of less than 100 bp, as maximum UNG efficiency requires the DNA molecule to be 150 bp (25).

An alternative to enzymatic inactivation is photochemical inactivation with isopsoralen. These compounds are added to the PCR mixture and intercalate between base pairs of the newly synthesized DNA molecules. After completion of the PCR, prior to opening of the reaction tubes, the tubes are exposed to long-wave UV light which cross-links the isopsoralens to the DNA. Any modified DNA that is carried over into a new PCR mixture is refractory to amplification because the polymerase molecule cannot extend the primer when the template DNA is cross-linked (16, 49). This method is easy to use and inexpensive, but several problems have been reported, including inhibition of amplification by isopsoralen compounds, changes in the apparent molecular weight of the product, and decreased hybridization efficiency (16, 25, 99). Most of these problems can be overcome with appropriate modifications of the reaction conditions. However, photochemical inactivation is difficult for DNA fragments less than 100 bp in length and those with high G+C contents (25).

Quality Control and Assurance

Verification and validation are terms that are often used interchangeably; however, they are very different processes. *Verification* is the process by which assay performance is determined; parameters such as sensitivity, specificity, positive and negative predictive values, and accuracy are established. The verification of an assay is completed before it is used for patient testing. *Validation* is the ongoing process of proving that the assay is performing as expected and achieves the intended results.

The verification of an assay includes analytical verification and clinical verification. The analytical verification provides information on the performance characteristics of the assay, while the clinical verification determines the clinical utility of the assay. Determining the clinical utility of a molecular assay can be difficult when the molecular assay is more sensitive than the gold standard. This was seen with the commercial assays designed to detect *C. trachomatis* in genital specimens. Molecular assays proved to be much more sensitive than the gold standard method of culture. An insensitive gold standard can make a molecular assay appear to have a falsely low specificity. In this situation, an expanded gold standard can be used. For *C. trachomatis* this included testing by direct fluorescent-antibody assay and/or another molecular method (32, 57, 102). There are additional challenges when determining the clinical utility of molecular assays that detect rare pathogens. These assays are usually developed in-house, and any given medical center may see very few cases of disease caused by such rare pathogens. In this situation it is important to inquire about assay verification, because it is possible that an assay could be brought into clinical use without an appropriate clinical verification. Moreover, standards and control material can be difficult to obtain for rare pathogens. Several companies now provide control material for the more common molecular assays such as those for *C. trachomatis*, *N. gonorrhoeae*, HIV-1, and HCV.

A positive control is designed to ensure that the test can consistently detect a concentration of target nucleic acid at or near the limit of detection of the assay. The positive control should be present at the lowest concentration that can be reproducibly amplified. A positive control present at a concentration that is significantly greater than the cutoff of the assay may not detect small decreases in amplification efficiency. In addition, large amounts of target DNA can increase problems with contamination in the laboratory. Depending on the availability of material, the positive control may be purified nucleic acid or lysed or intact organisms. An extraction control tests the ability of the nucleic acid extraction or purification method to successfully free nucleic acid from the organism. The extraction control, which should be intact organisms, can also serve as a positive control if it is used at the appropriate concentration.

Monitoring for the presence of inhibitors in a specimen is important, particularly for complex specimens such as blood or sputum. A wide range of substances can inhibit amplification reactions, including, but not limited to, heme, glycoproteins, heparin, phenol, urine crystals, and EDTA. Several methods can be used to control for inhibition. A commonly used method is to amplify two aliquots of a clinical specimen, one directly and the second spiked with an aliquot of positive control DNA. For a specimen to be considered negative for the target analyte, the test result for the specimen amplified directly must be negative and that for the spiked specimen must be positive. If an inhibitor of amplification were present, the spiked specimen would be negative. The concentration of positive control used for the spike must be near the limit of detection of the assay to ensure that low-level inhibition of amplification is detected.

Another approach to monitoring for inhibition of amplification is adding an internal control to the clinical specimen prior to nucleic acid extraction. This approach is commonly used with quantitative assays, but internal controls may also be used with qualitative assays. The internal control molecule may be designed with the same primer binding sites as the target molecule but modified with an insertion or deletion of a portion of the molecule internal to the primer binding sites or a rearrangement of a sequence internal to the primer binding sites. This allows the separate detection of the internal control on the basis of either size or the use of a sequence-specific probe. For quantitative assays that use an internal control, this molecule can serve as both the quantitation standard and an inhibition control. Some quantitative assays do not add a quantitation standard to the clinical specimen prior to specimen processing; rather, a standard curve is run in parallel with the clinical samples. In this situation there is no internal control to monitor the quality of specimen extraction or the presence of inhibitors of amplification. The same would be true for a qualitative assay that did not contain an internal control.

Amplification of a human housekeeping gene (β-globin, DQA) may also be used as an internal control, but the gene should not be present in amounts in vast excess of the amounts of the target molecule or inhibition of amplification of the target molecule can occur without evidence of inhibition of the housekeeping gene. Inhibition controls should be included in assays that use a new specimen extraction method or specimen type. However, a cost-effective approach is to discontinue the use of these controls once the inhibition rate is determined to be less than 1 to 2%.

Under certain conditions there may be a need to determine if there is adequate nucleic acid in a specimen. This may be important when determining if nucleic acid was adequately extracted from paraffin-embedded tissue or when evaluating the quality of a specimen. The formalin fixation step of tissue processing cross-links protein to nucleic acid, which can inhibit the subsequent amplification process. Also, prior to reporting of a negative result it may be important to assess the quality of the specimen. In both of these situations, amplification of housekeeping genes can be used to determine if the specimen contained human

DNA. The absence of amplifiable human DNA from the specimen raises concern about whether the specimen quality is adequate.

Negative controls should be included in all assays and should be processed in a manner similar to that used for the clinical specimens. The negative control should be taken through all steps of the assay, including the nucleic acid extraction process. However, a negative result for the negative control does not ensure that there is not contamination in the run, as contamination is often low level and sporadic. The inclusion of multiple negative controls in the run may provide additional assurance that there is no contamination, but this may be cost prohibitive. Ideally, the negative control should be a clinical specimen that does not contain the analyte of interest. These types of controls may be difficult to obtain, so water or buffer may be substituted.

Proficiency testing for molecular diagnostic laboratories remains a challenge. At this time adequate external proficiency programs are not available to cover the wide variety of molecular infectious disease tests. At present, the College of American Pathologists has the only Center for Medicare and Medicaid Services-approved proficiency program for molecular testing for infectious diseases. Testing is provided three times per year for detection of *C. trachomatis* and *N. gonorrhoeae* and quantitation of HIV-1 and HCV RNA. An additional panel that may include proficiency testing for detection of *Borrelia burgdorferi*, CMV, HSV, HCV (qualitative), HPV, the *mecA* gene, and *M. tuberculosis*; for HCV and HIV-1 genotyping; and for bacterial molecular typing is also available three times per year. Proficiency testing programs are also available from other sources. Recently, AcroMetrix (Berkeley, Calif.) has begun proficiency testing for HIV-1 genotyping that includes two challenges per year with five specimens per challenge. The Centers for Disease Control and Prevention also offers the Model Performance Evaluation Program for the detection of HIV-1 twice per year.

When formal external proficiency testing programs are not available, laboratories have several alternatives. These include split-sample testing with other laboratories, split-sample testing by an established in-house method, or clinical validation of the test result by clinical diagnosis. When laboratories exchange specimens for proficiency testing, it is important that both laboratories use the same method, particularly for quantitative methods. It has been well documented that for the currently available commercial assays for the quantitation of HIV-1 RNA, the viral loads will differ between the various assays. The differences in viral loads may vary from 2- to 3-fold (52) to as much as 10-fold for any given patient (118). The same is seen with CMV viral loads when different amplification methods are used (115).

Reporting and Interpretation of Results

Interpretation of the results of molecular assays requires a basic understanding of the strengths and limitations of the technology used. In interpreting the results of molecular assays, one may encounter unique problems that are not routinely encountered with traditional microbiological assays such as culture and serology. Some of the problems that may occur when interpreting the results of molecular assays include false-positive results, distinguishing viable from nonviable organisms, and correlating nucleic acid detection with the presence of disease. The increased sensitivities of molecular assays can provide several advantages, including

the ability to use a specimen that is collected in a less invasive manner or the need for a smaller amount of specimen for testing.

When interpreting a positive test result, the issues that need to be considered are assay specificity and contamination. The specificities of most molecular assays are established by the primers and probes used during amplification and detection steps. If primers cross-react with other pathogens, false-positive results are possible. For example, primers designed to detect *Mycoplasma pneumoniae* from respiratory specimens must not cross-react with organisms comprising the normal oral flora or other common respiratory pathogens, such as *S. pneumoniae*. Although uncommon, problems with primer specificity do occur; the primers designed to amplify the 5′ untranslated region of enteroviruses have been reported to cross-react with rhinoviruses (98). This would not be a problem when testing cerebrospinal fluid (CSF) specimens but would preclude use of the assay with respiratory specimens. Problems with primer specificity have also been reported for a commercially available PCR assay designed to detect *N. gonorrhoeae*. The primers used in that assay cross-react with *Neisseria subflava*, a nonpathogenic organism found in the oral pharynx (27). False-positive results can also be due to contamination, which may occur during specimen processing or as a result of carryover contamination of previously amplified products.

The interpretation of a negative result requires consideration of assay sensitivity, specimen quality, nucleic acid extraction efficacy, and amplification efficiency. Problems with any of these factors can lead to a false-negative result, which is why measures to control for each of these parameters should be included in assays whenever feasible.

Molecular assays detect pathogen nucleic acid but cannot determine whether that nucleic acid is found in a viable or a nonviable organism. Pathogen nucleic acid can be detected for long periods of time after appropriate treatment is initiated. For example, *C. trachomatis* DNA can be found in the urine of patients for up to 3 weeks after completion of a course of therapy (30). The FDA-approved molecular assays for the detection of *M. tuberculosis* from respiratory specimens should not be used for patients with a recent history of tuberculosis or those receiving therapy. Again, this is due to the persistence of nucleic acid for months after the initiation of effective therapy. Similar results have been reported for the detection of HSV DNA in the CSF of patients with encephalitis. DNA can persist for 2 weeks or longer after the initiation of acyclovir therapy (55). Due to the persistence of pathogen DNA after the initiation of therapy, qualitative molecular assays should not be used to monitor the response to therapy. One notable exception is the use of a qualitative HCV RNA RT-PCR assay to monitor the response to therapy with interferon and ribavirin. In this instance, the absence of detectable viral RNA from plasma is used to define the treatment response (22, 68, 88).

The detection of pathogen nucleic acid does not ensure that the organism is the cause of disease. The organism may be present as part of the normal flora, colonizing a particular area, or causing infection. Distinguishing between colonization and infection may be more difficult when one is using molecular techniques that are more sensitive than culture. Organisms that are present in very low concentrations and that might have gone undetected by routine culture methods may be detected by molecular techniques.

Distinguishing colonization from infection is easier when a specimen from a normally sterile site such as CSF or

TABLE 3 FDA-approved molecular diagnostic tests for infectious diseases

Test	Method/manufacturer
C. trachomatis detection	Hybridization/Gen-Probe; LCR/Abbott; PCR/Roche; Hybrid capture/Digene; SDA/Becton Dickinson
N. gonorrhoeae detection	Hybridization/Gen-Probe; LCR/Abbott; SDA/Becton Dickinson; Hybrid capture/Digene
C. trachomatis and N. gonorrhoeae multiplex	PCR/Roche; TMA/Gen-Probe
Culture confirmation for Mycobacterium spp.	Hybridization/Gen-Probe
Culture confirmation for fungi and bacteria[a]	Hybridization/Gen-Probe
Detection of group A streptococcus	Hybridization/Gen-Probe
HCV detection	RT-PCR/Roche
Methicillin-resistant S. aureus detection	Cycling probe technology/ID Biomedical
HIV quantitation (standard or ultrasensitive)	RT-PCR/Roche; NASBA/bioMérieux
HIV resistance genotyping	CLIP sequencing/Visible Genetics
HPV detection	Hybrid capture/Digene
M. tuberculosis detection	TMA/Gen-Probe; PCR/Roche
Gardnerella, Trichomonas, and Candida detection	Hybridization/Becton Dickinson
CMV detection	Hybrid capture/Digene; NASBA/bioMérieux

[a] Fungi include B. dermatitidis, C. immitis, Cryptococcus neoformans, and H. capsulatum. Bacteria include Campylobacter spp., Enterococcus spp., group A streptococcus, group B streptococcus, H. influenzae, N. gonorrhoeae, S. pneumoniae, S. aureus, and L. monocytogenes.

blood is tested; however, this alone does not ensure that the organism is a true pathogen. This is a concern with the detection of herpesviruses, which cause lifelong latent infections. An important example of this is monitoring of transplant recipients for CMV disease by molecular methods. Initial studies used very sensitive qualitative PCR assays (31, 78), and it was clear that CMV DNA could be detected in the blood of patients who never went on to develop symptomatic disease. Recent studies have shown that quantitative DNA assays and a qualitative assay that detects pp67 mRNA are useful in distinguishing active from latent CMV infection (1, 47, 80). The use of quantitative assays and the detection of mRNA to improve clinical specificity will likely be useful in distinguishing active infection from latent infection with other herpesviruses.

Reporting of the results of a qualitative molecular assay is usually straightforward; the nucleic acid is either present in the sample or absent from the sample. Several key parameters that may also be reported are the limit of detection of the assay, data pertaining to the rate of inhibition for a given sample type, and the amplification method used for testing.

Reporting of the results of quantitative assays is more complex and requires consideration of several parameters including dynamic range, units, and precision. The results of quantitative assays can be expressed as the number of copies, the weight (in nanograms or picograms), or the number of international units of the target nucleic acid in a defined volume, such as 1 ml of plasma or blood, 1 g of tissue, or a certain number of leukocytes. When the results of quantitative assays are reported, the precision of the assay needs to be considered. For the currently available HIV-1 viral load assays, the assay and biological variability are approximately 0.5 $\log_{10}$ (100). Therefore, changes in viral load must exceed 0.5 $\log_{10}$ (threefold) in order to represent a biologically significant change in viral replication. For these assays, values should be reported as $\log_{10}$ rather than integers to avoid the overinterpretation of small changes in viral load. Quantitative assays have a defined linear or

dynamic range. Values below the lower limit of quantification should be reported as less than the lower limit of the linear range rather than negative. Values above the upper limit of quantification should be reported as greater than the upper limit of the linear range. For values above the limit of detection but below the limit of quantitation, results may be reported as detectable, less than the lower limit of the linear range. For example, if the lower limit of quantitation of an HIV-1 viral load assay is 400 copies/ml, a value of 250 copies/ml could be reported as detectable, <400 copies/ml. The report should also include the amplification method used. This is particularly important for quantitative methods, as values between different assay types are not always comparable.

Regulatory and Reimbursement Issues

The medical needs for new molecular microbiology tests have exceeded the capacity of the diagnostic industry to provide FDA-cleared test kits to fill these needs. Table 3 lists the nucleic acid-based tests for infectious diseases that have been cleared by FDA at the time that this chapter was written. Absent from this list are tests that have become a standard of care for a variety of diseases such as HSV encephalitis, enteroviral meningitis, and pertussis. Many laboratories have developed tests to fill these unmet needs. These tests that have been developed in-house must be appropriately verified and validated, as specified in sections 493.1201 to 493.1285 of the Clinical Laboratory Improvement Amendments (CLIA) of 1988. The costs for such tests are eligible for reimbursement by Medicare and other payers if they are determined to be part of a standard of care or of proven clinical benefit.

FDA requires a disclaimer on reports for tests developed in-house with analyte-specific reagents (ASRs). ASRs are chemical substances that are used in diagnostic tests to detect another specific substance in a specimen and are purchased from manufacturers under this label. The FDA-required disclaimer for tests that use ASRs reads: "This test result was developed and its performance characteristics determined by (laboratory name). It has not been cleared or approved by the U.S. Food and Drug Administration." This disclaimer was not intended to cover tests that have been developed in-house but that do not use ASRs or to cover the off-label uses of FDA-cleared products.

A laboratory may want to include clarifying statements in the reporting of results of in-house-developed tests that use ASRs. These statements could point out that FDA clearance is not necessary for these tests and that they are used for clinical purposes. Additional information could include the fact that the laboratory is certified under CLIA of 1988 to perform high-complexity testing and that pursuant to the requirements of CLIA the laboratory has established and verified the test's accuracy and precision.

Correct Current Procedural Terminology (CPT) coding of molecular microbiology tests is essential to coverage and reimbursement by payers (2). In 1998, many analyte-specific codes for direct probe, amplified probe, and amplified probe with quantification assays were established in the microbiology section of the CPT Coding Manual. Prior to 1998, molecular microbiology tests were billed by using multiple-component CPTs selected from the molecular pathology section. Recently multianalyte codes, codes for HIV resistance genotyping and phenotyping, and HCV genotyping were established. These changes have simplified the coding process and in many cases have increased the levels of reimbursement for molecular microbiology procedures.

FUTURE DIRECTIONS

Nucleic acid testing will continue to be one of the leading growth areas in laboratory medicine. The number of applications of this technology in diagnostic microbiology will continue to increase, and the technology will increasingly be incorporated into routine clinical microbiology laboratories as it becomes less technically complex and more accessible. More clinical and financial outcome data will be needed to justify the use of this expensive technology in an era of declining reimbursement and increased cost-consciousness.

Molecular diagnostics will largely remain a cottage industry, with the proliferation of tests developed by individual laboratories to satisfy new medical needs not met by the diagnostic test industry. As a result, one of the biggest concerns for the future is the development of effective proficiency testing programs that will help ensure that the results of these tests are reliable and reproducible between laboratories.

To a great extent the future of molecular microbiology depends on automation. Many of the available tests are labor-intensive, with much of the labor devoted to tedious sample processing methods. Sample processing remains the greatest challenge to automation, but the recent development of fully automated systems for molecular diagnostics offers hope for the future. Perhaps the most exciting prospects for automation come from the biochip sector. With the currently available technology, it is not difficult to imagine the development in the near future of a small chip that could automate several functions of the microbiology laboratory.

The use of multiplex nucleic acid-based assays to screen at-risk patients for panels of probable pathogens remains a goal for molecular microbiology. Success to date has been limited by technical difficulties, but the development of such assays is key to providing molecular tests with the same broad diagnostic range provided by culture and other conventional methods.

Advances in human genomics will be exploited in the future to develop tests for immunogenetic factors that may influence the risk of becoming infected with certain pathogens or the progression of disease. Human gene expression profiling with microarrays may be important in defining patterns of host gene expression associated with different pathogens or disease states. Better understanding of pathogen genomics and gene expression analysis will lead to the discovery of new diagnostic and therapeutic targets.

REFERENCES

1. **Aitken, C., W. Barrett-Muir, C. Millar, K. Templeton, J. Thomas, F. Sheridan, D. Jeffries, M. Yaqoob, and J. Breuer.** 1999. Use of molecular assays in diagnosis and monitoring of cytomegalovirus disease following renal transplantation. *J. Clin. Microbiol.* **37:**2804–2807.
2. **American Medical Association.** 2001. *Current Procedural Terminology for Pathology and Laboratory Medicine,* 4th ed. American Medical Association Press, Chicago, Ill.
3. **Arnold, L. J., Jr., P. W. Hammond, W. A. Wiese, and N. C. Nelson.** 1989. Assay formats involving acridinium ester-labeled DNA probes. *Clin Chem.* **35:**1588–1594.
4. **Barany, F.** 1991. Genetic disease detection and DNA amplification using cloned thermostable ligase. *Proc. Natl. Acad. Sci. USA* **88:**189–193.
5. **Beutler, E., T. Gelbart, and W. Kuhl.** 1990. Interference of heparin with the polymerase chain reaction. *BioTechniques* **9:**166.
6. **Birkenmeyer, L. G., and L. K. Mushahwar.** 1991. DNA probe amplification methods. *J. Virol. Methods* **35:**117–126.
7. **Blin, N., and D. W. Stafford.** 1976. A general method for isolation of high molecular weight DNA from eukaryotes. *Nucleic Acids Res.* **3:**2303–2308.
8. **Boom, R., C. Sol, M. Salimans, C. Jansen, P. M. Wertheim-van Dillen, and J. van derNoordaa.** 1990. Rapid and simple method for purification of nucleic acids. *J. Clin. Microbiol.* **28:**495–503.
9. **Caliendo, A. M., K. St. George, S. Y. Kao, J. Allega, B. H. Tan, R. LaFontaine, L. Bui, and C. R. Rinaldo.** 2000. Comparison of quantitative cytomegalovirus (CMV) PCR in plasma and CMV antigenemia assay: clinical utility of the prototype AMPLICOR CMV MONITOR test in transplant recipients. *J. Clin. Microbiol.* **38:**2122–2127.
10. **Carmody, M. W., and C. P. Vary.** 1993. Inhibition of DNA hybridization following partial dUTP substitution. *BioTechniques* **15:**692–699.
11. **Chamberlain, J. S., R. A. Gibbs, J. E. Rainer, P. N. Nguyen, and C. T. Caskey.** 1988. Deletion screening of the Duchenne muscular dystrophy locus via multiplex DNA amplification. *Nucleic Acids Res.* **16:**11141–11156.
12. **Chang, Y., E. Cesarman, M. S. Pessin, F. Lee, J. Culpepper, D. M. Knowles, and P. S. Moore.** 1994. Identification of herpesvirus-like DNA sequences in AIDS-associated Kaposi's sarcoma. *Science* **266:**1865–1869.
13. **Cheng, J., E. L. Sheldon, L. Wu, A. Uribe, L. O. Gerrue, J. Carrino, M. J. Heller, and J. P. O'Connell.** 1998. Preparation and hybridization analysis of DNA/RNA from *E. coli* on microfabricated bioelectronic chips. *Nat. Biotechnol.* **16:**541–546.
14. **Chomczynski, P., and N. Sacchi.** 1987. Single-step method of RNA isolation by acid guanidinium thiocyanate-phenol-chloroform extraction. *Anal. Biochem.* **62:**156–159.
15. **Choo, Q. L., G. Kuo, A. J. Weiner, L. R. Overby, D. W. Bradley, and M. Houghton.** 1989. Isolation of a cDNA

clone derived from a blood-borne non-A, non-B viral hepatitis genome. *Science* **244:**359–362.

16. **Cimino, G. D., K. C. Metchette, J. W. Tessman, J. E. Hearst, and S. T. Isaacs.** 1991. Post-PCR sterilization: a method to control carryover contamination for the polymerase chain reaction. *Nucleic Acids Res.* **19:**99–107.

17. **Clementi, M., S. Menzo, P. Bagnarelli, A. Manzin, A. Valenza, and P. E. Varaldo.** 1993. Quantitative PCR and RT-PCR in virology. *PCR Methods Appl.* **2:**191–196.

18. **Cohen, C., H. Kessler, S. Hunt, M. Sension, C. Farthing, M. Conant, S. Jacobson, J. Nadler, W. Verbiest, K. Hertogs, M. Ames, A. Rinehart, and N. Graham.** 2000. Phenotypic resistance testing significantly improves response to therapy: final analysis of a randomized trial (VIRA3001). *Antivir. Ther.* **5:**67.

19. **Collins, M. L., C. Zayati, J. J. Detmer, B. Daly, J. A. Kolberg, T. Cha, B. D. Irvine, J. Tucker, and M. S. Urdea.** 1995. Preparation and characterization of RNA standards for use in quantitative branched-DNA hybridization assays. *Anal. Biochem.* **226:**120–129.

20. **Compton, J.** 1991. Nucleic acid sequence-based amplification. *Nature* **350:**91–92.

21. **Cope, J. J., A. Hildesheim, M. H. Schiffman, M. M. Manos, A. T. Lorincz, R. D. Burk, A. G. Glass, C. Greer, J. Burkland, K. Helgesen, D. R. Scott, M. E. Sherman, R. J. Kurman, and K.-L. Liaw.** 1997. Comparison of the hybrid capture tube test and PCR for detection of human papillomavirus DNA in cervical specimens. *J. Clin. Microbiol.* **35:**2262–2265.

22. **Davis, G. L., R. Esteban-Mur, V. Rustgi, J. Hoefs, S. C. Gordon, C. Trepo, M. L. Shiffman, S. Zeuzem, A. Craxi, M.-H. Ling, and J. Albrecht for the International Hepatitis Interventional Therapy Group.** 1998. Interferon alpha-2b alone or in combination with ribavirin for the treatment of relapse of chronic hepatitis C. *N. Engl. J. Med.* **339:**1493–1499.

23. **Durant, J., P. Clevenberg, P. Halfon, P. Delgiudice, S. Porsin, P. Simonet, N. Montagne, C. A. B. Boucher, J. M. Schapiro, and P. Dellamonica.** 1999. Drug-resistance genotyping in HIV-1 therapy: the VIRADAPT randomised controlled trial. *Lancet* **353:**2195–2199.

24. **Esch, R. K.** 1997. Basic nucleic acid procedures, p. 35–60. *In* W. B. Coleman and G. Tsongalis (ed.), *Molecular Diagnostics for the Clinical Laboratorian.* Humana Press, Totowa, N.J.

25. **Espy, M. J., T. F. Smith, and D. H. Persing.** 1993. Dependence of polymerase chain reaction product inactivation protocols on amplicon length and sequence composition. *J. Clin. Microbiol.* **31:**2361–2365.

26. **Fairfax, M. R., M. A. Metcalf, and R. W. Cone.** 1991. Slow inactivation of dry PCR templates by UV light. *PCR Methods Appl.* **1:**142–143.

27. **Farrell, D. J.** 1999. Evaluation of AMPLICOR *Neisseria gonorrhoeae* PCR using *cppB* nested PCR and 16S rRNA PCR. *J. Clin. Microbiol.* **37:**386–390.

28. **Felmlee, T. A., R. P. Oda, D. A. Persing, and J. P. Landers.** 1995. Capillary electrophoresis of DNA: potential utility for clinical diagnoses. *J. Chromatogr.* **A717:**127–137.

29. **Fong, W. K., Z. Modrusan, J. P. McNevin, J. Marostenmaki, B. Zin, and F. Bekkaoui.** 2000. Rapid solid-phase immunoassay for detection of methicillin-resistant *Staphylococcus aureus* using cycling probe technology. *J. Clin. Microbiol.* **38:**2525–2529.

30. **Gaydos, C. A., K. A. Crotchfelt, M. R. Howell, S. Kralian, P. Hauptman, and T. C. Quinn.** 1998. Molecular amplification assays to detect chlamydial infections in urine specimens from high school female students and to monitor the persistence of chlamydial DNA after therapy. *J. Infect. Dis.* **177:**417–424.

31. **Gerna, G., D. Zipeto, M. Parea, M. G. Revello, E. Silini, E. Percivalle, M. Zavattoni, P. Grossi, and G. Milanesi.** 1991. Monitoring of human cytomegalovirus infections and ganciclovir treatment in heart transplant recipients by determination of viremia, antigenemia, and DNAemia. *J. Infect. Dis.* **164:**488–498.

32. **Green, T. A., C. M. Black, and R. E. Johnson.** 1998. Evaluation of bias in diagnostic-test sensitivity and specificity estimates computed by discrepant analysis. *J. Clin. Microbiol.* **36:**375–381.

33. **Gross-Bellard, M., P. Oudet, and P. Chambon.** 1973. Isolation of high-molecular-weight DNA from mammalian cells. *Eur. J. Biochem.* **36:**32–38.

34. **Guatelli, J. C., K. M. Whitfield, D. Y. Kwoh, K. J. Barringer, D. D. Richman, and T. R. Gingeras.** 1990. Isothermal *in vitro* amplification of nucleic acids by multienzyme reaction modeled after retroviral replication. *Proc. Natl. Acad. Sci. USA* **87:**1874–1878.

35. **Haberhausen, G., J. Pinsl, C.-C. Kuhn, and C. Markert-Hahn.** 1998. Comparative study of different standardization concepts in quantitative competitive reverse transcription-PCR assays. *J. Clin. Microbiol.* **36:**628–633.

36. **Hankin, R. C.** 1992. In situ hybridization: principles and applications. *Lab. Med.* **23:**764–770.

37. **Haqqi, T. M., G. Sarkar, C. S. David, and S. S. Sommer.** 1988. Specific amplification with PCR of a refractory segment of genomic DNA. *Nucleic Acids Res.* **16:**11844.

38. **Heid, C., J. Stevens, K. J. Livak, and P. M. Williams.** 1996. Real time quantitative PCR. *Genome Res.* **6:**986–994.

39. **Hendricks, D. A., B. J. Stowe, B. S. Hoo, J. Kolberg, B. D. Irvine, P. D. Neuwald, M. S. Urdea, and R. P. Perrillo.** 1995. Quantitation of HBV DNA in human serum using a branched DNA (bDNA) signal amplification assay. *Am. J. Clin. Pathol.* **104:**537–546.

40. **Higuchi, R.** 1989. Simple and rapid preparation of samples for PCR, p. 31–38. *In* H. Erlich (ed.), *PCR Technology: Principles and Applications for DNA Amplification.* Stockton Press, New York, N.Y.

41. **Higuchi, R., C. Fockler, G. Dollinger, and R. Watson.** 1993. Kinetic PCR analysis: real-time monitoring of DNA amplification reactions. *Bio/Technology* **11:**1026–1030.

42. **Hirsch, M. S., F. Brun-Vezinet, R. D'Aquila, S. Hammer, V. Johnson, D. Kuritzkes, J. Mellors, B. Clotet, B. Conway, L. Demeter, S. Vella, D. Jacobsen, and D. Richman.** 2000. Antiretroviral drug resistance testing in adults with HIV infection: recommendations of an International AIDS Society-USA panel. *JAMA* **283:**2417–2426.

43. **Hirsch, M. S., B. Conway, R. T. D'Aquila, V. A. Johnson, F. Brun-Vezinet, B. Clotet, L. M. Demeter, S. M. Hammer, D. M. Jacobsen, D. R. Kuritzkes, C. Loveday, J. W. Mellors, S. Vella, and D. Richman for the International AIDS Society—USA Panel.** 1998. Antiretroviral drug resistance testing in adults with HIV infection: implications for clinical management. *JAMA* **279:**1984–1991.

44. **Hirschel, B., H. R. Chang, N. Mach, P. F. Piguet, J. Cox, J. D. Piguet, M. T. Silva, L. Larsson, P. R. Klatser, and J. E. Thole.** 1990. Fatal infection with a novel, unidentified mycobacterium in a man with the acquired immunodeficiency syndrome. *N. Engl. J. Med.* **323:**109–113.

45. **Holland, P. M., R. D. Abramson, R. Watson, and D. H. Gelfand.** 1991. Detection of specific polymerase chain reaction product by utilizing the $5' \rightarrow 3'$ exonuclease

activity of *Thermus aquaticus* DNA polymerase. *Proc. Natl. Acad. Sci. USA* **88:**7276–7280.

46. Holodniy, M., L. Mole, B. Yen-Lieberman, D. Margolis, C. Starkey, R. Carroll, T. Spahlinger, J. Todd, and J. B. Jackson. 1995. Comparative stabilities of quantitative human immunodeficiency virus RNA in plasma from samples collected in VACUTAINER CPT, VACUTAINER PPT, and standard VACUTAINER tubes. *J. Clin. Microbiol.* **33:**1562–1566.

47. Humar, A., D. Gregson, A. M. Caliendo, A. McGeer, G. Malkan, M. Krajden, P. Corey, P. Greig, S. Walmsley, G. Levy, and T. Mazzulli. 1999. Clinical utility of quantitative cytomegalovirus viral load determination for predicting cytomegalovirus disease in liver transplant recipients. *Transplantation* **68:**1305–1311.

48. Innis, M. A., K. B. Myambo, D. H. Gelfand, and M. A. Brow. 1998. DNA sequencing with *Thermus aquaticus* DNA polymerase and direct sequencing of polymerase chain reaction-amplified DNA. *Proc. Natl. Acad. Sci. USA* **85:**9436–9440.

49. Isaacs, S. T., J. W. Tessman, K. C. Metchette, J. E. Hearst, and G. D. Cimino. 1991. Post-PCR sterilization: development and application to an HIV-1 diagnostic assay. *Nucleic Acids Res.* **19:**109–116.

50. Izraeli, S., C. Pfleiderer, and T. Lion. 1991. Detection of gene expression by PCR amplification of RNA derived from frozen heparinized whole blood. *Nucleic Acids Res.* **19:**6051.

51. Kern, D., M. Collins, T. Fultz, J. Detmer, S. Hamren, J. J. Peterkin, P. Sheridan, M. Urdea, R. White, T. Yeghiazarian, and J. Todd. 1996. An enhanced-sensitivity branched-DNA assay for quantification of human immunodeficiency virus type 1 RNA in plasma. *J. Clin. Microbiol.* **34:**3196–3202.

52. Kirstein, L. M., J. W. Mellors, C. R. Rinaldo, Jr., J. B. Margolick, J. V. Giorgi, J. P. Phair, E. Dietz, P. Gupta, C. H. Sherlock, R. Hogg, J. S. Montaner, and A. Munoz. 1999. Effects of anticoagulant, processing delay, and assay method (branched DNA versus reverse transcriptase PCR) on measurement of human immunodeficiency virus type 1 RNA levels in plasma. *J. Clin. Microbiol.* **37:**2428–2433.

53. Kricka, L. J. 1999. Nucleic acid detection technologies—labels, strategies, and formats. *Clin. Chem.* **45:**453–458.

54. Kwoh, D. Y., G. R. David, K. M. Whitfield, H. L. Chapelle, L. J. DiMichele, and T. R. Gingeras. 1989. Transcription-based amplification system and detection of amplified human immunodeficiency virus type 1 with a bead-based sandwich hybridization format. *Proc. Natl. Acad. Sci. USA* **86:**1173–1177.

55. Lakeman, F. D., R. J. Whitley, and National Institute of Allergy and Infectious Diseases Collaborative Antiviral Study Group. 1995. Diagnosis of herpes simplex encephalitis: application of polymerase chain reaction to cerebrospinal fluid from brain-biopsied patients and correlation with disease. *J. Infect. Dis.* **171:**857–863.

56. Lay, M. J., and C. T. Wittwer. 1997. Real-time fluorescence genotyping of factor V Leiden during rapid cycle PCR. *Clin. Chem.* **43:**2262–2267.

57. Lee, H. H., M. A. Chernesky, J. Schachter, J. D. Burczak, W. W. Andrews, S. Muldoon G. Leckie, and W. E. Stamm. 1995. Diagnosis of *Chlamydia trachomatis* genitourinary infection in women by ligase chain reaction assay of urine. *Lancet* **345:**213–216.

58. Leone, G., H. van Schijndel, B. van Gemen, F. R. Kramer, and C. D. Schoen. 1998. Molecular beacon probes combined with amplification by NASBA enable homogeneous, real-time detection of RNA. *Nucleic Acids Res.* **26:**2150–2155.

59. Lieber, M. R. 1997. The FEN-1 family of structure-specific nucleases in eukaryotic DNA replication, recombination and repair. *Bioessays* **19:**233–240.

60. Little, M. C., J. Andrews, R. Moore, S. Bustos, L. Jones, C. Embres, G. Durmowicz, J. Harris, D. Berger, K. Yanson, C. Rostkowski, D. Yursis, J. Price, T. Fort, A. Walters, M. Collis, O. Llorin, J. Wood, F. Failing, C. O'Keefe, B. Scrivens, B. Pope, T. Hansen, K. Marino, and K. Williams. 1999. Strand displacement amplification and homogeneous real-time detection incorporated in a second-generation DNA probe system, BDProbeTecET. *Clin. Chem.* **45:**777–784.

61. Loeffelholz, M. J., C. A. Lewinski, S. R. Silver, A. Purohit, S. A. Herman, D. A. Buonagurio, and E. A. Dragon. 1992. Detection of *Chlamydia trachomatis* in endocervical specimens by polymerase chain reaction. *J. Clin. Microbiol.* **30:**2847–2851.

62. Longo, M. C., M. S. Berninger, and J. L. Hartley. 1990. Use of uracil DNA glycosylase to control carry-over contamination in polymerase chain reactions. *Gene* **93:**125–128.

63. Lyamichev, V., A. Mast, J. G. Hall, J. R. Prudent, M. W. Kaiser, T. Takova, R. W. Kwiatkowski, T. J. Sander, M. deArruda, D. A. Arco, B. P. Neri, and M. A. Brow. 1999. Polymorphism identification and quantitative detection from genomic DNA by invasive cleavage of oligonucleotide probes. *Nat. Biotechnol.* **17:**292–296.

64. Mahony, J., S. Chong, D. Jang, K. Luinstra, M. Faught, D. Dalby, J. Sellors, and M. Chernesky. 1998. Urine specimens from pregnant and nonpregnant women inhibitory to amplification of *Chlamydia trachomatis* nucleic acid by PCR, ligase chain reaction, and transcription-mediated amplification: identification of urinary substances associated with inhibition and removal of inhibitory activity. *J. Clin. Microbiol.* **36:**3122–3126.

65. Mantero, G., A. Zonaro, A. Albertini, P. Bertolo, and D. Primi. 1991. DNA enzyme immunoassay: general method for detecting products of polymerase chain reaction. *Clin. Chem.* **37:**422–429.

66. Mazzulli, T., L. W. Drew, B. Yen-Lieberman, D. Jekic-McMullen, D. J. Kohn, C. Isada, G. Moussa, R. Chua, and S. Walmsley. 1999. Multicenter comparison of the Digene hybrid capture CMV DNA assay (version 2.0), the pp65 antigenemia assay, and cell culture for detection of cytomegalovirus viremia. *J. Clin. Microbiol.* **37:**958–963.

67. McDonough, S. H., C. Giachettik, Y. Yang, D. P. Kolk, E. Billyard, and E. L. Mimm. 1998. High throughput assay for the simultaneous or separate detection of human immunodeficiency virus (HIV) and hepatitis type C virus (HCV). *Infusionther. Transfusionmed.* **25:**164–169.

68. McHutchinson, J. G., S. C. Gordon, E. R. Schiff, M. L. Shiffman, W. M. Lee, V. K. Rustgi, Z. D. Goodman, M.-H. Ling, S. Cort, and J. K. Albrecht for the Hepatitis Interventional Therapy Group. 1998. Interferon alfa-2b alone or in combination with ribavirin as initial treatment for chronic hepatitis C. *N. Engl. J. Med.* **339:**1485–1492.

69. Mellors, J. W., C. R. Rinaldo, Jr., P. Gupta, R. M. White, J. A. Todd, and L. A. Kingsley. 1996. Prognosis in HIV-1 infection predicted by the quantity of virus in plasma. *Science* **272:**1167–1170.

70. Mitchell, P. S., M. J. Espy, T. F. Smith, D. R. Toal, P. N. Rys, E. F. Berbari, D. R. Osmon, and D. H. Persing. 1997. Laboratory diagnosis of central nervous system infections with herpes simplex virus by PCR performed with cerebrospinal fluid specimens. *J. Clin. Microbiol.* **35:**2873–2877.

71. Modrusan, Z., C. Marlowe, D. Wheeler, M. Pirseyedi, and R. N. Bryan. 1999. Detection of vancomycin resis-

tant genes vanA and vanB by cycling probe technology. *Mol. Cell. Probes* **13:**223–231.

72. **Morrison, T., J. J. Weiss, and C. T. Wittwer.** 1998. Quantification of low copy transcripts by continuous SYBR green I dye monitoring during amplification. *BioTechniques* **24:**954–958.

73. **Myers, T. W., and D. H. Gelfand.** 1991. Reverse transcription and DNA amplification by a *Thermus thermophilus* DNA polymerase. *Biochemistry* **30:**7661–7666.

74. **NCCLS.** 1995. *Molecular Diagnostic Methods for Infectious Diseases: Approved Guideline.* NCCLS document MM3-A. NCCLS, Wayne, Pa.

75. **NCCLS.** 2001. *Quantitative Molecular Methods for Infectious Diseases: Proposed Guideline.* NCCLS document MM6P. NCCLS, Wayne, Pa.

76. **Nichols, S. T., C. F. Spiropoulou, S. Morzunov, P. E. Rollin, T. G. Ksiazek, H. Feldmann, A. Sanchez, J. Childs, S. Zaki, and C. J. Peters.** 1993. Genetic identification of a hantavirus associated with an outbreak of acute respiratory illness. *Science* **262:**914–917.

77. **Nolte, F. S.** 1999. Branched DNA signal amplification for direct quantitation of nucleic acid sequences in clinical specimens. *Adv. Clin. Chem.* **33:**201–235.

78. **Nolte, F. S., R. K. Emmens, C. Thurmond, P. S. Mitchell, C. Pascuzzi, S. M. Devine, R. Saral, and J. R. Wingard.** 1995. Early detection of human cytomegalovirus viremia in bone marrow transplant recipients by DNA amplification. *J. Clin. Microbiol.* **33:**1263–1266.

79. **Nycz, C. M., C. H. Dean, P. D. Haaland, C. A. Spargo, and G. T. Walker.** 1998. Quantitative reverse transcription strand displacement amplification; quantitation of nucleic acids using an isothermal amplification technique. *Anal. Biochem.* **259:**226–234.

80. **Oldenburg, N., K. M. Lam, M. A. Khan, B. Top, N. M. Tacken, A. McKie, G. W. Mikhail, J. M. Middeldorp, A. Wright, N. R. Banner, and M. Yacoub.** 2000. Evaluation of human cytomegalovirus gene expression in thoracic organ transplant recipients using nucleic acid sequence-based amplification. *Transplantation* **70:**1209–1215.

81. **Orita, M., H. Iwahana, H. Kanazawa, K. Hayashi, and T. Sekiya.** 1989. Detection of polymorphism of human DNA by gel electrophoresis as single-strand conformation polymorphisms. *Proc. Natl. Acad. Sci. USA* **86:**2766–2770.

82. **Pang, J., J. Modlin, and R. Yolken.** 1992. Use of modified nucleotides and uracil-DNA glycosylase (UNG) for the control of contamination in the PCR-based amplification of RNA. *Mol. Cell. Probes* **6:**251–256.

83. **Pease, A. C., D. Solas, E. J. Sullivan, M. T. Cronin, C. P. Holmes, and S. P. Fodor.** 1994. Light-generated oligonucleotide arrays for rapid DNA sequence analysis. *Proc. Natl. Acad. Sci. USA* **91:**5022–5026.

84. **Persing, D. H. (ed.).** 1996. *PCR Protocols for Emerging Infectious Diseases.* ASM Press, Washington, D.C.

85. **Persing, D. H., T. F. Smith, F. C. Tenover and T. J. White (ed.).** 1993. *Diagnostic Molecular Microbiology: Principles and Applications.* ASM Press, Washington, D.C.

86. **Piccirilli, J. A., T. Krauch, S. E. Moroney, and S. A. Benner.** 1990. Enzymatic incorporation of a new base pair into DNA and RNA extends the genetic alphabet. *Nature* **343:**33–37.

87. **Poljak, M., and K. Seme.** 1996. Rapid detection and typing of human papillomaviruses by consensus polymerase chain reaction and enzyme-linked immunosorbent assay. *J. Virol. Methods* **56:**231–238.

88. **Poynard, T., P. Marcellin, S. S. Lee, C. Niederau, G. S. Minuk, G. Ideo, V. Bain, J. Heathcote, S. Zeuzem, C. Trepo, and J. Albrecht for the International Hepatitis Interventional Therapy Group (IHIT).** 1998. Randomised trial of interferon α2b plus ribavirin for 48 weeks or for 24 weeks versus interferon α2b plus placebo for 48 weeks for treatment of chronic infection with hepatitis C virus. *Lancet* **352:**1426–1432.

89. **Poynard, T., J. McHutchison, Z. Goodman, M.-H. Ling, and J. Albrecht for the ALGOVIRC Project Group.** 2000. Is an "a la carte" combination interferon alfa-2b plus ribavirin regimen possible for the first line treatment in patients with chronic hepatitis C? *Hepatology* **31:**211–218.

90. **Prince, A. M., and L. Andrus.** 1992. PCR: how to kill unwanted DNA. *BioTechniques* **12:**358–360.

91. **Reid, R., M. Greenberg, A. B. Jensen, M. Husain, J. Willett, Y. Daoud, G. Temple, C. R. Stanhope, A. Sherman, and D. G. Phibbs.** 1987. Sexually transmitted papillomaviral infections. I. The anatomic distribution and pathologic grade of neoplastic lesions associated with different viral types. *Am. J. Obstet. Gynecol.* **156:**212–222.

92. **Relman, D. A.** 1999. The search of unrecognized pathogens. *Science* **284:**129–131.

93. **Relman, D. A., J. S. Loutit, T. M. Schmidt, S. Falkow, and L. S. Tompkins.** 1990. The agent of bacillary angiomatosis: an approach to the identification of uncultured pathogens. *N. Engl. J. Med.* **323:**1573–1580.

94. **Relman, D. A., T. M. Schmidt, R. P. MacDermott, and S. Falkow.** 1992. Identification of the uncultured bacillus of Whipple's disease. *N. Engl. J. Med.* **327:**293–301.

95. **Ririe, K., R. P. Rasmussen, and C. T. Wittwer.** 1997. Product differentiation by analysis of DNA melting curves during the polymerase chain reaction. *Anal. Biochem.* **245:**154–160.

96. **Rosetti, S., S. Englisch, E. Bresin, P. Franco Pignatti, and A. E. Turco.** 1997. Detection of mutations in human genes by a new rapid method: cleavage fragment length polymorphism analysis (CFLPA). *Mol. Cell. Probes* **11:**155–160.

97. **Rossau, R., H. Traore, H. De Beenhouwer, W. Mijs, G. Jannes, P. De Rijk, and F. Portaels.** 1997. Evaluation of the INNO-LiPA Rif. TB assay, a reverse hybridization assay for the simultaneous detection of *Mycobacterium tuberculosis* complex and its resistance to rifampin. *Antimicrob. Agents Chemother.* **41:**2093–2098.

98. **Rotbart, H. A.** 1991. Nucleic acid detection systems for enteroviruses. *Clin. Microbiol. Rev.* **4:**156–168.

99. **Rys, P. N., and D. H. Persing.** 1993. Preventing false positives: quantitative evaluation of three protocols for inactivation of polymerase chain reaction amplification products. *J. Clin. Microbiol.* **31:**2356–2360.

100. **Saag, M. S., M. Holodniy, D. R. Kuritzkes, W. A. O'Brien, R. Coombs, M. E. Poscher, D. M. Jacobsen, G. M. Shaw, D. D. Richman, and P. A. Volberding.** 1996. HIV viral load markers in clinical practice. *Nat. Med.* **2:**625–629.

101. **Saiki, R. K., D. H. Gelfand, S. Stoffel, S. J. Scharf, R. Higuchi, K. B. Mullis, G. Horn, and H. A. Ehrlich.** 1988. Primer-directed enzymatic amplification of DNA with a thermostable DNA polymerase. *Science* **239:**487–491.

102. **Schachter, J., W. E. Stamm, T. C., Quinn, W. W. Andrews, J. D. Burczak, and H. H. Lee.** 1994. Ligase chain reaction to detect *Chlamydia trachomatis* infection of the cervix. *J. Clin. Microbiol.* **32:**2540–2543.

103. **Schena, M., D. Shalon, R. Heller, A. Chai, P. O. Brown, and R. W. Davis.** 1996. Parallel human genome analysis: microarray-based expression monitoring of 1000 genes. *Proc. Natl. Acad. Sci. USA* **93:**10614–10619.

104. **Schiff, E. R., M. De Medina, and R. S. Kahn.** 1999. New perspectives in the diagnosis of hepatitis C. *Semin. Liver Dis.* **19:**3–15.

105. **Solomon, D., M. Schiffman, R. Tarone, for the ALTS Study Group.** 2001. Comparison of three management strategies for patients with atypical squamous cells of undetermined significance: baseline results from a randomized trial. *J. Natl. Cancer Inst.* **93:**293–299.

106. **Sosnowski, R. G., E. Tu, W. F. Butler, J. P. O'Connell, and M. J. Heller.** 1997. Rapid determination of single base mismatch mutations in DNA hybrids by direct electric field control. *Proc. Natl. Acad. Sci. USA* **94:**1119–1123.

107. **Sreevatsan, S., J. B. Bookout, F. M. Ringplis, M. R. Pottathil, D. J. Marshall, M. Dearruda, C. Murvine, L. Fors, R. M. Pottachil, and R. J. Barathur.** 1998. Algorithmic approach to high-throughput molecular screening for alpha interferon-resistant genotypes in hepatitis C patients. *J. Clin. Microbiol.* **36:**1895–1901.

108. **Stuyver, L., A. Wyseur, A. Rombout, J. Louwagie, T. Scarcez, C. Verhofstede, D. Rimland, R. F. Schinazi, and R. Rossau.** 1997. Line probe assay for rapid detection of drug-selected mutations in the human immunodeficiency virus type 1 reverse transcriptase gene. *Antimicrob. Agents Chemother.* **41:**284–291.

109. **Stuyver, L., A. Wyseur, W. van Arnhem, F. Hernandez, and G. Maertens.** 1996. Second-generation line probe assay for hepatitis C virus genotyping. *J. Clin. Microbiol.* **34:**2259–2266.

110. **Tang, Y. W., N. M. Ellis, M. K. Hopkins, D. H. Smith, D. E. Dodge, and D. H. Persing.** 1998. Comparison of phenotypic and genotypic techniques for identification of unusual aerobic pathogenic gram-negative bacilli. *J. Clin. Microbiol.* **36:**3674–3679.

111. **Telenti, A., P. Imboden, F. Marchesi, T. Schmidheini, and T. Bodmer.** 1993. Direct, automated detection of rifampin-resistant *Mycobacterium tuberculosis* by polymerase chain reaction and single-strand conformation polymorphism analysis. *Antimicrob. Agents Chemother.* **37:**2054–2058.

112. **Tenover, F. C.** 1988. Diagnostic deoxyribonucleic acid probes for infectious diseases. *Clin. Microbiol. Rev.* **1:**82–101.

113. **Tenover, F. C.** 1996. Genotypic detection of antimicrobial resistance. *In* D. H. Persing (ed.), *PCR Protocols for Emerging Infectious Diseases.* ASM Press, Washington, D.C.

114. **Thornton, C. G., J. L. Hartley, and A. Rashtchian.** 1992. Utilizing uracil DNA glycosylase to control carryover contamination in PCR: characterization of residual UDG activity following thermal cycling. *BioTechniques* **13:**180–184.

115. **Tong, C., L. Cuevas, H. Williams, and A. Bakran.** 2000. Comparison of two commercial methods for measurement of cytomegalovirus load in blood samples after renal transplantation. *J. Clin. Microbiol.* **38:**1209–1213.

116. **Tyagi, S., D. P. Bratu, and F. R. Kramer.** 1998. Multicolor molecular beacons for allele discrimination. *Nat. Biotechnol.* **16:**49–53.

117. **Urdea, M., T. Horn, T. J. Fultz, M. Anderson, J. A. Running, S. Hamren, V. Ahle, and C.-A. Chang.** 1991. Branched DNA amplification multimers for the sensitive, direct detection of human hepatitis virus. *Nucleic Acids Symp. Ser.* **24:**197–200.

118. **Vandamme, A.-M., J.-C. Schmit, S. Van Dooren, K. Van Laethem, E. Gobbers, W. Kok, P. Goubau, M. Witvrouw, W. Peetermans, E. De Clercq, and J. Desmyter.** 1996. Quantification of HIV-1 RNA in plasma: comparable results with the NASBA–HIV-1 RNA QT and the AMPLICOR HIV Monitor test. *J. Acquir. Immune Defic. Syndr. Hum. Retrovirol.* **13:**127–139.

119. **Walker, G. T., M. S. Fraiser, J. L. Schram, M. C. Little, J. G. Nadeau, and D. P. Malinowski.** 1992. Strand displacement amplification—an isothermal, in vitro DNA amplification technique. *Nucleic Acids Res.* **20:**1691–1696.

120. **Walker, G. T., M. C. Little, J. G. Nadeau, and D. D. Shank.** 1992. Isothermal in vitro amplification of DNA by a restriction enzyme/DNA polymerase system. *Proc. Natl. Acad. Sci. USA* **89:**392–396.

121. **Walsh, E. E., K. M. McConnochie, C. E. Long, and C. B. Hall.** 1997. Severity of respiratory syncytial virus infection is related to virus strain. *J. Infect. Dis.* **175:**814–820.

122. **Woese, C. R.** 1987. Bacterial evolution. *Microbiol. Rev.* **51:**221–271.

123. **Wu, D. Y., and R. B. Wallace.** 1989. The ligation amplification reaction (LAR)—amplification of specific DNA sequences using sequential rounds of template-dependent ligation. *Genomics* **4:**560–569.

Principles of Stains and Media

KIMBERLE C. CHAPIN AND PATRICK R. MURRAY

18

DIRECT EXAMINATION OF SPECIMENS

The first step in the processing of most clinical material is the microscopic examination of the specimen. Direct examination is a rapid and cost-effective diagnostic aid developed to reveal and enumerate microorganisms and eukaryotic cells. Visible microorganisms may denote the presumptive etiologic agent or a lack thereof, guiding the laboratory in the selection of the appropriate isolation media and the physician in the selection of the appropriate empirical antibiotic therapy. The quality of the specimen and the measure of the inflammatory response can also be evaluated. In addition, the direct smear serves as a quality control indicator for attempts to cultivate observed organisms. The principles of the staining methods used in the direct examination of specimens are discussed in the first part of this chapter. Tables 1 to 3 give brief overviews of all commonly performed staining methods noted in this Manual. Procedures for the performance of tests with the stains are available in the chapters Reagents, Stains and Media: Bacteriology (chapter 27), Virology (chapter 79), Mycology (chapter 113), and Parasitology (chapter 128).

MICROSCOPY: TECHNICAL ASPECTS

Microscopes allow objects not seen by the naked eye to be visible. With light or bright-field microscopes, visible light is passed through the object and through a series of lenses such that the reflected light allows magnification of the object. Three factors are necessary for viewing organisms microscopically: magnification, resolution, and contrast. Magnification for light microscopy is the product of the objective lens (usually $\times10$, $\times20$, $\times40$, or $\times100$) and the ocular lens or eyepiece ($\times10$). Thus, the appearance of objects observed at a low power, such as $\times10$, would be the product of 10 times 10 or 100 times the original size. Resolution, or the extent at which the detail of a magnified object is defined, is a necessary component as well since the resolving power of a microscope needs to allow two bacterial cells to appear as distinct objects to identify them. For light microscopes, resolving power is at its greatest when oil is placed between the objective lens and the smear to prevent the light rays from dispersing as they pass through the smear. The total magnification with the oil lens is 100 times 10 or 1,000 times the original magnification. This

magnification and resolving ability are necessary to view bacteria. Finally, contrast is necessary for differentiation of most bacteria from each other and background material. Contrast occurs most commonly by using dyes or stains (15). Interestingly, the area of field of view, which is determined by field diameter and the ocular lens, may vary as much as threefold, depending on the brand of ocular used (Alex von Graevenitz, personal communication). For example, the Zeiss standard microscope with a Kpl $\times10$ ocular has a field diameter of 1.6 mm and a resulting area of field of 2.01 mm^2, whereas the Olympus BH microscope, with an SWHK 10/26.5 ocular and a field diameter of 2.65 mm, has an area of field of 5.51 mm^2, a greater than twofold difference. The effects of such differences in fields of view on smear screening and interpretation have not been reported.

Phase-contrast microscopy alters the microscopic technique to achieve contrast. Whereas light microscopy uses a staining technique to achieve contrast, phase-contrast microscopy achieves contrast from beams of light passing through different thicknesses of microbial cells or cell structures, with the beams of light being slowed and deflected with various intensities. Phase-contrast microscopy is most commonly used to visualize viable organisms or for fungal identification from culture. Dark-field microscopy also alters the microscopic technique to achieve contrast. In dark-field microscopy the condenser only allows light that hits an object, such as a bacterium, to pass from below upward into the objective. All other light that hits the slide is directed at an oblique angle and not into the objective. This makes the object appear bright and the background dark. The method is used most commonly for organisms with very thin dimensions, such as spirochetes, that cannot be seen by light microscopy (4).

CHEMICAL BASIS OF STAINING

Simple wet mounts, consisting of clinical material in a drop of saline, allow determination of cellular composition, morphology, and motility. However, cellular material and organisms are usually transparent and best distinguished by the use of dyes or biological stains. Antonie van Leeuwenhoek was the first to attempt the differentiation of bacteria with the use of natural colored agents such as beet juice in 1719 (11). Staining procedures and the understanding of the chemical basis of staining developed extensively in the area of histology, where cellular constituents were desired to be more clearly demarcated. The specific chemical bases of many stains are described in detail in older histology texts, including modifications and names of stains that we rarely encounter today in either clinical microbiology or histology (7, 8, 18).

Metachromasia is a characteristic color change which natural dyes (aniline dyes or products of such natural products) exhibit when bound to certain substances either in tissue or in aqueous solution. With the exception of hematoxylin, natural dyes have for the most part been replaced by artificial dyes. Artificial dyes are products of chemical derivatives from substances in coal tar, especially benzene. Two other important chemical groups, the chromophore and auxochrome, complete the dye compound (7, 8).

Chromophoric groups are the group of atoms within a dye molecule responsible for its color. Benzene, an aromatic organic compound, undergoes substitution reactions with radicals to form these new compounds which constitute the dye resonance system. Some of the molecular changes result in a colored product. The most important chromophoric groups are C=C, C=O, C=S, C=N, N=N, N=O, and NO_2. The greater the number of chromophores in a compound, the deeper the color of the compound is. Benzene plus a chromophore group is a chromogen. Although the chromogen is colored and typically ionic, it does not have great affinity for bacteria or tissues, and washing or mechanical processes will readily remove the compound. Thus, this group does not in itself constitute a dye. The molecule must also possess an ionizing group called an auxochrome, which allows the dye molecule as a unit to have affinity (cationic or anionic) to a compound and to function as a dye. The auxochrome group gives the compound the property of electrostatic dissociation or the ability to form salt linkages with the ionizable radicals on proteins, glycoproteins, and lipoproteins on tissue or organism cellular components. This process can occur either directly or through a chelating action of a mordant (8). Commonly occurring auxochromes are amino groups ($-NH_2^+$), hydroxyl groups ($-OH$), sulfates ($-SO_3^-$), and carboxyl groups ($-COOH$). With the exception of the amino groups which ionize to produce a positive charge and are considered basic (cationic), all of these auxochromes ionize to produce negative charges and are acidic (anionic). Some dyes have more than one auxochrome. Even in combinations with basic and acid auxochromes, the negative charge typically predominates (18).

Dyes are usually sold as salts; thus, it is the auxochrome group that usually determines whether a dye is classified as cationic (basic) or anionic (acidic). Most dyes will retain their cationic or anionic properties throughout the pH range of staining (pH 3 to 9) and thus reliably stain those structures that are oppositely charged. For example, DNA phosphate groups and mucopolysaccharides, which are negatively charged and acidic, will be stained with a basic dye. Basic (positively charged) components in cytoplasm will stain with an acid dye. Crystal violet, methylene blue, and safranin are typical cationic (basic) dyes; and eosin, acid fuchsin, and picric acid are typical anionic (acid) dyes.

WET MOUNTS AND SINGLE-STAIN METHODS

Wet-mount preparations are used to determine the cellular composition of a specimen as well as the morphology of organisms, their gross structures, and their biologic activities including motility (Table 1). The specimens can be examined by bright-field, phase-contrast, or dark-field microscopy. True wet mounts do not involve fixation of the clinical material and are viewed immediately upon preparation. Methods performed with a single stain such as methylene blue or iodine enhance visualization of organisms by increasing the contrast of structures and can be performed either as a wet mount or with fixed material (M'Fadyean stain) (3, 12). All organisms and cellular components stain shades of a similar color.

DIFFERENTIAL STAINING

While direct visualization of specimens in various wet mounts is useful, differentially stained specimens are the most helpful for presumptive grouping of the majority of pathogens (Table 2). The Gram stain and acid-fast stain are examples of differential stains. In addition, fluorescent stains (see below) may aid in the identification of organisms when specific attachment of fluorochromes occurs with organism components; auramine, calcofluor white, and fluorescein isothiocyanate (FITC) bound to monoclonal antibodies or FITC bound to protein nucleic acids are examples (13).

In fixed differential smear preparations, four components are typically used in a progressive manner, the primary stain, a mordant, a decolorizing agent(s), and a secondary stain or a counterstain. The primary stain usually stains all cellular components and organisms in the specimen the same color, as seen in simple procedures with a single stain (e.g., methylene blue). The mordant aids in the attachment of a dye to cellular components. Heat, phenol, and iodine are examples of mordants. Decolorizing agents are typically acids and alcohols, such as the acetone and alcohol mixture used in the Gram stain and sulfuric acid used in the modified Kinyoun (modified acid-fast) stain. Removal of the primary stain with the decolorizing agent allows a secondary stain ("counterstain") to be taken up by any decolorized organisms and background material. The secondary stain differentiates between those cells that retain the primary stain and those that do not. Examples include the purple (primary stain) and pink (counterstain) organisms seen by the Gram staining procedure or a pink acid-fast organism (primary stain) seen in a blue-counterstained background.

Gram Stains

The Gram stain is the most commonly used differential fixed stain in microbiology. The Gram reaction, morphology, and arrangement of the organisms give the physician clues to the preliminary identification and significance of the organisms. Gram-positive organisms are thought to retain the crystal violet dye because of the increased number of cross-linked teichoic acids and the decreased permeabilities of their cell walls to organic solvents because they contain little lipid. While the gram-positive organisms take up the counterstain, their color is not altered. The cell walls of gram-negative organisms, because of the higher lipid content associated with the cell wall, show increased permeability to decolorizer, and these organisms lose the crystal violet dye and take up the counterstain dye, safranin (4).

Some enhancement techniques are basic modifications of more standard differential or single-stain methods. These include the use of tartrazine and light green (an enhanced Gram stain; Remel) in place of safranin in the Gram stain and the addition of basic fuchsin to methylene blue (Wayson stain). Many other combinations and manipulations

TABLE 1 Wet mounts and single-stain methods

Direct examination method	Application	Principle	Time required (min)	Advantages	Disadvantages
Wet mount	Direct clinical examination of stool, vaginal discharge, urine sediment, aspirates	Used to detect organism motility and morphology of parasitic forms and fungi	1	Rapid	Limited contrast and resolution; Brownian movement may be confused with motility; experienced microscopist required
10% KOH	Direct examinations of specimens for fungi, e.g., skin scrapings, fluid aspirates	Proteinaceous host cell components are partially digested by alkali; fungal cell walls stay intact	5–10	Rapid detection of fungi	Background material may cause confusion; experienced microscopist required
10% KOH with lactophenol cotton blue	Direct examination of specimens for fungi, e.g., skin scrapings, fluid aspirates	Adds contrast for detection of fungi	5–10	Dye enhances detection of fungi	Background material may cause confusion; experienced microscopist required
Colloidal carbon (Indian ink, nigrosin)	Direct examination of CSF[a] and other body fluids for *Cryptococcus neoformans*	Polysaccharide capsule excludes ink particles producing a halo appearance	1	Rapid; diagnostic in CSF when present	Not as sensitive as cryptococcal antigen; cells and artifacts may cause confusion; experienced microscopist required
Lugol's iodine	Direct examination of stool	Nonspecific contrast dye to help differentiate parasitic cysts from leukocytes; cysts retain dye and appear light brown	1	Rapid, enhances differentiation	Background material may cause confusion; experienced microscopist required
Methylene blue staining	Direct examination of stool for leukocytes; detection of bacteria, particularly poorly staining gram-negative organisms, spirochetes, and *Corynebacterium diphtheriae*	Leukocytes and bacteria stain blue	1 up to 10 min for *C. diphtheriae*	Rapid; enhances differentiation	Leukocytes may disintegrate if stool is not examined promptly; overstaining may mask granules
M'Fadyean staining	Fixed examination of clinical specimens from patients suspected to have anthrax	Methylene blue dye stains *Bacillus anthracis* deep blue and demarcated pink capsule zone	4	Rapid, enhances differentiation of capsule	Staining rarely performed

[a] CSF, cerebrospinal fluid.

exist. See Table 2. The main purpose of these stains is to make organisms that are normally difficult to detect by the Gram staining method stand out more prominently. Typically, these enhancement techniques are used for the better visualization of gram-negative organisms. This is done by two methods. One method is to simply use a stain that will make the organism a darker color so that the normally weakly staining gram-negative organisms are visible (3, 12, 17). A second method is to make the background inflammatory cells and mucus, which often mask gram-negative organisms, a different color than the usual red-pink. This method is used with the tartrazine-fast green stain, which makes the background gray or green and the organism easily visible. In this staining method the Gram reaction of the organisms is

preserved (J. Kee, A. Hill, and K. Chapin, *Abstr. 94th Gen. Meet. Am. Soc. Microbiol. 1994*, abstr. C-242, 1994).

Acid-Fast Stains

The cells of certain organisms contain long-chain (34- to 90-carbon) fatty acids (mycolic acids) that give them a coat impervious to crystal violet and other basic dyes. Heat or detergent must be used to allow penetration of the primary dye fuchsin into the bacterium. Once the dye has been forced into the cell, it cannot be decolorized by the usual acid-alcohol solvent. The acid-fast stain is useful for identification of a specific group of bacteria (e.g., *Mycobacterium*, *Nocardia*, *Rhodococcus*, *Tsukamurella*, *Gordona*, *Legionella micdadei*) and the oocysts of *Cryptosporidium*, *Isospora*,

TABLE 2 Differential fixed staining methods

Differential fixed staining method	Application	Principle	Time required	Advantages	Disadvantages
Gram staining (conventional or Atkins' modification)	Differential bacterial and yeast stains; used to assess suitability of specimen for bacterial culture	Gram-positive organisms retain crystal violet and stain blue; gram-negative organisms do not retain crystal violet and stain pink due to the counterstain safranin	3 min	Rapid; commonly performed; can aid in choice of antibiotic therapy; used to assess specimen for culture and compare smear result to culture result	Organisms with damaged cell walls will stain unpredictably; *Nocardia* and fungi may not take up crystal violet completely; background and cellular elements stain pink, often masking gram-negative organisms
Anaerobic Gram staining variation	Differential stain used to detect anaerobic organisms (especially gram-negative bacteria) not easily seen with regular Gram stain	Basic carbolfuchsin used as counterstain instead of safranin; enhances detection of gram-negative organisms	3 min	Darker staining of gram-negative anaerobes such as *Fusobacterium* as well as other slender gram-negative organisms such as *Helicobacter* and *Campylobacter*	
Tartrazine-fast green Gram staining variation	Differential bacterial stain that enhances detection of organisms because cellular background is green	Use of fast green and tartrazine before safranin counterstain allows significant suppression of red-pink color of the background material; organisms still stain purple (gram positive) or pink (gram negative)	3 min	Allows excellent enhancement of small gram-negative organisms and detection of mixed cultures	Slight change in color appearance of organisms compared with that by regular Gram staining may be confusing
Spore staining (Wirtz-Conklin)	Differential stain for detection of bacterial spores	Spores take up the malachite green stain and the cellular debris and bacteria appear pink from the safranin counterstain	Slides can be stained for 45 min or gently heated to steaming for 3–6 min	Facilitates detection of bacterial spores which may otherwise be difficult to observe; while a heating step is more cumbersome, it enhances uptake of the stain into the spore	Gentle heating of slide may be difficult to control
Wayson staining	Direct examination of CSF[a] and other specimens for bacteria and amebae	A mixture of the dyes basic fuchsin and methylene blue that results in contrast staining between bacteria that stain deep blue and other material light blue or purple	3 min	Rapid, enhances differentiation	Staining reagents unstable; slides cannot be restained with Gram stain
Acid-fast staining (Ziehl-Neelson, Kinyoun, modified Kinyoun)	Detection of acid-fast and weakly acid-fast organisms (e.g., *Mycobacterium*, *Nocardia*, *Legionella micdadei*, *Rhodococcus*, *Tsukamurella*, *Gordona*, *Cryptosporidium*, *Isospora*, *Cyclospora*, and *Sarcocystis*)	Presence of long-chain fatty acids (mycolic acids) in cell wall or cystic forms makes organisms resistant to decolorization; organisms retain the carbol fuchsin dye and appear pink	2 h	Used to detect acid-fast and partially acid-fast organisms; presence generally significant from direct specimens	Low organism number makes slide examination tedious; tissue homogenates often mask presence of organisms because of deeply staining background
Periodic acid-Schiff staining	Detection of fungi, specifically yeast cells and hyphae, in tissue specimens	Combination of acid hydrolysis and staining of cell wall carbohydrates; fungi stain pink-magenta or purple and background appears orange or green if picric acid or light green, respectively, is used as the counterstain	1 h	Most fungi stain	Time-consuming; respiratory specimens must be digested or mucin will also stain pink-magenta

(Continued on next page)

TABLE 2 (Continued)

Differential fixed staining method	Application	Principle	Time required	Advantages	Disadvantages
Toluidine blue O staining	Rapid examinations of lung biopsy imprints and respiratory specimens for *P. carinii*	Background material removed by sulfation reagent and appears light blue; *P. carinii* cysts stain reddish blue or dark purple against the lighter background	20 min	Rapid method for detection of *P. carinii* cysts from appropriate specimen, such as bronchoalveolar lavage specimen	Differentiation of *P. carinii* from yeast may be difficult; cysts often appear crescent shaped; trophozoites are not discernible
Wright-Giemsa staining	Detection of parasites from blood smears, viral and chlamydial inclusions, toxoplasmosis, *P. carinii* trophozoites, *Histoplasma* yeast forms in tissue, *Yersinia*, *Ehrlichia*, and *Rickettsia*	Differential staining of basophilic and acidophilic material; combination of stains allows uptake by multiple structures	10 min–1 h	Detection of multiple organisms and cellular inclusions	Not specific for inclusions (*Chlamydia* is the exception); cannot determine bacterial Gram reaction
Wheatley trichrome staining	Detection of intestinal protozoan cysts and trophozoites	Provides contrast between parasite cytoplasm (blue-green tinged) and internal structures (red or purplish red) and background debris (green to blue-green) by using chromotrope 2R and light green combination	1 h	Permits detection of diagnostic internal structures of protozoa	Helminth eggs are generally stained very dark; human cells, yeast, and artifacts may also stain
Modified trichrome staining (Weber-Green) (Ryan-Blue)	Detection of microsporidia spores	Increase in chromotrope 2R stain concentration and staining time permits detection of pink microsporidial spores	2 h	Permits detection of pink microsporidial spores against a green (Weber) or blue (Ryan) background	Time-consuming staining method
Iron hematoxylin staining (Delafield's)	Detection of microfilaria	Provides contrast so internal filarial structures can be visualized; hematein, an amphoteric dye, when combined with iron, which acts as a mordant, creates an ironically charged dye lake that has affinity for cellular component	45 min	Permits greater detection of nuclei and sheath of microfilaria compared to Giemsa or Wright's stains	Stain not available commercially and involves extensive aging process
Iron hematoxylin staining	Detection of intestinal protozoan cysts, inclusions, nuclei, and trophozoites	Provides contrast between parasites and background debris; cytoplasm will have a blue-gray color, sometimes with a tinge of black; cysts tend to be slightly darker; nuclei and inclusions have a dark gray-blue color; background is pale gray or blue	60 min	Permits detection of diagnostic structures of protozoa	Helminth eggs are generally stained too dark to discern specific structural differences

[a] CSF, cerebrospinal fluid.

Sarcocystis, and *Cyclospora*. A number of modifications have been developed from the original acid-fast stains described by Ziehl in 1882 and Neelsen in 1883. The modifications most commonly used are the Kinyoun and modified Kinyoun (modified acid-fast) stains, which change the dye uptake process and decolorizer, respectively, and are used to differentiate these various acid-fast organisms. The age of the organisms or slight differences in the fatty acids between species alter the stain choice (1, 9; June Brown [Centers for Disease Control and Prevention], personal communication).

FLUORESCENT MICROSCOPY: TECHNICAL ASPECTS

Fluorescent microscopy has become commonplace in most clinical laboratories because of its ease of use in smear interpretation (5, 6, 16). Fluorescence is dependent on the ability of fluorophores (naturally fluorescent substances) or fluorochromes (fluorescent dyes or optical brighteners) to absorb the energy of nonvisible UV and short visible wavelengths, become excited, and emit the energy in the form of longer visible wavelengths. Each fluorochrome has characteristic wavelengths of absorption and emission that yield maximum fluorescence. High-pressure gas lamps of mercury, halogen, and xenon are capable of emitting short-wavelength light that is used with fluorochromes. Halogen light sources have the least excitation power and are not recommended. A series of filters is placed between the light source and the eyepiece. These include a heat filter, a red stop filter that eliminates infrared waves, a wavelength selector or exciter filter that transmits the light of the desired wavelength but that obscures other incident visible light (UV or blue-violet [BV]), and a barrier filter. The color seen depends on the barrier filter(s) used. The type of excitation filter used (UV, visible, or BV light) influences the intensity but not the color. Most fluorescent microscopes use incident illumination or illumination from above that passes through the objective down to the object via a dichromatic mirror beam splitter. The dichromatic mirror has the capability of being able to transmit light of some wavelengths and reflect light of other wavelengths. The light passes through the filters, hits the mirror, and is directed through the objective onto the fluorochrome-stained smear. The longer wavelengths emitted from the fluorescing specimen pass through the objective and the mirror; light passes through the dichromatic mirror because it is now a different wavelength. This emitted light then passes through a barrier filter which blocks scattered excitation light and allows only the longer-emission wavelengths to reach the ocular to form an image. Areas that have bound fluorochrome fluoresce, and other areas appear dark. Fluorochromes in solution may be added directly to clinical specimens or be tagged to other components such as monoclonal antibodies or protein nucleic acids that will result in organism-specific fluorescence.

FLUORESCENT STAINING PROCEDURES
See Tables 3 and 4.

ANTIBODY STAINING METHODS
See chapter 16 on immunoassays.

HISTOLOGIC TISSUE SPECIMEN INTERPRETATION
The clinical microbiologist is often asked to consult on smear interpretation of blood and body fluid specimens and of histologically stained sections of tissue. It should be remembered that most fungi, parasites, viral inclusions, and bacteria in these preparations cannot be identified definitively. For instance, the stain typically used in the hematology laboratory for blood and body fluids is the Wright-Giemsa preparation, which uniformly stains all bacteria blue. Thus, one must not call a blue coccus a gram-positive coccus until Gram staining can be done to help in differentiation. In addition, in stained tissue preparations, pathogens may be significantly different in appearance owing to the staining and fixative practices used in the histology laboratory. For instance, vacuolated areas may give the

appearance of a capsule in a nonencapsulated organism. For the best outcome in the histologic diagnosis of infectious etiologies, good communication between the surgical pathologist, microbiologist, and primary physician will result in the securing of tissue for fixation as well as for culture, and the two methods together more often than not provide the definitive diagnosis.

Histologic preparations often stain organisms similarly to the stains used in microbiology but have been modified for tissue. The Brown-Brenn (Gram) stain and Fite-Faraco (acid-fast) stain are examples of tissue stains where the organisms retain the color appearance seen with their microbiology counterpart (2, 10). Other common tissue stains often viewed by microbiologists include silver stains and the Wright-Giemsa stain. The Wright-Giemsa stain does not stain bacteria or fungi reliably, with the important exception of *Histoplasma capsulatum*, which will stain by Wright staining of bone marrow and peripheral blood. These preparations also stain infected cell culture monolayers and aid in the visualization of viral and *Chlamydia* inclusion bodies and *Toxoplasma* in tissue. Silver stains provide a differential stain that is best for detection of fungi and *Pneumocystis corinii* cyst walls in tissue (14). However, the stain also can detect bacteria and parasites. Differentiation of various yeast forms of *P. carinii* is difficult, and interpretation should be done with caution and in conjunction with the use of other specific stains. Refer to the review by Woods and Walker (19) and older histology texts for a comprehensive summary of the use of cytologic and histologic stains for the detection of microorganisms (7, 8, 18).

PRINCIPLES OF MEDIA
The purposes and descriptions of the media used in bacteriology, virology, mycology, and parasitology are described in chapters 27, 79, 113, and 128, respectively. This chapter focuses on the principles of the media used mainly for the isolation of bacteria.

General Considerations
Many components optimize the growth of microorganisms on media. The basic requirements for a medium include a nutrient source, a solidifying agent (for solid media), a specific pH, and any number of specific additives. The nutritional requirements of most microorganisms are complex. Most utilize an array of nutrient sources including nitrogen, carbon, inorganic salts, minerals, and other diverse substances. While some organisms can utilize a very simple medium such as nitrate or ammonia, most require protein hydrolysates or peptones. Peptones are the most common nutrient additives in media and are water-soluble materials prepared by enzymatic or acid hydrolysis of animal tissues or products and vegetable substances. Meat infusions were the initial growth-supporting components in media, but because they are cumbersome to prepare and lack batch-to-batch consistency, they are not truly defined. However, meat infusions are still used in certain media today. Agar serves as the solidifying agent and is derived from red seaweed. The acidity or alkalinity (pH) of a medium is important because microorganisms have strict pH requirements, with most growing in the range of pH neutrality. Components may be added to a medium for purposes of evaluating the pH. These include dyes that change color at a specific pH secondary to the production of acid or alkaline by-products of the organism and buffers that allow determination of the hydrogen ion concentra-

TABLE 3 Fluorescent staining methods

Fluorescent stain	Application	Principle	Time required	Advantages	Disadvantages
Acridine orange stain	Detection of bacteria in blood cultures, CSF,[a] buffy coats, and corneal scrappings; detection of fungi	Fluorochrome intercalates in nucleic acid in both native and denatured states; bacterial and fungal DNAs fluoresce orange and mammalian DNA fluoresces green with UV excitation	3 min	Sensitive method of detection in blood, CSF, and tissues; detects organisms difficult to see with Gram stain and low numbers of organisms such as *Bartonella* and *Helicobacter*; thick or bloody smears can be used; can Gram stain same slide to confirm result	Cellular specimens with an abundance of DNA may be difficult to interpret; interobserver variability seen with some specimens (e.g., buffy coat smears)
Auramine-rhodamine stain	Detection of mycobacteria and other acid-fast organisms	Nonspecific fluorochromes that bind to mycolic acids and resist decolorization by acid-alcohol (identical to acid-fast stains); organisms fluoresce orange-yellow with UV excitation and use of the secondary potassium permanganate stain	30 min	Allows rapid screening of specimens at lower magnification; is more sensitive than other acid-fast stains; can use other acid-fast stains on the same slide to confirm suspicious organisms	Low numbers of organisms may be difficult to confirm by routine acid-fast procedures
Calcofluor white stain	Detection of fungi, *P. carinii* cysts, and parasites, such as microsporidia and cysts of free-living amebae in clinical specimens	Nonspecific fluorochrome that binds to cellulose and chitin; organisms fluoresce blue-white or green if a barrier filter is used; optimal fluorescence occurs with UV and BV excitation; for eye protection, barrier filters of 510–530 nm are recommended	KOH clearing if necessary, then immediate viewing after adding stain	Can be mixed with KOH to clear specimens such as hair, skin, and nails for dermatophytes; rapid, sensitive, and inexpensive screening test; smears can be restained with conventional stains such as Gram stain	Difficulty in interpretation with cellular specimens that contain fluorescing collagen and elastic fibers; variable fluorescence is seen with darkly pigmented fungi; use with Evans blue helps to suppress green background fluorescence and imparts a red color when BV excitation is used
Fluorescein-conjugated antibodies and probes	Identification of specific organisms in clinical material (*Staphylococcus aureus*); used to confirm specific organism identification from cultures (CMV,[b] *Erhlichia, Francisella*)	Monoclonal antibodies or probes bound to the fluorochrome FITC to detect antigens or nucleic acids for specific pathogens in clinical specimens; pathogens fluoresce apple green or red depending on barrier filters used	1–3 h	Specific organism identification; especially useful for commonly occurring blood culture isolates, *Bordetella, Legionella, Pneumocystis*, and viral identification	Adequate clinical specimen must be submitted if done with direct specimen

[a] CSF, cerebrospinal fluid.
[b] CMV, cytomegalovirus.

tion. Other selective agents, such as antibiotics, dyes, and other nutrient sources, can be incorporated into media for the isolation of a particular organism. Other considerations that allow optimal microorganism growth include the incubation temperature and the gas in the growth environ-ment. Most clinically significant organisms are mesophiles, which means that they will optimally grow at temperatures of between 25 and 40°C. In addition, most species grow optimally in ambient air, but others require CO_2 or the total removal of O_2. Liquid media require all of the ingre-

TABLE 4 Recommended filter sets for flurochrome stains[a]

Manufacturer	Filter set	Excitation (nm)	Emission (nm)	Fluorochrome stain(s)[b]
Leica	13	450–490	>515	AO,[c] AR,[c] FITC[c]
	H3	420–490	>515	AO, AR, FITC
	L4	450–490	515–560	FITC
	D	355–425	>470	CW[c]
Nikon	B-2A[d]	450–490	>520	AO,[c] AR[c]
	B-2H	450–490	>515	AO
	B-3A	420–490	>520	CW
	BV-2A	405–445	>475	CW[c]
	UV-2B	380–425	>460	CW
	B-1E	470–490	520–560	FITC
	B-1A	470–490	>520	FITC[c]
Olympus	B	450–490	>515	AO, AR,[c] FITC
	IB	460–490	>515	AO,[c] FITC[c]
	UV	330–385	>420	CW[c]
Carl Zeiss	01	359–371	>400	CW
	02	330–390	>420	CW
	05	400–440	>475	CW[c]
	09	450–490	>520	AO,[c] AR,[c] FITC[c]
	10	450–490	520–560	AO, AR, FITC
Omega	XF53	490–575	520–620	TR[c]

[a] Listing of manufacturers' recommended filter sets as of July 2002. Continued improvements in this technology will determine the filter sets available in the future. Data provided by Paul Millman, Chroma Technology Corp., Brattleboro, VT (800-824-7663) in collaboration with the individual microscope manufacturers. Users are recommended to call the manufacturers of specific microscopes for clarification. Use of quartz halogen filter is not recommended because of low energy output.

[b] AO, acridine orange; AR, auramine-rhodamine; FITC, fluorescein isothiocyanate; CW, calcofluor white, TR, Texas Red.

[c] Preferred filters, although filter selection is subjective, on the basis of the specific application and the prior staining experience of the microscopist.

[d] The Nikon B-2A filter set is commonly used for FITC, although the manufacturer does not specify this application.

dients and conditions described above but lack the amount of the solidifying agent seen in tube slants or plated media.

Medium Types

Transport Media and Preservatives

Transport media are used in the collection and transport of specimens and were devised initially because fastidious organisms would not survive transport from the bedside to inoculation in the laboratory. Now transport media are even more crucial in providing an appropriate environment for specimens as more and more specimens are transported from distant sites and for long periods of time.

Generally, bacterial transport media come packaged in a plastic tube sleeve or in tubes with a small amount of liquid medium. A single or a double swab attached to a cap is used for collection of the specimen, which is then placed into the tube and secured. The cap allows the swab(s) to be easily removed from the transport medium for inoculation. Generally, transport media provide a nonnutrient source that sustains the viability of both aerobic and anaerobic organisms without allowing significant growth. Most transport media have specific ingredients that accomplish these goals. These include a small amount of agar or sponge to allow a solid base to which the organisms can attach and to reduce desiccation, an indicator oxidation-reduction agent

which shows when oxidation has occurred, and reagents that maintain the pH. Other additives allow the survival of specific organisms, such as sodium thioglycolate for anaerobes or charcoal, which reduces the effects of toxic metabolic products and which subsequently enhances the growth of the pathogens. Other ingredients are added for specific purposes and will be noted below. Transport media generally allow stability of specimens for 6 to 12 h at ambient temperatures and should not be refrigerated since some organisms do not survive at colder temperatures. Refer to the specimen collection chapters for specific organisms (chapters 20, 77, 111, and 126). When the specimen arrives in the laboratory, it should be plated as soon as possible. The material in the swab is extracted and placed onto the medium of choice. Care should be taken to inoculate the material from the swab itself when it is extracted from the tube and not the material that may have been in the swab system, such as gel.

Viruses and chlamydia have different transport requirements. Viral and *Chlamydia* transport media are designed to provide an isotonic solution containing protein, antibiotics to control bacteria, and a buffer to control pH. The media come in 15-ml polypropylene centrifuge tubes that contain approximately 2 to 3 ml of medium, 1-dram freezer vials with up to 2 ml of medium, and a tube and swab form with a gel base. While separate transport media for both viral pathogens and *Chlamydia* exist, more often, laboratories are using systems that can accomplish the culture of both of these pathogens as well as the *Ureaplasma* and *Mycoplasma* groups. The antibiotics used in these media are not inhibitory to either of the bacterial pathogens desired or viruses.

Parasitology transport media are actually preservatives meant to maintain the integrity of the parasite and not to maintain viability. The reagents used in these preparations, as well as propagation and isolation media, are described in chapter 128.

General-Purpose, Enriched, Selective, Differential, and Specialized Media

General-purpose, enriched, selective, differential, and specialized are the general categories of media that are used for growth and cultivation of microorganisms. Each type of medium is not exclusive, e.g., many selective media are also differential media. An example is MacConkey agar, which is selective for gram-negative organisms but which is also differential in that it is used to identify lactose-fermenting organisms. Descriptions of each type of medium follow.

General Purpose

General-purpose media are those media capable of detecting most aerobic and facultatively anaerobic organisms. An example of a medium in this category is sheep blood agar, which is commonly used for the general isolation of organisms directly from primary specimens inoculated onto the agar.

Enriched

Enriched media are media that allow fastidious organisms to grow because of the presence of specific nutrient additives such as hemin. Fastidious organisms may not grow well on general media. An example in this category is the growth of *Francisella* on chocolate agar. *Francisella* does not typically grow on blood agar but does grow on chocolate agar because chocolate agar is supplemented with cysteine.

Selective

Selective media are media that contain additives that enhance the presence of the desired organism by inhibiting other organisms. Most commonly, selection is attained with a dye or with the addition of an antibiotic. Examples include MacConkey agar that contains crystal violet, which inhibits most gram-positive organisms, and colistin-nalidixic acid agar, which contains antibiotics that inhibit most gram-negative organisms. The effectiveness of selectivity varies and is not always complete. Thus, partial breakthrough growth or smaller colonies of the inhibited organisms will grow. In addition, the ingredients that make the medium of a high selective nature may actually inhibit the desired pathogen; e.g., a medium that is selective for *Neisseria gonorrhoeae* (gonococci [GC]) and that contains vancomycin may inhibit some strains of GC.

Differential

Differential media are media that aid in the presumptive identification of organisms based on the organism's appearance on the medium. This can be demonstrated by colony color or a precipitate that forms on or around the colony. Examples include the agars used for the isolation of enteric pathogens, such as MacConkey, Hektoen enteric, and xylose-lysine-desoxycholate agars. In the case of MacConkey agar, lactose fermentation by the organism and exhibition of a bright pink magenta color by the colony mean that the organism is utilizing lactose.

Specialized

Specialized media are those media developed with additives for the purpose of isolating a specific pathogen. Such media include buffered charcoal yeast extract medium (BCYE), which is designed for the purpose of isolating *Legionella* species. Specialized media typically include nutrients that the specific pathogen requires but that are not found in general-purpose or enriched media. In the case of BCYE, cystcine and ferric pyrophosphate are provided. Other examples include virology culture media with essential amino acids that are required for the maintenance of cell lines and growth of viruses and anaerobic media that typically include vitamin K, hemin, and reducing agents.

Anaerobic Media

All general-purpose nonselective anaerobic blood agar media have similar formulations and include peptones, yeast extract, vitamin K (which is required for some *Porphyromonas* spp.), hemin (which enhances the growth of some *Bacteroides* spp.), 5% sheep blood (which allows for the detection of hemolysis), and reducing agents. All allow the isolation and cultivation of both strictly anaerobic and fastidiously anaerobic organisms. The difference in each of the media is the small variation in the peptones used and the inclusion of dextrose in some media as an energy source. These differences may make some of the media better for gram-negative or gram-positive organisms with slight variations in colonial characteristics. However, the differences between media are minimal. Additives used with some of these media allow the media to have both selective and differential properties. Enrichment broths are available in a number of formulations but are increasingly less commonly used for the routine isolation of anaerobes.

Susceptibility Media

While those media used for susceptibility media have multiple uses, they are used for susceptibility testing because the nutritive components, hydrolysate of casein, and beef extract are low in thymidine and thymine contents. Excess amounts of thymine and thymidine can make organisms appear to be more susceptible to sulfonamides and trimethoprim. Adjustment of the concentrations of small ions may be necessary for correct susceptibility reporting. Calcium and magnesium ion concentrations are adjusted to allow correct interpretations of *Pseudomonas* susceptibility results with the aminoglycosides, colistin, and tetracycline.

Mycobacteriology Media

Most of the nonselective media used for the isolation and cultivation of mycobacteria are enriched media that are egg based or agar based and that contain additives with fatty acids essential for growth of the organism. Common additives include albumin, which protects the tubercle bacilli from toxic agents, inorganic salts essential for growth, glycerol as a carbon and an energy source, and malachite green, which partially inhibits contaminating bacteria other than mycobacteria and which acts as a pH indicator. Because malachite green is a photosensitive dye, a medium with this ingredient should be stored in the dark. Mycobacteria prefer moisture, and tubes of media should be tightly sealed before inoculation. Liquid media are used for the recovery of small numbers of organisms and for decreasing the time to the detection of mycobacteria. The broths are also used to subculture stock strains and for other tests, such as susceptibility testing and tests with DNA probes.

Often, when specimens are plated, use of a combination of media enhances the detection of a variety of pathogens. For instance, a sputum specimen for bacterial culture is typically inoculated onto a general-purpose blood agar, an enriched chocolate agar, and a selective and differential MacConkey agar. Knowledge of the specimen source and the patient's diagnosis or symptoms helps to determine the appropriate medium that should be inoculated.

Preparation of Media

When preparing media from dehydrated materials, the manufacturers' instructions should be followed closely. Chemically cleaned glassware and distilled and/or demineralized water should always be used unless specified otherwise. Care in terms of accuracy should be taken when measuring liquid and dry ingredients. Mixing and solubilization of ingredients are typically done on hot plates, with magnetic stir bars placed in the bottom of the flask or beaker. Excessive heating should be avoided. Autoclaving or filtration sterilizes the media. Autoclaving of volumes of up to 500 ml at 121°C for 15 min is adequate. Larger volumes may require up to 20 to 30 min. The stir bars should be removed before sterilization. For quality control of autoclaving, specialized tape or paper is placed on the medium flask at the time of autoclaving. Enrichments such as blood and other labile additives such as filter-sterilized antibiotics should be added aseptically after the base medium has cooled.

Quality Control

The National Committee for Clinical Laboratory Standards has specific requirements for quality assurance of commercially prepared media, as documented in standard M22-A2 (12a). However, these recommendations do not apply to all media. In addition, any medium that is prepared by the user requires its own specific quality control. Storage of media should be in the dark at 2 to 8°C. Storage in the dark is preferred because additives, such as dyes, will deteriorate faster in the light. The date that the medium was received in the laboratory and the medium expiration date should be marked and easily visible when stored. Media should be in use only up to the time of the expiration date. Prolonged or incorrect storage of media, including transport media, can lead to desiccation of the medium, changing the composition of nutrients and selective agents.

REFERENCES

1. **Balows, A., and W. Hausler.** 1988. *Diagnostic Procedures for Bacterial, Mycotic and Parasitic Infection*, 7th ed. American Public Health Association, Washington, D.C.

2. **Cherukian, C. J., and E. A. Schenk.** 1982. A method of demonstrating gram-positive and gram-negative bacteria. *J. Histotechnol.* **5:**127–128.

3. **Daly, J. A., W. M. Gooch III, and J. M. Matsen.** 1985. Evaluation of the Wayson variation of a methylene blue staining procedure for the detection of microorganisms in cerebrospinal fluid. *J. Clin. Microbiol.* **21:**919–921.

4. **Forbes, B. A., D. Sahm, and A. Weissfeld.** 1999. Role of microscopy in the diagnosis of infectious diseases, p. 134–146. *In Bailey and Scott's Diagnostic Microbiology*, 10th ed. The C.V. Mosby Co., St. Louis, Mo.

5. **Harrington, B. J., and G. J. Hague.** 1991. Calcofluor white tips for improving its use. *Clin. Microbiol. Newsl.* **3:**3–5.

6. **Henrickson, K. J., K. R. Powell, and D. H. Ryan.** 1988. Evaluation of acridine orange-stained buffy coat smears for identification of bacteremia in children. *J. Pediatr.* **112:**65–86.

7. **Lillie, R. D.** 1977. The general nature of dyes and their classification, p. 19–39. *In E. H. Stotz and V. M. Emmel (ed.), H. J. Conn's Biological Stains*, 9th ed. The Williams & Wilkins Co., Baltimore, Md.

8. **Lillie, R. D.** 1977. The mechanism of staining, p. 40–59. *In E. H. Stotz and V. M. Emmel (ed.), H. J. Conn's Biological Stains*, 9th ed. The Williams & Wilkins Co., Baltimore, Md.

9. **Luna, J. G.** 1968. *Manual of Histologic Staining Methods of the Armed Forces Institute of Pathology*, 3rd ed, p. 102. McGraw-Hill Book Co., New York, N.Y.

10. **Luna, J. G.** 1968. *Manual of Histologic Staining Methods of the Armed Forces Institute of Pathology*, 3rd ed., p. 217–218. McGraw-Hill Book Co., New York, N.Y.

11. **Marti-Ibanez, F.** 1962. Baroque medicine, p. 185–195. *In F. Marti-Ibanez (ed.), The Epic of Medicine*. Clarkson N. Potter, Inc., New York, N.Y.

12. **Mirrett, S., B. A. Lauer, G. A. Miller, and L. B. Rfeller.** 1982. Comparison of acridine orange, methylene blue, and Gram stains for blood cultures. *J. Clin. Microbiol.* **14:**562–566.

12a. **National Committee for Clinical Laboratory Standards.** 1996. *Quality Assurance for Commercially Prepared Microbiological Culture Media.* Standard M22-A2. National Committee for Clinical Laboratory Standards, Wayne, Pa.

13. **Oliveira, K., G. W. Procop, D. Wilson, J. Coull, and H. Stender.** 2002. Rapid identification of *Staphylococcus aureus* directly from blood cultures by fluorescence in situ hybridization with peptide nucleic acids. *J. Clin. Microbiol.* **40:**247–251.

14. **Paradis, L. L., C. Ross, A. Dekker, and J. Dauber.** 1990. A comparison of modified methenamine silver and toluidine blue stains for the detection of *Pneumocystis carinii* in bronchoalveolar lavage specimens from immunsuppressed patients. *Acta Cytol.* **34:**511–518.

15. **Rose, R. A.** 1982. Light microscopy, p. 1–19. *In J. D. Bancroft and A. Stevens (ed.), Theory and Practice of Histological Techniques*, 2nd ed. Churchill Livingstone, New York, N.Y.

16. **Strumpf, I. J., A. Y. Tsang, M. A. Schork, and J. G. Weg.** 1976. The reliability of gastric smears by auramine-rhodamine staining technique for the diagnosis of tuberculosis. *Am. Rev. Respir. Dis.* **114:**971–976.

17. **Summanen, P. E., E. J. Baron, D. M. Citron, C. Strong, H. M. Wexler, and S. M. Finegold.** 1993. *Wadsworth Anaerobic Bacteriology Manual*, 5th ed. Star Publishing Co., Belmont, Calif.

18. **Thompson, S. W.** 1966. *Selected Histochemical and Histopathological Methods*. Charles C Thomas, Publisher, Springfield, Ill.

19. **Woods, G. L., and D. H. Walker.** 1996. Detection of infection or infectious agents by use of cytologic and histologic stains. *Clin. Microbiol. Rev.* **9:**382–404.

BACTERIOLOGY

VOLUME EDITOR
ELLEN JO BARON

SECTION EDITORS
J. STEPHEN DUMLER, GUIDO FUNKE,
J. MICHAEL JANDA, AND
ALEXANDER von GRAEVENITZ

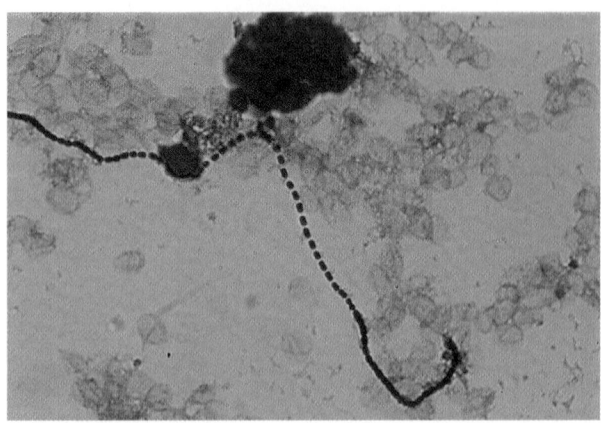

Streptococcus pyogenes.

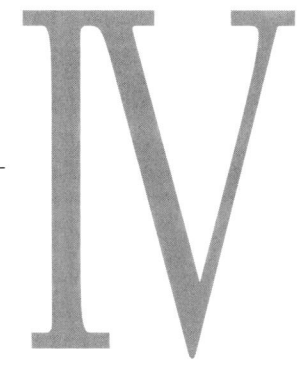

(continued)

Taxonomy and Classification of Bacteria*

PETER A. R. VANDAMME

19

Taxonomy is written by taxonomists for taxonomists; in this form the subject is so dull that few, if any, non-taxonomists are tempted to read it and presumably even fewer try their hand at it. It is the most subjective branch of any biological discipline, and in many ways is more of an art than a science.

With these words, S. T. Cowan introduced a sparkling essay on the sense and nonsense in bacterial taxonomy in 1971 (17). His contributions to the practice of bacterial taxonomy, written in the 1960s and 1970s (14–17), should be read by everyone interested in this field. Taxonomy is generally considered a synonym of systematics and is traditionally divided into classification (the orderly arrangement of organisms into taxonomic groups on the basis of similarity), nomenclature (the labeling of the units), and identification (the process of determining whether an unknown belongs to one of the units defined) (15). During the past decade, it became generally accepted that bacterial classification should reflect as much as possible the natural relationships between bacteria, which are considered the phylogenetic relationships encoded in highly conserved macromolecules such as 16S or 23S rRNA genes (61, 122).

It is true, of course, that every classification is artificial and that boundaries are made by humans. However, classification serves a very practical purpose, i.e., the recognition of organisms that were encountered before. In this era of whole-genome sequence analysis, it is more than ever obvious that the genomes of microbes may change, sometimes considerably. That does not alter our need to identify organisms, particularly in the context of epidemiological studies and surveillance, as identification bears a tremendous amount of accompanying information. Science indeed has a way of making itself useful, and the useful application of classification is identification (14).

CLASSIFICATION OF BACTERIA

The process of species delineation in bacterial systematics underwent drastic modifications as the species concept evolved in parallel with technical progress. Early classification systems used mainly morphological and biochemical

criteria to delineate the species of bacteria. This type of classification was monothetic, as it was based on a unique set of characteristics necessary and sufficient to delineate groups. This early classification concept was replaced by theories of so-called natural concepts, which were the phenetic and phylogenetic classifications (32). In the former, relationships between bacteria were based on the overall similarity of both phenotypic and genotypic characteristics. Phenetic classifications demonstrate the relationships between organisms as they exist without reference to ancestry or evolution. In phylogenetic classifications, relationships are described by ancestry, not according to their present properties.

Special-purpose and general-purpose classification systems are the main categories of classification systems. Special-purpose classification systems are objectively determined and do not fit a preconceived idea. For instance, the separation between the very closely related species *Escherichia coli* and *Shigella dysenteriae* does not conform to the general ideas of present-day species delineation (see below) but fits primarily a practical and historical purpose (32). Yet, nowadays, most taxonomists favor a general-purpose classification system that is stable, objective, and predictive and that can be applied to all bacteria. The classifications obtained with a general-purpose classification system do not fit a single purpose but attempt to reflect the natural diversity among bacteria. The best way to generate such general-purpose classifications is by combining the strengths of both phenetic and phylogenetic studies, a practice nowadays often referred to as polyphasic taxonomy (110).

Criteria for Species Delineation

The criteria used to delineate species have developed in parallel with technology. The early classifications were based on morphology and biochemical data. When evaluated by means of our present views, many of these early phenotype-based classifications generated extremely heterogeneous assemblages of bacteria. Individual species were characterized by a common set of phenotypic characters and differed from other species in one or a few characters which were considered important. The introduction of computer technology allowed comparison of large sets of characteristics for large numbers of strains, forming the basis for phenetic taxonomy (87, 91). Such numerical analyses of phenotypic characters yielded superior classifications

* This chapter contains information presented in chapter 14 by Patrick A. D. Grimont in the seventh edition of this Manual.

in terms of objectivity and stability. Gradually, chemotaxonomic and genotypic methods were introduced into classification systems. Numerous different chemical compounds were extracted from bacterial cells, and their suitability for use in the classification of bacteria and the definition of species has been analyzed.

In 1987, the Ad Hoc Committee on Reconciliation of Approaches to Bacterial Systematics (116) stated that taxonomy should be determined phylogenetically and that the complete genome sequence should therefore be the standard for species delineation. In present-day practice, whole-genome DNA-DNA hybridization analysis approaches the sequence standard and represents the best applicable procedure. A bacterial species was therefore defined as a group of strains, including the type strain, that share 70% or greater DNA-DNA relatedness with a ΔT_m of 5°C or less (T_m is the melting temperature of the hybrid, as determined by stepwise denaturation; ΔT_m is the difference in T_m [in degrees Celsius] between the homologous hybrid and the heterologous hybrid formed under standard conditions [116]). This species definition was based on a large amount of experience in combination with both DNA-DNA hybridization data and other characteristics. The designated type strain of a species serves as the name bearer of the species and as the reference specimen (95). It was also recommended that phenotypic and chemotaxonomic features should agree with this definition. Preferentially, several simple and straightforward tests should endorse the species delineation based on DNA-DNA hybridization values. Groups of strains which were delineated by means of DNA-DNA hybridization studies as distinct species but which could not be distinguished by phenotypic characteristics should not be named. The term "genomovar" was subsequently introduced for such phenotypically similar genomic species (103). However, the latter term may be somewhat misleading, as these taxa are given an infraspecific rank, whereas by definition they are to be considered species that cannot be reliably differentiated by phenotypic tests.

The level of DNA-DNA hybridization thus plays a key role in our present species concept as defined by Wayne et al. (116). Although that seems to suggest that the species definition became less vague, the practice of DNA-DNA hybridization is very complex (see below).

The Polyphasic Species Concept

A wide variety of cellular components have been used to study relationships between bacteria and to design classifications. The information present at the DNA level has been analyzed by estimations of the DNA base composition and the genome size, whole-genome DNA-DNA hybridization, restriction enzyme analysis, and, increasingly, direct sequence analysis of various genes. rRNA fractions have been studied intensively, particularly because they serve as phylogenetic markers (61). Various chemical compounds including fatty acids, mycolic acids, polar lipids, polysaccharides, sugars, polyamines, and respiratory quinones, as well as, again, a tremendous number of expressed features (data derived from, e.g., morphologic, serologic, and enzymologic studies), were all used to characterize bacteria. Several of these approaches have been applied to taxonomic analyses of virtually all bacteria. Others, such as amino acid sequencing, were performed on only a limited number of organisms because they are laborious, time-consuming, or technically demanding or because they were relevant only for a particular group.

The term "polyphasic taxonomy" was coined by Colwell (11) in 1970 and described the integration of all available genotypic, phenotypic, and phylogenetic information into a consensus type of general-purpose classification. It departs from the assumption that the overall biological diversity cannot be encoded in a single molecule and that the variability of characters is group dependent. Therefore, it integrates several generally accepted ideas for the classification and reclassification of bacteria. Polyphasic taxonomy as described by Vandamme et al. (110) is phylogeny based and uses sequence analysis and signature features of rRNA for the deduction of a phylogenetic framework for the classification of bacteria (39, 122). It is recognized that several other macromolecules such as the beta subunit of ATPase, elongation factor Tu, chaperonin, various ribosomal proteins, RNA polymerases, and tRNAs (39, 61) have similar potential. The next step in the process of classification is the delineation of individual species—and other taxa—within these phylogenetic branches. Despite its drawbacks, DNA-DNA hybridization forms the cornerstone of species delineation. However, the threshold value for species delineation should be allowed considerable variation. This polyphasic approach is pragmatic. For instance, *Bordetella pertussis*, *Bordetella parapertussis*, and *Bordetella bronchiseptica*, which share DNA-DNA hybridization levels of over 80%, are considered three distinct species because they differ in many phenotypic and chemotaxonomic aspects (107). In other genera which are phenotypically more homogeneous, such as *Acidovorax* (121), species are defined as groups of strains that have DNA-DNA hybridization levels of at least 40%. It is essential that the boundaries of species demarcation be flexible in order to achieve a classification scheme that facilitates identification.

The application of numerous other types of analyses of genotypic, chemotaxonomic, and phenotypic characteristics of bacteria to the delineation of bacteria at various hierarchical levels represents the third component of polyphasic taxonomy (110). The goal is to collect as much information as possible and to evaluate all results in relation to each other in order to draw useful conclusions. An additional advantage is that, once the taxonomic resolution of these approaches has been established for a particular group of bacteria through the analysis of a set of taxonomically well-characterized strains, they may be used as alternative tools to classify new isolates at different taxonomic levels. A typical example is the application of one-dimensional whole-cell protein electrophoresis as a replacement for DNA-DNA hybridization experiments for the species-level identification of *Helicobacter* species (109). It should be noted that the resolution of these alternative methods is often group dependent. For instance, cellular fatty acid analysis is useful for the accurate identification of strains of many bacterial species to the species level. In other bacterial groups, however, the cellular fatty acid profile may be indicative of the genus or a group of phylogenetically related genera but not of a particular species within one of these genera (110). Within the group of the gram-negative nonfermenting bacteria, this is nicely illustrated by the characteristic fatty acid profiles of members of the genera *Chryseobacterium*, *Empedobacter*, *Ornithobacterium*, and *Riemerella* (the last two genera are of veterinary interest), which are characterized by extremely high percentages (80 to 90% of the total fatty acid content) of saturated branched-chain fatty acids in the *iso* and *anteiso* configurations (111, 112).

The contours of a polyphasic bacterial species are obviously less clear than the ones defined by Wayne et al. (116), and this lack of a rigid definition has been contested as it allows too many interpretations (126). Polyphasic classification is empirical and contains elements from both phenetic and phylogenetic classifications. There are no strict rules or guidelines, and the approach integrates any significant information on the organisms, resulting in a consensus type of classification. Its main weakness is indeed that it relies on common sense to draw its conclusions. The bacterial species appears as a group of isolates in which a steady generation of genetic diversity resulted in clones characterized by a certain degree of phenotypic consistency, by a significant degree of DNA-DNA hybridization, and by a high level of 16S ribosomal DNA (rDNA) sequence homology (110).

Obviously, the species is the most important and, at the same time, the central element of bacterial taxonomy. There are at present no rules for the delineation of higher hierarchical ranks such as genus, family, and order. Although there is an expectation that at the generic level taxa should be supported by phenotypic descriptions (70), in practice, higher ranks are mostly delineated on the basis of 16S rDNA sequence comparisons and stability analyses of the clusters that are obtained. Undoubtedly, the latter has weakened the emphasis on phenotypic descriptions of taxa (126). In polyphasic taxonomy, attempts are made to endorse these phylogeny-driven demarcations by other data. An example is the subdivision of the former genus *Campylobacter* into the revised genus *Campylobacter* and the novel genera *Arcobacter* and *Helicobacter* (34, 108). Although this subdivision was mainly phylogeny based, it was supported by differences in respiratory quinone components and ultrastructural properties.

Major Groups of Bacteria

The tree of life based on comparative 16S rDNA studies comprises three lines of descent that are nowadays referred to as the domains *Bacteria*, *Archaea*, and *Eucarya* (122). The *Bacteria* have been grouped into 23 phyla, which are further subdivided into 28 classes (54). Three phyla, the *Proteobacteria*, the *Firmicutes* (gram-positive organisms with low G + C contents, including *Bacillus*, *Clostridium*, *Staphylococcus*, *Mycoplasma*, and the classical lactic acid bacteria such as *Enterococcus*, *Streptococcus*, and *Lactobacillus*), and the *Actinobacteria* (gram-positive organisms with high G + C contents, including *Bifidobacterium*, *Mycobacterium*, and *Corynebacterium*), comprise the large majority of the clinically relevant species. The *Bacteroidetes* (*Bacteroides*, flavobacteria, and sphingobacteria), the *Spirochaetes* (spirochetes and leptospiras), and the *Chlamydiae* (chlamydias) represent some of the other phyla. A more detailed overview is given by Krieg and Garrity (54) and Ludwig and Klenk (63) in their introductory chapters to the second edition of *Bergey's Manual of Systematic Bacteriology*. That edition is structured in an order based on the topology of the 16S rRNA phylogenetic tree.

The largest phylum by far is the *Proteobacteria*, which contains five main clusters (classes) of genera that are referred to with the Greek letters alpha, beta, gamma, delta, and epsilon (94). The *Proteobacteria* comprise the majority of the known gram-negative bacteria of medical, industrial, and agricultural significance. This phylum includes *Brucella*, *Ehrlichia*, and *Rickettsia* (*Alphaproteobacteria*); *Burkholderia*, *Bordetella*, and *Neisseria* (*Betaproteobacteria*); *Aeromonas*, *Legionella*, and *Vibrio* and the family

Enterobacteriaceae (*Gammaproteobacteria*); and *Campylobacter* and *Helicobacter* (*Epsilonproteobacteria*). The *Deltaproteobacteria* comprise a variety of mainly sulfate-reducing bacteria that have no clinical relevance.

Unculturable Bacteria

The classification and nomenclature of unculturable bacteria that are only minimally characterized by morphological characteristics or by differences in a molecular sequence (71) are outstanding challenges in bacterial classification. The members of the International Committee on Systematic Bacteriology have agreed to recognize a category that formally classifies incompletely described prokaryotes (72). This action was useful and timely because of the increasing involvement of sequencing technology in the characterization of prokaryotes that are difficult to cultivate. *Candidatus* is considered a taxonomic status for uncultured "candidate" species for which relatedness has been determined (for instance, for which phylogenetic relatedness has been determined by amplification and sequence analysis of prokaryotic RNA genes with universal prokaryotic primers) and authenticity has been verified by in situ probing or a similar technique for cell identification. In addition, it is also mandatory that information concerning phenotypic, metabolic, or physiological features be made available. The latter data may serve as a starting point for further investigation and eventual description and naming. A detailed list of items for inclusion in the codified record of a *Candidatus* taxon is provided elsewhere (72). With the increasing application of molecular methods to the assessment of the diversity of prokaryotic populations in nature and to the study of complex symbioses, it was anticipated that numerous *Candidatus* organisms would be recorded (72). There are several caveats. Information derived from 16S rRNA gene sequence analysis may not be sufficient to be sure that the uncultured organism represents a novel species (see below). Also, 16S rDNA sequences are not available for all known bacteria for comparison (this is particularly true, for instance, in the family *Enterobacteriaceae*). Alternatively, morphological characteristics, for example, may not be sufficiently reliable to conclude that uncultured cells represent a novel organism (110).

The practice of providing descriptive information for a *Candidatus* organism that leads to its successful cultivation is illustrated by *Campylobacter hominis* (57, 58). In a first study, the source of partial 16S rDNA sequences obtained by *Campylobacter* genus-specific PCR from human fecal samples was considered to be a new species that could not be cultured by the classical methods of culturing enteric campylobacters. Hence, "*Candidatus* Campylobacter hominis" was proposed (57). As phylogenetic analysis clustered this organism in a group of *Campylobacter* species, some of which prefer anaerobic conditions for optimal growth, application of anaerobic culture conditions in a subsequent study allowed the organism to be cultured and the classical binomial species name *Campylobacter hominis* was proposed (58). Proposing a *Candidatus* species is not required to delineate the appropriate culture conditions, as illustrated by the work of Teske et al. (101). Those investigators described molecular information about the composition of a coculture capable of sulfate reduction that was used to identify, delineate appropriate culture conditions, and, subsequently, isolate the components of the mixture in pure culture: a *Desulfovibrio* strain and an *Arcobacter* strain. However, having a clear working designation in many ways is more practical than having a set of accession numbers to discuss an uncultured bacterium.

CLASSIFICATION METHODS

In principle, all genotypic, phenotypic, and phylogenetic information can be used to classify bacteria. Genotypic information is derived from the nucleic acids (DNA and RNA) present in the cell, whereas phenotypic information is derived from proteins and their functions, different chemotaxonomic markers, and a wide range of other expressed features.

When working one's way through lists of methods, it is of primary interest to understand at which level these methods carry information and to realize their technical complexity, i.e., the amount of time and work required to analyze a certain number of isolates. The list of methods given below is not meant to be complete or to describe all of their aspects. It comprises the major categories of taxonomic techniques required to study bacteria at different taxonomic levels and roughly describes general concepts and applications of those techniques as well as some other considerations. Detailed descriptions of such methods can be found in handbooks such as those by Goodfellow and O'Donnell (32, 33) or Priest and Austin (81).

Genotypic Methods

DNA-DNA Hybridization Studies

At present, the bacterial species concept is generally accepted among taxonomists and DNA-DNA hybridization is acknowledged as the reference method for the establishment of relationships within and between species. As described above, Wayne et al. (116) defined a species as an entity which included "strains with approximately 70% or greater DNA-DNA relatedness and with 5°C or less ΔT_m." Both values were to be considered, and phenotypic characteristics had to agree with this definition. This DNA-DNA hybridization value is an indirect parameter of the sequence similarity between two entire genomes, and it is not yet possible to convert a DNA-DNA hybridization value into a percentage of whole-genome sequence similarity.

Different DNA-DNA hybridization procedures have been described: the hydroxyapatite method (4), the optical renaturation method (20), and the S1 nuclease method (18, 37) have mostly been used. The advantage of the optical renaturation method is that the DNA needs no label, but it has the inconvenience of not allowing ΔT_m determinations and to be insignificant below approximately 30% DNA-DNA binding. The hydroxyapatite method and the two procedures of the S1 nuclease method allow determination of the ΔT_m and were, to some extent, compared to each other (37). It has been shown that the results obtained by these methods give slightly different hybridization values but similar ΔT_m values. A linear correlation between the percent reassociation obtained by the spectrophotometric method and that obtained by the nitrocellulose filter method for hybridization values above 20 to 30% was also reported (44). These classical techniques, however, need considerable amounts of DNA and are time-consuming. New quick methods that consume less DNA have been described (7, 24, 47) and are replacing the classical methodologies (35). As long as DNA-DNA hybridization experiments form the cornerstone of methods for bacterial species definition, there will be a need for a new, more rapid, miniaturized, automated, and standardized method.

Many DNA-DNA hybridization protocols have been described, and it is often not clear if hybridizations were performed under optimal, stringent, or suboptimal conditions. The stringency of the reaction is determined by the salt and formamide concentrations and by the temperature and the mole percent G + C contents of the DNAs used. DNA-DNA hybridizations are often performed under standard conditions that are not necessarily optimal or stringent for all bacterial DNAs. As a standard, optimal conditions for hybridizations should be preferred because the optimal temperature curve for hybridization is rather broad (about 5°C) (110). DNA-DNA hybridization data obtained in different laboratories do not always correlate well, partly because different methodologies give different results (37), but also because hybridization data are not always obtained from studies performed under strictly comparable conditions (optimal, stringent, or suboptimal conditions). Examples of such a lack of correlation are found when one compares the results of DNA hybridization studies among campylobacters (for a review, see reference 110).

Obviously, quantitative comparisons of DNA hybridization values generated by different techniques should be handled with extreme caution. When different methodologies are used, it is safer to distinguish categories of DNA-DNA relatedness, such as "high DNA-DNA relatedness" (denoting relationships between strains of a single species), "low but significant DNA-DNA relatedness" (comprising the significant hybridization levels below the cutoff for a separate species; the depth of this range primarily depends on the technique used), and finally, "nonsignificant DNA-DNA relatedness" (denoting that the degree of DNA hybridization is too low to be measured by the method used).

rRNA Homology Studies

It is now generally accepted that rRNA is the best target for the study of phylogenetic relationships because it is present in all bacteria, it is functionally constant, and it is composed of highly conserved as well as more variable domains (39, 54, 63, 84, 92, 122). The components of the ribosome (rRNA and ribosomal proteins) have been the subjects of phylogenetic studies for several decades. The gradual development of molecular techniques enabled microbiologists to focus on the comparative study of rRNA molecules. Indirect comparison by either hybridization studies (21) or cataloguing of RNase T1-resistant oligonucleotides of 16S rRNA (27) revealed the natural relationships among and within a number of bacterial lineages (19, 122). Later, sequencing of the rRNA molecules gradually resulted in a database of 5S rRNA sequences (123). 5S rRNA was the first rRNA molecule to be sequenced for numerous bacteria because of its less complex primary and secondary structures. A limited number of 16S rRNA gene sequences became available by direct sequencing after cloning of the genes from the bulk of the DNA (62). Sequencing of 16S rRNA with conserved primers and reverse transcriptase (56) was an important advance in bacterial phylogeny and resulted in a spectacular increase in the number of 16S rRNA sequences sequenced.

Nowadays, these techniques have mostly been replaced by direct sequencing of parts or nearly entire 16S or 23S rDNA molecules by the PCR technique with a selection of appropriate primers. These sequences provide a phylogenetic framework that serves as the backbone for modern microbial taxonomy (54, 63). The results obtained and the dendrograms constructed with data obtained from the methods described above are more or less equivalent when one takes into account the specific resolution of each method. However, the larger the conserved elements, the more information they bear and the more reliable the conclusions become. International databases comprising all published and some unpublished partial or complete sequences have been constructed (74, 113). The presence of universal sequence motifs in the bacterial rRNA genes allowed taxonomists to classify unculturable organisms and to perform phylogenetic identifications and to detect individual cells in situ without cultivation (1).

More recently, however, it has been found that rRNA sequence analysis is no longer exclusively used to determine relationships between genera, families, and other higher ranks but often replaces DNA-DNA hybridization studies for the delineation of species in taxonomic practice. In many cases, such application of rRNA similarity data is not appropriate. In 1992, Fox et al. (28) reported that 16S rRNA sequence identity is not always sufficient to guarantee species identity. Indeed, three phenotypically similar *Bacillus* strains exhibited more than 99.5% rRNA sequence similarity (rRNA sequences are considered identical if they differ at less than 5 to 15 positions [28]), while DNA-DNA hybridization experiments indicated that they belonged to two distinct species. Stackebrandt and Goebel (92) reported on the place for 16S rRNA sequence analysis and DNA-DNA reassociation in the present species definition in bacteriology. Their extensive literature review revealed that organisms that share more than 97% rRNA similarity may or may not belong to a single species and that the level of resolution of 16S rRNA sequence analysis for determination of the similarity between closely related organisms is generally low. There is obviously no threshold value of 16S rRNA homology for species recognition (92). However, they reported that organisms with less than 97% 16S rRNA sequence homology will not give a DNA-DNA reassociation level of more than 60%, no matter which DNA-DNA hybridization method is used. In fact, rRNA sequence analysis seemed to rightfully replace DNA-DNA hybridization studies as part of the description of new species, provided that the rRNA similarity level was below 97% and provided that rRNA sequence data for all relevant taxa were available for comparison. However, more recent studies extended the observations on intraspecies 16S rDNA divergence considerably, as differences in 16S rDNA sequences of up to 4.5% were reported among strains of several species belonging to the *Epsilonproteobacteria* (42, 109).

Clearly, one should be prudent in drawing conclusions based on analysis of a single sequence. In 1995, Clayton and colleagues (8) presented a detailed comparison of duplicate rRNA sequences present in the GenBank database with remarkable results. Unexpectedly high levels of intraspecies variation (within and between strains) of 16S rRNA sequences were found. The variability was thought to represent interoperon variation within a single strain, strain-to-strain variations within a species, misidentification of strains, sequencing errors, or other laboratory errors. Critical selection and the use of sequences from databases are required. Alternatively, several other macromolecules have been examined for their potential as microbiological clocks. Among others, various ribosomal proteins (73), the beta subunit of ATPase (60, 63), elongation factor Tu (60, 63), chaperonin (114), and RNA polymerases (129) were shown to be valuable molecular chronometers in bacterial systematics. These alternative macromolecules should be universally distributed among bacteria, they should not be transmitted horizontally, and their molecular evolution

rates should be comparable to or somewhat higher than that of 16S rDNA, which would render them more suitable for differentiation of closely related organisms.

Other Applications of rRNA in Taxonomy
The interesting taxonomic properties of rRNA or rDNA molecules have been exploited in several alternative ways (36, 40, 43). An rRNA operon typically consists of the following components (5' to 3'): 16S, spacer, 23S, spacer, and 5S rRNA sequences. Amplification of part of this operon by PCR assays, followed by digestion of the amplicon with restriction enzymes and the electrophoretic separation of the resulting array of DNA fragments, is referred to as amplified rDNA restriction analysis or rDNA restriction fragment length polymorphism analysis (40). Depending on the target selected, the banding pattern is useful for species-level discrimination (for target sequences that are highly conserved) or for strain typing (for target sequences that are variable). The technique has most of the advantages inherent in the rRNA approach; in addition, it is clearly less expensive and more rapid than direct sequence analysis, and large numbers of strains can easily be examined. This not only renders the method a useful screening tool but also provides a better view of the intraspecies variability of the rRNA operon.

Another rRNA-based approach for the identification and classification of bacteria is ribotyping (3, 36). By this procedure, genomic DNA is digested with a restriction enzyme (or with a set of restriction enzymes). The digest is separated by electrophoresis, and the bands are transferred to a membrane and hybridized with a labeled rRNA probe. This probe may be based on 16S rRNA or 23S rRNA, or both, with or without the spacer region, or on a conserved fragment of one of the rRNA genes. Although designed and mostly used to determine interstrain relationships (36), a fully automated procedure for species-level identification of bacteria is commercially available (RiboPrinter; Du Pont Qualicon Inc., Wilmington, Del.).

Other Genotypic Methods for Bacterial Classification
A range of different genotypic techniques has been used to characterize bacteria at various taxonomic levels. The molar percentage of guanosine plus cytosine (the DNA base ratio or the percent G + C value) is one of the classical genotypic characteristics and is considered part of the standard description of bacterial taxa. Generally, the range observed within a species should be not more than 3%, and within a genus it should not be more than 10% (93). It varies between 24 and 76% in the bacterial world.

During the past decade, a tremendous number of molecular diagnostic methods, most of which are PCR based, have been developed. Most of these generate arrays of DNA fragments that are separated and detected in various ways, and appropriate software has been developed for pattern analysis and recognition and for database construction.

One of these DNA fingerprinting methods, amplified fragment length polymorphism (AFLP) analysis (127), was shown to be very useful for the classification of strains at the species and genus levels. The basic principle of AFLP analysis is restriction fragment length polymorphism analysis, but it uses a PCR-mediated amplification to select particular DNA fragments from the pool of restriction fragments. AFLP analysis screens for AFLPs by selective amplification of restriction fragments. The restriction is performed with two restriction enzymes, which yield DNA fragments with two different types of sticky ends that are randomly combined. To these ends, short oligonucleotides (adapters) are ligated to form templates for the PCR. The selective amplification reaction is performed by using two different primers that contain the same sequence as the adapters but whose sequences are extended to include one or more selective bases next to the restriction site of the primer. Only those fragments that completely match the primer sequence are amplified. The amplification process results in an array of about 30 to 40 DNA fragments, some of which are group specific, while others are strain specific (48).

PCR-based typing methods that use random or repetitive elements as primers have been applied to strain characterization of a wide variety of bacteria (64, 105, 118, 119). In several of these studies, species-specific DNA fragments or patterns have been generated (e.g., for species belonging to the genera *Campylobacter*, *Capnocytophaga*, *Enterococcus*, and *Naegleria* [22, 29]). These specific DNA fragments may be useful as probes for the rapid screening and identification of other isolates. Although primarily applied for infraspecies strain comparisons, these techniques are useful in classification as well.

Phenotypic Methods

Phenotypic methods comprise all those that are not directed toward DNA or RNA and therefore also include the chemical or chemotaxonomic techniques. As the introduction of chemotaxonomy is generally considered one of the essential milestones in the development of modern bacterial classification, it is often treated as a separate unit in taxonomic reviews. The classical phenotypic tests traditionally constituted the basis for the formal description of bacterial species and subspecies, genera, and families. While genotypic data are used to allocate taxa on a phylogenetic tree and to draw the major borderlines in classification systems, phenotypic consistency is required to generate useful classification systems and may therefore influence the depth of a hierarchical line (110, 116). The paucity or variability of phenotypic characteristics for certain bacterial groups regularly causes problems in describing or differentiating taxa. For such bacteria, alternative chemotaxonomic or genotypic methods are often required to reliably characterize strains.

The classical phenotypic characteristics of bacteria comprise morphological, physiological, and biochemical features. Individually, many of these characteristics were shown to be poor parameters for determination of genetic relatedness, yet as a whole, they provide descriptive information for the recognition of taxa. The morphology of a bacterium comprises both cellular characteristics (shape; the presence of an endospore, flagella, and inclusion bodies; and Gram staining characteristics) and colonial characteristics (color, dimensions, and form). The physiological and biochemical features comprise data on growth at different temperatures; growth in the presence of different pH values, salt concentrations, or atmospheric conditions; and growth in the presence of various substances such as antimicrobial agents and data on the presence or activities of various enzymes, utilization of compounds, etc. Very often, highly standardized procedures are required to obtain reproducible results within and between laboratories (e.g., see references 75 and 76).

In taxonomic practice, phenotypic characterization became compromised and sometimes more of a burden than a useful taxonomic activity. Frequently, phenotypic data are compared with data in the literature which were obtained by the use of other conditions or methods. The need for continued phenotypic characterization at every taxonomic level not only to delineate taxa and appreciate their phenotypic coherence but also to evaluate their physiological and ecological functions cannot be denied. A minimal phenotypic description is not only the identity card of a taxon but also a key to its biology. Although accepted as necessary, differential phenotypic characters are often hard to find with a reasonable amount of effort and time.

Numerical Analysis

Phenotypic data were the first to be analyzed by means of computer-assisted numerical comparison. In the 1950s, numerical taxonomy arose in parallel with the development of computers (87, 91) and allowed comparison of large numbers of phenotypic traits for large numbers of strains. Data matrices showing the degree of similarity between each pair of strains and cluster analyses resulting in dendrograms revealed a general picture of the phenotypic consistency of a particular group of strains. As such large numbers of characteristics reflect a considerable amount of genotypic information, it soon became evident that numerical analysis of large numbers of phenotypic characteristics was indeed taxonomically relevant.

Semiautomated Systems

A large number of miniaturized semiautomated phenotypic test systems are commercially available and partially replace classical phenotypic analyses. These microtest galleries can be used for both classification and identification (see chapter 14). They mostly contain a battery of dehydrated reagents. The reaction (growth, production of enzymatic activity, etc.) is initiated by adding a standardized inoculum. These galleries of phenotypic tests offer the advantages of being rapid, simple, and highly standardized. Often, reactions can be automatically read, data are processed, and the results are compared with a library as part of the identification protocol. The manufacturer typically gives recommendations for the age of the cells used in the inoculum, inoculum density, incubation conditions, and test interpretation. Properties of the cells present in the inoculum may be revealed directly within a few hours of incubation (e.g., revelation of preformed enzymes) or may be revealed only after additional growth and metabolism of reagents. Growth can be recorded as the generation of a visible layer of cells or as a color change induced by a pH or a redox change. It should be noted that the outcomes of a particular test obtained with a commercial system and by a classical procedure may be different. This, however, may occur with two classical procedures of the same test as well.

Chemical Methods

The term "chemotaxonomy" refers to the application of analytical methods to the collection of information on various chemical constituents of the cell to classify bacteria. As for the other phenotypic techniques and the genotypic techniques, some of the chemotaxonomic methods have been widely applied to vast numbers of bacteria, whereas others were so specific that their application was restricted to particular taxa.

Cellular Fatty Acid Analysis

Over 300 fatty acids and related compounds are present in bacterial cells. Polar lipids are the constituents of the lipid bilayer of bacterial membranes and have frequently been studied for classification and identification purposes. Other types of lipids, such as sphingophospholipids, occur in only a restricted number of taxa and were shown to have taxonomic value within these groups (49). Fatty acids are the major constituents of lipids and lipopolysaccharides and have been used extensively for taxonomic purposes. Variabilities in chain lengths, double-bond positions, and substituent groups are very useful for the characterization of bacterial taxa (97). Mostly, the total cellular fatty acid fraction is extracted, but particular fractions such as the fraction of polar lipids have also been analyzed.

The cellular fatty acid methyl ester composition is a stable parameter, provided that highly standardized culture conditions are used. The methylated fatty acids are typically separated by gas-liquid chromatography, and both the occurrence and the relative amounts of methylated fatty acids characterize bacterial fatty acid profiles. The procedure usually involves four steps: (i) growth of the cells under highly standardized conditions; (ii) saponification of the lipid components and methylation of the fatty acids in order to convert them into volatile derivatives; (iii) extraction of the methylated fatty acids into an organic solvent; and (iv) analysis of the extract by gas chromatography. The procedure is cheap and rapid and has reached a high degree of automation with a system developed by Microbial Identification Systems (MIDI, Inc., Newark, Del.). Isolates may be identified by using libraries supplied by the manufacturer.

Cellular fatty acid analysis offers many advantages over other phenotype-based identification methods; however, it has several limitations as well. First, the result of the analysis is culture dependent. The strains must be grown under identical conditions in order to compare their fatty acid compositions. Although the conditions recommended by the manufacturer allow cultivation of a large number of bacteria, different sets of conditions and databases are used for different groups of bacteria (e.g., aerobic bacteria, anaerobic bacteria, and mycobacteria). In addition, the level of resolution is organism dependent. Many bacteria may be adequately characterized and identified at the species level by means of their cellular fatty acid profiles. However, others are not, and often, species of the same genus or even different genera have highly similar fatty acid compositions. Whole-cell fatty acid analysis is increasingly used both in taxonomic studies and in identification analyses. The applications and restraints of the technique have been extensively discussed and documented by Welch (117). In the framework of polyphasic taxonomy, cellular fatty acid analysis is often very useful as a rapid and fairly inexpensive screening method. The method allows the comparison and clustering of large numbers of strains with minimal effort and yields descriptive information for characterization of the organisms.

Whole-Cell Protein Analysis

The comparison of whole-cell protein patterns obtained by a highly standardized procedure, sodium dodecyl sulfate-polyacrylamide gel electrophoresis, has proved to be extremely reliable for comparison and grouping of large numbers of closely related strains, and numerous studies document application of this procedure in taxonomic studies (13, 52, 80). Bacterial strains cultivated under highly standardized conditions have characteristic protein compositions that can be separated and visualized by electrophoretic techniques. Mostly, a high degree of similarity in whole-cell protein content is an indication of extensive DNA-DNA hybridization (13, 52, 80). Therefore, an obvious advantage of this technique is that once the correlation between percent similarity in whole-cell protein composition and DNA-DNA relatedness for a particular group has been established, it can replace DNA-DNA hybridization experiments. Provided that highly standardized conditions are used throughout the procedures of cultivation and electrophoresis, computer-assisted numerical comparisons of protein patterns are feasible, and databases can be created for identification purposes. This allows comparison of large numbers of strains and grouping of the strains in clusters of closely related strains (13, 52, 80). For some bacteria, numerical analysis is strongly hindered by the presence of distorted protein profiles or hypervariable (often immunogenic) dense protein bands. In these cases, visual comparison is essential to interpret the similarities of protein patterns.

Cell Wall Composition

The distinction between the gram-negative and the gram-positive types of bacteria is still one of the characteristics that is first analyzed in order to guide subsequent characterization and identification steps. The determination of the cell wall composition has traditionally been important for gram-positive bacteria. The peptidoglycan type of cell wall of gram-negative bacteria is rather uniform and provides little information. The cell walls of gram-positive bacteria, in contrast, contain various peptidoglycan types which may be genus or species specific (83, 97). The most valuable information is derived from the type and composition of the peptide cross-link between adjacent chains in the polymer network. A variable that received little attention is the degree of N and O acetylation of the amino sugars of the glycan chain. The analytical procedure is time-consuming, although a rapid screening method has been proposed. Membrane-bound teichoic acid is present in all gram-positive species, but cell wall-bound teichoic acid is present in only some gram-positive species. Teichoic acids can easily be extracted and purified and can be analyzed by gas-liquid chromatography (25).

Isoprenoid Quinones

Isoprenoid quinones occur in the cytoplasmic membranes of most prokaryotes and play important roles in electron transport, oxidative phosphorylation, and, possibly, active transport (10, 97). Two major structural groups, the naphthoquinones and the benzoquinones, are distinguished. The former can be further subdivided into two main types, the phylloquinones, which occur less commonly in bacteria, and the menaquinones. The large variability of the side chains (e.g., differences in length, saturation, and hydrogenation) can be used to characterize bacteria at different taxonomic levels (10).

Polyamines

Although the role of polyamines in the bacterial cell is not entirely clear, they seem to be important in bacterial metabolism (99). The observation of their universal character and quantitative and qualitative variabilities turned them into a suitable chemotaxonomic marker that can be examined by gas chromatography or high-performance liquid chromatography. Depending on the group of organisms studied, polyamine patterning has been used to trace relatedness at and above the genus level and at the species level.

Other Markers

A range of other chemical markers has been examined in bacterial classification. They include cytochromes, pigments, particular enzymes, sterols, and hopanoids (33). Very often, analytical difficulties have been the main restrictions to their wide-scale application. Novel generations of analytical methods are being developed, such as pyrolysis mass spectrometry, Fourier-transformation infrared spectrometry, UV resonance Raman spectrometry, electrospray mass spectrometry, and matrix-assisted laser desorption ionization–time of flight mass spectrometry (MALDI-TOF-MS) (65, 104). These are all sophisticated analytical techniques that examine the total chemical composition of bacterial cells and thus far have mostly found only restricted application (e.g., see reference 66). However, during the past decade one of these recently developed methods, MALDI-TOF-MS, has become a prominent technique in biological mass spectrometry and has found an increasing number of applications in diagnostic bacteriology. Surface or whole-cell components of a wide variety of gram-negative and gram-positive bacteria have been examined. This technique was shown to have considerable potential for identification of organisms at the genus, species, and strain levels. A comprehensive review of its present applications in bacteriology was recently published by van Baar (104).

IDENTIFICATION

Identification is part of taxonomy. It is the process whereby an organism is recognized as belonging to a known taxon (species, genus) and is designated accordingly. It relies on a comparison of the characters of an unknown with those of established units in order to name it appropriately. This implies that identification depends on adequate characterization.

Identification Strategy

In routine diagnostic laboratories, the majority of isolates are identified by classical biochemical tests and a combination of intuition and stepwise analysis of the results that are obtained. However, if an organism is not readily identified in a minimal amount of time and at a minimal expense, it often remains unidentified. Such strains must be identified without a clue to their phylogenetic affiliation, and this often occurs in the research setting. Undoubtedly, comparison of (nearly) entire 16S rDNA sequences is one of the most powerful tools for establishment of the phylogenetic neighborhood of an unknown organism, and commercial identification systems based on analysis of rRNA gene sequences have become available (e.g., MicroSeq 500 and 16S rDNA Bacterial Sequencing kit [Perkin-Elmer Applied Biosystems, Foster City, Calif.]). A fraction of the 5'-terminal region of 16S rDNA (positions 60 to 110 of the *Escherichia coli* numbering system) is one of the most informative or discriminating regions for the differentiation of closely related organisms (63). Similar variable regions (flanked by highly conserved regions) occur in the 23S rDNA (106). However, many taxonomic studies have revealed that this approach is often not sensitive enough to identify strains to the species level (see above). There is clearly a lack of knowledge not only of the strain-to-strain variation within a species but also of the interoperon variation within a single strain. Therefore, concluding that an unidentified isolate belongs to a particular species because it shares a high percentage of its 16S rRNA gene sequence

with that particular species or concluding that it represents a novel species because it occupies a unique position in the phylogenetic tree or because it shares only 97% of its 16S rDNA sequence with its closest neighbor is premature in the absence of appropriate complementary data. This is even more true for partial sequence data, as partial rRNA gene sequences carry only limited information about the molecule and different parts of the gene may carry information for different taxonomic levels (61, 63).

Alternative Approaches

As part of identification strategies, dichotomous keys based on morphological and biochemical characteristics have only partly been replaced by other methods. As described above, taxonomic analyses provided an impressive array of alternative techniques derived from analytical biochemistry and molecular biology for examination of numerous cellular compounds (32, 33, 81). Each of these parameters is useful for characterization and, hence, identification of bacteria. Databases of rRNA sequences, whole-cell fatty acid components, ribotyping profiles, or miniaturized series of phenotypic characteristics are available (see above and chapter 14) and allow identification of many isolates. Yet, the success of these databases also depends on the exactness of the methods and how carefully the individual entries have been delineated. The classification of new or unusual isolates will, however, often require a polyphasic approach, whereby an unknown is allocated to a certain phylogenetic neighborhood (typically by using 16S rDNA sequence analysis), followed by a comparison of characteristics of the unknown with those of its closest phylogenetic neighbors by using appropriate taxonomic tools in order to assign it a particular species rank.

Molecular Diagnostics

The information content of the rRNA cistrons and other genomic information have been used in several alternative ways for the identification of bacteria by the development of a range of DNA or RNA probes and amplification assays. Although the overall rRNA sequence similarity may be very high, the presence of variable regions in 16S or 23S RNA genes can provide the basis for specific and sensitive targets for identification purposes (e.g., see references 61, 85, and 106). During the last 20 years DNA technology has emerged and the tools of molecular biology are now used for the detection, characterization, and identification of bacteria. The first applications were labeled probes intended to hybridize with specific nucleic acid fragments. Later, in vitro nucleic acid amplification procedures were developed. It was thought that this enzymatic duplication and amplification of specific nucleic acid sequences would gradually replace culture-based approaches. However, it rapidly became clear that the molecular diagnostic approach has its own difficulties in terms of sensitivity, specificity, turnaround time, and cost. As a consequence, its application must be restricted to the solution of these problems in cases in which it is superior to the conventional approach (46). Molecular diagnostic techniques are indicated for the detection of organisms that cannot be grown in vitro or for which current culture techniques are too insensitive or for the detection of organisms that require sophisticated media or cell cultures and/or prolonged incubation times.

The basic principle of any molecular diagnostic test is the detection of a specific nucleic acid sequence by hybridization to a complementary sequence of DNA or RNA, a probe, followed by detection of the hybrid (61). There are two types of molecular diagnostic techniques: those in which the hybrids are not amplified prior to detection and those in which they are. With the probe technology not involving amplification, the probes used for the detection of complementary nucleic acid sequences are labeled with enzymes, chemiluminescent moieties, radioisotopes, or antigenic substrates (45). This technology was first applied in the field of infectious diseases for the detection of enterotoxigenic *E. coli* in stool samples by DNA hybridization after growth on MacConkey agar plates (68). This application illustrated the major advantage of the technology: in a mixture of pathogenic and nonpathogenic bacteria belonging to the same species present in the same specimen and difficult to distinguish by traditional culture and identification techniques, the former species could be easily detected and identified (45).

Alternatively, any DNA fragment can be copied by using a DNA polymerase, provided that some sequence data are known for the design of appropriate primers. In vitro DNA replication was made possible in 1959 when Kornberg (53) discovered DNA polymerase I, but only in 1986 did Mullis and coworkers (69) introduce the idea of PCR, i.e., reiteration of the process of DNA polymerization, leading to an exponential increase in the amount of nucleic acid. Alternative nucleic acid amplification techniques have been developed by using different enzymes and strategies, but they are all based on reiterative reactions. In most of these the target nucleic acid is amplified; in some, the probe is multiplied (12, 31, 38, 55, 115). The advantages of these amplification systems are obvious: they can be highly specific and rapid, and they have very high sensitivities. However, there are many practical problems as well (chapter 17; see also references 45 and 46).

Immunological Techniques

Immunoassays are procedures which measure antigen or antibody levels to determine whether patients are infected or are immunologically responding to infection or immunization. Two general approaches are distinguished: testing for specific microbial antigens and testing for specific microbial antigen-specific antibodies. These immunological techniques are described in detail in chapter 16. An important advantage of immunoassays is that they provide information even when culture and Gram staining results are negative for patients who received antimicrobial therapy.

Conclusion

At present, the scientifically and economically ideal identification technique remains beyond reach. Cowan's (14) intuitive approach (which is used when the identity of the unknown is anticipated) and the stepwise method (which involves the use of dichotomous keys) suffice for numerous isolates and require only simple, rapid, and cheap biochemical tests. Cowan's views are easily adapted to modern methodology. If this first-line approach fails, alternative procedures are required and available. At present, complete 16S rDNA sequence analysis is the most straightforward and obvious choice for establishment of a rough identity of an isolate, although in the present species concept, which is dominated by DNA-DNA hybridization levels, it fails to differentiate closely related species. Much of its superiority is based on its capacity to reveal the phylogenetic neighborhood of the organism studied, which is information not provided by any of the other current identification protocols. This information will direct the additional analyses required for final species-level identification.

NOMENCLATURE

Valid Publication of Bacterial Names

The International Code of Nomenclature of Bacteria (88) includes rules on how to name bacteria at different taxonomic ranks. The aim of nomenclature is that an organism is tagged with a unique name that carries valuable information. Prior to 1980, a proposal of a new bacterial taxon could be validly published in any microbiological book or journal, and the authors of the relevant sections of the successive editions of *Bergey's Manual of Determinative Bacteriology* had to attempt to give a complete list of the members of any particular genus or group of genera. The unavailability of type strains and the fact that microbiologists from different disciplines were not always familiar with each other's work caused great difficulty. All too often another worker would discover several years later that "his" or "her" organism had in fact been described earlier under a different name. This is nicely exemplified by the early taxonomic history of the organism now known as *Burkholderia cepacia*. This bacterium was first described as *Pseudomonas cepacia* by Walter Burkholder in 1950 as the phytopathogen responsible for bacterial rot of onions (5). In their seminal taxonomic study published in the 1960s, Stanier and colleagues (96) noted the extraordinary metabolic versatility of another novel pseudomonad for which they proposed the name *Pseudomonas multivorans*. The latter novel species was an environmental organism, mainly isolated from soil and water samples. A few years later Ballard and coworkers (2) reported on the synonymy between *P. cepacia* and *P. multivorans*. Nomenclatural priority was given to the former, as it was the oldest validly described species. In the same year, Jonsson (50) proposed the name *Pseudomonas kingii* for CDC group EO-1 (eugonic oxidizer group 1), an opportunistic human pathogen. Subsequent taxonomic analyses by Snell et al. (90) and Samuels et al. (82) again revealed that this novel organism was the same as *P. cepacia*, and nomenclatural priority was again given to the latter.

To overcome such problems and others, 1 January 1980 was chosen as a new starting date for bacterial nomenclature. At that time Approved Lists of Bacterial Names were published on behalf of the Judicial Commission of the International Committee on Systematic Bacteriology (86). Only those names included on these lists had standing in bacterial nomenclature, and names of taxa were to be included only if they were adequately described and if a type strain was available. From then onwards, all new names were validly published only in the *International Journal of Systematic Bacteriology* (now the *International Journal of Systematic and Evolutionary Microbiology*). Names could effectively be published in other journals and then validated subsequently by announcement in Validation Lists in the *International Journal of Systematic and Evolutionary Microbiology*. A number of organisms were involuntarily omitted from the Approved Lists and were revived later (for instance, see reference 78). After 1980, several updates of these lists were published in the form of Validation Lists, and in 1989, an update of all names validly published between 1 January 1980 and 1 January 1989 was published by Moore and Moore (67). Nowadays, complete overviews of validly published names can easily be obtained through Internet sites such as http://www.dsmz.de/bactnom/general.htm or http://www.bacterio.cict.fr/. Proposals of new taxa can continue to be made in any journal, but their names are only validated the moment that they are included in one of the Validation Lists, published regularly in the *International Journal of Systematic and Evolutionary Microbiology*. In case different names for the same organism are validly published, nomenclatural priority goes to the name that was validated first. As a result of this practice, all valid species in any particular group can easily be traced and reference strains are available.

Why Do Names Change?

There are, of course, more important causes for the modification of bacterial names than the occasional detection of synonymy. As described above, our present view on bacterial classification is phylogeny based. With the advent of rRNA-DNA hybridization and, subsequently, the various rDNA sequencing methods, taxonomists had a new framework in which they could revise classification schemes. The classical—and extreme—example is the revision of the taxonomy and nomenclature of the genus *Pseudomonas*, which has been proceeding painstakingly slowly for the past three decades. The most important reason for this slow progress is that through the work of De Vos and De Ley (23), it became clear that the genus *Pseudomonas* consisted not merely of five major species clusters (79) but that these clusters formed a polyphyletic part of a major group of bacteria now known as the *Proteobacteria*. Revision of the taxonomy of the pseudomonads had to consider the relationships of the various subbranches toward their numerous respective neighbors (51).

The modification of our view on classification is by far the most important reason for name changes. However, various forms of poor taxonomic practice also invoke many changes and, hence, irritation. As observed before (17), nomenclature often is "the generator of heat, bad temper and ill-will among taxonomists and every kind of microbiologists." The classification (and identification) of *Helicobacter* species represents a fine example of the difficulties encountered in our present-day view on taxonomy. Although often challenged, the level of DNA-DNA hybridization and not the level of 16S rRNA gene sequence similarity is the most critical parameter for species delineation. Relatively few laboratories have the experience required to perform DNA-DNA hybridization experiments in a highly standardized way. Yet, because of the tremendous clinical relevance of these bacteria, numerous investigators study all sorts of *Helicobacter*-like organisms from human and animal hosts. It is clear that the degree of biodiversity within the genus *Helicobacter* is very high and that there is a need for many DNA-DNA hybridization data to delineate the species. Regrettably, helicobacters mostly are fastidious organisms, and many are difficult (and some nearly impossible) to culture in vitro; in addition, the preparation of sufficient DNA for the hybridization experiments is a hardy, if not impossible, task. In practice, new species are often described on the basis of 16S rRNA gene sequence data and a limited number of phenotypic characteristics. A recent study that involved various taxonomic approaches, including DNA-DNA hybridization experiments, demonstrated that comparison of nearly complete 16S rDNA sequences combined with minimal biochemical characterization does not provide conclusive evidence for species-level identification and may prove highly misleading (109). Two presumed novel *Helicobacter* species were indeed identified as

Helicobacter cinaedi, which is one of the longest-known and most widely distributed *Helicobacter* species.

Another example is the gradual revision of the classification and nomenclature of group II pseudomonads. In 1992, Yabuuchi et al. (124) reclassified several rRNA group II pseudomonads as *Burkholderia* species. However, in that study only some of the rRNA group II pseudomonads were examined and the conclusions were based on data for only a limited set of strains. As a consequence, several additional rounds of name changes were required to reclassify the remaining rRNA group II pseudomonads as *Burkholderia* species (30, 102, 125, 128). This group of bacteria also serves as an example that illustrates two more causes for name changes: the lack of criteria for genus delineation (two of the *Burkholderia* species [*Burkholderia solanacearum* and *Burkholderia pickettii*] were again reclassified into the new genus *Ralstonia* [30, 125]) and the intrinsically inadequate description of species that comprise only a single isolate. The lack of precise guidelines for genus-level delineation was discussed recently by Young (126), who argued strongly for phenotypic coherence at the genus level that would have priority over phylogenetic information.

The so-called one-strain taxa (species or genera that are proposed on the basis of data for only one strain) have probably caused more problems than they solved, and this is definitely the case in the context of diagnostic microbiology. It is impossible to estimate the variability of the phenotype in the case of a species with one strain or in the case of a genus with one species and one strain, for which many recent examples exist. The question of whether such strains can be validly named has been the subject of many debates. There are different views, each with advantages and disadvantages. In diagnostic microbiology, it is well known that a species is characterized by a certain degree of variability. This variability can be measured by both phenotypic and genotypic criteria and may be revealed by simple biochemical testing or sophisticated genomic fingerprinting techniques. In the absence of sufficient strains for quantitation of the range of divergence within a species, it will be difficult or impossible to identify new isolates of this organism without DNA-DNA hybridization experiments. A classification based on results obtained with a single strain cannot be stable. Indeed, the detection of a second strain will inevitably necessitate revision of the original species description. The problem is best illustrated with a practical example. In 1994, the name *Burkholderia vandii* was proposed for a single isolate obtained from the roots of an orchid. DNA-DNA hybridization experiments were performed in two distinct studies: one reported a 57% level of hybridization to the *Burkholderia plantarii* type strain (102), and the second reported a value of 77% (9). In the first study, various phenotypic characteristics of the *B. plantarii* type strain were compared with those of the single orchid isolate. Several differences were found. The second study included several reference strains of *B. plantarii* and concluded that the differences in phenotypic characteristics that they detected were often among the characteristics that showed intraspecies variability. Moreover, the chemotaxonomic data did not reveal such differences.

Clearly, the examples of nomenclatural modifications described above could have been avoided, and that is the main reason why they jeopardize the credibility of taxonomists in the microbiology community. As a concluding remark, it should be mentioned that there is no "undo" function in bacterial nomenclature. A name that was validly published remains valid regardless of the number of modifications that it underwent thereafter. For instance, the changes of the name *Pseudomonas maltophilia* to *Xanthomonas maltophilia* (98) and, finally, *Stenotrophomonas maltophilia* (77) or the changes of the name *Pseudomonas acidovorans* to *Comamonas acidovorans* (100) and, finally, *Delftia acidovorans* (120) may be reasonable to some taxonomists, but the changes, particularly the most recent changes, have been refuted by many clinical microbiologists. As these six names were proposed and conform to the rules of bacterial nomenclature, they were all validated, and the use of each of them is correct and valid. Use of the original *Pseudomonas* names could imply that the user disagrees with the phylogenetic rationale for present-day genus-level classification. Use of the name *X. maltophilia* or *C. acidovorans* may simply indicate that one disagrees with the most recent modification, whether the reason is scientific, practical, or a simple statement of discord with successive and excessive name changes.

CONCLUSION

A much broader range of taxonomic studies of bacteria has gradually replaced the former reliance upon morphological, physiological, and biochemical characterizations. This polyphasic taxonomy takes into account all available phenotypic and genotypic information and integrates it in a consensus type of classification, framed in a general phylogeny derived from 16S rRNA sequence analysis. The bacterial species appears as a group of isolates which originated from a common ancestor population in which a steady generation of genetic diversity resulted in clones that had different degrees of recombination and that were characterized by a certain degree of phenotypic consistency, a significant degree of DNA-DNA hybridization, and a high degree of 16S rDNA sequence similarity (110).

The majority of bacteria in routine diagnostic laboratories will continue to be identified by classical methods, as these methods are adequate, cheap, readily available, and easy to handle. In the case of new or atypical isolates or in many research groups in which, for example, bacteria are isolated from new sources, a straightforward means of identification of microorganisms by a single method is often not possible and several methods are needed. The most direct approach is first to allocate such isolates in the phylogenetic framework and then to determine the finer relationships by means of a polyphasic approach. This tendency of identification to become polyphasic is an unavoidable reality.

In some cases, the consensus classification is a compromise that contains a minimum of contradictions. It is thought that the more parameters that become available in the future, the more polyphasic classification will gain stability. Although the idea is purely speculative at present, insight into the vast amount of data that are potentially available could be the basis for a perfectly reliable and stable classification system. However, already with our present data, it is sometimes unclear if it makes sense to order bacteria into a classification system. Undoubtedly, there is a huge amount of biodiversity which can be handled in a practical manner only if it is arrayed in an ordered structure, artificial or not, with appropriate terms for communication.

Our present view on classification reflects the best science of this time. The same was true in the past, when only data from morphological and biochemical analyses were available. The main perspective in bacterial taxonomy is that technological progress will dominate and drastically influence methodology, as it always has. More data will become available, more bacteria will be detected (whether they can be cultivated or not), there will be more automation, and bioinformatics will have to address the combination and linking of databases. Most importantly, we will have increasing access to whole-genome sequences, including sequences of highly conserved genes and others. This is a new type of information that is accessible to microbial taxonomy. It is encouraging that the phylogeny constructed by using the gene contents of some 12 completely sequenced bacteria correlated well with the phylogeny based on the 16S rDNA sequences from the same species (26). Comparative studies on overall gene content (89) and genome signatures (6) have begun to appear. These first studies revealed that horizontal gene transfer, although important for the microevolution of an individual clone, has only a limited role in determination of the overall gene contents of genomes. It was also shown that phylogenies based on sequences of genes participating in housekeeping functions may differ from those based on informational genes (such as transcription- and translation-related genes) (26, 41). In future taxonomic studies there will be a major role for DNA chip technology to cope with the need to examine many isolates within a single species (59).

It is a formidable challenge to use this information to evaluate classifications that have been carefully designed. It is not unlikely that microbial classification will change again when new and better insights are obtained.

REFERENCES

1. **Amann, R. I., W. Ludwig, and K.-H. Schleifer.** 1995. Phylogenetic identification and in situ detection of individual microbial cells without cultivation. *Microbiol. Rev.* **59:**143–169.
2. **Ballard, R. W., N. J. Palleroni, M. Doudoroff, and R. Y. Stanier.** 1970. Taxonomy of the aerobic pseudomonads: *Pseudomonas cepacia, P. marginata, P. alliicola* and *P. caryophylli. J. Gen. Microbiol.* **60:**199–214.
3. **Bingen, E. H., E. Denamur, and J. Elion.** 1994. Use of ribotyping in epidemiological surveillance of nosocomial outbreaks. *Clin. Microbiol. Rev.* **7:**311–327.
4. **Brenner, D. J., G. R. Fanning, A. V. Rake, and K. E. Johnson.** 1969. Batch procedure for thermal elution of DNA from hydroxyapatite. *Anal. Biochem.* **28:**447–459.
5. **Burkholder, W. H.** 1950. Sour skin, a bacterial rot of onion bulbs. *Phytopathology* **40:**115–117.
6. **Campbell, A., J. Mrazek, and S. Karlin.** 1999. Genome signature comparisons between prokaryote, plasmid, and mitochondrial DNA. *Proc. Natl. Acad. Sci. USA* **96:**9184–9189.
7. **Christensen, H., O. Angen, R. Mutters, J. E. Olsen, and M. Bisgaard.** 2000. DNA-DNA hybridization determined in micro-wells using covalent attachment of DNA. *Int. J. Syst. Evol. Microbiol.* **50:**1095–1102.
8. **Clayton, R. A., G. Sutton, P. S. Hinkle, C. Bult, and C. Fields.** 1995. Intraspecific variation in small-subunit rRNA sequences in GenBank: why single sequences may not adequately represent prokaryotic taxa. *Int. J. Syst. Bacteriol.* **45:**595–599.
9. **Coenye, T., B. Holmes, K. Kersters, J. R. W. Govan, and P. Vandamme.** 1999. *Burkholderia cocovenenans* (van Damme et al. 1960) Gillis et al. 1995 and *Burkholderia vandii* Urakami et al. 1994 are junior subjective synonyms of *Burkholderia gladioli* (Severini 1913) Yabuuchi et al. 1993 and *Burkholderia plantarii* (Azegami et al. 1987) Urakami et al. 1994, respectively. *Int. J. Syst. Bacteriol.* **49:**37–42.

10. **Collins, M. D.** 1994. Isoprenoid quinones, p. 265–311. *In* M. Goodfellow and A. G. O'Donnell (ed.) *Modern Microbial Methods. Chemical Methods in Prokaryotic Systematics.* John Wiley & Sons, Ltd., Chichester, United Kingdom.

11. **Colwell, R. R.** 1970. Polyphasic taxonomy of the genus *Vibrio*: numerical taxonomy of *Vibrio cholerae, Vibrio parahaemolyticus* and related *Vibrio* species. *J. Bacteriol.* **104:** 410–433.

12. **Compton, J.** 1991. Nucleic acid sequence-based amplification. *Nature (London)* **350:**91–92.

13. **Costas, M.** 1992. Classification, identification, and typing of bacteria by the analysis of their one-dimensional polyacrylamide gel electrophoretic protein patterns, p. 351–408. *In* A. Chambrach, M. J. Dunn, and B. J. Radola (ed.), *Advances in Electrophoresis,* vol. 5. VCH Verlagsgesellschaft, Weinheim, Germany.

14. **Cowan, S. T.** 1965. Principles and practice of bacterial taxonomy—a forward look. *J. Gen. Microbiol.* **39:**143–153.

15. **Cowan, S. T.** 1968. *A Dictionary of Microbial Taxonomic Usage.* Oliver & Boyd, Edinburgh, United Kingdom.

16. **Cowan, S. T.** 1970. Heretical taxonomy for bacteriologists. *J. Gen. Microbiol.* **61:**145–154.

17. **Cowan, S. T.** 1971. Sense and nonsense in bacterial taxonomy. *J. Gen. Microbiol.* **67:**1–8.

18. **Crosa, J. H., D. J. Brenner, and S. Falkow.** 1973. Use of a single-strand specific nuclease for analysis of bacterial and plasmid deoxyribonucleic acid homo- and heteroduplexes. *J. Bacteriol.* **115:**904–911.

19. **De Ley, J.** 1992. The *Proteobacteria:* ribosomal RNA cistron similarities and bacterial taxonomy, p. 2111–2140. *In* A. Balows, H. G. Trüper, M. Dworkin, W. Harder, and K.-H. Schleifer (ed.), *The Prokaryotes,* vol. 2, 2nd ed. Springer-Verlag, Berlin, Germany.

20. **De Ley, J., H. Cattoir, and A. Reynaerts.** 1970. The quantitative measurement of DNA hybridization from renaturation rates. *Eur. J. Biochem.* **12:**133–142.

21. **De Ley, J., and J. De Smedt.** 1975. Improvements of the membrane filter method for DNA:rRNA hybridization. *Antonie Leeuwenhoek J. Microbiol. Serol.* **41:**287–307.

22. **Descheemaeker, P., C. Lammens, B. Pot, P. Vandamme, and H. Goossens.** 1997. Evaluation of arbitrarily primed PCR analysis and pulsed-field gel electrophoresis of large genomic DNA fragments for identification of enterococci important in human medicine. *Int. J. Syst. Bacteriol.* **47:** 555–561.

23. **De Vos, P., and J. De Ley.** 1983. Intra- and intergeneric similarities of *Pseudomonas* and *Xanthomonas* ribosomal ribonucleic acid cistrons. *Int. J. Syst. Bacteriol.* **33:**487–509.

24. **Ezaki, T., Y. Hashimoto, and E. Yabuuchi.** 1989. Fluorometric deoxyribonucleic acid-deoxyribonucleic acid hybridization in microdilution wells as an alternative to membrane filter hybridization in which radioisotopes are used to determine genetic relatedness among bacterial strains. *Int. J. Syst. Bacteriol.* **39:**224–229.

25. **Fischer, W., P. Rösel, and H. U. Koch.** 1981. Effect of alanine ester substitution and other structural features of lipoteichoic acids on their inhibitory activity against autolysins of *Staphylococcus aureus. J. Bacteriol.* **146:**467–475.

26. **Fitz-Gibbon, S. T., and C. H. House.** 1999. Whole-genome based phylogenetic analysis of free-living microorganisms. *Nucleic Acids Res.* **27:**4218–4222.

27. **Fox, G. E., and E. Stackebrandt.** 1987. The application of 16S rRNA cataloguing and 5S rRNA sequencing in bacterial systematics. *Methods Microbiol.* **19:**406–458.

28. **Fox, G. E., J. D. Wisotzkey, and P. Jurtshuk.** 1992. How close is close: 16S rRNA sequence identity may not be sufficient to guarantee species identity. *Int. J. Syst. Bacteriol.* **42:**166–170.

29. **Giesendorf, B. A. J., W. G. V. Quint, P. Vandamme, and A. Van Belkum.** 1996. Generation of DNA probes for detection of microorganisms by polymerase chain reaction fingerprinting. *Zentbl. Bakteriol. Parasitenkd. Infektkrankh. Hyg. Abt. 1 Orig.* **283:**417–430.

30. **Gillis, M., T. V. Van, R. Bardin, M. Goor, P. Hebbar, A. Willems, P. Segers, K. Kersters, T. Heulin, and M. P. Fernandez.** 1995. Polyphasic taxonomy in the genus *Burkholderia* leading to an emended description of the genus and proposition of *Burkholderia vietnamiensis* sp. nov. for N₂-fixing isolates from rice in Vietnam. *Int. J. Syst. Bacteriol.* **45:**274–289.

31. **Gingeras, T. R., P. Prodanovich, T. Latimer, J. C. Guatelli, and D. D. Richman.** 1991. Use of self-sustained sequence replication amplification reaction to analyze and detect mutations in zidovudine-resistant human immunodeficiency virus. *J. Infect. Dis.* **164:**1066–1074.

32. **Goodfellow, M., and A. G. O'Donnell (ed.).** 1993. *Handbook of New Bacterial Systematics.* Academic Press, London, United Kingdom.

33. **Goodfellow, M., and A. G. O'Donnell (ed.).** 1994. *Modern Microbial Methods. Chemical Methods in Prokaryotic Systematics.* John Wiley & Sons, Ltd., Chichester, United Kingdom.

34. **Goodwin, C. S., J. A. Armstrong, T. Chilvers, M. Peters, M. D. Collins, L. Sly, W. McConnell, and W. E. S. Harper.** 1989. Transfer of *Campylobacter pylori* and *Campylobacter mustelae* to *Helicobacter* gen. nov. as *Helicobacter pylori* comb. nov. and *Helicobacter mustelae* comb. nov., respectively. *Int. J. Syst. Bacteriol.* **39:**397–405.

35. **Goris, J., K. Suzuki, P. De Vos, T. Nakase, and K. Kersters.** 1998. Evaluation of a microplate DNA-DNA hybridization method compared with the initial renaturation method. *Can. J. Microbiol.* **44:**1148–1153.

36. **Grimont, F., and P. Grimont.** 1986. Ribosomal ribonucleic acid gene restriction patterns as possible taxonomic tools. *Ann. Inst. Pasteur/Microbiol. (Paris)* **137B:**165–175.

37. **Grimont, P. A. D., M. Y. Popoff, F. Grimont, C. Coynault, and M. Lemelin.** 1980. Reproducibility and correlation study of three deoxyribonucleic acid hybridization procedures. *Curr. Microbiol.* **4:**325–330.

38. **Guatelli, J. C., K. M. Whitfield, D. Y. Kwoh, K. J. Barringer, D. D. Richman, and T. R. Gingeras.** 1990. Isothermal, *in vitro* amplification of nucleic acids by a multi enzyme reaction modelled after retroviral replication. *Proc. Natl. Acad. Sci. USA* **87:**1874–1878.

39. **Gupta, R. S.** 1998. Protein phylogenies and signature sequences: a reappraisal of evolutionary relationships among Archaebacteria, Eubacteria, and Eukaryotes. *Microbiol. Mol. Biol. Rev.* **62:**1435–1491.

40. **Gürtler, V., and V. A. Stanisich.** 1996. New approaches to typing and identification of bacteria using the 16S-23S rDNA spacer region. *Microbiology* **142:**3–16.

41. **Gürtler, V., and B. C. Mayal.** 2001. Genomic approaches to typing, taxonomy and evolution of bacterial isolates. *Int. J. Syst. Evol. Microbiol.* **51:**3–16.

42. **Harrington, C. S., and S. L. W. On.** 1999. Extensive 16S ribosomal RNA gene sequence diversity in *Campylobacter hyointestinalis* strains: taxonomic, and applied implications. *Int. J. Syst. Bacteriol.* **49:**1171–1175.

43. **Höfle, M. G.** 1990. Transfer RNAs as genotypic fingerprints of eubacteria. *Arch. Microbiol.* **153:**299–304.

44. **Huss, V. A. R., H. Festl, and K. H. Schleifer.** 1983. Studies on the spectrophotometric determination of DNA hybridization from renaturation rates. *Syst. Appl. Microbiol.* **4:**184–192.

45. **Ieven, M.** 1998. Detection. *Methods Microbiol.* **27:** 40–50.
46. **Ieven, M., and H. Goossens.** 1997. Relevance of nucleic acid amplification techniques for diagnosis of respiratory tract infections in the clinical laboratory. *Clin. Microbiol. Rev.* **10:**242–256.
47. **Jahnke, K.-D.** 1994. A modified method of quantitative colorometric DNA-DNA hybridization on membrane filters for bacterial identification. *J. Microbiol. Methods* **20:** 273–288.
48. **Janssen, P., R. Coopman, G. Huys, J. Swings, M. Bleeker, P. Vos, M. Zabeau, and K. Kersters.** 1996. Evaluation of the DNA fingerprinting method AFLP as a new tool in bacterial taxonomy. *Microbiology* **142:**1881–1893.
49. **Jones, D., and N. R. Krieg.** 1984. Serology and chemotaxonomy, p. 15–18. *In* N. R. Krieg and J. G. Holt (ed.), *Bergey's Manual of Systematic Bacteriology*, vol. 1. The Williams & Wilkins Co., Baltimore, Md.
50. **Jonsson, V.** 1970. Proposal of a new species *Pseudomonas kingii. Int. J. Syst. Bacteriol.* **20:**255–257.
51. **Kersters, K., W. Ludwig, M. Vancanneyt, P. De Vos, M. Gillis, and K.-H. Schleifer.** 1996. Recent changes in the classification of the pseudomonads: an overview. *Syst. Appl. Microbiol.* **19:**465–477.
52. **Kersters, K., B. Pot, D. Dewettinck, U. Torck, M. Vancanneyt, L. Vauterin, and P. Vandamme.** 1994. Identification and typing of bacteria by protein electrophoresis, p. 51–66. *In* F. G. Priest, A. Ramos-Cormenzana, and B. Tyndall (ed.), *Bacterial Diversity and Systematics.* Plenum Press, New York, N.Y.
53. **Kornberg, A.** 1959. Enzymic synthesis of desoxyribonucleic acid. *Harvey Lect.* **53:**83–112.
54. **Krieg, N. R., and G. M. Garrity.** 2001. On using the manual, p. 15–19. *In* D. R. Boone, R. W. Castenholz, and G. M. Garrity (ed.), *Bergey's Manual of Systematic Bacteriology*, vol. 2. Springer-Verlag, New York, N.Y.
55. **Kwoh, D. Y., G. R. Davis, K. M. Whitfield, H. L. Chapelle, L. J. DiMichele, and T. R. Gingeras.** 1989. Transcription based amplification system and detection of amplified human immunodeficiency virus type 1 with a bead-based sandwich hybridization format. *Proc. Natl. Acad. Sci. USA* **86:**1173–1177.
56. **Lane, D. J., B. Pace, G. J. Olsen, D. A. Stahl, M. Sogin, and N. R. Pace.** 1985. Rapid determination of 16S ribosomal RNA sequences for phylogenetic analysis. *Proc. Natl. Acad. Sci. USA* **82:**6955–6959.
57. **Lawson, A. J., D. Linton, and J. Stanley.** 1998. 16S rRNA gene sequences of 'Candidatus Campylobacter hominis,' a novel uncultivated species, are found in the gastrointestinal tract of humans. *Microbiology* **144:**2063–2071.
58. **Lawson, A. J., S. L. W. On, J. M. J. Logan, and J. Stanley.** 2001. *Campylobacter hominis* sp. nov., from the human gastrointestinal tract. *Int. J. Syst. Evol. Microbiol.* **51:**651–660.
59. **Lucchini, S., A. Thompson, and J. C. D. Hinton.** 2001. Microarrays for microbiologists. *Microbiology* **147:**1403–1414.
60. **Ludwig, W., J. Neumaier, N. Klugbauer, E. Brockmann, C. Roller, S. Jilg, K. Reetz, I. Schachtner, A. Ludvigsen, M. Bachleitner, U. Fisher, and K. H. Schleifer.** 1993. Phylogenetic relationships of bacteria based on comparative sequence analysis of elongation factor Tu and ATP-synthase beta subunit genes. *Antonie Leeuwenhoek J. Microbiol. Serol.* **64:**285–305.
61. **Ludwig, W., O. Strunk, S. Klugbauer, N. Klugbauer, M. Weienegger, J. Neumaier, M. Bachleitner, and K. H.** Schleifer. 1998. Bacterial phylogeny based on comparative sequence analysis. *Electrophoresis* **19:**554–568.
62. **Ludwig, W.** 1991. DNA sequencing in bacterial systematics, p. 69–94. *In* E. Stackebrandt and M. Goodfellow (ed.), *Nucleic Acid Techniques in Bacterial Systematics.* John Wiley & Sons, Ltd., Chichester, United Kingdom.
63. **Ludwig, W., and H.-P. Klenk.** 2001. Overview: a phylogenetic backbone and taxonomic framework for procaryotic systematics, p. 49–65. *In* D. R. Boone, R. W. Castenholz, and G. M. Garrity (ed.), *Bergey's Manual of Systematic Bacteriology*, vol. 2. Springer-Verlag, New York, N.Y.
64. **Lupski, J. R., and G. E. Weinstock.** 1992. Short, interspersed repetitive DNA sequences in prokaryotic genomes. *J. Bacteriol.* **174:**4525–4529.
65. **Magee, J.** 1994. Analysis of electrophoretic whole-organism protein fingerprints, p. 493–521. *In* M. Goodfellow and A. G. O'Donnell (ed.), *Modern Microbial Methods. Chemical Methods in Prokaryotic Systematics.* John Wiley & Sons, Ltd., Chichester, United Kingdom.
66. **Magee, J. T., J. M. Hindmarch, and C. W. I. Douglas.** 1997. A numerical taxonomic study of *Streptococcus sanguis*, *Streptococcus mitis*, and similar organisms using conventional tests and pyrolysis mass spectrometry. *Zentbl. Bakteriol. Parasitenkd. Infektkrankh. Hyg. Abt. 1 Orig.* **285:** 195–203.
67. **Moore, W. E. C., and L. V. H. Moore (ed.).** 1989. *Index of the Bacterial and Yeast Nomenclatural Changes Published in the* International Journal of Systematic Bacteriology *since the 1980 Approved Lists of Bacterial Names (1 January 1980 to 1 January 1989).* American Society for Microbiology, Washington, D.C.
68. **Moseley, S. L., I. Huq, A. R. Alim, M. So, M. Samadpour-Motalebi, and S. Falkow.** 1980. Detection of enterotoxigenic *Escherichia coli* by DNA colony hybridization. *J. Infect. Dis.* **142:**892–898.
69. **Mullis, K., F. Faloona, S. Scharf, R. Saiki, G. Horn, and H. Erlich.** 1986. Specific enzymatic amplification of DNA in vitro: the polymerase chain reaction. *Cold Spring Harbor Symp. Quant. Biol.* **51**(Pt. 1)**:**263–273.
70. **Murray, R. G. E., D. J. Brenner, R. R. Colwell, P. De Vos, M. Goodfellow, P. A. D. Grimont, N. Pfennig, E. Stackebrandt, and G. A. Zavarzin.** 1990. Report of the Ad Hoc Committee on Approaches to Taxonomy within the *Proteobacteria. Int. J. Syst. Bacteriol.* **40:**213–215.
71. **Murray, R. G. E., and K. H. Schleifer.** 1994. Taxonomic notes: a proposal for recording the properties of putative taxa of procaryotes. *Int. J. Syst. Bacteriol.* **44:**174–176.
72. **Murray, R. G. E., and E. Stackebrandt.** 1995. Taxonomic note: implementation of the provisional status *Candidatus* for incompletely described procaryotes. *Int. J. Syst. Bacteriol.* **45:**186–187.
73. **Ochi, K.** 1995. Comparative ribosomal protein sequence analyses of a phylogenetically defined genus, *Pseudomonas*, and its relatives. *Int. J. Syst. Bacteriol.* **45:**268–273.
74. **Olsen, G. J., G. Larsen, and C. R. Woese.** 1991. The ribosomal RNA database project. *Nucleic Acids Res.* **19**(Suppl.)**:**2017–2021.
75. **On, S. L. W., and B. Holmes.** 1991. Reproducibility of tolerance tests that are useful in the identification of campylobacteria. *J. Clin. Microbiol.* **29:**1785–1788.
76. **On, S. L. W., and B. Holmes.** 1992. Assessment of enzyme detection tests useful in identification of campylobacteria. *J. Clin. Microbiol.* **30:**746–749.
77. **Palleroni, N. J., and J. F. Bradbury.** 1993. *Stenotrophomonas*, a new bacterial genus for *Xanthomonas maltophilia* (Hugh 1980) Swings et al. 1983. *Int. J. Syst. Bacteriol.* **43:**606–609.

78. **Palleroni, N. J., and B. Holmes.** 1981. *Pseudomonas cepacia* sp. nov., nom. rev. *Int. J. Syst. Bacteriol.* **31:**479–481.

79. **Palleroni, N. J., R. Kunisawa, R. Contopoulou, and M. Doudoroff.** 1973. Nucleic acid homologies in the genus *Pseudomonas. Int. J. Syst. Bacteriol.* **23:**333–339.

80. **Pot, B., P. Vandamme, and K. Kersters.** 1994. Analysis of electrophoretic whole-organism protein fingerprints, p. 493–521. *In* M. Goodfellow and A. G. O'Donnell (ed.), *Modern Microbial Methods. Chemical Methods in Prokaryotic Systematics.* John Wiley & Sons, Ltd., Chichester, United Kingdom.

81. **Priest, F., and B. Austin.** 1993. *Modern Bacterial Taxonomy.* Chapman & Hall, London, United Kingdom.

82. **Samuels, S. B., C. W. Moss, and R. E. Weaver.** 1973. The fatty acids of *Pseudomonas multivorans* (*Pseudomonas cepacia*) and *Pseudomonas kingii. J. Gen. Microbiol.* **74:**275–279.

83. **Schleifer, K. H., and O. Kandler.** 1972. Peptidoglycan types of bacterial cell walls and their taxonomic implications. *Bacteriol. Rev.* **36:**407–477.

84. **Schleifer, K. H., and W. Ludwig.** 1989. Phylogenetic relationships of bacteria, p. 103–117. *In* B. Fernholm, K. Bremer, and H. Jörnvall (ed.), *The Hierarchy of Life.* Elsevier Science Publishers B.V., Amsterdam, The Netherlands.

85. **Schleifer, K. H., W. Ludwig, and R. Amann.** 1993. Nucleic acid probes, p. 463–510. *In* M. Goodfellow and A. G. O'Donnell (ed.), *Handbook of New Bacterial Systematics.* Academic Press, London, United Kingdom.

86. **Skerman, V. B. D., V. McGowan, and P. H. A. Sneath (ed.).** 1980. Approved lists of bacterial names. *Int. J. Syst. Bacteriol.* **30:**225–420.

87. **Sneath, P. H. A.** 1984. Numerical taxonomy, p. 111–118. *In* N. R. Krieg and J. G. Holt (ed.), *Bergey's Manual of Systematic Bacteriology,* vol. 1. The Williams & Wilkins Co., Baltimore, Md.

88. **Sneath, P. H. A. (ed.).** 1992. *International Code of Nomenclature of Bacteria,* 1990 revision. American Society for Microbiology, Washington, D.C.

89. **Snel, B., P. Bork, and M. A. Huynen.** 1999. Genome phylogeny based on gene content. *Nat. Genet.* **21:**108–110.

90. **Snell, J. J. S., L. R. Hill, S. P. Lapage, and M. A. Curtis.** 1972. Identification of *Pseudomonas cepacia* Burkholder and its synonymy with *Pseudomonas kingii* Jonsson. *Int. J. Syst. Bacteriol.* **22:**127–138.

91. **Sokal, R. R., and P. H. A. Sneath.** 1963. *Principles of Numerical Taxonomy.* W. H. Freeman & Co., San Francisco, Calif.

92. **Stackebrandt, E., and B. M. Goebel.** 1994. Taxonomic note: a place for DNA-DNA reassociation and 16S rRNA sequence analysis in the present species definition in bacteriology. *Int. J. Syst. Bacteriol.* **44:**846–849.

93. **Stackebrandt, E., and W. Liesack.** 1993. Nucleic acids and classification, p. 151–194. *In* M. Goodfellow and A. G. O'Donnell (ed.). *Handbook of New Bacterial Systematics.* Academic Press, London, United Kingdom.

94. **Stackebrandt, E., R. G. E. Murray, and G. H. Trüper.** 1988. *Proteobacteria* classis nov., a name for the phylogenetic taxon that includes the "purple bacteria and their relatives." *Int. J. Syst. Bacteriol.* **38:**321–325.

95. **Staley, J. T., and N. J. Krieg.** 1984. Classification of prokaryotic organisms: an overview, p. 1–3. *In* N. R. Krieg and J. G. Holt (ed.), *Bergey's Manual of Systematic Bacteriology,* vol. 1. The Williams & Wilkins Co., Baltimore, Md.

96. **Stanier, R. Y., N. J. Palleroni, and M. Doudoroff.** 1966. The aerobic pseudomonads: a taxonomic study. *J. Gen. Microbiol.* **43:**159–271.

97. **Suzuki, K., M. Goodfellow, and A. G. O'Donnell.** 1993. Cell envelopes and classification, p. 195–250. *In* M. Goodfellow and A. G. O'Donnell (ed.), *Handbook of New Bacterial Systematics.* Academic Press, London, United Kingdom.

98. **Swings, J., P. De Vos, M. Van den Mooter, and J. De Ley.** 1983. Transfer of *Pseudomonas maltophilia* Hugh 1981 to the genus *Xanthomonas* as *Xanthomonas maltophilia* (Hugh 1981) comb. nov. *Int. J. Syst. Bacteriol.* **33:**409–413.

99. **Tabor, C. W., and H. Tabor.** 1985. Polyamines in microorganisms. *Microbiol. Rev.* **49:**81–99.

100. **Tamaoka, J., D.-M. Ha, and K. Komagata.** 1987. Reclassification of *Pseudomonas acidovorans* den Dooren de Jong 1926 and *Pseudomonas testosteroni* Marcus and Talalay 1956 as *Comamonas acidovorans* comb. nov. and *Comamonas testosteroni* comb., nov. with an emended description of the genus *Comamonas. Int. J. Syst. Bacteriol.* **37:**52–59.

101. **Teske, A., P. Sigalevich, Y. Cohen, and G. Muyzer.** 1996. Molecular identification of bacteria from a coculture by denaturing gradient gel electrophoresis of 16S ribosomal DNA fragments as a tool for isolation in pure cultures. *Appl. Environ. Microbiol.* **62:**4210–4215.

102. **Urakami, T., C. Ito-Yoshida, H. Araki, T. Kijima, K.-I. Suzuki, and K. Komagata.** 1994. Transfer of *Pseudomonas plantarii* and *Pseudomonas glumae* to *Burkholderia* as *Burkholderia* spp. and description of *Burkholderia vandii* sp. nov. *Int. J. Syst. Bacteriol.* **44:**235–245.

103. **Ursing, J. B., R. A. Rossello-Mora, E. Garcia-Valdes, and J. Lalucat.** 1995. Taxonomic note: a pragmatic approach to the nomenclature of phenotypically similar genomic groups. *Int. J. Syst. Bacteriol.* **45:**604.

104. **van Baar, B. L.** 2000. Characterisation of bacteria by matrix-assisted laser desorption/ionisation and electrospray mass spectrometry. *FEMS Microbiol. Rev.* **24:**193–219.

105. **Van Belkum, A.** 1994. DNA fingerprinting of medically important microorganisms by use of PCR. *Clin. Microbiol. Rev.* **7:**174–184.

106. **Van Camp, G., S. Chapelle, and R. De Wachter.** 1993. Amplification and sequencing of variable regions in bacterial 23S ribosomal RNA genes with conserved primer sequences. *Curr. Microbiol.* **27:**147–151.

107. **Vancanneyt, M., P. Vandamme, and K. Kersters.** 1995. Differentiation of *Bordetella pertussis,* *B. parapertussis,* and *B. bronchiseptica* by whole-cell protein electrophoresis and fatty acid analysis. *Int. J. Syst. Bacteriol.* **45:**843–847.

108. **Vandamme, P., E. Falsen, R. Rossau, B. Hoste, P. Segers, R. Tytgat, and J. De Ley.** 1991. Revision of *Campylobacter,* *Helicobacter,* and *Wolinella* taxonomy: emendation of generic descriptions and proposal of *Arcobacter* gen. nov. *Int. J. Syst. Bacteriol.* **41:**88–103.

109. **Vandamme, P., C. S. Harrington, K. Jalava, and S. L. W. On.** 2000. Misidentifying helicobacters: the *Helicobacter cinaedi* example. *J. Clin. Microbiol.* **38:**2261–2266.

110. **Vandamme, P., B. Pot, M. Gillis, P. De Vos, K. Kersters, and J. Swings.** 1996. Polyphasic taxonomy, a consensus approach to bacterial classification. *Microbiol. Rev.* **60:**407–438.

111. **Vandamme, P., P. Segers, M. Vancanneyt, K. Van Hove, R. Mutters, J. Hommez, F. E. Dewhirst, B. J. Paster, K. Kersters, E. Falsen, L. A. Devriese, M. Bisgaard, K.-H. Hinz, and W. Mannheim.** 1994. *Ornithobacterium rhinotracheale* gen. nov., sp. nov., isolated from the avian respiratory tract. *Int. J. Syst. Bacteriol.* **44:**24–37.

112. **Vandamme, P., M. Vancanneyt, P. Segers, M. Ryll, B. Köhler, W. Ludwig, and K. H. Hinz.** 1999. *Coenonia anatina* gen. nov., sp. nov., a novel bacterium associated with respiratory disease in ducks and geese. *Int. J. Syst. Bacteriol.* **49:**867–874.

113. **Van de Peer, Y., J. Jansen, P. De Rijk, and R. De Wachter.** 1997. Database on the structure of small ribosomal subunit RNA sequences. *Nucleic Acids Res.* **25:** 111–116.

114. **Viale, A. M., A. K. Arakaki, F. C. Soncini, and R. G. Ferreyra.** 1994. Evolutionary relationships among eubacterial groups as inferred from GroEL (chaperonin) sequence comparisons. *Int. J. Syst. Bacteriol.* **44:**527–533.

115. **Walker, G. T., M. C. Little, J. G. Nadeau, and D. D. Shank.** 1992. Isothermal *in vitro* amplification of DNA by a restriction enzyme DNA polymerase system. *Proc. Natl. Acad. Sci. USA* **89:**392–396.

116. **Wayne, L. G., D. J. Brenner, R. R. Colwell, P. A. D. Grimont, P. Kandler, M. I. Krichevsky, L. H. Moore, W. E. C. Moore, R. G. E. Murray, E. Stackebrandt, M. P. Starr, and H. G. Trüper.** 1987. Report of the Ad Hoc Committee on Reconciliation of Approaches to Bacterial Systematics. *Int. J. Syst. Bacteriol.* **37:**463–464.

117. **Welch, D. F.** 1991. Applications of cellular fatty acid analysis. *Clin. Microbiol. Rev.* **4:**422–438.

118. **Welsh, J., and M. McClelland.** 1990. Fingerprinting genomes using PCR with arbitrary primers. *Nucleic Acids Res.* **18:**7213–7218.

119. **Welsh, J., and M. McClelland.** 1992. PCR-amplified length polymorphisms in tRNA intergenic spacers for categorizing staphylococci. *Mol. Microbiol.* **6:**1673–1680.

120. **Wen, A., M. Fegan, C. Hayward, S. Chakraborty, and L. I. Sly.** 1999. Phylogenetic relationships among members of the *Comamonadaceae*, and description of *Delftia acidovorans* (den Dooren de Jong 1926 and Tamaoka et al. 1987) gen. nov., comb. nov. *Int. J. Syst. Bacteriol.* **49:**567–576.

121. **Willems, A., E. Falsen, B. Pot, E. Jantzen, B. Hoste, P. Vandamme, M. Gillis, K. Kersters, and J. De Ley.** 1990. *Acidovorax*, a new genus for *Pseudomonas facilis, Pseudomonas delafieldii*, E. Falsen (EF) group 13, EF group 16, and several clinical isolates, with the species *Acidovorax facilis* comb. nov., *Acidovorax delafieldii* comb. nov., and *Acidovorax temperans* sp. nov. *Int. J. Syst. Bacteriol.* **40:** 384–398.

122. **Woese, C. R.** 1987. Bacterial evolution. *Microbiol. Rev.* **51:**221–271.

123. **Wolters, J., and A. Erdmann.** 1988. Compilation of 5S rRNA and 5S rRNA gene sequences. *Nucleic Acids Res.* **16**(Suppl.)**:**R1–R85.

124. **Yabuuchi, E., Y. Kosako, H. Oyaizu, I. Yano, H. Hotta, Y. Hashimoto, T. Ezaki, and M. Arakawa.** 1992. Proposal of *Burkholderia* gen. nov. and transfer of seven species of the genus *Pseudomonas* homology group II to the new genus, with the type species *Burkholderia cepacia* (Palleroni and Holmes 1981) comb. nov. *Microbiol. Immunol.* **36:**1251–1275.

125. **Yabuuchi, E., Y. Kosako, I. Yano, H. Hotta, and Y. Nishiuchi.** 1995. Transfer of two *Burkholderia* and an *Alcaligenes* species to *Ralstonia* gen. nov.: proposal of *Ralstonia pickettii* (Ralston, Palleroni and Doudoroff 1973) comb. nov., *Ralstonia solanacearum* (Smith 1896) comb. nov. and *Ralstonia eutropha* (Davis 1969) comb. nov. *Microbiol. Immunol.* **39:**897–904.

126. **Young, J. M.** 2001. Implications of alternative classifications and horizontal gene transfer for bacterial taxonomy. *Int. J. Syst. Evol. Microbiol.* **51:**945–953.

127. **Zabeau, M., and P. Vos.** 1993. *Selective Restriction Fragment Amplification: A General Method for DNA Fingerprinting.* Publication 0534858 A1. European Patent Office, Munich, Germany.

128. **Zhao, N., C. Qu, E. Wang, and W. Chen.** 1995. Phylogenetic evidence for the transfer of *Pseudomonas cocovenenans* (van Damme et al. 1960) to the genus *Burkholderia* as *Burkholderia cocovenenans* (van Damme et al. 1960) comb. nov. *Int. J. Syst. Bacteriol.* **45:**600–603.

129. **Zillig, W., H.-P. Klenk, P. Palm, G. Pühler, F. Gropp, R. A. Garret, and H. Leffers.** 1989. The phylogenetic relations of DNA-dependent RNA polymerases of archaebacteria, eukaryotes, and eubacteria. *Can. J. Microbiol.* **35:**73–80.

Specimen Collection, Transport, and Processing: Bacteriology*

RICHARD B. THOMSON, JR., AND J. MICHAEL MILLER

20

The use of specimens for bacteriologic analysis requires that specific clinical material be collected, stabilized, and transported according to exacting specifications to ensure valid results. Poor specimen quality contributes to misdiagnosis and inappropriate antimicrobial therapy. Communication between laboratory representative and clinician is essential to the proper selection of bacteriology tests and interpretation of their results. Laboratory personnel are responsible for monitoring and educating those collecting and transporting specimens. Laboratories are required by accrediting agencies to provide specimen collection and transport manuals. A useful alternative to printed manuals is an electronic version available over a local area network (88).

Specimens for bacteriologic culture should be collected as soon as possible after the onset of active disease and before the initiation of antimicrobial therapy. A second specimen may be necessary because of poor specimen quality or inadequate transport conditions that affected the first specimen but is otherwise rarely required for diagnosis of an acute infectious disease. Exceptions include the collection of multiple blood specimens for culture and the detection of fastidious or unusual pathogens not originally suspected.

SELECTION AND COLLECTION OF SPECIMENS

Material for bacteriologic testing should be collected from a site representative of the active disease process. Sites of an inflammatory process and free of contaminating flora are optimal. In practice, most specimen collection sites are contaminated with various quantities of commensal bacteria. As examples, vaginal and cervical floras contaminate endometrial specimens collected through the endocervix; the skin and environmental floras contaminate cutaneous fistulas and deep wounds that are open to skin or mucous membrane surfaces; the floras in the nasopharynx and nasal passages contaminate specimens from the nasal sinuses; and the flora in the upper respiratory tract contaminates sputum and other lower respiratory tract specimens. Table 1 lists

common diseases with appropriate and inappropriate clinical specimens (9, 195). General specimen selection and collection guidelines include the following (106).

1. Select the proper anatomic site from which to collect the specimen.
2. Avoid contamination with indigenous flora. Growth and reporting of members of the normal flora can be mistaken by the physician or caregiver as the cause of the infectious process. In addition, the flora can overgrow and obscure the true etiology.
3. Aspiration, irrigation with sterile nonbacteriostatic saline followed by aspiration, and biopsy of tissue are appropriate methods for specimen collection when anaerobic bacteria are suspected (Table 2). Collection with a swab is least desirable because of the relatively small amount of specimen sampled and the ease with which the swab can be contaminated with adjacent members of the normal flora. Specimens for anaerobic culture should be stored at room temperature, not refrigeration temperature, since oxygen diffuses into cold specimens more readily.
4. Collect a sufficient volume of material to enable all requested tests to be performed satisfactorily. Insufficient material may yield false-negative results.
5. Label each specimen with the patient's name, identification number, source of specimen, date and time of collection, and the initials of the collector.
6. Use a specimen container designed to promote survival of pathogenic bacteria, eliminate leakage of specimen, and allow safe handling during transportation and processing.

Specific specimen collection guidelines are summarized in Table 3.

TRANSPORTATION OF SPECIMENS

Specimens for bacterial culture should be transported to the laboratory immediately. Excessive delay or exposure to temperature extremes compromises results and must be avoided. General specimen transport guidelines include the following (9, 106).

1. Specimens must be transported promptly to the laboratory. If transport requires more than 2 h, a special

---

* This chapter contains information presented in chapter 4 by J. Michael Miller and Harvey T. Holmes and chapter 5 by Barbara S. Reisner, Gail L. Woods, Richard B. Thomson, Jr., Davise H. Larone, Lynne S. Garcia, and Robyn Y. Shimizu in the seventh edition of this Manual.

TABLE 1 Selection of common clinical specimens for bacterial culture[a]

Anatomic site	Clinical specimen	
	Appropriate	Inappropriate
Lower respiratory tract	Freshly expectorated mucus and inflammatory cells (pus), sputum	Saliva, oropharyngeal secretions, sinus drainage from nasopharynx
Sinus	Secretions collected by direct sinus aspiration or washes; curettage and biopsy material collected during endoscopy	Nasal or nasopharyngeal swab, nasopharyngeal secretions, sputum, and saliva
Urinary tract	Midstream urine, urine collected by "straight" catheterization, urine collected by suprapubic aspiration, urine collected during cystoscopy or other surgical procedure	Urine from Foley catheter collection bag
Superficial wound	Aspirations of pus or local irrigation fluid (nonbacteriostatic saline), swab of purulence originating from beneath the dermis	Swab of surface material or specimen contaminated with surface material, irrigation fluid with saline-containing preservative
Deep wound	Purulence, necrosis, or tissue from deep subcutaneous site	Specimen contaminated with surface material
Gastrointestinal tract	Freshly passed stool, washes or feces collected during endoscopy	Rectal swab, specimen for bacterial culture if diarrhea developed after patient was in hospital for >3 days
Venous blood	2 or 3 blood specimens collected from separate venipunctures, before initiation of antibiotics, each containing approximately 20 ml of blood for patient >90 lb (see Table 7 for pediatric volumes); antisepsis with iodine-containing compound or chlorhexidine	Clotted blood; one or more than three blood specimens collected within a 24-h period; vol of blood, <20 ml per culture (i.e., per venipuncture); antisepsis with alcohol only (adults)

[a] Reprinted from reference 169a with permission.

TABLE 2 Suitability of various specimens for anaerobic culture

Acceptable material (method of collection)	Unacceptable material (method of collection)
Aspirate (by needle and syringe)	Bronchoalveolar lavage washing
Bartholin's gland inflammation or secretions	Cervical secretions
Blood (venipuncture)	Endotracheal secretions (aspirate)
Bone marrow (aspirate)	Lochia secretions
Bronchoscopic secretions (protected specimen brush)	Nasopharyngeal swab
Culdocentesis fluid (aspirate)	Perineal swab
Fallopian tube fluid or tissue (aspirate/biopsy)	Prostatic or seminal fluid
IUD,[a] for *Actinomyces* spp.	Sputum (expectorated or induced)
Nasal sinus (aspirate)	Stool or rectal swabs samples
Placenta tissue (via cesarean delivery)	Tracheostomy secretions
Stool, for *Clostridium difficile*	Urethral secretions
Surgery (aspirate, tissue)	Urine (voided or from catheter)
Transtracheal aspirate	Vaginal or vulvar secretions (swab)
Urine (suprapubic aspirate)	

[a] IUD, intrauterine device.

holding medium or use of refrigeration temperature is required (Table 3).

2. Do not store specimens for bacterial culture for more than 24 h even with appropriate holding medium or refrigeration temperature.

3. Optimal transport times for clinical specimens for bacteriological culture depend on the volume of material obtained. Small volumes of fluid (<1 ml) or tissue (<1 cm³) should be submitted within 15 to 30 min to avoid evaporation, drying, and exposure to ambient conditions. Larger volumes and specimens in holding medium may be stored as long as 24 h.

4. Bacteria that are especially sensitive to ambient conditions include *Shigella* spp., *Neisseria gonorrhoeae*, *N. meningitidis*, *Haemophilus influenzae*, *Streptococcus pneumoniae*, and anaerobes. Reliable detection by culture of *Shigella* spp. requires immediate processing. *H. influenzae* is sensitive to low temperatures. Never refrigerate spinal fluid, genital, eye, or internal ear specimens.

5. Transportation of clinical specimens and infectious substances from one laboratory to another, regardless of the distance, requires strict attention to specimen packaging and labeling instructions. Materials for transport must be labeled properly, packaged, and protected during transport. Refer to the Centers for Disease Control and Prevention web site (www.cdc.gov/od/ohs/biosfty/shipdir.htm) for a complete description of packaging and shipping regulations mandated by the U.S. Department of Transportation.

Specific specimen transport guidelines are summarized in Table 3.

SPECIMENS FOR INFREQUENTLY ENCOUNTERED BACTERIA

Some bacteria cause infections that are infrequently encountered and require special transport conditions or holding media. In many instances, these specimens are shipped to reference laboratories; this necessitates relatively long transport times. Table 4 is a list of specimens and transport conditions for these bacteria (33).

PROCESSING OF SPECIMENS

Specimen processing includes detection of bacteria by staining and culturing, performing immunologic assays for microbial antigens, and use of molecular techniques that identify specific nucleic acid sequences. The recommendations that follow are neither all-inclusive nor applicable to all laboratory settings (Table 5). Gram-stained smears are recommended whenever (i) rapid stain results are necessary for patient care, (ii) analysis of cellularity is used to determine adequacy of specimen, or (iii) results are needed to help interpret culture findings by the laboratory technologist. Anaerobic culture should be included only when ordered with an appropriate specimen source (Table 2) and when the specimen was transported in an oxygen-free container free of contamination with normal skin and mucosal anaerobic floras. Gram-stained smear and culture interpretation may require the intervention and opinion of a laboratory director trained in medical microbiology or pathology and capable of reviewing clinical information with the patient's physician prior to report generation.

General Considerations

Safety
Refer to chapters 3 and 9 for a complete description of safety issues.

Processing
Specimens received for detection of bacteria by methods which include culture, staining, and antigen or nucleic acid detection must be processed in a timely manner. The lability of microorganisms and their antigens and nucleic acids mandates holding conditions and processing time limits. Improper handling prior to processing can result in death of pathogenic bacteria or overgrowth of contaminating bacteria. In addition, correct interpretations of culture results generally require a rough quantitation of bacterial densities in the clinical specimen. Allowing bacteria to multiply out of proportion to their original numbers may result in erroneous, sometimes detrimental, interpretations. General considerations for holding specimens and acceptable processing delays are summarized in Table 3 (106).

Processing at a Remote Site
Consolidation of laboratory services results in centralized microbiology laboratories located miles from the sites of specimen collection. Adhering to transportation and processing time limits developed for laboratories located within or adjacent to specimen collection (e.g., hospital) is impossible for remote laboratories. The best approach to location of a core laboratory and the amount of local processing that should be performed can be determined on the basis of guidelines proposed by the Infectious Disease Society of America (128). Refer to chapter 2 for a complete discussion of remote-site issues.

Specimen Labeling and Test Ordering Requirements
On arrival of specimens in the laboratory, the time and date of receipt should be recorded. Subsequently, the time of plating, which may differ substantially from the time of receipt, should be recorded. At the time of receipt, all specimens and requisitions should be carefully inspected. Specimens must be labeled and accompanied by a requisition reflecting the physician's order. Specimens are labeled with the patient's name and a description of the specimen source. The requisition must include the following information: patient name, age, sex, identifying number (such as social security number or unique registration/billing number), and location (hospital room, physician's office address, etc.); ordering physician's name; specimen source; date and time of collection; and test ordered. If the information is incomplete, laboratory personnel must call the collecting location and request the missing information. If a specimen is mislabeled or no patient name is provided, another specimen should be collected. Relabeling of a specimen is allowed only if another specimen cannot be collected, such as tissue collected during a surgical procedure. Laboratory procedures must clearly state the exceptions that are allowed, the steps needed to verify and document exceptions, and the individuals responsible for relabeling. When relabeling has occurred, the course of events must be outlined in the laboratory report so that the physician interpreting the results is aware of potential errors. Laws governing specimen labeling can be reviewed at the Centers for Medicare and Medicaid Services web site (http://www.hcfa.gov). Specimens from outpatient facilities require additional information for Medicare and Medicaid billing. Patient

TABLE 3 Bacteriology collection, transport, and storage guidelines[a]

Specimen type (reference)	Collection guidelines	Transport device and/or minimum vol	Transport[b] time and temp	Storage time	Replica limits	Comments
Abscess (14) General	Remove surface exudate by wiping with sterile saline or 70% alcohol					Tissue or fluid is always superior to a swab specimen. If swabs must be used, collect two, one for culture and one for Gram staining. Preserve swab material by placing in Stuart's or Amies medium.
Open	Aspirate if possible or pass a swab deep into the lesion to firmly sample the lesion's "fresh border"	Swab transport system	≤2 h, RT	≤24 h, RT	1/day/source	Samples of the base of the lesion and abscess wall are most productive.
Closed	Aspirate abscess material with needle and syringe; aseptically transfer *all* material into anaerobic transport device	Anaerobic transport system, ≥1 ml	≤2 h, RT	≤24 h, RT	1/day/source	Contamination with surface material will introduce colonizing bacteria not involved in the infectious process.
Bite wound	See Abscess					Do not culture animal bite wounds ≤12 h old (agents are usually not recovered) unless signs of infection are present.
Blood (139)	Disinfect culture bottle; apply 70% isopropyl alcohol or phenolic to rubber stoppers and wait 1 min	Blood culture bottles for bacteria; adult, ≥20 ml/set (higher vol most productive)	≤2 h, RT, or per instructions	≤2 h, RT, or per instructions	3 sets in 24 h	Acute febrile episode, antimicrobials to be started or changed immediately: 2 sets[c] from separate sites, all within 10 min (before antimicrobials). Nonacute disease, antimicrobials will not be started or changed immediately: 2 or 3 sets from separate sites all within 24 h at intervals no closer than 3 h (before antimicrobial[s]). Endocarditis, acute: 3 sets from 3 separate sites, within 1–2 h, before antimicrobials if possible.

(Continued on next page)

TABLE 3 Bacteriology collection, transport, and storage guidelines[a] (*Continued*)

Specimen type (reference)	Collection guidelines	Transport device and/or minimum vol	Transport[b] time and temp	Storage time	Replica limits	Comments
	Palpate vein before disinfection of venipuncture site					Endocarditis, subacute: 3 sets from 3 separate sites ≥1 h apart, within 24 h. If cultures are negative at 24 h, obtain 2–3 more sets.
						Fever of unknown origin: 2 or 3 sets from separate sites ≥1 h apart during a 24-h period. If negative at 24–48 h, obtain 2 or 3 more sets.
	Disinfection of venipuncture site: 1. Cleanse site with 70% alcohol 2. Swab concentrically, starting at the center, with an iodine preparation 3. Allow the iodine to dry 4. *Do not palpate vein at this point without sterile glove* 5. Collect blood 6. After venipuncture, remove iodine from the skin with alcohol	Infant and child, 1–20 ml/set depending on weight of patient				Some data indicate that an additional aerobic or fungal bottle is more productive than the anaerobic bottle. Pediatric: Collect immediately, rarely necessary to document continuous bacteremia with hours between cultures.
Bone marrow aspirate	Prepare puncture site as for surgical incision	Inoculate blood culture bottle or a lysis-centrifugation tube; plated specimen delivered to laboratory immediately	≤24 h, RT, if in culture bottle or tube	≤24 h, RT	1/day	Small volumes of bone marrow may be inoculated directly onto culture media. Routine bacterial culture of bone marrow is rarely useful.
Burn	Clean and debride the burn	Tissue is placed into a sterile screw-cap container; aspirate or swab exudate; transport in sterile container or swab transport system	≤24 h, RT	≤24 h, RT	1/day/source	A 3- to 4-mm punch biopsy specimen is optimum when quantitative cultures are ordered. Process for aerobic culture only. Quantitative culture may or may not be valuable. Cultures of surface samples of burns may be misleading.

Specimen	Collection procedure	Container and minimum volume	Transport	Storage	None	Comments
Catheter (96) i.v.	1. Cleanse the skin around the catheter site with alcohol 2. Aseptically remove catheter and clip 5 cm of distal tip directly into a sterile tube 3. Transport immediately to microbiology laboratory to prevent drying	Sterile screw-cap tube or cup	≤15 min, RT	≤2 h, 4°C	None	Acceptable i.v. catheters for semiquantitative culture (Maki method); central, CVP, Hickman, Broviac, peripheral, arterial, umbilical, hyperalimentation, Swan-Ganz.
Foley	Do not culture, since growth represents distal urethral flora					Not acceptable for culture.
Cellulitis, aspirate from area of (14)	1. Cleanse site by wiping with sterile saline or 70% alcohol 2. Aspirate the area of maximum inflammation (commonly the center rather than the leading edge) with a needle and syringe; irrigation with a small amount of sterile saline may be necessary 3. Aspirate saline into syringe, and expel into sterile screw-cap tube	Sterile tube (syringe transport not recommended)	≤15 min, RT	≤24 h, RT	None	Yield of potential pathogens in minority of specimens cultured.
CSF	1. Disinfect site with iodine preparation 2. Insert a needle with stylet at L3-L4, L4-L5, or L5-S1 interspace 3. Upon reaching the subarachnoid space, remove the stylet and collect 1–2 ml of fluid into each of 3 leakproof tubes	Sterile screw-cap tubes Minimum amt required: bacteria, ≥1 ml; AFB, ≥5 ml	Bacteria: never refrigerate; ≤15 min, RT	≤2 h, RT	None	Obtain blood for culture also. If only 1 tube of CSF is collected, it should be submitted to microbiology first; otherwise submit tube 2 to microbiology. Aspirate of brain abscess or a biopsy specimen may be necessary to detect anaerobic bacteria or parasites.

(Continued on next page)

TABLE 3 Bacteriology collection, transport, and storage guidelines[a] (*Continued*)

Specimen type (reference)	Collection guidelines	Transport device and/or minimum vol	Transport[b] time and temp	Storage time	Replica limits	Comments
Decubitus ulcer (14)	A swab is not the specimen of choice (see Comments) 1. Cleanse surface with sterile saline 2. If a sample biopsy is not available, aspirate inflammatory material from the base of the ulcer	Sterile tube (aerobic) or anaerobic system (for tissue)	≤2 h, RT	≤24 h, RT	1/day/source	Since a swab specimen of a decubitus ulcer provides no clinical information, it should not be submitted. A tissue biopsy sample or needle aspirate is the specimen of choice.
Dental culture: gingival, periodontal, periapical, Vincent's stomatitis	1. Carefully cleanse gingival margin and supragingival tooth surface to remove saliva, debris, and plaque 2. Using a periodontal scaler, carefully remove subgingival lesion material and transfer it to an anaerobic transport system 3. Prepare smear for staining with specimen collected in the same fashion	Anaerobic transport system	≤2 h, RT	≤24 h, RT	1/day	Periodontal lesions should be processed only by laboratories equipped to provide specialized techniques for the detection and enumeration of recognized pathogens.
Ear Inner (4)	Tympanocentesis reserved for complicated, recurrent, or chronic persistent otitis media 1. For intact eardrum, clean ear canal with soap solution and collect fluid via syringe aspiration technique (tympanocentesis) 2. For ruptured eardrum, collect fluid on flexible shaft swab via an auditory speculum	Sterile tube, swab transport medium, or anaerobic system	≤2 h, RT	≤24 h, RT	1/day/source	Results of throat or nasopharyngeal swab cultures are not predictive of agents responsible for otitis media and should not be submitted for that purpose.
Outer (4)	1. Use moistened swab to remove any debris or crust from the ear canal 2. Obtain a sample by firmly rotating the swab in the outer canal	Swab transport	≤2 h, RT	≤24 h, 4°C	1/day/source	For otitis externa, *vigorous* swabbing is required since surface swabbing may miss streptococcal cellulitis.

Specimen	Collection instructions	Container/transport device	Transport time/temp	Storage time/temp	Replicate limits	Comments
Eye						
Conjunctiva (2, 73)	1. Sample each eye with separate swabs (premoistened with sterile saline) by rolling over each conjunctiva 2. Medium may be inoculated at time of collection 3. Smear may be prepared at time of collection; roll swab over 1–2-cm area of slide	Direct culture inoculation: BAP and CHOC; laboratory inoculation: swab transport	Plates: ≤15 min, RT; swabs: ≤2 h, RT	≤24 h, RT	None	If possible, sample both conjunctiva, even if only one is infected, to determine the indigenous microflora. The uninfected eye can serve as a control with which to compare the agents isolated from the infected eye. If cost prohibits this approach, rely on the Gram stain to assist in interpretation of culture.
Corneal scrapings (2, 73)	1. Specimen collected by ophthalmologist 2. Using sterile spatula, scrape ulcers or lesions, and inoculate scraping directly onto medium 3. Prepare 2 smears by rubbing material from spatula onto 1–2-cm area of slide	Direct culture inoculations: BHI with 10% sheep blood, CHOC, and inhibitory mold agar	≤15 min, RT	≤24 h, RT	None	If conjunctival specimen is collected, do so before anesthetic application, which may inhibit some bacteria. Corneal scrapings are obtained after anesthesia. Include fungal media.
Vitreous fluid aspirates	Prepare eye for needle aspiration of fluid	Sterile screw-cap tube or direct inoculation of small amount of fluid onto media	≤15 min, RT	≤24 h, RT	1/day	Include fungal media. Anesthetics may be inhibitory to some etiologic agents.
Feces						
Routine culture (53)	Pass specimen directly into a clean, dry container; transport to microbiology laboratory within 1 h of collection or transfer to Cary-Blair holding medium	Clean, leak-proof, wide-mouth container or use Cary-Blair holding medium (>2 g)	Unpreserved: ≤1 h, RT Holding medium: ≤24 h, RT	≤24 h, 4°C ≤48 h, RT or 4°C	1/day	Do not perform routine stool cultures for patients whose length of hospital stay is >3 days and the admitting diagnosis was not gastroenteritis, without consultation with physician. Tests for *Clostridium difficile* should be considered for these patients. Swabs for routine pathogens are not recommended except for infants (see Rectal swabs).

(Continued on next page)

TABLE 3 Bacteriology collection, transport, and storage guidelines[a] (*Continued*)

Specimen type (reference)	Collection guidelines	Transport device and/or minimum vol	Transport[b] time and temp	Storage time	Replica limits	Comments
C. difficile culture (80)	Pass liquid or soft stool directly into a clean, dry container; soft stool is defined as stool assuming the shape of its container	Sterile, leak-proof, wide-mouth container, >5 ml	≤1 h, RT; 1–24 h, 4°C; >24 h, −20°C or colder	2 days, 4°C, for culture; 3 days at 4°C, or longer at −70°C for toxin test	1 or 2 specimens may be necessary to detect low toxin levels	Patients should be passing ≥5 liquid or soft stools per 24-h period. Testing of formed or hard stool is not recommended. Freezing at −20°C or above results in rapid loss of cytotoxin activity.
E. coli O157: H7 and other Shiga-toxin-producing serotypes (3, 44)	Pass liquid or bloody stool into a clean, dry container	Sterile, leak-proof, wide-mouth container, or Cary-Blair holding medium (>2 g)	Unpreserved: ≤1 h, RT Swab transport system: ≤24 h, RT or 4°C	≤24 h, 4°C ≤24 h, RT	1/day	Bloody or liquid stools collected within 6 days of onset among patients with abdominal cramps have the highest yield. Shiga toxin assay for all EHEC serotypes is better than sorbitol MacConkey culture for O157:H7 only.
Leukocyte detection (63) (not recommended for use with patients who have acute infectious diarrhea)	Pass feces directly into a clean, dry container; transport to microbiology laboratory within 1 h of collection, or transfer to ova and parasite transport system (10% formalin or PVA)	Sterile, leak-proof, wide-mouth container or 10% formalin and/or PVA; >2 ml	Unpreserved: ≤1 h, RT Formalin/PVA: indefinite, RT	≤24 h, 4°C Indefinite, RT	1/day	This procedure should be discouraged because it provides results of little clinical value. A Gram stain or simple methylene blue stain may be used to visualize leukocytes. Commercial detection methods are also available.
Rectal swab	1. Carefully insert a swab ca. 1 in. beyond the anal sphincter 2. Gently rotate the swab to sample the anal crypts 3. Feces should be visible on the swab for detection of diarrheal pathogens	Swab transport	≤2 h, RT	≤24 h, RT	1/day	Reserved for detecting *Neisseria gonorrhoeae*, *Shigella*, *Campylobacter*, and herpes simplex virus and anal carriage of group B *Streptococcus* and other beta-hemolytic streptococci, or for patients unable to pass a specimen.

Specimen	Collection guidelines	Transport device	Transport time	Storage	Replicate limits	Comments
Fistula	See Abscess					
Fluids: abdominal, amniotic, ascites, bile, joint, paracentesis, pericardial, peritoneal, pleural, synovial, thoracentesis (13)	1. Disinfect overlying skin with iodine preparation 2. Obtain specimen via percutaneous needle aspiration or surgery 3. Always submit as much fluid as possible; *never* submit a swab dipped in fluid	Anaerobic transport system, sterile screw-cap tube, or blood culture bottle for bacteria; transport immediately to laboratory. Bacteria, >1 ml	≤15 min, RT	≤24 h, RT; pericardial fluid and fluids for fungal cultures, ≤24 h, 4°C	None	Amniotic and culdocentesis fluids should be transported in an anaerobic system and need not be centrifuged prior to Gram staining. Other fluids are best examined by Gram staining of a cytocentrifuged preparation.
Gangrenous tissue	See Abscess					Discourage sampling of surface or superficial tissue. Tissue biopsy or aspiration should be performed.
Gastric Wash or lavage for mycobacteria (20)	Collect in early morning before patients eat and while they are still in bed. 1. Introduce a nasogastric tube into the stomach 2. Perform lavage with 25–50 ml of chilled, sterile distilled water 3. Recover sample and place in a leak-proof, sterile container	Sterile, leak-proof container	≤15 min, RT, or neutralize within 1 h of collection	≤24 h, 4°C	1/day	The specimen must be processed promptly, since mycobacteria die rapidly in gastric washings. Neutralize with sodium bicarbonate when holding for >1 h.
Biopsy for *H. pylori*	Collected by gastroenterologist during endoscopy	Sterile tube with transport medium	<1 h, RT	≤24 h, 4°C	None	Culture may be needed for antimicrobial testing.
Genital, female Amniotic fluid (182)	Aspirate via amniocentesis, or collect during cesarean delivery	Anaerobic transport system, ≥1 ml	≤2 h, RT	≤24 h, RT	None	Swabbing or aspiration of vaginal secretions is *not* acceptable because of the potential for contamination with the commensal vaginal flora.

(Continued on next page)

TABLE 3 Bacteriology collection, transport, and storage guidelines[a] (*Continued*)

Specimen type (reference)	Collection guidelines	Transport device and/or minimum vol	Transport[b] time and temp	Storage time	Replica limits	Comments
Bartholin gland secretions	1. Disinfect skin with iodine preparation 2. Aspirate fluid from ducts	Anaerobic transport system, ≥1 ml	≤2 h, RT	≤24 h, RT	1/day	
Cervical secretions (5)	1. Visualize the cervix using a speculum without lubricant 2. Remove mucus and secretions from the cervical os with swab, and discard the swab 3. Firmly yet gently sample the endocervical canal with a new sterile swab	Swab transport	≤2 h, RT	≤24 h, RT	1/day	See the text for collection and transport need for *Chlamydia trachomatis* and *Neisseria gonorrhoeae*.
Cul-de-sac fluid	Submit aspirate or fluid	Anaerobic transport system, >1 ml	≤2 h, RT	≤24 h, RT	1/day	
Endometrial tissue and secretions	1. Collect transcervical aspirate via a telescoping catheter 2. Transfer entire amount to anaerobic transport system	Anaerobic transport system, ≥1 ml	≤2 h, RT	≤24 h, RT	1/day	
Products of conception	1. Submit a portion of tissue in a sterile container 2. If obtained by cesarean delivery, immediately transfer to an anaerobic transport system	Sterile tube or anaerobic transport system	≤2 h, RT	≤24 h, RT	1/day	Do not process lochia, culture of which may give misleading results.
Urethral secretions (5)	Collect at least 1 h after patient has urinated 1. Remove old exudate from the urethral orifice 2. Collect discharge material on a swab by massaging the urethra; for females, massage the urethra against the pubic symphysis through the vagina	Swab transport	≤2 h, RT	≤24 h, RT	1/day	If no discharge can be obtained, wash the periurethral area with Betadine soap and rinse with water. Insert a small swab 2–4 cm into the urethra, rotate it, and leave it in place for at least 2 s to facilitate absorption.

Specimen	Collection procedure	Transport container	Transport	Storage	Frequency	Comments
Vaginal secretions (5)	1. Wipe away old secretions and discharge 2. Obtain secretions from the mucosal membrane of the vaginal wall with a sterile swab or pipette 3. If a smear is also needed, use a second swab	Swab transport	≤2 h, RT	≤24 h, RT	1/day	For intrauterine devices, place entire device into a sterile container and submit at RT. Gram stain, not culture, is recommended for the diagnosis of bacterial vaginosis.
Genital, female or male lesion	1. Clean with sterile saline, and remove lesion's surface with a sterile scalpel blade 2. Allow transudate to accumulate 3. While pressing the base of the lesion, *firmly* rub base with a sterile swab to collect fluid	Swab transport	≤2 h, RT	≤24 h, RT	1/day	For dark-field examination to detect *T. pallidum*, touch a glass slide to the transudate, add coverslip, and transport immediately to the laboratory in a humidified chamber (petri dish with moist gauze). *T. pallidum* cannot be cultured on artificial media.
Genital, male Prostate	1. Cleanse urethral meatus with soap and water 2. Massage prostate through rectum 3. Collect fluid expressed from urethra on a sterile swab	Swab transport or sterile tube for >1 ml of specimen	≤2 h, RT	≤24 h, RT	1/day	Pathogens in prostatic secretions may be identified by quantitative culture of urine before and after massage. Ejaculate may also be cultured.
Urethra	Insert a small swab 2–4 cm into the urethral lumen, rotate swab, and leave it in place for at least 2 s to facilitate absorption	Swab transport	≤2 h, RT	≤24 h, RT	1/day	
Pilonidal cyst	See Abscess					
Respiratory, lower Bronchoalveolar lavage, brush or wash, endotracheal aspirate	1. Collect washing or aspirate in a sputum trap 2. Place brush in sterile container with 1 ml of saline	Sterile container, >1 ml	≤2 h, RT	≤24 h, 4°C	1/day	A total of 40–80 ml of fluid is needed for quantitative analysis of BAL fluid. For quantitative analysis of brushings, place brush into 1.0 ml of saline.

(Continued on next page)

TABLE 3 Bacteriology collection, transport, and storage guidelines[a] (*Continued*)

Specimen type (reference)	Collection guidelines	Transport device and/or minimum vol	Transport[b] time and temp	Storage time	Replica limits	Comments
Sputum, expectorated (8)	1. Collect specimen under the direct supervision of a nurse or physician 2. Have patient rinse or gargle with water to remove excess oral flora. 3. Instruct patient to cough deeply to produce a lower respiratory specimen (not postnasal fluid) 4. Collect in a sterile container	Sterile container, >1 ml Minimum amount: bacteria, >1 ml	≤2 h, RT	≤24 h, 4°C	1/day	For pediatric patients unable to produce a sputum specimen, a respiratory therapist should collect a specimen via suction. The best specimen should have ≤10 squamous cells/100× field (10× objective and 10× ocular).
Sputum, induced (8)	1. Have patient rinse mouth with water after brushing gums and tongue 2. With the aid of a nebulizer, have patients inhale approximately 25 ml of 3–10% sterile saline 3. Collect in a sterile container.	Sterile container, >1 ml	≤2 h, RT	≤24 h, RT	1/day	Same as above for sputum, expectorated.
Respiratory, upper						
Oral	1. Remove oral secretions and debris from the surface of the lesion with a swab; discard this swab 2. Using a second swab, vigorously sample the lesion, avoiding any areas of normal tissue	Swab transport	≤2 h, RT	≤24 h, RT	1/day	Discourage sampling of superficial tissue for bacterial evaluation. Tissue biopsy specimens or needle aspirates are the specimens of choice.
Nasal	1. Insert a swab, premoistened with sterile saline, approximately 1–2 cm into the nares 2. Rotate the swab against the nasal mucosa	Swab transport	≤2 h, RT	≤24 h, RT	1/day	Anterior nose cultures are reserved for detecting staphylococcal carriers or for nasal lesions.

Specimen	Collection	Transport device or method	Transport time and temperature	Storage time and temperature	Replicate limit	Comments
Nasopharynx (4)	1. Gently insert a small swab (e.g., calcium alginate) into the posterior nasopharynx via the nose 2. Rotate swab slowly for 5 s to absorb secretions	Direct medium inoculation at bedside or examination table, swab transport	Plates: ≤15 min, RT; swabs: ≤2 h, RT	≤24 h, RT	1/day	
Throat or pharynx	1. Depress tongue with a tongue depressor 2. Sample the posterior pharynx, tonsils, and inflamed areas with a sterile swab	Swab transport	≤2 h, RT	≤24 h, RT	1/day	Throat swab cultures are contraindicated in patients with epiglottitis. Swabs for *Neisseria gonorrhoeae* should be placed in charcoal-containing transport medium and plated ≤12 h after collection. JEMBEC, Biobags, and the GonoPak are better for transport at RT.
Tissue	Collected during surgery or cutaneous biopsy procedure	Anaerobic transport system or sterile, screw-cap container; add several drops of sterile saline to keep small pieces of tissue moist	≤15 min, RT	≤24 h, RT	None	Always submit as much tissue as possible. If excess tissue is available, save a portion of surgical tissue at −70°C in case further studies are needed. Never submit a swab that has been rubbed over the surface of a tissue. For quantitative study, a sample of 1 cm³ is appropriate.
Urine Female, midstream (25)	1. While holding the labia apart, begin voiding 2. After several milliliters has passed, collect a midstream portion without stopping the flow of urine 3. The midstream portion is used for bacterial culture	Sterile, wide-mouth container, ≥1 ml, or urine transport tube with boric acid preservative	Unpreserved: ≤2 h, RT; preserved: ≤24 h, RT	≤24 h, 4°C	1/day	Chlamydial antigen detection in urine from women is less sensitive than in urine from men (148). Urine is toxic to cell lines and is therefore not the specimen of choice for chlamydial culture. Cleansing before voiding does not improve urine specimen quality; i.e., midstream urines are equivalent to clean-catch midstream urines (91, 132).

(Continued on next page)

TABLE 3 Bacteriology collection, transport, and storage guidelines[a] (*Continued*)

Specimen type (reference)	Collection guidelines	Transport device and/or minimum vol	Transport[b] time and temp	Storage time	Replica limits	Comments
Male, midstream (25)	1. While holding the foreskin retracted, begin voiding 2. After several milliliters has passed, collect a midstream portion without stopping the flow of urine 3. The midstream portion is used for culture	Sterile, wide-mouth container, ≥1 ml, or urine transport tube with boric acid preservative	Unpreserved: ≤2 h, RT	≤24 h, 4°C	1/day	First part of urine stream is used for probe tests and antigen test for chlamydia. Collect specimen for probe and antigen tests at least 2 h after last urination.
Straight catheter (25)	1. Thoroughly cleanse the urethral opening with soap and water 2. Rinse area with wet gauze pads 3. Aseptically, insert catheter into the bladder 4. After allowing approximately 15 ml to pass, collect urine to be submitted in a sterile container	Sterile, leak-proof container or urine transport tube with boric acid preservative	Unpreserved: ≤2 h, RT; preserved: ≤24 h, RT	≤24 h, 4°C	1/day	Catheterization may introduce members of the urethral flora into the bladder and increase the risk of iatrogenic infection.
Indwelling catheter	1. Disinfect the catheter collection port with 70% alcohol 2. Use needle and syringe to aseptically collect 5–10 ml of urine 3. Transfer to a sterile tube or container	Sterile leak-proof container or urine transport tube with boric acid preservative	Unpreserved: ≤2 h, RT; preserved: ≤24 h, RT	≤24 h, 4°C	1/day	Patients with indwelling catheters always have bacteria in their bladders. Do not collect urine from these patients unless they are symptomatic.
Wound	See Abscess					

[a] Abbreviations: AFB, acid-fast bacilli; BAP, blood agar plate; BHI, brain heart infusion; CHOC, chocolate agar; CVP, central venous pressure; i.v. intravenous; PVA, polyvinyl alcohol fixative; RT, room temperature.
[b] All specimens are to be transported in leak-proof plastic bags having a separate compartment for the requisition.
[c] One set refers to one culture with both aerobic and anaerobic broths.

TABLE 4 Specimen management for infrequently encountered organisms[a]

Organism (disease)	Specimen of choice	Transport issues	Comment
Bartonella sp. (cat scratch fever)	Blood, tissue, lymph node aspirate	1 wk at 4°C; indefinitely at −70°C	May see organisms in or on erythrocytes with Giemsa stain. Use Warthin-Starry silver stain for tissue. SPS is toxic.
Borrelia burgdorferi (Lyme disease)	Skin biopsy at lesion periphery, blood, CSF	Keep tissue moist and sterile; hand carry to laboratory if possible	Consider PCR in addition to culture. Culture yield is low. Warthin-Starry silver stain for tissue. AO and Giemsa for blood and CSF.
Borrelia sp. (relapsing fever)	Blood smear (blood)	Hand carry to laboratory if possible	Use direct wet mount in saline for dark-field microscopy. Stain with Wright's or Giemsa stain. Blood culture is unreliable.
Brucella sp.[b]	Blood, bone marrow	Transport at room temperature; pediatric lysis-centrifugation tube is helpful	Routine blood culture bottles are useful if held 30 days. Blind subculture may be necessary. Joint fluid culture in arthritis. Notify laboratory if *Brucella* suspected.
Klebsiella granulomatis (granuloma inguinale; donovanosis)	Tissue, subsurface scrapings	Transport at room temperature	Mostly a tropical disease. Stain with Wright's or Giemsa stain. Epithelium alone is inadequate. Organism cannot be cultured.
Coxiella (Q fever),[b] *Rickettsia* (spotted fevers; typhus)	Serum, blood, tissue	Blood and tissue are frozen at −70°C until shipped	Refer isolation to reference laboratory. Serologic diagnosis is preferred.
Ehrlichia sp.	Blood smear, skin biopsy, blood (with heparin or EDTA anticoagulant), CSF, serum	Material for culture sent on ice; keep tissue moist and sterile; hold at 4 to 20°C until tested or at −70°C for shipment; transport on ice or frozen for PCR test	Serologic diagnosis preferred. Fix smear in methanol. Tissue stained with FA or Gimenez stain. Refer isolate to reference laboratory. CSF for direct examination and PCR.
Francisella sp. (tularemia)[b]	Lymph node aspirate, scrapings, lesion biopsy, blood, sputum	Rapid transport to laboratory or freeze; ship on dry ice	Send to reference laboratory. Serologic testing helpful. Gram stain of tissue is not productive. IFA available. Culture effective 10% of the time.
Leptospira sp.	Serum, blood (citrate-containing anticoagulants should not be used), CSF (1st wk), urine (after 1st wk)	Blood, <1 h; urine, <1 h or dilute 1:10 in 1% bovine serum albumin and store at 4–20°C or neutralize with sodium bicarbonate	Serologic testing most helpful. Acidic urine is detrimental. Dark-field microscopy and direct FA available. Warthin-Starry silver stain for tissue.
Streptobacillus sp. (rat bite fever; Haverhill fever)	Blood, aspirates of joint fluid	High-volume bottle preferred	Do not refrigerate. Requires blood, serum, or ascitic fluid for growth. SPS is inhibitory. AO staining is helpful.

[a] Abbreviations: AO, acridine-orange; CSF, cerebrospinal fluid; EDTA, ethylenediaminetetraacetate; FA, fluorescent antibody; PCR, polymerase chain reaction; SPS, sodium polyanethol sulfonate. Data from reference 33.
[b] Laboratory safety hazard. Class II biologic safety cabinet required.

TABLE 5 Recommendations for Gram stain and plating media for bacteriology specimens[a,b]

Specimen or organism	Gram stain	Aerobic media	Anaerobic media	Comments
Body cavity fluids				Blood culture bottles should be used to incubate large volumes of specimens for all body cavity fluids
CSF (routine)	x	B C		
CSF (shunt)	x	B C Th		
Pericardial	x	B C	BBA	
Pleural	x	B C	BBA	
Peritoneal	x	B C Mac	BBA LKV BBE CNA	
CAPD	x	B C Th	BBA	
Synovial	x	B C		
Bone marrow	x	B C	BBA	
Catheter tip		B		
Ear external fluid/swab	x	B C Mac		
Ear internal fluid	x	B C	BBA	
Eye	x	B C		
Gastrointestinal tract				
Feces		B Mac HE Ca EB		C. jejuni/coli in 5% O_2–10% CO_2–85% N_2 at 42°C for all gastrointestinal tract specimens
Rectal swab		B Mac HE Ca EB		
Genital tract				
Vaginal/cervix		B TM		
Urethra/penis	x	TM		
Other	x	B C Mac TM	BBA LKV BBE CNA	
Group B streptococcal screen		Selective broth, subculture to B		
Lower respiratory tract				
Sputum	x	B C Mac		
Tracheal aspirate	x	B C Mac		
Bronchoalveolar lavage fluid	x	B C Mac		
Bronchoscopy brushing, washing	x	B C Mac	BBA LKV CNA	Protected bronchoscope brushing required for anaerobic culture
Tissue	x	B C Mac Th	BBA LKV BBE CNA	
Upper respiratory tract				
Nasopharynx		B C		
Nose		B		
Throat		B or SSA		Add chocolate agar for epiglottis
Urine		B Mac		
Wound or abscess				
Swab	x	B C Mac		Anaerobic culture not recommended for swab
Aspirate	x	B C Mac	BBA LKV BBE CNA	
Bordetella pertussis and B. parapertussis		Regan Lowe		
Brucella spp.		B C		
Corynebacterium diphtheriae		Cysteine-tellurite or Loeffler's serum		
Clostridium difficile		CCFA		
E. coli O157:H7 (EHEC)		Sorbitol-Mac		Shiga toxin EIA more sensitive
Francisella tularensis		C or BCYE		

(Continued on next page)

TABLE 5 *(Continued)*

Specimen or organism	Gram stain	Aerobic media	Anaerobic media	Comments
Group B *Streptococcus*		LIM broth		
Haemophilus ducreyi		C + vancomycin (3 µg/ml)		Gram stain resembling "school of fish"
Helicobacter pylori	x	B		*Campylobacter* gaseous atmosphere at 35–37°C
Legionella		BCYE		
Leptospira		Fletcher's medium or EMJH		30°C for up to 13 wk
Neisseria gonorrhoeae		TM		
Vibrio		TCBS		
Yersinia		CIN		

[a] CAPD, fluid from chronic ambulatory peritoneal dialysis; B, blood agar; C, chocolate blood agar; Mac, MacConkey agar; Th, thioglycolate broth; Ca, Campylobacter agar; HE, Hektoen enteric; EB, enrichment broth; SSA, group A *Streptococcus* selective agar; TM, Thayer-Martin; BCYE, buffered charcoal yeast extract; TCBS, thiosulfate citrate bile salt sucrose; CIN, cefsulodin-irgasan-novobiocin; BBA, brucella blood agar; LKV, laked blood with kanamycin and vancomycin; BBE, *Bacteroides* bile esculin; CNA, anaerobic colistin-nalidixic acid; CCFA, cycloserine-cefoxitin-fructose agar; EMJH, Ellinghausen-McCullough-Johnson-Harris medium.

[b] Set up anaerobic culture upon request, if specimen is collected and transported appropriately. Call physician if appropriate specimen does not have request for anaerobic culture.

diagnosis, in the form of an ICD-9 code, is required to confirm the need for a particular test. If a test is not deemed necessary for a specific diagnosis, the patient must sign an advanced beneficiary notice documenting that the test is not considered necessary and, if performed, the patient will be required to pay the test charge. Medicare and Medicaid compliance rules also can be reviewed at the Centers for Medicare and Medicaid Services web site.

Specimen Rejection

In spite of acceptable labeling, some specimen collection sites, transport containers, or transport conditions render the specimen unacceptable for processing (142). Table 3 lists acceptable criteria for specimen management based on collection or transport conditions and times. When specimens fall outside these limits, new specimens should be collected whenever possible. In addition, specimens may be rejected because of the quality of specimen material collected rather than the conditions of transport (Table 6). Specimen quality is evaluated by examining the quantity and cellular composition. Although the quantity of many specimens is limited by the collection method or physical size of the infected area, some specimens, such as urine, stool, and sputum, are available in abundance. If another specimen can be collected easily with a larger volume, it is appropriate and necessary to request new or additional material. If the specimen volume must be limited, small volumes of liquid specimens can be extended by adding 1 to 2 ml of sterile saline or a nutrient broth. It is important to add just enough liquid to provide specimen for all tests requested.

Examining the cellular composition of clinical material first requires a gross examination of the specimen. Infection gives rise to purulence (abundant polymorphonuclear cells), blood, necrosis, and mucus (mucous membrane specimens). In general, gross examination should identify yellow to tan purulence, red to rust-colored blood, clear and tenacious mucus, and brown to black discoloration of tissue denoting necrosis. Portions for smear and inoculation to culture media should be taken from these areas. Ideally, microscopic examination of smears, using a 10× microscope objective, should demonstrate many polymorphonuclear cells and few or no squamous epithelial cells indicating cutaneous or mucocutaneous contamination with the

normal bacterial flora. Specimens where tissue necrosis is present also may show elastin fibers in stained smears. Lower respiratory tract specimens are likely to show alveolar macrophages and Curschmann's spirals, indicating that secretions have originated from the distal airways. Curschmann's spirals are casts of bronchioles found in patients with chronic lung disease caused most commonly by asthma and cigarette smoking. Figures 1 and 2 illustrate elastin fibers and Curschmann's spirals, respectively. Although elastin fibers are present in noninfected surgical wounds and specimens from areas of tissue damage, they are also found in infected tissue where necrosis has occurred. Specimens determined to have gross bacterial contamination from the normal flora, indicated by an abundance of squamous epithelial cells, should be rejected. Specimens are rejected by contacting the patient's caregiver, explaining the reason for rejection, and requesting a replacement specimen of acceptable quality. Timely notification and collection of replacement specimen is necessary, especially in instances where antimicrobial therapy has been initiated. Specimen rejection criteria should be reviewed by appropriate laboratory and medical staff representatives before becoming policy. Examples of acceptable and unacceptable specimens are listed in Table 6.

Culture Interpretation

Following examination of the stained smear and culture incubation, agar culture plates are interpreted for bacterial growth by attempting to differentiate potential pathogens requiring identification and antimicrobial testing from contamination by colonizing members of the normal bacterial flora. This is accomplished by examining the relative quantities of each isolate, correlating culture results with Gram-stained smear results, and recognizing usual contaminants and pathogens from respective specimen sites. In general, when examining cultures of specimens from sites likely to be contaminated (e.g., sputum, urine, and superficial wounds), potential pathogens should outnumber the indigenous flora and should be seen in the direct Gram stain. When examining cultures of specimens from presumably sterile sites (e.g., cerebrospinal fluid [CSF], joint fluids, other body fluids, and deep tissue), potential pathogens occur in any quantity and may or may not be seen in the direct Gram-stained smear. Specific criteria for identifying

TABLE 6 Screening specimens requested for routine bacterial culture to ensure quality[a]

Specimen (reference)	Screening method	Results of screen[b]	
		Acceptable	Unacceptable
Sputum (119)	Microscopic examination of Gram-stained smear	<10 SEC/average 10× field	>10 SEC/average 10× field
Endotracheal aspirate (113)	Microscopic examination of Gram-stained smear	<10 SEC/average 10× field and bacteria detected in at least 1 of 20 fields (100×)	>10 SEC/average 10× field and no bacteria detected in 20 fields (100×)
Bronchoalveolar lavage fluid (174)	Microscopic examination of Gram-stained smear	<1% of cells present are SEC	>1% of cells present are SEC
Urine (186)	Urinalysis, Gram stain of urine sediment	<3+SEC by urinalysis; positive LE test result with >10 polymorphonuclear leukocytes/mm^3 from symptomatic patient (patients with asymptomatic bacteriuria may not have increased number of leukocytes)	≥3+SEC on urinalysis or more than 3 potential pathogens by Gram stain implies gross contamination
Superficial wound (155)	Microscopic examination of Gram-stained smear	<2+SEC, polymorphonuclear leukocytes present	>2+SEC and no polymorphonuclear neutrophils
Stool for bacterial pathogens (112)	Location of patient? Duration of hospitalization?	Outpatient or inpatient for ≤3 days	In hospital >3 days, or diarrhea developed while in hospital
Other specimens	Screening methods unavailable or unproven		

[a] Reprinted from reference 169a with permission.
[b] LE, leukocyte esterase; SEC, squamous epithelial cells.

FIGURE 1 (row 1, left) Gram stain of a surgical wound specimen, showing elastin fibers. Magnification, 10× ocular, 100× objective.

FIGURE 2 (row 1, right) Gram stain of a sputum specimen, showing Curschmann's spiral. Magnification, 10× ocular, 100× objective.

FIGURE 3 (row 2, left) Gram stain of vaginal secretions, showing clue cells. Magnification, 10× ocular, 100× objective.

FIGURE 4 (row 2, right) Gram stain of an unacceptable sputum specimen (grossly contaminated with oropharyngeal flora), showing >10 squamous epithelial cells per low-power field. Magnification, 10× ocular, 100× objective.

FIGURE 5 (row 3, left) Gram stain of an acceptable sputum specimen, showing <10 squamous epithelial cells per low-power field. Magnification, 10× ocular, 100× objective.

FIGURE 6 (row 3, right) Gram stain of urine, showing 4+ squamous epithelial cells, indicating gross contamination with vaginal or periurethral secretions and bacteria. Magnification, 10× ocular, 100× objective.

FIGURE 7 (row 4, left) Gram stain of urine, showing polymorphonuclear leukocytes and 4+ gram-negative bacilli. Magnification, 10× ocular, 100× objective.

FIGURE 8 (row 4, right) Gram stain of a wound specimen, showing polymorphonuclear leukocytes, mixed bacterial morphotypes suggesting aerobic and anaerobic bacteria, and both intra- and extracellular bacteria. This appearance suggests a mixed aerobic and anaerobic abscess or closed-space infection. Magnification, 10× ocular, 100× objective.

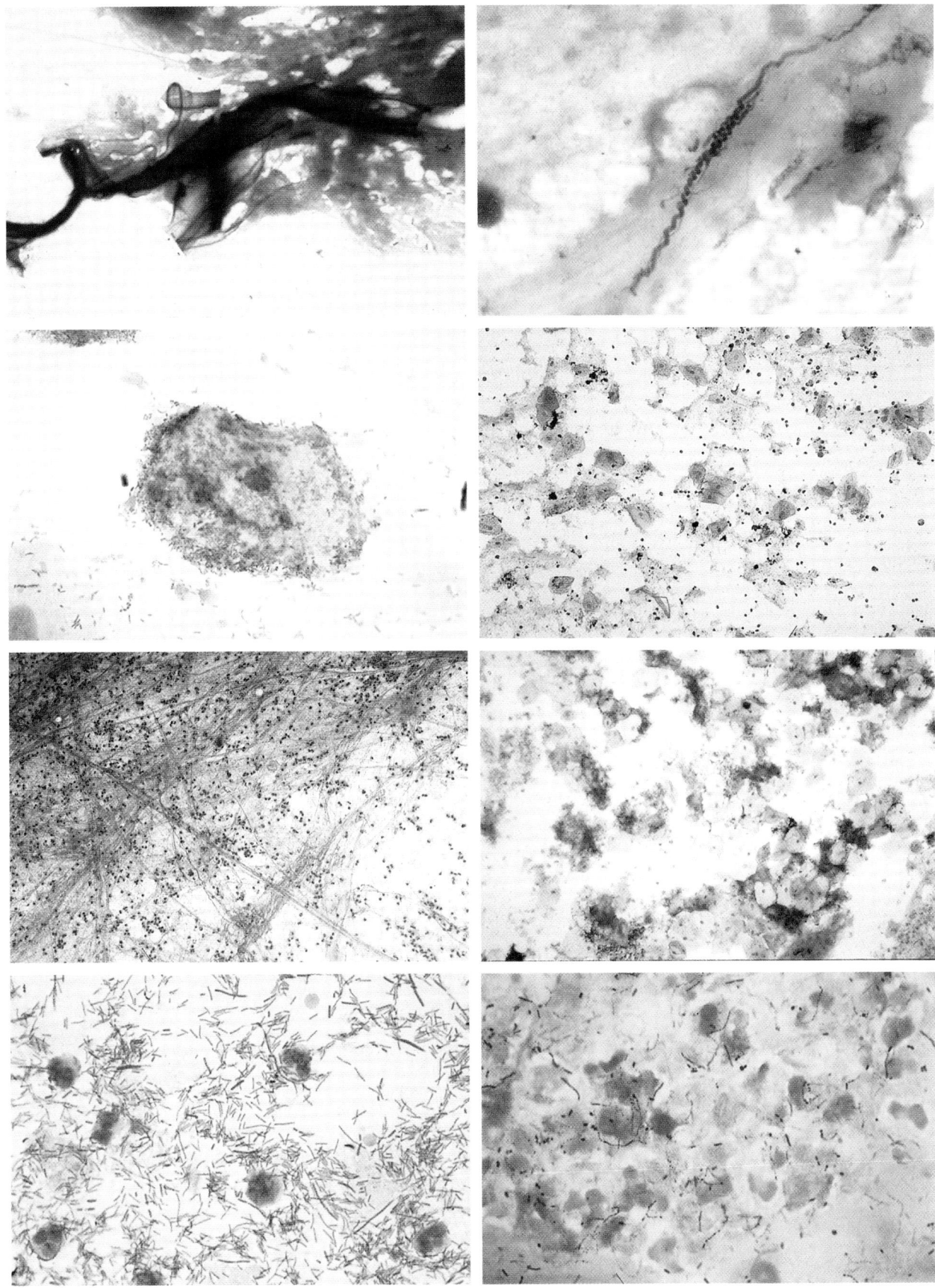

TABLE 7 Pediatric bacterial blood cultures: recommended blood volume[a]

Patient wt (lb)	Recommended blood vol/culture (ml)	Total blood vol for 2 cultures (ml)	Vol of blood equal to 1% of patient's total blood vol (ml)[b]
<19	1	2	2
18–30	3	6	6–10
30–60	5	10	10–20
60–90	10	20	20–30
90–120	15	30	30–40
>120	20	40	>40

[a] Data from reference 74.

[b] Blood volume calculated by assuming 85 ml/kg in newborns and 73 ml/kg in other patients. Two 20-ml blood specimens collected from an 80-kg adult (40 ml total) represent approximately 0.7% of the patient's total blood volume.

potentially significant isolates and contaminating members of the normal flora are addressed in the following sections of this chapter. It is a useful policy to save the culture plates for 1 week, allowing physicians the opportunity to call to request further identification or antimicrobial testing when clinically indicated

Critical Values in Microbiology

Many results in clinical microbiology can have an immediate impact on patient care. Although cultures require days to weeks to become positive, stained smear results, results of antigen or nucleic acid detection, and culture results from presumably sterile specimen sources may contain information necessitating important changes in therapy or care. Examples of medical emergencies that require immediate notification of the patient's health care provider include a positive blood culture, positive CSF Gram stain or culture, group A streptococcus detected in a surgical wound specimen, Gram stain suggesting gas gangrene or other systemic toxemia, and positive blood smear for malaria. Examples of results that require notification of physician or health care provider during a day shift, but not so immediate that calls are necessary during evening or overnight hours, include a positive acid-fast stain, new or unusual antimicrobial resistance, and the detection of highly significant or unusual microorganisms such as *Listeria*, *Legionella*, or *Brucella*. Most critical values are unique to individual medical centers and require laboratories to consult with medical staff representatives before compiling a call list for critical values (83, 95).

Blood and Intravascular Catheter Specimens

Blood is one of the most important specimens received by the laboratory for culture. In most cases, the presence of bacteria in blood (bacteremia) indicates an infection that has spread from a primary site such as the lungs (pneumonia). Such a bacteremia is referred to as a secondary bacteremia. In the absence of an identifiable infected source, the bacteremia is referred to as a primary bacteremia. Primary bacteremia can also result from "silent," subclinical passage of bacteria from contaminated areas of the body, such as mucous membranes, into the blood. Consequences of a clinically apparent primary or secondary bacteremia are sepsis, septic shock, or severe sepsis. Sepsis implies a bacteremia with signs and symptoms, such as fever, chills, and

tachycardia. Septic shock indicates the presence of hypotension with sepsis. Severe sepsis is characterized by septic shock with organ system failure and is associated with a 20 to 40% mortality rate (12).

A wide variety of bacteria are involved in bloodstream infections, the majority belonging to groups of bacteria, such as the streptococci/enterococci, staphylococci, or *Enterobacteriaceae*, that grow rapidly in culture (138, 191). It is important to recognize potential contaminants with similar growth patterns since treating contaminants as significant isolates is associated with unnecessary expense and dangers of antimicrobial misuse (10). Common contaminants included coagulase-negative staphylococci, corynebacteria, *Bacillus* spp., and propionibacteria. In general, single cultures positive for these bacteria represent contamination. Multiple, separate cultures growing one of these isolates are more likely to indicate a clinically significant bacteremia (77, 109, 190). Contamination is controlled by proper skin antisepsis before venipuncture. Iodine-containing antiseptics, including iodophors (iodine with a detergent) and tincture of iodine (iodine with alcohol), or chlorhexidine is needed to reduce the number of viable bacteria at the venipuncture site (93, 108). Contamination rates of less than 2 to 3% are desired (149). Higher rates should be investigated and corrected by educational efforts.

Bacteremic patients fall into many groups that determine specimen collection methods. Most patients are intermittently bacteremic, implying that bacteria are present in the blood for periods of time followed by nonbacteremic periods. Other patients who have intravascular sites of primary infection (such as endocarditis) are continuously bacteremic. All patients are likely to have very low levels of bacteria in the blood in spite of experiencing severe clinical symptoms. For these reasons, multiple blood cultures, each containing large volumes of blood, are required to detect bacteremia. As a rule for adults, two or three separate blood cultures, each inoculated with at least 20 ml of blood, are recommended per 24-h period (190). Pediatric recommendations are similar, except for the volumes of blood recommended (74). Adult and pediatric requirements for blood collection for culture are summarized in Tables 3 and 7.

It is best to collect blood directly into culture bottles during the venipuncture procedure rather than into transport tubes that are sent to the laboratory for subsequent transfer of blood into the culture bottles. Collection directly into culture bottles enables bacteria to begin growing immediately, decreases the amount of anticoagulant to which bacteria are exposed, and decreases the chances of needlestick accidents for health care personnel. The anticoagulant used in all blood culture systems is sodium polyanethanolsulfanate (SPS) and is known to be inhibitory to meningococci, gonococci, *Peptostreptococcus anaerobius*, *Streptobacillus moniliformis*, and *Gardnerella vaginalis* (137). Although few practical methods are available to avoid exposure of these bacteria in blood to SPS, it is advisable to diminish the total amount of SPS used by avoiding transport tubes that also include SPS.

Culture of blood is the most sensitive method available for the detection of bacteremia. Semiautomated blood culture systems are present in nearly every clinical laboratory. Refer to chapter 14 for a complete discussion of manual and automated blood culture systems. Occasionally, direct staining of blood collected by venipuncture can provide rapid, nearly immediate detection of bacteria in blood (135, 141). Gram staining a smear of peripheral blood or buffy coat layer may detect bacterial cells in the blood of patients with meningococcemia, *S. pneumoniae* infection, or overwhelming sepsis caused by other bacteria when the concentration of bacteria in blood is very high (approaching 10,000 bacterial cells per ml of blood). In spite of published reports documenting the occasional use of direct staining of blood, the likelihood of results impacting patient management does not warrant its use as a routine laboratory procedure.

Some bacteria, such as *Legionella* spp., mycobacteria, some *N. meningitidis* strains, and *N. gonorrhoeae*, fail to grow in routine commercial media and should be sought by using another method, such as lysis-centrifugation. Other bacteria may require prolonged incubation of media or the addition of adsorbents to bind antimicrobials or inhibitory substances. Chapter 14 provides a thorough description of blood culture systems and their use.

Positive blood culture bottles are evaluated initially by examining a Gram-stained smear of the broth. The report should include a description of the bacterial morphology and the Gram reaction. If a presumptive identification of the microorganism can be made, it may be added to the report. For example, a blood culture Gram stain report might state "Gram-positive cocci in clusters suggesting staphylococci." If a Gram stain fails to reveal organisms, an acridine orange stain may be more sensitive. Specimens in positive blood culture bottles should be subcultured to media based on the organism seen in the Gram-stained smear. In addition, since 5 to 10% of all bacteremias are polymicrobial (contain more than one bacterial type), the addition of a Columbia-colistin-nalidixic acid (CNA) or other gram-negative-bacterium-inhibitory agar medium to cultures showing gram-negative bacilli in the Gram stain or the addition of a MacConkey or related selective agar plate to cultures showing gram-positive bacteria is recommended. Anaerobic media and culture conditions should be used if the morphology of the organism seen in the Gram-stained smear is suggestive of an anaerobic bacterium or if the organism is recovered from an anaerobic culture bottle only.

Special Considerations

Anaerobes

Anaerobes have always accounted for a relatively small percentage of organisms recovered from blood. Over the past several years, some investigators have noted a decline in bloodstream infections by anaerobes (118). However, this is not the case in all hospitals (26). Therefore, laboratories should review their own data when deciding whether to include an anaerobic culture bottle as part of the routine workup of blood specimens. Anaerobic media available for use with the automated systems appear to perform adequately. It is important to note that if the anaerobic component of a blood culture is dropped, the inoculum should be added to an additional aerobic bottle to ensure that the full volume of blood is cultured.

Lysis Centrifugation

The Isolator lysis centrifugation system (Wampole Laboratories, Cranbury, N.J.) is a commercially available manual blood culture method (190). The system consists of a tube containing anticoagulant (SPS), EDTA, and saponin. After the tube is filled with blood during phlebotomy, the contents are mixed and centrifuged and the resulting pellet is inoculated onto agar media. The system effectively recovers aerobic and facultative bacteria and fungi. The Isolator System does not perform as well as other systems for recovering *S. pneumoniae*, other streptococci, *Pseudomonas aeruginosa*, and anaerobes (190). Advantages of the Isolator System are the ability to inoculate the pellet to specific agar media when attempting to detect unusual etiologies of bacteremia, such as *Legionella pneumophila*, *Francisella tularensis*, and *Bartonella* spp., and to provide colony counts, reported as CFU per milliliter of blood (34, 190). Disadvantages of the system are the labor involved in the initial processing and the potential for increased contamination that accompanies manipulation during processing (173).

Intravascular Catheter Tips

Culture of intravascular catheter tips is performed to determine the source of a bacteremia and should be performed only when concurrent blood cultures are obtained. Soft tissue infections around a catheter insertion site are diagnosed by culturing a wound specimen consisting of freshly expressed purulence that can be aspirated. The most common technique used to culture the intravascular portion of a catheter is the semiquantitative method, in which the 5-cm distal portion of the catheter is rolled across a blood agar plate four times (96). The catheter tip is discarded. Growth of more than 15 colonies is considered significant, i.e., implicating the catheter tip as the likely source of a bacteremia if a similar isolate is detected in a blood culture.

Other techniques have been described for the identification of catheter-related infections. A meta-analysis of data was reported concerning the use of three types of catheter segment culture and three blood culture methods to determine the sensitivity and specificity of each method (158). The three catheter segment cultures included qualitative, semiquantitative (e.g., catheter roll method), and quantitative (dilutions to determine bacterial quantities used), while the three blood culture methods included qualitative catheter blood culture (reported as positive or negative), quantitative catheter blood culture, and paired quantitative catheter and peripheral venipuncture blood cultures. Based on this analysis, a quantitative catheter segment culture was the most accurate method, with pooled sensitivity and specificity both exceeding 90%. The optimal method in all clinical settings for determining that an intravascular catheter is the source of a bacteremia has not been determined. Because the most serious manifestation of catheter infections is bacteremia, ordinary blood cultures may be the best way to determine which patients require therapy (136).

Sterile Body Fluid Specimens

Cerebrospinal Fluid

CSF is collected for the diagnosis of meningitis (58). Bacterial meningitis can be divided into acute and chronic clinical presentations (171). Acute meningitis with onset of symptoms within the previous 24 h is usually caused by pyogenic bacteria. Specific etiologies are related to the age of the patient and whether the disease is community or nosocomially acquired. Chronic meningitis, with symptoms lasting at least 4 weeks, can have a wide variety of causes (Table 8). As with all clinical specimens, even those collected from a presumably sterile site, growth of contaminants occasionally does occur.

CSF is usually obtained by lumbar spinal puncture. Although bacterial stain and culture can be performed with as little as 0.5 ml of fluid, larger volumes are preferred since culture methods are more sensitive when small numbers of

TABLE 8 Usual bacterial etiologies of infectious disease syndromes

Disease	Etiologies
Central nervous system infection	
Acute meningitis, neutrophilic pleocytosis	*Streptococcus pneumoniae*
	Neisseria meningitidis
	Listeria monocytogenes
	Streptococcus agalactiae
	Haemophilus influenzae
	Staphylococcus aureus
	Gram-negative bacilli[a]
	Anaerobic bacteria
	Bacillus anthracis
Acute meningitis, CSF shunt related	Coagulase-negative staphylococci
	Staphylococcus aureus
	Propionibacterium spp.
	Gram-negative enteric bacilli (e.g., *E. coli* and *Klebsiella* spp.)
	Gram-negative nonfermenting bacilli (e.g., *P. aeruginosa* and *Acinetobacter* spp.)
Chronic meningitis, predominantly lymphocytic pleocytosis	*Nocardia asteroides* complex
	Brucella species
	Leptospira interrogans
	Mycobacterium tuberculosis
	Treponema pallidum
	Borrelia burgdorferi
Gastrointestinal tract infection	
Infectious diarrhea[b]	*Salmonella*, many bioserovars
	Shigella spp.
	Campylobacter jejuni/coli
	Campylobacter spp. (other)
	EHEC serotypes
	C. difficile
	Vibrio spp.
	Aeromonas spp.
	Pleisomonas shigelloides
	Y. enterocolitica
	E. coli toxigenic, invasive, and effacing strains
	Listeria monocytogenes
	C. perfringens
	B. cereus
Ingestion of preformed toxin[c]	*S. aureus*
	B. cereus
	C. botulinum
Gastritis/gastric and duodenal ulcers	*Helicobacter pylori*
Genital tract infection	
Ulcers	*T. pallidum*
	H. ducreyi
	C. trachomatis (LGV)
	Klebsiella granulomatis
Urethritis	*N. gonorrhoeae*
	Ureaplasma urealyticum
Vulvovaginitis	*N. gonorrhoeae* and *C. trachomatis* in prepubescent girls
Bacterial vaginosis	Overgrowth of vaginal flora with anaerobic bacteria
Cervicitis	*N. gonorrhoeae*
	C. trachomatis
	U. urealyticum (controversial)
Endometritis	Enterobacteriaceae
	Streptococci (groups A and B)
	Enterococci
	Mixed anaerobic genera
Salpingitis/oophoritis	*N. gonorrhoeae*
	C. trachomatis
	Mixed aerobic and anaerobic flora

(Continued on next page)

TABLE 8 *(Continued)*

Disease	Etiologies
Pelvic abscess	Mixed aerobic and anaerobic flora
Epididymitis	*N. gonorrhoeae*
	C. trachomatis
	Enterobacteriacea
	P. aeruginosa
	Various gram-positive cocci
Ocular infections	
Conjunctivitis	*S. pneumoniae*
	S. aureus
	H. influenzae
	N. meningitidis
	C. trachomatis (inclusion conjunctivitis)
	C. trachomatis (trachoma)
	Others[d]
Keratitis	*S. aureus*
	S. pneumoniae
	P. aeruginosa
	Enterococci
	S. pyogenes (group A)
	Enterobacteriaceae
	P. multocida
	Others[e]
Endophthalmitis	*S. aureus*
	P. aeruginosa
	P. acnes
	B. cereus
	S. pneumoniae
	N. meningitidis
Periorbital cellulitis	*S. aureus*
	S. pyogenes (group A)
	S. pneumoniae
	H. influenzae
	Clostridium spp.
Otitis	
Otitis externa	*S. aureus*
	S. pyogenes (group A)
	P. aeruginosa
	Vibrio alginolyticus
Otitis media	*S. pneumoniae*
	H. influenzae
	M. catarrhalis
	S. aureus
	Rare pathogens
	Gram-negative bacilli
	Anaerobes
Respiratory tract infection	
Tracheitis, intubated patient	*Enterobacteriaceae*
	S. aureus
	P. aeruginosa
	Other nonfermenting gram-negative bacilli
Bronchitis, community acquired	*S. pneumoniae*
	H. influenzae (other *Haemophilus* spp.)
	M. catarrhalis
	S. aureus
	Chlamydophila pneumoniae
	M. pneumoniae
	B. pertussis
	S. pyogenes (group A)
	Less commonly, same as hospital acquired

(Continued on next page)

TABLE 8 Usual bacterial etiologies of infectious disease syndromes (*Continued*)

Disease	Etiologies
Bronchitis, hospital acquired	*Enterobacteriaceae* *S. aureus* *P. aeruginosa* Other nonfermenting gram-negative bacilli Less commonly, same as community acquired
Pneumonia, community acquired	*S. pneumoniae* *H. influenzae* *M. catarrhalis* *C. pneumoniae* *M. pneumoniae* *L. pneumophila* *N. asteroides* complex *P. multocida* Aspiration (anaerobes) Less commonly, same as hospital acquired
Pneumonia, hospital acquired	*Enterobacteriaceae* *S. aureus* *P. aeruginosa* *L. pneumophila* Other nonfermenting gram-negative bacilli Aspiration (anaerobes) Less commonly, same as community acquired
Lung abscess	*S. aureus* *Klebsiella pneumoniae* *P. aeruginosa* *S. pyogenes* (group A) Anaerobes (aspiration pneumonia) *N. asteroides* complex
Empyema	*S. pneumoniae* Anaerobes Viridans streptococci, especially *S. anginosus* group *S. aureus* *S. pyogenes* (group A) Gram-negative bacilli
Urinary tract infection Prostatitis	*Enterobacteriaceae* *P. aeruginosa* Enterococci
Urethral syndrome	Same as cystitis, but in lower numbers *C. trachomatis*/*N. gonorrhoeae* Unknown—negative culture (about 15% of this disease group)
Cystitis	*Enterobacteriaceae*, especially *E. coli* Enterococci *S. saprophyticus* (women of childbearing age) Nonfermenting gram-negative bacilli *Corynebacterium urealyticum* (patients with underlying urinary tract pathology)
Pyelonephritis	*Enterobacteriaceae* Enterococci Agents of bacteremia (descending infection), e.g., *S. aureus*

[a] Gram-negative bacilli including *Enterobacteriaceae*, *P. aeruginosa*, and other nonfermenting gram-negative bacilli.
[b] Disease caused by ingestion of bacterium followed by tissue invasion, toxin production, or other pathogenic mechanism.
[c] Disease caused by ingestion of preformed toxin.
[d] *C. diphtheriae*, *M. tuberculosis*, *F. tularensis*, *T. pallidum*, *B. henselae* (cat scratch), *P. multocida*, *B. thuringiensis*.
[e] *T. pallidum*, *N. gonorrhoeae*, *Moraxella* sp., *C. diphtheriae*, *Bacillus* spp., anaerobes, nontuberculous mycobacteria.

bacteria are concentrated by centrifugation before culture. A minimum of 5.0 ml and high-speed (3,000 × g) centrifugation are recommended for recovery of Mycobacterium tuberculosis, although the yield may still be low. Filtration through a 0.45-μm-pore-size filter results in better concentration of M. tuberculosis in CSF. Specimens should be transported to the laboratory immediately in a sterile container maintained at room temperature. All smears should be prepared by cytocentrifugation (153), and cultures should be inoculated with 0.5 ml of CSF or sediment resuspended in 0.5 ml of CSF following centrifugation (1,500 × g for 15 min) when more than 1 ml of fluid is received.

Smears should be Gram stained, and the results should be reported to the physician immediately. The results should include a description and semiquantitative enumeration of polymorphonuclear inflammatory cells and bacterial morphology. If the results are suggestive of a bacterial group, this too can be communicated. Rapid tests for bacterial antigens of group B streptococci, S. pneumoniae, N. meningitidis, E. coli, and H. influenzae type b are available by testing the supernatant of a centrifuged specimen or the unprocessed fluid. Data from several studies indicate that the sensitivity of these tests is lower than or equal to that of Gram staining (58, 78), except in cases of partially treated meningitis, where the antigen tests may be more sensitive. In addition, because clinical considerations mandate empirical therapy, the results of antigen testing of CSF have little if any effect on the care and management of the patient. For these reasons and because the cost of antigen testing is much higher than the cost of the Gram stain, the test should be considered only when direct communication with the clinical service documents a specific need, such as prior antimicrobial therapy. Media are inoculated in accordance with the recommendations in Table 5. Broth culture media are not necessary unless CSF is cultured from patients with a CSF shunt or external reservoir (103, 169).

Special Considerations

Anaerobic Bacteria

Anaerobic culture of CSF is not routinely necessary and should be added only when consultation provides evidence of chronic otitis media with mastoiditis, chronic sinusitis, or mixed aerobic and anaerobic soft tissue infection overlying the spine or the possibility of anaerobic brain abscess, subdural empyema, or epidural abscess (65, 67). Even when a parameningeal abscess contains anaerobes, detection of anaerobes by culture of CSF is unlikely to be helpful, since diagnosis and management are based on microbiological evaluation of the abscess.

Leptospira spp.

Leptospires can be detected in CSF during the first 10 days of acute illness. CSF should be collected before initiation of antimicrobial therapy and while the patient is febrile. Direct detection of leptospires is accomplished by dark-field examination of sediment from centrifuged CSF (1,500 × g for 30 min), although the sensitivity is very low, and by culture using semisolid media such as Fletcher's or Ellinghausen-McCullough-Johnson-Harris medium. An inoculum of 0.5 ml is recommended. Cultures should be incubated at room temperature for up to 13 weeks (33) (see chapter 59).

Other Body Fluids

Specimens include pericardial, pleural, peritoneal, peritoneal dialysis, and synovial fluids. A volume of 1 to 5 ml is adequate for the isolation of most bacteria. Fluid submitted on a swab can be accepted but is not optimal. Educational efforts should address the habits of physicians and caregivers who use swabs rather than adding aspirated fluid to an appropriate transport tube. Specimens for anaerobic culture should be transported in an oxygen-free tube. Specimens for the diagnosis of peritonitis associated with chronic ambulatory peritoneal dialysis should include at least 10 ml of fluid (185). All body fluids can be inoculated directly into blood culture bottles in the laboratory or at bedside. For the latter, 0.5 ml should be left in a separate sterile tube for preparation of a smear (11). Body fluids that may clot during transport should be transported in tubes containing anticoagulant. Because heparin, sodium citrate, and EDTA are inhibitory to some bacteria, SPS-containing tubes are recommended. Physicians should be made aware that SPS is inhibitory also and affects the growth of N. meningitidis, N. gonorrhoeae, Peptostreptococcus anaerobius, Streptobacillus moniliformis, and Gardnerella vaginalis (137).

In the laboratory, volumes greater than 1.0 ml for culture should be centrifuged at 1,500 × g for 15 min. The supernatant is removed, leaving about 0.5 ml in which to resuspend the sediment. The resuspended sediment is used to inoculate culture media. Cytocentrifugation of 0.5 ml or less (depending on turbidity of specimen) should be used to prepare smears for Gram staining before centrifugation to concentrate for culture. Alternatively, smears can be prepared from the same sediment used to inoculate the media; however, this method is less sensitive than cytocentrifugation (153).

Solid media used for culture of body fluid specimens should include chocolate and blood agar, as well as selective gram-positive and gram-negative agars if mixed infections are expected (e.g., when culturing abdominal fluids from patients with appendicitis) (Table 5). The inoculation of aerobic blood culture bottles with excess fluid is suggested for pericardial, pleural, and synovial fluids, in addition to peritoneal fluids from chronic ambulatory peritoneal dialysis patients, to enhance the detection of small numbers of bacteria that may be intracellular or inhibited by prior antimicrobial therapy (13). Cultures should be incubated at 35 to 37°C in the presence of 3 to 5% CO_2 for a minimum of 3 days before being discarded as negative. Blood culture bottles should be incubated for the usual 5- or 7-day protocol.

Some experts question the need to culture abdominal fluid from patients with intestinal tract perforation, since surgical drainage and broad-spectrum antimicrobials are effective in the majority of cases (121). Complications occur in this clinical setting when microorganisms other than the expected Enterobacteriaceae, anaerobes, and enterococci are involved. Standard empirical therapy may not adequately treat S. aureus, P. aeruginosa, Candida spp., or bacteria more resistant to antimicrobial agents than expected (57). A policy to refuse culture requests or limit the identification of isolates that do grow to an arbitrary number (such as three or fewer) may not apply uniformly to all patients.

Ear Specimens

Two types of ear specimens are received most commonly by the laboratory, swab specimens for the diagnosis of otitis externa and middle ear fluid specimens for the diagnosis of otitis media (Table 5). Potential pathogens at these two sites differ (Table 8) (16, 21, 145). Since anaerobic bacteria may be involved in middle ear infections, anaerobic culture should be performed on properly collected and transported specimens when requested. Direct examination of Gram-stained smears of middle ear fluid is helpful and is recommended with all culture requests.

External ear specimens may be contaminated with normal flora from the skin or ear canal. Isolates of coagulase-negative staphylococci, diphtheroids, and viridans streptococci may be listed as presumptive identifications without waiting for the results of antimicrobial testing. Middle ear fluid is less likely to be contaminated. All isolates should be reported, and, if requested, antimicrobial testing should be performed on strains with unpredictable susceptibility to antimicrobials.

Eye Specimens

Several types of specimens may be collected for the microbiological analysis of eye infections, including conjunctival scrapings obtained with a swab or sterile spatula for the diagnosis of conjunctivitis, corneal scrapings collected with a sterile spatula for the diagnosis of keratitis, vitreous fluid collected by aspiration for the diagnosis of endophthalmitis, and fluid material collected by aspiration or tissue biopsy for the diagnosis of periorbital cellulitis (194). Bacteria potentially present in these anatomic sites are listed in Table 8. Because the volume of specimen collected from corneal scrapings and vitreous fluid aspiration is very small, direct inoculation of agar culture plates and preparation of smears in the clinic or at the bedside is recommended (194). A close working association is needed between the laboratory and ophthalmologist to ensure a supply of appropriate culture media, correct inoculation technique of media, and rapid transport of plates and smears to the laboratory. Media should be inoculated by rubbing the specimen onto a small area of the agar plates. Plates are placed directly into the incubator without cross-streaking by laboratory personnel. This allows the plate reader to detect more easily any airborne contaminants that settle on the plate during inoculation procedures that occur outside controlled laboratory conditions.

Media needed for the detection of usual pathogens include chocolate agar for fastidious bacteria (Table 5). Media for other microorganisms (fungi, viruses, mycobacteria, etc.) should be inoculated if deemed appropriate by the ophthalmologist and microbiologist and specifically ordered. Incubation at 35 to 37°C in 3 to 5% CO_2 is necessary.

Special Considerations

Chlamydia trachomatis

Direct examination of conjunctival smears and detection of chlamydial antigen in conjunctival scrapings are useful in the diagnosis of inclusion conjunctivitis or trachoma (39). Chlamydial infection is diagnosed by direct fluorescent-antibody (DFA) staining with fluorescein-conjugated monoclonal antibodies or enzyme immunoassays (165). A less sensitive but readily available method involves the examination of Giemsa-stained conjunctival smears for intracytoplasmic perinuclear inclusions within epithelial cells. Cell culture for the isolation of C. trachomatis is sensitive but more time-consuming and more technically demanding than DFA or EIA. Conjunctival scrap-

ings and secretions for culture should be transported in 2SP medium (sucrose phosphate or sucrose phosphate glutamate) with bovine serum and antimicrobials (usually gentamicin, vancomycin, and nystatin or amphotericin B). Swabs with wooden shafts should be avoided since constituents of the wood are toxic to chlamydiae. Specimens for culture should be refrigerated during short delays or stored at −70°C for delays longer than 48 h. Molecular probes and PCR methods are available for the detection of C. trachomatis but are not Food and Drug Administration approved at this time for eye specimens (84).

Gastrointestinal Tract Specimens

Feces and in some cases rectal swab specimens are submitted to the microbiology laboratory to determine the etiologic agent of infectious diarrhea or food poisoning. Feces should be collected in a clean container with a tight lid and should not be contaminated with urine, barium, or toilet paper. Because intestinal pathogens can be killed by the metabolism of members of the fecal flora rapidly acidifying the specimen, specimens should be transferred to Cary-Blair transport medium soon after collection. Rectal swabs should be placed in a transport system containing an all-purpose medium such as Stuart's.

It should be standard practice in all laboratories to evaluate the appropriateness of stool culture requests. It is well established that patients who do not enter the hospital with diarrhea are unlikely to develop enteritis or colitis caused by bacterial agents other than Clostridium difficile (59, 111). For this reason, stool specimens for routine bacterial culture from patients who have been hospitalized for more than 3 days should not be processed without consultation and justification by the patient's physician or caregiver. Diarrhea that develops during hospitalization is likely to be caused by C. difficile or to occur for noninfectious reasons (51). A simple policy of rejecting stool specimens for routine bacterial culture from patients hospitalized for more than 3 days and offering C. difficile testing for nosocomial diarrhea is recommended. On the other hand, C. difficile colitis does occur as a community-acquired disease following hospital discharge or the use of outpatient antimicrobial therapy, and requests for diagnostic testing should not be rejected when ordered in the outpatient setting.

Fecal leukocyte examinations have been recommended for the differentiation of inflammatory diarrheas (fecal leukocyte positive) from secretory diarrheas (fecal leukocyte negative). Inflammatory diarrhea is likely to be caused by invasive bacteria, while secretory diarrhea results from toxin-producing bacteria, viruses, and protozoan pathogens (166). In practice, the detection and association of fecal leukocytes with specific etiologies are less clear (147). Fecal leukocyte morphology degrades in feces during transport and processing delays, making accurate recognition and quantitation difficult. In addition, invasive pathogens may result in fecal leukocytes being intermittently present or unevenly distributed in stool specimens. The former problem can be solved by using lactoferrin as a surrogate marker for fecal leukocytes (Leuco-Test; TechLab, Blacksburg, Va.), since lactoferrin is not degraded during normal transport and processing times. Lactoferrin-positive stool specimens are considered positive for fecal leukocytes. Although algorithms have been proposed depicting schemes for stool processing based on the use of a lactoferrin assay (53), they are not commonly used. The lactoferrin assay is used in the evaluation of patients with inflammatory bowel disease (46).

Usual gastrointestinal pathogens are listed in Table 8 (53). Inclusion of less frequently encountered pathogens should be considered when epidemiological factors suggest an increased likelihood. This may require periodic surveys of one's community to establish which pathogens are most common, especially when considering the addition of selective media or toxin assay for the routine detection of enterohemorrhagic E. coli, non-jejuni/coli Campylobacter, Vibrio spp., and Yersinia enterocolitica.

Selective and differential media are used to detect Salmonella and Shigella spp. (Table 5). These should include one that is differential but not selective for these pathogens, such as MacConkey agar, and one that is a mildly selective medium, such as Hektoen enteric or xylose-lysine desoxycholate agar. In some settings, a highly selective medium such as SS agar is also included. In addition, enrichment broth, such as Gram Negative (GN) broth or Selenite F broth, may increase the detection of Salmonella and is recommended for testing sensitive populations such as food handlers. Subculture of GN and Selenite F broths to a mildly selective and differential medium after 6 to 8 or 12 to 18 h of incubation, respectively, is necessary to prevent overgrowth by the normal flora and decreased usefulness of the broth (101). All agar plates should be incubated in air at 35 to 37°C for 2 days before being reported as negative. The decision whether to use a highly selective agar medium and an enrichment broth will vary from one laboratory to another. Optimally, additional media are used for a trial period to determine their value, which is measured by the detection of strains not present on the two standard media. In settings where such a trial is not possible, the use of MacConkey agar, Hektoen (HE) or xylose-lysine-deoxycholate (XLD) agar, and an enrichment broth is recommended (53).

Campylobacter jejuni and C. coli are detected with a medium such as Campylobacter agar with 10% sheep blood and selective antimicrobial agents (Table 5). Media are incubated at 42°C in a microaerophilic atmosphere of nitrogen (85%), carbon dioxide (10%), and oxygen (5%) for up to 3 days. Special enrichment broths are available for the recovery of Campylobacter; however, their routine use does not increase the number of Campylobacter-positive cultures significantly (1). Detection of other Campylobacter species may require media without antibiotics and incubation at 37°C (29).

Special Considerations

Other Enteric Pathogens

A physician order for Vibrio spp., Y. enterocolitica, Aeromonas spp., or Plesiomonas shigelloides may be needed in some geographic locations or epidemiologic situations, since the incidence of these bacteria is so low in most parts of the United States that the routine use of selective media is not justified. Media used for these enteric pathogens include thiosulfate citrate bile salts sucrose (TCBS) agar for vibrios, cefsulodin-irgasan-novobiocin (CIN) agar for Y. enterocolitica, and blood agar or selective blood agar to demonstrate hemolysis and provide a medium for oxidase testing for Aeromonas spp. and P. shigelloides (both oxidase positive) (53). All of these enteric pathogens grow on usual media, but detection is enhanced and simplified when specific selective media are used.

Enterohemorrhagic E. coli

The prevalence of enterohemorrhagic E. coli (EHEC) varies in different parts of the United States and the rest of the world. It has been established that in addition to E. coli O157:H7, other serotypes are implicated as enterohemorrhagic strains. In fact, in the United States approximately 50% of Shiga toxin-producing strains, those capable of causing hemorrhagic colitis and hemolytic-uremic syndrome, are not serotype O157:H7 (3, 44). For this reason, many laboratories have chosen to perform a Shiga toxin assay by EIA to detect all serotypes rather than using culture or antigen detection for O157:H7 strains only. Some Shiga toxin-producing strains may not harbor all the mechanisms needed to be fully pathogenic in humans. Additional data will emerge over the next few years. Strategies include testing all specimens year-round, testing all specimens only during the summer months when prevalence is highest, testing only specimens containing gross blood, testing only when ordered, or testing based on a combination of these factors. The best approach for a specific laboratory can be determined by a culture survey of all stool specimens during the summer months. Alternatively, one can contact neighboring hospital laboratories or local health departments, which may be able to provide prevalence data. Laboratories should check with public health authorities to see if EHEC-containing stools need to be forwarded for serotyping of toxin-producing E. coli strains.

Clostridium difficile

Approximately 15% of people who develop diarrhea following antimicrobial use have antibiotic-associated diarrhea caused by C. difficile. If use of the offending antimicrobial continues and disease remains undiagnosed and untreated, pathology may progress to more severe colitis, pseudomembranous colitis, and, possibly, death (6, 51). Nearly 100% of cases of pseudomembranous colitis are caused by C. difficile. Disease is caused by toxins (toxin A and toxin B) produced by C. difficile. The disease is diagnosed by detecting the organism or its toxins in stool. Cell culture cytotoxicity assay for the detection of toxin B, EIA for the detection of toxin A or toxins A and B, latex agglutination or EIA for the detection of glutamate dehydrogenase (an antigen associated with C. difficile and occasionally other bacterial species), and culture of C. difficile from stool specimens followed by toxin testing of the isolate are all methods used for diagnosis (6, 97). In practice, an EIA for toxin A or one that detects both toxins A and B is most practical since it requires minutes to hours to complete compared to 24 to 48 h for the cell culture cytotoxicity assay or 2 to 4 days for culture and toxin testing of the isolate. A single specimen detects 85 to 95% of specimens eventually proven to be toxin positive. Testing of a second specimen, after a single negative result, may be needed if symptoms persist and an alternative diagnosis has not been made (97).

Although C. difficile-associated gastrointestinal disease is most common in hospitalized patients, it can occur in any patient treated with antimicrobials, whether institutionalized or in the community. Testing should not be performed on formed stool (no diarrhea) or as a follow-up to therapy to confirm cure. Repeat testing is appropriate only if symptoms persist or recur (97). Symptoms in successfully treated patients will resolve over a few days, even though the patients may continue to carry C. difficile and may remain toxin positive for days or weeks (157). It is a faulty practice to require negative toxin or culture for *C. difficile* before allowing patients admission to long-term care facilities. Patients who do not have diarrhea and are not incontinent of stool are not a risk to other patients, even if they are carrying *C. difficile* and its toxins, when usual infection control measures are followed (6).

Rare and even fatal disease can be caused by toxin A-deficient strains (toxin B only produced), necessitating the occasional use of a toxin A-plus-B immunoassay or cell culture (72). For epidemiologic purposes, stool or rectal swabs placed in anaerobic transport medium may be cultured anaerobically to isolate *C. difficile*. The sample is inoculated to a selective medium such as cycloserine-cefoxitin-fructose agar (CCFA) and incubated anaerobically for 48 h (51).

Staphylococcus aureus and *Bacillus cereus*

Stool specimens or gastric contents collected from persons with short-incubation food poisoning (2 to 6 h) can be evaluated for *S. aureus* and *B. cereus*. In general, investigation is beneficial for the general public health rather than for a sick individual who recovers quickly, and it is best performed by public health laboratories rather than hospital clinical microbiology laboratories. Specimens should be examined by Gram stain, and because both of these organisms may be present normally in food, quantitative cultures must be performed. A series of dilutions (10^{-1} to 10^{-5}) of the specimen are prepared in buffered gelatin diluent, and 0.1-ml samples of the undiluted specimen and each of the dilutions are plated onto colistin nalidixic acid or phenylethyl alcohol blood agar. The presence of 10^5 CFU or more of *S. aureus* or *B. cereus* per g of specimen is of potential significance (18, 104).

Clostridium botulinum

The clinical diagnosis of food-borne and infant botulism may be confirmed by detecting botulinal toxin, *C. botulinum*, or both in feces (105). Optimally, 25 to 50 ml of stool, 15 to 20 ml of serum, and a sample of suspect food should be collected. Most clinical laboratories are not properly equipped to process specimens from persons with suspected botulism. In the United States, when a case of botulism is suspected, investigators at the Centers for Disease Control and Prevention should be notified to ensure appropriate diagnosis, treatment, and investigation of the potential outbreak. Botulism could be used as a biological weapon (see chapter 10). Unexpected numbers of cases or unusual presentations should be investigated.

Helicobacter pylori

H. pylori is an important cause of gastritis and peptic ulcer disease. The organism can be observed in tissue sections by using hematoxylin and eosin, Giemsa, or Warthin-Starry silver staining. In addition, organisms can be visualized in touch preparations of dissected tissue stained with the Gram stain. The presence of *H. pylori* in stomach or small bowel lesions can be confirmed by culture, antigen detection, urease detection, or the detection of exhaled bacterial metabolite (*H. pylori* breath test) (89, 179). Tissue biopsy specimens collected during endoscopy are used for culture and urease detection. Specimens for culture should be placed in transport medium (media containing 20% glycerol such as brucella broth are best for transport and storage) and transported to the laboratory immediately or refrigerated during delays (62). Lightly minced tissue is inoculated to freshly prepared blood agar and incubated in a humid microaerophilic atmosphere (5 to 10% carbon dioxide, 80 to 90% nitrogen, 5 to 10% oxygen) at 37°C for 7 days (Table 5). The addition of 5% hydrogen should improve the yield of *H. pylori*. Tissue for urease detection is placed as soon as possible into the detection system and processed as specified by the manufacturer. Stool for antigen detection should be handled as specified in the instructions included with the Premier Platinum HpSA test (Meridian Diagnostics, Inc., Cincinnati, Ohio) (55, 178). In some clinical situations, serologic testing for *H. pylori* antibody may be necessary. Serum should be collected and stored at refrigeration temperature for short periods (up to 1 week) or frozen at −70°C for longer periods (89).

Screening for Vancomycin-Resistant Enterococci or Beta-Hemolytic Streptococci

Detecting carriers of vancomycin-resistant enterococci for infection control purposes, group B streptococci in pregnant patients, and group A streptococci during investigations of outbreaks of necrotizing fasciitis or streptococcal toxic shock syndrome requires the collection of a rectal swab specimen. Carriers of vancomycin-resistant enterococci can be detected by culturing rectal swab or perirectal swab material (189). Specimens are inoculated to selective media such as colistin nalidixic acid blood agar containing 6 μg of vancomycin per ml. Carriers of group A streptococci can be detected by culturing rectal swab specimens on sheep blood agar or selective streptococcal agars used to detect patients with streptococcal pharyngitis. Carriers of group B streptococci are detected by culturing vaginal secretions and rectal swab material as discussed below (23).

Genital Tract Specimens

Genital tract specimens are sent to the microbiology laboratory to determine the etiology of various clinical syndromes, including vulvovaginitis, bacterial vaginosis, genital ulcers, urethritis, cervicitis, endometritis, salpingitis, and ovarian abscess in females and urethritis, epididymitis, prostatitis, and genital ulcers in males. These diseases and their etiologies are listed in Table 8 (5).

Many specimens are contaminated with normal skin or mucous membrane flora. Pathogens such as *Haemophilus ducreyi*, *Neisseria gonorrhoeae*, *Trichomonas vaginalis*, *Treponema pallidum*, and *Chlamydia trachomatis* are always significant. Other organisms such as *Staphylococcus aureus*, beta-hemolytic streptococci, members of the *Enterobacteriaceae* and anaerobes are pathogenic only in certain clinical situations. The specimen source, relative quantity of potential pathogen compared to normal flora, and Gram stain interpretation help the technologist determine which isolates require identification and antimicrobial testing. At a minimum, isolates from presumably sterile specimens and pure or predominant potential pathogens from specimens likely to be contaminated with the normal flora and containing polymorphonuclear neutrophils should be identified and reported. Mixtures of anaerobes do not require individual identification and listing in most cases. Laboratories should avoid isolating, identifying, and performing antimicrobial tests on every bacterial isolate from all specimens (5). In addition to the excessive cost of this approach, unnecessary reporting of bacterial species contributes to excessive treatment of patients. Exact protocols for workup and reporting may require discussion and mutual agreement with knowledgeable clinicians in each practice environment.

Special Considerations

N. gonorrhoeae and C. trachomatis

Nucleic acid probe and amplification methods are commercially available for the direct detection of *N. gonorrhoeae* and *C. trachomatis* in endocervical, urethral, and urine specimens. Users must pay close attention to the types of specimens approved for use with each kit. Specimens should be collected using the procedures and collection kits recommended by the manufacturer. In addition, false-positive reactions have been reported with some kits, necessitating confirmation of positive results (181).

Both EIA and DFA tests are commercially available for the direct detection of *C. trachomatis* in endocervical, urethral, and, with some EIA kits, urine specimens (148). If these kits are used, collection and processing must follow instructions provided by the manufacturer. Cell culture for *C. trachomatis* is recommended for use with specimens not approved for molecular or EIA kits. This is likely to include eye, rectal, and abscess specimens collected during surgery. In addition, culture is the only acceptable diagnostic procedure in some jurisdictions for medical-legal cases.

Culture for *N. gonorrhoeae* is optimal when the specimen is directly inoculated to a selective medium, such as modified Thayer-Martin medium, and incubated immediately (42). Transport of inoculated media to the laboratory must be carried out in an increased CO_2-containing environment. Swab specimens (cotton swabs should be avoided because they may be toxic) should be placed in a transport system containing Stuart's or Amies medium and delivered to the laboratory as quickly as possible. Specimens for *N. gonorrhoeae* culture should not be refrigerated; instead, they should be held at room temperature. As the transport time increases, recovery by culture decreases. Specimens requiring more than 24 h for transport are unacceptable. Detection by nonculture methods is recommended in most settings where the additional cost of testing by molecular techniques or immunoassay is not prohibitive (177).

Bacterial Vaginosis and Vaginitis

Bacterial vaginosis (BV) occurs when conditions result in overgrowth of the usual vaginal flora by various anaerobic genera including *Mobiluncus* and *Prevotella* (160). Although not characterized by a polymorphonuclear response, BV results in an increase in vaginal secretions that are relatively alkaline (pH > 4.5) compared to normal, the usual predominant flora of lactobacilli being replaced by anaerobes, and the presence of aromatic amines which are detected by adding 10% potassium hydroxide and noting a pungent, fishy odor. In addition, excessive growth of a facultative bacterium called *Gardnerella vaginalis* generally coincides with BV. Although *G. vaginalis* commonly is a member of the normal vaginal flora, the presence of increased concentrations that adhere to vaginal squamous epithelial cells, called clue cells, is pathognomonic of BV. Clue cells are squamous epithelial cells peppered with *G. vaginalis* bacteria, frequently showing heavier adherence toward the periphery of the cell and appearing like a donut (Fig. 3). As a result of these characteristic changes, BV is diagnosed best without culture (122). Wet mount or Gram-stained smears should be examined and interpreted as described in Table 9. In summary, BV should be diagnosed by performing a bedside pH and KOH "whiff test" and a laboratory Gram stain.

Candida and *Trichomonas* infections of the vulvovaginal areas are inflammatory conditions referred to as vaginitis

TABLE 9 Diagnosis of bacterial vaginosis, using a Gram-stained smear of vaginal secretions, by the Vaginal Infection and Prematurity study group criteria[a]

Score	Quantity of:		
	Lactobacillus morphotypes	Gardnerella and Bacteroides spp. morphotypes	Curved gram-variable rods (Mobiluncus spp. morphotypes)
0	4+	0	0
1	3+	1+	1+ or 2+
2	2+	2+	3+ or 4+
3	1+	3+	
4	0	4+	

[a] Quantity of morphotypes per average 100× oil immersion field: 0, no morphotypes present; 1+, less than 1 morphotype; 2+, 1 to 4 morphotypes; 3+, 5 to 30 morphotypes; 4+, 30 or more morphotypes. Total score = Lactobacillus morphotypes + Gardnerella and Bacteroides morphotypes + Mobiluncus morphotypes. A score of 0 to 10 is calculated for each person. A score of 7 to 10 indicates bacterial vaginosis, 4 to 6 is intermediate or indeterminate, and 0 to 3 is considered normal (no bacterial vaginosis). Adapted from reference 122.

rather than vaginosis. A combination probe assay (Affirm VPIII identification test; Becton Dickinson, Sparks, Md.) is commercially available for the simultaneous detection of *Candida* spp., *G. vaginalis*, and *Trichomonas vaginalis* in vaginal secretions (17). Specimens must be collected using procedures recommended by the manufacturer.

Screening for Group B Streptococcus

Carriers of group B streptococci are detected by culturing both vaginal secretions and rectal swab material. Swabs of the vaginal introitus and anorectum are collected and inoculated into a single enrichment broth such as Lim broth. This broth is incubated at 35°C or room temperature overnight and subcultured to a blood agar plate the following day (150).

Dark-Field Examination for *Treponema pallidum*

Dark-field examination of tissues, tissue exudates, and material collected from chancres can be used to confirm the diagnosis of syphilis. For dark-field microscopy, the specimen should be examined within 20 min of collection to ensure motility of treponemes and should not be exposed to temperature extremes during transport to a dark-field microscope. The test requires a microscope equipped with a dark-field condenser and experienced personnel who are able to recognize *T. pallidum* spirochetes based on the tightness and regularity of the spirals and on its characteristic corkscrew movement (86). A DFA stain can be performed on air-dried smears. The stability of the smear during transport and the easily identified, fluorescing treponemes make the DFA test an attractive alternative to dark-field microscopy (86). Unfortunately, reagents for the DFA test are not commercially or widely available; it may be performed at some Public Health Laboratories.

Haemophilus ducreyi

If infection with *H. ducreyi* is suspected, material from the base of the ulcer is collected and held at room temperature until needed for processing (90). One swab is used to prepare a smear for Gram staining. The presence of many small, pleomorphic, gram-negative bacilli and coccobacilli arranged in chains and groups (school of fish) suggests *H. ducreyi* but is rarely seen (sensitivity, 50% [see chapter 40]).

Recovery of the organisms by culturing on an enriched medium such as chocolate agar supplemented with Iso-VitaleX (Becton Dickinson Microbiology Systems) is necessary to confirm the diagnosis; culturing at 33°C yields better recovery than does culturing at 35°C.

Actinomyces spp.

Actinomyces spp. may cause pelvic inflammatory disease in women who use intrauterine contraceptive devices (IUD) (92). An IUD submitted for culture should be placed in a sterile liquid medium (preferably reduced, such as thioglycolate) and vortexed, and the liquid should be used to inoculate aerobic and anaerobic culture media. Inflammatory debris and tissue attached to the IUD should be removed and cultured aerobically and anaerobically. *Actinomyces* spp. produce small knots of intertwined bacterial filaments called grains, which may be 1 mm or more in diameter. These grains should be crushed on a slide, stained (Gram stain is acceptable), and cultured. The presence of branching gram-positive filaments suggests *Actinomyces* spp., which characteristically occur in mixed infections with other aerobic and anaerobic bacteria. Culture confirms the diagnosis.

Lower Respiratory Tract Specimens

Specimens from the lower respiratory tract are submitted to determine the etiology of airway disease (tracheitis and bronchitis), pneumonia, lung abscess, and empyema. Table 8 gives a list of lower respiratory tract diseases and their common etiologies. Usual specimens submitted consist of lower respiratory tract secretions and inflammation in the form of expectorated sputum; induced sputum; endotracheal tube aspirations (intubated patients); bronchial brushings, washes, or alveolar lavages collected during bronchoscopy; and pleural fluid (170). Specimens should be delivered to the laboratory promptly and processed without delay (within 1 h of collection). If delays are unavoidable, the specimen should be refrigerated.

Usual pathogens detected in lower respiratory tract secretions are present in specimens containing acute inflammatory cells (polymorphonuclear leukocytes) and in quantities greater than the contaminating respiratory flora. Frequently, pathogenic bacteria are present within the polymorphonuclear leukocytes. There are many ways to assess the quality of respiratory tract specimens. A simple screening method involves assessment of squamous epithelial cells only (119). Squamous epithelial cells are found in the oropharynx but not in the lower respiratory tract. Increased numbers (defined as more than 10 per 10× objective microscopic field) indicate gross contamination with oropharyngeal contents, which include the usual oral bacterial flora (Fig. 4 and 5). Most bacterial lower respiratory tract disease is caused by inapparent aspiration of oropharyngeal contents. It follows that the oropharyngeal flora includes the same bacteria that cause lower respiratory tract disease. Detection of a potential pathogen in a grossly contaminated specimen may represent contamination with members of the oropharyngeal flora. The lack of usefulness of data from contaminated specimens has resulted in policies for screening and rejecting grossly contaminated respiratory tract specimens. Table 6 lists respiratory tract specimens and the usual screening policies. Respiratory tract specimens for the detection of *Mycoplasma pneumoniae*, *Legionella* spp., dimorphic fungi, and *Mycobacterium tuberculosis* should not be screened for adequacy. All specimens

are considered acceptable for the detection of these microorganisms (30).

Once respiratory tract specimens have been deemed acceptable, Gram-stained smears should be examined further for inflammatory cells, bacteria, and other indicators of lower respiratory tract pathology, such as mucus, necrosis, intracellular bacteria, alveolar macrophages, and Curschmann's spirals (Fig. 2) (201). Tracheal and bronchial mucopurulence can be trapped behind an airway obstruction or within a lung abscess cavity or may pool in the bronchi or trachea, resulting in the death and disintegration of cells, reflected as necrosis and cell debris in stained smears. Intracellular bacteria can be differentiated from bacteria "lying" on top of polymorphonuclear leukocytes by their greater concentration within the phagocytic cell than in nearby extracellular areas. Phagocytosis is an active uptake process resulting in the concentration of bacteria within the cell. Alveolar macrophages are identified by their vacuolated cytoplasm and round eccentric nucleus, which is difficult to see in Gram-stained smears. Alveolar macrophages and Curschmann's spirals indicate areas within the smear that originated within the alveoli and distal airways (Fig. 2). Occasionally elastin fibers are seen in respiratory tract specimens (Fig. 1).

Bacteria should be reported when detected in Gram-stained smears if they are potential pathogens. Bacteria not present in sufficient quantity or not representative of morphotypes resembling potential pathogens should be lumped together and reported as normal respiratory flora. It is important to differentiate contaminating respiratory flora from respiratory flora causing aspiration pneumonia. Aspiration of relatively large amounts of oropharyngeal contents following loss of consciousness, paralysis of muscles involved with swallowing and breathing, or medical procedures such as intubation can result in infection of the airways with mixed respiratory flora, leading to lung abscess and empyema (98). Gram stain of sputum from patients with aspiration pneumonia can be highly suggestive of the diagnosis. Stained smears show many polymorphonuclear leukocytes and many mixed respiratory flora morphotypes, especially those suggesting streptococci and anaerobes. Much of the flora is intracellular. Aspiration pneumonia can be detected in hospitalized patients and those admitted directly from the community (7).

Cultures of respiratory tract material should include a selective gram-negative medium, such as MacConkey's agar, sheep blood agar, and chocolate agar, for the detection of *Haemophilus* spp. (Table 5). Culture plates should be incubated at 35°C in 3 to 5% CO_2 for 48 h before being reported as negative. Cultures are interpreted by examining the relative numbers and types of bacteria that grow. Table 10 summarizes the interpretative criteria used with respiratory tract specimens (172).

Special Considerations

Specimens Collected during Bronchoscopy

Bronchoalveolar lavage fluid and bronchial brush specimens from patients with suspected pneumonia should be cultured quantitatively to evaluate the significance of potential pathogens recovered (19). Bronchial brush specimens, which contain approximately 0.01 to 0.001 ml of secretions, should be placed in 1 ml of sterile nonbacteriostatic saline after collection. The specimen should be delivered to the laboratory immediately. In the laboratory, the specimen is agitated on a vortex mixer, a smear is prepared

TABLE 10 Interpretation of bacterial lower respiratory tract culture results[a]

Specimen (reference)	Likely to be significant	Not likely to be significant	Additional data suggesting isolate is significant
Sputum—coughed or induced	Predominant potential pathogen in Gram stain and culture. Neutrophils abundant.	Potential pathogen not present in Gram stain and only 1–2+ growth in culture. Neutrophils not abundant in Gram stain.	Potential pathogen within neutrophils (intracellular bacteria).
Endotracheal tube aspirate (99)	Predominant potential pathogen in Gram stain and culture. Neutrophils abundant.	Potential pathogen only 1–2+ growth in culture. Neutrophils not abundant in Gram stain.	Potential pathogen in quantities of >10⁶ CFU/ml. Potential pathogen within neutrophils (intracellular bacteria).
Bronchoalveolar lavage fluid	Predominant potential pathogen seen in every 100× field of Gram stain. Quantitative culture detects >10⁵ CFU of potential pathogen/ml.	Potential pathogen not seen in Gram stain. Quantitative culture detects <10⁴ CFU of potential pathogen/ml.	Potential pathogen within neutrophils (intracellular bacteria).

[a] Reprinted from reference 169a with permission.

by cytocentrifugation for staining with Gram stain, and 0.01 ml of specimen is inoculated to appropriate media by using a pipette or calibrated loop. Colony counts of more than 1,000 CFU of potential pathogens per ml (corresponding to 10^6 CFU/ml of original specimen) appear to correlate with disease. Bronchoalveolar lavage results in collection of 50 ml or more of saline from a larger lung volume. In the laboratory, a smear is prepared by cytocentrifugation and Gram stained (133). The Gram stain report should include a comment about the presence of squamous epithelial cells and intracellular bacteria. Grossly contaminated fluid (>1% of all cells are squamous epithelial cells) may have falsely elevated counts of potential pathogens. Intracellular bacteria are more likely to be potential pathogens. A 0.01- or 0.001-ml aliquot of bronchoalveolar fluid should be inoculated to agar media (Table 5). The recovery of <10,000 bacteria/ml suggests contamination. The recovery of >100,000 bacteria/ml suggests that the isolate is a potential pathogen. Detection of 10,000 to 100,000 bacteria per ml represents a "gray" zone (174). Counts of pathogens may be reduced by prior antimicrobial therapy or variations in "return" of lavage fluid during the bronchoscopy procedure (Table 10).

Legionella spp.

Legionella spp., especially *L. pneumophila*, are important causes of community- and hospital-acquired pneumonia (45). Legionellosis can be diagnosed by culture, DFA staining of smears of respiratory secretions, detection of antigens in urine, or serologic testing. Culture is preferred because, unlike other methods, it is not limited to the detection of certain species or serotypes. Before being cultured, respiratory samples should be diluted 10-fold in a bacteriologic broth, such as tryptic soy broth, or sterile water to dilute inhibitory substances that may be present in the specimen. Because legionellae grow slowly, optimal isolation from highly contaminated specimens, such as sputum, is achieved by decontaminating the specimens with acid before plating (187). The specimen is diluted 1:10 in KCl-HCl buffer (pH 2.2) and incubated for 4 min at room temperature. It is important not to incubate the specimen

for longer than 4 min because legionellae may themselves be killed by acid exposure. Specimens are inoculated onto buffered charcoal yeast extract agar with and without antimicrobial agents (e.g., vancomycin, polymyxin B, and anisomycin). The cultures are incubated in humidified air at 35°C for a minimum of 5 days. Using a dissecting microscope, small colonies with a ground-glass appearance, typical of *Legionella* spp., can be detected after 3 days of incubation.

Mycoplasma pneumoniae

M. pneumoniae is a common cause of pneumonia, referred to as primary atypical pneumonia. Because *M. pneumoniae* is fastidious and grows very slowly, a definitive diagnosis is often based on the results of serologic tests. When culture is required, the specimen of choice is a throat swab; however, sputum or other respiratory specimens are also acceptable. The specimen should be placed immediately into a transport medium containing protein, such as albumin, and penicillin to reduce the growth of contaminating bacteria. Specimens may be stored in the transport medium for up to 48 h at 4°C or frozen for longer periods at −70°C. PCR methods have been used successfully to detect *M. pneumoniae* directly in respiratory tract specimens. Molecular detection by PCR or a related technique may be the most sensitive method for the detection of *M. pneumoniae* (134).

Specimens from Patients with Cystic Fibrosis

Burkholderia cepacia is an important respiratory pathogen in persons with cystic fibrosis (54). This organism grows well on routine media; however, selective media such as PC (for *Pseudomonas cepacia*) and OFPBL (oxidative-fermentative polymyxin B-bacitracin-lactose) agars are useful for optimal recovery from respiratory secretions (27). Also see chapter 48.

Chlamydia and Chlamydophila spp.

Chlamydiae are important causes of respiratory illnesses in children and adults (123). *Chlamydia trachomatis* can cause serious respiratory disease in newborn infants.

Chlamydophila pneumoniae causes illness in all age groups, but most disease occurs in adolescents and young adults. *Chlamydophila psittaci* is primarily an animal pathogen but occasionally causes disease in humans exposed to sick animals. Lower respiratory tract secretions, in addition to nasopharyngeal washes, for the detection of chlamydiae are collected and transported to the laboratory immediately in a medium containing antimicrobial agents (e.g., gentamicin and nystatin). If delays in transport or processing occur, the specimen should be stored at 4°C for up to 48 h. Longer storage should be at −70°C or colder. Chlamydiae are detected by rapid cell culture techniques (shell vial) using McCoy cells for *C. trachomatis* and *C. psittaci* and HEp-2 cells for *C. pneumoniae*. As with *M. pneumoniae*, PCR may prove to be the most sensitive method for the detection of respiratory chlamydiae (134).

Nocardia asteroides Complex

Respiratory specimens for the detection of *N. asteroides* complex organisms (*N. asteroides*, *N. farcinica*, and *N. nova*) should be transported to the laboratory as soon as they are collected. For short delays, storage at 4°C is acceptable. Direct examination of a Gram-stained smear containing a *Nocardia* species shows thin, beaded gram-positive branching filaments. The filaments are also partially acid fast when stained by the modified Kinyoun method. There are no media used routinely for the specific recovery of *Nocardia* spp. since these organisms grow readily on many common media such as sheep blood and chocolate agar plates, Sabouraud's agar for fungi, Löwenstein-Jensen medium for mycobacteria, and charcoal yeast extract (CYE) agar for legionellae. Nocardiae survive mycobacterial decontamination procedures, but for culture from contaminated specimens, selective CYE agar is optimal (183). Although *Nocardia* spp. are detected commonly following 1 week of incubation, cultures are incubated for a total of 3 weeks at 35°C.

Upper Respiratory Tract

Upper respiratory tract specimens include the external nares, nasopharynx, throat, oral ulcerations, and inflammatory material from the nasal sinuses. Although few serious diseases involve these areas, many pathogens colonize or persist in these sites while causing symptomatic infection in deeper, less accessible sites (126).

Throat specimens are collected to diagnose pharyngitis caused by *Streptococcus pyogenes*. Swab specimens should be placed in a standard transport carrier containing Amies or modified Stuart's medium. Refrigeration is preferred if transport requires more than a few hours. Many rapid direct tests for group A streptococci are commercially available, including EIA, optical immunoassay, and nucleic acid-based probe assays (50, 164). The reported sensitivities of EIAs and an optical immunoassay vary between 60 and 95% but can be as low as 31% (21, 188). The nucleic acid-based assay has a sensitivity >90% (66, 69). When a rapid test is requested, two throat swabs should be collected. If only one swab is received, the culture plate should be inoculated first. Material remaining on the swab is used for the direct test. If the rapid test is positive, the second swab can be discarded, but if the rapid test is negative, the second swab must be used for culture to confirm the negative direct test. The nucleic acid-based probe test is considered sensitive and specific enough by many to obviate the need for confirmatory culture (69). A position paper by representatives of the American Academy of Family Physicians, the American College of Physicians-American Society of Internal Medicine, and the Centers for Disease Control and Prevention states that rapid tests do not require confirmatory culture when used with specimens from adult patients (28). This recommendation does not hold for specimens from children.

To culture group A streptococci, either sheep blood agar or selective blood agar may be used. Selective agar makes the organism easier to visualize by inhibiting the accompanying flora but may delay the appearance of colonies of *S. pyogenes*. Cultures should be incubated for 48 h at 35°C in an environment of reduced oxygen achieved by incubating anaerobically, in 5% CO_2, or in air with multiple "stabs" through the agar surface. Stabbing the agar surface with the inoculating loop pushes inoculum containing streptococci below the surface, where the oxygen concentration is reduced compared to ambient (21, 76). These culture conditions allow the recovery of group C and G streptococci, organisms which may cause pharyngitis but do not cause the serious sequelae associated with group A streptococci (176, 202).

Throat specimens also are used to detect patients infected with *Neisseria gonorrhoeae*. For best results, the specimen should be inoculated immediately to a selective medium, such as modified Thayer-Martin agar. Cultures are incubated for 72 h at 35°C in the presence of 5% CO_2.

The external nares can be cultured to detect carriers of *Staphylococcus aureus* by using a single swab to collect secretions from both the left and right nares. The usual carrier systems used for swab transport containing Amies or Stuart's medium are acceptable. In the laboratory, the specimen can be inoculated to a sheep blood agar plate; however, the use of selective media, such as colistin-nalidixic acid agar, or a selective and differential medium, such as mannitol salt agar, is helpful in differentiating *S. aureus* from coagulase-negative staphylococci and may be useful when interpreting large numbers of specimens (49, 192). Cultures should be incubated at 35°C for 2 days.

Nasopharyngeal secretions and cells are used to detect patients infected with *Bordetella* spp. and carriers of *N. meningitidis*. Specimens for the recovery of *B. pertussis* and *B. parapertussis* should be collected with a small-tip calcium alginate or Dacron swab. Rayon or cotton may be toxic to the organism. Swabs should be transported to the laboratory in special media. For delays of up to 24 h, Amies medium with charcoal can be used. If the transport time will exceed 24 h, Regan-Lowe transport medium should be used (71, 110). Culture, DFA staining, and PCR can be used for detection. PCR is the most sensitive for detecting *B. pertussis* (Dacron swabs are preferred for PCR tests) (94). Culture is performed using Regan-Lowe charcoal agar containing 10% horse blood and cephalexin. Because a few strains of *B. pertussis* do not grow in the presence of cephalexin, the use of Regan-Lowe medium with and without cephalexin is recommended for optimal recovery (68, 159). Cultures are incubated at 35°C for 5 to 7 days in a humid atmosphere. The DFA test has relatively low sensitivity and specificity for *Bordetella* but offers rapid results (94). Depending on the reagents used, either *B. pertussis* or *B. parapertussis* is detected.

Nasopharyngeal swab specimens are used to detect carriers of *N. meningitidis*. Transport in a swab container with Amies or Stuart's medium is acceptable. Specimens should be inoculated as quickly as possible to sheep blood or chocolate agar; however, selective agars for pathogenic *Neisseria* spp., such as modified Thayer-Martin agar, are necessary if interference by the normal flora is expected. Culture plates are incubated for 72 h in a humidified atmosphere at 35°C in the presence of 5% CO_2.

Vincent's angina is an oral infection characterized by pharyngitis, membranous exudate, fetid breath, and oral ulcerations. Sometimes referred to as fusospirochetal disease or necrotizing ulcerative gingivitis, it is caused by *Fusobacterium* spp., *Borrelia* sp., and other anaerobes. Diagnosis is made by direct examination of a smear of a swab specimen collected from the ulcerated lesions and stained with Gram stain (126). The presence of many spirochetes, fusiform bacilli, and polymorphonuclear leukocytes is presumptive evidence of this disease. Culture is not helpful. In addition, canker sores do not have a microbial etiology and should not be cultured.

Inflammatory material from the nasal sinuses should be cultured to detect the etiologies of sinusitis. Nearly all cases of bacterial sinusitis follow a primary upper respiratory tract viral infection. Bacteria are trapped in the sinus as a result of damage to the epithelial lining cells of the sinus, and inflammation and swelling narrow or close the nasal ostium, preventing normal drainage (60). Specimens collected during endoscopic procedures by physicians specializing in otorhinolaryngology are optimal since they are sampled directly from the infected sinus, avoiding contamination by the normal flora in the nasal passages. Aspirates, washes, scrapings or debridements, and biopsy material should be kept moist and sent in a sterile container to the laboratory (60). Examination of Gram-stained smears can provide a rapid, presumptive identification of likely pathogens. Aerobic culture is needed in all cases; anaerobic transport and culture may be needed in cases of chronic sinusitis. Ventilator-associated sinusitis occurs in fewer than 10% of patients with nasotracheal intubation. Members of the nosocomial flora are implicated. Endoscopic inspection is needed to obtain acceptable specimens for culture (193).

Special Considerations

Arcanobacterium haemolyticum

A. haemolyticum can cause pharyngitis and peritonsillar abscess (75). The organism can be recovered on media used to detect *S. pyogenes*. Colonies of *A. haemolyticum* are beta-hemolytic and easily confused with those of beta-hemolytic streptococci. Rapid differentiation can be accomplished with the Gram stain. *A. haemolyticum* is a diphtheroid-shaped gram-positive rod. Incubation of plates at 35°C for up to 72 h may be required for optimal detection.

Corynebacterium diphtheriae

Cultures of both throat and nasopharyngeal specimens are used in the diagnosis of diphtheria. When specimens are processed for culture without delay, no special transport medium or conditions are required. For transport to a reference laboratory, specimens should be sent dry in a container with desiccant (38). Alternatively, specimens collected on swabs may be placed in Stuart's or Amies medium for transport to the laboratory. Smears of specimens for *C. diphtheriae* can be stained with Gram stain and examined for pleomorphic (diphtheroid morphology) gram-positive rods. In addition, smears can be stained with Loeffler's methylene blue stain and examined for pleomorphic, beaded rods with swollen (club-shaped) ends and reddish-purple metachromatic granules. Bacteria with these characteristics are suggestive but not specific for *C. diphtheriae*. Specimens should

be inoculated to Loeffler's serum and potassium tellurite media for the recovery of *C. diphtheriae*. Cultures are incubated for 2 days at 35°C in 5% CO_2 before being reported as negative.

Epiglottitis

A throat swab specimen may be helpful in determining the etiology of epiglottitis, a rapidly progressing cellulitis of the epiglottis and adjacent structures with the potential for swollen tissues to cause airway obstruction. Epiglottitis is almost always caused by *H. influenzae* serotype b but is occasionally caused by other bacteria such as *S. pneumoniae* and *S. pyogenes* (175). The specimen should be collected by a physician only in a setting where emergency intubation can be performed immediately to secure a patent airway. Specimens should be inoculated onto enriched medium, such as chocolate agar, and incubated for 72 h at 35°C in an atmosphere of 5% CO_2. Nearly 100% of patients with epiglottitis caused by *H. influenzae* have a blood culture positive for the same bacterium.

Tissue Specimens

Tissue specimens are obtained during surgical procedures at significant risk and expense to the patient. Therefore, it is mandatory for the laboratory to receive sufficient specimen for both histopathologic and microbiological examination, bearing in mind that many microbiological tests and cultures may have been ordered. Histopathologic examination of the lesion serves to differentiate between infection and malignancy and also to distinguish between acute and chronic infectious processes (198). Swabs provide too little specimen and should be discouraged and eliminated through educational efforts.

Tissue should be transported in a sterile container that maintains moisture. To avoid drying, small pieces of tissue can be moistened with a few drops of sterile, nonbacteriostatic saline. Alternatively, very small pieces of tissue can be placed on a small square of moistened sterile gauze. This serves to maintain moisture and allow easy identification by those receiving and processing the specimen. Tissue should be gently minced or ground during processing to release microorganisms and to provide equal specimen for all media and smears. This can be accomplished by cutting with a sterile scalpel, grinding with a mortar and pestle or tissue grinder, or using a Stomacher (Seward Ltd., London, United Kingdom) (156). The resulting homogenate is used to prepare smears for staining and inoculate culture media. The Gram stain should be examined for the presence of polymorphonuclear leukocytes and bacteria. Grinding renders most cell morphology and tissue architecture difficult to recognize. Smears should be examined closely for intracellular bacteria, especially common with staphylococci and streptococci. For bacterial culture, processed tissue should be inoculated to enriched agar media. The use of a broth medium is controversial (112, 114). Anaerobic culture should be included when ordered and when tissue is transported in an oxygen-free environment. Large pieces of tissue, approximately 1 cm^3 or greater, maintain a reduced atmosphere in spite of brief aerobic transport. Oxygen-free transport may not be necessary in this circumstance, and absence of anaerobic transport should not disqualify large pieces of tissue from anaerobic culture. Routine, aerobic cultures are incubated for 72 h at 35°C in the presence of 5% CO_2.

Collecting and processing tissue offers an opportunity for exogenous contamination. Cultures growing small numbers of bacteria not commonly associated with infection, such as coagulase-negative staphylococci, corynebacteria, propionibacteria, and saprophytic *Neisseria* spp., may represent contamination rather than true "pathogens." In general, growth of these bacterial groups in broth culture only represents contamination, (112, 114). One or two bacterial colonies growing on a single plate, of many plates that have been inoculated, and not growing in broth culture (if used), generally represent contamination. Growth of one or two bacterial colonies on agar media not in the area of specimen inoculation or on streak lines in the second through fourth plate quadrants also is likely to represent contamination. In addition, it is assumed that bacteria considered contaminants were not detected in Gram-stained smears prepared from the original specimen. On the other hand, detection of the bacteria listed above as unlikely pathogens should always be reported when seen in the original Gram-stained smear, when present in quantities above a few colonies, and when detected on or in multiple media (36).

Special Considerations

Bone Marrow
Bone marrow aspirates can be submitted for culture in lysis centrifugation tubes (Isolator; Wampole Laboratories, Cranbury, N.J.). The "pediatric" tube holds a maximum of 1.5 ml of specimen. One or more of the 1.5-ml tubes can be used. Aspirates may also be submitted in a sterile container containing anticoagulant. Sterile tubes with anticoagulant are less desirable since they use heparin, sodium citrate, or EDTA as anticoagulant, all of which are more inhibitory than SPS (43, 144). Although SPS inhibits meningococci, gonococci, *Gardnerella vaginalis*, anaerobic cocci, and *Streptobacillus moniliformis*, these bacteria are unlikely to be detected in bone marrow aspirate specimens (137).

Although bone marrow aspirate cultures may be helpful in identifying disseminated fungal and mycobacterial diseases, they are unlikely to assist in the identification of usual bacterial diseases (184). Patients infected with human immunodeficiency virus may benefit from bone marrow culture when other specimen cultures have been unsuccessful (41). It is policy in some laboratories to consult with the ordering physician and suggest that routine bacterial culture is not necessary. In most cases, blood or other organ system culture is preferred for the identification of disseminated bacterial infections. Even if bone marrow culture is performed, direct Gram stain of bone marrow aspirates is not helpful and should not be a routine component of bacterial culture.

Lymph Nodes
Lymph node cultures in immunocompetent patients are positive only when there is a granuloma or acute inflammatory lesion, in which case the etiologies detected are limited to mycobacteria and fungi. Bacterial culture of lymph nodes in immunocompetent patients may not be necessary without specific clinical or epidemiological findings such as a patient with suspected tularemia (*Francisella tularensis*) (48).

Quantitative Tissue Culture
Tissue from a traumatic wound or burn injury may be submitted for quantitative culture, with results of $\geq 10^3$ CFU/ml being used to predict the likelihood of development of wound-related sepsis (102, 199). Limitations include the lack of reproducible results and the low predictive

value compared to histologic examination of tissue. To perform a quantitative culture, a portion of the specimen is weighed and homogenized in saline. The saline suspension is used to prepare serial dilutions for culture. Detailed procedures for quantitative tissue culture are given elsewhere (168).

Bartonella
Bartonella henselae is the agent of cat scratch disease in immunocompetent hosts and causes bacteremia, endocarditis, bacillary angiomatosis, and bacillary peliosis primarily in immunocompromised hosts. Optimal detection of the organism requires PCR (161). Culture is very difficult but can be attempted by inoculating blood collected using Isolator tubes (Wampole Laboratories) onto freshly prepared rabbit blood agar plates incubated in a moist environment for an extended period (15). Tissue culture may have a better yield than agar (see chapter 53). Lymph node tissue is macerated and inoculated into media directly. Because the detection of *B. henselae* is time-consuming and expensive, the diagnosis of cat scratch disease is most often made by clinical criteria and exclusion of other diseases. *B. henselae* can be observed in sections of fixed tissue stained with Warthin-Starry or Dieterle's silver stains (82, 107).

Urinary Tract Specimens
Diseases of the urinary tract include prostatitis, urethral syndrome, cystitis, and pyelonephritis. Etiologies are summarized in Table 8. Urine, prostatic secretion, or urethral cells/secretion specimens are needed to diagnose these diseases. Urine can be collected by midstream collection, catheterization (straight/in-out or indwelling), cystoscopic collection, or suprapubic aspiration. Foley catheter tips should not be submitted or accepted for culture since they are always contaminated with members of the urethral flora and quantitation is not possible. A first-voided morning urine is optimal, since in most cases bacteria have been multiplying in the bladder for several hours. Clean-catch urine, implying cleansing of periurethral areas, has not been shown to improve the quality of urine culture and is not recommended (91, 132).

Urine specimens should be transported to the laboratory immediately and processed within 2 h of collection. If a delay occurs, specimens may be refrigerated for up to 24 h. Transport tubes containing boric acid are available to stabilize the bacterial population at room temperature for 24 h if refrigeration is not available (87). Boric acid-preserved urines are acceptable for dipstick leukocyte esterase testing (200).

Urine culture is the most common test performed by most microbiology laboratories, and most urine cultures are negative; i.e., no specific potential pathogen is detected. Screening methods are available that attempt to rapidly separate specimens containing significant counts of bacteria from negative specimens. In general, screening methods perform well with specimens containing 10^5 CFU/ml of bacteria or more but perform poorly when colony counts are lower. Screening urine specimens by staining with the Gram stain is rapid and economical with regard to reagents but is labor-intense and requires a trained technologist. The presence of two or more bacteria of the same morphotype in each oil immersion field (100× objective lens) correlates with a count of 100,000 or greater by culture (140, 197). Commercially available dipstick tests that detect leukocyte esterase (an enzyme produced by neutrophils) and nitrite (the result of bacterial nitrate reductase acting on nitrate in the urine) are rapid, inexpensive, and simple to perform, but their sensitivity is low in some patient populations (124, 131, 152). False-negative dipstick screening occurs because frequent voiding dilutes the concentration of leukocyte esterase and nitrite in urine, enterococci and other less common urinary tract pathogens do not produce nitrate reductase, and many patients with asymptomatic bacteriuria do not have significant numbers of leukocytes in urine. In spite of this, outpatient screening algorithms have been proposed that incorporate enzyme screening in a "reflexive" urine test, i.e., urinalysis is performed, and if it is positive for leukocyte esterase or nitrate reductase a culture will be set up, whereas if it is negative a culture will not be done (24). Such screening works best in symptomatic patients, diabetics, and women older than 60 years (124, 131, 152).

Several automated urine screening systems are commercially available (129). The FiltraCheck-UTI colorimetric filtration system (Meridian Diagnostics, Inc.) involves forcing urine through a filter paper that retains cells, followed by a stain that is passed through the same filter. The intensity of the resulting color correlates with the number of cells, bacteria, and other particles adherent to the filter. The system provides rapid results and detects over 90% of all samples with bacterial counts of $\geq 10^5$ CFU/ml. Sensitivity decreases when detecting bacterial counts of $\geq 10^4$ CFU/ml (117, 130, 140, 162).

The UTI screen Bacterial ATP Assay (Coral Biotechnology, San Diego, Calif.) is a bioluminescence-based system that measures the reaction of ATP with luciferin and luciferase that produces light (162). By selectively releasing ATP from bacteria alone, the number of CFU per milliliter of urine is estimated with a luminometer. This procedure requires an incubation step, and so the results are not available for a few hours. The method has a sensitivity equal to that of other screening methods (>90% for counts of $\geq 10^5$ CFU/ml) but has higher specificity than filter methods (130, 140).

The Bac-T-Screen (bioMérieux Vitek, Hazelwood, Mo.) is an automated filtration device that detects >90% of urine samples containing bacteria in concentrations of $\geq 10^5$ CFU/ml. As with other filtration screening methods, the specificity is relatively low, resulting from the detection of polymorphonuclear and epithelial cells (117, 130, 162).

The Cellenium automated urine screening system (Trek Diagnostic Systems, Inc., Westlake, Ohio) uses fluorescence staining and video image analysis to perform rapid urine screening. Instrument algorithms are used to screen the specimens as positive or negative based on thresholds as low as 10^4 CFU/ml. Automation of the screening process allows screening of 70 specimens per h. Preliminary data suggest that the sensitivity of the Cellenium system for detecting urine pathogens at counts of $\geq 10^4$ CFU/ml is 92% or greater (M. T. Pezzlo, R. I. Baylon, G. L. Ton, K. D. Evans, and J. T. Shigei, Abstr. 99th Gen. Meet. Am. Soc. Microbiol. 1999, abstr. C-265, 1999).

The standard for quantitative bacterial culture of urine is the inoculation of 0.01 or 0.001 ml of specimen, using a calibrated plastic or wire loop, to appropriate media, usually sheep blood and MacConkey agars. The loop is dipped vertically into the well-mixed urine, just far enough to cover the loop, and the loopful of urine is spread over the surface of the agar plate by streaking from top to bottom in a vertical line and again from top to bottom perpendicular to this line in a back-and-forth fashion. Prior to plate inoculation, it is necessary to ensure that a film of urine fills the loop with no bubbles to alter the calibrated volume.

The inoculum of urine is spread over the entire agar surface to simplify counting of colonies after growth. Urine cultures are incubated at 35°C for 24 to 48 h. Although most urinary tract pathogens grow readily on the usual agar media, slowly growing pathogens and those inhibited by the presence of antimicrobials may not appear after overnight incubation (16 h). One approach uses the results of the leukocyte esterase and nitrite tests to determine which cultures are incubated for a full 48 h. Urine cultures that are negative after overnight incubation but that had one or both positive enzyme tests are incubated for an additional day. Those that had negative enzyme tests are reported as "no growth" in a final report (22, 116).

Contamination of urine is detected in approximately 5 to 40% of cultures. Contamination is not reduced by the use of central processing areas, refrigeration, urine-screening systems, specimen preservatives, and insulated specimen transport (180).

Agar paddles are available for urine culture in settings where inoculation and incubation of conventional agar plates are not convenient or possible (143). A standard film of urine is distributed over the agar-covered paddle, usually by dipping the paddle into a jar of urine. The paddle is then reinserted into its plastic container for incubation. Following incubation, the density of growth is estimated by comparing to photographs or drawings. A preliminary identification of gram positive or gram negative can be determined by colony color and morphology, and, when appropriate, the entire paddle can be forwarded to a reference laboratory for complete identification and antimicrobial testing of the isolate. Agar paddle culture of urine with approximate colony counts compares favorably with standard culture (143).

The urinary tract above the urethra is sterile in healthy humans, but the urethra is normally colonized with many different bacteria. Because of this, urine collected by midstream voiding techniques becomes contaminated during passage. Commensal bacteria are differentiated from potential pathogens by quantitative culture. Bacterial counts indicating "significant" bacteriuria (i.e., the isolate is a likely pathogen) vary with the host and type of infection. Table 11 summarizes significant counts for common clinical situations (163).

Severe urinary tract infection generally involves the kidneys (pyelonephritis) and results in bacteremia. Rapid diagnosis and administration of appropriate antimicrobial therapy is necessary. In this clinical setting, blood cultures are needed and a stat Gram stain of the urine can be useful. The Gram stain provides an immediate indication of the quality of the urine and a preliminary identification of the likely pathogen. Specimens containing large numbers of squamous epithelial cells are likely to be grossly contaminated with the periurethral or vaginal flora, and fresh samples should be collected immediately, before antimicrobials inhibit the growth of the true pathogen (Fig. 6). Gram stain identification of a potential pathogen confirms that empirical therapy is correct or may suggest a change based on an unexpected pathogen such as *S. aureus* (Fig. 7).

Special Considerations

Leptospires

Leptospira interrogans can be recovered from blood and CSF during the acute stages of disease and from urine after the first week of illness and for several months thereafter. Urine should be processed as soon as possible after collec-

TABLE 11 Interpretation of urine culture results[a]

Urine specimen and patient[b]	Likely to be significant[b]	Not likely to be significant[b]	Additional data suggesting isolate is significant
Midstream, female with cystitis	>10^2 CFU of potential pathogen/ml, urine LE is positive	Quantity of potential pathogen ≤ quantity of contaminating flora	
Midstream, female with pyelonephritis	>10^5 CFU of potential pathogen/ml, urine LE is positive	Quantity of potential pathogen ≤ quantity of contaminating flora	Gram stain demonstrates potential pathogen in neutrophils and/or casts
Midstream, asymptomatic bacteriuria	>10^5 CFU of potential pathogen/ml, urine LE is usually negative	<10^5 CFU of potential pathogen/ml; quantity of potential pathogen ≤ quantity of contaminating flora	Confirm by repeating test when clinically indicated
Midstream, male with UTI	>10^3 CFU of potential pathogen/ml, urine LE is positive	<10^3 CFU of potential pathogen/ml; quantity of potential pathogen ≤ quantity of contaminating flora	Gram stain demonstrates potential pathogen in neutrophils and/or casts
Straight catheter, all patients	>10^2 CFU of potential pathogen/ml, urine LE is positive in symptomatic patients.	<10^2 CFU of potential pathogen/ml; urine LE is negative	Gram stain demonstrates potential pathogen in neutrophils and/or casts
Indwelling catheter, all patients	>10^3 CFU of potential pathogens/ml (multiple pathogens may be present)	Bacteriuria detected in asymptomatic patients; urine LE is positive or negative	No reason to culture unless patient is symptomatic

[a] Reprinted from reference 169a with permission.
[b] LE, leukocyte esterase; UTI, urinary tract infection.

tion, because the acidity of urine harms the organisms. If a delay in processing is expected, urine should be neutralized with sodium bicarbonate, centrifuged (1,500 × g for 30 min), and resuspended in buffered saline before being used to inoculate media (see chapter 59). Alternatively, the urine may be diluted 1:10 in 1% bovine serum albumin and stored at 5 to 20°C. Undiluted urine and urine diluted 1:10, 1:100, and 1:1,000 in sterile buffered saline should be inoculated to Fletcher's or equivalent medium with and without neomycin (33). Cultures should be incubated at 30°C for at least 13 weeks (Table 5).

Bacterial Antigen Testing

Bacterial antigen testing kits, for the purpose of diagnosing bacterial meningitis, include procedures for use with urine specimens. In general, these kits should not be used with urine specimens for the diagnosis of bacterial meningitis. In addition, the Food and Drug Administration issued a product alert specifically cautioning against the use of the group B *Streptococcus* antigen kits with urine specimens because of the risk of both false-positive and false-negative results (47).

An EIA is commercially available for the detection of *Legionella pneumophila* serogroup 1 antigen in urine. The antigen may be detectable in urine for months following an infection. The assay has a sensitivity of 80% when performed on unconcentrated urine (61, 64). Sensitivity is increased when urine is concentrated. The drawback of this assay is that only disease caused by *L. pneumophila* serogroup 1 is detected. A new EIA has been evaluated that detects all *L. pneumophila* serogroup antigens in urine (sensitivity, 74% with unconcentrated urine and 92% with concentrated urine) (35).

Streptococcus pneumoniae antigen can be detected in urine using a commercially available EIA (NOW *S. pneumoniae* urinary antigen test; Binax, Portland, Maine) (115). Although the sensitivity for detecting urine antigen is 80% for patients with positive blood cultures and 52% for patients with positive sputum cultures, the specificity is high. This test may prove to be useful in settings where culture is not available, but at present it should be used in addition to, not in place of, culture.

Wound and Abscess Specimens

Abscess specimens should be collected by aspiration. Small amounts of purulence or wounds with nothing to aspirate can be irrigated with sterile, nonbacteriostatic saline to facilitate aspiration. In addition, wounds can be sampled by dissecting a small portion of infected tissue. Purulent specimens and wound specimens characterized by ulceration or necrosis, but with little moisture, can be collected with a swab, but this is generally inferior to aspiration or biopsy. Swab specimens contain less material, are more likely to be contaminated with the adjacent flora, and are not amenable to optimal anaerobic transport. When swabs are used for collection, two swabs should be used, one for culture and one for preparation of a smear. Deep lesions that communicate with the surface are most problematic. The cutaneous portion and sinus tract are contaminated with bacteria found at the surface. Surgical debridement and sampling are recommended. If surgery is not performed, an effort should be made to aspirate a "pocket" of infected material that is not open to the surface. As a last option, fresh specimen should be expressed from deep within the wound. A swab used to collect specimen from the surface overlying the draining wound is not acceptable. This is of particular importance when evaluating diabetic foot ulcers or infected pressure sores (146). Only deep specimens collected by aspiration or during debridement offer useful culture information (14).

Gram staining of wound and abscess specimens is very important. The Gram stain result provides rapid presumptive identification of etiology, it can be used to evaluate the quality of specimen submitted, and it guides the workup of culture results. Examination of a Gram-stained smear reveals bacterial morphotypes, acute inflammatory cells (polymorphonuclear neutrophils), intracellular bacteria, cell necrosis, and elastin fibers resulting from tissue necrosis. The quality of wound specimen can be evaluated by comparing the number of polymorphonuclear cells and squamous epithelial cells (Table 12) (155). Excess numbers of squamous epithelial cells suggest gross contamination with the cutaneous flora. It is acceptable to limit the workup of bacterial isolates when the specimen shows gross contamination. An example of a limited workup would be to list by Gram stain morphology the isolates encountered, with a comment explaining that the physician must call if a replacement specimen cannot be collected and further identification and antimicrobial testing are clinically warranted.

Special Circumstances

Cellulitis

Specimens from patients with cellulitis but without abscess are very difficult to collect. Recommendations have been made to inject a small volume of sterile, nonbacteriostatic saline into the infected tissue. The few drops that one can aspirate back should be sent for Gram stain and culture. Under the best of conditions, these specimens are unlikely to be positive (56, 70). Blood cultures from patients with cellulitis also are unlikely to be positive (125). In spite of the shortcomings of microbiology testing for patients with cellulitis, seriously ill patients may require biopsy and all should have blood collected for culture.

Necrotizing Fasciitis and Gas Gangrene

Necrotizing fasciitis and gas gangrene (myonecrosis) are medical emergencies requiring immediate diagnosis and therapy that may include antimicrobials, surgical debridement, and the use of immune globulin and immune medi-

ators to combat the fatal complications of severe septic shock (154, 167). Necrotizing fasciitis and gas gangrene are caused most commonly by toxin-producing *Streptococcus pyogenes*, other beta-hemolytic streptococci, *Staphylococcus aureus*, *Clostridium* spp., and mixed aerobic and anaerobic bacteria (40). The diagnosis is made by clinical examination of the patient and is confirmed by Gram stain and culture. Gram-stained smears generally show proteinaceous fluid, necrotic cell debris, rare or few polymorphonuclear leukocytes (because of cell lysis), and the bacterial etiology. Culture should confirm the etiology and provide antimicrobial test results where appropriate.

Anaerobic Abscess

Anaerobes characteristically produce purulent infections in areas adjacent to mucous membranes containing anaerobes from the normal flora. Specimens must be transported to the laboratory in sterile, oxygen-free containers (127). As reviewed above, aspirated fluid or excised tissue is the recommended specimen. Specimens should be stored at room temperature (not refrigerated) during transport and processing delays. Infections of the mouth and gums (and adjacent areas), aspiration pneumonia, empyema, intra-abdominal infections, deep tissue abscesses, infections of the female genital tract, infected pressure sores, and diabetic foot ulcers are generally caused by a mixture of aerobes and anaerobes. Because of the usual microscopic appearance of mixed aerobic-anaerobic abscesses, the Gram stain can rapidly identify these infectious processes (Fig. 8). The presence of many polymorphonuclear leukocytes, many bacteria with anaerobic morphotypes (thin gram-negative bacilli, thin and poorly staining gram-positive bacilli, boxcar-shaped gram-positive bacilli suggesting *Clostridium* spp.), and many intracellular bacteria suggests the presence of a mixed aerobic-anaerobic infectious process. Culture can determine the exact etiologies, characteristically a mixture of aerobes and anaerobes. However, the identity of most anaerobic bacteria and their susceptibility results are not necessary for the management of mixed infections. Aerobic and facultative bacteria present need full identification and antimicrobial testing results for proper therapeutic selection.

Specimens for anaerobic culture should be processed as soon as possible after arrival in the laboratory. Usual media

TABLE 12 Screening wound specimens to ensure quality[a]

		Quantity of cells per 10× (objective lens) microscopic field			
No. of neutrophils	Q-value for neutrophils	Q-value for squamous epithelial cells present in following no.[b]:			
		0	1–9	10–24	≥25
		0	−1	−2	−3
0	0	(1)	0	0	0
1–9	1+	1	0	−1	−2
10–24	2+	+2	+1	0	−1
≥25	3+	+3	+2	+1	0

[a] Attach Q-values to squamous cell and neutrophil quantities. Add the two Q-values together. Specimens with positive Q-values (+1 to +3) are more likely to contain increased numbers of potential pathogens and decreased numbers of potential contaminants. Specimens with negative Q-values (or a Q-value of zero) are likely to be contaminated with the local flora. Specimens with no squamous cells or neutrophils are scored as one (1), allowing neutropenic patients or those with necrotic or serous secretions to be processed as acceptable.

[b] The first row of numbers in the table is the Q-value for squamous epithelial cells only. The following four rows are the Q-values for the sum of the neutrophils and squamous epithelial cells.

include an anaerobic blood agar plate (CDC blood agar or brucella blood agar), a medium that inhibits gram-positive and facultative gram-negative bacilli such as KV blood agar (kanamycin-vancomycin), a differential or selective medium such as BBE (Bacteroides bile-esculin), and a gram-positive selective medium (colistin-nalidixic acid blood agar or phenylethyl alcohol blood agar) (Table 5). Media should be incubated in an anaerobic environment immediately after inoculation. Incubation in anaerobic containers, such as GasPak jars (Becton Dickinson Microbiology Systems, Cockeysville, Md.), AnaeroPack (Mitsubishi Gas Chemical America, Inc., New York, N.Y.), or Bio-Bag Anaerobic Culture Set (Becton Dickinson Microbiology Systems), or in an anaerobic chamber is acceptable (31, 32). Anaerobes grow more slowly than aerobic or facultative bacteria, necessitating a full 48 h of incubation before the colony size is large enough to interpret accurately. Negative anaerobic cultures should be held for 3 to 5 days before being reported as negative. Longer incubation is necessary for isolation of *Actinomyces* and some other fastidious anaerobes.

Autopsy Specimens

Microbiology testing as a component of the autopsy examination has been and continues to be controversial (100, 151, 196). Postmortem and agonal invasion of sterile tissues confuses the significance of positive culture results, prompting some to argue against microbiology testing. Others have found that the postmortem examination continues to uncover a significant number of infectious diagnoses, whether in the community or university hospital setting, which were missed by modern high-technology medicine (85). In addition, an important portion of missed diagnoses represents treatable diseases (120). The value of autopsy microbiology is further enhanced by its use to identify emerging diseases, community outbreaks, and antimicrobial resistance and to uncover the cause of death in organ transplant patients and others with immunocompromising conditions.

To minimize contamination of postmortem specimens, the body should be moved to a refrigerated locker (4 to 6°C) as soon as possible after death. Limited movement of the body has been shown to decrease the incidence of false-positive postmortem cultures (37). Although it has been shown that cultures of specimens collected from a refrigerated cadaver within 48 h of death did not show an increase in false-positive results, tissue and fluid specimens, as a rule, should be taken from refrigerated bodies within 15 h of death (81). This serves to diminish the likelihood of postmortem overgrowth of contaminants and improve the detection of true pathogens.

Specimens should be obtained by sterilizing the surface of the organ with a hot spatula or iron surface until the surface is thoroughly dry (37). Body fluids, including blood, should be collected first. For blood collection, the wall of the heart and large vessel should be seared and a sterile needle (18 to 20 gauge) should be inserted. A 20-ml volume (or as close to a 20-ml volume as possible) should be collected and injected directly into aerobic and anaerobic blood culture bottles. Blood culture results obtained before opening the chest cavity by percutaneous subxiphoid aspiration have been shown to have greater interpretive value (less contamination but detection of relevant organisms) (S. P. McClure and J. L. Staneck, Abstr. 81st Gen. Meet. Am. Soc. Microbiol. 1981, abstr. C-261, 1981). Solid viscera should be sampled by immediately cutting blocks of tissue from the center of the seared area. Samples should be

submitted to microbiology with a requisition providing a full explanation of the studies needed. Postmortem cultures can be very useful for detecting pathogens that are not considered members of the normal human flora, such as *Mycobacterium tuberculosis*, *Brucella* spp., *Bordetella pertussis*, some systemic fungi (*Histoplasma capsulatum*, *Coccidioides immitis*, etc.), parasitic helminths, and agents of biowarfare. Tissue samples should be transported to the microbiology laboratory immediately in sterile tubes. The use of transport media and laboratory processing methods should follow recommendations for premortem specimens. An efficient way to avoid unnecessary workup of contaminating microorganisms is to issue a preliminary report to the pathologist who performed the autopsy listing organisms detected by colony or Gram stain morphology, such as "lactose-fermenting gram-negative rod" or "gram-positive cocci in clusters." This is accompanied by a notation that further identification and antimicrobial testing will not be performed unless there is consultation with the laboratory director or technologist conducting the culture investigation. Plates can be held for 1 week and discarded if no additional information is requested.

Specimens for the Detection of Agents of Biological Warfare

An excellent review of the potential agents of biological warfare and their management in the clinical microbiology laboratory can be found in Cumitech 33 and chapter 10 of this Manual (52, 79).

REFERENCES

1. **Agulla, A., F. J. Merino, P. A. Villasante, J. V. Saz, A. Diaz, and A. C. Velasco.** 1987. Evaluation of four enrichment media for isolation of *Campylobacter jejuni*. J. Clin. Microbiol. **25:**174–175.
2. **Baker, A. S., B. Paton, and J. Haaf.** 1989. Ocular infections: clinical and laboratory considerations. Clin. Microbiol. Newsl. **11:**97–101.
3. **Banatvala, N., P. M. Griffin, K. D. Greene, T. J. Barrett, W. F. Bibb, J. H. Green, and J. G. Wells.** 2001. The United States National Prospective Hemolytic Uremic Syndrome Study: microbiologic, serologic, clinical, and epidemiologic findings. J. Infect. Dis. **183:**1063–1070.
4. **Bannatyne, R., C. Clausen, and L. R. McCarthy.** 1979. Cumitech 10, *Laboratory Diagnosis of Upper Respiratory Tract Infections*. Coordinating ed., I. B. R. Duncan. ASM Press, Washington, D.C.
5. **Baron, E., G. Cassell, L. Duffy, D. Eschenbach, J. R. Greenwood, S. Harvey, N. Madinger, E. Peterson, and K. Waites.** 1993. Cumitech 17A, *Laboratory Diagnosis of Female Genital Tract Infections*. Coordinating ed., S. J. Rubin. ASM Press, Washington, D.C.
6. **Bartlett, J. G.** 2002. Clinical practice. Antibiotic-associated diarrhea. N. Engl. J. Med. **346:**334–339.
7. **Bartlett, J. G., S. F. Dowell, L. A. Mandell, T. M. File, Jr., D. M. Musher, and M. J. Fine.** 2000. Practice guidelines for the management of community-acquired pneumonia in adults. Infect. Dis. Soc. Am. Clin. Infect. Dis. **31:**347–382.
8. **Bartlett, J. G., K. J. Ryan, T. F. Smith, and W. R. Wilson.** 1987. Cumitech 7A, *Laboratory Diagnosis of Lower Respiratory Tract Infections*. Coordinating ed., J. A. Washington II. ASM Press, Washington, D.C.
9. **Bartlett, R. C., M. Mazens-Sullivan, J. Z. Tetreault, S. Lobel, and J. Nivard.** 1994. Evolving approaches to management of quality in clinical microbiology. Clin. Microbiol. Rev. **7:**55–88.

10. Bates, D. W., L. Goldman, and T. H. Lee. 1991. Contaminant blood cultures and resource utilization. The true consequences of false-positive results. *JAMA* 265:365–369.

11. Blondeau, J. M., G. B. Pylypchuk, J. E. Kappel, B. Pilkey, and C. Lawler. 1998. Comparison of bedside- and laboratory-inoculated Bactec high- and low-volume resin bottles for the recovery of microorganisms causing peritonitis in CAPD patients. *Diagn. Microbiol. Infect. Dis.* 31:281–287.

12. Bone, R. C. 1991. The pathogenesis of sepsis. *Ann. Intern. Med.* 115:457–469.

13. Bourbeau, P., J. Riley, B. J. Heiter, R. Master, C. Young, and C. Pierson. 1998. Use of the BacT/Alert blood culture system for culture of sterile body fluids other than blood. *J. Clin. Microbiol.* 36:3273–3277.

14. Bowler, P. G., B. I. Duerden, and D. G. Armstrong. 2001. Wound microbiology and associated approaches to wound management. *Clin. Microbiol. Rev.* 14:244–269.

15. Brenner, S. A., J. A. Rooney, P. Manzewitsch, and R. L. Regnery. 1997. Isolation of *Bartonella (Rochalimaea) henselae*: effects of methods of blood collection and handling. *J. Clin. Microbiol.* 35:544–547.

16. Brook, I. 1998. Microbiology of common infections in the upper respiratory tract. *Primary Care* 25:633–648.

17. Brown, H. L., D. A. Fuller, T. E. Davis, J. R. Schwebke, and S. L. Hillier. 2001. Evaluation of the Affirm Ambient Temperature Transport System for the detection and identification of *Trichomonas vaginalis*, *Gardnerella vaginalis*, and *Candida* species from vaginal fluid specimens. *J. Clin. Microbiol.* 39:3197–3199.

18. Bryan, F. L. 1995. Procedures to use during outbreaks of food-borne disease, p. 209–226. *In* P. R. Murray, E. J. Baron, M. A. Pfaller, F. C. Tenover, and R. H. Yolken (ed.), *Manual of Clinical Microbiology*, 6th ed. ASM Press, Washington, D.C.

19. Cantral, D. E., T. G. Tape, E. C. Reed, J. R. Spurzem, S. I. Rennard, and A. B. Thompson. 1993. Quantitative culture of bronchoalveolar lavage fluid for the diagnosis of bacterial pneumonia. *Am. J. Med.* 95:601–607.

20. Carr, D. T., A. G. Karlson, and G. G. Stillwell. 1967. A comparison of cultures of induced sputum and gastric washings in the diagnosis of tuberculosis. *Mayo Clin. Proc.* 42:23–25.

21. Carroll, K., and L. Reimer. 1996. Microbiology and laboratory diagnosis of upper respiratory tract infections. *Clin. Infect. Dis.* 23:442–448.

22. Cavagnolo, R. 1995. Evaluation of incubation times for urine cultures. *J. Clin. Microbiol.* 33:1954–1956.

23. Centers for Disease Control and Prevention. 2000. From the Centers for Disease Control and Prevention: early-onset group B streptococcal disease—United States, 1998–1999. *JAMA* 284:1508–1510.

24. Chernow, B., G. P. Zaloga, S. Soldano, A. Quinn, P. Lyons, E. McFadden, D. Cook, and T. G. Rainey. 1984. Measurement of urinary leukocyte esterase activity: a screening test for urinary tract infections. *Ann. Emerg. Med.* 13:150–154.

25. Clarridge, J. E., M. T. Pezzlo, and K. L. Vosti. 1987. Cumitech 2A, *Laboratory Diagnosis of Urinary Tract Infections*, vol. 2A. Coordinating ed., A. S. Weissfeld. ASM Press, Washington, D.C.

26. Cockerill, F. R., III, J. G. Hughes, E. A. Vetter, R. A. Mueller, A. L. Weaver, D. M. Ilstrup, J. E. Rosenblatt, and W. R. Wilson. 1997. Analysis of 281,797 consecutive blood cultures performed over an eight-year period: trends in microorganisms isolated and the value of anaerobic culture of blood. *Clin. Infect. Dis.* 24:403–418.

27. Coenye, T., P. Vandamme, J. R. Govan, and J. J. LiPuma. 2001. Taxonomy and identification of the *Burkholderia cepacia* complex. *J. Clin. Microbiol.* 39:3427–3436.

28. Cooper, R. J., J. R. Hoffman, J. G. Bartlett, R. E. Besser, R. Gonzales, J. M. Hickner, and M. A. Sande. 2001. Principles of appropriate antibiotic use for acute pharyngitis in adults: background. *Ann. Emerg. Med.* 37:711–719.

29. Cornick, N. A., and S. L. Gorbach. 1988. *Campylobacter*. *Infect. Dis. Clin. North Am.* 2:643–654.

30. Curione, C. J., Jr., G. S. Kancko, J. L. Voss, F. Hesse, and R. F. Smith. 1977. Gram stain evaluation of the quality of sputum specimens for mycobacterial culture. *J. Clin. Microbiol.* 5:381–382.

31. Delaney, M. L., and A. B. Onderdonk. 1997. Evaluation of the AnaeroPack system for growth of clinically significant anaerobes. *J. Clin. Microbiol.* 35:558–562.

32. Doan, N., A. Contreras, J. Flynn, J. Morrison, and J. Slots. 1999. Proficiencies of three anaerobic culture systems for recovering periodontal pathogenic bacteria. *J. Clin. Microbiol.* 37:171–174.

33. Doern, G. V. 2000. Detection of selected fastidious bacteria. *Clin. Infect. Dis.* 30:166–173.

34. Doern, G. V. 1994. Manual blood culture systems and the antimicrobial removal device. *Clin. Lab. Med.* 14:133–147.

35. Domi, J., N. Gali, S. Blanco, P. Pedroso, C. Prat, L. Matas, and V. Ausina. 2001. Assessment of a new test to detect Legionella urinary antigen for the diagnosis of Legionnaires' disease. *Diagn. Microbiol. Infect. Dis.* 41:199–203.

36. Dow, G., A. Browne, and R. G. Sibbald. 1999. Infection in chronic wounds: controversies in diagnosis and treatment. *Ostomy Wound Manage.* 45:23–27, 29–40; quiz, 41–42.

37. du Moulin, G. C., and W. Love. 1988. The value of autopsy microbiology. *Clin. Microbiol. Newsl.* 10:165–167.

38. Efstratiou, A., K. H. Engler, I. K. Mazurova, T. Glushkevich, J. Vuopio-Varkila, and T. Popovic. 2000. Current approaches to the laboratory diagnosis of diphtheria. *J. Infect. Dis.* 181(Suppl. 1):S138–S145.

39. Elbagir, A., and P. A. Mardh. 1990. Evaluation of chlamydial tests in early trachoma. *APMIS* 98:276–280.

40. Elliott, D., J. A. Kufera, and R. A. Myers. 2000. The microbiology of necrotizing soft tissue infections. *Am. J. Surg.* 179:361–366.

41. Engels, E., P. W. Marks, and P. Kazanjian. 1995. Usefulness of bone marrow examination in the evaluation of unexplained fevers in patients infected with human immunodeficiency virus. *Clin. Infect. Dis.* 21:427–428.

42. Evangelista, A., and H. Beilstein. 1993. Cumitech 4A, *Laboratory Diagnosis of Gonorrhea*. Coordinating ed., C. Abramson. ASM Press, Washington, D.C.

43. Evans, G. L., T. Cekoric, Jr., and R. L. Searcy. 1968. Comparative effects of anticoagulants on bacterial growth in experimental blood cultures. *Am. J. Med. Technol.* 34:103–112.

44. Fey, P. D., R. S. Wickert, M. E. Rupp, T. J. Safranek, and S. H. Hinrichs. 2000. Prevalence of non-O157:H7 Shiga toxin-producing *Escherichia coli* in diarrheal stool samples from Nebraska. *Emerg. Infect. Dis.* 6:530–533.

45. File, T. M. 2000. The epidemiology of respiratory tract infections. *Semin. Respir. Infect.* 15:184–194.

46. Fine, K. D., F. Ogunji, J. George, M. D. Niehaus, and R. L. Guerrant. 1998. Utility of a rapid fecal latex agglutination test detecting the neutrophil protein, lactoferrin, for diagnosing inflammatory causes of chronic diarrhea. *Am. J. Gastroenterol.* 93:1300–1305.

47. **Food and Drug Administration.** 1997. *FDA Safety Alert: Risks of Devices for Direct Detection of Group B Streptococcal Antigen.* Food and Drug Administration, Washington, D.C.

48. **Freidig, E. E., S. P. McClure, W. R. Wilson, P. M. Banks, and J. A. Washington II.** 1986. Clinical-histologic-microbiologic analysis of 419 lymph node biopsy specimens. *Rev. Infect. Dis.* **8:**322–328.

49. **Gardam, M., J. Brunton, B. Willey, A. McGeer, D. Low, and J. Conly.** 2001. A blinded comparison of three laboratory protocols for the identification of patients colonized with methicillin-resistant *Staphylococcus aureus. Infect. Control Hosp. Epidemiol.* **22:**152–156.

50. **Gerber, M. A.** 1986. Diagnosis of group A beta-hemolytic streptococcal pharyngitis. Use of antigen detection tests. *Diagn. Microbiol. Infect. Dis.* **4:**5S–15S.

51. **Gerding, D. N., S. Johnson, L. R. Peterson, M. E. Mulligan, and J. Silva, Jr.** 1995. *Clostridium difficile*-associated diarrhea and colitis. *Infect. Control Hosp. Epidemiol.* **16:**459–477.

52. **Gilchrist, M. J. R., W. P. McKinney, J. M. Miller, and A. S. Weissfeld.** 2000. Cumitech 33, *Biological Agents Associated with Bioterrorism.* Coordinating ed., J. W. Snyder. ASM Press, Washington, D.C.

53. **Gilligan, P. H., J. M. Janda, M. A. Karmali, and J. M. Miller.** 1992. Cumitech 12A, *Laboratory Diagnosis of Bacterial Diarrhea.* Coordinating ed., F. S. Nolte. ASM Press, Washington, D.C.

54. **Gilligan, P. H.** 1991. Microbiology of airway disease in patients with cystic fibrosis. *Clin. Microbiol. Rev.* **4:**35–51.

55. **Gisbert, J. P., and J. M. Pajares.** 2001. Diagnosis of *Helicobacter pylori* infection by stool antigen determination: a systematic review. *Am. J. Gastroenterol.* **96:**2829–2838.

56. **Goldgeier, M. H.** 1983. The microbial evaluation of acute cellulitis. *Cutis* **31:**649–650, 653–654, 656.

57. **Gorbach, S. L.** 1993. Treatment of intra-abdominal infections. *J. Antimicrob. Chemother.* **31**(Suppl. A):67–78.

58. **Gray, L. D., and D. P. Fedorko.** 1992. Laboratory diagnosis of bacterial meningitis. *Clin. Microbiol. Rev.* **5:**130–145.

59. **Guerrant, R. L., T. Van Gilder, T. S. Steiner, N. M. Thielman, L. Slutsker, R. V. Tauxe, T. Hennessy, P. M. Griffin, H. DuPont, R. B. Sack, P. Tarr, M. Neill, I. Nachamkin, L. B. Reller, M. T. Osterholm, M. L. Bennish, and L. K. Pickering.** 2001. Practice guidelines for the management of infectious diarrhea. *Clin. Infect. Dis.* **32:**331–351.

60. **Gwaltney, J. M., Jr.** 1996. Acute community-acquired sinusitis. *Clin. Infect. Dis.* **23:**1209–1223; quiz, 1224–1225.

61. **Hackman, B. A., J. F. Plouffe, R. F. Benson, B. S. Fields, and R. F. Breiman.** 1996. Comparison of Binax Legionella Urinary Antigen EIA kit with Binax RIA Urinary Antigen kit for detection of *Legionella pneumophila* serogroup 1 antigen. *J. Clin. Microbiol.* **34:**1579–1580.

62. **Han, S. W., R. Flamm, C. Y. Hachem, H. Y. Kim, J. E. Clarridge, D. G. Evans, J. Beyer, J. Drnec, and D. Y. Graham.** 1995. Transport and storage of *Helicobacter pylori* from gastric mucosal biopsies and clinical isolates. *Eur. J. Clin. Microbiol. Infect. Dis.* **14:**349–352.

63. **Harris, J. C., H. L. Dupont, and R. B. Hornick.** 1972. Fecal leukocytes in diarrheal illness. *Ann. Intern. Med.* **76:**697–703.

64. **Harrison, T., S. Uldum, S. Alexiou-Daniel, J. Bangsborg, S. Bernander, V. Drasbrevear, J. Etienne, J. Helbig, D. Lindsay, I. Lochman, T. Marques, F. de Ory, I. Tartakovskii, G. Wewalka, and F. Fehrenbach.** 1998. A multicenter evaluation of the Biotest Legionella urinary antigen EIA. *Clin. Microbiol. Infect.* **4:**359–365.

65. **Hawkey, P. M., and L. A. Jewes.** 1985. How common is meningitis caused by anaerobic bacteria? *J. Clin. Microbiol.* **22:**325.

66. **Heelan, J. S., S. Wilbur, G. Depetris, and C. Letourneau.** 1996. Rapid antigen testing for group A *Streptococcus* by DNA probe. *Diagn. Microbiol. Infect. Dis.* **24:**65–69.

67. **Heerema, M. S., M. E. Ein, D. M. Musher, M. W. Bradshaw, and T. W. Williams, Jr.** 1979. Anaerobic bacterial meningitis. *Am. J. Med.* **67:**219–227.

68. **Heininger, U., G. Schmidt-Schlapfer, J. D. Cherry, and K. Stehr.** 2000. Clinical validation of a polymerase chain reaction assay for the diagnosis of pertussis by comparison with serology, culture, and symptoms during a large pertussis vaccine efficacy trial. *Pediatrics* **105:**E31.

69. **Heiter, B. J., and P. P. Bourbeau.** 1993. Comparison of the Gen-Probe Group A Streptococcus Direct Test with culture and a rapid streptococcal antigen detection assay for diagnosis of streptococcal pharyngitis. *J. Clin. Microbiol.* **31:**2070–2073.

70. **Ho, P. W., F. D. Pien, and D. Hamburg.** 1979. Value of cultures in patients with acute cellulitis. *South. Med. J.* **72:**1402–1403.

71. **Hoppe, J. E., and A. Weiss.** 1987. Recovery of *Bordetella pertussis* from four kinds of swabs. *Eur. J. Clin. Microbiol.* **6:**203–205.

72. **Johnson, S., S. A. Kent, K. J. O'Leary, M. M. Merrigan, S. P. Sambol, L. R. Peterson, and D. N. Gerding.** 2001. Fatal pseudomembranous colitis associated with a variant *Clostridium difficile* strain not detected by toxin A immunoassay *Ann. Intern. Med.* **135:**434–438.

73. **Jones, D. B., T. J. Liesegang, and N. M. Robinson.** 1981. Cumitech 13, *Laboratory Diagnosis of Ocular Infections.* Coordinating ed., J. A. Washington II. American Society for Microbiology, Washington, D.C.

74. **Kaditis, A. G., A. S. O'Marcaigh, K. H. Rhodes, A. L. Weaver, and N. K. Henry.** 1996. Yield of positive blood cultures in pediatric oncology patients by a new method of blood culture collection. *Pediatr. Infect. Dis. J.* **15:**615–620.

75. **Kain, K. C., M. A. Noble, R. L. Barteluk, and R. H. Tubbesing.** 1991. *Arcanobacterium hemolyticum* infection: confused with scarlet fever and diphtheria. *J. Emerg. Med.* **9:**33–35.

76. **Kellogg, J. A.** 1990. Suitability of throat culture procedures for detection of group A streptococci and as reference standards for evaluation of streptococcal antigen detection kits. *J. Clin. Microbiol.* **28:**165–169.

77. **Kim, S. D., L. C. McDonald, W. R. Jarvis, S. K. McAllister, R. Jerris, L. A. Carson, and J. M. Miller.** 2000. Determining the significance of coagulase-negative staphylococci isolated from blood cultures at a community hospital: a role for species and strain identification. *Infect. Control Hosp. Epidemiol.* **21:**213–217.

78. **Kiska, D. L., M. C. Jones, M. E. Mangum, D. Orkiszewski, and P. H. Gilligan.** 1995. Quality assurance study of bacterial antigen testing of cerebrospinal fluid. *J. Clin. Microbiol.* **33:**1141–1144.

79. **Klietmann, W. F., and K. L. Ruoff.** 2001. Bioterrorism: implications for the clinical microbiologist. *Clin. Microbiol. Rev.* **14:**364–381.

80. **Knoop, F. C., M. Owens, and I. C. Crocker.** 1993. *Clostridium difficile*: clinical disease and diagnosis. *Clin. Microbiol. Rev.* **6:**251–265.

81. **Koneman, E. W., T. M. Minckler, D. B. Shires, and D. S. De Jongh.** 1971. Postmortem bacteriology. II. Selection of cases for culture. *Am. J. Clin. Pathol.* **55:**17–23.

82. **Korbi, S., M. F. Toccanier, G. Leyvraz, J. Stalder, and Y. Kapanci.** 1986. Use of silver staining (Dieterle's stain) in the diagnosis of cat scratch disease. *Histopathology* **10:**1015–1021.

83. **Kost, G. J.** 1990. Critical limits for urgent clinician notification at US medical centers. *JAMA* **263:**704–707.

84. **Kowalski, R. P., M. Uhrin, M. Karenchak, R. L. Sweet, and Y. J. Gordon.** 1995. Evaluation of the polymerase chain reaction test for detecting chlamydial DNA in adult chlamydial conjunctivitis. *Ophthalmology* **102:** 1016–1019.

85. **Landefeld, C. S., M. M. Chren, A. Myers, R. Geller, S. Robbins, and L. Goldman.** 1988. Diagnostic yield of the autopsy in a university hospital and a community hospital. *N. Engl. J. Med.* **318:**1249–1254.

86. **Larsen, S. A.** 1989. Syphilis. *Clin. Lab. Med.* **9:**545–557.

87. **Lauer, B. A., L. B. Reller, and S. Mirrett.** 1979. Evaluation of preservative fluid for urine collected for culture. *J. Clin. Microbiol.* **10:**42–45.

88. **Lazinger, B., J. Steif, and E. Granit.** 1989. An online tests catalog for clinical laboratories. *J. Med. Syst.* **13:** 187–192.

89. **Leodolter, A., K. Wolle, and P. Malfertheiner.** 2001. Current standards in the diagnosis of *Helicobacter pylori* infection. *Dig. Dis.* **19:**116–122.

90. **Lewis, D. A.** 2000. Diagnostic tests for chancroid. *Sex. Transm. Infect.* **76:**137–141.

91. **Lifshitz, E., and L. Kramer.** 2000. Outpatient urine culture: does collection technique matter? *Arch. Intern. Med.* **160:**2537–2540.

92. **Lippes, J.** 1999. Pelvic actinomycosis: a review and preliminary look at prevalence. *Am. J. Obstet. Gynecol.* **180:**265–269.

93. **Little, J. R., P. R. Murray, P. S. Traynor, and E. Spitznagel.** 1999. A randomized trial of povidone-iodine compared with iodine tincture for venipuncture site disinfection: effects on rates of blood culture contamination. *Am. J. Med.* **107:**119–125.

94. **Loeffelholz, M. J., C. J. Thompson, K. S. Long, and M. J. Gilchrist.** 1999. Comparison of PCR, culture, and direct fluorescent-antibody testing for detection of *Bordetella pertussis*. *J. Clin. Microbiol.* **37:**2872–2876.

95. **Lum, G.** 1998. Critical limits (alert values) for physician notification: universal or medical center specific limits? *Ann. Clin. Lab. Sci.* **28:**261–271.

96. **Maki, D. G., C. E. Weise, and H. W. Sarafin.** 1977. A semiquantitative culture method for identifying intravenous-catheter-related infection. *N. Engl. J. Med.* **296:** 1305–1309.

97. **Manabe, Y. C., J. M. Vinetz, R. D. Moore, C. Merz, P. Charache, and J. G. Bartlett.** 1995. *Clostridium difficile* colitis: an efficient clinical approach to diagnosis. *Ann. Intern. Med.* **123:**835–840.

98. **Marik, P. E.** 2001. Aspiration pneumonitis and aspiration pneumonia. *N. Engl. J. Med.* **344:**665–671.

99. **Marquette, C. H., H. Georges, F. Wallet, P. Ramon, F. Saulnier, R. Neviere, D. Mathien, A. Rime, and A. B. Tonnel.** 1993. Diagnostic efficiency of endotracheal aspirates with quantitative bacterial cultures in intubated patients with suspected pneumonia. Comparison with the protected specimen brush. *Am. Rev. Respir. Dis.* **148:**138–144.

100. **McCurdy, B.** 2001. Cumitech 35, *Postmortem Microbiology*, vol. 35. Coordinating ed., B. W. McCurdy. ASM Press, Washington, D.C.

101. **McGowan, K. L., and M. T. Rubenstein.** 1989. Use of a rapid latex agglutination test to detect *Salmonella* and *Shigella* antigens from gram-negative enrichment broth. *Am. J. Clin. Pathol.* **92:**679–682.

102. **McManus, A. T., S. H. Kim, W. F. McManus, A. D. Mason, Jr., and B. A. Pruitt, Jr.** 1987. Comparison of quantitative microbiology and histopathology in divided burn-wound biopsy specimens. *Arch. Surg.* **122:**74–76.

103. **Meredith, F. T., H. K. Phillips, and L. B. Reller.** 1997. Clinical utility of broth cultures of cerebrospinal fluid from patients at risk for shunt infections. *J. Clin. Microbiol.* **35:**3109–3111.

104. **Messer, J. W., T. F. Midura, and J. T. Peeler.** 1993. Sampling plans, sample collection, shipment, and preparation for analysis, p. 25–49. *In* C. Vanderzaant and D. Splittstoesser (ed.), *Compendium of Methods for the Microbiological Examination of Foods*, 3rd ed. American Public Health Association, Washington, D.C.

105. **Midura, T. F.** 1996. Update: infant botulism. *Clin. Microbiol. Rev.* **9:**119–125.

106. **Miller, J. M.** 1998. *A Guide to Specimen Management in Clinical Microbiology*, 2nd ed. ASM Press, Washington, D.C.

107. **Miller-Catchpole, R., D. Variakojis, J. W. Vardiman, J. M. Loew, and J. Carter.** 1986. Cat scratch disease. Identification of bacteria in seven cases of lymphadenitis. *Am. J. Surg. Pathol.* **10:**276–281.

108. **Mimoz, O., A. Karim, A. Mercat, M. Cosseron, B. Falissard, F. Parker, C. Richard, K. Samii, and P. Nordmann.** 1999. Chlorhexidine compared with povidone-iodine as skin preparation before blood culture. A randomized, controlled trial. *Ann. Intern. Med.* **131:**834–837.

109. **Mirrett, S., M. P. Weinstein, L. G. Reimer, M. L. Wilson, and L. B. Reller.** 2001. Relevance of the number of positive bottles in determining clinical significance of coagulase-negative staphylococci in blood cultures. *J. Clin. Microbiol.* **39:**3279–3281.

110. **Morrill, W. E., J. M. Barbaree, B. S. Fields, G. N. Sanden, and W. T. Martin.** 1988. Effects of transport temperature and medium on recovery of *Bordetella pertussis* from nasopharyngeal swabs. *J. Clin. Microbiol.* **26:** 1814–1817.

111. **Morris, A. J., P. R. Murray, and L. B. Reller.** 1996. Contemporary testing for enteric pathogens: the potential for cost, time, and health care savings. *J. Clin. Microbiol.* **34:**1776–1778.

112. **Morris, A. J., L. K. Smith, S. Mirrett, and L. B. Reller.** 1996. Cost and time savings following introduction of rejection criteria for clinical specimens. *J. Clin. Microbiol.* **34:**355–357.

113. **Morris, A. J., D. C. Tanner, and L. B. Reller.** 1993. Rejection criteria for endotracheal aspirates from adults. *J. Clin. Microbiol.* **31:**1027–1028.

114. **Morris, A. J., S. J. Wilson, C. E. Marx, M. L. Wilson, S. Mirrett, and L. B. Reller.** 1995. Clinical impact of bacteria and fungi recovered only from broth cultures. *J. Clin. Microbiol.* **33:**161–165.

115. **Murdoch, D. R., R. T. Laing, G. D. Mills, N. C. Karalus, G. I. Town, S. Mirrett, and L. B. Reller.** 2001. Evaluation of rapid immunochromatographic test for detection of *Streptococcus pneumoniae* antigen in urine samples from adults with community-acquired pneumonia. *J. Clin. Microbiol.* **39:**3495–3498.

116. **Murray, P., P. Traynor, and D. Hopson.** 1992. Evaluation of microbiological processing of urine specimens: comparison of overnight versus two-day incubation. *J. Clin. Microbiol.* **30:**1600–1601.

117. **Murray, P. R., A. C. Niles, R. L. Heeren, and F. Pikul.** 1988. Evaluation of the modified Bac-T-Screen and FiltraCheck-UTI urine screening systems for detection of clinically significant bacteriuria. *J. Clin. Microbiol.* **26:** 2347–2350.

118. **Murray, P. R., P. Traynor, and D. Hopson.** 1992. Critical assessment of blood culture techniques: analysis of recovery of obligate and facultative anaerobes, strict aerobic bacteria, and fungi in aerobic and anaerobic blood culture bottles. *J. Clin. Microbiol.* **30:**1462–1468.

119. **Murray, P. R., and J. A. Washington.** 1975. Microscopic and bacteriologic analysis of expectorated sputum. *Mayo Clin. Proc.* **50:**339–344.

120. **Nichols, L., P. Aronica, and C. Babe.** 1998. Are autopsies obsolete? *Am. J. Clin. Pathol.* **110:**210–218.

121. **Nichols, R. L.** 1985. Intraabdominal infections: an overview. *Rev. Infect. Dis.* **7**(Suppl. 4)**:**S709–S715.

122. **Nugent, R. P., M. A. Krohn, and S. L. Hillier.** 1991. Reliability of diagnosing bacterial vaginosis is improved by a standardized method of Gram stain interpretation. *J. Clin. Microbiol.* **29:**297–301.

123. **Peeling, R. W., and R. C. Brunham.** 1996. Chlamydiae as pathogens: new species and new issues. *Emerg. Infect. Dis.* **2:**307–319.

124. **Pels, R. J., D. H. Bor, S. Woolhandler, D. U. Himmelstein, and R. S. Lawrence.** 1989. Dipstick urinalysis screening of asymptomatic adults for urinary tract disorders. II. Bacteriuria. *JAMA* **262:**1221–1224.

125. **Perl, B., N. P. Gottehrer, D. Raveh, Y. Schlesinger, B. Rudensky, and A. M. Yinnon.** 1999. Cost-effectiveness of blood cultures for adult patients with cellulitis. *Clin. Infect. Dis.* **29:**1483–1488.

126. **Peterson, L., and R. B. Thomson, Jr.** 1999. Use of the clinical microbiology laboratory for the diagnosis and management of infectious diseases related to the oral cavity. *Infect. Dis. Clin. North Am.* **13:**775–795.

127. **Peterson, L. R.** 1997. Effect of media on transport and recovery of anaerobic bacteria. *Clin. Infect. Dis.* **25**(Suppl. 2)**:**S134–S136.

128. **Peterson, L. R., J. D. Hamilton, E. J. Baron, L. S. Tompkins, J. M. Miller, C. M. Wilfert, F. C. Tenover, and R. B. Thomson, Jr.** 2001. Role of clinical microbiology laboratories in the management and control of infectious diseases and the delivery of health care. *Clin. Infect. Dis.* **32:**605–611.

129. **Pezzlo, M.** 1988. Detection of urinary tract infections by rapid methods. *Clin. Microbiol. Rev.* **1:**268–280.

130. **Pezzlo, M. T., V. Ige, A. P. Woolard, E. M. Peterson, and L. M. de la Maza.** 1989. Rapid bioluminescence method for bacteriuria screening. *J. Clin. Microbiol.* **27:**716–720.

131. **Pfaller, M. A., and F. P. Koontz.** 1985. Laboratory evaluation of leukocyte esterase and nitrite tests for the detection of bacteriuria. *J. Clin. Microbiol.* **21:**840–842.

132. **Prandoni, D., M. H. Boone, E. Larson, C. G. Blane, and H. Fitzpatrick.** 1996. Assessment of urine collection technique for microbial culture. *Am. J. Infect. Control* **24:**219–221.

133. **Prekates, A., S. Nanas, A. Argyropoulou, G. Margariti, T. Kyprianou, E. Papagalos, O. Paniara, and C. Roussos.** 1998. The diagnostic value of gram stain of bronchoalveolar lavage samples in patients with suspected ventilator-associated pneumonia. *Scand. J. Infect. Dis.* **30:**43–47.

134. **Ramirez, J. A., S. Ahkee, A. Tolentino, R. D. Miller, and J. T. Summersgill.** 1996. Diagnosis of *Legionella pneumophila, Mycoplasma pneumoniae,* or *Chlamydia pneumoniae* lower respiratory infection using the polymerase chain reaction on a single throat swab specimen. *Diagn. Microbiol. Infect. Dis.* **24:**7–14.

135. **Reik, H., and S. J. Rubin.** 1981. Evaluation of the buffy-coat smear for rapid detection of bacteremia. *JAMA* **245:**357–359.

136. **Reimer, L. G.** 1994. Catheter-related infections and blood cultures. *Clin. Lab. Med.* **14:**51–58.

137. **Reimer, L. G., and L. B. Reller.** 1985. Effect of sodium polyanetholesulfonate and gelatin on the recovery of *Gardnerella vaginalis* from blood culture media. *J. Clin. Microbiol.* **21:**686–688.

138. **Reimer, L. G., M. L. Wilson, and M. P. Weinstein.** 1997. Update on detection of bacteremia and fungemia. *Clin. Microbiol. Rev.* **10:**444–465.

139. **Reller, L. B., P. R. Murray, and J. D. MacLowry.** 1982. Cumitech 1A, *Blood Cultures II,* vol. 1A. Coordinating ed., J. A. Washington II. American Society for Microbiology, Washington, D.C.

140. **Rippin, K. P., W. C. Stinson, J. Eisenstadt, and J. A. Washington.** 1995. Clinical evaluation of the slide centrifuge (cytospin) gram's stained smear for the detection of bacteriuria and comparison with the FiltraCheck-UTI and UTIscreen. *Am. J. Clin. Pathol.* **103:**316–319.

141. **Ristuccia, P. A., R. A. Hoeffner, M. Digamon-Beltran, and B. A. Cunha.** 1987. Detection of bacteremia by buffy coat smears. *Scand. J. Infect. Dis.* **19:**215–217.

142. **Robinson, A.** 1994. Rationale for cost-effective laboratory medicine. *Clin. Microbiol. Rev.* **7:**185–199.

143. **Rosenberg, M., S. A. Berger, M. Barki, S. Goldberg, A. Fink, and A. Miskin.** 1992. Initial testing of a novel urine culture device. *J. Clin. Microbiol.* **30:**2686–2691.

144. **Rosett, W., and G. R. Hodges.** 1980. Antimicrobial activity of heparin. *J. Clin. Microbiol.* **11:**30–34.

145. **Sander, R.** 2001. Otitis externa: a practical guide to treatment and prevention. *Am. Fam. Physician* **63:**927–936, 941–942.

146. **Sapico, F. L., H. N. Canawati, J. L. Witte, J. Z. Montgomerie, F. W. Wagner, Jr., and A. N. Bessman.** 1980. Quantitative aerobic and anaerobic bacteriology of infected diabetic feet. *J. Clin. Microbiol.* **12:**413–420.

147. **Savola, K. L., E. J. Baron, L. S. Tompkins, and D. J. Passaro.** 2001. Fecal leukocyte stain has diagnostic value for outpatients but not inpatients. *J. Clin. Microbiol.* **39:**266–269.

148. **Schachter, J.** 1997. DFA, EIA, PCR, LCR and other technologies: what tests should be used for diagnosis of chlamydia infections? *Immunol. Investig.* **26:**157–161.

149. **Schifman, R. B., C. L. Strand, F. A. Meier, and P. J. Howanitz.** 1998. Blood culture contamination: a College of American Pathologists Q-Probes study involving 640 institutions and 497134 specimens from adult patients. *Arch. Pathol. Lab. Med.* **122:**216–221.

150. **Schrag, S., R. Gorwitz, K. Fultz-Butts, and A. Schuchat.** 2002. Prevention of perinatal group B streptococcal disease: revised guidelines from CDC. *Morb. Mortal. Wkly. Rep.* **51**(RR11)**:**1–22.

151. **Schwartz, D. A., and C. J. Herman.** 1996. The importance of the autopsy in emerging and reemerging infectious diseases. *Clin. Infect. Dis.* **23:**248–254.

152. **Semeniuk, H., and D. Church.** 1999. Evaluation of the leukocyte esterase and nitrite urine dipstick screening tests for detection of bacteriuria in women with suspected uncomplicated urinary tract infections. *J. Clin. Microbiol.* **37:**3051–3052.

153. **Shanholtzer, C. J., P. J. Schaper, and L. R. Peterson.** 1982. Concentrated Gram stain smears prepared with a cytospin centrifuge. *J. Clin. Microbiol.* **16:**1052–1056.

154. **Sharkawy, A., D. E. Low, R. Saginur, D. Gregson, B. Schwartz, P. Jessamine, K. Green, and A. McGeer.** 2002. Severe group A streptococcal soft-tissue infections in Ontario: 1992–1996. *Clin. Infect. Dis.* **34:**454–460.

155. **Sharp, S.** 1999. Algorithms for wound specimens. *Clin. Microbiol. Newsl.* **21:**118–120.

156. **Sharpe, A. N., and A. K. Johnson.** 1972. Stomaching: a new concept in bacteriological sample preparation. *Appl. Microbiol.* **24:**175–178.

157. **Shim, J. K., S. Johnson, M. H. Samore, D. Z. Bliss, and D. N. Gerding.** 1998. Primary symptomless colonisation by *Clostridium difficile* and decreased risk of subsequent diarrhoea. *Lancet* **351:**633–636.

158. **Siegman-Igra, Y., A. M. Anglim, D. E. Shapiro, K. A. Adal, B. A. Strain, and B. M. Farr.** 1997. Diagnosis of vascular catheter-related bloodstream infection: a meta-analysis. *J. Clin. Microbiol.* **35:**928–936.

159. **Sloan, L. M., M. K. Hopkins, P. S. Mitchell, E. A. Vetter, J. E. Rosenblatt, W. S. Harmsen, F. R. Cockerill, and R. Patel.** 2002. Multiplex LightCycler PCR assay for detection and differentiation of *Bordetella pertussis* and *Bordetella parapertussis* in nasopharyngeal specimens. *J. Clin. Microbiol.* **40:**96–100.

160. **Sobel, J. D.** 2000. Bacterial vaginosis. *Annu. Rev. Med.* **51:**349–356.

161. **Spach, D. H., and J. E. Kochler.** 1998. *Bartonella*-associated infections. *Infect. Dis. Clin. North Am.* **12:** 137–155.

162. **Stager, C. E., and J. R. Davis.** 1990. Evaluation of the FiltraCheck-UTI for detection of bacteriuria. *Diagn. Microbiol. Infect. Dis.* **13:**289–295.

163. **Stamm, W. E., and T. M. Hooton.** 1993. Management of urinary tract infections in adults. *N. Engl. J. Med.* **329:**1328–1334.

164. **Steed, L. L., E. K. Korgenski, and J. A. Daly.** 1993. Rapid detection of *Streptococcus pyogenes* in pediatric patient specimens by DNA probe. *J. Clin. Microbiol.* **31:**2996–3000.

165. **Stenberg, K., B. Herrmann, L. Dannevig, A. N. Elbagir, and P. A. Mardh.** 1990. Culture, ELISA and immunofluorescence tests for the diagnosis of conjunctivitis caused by *Chlamydia trachomatis* in neonates and adults. *APMIS* **98:**514–520.

166. **Stephen, J.** 2001. Pathogenesis of infectious diarrhea. *Can. J. Gastroenterol.* **15:**669–683.

167. **Stevens, D. L.** 2000. Streptococcal toxic shock syndrome associated with necrotizing fasciitis. *Annu. Rev. Med.* **51:**271–288.

168. **Strain, B.** 1992. Quantitative bacteriology: tissues and aspirates, p. 1.16a.1–1.16a.4. *In* H. D. Isenberg (ed.), *Clinical Microbiology Procedures Handbook.* American Society for Microbiology, Washington, D.C.

169. **Sturgis, C. D., L. R. Peterson, and J. R. Warren.** 1997. Cerebrospinal fluid broth culture isolates: their significance for antibiotic treatment. *Am. J. Clin. Pathol.* **108:** 217–221.

169a. **Tan, J. S. (ed.).** 2002. *Expert Guide to Infectious Diseases.* American College of Physicians, Philadelphia, Pa.

170. **Thomson, R. B., Jr., and L. Peterson.** 2001. Microbiology laboratory diagnosis of pulmonary infections, p. 541–559. *In* M. S. Niederman, G. A. Sarosi, and J. Glassroth (ed.), *Respiratory Infections,* 2nd ed. Lippincott Williams & Wilkins, Philadelphia, Pa.

171. **Thomson, R. B., Jr., and H. Bertram.** 2001. Laboratory diagnosis of central nervous system infections. *Infect. Dis. Clin. North Am.* **15:**1047–1071.

172. **Thomson, R. B., Jr., and L. R. Peterson.** 1998. Role of the clinical microbiology laboratory in the diagnosis of infections. *Cancer Treat. Res.* **96:**143–165.

173. **Thomson, R. B., Jr., S. J. Vanzo, N. K. Henry, K. L. Guenther, and J. A. Washington II.** 1984. Contamination of cultures processed with the isolator lysis-centrifugation blood culture tube. *J. Clin. Microbiol.* **19:**97–99.

174. **Thorpe, J. E., R. P. Baughman, P. T. Frame, T. A. Wesseler, and J. L. Staneck.** 1987. Bronchoalveolar lavage for diagnosing acute bacterial pneumonia. *J. Infect. Dis.* **155:**855–861.

175. **Trollfors, B., O. Nylen, C. Carenfelt, M. Fogle-Hansson, A. Freijd, A. Geterud, S. Hugosson, K. Prellner, E. Neovius, H. Nordell, A. Backman, B. Kaijser, T. Lagergard, M. Leinonen, P. Olcen, and J. Pilichowska-Paszkiet.** 1998. Aetiology of acute epiglottitis in adults. *Scand. J. Infect. Dis.* **30:**49–51.

176. **Turner, J. C., F. G. Hayden, M. C. Lobo, C. E. Ramirez, and D. Murren.** 1997. Epidemiologic evidence for Lancefield group C beta-hemolytic streptococci as a cause of exudative pharyngitis in college students. *J. Clin. Microbiol.* **35:**1–4.

177. **Uhrin, M.** 1997. Molecular diagnostics. The polymerase chain reaction and its use in the diagnosis of *Chlamydia trachomatis* and *Neisseria gonorrhoeae. Gac. Med. Mex.* **133:**133–137.

178. **Vaira, D., N. Vakil, M. Menegatti, B. van't Hoff, C. Ricci, L. Gatta, G. Gasbarrini, M. Quina, J. M. Pajares Garcia, A. van Der Ende, R. van Der Hulst, M. Anti, C. Duarte, J. P. Gisbert, M. Miglioli, and G. Tytgat.** 2002. The stool antigen test for detection of *Helicobacter pylori* after eradication therapy. *Ann. Intern. Med.* **136:** 280–287.

179. **Vakil, N., D. Rhew, A. Soll, and J. J. Ofman.** 2000. The cost-effectiveness of diagnostic testing strategies for *Helicobacter pylori. Am. J. Gastroenterol.* **95:**1691–1698.

180. **Valenstein, P., and F. Meier.** 1998. Urine culture contamination: a College of American Pathologists Q-Probes study of contaminated urine cultures in 906 institutions. *Arch. Pathol. Lab. Med.* **122:**123–129.

181. **Van Der Pol, B., D. H. Martin, J. Schachter, T. C. Quinn, C. A. Gaydos, R. B. Jones, K. Crotchfelt, J. Moncada, D. Jungkind, B. Turner, C. Peyton, J. F. Kelly, J. B. Weiss, and M. Rosenstraus.** 2001. Enhancing the specificity of the COBAS AMPLICOR CT/NG test for *Neisseria gonorrhoeae* by retesting specimens with equivocal results. *J. Clin. Microbiol.* **39:**3092–3098.

182. **Van Enk, R. A., and K. D. Thompson.** 1990. Microbiologic analysis of amniotic fluid. *Clin. Microbiol. Newsl.* **12:**169–172.

183. **Vickers, R. M., J. D. Rihs, and V. L. Yu.** 1992. Clinical demonstration of isolation of *Nocardia asteroides* on buffered charcoal-yeast extract media. *J. Clin. Microbiol.* **30:** 227–228.

184. **Volk, E. E., M. L. Miller, B. A. Kirkley, and J. A. Washington.** 1998. The diagnostic usefulness of bone marrow cultures in patients with fever of unknown origin. *Am. J. Clin. Pathol.* **110:**150–153.

185. **von Graevenitz, A., and D. Amsterdam.** 1992. Microbiological aspects of peritonitis associated with continuous ambulatory peritoneal dialysis. *Clin. Microbiol. Rev.* **5:**36–48.

186. **Walter, F. G., R. L. Gibly, R. K. Knopp, and D. J. Roe.** 1998. Squamous cells as predictors of bacterial contamination in urine samples. *Ann. Emerg. Med.* **31:**455–458.

187. **Ward, K. W.** 1992. Processing and interpretation of specimens for *Legionella* spp. 1. *Legionella* specimen processing, p. 1.12.1–1.12.8. *In* H. D. Isenberg (ed.), *Clinical Microbiology Procedures Handbook.* American Society for Microbiology, Washington, D.C.

188. **Wegner, D. L., D. L. Witte, and R. D. Schrantz.** 1992. Insensitivity of rapid antigen detection methods and single blood agar plate culture for diagnosing streptococcal pharyngitis. *JAMA* **267:**695–697.

189. **Weinstein, J. W., S. Tallapragada, P. Farrel, and L. M. Dembry.** 1996. Comparison of rectal and perirectal swabs for detection of colonization with vancomycin-resistant enterococci. *J. Clin. Microbiol.* **34:**210–212.

190. **Weinstein, M. P.** 1996. Current blood culture methods and systems: clinical concepts, technology, and interpretation of results. *Clin. Infect. Dis.* **23:**40–46.

191. **Weinstein, M. P., M. L. Towns, S. M. Quartey, S. Mirrett, L. G. Reimer, G. Parmigiani, and L. B. Reller.** 1997. The clinical significance of positive blood cultures in the 1990s: a prospective comprehensive evaluation of the microbiology, epidemiology, and outcome of bacteremia and fungemia in adults. *Clin. Infect. Dis.* **24:**584–602.

192. **Wenzel, R. P., D. R. Reagan, J. S. Bertino, Jr., E. J. Baron, and K. Arias.** 1998. Methicillin-resistant Staphylococcus aureus outbreak: a consensus panel's definition and management guidelines. *Am. J. Infect. Control* **26:**102–110.

193. **Westergren, V., L. Lundblad, H. B. Hellquist, and U. Forsum.** 1998. Ventilator-associated sinusitis: a review. *Clin. Infect. Dis.* **27:**851–864.

194. **Wilhelmus, K., T. Liesagang, M. Osato, and D. Jones.** 1994. Cumitech 13A, *Laboratory Diagnosis of Ocular Infections.* Coordinating ed., S. C. Specter. ASM Press, Washington, D.C.

195. **Wilson, M. L.** 1997. Clinically relevant, cost-effective clinical microbiology. Strategies to decrease unnecessary testing. *Am. J. Clin. Pathol.* **107:**154–167.

196. **Wilson, S. J., M. L. Wilson, and L. B. Reller.** 1993. Diagnostic utility of postmortem blood cultures. *Arch. Pathol. Lab. Med.* **117:**986–988.

197. **Winquist, A. G., M. A. Orrico, and L. R. Peterson.** 1997. Evaluation of the cytocentrifuge Gram stain as a screening test for bacteriuria in specimens from specific patient populations. *Am. J. Clin. Pathol.* **108:**515–524.

198. **Woods, G. L., and D. H. Walker.** 1996. Detection of infection or infectious agents by use of cytologic and histologic stains. *Clin. Microbiol. Rev.* **9:**382–404.

199. **Woolfrey, B. F., J. M. Fox, and C. O. Quall.** 1981. An evaluation of burn wound quantitative microbiology. I. Quantitative eschar cultures. *Am. J. Clin. Pathol.* **75:**532–537.

200. **Wright, D. N., R. Boshard, P. Ahlin, B. Saxon, and J. M. Matsen.** 1985. Effect of urine preservation on urine screening and organism identification. *Arch. Pathol. Lab. Med.* **109:**819–822.

201. **Yungbluth, M.** 1995. The laboratory diagnosis of pneumonia. The role of the community hospital pathologist. *Clin. Lab. Med.* **15:**209–234.

202. **Zwart, S., G. J. Ruijs, A. P. Sachs, W. J. van Leeuwen, J. W. Gubbels, and R. A. de Melker.** 2000. Beta-haemolytic streptococci isolated from acute sore-throat patients: cause or coincidence? A case-control study in general practice. *Scand. J. Infect. Dis.* **32:**377–384.

Algorithm for Identification of Aerobic Gram-Positive Cocci

KATHRYN L. RUOFF

21

Gram-positive cocci recovered from aerobic cultures can be differentiated by the tests shown in Tables 1 and 2. These organisms include "aerotolerant anaerobes," facultative anaerobes, microaerophiles, and obligate aerobes. The genera display variable colony morphologies and hemolytic and catalase (Tables 1 and 2) reactions. Their cellular morphologies as revealed in Gram stains of broth cultures are generally either streptococcal, consisting of gram-positive cocci or coccobacilli arranged in pairs and/or chains, or staphylococcal, in which cells appear as cocci arranged in pairs, tetrads, clusters, and irregular groups. No taxonomic kinship is implied by division of these bacteria into two groups based on cellular morphology. The reader is referred to the chapters noted in the tables for more detailed descriptions of these organisms.

TABLE 1 Characteristics of catalase-negative gram-positive cocci that grow aerobically and form cells arranged in pairs and chains[a]

PYR	LAP	6.5% NaCl	BE	Motility	45°C	Probe	HIP	Satellitism	10°C	Organism (chapter)
+	+	+	+	+	+					Enterococcus (30)
					−					Vagococcus (31)
				−		+				Enterococcus (30)
						−				Lactococcus (31)
			−				+	−		Facklamia spp.[b] (31)
							−	V		Ignavigranum (31)
		−	+	+						Vagococcus (31)
				−						Lactococcus (31)
			−					+		Abiotrophia, Granulicatella (31)
								−		Gemella spp.[c] (31)
	−	+								Globicatella (31)
		−								Dolosicoccus (31)
−	−									Leuconostoc[d] (31)
	+								+	Lactococcus (31)
									−	Streptococcus[e] (29)

[a] See chapters 27 and 29 to 31 for descriptions of the methods for performing the tests referred to in this table. Reactions shown are typical, but exceptions may occur. Abbreviations and symbols: PYR, production of pyrrolidonyl arylamidase; LAP, production of leucine aminopeptidase; 6.5% NaCl, growth in 6.5% NaCl; BE, hydrolysis of esculin in the presence of 40% bile; 45°C, growth at 45°C; Probe, reaction with commercially available nucleic acid probe for the genus Enterococcus; HIP, hydrolysis of hippurate; Satellitism, satelliting growth behavior; 10°C, growth at 10°C; +, most strains positive; −, most strains negative; V, variable reactions are observed.

[b] The reactions in this table are typical for F. hominis, F. sourekii, and F. ignava. F. languida cells tend to be arranged in clusters, and isolates are hippurate hydrolysis negative (Table 2).

[c] G. morbillorum, G. bergeriae, and G. sanguinis cells tend to be arranged in pairs and chains, in contrast to the cells of G. haemolysans, which are arranged in pairs, tetrads, and clusters (Table 2).

[d] Leuconostoc is distinguished from the other catalase-negative organisms in Table 1 by its ability to produce gas as an end product of glucose metabolism and its intrinsic resistance to vancomycin.

[e] Most streptococci are PYR negative, with the exception of S. pyogenes isolates and some strains of S. pneumoniae, which are PYR positive.

TABLE 2 Differentiating features of gram-positive cocci that grow aerobically and form cells arranged in clusters or irregular groups[a]

Catalase	Obligate aerobe	Oxidase	PYR	LAP	NaCl	ESC	Hemolysis	Vancomycin	BGUR	Organism (chapter)
+	+	+			+[b]					*Micrococcus* (28)
	−				+[c]					*Alloiococcus* (28)
	−	−			+[b]					*Staphylococcus* (28)
					−[b]					*Rothia mucilaginosa*[d] (28)
−	−		+	+	+[c]	+			−	*Dolosigranulum* (31)
									+	*Aerococcus sanguicola* (31)
						−			−	*Facklamia languida*[e] (31)
					−[c]	+				*Rothia mucilaginosa*[d] (28)
						−				*Gemella haemolysans*[f] (31)
				−			α			*Aerococcus viridans*[g] (31)
							γ			*Helcococcus*[g] (31)
			−	+				R		*Pediococcus* (31)
								S	+	*Aerococcus urinae* (31)
				−					+	*Aerococcus urinaehominis* (31)
									−	*Aerococcus christensenii* (31)

[a] See chapters 27, 28, and 31 for descriptions of the methods for performing the phenotypic tests referred to in this table. Reactions shown are typical; exceptions may occur. Abbreviations: PYR, production of pyrrolidonyl arylamidase; LAP, production of leucine aminopeptidase; NaCl, growth in the presence of either 5 or 6.5% NaCl (see footnotes *c* and *d*); ESC, esculin hydrolysis; BGUR, production of β-glucuronidase; +, most strains positive; −, most strains negative; V, variable reactions are observed; α, alpha-hemolysis on sheep blood agar; γ, nonhemolytic reaction on sheep blood agar; S, susceptible; R, resistant.

[b] Growth in the presence of 5% sodium chloride.

[c] Growth in the presence of 6.5% sodium chloride.

[d] *Rothia mucilaginosa* isolates are usually catalase negative or weakly positive but may be strongly catalase positive.

[e] *Ignavigranum ruoffiae* (Table 1) exhibits identical reactions to those of *F. languida* in the PYR, ESC, and NaCl tests. However, *I. ruoffiae* cells are arranged primarily in chains while *F. languida* cells usually form clusters. Other *Facklamia* species form cells arranged in pairs and chains (Table 1).

[f] *G. haemolysans* cells tend to be arranged in pairs, tetrads, and groups, in contrast to the cells of other *Gemella* species, which usually occur in pairs and short chains (Table 1).

[g] *Helcococcus* strains form tiny pinpoint nonhemolytic colonies on blood agar after 24 h of aerobic incubation at 35°C, while *Aerococcus viridans* isolates form larger alpha-hemolytic colonies under similar incubation conditions. In contrast to helcococci, *A. viridans* prefers aerobic incubation atmospheres.

Algorithm for Identification of Aerobic Gram-Positive Rods

GUIDO FUNKE

22

The aim of the algorithm for the identification of aerobic gram-positive rods described in this chapter is simply to guide the reader of this Manual to the appropriate chapter for further information. The algorithm emphasizes that Gram stain (performed on 24- to 48-h-old colonies from rich media) and macroscopic morphologies are the initial key features for the differentiation of aerobic gram-positive rods. All strains of aerobic gram-positive rods (except the non-rapidly growing mycobacteria) are initially grown on blood agar plates.

Regular rods are organisms with cells whose longitudinal edges are usually not curved but are parallel. If spore formation is not observed initially, it can be tested for on a nutritionally depleted medium. Catalase activity should be tested with media lacking heme groups. The type of metabolism can be checked in oxidative-fermentative media or in cystine Trypticase agar medium. Irregular rods are organisms with cells whose longitudinal edges are curved and not parallel. Diagnostic end products of glucose metabolism can be detected by chromatographic methods only. Slight beta-hemolysis is best observed when cells are incubated in a CO_2-enriched atmosphere. Yellow- or orange-pigmented rods are always irregular rods. Some genera that stain partially acid-fast (e.g., *Gordonia* and *Rhodococcus*) may also show a yellow-orange pigment. Rods exhibiting vegetative substrate filaments show branched hyphae, which either form spores or reproduce by fragmentation. It is obvious that vegetative substrate filaments might not be present initially (i.e., within 48 h), and so these organisms are prone to initial misidentification.

For the yellow-orange genera (e.g., *Microbacterium*, *Curtobacterium*, and *Leifsonia*), as well as the rods exhibiting vegetative substrate filaments, chemotaxonomic methods must very often be used for definitive identification to the genus level; for example, all partially acid-fast bacteria can be identified to the genus level by analysis of mycolic acids.

It is emphasized that genera which contain strict anaerobic gram-positive rods may also contain aerobically growing species. This is particularly true for the genus *Actinomyces* (as it is presently defined). *Clostridium tertium* (a strong gas producer) may also grow aerobically. Furthermore, it should also be mentioned that some aerobic gram-positive cocci (e.g., *Leuconostoc* spp. and *Streptococcus mutans*) might initially be misidentified as gram-positive rods because of their initial Gram stain appearance. Likewise, but less frequently, some gram-positive rods (e.g., *Rhodococcus* spp.) might initially be misidentified as gram-positive cocci because of their initial Gram stain appearance.

This algorithm should serve only as the basis of a very preliminary identification of an unknown aerobic gram-positive rod, and the reader is referred to the chapters given in Table 1 for further information.

TABLE 1 Algorithm for identification of aerobic gram-positive rods

Cellular morphology	Yellow-orange pigment	Vegetative substrate filaments	Spore formation	Catalase activity	H$_2$S in TSI	Other unusual Gram stain feature	Diagnostic end product of glucose metabolism[a]	Slight beta-hemolysis	Metabolism[b]	Slow acid production	Acid-fast stain	Partially acid-fast stain	Aerial vegetative filaments	Motility	Growth at 50°C	Organism (chapter)
Regular			+													Bacillus, including Paeni-, Brevi-, Aneurini-, and Virgibacillus (32)
			−	+												Listeria (33)
				−	+											Erysipelothrix (33)
					−											Lactobacillus (55)
				+		Club-shaped rods										Corynebacterium (34)
Irregular	−															
						Slim, long rods										Turicella (34)
						Very coccoid rods										Dermabacter (34)
						May show jointed rods										Arthrobacter (34)
						May show short rods										Brevibacterium (34)
						May show branching										Actinomyces (55), Propionibacterium (55), Rothia (28, 34)
				−		Coccoid rods, Gram variable										Gardnerella (34)

(Continued on next page)

TABLE 1 Algorithm for identification of aerobic gram-positive rods (*Continued*)

Cellular morphology	Yellow-orange pigment	Vegetative substrate filaments	Spore formation	Catalase activity	H₂S in TSI	Other unusual Gram stain feature	Diagnostic end product of glucose metabolism[a]	Slight beta-hemolysis	Metabolism[b]	Slow acid production	Acid-fast stain	Partially acid-fast stain	Aerial vegetative filaments	Motility	Growth at 50°C	Organism (chapter)
							S	+ −								*Arcanobacterium* (34), *Actinomyces* (55)
							A									*Bifidobacterium* (55)
							L									*Rothia* (28, 34)
	+	+														*Oerskovia, Cellulosimicrobium* (both 34)
		−		+					O	+						*Curtobacterium* (34)
										−						*Microbacterium, Leifsonia* (both 34)
									F							*Microbacterium, Cellulomonas, Exiguobacterium* (all 34)
				−												*Microbacterium* (34)
	−	+									⌐					*Mycobacterium* (36, 37)
											−	+	+			*Nocardia* (35)
													−			*Tsukamurella, Gordonia, Rhodococcus* (all 35)
												−		+		*Dermatophilus* (35)
													+	−		*Micromonospora, Actinomadura* (both 35)
													+		+	*Saccharomonospora, Saccharopolyspora, Thermoactinomyces* (all 35)
															−	*Actinomadura, Amycolata, Amycolatopsis, Nocardiopsis, Streptomyces* (all 35)

[a] S, succinic acid; A, acetic acid; L, lactic acid.
[b] O, oxidative; F, fermentative.

Algorithms for Identification of Aerobic Gram-Negative Bacteria*

PAUL C. SCHRECKENBERGER AND JANE D. WONG

23

These algorithms are meant to assist in the identification of organisms that are not readily identified by methods in place in most clinical laboratories. Microbiologists planning to identify an unknown gram-negative rod begin with colonies on an agar plate. Our definition of "good growth on blood agar plate (BAP)" is the presence of distinct colonies (approximately 1 mm) on tryptic soy agar with 5% sheep blood after 24 h of incubation at 35°C in room atmosphere. Poor growth indicates that more than 24 h of incubation is necessary for the development of distinct colonies. If an organism fails to grow on BAP after 72 h, it is considered to show "no growth." Morphological and phenotypic criteria were chosen not only for their discriminatory value but also because the methods are available in most laboratories. Cellular morphology is determined by using a Gram stain from a young colony on a BAP. The description of "tiny coccobacilli" used for *Brucella* and *Francisella* implies almost indiscernible cells resembling grains of sand. For many organisms with pleomorphic morphologies, we chose to represent the dominant shape.

The urea test refers to conventional Christensen's urea reaction after 24 h of incubation, whereas the rapid urea result is read after 4 h. Glucose fermentation refers to an acid reaction in the butt of a Kligler iron agar (KIA) or triple sugar iron agar (TSI) tube. "Glucose oxidized" refers to acid production in the upper portion of oxidative-fermentative (OF) media. "BHI + serum" refers to brain heart infusion agar with 10% (vol/vol) serum added. The oxidase test refers to results obtained with the N,N,N,N-tetramethyl-p-phenylenediamine dihydrochloride reagent. Mo-

tility is best observed by preparing a wet preparation from a young colony on a BAP. Decarboxylase reactions are determined by using an extremely turbid inoculum in Moeller's media (heavier than usual inoculum). Polymyxin B sensitivity is indicated by any zone of inhibition surrounding a 300-U disk on a BAP. For glucose-nonfermenting bacilli and other fastidious organisms, the indole test is performed using the Ehrlich's extraction method. "Esculin" refers to hydrolysis of esculin in media without bile.

These algorithms are dichotomous, since many organisms may fall into more than one group due to phenotypic variability of a given trait. The presence of two or more atypical traits or a major variation from the ideal phenotype depicted in these algorithms, due to antibiotic use, auxotrophy, or other reasons, may limit the algorithms' utility. These algorithms are intended as a guide to presumptive identification of an unknown isolate. The reference chapter describing the organism should be consulted to determine the definitive identification. To use the algorithms, start with Tables 1 through 3 for gram-negative bacteria that grow well on blood agar in 24 h at room atmosphere and Table 4 for fastidious gram-negative bacteria. In each case, begin in the upper left-hand column; if the test organism matches the given characteristic, then continue horizontally to the right to the next reaction. If the reaction in the box matches your test organism, continue moving horizontally until you reach the organisms listed in the right-hand column. When the reaction in the box does not match your test organism, move down the column vertically to find the reaction that matches. Repeat the process until you reach the right-hand column. Be sure to check all your reactions with the organism characteristics given in the referenced chapter.

---

* This chapter contains information presented in chapter 26 by Paul C. Schreckenberger, J. Michael Janda, Jane D. Wong, and Ellen Jo Baron in the seventh edition of this Manual.

TABLE 1 Identification algorithm no. 1 for gram-negative bacteria that grow well on blood agar, including glucose fermenters

Cell morphology	Glucose fermented	Pigmented colonies	Oxidase	6% NaCl	Motility	Sucrose fermented	H_2S in TSI	Indole	Glucose oxidized	Fluorescent pigment	Yellow-pigmented colonies	Polymyxin B	ONPG	Lysine decarboxylase	Arginine decarboxylase	Urea	Esculin	OF mannitol	OF maltose	Growth on MacConkey	Lactose, xylose, or trehalose fermented	Phenylalanine deaminase	H_2S in TSI	ONPG	Nitrate to gas	Organism group (chapter)
Rods	+	Purple																								Chromobacterium (39)
		Other	+	+																						Vibrio (46)
				−	+																					Aeromonas (45), Plesiomonas (44)
					−	+																				Pasteurella (39), Actinobacillus (39)
						−																				Pasteurella bettyae (39)
								+							+											EF4a (39)
								−							−											Pasteurella avium (39), Actinobacillus actinomycetemcomitans (39)
			−	+																						Vibrio metschnikovii (46)
				−																+	+					Enterobacteriaceae (41–44)
																					−	+				Providencia, Morganella (41, 44)
																						−	+			Edwardsiella (41, 44)
																							−			Pasteurella bettyae (39)
																				−						P. bettyae (39)
	−	Pink																								Methylobacterium, Roseomonas (49)
		Not pink	+		+		+																			Shewanella spp. (49)

Organism					
Balneatrix alpica (49)				−	+
Pseudomonas aeruginosa, P. fluorescens, P. putida (47)				+ +	
Agrobacterium yellow group, O-1, O-2, *Sphingomonas* spp. (49)			−	+	
Pseudomonas-like group 2 (49)	+		R +	−	
Burkholderia cepacia complex (48)	−		− +		
B. stabilis (48)		− +			
B. pseudomallei (48)		− +	− +		
Ralstonia mannitolytica (48)			−		
Pandoraea spp., *Ralstonia* spp. (48)		+	+		
Ochrobactrum anthropi, Achromobacter groups B and E (49)		−	+		
CDC Vb-3 (47), OFBA-1 (49)		+	S +		
Pseudomonas-like group 2, OFBA-1 (49), *Acidovorax* spp. (48)		− + +			
P. mendocina (47), CDC Ic, OFBA-1 (49)		−			
Rhizobium radiobacter (49)	+	−	+		
Ochrobactrum anthropi, Achromobacter group F, *Halomonas venusta* (49)	−	+	+		
P. stutzeri (47), *Ochrobactrum anthropi* (49)	+		−		
Pseudomonas-like group 2, *Herbaspirillum*, CDC halophilic nonfermenter group 1 (49)	−	−			
CDC group O-3 (49), *Brevundimonas vesicularis* (48)			+		
P. stutzeri (47), *A. xylosoxidans* subsp. *xylosoxidans* (49)	+	− +			
A. xylosoxidans subsp. *xylosoxidans* (49), *Brevundimonas diminuta* (48)	−				

TABLE 2 Identification algorithm no. 2 for gram-negative bacteria that grow well on blood agar, limited to oxidase-positive glucose nonfermenters

Cell morphology	Glucose fermented	Pigmented colonies	Oxidase	Motility	H_2S in TSI	Indole	Glucose oxidized	Yellow-pigmented colonies	Polymyxin B	Arginine decarboxylase	Rapid urea	NO_2 reduction	Acetamide	Esculin	OF mannitol	Urea	Growth in 6.5% NaCl	Gelatin	NO_3 to NO_2	Organism group (chapter)
Rod	−	Not pink	+	+	−	−	−		R											Pandoraea spp. (48)
									S	+										P. pseudoalcaligenes, P. alcaligenes, Pseudomonas species group 1 (47)
										−	+									Bordetella bronchiseptica, Oligella ureolytica (49), Ralstonia paucula (48)
											−	+							+	Pseudomonas sp. group 1 (47), Achromobacter xylosoxidans subsp. denitrificans (49)
																			−	Alcaligenes faecalis (49)
												−	+		+					Delftia acidovorans (48)
								+							−				+	Achromobacter piechaudii (49)
								−											−	Bordetella avium (49, 50)
													−				+			CDC halophilic group 1 (49)
																	−		+	P. pseudoalcaligenes (33), P. alcaligenes (47), Comamonas terrigena (48), C. testosteroni (48), A. piechaudii (49)
																			−	Brevundimonas diminuta (48), Brevundimonas vesicularis (48), Bordetella hinzii (49, 50), P. alcaligenes (47), Ralstonia gilardii (48)
				−		+	+													Chryseobacterium indologenes/gleum, Empedobacter brevis, CDC group IIi (49)
											+									Bergeyella zoohelcum (49)
														+	+					C. meningosepticum (49)
											−			−	−					CDC group IIc, IIh, IIi (49)
																		+		Weeksella virosa (49), E. brevis (49)
																		−		CDC group IIe, IIg (49)
						−								+	+					Sphingobacterium spiritivorum (49)
															−	+			+	Sphingobacterium thalpophilum (49)
																			−	Sphingobacterium multivorum (49)
																−				Sphingomonas paucimobilis (49), Sphingobacterium mizutaii (49)
																			+	EF-4b, EO-2, Psychrobacter immobilis (49)
							−							−					−	EO-3, EO-4 (49)
											+							+		Myroides spp. (49)
											−							+		Oligella ureolytica (49)
														+						Alishewanella fetalis (49)
														−						Neisseria weaveri, N. elongata, Gilardi rod group 1 (38, 49)

TABLE 3 Identification algorithm no. 3 for gram-negative bacteria that grow well on blood agar, including glucose-nonfermenting rods, cocci, and coccobacilli

Cell morphology	Glucose fermented	Pigmented colonies	Oxidase	Motility	Glucose oxidized	DNase	Urea	OF mannitol	Lysine decarboxylase or OF lactose	Lysine decarboxylase	OF maltose	Esculin	NO₂ reduced	NO₃ reduced	Brown diffusible pigment	Organism group (chapter)
Rods	–	Not pink	–	+	+			+	+							Burkholderia cepacia complex (48)
									Both negative		+	+				Pseudomonas luteola (47)
											–	–				Pseudomonas oryzihabitans (47)
											–					Burkholderia gladioli (48)
					–			–		+						Stenotrophomonas maltophilia (48)
										–						Sphingomonas paucimobilis (49)
					–							+				Massilia timonae (49)
												–				Bordetella trematum (49, 50)
				–	+											Acinetobacter baumannii, EO-5 (49)
					–		+									Bordetella parapertussis (49, 50)
														+		CDC NO-1 (49)
														–	+	Bordetella holmesii (49)
							–								–	Acinetobacter lwoffii (49)
Diplococci			+													Neisseria, Moraxella catarrhalis (38)
			–													Acinetobacter (49)
Coccobacilli			+	+												Oligella ureolytica (49)
				–	+									+		EF-4b, EO-2, Psychrobacter immobilis (saccharolytic) (49)
														–		EO-3, EO-4 (49)
					–	+										Moraxella canis, M. catarrhalis (38)
						–	+									Psychrobacter phenylpyruvica (49), Brucella spp. (51)
							–						+			Oligella urethralis (49)
													–	+		Moraxella lacunata, M. nonliquefaciens, M. osloensis, P. immobilis (asaccharolytic) (49)
														–		M. atlantae, M. lincolnii, M. osloensis, P. immobilis (asaccharolytic) (49)
				–	+											Acinetobacter baumannii, EO-5 (49)
					–		+									Bordetella parapertussis (49, 50)
														+		CDC NO-1 (49)
														–	+	Bordetella holmesii (49, 50)
			–				–								–	Acinetobacter lwoffii (49)

TABLE 4 Identification algorithm no. 4 for gram-negative bacteria with poor or no growth on blood agar

Growth on BAP	Growth only on:	Cellular morphology	Urea	Pigmented colonies	Oxidase	6% NaCl	H$_2$S in TSI	Cauliflower-like colonies	O-shaped cells	Require X ± V	Organism group (chapter)
Poor		Tiny coccobacilli	+								Brucella (51)
			−		+		+				Francisella philomiragia (51)
							−				Bordetella (50)
					−						Francisella (51)
		Rods		Pink							Methylobacterium, Roseomonas (49)
				Other				+			Bartonella (53)
								−			Haemophilus aphrophilus (40), various (39)
		Diplococci or coccobacilli							+		EO-2 (49)
									−		Neisseria (38), Moraxella (49)
None	Chocolate	Diplococci or coccobacilli									Neisseria (38)
		Fusiform rods									Capnocytophaga (39)
		Rods						+			Bartonella, Afipia (53)
								−		+	Haemophilus (40)
										−	Francisella (51)
	BCYE^a	Long gram-negative rods									Legionella (14)
		Regular rods			+						Bordetella (50)
					−						Francisella (51)
	BHI + serum	Pleomorphic, beaded filamentous rods									Streptobacillus (39)
		Small rods									Bartonella, Afipia (53)

^{a} BAP, blood agar plate; BCYE, buffered charcoal yeast extract agar; BHI, brain heart infusion agar.

Algorithm for Identification of Anaerobic Bacteria*

DIANE M. CITRON

24

Anaerobic bacteria are defined for the purposes of this algorithm as organisms displaying better growth when incubated in an anaerobic environment than in the presence of oxygen. The use of selective and differential agars for the primary setup of clinical specimens and prompt incubation in an anaerobic environment allow the rapid presumptive identification of important groups of anaerobes based on distinctive characteristics, such as bile resistance, pigmentation, a double zone of beta-hemolysis, or the presence of fusiform cells on Gram stain. Examples of such agars include Bacteroides-bile-esculin (BBE) agar for isolation and presumptive identification of the *Bacteroides fragilis* group and *Bilophila wadsworthia*. Brucella agar supplemented with laked blood, kanamycin, and vancomycin inhibits enteric and gram-positive organisms and is thus useful for isolation and characterization of *Bacteroides*, *Prevotella*, and some strains of fusobacteria. Pigmented *Prevotella* spp. produce pigment more rapidly and intensely on laked blood agar. Phenylethyl alcohol blood agar (PEA) and colistin nalidixic acid blood agar inhibit enteric organisms and swarming *Proteus* spp. but allow the growth and isolation of many gram-positive and gram-negative anaerobes. PEA also inhibits the swarming by *Clostridium septicum*, which can completely overgrow and contaminate other anaerobic organisms in a mixed culture. All media for culture of anaerobes should be supplemented with vitamin K_1 and hemin.

Simple tests such as tests for susceptibility (inhibition zone diameters, ≥ 10 mm) to the special potency disks with 1,000 μg of kanamycin, 5 μg of vancomycin, and 10 μg of colistin; tests for growth in the presence of 20% bile; the spot indole test; and tests for nitrate reduction, catalase and urease production, and lecithinase and lipase production on egg yolk medium are rapid and useful for initial grouping of many anaerobes (1).

The gram-positive non-spore-forming rods are difficult to group by simple tests. Nitrate-reducing strains include *Actinomyces*, *Propionibacterium*, and some of the *Eubacterium*-like group members. Most *Propionibacterium* spp. and some species of *Actinomyces* are catalase positive. Lactobacilli and bifidobacteria do not reduce nitrate and are catalase, urease, and indole negative.

The genus *Clostridium* includes the gram-positive spore-forming rods; however, many members of this group appear to be gram negative, and spores can be difficult to see under routine conditions. While many species require extensive testing for complete identification, some very clinically important species can be recognized by examination for easily observable characteristics.

Anaerobic bacteria are a diverse group of organisms and include members that often exhibit seemingly contradictory characteristics, such as gram-negative rods sensitive to vancomycin (certain clostridia, *Porphyromonas* spp.), gram-positive rods resistant to vancomycin (some lactobacilli), or rods that appear as cocci (some *Prevotella* and *Porphyromonas* spp.). The algorithm in Table 1 includes characteristics that should be helpful for suggesting the correct category for anaerobes encountered in clinical specimens.

REFERENCE

1. **Jousimies-Somer, H., P. Summanen, D. M. Citron, E. J. Baron, H. M. Wexler, and S. M. Finegold.** 2002. *Wadsworth-KTL Anaerobic Bacteriology Manual*, 6th ed. Star Publishing Co., Belmont, Calif.

* This chapter contains information presented in chapter 45 by Ellen Jo Baron and Diane M. Citron in the seventh edition of this Manual.

TABLE 1 Algorithm for identification of bacteria that grow better anaerobically than aerobically

Cellular morphology	Gram reaction	Growth on BBE agar	Pattern on kanamycin and vancomycin disk[a]	Pigment or red fluorescence	Nitrate	Catalase	Spores	Spreading, irregular, peaked, or large colony	Large boxcar-shaped cells, beta-hemolysis	Organism (chapter)
Rod or coccobacillus	−	+	R/R							B. fragilis group (56)
			S/R		−	−				Fusobacterium mortiferum-Fusobacterium varium group (56)
					+	+				Bilophila wadsworthia (56)
		−	R/S	+/−	−	+/−				Porphyromonas (56)
			R/R	+/−	−	−				Prevotella (56)
				−			Rare	+		Clostridium innocuum (54)
			S/S	+			Rare	−		Clostridium ramosum (54)
				−			Rare	−		Clostridium clostridioforme (54)
			S/R		+	−				Bacteroides ureolyticus, B. ureolyticus-like or Campylobacter spp. (56)
					−					Fusobacterium (56)
	+/variable		S/R							Lactobacillus (55)
			S/S	−	−	−				Lactobacillus, Bifidobacterium, or Eubacterium-like group (55)
				+/−	+	+/−				Actinomyces, Propionibacterium, Eubacterium-like group (55)
				+	−	−	Rare			Clostridium ramosum (54)
				−	+/−	−	+	+		Clostridium spp. (54)
						−	+		+	Clostridium perfringens (54)
Coccus	+		S/S							Peptostreptococcus-like group (55)
	−		S/R							Veillonella, Acidaminococcus, or Megasphaera (56)

[a] R, resistant; S, susceptible.

Algorithms for Identification of Curved and Spiral-Shaped Gram-Negative Rods*

JAMES VERSALOVIC

25

Curved and spiral-shaped bacteria have a common microscopic morphology but represent diverse bacterial pathogens. These organisms are curved, helical, or spiral-shaped gram-negative rods. Specific detection of these organisms requires a combination of tests including microscopy, biochemical tests, antigen tests, serologic tests, bacteriologic culture, and molecular approaches. The following tables and figure summarize the epidemiology of infections caused by the bacteria discussed in chapters 57 to 61 (Table 1) and the primary diagnostic strategies used for their detection (Table 2; Fig. 1).

REFERENCE

1. **Washburn, R. G.** 2002. Spirillum minus (rat-bite fever), p. 2518. *In* G. L. Mandell, J. E. Bennett, and R. Dolin (ed.), *Principles and Practice of Infectious Diseases*. Churchill Livingstone, Philadelphia, Pa.

---

* This chapter contains information presented in chapter 49 by Patrick R. Murray in the seventh edition of this Manual.

TABLE 1 Epidemiology of human infections with curved or spiral-shaped gram-negative rods

Organism	Primary disease	Animal reservoir	Vector or mode of transmission
Arcobacter butzleri	Gastroenteritis, bacteremia, endocarditis, peritonitis	Birds, cattle, horses, poultry, pigs, primates	Fecal-oral; ingestion of contaminated food or water
Arcobacter cryaerophilus	Gastroenteritis, bacteremia	Cattle, horses, pigs, poultry, sheep	Fecal-oral; ingestion of contaminated food or water
Borrelia afzelii	Lyme disease	Rodents	Tick borne (*Ixodes* spp.)
Borrelia burgdorferi	Lyme disease	Rodents	Tick borne (*Ixodes* spp.)
Borrelia garinii	Lyme disease	Rodents, birds	Tick borne (*Ixodes* spp.)
Borrelia recurrentis	Epidemic relapsing fever	Humans	Louse borne (*Pediculus humanus humanus*)
Borrelia spp.	Endemic relapsing fever	Chipmunks, squirrels, rodents, humans	Tick borne (*Ornithodoros* spp.)
Brachyspira aalborgi	Intestinal spirochetosis	Humans	Fecal-oral
Brachyspira (Serpulina) pilosicoli	Intestinal spirochetosis	Chickens, dogs, pigs, humans, rodents	Fecal-oral
Campylobacter coli	Gastroenteritis	Poultry	Fecal-oral; ingestion of contaminated food or water
Campylobacter fetus	Bacteremia, extraintestinal infections, gastroenteritis	Cattle, sheep	Fecal-oral; ingestion of contaminated food or water
Campylobacter jejuni	Gastroenteritis	Poultry, dogs	Ingestion of contaminated food or water
Campylobacter lari	Gastroenteritis	Birds (gulls), cats, dogs, chickens, seals, shellfish	Fecal-oral; ingestion of contaminated water
Campylobacter upsaliensis	Gastroenteritis	Cats, dogs, ducks, primates	Fecal-oral
Helicobacter canis	Gastroenteritis	Cats, dogs, humans	Contact with infected dogs
Helicobacter canadensis	Gastroenteritis	Humans	Fecal-oral
Helicobacter cinaedi	Gastroenteritis, arthritis, bacteremia, cellulitis	Hamsters, humans	Fecal-oral
Helicobacter fennelliae	Gastroenteritis, bacteremia	Humans	Fecal-oral
Helicobacter pullorum	Gastroenteritis	Poultry, humans	Fecal-oral; ingestion of contaminated food
Helicobacter pylori	Gastritis, peptic ulcer disease, gastric cancers	Humans, cats	Oral-oral; fecal-oral
Helicobacter winghamensis	Gastroenteritis	Humans	Fecal-oral
Leptospira spp.	Leptospirosis	Cattle, dogs, goats, horses, rodents, swine	Contact exposure to urine or tissue of infected animals
Spirillum minus[a]	Rat bite fever	Rat	Rat bites
Treponema carateum	Pinta	Humans	Contact exposure (skin lesions)
Treponema pallidum subsp. *pallidum*	Venereal syphilis	Humans	Sexual contact; intimate contact with an active lesion; transplacental
Treponema pallidum subsp. *endemicum*	Endemic syphilis (bejel)	Humans	Oral-oral (contact with infected mucous membranes)
Treponema pallidum subsp. *pertenue*	Yaws	Humans	Contact exposure (skin lesions)

[a] See reference 1.

TABLE 2 Diagnostic tests for detection and identification of curved or spiral-shaped gram-negative rods

Organism	Disease	Chapter	Diagnostic strategies[a]
Arcobacter spp.	Gastroenteritis	57	Specimen type: Stool Screening/Direct: NA Confirmation: Microaerobic culture
Borrelia afzelii, B. burgdorferi, B. garinii	Lyme disease	60	Specimen type: Peripheral blood Screening/Direct: Serologic testing (ELISA or IFA) Confirmation: IgG and IgM immunoblotting for specific serum antibodies
Borrelia spp.	Relapsing fever	60	Specimen type: Peripheral blood Screening/Direct: Blood smear (thin) with Wright-Giemsa, AO, dark-field microscopy Confirmation: Blood smear (thick)
Brachyspira spp.	Intestinal spirochetosis	61	Specimen type: Colonic biopsy Screening/Direct: Histopathology (H&E, silver stain) Confirmation: anaerobic culture; PCR using rRNA and/or NADH oxidase gene targets
Campylobacter spp.	Gastroenteritis	57	Specimen type: Stool Screening/Direct: Fecal smear (Gram stain) Confirmation: Microaerobic culture
Campylobacter fetus	Bacteremia/ sepsis	57	Specimen type: Peripheral blood Screening/Direct: Blood culture smear (Gram [carbol fuchsin] or AO stain) Confirmation: Microaerobic culture
Helicobacter pylori	Gastritis/Peptic ulcer	58	Specimen type: Peripheral blood, breath, gastric biopsy sample, stool Screening/Direct: IgG serologic testing, RUT Confirmation: Histopathology (special stains), fecal antigen (ELISA), urea breath test
Helicobacter spp.	Gastroenteritis	58	Specimen type: Stool Screening/Direct: NA Confirmation: Microaerobic culture
Leptospira spp.	Leptospirosis	59	Specimen type: Peripheral blood Screening/Direct: Blood smear (dark-field microscopy) or direct fluorescent-antibody testing Confirmation: Serologic testing (microscopic agglutination test)
Spirillum minus[b]	Rat bite fever		Specimen type: Peripheral blood, exudate Screening/Direct: Blood smear (Wright, Giemsa, dark-field microscopy) Confirmation: NA
Treponema carateum	Pinta	61	Specimen type: Skin lesion, peripheral blood Screening/Direct: Dark-field microscopy of lesion exudates, serologic testing (VDRL) Confirmation: Serologic testing (FTA-ABS)
Treponema pallidum (all subspecies)	Bejel, venereal syphilis, yaws	61	Specimen Type: Skin lesion, peripheral blood Screening/Direct: Dark-field microscopy of lesion exudates, serologic testing (RPR, VDRL) Confirmation: Serologic testing (FTA-ABS, TP-PA, specific EIAs)

[a] NA, not applicable; H&E, hematoxylin and eosin; AO, acridine orange; RUT, rapid urease testing; RPR, rapid plasma reagin test; VDRL, venereal disease research laboratory test; FTA-ABS, fluorescent treponemal antibody absorption test; TP-PA, *Treponema pallidum* particle agglutination test; DFA, direct fluorescent antibody.
[b] See reference 1.

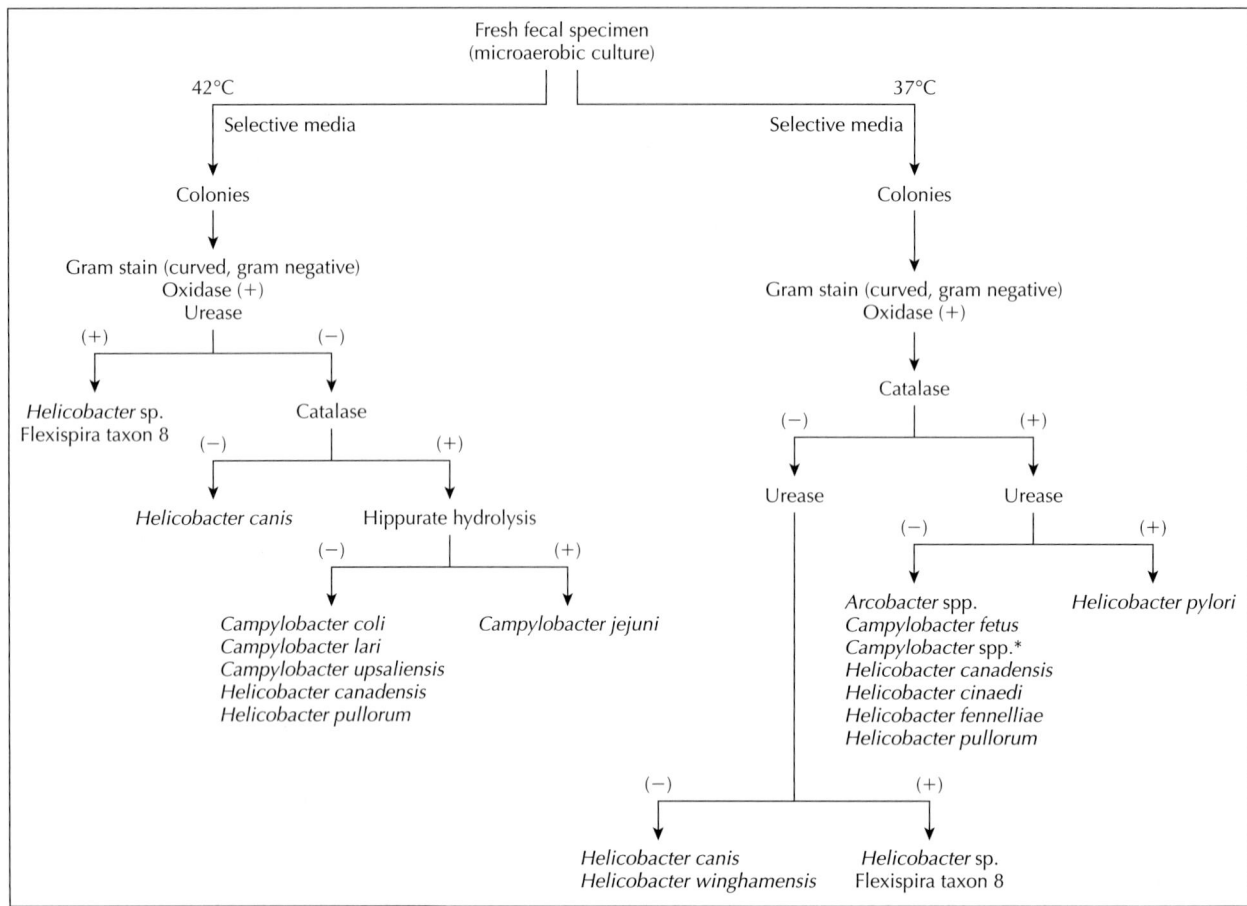

FIGURE 1 Flowchart of stool evaluation for patients suspected of having enteritis due to infection with curved gram-negative rods. *, Thermophilic *Campylobacter* species (*C. coli*, *C. jejuni*, *C. lari*, *C. upsaliensis*) may form colonies at 37°C.

Algorithms for Identification of *Mycoplasma, Ureaplasma,* and Obligate Intracellular Bacteria*

J. STEPHEN DUMLER

26

The bacteria discussed in chapters 62 to 66 differ from bacteria described in other parts of this Manual by several characteristics, including lack of efficient staining by the Gram stain method and, except for *Mycoplasma* and *Urea-plasma* species, the requirement for intracellular growth. Thus, the most frequently used tests in clinical microbiology laboratories, the Gram stain and culture on artificial media, are unable to detect these organisms in clinical samples. Diagnosis of infections caused by these bacteria has traditionally been accomplished by Romanowsky staining (Giemsa and Wright stains) of clinical samples or by detection of antibody responses to infection using a variety of serological tests. Molecular diagnostic tools and improved culture methods have significantly improved our ability to detect these agents and to diagnose the diseases that they cause and, for some, are becoming standard practice. The following tables summarize the epidemiology of these infections (Table 1) and the diagnostic tests most often used for the detection of the causative bacteria (Table 2).

---

* This chapter contains information presented in chapter 55 by Patrick R. Murray in the seventh edition of this Manual.

TABLE 1 Epidemiology and clinical disease of infections with *Anaplasma*, *Chlamydia*, *Chlamydophila*, *Coxiella*, *Ehrlichia*, *Mycoplasma*, *Rickettsia*, and *Ureaplasma*

Organism	Disease	Reservoir	Vector and mode of transmission
Anaplasma phagocytophila	Human granulocytic ehrlichiosis (HGE): fever, headache, myalgia, systemic involvement except for central nervous system	White-footed mouse, other small mammals, ruminants, deer	*Ixodes scapularis* (deer or black-legged tick), *I. pacificus* (western black-legged tick), *I. ricinus* (rabbit tick) bites
Chlamydia trachomatis	Endemic trachoma, inclusion conjunctivitis, lymphogranuloma venereum, urethritis, epididymitis, cervicitis, salpingitis, perihepatitis, pneumonia	Humans	Sexual contact, hand-eye contact, insect fomites, infected birth canal
Chlamydophila pneumoniae	Pneumonia, bronchitis, sinusitis, pharyngitis, chronic vascular infections	Humans	Inhalation of infected aerosols
Chlamydophila psittaci	Psittacosis (pneumonia), systemic infections	Birds, domestic animals	Inhalation of infected aerosols
Coxiella burnetii	Acute Q fever: self-limited febrile illness with or without pneumonia and hepatitis; chronic Q fever: endocarditis, endovascular infections	Cattle, sheep, goats, cats, rabbits, dogs, ticks	Inhalation of infected aerosols; ingestion of nonpasteurized dairy products
Ehrlichia chaffeensis	Human monocytotropic ehrlichiosis (HME): fever, headache, myalgia, systemic involvement including central nervous system	White-tailed deer, dogs and other canids, raccoons	*Amblyomma americanum* (Lone Star tick) and potentially *Dermacentor variabilis* (American dog tick) bites
Ehrlichia ewingii	"Ewingii" granulocytic ehrlichiosis: fever, headache, myalgia, predominantly in immunocompromised individuals	Dogs and other canids	*Amblyomma americanum* (Lone Star tick)
Mycoplasma hominis	Acute pyelonephritis, genital infections, systemic infections (?)	Humans	Sexual contact, vertical transmission in utero or intrapartum
Mycoplasma pneumoniae	Pneumonia, tracheobronchitis, pharyngitis, extrarespiratory complications (arthritis, etc.)	Humans	Contact with infectious aerosols or fomites
Orientia tsutsugamushi	Scrub typhus	Chiggers (larval mites)	*Leptotrombidium* spp. (chigger) bites
Rickettsia africae	African tick-bite fever	Not established	*Amblyomma variegatum* tick bites
Rickettsia akari	Rickettsialpox	Mice and other small mammals	*Allodermanyssus sanguineus* (mouse mite) bites
Rickettsia conorii	Boutonneuse fever or Mediterranean spotted fever	Small mammals and ticks	*Rhipicephalus sanguineus* (brown dog) tick bites
Rickettsia felis	Murine typhus-like illness	Fleas, opossums, cats, dogs	*Ctenocephalides felis* (cat fleas); contamination of infected flea feces into flea bite
Rickettsia prowazekii	Epidemic typhus	Humans, lice, flying squirrels	*Pediculus humanus* subsp. *corporis* (body louse); contamination of louse bite with infected louse feces
Rickettsia rickettsii	Rocky Mountain spotted fever	Ticks, small- and medium-size mammals	*Dermacentor variabilis* (American dog tick), *Dermacentor andersoni* (wood tick), *Amblyomma cajennense* (Central and South America), *Rhipicephalus sanguineus* (Central America)
Rickettsia typhi	Murine typhus	Rats and other rodents, opossums	*Xenopsylla cheopis* (rat fleas) and *Ctenocephalides felis* (cat fleas); contamination of flea bite with infected flea feces
Ureaplasma urealyticum	Urethritis, epididymitis, orchitis, urinary calculi, abortion, premature rupture of membranes	Humans	Sexual contact, in utero or peripartum vertical transmission

TABLE 2 Diagnostic tests for *Anaplasma, Chlamydia, Chlamydophila, Coxiella, Ehrlichia, Mycoplasma, Rickettsia,* and *Ureaplasma*

Organism	Diagnostic test[a]
Anaplasma phagocytophila	**Microscopy:** Giemsa or Wright stain of peripheral blood or buffy coat smears is positive in approximately 60% of infected persons. **Antigen tests:** None available. **Molecular tests:** EDTA-anticoagulated blood collected during the pretreatment acute phase of illness is used for PCR amplification. Species- and genus-specific tests are available. Current test of choice for diagnosis during active infection. **Culture:** EDTA-anticoagulated peripheral blood is inoculated onto HL-60, THP1, or other myelocytic cell lines. Positive cultures may be obtained between 3 and 30 days from many samples if inoculated within 24 h and if obtained before the start of antimicrobial therapy. Lack of timely results precludes frequent use. **Serologic tests:** IFA is the most frequently used test. A fourfold or greater rise in titer or a single peak titer of ≥80 in a patient with a typical clinical features of HGE confirms infection. Test sensitivity is between 90 and 100%; specificity is approximately 95%.
Chlamydia trachomatis	**Microscopy:** Organisms may be detected by Giemsa stain or DFA test. The DFA test is more sensitive, but neither test should be used alone. **Antigen tests:** Commercial EIAs vary in sensitivity, are only 97% specific, and are not suitable for use alone in screening. Confirmatory EIA may increase specificity to 99.5%. Point-of-care tests are only 60 to 70% sensitive compared to molecular tests. **Molecular tests:** Commercial hybridization and amplification tests (PCR, ligase chain reaction, strand displacement amplification, transcription-mediated amplification) are available and are the tests of choice for confirmation of *C. trachomatis* infections. Results of molecular tests for *C. trachomatis* are not admissible as evidence in U.S. courts. **Culture:** Recovered in many different cell cultures including McCoy, HeLa, HEp-2, HL, and monkey kidney. Test sensitivity is dependent on the quality of the submitted specimen. **Serologic tests:** MIF test is most sensitive and specific (test of choice). Diagnosis of acute *C. trachomatis* infection is confirmed by a fourfold or greater rise in antibody titer. Rising antibody titers may not be observed with chronic, repeated, or systemic infections. A single IgM titer of ≥32 supports a diagnosis of neonatal pneumonia.
Chlamydophila pneumoniae	**Microscopy:** Organisms may be detected by Giemsa stain or DFA test directed against LPS, but both tests are relatively insensitive. **Antigen tests:** Available EIAs directed against LPS detect all *Chlamydia* and *Chlamydophila* species but are licensed only for *C. trachomatis.* **Molecular tests:** None commercially available. **Culture:** Recovered best if inoculated onto HL cells or HEp-2 cells. **Serologic tests:** MIF test is most sensitive and specific (test of choice). Diagnosis confirmed by fourfold or greater rise in titer or single samples with IgM titer of ≥16 and/or IgG titer of ≥512.
Chlamydophila psittaci	**Microscopy:** Organisms may be detected by Giemsa stain or DFA test directed against LPS, but both tests are relatively insensitive. **Antigen tests:** Available EIA tests directed against LPS detect all *Chlamydia* and *Chlamydophila* species but are licensed only for *C. trachomatis.* **Molecular tests:** None commercially available. **Culture:** Recovered in many different cell cultures including McCoy, HeLa, HEp-2, HL, and monkey kidney. **Serologic tests:** MIF test is most sensitive and specific (test of choice).
Coxiella burnetii	**Microscopy:** DFA or immunohistochemistry may be performed but are insensitive and not widely available. **Antigen tests:** None commercially available. **Molecular tests:** PCR available only through reference laboratories; more sensitive than culture from frozen tissue, blood, or for chronic disease; less useful for serum. **Culture:** May be cultivated in a variety of cell lines, especially Vero cells and HEL cells, or by inoculation into embryonated chicken yolk sacs or laboratory animals. **Serologic tests:** Most frequently used diagnostic test. An IFA test is recommended. Acute Q fever is confirmed by a fourfold or greater rise in titer to phase II antigens or a single IgM titer of ≥50 and IgG titer of ≥200. Chronic Q fever is confirmed in a single serum sample with an IgG titer to phase I and phase II antigens of ≥1,600. A decreasing antibody titer suggests successful therapy.
Ehrlichia chaffeensis	**Microscopy:** Giemsa or Wright stain of peripheral blood or buffy coat smears is positive in up to 29% of infected persons. **Antigen tests:** None available. **Molecular tests:** EDTA-anticoagulated blood collected during the pretreatment acute phase of illness is used for PCR amplification. Species- and genus-specific tests are available. Current test of choice for diagnosis during active infection.

(Continued on next page)

TABLE 2 Diagnostic tests for *Anaplasma, Chlamydia, Chlamydophila, Coxiella, Ehrlichia, Mycoplasma, Rickettsia,* and *Ureaplasma* (Continued)

Organism	Diagnostic test[a]
Ehrlichia chaffeensis (Continued)	**Culture:** EDTA-anticoagulated peripheral blood or CSF is inoculated onto DH82, THP1, or other macrophage cell lines. Positive cultures may be obtained between 5 and 30 days from most samples if inoculated within 12 h and if obtained before the start of antimicrobial therapy. Lack of timely results precludes frequent use. **Serologic tests:** IFA is the most frequently used test. A fourfold or greater rise in titer or a single peak titer of ≥64 in a patient with a clinically compatible illness is considered evidence of infection. Test sensitivity is believed to be high.
Ehrlichia ewingii	**Microscopy:** Giemsa or Wright stain of peripheral blood or buffy coat smears is positive in approximately half of infected persons. **Antigen tests:** None available. **Molecular tests:** EDTA-anticoagulated blood collected during the pretreatment acute phase of illness is used for PCR amplification. Species- and genus-specific tests are available. Current tests of choice for diagnosis during active infection. **Culture:** Not yet cultivated in vitro. **Serologic tests:** No specific serologic test available. Antibodies to *E. ewingii* react with *E. chaffeensis* and may be detected by IFA. A fourfold or greater rise in titer or a single peak titer ≥64 in a patient with a clinically compatible illness is considered evidence of infection by an *Ehrlichia* species. Test sensitivity is believed to be high.
Mycoplasma hominis	**Microscopy:** Not useful. **Antigen tests:** None commercially available. **Molecular tests:** PCR tests have been developed but are less useful than culture. **Culture:** Organisms are isolated from a variety of clinical samples. Wood-shafted cotton swabs should be avoided. Mycoplasmas are extremely labile, and appropriate transport medium should be used. Can be recovered on SP4 glucose broth supplemented with arginine. Growth occurs within 2 to 4 days. **Serologic tests:** Not recommended for routine use.
Mycoplasma pneumoniae	**Microscopy:** Not useful. **Antigen tests:** A variety of tests (DFA, CIE, EIA, and immunoblotting) have been developed but lack sensitivity and specificity. **Molecular tests:** PCR amplification tests are highly sensitive and have unknown specificity, but clinical studies have yielded variable results compared with culture and serologic testing. Commercial kits are not currently available in the United States. **Culture:** Organisms are isolated from a variety of clinical samples. Wood-shafted cotton swabs should be avoided. Mycoplasmas are extremely labile, and appropriate transport medium should be used. Can be recovered on SP4 glucose broth supplemented with arginine. Growth occurs after 21 days. Widely considered insensitive for diagnosis confirmation. **Serologic tests:** EIAs are more sensitive and specific than CF; detection of seroconversion by demonstration of a fourfold increase in antibody titer is preferred, but detection of IgM antibodies in a single serum sample may be useful. The cold agglutinin test is approximately 50% sensitive and is not specific.
Orientia tsutsugamushi	**Microscopy:** DFA or immunohistochemistry on skin or other tissues may be performed, but tests are not widely available. **Antigen tests:** Not available. **Molecular tests:** PCR amplification performed on EDTA-anticoagulated blood, buffy coat leukocytes, plasma, or tissue samples obtained during acute phase of illness; available only through reference laboratories. **Culture:** Isolation is performed by intraperitoneal inoculation of mice. Performed only in reference and research laboratories. **Serologic tests:** With the IFA test in an area of endemic infection, a titer of ≥400 is 98% specific and 48% sensitive overall. Lower cutoffs are used in populations in areas where infection is not endemic. Indirect immunoperoxidase is also sensitive and specific, with diagnostic cutoffs of ≥128 for IgG and ≥32 for IgM. Dot EIA kits are available and have slightly lower sensitivity and specificity than IFA. Weil-Felix (*Proteus*) febrile agglutinin test is insensitive and nonspecific.
Rickettsia africae and *Rickettsia conorii*	**Microscopy:** DFA or immunohistochemistry on skin biopsy specimen of rash or eschar is sensitive and specific for spotted fever group rickettsiae. Antibodies are not commercially available. **Antigen tests:** Not available. **Molecular tests:** PCR amplification performed on EDTA-anticoagulated blood, buffy coat leukocytes, plasma, or tissue samples obtained during acute phase of illness; available only through reference laboratories. **Culture:** Heparin-anticoagulated blood plasma or buffy coat cells are inoculated into shell vials seeded with cell lines such as Vero, L-929, HEL, or MRC-5. Infected cells are detected by Giemsa, Gimenez, or fluorescent-antibody staining after 48 to 72 h. Sensitivity is approximately 60%. **Serologic tests:** IFA is sensitive using either *R. africae* or other spotted fever group rickettsial antigens (e.g., *R. rickettsii*), but sensitivity is low during the acute phase of illness. A fourfold increase in titer is generally considered most specific, but single titers of ≥128 for IgG and ≥32 for IgM are considered diagnostically significant. A dot EIA that is slightly less sensitive and specific is available for *R. conorii*.

(Continued on next page)

TABLE 2 *(Continued)*

Organism	Diagnostic test[a]
Rickettsia akari	**Microscopy:** DFA or immunohistochemistry on skin biopsy specimen of rash or eschar is sensitive and specific for spotted fever group rickettsiae. Antibodies are not commercially available. **Antigen tests:** Not available. **Molecular tests:** None described. **Culture:** Heparin-anticoagulated blood plasma or buffy coat cells are inoculated into shell vials seeded with cell lines such as Vero, L-929, HEL, or MRC-5. Infected cells are detected by Giemsa, Gimenez, or fluorescent-antibody staining after 48 to 72 h. Sensitivity is not known but is probably approximately 60%. **Serologic tests:** IFA is sensitive using either *R. akari* or other spotted fever group rickettsial antigens (e.g., *R. rickettsii*), but sensitivity is low during the acute phase of illness. A fourfold increase in titer is generally considered most specific, but single titers of ≥128 for IgG and ≥32 for IgM are considered diagnostically significant.
Rickettsia felis	**Microscopy:** Not available. **Antigen tests:** Not available. **Molecular tests:** PCR amplification performed on EDTA-anticoagulated blood, buffy coat leukocytes, plasma, or tissue samples obtained during acute phase of illness; available only through reference laboratories. **Culture:** Not available except through research laboratories. **Serologic tests:** No specific serologic test is available, but serum antibodies reactive with *R. prowazekii* and *R. typhi* may be detected.
Rickettsia prowazekii	**Microscopy:** Not available. **Antigen tests:** Not available. **Molecular tests:** PCR amplification performed on EDTA-anticoagulated blood, buffy coat leukocytes, plasma, or tissue samples obtained during acute phase of illness; available only through reference laboratories. **Culture:** Heparin-anticoagulated blood plasma or buffy coat cells are inoculated into shell vials seeded with cell lines such as Vero, L-929, HEL, or MRC-5. Infected cells are detected by Giemsa, Gimenez, or fluorescent-antibody staining after 48 to 72 h. Sensitivity is not known. **Serologic tests:** IFA is sensitive using either *R. prowazekii* or *R. typhi* as antigen. A fourfold increase in titer is generally considered most specific, but single titers of ≥128 for IgG and ≥32 for IgM are considered diagnostically significant.
Rickettsia rickettsii	**Microscopy:** DFA or immunohistochemistry on skin biopsy specimen of rash is 70% sensitive and 100% specific. Antibodies are not commercially available. **Antigen tests:** Not available. **Molecular tests:** PCR amplification performed on EDTA-anticoagulated blood, buffy coat leukocytes, plasma, or tissue samples obtained during acute phase of illness; available only through reference laboratories. **Culture:** Heparin-anticoagulated blood plasma or buffy coat cells are inoculated into shell vials seeded with cell lines such as Vero, L-929, HEL, or MRC-5. Infected cells are detected by Giemsa, Gimenez, or fluorescent-antibody staining after 48 to 72 h. Sensitivity is not known. **Serologic tests:** IFA is sensitive using *R. rickettsii* or other spotted fever group rickettsial antigens, but sensitivity is low during the acute phase of illness. A fourfold increase in titer is generally considered most specific, but single titers of ≥128 for IgG and ≥32 for IgM are considered diagnostically significant.
Rickettsia typhi	**Microscopy:** DFA or immunohistochemistry on skin biopsy specimen of rash is sensitive and specific. Antibodies are not commercially available. **Antigen tests:** Not available. **Molecular tests:** PCR amplification performed on EDTA-anticoagulated blood, buffy coat leukocytes, plasma, or tissue samples obtained during acute phase of illness; available only through reference laboratories. **Culture:** Heparin-anticoagulated blood plasma or buffy coat cells are inoculated into shell vials seeded with cell lines such as Vero, L-929, HEL, or MRC-5. Infected cells are detected by Giemsa, Gimenez, or fluorescent-antibody staining after 48 to 72 h. Sensitivity is not known. **Serologic tests:** IFA is sensitive using either *R. prowazekii* or *R. typhi* as antigen. A fourfold increase in titer is generally considered most specific, but single titers of ≥128 for IgG and ≥32 for IgM are considered diagnostically significant. A dot EIA that is slightly less sensitive and specific is available for *R. typhi*.
Ureaplasma urealyticum	**Microscopy:** Not useful. **Antigen tests:** None commercially available. **Molecular tests:** PCR tests have been developed but are less useful than culture. **Culture:** Organisms are isolated from a variety of clinical samples. Wood-shafted cotton swabs should be avoided. Ureaplasmas are extremely labile, and appropriate transport medium should be used. Can be recovered on Shepard's 10B urea broth and A8 urea agar. Growth occurs within 2 to 4 days. **Serologic tests:** Not recommended for routine use.

[a] Abbreviations: CF, complement fixation; CIE, counterimmunoelectrophoresis; CSF, cerebrospinal fluid; DFA, direct fluorescent antibody; EIA, enzyme immunoassay; IFA, indirect fluorescent antibody; Ig, immunoglobulin; LPS, lipopolysaccharide; M-IF, microimmunofluorescence.

Reagents, Stains, and Media: Bacteriology

KIMBERLE C. CHAPIN AND TSAI-LING LAUDERDALE

27

REAGENTS

The reagents listed in this chapter include those determined to be commonly used and a few highly specialized reagents. For information on specific reagents not included here, refer to the literature cited in the chapter in which the reagent is mentioned or the general references listed at the end of this chapter (34, 40). Reagents are listed in alphabetical order with a brief description of their intended use and ingredients. The test protocol is included where appropriate. A fresh 18- to 24-h pure broth culture or well-isolated colonies from nonselective medium should be used for testing. Many of these reagents and tests are available commercially individually or are incorporated into commercial identification kit systems.

Unless stated otherwise, the reagents listed in this section should be prepared by dissolving the reagent components in the stated liquid with a magnetic stirring bar. The standard sterilization technique of autoclaving at 121°C at 15 lb/in.² for 15 min should be used when needed. However, certain solutions such as those containing antibiotics or carbohydrates cannot be autoclaved because they will be denatured. These solutions are sterilized by filtration through a 0.22-μm-pore-size filter. Additionally, certain reagents require different heat sterilization times. Instructions for reagents that require special preparation or sterilization protocols are included in the discussion of the reagent.

It is critical that distilled, deionized water be used in the preparation of all components. Removal of contaminating pyrogens and minerals from water used for culture reagents is imperative, especially for the success of cell culture systems.

Storage of prepared reagents in sterile, airtight, screw-cap containers is recommended. Some reagents require storage in dark containers, and some need to be stored refrigerated (2 to 8°C) instead of at room temperature. Special storage instructions are given when appropriate.

Standard safety precautions should be taken when preparing the reagents. Follow the safety guidelines for the chemicals being used, in addition to the laboratory safety protocols. For reagents that are prepared in-house, proper quality control measures must be taken with appropriate positive and negative controls.

■ Acetoin (acetyl-methyl-carbinol)
See Voges-Proskauer test

■ N-Acetyl-L-cysteine-sodium hydroxide (NALC-NaOH)
NALC is a mucolytic agent used for digestion, and NaOH is a decontamination agent used in the processing of specimens for mycobacteriology. Sodium citrate is included in the mixture to exert a stabilizing effect on the acetylcysteine.

4% NaOH, sterile	50 ml
2.9% Sodium citrate, sterile	50 ml
NALC powder	0.5 g

Mix well in a sterile container. Use within 24 h of preparation.

■ Bile solubility (10% sodium deoxycholate)
The bile solubility test is used as a presumptive identification test for *Streptococcus pneumoniae*. Sodium deoxycholate is a surface-active bile salt. It acts upon the cell wall of pneumococci, resulting in cell lysis. The test is performed with alpha-hemolytic streptococcal colonies. Oxgall is a dehydrated bile that can be used, but sodium deoxycholate is preferred.

Sodium deoxycholate	1.0 g
Sterile distilled water	9.0 ml

The pH should be 7.0. Store refrigerated in a sterile dark bottle.

Tube method
Prepare a heavy suspension of the organism in 2 ml of buffered broth (pH 7.4) or physiologic saline (pH 7.0). The pH of the solution should not be below 6.8. Divide the organism suspension into two tubes. To one tube add a few drops of the 10% sodium deoxycholate solution. To the other tube add the same amount of sterile physiological saline. Incubate at 35°C. If the organism is bile soluble, the tube containing the bile salt will lose its turbidity in 5 to 15 min and show an increase in viscosity concomitant with clearing.

Agar colony test
Put a couple of drops of sodium deoxycholate on the suspected colonies. Incubate the plate right side up for 30 min

at 35°C. Pneumococcal colonies will be lysed, but viridans group streptococci will not.

■ Bovine albumin fraction V, 0.2%

The 0.2% bovine albumin solution is used to buffer specimens for mycobacterial culture following decontamination with NALC-NaOH.

Bovine albumin solution, 5%..............	40.0 ml
Sodium chloride	8.5 g
Distilled water	960.0 ml

Adjust to pH 6.8 ± 0.2 with 4% NaOH. Sterilize by filtration. Aliquot into sterile screw-cap tubes. Store refrigerated.

Following decontamination and concentration by centrifugation, the sedimented specimen is resuspended in 1 to 2 ml of sterile 0.2% bovine albumin fraction V. This suspension is then used to inoculate media and prepare microscopic smears.

■ Catalase

Hydrogen peroxide (H_2O_2) is used to determine if bacteria produce the enzyme catalase. H_2O_2 (3%) is commercially available.

Slide method

Transfer a test colony to a clean glass slide and add 1 drop of 3% H_2O_2. Development of bubbles is considered a positive result. Extreme care should be taken to avoid picking up any media from a blood-containing agar plate because catalase is present in erythrocytes and any carryover of blood cells can cause a false-positive reaction. Hydrogen peroxide solution for detection of catalase in anaerobes is typically 15%.

Tube method

Add 1.0 ml of 3% H_2O_2 to an overnight pure culture slant. (Do not use blood agar medium). Observe for immediate bubbling.

■ Cetylpyridinium chloride-sodium chloride (CPC-NaCL)

CPC-NaCl is used for decontamination of transported sputum specimens for mycobacteriology culture.

Cetylpyridinium chloride....................	1 g
Sodium chloride	2 g
Distilled water	100 ml

Mix and store in a sealed brown bottle at room temperature. If crystals form, the solution should be gently heated before use.

An equal amount of sputum and CPC-NaCl is mixed until the specimen is liquefied, and then the specimen can be shipped to the testing site. Specimens treated with CPC-NaCl must be cultured on egg-based media or else residual CPC will inhibit mycobacterial growth.

■ Coagulase

The coagulase test is used to detect free coagulase or bound coagulase (clumping factor) and differentiate coagulase-producing *Staphylococcus* from other *Staphylococcus* spp. De-

hydrated rabbit plasma reagent with EDTA is commercially available. Rehydrate and perform the test according to the manufacturer's directions. While human plasma is preferred for detection of clumping factor with *Staphylococcus lugdunensis* and *Staphylococcus schleiferi*, it is not recommended for routine testing because it may contain antibodies against staphylococcus.

Slide test

The slide test detects bound coagulase or clumping factor. Emulsify a heavy suspension of staphylococci in a small drop of water on a clean glass slide. If autoagglutination occurs, do not continue; instead, perform a tube test. Add 1 small drop of rabbit plasma reagent to the suspension. Mix with a continuous circular motion while observing for the formation of visible white clumps. Known positive and negative controls should be set up in parallel. Negative or delayed positive (20 to 60 s) results should be confirmed by the tube test.

Tube coagulase test

The tube coagulase test detects bound and free coagulase. Dispense 0.5 ml of rabbit plasma into a sterile tube. Inoculate a loopful of the test organism into the tube. Incubate the tube at 35°C for 4 h. Observe for clotting at intervals during the first 4 h because some staphylococci produce fibrolysin, which could lyse the clot. Do not shake or agitate the tube while checking for clotting. The formation of a clot is considered positive. The majority of coagulase-positive *Staphylococcus aureus* isolates will form a clot within 4 h. Incubate the tube at room temperature overnight if no visible clot is observed after 4 h. Some investigators have recommended incubation at 35°C.

■ Dyes and pH indicators

A variety of dyes and pH indicators are used in media and reagents. The most common are given in Table 1.

■ Efrotomycin test

The efrotomycin test is used to separate *Enterococcus casseliflavus* and *Enterococcus gallinarum* (resistant) from *Enterococcus*

TABLE 1 Dyes and pH indicators

Indicator	pH and color	
Acid fuchsin (Andrade's)	5.0, pink	8.0, pale yellow
Bromcresol green	3.8, yellow	5.4, blue
Bromcresol purple	5.2, yellow	6.8, purple
Bromphenol blue	3.0, yellow	4.6, blue
Bromthymol blue	6.0, yellow	7.6, dark blue
Chlorcresol green	4.0, yellow	5.6, blue
Chlorphenol red	5.0, yellow	6.6, red
Cresolphthalein	8.2, colorless	9.8, red
m-Cresol purple	7.4, yellow	9.0, purple
Cresol red	7.2, yellow	8.8, red
Methyl red	4.4, red	6.2, yellow
Neutral red	6.8, red	8.0, yellow
Phenolphthalein	8.3, colorless	10.0, red
Phenol red	6.8, yellow	8.4, red
Thymol blue	8.0, yellow	9.6, blue
Resazurin	Oxidized: blue, nonfluorescent	Reduced: red, fluorescent
Triphenyl-tetrazolium chloride	Oxidized: colorless	Reduced: red

faecium (susceptible). Dissolve 100 mg of efrotomycin (Merck Sharpe & Dohme) in 0.1 ml of dimethyl sulfoxide and dilute in 9.9 ml of sterile distilled water. Dispense 10 μl of this solution onto filter paper disks and dry in the dark at room temperature for 5 to 6 h. A heavy inoculum of bacteria is spread with a loop or swab over half of a Trypticase soy blood agar plate, the efrotomycin disk is then placed on the heavy inoculum, and the plate is incubated for 18 to 24 h at 35°C. Organisms with any growth inhibition are considered efrotomycin susceptible. The availability of this antibiotic may be limited. An alternative test is the 1-O-methyl-α-D-glucopyranoside test (see below).

■ **Ehrlich reagent**
See Indole test.

■ **Ferric ammonium citrate, 1%**
Hydrolysis of esculin to esculetin is detected when the product reacts with ferric ammonium citrate to form a brown or black complex.

Dissolve 1.0 g of ferric ammonium citrate in 100 ml of distilled water. Store in a dark bottle, refrigerated, for up to 1 year.

After esculin broth is inoculated with the test organism and incubated for 1 to 2 days, a few drops of ferric ammonium citrate are added. A brown-black color develops immediately in positive tests. This test can also be performed by incorporating an iron salt in esculin agar medium.

■ **Ferric chloride reagent**
Ferric chloride reagent is used in both the phenylalanine deaminase test and the sodium hippurate hydrolysis test.

Ferric chloride (FeCl$_3$ · 6H$_2$O)	12 g
Hydrochloric acid, 2%	100 ml

Hydrochloric acid (2%) is prepared by adding 5.4 ml of concentrated hydrochloric acid (37%) to 94.6 ml of distilled water.

Test procedure. The phenylalanine deaminase test is performed by adding 4 or 5 drops of ferric chloride reagent onto overnight growth on phenylalanine agar or broth. If phenylpyruvic acid has formed, a brown color develops in the medium (positive reaction). Ferric chloride reagent can also be added to inoculated broths (e.g., heart infusion broth or Todd-Hewitt broth) supplemented with hippurate. Hydrolysis of hippurate produces benzoic acid and glycine. An insoluble brown ferric benzoate precipitate will form in a positive hydrolysis reaction.

■ **Fildes enrichment**
Fildes enrichment is a source of growth factors used to supplement media for the isolation of fastidious organisms. Commercial preparations are available and include the following ingredients:

Pepsin	4.0 g
Sodium chloride	5.4 g
Sodium hydroxide	70.0 ml
Hydrochloride acid, concentrated	24.0 ml
Sheep blood	200 ml
Deionized water	600 ml

The pH should be 7.0 ± 0.2. Media should be supplemented to a final concentration of 5.0%.

■ **Formate-fumarate additive**
Supplementation of media with formate and fumarate has been used to characterize selected anaerobes (e.g., *Bacteroides ureolyticus* group)

Sodium formate	3.0 g
Fumaric acid	3.0 g
Distilled water	50.0 ml

To adjust the pH, add 20 pellets of NaOH, stirring until the pellets are dissolved and the fumaric acid is in solution. Bring the final pH to 7.0 with 4 N NaOH. Sterilize by filtration. Store refrigerated for up to 6 months. Add 0.5 ml of this solution to 10 ml of thioglycolate broth. Anaerobic growth in supplemented broth is then compared with the growth in unsupplemented broth.

■ **β-Galactosidase**
See *o*-nitrophenyl-β-D-galactopyranoside (ONPG).

■ **β-Glucuronidase (see also MUG)**
Detection of β-glucuronidase activity is useful for the rapid identification of *Escherichia coli*, *Streptococcus anginosus* group, and other bacteria. A solution of 0.1% (wt/vol) *p*-nitrophenyl-β-D-glucopyranoside (colorimetric substrate) in 0.067 M Sorensen phosphate buffer (pH 8.0) is prepared. Tubes containing 0.5 ml of the substrate solution are inoculated with a loopful of bacteria from an overnight culture. The tubes are incubated at 35°C and examined after 4 h for the appearance of a yellow color (liberated *p*-nitrophenol). The fluorometric substrate 4-methylumbelliferyl-β-D-glucuronide (see MUG) is commercially available and yields a fluorescent product when hydrolyzed by β-glucuronidase.

■ **Glycine-buffered saline**
Glycine-buffered saline (0.043 M glycine, 0.15 M NaCl [pH 9.0]) is used in some serological procedures and as a transport medium for enteric organisms.

Glycine	3.23 g
NaCl	8.77 g
Distilled water	1,000 ml

■ **Hemin solution, 5-mg/ml stock**
The hemin solution is one of the additives in thioglycolate and brucella base media that makes them enriched for fastidious organisms. Dissolve 0.5 g of hemin in 10 ml of 1 N NaOH. Bring the volume up to 100 ml with distilled water. Sterilize by autoclaving. Store refrigerated for up to 1 month. It is used at a final concentration of 5 μg/ml of medium.

■ **Hippurate test**
The hippurate test measures the hydrolysis of sodium hippurate. Hippurate is hydrolyzed to benzoic acid and glycine by the enzyme hippurate hydrolase (hippuricase), which is

produced by some bacteria including group B streptococci, some *Listeria* spp., *Gardnerella vaginalis*, *Campylobacter jejuni*, and *Legionella pneumophila*. The procedure described here detects the presence of glycine with the ninhydrin reagent. Ferric chloride reagents can also be used (see above).

Test procedure. A 1% (wt/vol) solution of sodium hippurate is prepared in 0.067 M Sorensen phosphate buffer (pH 6.4). Tubes containing 0.5 ml of this solution are inoculated and incubated at 35°C for 2 h, after which 0.2 ml of the ninhydrin reagent is added. Development of a deep blue-purple color within 5 min is a positive reaction.

For *Legionella pneumophila*, inoculate a 0.5-ml aliquot of 1% sodium hippurate solution with a loopful of organism and incubate at 35°C in ambient air for 18 to 20 h. Add 0.2 ml of ninhydrin reagent, mix well, and incubate for an additional 10 min at 35°C. Observe for 20 min for blue-purple color development.

Ninhydrin reagent, 3.5%

Ninhydrin	3.5 g
Acetone	50 ml
1-Butanol	50 ml

Mix acetone and butanol in a sterile dark container. Add ninhydrin, mix, and store at room temperature.

■ Indole test

The indole test is used for the determination of the organism's ability to produce indole from deamination of tryptophan by tryptophanase. Both the Ehrlich and Kovàcs reagents should be stored refrigerated away from light. For the Ehrlich and Kovàcs reagents, dissolve the aldehyde in alcohol and then slowly add acid to the mixture.

Ehrlich reagent

Ethyl alcohol, 95%	95 ml
p-Dimethylaminobenzaldehyde	1 g
Hydrochloric acid, concentrated	20 ml

Test procedure. Indole is first extracted with xylene. Add 1 ml of xylene to a 48-h tryptone broth or other tryptophan-containing broth medium. Shake the tube vigorously for 20 s and let stand for 1 to 2 min to allow the xylene extract to come to the top of the broth. Gently add 0.5 ml of the Ehrlich reagent down the side of the tube. Do not shake the tube. A red ring at the interface of the medium and the reagent phase within 5 min represents a positive test. Ehrlich's reagent is preferred for organisms that produce small amounts of indole, such as nonfermenters and anaerobes.

Kovàcs indole reagent

Pure amyl or isoamyl alcohol	150 ml
p-Dimethylaminobenzaldehyde	10 g
Hydrochloric acid, concentrated	50 ml

Test procedure. Add 5 drops of Kovàcs reagent to either 48-h-old 2% tryptone broth or an 18- to 24-h-old tryptophan broth culture. Do not shake the tube after the addition of reagent. A red color at the surface of the medium is a positive test.

Spot indole test

p-Dimethylaminocinnamaldehyde (DMACA)	200 mg
Hydrochloric acid, concentrated	2 ml
Distilled water	18 ml

Add the acid to the water, and let it cool before adding DMACA.

Test procedure. Moisten a piece of Whatman no. 3 paper with a couple drops of the reagent. Remove a well-isolated colony from an 18- to 24-h-old culture on a blood agar plate with a sterile inoculating loop or a wooden stick and smear it on the moistened filter paper. Observe for a blue to blue-green color within 2 min for a positive reaction. No color change or a pinkish tinge is considered negative. This test should only be conducted with colonies from media containing sufficient tryptophan and no glucose. Colonies from media containing dyes (e.g., MacConkey or eosin-methylene blue [EMB] agar) may cause misleading results and should not be used. Colonies from mixed cultures should not be used, as indole-positive colonies can cause indole-negative colonies to appear weakly positive.

■ LAP (leucine aminopeptidase or leucine arylamidase) test

The LAP test detects the presence of leucine aminopeptidase (LAP). The substrate leucine-α-naphthylamide is hydrolyzed by LAP to leucine and free α-naphthylamine. α-Naphthylamine reacts with *p*-dimethylaminocinnamaldehyde (DMACA) to form a red color. The LAP test along with pyrrolidonyl-α-naphthylamide hydrolysis is helpful in the presumptive characterization of catalase-negative, gram-positive cocci (streptococci, enterococci, and streptococcus-like organisms). Some commercial identification kits include an assay for this enzyme, and a commercial rapid disk test is also available.

■ Lysozyme solution

Lysozyme	50 mg
Hydrochloric acid, 0.01 N	50 ml

Mix and sterilize by filtration. Store refrigerated. It may be stored for only 1 week.

Test procedure. Add 5 ml of lysozyme solution to 95 ml of basal glycerol broth, dispense in 5-ml aliquots, and keep refrigerated. The growth of the test organism in the lysozyme-supplemented glycerol broth is compared with the growth in the unsupplemented glycerol broth.

■ Lysozyme test

The lysozyme test measures the ability of organisms, such as *Nocardia*, to grow in the presence of lysozyme.

Basal glycerol broth

Peptone	1.0 g
Beef extract	0.6 g
Glycerol	14.0 ml
Distilled water	200 ml

Mix well and autoclave to sterilize. Store refrigerated. It may be stored for up to 3 months.

■ McFarland standard

For different McFarland standards, mix the designated amounts of 1% anhydrous barium chloride ($BaCl_2$) and 1% (vol/vol) cold pure sulfuric acid (H_2SO_4), as shown in Table 2, in screw-cap tubes. Tightly seal the tubes. When the barium sulfate is shaken up well, the density in each tube corresponds approximately to the bacterial suspension listed in Table 2. Store the prepared standard tubes in the dark at room temperature. The absorbance of the 0.5 Mc-Farland standard should be 0.08 to 0.10 at 625 nm using a spectrophotometer with a 1-cm light path. The standard should be checked regularly to make sure the density is still accurate.

■ 1-*O*-Methyl-α-D-glucopyranoside (MGP) (α-methyl-D-glucoside)

The MGP test is used to separate *Enterococcus casselifla-vus* and *Enterococcus gallinarum* (positive) from *Enterococcus faecalis* and *Enterococcus faecium* (negative). Heart infusion broth is prepared with 1% MGP and 0.006% bromcresol purple indicator, distributed into 2-ml aliquots, and autoclaved for 10 min. The broth is inoculated with a drop of an overnight broth culture or several colonies from a blood agar plate and incubated for 1 day at 35°C. Prolonged incubation for up to 7 days may be necessary. Development of a yellow color indicates a positive reaction.

■ Methylumbelliferyl-β-D-glucuronidase (MUG) test (see also β-Glucuronidase)

The MUG test is a fluorogenic assay for β-glucuronidase. The enzyme hydrolyzes the substrate 4-methylumbelliferyl-β-D-glucuronide to yield 4-methylumbelliferyl, which fluoresces blue under long-wave UV light. The test is normally used for the presumptive identification of *Escherichia coli* and, more recently, streptococcal strains. The colorimetric test method is described under β-Glucuronidase.

Dissolve 50 mg of 4-methylumbelliferyl-β-D-glucuronide in 10 ml of 0.05 M Soresens phosphate buffer (pH 7.5). Dilute the stock 4-methylumbelliferyl-β-D-glucuronide solution 1:16 and add 1.25 ml to a vial containing 50 sterile

TABLE 2 McFarland standards protocol

Standard	Vol (ml)		Corresponding bacterial suspension (10^8 CFU/ml)
	1% $BaCl_2$	1% H_2SO_4	
0.5	0.05	9.95	1.5
1	0.1	9.9	3
2	0.2	9.8	6
3	0.3	9.7	9
4	0.4	9.6	12
5	0.5	9.5	15
6	0.6	9.4	18
7	0.7	9.3	21
8	0.8	9.2	24
9	0.9	9.1	27
10	1.0	9.0	30

paper disks. Allow the disks to be thoroughly saturated until no liquid remains in the vial. Spread the saturated disks out and allow them to dry completely. The disks can be stored in a dark bottle at −20°C for 1 year or at 4°C for 1 month.

Test procedure. Wet the disk with 1 drop of sterile water. Apply the organism to the disk with a wooden stick or loop and then incubate the disk for up to 2 h at 35°C. Shine a long-wave UV light on the disk. A positive reaction is indicated by blue fluorescence. A negative reaction is indicated by the lack of fluorescence.

■ Modified oxidase

The modified oxidase test is used for differentiation of *Micrococcus* and related organisms from most other aerobic gram-positive cocci. Six percent tetramethyl-*p*-phenylene-diamine dihydrochloride (the same chemical used in Ko-vàcs oxidase reagent) dissolved in dimethyl sulfoxide is used as the reagent. Keep the reagent away from light. A loopful of colonies from blood agar plates is smeared onto filter paper, and the reagent is dropped onto the bacterial growth. Development of a blue to purple-blue color in 2 min indicates a positive reaction. Commercially prepared discs are available (16).

■ Middlebrook enrichment (oleic acid-albumin-dextrose-catalase [OADC] and albumin-dextrose-catalase [ADC])

The Middlebrook enrichment is added to various Middle-brook media. The OADC enrichment contains oleic acid as a carbon source, and both supplements contain dextrose as a carbon source and bovine albumin fraction V and catalase as growth factors. WR 1339 Triton X-100 encourages cording in *Mycobacterium tuberculosis*. All the enrichments described below are prepared in 100 ml and added to 900 ml of preautoclaved medium that has been cooled to 50 to 55°C.

OADC enrichment

Bovine albumin fraction V	5.0 g
Dextrose	2.0 g
Sodium chloride..................	0.85 g
Oleic acid.......................	0.05 g
Catalase	4.0 mg (0.004 g)

Add all components to distilled and deionized water and bring the volume to 100 ml. Mix thoroughly and filter sterilize.

OADC enrichment with WR 1339

Add 0.25 g of WR 1339 Triton X-100 to the OADC ingredients listed above. Prepare as described above.

ADC enrichment

Bovine albumin fraction V	5.0 g
Dextrose	2.0 g
Catalase	4.0 mg (0.004 g)

Add all components to distilled and deionized water and bring the volume to 100 ml. Mix thoroughly and filter sterilize.

■ Nessler reagent

The Nessler reagent is used in the determination of acet-amide hydrolysis by some gram-negative bacteria.

Nessler reagent

Solution A

Dissolve 1 g of mercuric chloride in 6 ml of distilled water. Add 2 to 3 drops of concentrated hydrochloric acid (HCl) to dissolve the sediment.

Solution B

Dissolve 2.5 g of potassium iodide in 6 ml of distilled water completely. Add to solution A.

Solution C

Dissolve 6 g of potassium hydroxide in 6 ml of distilled water completely. Add to the mixture of solutions A and B. Add 13 ml of distilled water. Mix well. Filter with a sintered-glass funnel before use and store in a dark bottle. Note: do not use a Nalgene filter. The Nessler reagent solution may decompose at room temperature after several weeks and should therefore be checked with each use.

Test procedure. Inoculate 1 ml of mineral-based broth medium (carbon assimilation medium) supplemented with 0.1% acetamide. After incubation for 24 h at 30°C, add 1 drop of Nessler reagent. A positive reaction is indicated by a red-brown sediment due to the presence of ammonia from the action of acylamidase. Acetamide agar is available commercially.

■ Nitrate reduction

The nitrate reduction test is used to determine the ability of an organism to reduce nitrate to nitrite or free nitrogen gas.

Reagent A

N,N-Dimethyl-α-naphthylamine	0.6 ml
Acetic acid (5 N), 30%	100 ml

Reagent B

Sulfanilic acid	0.8 g
Acetic acid (5 N), 30%	100 ml

Store each reagent in a brown glass bottle in the refrigerator. Store away from light.

Test procedure. At the time of testing, mix an equal portion of each reagent and then add 10 drops to the overnight growth from the nitrate broth culture. A positive reaction is indicated by the development of a red color within 1 to 2 min, which means that nitrate has been reduced to nitrite. Negative reactions are confirmed by adding a pinch (approximately 20 mg) of zinc dust with development of red color within 5 to 10 min, which indicates that nitrate has not been reduced by the organism. If the tube remains clear, nitrate has been reduced to free nitrogen gas, and a clear tube is considered a positive reaction.

■ *o*-Nitrophenyl-β-D-galactopyranoside (ONPG)

The ONPG test is used to determine the ability of an organism to ferment lactose. It is especially useful for identification of members of the family *Enterobacteriaceae*. ONPG-impregnated tablets can be purchased commercially. Commercially prepared reagents are recommended because it is tedious and difficult to prepare the reagent in-house.

■ Oxalic acid, 5%

Oxalic acid is used as a decontamination agent for specimens that contain *Pseudomonas* spp. when culturing for mycobacteria. The reagent is especially helpful when processing respiratory specimens from cystic fibrosis patients.

Oxalic acid	50 g
Distilled water	1,000 ml

Autoclave to sterilize and store at room temperature. The solution has an expiration date of 1 year.

■ Oxidase, modified (see Modified oxidase test)

■ Oxidase test

The oxidase test detects the presence of a cytochrome oxidase system. Production of a dark blue-purple color on either a filter paper strip or disk indicates a positive test. A number of reagents can be used for this test.

Kovàcs oxidase reagent:
   1% tetramethyl-*p*-phenylenediamine dihydrochloride (in water)
Gordon and McLeod's reagent:
   1% dimethyl-*p*-phenylenediamine dihydrochloride (in water)
Gaby and Hadley (indolphenol oxidase) reagents:
   1% α-naphthol in 95% ethanol
   1% *p*-aminodimethylaniline HCl

Kovàcs reagent is less toxic and is more sensitive than the other reagents. Add a few drops of the reagent to a strip of filter paper (Whatman no. 2 or equivalent) and then smear a loopful of the organism on the paper with a platinum loop or wooden stick. A wire loop containing iron may give a false-positive reaction. The oxidase test should not be performed on colonies growing on medium containing a high concentration of glucose because the fermentation of glucose may inhibit oxidase activity. Only colonies from nonselective, nondifferential media should be used to detect oxidase. A positive reaction with the Kovàcs reagent develops within 10 to 15 s and is characterized by the development of a dark purple-black color. If the Kovàcs solution becomes blue due to autooxidation, it should be discarded. The dimethyl compound in Gordon and McLeod's reagent is more stable than the tetramethyl compound (Kovàcs reagent). A positive reaction is characterized by a blue color and develops within 10 to 30 min.

■ Phosphate-buffered saline (PBS)

10× stock solutions

1. 0.1 M NaH_2PO_4 (sodium phosphate, monobasic). Dissolve 13.9 g of NaH_2PO_4 in 1,000 ml of deionized water.
2. 0.1 M Na_2HPO_4 (sodium phosphate, dibasic). Dissolve 26.8 g of $Na_2HPO_4 \cdot 7H_2O$ in 1,000 ml of deionized water.
3. 8.5% NaCl (sodium chloride). Dissolve 85.0 g of NaCl in 1,000 ml of deionized water. Sterilize by autoclaving for 20 min or by filtration. Store refrigerated.

Working PBS
Prepare a solution of the desired pH by combining the 10× stocks.

0.1 M NaH$_2$PO$_4$	See Table 3
0.1 M Na$_2$HPO$_4$	See Table 3
8.5% NaCl..........................	100 ml
Deionized water......................	to 1,000 ml

■ Polysorbate 80
See Tween 80

■ Potassium chloride, 0.2 M (pH 2.2)
Potassium chloride (0.2 M; pH 2.2) is used to treat respiratory specimens for the recovery of *Legionella*.

Potassium chloride (0.2 M)	865.0 ml
Hydrochloric acid (0.2 M)	135.0 ml

Approximately 0.5 ml of specimen is mixed thoroughly with 4.5 ml of the 0.2 M potassium chloride (pH 2.2) solution, and the mixture is allowed to stand for 15 min at room temperature. The mixture is then neutralized to pH 7.0 with 0.1 N KOH and is inoculated onto isolation media.

■ Pyrrolidonyl-α-naphthylamide (PYR) hydrolysis
PYR is hydrolyzed by organisms that possess the enzyme pyrrolidonyl arylamidase (43). The PYR test is used for rapid presumptive identification of group A alpha-hemolytic streptococci (*Streptococcus pyogenes*), *Enterococcus* spp., and other gram-positive cocci that grow aerobically and form cells arranged in pairs and chains. A pure culture or isolated colony for testing is critical given the number of PYR-positive organisms with similar Gram stain morphology and hemolytic characteristics.

PYR substrate (L-pyrrolidonyl-α-naphthylamide)
First dissolve PYR in methyl alcohol and then dilute with sterile distilled water. Adjust the pH to 5.7 to 6.0. It is used at 0.01% in broth or agar media and at 0.02% in filter paper strips.

TABLE 3 Preparation of pH-specific 0.1 M sodium phosphate buffer[a]

pH	Vol (ml) A	Vol (ml) B	pH	Vol (ml) A	Vol (ml) B
5.7	93.5	6.5	6.9	45.0	55.0
5.8	92.0	8.0	7.0	39.0	61.0
5.9	90.0	10.0	7.1	33.0	67.0
6.0	87.7	12.3	7.2	28.0	72.0
6.1	85.0	15.0	7.3	23.0	77.0
6.2	81.5	18.5	7.4	19.0	81.0
6.3	77.5	22.5	7.5	16.0	84.0
6.4	73.5	26.5	7.6	13.0	87.0
6.5	68.5	31.5	7.7	10.5	89.5
6.6	62.5	37.5	7.8	8.5	91.5
6.7	56.5	43.5	7.9	7.0	93.0
6.8	51.0	49.0	8.0	5.3	94.7

[a] A, 0.1 M NaH$_2$PO$_4$; B, 0.1 M Na$_2$HPO$_4$.

PYR reagent (DMACA)

p-Dimethylaminocinnamaldehyde (DMACA).............................	200 mg
Hydrochloric acid, concentrated	2 ml
Distilled water	18 ml

Add the acid to the water, and let it cool before adding DMACA.

Tube method. Prepare PYR broth (Todd-Hewitt broth containing 0.01% of the PYR substrate). Autoclave to sterilize. Dispense 0.15 ml per tube. Emulsify colonies from a blood agar plate in the PYR broth to a turbidity of a McFarland no. 2 standard (milky suspension). Incubate at 35°C for 2 h. Add 1 drop of the PYR reagent to each tube with gentle shaking. Observe for development of a cherry red color after 2 min. Yellow orange or orange-pink colors are considered negative.

Spot paper strip method. Cut Whatman no. 3 filter paper into strips. Saturate the strips with 0.02% PYR substrate. Dry at room temperature and store desiccated at 2 to 6°C. Prior to testing, moisten the strip with sterile distilled water. With an inoculating loop or wooden stick, rub colonies onto the strip. Incubate for 10 min at 35°C. Then add the PYR reagent to the strip and observe for development of a red color change. A yellow, orange, or pink color is considered negative. For both methods, a positive reaction is indicated by a cherry red to a dark purple-red color. A negative reaction is indicated by an orange or yellow (no change) color. PYR media and strips are available commercially.

■ Saline
Saline is used as a diluent in a variety of procedures. Normal or physiologic saline is 0.85%.

Sodium chloride	8.5 g
Distilled water	1,000 ml

Other concentrations (e.g., 0.45%) are also used.

■ Skim milk, 20%
Skim milk is used to stabilize bacterial suspensions, particularly those containing anaerobes, for freezing.

Skim milk powder	20 g
Distilled water.............................	100 ml

After the skim milk is dissolved in the water, dispense 0.25 to 0.5 ml into 2-ml vials. Autoclave at 110°C for 10 min. The vials can be refrigerated for up to 6 months.

■ Sodium bicarbonate (NaHCO$_3$), 20 mg/ml
Sodium bicarbonate is added to thioglycolate broth to enrich it for the recovery of anaerobes. Dissolve 2 g of NaHCO$_3$ in 100 ml of distilled water. Filter sterilize and store refrigerated for up to 6 months. Add 0.5 ml to 10 ml of thioglycolate broth.

■ Sodium citrate (0.1 M), 2.9%

Sodium citrate, dihydrate	29.4 g
Distilled water	1,000 ml

Dissolve and autoclave. Store at room temperature. If a precipitate forms, discard and prepare a fresh solution.

■ Sodium hydroxide (1 N), 4%

Sodium hydroxide	40 g
Distilled water	1,000 ml

Dissolve and autoclave. Store at room temperature. If a precipitate forms, discard and prepare a fresh solution.

■ Sodium polyanetholesulfonate (SPS) disks

SPS disks are used to differentiate *Peptostreptococcus anaerobius* (which is inhibited by SPS) from other anaerobic cocci. Dissolve 5 g of SPS in 100 ml of distilled water, filter sterilize, and then dispense 2 μl onto 6-mm-diameter sterile filter paper disks. Allow the disks to dry at room temperature for 72 h. The dried disks are stable at room temperature for up to 6 months. A zone of inhibition of 12 mm indicates that the organism is susceptible.

■ Sorensen pH buffer solutions (M/15 phosphate buffer solutions)

Solution A
M/15 (0.067 M) sodium phosphate, dibasic. Dissolve 9.464 g of anhydrous Na_2HPO_4 in 1 liter of distilled water.

Solution B
M/15 (0.067 M) potassium phosphate, monobasic. Dissolve 9.073 g of anhydrous KH_2PO_4 in 1 liter of distilled water. Mix x ml of solution A and solution B as indicated in Table 4 for a buffer of the desired pH.

■ Tween 80 (Polysorbate 80), 10%

Tween 80 (Polysorbate 80)	10 ml
Distilled water	90 ml

Mix Tween 80 with water until it is dissolved. Autoclave at 121°C at 15 lb/in.^{2} for 10 min. Swirl the solution immediately after autoclaving and during cooling to resolubilize the Tween 80. Store refrigerated. The solution can be used

for 6 months. Add 0.5 ml of 10% Tween 80 to 10 ml of broth medium when it is used as a medium supplement.

■ Urease test
Rapid enzymatic tests are used to identify a number of organisms. The procedure for identifying *Haemophilus* spp. is described.

KH_2PO_4	0.1 g
K_2HPO_4	0.1 g
NaCl	0.5 g
Phenol red, 1:500	0.5 ml

Add all ingredients to 100 ml of distilled water. Adjust the pH to 7.0 with NaOH and add 10.4 ml of a 20% (wt/vol) aqueous solution of urea. To make 1:500 phenol red, dissolve 0.2 g of phenol red in NaOH and add distilled water to 100 ml. The development of a red color within 4 h after inoculation indicates urease activity.

■ Vitamin K, 10-mg/ml stock
Vitamin K (3-phytylmenadione) is added to enrich media for the recovery of anaerobes. Mix 0.2 g of vitamin K in 20 ml of 95% ethanol by aseptic technique. Vitamin K is a viscous liquid, and it may be hard to measure the exact amount. Adjust the amount of 95% ethanol accordingly to obtain a 10-mg/ml stock. Store refrigerated in a sterile dark bottle. The stock solution can be further diluted in sterile distilled water to obtain a 1-mg/ml working solution, which can be stored refrigerated in a dark bottle for up to 30 days.

■ Voges-Proskauer (VP) test
The VP test is used to detect acetoin (acetyl-methyl-carbinol), which is produced by certain microorganisms during growth in a buffered peptone-glucose broth (MR-VP broth). The VP test is commonly used to aid in the differentiation between genera (such as *Escherichia coli* from the *Klebsiella* and *Enterobacter* groups) and other species of the *Enterobacteriaceae* family. The test can be used as a differential test for other organism groups (viridans group streptococci).

Reagent A: 5% α-naphthol
Dissolve 5 g of α-naphthol in 100 ml of absolute ethanol. Store refrigerated in a brown glass bottle away from light.

Reagent B: 40% KOH
Dissolve 40 g of potassium hydroxide in 100 ml of distilled water.

Test procedure. Inoculate MR-VP broth and incubate until good growth is obtained. Add 0.6 ml of the α-naphthol solution and 0.2 ml of the 40% KOH solution to 2.5 ml of culture broth. Shake well after the addition of each reagent. A positive reaction, indicated by the formation of a pink-red product, occurs within 5 min. However, allow 15 min for color development before considering the test negative.

STAINS

Direct Examination of Specimens
The first step in the processing of most clinical material is the microscopic examination of the specimen. Direct ex-

TABLE 4 Sorensen pH buffer solutions

pH	Vol (ml)	
	Solution A	Solution B
5.29	0.25	9.75
5.59	0.5	9.5
5.91	1.0	9.0
6.24	2.0	8.0
6.47	3.0	7.0
6.64	4.0	6.0
6.81	5.0	5.0
6.98	6.0	4.0
7.17	7.0	3.0
7.38	8.0	2.0
7.73	9.0	1.0
8.04	9.5	0.5

amination is a rapid, cost-effective diagnostic aid. Methods for direct examination are designed to reveal and enumerate microorganisms and eukaryotic cells. Visible microorganisms may denote the presumptive etiologic agent, guiding the laboratory in the selection of the appropriate isolation media and the physician in the selection of the appropriate empirical antibiotic therapy. The quality of the specimen and the measure of the inflammatory response can also be evaluated. In addition, the direct smear serves as a quality control indicator for attempts to isolate observed organisms (18, 38, 42).

Smear Preparation

Smears may be made from clinical material, culture broths, or isolated colonies. These smears should be prepared on clean glass slides since dirt and grease may interfere with adhesion of the sample to the slide and with the staining process. The best smears are prepared after thoughtful selection of those portions of the sample most likely to reveal the etiologic agent (e.g., a purulent portion of sputum). Smears should contain enough material for an adequate survey of the specimen but should not be overly thick because thick smears may peel or flake off the slide during staining procedures. Thick smears also make the timing of decolorization harder to judge. Smears from swabs should be prepared by rolling the swab over the slide. This method of application helps to preserve host cell morphology and microorganism cell arrangements. Tissue smears may be prepared either by touching freshly exposed cut surfaces directly onto a slide or by first using a tissue grinder or stomacher to homogenize the sample. Smears from aspirates or body fluids may be prepared in several different ways, depending upon the amount of material and equipment available. When the quantity of a liquid sample is limited, a single drop placed on a slide will suffice. If more sample is available, the material should be centrifuged (1,500 × g for 15 min) to concentrate any cells, and the sediment can then be used to prepare the smear. An additional option for the preparation of smears from liquid samples is the use of cytocentrifugation. The cytocentrifuge method uses specimen funnels that are mounted with a slide and filter card and placed in the centrifuge. During centrifugation, the filter card absorbs the supernatant, while cells and microorganisms are centrifuged through a hole in the filter paper strip and are deposited in a continuous layering fashion onto a 6-mm-diameter circular area of the slide. The method is sensitive for the detection of pathogens from sterile body fluids, particularly cerebrospinal fluid (CSF) and peritoneal fluids (8, 49). The method has also been used for detection of acid-fast organisms and *Pneumocystis carinii* from respiratory specimens (19). The deposition of specimen in a discrete area and the ability to lyse erythrocytes during centrifugation are particularly advantageous characteristics that allow more rapid and enhanced resolution in a smear examination.

Samples are fixed to the slides with either heat or methanol. Methanol fixation is preferred since heating may produce artifacts, may create aerosols, and may not adhere the specimen adequately to the slide (35). Once dry, the fixed smear is ready for staining.

Smear Preparations and Staining Methods

The following staining methods and techniques are individual methods used most often in the clinical bacte-

riology laboratory. They are presented in the following categories: the wet mounts and single-stain, differential staining, acid-fast staining, and fluorescent staining methods. The stain method and significant characteristics are described. The principles of the stains used for all microorganisms are described in chapter 18. Readers are referred to chapters 79, 113, and 128 for those staining procedures most commonly performed in the specialties of virology, mycology, and parasitology, respectively, and other specific references (5, 13, 32, 35, 45, 50, 52, 54, 57).

Wet Mounts and Single-Stain Methods

■ **Colloidal carbon wet mounts (India ink, nigrosin) (see chapter 113)**

■ **KOH with and without lactophenol cotton blue (see chapter 113)**

■ **Lugol's iodine (see chapter 128)**

■ **Methylene blue stain**

Methylene blue is a simple direct stain used for a variety of purposes. The stain reveals the morphology of fusiform bacteria and spirochetes from oral infections (Vincent's angina). It may also establish the intracellular location of microorganisms such as *Neisseria*. Methylene blue is the stain of choice for identification of the metachromatic granules of diphtheria; however, one should be careful about overstaining, because this lessens the contrast between the bacteria and the granules. Methylene blue stains organisms or leukocytes a deep blue in a light gray background. *Corynebacterium diphtheriae* appears as a blue bacillus with prominent darker blue metachromatic granules.

Basic procedure

Fix the prepared slide in absolute methanol for 1 to 3 min or heat fix. Air dry the slide and then stain with 0.5 to 1.0% aqueous methylene blue for 30 to 60 s and up to 10 min for possible *C. diphtheriae* granules. Rinse in water, blot dry, and examine at ×100 to ×1,000 magnification.

■ **M'Fadyean stain**

The M'Fadyean stain is a modification of the methylene blue stain developed originally for detecting *Bacillus anthracis* in clinical specimens. The rectangular bacteria stain black-deep blue in chains of two to a few cells in number. Virulent *B. anthracis* rods will be surrounded by a clearly demarcated zone giving the appearance of a pink capsule ("M'Fadyean reaction").

Basic procedure

As *B. anthracis* is suspected, safety precautions must be taken throughout the procedure. All materials, including spent staining washes, should be discarded into disinfectant effective against endospores or autoclaved. See chapter 8. The staining reagent is prepared by dissolving 0.05 mg of methylene blue solution per ml in 20 mM potassium phosphate adjusted to pH 7.3. After the prepared slide is air dried, it is fixed in absolute methanol for 2 to 3 min. The slide is then dried and a large drop of the methylene blue solution is place on the slide for 1 min. Rinse the slide under water into a 10% hypochlorite solution, blot, and allow to dry. Examine at ×100 to ×1,000 magnification.

Differential Staining Methods

■ Gram staining

Gram staining is the single most useful test in the clinical microbiology laboratory. It is the differential staining procedure most commonly used for direct microscopic examination of specimens and bacterial colonies because it has a broad staining spectrum. First devised by Hans Christian Joachim Gram late in the 19th century, it has remained basically the same procedure and serves in dividing bacteria into two main groups: gram-positive organisms which retain the primary crystal violet dye and which appear deep blue or purple and gram-negative organisms which can be decolorized, thereby losing the primary stain and subsequently taking up the counterstain safranin and appearing red or pink. The staining spectrum includes almost all bacteria, many fungi, and parasites such as *Trichomonas, Strongyloides,* and miscellaneous protozoan cysts. The significant exceptions include organisms such as *Treponema, Mycoplasma, Chlamydia,* and *Rickettsia,* which are too small to visualize by light microscopy or which lack a cell wall. Mycobacteria are generally not seen by Gram staining; however, in smears illustrating heavy infections, the organism may give a beaded appearance that is somewhat similar to that of *Nocardia* spp. or may exhibit organism "ghosts" (17). Gram staining can also be used to differentiate epithelial and inflammatory cells, thus providing information about the state of infection and the quality of the specimen (7, 22, 38, 42).

The Gram reaction, morphology, and arrangement of the organisms give the physician clues to the preliminary identification and significance of the organisms. Problems with analysis of the Gram staining generally result from errors in preparation of the slide, such as a smear that is too thick, excessive heat fixing (which can distort organisms), improper decolorization, and inexperience. Overdecolorization results in an abundance of bacteria that appear to be gram negative, while underdecolorization results in too many bacteria that appear to be gram positive. If a chain of cocci resembling streptococci (normally gram positive) and epithelial cells appears to be gram negative, the slide is overdecolorized. Slides stained by Atkins' Gram staining method are less sensitive to decolorization because the mordant is more effective in retaining crystal violet. This allows better visualization of gram-positive organisms, especially those very sensitive to decolorization such as *Streptococcus pneumoniae* and *Bacillus* spp. Atkins' method does not offer a significant advantage over the conventional Gram staining procedure in visualizing gram-negative organisms, and in fact, such visualization may be more difficult with some specimens such as blood cultures. Laboratories should evaluate both Gram staining procedures and then institute one as the routine procedure.

Two methods of Gram staining are presented here. The first method is the conventional Gram staining method used by most laboratories. The second is an altered Gram staining method devised by Atkins (2) in 1920 that uses gentian violet, a different mordant, and acetone as the decolorizing agent.

Basic procedure—conventional Gram staining

The prepared slide is fixed in 95% methanol for 2 min. After the slide is air dried it is flooded with crystal violet (10 g of 90% dye in 500 ml of absolute methanol). After at least 15 s, the slide is washed with water and flooded with iodine (6 g of I_2 and 12 g of KI in 1,800 ml of H_2O). The slide is washed with water after 15 s, decolorized with acetone-alcohol (400 ml of acetone in 1,200 ml of 95% ethanol), washed immediately, and counterstained for at least 15 s with safranin (10 g of dye in 1,000 ml of H_2O). This slide is then washed, blotted dry, and examined at ×100 to ×1,000 magnification.

Basic procedure—Atkins' Gram staining

The primary stain is gentian violet (20 g of crystal violet is dissolved in 200 ml of 95% methanol, 8 g of ammonium oxalate is dissolved in 800 ml of distilled water, and the solutions are mixed together and filtered after 24 h). The mordant is Atkins' iodine (20 g of crystals is dissolved in 100 ml of 1 N NaOH; the mixture is then combined with 900 ml of distilled water and stored in a brown bottle at room temperature). Acetone is the decolorizer, and safranin is the counterstain. The staining procedure is the same as that used for the conventional Gram staining procedure.

There is some debate on the length of time that each staining component should be left on the slide. In actual practice, the two dyes and the mordant should each be allowed to remain on the slide for at least 15 s. More time has little effect. Most critical is the amount of time that the decolorizer is used. Unfortunately, the amount of decolorizer is directly related to the thickness of the specimen on the slide. The old benchmark that the slide should continue to receive decolorizer until no more crystal violet is seen to be washing away is still true but is difficult to attain in practice.

■ Spore stain (Wirtz-Conklin)

The Wirtz-Conklin spore stain is a differential stain for detection of spores. Spore-forming bacteria and cell debris will appear pink-red with green-staining spores.

Basic procedure

After the prepared slide is air dried and heat fixed, it is flooded with 5 to 10% aqueous malachite green. Stain is left on the slide for 45 min. Alternatively, the slide can be heated gently to steaming for 3 to 6 min. Heating to steaming enhances the uptake of the stain into the spores. The slide is then rinsed with tap water. Aqueous safranin (0.5%) is used as a counterstain for 30 s. Rinse in water, blot dry, and examine at ×400 to ×1,000 magnification.

■ Wayson stain

The Wayson stain is a modification of the methylene blue stain and is actually a mix of two stains. It has been used for screening CSF for bacteria and amoebae and examining specimens for *Yersinia pestis.* The advantage of this stain is that the contrast between organisms and proteinaceous background is good. Organisms stain dark blue, leukocytes stain light blue and purple, and the background is light blue. However, slides stained by this method cannot be restained with the Gram stain, and the tinctorial qualities of the stain deteriorate over time.

Basic procedure

The staining reagents are prepared by dissolving 0.2 g of basic fuchsin in 10 ml of 95% ethyl alcohol and 0.75 g of methylene blue in 10 ml of 95% ethyl alcohol. The two solutions are added together slowly into 200 ml of 5% phenol in distilled water. The stain is then filtered and stored in an opaque bottle at room temperature. After the prepared slide is air dried, it is methanol fixed for 2 min and stained for 1 min. Rinse in water, blot dry, and examine at ×100 to ×1,000 magnification.

Acid-Fast Staining Methods

The cells of certain organisms contain long-chain (30- to 90-carbon) fatty acids (mycolic acids) that give them a coat impervious to crystal violet and other basic dyes. Heat or detergent must be used to allow penetration of the primary dye into the bacterium. Once the dye has been forced into the cell, it cannot be decolorized by the usual solvent process. The acid-fast stains are useful for identification of a specific group of bacteria (e.g., *Mycobacterium, Nocardia, Rhodococcus, Tsukamurella, Gordona, Legionella micdadei*) and the oocysts of *Cryptosporidium, Isopora, Sarcocystis,* and *Cyclospora*. The Ziehl-Neelsen (Z-N) stain is one of the original acid-fast stains described. A number of modifications of the Z-N staining procedure have occurred to differentiate various acid-fast organisms as well as simplify the staining process (5, 33, 53).

■ Ziehl-Neelsen stain

Basic procedure

The prepared slide is heat fixed for 2 h at 70°C. The slide is then flooded with carbol-fuchsin (0.3 g of basic fuchsin is dissolved in 10 ml of 95% ethanol, 5 ml of phenol and 95 ml of water are added, and the solution is filtered before use). Heat the slide slowly to steaming and maintain for 3 to 5 min at 60°C. After the slide is cooled, wash the slide with water and decolorize it with acid-alcohol (97 ml of 95% ethanol in 3 ml of HCl). Wash and counterstain for 20 to 30 s with methylene blue (0.3 g of dye in 100 ml of H₂O). Wash, blot dry, and examine at ×400 to ×1,000 magnification.

An acid-fast organism stains red, and the background of cellular elements and other bacteria are blue, the color of the counterstain.

■ Kinyoun stain (Kinyoun modification of Z-N stain)

The basic difference between the Z-N and Kinyoun stains is the substitution of phenol in the primary stain process for steam. The primary stain consists of 4 g of basic fuchsin, 20 ml of 95% alcohol, 8 g of phenol, and 100 ml of distilled water. Both stains have the same sensitivity and specificity, yet the Kinyoun (cold) staining procedure is less time-consuming and is easier to perform.

■ Modified Kinyoun stain (modified acid-fast stain)

Another modification of acid-fast staining procedure has been the use of a weaker decolorizing agent (0.5 to 1.0% sulfuric acid) in place of the 3% acid-alcohol. This particular stain helps differentiate those organisms known to be partially or weakly acid fast, particularly *Nocardia, Rhodococcus, Tsukamurella,* and *Gordona*. These organisms do not stain well with the Z-N stain or the Kinyoun stain.

The acid-fast stains are important clinically and are relatively simple to use. Definitive identification of an acid-fast organism from a clinical specimen cannot be made by staining alone, but certain clues may be helpful. Mycobacteria often appear as slender, slightly curved rods and may show darker granules that give the impression of beading. *Mycobacterium tuberculosis* can appear as beaded bacilli arranged in parallel strands or "cords"; *Mycobacterium kansasii* may form long, often broad and banded cells; *Mycobacterium avium* complex cells appear as short, uniformly staining coccobacilli. *Nocardia* spp. often branch and almost always show a speckled appearance.

Difficulty in interpretation can result from smears that are too thick or insufficiently decolorized, yielding an acid-fast artifact. As a quality control measure, a known acid-fast organism such as nonpathogenic *M. tuberculosis* HRV 37 and a non-acid-fast organism such as *Streptomyces* spp. can be stained in parallel with the clinical specimen and compared.

Factors such as age and exposure to drugs and a particular acid-fast organism itself may vary the acid-fast presentation. For example, while *M. tuberculosis* is consistently acid fast (with the Z-N or Kinyoun stain), *Mycobacterium leprae* and *Nocardia* spp. are not. Therefore, use of the modified Kinyoun stain may be necessary for these organisms (33, 53; June Brown, [Centers for Disease Control and Prevention], personal communication). Other modifications used in tissue preparations such as the Fite-Faraco stain and the Pottz stain may be preferred for unusual isolates such as *M. leprae* (53).

Detection of small numbers of acid-fast organisms in clinical specimens is generally significant. However, the use of acid-fast stains for gastric aspirates in the interpretation of pulmonary disease in adults or for stool specimens from human immunodeficiency virus-positive patients in diagnosing *M. avium-Mycobacterium intracellulare* infection yields very poor specificity (false-positive smears with saprophytic organisms) as well as poor sensitivity (51). In addition, patients receiving adequate therapy may still have positive smears without positive cultures for a number of weeks. Rarely, small numbers of acid-fast organisms in a smear may represent transferred contamination or the use of reagents contaminated with nonviable saprophytic mycobacteria (e.g., *Mycobacterium gordonae*). All smear-positive but culture-negative specimens should be investigated carefully.

Fluorescent Staining Procedures

See chapter 18 for fluorochrome filter recommendations.

■ Acridine orange

Acridine orange is a fluorochrome that can be intercalated into nucleic acid in both the native and the denatured states (48). The staining procedure is rapid and is more sensitive than the Gram staining procedure in the detection of organisms in blood culture broths, CSF, and buffy coat preparations (23, 31, 36). Acridine orange is also useful in a series of miscellaneous infectious etiologies, such as *Acanthamoeba* infections, infectious keratitis, and *Helicobacter pylori* gastritis (21). Bacterial and fungal DNAs fluoresce orange under UV light, and mammalian DNA fluoresces green. Results for cellular specimens or heavily laden bacterial specimens may be difficult to interpret owing to excessive fluorescence, and some interobserver variability may be noted.

Basic procedure

After the prepared slide is fixed in methanol and air dried, it is flooded with the acridine orange solution (stock solution, 1 g of dye in 100 ml of H_2O; working solution, 0.5 ml of stock added to 5 ml of 0.2 M acetate buffer [pH 4.0]). After 2 min, rinse the slide with tap water, air dry, and examine with UV light at ×100 to ×1,000 magnification.

■ Auramine-rhodamine

Auramine and rhodamine are nonspecific fluorochromes that bind to mycolic acids and that are resistant to decolorization with acid-alcohol (18). Staining procedures with these fluorochromes are thus equivalent to the fuchsin-based acid-fast procedures. The stain has become commonplace in laboratories that routinely perform acid-fast examinations because it allows rapid screening of specimens and because the procedure is more sensitive than the traditional acid-fast procedures. Acid-fast organisms fluoresce orange-yellow in a black background. If the secondary stain is not used, the organisms fluoresce a yellow-green color. Smears with suspicious organisms may be confirmed directly with a Kinyoun stain. However, a single organism or a low number of organisms may be difficult to confirm.

Basic procedure
The prepared slide is fixed at 65°C for at least 2 h. It is then stained for 15 min with the auramine-rhodamine solution (1.5 g of auramine O, 0.75 g of rhodamine B, 75 ml of glycerol, 10 ml of phenol, and 50 ml of H_2O) and rinsed with water, followed by decolorization for 2 to 3 min with 0.5% HCl in 70% ethanol. After the slide is rinsed it is counterstained with 0.5% potassium permanganate for 2 to 4 min. The slide is rinsed, dried, and examined under UV light at ×100 to ×400 magnification.

Antibody Staining Methods
See chapter 16 on immunoassays.

MEDIA

This section reviews the basic components necessary in media for the growth and identification of organisms isolated in the clinical microbiology laboratory, specifically in bacteriology. Media for the major groups of microorganisms are listed alphabetically. Refer to chapter 18 for a discussion of the specific principles of different media. The specific intended use and significant components will be provided for each medium. Because media may be purchased from a number of suppliers and minor formulation variations exist for each medium, formulas as well as inoculation and incubation conditions, quality control, and limitations to the use of the media will not be specifically mentioned except in rare instances. Readers are referred to comprehensive references on microbiological media (4, 6, 12, 14, 15, 26, 28, 39, 46, 47, 56), including the *Handbook of Media for Clinical Microbiology*, 2nd edition (3), by R. M. Atlas and J. W. Snyder, and *The Difco Manual*, 10th edition (10) and 11th edition (11), from Becton Dickinson Biosciences. In addition, the package inserts with purchased specialized media offer excellent and specific descriptions. The formulations of a given medium from the different manufacturers do vary slightly and may have been modified from the original description of the medium in the literature. A typical comment from the manufacturer is that the "classical" formula has been adjusted to meet performance standards. Again, the package insert or the formula being prepared from a reference should be followed closely. Chapters in this Manual are noted when appropriate to describe a referenced method for a specific organism. Appendix 1 describes the additives commonly added to media. Refer to Appendix 2 for suppliers of media and reagents.

Preparation of Media
When preparing media from dehydrated materials, the manufacturers' instructions should be followed closely. Chemically cleaned glassware and distilled and/or demineralized water should always be used unless specified otherwise. Care in terms of accuracy should be taken when measuring liquid and dry ingredients. Mixing and solubilization of ingredients are typically done on hot plates, with magnetic stir bars placed in the bottom of the flask or beaker. Excessive heating should be avoided. Autoclaving or filtration sterilizes the media. Autoclaving of volumes of up to 500 ml at 121°C for 15 min is adequate. Larger volumes may require up to 20 to 30 min. The stir bars should be removed before sterilization. For quality control of autoclaving, specialized tape or paper is placed on the medium flask at the time of autoclaving. Enrichments such as blood and other labile additives such as filter-sterilized antibiotics should be added aseptically after the base medium has cooled.

Quality Control
The National Committee for Clinical Laboratory Standards (NCCLS) has specific requirements for quality assurance of commercially prepared media, as documented in standard M22-A2 (41). However, these recommendations do not apply to all media. In addition, any medium that is prepared by the user requires its own specific quality control. Storage of media should be in the dark at 2 to 8°C. Storage in the dark is preferred because additives, such as dyes, will deteriorate faster in the light. The date that the medium was received in the laboratory and the medium expiration date should be marked and easily visible when stored. Media should be in use only up to the time of the expiration date. Prolonged or incorrect storage of media, including transport media, can lead to desiccation of the medium, changing the composition of nutrients and selective agents.

Plating of Specimens on Media
Media should be warmed to room temperature before inoculation of specimens. In addition, a medium that has obvious contamination, such as colony growth or turbidity in broth medium, or that looks damaged in any way should not be used. Damage may include such things as a cracked petri dish and agar that has changed color, demonstrates precipitates, or is dehydrated.

Bacteriology Media

■ A7 and A8 agars
A7 and A8 agars are selective and differential media used for the cultivation, identification, and differentiation of *Ureaplasma* spp. and *Mycoplasma hominis*. Both media contain a soy and casein digest agar base and a supplement solution that contains yeast extract, horse serum, cysteine enrichment solution, and penicillin. Incorporation of urea aids in the identification of urease production to differentiate the organisms on the basis of the appearance of golden to dark brown colonies. There are two main differences between the agars: the use of manganous sulfate in A7 agar and putrescine dihydrochloride and calcium chloride in A8 agar for the detection and enhancement of growth of

urease-positive colonies. *Ureaplasma* colonies are small golden brown colonies that are usually identified at 72 h. *Mycoplasma* colonies have a fried egg appearance and may have a golden or amber color. Refer to the appendixes in chapter 62 for specific formulas.

■ Alkaline peptone water

Alkaline peptone water is an enrichment broth used for the isolation of small numbers of *Vibrio* and *Aeromonas* isolates from stool specimens. Adjustment of the broth to pH 8.4 and inclusion of sodium chloride at a concentration of 0.5 to 1.0% makes it selective for *Vibrio* species.

■ American Trudeau Society medium

American Trudeau Society medium is a nonselective enriched medium used for the isolation and cultivation of mycobacteria. The medium is an egg-based medium. The coagulated egg provides fatty acids essential for support of mycobacterial growth. Glycerol and potato flour provide other nutrients. Malachite green is a partially selective agent that inhibits bacteria. The concentration of malachite green is low, and no other antibiotics are present in this medium; thus, it is very susceptible to proteolytic damage caused by contaminating organisms. This medium is best for specimens not usually contaminated with other microorganisms, i.e., tissue biopsy specimens or CSF.

■ Amies transport medium with and without charcoal

Amies transport medium is a modification of Stuart's medium. The glycerol phosphate used to maintain the pH in Stuart's medium has been found to enhance the growth of certain organisms that utilize this as a nutrient and to allow overgrowth of potential contaminants. In Amies medium, phosphate buffer replaced the glycerol phosphate ingredient and other salts were added to control the permeability of bacterial cells. Amies medium with charcoal is preferred for the isolation of *Neisseria* spp. because the charcoal neutralizes metabolic products toxic to the organisms.

■ Anaerobic blood agar (CDC)

The Centers for Disease Control and Prevention (CDC) formulation of anaerobic blood agar is a general-purpose medium used for the isolation and cultivation of anaerobic bacteria. The nutritive base is tryptic soy agar supplemented with yeast extract, vitamin K, hemin, and sheep blood. This medium is best for the isolation of anaerobic gram-positive cocci and is inferior to brucella or Schaedler's agar.

■ 10B arginine broth

10B arginine broth is a medium used for the transport and growth of *Mycoplasma hominis* and *Ureaplasma urealyticum*. The medium contains nitrogenous components, amino acids, and other components necessary for growth; and cefoperazone is added to reduce bacterial contamination. Two primary compounds, namely, urea and arginine, as well as the phenol red indicator, aid in the identification of the organisms. *Ureaplasma* hydrolyzes urea and releases ammonia; *Mycoplasma* deaminates the arginine. Both reactions result in an alkaline pH shift and change the color of the medium from yellow to pink. *Ureaplasma* depletes urea in the medium quickly (<12 h), with subsequent death of the

culture. Thus, after the color changes, the cultures need to be subcultured quickly to a medium such as A8 or A7 agar that supports the organisms. Limitations of the medium are that other species of *Mycoplasma* and bacteria may also change the color of the medium. Refer to the appendixes in chapter 62 for the specific formula.

■ Ashdown agar

Ashdown agar is a selective and differential medium consisting of Trypticase soy agar with 4% glycerol, 0.005 mg of crystal violet per ml, 0.05 mg of neutral red per ml, and 0.004 mg of gentamicin per ml specifically designed for the isolation of *Pseudomonas pseudomallei*, the causative agent of melioidosis. Glycerol and neutral red allow differentiation from other pseudomonads since *P. pseudomallei* appears flat with rough wrinkled colonies due to the glycerol and absorbs the neutral red dye, whereas other pseudomonads do not. The medium is made selective by the addition of crystal violet, which inhibits gram-positive organisms, and gentamicin, which inhibits gram-negative organisms (1).

■ *Bacillus cereus* medium

Bacillus cereus medium is an enriched medium used for the isolation of *Bacillus cereus*. The base includes agar, yeast extract, and buffers. Mannitol combined with bromocresol purple as the indicator dye makes the medium differential. An egg yolk emulsion is added for the detection of the lecithinase activity seen with *B. cereus*.

■ BACTEC 12B radiometric medium

BACTEC 12B medium (Becton Dickinson Biosciences) is a liquid nonselective medium used for the isolation and identification of *Mycobacterium* species in conjunction with the BACTEC system. The medium consists of a 7H9 broth base. The radiometric BACTEC system also incorporates ^{14}C-labeled palmitic acid and detects radioactive carbon dioxide. An antibiotic enrichment supplement is added to the medium to make it selective for mycobacteria. This supplement includes the antibiotics polymyxin B, amphotericin B, nalidixic acid, trimethoprim, and aziocillin (PANTA) and polyoxylene stearate as a *Mycobacterium* growth enhancer. A total of 0.5 ml of processed specimen may be accommodated in the vial. The BACTEC 12B medium is most commonly used for susceptibility testing. Newer nonradiometric systems are available for monitoring for mycobacterial growth and/or are used for susceptibility testing. These include the 9200 series (Becton Dickinson Biosciences), MGIT (Becton Dickinson Biosciences), ESPII (TREK Diagnostic Systems), and MB BactAlert 3D (bioMérieux, Inc.). Manual medium systems also exist for the detection of mycobacteria, such as the Isolator (Wampole Laboratories) and Septi-Chek AFB (Becton Dickinson Biosciences) systems. The reader is referred to chapters 36 and 73 for specifics on the medium formulations and antibiotic supplements for each system.

■ BACTEC 13A radiometric medium

BACTEC 13A medium, like BACTEC 12A medium, is a liquid nonselective medium used for the isolation and identification of *Mycobacterium* species in conjunction with the BACTEC system. This medium is used specifically for bone marrow and blood specimens. The medium is a Middlebrook 7H13 broth with SPS, an anticoagulant. ^{14}C-labeled palmitic acid is incorporated into the medium used in conjunction with the radiometric system. The benefit of this medium is that a large volume of specimen, up to 5 ml, can be directly inoculated into the bottle.

■ *Bacteroides* bile esculin agar

Bacteroides bile esculin agar is an enriched, selective, and differential medium used for the isolation and presumptive identification of members of the *Bacteroides fragilis* group and *Bilophila wadsworthia*. The nutritive base includes casein and soybean peptones, hemin, and vitamin K. The differential characteristic of esculin hydrolysis is identified by the product, esculetin, which reacts with the ferric ammonium citrate to form a complex and produce a brown-black coloration around the colony. The selective agents include bile, which inhibits most gram-positive bacteria and anaerobic organisms other than members of the *B. fragilis* group, and gentamicin, which inhibits facultative anaerobes. Bile esculin agar with kanamycin and enriched with vitamin K and hemin is a formulation that is more enriched and selective than *Bacteroides* bile esculin agar for the isolation of the *B. fragilis* group. This medium includes beef extract and pancreatic digest of gelatin, vitamin K, and hemin as the nutritive base. Bile inhibits the same organisms described above, and kanamycin is inhibitory for facultatively anaerobic and aerobic gram-negative bacilli.

■ Baird Parker agar base

Baird Parker agar base is a beef extract, peptone, and yeast extract base used to prepare egg-tellurite-glycine-pyruvate agar (ETGPA). ETGPA is an enriched, selective, and differential agar used for the detection of coagulase-positive staphylococci (*Staphylococcus aureus*) from food and other nonclinical sources. Glycerol and lithium make the medium selective by inhibiting many bacteria. Tellurite is also inhibitory to bacteria. The egg yolk emulsion is an enrichment. Tellurite and the egg yolk emulsion also act as differential determinants. When *S. aureus* reduces tellurite, it imparts a black color to the colony, and lecithinase activity is demonstrated by a clearing around the colony. *S. aureus* appears as black-brown colonies with clear zones around the colony.

■ Bile esculin agar

Bile esculin agar is a selective and differential medium used for the isolation and differentiation of *Enterococcus* and *Streptococcus bovis* (group D *Streptococcus*) from non-group D *Streptococcus*. The nutritive base includes peptone and beef extract. The selective agent is bile (oxgall), which inhibits gram-positive organisms and most strains of streptococci except *S. bovis* and *Enterococcus*. Esculin hydrolysis is a characteristic that differentiates enterococci and *S. bovis* from other organisms. Esculin in the medium is hydrolyzed to esculetin and dextrose. A black-brown pigment forms when the iron salt (ferric citrate) is used as the color indicator of esculin hydrolysis and subsequent esculetin formation. *S. bovis* and *Enterococcus faecalis* grow on the medium and exhibit blackening around the colony.

■ Bile esculin agar plus vancomycin at 6 μg/ml

Bile esculin agar plus vancomycin is a selective and differential medium used to identify vancomycin-resistant strep-

tococci and enterococci. Colonies appear the same as they do on bile esculin agar. Growth of group D streptococci and enterococci occurs with esculin hydrolysis in the presence of bile, appearing as blackening of the medium.

■ Bile esculin azide agar and broth (Enterococcosel)

Bile esculin azide agar or broth is a selective and differential medium for *S. bovis* (group D *Streptococcus*) and enterococci. As with bile esculin agar, esculin is incorporated into the medium, and precipitation with ferric ions forms a brown-black pigment, which identifies these species. Bile esculin azide medium has a reduced percentage of bile and makes the medium less inhibitory to non-group D streptococci. Sodium azide is incorporated to inhibit gram-negative organisms. Addition of 6 μg of vancomycin per ml makes the medium selective for vancomycin-resistant enterococci. Incorporation of aztreonam subsequently increases the selectivity by inhibiting other organisms, especially gram-negative organisms, contaminating specimens.

■ Bismuth sulfite agar

Bismuth sulfite agar is a highly selective and differential medium used for the isolation of *Salmonella enterica* subsp. *enterica* serovar Typhi and other enteric bacilli. Beef extract, peptones, and dextrose are the nutritive base. Bismuth sulfite, a heavy metal, and brilliant green are selective agents which inhibit most commensal gram-positive and gram-negative organisms. Ferrous sulfate is an indicator for hydrogen sulfide production, which occurs when the hydrogen sulfide produced by *Salmonella* reacts with the iron salt. This reaction causes a black or green metallic colony and a black or brown precipitate. Colony morphology and color help differentiate *Salmonella* species. This medium may be inhibitory for some species of *Shigella*. Readers are referred to chapter 42 for other selective media for enteric organisms.

■ Blood agar (see Columbia agar with 5% sheep blood)

■ Blood culture media

All blood culture medium formulations are based on a nutrient peptone broth with variations due to hydrolysis or digestion of the source protein. Additives for neutralization of serum components and/or inactivation of antibiotics, such as SPS, chelators, or resins, vary with the manufacturer. The reader is referred to chapter 14 for specific formulations for specific blood culture media and various commercial systems.

■ Bordet-Gengou medium

Bordet-Gengou medium is an enriched medium used for the isolation and cultivation of *Bordetella pertussis* from clinical specimens. The medium contains potato infusion, glycerol, and peptones as the nutritive base. Sheep blood allows detection of hemolytic reactions and provides other nutrients for *Bordetella*. The medium can be supplemented with methicillin, which inhibits some of the normal oral flora that is obtained upon collection of the specimen. Culture plates should be held for no more than 7 days.

■ **Brain heart infusion agar**

Brain heart infusion agar is a general-purpose medium used for the isolation of a wide variety of pathogens, including yeast, molds, and bacteria, including *Nocardia* spp. The basic formula includes brain heart infusion from solids as well as meat peptones, yeast extract, and dextrose. One variation that exists is brain heart infusion agar with vitamin K and hemin for the enrichment of anaerobes. The anaerobic formulation may be optimal for the isolation of *Eubacterium* spp. but inferior for the isolation of other anaerobic gram-negative organisms, especially those that produce pigment.

■ **Brain heart infusion agar with 7% horse blood and brain heart infusion agar with 1% serum (see Brain heart infusion agar)**

Brain heart infusion agar with horse blood or serum enriches the medium for the isolation of *Helicobacter* spp.

■ **Brain heart infusion broth**

Brain heart infusion broth is a general-purpose clear liquid medium that is used to cultivate a wide variety of organisms. It is also used for the preparation of inocula for susceptibility tests and identification. The medium is especially useful as a blood culture medium. The main nutritive base includes infusion from brains and beef heart. Peptones, glucose, sodium chloride, and buffers are other additives. Sodium chloride acts as an osmotic agent, and disodium phosphate acts as a buffer. Formulations with 6.5% NaCl are used for the isolation of salt-tolerant streptococci, formulations with 0.1% agar that reduce O₂ tension favor anaerobes, and formulations with Fildes enrichment are used for the isolation of fastidious organisms such as *Haemophilus* and *Neisseria*.

Brain heart infusion broth is also used for the preparation of inocula for antimicrobial susceptibility testing and broth dilution MIC testing procedures. The medium contains infusions of brain, casein, and meat peptones.

■ **Brain heart infusion-vancomycin agar (see Brain heart infusion agar)**

Brain heart infusion-vancomycin agar is a selective medium used for the isolation of vancomycin-resistant enterococci. The base is brain heart infusion agar. Vancomycin is added at 6 μg/ml to select for vancomycin-resistant enterococci.

■ **Brilliant green agar**

Brilliant green agar is a highly selective and differential medium used for the isolation of *Salmonella* species except for *Salmonella* serovar Typhi. The nutritive base contains meat and casein peptones. Brilliant green dye at a high concentration is the selective agent and inhibits most gram-positive and gram-negative bacteria, including *Shigella* species and *Salmonella* serovar Typhi. Phenol red is the pH indicator. Yeast extract provides additional nutrients. Sugars included in the medium are sucrose and lactose. Acid production in the fermentation of these sugars produces yellow-green colonies with a yellow-green zone. Nonfermenters of sucrose and lactose may range in color from white to reddish pink with a red zone around the colony (*Salmonella*).

■ **Brucella agar**

Brucella agar is a medium designed originally for the purpose of isolating *Brucella* spp. from dairy products. Brucella agar with 5% horse blood can be used as a general-purpose medium for the isolation of both aerobic and anaerobic fastidious organisms. The nutritive base includes a peptone mix, including meat peptones, dextrose, and yeast extract.

■ **Brucella agar with cefoxitin and cycloserine**

Brucella agar with cefoxitin and cycloserine is a selective and differential sheep blood medium used for the isolation of *Clostridium difficile*. Brucella agar is the nutritive base. Vitamin K and sheep blood provide other growth enhancers. Cefoxitin and cycloserine inhibit most gram-positive and gram-negative organisms, respectively. *Enterococcus* is not inhibited. Another differential characteristic is that *C. difficile* colonies fluoresce yellow-green under UV light.

■ **Brucella agar with hemin and vitamin K**

Brucella agar with hemin and vitamin K is a general-purpose nonselective and enriched medium used for the isolation and cultivation of anaerobic bacteria. Casein peptones, dextrose, and yeast extract are the nutritive base. Hemin and vitamin K provide further enrichments. Defibrinated sheep blood allows determination of hemolytic reactions. Because of the high carbohydrate content, colonies with beta-hemolytic reactions may have a greenish hue. The medium is better for gram-negative organisms.

■ **Brucella agar with 5% horse blood**

Horse blood enriches brucella agar for fastidious organisms, such as *Helicobacter pylori*, by providing both hemin (factor X) and NAD (factor V) factors. The use of horse blood also allows determination of hemolytic reactions. However, for *Streptococcus* spp. hemolytic reactions on horse blood differ from those on media with sheep blood. Hemolytic patterns for *Haemophilus* also differ.

■ **Brucella broth**

Brucella broth is a liquid medium that is used to cultivate *Campylobacter* species and to identify the organisms to the species level. Brucella base that contains peptones, dextrose, and yeast extract is the nutritive base. Sodium bisulfite is a reducing agent.

■ **Buffered charcoal yeast extract medium (BCYE) (selective and nonselective)**

BCYE is a specialized enriched agar medium used for the isolation and cultivation of *Legionella* species from environmental and clinical specimens. *Legionella* species, especially *Legionella pneumophila*, require specific nutrients for growth. One is iron and the other is the amino acid L-cysteine. In BCYE these are provided by ferric pyrophosphate and L-cysteine hydrochloride. The nutritive base is yeast extract and α-ketoglutarate. N-2-Acetamido-2-aminoethane sulfonic acid buffer maintains the pH of the medium. Charcoal acts as a detoxifying agent and surface tension modifier. Antibiotics may also be added to the medium. Typically, manufacturers provide them in two combinations of three antibiotics. One is polymyxin B, anisomycin, and vancomycin, and the other is polymyxin B, anisomycin, and cefamandole (PAC). In these combinations polymyxin B inhibits gram-negative bacilli, anisomycin inhibits yeast, vancomycin inhibits gram-positive organisms, and cefamandole inhibits both gram-positive and gram-negative organisms. BCYE with PAC may be inhibitory to some strains of *Legionella micdadei*. Nonselective BCYE can support the growth of other fastidious organisms such as *Nocardia* and *Francisella*. BCYE can also be a differential medium with the addition of the dyes bromcresol purple and bromthymol blue. *L. pneumophila* produces light blue colonies with a pale green tint. This differential medium is also called Wadowsky-Lee medium and can be used for isolation of actinomycetes.

■ Buffered glycerol saline

Buffered glycerol saline is a multipurpose transport medium. The transport medium has been used for the isolation of bacteria, such as *Aeromonas* spp., as well as viruses. In addition, glycerol-containing media may also be used for long-term storage of isolates and transport and storage of biopsy specimens.

■ *Burkholderia cepacia* selective agar

Burkholderia cepacia selective agar is an enriched and selective medium used for the isolation of *Burkholderia cepacia*. Trypticase peptone, yeast extract, sodium chloride, sucrose, and lactose are the nutritive base. The medium is made selective by the addition of polymyxin B, gentamicin, vancomycin, and crystal violet. The medium supports the growth of *B. cepacia* and inhibits >90% of other isolates. This agar is more sensitive and more selective than *Pseudomonas cepacia* agar and oxidative-fermentative polymyxin B-bacitracin-lactose (OFPBL) medium (24).

■ *Campylobacter* blood agar

Campylobacter blood agar is an enriched selective blood agar medium used for the isolation of *Campylobacter* species. The nutritive base is brucella agar. Sheep blood provides heme and other growth factors. The selectivity of the medium comes from the incorporation of five antimicrobial agents. These agents inhibit normal stool flora such as members of the family *Enterobacteriaceae*, staphylococci, and yeast. Trimethoprim, vancomycin, amphotericin B, polymyxin B, and cephalothin are the five agents. Plates should be incubated in a microaerophilic environment. Due to the dextrose content of the brucella base, weak oxidase reactions may be exhibited. Some species of campylobacter, e.g., *Campylobacter fetus* subsp. *fetus* and *Campylobacter upsaliensis*, are inhibited by cephalosporins. Media with cephalothin have been shown to be more inhibitory than those with cefoperazone. See chapter 57 for additional selective media.

■ Campylobacter charcoal differential (CCD) agar

CCD agar is a blood free selective medium used for the isolation of *Campylobacter* from stool specimens. Cefoperazone replaces cephazolin in other selective agars. The nutritive base is Preston agar, which consists of beef extract and peptones. This agar has been shown to be less inhibitory than other campylobacter agars for all *Campylobacter*

species as well as more inhibitory to contaminating organisms (25).

■ *Campylobacter* thioglycolate medium

Campylobacter thioglycolate medium is a selective holding medium used for the isolation of *Campylobacter* species. The low concentration of agar in thioglycolate broth provides a reduced oxygen content. The selective agents include the same as those in *Campylobacter* agar: trimethoprim, vancomycin, polymyxin B, cephalothin, and amphotericin B.

■ Cary-Blair transport medium

Cary-Blair transport medium was specifically designed to enhance the survival of enteric bacterial pathogens. The medium has a low nutrient content, which allows organism survival without replication; sodium thioglycolate, which allows a low oxidation-reduction potential; and a high pH, which minimizes the destruction of bacteria when acid is produced.

■ Cefoperazone-vancomycin-amphotericin B (CVA) medium

CVA medium is a selective and enriched blood agar medium used for the isolation of *Campylobacter* species. The nutritive agar base is brucella agar. Sheep blood provides hemin and other growth nutrients. The antibiotics in this medium are vancomycin, amphotericin B, and cefoperazone, which inhibit gram-positive organisms, fungi, and aerobic and anaerobic gram-positive and gram-negative organisms, respectively. The limitations of this medium are that some campylobacters (e.g., *C. fetus* subsp. *fetus*) are inhibited and that weak oxidase reactions may occur due to the dextrose in the brucella agar base. CVA medium is a good medium to use if only a single selective medium for *Campylobacter* can be used.

■ Cefsulodin-irgasan-novobiocin (CIN) medium, *Yersinia* selective agar

CIN medium or *Yersinia* selective agar is a selective and differential medium used for the isolation and differentiation of *Yersinia enterocolitica* from clinical specimens and food sources. The nutritive base includes peptones and beef and yeast extracts. The selective agents are sodium desoxycholate, crystal violet, cefsulodin, irgasan (triclosan), and novobiocin. The medium is available with 4 and 8 μg of cefsulodin per ml. The lower concentration is recommended for better growth of clinically significant *Yersinia* spp. as well as growth of *Aeromonas* spp. Mannitol is the sugar, and neutral red is the indicator. Organisms that ferment mannitol in the presence of the neutral red dye cause a pH drop around the colony. The colony becomes transparent, with absorption of the red dye to form a red bulls-eye appearance in the center with *Yersinia*, and *Aeromonas* has a pink center with an uneven clear apron. Most other bacteria including other enteric mannitol fermenters are inhibited. Some *Yersinia* isolates may require cold enrichment at 4°C and subsequent subculture to CIN medium. See chapters 42 and 45.

■ Cetrimide agar

Cetrimide agar is a selective and differential medium used for the identification of *Pseudomonas aeruginosa*. Cetrimide is the selective agent and inhibits most bacteria by acting as a detergent. *Pseudomonas* produces a number of pigments. Two pigments can be detected with this medium. The magnesium chloride and potassium sulfate stimulate the blue-green pyocyanin pigment, and the fluorescent yellow-green pigment can be seen with a UV light. The low iron content of the medium stimulates pigment production.

■ Charcoal selective medium

Charcoal selective medium is an enriched selective medium used for the isolation of *Campylobacter* species. In this medium the nutritive base is a Columbia agar base, and charcoal is used to effectively replace blood components. The selective agents used in this medium include vancomycin, cefoperazone, and cycloheximide. Vancomycin and cefoperazone effectively inhibit gram-positive and gram-negative organisms, including *Pseudomonas*. Fungi are inhibited by cycloheximide. The limitation of this medium is that some *Campylobacter* species, e.g., *C. fetus* subsp. *fetus*, are inhibited by cephalosporins.

■ Chocolate agar

Chocolate agar is a general-purpose medium used for the isolation and detection of a wide variety of microorganisms, including fastidious species such as *Neisseria* and *Haemophilus*. Chocolate agar originated as a GC agar base which includes meat and casein peptones, phosphate buffer to maintain pH, and cornstarch to detoxify fatty acids in the medium. Hemoglobin is added to the medium to provide hemin or X factor. The appearance of hemin in dry powdered form is reddish brown. When hemoglobin is hydrated and added to the medium, it gives the agar base the "chocolate" appearance. Another enrichment added is a defined supplement, such as IsoVitaleX, which provides NAD or V factor. Both of these components added to the GC agar base make the enriched chocolate agar. Levinthal agar is a variation on chocolate agar. The medium is a selective and differential medium used for the isolation and identification of *Haemophilus influenzae* type b. The medium is a chocolate agar base that is made transparent by the removal of particulate matter either by centrifugation or by filtration through sterile filter paper. The medium contains bacitracin to inhibit respiratory flora and *H. influenzae* type b antiserum, allowing detection of an immunoprecipitation reaction. Colonies of encapsulated strains show a bright iridescence (red-blue-green-yellow) when light is transmitted from behind the clear medium.

■ Chopped meat glucose broth

Chopped meat glucose broth is an enriched medium that supports the growth of most anaerobes. It is most commonly used to isolate *Clostridium botulinum* from mixed bacterial growth. Beef heart, peptones, and dextrose supply the essential nutrients. The −SH groups from cooked and denatured muscle protein are the reducing agents in the medium. Vitamin K and hemin are additives used to maximize the growth of specific anaerobes.

■ CHROMAgars

CHROMAgars are microorganism-specific chromogenic culture media used for the isolation and identification of a variety of organisms. First-generation agars are monochromogenic. Second-generation agars are multicolor. Both are differential and selective. The nutritive agar base includes peptone and glucose. Different additives, proprietary chromogenic mixtures, and antibiotics have resulted in a series of media specific for such organisms as *Listeria*, *Staphylococcus aureus*, *Escherichia coli* O157, yeast, and other organisms.

■ Columbia agar with 5% sheep blood

Columbia agar with 5% sheep blood is a general-purpose medium used for the isolation of a variety of microorganisms including fastidious organisms. This medium contains meat and casein peptones and beef extract, yeast extract, and corn starch as the nutritive base. Sheep blood allows determination of hemolytic reactions and provides X factor. However, the substantial carbohydrate content may make beta-hemolytic streptococci appear to be alpha-hemolytic or take on a greenish hue. NADase enzyme in sheep blood destroys the V factor (NAD); thus, organisms that require this factor do not grow. Incorporation of horse or rabbit blood allows beta-hemolysis to be seen better, with some strains of gram-positive cocci infrequently isolated. See chapter 31.

■ Columbia broth

Columbia broth is a general-purpose clear liquid medium used especially for blood culture medium. The broth supports the growth of a wide range of microorganisms. The base is similar to Columbia agar with meat peptones, casein, and yeast extract. Salt and Tris buffers have been added to enhance the growth of microorganisms and increase the buffering capacity, respectively. For the purpose of blood culture medium, additional ingredients include carbon dioxide, which is stimulatory for many organisms; cysteine, which improves isolation of anaerobic and aerobic organisms from blood; SPS, a polyanionic anticoagulant which inactivates aminoglycosides and which interferes with the complement, lysozyme activity, and the phagocytic activity inherent in a blood specimen; and glucose, which provides a hypertonic medium for the isolation of cell wall-deficient forms.

■ Columbia-colistin-nalidixic acid agar with 5% sheep blood

Columbia-colistin-nalidixic acid agar with 5% sheep blood is a selective and differential medium commonly used in the isolation of gram-positive aerobic and anaerobic organisms from mixed clinical specimens. The base is Columbia agar with 5% sheep blood that allows the detection of hemolytic reactions and provides additional enrichment and X factor (heme). The medium is made selective by the inclusion of the antibiotics colistin and nalidixic acid, which inhibit gram-negative organisms. Swarming *Proteus* spp. are inhibited. Supplementation with glutathione and lead acetate allows a selective and differential medium for *Peptostreptococcus*.

■ Cycloserine-cefoxitin-fructose agar

Cycloserine-cefoxitin-fructose agar is a selective and differential agar medium used for the isolation of *Clostridium difficile*. The nutritive base includes animal peptones and fructose. The selective agents include cycloserine and cefoxitin. Cycloserine inhibits gram-negative organisms, especially *Escherichia coli*, and cefoxitin is a broad-spectrum antibiotic that is active against both gram-positive and gram-negative organisms. *Enterococcus* is not inhibited. The medium is differential by the addition of neutral red. *Clostridium* raises the pH of the medium and allows the neutral red indicator to change to yellow. Both the colony and the surrounding medium turn yellow. In addition, *C. difficile* colonies yield a gold-yellow fluorescence when viewed under long-wave UV light.

■ Cysteine-albumin broth with 20% glycerol

Cysteine-albumin broth with 20% glycerol is used for transport and storage of gastric biopsy specimens for the recovery of *Helicobacter pylori*.

■ Cystine glucose blood agar

Cystine glucose blood agar is an enriched medium used for the isolation of *Francisella* spp. The nutritive base is beef heart infusion, peptones, and glucose. *Francisella* requires cystine for growth. Rabbit blood provides hemoglobin enrichment.

■ Cystine-tellurite blood agar

Cystine-tellurite blood agar is a modification of Tinsdale agar and is both a selective and a differential medium used for the detection of *Corynebacterium diphtheriae*. Casein peptones, beef infusion, and yeast extract are the nutritive base. Potassium tellurite is both the selective and differential agent. Gram-negative organisms and most upper respiratory flora are inhibited; *Corynebacterium* spp. are the exception. The potassium tellurite also allows differentiation of *C. diphtheriae* from other biotypes by the dull metal gray or black colony appearance indicative of tellurite reductase activity and the brown halo around the colony consistent with cystinase activity. Other organisms such as staphylococci may reduce tellurite and produce black colonies. These are easily differentiated by Gram staining.

■ Diagnostic sensitivity agar

Diagnostic sensitivity agar is a medium used in the cultivation of organisms for susceptibility testing. The base is proteose peptone, veal infusion solids, agar, and glucose, with other additives. The medium is available as a premixed powder from Oxoid Unipath. See chapter 70 for specific uses.

■ DNA-toluidine blue agar

DNA-toluidine blue agar is a differential medium used most commonly for the detection and differentiation of *Staphylococcus* spp. The nutritive base is tryptic soy agar. Supplementation with DNA permits detection of the activity of DNase (or heat-stable staphylococcal nuclease), which has endo- and exonucleolytic properties and which can cleave the DNA or RNA produced by most coagulase-positive staphylococci. The medium is blue due to the toluidine blue O, and DNase activity is detected by a pink zone around the colony secondary to the metachromatic property of the dye.

■ Dubos Tween-albumin broth

Dubos Tween-albumin broth is a nonselective medium used for the isolation and cultivation of mycobacteria. Polysor-

bate 80 (Tween 80) is an oleic acid ester and acts as an essential fatty acid necessary for the growth of mycobacteria. In addition, Tween 80 acts as a dispersal agent and allows a small inoculum to grow as a more homogeneous growth. Casein peptone and asparagine provide other nutrients. Phosphates provide a buffering system, and albumin provides protection from toxic substances in the medium and a source of protein. Cultures of *Mycobacterium tuberculosis* may form cords in the medium, and other mycobacteria grow more diffusely.

■ Egg-tellurite-glycine-pyruvate agar (ETGPA) (see Baird-Parker agar base)

■ Egg yolk agar (modified McClung-Toabe agar)

Egg yolk agar medium (modified McClung-Toabe agar) is a selective and differential medium used for the isolation and differentiation of *Clostridium* spp. McClung and Toabe reported on the use of egg yolk medium for the identification of species of clostridia by the detection of lecithinase and lipase activities. Degradation of lecithin results in an opaque precipitate around the colony, and lipase destroys fats in the egg yolk, which results in an iridescent sheen on the colony surface. Proteolysis can also be determined with egg yolk agar, as indicated by a translucent clearing of the medium around the colony. The medium should be incubated anaerobically for a minimum of 48 h. It should be held for up to 7 days for the detection of lipase activity. Addition of neomycin makes the egg yolk agar moderately selective by inhibiting some facultative anaerobic gram-negative bacilli. Lecithinase positivity is also seen with some *Bacillus* spp. (see Chapter 23). Lipase and proteolytic activity can also be demonstrated with some anaerobes. See chapter 40.

■ Ellinghausen-McCullough/Johnson-Harris medium

Ellinghausen-McCullough/Johnson-Harris medium is an enriched semisolid medium used for the isolation and cultivation of *Leptospira*. Stuart's medium is the base to which multiple modifications for optimization of the recovery of *Leptospira* have been made since the original description. Bovine albumin and Tween provide lipids and long-chain fatty acids. B vitamins and ammonium ion provide essential vitamins and a nitrogen source. Lysed erythrocytes provide other essential supplements such as iron. The medium is made selective by adding 5-fluorouracil either alone or with fosfomycin and nalidixic acid.

■ Enterococcosel agar (see Bile esculin azide agar and broth)

■ Eosin-methylene blue agar

Eosin-methylene blue agar is a selective and differential medium used for the isolation and differentiation of enteric pathogens from contaminated clinical specimens. Pancreatic digest makes up the nutritive base. Eosin and methylene blue are the selective agents and inhibit gram-positive organisms. The sugars are lactose and, in certain modifications, sucrose. Organisms that ferment lactose bind to the dyes under acidic conditions and appear as blue-black colonies with a metallic sheen. Under less acidic conditions, other coliforms appear as mucoid and brown-pink colonies. Nonfermenters, such as *Salmonella, Shigella,* and *Proteus,* appear as the color of the medium (amber) or transparent and colorless. Eosin-methylene blue agar should be stored in the dark because of the loss of support of growth when it is exposed to visible light.

■ ESP Myco
ESP Myco medium is used with the ESPII culture system (TREK Diagnostic Systems) for the detection of mycobacterial growth. The medium is a Middlebrook 7H9 broth enriched with glycerol, Casitone, and cellulose sponge disks. OADC enrichment is added prior to use.

■ Fastidious anaerobic agar (*Fusobacterium* selective agar)
Fastidious anaerobic agar is an enriched sheep blood medium used for the isolation and cultivation of anaerobic organisms. Peptone, glucose, agar, and starch make up the solid base. Sheep blood, vitamin K, and hemin are enrichments for anaerobes. A larger amount of hemin is used in fastidious anaerobic agar than in other anaerobic media. This medium is used for the isolation of *Fusobacterium* spp. and formate-fumarate-requiring species.

■ Fletcher's medium
Fletcher's medium is an enriched semisolid medium used for the isolation and growth of *Leptospira*. The medium is a peptone and beef extract base with a 1.5% agar concentration. Rabbit serum supplies long-chain fatty acids and albumin and has been found to be superior to other serum sources for the isolation of *Leptospira*. 5-Fluorouracil may be added to select for *Leptospira*. Cultures should be incubated in air and at 28 to 30°C.

■ FlexTrans viral and chlamydia transport medium
FlexTrans viral and chlamydia transport medium is intended to be used as a transport medium for viruses and/or chlamydia. The medium consists of minimal essential medium, bovine serum albumin, glutamine, and sucrose with a phenol red indicator. Microbial growth is inhibited by the incorporation of the antibiotics amphotericin B, gentamicin, and streptomycin.

■ GC agar base
GC agar base is used for susceptibility testing of *Neisseria gonorrhoeae*. The agar base consists of a GC agar base which includes digest of casein, animal peptones, corn starch, NaCl, and buffers. A 1% defined growth supplement is added. The supplement contains a low concentration of cysteine to avoid activation of various beta-lactam antibiotics such as penems, carbapenems, and clavulanic acid. GC agar base with 5% fetal bovine serum and 10% CVA medium enrichment allows isolation of *Haemophilus ducreyi* (37) (see chapter 40).

■ GC-Lect, GonoPAK, and John E. Martin Biological Enrichment Chamber (JEMBEC) (Becton Dickinson Biosciences) transport medium systems
GC-Lect, GonoPAK, and JEMBEC are transport and inoculation media used for direct plating of specimens for the detection of *N. gonorrhoeae*. Thayer-Martin, modified Thayer-Martin, or Martin Lewis agar is the base. Each system is self-contained with a tablet that allows production of a CO_2 atmosphere and enhances recovery of the pathogen. The GonoPAK system can be transported at room temperature.

■ GN broth
GN broth is an enriched selective broth medium used for the isolation of gram-negative bacilli. Specifically, *Salmonella* and *Shigella* are isolated more effectively in GN broth than on solid medium alone. The nutritive base includes casein and meat peptones as well as mannitol and dextrose. The concentration of mannitol limits the growth of some other contaminating enteric organisms. Sodium desoxycholate and sodium citrate help to inhibit gram-positive organisms and some gram-negative organisms. Enteric organisms do not overgrow the pathogens in the first 6 h of incubation, at which time the broth should be subcultured.

■ Haemophilus test medium and broth
Haemophilus test medium is an enriched medium used for susceptibility testing of *Haemophilus* species. The medium contains beef and casein extracts. Yeast extract, hematin, and nicotinamide (NAD) provide necessary growth factors and enrichments. Antagonists to sulfonamides and trimethoprim are removed by thymidine phosphorylase. The advantage of the agar medium is that it is a clear agar base with which sharp growth endpoint interpretations can be made. The calcium and magnesium concentrations are adjusted to the concentrations recommended by NCCLS. The medium is also used as a broth for susceptibility testing by determination of MICs. See chapter 71 for the specific formulation.

■ Heart infusion agar and broth
Heart infusion agar and broth are general-purpose media used for the isolation of a variety of microorganisms. Heart muscle infusion, casein peptones, and yeast extract are the nutritive base. Fastidious organisms do not grow well on or in this medium because no additional enrichments or sheep blood is incorporated. Incorporation of 5% rabbit blood allows the detection of more fastidious *Actinomyces*.

■ Hektoen enteric agar
Hektoen enteric agar is a selective and differential medium used for the isolation and differentiation of enteric pathogens from contaminated clinical specimens. Animal peptones and yeast extract provide the nutritive base. Bile salts and the indicator dyes (bromthymol blue and acid fuchsin) in the medium are the selective agents and inhibit gram-positive organisms. Lactose, sucrose, and salicin are the carbohydrates incorporated to differentiate fermenters from nonfermenters. In addition, differentiation of species occurs with the use of sodium thiosulfate and ferric ammonium citrate, which allow the detection of hydrogen sulfide production. Organisms that produce hydrogen sulfide appear, with the formation of a black precipitate on the colony. Fermenters, such as *Escherichia coli*, produce colonies which are yellow-pink in color, *Shigella* colonies are green or transparent, and *Salmonella* colonies are green or transparent with black centers.

■ **Hemin-supplemented egg yolk agar (see Neomycin egg yolk agar)**

■ **Isolator or lysiscentrifugation tube (Wampole Laboratories)**

Isolator is a unique system used to recover organisms from blood through a simultaneous process of lysis and centrifugation. The tubes contain saponin, a lysing agent, and EDTA, an anticoagulant as well as a fluorocarbon that acts as a cushioning agent during centrifugation. The system creates a layer that is subsequently plated onto media appropriate for organism recovery. The system is especially good for the recovery of dimorphic fungi, yeasts, mycobacteria, and *Bartonella* spp. Recovery of anaerobes, *Haemophilus* spp., and pneumococci may be reduced if the tube is not processed within 8 h of inoculation.

■ **Iso-Sensitest agar and broth**

Iso-Sensitest agar and broth are media used for susceptibility testing in countries other than the United States. The base includes hydrolyzed casein, peptones, and glucose with other additives. The medium is available as a premixed powder from Oxoid Unipath. See chapter 70 for specific uses.

■ **Kanamycin-vancomycin laked sheep blood agar**

Kanamycin-vancomycin laked sheep blood agar is an enriched, selective, and differential medium used for the isolation and cultivation of anaerobic bacteria, especially slowly growing and fastidious anaerobes from clinical specimens, such as *Bacteroides* spp. and *Prevotella* spp. The base is CDC anaerobic blood agar. The selective agents are kanamycin and vancomycin (7.5 μg/ml) to prevent obligate facultative gram-negative and gram-positive bacteria and facultative anaerobic bacteria, respectively. Use of a medium with 2 μg of vancomycin per ml allows better growth of *Porphyromonas* spp. Laked blood is used to allow optimal pigmentation of anaerobes such as the pigmented *Prevotella* spp.

■ **Lactobacillus MRS broth**

Lactobacillus MRS (deMan, Rogosa, and Sharpe) broth is a nonselective liquid medium used for the isolation and cultivation of lactobacilli from clinical specimens and dairy and food products. The nutritive base includes peptones, yeast extract with buffers, and glucose. Polysorbate 80 (Tween 80) supplies fatty acids and magnesium for additional growth requirements. Sodium acetate and ammonium citrate may inhibit normal flora including gram-negative bacteria, oral flora, and fungi and improve the growth of the lactobacilli. The growth of lactobacilli is favored when the pH is adjusted to 6.1 to 6.6. Gas production can help identify leuconostocs from pediococci in conjunction with arginine degradation to differentiate these organisms from lactobacilli (9). See chapter 31.

■ **Levinthal agar with bacitracin and *Haemophilus influenzae* antiserum (see Chocolate agar)**

■ **Lim broth**

Lim broth is a modification of Todd-Hewitt broth and is an enriched selective liquid medium used for the isolation and cultivation of *Streptococcus agalactiae*. Peptones, salts, and dextrose provide the nutritional base. Yeast extract provides B vitamins and additional enrichment. The antibiotics colistin and nalidixic acid inhibit gram-negative organisms. Lim broth has shown better recovery of group B streptococcus than Todd-Hewitt with gentamicin and nalidixic acid (K. Fackrell and N. Dick, *Abstr. 101st Gen. Meet. Am. Soc. Microbiol.*, abstr. C-107, 2001).

■ **Lithium chloride-phenylethanol-moxalactam agar**

Lithium chloride-phenylethanol-moxalactam agar is an enriched and selective agar used for the isolation and cultivation of *Listeria monocytogenes*. Peptones and beef extract are the nutritive base. Phenylethyl alcohol, glycine anhydride, and lithium chloride suppress the growth of gram-positive and gram-negative organisms. Moxalactam makes the agar more selective by inhibiting gram-negative organisms such as *Pseudomonas* and additional gram-positive organisms. *Listeria* enriched in a broth for 24 h is subsequently subcultured onto the selective medium for isolation when trying to isolate the organism from contaminated sites. The medium is not differential, but use of oblique lighting may show *Listeria* colonies to be blue.

■ **Loeffler's medium**

Loeffler's medium is an enriched nonselective medium used for the cultivation of corynebacteria, especially *Corynebacterium diphtheriae*. The nutritive base is heart infusion and peptones with dextrose. Horse serum and egg cause the medium to coagulate during sterilization and provide other nutritive proteins. The medium enhances the production of metachromatic granules within the cells of the organisms. These granules are seen when smears of the organism are viewed with the methylene blue stain.

■ **Lombard-Dowell egg yolk agar (see Neomycin egg yolk agar)**

■ **Lowenstein-Jensen medium**

Lowenstein-Jensen medium is an enriched nonselective medium used for the isolation and cultivation of mycobacteria. It is similar to American Trudeau Society medium in its content and its ability to grow mycobacteria. Lowenstein-Jensen medium is an egg-based medium with glycerol and potato flour. The concentration of malachite green is twice that in American Trudeau Society medium, and thus, the malachite green is somewhat more inhibitory for contaminating organisms. Inorganic salts may make the medium more enriched for mycobacteria.

■ **Lowenstein-Jensen medium (Gruft modification)**

The Gruft modification of Lowenstein-Jensen medium is an enriched selective medium used for the isolation of mycobacteria. Penicillin and nalidixic acid are added to the medium and inhibit gram-positive and gram-negative organisms, respectively. RNA is added as a growth stimulant.

■ **Lowenstein-Jensen medium (Mycobactosel modification)**

The Mycobactosel modification of Lowenstein-Jensen medium is an enriched selective medium used for the isolation of mycobacteria. Antibiotics different from those used in the Gruft modification are added to make the medium more selective against bacteria. Cycloheximide, lincomycin, and nalidixic acid inhibit saprophytic fungi, gram-positive organisms, and gram-negative organisms, respectively. No RNA is added.

■ Lowenstein-Jensen medium with 1% ferric ammonium citrate

Lowenstein-Jensen medium with 1% ferric ammonium citrate is an enriched and selective egg-based medium used for the recovery of *Mycobacterium haemophilum*. Ferric ammonium citrate is the additive which allows this organism to grow.

■ Lowenstein-Jensen medium with 5% NaCl

Lowenstein-Jensen medium with 5% NaCl is an enriched selective medium used to differentiate sodium chloride-tolerant strains of *Mycobacterium*. Most rapid growers, i.e., the *Mycobacterium fortuitum* complex, as well as the more slowly growing organism *Mycobacterium triviale*, grow on this medium. The exception is the more resistant organism *Mycobacterium chelonae*, which does not grow on this medium.

■ Lysis-centrifugation tube (see Isolator)

■ MacConkey agar

MacConkey agar is a selective and differential medium used for the isolation of gram-negative organisms. The nutritive base includes a variety of peptones. The medium is made selective by the incorporation of bile (although at levels less than those used in other enteric media) and crystal violet, which inhibit gram-positive organisms, especially enterococci and staphylococci. An agar concentration greater than that described in the original reference helps to inhibit swarming *Proteus*. The medium is differential by use of the combination of neutral red and lactose. When an organism ferments lactose, the drop in pH causes the colony to take on a pink-red appearance.

■ MacConkey agar with sorbitol (SMAC)

SMAC is a selective and differential medium used for the isolation and differentiation of sorbitol-negative *E. coli*. Shiga toxin-producing strains of *E. coli*, such as *E. coli* O157:H7, which may cause hemorrhagic colitis, are indistinguishable from other *E. coli* serotypes on routine stool isolation media such as MacConkey agar because they all ferment lactose. SMAC has D-sorbitol instead of the lactose in the MacConkey agar formulation. Shiga toxin-producing strains of *E. coli* do not ferment sorbitol and appear as colorless colonies. Sorbitol-fermenting strains are pink. The medium inhibits enterococci with crystal violet and other gram-positive organisms with bile salts. SMAC with cefixime and tellurite has been used to increase selection of *E. coli*. However, some strains may be inhibited.

■ MacConkey broth

MacConkey broth is a differential medium containing the indicator bromocresol purple used for the detection of coliform organisms from contaminated food, water, or stools. The broth contains peptone, lactose, bile salts, and sodium chloride. Bromcresol purple is less inhibitory than neutral red for coliforms. The color change from purple to yellow is a more sensitive and definitive indication of acid formation.

■ Mannitol-egg yolk-polymyxin B agar

Mannitol-egg yolk-polymyxin B agar is an enriched, selective, and differential medium used for the isolation of *B. cereus* from mixed clinical specimens. The nutritive base includes peptone and beef extract. Egg yolk emulsion is added for the detection of lecithinase activity, which is usually limited to *B. cereus*. Phenol red and mannitol are combined to make the medium differential. Contaminating gram-negative organisms are inhibited by the polymyxin B.

■ Mannitol salt agar

Mannitol salt agar is a selective and differential medium used for the isolation of *S. aureus*. The nutritive base includes peptones, beef extract, and mannitol. Phenol red is the indicator. The selective nature of the medium is the high salt content (7.5% NaCl), which inhibits most organisms except staphylococci. The differential component for identification of *S. aureus* is the combination of mannitol and phenol red. The color change around the colony from red to yellow upon the fermentation of mannitol and the subsequent drop in the pH of the medium identifies the staphylococcus.

■ Martin-Lewis agar

Martin-Lewis agar is an enriched and selective medium for the isolation of *N. gonorrhoeae*, (27). Martin-Lewis agar is a modification of the modified Thayer-Martin formulation. The nutritive base is chocolate agar. The specific differences from the modified Thayer-Martin formulation are the use of a higher concentration of vancomycin (4.0 versus 3.0 μg/ml), which inhibits more gram-positive organisms, and the replacement of nystatin with anisomycin, which improves the inhibition of *Candida* species. Trimethoprim and colistin are incorporated as well for inhibition of other commensal organisms. Some strains of pathogenic *Neisseria* have been reported to be inhibited by vancomycin and trimethoprim.

■ MB/BacT ALERT

The MB/BacT ALERT contains a modified Middlebrook 7H9 medium supplemented with casein, bovine serum albumin, and catalase. It is used with the MB/BacT ALERT 3D system (bioMérieux, Inc.) for the cultivation and detection of mycobacterial growth.

■ Middlebrook 7H10 agar

Middlebrook 7H10 agar is an enriched nonselective agar-based medium used for the isolation and cultivation of *Mycobacterium* species. Essential ingredients include inorganic salts, glycerol, and an OADC enrichment. The OADC enrichment includes oleic acid, which is a fatty acid used in the metabolism of mycobacteria; albumin, which protects against toxic agents and which is a source of protein; dextrose, which is used as a source of energy; and catalase, which destroys toxic peroxides in the medium.

■ **Middlebrook 7H11 agar**

Middlebrook 7H11 agar is a nonselective agar-based medium used for the isolation and cultivation of *Mycobacterium* species. The formulation is identical to that of Middlebrook 7H10 medium except for the addition of casein hydrolysate. Casein hydrolysate is added as a growth stimulant for drug-resistant strains of *M. tuberculosis*. The formulation of Middlebrook 7H11 thin pour agar is identical to that of Middlebrook 7H11 agar except that the agar plate has a reduced volume. The plates are sealed and every 2 days are examined along the isolation streak lines for evidence of microcolonies. This technique allows for faster detection on solid medium than in standard tube media or on thick media on plates.

■ **Middlebrook 7H9 broth with glycerol**

Middlebrook 7H9 broth with glycerol is an enriched nonselective broth for the isolation of *Mycobacterium* species. Glycerol, inorganic compounds, and cations supply essential nutrients and stimulate growth. ADC enrichment is added to the broth. ADC enrichment includes albumin, which binds to free fatty acids that are toxic to *Mycobacterium* species; dextrose, which supplies energy; and catalase, which destroys toxic peroxides which may be present in the medium.

■ **Mitchison 7H11 selective agar**

Mitchison 7H11 selective agar is an enriched selective agar-based medium used for the isolation of *Mycobacterium* species. The basic formulation is Middlebrook 7H11 agar: glycerol, inorganic salts, casein hydrolysate, malachite green, and OADC enrichment. Antibiotics are added to make the medium very selective for mycobacteria. Carbenicillin and polymyxin B, amphotericin B, and trimethoprim are active against most members of the family *Enterobacteriaceae*, yeast, and *Proteus* species, respectively.

■ **Modified irgasan-ticarcillin-potassium chromate broth**

Modified irgasan-ticarcillin-potassium chromate broth is a selective broth used for the isolation of *Yersinia enterocolitica*. The base is the modified Rappaport-Vassiliadis enrichment broth with minor alterations. Irgasan and ticarcillin replace the carbenicillin. The chromate makes the medium more selective by inhibiting members of the family *Enterobacteriaceae*. *Enterobacteriaceae* have A nitrase activity which splits chlorate to toxic by-products. *Yersinia* spp. have B nitrase activity which cannot split the chlorate.

■ **Modified Thayer-Martin agar**

Modified Thayer-Martin agar is an enriched and selective agar for the isolation of pathogenic *Neisseria* species from clinical specimens with mixed flora. The nutritive base is chocolate agar. Modified Thayer-Martin agar has three significant changes from the original Thayer-Martin medium. The medium has less agar and less dextrose, and these characteristics allow the improved growth of *Neisseria*. The third change was the addition of trimethoprim, which inhibits swarming *Proteus* spp. Vancomycin and colistin inhibit gram-positive and gram-negative bacteria, respectively. This medium is recommended over the original

formulation for the isolation of pathogenic *Neisseria*. Some strains of pathogenic *Neisseria* have been reported to be inhibited by vancomycin and trimethoprim.

■ **Mueller-Hinton agar with and without 5% sheep blood**

Mueller-Hinton agar is the agar recommended by NCCLS for the routine susceptibility testing of nonfastidious microorganisms by the Kirby-Bauer disk diffusion susceptibility method. Mueller-Hinton agar with 5% sheep blood is used for susceptibility testing of *Streptococcus pneumoniae*. Beef and casein extracts and soluble starch in an agar base make up the nutritive base of the medium. Starch protects the organism from toxic materials that may be in the medium. Calcium and magnesium concentrations are controlled.

■ **Mueller-Hinton agar with 2% NaCl**

Mueller-Hinton agar with 2% NaCl is a selective medium used for testing the susceptibility of *Staphylococcus* to the penicillinase-resistant penicillins methicillin, nafcillin, and oxacillin by agar dilution or with the gradient-based system (E test). The sodium chloride added to the medium enhances the growth of staphylococci. Heteroresistant methicillin-resistant strains are more easily detected with this medium by increasing the incubation time to 24 h and by incubation at cooler temperatures (35°C).

■ **Mueller-Hinton agar with 4% NaCl and 6 μg of oxacillin per ml**

Mueller-Hinton agar with 4% NaCl and 6 μg of oxacillin per ml is selective and is the differential medium used to screen *S. aureus* for resistance to penicillinase-resistant penicillins (e.g., nafcillin, methacillin, and oxacillin). Incubation for 24 h at 35°C in ambient air is recommended before interpretation of growth. Use transmitted light.

■ **Mueller-Hinton broth**

Mueller-Hinton broth is a magnesium and calcium cation-adjusted liquid medium used in procedures for the susceptibility testing of aerobic gram-positive and gram-negative organisms by both macrodilution and microdilution methods. The nutritive base includes beef extract and peptones. Starch is a detoxifying agent.

■ **Multiprobe medium**

Multiprobe medium (M4) is a collection and transport medium used for viral, chlamydial, and mycoplasma organisms. The medium is a supplemented Hanks' balanced salt solution buffered with HEPES buffer and with phenol red as the pH indicator. The antibiotics vancomycin, amphotericin B, and colistin are added to inhibit bacterial organisms, and as such, the medium cannot be used for bacterial culture.

■ **Mycobacteria growth indicator tube (MGIT)**

MGIT (Becton Dickinson Microbiology Systems) is a Middlebrook 7H9-based broth system that contains a fluorescence indicator, which is used for the detection of mycobacterial growth. Middlebrook 7H9 broth is supplemented with multiple growth enrichments prior to use. The chapter on *Mycobacterium* (chapter 36) describes and compares this system with the BACTEC system in much more detail.

■ Mycobactosel agar

Mycobactosel is a BBL trade name for an enriched selective agar-based medium used for the isolation of *Mycobacterium* species. The medium is called by other names, depending on the manufacturer. The basic formulation is a Middlebrook 7H11 base, glycerol, inorganic salts, casein hydrolysate, malachite green, and OADC enrichment. Antibiotics are added to make the medium selective. The principle used for the Middlebrook 7H11 formulation to which antibiotics are added is the same as that used for Mitchison 7H11 medium. The antibiotics differ between Mycobactosel agar and Mitchison 7H11 medium. The antibiotics in Mycobactosel agar are cycloheximide, lincomycin, and nalidixic acid, which inhibit saprophytic fungi, gram-positive organisms, and gram-negative organisms, respectively.

■ NAG medium

NAG medium is an enriched and selective medium used for the isolation and cultivation of *Haemophilus* species from clinical specimens with mixed flora. The agar base is blood agar with *N*-acetyl-D-glucosamine (NAG), hemin, and NAD. NAG medium allows spheroblastic *Haemophilus influenzae* to revert morphologically. Spheroblastic forms may be seen in patients receiving beta-lactam antibiotics. Bacitracin makes the medium selective by inhibiting gram-positive organisms that occur as normal respiratory flora. This medium has been found to be especially helpful in isolating *H. influenzae* from respiratory specimens from cystic fibrosis patients. Placement of cefsulodin disks on the primary streak helps to inhibit *Pseudomonas* spp. to make the medium more selective.

■ Neomycin egg yolk agar

Neomycin egg yolk agar is a selective and differential medium used for the differentiation of anaerobic organisms that are lipase positive, including *Clostridium* spp., *Prevotella intermedia*, *Fusobacterium necrophorum*, and some strains of *Prevotella loescheii*. The nutritive base includes peptones and yeast extract. Vitamin K and L-cystine make the medium optimal for the isolation of anaerobes. Egg emulsion adds enrichment and makes the medium differential by detecting lipase activity. Neomycin makes the medium selective by inhibiting both gram-positive and gram-negative organisms and differential by the fermentation of lactose.

■ Neomycin-vancomycin agar

Neomycin-vancomycin agar is an enriched and selective medium that is particularly good for the isolation and cultivation of *Fusobacterium* from clinical specimens. The nutritive base is fastidious anaerobe agar with 5% sheep blood. The selective agents include neomycin and vancomycin, which inhibit gram-negative and gram-positive organisms, respectively.

■ New York City medium

New York City medium is an enriched and selective medium for the isolation of pathogenic *Neisseria* from clinical specimens. It also supports the growth of large-colony mycoplasmas and *U. urealyticum*. The medium is a clear peptone-corn starch agar base with lysed horse erythrocytes, horse plasma, and yeast dialysate, which are used instead of the hemoglobin and the supplements used for the other enriched and selective media for *Neisseria*. The antibiotics that make the medium selective include vancomycin, colistin, and amphotericin B, which inhibit gram-positive bacteria, gram-negative bacteria, and fungi, respectively. While human blood products can replace the horse blood products, sheep blood cannot be used.

■ Nucleic acid transport (NAT) (Medical Packaging Corporation)

NAT is a nucleic acid transport device that has been cleared by the Food and Drug Administration for use with multiple amplification and hybridization testing formats.

■ Oxford agar

Oxford agar is an enriched and selective medium used for the isolation of *Listeria monocytogenes*. Columbia agar is the base, and it is supplemented with esculin and ferric ammonium citrate for the detection of esculin hydrolysis by listeriae. Suppression of contaminants is accomplished by the addition of lithium, cycloheximide, colistin, acriflavine, cefotetan, and fosfomycin. A modified Oxford agar replaces cycloheximide, acriflavine, cefotetan, and fosfomycin with moxalactam. Listerias appear black with a black halo.

■ Oxidative-fermentative polymyxin B-bacitracin-lactose agar

Oxidative-fermentative polymyxin B-bacitracin-lactose medium is a selective and differential medium used for the isolation of *Burkholderia cepacia* from respiratory specimens from patients with cystic fibrosis. The nutritive base is an oxidative-fermentative medium with peptones. When acid is produced from the utilization of the lactose sugar, as occurs with *B. cepacia*, the bromthymol blue indicator changes the colony from green to yellow. Polymyxin B and bacitracin are the selective agents and inhibit some gram-negative and gram-positive organisms, respectively. Other organisms seen in cystic fibrosis patients may grow on this medium and are differentiated by the inability to produce acid from lactose.

■ P agar

P agar is an enriched medium used for cultivation and isolation of staphylococci. The agar base includes peptone, yeast extract, NaCl, and glucose.

■ Peptone yeast extract broth

Peptone yeast extract broth is a controlled medium used in the analysis of metabolic products by gas-liquid chromatography because there is negligible acid volatility within the medium.

■ Petragnani medium

Petragnani medium is an egg-based medium. It contains more than twice the concentration of malachite green in the Lowenstein-Jensen medium and is most commonly used for the isolation and cultivation of mycobacteria from heavily contaminated specimens. It is also used for the cultivation and maintenance of *Mycobacterium smegmatis*.

■ Phenylethyl alcohol (PEA) agar

PEA agar is an enriched and selective blood agar medium used for the detection and isolation of anaerobic organisms, particularly fastidious and slowly growing bacteria, from clinical specimens with mixed flora. The base is Trypticase soy agar with yeast extract, vitamin K, cystine, and hemin. The medium is selective as a result of the incorporation of phenylethyl alcohol, which reversibly inhibits DNA synthesis and thus inhibits facultative anaerobic gram-negative bacteria, such as members of the family *Enterobacteriaceae*. PEA agar inhibits swarming by *Proteus* spp. and *Clostridium septicum*.

■ PLM-5 TM

PLM-5 TM is a proprietary medium formulation similar to Ellinghausen-McCullough/Johnson-Harris medium that is used for the isolation and cultivation of *Leptospira*.

■ Polymyxin B-acriflavine-lithium chloride-ceftazidime-esculin-mannitol (PALCAM) agar

PALCAM agar is an enriched, differential, and selective agar medium used for the isolation of *L. monocytogenes*. Columbia agar supplemented with glucose, mannitol, and yeast extract is the nutritive base. Esculin and ferric ammonium citrate are added to detect esculin hydrolysis by listeriae. Fermentation of mannitol is detected with the indicator dye phenol red. Lithium, acriflavine, ceftazidime, and polymyxin B are added as selective agents. For contaminated specimens an enriched broth is inoculated and incubated for 24 h. Subsequently, 0.1 ml is subcultured onto PALCAM agar. Listeria colonies appear gray-green with a sunken black center.

■ Polymyxin B-lysozyme-EDTA-thallous acetate agar

Polymyxin B-lysozyme-EDTA-thallous acetate agar is a selective agar used for the isolation of *Bacillus anthracis* from environmental specimens. Heart infusion agar is the base. Thallous acetate and EDTA are additional additives speculated to have advantages for the recovery of *B. anthracis*. Lysozyme is an additive which inhibits *Bacillus* spp. other than *B. cereus* and *B. anthracis*. The addition of thallous acetate, EDTA, and lysozyme together has an additive effect which results in the inhibition of most non-*B. anthracis* species. Polymyxin B inhibits gram-negative organisms. Colonies of *B. anthracis* grown on polymyxin B-lysozyme-EDTA-thallous acetate agar are smaller and smoother than those grown on plain heart infusion agar and are creamy white with a ground-glass texture. *B. cereus* is usually inhibited (30).

■ Polymyxin B-pyruvate-egg yolk-mannitol-bromthymol blue agar

Polymyxin B-pyruvate-egg yolk-mannitol-bromthymol blue agar is an enriched, selective, and differential medium used for the isolation of *Bacillus cereus*. The nutritive agar base includes peptones, agar, and buffers. Egg yolk emulsion allows detection of lecithinase activity, which is unique to

B. cereus. Sodium pyruvate is added to reduce the size of the colonies, which may be important when performing plate counts. Bromthymol blue and mannitol combine to make the medium differential. *B. cereus* does not produce acid from mannitol and has a distinctive bright blue color. Polymyxin B inhibits contaminating gram-negative organisms from clinical specimens with mixed flora, such as stool specimens. Mannitol-egg yolk-polymyxin B agar is similarly used for the isolation of *B. cereus*.

■ Polysorbate 80 medium (see Ellinghausen-McCullough/Johnson-Harris medium)

■ *Pseudomonas cepacia* (PC) agar

PC agar is a selective medium used for the isolation of *Burkholderia cepacia* (formerly *Pseudomonas cepacia*) from respiratory specimens from cystic fibrosis patients. The medium was originally derived from a holding medium containing salts, phenol red, and agar in a phosphate buffer. Selective agents include crystal violet, ticarcillin, and polymyxin B, which inhibit many gram-positive and gram-negative organisms. PC agar may inhibit *B. cepacia* as well (20, 24, 55).

■ Rappaport-Vassilladis enrichment broth

Rappaport-Vassiliadis enrichment broth is a selective and enriched broth used for the isolation and cultivation of *Salmonella* spp. from food and environmental specimens. A modified Rappaport-Vassiliadis broth is a more selective broth used for the isolation and cultivation of *Yersinia enterocolitica* from foods. Basic Rappaport-Vassiliadis medium contains soybean peptone digest with salts and malachite green. Malachite green suppresses the growth of contaminating bacteria. The modified Rappaport-Vassiliadis broth uses pancreatic digest of casein with salts, malachite green, and carbenicillin.

■ Regan-Lowe medium

Regan-Lowe medium is an enriched and selective medium used for the isolation of *Bordetella pertussis*. Beef extract, pancreatic digest, horse blood, and niacin are the nutritional base. Starch and charcoal neutralize toxic substances such as fatty acids and peroxides that are toxic to *Bordetella*. Cephalexin is added to inhibit the normal flora in the nasopharynx. Regan-Lowe transport medium contains half-strength charcoal and horse blood.

■ Salmonella-shigella agar

Salmonella-shigella agar is a selective and differential medium used for the isolation and differentiation of *Salmonella* and *Shigella* from clinical specimens and other sources. The nutritive base contains animal and casein peptones and beef extract. The selective agents are bile salts, citrates, and brilliant green dye, which inhibit gram-positive organisms. The high degree of selectivity of the medium results in the inhibition of some strains of *Shigella*, and the medium is not recommended as a primary medium for isolation of this species. The medium contains only lactose and thus differentiates organisms on the basis of lactose fermentation. The formation of acid on fermentation of lactose causes the neutral red indicator to make red colonies. Non-lactose-fermenting organisms are clear on the medium. As with Hektoen enteric agar, sodium thiosulfate and ferric ammonium citrate allow the differentiation of organisms that produce hydrogen sulfide. Lactose fermenters, such as *E. coli*, have colonies which are pink with a precipitate, *Shigella* appears transparent or amber, and *Salmonella* appears transparent or amber with black centers. Some strains of *Shigella dysenteriae* are inhibited.

■ **Schaedler's agar**

Schaedler's agar is a general-purpose medium used for the isolation and cultivation of anaerobic bacteria. The nutritive base includes vegetable and meat peptones, dextrose, and yeast extract. Sheep blood, vitamin K, and hemin provide other additives that stimulate the growth of fastidious anaerobes. Because of the high carbohydrate content, colonies with beta-hemolytic reactions may have a greenish hue. This medium may be better than other nonselective anaerobic media for the isolation of fastidious anaerobic organisms.

■ **Schleifer-Kramer agar**

Schleifer-Kramer agar is a selective medium used for the isolation of *Staphylococcus* from heavily contaminated specimens such as feces. The nutritional base includes casein peptones with beef and yeast extracts, glycine, and sodium pyruvate. Sodium azide at 0.45% makes the medium selective for staphylococci and some other gram-positive organisms by inhibiting gram-negative organisms.

■ **Selenite broth**

Selenite broth is an enrichment broth medium used for the isolation of *Salmonella* and *Shigella* species. Casein and meat peptones provide nutrients. Selenite inhibits enterococci and coliforms that are part of the normal flora if they are subcultured within 12 to 18 h. However, reduction of selenite produces an alkali condition that may inhibit the recovery of *Salmonella*. Lactose and phosphate buffers are added to allow stability of the pH. When fermenting organisms produce acid, the acid neutralizes the effect of the selenite reduction and subsequent alkalinization. Cystine added to selenite broth enhances the recovery of *Salmonella*.

■ **Sensitest agar**

Sensitest agar is a medium used in susceptibility testing outside of the United States. The base is pancreatic digest of casein, peptones, and glucose with other additives. The medium is available as a premixed powder from Oxoid Unipath. See chapter 70 for specific uses.

■ **Septic-Chek biphasic mycobacterial media**

The Septic-Chek system (Becton Dickinson Microbiology Systems) is a mycobacterial culture system which contains modified 7H9 broth and three types of solid media, modified Lowenstein-Jensen, Middlebrook 7H11, and chocolate agars, with various supplements. This medium is described in detail in the chapter on *Mycobacterium* (chapter 36).

■ **Skim milk-tryptone-glucose-glycerin (STGG) medium**

STGG medium is a transport medium that has been used for collection of nasopharyngeal swabs for the purposes of isolation and preservation of *Streptococcus pneumoniae*. Collection and storage of nasopharyngeal swabs on STGG medium at −70 or −20°C were shown to be equal to collection and storage of nasopharyngeal swabs directly on selective medium (44).

■ **Skirrow medium**

Skirrow medium is an enriched selective blood agar medium used for the isolation of *Campylobacter* spp. from specimens with mixed flora. The nutritive agar base is brucella agar. Hematin is provided by sheep blood. The selective agents are trimethoprim, vancomycin, and polymyxin B, which inhibit the normal flora found in fecal specimens.

■ **Storage media (see chapter 7)**

■ **Streptococcus selective agar**

Streptococcus selective agar is a selective medium for detection of streptococci. The agar base is Columbia agar. Various antibiotic supplements have been used to make the medium selective for streptococci and to reduce the numbers of gram-negative organisms. Colistin and oxolinic acid are one combination less detrimental to *Streptococcus* spp. (29).

■ **Stuart's transport media with and without charcoal**

Stuart's transport medium is an early transport medium first described in 1948. This medium uses glycerol phosphate to maintain the specimen as well as maintain the pH, agar, methylene blue as a redox indicator, and sodium thioglycolate to allow the survival of anaerobes. The glycerol phosphate has also been found to be used as an energy source by certain contaminants which may overgrow the desired pathogen. Charcoal may be added and acts as a detoxifying agent.

■ **Sucrose-phosphate-glutamate transport medium**

Sucrose-phosphate-glutamate transport medium is used for the maintenance and transport of *Chlamydia* species and viruses. Sucrose and two buffer solutions are the base. Bovine serum and glutamic acid are additives. Glutamic acid is a stabilizing agent that is especially useful for enveloped viruses. The antibiotic combination may be the same or slightly different from that in 2-sucrose-phosphate. Most commonly the antibiotic combination is vancomycin, streptomycin, and nystatin, which inhibit both gram-positive and gram-negative organisms, as well as yeast.

■ **2-Sucrose-phosphate transport medium**

2-Sucrose-phosphate medium is used for the transport of specimens for the purposes of culturing *Chlamydia trachomatis* and *Mycoplasma* spp. Sucrose (0.2 M) and two potassium phosphate buffers are the base. Fetal bovine serum allows the *Chlamydia* to maintain infectivity, and the antibiotics nystatin and gentamicin are added to inhibit yeast and bacteria.

■ Tetrathionate broth base

Tetrathionate broth base is an enriched liquid medium used for the isolation of *Salmonella* species from contaminated clinical specimens and other products. The nutritive base includes pancreatic digest of casein and peptic digest of animal tissue with sodium thiosulfate. Bile salts inhibit gram-positive organisms and tetrathionate, which is formed when an iodine-potassium iodide solution is added and which is inhibitory to other normal intestinal flora. Addition of brilliant green inhibits gram-negative and gram-positive organisms, including some *Salmonella* spp.

■ Thayer-Martin agar

Thayer-Martin agar is an enriched and selective medium used for the isolation of *Neisseria* from clinical specimens with mixed flora. The nutritive base is chocolate agar, which is a GC agar base with casein and meat peptones, cornstarch for the neutralization of fatty acids, and phosphate buffer for control of the pH. The chocolate agar occurs with the addition of hemoglobin, which provides hemin or X factor, and IsoVitaleX enrichment, which provides NAD, vitamins, and other nutrients, to improve the growth of pathogenic *Neisseria*. The medium is made selective by the addition of vancomycin, colistin, and nystatin, which inhibit the normal flora of gram-positive bacteria, gram-negative bacteria, and fungi, respectively. Some strains of pathogenic *Neisseria* have been reported to be inhibited by vancomycin and trimethoprim.

■ Thioglycolate with hemin and vitamin K

Thioglycolate broth with hemin and vitamin K is an enriched liquid medium used to support the growth of microaerophillic and anaerobic organisms, including fastidious organisms. Casein and soy peptones supply the basic nutrients. Sodium thioglycolate and L-cystine are the reducing agents in the medium, while hemin and vitamin K are additional additives that allow more fastidious anaerobes to thrive. A small amount of agar helps to slow the diffusion of oxygen and is more suitable for anaerobic organisms.

■ Thiosulfate citrate bile salt sucrose (TCBS)

TCBS is a highly selective and differential medium for the recovery of *Vibrio* spp. except *V. hollisae* and *V. cincinnatiensis*. The medium is inhibitory to gram-positive organisms by incorporation of oxgall, a naturally occurring substance containing a mixture of bile salts and sodium cholate, a pure bile salt. Peptic and casein digests are the nutritive base, and sucrose is a fermentable carbohydrate for the metabolism of vibrios. Sodium thiosulfate provides a sulfur source, and ferric citrate detects hydrogen sulfide production. Bromthymol blue and thymol blue are the pH indicators. Alkaline pH enhances the recovery of *V. cholerae*. The color that appears on the agar is dependent on the species. See chapter 46.

■ Tinsdale agar (see Cystine-tellurite blood agar)

■ Todd-Hewitt broth with gentamicin and nalidixic acid

Todd-Hewitt broth is used for the isolation of beta-hemolytic streptococci from mixed flora, especially group B streptococci from vaginal specimens. Beef heart infusion and peptone are the nutritive base, dextrose is the energy source, and sodium-based buffers protect the hemolysin from inactivation. The antibiotics make the medium selective by inhibiting gram-negative bacilli.

■ Tryptic or Trypticase soy agar base with 5% sheep blood

Tryptic or Trypticase soy agar base with 5% sheep blood is a general-purpose medium used for the isolation of a wide variety of organisms. The medium contains soybean and casein peptones as the nutritive base. The addition of sheep blood enriches the medium, and the sheep blood allows the growth of more fastidious organisms by providing hemin (X factor). V factor (NAD) is inactivated by enzymes in the sheep blood and thus does not allow the growth of organisms that require the NAD additive, such as *Haemophilus influenzae*. The use of sheep blood provides an excellent means of interpretation of hemolytic reactions, especially those of *Streptococcus* spp.

■ Tryptic or Trypticase soy broth

Tryptic or Trypticase soy broth is a general-purpose clear liquid medium used for the cultivation of a wide variety of organisms. It is also recommended by NCCLS for preparation of an inoculum for Kirby-Bauer disk diffusion susceptibility testing and is the NCCLS choice as a sterility testing medium. The base includes digests of casein and soybean, with additional additives of glucose, sodium chloride to maintain osmotic equilibrium, and buffers. For the purpose of a blood culture medium, additional additives include carbon dioxide to enhance the growth of microorganisms and SPS, an anticoagulant, to inactivate blood components and aminoglycosides. Formulations with 6.5% NaCl exist for the purposes of differentiating enterococcal species or salt-tolerant streptococci. Fildes enrichment is added to cultivate fastidious organisms such as *Haemophilus* spp.

■ Trypticase soy agar with horse or rabbit blood

Trypticase soy agar with horse or rabbit blood medium is used for the isolation of *Haemophilus* species. The nutritive base is a combination of soy and casein peptones. The medium provides smaller but adequate amounts of X (hemin) and V (NAD) factors compared to the amounts in sheep blood and is used for the isolation of *Haemophilus* species. In addition, the medium with horse or rabbit blood allows determination of hemolytic reactions.

■ University of Vermont modified Listeria enrichment broth

University of Vermont modified Listeria enrichment broth is an enriched and selective liquid medium used for the isolation of *Listeria monocytogenes*. The nutritive base contains pancreatic digest of casein and animal tissue and beef and yeast extract and is supplemented with esculin, acriflavine, and nalidixic acid.

■ VACC III medium

VACC III medium is a transport and collection medium specifically designed to maintain the viability of mixed anaerobes from peridontal and endodontal sites. The medium is particularly useful for transport of paper points that are placed in gingival crevices to soak up secretions. Prereduced, buffered salt suspension (0.5 to 2.0 ml) is placed into a tube with a similar total volume (2 ml) with or without six to eight glass beads (diameter, 0.1 to 1.5 mm). The beads aid in dispersing the polysaccharide matrices that occur with gingival plaques and granular aggregates (52).

■ V agar

V agar is an enriched and selective medium used for the isolation of *Haemophilus ducreyi* from clinical specimens. The nutritive base is GC agar. The addition of 2% hemoglobin, 5% fetal bovine serum, and a supplement containing NAD enhances the recovery of the organism. Vancomycin at 3 μg/ml is added to the medium to make it selective for the pathogen and to inhibit contaminating bacteria. Many formulations with the GC agar base, the enrichments, and vancomycin exist.

■ Wadowsky-Yee medium (see Buffered charcoal yeast extract medium)

■ Wilkins-Chalgren broth and agar

Wilkins-Chalgren medium is recommended for susceptibility testing with anaerobic organisms. The medium contains specific nutrients that support the growth of anaerobes such as yeast extract, vitamin K, hemin, and arginine. The use of peptones allows a more standardized medium.

■ Xylose-lysine-desoxycholate agar

Xylose-lysine-desoxycholate agar is a selective and differential medium used for the isolation and differentiation of enteric pathogens from clinical specimens. The nutritive base includes carbohydrates and yeast extract. This medium is more supportive of fastidious enteric organisms such as *Shigella*. The selective agent is desoxycholate, which inhibits gram-positive organisms. Phenol red is the color indicator. As with Hektoen enteric and Salmonella-Shigella agars, ferric ammonium citrate (indicator) and sodium thiosulfate (sulfur source) allow identification of organisms that produce H_2S with the appearance of colonies with a black center. The medium contains xylose, which most enteric organisms ferment. The most important exception is *Shigella*, the colonies of which appear to be transparent or the color of the red media. The lysine in the medium is utilized by the enteric organisms that contain the lysine decarboxylase enzyme. For *Salmonella*, which contains the lysine enzyme, this reaction reverts the pH to an alkaline state and the colony appears to be transparent or red with a black center. The lactose and sucrose in the medium help to differentiate other enteric organisms. When other enteric organisms ferment these sugars, they maintain the pH at an acidic condition and the colonies appear yellow or yellow-red.

■ Yersinia selective agar (see Cefsulodin-irgasan-novobiocin medium)

APPENDIX 1
Medium Additives

N-2-Acetamido-2-aminoethane sulfonic acid (ACES): allows optimal pH buffering capacity without inhibition of bacteria as seen with other inorganic buffers

Acriflavine: selective agent, suppresses gram-positive organisms

ADC enrichment: a supplement added to mycobacteriology media that includes albumin, dextrose, catalase, and sodium chloride; catalase destroys peroxides that may be in the medium

Agar used in broth medium (0.05 to 0.1%): used to reduce O_2 tension

Albumin: protects against toxic by-products in medium; binds free fatty acids

Antibiotics: one or many may be added to make a medium selective; inhibitory capacity may vary depending on the concentration used

Bismuth sulfite: heavy metal that is inhibitory to commensal organisms

Carbohydrates: energy source; used to make medium differential when combined with an indicator

Cetrimide: acts as a quaternary ammonium cationic detergent that causes nitrogen and phosphorus to be released from bacterial cells other than *Pseudomonas aeruginosa*

Charcoal: detoxifying agent, surface tension modifier, scavenger of radicals and peroxides

Cornstarch: works as a detoxifying agent; may provide additional nutrients as an energy source

Dextrose: makes the medium hypertonic, energy source

Egg yolk: used to demonstrate lecithinase, lipase, and proteolytic activities and fatty acids

Ferric ammonium citrate: iron salt used in combination with other agents (esculin, sodium thiosulfate) to make medium differential by producing a black precipitate

Fildes: peptic digest of sheep blood that provides a rich source of nutrients including X (hemin) and V (NAD) factors

Glycerol: a purified alcohol and an abundant source of carbon; used in culture, transport, and storage media and reagent preparation

Glycine: a selective agent that is inhibitory to organisms

IsoVitaleX (BBL): provides V factor (NAD) and additional nutritive ingredients, such as vitamins, amino acids, ferric ion, and dextrose, to stimulate growth of fastidious organisms

Laked blood: created by freeze-thaw cycles of blood; enhances pigment production of anaerobes

Lithium chloride: a selective agent that inhibits organisms

Malachite green: a dye that partially inhibits bacteria

NAD (V factor): necessary for growth of some fastidious organisms

OADC enrichment: a supplement added to mycobacteriology media that includes oleic acid, albumin, dextrose, catalase, and sodium chloride; the oleic acid provides fatty acids utilized by mycobacteria, and the catalase destroys peroxides that may be in the medium

Oxgall (bile): inhibits specific organisms; allows medium to be selective

Peptones: carbohydrate-free source of nutrients

Phenylethyl alcohol: reversibly inhibits DNA synthesis; results in inhibition of facultative anaerobic gram-negative organisms

Pyridoxal: liquid supplement added to media for isolation of fastidious organisms; also comes in the form of a disk to be used in satellite tests.

Rabbit blood: enhances pigment production of anaerobes; hemolytic reactions of streptococci are "correct"

Serum: albumin, fatty acids

Sheep blood and human blood: provide hemin and other nutrients; allow true hemolytic reactions of streptococci; NADase enzyme inactivates the NAD in the sheep blood and is not available for organisms

Sodium azide: a selective agent that inhibits gram-negative organisms

Sodium bicarbonate: neutralization agent used with gastric wash or lavage specimens for recovery of acid-fast organisms.

Sodium bisulfite: disinfectant, antioxidant, or reducing agent

Sodium chloride: maintains osmotic equilibrium; when added at a high concentration it may be a selective agent

Sodium citrate: a selective agent, inhibitory to organisms

Sodium desoxycholate: a salt of bile acid and a selective agent that inhibits gram-positive and spore-forming organisms

Sodium polyanethole sulfonate (SPS): a polyanionic anticoagulant that inactivates aminoglycosides, interferes with the complement cascade, lysozyme activity, and phagocytic activity inherent in blood; may be inhibitory to *Neisseria*, *Gardnerella*, *Streptobacillus*, *Peptostreptococcus*, *Francsella* and *Moraxella* spp.

Sodium pyruvate: growth stimulant

Sodium selenite: a selective agent that inhibits coliforms

Sodium thioglycolate: a reducing agent

Starch: a polysaccharide and detoxifying agent; incorporated into some media as a differential agent

Tellurite: is toxic to egg-clearing strains of bacteria; imparts black color to colony

Tween 80 (polysorbate 80): an oleic acid ester that stimulates growth and provides fatty acids as well as acts as a dispersal agent

Vitamin K: ingredient required for optimal growth of certain obligate anaerobes, such as the *Bacteroides* group

Yeast extract: water-soluble product that provides B vitamins and proteins

APPENDIX 2
Product Suppliers and Manufacturers of Reagents, Stains, Microscopes, and Media

1. Anaerobe Systems
   15906 Concord Circle
   Morgan Hill, CA 95037
2. Applied Biosystems
   850 Lincoln Centre Drive
   Foster City, CA 94404
3. BBL/Difco (see Becton Dickinson Microbiology Systems)
4. Becton Dickinson Microbiology Systems
   7 Loveton Circle
   Sparks, MD 21152
   800-638-8663
   www.bd.com/microbiology
5. Carl Zeiss, Inc., Microscopy
   & Imaging Systems
   One Zeiss Drive
   Thorwood, NY 10594
   www.zeiss.com/micro
6. Carr-Scarbourough (see Remel)
7. Chromager
   4, place du 18 Juin 1940
   Paris, F-75006
   France
   www.chromager.com
8. Copan Diagnostics, Inc.
   2175 Sampson Avenue, Suite 124
   Corona, CA 92879
   www.Copanusa.com
9. Hardy Diagnostics
   1430 West McCoy Lane
   Santa Monica, CA 93455
   www.Hardydignostics.com
10. Lab M
    35888 Center Ridge Road
    North Ridgeville, OH 44039
    www.idgplc.com
11. Marcor Development Corporation
    341 Mechele Place
    Carlstadt, NJ 07072
12. Medical Chemical Corporation
    19430 Van Ness Avenue
    Torrance, CA 90501
13. Medical Packaging Corporation
    941 Avenido Acaso
    Carnarillo, CA 93012
14. Medical Wire & Equipment-MWE
    Leafield Industrial Estate
    Corsham, Wiltshire, SN13 9RT
    England
    www.mwe.co.uk
15. Nikon Instruments, Inc.
    1300 Walt Whitman Road
    Melville, NY 11747
    www.nikonusa.com
16. Northeast Laboratory Services
    P.O. Box 788
    Rt. 137 China Rd.
    Waterville, ME 04903
    800-244-8378
17. Olympus America, Inc.
    Two Corporate Center Drive
    Melville, NY 11747
    www.olympus.com
18. Oxoid, Inc.
    800 Proctor Avenue
    Ogdensburg, NY 13669
    www.oxoid.ca
19. PML Microbiologicals
    27120 SW 95th Avenue
    Wilsonville, OR 97070
    www.Pmlmicro.com
20. Remel, Inc.
    12076 Santa Fe Drive
    Lenexa, KS 66215
    www.remelinc.com
21. Starplex Scientific, Inc.
    50 Steinway Boulevard
    Etobicoke, Ontario M9W 6Y3
    Canada
    www.starplexscientific.com

REFERENCES

1. **Ashdown, L. R.** 1979. An improved screening technique for isolation of Pseudomonas pseudomallei from clinical specimens. *Pathology* **11:**293–297.
2. **Atkins, K. N.** 1920. Report of committee on descriptive chart. Part III. A modification of the Gram stain. *J. Bacteriol.* **5:**321–324.
3. **Atlas, R. M., and J. W. Snyder.** 1995. *Handbook of Media for Clinical Microbiology*, 2nd ed. CRC Press, Inc., Boca Raton, Fla.
4. **Atlas, R. M., and L. C. Parks.** 1997. *Microbiological Media*. CRC Press, Inc., Boca Raton, Fla.
5. **Balows, A., and W. Hausler.** 1988. *Diagnostic Procedures for Bacterial, Mycotic and Parasitic Infection*, 7th ed. American Public Health Association, Washington, D.C.

6. **Balows, A., W. J. Hausler, Jr., K. L. Herrmann, H. D. Isenberg, and H. J. Shadomy (ed.).** 1991. *Manual of Clinical Microbiology,* 5th ed. American Society for Microbiology, Washington, D.C.

7. **Bartlett, J. G., K. J. Ryan, T. F. Smith, and W. R. Wilson.** 1987. *Cumitech 7A, Laboratory Diagnosis of Lower Respiratory Tract Infections.* Coordinating ed., J. A. Washington II. American Society for Microbiology, Washington, D.C.

8. **Chapin-Robertson, K., S. E. Dahlberg, and S. C. Edberg.** 1992. Clinical and laboratory analyses of cytospin-prepared Gram stains for recovery and diagnosis of bacteria from sterile body fluids. *J. Clin. Microbiol.* **30:**377–380.

9. **DeMan, J. C., M. Rogosa, and M. E. Sharpe.** 1960. A medium for the cultivation of lactobacilli. *J. Appl. Bacteriol.* **23:**130–135.

10. **Difco Laboratories.** 1985. Dehydrated culture media and reagents for microbiology, p. 9–25. *In The Difco Manual,* 10th ed. Difco Laboratories, Detroit, Mich.

11. **Difco Laboratories.** 1998. *The Difco Manual,* 11th ed. Difco Laboratories, Division of Becton Dickinson, Sparks, Md.

12. **Doern, G. V., and R. N. Jones.** 1991. Antimicrobial susceptibility test: fastidious and unusual bacteria, p. 1130. *In* A. Balows, W. J. Hausler, Jr., K. L. Herrmann, H. D. Isenberg, and H. J. Shadomy (ed.), *Manual of Clinical Microbiology,* 5th ed. American Society for Microbiology, Washington, D.C.

13. **Emmons, C., C. Binford, K. J. Kwon-Chung, and J. Utz.** 1977. *Medical Mycology,* 3rd ed. Lea & Febiger, Philadelphia, Pa.

14. **Engelkirk, P. G., J. Duben-Engelkirk, and V. R. Dowell.** 1992. *Principles and Practice of Clinical Anaerobic Bacteriology.* Star Publishing Co., Belmont, Calif.

15. **Ewing, W. H.** 1986. *Edwards and Ewing's Identification of Enterobacteriaceae,* 4th ed. Elsevier, New York, N.Y.

16. **Faller, A., and K.-H. Schleifer.** 1981. Modified oxidase and benzidine tests for separation of staphylococci from micrococci. *J. Clin. Microbiol.* **13:**1031–1035.

17. **Fisher, J. F., M. Ganapathy, B. H. Edwards, and C. L. Newman.** 1990. Utility of Gram's and Giemsa stains in the diagnosis of pulmonary tuberculosis. *Am. Rev. Respir. Dis.* **141:**511–513.

18. **Forbes, B. A., D. F. Sahm, and A. S. Weissfeld.** 1999. Role of microscopy in the diagnosis of infectious disease, 134–149. *In Bailey and Scott's Diagnostic Microbiology,* 10th ed. The C.V. Mosby Co., St. Louis, Mo.

19. **Gill, V. J., N. A. Nelson, F. Stock, and G. Evans.** 1988. Optimal use of the cytocentrifuge for recovery and diagnosis of *Pneumocystis carinii* in bronchoalveolar lavage and sputum specimens. *J. Clin. Microbiol.* **26:**1641–1644.

20. **Gilligan, P. H., P. A. Gage, L. M. Bradshaw, D. V. Schidlow, and B. T. DeCicco.** 1985. Isolation medium for the recovery of *Pseudomonas cepacia* from respiratory secretions of patients with cystic fibrosis. *J. Clin. Microbiol.* **22:**5–8.

21. **Groden, L. R., J. Rodnite, J. H. Brinser, and G. I. Genvert.** 1990. Acridine orange and Gram stains in infectious keratitis. *Cornea* **9:**122–124.

22. **Heineman, H. S., J. K. Chawla, and W. M. Lofton.** 1977. Misinformation from sputum cultures without microscopic examination. *J. Clin. Microbiol.* **6:**518–527.

23. **Henrickson, K. J., K. R. Powell, and D. H. Ryan.** 1988. Evaluation of acridine orange-stained buffy coat smears for identification of bacteremia in children. *J. Pediatr.* **112:** 65–86.

24. **Henry, D., M. Campbell, C. McGimpsey, A. L. Clarke, L. Louden, J. L. Burns, M. H. Roe, P. Vandamme, and D. Speert.** 1999. Comparison of isolation media for recovery of *Burkholderia cepacia* complex from respiratory secretions of patients with cystic fibrosis. *J. Clin. Microbiol.* **37:**1004–1007.

25. **Hutchinson, D. H., and F. J. Bolton.** 1984. Improved blood free selective medium for the isolation of Campylobacter jejuni from faecal specimens. *J. Clin. Pathol.* **37:** 956–957.

26. **Isenberg, H. D. (ed. in chief).** 1992. *Clinical Microbiology Procedures Handbook.* American Society for Microbiology, Washington, D.C.

27. **Kellogg, D. S., Jr., K. K. Holmes, and G. A. Hill.** 1976. *Cumitech 4, Laboratory Diagnosis of Gonorrhea.* Coordinating ed., S. Marcus and J. C. Sherris. American Society for Microbiology, Washington, D.C.

28. **Kent, P. T., and G. P. Kubica.** 1985. *Public Health Mycobacteriology—A Guide for the Level III Laboratory.* Centers for Disease Control, Atlanta, Ga.

29. **Kirby, R., and K. L. Ruoff.** 1995. Cost-effective, clinically relevant method for rapid identification of beta-hemolytic streptococci and enterococci. *J. Clin. Microbiol.* **33:**1154–1157.

30. **Knisely, R. F.** 1966. Selective medium for *Bacillus anthracis. J. Bacteriol.* **92:**784–786.

31. **Lauer, B. A., L. B. Reller, and S. Mirrett.** 1981. Comparison of acridine orange and Gram stains for detection of microorganisms in cerebrospinal fluid and other clinical specimens. *J. Clin. Microbiol.* **14:**201–205.

32. **Lillie, R. D.** 1977. The general nature of dyes and their classification, p. 19–39. *In* E. H. Stotz and V. M. Emmel (ed.), *H. J. Conn's Biological Stains,* 9th ed. The Williams & Wilkins Co., Baltimore, Md.

33. **Luna, J. G.** 1968. *Manual of Histologic Staining Methods of the Armed Forces Institute of Pathology,* 3rd ed., p. 102. McGraw-Hill Book Co., New York, N.Y.

34. **MacFaddin, J. F.** 2000. *Biochemical Tests for Identification of Medical Bacteria,* 3rd ed. Lippincott Williams & Wilkins, Philadelphia, Pa.

35. **Mangels, J. I., M. E. Cox, and L. H. Lindberg.** 1984. Methanol fixation: an alternative to heat fixation of smears before staining. *Diagn. Microbiol. Infect. Dis.* **2:**129.

36. **Mirrett, S., B. A. Lauer, G. A. Miller, and L. B. Rfeller.** 1982. Comparison of acridine orange, methylene blue, and Gram stains for blood cultures. *J. Clin. Microbiol.* **14:**562–566.

37. **Morse, S.** 1989. Chancroid and *Haemophilus ducreyi. Clin. Microbiol. Rev.* **2:**137–157.

38. **Murray, P. R., and J. A. Washington II.** 1975. Microscopic and bacteriologic analysis of expectorated sputum. *Mayo Clinic Proc.* **50:**339–344.

39. **National Committee for Clinical Laboratory Standards.** 1997. *Methods for Antimicrobial Susceptibility Testing of Anaerobic Bacteria: Approved Standard, M11-A4,* 4th ed. National Committee for Clinical Laboratory Standards, Wayne, Pa.

40. **National Committee for Clinical Laboratory Standards.** 2000. *Abbreviated Identification of Bacteria and Yeast: Proposed Guideline M35-P.* National Committee for Clinical Laboratory Standards, Wayne, Pa.

41. **National Committee for Clinical Laboratory Standards.** 1996. *Quality Assurance for Commercially Prepared Microbiological Culture Media: Standard M22-A2.* National Committee for Clinical Laboratory Standards, Wayne, Pa.

42. **Nugent, P. P., N. A. Krohn, and S. L. Hillier.** 1991. Reliability of diagnosing bacterial vaginosis is improved by a standardized method of Gram stain interpretation. *J. Clin. Microbiol.* **29:**297–301.

43. **Oberhofer, T. R.** 1986. Value of the L-pyrrolidonyl-α-naphthylamide hydrolysis test for identification of select gram-positive cocci. *Diagn. Microbiol. Infect. Dis.* **4:**43–47.

44. O'Brien, K. L., M. A. Bronsdon, R. Dagan, P. Yagupsky, J. Janco, J. Elliott, C. G. Whitney, Y.-H. Yang, L. E. Robinson, B. Schwartz, and G. M. Carlone. 2001. Evaluation of a medium (STGG) for transport and optimal recovery of *Streptococcus pneumoniae* from nasopharyngeal secretions collected during field studies. *J. Clin. Microbiol.* **39:**1020–1024.

45. Paradis, I. L., C. Ross, A. Dekker, and J. Dauber. 1990. A comparison of modified methenamine silver and toluidine blue stains for the detection of *Pneumocystis carinii* in bronchoalveolar lavage specimens from immunsuppressed patients. *Acta Cytol.* **34:**511–518.

46. Power, D. A., and P. J. McCuen. 1988. *Manual of BBL Products and Laboratory Procedures,* 6th ed. Becton Dickinson Microbiology Systems, Cockeysville, Md.

47. Remel Microbiology Products. 2000. *Technical Manual.* Remel Microbiology Products, Lenexa, Kans.

48. Rose, R. A. 1982. Light microscopy, p. 1–19. *In* J. D. Bancroft and A. Stevens (ed.), *Theory and Practice of Histological Techniques,* 2nd ed. Churchill Livingstone, New York, N.Y.

49. Shanholtzer, C. J., P. J. Schaper, and L. R. Peterson. 1982. Concentrated Gram stain smears prepared with a cytospin centrifuge. *J. Clin. Microbiol.* **16:**1052–1056.

50. Spencer, F. M., and L. S. Monroe. 1976. *The Color Atlas of Intestinal Parasites,* 2nd ed. Charles C Thomas, Publisher, Springfield, Ill.

51. Strumpf, I. J., A. Y. Tsang, M. A. Schork, and J. G. Weg. 1976. The reliability of gastric smears by auramine-rhodamine staining technique for the diagnosis of tuberculosis. *Am. Rev. Respir. Dis.* **114:**971–976.

52. Summanen, P., E. J. Baron, D. M. Citron, C. Strong, H. M. Wexler, and S. M. Finegold. 1993. *Wadsworth Anaerobic Bacteriology Manual,* 5th ed. Star Publishing Co., Belmont, Calif.

53. Thompson, S. W. 1960. *Selected Histochemical and Histopathological Methods.* Charles C Thomas, Publisher, Springfield, Ill.

54. Tompkins, V. N., and J. K. Miller. 1947. Staining intestinal protozoa with iron-hematoxylin-phosphotungstic acid. *Am. J. Clin. Pathol.* **17:**755–758.

55. Welch, D. F., M. J. Muszynski, H. P. Chik, M. J. Marcon, M. M. Hribar, P. H. Gilligan, J. M. Matsen, P. A. Ahlin, B. C. Hilman, and S. A. Chartrand. 1987. Selective and differential medium for recovery of *Pseudomonas cepacia* from the respiratory tracts of patients with cystic fibrosis. *J. Clin. Microbiol.* **25:**1730–1734.

56. Weyant, R. S., C. W. Moss, R. E. Weaver, D. G. Hollis, J. G. Jordan, E. C. Cook, and M. I. Daneshvar. 1995. *Identification of Unusual Pathogenic Gram-Negative Aerobic and Facultative Anaerobic Bacteria,* 2nd ed. The Williams & Wilkins Co., Baltimore, Md.

57. Wheatley, W. 1951. A rapid staining procedure for intestinal amoebae and flagellates. *Am. J. Clin. Pathol.* **21:**990–991.

Staphylococcus, Micrococcus, and Other Catalase-Positive Cocci That Grow Aerobically*

TAMMY L. BANNERMAN

28

TAXONOMY

Members of the genera *Staphylococcus* and *Micrococcus* are catalase-positive, gram-positive cocci and were placed together with *Stomatococcus* and *Planococcus* in the family *Micrococcaceae* (158). However, the results of DNA base composition (164), DNA-rRNA hybridization (85), and comparative oligonucleotide cataloguing of 16S rRNA (119, 172) have indicated that the genera *Staphylococcus* and *Micrococcus* are not closely related. The genus *Staphylococcus* is most closely related to the newly described genus *Macrococcus* (90), but it also has a relatively close relationship to the genera *Bacillus, Brochothrix, Gemella, Listeria,* and *Planococcus.* These genera have been tentatively arranged together with staphylococci and several other genera in a family *Bacillaceae* (24) of the broad *Bacillus-Lactobacillus-Streptococcus* cluster (120, 171) or order *Bacillales* (24). On the other hand, the genus *Micrococcus* is most closely related to the genus *Arthrobacter* of the coryneform or actinomycete group (170, 172). The genus *Micrococcus* has been dissected into the six genera *Micrococcus* (containing the species *Micrococcus luteus, Micrococcus lylae,* and newly described *Micrococcus antarcticus), Kocuria* (containing the former species *Micrococcus roseus, Micrococcus varians,* and *Micrococcus kristinae), Kytococcus* (the former *Micrococcus sedentarius), Nesterenkonia* (the former *Micrococcus halobius), Dermacoccus* (the former *Micrococcus nishinomiyaensis),* and *Arthrobacter* (the former *Micrococcus agilis,* a member of the "*Arthrobacter globiformis-Arthrobacter citreus* group") (102, 116, 169). The genus *Kocuria* is more closely related to the genus *Rothia* than to other actinomycetes, and the genus *Kytococcus* is most closely related to the genus *Dermacoccus* (169). Additional catalase-positive, gram-positive cocci include *Alloiococcus otitis* (1, 49), *Rothia mucilaginosa* (12, 35), and on occasion *Aerococcus. Aerococcus* is discussed in chapter 31.

DESCRIPTION OF THE GENERA

Members of the genus *Staphylococcus* are gram-positive cocci (0.5 to 1.5 μm in diameter) that occur singly and in pairs, tetrads, short chains (three or four cells), and irregular "grape-like" clusters. They are nonmotile, nonsporeforming, usually catalase positive, and typically unencapsulated or with limited capsule formation. The species are facultative anaerobes, except for *Staphylococcus saccharolyticus* and *S. aureus* subsp. *anaerobius,* which are anaerobic and catalase negative and do not form gas from carbohydrates. Some uncommon strains of staphylococci may require the presence of CO_2 or other metabolites (hemin, menadione, etc.) (167) or a hypertonic medium for growth (150). The cellular fatty acid compositions of staphylococci consist mainly of iso- and anteiso-$C_{15:0}$, anteiso-$C_{17:0}$, $C_{18:0}$, and $C_{20:0}$ (195). The genome size is in the range of 2,000 to 3,000 kb (55, 90, 147).

Members of the genus *Micrococcus* are gram-positive cocci (1 to 1.8 μm in diameter), occurring mostly in pairs, tetrads, and irregular clusters. Cohn (34) introduced the genus *Micrococcus* to represent small spherical bacteria such as staphylococci, micrococci, and streptococci as well as some other groups. Micrococci and staphylococci have been confused with one another for more than a century on the basis of their rather similar cellular morphologies, Gram-staining results, and positive catalase activities. Both genera are commonly found living on mammalian skin and may be present in various human and veterinary clinical specimens, although micrococci are found less frequently than staphylococci and are generally regarded as saprophytic rather than as opportunistic pathogens. By the mid-1960s, a clear distinction could be made between staphylococci and micrococci on the basis of their DNA base composition (165). Members of the genus *Staphylococcus* have a G+C content of 30 to 39 mol%, whereas members of the *Micrococcus* and related genera have a G+C content within the range of 66 to 75 mol%. In the clinical laboratory, staphylococci can be easily distinguished from micrococci on the basis of the former's resistance to bacitracin and susceptibility to furazolidone (7, 8). Micrococci are oxidase positive, while staphylococci are oxidase negative, with the exception of *S. lentus, S. sciuri,* and *S. vitulus.* The cellular fatty acid composition consists mainly of $C_{15:0}$ (195).

Alloiococci are aerobic, weakly catalase-positive, gram-positive cocci, occurring mostly in pairs and clusters. The G+C content is 44 to 45 mol%. This organism can be easily distinguished from the aerobic micrococci by its

---

* This chapter contains information presented in chapter 16 by Wesley E. Kloos and Tammy L. Bannerman in the seventh edition of this Manual.

negative oxidase reaction. The cellular fatty acid composition consists mainly of $C_{16:0}$, $C_{18:1}$, $C_{18:2}$, and $C_{18:0}$ (18). *R. mucilaginosa* is a facultative anaerobe, catalase-variable, gram-positive coccus, occurring mostly in clusters. The G+C content is 56 to 60.4 mol%. *R. mucilaginosa* can easily be distinguished from staphylococci and micrococci by its inability to grow on 5% NaCl agar. The cellular fatty acid composition consists mainly of anteiso-C_{15}, iso-C_{16}, and iso-C_{14} (35).

Members of the genus *Macrococcus* (including the species *Macrococcus caseolyticus* [formerly *Staphylococcus caseolyticus*], *Macrococcus equipercicus*, *Macrococcus bovicus*, and *Macrococcus carouselicus*) can be distinguished from staphylococci on the basis of their generally higher G+C DNA percents (38 to 45 mol%), absence of cell wall teichoic acids (with the possible exception of M. *caseolyticus*), smaller genome size of approximately 1,500 to 1,800 kb, larger Gram-stained cell size of 1.3 to 2.5 μm in diameter, and unique ribotype and macrorestriction patterns (90). Macrococci can be distinguished from most species of staphylococci (except S. *sciuri*, S. *lentus*, and S. *vitulinus*) by the former's oxidase activity. They are susceptible to a wide range of antibiotics and do not exhibit the antibiotic resistance profiles characteristic of many staphylococcal species. However, like staphylococci, macrococci have a cell wall peptidoglycan that has L-lysine as the diamino acid and that has an interpeptide bridge that is susceptible to the action of lysostaphin. Since the clinical significance of macrococci has yet to be established and the genus has a rather restricted host range of only whales and related aquatic mammals and hoofed animals, they will not be described further in this chapter. The main characteristics used for differentiating staphylococci from micrococci and other gram-positive cocci encountered in the clinical laboratory are listed in Table 1.

The genus *Staphylococcus* is currently composed of 35 species (89, 111, 148, 185) and 17 subspecies (89, 148), as depicted in Table 2. The genus *Micrococcus* is currently composed of three species (103, 116, 169). M. *luteus* is the most common micrococcal species found in nature and in clinical specimens. The more distantly related species *Kocuria varians*, *Kocuria kristinae*, and *Kytococcus sedentarius* are occasionally found in clinical specimens and can be distinguished from micrococci on the basis of their cellular fatty acid compositions and by several simple tests listed below in the section on the identification of *Micrococcus* species (103, 169).

NATURAL HABITATS

Staphylococci are widespread in nature, although they are mainly found living on the skin, skin glands, and mucous membranes of mammals and birds. They may be found in the mouth, blood, mammary glands, and intestinal, genitourinary, and upper respiratory tracts of these hosts. Staphylococci generally have a benign or symbiotic relationship with their host; however, they may develop the life-style of a pathogen if they gain entry into the host tissue through trauma of the cutaneous barrier, inoculation by needles, or direct implantation of medical devices (foreign bodies). Infected tissues of the host may support large populations of staphylococci, and in some situations, they may persist for long periods. The presence of enterotoxigenic strains of staphylococci (most notably, certain strains of S. *aureus*) in various food products is regarded as a public health hazard because of the ability of these strains to produce intoxication or food poisoning.

Staphylococci found on humans and other primates include S. *aureus*, S. *epidermidis*, S. *capitis*, S. *caprae*, S. *saccharolyticus*, S. *warneri*, S. *pasteuri*, S. *haemolyticus*, S. *hominis*, S. *lugdunensis*, S. *auricularis*, S. *saprophyticus*, S. *cohnii*, S. *xylosus*, and S. *simulans* (87, 89, 99). Most of the species listed above produce resident populations on humans. However, S. *xylosus* and S. *simulans* are usually transients on humans and are primarily acquired from domestic animals and their products. On the other hand, some of the human staphylococcal species are transients or temporary residents on domestic animals. S. *aureus* is a major species of primates, although specific ecovars or biotypes can be found occasionally living on different domestic animals or birds (42, 86). S. *schleiferi*, S. *intermedius*, and S. *felis* are commonly found living on carnivora (89, 99). However, S. *schleiferi* may produce serious infections in humans (51, 72, 78) and S. *intermedius* may produce infections in humans as a result of dog bites (175). S. *lutrae* has recently been isolated from the European otter, a carnivore (53). S. *xylosus*, S. *kloosii*, and S. *sciuri* are common residents on a variety of rodents (89). S. *hyicus*, S. *chromogenes*, S. *sciuri*, S. *lentus*, and S. *vitulinus* are common residents of ungulates and, in addition, may be isolated from their food products (43, 91, 192). The last three species are also common residents of whales and related aquatic mammals. Other staphylococci associated with food products include S. *fleurettii*, S. *condimenti*, S. *carnosus*, and S. *piscifermentans* (148, 177, 185).

Some *Staphylococcus* species demonstrate habitat or niche preferences on their particular hosts (87). For example, S. *capitis* subsp. *capitis* is found as large populations on the adult human head, especially the scalp and forehead, where sebaceous glands are numerous and well developed. S. *capitis* subsp. *urealyticus* is also found on the head but may produce relatively large populations in the axillae of some individuals (9). S. *auricularis* has a strong preference for the external auditory meatus. S. *hominis* and S. *haemolyticus* generally produce larger populations in areas of the skin where apocrine glands are numerous, such as the axillae and pubic areas (86). S. *aureus* prefers the anterior nares as a habitat, especially in the adult human. The novobiocin-resistant staphylococci, particularly S. *cohnii*, are found in large populations on the human feet. S. *saprophyticus* appears in large numbers in females between the ages of 10 and 29 years (154).

Certain *Staphylococcus* species are found frequently as etiologic agents of a variety of human and animal infections. In this chapter, we are concerned primarily with the identification of S. *aureus*, S. *epidermidis*, S. *haemolyticus*, S. *lugdunensis*, and S. *saprophyticus*, species most commonly associated with human infections, and S. *intermedius* and S. *hyicus*, species of especial veterinary interest. S. *schleiferi* has been considered a significant pathogen in some European countries but has seldom been isolated from infections in the United States.

Micrococci are widespread in nature and are commonly found on the skin of humans and other mammals (95, 100, 103). They are generally believed to be temporary residents and are most frequently found on the exposed skin of the face, arms, hands, and legs. Alloiococci are isolated from human middle ear fluid (1, 49), and *R. mucilaginosa* is probably a normal inhabitant of the mouth and upper respiratory tract (12).

TABLE 1 Differentiation of members of the genus *Staphylococcus* from other gram-positive cocci[a]

Genus and exceptional species	G+C content of DNA (mol%)	Strict aerobe	Facultative anaerobe or microaerophil	Strict anaerobe	Tetrad cell arrangement	Strong adherence on agar	Motility	Growth on: 5% NaCl agar	6.5% NaCl agar	12% NaCl agar	P agar in 18 h [b]	Catalase [c]	Benzidine test [d]	Modified oxidase test [e]	Anaerobic acid from glucose [f]	Aerobic acid from glycerol	Growth on Schleifer-Kramer agar [g]	Resistance to: Lysostaphin (200 µg/ml)	Erythromycin (0.4 µg/ml)	Bacitracin (0.04 U) [h]	Furazolidone (100 µg) [i]
Staphylococcus	30–39	−	d	−	d	−[j]	−	+	+	d	+	+	+	−	d	+	+	−	+	+	−
S. aureus subsp. anaerobius		−	±	±	−	−	−	+	+	d	−	−	−	−	+	+	ND	−	+	ND	−
S. saccharolyticus		−	±	±	+	−	−	+	+	±	−	−	±	−	+	+	ND	−	+	ND	−
S. hominis		±[k]	±	−	+	−	−	+	+	±	+	+	+	−	+	+	+	−	+	+	−
S. auricularis		−	+	−	+	−	−	+	+	±	−	+	+	−	+	+	ND	−	+	+	−
S. saprophyticus, S. cohnii, S. xylosus		d	d	−	−	−	−	+	+	±	+	+	+	−	−	+	+	−	+	+	−
S. kloosii, S. equorum, S. arlettae		±	±	−	−	−	−	+	+	±	d	+	+	−	−	+	+	−	+	+	−
S. intermedius		−	+	−	−	−	−	+	+	+	+	+	+	−	+	+	±	−	+	+	−
S. sciuri, S. lentus, S. vitulinus		±	±	−	d	−	−	+	+	d	d	+	+	+	−	+	+	−	+	+	−
Macrococcus[l]	38–45	±	±	−	d	−	−	+	+	±	d	+	+	+	−	d	ND	−	+	+	
Enterococcus	34–42	−	+	−	−	−	d	+	+	(±)	±	−	−	−	+	d	(±)	+	+	+	−
Streptococcus	34–46	−	+	d	−	−	−	d	d	−	−	−	−	−	(+)	d	−	+	ND	d	−
Aerococcus	35–40	−	+	−	+	−	−	+	+	+	−	−	−	−	(+)	ND	ND	+	ND	−	−
Planococcus	39–52	+	−	−	d	−	+	+	+	+	−	+	+	ND	+	−	ND	−	ND	ND	−
Alloiococcus	44–45	+	−	−	−	−	−	+	+	ND	ND	±	+	−	ND	−	ND	ND	ND	ND	ND
Rothia mucilaginosa	56–60	−	+	−	d	+	−	−	−	−	−	±	+	−	+	d	ND	+	ND	−	d
Micrococcus and related genera	66–75	+	−	−	+	−	−	+	+	d	−	+	+	+	−	−	−	+	−[m]	−	+
Kocuria kristinae	67	±	±	−	+	−	−	+	+	±	−	+	+	+	(+)	+	(±)	+	−	−	+

[a] Symbols and abbreviations: +, 90% or more species or strains positive; ±, 90% or more species or strains weakly positive; −, 90% or more species or strains negative; d, 11 to 89% of species or strains positive; ND, not determined; parentheses indicate a delayed reaction.

[b] Growth on P agar is under aerobic conditions and at 35 to 37°C. Positive growth is indicated for detectable colony formation of at least 1 mm diameter; ± indicates detectable colony formation between 0.5 and 1 mm diameter. Growth on sheep or bovine blood agar is slightly greater but less discriminative between staphylococci and other genera.

[c] Sometimes a weak catalase or pseudocatalase reaction can be observed in certain strains of species designated catalase negative. In some species, catalase activity may be activated by hemin supplementation.

[d] The benzidine test detects the presence of cytochromes. Some strains of benzidine test-negative species can synthesize cytochromes on aerobic media supplemented with hemin (50).

[e] See reference 159.

[f] Standard oxidation-fermentation test (48, 159).

[g] Growth is under aerobic conditions and at 35 to 37°C for 24 to 48 h. Positive growth is indicated for a number of CFU on selective medium comparable to that on plate count agar and a colony 0.5 mm in diameter; ± indicates a significant reduction in CFU on the selective medium compared to that on plate count agar, and parentheses indicate a colony of pinpoint size to 0.5 mm in diameter (160).

[h] A disk is used. Positive indicates resistance and no zone of inhibition. *Micrococcus*, *Kocuria*, *Kytococcus*, *Stomatococcus*, and *Aerococcus* spp. are susceptible and have an inhibition zone of 10 to 25 mm in diameter.

[i] A disk is used. Positive indicates resistance and a zone of inhibition of 0 to 9 mm. Susceptible species have a zone size of 15 to 35 mm in diameter (68).

[j] Some strains of *S. epidermidis* adhere tenaciously to the surface of agar, and this property is correlated with heavy slime production.

[k] *S. hominis* does not demonstrate growth in the anaerobic portion of thioglycolate medium within 24 h and may produce only very poor growth in this portion following 3 to 5 days of incubation. However, it will grow and ferment glucose anaerobically (standard oxidation-fermentation test). Failure to grow anaerobically in thioglycolate may be due in part to inhibition by the ingredients.

[l] *Macrococcus* species can also be differentiated from *Staphylococcus* species on the basis of their generally larger Gram-stained cell size (≥2 µm) and larger number of chromosome fragments produced by digestion with *Not*I (12 to 36 fragments) (90).

[m] A few *Micrococcus* strains demonstrate high-level (MIC ≥50 µg/ml) erythromycin resistance.

CLINICAL SIGNIFICANCE

Staphylococcus

The coagulase-positive species S. aureus is well documented as a human opportunistic pathogen. As a nosocomial pathogen, S. aureus has been a major cause of morbidity and mortality. S. aureus infections are often acute and pyogenic and, if untreated, may spread to surrounding tissue or via bacteremia to metastatic sites (involving other organs). Some of the infections caused by S. aureus involve the skin; these include furuncles or boils, cellulitis, impetigo, and postoperative wound infections of various sites. Some of the more serious infections produced by S. aureus are bacteremia, pneumonia, osteomyelitis, acute endocarditis, myocarditis, pericarditis, cerebritis, meningitis, chorioamnionitis (137), scalded skin syndrome, and abscesses of the muscle, urogenital tract, central nervous system, and various intra-abdominal organs. Small-colony variants (SCVs) of S. aureus are a naturally occurring subpopulation which grows slowly and produces small colonies on routine media. This population of S. aureus is most common in patient populations with unusually persistent infections, such as cystic fibrosis or chronic osteomyelitis, and who are chronically exposed to aminoglycosides and trimethoprim-sulfamethoxazole (117, 150). Although S. aureus infection in children or adults with cystic fibrosis does not significantly affect respiratory function (129, 179), the continuous use of antistaphylococcal antimicrobial therapy increases the risk of colonization with Pseudomonas aeruginosa (153).

The presence of S. aureus in foods can present a potential public health hazard since many strains of S. aureus produce enterotoxins (46). The most common symptoms of staphylococcal food poisoning include vomiting and diarrhea, which occur 2 to 4 h after ingestion of the toxin. The illness may be relatively mild (lasting only a few hours), but some cases may require hospitalization. Foods commonly associated with staphylococcal food poisoning are meat, meat products, salads, cream-filled bakery products, and dairy products.

Toxic shock syndrome (TSS), a community-acquired disease, has also been attributed to infection or colonization with S. aureus. A single clone has been shown to cause the majority of the cases (134). TSS was prevalent in young, menstruating females who used certain types of highly absorbent tampons (181). TSS-associated nongenital S. aureus has also been found in men and nonmenstruating women. TSS is associated with strains that produce and secrete the exotoxin toxic shock syndrome toxin 1 (TSST-1) (161). TSST-1 is a member of a superantigen family that has the ability to stimulate T cells (32) and induce tumor necrosis factor (143) and the cytokine interleukin-1 (144). Methods for recognizing TSST-1 production include radioimmunoassay, enzyme-linked immunosorbent assay (131), reversed passive latex agglutination (Oxoid, Ogensburg, N.Y.) (47, 197), and PCR (11, 79, 127, 133, 162).

Methicillin-resistant S. aureus (MRSA) emerged in the 1980s as a major clinical and epidemiologic problem in hospitals. Presently, hospitals of all sizes are facing the MRSA problem. Recommendations for the management or control of the spread of MRSA have been made available (19, 20, 196). Nasal carriage of S. aureus or MRSA has been suggested as a risk factor for the development of infections. Strategies for eliminating the nasal carriage of this species,

thus reducing the infection rate, have been proposed by Kluytmans et al. (101). MRSA is beginning to spread out of the hospitals and into communities. High-risk groups, including intravenous drug users, persons with a serious underlying disease, persons receiving antimicrobial therapy, and persons recently discharged from the hospital, have accounted for the first reports of MRSA in the community (115, 157). However, more recently, cases have been reported in which these risk factors are absent (73). One trait shared by many community-acquired strains is their susceptibility to antimicrobials (27, 73). MRSA is emerging as a major threat in the community since its prevalence may be as high as 25% within the next 5 to 10 years (29).

The coagulase-negative Staphylococcus (CoNS) species as a group constitute a major component of the normal microflora of humans. The role of CoNS species in causing nosocomial infections has been recognized and well documented over the last two decades, especially for the species S. epidermidis. The infection rate has been correlated with the increase in the use of prosthetic and indwelling devices and the growing number of immunocompromised patients in hospitals. The need exists for the accurate identification of CoNS to enable precise delineation of the clinical disease produced by this group of bacteria and determination of the etiologic agent. A review of CoNS has summarized factors that are helpful in associating the staphylococci as the etiologic agent (92). These results included (i) the isolation of a strain in pure culture from the infected site or body fluid (most contaminated clinical specimens produce mixed cultures of different strains and/or species; however, some infections may be the consequence of more than one strain or species) and (ii) the repeated isolation of the same strain or combination of strains over the course of the infection. S. epidermidis has been documented as a pathogen in numerous cases of bacteremia, native- and prosthetic-valve endocarditis, surgical wounds, and urinary tract, cerebrospinal fluid, prosthetic joint, peritoneal dialysis-related, ophthalmologic, and intravascular catheter-related infections (39, 156). S. saprophyticus is an important opportunistic pathogen in human urinary tract infections, especially in young, sexually active females. It has been proposed as an agent of nongonococcal urethritis in males or a cause of other sexually transmitted diseases, prostatitis, wound infections, and septicemia. S. haemolyticus, the second most frequently encountered CoNS species associated with human infections, has been implicated in native-valve endocarditis, septicemia, peritonitis, urinary tract infections, and wound, bone, and joint infections (92, 156). S. lugdunensis has been reported as a frequent cause of endocarditis (184). The aggressive nature of these infections, the need for valve replacement, and the high mortality suggest that quick recognition of S. lugdunensis is needed so that appropriate antimicrobial therapy can be administered for a better patient outcome. S. lugdunensis has also been implicated in arthritis, bacteremia, catheter infections, prosthetic joint infections, and urinary tract infections.

Other CoNS species have been implicated in a variety of infections. For example, S. capitis, S. caprae, S. saccharolyticus, S. simulans, and S. warneri have been implicated in endocarditis; S. capitis, S. hominis, S. schleiferi, S. simulans, and S. warneri have been implicated in septicemia; S. warneri and S. simulans have been implicated in osteomyelitis; S. cohnii has been implicated in native-valve endocarditis and pneumonia; S. cohnii, S. xylosus, S. schleiferi, S. hominis, and S. caprae have been implicated in urinary tract infections; S. caprae and S. cohnii have been implicated in

TABLE 2 Differentiation of *Staphylococcus* species

Species	Colony size (large)[b]	Colony pigment[c]	Anaerobic growth[d]	Aerobic growth[e]	Staphylocoagulase	Clumping factor[f]	Heat-stable nuclease	Hemolysins[g]	Catalase[h]	Oxidase[i]	Alkaline phosphatase	Arginine arylamidase	Pyrrolidonyl arylamidase[j]	Ornithine decarboxylase	Urease[j]	β-Glucosidase[j]	β-Glucuronidase[j]	β-Galactosidase[j]	Arginine utilization[j]	Acetoin production	Nitrate reduction	Esculin hydrolysis	Novobiocin resistance[k]	Polymyxin B resistance[l]	D-Trehalose	D-Mannitol	D-Mannose	D-Turanose	D-Xylose	D-Cellobiose	L-Arabinose	Maltose	α-Lactose	Sucrose	N-Acetylglucosamine	Raffinose
S. aureus subsp. *aureus*	+	+	+	+	+	+	+	+	+	−	+	−	−	−	d	+	−	−	+	+	+	−	−	+	+	+	+	+	−	−	−	+	+	+	+	−
S. aureus subsp. *anaerobius*	−	−	(+)	(±)	+	−	+	+	−	−	+	ND	ND	ND	ND	−	−	−	ND	+	−	−	−	ND	−	ND	−	ND	−	−	−	+	−	+	−	−
S. epidermidis	−	−	+	+	−	−	−	(d)	+	−	+[m]	−	−	(d)	+	(d)	−	−	d	+	+	−	−	−	−	−	(+)	(d)	−	−	−	+	d	+	−	−
S. capitis subsp. *capitis*	−	−	(+)	+	−	−	−	(d)	+	−	−	−	−	−	+	−	−	−	d	d	d	−	−	−	−	+	+	−	−	−	−	+	(d)	+	−	−
S. capitis subsp. *ureolyticus*	d	(d)	(+)	(±)	−	−	−	(d)	+	−	(+)	−	d	−	+	−	−	−	+	ND	+	ND	−	−	(+)	d	+	−	−	−	−	(d)	+	+	ND	−
S. caprae	−	−	+	+	−	−	−	(d)	+	−	(+)	−	p	+	+	−	−	−	+	ND	+	−	−	−	(+)	d	+	−	−	−	−	(d)	+	+	ND	−
S. saccharolyticus	−	−	+	−	−	−	−	−	−	−	p	−	ND	ND	ND	ND	p	ND	+	ND	+	−	−	−	−	d	(+)	ND	−	−	−	−	d	−	ND	−
S. warneri	d	d	+	+	−	−	−	(d)	+	−	−	−	−	(d)	+	+	p	−	d	+	d	−	−	−	+	d	−	(d)	−	−	−	(+)	d	+	p	−
S. pasteuri[n]	d	d	+	+	−	−	−	(d)	+	−	−	−	−	(d)	+	+	+	−	d	d	d	−	−	ND	+	d	−	(d)	−	−	−	(d)	d	+	+	−
S. haemolyticus	+	d	+	+	−	−	−	(+)	+	−	−	−	+	−	+	p	p	−	d	d	+	−	−	−	+	d	−	+	−	−	−	+	d	(+)	p	−
S. hominis subsp. *hominis*	−	d	−	+	−	−	−	−	+	−	−	−	−	−	+	−	−	−	−	d	d	−	+	−	−	−	−	−	−	−	−	+	d	(+)	−	−
S. hominis subsp. *novobiosepticus*[o]	−	−	+	+	−	(+)	+	(+)	+	−	−	ND	+	−	d	+	−	(+)	−	+	+	−	+	d	+	−	+	−	−	−	−	+	+	+	+	−
S. lugdunensis	d	−	+	+	−	+	+	(+)	+	−	+	−	+	+	d	+	−	−	+	+	+	−	−	p	+	−	+	(d)	−	−	−	−	+	+	(+)	−
S. schleiferi subsp. *schleiferi*	−	−	+	+	−	+	+	(+)	+	−	+	+	+	−	−	−	−	−	d	+	+	−	−	−	d	−	+	−	−	−	−	−	−	d	ND	−
S. schleiferi subsp. *coagulans*	d	−	+	+	+	−	+	(+)	+	−	+	−	+	−	+	−	−	ND	−	+	+	ND	−	ND	+	−	+	ND	−	−	−	−	−	d	ND	−
S. muscae	d	−	+	(±)	−	−	−	(+)	+	−	+	ND	ND	ND	−	ND	ND	(d)	−	−	ND	−	−	ND	+	−	−	(d)	+	−	−	(+)	−	+	ND	−
S. auricularis	−	−	(±)	(+)	−	−	−	−	+	−	−	+	−	−	−	−	ND	+	d	−	(d)	−	−	−	(+)	−	−	+	−	−	−	+	−	+	p	−
S. saprophyticus subsp. *saprophyticus*	+	d	(+)	+	−	−	+	−	+	−	−	+	+	ND	d	p	−	p	−	−	−	−	+	ND	+	−	−	+	−	−	−	+	−	+	−	−
S. saprophyticus subsp. *bovis*	−	+	+	−	−	−	−	−	+	−	−	−	+	−	+	d	−	d	−	d	−	−	+	ND	+	−	−	+	−	−	−	+	−	+	+	−
S. cohnii subsp. *cohnii*	d	−	d	+	−	−	−	(d)	+	−	−	−	d	−	+	d	−	p	−	d	−	−	+	−	+	d	(d)	−	−	−	−	(d)	−	−	−	−
S. cohnii subsp. *ureolyticus*	+	d	(+)	+	−	−	−	(d)	+	−	+	−	d	−	+	−	+	+	−	d	−	−	+	−	+	d	+	−	−	−	−	(+)	+	+	d	−
S. xylosus	+	d	d	+	−	−	−	−	+	−	d	−	d	−	+	+	+	+	−	d	d	d	+	−	+	+	+	d	−	−	d	+	d	+	+	d

S. kloosii
S. equorum
S. arlettae
S. gallinarum
S. succinus
S. simulans
S. carnosus subsp. *carnosus*
S. carnosus subsp. *utilis*
S. piscifermentans
S. condimenti
S. felis
S. lutrae
S. intermedius
S. delphini
S. hyicus
S. chromogenes
S. sciuri subsp. *sciuri*
S. sciuri subsp. *carnaticus*
S. sciuri subsp. *rodentium*
S. lentus
S. fleurettii
S. vitulinus

[a] Symbols and abbreviations (unless otherwise indicated): +, 90% or more strains positive; ±, 90% or more strains weakly positive; −, 90% or more strains negative; d, 11 to 89% of strains positive; ND, not determined; parentheses indicate a delayed reaction.

[b] Positive is defined as a colony diameter of ≥6 mm after incubation on P agar at 34 to 35°C for 3 days and at room temperature (ca. 25°C) for an additional 2 days; exceptions for S. *succinus* (4 to 6 mm on tryptic soy agar) and S. *fleuretti* (8 to 12 mm on tryptic soy agar).

[c] Positive is defined as the visual detection of carotenoid pigments (e.g., yellow, yellow-orange, or orange) during colony development at normal incubation or room temperatures. Pigments may be enhanced by the addition of milk, fat, glycerol monoacetate, or soaps to P agar.

[d] Growth is measured in a semisolid thioglycolate medium. Symbols: +, moderate or heavy growth down the tube within 18 to 24 h; ±, heavier growth in the upper portion of the tube and weaker growth in the lower, anaerobic portion of tube; −, no visible growth within 48 h but very weak diffuse growth or a few scattered, small colonies in the lower portion of tube by 72 to 96 h. Parentheses indicate delayed growth appearing within 24 to 72 h, sometimes noted as large discrete colonies in the lower portion of tube.

[e] Growth is measured on P agar or bovine, sheep, or human blood agar at 34 to 37°C. S. *equorum* grows slowly at 35 to 37°C; its optimum growth temperature is 30°C. The anaerobic species S. *saccharolyticus* and S. *aureus* subsp. *anaerobius* grow very slowly in the presence of air. Aerobic growth may be increased slightly by subculture in the presence of air. S. *aureus* subsp. *anaerobius* requires the addition of blood, serum, or egg yolk for growth on primary isolation medium. S. *auricularis*, S. *lentus*, and S. *vitulus* produce just detectable colonies on P agar in 24 to 36 h, and these colonies remain very small (1 to 2 mm in diameter).

[f] Clumping factor is detected in rabbit or human plasma (slide coagulase test). Human plasma is preferred for the detection of clumping factor with S. *lugdunensis* and S. *schleiferi*. Latex agglutination is somewhat less reliable for detection of clumping factor or fibrinogen affinity factor in S. *lugdunensis*.

[g] Hemolysis is detected on bovine blood agar. Symbols and abbreviations: +, wide zone of hemolysis within 24 to 36 h; (+), delayed moderate to wide zone of hemolysis within 48 to 72 h; (d), no or delayed hemolysis; −, no or only very narrow zone (1 mm) of hemolysis within 72 h. Some of the strains designated negative may produce a slight greening or browning of blood agar.

[h] Catalase and cytochrome synthesis cannot be induced in S. *aureus* subsp. *anaerobius* by the addition of H_2O_2 or hemin to the culture medium. Catalase can be induced in S. *saccharolyticus* by hemin supplementation. In this species, cytochromes a and b are present in small quantities.

[i] Oxidase is determined by the modified oxidase test to detect the presence of cytochrome c (50).

[j] These activities are determined primarily by commercial rapid-identification tests (see the text).

[k] Positive is defined as an MIC of 1.6 μg/ml or a growth inhibition zone diameter of ≥16 mm with a 5-μg novobiocin disk.

[l] Positive is defined as a growth inhibition zone diameter of <10 mm with a 300-U polymyxin B disk.

[m] Alkaline phosphatase activity is negative for approximately 6 to 15% of strains of S. *epidermidis*, depending on the population sampled. A small but significant number of clinical isolates have been phosphatase negative.

[n] rRNA gene restriction site polymorphism using pBA2 as a probe can distinguish this species from other staphylococcal species, including S. *warneri* (30).

[o] All strains tested were resistant also to penicillin G, methicillin, oxacillin, gentamicin, and streptomycin.

[p] Positive reactions are with the Staph Latex agglutination test (Remel) that detects clumping factor and/or protein A.

arthritis; *S. schleiferi* and *S. caprae* have been implicated in wound and joint infections and osteomyelitis; and *S. capitis*, *S. schleiferi*, and *S. warneri* have been implicated in catheter infections (23, 92, 156). *S. hominis* subsp. *novobiosepticus* has been isolated from human blood cultures, and has been associated with clinically significant septicemia (94, 193). *S. sciuri* has been isolated from wounds, skin, and soft tissue infections (124). In many cases patients with infections caused by these CoNS have predisposing or underlying diseases affecting the immune system and had also experienced surgery or intravascular manipulations.

The coagulase-positive species *S. intermedius* and the coagulase-variable species *S. hyicus* are of particular importance in veterinary infections. *S. aureus* and these two coagulase-positive species are serious opportunistic pathogens of animals. *S. intermedius* has been associated with a variety of canine infections including cellulitis, otitis, externa, pyoderma, abscesses, reproductive tract infections, mastitis, and wound infections (44, 56, 99). *S. intermedius* infections in humans are usually associated with animal bites (175). This species has been implicated in a food-poisoning outbreak involving butter-blend products (84). *S. hyicus* has been implicated in infectious exudative epidermitis and septic polyarthritis in pigs and mastitis in cows (44, 99). *S. schleiferi* subsp. *coagulans* has been isolated from dogs with external-ear otitis (77).

Micrococcus, Alloiococcus, and *Rothia mucilaginosa*

Members of the genus *Micrococcus* and the related coccal genera *Kocuria* and *Kytococcus* are generally considered to be harmless saprophytes that inhabit or contaminate the skin, mucosa, and perhaps also the oropharynx; however, they can be opportunistic pathogens in certain immunocompromised patients. *M. luteus* has been implicated as the causative agent in cases of intracranial abscesses, pneumonia, septic arthritis, endocarditis, and meningitis (93, 103, 164). *K. sedentarius* has been associated with prosthetic-valve endocarditis (140) and is often associated with pitted keratolysis (139). Other infections associated with micrococci and their relatives include bacteremia, continuous ambulatory peritoneal dialysis peritonitis, and the infection of a cerebrospinal fluid shunt (122).

Significant levels of inflammatory cells along with the observation of intracellular *Alloiococcus* led Faden and Dryja (49) to suggest that this organism plays a pathogenic role in persistent otitis media. Additional studies employing either culture (60) or PCR (13, 70, 71) have supported the role of alloiococci in chronic otitis media. *R. mucilaginosa* has been implicated in numerous reports of infection since the mid- to late-1980s. This organism has been isolated from cases of bacteremia, endocarditis, endophthalmitis, intravascular catheter and central nervous system infections, pneumonia, peritonitis, and septicemia (6, 58, 62, 112, 126, 138, 176).

COLLECTION, TRANSPORT, AND STORAGE OF SPECIMENS

The general principles of collection, transport, and storage of specimens as described in chapters 6, 7, and 20 of this Manual are applicable to the organisms listed in this chapter. No special methods or precautions are usually required for these organisms because they are easily obtained from clinical material of most infection sites and are relatively resistant to drying and to moderate temperature changes. Some strains of staphylococci may require anaerobic conditions or CO_2 supplementation for satisfactory growth, but they survive transport and limited storage in air.

DIRECT EXAMINATION

The direct microscopic examination of normally sterile fluids such as cerebrospinal fluid and joint aspirates may be useful. Direct examination of certain nonsterile fluids may also be very useful if the microscopist carefully evaluates the specimen by noting the presence of inflammatory cells versus epithelial cells. Even if large numbers of gram-positive cocci are present, only a presumptive report of "gram-positive cocci resembling staphylococci (or micrococci)" should be made. Culture and appropriate identification techniques must confirm this report. It must also be emphasized that microscopy by itself cannot adequately differentiate various species of staphylococci or micrococci from one another or from planococci, some streptococci, aerococci, various anaerobic cocci, or other cocci related to micrococci.

ISOLATION PROCEDURES

Considering the widespread distribution of staphylococci and micrococci over the body surface, careful and thoughtful procedures should be used to isolate organisms from the focus or foci of infection without collecting any members of the surrounding normal flora (92). Distinguishing contaminants from the infecting staphylococci and micrococci continues to be a challenge for the clinical microbiology laboratory.

The basic procedures for culture and isolation described in chapter 20 of this Manual should be followed. Every specimen should be plated onto blood agar (preferably sheep blood agar) and other media as indicated. On blood agar, abundant growth of most staphylococcal species occurs within 18 to 24 h and abundant growth of micrococci occurs within 36 to 48 h. Although most CoNS colony morphologies cannot be distinguished from one another, preliminary identification testing should begin after overnight incubation. Colonies should be allowed to grow for at least an additional 2 days to 3 days before the primary isolation plate is confirmed for species or strain composition (97, 98). This growth period is particularly important if it is necessary to sample more than one colony to obtain sufficient inocula and to determine the predominant organism or a pure culture. Failure to hold plates for 72 h can result in (i) selection of more than one species or strain if two or more colonies are sampled to produce an inoculum, (ii) selection of an organism(s) not producing the infection if the specimen contains two or more different species or strains, and (iii) incorrect labeling of a mixed culture as a pure culture. Colonies should be Gram stained, subcultured, and tested for genus, species, and, when applicable, strain properties. Most staphylococci of major medical interest produce growth in the upper as well as the lower anaerobic portions of the thioglycolate broth or semisolid agar (98).

Specimens from heavily contaminated sources such as feces should also be streaked onto a selective medium: Schleifer-Krämer agar (160), mannitol-salt agar, Columbia colistin-nalidixic acid agar, lipase-salt-mannitol agar (Remel, Lenexa, Kans.), or phenylethyl alcohol agar. These media inhibit the growth of gram-negative organisms but allow staphylococci and certain other gram-positive cocci to grow. On selective media, incubation should be extended to at least 48 to 72 h for discernible colony development.

IDENTIFICATION

Staphylococcus Species

Staphylococcus species can be identified on the basis of a variety of conventional phenotypic characters (88, 93, 99) (Table 2). The most clinically significant species can be identified on the basis of several key characteristics (Table 3). In addition, species can be identified on the basis of molecular phenotypic properties such as cellular fatty acids (105), multilocus enzyme electrophoresis (201), and whole-cell polypeptides (33) and genotypic properties such as chromosome restriction fragments (14), macrorestriction patterns (10, 55), ribotypes (41, 192), amplification of DNA regions (57, 121, 128, 199), and *hsp60* sequencing (108). Most of the molecular methods are currently confined to the reference or research laboratory.

Some laboratories may choose to restrict complete species identification of the CoNS to isolates from normally sterile sites such as blood (when considered to be clinically significant) or joint or cerebrospinal fluid and to distinguish routinely (i) *S. saprophyticus* from other CoNS isolated from urine; (ii) *S. epidermidis*, *S. lugdunensis*, and *S. schleiferi* isolated from colonized shunts, catheters, or prosthetic devices; and (iii) *S. epidermidis*, *S. lugdunensis*, and *S. haemolyticus* isolated from soft tissue infections or endocarditis.

Colonial Appearance

On nonselective blood agar, nutrient agar, tryptic soy agar, brain heart infusion agar, or P agar, isolated colonies of most staphylococci are 1 to 3 mm in diameter within 24 h and 3 to 8 mm in diameter by 3 days of incubation in air at 34 to 37°C, depending on the species (99). The exceptional species *S. aureus* subsp. *anaerobius*, *S. saccharolyticus*, *S. auricularis*, *S. equorum*, *S. vitulinus*, and *S. lentus* grow more slowly than other staphylococci and usually require 24 to 36 h for detectable colony development. The typical 24-h *S. aureus* colonies are pigmented, smooth, entire, slightly raised, and hemolytic on routine blood agar. The typical 24-h CoNS colony is unpigmented, smooth, entire, glistening, slightly raised to convex, and opaque. Colony morphology can be a useful supplementary characteristic in the identification of species. In order for differences to be observed, the isolated colonies need to develop for several days at 34 to 37°C and then grow for 2 days at room temperature.

Colonies of *S. aureus* are usually large (6 to 8 mm in diameter), smooth, entire, slightly raised, and translucent. On P agar, they become nearly transparent by 3 to 5 days of incubation. The colonies of most strains are pigmented, ranging from cream-yellow to orange. Rare strains with relatively large capsules produce colonies that are smaller and more convex than those of unencapsulated strains and have a glistening, wet appearance. SCVs of *S. aureus* might be isolated from patients with persistent or recurrent infections, e.g., chronic osteomyelitis and cystic fibrosis. These colonies are pinpoint in size, nonhemolytic, and nonpigmented. Typically, normal growth can be restored if the isolate is allowed to grow in the presence of menodione, hemin, and/or CO_2 supplementation (151, 189). *S. epidermidis* colonies are relatively small and range from 2.5 to 6 mm in diameter, depending on the strain. Pigment is not

usually detected. Some of the slime-producing strains are extremely sticky and adhere to the agar surface. Colonies of *S. haemolyticus* are usually larger than those of *S. epidermidis* and *S. hominis* and are 5 to 9 mm in diameter. They are smooth, butyrous, and opaque, like those of the related species *S. hominis*, and may be unpigmented or cream to yellow-orange. Colonies of *S. lugdunensis* are usually 4 to 7 mm in diameter, smooth, and glossy and may be unpigmented or cream to yellow-orange. The edge is entire and rather flat, while the center is slightly domed. They are sometimes confused with colonies of *S. warneri*. *S. schleiferi* colonies are usually 3 to 5 mm in diameter and unpigmented. They are smooth, glossy, and slightly convex with entire edges. Colonies of *S. saprophyticus* are large (5 to 8 mm in diameter), entire, very glossy, opaque, smooth, butyrous, and more convex than the colonies of the aforementioned species. Approximately one-half of the strains are pigmented, ranging from cream to yellow-orange. Colonies of *S. intermedius* and *S. hyicus* are relatively large, usually 5 to 8 mm in diameter. They are slightly convex, entire, smooth, glossy, and usually unpigmented. Colonies of *S. intermedius* are translucent. Those of *S. hyicus* are more opaque, becoming translucent with prolonged incubation.

Coagulase Production

The ability to clot plasma continues to be the most widely used and generally accepted criterion for the identification of pathogenic staphylococci associated with acute infections, i.e., *S. aureus* in humans and animals and *S. intermedius* and *S. hyicus* in animals. Two different coagulase tests can be performed: a tube test for free coagulase and a slide test for bound coagulase or clumping factor (93). While the tube test is definitive, the slide test may be used as a rapid screening technique to identify *S. aureus*. However, 10 to 15% of *S. aureus* strains may yield a negative result. A positive slide test may also aid in the identification of the new species *S. lugdunensis* and *S. schleiferi* (Table 3). A variety of plasmas may be used for either test; however, dehydrated rabbit plasma containing EDTA is commercially available and most satisfactory with the exception that human plasma is somewhat more satisfactory for the identification of *S. lugdunensis* and *S. schleiferi*. Human plasma should not be used unless it has been carefully tested for clotting capability and lack of infectious agents.

The tube coagulase test is best performed by mixing 0.1 ml of an overnight culture in brain heart infusion broth with 0.5 ml of reconstituted plasma (preferably in a glass tube), incubating the mixture at 37°C in a water bath or heat block for 4 h, and observing the tube for clot formation by slowly tilting it 90° from the vertical. Alternatively, a large, well-isolated colony on a noninhibitory agar can be transferred into 0.5 ml of reconstituted plasma and incubated as describe above. Any degree of clotting constitutes a positive test. However, a flocculent or fibrous precipitate is not a true clot and should be recorded as a negative result. Incubation of the test overnight has also been recommended for *S. aureus*, since a small number of strains may require longer than 4 h for clot formation. For veterinary clinical laboratories, it is important to note that some strains of *S. intermedius* and most coagulase-producing strains of *S. hyicus* require more than 4 h for a positive coagulase test. Clot formation by these species may require 12 to 24 h of incubation. If the incubation time exceeds 4 h, the following points must be considered: (i) staphylokinase produced by some strains may lyse the clot after prolonged incubation, yielding false-negative results; (ii) if

TABLE 3 Key tests for identification of the most clinically significant *Staphylococcus* species

Species	Test[a]								
	Colony pigment[b]	Staphylo-coagulase	Clumping factor[b]	Heat-stable nuclease	Alkaline phosphatase	Pyrrolidonyl arylamidase[b]	Ornithine decarboxylase	Urease[b]	β-Galactosidase[b]
S. aureus subsp. *aureus*	+	+	+	+	+	−	−	d	−
S. epidermidis	−	−	−	−	+	−	(d)	+	−
S. haemolyticus	d	−	−	−	−	+	−	−	−
S. hyicus (veterinary)	−	d	−	+	+	−	−	d	−
S. intermedius (veterinary)	−	+	d	+	+	+	−	+	+
S. lugdunensis	d	−	(+)	−	−	+	+	d	−
S. schleiferi subsp. *schleiferi*	−	−	+	+	+	+	−	−	(+)
S. saprophyticus subsp. *saprophyticus*	d	−	−	−	−	−	−	+	+

[a] Symbols: +, 90% or more species or strains positive; ±, 90% or more species or strains weakly positive; −, 90% or more species or strains negative; d, 11 to 89% of species or strains positive; parentheses indicate a delayed reaction.
[b] Descriptions are the same as those in Table 2.

the plasma used is not sterile (and some are not), either false-positive or false-negative results may occur; and (iii) an inoculum from an agar-grown colony may not be pure, and a contaminant may produce false results after prolonged incubation. For those uncommon *S. aureus* strains requiring a longer clotting period, other characteristics (Table 3) should also be tested to confirm identity. Additional characteristics are required to identify rare CoNS mutants and some encapsulated strains.

The slide coagulase test is performed by making a heavy uniform suspension of growth in distilled water, stirring the mixture to a homogeneous composition so as not to confuse clumping with autoagglutination, adding 1 drop of plasma, and observing for clumping within 10 s. The slide test is very rapid and more economical of plasma than the tube test. Slide tests must be read quickly because false-positive results may appear with reaction times longer than 10 s. In addition, colonies for testing must not be picked from media containing high concentrations of salt (e.g., mannitol-salt agar) because autoagglutination and false-positive results may occur. Some uncommon strains of *S. intermedius* may give a positive slide test result. Alternative methods for the slide test include commercial hemagglutination slide tests for clumping factor and latex agglutination tests that detect clumping factor and protein A and/or surface antigens, although latex agglutination tests may not always yield the same reaction as the slide test. Latex agglutination tests often have a higher specificity and sensitivity than the conventional slide test for the identification of *S. aureus*, although they are generally less reliable for the identification of *S. lugdunensis*. Some members of the *S. saprophyticus* and *S. sciuri* species groups and *Macrococcus* species may produce positive results in latex agglutination tests, but they are usually negative for the slide test. Due to the low levels of bound coagulase and protein A in MRSA strains, the detection of MRSA by rapid agglutination tests requires the incorporation of antibodies against staphylococcal capsular polysaccharides. Latex agglutination tests that detect

both serotype 5 and serotype 8 capsular polysaccharides of methicillin-susceptible *S. aureus* and MRSA strains are available (54); however, false-positive reactions can occur (17, 63, 183). When the organism being tested is suspected of being *S. aureus*, negative slide tests should be confirmed by the tube coagulase test. Commercial latex agglutination kits can be acquired from various manufacturers, including the Slidex Staph (bioMérieux Vitek, Hazelwood, Mo.), BBL Staphyloslide (Becton Dickinson Biosciences, Sparks, Md.), Staphaurex (Murex Diagnostics Inc., Norcross, Ga.), and Bacti Staph Latex (Remel).

Heat-Stable Nuclease

A heat-stable staphylococcal nuclease (thermonuclease [TNase]) that has endo- and exonucleolytic properties and can cleave DNA or RNA is produced by most strains of *S. aureus*, *S. schleiferi*, *S. intermedius*, and *S. hyicus*. Some strains of *S. epidermidis*, *S. simulans*, and *S. carnosus* demonstrate a weak TNase activity. TNase can be detected by using a metachromatic-agar diffusion procedure and DNase-toluidine blue agar (109). A seroinhibition test has been developed to distinguish *S. aureus* TNase from those of other species (110). A commercial TNase test with toluidine blue agar is available (Remel) and can be interpreted in 4 h.

Phosphatase Activity

Phosphatase activity based on the hydrolysis of *p*-nitrophenylphosphate into P_i and *p*-nitrophenol by alkaline phosphatase has been incorporated into several of the commercial biochemical test systems for staphylococcal species identification. Phosphatase activity is indicated by the release of yellow *p*-nitrophenol from the colorless substrate. Key Scientific Co. (Roundrock, Tex.) manufactures an alkaline phosphatase tablet that may detect activity in staphylococci, although it has not yet been widely accepted because it has a small database.

Acetoin production	Novobiocin resistance[b]	Polymyxin B resistance[b]	Acid (aerobically) from:							
			D-Trehalose	D-Mannitol	D-Mannose	D-Turanose	D-Xylose	D-Cellobiose	Maltose	Sucrose
+	−	+	+	+	+	+	−	−	+	+
+	−	+	−	−	(+)	(d)	−	−	+	+
+	−	−	+	d	−	(d)	−	−	+	+
−	−	+	+	−	+	−	−	−	−	+
−	−	−	+	(d)	+	d	−	−	(±)	+
+	−	d	+	−	+	(d)	−	−	+	+
+	−	−	d	−	+	−	−	−	−	−
+	+		+	d	−	+	−	−	+	+

Strains of *S. aureus*, *S. schleiferi*, *S. intermedius*, and *S. hyicus* and most strains of *S. epidermidis* are alkaline phosphatase positive. Phosphatase-negative strains of *S. epidermidis* can be distinguished from the related species *S. hominis* on the basis of their strong anaerobic growth in thioglycolate within 18 to 24 h or resistance to a 300-U disk of polymyxin B (see below).

Pyrrolidonyl Arylamidase Activity

Pyrrolidonyl arylamidase (pyrrolidonase) activity can be determined by the hydrolysis of pyroglutamyl-β-naphthylamide (L-pyrrolidonyl-β-naphthylamide [PYR]) into L-pyrrolidone and β-naphthylamine, which combines with a PYR reagent (p-dimethylaminocinnamaldehyde) to produce a red color. A commercial kit containing PYR broth and PYR reagent (Remel), recommended for the identification of streptococci, is useful for distinguishing certain staphylococcal species. A loopful of a 24-h agar slant culture or several well-isolated colonies are dispersed in the PYR broth (containing 0.01% PYR) to a turbidity of a McFarland no. 2 standard. The suspension is incubated at 35°C for 2 h. After incubation, 2 drops of PYR reagent are added to each tube without mixing. The development of a red color within 2 min is indicative of positive activity. A yellow, orange, or pink color is considered a negative result. Alternatively, the basic features of the test have been incorporated into several of the commercial biochemical test panels for the identification of staphylococcal species. *S. haemolyticus*, *S. lugdunensis*, *S. schleiferi*, and *S. intermedius* are usually pyrrolidonase positive.

Ornithine Decarboxylase Activity

A positive ornithine decarboxylase activity can identify the species *S. lugdunensis* with considerable accuracy. Ornithine decarboxylase activity can be determined by a slight modification of the test described by Moeller (132). Decarboxylase basal medium (Becton Dickinson Biosciences) is prepared as specified by the manufacturer, 1% (wt/vol)

L-ornithine dihydrochloride is added, and the final medium is adjusted to pH 6 with 1 N sodium hydroxide before sterilization. The medium is dispensed in 3- to 4-ml amounts in small (13- by 100-mm) screw-cap tubes and autoclaved at 121°C for 10 min. A loopful of an overnight agar slant culture or several well-isolated colonies are dispersed in the test broth, and then the contents of each tube are overlaid with 4 to 5 mm of sterile mineral oil. Inoculated tubes should be incubated at 35 to 37°C for up to 24 h. They can be read initially as early as 8 h for the positive identification of most strains of *S. lugdunensis*; at this time, *S. epidermidis* will produce negative results. A positive reaction is indicated by alkalinization of the medium, with a change in the initial grayish color or slight yellowing (caused by the initial fermentation of glucose) to violet (caused by decarboxylation of L-ornithine). A yellow color at 24 h indicates a negative result.

Urease Activity

Conventional urea broth or agar (Becton Dickinson Biosciences; Oxoid) has been used to detect urease activity in staphylococcal species. The test detects the release of ammonia from urea, resulting in an increase in pH that is shown by the phenol red indicator changing from yellow to red or cerise. A miniaturization of the broth urease test has been incorporated into several of the commercial biochemical test systems for species identification of staphylococci. *S. epidermidis*, *S. intermedius*, and most strains of *S. saprophyticus* are usually urease positive.

β-Galactosidase Activity

Detection of high levels of β-galactosidase activity for the differentiation of certain staphylococcal species can be accomplished by commercial biochemical test systems that use 2-naphthol-β-D-galactopyranoside as a substrate. Fast blue BB salt in 2-methoxyethanol is added to the test well after an appropriate incubation period to detect free β-naphthol released by β-galactosidase. A positive activity is indicated by a plum purple color. By this assay, *S. intermedius* and most strains of *S. saprophyticus* are β-galactosidase positive and *S. schleiferi* is delayed or weakly positive.

Acetoin Production

Acetoin production from glucose or pyruvate is a useful alternative characteristic to distinguish *S. aureus* (positive) from another coagulase-positive species, *S. intermedius* (negative) and coagulase-positive strains of *S. hyicus* (negative). A conventional Voges-Proskauer test tube method with an incubation of 72 h or the more rapid paper disk method of Davis and Hoyling (40) is recommended for this test. The accuracy of the disk test is comparable to that of conventional Voges-Proskauer tests requiring longer incubation. Alternatively, acetoin production can be determined by using a Key Scientific Products tablet or by a miniaturized Voges-Proskauer test as incorporated into several of the commercial biochemical test systems for staphylococcal species identification.

Novobiocin Resistance

A simple disk diffusion test for estimating novobiocin susceptibility and distinguishing *S. saprophyticus* from other clinically important species can be performed by use of a 5-μg novobiocin disk on either P agar (98), Mueller-Hinton agar (4), or tryptic soy sheep blood agar (59). With an inoculum suspension equivalent in turbidity to a 0.5 McFarland opacity standard and incubation at 35 to 37°C for overnight to 24 h, novobiocin resistance is indicated by an inhibition zone diameter of ≤16 mm with any of these media. Rapid disk elution procedures with either manual or automated instrument interpretation have also been reported to predict novobiocin resistance reliably after only 4 to 5 h of incubation (67). Novobiocin resistance is intrinsic to *S. saprophyticus* and several other species (Table 2) but uncommon in the other clinically important species.

Polymyxin B Resistance

A simple disk diffusion test for estimating polymyxin B susceptibility to distinguish several of the clinically important species can be done by using a 300-U polymyxin B (Becton Dickinson) disk (69). The test can be performed on any of the media mentioned above for estimation of novobiocin resistance. However, the largest database has been obtained with the use of tryptic soy sheep blood agar. Test conditions should be similar to those described above for novobiocin resistance. The 5-μg novobiocin disk and the 300-U polymyxin B disk can be tested on the same inoculated plate. Polymyxin B resistance is indicated by an inhibition zone diameter of <10 mm. *S. aureus*, *S. epidermidis*, *S. hyicus*, and *S. chromogenes* are usually resistant. Some strains of *S. lugdunensis* are also resistant (68).

Acid Production from Carbohydrates

Acid production from carbohydrates can be easily detected by using the agar plate method of Kloos and Schleifer (98). Carbohydrate reactions are also incorporated into several of the commercial biochemical test systems for staphylococcal species identification. These systems use a more acid-sensitive indicator than the bromcresol purple (pH ≤ 5.2) in the agar plate method. For this and other reasons, the results of conventional carbohydrate tests (Tables 2 and 3) may be slightly different from those obtained from rapid commercial biochemical test systems.

Its production of acid from maltose and sucrose and absence of acid production for trehalose and mannitol can distinguish *S. epidermidis* from other novobiocin-susceptible species. Some uncommon strains of this species may produce acid from trehalose. These isolates can be distinguished from other species on the basis of phosphatase activity, anaerobic growth in thioglycolate, polymyxin B resistance, colonial morphology, and absence of ornithine decarboxylase and pyrrolidonase activities. Production of acid from trehalose, mannose, maltose, and sucrose and absence of acid production from mannitol can identify *S. lugdunensis*. *S. schleiferi* produces acid from mannose and sometimes from trehalose but does not produce acid from mannitol, maltose, or sucrose. Its production of acid from sucrose and turanose and absence of acid production from mannose, xylose, cellobiose, arabinose, and raffinose can distinguish *S. saprophyticus* from other novobiocin-resistant species.

Identification of Species by Using Commercial Biochemical or Nucleic Acid Test Systems

Several manufacturers of commercial kit identification systems (see chapter 14 of this Manual) and automated instruments have released products that can identify a number of the *Staphylococcus* species with an accuracy of 70 to >90% with relative speed and simplicity (92, 146). Since their introduction, systems have been improved and expanded to include more species. Their reliability will continue to increase as the result of a growing database and development of more discriminating tests. *S. aureus*, *S. epidermidis*, *S. capitis*, *S. haemolyticus*, *S. saprophyticus*, *S. simulans*, and *S. intermedius* can be identified reliably by most of the commercial systems now available. For some systems, reliability depends on additional testing as suggested by the manufacturer. Additional testing might include determining coagulase, clumping factor, or ornithine decarboxylase activity, anaerobic growth in thioglycolate, or novobiocin resistance. If one or more of these key tests are not included in the particular manufacturer's product, identification could be uncertain with respect to some species. Identification systems now available include RAPI-DEC Staph (identification of *S. aureus*, *S. epidermidis*, and *S. saprophyticus*) and API STAPH (bioMérieux Vitek, Inc., Hazelwood, Mo.); VITEK, a fully automated microbiology system that uses a Gram Positive Identification (GPI) Card (bioMérieux Vitek); MicroScan Pos ID panel (read manually or on MicroScan instrumentation) and MicroScan Rapid Pos ID panel (read by the WalkAway systems; in addition, the ID panels are available with antimicrobial agents for susceptibility testing) (Dade MicroScan, Inc., West Sacramento, Calif.); Crystal Gram-Positive Identification System, Crystal Rapid Gram-Positive Identification System, Pasco MIC/ID Gram-Positive Panel, and Phoenix, an automated identification system (Becton Dickinson Biosciences); GP MicroPlate test panel (read manually using the Biolog MicroLog system, or automatically with the Biolog MicroStation system) (Biolog, Hayward, Calif.); MIDI Sherlock Identification System Microbial Identification System (MIS), which automates microbial identification by combining cellular fatty acid analysis with computerized high-resolution gas chromatography (MIDI, Newark, Del.); and RiboPrinter Microbial Characterization System (Qualicon, Inc. Wilmington, Del.), based on ribotype pattern analysis. Rapid identification of the species *S. aureus* can be made using the AccuProbe culture identification test for *S. aureus* (Gen-Probe, Inc., San Diego, Calif.). This test is a DNA probe assay directed against rRNA and is very accurate (≥95% specificity) (3, 166). Tube coagulase-negative and slide test-negative strains of *S. aureus* should be identified correctly by the AccuProbe test.

Micrococcus and Related Species, *Alloiococcus*, and *Rothia mucilaginosa*

Pigment production and colony morphology may be used as simple tests in the presumptive identification of *Micrococcus* species and other related gram-positive cocci (100, 103). Several other phenotypic characters can be used to identify micrococci in the clinical laboratory (103, 169). *M. lylae* can be distinguished from *M. luteus* by its cream-white or nonpigmented colonies, lack of growth on organic nitrogen agar, and lysozyme resistance. However, a small percentage of *M. luteus* strains produce cream-white colonies. *Micrococcus* species can be distinguished from the genus *Kocuria* on the basis of their inability to produce acid aerobically from D-glucose and β-D-fructose. Furthermore, the species *K. varians* and *K. rosea* can be distinguished from micrococci by showing nitrate reduction and negative or only weak oxidase activity, and *K. kristinae* can be distinguished from micrococci by showing production of acid, aerobically, from glycerol and D-mannose, production of acetoin, and hydrolysis of esculin. The orange-pigmented species *Dermacoccus nishinomiyaensis* can be distinguished from micrococci by showing small pale orange colonies, nitrate reduction, and lack of growth on 7.5% NaCl agar. *K. sedentarius* differs from other micrococci by being resistant to penicillin and methicillin and exhibiting arginine dihydrolase activity. Colonies of this species may produce a brownish water-soluble pigment and may grow more slowly than those of micrococci. *Nesterenkonia halobia* can easily be separated from micrococci because it requires at least 5% NaCl for growth.

Alloiococci form small alpha-hemolytic colonies on blood agar after 48 h of incubation. Isolates can be distinguished from other similar organisms by their inability to utilize carbohydrates, their obligate aerobic nature, and their negative oxidase test. On routine blood agar, colonies of *R. mucilaginosa* are mucoid or sticky, transparent to white, and nonhemolytic and often adhere to the agar. This organism is distinguished from similar organisms by its inability to grow in the presence of 5% NaCl and its ability to hydrolyze gelatin and esculin.

Strain Identification

Members of a bacterial strain constitute a population of cells descended from a common ancestor at a relatively recent point in time. In the most recent examples, a strain represents a clonal population with each of its members being genetically identical (isogenic) and demonstrating identical phenotypic characteristics (88). It is also reasonable to define a strain as representing a clonal population in which some of its members differ from one another on the basis of only one or a few mutations or the loss or acquisition of an extrachromosomal element (e.g., phage, plasmid, or transposon). Strain identification is very important in distinguishing contaminants from the etiologic agent. Multiple isolations of the same strain demonstrate a high likelihood that the strain is clinically significant. Strain delineation is important in examining isolates from individual patients as well as those in outbreak situations. General considerations for epidemiologic typing of bacteria are discussed in chapter 12 of this Manual.

Strain typing may be accomplished by a variety of methods, including the examination of phenotypic and genotypic characters. Most tests require special media, techniques, and/or instrumentation and would be better performed in a reference laboratory. Nevertheless, some approaches to strain identification, such as the description of colonial morphology and the development of biotype profiles and antibiograms, can be used by the small clinical laboratory. Colonial morphology is a character that can identify individual strains in many of the staphylococcal species. In general, colony recognition has little impact on patient care associated with the treatment of acute illness caused by *S. aureus*. However, strain colony recognition is useful when a CoNS species or *Micrococcus* species is suspected in situations involving chronic infections and treatment failure. Colonies should be allowed to develop on the primary isolation medium for 3 to 4 days at 35 to 37°C and then for 2 days at room temperature for an initial screening. Colonies of the same strain generally exhibit similar features of size, consistency, edge, profile, lustre, and color on nonselective media commonly used for the culture of staphylococci or micrococci. Certain strains may exhibit variant morphotypes, and in these situations chromosomal analyses should help to clarify the mutual relationship of each morphotype. At least one colony of each morphotype should be selected from the primary isolation plate for subsequent analyses. Members of the same strain usually have the same biotype profile. However, further differentiation may be necessary if the strain has a common biotype profile. Antibiograms are commonly determined in the laboratory, and highly standardized procedures have been established. A unique susceptibility pattern can serve as a valuable marker. The more common patterns will provide some support for identification if testing is confined to a small area or community. On occasion, a strain may demonstrate variation in pattern due to the acquisition or loss of antibiotic resistance genes or their activity, making identification more difficult.

Most *Staphylococcus* species contain a variety of different plasmids (96). Consequently, plasmid composition can serve as a valuable typing tool for strain identification. In most staphylococcal species there is a relationship between antibiotic resistance pattern and the presence of certain plasmids carrying resistance genes. In this regard, plasmid composition may not be entirely independent of the antibiogram. For plasmids of identical size, restriction endonuclease fragment analysis may provide additional information for determining the identity. Such plasmids are considered to be different if their fragment patterns are different. Unfortunately, some common plasmids are highly conserved (e.g., small tetracycline [*tetK*] resistance plasmids or small erythromycin [*ermC*] resistance plasmids) and often have identical fragment patterns irrespective of the strain or species carrying them. Some strains exhibit clonal variation in their plasmid profiles. The addition or deletion of an entire plasmid or a restriction fragment within a plasmid most often represents this variation, although different recombinant plasmids are occasionally observed.

Cellular fatty acid profiling may be useful as a screening tool in epidemiologic studies, in addition to its use in the identification of *Staphylococcus* species and subspecies. Electrophoretic analysis of multilocus enzymes has proved to be useful in distinguishing stains of *S. aureus* isolated from various sources. Molecular typing techniques that examine the chromosome, such as pulsed-field gel electrophoresis of SmaI-digested genomic DNA (10, 55) and ribotyping (65, 180), have successfully delineated staphylococcal strains. Although we would expect restriction fragment patterns to be quite stable and similar among members of the same strain, some clonal variation has been observed with certain strains with respect to the size and number of fragments present. The acquisition or loss of prophages, transposition events, and/or recombination events with resident extra-chromosomal DNA might explain such variation. PCR is being investigated for its role as a rapid strain-screening method for staphylococcal epidemiologic studies. Target sequences include the coagulase gene (31, 74), protein A gene (141), 16S–23S rRNA intergenic spacer region (64, 104, 106, 186), and randomly amplified polymorphic DNA (16, 142, 182).

ANTIBIOTIC SUSCEPTIBILITIES

Nosocomial infections caused by methicillin resistant staphylococci pose a serious problem for health care institutions. The detection of resistance in these isolates has been hampered due to the variability in standard techniques used in determining methicillin resistance. The resistant strains are often heteroresistant to β-lactam antibiotics in that two subpopulations (one susceptible and the other resistant) coexist within a culture (28). Each cell in the population may carry the genetic information for resistance, but only a small fraction (10^{-8} to 10^{-4}) can actually express the resistant phenotype under in vitro testing conditions. The resistant subpopulation usually grows much more slowly than the susceptible subpopulation and therefore may be missed when in vitro testing is performed. The successful detection of heteroresistant strains depends largely on promoting the growth of the resistant subpopulations, which is favored by neutral pH, lower temperatures (30 to 35°C), the presence of NaCl (2 to 4%), and possible prolonged incubation (up to 48 h) (22, 36, 125). Oxacillin resistance in staphylococci can be detected by the methods recommended by the National Committee for Clinical Laboratory Standards (NCCLS) guidelines (136) and those described in chapters 70 and 74 of this Manual. To increase the accuracy of methicillin susceptibilities, recent NCCLS guidelines have given S. aureus and CoNS isolates different susceptibility breakpoints (136). A study by Gradelski et al. (61) confirmed the accuracy of the new breakpoints for S. aureus, S. epidermidis, and S. haemolyticus. However, the breakpoints have produced errors for other CoNS species. Difficulties in the differentiation of MRSA isolates from borderline oxacillin-resistant strains of S. aureus (BORSA), which are resistant due to hyperproduction of β-lactamase and not the presence of the mecA determinant, may be problematic to many clinical laboratories not routinely utilizing PCR as their standard method of detecting MRSA. However, to date there have been no reports of treatment failure during therapy with penicillinase-resistant penicillins in infections by these organisms.

Rapid detection of the mecA gene in S. aureus by DNA amplification and hybridization, commercially available fluorescence tests (76, 152, 155), and the slide latex agglutination test (25, 135, 155) has been found to be accurate and provides results more quickly than do standard susceptibility tests. Accurate differentiation of MRSA isolates from BORSA isolates has been reported through the use of the slide latex agglutination test (118). Caution should be taken in the use of DNA probes in antibiotic susceptibility testing, since the probes only indicate gene sequences and the potential of the bacterium to demonstrate antibiotic resistance. They do not necessarily discriminate between functional and nonfunctional genes. Furthermore, the widespread animal staphylococcal species S. sciuri has a native mecA homolog that is different from the homolog found in MRSA and other methicillin-resistant staphylococci (37, 91, 94). The two mecA homologs have about 79 to 80% base pair similarity and appear to be rather similar by DNA hybridization; however, they can be distinguished by PCR conducted under different conditions of stringency and they are expressed differently. Typical S. sciuri strains carrying the native mecA homolog are susceptible or express uniform borderline resistance to methicillin, whereas staphylococci carrying the MRSA mecA homolog express heterogeneous resistance to methicillin. Human isolates of S. sciuri have been described that carry both the native mecA gene and the MRSA mecA gene (38). S. sciuri, however, is rarely isolated from human infections.

Antimicrobic susceptibility testing of SCVs of S. aureus presents a challenge for the clinical microbiology laboratory. Since SCVs have only minimal amounts of ATP available, they cannot effectively transport aninoglycosides into the cell; therefore, resistance to gentamicin and other aminoglycosides can be expected (150). Resistance to trimethoprim-sulfamethoxazole is observed in thymidine auxotrophs (149). The slow growth of SCVs limits the usefulness of antimicrobials directed against the cell wall. No approved method has been developed to determine the susceptibility of SCVs. However, susceptibility profiles have been determined by broth or agar dilution MIC methods using low levels of auxotroph supplements (83, 149), disk diffusion under NCCLS guidelines with Mueller-Hinton (MH) agar supplemented with blood (83), and E test (AB Biodisk, Piscataway, N.J.) on MH agar supplemented with blood (83).

With the increase in methicillin resistance in Staphylococcus species, other antibiotics have been used in the treatment of serious infections caused by this group of bacteria. The glycopeptide vancomycin has been regarded as the drug of choice for the treatment of infections due to methicillin-resistant staphylococci. However, the appearance of vancomycin-intermediate isolates (MICs, 8 to 16 μg/ml) of S. aureus (VISA), resistant CoNS, and the potential for the development of resistance require the need for prudent use of the drug (15, 163, 178, 194). With the continued observance of VISA isolates, clinical laboratories need to incorporate an algorithm for the detection and reporting of VISA isolates (123). The detection of vancomycin-heteroresistant populations of staphylococci appears to be a similar challenge as seen for methicillin heteroresistant populations. A recent evaluation of methods used to detect staphylococcal isolates with reduced susceptibility to glycopeptides suggests that the E test with an inoculum of 2.0 McFarland onto brain heart infusion (BHI) agar yielded the highest sensitivity and specificity of 88 and 88%, respectively (191). The Centers for Disease Control and Prevention (CDC) has adopted three criteria that must all be met for the verification of VISA: broth microdilution vancomycin MICs of 8 to 16 μg/ml, E test vancomycin MICs of ≥6 μg/ml, and growth within 24 h on commercial BHI agar screen plates containing 6 μg of vancomycin per ml (178). Interim guidelines have been established to prevent and control staphylococcal infections associated with reduced susceptibility to vancomycin (26).

Reviews have summarized the antimicrobial susceptibilities of staphylococcal isolates to various drugs (89, 114). Multidrug resistance is more frequent in S. haemolyticus, S. epidermidis, S. hominis, and S. aureus than in other staphylococcal species isolated in the clinical laboratory. Increased levels of resistance to antimicrobial agents used for therapy including aminoglycosides, glycopeptides, quinolones, tetracyclines, macrolides, lincosamides, and trimethoprim-sulfamethoxazole make the treatment of multidrug-resistant staphylococcal infections difficult. Prevention of the initial infection through the eradication of *S. aureus* on colonized patients has met with moderate success. Mupirocin has been used to eradicate nasal carriage of *S. aureus*, but resistance has been observed (21, 200). A variety of new compounds being investigated or utilized for effective therapy include daptomycin (2, 198), an everninomicin antibiotic (52, 82), a new semisynthetic glycopeptide (5, 66, 145), glycylcycline (80, 174), oxazolidinones (45), and quinupristin/dalfopristin (81, 113, 168, 190).

Micrococci appear to be susceptible to most antibiotics. Successful treatment has been accomplished using vancomycin, penicillin, gentamicin, clindamycin, or a combination of these antibiotics (122). Strains of alloiococci show resistance to both erythromycin and trimethoprim-sulfamethoxazole and relative resistance to beta-lactams (18). *R. mucilaginosa* appears to be variable in its antimicrobial susceptibility (126, 130, 187, 188). The observation that *R. mucilaginosa* exhibits poor to no growth on MH agar and MH agar with sheep blood may make susceptibility testing a challenge for clinical microbiology laboratories (126, 130).

EVALUATION, INTERPRETATION, AND REPORTING OF RESULTS

Considering the frequency of the species, it is prudent to consider *S. aureus* the etiologic agent when it is isolated from a clinical specimen. The identities of suspected isolates should be confirmed on the basis of coagulase testing and also preferably on the basis of biochemical profile using a commercial identification system. At a significant but reasonable initial cost, the AccuProbe culture identification test for *S. aureus* (Gen-Probe) may be used to accurately identify the uncommon tube coagulase-negative or slide test-negative strains of *S. aureus* and could be used for the routine identification of the species. Strains of *S. aureus* should be monitored in the event of outbreaks in nosocomial and community populations. With the completion of whole-genome sequencing of an MRSA strain with vancomycin resistance, new insights into its pathogenic mechanisms are available (107). Hopefully, this research will provide information for the development of future treatment and prevention measures for this important staphylococcal pathogen.

It is a common practice to consider *S. epidermidis* the etiologic agent when it is isolated from colonized shunts or catheters in association with bacteremia or from prosthetic devices in association with clinical and pathologic evidence. *S. saprophyticus* is considered an etiologic agent when it is isolated from patients with urinary tract infections. Although these assessments are not always accurate, they are based on the known pathogenic potential of these species. Traditionally, colony counts of ≥100,000 CFU/ml in two or more cultures of midstream urine in females indicate a significant bacteriuria or urinary tract infection. Since staphylococci grow relatively slowly in urine, it has been suggested that lower colony counts of 100 to 10,000 CFU/ml should be considered an appropriate range for significant bacteriuria in the presence of pyuria (75, 173). Repeated isolation of a predominant strain or a strain in pure culture is quite convincing when attempting to determine the etiologic agent. For many of the other staphylo-

coccal and microccocal species, it is imperative that individual strains be identified and monitored, preferably over the course of the infection, before their etiology can be evaluated. In the small clinic or small community hospital laboratory, CoNS isolates are seldom identified to species, although isolates of interest are sometimes sent to private or other reference laboratories for identification to the species, subspecies, or strain level. When it is deemed necessary to identify the etiologic agent, e.g., as a result of treatment failure or during an outbreak, it is important that one or more aged (≥72-h) colonies of a particular morphotype be isolated from the primary plate of each culture to be identified. The practice of pooling two or more young (24- to 48-h) colonies in the preparation of an inoculum or culture carries with it the risk of producing a mixed culture, resulting in an erroneous identification and accompanying antibiogram. Selecting only one young colony from a primary isolation plate carries with it the risk of missing the actual etiologic agent.

At many large community and teaching hospitals, state health departments, and the CDC, both conventional and molecular methods are being performed for the complete identification of staphylococci. CoNS species and subspecies are usually identified on the basis of their phenotypic characters by commercial rapid identification systems and some supplemental conventional methods, as discussed above. Any isolation of the species *S. aureus* should be considered suspect and processed for a confirmed identification together with an antibiogram. The role of SCVs in clinical disease and the most appropriate means for identifying these isolates and obtaining accurate antimicrobial susceptibility profiles remain to be determined. However, SCVs are linked to patients with persistent and recurrent infections. In general, a combination of two or more conventional typing techniques is used for strain identification. Ribotyping and pulsed-field gel electrophoresis appear to be the most objective and discriminatory molecular techniques currently available.

REFERENCES

1. **Aguirre, M., and M. D. Collins.** 1992. Phylogenetic analysis of *Alloiococcus otitis* gen. nov., sp. nov., an organism from human middle ear fluid. *Int. J. Syst. Bacteriol.* **42:**79–83.
2. **Akins, R. L., and M. J. Rybak.** 2001. Bactericidal activities of two daptomycin regimens against clinical strains of glycopeptide intermediate-resistant *Staphylococcus aureus*, vancomycin-resistant *Enterococcus faecium*, and methicillin-resistant *Staphylococcus aureus* isolates in an in vitro pharmacodynamic model with simulated endocardial vegetations. *Antimicrob. Agents Chemother.* **45:**454–459.
3. **Allaouchiche, B., H. Meugnier, J. Freney, J. Fleurette, and J. Motin.** 1996. Rapid identification of *Staphylococcus aureus* in bronchoalveolar lavage fluid using a DNA probe (Accuprobe). *Intensive Care Med.* **22:**683–687.
4. **Almeida, R. J., and J. H. Jorgensen.** 1982. Use of Mueller-Hinton agar to determine novobiocin susceptibility of coagulase-negative staphylococci. *J. Clin. Microbiol.* **16:**1155–1156.
5. **Al-Nawas, B., and P. M. Shah.** 1998. Intracellular activity of vancomycin and LY333328, a new semisynthetic glycopeptide, against methicillin-resistant *Staphylococcus aureus*. *Infection* **26:**165–167.
6. **Ascher, D. P., C. Zbick, C. White, and G. W. Fischer.** 1991. Infections due to *Stomatococcus mucilaginosus*: 10 cases and review. *Rev. Infect. Dis.* **13:**1048–1052.

7. **Baker, J. S.** 1984. Comparison of various methods for differentiation of staphylococci and micrococci. *J. Clin. Microbiol.* **19:**875–879.

8. **Baker, J. S., M. F. Hackett, and D. J. Simard.** 1986. Variations in bacitracin susceptibility in *Staphylococcus* and *Micrococcus* species. *J. Clin. Microbiol.* **23:**963–964.

9. **Bannerman, T. L., and W. E. Kloos.** 1991. *Staphylococcus capitis* subsp. *urealyticus* subsp. nov. from human skin. *Int. J. Syst. Bacteriol.* **41:**144–147.

10. **Bannerman, T. L., G. A. Hancock, F. C. Tenover, and J. M. Miller.** 1995. Pulsed-field gel electrophoresis as a replacement for bacteriophage typing of *Staphylococcus aureus*. *J. Clin. Microbiol.* **33:**551–555.

11. **Becker, K., R. Roth, and G. Peters.** 1998. Rapid and specific detection of toxigenic *Staphylococcus aureus*: use of two multiplex PCR enzyme immunoassays for amplification and hybridization of staphylococcal enterotoxin genes, exfoliative toxin genes, and toxic shock syndrome toxin 1 gene. *J. Clin. Microbiol.* **36:**2548–2553.

12. **Bergan, T., and M. Kocur.** 1982. *Stomatococcus mucilaginosus* gen. nov., sp. nov., ep. rev., a member of the family *Micrococcaceae*. *Int. J. Syst. Bacteriol.* **32:**374–377.

13. **Beswick, A. J., B. Lawley, A. P. Fraise, A. L. Pahor, and N. L. Brown.** 1999. Detection of *Alloiococcus otitis* in mixed bacterial populations from middle-ear effusions of patients with otitis media. *Lancet* **354:**386–389.

14. **Bialkowska-Hobrzanska, H., D. Jaskot, and O. Hammerberg.** 1990. Evaluation of restriction endonuclease fingerprinting of chromosomal DNA and plasmid profile analysis for characterization of multiresistant coagulase-negative staphylococci in bacteremic neonates. *J. Clin. Microbiol.* **28:**269–275.

15. **Biavasco, F., C. Vignaroli, and P. E. Varaldo.** 2000. Glycopeptide resistance in coagulase-negative staphylococci. *Eur. J. Clin. Microbiol. Infect. Dis.* **19:**403–417.

16. **Bingen, E., M. C. Barc, N. Brahimi, E. Vilmer, and F. Beaufils.** 1995. Randomly amplified polymorphic DNA analysis provides rapid differentiation of methicillin-resistant coagulase-negative staphylococci. *J. Clin. Microbiol.* **32:**2113–2119.

17. **Blake, J. E., and M. A. Metcalfe.** 2001. A shared noncapsular antigen is responsible for false-positive reactions by *Staphylococcus epidermidis* in commercial agglutination tests for *Staphylococcus aureus*. *J. Clin. Microbiol.* **39:**544–550.

18. **Bosley, G. S., A. M. Whitney, J. M. Pruckler, C. W. Moss, M. Daneshvar, T. Sih, and D. F. Talkington.** 1995. Characterization of ear fluid isolates of *Alloiococcus otitidis* from patients with recurrent otitis media. *J. Clin. Microbiol.* **33:**2876–2880.

19. **Boyce, J. M.** 1991. Should we vigorously try to contain and control methicillin-resistant *Staphylococcus aureus*? *Infect. Control Hosp. Epidemiol.* **12:**46–54.

20. **Boyce, J. M.** 1995. Strategies for controlling methicillin-resistant *Staphylococcus aureus* in hospitals. *J. Chemother.* **7**(Suppl. 3):81–85.

21. **Bradley, S. F., M. A. Ramsey, T. M. Morton, and C. A. Kauffman.** 1995. Mupirocin resistance: clinical and molecular epidemiology. *Infect. Control Hosp. Epidemiol.* **16:**354–358.

22. **Brown, D. F. J.** 2001. Detection of methicillin/oxacillin resistance in staphylococci. *J. Antimicrob. Chemother.* **48**(Suppl. S1):65–70.

23. **Calvo, J., J. L. Hernandez, M. C. Farinas, D. Garcia-Palomo, and J. Aguero.** 2000. Osteomyelitis caused by *Staphylococcus schleiferi* and evidence of misidentification of this *Staphylococcus* species by an automated bacterial identification system. *J. Clin. Microbiol.* **38:**3887–3889.

24. **Cato, E. P., and E. Stackebrandt.** 1989. Taxonomy and phylogeny, p. 1–26. *In* N. P. Minton and D. J. Clarke (ed.), *Clostridia*. Plenum Press, New York, N.Y.

25. **Cavassini, M., A. Wenger, K. Jaton, D. S. Blanc, and J. Bille.** 1999. Evaluation of MRSA-Screen, a simple anti-PBP 2a slide latex agglutination kit, for rapid detection of methicillin resistance in *Staphylococcus aureus*. *J. Clin. Microbiol.* **37:**1591–1594.

26. **Centers for Disease Control and Prevention.** 1997. Interim guidelines for the prevention and control of staphylococcal infections associated with reduced susceptibility to vancomycin. *Morb. Mortal. Wkly. Rep.* **46:**626–628, 635–636.

27. **Centers for Disease Control and Prevention.** 1999. Four pediatric deaths from community-acquired methicillin-resistant *Staphylococcus aureus*—Minnesota and North Dakota, 1997–1999. *Morb. Mortal. Wkly. Rep.* **48:**707–710.

28. **Chambers, H. F.** 1988. Methicillin-resistant staphylococci. *Clin. Microbiol. Rev.* **1:**173–186.

29. **Chambers, H. F.** 2001. The changing epidemiology of *Staphylococcus aureus*? *Emerg. Infect. Dis.* **7:**178–182.

30. **Chesneau, O., A. Morvan, F. Grimont, H. Labischinski, and N. El Solh.** 1993. *Staphylococcus pasteuri* sp. nov., isolated from human, animal, and food specimens. *Int. J. Syst. Bacteriol.* **43:**237–244.

31. **Chiou, C. S., H. L. Wei, and L. C. Yang.** 2000. Comparison of pulsed-field gel electrophoresis and coagulase gene restriction profile analysis techniques in the molecular typing of *Staphylococcus aureus*. *J. Clin. Microbiol.* **38:**2186–2190.

32. **Choi, Y., B. Kotzin, L. Herron, J. Callahan, P. Marrack, and J. Kappler.** 1989. Interaction of *Staphylococcus aureus* toxin "superantigens" with human T cells. *Proc. Natl. Acad. Sci. USA* **86:**8941–8945.

33. **Clink, J., and T. H. Pennington.** 1987. Staphylococcal whole-cell polypeptide analysis: evaluation as a taxonomic and typing tool. *J. Med. Microbiol.* **23:**41–44.

34. **Cohn, F.** 1872. Untersuchungen über Bacterien. *Beitr. Biol. Pflanz.* Bd. 1, Heft **2:**127–224.

35. **Collins, M. D., R. A. Hutson, V. Båverud, and E. Falsen.** 2000. Characterization of a *Rothia*-like organism from a mouse: description of *Rothia nasimurium* sp. nov. and reclassification of *Stomatococcus mucilaginosus* as *Rothia mucilaginosa* comb. nov. *Int. J. Syst. Evol. Microbiol.* **50:**1247–1251.

36. **Coudron, P. E., D. L. Jones, H. P. Dalton, and G. L. Archer.** 1986. Evaluation of laboratory tests for detection of methicillin-resistant *Staphylococcus aureus* and *Staphylococcus epidermidis*. *J. Clin. Microbiol.* **24:**764–769.

37. **Couto, I., H. De Lencastre, E. Severina, W. E. Kloos, J. A. Webster, R. J. Hubner, I. Santos Sanches, and A. Tomasz.** 1996. Ubiquitous presence of a *mecA* homologue in natural isolates of *Staphylococcus sciuri*. *Microb. Drug Resist.* **2:**377–391.

38. **Couto, I., I. Santos Sanches, R. Sá-Leão, and H. de Lencastre.** 2000. Molecular characterization of *Staphylococcus sciuri* strains isolated from humans. *J. Clin. Microbiol.* **38:**1136–1143.

39. **Crossley, K. B., and G. L. Archer (ed.).** 1997. *The Staphylococci in Human Disease*. Churchill Livingstone, Inc., New York, N.Y.

40. **Davis, G. H. G., and B. Hoyling.** 1973. Use of a rapid acetoin test in the identification of staphylococci and micrococci. *Int. J. Syst. Bacteriol.* **23:**281–282.

41. **DeBuyser, M.-L., A. Morvan, S. Aubert, F. Dilasser, and N. El Solh.** 1992. Evaluation of ribosomal RNA gene probe for the identification of species and subspecies within the genus *Staphylococcus*. *J. Gen. Microbiol.* **138:**889–899.

42. **Devriese, L. A.** 1984. A simplified scheme for biotyping *Staphylococcus aureus* strains isolated from different animal species. *J. Appl. Bacteriol.* **56:**215–220.

43. **Devriese, L. A.** 1986. Coagulase-negative staphylococci in animals, p. 51–57. *In* P.-A. Mårdh and K. H. Schleifer (ed.), *Coagulase-Negative Staphylococci.* Almqvist & Wiksell International, Stockholm, Sweden.

44. **Devriese, L. A.** 1990. Staphylococci in healthy and diseased animals. *J. Appl. Bacteriol. Symp. Suppl.* **69:**71S–80S.

45. **Diekema, D. I., and R. N. Jones.** 2000. Oxazolidinones: a review. *Drugs* **59:**7–16.

46. **Downes, F. P., and K. Ito (ed.).** 2001. *Compendium of Methods for the Microbiological Examination of Foods,* 4th ed. American Public Health Association, Washington, D.C.

47. **Espersen, F., L. Baek, P. Kjaeldgaard, and V. T. Rosdahl.** 1988. Detection of staphylococcal toxic shock syndrome toxin 1 by a latex agglutination kit. *Scand. J. Infect. Dis.* **20:**449–450.

48. **Evans, J. B., W. L. Bradford, Jr., and C. F. Niven.** 1955. Comments concerning the taxonomy of the genera *Micrococcus* and *Staphylococcus. Int. Bull. Bacteriol. Nomencl. Taxon.* **5:**61–66.

49. **Faden, H., and D. Dryja.** 1989. Recovery of a unique bacterial organism in human middle ear fluid and its possible role in chronic otitis media. *J. Clin. Microbiol.* **27:**2488–2491.

50. **Faller, A., and K. H. Schleifer.** 1981. Modified oxidase and benzidine tests for separation of staphylococci from micrococci. *J. Clin. Microbiol.* **13:**1031–1035.

51. **Fleurette, J., M. Bes, Y. Brun, J. Freney, F. Forey, M. Coulet, M. E. Reverdy, and J. Etienne.** 1989. Clinical isolates of *Staphylococcus lugdunensis* and *S. schleiferi:* bacteriological characteristics and susceptibility to antimicrobial agents. *Res. Microbiol.* **140:**107–118.

52. **Foster, D. R., and M. J. Rybak.** 1999. Pharmacologic and bacteriologic properties of SCH-27899 (Ziracin), an investigational antibiotic from the everninomicin family. *Pharmocotherapy* **19:**1111–1117.

53. **Foster, G., H. M. Ross, R. A. Hutson, and M. D. Collins.** 1997. *Staphylococcus lutrae* sp. nov., a new coagulase-positive species isolated from otters. *Int. J. Syst. Bacteriol.* **47:**724–726.

54. **Fournier, J.-M., A. Bouvet, D. Mathieu, F. Nato, A. Boutonnier, R. Gerbal, P. Brunengo, C. Saulnier, N. Sagot, B. Slizewicz, and J.-C. Mazie.** 1993. New latex reagent using monoclonal antibodies to capsular polysaccharide for reliable identification of both oxacillin-susceptible and oxacillin-resistant *Staphylococcus aureus. J. Clin. Microbiol.* **31:**1342–1344.

55. **George, C. G., and W. E. Kloos.** 1994. Comparison of the *SmaI*-digested chromosomes of *Staphylococcus epidermidis* and the closely related species *Staphylococcus capitis* and *Staphylococcus caprae. Int. J. Syst. Bacteriol.* **44:**404–409.

56. **Girard, C., and R. Higgins.** 1999. *Staphylococcus intermedius* cellulitis and toxic shock in a dog. *Can. Vet. J.* **40:**501–502.

57. **Goh, S. H., Z. Santucci, W. E. Kloos, M. Faltyn, C. G. George, D. Driedger, and S. M. Hemmingsen.** 1997. Identification of *Staphylococcus* species and subspecies by the chaperonin 60 gene identification method and reverse checkerboard hybridization. *J. Clin. Microbiol.* **35:**3116–3121.

58. **Goldman, M., U. B. Chaudhary, A. Greist, and C. A. Fausel.** 1998. Central nervous system infections due to *Stomatococcus mucilaginosus* in immunocompromised hosts. *Clin. Infect. Dis.* **27:**1241–1246.

59. **Goldstein, J., R. Schulman, E. Kelly, G. McKinley, and J. Fung.** 1983. Effect of different media on determination

60. **Gomez-Hernando, C., C. Toro, M. Gutierrez, A. Enriquez, and M. Baquero.** 1999. Isolation of *Alloiococcus otitidis* from the external ear in children. *Eur. J. Clin. Microbiol. Infect. Dis.* **18:**69–70.

61. **Gradelski, E., L. Valera, L. Aleksunes, D. Bonner, and J. Fung-Tomc.** 2001. Correlation between genotype and phenotype categorization of staphylococci based on methicillin susceptibility and resistance. *J. Clin. Microbiol.* **39:**2961–2963.

62. **Granlund, M., M. Linderholm, M. Norgren, C. Olofsson, A. Wahlin, and S. E. Holm.** 1996. *Stomatococcus mucilaginosus* septicemia in leukemic patients. *Clin. Microbiol. Infect.* **2:**179–185.

63. **Gupta, H., N. McKinnon, L. Louie, M. Louie, and A. E. Simor.** 1998. Comparison of six rapid agglutination tests for the identification of *Staphylococcus aureus,* including methicillin-resistant strains. *Diagn. Microbiol. Infect. Dis.* **31:**333–336.

64. **Gurtler, V., and H. D. Barrie.** 1995. Typing of *Staphylococcus aureus* strains by PCR-amplification of variable length 16S–23S rDNA spacer regions: characterization of spacer sequences. *Microbiology* **141:**1255–1265.

65. **Hadorn, K., W. Lenz, F. H. Kayser, I. Shalit, and C. Krasemann.** 1990. Use of a ribosomal RNA gene probe for epidemiological study of methicillin and ciprofloxacin resistant *Staphylococcus aureus. Eur. J. Clin. Microbiol. Infect. Dis.* **9:**649–653.

66. **Harland, S., S. E. Tebbs, and T. S. J. Elliott.** 1998. Evaluation of the in-vitro activity of the glycopeptide antibiotic LY333328 in comparison with vancomycin and teicoplanin. *J. Antimicrobiol. Chemother.* **41:**273–276.

67. **Harrington, B. J., and J. M. Gaydos.** 1984. Five-hour novobiocin test for differentiation of coagulase-negative staphylococci. *J. Clin. Microbiol.* **19:**279–280.

68. **Hébert, G. A.** 1990. Hemolysins and other characteristics that help differentiate and biotype *Staphylococcus lugdunensis* and *Staphylococcus schleiferi. J. Clin. Microbiol.* **28:**2425–2431.

69. **Hébert, G. A., C. G. Crowder, G. A. Hancock, W. R. Jarvis, and C. Thornsberry.** 1988. Characteristics of coagulase-negative staphylococci that help differentiate these species and other members of the family *Micrococcaceae. J. Clin. Microbiol.* **26:**1939–1949.

70. **Hendolin, P. H., U. Karkkainen, T. Himi, A. Markkanen, and J. Ylikoski.** 1999. High incidence of *Alloiococcus otitis* in otitis media with effusion. *Pediatr. Infect. Dis. J.* **18:**860–865.

71. **Hendolin, P. H., A. Markkanen, J. Ylikoski, and J. J. Wahlfors.** 1997. Use of multiplex PCR for simultaneous detection of four bacterial species in middle ear effusions. *J. Clin. Microbiol.* **35:**2854–2858.

72. **Hernández, J. L., J. Calvo, R. Sota, J. Agüero, J. D. García-Palomo, and M. C. Fariñas.** 2001. Clinical and microbiological characteristics of 28 patients with *Staphylococcus schleiferi* infection. *Eur. J. Clin. Microbiol. Infect. Dis.* **20:**153–158.

73. **Herold, B. C., L. C. Immergluck, M. C. Maranan, D. S. Lauderdale, R. E. Gaskin, S. Boyle-Vavra, C. D. Leitch, and R. S. Daum.** 1998. Community-acquired methicillin-resistant *Staphylococcus aureus* in children with no identified predisposing risk. *JAMA* **279:**593–598.

74. **Hookey, J. V., J. F. Richardson, and B. D. Cookson.** 1998. Molecular typing of *Staphylococcus aureus* based on PCR restriction fragment length polymorphism and DNA sequence analysis of the coagulase gene. *J. Clin. Microbiol.* **36:**1083–1089.

75. **Hovelius, B.** 1986. Epidemiological and clinical aspects of urinary tract infections caused by *Staphylococcus saprophyticus*, p. 195–202. *In* P.-A. Mårdh and K. H. Schleifer (ed.), *Coagulase-Negative Staphylococci*. Almqvist & Wiksell International, Stockholm, Sweden.

76. **Ieven, M., H. Jansens, D. Ursi, J. Verhoeven, and H. Goossens.** 1995. Rapid detection of methicillin resistance in coagulase-negative staphylococci by commercially available fluorescence test. *J. Clin. Microbiol.* **33:**2183–2185.

77. **Igimi, S., E. Takahashi, and T. Mitsuoka.** 1990. *Staphylococcus schleiferi* subsp. *coagulans* subsp. nov., isolated from the external auditory meatus of dogs with external ear otitis. *Int. J. Syst. Bacteriol.* **40:**409–411.

78. **Jean-Pierre, H., H. Darbas, A. Jean-Roussenq, and G. Boyer.** 1989. Pathogenicity in two cases of *Staphylococcus schleiferi*, a recently described species. *J. Clin. Microbiol.* **27:**2110–2111.

79. **Johnson, W. M., and S. D. Tayler.** 1993. PCR detection of genes for enterotoxins, exfoliative toxins, and toxic shock syndrome toxin-1 in *Staphylococcus aureus*, p. 294–299. *In* D. H. Persing, T. F. Smith, F. C. Tenover, and T. J. White (ed.), *Diagnostic Molecular Microbiology: Principles and Applications*. American Society for Microbiology, Washington, D.C.

80. **Jones, R. N.** 1999. Disk diffusion susceptibility test development for the new glycylcycline, GAR-936. *Diagn. Microbiol. Infect. Dis.* **35:**249–252.

81. **Jones, R. N., C. H. Ballow, D. J. Biedenbach, J. A. Deinhart, and J. J. Schentag.** 1998. Antimicrobial activity of quinupristin-dalfopristin (RP 59500, Synercid) tested against over 28,000 recent clinical isolates from 200 medical centers in the United States and Canada. *Diagn. Microbiol. Infect. Dis.* **31:**437–451.

82. **Jones, R. N., S. A. Marshall, M. E. Erwin, and the Quality Control Study Group.** 1999. Antimicrobial activity and spectrum of SCH27899 (Ziracin®) tested against gram-positive species including recommendations for routine susceptibility testing methods and quality control. *Diagn. Microbiol. Infect. Dis.* **34:**103–110.

83. **Kahl, B., H. Herrmann, A. S. Everding, H. G. Koch, K. Becker, E. Harms, R. A. Proctor, and G. Peters.** 1998. Persistent infection with small colony variant strains of *Staphylococcus aureus* in patients with cystic fibrosis. *J. Infect. Dis.* **177:**1023–1029.

84. **Khambaty, F. M., R. W. Bennet, and D. B. Shah.** 1994. Application of pulsed-field gel electrophoresis to epidemiological characterization of *Staphylococcus intermedius* implicated in a food-related outbreak. *Epidemiol. Infect.* **113:**75–81.

85. **Kilpper, R., U. Buhl, and K. H. Schleifer.** 1980. Nucleic acid homology studies between *Peptococcus saccharolyticus* and various anaerobic and facultative anaerobic Gram-positive cocci. *FEMS Microbiol. Lett.* **8:**205–210.

86. **Kloos, W. E.** 1980. Natural populations of the genus *Staphylococcus*. *Annu. Rev. Microbiol.* **34:**559–592.

87. **Kloos, W. E.** 1986. Ecology of human skin, p. 37–50. *In* P.-A. Mårdh and K. H. Schleifer (ed.), *Coagulase-Negative Staphylococci*. Almqvist & Wiksell International, Stockholm, Sweden.

88. **Kloos, W. E.** 1990. Systematics and the natural history of staphylococci. 1. *J. Appl. Bacteriol. Symp. Suppl.* **69:**25S–37S.

89. **Kloos, W. E.** 1998. *Staphylococcus* p. 577–632. *In* L. Collier, A. Balows, and M. Sussman (ed.), *Topley & Wilson's Microbiology and Microbial Infections*, vol. 2, 9th ed. Edward Arnold, London, United Kingdom.

90. **Kloos, W. E., D. N. Ballard, C. G. George, J. A. Webster, R. J. Hubner, W. Ludwig, K. H. Schleifer, F.** Fiedler, and K. Schubert. 1998. Delimiting the genus *Staphylococcus* through description of *Macrococcus caseolyticus* gen. nov., comb. nov., *Macrococcus bovicus* sp. nov., and *Macrococcus carouselicus* sp. nov. *Int. J. Syst. Bacteriol.* **48:**859–877.

91. **Kloos, W. E., D. N. Ballard, J. A. Webster, R. J. Hubner, A. Tomasz, I. Couto, G. L. Sloan, H. P. DeHart, F. Fiedler, K. Schubert, H. De Lencastre, I. Santos Sanches, H. E. Heath, P. A. LeBlanc, and Å. Ljungh.** 1997. Ribotype delineation and description of *Staphylococcus sciuri* subspecies and their potential as reservoirs of methicillin resistance and staphylolytic enzyme genes. *Int. J. Syst. Bacteriol.* **47:**313–323.

92. **Kloos, W. E., and T. L. Bannerman.** 1994. Update on clinical significance of coagulase-negative staphylococci. *Clin. Microbiol. Rev.* **7:**117–140.

93. **Kloos, W. E., and T. L. Bannerman.** 1995. *Staphylococcus* and *Micrococcus*, p. 282–298. *In* P. R. Murray, E. J. Baron, M. A. Pfaller, F. C. Tenover, and R. H. Yolken (ed.), *Manual of Clinical Microbiology*, 6th ed. American Society for Microbiology, Washington, D.C.

94. **Kloos, W. E., C. G. George, J. S. Olgiati, L. Van Pelt, M. L. McKinnon, B. L. Zimmer, E. Muller, M. P. Weinstein, and S. Mirrett.** 1998. *Staphylococcus hominis* subsp. *novobiosepticus* subsp. nov., a novel trehalose- and N-acetyl-D-glucosamine-negative, novobiocin- and multiple antibiotic-resistant subspecies isolated from human blood cultures. *Int. J. Syst. Bacteriol.* **48:**799–812.

95. **Kloos, W. E., and M. S. Musselwhite.** 1975. Distribution and persistence of *Staphylococcus* and *Micrococcus* species and other aerobic bacteria on human skin. *Appl. Microbiol.* **30:**381–395.

96. **Kloos, W. E., B. S. Orban, and D. D. Walker.** 1981. Plasmid composition of *Staphylococcus* species. *Can. J. Microbiol.* **27:**271–278.

97. **Kloos, W. E., and K. H. Schleifer.** 1975. Isolation and characterization of staphylococci from human skin. II. Descriptions of four new species: *Staphylococcus warneri*, *Staphylococcus capitis*, *Staphylococcus hominis*, and *Staphylococcus simulans*. *Int. J. Syst. Bacteriol.* **25:**62–79.

98. **Kloos, W. E., and K. H. Schleifer.** 1975. Simplified scheme for routine identification of human *Staphylococcus* species. *J. Clin. Microbiol.* **1:**82–88.

99. **Kloos, W. E., K. H. Schleifer, and F. Götz.** 1991. The genus *Staphylococcus*, p. 1369–1420. *In* A. Balows, H. G. Trüper, M. Dworkin, W. Harder, and K. H. Schleifer (ed.), *The Prokaryotes*, 2nd ed. Springer-Verlag, New York, N.Y.

100. **Kloos, W. E., T. G. Tornabene, and K. H. Schleifer.** 1974. Isolation and characterization of micrococci from human skin, including two new species: *Micrococcus lylae* and *Micrococcus kristinae*. *Int. J. Syst. Bacteriol.* **24:**79–101.

101. **Klutymans, J., A. van Belkum, and H. Verbrugh.** 1997. Nasal carriage of *Staphylococcus aureus*: epidemiology, underlying mechanisms, and associated risks. *Clin. Microbiol. Rev.* **10:**505–520.

102. **Koch, C., and E. Stackebrandt.** 1995. Reclassification of *Micrococcus agilis* (Ali-Cohen 1889) to *Arthrobacter* as *Arthrobacter agilis* comb. nov. and emendation of the genus *Arthrobacter*. *Int. J. Syst. Bacteriol.* **45:**837–839.

103. **Kocur, M., W. E. Kloos, and K. H. Schleifer.** 1991. The genus *Micrococcus*, p. 1300–1311. *In* A. Balows, H. G. Trüper, M. Dworkin, W. Harder, and K. H. Schleifer (ed.), *The Prokaryotes*, 2nd ed. Springer-Verlag, New York, N.Y.

104. **Kostman, J. R., M. B. Alden, M. Mair, T. D. Edlind, J. J. LiPuma, and T. L. Stull.** 1995. A universal approach to bacterial molecular epidemiology by polymer-

ase chain reaction ribotyping. *J. Infect. Dis.* **171:**204–208.

105. **Kotilainen, P., P. Huovinen, and E. Eerola.** 1991. Application of gas-liquid chromatographic analysis of cellular fatty acids for species identification and typing of coagulase-negative staphylococci. *J. Clin. Microbiol.* **29:** 315–322.

106. **Kumari, D. N., V. Keer, P. M. Hawkey, P. Parnell, N. Joseph, J. F. Richardson, and B. Cookson.** 1997. Comparison and application of ribosome spacer DNA amplicon polymorphisms and pulsed-field gel electrophoresis for differentiation of methicillin-resistant *Staphylococcus aureus* strains. *J. Clin. Microbiol.* **35:**881–885.

107. **Kuroda, M., T. Ohta, I. Uchiyama, T. Baba, H. Yuzawa, I. Kobayashi, L. Cui, A. Oguchi, K. Aoki, Y. Nagai, J. Lian, T. Ito, M. Kanamori, H. Matsumaru, A. Maruyama, H. Murakami, A. Hosoyama, Y. Mizutani-Ui, N. K. Takahashi, T. Sawano, T. Inoue, C. Kaito, K. Sekimizu, H. Hirakawa, S. Kuhara, S. Goto, J. Yabuzaki, M. Kanehisa, A. Yamashita, K. Oshima, K. Furuya, C. Yoshino, T. Shiba, M. Hattori, N. Ogasawara, H. Hayashi, and K. Hiramatsu.** 2001. Whole genome sequencing of methicillin-resistant *Staphylococcus aureus*. *Lancet* **357:**1225–1240.

108. **Kwok, A. Y. C., S.-C. Su, R. P. Reynolds, S. J. Bay, Y. Av-Gay, N. J. Dovichi, and A. W. Chow.** 1999. Species identification and phylogenetic relationships based on partial *hsp60* gene sequences within the genus *Staphylococcus. Int. J. Syst. Bacteriol.* **49:**1181–1192.

109. **Lachica, R. V. F., P. D. Hoeprich, and C. Genigeorgis.** 1972. Metachromatic agar-diffusion microslide technique for detecting staphylococcal nuclease in foods. *Appl. Microbiol.* **23:**168–169.

110. **Lachica, R. V. F., S. S. Jang, and P. D. Hoeprich.** 1979. Thermonuclease seroinhibition test for distinguishing *Staphylococcus aureus* and other coagulase-positive staphylococci. *J. Clin. Microbiol.* **9:**141–143.

111. **Lambert, L. H., T. Cox, K. Mitchell, R. A. Rosselló-Mora, C. del Cueto, D. E. Dodge, P. Orkand, and R. J. Cano.** 1998. *Staphylococcus succinus* sp. nov., isolated from Dominican amber. *Int. J. Syst. Bacteriol.* **48:**511–518.

112. **Lambotte, O., T. Debord, C. Soler, and R. Roue.** 1999. Pneumonia due to *Stomatococcus mucilaginosus* in an AIDS patient: case report and literature review. *Clin. Microbiol. Infect.* **5:**112–114.

113. **Larkin, J., L. Busciglio, H. Fontanet, and G. Gamouras.** 1998. *Staphylococcus epidermidis* endocarditis treated with RP 59500 (quinupristin/dalfopristin). *Clin. Infect. Dis.* **26:**1239–1240.

114. **Laverdiere, M., K. Weiss, R. Rivest, and J. Delorme.** 1998. Trends in antibiotic resistance of staphylococci over an eight-year period: differences in the emergence of resistance between coagulase-positive and coagulase-negative staphylococci. *Microb. Drug Resist.* **4:**119–122.

115. **Layton, M. C., W. J. Hierholzer, and J. E. Patterson.** 1995. The evolving epidemiology of methicillin-resistant *Staphylococcus aureus* at a university hospital. *Infect. Control Hosp. Epidemiol.* **16:**12–17.

116. **Liu, H., Y. Xu, Y. Ma, and P. Zhou.** 2000. Characterization of *Micrococcus antarcticus* sp. nov., a psychrophilic bacterium from Antarctica. *Int. J. Syst. Evol. Microbiol.* **50:**715–719.

117. **Looney, W. J.** 2000. Small-colony variants of *Staphylococcus aureus. Br. J. Biomed. Sci.* **57:**317–322.

118. **Louie, L., S. O. Matsumura, E. Choi, M. Louie, and A. E. Simor.** 2000. Evaluation of three rapid methods for detection of methicillin resistance in *Staphylococcus aureus. J. Clin. Microbiol.* **38:**2170–2173.

119. **Ludwig, W., K. H. Schleifer, G. E. Fox, E. Seewaldt, and E. Stackebrandt.** 1981. A phylogenetic analysis of staphylococci, *Peptococcus saccharolyticus* and *Micrococcus mucilaginosus. J. Gen. Microbiol.* **125:**357–366.

120. **Ludwig, W., E. Seewaldt, R. Kilpper-Bälz, K. H. Schleifer, L. Magrum, C. R. Woese, G. F. Fox, and E. Stackebrandt.** 1985. The phylogenetic position of *Streptococcus* and *Enterococcus. J. Gen. Microbiol.* **131:** 543–551.

121. **Maes, N., Y. de Gheldre, R. de Ryck, M. Vaneechoutte, H. Meugnier, J. Etienne, and M. J. Struelens.** 1997. Rapid and accurate identification of *Staphylococcus* species by tRNA intergenic spacer length polymorphism analysis. *J. Clin. Microbiol.* **35:**2477–2481.

122. **Magee, J. T., I. A. Burnett, J. M. Hindmarch, and R. C. Spencer.** 1990. *Micrococcus* and *Stomatococcus* spp. from human infections. *J. Infect.* **16:**67–73.

123. **Marlowe, E. M., M. D. Cohen, J. F. Hindler, K. W. Ward, and D. A. Bruckner.** 2001. Practical strategies for detecting and confirming vancomycin-intermediate *Staphylococcus aureus:* a tertiary-care hospital laboratory's experience. *J. Clin. Microbiol.* **39:**2637–2639.

124. **Marsou, R., M. Bes, M. Boudouma, Y. Brun, H. Meugnier, J. Freney, F. Vandenesch, and J. Etienne.** 1999. Distribution of *Staphylococcus sciuri* subspecies among human clinical specimens, and profile of antibiotic resistance. *Res. Microbiol.* **150:**531–541.

125. **McDougal, L. K., and C. Thornsberry.** 1984. New recommendations for disk diffusion antimicrobial susceptibility tests for methicillin-resistant (heteroresistant) staphylococci. *J. Clin. Microbiol.* **19:**482–488.

126. **McWhinney, P. H. M., C. C. Kibbler, S. H. Gillespie, S. Patel, D. Morrison, A. V. Hoffbrand, and H. G. Prentice.** 1992. *Stomatococcus mucilaginosus:* an emerging pathogen in neutropenic patients. *Clin. Infect. Dis.* **14:** 641–646.

127. **Mehrotra, M., G. Wang, and W. M. Johnson.** 2000. Multiplex PCR for detection of genes for *Staphylococcus aureus* enterotoxins, exfoliative toxins, toxic shock syndrome toxin 1, and methicillin resistance. *J. Clin. Microbiol.* **38:**1032–1035.

128. **Mendoza, M., H. Meugnier, M. Bes, J. Etienne, and J. Freney.** 1998. Identification of *Staphylococcus* species by 16S–23S rDNA intergenic spacer PCR analysis. *Int. J. Syst. Bacteriol.* **48:**1049–1055.

129. **Miall, L. S., N. T. McGinley, K. G. Brownlee, and S. P. Conway.** 2001. Methicillin resistant *Staphylococcus aureus* (MRSA) infections in cystic fibrosis. *Arch. Dis. Child.* **84:**160–162.

130. **Mitchell, P. S., B. J. Huston, R. N. Jones, L. Holcomb, and F. P. Koontz.** 1990. *Stomatococcus mucilaginosus* bacteremias; typical case presentations, simplified diagnostic criteria, and a literature review. *Diagn. Microbiol. Infect. Dis.* **13:**521–525.

131. **Miwa, K., M. Fukuyama, R. Sakai, S. Shimizu, N. Ida, M. Endo, and H. Igarashi.** 2000. Sensitive enzyme-linked immunosorbent assays for the detection of bacterial superantigens and antibodies against them in human plasma. *Microbiol. Immunol.* **44:**519–523.

132. **Moeller, V.** 1955. Simplified tests for some amino acid decarboxylases and for the arginine dihydrolase system. *Acta Pathol. Microbiol. Scand.* **36:**158–172.

133. **Monday, S. R., and G. A. Bohach.** 1999. Use of multiplex PCR to detect classical and newly described pyrogenic toxin genes in staphylococcal isolates. *J. Clin. Microbiol.* **37:**3411–3414.

134. **Musser, J. M., P. M. Schlievert, A. W. Chow, P. Ewan, B. N. Kreiswirth, V. T. Rosdahl, A. S. Naidu, W. White, and R. K. Selander.** 1990. A single clone of *Staphylococcus aureus* causes the majority of cases of toxic shock syndrome. *Proc. Natl. Acad. Sci. USA* **87:**225–229.

135. **Nakatomi, Y., and J. Sugiyama.** 1998. A rapid latex agglutination assay for the detection of penicillin-binding protein 2'. *Microbiol. Immunol.* **42:**739–743.

136. **National Committee for Clincal Laboratory Standards.** 2001. *Performance Standards for Antimicrobial Susceptibility Testing.* Document M100-S10. National Committee for Clinical Laboratory Standards, Wayne, Pa.

137. **Negishi, H., T. Matsuda, K. Okuyama, S. Sutoh, Y. Fujioka, and S. Fujimoto.** 1998. *Staphylococcus aureus* causing chorioamnionitis and fetal death with intact membranes at term. A case report. *J. Reprod. Med.* **43:**397–400.

138. **Nielsen, H.** 1994. Vertebral osteomyelitis with *Stomatococcus mucilaginosus*. *Eur. J. Clin. Microbiol. Infect. Dis.* **13:**775–776.

139. **Nordstrom, K. M., K. J. McGinley, L. Cappiello, J. M. Zechman, and J. J. Leyden.** 1987. Pitted keratolysis. The role of *Micrococcus sedentarius*. *Arch. Dermatol.* **123:**1320–1325.

140. **Old, D. C., and G. P. McNeill.** 1979. Endocarditis due to *Micrococcus sedentarius* incertae sedis. *J. Clin. Pathol.* **32:**951–952.

141. **Oliveira, D. C., I. Crisóstomo, I. Santos-Sanches, P. Major, C. R. Alves, M. Aires-de-Sousa, M. K. Thege, and H. de Lencastre.** 2001. Comparison of DNA sequencing of the protein A gene polymorphic region with other molecular typing techniques for typing epidemiologically diverse collections of methicillin-resistance *Staphylococcus aureus*. *J. Clin. Microbiol.* **39:**574–580.

142. **Olmos, A., J. J. Camarena, J. M. Nogueira, J. C. Navarro, J. Risen, and R. Sánchez.** 1998. Application of an optimized and highly discriminatory method based on arbitrarily primed PCR for epidemiologic analysis of methicillin-resistant *Staphylococcus aureus* nosocomial infections. *J. Clin. Microbiol.* **36:**1128–1134.

143. **Parsonnet, J., and Z. A. Gillis.** 1988. Production of tumor necrosis factor by human monocytes in response to toxic shock syndrome toxin-1. *J. Infect. Dis.* **158:**1026–1033.

144. **Parsonnet, J., R. K. Hickman, D. D. Eardley, and G. B. Pier.** 1985. Induction of human interleukin-1 by toxic shock syndrome toxin-1. *J. Infect. Dis.* **151:**514–522.

145. **Patel, R., M. S. Rouse, K. E. Piper, F. R. Cockerill III, and J. M. Steckelberg.** 1998. In vitro activity of LY333328 against vancomycin-resistant enterococci, methicillin-resistant *Staphylococcus aureus*, and penicillin-resistant *Streptococcus pneumoniae*. *Diagn. Microbiol. Infect. Dis.* **30:**89–92.

146. **Pfaller, M. A., and L. A. Herwaldt.** 1988. Laboratory, clinical, and epidemiological aspects of coagulase-negative staphylococci. *Clin. Microbiol. Rev.* **1:**281–299.

147. **Prevost, G., B. Jaulhac, and Y. Piemont.** 1992. DNA fingerprinting by pulsed-field gel electrophoresis is more effective than ribotyping in distinguishing among methicillin-resistant *Staphylococcus aureus* isolates. *J. Clin. Microbiol.* **30:**967–973.

148. **Probst, A. J., C. Hertel, L. Richter, L. Wassill, W. Ludwig, and W. P. Hammes.** 1998. *Staphylococcus condimenti* sp. nov., from soy sauce mash, and *Staphylococcus carnosus* (Schleifer and Fischer 1982) subsp. *utilis* subsp. nov. *Int. J. Syst. Bacteriol.* **48:**651–658.

149. **Proctor, R. A., B. Kahl, C. von Eiff, P. E. Vandaux, D. P. Lew, and G. Peters.** 1998. Staphylococcal small-colony variants have novel mechanisms for antibiotic resistance. *Clin. Infect. Dis.* **27**(Suppl. 1):S68–S74.

150. **Proctor, R. A., and G. Peters.** 1998. Small colony variants in staphylococcal infections: diagnostic and therapeutic implications. *Clin. Infect. Dis.* **27:**419–423.

151. **Proctor, R. A., P. van Langevelde, M. Kristjansson, J. M. Maslow, and R. D. Arbeit.** 1995. Persistent and relapsing infections associated with small-colony variants of *Staphylococcus aureus*. *Clin. Infect. Dis.* **20:**95–102.

152. **Qadri, S. M. H., Y. Ueno, H. Imambaccus, and E. Almodovar.** 1994. Rapid detection of methicillin-resistant *Staphylococcus aureus* by Crystal MRSA ID System. *J. Clin. Microbiol.* **32:**1830–1832.

153. **Ratjen, F., G. Comes, K. Paul, H. G. Posselk, T. O. Wagner, K. Harms, and the German Board of the European Registry for Cystic Fibrosis (ERCF).** 2001. Effect of continuous antistaphylococcal therapy on the rate of *P. aeruginosa* acquisition in patients with cystic fibrosis. *Pediatr. Pulmonol.* **31:**13–16.

154. **Reuther, J. W. A., and W. C. Noble.** 1993. An ecological niche for *Staphylococcus saprophyticus*. *Microbial Ecol. Health Dis.* **6:**209–212.

155. **Rohrer, M., M. Tschierske, R. Zbinden, and B. Berger-Bächi.** 2001. Improved methods for detection of methicillin-resistant *Staphylococcus aureus*. *Eur. J. Clin. Microbiol. Infect. Dis.* **20:**267–270.

156. **Rupp, M. E., and G. L. Archer.** 1994. Coagulase-negative staphylococci: pathogens associated with medical progress. *Clin. Infect. Dis.* **19:**231–245.

157. **Saravolatz, L. D., D. J. Pohlod, and L. M. Arking.** 1982. Community-acquired methicillin-resistant *Staphylococcus aureus* infections: a new source for nosocomial outbreaks. *Ann. Intern. Med.* **97:**325–329.

158. **Schleifer, K. H.** 1986. Gram-positive cocci, p. 999–1002. *In* J. G. Holt, P. H. A. Sneath, N. S. Mair, and M. S. Sharpe (ed.), *Bergey's Manual of Systematic Bacteriology*, vol. 2. The Williams & Wilkins Co., Baltimore, Md.

159. **Schleifer, K. H.** 1986. Taxonomy of coagulase-negative staphylococci, p. 11–26. *In* P.-A. Mårdh and K. H. Schleifer (ed.), *Coagulase-Negative Staphylococci*. Almqvist & Wiksell International, Stockholm, Sweden.

160. **Schleifer, K. H., and E. Krämer.** 1980. Selective medium for isolating staphylococci. *Zentbl. Bakteriol. Hyg. Abt. 1 Orig. Reihe C* **1:**270–280.

161. **Schlievert, P. M., K. N. Shands, B. B. Dan, G. P. Schmid, and R. D. Nishimura.** 1981. Identification and characterization of an exotoxin from *Staphylococcus aureus* associated with toxic shock syndrome. *J. Infect. Dis.* **143:**509–516.

162. **Schmitz, F. J., M. Steiert, B. Hofmann, J. Verhoef, U. Hadding, H. P. Heinz, and K. Kohrer.** 1998. Development of a multiplex-PCR for direct detection of the genes for enterotoxin B and C, and toxic shock syndrome toxin-1 in *Staphylococcus aureus* isolates. *J. Med. Microbiol.* **47:**335–340.

163. **Schwalbe, R. S., J. T. Stapleton, and P. H. Gilligan.** 1987. Emergence of vancomycin resistance in coagulase-negative staphylococci. *N. Engl. J. Med.* **316:**927–931.

164. **Seifert, H., M. Kaltheuner, and F. Perdreau-Remington.** 1995. *Micrococcus luteus* endocarditis: case report and review of literature. *Zentbl. Bakteriol.* **282:**431–435.

165. **Silvestri, L. G., and L. R. Hill.** 1965. Agreement between deoxyribonucleic acid base composition and taxonomic classification of gram-positive cocci. *J. Bacteriol.* **90:**136–140.

166. Skulnick, M., A. E. Simor, M. P. Patel, H. E. Simpson, K. J. O'Quinn, D. E. Low, and A. M. Phillips. 1994. Evaluation of three methods for the rapid identification of *Staphylococcus aureus* in blood cultures. *Diagn. Microbiol. Infect. Dis.* **19:**5–8.

167. Slifkin, M., L. P. Merkow, S. A. Kreuzberger, C. Engwall, and M. Pardo. 1971. Characterization of CO$_2$ dependent microcolony variants of *Staphylococcus aureus.* *Am. J. Clin. Pathol.* **56:**584–592.

168. Speciale, A., K. La Ferla, F. Caccamo, and G. Nicoletti. 1999. Antimicrobial activity of quinupristin/dalfopristin, a new injectable streptogramin with a wide Gram-positive spectrum. *Int. J. Antimicrob. Agents* **13:**21–28.

169. Stackebrandt, E., C. Koch, O. Gvozdiak, and P. Schumann. 1995. Taxonomic dissection of the genus *Micrococcus: Kocuria,* gen. nov., *Nesterenkonia* gen. nov., *Kytococcus* gen. nov., *Dermacoccus* gen. nov., and *Micrococcus* Cohn 1872 gen. emend. *Int. J. Syst. Bacteriol.* **45:**682–692.

170. Stackebrandt, E., B. J. Lewis, and C. R. Woese. 1980. The phylogenetic structure of the coryneform group of bacteria. *Zentbl. Bakteriol. Parasitenkd. Infektionskr. Hyg. Abt. 1 Orig. Reihe C* **2:**137–149.

171. Stackebrandt, E., and M. Teuber. 1988. Molecular taxonomy and phylogenetic position of lactic acid bacteria. *Biochimie* **70:**317–324.

172. Stackebrandt, E., and C. R. Woese. 1979. A phylogenetic dissection of the family *Micrococcaceae. Curr. Microbiol.* **2:**317–322.

173. Stamm, W. E. 1988. Protocol for diagnosis of urinary tract infection: reconsidering the criterion for significant bacteriuria. *Urology.* **32**(Suppl.):6–10.

174. Sum, P. E., V. J. Lee, R. T. Testa, J. J. Hlavka, G. A. Ellestad, J. D. Bloom, Y. Gluzman, and F. P. Tally. 1994. Glycylcyclines. 1. A new generation of potent antibacterial agents through modification of 9-aminotetracyclines. *J. Med. Chem.* **37:**184–188.

175. Talan, D., D. Staatz, A. Staatz, E. J. Goldstein, K. Singer, and G. Overturf. 1989. *Staphylococcus intermedius* in canine gingiva and canine-inflicted human wound infections: laboratory characterization of a newly recognized zoonotic pathogen. *J. Clin. Microbiol.* **27:**78–81.

176. Tan, R., V. White, G. Servais, and E. A. Bryce. 1994. Postoperative endophthalmitis caused by *Stomatococcus mucilaginosus. Clin. Infect. Dis.* **18:**492–493.

177. Tanasupawat, S., Y. Hasimoto, T. Ezaki, M. Kozaki, and K. Komagata. 1992. *Staphylococcus piscifermentans* sp. nov., from fermented fish in Thailand. *Int. J. Syst. Bacteriol.* **42:**577–581.

178. Tenover, F. C., J. W. Biddle, and M. V. Lancaster. 2001. Increasing resistance to vancomycin and other glycopeptides in *Staphylococcus aureus. Emerg. Infect. Dis.* **7:**327–332.

179. Thomas, S. R., K. M. Gyi, H. Gaya, and M. E. Hodson. 1998. Methicillin-resistant *Staphylococcus aureus:* impact at a national cystic fibrosis centre. *J. Hosp. Infect.* **40:**203–209.

180. Thomson-Carter, F. M., P. E. Carter, and T. H. Pennington. 1989. Differentiation of staphylococcal species and strains by ribosomal RNA gene restriction patterns. *J. Gen. Microbiol.* **135:**2093–2097.

181. Tierno, P. M., Jr., and B. A. Hanna. 1989. Ecology of toxic shock syndrome: amplification of toxic shock syndrome toxin 1 by materials of medical interest. *Rev. Infect. Dis.* **11**(Suppl. 1):S182–S186.

182. Van Belkum, A., J. Kluytmans, W. van Leeuwen, R. Bax, W. Quint, E. Peters, A. Fluit, C. Vandenbroucke-Grauls, A. van den Brule, H. Koeleman, W. Melchers,

J. Meis, A. Elaichouni, M. Vaneechoutte, F. Moonens, N. Maes, M. Struelens, F. Tenover, and H. Verbrugh. 1995. Multicenter evaluation of arbitrarily primed PCR for typing of *Staphylococcus aureus* strains. *J. Clin. Microbiol.* **33:**1537–1547.

183. Van Griethuysen, A., M. Bes, J. Etienne, R. Zbinden, and J. Kluytmans. 2001. International multicenter evaluation of latex agglutination tests for identification of *Staphylococcus aureus. J. Clin. Microbiol.* **39:**86–89.

184. Vandenesch, F., J. Etienne, M. E. Reverdy, and S. J. Eykyn. 1993. Endocarditis due to *Staphylococcus lugdunensis:* report of 11 cases and review. *Clin. Infect. Dis.* **17:**871–876.

185. Vernozy-Rozand, C., C. Mazuy, H. Meugnier, M. Bes, Y. Lasne, F. Fiedler, J. Etienne, and J. Freney. 2000. *Staphylococcus fleurettii* sp. nov., isolated from goat's milk cheese. *Int. J. Syst. Evol. Microbiol.* **50:**1521–1527.

186. Villard, L., A. Kodjo, E. Borges, F. Maurin, and Y. Richard. 2000. Ribotyping and rapid identification of *Staphylococcus xylosus* by 16–23S spacer amplification. *FEMS Microbiol. Lett.* **185:**83–87.

187. von Eiff, C., M. Herrmann, and G. Peters. 1995. Antimicrobial susceptibilities of *Stomatococcus mucilaginosus* and of *Micrococcus* spp. *Antimicrob. Agents Chemother.* **39:**268–270.

188. von Eiff, C., and G. Peters. 1998. In vitro activity of ciprofloxacin, ofloxacin, and levofloxacin against *Micrococcus* species and *Stomatococcus mucilaginosus* isolated from healthy subjects and neutropenic patients. *Eur. J. Clin. Microbiol. Infect. Dis.* **17:**890–892.

189. von Eiff, C., R. A. Proctor, and G. Peters. 2000. Small colony variants of staphylococci: link to persistent infections. *Berl. Munch. Tierarztl. Wochenschr.* **113:**321–325.

190. von Eiff, C., R. R. Reinert, M. Kresken, J. Brauers, J. Hafner, and G. Peters. 2000. Nationwide German multicenter study on prevalence of antibiotic resistance in staphylococcal bloodstream isolates and comparative in vitro activities of quinupristin-dalfopristin. *J. Clin. Microbiol.* **38:**2819–2823.

191. Walsh, T. R., A. Bolmström, A. Qwärnström, P. Ho, M. Wootton, R. A. Howe, A. P. MacGowen, and D. Diekema. 2001. Evaluation of current methods for detection of staphylococci with reduced susceptibility to glycopeptides. *J. Clin. Microbiol.* **39:**2439–2444.

192. Webster, J. A., T. L. Bannerman, R. Hubner, D. N. Ballard, E. Cole, J. Bruce, F. Fiedler, K. Schubert, and W. E. Kloos. 1994. Identification of the *Staphylococcus sciuri* species group with EcoRI fragments containing rRNA sequences and description of *Staphylococcus vitulus* sp. nov. *Int. J. Syst. Bacteriol.* **44:**454–460.

193. Weinstein, M. P., S. Mirrett, L. Van Pelt, M. McKinnon, B. L. Zimmer, W. E. Kloos, and L. B. Reller. 1998. Clinical importance of identifying coagulase-negative staphylococci isolated from blood cultures: evaluation of MicroScan Rapid and Dried Overnight Gram-Positive panels versus a conventional reference method. *J. Clin. Microbiol.* **36:**2089–2092.

194. Weiss, K., D. Rouleau, and M. Laverdiere. 1996. Cystitis due to vancomycin-intermediate *Staphylococcus saprophyticus. J. Antimicrob. Chemother.* **37:**1039–1040.

195. Welch, D. F. 1991. Applications of cellular fatty acid analysis. *Clin. Microbiol. Rev.* **4:**422–438.

196. Wenzel, R. P., D. R. Reagen, J. S. Bertino, E. J. Baron, and K. Arias. 1998. Methicillin-resistant *Staphylococcus aureus* outbreak: a consensus panel's definition and management guidelines. *Am. J. Infect. Control* **26:**102–110.

197. **Wieneke, A. A.** 1988. The detection of enterotoxin and toxic shock syndrome toxin-1 production by strains of *Staphylococcus aureus. Int. J. Food Microbiol.* **7:**25–30.

198. **Wise, R., J. M. Andrews, and J. P. Ashby.** 2001. Activity of daptomycin against gram-positive pathogens: a comparison with other agents and the determination of a tentative breakpoint. *J. Antimicrob. Chemother.* **48:**563–567.

199. **Yugueros, J., A. Temprano, B. Berzal, M. Sánchez, C. Hernanz, J. M. Luengo, and G. Naharro.** 2000. Glyceraldehyde-3-phosphate dehydrogenase-encoding gene as a useful taxonomic tool for *Staphylococcus* spp. *J. Clin. Microbiol.* **38:**4351–4355.

200. **Zakrzewska-Bode, A., H. L. Muytjens, and K. D. Liem.** 1995. Mupirocin resistance in coagulase-negative staphylococci, after topical prophylaxis for the reduction of colonization of central venous catheters. *J. Hosp. Infect.* **31:**189–193.

201. **Zimmerman, R. J., and W. E. Kloos.** 1976. Comparative zone electrophoresis of esterases of *Staphylococcus* species isolated from mammalian skin. *Can. J. Microbiol.* **22:** 771–779.

Streptococcus

KATHRYN L. RUOFF, R. A. WHILEY, AND D. BEIGHTON

29

TAXONOMY

Molecular taxonomic studies of the genus *Streptococcus* have contributed to broad changes in the classification of these organisms over the last two decades. The enterococci (previously considered group D streptococci) and the lactococci (previously classified as group N streptococci) now reside in their own genera, *Enterococcus* and *Lactococcus*, respectively (95). Although traditional phenotypic criteria (hemolytic reactions, Lancefield serologic groups) for classification of the streptococci are still useful in certain circumstances, the older classification schemes have been tempered by new taxonomic knowledge. For beta-hemolytic streptococci, we now realize that unrelated species may produce identical Lancefield antigens and that strains genetically related at the species level may have heterogeneous Lancefield antigens.

In spite of these exceptions to the traditional rules of streptococcal taxonomy, hemolytic reactions and Lancefield serologic tests can still be used to divide the streptococci into broad categories as a first step in identification of clinical isolates. Beta-hemolytic isolates from humans with Lancefield group A, C, or G antigen can be subdivided into two groups: large-colony (>0.5 mm in diameter) and small-colony (<0.5 mm in diameter) formers. Large-colony-forming group A (*Streptococcus pyogenes*), C, and G strains are "pyogenic" streptococci, replete with a variety of effective virulence mechanisms. Strains of large-colony-forming beta-hemolytic group C and G streptococci are currently classified in the same subspecies, *Streptococcus dysgalactiae* subsp. *equisimlis* (110). A recent report, however, described three *S. dysgalactiae* subsp. *equisimilis* blood culture isolates with Lancefield's group A, but not C or G, antigen (19), further illustrating the inadequacy of serologic testing alone for accurate identification of beta-hemolytic streptococci. Other group C, G, and L streptococci normally isolated from animals and infrequently isolated from human infection have been classified in the species *Streptococcus dysgalactiae* subsp. *dysgalactiae*, *Streptococcus canis*, *Streptococcus equi* subsp. *equi*, and *Streptococcus equi* subsp. *zooepidemicus* (29, 43).

The small-colony-forming beta-hemolytic strains with group A, C, or G Lancefield antigens are genetically different from the "pyogenic" strains and belong to the anginosus or "*Streptococcus milleri*" species group, composed of *Streptococcus anginosus*, *Streptococcus constellatus*, and *Streptococcus intermedius*. In spite of the existence of these groupable beta-hemolytic strains, members of the anginosus species group are considered to be viridans group streptococci, the majority of which display alpha-hemolytic or nonhemolytic reactions. Although the small-colony-forming strains may participate in infection (notably abscesses), they are also found as commensals whose pathogenic abilities appear to be much more subtle than those of the pyogenic streptococci. *Streptococcus agalactiae*, a large-colony-forming species, is still identified reliably by its production of Lancefield group B antigen or other phenotypic traits.

Among non-beta-hemolytic streptococcal strains, alpha-reacting isolates can be separated into the species *Streptococcus pneumoniae* (optochin and bile susceptible) and the viridans division, composed of a number of species groups. Kawamura et al. (66) examined 16S rRNA sequences among streptococcal strains and found a close phylogenetic relationship between *S. pneumoniae* and viridans group streptococci, suggesting that *S. pneumoniae* be included as a member of the mitis species group. Recently the names of several species, some long established, within the viridans group streptococci were changed on the basis of correct grammar according to rule 12c of the International Code of Nomenclature of Bacteria (107, 108). Those species affected included *Streptococcus cricetus*, *S. crista*, *S. rattus*, *S. sanguis*, and *S. parasanguis*, which were amended to *S. criceti*, *S. cristatus*, *S. ratti*, *S. sanguinis*, and *S. parasanguinis*, respectively. This has been challenged as unnecessary and potentially confusing (72), although some authors have already adopted the emended nomenclature. The Judicial Commission of the International Committee on Systematic Bacteriology recently ruled (minutes of the meeting published in vol. 50, p. 2239, of the *International Journal of Systematic and Evolutionary Microbiology*, 2000) that priority be given to the stabilization of nomenclature over orthographic correctness and that names on the Approved Lists of Bacterial Names, the Validation Lists, and the Notification Lists should not be changed on grammatical grounds. We have used the names of species as originally validly published and have not adopted the name changes proposed by Trüper and De' Clari (107, 108) in this chapter.

Organisms formerly known as the nutritionally variant streptococci currently occupy two newly described genera, *Abiotrophia* and *Granulicatella* (see chapter 31). Streptococci with Lancefield's group D antigen include the non-hemolytic species *Streptococcus bovis*. Organisms previously thought to be anaerobic streptococci have been shown to be unrelated to members of the genus *Streptococcus* (78).

DESCRIPTION OF THE GENUS

Bergey's Manual of Systematic Bacteriology (55) describes streptococci as gram-positive, catalase-negative facultatively anaerobic bacteria forming spherical or ovoid cells less than 2 μm in diameter. The G+C content of the DNA of members of the genus ranges from 34 to 46 mol%. Although the streptococci grow in the presence of oxygen, they are unable to synthesize heme compounds and are therefore incapable of respiratory metabolism. Some strains of *S. pneumoniae* and certain viridans species require elevated (5%) CO_2 levels for growth; the growth of many streptococcal isolates is stimulated in a CO_2-enriched atmosphere. Streptococci are nutritionally fastidious with variable nutritional requirements, and growth on complex media is enhanced by the addition of blood or serum. Glucose and other carbohydrates are metabolized fermentatively with the production of lactic acid as the major metabolic end product. Gas is not produced as a result of glucose metabolism. Isolates of streptococci produce the enzyme leucine aminopeptidase (LAP), but production of pyrrolidonyl arylamidase (PYR) is rare among streptococci, occurring only in isolates of *S. pyogenes* and some strains of pneumococci.

NATURAL HABITATS

Streptococci are usually found as parasites of humans and other animals. While some streptococci function as virulent pathogens, other strains live harmoniously with their hosts as normally avirulent commensals. Streptococci are transient colonizers of skin and resident colonizers of mucous membranes. They can be isolated as part of the normal flora of the alimentary, respiratory, and genital tracts. The viridans streptococci are well characterized as residents of the oral cavity, where some strains form part of the normal dental plaque flora.

CLINICAL SIGNIFICANCE

Streptococcus pyogenes

Beta-hemolytic, bacitracin-susceptible, PYR-positive, large-colony-forming streptococci with Lancefield's group A antigen are included in the species *S. pyogenes* and represent one of the most impressive human pathogens. The numerous virulence factors of *S. pyogenes* (M protein, encoded by the *emm* genes; pyrogenic exotoxins, encoded by the *spe* genes; hyaluronic acid capsule; hemolysins; and other factors) allow it to cause a wide array of serious infections including pharyngitis, respiratory infection, skin (impetigo and erysipelas) and soft tissue infections, endocarditis, meningitis, puerperal sepsis, and arthritis. Infection with toxin-producing strains can result in scarlet fever or more serious toxic shock-like symptoms.

S. pyogenes pharyngitis is characterized by pharyngeal pain, swelling, and erythema accompanied by fever and anterior cervical adenopathy. Suppurative sequelae of streptococcal pharyngitis may ensue from spread of infection to contiguous tissue or by bacteremic dissemination. Nonsuppurative sequelae include rheumatic fever and acute glomerulonephritis. While either of these conditions may follow pharyngitis, only glomerulonephritis is linked to *S. pyogenes* infections of the skin.

In recent years there has been an increase in the number of reports of severe *S. pyogenes* infection, including necrotizing fasciitis and infections associated with a toxic shock-like syndrome. Many of the streptococcal isolates from such cases produce M protein type 1 or 3, but current hypotheses suggest that streptococcal pyrogenic exotoxins are more directly involved in the production of severe infection with shock. The ability of pyrogenic exotoxins to act as superantigens, like the staphylococcal toxic shock toxin, is thought to contribute to the production of shock in these infections (40, 99).

Streptococcus agalactiae

Beta-hemolytic streptococci with Lancefield's group B antigen (*S. agalactiae*) are an important cause of serious neonatal infection characterized by sepsis and meningitis. Colonization of the maternal genital tract is associated with colonization of infants and risk of neonatal disease. Early-onset infection occurs within the first few days after delivery and often is associated with pneumonia, while late-onset disease usually appears after 1 week of age. *S. agalactiae* is also associated with postpartum infections. Conditions that predispose nonpregnant adults to *S. agalactiae* infection include diabetes mellitus, cancer, and human immunodeficiency virus infection. Adult *S. agalactiae* infections include bacteremia, endocarditis, skin and soft tissue infection, pneumonia, and osteomyelitis (96).

Other Beta-Hemolytic Streptococci

Human isolates of group C and G streptococci that form large colonies belong to the subspecies *S. dysgalactiae* subsp. *equisimilis* and are pyogenic streptococci similar to *S. pyogenes* with respect to virulence traits. They cause a wide range of serious infections such as bacteremia, endocarditis, meningitis, septic arthritis, and infections of the respiratory tract and skin. The clinical symptoms of pharyngeal infection caused by these streptococci are similar to those of *S. pyogenes* pharyngitis, except for the strong association of *S. pyogenes* with nonsuppurative sequelae. Poststreptococcal glomerulonephritis has, however, also been rarely associated with outbreaks of group C pharyngitis (6, 39). Strains of large-colony-forming group C and G streptococci normally isolated from animals have also been noted infrequently as agents of human infection (see "Other Streptococci Isolated Infrequently from Human Clinical Specimens" below).

Small-colony-forming beta-hemolytic streptococcal strains may express Lancefield group A, C, F, or G antigen or may be nongroupable. These streptococci are usually identified as members of the anginosus or "*S. milleri*" group of species (see "Viridans Group Streptococci" below). Although these organisms can be isolated from pyogenic infections (notably abscesses), they may reside in the pharynx as commensals. Turner et al. (109) found no association between these streptococci and pharyngitis, but Whiley et al. (119) proposed that some small-colony-forming beta-hemolytic group C strains classified as *S. constellatus* subsp. *pharyngis* appear to be associated with throat infection.

Streptococcus pneumoniae

Despite its close phylogenetic relationship to members of the relatively avirulent viridans group streptococci (*S. pneumoniae* is considered a member of the mitis species group), the pneumococcus is an important agent of community-acquired pneumonia that may be accompanied by bacteremia. Oropharyngeal carriage of pneumococci is common and contributes to the difficulty of interpreting the significance of pneumococci in cultures of expectorated sputum. Other pneumococcal infections include otitis media, sinusitis, meningitis, and endocarditis. Vaccines designed to protect against infection by pneumococci with predominant capsular polysaccharide types (4, 6B, 9V, 14, 18C, 19F, 23F, and additional serotypes depending on the vaccine) are available.

Viridans Group Streptococci

Viridans group streptococci are normal inhabitants of the oral cavity, gastrointestinal tract, and female genital tract, and they are often considered to be contaminants when isolated from blood cultures, where they may be found as transients in the bloodstream. However, their presence may be associated with subacute bacterial endocarditis, especially in patients with prosthetic heart values, with S. *sanguis*, S. *mitis*, S. *oralis*, and S. *gordonii* being frequently isolated (18, 35). Members of the mutans group are associated with dental caries in humans and animals, with S. *mutans* and S. *sobrinus* being the species most frequently isolated from carious lesions and dental plaque. S. *mutans* may also be isolated from patients with endocarditis. S. *intermedius* is often isolated among the polymicrobial flora of deep-seated abscesses, notably in the liver and brain (117). Other members of the anginosus group may be isolated from oral abscesses, with S. *anginosus* also being isolated from female genital infections. The clinical significance, if any, of the mannitol-fermenting S. *anginosus* strains frequently isolated from the female genitourinary tract is uncertain. Strains of S. *constellatus* have been isolated relatively frequently from thoracic sites and the respiratory tract, although anatomical associations in infections are less clear than for other anginosus group species. The viridans group streptococci are assuming an increasing role in infections in neutropenic patients (15). Complications associated with bacteremia in these patients include endocarditis, acute respiratory distress syndrome, and shock (16, 41). The major species causing infections in neutropenic patients are S. *oralis*, S. *mitis*, and S. *salivarius* (8, 63). The use of commercial kits to identify the viridans group streptococci has meant that in many studies S. *oralis* is identified incorrectly as "S. *mitis*."

Streptococcus bovis

Bacteremia caused by S. *bovis* isolates, particularly biotype I, is associated with malignancies of the gastrointestinal tract (93). These organisms are also agents of endocarditis and have been isolated from patients with meningitis (88).

Other Streptococci Isolated Infrequently from Human Clinical Specimens

A few streptococcal species that appear to be pathogens primarily in animals have been documented as agents of human infection. These include some of the large-colony-forming strains with group C (S. *dysgalactiae* subsp. *dysgalactiae*, S. *equi* subsp. *equi*, and S. *equi* subsp. *zooepidemicus*) or G (S. *canis*) antigens. S. *suis*, a pathogen of swine, has been noted as an agent of meningitis in humans (100). Some S. *suis* strains can produce a beta-hemolytic reaction on horse blood agar, but all are alpha-hemolytic on agars containing sheep blood. These organisms are serologically

heterogeneous, with strains expressing Lancefield group R, S, or T antigen and a variety of capsular antigens (101). S. *porcinus*, also a pathogen of pigs, has been identified occasionally as an agent of human infection (42). Strains of this species are beta-hemolytic on sheep blood agar, may produce Lancefield group E, P, U, or V antigen, and, while positive for production of PYR like S. *pyogenes*, are bacitracin resistant. S. *porcinus* strains produce a positive CAMP reaction and may react with commercially available group B agglutination reagents (103), but they are differentiated from S. *agalactiae* by virtue of their ability to produce PYR.

S. *iniae*, a fish pathogen, has been associated with cellulitis, bacteremia, endocarditis, and meningitis in humans with a history of handling fish (often tilapia, a freshwater fish) while suffering from percutaneous injuries. Molecular typing evidence suggested that an invasive clone of the organism was responsible for causing observed cases of disease in humans as well as fish. S. *iniae* strains form a narrow zone of beta-hemolysis surrounded by a larger alpha-hemolytic zone and are sometimes mistakenly characterized as alpha-hemolytic. Beta-hemolysis is reliably observed in anaerobically incubated cultures. S. *iniae* strains are PYR positive and Voges-Proskauer negative and show variable suceptibilies to bacitracin, making some isolates physiologically similar to S. *pyogenes*. They do not, however, react with Lancefield group A or other group antisera (112, 113).

COLLECTION, TRANSPORT, AND STORAGE OF SPECIMENS

Specimens suspected of harboring streptococci should be collected by methods outlined elsewhere (see chapters 6 and 20). In general, a transport system need not be used if the transport time is less than 2 h. Although some streptococci (e.g., S. *pyogenes*) can survive desiccation and refrigeration, others (e.g., pneumococci) are fairly fragile, and thus every effort should be made to process specimens as soon as possible. A recent report notes that STGG (skim milk, tryptone, glucose, and glycerin) medium (see chapter 27) is useful for transport and storage of nasopharyngeal specimens collected for isolation of pneumococci (83).

Recommendations have been formulated by the Centers for Disease Control and Prevention for collection of specimens used to establish carriage of group B streptococci in pregnant women (22). Pregnant women should be cultured at 35 to 37 weeks gestation. Rectal and vaginal swabs should be collected and placed together into a nonnutritive moist swab transport system. The specimens may be held under refrigeration or at room temperature for up to 4 days before being cultured in a selective broth medium (see "Special Procedures for Group B Streptococci" below).

ISOLATION PROCEDURES

General Procedures

Many commonly used nonselective laboratory media support the growth of streptococci; complex media enriched with blood are desirable because the hemolytic reaction of the streptococcal isolate may be determined early in the identification process. Hemolytic patterns may vary with the source of animal blood or type of basal medium used in blood agars. Media selective for gram-positive bacteria (e.g., phenylethyl alcohol agar or Columbia agar with colistin and nalidixic acid) will also support the growth of streptococci. Columbia agar with sheep blood and gentamicin has been described as superior to sheep blood agar for isolation of *S. pneumoniae* from middle ear fluid specimens (85), and other selective media may be used for the isolation of groups A and B streptococci from sites containing normal flora (see "Special Procedures for Throat Cultures" and "Special Procedures for Group B Streptococci" below).

Cultures for isolation of streptococci should be incubated at 35 to 37°C. Ambient atmospheres are suitable for many streptococci, but since pneumococci and some viridans strains require elevated CO_2 concentrations, incubation in an atmosphere containing 5% CO_2 or in a candle jar will enhance the recovery of streptococcal isolates. Streptococci grow well in anaerobic atmospheres, but their facultative nature makes anaerobic incubation unnecessary for isolation.

Special Procedures for Throat Cultures

Complex media containing 5% sheep blood are usually recommended for the culture of throat specimens because NADase activity in sheep blood reduces the NAD content to levels insufficient for growth of *Haemophilus haemolyticus*, a commensal that forms colonies that might be confused with those of beta-hemolytic streptococci. Throat swabs should be rolled firmly over one-sixth of the plate to deposit the specimen. A loop is used to carefully streak the inoculum over the surface of the plate. The loop is then used (without sterilization) to stab the agar several times in an area of the plate that has not been streaked, in an effort to deposit beta-hemolytic streptococci beneath the agar surface. Subsurface growth will display the most reliable hemolytic reactions due to the activity of both oxygen-stable and oxygen-labile streptolysins.

In a coherent review of methods designed to improve the recovery of beta-hemolytic streptococci from throat specimens, Kellogg (70) concluded that 90 to 95% of *S. pyogenes* isolates from symptomatic patients should be detected by any of the following methods: sheep blood agar incubated anaerobically for 48 h, sheep blood agar incubated aerobically without CO_2 supplementation for 48 h (a coverglass may be placed over the primary inoculation area to reduce oxygen tension and enhance hemolysis), and sheep blood agar containing trimethoprim-sulfamethoxazole incubated anaerobically for 48 h. Cultures should be examined after 18 to 24 h of incubation and reincubated if negative, with a final examination at 48 h. Increased isolations of group A streptococci on sheep blood agar during the second 24 h of incubation have ranged from 2 to 46% in published studies. Incubation of throat culture plates in a CO_2-enriched atmosphere seems to encourage the recovery of non-group A beta-hemolytic streptococci.

Special Procedures for *S. agalactiae* (Group B Streptococci)

Detection of group B streptococci in the genital and gastrointestinal tracts of expectant mothers can identify infants at risk for infection and guide intrapartum administration of antibiotics. As described above, vaginal and rectal swabs, or a single swab inserted into the vagina and then the rectum, should be collected at 35 to 37 weeks gestation and inoculated into a selective broth medium. The Centers for Disease Control and Prevention recommend the use of Todd-Hewitt broth containing either 10 μg of colistin per ml and 15 μg of nalidixic acid per ml (Lim broth; Becton Dickinson, Cockeysville, Md.) or 8 μg of gentamicin per ml and 15 μg of nalidixic acid per ml

(Hardy Diagnostics, Santa Maria, Calif.). Selective media should be incubated at room temperature for 18 to 24 h before being subcultured to sheep blood agar. The blood agar subcultures should be examined for group B streptococci after 24 h of incubation at 35 to 37°C in an atmosphere containing 5% CO_2 and, if negative at the first observation, should be reexamined after a second 24-h incubation (22). Studies suggest that other formulations of selective media (Granada agar; Hardy Diagnostics) are highly sensitive for detecting group B streptococcal colonization in pregnant women (46, 90).

IDENTIFICATION

Direct Detection

Direct detection of streptococci via Gram stains is most useful when applied to specimens that are normally devoid of indigenous streptococcal flora. The Quellung test is a more specific method for microscopic detection of pneumococci in specimens and relies on the visual enhancement of the pneumococcal capsule after reaction of the streptococci with anticapsular antisera (Statens Seruminstitut, Copenhagen, Denmark). A drop of specimen is mixed with a loopful of antiserum and a loopful of saturated aqueous methylene blue and examined under a coverslip after 10 min. Encapsulated pneumococcal cells will appear to be surrounded by a halo. Immunofluorescent stains may also be used for direct detection of streptococci. Conjugated antibody for detection of group A streptococci is commercially available (Becton Dickinson).

Direct detection of streptococcal antigens has been used to identify group A streptococci in throat specimens. The sensitivities of these techniques depend not only on the method used but also on the numbers of streptococci present in the sample. These tests display excellent specificity, in spite of the rarely encountered non-*S. pyogenes* streptococcal strains with group A antigen. In general, streptococci are transferred from the swab containing the specimen to a chemical (e.g., nitrous acid) or enzymatic (e.g., pronase) extraction solution. After a short incubation period, antigen in the suspension is detected via agglutination methods (47), enzyme immunoassay (38, 58), or other methods (48, 54). While antigen detection methods are rapid and specific, false-negative results may occur with specimens containing small numbers of streptococci. Since the presence of low counts of streptococci may be clinically significant, negative antigen detection tests should be followed up with culture (47).

Antigen detection techniques have also been used for rapid identification of group B streptococci in urogenital specimens. In most evaluations of methods involving direct detection from specimens, latex agglutination assays (50), enzyme immunoassay methods (49, 89, 122), and optical immunoassay methods (21) have not proven sensitive enough to detect low levels of colonization and are consequently not recommended for screening pregnant women for group B streptococcal carriage. These methods do, however, seem to be effective in identifying heavily colonized women. Protocols involving incubation of specimens in a selective medium for 5 to 20 h before antigen testing via agglutination will reveal even light colonization (77, 84). In a recent study, intrapartum screening by an optical immunoassay method identified more at-risk infants than did screening cultures at 28 weeks gestation or identification of clinical risk factors (11).

Normally sterile body fluids may also be tested directly for streptococcal antigens. Commercially available products that detect the Lancefield antigen of group B streptococci and the capsular polysaccharide antigen of pneumococci may be used to determine the presence of these organisms in cerebrospinal fluid and in blood cultures. The clinical usefulness of these rapid bacterial antigen detection tests has, however, been debated (102). As of this writing, a commercially available rapid test for detection of pneumococcal C polysaccharide antigen in urine (Binax, Portland, Maine) was found not to be useful for distinguishing between patients with pneumococcal pneumonia and those who are colonized with pneumococci in a pediatric population (37). One study performed on adults, who tend to show lower frequencies of pneumococcal carriage than children, suggested that this method may prove useful in diagnosis of pneumococcal pneumonia (34).

A nucleic acid probe-based test for direct detection of group A streptococci in throat swabs is commercially available (GASD; GenProbe, San Diego, Calif.) (56). Additional evaluation of this or similar products is necessary before their true utility and cost-effectiveness can be established. The use of commercially available nucleic acid probe tests for the direct detection of *S. pneumoniae* and group B streptococci from positive blood cultures has also been described (AccuProbe; GenProbe) (26), along with probe-based detection (17, 75, 121) and real-time, rapid PCR assays (13) for group B streptococci in genital specimens. These methods have not yet gained wide acceptance.

Hemolytic Reactions on Culture Media

Beta-hemolysis appears as complete clearing (lysis of red blood cells) of the medium. This reaction may be obscured by the inhibition of streptolysin O by oxygen or by the production of peroxide by streptococci growing in air or in the presence of increased CO_2 levels; thus, anaerobic incubation or observation of hemolysis in the area of stabs in the agar is optimal for accurate determination of beta-hemolytic reactions. In the alpha-hemolytic reaction, red blood cells are not completely lysed but growth is surrounded by greenish discoloration of the agar due to streptococcal action on hemoglobin. Nonhemolytic or gamma-hemolytic streptococci have no effect on blood agar.

Description of Colonies

Streptococcal colonies vary in color from gray to whitish and are usually glistening in appearance, although dry colonies are also observed. The beta-hemolytic pyogenic streptococci of groups A, C, and G form relatively large colonies (>0.5 mm in diameter after 24 h of incubation) compared with the pinpoint colonies of the small-colony-forming beta-hemolytic strains of the anginosus or "*S. milleri*" group. Occasional strains of *S. pyogenes* may form mucoid colonies.

Cultures of the small-colony-forming beta-hemolytic streptococci and other anginosus group strains may produce a distinct odor, which has been described as buttery or caramel-like and has been attributed to the production of diacetyl by these bacteria (23). Colonies of group B streptococci tend to be larger and have less pronounced zones of beta-hemolysis compared to other beta-hemolytic strains; some group B strains are nonhemolytic.

Alpha-hemolytic colonies with depressions in their centers are characteristic of pneumococci, while viridans group streptococcal colonies have a domed appearance. Pneumococci may also produce various amounts of capsular polysaccharide, contributing to a mucoid colonial appearance.

Some viridans group streptococcal strains, along with *S. bovis*, form nonhemolytic, grayish colonies.

Catalase Test Reaction

Streptococci are catalase negative when tested with 3% hydrogen peroxide. To perform the test, a loopful of growth is transferred from an agar plate culture to a glass microscope slide or an empty petri dish. No reaction (no evolution of bubbles) on addition of a drop of 3% H_2O_2 signifies a negative result. False-positive reactions may occur when growth for a test is taken from blood-containing media. Isolates with streptococcal cellular morphology that test positive for catalase should be subcultured to a medium devoid of blood and retested.

Identification of Beta-Hemolytic Isolates: Serologic Tests

Numerous products using rapid antigen extraction methods and agglutination techniques for antigen detection are available commercially for the Lancefield grouping of beta-hemolytic isolates. The presence of the group B antigen seems to correlate closely with a strain's identity as *S. agalactiae*, and most group F beta-hemolytic small-colony-forming strains appear to be members of the anginosus or "*S. milleri*" group of species. Lancefield antigens of groups A, C, and G, however, are not specific for a single streptococcal species. Organisms with these antigens can be differentiated by biochemical tests, as summarized in Table 1. When beta-hemolytic isolates that fail to react with Lancefield group A, B, C, F, or G antisera are encountered, physiological characterization may aid in identification.

Identification of Streptococci by Using Commercially Available Products

A number of streptococcal identification products incorporating batteries of physiological tests have been made commercially available over the last 2 decades (see chapter 14). In general, these products perform well with commonly isolated streptococci but may lack accuracy for identifying streptococci of the viridans group, which has undergone many recent taxonomic and nomenclatural changes. For the bulk of pathogenic streptococci isolated in clinical laboratories (e.g., *S. pyogenes*, group B streptococci, and *S. pneumoniae*), serologic or presumptive physiological tests (as described below) offer an acceptable alternative to commercially available identification systems.

Identification of Beta-Hemolytic Isolates: Physiological Tests

PYR Test

The PYR test determines activity of pyrrolidonyl arylamidase, also called pyrrolidonyl aminopeptidase, an enzyme produced by *S. pyogenes* but not by other beta-hemolytic streptococci except for the rarely encountered animal-associated species *S. porcinus* and *S. iniae* (see "Other Streptococci Isolated Infrequently from Human Clinical Specimens" above). Products employing rapid methods for performance of the PYR test are commercially available. Since other organisms that may be isolated along with *S. pyogenes* may also give a positive PYR reaction, only pure cultures or isolated colonies of beta-hemolytic streptococci should be tested. Beta-hemolytic strains of enterococci might be confused with *S. pyogenes*, since both organisms are PYR positive. Differences in colony size and morphol-

TABLE 1 Differentiating characteristics of beta-hemolytic streptococci of human origin[a]

Lancefield group	Colony size	Species	PYR	VP[b]	CAMP	BGUR
A	Large	S. pyogenes	+	−	−	NA
A	Small	Anginosus group[c]	−	+	−	NA
B		S. agalactiae	−	NA	+	NA
C	Large	S. dysgalactiae subsp. equisimilis[d]	−	−	−	+
C	Small	Anginosus group[c]	−	+	−	−
F	Small	Anginosus group[c]	−	+	−	NA
G	Large	S. dysgalactiae subsp. equisimilis[d]	−	−	−	+
G	Small	Anginosus group[c]	−	+	−	−
Nongroupable	Small	Anginosus group[c]	−	+	−	NA

[a] Symbols and abbreviation: +, positive; −, negative; NA, data not available.

[b] VP test results for group B streptococci (S. agalactiae) have been omitted from the table due to conflicting reports in the literature, which may have resulted from the use of different test methods. The VP test result is not critical for the identification of group B streptococci.

[c] Also called the "S. milleri" group.

[d] Current data suggest that large-colony-forming group C and G beta-hemolytic strains of human origin are related at the species level. The name S. dysgalactiae subsp. equisimilis has been proposed for these streptococci (110). The ability to ferment trehalose and sorbitol was used in the past to differentiate group C beta-hemolytic streptococci into the species S. equi, S. equisimilis, and S. zooepidemicus. See the text and Table 2 for the current classification of group C and G streptococci.

ogy and other traits should allow for differentiation of these bacteria (see chapter 30).

Bacitracin Susceptibility

Although S. pyogenes can be identified rapidly by antigenic methods or the PYR test, a test for bacitracin susceptibility can be helpful in differentiating S. pyogenes from small-colony-forming group A strains or from other PYR-positive beta-hemolytic species (see "Other Streptococci Isolated Infrequently from Human Clinical Specimens" above). A 0.04-U bacitracin disk is applied to a sheep blood agar plate that has been heavily inoculated with three or four colonies of a pure culture of the streptococcus to be tested. After overnight incubation at 35°C, any zone of inhibition around the disk is interpreted as indicating susceptibility.

VP Test

The Voges-Proskauer (VP) test for acetoin production will differentiate small-colony-forming beta-hemolytic anginosus ("S. milleri") group strains with Lancefield group A, C, or G antigens from large-colony-forming pyogenic strains with the same Lancefield antigens (Table 1). Facklam and Washington, in a previous edition of the Manual, described a version of this test for streptococci in which overnight growth from an entire agar plate culture is used to inoculate 2 ml of VP broth. After 6 h of incubation at 35°C, a few drops each of Coblentz reagents A and B (see chapter 27) are added and the tube is shaken and incubated at room temperature for 30 min. A positive test is indicated by the development of a cherry red (or even slightly pink) color.

BGUR Test

The BGUR test assays for the action of β-D-glucuronidase, an enzyme produced by human isolates of large-colony-forming beta-hemolytic group C and G streptococci but not by their small-colony-forming anginosus group ("S. milleri") counterparts (Table 1). Rapid methods for the BGUR test are commercially available (Becton Dickinson, Hardy Diagnostics, and other sources). In addition, the use of methylumbelliferyl-β-D-glucuronide (MUG)-containing MacConkey agar, normally used for the isolation and presumptive identification of Escherichia coli, in a rapid fluorogenic assay for BGUR in streptococcal strains has been described (74).

Differentiation of Large-Colony-Forming Group C and G Isolates by Carbohydrate Fermentation Tests

Traditionally, large-colony-forming group C isolates have been differentiated into species based on their ability to ferment various carbohydrates. Studies of the genetic relatedness of group C and G streptococci have, however, shown that human isolates classified in the traditional group C species S. equisimilis are genetically similar enough to group G large-colony-forming human isolates to be classified in the same species, which was given the name S. dysgalactiae. Strains formerly classified as S. zooepidemicus were considered, on the basis of genetic data, to form a subspecies of S. equi (43). A subsequent study of these organisms proposed the division of S. dysgalactiae into two subspecies, S. dysgalactiae subsp. equisimilis to accommodate beta-hemolytic large-colony-forming group C and G strains isolated from humans and S. dysgalactiae subsp. dysgalactiae as the name for beta-, alpha-, and nonhemolytic animal strains with group C or L antigen (110). S. canis, an additional species composed of beta-hemolytic group G streptococci normally isolated from animals, has been noted as an infrequent cause of human infection (14).

Table 2 displays some differentiating features of the currently recognized species of large-colony-forming beta-hemolytic streptococci that may express Lancefield group C or G antigen. The table includes their reactions in trehalose and sorbitol fermentation broths, media that have traditionally been used to differentiate among strains isolated from human clinical infections. Carbohydrate fermentation broths (heart infusion broth containing 1.0% carbohydrate and bromcresol purple as an indicator [see chapter 27]) can be used for characterization of these bacteria if differentiation beyond the level of Lancefield serologic characteristics is desired. Strains of group C and G streptococci that are normally isolated from domesticated animals are occasionally reported as agents of human infection.

CAMP Test

The majority of group B streptococci produce a diffusable extracellular protein (CAMP factor, named for Christie, Atkins, and Munch-Peterson, who first described it) that acts synergistically with staphylococcal beta-lysin to cause lysis of red blood cells. Single straight streaks of the streptococcus to be tested and a beta-lysin-producing Staphylo-

TABLE 2 Differentiating features of human and animal strains of large-colony-forming beta-hemolytic streptococci with Lancefield's group C or G antigen[a]

Species	Lancefield antigen(s)	Hosts	Trehalose	Sorbitol
S. dysgalactiae subsp. equisimilis[b]	C, G	Humans	+	−
S. dysgalactiae subsp. dysgalactiae[b]	C, L	Animals	+	−[c]
S. equi subsp. equi	C	Animals	−	−
S. equi subsp. zooepidemicus	C	Animals	−	+
S. canis[d]	G	Animals	−	−[c]

[a] Symbols: +, positive; −, negative.

[b] S. dysgalactiae subsp. equisimilis, characteristically isolated from humans, exhibits proteolytic activity on human fibrin and streptokinase activity on human plasminogen. Both activities are lacking in S. dysgalactiae subsp. dysgalactiae strains, which are normally isolated from animals and may be alpha- or nonhemolytic as well as beta-hemolytic and may produce Lancefield group C or L antigen (110).

[c] Exceptions may occur.

[d] Most strains of S. canis are negative for production of BGUR, in contrast to most other strains of large-colony-forming beta-hemolytic group C or G streptococci.

coccus aureus strain are made perpendicular to each other and about 3 to 4 mm apart on the surface of a sheep blood agar plate. After overnight incubation in ambient atmosphere at 35°C, a positive test will appear as an arrowhead-shaped zone of complete hemolysis in the area into which both staphylococcal beta-lysin and CAMP factor have diffused. An alternative method involving beta-lysin-containing disks has also been described (120).

Hippurate Hydrolysis Test

The ability to hydrolyze hippurate is an alternate test for the presumptive identification of group B streptococci. A rapid version of this test can be performed by incubating a turbid suspension of cells in 0.4 ml of 1% aqueous sodium hippurate for 2 h at 35°C. Glycine formed as an end product of hippurate hydrolysis is detected by adding 5 drops of ninhydrin reagent, reincubating for 10 min, and observing the development of a deep purple color, which signifies a positive reaction (see chapter 27) (60).

Identification of Beta-Hemolytic Isolates: Nucleic Acid Probe Tests

Nucleic acid probes for identification of cultured isolates of group A S. pyogenes and B streptococci are currently available (GenProbe) (25, 26).

Identification of Non-Beta-Hemolytic Isolates: Serologic Tests

Commercially available agglutination reagents (Becton Dickinson and other sources) can aid in the identification of non-beta-hemolytic strains of group B streptococci and pneumococci. Reagents specific for the Lancefield group D antigen may be useful in the identification of S. bovis, but the group D antigen is not easily demonstrated in some strains. Moreover, the group D antigen is fairly nonspecific, being produced by certain streptococci and by members of the genera Enterococcus and Pediococcus. Physiological testing is generally more reliable than serologic methods for identifying non-beta-hemolytic isolates.

Identification of Non-Beta-Hemolytic Streptococci: Physiological Tests

Table 3 summarizes the physiological characteristics of non-beta-hemolytic (alpha- and nonhemolytic) streptococci. It should be remembered that non-beta-hemolytic strains of group B streptococci can be differentiated from the streptococci mentioned below by the CAMP test or serologic testing. The optochin and bile solubility tests are

used to differentiate pneumococci from viridans group streptococci, although strains with atypical reactions in these tests may be encountered (81). Viridans group streptococci can be further characterized to the species or species group level by using physiological testing and identification kits [see "Identification of Viridans Group and Group D Streptococci (S. bovis)" below].

The nonhemolytic streptococci may belong to the species S. bovis or to various viridans group species. The ability of S. bovis to hydrolyze glycoside esculin in the presence of 40% bile distinguishes it from the majority of viridans group strains. S. bovis can be completely characterized to the biotype level with commercially available products, including API 20 Strep (bioMérieux Vitek, Hazelwood, Mo.) (93). The CAMP test may be of use for testing isolates suspected of being non-beta-hemolytic group B streptococci.

Optochin Test

Commercially available optochin disks are applied to a quarter of a blood agar plate that has been streaked with a few colonies of the organism to be tested. After overnight incubation at 35°C in either a candle jar or CO_2 incubator, inhibition zones are measured. Zones of >14 mm with a 6-mm disk or >16 mm with a 10-mm disk are indicative of inhibition and identify the isolate as S. pneumoniae. Isolates displaying smaller zones of inhibition should be subjected to an additional test for bile solubility to confirm their identity.

Bile Solubility Test

Aliquots containing 0.5 ml of a 0.5 to 1.0 McFarland saline suspension of the organisms to be tested are added to each

TABLE 3 Differentiation of non-beta-hemolytic streptococci[a]

Streptococcus	Optochin susceptible	Bile soluble	Bile esculin
S. pneumoniae[b]	+	+	−
S. bovis	−	−	+
Other viridans group streptococci	−	−	−[c]

[a] Symbols: +, positive; −, negative. Strains of group B streptococci (S. agalactiae) may be non-beta-hemolytic; serologic methods, the CAMP test or the hippurate hydrolysis test should be used to rule out possible group B strains.

[b] Some strains of S. pneumoniae may be PYR positive.

[c] Occasional strains of viridans streptococci produce weakly positive bile esculin reactions.

of two small (13- by 100-mm) test tubes. An equal amount (0.5 ml) of 2% sodium deoxycholate (bile) is added to one tube, while 0.5 ml of saline added to the second tube serves as a control. A positive bile solubility test (indicative of pneumococci) appears as clearing in the presence of deoxycholate but not in the control tube after incubation at 35°C for up to 2 h. In some reports, 10% sodium deoxycholate has been used in this procedure, resulting in a final deoxycholate concentration of 5% instead of 1%.

In a plate method for testing bile solubility, 1 drop of a solution of 10% sodium deoxycholate is placed directly on a colony of the strain to be tested. The plate can be kept at room temperature or placed into an aerobic incubator at 35°C for approximately 15 min until the reagent dries, but it must be kept level to prevent the reagent from running over the plate and washing away the colony. Pneumococcal colonies will disappear or be flattened, while bile-resistant streptococcal colonies will be unaffected (7). The use of 2% sodium deoxycholate in this method has been documented in older reports in the literature.

Bile Esculin Test

Bile esculin medium (available from commercial sources) in either plates or slants should be inoculated with one to three colonies of the organism to be tested and incubated at 35°C in an ambient atmosphere for up to 48 h. A definitive blackening of plated media or blackening of at least half of an agar slant is considered a positive test, indicative of S. bovis. Occasional viridans group strains are positive in this test or display weakly positive reactions that are difficult to interpret (92). Isolates from patients with serious infections (e.g., endocarditis) should be more completely characterized (see below) as opposed to being identified as S. bovis on the basis of the bile esculin test alone.

Identification of Non-Beta-Hemolytic Isolates: Nucleic Acid Probe Tests

A nucleic acid probe test for identification of pneumococcal isolates is now commercially available (AccuProbe; GenProbe). Although this test is relatively expensive compared to traditional pneumococcal identification tests, its superior specificity makes it useful as a backup test for strains with atypical reactions in the bile solubility and optochin susceptibility tests (27).

Identification of Viridans Group and Group D Streptococci (S. bovis)

Viridans group streptococci have traditionally been difficult to identify (97). Application of chemotaxonomic and genome-based techniques, particularly DNA-DNA reassociation, has led to a considerable increase in the number of species recognized and to the inclusion of S. bovis within the viridans group. However, improved identification schemes have been developed that provide a means by which the currently recognized viridans group species may be identified (9, 73). Commercially available identification kits have also begun to adjust to this increase in the number of species by expanding their repertoire of tests (45, 71) but still lag behind the number of species currently recognized in the literature. It should be noted that the nomenclature systems used among these products are not always uniform (57).

Alternative approaches to identifying oral streptococci have been described that include the use of whole-cell-derived protein patterns by sodium dodecyl sulfate-poly-acrylamide gel electrophoresis (111), pyrolysis mass spectrometry (79), monoclonal antibodies (28), and DNA-based methods taking advantage of the considerable potential offered by PCR amplification of species-specific gene signatures (2, 68, 91, 106). Despite the promise that these molecular approaches offer, a strategy that enables all oral streptococcal species to be recognized has yet to be described.

In a study of the genus Streptococcus based on sequence comparisons of the small-subunit (16S) rRNA gene, a total of six species groups were demonstrated, the pyogenic (beta-hemolytic, large-colony formers) group and the five additional groups which include the species considered in this section. The nonpyogenic groups were designated (i) the mitis group, (ii) the anginosus group, (iii) the mutans group, (iv) the salivarius group, and (v) the bovis group (66). Two alpha-hemolytic species, S. acidominimus and S. suis (the latter is beta-hemolytic on horse blood), remained ungrouped in this study and also in a similar, previous study (12), while S. ferus, a rat isolate and a candidate for inclusion in the mutans group of species, has yet to be unequivocally classified. The members of these species groups commonly isolated from humans and their differential physiological traits are shown in Tables 4 to 6. Brief descriptions of these species are given below.

Mitis Group

The mitis group includes S. mitis, S. sanguis, S. parasanguis, S. gordonii, S. crista, and S. oralis, together with S. pneumoniae. This group of alpha-hemolytic streptococci includes several species of known clinical significance, together with others for which few or no clinical data have been collected. These species form a group whose classification and nomenclature have been a source of considerable confusion in the past. Current species descriptions for S. sanguis, S. gordonii, S. oralis, and S. mitis, all of which are found in mature dental plaque, are those of Kilian et al. (73), who provide a comprehensive review and discussion of the history of these species epithets and the taxa to which they have been applied. Both S. parasanguis and S. crista have been described more recently (53, 116). Strains produce extracellular polysaccharide (dextran) from sucrose to give hard, adherent, smooth colonies. The majority of strains react with Lancefield group H antiserum raised against strain Blackburn (British group H). Subdivision of S. sanguis on the basis of biochemical characters has been put forward, although it is difficult to equate the biovars of one study (73) with the biotypes of another (9); the clinical relevance of these is unknown. The majority of strains of S. gordonii produce colonies like S. sanguis on sucrose agar. Strains of this species frequently react with Lancefield group H antiserum raised against strain F90A (ATCC 12396) or against strain Blackburn. One point of confusion with these streptococci has been that the previous type strain of S. mitis prior to the emended description of this species by Kilian et al. (73) was strain NCTC 3165, which has since been replaced by a new type strain, NCTC 12261T. NCTC 3165 was subsequently included within S. gordonii. S. oralis and S. mitis are both characterized by an unusual cell wall type, which contains ribitol teichoic acid and lacks significant amounts of rhamnose. Extracellular polysaccharide production is a variable characteristic of S. oralis and is negative in S. mitis. S. parasanguis and S. crista are two additions to the mitis group, and little clinical information about them is currently available. S. parasan-

guis has been isolated from clinical specimens (throats, blood, and urine), while *S. crista* strains originated from the mouth and upper respiratory tract (dental plaque, periodontal abscess, and throat). Both are alpha-hemolytic and hydrolyze arginine but not esculin. Extracellular polysaccharide production is negative for *S. parasanguis* and is a variable characteristic of *S. crista*. The latter species is also characterized by the presence of lateral tufts of fibrils on the cell surface. *S. peroris* and *S. infantis* are alpha-hemolytic species that were isolated from the human pharynx and teeth (67). Oral streptococci that carry tufted fibrils on their surface and are unable to hydrolyze arginine or esculin, which were originally referred to as tufted *Streptococcus sanguis* biotype II or "tufted mitior" (52), have been shown to belong to the mitis group and to constitute a further taxon at the species level (69). However, these streptococci cannot be biochemically separated from *S. mitis* and thus currently remain unidentifiable. Differential characteristics of species in the mitis group are shown in Table 4.

Anginosus Group

The anginosus group includes *S. anginosus*, *S. constellatus*, and *S. intermedius*. A confused nomenclatural history surrounds this group, which now includes streptococci previously referred to as *Streptococcus*-MG, hemolytic and non-hemolytic streptococci possessing the type antigens of Lancefield group F, the minute-colony-forming streptococci of Lancefield groups F and G, *S. milleri*, the "*S. milleri*" group, *Streptococcus*-MG-intermedius, *S. anginosus-constellatus*, *S. anginosus*, *S. constellatus*, and *S. intermedius*. Currently the group is divided into three distinct, closely related species that have retained the names *S. anginosus*, *S. constellatus*, and *S. intermedius*, albeit with emended descriptions (115). Strains may be non-, alpha-, or beta-hemolytic on blood agar, although a higher proportion of *S. intermedius* strains are nonhemolytic. Growth is frequently enhanced in the presence of 5% CO_2, with some strains requiring anaerobic conditions. No extracellular polysaccharide is produced. *S. anginosus* strains may possess Lance-

TABLE 4 Differentiation of species in the mitis group[a]

Test	S. sanguis			S. parasanguis	S. gordonii	S. crista	S. oralis	S. mitis	S. peroris	S. infantis
	Biotype 1[b]	Biotype 2[b]	Biotype 3[b]							
Enzyme activity										
β-D-Fucosidase	−	+	+	V	−	−	−	−	−	V
β-D-Acetylgal[c]	−	−	−	+	V	+	+	−	NT	NT
Neuraminidase	−	−	−	−	−	−	+	V	NT	NT
α-L-Fucosidase	−	−	−	V	+	+	−	−	NT	NT
β-D-Acetylglu[d]	−	V	+	+	+	+	+	−	−	V
α-D-Glucosidase[e]	−	−	−	+	V	−	+	+	NT	NT
β-D-Glucosidase[e]	V	+	V	V	+	−	−	−	−	−
α-Arabinosidase	−	−	−	V	−	−	−	−	NT	NT
α-D-Galactosidase[e]	V	+	−	+	−	−	V	V	−	−
β-D-Galactosidase[e]	−	V	+	+	V	V	V	V	−	+
Acid from:										
Amygdalin	−	+	−	V	+	−	−	−	−	−
Inulin	V	V	V	−	+	−	−	−	−	V
Mannitol	−	−	−	−	−	−	−	−	NT	NT
N-Acetylglu[f]	+	+	+	+	+	+	+	+	NT	−
Raffinose	+	+	−	V	−	−	V	+	−	−
Sorbitol	V	V	−	−	−	−	−	−	−	−
Arbutin	+	+	V	V	+	+	−	−	−	+
Lactose	+	+	+	+	+	V	+	V	+	−
Melibiose	+	V	−	V	−	−	V	+	−	+
Tagatose	NT	NT	NT	V	V	V	V	−	−	+
Hydrolysis of:										
Arginine	+	+	+	+	+	V	−	−	−	−
Esculin	+	+	−	V	+	−	V	−	−	−
Production of:										
Acetoin (VP)	−	−	−	−	−	−	−	−	−	−
Urease	−	−	−	−	−	−	−	−	−	−
Hyaluronidase	−	−	−	−	−	−	−	−	NT	NT
Alkaline phosphatase	NT	NT	NT	V	+	−	V	V	V	−

[a] Symbols and abbreviations: +, positive; −, negative; V, variable; NT, not tested.
[b] Biotypes are those of Beighton et al. (9).
[c] β-D-Acetylgal, β-D-acetylgalactosaminidase.
[d] β-D-Acetylglu, β-D-acetylglucosaminidase.
[e] The percentage of strains giving positive reactions may vary depending on the exact methods used.
[f] N-Acetylglu, N-acetylglucosamine.

field group A, C, F, or G antigens or be nongroupable. *S. constellatus* strains are frequently beta-hemolytic and possess mainly Lancefield group F antigens or are nongroupable, although some strains may be of group A, C, or G. *S. intermedius* seems to be less serologically diverse with respect to Lancefield group antigens than are the other group members, with strains being either nongroupable or of group F.

Further taxonomic proposals have been made for beta-hemolytic Lancefield group C strains of *S. constellatus* (118, 119). These are to the effect that *S. constellatus* constitutes two subspecies: *S. constellatus* subsp. *constellatus*, which is isolated from a relatively broad clinical background, and *S. constellatus* subsp. *pharyngis*, which shows a marked association with the human throat and pharyngitis. Two DNA homology groups have also been shown within *S. anginosus* strains of the same phenotype, although discriminating biochemical tests for identification are needed before taxonomic proposals can be made regarding further subdivision of *S. anginosus*. Other studies support the recognition of *S. anginosus*, *S. constellatus*, and *S. intermedius* within the anginosus group (12, 66) and further centers of taxonomic variation within them (61, 62). Differential characteristics of the species in the anginosus group are shown in Table 5.

Mutans Group

The mutans group includes *S. mutans*, *S. sobrinus*, *S. criceti*, *S. rattus*, *S. downei*, and *S. macacae*. These species are characterized by the production of water-soluble and -insoluble extracellular polysaccharides from sucrose and by the ability to produce acid from a relatively wide range of carbohydrates. *S. mutans* cells may form short rods on solid media or in broth culture under acidic conditions. On blood agar, colonies are often hard and adherent and are usually alpha-hemolytic, with occasional strains giving beta-hemolysis. *S. sobrinus* strains are mostly nonhemolytic or occasionally alpha-hemolytic. On sucrose-containing agar, colonies are rough, heaped, and surrounded by liquid containing glucan. *S. rattus* colonies are rubbery on sucrose agar or, as with *S. criceti*, may be rough and heaped with surrounding liquid glucan. Differential characteristics of *S. mutans* and *S. sobrinus* are shown in Table 6.

Salivarius Group

The salivarius group includes *S. salivarius*, *S. vestibularis*, and *S. thermophilus*. *S. salivarius* and *S. vestibularis* both inhabit the human oral cavity, in contrast to the third member of the group, *S. thermophilus*, which is isolated from dairy sources. *S. salivarius* is isolated from most areas within

TABLE 5 Differentiation of species in the anginosus group[a]

Test	S. anginosus	S. constellatus subsp. constellatus	S. constellatus subsp. pharyngis	S. intermedius
Enzyme activity				
β-D-Fucosidase	−	−	+	+
β-D-Acetylgal[b]	−	−	+	+
Neuraminidase	−	−	−	+
α-L-Fucosidase	−	−	−	−
β-D-Acetylglu[c]	−	−	+	+
α-D-Glucosidase	V	+	+	+
β-D-Glucosidase	+	−	+	V
α-Arabinosidase	V	−	−	−
α-D-Galactosidase	V	−	−	−
β-D-Galactosidase	V	V	+	+
Acid from:				
Amygdalin	+	V	+	V
Inulin	−	−	−	−
Mannitol	−	−	−	−
N-Acetylglu[d]	V	V	+	+
Raffinose	V	−	−	−
Sorbitol	−	−	−	−
Arbutin	+	+	+	+
Lactose	+	V	+	+
Melibiose	V	V	−	V
Hydrolysis of:				
Arginine	+	+	+	+
Esculin	+	V	+	+
Production of:				
Acetoin (VP)	+	+	+	+
Urease	−	−	−	−
Hyaluronidase	−	+	V	+

[a] Symbols and abbreviation: +, positive; −, negative; V, variable.
[b] β-D-Acetylgal, β-D-acetylgalactosaminidase.
[c] β-D-Acetylglu, β-D-acetylglucosaminidase.
[d] N-Acetylglu, N-acetylglucosamine.

TABLE 6 Biochemical characteristics of *S. mutans*, *S. sobrinus*, *S. salivarius*, *S. vestibularis*, and *S. bovis*[a]

Test	S. mutans	S. sobrinus	S. salivarius	S. vestibularis	S. bovis
Enzyme activity					
β-D-Fucosidase	−	−	V	−	NA
β-D-Acetylgal[b]	−	−	−	−	NA
Neuraminidase	−	−	−	−	NA
α-L-Fucosidase	−	−	−	−	NA
β-D-Acetylglu[c]	−	−	−	−	−
α-D-Glucosidase	+	+	V	V	NA
β-D-Glucosidase	+	−	V	−	+
α-Arabinosidase	−	−	+	+	NA
α-D-Galactosidase	V	−	−	−	V
β-D-Galactosidase	+	+	+	+	−[V d]
Acid from:					
Amygdalin	+	−	V	V	V
Inulin	+	−	V	−	+
Mannitol	+	+	−	−	+[−d]
N-Acetylglu[e]	+	−	V	V	+
Raffinose	+	−	V	−	+
Sorbitol	+	V	−	−	−
Arbutin	V	−	+	V	V
Lactose	+	+	+	V	+
Melibiose	+	−	−	−	+
Hydrolysis of:					
Arginine	−	−	−	−	−
Esculin	V	−	+	V	+
Production of:					
Acetoin (VP)	+	+	+	−	+
Urease	−	−	V	+	−
Hyaluronidase	−	−	−	−	−

[a] Symbols: +, positive; −, negative; V, variable; NA, data not available.
[b] β-D-Acetylgal, β-D-acetylgalactosaminidase.
[c] β-D-Acetylglu, β-D-acetylglucosaminidase.
[d] Test scores in superscript are for "variant" strains (see text). Variant strains are also variable (V) for glucuronidase and do not produce extracellular polysaccharides.
[e] N-Acetylglu, N-acetylglucosamine.

the mouth, especially the tongue, mucosal surfaces, and saliva. *S. vestibularis* was initially isolated from the oral vestibule, although the full extent of its colonization of the oral surfaces has not been determined. Neither species is considered to be an important pathogen, although *S. salivarius* occasionally causes septicemia in neutropenic patients. *S. salivarius* strains are usually non- or alpha-hemolytic on blood agar and form distinctive colonies on sucrose agar due to the production of extracellular polysaccharide, resulting in large mucoid colonies (soluble fructan or levan) or large hard colonies that may pit the agar (insoluble glucan or dextran). A high proportion of *S. salivarius* strains react with Lancefield group K antiserum. Urease production is a characteristic of approximately half (proportions vary among studies) of the *S. salivarius* strains isolated. *S. vestibularis* is alpha-hemolytic and urease positive and does not produce extracellular polysaccharide from sucrose. Differential characteristics of *S. salivarius* and *S. vestibularis* are shown in Table 6.

Bovis Group

The bovis group includes *S. bovis*, *S. alactolyticus*, and *S. equinus*. Despite the clinical significance of *S. bovis* in endocarditis and colonic cancer, the confusing array of biotypes presented by human and bovine strains has hin-dered the classification and identification of this group of streptococci. DNA-DNA reassociation studies have revealed considerable heterogeneity (24, 44, 82), with the most recent studies showing a clear separation of human strains of *S. bovis* from animal strains and the division of the latter into two distinct homology groups. *S. bovis* strains from humans are described as being "typical" (biotype I, able to ferment mannitol and produce copious amounts of an extracellular polysaccharide, glucan, from sucrose) or "variant" (biotype II, unable to ferment mannitol or produce glucan). Commercial kits (Rapid ID STREP; bio-Mérieux, Marcy l'Etoile, France) may differentiate between biotypes II/1 and II/2 on the basis of the production of both β-glucuronidase and β-galactosidase and the production of acid from trehalose but not from glycogen by the latter. *S. bovis* and *S. mutans* strains may resemble each other due to the production of glucan, fermentation of mannitol, and growth on bile esculin agar. However, *S. bovis* does not ferment sorbitol, is able to ferment starch or glycogen, and gives a Lancefield group D serologic reaction. The differentiation of *S. bovis* from *S. salivarius* strains has been suggested on the basis of the Lancefield group D reaction; ability to grow on bile esculin agar; fermentation of mannitol, inulin, and starch; and urease production (92). *S. bovis* strains are virtually always β-galactosidase negative and α-galactosidase positive, in contrast to *S. salivarius*. In addition, β-glucuronidase production by *S. bovis* biotype II/2 may be a useful test. The biochemical characteristics of *S. bovis* are shown in Table 6.

Identification of Viridans Group Streptococci: Physiological Tests

Fluorogenic Substrates

The enzymatic activities listed in Tables 4 to 6 can be assayed with fluorogenic substrate reagents (see chapter 27). Colonies from Columbia blood agar containing 5% (vol/vol) defibrinated horse blood are suspended in TES buffer (see chapter 27) to approximately 10^8 organisms/ml (optical density at 620 nm, 0.1), and 50 μl of bacterial suspension is added to 20 μl of fluorogenic substrate solution in a flat-bottom microtiter tray well. After incubation at 37°C for 3 h, substrate degradation is visualized as bright blue fluorescence when viewed under long-wave UV light. This test format may be scored qualitatively on a UV transilluminator by using a UV lamp or quantitatively in a UV plate reader. Standardized conditions for incubation should be used to obtain consistent results with these substrates (1).

Carbohydrate Fermentation

The microtiter plate method may also be used to assess the ability of strains to acidify the carbohydrates listed in Tables 4 to 6. Three drops of carbohydrate solution (see chapter 27) per well is inoculated with 1 drop of an overnight culture in Todd-Hewitt broth (Oxoid, Basingstoke, United Kingdom; Becton Dickinson). Incubation is carried out at 37°C for 24 h anaerobically. Acid production is indicated by the formation of a yellow color (76).

Arginine Hydrolysis

Arginine hydrolysis is a key reaction in the identification of viridans streptococci, and several test methods have been published. Discrepancies can occur between them (114). Two commonly used methods are detailed here.

1. Moeller's decarboxylase broth containing arginine (Becton Dickinson and other sources) should be inoculated with the test organism, overlaid with mineral oil, and incubated at 35 to 37°C for up to 7 days. Degradation of arginine results in an increase in pH, indicated by development of a purple color. Negative results are indicated by a yellow color, which is due to acid accumulation from metabolism of glucose only.

2. A microtiter plate method employs the broth described in chapter 27. Three drops of the arginine-containing reagent are inoculated with 1 drop of an overnight Todd-Hewitt broth culture and incubated for 24 h at 37°C anaerobically. Production of ammonia is detected by the appearance of an orange color on addition of 1 drop of Nessler's reagent (10).

Urea Hydrolysis Test

Christensen urea agar (Becton Dickinson, other sources) is inoculated and incubated aerobically at 35°C for up to 7 days. Development of a pink color indicates a positive reaction. An alternative format is to dispense Christensen's medium made up without agar into a microtiter tray well and, after inoculation, overlay it with oil prior to incubation.

VP Test

For a rapid version of the VP test, see "Identification of Beta-Hemolytic Isolates: Physiological Tests" (above). A more standard method for performing the VP test, requiring extended incubation, is described in chapter 27.

Esculin Hydrolysis

Esculin agar slants (Becton Dickinson, other sources) are inoculated and incubated for up to 1 week. A positive reaction appears as a blackening of the medium; no change in color indicates a negative esculin hydrolysis test. A version of the esculin hydrolysis test involving broth is described in chapter 27.

Hyaluronidase Production

Hyaluronidase activity can be detected on agar plates by the method of Smith and Willett (98), as described in chapter 27. The strains to be tested are inoculated by stabbing into the agar and incubated anaerobically at 37°C overnight. After the plate is flooded with 2 M acetic acid, hyaluronidase activity is indicated by the appearance of a clear zone around the stab. Homer et al. (59) have also described a quantitative method of determining hyaluronidase activity that is carried out in microtiter trays.

Production of Extracellular Polysaccharide

Strains are streaked out for single colonies on sucrose containing agar. The two most commonly used media are (i) mitis-salivarius agar containing 0.001% (wt/vol) potassium tellurite (Becton Dickinson) and (ii) tryptone-yeast-cystine agar (Lab M, Bury, United Kingdom). Incubation may be carried out for up to 5 days at 37°C.

Two other tests found to be useful, particularly in helping to discriminate among the oralis group species, are production of immunoglobulin A protease (73) and amylase binding (36). However, these tests are unlikely to be used in routine clinical microbiology laboratories at present.

SEROLOGIC TESTS

Serologic tests are available to detect immune responses in patient sera to both extracellular products (streptolysin O, hyaluronidase, DNase B, NADase, and streptokinase) and cellular components (M protein and group A antigen) of *S. pyogenes*. These tests are useful in demonstrating antecedent streptococcal infection in patients who lack documentation of recent infection but who present with nonsuppurative sequelae (rheumatic fever or glomerulonephritis). Ayoub and Harden (4) provide a further discussion and describe methods for performing these tests.

ANTIBIOTIC SUSCEPTIBILITIES

In spite of reports of resistance in certain isolates, penicillin remains the drug of choice for treatment of infections caused by most streptococci, while narrow-spectrum cephalosporins, erythromycin (or neomacrolides like azithromycin, clarithromycin, and dirythromycin), or vancomycin serve as alternative choices for treatment (80). An increase in erythromycin resistance in *S. pyogenes* was noted during the 1990s in numerous locations worldwide. High rates of resistance (20 to 40% of isolates tested) have been documented in various geographical locations. Although the streptococci are, as of this writing, considered susceptible to vancomycin, one report described the isolation of a vancomycin-resistant *S. bovis* strain during routine screening of stool specimens for vancomycin-resistant enterococci (87).

Penicillin treatment failures have been ascribed to tolerance, a situation in which bacterial growth is inhibited by penicillin but the bactericidal activity of the drug is greatly reduced. Another possible explanation for treatment failure, especially in pharyngitis, is the presence of β-lactamase-producing bacteria at the site of infection (20) or poor patient compliance with dosing regimens. Concern about the efficacy of penicillin alone for effective treatment of life-threatening infections has led to the use of synergistic combinations of drugs (e.g., penicillin and gentamicin) for treatment of severe group B disease and for endocarditis due to viridans group streptococci that are relatively resistant to penicillin (MIC, >0.1 to 0.2 μg/ml [31]).

The most notable trends in changing antimicrobial susceptibility patterns among the streptococci are penicillin resistance and multiple resistance in pneumococci and increasing frequencies of penicillin resistance in viridans group streptococci. Approximately 34% of viridans group streptococcal bloodstream isolates collected during a 1997 to 1999 surveillance study in the United States, Canada, and Latin America were not susceptible to penicillin. Penicillin-nonsusceptible strains were also less susceptible to other non-β-lactam agents and were found more often in cancer patients than in patients without cancer (30). *S. mitis* isolates are notable for displaying penicillin resistance, and South African workers have also observed high-level gentamicin resistance (and absence of a synergistic β-lactam/aminoglycoside effect) in *S. mitis* strains (86). It should be remembered that viridans group strains identified as "*S. mitis*" will include a significant proportion of strains that would be identified as *S. oralis* if more discriminatory tests were applied. While anginosus ("*S. milleri*") group isolates have been found to be generally penicillin susceptible by some workers (33, 64, 105), there are also reports that suggest the impending emergence of penicillin resistance in these organisms (5).

Penicillin resistance in pneumococci has been reported in areas all over the world, and its incidence appears to be increasing. The reported frequencies of penicillin-resistant pneumococcal strains are variable, depending on the geographical location (32, 94). Extended-spectrum cephalosporins (e.g., cefriaxone or cefotaxime) have been used successfully to treat serious infections caused by penicillin-resistant pneumococci, but resistance to these agents also seems to be increasing. Pneumococcal strains displaying resistance to a variety of other antibiotics (erythromycin, tetracycline, chloramphenicol, and trimethoprim-sulfamethoxazole) have been encountered. Multiple resistance (resistance to three or more classes of antibiotics) may occur in the presence or absence of penicillin resistance (3).

The evolving antimicrobial resistance patterns of streptococci make accurate assessment of susceptibility in these organisms an important function of the clinical microbiology laboratory. Chapters 70 and 71 of this Manual should be consulted for information on performance of susceptibility testing. Various commercially available systems (see chapter 15) may also be used for determining streptococcal antimicrobial susceptibilities. In general, these systems perform satisfactorily with *S. pneumoniae* isolates (51, 65, 104).

EVALUATION, INTERPRETATION, AND REPORTING OF RESULTS

Beta-hemolytic streptococci and pneumococci are virulent pathogens, and consequently the detection and reporting of these organisms from all types of specimens have been emphasized in the clinical laboratory. Timely evaluation and reporting of throat specimens positive for *S. pyogenes* will allow prompt antibiotic treatment, reducing the risk of nonsuppurative sequelae. While large-colony-forming group C and G streptococci (*S. dysgalactiae* subsp. *equisimilis*) have been documented as agents of pharyngitis, small-colony-forming beta-hemolytic streptococci (anginosus or "*S. milleri*" group) seem to represent constituents of the normal throat flora (109), although a role in pharyngitis for certain small-colony-forming strains with the group C antigen has been suggested (119). Small-colony-forming beta-hemolytic strains are, however, well documented as pathogens in infections other than pharyngitis.

The identification of viridans group streptococci to the species or group level should be reserved for isolates from patients with serious infections, particularly endocarditis, abscesses, and infections in neutropenic patients. Since viridans group streptococci are causative agents of shock, endocarditis, and pulmonary infections in neutropenic patients (16, 41), careful evaluation of the significance of these streptococci in blood cultures from members of this patient population is required. Viridans group streptococci from blood cultures in neutropenic patients should be identified since this may assist in the treatment of complications, which may be common in these patients. It should be remembered that anginosus ("*S. milleri*") group organisms recovered from abscess or wound specimens, even when other organisms are present, are likely to be pathogens and not contaminants. As mentioned above, *S. bovis* biotyping may be useful because of a correlation between biotype I and endocarditis and gastrointestinal malignancy.

We acknowledge the significant contributions to this chapter made by R. R. Facklam and J. A. Washington in the fifth edition of this Manual.

REFERENCES

1. **Ahmet, Z., M. Warren, and E. T. Houang.** 1995. Species identification of members of the *Streptococcus milleri* group isolated from the vagina by ID 32 Strep system and differential phenotypic characteristics. *J. Clin. Microbiol.* **33:** 1592–1595.
2. **Alam, S., S. R. Brailsford, R. A. Whiley, and D. Beighton.** 1999. PCR-based methods for genotyping viridans group streptococci. *J. Clin. Microbiol.* **37:**2772–2776.
3. **Applebaum, P. C.** 1996. Epidemiology and in vitro susceptibility of drug-resistant *Streptococcus pneumoniae*. *Pediatr. Infect. Dis. J.* **15:**932–939.
4. **Ayoub, E. M., and E. Harden.** 1997. Immune response to streptococcal antigens: diagnostic methods, p. 450–457. *In* N. R. Rose, E. Conway de Macario, J. D. Folds, H. C. Lane, and R. M. Nakamura (ed.), *Manual of Clinical Laboratory Immunology*, 5th ed. American Society for Microbiology, Washington, D.C.
5. **Bantar, C., L. Fernandez Canigia, S. Relloso, A. Lanza, H. Bianchini, and J. Smayevsky.** 1996. Species belonging to the "*Streptococcus milleri*" group: antimicrobial susceptibility and comparative prevalence in significant clinical specimens. *J. Clin. Microbiol.* **34:**2020–2022.
6. **Barnham, M., T. J. Thornton, and K. Lange.** 1983. Nephritis caused by *Streptococcus zooepidemicus* (Lancefield group C). *Lancet* **i:**945–948.

7. Baron, E. J., L. R. Peterson, and S. M. Finegold. 1994. Conventional and rapid microbiological methods for identification of bacteria and fungi, p. 97–122. In E. J. Baron, L. R. Peterson, and S. M. Finegold (ed.), Bailey and Scott's Diagnostic Microbiology, 9th ed. The C. V. Mosby Co., St. Louis, Mo.

8. Beighton, D., A. D. Carr, and B. A. Oppenheim. 1994. Identification of viridans streptococci associated with bacteraemia in neutropaenic cancer patients. J. Med. Microbiol. 40:202–204.

9. Beighton, D., J. M. Hardie, and R. A. Whiley. 1991. A scheme for the identification of viridans streptococci. J. Med. Microbiol. 35:367–372.

10. Beighton, D., R. R. B. Russell, and H. Hayday. 1981. The isolation and characterisation of Streptococcus mutans serotype h from dental plaque of monkeys (Macaca fascicularis). J. Gen. Microbiol. 124:271–279.

11. Benitz, W. E., J. B. Gould, and M. L. Druzin. 1999. Risk factors for early-onset group B streptococcal sepsis: estimation of odds ratios by critical literature review. Pediatrics 103:1–14.

12. Bentley, R. W., J. A. Leigh, and M. D. Collins. 1991. Intrageneric structure of Streptococcus based on comparative analysis of small subunit rRNA sequences. Int. J. Syst. Bacteriol. 41:487–494.

13. Bergeron, M. G., D. Ke, C. Menard, F. J. Picard, M. Gagnon, M. Bernier, M. Ouellette, P. H. Roy, S. Marcoux, and W. D. Fraser. 2000. Rapid detection of group B streptococci in pregnant women at delivery. N. Engl. J. Med. 343:175–179.

14. Bert, F., and N. Lambert-Zechovsky. 1997. Septicemia caused by Streptococcus canis in a human. J. Clin. Microbiol. 35:777–779.

15. Bochud, P. Y., T. Calandra, and P. Francioli. 1994. Bacteremia due to viridans streptococci in neutropenic patients: a review. Am. J. Med. 97:256–264.

16. Bochud, P. Y., P. Eggiman, T. Calandra, G. van Melle, L. Saghafi, and P. Francioli. 1994. Bacteremia due to viridans streptococcus in neutropenic patients with cancer: clinical spectrum and risk factors. Clin. Infect. Dis. 20:469–470.

17. Bourbeau, P. P., B. J. Heiter, and M. Figdore. 1997. Use of Gen-Probe AccuProbe Group B Streptococcus Test to detect group B streptococci in broth cultures of vaginal-anorectal specimens from pregnant women: comparison with traditional culture method. J. Clin. Microbiol. 35:144–147.

18. Bouvet, A., A. Durand, C. Devine, J. Etienne, C. Leport, and the Groupe d'Enquête sur l'Endocardite en France 1990–1991. 1994. In vitro susceptibility to antibiotics of 200 strains of streptococci and enterococci isolated during infective endocarditis, p. 72–73. In A. Totalian (ed.), Pathogenic Streptococci: Present and Future. Lancer Publications, St. Petersburg, Russia.

19. Brandt, C. M., G. Haase, N. Schnitzler, R. Zbinden, and R. Lütticken. 1999. Characterization of blood culture isolates of Streptococcus dysgalactiae subsp. equisimilis possessing Lancefield's group A antigen. J. Clin. Microbiol. 37:4194–4197.

20. Brook, I., and A. E. Gober. 1995. Role of bacterial interference and beta-lactamase-producing bacteria in the failure of penicillin to eradicate group A streptococcal pharyngotonsillitis. Arch. Otolaryngol. Head Neck Surg. 121:1405–1409.

21. Carroll, K. C., D. Ballou, M. Varner, H. Chun, R. Traver, and J. Salyer. 1996. Rapid detection of group B streptococcal colonization of the genital tract by a commercial optical immunoassay. Eur. J. Clin. Microbiol. Infect. Dis. 15:206–210.

22. Centers for Disease Control and Prevention. 1996. Prevention of perinatal group B streptococcal disease: a public health perspective. Morb. Mortal. Wkly. Rep. 45(RR-7): 1–24.

23. Chew, T. A., and J. M. B. Smith. 1992. Detection of diacetyl (caramel odor) in presumptive identification of the "Streptococcus milleri" group. J. Clin. Microbiol. 30: 3028–3029.

24. Coykendall, A. L., and K. B. Gustafson. 1985. Deoxyribonucleic acid hybridizations among strains of Streptococcus salivarius and Streptococcus bovis. Int. J. Syst. Bacteriol. 35:274–280.

25. Daly, J. A., N. L. Clifton, K. C. Seskin, and W. M. Gooch III. 1991. Use of rapid, nonradioactive DNA probes in culture confirmation tests to detect Streptococcus agalactiae, Haemophilus influenzae, and Enterococcus spp. from pediatric patients with significant infections. J. Clin. Microbiol. 29:80–82.

26. Davis, T. E., and D. D. Fuller. 1991. Direct identification of bacterial isolates in blood cultures by using a DNA probe. J. Clin. Microbiol. 29:2192–2196.

27. Denys, G. A., and R. B. Carey. 1992. Identification of Streptococcus pneumoniae with a DNA probe. J. Clin. Microbiol. 30:2725–2727.

28. De Soet, J. J., and J. De Graaff. 1990. Monoclonal antibodies for enumeration and identification of mutans streptococci in epidemiological studies. Arch. Oral Biol. 35:165S–168S.

29. Devriese, L. A., J. Hommez, R. Kilpper-Balz, and K. H. Schleifer. 1986. Streptococcus canis sp. nov.: a species of group G streptococci from animals. Int. J. Syst. Bacteriol. 36:422–425.

30. Diekema, D. J., M. L. Beach, M. A. Pfaller, R. N. Jones, and the SENTRY Participants Group. 2001. Antimicrobial resistance in viridans streptococci among patients with and without the diagnosis of cancer in the USA, Canada and Latin America. Clin. Microbiol. Infect. 7:152–157.

31. Dinubile, M. J. 1990. Treatment of endocarditis caused by relatively resistant nonenterococcal streptococci: is penicillin enough? Rev. Infect. Dis. 12:112–117.

32. Doern, G. V., A. B. Brueggemann, H. Huynh, E. Wingert, and P. Rhomberg. 1999. Antimicrobial resistance with Streptococcus pneumoniae in the United States, 1997–98. Emerg. Infect. Dis. 5:757–765.

33. Doern, G. V., M. J. Ferraro, A. B. Brueggemann, and K. L. Ruoff. 1996. Emergence of high rates of antimicrobial resistance among viridans group streptococci in the United States. Antimicrob. Agents Chemother. 40:891–894.

34. Dominguez, J., N. Gali, S. Blanco, P. Pedroso, C. Prat, L. Matas, and V. Ausina. 2001. Detection of Streptococcus pneumoniae antigen by a rapid immunochromatographic assay in urine samples. Chest 111:9–11.

35. Douglas, C. W. I., J. Heath, K. K. Hampton, and F. E. Preston. 1993. Identity of viridans streptococci isolated from cases of infective endocarditis. J. Med. Microbiol. 39:179–182.

36. Douglas, C. W. I., A. A. Pease, and R. A. Whiley. 1990. Amylase-binding as a discriminator among oral streptococci. FEMS Microbiol. Lett. 66:193–198.

37. Dowell, S. F., R. L. Garman, G. Liu, O. S. Levine, and Y. Yang. 2001. Evaluation of Binax NOW, an assay for the detection of pneumococcal antigen in urine samples, performed among pediatric patients. Clin. Infect. Dis. 32: 824–825.

38. Drulak, M., W. Bartholomew, L. LaScolea, D. Amsterdam, N. Gunnersen, J. Yong, C. Fijalkowski, and S. Winston. 1991. Evaluation of the modified Visuwell

Strep-A enzyme immunoassay for detection of group-A *Streptococcus* from throat swabs. *Diagn. Microbiol. Infect. Dis.* **14**:281–285.

39. **Duca, E., G. Teodorovici, C. Radu, A. Vita, P. Talasman-Niculescu, E. Bernescu, C. Feldi, and V. Rosca.** 1969. A new nephritogenic streptococcus. *J. Hyg. Camb.* **67**:691–698.

40. **Efstratiou, A.** 2000. Group A streptococci in the 1990s. *J. Antimicrob. Chemother.* **45**(Topic T1):3–12.

41. **Elting, L. S., G. P. Bodey, and B. H. Keefe.** 1992. Septicemia and shock syndrome due to viridans streptococci: a case-control study of predisposing factors. *Clin. Infect. Dis.* **14**:1201–1207.

42. **Facklam, R., J. Elliott, N. Pigott, and R. Franklin.** 1995. Identification of *Streptococcus porcinus* from human sources. *J. Clin. Microbiol.* **33**:385–388.

43. **Farrow, J. A. E., and M. D. Collins.** 1984. Taxonomic studies on streptococci of serological groups C, G and L and possibly related taxa. *Syst. Appl. Microbiol.* **5**:483–493.

44. **Farrow, J. A. E., J. Kruze, B. A. Phillips, A. J. Bramley, and M. D. Collins.** 1984. Taxonomic studies on *Streptococcus bovis* and *Streptococcus equinus*: description of *Streptococcus alactolyticus* sp. nov. and *Streptococcus saccharolyticus*. sp. nov. *Syst. Appl. Microbiol.* **5**:467–482.

45. **Freney, J., S. Bland, J. Etienne, M. Desmonceux, J. M. Boeufgras, and J. Fleurette.** 1992. Description and evaluation of the semiautomated 4-hour Rapid ID 32 Strep method for identification of streptococci and members of related genera. *J. Clin. Microbiol.* **30**:2657–2661.

46. **Garcia Gil, E., M. C. Rodriguez, R. Bartolome, B. Berjano, L. Cabero, and A. Andreu.** 1999. Evaluation of the Granada agar plate for detection of vaginal and rectal group B streptococci in pregnant women. *J. Clin. Microbiol.* **37**:2648–2651.

47. **Gerber, M. A.** 1986. Diagnosis of group A beta-hemolytic streptococcal pharyngitis, use of antigen detection tests. *Diagn. Microbiol. Infect. Dis.* **4**:5S–15S.

48. **Gerber, M. A., M. F. Randolph, and K. K. DeMeo.** 1990. Liposome immunoassay for rapid identification of group A streptococci directly from throat swabs. *J. Clin. Microbiol.* **28**:1463–1464.

49. **Granato, P. A., and M. T. Petosa.** 1991. Evaluation of a rapid screening test for detecting group B streptococci in pregnant women. *J. Clin. Microbiol.* **29**:1536–1538.

50. **Green, M., B. Dashefsky, E. R. Wald, S. Laifer, J. Harger, and R. Guthrie.** 1993. Comparison of two antigen assays for rapid intrapartum detection of vaginal group B streptococcal colonization. *J. Clin. Microbiol.* **31**:78–82.

51. **Guthrie, L. L., S. Banks, W. Setiawan, and K. B. Waites.** 1999. Comparison of MicroScan, MICroStrep, PASCO, and Sensititre MIC panels for determining antimicrobial susceptibilities of *Streptococcus pneumoniae*. *Diagn. Microbiol. Infect. Dis.* **33**:267–273.

52. **Handley, P. S., P. L. Carter, J. E. Wyatt, and L. M. Hesketh.** 1985. Surface structures (peritrichous fibrils and tufts of fibrils) found on *Streptococcus sanguis* strains may be related to their ability to coaggregate with other oral genera. *Infect. Immun.* **47**:217–227.

53. **Handley, P., A. Coykendall, D. Beighton, J. M. Hardie, and R. A. Whiley.** 1991. *Streptococcus crista* sp. nov., a viridans streptococcus with tufted fibrils, isolated from the human oral cavity and throat. *Int. J. Syst. Bacteriol.* **41**:543–547.

54. **Harbeck, R. J., J. Teague, G. R. Crossen, D. M. Maul, and P. L. Childers.** 1993. Novel, rapid optical immunoassay technique for detection of group A streptococci from pharyngeal specimens: comparison with standard culture methods. *J. Clin. Microbiol.* **31**:839–844.

55. **Hardie, J. M.** 1986. Genus *Streptococcus* Rosenbach 1884, 22[AL], p. 1043–1071. *In* P. H. A. Sneath, N. S. Mair, M. E. Sharpe, and J. G. Holt (ed.), *Bergey's Manual of Systematic Bacteriology*, vol. 2. The Williams & Wilkins Co., Baltimore, Md.

56. **Heelan, J. S., S. Wilbur, G. Depetris, and C. Letourneau.** 1996. Rapid antigen testing for group A streptococcus by DNA probe. *Diagn. Microbiol. Infect. Dis.* **24**:65–69.

57. **Hinnebusch, C. J., D. M. Nikolai, and D. A. Bruckner.** 1991. Comparison of API Rapid STREP, Baxter Microscan Rapid Pos ID Panel, BBL Minitek Differential Identification System, IDS RapID STR System, and Vitek GPI to conventional biochemical tests for identification of viridans streptococci. *Am. J. Clin. Pathol.* **96**:459–463.

58. **Hoffman, S.** 1990. Detection of group A streptococcal antigen from throat swabs with five diagnostic kits in general practice. *Diagn. Microbiol. Infect. Dis.* **13**:209–215.

59. **Homer, K. A., L. Denbow, R. A. Whiley, and D. Beighton.** 1993. Chondroitin sulfate depolymerase and hyaluronidase activities of viridans streptococci determined by a sensitive spectrophotometric assay. *J. Clin. Microbiol.* **31**:1648–1651.

60. **Hwang, M. N., and G. M. Ederer.** 1975. Rapid hippurate hydrolysis method for presumptive identification of group B streptococci. *J. Clin. Microbiol.* **1**:114–115.

61. **Jacobs, J. A., C. S. Schot, A. E. Bunschoten, and L. M. Schouls.** 2000. Rapid species identification of "*Streptococcus milleri*" strains by line blot hybridization: identification of a distinct 16S rRNA population closely related to *Streptococcus constellatus*. *J. Clin. Microbiol.* **34**:1717–1721.

62. **Jacobs, J. A., L. M. Schouls, and R. A. Whiley.** 2000. DNA-DNA reassociation studies of *S. constellatus* strains with unusual 16S RNA sequences within the anginosus group of *Streptococcus*. *Int. J. Syst. Evol. Microbiol.* **50**:247–249.

63. **Jacobs, J. A., H. C. Schouten, E. E. Stobberingh, and P. B. Soeters.** 1995. Viridans streptococci isolated from the bloodstream. Relevance of species identification. *Diagn. Microbiol. Infect. Dis.* **22**:267–273.

64. **Jacobs, J. A., and E. E. Stobberingh.** 1996. In-vitro antimicrobial susceptibility of the '*Streptococcus milleri*' group (*Streptococcus anginosus*, *Streptococcus constellatus* and *Streptococcus intermedius*). *J. Antimicrob. Chemother.* **37**:371–375.

65. **Jorgensen, J. H., A. L. Barry, M. M. Traczewski, D. F. Sahm, M. L. McElmeel, and S. A. Crawford.** 2000. Rapid automated antimicrobial susceptibility testing of *Streptococcus pneumoniae* by use of the bioMerieux VITEK 2. *J. Clin. Microbiol.* **38**:2814–2818.

66. **Kawamura, Y., X.-G. Hou, F. Sultana, H. Miura, and T. Ezaki.** 1995. Determination of 16S rRNA sequences of *Streptococcus mitis* and *Streptococcus gordonii* and phylogenetic relationships among members of the genus *Streptococcus*. *Int. J. Syst. Bacteriol.* **45**:406–408.

67. **Kawamura, Y., X.-G. Hou, Y. Todome, F. Sultana, K. Hirose, S.-E. Shu, T. Ezaki, and H. Ohkuni.** 1998. *Streptococcus peroris* sp. nov. and *Streptococcus infantis* sp. nov., new members of the *Streptococcus mitis* group, isolated from human clinical specimens. *Int. J. Syst. Bacteriol.* **48**:921–927.

68. **Kawamura, Y., R. A. Whiley, S.-E. Shu, T. Ezaki, and J. M. Hardie.** 1999. Genetic approaches to the identification of the mitis group within the genus *Streptococcus*. *Microbiology* **145**:2605–2613.

69. **Kawamura, Y., R. A. Whiley, L. Zhao, T. Ezaki, and J. M. Hardie.** 2000. Taxonomic study of 'tufted mitior' strains of streptococci (*Streptococcus sanguinis* biotype II):

recognition of a new genospecies. *Syst. Appl. Microbiol.* **23:**245–250.

70. **Kellog, J.** 1990. Suitability of throat culture procedures for detection of group A streptococci and as reference standards for evaluation of streptococcal antigen detection kits. *J. Clin. Microbiol.* **28:**165–169.

71. **Kikuchi, K., T. Enari, K.-I. Totsuka, and K. Shimizu.** 1995. Comparison of phenotypic characteristics, DNA-DNA hybridisation results, and results with a commercial rapid biochemical and enzymatic reaction system for identification of viridans group streptococci. *J. Clin. Microbiol.* **33:**1215–1222.

72. **Kilian, M.** 2001. Recommended conservation of the names *Streptococcus sanguis*, *Streptococcus rattus*, *Streptococcus cricetus* and seven other names included in the Approved Lists of Bacterial Names. Request for an opinion. *Int. J. Syst. Evol. Microbiol.* **51:**723–724.

73. **Kilian, M., L. Mikkelsen, and J. Henrichsen.** 1989. Taxonomic study of viridans streptococci: description of *Streptococcus gordonii* sp. nov. and emended descriptions of *Streptococcus sanguis* (White and Niven 1946), *Streptococcus oralis* (Bridge and Sneath 1982), and *Streptococcus mitis* (Andrewes and Horder 1906). *Int. J. Syst. Bacteriol.* **39:**471–484.

74. **Kirby, R., and K. L. Ruoff.** 1995. Cost-effective, clinically relevant method for rapid identification of beta-hemolytic streptococci and enterococci. *J. Clin. Microbiol.* **33:**1154–1157.

75. **Kircher, S. M., M. P. Meyer, and J. A. Jordan.** 1996. Comparison of a modified DNA hybridization assay with standard culture enrichment for detecting group B streptococci in obstetric patients. *J. Clin. Microbiol.* **34:**342–344.

76. **Kral, T. A., and L. Daneo-Moore.** 1981. Biochemical differentiation of certain oral streptococci. *J. Dent. Res.* **60:**1713–1718.

77. **Lim, D. V., W. J. Morales, and A. F. Walsh.** 1987. Lim group B strep broth and coagglutination for rapid identification of group B streptococci in preterm pregnant women. *J. Clin. Microbiol.* **25:**452–453.

78. **Ludwig, W., M. Weizenegger, R. Kilpper-Balz, and K. H. Schleifer.** 1988. Phylogenetic relationships of anaerobic streptococci. *Int. J. Syst. Bacteriol.* **38:**15–18.

79. **Magee, J. T., J. M. Hindmarch, and C. W. I. Douglas.** 1997. A numerical taxonomic study of *Streptococcus sanguis*, *S. mitis* and similar organisms using conventional and pyrolysis mass spectrometry. *Zentbl. Bakteriol.* **285:**195–203.

80. **Moellering, R. C., Jr.** 2000. Principles of anti-infective therapy, p. 223–235. *In* G. L. Mandell, J. E. Bennett, and R. Dolin (ed.), *Mandell, Douglas and Bennett's Principles and Practice of Infectious Diseases*, 5th ed. Churchill Livingstone, Inc., New York, N.Y.

81. **Mundy, L. S., E. N. Janoff, K. E. Schwebke, C. J. Shanholtzer, and K. E. Willard.** 1998. Ambiguity in the identification of *Streptococcus pneumoniae*. Optochin, bile solubility, quellung and the AccuProbe DNA probe test. *Am. J. Clin. Pathol.* **109:**55–61.

82. **Nelms, L. F., D. A. Odelson, T. R. Whitehead, and R. B. Hespell.** 1995. Differentiation of ruminal and human *Streptococcus bovis* strains by DNA homology and 16S rRNA probes. *Curr. Microbiol.* **31:**294–300.

83. **O'Brien, D. L., M. A. Bronsdon, R. Dagan, P. Yagupsky, J. Janco, J. Elliott, C. G. Whitney, Y. Yang, and G. M. Carlone.** 2001. Evaluation of a medium (STGG) for transport and optimal recovery of *Streptococcus pneumoniae* from nasopharyngeal secretions collected during field studies. *J. Clin. Microbiol.* **39:**1021–1024.

84. **Park, C. H., N. M. Vandel, D. K. Ruprai, E. A. Martin, K. M. Gates, and D. Coker.** 2001. Detection of group B streptococcal colonization in pregnant women using direct

85. **Peled, N., and P. Yagupsky.** 1999. Improved detection of *Streptococcus pneumoniae* in middle-ear fluid cultures by use of a gentamicin-containing medium. *J. Clin. Microbiol.* **37:**3415–3416.

86. **Potgieter, E., M. Carmichael, H. J. Koornhof, and L. J. Chalkley.** 1992. In vitro antimicrobial susceptibility of viridans streptococci isolated from blood cultures. *Eur. J. Clin. Microbiol. Infect. Dis.* **11:**543–546.

87. **Poyart, C., C. Pierre, G. Quesne, B. Pron, P. Berche, and P. Trieu-Cuot.** 1997. Emergence of vancomycin resistance in the genus *Streptococcus*: characterization of a *vanB* transferable determinant in *Streptococcus bovis*. *Antimicrob. Agents Chemother.* **41:**24–29.

88. **Purdy, R. A., B. Cassidy, and T. J. Marrie.** 1990. *Streptococcus bovis* meningitis: report of 2 cases. *Neurology* **40:**1782–1784.

89. **Raymond, J., C. Sauvestre, M. Bergeret, F. Lewin, C. Francoual, J. Chavinie, and J. LePerq.** 1997. Group B streptococcus: rapid intrapartum detection and influence of density of maternal colonization on vertical transmission. *Clin. Microbiol. Infect.* **3:**507–509.

90. **Rosa-Fraile, M., J. Rodriguez-Granger, M. Cueto-Lopez, A. Sampedro, E. B. Gaye, J. M. Haro, and A. Andreu.** 1999. Use of Granada medium to detect group B streptococcal colonization in pregnant women. *J. Clin. Microbiol.* **37:**2674–2677.

91. **Rudney, J. D., and C. J. Larson.** 1993. Species identification of the oral streptococci by restriction fragment polymorphism analysis of rRNA genes. *J. Clin. Microbiol.* **31:**2467–2473.

92. **Ruoff, K. L., M. J. Ferraro, J. Holden, and L. J. Kunz.** 1984. Identification of *Streptococcus bovis* and *Streptococcus salivarius* in the clinical laboratory. *J. Clin. Microbiol.* **20:**223–226.

93. **Ruoff, K. L., S. I. Miller, C. V. Garner, M. J. Ferraro, and S. B. Calderwood.** 1989. Bacteremia with *Streptococcus bovis* and *Streptococcus salivarius*: clinical correlates of more accurate identification of isolates. *J. Clin. Microbiol.* **27:**305–308.

94. **Sahm, D. F., M. E. Jones, M. L. Hickey, D. R. Diakun, S. V. Mani, and C. Thornsberry.** 2000. Resistance surveillance of *Streptococcus pneumoniae*, *Haemophilus influenzae* and *Moraxella catarrhalis* isolated in Asia and Europe, 1997–98. *J. Antimicrob. Chemother.* **45:**457–466.

95. **Schleifer, K. H., and R. Kilpper-Balz.** 1987. Molecular and chemotaxonomic approaches to the classification of streptococci, enterococci and lactococci: a review. *Syst. Appl. Microbiol.* **10:**1–19.

96. **Schuchat, A.** 1999. Group B streptococcus. *Lancet* **353:**51–56.

97. **Sherman, J. M.** 1937. The streptococci. *Bacteriol. Rev.* **1:**3–97.

98. **Smith, R. F., and N. P. Willett.** 1968. Rapid plate method for screening hyaluronidase and chondroitin sulfatase-producing microorganisms. *Appl. Microbiol.* **16:**1434–1436.

99. **Stevens, D. L.** 1995. Streptococcal toxic-shock syndrome: spectrum of disease, pathogenesis, and new concepts in treatment. *Emerg. Infect. Dis.* **3:**69–78.

100. **Tambyah, P. A., G. Kumarasinghe, H. L. Chan, and K. O. Lee.** 1997. *Streptococcus suis* infection complicated by purpura fulminans and rhabdomyolysis: case report and review. *Clin. Infect. Dis.* **24:**710–712.

101. **Tarradas, C., A. Arenas, A. Maldonado, I. Luque, A. Miranda, and A. Perea.** 1994. Identification of *Streptococcus suis* isolated from swine: proposal for biochemical parameters. *J. Clin. Microbiol.* **32:**578–580.

102. **Thomas, J. G.** 1994. Routine CSF antigen detection for agents associated with bacterial meningitis: another point of view. *Clin. Microbiol. Newsl.* **16:**89–95.

103. **Thompson, T., and R. R. Facklam.** 1997. Cross-reactions of reagents from streptococcal grouping kits with *Streptococcus porcinus. J. Clin. Microbiol.* **35:**1885–1886.

104. **Thorvilson, J., P. Kohner, N. Henry, and F. Cockerill.** 1997. Comparison of agar dilution, broth dilution, disk diffusion, and the E-test for susceptibility testing of penicillin-susceptible and penicillin-resistant *Streptococcus pneumoniae. Eur. J. Clin. Microbiol. Infect. Dis.* **16:**391–394.

105. **Tracy, M., A. Wanahita, Y. Shuhatovich, E. A. Goldsmith, J. E. Clarridge III, and D. M. Musher.** 2001. Antibiotic susceptibilities of genetically characterized *Streptococcus milleri* group strains. *Antimicrob. Agents. Chemother.* **45:**1511–1514.

106. **Truong, T. L., C. Menard, C. Mouton, and L. Trahan.** 2000. Identification of mutans and other oral streptococci by random amplified polymorphic DNA analysis. *J. Med. Microbiol.* **49:**63–71.

107. **Trüper, H. G., and L. De' Clari.** 1997. Taxonomic note: necessary correction of specific epithets formed as substantives (nouns) "in apposition." *Int. J. Syst. Bacteriol.* **47:**908–909.

108. **Trüper, H. G., and L. De' Clari.** 1998. Taxonomic note: erratum and correction of further specific epithets formed as substantives (nouns) "in apposition." *Int. J. Syst. Bacteriol.* **48:**615.

109. **Turner, J. C., A. Fox, K. Fox, C. Addy, C. Z. Garrison, B. Herron, C. Brunson, and G. Betcher.** 1993. Role of group C beta-hemolytic streptococci in pharyngitis: epidemiologic study of clinical features associated with isolation of group C streptococci. *J. Clin. Microbiol.* **31:**808–811.

110. **Vandamme, P., B. Pot, E. Falsen, K. Kersters, and L. A. DeVries.** 1996. Taxonomic study of Lancefield streptococcal groups C, G, and L (*Streptococcus dysgalactiae*) and proposal of S. *dysgalactiae* subsp. *equisimilis* subsp. nov. *Int. J. Syst. Bacteriol.* **46:**774–781.

111. **Vandamme, P., U. Torck, E. Falsen, B. Pot, H. Goossens, and K. Kersters.** 1998. Whole-cell protein electrophoretic analysis of viridans streptococci: evidence for heterogeneity among *Streptococcus mitis* biovars. *Int. J. Syst. Bacteriol.* **48:**117–125.

112. **Weinstein, M. R., M. Litt, D. A. Kertesz, P. Wyper, D. Rose, M. Coulter, A. McGeer, R. Facklam, C. Ostach, B. M. Willey, A. Borczyk, and D. E. Low.** 1997. Invasive infections due to a fish pathogen, *Streptococcus iniae. N. Engl. J. Med.* **337:**589–594.

113. **Weinstein, M., D. E. Low, A. McGeer, B. Willey, D. Rose, M. Coulter, P. Wyper, A. Borczyk, and M. Lovgren.** 1996. Invasive infection with *Streptococcus iniae*-Ontario, 1995–1996. *Morb. Mortal. Wkly. Rep.* **45:** 650–653.

114. **West, P. W. J., H. A. Foster, Q. Electricwala, and A. Alex.** 1996. Comparison of five methods for the determination of arginine hydrolysis by viridans streptococci. *J. Med. Microbiol.* **45:**501–504.

115. **Whiley, R. A., and D. Beighton.** 1991. Emended descriptions and recognition of *Streptococcus constellatus*, *Streptococcus intermedius*, and *Streptococcus anginosus* as distinct species. *Int. J. Syst. Bacteriol.* **41:**1–5.

116. **Whiley, R. A., H. Y. Fraser, C. W. I. Douglas, J. M. Hardie, A. M. Williams, and M. D. Collins.** 1990. *Streptococcus parasanguis* sp. nov., an atypical viridans streptococcus from human clinical specimens. *FEMS Lett.* **68:**115–122.

117. **Whiley, R. A., H. Fraser, J. M. Hardie, and D. Beighton.** 1990. Phenotypic differentiation of *Streptococcus intermedius*, *Streptococcus constellatus* and *Streptococcus anginosus* strains within the "*Streptococcus milleri* groups." *J. Clin. Microbiol.* **28:**1497–1501.

118. **Whiley, R. A., L. M. C. Hall, J. M. Hardie, and D. Beighton.** 1997. Genotypic and phenotypic diversity within *Streptococcus anginosus. Int. J. Syst. Bacteriol.* **47:** 645–650.

119. **Whiley, R. A., L. M. C. Hall, J. M. Hardie, and D. Beighton.** 1999. A study of small colony beta-haemolytic, Lancefield group C streptococci within the anginosus group: description of *Streptococcus constellatus* subsp. *pharyngis* subsp. nov., associated with the human throat and pharyngitis. *Int. J. Syst. Bacteriol.* **49:**1443–1449.

120. **Wilkinson, H. W.** 1977. CAMP-disk test for presumptive identification of group B streptococci. *J. Clin. Microbiol.* **6:**42–45.

121. **Williams-Bouyer, N., B. S. Reisner, and G. L. Woods.** 2000. Comparison of Gen-Probe AccuProbe group B streptococcus culture identification test with conventional culture for the detection of group B streptococci in broth cultures of vaginal-anorectal specimens from pregnant women. *Diagn. Microbiol. Infect. Dis.* **36:**159–162.

122. **Wust, J., G. Hebisch, and K. Peters.** 1993. Evaluation of two enzyme immunoassays for rapid detection of group B streptococci in pregnant women. *Eur. J. Clin. Microbiol. Infect. Dis.* **12:**124–127.

Enterococcus*

LÚCIA MARTINS TEIXEIRA AND RICHARD R. FACKLAM

30

TAXONOMIC ASPECTS

Microorganisms that are now included in the genus *Enterococcus* were mainly related to the "streptococci of fecal origin" or "enterococci." They were considered for a long time to be a major division of the genus *Streptococcus*, differentiated by their higher resistance to chemical and physical agents and accommodating most of the serologic group D streptococci. In the last decades, however, the enterococci have undergone considerable changes in taxonomy, which started with the splitting of the genus *Streptococcus* and the recognition of *Enterococcus* as a separate genus (93). Definite evidence that *Streptococcus faecalis* and *Streptococcus faecium* were sufficiently different from the other members of the genus to merit allocation into a separate genus was provided by studies using molecular approaches (93). The other enterococcal species were then transferred to the new genus, and several new species were described and proposed for inclusion in the genus *Enterococcus* (12–15, 18, 19, 21, 30, 61, 86, 97, 99, 107, 109, 115).

The phylogenetic analysis of genera of catalase-negative gram-positive cocci based on the comparison of the 16S rRNA gene sequences has revealed that *Enterococcus* is more closely related to *Vagococcus*, *Tetragenococcus*, and *Carnobacterium* than to *Streptococcus* and *Lactococcus*, genera with which it has been phenotypically associated (20, 27).

Current criteria for inclusion in the genus *Enterococcus* include a combination of DNA-DNA reassociation values, 16S rRNA gene sequencing, whole-cell protein analysis, and conventional phenotypic tests. While DNA-DNA reassociation is considered the "gold standard" for species definition, 16S rRNA gene sequencing and whole-cell protein analysis correlate very well with this gold standard (65, 76, 101, 102, 107). The long-chain fatty acid composition of enterococcal cells, as revealed by gas-liquid chromatography, is also of taxonomic value and has been used to discriminate species (42, 93, 107). The use of these techniques has shown that some of the proposed species have not been validated as new *Enterococcus* species. *Enterococcus seriolicida* was shown to be homologous to *Lactococcus garvieae* (103). Since *L. garvieae* was named first, it was retained as the species name. *Enterococcus casseliflavus* and *Enterococcus flavescens* were also shown to be related at the species level (101), with *E. casseliflavus* being retained as the species denomination. *Enterococcus solitarius* was shown to be more closely related to the genus *Tetragenococcus* than to any species of *Enterococcus* by 16S rRNA gene sequence analysis (116). Recently, DNA-DNA reassociation studies have demonstrated that *E. solitarius* and *Tetragenococcus halophilus* constitute a single species (L. M. Teixeira, unpublished results).

DESCRIPTION OF THE GENUS

The members of the genus *Enterococcus* are catalase-negative gram-positive cocci that occur singly or arranged in pairs or as short chains. Cells are sometimes coccobacillary when Gram stains are prepared from growth on solid medium, but they tend to be ovoid and in chains when grown in thioglycolate broth. Enterococci are facultative anaerobes that grow at temperatures ranging from 10 to 45°C, with optimum growth at 35°C. They grow in broth containing 6.5% NaCl, and they hydrolyze esculin in the presence of 40% bile salts (bile-esculin [BE] medium). Some species are motile. Most enterococci, apart from *E. cecorum*, *E. columbae*, *E. pallens*, and *E. saccharolyticus*, hydrolyze L-pyrrolidonyl-β-naphthylamide (PYR) by producing pyrrolidonyl arylamidase (pyrrolidonase [PYRase]); all strains hydrolyze leucine-β-naphthylamide by producing leucine aminopeptidase (LAPase). Enterococci are not able to synthesize porphyrins and therefore do not produce cytochrome enzymes (20, 43). However, a pseudocatalase is sometimes produced when strains of *E. faecalis* are grown on blood-containing media, and a weak effervescence is observed in the catalase test. Nearly all strains are fermentative, gas is not produced, and lactic acid is the end product of glucose fermentation. Most strains produce a cell wall-associated glycerol teichoic acid that is identified as Lancefield's serologic group D antigen. The G+C content of the DNA ranges from 37 to 45 mol% (93).

The other genera of catalase-negative gram-positive cocci and the characteristics that distinguish them from the enterococci are discussed in chapters 29 and 31. Accurate presumptive identification of a catalase-negative gram-pos-

* This chapter contains information presented in chapter 18 by Richard R. Facklam, Daniel F. Sahm, and Lúcia Martins Teixeira in the seventh edition of this Manual.

itive coccus as an *Enterococcus* can be accomplished by demonstrating that the unknown strain is positive in the BE, PYR, and LAP tests and grows in the presence of 6.5% NaCl and at 45°C. Because strains of *Lactococcus, Leuconostoc, Pediococcus,* and *Vagococcus* with phenotypic similarities have been isolated from human infections (29, 100), the presumptive identification of enterococci based only on the BE reaction and growth in 6.5% NaCl broth can be erroneous. Demonstrating the presence of group D antigen by serologic reaction may be helpful in the identification, although antigen is detected in only about 80% of the enterococcal strains. On the other hand, pediococci and leuconostocs (29), as well as some vagococcal strains (100), can also react with anti-group D serum. Reactivity with the AccuProbe *Enterococcus* genetic probe manufactured by GenProbe, Inc. (San Diego, Calif.), can also be used to confirm an unknown strain as *Enterococcus.* Strains of all known *Enterococcus* species, except the type strains of *E. cecorum, E. columbae, E. pallens,* and *E. saccharolyticus* react with this probe. However, *Vagococcus* strains also react (100).

NATURAL HABITATS

Several intrinsic characteristics of the enterococci allow them to grow and survive in harsh environments and to persist almost everywhere. Enterococci are widespread in nature and can be found in soil, water, food, plants, and in animals, including mammals, birds, and insects (5, 20). In humans, as in other animals, they are predominantly inhabitants of the gastrointestinal tract and are less common in other sites, such as in the genitourinary tract and the oral cavity. The prevalence of the different enterococcal species appears to vary according to the host and is also influenced by age, diet, and other factors that may be related to changes in physiologic conditions, such as underlying diseases and prior antimicrobial therapy (20). *E. faecalis* is one of the most common bacteria isolated from the human gastrointestinal tract. It is likely that *E. faecium, E. casseliflavus,* and *E. gallinarum* are also found in variable proportions in the human gastrointestinal tract (20, 25, 44, 95). The available limited information on the distribution of distinct enterococcal species in other sources indicates that there are differences from the distribution in humans (20, 94). Several aspects of the ecology of the enterococci merit further evaluation, especially in the light of the changing classification and taxonomic approaches of the genus.

CLINICAL SIGNIFICANCE

The enterococci are commensal microorganisms that act as opportunistic pathogens, particularly in elderly patients with serious underlying diseases and in other immunocompromised patients who have been hospitalized for prolonged periods, use invasive devices, and/or have received broad-spectrum antimicrobial therapy. Several potential virulence factors have been identified in enterococci, as reviewed recently (24, 40, 43, 47, 68, 95), but none has been established as having a major contribution to virulence in humans. Although the enterococci can be a cause of infections in humans in the community and in the hospital, these microorganisms began to be recognized with increasing frequency as common causes of hospital-acquired infections in the late 1970s, paralleling the increasing resistance to most currently used antimicrobial agents. As a result,

enterococci have emerged as one of the leading therapeutic challenges when associated with serious or life-threatening infections. This trend is likely to continue as the overall population ages and more people become at risk for infection (63). The ubiquitous presence of enterococci, however, requires caution in establishing the clinical significance of a particular isolate. This is especially important regarding in vitro susceptibility testing decisions (see "Susceptibility to Antimicrobial Agents" below).

The variety of infections in which enterococci are involved has been thoroughly reviewed and summarized (40, 69, 95). Although the spectrum of infections has remained relatively unchanged since the extensive review by Murray in 1990 (69), the prevalence of these organisms as nosocomial pathogens is clearly increasing. Enterococci have become the second most common agent recovered from nosocomial urinary tract infections (UTIs) and wound infections and the third leading cause of nosocomial bacteremia in the United States (40, 66, 69, 92). UTIs are the most common of the enterococcal infections: enterococci have been implicated in approximately 10% of all UTIs (31) and in 16% of nosocomial UTIs (92). Enterococcal bacteriuria usually occurs in patients with underlying structural abnormalities and/or in those who have undergone urologic manipulations (66). Intra-abdominal and pelvic infections are the next most commonly encountered infections. However, cultures from patients with peritonitis, intra-abdominal or pelvic abscesses, biliary tract infections, surgical site infections, and endomyometritis are frequently polymicrobial, and the role of enterococci in this setting remains controversial. Enterococci have been considered an important cause of endocarditis since early descriptions and are estimated to account for about 20% of the cases of native-valve bacterial endocarditis and for about 6 to 7% of prosthetic-valve endocarditis (40, 63). Whereas endocarditis is a serious enterococcal infection, it is less common than bacteremia. Enterococcal infections of the respiratory tract or the central nervous system, as well as otitis, sinusitis, septic arthritis, and endophthalmitis, may occur but are rare (40, 69, 95). There is evidence for a role in dental infections (96). The significance of isolates from some of these sites should be carefully evaluated before any clinical decisions are made.

E. faecalis is usually the most frequent enterococcal species recovered from human clinical specimens, representing 80 to 90% of the isolates, followed by *E. faecium,* which is found in 5 to 10% of enterococcal infections (7, 28, 36, 94). In one recent report, the ratio of *E. faecalis* to *E. faecium* from clinical specimens was 4:1 (43). The other enterococcal species are identified less frequently. However, clusters of infections with *E. casseliflavus* (73) and *E. raffinosus* (112) have been reported. Although less frequently or even rarely, several of the other enterococcal species, including *E. avium, E. cecorum, E. dispar, E. durans, E. gallinarum, E. gilvus, E. hirae, E. mundtii, E. pallens,* and *E. faecalis* variant strains, have also been isolated from human sources (15, 28, 36, 42, 94, 107). *E. columbae, E. haemoperoxidans, E. malodoratus, E. moraviensis, E. porcinus, E. pseudoavium, E. ratti, E. saccharolyticus,* and *E. sulfureus* have not been isolated from human sources.

COLLECTION, TRANSPORT, AND STORAGE OF SPECIMENS

The standard methods of collecting blood, urine, wound secretions, and other secretions or swab specimens are adequate (see chapters 6 and 20). No special methods or procedures are usually necessary for transporting clinical specimens containing enterococci. Transport can be performed on almost any transport media or on swabs that are kept dry. Like most clinical samples, the material should be cultured as soon as possible, preferably within 1 h.

Enterococcal strains can be stored indefinitely when lyophilized. In our experience, cultures frozen at −70°C or below can be stored for several years as heavy cell suspensions made directly in defibrinated sheep or rabbit blood or in a (10%) skim milk solution containing 10% glycerol. Most strains of enterococci survive several months at 4°C on ordinary agar slants.

ISOLATION PROCEDURES

Trypticase soy–5% sheep blood agar, brain heart infusion–5% sheep blood agar, or any blood agar base containing 5% animal blood supports the growth of enterococci. Some strains of E. faecalis are beta-hemolytic on agar bases containing rabbit, horse, or human blood but non-beta-hemolytic on the same base media containing sheep blood. Some strains of E. durans are beta-hemolytic regardless of the type of blood used. The other species are usually alpha-hemolytic or nonhemolytic. Enterococci grow at 35 to 37°C and do not require an atmosphere containing increased levels of CO_2, although some strains grow better in this atmosphere. If the sample to be cultured is likely to contain gram-negative bacteria, BE azide, Pfizer selective enterococcus, and some other commercially prepared media containing azide are excellent primary isolation media. The use of selective media for the isolation of enterococci has been previously reviewed (20, 26, 87). Since then, several new media have been described, including those containing chromogenic substrates for the isolation and presumptive identification of enterococci from urine (64) and the cephalexin-aztreonam-arabinose agar for the isolation of E. faecium from heavily contaminated sites (33).

The increasing incidence of vancomycin resistance among the enterococci has raised the importance of selective isolation of vancomycin-resistant enterococci (VRE). Early identification of VRE is necessary for controlling the spread of these organisms (41). Several different selective agar and/or broth media have been used for the isolation of VRE from sources containing normal flora, such as stool samples and rectal swabs (44, 53, 89, 90). Although there is no single generally accepted screening method at this point, the use of a selective-enrichment broth to enhance the recovery of VRE seems the most effective procedure. Enterococcosel broth (a BE azide medium supplied by Becton Dickinson Microbiology Systems, Cockeysville, Md.) has been used in a number of studies as the base medium supplemented with different concentrations of vancomycin, with 6 μg/ml being the most common concentration. In some of these studies, vancomycin and other antimicrobials, such as aztreonam and clindamycin, have been used in the enrichment broth as well as in the subculture medium. It would be prudent, however, to use a nonselective agar as well for subculturing from a selective-enrichment broth, since some strains may be inhibited to the point of very poor or no growth. Satake et al. (90) have evaluated several selective media for the isolation of VRE from fecal specimens before and after broth enrichment. They found that culturing with Enterococcosel agar containing 6 μg of vancomycin/ml after enrichment in supplemented Colum-

bia colistin-nalidixic acid broth at 35°C was the most sensitive method.

In some circumstances, it may be necessary to recover VRE from environmental surfaces for epidemiologic studies. The organisms are isolated from these surfaces by swabbing the surfaces with premoistened swabs and placing them either into an enrichment broth or onto agar plates. Alternatively the Rodac imprint method may be used by applying the agar surface directly to the environmental surface to be cultured (38).

Because a laboratory report of VRE can initiate a cascade of infection control events that are time-consuming and costly (9, 41), laboratories must be certain of the epidemiologic importance of any suspected VRE isolate. The transferable and high-level VanA and VanB resistance associated with E. faecalis and E. faecium is the intended focus of infection control efforts. In contrast, the intrinsic low level VanC resistance, which is not transferable and is not associated with wide dissemination of resistant strains, is much less likely to be of importance to the surveillance efforts of infection control personnel (9, 43, 89, 90). Therefore, while the use of sensitive methods for isolating VRE from surveillance specimens is important, the need for establishing protocols to rapidly determine the likely underlying mechanism of resistance associated with the different genetic determinants (e.g., vanA, vanB, and vanC [see chapter 68]) is equally important (46, 89, 90).

IDENTIFICATION OF ENTEROCOCCUS SPECIES

Identification by Conventional Physiological Testing

Once it is established that an unknown catalase-negative gram-positive coccus is a member of Enterococcus or a closely related genus (Lactococcus or Vagococcus), the conventional tests (see reference 29 and chapters 29 and 31 for methods) listed in Table 1 can be used to identify the species. It should be pointed out that most of the information presented here is related to the phenotypic characteristics of strains isolated from humans. Strains isolated from nonhuman sources may be different. Enterococcal species are separated into five physiological groups based on acid formation from mannitol and sorbose and on hydrolysis of arginine (Table 1). The species of each group are then identified according to additional testing. The grouping is based on key phenotypic tests that can be performed in any diagnostic laboratory. Identification of enterococcal species by conventional tests is not rapid and may require incubation for up to 10 days. However, most identifications can be made after 2 days of incubation.

Group I consists of E. avium, E. malodoratus, E. pseudoavium, E. raffinosus, E. saccharolyticus, E. gilvus, and E. pallens. These species form acid from mannitol and sorbose but do not hydrolyze arginine. They are differentiated by reactions in arabinose and raffinose tests, the capacity to utilize pyruvate, and whether or not the strains are pigmented (Table 1). Production of acid from methyl-α-D-glucopyranoside (MGP) also helps to differentiate some of these species from each other.

Group II comprises E. faecalis, E. faecium, E. casseliflavus, E. gallinarum, and E. mundtii. These species form acid from mannitol and hydrolyze arginine but fail to form acid from sorbose. Atypical strains fail to hydrolyze arginine or form acid from mannitol. Lactococcus sp. is also listed in this

TABLE 1 Phenotypic characteristics used for the identification of *Enterococcus* species and some physiologically related species of other gram-positive cocci

Species	MAN	SOR	ARG	ARA	SBL	RAF	TEL	MOT	PIG	SUC	PYU	MGP
Group I												
E. avium	+	+	−	+	+	−	−	−	−	+	+	V
E. gilvus	+	+	−	−	+	+	−	−	+	+	+	−
E. malodoratus	+	+	−	−	+	+	−	−	−	+	+	V
E. pallens	+	+	−	−	+	+	−	−	+	+	−	+
E. pseudoavium	+	+	−	−	+	−	−	−	−	+	+	+
E. raffinosus	+	+	−	+	+	+	−	−	−	+	+	V
E. saccharolyticus[b]	+	+	−	−	+	+	−	−	−	+	−	+
Group II												
E. faecalis	+[d]	−	+[d]	−	+	−	+	−	−	+[d]	+	−
Lactococcus sp.	+	−	+	−	−	−	−	−	−	V	−	−
E. faecium	+[d]	−	+	+	V	V	−	−	−	+[d]	−	−
E. casseliflavus	+	−	+[d]	+	V	+	−[d]	+[d]	+[d]	+	V	+
E. gallinarum	+	−	+[d]	+	−	+	−	+[d]	−	+	−	+
E. mundtii	+	−	+	+	V	+	−	−	+	+	−	+
Group III												
E. dispar	−	−	+	−	−	+	−	−	−	+	+	+
E. durans	−	−	+	−	−	−	−	−	−	−	−	−
E. hirae	−	−	+	−	−	+	−	−	−	+	−	−
E. porcinus[c]	−	−	+	−	−	−	−	−	−	−	−	−
E. ratti	−	−	+	−	−	−	−	−	−	−	−	−
Group IV												
E. asini[b]	−	−	−	−	−	−	−	−	−	+	−	−
E. cecorum[b]	−	−	−	−	+	+	−	−	−	+	+	−
E. sulfureus	−	−	−	−	−	+	−	−	+	+	−	+
Group V												
E. columbae[b]	+	−	−	+	+	+	−	−	−	+	+	−
Vagococcus sp.	+	−	−	−	+	−	−	+	−	+	−	+

[a] Abbreviations and symbols: MAN, mannitol; SOR, sorbose; ARG, arginine; ARA, arabinose; SBL, sorbitol; RAF, raffinose; TEL, 0.04% tellurite; MOT, motility; PIG, pigment; SUC, sucrose; PYU, pyruvate; MGP, methyl-α-D-glucopyranoside; +, 90% or more of the strains are positive; −, 10% or less of the strains are positive; V, variable (11 to 89% of the strains are positive).
[b] Phenotypic characteristics based on data from type strains.
[c] The phenotypic characteristics of *E. porcinus* are identical to those of *E. villorum*. These two recently described species correspond to a single taxon.
[d] Occasional exceptions occur (<3% of strains show aberrant reactions).

group because the phenotypic characteristics of some strains can lead to misidentification as an *Enterococcus*. If nonmotile variants of *E. casseliflavus* and *E. gallinarum* are encountered, production of acid from MGP can be used to help in the identification of these species. *E. casseliflavus* and *E. gallinarum* form acid from MGP, while *E. faecium* and *E. mundtii* do not. In all likelihood, the mannitol-positive strains of *E. haemoperoxidus*, a recently described species (97), will also fall into group II.

Group III enterococci hydrolyze arginine but do not form acid from mannitol or sorbose. This group consists of *E. dispar*, *E. durans*, *E. hirae*, and two new species, *E. ratti* and *E. villorum* (*E. porcinus*) (99, 109). Phenotypic characteristics of *E. porcinus* are identical to those of *E. villorum*, and there is evidence that they constitute a single species. Two independent groups of investigators examined the taxonomy of these strains and named the species differently. The new species in this group are difficult to identify and differentiate from *E. durans*. *E. durans*, *E. porcinus*, and *E. ratti* have very similar phenotypic profiles

in the tests listed in Table 1. They can be differentiated by reactions in litmus milk, hydrolysis of hippurate, and acid formation from trehalose and xylose. *E. durans* forms acid and clots litmus milk, *E. porcinus* forms acid but no clot, and *E. ratti* does not form acid or clot. *E. durans* hydrolyzes hippurate, while *E. porcinus* does not. *E. ratti* is variable in the hippurate hydrolysis test. *E. durans* forms acid from trehalose but not from xylose, *E. porcinus* forms acid from both trehalose and xylose, and *E. ratti* does not form acid from either trehalose or xylose. The other members of this group are easily identified by the reactions in the pyruvate, arabinose, raffinose, and sucrose tests. Uncommon mannitol-negative variant strains of *E. faecalis* and *E. faecium* resemble species in this group. However, *E. faecalis* strains are positive in the pyruvate test but do not form acid from arabinose, raffinose, or sucrose, and *E. faecium* variant strains form acid from arabinose. If the results of conventional tests compare to the results of testing with the API system originally reported (97), the mannitol-negative strains of *E. haemoperoxidus*, a recently described species, will be grouped with the enterococci in group III. In addition, it appears that the mannitol-negative strains of *E. haemoperoxidus*, although similar to *E. dispar*, can be differentiated from the other group III enterococci.

Group IV is composed of three species (*E. asini*, *E. cecorum*, and *E. sulfureus*) that do not form acid from mannitol or sorbose and fail to hydrolyze arginine. These three species can be differentiated by acid formation from raffinose and sorbitol and by the pigmentation test (Table 1). *E. sulfureus* is the only member of this group to form acid from MGP.

Group V consists of *E. columbae* and *Vagococcus*. Variant strains of *E. casseliflavus*, *E. gallinarum*, and *E. faecalis* that fail to hydrolyze arginine resemble the microorganisms included in this group. However, these variant strains have characteristics similar to the strains that hydrolyze arginine and can be differentiated by these same phenotypic tests. *Vagococcus* spp. are listed here because the phenotypic characteristics of *V. fluvialis* are very similar to those of the genus *Enterococcus* and some strains may be identified as enterococci (100, 101). It appears that *E. moraviensis*, another newly described species, will fall into group V enterococci; if the results of conventional tests are similar to those of the API testing originally reported (97), *E. moraviensis* will be easily differentiated from the other group V enterococci.

Since 1995, we have tested more than 400 strains of enterococci for species identification, and at this time we have not been able to identify 4 strains to the species level. Since many of the strains we are asked to identify are atypical, we expect that 99% of the strains can be identified to the species level by conventional phenotypic tests in a routine clinical laboratory.

Identification by Commercial Systems or by Molecular Methods

There are several commercially available miniaturized, manual, semiautomated, and automated identification systems for the identification of *Enterococcus* species. Since their introduction, these systems have been updated to improve their performance characteristics and expand their identification capabilities as investigators have become more aware of inaccuracies (16, 34, 39, 112). In general, these systems are reliable for the identification of *E. faecalis* and, to a lesser extent, *E. faecium*. Accurate identification of other species by most systems depends on additional testing, although improvements have been observed with updated formats and data banks. Commercial systems now available for the identification of enterococcal species include the API 20S and API Rapid ID32 STREP systems (bioMérieux, Hazelwood, Mo.), the Crystal Gram-Positive and Crystal Rapid Gram-Positive identification systems (Becton Dickinson Microbiology Systems), the Gram Positive Identification Card of the Vitek system (bioMérieux), and the Gram-Positive Identification panel of the MicroScan Walk/Away system (Dade MicroScan, West Sacramento, Calif.). The accuracy of identification by some of these systems in comparison to identification by molecular techniques was recently reported (1). In general, approximately 80% of all enterococcal isolates will be accurately identified by any one of these systems; however, the accuracy will be dependent on the distribution of species found in each specific setting. Identification of unusual species by a commercial system should be confirmed by a reference method before being reported.

Molecular methods such as DNA-DNA hybridization and sequencing of the 16S rRNA genes have been used primarily for taxonomic purposes in special laboratories. In the past 10 years, however, the application of molecular techniques for the identification of *Enterococcus* species has expanded dramatically. The range of molecular procedures proposed for the identification of enterococcal species was recently reviewed and summarized (27). They include analysis of whole-cell protein (WCP) profiles by sodium dodecyl sulfate-polyacrylamide gel electrophoresis; vibrational spectroscopic analysis; proton magnetic resonance spectroscopic analysis; randomly amplified polymorphic DNA (RAPD) analysis; sequencing analysis of the 16S rRNA gene; fragment length polymorphism analysis of amplified 16S rDNA; broad-range PCR amplification of the 16S rDNA; sequencing of domain V of the 23S rRNA gene; amplification of the tRNA or the rRNA intergenic spacers or of the D-Ala:D-Ala ligases (*ddl*) and the vancomycin resistance (*van*) genes; sequencing of the *ddl* genes or of the manganese-dependent superoxide dismutase (*sodA*$_{int}$) gene; sequencing and hybridization of the chaperonin 60 (*cpn*60) gene; amplification and probing of the *Enterococcus* protein A (*efaA*) gene or of the *E. faecalis* adhesin for collagen (*ace*) gene; and amplification of the elongation factor EF-Tu (*tuf*) gene or the pEM1225 gene.

Among the molecular techniques proposed to identify the enterococcal species, sodium dodecyl sulfate-polyacrylamide gel electrophoresis analysis of WCP profiles is the only one that has been extensively evaluated and is recommended for general use. This method was shown to be reliable for the differentiation and identification of typical and atypical *Enterococcus* strains, since WCP profiles are species specific (65, 101, 102). Apart from minor qualitative and/or quantitative differences among strains, each of the known enterococcal species corresponds to a unique WCP profile. WCP profiles of related species of *Lactococcus* and *Vagococcus* are also unique and different from those of the enterococci (100–103). Table 1, depicting the phenotypic characteristics of the *Enterococcus* species in this chapter, is based on correlations between the WCP profiles and the phenotypic tests, sometimes in conjunction with DNA-DNA reassociation experiments. The introduction of the use of computer programs to aid in the analysis and interpretation of the gel images is contributing to a broader application of this technique. Sequencing of the 16S RNA gene has been performed for all species of enterococci, and the sequences are available via GenBank for comparison purposes. We would urge caution in the use of this technique because the criteria for sequence differences have not been followed. Some species differ by only 2 or 3 bases over the 1,400-base span of the gene. Among the other molecular methods, only a few have been performed in more than one laboratory or have been evaluated for the majority of *Enterococcus* species. Some do not appear to be practical for routine use in clinical laboratories. On the other hand, some of these recently developed molecular procedures deserve consideration for expanded testing and future improvement.

TYPING METHODS

The increasing documentation of *Enterococcus* as a leading nosocomial pathogen, as well as the evidence supporting the concept of exogenous acquisition of enterococcal infections, has generated an additional need for typing the isolates as a means of assisting infection control and for performing epidemiologic studies. Therefore, the investigation of nosocomial outbreaks, along with the dissemination of enterococcal strains harboring antimicrobial resistance markers, is of major interest, particularly in the light of the increasing occurrence of VRE. Early epidemiologic investigations of enterococcal infections were based on phenotypic characteristics and have been hampered by the lack of simple, highly reproducible, and sufficiently discriminatory typing systems. Classic phenotypic methods used to investigate the diversity among isolates of a given enterococcal species have frequently failed to adequately discriminate among strains, and they have limited value in epidemiologic studies. However, the use of phenotypic typing methods in association with more recent molecular techniques can contribute valuable information (51, 67, 114).

The introduction of various molecular techniques has substantially improved our ability to discriminate among enterococcal isolates and has provided critical insights into epidemiologic aspects of enterococcal infections. As a result of the use of more discriminatory typing methods, it has been possible to demonstrate that strains can be exogenously acquired by direct and indirect contact among patients (57, 78, 114, 117, 118). Intrahospital transmission and interhospital spread have also been documented for antimicrobial-resistant enterococci (10, 88, 114).

The first molecular techniques developed for typing of enterococci were the analysis of plasmid profiles and the restriction enzyme analysis of genomic DNA by conventional electrophoresis (52, 58, 84, 91). These techniques may be helpful in some instances, but problems have been encountered with their use. A remarkable contribution to our ability to discriminate among enterococcal strains was the use of techniques involving the analysis of chromosomal DNA restriction endonuclease profiles by pulsed-field gel electrophoresis (PFGE) by either field inversion gel electrophoresis (37) or, ideally, counter-clamped homogeneous electric field electrophoresis (35, 37, 71, 78, 80, 81), which is the basis for most of the recent PFGE studies. Multilocus enzyme electrophoresis (8, 106), ribotyping (25, 35, 51, 81, 117), and PCR-based typing methods, such as the RAPD-PCR assay and repetitive-element sequence PCR, have also been used to investigate the genetic relationship among enterococcal strains (3, 17, 45, 60). Sequencing of PCR products and restriction fragment length polymorphism analysis of PCR products have been used to trace and to determine differences among specific resistance genes in enterococci; they therefore represent additional tools for typing resistant strains (22, 50, 56, 77, 113).

Results from a number of investigations indicate that analysis of SmaI restriction digests of genomic DNA by PFGE is widely useful for studying enterococcal species (2, 4, 8, 10, 11, 17, 35, 60, 70, 78, 80, 81, 85, 105, 106), showing definite advantages in strain discrimination. PFGE is currently the single most useful and reliable typing method and is considered the "gold standard" for the epidemiologic analysis of enterococcal infections. However, the need for specialized equipment, as well as the lack of standardized conditions for electrophoresis and criteria for interpreting PFGE banding profiles, still limits a more extensive application of the technique, particularly for long-term studies. In addition, comparison of results is often difficult due to the use of different procedures, particularly in relation to electrophoresis parameters. The development of standardized protocols as a result of collaborative studies is needed to allow interlaboratory comparison in future investigations. Several protocols for performing PFGE analysis of enterococcal strains have been published. Most of the information accumulated over the last years is related to *E. faecium* (4, 67, 74, 81, 83, 85, 113) and *E. faecalis* (2, 59, 83, 105). Although PFGE has been more discriminatory than other methods, epidemiologic interpretation of PFGE profiles is not always clear-cut. The occurrence of genetic events can be associated with substantial changes in the PFGE profiles, leading to problems in clonality assessment (50, 67, 91). The more appropriate interpretation in such cases remains a controversial issue, since it may be difficult to define which level of polymorphism is acceptable. In consequence, there is no single definitive typing technique for enterococci: however, a strong match of the results of several typing techniques, particularly those based on different genomic polymorphism, can be used as indicative of high relatedness. The use of PFGE in conjunction with at least an additional typing technique or independent PFGE analysis using different restriction enzymes is highly recommended to help in clarifying the epidemiologic interpretation. General principles proposed for the interpretation of molecular typing data, based on fragment differences (104), are usually applied to interpret PFGE profiles obtained for enterococcal strains. The use of well-characterized control strains along with the unknown isolates being tested is recommended. Two reference strains, *E. faecalis* OG1RF (SS 1351) and *E. faecium* GE1 (SS 1350), have been proposed (104).

SUSCEPTIBILITY TO ANTIMICROBIAL AGENTS AND EVALUATION, INTERPRETATION, AND REPORTING OF RESULTS

Resistance to several commonly used antimicrobial agents is a remarkable characteristic of most of the enterococcal species. Moreover, most of this information is based on studies with *E. faecalis* and *E. faecium*, the two species most frequently associated with human infections. Antimicrobial resistance can be classified as either intrinsic or acquired. Intrinsic resistance is related to inherent or natural chromosomally encoded characteristics present in all or most of the enterococci. Furthermore, certain specific mechanisms of intrinsic resistance to some antimicrobial agents are typically associated with a particular enterococcal species or group of species. In contrast, the occurrence of acquired resistance is more variable, resulting from either mutation in existing DNA or acquisition of new genetic determinants found in plasmids or transposons (43, 54, 69, 70, 95). Enterococcal intrinsic resistance involves two major groups of antimicrobial therapeutic drugs: the aminoglycosides and the β-lactams. Because of the poor activity of several antimicrobial agents against enterococci as a result of intrinsic resistance, the recommended therapy for serious infections (i.e., endocarditis, meningitis, and other systemic infections, especially in immunocompromised patients) includes a combination of a cell wall-active agent, such as a β-lactam (usually penicillin) or vancomycin, combined with an aminoglycoside (usually gentamicin or streptomycin) (43, 69, 70, 95). These combinations overcome the intrinsic resistance exhibited by the enterococci, and a synergistic bactericidal effect is generally achieved.

In addition to the intrinsic resistance traits, enterococci have acquired different genetic determinants that confer resistance to several classes of antimicrobials, including chloramphenicol, tetracyclines, macrolides, lincosamides and streptogramins, aminoglycosides, β-lactams, glycopeptides, and, more recently, quinolones. Over the last decades, the occurrence of acquired antimicrobial resistance among enterococci, especially high-level resistance (HLR) to aminoglycosides and β-lactams and resistance to glycopeptides (especially vancomycin), has been increasingly reported. Isolates that are resistant to the cell wall-active agent or have HLR to aminoglycosides are resistant to the synergistic effects of combination therapy and constitute an even more serious problem for the effective management of enterococcal infections. Therefore, detection of resistance to these groups of antimicrobial agents is important. Enterococcal isolates exhibiting HLR to one or more aminoglycosides have been described with increasing frequency (2, 43, 54, 69, 70, 94, 95) and now make up large proportions of isolates in several geographic areas. Strains expressing acquired HLR to aminoglycosides are frequently associated with aminoglycoside MICs of >2,000 μg/ml and cannot be detected by diffusion tests with conventional disks. Special tests using high-content gentamicin and streptomycin disks, as well as a single-dilution method, were developed to screen for this type of resistance (98) (see chapter 74). Strains exhibiting high-level resistance to penicillin and ampicillin as a result of containing altered penicillin-binding proteins have also disseminated widely in the last several years (6, 43, 69, 70, 95), and strains producing β-lactamase have been identified (36, 69).

The emergence of vancomycin resistance as a therapeutic problem in enterococcal strains was first documented in Western Europe and in the United States (48, 55, 108). Since then, the isolation of VRE has been continuously reported in diverse locations (9, 43, 70). VRE strains have been classified into phenotypes and genotypes. Six types of glycopeptide resistance have already been described among enterococci. Three of them are the most common: the VanA phenotype, associated with inducible high-level resistance to vancomycin as well as to teicoplanin, encoded by the *vanA* gene; the VanB phenotype, associated with variable (moderate to high) levels of inducible resistance to vancomycin only, encoded by the *vanB* gene; and the VanC phenotype, associated with noninducible low-level resistance to vancomycin. The VanA and VanB phenotypes are considered the most clinically relevant and are usually associated with *E. faecium* and *E. faecalis* strains, while VanC-mediated resistance is an intrinsic characteristic of *E. gallinarum* (*vanC1* genotype) and *E. casseliflavus* (*vanC2* and *vanC3* genotypes) strains (9, 11, 43, 70). The remaining three types of enterococcal glycopeptide resistance seem to occur rarely and are encoded by genetic determinants that were recently recognized, *vanD* (74, 79), *vanE* (32), and *vanG* (62).

The diversity and, in some cases, species specificity of emerging antimicrobial resistance traits among enterococcal isolates created an additional need for accurate identification at the species level and for in vitro evaluation of susceptibility to antimicrobial agents. The significance of a particular enterococcal isolate is a major factor in determining when antimicrobial testing should be done. Once the need to test a particular isolate has been established, selection of the appropriate antimicrobial agents for testing must be considered on the basis of the site of infection. Testing of antimicrobials to which enterococci are intrinsically resistant is contraindicated. The drugs that should not be tested for include aminoglycosides at standard concentrations, aztreonam, cephalosporins, clindamycin, methicillin (or oxacillin), and trimethoprim-sulfamethox-

azole; they may appear active against enterococci in vitro but are not effective clinically, and isolates should not be reported as susceptible. Due to difficulties with some phenotypic methods for detection of HLR to aminoglycosides and resistance to vancomycin, updated guidelines for the selection of antimicrobial agents should be followed for routine testing and reporting. Standards for performance and interpretative criteria for susceptibility testing of enterococci have been published by the National Committee for Clinical Laboratory Standards (72) and are discussed in detail in chapter 70.

As already mentioned, susceptibility testing for resistance to synergy should be done with any enterococcal isolate implicated in infections for which combination therapy is indicated, e.g., those associated with systemic infections. Enterococci are also frequently encountered in polymicrobial infections associated with the gastrointestinal tract or superficial wounds of hospitalized patients. Their pathogenic significance in such settings is uncertain, but susceptibility testing is warranted when predominant or heavy growth is observed (66). Testing of enterococcal isolates from UTIs from the lower urinary tract is optional, since these infections usually respond to therapy with ampicillin. However, many hospital infection control programs require routine testing as a means of surveillance for VRE. For instances when testing a urinary tract isolate is appropriate, ciprofloxacin, levofloxacin, nitrofurantoin, norfloxacin, or tetracycline could be selected, in addition to ampicillin (43, 95). In cases of treatment failure, testing is always warranted.

Although β-lactams other than penicillin or ampicillin (e.g., mezlocillin, piperacillin, azlocillin, amoxicillin-clavulanate, ampicillin-sulbactam, and imipenem) do not offer any significant advantages over ampicillin when they are used against enterococci, they may be of interest for use against polymicrobial infections involving enterococci and gram-negative bacilli. Ampicillin testing, along with a test for β-lactamase production, can be used to predict resistance to these other β-lactam antibiotics. Testing these other drugs is rarely necessary. A positive test for β-lactamase production (see chapter 74) indicates resistance to ampicillin and the acylureidopenicillins (i.e., azlocillin, mezlocillin, or piperacillin). Resistance to ampicillin revealed by disk diffusion or dilution methods indicates penicillin-binding protein-mediated resistance to these agents, as well as to β-lactam–β-lactamase inhibitor combinations and imipenem (69, 72, 95, 110).

While in vitro methods for detecting vancomycin resistance are discussed in detail in chapter 74, some aspects of VanC-containing species (i.e., *E. gallinarum* and *E. casseliflavus*) need to be emphasized. Resistance usually associated with *vanC* genotypes is not detected by disk diffusion, but VanC strains usually grow on vancomycin agar screen tests. Because the clinical significance of the VanC resistance is still uncertain, the implications of these two in vitro testing issues for patient management are uncertain. However, the need to differentiate VanA or VanB strains from VanC strains is quite evident for therapeutic, infection control, and surveillance reasons. Because growth on vancomycin agar screen fails to help make this important distinction, species identification is necessary. VanC resistance has yet to be described in *E. faecalis* or *E. faecium*, so growth of either of these species on the screening agar is likely to be due to VanA or VanB resistance. Although rare, the occurrence of the other kinds of vancomycin resistance may also be considered. Additionally, VanA resistance together with VanC resistance has been described in *E. gallinarum*, so identification of an organism to a species that usually harbors only VanC resistance does not completely rule out the presence of higher-level vancomycin resistance. In this regard, determining vancomycin MICs is useful since VanC resistance frequently results in MICs of <16 μg/ml whereas VanA and VanB resistances usually result in MICs of >32 μg/ml. Resistance to other agents such as ampicillin and aminoglycosides also is uncommon among VanC isolates. Because of limited alternatives, chloramphenicol, erythromycin, tetracycline (or doxycycline or minocycline), and rifampin may be tested for use against VRE. Testing of quinupristin-dalfopristin or linezolide, antimicrobials recently licensed for clinical use, is recommended for use against vancomycin-resistant *E. faecium*.

Of importance is that while enterococci as a group are often discussed in terms of the multiple drug resistance they can express, two of the most problematic resistance profiles, ampicillin and vancomycin resistance, are associated with *E. faecium* far more commonly than with other species (9, 68, 70). This is important in terms of resistance surveillance. Because ampicillin resistance and vancomycin resistance in *E. faecalis* are relatively uncommon compared to that in *E. faecium*, widespread emergence and dissemination of these resistances in *E. faecalis* would significantly add to the current problem of multiply resistant enterococci. Therefore, enterococcal species identification is important for the purposes of therapy and meaningful surveillance.

Molecular methods (see chapter 75) have been used to detect specific antimicrobial drug resistance genes (11, 23, 25, 46, 49, 74, 75, 77, 82, 89, 90, 98, 111) and have substantially contributed to our understanding of the spread of acquired enterococcal resistance, especially resistance to vancomycin. However, because of their high specificity, molecular methods will not detect antimicrobial resistance due to a mechanism that is not included in the testing and will not detect resistance due to emerging resistance mechanisms.

REFERENCES

1. **Angeletti, S., G. Lorino, G. Gherardi, F. Battistoni, M. D. Cesaris, and G. Dicuonzo.** 2001. Routine molecular identification of enterococci by gene-specific PCR and 16S ribosomal DNA sequencing. *J. Clin. Microbiol.* **39:** 794–797.
2. **Antalek, M. D., J. M. Mylotte, A. J. Lesse, and J. A. Sellick, Jr.** 1995. Clinical and molecular epidemiology of *Enterococcus faecalis* bacteremia, with special reference to strains with high-level resistance to gentamicin. *Clin. Infect. Dis.* **20:**103–109.
3. **Barbier, N., P. Sauinier, E. Chachaty, S. Dumontier, and A. Andremont.** 1996. Random amplified polymorphic DNA typing versus pulsed-field gel electrophoresis for epidemiologic typing of vancomycin-resistant enterococci. *J. Clin. Microbiol.* **34:**1096–1099.
4. **Bischoff, W. E., T. M. Reynolds, G. O. Hall, R. P. Wenzel, and M. B. Edmond.** 1999. Molecular epidemiology of vancomycin-resistant *Enterococcus faecium* in a large urban hospital over a 5-year period. *J. Clin. Microbiol.* **37:**3912–3916.
5. **Blaimont, B., J. Charlier, and G. Wauters.** 1995. Comparative distribution of *Enterococcus* species in faeces and clinical samples. *Microb. Ecol. Health Dis.* **8:**87–92.
6. **Boyce, J. M., S. M. Opal, G. Potter-Bynoe, R. G. La-Forge, M. J. Zervos, G. Furtado, G. Victor, and A. A. Medeiros.** 1992. Emergence and nosocomial transmission of ampicillin-resistant enterococci. *Antimicrob. Agents Chemother.* **36:**1032–1039.
7. **Buschelman, B. J., M. J. Bale, and R. N. Jones.** 1993. Species identification and determination of high-level aminoglycoside resistance among enterococci. Comparison study of sterile body fluid isolates, 1985–1991. *Diagn. Microbiol. Infect. Dis.* **16:**119–122.
8. **Carvalho, M. G. S., M. C. E. Vianni, J. A. Elliott, M. Reeves, R. R. Facklam, and L. M. Teixeira.** 1997. Molecular analysis of *Lactococcus garvieae* and *Enterococcus gallinarum* isolated from water buffalos with subclinical mastitis. *Adv. Exp. Med. Biol.* **418:**401–404.
9. **Cetinkaya, Y., P. Falk, and C. G. Mayhall.** 2000. Vancomycin-resistant enterococci. *Clin. Microbiol. Rev.* **13:** 686–707.
10. **Chow, J. W., A. Kuritza, D. M. Shlaes, M. Green, D. F. Sahm, and M. J. Zervos.** 1993. Clonal spread of vancomycin-resistant *Enterococcus faecium* between patients in three hospitals in two states. *J. Clin. Microbiol.* **31:**1609–1611.
11. **Clark, N. C., L. M. Teixeira, R. R. Facklam, and F. C. Tenover.** 1998. Detection and differentiation of the *vanC-1, vanC-2,* and *vanC-3* glycopeptide resistance genes in enterococci. *J. Clin. Microbiol.* **36:**2294–2297.
12. **Collins, M. D., R. R. Facklam, J. A. E. Farrow, and R. Williamson.** 1989. *Enterococcus raffinosus* sp. nov., *Enterococcus solitarius* sp. nov. and *Enterococcus pseudoavium* sp. nov. *FEMS. Microbiol. Lett.* **57:**283–288.
13. **Collins, M. D., J. A. E. Farrow, and D. Jones.** 1986. *Enterococcus mundtii* sp. nov. *Int. J. Syst. Bacteriol.* **36:**8–12.
14. **Collins, M. D., D. Jones, J. A. E. Farrow, R. Kilpper-Balz, and K. H. Schleifer.** 1984. *Enterococcus avium* nom. rev., comb. nov.; *E. casseliflavus* nom. rev.; *E. durans* nom. rev., comb. nov.; *E. gallinarum* comb. nov.; and *E. malodoratus* sp. nov. *Int. J. Syst. Bacteriol.* **34:**220–223.
15. **Collins, M. D., U. M. Rodrigues, N. E. Pigott, and R. R. Facklam.** 1991. *Enterococcus dispar* sp. nov., a new *Enterococcus* species from human sources. *Lett. Appl. Microbiol.* **12:**95–98.
16. **d'Azevedo, P. A., C. A. G. Dias, A. L. S. Goncalves, F. Rowe, and L. M. Teixeira.** 2001. Evaluation of an automated system for the identification and antimicrobial susceptibility testing of enterococci. *Diagn. Microbiol. Infect. Dis.* **42:**157–161.
17. **Descheemaeker, P., C. Lammens, B. Pot, P. Vandamme, and H. Goossens.** 1997. Evaluation of arbitrarily primed PCR analysis and pulsed-field gel electrophoresis of large genomic DNA fragments for identification of enterococci important in human medicine. *Int. J. Syst. Bacteriol.* **47:** 555–561.
18. **De Vaux, A., G. Laguerre, C. Divies, and H. Prevost.** 1998. *Enterococcus asini* sp. nov. isolated from the caecum of donkeys (*Equus asinus*). *Int. J. Syst. Bacteriol.* **48:**383–387.
19. **Devriese, L. A., K. Ceyssens, U. M. Rodrigues, and M. D. Collins.** 1990. *Enterococcus columbae*, a species from pigeon intestines. *FEMS Microbiol. Lett.* **71:**247–252.
20. **Devriese, L. A., M. D. Collins, and R. Wirth.** 1992. The genus *Enterococcus*, p. 1465–1481. *In* A. Balows, H. G. Trüper, M. Dworkin, W. Harder, and K. H. Schleifer (ed.), *The Prokaryotes. A Handbook on the Biology of Bacteria: Ecophysiology, Isolation, Identification, Applications,* 2nd ed. Springer-Verlag, New York, N.Y.
21. **Devriese, L. A., G. N. Dutta, J. A. E. Farrow, A. Van de Kerckhove, and B. A. Phillips.** 1983. *Streptococcus ceco-*

rum, a new species isolated from chickens. *Int. J. Syst. Bacteriol.* **33:**772–776.

22. **Donabedian, S., E. Hershberger, L. A. Thal, J. W. Chow, D. B. Clewell, B. Robinson-Dunn, and M. J. Zervos.** 2000. PCR fragment length polymorphism analysis of vancomycin-resistant *Enterococcus faecium. J. Clin. Microbiol.* **38:**2885–2888.

23. **Duh, R.-W., K. V. Singh, K. Malathum, and B. E. Murray.** 2001. *In vitro* activity of 19 antimicrobial agents against enterococci from healthy subjects and hospitalized patients and use of an ace gene probe from *Enterococcus faecalis* for species identification. *Microb. Drug Resist.* **7:**39–46.

24. **Eaton, T. J., and M. J. Gasson.** 2001. Molecular screening of *Enterococcus* virulence determinants and potential for genetic exchange between food and medical isolates. *Appl. Environ. Microbiol.* **67:**1628–1635.

25. **Endtz, H. P., N. van den Braak, A. van Belkum, J. A. J. W. Kluytmans, J. G. M. Koeleman, L. Spanjaard, A. Voss, A. J. L. Weersink, C. M. J. E. Vandenbroucke-Grauls, A. G. M. Buiting, A. van Duin, and H. A. Verbrugh.** 1997. Fecal carriage of vancomycin-resistant enterococci in hospitalized patients and those living in the community in the Netherlands. *J. Clin. Microbiol.* **35:**3026–3031.

26. **Facklam, R. R.** 1976. A review of the microbiological techniques for the isolation and identification of streptococci. *Crit. Rev. Clin. Lab. Sci.* **6:**287–317.

27. **Facklam, R. R., M. D. G. S. Carvalho, and L. M. Teixeira.** 2002. History, taxonomy, biochemical characteristics, and antibiotic susceptibility testing of enterococci, p. 1–54. *In* M. S. Gilmore, D. B. Clewell, P. Courvalin, G. M. Dunny, B. E. Murray, and L. B. Rice (ed.), *The Enterococci: Pathogenesis, Molecular Biology, and Antibiotic Resistance.* ASM Press, Washington, D.C.

28. **Facklam, R. R., and M. D. Collins.** 1989. Identification of *Enterococcus* species isolated from human infections by a conventional test scheme. *J. Clin. Microbiol.* **27:**731–734.

29. **Facklam, R. R., and J. A. Elliott.** 1995. Identification, classification, and clinical relevance of catalase-negative, gram-positive cocci, excluding the streptococci and enterococci. *Clin. Microbiol. Rev.* **8:**479–495.

30. **Farrow, J. A. E., and M. D. Collins.** 1985. *Enterococcus hirae*, a new species that includes amino acid assay strain NCDO 1258 and strains causing growth depression in young chickens. *Int. J. Syst. Bacteriol.* **35:**73–75.

31. **Felmingham, D., A. P. R. Wilson, A. I. Quintana, and R. N. Gruneberg.** 1992. *Enterococcus* species in urinary tract infection. *Clin. Infect. Dis.* **15:**295–301.

32. **Fines, M., B. Perichon, P. Reynolds, D. F. Sahm, and P. Courvalin.** 1999. VanE, a new type of acquired glycopeptide resistance in *Enterococcus faecalis* BM4405. *Antimicrob. Agents Chemother.* **43:**2161–2164.

33. **Ford, M., J. D. Perry, and F. K. Gould.** 1994. Use of cephalexin-aztreonam-arabinose agar for selective isolation of *Enterococcus faecium. J. Clin. Microbiol.* **32:**2999–3001.

34. **Garcia-Garrote, F., E. Cercenado, and E. Bouza.** 2000. Evaluation of a new system, VITEK 2, for identification and antimicrobial susceptibility testing of enterococci. *J. Clin. Microbiol.* **38:**2108–2111.

35. **Gordillo, M. E., K. V. Singh, and B. E. Murray.** 1993. Comparison of ribotyping and pulsed-field gel electrophoresis for subspecies differentiation of strains of *Enterococcus faecalis. J. Clin. Microbiol.* **31:**1570–1574.

36. **Gordon, S., J. S. Swenson, B. C. Hill, N. E. Pigott, R. R. Facklam, R. C. Cooksey, C. Thornsberry, the Enterococcal Study Group, W. R. Jarvis, and F. C. Tenover.** 1992. Antimicrobial susceptibility patterns of common

and unusual species of enterococci causing infections in the United States. *J. Clin. Microbiol.* **30:**2373–2378.

37. **Green, M., K. Barbadora, S. Donabedian, and M. J. Zervos.** 1995. Comparison of field inversion gel electrophoresis with contour-clamped homogeneous electric field electrophoresis as a typing method for *Enterococcus faecium. J. Clin. Microbiol.* **33:**1554–1557.

38. **Hacek, D. M., W. E. Trick, S. M. Collins, G. A. Noskin, and L. R. Peterson.** 2000. Comparison of the Rodac imprint method to selective enrichment broth for recovery of vancomycin-resistant enterococci and drug-resistant *Enterobacteriaceae* from environmental surfaces. *J. Clin. Microbiol.* **38:**4646–4648.

39. **Hamilton-Miller, J. M. T., and S. Shah.** 1999. Identification of clinically isolated vancomycin-resistant enterococci: comparison of API and BBL Crystal systems. *J. Med. Microbiol.* **48:**695–696.

40. **Hancock, L. E., and M. S. Gilmore.** 2000. Pathogenicity of enterococci, p. 251–258. *In* V. A. Fischetti, R. P. Novick, J. J. Ferretti, D. A. Portnoy, and J. I. Rood (ed.), *Gram-Positive Pathogens.* ASM Press, Washington, D.C.

41. **Hospital Infection Control Practices Advisory Committee.** 1995. Recommendations for preventing the spread of vancomycin resistance. *Infect. Control Hosp. Epidemiol.* **16:**105–113.

42. **Hsueh, P. R., L. J. Teng, Y. C. Chen, P. C. Yang, S. W. Ho, and K. T. Luh.** 2000. Recurrent bacteremic peritonitis caused by *Enterococcus cecorum* in patients with liver cirrhosis. *J. Clin. Microbiol.* **38:**2450–2452.

43. **Huycke, M. M., D. F. Sahm, and M. S. Gilmore.** 1998. Multiple-resistant enterococci: the nature of the problem and an agenda for the future. *Emerg. Infect. Dis.* **4:**239–249.

44. **Ieven, M., E. Vercauteren, P. Descheemaeker, F. Van Laer, and H. Goossens.** 1999. Comparison of direct plating and broth enrichment culture for the detection of intestinal colonization by glycopeptide-resistant enterococci among hospitalized patients. *J. Clin. Microbiol.* **37:**1436–1440.

45. **Issack, M. J., E. G. M. Power, and G. L. French.** 1996. Investigation of an outbreak of vancomycin-resistant *Enterococcus faecium* by random amplified polymorphic DNA (RAPD) assay. *J. Hosp. Infect.* **33:**191–200.

46. **Jayaratne, P., and C. Rutherford.** 1999. Detection of clinically relevant genotypes of vancomycin-resistant enterococci in nosocomial surveillance specimens by PCR. *J. Clin. Microbiol.* **37:**2090–2092.

47. **Jett, B. D., M. M. Huycke, and M. S. Gilmore.** 1994. Virulence of enterococci. *Clin. Microbiol. Rev.* **7:**462–478.

48. **Kaplan, A. H., P. H. Gilligan, and R. R. Facklam.** 1988. Recovery of resistant enterococci during vancomycin prophylaxis. *J. Clin. Microbiol.* **26:**1216–1218.

49. **Kariyama, R., R. Mitsuhata, J. W. Chow, D. B. Clewell, and H. Kumon.** 2000. Simple and reliable multiplex PCR assay for surveillance of isolates of vancomycin-resistant enterococci. *J. Clin. Microbiol.* **38:**3092–3095.

50. **Kawalec, M., M. Gniadkowski, and W. Hryniewicz.** 2000. Outbreak of vancomycin-resistant enterococci in a hospital in Gdansk, Poland, due to horizontal transfer of different Tn1546-like transposon variants and clonal spread of several strains. *J. Clin. Microbiol.* **38:**3317–3322.

51. **Kühn, I., L. G. Burman, S. Haeggman, K. Tullus, and B. E. Murray.** 1995. Biochemical fingerprinting compared with ribotyping and pulsed-field gel electrophoresis of DNA for epidemiological typing of enterococci. *J. Clin. Microbiol.* **33:**2812–2817.

52. **Lacoux, P. A., J. Z. Jordens, C. M. Fentin, M. Guiney, and T. H. Pennington.** 1992. Characterization of entero-

coccal isolates by restriction enzyme analysis of genomic DNA. *Epidemiol. Infect.* **109:**69–80.

53. **Landman, D., J. M. Quale, E. Oydna, B. Willey, V. Ditore, M. Zaman, K. Patel, G. Saurina, and W. Huang.** 1996. Comparison of five selective media for identifying fecal carriage of vancomycin-resistant enterococci. *J. Clin. Microbiol.* **34:**751–752.

54. **Leclercq, R.** 1997. Enterococci acquire new kinds of resistance. *Clin. Infect. Dis.* **24:**S80–S84.

55. **Leclercq, R., E. Derlot, J. Duval, and P. Courvalin.** 1988. Plasmid-mediated resistance to vancomycin and teicoplanin in *Enterococcus faecium. N. Engl. J. Med.* **319:** 157–161.

56. **Lee, W. G., J. A. Jernigan, J. K. Rasheed, G. J. Anderson, and F. C. Tenover.** 2001. Possible horizontal transfer of the *vanB2* gene among genetically diverse strains of vancomycin-resistant *Enterococcus faecium* in a Korean hospital. *J. Clin. Microbiol.* **39:**1165–1168.

57. **Livornese, L. L., Jr., S. Dias, C. Samel, B. Romanowski, S. Taylor, P. May, P. Pitsakis, G. Woods, D. Kaye, M. E. Levison, and C. C. Johnson.** 1992. Hospital-acquired infection with vancomycin-resistant *Enterococcus faecium* transmitted by electronic thermometers. *Ann. Intern. Med.* **117:**112–116.

58. **Luginbuhl, L. M., H. A. Rotbart, R. R. Facklam, M. H. Roe, and J. A. Elliott.** 1987. Neonatal enterococcal sepsis: case-control study and description of an outbreak. *Pediatr. Infect. Dis. J.* **6:**1022–1030.

59. **Ma, X., K. Michiaki, A. Takahashi, K. Tanimoto, and Y. Ike.** 1998. Evidence of nosocomial infection in Japan caused by high-level gentamicin-resistant *Enterococcus faecalis* and identification of the pheromone-responsive conjugative plasmid encoding gentamicin resistance. *J. Clin. Microbiol.* **36:**2460–2464.

60. **Malathum, K., K. V. Singh, G. M. Weinstock, and B. E. Murray.** 1998. Repetitive sequence-based PCR versus pulsed-field gel electrophoresis for typing of *Enterococcus faecalis* at the subspecies level. *J. Clin. Microbiol.* **36:**211–215.

61. **Martinez-Murcia, A. J., and M. D. Collins.** 1991. *Enterococcus sulfureus,* a new yellow-pigmented *Enterococcus* species. *FEMS Microbiol. Lett.* **80:**69–74.

62. **McKessar, S. J., A. M. Berry, J. M. Bell, J. D. Turnidge, and J. C. Paton.** 2000. Genetic characterization of *vanG,* a novel vancomycin resistance locus of *Enterococcus faecalis. Antimicrob. Agents Chemother.* **44:**3224–3228.

63. **Megran, D. W.** 1992. Enterococcal endocarditis. *Clin. Infect. Dis.* **15:**63–71.

64. **Merlino, J., S. Siarakas, G. J. Robertson, G. R. Funnel, T. Gottlieb, and R. Bradbury.** 1996. Evaluation of CHROMagar Orientation for differentiation and presumptive identification of gram-negative bacilli and *Enterococcus* species. *J. Clin. Microbiol.* **34:**1788–1793.

65. **Merquior, V. L. C., J. M. Peralta, R. R. Facklam, and L. M. Teixeira.** 1994. Analysis of electrophoretic whole-cell protein profiles as a tool for characterization of *Enterococcus* species. *Curr. Microbiol.* **28:**149–153.

66. **Moellering, R. C., Jr.** 1992. Emergence of *Enterococcus* as a significant pathogen. *Clin. Infect. Dis.* **14:**1173–1178.

67. **Morrison, D., N. Woodford, S. P. Barrett, P. Sisson, and B. D. Cookson.** 1999. DNA banding pattern polymorphism in vancomycin-resistant *Enterococcus faecium* and criteria for defining strains. *J. Clin. Microbiol.* **37:**1084–1091.

68. **Mundy, L. M., D. F. Sahm, and M. Gilmore.** 2000. Relationships between enterococcal virulence and antimicrobial resistance. *Clin. Microbiol. Rev.* **13:**513–522.

69. **Murray, B. E.** 1990. The life and times of the *Enterococcus. Clin. Microbiol. Rev.* **3:**46–65.

70. **Murray, B. E.** 1998. Diversity among multidrug-resistant enterococci. *Emerg. Infect. Dis.* **4:**37–47.

71. **Murray, B. E., K. V. Singh, J. D. Heath, B. R. Sharma, and G. M. Weinstock.** 1990. Comparison of genomic DNAs of different enterococcal isolates using restriction endonucleases with infrequent recognition sites. *J. Clin. Microbiol.* **28:**2059–2063.

72. **National Committee for Clinical Laboratory Standards.** 2001. *Performance Standards for Antimicrobial Susceptibility Testing. Eleventh Informational Supplement.* NCCLS document M100-S11. NCCLS, Wayne, Pa.

73. **Nauschuetz, W. F., S. B. Trevino, L. S. Harrison, R. N. Longfield, L. Fletcher, and W. G. Wortham.** 1993. *Enterococcus casseliflavus* as an agent of nosocomial bloodstream infections. *Med. Microbiol. Lett.* **2:**102–108.

74. **Ostrowsky, B. E., N. C. Clark, C. Thauvin-Eliopoulos, L. Venkataraman, M. H. Samore, F. C. Tenover, G. M. Eliopoulos, R. C. Moellering, Jr., and H. S. Gold.** 1999. A cluster of VanD vancomycin-resistant *Enterococcus faecium*: molecular characterization and clinical epidemiology. *J. Infect. Dis.* **180:**1177–1185.

75. **Papaparaskevas, J., A. Vatopoulos, P. T. Tassios, A. Avlami, N. J. Legakis, and V. Kalapothaki.** 2000. Diversity among high-level aminoglycoside-resistant enterococci. *J. Antimicrob. Chemother.* **45:**277–283.

76. **Patel, R., K. E. Piper, M. S. Rouse, J. M. Steckelberg, J. R. Uhl, P. Kohner, M. K. Hopkins, F. R. Cockerill, and B. C. Kline.** 1998. Determination of 16S rRNA sequences of enterococci and application to species identification of nonmotile *Enterococcus gallinarum* isolates. *J. Clin. Microbiol.* **36:**3399–3407.

77. **Patel, R., J. R. Uhl, P. Kohner, K. K. Hopkins, and F. R. Cockerill III.** 1997. Multiplex PCR detection of *vanA, vanB, vanC-1,* and *vanC-2/3* genes in enterococci. *J. Clin. Microbiol.* **35:**703–707.

78. **Pegues, D. A., C. F. Pegues, P. L. Hibberd, D. S. Ford, and D. C. Hooper.** 1997. Emergence and dissemination of a high vancomycin-resistant *vanA* strains of *Enterococcus faecium* at a large teaching hospital. *J. Clin. Microbiol.* **35:**1565–1570.

79. **Perichon, B., P. Reynolds, and P. Courvalin.** 1997. VanD-type glycopeptide-resistant *Enterococcus faecium* BM4339. *Antimicrob. Agents Chemother.* **41:**2016–2018.

80. **Perlada, D. E., G. A. Smulian, and M. T. Cushion.** 1997. Molecular epidemiology and antibiotic susceptibility of enterococci in Cincinnati, Ohio: a prospective citywide survey. *J. Clin. Microbiol.* **35:**2342–2347.

81. **Plessis, P., T. Lamy, P. Y. Donnio, F. Autuly, I. Grulois, P. Y. Le Prise, and J. L. Avril.** 1995. Epidemiologic analysis of glycopeptide-resistant *Enterococcus* strains in neutropenic patients receiving prolonged vancomycin administration. *Eur. J. Clin. Microbiol. Infect. Dis.* **14:**959–963.

82. **Portillo, A., F. Ruiz-Larrea, M. Zarazaga, A. Alonzo, J. L. Martinez, and C. Torres.** 2000. Macrolide resistance genes in *Enterococcus* spp. *Antimicrob. Agents Chemother.* **44:**967–971.

83. **Privitera, O., A. Agodi, M. Puntorieri, A. Primavera, M. Santagati, A. Privitera, M. L. Mezzatesta, E. Giuffrida, and S. Stefani.** 1995. Molecular epidemiology of enterococci with high-level resistance to aminoglycosides. *Microb. Drug Resist.* **1:**293–297.

84. **Quednau, M., S. Ahrnè, and G. Molin.** 1999. Genomic relationships between *Enterococcus faecium* strains from different sources and with different antibiotic resistance profiles evaluated by restriction endonuclease analysis of total chromosomal DNA using *Eco*RI and *Pvu*II. *Appl. Environ. Microbiol.* **65:**177–180.

85. **Reinert, R. R., G. Conrads, J. J. Schlaeger, G. Werner, W. Witt, R. Lutticken, and I. Klare.** 1999. Survey of antibiotic resistance among enterococci in North Rhine-Westphalia, Germany. *J. Clin. Microbiol.* **37:**1638–1641.

86. **Rodrigues, U., and M. D. Collins.** 1990. Phylogenetic analysis of *Streptococcus saccharolyticus* based on 16S rRNA sequencing. *FEMS Microbiol. Lett.* **71:**231–234.

87. **Sabbaj, J., V. L. Sutter, and S. M. Finegold.** 1971. Comparison of selective media for isolation of presumptive group D streptococci from human feces. *Appl. Microbiol.* **22:**1008–1011.

88. **Sader, H. S., M. A. Pfaller, F. C. Tenover, R. J. Hollis, and R. N. Jones.** 1994. Evaluation and characterization of multiresistant *Enterococcus faecium* from 12 U.S. medical centers. *J. Clin. Microbiol.* **32:**2840–2842.

89. **Sahm, D. F., L. Free, C. Smith, M. Eveland, and L. M. Mundy.** 1997. Rapid characterization schemes for surveillance isolates of vancomycin-resistant enterococci. *J. Clin. Microbiol.* **35:**2026–2030.

90. **Satake, S., N. Clark, D. Rimland, F. S. Nolte, and F. C. Tenover.** 1997. Detection of vancomycin-resistant enterococci in fecal samples by PCR. *J. Clin. Microbiol.* **35:**2325–2330.

91. **Savor, C., M. A. Pfaller, J. A. Kruszynski, R. J. Hollis, G. A. Noskin, and L. R. Peterson.** 1998. Comparison of genomic methods for differentiating strains of *Enterococcus faecium*: assessment using clinical epidemiologic data. *J. Clin. Microbiol.* **36:**3327–3331.

92. **Schaberg, D. R., D. H. Culver, and R. P. Gaynes.** 1991. Major trends in the microbial etiology of nosocomial infection. *Am. J. Med.* **91:**79S–82S.

93. **Schleifer, K. H., and R. Kilpper-Balz.** 1984. Transfer of *Streptococcus faecalis* and *Streptococcus faecium* to the genus *Enterococcus* nom. rev. as *Enterococcus faecalis* comb. nov. and *Enterococcus faecium* comb. nov. *Int. J. Syst. Bacteriol.* **34:**31–34.

94. **Stern, C. S., M. G. S. Carvalho, and L. M. Teixeira.** 1994. Characterization of enterococci isolated from human and nonhuman sources in Brazil. *Diagn. Microbiol. Infect. Dis.* **20:**61–67.

95. **Strausbaugh, L. J., and M. S. Gilmore.** 2000. Enterococcal infections, p. 280–301. *In* D. L. Stevens and E. L. Kaplan (ed.) *Streptococcal Infections: Clinical Aspects, Microbiology, and Molecular Pathogenesis.* Oxford University Press, Inc., New York, N.Y.

96. **Sundqvist, G., D. Figdor, S. Persson, and U. Sjogren.** 1998. Microbiologic analysis of teeth with failed endodontic treatment and the outcome of conservative retreatment. *Oral Surg. Oral Med. Oral Pathol.* **85:**86–93.

97. **Svec, P., L. A. Devriese, I. Sedlacek, M. Baele, M. Vancanneyt, F. Haesbrouck, J. Swings, and J. Doskar.** 2001. *Enterococcus haemoperoxidus* sp. nov. and *Enterococcus moraviensis* sp. nov., isolated from water. *Int. J. Syst. Evol. Microbiol.* **51:**1567–1574.

98. **Swenson, J. M., M. J. Ferraro, D. F. Sham, N. C. Clark, D. H. Culver, F. C. Tenover, and the National Committee for Clinical Laboratory Standard Working Group on Enterococci.** 1995. Multilaboratory evaluation of screening methods for detection of high-level aminoglycoside resistance in enterococci. *J. Clin. Microbiol.* **33:**3008–3018.

99. **Teixeira, L. M., M. G. S. Carvalho, M. M. B. Espinola, A. G. Steigerwalt, M. P. Douglas, D. J. Brenner, and R. R. Facklam.** 2001. *Enterococcus porcinus* sp. nov. and *Enterococcus ratti* sp. nov. associated with enteric disorders in animals. *Int. J. Syst. Evol. Microbiol.* **51:**1737–1743.

100. **Teixeira, L. M., M. G. S. Carvalho, V. L. Merquior, A. G. Steigerwalt, D. J. Brenner, and R. R. Facklam.** 1997. Phenotypic and genotypic characterization of *Vagococcus fluvialis*, including strains isolated from human sources. *J. Clin. Microbiol.* **35:**2778–2781.

101. **Teixeira, L. M., M. G. S. Carvalho, V. L. Merquior, A. G. Steigerwalt, M. G. M. Teixeira, D. J. Brenner, and R. R. Facklam.** 1997. Recent approaches on the taxonomy of the enterococci and some related microorganisms. *Adv. Exp. Med. Biol.* **418:**397–400.

102. **Teixeira, L. M., R. R. Facklam, A. G. Steigerwalt, N. E. Pigott, V. L. C. Merquior, and D. J. Brenner.** 1995. Correlation between phenotypic characteristics and DNA relatedness with *Enterococcus faecium* strains. *J. Clin. Microbiol.* **33:**1520–1523.

103. **Teixeira, L. M., V. L. C. Merquior, M. C. E. Vianni, M. G. S. Carvalho, S. E. L. Fracalanzza, A. G. Steigerwalt, D. J. Brenner, and R. R. Facklam.** 1996. Phenotypic and genotypic characterization of atypical *Lactococcus garvieae* strains isolated from water buffalos with subclinical mastitis and confirmation of *L. garvieae* as a senior subjective synonym of *Enterococcus seriolicida.* *Int. J. Syst. Bacteriol.* **46:**664–668.

104. **Tenover, F. C., R. D. Arbeit, R. V. Goering, P. A. Mickelsen, B. E. Murray, D. H. Persing, and B. Swaminathan.** 1995. Interpreting chromosomal DNA restriction patterns produced by pulsed-field gel electrophoresis: criteria for bacterial strain typing. *J. Clin. Microbiol.* **33:**2233–2239.

105. **Thal, L. A., J. W. Chow, J. E. Patterson, M. B. Perri, S. Donabedian, D. B. Clewell, and M. J. Zervos.** 1993. Molecular characterization of highly gentamicin-resistant *Enterococcus faecalis* isolates lacking high-level streptomycin resistance. *Antimicrob. Agents Chemother.* **37:**134–137.

106. **Tomayko, J. F., and B. E. Murray.** 1995. Analysis of *Enterococcus faecalis* isolates from intercontinental sources by multilocus enzyme electrophoresis and pulsed-field gel electrophoresis. *J. Clin. Microbiol.* **33:**2903–2907.

107. **Tyrrell, G. J., L. Turnbull, L. M. Teixeira, J. Lefebvre, M. G. S. Carvalho, R. R. Facklam, and M. Lovgren.** 2002. *Enterococcus gilvus* sp. nov. and *Enterococcus pallens* sp. nov. isolated from human clinical specimens. *J. Clin. Microbiol.* **40:**1140–1145.

108. **Uttley, A. H. C., C. H. Collins, J. Naidoo, and R. C. George.** 1988. Vancomycin-resistant enterococci. *Lancet* **i:**57–58.

109. **Vancanneyt, M., C. Snauwaert, I. Cleenwerck, M. Baele, P. Descheemaeker, H. Goossens, B. Pot, P. Vandamme, J. Swings, F. Hasebrouck, and L. A. Devriese.** 2001. *Enterococcus villorum* sp. nov., an enteroadherent bacterium associated with diarrhoea in piglets. *Int. J. Syst. Evol. Microbiol.* **51:**393–400.

110. **Weinstein, M. P.** 2001. Comparative evaluation of penicillin, ampicillin, and imipenem MICs and susceptibility breakpoints for vancomycin-susceptible and vancomycin-resistant *Enterococcus faecalis* and *Enterococcus faecium.* *J. Clin. Microbiol.* **39:**2729–2731.

111. **Werner, G., I. Klare, H. Heier, K. H. Hinz, G. Bohme, M. Wendt, and W. Witte.** 2000. Quinupristin/dalfopristin-resistant enterococci of the *satA* (*vatD*) and *satG* (*vatE*) genotypes from different ecological origins in Germany. *Microb. Drug Resist.* **6:**37–47.

112. **Wilke, W. W., S. A. Marshall, S. L. Coffman, M. A. Pfaller, M. B. Edmund, R. P. Wenzel, and R. N. Jones.** 1997. Vancomycin-resistant *Enterococcus raffinosus*: molecular epidemiology, species identification error, and frequency of occurrence in national resistance surveillance program. *Diagn. Microbiol. Infect. Dis.* **28:**43–49.

113. **Willems, R. J. L., J. Top, N. van den Braak, A. van Belkum, A. van den Bogaard, and J. D. A. van Embden.** 2000. Host specificity of vancomycin-resistant *Enterococcus faecium*. *J. Infect. Dis.* **182:**816–823.

114. **Willey, B. M., A. J. McGree, M. A. Ostrowski, B. N. Kreiswirth, and D. E. Low.** 1994. The use of molecular typing techniques in the epidemiologic investigation of resistant enterococci. *Infect. Control Hosp. Epidemiol.* **15:** 548–556.

115. **Williams, A. M., J. A. E. Farrow, and M. D. Collins.** 1989. Reverse transcriptase sequencing of 16S ribosomal RNA from *Streptococcus cecorum*. *Lett. Appl. Microbiol.* **8:**185–189.

116. **Williams, A. M., U. M. Rodrigues, and M. D. Collins.** 1991. Intrageneric relationships of enterococci as determined by reverse transcriptase sequencing of small-subunit rRNA. *Res. Microbiol.* **142:**67–74.

117. **Woodford, N., D. Morrison, A. P. Johnson, V. Briant, R. C. George, and B. Cookson.** 1993. Application of DNA probes for rRNA and *vanA* genes to investigation of a nosocomial cluster of vancomycin-resistant enterococci. *J. Clin. Microbiol.* **31:**653–658.

118. **Zervos, M. J., S. Dembinski, T. Mikesell, and D. R. Schaberg.** 1986. High-level resistance to gentamicin in *Streptococcus faecalis*: risk factors and evidence for exogenous acquisition of infection. *J. Infect. Dis.* **153:**1075–1083.

Aerococcus, Abiotrophia, and Other Infrequently Isolated Aerobic Catalase-Negative, Gram-Positive Cocci

KATHRYN L. RUOFF

31

TAXONOMY

The bacteria included in this chapter are taxonomically diverse catalase-negative, gram-positive cocci. All, however, share the characteristic of being infrequent clinical isolates found as opportunistic agents of infection in hosts who are usually compromised. Most of these organisms resemble other more-well-known clinical isolates (i.e., streptococci and enterococci) and consequently may be mistaken for members of those genera. These bacteria may have been misidentified or overlooked in clinical cultures in the past or may represent emerging pathogens in compromised patient populations. Table 1 lists the organisms included here along with some of their basic characteristics.

Most organisms discussed in this chapter exhibit fairly low G + C contents (30 to 45 mol%) and are not currently affiliated with taxa above the genus level. Two additional infrequently isolated gram-positive cocci (*Rothia mucilaginosa* and *Alloiococcus*) can display positive catalase reactions. The catalase-variable *Rothia mucilaginosa* (23), formerly called *Stomatococcus mucilaginosus* (55 to 60 mol% G + C), was historically included with staphylococci in the family *Micrococcaceae* (81). The sole species of the catalase-positive genus *Alloiococcus* was originally named *Alloiococcus otitis* (1), but von Graevenitz recommended that it be renamed *Alloiococcus otitidis*, in keeping with the rules of the *Bacteriological Code* (92). The reader is referred to chapter 28 for information on these microorganisms.

The genus *Lactococcus* is composed of organisms formerly classified as Lancefield group N streptococci (82). Motile *Lactococcus*-like organisms with the Lancefield group N antigen (a teichoic acid antigen) have been classified in the genus *Vagococcus* (20, 93). The vagococci also resemble the enterococci, and Facklam and Elliott (43) reported that *Vagococcus* isolates examined at the Centers for Disease Control and Prevention (CDC) gave positive reactions in a commercially available nucleic acid probe test (Gen Probe, San Diego, Calif.) for enterococci.

The genera *Abiotrophia* and *Granulicatella* have been proposed to accommodate organisms previously known as nutritionally variant or satelliting streptococci (28, 57). These bacteria were initially considered to be nutritional mutants of viridans streptococcal strains, most notably of the species *Streptococcus mitis*. The work of Bouvet et al. (11) suggested that these organisms were really members of

two novel streptococcal species given the names *Streptococcus defectivus* and *Streptococcus adjacens*. A comparative analysis of 16S rRNA sequences led Kawamura et al. to propose the creation of a new genus, *Abiotrophia*, containing two species, *Abiotrophia defectiva* and *Abiotrophia adiacens*, to accommodate these bacteria (57). A third species from human sources, *Abiotrophia elegans*, was described in 1998 (78). Kanamoto et al. noted the heterogeneity among *Abiotrophia* strains and described a fourth species, *Abiotrophia para-adiacens* (56). Most recently, Collins and Lawson proposed a new genus, *Granulicatella*, with *Granulicatella adiacens* and *Granulicatella elegans* representing strains formerly called *A. adiacens* and *A. elegans*. *A. defectiva* remains as the sole *Abiotrophia* species (28).

Taxonomic changes among the intrinsically vancomycin-resistant catalase-negative gram-positive cocci include the formation of the new genus *Weissella* to accommodate the former *Leuconostoc paramesenteroides* and related species (32). The vancomycin-susceptible species *Pediococcus halophilus*, formerly included in the otherwise intrinsically vancomycin-resistant *Pediococcus* genus, was reclassified in the genus *Tetragenococcus* (33). Tetragenococci have not, however been isolated from human clinical specimens.

The organism we now know as *Gemella morbillorum* was noted in 1917 by Tunicliff (88), who was searching for the etiologic agent of measles. The organism she isolated from the blood cultures of numerous measles patients was originally named *Diplococcus rubeolae*. This bacterium has also been known as *Diplococcus morbillorum*, *Peptostreptococcus morbillorum*, and *Streptococcus morbillorum*; a proposal to include it in the genus *Gemella* was made in 1988 (59). *Gemella haemolysans* was originally classified as a *Neisseria* species owing to its gram-variable or even gram-negative nature and its cellular morphology (diplococci with flattened adjacent sides). Collins et al. recently described two additional *Gemella* species isolated from human sources, *Gemella bergeriae* (25) and *Gemella sanguinis* (26). The genus *Dolosigranulum* shows phenotypic similarities to *Gemella*, although it is not phylogenetically closely related to *Gemella* strains (3, 63).

Aerococcus urinae, described in 1992, is pyrrolidonyl arylamidase (PYR) negative and leucine aminopeptidase (LAP) positive, showing reactions opposite those of *Aerococcus viridans* in these important identification tests (2). In spite of these phenotypic differences, molecular taxonomic

TABLE 1 Basic phenotypic characteristics of catalase-negative gram-positive cocci[a]

Organism (reference[s])	PYR	LAP	NaCl	BE	ESC	MOT	HIP	SAT	ARG	BGUR	MORPH	VAN
Abiotrophia defectiva (28, 57)	+	+	−	−	−	−	ND	+	−	−	Chains	S
Aerococcus christensenii (27)	−	ND	+	ND	ND	−	+	−	−	−	Clusters	S
Aerococcus sanguicola (66)	+	+	+	+	+	ND	+	−	+	+	Clusters	ND
Aerococcus urinae (17, 18)	−	+	+	−	V	−	+	−	−	+	Clusters	S
Aerococcus urinaehominis (65)	−	−	ND	ND	ND	ND	+	−	−	+	Clusters	ND
Aerococcus viridans[b] (43)	+	−	+	V	ND	−	ND	−	ND	ND	Clusters	S
Dolosicoccus (31)	+	−	−	ND	ND	−	ND	−	ND	ND	Chains	S
Dolosigranulum (3, 63)	+	+	+	ND	+[c]	−	ND	−	ND	−	Clusters	S
Enterococcus[d,e] (43)	+	+	+	+	+	V	ND	−	ND	ND	Chains	S/R
Facklamia languida[f] (63, 64)	+	+	+	ND	−	−	−	−	ND	−	Clusters	S
Facklamia spp.[f] (22, 24, 29, 63)	+	+	+	ND	−	−	+	−	ND	ND	Chains	S
Gemella haemolysans[g] (43)	+	+	−	−	−	−	ND	−	ND	ND	Clusters	S
Gemella spp.[g] (25, 26, 43)	+	+	−	−	ND	−	ND	−	ND	ND	Chains	S
Globicatella (19, 43)	+	−	+	V	ND	−	ND	−	ND	ND	Chains	S
Granulicatella adiacens[h] (28, 57)	+	+	−	−	ND	−	ND	+	−	+	Chains	S
Granulicatella elegans[h] (28, 57)	+	+	−	−	ND	−	ND	+	+	−	Chains	S
Helcococcus[b] (21, 43)	+	−	+	−	ND	−	ND	−	ND	ND	Clusters	S
Ignavigranum (30, 63)	+	+	+	ND	−	−	−	V	ND	ND	Chains	S
Lactococcus[e,i] (43)	V	+	V	+	+	−	ND	−	ND	ND	Chains	S
Leuconostoc (43)	−	−	+	V	ND	−	ND	−	ND	ND	Chains	R
Pediococcus (43)	−	+	V	+	ND	−	ND	−	ND	ND	Clusters	R
Streptococcus[i,j] (43)	V	+	V	V	V	−	ND	−	ND	ND	Chains	S
Tetragenococcus (43)	−	+	+	+	ND	−	ND	ND	ND	ND	Clusters	S
Vagococcus[d] (43)	+	+	V	+	+	+	ND	−	ND	ND	Chains	S

[a] Abbreviations and symbols: PYR, production of pyrrolidonyl arylamidase; LAP, production of leucine aminopeptidase; NaCl, growth in 6.5% NaCl; BE, hydrolysis of esculin in the presence of 40% bile; ESC, hydrolysis of esculin; MOT, motility; HIP, hydrolysis of hippurate; SAT, satelliting behavior; ARG, hydrolysis of arginine; BGUR, production of β-glucuronidase; MORPH, cellular arrangement; VAN, susceptibility to vancomycin. +, ≥90% of strains positive; −, ≤10% of strains positive; V, variable (10 to 90% of strains positive); ND, no data; chains, cells arranged primarily in pairs and chains; clusters, cells arranged primarily in clusters, tetrads, or irregular groups; S, susceptible; R, resistant.

[b] A. viridans prefers an aerobic growth atmosphere and is alpha-hemolytic. The phenotypically similar H. kunzii is facultative and usually nonhemolytic.

[c] LaClaire and Facklam (63) note that strains of Dolosigranulum are esculin hydrolysis positive when tested on conventional media, but the original description of this organism notes a lack of esculin hydrolysis activity (2).

[d] Most enterococcal strains are capable of growth at 45°C, differentiating them from vagococci, which may be phenotypically similar. Strains of vagococci have been reported as testing positive with a commercially available nucleic acid probe for members of the genus Enterococcus.

[e] Phenotypically similar strains of enterococci and lactococci can be differentiated by using a commercially available nucleic acid probe for members of the genus Enterococcus.

[f] F. languida cells are characteristically arranged in pairs and chains, while cells of other Facklamia species are arranged in clusters.

[g] G. haemolysans cells are arranged in pairs and clusters, while the cells of other Gemella species are arranged in pairs and chains.

[h] Formerly classified as members of the genus Abiotrophia.

[i] Most lactococcal strains are capable of growth at 10°C, differentiating them from streptococci, which may be phenotypically similar.

[j] Streptococcus pyogenes and some strains of Streptococcus pneumoniae are PYR positive.

studies suggest that *A. urinae* should remain in the *Aerococcus* genus. Organisms currently included in the *A. urinae* species are fairly heterogeneous and can probably be subdivided into at least two subspecies (18). *Aerococcus christensenii*, isolated from the human genitourinary tract, was described by Collins et al. in 1999 (27) and has been recently joined by the new species *Aerococcus sanguicola* (66) and *Aerococcus urinaehominis* (65).

Three recently described catalase-negative genera (*Facklamia*, *Ignavigranum*, and *Dolosicoccus*) are related to but distinct from *Globicatella sanguinis*, an organism initially named *Globicatella sanguis*, which was described in 1992 (19). *Facklamia* currently contains four species isolated from human sources: *Facklamia hominis* (22), *Facklamia sourekii* (24), *Facklamia ignava* (29), and *Facklamia languida* (64). The genus *Ignavigranum*, currently consisting of a single species, *Ignavigranum ruoffiae*, was recently described by Collins et al. (30), along with the genus *Dolosicoccus* and its single species *Dolosicoccus paucivorans* (31).

The examination of gram-positive cocci by molecular taxonomic methods has encouraged the delineation of these new groups of organisms and the refinement of a genetically based taxonomy for the catalase-negative gram-positive cocci.

DESCRIPTION OF THE GENERA

The organisms included in this chapter form gram-positive coccoid cells, but *G. haemolysans* may appear gram variable or gram negative due to the ease with which its cells are decolorized. Cell shape and arrangement can aid in dividing these organisms into two broad groups: those with a "streptococcus-like" Gram stain (coccobacilli in pairs and chains) and those with a "staphylococcus-like" Gram stain (more spherical cocci in pairs, tetrads, or clusters). Members of the genera *Abiotrophia* and *Granulicatella* (formerly the nutritionally variant streptococci) form coccobacilli arranged in pairs and chains, but these organisms may also appear pleomorphic, especially when grown under less than optimal nutritional conditions. Dividing these diverse bacteria into two groups based on cellular shape and arrangement serves only as an aid in identification; no relatedness of organisms is implied by this grouping. With the exception of the infrequently isolated vagococci, these organisms are nonmotile.

Most of the genera are catalase-negative facultative anaerobes, but *Aerococcus viridans* is classified as a microaerophile that grows poorly if at all under anaerobic conditions. Some strains of *Aerococcus* exhibit weakly positive catalase reactions due to nonheme catalase activity. None of the genera are beta-hemolytic on routinely employed blood agars, but *G. haemolysans* is described as producing beta-hemolysis on agars supplemented with rabbit or horse blood (76) and some strains of *G. bergeriae* and *G. sanguinis* may exhibit hemolytic reactions on horse blood agar (25, 26).

NATURAL HABITATS

Some of the genera discussed here are members of the normal flora of the oral cavity or upper respiratory tract (*Gemella*, *Abiotrophia*, and *Granulicatella*) or colonize the skin (*Helcococcus*). Foods and vegetation are normal habitats for lactococci, pediococci, and leuconostocs (48, 49); these genera may also be found as members of the normal flora of the alimentary tract, but thorough data supporting this contention are lacking. Aerococci are environmental isolates that can also be found on human skin. Although they have been isolated from human sources, the natural habitats of many of the organisms mentioned here are not well characterized.

CLINICAL SIGNIFICANCE

Although the organisms included in this chapter may be present as contaminants in clinical cultures, they are also isolated infrequently as opportunistic pathogens. These bacteria appear to be of low virulence and are usually pathogenic only in compromised hosts. Infection often occurs in previously damaged tissues (e.g., heart valves) or may be nosocomial and associated with prolonged hospitalization, antibiotic treatment, invasive procedures, and the presence of foreign bodies. Specimens likely to yield significant isolates of these bacteria are blood, cerebrospinal fluid, urine, and wounds.

Lactococcus

Difficulties in distinguishing lactococci from either streptococci or enterococci have probably led to the misidentification of clinical *Lactococcus* isolates in the past and may have contributed to the paucity of reports concerning the clinical role of these bacteria. Elliott et al. (38) studied the phenotypic characteristics of a number of lactococcal strains isolated from blood, urinary tract infections, and an eye wound culture. The authors observed that three of the blood culture isolates were from patients diagnosed with prosthetic valve endocarditis. Other reports have noted cases of lactococcal native-valve endocarditis (46, 67, 75), septicemia in an immunosuppressed patient (69), and osteomyelitis (54).

Vagococcus

To date, only a handful of *Vagococcus* isolates from human sources have been reported in the literature. Teixeira et al. (87) described strains isolated from blood, peritoneal fluid, and a wound. Vagococci are motile organisms that, like lactococci, elaborate the Lancefield group N antigen (43). Difficulties encountered in identifying vagococci may par-

tially account for their infrequent recognition in clinical cultures.

Abiotrophia and Granulicatella

Organisms formally known as nutritionally variant streptococci are normal residents of the oral cavity but have been identified as agents of endocarditis involving both native and prosthetic valves. These organisms have also been isolated from ophthalmic infections (70, 72), a brain abscess following neurosurgery (10), and a case of iatrogenic meningitis following myelography (80).

Leuconostoc and Pediococcus

The vancomycin-resistant genera *Leuconostoc* and *Pediococcus* have been recognized in clinical specimens since the mid-1980s. Handwerger et al. (53) noted host defense impairment, invasive procedures breaching the integument, gastrointestinal symptoms, and prior antibiotic treatment as common features among adult patients infected with *Leuconostoc*. They also observed a predisposition to *Leuconostoc* bacteremia among neonates, suggesting that during delivery, infants may become colonized by leuconostocs inhabiting the maternal genital tract. In addition to causing bacteremia, leuconostocs have been isolated from cerebrospinal fluid, peritoneal dialysate fluid, and wounds.

The clinical significance of *Pediococcus* is less well documented. Mastro et al. (68) could find no clearly defined syndrome associated with isolation of *Pediococcus acidilactici* from blood cultures in nine cases they reviewed. They concluded that while this organism may be an opportunist in severely compromised patients, further data were needed to clarify its clinical significance. Later reports described *P. acidilactici* as an agent of septicemia and hepatic abscess (50, 84).

Gemella

G. haemolysans has been isolated as a pathogen in patients with endocarditis (16), meningitis (47), and a total knee arthroplasty (37). *G. morbillorum* has been isolated (when still classified as a streptococcus [see "Taxonomy" above]) from blood, respiratory, genitourinary, wound, and abscess cultures (42). This *Gemella* species has been implicated in cases of empyema and lung abscess (35), septic shock (91), osteomyelitis (90), endocarditis (45), and infection in an arteriovenous shunt (4). The clinical significance of *G. bergeriae* and *G. sanguinis* is not well described, but strains of these species have been isolated from blood cultures and may also function as agents of endocarditis (25, 26).

Dolosigranulum

Little is known about the clinical significance of *Dolosigranulum*, a genus that is phenotypically similar but not closely related to *Gemella* (3). Strains of *D. pigrum*, the sole species in the genus, have been isolated from blood, ocular, and respiratory specimens (61), and this organism has been cited as a probable agent in a case of synovitis (52).

Aerococcus

Although aerococci appear as contaminants in clinical cultures, occasional reports have noted a clinically significant role for these organisms in cases of endocarditis and bacteremia (34, 58, 73). Until the early 1990s, *A. viridans* was the only species isolated from human specimens, but it has been joined more recently by four newly described species. *A. urinae* (2) has been implicated as a urinary tract pathogen in patients predisposed to infection (17) and also as an agent of endocarditis (60, 85). Little is currently known about the clinical significance of *A. christensenii* (isolated from vaginal specimens [27]), *A. urinaehominis* (isolated from urine [65]), and *A. sanguicola* (isolated from blood [66]).

Globicatella

Globicatella sanguinis (originally named *Globicatella sanguis*), the sole species in the genus, has been isolated from cases of bacteremia, urinary tract infection, and meningitis (19).

Facklamia

Members of the recently described *Facklamia* genus are closely related to but phenotypically and phylogenetically distinct from *Globicatella* (22). Strains of the four *Facklamia* species isolated from humans have been recovered from blood, wound, and genitourinary sites (22, 24, 29, 64).

Ignavigranum

Only a few strains of *Ignavigranum ruoffiae*, the sole species in the genus, have been described to date. Sites of isolation include a wound and an ear abscess (30).

Dolosicoccus

The single reported strain of *Dolosicoccus paucivorans*, the only species currently included in the genus, was isolated from a blood culture from an elderly patient with pneumonia (31).

Helcococcus

Helcococcus kunzii, the only species of *Helcococcus* isolated from human sources to date, has been recovered from intact skin of the lower extremities (51), as well as from wound cultures (notably foot ulcers) containing mixtures of bacteria (21). Consequently, the clinical significance of this organism is difficult to interpret, since it may be present merely as a colonizer of the wound site. The ability of this species to function as an opportunist was, however, suggested by its isolation in pure culture from an infected sebaceous cyst (74) and a breast abscess (15).

COLLECTION, TRANSPORT, AND STORAGE OF SPECIMENS

The organisms described in this chapter have all been isolated from routine cultures of clinical specimens, and special requirements for collection and processing of specimens have not been described. Since these bacteria are facultative anaerobes or microaerophiles, aerobic collection, transport, and storage methods as described in chapter 6 should allow their isolation.

ISOLATION PROCEDURES

Generally, there are no special requirements for isolation of the group of bacteria discussed here: general recommendations for the culture of blood, body fluids, and other specimens should be followed (see chapter 6). These organisms are likely to be isolated on rich, nonselective media (e.g., blood or chocolate agar, thioglycolate broth) since they are nutritionally fastidious. If selective isolation of the vancomycin-resistant genera *Leuconostoc* and *Pediococcus* is desired, Thayer-Martin medium may be used to inhibit members of the normal flora or other contaminating microorganisms (79). Some of the genera (e.g., *Helcococcus*)

grow slowly, forming tiny colonies that may not be visible unless extended incubation (48 to 72 h) is employed. The recovery of many of the genera described in this chapter may be enhanced by CO_2 enrichment of the incubation atmosphere.

Members of the genera *Abiotrophia* and *Granulicatella* usually grow on chocolate agar, on brucella agar with 5% horse blood, and in thioglycolate broth, but not on Trypticase soy agar with 5% sheep blood. These organisms can be cultured on nonsupportive media that have been appropriately supplemented (see "*Abiotrophia* and *Granulicatella*" below).

IDENTIFICATION

The suggestions for identification presented in this section reflect currently available information on the infrequently isolated catalase-negative gram-positive cocci that grow aerobically. Additional taxonomic studies and observations on clinical isolates may alter future protocols and introduce additional organisms into the identification schemes presented here. Although Gram stain morphology is prone to subjective interpretation, it has been used as a major decision point in the identification protocols, with two general categories: Gram stain morphology resembling that of streptococci, meaning cocci or coccobacilli in pairs and chains, versus staphylococcal morphology, consisting of coccoid cells arranged in pairs, clusters, or tetrads. Broth-grown cells (thioglycolate broth is suitable) should be used for making morphological determinations. The flow diagrams in this chapter (Fig. 1 and 2) should not be used for definitive identification. In most cases, additional procedures (Table 1) are recommended before identification to the genus level is made. Identifications of unfamiliar organisms from important specimens should be confirmed by a reference laboratory.

Procedures for Initial Differentiation of Genera with Negative Catalase Reactions

Initial testing of catalase-negative isolates with "streptococcal" (Fig. 1) or "staphylococcal" (Fig. 2) Gram stain morphology is represented in the flow diagrams. Note that *Gemella* and *Facklamia* strains may display either type of cellular morphology, depending on species (see "Additional Procedures for Characterization of **Selected** Genera with Negative Catalase Reactions" below). Descriptions of tests for these organisms follow.

Catalase Test

If a positive or weakly positive catalase reaction is observed with growth from blood-containing medium, growth from a medium devoid of blood (e.g., brain heart infusion agar) should be used to repeat the catalase test. A loopful of growth is transferred to a microscope slide or an empty petri dish and observed for the evolution of bubbles after addition of a drop of 3% H_2O_2. It may be necessary to use a hand lens to detect weakly positive reactions.

PYR Test

See "Identification of Beta-Hemolytic Isolates: Physiological Tests" in chapter 29 for a description of the PYR test. Rapid disk tests are commercially available (43).

LAP Test

The LAP test determines the presence of the enzyme leucine aminopeptidase (LAP), also called leucine arylami-

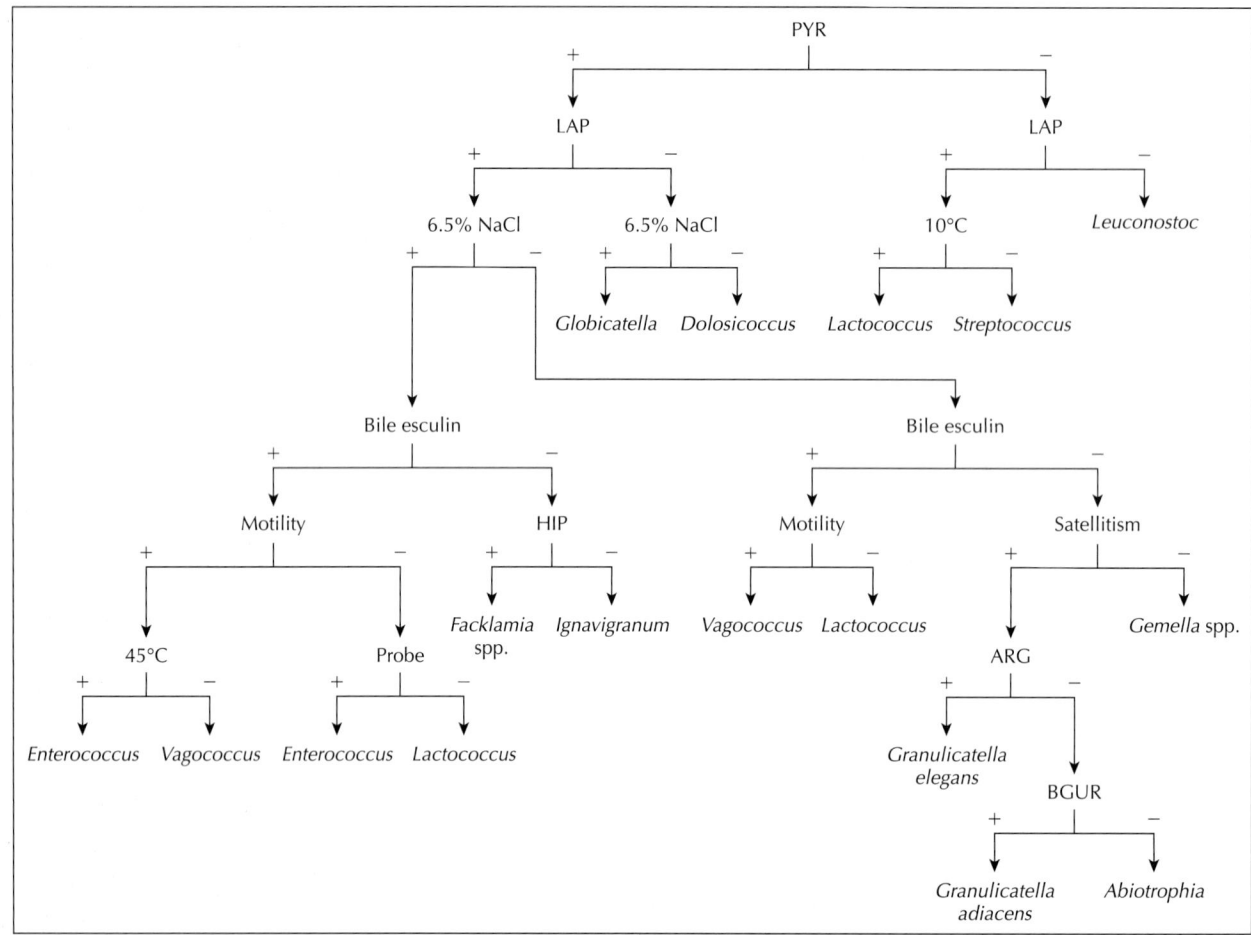

FIGURE 1 Identification of catalase-negative gram-positive cocci that grow aerobically with cells arranged in pairs or chains. Abbreviations: PYR, pyrrolidonyl arylamidase activity; LAP, leucine aminopeptidase activity; 6.5% NaCl, growth in broth containing 6.5% NaCl; Bile esculin, hydrolysis of esculin in the presence of 40% bile; Motility, motility in motility test medium; 45°C, growth at 45°C; 10°C, growth at 10°C; Probe, reaction with commercially available nucleic acid probe for the genus *Enterococcus*; HIP, hydrolysis of hippurate; Satellitism, satelliting growth behavior; ARG, arginine hydrolysis activity; BGUR, β-glucuronidase activity.

dase. An assay for this enzyme is contained in some commercially available identification kits (e.g., API 20Strep [BioMérieux, Hazelwood, Mo.]); alternatively, a rapid disk test for LAP is available commercially (Carr-Scarborough Microbiologicals, Inc., Stone Mountain, Ga.; BD Diagnostic Systems, Sparks, Md.; Remel, Lenexa, Kans.). The manufacturer's instructions should be followed when performing the test (44).

Growth in 6.5% NaCl
Heart infusion broth supplemented with 6.0% NaCl, with or without the acid-base indicator bromcresol purple, may be used for this test. The broth is inoculated with two or three colonies of the organism to be tested and incubated at 35°C for up to 72 h. Turbidity with or without a color change from purple to yellow (due to production of acid) indicates growth (43, 44).

Bile Esculin Test
The ability to hydrolyze esculin in the presence of 40% bile is tested by culturing the test organism on bile esculin agar

in an ambient atmosphere incubator at 35°C for up to 48 h. Blackening of the agar indicates a positive reaction (44).

Motility Test
The motility test is performed by stab-inoculating modified motility test medium and incubating the culture at 30°C (instead of 35°C) for up to 48 h, as described by Facklam and Elliott (43).

Hippurate Hydrolysis Test
Facklam and Elliott recommend a conventional broth medium for determining hippurate hydrolysis (43). This test may also be contained in commercially available identification kits.

Satellitism Test
In a test for satelliting behavior, the strain to be examined is streaked for confluent growth on a medium that fails to support growth or supports only weak growth (e.g., sheep blood agar or brain heart infusion agar). A single cross streak of *Staphylococcus aureus* (ATCC 25923 or another

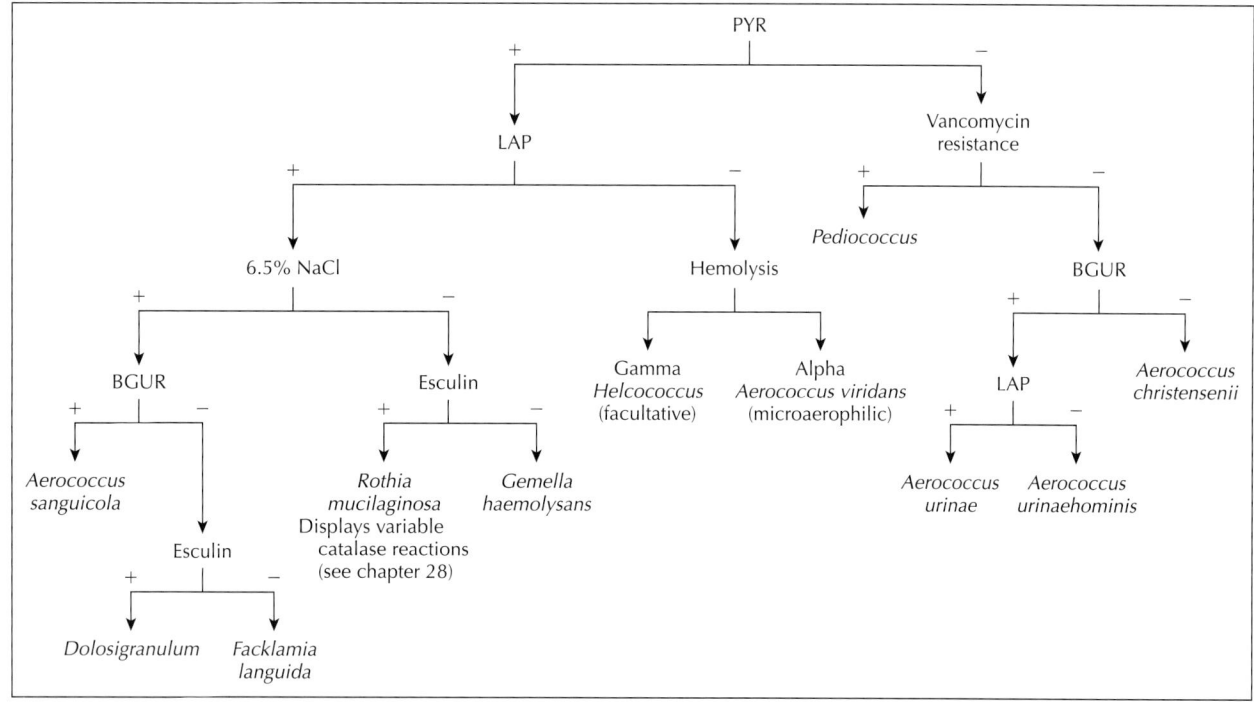

FIGURE 2 Identification of catalase-negative gram-positive cocci that grow aerobically with cells arranged in pairs, tetrads, clusters, or irregular groups. Abbreviations: PYR, pyrrolidonyl arylamidase activity; LAP, leucine aminopeptidase activity; 6.5% NaCl, growth in broth containing 6.5% NaCl; Esculin, hydrolysis of esculin; BGUR, β-glucuronidase activity.

suitable strain) is applied to the inoculated area. After incubation at 35°C in an atmosphere containing an elevated CO_2 concentration, strains of *Abiotrophia* or *Granulicatella* will grow only in the vicinity of the staphylococcal growth. Alternatively, the medium can be supplemented with pyridoxal in the form of an aqueous stock solution of filter-sterilized 0.01% pyridoxal hydrochloride. This solution, which can be stored frozen, should be added to the medium to achieve a final concentration of 0.001%. Disks containing pyridoxal may also be used in the satelliting test and are commercially available (Remel). Some strains of *Ignavigranum* may show satelliting behavior (30).

Arginine Hydrolysis Test

The arginine hydrolysis test can be performed with Moeller's decarboxylase broth containing arginine, as described in "Identification of Viridans Streptococci: Physiological Tests" in chapter 29 (43).

β-Glucuronidase Test

A test for β-glucuronidase is included in a number of commercially available identification products or may be performed using commercially prepared disks.

Vancomycin Susceptibility Test

Several colonies are streaked over half of a plate containing trypticase soy agar with 5% sheep blood. After a 30-μg vancomycin disk is placed in the center of the inoculated area, the plate is incubated overnight in a CO_2-enriched atmosphere at 35°C. Any zone of inhibition indicates susceptibility, while resistant strains exhibit no inhibition zone (43, 44).

Esculin Hydrolysis Test

Esculin agar slants (heart infusion agar containing 0.1% esculin and 0.5% ferric citrate) are used. After inoculation, the slants are incubated at 35°C for up to 7 days. Partial or complete blackening of the agar indicates a positive reaction (43).

Additional Procedures for Characterization of Selected Genera with Negative Catalase Reactions

Lactococcus

Facklam et al. (43, 44) recommended growth temperature tests for distinguishing lactococci from streptococci and enterococci. Consult Fig. 1 for growth temperature characteristics of each genus. Broths (heart infusion broth containing 1% glucose and bromcresol purple indicator) are inoculated with a single colony or drop of broth culture of the test strain and incubated at 35°C for up to 7 days. A water bath is recommended for incubation of cultures at 45°C. Turbidity with or without a change in the broth's indicator to yellow indicates a positive test.

If it is important to rule out enterococci, suspicious isolates can be tested by a commercially available nucleic acid probe test for the genus *Enterococcus*. *Lactococcus lactis* and *Lactococcus garvieae* are the species most commonly isolated from clinical specimens. Further information on the differentiation of *Lactococcus* isolates to the species level may be found elsewhere (38, 40, 82).

Abiotrophia and Granulicatella

Compilations of additional phenotypic traits for *Abiotrophia* and *Granulicatella* species can be found elsewhere (7, 12,

28). Davis and Peel (36) reported that the API 20 Strep system (bioMérieux, Marcy l'Etoile, France) was superior to the rapid ID32 Strep system (bioMérieux) for identification of these organisms. They found that accurate results were obtained when a dense inoculum (confluent growth from two blood agar plates) was used.

Leuconostoc and Pediococcus

Members of the genera *Leuconostoc* and *Pediococcus* produce small alpha-hemolytic or nonhemolytic colonies on blood agar; these colonies can appear similar to those of viridans streptococci. In addition to differing cellular morphologies (Table 1), these vancomycin-resistant genera, along with vancomycin-resistant strains of lactobacilli that form short coccoid cells, may be separated by tests for gas production from glucose and arginine hydrolysis. Leuconostocs produce gas and are always arginine negative. Lactobacilli are variable in both tests, but a positive arginine test in a gas-producing strain would rule out the identity of the organism as a leuconostoc. Pediococci are gas production negative and show variable reactions in the arginine test, although *P. acidilactici* and *P. pentosaceus*, the two species commonly found in clinical material, are arginine positive.

Gas production is measured by inoculating MRS (deMan, Rogosa, and Sharpe) broth (BD Diagnostic Systems; Hardy Diagnostics, Santa Maria, Calif.) with the test organism, sealing the culture with melted petrolatum, and incubating it for up to 7 days at 35°C. Gas production is evidenced by displacement of the petrolatum plug (43, 44). The arginine hydrolysis test can be performed with Moeller's decarboxylase broth containing arginine, as described above. Lancefield group D antigen can be detected in pediococci (44). References 5, 6, 39, 43, 44, and 77 should be consulted for further information on the identification of *Leuconostoc* and *Pediococcus* to the species level.

The organism formerly known as *P. halophilus* was recently reclassified as *Tetragenococcus halophilus* (33). Although this organism shares some phenotypic characteristics with pediococci, it is vancomycin susceptible. Although there are no current reports of clinical isolates of *T. halophilus*, this species should be suspected if vancomycin-susceptible *Pediococcus*-like strains are encountered.

Gemella

Facklam and Washington (44) state that all *Gemella* species are PYR positive but that G. *morbillorum* displays a weakly positive reaction. Earlier studies (8, 9) generally support these data but record some isolates of both G. *haemolysans* and G. *morbillorum* as negative in the PYR test. Facklam and Washington note that a large inoculum must be used when testing these bacteria for the PYR enzyme. LAP is usually absent in isolates of G. *haemolysans* but present in strains of G. *morbillorum* (8, 9). On sheep blood agar media, gemellas form small colonies that are similar in appearance to those of viridans streptococci. Slow growth of some *Gemella* strains may lead to confusion of these organisms with *Abiotrophia* or *Granulicatella* (formerly called nutritionally variant streptococci). A test for satelliting behavior will separate these two groups of bacteria (44).

Cells of G. *haemolysans* are easily decolorized and resemble those of neisserias, since they occur in pairs with the adjacent sides flattened. G. *haemolysans* prefers an aerobic growth atmosphere. G. *morbillorum* cells are gram positive and are arranged in pairs and short chains; individual cells in a given pair may be of unequal sizes. G. *morbillorum* is described as favoring anaerobic growth conditions. Only a

small number of strains of G. *bergeriae* and G. *sanguinis* have been reported to date. Information on the phenotypic characteristics of these *Gemella* species can be found in references 25 and 26.

Aerococcus

In addition to the traits listed in Table 1, *A. viridans* is characterized by displaying weak or no growth when incubated in an anaerobic atmosphere (41). This trait can be tested by incubating duplicate blood agar plate cultures of the organism in question in an anaerobic and an aerobic atmosphere and comparing growth after 24 to 48 h. When grown aerobically, *A. viridans* forms alpha-hemolytic colonies that, depending on the observer, could be confused with those of either viridans streptococci or enterococci. *A. urinae* forms small (0.5 mm in diameter after 24 h of incubation) alpha-hemolytic, convex, shiny, transparent colonies on blood agar media. *A. urinae* is PYR negative and LAP positive, in contrast to *A. viridans* (2). Additional information on the identifying characteristics of *A. urinae* can be found elsewhere (17), and a second biotype (esculin hydrolysis-positive) of this species has been described (18). Information on the phenotypic traits of the recently described species *A. christensenii*, *A. sanguicola*, and *A. urinaehominis* is given in Table 1 (27, 65, 66).

Helcococcus

In addition to the characteristics shown in Table 1, most isolates of the slowly growing *Helcococcus* produce an API 20Strep (BioMéreux, Hazelwood, Mo.) profile of 4100413, corresponding to an identification of "doubtful" *A. viridans*. Colony morphology (tiny gray, usually slightly alpha-hemolytic colonies), good growth under anaerobic conditions, and stimulation of growth by the addition of 1% horse serum or 0.1% Tween 80 to the medium differentiate *H. kunzii* from aerococci (21).

ANTIBIOTIC SUSCEPTIBILITIES

The lack of standardized methods and interpretation criteria for susceptibility testing results, along with relatively small collections of clinical isolates for some of the genera discussed in this chapter, makes it difficult to accurately assess antimicrobial susceptibility patterns. With the exception of *Leuconostoc* and *Pediococcus*, all of the genera display susceptibility to vancomycin. Since many of the bacteria dealt with here are fairly fastidious, investigators have often used blood-supplemented Mueller-Hinton medium and, if necessary for good growth, incubation in a CO_2-enriched atmosphere. Pyridoxal hydrochloride (0.001%) should also be added to blood-supplemented media for testing strains of *Abiotrophia* and *Granulicatella*. Most studies have employed streptococcal (other than *Streptococcus pneumoniae*) interpretative criteria for determining susceptibility. Details of susceptibility testing methods and interpretive criteria referred to above can be found elsewhere (71).

Limited information on the in vitro antimicrobial susceptibility of *Lactococcus lactis* and *Lactococcus garvieae* strains isolated from humans suggests that *L. garvieae* isolates are less susceptible to penicillin and cephalothin than are strains of *L. lactis*. The uniform resistance of *L. garvieae* to clindamycin, in contrast to the uniform susceptibility of the *L. lactis* strains examined by Elliott and Facklam (40), led them to propose a test for clindamycin susceptibility as an aid in differentiation of these two species. In clinical practice, cases of lactococcal endocarditis have been successfully treated with either penicillin alone or penicillin and gentamicin (67, 75).

Teixeira et al. examined a small collection of *Vagococcus* isolates and observed that all strains tested were susceptible to ampicillin, cefotaxime, and trimethoprim-sulfamethoxazole. All strains were resistant to clindamycin, lomefloxacin, and ofloxacin. Variable results were observed with other antimicrobial agents (87).

The vancomycin-resistant genera *Leuconostoc* and *Pediococcus* are also resistant to teicoplanin. Although these organisms are usually susceptible to imipenem, minocycline, chloramphenicol and gentamicin, their penicillin MICs correspond to the moderately susceptible category (86).

Abiotrophia and *Granulicatella* isolates display a range of penicillin MICs, with the majority of strains classified as either susceptible or relatively resistant. There is also variability in susceptibility to aminoglycosides, but no cases of high-level resistance have been reported. A synergistic effect between β-lactam agents and aminoglycosides has been demonstrated for isolates of *Abiotrophia* (55). Tuohy et al. examined a collection of 27 *G. adiacens* and 12 *A. defectiva* strains and noted that all isolates were susceptible to clindamycin, rifampin, levofloxacin, ofloxacin, and quinupristin-dalfopristin (89). These authors noted that the susceptibilities of G. *adiacens* and A. *defectiva*, respectively, to other agents tested were as follows: penicillin, 55 and 8%; amoxicillin, 81 and 92%; ceftriaxone, 63 and 83%; and meropenem, 96 and 100% (89).

A. viridans and *G. haemolysans* appear to be susceptible to penicillin and display a low level of resistance to aminoglycosides (13, 14). Buu-Hoi et al. (13) noted that while A. *viridans* seems to be naturally susceptible to macrolides, tetracyclines, and chloramphenicol, resistance to these agents has been observed. A. *urinae* has been described as susceptible to penicillin, amoxicillin, and nitrofurantoin but resistant to sulfonamides and netilmicin. Isolates display variable susceptibility to trimethoprim and co-trimoxazole (17, 83). Buu-Hoi et al. (14) demonstrated a synergistic effect of penicillin and gentamicin against G. *haemolysans*.

A collection of 27 clinical isolates of *D. pigrum* studied by LaClaire and Facklam (61) all exhibited susceptibility to penicillin, amoxicillin, cefotaxime, cefuroxime, clindamycin, levofloxacin, meropenem, quinupristin-dalfopristin, rifampin, and tetracycline. Variable susceptibility to erythromycin was noted, and 1 of the 27 strains was resistant to trimethoprim-sulfamethoxazole. The small number of *Helcococcus* isolates examined displayed susceptibility to penicillin and clindamycin, and most strains were resistant to erythromycin (15, 74). Strains of *Facklamia* exhibit variable susceptibility to a variety of antibiotics (62).

EVALUATION, INTERPRETATION, AND REPORTING OF RESULTS

Since the gram-positive cocci discussed in this chapter may appear in clinical cultures as contaminants or part of the normal flora, efforts to identify them should be made only when isolates are considered to be clinically significant (i.e., isolated repeatedly, in pure culture, or from normally sterile sites). It should be remembered that these bacteria are opportunists: isolation from an immunocompetent patient may not have the same significance as isolation from a compromised host. Communication with clinicians should

guide the microbiology laboratory in evaluating the significance of these infrequently isolated organisms.

Vancomycin susceptibility testing should be performed routinely on significant isolates. Documenting resistance to this antibiotic will not only guide therapy but also aid in identification of the isolate. The method mentioned in this chapter, using a nonstandardized inoculum, seems to be fairly reliable for determining susceptibility to this drug for identification purposes. Since general standardized susceptibility testing methods do not exist for these infrequently isolated gram-positive cocci, caution should be observed in interpretation of in vitro susceptibility test results. A reference laboratory should be consulted for identification or confirmation of the identity of unfamiliar organisms.

REFERENCES

1. **Aguirre, M., and M. D. Collins.** 1992. Phylogenetic analysis of *Alloiococcus otitis* gen. nov., sp. nov., an organism from human middle ear fluid. *Int. J. Syst. Bacteriol.* **42:** 79–83.
2. **Aguirre, M., and M. D. Collins.** 1992. Phylogenetic analysis of some *Aerococcus*-like organisms from urinary tract infections: description of *Aerococcus urinae* sp. nov. *J. Gen. Microbiol.* **138:**401–405.
3. **Aguirre, M., D. Morrison, B. D. Cookson, F. W. Gay, and M. D. Collins.** 1993. Phenotypic and phylogenetic characterization of some *Gemella*-like organisms from human infections: description of *Dolosigranulum pigrum* gen. nov., sp. nov. *J. Appl. Bacteriol.* **75:**608–612.
4. **Bannatyne, R. M., and I. W. Fong.** 1992. *Gemella morbillorum* infection in an arteriovenous shunt. *Clin. Microbiol. Newsl.* **14:**7–8.
5. **Barreau, C., and G. Wagener.** 1990. Characterization of *Leuconostoc lactis* strains from human sources. *J. Clin. Microbiol.* **28:**1728–1733.
6. **Barros, R. R., M. D. Carvalho, J. M. Peralta, R. R. Facklam, and L. M. Teixeira.** 2001. Phenotypic and genotypic characterization of *Pediococcus* strains isolated from human clinical sources. *J. Clin. Microbiol.* **39:**1241–1246.
7. **Beighton, D., K. A. Homer, A. Bouvet, and A. R. Storey.** 1995. Analysis of enzymatic activities for differentiation of two species of nutritionally variant streptococci, *Streptococcus defectivus* and *Streptococcus adjacens*. *J. Clin. Microbiol.* **33:**1584–1587.
8. **Berger, U.** 1985. Prevalence of *Gemella haemolysans* on the pharyngeal mucosa of man. *Med. Microbiol. Immunol.* **174:**267–274.
9. **Berger, U., and A. Pervanidis.** 1986. Differentiation of *Gemella haemolysans* (Thjotta and Boe 1938) Berger 1960 from *Streptococcus morbillorum* (Prevot 1933) Holdeman and Moore 1974. *Zentbl. Bakteriol. Mikrobiol. Ser. Hyg.* **261:**311–321.
10. **Biermann, C., G. Fries, P. Jehnichen, S. Bhakdi, and M. Husmann.** 1999. Isolation of *Abiotrophia adiacens* from a brain abscess which developed in a patient after neurosurgery. *J. Clin. Microbiol.* **37:**769–771.
11. **Bouvet, A., F. Grimont, and P. A. D. Grimont.** 1989. *Streptococcus defectivus* sp. nov. and *Streptococcus adjacens* sp. nov., nutritionally variant streptococci from human clinical specimens. *Int. J. Syst. Bacteriol.* **39:**290–294.
12. **Bouvet, A., F. Villeroy, F. Cheng, C. Lamesch, R. Williamson, and L. Gutmann.** 1985. Characterization of nutritionally variant streptococci by biochemical tests and penicillin-binding proteins. *J. Clin. Microbiol.* **22:**1030–1034.

13. **Buu-Hoi, A., C. LeBouguenec, and T. Horaud.** 1989. Genetic basis of antibiotic resistance in *Aerococcus viridans. Antimicrob. Agents Chemother.* **33:**529–534.

14. **Buu-Hoi, A., A. Sapoetra, C. Branger, and J. F. Acar.** 1982. Antimicrobial susceptibility of *Gemella haemolysans* isolated from patients with subacute endocarditis. *Eur. J. Clin. Microbiol.* **1:**102–106.

15. **Chagla, A. H., A. A. Borczyk, R. R. Facklam, and M. Lovgren.** 1998. Breast abscess associated with *Helcococcus kunzii. J. Clin. Microbiol.* **36:**2377–2379.

16. **Chatelain, R., J. Croize, P. Rouge, C. Massot, H. Dabernat, J. C. Auvergnat, A. Buu-Hoi, J. P. Stahl, and F. Bimet.** 1982. Isolment de *Gemella haemolysans* dans trois cas d'endocardites bacteriennes. *Med. Mal. Infect.* **12:**25–30.

17. **Christensen, J. J., H. Vibits, J. Ursing, and B. Korner.** 1991. *Aerococcus*-like organism, a newly recognized potential urinary tract pathogen. *J. Clin. Microbiol.* **29:**1049–1053.

18. **Christensen, J. J., A. M. Whitney, L. M. Teixeira, A. G. Steigerwalt, R. R. Facklam, B. Korner, and D. J. Brenner.** 1997. *Aerococcus urinae:* intraspecies genetic and phenotypic relatedness. *Int. J. Syst. Bacteriol.* **47:**28–32.

19. **Collins, M. D., M. Aguirre, R. R. Facklam, J. Shallcross, and A. M. Williams.** 1992. *Globicatella sanguis* gen. nov., sp. nov., a new Gram-positive catalase negative bacterium from human sources. *J. Appl. Bacteriol.* **73:**433–437.

20. **Collins, M. D., C. Ash, J. A. E. Farrow, S. Wallbanks, and A. M. Williams.** 1989. 16S ribosomal ribonucleic acid sequence analyses of lactococci and related taxa. Description of *Vagococcus fluvialis* gen. nov., sp. nov. *J. Appl. Bacteriol.* **67:**453–460.

21. **Collins, M. D., R. R. Facklam, U. M. Rodrigues, and K. L. Ruoff.** 1993. Phylogenetic analysis of some *Aerococcus*-like organisms from clinical sources: description of *Helcococcus kunzii* gen. nov., sp. nov. *Int. J. Syst. Bacteriol.* **43:**425–429.

22. **Collins, M. D., E. Falsen, J. Lemozy, E. Åkervall, B. Sjödén, and P. A. Lawson.** 1997. Phenotypic and phylogenetic characterization of some *Globicatella*-like organisms from human sources: description of *Facklamia hominis* gen. nov., sp. nov. *Int. J. Syst. Bacteriol.* **47:**880–882.

23. **Collins, M. D., R. A. Hutson, V. Baverud, and E. Falsen.** 2000. Characterization of a *Rothia*-like organism from a mouse: description of *Rothia nasimurium* sp. nov. and reclassification of *Stomatococcus mucilaginosus* as *Rothia mucilaginosa* comb. nov. *Int. J. Syst. Evol. Microbiol.* **50:**1247–1251.

24. **Collins, M. D., R. A. Hutson, E. Falsen, and B. Sjoden.** 1999. *Facklamia sourekii* sp. nov., isolated from human sources. *Int. J. Syst. Bacteriol.* **49:**635–638.

25. **Collins, M. D., R. A. Hutson, E. Falsen, B. Sjoden, and R. R. Facklam.** 1998. *Gemella bergeriae* sp. nov., isolated from human clinical specimens. *J. Clin. Microbiol.* **36:**1290–1293.

26. **Collins, M. D., R. A. Hutson, E. Falsen, B. Sjoden, and R. R. Facklam.** 1998. Description of *Gemella sanguinis* sp. nov., isolated from human clinical specimens. *J. Clin. Microbiol.* **36:**3090–3093.

27. **Collins, M. D., M. R. Jovita, R. A. Hutson, M. Ohlen, and E. Falsen.** 1999. *Aerococcus christensenii* sp. nov., from the human vagina. *Int. J. Syst. Bacteriol.* **49:**1125–1128.

28. **Collins, M. D., and P. A. Lawson.** 2000. The genus *Abiotrophia* (Kawamura et al.) is not monophyletic: proposal of *Granulicatella* gen. nov., *Granulicatella adiacens* comb. nov., *Granulicatella elegans* comb. nov. and *Granulicatella balaenopterae* comb. nov. *Int. J. Syst. Evol. Microbiol.* **50:**365–369.

29. **Collins, M. D., P. A. Lawson, R. Monasterio, E. Falsen, B. Sjoden, and R. R. Facklam.** 1998. *Facklamia ignava* sp. nov., isolated from human clinical specimens. *J. Clin. Microbiol.* **36:**2146–2148.

30. **Collins, M. D., P. A. Lawson, R. Monasterio, E. Falsen, B. Sjoden, and R. R. Facklam.** 1999. *Ignavigranum ruoffiae* sp. nov., isolated from human clinical specimens. *Int. J. Syst. Bacteriol.* **49:**97–101.

31. **Collins, M. D., M. Rodriguez Jovita, R. A. Hutson, E. Falsen, B. Sjoden, and R. R. Facklam.** 1999. *Dolosicoccus paucivorans* gen. nov., sp. nov., isolated from human blood. *Int. J. Syst. Bacteriol.* **49:**1439–1442.

32. **Collins, M. D., J. Samelis, J. Metaxopoulos, and S. Wallbanks.** 1993. Taxonomic studies on some leuconostoc-like organisms from fermented sausages: description of a new genus *Weissella* for the *Leuconostoc paramesenteroides* group of species. *J. Appl. Bacteriol.* **75:**595–603.

33. **Collins, M. D., A. M. Williams, and S. Wallbanks.** 1990. The phylogeny of *Aerococcus* and *Pediococcus* as determined by 16S rRNA sequence analysis: description of *Tetragenococcus* gen. nov. *FEMS Microbiol. Lett.* **70:**255–262.

34. **Colman, G.** 1967. *Aerococcus*-like organisms isolated from human infections. *J. Clin. Pathol.* **20:**294–297.

35. **da Costa, C. T., C. Porter, K. Parry, A. Morris, and A. H. Quoraishi.** 1996. Empyema thoracis and lung abscess due to *Gemella morbillorum. Eur. J. Clin. Microbiol. Infect. Dis.* **15:**75–77.

36. **Davis, J. M., and M. M. Peel.** 1994. Identification of ten clinical isolates of nutritionally variant streptococci by commercial streptococcal identification systems. *Aust. J. Med. Sci.* **15:**52–55.

37. **Eggelmeijer, F., P. Petit, and B. A. C. Dijkmans.** 1992. Total knee arthroplasty infection due to *Gemella haemolysans. Br. J. Rheumatol.* **31:**67–69.

38. **Elliott, J. A., M. D. Collins, N. E. Pigott, and R. R. Facklam.** 1991. Differentiation of *Lactococcus lactis* and *Lactococcus garvieae* from humans by comparison of whole-cell protein patterns. *J. Clin. Microbiol.* **29:**2731–2734.

39. **Elliott, J. A., and R. R. Facklam.** 1993. Identification of *Leuconostoc* spp. by analysis of soluble whole-cell protein patterns. *J. Clin. Microbiol.* **31:**1030–1033.

40. **Elliott, J. A., and R. R. Facklam.** 1996. Antimicrobial susceptibilities of *Lactococcus lactis* and *Lactococcus garvieae* and a proposed method to discriminate between them. *J. Clin. Microbiol.* **34:**1296–1298.

41. **Evans, J. B.** 1986. Genus *Aerococcus* Williams, Hirch and Cowan 1953, 475[AL], p. 1080. *In* P. H. A. Sneath, N. S. Mair, M. E. Sharpe, and J. G. Holt (ed.), *Bergey's Manual of Systematic Bacteriology,* vol. 2. The Williams & Wilkins Co., Baltimore, Md.

42. **Facklam, R. R.** 1977. Physiological differentiation of viridans streptococci. *J. Clin. Microbiol.* **5:**184–201.

43. **Facklam, R., and J. A. Elliott.** 1995. Identification, classification, and clinical relevance of catalase-negative, gram-positive cocci, excluding the streptococci and enterococci. *Clin. Microbiol. Rev.* **8:**479–495.

44. **Facklam, R. R., and J. A. Washington II.** 1991. *Streptococcus* and related catalase-negative gram-positive cocci, p. 238–257. *In* A. Balows, W. J. Hausler, Jr., K. L. Herrmann, H. D. Isenberg, and H. J. Shadomy (ed.), *Manual of Clinical Microbiology,* 5th ed. American Society for Microbiology, Washington, D.C.

45. **Farmaki, E., E. Roilides, E. Darilis, M. Tsivitanidou, C. Panteliadis, and D. Sofianou.** 2000. *Gemella morbillorum* endocarditis in a child. *Pediatr. Infect. Dis. J.* **19:**751–753.

46. **Fefer, J. J., K. R. Ratzan, S. E. Sharp, and E. Saiz.** 1998. *Lactococcus garvieae* endocarditis: report of a case and re-

view of the literature. *Diagn. Microbiol. Infect. Dis.* **32:** 127–130.

47. **Garcia-Marcos, J. A., M. Meseguer, and F. Baquero.** 1992. Meningitis due to *Gemella haemolysans. Clin. Microbiol. Newsl.* **14:**142–143.

48. **Garvie, E. I.** 1986. Genus *Leuconostoc* van Tieghem 1878, 198^AL emend mut. char. Hucker and Pederson 1930, 66^AL, p. 1071–1075. *In* P. H. A. Sneath, N. S. Mair, M. E. Sharpe, and J. G. Holt (ed.), *Bergey's Manual of Systematic Bacteriology,* vol. 2. The Williams & Wilkins Co., Baltimore, Md.

49. **Garvie, E. I.** 1986. Genus *Pediococcus* Claussen 1903, 68^AL, p. 1075–1079. *In* P. H. A. Sneath, N. S. Mair, M. E. Sharpe, and J. G. Holt (ed.), *Bergey's Manual of Systematic Bacteriology,* vol. 2. The Williams & Wilkins Co., Baltimore, Md.

50. **Golledge, C. L., N. Stingemore, M. Aravena, and K. Joske.** 1990. Septicemia caused by vancomycin-resistant *Pediococcus acidilactici. J. Clin. Microbiol.* **28:**1678–1679.

51. **Haas, J., S. L. Jernick, R. J. Scardina, J. Teruya, A. M. Caliendo, and K. L. Ruoff.** 1997. Colonization of skin by *Helcococcus kunzii. J. Clin. Microbiol.* **35:**2759–2761.

52. **Hall, G. S., S. Gordon, S. Schroeder, K. Smith, K. Anthony, and G. W. Procop.** 2001. Case of synovitis potentially caused by *Dolosigranulum pigrum. J. Clin. Microbiol.* **39:**1202–1203.

53. **Handwerger, S., H. Horowitz, K. Coburn, A. Kolokathis, and G. P. Wormser.** 1990. Infection due to *Leuconostoc* species: six cases and review. *Rev. Infect. Dis.* **12:**602–610.

54. **James, P. R., S. M. Hardman, and D. L. Patterson.** 2000. Osteomyelitis and possible endocarditis secondary to *Lactococcus garvieae*: a first case report. *Postgrad. Med. J.* **76:**301–303.

55. **Johnson, C. C., and A. R. Tunkel.** 1995. Viridans streptococci and groups C and G streptococci, p. 1845–1861. *In* G. L. Mandell, J. E. Bennett, and R. Dolin (ed.), *Mandell, Douglas and Bennett's Principles and Practice of Infectious Diseases,* 4th ed. Churchill Livingstone, Inc., New York, N.Y.

56. **Kanamoto, T., S. Sato, and M. Inoue.** 2000. Genetic heterogeneities and phenotypic characteristics of strains of the genus *Abiotrophia* and proposal of *Abiotrophia para-adiacens* sp. nov. *J. Clin. Microbiol.* **38:**492–498.

57. **Kawamura, Y., X. Hou, F. Sultana, S. Liu, H. Yamamoto, and T. Ezaki.** 1995. Transfer of *Streptococcus adjacens* and *Streptococcus defectivus* to *Abiotrophia* gen. nov. as *Abiotrophia adiacens* comb. nov. and *Abiotrophia defectiva* comb. nov., respectively. *Int. J. Syst. Bacteriol.* **45:**798–803.

58. **Kern, W., and E. Vanek.** 1987. *Aerococcus* bacteremia associated with granulocytopenia. *Eur. J. Clin. Microbiol.* **6:**670–673.

59. **Kilpper-Balz, R., and K. H. Schleifer.** 1988. Transfer of *Streptococcus morbillorum* to the genus *Gemella* as *Gemella morbillorum* comb. nov. *Int. J. Syst. Bacteriol.* **38:**442–443.

60. **Kristensen, B., and G. Nielsen.** 1995. Endocarditis caused by *Aerococcus urinae*, a newly recognized pathogen. *Eur. J. Clin. Microbiol. Infect. Dis.* **14:**49–51.

61. **LaClaire, L., and R. Facklam.** 2000. Antimicrobial susceptibility and clinical sources of *Dolosigranulum pigrum* cultures. *Antimicrob. Agents Chemother.* **44:**2001–2003.

62. **LaClaire, L., and R. Facklam.** 2000. Antimicrobial susceptibilities and clinical sources of *Facklamia* species. *Antimicrob. Agents Chemother.* **44:**2130–2132.

63. **LaClaire, L. L., and R. R. Facklam.** 2000. Comparison of three commercial rapid identification systems for the unusual gram-positive cocci *Dolosigranulum pigrum, Ignavigra-*

num *ruoffiae,* and *Facklamia* species. *J. Clin. Microbiol.* **38:**2037–2042.

64. **Lawson, P. A., M. D. Collins, E. Falsen, B. Sjoden, and R. R. Facklam.** 1999. *Facklamia languida* sp. nov., isolated from human clinical specimens. *J. Clin. Microbiol.* **37:** 1161–1164.

65. **Lawson, P. A., E. Falsen, M. Ohlen, and M. D. Collins.** 2001. *Aerococcus urinaehominis* sp. nov., isolated from human urine. *Int. J. Syst. Evol. Microbiol.* **51:**683–686.

66. **Lawson, P. A., E. Falsen, K. Truberg-Jensen, and M. D. Collins.** 2001. *Aerococcus sanguicola* sp. nov., isolated from a human clinical source. *Int. J. Syst. Evol. Microbiol.* **51:**475–479.

67. **Mannion, P. T., and M. M. Rothburn.** 1990. Diagnosis of bacterial endocarditis caused by *Streptococcus lactis. J. Infect.* **21:**317–318.

68. **Mastro, T. D., J. S. Spika, P. Lozano, J. Appel, and R. R. Facklam.** 1990. Vancomycin-resistant *Pediococcus acidilactici*: nine cases of bacteremia. *J. Infect. Dis.* **161:**956–960.

69. **Mofredj, A., D. Baraka, G. Kloeti, and J. L. Dumont.** 2000. *Lactococcus garvieae* septicemia with liver abscess in an immunosuppressed patient. *Am. J. Med.* **109:**513–514.

70. **Namdari, H., K. Kintner, B. A. Jackson, S. Namdari, J. L. Hughes, R. R. Peairs, and D. J. Savage.** 1999. *Abiotrophia* species as a cause of endophthalmitis following cataract extraction. *J. Clin. Microbiol.* **37:**1564–1566.

71. **National Committee for Clinical Laboratory Standards.** 2000. *Methods for Dilution Antimicrobial Susceptibility Tests for Bacteria That Grow Aerobically,* 5th ed. Approved standard M7-A5. National Committee for Clinical Laboratory Standards, Wayne, Pa.

72. **Ormerod, L. D., K. L. Ruoff, D. M. Meisler, P. J. Wasson, J. C. Kinter, S. P. Dunn, J. H. Lass, and I. Van de Rijn.** 1991. Infectious crystalline keratopathy. Role of nutritionally variant streptococci and other bacterial factors. *Ophthalmology* **98:**159–169.

73. **Parker, M. T., and L. C. Ball.** 1976. Streptococci and aerococci associated with systemic infection in man. *J. Med. Microbiol.* **9:**275–302.

74. **Peel, M. M., J. M. Davis, K. J. Griffin, and D. L. Freedman.** 1997. *Helcococcus kunzii* as sole isolate from an infected sebaceous cyst. *J. Clin. Microbiol.* **35:**328–329.

75. **Pellizzer, G., P. Benedetti, F. Biavasco, V. Manfrin, M. Franzetti, M. Scagnelli, C. Scarparo, and F. de Lalla.** 1996. Bacterial endocarditis due to *Lactococcus lactis* subsp. *cremoris*: case report. *Clin. Microbiol. Infect.* **2:**230–232.

76. **Reyn, A.** 1986. Genus *Gemella* Berger 1960, 253^AL, p. 1081–1082. *In* P. H. A. Sneath, N. S. Mair, M. E. Sharpe, and J. G. Holt (ed.), *Bergey's Manual of Systematic Bacteriology,* vol. 2. The Williams & Wilkins Co., Baltimore, Md.

77. **Riebel, W. J., and J. A. Washington.** 1990. Clinical and microbiologic characteristics of pediococci. *J. Clin. Microbiol.* **28:**1348–1355.

78. **Roggenkamp, A., M. Abele-Horn, K-H. Trebesius, U. Tretter, I. B. Autenrieth, and J. Heesemann.** 1998. *Abiotrophia elegans* sp. nov., a possible pathogen in patients with culture-negative endocarditis. *J. Clin. Microbiol.* **36:** 100–104.

79. **Ruoff, K. L., D. R. Kuritzkes, J. S. Wolfson, and M. J. Ferraro.** 1988. Vancomycin-resistant gram-positive bacteria isolated from human sources. *J. Clin. Microbiol.* **26:** 2064–2068.

80. **Schlegel, I., C. Merlet, J. M. Laroche, A. Fremaux, and P. Geslin.** 1999. Iatrogenic meningitis due to *Abiotrophia defectiva* after myelography. *Clin. Infect. Dis.* **28:**155–156.

81. **Schleifer, K. H.** 1986. Family I. *Micrococcaceae* Prevot 1961, 31^AL, p. 1003–1035. *In* P. H. A. Sneath, N. S. Mair, M. E. Sharpe, and J. G. Holt (ed.), *Bergey's Manual of*

Systematic Bacteriology, vol. 2. The Williams & Wilkins Co., Baltimore, Md.

82. **Schleifer, K. H., J. Kraus, C. Dvorak, R. Kilpper-Balz, M. D. Collins, and W. Fischer.** 1985. Transfer of *Streptococcus lactis* and related streptococci to the genus *Lactococcus* gen. nov. *Syst. Appl. Microbiol.* **6:**183–195.

83. **Schurr, P. M. H., M. E. E. van Kasteren, L. Sabbe, M. C. Vos, M. M. P. C. Janssens, and A. G. M. Buiting.** 1997. Urinary tract infections with *Aerococcus urinae* in the south of the Netherlands. *Eur. J. Clin. Microbiol. Infect. Dis.* **16:**871–875.

84. **Sire, J. M., P. Y. Donnio, R. Mensard, P. Pouedras, and J. L. Avril.** 1992. Septicemia and hepatic abscess caused by *Pediococcus acidilactici. Eur. J. Clin. Microbiol. Infect. Dis.* **11:**623–625.

85. **Skov, R. L., M. Klarlund, and S. Thorsen.** 1995. Fatal endocarditis due to *Aerococcus urinae. Diagn. Microbiol. Infect. Dis.* **21:**219–221.

86. **Swenson, J. M., R. R. Facklam, and C. Thornsberry.** 1990. Antimicrobial susceptibility of vancomycin-resistant *Leuconostoc, Pediococcus,* and *Lactobacillus* species. *Antimicrob. Agents Chemother.* **34:**543–549.

87. **Teixeira, L. M., M. G. Carvalho, V. L. Merquior, A. G. Steigerwalt, D. J. Brenner, and R. R. Facklam.** 1997. Phenotypic and genotypic characterization of *Vagococcus*

fluvialis, including strains isolated from human sources. *J. Clin. Microbiol.* **35:**2778–2781.

88. **Tunicliff, R.** 1917. The cultivation of a micrococcus from blood in pre-eruptive and eruptive stages of measles. *JAMA* **68:**1028–1030.

89. **Tuohy, M. J., G. W. Procop, and J. A. Washington.** 2000. Antimicrobial susceptibility of *Abiotrophia adiacens* and *Abiotrophia defectiva. Diagn. Microbiol. Infect. Dis.* **38:**189–191.

90. **van Dijk, M., B. J. van Royen, P. I. Wuisman, T. A. Hekker, and C. van Guldener.** 1999. Trochanter osteomyelitis and ipsilateral arthritis due to *Gemella morbillorum. Eur. J. Clin. Microbiol. Infect. Dis.* **18:**600–602.

91. **Vasishtha, S., H. D. Isenberg, and S. K. Sood.** 1996. *Gemella morbillorum* as a cause of septic shock. *Clin. Infect. Dis.* **22:**1084–1086.

92. **von Graevenitz, A.** 1993. Revised nomenclature of *Alloiococcus otitis. J. Clin. Microbiol.* **31:**472.

93. **Wallbanks, S., A. J. Martinez-Murcia, J. L. Fryer, B. A. Phillips, and M. D. Collins.** 1990. 16S rRNA sequence determination for members of the genus *Carnobacterium* and related lactic acid bacteria and description of *Vagococcus salmoninarum* sp. nov. *Int. J. Syst. Bacteriol.* **40:**224–230.

Bacillus and Other Aerobic Endospore-Forming Bacteria

NIALL A. LOGAN AND PETER C. B. TURNBULL

32

TAXONOMY

Bacillus has been divided into more manageable and better-defined groups on the basis of 16S rRNA sequencing studies. So far, nine new genera have been proposed: *Alicyclobacillus* (64), which contains four species of thermoacidophiles; *Paenibacillus* (2), containing 27 species and including organisms formerly called *B. polymyxa*, *B. macerans*, *B. alvei*, and the honeybee pathogens *B. larvae* and *B. pulvifaciens* (now both subspecies of *P. larvae*); *Brevibacillus* (51), containing 10 species and including organisms formerly called *B. brevis* and *B. laterosporus*; *Aneurinibacillus* (51), with *A. aneurinilyticus* and two other species; *Virgibacillus* (27), with *V. pantothenticus* and one other species; *Gracilibacillus* and *Salibacillus* (63), which each contain two species of halophiles; *Geobacillus* (47), with eight species of thermophiles including *B. stearothermophilus*; and *Ureibacillus* (20), with two round-spored, thermophilic species.

Sporosarcina contains the motile, spore-forming coccus *S. ureae*, which is closely related to *B. sphaericus*, and four rod-shaped, round-spored species, including *Bacillus pasteurii*, that have now been placed in this genus (65). Other genera of aerobic endospore formers are *Sulfobacillus*, *Amphibacillus*, *Halobacillus*, *Ammoniphilus*, and *Thermobacillus* (21, 48, 53, 55, 66).

Bacillus continues to accommodate the best-known species such as *B. subtilis* (the type species), *B. anthracis*, *B. cereus*, *B. licheniformis*, *B. megaterium*, *B. pumilus*, *B. sphaericus*, and *B. thuringiensis*. It still remains a large genus, with 70 species, since losses of species to other genera have been balanced by proposals for new *Bacillus* species. Members of the *B. cereus* group, *B. anthracis*, *B. cereus*, and *B. thuringiensis*, are really pathovars of a single species (58). New species and subspecies of aerobic endospore formers are regularly described (22 between 1999 and mid-2001, during which period no proposals for merging species had been made) but often on the basis of very few strains.

DESCRIPTIONS OF THE GENERA

Although the production of resistant endospores in the presence of oxygen remains the defining feature for *Bacillus* and the new genera derived from it, the definition was undermined by the discovery of *Bacillus infernus*, which is strictly anaerobic (7).

The members likely to be isolated in a clinical laboratory are gram-positive (in young cultures) but sometimes gram-variable or frankly gram-negative, rod-shaped, endospore-forming organisms which may be aerobic or facultatively anaerobic. They are mostly catalase positive and may be motile by means of peritrichous flagella. Most species are mesophilic, but *Bacillus* contains some thermophiles and psychrophiles and *Paenibacillus* contains one psychrophilic species. *Alicyclobacillus*, *Ammoniphilus*, *Amphibacillus*, *Gracilibacillus*, *Halobacillus*, *Salibacillus*, *Sulfobacillus*, *Thermobacillus*, and *Ureibacillus* strains are unlikely to be encountered in a clinical laboratory, and clinical isolates of *Geobacillus* and *Sporosarcina* have not been reported, so these genera are not considered further.

Unfortunately, taxonomic progress has not revealed readily determinable features characteristic of each genus. They show wide ranges of sporangial morphologies and phenotypic test patterns. Many recently described species represent genomic groups disclosed by DNA-DNA pairing experiments, and routine phenotypic characters for distinguishing some of them are very few and of unproven value.

NATURAL HABITATS

Most aerobic endospore formers are saprophytes widely distributed in the natural environment, but some species are opportunistic or obligate pathogens of animals, including humans, other mammals, and insects. The main habitats are soils of all kinds, ranging from acidic to alkaline, hot to cold, and fertile to desert, and the water columns and bottom deposits of freshwater bodies and marine waters. Their spores readily survive distribution in soils, dusts, and aerosols from these natural environments to a wide variety of other habitats. Dried foods such as spices, milk powders, and farinaceous products are often quite heavily contaminated with spores. *B. anthracis* is, to all intents and purposes, an obligate pathogen of animals and humans; if it ever multiplies in the environment, it probably does so only rarely. Its close relative, *B. cereus*, is now well established as an opportunistic pathogen, and other aerobic endospore formers can also, from time to time, be opportunistic pathogens. Six organisms are important as insect pathogens: *B. thuringiensis* (another close relative of *B. anthracis*), *B. popilliae*, *B. lentimorbus*, *B. sphaericus*, and the two *P. larvae* subspecies.

CLINICAL SIGNIFICANCE

The majority of aerobic endospore-forming species apparently have little or no pathogenic potential and are rarely associated with disease in humans and other animals. The principal exceptions to this are *B. anthracis*, the agent of anthrax, and *B. cereus*, but a number of other species, particularly *B. licheniformis*, have been implicated in food poisoning and other human and animal infections. The resistance of the spores to heat, radiation, disinfectants, and desiccation also results in aerobic endospore formers being troublesome contaminants in the operating room, on surgical dressings, in pharmaceutical products, and in foods.

On the positive side, several of the species are of clinical or health importance in a variety of ways: in the production of antibiotics (particularly bacitracin from *B. licheniformis* or *B. subtilis* and polymyxin from *P. polymyxa*) or vitamins (e.g., vitamins B_{12} and B_2 from *B. megaterium* and biotin and riboflavin from *B. subtilis*); as the bases of antibiotic assays (*B. cereus*, *B. circulans*, *B. megaterium*, *B. pumilus*, *B. subtilis*, *G. stearothermophilus*); in the validation of disinfectants (*B. cereus*) and the monitoring of fumigation (*B. subtilis*), heat sterilization (*G. stearothermophilus*), and radiation (*B. pumilus*) processes; and in various clinical tests (such as a uric acid assay utilizing *B. fastidiosus*, a *Chlamydia* detection assay utilizing a variant of subtilisin from *B. subtilis*, and a blood-screening test for phenylketonuria-utilizing *B. subtilis*). The restriction endonucleases and DNA polymerases of several *Bacillus* species are of considerable importance as research tools for better understanding of disease and improved diagnosis. *Bacillus* species lend themselves well to host-vector systems for production of bioengineered therapeutic products. A number of *Bacillus* species are the active ingredients of probiotics for animals and humans.

Bacillus anthracis

Anthrax remains the best-known clinical condition caused by a *Bacillus* species. It is primarily a disease of herbivores; before an effective veterinary vaccine became available in the late 1930s, anthrax was one of the foremost causes worldwide of mortality in cattle, sheep, goats, and horses. Humans almost invariably contract anthrax directly or indirectly from animals. The development and application of veterinary and human vaccines, together with improvements in factory hygiene and sterilization procedures for imported animal products and the increased use of manmade alternatives to animal hides and hair, have resulted over the past half century in a marked decline in the incidence of the disease in both animals and humans. Nevertheless, the disease continues to be endemic in many countries, particularly those that lack an efficient vaccination policy. Because anthrax spores remain viable in soil for many years and their persistence does not depend on animal reservoirs, *B. anthracis* is exceedingly difficult to eradicate from an area of endemic infection; regions where the infection is not endemic must be constantly on the alert for the arrival of *B. anthracis* in imported products of animal origin. The disease is of the point source type, and direct human-to-human transmission is exceedingly rare. Direct animal-to-animal transmission within a species (i.e., excluding the case of carnivorous scavengers feeding on meat from anthrax-infected carcasses) is also very rare.

Circumstantial evidence shows that, compared with obligate herbivores, humans are moderately resistant to anthrax. Human anthrax is traditionally classified as either (i) nonindustrial, resulting from close contact with infected animals or their carcasses after death from the disease, or (ii) industrial, acquired by those employed in processing wool, hair, hides, bones, or other animal products. Nonindustrial cases are usually cutaneous, but *B. anthracis* meningitis and intestinal anthrax are occasionally reported. Industrial anthrax is also usually cutaneous but has a higher probability than nonindustrial anthrax of taking the inhalational form from inhaling spore-laden dust. A few reports exist of laboratory-acquired infections, although not in recent years (14). A substantial outbreak of anthrax occurred in April 1979 in the city of Sverdlovsk, former USSR (now Yekaterinburg, Russia), in the Urals as a result of the accidental release of spores from a military production facility (45).

B. anthracis has been subjected to military research, development, and occasional deployment in several different countries over many years, following attacks on livestock during the First World War (12), and it has remained high on the list of potential agents in discussions of biological warfare or bioterrorism (32). Unfortunately, this has given an unjustified doomsday image to the natural disease, since nature cannot remotely emulate the overwhelmingly massive exposures that could be created artificially. The natural disease is readily controllable, in contrast to outbreaks following acts of biowarfare or bioterrorism. However, in public consciousness, *B. anthracis* is associated more with warfare and terrorism than with a disease of herbivores, and, as the attacks in the United States in late 2001 attest (35), it is feared accordingly (see chapter 10).

Cutaneous cases account for about 99% of all human cases of naturally acquired anthrax worldwide. *B. anthracis* is not invasive, and cutaneous infection occurs through a break in the skin; therefore, the lesions generally occur on exposed regions of the body. Before the availability of antibiotics and vaccines, 10 to 20% of untreated cases of cutaneous anthrax were fatal. The rare fatalities seen today are due to obstruction of the airways by the edema that accompanies lesions on the face or neck and to sequelae of secondary cellulitis or meningitis.

Intestinal and inhalational (pulmonary) forms are more often fatal, because they go unrecognized until too late for effective therapy. Pharyngeogastrointestinal anthrax is not uncommon in countries with endemic infection where socioeconomic conditions are poor and people eat the meat of animals that have died suddenly (1, 17); asymptomatic infections and symptomatic infections with recovery may not be uncommon (11, 57). The number of recorded cases of naturally acquired inhalational anthrax in the United States since 1900 and up until the bioterrorist attack of 2001 was just 18, with 16 (88.9%) of them being fatal (8); figures in the United Kingdom show a similar picture. In 10 confirmed cases of inhalational anthrax that followed the bioterrorist attack in the United States, in which spores were delivered in mailed letters and packages, early recognition and treatment helped to achieve a survival level of 60% (30). At the time of going to press in early 2002, a total of 22 cases of anthrax had been identified in relation to the bioterrorist events of the last 4 months of 2001; 11 were confirmed as inhalational anthrax, and 11 (7 confirmed and 4 suspected) were cutaneous.

The incubation period in cutaneous anthrax is generally 2 to 3 days (with extremes of approximately 12 h to 2 weeks). A small pimple or papule appears, and over the next 24 h a ring of vesicles develops around it, and it ulcerates, dries, and blackens into the characteristic eschar.

This enlarges, becoming thick and adherent to underlying tissues over the ensuing week, and is surrounded by edema, which may be very extensive. Pus and pain are normally absent; their presence, or the presence of marked lymphangitis and fever, probably indicates secondary bacterial infection. Historical records show a mortality rate of approximately 20% in untreated cutaneous cases. Intestinal anthrax is essentially cutaneous anthrax occurring on the intestinal mucosa. Symptoms of gastroenteritis may occur prior to onset of systemic symptoms.

In inhalational anthrax the inhaled spores are carried by macrophages from the lungs, where there is no overt infection, to the lymphatic system, where the infection progresses. Germination and initial multiplication begin within the macrophages while in transit to the lymph nodes (25). The vegetative cells kill the macrophages and are released into the bloodstream, where they continue to multiply and lead to fatal septicemia. Undiagnosed low-grade inhalational infections with recovery may occur. The replacement of the older name for this form of the disease, "pulmonary anthrax" with the newer name "inhalational anthrax" is a reflection of the fact that active infection occurs in the lymph nodes, rather than the lungs themselves. Analysis of 10 of the cases associated with the bioterrorist events of 2001 (30) revealed a median incubation period of 4 days (range, 4 to 6 days) and a variety of symptoms at initial presentation including fever or chills ($n = 10$), sweats ($n = 7$), fatigue or malaise ($n = 10$), minimal or nonproductive cough ($n = 9$), dyspnea ($n = 8$), and nausea or vomiting ($n = 9$). All patients had abnormal chest X rays with infiltrates ($n = 7$), pleural effusion ($n = 8$), and mediastinal widening ($n = 7$). Mediastinal lymphadenopathy was present in seven patients.

In fatal cases of any of the forms, the generalized symptoms, which may be mild (fatigue, malaise, fever, and/or gastrointestinal symptoms), are followed by sudden onset of acute illness characterized by dyspnea, cyanosis, severe pyrexia, and disorientation followed by circulatory failure, shock, coma, and death, all within a few hours. Depending on the host, there is a rapid buildup of the bacteria in the blood over the last few hours to terminal levels of 10^7 to 10^9/ml in the most susceptible species. Considerable progress is being made in deciphering the manner in which the toxin of *B. anthracis* produces the signs and symptoms of the disease (24).

Opportunistic Pathogens
Opportunistic infections with *Bacillus* species other than *B. anthracis* have been reported since the late 19th century. It is important to assess isolates of *Bacillus* in the light of any other species cultured and the clinical context and to be cautious or wary of dismissing them as mere contaminants. In the case of posttraumatic endophthalmitis, *Bacillus* species, particularly *B. cereus*, may be the second most commonly isolated organisms after *Staphylococcus epidermidis* (16). For relevant reviews, see references 4 and 39.

Bacillus cereus Group
Bacillus cereus is next in importance to *B. anthracis* as a pathogen of humans (and other animals), causing food-borne illness and opportunistic infections, and its ubiquity ensures that cases are not uncommon.

In relation to food-borne illness, *B. cereus* is the etiological agent of two distinct food-poisoning syndromes (34): (i) the diarrheal type, characterized by abdominal pain with diarrhea 8 to 16 h after ingestion of the contam-

inated food and associated with a diversity of foods from meats and vegetable dishes to pastas, desserts, cakes, sauces, and milk, and (ii) the emetic type, characterized by nausea and vomiting 1 to 5 h after eating the offending food, predominantly oriental rice dishes, although occasionally other foods such as pasteurized cream, milk pudding, pastas, and reconstituted formulas have been implicated. One outbreak followed the mere handling of contaminated rice in a children's craft activity (9), and fulminant liver failure associated with the emetic toxin has been reported (43). Both syndromes arise as a direct result of the fact that *B. cereus* spores can survive normal cooking procedures; under conditions of improper storage after cooking, the spores germinate and the vegetative cells multiply. Strains of *B. thuringiensis*, which are close relatives of *B. cereus*, may also produce the diarrheal toxin, and *B. thuringiensis* has indeed been implicated in cases of gastroenteritis (15).

The toxigenic basis of *B. cereus* food poisoning and other *B. cereus* infections has begun to be elucidated, and a complex picture is emerging (3). A toxin possibly associated with *B. licheniformis* food poisoning has been identified (46), but, in general, toxins or virulence factors widely accepted as responsible for symptoms periodically associated with *Bacillus* species other than those in the *B. cereus* group have not been identified.

B. cereus is also a destructive ocular pathogen. Endophthalmitis may follow penetrating trauma of the eye or hematogenous spread, evolving very rapidly. Loss both of vision and the eye is likely if appropriate treatment is instituted too late (16). Other *B. cereus* infections occur mainly, although not exclusively, in persons predisposed by neoplastic disease, immunosuppression, alcoholism and other drug abuse, or some other underlying condition, and fatalities occasionally result. Reported conditions include bacteremia, septicemia, fulminant sepsis with hemolysis, meningitis, brain hemorrhage, ventricular shunt infections, endocarditis, pneumonia, empyema, pleurisy, lung abscess, brain abscess, osteomyelitis, salpingitis, urinary tract infection, and primary cutaneous infections. Wound infections, mostly in otherwise healthy persons, have been reported following surgery, road traffic and other accidents, scalds, burns, plaster fixation, drug injection, and close-range gunshot and nail bomb injuries; some became necrotic and gangrenous. A fatal inflammation was caused by a blank firearm injury; blank cartridge propellants are commonly contaminated with the organism (50). Neonates also appear to be particularly susceptible to *B. cereus*, especially with umbilical stump infections; respiratory tract infections associated with contaminated ventilation systems have also occurred (61). There have been reports of wound, burn, and ocular infections with *B. thuringiensis* (15), but there is as yet no evidence of infections associated with the use of this organism as an insecticide.

B. cereus also causes infections in domestic animals. It is a well-recognized agent of mastitis and abortion in cattle and can cause these conditions in other livestock (5).

Other Species
Reports of infections with non-*B. cereus* group species are comparatively rare but very diverse (4, 39), and several hospital pseudoepidemics have been associated with contaminated blood culture systems. *B. licheniformis* has been reported from ventriculitis following the removal of a meningioma, cerebral abscess after penetrating orbital injury, septicemia following arteriography, bacteremia associated with indwelling central venous catheters (6), bacteremia

during pregnancy with eclampsia and acute fibrinolysis, peritonitis in a chronic ambulatory peritoneal dialysis patient and in a patient with volvulus and small-bowel perforation, and ophthalmitis and corneal ulcer after trauma. There have also been reports of L-form organisms, phenotypically similar to *B. licheniformis*, occurring in human blood and other body fluids (39). *B. licheniformis* can cause food-borne diarrheal illness and has been associated with an infant fatality (46). This organism is frequently associated with bovine abortion and occasionally with bovine mastitis (5); these types of *B. licheniformis* and *B. cereus* infections are associated with wet and dirty conditions during winter housing, particularly when the animals lie in spilled silage (5).

The name *B. subtilis* was often used to mean any aerobic, endospore-forming organism, but since 1970 there have been reports of infection in which identification of this species appears to have been made accurately. They include cases associated with neoplastic disease: fatal pneumonia and bacteremia, a septicemia, and an infection of a necrotic axillary tumor in breast cancer patients; breast prosthesis and ventriculoatrial shunt infections; endocarditis in a drug abuser; meningitis following a head injury; cholangitis associated with kidney and liver disease; and isolations from surgical wound drainage sites. Administration of a probiotic preparation of this species, marketed for the treatment or prevention of intestinal disorders, led to a fatal septicemia in an immunocompromised patient (49). *B. subtilis* has also been implicated in food-borne illness and in cases of bovine mastitis and of ovine abortion (4, 39).

Organisms identified as *B. circulans* have been isolated from cases of meningitis, a cerebrospinal fluid shunt infection, endocarditis, endophthalmitis (54), a wound infection in a cancer patient, and a bite wound; and *B. coagulans* has been isolated from corneal infection, bacteremia, and bovine abortion. *B. pumilus* has been found in cases of pustule and rectal fistula infection and in association with bovine mastitis. *B. sphaericus* has been implicated in a fatal lung pseudotumor and in meningitis (4, 39).

B. brevis has been isolated from corneal infection and has been implicated in several incidents of food poisoning; since these reports, the species was split (see "Taxonomy" above) and transferred to the new genus *Brevibacillus*. Strains of the new species, *Brevibacillus agri*, have been isolated in association with an outbreak of waterborne illness in Sweden, and other *Brevibacillus* species have been found in human blood and bronchoalveolar lavage fluid specimens. *Brevibacillus laterosporus* has been reported in association with a severe case of endophthalmitis (4, 39).

Paenibacillus alvei has been isolated from cases of meningitis, a prosthetic hip infection in a patient with sickle cell anemia, a wound infection, and, in association with *Clostridium perfringens*, a case of gas gangrene. *P. macerans* has been isolated from a wound infection following removal of a malignant melanoma and from bovine abortion, and *P. polymyxa* has been isolated from ovine abortion (39).

COLLECTION, TRANSPORT, AND STORAGE OF SPECIMENS

Clinical specimens for isolation of *Bacillus* species other than *B. anthracis* can be handled without special precautions. *Bacillus* species normally survive transport in freshly collected specimens or in a standard transport medium.

Safety Aspects in Relation to Anthrax

Anthrax is not highly contagious. Cutaneous anthrax is readily treated and is life-threatening only in exceptional cases; the infectious doses in the human inhalational and intestinal forms (also treatable if recognized) are generally very high (50% lethal dose, >10,000 spores). Precautions, therefore, need to be sensible, not extreme. When collecting specimens related to suspected anthrax, disposable gloves, disposable apron or overalls, and boots which can be disinfected after use should be worn; for dusty samples that might contain many spores, the use of headgear and dust masks should be considered.

Disposable items should be discarded into suitable containers for autoclaving followed by incineration. Nonautoclavable items should be immersed overnight in 10% formalin (5% formaldehyde solution). Glutaraldehyde (5%) is also effective. Items that cannot be immersed should be bagged and sent for formaldehyde fumigation. Ethylene oxide and hydrogen peroxide vapor are also effective fumigants, but the latter is inappropriate if organic matter is being treated. The best disinfectant for specimen spillages is again formalin; where this is considered impractical, 10% hypochlorite solution can be used, although its limitations should be appreciated: it is rapidly neutralized by organic matter, and it corrodes metals. Other strong oxidizing agents, such as hydrogen peroxide (5%) and peracetic acid (1%), are also effective but with the same organic matter limitations. For further discussion, see reference 59 and the websites www.bt.cdc.gov and www.hopkins-biodefense.org.

DIAGNOSIS OF ANTHRAX

Human Anthrax

In all cases, specimens from possible sources of the infection (carcass, hides, hair, bones, etc.) should be sought in addition to specimens from the patients themselves.

Cutaneous Anthrax

Swabs are appropriate for collecting vesicular fluid. Adequate material should be submitted for both culture and a smear to visualize the capsule.

Intestinal Anthrax

Anthrax will be suspected only if an adequate history of the patient is known. If the patient is not severely ill, a fecal specimen may be collected. However, isolation of *B. anthracis* may not be successful. If the patient is severely ill, blood should also be cultured, although isolation may not be possible after antimicrobial treatment. Treatment should not await laboratory results. A blood smear may reveal the encapsulated bacilli or, if treatment has started, capsule "ghosts."

Postmortem blood collected by venipuncture (a characteristic of anthrax is nonclotting blood at death) should be examined by smear (for capsule) and culture. Any hemorrhagic fluid from the nose, mouth or anus should be cultured. If these are positive, no further specimens are needed. If they are negative, specimens of peritoneal fluid, spleen, and/or mesenteric lymph nodes, aspirated by techniques avoiding spillage of fluids, may be collected for smear and culture. Histologic testing is only of academic interest.

Inhalational (Pulmonary) Anthrax

As with the intestinal form, anthrax will be suspected only if the patient's history suggests the possibility. If the patient is not severely ill, immediate specimen collection is likely to be unfruitful, and the person should be treated and simply observed; paired sera (when first seen and at least 10 days later) may be useful for confirmation of the diagnosis. In the severely ill patient, blood smear and culture should be done. Again, results will depend somewhat on previous treatment. Postmortem, the approach described for intestinal anthrax should be followed.

Gram Stain

Inevitably, the first examination of smears and cultures is with the Gram stain. In the past, Gram stains have been regarded of limited value in anthrax diagnosis, because they do not reveal the capsule. Clearly, in recent bioterrorism cases, Gram-stained preparations were considered of high value (Fig. 1), but some caution still needs to be urged. In a well-developed country such as the United States, it is unlikely that large numbers of gram-positive bacteria in the blood at death are anything but *B. anthracis*, particularly when this is supported by the recent history of events. In other circumstances, and in animals in particular, the blood or other specimen may not be collected soon after death and before putrefactive organisms quickly appear, and *B. anthracis* may be indistinguishable without the use of the proper capsule stain. India ink stain results are inconsistent.

Further laboratory criteria for confirming cases as anthrax are given under "Identification" (below).

Potential Bioterrorism Specimens

A Laboratory Response Network (LRN) has been established by the Centers for Disease Control and Prevention in Atlanta to provide the appropriate laboratory response to acts of bioterrorism. A microbiology laboratory in the United States receiving specimens associated with a potential bioterrorist event should contact a laboratory within this network for instructions as to how to proceed. State Health Laboratories are part of the LRN and will be able to provide guidance, or the LRN can be accessed using the internet.

Guidelines relating to the specimens that might be collected and received and their examination procedures for *B. anthracis* (and other possible select agents) can be found at www.phppo.cdc.gov/nltn/btp.asp and on www.bt.cdc.gov (click on Laboratory Issues). The 24-h hotline number for urgent advice is (770) 488-7100.

Guidelines on responsibilities to notify local infection control personnel, health care facilities, local and state health departments, local police, the FBI field office, and medical emergency services can be found on www.bt.cdc.gov (click on Planning Guidance).

In general, the laboratory examination of clinical specimens will be as described above for cases of naturally acquired anthrax. Nonclinical materials associated with attempts at deliberate release may be very hazardous, and no attempt to process them should be made without the appropriate instructions from the correct authorities (see also chapter 10).

Novel Tests

The M'Fadyean polychrome methylene blue staining test dates from 1903 and has proved a remarkably successful rapid diagnostic test over the decades. However, reliable stain and adequate quality control of its performance are becoming hard to guarantee. A rapid immunochromatographic on-site test has been developed but is not commercially available (10). PCR methods are available for con-

firmation of virulent isolates, but, as yet, procedures for direct diagnosis have not been fully developed.

Animal Anthrax

Anthrax should be considered as the possible cause of death in herbivorous animals which have died suddenly and unexpectedly, particularly if hemorrhage from the nose, mouth, or anus has occurred and if death has taken place at a site with a history of anthrax (perhaps several decades previously).

Carcasses 1 to 2 Days Old

Due to the nonclotting nature of blood in anthrax victims, it is usually possible to aspirate a few drops of blood from a vein for (i) M'Fadyean-stained smear and (ii) direct plate culture on blood agar.

Pigs frequently do not develop the enormous terminal bacteremia seen in herbivores, and the encapsulated rods may not be visible in blood smears. When cervical edema is present, smears and cultures should be made of fluid aspirated from the enlarged mandibular and suprapharyngeal lymph nodes. In porcine intestinal anthrax, possibly only obvious at necropsy, bacilli are usually visible in stained smears made from mesenteric lymph nodes.

Older Putrefying Carcasses

B. anthracis competes poorly with putrefactive organisms and may not be seen in smears after 2 to 3 days, so that culture is necessary for diagnostic confirmation. Sections of tissue, or any blood-stained material, should be collected. If the animal has been opened, spleen or lymph node specimens should be taken. With putrefied and very old carcasses, swabs of the nostrils and eye sockets are likely to yield *B. anthracis*, but the best specimens may be samples of contaminated soil from beneath the nose and anus.

Other Specimens

Tests for the presence of *B. anthracis* may be requested on a variety of specimens such as animal products (e.g., wool, hides, hair, and bonemeal) from regions of endemic infection, soil or other materials from old burial sites or from sites of tanneries or laboratories due for redevelopment, or other environmental materials associated with outbreaks (e.g., sewage sludge). At present, culture by the selective agar techniques described below is the only available approach. Suitably equipped laboratories are beginning to use PCR techniques for rapid detection of *B. anthracis* in such samples, but at present it is advisable to confirm positive results by conventional methods.

ISOLATION PROCEDURES

All the clinically significant isolates reported to date are of species that grow, and often sporulate, on routine laboratory media at 37°C. It seems unlikely that many clinically important but more fastidious strains are being missed for the want of special media or growth conditions. Maintenance is simple if spores can be obtained, but it is a mistake to assume that a primary culture or subculture on blood agar will automatically yield spores if stored on the bench or in the incubator. It is best to grow the organism for a few days on nutrient agar containing 5 mg of manganese sulfate per liter and refrigerate when microscopy shows that most cells have sporulated. For most species, sporulated cultures on slants of this medium, sealed after incubation, can survive

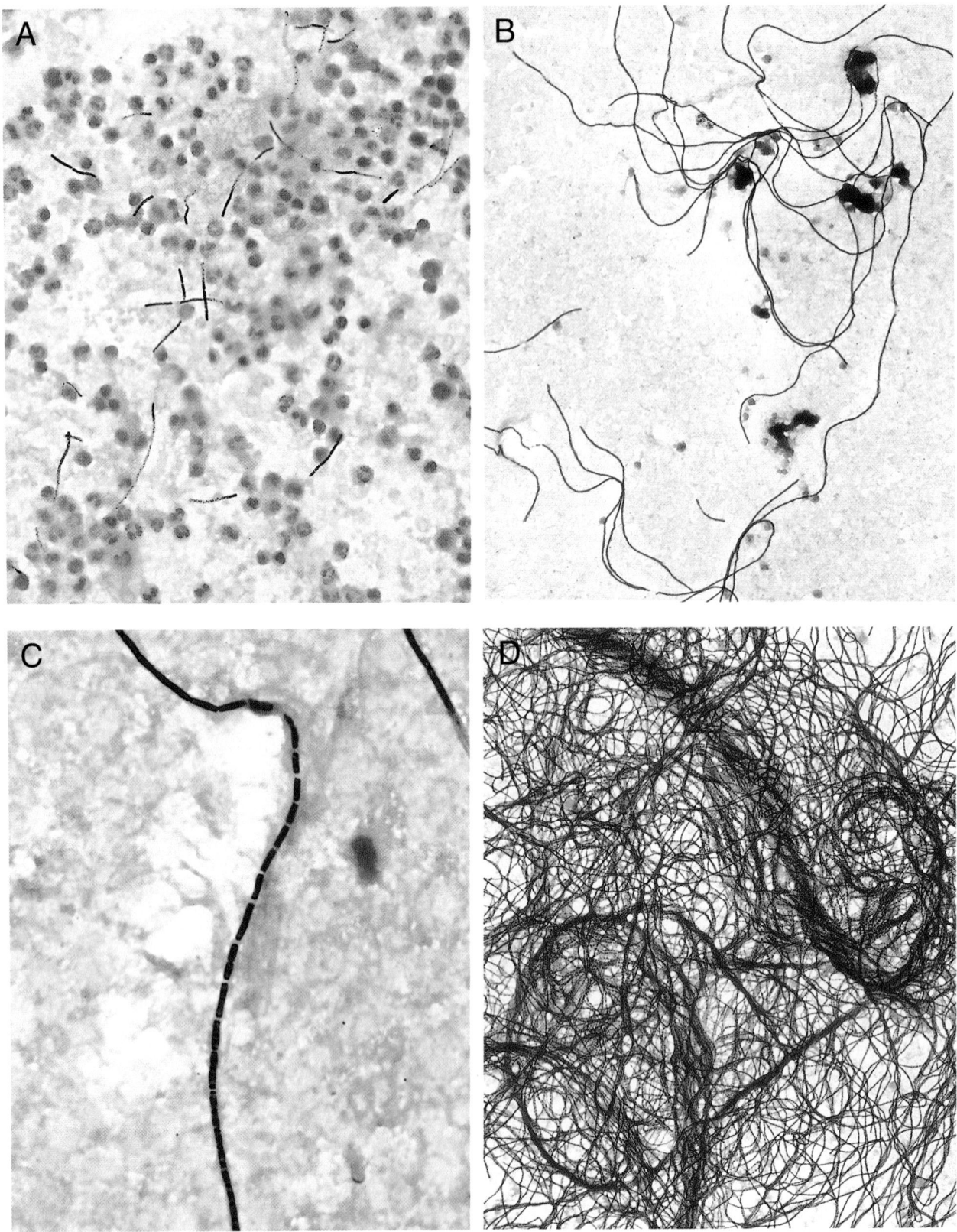

FIGURE 1 Gram stains of *B. anthracis* associated with a bioterrorism attack. (A) Gram-positive rods in peripheral blood buffy coat of an infected patient (magnification, ×400). (B to D) Appearance of gram-positive rods in blood culture broth after a 1-h incubation (magnification, ×200) (B), after a 1-h incubation (magnification, ×1,000) (C), and after a 24-h incubation (magnification, ×200) (D). Photographs courtesy of H. Masur.

in a refrigerator for years. Alternatively, cultures (preferably sporulated) can be frozen or lyophilized.

Safety Considerations

Isolation and presumptive identification of *B. anthracis* can be performed safely in the routine clinical microbiology laboratory, provided that normal good laboratory practice is observed; vaccination is not required for minimal handling of the organism (29). If aerosols are likely to be generated, the work should be performed in a safety cabinet. Further information, especially relevant to the use of anthrax as a weapon, can be found at www.bt.cdc.gov and www. hopkins-biodefense.org. All of the other species of aerobic endospore-forming bacteria that may be isolated from clinical specimens can be handled safely on the open bench.

Specimens with Mixed Microflora

In specimens submitted for food-poisoning investigations or for isolation of *B. anthracis* from old carcasses, animal products, or environmental specimens, the organisms are present mostly as spores. Heating at 62.5°C for 15 min both heat shocks the spores and effectively destroys non-spore-forming contaminants (solid samples should first be emulsified in sterile, deionized water, 1:2 [wt/vol]). Direct plate cultures are made on blood, nutrient, or selective agars, as appropriate, by spreading up to 250-μl volumes from undiluted and 10- and 100-fold diluted treated samples.

Enrichment procedures are generally inappropriate for isolations from clinical specimens, but when searching for *B. cereus* in stools 3 days or more after a food-poisoning episode, nutrient or tryptic soy broth with polymyxin (100,000 U/liter) may be added to the heat-treated specimen. There is no effective enrichment method for *B. anthracis* in old animal specimens or environmental samples; isolation from these is best done with polymyxin-lysozyme EDTA-thallous acetate (PLET) agar (33; see chapter 27). Aliquots (250 μl) of the undiluted and 1:10- and 1:100-diluted heat-treated suspension of the specimen are spread across PLET plates, which are read after incubation for 36 to 40 h at 37°C. Roughly circular, creamy-white colonies, 1 to 3 mm in diameter, with a ground-glass texture are subcultured on (i) blood agar plates to test for gamma phage and penicillin susceptibility and for hemolysis and (ii) directly or subsequently in blood to look for capsule production by using M'Fadyean's stain. PCR-based methods are being used increasingly for confirming the identity of isolates (59).

Several media have been designed for isolation, identification, and enumeration of *B. cereus* organisms. They exploit the organism's egg yolk reaction positivity and acid-from-mannitol negativity; pyruvate and polymyxin may be included for selectivity. Three satisfactory formulations are MEYP (mannitol, egg yolk, polymyxin B agar), PEMBA (polymyxin B, egg yolk, mannitol, bromthymol blue agar), and BCM (*Bacillus cereus* medium) (62). There are no selective media for other bacilli, but spores can be selected for by heat treating part of the specimen, as described above; the vegetative cells of both spore formers and non-spore formers are killed, but the heat-resistant spores not only survive but also may be heat shocked into subsequent germination. The other part of the specimen is cultivated without heat treatment in case spores are very heat sensitive or absent.

Heat treatment is not appropriate for fresh clinical specimens, where spores are usually sparse or absent.

IDENTIFICATION

These organisms do not always stain gram positive. Before attempting to identify an isolate to species level, it is important to establish that the isolate really is an aerobic endospore former and that other inclusions are not being mistaken for spores. A Gram-stained smear showing cells with unstained areas suggestive of spores can be stripped of oil with acetone-alcohol, washed, and then stained for spores. Spores are stained in heat-fixed smears by flooding with 10% aqueous malachite green for up to 45 min (without heating) followed by washing and counterstaining with 0.5% aqueous safranin for 30 s; spores are green within pinkish red cells at a magnification of ×1,000 (Fig. 2). Phase-contrast microscopy (at a magnification of ×1,000) should be used if available, since it is superior to spore staining and more convenient. Spores are larger, more phase-bright, and more regular in shape, size, and position than other kinds of inclusion such as polyhydroxybutyrate (PHB) granules (Fig. 3d), and sporangial appearance is valuable in identification (Fig. 3).

Members of the *B. cereus* group (see above) and *B. megaterium* produce large amounts of storage material when grown on carbohydrate media, but on routine media this vacuolate or foamy appearance is rarely sufficiently pronounced to cause confusion. Isolates of other organisms have often been submitted to reference laboratories as *Bacillus* species because they were large, aerobic gram-positive rods, even though sporulation had not been observed, or because PHB granules or other storage inclusions had been mistaken for spores.

Bacillus contains facultative anaerobes as well as strict aerobes, which can be a valuable characteristic in identification. For example, *B. licheniformis* and *B. subtilis*, which have very similar colonial (Fig. 4j) and microscopic (Fig. 3e) morphologies, are facultatively anaerobic and strictly aerobic, respectively; likewise, the two large-celled species *B. cereus* and *B. megaterium* (Fig. 3b and d) are facultatively anaerobic and strictly aerobic, respectively.

The most widely used diagnostic schemes involve traditional phenotypic tests (22) or miniaturized tests in the API

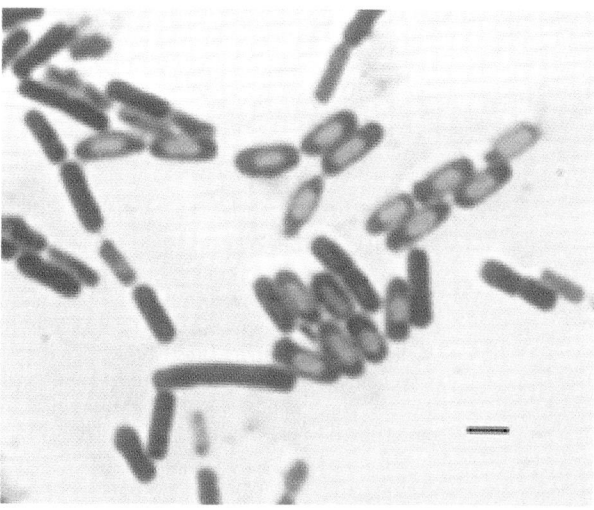

FIGURE 2 Photomicrograph of a spore-stained preparation of *B. cereus* sporangia, viewed by bright-field microscopy. Spores are stained green, and vegetative cells are counterstained red. Bar, 2 μm. (Courtesy of M. Rodriguez-Diaz.)

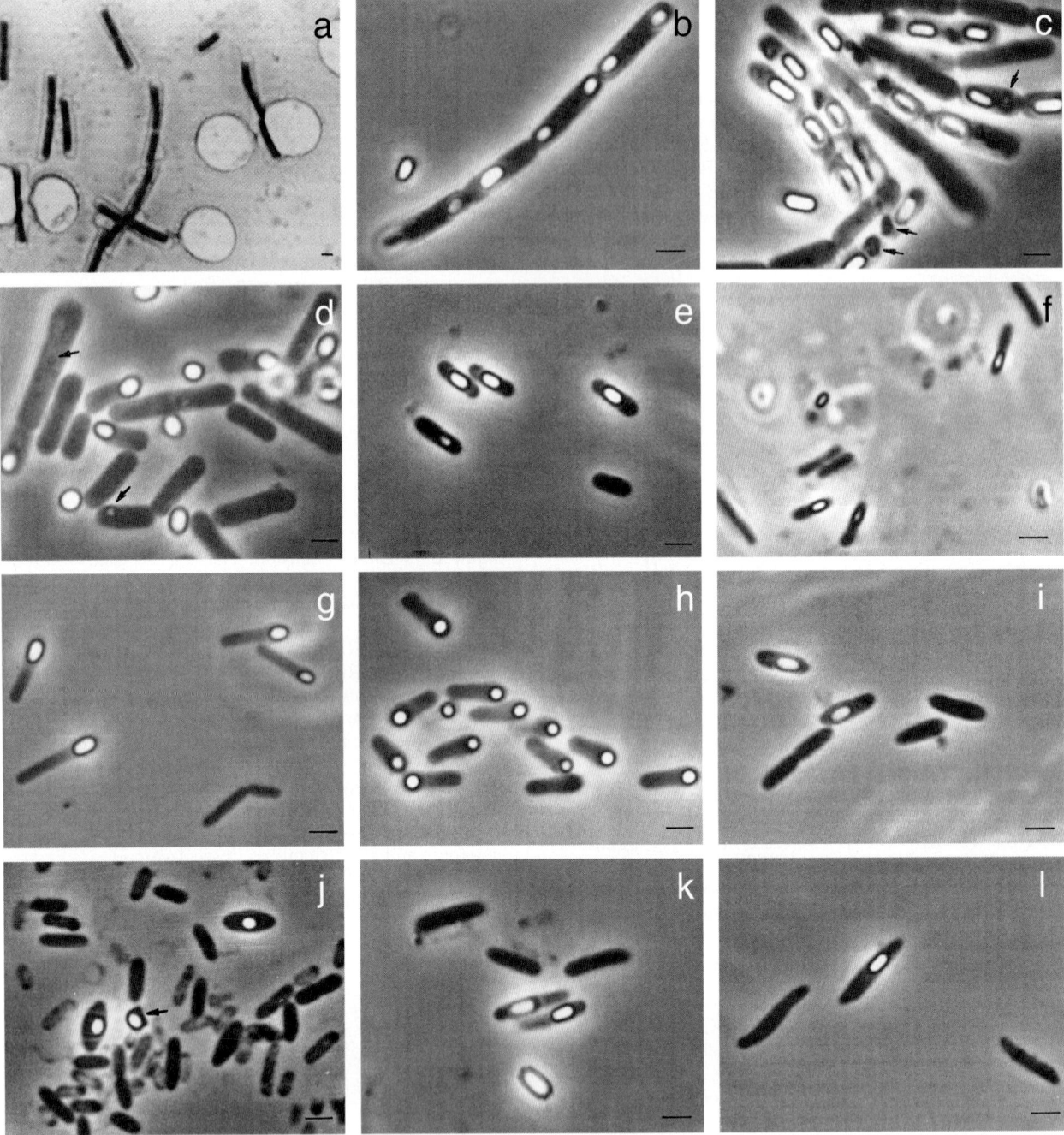

FIGURE 3 Photomicrographs of endospore-forming bacteria viewed by bright-field (a) and phase-contrast (b to l) microscopy. Bars, 2 μm. (a) *B. anthracis*, M'Fadyean stain showing capsulate rods in guinea pig blood smear; (b) *B. cereus*, broad cells with ellipsoidal, subterminal spores, not swelling the sporangia; (c) *B. thuringiensis*, broad cells with ellipsoidal, subterminal spores, not swelling the sporangia, and showing parasporal crystals of insecticidal toxin (arrowed); (d) *B. megaterium*, broad cells with ellipsoidal and spherical, subterminal and terminal spores, not swelling the sporangia, and showing PHB inclusions (arrows); (e) *B. subtilis*, ellipsoidal, central and subterminal spores, not swelling the sporangia; (f) *B. pumilus*, slender cells with cylindrical, subterminal spores, not swelling the sporangia; (g) *B. circulans*, ellipsoidal, subterminal spores, swelling the sporangia; (h) *B. sphaericus*, spherical, terminal spores, swelling the sporangia; (i) *Brevibacillus brevis*, ellipsoidal, subterminal spores, one swelling its sporangium slightly; (j) *Brevibacillus laterosporus*, ellipsoidal, central spores with thickened rims on one side (arrowed), swelling the sporangia; (k) *Paenibacillus polymyxa*, ellipsoidal, paracentral to subterminal spores, swelling the sporangia slightly; (l) *Paenibacillus alvei*, cells with tapered ends, ellipsoidal, paracentral to subterminal spores, not swelling the sporangium.

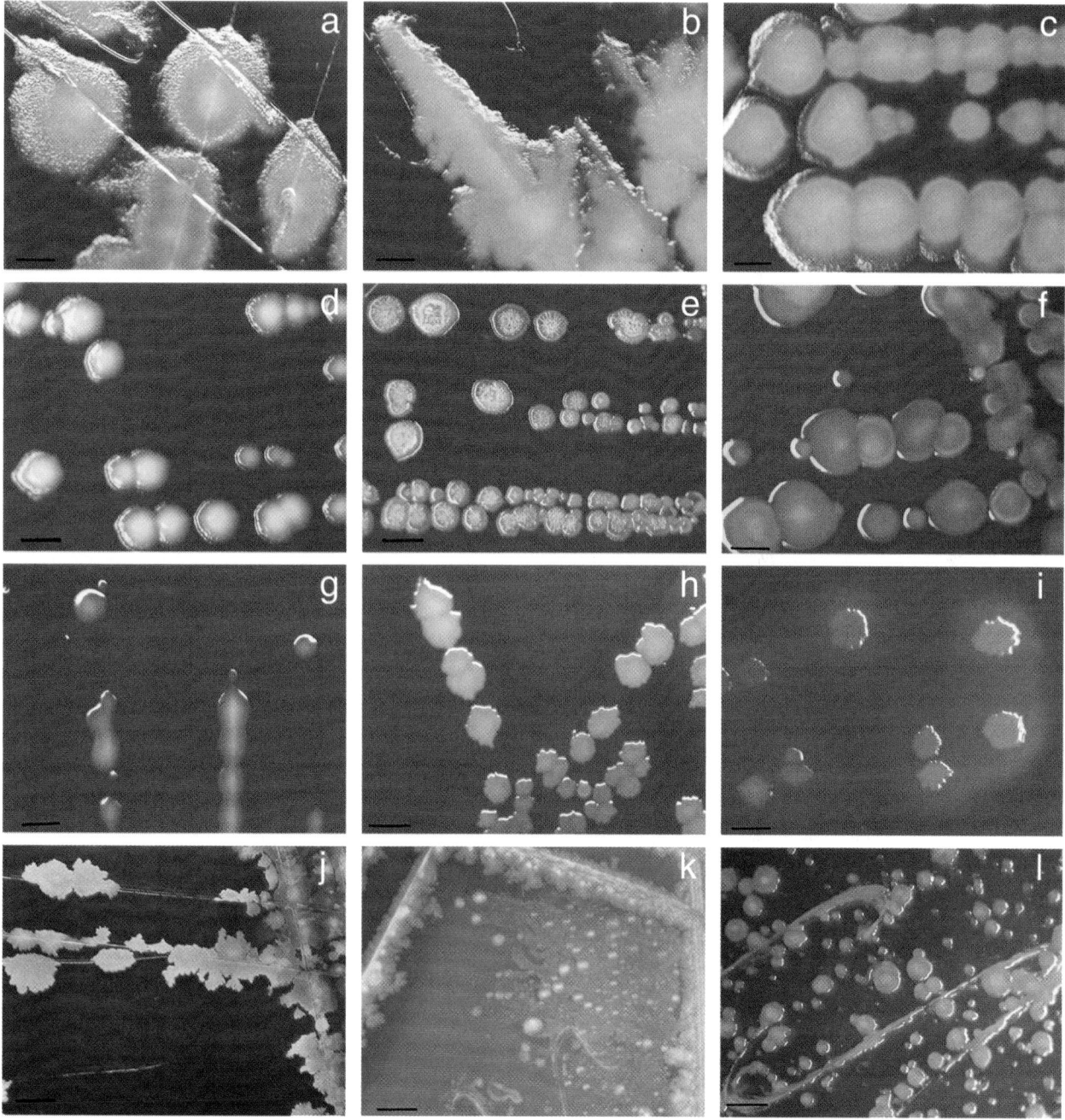

FIGURE 4 Colonies of endospore-forming bacteria on blood agar (a to i) and nutrient agar (j to l) after 24 to 36 h at 37°C. Bars, 2 mm. (a) *B. anthracis*; (b) *B. cereus*; (c) *B. thuringiensis*; (d) *B. megaterium*; (e) *B. pumilus*; (f) *B. sphaericus*; (g) *Brevibacillus brevis*; (h) *Brevibacillus laterosporus*; (i) *Paenibacillus polymyxa*; (j) *B. subtilis*; (k) *B. circulans*; (l) *Paenibacillus alvei*.

20E and 50CHB systems (bioMérieux, Marcy l'Etoile, France) (41, 42). The API 20E/50CHB kits can be used for the presumptive distinction of *B. anthracis* from other members of the *B. cereus* group within 48 h. bioMérieux also offers a *Bacillus* card for the Vitek automated identification system. Since many new species have been proposed since these schemes were established, updated API and Vitek databases need to be prepared. Biolog Inc. (Hayward, Calif.) also offers a *Bacillus* database. The effectiveness of such kits can vary with the genera and species of aerobic endospore formers concerned, but they are improving with continuing development and more extensive databases (41). It is stressed that their use should always be preceded by the basic characterization tests described below.

Other approaches include chemotaxonomic fingerprinting by fatty acid methyl ester profiling, polyacrylamide gel electrophoresis analysis, pyrolysis mass spectrometry, and Fourier-transform infrared spectroscopy. All these approaches have been successfully applied either across the genera or to small groups. As with genotypic profiling

TABLE 1 Characters for differentiating reactive *Bacillus*, *Paenibacillus*, and *Virgibacillus* species[a]

| Character[b] | Bacillus | | | | | | | | B. megaterium |
| | B. subtilis group | | | | B. cereus group | | | | |
	B. subtilis	B. amyloliquefaciens	B. licheniformis	B. pumilus	B. cereus[c]	B. anthracis	B. thuringiensis	B. mycoides	
Rod mean diameter (μm)	0.8	0.8	0.8	0.7	1.4	1.3	1.4	1.3	1.5
Chains of cells	(−)	(+)	(+)	−	+	+	+	+	+
Motility	+	+	+	+	+	−	+	−	+
Sporangia[d]									
Spore shape	E	E	E(C)	C, E	E(C) [E]	E	E(C)	E	E, S
Spore position	S, C	S, T	S, C	S, C	S, C	S	S	S(C)	S, C
Sporangium swollen	−	−	−	−	−	−	−	−	−
Parasporal crystals	−	−	−	−	−	−	+	−	−
Parasporal bodies	−	−	−	−	−	−	−	−	−
Anaerobic growth	−	−	+	−	+	+	+	+	−
Growth at:									
50°C	v	v	+	v	−	−	−	−	−
65°C	−	−	−	−	−	−	−	−	−
Egg yolk reaction	−	−	−	−	+	+	+	+	−
Casein hydrolysis	+	+	+	+	+	+	+	+	+
Starch hydrolysis	+	+	+	−	+	+	+	+	+
Arginine dihydrolase	−	−	+	−	v[(−)]	−	+	v	−
Indole production	−	−	−	−	−	−	−	−	−
Gelatin hydrolysis	+	+	+	+	+	(+)	+	+	+
Nitrate reduction	+	+	+	−	(+)[+]	+	+	(+)	−
Gas from carbohydrates	−	−	−	−	−	−	−	−	−
Acid from:									
D-Arabinose	−	−	−	−	−	−	−	−	−
Glycerol	+	+	+	ǀ	+[v]	−	+	+	+
Glycogen	+	+	+	−	+[−]	+	+	+	+
Inulin	(+)	−	v	−	−	−	−	−	+
Mannitol	+	+	+	+	−	−	−	−	+
Salicin	+	+	+	+	+[−]	−	(+)	(+)	+
D-Trehalose	+	+	+	+	+	+	+	+	+

[a] Symbols and abbreviations: +, >85% positive; (+), 75 to 84% positive; v, variable (26 to 74% positive); (−), 16 to 25% positive; −, 0 to 15% positive.
[b] Arginine dihydrolase, indole production, gelatin hydrolysis, and nitrate reduction reactions were determined using tests in the API 20E strip. Acid from carbohydrate reactions were determined using the API 50CHB system.

methods, large databases of authentic strains are necessary; some of these are commercially available, such as the Microbial Identification System software (Microbial ID. Inc., Newark, Del.) database for fatty acid methyl ester analysis.

For diagnostic purposes, the aerobic endospore formers comprise two groups, the reactive ones, which give positive results in various routine biochemical tests and which are therefore easier to identify, and the nonreactive ones, which give few if any positive results in such tests. Nonreactive isolates tend to dominate the identification requests sent to reference laboratories. Tables 1 and 2 show reactions for some species belonging to both of these groups, and the phenotypic test schemes (22, 42) outlined above may be used in conjunction with them. Characters for identifying other species may be found in references 13, 26, 28, and 42.

Bacillus cereus Group: Identification of *B. anthracis*

Colonies of *B. cereus* and relatives are very variable but readily recognized (Fig. 4a to c): they are characteristically large (2 to 7 mm in diameter) and vary in shape from circular to irregular, with entire to undulate, crenate, or fimbriate edges; they have matt or granular textures. Smooth and moist colonies are not uncommon, however. The optimum growth temperature is about 37°C, with minima and maxima of 15 to 20°C and 40 to 45°C, respectively. Although colonies of *B. anthracis* and *B. cereus* can be similar in appearance, those of the former are generally smaller and nonhemolytic, may show more spiking or tailing along the lines of inoculation streaks, and are very tenacious compared with the usually more butyrous consistency of *B. cereus* and *B. thuringiensis* colonies, so that they may be pulled into standing peaks with a loop. *B. mycoides* produces characteristic rhizoid or hairy-looking, adherent colonies which readily cover the whole agar surface.

It is generally easy to distinguish virulent *B. anthracis* from other members of the *B. cereus* group. An isolate with the correct colonial morphology (Fig. 4a), white or gray in color, nonhemolytic or only weakly hemolytic, nonmotile, susceptible to the diagnostic gamma phage (inquiries about gamma phage should be addressed to the Diagnostic Systems Division, USAMRIID, Fort Detrick, Frederick, MD 21702-5011) and penicillin, and able to produce the characteristic capsule (as shown by M'Fadyean staining; Fig. 3a) is *B. anthracis*.

Bacillus						Paenibacillus				Virgibacillus pantothenticus
B. circulans group			B. coagulans	B. stearothermophilus	B. thermodenitrificans	P. polymyxa	P. alvei	P. macerans	P. validus	
B. circulans	B. firmus	B. lentus								
0.8	0.8	0.8	0.8	0.9	0.8	0.9	0.8	0.7	0.80	0.6
−	−	(+)	v	−	v	−	(−)	−	−	+
+	+	+	+	+	−	+	+	+	+	+
E	E	E	E	E	E	E	E(C)	E	E	E, S
S, T	S(C)	S, C	S, T	S, T	S	S, C	S, C	S, T	S, T	S, T
+	v	v	+	+	−	+	+	+	+	+
−	−	−	−	−	−	−	−	−	−	−
−	−	−	−	−	−	−	−	−	−	−
+	−	−	+	−	−	+	+	+	−	+
−	−	−	+	+	+	−	−	v	v	v
−	−	−	−	+	+	−	−	−	−	−
−	−	−	−	−	−	−	+	−	−	−
−	+	v	v	(+)	(−)	+	+	−	−	+
+	+	+	+	+	+	+	+	+	+	+
(−)	−	−	v	−	−	−	−	−	−	(−)
−	−	−	−	−	−	−	+	−	−	−
−	v	v	−	+	+	+	+	v	−	+
v	(+)	(+)	(−)	v	(+)	v	−	−	v	v
−	−	−	−	−	−	+	−	+	−	−
−	−	−	−	−	−	−	−	+	−	+
v	−	v	+	(+)	v	+	+	+	+	+
+	−	v	−	+	−	+	v	+	v	−
(+)	−	(−)	−	−	−	+	−	+	v	−
+	v	(+)	v	−	v	+	−	+	+	−
+	−	+	+	(−)	v	+	v	+	−	+
+	v	(+)	+	+	+	+	v	+	+	+

^{c} Reactions shown in brackets are for the biotype isolated particularly in connection with outbreaks of emetic-type food poisoning and for strains of serovars 1, 3, 5, and 8, which are commonly associated with such outbreaks.

^{d} Spore shape: C, cylindrical; E, ellipsoidal; S, spherical. Spore position: C, central or paracentral; S, subterminal; T, terminal. The most-common shapes and positions are listed first, and those shown in parentheses are infrequently observed.

An isolate showing the characteristic phenotype but unable to produce capsules may be an avirulent form lacking either or both capsule or toxin genes (60) and should be referred to a specialist laboratory; such isolates are generally found in environmental samples and are frequently identified in routine laboratories as *B. cereus* and discarded. Primer sequences are now available for confirming the presence of the toxin and capsule genes (29) and hence the virulence of an isolate. Molecular studies are giving valuable insights into genetic profiles among the *B. cereus* group (31, 58).

The capsule of virulent *B. anthracis* can be demonstrated on nutrient agar plus 0.7% sodium bicarbonate incubated overnight under 5 to 7% CO_2 (candle jars perform well). Colonies of the encapsulated *B. anthracis* appear mucoid, and the capsule can be visualized by staining smears with M'Fadyean's polychrome methylene blue or India ink (59) or by indirect fluorescent-antibody staining (inquiries about fluorescent-antibody capsule staining should be addressed to USAMRIID at the above address). More simply, 2.5 ml of blood (defibrinated horse blood seems best; horse and fetal calf serum are quite good) can be inoculated with a pinhead quantity of growth from the suspect colony, incu-bated statically for 6 to 18 h at 37°C, and M'Fadyean stained (Fig. 3a). The M'Fadyean stain is preferable to other capsule-staining methods, since it is more specific for *B. anthracis* capsules.

The key characteristics for recognizing and distinguishing the *B. cereus* group are colonial morphology (Fig. 4a to c); large cells often in chains, producing ellipsoidal spores not swelling the sporangia (Fig. 3b and c), usually within 48 h and often apparent after 24 h; facultative anaerobes; and egg yolk reaction (i.e., lecithinase) positive. Negative or very weak hemolysis and lack of motility (hanging-drop or tubed medium) distinguish *B. anthracis* and *B. mycoides* from *B. cereus* and *B. thuringiensis*. *B. cereus*, *B. mycoides*, *B. thuringiensis*, and, to a lesser extent, *B. anthracis* synthesize lecithinases, forming opaque zones of precipitation around colonies on egg yolk agar as the colonies grow (i.e., usually after overnight or perhaps 24-h incubation). Recognition of *B. thuringiensis* is largely dependent on observation of its cuboid or diamond-shaped parasporal crystals in sporulated cultures (after 2 to 5 days) by phase-contrast microscopy (Fig. 3c) or by staining with malachite green.

TABLE 2 Characters for differentiating nonreactive *Bacillus*, *Aneurinibacillus*, and *Brevibacillus* species[a]

Character[b]	Bacillus		Aneurinibacillus aneurinilyticus	Brevibacillus		
	B. sphaericus	*B. badius*		*B. brevis*	*B. agri*	*B. laterosporus*
Rod mean diameter (μm)	1.0	0.9	0.8	0.9	0.9	0.9
Chains of cells	−	+	−	−	−	−
Motility	+	+	+	+	+	+
Sporangia[c]						
Spore shape	S(E)	E	E	E	E	E
Spore position	S, T	S, C, T	S, C	S, C	S, C	S, C
Sporangium swollen	+	−	+	+	+	+
Parasporal crystals	−	−	−	−	−	−
Parasporal bodies	−	−	−	−	−	+
Anaerobic growth	−	−	−	−	−	+
Growth at:						
50°C	−	+	+	−	v	−
65°C	−	−	−	−	−	−
Casein hydrolysis	v	+	−	+	+	+
Gelatin hydrolysis	−	+	−	+	+	+
Nitrate reduction	−	−	+	+	−	+
Acid from:						
Glycerol	−	−	+	v	−	+
Mannitol	−	−	−	v	+	+
D-Trehalose	−	−	−	−	v	+
Assimilation of:						
D-Fructose	(−)	−	−	+	+	+
D-Gluconate	+	−	v	+	+	−
D-Glucosamine	(−)	−	−	+	−	−
Glutarate	(−)	+	+	−	−	−
DL-Lactate	+	+	+	−	+	−
Putrescine	(−)	+	+	−	+	−
D-Trehalose	−	−	−	+	+	+

[a] Symbols and abbreviations: +, >85% positive; (+), 75 to 84% positive; v, variable (26 to 74% positive); (−), 16 to 25% positive; −, 0 to 15% positive.

[b] Gelatin hydrolysis and nitrate reduction reactions were determined using tests in the API 20E strip. Acids from carbohydrate reactions were determined using the API 50CHB system, and assimilation reactions were determined using the API Biotype 100 system; both kinds of reactions may also be investigated using the media described in reference 40, along with appropriate reference strains.

[c] Spore shape: C, cylindrical; E, ellipsoidal; S, spherical. Spore position: C, central or paracentral; S, subterminal; T, terminal. The most-common shapes and positions are listed first, and those shown in parentheses are infrequently observed.

Other Species

Other species show a very wide range of colonial morphologies, both within and between species, after 24 to 48 h (Fig. 4). They vary from moist and glossy (Fig. 4f to i) through granular to wrinkled (Fig. 4e); their shape varies from round to irregular (Fig. 4d to j), sometimes spreading (Fig. 4k and l), with entire through undulate or crenate to fimbriate edges (Fig. 4d to j); sizes range from 1 to 5 mm; color commonly ranges from buff or creamy grey to off-white, but some strains produce orange pigment; hemolysis may be absent, slight or marked, and partial or complete (Fig. 4h); elevations range from effuse through raised to convex; consistency is usually butyrous, but mucoid and dry, and adherent colonies are not uncommon. Despite this diversity, *Bacillus* colonies are not generally difficult to recognize, and some species have characteristic yet seemingly infinitely variable colonial morphologies, as does the *B. cereus* group (Fig. 4a to c).

B. subtilis and *B. licheniformis* produce similar colonies, which are exceptionally variable in appearance and often appear to be mixed cultures (Fig. 4j); colonies are irregular in shape and of moderate diameter (2 to 4 mm) and range from moist and butyrous or mucoid (with margins varying from undulate to fimbriate) through membranous with an underlying mucoid matrix, with or without mucoid bead-ing at the surface, to rough and crusty as they dry. The "licheniform" colonies of *B. licheniformis* tend to be quite adherent.

Rotating and migrating microcolonies, which may show spreading growth (Fig. 4k), have been observed macroscopically in about 13% of strains received as *B. circulans*, but this very heterogeneous species continues to undergo radical taxonomic revision, with many spreading strains being assigned to other species. Motile, spreading microcolonies, which commonly have an unpleasant smell, are more typical of *Paenibacillus alvei* (Fig. 4l).

Other species that have been encountered in the clinical laboratory include *B. coagulans*, *B. megaterium*, *B. pumilus*, and *B. sphaericus*; *B. brevis* and *B. laterosporus* (now both *Brevibacillus*); and *B. macerans* and *B. polymyxa* (now both *Paenibacillus*); they do not produce particularly distinctive growth (Fig. 4d to i).

Microscopic morphologies, particularly of sporangia (Fig. 3), are much more helpful for distinguishing between species. Vegetative cells are usually round ended, but those of *P. alvei* may be tapered (Fig. 3l). The large cells of *B. megaterium* may accumulate PHB (Fig. 3d) and appear vacuolate or foamy when grown on glucose nutrient agar. Overall, cell widths vary from about 0.5 to 1.5 μm, and lengths vary from 1.5 to 8 μm. Most strains of these species are motile. Spore shapes vary from cylindrical (Fig. 3f) through ellipsoidal (Fig. 3b, c to e, g, i to l) to spherical (Fig. 3d and h); bean or kidney-shaped, curved-cylindrical, and pear-shaped spores are also seen occasionally. Spores may be terminally (Fig. 3h), subterminally (Fig. 3b, c, f, g, and i), or centrally (Fig. 3e and j) positioned within sporangia and may distend them (Fig. 3g to k). Despite within-species and within-strain variation, sporangial morphologies tend to be characteristic of species and may allow tentative identification by the experienced worker. One species, *Brevibacillus laterosporus*, produces very distinctive ellipsoidal spores which have thickened rims on one side, so that they appear to be laterally displaced in the sporangia (Fig. 3j).

All these species are mesophilic and grow well between 30 and 37°C. Minimum temperatures for growth lie mostly between 5 and 20°C, and maxima lie mostly between 35 and 50°C. Strains of *B. coagulans* may show slight thermophily and grow up to 55 to 60°C.

SEROLOGICAL TESTS

Species and Strain Differentiation

Initial attempts to develop simple serological differentiation systems for *Bacillus* species were dogged by cross-reacting antigens and autoagglutination of the hydrophobic spores. Monoclonal antibody tests based on specific spore cortex or cell wall epitopes, for reliable differentiation of *B. anthracis* from close relatives, are not yet available. Breakthroughs have recently been made in the long-standing problem of differentiating strains of *B. anthracis* for epidemiological and strategic purposes by using amplified fragment length polymorphism analysis (29, 31).

A strain differentiation system for *B. cereus* based on flagellar (H) antigens is available at the Food Hygiene Laboratory, Central Public Health Laboratory, Colindale, London, United Kingdom, for investigations of food-poisoning outbreaks or other *B. cereus*-associated clinical problems (34).

B. thuringiensis strains are classified on the basis of their flagellar antigens; 82 serovars have been recognized (36). This is done at the Pasteur Institute, Paris, France, and at Abbott Laboratories, North Chicago, Ill.

Toxin and Antitoxin Detection

The three protein components of anthrax toxin (protective antigen [PA], lethal factor [LF], and edema factor [EF]) and antibodies to them can be used in enzyme immunoassay systems. For routine confirmation of anthrax infection or for monitoring responses to anthrax vaccines, antibodies against protective antigen alone appear to be satisfactory; they have proved useful for epidemiological investigations in humans and animals. In human anthrax, however, early treatment sometimes prevents antibody development (57). The current human vaccine in the United States is an aluminium hydroxide-adsorbed vaccine strain culture filtrate containing a relatively high proportion of PA and relatively small amounts of LF and EF (56).

In countries of the former USSR, a skin test utilizing Anthraxin (trade mark), a heat-stable extract from a noncapsulate strain of *B. anthracis*, which has been licensed for human and animal use since 1962 is widely acclaimed for the retrospective diagnosis of anthrax (52). The delayed-type hypersensitivity is interpreted as indicating cell-mediated immunity to anthrax and can be used to diagnose

anthrax retrospectively or to evaluate the vaccine-induced immune status after several years. Anthraxin does not contain highly specific anthrax antigens and depends on the nature of anthrax rather than the specificity of the antigens involved. This is also true of the Ascoli test, which, dating from 1911, must be one of the oldest antigen detection tests in microbiology. It is a precipitin test using hyperimmune serum raised to *B. anthracis* whole-cell antigen to provide rapid retrospective evidence of anthrax infection in an animal from which the material being tested was derived. The test is still in use in eastern Europe and central Asia.

The enterotoxin complex responsible for the diarrheal type of *B. cereus* food poisoning has been increasingly well characterized (23). Two commercial kits are available for its detection in foods and feces, the BCET-RPLA (Oxoid Ltd., Basingstoke, United Kingdom; product code TD950) and the VIA (TECRA Diagnostics, Roseville, NSW, Australia; product code BDEVIA48). However, these kits detect different antigens, and there is some controversy about their reliabilities. Other assays, based on tissue culture, have also been developed (19). The emetic toxin of *B. cereus* has been identified as a dodecadepsipeptide, and it may be assayed in food extracts or culture filtrates using HEp-2 cells (18).

STRAIN DIFFERENTIATION FOR *BACILLUS ANTHRACIS*

As a species, *B. anthracis* is highly monomorphic, and it is only very recently that strain differentiation has become possible by means of molecular methods. Particular success has now been achieved by means of multilocus variable-number tandem repeat analysis (31). This is, however, a technique currently confined to the specialist laboratory. Inquiries about strain typing should be addressed to Dr. Paul Keim, Department of Biological Sciences, Northern Arizona University, P.O. Box 5640, Flagstaff, AZ 86011.

ANTIMICROBIAL SUSCEPTIBILITIES

B. anthracis is almost invariably susceptible to penicillin; only five published reports of resistant isolates appear to exist. It is susceptible to gentamicin, erythromycin, and chloramphenicol, and tests in primates and guinea pigs have shown that infection responds to ciprofloxacin and doxycycline. It is normally susceptible to streptomycin but resistant to cephalosporins. Combination therapy, begun early, with a fluoroquinolone such as ciprofloxacin and at least one other antibiotic to which the organism is sensitive, appears to improve survival (30).

B. cereus and *B. thuringiensis* produce a broad-spectrum β-lactamase and are thus resistant to penicillin, ampicillin, and cephalosporins. They are also resistant to trimethoprim but almost always susceptible to clindamycin, erythromycin, chloramphenicol, vancomycin, and the aminoglycosides and usually sensitive to tetracycline and sulfonamides. However, a fulminant meningitis which did not respond to chloramphenicol has been reported (44). Oral ciprofloxacin has been used successfully in the treatment of *B. cereus* wound infections. Clindamycin with gentamicin, given early, appears to be the best treatment for ophthalmic infections caused by *B. cereus*, and experiments with rabbits suggest that intravitreal corticosteroids and antibiotics may be effective in such cases (38).

Information is sparse on treatment of infections by other *Bacillus* species. Gentamicin was effective in treating a case of *B. licheniformis* ophthalmitis, and cephalosporin was effective against *B. licheniformis* bacteremia and septicemia. *B. subtilis* endocarditis in a drug abuser was successfully treated with cephalosporin, and gentamicin was successful against a *B. subtilis* septicemia. Penicillin, its derivatives, or cephalosporins probably form the best first choices for treatment of infections attributed to other *Bacillus* species. Strains of *B. cereus*, other *Bacillus* species, and *Paenibacillus* showing vancomycin resistance have been isolated from clinical specimens (37; A. von Gottberg and W. van Nierop, personal communication).

EVALUATION, INTERPRETATION, AND REPORTING OF RESULTS

Apart from *B. anthracis*, the majority of *Bacillus* species are common environmental contaminants, and isolation from a single clinical specimen is generally not a sufficient basis for incriminating one of these organisms as the etiological agent. Moderate or heavy growth of aerobic endospore formers from wounds is usually significant, however, and *B. cereus* infections of the eye are emergencies which should always be taken seriously and reported to the physician immediately.

In the clinical laboratory, the most important questions to ask about an aerobic spore-forming isolate are the following. Was it isolated in pure culture or at least apparently dominating the flora? Was it isolated in large numbers? Was it isolated more than once? A repeatedly isolated aerobic endospore former, found in large numbers in pure culture, particularly from blood cultures, is unlikely to be a mere contaminant. Histopathology and tests on the toxigenicity of the isolate may also help decide the relevance of the isolate.

Low-level contamination of foodstuffs by aerobic endospore formers is common, as is asymptomatic transient fecal carriage by human and animal populations. Therefore, in food-borne illness investigations, qualitative isolation tests are insufficient. The ideal criteria for establishing that an aerobic endospore former is the etiological agent are the isolation of significant numbers ($>10^5$ CFU/g) of the organism from the epidemiologically incriminated food (and, in the case of suspected *B. cereus* food poisoning, detection of emetic toxin and/or enterotoxin) together with recovery of the same strain (biovar, serovar, phage type, plasmid type, etc.) in significant numbers from acute-phase specimens (feces or vomitus) from the patients. In practice, it is rare that these ideal criteria can be met. A complete set of the appropriate food and clinical specimens is seldom available, and the epidemiological aspects of the outbreak, such as incubation times, clinical symptoms, the types of food implicated, the time lapse between the episode and specimen collection, and the manner in which the food was stored during this period, must all be considered along with the laboratory findings in forming conclusions about the etiology.

B. anthracis continues to be generally regarded as an obligate pathogen; its continued existence in the ecosystem appears to depend on a periodic multiplication phase within an animal host, and its environmental presence reflects contamination from an animal source at some time rather than self-maintenance within the environment. When human and animal specimens are tested, it is usually sought only when the case history suggests that it is reasonable to suspect anthrax. Demonstration of encapsulating *B. anthracis* cells, even in small numbers, confirms the clinical suspicion of anthrax, because the bacterium is rapidly destroyed by putrefactive processes after the host's death.

REFERENCES

1. **Anonymous** 1994. Anthrax control and research, with special reference to national programme development in Africa: Memorandum from a WHO meeting. *Bull. W. H. O.* **72:**13–22.
2. **Ash, C., F. G. Priest, and M. D. Collins.** 1993. Molecular identification of rRNA group 3 bacilli (Ash, Farrow, Wallbanks and Collins) using a PCR probe test. *Antonie Leeuwenhoek* **64:**253–260.
3. **Beecher, D. J.** 2002. The *Bacillus cereus* group, p. 1161–1190. *In* M. Sussman (ed.), *Molecular Medical Microbiology.* Academic Press, Ltd., London, United Kingdom.
4. **Berkeley, R. C. W., and N. A. Logan.** 1997. *Bacillus, Alicyclobacillus* and *Paenibacillus,* p. 185–204. *In* A. M. Emmerson, P. M. Hawkey, and S. H. Gillespie (ed.), *Principles and Practice of Clinical Bacteriology.* John Wiley & Sons, Ltd., Chichester, United Kingdom.
5. **Blowey, R., and P. Edmondson.** 1995. *Mastitis Control in Dairy Herds. An Illustrated and Practical Guide.* Farming Press Books, Ipswich, United Kingdom.
6. **Blue, S. R., V. R. Singh, and M. A. Saubolle.** 1995. *Bacillus licheniformis* bacteremia: five cases associated with indwelling central venous catheters. *Clin. Infect. Dis.* **20:**620–633.
7. **Boone, D. R., Y. Liu, Z.-J. Zhao, D. L. Balkwill, G. R. Drake, T. O. Stevens, and H. C. Aldrich.** 1995. *Bacillus infernus* sp. nov., an Fe(III)- and Mn(IV)-reducing anaerobe from the deep terrestrial subsurface. *Int. J. Syst. Bacteriol.* **45:**441–448.
8. **Brachman, P., and A. Kaufmann.** 1998. Anthrax, p. 95–107. *In* A. Evans and P. Brachman (ed.), *Bacterial Infections of Humans.* Plenum Medical Book Co., New York, N.Y.
9. **Briley, R. T., J. H. Teel, and J. P. Fowler.** 2001. Nontypical *Bacillus cereus* outbreak in a child care center. *J. Environ. Health* **63:**9–11.
10. **Burans, J., A. Keleher, T. O'Brien, J. Hager, A. Plummer, and C. Morgan.** 1996. Rapid method for the diagnosis of *Bacillus anthracis* infection in clinical samples using a hand-held assay. *Salisbury Med. Bull.* **87** (Spec. Suppl.):36–37.
11. **Centers for Disease Control and Prevention.** 2000. Human ingestion of *Bacillus anthracis*-contaminated meat—Minnesota, August 2000. *JAMA* **284:**1644–1646.
12. **Christopher, G. W., T. J. Cieslak, J. A. Pavlin, and E. M. Eitzen.** 1997. Biological warfare; a historical perspective. *JAMA* **278:**412–417.
13. **Claus, D., and R. C. W. Berkeley.** 1986. Genus *Bacillus* Cohn 1872, p. 1105–1139. *In* P. H. A. Sneath, N. S. Mair, M. E. Sharpe, and J. G. Holt (ed.), *Bergey's Manual of Systematic Bacteriology,* vol. 2. The Williams & Wilkins Co., Baltimore, Md.
14. **Collins, C. H.** 1988. *Laboratory Acquired Infections,* 2nd ed., p. 16. Butterworths, London, United Kingdom.
15. **Damgaard, P. H., P. E. Granum, J. Bresciani, M. V. Torregrossa, J. Eilenberg, and L. Valentino.** 1997. Characterization of *Bacillus thuringiensis* isolated from infections in burn wounds. *FEMS Immunol. Med. Microbiol.* **18:**47–53.
16. **Davey, R. T., Jr., and W. B. Tauber.** 1987. Posttraumatic endophthalmitis: the emerging role of *Bacillus cereus* infection. *Rev. Infect. Dis.* **9:**110–123.

17. **Dietvorst, D. C. E.** 1996. Farmers' attitudes towards the control and prevention of anthrax in Western Province, Zambia. *Salisbury Med. Bull.* **87** (Spec. Suppl.):102–103.

18. **Finlay, W. J. J., N. A. Logan, and A. D. Sutherland.** 1999. Semiautomated metabolic staining assay for *Bacillus cereus* emetic toxin. *Appl. Environ. Microbiol.* **65:**1811–1812.

19. **Fletcher, P., and N. A. Logan.** 1999. Improved cytotoxicity assay for *Bacillus cereus* diarrhoeal enterotoxin. *Lett. Appl. Microbiol.* **28:**394–400.

20. **Fortina, M. G., R. Pukall, P. Schumann, D. Mora, C. Parini, P. L. Manachini, and E. Stackebrandt.** 2001. *Ureibacillus* gen. nov., a new genus to accommodate *Bacillus thermosphaericus* (Andersson *et al.* 1995), emendation of *Ureibacillus thermosphaericus* and description of *Ureibacillus terrenus* sp. nov. *Int. J. Syst. Evol. Microbiol.* **51:**447–455.

21. **Golovacheva, R. S., and G. I. Karavaiko.** 1978. A new genus of thermophilic spore-forming bacteria, *Sulfobacillus*. *Microbiologya* **47:**658–665.

22. **Gordon, R. E., W. C. Haynes, and C. H.-N. Pang.** 1973. *The Genus* Bacillus. Agriculture Handbook 427. U.S. Department of Agriculture, Washington, D.C.

23. **Granum, P. E.** 2002. *Bacillus cereus* and food poisoning, p. 37–46. *In* R. C. W. Berkeley, M. Heyndrickx, N. A. Logan, and P. de Vos (ed.), *Applications and Systematics of* Bacillus *and Relatives.* Blackwell Science, Oxford, United Kingdom.

24. **Hanna, P.** 1999. Lethal toxin actions and their consequences. *J. Appl. Microbiol.* **87:**285–287.

25. **Hanna, P. C., and J. A. W. Ireland.** 1999. Understanding *Bacillus anthracis* pathogenesis. *Trends Microbiol.* **7:**180–182.

26. **Heyndrickx, M., K. Vandemeulebroecke, P. Scheldeman, K. Kersters, P. De Vos, N. A. Logan, A. M. Aziz, N. Ali, and R. C. W. Berkeley.** 1996. A polyphasic reassessment of the genus *Paenibacillus*, reclassification of *Bacillus lautus* (Nakamura 1984) as *Paenibacillus lautus* comb. nov. and of *Bacillus peoriae* (Montefusco et al. 1993) as *Paenibacillus peoriae* comb. nov. Emended descriptions of *P. lautus* and of *P. peoriae*. *Int. J. Syst. Bacteriol.* **46:**988–1003.

27. **Heyndrickx, M., L. Lebbe, M. Vancanneyt, K. Kersters, P. De Vos, G. Forsyth, and N. A. Logan.** 1998. *Virgibacillus:* a new genus to accommodate *Bacillus pantothenticus* (Proom and Knight 1950). Emended description of *Virgibacillus pantothenticus*. *Int. J. Syst. Bacteriol.* **48:**99–106.

28. **Heyndrickx, M., L. Lebbe, M. Vancanneyt, K. Kersters, P. De Vos, N. A. Logan, G. Forsyth, S. Nazli, N. Ali, and R. C. W. Berkeley.** 1997. A polyphasic reassessment of the genus *Aneurinibacillus*, reclassification of *Bacillus thermoaerophilus* (Meier-Stauffer *et al.* 1996) as *Aneurinibacillus thermoaerophilus* comb. nov. and emended descriptions of *A. aneurinolyticus*, of *A. migulanus* and of *A. thermoaerophilus*. *Int. J. Syst. Bacteriol.* **47:**808–817.

29. **Jackson, P. J., M. E. Hugh-Jones, D. M. Adair, G. Green, K. K. Hill, C. R. Kuske, L. M. Grinberg, F. A. Abramova, and P. Keim.** 1998. PCR analysis of tissue samples from the 1979 Sverdlovsk anthrax victims: the presence of multiple *Bacillus anthracis* strains in different victims. *Proc. Natl. Acad. Sci. USA* **95:**1224–1229.

30. **Jernigan, J. A., D. S. Stephens, D. A. Ashford, C. Omenaca, M. S. Topiel, M. Galbraith, M. Tapper, T. L. Fisk, S. Zaki, T. Popovic, R. F. Meyer, C. P. Quinn, S. A. Harper, S. K. Fridkin, J. J. Sejvar, C. W. Shepard, M. McConnell, J. Guarner, W.-J. Shieh, J. M. Malecki, J. L. Gerberding, J. M. Hughes, and B. A. Perkins.** 2001. Bioterrorism-related inhalational anthrax: the first 10 cases reported in the United States. *Emerg. Infect. Dis.* **7:**933–944. [Online.]

31. **Keim, P., L. B. Price, A. M. Klevytska, K. L. Smith, J. M. Schupp, R. Okinaka, P. J. Jackson, and M. E. Hugh-Jones.** 2000. Multiple-locus variable-number tandem repeat analysis reveals genetic relationships within *Bacillus anthracis*. *J. Bacteriol.* **182:**2928–2936.

32. **Klietmann, W. F., and K. L. Ruoff.** 2001. Bioterrorism: implications for the clinical microbiologist. *Clin. Microbiol. Rev.* **14:**364–381.

33. **Knisely, R. F.** 1966. Selective medium for *Bacillus anthracis*. *J. Bacteriol.* **92:**784–786.

34. **Kramer, J. M., and R. J. Gilbert.** 1992. *Bacillus cereus* gastroenteritis, p. 119–153. *In* A. T. Tu (ed.), *Food Poisoning. Handbook of Natural Toxins*, vol. 7. Marcel Dekker, Inc., New York, N.Y.

35. **Lane, H. C., and A. S. Fauci.** 2001. Bioterrorism on the home front: a new challenge for American medicine. *JAMA* **286:**2595–2597.

36. **Lecadet, M.-M., E. Frachon, V. Cosmao Dumanoir, H. Ripouteau, S. Hamon, P. Laurent, and I. Thiéry.** 1999. Updating the H-antigen classification of *Bacillus thuringiensis*. *J. Appl. Microbiol.* **86:**660–672.

37. **Ligozzi, M., G. L. Cascio, and R. Fontana.** 1998. *vanA* gene cluster in a vancomycin-resistant clinical isolate of *Bacillus circulans*. *Antimicrob. Agents Chemother.* **42:**2055–2059.

38. **Liu, S. M., T. Way, M. Rodrigues, and S. M. Steidl.** 2000. Effects of intravitreal corticosteroids in the treatment of *Bacillus cereus* endophthalmitis. *Arch. Ophthalmol.* **118:**803–806.

39. **Logan, N. A.** 1988. *Bacillus* species of medical and veterinary importance. *J. Med. Microbiol.* **25:**157–165.

40. **Logan, N. A.** 1989. Numerical taxonomy of violet-pigmented, gram-negative bacteria and description of *Iodobacter fluviatile* gen. nov., comb. nov. *Int. J. Syst. Bacteriol.* **40:**297–301.

41. **Logan, N. A.** 2002. Modern identification methods, p. 123–140. *In* R. C. W. Berkeley, M. Heyndrickx, N. A. Logan, and P. de Vos (ed.), *Applications and Systematics of* Bacillus *and Relatives.* Blackwell Science, Oxford, United Kingdom.

42. **Logan, N. A., and R. C. W. Berkeley.** 1984. Identification of *Bacillus* strains using the API system. *J. Gen. Microbiol.* **130:**1871–1882.

43. **Mahler, H., A. Pasi, J. M. Kramer, P. Schulte, A. C. Scoging, W. Bär, and S. Krähenbühl.** 1997. Fulminant liver failure in association with the emetic toxin of *Bacillus cereus*. *N. Engl. J. Med.* **336:**1142–1148.

44. **Marshman, L. A. G., C. Hardwidge, and P. M. W. Donaldson.** 2000. *Bacillus cereus* meningitis complicating cerebrospinal fluid fistula repair and spinal drainage. *Br. J. Neurosurg.* **14:**580–582.

45. **Meselson, M., J. Guillemin, M. Hugh-Jones, A. Langmuir, I. Popova, A. Shelokov, and O. Yampolskaya.** 1994. The Sverdlovsk anthrax outbreak of 1979. *Science* **266:**1202–1208.

46. **Mikkola, R., M. Kolari, M. A. Andersson, J. Helin, and M. S. Salkinoja-Salonen.** 2000. Toxic lactonic lipopeptide from food poisoning isolates of *Bacillus licheniformis*. *Eur. J. Biochem.* **267:**4068–4074.

47. **Nazina, T. N., T. P. Tourova, A. B. Poltaraus, E. V. Novikova, A. A. Grigoryan, A. E. Ivanova, A. M. Lysenko, V. V. Petrunyaka, G. A. Osipov, S. S. Belyaev, and M. V. Ivanov.** 2001. Taxonomic study of aerobic thermophilic bacilli: descriptions of *Geobacillus subterraneus* gen. nov., sp. nov. and *Geobacillus uzenensis* sp. nov. from petroleum reservoirs and transfer of *Bacillus stearothermophilus, Bacillus thermocatenulatus, Bacillus thermoleo-*

vorans, Bacillus kaustophilus, Bacillus thermoglucosidasius, Bacillus thermodenitrificans to *Geobacillus* as *Geobacillus stearothermophilus, Geobacillus thermocatenulatus, Geobacillus thermoleovorans, Geobacillus kaustophilus, Geobacillus thermoglucosidasius, Geobacillus thermodenitrificans. Int. J. Syst. Evol. Microbiol.* **51**:433–446.

48. **Niimura, Y., E. Koh, F. Yanagida, K.-I. Suzuki, K. Komagata, and M. Kozaki.** 1990. *Amphibacillus xylanus* gen. nov., sp. nov., a facultatively anaerobic sporeforming xylan-digesting bacterium which lacks cytochrome, quinone, and catalase. *Int. J. Syst. Bacteriol.* **40**:297–301.

49. **Oggioni, M., G. Pozzi, P. E. Valensis, P. Galieni, and C. Bigazzi.** 1998. Recurrent septicemia in an immunocompromised patient due to probiotic strains of *Bacillus subtilis. J. Clin. Microbiol.* **36**:325–326.

50. **Rothschild, M. A., and O. Leisenfeld.** 1996. Is the exploding powder from blank cartridges sterile? *Forensic Sci. Int.* **83**:1–13.

51. **Shida, O., H. Takagi, K. Kadowaki, and K. Komagata.** 1996. Proposal for two new genera, *Brevibacillus* gen. nov. and *Aneurinibacillus* gen. nov. *Int. J. Syst. Bacteriol.* **46**: 939–946.

52. **Shlyakhov, E., and E. Rubinstein.** 1994. Human live anthrax vaccine in the former USSR. *Vaccine* **12**:727–730.

53. **Spring, S., W. Ludwig, M. C. Marquez, A. Ventosa, and K.-H. Schleifer.** 1996. *Halobacillus* gen. nov., with descriptions of *Halobacillus litoralis* sp. nov. and *Halobacillus trueperi* sp. nov., and transfer of *Sporosarcina halophila* to *Halobacillus halophilus* comb. nov. *Int. J. Syst. Bacteriol.* **46**:492–496.

54. **Tandon, A., M. L. Tay-Kearney, C. Metcalf, and I. McAllister.** 2001. *Bacillus circulans* endophthalmitis. *Clin. Exp. Ophthalmol.* **29**:92–93.

55. **Touzel, J. P., M. O'Donohue, P. Debeire, E. Samain, and C. Breton.** 2000. *Thermobacillus xylanilyticus* gen. nov., sp. nov., a new aerobic thermophilic xylan-degrading bacterium isolated from soil. *Int. J Syst. Evol. Microbiol.* **50**: 315–320.

56. **Turnbull, P. C. B.** 2000. Current status of immunization against anthrax: old vaccines may be here to stay for a while. *Curr. Opin. Infect. Dis.* **13**:113–120.

57. **Turnbull, P. C. B., M. Doganay, P. M. Lindeque, B. Aygen, and J. McLaughlin.** 1992. Serology and anthrax in humans, livestock and Etosha National Park wildlife. *Epidemiol. Infect.* **108**:299–313.

58. **Turnbull, P. C. B., P. J. Jackson, K. K. Hill, A.-B. Kolstø, P. Keim, and D. J. Beecher.** 2002. Longstanding taxonomic enigmas with the 'Bacillus cereus group' are on the verge of being resolved by far-reaching molecular developments. Forecasts on the possible outcome by an *ad hoc* team, p. 23–36. *In* R. C. W. Berkeley, M. Heyndrickx, N. A. Logan, and P. de Vos (ed.), *Applications and Systematics of* Bacillus *and Relatives.* Blackwell Science, Oxford, United Kingdom.

59. **Turnbull, P. C. B., R. Böhm, O. Cosivi, M. Doganay, M. E. Hugh-Jones, D. D. Joshi, M. K. Lalitha, and V. de Vos.** 1998. *Guidelines for the Surveillance and Control of Anthrax in Humans and Animals.* WHO/EMC/ZDI/98.6, World Health Organization, Geneva, Switzerland.

60. **Turnbull, P. C. B., R. A. Hutson, M. J. Ward, M. N. Jones, C. P. Quinn, N. J. Finnie, C. J. Duggleby, J. M. Kramer, and J. Melling.** 1992. *Bacillus anthracis* but not always anthrax. *J. Appl. Bacteriol.* **72**:21–28.

61. **Van der Zwet, W. C., G. A. Parlevliet, P. H. Savelkoul, J. Stoof, A. M. Kaiser, A. M. Van Furth, and C. M. Vandenbroucke-Grauls.** 2000. Outbreak of *Bacillus cereus* infections in a neonatal intensive care unit traced to balloons used in manual ventilation. *J. Clin. Microbiol.* **38**:4131–4136.

62. **van Netten, P., and J. M. Kramer.** 1992. Media for the detection and enumeration of *Bacillus cereus* in foods: a review. *Int. J. Food Microbiol.* **17**:85–99.

63. **Wainø, M., B. J. Tindall, P. Schumann, and K. Ingvorsen.** 1999. *Gracilibacillus* gen. nov., with description of *Gracilibacillus halotolerans* gen. nov., sp. nov.: transfer of *Bacillus dipsosauri* to *Gracilibacillus dipsosauri* comb. nov., and *Bacillus salexigens* to the genus *Salibacillus* gen. nov., as *Salibacillus salexigens* comb. nov. *Int. J. Syst. Bacteriol.* **49**:821–831.

64. **Wisotzkey, J. D., P. Jurtshuk, Jr., G. E. Fox, G. Deinhard, and K. Poralla.** 1992. Comparative sequence analyses on the 16S rRNA (rDNA) of *Bacillus acidocaldarius, Bacillus acidoterrestris,* and *Bacillus cycloheptanicus* and proposal for creation of a new genus, *Alicyclobacillus* gen. nov. *Int. J. Syst. Bacteriol.* **42**:263–269.

65. **Yoon, J.-H., K.-C. Lee, N. Weiss, Y. H. Kho, K. H. Kang, and Y.-H. Park.** 2001. *Sporosarcina aquimarina* sp. nov., a bacterium isolated from seawater in Korea, and transfer of *Bacillus globisporus* (Larkin and Stokes 1967), *Bacillus psychrophilus* (Nakamura 1984), and *Bacillus pasteurii* (Chester 1898) to the genus *Sporosarcina* as *Sporosarcina globispora* comb. nov., *Sporosarcina psychrophila* comb. nov. and *Sporosarcina pasteurii* comb. nov., and emended description of the genus *Sporosarcina. Int. J. Syst. Evol. Microbiol.* **51**:1079–1086.

66. **Zaitsev, G., I. V. Tsitko, F. A. Rainey, Y. A. Trotsenko, J. S. Uotila, E. Stackebrandt, and M. S. Salkinoja-Salonen.** 1998. New aerobic ammonium-dependent obligately oxalotrophic bacteria: description of *Ammoniphilus oxalaticus* gen. nov., sp. nov. and *Ammoniphilus oxalivorans* gen. nov., sp. nov. *Int. J. Syst. Bacteriol.* **48**:151–163.

Listeria and Erysipelothrix

JACQUES BILLE, JOCELYNE ROCOURT,
AND BALA SWAMINATHAN

33

LISTERIA

Taxonomy

Listeria and *Brochothrix* form one of several sublines within the *Clostridium* subdivision. The *Listeria-Brochothrix* subline is approximately equidistant from the *Bacillus* and *Enterococcus-Carnobacterium* sublines. On the basis of 23S rRNA sequences, *Listeria* is most similar to *Bacillus* and *Staphylococcus*. Phylogenetically, *Listeria* is sufficiently remote from *Lactobacillus* to justify its exclusion from the family *Lactobacillaceae* and formation of a separate *Listeria-Brochothrix* family (20). The phylogenetic position of *Listeria* is consistent with the low G+C content of its DNA (36 to 42 mol%) (20, 45, 73).

Listeria monocytogenes is the type species and one of six species in the genus *Listeria*. The other species are *L. ivanovii*, *L. innocua*, *L. seeligeri*, *L. welshimeri*, and *L. grayi* (81). Two subspecies of *L. ivanovii* have been described: *L. ivanovii* subsp. *ivanovii* and *L. ivanovii* subsp. *londoniensis*. Based on the results of DNA-DNA hybridization, multilocus enzyme analysis, and 16S rRNA sequencing, the six species in the genus *Listeria* are divided into two lines of descent: (i) *L. monocytogenes* and its closely related species, namely, *L. innocua*, *L. ivanovii* (subspecies *ivanovii* and *londoniensis*), *L. welshimeri*, and *L. seeligeri*, and (ii) *L. grayi* (14, 15, 20, 64, 67). Within the genus *Listeria*, only *L. monocytogenes* and *L. ivanovii* are considered to be pathogenic, as evidenced by their 50% lethal dose in mice and their ability to grow in mouse spleen and liver. *L. monocytogenes* is a human pathogen of high public health concern; *L. ivanovii* is primarily an animal pathogen.

Description of the Genus

Members of the genus *Listeria* are asporogenous, nonbranching, regular, short (0.5 to 2 by 0.4 to 0.5 μm) gram-positive rods that occur singly or in short chains. Filaments 6 to 20 μm long may occur in older or rough cultures. The organisms are motile at 28°C by means of one to five peritrichous flagella but are much less motile at 37°C. Colonies are small (1 to 2 mm after 1 or 2 days of incubation at 37°C), smooth, and blue-gray on nutrient agar when examined with obliquely transmitted light. The optimum growth temperature is between 30 and 37°C, but growth occurs at 4°C within a few days. *Listeria* spp. are facultatively anaerobic. Catalase is produced except in a few strains (23), and the oxidase test is negative. Acid is produced from D-glucose and other sugars. The Voges-Proskauer and methyl red tests are positive. Esculin is hydrolyzed in a few hours. Urea and gelatin are not hydrolyzed. Neither indole nor H_2S is produced. The cell wall contains a directly cross-linked peptidoglycan based on *meso*-diaminopimelic acid, as well as lipoteichoic acid, but no mycolic acid; the major menaquinone (MK-7) contains seven isoprene units. The G+C content of the DNA is 36 to 42 mol% (73). The two predominant cellular fatty acids are $C_{ai15:0}$ and $C_{ai17:0}$ (branched-chain type) (7).

Natural Habitats

Listeria species are widely distributed in the environment. They have been isolated from soil, decaying vegetable matter, silage, sewage, water, animal feed, fresh and frozen poultry, fresh and processed meats, raw milk, cheese, slaughterhouse waste, and asymptomatic human and animal carriers (25). *L. monocytogenes* has been isolated from numerous species of mammals, birds, fish, crustaceans, and insects (24). Nevertheless, the primary habitats of *L. monocytogenes* are considered to be the soil and decaying vegetable matter, in which it survives and grows saprophytically. Because of its widespread occurrence, *L. monocytogenes* has many opportunities to enter food production and processing environments, and because of its ability to grow at 4°C, it can cause disease in persons ingesting colonized food (24, 65).

Clinical Significance

In nonpregnant human adults, *L. monocytogenes* causes primarily meningitis, encephalitis, and/or septicemia (53, 71). Elderly patients or persons with predisposing conditions that lower cell-mediated immunity, such as transplants, lymphomas, and AIDS, are especially susceptible. On rare occasions, patients have no known predisposing conditions. The tropism of *L. monocytogenes* for the central nervous system leads to severe disease, often with high mortality (20 to 50%) or with neurologic sequelae among survivors (18). In pregnant women, *L. monocytogenes* often causes an influenza-like bacteremic illness that, if untreated, may lead to placentitis and/or amnionitis and infection of the fetus, resulting in abortion, stillbirth, or premature birth because it is able to cross the placenta. Early diagnosis can be made in some cases by detecting *L.*

461

monocytogenes in maternal blood cultures; at birth, the diagnosis is made by detecting the organism in cerebrospinal fluid (CSF), blood, amniotic fluid, respiratory secretions, placental or cutaneous swabs, gastric aspirate, or meconium of the neonate. Direct microscopic visualization of gram-positive rods in these specimens could be invaluable in early diagnosis of the disease.

Focal infections rarely occur after an episode of bacteremia. However, primary cutaneous listeriosis with or without bacteremia has been reported among veterinarians and abattoir workers, who acquire the illness through contact with infected animal tissues (50). Endocarditis, arthritis, osteomyelitis, intra-abdominal abscesses, endophthalmitis, and pleuropulmonary infections have been described infrequently (44).

The incubation period and infective dose have not been firmly established. Reported incubation times vary from a few days to 2 to 3 months. Gastrointestinal symptoms such as diarrhea have been observed in some individuals with systemic listeriosis. A transient healthy carrier state exists in 2 to 20% of animals and humans (24). In the past decade, several outbreaks of febrile gastroenteritis caused by *L. monocytogenes* have been documented (34). These gastroenteritis outbreaks differ from the invasive outbreaks in several respects. They affect persons with no known predisposing risk factors for listeriosis. The infectious dose appears to be higher (1.9×10^5 to 1×10^9 CFU/g or ml) than that for typical invasive listeriosis in the susceptible population. Finally, the symptoms appear within several hours (18 to 27 h) of exposure (similar to other bacterial enteric infections) in gastrointestinal listeriosis, in contrast to the several weeks of incubation observed for invasive listeriosis (3, 21, 32, 68). Therefore, the possibility of infection with *L. monocytogenes* should be considered in investigations of gastroenteritis in which routine enteric pathogens have been ruled out. Cervicovaginal carriage in women (including pregnant ones) seems to be nonexistent.

Listeriosis is observed mainly in industrialized countries. It can occur sporadically or epidemically; in both, contaminated foods are the primary mode of transmission. A few limited, non-food-related nosocomial outbreaks, mainly in nurseries, have been described (48). The number of sporadic cases of listeriosis in countries that report the illness is typically in the range of 0.5 to 0.8 cases per 100,000 persons (66); during food-borne-disease outbreaks, the incidence may rise to 5 cases per 100,000 persons (10). Foods implicated as vehicles of infection are ready-to-eat food stored at refrigeration temperature and able to sustain *Listeria* growth, including coleslaw (cabbage), soft cheeses, paté, poultry, turkey frankfurters, mushrooms, milk, pork tongue in jelly, and smoked fish. Large numbers of organisms ($>10^3$ CFU/g) were detected in foods quantitatively assayed for the organism (24).

The pathogenesis of *L. monocytogenes* in human infections is unclear. However, after contaminated food has been ingested, the development of an invasive infection in some individuals depends on several factors: host susceptibility, gastric acidity, inoculum size, virulence factors of the organism, and the type of food. After penetrating the epithelial barrier of the intestinal tract, *L. monocytogenes* can grow within hepatic and splenic macrophages, due to a number of virulence factors (74), and then spread to the central nervous system or pregnant uterus. Immunity to listeriosis relies mainly on T-cell-mediated activation of macrophages by lymphokines; the role of humoral defenses is not fully understood (65).

Determination of Pathogenicity

Methods using laboratory animals for evaluation of the virulence potential of *Listeria* isolates are available but are not used routinely. Such tests include intraperitoneal inoculation of mice, inoculation of the chorioallantoic membrane of embryonated eggs, and inoculation of the conjunctivas of rabbits (Anton test). A sensitive immunocompromised-mouse model in which relatively low numbers of virulent listeriae cause the deaths of these immunosuppressed animals within 3 days has been developed (75). Also, cell culture cytotoxicity assays using the human intestinal epithelial cell line Caco-2 have been developed to determine the virulence potential of *Listeria* isolates in vitro (65). While the results generally agree with those of animal tests, cytotoxicity assays do not provide as quantitative a measure of virulence as the animal tests do (50% lethal dose). Also, some outbreak-associated *L. monocytogenes* isolates show very little cytotoxicity in the Caco-2 cell assays (61).

Collection, Transportation, and Storage of Specimens

Laboratory Safety

The infectious dose for listeriosis has not been determined, and it may depend, in part, on the susceptibility of the host. Therefore, laboratorians working with *L. monocytogenes* should be made aware of this potential risk and advised to be particularly cautious when working with this organism (39). Because *L. monocytogenes* takes advantage of the localized immunosuppression at the maternal-fetal interface and attacks the fetus with devastating consequences (stillbirths and abortions) while only causing mild, flu-like symptoms in the mother, pregnant women should be particularly careful working in a laboratory where *L. monocytogenes* is propagated or handled.

Specimens

Clinical

L. monocytogenes is readily isolated from clinical specimens obtained from normally sterile sites (blood, CSF, amniotic fluid, placenta, or fetal tissue). These specimens should be immediately cultured at 35°C or stored at 4°C for up to 48 h. Stool specimens are more productive than rectal swabs when epidemiologic studies of carriage rates are undertaken. One gram of stool can be inoculated into 100 ml of a selective enrichment broth (University of Vermont [UVM] enrichment broth or polymyxin-acriflavin-lithium chloride-ceftazidime esculin-mannitol [PALCAM]) (see chapter 27) and then shipped at room temperature by overnight mail. If this is not possible, stools should be shipped frozen on dry ice by overnight mail. Other nonsterile site specimens may be stored at 4°C for 24 to 48 h. To avoid overgrowth of *L. monocytogenes* by contaminating microflora during longer periods of storage, freezing of specimens at −20°C is recommended. Routine stool cultures performed in clinical laboratories should not include *Listeria* detection.

Foods

Food samples must be collected aseptically in sterile containers. Whenever possible, foods packaged in original containers must be collected. Attempts should be made to collect at least 100 g of a sample. Samples may be placed in sterile bags and shipped on ice by overnight mail. Ice cream and other frozen products are best transported in the frozen state in the original container and must be thawed immediately before analysis. Although *L. monocytogenes* is relatively resistant to freezing, repeated freezing and thawing may adversely affect the viability of the bacteria.

Isolates

Cultures of *Listeria* spp. may be shipped to a distant laboratory on a non-glucose-containing agar slant (such as heart infusion agar or tryptic soy agar) packaged to conform with the requirements for interstate shipment of etiologic agents (e.g., U.S. Code of Federal Regulations, 42CFR, part 72).

Isolation Procedures

Culture

Clinical specimens from normally sterile sites can be directly plated on tryptic soy agar containing 5% sheep, horse, or rabbit blood. Samples for blood culture can be inoculated into conventional blood culture broth. Clinical specimens obtained from nonsterile sites and foods and environmental specimens should be selectively enriched for *Listeria* spp. before being plated.

The U.S. Department of Agriculture (USDA) method and the Netherlands Government Food Inspection Service (NGFIS) method are used together at the Centers for Disease Control and Prevention to isolate *L. monocytogenes* from non-sterile-site clinical specimens and foods (31). Individually, the two methods are approximately 75% sensitive; in conjunction with each other, they are 90% sensitive. The USDA method involves enrichment of the specimen in UVM primary selective enrichment broth (1 part sample plus 9 parts of broth) at 30°C. After 24 h, 0.1 ml of the enrichment culture is plated on lithium chloride-phenylethanol-moxalactam (LPM) agar and Oxford or modified Oxford agar (see chapter 27). Another 0.1 ml of the enrichment culture is added to 10 ml of UVM secondary selective enrichment broth, which is then incubated for an additional 24 h. The secondary enrichment culture is plated as described above. The plates are incubated at 35°C and examined after 24 and 48 h. All of the media named above are described in the compendium by Atlas and Parks (2), in chapter 27, and in the fifth edition of this Manual (52).

The NGFIS method involves enrichment of the specimen in liquid PALCAM-egg yolk broth (see chapter 27) (79) at 30°C and plating of the enrichment culture on PALCAM agar at 24 and 48 h. PALCAM agar is incubated at 30°C for 48 h under microaerobic conditions (5% oxygen, 7.5% carbon dioxide, 7.5% hydrogen, and 80% nitrogen).

LPM agar (43) was developed as a highly selective but nondifferential medium for the isolation of *Listeria* species. Colonies on LPM agar are examined under a stereozoom microscope (magnification, ×15 to ×25), with oblique lighting directed to the microscope stage by a concave mirror positioned at a 45° angle to the incident light (Henry illumination). *Listeria* colonies appear blue, while colonies of other bacteria appear yellowish or orange.

Oxford and PALCAM agars contain selective differential chemicals that eliminate the need for examination under oblique lighting. On Oxford and modified Oxford agars, *Listeria* colonies appear black, are 1 to 3 mm in diameter, and are surrounded by a black halo after 24 to 48 h of incubation at 37°C. Color formation is due to the hydrolysis of esculin by *Listeria* spp. and the formation of black iron-phenol compounds in the medium. On PALCAM agar, *Listeria* colonies appear gray-green, are approximately 2 mm in diameter, and have black sunken centers; esculin, ferric iron, D-mannitol, and phenol red contribute to this color formation. CHROMagar *Listeria* (CHROMagar, Paris, France) is a newly introduced medium to discriminate between *L. monocytogenes* and other *Listeria* spp. On this medium, *L. monocytogenes* colonies appear blue with a white halo (due to the activity of a specific phospholipase), while the other bacteria appear blue or colorless or are inhibited. Suspect colonies (3 to 10 colonies per plate) are transferred to tryptic soy agar with 5% sheep blood and incubated for 18 h at 35°C for further workup.

Rapid Detection

Commercially available tests for the rapid detection of *Listeria* species in selective enrichment broths from food samples are based on immunoassays that use monoclonal antibodies (Listeria-Tek [Organon-Teknika, Turnhoout, Belgium], Listeria immunoenzymatic detection kit [Transia, Paris, France], Listeria visual immunoassay [Tecra, Sydney, Australia], Vidas-Lis [bioMérieux, Marcy-l'Etoile, France], Listeria Rapid Test [Unipath/Oxoid Clearview, Basingstoke, United Kingdom], and Vidas-Lis [bioMérieux]). These tests are genus specific. Lister Test (VICAM, Watertown, N.Y.), Vidas-LMO, and a DNA probe *L. monocytogenes* assay (Gene-Trak, Naperville, Iowa) are *L. monocytogenes* specific (8). These kits are for use with food products only; they are not designed for the analysis of clinical specimens, for diagnosis, or for treatment.

L. monocytogenes DNA in CSF and tissue (fresh or in paraffin blocks) can be specifically detected by PCR-based tests (37, 70). The PCR assay is highly sensitive and specific and could be particularly useful when prior administration of antimicrobial agents compromises culture.

Identification

Genus Identification

A simplified identification is based on the following tests: Gram stain, observation of tumbling motility in a wet mount, positive catalase reaction, and esculin hydrolysis. Acid production from D-glucose and positive Voges-Proskauer and methyl red reactions are confirmatory tests.

Differentiation of the Genus *Listeria* from Other Genera

Because they share some characteristics, *Listeria* spp. and some other gram-positive bacteria may be confused. *Streptococcus* spp. may be differentiated from *Listeria* spp. on the basis of Gram stain morphology, motility, and catalase activity. *Erysipelothrix* spp. differ from *Listeria* spp. in motility, catalase reaction, and ability to grow at 4°C (*Erysipelothrix* spp. do not grow at that temperature). Among background microflora of foods, *Lactobacillus* spp. are usually nonmotile and catalase negative, *Brochothrix* spp. are unable to grow at 37°C, and *Kurthia* spp. are strictly aerobic and esculin negative.

Species Identification

The scheme for identification of *Listeria* species is shown in Table 1. Identification of *Listeria* isolates to species level is crucial, because all species can contaminate foods, but only *L. monocytogenes* is of public health concern. Identification is based on a limited number of biochemical markers, among which hemolysis is essential to differentiating be-

TABLE 1 Biochemical differentiation of species in the genus *Listeria*[a]

Characteristic	*L. grayi*	*L. innocua*	*L. ivanovii*	*L. ivanovii* subsp. *londoniensis*	*L. monocytogenes*	*L. seeligeri*	*L. welshimeri*
Beta-hemolysis	−	−	++[b]	++	+	+	−
CAMP[c] test reaction							
S. aureus	−	−	−	−	+	+	−
R. equi	−	−	+	+	V	−	−
Acid production from:							
Mannitol	+	−	−	−	−	−	−
α-Methyl-D-mannoside	+	+	−	−	+	−	+
L-Rhamnose	V	V	−	−	+	−	V
Soluble starch	+	−	−	−	−	ND	ND
D-Xylose	−	−	+	+	−	+	+
Ribose	V	−	+	−	−	−	−
N-Acetyl-β-D-mannosamine	ND	ND	V	+	ND	ND	ND
Hippurate hydrolysis	−	+	+	+	+	ND	ND
Reduction of nitrate	V	−	−	−	−	ND	ND
Associated serovar(s)	S	4ab, US, 6a, 6b	5	5	1/2a, 1/2b, 1/2c, 3a, 3b, 3c, 4a, 4ab, 4b, 4c, 4d, 4e, 7	1/2a, 1/2b, 1/2c, US, 4b, 4d, 6b	1/2b, 4c, 6a, 6b, US

[a] See references 15 and 73. Symbols and abbreviations: +, ≥90% of strains are positive; −, ≥90% of strains are negative; ND, not determined; V, variable; US, undesignated serotype; S, specific.
[b] ++, usually a wide zone or multiple zones.
[c] See text and Fig. 2.

tween *L. monocytogenes* and the most frequently isolated nonpathogenic *Listeria* species, *L. innocua*.

Hemolysis

Only three species, *L. monocytogenes*, *L. seeligeri*, and *L. ivanovii*, are hemolytic on sheep blood agar plates. Recent studies indicated hemolysin to be the major virulence factor of *L. monocytogenes*; however, hemolysis alone cannot be used as an indicator of the presence of a virulent species because *L. seeligeri* is hemolytic but nonpathogenic. *L. monocytogenes* and *L. seeligeri* produce narrow zones of hemolysis that frequently do not extend much beyond the edge of the colonies, whereas *L. ivanovii* exhibits a wide zone of hemolysis (Fig. 1).

The CAMP (Christie, Atkins, Munch-Peterson) test uses a β-lysin-producing *Staphylococcus aureus* or *Rhodococ-*

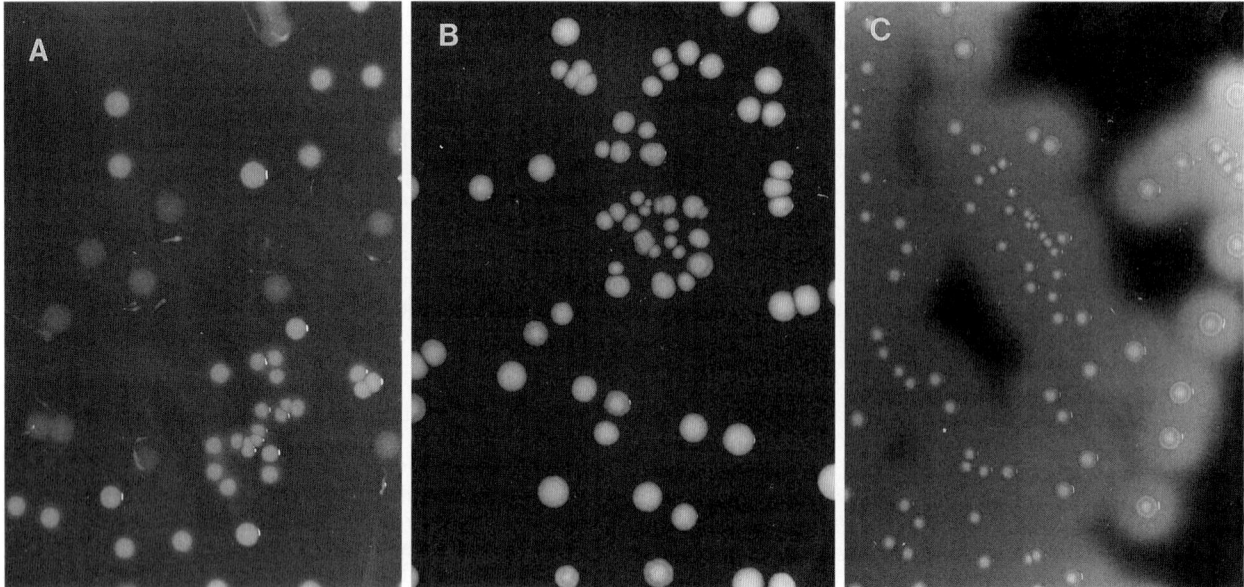

FIGURE 1 Macroscopic view of colonies on 5% human blood agar plates after 24 h of incubation. (A) *L. monocytogenes:* discrete zone of beta-hemolysis under the removed colonies. (B) *L. innocua:* no hemolysis. (C) *L. ivanovii:* wide zone of beta-hemolysis around the colonies.

cus equi strain streaked in one direction on a sheep blood agar plate and test cultures of *Listeria* spp. streaked at right angles to (but not touching) the *S. aureus* and *R. equi* lines. According to *Bergey's Manual of Systematic Bacteriology* (73), hemolysis of *L. monocytogenes* and *L. seeligeri* is enhanced in the vicinity of the *S. aureus* streak, and *L. ivanovii* hemolysis is enhanced in the vicinity of *R. equi* (resulting in a shovel shape [Fig. 2]). However, because many investigators have reported observing a synergistic hemolysis reaction between *L. monocytogenes* and *R. equi* this CAMP reaction must be interpreted with caution. A β-lysin disk (Remel, Lenexa, Kans.) could be used to ob-

serve enhancement of *L. monocytogenes* hemolysis with β-lysin from *S. aureus*.

Acid Production from Carbohydrates

L. monocytogenes is always D-xylose negative and α-methyl-D-mannoside positive. Rare atypical strains may be L-rhamnose negative. Test tubes are incubated for 7 days at 37°C in an aerobic incubator.

Miniaturized Biochemical Tests

The API-Listeria test (bioMérieux Vitek, Inc., Hazelwood, Mo.) was specifically designed for this genus and includes 10 biochemical differentiation tests in a microtube format. It includes a patented "DIM" test, based on the absence or presence of arylamidase, which distinguishes between *L. monocytogenes* (positive) and *L. innocua* (negative), without further tests for hemolytic activity (11). Another system based on 15 biochemical tests (Micro-ID Listeria [Organon-Teknika]) performs equally well but needs an additional test for hemolytic activity to differentiate *L. monocytogenes* from *L. innocua* (5). Similar performances are obtained with the API Coryne System (bioMérieux), which correctly identifies *Listeria* isolates to the genus level (42).

DNA Probe Assay for Colony Confirmation

A 30-min chemiluminescence DNA probe assay is available (Gen-Probe, San Diego, Calif.) for the rapid confirmation of *L. monocytogenes* from colonies on primary isolation plates. This assay was highly specific for *L. monocytogenes* in two independent evaluations (54, 59).

Typing Techniques

Serotyping

Strains of *Listeria* species are divided into serotypes on the basis of somatic (O) and flagellar (H) antigens (72). Thirteen serotypes (1/2a, 1/2b, 1/2c, 3a, 3b, 3c, 4a, 4ab, 4b, 4c, 4d, 4e, and 7) of *L. monocytogenes* are known; 4bX, a variant of serotype 4b, was implicated in a listeriosis outbreak traced to contaminated paté in England (49). Serotyping antigens are shared among *L. monocytogenes*, *L. innocua*, *L. seeligeri*, and *L. welshimeri*. Most human disease is caused by serotypes 1/2a, 1/2b, and 4b; therefore, serotyping alone is not sufficiently discriminating for subtyping purposes. Nevertheless, serotyping is useful as a first-level discriminator. Also, unlike other subtyping methods, serotype designations are universal. Determination of the serotype also facilitates selection of appropriate controls for molecular subtyping methods. A recently introduced commercial kit for serotyping *Listeria* is available (Denka Seiken, Tokyo, Japan).

Phage Typing

Because of the poor discriminating ability of serotyping, phage typing was the only means of distinguishing strains of the same serotype before the introduction of molecular methods (63). Marquet-Van der Mee and Audurier (47) have proposed the inclusion of seven new experimental phages to the international phage set for subtyping *L. monocytogenes* to improve overall typeability and the discriminating power of the system. However, despite its usefulness, phage typing is hampered by the nontypeability of some strains and has been replaced now by molecular methods (especially DNA macrorestriction pattern analysis).

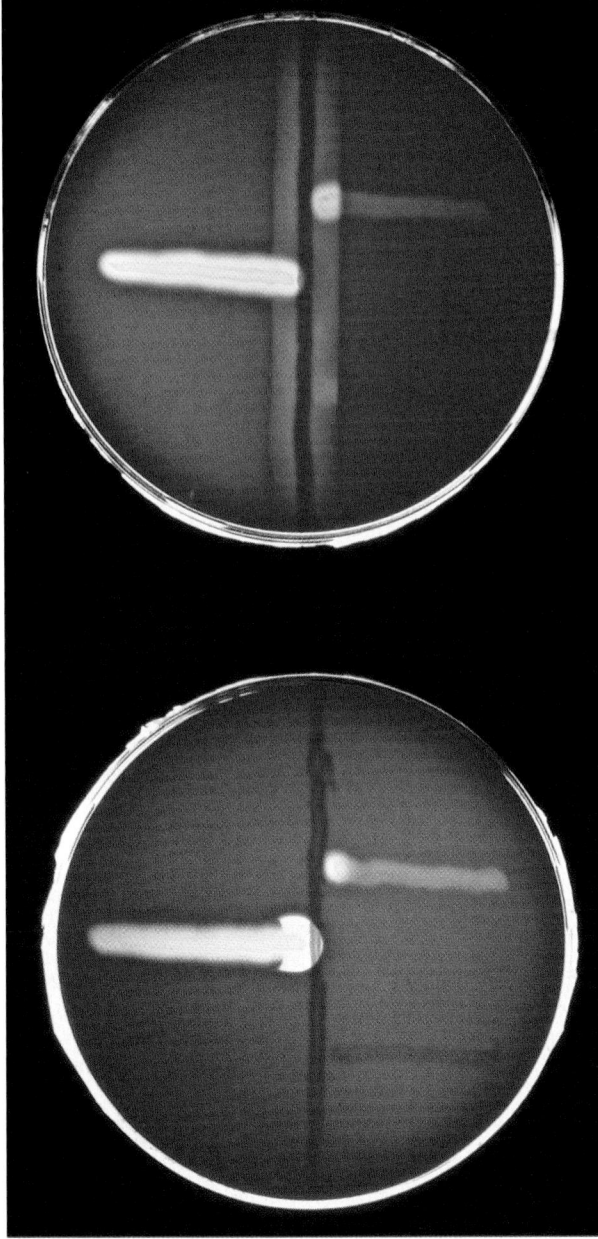

FIGURE 2 CAMP test done with *S. aureus* CIP 5710 (top plate) and *R. equi* CIP 5869 (bottom plate) after 24 h of incubation. Upper right, *L. monocytogenes*; lower right, *L. innocua*; middle left, *L. ivanovii*.

MLEE

Typically, 10 to 25 enzyme loci are examined by multilocus enzyme electrophoresis (MLEE) for each strain. Each unique mobility variant of an enzyme is given a unique numeric allele designation. Each strain is defined by a string of numerical values for the alleles examined (electrophoretic type). MLEE has been extremely useful for taxonomic studies and for characterizing the evolution of strains within the species (9, 13, 14, 60, 70); however, it does not have adequate discriminatory power for use as the sole subtyping method for epidemiologic investigations.

DNA Microrestriction Pattern Analysis

Characterization of chromosomal DNA by restriction endonuclease analysis or ribosomal DNA gene restriction patterns (ribotyping) has been used to differentiate *L. monocytogenes* strains in different serotypes and within a given serotype, in particular serotype 4b, which is most frequently involved in outbreaks. Microrestriction patterns generated by high-frequency-cutting restriction enzymes (e.g., *Eco*RI) have proved useful in epidemiologic investigations (4, 55), although the complexity of patterns makes it difficult to compare the patterns of several strains. Ribotyping simplifies the microrestriction patterns by rendering visible only the DNA fragments containing part or all of the ribosomal genes, but its discriminating ability, particularly for serotype 4b, may not be adequate (4, 28, 35, 36, 56). A completely automated RiboPrinter system (Qualicon, Wilmington, Del.) facilitates rapid and easy subtyping of *L. monocytogenes* within 8 h. Although ribotyping alone does not have adequate discriminating power for epidemiologic investigations of outbreaks, the automated RiboPrinter is invaluable for preliminary recognition of disease clusters and for identification of transient and long-term resident strains of *L. monocytogenes* in food processing plants and their environments (22, 57).

DNA Macrorestriction PFGE Pattern Analysis

Brosch et al. (17) evaluated the pulsed-field gel electrophoresis (PFGE) method for the World Health Organization (WHO) multicenter international typing study of *L. monocytogenes*. Four laboratories participated in using PFGE to analyze 80 coded strains. Two restriction endonucleases (*Apa*I and *Sma*I) were used by all laboratories; one laboratory used an additional restriction endonuclease (*Asc*I). Agreement of typing data among the four laboratories ranged from 79 to 90%. Sixty-nine percent of the strains were placed in exactly the same genomic group by all four laboratories; most of the epidemiologically related strains were correctly identified by all four laboratories. This study validated the previous claims that PFGE is a highly discriminating and reproducible method for subtyping *L. monocytogenes* and is particularly useful for subtyping serotype 4b isolates, which are not typed satisfactorily by most other typing methods.

In the United States, the Centers for Disease Control and Prevention has established a network (PulseNet) of public health and food regulatory laboratories that routinely subtype food-borne pathogenic bacteria to rapidly detect food-borne disease clusters that may have a common source. PulseNet laboratories use highly standardized protocols for subtyping of bacteria by PFGE and are able to quickly compare PFGE patterns of food-borne pathogens from different locations within the country via the Internet (76) (PFGE@cdc.gov). A 1-day standardized protocol for PFGE subtyping of *L. monocytogenes* was added to PulseNet

in 1998 (29). Routine and timely subtyping of *L. monocytogenes* by participating PulseNet laboratories has significantly enhanced the ability to recognize and investigate outbreaks.

RAPD

Boerlin et al. (16) performed an extensive evaluation of random amplification of polymorphic DNA (RAPD) by typing 100 *L. monocytogenes* isolates which had been characterized by serotyping, phage typing, MLEE analysis, restriction endonuclease analysis, and ribotyping. They found RAPD to be highly discriminating. O'Donoghue et al. (58) found RAPD to be useful for typing serogroup 1/2; also, they found that the method distinguished serotype 4bX strains involved in a paté-associated outbreak from other serotype 4b isolates. Wernars et al. (82) evaluated RAPD for the WHO collaborative study. Six laboratories participated in the study. By use of three different 10-mer primers, the median reproducibility of the RAPD results obtained by the six participants was 86.5% (range, 0 to 100%). Failure in reproducibility was due mainly to results obtained with one particular primer. They concluded that RAPD analysis is a rapid and relatively simple technique for epidemiological typing of *L. monocytogenes* isolates and that reproducible and useful results can be obtained. Despite the simplicity and high discriminating ability of RAPD, much more work is needed to make RAPD typing a standard technique for general and widespread use. Its primary drawback is the inconsistent reproducibility of patterns.

Present Status of Subtyping

The vast majority of *L. monocytogenes* strains causing sporadic infections or outbreaks belong to serotypes 1/2a, 1/2b, and 4b. Strains of serotype 1/2a are highly heterogeneous and thus are easily differentiated by any of the molecular methods and by phage typing when the strains are phage typeable. In contrast, strains of serotype 4b are more closely related and probably necessitate the combined use of several methods to be optimally differentiated. This has been confirmed by the first results of an international multicenter study aimed at evaluating the different subtyping methods for *L. monocytogenes* and at standardizing the most promising one (12).

Serodiagnosis

Serologic responses to whole-cell antigens cannot be used for diagnosis because of antigenic cross-reactivity between *L. monocytogenes* and other gram-positive bacteria such as staphylococci, enterococci, and *Bacillus* species. Furthermore, patients with culture-confirmed listeriosis have had undetectable antibody levels (71). Determination of levels of antibody to listeriolysin O may be of value both for invasive listeriosis and for febrile gastroenteritis (6). Although a serologic method based on the detection of antibodies against recombinant truncated forms of listeriolysin O may be more specific (26), serological tests are not recommended at the present time.

Antimicrobial Susceptibilities

The pattern of antimicrobial susceptibility and resistance of *L. monocytogenes* has been relatively stable for many years (78). In vitro, the organism is susceptible to penicillin, ampicillin, gentamicin, erythromycin, tetracycline, rifampin, and chloramphenicol (69, 83) but only moderately susceptible to quinolones (33). However, many of these antimicrobial agents are only bacteriostatic. Penicillin or ampicillin with or without an aminoglycoside is usually recommended for the treatment of listeriosis. Studies in vitro and in animal models have shown that an aminoglycoside enhances the antimicrobial (bactericidal) activity of penicillin against *L. monocytogenes* (51). Trimethoprim-sulfamethoxazole and aminoglycosides are among the few anti-infective agents that are bactericidal to *L. monocytogenes*; only trimethoprim-sulfamethoxazole has been used occasionally with success. Resistance plasmids conferring resistance to chloramphenicol, macrolides, and tetracyclines have been found in several clinical isolates of *L. monocytogenes* and have raised concern for the future (30). Cephalosporins are ineffective in vitro, although in vitro tests may indicate susceptibility, and should never be administered when listeriosis is suspected.

Evaluation, Interpretation, and Reporting of Results

Colonies from blood, CSF, or other normally sterile-site specimens that show subdued beta-hemolysis on blood agar should be subjected to motility tests, Gram staining, catalase testing, and esculin hydrolysis to confirm identification. They may resemble group B streptococcal colonies on blood agar plates. The CAMP test is not necessary on a routine basis, and the β-lysin test may be substituted for it. Use of the API-Listeria test may eliminate the need for enhanced hemolysis testing altogether. If *L. monocytogenes* is present in low numbers in CSF, the direct examination of Gram-stained clinical specimens may be of little or no value. Also, Gram-stained *Listeria* cells closely resemble other gram-positive bacteria, such as streptococci, enterococci, or corynebacteria. If antimicrobial therapy was initiated before a CSF specimen was obtained, culture results may be negative. In these instances, Gram staining may be useful, but additional confirmation by methods such as PCR (for laboratories that have the capability) may be needed.

ERYSIPELOTHRIX

Taxonomy

Included at one time in the coryneform group, *Erysipelothrix* is now classified within the regular non-spore-forming gram-positive rods, a group that comprises the genera *Listeria* and *Lactobacillus*. The genus *Erysipelothrix* has two species, *E. rhusiopathiae* and *E. tonsillarum* (77). *E. rhusiopathiae*, which is widely distributed in nature and can be carried by a variety of animals, has been recognized for more than 100 years as the agent of swine erysipelas and occasionally causes erysipeloid, a human cutaneous infection usually localized to the hands and fingers (62).

Description of the Genus

Erysipelothrix organisms are mesophilic, facultatively anaerobic, non-spore-forming, non-acid-fast, gram-positive bacteria that appear microscopically as short rods (0.2 to 0.5 μm by 0.8 to 2.5 μm) with rounded ends and occur singly, in short chains, or in long nonbranching filaments (60 μm or more in length). They are nonmotile and grow in complex media at a wide range of temperatures (5 to 42°C; optimum, 30 to 37°C) and at an alkaline pH (6.7 to 9.2; optimum, 7.2 to 7.6). Like *Listeria* organisms, they can grow in the presence of high concentrations of sodium chloride (up to 8.5%). Metabolically, *Erysipelothrix* organisms are catalase negative and oxidase negative, do not hydrolyze esculin, and weakly ferment glucose without the production of gas. They are methyl red and Voges-Proskauer negative

and do not produce indole or hydrolyze urea but distinctively produce H$_2$S in triple sugar iron agar (38). Key fatty acids are C$_{16:0}$ and C$_{18:cis9}$ (7).

Natural Habitat

E. rhusiopathiae is widespread in nature and is remarkably persistent under environmental conditions such as low temperature and alkaline pH and within organic matter favoring survival. The organism is parasitic on mammals, birds, and fish but is most frequently associated with pigs. Contamination of water and soil from the feces and urine of sick and asymptomatic animals often occurs.

E. tonsillarum has been recovered from water and from the tonsils of healthy swine.

Clinical Significance

Infection with *E. rhusiopathiae* is a zoonosis. Many animal species, especially turkeys and swine, carry the organism in their digestive tracts or tonsils. *E. rhusiopathiae* causes chronic or acute swine erysipelas. Erysipelas can present in several clinical manifestations: skin infection, arthritis, septicemia, and endocarditis. Other domestic and wild animals and birds also can be affected, in particular sheep, rabbits, cattle, and turkeys. Infection is most likely acquired by ingestion of contaminated matter (62).

In humans, *E. rhusiopathiae* mostly causes erysipeloid, a localized cellulitis developing within 2 to 7 days around the inoculation site. The disease is contracted through skin abrasion, injury, or a bite on the hands or arms of individuals handling animals or animal products. Erysipeloid is an occupational disease, occurring most frequently among veterinarians, butchers, and particularly fish handlers. The lesion usually is violaceous and painful, indurated with edema and inflammation but without suppuration, and clearly delineated at the border. Regional lymphangitis may be present, as well as an adjacent arthritis. Dissemination and endocarditis can occur, especially in immunocompromised patients; their prognosis is generally poor (27). Healing usually takes 2 to 4 weeks, sometimes months, and relapses are common. No apparent immunity develops after an episode of erysipeloid.

E. tonsillarum has not yet been recovered from humans.

Collection, Transport, and Storage of Specimens

Biopsy specimens from erysipeloid lesions are the best source of *E. rhusiopathiae*. Care should be taken to cleanse and disinfect the skin before sampling. The organisms typically are located deep in the subcutaneous layer of the leading edge of the lesion; hence, a biopsy of the entire thickness of the dermis at the periphery of the lesion should be taken for Gram stain and culture. Swabs from the surface of the skin are not useful. In disseminated disease, the organism can be cultured from blood without special procedures.

Isolation Procedures

Microscopic Examination

Generally, direct examination of Gram-stained biopsy specimens is of little value. However, the presence of long, slender, gram-positive rods in tissue from an individual with a consonant history is suggestive of erysipeloid.

Culture

Biopsy specimens should be plated on blood agar or chocolate blood agar, placed in tryptic soy or Schaedler broth (see chapter 27), and incubated at 35°C aerobically or in 5% CO_2 for 7 days. Blood from patients with septicemia or endocarditis can be plated directly onto blood agar plates for primary isolation or inoculated in commercial blood culture systems. *E. rhusiopathiae* colonies generally develop in 1 to 3 days, being pinpoint (<0.1 to 0.5 mm in diameter) on blood agar plates after 24 h of incubation; at 48 h, two distinct colony types can be observed. The smaller, smooth colonies are 0.3 to 1.5 mm in diameter, transparent, convex, and circular with entire edges. Larger, rough colonies are flatter and more opaque and have a matt surface and an irregular, fimbriated edge. A zone of greenish discoloration frequently develops underneath the colonies on blood agar plates after 2 days of incubation (38).

Rapid Detection

A genus-specific PCR amplification system using a DNA sequence coding for the 16S rRNA gene has been used with pig samples (46).

Identification

Gram Staining of Colonies from a 24-h Blood Agar Plate

Cells stain gram positive but can decolorize and appear gram negative, with gram-positive granules giving a beaded effect. Cells from smooth colonies appear as rods or coccobacilli, sometimes in short chains. Cells from rough colonies appear as long filaments, often more than 60 μm.

Biochemical Identification of *E. rhusiopathiae*

E. rhusiopathiae is catalase negative, lactose and H_2S positive, and nitrate, urease, esculin, gelatin, xylose, mannose, maltose, and sucrose negative. *E. tonsillarum* differs biochemically from *E. rhusiopathiae* by being sucrose positive. Vitek automated systems, as well as API Coryne, usually identify *E. rhusiopathiae* correctly.

Differentiation of *Erysipelothrix* from Related Genera

Genera that have morphological and physiological characteristics in common with *Erysipelothrix* include *Lactobacillus*, *Listeria*, *Brochothrix*, and *Kurthia*. All are regular nonpigmented, non-spore-forming, gram-positive rods (40). A major discriminatory test is that *E. rhusiopathiae* produces H_2S in triple sugar iron, whereas other genera do not. Furthermore, *Listeria*, *Brochothrix*, and *Kurthia* species are catalase positive. In addition, *Listeria* isolates are motile, are esculin positive, and are not alpha-hemolytic. *Brochothrix* isolates strongly ferment carbohydrates, are Voges-Proskauer positive, and do not grow above 30°C. *Kurthia* species are strict aerobes, motile, and nonhemolytic (41). Corynebacteria and streptococci also can be confused with *E. rhusiopathiae*, but careful examination of cell morphology should facilitate the distinction. The production of H_2S in triple sugar iron by a gram-positive bacterium is usually indicative of *E. rhusiopathiae* because very few gram-positive bacteria of clinical origin produce H_2S. Exceptions include some *Bacillus* strains, but they are easily differentiated from *E. rhusiopathiae* by cellular morphology, spore formation, and catalase reaction. An additional trait highly characteristic of *E. rhusiopathiae* is its "pipe cleaner" pattern of growth in gelatin stab cultures incubated at 22°C (38, 80).

Typing Systems

Twenty-two serovars of *E. rhusiopathiae* have been identified on the basis of heat-stable somatic antigens. Although most isolates are serovar 1 or 2, no serotyping schemes are available for routine use in clinical laboratories (38). Both MLEE and ribotyping methods have been applied to *Erysipelothrix* strains and have shown an important genetic diversity (1, 19). In these studies, serotyping was unreliable for use as an epidemiologic tool.

Pathogenicity Testing

Most strains of *E. rhusiopathiae* are virulent for mice in a mouse protection test.

Serological Tests

Since humans apparently do not develop immunity after an episode of erysipeloid, there are no serological tests for routine use to demonstrate antibodies to *E. rhusiopathiae*. Active immunization of animals with a live attenuated vaccine protects against erysipelas (62); however, a natural infection of erysipeloid in humans does not prevent relapses or reinfection from occurring.

Antibiotic Susceptibility

E. rhusiopathiae isolates are generally susceptible to penicillin, cephalosporins, clindamycin, imipenem, tetracycline, chloramphenicol, erythromycin, and the fluoroquinolones; they are usually resistant to aminoglycosides, sulfonamides, and vancomycin. Penicillin is the treatment of choice for both localized and systemic infections (27).

REFERENCES

1. **Ahrné, S., I.-M. Stenström, N. E. Jensen, B. Pettersson, M. Uhlén, and G. Molin.** 1995. Classification of *Erysipelothrix* strains on the basis of restriction fragment length polymorphisms. *Int. J. Syst. Bacteriol.* **45:**382–385.
2. **Atlas, R. M., and L. C. Parks (ed.).** 1993. *Handbook of Microbiological Media.* CRC Press, Inc., Boca Raton, Fla.
3. **Aureli, P., G. C. Fiorucci, D. Caroli, G. Marchiaro, O. Novara, L. Leone, and S. Salmaso.** 2000. An outbreak of febrile gastroenteritis associated with corn contaminated by *Listeria monocytogenes*. *N. Engl. J. Med.* **342:**1236–1241.
4. **Baloga, A. O., and S. K. Harlander.** 1991. Comparison of methods for discrimination between strains of *Listeria monocytogenes* from epidemiological surveys. *Appl. Environ. Microbiol.* **57:**2324–2331.
5. **Bannerman, E., M.-N. Yersin, and J. Bille.** 1992. Evaluation of the Organon-Teknika MICRO-ID LISTERIA System. *Appl. Environ. Microbiol.* **58:**2011–2015.
6. **Berche, P., K. A. Reich, M. Bonnichon, J.-L. Beretti, C. Geoffroy, J. Raveneau, P. Cossart, J.-L. Gaillard, P. Geslin, H. Kreis, and M. Véron.** 1990. Detection of anti-listeriolysin O for serodiagnosis of human listeriosis. *Lancet* **ii:**624–627.
7. **Bernard, K. A., M. Bellefeuille, and E. P. Ewan.** 1991. Cellular fatty acid composition as an adjunct to the identification of asporogenous, aerobic Gram-positive rods. *J. Clin. Microbiol.* **29:**83–89.
8. **Beumer, R. R., M. C. te Giffel, M. T. C. Kok, and F. M. Rombouts.** 1996. Confirmation and identification of *Listeria* spp. *Lett. Appl. Microbiol.* **22:**448–452.
9. **Bibb, W. F., B. G. Gellin, R. Weaver, B. Schwartz, B. D. Plikaytis, M. W. Reeves, R. W. Pinner, and C. V. Broome.** 1990. Analysis of clinical and food-borne isolates of *Listeria monocytogenes* in the United States by multilo-

cus enzyme electrophoresis and application of the method to epidemiologic investigations. *Appl. Environ. Microbiol.* **56:**2133–2141.

10. Bille, J. 1990. Epidemiology of human listeriosis in Europe, with special reference to the Swiss outbreak, p. 71–74. *In* A. J. Miller, J. L. Smith, and G. A. Somkuti (ed.), *Food-borne Listeriosis.* Elsevier, Amsterdam, The Netherlands.

11. Bille, J., B. Catimel, E. Bannerman, C. Jacquet, M.-N. Yersin, I. Caniaux, D. Monget, and J. Rocourt. 1992. API-Listeria, a new and promising one-day system to identify *Listeria* isolates. *Appl. Environ. Microbiol.* **58:**1857–1860.

12. Bille, J., and J. Rocourt. 1996. WHO international multicenter *Listeria monocytogenes* subtyping study—rationale and set-up of the study. *Int. J. Food Microbiol.* **32:**251–262.

13. Boerlin, P., and J.-C. Piffaretti. 1991. Typing of human, animal, food, and environmental isolates of *Listeria monocytogenes* by multilocus enzyme electrophoresis. *Appl. Environ. Microbiol.* **57:**1624–1629.

14. Boerlin, P., J. Rocourt, and J.-C. Piffaretti. 1991. Taxonomy of the genus *Listeria* by using multilocus enzyme electrophoresis. *Int. J. Syst. Bacteriol.* **41:**59–64.

15. Boerlin, P., J. Rocourt, F. Grimont, P. A. D. Grimont, C. Jacquet, and J.-C. Piffaretti. 1992. *Listeria ivanovii* subsp. *londoniensis* subsp. nov. *Int. J. Syst. Bacteriol.* **42:**69–73.

16. Boerlin, P., E. Bannerman, F. Ischer, J. Rocourt, and J. Bille. 1995. Typing of *Listeria monocytogenes:* a comparison of random amplification of polymorphic DNA with 5 other methods. *Res. Microbiol.* **146:**35–49.

17. Brosch, R., M. Brett, B. Catimel, J. B. Luchansky, B. Ojeniyi, and J. Rocourt. 1996. Genomic fingerprinting of 80 strains from the WHO multicenter international typing study of *Listeria monocytogenes* via pulsed-field gel electrophoresis (PFGE). *Int. J. Food Microbiol.* **32:**343–355.

18. Büla, C. J., J. Bille, and M. P. Glauser. 1995. An epidemic of food-borne listeriosis in Western Switzerland: description of 57 cases involving adults. *Clin. Infect. Dis.* **20:**66–72.

19. Chooromoney, K. N., D. J. Hampson, G. J. Eamens, and M. J. Turner. 1994. Analysis of *Erysipelothrix rhusiopathiae* and *Erysipelothrix tonsillarum* by multilocus enzyme electrophoresis. *J. Clin. Microbiol.* **32:**371–376.

20. Collins, M. D., S. Wallbanks, D. J. Lane, J. Shah, R. Nietupski, J. Smida, M. Dorsch, and E. Stackebrandt. 1991. Phylogenetic analysis of the genus *Listeria* based on reverse transcriptase sequencing of 16S rRNA. *Int. J. Syst. Bacteriol.* **41:**240–246.

21. Dalton, C. B., C. C. Austin, J. Sobel, P. S. Hayes, W. F. Bibb, L. M. Graves, B. Swaminathan, M. E. Proctor, and P. M. Griffin. 1997. An outbreak of gastroenteritis and fever due to *Listeria monocytogenes* in milk. *N. Engl. J. Med.* **336:**100–105.

22. De Cesare, A., J. L. Bruce, T. R. Dambaugh, M. E. Guerzoni, and M. Wiedmann. 2001. Automated ribotyping using different enzymes to improve discrimination of *Listeria monocytogenes* isolates, with a particular focus on serotype 4b strains. *J. Clin. Microbiol.* **39:**3002–3005.

23. Elsner, H.-A., I. Sobottka, A. Bubert, H. Albrecht, R. Laufs, and D. Mack. 1996. Catalase-negative *Listeria monocytogenes* causing lethal sepsis and meningitis in an adult hematologic patient. *Eur. J. Clin. Microbiol. Infect. Dis.* **15:**965–967.

24. Farber, J. M., and P. I. Peterkin. 1991. *Listeria monocytogenes*, a food-borne pathogen. *Microbiol. Rev.* **55:**476–511.

25. Fenlon, D. R. 1999. *Listeria monocytogenes* in the natural environment, p. 30–40. *In* E. T. Ryser and E. H. Marth (ed.), Listeria, *Listeriosis, and Food Safety,* 2nd ed. Marcel Dekker, Inc., New York, N.Y.

26. Gholizadeh, Y., C. Poyart, M. Juvin, J.-L. Beretti, J. Croizé, P. Berche, and J.-L. Gaillard. 1996. Serodiagnosis of listeriosis based upon detection of antibodies against recombinant truncated forms of listeriolysin O. *J. Clin. Microbiol.* **34:**1391–1395.

27. Gorby, G. L., and J. E. Peacock, Jr. 1988. *Erysipelothrix rhusiopathiae* endocarditis: microbiologic, epidemiologic, and clinical features of an occupational disease. *Rev. Infect. Dis.* **10:**317–325.

28. Graves, L. M., B. Swaminathan, M. W. Reeves, and J. Wenger. 1991. Ribosomal DNA fingerprinting of *Listeria monocytogenes* using a digoxigenin-labeled DNA probe. *Eur. J. Epidemiol.* **7:**77–82.

29. Graves, L. M., and B. Swaminathan. 2001. PulseNet standardized protocol for subtyping *Listeria monocytogenes* by macrorestriction and pulsed-field gel electrophoresis. *Int. J. Food Microbiol.* **65:**55–62.

30. Hadorn, K., H. Hächler, A. Schaffner, and F. H. Kayser. 1993. Genetic characterization of plasmid-encoded multiple antibiotic resistance in a strain of *Listeria monocytogenes* causing endocarditis. *Eur. J. Clin. Microbiol. Infect. Dis.* **12:**928–937.

31. Hayes, P. S., L. M. Graves, B. Swaminathan, G. W. Ajello, G. B. Malcolm, R. E. Weaver, R. Ransom, K. Deaver, B. D. Plikaytis, A. Schuchat, J. D. Wenger, R. W. Pinner, C. V. Broome, and The Listeria Study Group. 1992. Comparison of three selective enrichment methods for the isolation of *Listeria monocytogenes* from naturally contaminated foods. *J. Food Prot.* **55:**952–959.

32. Heitmann, M., P. Gerner-Smidt, and O. Heltberg. 1997. Gastroenteritis caused by *Listeria monocytogenes* in a private day-care facility. *Pediatr. Infect. Dis. J.* **16:**827–828.

33. Hof, H., T. Nichterlein, and M. Kretschmar. 1997. Management of listeriosis. *Clin. Microbiol. Rev.* **10:**345–357.

34. Hof, H. 2001. *Listeria monocytogenes:* a causative agent of gastroenteritis? *Eur. J. Clin. Microbiol. Infect. Dis.* **20:**369–373.

35. Jacquet, C., S. Aubert, N. El Sohl, and J. Rocourt. 1992. Use of rRNA gene restriction patterns for the identification of *Listeria* species. *Syst. Appl. Microbiol.* **15:**42–46.

36. Jacquet, C., J. Bille, and J. Rocourt. 1992. Typing of *Listeria monocytogenes* by restriction fragment length polymorphism of the ribosomal ribonucleic acid gene region. *Zentbl. Bakteriol. Hyg. A* **276:**356–365.

37. Jaton, K., R. Sahli, and J. Bille. 1992. Development of polymerase chain reaction assays for detection of *Listeria monocytogenes* in clinical cerebrospinal fluid samples. *J. Clin. Microbiol.* **30:**1931–1936.

38. Jones, D. 1986. Genus *Erysipelothrix* Rosenbach 1909, 367AL, p. 1245–1249. *In* P. H. A. Sneath, N. S. Mair, M. E. Sharpe, and J. G. Holt (ed.), *Bergey's Manual of Systematic Bacteriology,* vol. 2. Williams & Wilkins, Baltimore, Md.

39. Jones, G. L. (ed.). 1989. *Isolation and Identification of* Listeria monocytogenes. Centers for Disease Control, Atlanta, Ga.

40. Kandler, O., and N. Weiss. 1986. Regular, nonsporing Gram-positive rods, p. 1208–1209. *In* P. H. A. Sneath, N. S. Mair, M. E. Sharpe, and J. G. Holt (ed.), *Bergey's Manual of Systematic Bacteriology,* vol. 2. Williams & Wilkins, Baltimore, Md.

41. Keddie, R. M., and S. Shaw. 1986. Genus *Kurthia* Trevisan 1885, 92AL, p. 1255–1257. *In* P. H. A. Sneath, N. S. Mair, M. E. Sharpe, and J. G. Holt (ed.), *Bergey's Manual of Systematic Bacteriology,* vol. 2. Williams & Wilkins, Baltimore, Md.

42. **Kerr, K. G., P. M. Hawkey, and R. W. Lacey.** 1993. Evaluation of the API Coryne System for identification of *Listeria* species. *J. Clin. Microbiol.* **31:**749–750.

43. **Lee, W. H., and D. McClain.** 1986. Improved *Listeria monocytogenes* selective agar. *Appl. Environ. Microbiol.* **52:**1215–1217.

44. **Lorber, B.** 2000. *Listeria monocytogenes*, p. 2208–2215. *In* G. L. Mandell, R. Douglas, and J. E. Bennett (ed.), *Principles and Practice of Infectious Diseases*, 5th ed. Churchill Livingstone, New York, N.Y.

45. **Ludwig, W., K.-H. Schleifer, and E. Stackebrandt.** 1984. 16S rRNA analysis of *Listeria monocytogenes* and *Brochothrix thermosphacta*. *FEMS Microbiol. Lett.* **25:**199–204.

46. **Makino, S.-I., Y. Okada, T. Maruyama, K. Ishikawa, T. Takahashi, M. Nakamura, T. Ezaki, and H. Morita.** 1994. Direct and rapid detection of *Erysipelothrix rhusiopathiae* DNA in animals by PCR. *J. Clin. Microbiol.* **32:**1526–1531.

47. **Marquet-Van der Mee, N., and A. Audurier.** 1995. Proposals for optimization of the international phage typing system for *Listeria monocytogenes*: combined analysis of phage lytic spectrum and variability of typing results. *Appl. Environ. Microbiol.* **61:**303–309.

48. **McLauchlin, J., and P. N. Hoffman.** 1989. Neonatal cross-infection from *Listeria monocytogenes*. *Commun. Dis. Rep.* **16:**3–4.

49. **McLauchlin, J., S. M. Hall, S. K. Velani, and R. J. Gilbert.** 1991. Human listeriosis and paté: a possible association. *Br. Med. J.* **303:**773–775.

50. **McLauchlin, J., and J. C. Low.** 1994. Primary cutaneous listeriosis in adults: an occupational disease of veterinarians and farmers. *Vet. Rec.* **135:**615–617.

51. **Moellering, R. C., G. Medoff, I. Leech, C. Wennersten, and L. J. Kunz.** 1972. Antibiotic synergism against *Listeria monocytogenes*. *Antimicrob. Agents. Chemother.* **1:**30–34.

52. **Nash, P., and M. M. Krenz.** 1991. Culture media, p. 1226–1288. *In* A. Balows, W. J. Hausler, Jr., K. L. Herrmann, H. D. Isenberg, and H. J. Shadomy (ed.), *Manual of Clinical Microbiology*, 5th ed. American Society for Microbiology, Washington, D.C.

53. **Nieman, R. E., and B. Lorber.** 1980. Listeriosis in adults, a changing pattern: report of eight cases and a review of the literature, 1968–1978. *Rev. Infect. Dis.* **2:**207–227.

54. **Ninet, B., E. Bannerman, and J. Bille.** 1992. Assessment of the Accuprobe *Listeria monocytogenes* culture identification reagent kit for rapid colony confirmation and its application in various enrichment broths. *Appl. Environ. Microbiol.* **58:**4055–4059.

55. **Nocera, D., E. Bannerman, J. Rocourt, K. Jaton Ogay, and J. Bille.** 1990. Characterization by DNA restriction endonuclease analysis of *Listeria monocytogenes* strains related to the Swiss epidemic of listeriosis. *J. Clin. Microbiol.* **28:**2259–2263.

56. **Nocera, D., M. Altwegg, G. Martinetti Lucchini, E. Bannerman, F. Ischer, J. Rocourt, and J. Bille.** 1993. Characterization of *Listeria* strains from a foodborne listeriosis outbreak by rDNA gene restriction patterns compared to four other typing methods. *Eur. J. Clin. Microbiol. Infect. Dis.* **12:**162–169.

57. **Norton, D. M., M. A. McCamey, K. L. Gall, J. M. Scarlett, K. J. Boor, and M. Wiedmann.** 2001. Molecular studies on the ecology of *Listeria monocytogenes* in the smoked fish processing industry. *Appl. Environ. Microbiol.* **67:**198–205.

58. **O'Donoghue, K., K. Bowker, J. McLauchlin, D. S. Reeves, P. M. Bennett, and A. P. MacGowan.** 1995. Typing of *Listeria monocytogenes* by random amplified polymorphic DNA (RAPD) analysis. *Int. J. Food Microbiol.* **27:**245–252.

59. **Okwumabua, O., B. Swaminathan, P. Edmonds, J. Wenger, J. Hogan, and M. Alden.** 1992. Evaluation of a chemiluminescent DNA probe assay for the rapid confirmation of *Listeria monocytogenes*. *Res. Microbiol.* **143:**183–189.

60. **Piffaretti, J.-C., H. Kressebuch, M. Aeschbacher, J. Bille, E. Bannerman, J. M. Musser, R. K. Selander, and J. Rocourt.** 1989. Genetic characterization of clones of the bacterium *Listeria monocytogenes* causing epidemic disease. *Proc. Natl. Acad. Sci. USA* **86:**3818–3822.

61. **Pine, L., S. Kathariou, F. Quinn, V. George, J. D. Wenger, and R. E. Weaver.** 1991. Cytopathogenic effects in enterocytelike Caco-2 cells differentiate virulent from avirulent *Listeria* strains. *J. Clin. Microbiol.* **29:**990–996.

62. **Reboli, A. C., and W. E. Farrar.** 1989. *Erysipelothrix rhusiopathiae*: an occupational pathogen. *Clin. Microbiol. Rev.* **2:**354–359.

63. **Rocourt, J., A. Audurier, A. L. Courtieu, J. Durst, S. Ortel, A. Schrettenbrunner, and A. G. Taylor.** 1985. A multicenter study on the phage typing of *Listeria monocytogenes*. *Zentbl. Bakteriol. Hyg. A* **259:**489–497.

64. **Rocourt, J., P. Boerlin, F. Grimont, C. Jacquet, and J.-C. Piffaretti.** 1992. Assignment of *Listeria grayi* and *Listeria murrayi* to a single species, *Listeria grayi*, with a revised description of *Listeria grayi*. *Int. J. Syst. Bacteriol.* **42:**171–174.

65. **Rocourt, J., and P. Cossart.** 1997. *Listeria monocytogenes*, p. 337–352. *In* M. P. Doyle, L. R. Beuchat, and T. J. Montville (ed.), *Food Microbiology: Fundamentals and Frontiers*. ASM Press, Washington, D.C.

66. **Rocourt, J., C. Jacquet, and J. Bille.** 1997. *Human Listeriosis, 1991–1992.* WHOFNU/FOS/97.1.1997. Food Safety Unit Division of Food and Nutrition, World Health Organization, Geneva, Switzerland.

67. **Rocourt, J.** 1999. The genus *Listeria* and *Listeria monocytogenes*: phylogenetic position, taxonomy, and identification, p. 1–20. *In* E. T. Ryser and E. H. Marth (ed.), *Listeria, Listeriosis, and Food Safety*, 2nd ed. Marcel Dekker, New York, N.Y.

68. **Salamina, G., E. Dalle Donne, A. Niccolini, G. Poda, D. Cesaroni, M. Bucci, R. Fini, M. Maldini, A. Schuchat, B. Swaminathan, W. Bibb, J. Rocourt, N. Binkin, and S. Salmaso.** 1996. A foodborne outbreak of gastroenteritis involving *Listeria monocytogenes* in Northern Italy. *Epidemiol. Infect.* **117:**429–436.

69. **Scheld, W. M.** 1983. Evaluation of rifampin and other antibiotics against *Listeria monocytogenes* in vitro and in vivo. *Rev. Infect. Dis.* **5**(Suppl. 3)**:**S593–S599.

70. **Schuchat, A., C. Lizano, C. V. Broome, B. Swaminathan, C. Kim, and K. Winn.** 1991. Outbreak of neonatal listeriosis associated with mineral oil. *Pediatr. Infect. Dis.* **10:**183–189.

71. **Schuchat, A., B. Swaminathan, and C. V. Broome.** 1991. Epidemiology of human listeriosis. *Clin. Microbiol. Rev.* **4:**169–183.

72. **Seeliger, H. P. R., and K. Hohne.** 1979. Serotyping of *Listeria monocytogenes* and related species. *Methods Microbiol.* **13:**31–49.

73. **Seeliger, H. P. R., and D. Jones.** 1986. Genus *Listeria* Pirie, 1940, 383[AL], p. 1235–1245. *In* P. H. A. Sneath, N. S. Mair, M. E. Sharpe, and J. G. Holt (ed.), *Bergey's Manual of Systematic Bacteriology*, vol. 2. Williams & Wilkins, Baltimore, Md.

74. **Shehnan, B., C. Kocks, S. Drami, A. D. Klarsfeld, J. Mengaud, and P. Cossart.** 1994. Molecular and genetic determinants of the *Listeria monocytogenes* infectious process. *Curr. Top. Microbiol. Immunol.* **192:**187–216.

75. **Stelma, G. N., A. L. Reyes, J. T. Peeler, D. W. Francis, J. M. Hunt, P. L. Spaulding, C. H. Johnson, and J.**

Lovett. 1987. Pathogenicity test for *Listeria monocytogenes* using immunocompromised mice. *J. Clin. Microbiol.* **25:** 2085–2089.

76. **Swaminathan, B., T. J. Barrett, S. B. Hunter, and R. V. Tauxe.** 2001. PulseNet: the molecular subtyping network for foodborne bacterial disease surveillance, United States. *Emerg. Infect. Dis.* **7:**382–389.

77. **Takahashi, T., T. Fujisawa, Y. Tamura, S. Suzuki, M. Muramatsu, T. Sawada, Y. Benno, and T. Mitsuoka.** 1992. DNA relatedness among *Erysipelothrix rhusiopathiae* strains representing all twenty-three serovars and *Erysipelothrix tonsillarum.* *Int. J. Syst. Bacteriol.* **42:**469–473.

78. **Troxler, R., A. von Graevenitz, G. Funke, B. Wiedemann, and I. Stock.** 2000. Natural antibiotic susceptibility of *Listeria* species: *L. grayi, L. innocua, L. ivanovii, L. monocytogenes, L. seeligeri,* and *L. welshimeri* strains. *Clin. Microbiol. Infect.* **6:**525–535.

79. **van Netten, P., I. Perales, A. van de Moosdijk, G. D. W. Curtis, and D. A. A. Mossel.** 1989. Liquid and solid differential media for the detection and enumeration of *Listeria monocytogenes* and other *Listeria* spp. *Int. J. Food Microbiol.* **8:**299–316.

80. **Weaver, R. E.** 1985. *Erysipelothrix,* p. 209–210. *In* E. H. Lennette, A. Balows, W. J. Hausler, Jr., and H. J. Shadomy (ed.), *Manual of Clinical Microbiology,* 4th ed. American Society for Microbiology, Washington, D.C.

81. **Welshimer, H. J., and A. L. Meredith.** 1971. *Listeria murrayi:* a nitrate-reducing mannitol-fermenting *Listeria. Int. J. Syst. Bacteriol.* **21:**3–7.

82. **Wernars, K., P. Boerlin, A. Audurier, E. G. Russell, G. D. W. Curtis, L. Herman, and V. van der Mee-Marquet.** 1996. The WHO multicenter study on *Listeria monocytogenes* subtyping: random amplification of polymorphic DNA (RAPD). *Int. J. Food Microbiol.* **32:**325–341.

83. **Wiggins, G. L., W. L. Albritton, and J. C. Feeley.** 1978. Antibiotic susceptibility of clinical isolates of *Listeria monocytogenes. Antimicrob. Agents Chemother.* **12:** 854–860.

Coryneform Gram-Positive Rods

GUIDO FUNKE AND KATHRYN A. BERNARD

34

This chapter deals with aerobically growing, asporogenous, irregularly shaped, non-partially acid-fast, gram-positive rods generally called coryneforms. The term "coryneform" is actually somewhat misleading since only true *Corynebacterium* spp. exhibit a typical club-shaped ("*coryne*," meaning "club" in ancient Greek) morphology whereas all the other bacteria discussed in this chapter show an irregular morphology. However, in our experience, the term "coryneforms" is a common and convenient expression used by many clinical microbiologists, and, therefore, the term will be used in this chapter.

The coryneform bacteria which were, for didactical reasons, not included in this chapter comprise *Actinomyces* spp. (in particular, the most frequently encountered species on aerobic plates, *A. europaeus, A. neuii, A. radingae,* and *A. turicensis*), the newly described genus *Actinobaculum, Propionibacterium* spp. (*P. acnes, P. avidum,* and *P. granulosum*), and *Propioniferax innocua* (see in chapter 55), whereas *Arcanobacterium* spp. are included. *Gardnerella vaginalis* is included in this chapter but is discussed separately. Regularly shaped aerobically growing gram-positive rods (*Bacillus, Listeria* and *Erysipelothrix, Clostridium tertium,* and *Lactobacillus*) are covered in chapters 32, 33, 54, and 55, respectively. Taxa which might be initially misidentified as coryneform bacteria also include partially acid-fast bacteria and other actinomycetes (see chapter 35) as well as rapidly growing mycobacteria (see chapter 37).

GENERAL TAXONOMY

The bacteria discussed in this chapter all belong to the class *Actinobacteria,* whose genera are characterized by specific 16S rDNA signature nucleotides (119). All the genera described in this chapter except *Exiguobacterium* and *Gardnerella* belong to the lineage of the gram-positive bacteria with high guanine-plus-cytosine (G+C) content. The coryneform bacteria are most diverse and are differentiated by chemotaxonomic features (Table 1). Phylogenetic investigations, in particular 16S rRNA gene sequencing, have, in general, confirmed the framework set by chemotaxonomic investigations. The 16S rRNA gene sequencing data demonstrate that the genera *Corynebacterium* and *Turicella* are more closely related to the partially acid-fast bacteria and to the genus *Mycobacterium* than to the other coryneform organisms covered in this chapter (61, 91, 110).

The genus *Arthrobacter,* which contains rods, is phylogenetically intermixed with the genus *Micrococcus* (and genera formerly called *Micrococcus*), which contains cocci (44, 72). The genus *Rothia* contains both rod-forming organisms, represented by *Rothia dentocariosa,* and a coccus-forming species, *Rothia mucilaginosa,* the former *Stomatococcus mucilaginosus* (21). Other genera which are phylogenetically closely related include *Oerskovia, Cellulosimicrobium,* and *Cellulomonas* (54, 112), as well as *Arcanobacterium* and *Actinomyces* (92). The genus *Dermabacter* is loosely associated with the genera *Arthrobacter* and *Micrococcus,* whereas the genus *Brevibacterium* forms a distinct line of descent (8).

DESCRIPTIONS OF THE GENERA

Genus *Corynebacterium*

The genus *Corynebacterium* is presently composed of 59 species (and two taxon groups), 36 (and the two taxon groups) of which are medically relevant. The species which are not known to be isolated from humans or to cause diseases in humans are *C. ammoniagenes, C. auriscanis, C. bovis, C. callunae, C. camporealensis, C. capitovis, C. casei, C. cystitidis, C. efficiens, C. felinum, C. flavescens, C. glutamicum, C. kutscheri, C. mastitidis, C. mooreparkense, C. mycetoides, C. phocae, C. pilosum, C. renale, C. testudinoris, C. terpenotabidum, C. variabile,* and *C. vitaeruminis.* Fourteen of the *Corynebacterium* species have been defined since the last edition of this Manual (Table 2).

The cell wall of corynebacteria contains *meso*-diaminopimelic acid (*m*-DAP) as the diamino acid as well as short-chain mycolic acids with 22 to 36 carbon atoms (16). *C. amycolatum* and *C. kroppenstedtii* are the only genuine *Corynebacterium* species which do not possess mycolic acids (15, 17). The corynebacterial cell wall also contains arabinose and galactose (16), but their detection is not recommended for the routine clinical laboratory. Palmitic ($C_{16:0}$), oleic ($C_{18:1\omega9c}$), and stearic ($C_{18:0}$) acids are the main cellular fatty acids (CFAs) in all corynebacteria, and tuberculostearic acid (TBSA) can also be found in some species like *C. urealyticum* and *C. confusum* (4, 51). The G+C content of *Corynebacterium* spp. varies from 46 mol% (in *C. kutscheri*) to 74 mol% (in *C. auris*) (47), indicating the enormous diversity within this genus. The phylogenetic relationships within the genus *Corynebacte-*

TABLE 1 Some chemotaxonomic features of the bacteria covered in this chapter

Genus	Major CFAs	Mycolic acids	Peptidoglycan diamino acid[a]	Acyl type
Corynebacterium	18:1ω9c, 16:0, 18:0	+[b]	m-DAP	Acetyl
Turicella	18:1ω9c, 16:0, 18:0	−	m-DAP	Glycolyl
Arthrobacter	15:0ai, 17:0ai, 15:0i	−	LYS	Acetyl
Brevibacterium	15:0ai, 17:0ai, 15:0i	−	m-DAP	Acetyl
Dermabacter	17:0ai, 15:0ai, 16:0i	−	m-DAP	ND[c]
Rothia	15:0ai, 17:0ai, 16:0i	−	LYS	ND
Exiguobacterium	17:0ai, 15:0ai, 16:0, 13:0i	−	LYS	ND
Oerskovia	15:0ai, 15:0i, 17:0ai	−	LYS	Acetyl
Cellulomonas	15:0ai, 16:0, 17:0ai	−	ORN	Acetyl
Cellulosimicrobium	15:0ai, 15:0i, 17:0ai	−	LYS	Acetyl
Microbacterium	15:0ai, 17:0ai, 16:0i	−	LYS, ORN	Glycolyl
Curtobacterium	15:0ai, 17:0ai, 16:0i	−	ORN	Acetyl
Leifsonia	17:0ai, 15:0ai, 16:0i	−	DAB	ND
Arcanobacterium	18:1ω9c, 16:0, 18:0	−	LYS	ND
Gardnerella	16:0, 18:1ω9c, 14:0	−	LYS	ND

[a] m-DAP, meso-diaminopimelic acid; LYS, lysine; ORN, ornithine; DAB, diaminobutyric acid.
[b] Exceptions: C. amycolatum and C. kroppenstedtii.
[c] ND, no data.

rium have been outlined (91, 110) and create an extensive and reliable database for future comparative 16S rRNA gene studies, e.g., for the delineation of new species.

Gram staining of corynebacteria shows slightly curved, gram-positive rods with sides not parallel and sometimes slightly wider ends, giving some of the bacteria a typical club shape (Fig. 1a). Corynebacteria whose morphologies differ from this morphology include C. durum, C. matruchotii, and C. sundsvallense (see below under each species). Cells infrequently stain unevenly. If Corynebacterium cells are taken from fluid media, they are arranged as single cells, in pairs, in V forms, in palisades, or in clusters with a so-called Chinese letter appearance. It is again emphasized that the club-shaped form of the rods is observed only for true Corynebacterium spp. Corynebacteria are always catalase positive, and the medically relevant species are all nonmotile. The genus Corynebacterium includes both fermenting and nonfermenting species.

Genus *Turicella*

The genus Turicella is phylogenetically closely related to Corynebacterium but contains T. otitidis as the only species.

The cell wall contains m-DAP, but mycolic acids are not present (61). The main CFAs for T. otitidis are the same as those for Corynebacterium spp., but all T. otitidis strains also contain significant amounts of TBSA (2 to 10% of all CFAs) (61). T. otitidis is the only coryneform bacterium that has a polar lipid profile without glycolipids (102). The G+C content varies between 65 and 72 mol% (61).

Gram staining shows relatively long gram-positive rods (Fig. 1b). T. otitidis is catalase positive, nonmotile, and an oxidizer.

Genus *Arthrobacter*

The genera Arthrobacter and Micrococcus are so closely related phylogenetically that it has been stated that micrococci are, in fact, arthrobacters which are unable to express rod forms (72). Presently, the genus Arthrobacter contains over 20 species, of which only a few have been recovered from human clinical specimens (44, 69, 132). Lysine is the diamino acid of the cell wall, and $C_{15:0ai}$ is the overall dominating CFA, which represents more than 50% of all CFAs in most Arthrobacter species. The G+C content

TABLE 2 Chronology of recently proposed or reclassified medically and non-medically relevant coryneform bacteria since publication of the previous edition of this Manual

Yr of definition	Human isolates (reference)	Veterinary or environmental isolates (reference)
1998	Arthrobacter creatinolyticus (69), Microbacterium spp. (121)	
1999		Brevibacterium avium (90), Corynebacterium auriscanis (20), Corynebacterium terpenotabidum (122)
2000	Arthrobacter albus (132), Arthrobacter luteolus (132), Corynebacterium simulans (131), Leifsonia aquatica (35), Rothia mucilaginosa (21)	Cellulomonas humilata (22), Rothia nasimurium (21)
2001	Brevibacterium paucivorans (133), Cellulosimicrobium cellulans (112), Corynebacterium freneyi (101), Corynebacterium matruchotii-like (98), Corynebacterium "nigricans" (113), Microbacterium resistens (2)	Arcanobacterium pluranimalium (76), Corynebacterium capitovis (18), Corynebacterium casei (6), Corynebacterium felinum (19), Corynebacterium mooreparkense (6), Corynebacterium testudinoris (19), further Microbacterium spp. (2)
2002	Corynebacterium aurimucosum (136), Corynebacterium sanguinis (Funke, Hoyle, and Collins, submitted)	Corynebacterium efficiens (38)

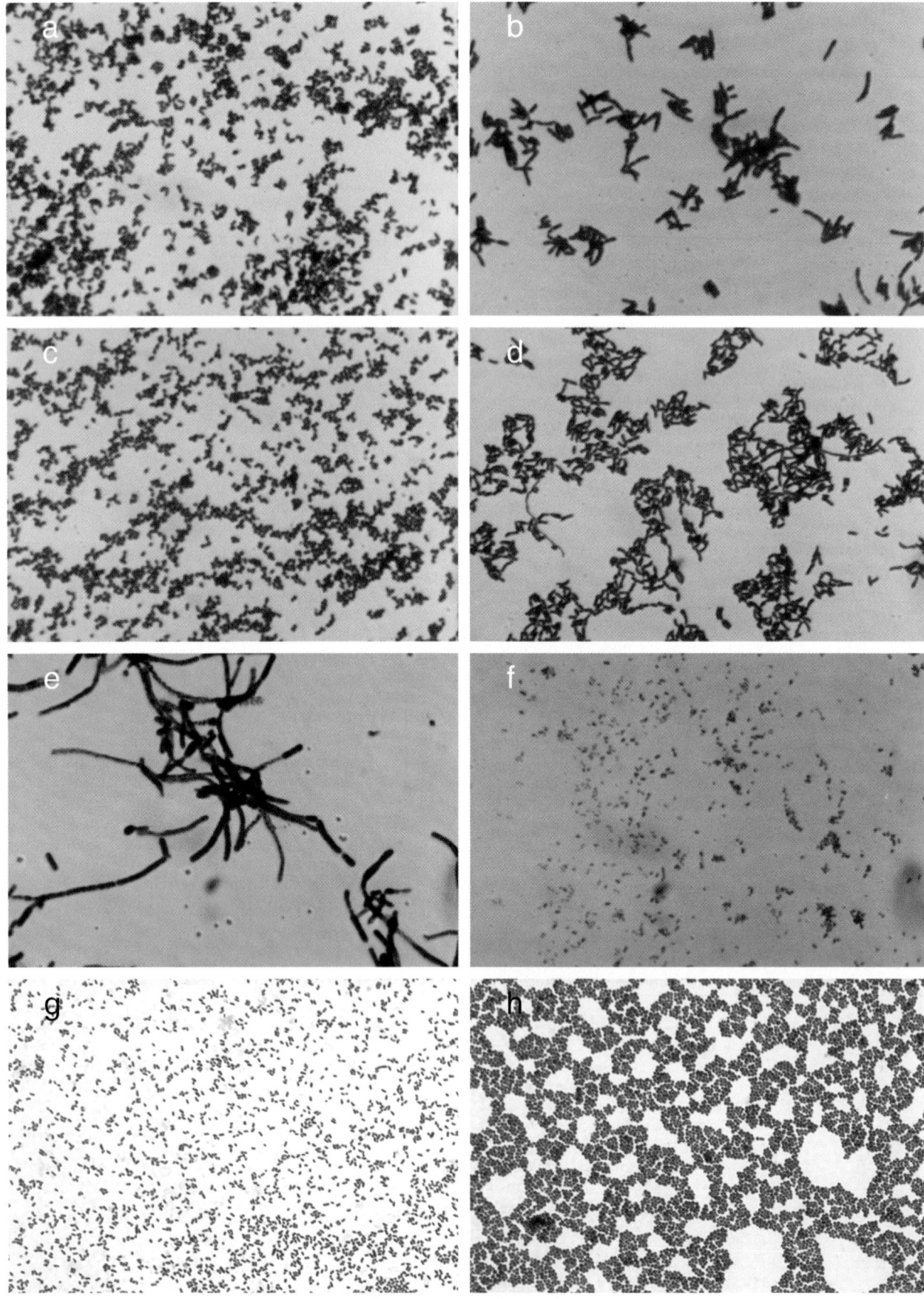

varies between 59 and 70 mol%, indicating the diversity within this genus.

Gram staining may demonstrate a rod-coccus cycle (i.e., rod forms in younger cultures and cocci in older colonies) when cells are grown on rich media (e.g., Columbia base agar). Jointed rods (i.e., rods in a rectangular form, which contributed to the designation of this genus as "*arthros*," meaning "joint" in ancient Greek) may also be observed in younger cultures (i.e., after 24 h) but may not be demonstrable for every species. Arthrobacters are catalase positive, motility is variable, and they are always oxidizers.

Genus *Brevibacterium*

The genus *Brevibacterium* presently comprises eight species (41, 90, 133). m-DAP is the diamino acid of the cell wall. $C_{15:0ai}$ and $C_{17:0ai}$ usually represent more than 75% of all CFAs (41). The G+C content varies between 60 and 67 mol%.

Gram staining demonstrates relatively short rods, which may develop into cocci when cultures are getting older (after 3 days). Brevibacteria are catalase positive, nonmotile, and oxidizers.

Genus *Dermabacter*

The genus *Dermabacter* presently comprises only one species, *D. hominis*. m-DAP is the diamino acid of the cell wall, and $C_{15:0ai}$ and $C_{17:0ai}$ usually account for 40 to 60% of all CFAs. The G+C content range is between 60 and 62 mol% (70).

Gram staining shows very short rods (Fig. 1c), which are often initially misinterpreted as cocci. *D. hominis* strains are catalase positive and nonmotile and possess a fermentative metabolism as demonstrated by glucose fermentation.

Genus *Rothia*

For didactical reasons, the genus *Rothia* is also included in this chapter because some species are rod-like. Collins et al. have recently reclassified *Stomatococcus mucilaginosus* as *Rothia mucilaginosa* (21). The genus *Rothia* belongs to the family *Micrococcaceae*. Since *Rothia mucilaginosa* exhibits coccoid forms in the Gram stain, the genus *Rothia* is also covered in chapter 28 (on the catalase-positive grampositive cocci). However, the species *R. dentocariosa* clearly exhibits mainly rod forms and is therefore covered in this chapter.

Lysine is the diamino acid of the cell wall, and $C_{15:0ai}$ and $C_{17:0ai}$ usually represent 40 to 60% of all CFAs. The G+C content ranges between 47 and 56 mol%. *Rothia* strains can be quite pleomorphic by Gram staining, but filamentous forms are normally not observed. They have a variable catalase reaction, are nonmotile, and exhibit a fermentative metabolism.

Genus *Exiguobacterium*

The genus *Exiguobacterium* is phylogenetically related to the so-called group 2 bacilli (36). Presently, *E. aurantiacum* and *E. acetylicum* (the former *Brevibacterium acetylicum*)

(36) are the only two species described for this genus, but *E. aurantiacum* has not been mentioned in any publication as being isolated from human clinical material. Lysine is the diamino acid of the cell wall, and $C_{15:0ai}$ and $C_{17:0ai}$ comprise only about 30 to 40% of the total CFAs. *E. acetylicum* contains significant amounts of $C_{13:0i}$ and $C_{13:0ai}$, which are not found in any other coryneform taxon (4). The G+C content is about 47 mol%.

Exiguobacteria are found as relatively short rods in young cultures. Strains are catalase positive and motile and have a fermentative metabolism.

Genus *Oerskovia*

In older textbooks, oerskoviae were assigned to the nocardioform group of organisms due to their morphological features. This includes extensive branching, vegetative hyphae, and penetration into agar, but they have no aerial hyphae. However, there is now phylogenetic evidence that *Oerskovia*, with the only presently described species, *O. turbata*, is more closely related to genera like *Cellulomonas* than to the mycolic acid-containing genera like *Nocardia*. Lysine is the diamino acid of the cell wall, and $C_{15:0ai}$ and $C_{15:0i}$ are the main CFAs in oerskoviae, comprising about 40 to 60% of all CFAs. The G+C content is 70 to 75 mol%.

Gram staining shows coccoid to rod-shaped bacteria which originate from the breaking up of mycelia. *O. turbata* strains are catalase positive, motility is variable, and they are fermentative.

Genus *Cellulomonas*

The genus *Cellulomonas* presently comprises nine species, of which only *C. hominis* has been described as being isolated from humans (22, 54, 112). Ornithine is the diamino acid of the cell wall, and $C_{15:0ai}$ and $C_{16:0}$ are the main CFAs. The G+C content is 71 to 76 mol%.

Gram staining shows small, thin rods. All *Cellulomonas* spp., except *C. fermentans* and *C. humilata*, are catalase positive, their motility is variable, all except *C. hominis* are cellulolytic (*C. hominis* did not hydrolyze cellulose in the test system used [54]), and they have a fermentative metabolism.

Genus *Cellulosimicrobium*

The genus *Cellulosimicrobium* comprises only one species, *C. cellulans*, which had been designated *Cellulomonas cellulans* or *Oerskovia xanthineolytica* in the past (112). The reason for removing *C. cellulans* from the genus *Cellulomonas* was that the topology of the 16S rDNA dendrogram indicated that the branching point of this taxon was outside *Cellulomonas* proper (112). In addition, the chemotaxonomic characteristic with lysine as the diamino acid supported the reclassification. Predominant CFAs include $C_{15:0ai}$ and $C_{15:0i}$. The major menaquinone (MK) is MK-9(H_4), and the G+C content is 74 mol%. It should be noted that the genus *Cellulosimicrobium* is closely related to the genus *Oesrkovia* but nevertheless distinct.

FIGURE 1 Gram stain morphologies of *Corynebacterium diphtheriae* ATCC 14779 after 48 h of incubation (a), *Turicella otitidis* DSM 8821 (48 h) (b), *Dermabacter hominis* ATCC 51325 (48 h) (c), *Corynebacterium durum* DMMZ 2544 (72 h) (d), *Corynebacterium matruchotii* ATCC 14266 (24 h) (e), *Gardnerella vaginalis* ATCC 14018 (48 h) (f), black-pigmented *Corynebacterium* "nigricans" HC-NML 91-0032 (24 h) (g), and a black-pigmented *Rothia*-like CDC coryneform group 4 strain HC-NML 77-0298 (24 h) (h). Panels g and h were kindly provided by J. Koenig, Health Canada.

In young cultures, a mycelium is produced that fragments later into irregular, curved, and club-shaped rods. Catalase activity is detected, and strains are nonmotile. All strains show a fermentative metabolism.

Genus *Microbacterium*

It had been known since the mid-1990s that the genera *Microbacterium* and *Aureobacterium* are phylogenetically intermixed (97). The diamino acid in the third position of the tetrapeptide of the peptidoglycan was considered one of the most important chemotaxonomical markers. L-Lysine is present in microbacteria, and D-ornithine is present in the former aureobacteria. Because in some particular genera (e.g., *Propionibacterium* and *Bifidobacterium*) there is not a good correlation between the type of the diamno acid in their peptidoglycan and their phylogenetic trees and because a set of signature nucleotides within the 16S rDNA of both microbacteria and aureobacteria was demonstrated, it has been proposed to unify both genera in a redefined genus, *Microbacterium* (120).

Over 40 *Microbacterium* species have been validated to date, but only a minority of them have been demonstrated to be of clinical importance. Microbacteria are frequently encountered in environmental specimens (e.g., soil). However, it is most likely that a plethora of new microbacteria isolated from human clinical specimens will be established in the near future. $C_{15:0ai}$ and $C_{17:0ai}$ are the two main CFAs, often representing up to 75% of the total CFAs (43, 63, 120). The G+C content of *Microbacterium* spp. is 65 to 76 mol%, indicating the diversity within the genus.

Gram staining often shows thin or short rods with no branching. Catalase activity and motility are variable. Microbacteria can be either fermenters or oxidizers.

Genus *Curtobacterium*

Curtobacterium spp., like microbacteria, belong to the peptidoglycan type B actinomycetes (i.e., cross-linkage between positions 2 and 4 of the two peptide subunits). Ornithine is the diamino acid and is the only amino acid composing the interpeptide bridge. Curtobacteria have an acyl-type acetyl peptidoglycan and menaquinone MK-9 as major MK, whereas microbacteria possess a glycolyl type and MK-11,12 (Table 1). $C_{15:0ai}$ and $C_{17:0ai}$ represent more than 75% of all CFAs (G. Funke, M. Aravena-Roman, N. Weiss, and P. A. Lawson, submitted for publication). The G+C contents range from 68 to 75 mol%. Six *Curtobacterium* species are validly described.

Gram staining shows small and short rods with no branching. Catalase activity is positive, motility is observed in most strains, and all strains show a respiratory metabolism which proceeds slowly in oxidizing carbohydrates.

Genus *Leifsonia*

The former "*Corynebacterium aquaticum*" has been recently transferred into the new genus *Leifsonia* as *L. aquatica* (35). This species is the only medically relevant species in this genus. *L. aquatica* strains belong to the peptidoglycan B-type actinomycetes and therefore cannot be true corynebacteria, which actually possess an A type of peptidoglycan (i.e., cross-linkage between positions 3 and 4 of the two peptide subunits). Diaminobutyric acid is the diamino acid of the cell wall peptidoglycan, and $C_{15:0ai}$ and $C_{17:0ai}$, as in microbacteria, are the main CFAs but represent <75% of all CFAs (63). The G+C content is about 70 mol%.

Gram staining shows thin rods. The strains are catalase and oxidase positive (the latter is an atypical feature for coryneform bacteria), always motile, and oxidizers.

Genus *Arcanobacterium*

The genus *Arcanobacterium* contains five species, of which *A. haemolyticum*, *A. bernardiae*, and *A. pyogenes* have been recovered from human clinical specimens. *A. pyogenes*, as well as *A. phocae* and *A. pluranimalium*, has been isolated from veterinary material. Lysine is the diamino acid of the cell wall, whereas lysine or ornithine is found in the phylogenetically closely related *Actinomyces* spp. Arcanobacteria contain MKs of the MK-9(H_4) type, whereas the *Actinomyces* spp. examined so far have MK-10(H_4). The main CFAs of arcanobacteria are $C_{16:0}$, $C_{18:1\omega9c}$, and $C_{18:0}$ (as in *Corynebacterium* spp. and *T. otitidis*), but in contrast to corynebacteria, significant amounts of $C_{10:0}$, $C_{12:0}$, and $C_{14:0}$ may also be detected (4). The G+C content is 48 to 52 mol%.

Gram staining of arcanobacteria shows irregular grampositive rods. All arcanobacteria except *A. phocae* and *A. pluranimalium* (76) are catalase negative, and they are nonmotile and fermentative.

NATURAL HABITAT

Many species of the corynebacteria are part of the normal flora of the skin and mucous membranes in humans and mammals. The habitat for a minority of the species (e.g., *C. callunae* and *C. terpenotabidum*) is the environment. It is noteworthy that not all corynebacteria are equally distributed over skin and mucous membranes but many of them occupy a specific niche. *C. diphtheriae* can be isolated from the nasopharynx as well as from skin lesions, which actually represent a reservoir for the spread of diphtheria. Important opportunistic pathogens like *C. amycolatum*, *C. striatum*, and *D. hominis* are part of the normal human skin flora but have thus far not been recovered from throat swabs from healthy individuals (129). Coryneform bacteria prominent in the oropharynx include *C. durum* and *R. dentocariosa* (129). *C. auris* and *T. otitidis* seem to have an almost exclusive preference for the external auditory canal (G. Funke, unpublished observation). In nearly every instance that *C. macginleyi* has been isolated, it has been recovered from eye specimens (52, 71). In addition, the normal corynebacterial flora of the conjunctiva is lipophilic (130). Another *Corynebacterium* species with a distinctive niche is *C. glucuronolyticum*, which is almost exclusively isolated from genitourinary specimens from humans (40) and, as recently shown, also from animals (26). *C. urealyticum*, another genitourinary pathogen, has, like *C. jeikeium*, also been cultured from the inanimate hospital environment (88).

The natural habitat of arcanobacteria is not fully understood, but *A. haemolyticum* is recovered from throat as well as from wound swabs (11, 79) whereas *A. bernardiae* has been found mainly in abscesses adjacent to skin (Funke, unpublished). It is unclear whether the two species are part of the normal skin and/or the gastrointestinal flora. *A. pyogenes* is found on mucous membranes of cattle, sheep, and swine. Brevibacteria can be found on dairy products (e.g., cheese) but are also inhabitants of the human skin (41). Arthrobacters are some of the most frequently isolated bacteria when soil samples are cultured, but *Arthrobacter cumminsii* also seems to be present on human skin (53). Members of the genera *Exiguobacterium*, *Oerskovia*, *Cellu-*

lomonas, *Cellulosimicrobium*, and *Microbacterium* have their habitats in the inanimate environment (e.g., soil and activated sludge). *Microbacterium* spp. have also been recovered from hospital environments (43). Curtobacteria are primarily plant pathogens (Funke, Aravena-Roman, et al., submitted).

CLINICAL SIGNIFICANCE

Estimation of the clinical significance of coryneform bacteria isolated from clinical specimens is often confusing for clinical microbiologists. This is in part due to the natural habitat of coryneform bacteria, which may lead to their recovery if specimens were not taken correctly. The reader is referred to the guidelines on minimal microbiological requirements in publications on disease associations of coryneform bacteria (62).

Coryneform bacteria should be identified to the species level if they are isolated (i) from normally sterile body sites, e.g., blood (unless only one of multiple specimens became positive); (ii) from adequately collected clinical material if they are the predominant organisms; and (iii) from urine specimens if they are the only bacteria encountered and the bacterial count is $>10^4$/ml or if they are the predominant organisms and the total bacterial count is $>10^5$/ml.

The clinical significance of coryneform bacteria is strengthened by the following findings: (i) multiple specimens are positive for the same coryneform bacteria; (ii) coryneform bacteria are seen in the direct Gram stain, and a strong leukocyte reaction is also observed; and (iii) other organisms recovered from the same material are of low pathogenicity.

For a comprehensive summary of case reports on individual coryneform bacteria, the reader is referred to a review article (62). The most frequently reported coryneforms, as well as their established disease associations, are listed in Table 3.

Historically, diphtheria caused by *C. diphtheriae* (or *C. ulcerans*) is the most prominent infectious disease for which coryneform bacteria are responsible. Therefore, special attention is given to that disease in this chapter. As a result of immunization programs, the disease has nearly disappeared in countries with high socioeconomic standards. However, it is still endemic in some subtropical and tropical countries as well as among individuals of certain ethnic groups (e.g., indigenous peoples in the Americas and Australia). In the 1990s, diphtheria reemerged in the states of the former Soviet Union. However, despite increased global travel activities, only a few imported cases have been reported by countries with well-developed health care systems.

The main manifestation of diphtheria is an upper respiratory tract illness with sore throat, dysphagia, lymphadenitis, low grade-fever, malaise, and headache. A nasopharyngeal adherent membrane which occasionally leads to obstruction is characteristic. The severe systemic effects of diphtheria include myocarditis, neuritis, and kidney damage caused by the *C. diphtheriae* exotoxin, which is encoded by a bacteriophage carrying the *tox* gene. *C. diphtheriae* may also cause cutaneous diphtheria or endocarditis (with either toxin-positive or toxin-negative strains). Some people with poor hygienic standards (e.g., drug and alcohol abusers) are prone to colonization (on the skin more often than in the pharynx) by *C. diphtheriae* strains, which are often nontoxigenic.

COLLECTION, TRANSPORT, AND STORAGE OF SPECIMENS

In general, coryneform bacteria do not need special handling when samples are collected.

C. diphtheriae

The diagnosis of diphtheria is primarily a clinical one. The physician should notify the receiving laboratory immediately of suspected diphtheria. In case of respiratory diphtheria, material for culture should be obtained on a swab (either a cotton- or a polyester-tipped swab) from the inflamed areas in the nasopharynx. Multisite sampling (nasopharynx) is thought to increase sensitivity. If membranes are present and can be removed (swabs from beneath the membrane are most valuable), they should also be sent to the microbiology laboratory (although *C. diphtheriae* might not be culturable from those in every instance). Nasopharyngeal swabs should be obtained from suspected carriers. It is preferable that the swabs be immediately transferred to the microbiology laboratory for culturing. If the swabs must be sent to the laboratory, semisolid transport media (e.g., Amies [see chapters 6 and 20]) ensure the maintenance of the bacteria. All coryneform bacteria are relatively resistant to drying and moderate temperature changes. Material from patients with suspected cases of wound diphtheria can be obtained by swab or aspiration.

After the appropriate isolation media have been inoculated (see "Isolation Procedures and Incubation" below), the swabs taken from diphtheritic membranes may be subjected to Neisser or Loeffler methylene blue staining. However, it is noteworthy that the sensitivity of the microscopic examination is limited.

A PCR-based direct detection system for diphtheria toxin has been described by the Centers for Disease Control and Prevention (CDC) (84). Their system had the highest sensitivity when Dacron polyester-tipped swabs were used and when silica gel packages were stored at 4°C rather than at room temperature. CDC accepts swabs, pieces of diphtheria membranes, or biopsy tissue for this assay (K. M. Bisgard, C. Vitek, A. Golaz, T. Popovic, and M. Wharton, Diphtheria [http://www.cdc.gov/nip/publications/surv-manual/dip.pdf]). This approach was successfully used for a retrospective study for which only formalin-fixed clinical specimens were available (73). However, direct detection for diphtheria toxin as the sole, primary test for clinical specimens has not been recommended, and microbiological culture is essential for confirming diphtheria (29).

Long-term preservation in skim milk at −70°C is applicable to all coryneform bacteria. The same skim milk tube except for those containing lipophilic corynebacteria can be thawed and put into the freezer again, and this can be done several times (Funke, unpublished). For nonlipophilic coryneforms, good results were also observed with Microbank tubes (Pro Lab Diagnostics, Austin, Tex.) (Funke, unpublished). The advantage of using these tubes is that individual beads can be taken out of the tube. Coryneform bacteria can also be stored for decades when they are kept lyophilized in an appropriate medium (e.g., 0.9% NaCl containing 2% bovine serum albumin).

ISOLATION PROCEDURES AND INCUBATION

Coryneform bacteria including *C. diphtheriae* can be readily isolated from a 5% sheep blood agar (SBA)-based selective

TABLE 3 Most frequently reported disease associations of coryneform bacteria in humans

Taxon	Disease or disease association	Reference(s)[a]
C. amycolatum	Wound infections, foreign body infections, bacteremia, sepsis, urinary tract infections, respiratory tract infections	46, 75
CDC group F-1	Urinary tract infections	
CDC group G	Catheter infections, bacteremia, endocarditis, wound infections, eye infections	
C. diphtheriae (toxigenic)	Throat diphtheria, cutaneous diphtheria	30; http://www.cdc.gov/nip/publications/surv-manual/dip.pdf
C. diphtheriae (nontoxigenic)	Endocarditis, foreign body infections, pharyngitis	3, 39, 99
C. glucuronolyticum	Genitourinary tract infections (mainly males)	40
C. jeikeium	Endocarditis, bacteremia, foreign body infections, wound infections	103
C. macginleyi	Eye infections	52, 71
C. minutissimum	Wound infections, urinary tract infections, respiratory tract infections	139
C. "nigricans"	Genitourinary tract infections (mainly females)	113; Bernard et al., submitted
C. pseudodiphtheriticum	Respiratory tract infections, endocarditis	
C. pseudotuberculosis	Lymphadenitis (occupational)	93
C. riegelii	Urinary tract infections (females)	49
C. striatum	Wound infections, respiratory tract infections, foreign body infections	
C. ulcerans (toxigenic)	Respiratory diphtheria	
C. urealyticum	Urinary tract infections, bacteremia, wound infections	116
Arthrobacter spp.	Bacteremia, foreign body infections, urinary tract infections	44, 53, 69, 132
Brevibacterium spp.	Bacteremia, foreign body infections, malodorous feet	41
D. hominis	Wound infections, bacteremia	60, 64
Rothia spp.	Endocarditis, bacteremia, respiratory tract infections	
Oerskovia sp.	Foreign body infections, bacteremia	
Cellulomonas spp.	Bacteremia, wound infections	54
Cellulosimicrobium sp.	Foreign body infections, bacteremia	
Microbacterium spp.	Bacteremia, foreign body infections, wound infections	43, 63
A. bernardiae	Abscess formation (together with mixed anaerobic flora)	56
A. haemolyticum	Pharyngitis in older children, wound and tissue infections	11, 79
A. pyogenes	Abscess formation, wound and soft tissue infections	
G. vaginalis	Bacterial vaginosis, endometritis, postpartum sepsis	12

[a] References for taxa without references are our observations. For further information, see reference 62.

medium containing 100 μg of fosfomycin per ml (plus 12.5 μg of glucose-6-phosphate per ml) since nearly all coryneforms (except *Actinomyces* spp. and *D. hominis*) are highly resistant to this compound (125, 129). It is also possible to put disks containing 50 μg of fosfomycin (plus 50 μg of glucose-6-phosphate [already incorporated in the disk]) (BD Diagnostics, Sparks, Md.) on an SBA plate and then examine the colonies which grow around the disk. Selective media for coryneform bacteria containing 50 to 100 μg of furazolidone (Sigma, St. Louis, Mo.) per ml have also been described. If lipophilic corynebacteria like *C. jeikeium* or *C. urealyticum* are sought, then 0.1 to 1.0% Tween 80 (Merck, Darmstadt, Germany) should be added to an SBA plate (before pouring the medium). It is also possible to streak sterile filtered Tween 80 with a cotton swab onto SBA plates. Coryneform bacteria do not grow on Mac-Conkey agar. However, if "coryneform" bacteria are recovered from this medium, they should be examined carefully to rule out rapidly growing mycobacteria.

With very few exceptions (some arthrobacters, microbacteria, and curtobacteria, which have optimal growth temperatures between 30 and 35°C), the medically relevant coryneform bacteria all grow at 37°C. It is desirable to culture specimens for coryneform bacteria in a CO_2-enriched atmosphere since some taxa, e.g., *Rothia* and *Arcanobacterium* spp., grow much better under those conditions. Nearly all medically relevant coryneform bacteria grow within 48 h, and so primary culture plates should not be incubated longer than that. However, if liquid media are used (e.g., for specimens from normally sterile body sites), these should be checked after 5 days by Gram staining for the presence of coryneform bacteria (only if growth is observed with the naked eye) before they are discarded.

It is recommended that urine specimens be incubated for longer than 24 h to check for the presence of *C. urealyticum* but only when patients are symptomatic or have alkaline urine or struvite crystals in their urine sediment (116).

C. diphtheriae

The primary plating medium for the cultivation of *C. diphtheriae* should be SBA plus one selective medium (e.g., Cystine-Tellurite blood agar [CTBA] or freshly prepared Tinsdale medium) (29, 30). If silica gel is used as a transport medium, the desiccated swabs should be additionally incubated overnight in broth (supplemented with either plasma or blood), which should then be streaked onto the primary plating medium. The plates are read after 18 to 24 h of incubation at 37°C, preferably in a 5% CO_2-enriched atmosphere. Tellurite inhibits the growth of many noncoryneform bacteria, but even a few *C. diphtheriae* strains are sensitive to potassium tellurite and will therefore not grow on CTBA but may grow on SBA. It is noteworthy that growth on CTBA and tellurite reduction are not specific for *C. diphtheriae*, since many other coryneforms may also produce black (albeit smaller) colonies. The best medium for direct culturing of *C. diphtheriae* is probably Tinsdale medium (30). However, the limitations of Tinsdale medium are its relatively short shelf life (<4 weeks) and the necessity to add horse serum to it. On Tinsdale plates, both tellurite reductase activity (as shown by black colonies) and cystinase activity (as shown by a brown halo around the colonies) can be observed (see Fig. 3i). If neither CTBA nor Tinsdale medium is available, colistin-nalidixic acid blood agar (CNA) plates are recommended for the isolation of *C. diphtheriae* or any other coryneform bacterium. It is necessary to pick multiple colonies from CNA plates to rule out *C. diphtheriae* (first Gram staining, then subculturing, and then biochemical testing). Nonselective Loeffler serum slants are no longer recommended for the primary isolation of *C. diphtheriae* because of overgrowth by other bacteria (but *C. diphtheriae* cells with polar bodies are produced on Loeffler or Pai slants only).

IDENTIFICATION AND TYPING SYSTEMS

Basic tests available in every microbiology laboratory are of great value for the identification of coryneform bacteria. The Gram staining morphology of the cells can exclude the assignment to many genera and may even lead to the assignment to the correct genus (e.g., to the genus *Corynebacterium*, *Turicella*, or *Dermabacter*) (Fig. 1). Morphology, size, pigment, odor, and hemolysis of colonies are also valuable criteria in the differential diagnosis of coryneform bacteria.

von Graevenitz and Funke (128) had outlined a biochemical identification system for coryneform bacteria which was based on previous results from CDC Special Bacteriology Reference Laboratory (66; D. G. Hollis, Handout, 92nd Gen. Meet. Am. Soc. Microbiol. 1992). This system includes the following reactions: catalase, test for fermentation or oxidation (in our experience, this is best observed in semisolid cystine Trypticase agar [CTA] medium [rather than on triple sugar iron or oxidation-fermentation media], with fermentation indicated by acid

or alkali production in the entire tube and oxidation found at the surface of the tube); motility; nitrate reduction (24-h incubation); urea hydrolysis (24-h incubation); esculin hydrolysis (up to 48-h incubation); acid production from glucose, maltose, sucrose, mannitol, and xylose (48-h incubation); CAMP reaction (24-h incubation) with a beta-hemolysin-producing strain of *Staphylococcus aureus* (e.g., strain ATCC 25923), i.e., positive reaction indicated by an augmentation of the effect of *S. aureus* beta-hemolysin on erythrocytes, resulting in a complete hemolysis in an arrowhead configuration (Fig. 2); and a test for lipophilia (24-h incubation), which is performed only for catalase-positive colonies <0.5 mm in diameter. For the test for lipophilia, colonies are subcultured onto ordinary SBA and onto a 0.1 to 1% Tween 80-containing SBA plate. Lipophilic corynebacteria develop colonies up to 2 mm in diameter after 24 h on Tween-supplemented agar. It has also been suggested that growth in brain heart infusion broth with and without supplementation of 1% Tween 80 be compared and strains which grow only in the supplemented broth can be called lipophilic. The identification protocols given in this chapter are, in principle, based on

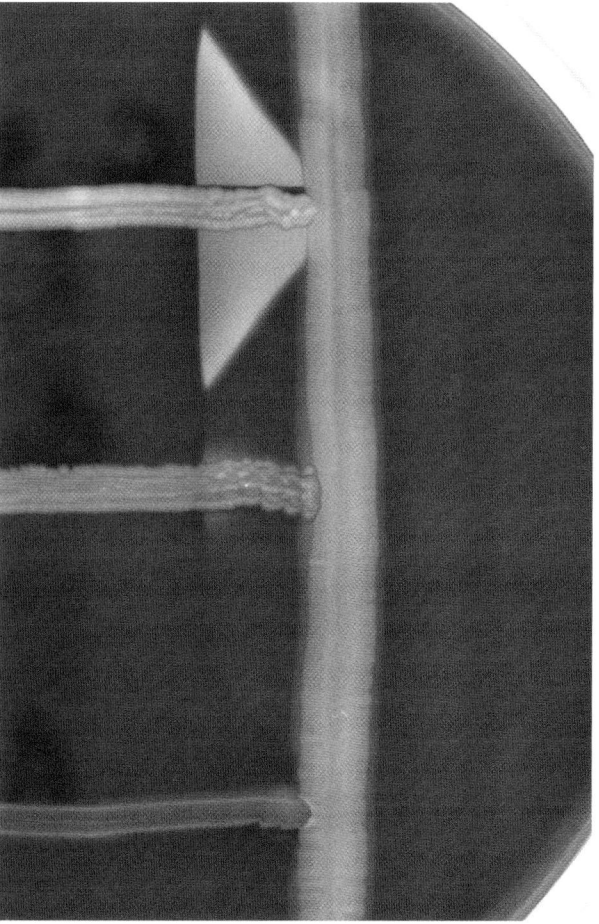

FIGURE 2 CAMP reactions of different coryneform bacteria after 24 h. (Top) *C. glucuronolyticum* DMMZ 891 (positive reaction). (Middle) *C. diphtheriae* ATCC 14779 (negative reaction). (Bottom) *A. haemolyticum* ATCC 9345 (CAMP inhibition reaction). The vertical streak is *S. aureus* ATCC 25923.

the identification system of von Graevenitz and Funke (128) mentioned above (Tables 4 and 5).

The presently available commercial identification systems include the API (RAPID) Coryne system (bioMérieux, Marcy l'Etoile, France), the RapID CB Plus system (Remel, Lenexa, Kans.), the Biolog GP plate (Biolog, Hayward, Calif.), the MicroScan panel (Dade Behring, Sacramento, Calif.), the BBL Crystal GP system (BD, Sparks, Md.), and the MCN GP plate (Merlin Diagnostics, Bornheim-Hersel, Germany). So far, evaluations have been published only for the first three systems (57, 59, 78). The API Coryne system contains 49 taxa in its present database (version 2.0). In a comprehensive multicenter study it was found that 90.5% of the strains belonging to the taxa included were correctly identified, with additional tests needed for correct identification for 55.1% of all strains tested (59). The results were highly reproducible if the manufacturer's recommendations for use were rigorously followed. It was concluded that the system is a useful tool for the identification of the diverse group of coryneform bacteria encountered in the routine clinical laboratory. The RapID CB Plus system correctly identified 80.9% of the strains to the genus and species levels and an additional 12.2% to the genus level but with less accurate species designations; it was also concluded that this system may perform well under the conditions of a routine clinical laboratory (57). The Biolog GP plate system (database version 3.50) identified only about 60% of all strains tested to the correct genus level or to the correct species level (78). However, in the meantime the company has significantly improved both the technology and the database, but published evaluations of the revised system are still pending. The latter is also true for the three other commercial identification systems. The Vitek system (see chapter 14) still has the disadvantage of a relatively limited database for coryneform bacteria. It is always important to question critically the identifications provided by any commercial identification system and to correlate the results with simple basic characteristics such as macroscopic morphology and Gram stain results.

For some identifications the commercial API 50CH system (bioMérieux) has been found to be useful. For example, when applying the AUX medium (usually attached to the kit for gram-negative nonfermenters [bioMérieux]) to the API 50CH system, utilization reactions which allow the differentiation of *Brevibacterium* spp. or some *Arthrobacter* spp. can be observed (41, 44).

A reference laboratory would also use chromatographic techniques for further characterization of coryneform bacteria. The presence of mycolic acids and their chain lengths can be detected by either thin-layer chromatography (TLC), gas chromatography and mass spectrometry, or high-performance liquid chromatography (25). These methods can be useful for the differentiation of *Corynebacterium* spp. (mycolic acids of 22 to 36 carbon atoms) from the partially acid-fast bacteria (mycolic acids of 30 to 78 carbon atoms) but may also provide evidence that a coryneform bacterium is not a *Corynebacterium* species (exceptions are *C. amycolatum* and *C. kroppenstedtii*) if mycolic acids are not detected. The detection of the diamino acid of the peptidoglycan by one-dimensional TLC is of certain value for determining the genus to which a particular strain belongs (Table 1). In some cases, partial hydrolysates of the peptidoglycan are separated by two-dimensional TLC to reveal the interpeptide bridge of the peptidoglycan in order to distinguish between genera with the same diamino acid

in the peptide moiety. For example, some of the yellow-pigmented microbacteria and all curtobacteria have ornithine as their diamino acids, but microbacteria have (glycine)-ornithine as the interpeptide bridge whereas curtobacteria possess ornithine only.

The analysis of CFAs by means of gas-liquid chromatography with the Sherlock system (MIDI Inc., Newark, Del.) is an extremely useful method for the identification of coryneform bacteria. This system is, in general, able to identify coryneform bacteria to the genus level, but identification to the species level is impossible in most cases, although the commercial database suggests that it is possible. This is because of the very closely related CFA profiles of coryneform bacteria belonging to the same genus (4) and because the quantitative profiles observed depend strongly on the incubation conditions. When a laboratory creates its individual database based on its own entries, species identification becomes possible in some cases (K. A. Bernard, unpublished observation). The mycolic acids of some corynebacteria (e.g., *C. auris*) are cleaved at the temperature (300°C) produced in the injection port of the system, resulting in fatty acids which were identified as, e.g., $C_{17:1\omega6c}$ to $C_{\omega9c}$, by the Sherlock system (47).

Molecular genetic-based identification systems for coryneform bacteria have been outlined in recent years. Restriction fragment length polymorphism analysis of the partly amplified and digested 16S rRNA gene has been demonstrated to be of use for the identification of species within the genera *Corynebacterium* and *Brevibacterium* (9,126). Some corynebacteria may also be identified to the species level by examination of the length of the 16S–23S rRNA intergenic spacer region (1). rRNA gene restriction fragment polymorphism analysis (ribotyping) has recently been demonstrated to allow the identification of corynebacteria if three different restriction enzymes (BstEII, SmaI, and SphII) are used (5). In particular, potentially new corynebacterial species can be checked by this method for clustering with already established species. For pure taxononomic investigations of coryneform bacteria, full-length 16S rRNA gene sequencing and, in selected cases, quantitative DNA-DNA hybridizations might be necessary but will be restricted to the reference laboratory.

The commercial MicroSeq 500 16S bacterial sequencing kit (Perkin-Elmer, Foster City, Calif.) has been applied to the identification of coryneform bacteria, but discordant results (extensive phenotyping as gold standard) were observed for >30% of the *Corynebacterium* isolates, mainly due to the present database of the commercial system (123). However, due to the short running time (approximately 15 to 19 h), this and other similar systems will further spread to the routine clinical laboratory, in which case direct costs should drop from >$80 per test and databases will be improved.

It is emphasized that unidentifiable, clinically significant coryneform bacteria should be sent to an established reference laboratory experienced in corynebacterial identification.

DESCRIPTIONS OF GENERA AND SPECIES

Genus *Corynebacterium*

C. accolens

C. accolens (87) is found in specimens from the eyes, ears, nose, and oropharynx. Endocarditis of native aortic and

TABLE 4 Identification of medically relevant *Corynebacterium* spp.[a]

Species	Fermentation/ oxidation	Lipophilism	Nitrate reduction	Urease	Esculin hydrolysis	Pyrazin-amidase	Alkaline phos-phatase	Acid production from:					CAMP reaction	Other traits
								Glucose	Maltose	Sucrose	Mannitol	Xylose		
C. accolens	F	+	+	−	−	V	−	+	−	V	V	−	−	
C. afermentans subsp. afermentans	O	−	−	−	−	+	+	−	−	−	−	−	V	
C. afermentans subsp. lipophilum	O	+	−	−	−	+	+	−	−	−	−	−	V	
C. amycolatum	F	−	V	V	−	+	+	+	V	V	−	−	−	Most 0/129 resistant, propionic acid detected[b]
C. argentoratense	F	−	−	−	−	+	V	+	−	−	−	−	−	Chymotrypsin may be positive; propionic acid detected
C. aurimucosum	F	−	−	−	−	+	+	+	+	+	−	−	ND	Sticky colonies, slightly yellowish
C. auris	O	−	−	−	−	+	+	−	−	−	−	−	+	Slight adherence to agar, cleaved mycolics
C. bovis[c]	F	+	−	−	−	−	+	+	−	−	−	−	−	TBSA positive; fructose positive
C. confusum	F	−	+	−	−	+	+	(+)	−	−	−	−	−	Tyrosine negative, propionic acid detected
C. coyleae	F	−	−	−	−	+	+	(+)	−	+	−	−	+	
CDC group F-1	F	+	V	+	−	+	−	+	+	+	−	−	−	
CDC group G	F	+	V	−	−	+	+	+	V	V	−	−	−	Fructose positive, anaerobic growth positive
C. diphtheriae biotype gravis	F	−	+	−	−	−	−	+	+	−	−	−	−	Glycogen positive, propionic acid detected
C. diphtheriae biotype intermedius	F	+	+	−	−	−	−	+	+	−	−	−	−	Propionic acid detected
C. diphtheriae biotype mitis and belfanti	F	−	±[d]	−	−	−	−	+	+	−	−	−	−	Glycogen negative, propionic acid detected
C. durum	F	−	+	(V)	(V)	+	−	+	+	+	V	−	−	Adherent to agar, propionic acid detected
C. falsenii	F	−	−	(+)	−	(+)	+	(+)	V	−	−	−	+	Yellowish
C. freneyi	F	−	V	−	−	+	+	+	+	+	−	−	ND	α-Glucosidase positive, grows at 20°C and 42°C
C. glucuronolyticum	F	−	V	V	V	+	V	+	V	+	−	V	+	β-Glucuronidase positive, propionic acid detected
C. imitans	F	−	V	−	−	(+)	+	+	+	(+)	−	−	+	Tyrosine negative, 0/129 resistant
C. jeikeium	O	+	−	−	−	+	+	+	V	−	−	−	−	Fructose negative, anaerobic growth negative

(Continued on next page)

481

TABLE 4 Identification of medically relevant *Corynebacterium* spp.[a] *(Continued)*

Species	Fermentation/ oxidation	Lipophilism	Nitrate reduction	Urease	Esculin hydrolysis	Pyrazin- amidase	Alkaline phos- phatase	Acid production from:					CAMP reaction	Other traits
								Glucose	Maltose	Sucrose	Mannitol	Xylose		
C. kroppenstedtii	F	+	−	−	+	+	−	+	V	+	−	−	−	Lacking mycolic acids, propionic acid detected
C. lipophiloflavum	O	+	−	−	−	+	+	−	−	−	−	−	−	Yellow
C. macginleyi	F	+	+	−	−	−	+	+	−	+	V	−	−	
C. matruchotii	F	−	+	−	V	+	−	+	+	+	−	−	−	"Whip handle" (upon Gram staining); propionic acid detected
C. minutissimum	F	−	−	−	−	+	+	+	+	V	V	−	−	Tyrosine positive
C. mucifaciens	O	−	−	−	−	+	+	+	−	V	−	−	−	Very mucoid yellowish colonies
C. "nigricans"[e]	F	−	−	−	−	V	V	+	+	(+)	−	−	−	Black-pigmented colonies, adherent
C. propinquum	O	−	+	−	−	V	V	−	−	−	−	−	−	Tyrosine positive
C. pseudodiphtheriticum	O	−	+	+	−	+	V	−	−	−	−	−	−	
C. pseudotuberculosis	F	−	V	+	−	−	V	+	+	V	−	−	REV	Propionic acid detected
C. riegelii	F	−	−	+	−	V	V	(+)	(+)	−	−	−	−	
C. sanguinis	F	−	−	−	−	+	+	+	+	−	−	−	−	Yellowish
C. singulare	F	−	+	+	−	V	+	+	+	+	−	−	−	Tyrosine positive
C. simulans[f]	F	−	+	−	−	V	+	+	−	+	−	−	−	Reduces nitrite
C. striatum	F	−	+	−	−	V	V	+	−	V	−	−	V	Tyrosine positive
C. sundsvallense	F	−	−	+	−	V	V	+	+	+	−	−	−	Sticky colonies
C. thomssenii	F	−	−	+	−	+	+	+	+	+	−	−	−	N-Acetyl-β-glucosaminidase positive, sticky colonies
C. ulcerans	F	−	−	+	−	+	+	+	+	−	−	−	REV	Glycogen positive, propionic acid detected
C. urealyticum	O	+	−	+	−	+	V	−	−	−	−	−	−	
C. xerosis	F	−	V	−	−	+	+	+	+	+	−	−	−	0/129 susceptible, propionic acid not detected

[a] Abbreviations and symbols: F, fermentation; O, oxidation; +, positive; −, negative; V, variable; (), delayed or weak reaction; ND, no data; REV, CAMP inhibition reaction.

[b] Propionic acid as a glucose fermentation product.

[c] Blood culture isolate (Bernard et al., submitted) was also ONPG positive, oxidase positive, weakly maltose positive but negative by API Coryne, propionic acid was not detected; β-galactosidase was not observed using two methods (API Coryne, API Zym); API Coryne code obtained 0101104.

[d] *C. diphtheriae* biotype *mitis* is nitrate reductase positive, and *C. diphtheriae* biotype *belfanti* is nitrate reductase negative.

[e] At the time of writing, not a valid species name. Strain of C. "nigricans" described in reference 113 as being pyrazinamidase and alkaline phosphatase positive, but strains in Bernard et al. (submitted) were negative for these enzymes, using an API Coryne strip, giving rise to the code 0000125.

[f] *C. simulans* (131) is a strong nitrite reducer at low and high concentrations; nitrate reduction may appear to be negative unless further tested using zinc dust; one strain was catalase negative (Bernard et al., submitted).

TABLE 5 Identification of medically relevant coryneform bacteria other than *Corynebacterium* spp.[a]

Taxon	Catalase	Fermentation/ oxidation	Motility	Nitrate reduction	Urease	Esculin hydrolysis	Glucose	Maltose	Sucrose	Mannitol	Xylose	Other traits
Turicella otitidis	+	O	−	−	−	−	−	−	−	−	−	CAMP reaction positive, long rods
Arthrobacter spp.	+	O	V	V	V	V	V	V	V	−	−	
Brevibacterium spp.	+	O	−	V	−	−	V	V	V	−	V	Odor cheese-like
Dermabacter hominis	+	F	−	−	−	+	+	+	+	−	−	Small rods
Rothia dentocariosa	V	F	−	+	−	+	+	+	+	−	+	Some strains adherent
Exiguobacterium acetylicum	+	F	+	V	−	+	+	+	+	+	+	
Oerskovia turbata	+	F	V	+	−	+	+	+	+	−	+	Xanthine not hydrolyzed
Cellulomonas spp.	+	F	V	+	−	+	+	+	+	V	+	
Cellulosimicrobium cellulans	+	F/O	−	+	−	+	+	+	+	−	+	Hydrolysis of xanthine
Microbacterium spp.	V	F/O	V	V	V	V	+	V	V	V	V	
Curtobacterium spp.	+	O	V	−	−	+	+	V	V	V	+	
Leifsonia aquatica	+	O	+	V	−	V	+	+	+	+	+	
Arcanobacterium haemolyticum	−	F	−	−	−	−	+	+	V	−	−	CAMP inhibition reaction
Arcanobacterium pyogenes	−	F	−	−	−	V	+	V	V	V	+	
Arcanobacterium bernardiae	−	F	−	−	−	−	+	+	−	−	−	
Gardnerella vaginalis	−	F	−	−	−	−	+	+	V	−	−	Decolorized cells in Gram stain

[a] Abbreviations and symbols: +, positive reaction; −, negative reaction; V, variable reaction; O, oxidation; F, fermentation.

mitral valves due to this agent has been described. Colonies are, as for all other lipophilic corynebacteria, convex, smooth, and <0.5 mm in diameter on SBA. *C. accolens* strains had initially been described as exhibiting satellitism in the vicinity of *S. aureus* strains, attributable to its lipophilism (for the recommended method to demonstrate lipophilism, see "Identification and Typing Systems" above). *C. accolens* has a variable pyrazinamidase reaction but is negative for alkaline phosphatase, thus differentiating it from the morphologically and biochemically closely related CDC group G bacteria (Table 4). The API Coryne and RapiD CB Plus systems correctly identify *C. accolens* (57, 59). *C. accolens* strains are susceptible to a broad spectrum of antibiotics.

C. afermentans subsp. afermentans

C. afermentans subsp. *afermentans* (104) is part of the normal human skin flora and has so far been isolated mainly from blood cultures. Colonies are whitish, convex with regular edges, creamy, and about 1 to 1.5 mm in diameter after 24 h of incubation. *C. afermentans* subsp. *afermentans* has an oxidative metabolism. The API Coryne system provides the numerical code of 2100004 for this species. About 60% of all strains of this taxon are CAMP reaction positive. *C. afermentans* subsp. *afermentans* can be differentiated from *C. auris* and *T. otitidis* (both of which give the same API numerical code) by the consistency of its colonies (*C. auris* is slightly adherent to agar) and morphology on Gram staining (*T. otitidis* has longer cells). Further differential reactions include the carbohydrate utilization reactions tested with either the Biolog GP plate or the bioMérieux biotype 100 gallery (61, 102). By chemotaxonomic means, both *C. afermentans* subspecies and *C. auris* contain mycolates whereas *T. otitidis* lacks them, but these techniques are not applicable in a routine clinical laboratory. *C. afermentans* subsp. *afermentans* is generally susceptible to β-lactam antibiotics.

C. afermentans subsp. lipophilum

Strains belonging to the species *C. afermentans* subsp. *lipophilum* (104) have been isolated mainly from blood cultures as well as from superficial wounds. Colonies are, typically for lipophilic corynebacteria, convex, smooth, and <0.5 mm in diameter after 24 h. *C. afermentans* subsp. *lipophilum* has an oxidative metabolism and does not produce acid from any of the carbohydrates usually tested (Table 4). It is the only species of lipophilic corynebacteria which may exhibit a positive CAMP reaction. *C. afermentans* subsp. *lipophilum* is not included in the API Coryne database. The numerical profile observed for the species is 2100004, and so by that method it cannot be discerned from the more robustly growing *C. afermentans* subsp. *afermentans*, *C. auris*, or *T. otitidis*. Strains are usually susceptible to β-lactam antibiotics.

C. amycolatum

C. amycolatum is part of the normal human skin flora but was not recovered from throat swabs from healthy persons (129). *C. amycolatum* is the most frequently encountered *Corynebacterium* species in human clinical material (62). It is also the most frequently isolated non-lipophilic *Corynebacterium* in dairy cows with mastitis (68). *C. amycolatum* strains are often multidrug resistant (58). Colonies are very typically dry, waxy, and grayish white with irregular edges and are 1 to 2 mm in diameter after 24 h of incubation (Fig.

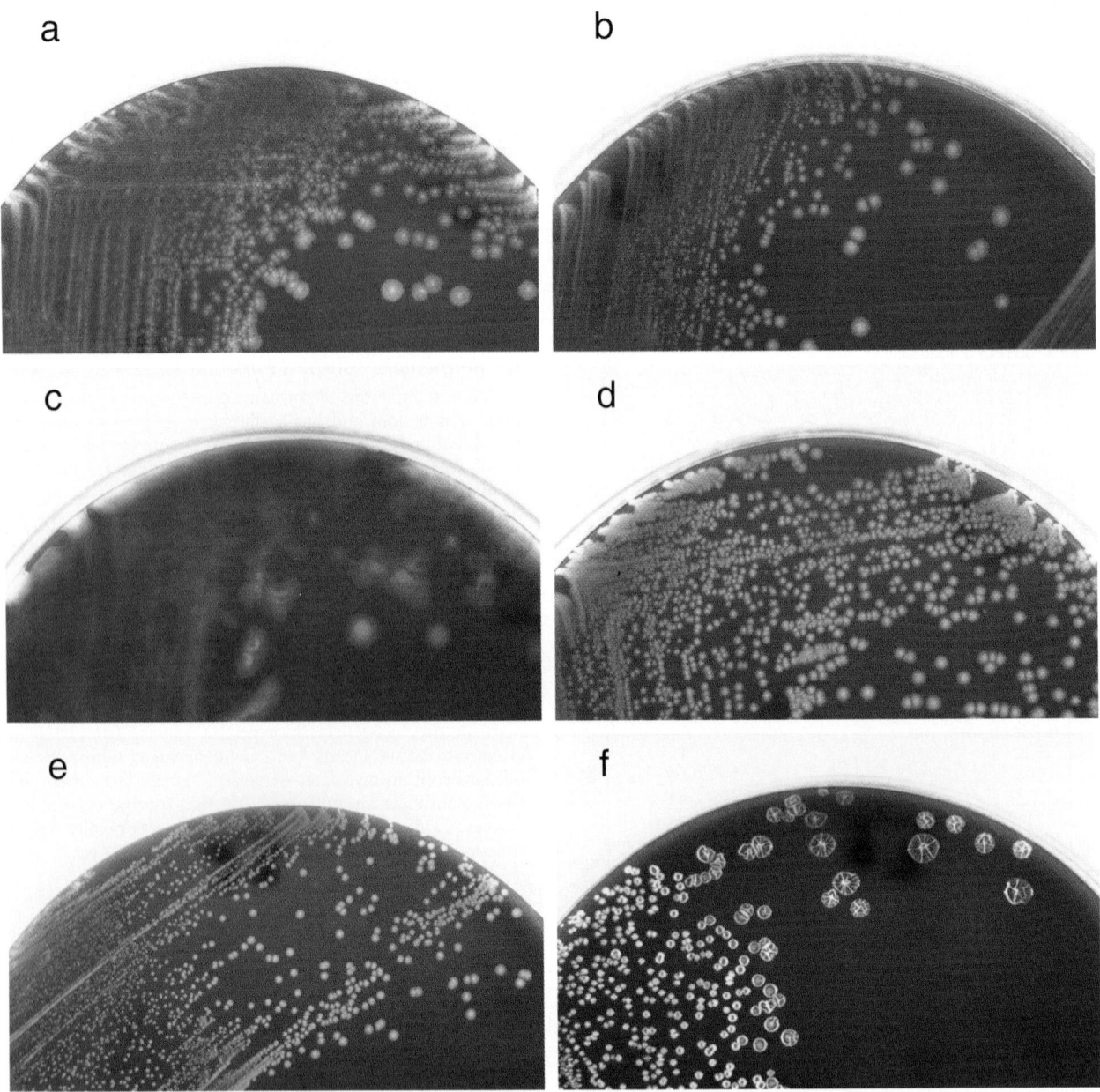

FIGURE 3 Colony morphologies of different coryneform bacteria after 48 h of incubation on SBA. (a) *C. amycolatum* LCDC 91-0077; (b) *C. diphtheriae* ATCC 14779; (c) *C. mucifaciens* LCDC 97-0202; (d) *C. striatum* ATCC 6940; (e) *D. hominis* ATCC 51325; (f) *R. dentocariosa* LCDC 95-0154; (g) black-pigmented *C. "nigricans"* HC-NML 91-0032 (after 96 h); (h) black-pigmented *Rothia*-like CDC coryneform group 4 strain HC-NML 77-0298 (after 96 h); (i) *C. diphtheriae* biotype *gravis* colonies on a Tinsdale agar plate. Panels g and h are photos by K. Bernard. Panel i was kindly provided by C. Hinnebusch and M. Cohen, UCLA School of Medicine, Los Angeles, Calif.

3a). *C. amycolatum* actually has a fermentative metabolism, but when CTA media are used for the observation of acid production from carbohydrates, *C. amycolatum* appears to resemble an oxidizer (i.e., the main acid production is at the surface of the medium). Strains of *C. amycolatum* are remarkable for their variability in basic biochemical reactions (Table 4) and have often been misidentified in the past as the biochemically similar species *C. xerosis*, *C. striatum*, or

C. minutissimum (46, 134, 139). These four species can be differentiated by the following reactions: *C. amycolatum* and *C. minutissimum* do not grow at 20°C but *C. xerosis* and *C. striatum* do; in addition, *C. xerosis* does not ferment glucose at 42°C whereas the other three species do, and *C. minutissimum* and *C. striatum* produce alkali from formate but *C. amycolatum* and *C. xerosis* do not (133). When tested on Mueller-Hinton agar supplemented with 5%

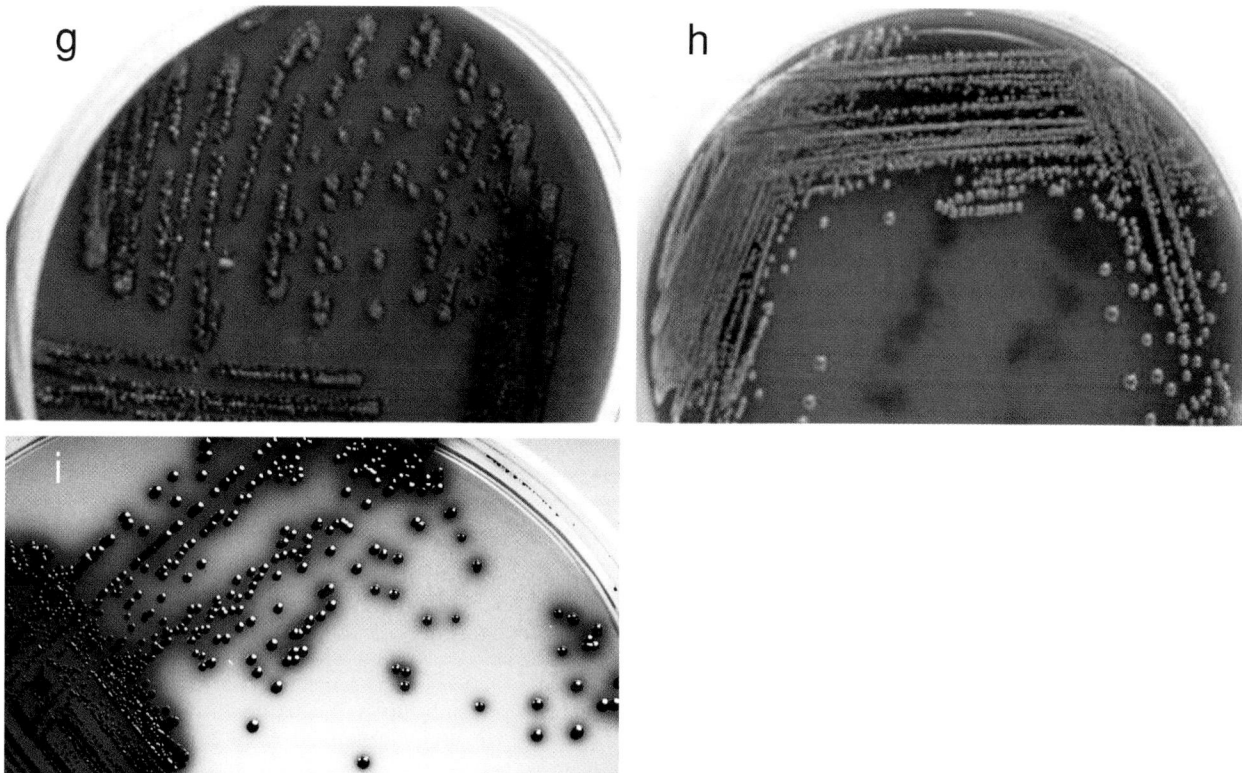

FIGURE 3 (*Continued*)

sheep blood, nearly all *C. amycolatum* strains were resistant to the vibriocidal compound 0/129 (150-μg disks) (Oxoid, Basingstoke, United Kingdom), as indicated by no zone of inhibition around the disk (46). In contrast, only 4% of all *C. amycolatum* strains were resistant to 0/129 when tested on Mueller-Hinton agar with 5% horse blood (75). The API Coryne system identifies this species very well, but in every case additional reactions must be carried out to confirm the identification of *C. amycolatum* (59). All *C. amycolatum* strains produce propionic acid as the major end product of glucose metabolism. In contrast to many other corynebacteria, *C. amycolatum* exhibits only weak or no leucine arylamidase activity. The identification may also be suggested by the absence of mycolic acids. In addition, it may be shown that acyl phosphatidylglycerol is a major phospholipid in *C. amycolatum,* in contrast to other *Corynebacterium* spp., in which other phospholipids are predominant.

C. argentoratense

C. argentoratense (106) has been isolated from the human throat as well as in one case, from a blood culture (K. A. Bernard, C. Munro, D. Wiebe, and E. Ongsansoy, submitted for publication). Colonies are cream colored, nonhemolytic, slightly rough, and 2 mm in diameter after 48 h of incubation. Phenotypically, *C. argentoratense* may appear to be very similar to (rare) ribose-negative strains of *C. coyleae*. However, glucose fermentation by *C. argentoratense*

is quite rapid, compared to the slowly fermenting species *C. coyleae*. As well, CAMP-negative *C. argentoratense* produces propionic acid as a fermentation product but CAMP-positive *C. coyleae* does not (55; Bernard et al., submitted). *C. argentoratense* is the only medically relevant *Corynebacterium* species expressing α-chymotrypsin activity, which can be observed in the API ZYM (bioMérieux) system; however, the blood culture isolate was not observed to produce that enzyme (Bernard et al., submitted). Although *C. argentoratense* is phylogenetically closely related to *C. diphtheriae*, it does not harbor the *tox* gene coding for the diphtheria toxin.

C. aurimucosum

C. aurimucosum was described recently, and the characteristics outlined are based on a single strain isolated from a human clinical specimen (136). On 5% SBA plates, colonies are 1 to 2 mm in diameter after 24 h, slightly yellow, and sticky, but on Trypticase soy agar without blood, they appear colorless and slimy. The basic biochemical profile (Table 4) is similar to that of *C. minutissimum.*

C. auris

C. auris (47) has been isolated almost exclusively from the ear region. Colonies are dryish, are slightly adherent to but do not penetrate agar, become slightly yellowish with time, and have diameters ranging from 1 to 2 mm after 48 h of incubation. *C. auris* does not produce acid from any carbohydrates usually tested. However, utilization reactions applying either the Biolog GP plate or the bioMérieux biotype

100 system may help in distinguishing *C. auris* from *C. afermentans* subsp. *afermentans* and *T. otitidis*, but in the clinical routine laboratory this can also be achieved by morphologic differentiation (see "*C. afermentans* subsp. *afermentans*" above). All *C. auris* strains are strongly CAMP test positive. The API Coryne system provides the numerical code 2100004 for this species. Abundant degradation products of mycolic acids are indirectly observed when CFA patterns are determined with the Sherlock system (47). It is noteworthy that the MICs of β-lactam antibiotics for *C. auris* strains are elevated, but the molecular mechanism for this is not known at present (58).

C. bovis

Occasionally, but not in the recent era, human infections had been attributed to the lipophilic bovine species, *C. bovis*. Characterization of lipophilic-appearing corynebacteria based solely on the use of phenotypic tests was probably incorrect in the absence of modern polyphasic methods or identification schemes such as those found in Table 4. This species had not been definitively recovered for many years from human clinical material, as previously reviewed (62). Recently, however, a human blood culture isolate of *C. bovis* was identified based on a polyphasic approach, including phenotypic, chemotaxonomic, and genotypic characteristics, with an API Coryne code of 0101104 (Bernard et al., submitted). Therefore, clinical microbiologists should be aware that this bacterium may be very rarely recovered from human specimens.

C. confusum

C. confusum has been isolated from patients with foot infections, a blood culture (51), and breast abscess (Bernard et al., submitted). Colonies are whitish, glistening, convex, creamy, and up to 1.5 mm in diameter after 48 h. Acid from glucose is produced only very weakly, becoming visible in the API Coryne or the API 50CH gallery only after 48 to 72 h. Weak growth under anaerobic conditions corresponds to slow fermentative acid production. It is advisable to incubate the API Coryne system after 24 h for another day in cases in which the results for acid production are ambiguous (i.e., only a slight change in the color of the indicator). After 48 h of incubation, the API Coryne system provides the numerical code 3100304 for this species; the breast abscess strain had a code of 3100104. Interestingly, the breast abscess strain was also CAMP positive, making it potentially more difficult to distinguish from *C. coyleae* isolates (Bernard et al., submitted). *C. confusum* is correctly identified by the RapID CB Plus system (57). If glucose fermentation is judged to be negative, *C. confusum* strains can be misidentified as *C. propinquum*. However, in contrast to that species, *C. confusum* does not hydrolyze tyrosine and contains small amounts of TBSA (1 to 3%) whereas *C. propinquum* hydrolyzes tyrosine but does not contain TBSA. *C. confusum* is differentiated from *C. coyleae* and *C. argentoratense* by its ability to reduce nitrate.

C. coyleae

C. coyleae (55) has been isolated mainly from cultures of blood and other normally sterile body fluids, but it may also be recovered from genitourinary specimens (Bernard et al., submitted; Funke, unpublished). Colonies are whitish and slightly glistening with entire edges and are about 1 mm in diameter after 24 h. The consistency of the colonies is either creamy or sticky. A slow fermentative acid production from glucose and a strongly positive CAMP reaction are the most significant phenotypic characteristics. *C. coyleae* is positive for cystine arylamidase, which is not observed for many other corynebacteria. Various API Coryne numerical codes have been observed, especially 2100304 and 6100304. *C. coyleae* is always positive for ribose fermentation, whereas the biochemically similar species *C. argentoratense* is variable for this reaction. The API Coryne database lists only 6% glucose-fermenting *C. coyleae* strains, and therefore, when applying this commercial identification system, the clinical microbiologist may not receive a correct identification (59). However, the two numerical profiles given above, combined with a positive CAMP reaction, are highly indicative of *C. coyleae*. This species is correctly identified by the RapID CB Plus system (57).

CDC Group F-1 Bacteria

CDC group F-1 bacteria (107) have not been given a species name. Although they are genetically distinct, no distinguishing phenotypic markers which clearly allow their separation from other defined *Corynebacterium* spp. have been found. The characteristics of the CDC group F-1 bacteria are consistent with the definition of the genus *Corynebacterium* in all respects. The strains are lipophilic and are the only lipophilic fermentative *Corynebacterium* species able to hydrolyze urea. Of note is the negative alkaline phosphatase reaction (Table 4). CDC group F-1 strains are usually susceptible to penicillin but are often resistant to macrolides.

CDC Group G Bacteria

CDC group G bacteria possess all chemotaxonomic features of true corynebacteria but cannot be given a species name since it has so far been impossible to find phenotypic traits allowing for a unanimous definition (107). These lipophilic strains can be separated from *C. jeikeium* by their anaerobic growth and fermentative acid production from fructose (103). Further biochemical features of CDC group G bacteria are given in Table 4. The API Coryne system correctly identifies CDC group G bacteria. They might be multidrug resistant, but the most frequently observed resistance is to macrolides and lincosamides.

C. diphtheriae

C. diphtheriae is commonly divided into four biotypes, *gravis*, *mitis*, *belfanti*, and *intermedius*; biotype differentiation is recommended by the World Health Organization (WHO) and CDC (29, 30) (http://www.cdc.gov/nip/publications/surv-manual/dip.pdf), although biotypes cannot be assigned separate subspecies status (108), nor is biotyping satisfactory for epidemiologic tracking. Initially, these biotypes were defined by differences in colony morphology and biochemical reactions (Table 4). However, only *C. diphtheriae* biotype *intermedius* can be identified on the basis of colonial morphology (small, gray, or translucent lipophilic colonies) (24) as well as positive dextrin fermentation. Other *C. diphtheriae* biotypes produce larger (up to 2 mm after 24 h) white or opaque colonies (Fig. 3b) which are indistinguishable from each other. The lipophilic *C. diphtheriae* biotype *intermedius* occurs only rarely in clinical infections, and *C. diphtheriae* biotype *belfanti* strains almost never harbor the diphtheria toxin gene.

Presumptive identification of *C. diphtheriae* (as well as of *C. pseudotuberculosis* and *C. ulcerans*) may be made by testing suspicious gram-positive rods for the presence of cystinase (as detected by using Tinsdale medium or diagnostic tablets [Rosco, Taastrup, Denmark]) and the absence of pyrazinamidase (diagnostic tablets are available from Key Scientific Products, Round Rock, Tex.). The API Coryne system identifies *C. diphtheriae* strains, with additional tests needed for the differentiation of *C. diphtheriae* biotype *mitis*, *C. diphtheriae* biotype *belfanti*, and *C. diphtheriae* biotype *intermedius* (59). Large amounts of propionic acid are produced as the end product of glucose metabolism (37). *C. diphtheriae* strains are distinct from all other coryneform bacteria (except *C. pseudotuberculosis* and *C. ulcerans*) in their CFA patterns because of the presence of a large volume of $C_{16:1\omega7c}$ (4).

Diphtheria Toxin Testing

It is recommended that at least 10 colonies of *C. diphtheriae* and related species be tested for diphtheria toxin by the Elek method, modified as described by Engler et al. (32), in a laboratory with skill in performing the test and in interpreting the test results. The modified Elek method described by the WHO Diphtheria Reference Unit was initially used to characterize strains from the 1990s epidemic in Russia and Ukraine and was found to be faster and less technically problematic than the original version. Antitoxins from various suppliers (e.g., Swiss Serum and Vaccine Institute, Bern, Switzerland; Pasteur Mérieux, Lyon, France; CDC Biological Products Division, Atlanta, Ga.), applied to blank filter disks at 10 IU/disk, have been successfully used with the modified Elek test (29), and precipitin lines can be read as early as 24 h (32) (Fig. 4). A similar modification of the Elek test, which can test up to 24 isolates on the same plate, has been described (100). A 3-h enzyme-linked immunosorbent assay for the detection of diphtheria toxin from clinical isolates of *Corynebacterium* spp. has been developed by the WHO Diphtheria Reference Unit (33). A rapid and simple test for detecting diphtheria toxin, called the immunochromatographic strip (ICS) assay, has been developed by the Program for Appropriate Technology in Health (PATH, Seattle, Wash.) and the WHO Reference Center (31). In this test, pure cultures of toxigenic diphtheria strains may be identified within 10 to 15 min after a 3-h incubation in an enrichment broth or detected in 4 to 6 h after clinical specimens containing toxigenic strains had been previously incubated in an enrichment broth for 16 h. Validation studies suggest that it has 98 to 100% specificity and 95 to 100% sensitivity for strains otherwise found to be toxigenic by two or more methods (the modified Elek and *tox* gene assay [described below]). Positive results were not seen for nontoxigenic *C. diphtheriae* or *C. ulcerans* strains, for other *Corynebacterium* species, or for other bacteria normally found in the throat (31). Colonies from a pure culture are emulsified in enrichment broth containing an ICS strip, and a diagnostic band will appear if the strain is toxigenic, in parallel to a positive control band (Fig. 5). The strips are thought to be stable for months at ambient temperatures and require minimal expertise to use and interpret. At the time of writing, commercial development of this product was under way but is not yet complete.

PCR-based methods for the detection of the diphtheria toxin gene (*tox*) in isolated bacteria have been developed and validated (29, 65). In addition, *tox* PCR assays applied directly to clinical specimens are accepted by CDC (http://www.cdc.gov/nip/publications/surv-manual/dip.pdf),

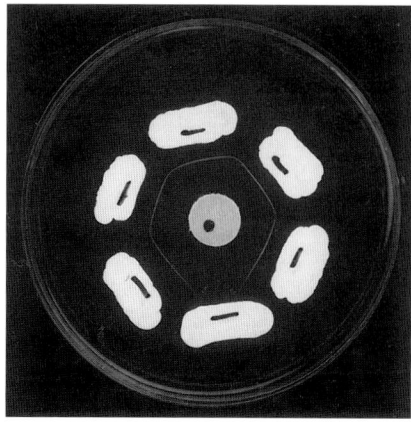

FIGURE 4 Modified Elek test (see the text) with antitoxin disk in the center. Strains are (clockwise starting at noon) NCTC 3984 (weakly toxin-positive *C. diphtheriae* biotype *gravis*), NCTC 10648 (strongly toxin-positive *C. diphtheriae* biotype *gravis*), a test strain (which was found to be a toxin producer), NCTC 10356 (nontoxigenic *C. diphtheriae* biotype *belfanti*), another test strain (also a toxin producer), and (again) NCTC 10648. The photo was kindly supplied by K.-H. Engler (WHO Diphtheria Reference Unit, Central Public Health Laboratory, London, United Kingdom).

particularly because isolation is not always possible for patients already receiving antibiotics. However, a PCR-positive patient from whom bacteria are not isolated or without a histopathologic diagnosis and without an epidemiologic linkage to a patient with a laboratory-confirmed case of diphtheria should be classified as having a "probable case" of diphtheria, since to date there are insufficient data to conclude that a PCR-positive result always implies diphtheria. Also, detection of the toxin gene in samples by PCR cannot automatically be attributed to one species, because *C. diphtheriae* as well as *C. ulcerans* and *C. pseudotuberculosis* may harbor the bacteriophage which carries the diphtheria toxin gene. Furthermore, *tox*-containing nontoxigenic isolates have been described and characterized further (13). A comprehensive history of the biology and molecular epidemiology of the diphtheria toxin has been reviewed by Holmes (67). Nontoxigenic strains of *C. diphtheriae*, i.e., those which do not express toxin in the Elek test or those which lack a detectable diphtheria toxin gene by PCR, have caused serious disease such as cases or outbreaks of skin disease or endocarditis, associated with occasional mortality, among homeless people, alcoholics, and intravenous drug abusers (3, 39, 62, 99).

Typing Methods

Outbreaks of *C. diphtheriae* in the states of the former Soviet Union and other locations have been studied by whole-cell peptide analysis, whole-genome restriction fragment length polymorphism analysis, ribotyping, pulsed-field gel electrophoresis, PCR single-strand conformation polymorphism analysis of *tox* and *dtxR* (i.e., the regulatory element of the diphtheria toxin) as well as of the 16S–23S rRNA gene spacer region, amplified fragment length polymorphisms, random amplification of polymorphic DNA (RAPD), and multilocus enzyme electrophoresis (27, 28, 81, 85, 96). Sequencing studies with *C. diphtheriae*

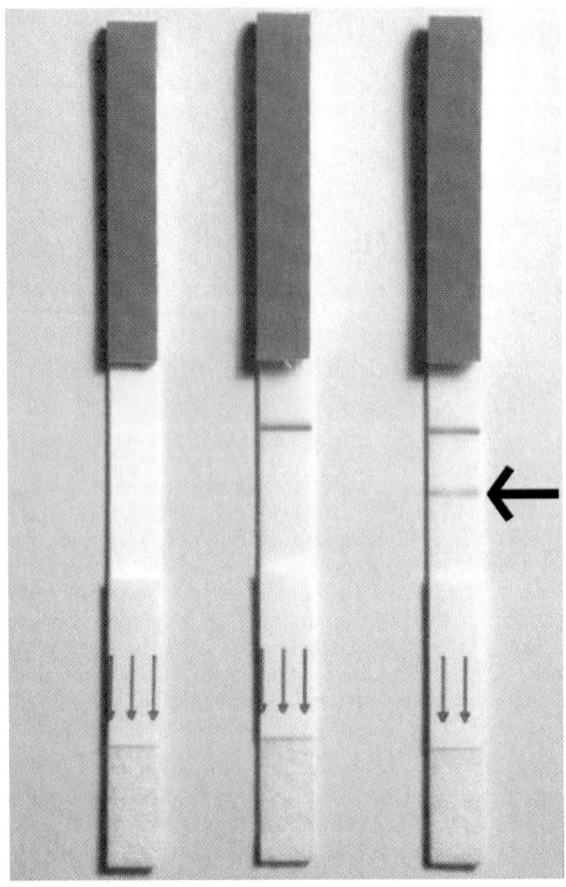

FIGURE 5 ICS strip for diphtheria toxin detection. (Left) Unused control; (middle), single control line on top, indicating a presumptively nontoxigenic strain; (right), two lines present (second line indicated by arrow, whether strong or faint), indicating that a strain is positive for diphtheria toxin. The photo was kindly provided by K. H. Engler (WHO Diphtheria Reference Unit, Central Public Health Laboratory, London, United Kingdom).

strains from the recent epidemic in the former Soviet Union have shown that point mutations within the *tox* gene were silent mutations whereas multiple point mutations (which even led to amino acid substitutions) were observed for the *dtxR* gene, corresponding to the heterogeneity of outbreak strains as revealed by PCR single-strand conformation polymorphism analysis (83). Molecular epidemiologic studies using RAPD have been used to rapidly screen a large number of *C. diphtheriae* strains to identify the epidemic clonal group associated with the outbreak in the former Soviet Union. Isolates derived from specific populations in the United States and Canada, and characterized using multilocus enzyme electrophoresis ribotyping, and RAPD, were found to be members of persistent endemic strains rather than being imported from other countries where diphtheria is endemic (81, 95).

Antibiotic treatment is required to eliminate *C. diphtheriae* and prevent its spread; however, it is not a substitute for antitoxin prevention. The antibiotics of choice are penicillins or macrolides. Sporadic isolates of *C. diphtheriae* resistant to erythromycin or rifampin have been reported.

Penicillin and some of the newer ketolides were tested against a large collection of geographically diverse strains and were found to generally demonstrate significant efficacy against *C. diphtheriae* but reduced ketolide activity against some Southeast Asian strains (34). It is believed that between 20 and 60% of adults in the United States lack protective antibodies to diphtheria toxin, which could pose a potentially significant public health risk and could result in the reemergence of this disease (81).

C. durum

C. durum (105) was originally described as being isolated exclusively from respiratory tract specimens. Well-characterized isolates have now been recovered from additional sites, including the gingiva, blood cultures and abscesses (98). *C. durum* strains were originally isolated after 2 to 3 days from nonselective charcoal-buffered yeast extract plates inoculated with sputa or bronchial washings. *C. durum* is the most frequent *Corynebacterium* species isolated from throat swabs of healthy persons (129). Its pathogenic potential is unclear at present. It is a peculiar nonlipophilic organism that forms colonies of only 0.5 to 1 mm in diameter after aerobic incubation for 72 h. Original description of this bacterium cited beige and rough colonies with convolutions, an irregular margin, and strong adherence to agar if grown under aerobic conditions (105). However, strains described in a later publication were found to be sometimes smoother and not necessarily adherent to agar (98). Gram staining of aerobic cultures shows long and filamentous rods with occasional "bulges," but true *C. durum* isolates do not have *C. matruchotii*-like "whip handles" (Fig. 1d and e). Long forms are not otherwise found among other *Corynebacterium* species, nor are they observed for *C. durum* when cells are grown in a 10% CO_2-enriched atmosphere (105). Strains grow only weakly under anaerobic conditions. They always reduce nitrate, and some may exhibit weak and delayed urease and esculinase activities. Most (but not all [129]) *C. durum* strains ferment mannitol, which is another very unusual feature for true corynebacteria (Table 4). API Coryne codes observed for *C. durum* include 3000135, 3001135, 3040135, 3400115, 3400135, 3400305, 3400325, and 3400335 (105), as well as 3040325, 3040335, 3440335, and 3441335 (98). This suggests that most strains are negative for alkaline phosphatase and all appear to be negative for pyrrolidonyl arylamidase. Only a small number of *C. durum* strains have been tested with the RapID system, and all were correctly identified (57). It is most likely that some strains identified as *C. matruchotii* in the past may actually have been *C. durum* strains and that differentiation can be difficult if phenotypic methods alone are used. Both species produce propionic acid as a fermentation product (Bernard et al., submitted). *C. durum* usually ferments galactose and very often mannitol, whereas *C. matruchotii* is usually negative for those sugars. The *C. matruchotii* type strain exhibits α-glucosidase activity, which is not observed in *C. durum* (105). It has recently been shown that some *C. durum* strains also express β-galactosidase activity and ferment ribose (129).

C. falsenii

C. falsenii strains (115) have so far been isolated only from sterile body fluids. Colonies are whitish, glistening, and smooth with entire edges and are 1 to 2 mm in diameter after 24 h. After 72 h, most strains described to date exhibit a yellowish pigment, which becomes even more intense after 120 h. This pigment is not observed in any other nonlipophilic *Corynebacterium* species encountered in clinical specimens, except in the rarely isolated species *C. aurimucosum* and *C. sanguinis* and the rarely found species *C. xerosis* (the colonies of the latter are dry, in contrast to *C. falsenii* colonies). The most characteristic biochemical features of *C. falsenii* are a slow but fermentative acid production from glucose, a weak pyrazinamidase reaction, and a weak urease activity which becomes visible in either Christensen's urea broth or the API Coryne system after overnight incubation only. API Coryne codes observed for *C. falsenii* are 2101104 and 2101304 (115; Bernard et al., submitted).

C. freneyi

C. freneyi has been outlined recently based on the study of three strains (101). All these strains had been isolated from skin-related material. *C. freneyi* is phylogenetically closely related to *C. xerosis*. Colonies of *C. freneyi* are whitish, dry, and rough; have irregular edges; and are 0.5 to 1 mm in diameter after a 48-h incubation. However, *C. freneyi* strains are nonlipophilic. The basic biochemical profile (Table 4) is also similar to that of *C. xerosis*. All *C. freneyi* strains studied so far exhibit α-glucosidase activity, which is not frequently observed in other *Corynebacterium* species (very few *C. amycolatum* and all *C. xerosis* strains express this enzyme). *C. freneyi* can be differentiated from *C. xerosis* by glucose fermentation at 42°C and growth at 20°C, whereas *C. xerosis* is negative for the last two reactions.

C. glucuronolyticum

C. seminale is a junior synonym of *C. glucuronolyticum* (26, 40). This species is probably part of the normal genitourinary flora of males, while its presence in females is uncertain. Colonies are whitish-yellowish, convex, and creamy and measure 1 to 1.5 mm in diameter after 24 h. The fermentative species *C. glucuronolyticum* is remarkable for its variability in basic biochemical reactions (Table 4). It is the only medically relevant *Corynebacterium* species exhibiting β-glucuronidase activity. When urease activity is present, it is abundant in Christensen's urea broth, becoming positive after only 5 min of incubation at room temperature (40). *C. glucuronolyticum* is also one of the very few corynebacteria which are able to hydrolyze esculin. All *C. glucuronolyticum* strains are CAMP reaction positive (Fig. 2). With the exception of strains which are alkaline phosphatase positive, the API Coryne strip identifies *C. glucuronolyticum* well (59), although the profiles obtained from human strains may differ from those for animal isolates (26). Propionic acid is one of the major end products of glucose metabolism. *C. glucuronolyticum* strains are often tetracycline resistant and may also exhibit resistance to macrolides and lincosamides (58). 16S rRNA gene sequences derived from fluids of patients with prostatitis are homologous to sequences derived for this species, indicating that *C. glucuronolyticum* might be involved in selected cases of prostatitis (124).

C. imitans

C. imitans was originally isolated from a nasopharyngeal specimen of a child suspected of having throat diphtheria, as well as from three adult contacts (42). This was the first well-documented case of person-to-person transmission of a *Corynebacterium* other than *C. diphtheriae* in a nonhospital setting. Additional strains of *C. imitans* have been recovered from blood cultures (Bernard et al., submitted). Colonies are whitish-grayish and glistening, with entire edges; are creamy; and measure 1 to 2 mm in diameter. The strain did not produce a brown halo on Tinsdale medium but was tellurite reductase positive. Interestingly, Neisser staining was positive for polar bodies. Pyrazinamidase activity was weak only, as was fermentation of sucrose, which may lead to the initial misidentification as an atypical *C. diphtheriae* strain. It is not unlikely that *C. imitans* may also have been misidentified as *C. minutissimum* in the past since the basic biochemical reactions of the two taxa are quite similar (Table 4). However, *C. imitans* is CAMP reaction positive and does not hydrolyze tyrosine, whereas the opposite reactions are observed for *C. minutissimum*. The API Coryne system provided the numerical codes 1100325, 2100324, and 3100325 for *C. imitans*, indicating a negative α-glucosidase reaction, whereas all *C. diphtheriae* strains express this enzyme. *C. imitans* strains do not produce propionic acid as a fermentation product, unlike *C. diphtheriae* (Bernard et al., submitted), and the CFA composition profiles for each species differ qualitatively, since *C. diphtheriae* and closely related species have a unique pattern among the *Corynebacterium* spp. (4). Diphtheria toxin assay using the Elek test or the ICS strip or by assaying for *tox* gene by PCR were all negative for *C. imitans* strains (42; Bernard et al., submitted). *C. imitans* is resistant to 0/129, while *C. diphtheriae* is not.

C. jeikeium

C. jeikeium is one of the most frequently encountered corynebacteria in clinical specimens (62). Nosocomial transmission has been described. It is often resistant to multiple antibiotics (including penicillin and gentamicin), but this cannot be used as a taxonomic characteristic because the phenotypically closely related CDC group G bacteria may also demonstrate multidrug resistance. Quantitative DNA-DNA hybridization experiments had shown that *C. jeikeium* includes two genomospecies for which the penicillin and gentamicin MICs are low, but since they could otherwise not be differentiated phenotypically from the resistant *C. jeikeium* strains, they were not proposed as independent species (103). Colonies of *C. jeikeium* are tiny, low, entire, and grayish white. *C. jeikeium* is a strict aerobe which may oxidatively produce acid from glucose and sometimes from maltose but not from fructose (CDC group G bacteria are positive for acid production from fructose). The RapID CB Plus system correctly identifies *C. jeikeium*, as does the API Coryne system if ancillary tests are used (57, 59). As for all other lipophilic corynebacteria, imperfectly cleaved mycolic acids coeluting with CFAs at or near equivalent chain lengths of 14.966 to 15.000 or equivalent chain lengths of 16.7 to 16.8 have never been observed among *C. jeikeium* strains (4; Bernard, unpublished).

C. kroppenstedtii

C. kroppenstedtii (17) is a rarely recovered species originally isolated from the sputum of a patient with pulmonary disease. Additional strains have been isolated from a breast abscess, open-lung biopsy specimen, and sputum (Bernard et al., submitted). Apart from *C. amycolatum*, it is the only *Corynebacterium* species lacking mycolic acids. Colonies are grayish, translucent, slightly dry, and less than 0.5 mm in diameter after 24 h of incubation at 37°C. *C. kroppenstedtii* is lipophilic and is one of the few medically relevant *Corynebacterium* species exhibiting esculinase activity. Other biochemical characteristics are given in Table 4. It can be separated from *C. durum*, *C. matruchotii*, and *C. glucuronolyticum* by its colony morphology and from *C. glucuronolyticum* also by its negative CAMP reaction.

C. lipophiloflavum

C. lipophiloflavum (45) is represented by only a single strain, which has been isolated from vaginal discharge from a patient with bacterial vaginosis. It has the same biochemical screening pattern as *C. urealyticum*, except that it exhibits a strong yellow pigment and weaker urease activity (Table 4). In contrast to most *C. urealyticum* strains, the *C. lipophiloflavum* strain observed was not multidrug resistant.

C. macginleyi

C. macginleyi (107) has been isolated almost exclusively from eye specimens, from both diseased (52, 71) and healthy (130) conjunctiva. Colonies are typical for lipophilic corynebacteria (see above). When grown on Tween 80-SBA plates (better growth is usually found on plates supplemented with 0.1% Tween 80 than on those supplemented with 1.0% Tween 80), some *C. macginleyi* strains exhibit a rose pigment, which is not seen for any other lipophilic *Corynebacterium* species. *C. macginleyi* is one of the very few *Corynebacterium* species not expressing pyrazinamidase activity (Table 4). Most *C. macginleyi* strains ferment mannitol, while the majority of other corynebacteria are unable to do so. The API Coryne system correctly identifies *C. macginleyi* (59). Strains belonging to this species are susceptible to a broad spectrum of antibiotics (52).

C. matruchotii

C. matruchotii is thought to be a natural inhabitant of the oral cavity, particularly on calculus and plaque deposits, and so has been much studied by oral microbiologists (98). Otherwise it is a very rare human pathogen. Microcolonies appear flat, filamentous, and spider-like, but macrocolonies have a variable appearance. *C. matruchotii* demonstrates a very unusual appearance on Gram staining, in that so-called "whip handles" (i.e., filamentous bacteria with a single short bacillus adjacent to the end of the filament, creating the illusion of a whip) are observed (Fig. 1e). This microscopic presentation is consistent even when isolates which have been preserved for many years in a culture collection are stained. It has recently been demonstrated that heterogeneity existed among *C. matruchotii* strains obtained from international culture collections and that some strains represented were misidentified *C. durum* isolates (98). *C. matruchotii* strains are consistently negative for galactose, whereas *C. durum* strains can be positive. The API Coryne system database does not contain *C. matruchotii*; the numerical codes observed for *C. matruchotii* include 7000325, 7010325, and 7050325.

C. matruchotii-Like Strain

The *C. matruchotii* species is represented by a single strain, ATCC 43833 (98). It had been deposited in ATCC as *C. matruchotii*, but it is a distinct species as revealed by dot-blot hybridization and 16S rDNA sequencing data. Colonies are pinpoint to 0.1 mm in diameter, grayish-white, with a smooth, nonadherent texture. Biochemical screening reactions are similar to *C. minutissimum*, except that

strain ATCC 43833 exhibits esculinase activity in the API Coryne system. The numerical API Coryne profile for this unvalidated taxon is 2140325.

C. minutissimum

C. minutissimum is a member of the normal human skin flora. Its association with erythrasma is highly questionable (139). Colonies of *C. minutissimum* are whitish-grayish, shiny and moist, convex, and circular; have entire edges; and are about 1 to 1.5 mm in diameter after 24 h. Most of the colonies are creamy, but some may also have a sticky consistency. *C. minutissimum* strains have a fermentative metabolism and produce acid from sucrose variably. Very few *C. minutissimum* strains are also able to produce acid from mannitol (139). The API Coryne system identifies *C. minutissimum*, with additional tests being necessary for most of the strains (59). Many *C. minutissimum* strains are pyrrolidonyl arylamidase positive. *C. minutissimum* strains exhibit DNase activity (139), and nearly all strains hydrolyze tyrosine, whereas only a very few strains exhibit a positive CAMP reaction. Lactic and succinic acids are the major end products of glucose metabolism (37, 139). Some isolates possess TBSA in their cell membranes. Nearly all *C. minutissimum* strains are susceptible to O/129 (150-μg disk); i.e., they exhibit an inhibition zone around the disk (usually between 20 and 35 mm in diameter).

C. mucifaciens

C. mucifaciens (48) has been isolated mainly from blood cultures and other sterile body fluids, but it has also been recovered from abscesses, soft tissue, and dialysate (Bernard et al., submitted). Colonies are very distinct because they are slightly to overtly yellow and very mucoid (Fig. 3c). *C. mucifaciens* is the only presently known *Corynebacterium* species exhibiting such mucoid colonies; this characteristic strongly reminds the bacteriologist of *Rhodococcus equi* colonies. An extracellular substance (probably polysaccharides) causing connective filaments between the cells has been demonstrated as the ultrastructural correlate of the mucoid colonies. Colonies are about 1 to 1.5 mm after 24 h of incubation and have entire edges. They appear less mucoid after extended incubation for 96 h. One aberrant isolate from a blood culture did not exhibit yellowish pigment or the mucoidal characteristic and so was initially difficult to identify (Bernard et al., submitted). *C. mucifaciens* has an oxidative metabolism. It consistently produces acid from glucose, but acid production from sucrose is variable. The API Coryne numerical codes 2000004, 2000104, 2000105, 2100104, 2100105, 6000004, 6100104, and 6100105 have been observed for *C. mucifaciens*, suggesting that glucose oxidation is occasionally too slow to be observed by that method. *C. mucifaciens* is enzymatically less active than *R. equi*, which exhibits α- and β-glucosidase activities not observed for *C. mucifaciens*. In addition, *C. mucifaciens* produces acid from fructose and may produce acid from glycerol and mannose, but acid production from these sugars is not seen in *R. equi* strains. Tuberculostearic acid can be detected in amounts of 1 to 2% of the total CFAs. β-Lactam antibiotics and aminoglycosides show very good activities against *C. mucifaciens*.

C. "nigricans"

C. "nigricans" is an unusual black-pigmented *Corynebacterium* (Fig. 3g) that was isolated from the vaginal sample of a woman with spontaneous abortion, but a disease association could not be established (113). Two additional strains were isolated from the vagina and a vulval ulcer (Bernard et al., submitted). *C. "nigricans"* has not been formally described and validated so far. This taxon would probably require differentiation from the black-grayish-pigmented CDC coryneform group 4 bacteria (Hollis, ASM Meeting handout), which biochemically and chemotaxonomically are otherwise *Rothia*-like (Bernard, unpublished). Its basic biochemical profile (Table 4) is similar to that of *C. minutissimum*, but the black-pigmented *Corynebacterium* also pits the agar and has a strong adhesion to agar. Another unusual feature of this bacterium is that some strains can ferment glycogen (which is seen in very few true corynebacteria like some *C. diphtheriae*). It is not unlikely that the genitourinary tract might be the habitat of *C. "nigricans"* as well as for some CDC coryneform group 4 strains.

C. propinquum

C. propinquum is the closest phylogenetic relative of *C. pseudodiphtheriticum* (91, 110) and has the same niche (i.e., the oropharynx) as *C. pseudodiphtheriticum*. Colonies are whitish and somewhat dryish with entire edges and are 1 to 2 mm in diameter after 24 h of incubation. This species reduces nitrate and hydrolyzes tyrosine but does not hydrolyze urea (Table 4). The API Coryne system and the RapID CB Plus system correctly identify *C. propinquum* strains (57, 59).

C. pseudodiphtheriticum

C. pseudodiphtheriticum is part of the normal oropharyngeal flora. As described in Table 3, this species has been well documented to cause pneumonia in various patient populations. In one instance, an isolate caused diphtheria-like disease including the formation of a pseudomembrane and so triggered an extensive outbreak control response. Colonies are whitish, slightly dry with entire edges, and 1 to 2 mm in diameter after 48 h of incubation. This nonfermenting species reduces nitrate and hydrolyzes urea but does not produce acid from any of the commonly tested carbohydrates (Table 4). Some strains hydrolyze tyrosine. The API Coryne system and the RapiD CB Plus system correctly identify *C. pseudodiphtheriticum* strains (57, 59). For this species, imperfectly cleaved mycolic acids coeluting with CFAs have been demonstrated (4). *C. pseudodiphtheriticum* strains are susceptible to β-lactam antibiotics, but resistance to macrolides and lincosamides has been observed.

C. pseudotuberculosis

C. pseudotuberculosis is phylogenetically closely related to *C. diphtheriae* (91, 110), may harbor the diphtheria toxin gene, produces propionic acid as a fermentation product, and contains large amounts of the CFA $C_{16:1\omega7c}$ (4). Colonies are yellowish white, opaque, convex, and about 1 mm in diameter after 24 h. Like *C. ulcerans*, *C. pseudotuberculosis* is positive for urease and the CAMP inhibition test (complete inhibition of the effect of *S. aureus* β-hemolysin on sheep erythrocytes is achieved by streaking the presumed *C. pseudotuberculosis* strain at a right angle toward *S. aureus* and incubating overnight; a beta-hemolysin inhibition zone in the form of a triangle is observed, as is the case for *A. haemolyticum* [Fig. 2]). *C. pseudotuberculosis* is not susceptible to 0/129, whereas *C. ulcerans* strains are (68). *C. pseudotuberculosis* is variable for both nitrate reduction and sucrose fermentation. The API Coryne system and the RapiD CB Plus panel correctly identify this species (57, 59). Pulsed-field gel electrophoresis using the restriction enzyme *Sfi*I has been applied to characterize epidemiologically linked veterinary isolates (23).

C. riegelii

C. riegelii strains were originally described as being isolated from females with urinary tract infections (49), but additional strains have been recovered from blood cultures, including cord blood (Bernard et al., submitted). Colonies are whitish, glistening, and convex with entire margins and are up to 1.5 mm in diameter after 48 h of incubation. Some colonies are of a creamy consistency, whereas others are sticky. *C. riegelii* strains exhibit a very strong urease activity with Christensen's urea broth, becoming positive within 5 min at room temperature after inoculation. A very peculiar characteristic of *C. riegelii* is the slow fermentation of maltose but not glucose. No other defined *Corynebacterium* species exhibits this feature (Table 4). The weak anaerobic growth of *C. riegelii* corresponds to the weak fermentative metabolism. The API Coryne system codes observed for *C. riegelii* include 0101224, 2001224, and 2101224.

C. sanguinis

The presently known strain of *C. sanguinis* was isolated from a blood culture (G. Funke, L. Hoyle, and M. D. Collins, submitted for publication). Colonies are yellowish, smooth, slightly dryish, and up to 1.5 mm in diameter after 48 h of incubation. Slow fermentative acid production from glucose but not from maltose or sucrose and the presence of small amounts of TBSA (2 to 3%) are the most significant phenotypic features. *C. sanguinis* can be differentiated from *C. coyleae* by its negative CAMP reaction, from *C. falsenii* by its negative urease reaction, and from *C. confusum* by its yellow pigment and an inability to reduce nitrate. *C. argentoratense* produces acid from glucose more rapidly than *C. sanguinis* and also exhibits larger colonies after 24 h of incubation. The numerical API Coryne system code for *C. sanguinis* is 6100304.

C. simulans

C. simulans has been delineated recently from some *C. striatum*-like strains (131). The three strains described in the original publication came from skin-related specimens (foot abscess, lymph node biopsy specimen, and boil). Two additional strains have been characterized, one from bile and one from a blood culture (Bernard et al., submitted). Colonies of *C. simulans* (grayish-white, glistening, creamy, 1 to 2 mm in diameter) are very similar to *C. minutissimum*, *C. singulare*, and *C. striatum*, all of which are the closest phylogenetic neighbors. *C. simulans* is the only valid *Corynebacterium* species described to date which reduces nitrite. Further characteristics which separate *C. simulans* from the closely related nonlipophilic, fermentative corynebacteria are its inability to acidify ethylene glycol and to grow at 20°C (in contrast to *C. striatum*). API Coryne profiles include 0100305, 2100105, 2100301, 2100305, and 3000125 (including the falsely negative nitrate reduction reaction because of the strong nitrite reduction). The blood culture isolate (code 2100301) was repeatedly catalase negative, making its identification difficult except when polyphasic characterization is done at a reference center (Bernard et al., submitted).

C. singulare

Two strains of *C. singulare* have been described to date (109): one strain from semen and one from a blood culture. Colonies are circular and slightly convex with entire margins and are of a creamy consistency, as observed for *C. minutissimum* and *C. striatum*. Key biochemical reactions are like those for *C. minutissimum*, except that urease activity is observed (Table 4). The numerical API Coryne system profile is 6101125, indicative that pyrrolidonyl aryl-amidase activity is observed. Like *C. minutissimum* and *C. striatum*, *C. singulare* also hydrolyzes tyrosine. *C. singulare* can be differentiated from *C. minutissimum* with use of the bioMérieux biotype 100 gallery, but this is not a usual clinical microbiology laboratory test. *C. singulare* does not produce propionic acid as a fermentation product, differentiating it from *C. amycolatum*.

C. striatum

C. striatum is part of the normal human skin flora. Nosocomial transmission of *C. striatum* has been documented (77). Colonies are convex, circular, shiny, moist, and creamy with entire edges and are about 1 to 1.5 mm in diameter after 24 h of incubation (Fig. 3d). Some investigators have described *C. striatum* colonies as somewhat like those of small coagulase-negative staphylococci. *C. striatum* has a fermentative metabolism, and acid production from sucrose is variable. The API Coryne system identifies *C. striatum*, but with additional tests needed in most cases (59). A few *C. striatum* strains might also be nitrate reductase negative (Funke, unpublished). All *C. striatum* strains hydrolyze tyrosine, and some strains are CAMP reaction positive; however, the CAMP reaction of *C. striatum* strains is usually not as strong as that of other CAMP test-positive species (e.g., *C. auris* or *C. glucuronolyticum*). Lactic and succinic acids are the major end products of glucose metabolism (37). All *C. striatum* strains are susceptible to 0/129. Resistance to macrolides and lincosamides due to the presence of an rRNA methylase has been described. *C. striatum* may also be resistant to quinolones and tetracyclines.

C. sundsvallense

C. sundsvallense (14; Bernard et al., submitted) is a newly described species that has been isolated from blood cultures, a vaginal swab, and a sinus drainage from an infected groin. Colonies of this nonlipophilic species are buff or slightly yellowish and adherent to agar and have a sticky consistency. Gram staining shows bulges or knobs at the ends of some rods, and these are not seen in any other corynebacteria. Fermentation of glucose, lactose, and sucrose is slow (Table 4). *C. sundsvallense* can be separated from *C. durum* by its positive α-glucosidase reaction and its inability to ferment galactose. It is further differentiated from *C. matruchotii* by expressing urease but not nitrate reductase activity and by not producing propionic acid as an end product of glucose metabolism (14; Bernard et al., submitted).

C. thomssenii

C. thomssenii (138) is a rare species; it was originally repeatedly isolated from a patient with pleural effusion and a second strain was recovered from the environment in Canada (Bernard et al., submitted). This species is fastidious and slowly growing, resulting in colonies of <0.5 mm after 48 h, but it is not lipophilic. After 96 h, colonies are molar tooth-like, very sticky, and slightly adherent to agar. The clinical strain of *C. thomssenii* is the only *Corynebacterium* species expressing N-acetyl-β-glucosaminidase activity, which can be observed in either the API Coryne or API ZYM systems. Acid is slowly and fermentatively produced

from glucose, maltose, and sucrose, and the resulting API Coryne code for *C. thomssenii* is 2121125.

C. ulcerans

Phylogenetically, *C. ulcerans* (108) is, together with *C. pseudotuberculosis*, the closest relative of *C. diphtheriae* (91, 110), can harbor the diphtheria toxin gene, and contains significant amounts of $C_{16:1\omega7c}$. Disease associated with this bacterium is rare, but if the organism is recovered from pseudomembranous material, the infection must be treated like a case of diphtheria (29, 30). Colonies are somewhat dry and waxy and gray-white with light hemolysis, being 1 to 2 mm in diameter after 24 h. *C. ulcerans* may be differentiated from *C. diphtheriae* by urease activity and a CAMP inhibition reaction (Table 4). Strains of *C. ulcerans* are positive for glycogen, starch, and trehalose fermentation. The API Coryne system and the RapID CB Plus identification strip correctly identify *C. ulcerans* (57, 59).

C. urealyticum

C. urealyticum is one of the more frequently isolated clinically significant corynebacteria from clinical specimens (62). It is strongly associated with urinary tract infections. Recovery of this bacterium is often associated with alkaline urine, resulting in the production of struvite crystals. As with all other lipophilic corynebacteria, colonies are pinpoint, convex, smooth, and whitish-grayish on regular SBA. *C. urealyticum* is a strict aerobe and has very strong urease activity (Table 4). Commercial identification systems correctly identify *C. urealyticum*. A PCR-based assay for detection of *C. urealyticum* has recently been described (114). *C. urealyticum* is almost always multidrug resistant (62, 116), but rare penicillin-susceptible strains have also been described.

C. xerosis

The natural habitat of *C. xerosis* is unknown, although it has recently been isolated from vaginal swabs (Funke, unpublished). Colonies are dry, granular, and yellowish with irregular edges and are 1 to 1.5 mm in diameter after 24 h. It must be emphasized that nearly all "*C. xerosis*" strains which appeared in the literature before 1996 may have been misidentified *C. amycolatum* strains (46). *C. striatum* strains were also misidentified as *C. xerosis* in the past. *C. xerosis* has a fermentative metabolism, is variable for the presence of nitrate reductase, but always expresses α-glucosidase as well as leucine arylamidase activities. Because *C. xerosis* was thought to be rarely encountered in clinical specimens, it was not included in the API Coryne system version 2.0 database. The numerical profiles observed for *C. xerosis* strains include 2110325 and 3110325. The RapID CB Plus system correctly identifies *C. xerosis* (57). Lactic acid is the major end product of glucose metabolism, and strains are susceptible to 0/129.

Biochemical Reactions for Other Genera

The key biochemical reactions for the genera other than *Corynebacterium* are given in Table 5.

Genus *Turicella*

T. otitidis is almost exclusively isolated from clinical specimens from the ear region, but it does not cause otitis media with effusion in children (Funke, unpublished). Colonies are whitish, convex, and creamy with entire edges and are 1 to 1.5 mm in diameter after 48 h of incubation. Some young colonies show a greenish appearance when taken away from the plates with a swab. The distinctive Gram stain morphology of *T. otitidis* is shown in Fig. 1b. Differentiation from *C. auris* and *C. afermentans* subsp. *afermentans* is readily achieved on the basis of morphologic features, but utilization reactions may also assist in the differentiation of these taxa (47, 102). All *T. otitidis* strains are strongly CAMP reaction positive and give the numerical code 2100004 in the API Coryne system. The MICs of β-lactam antibiotics for many strains are very low; some strains might be resistant to macrolides and clindamycin (58).

Genus *Arthrobacter*

Arthrobacter spp. might be members of the indigenous normal human flora, but their main habitat is soil. *A. cumminsii* seems to be a normal commensal in humans and has been demonstrated to be the most frequently isolated *Arthrobacter* species in human clinical specimens (53, 132). *Arthrobacter* colonies are usually whitish-grayish, slightly glistening, creamy, and 2 mm or more in diameter after 24 h. *A. cumminsii* is slightly smaller than the other arthrobacters and may also exhibit a sticky consistency (53). *Arthrobacter* spp. usually do not oxidize any of the carbohydrates routinely tested and do not express a cheese-like smell, as is often found for the phenotypically closely related brevibacteria. Some arthrobacters are motile, whereas brevibacteria are always nonmotile. Like brevibacteria, *Arthrobacter* spp. express DNase and have gelatinase activity (44). The identification of arthrobacters at the species level might be achieved by carbohydrate utilization tests, but this is recommended for the reference laboratory only. For the near future, it is expected that numerous other *Arthrobacter* species, some of which represent new species, will be described as having been recovered from clinical material. *A. creatinolyticus*, *A. luteolus*, and *A. albus* are examples of recently validated species (69, 132). *A. albus* is phylogenetically closely related to *A. cumminsii* but might be differentiated phenotypically by being resistant to desferrioxamine whereas *A. cumminsii* is susceptible (132). *A. cumminsii* has a distinctive CFA pattern, with $C_{14:0i}$ and $C_{14:0}$ each representing 2 to 4% of all CFAs (53). The penicillin MICs for most *Arthrobacter* strains are low (44). Aminoglycosides and quinolones show only very weak activities against *A. cumminsii* strains (53).

Genus *Brevibacterium*

Some *Brevibacterium* spp. are members of the normal human skin flora. Colonies are whitish-grayish, convex, mostly creamy, and 2 mm or more in diameter after 24 h. *B. mcbrellneri* colonies have a more granular appearance and are drier than those of other brevibacteria. Some brevibacteria may develop a yellowish or greenish pigment after prolonged incubation. Many *Brevibacterium* strains isolated from human clinical material give off a distinctive cheese-like odor. Brevibacteria are nonmotile and halotolerant (6.5% NaCl) and form methanethiol from methionine, but this test is specific for brevibacteria only when it is read within 2 h (41). Brevibacteria can be identified to the species level by carbohydrate utilization tests. More than 90% of all clinical *Brevibacterium* isolates are *B. casei* (41). The MICs of β-lactam antibiotics for brevibacteria are often elevated (58, 125).

Genus *Dermabacter*

D. hominis strains are part of the normal skin flora. Colonies are whitish, convex, of a creamy or sticky consistency, and 1 to 1.5 mm in diameter after 48 h (Fig. 3e). *D. hominis* strains are sometimes mistaken for small-colony coagulase-negative staphylococci. The Gram stain result is distinctive, with coccobacillary or coccoidal forms (Fig. 1c). The key biochemical reactions are given in Table 5. *D. hominis* is one of the few coryneform bacteria with a variable reaction for xylose fermentation. It is the only catalase-positive coryneform bacterium (except *Actinomyces neuii* [37]) that is able to decarboxylate lysine and ornithine (60; Hollis, ASM Meeting handout). The API Coryne system and the RapID CB Plus panel correctly identify this species (57, 59). *D. hominis* strains may be resistant to aminoglycosides (60, 125).

Genus *Rothia*

The genus *Rothia* presently comprises three validated species, namely, *R. dentocariosa* (the type species), *R. mucilaginosa* (formerly designated *Stomatococcus mucilaginosus*), and *R. nasimurium* (isolated from a mouse), as well as *R. dentocariosa* genomovar II (21, 74). The latter has not been formally named because it has not been possible to biochemically distinguish it from authentic *R. dentocariosa* sensu stricto (genomovar I) (74). Some of the CDC coryneform group 4 bacteria (Fig. 3h) were also shown phenotypically and by CFA composition to be closely related to *R. dentocariosa* (4; K. A. Bernard and G. Funke, unpublished observation) whereas other members of the original CDC coryneform group 4 bacteria are probably representatives of *C. "nigricans."*

Colonies of *R. dentocariosa* are whitish, raised, and smooth or rough or have a "spoke-wheel" form (Fig. 3f), and they are up to 2 mm in diameter after 48 h. *Rothia* strains usually grow better in a CO_2-enriched atmosphere. The biochemical features of *R. dentocariosa* are given in Table 5. The API Coryne system correctly identifies *R. dentocariosa* (59). Its CFA composition is of the branched-chain type (4), which allows differentiation from the biochemically similar species *C. durum*, *C. matruchotii*, and *Actinomyces viscosus* (see chapter 55), all of which also occupy the oropharynx. *R. dentocariosa* may also be confused with *D. hominis* and *Propionibacterium avidum* (see chapter 55), both of which, in contrast, always exhibit smooth colonies. As shown in a study of the pharyngeal bacterial flora of healthy adults, one-third of all *R. dentocariosa* strains isolated were negative for the key biochemical reaction catalase (129). The MICs of aminoglycosides for some *R. dentocariosa* strains are elevated, whereas penicillins usually show good in vitro activities against *Rothia* strains (Funke, unpublished).

Genus *Exiguobacterium*

It is not known whether exiguobacteria are members of the indigenous bacterial flora of humans. Colonies of *E. acetylicum* are plain, golden-yellow to orange, and up to 2 mm in diameter after 24 h of incubation. Acid from carbohydrates is rapidly produced by fermentative metabolism. Exiguobacteria are motile and often oxidase positive. They might be confused with microbacteria, but CFA analysis provides a clear-cut distinction between the two genera (Table 1). The pathogenic potential of *E. acetylicum* seems to be rather low, since it has been isolated from different sources (e.g., skin, wounds, and cerebrospinal fluid [66]), but case reports on infectious diseases due to *E. acetylicum* are not extant. Cases of pseudobacteremia due to *E. acetylicum* have been observed.

Genus *Oerskovia*

O. turbata is usually acquired from the environment (e.g., soil). Colonies are pale yellow to phosphorous yellow, convex, and creamy; they penetrate agar; and they are approximately 1 to 2 mm in diameter after 24 h. *O. turbata* rapidly produces acid from sugars by fermentation; it also exhibits a very strong esculin reaction. The genus is well identified by the API Coryne system (59). *O. turbata* does not hydrolyze xanthine or hypoxanthine, whereas the related *C. cellulans* is able to do so.

Genus *Cellulomonas*

Cellulomonas strains are usually acquired from the environment. Colonies are first whitish or pale or bright yellow, but after 7 days nearly all *Cellulomonas* strains are somewhat yellow. Colonies vary between 0.5 and 1.5 mm in diameter after 24 h, are convex and creamy, and have entire edges. *Cellulomonas* spp. are variable for the fermentation of mannitol. Other key biochemical reactions of *Cellulomonas* spp. are given in Table 5. The majority of *Cellulomonas* strains express cellulase activity, demonstrated by incubating a heavy bacterial suspension (McFarland no. 6 standard) with a piece of sterile copy paper in a 0.9% NaCl solution for 10 days, resulting in dissolution of the paper (54).

Genus *Cellulosimicrobium*

Colonies of *C. cellulans* are similar to *O. turbata* (see above) and also pit agar. In addition, *C. cellulans* exhibits a biochemical screening profile which is very similar to that of *O. turbata* (Table 5). However, *C. cellulans* hydrolyzes either xanthine or hypoxanthine whereas *O. turbata* does not and *O. turbata* strains might be motile whereas *C. cellulans* strains are not (66, 112).

Genus *Microbacterium*

Microbacteria account for the majority of yellow-pigmented coryneform bacteria isolated from clinical specimens. All shades of yellow pigment are observed, ranging from pale to bright yellow and orange. Most of the strains are catalase positive, but catalase-negative strains might be observed. Some microbacteria grow under anaerobic conditions but only weakly. Some microbacteria are nitrate reductase negative, which separates them from the phenotypically closely related genus *Cellulomonas*, all of whose presently defined members are nitrate reductase positive (Table 5). Microbacteria may ferment mannitol but not xylose, whereas the lack of xylose fermentation has not been observed for *Cellulomonas* strains described so far.

Species identification is almost impossible since for many defined *Microbacterium* species the type strain is the only representative, preventing the creation of a comprehensive database. Final identification to the species level is best achieved by chemotaxonomic (interpeptide bridges) and molecular genetic (e.g., 16S rRNA gene sequencing) investigations. It is most likely that a plethora of new *Microbacterium* species, also isolated from human clinical specimens, might be proposed in the next few years.

Microbacteria are usually susceptible to vancomycin (except *M. resistens* [2, 50]), but susceptibility to other antimicrobial agents is unpredictable (in particular, resistance to aminoglycosides has been observed [43]); therefore, every individual clinically significant strain must be tested.

Genus *Curtobacterium*

Curtobacteria are infrequently isolated yellow- or yellow-orange-pigmented oxidative coryneform bacteria. In contrast to most microbacteria, they produce acid from carbohydrates very slowly (within 4 to 7 days) (Funke, Aravena-Roman, et al., submitted). Curtobacteria are usually nitrate reductase negative but strongly hydrolyze esculin (Table 5). *C. pusillum* and related strains have a most unusual CFA composition, which is not observed in any other coryneform bacteria, with feature 7 ($C_{18:1\omega9c/\omega12t/\omega7c}$) representing more than 50% of all CFAs (Funke, Aravera-Roman, et al., submitted). Again, the differentiation of curtobacteria is very difficult and should be performed only in a reference laboratory. The MICs of macrolides and rifampin for curtobacteria are very low.

Genus *Leifsonia*

Leifsonia aquatica is very rarely encountered in clinical specimens. It is always motile, does not hydrolyze either gelatin or casein, and has a stronger DNase activity than most microbacteria (63). *L. aquatica* is the only species within the genus *Leifsonia* which is able to grow in broth enriched with 5% NaCl (35). Its yellow pigment develops relatively slowly within 3 to 4 days. The MICs of vancomycin for some *L. aquatica* strains were shown to be elevated (8 μg/ml) (63), but the precise mechanism of this resistance is not known.

Genus *Arcanobacterium*

The genus *Arcanobacterium* comprises five species, all of which except *A. pluranimalium* exhibit beta-hemolysis on SBA. The three medically relevant species, *A. haemolyticum*, *A. pyogenes*, and *A. bernardiae*, are all catalase negative, whereas the two species recovered from animals, *A. phocae* and *A. pluranimalium*, are catalase positive. All species show a fermentative glucose metabolism, with succinic and lactic acids as their major end products. All arcanobacteria grow and express hemolysis best in a CO_2-enriched atmosphere.

The colonies of the type species, *A. haemolyticum*, are 0.5 mm in diameter after 48 h of incubation at 37°C, and two morphotypes have been described: one rough type isolated mainly from the respiratory tract and one smooth type isolated mainly from wounds (11). The biochemical reactions of *A. haemolyticum* are given in Table 5. Of major value for the identification of *A. haemolyticum* is the so-called CAMP inhibition test (see the description of the CAMP inhibition test in the section on *C. pseudotuberculosis*) (Fig. 2). The protein responsible for this phenomenon is a phospholipase D excreted by *A. haemolyticum*, and this protein is genetically and functionally similar to the ones expressed by *C. ulcerans* and *C. pseudotuberculosis*. *A. haemolyticum*, as well as the two other medically relevant arcanobacteria, is correctly identified by the API Coryne system (59).

A. pyogenes colonies are the largest of all arcanobacteria colonies, with diameters of up to 1 mm after 48 h of incubation. Of all the arcanobacteria, this species also shows the sharpest zone of beta-hemolysis on SBA. The protein responsible for hemolysis, named pyolysin, is also an important virulence factor in vivo. Gram stains may show some branching rods. *A. pyogenes* is the only *Arcanobacterium* species of medical relevance that expresses β-glucuronidase activity and that is capable of fermenting xylose.

A. bernardiae (56, 92) has glassy, whitish colonies of <0.5 mm in diameter after 48 h. Some colonies have a creamy consistency, whereas others are sticky. Gram staining shows relatively short rods without branching. Most *A. bernardiae* strains belong to the very few coryneform bacteria that are able to ferment glycogen. Another peculiar feature of *A. bernardiae* strains is their ability to produce acid faster from maltose than from glucose.

The MICs of all β-lactams, rifampin, and tetracycline for arcanobacteria are very low, whereas aminoglycosides and quinolones have reduced activities against arcanobacteria (Funke, unpublished). Macrolides also exhibit excellent activities against arcanobacteria and are an alternative to β-lactam antibiotics for the treatment of infections, since treatment failures due to β-lactam antibiotics because of the inability of β-lactam antibiotics to act intracellularly have been reported.

ANTIMICROBIAL SUSCEPTIBILITIES

The susceptibility patterns for each taxon were given with the individual descriptions (see above). Since the antimicrobial susceptibility of coryneform bacteria is not predictable in every case, susceptibility testing should always be performed with clinically significant isolates (see "Clinical Significance" above). Due to the emergence of vancomycin-resistant gram-positive organisms, it has become inappropriate to recommend glycopeptides as first-line drugs for the treatment of infections caused by coryneform bacteria. It is also noteworthy that some coryneform bacteria (e.g., *Microbacterium resistens*) are intrinsically vancomycin resistant.

The National Committee for Clinical Laboratory Standards (NCCLS) has not explicitly published guidelines for the susceptibility testing of coryneform bacteria. However, clinical laboratories are often asked to carry out susceptibility testing with coryneform bacteria. A pragmatic approach includes disk diffusion testing on Mueller-Hinton agar supplemented with 5% sheep blood. Incubation is at 35°C in ambient air for 24 h; for a very few strains (e.g., lipophilic corynebacteria) 48 h may be required. Lipophilic corynebacteria, *Rothia* spp., and *Arcanobacterium* spp. should be incubated in a 5% CO_2-enriched atmosphere to obtain better growth. The presently recommended interpretation criteria are those established for streptococci (135). The laboratory report should indicate which interpretive criteria have been used.

MICs can be determined by either the E test (AB Biodisk, Solna, Sweden) or the agar dilution or broth microdilution method. The results of the E test have been shown to correlate well with those of both the broth microdilution and the agar dilution methods for *Corynebacterium* spp. (80, 137), as well as with the agar dilution method for *A. haemolyticum* (10). The E test should be carried out on Mueller-Hinton agar supplemented with 5% sheep blood. The same medium is used for the agar dilution method (58), but this method is not applicable in the routine laboratory; rather, it should be used in studies with individual antimicrobial agents. MICs should be reported without interpretive criteria, but if required by the clinician, the criteria applied should be mentioned and the report should indicate that there are presently no established standards for coryneform bacteria.

EVALUATION, INTERPRETATION, AND REPORTING OF RESULTS

The guidelines related to when coryneform bacteria should be identified to the species level (see "Clinical Significance" above) are also applicable for evaluating and interpreting culture results; i.e., whenever coryneform bacteria are identified to the species level, the results should be reported.

In the rare case of microscopically suspected *C. diphtheriae* (i.e., a positive Neisser staining result), the physician in charge of the patient should be notified immediately, although culture results and toxin testing results become available only later.

It is evident that repeated isolation of a predominant strain of a coryneform bacterium or a coryneform bacterium growing in pure culture suggests an etiological relationship to the patient's disease. If coryneform bacteria are present in blood cultures, the physician in charge should be notified immediately, and it should be emphasized when reporting that the clinical significance of the coryneform bacteria must be carefully examined by cooperation between the microbiology laboratory and the physician. In our experience, one positive blood culture out of two or three aerobically and anaerobically incubated pairs of blood cultures is hardly ever clinically significant (except in cases of treated endocarditis). Care must be taken in interpretation of the results for patients for whom half or more of the blood specimens taken for culture become positive for coryneform bacteria, in particular when lipophilic corynebacteria are cultured, since not all blood samples taken from patients with endocarditis due to lipophilic corynebacteria may eventually become positive.

On the other hand, coryneform bacteria should be reported as "normal flora" when they are grown in equal or smaller numbers from nonsterile sites together with other members of the resident flora. It is suggested that the primary isolation plates be retained for at least 72 h before they are discarded in order to have the opportunity to assess the bacterial population retrospectively.

APPENDIX 1
Genus *Gardnerella*

The genus *Gardnerella* does not have a particular phylogenetic relationship to any of the established genera described in this chapter. It is remotely related to the genus *Bifidobacterium* (82, 127), and these genera share some important features, such as production of acetic and lactic acids as fermentation products. A 16S rRNA gene PCR product selected for detection of a *G. vaginalis*-specific sequence was found to have some less-than-specific homology to several *Bifidobacterium* species (86). *G. vaginalis* is the only species belonging to the genus *Gardnerella*. Studies on the ultrastructure of the cell wall of *G. vaginalis* have demonstrated that it has a cell wall similar to but much thinner than the cell walls of other gram-positive bacteria (i.e., there is a smaller peptidoglycan layer) (111). Lysine is the diamino acid of the cell wall, and the CFAs are similar to those detected in *Actinomyces* spp., *Arcanobacterium* spp., and *Corynebacterium* spp., with $C_{16:0}$ and $C_{18:1\omega9c}$ predominating. The G+C content of 42 to 44 mol% is lower than that of every other genus described in this chapter.

Gram stains show thin gram-variable rods or coccobacilli (Fig. 1f). Catalase is not produced, and cells are nonmotile and have a slow fermentative metabolism.

Natural habitat

G. vaginalis can be found in the anorectal flora of healthy adults of both sexes as well as in that of children (12). It is also part of the endogenous vaginal flora in women of reproductive age. The optimal pH for the growth of G. *vaginalis* is between 6 and 7. The organism can also be recovered from the urethras of the male partners of women with bacterial vaginosis (BV) (12).

Clinical significance

G. *vaginalis* is associated with BV; its causative role in the syndrome is controversial (117, 118). Recurrent BV is due to reinfection rather than to relapse (i.e., overgrowth of the previously colonizing biotype). In pregnant women, BV may lead to preterm birth, premature rupture of membranes, and chorioamnionitis (12). G. *vaginalis* may also be recovered from cultures of blood from patients with postpartum or postabortal fevers and may also cause infections in newborns. Although it might be recovered from the urethras of males, its disease association in males is questionable. Serious infections in sites other than those associated with the genital tract or obstetrics are rare, but have been reported.

Collection, transport, and storage of specimens

Vaginal and extravaginal specimens can be collected with cotton-tipped swabs. It is best to take one swab for direct examination and to take another swab for culture if necessary, such as for epidemiologic studies. If culture media cannot be directly inoculated, the swab should be placed in a transport medium (e.g., Amies) and culture should be done within 24 h. It is noteworthy that G. *vaginalis* is susceptible to sodium polyanethol sulfonate (SPS), so an SPS-free medium (or an SPS medium supplemented with gelatin) should be used for optimal recovery of G. *vaginalis* from blood culture systems whenever G. *vaginalis* is suspected.

Isolation and identification

The "gold standard" for the diagnosis of BV is direct examination of vaginal secretions and not the culture of G. *vaginalis*, since G. *vaginalis* can also be recovered from healthy women. A bedside test for BV is examination of the vaginal discharge to detect the typical "fishy" trimethylamine odor, which is enhanced after alkalinization with 10% KOH. The typical smear of vaginal discharge from BV patients shows "clue cells" (bacteria covering epithelial cell margins) together with a mixed flora consisting of large numbers of small gram-negative (predominantly *Prevotella* and *Porphyromonas* spp.) and gram-variable (G. *vaginalis*) rods and coccobacilli, whereas lactobacilli are almost always absent. It is recommended that a standardized Gram staining interpretative scheme be used to improve the reproducibility of this method (89, 118). Detection of G. *vaginalis* in vaginal specimens processed using a DNA probe-based system, Affirm VPIII (BD), has been reported to be useful as a surrogate for wet mount cell examination (7). Although not recommended for routine laboratory procedures, the isolation of G. *vaginalis* can support the diagnosis of BV. Vaginal swabs are cultured on Vaginalis agar (see chapter 27 for the preparation) and should be semiquantitatively streaked out with a loop. Incubation is carried out at 35 to 37°C in a 5% CO$_2$-enriched atmosphere or in a candle jar. Beta-hemolysis is observed on human or rabbit blood-containing media but not on SBA. Plates may be checked for the growth of diffuse beta-hemolytic colonies of <0.5 mm in diameter after 24 h, but very often G. *vaginalis* is best observed after 48 h. Gram staining of the suspected colonies confirms the diagnosis of G. *vaginalis*.

Eight G. *vaginalis* biotypes had been proposed on the basis of the reactions for lipase, β-galactosidase, and hippurate hydrolysis (94), with biotypes 1, 5, and 6 being the most common. The diagnostic value of these biotypes is questionable since they have not been demonstrated to be associated with certain diseases or certain forms of disease. They may have some value for longitudinal studies, but molecular genetic typing methods are likely to be superior to biotyping. G. *vaginalis* strains are consistently α-glucosidase and starch hydrolysis positive, but only 90% of G. *vaginalis* strains hydrolyze hippurate. The API Coryne system identifies G. *vaginalis* well (59). The identification of G. *vaginalis* can also be confirmed by antimicrobial agent disk inhibition tests with 50 μg of metronidazole (inhibition present), 5 μg of trimethoprim (inhibition present), and 1 mg of sulfonamide (inhibition absent).

"G. *vaginalis*-like" organisms recovered from patients with BV have been demonstrated to represent *Actinomyces turicensis* strains (127). G. *vaginalis* can be differentiated from these organisms in that it has acetic acid as the main end product of glucose fermentation and is unable to produce acid from xylose, whereas *A. turicensis* strains have succinic acid as the end product and produce acid from xylose.

Antimicrobial susceptibilities

Metronidazole is the drug of choice both for local therapy of BV and for systemic therapy of extravaginal infections caused by BV-associated flora. Systemic infections due to G. *vaginalis* alone can be treated with ampicillin or amoxicillin, since β-lactamase-producing G. *vaginalis* strains have not been observed so far. Susceptibility testing for G. *vaginalis* is not recommended, and no specific NCCLS guidelines are extant.

REFERENCES

1. **Aubel, D., F. N. R. Renaud, and J. Freney.** 1997. Genomic diversity of several *Corynebacterium* species identified by amplification of the 16S–23S rRNA gene spacer regions. *Int. J. Syst. Bacteriol.* **47:**767–772.
2. **Behrendt U., A. Ulrich, and P. Schumann.** 2001. Description of *Microbacterium foliorum* sp. nov. and *Microbacterium phyllosphaerae* sp. nov., isolated from the phyllospheres of grasses and the surface litter after mulching the sward, and reclassification of *Aureobacterium resistens* (Funke et al. 1998) as *Microbacterium resistens* comb. nov. *Int. J. Syst. Evol. Microbiol.* **51:**1267–1276.
3. **Belko J., D. L. Wessel, and R. Malley.** 2000. Endocarditis caused by *Corynebacterium diphtheriae*: case report and review of the literature. *Pediatr. Infect. Dis. J.* **19:**159–163.
4. **Bernard, K. A. M. Bellefeuille, and E. P. Ewan.** 1991. Cellular fatty acid composition as an adjunct to the identification of asporogenous, aerobic gram-positive rods. *J. Clin. Microbiol.* **29:**83–89.
5. **Björkroth, J., H. Korkeala, and G. Funke.** 1999. rRNA gene RFLP as an identification tool for *Corynebacterium* species. *Int. J. Syst. Bacteriol.* **49:**983–989.
6. **Brennan, N. M., R. Brown, M. Goodfellow, A. C. Ward, T. P. Beresford, P. J. Simpson, P. F. Fox, and T. M. Cogan.** 2001. *Corynebacterium mooreparkense* sp. nov. and *Corynebacterium casei* sp. nov., isolated from the surface of a smear-ripened cheese. *Int. J. Syst. Evol. Microbiol.* **51:**843–852.
7. **Briselden, A. M., and S. L. Hillier.** 1994. Evaluation of Affirm VP Microbial Identification test for *Gardnerella vaginalis* and *Trichomonas vaginalis*. *J. Clin. Microbiol.* **32:**148–152.
8. **Cai, J., and M. D. Collins.** 1994. Phylogenetic analysis of species of the *meso*-diaminopimelic acid-containing genera *Brevibacterium* and *Dermabacter*. *Int. J. Syst. Bacteriol.* **44:**583–585.
9. **Carlotti, A., and G. Funke.** 1994. Rapid distinction of *Brevibacterium* species by restriction analysis of rDNA generated by polymerase chain reaction. *Syst. Appl. Microbiol.* **17:**380–386.
10. **Carlson, P.** 2000. Comparison of the E test and agar dilution methods for susceptibility testing of *Arcanobacterium haemolyticum*. *Eur. J. Clin. Microbiol. Infect. Dis.* **19:**891–893.
11. **Carlson, P., K. Lounatmaa, and O. V. Renkonen.** 1994. Biotypes of *Arcanobacterium haemolyticum*. *J. Clin. Microbiol.* **32:**1654–1657.
12. **Catlin, B. W.** 1992. *Gardnerella vaginalis*: characteristics, clinical considerations, and controversies. *Clin. Microbiol. Rev.* **5:**213–237.

13. **Cianciotto, N. P., and N. B. Groman.** 1997. Characterization of bacteriophages from *tox*-containing, nontoxigenic isolates of *Corynebacterium diphtheriae*. *Microb. Pathog.* **22:**343–351.

14. **Collins, M. D., K. A. Bernard, R. A. Hutson, B. Sjöden, A. Nyberg, and E. Falsen.** 1999. *Corynebacterium sundsvallense* sp. nov., from human clinical specimens. *Int. J. Syst. Bacteriol.* **49:**361–366.

15. **Collins, M. D., R. A. Burton, and D. Jones.** 1988. *Corynebacterium amycolatum* sp. nov. a new mycolic acid-less *Corynebacterium* species from human skin. *FEMS Microbiol. Lett.* **49:**349–352.

16. **Collins, M. D., and C. S. Cummins.** 1986. Genus *Corynebacterium*, p. 1266–1276. *In* P. H. A. Sneath, N. S. Mair, M. E. Sharpe, and J. G. Holt (ed.), *Bergey's Manual of Systematic Bacteriology*, vol. 2. The Williams & Wilkins Co., Baltimore, Md.

17. **Collins, M. D., E. Falsen, E. Akervall, B. Sjöden, and A. Alvarez.** 1998. *Corynebacterium kroppenstedtii* sp. nov., a novel corynebacterium that does not contain mycolic acids. *Int. J. Syst. Bacteriol.* **48:**1449–1454.

18. **Collins, M. D., L. Hoyles, G. Foster, B. Sjöden, and E. Falsen.** 2001. *Corynebacterium capitovis* sp. nov., from a sheep. *Int. J. Syst. Evol. Microbiol.* **51:**857–860.

19. **Collins, M. D., L. Hoyles, R. A. Hutson, G. Foster, and E. Falsen.** 2001. *Corynebacterium testudinoris* sp. nov., from a tortoise, and *Corynebacterium felinum* sp. nov., from a Scottish wild cat. *Int. J. Syst. Evol. Microbiol.* **51:**1349–1352.

20. **Collins, M. D., L. Hoyles, P. A. Lawson, E. Falsen, R. L. Robson, and G. Foster.** 1999. Phenotypic and phylogenetic characterization of a new *Corynebacterium* species from dogs: description of *Corynebacterium auriscanis* sp. nov. *J. Clin. Microbiol.* **37:**3443–3447.

21. **Collins, M. D., R. A. Hutson, V. Baverud, and E. Falsen.** 2000. Characterization of a *Rothia*-like organism from a mouse: description of *Rothia nasimurium* sp. nov. and reclassification of *Stomatococcus mucilaginosus* as *Rothia mucilaginosa* comb. nov. *Int. J. Syst. Evol. Bacteriol.* **50:**1247–1251.

22. **Collins, M. D., and C. Pascual.** 2000. Reclassification of *Actinomyces humiferus* (Gledhill and Casida) as *Cellulomonas humilata* nom. corrig., comb. nov. *Int. J. Syst. Evol. Microbiol.* **50:**661–663.

23. **Connor, K. M., M. M. Quirie, G. Baird, and W. Donachie.** 2000. Characterization of United Kingdom isolates of *Corynebacterium pseudotuberculosis* using pulsed-field gel electrophoresis. *J. Clin. Microbiol.* **38:**2633–2637.

24. **Coyle, M. B., D. J. Nowowiejski, J. Q. Russell, and N. B. Groman.** 1993. Laboratory review of reference strains of *Corynebacterium diphtheriae* indicated mistyped *intermedius* strains. *J. Clin. Microbiol.* **31:**3060–3062.

25. **de Briel, D., F. Couderc, P. Riegel, F. Jehl, and R. Minck.** 1992. High-performance liquid chromatography of corynomycolic acids as a tool in identification of *Corynebacterium* species and related organisms. *J. Clin. Microbiol.* **30:**1407–1417.

26. **Devriese, L. A., P. Riegel, J. Hommez, M. Vaneechoutte, T. de Baere, and F. Haesebrouck.** 2000. Identification of *Corynebacterium glucuronolyticum* strains from urogenital tract of humans and pigs. *J. Clin. Microbiol.* **38:**4657–4659.

27. **De Zoysa, A., and A. Efstratiou.** 2000. Use of amplified fragment length polymorphisms for typing *Corynebacterium diphtheriae*. *J. Clin. Microbiol.* **38:**3843–3845.

28. **De Zoysa, A. S., and A. Efstratiou.** 1999. PCR typing of *Corynebacterium diphtheriae* by random amplification of polymorphic DNA. *J. Med. Microbiol.* **48:**335–340.

29. **Efstratiou, A., K. H. Engler, I. K. Mazurova, T. Glushkevich, J. Vuopio-Varkila, and T. Popovic.** 2000. Current approaches to the laboratory diagnosis of diphtheria. *J. Infect. Dis.* **181**(Suppl. 1)**:**S138–S145.

30. **Efstratiou, A., and R. C. George.** 1999. Laboratory guidelines for the diagnosis of infections caused by *Corynebacterium diphtheriae* and *C. ulcerans*. World Health Organization. *Commun. Dis. Public Health.* **2:**250–257.

31. **Engler K. H., A. Efstratiou, D. Norn, R. S. Kozlov, I. Selga, T. G. Glushkevich, M. Tam, V. G. Melnikov, I. K. Mazurova, G. Y. Tseneva, L. P. Titov, and R. C. George.** 2002. Immunochromatographic strip test for rapid detection of diphtheria toxin: description and multicenter evaluation in areas of low and high prevalence of diphtheria. *J. Clin. Microbiol.* **40:**80–83.

32. **Engler, K. H., T. Glushkevich, I. K. Mazurova, R. C. George, and A. Efstratiou.** 1997. A modified Elek test for detection of toxigenic corynebacteria in the diagnostic laboratory. *J. Clin. Microbiol.* **35:**495–498.

33. **Engler, K. H., and A. Efstratiou.** 2000. Rapid enzyme immunoassay for determination of toxigenicity among clinical isolates of corynebacteria. *J. Clin. Microbiol.* **38:** 1385–1389.

34. **Engler, K. H., M. Warner, and R. C. George.** 2001. In vitro activity of ketolides HMR 3647 and seven other antimicrobial agents against *Corynebacterium diphtheriae*. *J. Antimicrob. Chemother.* **47:**27–31.

35. **Evtushenko, L. I., L. V. Dorofeeva, S. A. Subbotin, J. R. Cole, and J. M. Tiedje.** 2000. *Leifsonia poae* gen. nov., sp. nov., isolated from nematode gall on *Poa annua*, and reclassification of 'Corynebacterium aquaticum' Leifson 1962 as *Leifsonia aquatica* (ex Leifson 1962) gen. nov., nom. rev., comb. nov., and *Clavibacter xyli* Davis et al. 1984 with two subspecies as *Leifsonia xyli* (Davis et al. 1984) gen. nov., comb. nov. *Int. J. Syst. Evol. Microbiol.* **50:**371–380.

36. **Farrow, J. A. E., S. Wallbanks, and M. D. Collins.** 1994. Phylogenetic interrelationships of round-spore-forming bacilli containing cell walls based on lysine and the non-spore-forming genera *Caryophanon*, *Exiguobacterium*, *Kurthia*, and *Planococcus*. *Int. J. Syst. Bacteriol.* **44:**74–82.

37. **Früh, M., A. von Graevenitz, and G. Funke.** 1998. Use of second-line biochemical and susceptibility tests for the differential diagnosis of coryneform bacteria. *Clin. Microbiol. Infect.* **4:**332–338.

38. **Fudou, R., Y. Jojima, A. Seto, K. Yamada, E. Kimura, T. Nakamatsu, A. Hiraishi, and S. Yamanaka.** 2002. *Corynebacterium efficiens* sp. nov., a glutamic-acid-producing species from soil and vegetables. *Int. J. Syst. Evol. Microbiol.* **52:**1127–1131.

39. **Funke, G., M. Altwegg, L. Frommelt, and A. von Graevenitz.** 1999. Emergence of related nontoxigenic *C. diphtheriae* biotype *mitis* strains in Western Europe. *Emerg. Infect. Dis.* **5:**477–480.

40. **Funke, G., K. A. Bernard, C. Bucher, G. E. Pfyffer, and M. D. Collins.** 1995. *Corynebacterium glucuronolyticum* sp. nov. isolated from male patients with genitourinary infections. *Med. Microbiol. Lett.* **4:**204–215.

41. **Funke, G., and A. Carlotti.** 1994. Differentiation of *Brevibacterium* spp. encountered in clinical specimens. *J. Clin. Microbiol.* **32:**1729–1732.

42. **Funke, G., A. Efstratiou, D. Kuklinska, R. A. Hutson, A. de Zoysa, K. H. Engler, and M. D. Collins.** 1997. *Corynebacterium imitans* sp. nov. isolated from patients with suspected diphtheria. *J. Clin. Microbiol.* **35:**1978–1983.

43. **Funke, G., E. Falsen, and C. Barreau.** 1995. Primary identification of *Microbacterium* spp. encountered in clinical specimens as CDC coryneform group A-4 and A-5 bacteria. *J. Clin. Microbiol.* **33:**188–192.

44. **Funke, G., R. A. Hutson, K. A. Bernard, G. E. Pfyffer, G. Wauters, and M. D. Collins.** 1996. Isolation of *Arthrobacter* spp. from clinical specimens and description of *Arthrobacter cumminsii* sp. nov. and *Arthrobacter woluwensis* sp. nov. *J. Clin. Microbiol.* **34:**2356–2363.

45. **Funke, G., R. A. Hutson, M. Hilleringmann, W. R. Heizmann, and M. D. Collins.** 1997. *Corynebacterium lipophiloflavum* sp. nov. isolated from a patient with bacterial vaginosis. *FEMS Microbiol. Lett.* **150:**219–224.

46. **Funke, G., P. A. Lawson, K. A. Bernard, and M. D. Collins.** 1996. Most *Corynebacterium xerosis* strains identified in the routine clinical laboratory correspond to *Corynebacterium amycolatum.* *J. Clin. Microbiol.* **34:**1124–1128.

47. **Funke, G., P. A. Lawson, and M. D. Collins.** 1995. Heterogeneity within Centers for Disease Control and Prevention coryneform group ANF-1-like bacteria and description of *Corynebacterium auris* sp. nov. *Int. J. Syst. Bacteriol.* **45:**735–739.

48. **Funke, G., P. A. Lawson, and M. D. Collins.** 1997. *Corynebacterium mucifaciens* sp. nov., an unusual species from human clinical material. *Int. J. Syst. Bacteriol.* **47:** 952–957.

49. **Funke, G., P. A. Lawson, and M. D. Collins.** 1998. *Corynebacterium riegelii* sp. nov., an unusual species isolated from female patients with urinary tract infections. *J. Clin. Microbiol.* **36:**624–627.

50. **Funke, G., P. A. Lawson, F. S. Nolte, N. Weiss, and M. D. Collins.** 1998. *Aureobacterium resistens* sp. nov. exhibiting vancomycin resistance and teicoplanin susceptibility. *FEMS Microbiol. Lett.* **158:**89–93.

51. **Funke, G., C. R. Osorio, R. Frei, P. Riegel, and M. D. Collins.** 1998. *Corynebacterium confusum* sp. nov., isolated from human clinical specimens. *Int. J. Syst. Bacteriol.* **48:**1291–1296.

52. **Funke, G., M. Pagano-Niederer, and W. Bernauer.** 1998. *Corynebacterium macginleyi* has to date been isolated exclusively from conjunctival swabs. *J. Clin. Microbiol.* **36:** 3670–3673.

53. **Funke, G., M. Pagano-Niederer, B. Sjöden, and E. Falsen.** 1998. Characteristics of *Arthrobacter cumminsii*, the most frequently encountered *Arthrobacter* species in human clinical specimens. *J. Clin. Microbiol.* **36:**1539–1543.

54. **Funke, G., C. Pascual Ramos, and M. D. Collins.** 1995. Identification of some clinical strains of CDC coryneform group A-3 and group A-4 bacteria as *Cellulomonas* species and proposal of *Cellulomonas hominis* sp. nov. for some group A-3 strains. *J. Clin. Microbiol.* **33:**2091–2097.

55. **Funke, G., C. Pascual Ramos, and M. D. Collins.** 1997. *Corynebacterium coyleae* sp. nov., isolated from human clinical specimens. *Int. J. Syst. Bacteriol.* **47:**92–96.

56. **Funke, G., C. Pascual Ramos, J. Fernandez-Garayzabal, N. Weiss, and M. D. Collins.** 1995. Description of human-derived Centers for Disease Control coryneform group 2 bacteria as *Actinomyces bernardiae* sp. nov. *Int. J. Syst. Bacteriol.* **45:**57–60.

57. **Funke, G., K. Peters, and M. Aravena-Roman.** 1998. Evaluation of the RapID CB Plus system for identification of coryneform bacteria and *Listeria* spp. *J. Clin. Microbiol.* **36:**2439–2442.

58. **Funke, G., V. Pünter, and A. von Graevenitz.** 1996. Antimicrobial susceptibility patterns of some recently established coryneform bacteria. *Antimicrob. Agents Chemother.* **40:**2874–2878.

59. **Funke, G., F. N. R. Renaud, J. Freney, and P. Riegel.** 1997. Multicenter evaluation of the updated and extended API (RAPID) Coryne database 2.0. *J. Clin. Microbiol.* **35:**3122–3126.

60. **Funke, G., S. Stubbs, G. E. Pfyffer, M. Marchiani, and M. D. Collins.** 1994. Characteristics of CDC group 3 and group 5 coryneform bacteria isolated from clinical specimens and assignment to the genus *Dermabacter. J. Clin. Microbiol.* **32:**1223–1228.

61. **Funke, G., S. Stubbs, G. E. Pfyffer, M. Marchiani, and M. D. Collins.** 1994. *Turicella otitidis* gen. nov., sp. nov., a coryneform bacterium isolated from patients with otitis media. *Int. J. Syst. Bacteriol.* **44:**270–273.

62. **Funke, G., A. von Graevenitz, J. E. Clarridge III, and K. A. Bernard.** 1997. Clinical microbiology of coryneform bacteria. *Clin. Microbiol. Rev.* **10:**125–159.

63. **Funke, G., A. von Graevenitz, and N. Weiss.** 1994. Primary identification of *Aureobacterium* spp. isolated from clinical specimens as "*Corynebacterium aquaticum.*" *J. Clin. Microbiol.* **32:**2686–2691.

64. **Gomez-Garces, J. L., J. Oteo, G. Garcia, B. Aracil, J. I. Alos, and G. Funke.** 2001. Bacteremia by *Dermabacter hominis*, a rare pathogen. *J. Clin. Microbiol.* **39:**2356–2357.

65. **Hauser, D., M. R. Popoff, M. Kiredjian, P. Boquet, and F. Bimet.** 1993. Polymerase chain assay for diagnosis of potentially toxigenic *Corynebacterium diphtheriae* strains: correlation with ADP-ribosylation activity assay. *J. Clin. Microbiol.* **31:**2720–2723.

66. **Hollis, D. G., and R. E. Weaver.** 1981. *Gram-Positive Organisms: a Guide to Identification.* Special Bacteriology Section, Centers for Disease Control, Atlanta, Ga.

67. **Holmes, R. K.** 2000. Biology and molecular epidemiology of diphtheria toxin and the *tox* gene. *J. Infect. Dis.* **181**(Suppl. 1)**:**S156–S167.

68. **Hommez, J., L. A. Devriese, M. Vaneechoutte, P. Riegel, P. Butaye, and F. Haesebrouck.** 1999. Identification of nonlipophilic corynebacteria isolated from dairy cows with mastitis. *J. Clin. Microbiol.* **37:**954–957.

69. **Hou, X.-G., Y. Kawamura, F. Sultana, S. Shu, K. Hirose, K. Goto, and T. Ezaki.** 1998. Description of *Arthrobacter creatinolyticus* sp. nov., isolated from human urine. *Int. J. Syst. Bacteriol.* **48:**423–429.

70. **Jones, D., and M. D. Collins.** 1988. Taxonomic studies on some human cutaneous coryneform bacteria: description of *Dermabacter hominis* gen. nov. sp. nov. *FEMS Microbiol. Lett.* **123:**167–172.

71. **Joussen, A. M., G. Funke, F. Joussen, and G. Herbertz.** 2000. *Corynebacterium macginleyi*: a conjunctiva specific pathogen. *Br. J. Ophthalmol.* **84:**1420–1422.

72. **Koch, C., F. A. Rainey, and E. Stackebrandt.** 1994. 16S rDNA studies on members of *Arthrobacter* and *Micrococcus*: an aid for their future taxonomic restructuring. *FEMS Microbiol. Lett.* **123:**167–172.

73. **Komiya, T., N. Shibata, M. Ito, M. Takahashi, and Y. Arakawa.** 2000. Retrospective diagnosis of diphtheria by detection of *Corynebacterium diphtheriae tox* gene in a formaldehyde-fixed throat swab using PCR and sequencing analysis. *J. Clin. Microbiol.* **38:**2400–2402.

74. **Kronvall, G., M. Lanner-Sjöberg, L. V. von Stedingk, H.-S. Hanson, B. Pettersson, and E. Falsen.** 1998. Whole cell protein and partial 16S rRNA gene sequence analysis suggest the existence of a second *Rothia* species. *Clin. Microbiol. Infect.* **4:**255–263.

75. **Lagrou, K., J. Verhaegen, M. Janssens, G. Wauters, and L. Verbist.** 1998. Prospective study of catalase-positive coryneform organisms in clinical specimens: identifica-

tion, clinical relevance, and antibiotic susceptibility. *Diagn. Microbiol. Infect. Dis.* **30:**7–15.

76. **Lawson, P. A., E. Falsen, G. Foster, E. Eriksson, N. Weiss, and M. D. Collins.** 2001. *Arcanobacterium pluranimalium* sp. nov., isolated from porpoise and deer. *Int. J. Syst. Evol. Microbiol.* **51:**55–59.

77. **Leonard, R. B., D. J. Nowowiejski, J. J. Warren, D. J. Finn, and M. B. Coyle.** 1994. Molecular evidence of person-to-person transmission of a pigmented strain of *Corynebacterium striatum* in intensive care units. *J. Clin. Microbiol.* **32:**164–169.

78. **Lindenmann, K., A. von Graevenitz, and G. Funke.** 1995. Evaluation of the Biolog system for the identification of asporogenous, aerobic gram-positive rods. *Med. Microbiol. Lett.* **4:**287–296.

79. **Mackenzie, A., L. A. Fuite, F. T. H. Chan, J. King, U. Allen, N. MacDonald, and F. Diaz-Mitoma.** 1995. Incidence and pathogenicity of *Arcanobacterium haemolyticum* during a 2-year study in Ottawa. *Clin. Infect. Dis.* **21:**177–181.

80. **Martinez-Martinez, L., M. C. Ortega, and A. I. Suarez.** 1995. Comparison of E-test with broth microdilution and disk diffusion for susceptibility testing of coryneform bacteria. *J. Clin. Microbiol.* **33:**1318–1321.

81. **Marston, C. K., F. Jamieson, F. Cahoon, G. Lesiak, A. Golaz, M. Reeves, and T. Popovic.** 2001. Persistence of a distinct *Corynebacterium diphtheriae* clonal group within two communities in the United States and Canada where diphtheria is endemic. *J. Clin. Microbiol.* **39:**1586–1590.

82. **Miyake T., K. Watanabe, T. Watanabe, and H. Oyaizu.** 1998. Phylogenetic analysis of the genus *Bifidobacterium* and related genera based on 16S rDNA sequences. *Microbiol. Immunol.* **42:**661–667.

83. **Nakao, H., I. K. Mazurova, T. Glushkevich, and T. Popovic.** 1997. Analysis of heterogeneity of *Corynebacterium diphtheriae* toxin gene, *tox*, and its regulatory element, *dtxR*, by direct sequencing. *Res. Microbiol.* **148:**45–54.

84. **Nakao, H., and T. Popovic.** 1997. Development of a direct PCR assay for detection of the diphtheria toxin gene. *J. Clin. Microbiol.* **35:**1651–1655.

85. **Nakao, H., and T. Popovic.** 1998. Development of a rapid ribotyping method for *Corynebacterium diphtheriae* by using PCR single-strand conformation polymorphism: comparison with standard ribotyping. *J. Microbiol. Methods* **31:**127–134.

86. **Nath, K., J. W. Sarosy, and S. P. Stylianou.** 2000. Suitability of a unique 16S rRNA gene PCR product as an indicator of *Gardnerella vaginalis*. *BioTechniques* **28:**222–226.

87. **Neubauer, M., J. Sourek, M. Ryc, J. Bohacek, M. Mara, and J. Mnukova.** 1991. *Corynebacterium accolens* sp. nov., a gram-positive rod exhibiting satellitism, from clinical material. *Syst. Appl. Microbiol.* **14:**46–51.

88. **Nieto, E., J. Zapardiel, and F. Soriano.** 1996. Environmental contamination by *Corynebacterium urealyticum* in a teaching hospital. *J. Hosp. Infect.* **32:**78–79.

89. **Nugent, R. P., M. A. Krohn, and S. L. Hillier.** 1991. Reliability of diagnosing bacterial vaginosis is improved by a standardized method of Gram stain interpretation. *J. Clin. Microbiol.* **29:**297–301.

90. **Pascual, C., and M. D. Collins.** 1999. *Brevibacterium avium* sp. nov., isolated from poultry. *Int. J. Syst. Bacteriol.* **49:**1527–1530.

91. **Pascual, C., P. A. Lawson, J. A. E. Farrow, M. Navarro Gimenez, and M. D. Collins.** 1995. Phylogenetic analysis of the genus *Corynebacterium* based on 16S rRNA gene sequences. *Int. J. Syst. Bacteriol.* **45:**724–728.

92. **Pascual Ramos, C., G. Foster, and M. D. Collins.** 1997. Phylogenetic analysis of the genus *Actinomyces* based on 16S rRNA gene sequences: description of *Arcanobacterium phocae* sp. nov., *Arcanobacterium bernardiae* comb. nov., and *Arcanobacterium pyogenes* comb. nov. *Int. J. Syst. Bacteriol.* **47:**46–53.

93. **Peel, M. M., G. G. Palmer, A. M. Stacpoole, and T. G. Kerr.** 1997. Human lymphadenitis due to *Corynebacterium pseudotuberculosis*: report of ten cases from Australia and review. *Clin. Infect. Dis.* **24:**185–191.

94. **Piot, P., E. van Dyck, M. Peeters, J. Hale, P. A. Totten, and K. K. Holmes.** 1984. Biotypes of *Gardnerella vaginalis*. *J. Clin. Microbiol.* **20:**677–679.

95. **Popovic, T., C. Kim, J. Reiss, M. Reeves, H. Nakao, and A. Golaz.** 1999. Use of molecular subtyping to document long-term persistence of *Corynebacterium diphtheriae* in South Dakota. *J. Clin. Microbiol.* **37:**1092–1099.

96. **Popovic, T., I. K. Mazurova, A. Efstratiou, J. Vuopio-Varkila, M. W. Reeves, A. de Zoysa, T. Glushkevich, and P. Grimont.** 2000. Molecular epidemiology of diphtheria. *J. Infect. Dis.* **181**(Suppl. 1)**:**S168–S177.

97. **Rainey, F., N. Weiss, H. Prauser, and E. Stackebrandt.** 1994. Further evidence for the phylogenetic coherence of actinomycetes with group B-peptidoglycan and evidence for the phylogenetic intermixing of the genera *Microbacterium* and *Aureobacterium* as determined by 16S rDNA analysis. *FEMS Microbiol. Lett.* **118:**135–140.

98. **Rassoulian Barrett, S. L., B. T. Cookson, L. C. Carlson, K. A. Bernard, and M. B. Coyle.** 2001. Diversity within reference strains of *Corynebacterium matruchotii* includes *Corynebacterium durum* and a novel organism. *J. Clin. Microbiol.* **39:**943–948.

99. **Reacher M., M. Ramsay, J. White, A. De Zoysa, A. Efstratiou, G. Mann, A. Mackay, and R. C. George.** 2000. Nontoxigenic *Corynebacterium diphtheriae*: an emerging pathogen in England and Wales? *Emerg. Infect. Dis.* **6:**640–645.

100. **Reinhardt, D. J., A. Lee, and T. Popovic.** 1998. Antitoxin-in-membrane and antitoxin-in-well assays for detection of toxigenic *Corynebacterium diphtheriae*. *J. Clin. Microbiol.* **36:**207–210.

101. **Renaud, F. N. R., D. Aubel, P. Riegel, H. Meugnier, and C. Bollet.** 2001. *Corynebacterium freneyi* sp. nov., alpha-glucosidase-positive strains related to *Corynebacterium xerosis*. *Int. J. Syst. Evol. Microbiol.* **51:**1723–1728.

102. **Renaud, F. N. R., A. Gregory, C. Barreau, D. Aubel, and J. Freney.** 1996. Identification of *Turicella otitidis* isolated from a patient with otorrhea associated with surgery: differentiation from *Corynebacterium afermentans* and *Corynebacterium auris*. *J. Clin. Microbiol.* **34:**2625–2627.

103. **Riegel, P., D. de Briel, G. Prevost, F. Jehl, and H. Monteil.** 1994. Genomic diversity among *Corynebacterium jeikeium* strains and comparison with biochemical characteristics. *J. Clin. Microbiol.* **32:**1860–1865.

104. **Riegel, P., D. de Briel, G. Prevost, F. Jehl, H. Monteil, and R. Minck.** 1993. Taxonomic study of *Corynebacterium* group ANF-1 strains: proposal of *Corynebacterium afermentans* sp. nov. containing the subspecies C. afermentans subsp. afermentans subsp. nov. and C. afermentans subsp. lipophilum subsp. nov. *Int. J. Syst. Bacteriol.* **43:**287–292.

105. **Riegel, P., R. Heller, G. Prevost, F. Jehl, and H. Monteil.** 1997. *Corynebacterium durum* sp. nov., from human clinical specimens. *Int. J. Syst. Bacteriol.* **47:**1107–1111.

106. **Riegel, P., R. Ruimy, D. de Briel, G. Prevost, F. Jehl, F. Bimet, R. Christen, and H. Monteil.** 1995. *Corynebacterium argentoratense* sp. nov., from human throat. *Int. J. Syst. Bacteriol.* **45:**533–537.

107. **Riegel, P., R. Ruimy, D. de Briel, G. Prevost, F. Jehl, R. Christen, and H. Monteil.** 1995. Genomic diversity and phylogenetic relationships among lipid-requiring diphtheroids from humans and characterization of *Corynebacterium macginleyi* sp. nov. *Int. J. Syst. Bacteriol.* **45:**128–133.

108. **Riegel, P., R. Ruimy, D. de Briel, G. Prevost, F. Jehl, R. Christen, and H. Monteil.** 1995. Taxonomy of *Corynebacterium diphtheriae* and related taxa, with recognition of *Corynebacterium ulcerans* sp. nov., nom. rev. *FEMS Microbiol. Lett.* **126:**271–276.

109. **Riegel, P., R. Ruimy, F. N. R. Renaud, J. Freney, G. Prevost, F. Jehl, R. Christen, and H. Monteil.** 1997. *Corynebacterium singulare* sp. nov., a new species for urease-positive strains related to *Corynebacterium minutissimum. Int. J. Syst. Bacteriol.* **47:**1092–1096.

110. **Ruimy, R., P. Riegel, P. Boiron, H. Monteil, and R. Christen.** 1995. Phylogeny of the genus *Corynebacterium* deduced from analyses of small-subunit ribosomal DNA sequences. *Int. J. Syst. Bacteriol.* **45:**740–746.

111. **Sadhu, K., P. A. G. Domingue, A. W. Chow, J. Nelligan, N. Cheng, and J. W. Costerton.** 1989. *Gardnerella vaginalis* has a gram-positive cell-wall ultrastructure and lacks classical cell-wall lipopolysaccharide. *J. Med. Microbiol.* **29:**229–235.

112. **Schumann, P., N. Weiss, and E. Stackebrandt.** 2001. Reclassification of *Cellulomonas cellulans* (Stackebrandt and Keddie 1986) as *Cellulosimicrobium cellulans* gen. nov., comb. nov. *Int. J. Syst. Evol. Microbiol.* **51:**1007–1010.

113. **Shukla, S. K., D. N. Vevea, D. N. Frank, N. R. Pace, and K. D. Reed.** 2001. Isolation and characterization of a black-pigmented *Corynebacterium* sp. from a woman with spontaneous abortion. *J. Clin. Microbiol.* **39:**1109–1113.

114. **Simoons-Smit, A. M., P. H. M. Savelkoul, D. W. W. Newling, and C. M. J. Vandenbroucke-Grauls.** 2000. Chronic cystitis caused by *Corynebacterium urealyticum* detected by polymerase chain reaction. *Eur. J. Clin. Microbiol. Infect. Dis.* **19:**949–952.

115. **Sjöden, B., G. Funke, A. Izquierdo, E. Akervall, and M. D. Collins.** 1998. Description of some coryneform bacteria isolated from human clinical specimens as *Corynebacterium falsenii* sp. nov. *Int. J. Syst. Bacteriol.* **48:**69–74.

116. **Soriano, F., J. M. Aguado, C. Ponte, R. Fernandez-Roblas, and J. L. Rodriguez-Tudela.** 1990. Urinary tract infection caused by *Corynebacterium* group D2: report of 82 cases and review. *Rev. Infect. Dis.* **12:**1019–1034.

117. **Spiegel, C. A.** 1991. Bacterial vaginosis. *Clin. Microbiol. Rev.* **4:**485–502.

118. **Spiegel, C. A.** 1999. Bacterial vaginosis: changes in laboratory practice. *Clin. Microbiol. Newsl.* **21:**33–37.

119. **Stackebrandt, E., F. Rainey, and N. L. Ward-Rainey.** 1997. Proposal for a new hierarchic classification system, *Actinobacteria* classis nov. *Int. J. Syst. Bacteriol.* **47:**479–491.

120. **Takeuchi, M., and K. Hatano.** 1998. Union of the genera *Microbacterium* Orla-Jensen and *Aureobacterium* Collins et al. in a redefined genus *Microbacterium. Int. J. Syst. Bacteriol.* **48:**739–747.

121. **Takeuchi, M., and K. Hatano.** 1998. Proposal of six new species in the genus *Microbacterium* and transfer of *Flavobacterium marinotypicum* ZoBell and Upham to the genus *Microbacterium* as *Microbacterium marinotypicum* comb. nov. *Int. J. Syst. Bacteriol.* **48:**973–982.

122. **Takeuchi, M., T. Sakane, T. Nihira, Y. Yamada, and K. Imai.** 1999. *Corynebacterium terpenotabidum* sp. nov., a bacterium capable of degrading squalene. *Int. J. Syst. Bacteriol.* **49:**223–229.

123. **Tang, Y.-W., A. von Graevenitz, M. G. Waddington, M. K. Hopkins, D. H. Smith, H. Li, C. P. Kolbert, S. O. Montgomery, and D. H. Persing.** 2000. Identification of coryneform bacterial isolates by ribosomal DNA sequence analysis. *J. Clin. Microbiol.* **38:**1676–1678.

124. **Tanner, M. A., D. Shoskes, A. Shahed, and N. R. Pace.** 1999. Prevalence of corynebacterial 16S rRNA sequences in patients with bacterial and "nonbacterial" prostatitis. *J. Clin. Microbiol.* **37:**1863–1870.

125. **Troxler, R., G. Funke, A. von Graevenitz, and I. Stock.** 2001. Natural antibiotic susceptibility of recently established coryneform bacteria. *Eur. J. Clin. Microbiol. Infect. Dis.* **20:**315–323.

126. **Vaneechoutte, M., P. Riegel, D. de Briel, H. Monteil, G. Verschraegen, A. De Rouck, and G. Claeys.** 1995. Evaluation of the applicability of amplified rDNA-restriction analysis (ARDRA) to identification of species of the genus *Corynebacterium. Res. Microbiol.* **146:**633–641.

127. **van Esbroeck, M., P. Vandamme, E. Falsen, M. Vancanneyt, E. Moore, B. Pot, F. Gavini, K. Kersters, and H. Goossens.** 1996. Polyphasic approach to the classification and identification of *Gardnerella vaginalis* and unidentified *Gardnerella vaginalis*-like coryneforms present in bacterial vaginosis. *Int. J. Syst. Bacteriol.* **46:**675–682.

128. **von Graevenitz, A., and G. Funke.** 1996. An identification scheme for rapidly and aerobically growing gram-positive rods. *Zentbl. Bakteriol. Parasitenkd. Infektionskr. Hyg. Abt. 1 Orig.* **284:**246–254.

129. **von Graevenitz, A., V. Pünter-Streit, P. Riegel, and G. Funke.** 1998. Coryneform bacteria in throat cultures of healthy individuals. *J. Clin. Microbiol.* **36:**2087–2088.

130. **von Graevenitz, A., U. Schumacher, and W. Bernauer.** 2001. The corynebacterial flora of the normal human conjunctiva is lipophilic. *Curr. Microbiol.* **42:**372–374.

131. **Wattiau, P., M. Janssens, and G. Wauters.** 2000. *Corynebacterium simulans* sp. nov., a non-lipophilic, fermentative *Corynebacterium. Int. J. Syst. Evol. Microbiol.* **50:**347–353.

132. **Wauters, G., J. Charlier, M. Janssens, and M. Delmee.** 2000. Identification of *Arthrobacter oxydans*, *Arthrobacter luteolus* sp. nov., and *Arthrobacter albus* sp. nov., isolated from human clinical specimens. *J. Clin. Microbiol.* **38:**2412–2415.

133. **Wauters, G., J. Charlier, M. Janssens, and M. Delmee.** 2001. *Brevibacterium paucivorans* sp. nov., from human clinical specimens. *Int. J. Syst. Evol. Bacteriol.* **51:**1703–1707.

134. **Wauters, G., B. van Bosterhaut, M. Janssens, and J. Verhaegen.** 1998. Identification of *Corynebacterium amycolatum* and other nonlipophilic fermentative corynebacteria of human origin. *J. Clin. Microbiol.* **36:**1430–1432.

135. **Weiss, K., M. Laverdiere, and R. Rivest.** 1996. Comparison of antimicrobial susceptibilities of *Corynebacterium* species by broth microdilution and disk diffusion methods. *Antimicrob. Agents Chemother.* **40:**930–933.

136. **Yassin, A. F., U. Steiner, and W. Ludwig.** 2002. *Corynebacterium aurimucosum* sp. nov. and emended description of *Corynebacterium minutissimum* Collins and Jones (1983). *Int. J. Syst. Evol. Microbiol.* **52:**1001–1005.

137. **Zapardiel, J., E. Nieto, M. I. Gegundez, I. Gadea, and F. Soriano.** 1994. Problems in minimum inhibitory concentration determinations in coryneform organisms—comparison of an agar dilution and the Etest. *Diagn. Microbiol. Infect. Dis.* **19:**171–173.

138. **Zimmermann, O., C. Spröer, R. M. Kroppenstedt, E. Fuchs, H. G. Köchel, and G. Funke.** 1998. *Corynebacterium thomssenii* sp. nov., a *Corynebacterium* with *N*-acetyl-β-glucosaminidase activity from human clinical specimens. *Int. J. Syst. Bacteriol.* **48:**489–494.

139. **Zinkernagel, A. S., A. von Graevenitz, and G. Funke.** 1996. Heterogeneity within *Corynebacterium minutissimum* strains is explained by misidentified *Corynebacterium amycolatum* strains. *Am. J. Clin. Pathol.* **106:**378–383.

Nocardia, Rhodococcus, Gordonia, Actinomadura, Streptomyces, and Other Aerobic Actinomycetes*

JUNE M. BROWN AND MICHAEL M. McNEIL

35

TAXONOMY

The systematics of the aerobic actinomycetes began as a largely intuitive discipline based on microscopic morphology but has become increasingly objective with the introduction and application of modern taxonomic procedures, notably chemosystematic, molecular systematic, and numerical taxonomic methods. Although the attribute of branched, filamentous hyphae that either form spores or reproduce by fragmentation remains central to the definition of an actinomycete, it is clear that many actinomycete genera are only distantly related phylogenetically (147, 159, 160). Although more than 40 genera are currently described as aerobic actinomycetes, only 16 appear to be relevant to human and veterinary medicine. The medically important genera are *Actinomadura, Corynebacterium, Dermatophilus, Gordonia, Mycobacterium, Nocardia, Rhodococcus, Streptomyces, Saccharomonospora, Saccharopolyspora, Thermoactinomyces, Tropheryma* (only one species, *T. whipplei*, the recently validated agent of Whipple's disease) (99), *Tsukamurella*, and, to a lesser extent, *Amycolatopsis, Micromonospora*, and *Nocardiopsis*. The main characteristics used for identification of the clinically important aerobic actinomycetes to the genus level are given in Table 1.

The mycolic acid-containing actinomycetes or mycolata, notably corynebacteria, mycobacteria, and nocardiae, have a set of chemical markers in common (i.e., the cell wall components *meso*-diaminopimelic acid [*meso*-DAP], arabinose and galactose, and mycolic acids) that characterizes them as the mycolata genera. On the basis of these chemical markers, along with complementary 16S rRNA gene sequence data, Chun et al. (37) classified the mycolata genera into two genetic clusters: the family *Corynebacteriaceae*, which encompasses the genera *Corynebacterium* and *Dietzia*, and the family *Mycobacteriaceae*, which includes the genera *Gordonia, Mycobacterium, Nocardia, Rhodococcus, Skermania*, and *Tsukamurella*. Although *Corynebacterium amycolatum* and *Corynebacterium kroppenstedtii* lack mycolic acids, they have a close phylogenetic relationship with other species of *Corynebacterium* (39). Phylogenetic investigations of 16S rRNA gene sequence clustering and the presence of unique signature nucleotides proposed by Stackebrandt et al. (187) generated an alternate classification system for the genera described in this chapter: the closely related genera *Corynebacterium* and *Turicella* are classified in an emended family *Corynebacteriaceae*, the genus *Mycobacterium* is classified in the family *Mycobacteriaceae*, and the genera *Dietzia, Gordonia*, and *Tsukamurella* are classified in the new families *Dietziaceae, Gordoniaceae*, and *Tsukamurellaceae*, respectively. These taxa, along with the genera *Nocardia* and *Rhodococcus* in the family *Nocardiaceae*, are in the lineage of the class *Actinobacteria*, order *Actinomycetales*, and suborder *Corynebacterineae*. Additionally, the reclassification of *Nocardia pinensis* to the genus *Skermania* (36) and the description of the genus *Williamsia* (82) elevate the mycolata genera to nine, although *Skermania, Williamsia*, and *Dietzia* have not been reported to be of human medical importance. The distinguishing characteristics of the mycolic acid-containing genera are given in Table 2.

DESCRIPTION OF THE GENERA

Nocardia

The genus *Nocardia* is currently composed of 22 validly described species (64, 65, 72, 74, 233, 237; B. A. Brown, R. W. Wilson, V. A. Steingrube, Z. Blacklock, and R. J. Wallace, Jr., *Abstr. 97th Gen. Meet. Am. Soc. Microbiol. 1997*, abstr. C-65, p. 131, 1997). However, despite recent taxonomic changes, there is evidence that there are other species to be described, in particular, the *Nocardia asteroides* complex, *N. brevicatena, N. carnea, N. nova*, and *N. pseudobrasiliensis* (41, 64). The species that are not clinically significant include *N. crassostreae, N. cummidelens, N. flavorosea, N. fluminea, N. salmonicida, N. seriolae, N. soli, N. uniformis*, and *N. vaccinii* (64, 118). The distinguishing characteristics of the 13 medically relevant species are given in Table 3. Members of the genus *Nocardia* form extensively branched hyphae that fragment into rod-shaped to coccoid, nonmotile elements and usually form aerial hyphae, which at times are visible only microscopically (65). Nocardiae are characterized by the presence of *meso*-DAP, arabinose, and galactose in their wall peptidoglycan (wall chemotype IV) (103), having muramic acid in the

* This chapter contains information presented in chapter 24 by June M. Brown, Michael M. McNeil, and Edward P. Desmond in the seventh edition of this Manual.

TABLE 1 Tests used for the presumptive identification of the medically important aerobic actinomycetes to the genus level[a,b]

Genus	Vegetative filaments		Conidia	Acid-fast nature	Presence[c] in whole cells of:		Mycolic acids	Metabolism of glucose	Growth at 50°C	Arylsulfatase	Growth in lysozyme
	Substrate	Aerial			DAP	Sugars					
Actinomadura	+	V	V	−	meso	Mad	−	O	−	−	−
Amycolatopsis	+	+	V	−	meso	Arab, Gal	−	O	−	−	−
Corynebacterium	+	−	−	−	meso	Arab, Gal	+	O, F	−	−	−
Dermatophilus[d]	+	−	−	−	meso	Mad	−	F	−	−	NT
Gordona	+	−	−	W	meso	Arab, Gal	+	O	−	−	V
Micromonospora	+	−	+	−	meso	Arab, Xyl	−	O	−	−	−
Mycobacterium	+	−	−	+	meso	Arab, Gal	+	O	−	+	−
Nocardia	+	+	V	W	meso	Arab, Gal	+	O	−	−[e]	+
Nocardiopsis	+	+	+	−	meso	None	−	O	−	−	−
Rhodococcus	+	−	−	W	meso	Arab, Gal	+	O	−	−	V
Saccharomonospora	+	+	+	−	meso	Arab, Gal	−	O	+	−	−
Saccharopolyspora	+	+	+	−	meso	Arab, Gal	−	O	+	−	V
Streptomyces	+	+	+	−	L	None	−	O	−	−	−
Thermoactinomyces	+	+	+	−	meso	Arab, Gal	−	O	+	−	+
Tsukamurella	+	−	−	W	meso	Arab, Gal	+	O	−	−	+

[a] Data adapted from reference 127.
[b] Symbols and abbreviations: +, 90% or more of strains are positive; −, 90% or more of the strains are negative; V, 11 to 89% of the strains are positive; O, oxidative; F, fermentative; NT, not tested; Mad, madurose; Arab, arabinose; Gal, galactose; Xyl, xylose; W, weakly or partially acid fast.
[c] As determined by the method of Becker et al. (13) for whole-cell DAP and sugars.
[d] Genus is motile.
[e] *N. nova* isolates (75%) are arylsulfatase positive in 14 days (213); the type strain of *N. africana* is positive in 3 days when tested in the CDC Actinomycete Reference Laboratory.

N-glycolated form, having diphosphatidylglycerol, phosphatidylethanolamine, phosphatidylinositol, and phosphatidylinositol mannosides as their major phospholipids; having major amounts of straight-chain, unsaturated, and tuberculostearic acids; having mycolic acids with 40 to 60 carbon atoms; and having DNAs that are rich in guanine-plus-cytosine (G+C) content (64 to 72 mol%) (72). The differentiation of the genus *Nocardia* from related genera is given in Table 2. The differential characteristics of relevant species within the genus *Nocardia* are given in Table 3.

Rhodococcus

At present, the genus contains 12 validly described species (15, 62, 63, 90, 125, 193). The members of the genus *Rhodococcus* consist of a diverse group of organisms that are quite variable in their morphology, biochemical characteristics, growth patterns, and capacity to cause disease. *R. equi* is the major species of *Rhodococcus* of medical importance. The other three species, *R. erythropolis*, *R. rhodnii*, and *R. rhodochrous*, have only infrequently been implicated as the causative agents of disease. The differential characteristics of these four medically important *Rhodococcus* species are given in Table 4. The differentiation of the genus *Rhodococcus* from related genera is given in Table 2.

Gordonia

In 1988, Stackebrandt et al. reintroduced the genus *Gordonia* (formerly *Gordona*) to accommodate microorganisms previously considered to be rhodococci based on comparative analyses of genes coding for 16S rRNA (188). In 1997, Stackebrandt et al. (187) redefined the genus to include 13 validly described species; however, only 5 of these species, *Gordonia aichiensis*, *G. bronchialis*, *G. rubropertincta*, *G. sputi*, and *G. terrae*, are of medical importance. Two taxa,

Nocardia amarae and *Rhodococcus aichiensis*, have been transferred to the genus *Gordonia* as *G. amarae* and *G. aichiensis*, respectively (91). Eight species, *G. alkanivorans*, *G. amarae*, *G. amicalis*, *G. desulfuricans*, *G. hydrophobica*, *G. hirsuta*, *G. polyisoprenivorans*, and *G. rhizophera*, have not been isolated from clinical specimens (16, 64, 87, 88, 90, 93, 110, 196). The differentiation of the genus *Gordonia* from related genera is given in Table 2. The differential characteristics of the five medically important members of the genus *Gordonia* are given in Table 5.

Tsukamurella

Tsukamurella paurometabola was first described as *Gordonia aurantiaca* in humans in 1971 by Tsukamura and Mizuma and was isolated from sputum of patients with tuberculosis (203). *T. paurometabola* was referred to variously as *Gordonia aurantiaca* and *Rhodococcus aurantiacus* until Collins et al. found it to be identical to *Corynebacterium paurometabolum* by 16S rRNA gene sequence analysis, renamed the genus *Tsukamurella* with *Tsukamurella paurometabola* as the type species, and assigned a new type strain (40). Recently, five additional species have been assigned to this genus: *T. inchonensis*, *T. pulmonis*, *T. strandjordae*, *T. tyrosinosolvens*, and *T. wratislaviensis* (66, 85, 231, 232, 234). Yassin et al. have clearly shown that > 99% 16S rRNA gene sequence similarity exists between *Tsukamurella* strains, but this high similarity does not indicate membership in the same species (231, 232, 234). The major chemotaxonomic characteristics that distinguish the genus *Tsukamurella* from other mycolic acid-containing taxa are summarized in Table 2. The characteristics that differentiate the members within the genus *Tsukamurella* are given in Table 6.

TABLE 2 Differential characteristics of the mycolic acid-containing genera[a,b]

| Genus | Acid-fast nature | Macroscopic aerial filaments | Arylsulfatase production in 14 days | Range of carbon atoms in mycolic acids | Presence of: | | | Major menaquinone | Glycolated muramic acid | G+C content of DNA (mol%) |
					Tuberculostearic acid	Phosphatidylethanolamine	Phosphatidylinositol and phosphatidylinositol mannosides			
Corynebacterium	–	–	–	22–38	–	–[c]	+	MK-8 (H$_2$), MK-9 (H$_2$)	–[d]	51–67
Dietzia	W	–	–	34–38	+	–	–	MK-8 (H$_2$)	–[d]	73
Gordonia	W	–	–	54–66	+	+	+	MK-9 (H$_2$)	+	63–69
Mycobacterium	+	–	+	70–90	+	+	+	MK-9 (H$_2$)	+	62–70
Nocardia	W	+	–[e]	50–62	+	+	+	MK-8 (H$_4$-ω-cycl)	+	64–72
Rhodococcus	W	–	–	34–54	+	+	+	MK-8 (H$_2$)	+	63–73
Skermania	–	+	ND	58–64	+	+	+	MK-8 (H$_4$-ω-cycl)	+	68
Tsukamurella	W	–	–	64–78	+	+	+	MK-9	+	67–68
Williamsia	–	–	ND	50–56	+	+	+	MK-9 (H$_2$)	+	64–65

[a] Data taken from references 36, 63, 64, and 160.
[b] Symbols: –, 90% or more of the strains are negative; +, 90% or more of the strains are positive; W, weakly or partially acid fast; ND, not determined.
[c] Some *Corynebacterium* species contain phosphatidylethanolamine (160).
[d] These genera contain acetylated muramic acid (63).
[e] *N. nova* isolates (75%) are arylsulfatase positive in 14 days (213); the type strain of *N. africana* is positive in 3 days when tested in the CDC Actinomycete Reference Laboratory.

Actinomadura

Actinomadura madurae was first recognized in 1894 by Vincent, who named the organism "*Streptothrix madurae*" and described it as the causative agent of "Madura foot" (209). Subsequently, the taxonomy of the genus *Actinomadura* has undergone numerous revisions based on the application of chemical, numerical phenetic, and molecular systematic methods (83). The genus is now well defined and is composed of 27 validly described species (83). Three of these *Actinomadura* species, *A. latina*, *A. madurae*, and *A. pelletieri*, are clinically significant (200). *A. latina*, described in 1997 by Trujillo and Goodfellow (200), included some strains previously identified as *A. pelletieri*. Members of the genus *Actinomadura* are gram-positive, nonfragmenting bacilli that have branched substrate and sparse aerial hyphae that each carry up to 15 arthrospores. Phenotypic characteristics of each of the medically important species, along with other agents of actinomycetoma, are given in Table 7. The major characteristics that separate this genus from other aerobic actinomycetes are given in Table 1.

Streptomyces

Streptomyces somaliensis was first described by Brumpt in 1906 as "*Indiella somaliensis*" and was isolated from patients affected with mycetomas in French Somaliland (28). The taxonomy of the genus *Streptomyces* has undergone many revisions due to the application of chemical, numeric taxonomic, and molecular systematic methods; however, this genus has species yet to be described and identification to the species level remains difficult and is impossible using phenotypic methods alone (127). Despite limitations in the ability to accurately identify these species, there are reports that species other than *S. somaliensis* may be of medical importance. These include *Streptomyces albus*, *Streptomyces anulatus* (formerly *S. griseus*), *Streptomyces lavendulae*, *Streptomyces rimosus*, and *Streptomyces violaceoruber* (127). Phenotypic differences between *S. somaliensis* and other medically important agents of actinomycetoma are given in Table 7. Since the study by Pridham et al. in 1958 that described more than 1,000 species of *Streptomyces* (156), the taxonomy of this genus has been evaluated and re-evaluated (4, 98, 220). There have been several studies based on phylogenetic analyses with 16S rRNA sequence data and on the ribosomal AT-L30 protein and N-terminal acid sequences (147, 226), numerical phenetic studies with 329 miniaturized tests (84), sodium dodecyl sulfate-polyacrylamide gel electrophoresis (119), and DNA fingerprinting with pulsed-field gel electrophoresis (19). The taxonomy of this genus will continue to be uncertain until a comprehensive DNA-DNA hybridization study that includes type strains of all validly described species is performed. The major characteristics that separate this genus from other aerobic actinomycetes are given in Table 1.

Tropheryma whipplei

T. whipplei was named after George Whipple, who described the first patient with Whipple's disease in 1907 (219). In 1991, Wilson et al. identified the uncultivated agent of Whipple's disease as an actinomycete based on a partial sequence of the 16S rRNA gene (223). The following year, Relman et al. characterized and provisionally named the putative agent "*Tropheryma whippelii*" based on almost the entire 16S rRNA gene sequence (166). In 2001, La Scola et al. isolated the Whipple's disease bacillus from the cardiac valve of a patient with endocarditis and proposed the organism's name to be validated as *Tropheryma*

whipplei (99, 163). This strain was cultured and maintained on human embryonic lung fibroblast monolayers; however, it has not been subcultured on artificial media in the laboratory. The phylogenetic position of *T. whipplei* has been reassessed by additional sequencing of the 16S rRNA gene (114). On this basis, it was placed in the actinomycetes clade in the class *Actinobacteria* closely similar to actinomycetes with group B peptidoglycan and members of the genus *Cellulomonas*. Its DNA G+C content was determined to be 59.4 mol%, within the range of gram-positive bacteria (99).

Other Aerobic Actinomycetes

The genus *Nocardiopsis* was described by Meyer (134) for microorganisms previously designated "*Streptothrix dassonvillei*," "*Nocardia dassonvillei*," or "*Actinomadura dassonvillei*." Currently, the genus *Nocardiopsis* consists of eight validly described species in the family *Nocardiopsaceae*: *N. alba* (235), *N. dassonvillei* (134), *N. halophila* (1), *N. kunsanensis* (35), *N. listeri* (71), *N. lucentensis* (230), and *N. prasina* and *N. synnemataformans* (235). Only *N. dassonvillei* and *N. synnemataformans* have been reported as being isolated from humans. Members of the genus *Nocardiopsis* exhibit fragmentation of substrate and aerial hyphae into zigzag chains of arthrospores that are characteristic for this genus (134). These microorganisms contain *meso*-DAP but no diagnostically important carbohydrate (cell wall chemotype III) (103). Other features include lack of mycolic acids, the presence of muramic acid of the acetyl type, and a DNA G+C content between 64 and 69 mol% (161, 235). The current differentiation of the *Nocardiopsis* species is based on the color of the hyphae and physiological characteristics. The major characteristics that separate this genus from other aerobic actinomycetes are given in Table 1.

Amycolatopsis orientalis ("*Nocardia orientalis*," "*Streptomyces orientalis*") is known primarily for the production of the antimicrobial agent vancomycin (152). Although isolates of this species have a cell wall composition similar to that of the true nocardiae (presence of *meso*-DAP, arabinose, and galactose), they do not contain mycolic acids (105).

The genus *Micromonospora* is known primarily as the microbiologic source of clinically significant antimicrobial agents, especially the aminoglycosides and macrolides. The characteristics that separate the genus *Micromonospora* from other actinomycetes are given in Table 1.

Dermatophilosis was first recognized as an infectious disease in 1915 by Van Saceghem, who described the disease in cattle in the former Belgian Congo (206). In 1995, Masters et al. described a new species, *Dermatophilus chelonae*, from chelonids (two turtles and one tortoise) (123). Members of the genus *Dermatophilus* are characterized by a unique life cycle, at the beginning and end of which are motile zoospores of 0.5 μm in diameter. The characteristics that separate the genus *Dermatophilus* from other actinomycetes are given in Table 1.

Three genera of thermophilic actinomycetes are considered of medical importance: *Saccharomonospora*, *Saccharopolyspora* (or *Faenia*), and *Thermoactinomyces*. Within these three genera, there is one important species of *Saccharomonospora* (*S. viridis*), one important species of *Saccharopolyspora* (*S. rectivirgula* [*Faenia rectivirgula*]), and three important species of *Thermoactinomyces* (*T. thalpophilus*, *T. sacchari*, and *T. vulgaris*). Thermotolerance to 50°C or above is a pathognomonic characteristic for all of the thermophilic species. In addition, all these species form

TABLE 3 Characteristics differentiating the medically important species of the genus *Nocardia*[a,b]

Characteristic	N. abscessus	N. africana	N. asteroides sensu stricto type VI	N. brasiliensis	N. brevicatena complex	N. carnea	N. farcinica[c]
Hydrolysis of:							
Acetamide	−	−	V	−	−	NT	+
Adenine	−	−	−	−	−	−	−
Casein	−	+	−	+	−	−	−
Esculin	−	−	−	+	+	+	+
Hypoxanthine	−	−	−	+	−	−	−
Tyrosine	−	−	−	+	−	−	−
Xanthine	−	−	−	−	−	−	−
Utilization as sole carbon source of:							
Adonitol (ribitol)	−	−	−	−	−	−	−
L-Arabinose	−	−	−	−	−	−	−
Citrate	+	+	V	+	−	−	−
i-Erythritol	−	−	−	−	−	−	+
D-Galactose	−	−	V	+	−	−	−
D-Glucose	+	+	+	+	−	−	+
i-myo-Inositol	−	−	−	+	−	−	−
D-Mannitol	−	−	−	+	−	+	−
L-Rhamnose	V	−	V	−	V	−	+
D-Sorbitol (D-glucitol)	−	−	−	−	−	+	−
D-Trehalose	V	−	V	+	V	−	−
Growth at or in:							
45°C	V	+	V	−	V	−	+
Lysozyme broth	+	+	+	+	V	+	+
Production of arylsulfatase	−	NG	−	−	−	−	−
Resistance to:							
Amikacin (MIC, >16 μg/ml)	−	−	−	−	−	NT	−
Gentamicin[d] (zone, ≤10 mm)	−	+	−	NT	V	NT	+
Kanamycin (MIC, >16 μg/ml)	−	+	V	NT	−	NT	+
Tobramycin[d] (zone, <20 mm)	−	NT	−	NT	+	NT	+
Ciprofloxacin (MIC, >4 μg/ml)	+	NT	−	+	−	NT	−
Ampicillin (MIC, >4 μg/ml)	I	−	+	V	V	NT	+
Amox-clav (MIC, ≥64/32 μg/ml)	NT	NT	NT	−	V	NT	−
Cefamandole[d] (zone, <20 mm)	−	NT	−	V	V	NT	+
Cefotaxime (MIC, ≥64 μg/ml)	−	NT	−	V	−	NT	+
Ceftriaxone (MIC, ≥64 μg/ml)	−	NT	−	V	−	NT	+
Erythromycin[d] (zone, <30 mm)	+	−	I	−	+	NT	+

[a] Data derived from references 72, 74, 171, 213, 217, 224, 233, and 236 and Brown et al., *Abstr. 97th Gen. Meet. Am. Soc. Microbiol. 1997.*

[b] Abbreviations and symbols: −, 90% or more of the strains are negative; +, 90% or more of the strains are positive; V, 11 to 89% of the strains are positive; NT, not tested; NG, not given; I, intermediate; amox-clav, amoxicillin-clavulanate.

[c] *N. farcinica* has the capacity to opacify Middlebrook 7H10 agar (55).

meso-DAP and lack mycolic acids in their cell walls. Although the first practical scheme for identifying the thermophilic actinomycetes was developed in 1975 by Kurup and Fink and has remained clinically useful (94), this group of microorganisms has undergone numerous taxonomic changes (204).

NATURAL HABITATS

The aerobic actinomycetes are ubiquitous in the environment; they have been isolated worldwide from soil, freshwater, marine water, and organic matter (61). *Nocardia* spp. and related bacteria are considered saprophytic soil microorganisms, primarily responsible for the decomposition of organic plant material (148, 153). Although *N. asteroides* appears to be geographically widespread, most cases of *N. brasiliensis* infection in the United States have originated in the Southeast or Southwest (186). No environmental source for *N. transvalensis* has yet been identified. However, as has been found for *N. asteroides*, soil is a probable reservoir for this unusual actinomycete.

The species of *Rhodococcus* are widely distributed in the environment: *R. coprophilus*, *R. equi*, *R. erythropolis*, *R. fascians*, *R. globerulus*, *R. rhodochrous*, and *R. ruber* have been isolated from soil; *R. coprophilus* and *R. equi* have been isolated from herbivore dung; *R. fascians* has been isolated from plants and the intestinal tract of carp; *R. marinonascens* has been isolated from the uppermost layer of marine

N. nova	N. otitidiscaviarum	N. paucivorans	N. pseudobrasiliensis	N. transvalensis (N. asteroides type IV)	N. transvalensis (sensu stricto)	N. transvalensis (new taxon I)	N. transvalensis (new taxon II)	N. veterana
–	–	–	+	–	–	–	–	–
–	–	–	+	–	–	–	–	–
–	–	–	+	–	–	–	–	–
–	+	V	+	–	–	–	–	–
–	+	–	+	+	+	+	+	–
–	–	–	+	–	–	–	–	–
–	+	–	–	–	–	–	–	–
–	–	–	–	–	+	+	+	NG
–	V	–	–	–	–	–	–	NG
–	–	–	+	+	+	+	+	–
–	–	–	–	+	+	V	V	NG
–	–	–	+	–	+	+	V	–
+	+	–	+	+	+	V	V	NG
–	+	–	+	–	+	+	–	+
–	V	–	+	–	V	+	V	NG
–	–	–	–	–	–	–	–	+
–	–	–	–	–	+	+	–	NG
V	V	+	+	+	+	+	+	NG
–	V	NT	–	NT	NT	NT	NT	NT
+	+	+	+	+	+	+	+	+
V	–	–	–	–	–	–	–	–
–	–	NT	–	+	+	V	V	NT
V	NT	NT	NT	+	+	+	+	NT
V	NT	NT	NT	+	+	+	+	NT
V	NT	NT	–	+	+	+	+	NT
+	NT	NT	–	NT	NT	NT	NT	NT
–	+	NT	V	NT	NT	NT	NT	NT
+	+	NT	V	V	+	V	–	NT
–	NT	NT	NT	NT	NT	NT	NT	NT
–	V	NT	NT	NT	NT	NT	NT	NT
–	V	NT	NT	NT	NT	NT	NT	NT
–	+	NT	–	+	+	+	+	NT

[d] Disk content (micrograms) was as follows: gentamicin, 10 μg; tobramycin, 10 μg; cefamandole, 30 μg; and erythromycin, 30 μg. The method was adapted from reference 215. Briefly, the inoculum was adjusted to a turbidity equivalent to that of a 0.5 McFarland barium sulfate standard and was streaked onto a Mueller-Hinton agar plate, the plate was inoculated at 35°C, and the zone of inhibition was read at 48 h.

sediments; and *R. rhodnii* has been isolated from the intestine of the reduvid bug (62, 64). In 1984, Barton and Hughes detected *R. equi* in 54% of soil samples examined and from intestinal contents, feces from the rectum, and dung of all grazing herbivorous species examined (9).

Members of the genus *Gordonia* are widely distributed: *G. aichiensis* has been isolated from human sputum (62); *G. bronchialis*, *G. rubropertincta*, *G. sputi*, and *G. terrae* have been isolated from sputa and soil (62, 201); *G. amarae* has been isolated from foam formed on the surface of aeration tanks in activated-sludge sewage treatment plants (64); *G. hirsuta* and *G. hydrophobica* have been isolated from biofilters for waste gas treatment (16, 90); and *G. polyisoprenivorans* has been isolated from soil (110).

Members of the genus *Tsukamurella* are found naturally in soil, sludge, and arthropods (66).

The natural habitat of the pathogenic actinomadurae is thought to be the environment; these agents are inhabitants of the surface layers of the soil, and they may be introduced by percutaneous trauma and most commonly cause mycetomatous involvement of the lower extremity, although other sites of the human body may also be affected. *A. madurae* seems to be widespread in soil, whereas to date, *A. latina* and *A. pelletieri* have been found only in clinical specimens (200).

Very little is known about the role of *Streptomyces* species in natural environments, although evidence for their occurrence is extensive. Streptomycetes are widely distrib-

TABLE 4 Differential characteristics of the medically important *Rhodococcus* species[a,b]

Characteristic	*R. equi*	*R. erythropolis*	*R. rhodnii*	*R. rhodochrous*
Morphogenetic sequence	R-C	RB-R-C	RB-R-C	RB-R-C
Pigment	Pink	Orange to red	Red	Rose
Decomposition of:				
Adenine	+	+	−	V
Tyrosine	−	V	V	V
Utilization of:				
D-Galactose	+	V	+	V
i-*myo*-Inositol	−	+	−	−
D-Mannitol	−	+	+	+
L-Rhamnose	V	−	−	−
D-Sorbitol	−	+	−	+
D-Sucrose	−	+	−	V
Citrate	−	+	V	V

[a] Data adapted from references 62 and 63.
[b] Symbols: R-C, rod-coccus; RB-R-C, rudimentary branching-rod-coccus; +, positive; −, negative; V, variable.

uted in terrestrial and aquatic habitats. Most are strict saprophytes, but some form parasitic associations with plants and animals. *S. somaliensis*, a well-established causal agent of actinomycetoma, is rarely reported in the United States but has been reported in Mexico as well as African countries (77).

The natural habitat of *T. whipplei* has not been identified; however, evidence from PCR studies has suggested that the bacterium is more widespread than previously realized. The demonstration by PCR of *T. whipplei* DNA in saliva, dental plaque, duodenal biopsy specimens, gastric juice, and feces from healthy persons implies that it is a commensal in the gastrointestinal tract (48, 50, 113, 194). The detection of *T. whipplei* DNA by PCR in sewage samples in Germany may reflect fecal shedding of the bacillus or may suggest an environmental source (116). On the other hand, PCR detection of *T. whipplei* DNA by PCR in feces of patients diagnosed with Whipple's disease may be a good alternative to duodenal biopsies in screening suspected patients (69, 113).

The natural reservoir for *D. congolensis* is currently unknown; however, contaminated soil is a likely source (104). These organisms have a worldwide distribution but are most prevalent in the tropics and subtropics (238).

Thermophilic microorganisms are ubiquitous and can be found in water, air, soil, and compost piles; home and industrial air-conditioning systems; and house dusts, hay, and bagasse (solid plant residue left after sugar cane has been crushed to extract sugar) (96).

CLINICAL SIGNIFICANCE

Nocardia

Nocardial infections are rare in humans, occurring most frequently in patients who are severely immunocompromised (127). *Nocardia* infection is usually acquired by inhalation, but, rarely, direct skin inoculation is implicated.

Nocardiosis appears to have a slight predilection for males and usually affects adults in the third and fourth decades. Most clinical infections in temperate countries have been caused by *N. asteroides* complex, *N. brasiliensis*, and, rarely, *N. otitidiscaviarum*. *N. asteroides* complex (including *N. abscessus*, *N. asteroides* sensu stricto type VI, *N. farcinica*, and *N. nova*) has been considered to be responsible for the majority of serious invasive infections. It appears that the *N. asteroides* complex remains a heterogeneous group of organisms and, of high importance, has variable antibiotic susceptibilities (216). Until recently, *N. abscessus*, *N. farcinica*, and *N. nova* were not distinguished from *N. asteroides* in reported series, but they have now been recognized as distinct species with individual biochemical and antimicrobial susceptibility profiles (213, 216, 217). *N. brasiliensis* has been associated particularly with subcutaneous infections and is predominant in tropical countries (186). The new taxon *N. pseudobrasiliensis*, which was recently separated from *N. brasiliensis*, appears to be generally associated with noncutaneous (pulmonary, central nervous system, or systemic) nocardiosis (171, 212).

Although nocardiosis is most often considered a late-presenting, community-acquired infection, nosocomial outbreaks of nocardiosis in immunocompromised patients have been reported and were attributed to airborne and/or person-to-person transmission (53, 175, 218). The clinical manifestations, severity, and prognosis of disease in the infected patient are extremely variable and may be determined by factors such as the route of infection and the presence or absence of a properly functioning immune system. In immunocompetent hosts, localized subcutaneous infection may result from inoculation of these microorganisms at the time of surgery or from traumatic percutaneous inoculation as a result of outdoor activities. Although other *Nocardia* species may cause primary cutaneous infections, *N. brasiliensis* is the predominant causative agent (186). In severely immunocompromised patients, the principal predisposing factors include immunosuppressive therapy, particularly steroid drugs, neoplastic diseases, solid-organ and bone marrow transplantation, chronic bronchopulmonary diseases, and AIDS. The most common clinical presentations are invasive pulmonary infection and disseminated disease (10, 11, 127). However, invasive disease may also occur in immunocompetent patients. In addition, underlying pulmonary disorders (e.g., cancer or tuberculosis) may predispose to respiratory tract colonization with *Nocardia*.

TABLE 5 Differential physiological characteristics of the medically important *Gordonia* species[a,b]

Characteristic	*G. aichiensis*	*G. bronchialis*	*G. rubropertincta*	*G. sputi*	*G. terrae*
Utilization of[c]:					
D-Galactose	+	−	+	+	+
i-*myo*-Inositol	−	+	−	−	−
D-Mannitol	−	−	+	+	+
Raffinose	−	−	−	+	+
L-Rhamnose	−	−	−	−	+
D-Sorbitol	−	−	+	+	+
Citrate	+	−	+	−	+

[a] Data adapted from references 16 and 62.
[b] Symbols: +, ≥90% of the strains are positive; −, ≥90% of the strains are negative.
[c] The concentration used to determine carbon source utilization was 1.0% except for growth on citrate, which was tested at 0.1%.

TABLE 6 Differential characteristics of the genus *Tsukamurella*[a,b]

Characteristic	T. inchonensis	T. paurometabola	T. pulmonis	T. strandjordae	T. tyrosinosolvens	T. wratislaviensis
Decomposition of:						
Hypoxanthine	+	−	−	−	+	+
Xanthine	−	−	−	−	+	+
Tyrosine	−	−	−	−	+	+
Utilization as sole carbon source:						
Cellobiose	+	−	−	NT[c]	−	−
Maltose	+	−	−	+	+	+
i-myo-Inositol	+	−	−	+	+	+
D-Mannitol	+	−	+	+	+	+
D-Sorbitol	+	−	+	+	+	+
Citrate	+	+	−	+	V	−
Utilization of acetamide as sole carbon and nitrogen source	+	−	+	NT	+	−
Growth at 45°C	+	−	−	−	−	NT

[a] Data adapted from references 40, 85, 231, 232, and 234.
[b] Symbols: +, positive; −, negative; V, variable; NT, not tested.
[c] Data obtained with API 50 CH (bioMérieux Vitek, Hazelwood, Mo.) (85).

Nocardia spp. have also rarely been implicated to cause mild clinical infections in humans, including pharyngitis, bronchitis, and otitis media (106).

Cutaneous nocardiosis may be subdivided into four clinical types: mycetoma, lymphocutaneous infection, superficial skin infection (abscess or cellulitis), and secondary cutaneous involvement with disseminated disease. In North and South America, Mexico, and Australia, *N. brasiliensis* is the chief cause of actinomycetoma. In India, *A. madurae* is the major pathogen, whereas *A. pelletieri* and

S. somaliensis predominate in the African continent (106). These infections most commonly affect patients in rural areas in developing countries. Patients with these chronic infections may give a history of specific minor localized traumatic injury. The foot is the most common site of involvement; however, the hand, face, and neck may also be affected (127).

Pulmonary nocardiosis may be associated with nonspecific clinical findings; however, immunocompetent patients may have a chronic course, as opposed to the progressive,

TABLE 7 Differential characteristics of the major agents of actinomycetoma[a,b]

Characteristic	Actinomadura			Nocardia brasiliensis	Streptomyces somaliensis
	A. latina	A. madurae	A. pelletieri		
Presence in whole cell of:					
meso-DAP	+	+	+	+	−
L-DAP	−	−	−	−	+
Arabinose	−	−	−	+	−
Galactose	+	+	+	+	−
Madurose	+	+	+	−	−
Mycolic acids	−	−	−	+	−
Decomposition of:					
Esculin	+	+	−	+	−
Hypoxanthine	V	+	+	+	+
Carbon utilization of:					
Adonitol	−	+	−	−	ND
L-Arabinose	+	+	−	+	−
D-Mannitol	+	+	−	−	−
L-Rhamnose	−	+	−	−	−
D-Xylose	−	+	−	−	−
Granules					
Color	ND	White to yellow, or red	Red	White to yellow	Yellow to brown
Size	ND	1–5 mm	0.3–0.5 mm	<1 mm	1–2 mm

[a] Data derived from references 77 and 200.
[b] Abbreviations and symbols: DAP, diaminopimelic acid; +, positive; −, negative; V, variable; ND, not determined.

disseminated, and life-threatening infection seen in severely immunocompromised patients. The most frequent clinical presentation may be as a subacute or chronic, often necrotizing pneumonia, which is frequently associated with cavitation (59, 127). Local complications of invasive Nocardia pulmonary infections include pleural effusion, empyema, pericarditis, mediastinitis, superior vena cava obstruction, and, rarely, development of local chest wall and neck abscesses. Metastatic infective foci may be present but unrecognized at the time of the patient's initial presentation with pulmonary nocardiosis, and infection in these sites may not become clinically evident until after the patient has begun receiving antimicrobial therapy.

Disseminated nocardiosis is often a late-presenting, difficult-to-diagnose, and potentially life-threatening infection. From an initial pulmonary or cutaneous infection, nocardial infection can disseminate to other organ systems, most commonly the central nevous system, skin, and subcutaneous tissue (127, 222).

N. farcinica may cause a variety of clinical presentations, including cerebral abscess, keratitis, bacteremia, and pulmonary, kidney, and cutaneous infections (49, 133, 177). It is clearly important to differentiate between N. farcinica and other members of N. asteroides complex. N. farcinica has a high degree of resistance to various antibiotics, especially to broad-spectrum cephalosporins, which may make treatment of the infection difficult (176, 217), and mouse pathogenicity studies have demonstrated that this may be a more virulent species than the other N. asteroides complex species (43). N. farcinica occurs more frequently than was previously recognized (175, 197, 198). This can be attributed to recent developments in diagnostic methods and possibly also to a change in the spectrum of human nocardiosis in countries such as Germany, where N. farcinica is the prevailing species (176). Other reports from France, Germany, and the United States have implicated N. farcinica as the cause of postoperative wound infections in patients undergoing cardiac and other vascular surgeries (23, 53, 218).

The clinical diseases associated with N. nova isolates are similar to those previously described for diseases due to N. farcinica and N. asteroides complex microorganisms. The reasons for identifying these microorganisms include their susceptibility to erythromycin and broad-spectrum cephalosporins and resistance to amoxicillin-clavulanate (178). Also, as suggested for N. farcinica infections, infection with N. nova may be more common than is currently suspected; however, the successful detection of these newly recognized species is dependent on the performance of appropriate isolation and characterization techniques as well as increased clinical and microbiological awareness (213).

Infections with N. transvalensis have been reviewed by McNeil et al. (129). Initially recognized as a cause of mycetoma, N. transvalensis infections have also been reported to cause life-threatening invasive pulmonary and disseminated infections in severely immunocompromised patients (7, 127, 129, 131). Importantly, clinical isolates of this unusual species may demonstrate a high level of inherent resistance to amikacin and aminoglycosides in general. In addition, therapy with trimethoprim-sulfamethoxazole (TMP-SMX) may not always be effective for this infection (127, 224). In the recent study by Wilson et al. (224), N. transvalensis complex isolates showed a difference in geographic distribution of the designated subgroups. No isolates of the former N. asteroides complex type IV (now considered a member of the N. transvalensis complex) were

identified among the clinical isolates identified in Queensland, Australia. However, the majority (75%) of N. transvalensis isolates of the new taxon I were from that location (224).

The four most recently identified Nocardia species, N. abscessus, N. africana, N. paucivorans, and N. veterana, have only rarely been encountered as agents of disease (72, 74, 233, 236). N. abscessus has been isolated from patients with abscesses of knee joint, fibula, and leg (236); N. africana has been isolated from patients with pulmonary infections (74); N. paucivorans has been isolated from the sputa and bronchial secretions of a patient with chronic lung disease (233); and N. veterana has been isolated from bronchial lavage of a patient with upper lobe lesions (the strain was thought not to be of medical importance) (72).

Rhodococcus

Rhodococci have rarely been associated with human infection. Rhodococcus equi is a rare opportunistic pathogen found in severely immunocompromised patients and, most commonly in recent years, in human immunodeficiency virus (HIV)-infected persons (109, 155). Most often, patients have a slowly progressive granulomatous pneumonia with lobar infiltrates, frequently progressing to cavitating lesions visible on a chest radiograph. Other manifestations of infection include abscesses of the central nervous system, pelvis, and subcutaneous tissue and lymphadenitis (181). Cases of lung infection caused by inhalation and cutaneous lesions caused by wound contamination have been documented; the latter are almost the only R. equi infections reported in healthy persons, frequently children (207). Despite increased awareness of this organism as an opportunistic pathogen in humans, delays in accurate diagnosis of R. equi are still common (127, 181). Factors responsible may include the insidious onset of disease; the clinical resemblance of the infection to other related actinomycotic, fungal, and mycobacterial infections; and the relatively unremarkable bacteriologic profile of R. equi (45). Morphology, partial acid fastness, and a distinctive histopathologic profile in bronchial specimens contribute to an accurate clinical diagnosis. Histopathologic examination may reveal polymorphonuclear leukocytes with intracellular pleomorphic gram-positive bacteria, microabscesses, pseudotumors, and malakoplakia (181, 207). Malakoplakia is a relatively rare granulomatous inflammation not typically associated with histology of lung infection and can be a marker for this infection (181, 195). However, a conclusive diagnosis and differentiation from similar pathogens require the isolation and identification of R. equi from clinical specimens including sputum, bronchial lavage fluid, and open-lung biopsy specimens. Blood cultures from severely immunocompromised patients with R. equi infection often contain the organism. Patient's blood cultures may be positive in 65% of cases that occur secondary to HIV infection (195). AIDS patients with documented R. equi pneumonia can have a >50% mortality and a course punctuated by multiple relapses, which are common even when successful treatment is ultimately achieved (46, 109).

There have been reports of human infections caused by other rhodococci (not R. equi) (14, 15, 64, 127). Although such reports are very rare, these infections may be more common and go undetected because of the difficulties in identifying rhodococci by traditional methods and a lack of recognition of their potential pathogenicity. Reports of Rhodococcus species isolated from immunosuppressed patients have included *R. erythropolis* isolated from an HIV-positive patient and a peritoneal dialysis patient, and *R. rhodochrous* from a chronic corneal ulcer (15). Also, *Rhodococcus* organisms unspecified to species level have been isolated from patients with meningitis, pulmonary disease, and skin infections (14, 42).

Gordonia

Included at one time in the genus *Rhodococcus, Gordonia* species are difficult to identify by traditional methods and impossible to separate from each other and the related rhodococci; therefore, reports of infection with this species may not identify the species. Sternal wound infections, catheter-associated sepsis, and brain, cutaneous, and pulmonary infections have all been described as infections in which a *Gordonia* sp. was the suspected etiologic agent (29, 31, 47, 95, 107, 122, 168, 170).

Tsukamurella

The first description of the organism now classified as *Tsukamurella paurometabola* was in 1971 by Tsukamura and Mizuno (203). The organism was isolated from the sputum of patients with tuberculosis in Japan. This microorganism appears to be pathogenic only in specific circumstances, such as immunosuppression, presence of an indwelling foreign body, or a patient with chronic infection such as tuberculosis. Rare human infections with *Tsukamurella* have been described, including chronic lung infections (203), subcutaneous abscesses and necrotizing tenosynovitis (202), cutaneous lesions (68), meningitis in a patient with hairy cell leukemia (157), peritonitis (32), catheter-related bacteremia in patients with cancer (97, 183), acute myelogenous leukemia (38), and a patient with renal failure undergoing hemodialysis (R. S. Jones, T. Fekete, A. L. Truant, and V. Satishchandran, Letter, *Clin. Infect. Dis.* 18:830–832, 1994). In addition, this organism has been isolated from an HIV-infected patient, although it was thought to represent colonization and not a true infection (167). Although it is clear that all these isolates are species of *Tsukamurella*, most probably they are not *T. paurometabola* as this species is currently defined (40). *T. inchonensis* was isolated from multiple blood cultures obtained from a patient who had ingested hydrochloric acid and from necrotic lung tissue of another patient (231); *T. pulmonis* was isolated from the sputum of a patient with mycobacterial lung infection (232); and *T. tyrosinosolvens* strains were isolated from blood cultures from two patients with cardiac pacemakers implanted and from a patient with chronic lung infection (234). The most recently described species, *T. strandjordae*, was isolated from cultures of blood from a child with leukemia (85).

Actinomadura

Actinomadura madurae is a frequent cause of actinomycotic mycetomas. In mycetomas, the etiologic agents occur in the form of granules. The majority of the reports of infection caused by this species are from tropical and subtropical countries. However, the higher prevalence of such infections in warm climates may also only be a reflection of patients' increased tendency for exposure by walking barefoot (25). A review of the species of aerobic actinomycetes identified by the Actinomycete Laboratory of the Centers for Disease Control and Prevention from October 1985 through February 1988 from clinical specimens found that *A. madurae* accounted for 42 (11.5%) of the total of 366 referred isolates, and that this species was second in fre-

quency only to *N. asteroides*, which accounted for 98 (26.8%) of these isolates (130). The majority of isolates in this study were from sputum (24 isolates; 57.1%) and wounds (13 isolates; 31%). However, 1 (2.4%) of the 42 isolates was a blood isolate, which suggests a potential role for *A. madurae* as a colonizing and/or infecting microorganism in some patients. The new clinically important species, *A. latina*, has been isolated only from mycetoma (200). There are a few recent reports of nonmycetomic infections with *Actinomadura*. *A. madurae* peritonitis developed in a patient undergoing long-term ambulatory peritoneal dialysis who had no history of travel to tropical regions (229). Interestingly, this patient's infection responded to intraperitoneal therapy with amikacin. In addition in 1992, the first AIDS patient with pneumonia caused by *A. madurae* was reported (132).

Streptomyces

Because most of the members of the genus *Streptomyces* are saprophytes, it has been traditional to minimize their significance in clinical microbiology. One species, *S. somaliensis*, has been identified as one of the etiologic agents of actinomycotic mycetoma occurring in many countries, including Algeria, India, Malaysia, Mexico, Niger, Nigeria, Saudi Arabia, Somalia, South Africa, Sudan, the United States, and Venezuela (8, 25, 51). In these countries, this species has been associated in particular with mycetomas affecting the head and neck. The only case of nonmycetomic *S. somaliensis* infection was reported in 1970 in a patient with a perforated peritoneum (70). Several recent reviews suggest that it is no longer acceptable to consider this species the only human pathogen of this genus. Non-*somaliensis Streptomyces* spp. have been identified from clinical human and animal specimens (17, 127, 137, 140) including two cases where large numbers of organisms were observed in histopathologic sections from a patient with chronic pericarditis and a patient with a traumatic wound infection (182, 239). All of these species are considered to be of potential medical importance. In two of these studies, most of the *Streptomyces* isolates (sputum, wound, blood, and brain) were identified as *Streptomyces anulatus* (previously "*Streptomyces griseus*") (130, 137). In these reports, the assignment to species was based only on phenotypic characteristics and chemotaxonomic cell wall studies and not on the newer molecular methods. There is a discrepancy between the large number of *S. anulatus* strains identified in clinical reference laboratories and the relatively small number of publications claiming a disease association.

Other Actinomycetes

Tropheryma whipplei (formerly "*Tropheryma whippelii*," a nonvalidated taxon) is the putative causal agent of Whipple's disease (99). First described in 1907 by George Whipple as "intestinal lipodystrophy" (219), this disease is a rare multisystemic bacterial infection with variable clinical manifestations. "Classical" patients usually present with malabsorption and significant weight loss; however, extraintestinal involvement including the central nervous, cardiovascular, lymphatic, and pulmonary systems and arthralgias are not uncommon and may persist for years even in the absence of gastrointestinal manifestations (44, 54, 115, 165, 169). The various clinical manifestations of Whipple's disease have often been assumed to represent immunologic differences among patients, although such host factors still remain to be shown (120, 121). On the other hand, the range of different symptoms may represent heterogeneity among strains of *T. whipplei*; further molecular epidemiologic investigations are clearly needed to establish such correlations (79, 117). Whipple's disease is fatal if untreated, and antibiotics may be administered for at least 1 year to prevent relapses (136, 164).

Dermatophilosis may infect both wild and domestic animals and is usually manifest as severe skin lesions (3). In addition to cattle, the disease has been reported mainly in horses, goats, and sheep. Recently, *Dermatophilus congolensis* or *Dermatophilus*-like infections have been reported in camels, crocodiles, and beluga whales (30, 60, 135). Less commonly, the disease has been described in humans. Acquisition of *D. congolensis* by humans is usually the result of contact with tissues of infected animals or contaminated animal products (60, 199). Occupational groups that have the greatest risk for acquiring the infection include abattoir workers, butchers, dairy farmers, hunters, and veterinarians (237, 238). Infection of an HIV-infected animal handler with "hairy" leukoplakia has been reported (31). Microorganisms indistinguishable from *D. congolensis* have been seen and isolated from patients with pitted keratolysis, which characteristically attacks the soles of the feet (227). Such involvement of human keratinized tissue is not surprising since the microorganism is known to liberate significant amounts of keratinase when cultured on appropriate substrate media (75).

The first clinical isolation of *Nocardiopsis dassonvillei* was in 1911, by Liegard and Landrieu from a patient with conjunctivitis (108). Although there have been infrequent reports of clinical disease caused by *Nocardiopsis* species, *N. dassonvillei* has been associated with various human infections, including bacteremia (12), mycetomas (184), skin infections (152; S. M. Singh, J. Naidu, S. Mukerjee, and A. Malkani, *Program Abstr. XI Confr. Int. Soc. Hum. Anim. Mycol.*, abstr. PS1.91, p. 85, 1991), and extrinsic alveolitis (18). In 1997, Yassin et al. described a new species, *N. synnemataformans*, which was isolated from the sputum of a kidney transplant patient (235).

Of the 21 isolates of *Amycolatopsis orientalis* studied by Gordon et al. in 1978, most were isolated from soil and vegetable matter; however, the site of isolation for two isolates was reported to be cerebrospinal fluid (CSF) and an unknown clinical source (67). Nothing more is known about the pathogenicity of this microorganism.

Organisms of the genus *Micromonospora* have rarely been encountered in human clinical specimens. In a recent review of the clinical isolates received in the Actinomycete Laboratory at the Centers for Disease Control and Prevention (CDC) during a 29-month study period, only 6 of 366 were identified as members of this genus (130). In addition, to our knowledge, no case descriptions of human infections have been published.

Relatively few species of thermophilic actinomycetes have been recognized to cause human disease. Repeated inhalation of dusts containing these microorganisms or their spores may result in hypersensitivity pneumonitis/extrinsic allergic alveolitis, a serious, disabling, immunologically mediated pulmonary disease that may affect agricultural, office, and industrial workers. Various names have been given to different forms of hypersensitivity pneumonitis. These names indicate either the high-risk occupational group affected, the substrate that gives rise to the particular antigen, or a specific type of environmental exposure. In 1963, the predominant allergin from dust of moldy hay was identified to be *Saccharopolyspora rectivirgula* (151); however, another species, *Thermoactinomyces vul-*

garis, may also be present and induce the best characterized form of the disease, farmer's lung. Other forms of the disease and their associated allergens include mushroom worker's lung, induced by exposure to moldy compost (*S. rectivirgula* and *T. vulgaris*); bagassosis, induced by exposure to moldy sugar cane (*T. sacchari* and *T. vulgaris*); air conditioner-associated lung disease, resulting from contaminated ventilation ducts (*S. viridis* and *T. vulgaris*); and humidification system-induced disease, caused by contamination of the system's reservoir (*T. vulgaris*). Importantly, in addition to dusts containing the actinomycetes, hypersensitivity pneumonitis may result from inhalation of dusts containing various fungi, avian serum proteins, and other substances. All of these particulate allergens are characterized by a small particle size (1 to 5 μm) that facilitates their penetration to the lung alveoli, where they can impinge and persist for long periods (99). Despite the variety of settings and multiple possible etiologies, similar presenting symptoms and signs in these patients and the typical findings on histopathologic examination of pulmonary tissues are consistent with a singular pathologic process or disease entity, which has been termed hypersensitivity pneumonitis.

COLLECTION, TRANSPORT, AND STORAGE OF SPECIMENS

General guidelines for the handling of clinical specimens and cultures suspected of containing actinomycetes (biosafety level 2 microorganisms) are discussed in chapter 6.

The general principles of collection, transport, and storage are applicable to most aerobic actinomycetes. However, if samples are suspected of containing nocardiae, they should not be refrigerated or placed on ice before being transported. Some strains of *Nocardia* lose their viability after exposure to near-freezing temperatures. Since the respiratory tract is the most common portal of entry for the nocardiae, most specimens from patients with suspected nocardiosis are sputum, bronchoalveolar lavage fluid, transtracheal aspirates, or lung biopsy tissue. Of importance, in some cases of pulmonary nocardiosis, oft-repeated sputum cultures may not yield nocardial isolates; invasive procedures may be needed to make the diagnosis (127). The diagnostic yield of cultures of specimens obtained by invasive procedures such as transtracheal aspiration, bronchoscopic biopsy, and fine-needle aspiration has been reported to range between 85 and 90% (127). Therefore, particularly in the management of high-risk patients, clinicians must maintain a high degree of clinical suspicion for the diagnosis and, as indicated, perform invasive procedures on these patients. If necessary, clinicians should alert clinical microbiology and pathology laboratory personnel to use special methods to look for and identify microorganisms suspected to be *Nocardia* spp. (127). Tissue specimens may be from extrapulmonary sites that also may be infected (e.g., subcutaneous and/or brain biopsy specimens) as well as body fluids (e.g., blood and CSF). Normally sterile fluids and tissues should be transported to the laboratory promptly, especially if their collection required an invasive procedure. Invasive procedures are usual for brain infections, since the CSF is usually negative for nocardiae even though the patient may have extensive brain lesions. CSF should be cultured for nocardiae only in circumstances where meningitis due to these organisms is suspected clinically, and these cultures should be held for 2 to 3 weeks (73).

Depending on the clinical presentation, the specimens that may yield rhodococci, gordoniae, or tsukamurellae include blood, lower respiratory tract secretions, and intravascular catheter tips. Collection and transport techniques should follow submission protocols commonly used for routine microbiologic isolation studies (see chapter 20).

If actinomycotic mycetoma is suspected, aspirates, if possible, rather than swabs of sinus tracts should be collected for the isolation of *Actinomadura* species, *N. brasiliensis*, and *Streptomyces* species. If granules are present in this drainage material, they should be washed repeatedly in sterile saline to remove contaminating bacteria or fungi before shipping to a reference laboratory for study. If drainage is absent or minimal, biopsy of deeper tissue is necessary, or, alternatively, specimens may include scrapings or aspirates from draining lesions (73).

DIRECT EXAMINATION

In patients with suspected nocardial infection and a compatible clinical picture, a definitive diagnosis usually depends on the demonstration of the organisms in smears or sections examined microscopically, together with isolation and identification by microbiologic culture. The importance of direct microscopic examination of stained preparations of clinical specimens in the diagnosis of aerobic actinomycotic infections cannot be overemphasized. The specimens most frequently received in the clinical microbiology laboratory for evaluation include sputum, bronchial lavage fluid, exudate, or CSF. If possible, the material should be spread out in a petri dish and observed for clumps of the microorganisms, which may resemble granules. If clumps or granules are present, they should be selectively removed and crushed between two glass microscope slides for microscopic examination. In addition, duplicate direct smears of the clinical material should always be prepared for staining; one smear should be stained with Gram's stain, and the other should be stained with the modified Kinyoun acid-fast stain. The method for the modified Kinyoun acid-fast stain is given in chapter 27 (112). On Gram-stained smears, gram-positive branched filamentous hyphae (Fig. 1) are seen that are similar to the appearance of nocardiae in cultures (Fig. 2): they measure 0.5 to 1 μm in diameter and as much as 20 μm in length. To be of diagnostic value, the hyphae must branch at right angles. Although the hyphae of nocardiae may resemble those of *Actinomyces* species in width, they are usually much longer and more widely scattered throughout purulent material and in the walls of the abscesses. In mycetoma, compact granules are formed, similar to those observed for the anaerobic actinomycetes. Very rarely, clubbing has been seen with *N. asteroides* (124), but often granules with clubbing are seen with *N. brasiliensis* and *N. otitidiscaviarum* (185). The hematoxylin and eosin stain is very useful for staining the tissue and the granules but does not stain the individual filaments (33) (Fig. 3). A tissue Gram stain such as the modified Brown and Brenn procedure (see chapter 27) is recommended for demonstration of the gram-positive filaments of nocardiae (34). The Gomori methenamine silver stain may also be useful. However, in both of these procedures, the filaments may not stain uniformly. Acid-fast stains are also of value in the histopathologic diagnosis of infections caused by *N. asteroides*, *N. brasiliensis*, and *N. otitidiscaviarum*. These species are frequently, but not always, acid-fast in tissue sections stained by both the modified Kinyoun or the Fite-Faraco (see chapter 27) staining methods (112). *Actinomyces* and

related species are usually not acid fast. These examinations provide a rapid presumptive diagnosis of the patient's infection, and the information they yield may critically influence the clinician's choice of initial antimicrobial therapy.

In stained smears of clinical specimens, in particular purulent material and tissue (obtained by biopsy, surgery, and autopsy), the coccoid or coccobacillary form of *R. equi* is usually seen intracellularly in macrophages and extracellularly (Fig. 4). However, bacillary *R. equi* forms have been found in clinical specimens such as blood, bronchial lavage fluid, and sputum (45). In contrast, in all reported cases of non-*R. equi* rhodococcal infection, the direct smears prepared from clinical material have shown gram-positive coccobacilli, and in smears prepared from sputum they were more filamentous than reported for *R. equi* (127, 149).

Previously, the diagnosis of Whipple's disease was characteristically made only by histopathologic demonstration of "foamy" macrophages infiltrating the lamina propria of the small intestine, which contain periodic acid-Schiff (PAS)-positive bacilli ("Whipple's bacilli") that may also be found extracellularly (44). The small size (0.25 by 1 to 2 μm) of the bacterium in infected tissue makes it difficult to see unless visualized by electron microscopy. This bacterium contains a distinct trilamellar cell wall that is more typically seen in gram-negative bacteria (54). In 2001, Fredricks and Relman visualized *T. whipplei* 16S rRNA in tissue by fluorescent in situ hybridization (56). Thus, they provided the evidence that the Whipple's bacterium was growing extracellularly and suggested that the bacterium was not an obligate intracellular pathogen as previously thought.

Although *D. congolensis* may be seen at any stage of development in direct examination of clinical materials, the appearance of branched filaments divided in their transverse and longitudinal planes is seen most frequently and is pathognomonic (238). These microorganisms may be seen in wet mounts or in smears of clinical material stained with methylene blue or by the Giemsa method (Fig. 5). A Gram-stained preparation is not likely to be helpful for visualizing these microorganisms because it is too dark and obscures crucial morphologic detail.

ISOLATION

Since the aerobic actinomycetes are slowly growing microorganisms, their isolation from cultures of samples obtained from normally sterile sites, such as blood or CSF, typically requires a prolonged incubation time (i.e., approximately 2 weeks). Isolation from tissue samples may take even longer (i.e., up to 3 weeks). These microorganisms grow satisfactorily on most of the nonselective media used for the isolation of bacteria, mycobacteria, and fungi. Blood specimens for culture may be inoculated into either conventional two-bottle broth blood culture systems, biphasic blood culture bottles, or automated radiometric or nonradiometric blood culture systems; each of these systems supports the growth of *Nocardia* microorganisms (205). However, satisfactory isolation of these microorganisms by these methods must still take into account factors such as maintaining the incubating cultures for up to 2 weeks and performing frequent and terminal subcultures (205). Blood specimens processed by lysis-centrifugation, exudates, joint and CSF specimens, and homogenized tissue specimens are inoculated directly into media such as thioglycolate broth, Trypticase soy broth, or chopped-meat glucose broth. The

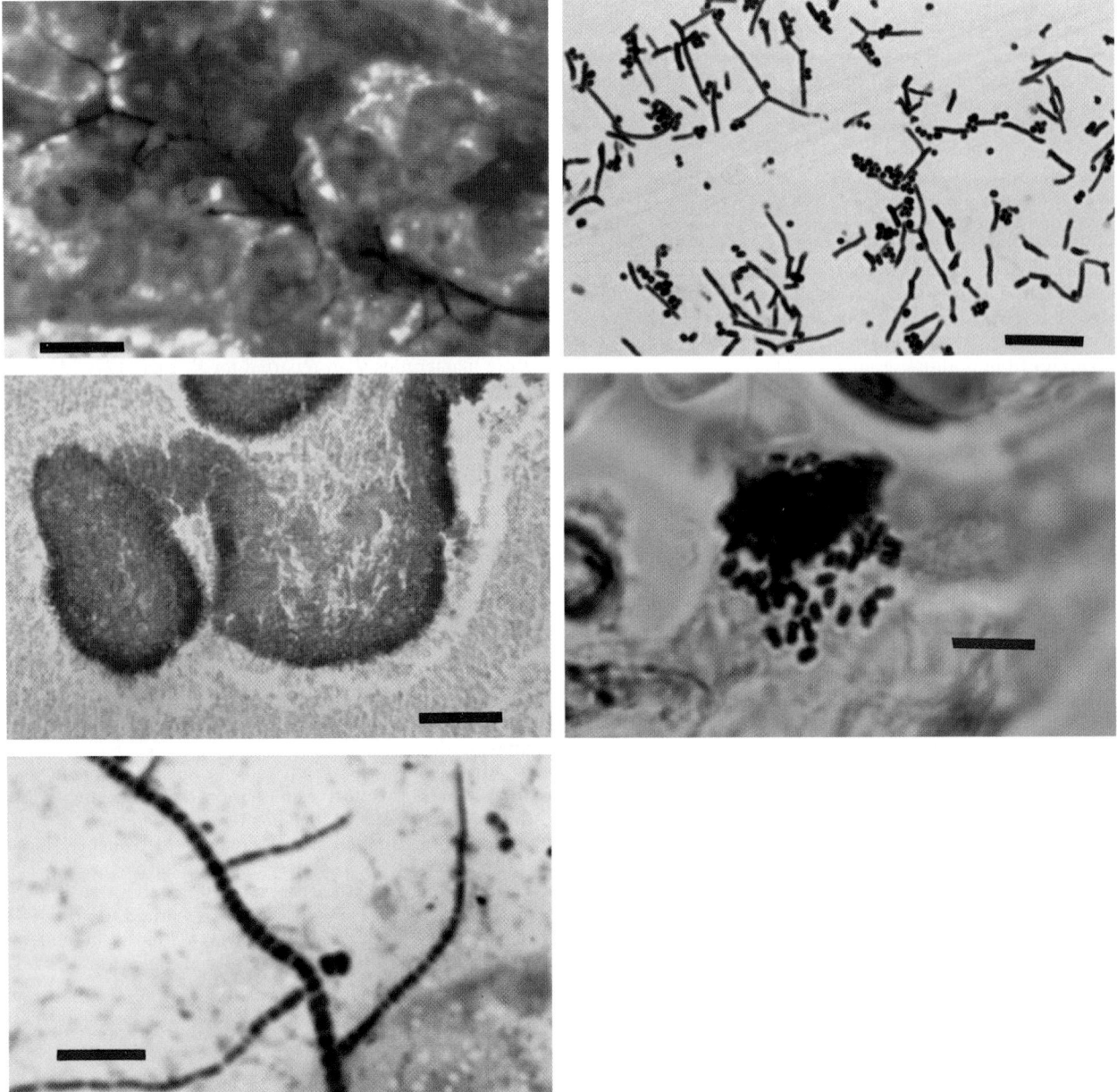

FIGURE 1 (top left) *Nocardia asteroides:* branched, beaded hyphae in a direct smear of sputum (Gram stain). Bar, 10 μm.

FIGURE 2 (top right) *Nocardia farcinica:* branched hyphae, coccobacilli, and bacillary forms. A direct preparation from culture is shown (Gram stain). Bar, 10 μm.

FIGURE 3 (middle left) *Nocardia brasiliensis:* granule in a section from a human mycetoma. No microorganisms are visible (hematoxylin and eosin stain). Bar, 40 μm.

FIGURE 4 (middle right) *Rhodococcus equi:* coccobacillary forms in a section of human lung tissue (Brown and Brenn Gram stain). Bar, 10 μm.

FIGURE 5 (bottom left) *Dermatophilus congolensis:* branched filaments divided in transverse and longitudinal planes with tapered fine hyphae. A direct preparation from infected subcutaneous tissue is shown (Giemsa stain). Bar, 10 μm.

thioglycolate broth media, in addition to supporting the growth of aerobic actinomycetes, support the growth of anaerobic actinomycetes if these are present (174). Although the optimal blood culture method has not been defined, the use of the Isolator lysis centrifugation system (Wampole Laboratories, Cranburg, N.J.) is recommended as a reliable method (52). All specimens from sterile sites may be inoculated directly onto solid media; however, the plates must be sealed in a manner to prevent dehydration.

The isolation of aerobic actinomyces from the complex mixed flora of the soil and clinical specimens that are from normally nonsterile sites (e.g., samples from the respiratory tract and mycetomas) requires selective enrichment in a broth supplemented with 5% sodium chloride alone or in combination with 0.5 mg of cycloheximide per ml of medium, or a pretreatment with low-pH KCl-HCl before these specimens are plated on selective isolation media (127, 208). Because slow growth over 2 days to 2 weeks on routine culture media allows bacterial overgrowth to obscure the *Nocardia* colonies, isolation of *Nocardia* from soil and nonsterile sites may be difficult. Additionally, *Nocardia* often does not survive specimen digestive procedures used in mycobacterial culture techniques. The observation that some nocardial isolates may not survive in respiratory specimens has prompted studies of procedures to facilitate the recovery of aerobic actinomycetes from these sources (127). In 1987, Murray et al. demonstrated that digestion-decontamination of respiratory tract specimens with N-acetyl-L-cysteine, sodium hydroxide, and benzalkonium was toxic to *Nocardia* (142). These investigators also studied Thayer-Martin medium containing colistin, nystatin, and vancomycin, a selective medium commonly used in clinical laboratories for the isolation of *Neisseria* species from contaminated specimens. Although this medium was not evaluated with clinical specimens, the successful results of this study with seeded sputum specimens encouraged further studies (142). Another promising medium is buffered charcoal-yeast extract (BCYE) agar and selective BCYE that contains anisomycin, polymyxin, and vancomycin; these media are commonly used in clinical microbiology laboratories for the isolation of *Legionella* species from respiratory specimens (57, 208). However, one of these investigators found that pretreatment of the specimens with a low-pH (pH 2.2) KCl-HCl solution for 4 min was necessary (208). No optimal method for isolating the aerobic actinomycetes from potentially contaminated specimens exists; however, the methods discussed represent an improvement over the direct plating of these specimens on conventional media, such as Sabouraud dextrose agar (SDA), brain heart infusion agar, blood agar, or Lowenstein-Jensen medium.

After initial isolation, subcultures must be incubated at 25, 35, and 45°C to determine the optimal temperature for growth of the microorganisms. Most isolates of *N. asteroides* complex grow best at 35°C, while most isolates of *Streptomyces* grow best at 25°C. Any specimen suspected of containing a thermophilic actinomycete must also be incubated at 50°C since thermophiles grow at this elevated temperature. With the exception of *D. congolensis*, enhancement with a CO_2 atmosphere is not necessary for the growth of the aerobic actinomycetes (238).

Isolation of *R. equi* requires selective media if the organisms are from soil or feces of grazing herbivores. Recently, a new selective medium for *R. equi*, containing ceftazidime (20 mg/liter) and novobiocin (25 mg/liter) in a Mueller-Hinton agar base, was described (210). This selective medium proved to be less inhibitory for *R. equi* than did

selective media devised in earlier studies and grew very few other nocardioforms.

Although numerous attempts to reproducibly cultivate the Whipple's bacillus on artificial media in the laboratory have failed, propagation in human interleukin-treated macrophage cultures (179) and propagation in human fibroblasts have been achieved in reference laboratories (54, 163). Although *T. whipplei* was propagated from cardiac valves in human macrophages, this culture no longer exists (179). Raoult et al. were able to propagate and subculture the bacillus in a human fibroblast cell line and have estimated its doubling time as about 17 days (163).

Isolation of *D. congolensis* may be difficult. Clinical materials, preferably the underside of scabs, should be streaked onto a blood plate and incubated aerobically and in 5 to 10% CO_2 at 35 to 37°C. Highly contaminated specimens may require animal passage for successful isolation; crusts and scabs are ground and applied to the shaved and scarified skin of a rabbit (238). Cutaneous lesions develop in the animal within 2 to 7 days. The microorganism may then be isolated in pure culture from these infected sites.

IDENTIFICATION

Until recently, very little attention has been paid to the correct taxonomic assignment of clinically significant actinomycetes. The actinomycetes can be identified to the genus level on the basis of a variety of conventional phenotypic characteristics including microscopic (Gram and acid-fast staining) and colonial morphology, growth requirements, metabolism of glucose, arylsulfatase production, growth in lysozyme, and phenotypic molecular characteristics including whole-cell isomers of DAP and mycolic acid composition (Table 1). Some of these tests are beyond the capabilities of most clinical laboratories. However, both microscopic and colonial morphology, combined with a few physiologic tests, can give a presumptive identification to genus or species level. A schematic flowchart for the tentative identification of medically important aerobic actinomycetes and related genera is given in Fig. 6. Unfortunately the determination of isomers of DAP is the only method to separate *Streptomyces* species from related genera. In addition to *Streptomyces* species, the definitive identification of the genera *Actinomadura* and *Nocardiopsis* requires referral of an isolate to a reference laboratory. As newer molecular techniques are applied to these organisms, many genera and species are being redefined. These genotypic methods include PCR-based methods, DNA hybridization, and sequencing of 16S rRNA.

On primary isolation, typical colonial growth may be slow to appear. Cultures should be held for 2 weeks before being discarded as negative (127).

Microscopic Morphology

The well-known acid fastness of *Nocardia* spp. is often more pronounced in clinical than in cultured material. With the modified Kinyoun technique, *Nocardia* spp. may be partially acid fast (showing both acid-fast and non-acid-fast bacilli and filaments). The presence of acid-fast branched filaments may be indicative of *Nocardia* spp.; however, in clinical material the result of acid-fast staining may be variable. Most isolates of *Nocardia* spp. in culture are weakly acid fast by the modified Kinyoun procedure when 1% sulfuric acid is used as a decolorizing agent (Fig. 7) (17). However, interpretation of the acid-fast stain is frequently

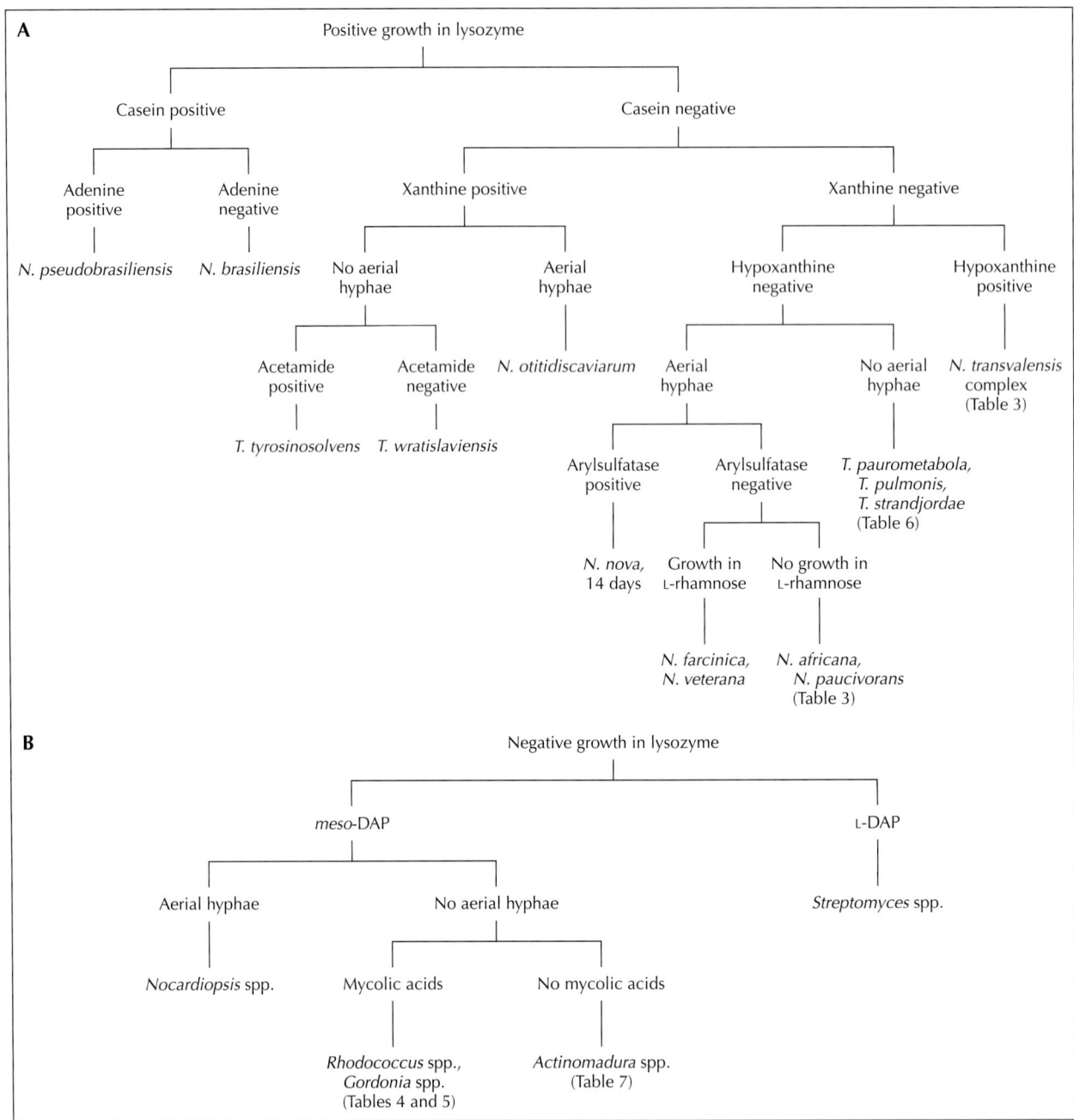

FIGURE 6 Schematic flowcharts for the tentative identification of major medically important aerobic actinomycetes with positive (A) and negative (B) growth in lysozyme.

difficult. Variations in results may be dependent on the type of growth medium (high-lipid-containing media such as Lowenstein-Jensen or Middlebrook 7H10 are best for demonstrating acid fastness). Of importance, isolates of *Streptomyces* spp. must be distinguished and may have acid-fast coccoid forms and non-acid-fast hyphae but are considered non-acid fast.

The acid-fast stain, long considered of primary importance in the identification of *Nocardia* spp., is a difficult test to standardize, and this may affect its interpretation. For example, if the entire acid-fast-stained smear appears bluish pink, the stain must be repeated: there must be a contrast

between the carbol fuchsin and the counterstain. Also, the demonstration of acid fastness by microorganisms grown in culture should be used only in conjunction with other tests as a supportive but not absolute diagnostic test (17).

In cultures, the microscopic morphology of nocardial cells is similar to that demonstrated in clinical material. They are gram positive, with short to extensively branched vegetative hyphae less than 1 μm in diameter that may fragment into bacillary or coccoid nonmotile forms. Short chains of conidia (two to three) may be found on the aerial hyphae but are rarely seen on the substrate hyphae. The most satisfactory method for demonstrating the micromor-

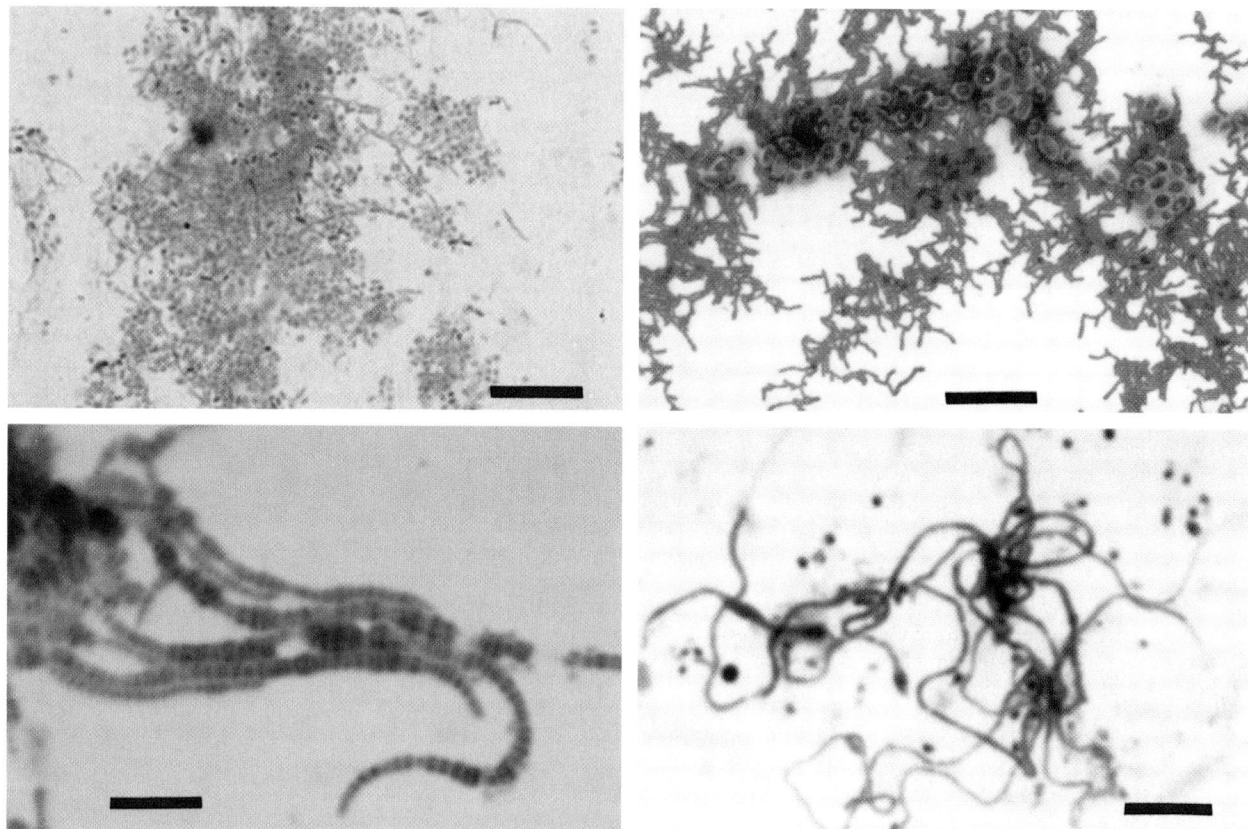

FIGURE 7 (top left) *Nocardia farcinica:* rare acid-fast organisms from a smear of a Lowenstein-Jensen agar slant grown for 3 days (modified Kinyoun stain). Bar, 10 μm.

FIGURE 8 (top right) *Rhodococcus rhodochrous:* the coccobacilli are arranged in a zigzag fashion. A slide culture preparation was grown on cornmeal agar without dextrose and was incubated for 1 week at 25°C (lactofuchsin stain). Bar, 10 μm.

FIGURE 9 (bottom left) *Dermatophilus congolensis:* branched filaments divided in transverse and longitudinal planes with tapered fine hyphae. A direct preparation from culture is shown (Giemsa stain). Bar, 10 μm.

FIGURE 10 (bottom right) *Micromonospora* species: fine branched hyphae with single spores. A direct preparation from culture is shown (Gram stain). Bar, 10 μm.

phology of the nocardial culture is by direct in situ observation of a slide culture containing undisturbed colonies of the microorganism grown on a minimal medium such as tap water agar or cornmeal without dextrose (73). Culture preparations on these minimal media are incubated at 25°C and examined periodically for 2 to 3 weeks. In examining slide cultures under the microscope, it is important to recognize true branched substrate hyphae, aerial hyphae, and sporulation. The substrate hyphae of *Nocardia* spp. appear as very fine, dichotomously branched filaments. Movement of the objective up and down through several planes will reveal aerial hyphae. The presence of aerial hyphae differentiates *Nocardia* spp. from other related genera such as *Corynebacterium, Gordonia, Mycobacterium, Rhodococcus,* and *Tsukamurella.* The rapidly growing mycobacteria, which phenotypically resemble the nocardiae, have simple, relatively short substrate hyphae that branch at acute angles, in contrast to the complex hyphae of the nocardiae, which branch at right angles and usually have secondary branches.

Rhodococci grow as coccobacilli arranged in a zigzag fashion (Fig. 8) on in situ slide cultures. The microscopic morphology of *R. equi* in culture is cyclic, varying from bacillary to coccoid depending on incubation time and growth conditions. At 6 h on heart infusion agar (HIA) incubated at 35°C, these microorganisms are completely bacillary, but at 24 h they become completely coccoid. Gram-positive rudimentary branched filaments have been reportedly observed from cultures in liquid medium, especially from young cultures. The microscopic morphology of the other *Rhodococcus* species is also cyclic, varying from a simple rod-coccus cycle in some species similar to *R. equi* to a more complex hypha-rod-coccus cycle in others (*R. coprophilus, R. fascians, R. marinonascens,* and *R. ruber*). *R. coprophilus, R. erythropolis, R. globerulus, R. rhodnii,* and *R. rhodochrous* are differentiated further into elementary branched hypha-rod-coccus cyclic forms (62, 64). The branched hyphae may be rudimentary, highly transitory, or extensive. All of the rhodococci from clinical specimens and from colonies in culture are generally weakly acid fast when stained by either the modified Kinyoun or Ziehl-Neelsen method (62).

Members of the genus *Gordonia* are aerobic, gram-positive, slightly acid-fast, nonmotile short rods (0.5 to 0.2 μm in diameter) that have a rod-coccus growth cycle. The cells do not form spores or capsules or produce aerial hyphae.

Tsukamurellae are aerobic and gram positive and stain as slightly acid-fast bacilli with modified Kinyoun (17). Most cells are long rods that fragment into three parts, which then separate and grow independently. The cells do not form spores or capsules or produce aerial hyphae.

The microscopic morphology of *D. congolensis* in culture is similar to that observed in clinical specimens. Depending on the age of the isolate and the type of medium used for culture, one may see completely coccal elements, many with flagella or irregularly arranged cells in packets; germinating spores; or branched segmented or nonsegmented filaments (Fig. 9). Motility is usually evident in isolates from fresh cultures. If cocci only are seen and *D. congolensis* is suspected, younger cultures should be examined for hyphae (238).

The *Nocardiopsis* spp. produce hyphae that are long and branched and fragment completely into zigzag chains of arthroconidia, which are characteristic of this species (134). The sporulation process was studied in detail by Williams et al. (221). They observed that the process is initiated by a single ingrowth of the hyphae wall, resulting in a cross-wall. The first elements delimited are often long and sometimes subdivided by further cross-wall formation. The process is completed by the disruption of the sheath between the spores. From these observations, it seems that the characteristic zigzag arrangement of developing spore chains is caused by lateral displacement of spores within the sheath (221).

The thermophilic actinomycetes are gram positive and non-acid fast. Individual thermophilic species are differentiated on the basis of their microscopic and macroscopic morphology—in particular, their number of spores and the type of spore production. *S. rectivirgula* has short chains of spores that are on substrate and aerial hyphae; *S. viridis* has single spores only on aerial hyphae; and the three *Thermoactinomyces* species all produce endospores. *T. vulgaris* has single endospores on sporophores on both aerial and substrate hyphae; *T. thalpophilus* has single endospores sessile on aerial and substrate hyphae; and *T. sacchari* has single endospores on sphorophores on both aerial and substrate hyphae.

Colonies of *Micromonospora* produce single spores on the substrate hyphae, which is one of the well-defined characteristics of this genus (Fig. 10).

Microscopically, colonies of *A. orientalis* may produce aerial hyphae that form cylindrical, occasionally ovoid conidia in straight to flexuous chains. The substrate hyphae branch frequently and appear to zigzag in places.

Colonial Appearance

Aerial hyphae may be seen macroscopically in cultures, but in the early stages of growth they are seen only with the microscope. A stereomicroscope microscope with ×10 to ×50 magnification is useful for this purpose. Macroscopic aerial hyphae may be lacking, sparse, or very abundant in *Nocardia* cultures; therefore, colonies may have a smooth appearance or, more commonly, a chalky white appearance reflecting the growth of aerial hyphae (Fig. 11). The gross morphology of the nocardiae is extremely variable and may

differ depending on the growth medium or the incubation temperature used. The color of most colonies of *N. asteroides* complex varies from salmon pink to orange on SDA and HIA agar slants upon maturity (1 to 2 weeks) at 25 to 35°C (it is often more pronounced at 25°C). The opacification of Middlebrook 7H10 agar with all isolates of *N. farcinica* studied is a useful adjunct for the identification of *N. farcinica* (55). *N. brasiliensis* colonies are usually orange-tan; in contrast, *N. otitidiscaviarum* colonies are usually pale tan. *N. transvalensis* colonies may vary in color from pale tan to violet.

The genus *Rhodococcus* consists of a diverse group of organisms that are quite variable in their colonial morphology. These bacteria may produce rough, smooth, or mucoid and pigmented buff, coral, orange, or deep rose colonies after several days of incubation. Growth occurs at 28 and 35°C but not at 45°C. *R. coprophilus* and *R. ruber* may demonstrate a few aerial hyphae, whereas none of the other *Rhodococcus* species form aerial hyphae. The colonial morphology of *R. equi* is diverse and consists of three major varieties. The classic colony type is pale pink and slimy in 2 to 4 days on HIA or on HIA containing 5% rabbit or sheep blood incubated aerobically at 35°C (Fig. 12). The second most frequent colony type is coral and nonslimy when grown on the same media under similar incubation conditions. The third and least common colony type is pale yellow, nonslimy, more opaque than the classical slimy type of colony, and identical to that of the *R. equi* type strain (ATCC 6939). Colorless colonial variants may also occur, particularly in *R. equi*.

Colonies of *G. sputi* are less pigmented than the other *Gordonia* species; they are smooth, mucoid, and adherent to the media. *G. amarae* may produce rudimentary microscopically visible hyphae, and *G. bronchialis* may produce aerial synnemata consisting of unbranched filaments that coalesce and project upward and that may be confused with aerial hyphae. *G. sputi* and *G. bronchialis* produce dry, raised, beige colonies on rabbit or sheep blood agar that become salmon colored after several days of culture (Fig. 13 and 14), whereas the colonies of *G. amarae* and *G. hydrophobica* remain beige. Growth occurs at 28 and 35°C but not at 45°C.

At 24 h on HIA containing 5% rabbit or sheep blood, colonies of the species *Tsukamurella* are usually 0.5 to 2.0 mm in diameter. These colonies are circular, usually have entire edges but may have rhizoid edges, are dry but easily emulsified, and are white to creamy to orange. Rough colonies are produced after prolonged incubation for up to 7 days. They are characteristically cerebriform and do not produce aerial hyphae (Fig. 15). These colonies superficially resemble the rapidly growing mycobacteria, especially when cream in color. However, the mycobacteria can be differentiated from the genus *Tsukamurella* by arylsulfatase production within 14 days.

Colonies of *Actinomadura* species may be white to pink to red, are usually mucoid, and have a molar tooth appearance. Rare aerial hyphae are produced. *Actinomadura* species grow more slowly than other actinomycetes.

Colonies of *Streptomyces* species produce a wide variety of pigments that are responsible for coloration of the substrate and aerial hyphae: soluble pigments also may be produced (Fig. 16). Many strains of *Streptomyces* do not produce aerial hyphae.

D. congolensis has tiny (0.5 to 1.0 mm), round colonies at 24 h on HIA containing horse, sheep, or rabbit blood at 35 to 37°C. The appearance of these colonies may vary, but

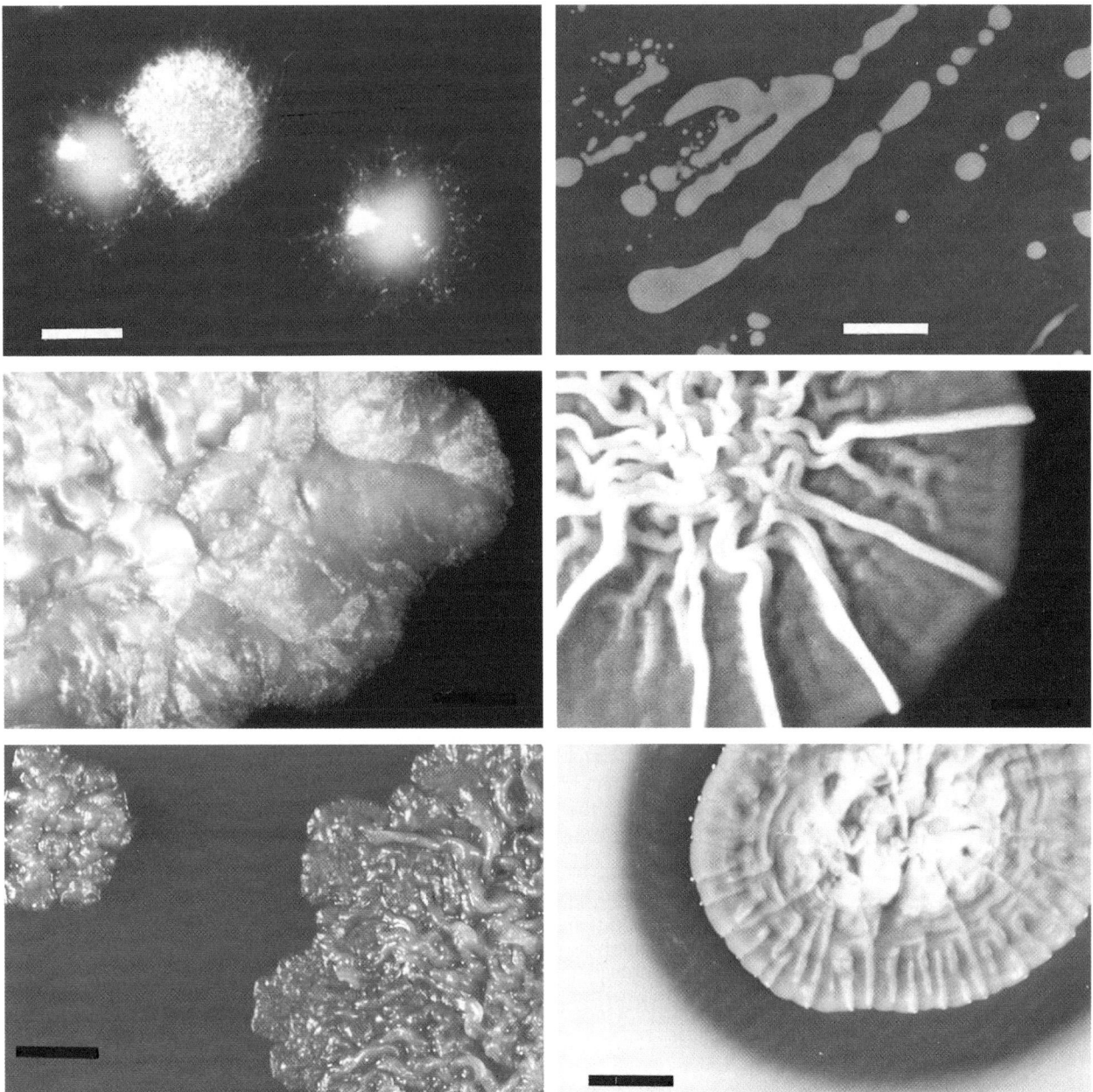

FIGURE 11 (top left)   *Nocardia farcinica:* colonies with and without aerial hyphae grown for 5 days on HIA. Bar, 100 μm.

FIGURE 12 (top right)   *Rhodococcus equi:* classical pink, slimy colonies grown for 5 days on an HIA plate with 5% rabbit blood. Bar, 100 μm.

FIGURE 13 (middle left)   *Gordonia terrae:* colony grown for 5 days on an HIA plate with 5% rabbit blood. Bar, 100 μm.

FIGURE 14 (middle right)   *Gordonia bronchialis:* colony grown for 5 days on an HIA plate with 5% rabbit blood. Bar, 100 μm.

FIGURE 15 (bottom left)   *Tsukamurella tyrosinosolvens:* colony grown for 5 days on an HIA plate with 5% rabbit blood. Bar, 100 μm.

FIGURE 16 (bottom right)   *Streptomyces* species: colony grown for 10 days on casein decomposition plate. Bar, 100 μm.

they are usually gray-white and adherent and pit the medium. Later, in 2 to 5 days, they develop an orange pigment. Frequently, there is beta-hemolysis, which is enhanced with increased concentrations of carbon dioxide. This beta-hemolysis is also more prominent in areas of the medium where colonies are crowded. There is no growth on SDA.

The colonies of *N. dassonvillei* on organic media are abundant, coarsely wrinkled, and folded with a well-developed substrate mycelium and range in color from yellow to orange to brown; the colonies of *N. lucentensis* range from yellow to brown; the colonies of *N. synnemataformans* are deeply pimento colored; and the colonies of *N. alba*, *N. halophila*, *N. listeri*, and *N. prasina* are colorless (1, 71, 230, 235).

The color of the colonies of *Micromonospora* on agar media is initially pale yellow to light orange. With maturity, the colonies become progressively darker with the production of brown to black spores on some media, for example, SDA. Although some species have been reported to have maroon-purple and blue-green pigments in research laboratories, they have not been observed in cultures from clinical specimens.

The colonies of *S. rectivirgula* (*Faenia rectivirgula*) are usually yellow, and the colonies of *S. viridis* are blue-green. All the colonies of *T. sacchari*, *T. thalpophilus*, and *T. vulgaris* are colorless to white.

The colonies of *A. orientalis* are cream or peach.

The colonies of *A. autotrophica* have cream-colored aerial hyphae and yellow to brown substrate hyphae.

Acid Production or Utilization of Carbohydrates

Two principal systems for testing the physiology of *Nocardia* spp. are the "Gordon" and "Goodfellow" methods. The former method, summarized by Berd (17) and Mishra et al. (137), is useful in differentiating the actinomycetes to the generic level on the basis of about 40 tests. However, Goodfellow, using 140 characters, found that some of the taxa recognized by Gordon were heterogeneous, in particular, the *N. asteroides* complex (65). Acid production of carbohydrates is used in the Gordon method and utilization of carbohydrates is used in the Goodfellow method for the differentiation of the actinomycetes. Tables 3 through 7 compare the utilization of carbohydrates for differentiating the medically important species within the genera *Actinomadura*, *Gordonia*, *Nocardia*, and *Tsukamurella* (66, 171, 200, 213, 217, 224, 230–236). For the oxidative acid production from carbohydrates using Gordon's method, a basal medium is used: 1.00 g of $(NH_4)_2HPO_4$, 0.02 g of KCl, 0.20 g of $MgSO_4 \cdot 7H_2O$, 15.00 g of agar, and 1,000 ml of distilled H_2O. Then 15 ml of a 4.0% solution of bromcresol purple is added to each liter of the basal medium, and the pH is adjusted to 7.0. To a 90-ml aliquot of basal medium, 10 ml of 10% carbohydrate solution is added and the solution is autoclaved for 10 min. A 5-ml volume of the medium is dispensed into 15- by 125-mm screw-cap tubes and slanted. Autoclavable sugars include adonitol, dulcitol, i-erythritol, D-galactose, D-glucose, glycerol, i-myo-inositol, D-mannitol, D-mannose, melibiose, raffinose, salicin, D-sorbitol, and trehalose. For the nonautoclavable carbohydrates, 10 ml of 10% Seitz-filtered carbohydrate solution is aseptically added to 90 ml aliquots of autoclaved basal medium cooled to 45°C, and 5 ml is dispensed into 15- by 125-mm tubes and slanted. Seitz-filtered carbohydrates include L-arabinose, cellobiose, fructose, lactose, maltose, L-rhamnose, sucrose, and D-xylose. The tubes are inoculated with several drops of a dense broth culture suspension

(Trypticase soy broth or Middlebrook 7H9 broth) with a capillary pipette and incubated at 25 or 35°C for 3 weeks. An acid reaction, indicated by the appearance of a yellow color, is considered positive (17). For carbon utilization of carbohydrates, the methods are a modification of the method described by Yassin et al. (231). A basal medium [3.0 g of KH_2PO_4, 1.0 g of $MgSO_4$, 0.2 g of $CaCl_2$, 10.0 g of $(NH_4)_2SO_4$, 1.0 g of KNO_3, 3.0 g of NaCl, 1,000 ml of distilled H_2O] supplemented with 4 ml of a trace salt solution (100.0 mg of H_3BO_3 [boric acid], 48.0 mg of $CuSO_4$, 20.0 mg of KI, 100.0 mg of $FeCl_3$, 80.0 mg of $MnSO_4$, 80.0 mg of $ZnSO_4$, 100.0 ml of distilled H_2O) is used. After autoclaving, this basal medium is adjusted to pH 7.2 with sterile 0.1 N NaOH solution. To this 100-ml solution, a filter-sterilized carbon source (final concentration, 0.01 M) and 0.2 ml of a filter-sterilized vitamin solution (0.2 mg of biotin, 10.0 mg of calcium pantothenate, 10.0 mg of *p* aminobenzoic acid, 20.0 mg of thiamine hydrochloride, and 100.0 ml of distilled H_2O) are added aseptically. A 2-ml volume of the medium is dispensed into 15- by 125-mm screw-cap tubes. The tubes are inoculated with one drop of a broth culture suspension with a capillary pipette and incubated at 25 or 35°C for 3 weeks. Tests are considered positive for carbon utilization if growth was greater in the basal medium plus carbon than in the control basal medium without carbon. Problems may occur with some organisms such as some *Streptomyces* species grown in the control basal medium without carbon supplements. Usually acid production of carbohydrates is comparable to carbohydrate utilization; however, early readings (<1 week) of acid production from some carbohydrates are important, since some carbohydrates (L-rhamnose and cellobiose) revert to negative reactions on prolonged incubation (175).

The new species of *Nocardiopsis*, *N. synnemataformans*, differs from *N. dassonvillei* by its ability to utilize i-myo-inositol, D-mannitol, and D-xylose and its inability to utilize trehalose.

D. congolensis produces acid but no gas in fermentative basal medium from glucose in 48 h; however, it may produce acid transiently from galactose (acid in 48 h; negative in 2 weeks) (238). In addition, some strains produce acid from maltose in 1 to 2 weeks. No acid is produced from dulcitol, lactose, D-mannitol, salicin, D-sorbitol, sucrose, or D-xylose.

Decomposition of Substrates

The ability or inability of the aerobic actinomycetes to decompose adenine, casein, hypoxanthine, tyrosine, and xanthine continues to be a major and generally accepted criterion for the tentative identification of *N. brasiliensis*, *N. pseudobrasiliensis*, *N. otitidiscaviarum*, *N. transvalensis*, *Actinomadura* species, *Nocardiopsis* species, *Streptomyces* species, and *Tsukamurella* species. These tests are not useful for separating *N. abscessus*, *N. asteroides* sensu stricto type VI, *N. brevicatena*, *N. farcinica*, *N. nova*, *N. paucivorans*, and *N. veterana* from each other and from the related genera *Corynebacterium*, *Gordonia*, *Mycobacterium*, and *Rhodococcus*. These tests are performed by inoculating growth onto the surface of quadrant plates of adenine, hypoxanthine, tyrosine, xanthine (0.4 g of each added to 100 ml of basal medium that contains 5 g of peptone, 3 g of beef extract, 15 g of agar, and 1,000 ml of distilled water), and casein (10 g of skim milk powder in 100 ml of distilled water and 2 g of agar in 100 ml are autoclaved separately, mixed, and poured into quadrant plates) and incubated at 35°C (or

25°C if the isolate does not grow well at 35°C). The casein plates are observed at 7 and 14 days for clearing beneath and around the growth. The adenine, hypoxanthine, and tyrosine plates are observed weekly for 4 weeks and the xanthine plates are observed weekly for 3 weeks for clearing of the crystals (17). Isolates of *D. congolensis* may take up to 7 days to decompose casein. Hypoxanthine, tyrosine, and xanthine are not decomposed.

The thermophilic actinomycetes are separated by decomposition of adenine, casein, hypoxanthine, tyrosine, and xanthine (94, 96).

Most isolates of *Micromonospora* are strongly proteolytic; all isolates from human clinical specimens have decomposed casein and 75% have decomposed tyrosine (17). No isolates decompose hypoxanthine or xanthine.

Growth in Lysozyme

Growth in lysozyme is one of the most valuable tests for differentiating between nocardiae and other aerobic actinomycetes. The preparation of the lysozyme is as follows: 95 ml of sterile glycerol broth (5 g of peptone, 70 ml of glycerol, and 1,000 ml of distilled water) are mixed with 5 ml of lysozyme solution (100 mg of lysozyme [Sigma Chemical Co., St. Louis, Mo.] in 100 ml of 0.01 N hydrochloric acid sterilized by filtration), and the mixture is dispensed into test tubes. These tubes and controls containing glycerol broth without lysozyme are inoculated with 1 drop of culture suspension using a Pasteur pipette and are observed weekly for 4 weeks. The test is considered positive if good growth is noted in both tubes and negative if growth is good in the control tube but poor or absent in the tube containing the lysozyme (17). Except for 10 lysozyme-susceptible isolates of the *N. brevicatena* complex, all other *N. brevicatena* complex isolates and all *Nocardia* species grow in the presence of lysozyme (Brown et al., Abstr. 97th Gen. Meet. Am. Soc. Microbiol. 1997).

Arylsulfatase Production

Arylsulfatase production can be determined by using a modification of the technique of Kubica, in which a 0.008 M phenolphthalein disulfate solution in Middlebrook 7H-9 (2.5 ml of 0.08 M phenolphthalein disulfate stock added to 200 ml of Middlebrook 7H-9) is used as the substrate. Color is developed by the addition of 2 N sodium carbonate. Arylsulfatase activity is indicated by the development of a deep pink color (92). Rapidly growing *Mycobacterium* strains are usually positive within 3 days, as is the type strain of *N. africana* when the test is performed in the CDC Actinomycete Laboratory; most strains of *N. nova* are positive within 14 days. Arylsulfatase-positive strains of *N. nova* can be distinguished from the *Mycobacterium* species by the presence of aerial hyphae. Arylsulfatase-positive strains of *N. nova* can be distinguished from the *Mycobacterium* species by the presence of aerial hyphae. *N. africana* can be distinguished from the *Mycobacterium* species by the presence of aerial hyphae and the hydrolysis of casein.

Antibiogram

Wallace and colleagues have shown that the determination of antimicrobial susceptibility results using a combination of broth microdilution and disk diffusion methods for amikacin, amoxicillin-clavulanate, ampicillin, cefotaxime, ciprofloxacin, erythromycin, and minocycline may be useful for species identification within the genus *Nocardia* (Table 3). *N. abscessus* is characterized by susceptibility to amikacin, cefotaxime, ciprofloxacin, and minocycline; interme-

diate resistance to ampicillin; and resistance to erythromycin and amoxicillin-clavulanate. *N. asteroides* sensu stricto (unnamed taxon group VI) is characterized by susceptibility to amikacin, cefotaxime, ciprofloxacin, and minocycline; intermediate resistance to erythromycin; and resistance to ampicillin and amoxicillin-clavulanate. *N. farcinica* is characterized by susceptibility to amikacin, amoxicillin-clavulanate, ciprofloxacin, and minocycline and resistance to ampicillin, cefotaxime, and erythromycin. *N. nova* is characterized by susceptibility to amikacin, ampicillin, erythromycin, and minocycline and resistance to amoxicillin-clavulanate and ciprofloxacin (213, 215, 217).

Cell Wall Composition

Although the actinomycetous nature of a suspected aerobic isolate is often immediately obvious, particularly if aerial hyphae are present, reliable differentiation of aerobic actinomycetes to the generic level is usually possible only when chemotaxonomic techniques are used. These include examination of diagnostic cell wall components and testing for the presence or absence of mycolic acids, metabolism of glucose, and growth in lysozyme. The determination of certain diagnostic cell wall components provides especially useful data. In whole microorganism hydrolysates, the presence or absence of 2,6-DAP and the differentiation of its isomers are of great diagnostic relevance. In addition, such hydrolysates may contain diagnostic sugars, which are also of value in the definitive identification of these microorganisms. The cell wall components that differentiate the major groups of the actinomycetes are given in Table 1. In routine work, the simplified techniques of Becker et al. (13), Lechevalier et al. (103), Berd (17), and Staneck and Roberts (189) are recommended for the detection of diagnostic amino acids and sugars. Before the analysis of whole-cell hydrolysates was introduced as a diagnostic tool, many *Micromonospora* isolates were probably discarded as unidentified actinomycetes. The application of this test, together with the characteristic formation of orange colonies that turn black and the production of single spores, may result in more frequent identification of this rare species in the clinical laboratory (17).

The presence or absence of mycolic esters is one of the major tests used in the presumptive identification to the genus level (Table 2). Nishiuchi et al. analyzed the genera *Dietzia, Gordonia, Mycobacterium, Nocardia,* and *Rhodococcus* using capillary gas-liquid chromatography and mass spectrometry (144, 145). Although there was some degree of overlap, these investigators were able to divide these five genera into six groups based on the number of double bonds and the average chain length of carbons. *Rhodococcus* species are clearly divided into two groups based on their mycolic acid profiles and degree of unsaturation. This finding suggests the possibility that the genus *Rhodococcus* actually consists of two genera. It also correlates with recent 16S rRNA gene sequence data reported by Goodfellow et al. (64). In this study, Goodfellow et al. suggested that there are three significant groups: (i) *Nocardia*; (ii) subgroup *R. rhodochrous*, which includes *R. coprophilus, R. rhodochrous, R. ruber,* and *R. zopfii*; and (iii) the *R. erythropolis* subgroup, which consists of *R. erythropolis, R. fascians, R. globerulus, R. marinonascens, R. opacus, R. percolatus,* and *T. wraitislaviensis* (64). McNabb et al. studied an additional chemotaxonomic tool, fatty acid analysis, in a study of 568 type and reference strains of pathogenic aerobic actinomycetes by using the Microbial Identification System (MIS; Microbial Identification Inc., Newark, Del.) (126). This approach of characterizing actinomycetes has met with limited success. When compared with the 39 type strains, only 117 of 529 (33.5%) isolates were identified as valid species. As further taxonomic revisions of the actinomycetes occur, fatty acid analysis may become one of the most practical methods for the rapid identification of this group of organisms.

Identification Using Commercial Biochemical or Miniaturized Test Systems

In contrast to the use of conventional, growth-dependent procedures for identifying bacteria, the use of chromogenic enzyme substrates can rapidly detect constitutive enzymes produced by microorganisms.

The API ZYM system (bioMérieux Vitek, Inc., Marcy L'Etoile, France) was evaluated for the rapid identification of *Actinomycetaceae* and related bacteria by Kilian (86). In combination with the β-xylosidase test, catalase activity, and oxygen requirements, 12 of 19 enzymes screened proved to be of value for differentiating species of the family *Actinomycetaceae* and some related species within 4 h. Although the reactions of 12 strains of *N. asteroides* were consistent, the author recommended that additional strains of *N. brasiliensis*, *N. otitidiscaviarum*, and *A. pelletieri* be evaluated before this method is used for the identification of these taxa. In 1990, Boiron and Provost further evaluated the API ZYM system for detection of constitutive enzymes by chromogenic substrates (24). The results of this study were consistent with those of Kilian's study (86), except for two enzymatic reactions with *N. brasiliensis*. However, these studies used different media for growth of the inocula and different incubation times.

A related application of rapid chromogenic substrate tests is the fluorogenic enzyme method described by Goodfellow et al. to study the numerical taxonomy of *Rhodococcus* species (64). Fluorescence is a much more sensitive method for the detection of enzymatic activity than the chromogenic method, and the instrument detection systems are highly sensitive to low levels of fluorescence. Prolonged incubation of unknown bacteria to produce a detectable end point is not required, and readings are possible in as soon as 2 h.

Other miniaturized methods include two Microscan products (Dade MicroScan Inc., West Sacramento, Calif.), Rapid Anaerobe Identification and *Haemophilus-Neisseria* panels that test for preformed enzymes (20); bioMérieux ID 32C Yeast Identification System (bioMérieux Vitek) (141); and another system based on 273 phenotypic tests (84). However, the last approach, using numerous tests, is not applicable in the routine clinical laboratory and may be more suitable to specialized reference or research laboratories. The "Biotype-100" strips (bioMérieux, La Balme-Les-Grottes, France) were evaluated for their ability to distinguish species of *Dietzia*, *Gordonia*, and *Rhodococcus* based on carbon utilization in comparison with conventional methods (22). In 2001, Kattar et al. (85) utilized five miniaturized identification systems: API Coryne system (version 2.0); the API 20C AUX system, the API 50 CH system, and the APIZYM system (bioMérieux Vitek, Hazelwood, Mo.); and the RapID CB Plus system (Remel, Lenexa, Kans.) to characterize a new species, *T. strandjordae*, and to differentiate it from related species of *Tsukamurella*. The API 50 CH system was the best system for carbon utilization studies and gave comparable results to those of traditional carbon utilization studies (85).

Although these rapid, miniaturized methods can be helpful for identifying well-defined aerobic actinomycete species, many of these organisms do not fit into established genera, so these systems are more suitable for use in specialized reference or research laboratories.

Identification Using Nucleic Acid Systems and Other Novel Methods

Recent advances in molecular techniques have shown promise as rapid and specific aids in the identification of many difficult-to-identify bacteria.

After DNA amplification of the 439-bp segment of the *hsp* gene, a PCR based identification schema using the restriction enzymes *Msp*I and *Hinf*I identified 16 of 20 taxa of aerobic actinomycetes, including *Actinomadura*, *Gordonia*, *Nocardia*, *Rhodococcus*, *Streptomyces*, and *Tsukamurella* (190, 192, 224, 225). However, multiple restriction fragment length polymorphism patterns were seen with these enzymes with G. *bronchialis*, *N. asteroides* sensu stricto group VI, *N. otitidiscaviarum*, *N. transvalensis*, and *Streptomyces* spp. Further differentiation of *N. transvalensis* into four subgroups was accomplished with the enzymes *Hae*III, *Nar*I, and *Xho*I (224). Recently, after DNA amplification of a portion of the 16S rRNA gene, PCR-restriction analysis was useful in identification of the *Nocardia* species with the enzymes *Hin*PII, *Dpn*II, *Sph*I, and *Bst*EII (41) and several *Rhodococcus* species with the enzymes *Kpn*I and *Sac*II (14). Using a similar approach, Laurent et al. were able to identify the medically important *Nocardia* spp. with the 16S rRNA gene PCR (102). All of these methods were as sensitive as traditional methods, less time-consuming (2 to 5 working days), and less labor-intensive (225). Beyazova and Lechevalier were able to identify *Streptomyces* species by restriction endonuclease digestion of large DNA fragments (19). Although more time-consuming, ribotyping using a 16S rRNA gene probe was used for the identification of four different species within the *N. asteroides* complex (101) and isolates of the genera *Rhodococcus* and *Gordonia* (100). Recently, 16S rRNA gene sequencing was useful in identifying *N. dassonvillei* (12).

Diagnostic histopathology continues to be an essential counterpart of clinical microbiology. Application of in situ hybridization methods may be particularly beneficial when putative microorganisms are rare, are unculturable as *T. whipplei* (56), or have a nonspecific (coccoid) morphology as seen with *R. equi* (J. Brown, M. McNeil, P. Greer, B. Lasker, R. Bluth, W. Schaffner, D. Oblack, J. Jahre, and S. Zaki, Abstr. 91st Gen. Meet. Am. Soc. Microbiol. 1991, abstr. D-26, p. 82, 1991) and other rhodococci (64). An important and even more recent technological advance has been the PCR analysis of 16S rRNA gene sequence from tissue, which has further increased the sensitivity of detection of microorganisms that cannot be cultured on artificial media (162, 166, 223).

Traditionally, *T. whipplei* is identified by routine histopathologic analysis with PAS-positive tissues (usually intestinal) and clinical diagnosis. Although electron microscopy is time-consuming and may be available in reference laboratories only, it allows one to demonstrate the characteristic trilamellar cell wall ultrastructure of the Whipple's bacillus and is recommended especially for extraintestinal sites (44). On the basis of sequence analysis of the 16S rRNA gene, several diagnostic PCR assays have recently been established (54, 58). Well-optimized PCR assays are capable of detecting small numbers of 16S rRNA genes, and PCR analysis of histopathologically confirmed Whipple's disease is usually positive. PCR methods are more sensitive than traditional microscopic methods; thus, PCR facilitates the diagnosis of histopathologically negative or inconclusive cases and helps with monitoring typical and atypical cases of Whipple's disease (52).

Because PCR products of the presumably appropriate size may be derived from organisms other than *T. whipplei* (76, 143), an additional test is recommended to confirm the PCR results, especially in the absence of histopathologic evidence. Although hybridization and sequencing of amplicons may provide further evidence for the presence of *T. whipplei* DNA, these techniques are rather tedious and time-consuming and do not reliably exclude the possibility of amplicon carryover contamination. In contrast, additional *T. whipplei*-specific PCR assays targeting an independent region, such as analogous portions of 23S rRNA or hsp65 genes, may provide the necessary confirmation in a timely manner (78, 79, 139). However, *T. whipplei* DNA has also been found in patients without clinical signs of Whipple's disease (48, 50, 194). Therefore, positive PCR results in PAS-inconclusive specimens should always be interpreted taking into consideration clinical features.

In 1995, Provost et al. utilized the yeast killer system to separate species within the *N. asteroides* complex (158). Briefly, self-immune killer yeasts [*Pichia mrakii* (K9) and *Pichia lynferdii* (K76)] secrete extracellular glycoproteins or killer toxins that produce different patterns of inhibition zones against three species of the *N. asteroides* complex. This method was relatively rapid (results were available within 5 days of incubation), economic, and feasible compared with traditional methods, which may take up to 3 weeks.

Comparative studies of the available phenetic and genetic methods, which include well-characterized clinical and reference isolates, are needed to determine which technique is best for identification of each major pathogen.

Strain Identification

Molecular subtyping techniques have been successfully applied in the investigation of several nosocomial pseudo-outbreaks and nosocomial outbreaks as well as the evaluation of multiple, related isolates of the *N. asteroides* complex (111, 150), *N. farcinica* (23, 53, 133, 218), *N. brasiliensis* (191), *G. bronchialis* (168), *Rhodococcus* spp. (100), *T. paurometabola* (6), and *T. whipplei* (79, 80, 114, 115). The methods include *Pvu*II-, *Pst*I-, and *Sal*I-digested genomic DNA (6, 100, 133, 150, 168, 218), pulsed-field gel electrophoresis (23, 111, 191), randomly amplified polymorphic DNA PCR (53, 111), ribotyping (6, 53, 133, 218), and plasmid analysis (81).

In 1988, Morace et al. (138) described a biotyping method that has promise as a highly discriminative epidemiologic tool. They found that nine killer yeasts, grouped into triplets, selected from a panel of 44 yeasts belonging to the genera *Candida*, *Kluyveromyces*, *Pichia*, and *Saccharomyces* differentiated eight *Nocardia* test strains. However, this technique has yet to be evaluated using a significant number of epidemiologically related *Nocardia* strains. Until such a study is performed, the usefulness of this method is unclear.

PCR amplification of *T. whipplei* DNA and sequencing of the 16S–23S rDNA intergenic spacer region with specific primers (78, 114, 115) and sequencing of domain III of the 23 rRNA gene with specific primers (79, 80, 115) have identified six subtypes of *T. whipplei*.

SEROLOGY

Most serologic tests for the actinomycetes have been hampered by lack of specificity and sensitivity and are complicated further by the lack of antigenic homogeneity or the inability of some clinical isolates to secrete the antigen under study. A number of antigens have been proposed for serologic testing, including the 24- and 26-kDa proteins (173), the 55-kDa protein (5), and the 36-, 55-, and 62-kDa proteins (89); culture filtrates, cytoplasmic extracts, cord factor (trehalose dimycolate), and whole cells for the nocardiae (89); a soluble culture filtrate for *R. equi* (211); cell extracts for *Actinomadura* spp. (127); and culture extracts of the thermophilic actinomycetes (96). The serologic testing methods evaluated included mostly enzyme-linked immunosorbent assay and Western blot techniques; however, immunodiffusion and indirect immunofluorescence methods have also been studied. Except for certain value in the diagnosis of hypersensitivity pneumonitis, most of these serologic tests are experimental with some potential diagnostic value and may be useful as indicators of response to therapy (25, 173). Recently, the presence of anti-*N. brasiliensis* antibodies in humans has been helpful in serodiagnosis and has been introduced into routine clinical laboratories (172). Five *N. brasiliensis* mycetoma patients tested positive in this assay, and it showed a cross-reactivity only in patients with *N. asteroides*. More studies are needed to evaluate the usefulness of this test in the diagnosis of systemic infections caused by *N. asteroides* (175).

ANTIMICROBIAL THERAPY

Recent in vitro and in vivo studies, clinical observations, and taxonomic developments indicate that antimicrobial therapy must be adjusted to the particular species of *Nocardia* present, to individual strain antimicrobial susceptibility patterns, and to the site and type of infection (10, 11, 106, 127, 128). Sulfonamides alone or in combination with trimethoprim (TMP-SMX) are the therapy of choice for nocardiosis. However, in patients with disease disseminated to the central nervous system or with depressed cell-mediated immunity, such as occurs in renal transplant recipients and HIV-infected patients, therapy may be complicated. The frequent use of TMP-SMX for this infection may not be related as much to properties of synergism or improved efficacy compared with that of sulfonamide treatment alone as to favorable pharmacokinetics (effective CSF penetration) and general familiarity among clinicians. Patient intolerance to TMP-SMX is a problem encountered frequently in the therapy of HIV-infected patients (197).

Antimicrobial therapy for pulmonary and/or systemic *R. equi* infections is problematic since the majority of patients relapse in spite of treatment and the attributable mortality is high, especially among AIDS patients (109). Careful and repeated culture and susceptibility testing during treatment are essential to detect acquired resistance (146). One proposed regimen involves a parenteral glycopeptide plus imipenem for at least 3 weeks followed by an oral combination of rifampin plus either macrolides or tetracycline (109).

Therapeutic guidance for patients with infections due to other aerobic actinomycetes concerning the most appropriate drug treatment and duration of therapy is undefined. Thus, antimicrobial susceptibility testing of clinically significant isolates is needed and should be done at a specialized reference laboratory (109).

Recently, the method of serial twofold broth microdilution in cation-supplemented Mueller-Hinton broth has been approved by the National Committee for Clinical Laboratory Standards (NCCLS) for antimicrobial susceptibility testing of the aerobic actinomycetes (228). Over the years, a few investigators have evaluated conventional susceptibility studies for these microorganisms, including the agar dilution (21, 180), broth dilution (21, 214, 216), and disk diffusion (21, 214) methods. Recently, two newer methods, the epsilometer test (E test [AB Biodisk, Solna, Sweden]) (21) and the radiometric broth method (180), have been evaluated. In 1997, Ambaye et al. studied isolates of the members of the N. asteroides complex, comparing the three conventional methods (agar dilution, broth dilution, and disk diffusion) with the E test and the radiometric methods for a panel of nine antimicrobial agents: amikacin, amoxicillin-clavulanate, ampicillin, ceftriaxone, ciprofloxacin, erythromycin, imipenem, minocycline, and TMP-SMX (2). These investigators determined that the radiometric broth method had the highest level of agreement when the results were combined for all antimicrobial agents tested; the agar dilution test method had the lowest level of agreement with the consensus interpretative results (2). Linezolid, an oxazolidinone that is one of the new synthetic classes of antibiotics and is available as an oral antimicrobial agent, was recently tested by broth microdilution against 140 clinical isolates belonging to seven species of Nocardia (27). Linezolid is the first antimicrobial agent that has demonstrated activity against all Nocardia species including the multidrug-resistant N. farcinica and N. transvalensis (27).

EVALUATION, INTERPRETATION, AND REPORTING OF RESULTS

The limited availability of laboratories with appropriate capabilities for identification of the actinomycetes is a problem. However, modern communication networks and the ability to rapidly ship specimens have made the services of a few reference laboratories more widely available.

Determining whether a particular strain of Streptomyces is involved in a disease process can sometimes be difficult because most of these actinomycetes may be recovered from clinical specimens as contaminants. Many published case reports of disease associated with Streptomyces species are often cited, although they repeatedly provide minimal or erroneous laboratory data on the identification of the infecting organism. Therefore, we propose the following criteria to aid in validating the microbiologic identification of Streptomyces species in published case reports and consequently validating the association of disease with a particular Streptomyces species: (i) microscopic description of Gram stain of the clinical material as well as the bacterial culture; (ii) macroscopic description of the size, pigment, odor, and hemolysis of colonies; (iii) physiological reactions that include temperature requirements, decomposition of the substrates adenine, casein, hypoxanthine, tyrosine, and xanthine, and utilization of carbohydrates; (iv) chemotaxonomic investigations (e.g., cellular fatty acids, presence or absence of mycolic acids, and cell wall analysis [the presence of L-DAP must be determined]); and (v) molecular analysis (e.g., 16S rRNA gene sequence); and pure culture or repeated isolation from a normally sterile site.

REFERENCES

1. **Al-tai, A. M., and J.-S. Ruan.** 1994. *Nocardiopsis halophila* sp. nov., a new halophilic actinomycete isolated from soil. *Int. J. Syst. Bacteriol.* **44**:474–478.

2. **Ambaye, A., P. C. Kohner, P. C. Wollan, K. L. Roberts, G. D. Roberts, and F. R. Cockerill III.** 1997. Comparison of agar dilution, broth microdilution, disk diffusion, E-test, and BACTEC radiometric methods for antimicrobial susceptibility testing of clinical isolates of the *Nocardia asteroides* complex. *J. Clin. Microbiol.* **35**:847–852.

3. **Ambrose, N. C.** 1996. The pathogenesis of dermatophilosis. *Trop. Anim. Health Prod.* **28**:29S–37S.

4. **Anderson, A. S., and E. M. H. Wellington.** 2001. The taxonomy of *Streptomyces* and related genera. *Int. J. Syst. Evol. Microbiol.* **51**:797–814.

5. **Angeles A. M., and A. M. Sugar.** 1987. Identification of a common immunodominant protein in culture filtrates of three *Nocardia* species and use in etiologic diagnosis of mycetoma. *J. Clin. Microbiol.* **25**:2278–2280.

6. **Auerbach, S. B., M. M. McNeil, J. M. Brown, B. A. Lasker, and W. R. Jarvis.** 1992. Outbreak of pseudoinfection with *Tsukamurella paurometabolum* traced to laboratory contamination: efficacy of a joint epidemiological and laboratory investigation. *Clin. Infect. Dis.* **14**:1015–1022.

7. **Baghdadlian, H., S. Sorger, K. Knowles, M. McNeil, and J. Brown.** 1989. *Nocardia transvalensis* pneumonia in a child. *Pediatr. Infect. Dis. J.* **8**:470–471.

8. **Baril, L., P. Boiron, V. Manceron, S. O. Ely, P. Jamet, E. Favre, E. Caumes, and F. Bricaire.** 1999. Refractory craniofacial actinomycetoma due to *Streptomyces somaliensis* that required salvage therapy with amikacin and imipenem. *Clin. Infect. Dis.* **29**:460–461.

9. **Barton, M. D., and K. L. Hughes.** 1984. Ecology of *Rhodococcus equi*. *Vet. Microbiol.* **9**:65–76.

10. **Beaman, B. L., and L. Beaman.** 1994. *Nocardia* species: host-parasite relationships. *Clin. Microbiol. Rev.* **7**:213–264.

11. **Beaman, B. L., P. Boiron, L. Beaman, G. H. Brownell, K. Schaal, and M. E. Gombert.** 1992. *Nocardia* and nocardiosis. *J. Med. Vet. Mycol.* **30**:317–331.

12. **Beau, F., C. Bollet, T. Coton, E. Garnotel, and M. Drancourt.** 1999. Molecular identification of a *Nocardiopsis dassonvillei* blood isolate. *J. Clin. Microbiol.* **37**:3366–3368.

13. **Becker, B., P. Lechevalier, R. E. Gordon, and H. A. Lechevalier.** 1964. Rapid differentiation between *Nocardia* and *Streptomyces* by paper chromatography of whole-cell hydrolysates. *Appl. Microbiol.* **12**:421–423.

14. **Bell, K. S., M. S. Kuyukina, S. Heidbrink, J. C. Philp, D. W. Aw, I. B. Ivshina, and N. Christofi.** 1999. Identification and environmental detection of *Rhodococcus* species by 16S rDNA-targeted PCR. *J. Appl. Microbiol.* **87**:472–480.

15. **Bell, K. S., J. C. Philp, D. W. Aw, and N. Christofi.** 1998. The genus *Rhodococcus*. *J. Appl. Microbiol.* **85**:195–210.

16. **Bendinger, B.** 1995. *Gordona hydrophobica* sp. nov., isolated from biofilters for waste gas treatment. *Int. J. Syst. Bacteriol.* **45**:544–548.

17. **Berd, D.** 1973. Laboratory identification of clinically important aerobic actinomycetes. *Appl. Microbiol.* **25**:665–681.

18. **Bernatchez, H., and E. Lebreux.** 1991. *Nocardiopsis dassonvillei* recovered from a lung biopsy and a possible cause of extrinsic alveolitis. *Clin. Microbiol. Newsl.* **13**:174–175.

19. **Beyazova, M., and M. P. Lechevalier.** 1993. Taxonomic utility of restriction endonuclease fingerprinting of large DNA fragments from *Streptomyces* strains. *Int. J. Bacteriol.* **43**:674–682.

20. **Biehle, J. R., S. J. Cavalieri, T. Felland, and B. L. Zimmer.** 1996. Novel method for rapid identification of

Nocardia species by detection of preformed enzymes. *J. Clin. Microbiol.* **34:**103–107.

21. **Biehle, J. R., S. J. Cavalieri, M. A. Saubolle, and L. J. Getsinger.** 1994. Comparative evaluation of the E test for susceptibility testing of *Nocardia* species. *Diagn. Microbiol. Infect. Dis.* **19:**101–110.

22. **Bizet, C., C. Barreau, C. Harmant, M. Nowakowski, and A. Pietfroid.** 1997. Identification of *Rhodococcus, Gordona* and *Dietzia* species using carbon source utilization tests ("Biotype-100" strips). *Res. Microbiol.* **148:**799–809.

23. **Blumel, J., E. Blumel, A. F. Yassin, H. Schmidt-Rotte, and K. P. Schaal.** 1998. Typing of *Nocardia farcinica* by pulsed-field gel electrophoresis reveals an endemic strain as source of hospital infections. *J. Clin. Microbiol.* **36:**118–122.

24. **Boiron, P., and F. Provost.** 1990. Enzymatic characterization of *Nocardia* spp. and related bacteria by API ZYM profile. *Mycopathologia* **110:**51–56.

25. **Boiron, P., R. Locci, M. Goodfellow, S. A. Gumaa, K. Isik, B. Kim, M. M. McNeil, M. C. Salinas-Carmona, and H. Shojaei.** 1998. *Nocardia*, nocardiosis and mycetoma. *Med. Mycol.* **36**(Suppl. 1)**:**26–37.

26. **Briglia, M., F. A. Rainey, E. Stackebrandt, G. Schraa, and M. S. Salkinoja-Salonen.** 1996. *Rhodococcus percolatus* sp. nov., a bacterium degrading 2,4,6-trichlorophenol. *Int. J. Syst. Bacteriol.* **46:**23–30.

27. **Brown-Elliott, B. A., S. C. Ward, C. J. Crist, L. B. Mann, R. W. Wilson, and R. J. Wallace, Jr.** 2001. In vitro activities of linezolid against multiple *Nocardia* species. *Antimicrob. Agents Chemother.* **45:**1295–1297.

28. **Brumpt, E.** 1906. Les mycetomes. *Arch. Parasitol.* **10:**489–527.

29. **Buchman, A. L., M. M. McNeil, J. M. Brown, B. A. Lasker, and M. E. Ament.** 1992. Central venous catheter sepsis caused by unusual *Gordona (Rhodococcus)* species: identification with a digoxigenin-labeled rDNA probe. *Clin. Infect. Dis.* **15:**694–697.

30. **Buenviaje, G. N., R. G. Hirst, P. W. Ladds, and J. M. Millan.** 1997. Isolation of *Dermatophilus* sp. from skin lesions in farmed saltwater crocodiles (*Crocodylus porosus*). *Aust. Vet. J.* **75:**365–367.

31. **Bunker, M. L., L. Chewning, S. E. Wang, and M. A. Gordon.** 1988. *Dermatophilus congolensis* and "hairy" leukoplakia. *J. Clin. Pathol.* **89:**683–687.

32. **Casella, P., A. Tommasi, and A. M. Tortorano.** 1987. Peritonite da *Gordona aurantiaca (Rhodococcus aurantiacus)* in dialisi peritoneale ambulatore continua. *Microbiologia* **2:**47–48.

33. **Chandler, F. W., W. Kaplan, and L. Ajello.** 1980. A *Color Atlas and Textbook of Histopathology of Mycotic Diseases,* p. 85, 243. Wolfe Medical Publications, London, United Kingdom.

34. **Cherukian, C. J., and E. A. Schenk.** 1982. A method of demonstrating gram-positive and gram-negative bacteria. *J. Histotechnol.* **5:**127–128.

35. **Chun, J., K. S. Bae, E. Y. Moon, S. O. Jung, H. K. Lee, and S. J. Kim.** 2000. *Nocardiopsis kunsanensis* sp. nov., a moderately halophilic actinomycete isolated from a saltern. *Int. J. Syst. Evol. Microbiol.* **50:**1909–1913.

36. **Chun, J., L. L. Blackall, S. O. Kang, Y. C. Hah, and M. Goodfellow.** 1997. A proposal to reclassify *Nocardia pinensis* Blackall et al. as *Skermania piniformis* gen. nov., comb. nov. *Int. J. Syst. Bacteriol.* **47:**127–131.

37. **Chun, J., S. O. Kang, Y. C. Hah, and M. Goodfellow.** 1996. Phylogeny of mycolic acid-containing actinomycetes. *J. Ind. Microbiol.* **17:**205–213.

38. **Clausen, C., and C. K. Wallis.** 1994. Bacteremia caused by *Tsukamurella* species. *Clin. Microbiol. Newsl.* **16:**6–8.

39. **Collins, M. D., E. Falsen, E. Akervall, B. Sjoden, and A. Alvarez.** 1998. *Corynebacterium kroppenstedtii* sp. nov., a novel corynebacterium that does not contain mycolic acids. *Int. J. Syst. Bacteriol.* **48:**1449–1454.

40. **Collins, M. D., J. Smida, M. Dorsch, and E. Stackebrandt.** 1988. *Tsukamurella* gen. nov., harboring *Corynebacterium paurometabolum* and *Rhodococcus aurantiacus. Int. J. Syst. Bacteriol.* **38:**385–391.

41. **Conville, P. S., S. H. Fischer, C. P. Cartwright, and F. G. Witebsky.** 2000. Identification of *Nocardia* species by restriction endonuclease analysis of an amplified portion of the 16S rRNA gene. *J. Clin. Microbiol.* **38:**158–164.

42. **DeMarais, P. I., and F. E. Kocka.** 1995. *Rhodococcus* meningitis in an immunocompetent host. *Clin. Infect. Dis.* **20:**167–169.

43. **Desmond, E. P., and M. Flores.** 1993. Mouse pathogenicity studies of *Nocardia asteroides* complex species and clinical correlations with human isolates. *FEMS Microbiol. Lett.* **110:**281–284.

44. **Dobbins, W. O., III.** 1995. The diagnosis of Whipple's disease. *N. Engl. J. Med.* **332:**390–392.

45. **Doig, C., M. J. Gill, and D. L. Church.** 1991. *Rhodococcus equi*—an easily missed opportunistic pathogen. *Scand. J. Infect. Dis.* **23:**1–6.

46. **Donisi, A., M. G. Suardi, S. Casari, M. Longo, G. P. Cadeo, and G. Carosi.** 1996. *Rhodococcus equi* infection in HIV-infected patients. *AIDS* **10:**359–362.

47. **Drancourt, M., M. M. McNeil, J. M. Brown, B. A. Lasker, M. Maurin, M. Choux, and D. Raoult.** 1994. Brain abscess due to *Gordona terrae* in an immunocompromised child: case report and review of infections caused by *G. terrae. Clin. Infect. Dis.* **19:**258–262.

48. **Dutly, F., H. P. Hinrikson, T. Seidel, S. Morgenegg, M. Altwegg, and P. Bauerfeind.** 2000. *Tropheryma whippelii* DNA in saliva of patients without Whipple's disease. *Infection* **28:**219–222.

49. **Eggink, C. A., P. Wesseling, P. Boiron, and J. F. Meis.** 1997. Severe keratitis due to *Nocardia farcinica. J. Clin. Microbiol.* **35:**999–1001.

50. **Ehrbar, H. U., P. Bauerfeind, F. Dutly, H. R. Koelz, and M. Altwegg.** 1999. PCR-positive tests for *Tropheryma whippelii* in patients without Whipple's disease. *Lancet* **353:**2214.

51. **el Hassan, A. M., A. H. Fahal, A. O. Ahmed, A. Ismail, and B. Veress.** 2001. The immunopathology of actinomycetoma lesions caused by *Streptomyces somaliensis. Trans. R. Soc. Trop. Med. Hyg.* **95:**89–92.

52. **Esteban, J., J. M. Ramos, M. L. Fernandez-Guerrero, and F. Soriano.** 1994. Isolation of *Nocardia* sp. from blood cultures in a teaching hospital. *Scand. J. Infect. Dis.* **26:**693–696.

53. **Exmelin, L., B. Malbruny, M. Vergnaud, F. Prosvost, P. Boiron, and C. Morel.** 1996. Molecular study of nosocomial nocardiosis outbreak involving heart transplant recipients. *J. Clin. Microbiol.* **34:**1014–1016.

54. **Fenollar, F., and D. Raoult.** 2001. Whipple's disease. *Clin. Diagn. Lab. Immunol.* **8:**1–8.

55. **Flores, M., and E. Desmond.** 1993. Opacification of Middlebrook agar as an aid in identification of *Nocardia farcinica. J. Clin. Microbiol.* **31:**3040–3041.

56. **Fredricks, D. N., and D. A. Relman.** 2001. Localization of *Tropheryma whippelii* rRNA in tissues from patients with Whipple's disease. *J. Infect. Dis.* **183:**1229–1237.

57. **Garratt, M. A., H. T. Holmes, and F. S. Nolte.** 1992. Selective buffered charcoal-yeast-extract medium for isolation of nocardiae from mixed cultures. *J. Clin. Microbiol.* **30:**1891–1892.

58. **Geissdorfer, W., I. Wittmann, G. Seitz, R. Cesnjevar, M. Rollinghoff, C. Schoerner, and C. Bogdan.** 2001. A case of aortic valve disease associated with *Tropheryma whippelii* infection in the absence of other signs of Whipple's disease. *Infection* **29:**44–47.

59. **Georghiou, P. R., and Z. M. Blacklock.** 1992. Infection with *Nocardia* species in Queensland. A review of 102 clinical isolates. *Med. J. Aust.* **156:**692–697.

60. **Gitao, C. G., H. Agab, and A. J. Khalifalla.** 1998. Outbreaks of *Dermatophilus congolensis* infection in camels (*Camelus dromedarius*) from the Butana region in eastern Sudan. *Rev. Sci. Technol.* **17:**743–748.

61. **Goodfellow, M.** 1983. Ecology of actinomycetes. *Annu. Rev. Microbiol.* **37:**189–216.

62. **Goodfellow, M.** 1989. Genus *Rhodococcus* Zopf 1891^{AL}, p. 2362–2371. *In* S. T. Williams, M. E. Sharpe, and J. G. Holt (ed.), *Bergey's Manual of Systematic Bacteriology*, vol. 4. The Williams & Wilkins Co., Baltimore, Md.

63. **Goodfellow, M., G. Alderson, and J. Chun.** 1999. Rhodococcal systematics: problems and developments. *Antonie Leeuwenhoek* **74:**3–20.

64. **Goodfellow, M., K. Isik, and E. Yates.** 1999. Actinomycete systematics: an unfinished synthesis. *Nova Acta Leopold.* **80:**47–82.

65. **Goodfellow, M., and M. P. Lechevalier.** 1989. Genus *Nocardia* Trevisan 1889, 9^{AL}, p. 2350–2361. *In* S. T. Williams, M. E. Sharpe, and J. G. Holt (ed.), *Bergey's Manual of Systematic Bacteriology*, vol. 4. The Williams & Wilkins Co., Baltimore, Md.

66. **Goodfellow, M., J. Zakrzewska-Czerwinska, E. G. Thomas, M. Mordarski, A. C. Ward, and A. L. James.** 1991. Polyphasic taxonomic study of the genera *Gordona* and *Tsukamurella* including the description of *Tsukamurella wratislaviensis* sp. nov. *Zentbl. Bakteriol.* **275:**162–178.

67. **Gordon, R. E., S. K. Mishra, and D. A. Barnett.** 1978. Some bits and pieces of the genus *Nocardia: N. carnea, N. vaccinii, N. transvalensis, N. orientalis* and *N. aerocoligenes.* *J. Gen. Microbiol.* **109:**69–78.

68. **Granel, F., A. Lozniewski, A. Barbaud, C. Lion, M. Dailloux, M. Weber, and J. L. Schmutz.** 1996. Cutaneous infection caused by *Tsukamurella paurometabolum. Clin. Infect. Dis.* **23:**839–840.

69. **Gross, M., C. Jung, and W. G. Zoller.** 1999. Detection of *Tropheryma whippelii* DNA (Whipple's disease) in faeces. *Ital. J. Gastroenterol. Hepatol.* **31:**70–72.

70. **Gruet, M., L. Maydat, and R. Ferro.** 1970. Peritonite a *Streptomyces somaliensis. Bull. Soc. Med. Afr. Noire* **15:**609–610.

71. **Grund, E., and R. M. Kroppenstedt.** 1990. Chemotaxonomy and numerical taxonomy of the genus *Nocardiopsis. Int. J. Syst. Bacteriol.* **40:**5–11.

72. **Gurtler, R., R. Smith, B. C. Mayall, G. Potter-Reinemann, E. Stackebrandt, and R. M. Kroppenstedt.** 2001. *Nocardia veterana* sp. nov., isolated from human bronchial lavage. *Int. J. Syst. Evol. Microbiol.* **51:**933–936.

73. **Haley, L. D., and C. S. Callaway.** 1978. *Laboratory Methods in Medical Mycology*, p. 29–44. CDC publication 78-8361. U.S. Government Printing Office, Washington, D.C.

74. **Hamid, M. E., L. Maltonado, G. S. Sharaf Eldin, M. F. Mohamed, N. S. Saeed, and M. Goodfellow.** 2001. *Nocardia africana* sp. nov., a new pathogen isolated from patients with pulmonary infections. *J. Clin. Microbiol.* **39:**625–630.

75. **Hanel, H., J. Kalisch, M. Keil, W. C. Marsch, and M. Buslau.** 1991. Quantification of keratolytic activity from *Dermatophilus congolensis. Med. Microbiol. Immunol.* **180:**45–51.

76. **Harmsen, D., J. Heesemann, T. Brabletz, T. Kirchner, and H. K. Muller-Hermelink.** 1994. Heterogeneity among Whipple's-disease-associated bacteria. *Lancet* **343:**1288.

77. **Hay, R. J., E. S. Mahgoub, G. Leon, S. Al-Sogair, and O. Welsh.** 1992. Mycetoma. *J. Med. Vet. Mycol.* **30:**41–49.

78. **Hinrikson, H. P., F. Dutly, and M. Altwegg.** 2000. Analysis of the actinobacterial insertion in domain III of the 23S rRNA gene of uncultured variants of the bacterium associated with Whipple's disease using broad-range and 'Tropheryma whippelii'-specific PCR. *Int. J. Syst. Evol. Microbiol.* **50:**1007–1011.

79. **Hinrikson, H. P., F. Dutly, and M. Altwegg.** 2000. Evaluation of a specific nested PCR targeting domain III of the 23S rRNA gene of "Tropheryma whippelii" and proposal of a classification system for its molecular variants. *J. Clin. Microbiol.* **38:**595–599.

80. **Hinrikson, H. P., F. Dutly, S. Nair, and M. Altwegg.** 1999. Detection of three different types of 'Tropheryma whippelii' directly from clinical specimens by sequencing, single-strand conformation polymorphism (SSCP) analysis and type-specific PCR of their 16S–23S ribosomal intergenic spacer region. *Int. J. Syst. Bacteriol.* **49:**1701–1706.

81. **Jonsson, S., R. J. Wallace, Jr., S. I. Hull, and D. M. Musher.** 1986. Recurrent *Nocardia* pneumonia in an adult with chronic granulomatous disease. *Am. Rev. Respir. Dis.* **133:**932–934.

82. **Kampfer, P., M. A. Andersson, F. A. Rainey, R. M. Kroppenstedt, and M. Salkinoja-Salonen.** 1999. *Williamsia muralis* gen. nov., sp. nov., isolated from the indoor environment of a children's day care centre. *Int. J. Syst. Bacteriol.* **49:**681–687.

83. **Kampfer, P., W. Dott, and R. M. Kroppenstedt.** 1990. Numerical classification and identification of some nocardioform bacteria. *J. Gen. Appl. Microbiol.* **36:**309–331.

84. **Kampfer, P., R. M. Kroppenstedt, and W. Dott.** 1991. A numerical classification of the genera *Streptomyces* and *Streptoverticillium* using miniaturized physiological tests. *J. Gen. Microbiol.* **137:**1831–1891.

85. **Kattar, M. M., B. T. Cookson, L. C. Carlson, S. K. Stiglich, M. A. Schwartz, T. T. Nguyen, R. Daza, C. K. Wallis, S. L. Yarfitz, and M. B. Coyle.** 2001. *Tsukamurella strandjordae* sp. nov., a proposed new species causing sepsis. *J. Clin. Microbiol.* **39:**1467–1476.

86. **Kilian, M.** 1978. Rapid identification of *Actinomycetaceae* and related bacteria. *J. Clin. Microbiol.* **57:**127–133.

87. **Kim, S. B., R. Brown, C. Oldfield, S. C. Gilbert, and M. Goodfellow.** 1999. *Gordonia desulfuricans* sp. nov., a benzothiophene-desulphurizing actinomycete. *Int. J. Syst. Bacteriol.* **49:**1845–1851.

88. **Kim, S. B., R. Brown, C. Oldfield, S. C. Gilbert, S. Iliarionov, and M. Goodfellow.** 2000. *Gordonia amicalis* sp. nov., a novel dibenzothiophene-desulphurizing actinomycete. *Int. J. Syst. Evol. Microbiol.* **50:**2031–2036.

89. **Kjelstrom, J. A., and B. L. Beaman.** 1993. Development of a serologic panel for the recognition of nocardial infections in a murine model. *Diagn. Microbiol. Infect. Dis.* **16:**291–301.

90. **Klatte, S., R. M. Kroppenstedt, and F. A. Rainey.** 1994. *Rhodococcus opacus* sp. nov. *Syst. Appl. Bacteriol.* **17:**355–360.

91. **Klatte, S., F. A. Rainey, and R. M. Kroppenstedt.** 1994. Transfer of *Rhodococcus aichiensis* Tsukamura 1982 and *Nocardia amarae* Lechevalier and Lechevalier 1974 to the genus *Gordona* as *Gordona aichiensis* comb. nov. and *Gordona amarae* comb. nov. *Int. J. Syst. Bacteriol.* **44:**769–773.

92. **Kubica, G. B., and A. L. Ridgeon.** 1961. The arylsulfatase activity of acid-fast bacilli. III. Preliminary investigation of rapidly growing acid-fast bacilli. *Am. Rev. Respir. Dis.* **83:**737–740.

93. **Kummer, C., P. Schumann, and E. Stackebrandt.** 1999. *Gordonia alkanivorans* sp. nov. isolated from tar-contaminated soil. *Int. J. Syst. Bacteriol.* **49:**1513–1522.

94. **Kurup, V. P., and J. N. Fink.** 1975. A scheme for the identification of thermophilic actinomycetes associated with hypersensitivity pneumonitis. *J. Clin. Microbiol.* **2:**55–61.

95. **Kuwabara, M., T. Onitsuka, K. Nakamura, M. Shimada, S. Ohtaki, and Y. Mikami.** 1999. Mediastinitis due to *Gordona sputi* after CABG. *J. Cardiovasc. Surg.* **40:**675–677.

96. **Lacey, J.** 1989. Genus *Faenia* Kurup and Agre 1983, 664^{VP} (*Micropolyspora* Lechevalier, Soltorovsky and McDermont 1961, 11^{AL}), p. 2387–2392. *In* S. T. Williams, M. E. Sharpe, and J. G. Holt (ed.), *Bergey's Manual of Systematic Bacteriology*, vol. 4. The Williams & Wilkins Co., Baltimore, Md.

97. **Lai, K. K.** 1993. A cancer patient with central venous catheter-related sepsis caused by *Tsukamurella paurometabolum* (*Gordona aurantiaca*). *Clin. Infect. Dis.* **17:**285–287.

98. **Langham, C. D., S. T. Williams, P. H. Sneath, and A. M. Mortimer.** 1989. New probability matrices for identification of *Streptomyces*. *J. Gen. Microbiol.* **135:**121–133.

99. **La Scola, B., F. Fenollar, P. E. Fournier, M. Altwegg, and D. Raoult.** 2001. Description of *Tropheryma whipplei* gen. nov. sp. nov., the Whipple's disease bacillus. *Int. J. Syst. Evol. Microbiol.* **51:**1471–1479.

100. **Lasker, B. A., J. M. Brown, and M. M. McNeil.** 1992. Identification and epidemiological typing of clinical and environmental isolates of the genus *Rhodococcus* with use of a digoxigenin-labeled rDNA gene probe. *Clin. Infect. Dis.* **15:**223–233.

101. **Laurent, F., A. Carlotti, P. Boiron, J. Villard, and J. Freney.** 1996. Ribotyping: a tool for taxonomy and identification of the *Nocardia asteroides* complex species. *J. Clin. Microbiol.* **34:**1079–1082.

102. **Laurent, F. J., F. Provost, and P. Boiron.** 1999. Rapid identification of clinically relevant *Nocardia* species to genus level by 16S rRNA gene PCR. *J. Clin. Microbiol.* **37:**99–102.

103. **Lechevalier, H. A., M. P. Lechevalier, and B. Becker.** 1966. Comparison of the chemical composition of cell walls of nocardiae with that of other aerobic actinomycetes. *Int. J. Syst. Bacteriol.* **16:**151–166.

104. **Lechevalier, M. P.** 1989. Actinomycetes with multilocular sporangia, p. 2405–2417. *In* S. T. Williams, M. E. Sharpe, and J. G. Holt (ed.), *Bergey's Manual of Systematic Bacteriology*, vol. 4. The Williams & Wilkins Co., Baltimore, Md.

105. **Lechevalier, M. P., H. Prauser, D. P. Labeda, and J. S. Ruan.** 1986. Two new genera of nocardioform actinomycetes: *Amycolata* gen. nov. and *Amycolatopsis* gen. nov. *Int. J. Syst. Bacteriol.* **36:**29–37.

106. **Lerner, P. I.** 1996. Nocardiosis. *Clin. Infect. Dis.* **22:**891–903.

107. **Lesens, O., Y. Hansmann, P. Riegel, R. Heller, M. Benaissa-Djellouli, M. Martinot, H. Petit, and D. Christmann.** 2000. Bacteremia and endocarditis caused by a *Gordonia* species in a patient with a central venous catheter. *Emerg. Infect. Dis.* **6:**382–385.

108. **Liegard, H., and M. Landrieu.** 1911. Un cas de mycose conjonctivale. *Ann. Ocul.* **146:**418–426.

109. **Linder, R.** 1997. *Rhodococcus equi* and *Arcanobacterium haemolyticum*: two "coryneform" bacteria increasingly recognized as agents of human infection. *Emerg. Infect. Dis.* **3:**145–153.

110. **Linos, A., A. Steinbuchel, C. Sproer, and R. M. Kroppenstedt.** 1999. *Gordonia polyisoprenivorans* sp. nov., a rubber-degrading actinomycete isolated from an automobile tyre. *Int. J. Syst. Bacteriol.* **49:**1785–1791.

111. **Louie, L., M. Louie, and A. E. Simor.** 1997. Investigation of a pseudo-outbreak of *Nocardia asteroides* infection by pulsed-field gel electrophoresis and randomly amplified polymorphic DNA PCR. *J. Clin. Microbiol.* **35:**1582–1584.

112. **Luna, J. G.** 1968. *Manual of Histologic Staining Methods of the Armed Forces Institute of Pathology*, 3rd ed., p. 217–218. McGraw-Hill Book Co., New York, N.Y.

113. **Maibach, R., F. Dutley, and M. Altwegg.** 1999. Detection of *Tropheryma whippelii* DNA in feces by PCR using a target capture method. *J. Microbiol. Methods* **38:**200.

114. **Maiwald, M., H. J. Ditton, A. von Herbay, F. A. Rainey, and E. Stackebrandt.** 1996. Reassessment of the phylogenetic position of the bacterium associated with Whipple's disease and determination of the 16S-23S ribosomal intergenic spacer sequence. *Int. J. Syst. Bacteriol.* **46:**1078–1082.

115. **Maiwald, M., and D. Relman.** 2001. Whipple's disease and *Tropheryma whippelii*: secrets slowly revealed. *Clin. Infect. Dis.* **32:**457–463.

116. **Maiwald, M., F. Schuhmacher, H. J. Ditton, and A. von Herbay.** 1998. Environmental occurrence of the Whipple's disease bacterium (*Tropheryma whippelii*). *Appl. Environ. Microbiol.* **64:**760–762.

117. **Maiwald, M., A. von Herbay, P. W. Lepp, and D. A. Relman.** 2000. Organization, structure, and variability of the rRNA operon of the Whipple's disease bacterium (*Tropheryma whippelii*). *J. Bacteriol.* **182:**3292–3297.

118. **Maldonado, L., J. V. Hookey, A. C. Ward, and M. Goodfellow.** 2000. The *Nocardia salmonicida* clade, including descriptions of *Nocardia cummidelens* sp. nov., *Nocardia fluminea* sp. nov. and *Nocardia soli* sp. nov. *Antonie Leeuwenhoek* **78:**367–377.

119. **Manchester, L., B. Pot, K. Kersters, and M. Goodfellow.** 1990. Classification of *Streptomyces* and *Streptoverticillium* species by numerical analysis of electrophoretic protein patterns. *Syst. Appl. Microbiol.* **13:**333–337.

120. **Marth, T., M. Neurath, B. A. Cuccherini, and W. Strober.** 1997. Defects of monocyte interleukin 12 production and humoral immunity in Whipple's disease. *Gastroenterology* **113:**442–448.

121. **Marth, T., and W. Strober.** 1996. Whipple's disease. *Semin. Gastrointest. Dis.* **7:**41–48.

122. **Martin, T., D. J. Hogan, F. Murphy, I. Natyshak, and E. P. Ewan.** 1991. *Rhodococcus* infection of the skin with lymphadenitis in a nonimmunocompromised girl. *J. Am. Acad. Dermatol.* **24:**328–332.

123. **Masters, A. M., T. M. Ellis, J. M. Carsons, S. S. Sutherland, and A. R. Gregory.** 1995. *Dermatophilus chelonae* sp. nov., isolated from chelonids in Australia. *Int. J. Syst. Bacteriol.* **45:**50–56.

124. **McClung, N. M.** 1960. Isolation of *Nocardia asteroides* from soils. *Mycologia* **52:**154–156.

125. **McMinn, E. J., G. Alderson, H. I. Dodson, M. Goodfellow, and A. C. Ward.** 2000. Genomic and phenomic differentiation of *Rhodococcus equi* and related strains. *Antonie Leeuwenhoek* **78:**331–340.

126. **McNabb, A., R. Shuttleworth, R. Behme, and W. D. Colby.** 1997. Fatty acid characterization of rapidly growing pathogenic aerobic actinomycetes as a means of identification. *J. Clin. Microbiol.* **35:**1361–1368.

127. **McNeil, M. M., and J. M. Brown.** 1994. The medically important aerobic actinomycetes: epidemiology and microbiology. *Clin. Microbiol. Rev.* **7:**357–417.

128. **McNeil, M. M., and J. M. Brown.** 1999. *Nocardia,* p. 310–323. *In* V. L. Yu, T. C. Merigan, and S. L. Barriere (ed.), *Antimicrobial Therapy and Vaccines.* The Williams & Wilkins Co., Baltimore, Md.

129. **McNeil, M. M., J. M. Brown, P. R. Georghiou, A. M. Allworth, and Z. M. Blacklock.** 1992. Infections due to *Nocardia transvalensis:* clinical spectrum and antimicrobial therapy. *Clin. Infect. Dis.* **15:**453–463.

130. **McNeil, M. M., J. M. Brown, W. R. Jarvis, and L. Ajello.** 1990. Comparison of species distribution and antimicrobial susceptibility of aerobic actinomycetes from clinical specimens. *Rev. Infect. Dis.* **12:**778–783.

131. **McNeil, M. M., J. M. Brown, C. H. Magruder, K. T. Shearlock, R. A. Saul, D. P. Allred, and L. Ajello.** 1992. Disseminated *Nocardia transvalensis* infection: an unusual opportunistic pathogen in severely immunocompromised patients. *J. Infect. Dis.* **165:**175–178.

132. **McNeil, M. M., J. M. Brown, G. Scalise, and C. Piersimoni.** 1992. Nonmycetomic *Actinomadura madurae* infection in a patient with AIDS. *J. Clin. Microbiol.* **30:**1008–1010.

133. **McNeil, M. M., S. Ray, P. E. Kozarsky, and J. M. Brown.** 1997. *Nocardia farcinica* pneumonia in a previously healthy woman: species characterization with use of a digoxigenin-labeled cDNA probe. *Clin. Infect. Dis.* **25:**933–934.

134. **Meyer, J.** 1976. *Nocardiopsis,* a new genus of the order *Actinomycetales. Int. J. Syst. Bacteriol.* **26:**487–493.

135. **Mikaelian, I., J. M. Lapointe, P. Labelle, R. Higgins, M. Paradis, and D. Martineau.** 2001. *Dermatophilus*-like infection in beluga whales, *Delphinapterus leucas,* from the St. Lawrence estuary. *Vet. Dermatol.* **12:**59–62.

136. **Misbah, S. A., and N. P. Mapstone.** 2000. Whipple's disease revisited. *J. Clin. Pathol.* **53:**50–55.

137. **Mishra, S. K., R. E. Gordon, and D. A. Barnett.** 1980. Identification of nocardiae and streptomycetes of medical importance. *J. Clin. Microbiol.* **11:**728–736.

138. **Morace, G., G. Dettori, M. Sanguinetti, S. Manzara, and L. Polonelli.** 1988. Biotyping of aerobic actinomycetes by modified killer system. *Eur. J. Epidemiol.* **4:**99–103.

139. **Morgenegg, S., F. Dutly, and M. Altwegg.** 2000. Cloning and sequencing of a part of the heat shock protein 65 gene (*hsp65*) of "*Tropheryma whippelii*" and its use for detection of "*T. whippelii*" in clinical specimens by PCR. *J. Clin. Microbiol.* **38:**2248–2253.

140. **Mossad, S. B., J. W. Tomford, R. Stewart, N. B. Ratliff, and G. S. Hall.** 1995. Case report of *Streptomyces* endocarditis of a prosthetic aortic valve. *J. Clin. Microbiol.* **33:**335–337.

141. **Muir, D. B., and R. C. Pritchard.** 1997. Use of bioMerieux ID 32C yeast identification system for identification of aerobic actinomycetes of medical importance. *J. Clin. Microbiol.* **35:**3240–3243.

142. **Murray, P. R., R. L. Heeren, and A. C. Niles.** 1987. Effect of decontamination procedures on recovery of *Nocardia* spp. *J. Clin. Microbiol.* **25:**2010–2011.

143. **Neumann, K., V. Neumann, S. Zierz, and R. Lahl.** 1997. Coinfection with *Tropheryma whippelii* and a Whipple's disease-associated bacterial organism detected in a patient with central nervous system Whipple's disease. *J. Clin. Microbiol.* **35:**1645.

144. **Nishiuchi, Y., T. Baba, and I. Yano.** 2000. Mycolic acids from *Rhodococcus, Gordonia,* and *Dietzia. J. Microbiol. Methods* **40:**1–9.

145. **Nishiuchi, Y., T. Baba, H. H. Hotta, and I. Yano.** 1999. Mycolic acid analysis in *Nocardia* species. The mycolic acid compositions of *Nocardia asteroides, N. farcinica,* and *N. nova. J. Microbiol. Methods* **37:**111–122.

146. **Nordmann, P.** 1995. Antimicrobial susceptibility of human isolates of *Rhodococcus equi. Med. Microbiol. Lett.* **4:**277–286.

147. **Ochi, K.** 1995. Phylogenetic analysis of mycolic acid-containing wall-chemotype IV actinomycetes and allied taxa by partial sequencing of ribosomal protein AT-L30. *Int. J. Syst. Bacteriol.* **45:**507–514.

148. **Orchard, V. A., and M. Goodfellow.** 1980. Numerical classification of some named strains of *Nocardia asteroides* and related isolates from soil. *J. Gen. Microbiol.* **118:**295–312.

149. **Osoagbaka, O. U.** 1989. Evidence for the pathogenic role of *Rhodococcus* species in pulmonary diseases. *J. Appl. Bacteriol.* **66:**497–506.

150. **Patterson, J. E., K. Chapin-Robertson, S. Waycott, P. Farrel, A. McGeer, M. M. McNeil, and S. C. Edberg.** 1992. Pseudoepidemic of *Nocardia asteroides* associated with a mycobacterial culture system. *J. Clin. Microbiol.* **30:**1357–1360.

151. **Pepys, J., P. A. Jenkins, G. N. Festenstein, P. H. Gregory, M. Lacey, and F. A. Skinner.** 1963. Thermophilic actinomycetes as a source of farmer's lung hay antigen. *Lancet* **ii:**607–611.

152. **Philip, A., and G. D. Roberts.** 1984. *Nocardiopsis dassonvillei* cellulitis of the arm. *Clin. Microbiol. Newsl.* **6:**14–15.

153. **Pier, A. C., and R. E. Fichtner.** 1981. Distribution of serotypes of *Nocardia asteroides* from animal, human, and environmental sources. *J. Clin. Microbiol.* **13:**548–553.

154. **Pittenger, R. C., and R. B. Brigham.** 1956. *Streptomyces orientalis* nov. sp., the source of vancomycin. *Antibiot. Chemother.* **6:**642–647.

155. **Prescott, J. F.** 1991. *Rhodococcus equi:* an animal and human pathogen. *Clin. Microbiol. Rev.* **4:**20–34.

156. **Pridham, T. G., C. W. Hesseltine, and R. G. Benedict.** 1958. A guide for the classification of streptomycetes according to selected groups. *Appl. Microbiol.* **6:**52–79.

157. **Prinz, G., E. Ban, S. Fekete, and Z. Szabo.** 1985. Meningitis caused by *Gordona aurantiaca* (*Rhodococcus aurantiacus*). *J. Clin. Microbiol.* **22:**472–474.

158. **Provost, F., L. Polonelli, S. Conti, P. Fisicaro, M. Gerloni, and P. Boiron.** 1995. Use of yeast killer system to identify species of the *Nocardia asteroides* complex. *J. Clin. Microbiol.* **33:**8–10.

159. **Rainey, F. A., J. Burghardt, R. M. Kroppenstedt, S. Klatte, and E. Stackebrandt.** 1995. Phylogenetic analysis of the genera *Rhodococcus* and *Nocardia* and evidence for the evolutionary origin of the genus *Nocardia* from within the radiation of *Rhodococcus* species. *Microbiology* **141:**523–528.

160. **Rainey, F. A., S. Klatte, R. M. Kroppenstedt, and E. Stackebrandt.** 1995. *Dietzia,* a new genus including *Dietzia maris* comb. nov., formerly *Rhodococcus maris. Int. J. Syst. Bacteriol.* **45:**32–36.

161. **Rainey, F. A., N. Ward-Rainey, R. M. Kroppenstedt, and E. Stackebrandt.** 1996. The genus *Nocardiopsis* represents a phylogenetically coherent taxon and a distinct actinomycete lineage: proposal of *Nocardiopsaceae* fam. nov. *Int. J. Syst. Bacteriol.* **46:**1088–1092.

162. **Ramzan, N. N., E. Loftus, Jr., L. J. Burgart, M. Rooney, K. P. Batts, R. H. Wiesner, D. N. Fredricks, D. A. Relman, and D. H. Persing.** 1997. Diagnosis and monitoring of Whipple disease by polymerase chain reaction. *Ann. Intern. Med.* **126:**520–527.

163. **Raoult, D., M. L. Birg, B. La Scola, P. E. Fournier, M. Enea, H. Lepidi, V. Roux, J. C. Piette, F. Vandenesch, D. Vital-Durand, and T. J. Marrie.** 2000. Cultivation of the bacillus of Whipple's disease. *N. Engl. J. Med.* **342:**620–625.

164. **Ratnaike, R. N.** 2000. Whipple's disease. *Postgrad. Med. J.* **76:**760–766.

165. **Relman, D. A.** 1997. Emerging infections and newly-recognised pathogens. *Neth. J. Med.* **50:**216–220.

166. **Relman, D. A., T. M. Schmidt, R. F. MacDermott, and S. Falkow.** 1992. Identification of the uncultured bacillus of Whipple's disease. *N. Engl. J. Med.* **327:**293–301.

167. **Rey, D., D. De Briel, R. Heller, P. Fraisse, M. Partisani, M. Leiva-Mena, and J. M. Lang.** 1995. *Tsukamurella* and HIV infection. *AIDS* **9:**1379.

168. **Richet, H. M., P. C. Craven, J. M. Brown, B. A. Lasker, C. Cox, M. M. McNeil, A. D. Tice, W. R. Jarvis, and O. C. Tablan.** 1991. A cluster of *Rhodococcus (Gordona) bronchialis* sternal-wound infections after coronary-artery bypass surgery. *N. Engl. J. Med.* **324:**104–109.

169. **Rickman, L. S., W. R. Freeman, W. R. Green, S. T. Feldman, J. Sullivan, V. Russack, and D. A. Relman.** 1995. Brief report: uveitis caused by *Tropheryma whippelii* (Whipple's bacillus). *N. Engl. J. Med.* **332:**363–366.

170. **Riegel, P., R. Ruimy, D. De Briel, F. Eichler, J. P. Bergerat, R. Christen, and H. Monteil.** 1996. Bacteremia due to *Gordona sputi* in an immunocompromised patient. *J. Clin. Microbiol.* **34:**2045–2047.

171. **Ruimy, R., P. Riegel, A. Carlotti, P. Boiron, G. Bernardin, H. Monteil, R. J. Wallace, Jr., and R. Christen.** 1996. *Nocardia pseudobrasiliensis* sp. nov., a new species of *Nocardia* which groups bacterial strains previously identified as *Nocardia brasiliensis* and associated with invasive diseases. *Int. J. Syst. Bacteriol.* **46:**259–264.

172. **Salinas-Carmona, M. C., M. A. Castro-Corona, J. Sepulveda-Saavedra, and L. I. Perez.** 1997. Monoclonal antibodies to P24 and P61 immunodominant antigens from *Nocardia brasiliensis. Clin. Diagn. Lab. Immunol.* **4:**133–137.

173. **Salinas-Carmona, M. C., O. Welsh, and S. M. Casillas.** 1993. Enzyme-linked immunosorbent assay for serological diagnosis of *Nocardia brasiliensis* and clinical correlation with mycetoma infections. *J. Clin. Microbiol.* **31:** 2901–2906.

174. **Schaal, K. P.** 1984. Laboratory diagnosis of actinomycete diseases, p. 441–456. *In* M. Goodfellow, M. Mordarski, and S. T. Williams (ed.), *The Biology of the Actinomycetes.* Academic Press, Ltd., London, United Kingdom.

175. **Schaal, K. P.** 1991. Medical and microbiological problems arising from airborne infection in hospitals. *J. Hosp. Infect.* **18:**451–459.

176. **Schaal, K. P., and H. J. Lee.** 1992. Actinomycete infections in humans—a review. *Gene* **15:**201–211.

177. **Schiff, T. A., M. M. McNeil, and J. M. Brown.** 1993. Cutaneous *Nocardia farcinica* infection in a nonimmunocompromised patient: case report and review. *Clin. Infect. Dis.* **16:**756–760.

178. **Schiff, T. A., M. Sanchez, J. Moy, D. Klirsfeld, M. M. McNeil, and J. M. Brown.** 1993. Cutaneous nocardiosis caused by *Nocardia nova* occurring in an HIV-infected individual: a case report and review of the literature. *J. Acquir. Immune Defic. Syndr.* **6:**849–851.

179. **Schoedon, G., D. Goldenberger, R. Forrer, A. Gunz, F. Dutly, M. Hochli, M. Altwegg, and A. Schaffner.** 1997. Deactivation of macrophages with interleukin-4 is the key to the isolation of *Tropheryma whippelii. J. Infect. Dis.* **176:**672–677.

180. **Scopetti, F., E. Iona, L. Fattorini, A. Goglio, N. Franceschini, G. Amicosante, and G. Orefici.** 1994. Activity of antimicrobial drugs evaluated by agar dilution and radiometric methods against strains of *Nocardia asteroides* isolated in Italy from immunocompromised patients. *J. Chemother.* **6:**29–34.

181. **Scott, M. A., B. S. Graham, R. Verrall, R. Dixon, W. Schaffner, and K. T. Tham.** 1995. *Rhodococcus equi*—an increasingly recognized opportunistic pathogen. Report of 12 cases and review of 65 cases in the literature. *Am. J. Clin. Pathol.* **103:**649–655.

182. **Shanley, J. D., K. Synder, and J. S. Child.** 1979. Chronic pericarditis due to *Streptomyces* species. *Am. J. Clin. Pathol.* **72:**107–110.

183. **Shapiro, C. L., R. F. Haft, N. M. Gantz, G. V. Doern, J. C. Christenson, R. O'Brien, J. C. Overall, B. A. Brown, and R. J. J. Wallace.** 1992. *Tsukamurella paurometabolum:* a novel pathogen causing catheter-related bacteremia in patients with cancer. *Clin. Infect. Dis.* **14:**200–203.

184. **Sindhuphak, W., E. MacDonald, and E. Head.** 1985. Actinomycetoma caused by *Nocardiopsis dassonvillei. Arch. Dermatol.* **121:**1332–1334.

185. **Slack, J. M., and M. A. Gerencser.** 1975. Actinomyces, *Filamentous Bacteria.* Burgess Publishing Co., Minneapolis, Minn.

186. **Smego, R. A., Jr., and H. A. Gallis.** 1984. The clinical spectrum of *Nocardia brasiliensis* infection in the United States. *Rev. Infect. Dis.* **6:**164–180.

187. **Stackebrandt, E., F. A. Rainey, and N. L. Ward-Rainey.** 1997. Proposal for a new hierarchic classification system, *Actinobacteria* classis nov. *Int. J. Syst. Bacteriol.* **47:**479–491.

188. **Stackebrandt, E., J. Smida, and M. Collins.** 1988. Evidence of phylogenetic heterogeneity within the genus *Rhodococcus:* revival of the genus *Gordona* (Tsukamura). *J. Gen. Microbiol.* **35:**364–368.

189. **Staneck, J. L., and G. D. Roberts.** 1974. Simplified approach to identification of aerobic actinomycetes by thin-layer chromatography. *Appl. Microbiol.* **28:**226–231.

190. **Steingrube, V. A., B. A. Brown, J. L. Gibson, R. W. Wilson, J. Brown, Z. Blacklock, K. Jost, S. Locke, R. F. Ulrich, and R. J. Wallace, Jr.** 1995. DNA amplification and restriction endonuclease analysis for differentiation of 12 species and taxa of *Nocardia,* including recognition of four new taxa within the *Nocardia asteroides* complex. *J. Clin. Microbiol.* **33:**3096–3101.

191. **Steingrube, V. A., R. J. Wallace, Jr., B. A. Brown, Y. Pang, B. Zeluff, L. C. Steele, and Y. Zhang.** 1991. Acquired resistance of *Nocardia brasiliensis* to clavulanic acid related to a change in beta-lactamase following therapy with amoxicillin-clavulanic acid. *Antimicrob. Agents Chemother.* **35:**524–528.

192. **Steingrube, V. A., R. W. Wilson, B. A. Brown, K. C. Jost, Jr., Z. Blacklock, J. L. Gibson, and R. J. Wallace, Jr.** 1997. Rapid identification of clinically significant species and taxa of aerobic actinomycetes, including *Actinomadura, Gordona, Nocardia, Rhodococcus, Streptomyces,* and *Tsukamurella* isolates, by DNA amplification and restriction endonuclease analysis. *J. Clin. Microbiol.* **35:** 817–822.

193. **Stoecker, M. A., R. P. Herwig, and J. T. Staley.** 1994. *Rhodococcus zopfii* sp. nov., a toxicant-degrading bacterium. *Int. J. Syst. Bacteriol.* **44:**106–110.

194. **Street, S., H. D. Donoghue, and G. H. Neild.** 1999. *Tropheryma whippelii* DNA in saliva of healthy people. *Lancet* **354:**1178–1179.

195. **Sutor, G. C., C. Fibich, P. Kirscher, M. Kuske, R. E. Schmidt, I. Schedel, and H. Deicher.** 1996. Poststenotic cavitating pneumonia due to *Rhodococcus equi* in HIV infection. *AIDS* **10:**339–340.

196. **Takeuchi, M., and K. Hatano.** 1998. *Gordonia rhizosphera* sp. nov. isolated from the mangrove rhizosphere. *Int. J. Syst. Bacteriol.* **48:**907–912.

197. **Telzak, E. E., J. Hii, B. Polsky, T. E. Kiehn, and D. Armstrong.** 1989. *Nocardia* infection in the acquired immunodeficiency syndrome. *Diagn. Microbiol. Infect. Dis.* **12:**517–519.

198. **Torres, O. H., P. Domingo, R. Pericas, P. Boiron, J. A. Montiel, and G. Vazquez.** 2000. Infection caused by *Nocardia farcinica:* case report and review. *Eur. J. Clin. Microbiol. Infect. Dis.* **19:**205–212.

199. **Towersey, L., E. D. Martins, A. T. Londero, R. J. Hay, P. J. Soares Filho, C. M. Takiya, C. C. Martins, and O. F. Gompertz.** 1993. *Dermatophilus congolensis* human infection. *J. Am. Acad. Dermatol.* **29:**351–354.

200. **Trujillo, M. E., and M. Goodfellow.** 1997. Polyphasic taxonomic study of clinically significant actinomadurae including the description of *Actinomadura latina* sp. nov. *Zentbl. Bakteriol.* **285:**212–233.

201. **Tsukamura, M.** 1978. Numerical classification of *Rhodococcus* (formerly *Gordona*) organisms recently isolated from sputa of patients: description of *Rhodococcus sputi* Tsukamura sp. nov. *Int. J. Syst. Bacteriol.* **28:**169–181.

202. **Tsukamura, M., K. Hikosaka, K. Nishimura, and S. Hara.** 1988. Severe progressive subcutaneous abscesses and necrotizing tenosynovitis caused by *Rhodococcus aurantiacus. J. Clin. Microbiol.* **26:**201–205.

203. **Tsukamura, M., and S. Mizuno.** 1971. A new species *Gordona aurantiaca* occurring in sputa of patients with pulmonary disease. *Kekkaku* **46:**93–98.

204. **Unsworth, B. A., and T. Cross.** 1980. Thermophilic actinomycetes implicated in farmer's lung; numerical taxonomy of *Thermoactinomyces* species, p. 389–390. *In* M. Goodfellow and R. G. Broad (ed.), *Microbiological Classification and Identification.* Academic Press, Ltd., London, United Kingdom.

205. **Vannier, A. M., B. H. Ackerman, and L. F. Hutchins.** 1992. Disseminated *Nocardia asteroides* diagnosed by blood culture in a patient with disseminated histoplasmosis. *Arch. Pathol. Lab. Med.* **4:**537–539.

206. **Van Saceghem, R.** 1915. Dermatose contagieuse (impetigo contagieux). *Bull. Soc. Pathol. Exot. Fil.* **8:**354–359.

207. **Verville, T. D., M. M. Huycke, R. A. Greenfield, D. P. Fine, T. L. Kuhls, and L. N. Slater.** 1994. *Rhodococcus equi* infections of humans. 12 cases and a review of the literature. *Medicine* **73:**119–132.

208. **Vickers, R. M., J. D. Rihs, and V. L. Yu.** 1992. Clinical demonstration of isolation of *Nocardia asteroides* on buffered charcoal-yeast extract media. *J. Clin. Microbiol.* **30:**227–228.

209. **Vincent, M. H.** 1894. Etude sur le parasite du "pied de madura." *Ann. Inst. Pasteur* **8:**129–151.

210. **von Graevenitz, A., and V. Punter-Streit.** 1995. Development of a new selective plating medium for *Rhodococcus equi. Microbiol. Immunol.* **39:**283–284.

211. **Vullo, V., C. M. Mastroianni, M. Lichtner, F. Mengoni, E. Chiappini, C. D'Agostino, and S. Delia.** 1996. Serologic responses to *Rhodococcus equi* in individuals with and without human immunodeficiency virus infection. *Eur. J. Clin. Microbiol. Infect. Dis.* **15:**588–594.

212. **Wallace, R. J., Jr., B. A. Brown, Z. Blacklock, R. Ulrich, K. Jost, J. M. Brown, M. M. McNeil, G. Onyi, V. A. Steingrube, and J. Gibson.** 1995. New *Nocardia* taxon among isolates of *Nocardia brasiliensis* associated with invasive disease. *J. Clin. Microbiol.* **33:**1528–1533.

213. **Wallace, R. J., Jr., B. A. Brown, M. Tsukamura, J. M. Brown, and G. O. Onyi.** 1991. Clinical and laboratory features of *Nocardia nova. J. Clin. Microbiol.* **29:**2407–2411.

214. **Wallace, R. J., Jr., E. J. Septimus, D. M. Musher, and R. R. Martin.** 1977. Disk diffusion susceptibility testing of *Nocardia* species. *J. Infect. Dis.* **35:**568–576.

215. **Wallace, R. J., Jr., and L. C. Steele.** 1988. Susceptibility testing of *Nocardia* species for the clinical laboratory. *Diagn. Microbiol. Infect. Dis.* **9:**155–166.

216. **Wallace, R. J., Jr., L. C. Steele, G. Sumter, and J. M. Smith.** 1988. Antimicrobial susceptibility patterns of *Nocardia asteroides. Antimicrob. Agents Chemother.* **32:**1776–1779.

217. **Wallace, R. J., Jr., M. Tsukamura, B. A. Brown, J. Brown, V. A. Steingrube, Y. S. Zhang, and D. R. Nash.** 1990. Cefotaxime-resistant *Nocardia asteroides* strains are isolates of the controversial species *Nocardia farcinica. J. Clin. Microbiol.* **28:**2726–2732.

218. **Wenger, P. N., J. M. Brown, M. M. McNeil, and W. R. Jarvis.** 1998. *Nocardia farcinica* sternotomy site infections in patients following open heart surgery. *J. Infect. Dis.* **178:**1539–1543.

219. **Whipple, G. H.** 1907. A hitherto undescribed disease characterized anatomically by deposits of fat and fatty acids in the intestinal and mesenteric lymphatic tissues. *Johns Hopkins Hosp. Bull.* **18:**382–391.

220. **Williams, S. T., M. Goodfellow, and G. Alderson.** 1989. Genus *Streptomyces* Waksman and Henrici 1943, 339[AL], p. 2453–2492. *In* S. T. Williams, M. E. Sharpe, and J. G. Holt (ed.), *Bergey's Manual of Systematic Bacteriology*, vol. 4. The Williams & Wilkins, Co., Baltimore, Md.

221. **Williams, S. T., G. P. Sharples, and R. M. Bradshaw.** 1974. Spore formation in *Actinomadura dassonvillei* (Brocq-Rousseau) Lechevalier and Lechevalier. *J. Gen. Microbiol.* **84:**415–419.

222. **Wilson, J. P., H. R. Turner, K. A. Kirchner, and S. W. Chapman.** 1989. Nocardial infections in renal transplant recipients. *Medicine* **68:**38–57.

223. **Wilson, K. H., R. Blitchington, R. Frothingham, and J. A. Wilson.** 1991. Phylogeny of the Whipple's-disease-associated bacterium. *Lancet* **338:**474–475.

224. **Wilson, R. W., V. A. Steingrube, B. A. Brown, Z. Blacklock, K. C. Jost, A. McNabb, W. D. Colby, J. R. Biehle, J. L. Gibson, and R. W. Wallace, Jr.** 1997. Recognition of a *Nocardia transvalensis* complex by resistance ot aminoglycosides, including amikacin, and PCR-restriction fragment length polymorphism analysis. *J. Clin. Microbiol.* **35:**2235–2242.

225. **Wilson, R. W., V. A. Steingrube, B. A. Brown, and R. J. Wallace, Jr.** 1998. Clinical application of PCR-restriction enzyme pattern analysis for rapid identification of aerobic actinomycete isolates. *J. Clin. Microbiol.* **36:**148–152.

226. **Witt, D., and E. Stackebrandt.** 1990. Unification of the genera *Streptoverticillium* and *Streptomyces*, and amendation of *Streptomyces* Waksman and Henrici 1943[AL]. *Syst. Appl. Microbiol.* **13:**361–371.

227. **Woodger, A. J., M. Baxter, F. M. Rush-Munro, J. Brown, and W. Kaplan.** 1985. Isolation of *Dermatophilus congolensis* from two New Zealand cases of pitted keratolysis. *Australas. J. Dermatol.* **26:**29–35.

228. **Woods, G. L., B. A. Brown-Elliott, E. P. Desmond, G. S. Hall, L. Heifets, G. E. Pfyffer, M. R. Plaunt, J. C. Ridderhof, R. J. Wallace, Jr., N. G. Warren, and F. G. Witebsky.** 2001. *Susceptibility Testing of Mycobacteria, Nocardia, and Other Actinomycetes.* Tentative standard, 2nd ed. NCCLS 20 (26); M24-T2. NCCLS, Wayne, Pa.

229. **Wust, J., H. Lanzendorfer, A. von Graevenitz, H. J. Gloor, and B. Schmid.** 1990. Peritonitis caused by *Actinomadura madurae* in a patient on CAPD. *Eur. J. Clin. Microbiol. Infect. Dis.* **9:**700–701.

230. **Yassin, A. F., E. A. Galinski, A. Wohlfarth, K. Jahnke, K. P. Schaal, and H. G. Truper.** 1993. A new actinomycete species. *Nocardiopsis lucentensis* sp. nov. *Int. J. Syst. Bacteriol.* **43:**266–271.

231. **Yassin, A. F., F. A. Rainey, H. Brzezinka, J. Burghardt, H. J. Lee, and K. P. Schaal.** 1995. *Tsukamurella inchonensis* sp. nov. *Int. J. Syst. Bacteriol.* **45:**522–527.

232. **Yassin, A. F., F. A. Rainey, H. Brzezinka, J. Burghardt, M. Rifai, P. Seifert, K. Feldmann, and K. P. Schaal.** 1996. *Tsukamurella pulmonis* sp. nov. *Int. J. Syst. Bacteriol.* **46:**429–436.

233. **Yassin, A. F., F. A. Rainey, J. Burghardt, H. Brzezinka, M. Mauch, and K. P. Schaal.** 2000. *Nocardia paucivorans* sp. nov. *Int. J. Syst. Evol. Microbiol.* **50:**803–809.

234. **Yassin, A. F., F. A. Rainey, J. Burghardt, H. Brzezinka, S. Schmitt, P. Seifert, O. Zimmermann, H. Mauch, D. Gierth, I. Lux, and K. P. Schaal.** 1997. *Tsukamurella tyrosinosolvens* sp. nov. *Int. J. Syst. Bacteriol.* **47:**607–614.

235. **Yassin, A. F., F. A. Rainey, J. Burghardt, D. Gierth, J. Ungerechts, I. Lux, P. Seifert, C. Bal, and K. P. Schaal.** 1997. Description of *Nocardiopsis synnemataformans* sp. nov., elevation of *Nocardiopsis alba* subsp. *prasina* to *Nocardiopsis prasina* comb. nov., and designation of *Nocardiopsis antarctica* and *Nocardiopsis alborubida* as later subjective synonyms of *Nocardiopsis dassonvillei*. *Int. J. Syst. Bacteriol.* **47:**983–988.

236. **Yassin, A. F., F. A. Rainey, U. Mendrock, H. Brzezinka, and K. P. Schaal.** 2000. *Nocardia abscessus* sp. nov. *Int. J. Syst. Evol. Microbiol.* **50:**1487–1493.

237. **Yeruham, I., A. Hadani, and D. Elad.** 1991. Human dermatophilosis *Dermatophilus congolensis* in dairymen in Israel. *Isr. J. Vet. Med.* **46:**114–116.

238. **Zaria, L. T.** 1993. *Dermatophilus congolensis* infection (dermatophilosis) in animals and man. An update. *Comp. Immunol. Microbiol. Infect. Dis.* **16:**179–222.

239. **Zbinden, R., A. Zimmerman, and P. Boiron.** 1995. *Streptomyces* spp. as a cause of a wound infection. *Clin. Microbiol. Newsl.* **17:**167–168.

Mycobacterium: General Characteristics, Isolation, and Staining Procedures*

GABY E. PFYFFER, BARBARA A. BROWN-ELLIOTT,
AND RICHARD J. WALLACE, JR.

36

Many species within the genus *Mycobacterium* are prominent pathogens, e.g., the members of *Mycobacterium tuberculosis* complex and *M. leprae*. In addition, numerous species of environmental mycobacteria called nontuberculous mycobacteria (NTM) (formerly "atypical mycobacteria" or "mycobacteria other than tubercle bacilli") are responsible for various kinds of mycobacterioses.

Tuberculosis remains a major global public health problem. In 1997, there were 8 million estimated new cases including 3.5 million cases of smear-positive (and hence highly infectious) pulmonary tuberculosis. Nearly 2 million people died of tuberculosis, with a global case fatality rate of 23% but reaching >50% in some African countries due to high rates of coexisting human immunodeficiency virus (HIV) infection. The actual global prevalence of *M. tuberculosis* infection is 32%, corresponding to approximately 1.9 billion people (46). If control of tuberculosis is not further strengthened in the future, the World Health Organization (WHO) estimates that between 2000 and 2020, nearly one billion people will be newly infected, 200 million people will become sick, and another 35 million people will die from tuberculosis (209).

On the other hand, between 1953 and 1985, the number of cases reported annually in the United States dropped by 74% from 84,304 to 22,201. Subsequently, the downward trend stopped. Factors facilitating the resurgence of tuberculosis in the United States included (i) the advent of the AIDS epidemic, (ii) immigration from high-prevalence countries, (iii) transmission in high-risk settings (e.g., hospitals and prisons), and (iv) the coincident increase in the number of cases of multidrug-resistant tuberculosis. Since 1992, the number of reported cases has again decreased (case rate, 6.8/100,000), reflecting the effectiveness of prevention strategies and control measures implemented by the health authorities, including the use of more rapid and efficient laboratory algorithms to detect *M. tuberculosis* and susceptibility testing against antituberculosis drugs. In this context, the clinical mycobacteriology laboratory plays an important role (70).

With the advent of new laboratory techniques, new NTM species are being discovered, some of which are sources of diseases in humans. Rapid and reliable identification of NTM is thus mandatory but is becoming increasingly complex. The level of service and the choice of methods should be determined by the patient population served by the laboratory and by the resources available.

TAXONOMY AND DESCRIPTION OF THE GENUS

The genus *Mycobacterium* is the only genus in the family *Mycobacteriaceae* (198) and is related to other mycolic acid-containing genera. The high G+C content of the DNA of *Mycobacterium* species (61 to 71 mol%, except for *M. leprae* [55%]) (60) is within the range of those of the other mycolic acid-containing genera, *Gordonia* (63 to 69 mol%), *Tsukamurella* (68 to 74 mol%), *Nocardia* (64 to 72 mol%), and *Rhodococcus* (63 to 73 mol%) (61).

Mycobacteria are aerobic (although some species are able to grow under a reduced-O_2 atmosphere), non-spore-forming, nonmotile, slightly curved or straight rods, measuring 0.2 to 0.6 μm by 1.0 to 10 μm, which may branch. Colony morphology varies among the species, ranging from smooth to rough and from nonpigmented (nonphotochromogens) to pigmented. Colonies of the latter are regularly or variably yellow, orange, or, rarely, pink, usually due to carotenoid pigments. Some species require light to form pigment (photochromogens), while other species form pigment in either the light or the dark (scotochromogens). Aerial filaments are very rarely formed and are never visible without magnification. Filamentous or mycelium-like growth sometimes occurs but, on slight disturbance, easily fragments into rods or coccoid elements (60).

The cell wall peptidoglycolipid contains *meso*-diaminopimelic acid, alanine, glutamic acid, glucosamine, muramic acid, arabinose, and galactose. Mycolic acids (number of carbon atoms ranging from 60 to 90), together with free lipids (e.g., trehalose-6,6′-dimycolate), provide a hydrophobic permeability barrier (18, 22). Other important fatty acids are waxes, phospholipids, mycoserosic, and phthienoic acids. Various patterns of cellular fatty acids (number of carbon atoms ranging from 10 to 20) are found as well, including tuberculostearic (10-*R*-methyloctadecanoic) acid, a

* This chapter contains information presented in chapter 25 by Beverly G. Metchock, Frederick S. Nolte, and Richard J. Wallace, Jr., in the seventh edition of this Manual.

unique cell component for a number of members of the *Actinomycetales* (18).

The high content of complex lipids of the cell wall prevents access by common aniline dyes. Although not readily stained by Gram's method, mycobacteria are usually considered gram positive. They may appear as clear zones or "ghosts" in Gram-stained smears. Once stained with special procedures, however, mycobacteria are not easily decolorized, even with acid-alcohol; i.e., they are acid-fast. However, acid fastness can be partly or completely lost at some stage of growth by a proportion of the cells of some species, particularly the rapidly growing ones.

A natural division exists between slowly and rapidly growing species of mycobacteria. Slow growers require more than 7 days to produce colonies on solid media from a dilute inoculum under ideal culture conditions. Rapid growers, by definition, require less than 7 days when subcultured on Löwenstein-Jensen (L-J) medium but may also take several weeks to appear on primary culture from clinical specimens.

NUTRITIONAL REQUIREMENTS AND GROWTH

Most species adapt readily to growth on relatively simple substrates, using ammonia or amino acids as nitrogen sources and glycerol as a carbon source in the presence of mineral salts. A few species (e.g., M. *genavense* and M. *haemophilum*) are fastidious and require supplements such as mycobactin, hemin, or other iron compounds. To date, M. *leprae* has not been cultured outside living cells. Growth of mycobacteria is stimulated by carbon dioxide and by fatty acids, which may be provided in the form of egg yolk or oleic acid, even though the latter is toxic in higher concentrations ($\geq$1%) and has to be neutralized by albumin. Optimum temperatures for growth vary widely among species (from <30 to 45°C). Compared to other bacteria, growth of most mycobacterial species is slow, with generation times up to approximately 20 h on commonly used media. Depending on the species, visible colonies may appear after a few days to 6 weeks of incubation under optimum conditions.

SUSCEPTIBILITY TO PHYSICAL AND CHEMICAL AGENTS

Mycobacteria are able to survive for weeks to months on inanimate objects if protected from sunlight. M. *tuberculosis* complex, for instance, survives for several months on surfaces or in soil or cow dung, from which other animals may be infected (111). Mycobacteria are easily killed by heat (>65°C for at least 30 min) and by UV (sun) light but not by freezing or desiccation. They are more resistant to acids, alkalis, and some chemical disinfectants than are most other non-spore-forming bacteria. Malachite green, quaternary ammonium compounds, hexachlorophene, and chlorhexidine are bacteriostatic at best. Other commonly used sterilants, such as ethylene oxide and formaldehyde vapor, as well as disinfectants such as chlorine compounds, 70% ethanol, 2% alkaline glutaraldehyde, peracetic acid, and stabilized hydrogen peroxide are effective in killing M. *tuberculosis*. However, agents that are inactivated in the presence of organic matter (e.g., alcohols) cannot be relied on to disinfect sputum and other protein-containing materials. With iodophors, the bactericidal effect depends on the content of available iodine as well as on the presence of organic matter (19).

HABITATS

The genus *Mycobacterium* includes obligate pathogens, opportunistic pathogens, and saprophytes. M. *tuberculosis* complex and M. *leprae* are incapable of replication in the inanimate environment; their major ecological niche is tissues of humans and warm-blooded animals. In contrast, the NTM are free-living mycobacteria and are usually found in association with watery habitats such as lakes, rivers, and wet soil. Some human pathogenic NTM species, however, have yet to be recovered from soil or water, e.g., M. *ulcerans*, M. *haemophilum*, M. *asiaticum*, M. *shimoidei*, and M. *szulgai* (6). Some other NTM species have been recovered only rarely from natural waters or soils but readily from tap water in settings where disease due to NTM was frequent or cultures from clinical specimens were often positive. Examples are M. *kansasii*, M. *xenopi*, M. *malmoense*, and M. *simiae* (6). M. *avium* complex, M. *gordonae*, M. *fortuitum*, M. *chelonae*, M. *abscessus*, M. *peregrinum*, M. *mucogenicum*, and M. *genavense* have been recovered from tap water and also occur in nosocomial disease or pseudo-outbreaks (6, 80, 187). Although not components of the normal bacterial flora of humans or animals, NTM may be isolated from the skin, upper respiratory tract, intestinal tract, and genital tract in asymptomatic individuals (49). Due to their ubiquitous nature, the question of their clinical significance is therefore important but is not always easy to answer (6).

Well-known sources of positive cultures are bronchoscopes and related devices. Organisms isolated were M. *tuberculosis* (2), M. *xenopi* (16), M. *chelonae* (58), and other NTM.

CLINICAL SIGNIFICANCE AND DESCRIPTION OF SPECIES

With the advent of better biochemical and molecular techniques for culture and identification, close to 100 mycobacterial species have now been described.

M. tuberculosis Complex

M. *tuberculosis* complex includes M. *tuberculosis*, M. *bovis* (including M. *bovis* BCG), M. *africanum*, M. *microti*, and M. *canettii*, which form a tight, discrete group of organisms that display >95% DNA-DNA homology. Recent comparative genomics using the complete DNA sequence of M. *tuberculosis* has provided information on regions of the genome that are deleted in other members of the complex (62). Identification to the species level is justified for epidemiologic, public health, and therapeutic reasons.

Mycobacterium tuberculosis

In the industrialized world, a higher prevalence of tuberculosis occurs in the medically underserved ethnic minorities, the urban poor, homeless persons, prison inmates, alcoholics, intravenous drug users, the elderly in general, foreign-born persons from areas of high prevalence, and contacts of persons with active tuberculosis. Today, HIV infection is the greatest known risk factor for progression of latent infection to active tuberculosis. Combined HIV and tuberculosis infections, especially in combination with drug resistance, have caused outbreaks with extremely high mortality rates (30, 31). Groups with a higher likelihood of progression also include individuals with underlying medical conditions, persons who have been infected within the past 2 years, children $\leq$4 years old, and persons with fibrotic and cancerous lesions on chest radiographs.

M. *tuberculosis* is carried in airborne particles (droplet nuclei) generated when patients with pulmonary tuberculosis cough. These particles, 1 to 5 μm in size, are kept "suspended" by normal air currents. Infection occurs when a susceptible person inhales the droplet nuclei. Once in the alveoli, the organisms are engulfed by alveolar macrophages. Usually, the host cell-mediated immune response limits the multiplication and spread of M. *tuberculosis*. However, some bacilli can remain viable but dormant for many years after the initial infection. Patients latently infected with M. *tuberculosis* usually have a positive purified protein derivative (PPD) skin test but are asymptomatic and not infectious. In general, persons with a latent infection have a 10% risk during their lifetime for development of active tuberculosis. By contrast, patients with HIV infection have a 10 to 15% risk per year for progression to manifest disease (4).

Tuberculosis in adults is a slowly progressive process characterized by chronic inflammation and caseation and by formation of cavities. These foci may rupture into the bronchi, allowing very large numbers of organisms to spread to other areas of the lungs and to be aerosolized by coughing, hence infecting other persons. The clinical features of pulmonary tuberculosis are cough, weight loss, night sweat, low-grade fever, dyspnea, and chest pain. Extrapulmonary manifestations of M. *tuberculosis* infection include cervical lymphadenitis, pleuritis, pericarditis, synovitis, meningitis, and infections of the skin, joints, bones, and internal organs. With respect to the ordinary clinical picture of tuberculosis, pulmonary disease in AIDS patients often differs in radiologic findings, is usually more rapidly progressive, and disseminates more frequently, sometimes even without the formation of granulomas.

In culture, colonies of M. *tuberculosis* are off-white and rough on solid medium (Fig. 1), although on moist media they may tend to be smoother. In addition to the classical M. *tuberculosis*, there exists an Asian variant, which is susceptible to thiophene-2-carboxylic acid hydrazide. In

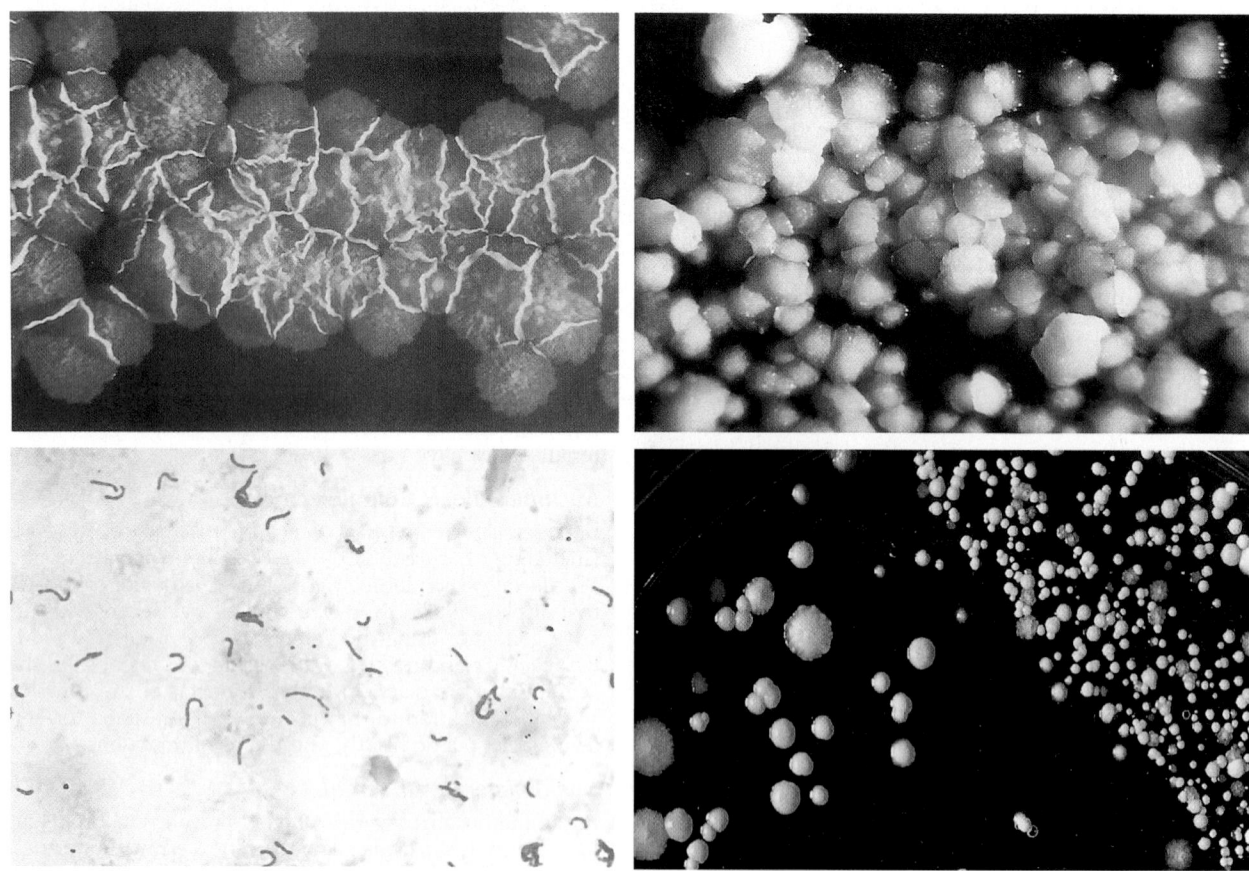

FIGURE 1 (top left) *Mycobacterium tuberculosis* on Middlebrook 7H10 agar. Note the dry and rough colonies, sometimes with a nodular or wrinkled surface.

FIGURE 2 (top right) *Mycobacterium bovis* BCG on Middlebrook 7H10 agar. Colonies may be flat as well as round with irregular edges.

FIGURE 3 (bottom left) Acid-fast staining (Ziehl-Neelsen) of *Mycobacterium microti*. Note the characteristic curved ("croissant-like") microscopic morphology. (Photograph kindly provided by D. van Soolingen.)

FIGURE 4 (bottom right) *Mycobacterium canettii* on Middlebrook 7H10 agar. Note the heterogeneous colony morphology consisting of some flat and smooth but predominantly domed and glossy colonies. (Photograph kindly provided by D. van Soolingen.)

contrast to M. *tuberculosis*, these strains often contain a few to none IS*6110* elements in their genome (see chapter 37). Another subspecies of M. *tuberculosis* isolated from goats has recently been characterized by molecular techniques as M. *tuberculosis* subsp. *caprae* (7).

M. bovis

M. *bovis* causes tuberculosis in warm-blooded animals such as cattle, dogs, cats, pigs, parrots, badgers, and some birds of prey, but also in primates and humans. Human disease is very similar to that caused by M. *tuberculosis* and is treated accordingly, except that pyrazinamide is inefficient due to the inherent resistance of most M. *bovis* strains against that drug. The organism grows poorly on L-J medium, but growth is stimulated if glycerol is replaced by pyruvate. In contrast to most members of M. *tuberculosis* complex, M. *bovis* is able to grow in a reduced-O_2 atmosphere. Colonies on egg-based media are small and rounded, with irregular edges and a granular surface; on agar media colonies are small and flat (198).

M. bovis BCG

In many parts of the world, bacillus Calmette-Guérin (BCG) is still used for vaccine purposes. It was distributed by Calmette in 1924 to laboratories around the world and has been maintained in vitro by serial passages. Today, there exists a genetically heterogeneous conglomerate of BCG strains (Fig. 2) (15, 165) which predominantly conform to the properties described for M. *bovis* except that they are more attenuated in virulence. In rare instances, BCG may disseminate as a complication of intravesical BCG immunostimulation against bladder cancer (1).

M. africanum

M. *africanum* is a cause of human tuberculosis in tropical Africa (13). Its colonies resemble those of M. *tuberculosis*, and its physiological and biochemical properties position it between M. *tuberculosis* and M. *bovis* (66). The definition of M. *africanum* is not simple, and its validity is questioned by some authors. However, recent genotypic analyses based on variable numbers of tandem repeats and other molecular characteristics have set M. *africanum* apart from other members of the M. *tuberculosis* complex (55, 185).

M. microti

Originally isolated from rodents such as voles and shrews, M. *microti* causes naturally acquired tuberculosis in guinea pigs, rabbits, llamas, cats, and other warm-blooded animals. It has recently been identified as a causative agent of tuberculosis in both immunocompetent and immunosuppressed humans (183). Usually revealing a characteristic, "croissant-like" morphology in stained smears (Fig. 3), the organism normally fails to grow in culture. At least the vole type of M. *microti* can easily be recognized upon spacer oligotyping (see chapter 37), since it contains an exceptionally short genomic direct repeat region, resulting in identical two-spacer sequence reactions (183).

M. canettii

The youngest member of the M. *tuberculosis* complex was described by Canetti in 1969 and in the late 1990s by van Soolingen et al. (184) and Pfyffer et al. (126). In the last two reports, it was the etiological agent of lymphadenitis in a child and of generalized tuberculosis in an HIV-positive patient, respectively. Its natural reservoir is unknown. The facts that both patients were exposed in Africa and that five more cases of cervical lymphadenitis have been reported from Djibouti (P. Gérome, J. L. Koeck, T. Bernatas, M. Fabre, V. Hervé, A. Varnerot, and V. Vincent, *Abstr. 21st Annu. Congr. Eur. Soc. Mycobacteriol.*, abstr. OTu 24, 2000), support the hypothesis that M. *canettii* might be more abundant on the African continent. With its smooth, round, and glossy colonies (Fig. 4), it differs considerably from all other members of the M. *tuberculosis* complex and can even be mistaken for an NTM.

M. leprae

Estimates from the WHO put the global prevalence of leprosy (Hansen's disease) at 11 million persons, with the majority of cases occurring in South and Southeast Asia, Africa, and Latin America (181, 208). In the past centuries, leprosy also occurred on a large scale in Europe. Even though the disease has remained endemic in small pockets in the United States (Texas, California, Louisiana, Hawaii, and Puerto Rico) (106), the majority of infections now seen in North America have been acquired abroad. These imported cases appear to present a negligible risk for transmission within the United States.

Leprosy is a chronic, granulomatous, and debilitating disease (75). Its principal manifestations include anesthetic skin lesions and peripheral neuropathy with nerve thickening. It illustrates a continuous spectrum of disease with very few demonstrable bacilli (tuberculoid leprosy) to a progressive, widespread form of the disease with massive numbers of organisms due to the absence of cell-mediated immunity (lepromatous leprosy). The majority of leprosy patients show manifestations between these two polar forms and are clinically unstable. Medical complications arise from nerve damage and immune reactions (75).

Shedding from the nose, rather than from skin lesions, is important for transmission, which most probably results from prolonged and intimate contact with a person with multibacillary disease. The natural reservoir for M. *leprae* is not well established, but naturally occurring infections in the nine-banded armadillo (*Dasypus novemcinctus*) have been documented in Texas and Louisiana.

M. *leprae* differs from all other mycobacteria in that it cannot be cultured in vitro. There is, to date, only one report where M. *leprae* was claimed to show sparse growth in a special medium at 32°C (118). By tradition, the diagnosis of leprosy is essentially a clinical one, based on finding one or more signs of disease which are supported by the presence of acid-fast bacilli (AFB) on slit skin smears or in skin biopsy specimens. In the case of lepromatous disease, nodules and plaques are the preferred sites for biopsies, which will reveal numerous AFB. Conversely, in patients with tuberculoid leprosy, the rims of lesions, where usually only a few or no AFB are found, should be biopsied. A number of PCR assays have been established to conclusively identify the organism (135). When the disease is treated adequately, infectiousness is generally lost after 3 days of treatment (106).

Nontuberculous Mycobacteria Frequently Involved in Human Disease

Slowly Growing Species

M. avium Complex

M. *avium* complex (MAC) organisms have been isolated from water, soil, plants, and other environmental sources. They are important pathogens of poultry and swine but were not recognized as a cause of human disease until the 1940s. Generally, these organisms are of low pathogenicity. Single positive specimens with small numbers of AFB as colonizers are not infrequently observed in individuals without apparent disease. This complicates the interpretation of culture results, particularly from specimens of the respiratory tract (6, 49). However, as a result of the AIDS pandemic, MAC has become the most common environmental NTM causing disease in humans.

Before the advent of AIDS, the most common presentation of MAC infection was pulmonary disease showing several different clinical patterns, i.e., tuberculosis-like infiltrates, nodular bronchiectasis, solitary nodules, and diffuse infiltrates in immunocompromised patients (167, 192). Tuberculosis-like upper-lobe fibrocavitary disease due to MAC typically occurs in white men 45 to 60 years of age who are heavy smokers, many of whom abuse alcohol, and some of whom have preexisting lung disease. The clinical presentation is similar to that of tuberculosis. Nodular bronchiectasis usually occurs in elderly nonsmoking women with no predisposing disorders of the lungs or immune system other than associated bronchiectasis. These patients usually present with persistent cough only. MAC is also isolated from up to 20% of young adults with cystic fibrosis, particularly in the southeastern United States, but its contribution to the disease process has not been established (97). Further, it is also the leading cause of localized mycobacterial lymphadenitis in children, especially in those aged 1 to 5 years (205); this lymphadenitis is usually unilateral and involves lymph nodes in the submandibular, submaxillary, or periauricular areas. Less frequent are thoracic infections in otherwise healthy children (51).

While disseminated MAC infections in non-AIDS patients are extremely rare (84), patients with AIDS may present with disseminated or focal infections (85). Disseminated infection occurs mostly when the CD4 count is below 100 cells/mm^3. Bacteremia occurs in almost all those patients, its magnitude ranging from <1 to 10^2 CFU/ml. The organism is found almost exclusively in circulating monocytes. Almost any organ (e.g., lungs and intestines) may be involved, with levels of mycobacteria as high as 10^{10} CFU/g of tissue. Focal infections commonly involve the lungs or the gastrointestinal tract and occasionally also peripheral lymph nodes (87).

MAC organisms are well known for their heterogeneous colony morphology. Glossy, whitish colonies may often occur together with smaller translucent colonies. A third, less frequent morphology resembles the dry and flat colonies of M. tuberculosis. Some MAC strains may develop a yellowish pigment with age. Traditionally, MAC has consisted of 28 serotypes (referred to as serovars) of two distinct species, M. avium and M. intracellulare. Serovars 1 to 6, 8 to 11, and 21 are M. avium, while serovars 7, 12 to 20, and 22 to 28 are M. intracellulare. Inclusion of M. scrofulaceum (serovars 41 to 43) in the group as M. avium-M. intracellulare-M. scrofulaceum (MAIS complex) is no longer appropriate, given the advances in mycobacterial systematics (196, 197). M. avium and M. intracellulare are easily distinguishable by genetic methods, such as DNA probes, 16S rRNA gene sequencing, and analysis of the restriction enzyme patterns of the 65-kDa heat shock protein gene (hsp) (168). There is evidence for a third species within MAC which is generally referred to as the MAC-X strain (197). Those strains are recognized by the commercial DNA MAC Accuprobe (Gen-Probe, San Diego, Calif.), but are negative with the M. avium and M. intracellulare

probes. More than 90% of MAC strains isolated from AIDS patients are M. avium (as are most of the pathogenic isolates from pigs and cattle). In these patients relatively few serovars of M. avium account for the majority of infections.

Based on phenotypic and genetic characteristics, three subspecies of M. avium have been proposed: subsp. avium, subsp. paratuberculosis, and subsp. silvaticum (170).

M. genavense

M. genavense is a slow-growing NTM that was isolated in 1991 from the blood of an AIDS patient in Geneva, Switzerland (21), and subsequently in the United States and in several other European countries (38, 49, 177). It has been associated with enteritis and genital and soft tissue infections in HIV-positive and HIV-negative immunocompromised individuals. Clinically, disseminated disease in HIV-positive patients is similar to that caused by MAC. However, stool specimens were more often smear positive in M. genavense infections (119). M. genavense is also the most common cause of mycobacterial disease in a variety of pet birds including parrots and parakeets (83, 134).

Analysis of the 16S rRNA sequences indicates that this species is most closely related to M. simiae. The organism was first isolated in BACTEC 13A medium, but only after extended incubation (6 to 8 weeks). It fails to grow on L-J, 7H11 agar, or other media commonly used for the isolation of mycobacteria. Middlebrook 7H11 agar supplemented with mycobactin J (Allied Monitor, Fayette, Mo.), however, supports the growth of M. genavense (38), as do microaerophilic conditions (137), the radiometric BACTEC 7H12 PZA test medium (178), or addition of blood and charcoal to acidified Middlebrook agar (136).

M. haemophilum

M. haemophilum was first isolated in 1978 from a subcutaneous lesion in a patient with Hodgkin's disease (147). Approximately 50% of infections have been in patients with AIDS, with a relatively large number reported from New York City (29). The other cases have been in other immunosuppressed individuals (147) but also in immunocompetent pediatric patients with localized cervical lymphadenopathy (146) or with a pulmonary nodule (200). The classical clinical presentation is that of multiple skin nodules in clusters with or without a definite pattern, commonly involving the extremities, and occasionally associated with abscesses, draining fistulas, cellulitis, and osteomyelitis (49).

M. haemophilum infections may be underrecognized because of the predilection of this species for a low incubation temperature (30°C) and its unique requirement for ferric ammonium citrate or hemin for growth. If M. haemophilum is suspected in a clinical specimen but the culture remains negative, the organism may be recovered simply by using a chocolate agar plate.

M. kansasii

In the United States and many other countries, M. kansasii is second only to MAC as a cause of NTM lung disease (6, 49). The organism has been cultured from tap water in municipalities around the world where clinical disease occurs. It is common in mine workers in both the United Kingdom and South Africa (36) and differs from MAC in that the response to chemotherapy is much better (6).

Chronic pulmonary disease resembling classical tuberculosis is the most common manifestation of M. *kansasii*; it often involves the upper lobes. Extrapulmonary infections are uncommon and include cervical lymphadenitis in children (211), cutaneous and soft tissue infections (34, 150), and musculoskeletal disease (17, 131). M. *kansasii* rarely disseminates, except in patients with severely impaired cellular immunity (e.g., due to organ transplants) or in patients with AIDS (6).

M. *kansasii* is a photochromogenic species. Studies of the base sequences of the 16S rRNA suggest that phylogenetically it is closely related to the slowly growing, nonpigmented species M. *gastri*. Molecular studies have defined five genotypes of M. *kansasii*, all of which are able to cause human disease (128).

M. malmoense

The species name M. *malmoense* is derived from the city of Malmö in Sweden, where the first strains were isolated from patients in 1977. Disease due to this organism was later found in other European countries (6, 79, 176). It remains rare in the United States (24), Canada (5), and other areas of the world. However, in these countries M. *malmoense* infection may be more common than suspected, because 8 to 12 weeks may be needed to isolate some strains, which is longer than many laboratories in North America hold mycobacterial cultures.

Patients with M. *malmoense* infection are usually young children with cervical lymphadenitis or adults with chronic pulmonary disease (6, 49), mostly middle-aged men with previously documented pneumoconiosis. Extrapulmonary and disseminated infections have rarely been reported. The species has been recovered from soil and water (6).

M. marinum

M. *marinum* causes cutaneous infections as a result of trauma to the skin and subsequent exposure to contaminated freshwater fish tanks ("fish tank granuloma") or saltwater. The disease occurs worldwide. In the United States, it is most common in southern coastal states (90). The more typical presentation is a single papulonodular lesion confined to one extremity, usually the elbow, knee, foot, toe, or finger. It appears 2 to 3 weeks after inoculation and, with time, may become verrucous or ulcerated (49). A second type resembles cutaneous sporotrichosis, in which the primary inoculation is followed by spread along the lymphatics. More severe complications include tenosynovitis, arthritis, bursitis, and osteomyelitis. Disseminated infections, including infections in patients with AIDS or persons undergoing systemic steroid therapy, have been rare (81). M. *marinum* is photochromogenic and requires incubation at 28 to 30°C on primary isolation.

M. simiae

M. *simiae* was first isolated in 1965 from monkeys. Clinical isolates have come from a few geographic areas, including the southwestern United States (6, 143), Israel (86), and the Caribbean (6). The organism has been recovered from tap water in some of these areas, and most positive cultures from humans came from single positive specimens with low colony counts, suggesting that most isolates represent environmental contamination. Clinical manifestations such as osteomyelitis and chronic pulmonary and disseminated disease are rare (see reference 49 and references therein). Cases of M. *simiae* infection mimicking MAC in AIDS patients have been reported (86). M. *simiae*

is one of the very few NTM that synthesize niacin. Unless tested for pigment production under the influence of light, it may be misidentified as M. *tuberculosis* by inexperienced observers.

M. szulgai

M. *szulgai* was first described as a distinct species in 1972. Its distribution appears to be worldwide, but the natural reservoir is unknown. Patients were almost exclusively middle-aged men presenting with chronic pulmonary disease indistinguishable from tuberculosis (175). The remaining presentations included rare cases of bursitis, cervical adenitis, tenosynovitis, cutaneous infections, and osteomyelitis (6, 49). Cases of M. *szulgai* infection in AIDS patients and disseminated disease in an immunocompetent patient have been reported as well (50).

Although M. *szulgai* is closely related to M. *malmoense* based on the 16S rRNA gene sequences, phenotypic distinction between the two species is easy. The organism is scotochromogenic at 37°C and photochromogenic at 25°C (94).

M. ulcerans

The frequency of M. *ulcerans* infection has long been underestimated due to difficulties in isolating the pathogen. Today, M. *ulcerans* infection is the third most frequent mycobacterial disease in humans after tuberculosis and leprosy. In Africa the disease is known as Buruli ulcer, and in Australia it is known as Bairnsdale ulcer (6, 49, 63). Closely associated with tropical wetlands, M. *ulcerans* most probably proliferates in mud beneath stagnant waters. Disease probably occurs via direct contact with a contaminated environment or via water-dwelling fauna such as insects. It typically begins as a painless lump under the skin at the site of previous trauma on the lower extremities. After a few weeks, a shallow ulcer develops at the site of the lump. M. *ulcerans* produces a toxin that causes necrosis (182). The type of disease ranges from a localized nodule or ulcer to widespread ulcerative or nonulcerative disease including osteomyelitis. If untreated, severe limb deformities with contractures and scarring are common. There is growing evidence that M. *ulcerans* also produces disease in wild animals such as lizards, opossums, koala bears, armadillos, rats, mice, and cattle (133).

Failure to cultivate this organism in the past was due to its fastidious, heat-sensitive nature (temperature optimum, 30°C), as well as to a long generation time relative to that of other environmental mycobacteria. Many conventional decontamination protocols used in mycobacteriology interfere with the viability of M. *ulcerans* (121). Treatment with mild hydrochloric acid (final concentration, 0.03 N) as a decontamination agent provides the best results. A mixture of polymyxin B, amphotericin B, nalidixic acid, trimethoprim, and azlocillin (PANTA) may control secondary contamination. Supplementation with egg yolk or reduced oxygen tension enhances the rate of recovery in the BACTEC 460TB System (120). Molecular techniques have been developed which may help to lead to more rapid diagnosis (132).

M. xenopi

M. *xenopi* was first isolated in 1957 from skin lesions on an African toad (*Xenopus laevis*), but it was not recognized as a human pathogen until 1965. By 1979, 50 cases of M. *xenopi* infection in humans had been reported, primarily from the United Kingdom, France, Denmark, Australia, and the United States (6, 49). In some areas such as Canada and southeast England, M. *xenopi* is second only to MAC as an NTM clinical isolate (6). Increased isolation of M. *xenopi* from clinical specimens may, however, also be due to improved laboratory techniques (45). The optimum growth temperature for the species is 45°C, and it seems to occur frequently in hot water systems. Nosocomial infection and pseudoinfection via water storage tanks in hospitals have been described (155).

Pulmonary disease is the most common manifestation of infection (6, 91), usually occurring in male adult patients with underlying lung disease such as chronic obstructive pulmonary disease or bronchiectasis. Extrapulmonary infections such as septic arthritis (93), spondylitis (39), and dissemination (95) have also been described in immunocompromised individuals.

Rapidly Growing Mycobacteria

Because the two rapidly growing species M. *fortuitum* and M. *chelonae* (formerly M. *chelonei*) share a number of characteristics and are associated with similar types of infections, they were historically referred to collectively as the M. *fortuitum* complex (149). This taxonomic grouping has become less satisfactory with the recognition of additional species and taxa within the complex (e.g., M. *peregrinum*, M. *abscessus*, and M. *immunogenum* [49, 103, 190, 203]), all of which differ in drug susceptibilities and in the type of clinical disease caused. Rapidly growing mycobacteria (RGM) differ from slow-growing species in that they grow readily on blood agar or chocolate agar in 3 to 5 days and <7 days on L-J medium when subcultured (with the optimal incubation temperature).

M. *fortuitum* Group

Members of the M. *fortuitum* group are responsible for a number of different types of sporadic infections including osteomyelitis, cellulitis, surgical wound and posttraumatic wound infections, central catheter-related infections, and, rarely, chronic pulmonary disease (187). M. *fortuitum* and M. *abscessus* have been the most common RGM species associated with outbreaks and pseudo-outbreaks (187). M. *fortuitum* and M. *peregrinum* have been isolated from natural and tap water, and M. *fortuitum* and the unnamed third biovariant have also been isolated from soil, dust, and/or mud (188).

The M. *fortuitum* group traditionally consists of three species/taxa: M. *fortuitum*, M. *peregrinum*, and the unnamed third biovariant complex. Additional species proposed as members include M. *septicum*, M. *mageritense*, M. *alvei*, and M. *senegalense* (see below). The third biovariant complex has been subdivided into sorbitol-positive and sorbitol-negative subgroups. Studies in progress suggest that these two subgroups consist of at least six different species (M. Schinsky, J. Brown, et al., unpublished data) which show minimal differences in susceptibility to antimicrobial agents and produce similar clinical diseases. Separation of these species and taxa can only be done with carbohydrate utilization, restriction fragment length polymorphism (RFLP) of the *hsp* gene encoding the 65-kDa HSP (147, 162), or 16S rDNA sequencing.

M. *abscessus*

The nonpigmented organism M. *abscessus* is closely related to M. *chelonae*. It is responsible for almost 90% of chronic lung disease due to RGM (65) and has caused posttraumatic wound infections (191), >90% of cases of otitis media following tympanostomy tube placement (54), and disseminated cutaneous disease similar to M. *chelonae* infection in immunosuppressed patients. The organism is present in tap water and has been associated with injection-related nosocomial outbreaks and sporadic cases of sternal and mammoplasty wound infections, as well as bacteremia associated with central venous, arterial, and hemodialysis catheters.

M. *chelonae*

M. *chelonae* is the RGM most likely to be encountered in immunosuppressed patients. The most common clinical picture is a disseminated nodular skin disease with draining lesions but minimal symptoms in patients on steroids or otherwise immunosuppressed. Intravenous catheter infections and posttraumatic wound infections also occur (6). The environmental reservoir for this species is unknown; it is relatively rare in tap water.

M. *chelonae* is the slowest growing member of the complex and generally requires 28 to 30°C for primary isolation. It is most closely related to M. *abscessus* but can be separated from it by its ability to utilize citrate as a sole carbon source (149), by drug susceptibility patterns, or by the RFLP pattern of the *hsp* gene encoding the 65-kDa HSP. NaCl tolerance is generally too unreliable to separate the two species.

M. *mucogenicum*

Recognized in 1995 on the basis of 16S rRNA gene sequence differences to other RGM (158), M. *mucogenicum* was previously grouped within the M. *chelonae*-M. *abscessus* taxon. Because of different phenotypic characteristics and a 16S rDNA sequence more closely related to the M. *fortuitum* group, it should now be added to that group. Its name reflects a mucoid morphology (158, 187), but it was first called an "M. *chelonei*-like organism" when reported as the etiologic agent of an outbreak of peritonitis in a dialysis unit (190). It has been recovered mainly from tap water and is frequently isolated from single samples of sputum, in which its presence usually results from contamination. Clinical disease has been associated with intravenous catheter and posttraumatic wound infections (190).

Nontuberculous Mycobacteria Rarely Recovered or Rarely Causing Human Disease

Slowly Growing Species

Several species of slowly growing mycobacteria including M. *gordonae*, M. *scrofulaceum*, and M. *terrae* complex are not infrequently recovered but are rarely associated with human disease. Some of the case reports of infections attributable to these mycobacteria, especially from the era before the introduction of molecular laboratory techniques, lack sufficient documentation of identification or disease association. Other species (such as M. *asiaticum* or M. *shimoidei*) are so rarely recovered that most laboratories will never see them.

M. *asiaticum*

M. *asiaticum* was not recognized as a distinct species until 1971, although it had previously been isolated from monkeys. The first published report of human disease described five patients with pulmonary disease in Australia (20). The organism has since infrequently been isolated from patients with respiratory disease in the United States and elsewhere (166). Cases of bursitis (40) and tenosynovitis (53) have been described. Colony morphology is similar to that of M. *gordonae*, differing primarily in that M. *gordonae* is scotochromogenic whereas M. *asiaticum* is photochromogenic (196).

M. celatum
First described in 1993 (26), M. *celatum* has been isolated from diverse geographic areas, i.e., throughout the United States, Finland, and Somalia, and mostly from respiratory tract specimens but also from stool and blood. In one series, 32% of the patients from whom it was isolated were infected with HIV (26, 59). M. *celatum* has also been isolated from immunocompetent patients, e.g., from a child suffering from lymphadenitis (69) and an elderly female patient with a fatal pulmonary infection (27).

M. *celatum* shares morphological and biochemical characteristics with MAC, M. *malmoense*, and M. *shimoidei* and can therefore not be identified by conventional tests. Within the bacterial chromosome, M. *celatum* has two copies of the 16S rRNA gene (139). Several subgroups have been identified, with the use of RFLP of the gene encoding the 65-kDa HSP (129). Due to high similarities in the 16S rRNA gene sequence to that of M. *tuberculosis*, a few strains were misidentified as M. *tuberculosis* complex when a commercially available DNA probe was used (172).

M. gastri
As opposed to M. *gordonae*, M. *gastri* is infrequently encountered in the clinical laboratory. In the light of modern identification, none of the reports gave sufficient details of the properties of the organisms to conclusively identify them as M. *gastri*.

M. gordonae
M. *gordonae* is the most commonly encountered "nonpathogenic" species in clinical mycobacteriology laboratories. This scotochromogenic species is widely distributed in soil and water. A pseudo-outbreak associated with drinking water in a French hospital underlined the necessity for proper maintenance of water supply equipment (104). In only 1 of 38 published reports of M. *gordonae* infection was there convincing evidence that the organism played a role in disease (196). There are also reports of peritonitis in patients undergoing continuous ambulatory peritoneal dialysis (73). Recently, Eckburg et al. (47) have reviewed clinical and chest radiographic findings among persons with sputum culture positive for M. *gordonae* and concluded that it is a nonpathogenic colonizing organism, even among persons with local or general immune suppression and abnormal chest X-ray findings.

M. scrofulaceum
The name was derived from scrofula, a historical term used to describe mycobacterial infections of the cervical lymph glands. Until the 1980s, M. *scrofulaceum* was the most common cause of mycobacterial cervical lymphadenitis in children. It has been replaced primarily by MAC (205). Other types of clinical disease are rare. They include pulmonary disease, conjunctivitis, osteomyelitis, meningitis, granulomatous hepatitis, and disseminated disease (see reference 49 and references therein). M. *scrofulaceum* accounted for 14% of the isolates tested in respiratory specimens collected from South African miners (36).

M. shimoidei
M. *shimoidei* was first described in 1988 in a Japanese patient with chronic cavitary lung disease. Only a few clinical cases have been reported since then (107). It is a thermophilic organism, growing well at 45°C. Biochemically, the organism is similar to M. *terrae* complex but can be separated from it by catalase and β-galactosidase tests. The unique sequence of the 16S rRNA gene and the 16S–23S rDNA spacer region allow unambiguous identification of the organism (101).

M. terrae Complex
M. *terrae* complex consists of three species, M. *terrae*, M. *nonchromogenicum*, and M. *triviale*. Clinical disease due to M. *terrae* is generally limited to tenosynovitis of the hand following local trauma and pulmonary disease (152). M. *nonchromogenicum*, ubiquitous in the aquatic environment, has recently been the cause of bacteremia in an AIDS patient (108). Separation of the members of the complex, especially M. *terrae* from M. *nonchromogenicum*, requires molecular methods.

Rapidly Growing Mycobacteria

M. senegalense
Originally described in 1973 as a subspecies of M. *farcinogenes*, M. *senegalense* was later recognized as a different species by 16S rDNA sequence analysis (33). It is a causative agent of farcy, a disease of skin and superficial lymphatics in African bovines, and has not been reported from the United States or Europe.

M. smegmatis Group
The M. *smegmatis* group is composed of three species, M. *smegmatis* sensu stricto, M. *goodii*, and M. *wolinskyi* (23). Clinical diseases caused by M. *smegmatis* sensu stricto include cellulitis, localized abscesses, osteomyelitis following a traumatic event, and intravenous catheter and postsurgical infections (23, 188).

High-pressure liquid chromatography mycolic acid profiles of the M. *smegmatis* group are similar to those of M. *fortuitum*, as are other biochemical characteristics, except that its members have a negative 3-day arylsulfatase test result. Also, M. *smegmatis* and M. *goodii* often have a late yellow-orange pigment on 7H10 agar after 7 to 10 days.

New Species of Nontuberculous Mycobacteria
Most of the new NTM species have been described within the last 5 to 10 years. Much less is known about these species than about those mentioned above, and the numbers of clinical cases are very limited.

Slowly Growing Species

M. bohemicum
M. *bohemicum* is a bright yellow species originally described in 1998 in a patient with Down's syndrome and tuberculosis (138). Rare cases of cervical lymphadenitis in children (174) have been reported as well. Isolates have been recovered from veterinary (goat) and environmental (freshwater) sources (173). For identification, analysis of the 16S rRNA gene sequence is required (138, 174).

M. branderi
M. *branderi* was first described in 1992 in 14 respiratory isolates collected in Finland. Since then, M. *branderi* has

also been isolated from an infected wound on the hand (204). Identification of the organism requires 16S rRNA gene sequence analysis (100, 204), which shows that the species is most closely related to M. celatum, M. cookii, and M. xenopi.

M. conspicuum

M. conspicuum was first isolated in 1995 from two AIDS patients with disseminated disease (159). The organism grew at 22 to 31°C and produced pale yellow colonies on solid media. Unusually, the strains do not grow at 37°C except in BACTEC 12B medium. Based on its 16S rRNA gene sequence, it is most closely related to M. asiaticum and M. gordonae (159).

M. heckeshornense

M. heckeshornense was described in 2000 as a scotochromogenic species (140, 142) recovered in multiple cultures from the lungs of an immunocompetent patient with severe bilateral cavitary disease. On the basis of its unique 16S rRNA and 16S–23S spacer gene sequences, it appears to be a new species (140, 142).

M. heidelbergense

The nonphotochromogenic organism M. heidelbergense was described in 1997 as an isolate from a child with recurrent cervical lymphadenitis (67). An M. heidelbergense infection was also found to mimic a lung tumor in a previously healthy woman (127). Biochemically, M. heidelbergense is indistinguishable from M. malmoense but unable to grow under microaerophilic conditions. Sequencing of the 16S rRNA gene, however, positions the organism on a branch separate from M. malmoense but within a group of slowly growing mycobacteria with a high degree of similarity to M. simiae (67).

M. interjectum

M. interjectum was recovered from children with chronic lymphadenitis (11, 160) and from an AIDS patient with diarrhea (64). Colonies are smooth and scotochromogenic. Visible growth is produced within 21 to 28 days. Fatty acid patterns by gas-liquid chromatography were similar to those of M. scrofulaceum. By 16S rDNA sequencing, the organism is most closely related to M. simiae (160).

M. intermedium

The photochromogenic species M. intermedium was repeatedly isolated from a patient with chronic pulmonary disease and can be easily confused with M. asiaticum, although differences exist in colony morphology (109).

M. lentiflavum

M. lentiflavum was first described in 1996 as a cluster of slowly growing pigmented organisms (158). The majority of the isolates were from respiratory specimens. The organism has been reported as an etiological agent of cervical lymphadenitis (68) and of disseminated infection in an HIV-positive patient (117). It does not grow at 45°C (161). The organism usually has a bright yellow pigment and distinct patterns of mycolic acids and cellular fatty acids.

M. triplex

M. triplex was characterized in 1996 as an unusual cluster of slowly growing mycobacteria that strongly resembled MAC (52) but were DNA MAC probe negative. The majority were from either lymph nodes or respiratory sam-
ples. M. triplex has caused disseminated mycobacteriosis in an HIV-positive patient during antiretroviral therapy (35) and in a liver transplant patient (82). By 16S rDNA sequencing, the organism is most closely related to M. genavense and M. simiae. It differs from M. simiae in not producing any pigment and from M. genavense in growing easily on solid media (52).

M. tusciae

The yellow-pigmented organism M. tusciae, first described in 1999, has been found in tap water but also in a few clinical specimens, e.g., in a lymph node of an immunocompromised child and in a respiratory specimen of a patient with cystic fibrosis (179).

Rapidly Growing Species

M. alvei

M. alvei, a nonphotochromogenic species first described in 1992 (11), has been recovered from samples from a river and from riverbed soil in Spain and from human sputa. The authors of this chapter claim to have evidence (unpublished) for a causative role in clinical disease.

M. goodii

M. goodii, a mycobacterium of the M. smegmatis group, was named after Robert Good in 1999 (23). Isolates have been recovered from patients with cellulitis and osteomyelitis following open fracture or penetrating trauma. The majority of cases of respiratory disease have been associated, like M. smegmatis sensu stricto (189), with underlying exogenous lipid pneumonia and achalasia with pulmonary infiltrates (23).

M. immunogenum

M. immunogenum is a nonpigmented species described in 2001 and first recognized in a study involving an outbreak of hypersensitivity pneumonitis among workers in an industrial plant (112). Isolates have also been recovered from nosocomial pseudo-outbreaks involving contaminated automated endoscope washers, from blood in catheter- and pacemaker-related infections, from the skin of a liver transplant patient with disseminated disease, and from an infant with severe combined immunodeficiency syndrome (203). On the basis of a unique RFLP pattern of the hsp gene encoding the 65-kDa HSP and subsequent 16S rDNA sequence analysis, the isolates were proposed to belong to a new species, M. immunogenum (203).

M. mageritense

The first isolates of M. mageritense were isolated in 1997 from sputum cultures from two hospitals in Spain but were not considered clinically significant (44). Recently, however, two isolates have been recovered from two different patients in Texas (R. J. Wallace, Jr., and B. A. Brown-Elliott, unpublished data). Like most of the newer species, organism recognition requires molecular methods such as RFLP restriction analysis of the hsp gene encoding the 65-kDa HSP or 16S rDNA sequencing.

M. septicum

M. septicum was recovered from blood cultures and a central venous catheter tip in a child with metastatic hepatoblastoma (148). Recent analyses of the 16S rRNA gene sequence and of mycolic acids by HPLC showed a close relationship to M. *peregrinum*, M. *senegalense*, and M. *fortuitum*. No other cases have been reported to date.

M. *wolinskyi*

Described in 1999 (23), M. *wolinskyi* is a nonpigmented species within the M. *smegmatis* group and was named after Emanuel Wolinsky. Of the seven isolates reported, three were recovered from surgical wound infections while the remaining four came from posttraumatic wound infections; some of them were erroneously identified as M. *smegmatis* (23).

Other RGM Species

Other RGM species have been recovered from clinical samples, and some appear to be disease-producing. These include M. *aichiense*, M. *aurum*, M. *brumae*, M. *chubuense*, M. *confluentis*, M. *flavescens*, M. *gadium*, M. *hassiacum*, M. *neoaurum*, M. *novocastrense*, M. *phlei*, M. *thermoresistibile*, and M. *vaccae*. In general, too few strains have been studied to be certain of the pathogenic potential of these species and their uniqueness (especially by genetic studies).

"No-Name" Mycobacteria

There are quite a few reports of novel NTM that cause disease in humans but have not been assigned to a particular species yet. For instance, a mycobacterium resembling M. *kansasii*, although nonphotochromogenic, was isolated from an AIDS patient with acute lymphadenitis (12). Evoking the same clinical manifestation in a child, another novel mycobacterium related to M. *triplex* was described by Hazra et al. (78).

SAFETY AND TRANSPORT ISSUES

Laboratory Safety Procedures

Nosocomial transmission of M. *tuberculosis* from patients or specimens is of major concern to health care workers (28). Because of the low infective dose of M. *tuberculosis* for humans (50% infective dose, <10 bacilli), specimens from persons with suspected or known cases of tuberculosis must be considered potentially infectious and handled with appropriate precautions (32). Control of aerosols and other forms of mycobacterial contamination is achieved in the laboratory by the use of properly functioning biological safety cabinets (BSC), centrifuges with safety carriers, and meticulous processing techniques (see also chapter 9).

Classification of mycobacteriology laboratory practices should be based on risk assessment (i.e., volume of tests, types of testing, prevalence of tuberculosis, rate of multidrug-resistant M. *tuberculosis*). Biosafety level 2 practices and facilities are required for laboratory work assessed as low risk. Aerosol-generating manipulations should be conducted in a class I or II BSC. More rigorous biosafety level 3 practices and facilities are required for laboratories assessed as being associated with higher risk. These laboratories process specimens for mycobacterial culture and propagate and manipulate cultures of M. *tuberculosis* (e.g., perform identification and susceptibility testing). Such practices require that laboratory access be restricted, that directional airflow be used to maintain the laboratory under negative pressure, and that workers wear special laboratory clothing and gloves. Biosafety level 3 practices and facilities are required for laboratories growing M. *tuberculosis* to high volumes, working with large numbers of resistant isolates,

or performing tests with unknown risk. For a detailed description of safety requirements in the mycobacteriology laboratory, refer to the CDC/NIH biosafety guide for laboratories (32).

All respiratory protective devices (respirators) used in the workplace should be certified by the National Institute for Occupational Safety and Health (NIOSH) (115). Respirators that contain a NIOSH-certified N-series filter with a 95% efficiency (N-95) rating are appropriate for use. They meet the recommendations from the CDC for selection of respirators for protection against M. *tuberculosis*, i.e., (i) the unloaded filter must filter particles 0.3 μm in size with an efficiency of 95% at flow rates up to 50 liters/min; (ii) the respirator must be qualitatively or quantitatively fit tested to obtain a face seal leakage rate of no more than 10%; (iii) it must fit different facial sizes and characteristics, which is attained by making the respirators available in at least three sizes; and (iv) it must be checked for face piece fit by the person wearing the respirator each time it is worn, in accordance with Occupational Safety and Health Administration (OSHA) standards. Surgical masks are not NIOSH-certified respirators and must not be worn to provide respiratory protection.

The determination of when and if to use respiratory protective devices in the laboratory should be based on risk assessment. A respirator program should be implemented by the laboratory and should include a written protocol describing when respirator use is necessary and procedures addressing (i) selection of the appropriate respirator, (ii) how to conduct fit testing, and (iii) training of personnel in the use, fit checking, and storage of the respirator.

All work involving specimens or cultures, such as making smears, inoculating media, adding reagents to biochemical test mixtures, opening centrifuge cups, and sonication, must be performed in a BSC. The handling of all specimens suspected of containing mycobacteria (including specimens processed for other microorganisms), with the exception of centrifugation for concentration purposes, must be done within the BSC. Specimens that are to be taken out of the BSC should be covered before transport. All work surfaces, including bench tops and the inside of the BSC, should be cleaned with an appropriate disinfectant before and after work. Effective disinfectants include Amphyl (Reckitt Benckiser North America, Wayne, N.J.) or other phenol-soap mixtures and 0.05 to 0.5% sodium hypochlorite (the concentration varies according to the nature of the contaminated surface); 5% phenol is no longer recommended as a surface disinfectant due to the documented toxicity of this compound to personnel. UV light is a useful adjunct for surface decontamination and may be used to radiate the work area when it is not in use. Centrifuges should be used with aerosol-free safety carriers to contain debris in the event that tubes break. Use of electric incinerators rather than open flames is recommended. The excess inoculum from inoculating loops, wire, or spades may be removed by dipping the tool into a container of 95% ethanol in washed sand prior to insertion in an incinerator. Disposable inoculating loops are recommended, as are syringes with permanently attached needles if needles are required. An autoclave should be available in an easily accessible area and should be used to decontaminate infectious waste before removal to disposal areas.

Personnel should be regularly monitored with the Mantoux PPD skin test (annually, and more often if a conversion in the laboratory or the institution has been documented [32]) to demonstrate conversions. Those with positive skin tests should be evaluated for active tuberculosis with a chest X ray and clinical evaluation. Physical examinations should be performed when necessary. New converters should be referred to the Employee Health and the Infection Control Departments for epidemiological evaluation. Laboratories should have written protocols describing procedures for handling laboratory accidents. In case of a laboratory accident with possible formation of aerosols, personnel should hold their breath as much as possible, make sure BSCs are on and centrifuges are turned off, and then leave the room and stay outside with the door closed for at least 30 min (the length of time depends on the type of accident and the degree of risk). Using appropriate respiratory protection devices, personnel can return to the accident area to clean the spill. PPD-negative personnel should be skin tested at 3 and 6 months after the accident. Persons who are immunocompromised should be discouraged from working in the mycobacteriology laboratory (32).

Transportation and Transfer of Biological Agents

Mycobacteria are on the list of the wide variety of infectious agents being regulated for shipping and transfer. Recent more stringent regulations on the transportation of biological agents have been enacted in the United States to ensure that the public and workers in the transportation chain are protected from exposure to any infectious agents (for other countries, please consult the specific regulations). Protection is achieved through (i) the requirements of rigorous packaging that will withstand rough handling and contain all liquid material within the package without leakage to the outside; (ii) appropriate labeling of the package with the biohazard symbol and other labels to alert the workers in the transportation chain to the hazardous contents of the package; (iii) documentation of the hazardous contents of the package, should such information be necessary in an emergency situation; and (iv) training of workers in the transportation chain to familiarize them with the hazardous contents in order to be able to respond to emergency situations.

The reader is referred to the following regulatory documents for further information:

Public Health Service 42. CFR part 72. *Interstate Transportation of Etiologic Agents*. This regulation is in revision to harmonize it with the other U.S. and international regulations. A copy of the current regulation may be obtained from the Internet at http://www.cdc.gov/od/ohs/biosfty/shipregs.htm.

Department of Transportation. 49 CFR Parts 171–178. *Hazardous Materials Regulations*. Applies to the shipment of both biological agents and clinical specimens. Information may be obtained from the Internet at http://www.access.gpo.gov/cgi-bin/cfrassemble. cgi?title=199849.

U.S. Postal Service. 39 CFR Part 111. *Mailability of Etiologic Agents*. Codified in *Domestic Mail Manual 124:38: Etiologic Agents Preparations*. A copy of the *Domestic Mail Manual* may be obtained from the Government Printing Office by calling 1-202-512-1800 or from the Internet at http://www.access.gpo.gov/cgi-bin/cfrassemble.cgi?title=199839.

OSHA. 29 CFR Part 1910.1030. *Occupational Exposure to Bloodborne Pathogens*. Provides minimal packaging and labeling requirements for transport of blood and body fluids. Information may be obtained from your local OSHA office or from the Internet at http://www.osha-slc.gov/OshStd_data/1910_1030.html.

International Air Transport Association (IATA). *Dangerous Goods Regulations (DGR)*. These regulations provide packaging and labeling requirements for infectious substances and materials, as well as for clinical specimens with a low probability of containing an infectious substance. A copy of the DGR may be obtained by calling 1-800-716-6326 or through the Internet at http://www.iata.org/cargo/dg/index.htm.

Permits *must* be obtained for importation and exportation of biological and infectious agents. These are obtained by contacting the CDC, Atlanta, Ga. (www.cdc.gov).

COLLECTION AND STORAGE OF SPECIMENS

General Rules

Many different types of clinical specimens may be collected for mycobacteriological analyses (88). The majority originate from the respiratory tract (sputum, tracheal, and bronchial aspirates; bronchoalveolar lavage fluid specimens), but urine, gastric aspirates, tissues, biopsy specimens, and normally sterile body fluids (such as cerebrospinal fluid and pleural and pericardial aspirates) are other commonly submitted specimens. Blood and fecal specimens are usually submitted from immunocompromised patients only.

Specimens should always be collected and submitted in sterile, leak-proof, disposable, appropriately labeled laboratory-approved containers without any fixatives. Waxed containers must not be used because they may yield false-positive AFB smear results (94). Generally, transport media or preservatives are not necessary owing to the robust nature of mycobacteria. Minute quantities of biopsy material (e.g., fine-needle aspirates) may be immersed in a small amount of sterile physiological saline. Collection should bypass areas of possible contamination, e.g., tap water, as much as possible since the presence of environmental mycobacteria may result in false-positive smear and/or culture results (187). In general, swabs are not optimal for the recovery of AFB since they provide limited material and the hydrophobicity of the mycobacterial cell envelope often compromises a transfer from swabs onto solid or into broth media. If transport to the laboratory is delayed more than 1 h, specimens (except blood) should be refrigerated at 4°C. Likewise, on arrival in the laboratory, specimens should be refrigerated until processed (see chapters 6 and 20 for additional information on specimen collection).

Sputum

Sputum, expectorated or induced, is the principal specimen obtained for the diagnosis of pulmonary tuberculosis. An early-morning specimen should be collected on three consecutive days. Pooled sputum specimens are unacceptable for mycobacterial processing because they are associated with increased contamination (94). Since the yield of culture from smear-positive specimens is high, two AFB smear-positive specimens are considered sufficient for the initial evaluation of pulmonary tuberculosis (164). Nelson et al. (116) demonstrated that the majority of culture-proven pulmonary tuberculosis cases are diagnosed from the first or second sputum specimen and that only rarely is a third specimen of diagnostic value. A more recent study, however, still concluded that three respiratory specimens are needed despite the availability of highly sensitive culture techniques (74). Follow-up cultures should be considered because it is culture (and not smear) which yields a definite answer about whether chemotherapy has been effective (110). Children may have difficulties producing sputum. In this age group, a gastric aspirate is usually the specimen of choice for the diagnosis of pulmonary tuberculosis.

Bronchial Aspirates, Bronchoalveolar Lavage Specimens, Fine-Needle Aspirates, and Lung Biopsy Specimens

In some patients unable to produce sputum, invasive collection techniques such as bronchoscopy may be necessary to diagnose pulmonary tuberculosis or mycobacteriosis. Special care is imperative for cleansing the bronchoscope to avoid cross-contamination with AFB from a preceding patient who underwent bronchoscopy (2, 16, 58). Also, the bronchoscope should not be in contact with tap water, which may contain environmental mycobacteria. Specimens collected by other invasive techniques such as fine-needle aspiration and open-lung biopsy may be submitted in difficult-to-diagnose cases.

Gastric Lavage Fluids

Aspiration of swallowed sputum from the stomach by gastric lavage may be necessary for infants, young children, and the obtunded. Fasting, early-morning specimens are recommended to obtain sputum swallowed during sleep. Samples of 5 to 10 ml, adjusted to neutral pH, should be collected on three consecutive days. If they cannot be processed within 4 h, the laboratory should provide sterile disposable containers with 100 mg of sodium carbonate for collection. Nonneutralized specimens are not acceptable because long-term exposure to acid is detrimental to mycobacteria.

Urine

The first morning specimen should be collected on three consecutive days by midstream (clean catch) voiding into a sterile container. The first morning specimen provides the best results because organisms accumulate in the bladder overnight. A minimum of 40 ml of urine is usually required for culture. Twenty-four-hour pooled specimens and small-volume specimens (unless a larger volume is not obtainable) are unacceptable. Catheterization should be used only if a midstream sample cannot be obtained.

Body Fluids

As much body fluid as possible (e.g., cerebrospinal, pleural, peritoneal, pericardial, and synovial fluid) is aseptically collected by aspiration or during surgical procedures. Bloody specimens may be anticoagulated with sodium polyanethole sulfonate. Because certain body fluids (such as cerebrospinal fluid [CSF] and peritoneal dialysis effluent) may contain very small numbers of mycobacteria, it is advisable to submit larger specimen volumes (e.g., >3 ml for CSF) to increase culture yields and the chance to detect mycobacterial organisms.

Tissues (Lymph Node, Skin, Other Biopsy Material)

At least 1 g of tissue, if possible, should be aseptically collected into a sterile container. It must not be immersed in saline or other liquid or wrapped in gauze. For cutaneous ulcers, biopsy material should be collected from the periphery of the lesion. Specimens submitted in formalin are unacceptable for smear and culture. Minute amounts of biopsy material may be immersed in a small amount of sterile saline.

Abscess Contents, Aspirated Pus, and Wounds

As much material as possible should be aspirated aseptically. In cutaneous lesions, material is aspirated from beneath the margin of the lesion. Also, for this type of specimen, a second set of cultures has to be incubated at 30°C since one of the organisms with a lower temperature optimum (M. haemophilum, M. marinum, or M. ulcerans) may be the infectious agent.

Blood

The majority of disseminated mycobacterial infections are due to MAC; therefore, if this organism is isolated from blood, it is always associated with clinical disease (77). If blood has to be transported before inoculation of the medium, sodium polyanethole sulfonate, heparin, or citrate may be used as anticoagulants; blood collected in EDTA and coagulated blood are not acceptable. Direct inoculation of blood onto a solid medium is not recommended (3). MAC survives for prolonged periods in Isolator lysis-centrifugation tubes (Wampole Laboratories, Cranbury, N.J.). Therefore, processing of Isolator tubes can be delayed for 24 h if absolutely necessary (76). If blood cannot be immediately processed by the laboratory, it should be stored at room temperature.

For many years, the Isolator system and the radiometric BACTEC 13A blood culture bottle (Becton Dickinson Microbiology Systems, Sparks, Md.) were the only reliable and therefore recommended systems for mycobacterial blood cultures (3, 8). Today, blood can also be cultivated by inoculating nonradiometric liquid media such as BACTEC Myco/F lytic medium (Becton Dickinson Microbiology Systems) (8), ESP Myco (Trek Diagnostic Systems, Westlake, Ohio) (186), or MB/BacT ALERT 3D (BioMérieux, Marcy l'Etoile, France) (131). (For culture media and systems, see below.)

Isolator tubes contain saponin, which lyses cells and releases intracellular mycobacteria. The BACTEC 13A bottle contains a lysing agent, is designed specifically for the recovery of mycobacteria from blood, and can directly be inoculated with 5 ml of blood without the potential hazards associated with the lysis-centrifugation procedure. A potential disadvantage of using the BACTEC 13A medium is the inability to determine the number of CFU per volume of blood, which can be determined with the Isolator System. However, the significance and necessity of obtaining quantitative data with each blood culture are unclear. The use of Isolator blood sediments to inoculate BACTEC 12B medium is contraindicated because one of the components, polypropylene glycol, is inhibitory to mycobacteria in the BACTEC 12B System (194). An identical effect on the growth of mycobacteria has also been reported with the Septi-Chek AFB liquid medium and the MGIT broth (56), but this is controversial (72).

Stool Specimens

Stool specimens (>1 g) have been used for detection of MAC from the gastrointestinal tracts of patients with AIDS, in conjunction with specimens from other sites. Past recommendations have been that stool be cultured for mycobacteria only if the direct smear of unprocessed stool is positive for AFB. The sensitivity of the stool smear, however, is only 32 to 34% (114), suggesting that its results should not determine whether a culture for mycobacteria be performed. Screening with smears is therefore not an effective way to identify patients at risk for developing disseminated MAC infection (76).

Inadequate Specimens

Processing of inappropriate clinical specimens for mycobacteria is a waste of both financial and personnel resources. There are quite a few reasons why a specimen should not be accepted (and the clinician should be notified), e.g., (i) too small an amount submitted, (ii) specimens consisting of saliva, (iii) dried swabs (biopsy is preferable), (iv) pooled sputum or urine, (v) broken sample containers, and (vi) interval too long (>7 days) between specimen collection and processing (122). Clinical staff must be properly trained to prevent the submission of unacceptable specimens.

ISOLATION PROCEDURES

Because mycobacteria usually grow slowly and require long incubation times, a variety of microorganisms other than mycobacteria can overgrow cultures of specimens obtained from nonsterile sites. Appropriate pretreatment and processing procedures (homogenization, decontamination, and concentration [88, 94]), culture media, and conditions of incubation must be selected to facilitate optimal recovery of mycobacteria (see also chapter 37). In particular, pretreatment of specimens has to be done carefully, i.e., by eliminating contaminants as much as possible while not seriously affecting the viability of mycobacteria.

Processing of Specimens

Decontamination of a specimen should be attempted only if it is thought to be contaminated. Tissues or body fluids collected aseptically usually do not require pretreatment. If the need to decontaminate a specimen is not clear, the specimen may be refrigerated until routine bacteriologic cultures are checked the next day. It may, however, be easier to initially inoculate a chocolate agar plate to check for sterility before a sample is processed for mycobacteria.

Normally Sterile Specimens

Normally sterile tissue samples may be ground in sterile 0.85% saline or 0.2% bovine albumin and then inoculated directly to the media. Because body fluids commonly contain only small numbers of mycobacteria, they should be concentrated to maximize the yield of mycobacteria before inoculation of media, i.e., centrifuged at ≥3,000 × g for 15 min prior to inoculation of the sediment. If the volume of fluid submitted for culture is small and the specimen cannot be obtained again, it may be added directly to liquid media.

Contaminated Specimens

The majority of specimens submitted for mycobacterial culture consist of a complex organic matrix contaminated with a variety of organisms. Mucin may trap mycobacterial cells and protect contaminating bacteria from the action of decontaminating agents. Thus, mycobacteria are recovered optimally from clinical specimens through the use of procedures which reduce or eliminate contaminating bacteria while releasing mycobacteria trapped in mucin and cells. Liquefaction of certain specimens, particularly sputum, is often necessary. Mycobacteria are then concentrated to enhance detection in stained smears and by culture.

Digestion and Decontamination Methods

Sodium hydroxide, the most commonly used decontaminant, also serves as a mucolytic agent but must be used cautiously because it is only somewhat less harmful to tubercle bacilli than to the contaminating organisms. The stronger the alkali, the higher its temperature during the time it acts on the specimen, and the longer it is allowed to act, the greater will be the killing action on both contaminants and mycobacteria (102). Harsh decontamination can kill 20 to 90% of the mycobacteria in a clinical specimen (94). Homogenization should occur by centrifugal swirling, and this swirling should not be vigorous enough to allow material to rise to the cap. After agitation, there should be at least a 15-min delay before opening the tube to allow any fine aerosol droplets formed during the mixing to settle. All such procedures should be carried out in a class II BSC.

Most commonly, a combination liquefaction-decontamination mixture is used. N-Acetyl-L-cysteine (NALC), dithiothreitol, and several enzymes effectively liquefy sputum. These agents have no direct inhibitory effect on bacterial cells; however, their use permits treatment with lower concentrations of sodium hydroxide, thereby indirectly improving the recovery of mycobacteria. Addition of cetylpyridinium chloride (see Appendix 1) to specimens mailed from remote collection stations to a central processing station has yielded a good recovery of M. tuberculosis without overgrowth by contaminating bacteria (154), but, based on our experience, this agent seriously compromises culture in the BACTEC 460TB System.

Under field conditions, liquefaction and concentration of sputum for acid-fast staining may be conducted by treating the specimens with an equal volume of 5% sodium hypochlorite solution (undiluted household bleach) and waiting 15 min before centrifugation (94, 144). Such a treated specimen, however, cannot be cultured because this chemical seriously affects the viability of AFB. The major limitation is therefore that a second specimen must be collected for culture. However, this method is very useful for rapid smear preparation and interpretation in laboratories that do not process specimens for culture or that do not have a BSC.

No single method of digestion and decontamination is ideal for all clinical specimens, all laboratories, and all circumstances. The laboratorian must be aware of the inherent limitations of the various methods used. Even under the best of conditions, all currently available procedures are toxic for mycobacteria to some extent. Thus, the best yield of mycobacteria may be expected to result from the use of the mildest decontamination procedure that sufficiently controls contaminants. Strict adherence to specimen processing is mandatory to ensure survival of the maximal number of mycobacteria. Most laboratories process specimens in batches; current recommendations suggest that specimen batches should be processed daily (169). The most widely used digestion-decontamination method is the NALC–2% NaOH method (94) (see Appendix 1), which is compatible with the radiometric BACTEC 460TB System and other commercially available newer broth culture systems. Pretreatment of clinical specimens with sodium dodecyl (lauryl) sulfate-NaOH is, by contrast, not suitable for the Mycobacteria Growth Indicator Tube (MGIT) cultivation method (124) since it results in poor recovery of mycobacteria and a delayed mean time to detection of AFB. Sodium hydroxide, oxalic acid, and to a lesser extent mild

HCl have a detrimental impact on the viability of *M. ulcerans* (121). A novel procedure for processing respiratory specimens utilizing C_{18}-carboxypropylbetaine (CB-18) has been described recently (171). Although culture and smear sensitivity were significantly improved compared to the NALC-NaOH procedure, the contamination rate was extremely high (20.8%).

Commonly used digestion-decontamination methods are described with step-by-step instructions in the guide by Kent and Kubica (94), the *Clinical Microbiology Procedures Handbook* (88), and Appendix 1. In general, the specimen is diluted with an equal volume of digestant and allowed to incubate for some time. A neutralizing buffer is added, and the specimen is centrifuged to sediment any AFB present. Centrifugation should be carried out at ≥3,000 × *g* for 15 min to obtain maximum recovery. The sediment is then inoculated onto the appropriate liquid and solid media.

Whatever method is used, care must be taken to prevent aerosol-mediated laboratory cross-contamination of patient specimens during processing (9, 25, 151). A single false-positive culture for *M. tuberculosis* could easily be the basis of a diagnosis of tuberculosis, with profound consequences for clinical management, epidemiologic investigations, and public health control measures (see chapter 2).

Optimization of Decontamination Procedures

While no contamination or very low rates of contamination indicate that the pretreatment conditions were too harsh and eliminated not only bacteria and fungi but also mycobacteria, a rate exceeding 5% of all digested and decontaminated specimens cultured is generally defined as excessive contamination. A high contamination rate (88, 94) suggests either too weak a decontamination or incomplete digestion. One or a combination of several of the following measures may be used to help decrease the contamination rate.

1. Cautiously and slightly increase the strength of the alkali treatment. Be aware that 4% NaOH will in time probably kill most tubercle bacilli.

2. Use a selective medium (one containing antibiotics) in addition to a nonselective primary culture medium to inhibit the growth of bacterial and fungal contaminants. Selective 7H11 agar (Mitchison medium), Mycobactosel agar (BBL Microbiology Systems, Cockeysville, Md.), or the Gruft modification of L-J medium should be considered. The most useful media for recovering MAC from stool specimens have been Mitchison's selective 7H11 agar and Mycobactosel L-J medium (210).

3. Make sure specimens are completely digested; partially digested specimens may not be completely decontaminated. Increase the NALC concentration to digest thick, mucoid specimens.

4. Use an alternative digestion-decontamination procedure for problem specimen types. Respiratory secretions from patients with cystic fibrosis, often overgrown with pseudomonads, can successfully be decontaminated with NALC-NaOH followed by the addition of 5% oxalic acid to the concentrated sediment (101).

To determine the decontaminating capabilities of each new batch of reagents, the laboratory may wish to inoculate blood agar plates with four to six decontaminated sputum specimens in addition to inoculating mycobacterial media. Numbers of contaminants that grow after 48 h of incubation at 35°C should be minimal to none (94).

Acid-Fast Stain Procedures

Smear microscopy is still one of the most rapid and inexpensive ways to diagnose tuberculosis. In parallel, it is a rapid means of identifying the most contagious patients. Normally, its predictive value for *M. tuberculosis* in expectorated sputum is >90% (105).

The common Gram stain is not suitable for mycobacteria. They may be gram-invisible, may appear as clear zones or "ghosts," or may appear as beaded gram-positive rods, particularly RGM (180). Special acid-fast staining procedures are necessary to promote the uptake of dyes. Although the exact nature of the acid-fast staining reaction is not completely understood, phenol allows penetration of the stain, which is facilitated by higher temperatures as applied, for instance, with Ziehl-Neelsen staining. Mycobacteria are able to form stable complexes with certain arylmethane dyes such as fuchsin and auramine O. The cell wall mycolic acid residues retain the primary stain even after exposure to acid-alcohol or strong mineral acids. This resistance to decolorization is required for an organism to be termed acid-fast. Certain staining protocols include a counterstain to highlight the stained organisms for easier microscopic recognition. Information about specific staining procedures (carbol fuchsin and fluorochrome) is given in chapter 27.

Because acid-fast artifacts may be present in a smear, it is necessary to view the cell morphology carefully. AFB are approximately 1 to 10 μm long and typically are slender rods, 0.2 to 0.6 μm wide, which may appear curved or bent. Individual bacilli may display heavily stained areas and areas of alternating stain, producing a beaded appearance. Assessment of AFB morphology for presumptive identification of mycobacterial species has to be done with caution and needs ample training and experience of the laboratory personnel. In liquid medium, *M. tuberculosis* often exhibits serpentine cording, but cords are also seen with some NTM species (113). NTM may appear pleomorphic, appearing as long filaments or coccoid forms, with uniform staining properties. *M. kansasii* organisms can often be suspected in stained sputum smears by their large size and cross-banding appearance (10). Cells of rapidly growing mycobacteria may be <10% acid fast and may not stain with the fluorochrome stain (92). If the presence of a rapid grower is suspected and acid-fast stains, in particular fluorochrome stains, are negative, it may be worthwhile to stain the smear with carbol fuchsin and use a weaker decolorizing process. Organisms that are truly acid fast are difficult to over-decolorize. The laboratory must be aware that there are nonmycobacterial organisms with various degrees of acid fastness, such as *Rhodococcus* species, *Nocardia* species, and *Legionella micdadei*, as well as the oocysts of *Cryptosporidium, Isospora,* and *Cyclospora.* Based on a recent study, Kinyoun's cold carbol fuchsin method is inferior to both the Ziehl-Neelsen and fluorochrome methods (156).

Each slide made from a clinical specimen should be thoroughly examined for the presence of AFB. When a carbol fuchsin-stained smear is read, a minimum of 300 fields should be examined (magnification, ×1,000) before the smear is reported as negative (88, 94). The fluorochrome stain is read at a lower power (×250) than the carbol fuchsin stain; therefore, more material can be examined in a given period. At the lower magnification, a minimum of 30 fields of view should be examined. This requires as little as 90 s. This ease of detection of AFB with the fluorochrome stain makes it the preferred staining method for clinical specimens, although an inexperienced observer may misinterpret fluorescent debris as bacilli.

All smears in which no AFB have been seen should be reported as negative. Conversely, when acid-fast organisms are detected on a smear, the smear should be reported as AFB positive and the staining method should be specified. It is best to confirm positive smears by having them reviewed by another experienced reader. Ideally, all positive fluorochrome-stained smears should be confirmed by a carbol fuchsin-based staining method, e.g., Ziehl-Neelsen, and slides should be stored for future reference (94). Information about the quantity of AFB observed on the smear should be provided. The recommended interpretations and reporting of smear results are given in Table 1. If only one or two organisms are seen on an entire smear, this should be noted but not reported. Confirmation of this finding should be attempted by preparation of additional smears from the same specimen or, if possible, smears prepared from a new specimen. Observations made with the fluorochrome smears should be converted to a format that equates these observations with those made with a 100× oil immersion objective.

However, the reliability of smear microscopy is highly dependent not only on the experience of the laboratory technician but also on the number of AFB present in the specimen. While 10^6 AFB/ml of specimen usually result in a positive smear, only 60% of the smears are positive if 10^4 AFB/ml are present (48). The overall sensitivity of the smear has been reported to range from 22 to 80% (105). An important factor influencing sensitivity is the minimum amount of sputum submitted to the laboratory. In a long-term study, the sensitivity of a concentrated smear from >5 ml of sputum was significantly greater than the sensitivity of a smear processed regardless of volume (193). Other factors influencing smear sensitivity include the type of specimens examined, staining techniques, the experience of the reader, the patient population being evaluated, and whether the smear has been done with or without pretreatment (indirect versus direct smear). Respiratory specimens yield the highest smear positivity rate (105). In practice, the fluorochrome stain is more sensitive than the carbol fuchsin stain, even when read at lower magnification, probably because the fluorochrome-stained smears are easier to read.

The specificity of the smear for the detection of mycobacteria is very high. Prolonged or very harsh specimen decontamination and short incubation of cultures may account for smear-positive but culture-negative results. Patients with pulmonary tuberculosis may have positive smears with negative cultures (for 2 to 10 weeks on average) during a course of appropriate treatment (98).

Cytocentrifugation of sputum has resulted in controversial results concerning the sensitivity of smear microscopy (144, 205). Concentration of sputum by centrifugation after liquefaction with 5% sodium hypochlorite is a possible means of increasing smear sensitivity, in particular in developing countries.

The diagnostic yield of acid-fast stains of body fluids is lower than for respiratory specimens because the number of mycobacteria is usually smaller. A variety of techniques have been used to concentrate mycobacteria from CSF and other body fluids, but comparative data are lacking. Centrifugation is not an effective way to concentrate mycobacteria in body fluids since mycobacteria have a buoyant density of approximately 1; therefore, many organisms remain in the supernatant (99). Sequential layering of several drops of uncentrifuged fluid on a slide or polycarbonate membrane filtration is probably the most effective means of concentrating mycobacteria for microscopy (153).

With each new batch of staining reagents, good laboratory practice includes the preparation of a positive and a negative smear for internal quality assessment. Smears containing M. tuberculosis or an NTM (positive control) and a gram-positive organism, preferably a Nocardia strain which is not totally acid fast (negative control), may be prepared in advance. Cross-contamination of slides during the staining process and the use of water contaminated with NTM during staining procedures are potential sources of false-positive results (43, 187). Staining jars or dishes should not be used. Transfer of AFB in the oil used for microscopy may also occur. Troubleshooting protocols to prevent false-positive and false-negative smear results have been established by the Association of State and Territorial Public Health Laboratory Directors (ASTPHLD) and CDC (9) (see chapter 2).

Culture

In detecting as few as 10^1 to 10^2 viable organisms/ml, specimen culture is more effective than smear. Media available for the recovery of mycobacteria (94) include nonselective and selective ones, the latter containing one or more antibiotics to prevent overgrowth by contaminating bacteria or fungi. Broth media are preferred for a rapid initial isolation of mycobacteria.

TABLE 1 Acid-fast smear evaluation and reporting[a]

Report	No. of AFB seen by staining method and magnification		
	Fuchsin stain	Fluorochrome stain	
	×1,000	×250	×450
No AFB seen	0	0	0
Doubtful; repeat	1–2/300 F[b] (3 sweeps)[c]	1–2/30 F (1 sweep)	1–2/70 F (1.5 sweeps)
1+	1–9/100 F (1 sweep)	1–9/10 F	2–18/50 F (1 sweep)
2+	1–9/10 F	1–9/F	4–36/10 F
3+	1–9/F	10–90/F	4–36/F
4+	>9/F	>90/F	>36/F

[a] Adapted from reference 94.
[b] F, microscope fields.
[c] In all cases, one full sweep refers to scanning the full length (2 cm) of a smear 1 cm wide by 2 cm long.

Solid Media

Egg-Based Media

Egg-based media contain whole eggs or egg yolk, potato flour, salts, and glycerol and are solidified by inspissation. These media have a good buffer capacity and a long shelf life (several months when refrigerated) and support good growth of most mycobacteria. Also, materials in the inoculum or medium that are toxic to mycobacteria are neutralized. Disadvantages of these media include variations from batch to batch depending on the quality of the eggs used, difficulties in discerning colonies from debris, and the inability to achieve accurate and consistent drug concentrations for susceptibility testing. When egg-based media become contaminated, they may liquefy.

Of the egg-based media, L-J medium is most commonly used in clinical laboratories. In general, it recovers M. *tuberculosis* well but is not as reliable for the recovery of other species. Petragnani medium contains about twice as much malachite green as does L-J medium and is most commonly used for recovery of mycobacteria from heavily contaminated specimens. American Trudeau Society medium contains a lower concentration of malachite green than does L-J medium and is therefore more easily overgrown by contaminants, but growth of mycobacteria is less inhibited, resulting in earlier growth of larger colonies.

Agar-Based Media

In contrast to egg-containing media, agar-based media are chemically well defined. Agar-based media are transparent and provide a ready means of detecting early growth of microscopic colonies easily distinguished from inoculum debris. Colonies may be observed in 10 to 12 days, in contrast to 18 to 24 days with egg-based media. Microscopic examination can be performed by simply turning over the plate and examining it by focusing on the agar surface through the bottom of the plate at ×10 to ×100 magnification. This may provide both earlier detection of growth than unaided visual examination and presumptive identification of the species of mycobacteria present. The use of thinly poured 7H11 agar plates (10 by 90 mm) (Remel, Lenexa, Kans.) facilitates this process since microcolonies are visible after 11 days (199). This method is an alternative to broth cultures for some laboratories. Agar-based media can be used for susceptibility testing. They do not readily support the growth of contaminants (94); however, the plates are expensive to prepare and their shelf life is relatively short (1 month in the refrigerator). Care should be exercised in preparation, incubation, and storage of the media, because excessive heat or light exposure may result in deterioration and in the release of formaldehyde, which is toxic to mycobacteria.

Middlebrook medium contains 2% glycerol, which enhances the growth of MAC. Nonantibiotic supplements may be helpful for the recovery of other mycobacteria and in special situations. Addition of 0.2% pyruvic acid is recommended if M. *bovis* is suspected (42), and 0.25% L-asparagine or 0.1% potassium aspartate added to 7H10 agar maximizes the production of niacin (96). Addition of 0.1% enzymatic hydrolysate of casein to the Middlebrook 7H11 formulation (the only difference from 7H10) improves the recovery of isoniazid-resistant strains of M. *tuberculosis.*

Selective Media

The addition of antimicrobial agents may be helpful in eliminating the growth of contaminating organisms. If a selective medium is used for a particular specimen, it should not be used alone but should be used in conjunction with a nonselective agar- or egg-based medium. Egg-based selective media include L-J Gruft with penicillin and nalidixic acid and Mycobactosel L-J medium with cycloheximide, lincomycin, and nalidixic acid. Mitchison selective 7H11 (7H11S) medium and its modifications contain carbenicillin (especially useful for inhibiting pseudomonads), polymyxin B, trimethoprim lactate, and amphotericin B.

Heme-Containing Medium for the Growth of M. *haemophilum*

M. *haemophilum* grows on egg- or agar-based media only if they are supplemented with hemin, hemoglobin, or ferric ammonium citrate (147). Thus, specimens from skin lesions, joints, or bone should be inoculated not only on chocolate agar but also on Middlebrook 7H10 agar with hemolyzed sheep erythrocytes, hemin, or a factor X disk or on L-J medium containing 1% ferric ammonium citrate, to enhance recovery of this organism. Broth media should be similarly supplemented. M. *haemophilum* can also be isolated from radiometric BACTEC 12B medium as well as from MB Redox broth (146).

Biphasic Media

The Septi-Chek System (Becton Dickinson Microbiology Systems) is a mycobacterial culture system consisting of a capped bottle containing 20 ml of modified 7H9 broth in an enhanced (20%) CO_2 atmosphere and a paddle containing three types of solid media, i.e., modified L-J, Middlebrook 7H11 agar, and chocolate agar, encased in a plastic tube. Bacterial contamination is detected on the chocolate agar. Cultures are inoculated by removing the bottle cap, adding the processed specimen, and then attaching the paddle to the bottle. Solid media are inoculated after 24 h of incubation in an upright position by inverting the bottles. A supplement containing glucose, glycerol, oleic acid, pyridoxal HCl, catalase, albumin, and antibiotics (PANTA) is added to the culture bottle before inoculation. During the incubation period, the bottles are periodically tipped to reinoculate the solid media as cultures are being read. The sensitivity of this system is comparable to that of the BACTEC 460TB System (89). Although the average time to detection of growth is longer than with the radiometric BACTEC medium, it is shorter than with conventional media.

Liquid Media

Broth media may be used for both primary isolation and subculturing of mycobacteria. Cultures based on liquid media yield significantly more rapid results than do those based on solid media. Also, isolation rates for mycobacteria are higher. Middlebrook 7H9 and Dubos Tween albumin broths are commonly used for subculturing stock strains of mycobacteria and preparing the inoculum for drug susceptibility tests and other in vitro tests. 7H9 broth is used as the basal medium for several biochemical tests. Tween 80 can be added to liquid media and acts as a surfactant which allows the dispersal of clumps of mycobacteria, resulting in a more homogeneous growth.

At present, a number of elaborate culture systems marketed for the isolation of mycobacteria are available commercially; they range from simple bottles and tubes such as MGIT (Becton Dickinson Microbiology Systems) and MB Redox (Heipha Diagnostica Biotest, Heidelberg, Germany) to semiautomated systems (BACTEC 460TB System; Becton Dickinson) and fully automated systems (e.g., BACTEC 9000 MB and BACTEC MGIT 960 [Becton Dickinson], ESP Culture System II [Trek Diagnostic Systems], and MB/BacT ALERT 3D System [BioMérieux]).

MB Redox

MB Redox (Heipha Diagnostica Biotest) is a nonradiometric medium based on a modified Kirchner medium enriched with growth-promoting additives, antibiotic compounds, and a colorless tetrazolium salt as a redox indicator, which is reduced to colored formazan by actively growing mycobacteria. With the naked eye, AFB are detected in the medium as pink to purple pinhead-sized particles. Recovery rates are similar to those observed for other liquid systems (157). Overall, it is a cost-efficient alternative with the disadvantage that it requires much handling during visual reading.

Mycobacterial Growth Indicator Tube (MGIT)

The MGIT (Becton Dickinson) contains a modified Middlebrook 7H9 broth in conjunction with a fluorescence quenching-based oxygen sensor (silicon rubber impregnated with a ruthenium pentahydrate) to detect the growth of mycobacteria. The large amount of oxygen initially present in the medium quenches the fluorescence of the sensor. Growth of mycobacteria or other microorganisms in the broth depletes the oxygen, and the indicator fluoresces brightly when the tubes are illuminated with UV light at 365 nm. For the manual version, a Wood's lamp or transilluminator can be used as the UV light source, while in the automated BACTEC MGIT 960 System (see below), tubes are continuously monitored by the instrument. Prior to use, the 7H9 broth is supplemented with oleic acid-albumin-dextrose to promote the growth of mycobacteria and with PANTA to suppress the growth of contaminants.

Overall, the sensitivity and time to growth detection of the MGIT System are similar to those of the BACTEC 460TB System and have been superior to solid media in clinical evaluations (37, 125). However, contamination rates for the MGIT System are currently higher than for the BACTEC 460TB System, probably owing to the enrichments added to the MGIT broth, which enhance the growth of both mycobacteria and nonmycobacterial organisms.

The principal advantages of the manual MGIT System over the BACTEC 460 TB System include reduced opportunity for cross-contamination of cultures, no need for needle inoculation, no radioisotopes, and no need for special instrumentation other than the UV light source. Its limitations include higher contamination rates, masking of fluorescence by blood or grossly bloody specimens, and possible lack of compatibility with some methods of digestion and decontamination of specimens (124). For susceptibility testing of primary drugs, MGIT is an equivalent replacement for the BACTEC 460TB System, in both the manual and automated versions (see chapter 73).

BACTEC 460TB System

[^{14}C]palmitic acid as a carbon source in the medium is metabolized by microorganisms to $^{14}CO_2$, which is monitored by the instrument. The amount of $^{14}CO_2$ and the rate at which the gas is produced are directly proportional to the growth rate of the organism in the medium.

An antimicrobial mixture/growth-promoting supplement (PANTA [see above]) is added to BACTEC 12B medium inoculated with decontaminated specimens in order to suppress residual contaminants. To potentially sterile specimens, polyoxyethylene stearate (POES) is added to enhance mycobacterial growth. For pretreatment of nonsterile specimens, the NALC-NaOH protocol is the method of choice, although some other procedures such as the sodium dodecyl sulfate-NaOH method are compatible with the BACTEC 460TB System as well (145). However, specimens processed by the Zephiran-trisodium phosphate, benzalkonium chloride, or cetylpyridinium chloride method cannot be used with the BACTEC 460TB System because residual quantities of these substances in the inoculum inhibit mycobacterial growth. BACTEC 13A medium is used for blood and bone marrow aspirate specimens. An enrichment fluid is added to a 13A vial before or after specimen inoculation. Caution has to be used with highly cellular clinical specimens since they may give false-positive results soon after inoculation, due to the metabolic activity of the cells.

The use of the BACTEC 460TB method has significantly improved recovery rates and times of mycobacterial isolation from respiratory secretions and other specimens (141). Smear-positive specimens usually grow within a few days. The average detection time is 5 to 14 days for M. tuberculosis and <7 days for NTM. This is also obvious with smear-negative specimens and specimens from treated patients. Limitations of the BACTEC 460TB System include inability to observe colony morphology, difficulty in recognizing mixed cultures, overgrowth by contaminants, cost, radioisotope disposal, and extensive use of syringes with the potential for needle punctures among laboratory technicians. Since the method is only semiautomated, vials have to be transferred to the incubator once the growth index has been read by the instrument.

The BACTEC 460TB System allows efficient antimicrobial susceptibility testing as well (see chapter 73). Generally, the initial positive vial can be used directly for identification and drug susceptibility testing. It is good laboratory practice to confirm acid fastness and to subculture positive BACTEC vials to a chocolate agar to check for potential contaminants or, if suspected, for mixed cultures.

Automated, Continuously Monitoring Systems

Several automated, continuously monitored systems have recently been developed for growth and detection of mycobacteria, i.e., the BACTEC 9000 MB (Becton Dickinson), the BACTEC MGIT 960 (Becton Dickinson), ESP Culture System II (Trek Diagnostic Systems), and the MB/BacT ALERT 3D (bioMérieux). All have in common that they are no longer based on the use of radioisotopes. The BACTEC 9000 MB System uses the same fluorescence quenching-based oxygen sensor as the MGIT System to detect growth. The technology used in ESP Culture System II is based on detection of pressure changes in the headspace above the broth medium in a sealed bottle as a result of gas production or consumption due to growth of microorganisms. The MB/BacT ALERT 3D System employs a colorimetric carbon dioxide sensor in each bottle to detect the growth of mycobacteria. Each of the systems includes a broth similar to 7H9 supplemented with a variety of growth factors and antimicrobial agents.

These systems have similar performance and operational characteristics. In clinical evaluations, recovery rates were similar to those of the BACTEC 460TB System and superior to those of conventional solid media (BACTEC 9000 MB [123]; BACTEC MGIT 960 [71, 202]; ESP Culture System II [207]; MB/BacT ALERT 3D [130, 202]). Time to detection of mycobacteria is almost the same as for the radiometric BACTEC 460TB technique. Throughout, contamination rates reported have been higher with these new systems than with the BACTEC 460TB System. All share the advantages over the radiometric broth system of having no potential for cross-contamination by the instrument, being less labor-intensive, having continuous monitoring, using no radioisotopes, addressing safety more appropriately, and offering electronic data management. Since these systems are monitoring continuously, bottles are incubated in the instruments for their entire life in the laboratory. As a consequence, these systems are both instrument and space intensive. Some automated systems also lack the versatility of the BACTEC 460TB System, in that direct inoculation of blood is, so far, not possible. The same holds for the incubation of cultures harboring mycobacteria with a lower temperature optimum such as M. *haemophilum*, M. *marinum*, or M. *ulcerans*. Except for the BACTEC 9000 MB System, susceptibility testing applications for the primary antituberculosis drugs including pyrazinamide (in some systems) are available (see chapter 73).

Medium Selection

Medium selection for the isolation of mycobacteria and culture reading schedules are usually based on personal preferences and/or laboratory tradition. Both should be optimized for the most rapid detection of positive cultures and identification of mycobacterial isolates. The variety of media and methods available today is sufficient to permit laboratories to develop an algorithm that is optimal for their patient population and administrative needs. However, workload, financial resources, and, in particular, the limited amounts of processed sediments are restraining factors in working with too many different types of media. Thus, cultivation of mycobacteria always involves a compromise.

Today, it is generally accepted that the use of a liquid medium in combination with at least one solid medium is essential for good laboratory practice in the isolation of mycobacteria. Addition of a solid medium is advantageous for the detection of strains which occasionally do not grow in liquid medium, aids in the detection of mixed mycobacterial infections, and can serve as a back-up for broth cultures, if contaminated. All positive cultures, even if identified directly from the broth, must be subcultured to solid media to detect mixed cultures and to correlate direct identification results with colony morphology. The biphasic Septi-Chek System can be used as a stand-alone system. In contrast, the radiometric BACTEC 460TB System and the new, nonradiometric growth systems such as BACTEC 9000, BACTEC MGIT 960, ESP Culture System II, and MB/BacT ALERT 3D cannot serve as stand-alone culture systems for mycobacteria for the reasons stated above.

Detection of colonies on solid medium certainly offers several advantages over detection of growth in broth, because colonial morphology can provide clues to identification and facilitate the selection of confirmatory tests including DNA probe tests. However, smears from broth-based systems can sometimes provide microscopic clues such as cord formation (see above), and it is possible to use the sediment from such cultures for confirmation by gene probes before growth is detected on solid media. The reli-

ability of the criterion of cord formation for presumptive identification of M. *tuberculosis* should be applied with caution since the phenomenon is also observed with some NTM species (10, 113).

Incubation

Temperature

The optimum incubation temperature for most cultures is 35 to 37°C. Exceptions include cultures obtained from skin and soft tissue specimens suspected to contain M. *marinum*, M. *ulcerans*, M. *chelonae*, or M. *haemophilum*, which have a lower temperature optimum. For such specimens, a second set of media should be inoculated and incubated at 25 to 33°C. BACTEC 460TB vials should be incubated at 36 to 38°C because optimum metabolism of the radiolabeled substrate occurs at 37 to 37.5°C for most species. Lower temperatures increase the detection time. The newer liquid medium-based automated culture systems do not offer the possibility of incubation at temperatures lower than 36 ± 1°C.

Atmosphere

An atmosphere of 5 to 10% CO_2 in air stimulates the growth of mycobacteria in primary isolation cultures using conventional media (14). Middlebrook agar requires a CO_2 atmosphere to ensure growth, while it is necessary to incubate egg media under CO_2 for only the first 7 to 10 days after inoculation, i.e., the log phase of growth. Subsequently, L-J cultures can be removed to ambient-air incubators if space is limited. In the absence of CO_2 incubators, plates may be incubated in commercially available bags with CO_2-generating tablets. Candle extinction jars are unacceptable for use in the mycobacteriology laboratory because the oxygen tension is lower than that required for growth of mycobacteria. Broth systems usually do not require incubation at increased CO_2 concentrations.

Time

Mycobacterial cultures on solid and in liquid media are generally held for 6 to 8 weeks before being discarded as negative. Specimens with positive smears that are culture negative should be held for an additional 4 weeks. The same should be done for culture-negative specimens which were positive for mycobacteria by one of the nucleic acid-based amplification assays or for patients with a persistent suspicion of tuberculosis. Plates should be incubated with the medium side down until the entire inoculum has been absorbed. Once this has happened, they should be incubated inverted in CO_2-permeable polyethylene bags or sealed with CO_2-permeable shrink-seal or cellulose bands to prevent the media from drying up during the incubation period. Tubed media should be incubated in a slanted position with the screw caps loose for at least a week until the inoculum has been absorbed; they can then be incubated upright if space is at a premium. Caps on the tubes should be tightened at 2 to 3 weeks to prevent desiccation of the media. Specimens from skin lesions should be incubated for 8 to 12 weeks if M. *ulcerans* is suspected.

Reading Schedule

Mycobacteria are relatively slowly growing organisms, and thus cultures can be examined less frequently than routine bacteriologic cultures. All solid media should be examined within 3 to 5 days after inoculation to permit early detection of rapidly growing mycobacteria and to enable the prompt removal of contaminated cultures. Young cultures (up to 4 weeks of age) should be examined twice a week, whereas older cultures could be examined at weekly intervals. Use of a hand lens for opaque media and a microscope for agar media will facilitate early detection of microcolonies.

Septi-Chek and the manual MGIT systems may be inspected for growth several times per week or daily for the first 1 to 2 weeks; Septi-Chek bottles should be inverted for reinoculation of the agar medium if growth is not observed. Afterward, these systems are inspected twice weekly or weekly for growth.

For BACTEC 460TB vials the reading schedule varies according to the laboratory workload. Low-volume laboratories may read cultures three times a week for the first 2 or 3 weeks and weekly thereafter for a total of 6 weeks, while high-volume laboratories may read cultures twice a week for the first 2 weeks and weekly thereafter. Some laboratories prioritize smear-positive specimens by separating them from smear-negative specimens and test the former more frequently. In addition, separation of "probable positive" cultures from negative ones will decrease the possibility of vial cross-contamination by the instrument. With more frequent testing of all specimens, however, earlier detection of positive cultures is expected. Readings of negative cultures in 12B medium usually remain below a growth index (GI) of 10; a GI of 10 or more is considered presumptively positive. At this point, the vials should be separated and tested daily. An acid-fast stain is performed when the GI is >50 to determine whether the culture contains mycobacteria. The morphology of mycobacteria seen in smears from 12B medium may be used for presumptive identification of *M. tuberculosis* complex by experienced laboratory personnel and to decide how to proceed with identification methods (10, 113). In addition, a smear of the broth from the vial may be Gram stained and/or the broth may be subcultured onto a sheep blood agar or chocolate agar plate to determine whether contamination is present. When the GI is 500 or more, BACTEC 460TB antimicrobial susceptibility testing can be performed (see below). Negative BACTEC 13A vials usually show a GI of 10 to 15. If the GI reaches 20 or more, the culture is considered presumptively positive. A smear is prepared at this point and stained for AFB. If the smear is positive, the vial is incubated further or subcultured for subsequent testing. If the smear is negative, incubation and testing are continued.

When using one of the new continuously monitoring systems (BACTEC 9000, BACTEC MGIT 960, ESP Culture System II, and MB/BacT ALERT 3D) technicians are automatically alerted by the instrument if a specimen turns positive. Irrespective of the system used, the acid fastness of the organism has to be confirmed by smear staining. Also, it is highly advisable to subculture the broth on a sheep blood or chocolate agar plate to rule out contaminants. Once growth of AFB is detected, susceptibility testing can be performed, always following the instructions specified by the manufacturers.

Laboratory Cross-Contamination

With the advent of molecular techniques designed for molecular epidemiology, cross-contamination linked either to laboratory procedures or, more rarely, to contaminated bronchoscopes can easily be proven (2, 16, 58). False-positive results may be generated at any step between specimen collection and reading of cultures (9). Laboratory personnel should be alerted for a possible laboratory error if

(i) the culture result is not compatible with the clinical picture, (ii) there is a late-appearing cluster of cultures which have scanty growth (<10 colonies on solid medium) or a significant delay in recovering mycobacteria from a liquid system, (iii) there is a large number of isolates of a particular species that is usually rare in the laboratory or of an organism that is normally considered an environmental contaminant, or (iv) there is only one positive culture from multiple specimens submitted from a single patient. Practices which can lead to false-positive culture results are numerous and include inadequate sterilization of instruments or equipment (such as bronchoscopes), use of contaminated water for specimen collection or for laboratory procedures, transfer of organisms from one specimen to another through direct contact or via common reagents or equipment, mixup of testing samples or lids of specimen containers, failure to take precautions which minimize the production of aerosols, etc. (see chapter 2).

APPENDIX 1
Commonly Used Digestion-Decontamination Methods

Refer to references 88 and 94 for details.

NALC-NaOH method

Reagents

Digestant: For each 100 ml, combine 50 ml of sterile 0.1 M (2.94%) trisodium citrate with 50 ml of 4% NaOH. The NaOH and citrate mixtures can be mixed, sterilized, and stored for future use. To this solution, add 0.5 g of powdered NALC just before use. Use within 24 h of addition of the NALC because the mucolytic action of NALC is inactivated on exposure to air.

Phosphate buffer: The buffer is 0.067 M and pH 6.8. Mix 50 ml of solution A (9.47 g of anhydrous Na_2HPO_4 in 1 liter of distilled water) and 50 ml of solution B (9.07 g of KH_2PO_4 in 1 liter of distilled water). If the final buffer requires pH adjustment, add solution A to raise the pH or solution B to lower it.

BSA (optional): Use sterile 0.2% bovine serum albumin (BSA) fraction V (pH 6.8).

Procedure

1. Transfer up to 10 ml of specimen to a sterile, graduated, 50-ml plastic centrifuge tube labeled with appropriate identification. The tube should have a leakproof, aerosol-free screw cap. Add an equal volume of the NALC-NaOH solution. The final concentration of NaOH in the tube is 1%.

2. Tighten the cap completely. Invert the tube so that the NALC-NaOH solution contacts all the inside surfaces of the tube and cap, and then mix the contents for approximately 20 s on a Vortex mixer. If liquefaction is not complete after this step, agitate the solution at intervals during the following decontamination period.

3. Allow the mixture to stand for 15 min at room temperature with occasional gentle shaking by hand. Avoid movement that causes aeration of the specimen. A small pinch of crystalline NALC may be added to viscous specimens for better liquefaction. Specimens should remain in contact with the decontaminating agent for only 15 min, since overprocessing results in reduced recovery of mycobacteria. If more active decontamination is needed, slightly increase the concentration of NaOH.

4. Add phosphate buffer (pH 6.8) up to the 50-ml mark on the tube.

5. Centrifuge the solution for at least 15 min at ≥3,000 × *g*.

6. Decant the supernatant fluid into a splashproof discard container containing a suitable disinfectant. Do not touch the lip of the tube to the discard container. Wipe the lip of each tube with disinfectant-soaked gauze (separate piece for each tube) to absorb drips, and recap.

7. Using a separate sterile pipette for each tube, add to the sediment 1 to 2 ml of sterile, 0.2% BSA fraction V (pH 6.8) or 1

to 2 ml of phosphate buffer (pH 6.8), and resuspend the sediment with the pipette or by shaking the tube gently by hand. BSA may have a buffering and detoxifying effect on the sediment and increases the adhesion of the specimen to solid media; however, it may lengthen detection times (for instance in the BACTEC 460TB System).

8. Inoculate the specimens onto appropriate solid culture media and into broth media. Use a separate disposable capillary pipette for each specimen to deliver 3 drops to solid medium.

9. Prepare a smear for acid-fast staining. Use a sterile disposable pipette to place 1 drop of the sediment onto a clean, properly labeled microscope slide, covering an area approximately 1 by 2 cm. Place the smears on an electric slide warmer at 65 to 75°C for 2 h to dry and fix them. Alternatively, air dry the smears and fix them by passing the slide three or four times through the blue cone of a flame (heat fixing does not always kill mycobacteria, and the slides are potentially infectious).

10. Refrigerate the remaining sediment for later use if needed (direct susceptibility testing, further treatment if specimen is contaminated, etc.).

The NALC-NaOH method can be used to process gastric lavage specimens, tissues, stool, urine, and other body fluids. For neutralized gastric lavage specimens and other body fluids (≥10 ml), centrifuge at ≥3,000 × g for 30 min in sterile screw-cap 50-ml centrifuge tubes, decant the supernatants, resuspend the sediments in 2 to 5 ml of sterile distilled water, and proceed as for sputum. If a gastric lavage specimen is mucopurulent, add 50 mg of NALC powder per 50 ml of lavage fluid and vortex before centrifugation. Tissue that is not collected aseptically can be ground, placed in a tube, homogenized by vortexing, and processed as for sputum. For stool specimens, place approximately 1 g of a formed specimen or 1 to 5 ml of a liquid specimen in a total volume of 10 ml of 7H9 broth, sterile water, or sterile saline; vortex vigorously for 30 s; and then allow large particles to settle to the bottom of the tube for 15 min. Remove 7 to 8 ml of supernatant, place into a 50-ml centrifuge tube, and process as for sputum.

Sodium hydroxide method

Reagents

Digestant: NaOH solution (2 to 4%). Sterilize by autoclaving.
2 N HCl: Dilute 33 ml of concentrated HCl to 200 ml with water. Sterilize by autoclaving.
Phenol red indicator: Combine 20 ml of phenol red solution (0.4% in 4% NaOH) and 85 ml of concentrated HCl with distilled water to make 1,000 ml.
Phosphate buffer: The buffer is 0.067 M and pH 6.8. See the NALC-NaOH procedure for buffer preparation.

Procedure

Follow the steps described for the NALC-NaOH method, substituting 2% NaOH for the NALC-alkali digestant.

1. Transfer a maximum volume of 10 ml of specimen to a sterile 50-ml screw-cap plastic centrifuge tube. Add an equal volume of NaOH.

2. With the cap tightened, invert the tube and then agitate the mixture vigorously for 15 min on a mechanical mixer, or vortex vigorously and let stand for exactly 15 min. If it is necessary to reduce excessive contamination, the NaOH concentration can be increased to 3 or 4%.

3. Add phosphate buffer (pH 6.8) up to the 50-ml mark on the tube. Recap the tube, and swirl by hand to mix well.

4. Centrifuge the specimen at ≥3,000 × g for 15 min, decant the supernatant, and add a few drops of phenol red indicator to the sediment. Neutralize the sediment with HCl. Thoroughly mix the contents of the tube. Stop acid addition when the solution is persistently yellow.

5. Resuspend the sediment in 1 to 2 ml of phosphate buffer or sterile 0.1% BSA fraction V.

6. Inoculate the resuspended sediment to the appropriate culture media, and prepare a smear.

Zephiran-trisodium phosphate method

Principle and Indications

This system can be used when the laboratory cannot monitor the exposure time to the decontaminating agent, since the timing of this digestion-decontamination process is not critical. Benzalkonium chloride (Zephiran), a quaternary ammonium compound, together with trisodium phosphate selectively destroys many contaminants while having little activity on tubercle bacilli. Zephiran is bacteriostatic to mycobacteria, and so the digested, centrifuged sediment must be neutralized with buffer before being inoculated onto agar medium. The phospholipids of egg medium neutralize this compound. It is incompatible with the BACTEC 460TB System.

Reagents

Zephiran-trisodium phosphate digestant: Dissolve 1 kg of trisodium phosphate (Na$_3$PO$_4$·12H$_2$O) in 4 liters of hot distilled water. Add 7.5 ml of Zephiran concentrate (17% benzalkonium chloride [Winthrop Laboratories, New York, N.Y.]), and mix. Store at room temperature.
Neutralizing buffer: Neutralizing buffer has a pH of 6.6. Add 37.5 ml of 0.067 M disodium phosphate buffer and 62.5 ml of 0.067 M monopotassium phosphate buffer (for preparation of buffer solutions, see the NALC-NaOH procedure).

Procedure

1. Transfer a maximum volume of 10 ml of specimen to a sterile, 50-ml screw-cap plastic centrifuge tube. Add an equal volume of the Zephiran-trisodium phosphate digestant.

2. Tighten the cap, invert the tube, and then agitate the mixture vigorously for 30 min on a mechanical shaker. Permit the material to stand, without shaking, for an additional 20 to 30 min at room temperature.

3. Centrifuge the specimen at ≥3,000 × g for 15 min, decant the supernatant, and add 20 ml of neutralizing buffer. Vortex for 30 s to thoroughly suspend the sediment in the buffer (the neutralizing buffer serves to inactivate traces of Zephiran in the sediment, which is critical if inoculation of an agar-based medium is intended).

4. Centrifuge the specimen again for 15 min.

5. Decant the supernatant, retaining some fluid to resuspend the sediment.

6. Inoculate egg-based medium, and make a smear. The phospholipids of egg medium provide neutralization for this quaternary compound.

Oxalic acid method

Indications

The oxalic acid method is superior to alkali methods for processing specimens consistently contaminated with *Pseudomonas* species and certain other contaminants. Specimens processed by this method may be used with the BACTEC 460TB System. It can also be used to decontaminate a previously processed sediment when cultures are contaminated with *Pseudomonas*.

Reagents

5% oxalic acid
Physiological saline (0.85%)
4% NaOH
Phenol red indicator or pH paper

Procedure

1. Add an equal volume of 5% oxalic acid to 10 ml or less of specimen in a 50-ml centrifuge tube (1:1, vol/vol).

2. Vortex the solution, and allow it to stand at room temperature for 30 min with occasional shaking.

3. Add sterile saline to the 50-ml mark on the centrifuge tube. Recap the tube, and invert it several times to mix the contents.

4. Centrifuge for 15 min at ≥3,000 × g, decant the supernatant fluid, and add a few drops of phenol red indicator to the sediment. Alternatively, use pH paper.

5. Neutralize with 4% NaOH.

6. Resuspend the sediment, inoculate it to media, and make smear.

CPC method

Principle and Indications

Cetylpyridinium chloride (CPC), a quaternary ammonium compound, is used to decontaminate specimens, while sodium chloride effects liquefaction. CPC is bacteriostatic for mycobacteria inoculated onto agar-based media. This effect is not neutralized in the digestion process, and thus sediments from specimens treated with CPC should be inoculated only on egg-based media. This method is incompatible with the BACTEC 460TB System.

This method is a means of digesting and decontaminating specimens in transit (>24 h). Mycobacteria remain viable for 8 days in the solution.

Reagents

CPC digestant-decontaminant: Dissolve 10 g of CPC and 20 g of NaCl in 1,000 ml of distilled water. The solution is self-sterilizing and remains stable if protected from light, extreme heat, and evaporation. Dissolve with gentle heat any crystals that might form in the working solution. Other reagents used in processing include sterile water and sterile saline or 0.2% sterile BSA fraction V.

Procedure

1. Collect 10 ml or less of sputum in a 50-ml screw-cap centrifuge tube.

2. Inside a BSC, add an equal volume of CPC-NaCl, cap securely, and shake by hand until the specimen liquefies.

3. Package the specimen appropriately as specified by current postal regulations, and send it to a processing laboratory.

4. Upon receipt in the processing laboratory (allow at least 24 h for digestion-decontamination to be completed), dilute the digested-decontaminated specimen to the 50-ml mark with sterile distilled water and recap securely. Invert the tube several times to mix the contents.

5. Centrifuge at ≥3,000 × g for 15 min, decant the supernatant fluid, and suspend the sediment in 1 to 2 ml of sterile water, saline, or 0.2% BSA fraction V.

6. Inoculate the resuspended sediment onto egg medium, and make a smear.

Sulfuric acid method

Indications

The sulfuric acid method may be useful for urine and other body fluids that yield contaminated cultures when processed by one of the alkaline digestants.

Reagents

4% sulfuric acid
4% sodium hydroxide
Sterile distilled water
Phenol red indicator

Procedure

1. Centrifuge the entire specimen for 30 min at ≥3,000 × g. This may require several tubes.

2. Decant the supernatant fluids; pool the sediments if several tubes were used for a single specimen.

3. Add an equal volume of 4% sulfuric acid to the sediment.

4. Vortex, and let stand for 15 min at room temperature.

5. Fill the tube to the 50-ml mark with sterile water.

6. Centrifuge at ≥3,000 × g for 15 min, and decant the supernatant.

7. Add 1 drop of phenol red indicator, and neutralize with 4% NaOH until a persistent pale pink color forms.

8. Inoculate the media, and make a smear.

REFERENCES

1. **Abramowsky, C., B. Gonzalez, and R. U. Sorensen.** 1993. Disseminated bacillus Calmette-Guérin infections in patients with primary immunodeficiencies. *Am. J. Clin. Pathol.* **100:**52–56.

2. **Agerton, T., S. Valway, B. Gore, C. Pozsik, B. Plikaytis, C. Woodley, and I. Onorato.** 1997. Transmission of a highly drug-resistant strain (strain W1) of *Mycobacterium tuberculosis. JAMA* **278:**1073–1077.

3. **Agy, M. B., C. K. Wassis, J. J. Plorde, L. C. Carlson, and M. B. Coyle.** 1989. Evaluation of four mycobacterial blood culture media: BACTEC 13A, Isolator/BACTEC 12B, Isolator/Middlebrook Agar and a biphasic medium. *Diagn. Microbiol. Infect. Dis.* **12:**303–308.

4. **Allen, S., J. Batungwanayo, K. Kerlikowske, A. R. Lifson, W. Wolf, R. Granich, H. Taelman, P. van de Perre, A. Serufilira, J. Bogaerts, et al.** 1993. Two-year incidence of tuberculosis in cohorts of HIV-infected and uninfected urban Rwandan women. *Am. Rev. Respir. Dis.* **146:**1439–1444.

5. **Al-Moamary, M. A., W. Black, and K. Elwood.** 1998. Pulmonary disease due to *Mycobacterium malmoense* in British Columbia. *Can. Respir. J.* **5:**135–138.

6. **American Thoracic Society.** 1997. Diagnosis and treatment of disease caused by nontuberculous mycobacteria. *Am. J. Respir. Crit. Care Med. Suppl.* **156:**S1–S25.

7. **Aranaz, A., E. Liebana, E. Gomez-Mampaso, J. C. Galan, D. Cousins, A. Ortega, J. Blazquez, F. Baquero, A. Mateos, G. Suarez, and L. Dominguez.** 1999. *Mycobacterium tuberculosis* subsp. *caprae* subsp. nov.: a taxonomic study of the *Mycobacterium tuberculosis* complex isolated from goats in Spain. *Int. J. Syst. Bacteriol.* **49:**1263–1273.

8. **Archibald, L. K., L. C. McDonald, R. M. Addison, C. McKnight, T. Byrne, H. Dobbie, O. Nwanyanwu, P. Kezembe, L. B. Reller, and W. R. Jarvis.** 2000. Comparison of BACTEC MYCO/F LYTIC and WAMPOLE ISOLATOR 10 (lysis-centrifugation) systems for detection of bacteremia, mycobacteremia, and fungemia in a developing country. *J. Clin. Microbiol.* **38:**2994–2997.

9. **Association of State and Territorial Public Health Laboratory Directors (ASTPHLD), and Centers for Disease Control and Prevention (CDC).** 1997. *Recognition and Prevention of False-Positive Test Results in Mycobacteriology. A Laboratory Training Program.* Centers for Disease Control and Prevention, Atlanta, Ga.

10. **Attorri, S., S. Dunbar, and J. E. Clarridge III.** 2000. Assessment of morphology for rapid presumptive identification of *Mycobacterium tuberculosis* and *Mycobacterium kansasii. J. Clin. Microbiol.* **38:**1426–1429.

11. **Ausina, V., M. Luquin, M. G. Barceló, M. A. Lanéelle, V. Lévy-Frébault, F. Belda, and G. Prats.** 1992. *Mycobacterium alvei* sp. nov. *Int. J. Syst. Bacteriol.* **42:**529–535.

12. **Bajolet, O., I. Beguinot, L. Brasme, R. Jaussard, D. Ingrand, and V. Vincent.** 2001. Isolation of an unusual *Mycobacterium* species from an AIDS patient with acute lymphadenitis. *J. Clin. Microbiol.* **39:**2018–2020.

13. **Baril, L., E. Caumes, C. Truffot-Pernot, F. Bricaire, J. Grosset, and M. Gentilini.** 1995. Tuberculosis caused by *Mycobacterium africanum* associated with involvement of the upper and lower respiratory tract, skin, and mucosa. *Clin. Infect. Dis.* **21:**653–655.

14. **Beam, E. R., and G. P. Kubica.** 1968. Stimulatory effects of carbon dioxide on the primary isolation of tubercle bacilli on agar containing medium. *Am. J. Clin. Pathol.* **50:**395–397.

15. **Behr, M. A., and P. M. Small.** 1999. A historical and molecular phylogeny of BCG strains. *Vaccine* **17:**915–922.
16. **Bennett, S. N., D. E. Peterson, D. R. Johnson, W. N. Hall, B. Robinson-Dunn, and S. Dietrich.** 1994. Bronchoscopy-associated *Mycobacterium xenopi* pseudoinfections. *Am. J. Respir. Crit. Care Med.* **150:**245–250.
17. **Bernard, L., V. Vincent, O. Lortholary, I. Raskine, C. Vettier, D. Colaitis, D. Mechali, F. Bricaire, E. Bouvet, F. B. Sadr, V. Lalande, and C. Perronne.** 1999. *Mycobacterium kansasii* septic arthritis: French retrospective study of 5 years and review. *Clin. Infect. Dis.* **29:**1455–1460.
18. **Besra, G. S., and D. Chatterjee.** 1994. Lipids and carbohydrates of *Mycobacterium tuberculosis,* p. 285–306. *In* B. R. Bloom (ed.), *Tuberculosis: Pathogenesis, Protection, and Control.* ASM Press, Washington, D.C.
19. **Best, M., S. A. Sattar, V. S. Springthorpe, and M. E. Kennedy.** 1990. Efficacies of selected disinfectants against *Mycobacterium tuberculosis. J. Clin. Microbiol.* **28:**2234–2239.
20. **Blacklock, Z., D. Dawson, D. Kane, and D. McEvoy.** 1983. *Mycobacterium asiaticum* as a potential pulmonary pathogen for humans. A clinical and bacteriologic review of five cases. *Am. Rev. Respir. Dis.* **127:**241–244.
21. **Böttger, E. C., A. Teske, P. Kirschner, S. Bost, H. R. Chang, V. Beer, and B. Hirschel.** 1991. Disseminated "*Mycobacterium genavense*" infection in patients with AIDS. *Lancet* **340:**76–80.
22. **Brennan, P. J.** 1994. Ultrastructure of *Mycobacterium tuberculosis.* p. 271–284. *In* B. R. Bloom (ed.), *Tuberculosis: Pathogenesis, Protection, and Control.* ASM Press, Washington, D.C.
23. **Brown, B. A., B. Springer, V. A. Steingrube, R. W. Wilson, G. E. Pfyffer, M. J. Garcia, M. C. Menendez, B. Rodriguez-Salgado, K. C. Jost, S. H. Chiu, G. Onyi, E. C. Böttger, and R. J. Wallace, Jr.** 1999. Description of *Mycobacterium wolinskyi* and *Mycobacterium goodii,* two new rapidly growing species related to *Mycobacterium smegmatis* and associated with human wound infections: a cooperative study from the International Working Group on Mycobacterial Taxonomy. *Int. J. Syst. Bacteriol.* **49:**1493–1511.
24. **Buchholz, U. T., M. M. McNeil, L. E. Keyes, and R. C. Good.** 1998. *Mycobacterium malmoense* infections in the United States, January 1993 through June 1995. *Clin. Infect. Dis.* **27:**551–558.
25. **Burman, W. J., and R. R. Reves.** 2000. Review of false-positive cultures for *Mycobacterium tuberculosis* and recommendations for avoiding unnecessary treatment. *Clin. Infect. Dis.* **31:**1390–1395.
26. **Butler, W. R., S. P. O'Connor, M. A. Yakrus, R. W. Smithwick, B. B. Plikaytis, C. W. Moss, M. M. Floyd, C. L. Woodley, J. O. Kilburn, F. S. Vadney, and W. M. Gross.** 1993. *Mycobacterium celatum. Int. J. Syst. Bacteriol.* **43:**539–548.
27. **Bux-Gewehr, I., H. P. Hagen, S. Rüsch-Gerdes, and G. E. Feurle.** 1998. Fatal pulmonary infection with *Mycobacterium celatum* in an apparently immunocompetent patient. *J. Clin. Microbiol.* **36:**587–588.
28. **Castro, K. G., and S. W. Dooley.** 1993. *Mycobacterium tuberculosis* transmission in healthcare settings: is it influenced by coinfection with human immunodeficiency virus? *Infect. Control Hosp. Epidemiol.* **14:**65–66.
29. **Centers for Disease Control.** 1991. *Mycobacterium haemophilum* infections, New York City Metropolitan Area, 1990–1991. *Morb. Mortal. Wkly. Rep.* **40:**636–643.
30. **Centers for Disease Control and Prevention.** 1997. USPHS/IDSA guidelines for the prevention of opportunistic infections in persons infected with human immuno-deficiency virus. *Morb. Mortal. Wkly. Rep.* **46**(RR-12)**:**1–46.
31. **Centers for Disease Control and Prevention.** 1998. Tuberculosis morbidity—United States, 1997. *Morb. Mortal. Wkly. Rep.* **47:**253–257.
32. **Centers for Disease Control and Prevention—National Institutes of Health.** 1999. *Biosafety in Microbiological and Biomedical Laboratories,* 4th ed. HHS publication (CDC) 017-040-00547-4. U.S. Government Printing Office, Washington, D.C. Available at www.cdc.gov/od/ohs/biosfty/bmbl4.
33. **Chamoiseau, G.** 1979. Etiology of farcy in African bovines: nomenclature of the causal organisms *Mycobacterium farcinogenes* Chamoiseau and *Mycobacterium senegalense* (Chamoiseau) comb. nov. *Int. J. Syst. Bacteriol.* **29:**407–410.
34. **Chaves, A., A. Torrelo, I. G. Mediero, M. Mendez-Rivas, A. Ortega-Calderon, and A. Zambrano.** 2001. Primary cutaneous *Mycobacterium kansasii* infection in a child. *Pediatr. Dermatol.* **18:**131–134.
35. **Cingolani, A., M. Sanguinetti, A. Antinori, L. M. Larocca, F. Ardito, B. Posteraro, G. Federico, G. Fadda, and L. Ortona.** 2000. Disseminated mycobacteriosis caused by drug-resistant *Mycobacterium triplex* in a human immunodeficiency virus-infected patient during highly active antiretroviral therapy. *Clin. Infect. Dis.* **31:**177–179.
36. **Corbett, E. L., M. Hay, G. J. Churchyard, T. Clayton, B. G. Williams, D. Hayes, D. Mulder, and K. M. de Cock.** 1999. *Mycobacterium kansasii* and *M. scrofulaceum* isolates from HIV-negative South African gold miners: incidence, clinical significance and radiology. *Int. J. Tuberc. Lung Dis.* **3:**501–507.
37. **Cornfield, D. B., K. G. Beavis, J. A. Greene, M. Bojac, and J. Bondi.** 1997. Mycobacterial growth and bacterial contamination in the Mycobacteria Growth Indicator Tube and BACTEC 460 culture systems. *J. Clin. Microbiol.* **35:**2068–2071.
38. **Coyle, M. B., L. Carlson, C. Wallis, R. Leonard, V. Raisys, J. Kilburn, M. Samadpour, and E. Böttger.** 1992. Laboratory aspects of *Mycobacterium genavense,* a proposed species isolated from AIDS patients. *J. Clin. Microbiol.* **30:**3206–3212.
39. **Danesh-Clough, T., J. C. Theis, and A. van der Linden.** 2000. *Mycobacterium xenopi* infection of the spine: a case report and literature review. *Spine* **25:**626–628.
40. **Dawson, D. J., Z. M. Blacklock, L. R. Ashidown, and E. C. Böttger.** 1995. *Mycobacterium asiaticum* as the probable causative agent in a case of olecranon bursitis. *J. Clin. Microbiol.* **33:**1042–1043.
41. **De Baere, T., M. Moerman, L. Rigouts, C. Dhooge, H. Vermeersch, G. Verschraegen, and M. Vaneechoutte.** 2001. *Mycobacterium interjectum* as causative agent of cervical lymphadenitis. *J. Clin. Microbiol.* **39:**725–727.
42. **Dixon, J. M. S., and E. H. Cuthbert.** 1967. Isolation of tubercle bacilli from uncentrifuged sputum on pyruvic acid medium. *Am. Rev. Respir. Dis.* **96:**119–122.
43. **Dizon, D., C. Mihailescu, and H. C. Bae.** 1976. Simple procedure for detection of *Mycobacterium gordonae* in water causing false-positive acid-fast smears. *J. Clin. Microbiol.* **3:**211.
44. **Domenech, P., M. S. Jimenez, M. C. Menendez, T. J. Bull, S. Samper, A. Manrique, and M. J. Garcia.** 1997. *Mycobacterium mageritense* sp. nov. *Int. J. Syst. Bacteriol.* **47:**535–540.
45. **Donnabella, V., J. Salazar-Schicchi, S. Bonk, B. Hanna, and W. N. Rom.** 2000. Increasing incidence of *Mycobacterium xenopi* at Bellevue Hospital: an emerging pathogen or a product of improved laboratory methods? *Chest* **118:**1365–1370.

46. **Dye, C., S. Scheele, P. Dolin, V. Pathania, and M. C. Raviglione.** 1999. Global burden of tuberculosis. Estimated incidence, prevalence, and mortality by country. *JAMA* **282:**677–686.

47. **Eckburg, P. B., E. O. Buadu, P. Stark, P. S. A. Sarinas, R. K. Chitkara, and W. G. Kuschner.** 2000. Clinical and chest radiographic findings among persons with sputum culture positive for *Mycobacterium gordonae*. *Chest* **117:**96–102.

48. **European Society of Mycobacteriology.** 1991. Decontamination, microscopy and isolation, p. 57–64. *In* M. D. Yates and D. G. Groothuis (ed.), *Diagnostic Public Health Mycobacteriology*. Bureau of Hygiene and Tropical Disease, London, United Kingdom.

49. **Falkinham, J. O.** 1996. Epidemiology of infection by nontuberculous mycobacteria. *Clin. Microbiol. Rev.* **9:**178–215.

50. **Fang, C.-T., S.-C. Chang, K.-T. Luh, Y.-L. Chang, P.-R. Hsueh, and W.-C. Hsieh.** 1999. Successful treatment of disseminated *Mycobacterium szulgai* infection with ciprofloxacin, rifampicin, and ethambutol. *J. Infect.* **38:**195–204.

51. **Fergie, J. E., T. W. Milligan, B. M. Henderson, and W. W. Stafford.** 1997. Intrathoracic *Mycobacterium avium* complex infection in immunocompetent children: case report and review. *J. Infect. Dis.* **24:**250–253.

52. **Floyd, M. M., L. S. Guthertz, V. A. Silcox, P. S. Duffey, Y. Jang, E. P. Desmond, J. T. Crawford, and W. R. Butler.** 1996. Characterization of an SAV organism and proposal of *Mycobacterium triplex* sp. nov. *J. Clin. Microbiol.* **34:**2963–2967.

53. **Foulkes, G. D., J. C. Floyd, and J. L. Stephens.** 1998. Flexor tenosynovitis due to *Mycobacterium asiaticum*. *J. Hand Surg.* **23:**753–756.

54. **Franklin, D. J., J. R. Starke, M. T. Brady, B. A. Brown, and R. J. Wallace, Jr.** 1994. Chronic otitis media after tympanostomy tube placement caused by *Mycobacterium abscessus*: a new clinical entity? *Am. J. Otol.* **15:**313–320.

55. **Frothingham, R., P. L. Strickland, G. Bretzel, S. Ramaswamy, J. M. Musser, and D. L. Williams.** 1999. Phenotypic and genotypic characterization of *Mycobacterium africanum* isolates from West Africa. *J. Clin. Microbiol.* **37:**1921–1926.

56. **Gamboa, F., Z. de la Rosa, J. Bustillo, M. P. Mora, I. Hernandez, and F. Mirque.** 2000. Negative effect of the components of the lysis-centrifugation system in the growth of mycobacteria in MGIT and Septi-Chek AFB liquid media. *Enferm. Infecc. Microbiol. Clin.* **18:**439–444.

57. **Gascogne-Binzi, D. M., R. E. L. Barlow, R. Frothingham, G. Robinson, T. A. Collyns, R. Gelletlie, and P. M. Hawkes.** 2001. Rapid identification of laboratory contamination with *Mycobacterium tuberculosis* using variable number tandem repeat analysis. *J. Clin. Microbiol.* **39:**69–74.

58. **Gillespie, T. G., L. Hogg, E. Budge, A. Duncan, and J. E. Coia.** 2000. *Mycobacterium chelonae* isolated from rinse water within an endoscope washer-disinfectant. *J. Hosp. Infect.* **45:**332–334.

59. **Golizadeh, Y., A. Varnerot, C. Maslo, B. Salauze, H. Badaoui, V. Vincent, and A. Bure-Rossier.** 1998. *Mycobacterium celatum* infection in two HIV-infected patients treated prophylactically with rifabutin. *Eur. J. Clin. Microbiol. Infect. Dis.* **17:**278–281.

60. **Good, R. C., and T. M. Shinnick.** 1998. *Mycobacterium*, p. 549–576. *In* L. Collier, A. Balows, and M. Sussman (ed.), *Topley & Wilson's Microbiology and Microbial Infections, Systematic Bacteriology*, 9th ed., vol. 2. Edward Arnold, London, United Kingdom.

61. **Goodfellow, M.** 1998. *Nocardia* and related genera, p. 463–489. *In* L. Collier, A. Balows, and M. Sussman (ed.), *Topley & Wilson's Microbiology and Microbial Infections, Systematic Bacteriology*, 9th ed., vol. 2. Edward Arnold, London, United Kingdom.

62. **Gordon, S. V., R. Brosch, A. Billault, T. Garnier, K. Eigelmeier, and S. Cole.** 1999. Identification of variable regions in the genomes of tubercle bacilli using bacterial artificial chromosome arrays. *Mol. Microbiol.* **32:**643–655.

63. **Goutzamanis, J. J., and G. L. Gilbert.** 1995. *Mycobacterium ulcerans* infection in Australian children: report of eight cases and review. *Clin. Infect. Dis.* **21:**1186–1192.

64. **Green, B. A., and B. Afessa.** 2000. Isolation of *Mycobacterium interjectum* in an AIDS patient with diarrhea. *AIDS* **16:**1282–1284.

65. **Griffith, D. E., W. M. Girard, and R. J. Wallace, Jr.** 1993. Clinical features of pulmonary disease caused by rapidly growing mycobacteria: an analysis of 154 patients. *Am. Rev. Respir. Dis.* **147:**1271–1278.

66. **Haas, W. H., G. Bretzel, B. Amthor, K. Schilke, G. Krommes, S. Rüsch-Gerdes, V. Sticht-Groh, and H. J. Bremer.** 1997. Comparison of DNA fingerprint patterns of isolates of *Mycobacterium africanum* from east and west Africa. *J. Clin. Microbiol.* **35:**663–666.

67. **Haas, W. H., W. R. Butler, P. Kirschner, B. B. Plikaytis, M. B. Coyle, B. Amthor, A. G. Steigerwalt, D. J. Brenner, M. Salfinger, J. T. Crawford, E. C. Böttger, and H. J. Bremer.** 1997. A new agent of mycobacterial lymphadenitis in children: *Mycobacterium heidelbergense* sp. nov. *J. Clin. Microbiol.* **35:**3203–3209.

68. **Haase, G., H. Kentrup, H. Skopnik, B. Springer, and E. C. Böttger.** 1997. *Mycobacterium lentiflavum*: an etiologic agent of cervical lymphadenitis. *Clin. Infect. Dis.* **25:**1245–1246.

69. **Haase, G., H. Skopnik, S. Bätge, and E. C. Böttger.** 1994. Cervical lymphadenitis caused by *Mycobacterium celatum*. *Lancet* **344:**1020–1021.

70. **Hale, Y. M., G. E. Pfyffer, and M. Salfinger.** 2001. Laboratory diagnosis of mycobacterial infections: new tools and lessons learned. *Clin. Infect. Dis.* **33:**834–846.

71. **Hanna, B. A., A. Ebrahimzadeh, L. B. Elliott, M. A. Morgan, S. M. Novak, S. Rüsch-Gerdes, M. Acio, D. F. Dunbar, T. M. Holmes, C. H. Rexer, C. Savthyakumar, and A. M. Vannier.** 1999. Multicenter evaluation of the BACTEC MGIT 960 System for recovery of mycobacteria. *J. Clin. Microbiol.* **37:**748–752.

72. **Hanna, B. A., S. B. Walters, S. J. Bonk, and L. J. Tick.** 1995. Recovery of mycobacteria from blood in Mycobacteria Growth Indicator Tube and Löwenstein-Jensen slant after lysis-centrifugation. *J. Clin. Microbiol.* **33:**3315–3316.

73. **Harro, C., G. L. Braden, A. B. Morris, G. S. Lipkowitz, and R. L. Madden.** 1997. Failure to cure *Mycobacterium gordonae* peritonitis associated with continuous ambulatory peritoneal dialysis. *Clin. Infect. Dis.* **24:**955–957.

74. **Harvell, J. D., W. K. Hadley, and V. L. Ng.** 2000. Increased sensitivity of the BACTEC 460 mycobacterial radiometric broth culture system does not decrease the number of respiratory specimens required for a definite diagnosis of pulmonary tuberculosis. *J. Clin. Microbiol.* **38:**3608–3611.

75. **Hastings, R. C., T. P. Gillis, J. L. Krahenbuhl, and S. G. Franzblau.** 1988. Leprosy. *Clin. Microbiol. Rev.* **1:**330–348.

76. **Havlik, J. A., B. Metchock, S. E. Thompson III, K. Barrett, D. Rimland, and C. R. Horsburgh, Jr.** 1993. A prospective evaluation of *Mycobacterium avium* complex colonization of the respiratory and gastrointestinal tracts of persons with human immunodeficiency virus infection. *J. Infect. Dis.* **168:**1045–1048.

77. Havlik, J., C. Horsburgh, B. Metchock, P. William, S. Fan, and S. Thompson. 1992. Disseminated *Mycobacterium avium* complex infection: clinical identification and epidemiologic trends. *J. Infect. Dis.* **165**:577–580.

78. Hazra, R., M. M. Floyd, A. Sloutsky, and R. N. Husson. 2001. Novel mycobacterium related to *Mycobacterium triplex* as a cause of cervical lymphadenitis. *J. Clin. Microbiol.* **39**:1227–1230.

79. Henriques, B., S. E. Hoffner, B. Petrini, I. Juhlin, P. Wahlen, and G. Källenius. 1994. Infection with *Mycobacterium malmoense* in Sweden: report of 221 cases. *Clin. Infect. Dis.* **18**:596–600.

80. Hillebrand-Haverkort, M. E., A. H. Kolk, L. F. Kox, J. J. ten Velden, and J. H. ten Veen. 1999. Generalized *Mycobacterium genavense* infection in HIV-infected patients: detection of the mycobacterium in hospital tap water. *Scand. J. Infect. Dis.* **31**:63–68.

81. Ho, P. L., B. K. Fung, W. Y. Ip, and S. S. Wong. 2001. A case of disseminated *Mycobacterium marinum* infection following systemic steroid therapy. *Scand. J. Infect. Dis.* **33**:232–233.

82. Hoff, E., M. Sholtis, G. Procop, C. Sabella, J. Goldfarb, R. Wyllie, R. Cunningham, L. Stockman, and G. Hall. 2001. *Mycobacterium triplex* in a liver transplant patient. *J. Clin. Microbiol.* **39**:2033–2034.

83. Hoop, R. K., E. C. Böttger, and G. E. Pfyffer. 1996. Etiological agents of mycobacterioses in pet birds between 1986 and 1995. *J. Clin. Microbiol.* **34**:991–992.

84. Horsburgh, C. R., Jr., U. G. Mason III, D. C. Farhi, and M. D. Iseman. 1985. Disseminated infection with *Mycobacterium avium-intracellulare.* A report of 13 cases and review of the literature. *Medicine* **64**:36–48.

85. Horsburgh, C., B. Metchock, J. McGowan, Jr., and S. Thompson. 1992. Clinical implications of recovery of *Mycobacterium avium* complex from the stool or respiratory tract of HIV-infected individuals. *AIDS* **6**:512–514.

86. Huminer, D., S. Dux, Z. Samra, L. Kaufman, A. Lavy, C. S. Block, and S. D. Pitlik. 1993. *Mycobacterium simiae* infection in Israeli patients with AIDS. *Clin. Infect. Dis.* **17**:508–509.

87. Inderlied, C., C. Kempler, and L. Bermudez. 1993. The *Mycobacterium avium* complex. *Clin. Microbiol. Rev.* **6**:266–310.

88. Isenberg, H. D. (ed.). 1993. *Clinical Microbiology Procedures Handbook,* vol. 1, p. 3.1.1–3.10.1. American Society for Microbiology, Washington, D.C.

89. Isenberg, H. D., R. F. D'Amato, L. Heifets, P. R. Murray, M. Scardamaglia, M. C. Jacobs, P. Alperstein, and A. Niles. 1991. Collaborative feasibility study of a biphasic system (Roche Septi-Chek AFB) for rapid detection and isolation of mycobacteria. *J. Clin. Microbiol.* **29**:1719–1722.

90. Jernigan, J. A., and B. M. Farr. 2000. Incubation period and sources for cutaneous *Mycobacterium marinum* infection: case report and review of the literature. *Clin. Infect. Dis.* **31**:439–443.

91. Jiva, T. M., H. M. Jacoby, L. A. Weymouth, D. A. Kaminski, and A. C. Portmore. 1997. *Mycobacterium xenopi:* innocent bystander or emerging pathogen? *Clin. Infect. Dis.* **24**:226–232.

92. Joseph, S., E. Vaichulis, and V. Houk. 1967. Lack of auramine-rhodamine fluorescence of Runyon group IV mycobacteria. *Am. Rev. Respir. Dis.* **95**:114–115.

93. Kelly, M., L. Thibert, and C. Sinave. 1999. Septic arthritis in the knee due to *Mycobacterium xenopi* in a patient undergoing hemodialysis. *Clin. Infect. Dis.* **29**:1342–1343.

94. Kent, P. T., and G. P. Kubica. 1985. *Public Health Mycobacteriology: a Guide for the Level III Laboratory.* U.S. Department of Health and Human Services, Centers for Disease Control, Atlanta, Ga.

95. Kesten, S., and C. Chaparro. 1999. Mycobacterial infections in lung transplant recipients. *Chest* **115**:741–745.

96. Kilburn, J. O., K. D. Stottmeier, and G. P. Kubica. 1968. Aspartic acid as a precursor for niacin synthesis by tubercle bacilli grown on 7H10 agar medium. *Am. J. Clin. Pathol.* **50**:582–586.

97. Kilby, J., P. Gilligan, J. Yankaskas, W. Highsmith, Jr., L. Edwards, and M. Knowles. 1992. Nontuberculous mycobacteria in adult patients with cystic fibrosis. *Chest* **102**:70–75.

98. Kim, T. C., R. S. Blackman, K. M. Heatwole, T. Kim, and D. F. Rochester. 1984. Acid-fast bacilli in sputum smears of patients with pulmonary tuberculosis. Prevalence and significance of negative smears pretreatment and positive smears post-treatment. *Am. Rev. Respir. Dis.* **129**:264–268.

99. Klein, G. C., M. M. Cummings, and C. H. Fish. 1952. Efficiency of centrifugation as a method of concentrating tubercle bacilli. *Am. J. Clin. Pathol.* **22**:581–585.

100. Koukila-Kähkölä, P., B. Springer, E. C. Böttger, L. Paulin, E. Jantzen, and M. L. Katila. 1995. *Mycobacterium branderi* sp. nov., a new potential human pathogen. *Int. J. Syst. Bacteriol.* **45**:549–553.

101. Koukila-Kähkölä, P., L. Paulin, E. Brander, E. Jantzen, M. Eho-Remes, and M. L. Katila. 2000. Characterization of a new isolate of *Mycobacterium shimoidei* from Finland. *J. Med. Microbiol.* **49**:937–940.

102. Krasnow, L., and L. G. Wayne. 1969. Comparison of methods for tuberculosis bacteriology. *Appl. Microbiol.* **18**:915–917.

103. Kusunoki, S., and T. Ezaki. 1992. Proposal of *Mycobacterium peregrinum* sp. nov., nom. rev., and elevation of *Mycobacterium chelonae* subsp. *abscessus* (Kubica et al.) to species status: *Mycobacterium abscessus* comb. nov. *Int. J. Syst. Bacteriol.* **42**:240–245.

104. Lalande, V., F. Barbut, A. Vernerot, M. Febvre, D. Nesa, S. Wadel, V. Vincent, and J. C. Petit. 2001. Pseudo-outbreak of *Mycobacterium gordonae* associated with water from refrigerated fountains. *J. Hosp. Infect.* **48**:76–79.

105. Lipsky, B. A., J. Gates, F. C. Tenover, and J. J. Plorde. 1984. Factors affecting the clinical value of microscopy for acid-fast bacilli. *Rev. Infect. Dis.* **6**:214–222.

106. Mastro, T. D., S. C. Redd, and R. F. Breiman. 1992. Imported leprosy in the United States, 1978 through 1988: an epidemic without secondary transmission. *Am. J. Public Health* **82**:1127–1130.

107. Mayall, B., V. Gurtler, L. Irving, A. Marzee, and D. Leslie. 1999. Identification of *Mycobacterium shimoidei* by molecular techniques: case report and summary of the literature. *Int. J. Tuberc. Lung Dis.* **3**:169–173.

108. Mayo, J., J. Collazos, and E. Martinez. 1998. *Mycobacterium nonchromogenicum* bacteremia in an AIDS patient. *Emerg. Infect. Dis.* **4**:124–125.

109. Meier, A., P. Kirschner, K.-H. Schröder, J. Wolters, R. M. Kroppenstedt, and E. C. Böttger. 1993. *Mycobacterium intermedium* sp. nov. *Int. J. Syst. Bacteriol.* **43**:204–209.

110. Migliori, G. B., M. C. Raviglione, T. Schaberg, P. D. Davies, J. P. Zellweger, M. Grzemska, T. Mihaescu, L. Clancy, and L. Casali. 1999. Tuberculosis management in Europe. Task Force of the European Respiratory Society (ERS), the World Health Organization (WHO) and the International Union Against Tuberculosis and Lung Diseases (IUATLD) Europe Region. *Eur. Respir. J.* **14**:978–992.

111. **Mitscherlich, E., and E. H. Marth.** 1984. *Microbial Survival in the Environment*, p. 232–266. Springer-Verlag, New York, N.Y.

112. **Moore, J. S., M. Christensen, R. W. Wilson, R. J. Wallace, Jr., Y. Zhang, D. R. Nash, and B. Shelton.** 2000. Mycobacterial contamination of metal working fluids: involvement of a possible new taxon of rapidly growing mycobacteria. *Am. Ind. Hyg. Assoc. J.* **61:**205–213.

113. **Morris, A. J., and L. B. Reller.** 1993. Reliability of cord formation in BACTEC media for presumptive identification of mycobacteria. *J. Clin. Microbiol.* **31:**2533–2534.

114. **Morris, A., L. B. Reller, M. Salfinger, K. Jackson, A. Sievers, and B. Dwyer.** 1993. Mycobacteria in stool specimens: the nonvalue of smears for predicting culture results. *J. Clin. Microbiol.* **31:**1385–1387.

115. **National Institute of Occupational Safety and Health.** 1995. *Respiratory Protective Devices: Final Rules and Notice.* 42 CFR part 84. *Fed. Regist.* **60:**30335–30398.

116. **Nelson, S. M., M. A. Deike, and C. P. Cartwright.** 1998. Value of examining multiple sputum specimens in the diagnosis of pulmonary tuberculosis. *J. Clin. Microbiol.* **36:**467–469.

117. **Niobe, S. N., C. M. Bebear, M. Clere, J. L. Pellegrin, C. Bebear, and J. Maugein.** 2001. Disseminated *Mycobacterium lentiflavum* infection in a human immunodeficiency virus-infected patient. *J. Clin. Microbiol.* **39:**2030–2032.

118. **Osawa, N.** 1997. Growth of *Mycobacterium leprae* in vitro. *Proc. Jpn. Acad. Ser. B* **73:**144–149.

119. **Ostergaard Thompson, V., U. B. Dragsted, J. Bauer, K. Fuursted, and J. Lundgren.** 1999. Disseminated infection with *Mycobacterium genavense*: a challenge to physicians and mycobacteriologists. *J. Clin. Microbiol.* **37:**3901–3905.

120. **Palomino, J. C., A. M. Obiang, L. Realini, W. M. Meyers, and F. Portaels.** 1998. Effect of oxygen on growth of *Mycobacterium ulcerans* in the BACTEC system. *J. Clin. Microbiol.* **36:**3420–3422.

121. **Palomino, J. C., and F. Portaels.** 1998. Effects of decontamination methods and culture conditions on viability of *Mycobacterium ulcerans* in the BACTEC system. *J. Clin. Microbiol.* **36:**402–408.

122. **Paramasivan, C. N., A. S. L. Narayana, R. Prabhakar, M. S. Rajagopal, P. R. Somasundaram, and S. P. Tripathy.** 1983. Effect of storage of sputum specimens at room temperature on smear and culture results. *Tubercle* **64:**119–124.

123. **Pfyffer, G. E., C. Cieslak, H. M. Welscher, P. Kissling, and S. Rüsch-Gerdes.** 1997. Rapid detection of mycobacteria in clinical specimen by using the automated BACTEC 9000 MB System and comparison with radiometric and solid-culture systems. *J. Clin. Microbiol.* **35:**2229–2234.

124. **Pfyffer, G. E., H. M. Welscher, and P. Kissling.** 1997. Pretreatment of clinical specimens with sodium dodecyl (lauryl) sulfate is not suitable for the Mycobacteria Growth Indicator Tube cultivation method. *J. Clin. Microbiol.* **35:**2142–2144.

125. **Pfyffer, G. E., H. M. Welscher, P. Kissling, C. Cieslak, M. J. Casal, J. Gutierrez, and S. Rüsch-Gerdes.** 1997. Comparison of the Mycobacteria Growth Indicator Tube (MGIT) with radiometric and solid culture for recovery of acid-fast bacilli. *J. Clin. Microbiol.* **35:**364–368.

126. **Pfyffer, G. E., R. Auckenthaler, J. D. A. van Embden, and D. van Soolingen.** 1998. *Mycobacterium canettii*, the smooth variant of M. *tuberculosis*, isolated from a Swiss patient exposed in Africa. *Emerg. Infect. Dis.* **4:**631–634.

127. **Pfyffer, G. E., W. Weder, A. Strässle, and E. W. Russi.** 1998. *Mycobacterium heidelbergense* species nov. infection mimicking a lung tumor. *Clin. Infect. Dis.* **27:**649–650.

128. **Picardeau, M., G. Prod'hom, L. Raskine, M. P. LePennec, and V. Vincent.** 1997. Genotypic characterization of five subspecies of *Mycobacterium kansasii.* *J. Clin. Microbiol.* **35:**25–32.

129. **Picardeau, M., T. J. Bull, G. Prod'hom, A. L. Pozniak, D. C. Shanson, and V. Vincent.** 1997. Comparison of a new insertion element, IS1407, with established molecular markers for the characterization of *Mycobacterium celatum. Int. J. Syst. Bacteriol.* **47:**640–644.

130. **Piersimoni, C., C. Scarparo, A. Callegaro, C. Passerini Tosi, D. Nista, S. Bornigia, M. Scagnelli, A. Rigon, G. Ruggiero, and A. Goglio.** 2001. Comparison of MB/BacT ALERT 3D System with radiometric BACTEC System and Löwenstein-Jensen medium for recovery and identification of mycobacteria from clinical specimen: a multicenter study. *J. Clin. Microbiol.* **39:**651–657.

131. **Pintado, V., J. Fortun, J. L. Casado, and E. Gomez-Mampaso.** 2001. *Mycobacterium kansasii* pericarditis as a presentation of AIDS. *Infection* **29:**48–50.

132. **Portaels, F., J. Aguiar, K. Fissette, P. A. Fonteyne, H. De Beenhouwer, P. de Rijk, A. Guédénon, R. Lemans, C. Steunou, C. Zinsou, J. M. Dumonceau, and W. M. Meyers.** 1997. Direct detection and identification of *Mycobacterium ulcerans* in clinical specimens by PCR and oligonucleotide-specific capture plate hybridization. *J. Clin. Microbiol.* **35:**1097–1100.

133. **Portaels, F., K. Chemlal, P. Elsen, P. D. R. Johnson, J. A. Hayman, J. Hibble, R. Kirkwood, and W. M. Meyers.** 2001. *Mycobacterium ulcerans* in wild animals. *Rev. Sci. Technol. Off. Int. Epizoot.* **20:**252–264.

134. **Portaels, F., L. Realini, L. Bauwens, H. Hirschel, W. M. Meyers, and W. De Meurichy.** 1996. Mycobacteriosis caused by *Mycobacterium genavense* in birds kept in a zoo: 11-year survey. *J. Clin. Microbiol.* **34:**319–323.

135. **Rastogi, N., K. Seng Gho, and M. Berchel.** 1999. Species-specific identification of *Mycobacterium leprae* by PCR-restriction fragment length polymorphism analysis of the *hsp65* gene. *J. Clin. Microbiol.* **37:**2016–2019.

136. **Realini, L., K. de Ridder, B. Hirschel, and F. Portaels.** 1999. Blood and charcoal added to acidified agar media promote growth of *Mycobacterium genavense. Diagn. Microbiol. Infect. Dis.* **34:**45–50.

137. **Realini, L., K. de Ridder, J. Palomino, B. Hirschel, and F. Portaels.** 1998. Microaerophilic conditions promote growth of *Mycobacterium genavense. J. Clin. Microbiol.* **36:**2565–2570.

138. **Reischl, U., S. Emler, Z. Horak, J. Kaustova, R. M. Kroppenstedt, N. Lehn, and L. Naumann.** 1998. *Mycobacterium bohemicum* sp. nov., a new slowly-growing scotochromogenic mycobacterium. *Int. J. Syst. Bacteriol.* **48:**1349–1355.

139. **Reischl, U., K. Feldmann, L. Naumann, B. J. Gaugler, B. Ninet, B. Hirschel, and S. Emler.** 1998. 16S rRNA sequence diversity in *Mycobacterium celatum* strains caused by the presence of two different copies of 16S rRNA gene. *J. Clin Microbiol.* **36:**1761–1764.

140. **Richter, E., S. Niemann, S. Rüsch-Gerdes, and D. Harmsen.** 2001. Description of *Mycobacterium heckeshornense* sp. nov. *J. Clin. Microbiol.* **39:**3023–3024.

141. **Roberts, G. D., N. L. Goodman, L. Heifets, H. W. Larsh, T. H. Lindner, J. K. McClatchy, M. R. McGinnis, S. H. Siddiqi, and P. Wright.** 1983. Evaluation of the BACTEC radiometric method for recovery of myobacteria and drug susceptibility testing of *Mycobacterium tuberculosis* from acid-fast smear-positive specimens. *J. Clin. Micobiol.* **18:**689–696.

142. **Roth, A., U. Reischl, N. Schönfeld, L. Naumann, S. Emler, M. Fischer, H. Mauch, R. Loddenkemper, and R. Kroppenstedt.** 2000. *Mycobacterium heckeshornense* sp. nov., a new pathogenic slowly growing *Mycobacterium* sp. causing cavitary lung disease in an immunocompetent patient. *J. Clin. Microbiol.* **38:**4102–4107.

143. **Rynkiewicz, D. L., G. D. Cage, W. R. Butler, and N. M. Ampel.** 1998. Clinical and microbiological assessment of *Mycobacterium simiae* isolates from a single laboratory in southern Arizona. *Clin. Infect. Dis.* **26:**625–630.

144. **Saceanu, C., N. Pfeiffer, and T. McLean.** 1993. Evaluation of sputum smears concentrated by cytocentrifugation for detection of acid-fast bacilli. *J. Clin. Microbiol.* **31:**2371–2374.

145. **Salfinger, M., and F. Kafader.** 1987. Comparison of two pretreatment methods for the detection of mycobacteria of BACTEC and Löwenstein-Jensen slants. *J. Microbiol. Methods* **6:**315–321.

146. **Samra, Z., L. Kaufman, A. Zeharia, S. Ashkenazi, J. Amir, J. Bahar, U. Reischl, and L. Naumann.** 1999. Optimal detection and identification of *Mycobacterium haemophilum* in specimens from pediatric patients with cervical lymphadenopathy. *J. Clin. Microbiol.* **37:**832–834.

147. **Saubolle, M. A., T. E. Kiehn, M. H. White, M. F. Rudinsky, and D. Armstrong.** 1996. *Mycobacterium haemophilum:* microbiology and expanding clinical and geographic spectra of diseases in humans. *Clin. Microbiol. Rev.* **9:**435–447.

148. **Schinsky, M. F., M. M. McNeil, A. M. Whitney, A. G. Steigerwalt, B. A. Lasker, M. M. Floyd, G. G. Hogg, D. J. Brenner, and J. M. Brown.** 2000. *Mycobacterium septicum* sp. nov. a new rapidly growing species associated with catheter-related bacteraemia. *Int. J. Syst. Evol. Microbiol.* **50:**575–581.

149. **Silcox, V. A., R. A. Good, and M. M. Floyd.** 1981. Identification of clinically significant *Mycobacterium fortuitum* complex isolates. *J. Clin. Microbiol.* **14:**686–691.

150. **Simms, V., and D. M. Musher.** 1998. Psoas muscle abscess due to *Mycobacterium kansasii* in an apparently immunocompetent adult. *Clin. Infect. Dis.* **27:**893–894.

151. **Small, P., N. McClenny, S. Sigh, G. Schoolnik, L. Tompkins, and P. Mickelsen.** 1993. Molecular strain typing of *Mycobacterium tuberculosis* to confirm cross-contamination in the mycobacteriology laboratory and modification of procedures to minimize occurrence of false-positive cultures. *J. Clin. Microbiol.* **31:**1677–1682.

152. **Smith, D. S., P. Lindholm-Levy, G. A. Huitt, L. B. Heifets, and J. L. Cook.** 2000. *Mycobacterium terrae:* case reports, literature review, and in vitro antibiotic susceptibility testing. *Clin. Infect. Dis.* **30:**444–453.

153. **Smithwick, R. W., and C. B. Stratigos.** 1981. Acid-fast microscopy on polycarbonate membrane filter sputum sediments. *J. Clin. Microbiol.* **13:**1109–1113.

154. **Smithwick, R. W., C. B. Stratigos, and H. L. David.** 1975. Use of cetylpyridinium chloride and sodium chloride for the decontamination of sputum specimens that are transported to the laboratory for the isolation of *Mycobacterium tuberculosis. J. Clin. Microbiol.* **1:**411–413.

155. **Sniadack, D. H., S. M. Ostroff, M. A. Karlix, R. W. Smithwick, B. Schwartz, M. A. Sprauer, V. A. Silcox, and R. C. Good.** 1993. A nosocomial pseudo-outbreak of *Mycobacterium xenopi* due to a contaminated potable water supply: lessons in prevention. *Infect. Control Hosp. Epidemiol.* **14:**636–641.

156. **Somoskövi, A., J. E. Hotaling, M. Fitzgerald, D. O'Donnell, L. M. Parsons, and M. Salfinger.** 2001. Lessons from a proficiency testing event for acid-fast microscopy. *Chest* **120:**250–257.

157. **Somoskövi, A., and P. Magyar.** 1999. Comparison of the Mycobacteria Growth Indicator Tube with MB Redox, Löwenstein-Jensen, and Middlebrook 7H11 media for recovery of mycobacteria in clinical specimens. *J. Clin. Microbiol.* **37:**1366–1369.

158. **Springer, B., E. C. Böttger, P. Kirschner, and R. J. Wallace, Jr.** 1995. Phylogeny of the *Mycobacterium chelonae*-like organism based on partial sequencing of the 16S rRNA gene and proposal of *Mycobacterium mucogenicum* sp. nov. *J. Clin. Microbiol.* **45:**262–267.

159. **Springer, B., E. Tortoli, I. Richter, R. Grünewald, S. Rüsch-Gerdes, K. Uschmann, F. Suter, M. D. Collins, R. M. Kroppenstedt, and E. C. Böttger.** 1995. *Mycobacterium conspicuum* sp. nov., a new species isolated from patients with disseminated infections. *J. Clin. Microbiol.* **33:**2805–2811.

160. **Springer, B., P. Kirschner, G. Rost-Meyer, K.-H. Schröder, R. M. Kroppenstedt, and E. C. Böttger.** 1993. *Mycobacterium interjectum*, a new species isolated from a patient with chronic lymphadenitis. *J. Clin. Microbiol.* **31:**3083–3089.

161. **Springer, B., W.-K. Wu, T. Bodmer, G. Haase, G. E. Pfyffer, R. M. Kroppenstedt, K.-H. Schröder, S. Emler, J. O. Kilburn, P. Kirschner, A. Telenti, M. B. Coyle, and E. C. Böttger.** 1996. Isolation and characterization of a unique group of slowly growing mycobacteria: description of *Mycobacterium lentiflavum* sp. nov. *J. Clin. Microbiol.* **34:**1100–1107.

162. **Steingrube, V. A., J. L. Gibson, B. A. Brown, Y. Zhang, R. W. Wilson, M. Rajagopalan, and R. J. Wallace, Jr.** 1995. PCR amplification and restriction endonuclease analysis of a 65-kilodalton heat shock protein gene sequence for taxonomic separation of rapidly growing mycobacteria. *J. Clin. Microbiol.* **33:**149–153. (Erratum, **33:**1686.)

163. **Reference deleted.**

164. **Stone, B. L., W. J. Burman, M. V. Hildred, E. A. Jarboe, R. R. Reves, and M. L. Wilson.** 1997. The diagnostic yield of acid-fast bacillus smear-positive specimens. *J. Clin. Microbiol.* **35:**1030–1031.

165. **Supply, P., E. Manzars, S. Lesjean, V. Vincent, B. Gicquel, and C. Locht.** 2000. Variable human minisatellite-like regions in the *Mycobacterium tuberculosis* genome. *Mol. Microbiol.* **36:**762–771.

166. **Taylor, L. Q., A. J. Williams, and S. Santiago.** 1990. Pulmonary disease caused by *Mycobacterium asiaticum. Tubercle* **71:**303–305.

167. **Teirstein, A., B. Damsker, P. Kirschner, D. Krellenstein, R. Robinson, and M. Chuang.** 1990. Pulmonary infection with MAI: diagnosis, clinical patterns, treatment. *Mt. Sinai J. Med.* **57:**209–215.

168. **Telenti, A., F. Marchesi, M. Balz, F. Bally, E. C. Böttger, and T. Bodmer.** 1993. Rapid identification of mycobacteria to the species level by polymerase chain reaction and restriction enzyme analysis. *J. Clin. Microbiol.* **31:**175–178.

169. **Tenover, F., J. Crawford, R. Huebner, L. Getter, C. R. Horsburgh, Jr., and R. C. Good.** 1993. The resurgence of tuberculosis: is your laboratory ready? *J. Clin. Microbiol.* **32:**767–770.

170. **Thorel, M.-F., M. Krichevsky, and V. Levy-Frébault.** 1990. Numerical taxonomy of mycobactin-dependent mycobacteria, emended description of *Mycobacterium avium*, and description of *Mycobacterium avium* subsp. *avium* subsp. nov., *Mycobacterium avium* subsp. *paratuberculosis* subsp. nov., and *Mycobacterium avium* subsp. *silvaticum* subsp. nov. *Int. J. Syst. Bacteriol.* **40:**254–260.

171. Thornton, C. G., K. M. McLellan, T. L. Brink, Jr., D. E. Lockwood, M. Romagnoli, J. Turner, W. G. Merz, R. S. Schwalbe, M. Moody, Y. Lue, and S. Passen. 1998. Novel method for processing respiratory specimens for detection of mycobacteria by using C_{18}-carboxypropylbetaine: blinded study. *J. Clin. Microbiol.* **36:** 1996–2003.

172. Tjhie, J. H. T., A. F. van Belle, M. Dessenkroon, and D. van Soolingen. 2001. Misidentification and diagnostic delay caused by a false-positive Amplified Mycobacterium Direct Test in an immunocompetent patient with a *Mycobacterium celatum* infection. *J. Clin. Microbiol.* **39:** 2311–2312.

173. Torkko, P., S. Suomalainen, E. Iivanainen, M. Suutari, L. Paulin, E. Rudback, E. Tortoli, V. Vincent, R. Mattila, and M. L. Katila. 2001. Characterization of *Mycobacterium bohemicum* isolated from human, veterinary, and environmental sources. *J. Clin. Microbiol.* **39:** 207–211.

174. Tortoli, E., A. Bartoloni, V. Manfrin, A. Mantella, C. Scarparo, and E. C. Böttger. 2000. Cervical lymphadenitis due to *Mycobacterium bohemicum. Clin. Infect. Dis.* **30:**210–211.

175. Tortoli, E., G. Besozzi, C. Lacchini, V. Penati, M. T. Simonetti, and S. Emler. 1998. Pulmonary infection due to *Mycobacterium szulgai* case report and review of the literature. *Eur. Respir. J.* **11:**975–977.

176. Tortoli, E., C. Piersimoni, A. Bartoloni, C. Burrini, A. P. Callegaro, G. Caroli, D. Colombri, A. Goglio, A. Mantella, C. P. Tosi, and M. T. Simonetti. 1997. Mycobacterium malmoense in Italy: the modern Norman invasion? *Eur. J. Epidemiol.* **13:**314–316.

177. Tortoli, E., F. Brunello, A. E. Cagni, D. Colombrita, D. Dionisio, L. Grisendi, V. Manfrin, M. Moroni, C. Passerini Tosi, G. Pinsi, C. Scarparo, and M. Tullia Simonetti. 1998. Mycobacterium genavense in AIDS patients, report of 24 cases in Italy and review of the literature. *Eur. J. Epidemiol.* **14:**219–224.

178. Tortoli, E., M. Tullia Simonetti, D. Dionisio, and M. Meli. 1994. Cultural studies on two isolates of *Mycobacterium genavense* from patients with acquired immunodeficiency syndrome. *Diagn. Microbiol. Infect. Dis.* **18:**7–12.

179. Tortoli, E., R. M. Kroppenstedt, A. Bartoloni, G. Caroli, I. Jan, J. Pawlowski, and S. Emler. 1999. Mycobacterium tusciae sp. nov. *Int. J. Syst. Bacteriol.* **49:** 1839–1844.

180. Trifiro, S., A.-M. Bourgault, F. Lebel, and P. René. 1990. Ghost mycobacteria on Gram stain. *J. Clin. Microbiol.* **28:**146.

181. van Baers, S. M., M. Y. L. de Witt, and P. R. Klatser. 1996. The epidemiology of *Mycobacterium leprae*: recent insight. *FEMS Microbiol. Lett.* **136:**221–230.

182. van der Werf, T. S., W. T. A. van der Graaf, J. W. Tappero, and K. Asiedu. 1999. Mycobacterium ulcerans infection. *Lancet* **354:**1013–1018.

183. van Soolingen, D., A. G. M. van der Zanden, P. E. W. de Haas, G. T. Noordhoek, A. Kiers, N. A. Foudraine, F. Portaels, A. H. J. Kolk, K. Kremer, and J. D. A. van Embden. 1998. Diagnosis of *Mycobacterium microti* infections among humans by using novel genetic markers. *J. Clin. Microbiol.* **36:**1840–1845.

184. van Soolingen, D., T. Hoogenboezem, P. E. W. de Haas, P. W. M. Hermans, M. A. Koedam, K. S. Teppema, P. J. Brennan, G. S. Besra, F. Portaels, J. Top, L. M. Schouls, and J. D. van Embden. 1997. A novel pathogenic taxon of the *Mycobacterium tuberculosis* complex, Canettii: characterization of an exceptional isolate from Africa. *Int. J. Syst. Bacteriol.* **47:**1236–1245.

185. Viana-Niero, C., C. Gutierrez, C. Sola, I. Filliol, F. Boulahbal, V. Vincent, and N. Rastogi. 2001. Genetic diversity of *Mycobacterium africanum* clinical isolates based on IS6110-restriction fragment length polymorphism analysis, spoligotyping, and variable number of tandem DNA repeats. *J. Clin. Microbiol.* **39:**57–65.

186. Waite, R. T., and G. L. Woods. 1998. Evaluation of BACTEC MYCO/F Lytic Medium for recovery of mycobacteria and fungi from blood. *J. Clin. Microbiol.* **36:** 1176–1179.

187. Wallace, R. 1987. Nontuberculous mycobacteria and water: a love affair with increasing clinical importance. *Infect. Dis. Clin. North Am.* **1:**677–686.

188. Wallace, R. J., Jr., B. A. Brown, V. A. Silcox, M. Tsukamura, D. R. Nash, L. C. Steele, V. A. Steingrube, J. Smith, G. Sumter, Y. Zhang, and Z. Blacklock. 1991. Clinical disease, drug suceptibility, and biochemical patterns of the unnamed third biovariant complex of *Mycobacterium fortuitum. J. Infect. Dis.* **163:**598–603.

189. Wallace, R. J., Jr., D. R. Nash, M. Tsukamura, Z. M. Blacklock, and V. A. Silcox. 1988. Human disease due to *Mycobacterium smegmatis. J. Infect. Dis.* **158:**52–59.

190. Wallace, R. J., Jr., V. A. Silcox, M. Tsukamura, B. A. Brown, J. O. Kilburn, W. R. Butler, and G. O. Onyi. 1993. Clinical significance, biochemical features, and susceptibility patterns of sporadic isolates of the *Mycobacterium chelonae*-like organism. *J. Clin. Microbiol.* **31:** 3231–3239.

191. Wallace, R. J., Jr., J. M. Swenson, V. Silcox, R. Good, J. A. Tschen, and M. S. Stone. 1983. Spectrum of disease due to rapidly growing mycobacteria. *Rev. Infect. Dis.* **5:**657–679.

192. Wallace, R. J., Jr., Y. Zhang, B. A. Brown, D. Dawson, D. T. Murphy, R. Wilson, and D. Griffith. 1998. Polyclonal *Mycobacterium avium* complex infections in patients with nodular bronchiectasis. *Am. J. Respir. Crit. Care Med.* **158:**1235–1244.

193. Warren, J. R., M. Bhattacharya, K. N. De Almeida, K. Trakas, and L. R. Peterson. 2000. A minimum 5.0 ml of sputum improves the sensitivity of acid-fast smear for *Mycobacterium tuberculosis. Am. J. Respir. Crit. Care Med.* **161:**1559–1562.

194. Wasilauskas, B. L., and R. M. Morrell, Jr. 1997. Isolator component responsible for inhibition of *Mycobacterium avium-M. intracellulare* in BACTEC 12B medium. *J. Clin. Microbiol.* **35:**588–590.

195. Wayne, L. 1985. The "atypical" mycobacteria: recognition and disease association. *Crit. Rev. Microbiol.* **12:** 185–222.

196. Wayne, L., and H. Sramek. 1992. Agents of newly recognized or infrequently encountered mycobacterial diseases. *Clin. Microbiol. Rev.* **5:**1–25.

197. Wayne, L., R. Good, M. Krichevsky, Z. Blacklock, H. David, D. Dawson, W. Gross, J. Hawkins, V. Levy-Frebault, C. McManus, F. Portaels, S. Rüsch-Gerdes, K. Schröder, V. Silcox, M. Tsukamura, L. Van den Breen, and M. Yakrus. 1991. Fourth report of the cooperative open-ended study of slowly growing mycobacteria of the International Working Group on Mycobacterial Taxonomy. *Int. J. Syst. Bacteriol.* **41:**463–472.

198. Wayne, L. G., and G. P. Kubica. 1986. Mycobacteria, p. 1435–1457. *In* P. H. A. Sneath, (ed.), *Bergey's Manual of Systematic Bacteriology*, vol. 2. The Williams & Wilkins Co., Baltimore, Md.

199. Welch, D., A. Guruswamy, S. Sides, C. Shaw, and M. Gilchrist. 1993. Timely culture of mycobacteria which utilizes a microcolony method. *J. Clin. Microbiol.* **31:** 2178–2184.

200. **White, D. A., T. E. Kiehn, A. Y. Bondoc, and S. A. Massarella.** 1999. Pulmonary nodule due to *Mycobacterium haemophilum* in an immunocompetent host. *Am. J. Respir. Crit. Care Med.* **160:**1366–1368.

201. **Whittier, S., K. Olivier, P. Gilligan, M. Knowles, P. Della-Latta, and The Nontuberculous Mycobacteria in Cystic Fibrosis Study Group.** 1997. Proficiency testing of clinical microbiology laboratories using modified decontamination procedures for detection of nontuberculous mycobacteria in sputum samples from cystic fibrosis patients. *J. Clin. Microbiol.* **35:**2706–2708.

202. **Whyte, T., B. Hanahoe, T. Collins, G. Corbett-Feeney, and M. Cormican.** 2000. Evaluation of the BACTEC MGIT 960 and MB/BacT Systems for routine detection of *Mycobacterium tuberculosis. J. Clin. Microbiol.* **38:**3131–3132.

203. **Wilson, R. W., V. A. Steingrube, E. C. Böttger, B. Springer, B. A. Brown-Elliott, V. Vincent, K. C. Jost, Jr., Y. Zhang, M. J. Garcia, S. H. Chiu, G. O. Onyi, H. Rossmore, D. R. Nash, and R. J. Wallace, Jr.** 2001. *Mycobacterium immunogenum* sp. nov., a novel species related to *Mycobacterium abscessus* and associated with clinical disease, pseudo-outbreaks and contaminated metalworking fluids: an international cooperative study on mycobacterial taxonomy. *Int. J. Syst. Evol. Microbiol.* **51:**1751–1764.

204. **Wolfe, J., C. Turenne, M. Alfa, G. Harding, L. Thibert, and A. Kabani.** 1999. *Mycobacterium branderi* from both a hand infection and a case of pulmonary disease. *J. Clin. Microbiol.* **38:**3896–3899.

205. **Wolinsky, E.** 1995. Mycobacterial lymphadenitis in children: a prospective study of 105 nontuberculous cases with long-term follow-up. *Clin. Infect. Dis.* **20:**954–963.

206. **Woods, G. L., E. Pentony, M. J. Boxley, and A. M. Gatson.** 1995. Concentration of sputum by cytocentrifugation for preparation of smears for detection of acid-fast bacilli does not increase sensitivity of the fluorochrome stain. *J. Clin. Microbiol.* **33:**1915–1916.

207. **Woods, G. L., G. Fish, M. Plaunt, and T. Murphy.** 1997. Clinical evaluation of Difco ESP Culture System II for growth and detection of mycobacteria. *J. Clin. Microbiol.* **35:**121–124.

208. **World Health Organization Study Group.** 1985. Epidemiology of leprosy in relation to control. *W. H. O. Tech. Rep. Ser.* **716:**1–60.

209. **World Health Organization.** 2001. *Tuberculosis.* Fact sheet 104. World Health Organization, Geneva, Switzerland.

210. **Yajko, D. M., P. S. Nassos, C. A. Sanders, P. C. Gonzalez, A. L. Reingold, C. R. Horsburgh, P. Hopewell, D. P. Chin, and W. K. Hadley.** 1993. Comparison of four decontamination methods for recovery of *Mycobacterium avium* complex from stools. *J. Clin. Microbiol.* **31:**302–306.

211. **Yamauchi, T., P. Ferrieri, and B. F. Anthony.** 1980. The etiology of acute cervical adenitis in children: serological and bacteriological studies. *J. Med. Microbiol.* **13:**37–43.

Mycobacterium: Phenotypic and Genotypic Identification*

VÉRONIQUE VINCENT, BARBARA A. BROWN-ELLIOTT, KENNETH C. JOST, JR., AND RICHARD J. WALLACE, JR.

37

IDENTIFICATION OF MYCOBACTERIA

Mycobacteria should always be identified to the species level if possible. They are usually preliminarily identified by traits such as growth rate and pigmentation, which will direct the selection of key biochemical tests to further characterize them (75). Unfortunately, different species may present convergent biochemical profiles and morphological features (Table 1). Similarly, variation occurs among strains, and their properties may not match those of the type strain. Traditional methods are well established, standardized, reproducible, and relatively inexpensive but limited in scope to the species for which large numbers of strains have been studied. Thus, identification errors may result, especially because no characteristic phenotype has been identified in several recently described species recognized on the basis of new 16S rRNA sequences.

Alternative laboratory methods for mycobacterial identification include analysis of mycolic acids by chromatography and genetic investigations using nucleic acid probes, nucleic acid amplification, and nucleic acid sequencing. It is now recommended to undertake mycobacterial identification with a strategy combining phenotypic and genotypic tests. For obvious reasons, all laboratories should perform identification of the *Mycobacterium tuberculosis* complex (MTBC) using a rapid method (135) to facilitate prompt identification and reporting of results to physicians.

Phenotypic Tests

Tables 1 and 2 show characteristic test results for the most commonly encountered species. Detailed descriptions of methods, procedures, and controls can be found elsewhere (63, 75).

Growth Rate and Preferred Growth Temperature

Growth rate refers to the length of time required to form mature, isolated colonies visible without magnification on solid media. Mycobacteria forming colonies within 7 days are termed rapid growers, while those requiring longer periods are termed slow growers. Genome analyses support this separation, since slowly growing mycobacteria have been shown to have only one copy of the genes encoding rRNA whereas rapidly growing mycobacteria (RGM), except for *M. chelonae* and *M. abscessus*, have two sets of those genes (8). Moreover, comparative 16S rDNA sequencing data clearly separate the RGM from the slowly growing species (128).

Isolated colonies are observed after media are inoculated with 0.1 ml of a 10^{-4} dilution of a standard culture suspension (SCS) prepared at an optical density at 580 nm of 0.25 using a tube with a 2-cm diameter; this roughly corresponds to a suspension of 1 mg (wet weight) of bacilli per ml (153). The cultures are incubated at 35 to 37°C. Some species have special nutrient or temperature requirements for growth (see chapter 36 for details). Cultures are observed at 5 to 7 days and weekly thereafter for visible colonies. Growth in relation to temperature can usually be adequately determined by observing cultures at 37 and 30°C. When more definitive identification is needed, isolates should be incubated at 28, 30, 35 to 37, and 42 or 45°C.

Pigmentation and Photoreactivity

Mycobacteria are classified into three groups based on the production of pigments. Photochromogens produce nonpigmented colonies when grown in the dark and pigmented colonies only after exposure to light. Scotochromogens produce deep yellow to orange pigmented colonies when grown in either the light or the dark (some strains show an increased pigment production on continuous exposure to light). Nonchromogens are nonpigmented in both the light and dark or have only a pale yellow, buff, or tan pigment that does not intensify after light exposure. These responses to light exposure were originally delineated to aid in the identification of nontuberculous mycobacteria (NTM). Members of the MTBC, however, are considered nonchromogens, and pigmented mycobacteria may be preliminarily reported as NTM.

Testing for pigment production should be done on isolated colonies from young cultures. Three tubes of media are inoculated with a standard culture suspension diluted to yield isolated colonies as described above. Two tubes are wrapped to be shielded from light, and the third is left uncovered. When growth is detected in the unshielded tube, one of the wrapped tubes should be examined. If colonies are not pigmented, the newly unshielded tube with

* This chapter contains information presented in chapter 25 by Beverly G. Metchock, Frederick S. Nolte, and Richard J. Wallace, Jr., in the seventh edition of this Manual.

TABLE 1 Distinctive properties of cultivable mycobacteria encountered in clinical specimens[a]

Descriptive term	Species	Optimal temp (°C)	Usual colony morphology[b]	Pigmentation[c]	Niacin	Growth on T2H (10 μg/ml)	Nitrate reduction	Semiquantitative catalase (mm of bubbles)	68°C catalase	Tween hydrolysis	Tellurite reduction	Tolerance to 5% NaCl	Iron uptake	Aryl-sulfatase, 3 days	16S rDNA ref. no.	Urease	Pyrazinamidase, 4 day	Nucleic acid probes available
Slow growers																		
TB complex	M. tuberculosis	37	R	N (100)	+(95)	+	+(97)	<45 (89)	-(1)	±(68)	±(36)	-(0)	-	-(0)	X58890	±(64)	+	+[d]
	M. africanum	37	R	N	V	V	V	<45	-	-	-	-	-	-	IDEM	+	-	+[d]
	M. bovis	37	Rt	N (100)	-(4)	-	-(9)	<45 (69)	-(2)	-(21)	ND	-(0)	-	-(0)	IDEM	±(50)	-	+[d]
	M. bovis BCG	37	R	N	-	-	-	<45	-	±	ND	ND	-	-	IDEM	+	-	+[d]
	M. canettii	37	Sm	N	+	+	+	ND	-	-	ND	ND	-	-	IDEM	ND	+	-
Nonchromogens	M. avium	35–37	Smt/R	N	-	+	-	<45	±	-	+	-	-	-	X52198	-	+	+[k]
	M. intracellulare	35–37	Smt/R	N	-	+	-	<45	±	-	+	-	-	-	X52927	-	+	+[k]
	M. haemophilum[e]	30	R	N	ND	+	-	<45	±	-	+	-	-	-	X88923	-	+	-
	M. malmoense	30	Sm	N (88)	-(0)	+	-(1)	<45 (99)	-/+	+(99)	+(74)	-(0)	-	-(0)	X52930	-(9)	+	-
	M. shimoidei	37	R	N	-	+	-	<45	+	+	ND	ND	-	-	AJ005005	-	+	-
	M. genavense	37	Smt	N	-	+	-	>45	+	+	ND	ND	-	-	X60070	+	+	-
	M. celatum	35	Sm/Smt	N (100)	-	+	-(0)	<45 (100)	+(100)	-(0)	+(100)	-(0)	-(0)	+(100)	L08170, L08169	-(0)	+(100)	-
	M. ulcerans	30	R	N	-	+	-	<45	+	-	ND	-	ND	-	X58954	V	-	-
	M. terrae complex	35	Sm/R	N (93)	-(1)	+	±(67)	>45 (93)	+(92)	+(99)	-/+(46)	-(2)	-	-(2)	X52925 (M. terrae)	-(13)	V	-
	M. triviale	37	R	N (100)	-(0)	+	+(89)	>45 (100)	+(100)	+(100)	-(25)	+(100)	-	±(56)	X88924	-/+(33)	V	-
	M. gastri	35	Sm/SR/R	N (100)	-(0)	+	-(0)	<45 (100)	-(11)	+(100)	±(50)	-(0)	-	-(0)	X52919	-/+(44)	-	-
	M. branderi	35	Sm	N (100)	-	ND	-	-	-	-	ND	ND	ND	-[f]	X82234	-	-	-
	M. heidelbergense	35	Sm	N (100)	-	ND	-	-	+	+	-	ND	ND	-	X70960	+	+	-
	M. triplex	35	Sm	N (100)	-(0)	+(100)	+(100)	>45 (100)	+(100)	-(0)	ND	ND	ND	-(0) +(50)[f]	U57632	+(100)	ND	-
Chromogens	M. kansasii	35	Sm/SR/R	P (96)	-(4)	+	+(99)	>45 (93)	+(91)	+(99)	-/+(31)	-(0)	-	-(0)	X15916	-/+(49)	-	+
	M. marinum	30	Sm/SR/R	P (100)	-/+(21)	+	-(0)	<45	-(30)	+[97]	-/+(39)	-(0)	-	-/+(41)[f]	X52920	+(83)	+	-
	M. avium	35–37	Sm/R	S	-	+	-	<45	±	-(9)	+	-	-	-	X52198	-	+	+
	M. intracellulare	35–37	Sm/R	S	-	+	-	<45	±	+(95)	+	-	-	-	X52927	-	+	+
	M. simiae	37	Sm	P (90)	±(63)	+	-(28)	>45 (93)	+(95)	-(9)	+(82)	-(0)	-	-(0)	X52931	±(69)	+	-
	M. asiaticum	37	Sm	P (86)	-(0)	+	-(5)	>45 (95)	+(95)	+(95)	-(20)	-(0)	-	-(0)	X55604	-(10)	-	-
	M. xenopi	42	Sm	N/S[g]	-	+	-	<45	+/-	+(97)	ND	-	+	+	X52929	ND	ND	-
	M. gordonae	37	Sm	S (99)	-(0)	+	-(1)	>45 (90)	+(96)	+(100)	-(29)	-(0)	-	V	X52923	V (31)	-/+	+

(Continued on next page)

TABLE 1 Distinctive properties of cultivable mycobacteria encountered in clinical specimens[a] (Continued)

Descriptive term	Species	Optimal temp (°C)	Usual colony morphology[b]	Pigmentation[c]	Niacin	Growth on T2H (10 μg/ml)	Nitrate reduction	Semiquantitative catalase (mm of bubbles)	68°C catalase	Tween hydrolysis	Tellurite reduction	Tolerance to 5% NaCl	Iron uptake	Arylsulfatase, 3 days	16S rDNA ref. no.	Urease	Pyrazinamidase, 4 day	Nucleic acid probes available
	M. scrofulaceum	37	Sm	S (97)	−(0)	+	−(5)	>45 (84)	+(94)	−(2)	±(64)	−(0)	−	V	X52924	V (31)	±	−
	M. szulgai	37	Sm or R	S/P (93)	−(0)	+	+(100)	>45 (98)	+(93)	−/+(49)	±(53)	−(0)	−	V	X52926	+(72)	+	−
	M. flavescens	37	Sm	S (100)[g]	−(0)	+	+(92)	>45 (94)	+(100)	+(100)	−/+(44)	±(62)	−	−(0)	X52932	+(72)	−	−
	M. intermedium	35	Sm	P	−	ND	−	ND	+	+	ND	ND	ND	+[i]	X67847	+/−(V)	±(V)	−
	M. lentiflavum	35	Sm	P	−	ND	−	±(V)	±(V)	−	ND	ND	ND	−[j]	AF317658	ND	±(V)	−
	M. interjectum	35	Sm	S	−	ND	−	V	V	−	ND	−	ND	V	X70961	+	+	−
	M. bohemicum	37–40	Sm	S	−	ND	−	−	+	−	−	−	ND	−[j]	U84502	weak	−	−
	M. conspicuum	30	Sm	S	−	+	−	<45	−(100)	+	−	−	ND	+[i]	X88922	−	−	−
	M. tusciae	30	R	S	−	+	+	−	−	+(10d)	ND	−	ND	−[f]	AF058299	+	ND	−
	M. heckeshornense	35	Sm	S	−	ND	−	−	+	−	ND	−	ND	−	AF174290	−	−	−
Rapid growers Nonchromogens	M. fortuitum group[h]	28–30	R/Sm	N (100)	−	+	+(100)	>45 (93)	+(90)	−/+(43)	+(92)	+(85)	+	+(97)	X52921	+(70)	+	−
	M. septicum	28–35	R	N (100)	−	ND	+	ND	ND	ND	ND	+	+	V	AF111809	ND	ND	−
	M. chelonae	28–30	Sm/R	N (100)	−/+	+	−(1)	>45 (92)	±(53)	−/+(39)	+(89)	V	−	+(95)	X82236	+(89)	+	−
	M. senegalense	30	R	N	−	ND	+	ND	ND	ND	+	−	−	+	M29567	+	ND	−
	M. abscessus	28–30	Sm/R	N (100)	−	ND	−	>45	ND	V	ND	±	ND	+	X82235	+	ND	−
	M. immunogenum	30–35	R/Sm	N (100)	−	ND	−(100)	ND	ND	ND	ND	−	−(100)	+(100)	AJ011771	ND	ND	−
	M. mucogenicum	28–30	Sm	N (100)	−	ND	V	>45	−(12)	+	−	−	Tan	+(84)	X80771	+	ND	−
	M. smegmatis	28–35	Sm/R	LS (95)	−	+	+(95)	<45 (87)	−(0)	+	+	+(100)	+(67)	−(5)	X52922	ND	ND	−
	M. wolinskyi	28–35	Sm	N (100)	−	ND	+(100)	<45 (89)	−/+(100)	ND	ND	+(100)	+	−(5)	Y12871	ND	ND	−
	M. goodii	28–35	Sm/R	LS (78)	−	ND	+(100)	<45 (50)	−(7)	ND	ND	+(88)	+	−(0)	Y12872	ND	ND	−
	M. mageritense	30–37	Sm	N (100)	ND	ND	+(70)	ND	−(0)	−(100)	ND	+(80)	+(40)	+(80)	X99838	+(60)	+(100)	−
Chromogens	M. phlei	30	R	S	−	+	+	>45	+	+	+	+	+	−	M29566	ND	ND	−
	M. vaccae	30	Sm	S	−	+	+	>45	+	+	+	V	+	−	X55601	ND	ND	−

[a] Modified from references 63 and 75. Plus and minus signs indicate the presence and absence, respectively, of the feature; V, variable; ±, usually present; −/+, usually absent; ND = not determined, Ref. No., reference number. The percentage of strains positive in each test is given in parentheses, and the test result is based on these percentages.
[b] R, rough; Sm, smooth; SR, intermediate in roughness; t, thin or transparent; f, filamentous extensions; Smt, smooth and transparent; Rt, rough and thin, or transparent; LS, late Scoto (7 to 10 days) on 7H10 agar.
[c] P, photochromogenic; S, scotochromogenic; N, nonchromogenic; (M. szulgai is scotochromogenic at 37°C and photochromogenic at 24°C).
[d] Probe identifies M. tuberculosis complex.
[e] Requires hemin as growth factor.
[f] Arylsulfatase reaction at 14 days is positive; number in parentheses = day.
[g] Young cultures may be nonchromogenic or possess only pale pigment that may intensify with age.
[h] Includes M. fortuitum, M. peregrinum, and M. fortuitum third biovariant complex.
[i] Results for 3-day arylsulfatase not available; 10-day arylsulfatase positive.
[j] Results for 3-day arylsulfatase not available; 10-day arylsulfatase negative.
[k] A MAC nucleic acid probe that recognizes M. avium, M. intracellulare, and the "X" strains is commercially available.

TABLE 2 Carbohydrate utilization tests of common rapidly growing mycobacteria[a]

Species or complex	Citrate	Mannitol	Inositol	Sorbitol
M. abscessus	−	−	−	−
M. chelonae	+	−	−	−
M. fortuitum	−	−	−	−
M. peregrinum	−	+	−	−
M. fortuitum third biovariant complex				
Sorbitol (+)	−	+	+	+
Sorbitol (−)	−	+	+	−
M. mucogenicum	+	+	−	−
M. smegmatis sensu stricto	V	+	+	+
M. wolinskyi	V	+	+	+
M. goodii	V	+	+	+

[a] Data from references 17 and 156. +, ≥80%; −, ≤20%; V, ≥21 to 79%.

its cap loosened is exposed to light (100-W tungsten bulb or fluorescent equivalent, placed 20 cm from the culture) for 1 to 5 h. Maximal oxygenation of the culture (loose cap, isolated colonies) is necessary for induction of the pigment, which is controlled by an oxygen-dependent, photoinducible enzyme. The tube is then reshielded and reincubated, and the colonies in the light-exposed tube are compared with those in the shielded tube after 24 h. Variations within species occur. Many M. avium and M. intracellulare isolates are pigmented. M. szulgai is a scotochromogen at 37°C but a photochromogen at 25°C.

Colony Morphology

Colony morphology of mycobacteria can be evaluated, according to the scheme developed by Runyon (111), by microscopically observing young (5- to 14-day-old) isolated colonies on plates inverted under the 10× power objective of a stereomicroscope with transmitted light. The best medium is a clear solid one like Middlebrook 7H10 or 7H11 agar. The large numbers of NTM species have made it increasingly difficult to provide a tentative identification of an NTM species by this method, and so the information gained by this technique is often used to direct the diagnostic procedure to other, more specific tests. The morphology of M. tuberculosis usually allows for a tentative identification of this species. Examination of the morphology of colonies is also important for the detection of mixed cultures. Figures 1 and 2 show the colony types of some frequently isolated species.

Arylsulfatase

Arylsulfatase hydrolyzes the bond between the sulfate group and the aromatic ring of tripotassium phenolphthalein disulfate to form free phenolphthalein, which is easily detected by a red color when alkali is added. Arylsulfatase activity can be detected in all mycobacteria after prolonged incubation. After a 3-day incubation, the test helps in identifying several species, mainly the most common clinically significant RGM species (i.e., the M. fortuitum complex which includes M. fortuitum, M. chelonae, and M. abscessus) and some slow-growing mycobacteria such as M. xenopi, M. triviale, and M. celatum.

Cultures in Dubos liquid medium (2 ml) containing 0.08 M phenolphthalein disulfate (tripotassium salt) are tested after 3 days of incubation by adding 0.3 ml of 1 M Na_2CO_3. The development of a pink color indicates a positive reac-

tion. M. fortuitum and M. avium (or M. intracellulare) can be used as positive and negative controls, respectively.

Catalase

Catalase is an intracellular, soluble enzyme capable of degrading hydrogen peroxide to water and oxygen. Two tests are used to detect catalase activity, a semiquantitative test that reflects differences in enzyme kinetics and a heat tolerance test. The enzyme is detected by adding H_2O_2 to a culture and observing for the formation of bubbles in the reaction mixture.

The semiquantitative test divides the mycobacteria into two groups, those producing a "low catalase" and those producing a "high catalase" based on the column of bubbles produced (less or more than 45 mm). A butt (not slant) of a Löwenstein-Jensen (L-J) medium tube (16 by 150 mm) is inoculated with 0.2 ml of an SCS prepared as described above for growth rate determination. The tubes are incubated for 2 weeks at 35°C with the cap loosened. Then 1 ml of reagent consisting of a 1:1 mixture of 10% Tween 80 and 30% H_2O_2 is added. The column of bubbles yielded is measured (in millimeters) after the tube has stood upright for 5 min at room temperature. M. tuberculosis H37Ra and M. kansasii can be used as controls for low and high catalase, respectively.

For the heat tolerance test, a loopful of colonies is suspended in 0.5 ml of 0.067 M phosphate buffer (pH 7) in a screw cap tube and incubated at 68°C for 20 min. Once it has cooled to room temperature, 0.5 ml of the Tween-H_2O_2 mixture is added. Formation of oxygen bubbles (positive test) is scored 20 min later. M. kansasii and M. tuberculosis H37Ra can be used as positive and negative controls, respectively.

Iron Uptake

The iron uptake test is used to detect rapid growers capable of converting ferric ammonium citrate to an iron oxide which is visible as a reddish brown color in the colonies. Iron uptake is useful in distinguishing M. chelonae and M. abscessus, commonly negative, from most other clinically significant RGM that are positive. Isolates of M. mucogenicum produce a less noticeable tan color. Slow growers are not capable of accumulating iron oxides.

An L-J slant is inoculated with 0.2 ml of SCS and incubated at 37°C until growth is visible. One drop of 20% aqueous ferric ammonium citrate is added for each milliliter of the L-J medium. After incubation at 37°C for up to 21 days, a reddish brown color in the colonies and a tan discoloration of the medium indicate a positive result. M. fortuitum and M. chelonae or M. abscessus can be used as positive and negative controls, respectively.

Niacin Accumulation Test

Niacin (nicotinic acid) functions as a precursor in the biosynthesis of coenzymes NAD and NADP. Although all mycobacteria produce nicotinic acid, some have a block in the NAD-scavenging pathway and excrete niacin. The niacin accumulated in the culture medium is then detected by its reaction with a cyanogen halide in the presence of a primary amine. Niacin-negative M. tuberculosis isolates are extremely rare. A positive niacin test should not be used alone to identify M. tuberculosis, however, because some strains of M. simiae and other mycobacteria, although infrequently encountered, also accumulate niacin. Performance of the supportive tests of nitrate reduction and 68°C

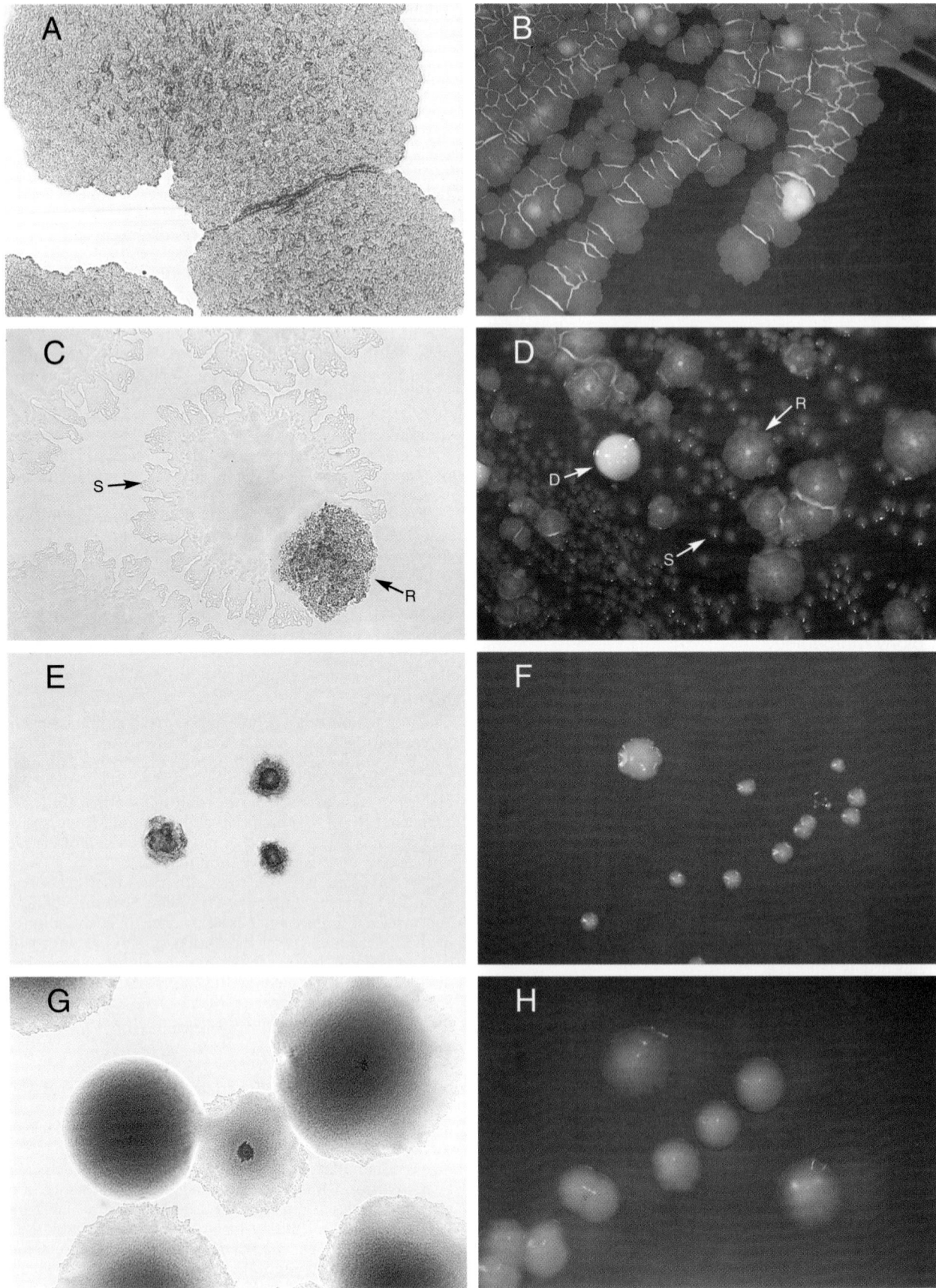

catalase are necessary for confirming the identification of *M. tuberculosis*.

A niacin paper strip version is available commercially (Becton Dickinson Microbiology Systems, Sparks, Md., and Remel Inc., Lenexa, Kans.). Manufacturer's recommendations should be followed. A heavily grown L-J culture medium is covered with 1 ml of distilled water, and the tube is placed horizontally to allow extraction for 20 min. Then 0.5 ml of the liquid is transferred to a tube. The strip is inserted, and the tube is sealed immediately. After 15 min at room temperature, a yellow color of the liquid (not on the strip) indicates a positive test. *M. tuberculosis* H37Ra and *M. avium* can be used as positive and negative controls, respectively.

Nitrate Reduction

Mycobacteria differ quantitatively in their abilities to reduce nitrate to nitrite. The nitrate reduction test is performed by adding 2 ml of $NaNO_3$ substrate to bacterial heavy suspension prepared with two loopfuls of bacteria emulsified in 0.2 ml of distilled water. The tube is shaken manually and incubated upright for 2 h in a 37°C water bath. After the tube is removed from the bath, 1 drop of reagent 1 (50 ml of HCl in 50 ml of H_2O), 2 drops of reagent 2 (0.2 g of sulfanilamide in 100 ml of H_2O), and 2 drops of reagent 3 (0.1 g of N-napthylthylenediamine dihydrochloride in 100 ml of H_2O) are added to the SCS. Immediate development of a pink-toned color is considered positive. *M. tuberculosis* H37Ra and *M. avium* can be used as positive and negative controls, respectively.

Pyrazinamidase

The enzyme pyrazinamidase hydrolyzes pyrazinamide (PZA) to ammonia and pyrazinoic acid, which can be detected by the addition of ferric ammonium sulfate. This test is most useful in separating *M. marinum* from *M. kansasii* and *M. bovis* from *M. tuberculosis*. In addition, one mechanism of PZA resistance of *M. tuberculosis* appears to be the inability of the organism to produce pyrazinoic acid, which is assumed to be the active component of the drug PZA. A pyrazinamidase-negative *M. tuberculosis* isolate is assumed to be PZA resistant as well.

The test medium consists of Dubos broth base containing 0.1 g of PZA, 2.0 g of pyruvic acid, and 15.0 g of agar per liter. The medium is dispensed in 5-ml amounts, autoclaved, and solidified in an upright position. The agar medium is heavily inoculated with growth from the culture

so that the inoculum should be visible. After incubation at 37°C for 4 days, 1 ml of 1% ferrous ammonium sulfate is added. The preparation is observed for up to 4 h for a pink band in the agar, which indicates a positive test. *M. avium* (or *M. intracellulare*) and uninoculated medium are used as positive and negative controls, respectively.

Sodium Chloride Tolerance

Few mycobacteria are able to grow in the presence of, or tolerate, 5% sodium chloride. *M. triviale* is the only slowly growing mycobacteria to do so. Pathogenic RGM, except *M. mucogenicum* and most isolates of *M. chelonae*, also grow in 5% NaCl.

L-J medium containing 5% NaCl or without salt is inoculated with 0.2 ml of SCS and incubated at 30 or 35°C. Growth or no growth is scored at 4 weeks. *M. fortuitum* and *M. tuberculosis* H37Ra can be used as positive and negative controls, respectively.

Inhibition by Thiophene-2-Carboxylic Acid Hydrazide

Inhibition by thiophene-2-carboxylic acid hydrazide (T2H) is used to distinguish niacin-positive *M. bovis* from *M. tuberculosis* and other nonchromogenic slowly growing mycobacteria. Most *M. bovis* isolates are susceptible to T2H, whereas *M. tuberculosis* and most other slowly growing mycobacteria are resistant.

Middlebrook 7H11 medium containing 10 µg of T2H (Aldrich Chemical Co., Milwaukee, Wis.) per ml is dispensed in 5-ml amounts onto slants. Tubes with and without T2H are inoculated with 0.2 ml of the 10^{-2} and 10^{-4} SCS dilutions. When growth is visible on the control tubes, the colonies are counted. The organism is recorded as resistant if growth on the T2H medium is > 1% of the growth on the control. *M. tuberculosis* H37Ra and *M. bovis* can be used as positive and negative controls, respectively.

Tellurite Reduction

Tellurite reductase reduces colorless potassium tellurite to a black metallic tellurium precipitate. The test is used to separate *M. avium* and *M. intracellulare* from most other nonchromogens. Some rapid growers can similarly present a positive tellurite test.

Two drops of 0.2% aqueous solution of potassium tellurite are added to 5-ml cultures (7 days old) of Middlebrook 7H9. The cultures are incubated and examined daily for 4 days or more. A positive test is shown by a jet black

FIGURE 1   (A) *M. tuberculosis* growth after 15 days. Thin, nonpigmented, rough colonies are seen on 7H11 agar; cording is apparent. Magnification, ×23,500. (B) *M. tuberculosis* growth after 10 days. Dry, buff, wrinkled colonies are visible on 7H11 agar. Magnification, ×587.5. (C) *M. avium* growth after 10 days. Flat, nonpigmented, smooth (S) colony with irregular edge and compact, nonpigmented rough (R) colony are seen on 7H11 agar. Magnification, ×23,500. (D) *M. avium* growth after 10 days. Nonpigmented colony variants are visible on 7H11 agar; smooth-flat (S), dome (D), and rough (R) variants are indicated. Magnification, ×587.5. (E) *M. xenopi* growth after 15 days. Nonpigmented, compact, rough colonies with an irregular periphery are seen on 7H11 agar; the colonies resemble a bird's nest. Magnification, ×23,500. (F) *M. xenopi* growth after 15 days. Smooth, dome shaped, and slight yellow colonies are visible on 7H11 agar. Magnification, ×705. (G) *M. gordonae* growth after 10 days. Orange smooth opaque entire colonies and orange smooth opaque colonies with irregular edge tint are seen on 7H11 agar. Magnification, ×23,500. (H) *M. gordonae* growth after 10 days. Smooth, orange, hemispheric colonies are seen on 7H11 agar. Magnification, ×705. (Photographs courtesy of Daniel Fedorko and Yvonne Shea, Department of Laboratory Medicine, Microbiology Service, National Institutes of Health, 2002.)

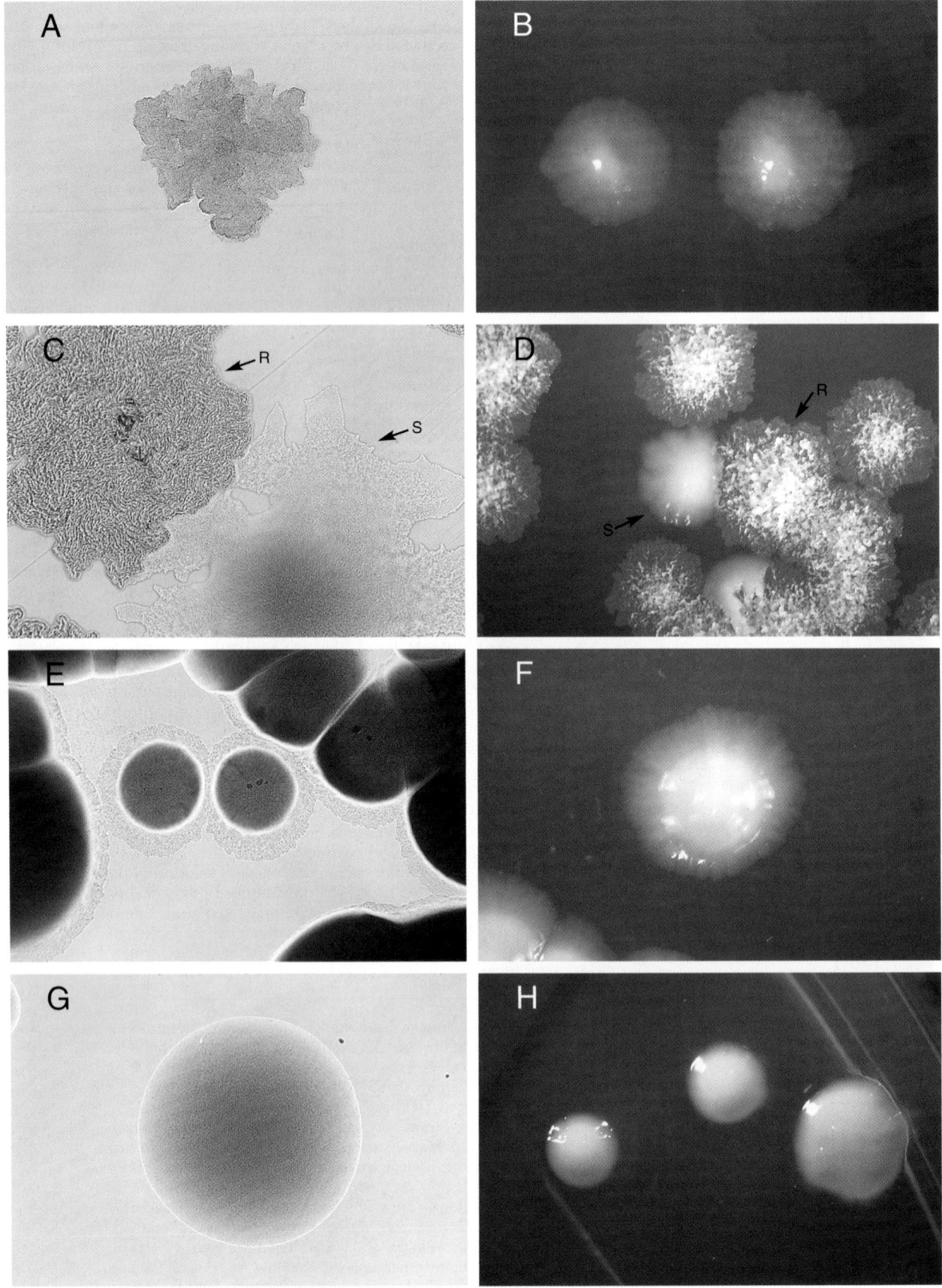

precipitate. M. avium and M. kansasii can be used as positive and negative controls, respectively.

Tween 80 Hydrolysis

Lipases produced by some mycobacterial species hydrolyze the detergent polyoxyethylene sorbitan monooleate (Tween 80) into oleic acid and polyoxyethylene sorbitol. Neutral red in the pH 7 test medium is bound by Tween 80 and has an amber color at a neutral pH. If Tween 80 is hydrolyzed, however, neutral red is no longer bound and reverts to its usual red color at pH 7. The test allows for differentiation among the slow-growing NTM species.

The substrate solution consists of 0.5 ml of Tween 80 in 100 ml of 0.067 M phosphate buffer (pH 7.0) to which 2 ml of a 1% aqueous solution of neutral red is added. The solution is dispensed in screw cap tubes in 4-ml amounts and autoclaved. A loopful of bacteria is suspended in a tube and incubated at 37°C. A change in color from amber to pink or red is recorded after 24 h and 5 and 10 days of incubation as a positive reaction. M. kansasii and M. avium can be used as positive and negative controls, respectively.

Urease

The ability of an isolate to hydrolyze urea to ammonia and CO_2 is useful in identifying both scotochromogens and nonchromogens. M. scrofulaceum is urease positive, whereas M. avium and M. intracellulare organisms are urease negative. The urease test is particularly helpful in the recognition of pigmented strains of M. avium.

The test medium is prepared by mixing 1 part of urea agar base concentrate with 9 parts of distilled water and dispensed in 4-ml amounts into tubes. A loopful of bacteria is emulsified in a test tube and incubated at 37°C for 3 days. A positive reaction is indicated by a pink to red color. M. scrofulaceum and M. gordonae can be used as positive and negative controls, respectively.

Mycolic Acid Analysis

Mycolic acid analysis has been recommended as one of several minimal criteria for the description of new mycobacterial species (153). Mycolic acids are high-molecular-weight (20 to 90 carbon atoms) alpha-substituted, beta-hydroxy fatty acids found in the cell wall of several bacterial genera: Corynebacterium, Rhodococcus, Gordonia, Skermania, Dietzia, Nocardia, Tsukamurella, and Mycobacterium (34).

High-pressure liquid chromatography (HPLC) of mycolic acid esters has been demonstrated to be a rapid and reliable method for identification of many Mycobacterium species (17, 23). A standardized method is available that describes sample preparation and chromatographic analysis (21). One to two loopfuls of cells grown on solid medium are suspended in a methanolic potassium hydroxide solution and saponified by heating. After acidification and extraction with chloroform, free mycolic acids are derivatized to p-bromophenacyl esters. Internal-standard molecular weight markers are added, and the sample is injected. The mycolic acid esters are separated on a reversed-phase C_{18} column by a methanol-methylene chloride gradient elution and detected by UV spectrophotometry (UV-HPLC). An extract prepared from M. intracellulare ATCC 13950 is used as a positive control and provides an external standard peak naming reference. The high biomass requirement of UV-HPLC can be reduced at least 200-fold by derivatizing mycolic acids to 6,7-dimethoxy-4-coumarinyl-methyl esters, which are measured by fluorescence detection HPLC (FL-HPLC). The increased analytical sensitivity of FL-HPLC allows the identification of acid-fast bacilli (AFB) from smear-positive clinical specimens, liquid medium cultures, and minute amounts of biomass from solid medium (17, 67). MTBC identification by FL-HPLC has been reported to achieve a sensitivity of 99% from BACTEC 12B medium with a growth index of ≥ 50 (67); a sensitivity of 85.3 to 92.6% has been described (E. R. Harrington, R. Nabi, and M. A. Lewinski, Abstr. 101st Gen. Meet. Am. Soc. Microbiol. 2001, abstr. C-365, p. 236, 2001; K. C. J. Jost, S. H. Chiu, T. Kenney, D. F. Dunbar, and L. B. Elliott, Abstr. 97th Gen. Meet. Am. Soc. Microbiol. 1997, abstr. U-143, p. 568, 1997) for direct analysis of moderately to strongly smear-positive clinical specimens.

HPLC patterns can be identified to the species or group level by visual or mathematical means. Recently, a pattern atlas derived from a multicenter study of more than 350 strains, representing 23 species, was published that illustrates species patterns (22). Additionally, pattern overlays of closely related species were presented along with pattern variations produced by strains of a single species. However, M. tuberculosis and M. bovis produce indistinguishable patterns.

Several mathematical models for pattern recognition have been described. Dichotomous keys using peak height ratios have been described for the identification of the M. avium complex (MAC) and related species (25) and for slow-growing species that produce a single mycolic acid cluster, including MTBC (23). The standardized method (21) recommends a visual comparison of a sample HPLC

FIGURE 2 (A) M. kansasii growth after 10 days in the dark. Nonpigmented, rough colonies are seen on 7H11 agar; stranding of bacilli is seen (similar to cording). Magnification, ×23,500. (B) M. kansasii growth after 15 days. Smooth colony with center elevated and thickened with thin rough periphery is seen on 7H11 agar; it is orange after light exposure. Magnification, ×470. (C) M. abscessus growth after 3 days. Rough (R) colonies having an irregular edge demonstrating stranding of bacilli and smooth (S), opaque, entire colonies are seen on 7H11 agar. Magnification, ×23,500. (D) M. abscessus off-white, rough (R), wrinkled colonies and off-white, rounded, smooth (S) colonies are visible on 7H11 agar. Magnification, ×352.5. (E) M. chelonae smooth domed colonies with narrow, thin irregular edges are visible on 7H11 agar. Magnification, ×23,500. (F) M. chelonae off-white, smooth-domed colonies with thin irregular edges are visible on 7H11 agar. Magnification, ×399.5. (G) M. mucogenicum nonpigmented, smooth, hemispheric, entire colonies are seen on 7H11 agar. Magnification, ×23,500. (H) M. mucogenicum nonpigmented, smooth, mucoid colonies are visible on 7H11 agar. Magnification, ×235. (Photographs courtesy of Daniel Fedorko and Yvonne Shea, Department of Laboratory Medicine, Microbiology Service, National Institutes of Health, 2002.)

pattern to an atlas of reference strain patterns in combination with the use of peak height ratios. This approach was reported to achieve an accuracy of 96.1% (136). Sophisticated multivariate pattern recognition models have been developed for mycobacterial identification methods. A Centers for Disease Control and Prevention (CDC)-developed library with models for 45 species has been described that achieved ≥97% overall accuracy (53), but this library is no longer available. An enhanced version of this library that reports both an identification and the quality of a match is commercially available (Pirouette and INSTEP software; Infometrix Inc., Woodinville, Wash.). Recently, a fully integrated automated FL-HPLC system, SMIS (Sherlock Mycobacteria Identification System; MIDI, Inc., Newark, Del.), was developed that combines the use of external and internal standards, chromatographic suitability software for overall system quality control, and pattern recognition models. A SMIS library version with entries for 26 mycobacterial species or groups was evaluated and demonstrated an overall accuracy of 85 to 90.6% (74). An enhanced version of the SMIS is under development.

HPLC is an attractive method for mycobacterial identification in the clinical laboratory. Although the initial equipment costs are high (approximately $50,000) and considerable expertise is required to operate nonautomated systems, material costs per test are economical compared with commercial probes. Sample preparation is simple, and many mycobacterial species or groups can be identified rapidly and accurately in a single analysis. The combination of automated quality control and pattern recognition software with a rapid and analytically sensitive method promises to be a powerful diagnostic tool for the mycobacteriology laboratory.

Mycobacterial Genomes

Genome sequences are available or being determined for several mycobacteria. Invaluable information is now available on the agents of tuberculosis and leprosy.

The complete genome sequence of M. tuberculosis H37Rv comprises 4,411,529 bp and contains approximately 4,000 genes encoding proteins and 50 genes coding for RNA (37). The genome is characterized by the abundance of genes encoding enzymes involved in fatty acid metabolism (more than 250, compared to 50 in Escherichia coli) and by extensive functional redundancy due to gene duplication events. Moreover, M. tuberculosis has an extremely clonal population structure, with genomic variation caused largely by insertion sequence movement rather than point mutation, suggesting that this pathogen is evolutionarily young (16, 72, 127). DNA-DNA hybridization studies showed that M. bovis and M. tuberculosis have more than 99% identity (62). Although they are members of a single genomic species, the strains may be differentiated on the basis of conventional identification tests (Table 1) as well as host range and virulence. Whole-genome comparisons within the MTBC using bacterial artificial chromosome arrays allowed the identification of M. bovis- and M. tuberculosis-specific deletion regions, which contribute to a more reliable identification of both species (54).

The M. leprae complete genome sequence has a genome size of 3.27 Mb, much smaller than that of M. tuberculosis (4.41 Mb) (38). Comparative proteome analysis revealed an extreme reductive evolution, since only 391 soluble proteins could be detected (versus 1,800 in M. tuberculosis) instead of the 3,000 proteins predicted if all the genes were active. Restriction fragment length polymorphism (RFLP)

analysis of genomes of M. leprae isolates from patients in geographically distinct regions and from animals (monkeys and armadillos) showed a high conservation of genomic sequences within the species, preventing further molecular epidemiological studies (35, 162).

More information can be found at the websites http://genolist.pasteur.fr/TubercuList for M. tuberculosis H37Rv, http://www.tigr.org/tdb/CMR/gmt/htmls/SplashPage.html for M. tuberculosis CDC1551, http://www.sanger.ac.uk/Projects/M_bovis for M. bovis, and http://genolist.pasteur.fr/Leproma for M. leprae.

Genotypic Identification of Mycobacterial Strains

PCR and Restriction Endonuclease Analysis

In 1992, Plikaytis and colleagues developed a PCR-restriction endonuclease analysis (PRA) method for the rapid identification of mycobacteria to the species level. This technique was based on PCR of a sequence of the gene encoding the 65-kDa heat shock protein (hsp65), followed by restriction enzyme digestion (99). In 1993, Telenti et al. presented a modification of this method using a smaller fragment (439 bp) and only two restriction endonucleases, BstEII and HaeIII (133). The method has been extensively used for mycobacterial identification (18, 43, 129, 133). M. tuberculosis is easily differentiated from the NTM by a characteristic band on HaeIII restriction endonuclease digestion. However, members of the MTBC are not discriminated by PRA. By contrast, most NTM can be recognized by their PRA patterns. Several alleles have been identified in M. gordonae (70), M. kansasii (2, 94), M. abscessus, M. chelonae, and M. peregrinum (105), indicating that the molecular clock of the hsp65 gene is faster than that of 16S rDNA. A study including 129 reference and clinical strains of nonpigmented RGM showed that 60% of the strains were differentiated by HaeIII digestion alone (129). Single unique patterns were seen with HaeIII and/or BstEII for all (100%) of M. fortuitum, M. smegmatis, M. mucogenicum, and sorbitol-negative third biovariant strains of M. fortuitum, and for 94 and 96% of M. chelonae and M. abscessus isolates studied, respectively (129).

Some authors have used other gene sequences for PRA. These include the rpoB gene that mediates rifampin resistance, the dnaJ gene, and the 16S-23S rRNA gene spacer (77, 91, 132). None have been studied as extensively as hsp65.

The advantages of PRA are that identification is largely independent of growth rate and requirements, equipment is not very expensive, and the method is relatively rapid and identifies most mycobacterial species including some not identified by phenotypic methods and/or HPLC. It also identifies most of the closely related aerobic actinomycetes such as Nocardia. The disadvantages are that it requires knowledge of PCR and is a relatively complex procedure. Furthermore, it is not commercialized or Food and Drug Administration (FDA) approved, and it requires a significant amount of in-house validation. A useful website is available for determining likelihood of species identification when band patterns are entered (http://www.hospvd.ch/prasite).

Commercially Available Identification Probes

AccuProbe

Acridinium ester-labeled DNA probes based on the detection of rRNA (GenProbe Inc., San Diego, Calif.) specific for MTBC, MAC (as well as separate probes for *M. avium* and *M. intracellulare*), *M. kansasii*, and *M. gordonae* are FDA approved and commercially available. The current total test time for the assay is within 2 h (32, 83). Briefly, target 16S rRNA is released from the organism by sonication. The labeled DNA probe combines with the organism's rRNA to form a DNA-rRNA hybrid. The labeled product is detected in a luminometer.

Tests with DNA probes can be performed using isolates from solid media or from broth cultures. Combining the probes with a broth culture system has the advantage of optimizing rapid detection and identification of mycobacteria present in clinical samples (32, 69). Procedural modifications are necessary when testing isolates recovered from BACTEC 12B or 13A medium. An aliquot of the BACTEC 12B broth culture is removed after a suitable growth index is attained. AFB are concentrated by centrifugation. The supernatant is decanted, and the pellet is resuspended in culture identification reagent. Testing then follows the procedure for testing colonies from solid media (as described in the AccuProbe technical insert). To eliminate high nonspecific chemiluminescence, BACTEC 13A broth medium containing blood is pretreated with 100 μl of 10% sodium dodecyl sulfate–50 mM EDTA (pH 7.2) before microcentrifugation to allow lysis of the erythrocytes and sorbitolization of the membranes. Pellets are washed with 1.0 to 1.5 ml of sterile water, centrifuged, and processed as indicated above. Appropriate positive and negative control organisms should be included in each assay run.

It has been shown that specificity is 100% when testing mycobacterial colonies. Sensitivity, however, varies with the species or species complexes: 95.2 to 97.2% for MAC, 100% for MTBC, 100% for *M. gordonae*, and 97.4 to 100% for *M. kansasii* (55, 83, 104, 141). Later studies using AccuProbe on more than 11,000 positive BACTEC (Becton Dickinson) cultures also showed 100% specificity and >85 to 100% sensitivity for all species tested (32, 103).

Advantages of this test include the simplicity and rapidity with which mycobacteria can be identified. The use of a nonradioactive procedure and the extended shelf life of the chemiluminescent probes offer the potential for widespread application in most clinical laboratory settings (55, 83). The procedure can also be used to test isolates recovered from newer broth culture instrumentation such as ESPII (Trek Diagnostics, Columbus, Ohio) and the BacT/Alert (bio-Mérieux, Marcy l'Étoile, France) and MGIT (Becton Dickinson).

A few limitations have been described when using AccuProbe. These include misidentification of *M. celatum* as MTBC (125) due to the similarity of the 16S rDNAs of these two species in the probe region (24). Additionally, probes do not differentiate among *M. tuberculosis*, *M. bovis*, *M. bovis* BCG, *M. africanum*, and *M. microti*. The specificity of the MTBC probe has been increased by extending the length of the selection reagent incubation step to 10 min. The temperature of the heating block has been shown to affect the specificity of the probe reaction. A temperature of 60 to 61°C is recommended to eliminate cross-reactivity with other species including *M. terrae* and *M. celatum* (125). Greater biomass in the test suspensions may also result in decreased specificity of the test (125). As with all laboratory tests, the user is reminded that the probe should be repeated or the results should be confirmed by an alter-

nate method if the results do not correlate with clinical or cultural observations.

INNO-LiPA Tests

In mycobacteria, the internal transcribed spacer region (ITS) of approximately 280 bp which separates the 16S and 23S rDNAs presents species-specific polymorphisms, with intraspecies polymorphisms in some species (50, 91, 109). A kit (INNO-LiPA Mycobacteria; Innogenetics, Ghent, Belgium), available only in Europe at present, includes ITS probes of several species. It is based on the reverse hybridization principle, in which the mycobacterial 16S-23S ITS is amplified by PCR. Biotinylated amplicons are subsequently hybridized with probes immobilized as parallel lines on a membrane strip. The addition of streptavidin labeled with alkaline phosphatase and a chromogenic substrate results in a purple-brown precipitate on hybridized lines. The kit may be applied to strains subcultured on solid or in liquid media. Lines on the strip include probes for the *Mycobacterium* genus, MTBC, *M. kansasii* (three probes: MKA-1, MKA-2, and MKA-3), *M. xenopi*, *M. gordonae*, *M. avium*, *M. intracellulare*, *M. scrofulaceum*, and *M. chelonae* (three probes: MCH-1, MCH-2, and MCH-3). An additional probe, designated MAIS, reacts with *M. avium*, *M. intracellulare*, and *M. scrofulaceum* and also with *M. malmoense*, *M. haemophilum*, and the so-called MAI-X isolates (or "intermediate" MAC, defined by positive hybridization with MAC AccuProbe and negative reaction with both the *M. avium* and *M. intracellulare* probes) (151). Moreover, the manufacturer warns against cross-reactions with other probes. Whereas the MKA-1 and MKA-2 probes react with *M. kansasii* only, the MKA-3 probe reacts with *M. kansasii* and *M. gastri* as well. *M. abscessus* isolates hybridize with one or two of the probes designed for *M. chelonae*.

The main advantage of the kit is that a range of several species can be identified by a single PCR assay and, unlike the AccuProbe, it does not require a tentative selection of the adequate probe. According to two studies performed on a total of 298 mycobacterial isolates, all isolates reacted positively with the genus probe. The specificity and sensitivity of probes for the *M. tuberculosis* complex, *M. xenopi*, *M. scrofulaceum*, *M. avium*, and *M. gordonae*, were excellent. However, some genuine *M. intracellulare* isolates were not detected with the MIN probe, designed for *M. intracellulare*, but were detected with the MAIS probe only (86, 140). Further evaluation is necessary to ascertain the specificity and sensitivity of the kit with respect to nonmycobacterial and mycobacterial species.

The test is performed in 6 h, including the preliminary PCR amplification. It requires several time-consuming washes. An automated machine, Auto-LiPA (Tecan Trading AG, Männedorf, Switzerland), which runs the washes and ensures the gentle shaking necessary for several steps of the procedure greatly contributes to time saving and ease of application in clinical laboratories. However, the cost of this apparatus may hamper its introduction into laboratories.

DNA Sequencing

The availability of DNA-sequencing technologies constituted a great benefit for mycobacterial identification, owing to the peculiar slow growth of these organisms. Recent improvements in automation of target amplification and sequence analysis led to practical implementation of DNA sequencing in the clinical laboratory. Manual sequencing should be discouraged. Sequencing the entire 16S rDNA (*rrs* gene, approximately 1,500 bp) or *hsp65* gene (approximately 4,400 bp) cannot be done in a routine clinical laboratory. However, identification of species-specific signatures within variable regions of these highly conserved genes allowed the design of simple PCR protocols followed by the direct sequencing of the PCR amplified products. Catalogues of sequences of mycobacterial species may be retrieved from databases (GenBank/EMBL website at http://www.ncbi.nlm.nih.gov) and conveniently imported and stored in a file in the laboratory. It may be cost-effective to run the specific amplification of the mycobacterial targets in the clinical laboratory and refer to a sub-contractor for sequencing. However, it is recommended that interpretation of the electropherograms and sequence analysis including alignment and comparison of the sequences for homology be performed in the laboratory since the user's decisions are required at the different steps of the analysis process. This strategy allows a laboratory to have access to sequencing technology and neither buy nor maintain an automated DNA sequencer. Liquid cultures or colonies from solid medium may be used for DNA extraction by boiling the sample without any further purification. The polymorphism of several conserved genes has been investigated for identifying mycobacterial species, such as the gene encoding the 32-kDa protein (123), the *dnaJ* gene (132), the *sod* gene encoding the superoxide dismutase (170), the *gyrB* gene coding for the gyrase subunit B (71), the *rpoB* gene coding for the RNA polymerase (77), and the ITS 16S–23S sequence (91, 109, 110). The most widely used targets are the *hsp65* gene and 16S rDNA (*rrs* gene).

The strategy for sequencing and identification of the signature sequences in 16S rDNA has been extensively described (78). Specific primers for mycobacteria (Table 3) have been designed for the amplification of the 16S rDNA to avoid contamination and enhance specificity. Amplification of a 1,030-bp region encompassing the 16S rDNA sequence is performed with primers 285 and 264. Sequencing reactions are performed with primer 244 or primer 259, using sequencing kits for automated DNA sequencers to characterize the two hypervariable regions, A and B, respectively. Both regions are located on the 5′ side of the *rrs* gene, corresponding to *E. coli* 16S rDNA positions 129 to 267 (region A) and 430 to 500 (region B). Determination of the sequence of hypervariable region A is the standard approach for routine identification of mycobacteria, whereas region B is more suited for strains which cannot be identified by sequence determination of region A and may represent isolates of hitherto undescribed taxa (126). 16S rRNA genes reflect a limited conserved region of the entire genome, and the molecular clock of the marker is rather slow. Species of recent divergence thus may contain 16S rRNA gene sequences that are highly similar. Moreover, no single 16S rDNA interstrain nucleotide sequence difference value that unequivocally defined species boundaries has been established for the genus *Mycobacterium* (160). For instance, M. *szulgai* and M. *malmoense* present a 2-nucleotide difference only in the 1,384-nucleotide segment examined whereas some M. *intracellulare* serotypes reveal microheterogeneity with 1 to 7 different nucleotides in a 782-nucleotide segment (160). However, it is well established that M. *malmoense* and M. *szulgai* are distinct species and that the serotypes referred to above belong to a single species. For routine identification, strains should be identified according to a 16S rDNA hypervariable region A matching the type strain sequence. Additional investigation using another molecular marker (e.g., *hsp65*) may be required for accurate identification since hypervariable region A cannot discriminate between some species encountered in clinical specimens, e.g., M. *kansasii* and M. *gastri*, M. *ulcerans* and M. *marinum*, M. *shimoidei* and M. *triviale*, and M. *abscessus* and M. *chelonae* (78). In addition, no polymorphisms are present among the different species in the M. *tuberculosis* complex.

Partial sequencing of the *hsp65* gene is performed using primers Tb11 and Tb12 (70) (Table 3) for the amplification of a 441-bp region (nucleotides 396 to 836 according to the numbering of the M. *tuberculosis hsp65* gene) (116). As indicated above for the PRA method, several *hsp65* alleles may be identified within a species. The polymorphism in *hsp65* gene allows unambiguous identification of species with close 16S rDNA sequences such as M. *gastri* and M. *kansasii* as well as the RGM M. *abscessus* and M. *chelonae* (70, 105). As with the 16S rRNA gene, all M. *tuberculosis* complex members have the same *hsp65* allele.

Genotypic Markers for Species Identification within the *M. tuberculosis* Complex

Several markers have been described for the identification of M. *tuberculosis* sensu stricto, M. *bovis*, M. *africanum*, M. *microti*, and the recently described M. *canettii* and M. *tuberculosis* subsp. *caprae*. As mentioned below and shown in Table 4, spoligotypes represent a useful way to precisely identify the species. However, PCR tests targeting independent, additional markers also provide a reliable, differential identification (Table 5). The *mtp40* gene coding for phospholipase C was the first genomic marker described for the differential identification of MTBC. Although *mtp40* was originally considered to be present in M. *tuberculosis* and absent in M. *bovis* (92), it was later shown that not all M. *tuberculosis* strains harbor the gene (161). The intraspecific sequence polymorphism of the *oxyR* and *pncA* genes led to the development of allele-specific PCR tests which allow a rapid differentiation between M. *tuberculosis* and M. *bovis* (45). The *oxyR* gene has an adenine at nucleotide 285 in M. *bovis* and a guanine in M. *tuberculosis*. The *pncA* gene has a guanine nucleotide at position 169 in M. *bovis* and a cytosine in M. *tuberculosis*. However, these tests do not differentiate between M. *tuberculosis* and M. *africanum*, M. *microti*, or M. *canettii* (Table 5). M. *tuberculosis* subsp. *caprae* is characterized by a polymorphism characteristic of M. *tuberculosis* in *pncA* and characteristic of M. *bovis* in *oxyR* (4). Moreover, as discussed below, spoligotypes confirm the specific identification (Table 4). Although still under evaluation, the PCR tests for the distribution of deletions (RD sequences) among the tubercle bacilli may

TABLE 3 Oligonucleotides used for mycobacterial identification by DNA sequencing

Target	Primer[a]	Sequence	Position[b]
rrs	285	5′ GAGAGTTTGATCCTGGCTCAG 3′	9–29
rrs	264	5′ TGCACACAGGCCACAAGGGA 3′	1046–1027
rrs	244	5′ CCCACTGCTGCCTCCCGTAG 3′	361–342
rrs	259	5′ TTTCACGAACAACGCGACAA 3′	609–590
hsp65	Tb11	5′ ACCAACGATGGTGTGTCCAT 3′	396–415
hsp65	Tb12	5′ CTTGTCGAACCGCATACCCT 3′	836–817

[a] Primers are described in references 70 and 78.
[b] "Position" refers to the *E. coli* 16S rDNA numbering for the *rrs* gene and to the M. *tuberculosis* numbering for the *hsp65* gene.

TABLE 4 Characteristic spoligotypes of some MTBC members

Strain	Spoligotype[a]						Reference
	1	9	19	29	39	43	
M. tuberculosis H37Rv	■■■■■■■■■■■■■■■■■□□■■■■■■■■■■■■■■■□■□□□■■■■■■■						68
M. bovis BCG Pasteur	■■□■■■■■□■■■■■■■■■□■■■■■■■■■■■■■■■■■■□□□□□						68
M. tuberculosis Beijing or W	□□□□□□□□□□□□□□□□□□□□□□□□□□□□□□□□□□□□□■■■■■■■■■						146
M. tuberculosis subsp. caprae	□■□□□□□□□□□□□□□□□□□□■■■■■■■■■■□■□□□□□■■■■■□□□□						4
M. canettii	□□□□□□□□□□□□□□□□□□□□□□□□□□□□□□□■□□□□□□■□□□□□□□						148
M. microti	□□■■□□□□□						149

[a] ■, positive hybridization; □, negative hybridization. Refer to the text for further comments and details on M. tuberculosis, M. bovis, and M. africanum spoligotypes.

contribute to the identification of M. tuberculosis, specifically RD9 for its differentiation from M. africanum and RD4 for its differentiation from M. microti (54).

These tests should be used for strains with phenotypes which do not fully match the type strain. For example, strains which hybridize with the M. tuberculosis complex probe and do not yield rough, cream, cauliflower-like colonies or do not produce niacin or nitrate reductase should be tested by oxyR/pncA allele-specific PCR tests, possibly by PCR tests targeting the RD sequences, or by spoligotyping. If these tests are not available in the laboratory, strains should be sent to a reference laboratory. Although M. tuberculosis is the most prevalent species isolated in clinical laboratories, identification of other members of the MTBC complex is of the utmost epidemiological importance and may govern the management of contact-tracing investigations and/or treatment.

Direct Amplification Tests

Direct amplification tests are designed to identify cultures positive for MTBC directly from patient specimens by using commercially available kits.

Amplified *Mycobacterium tuberculosis* Direct Test

The Gen-Probe amplified *Mycobacterium tuberculosis* direct test (MTD) is a rapid rRNA amplification assay for the detection of M. tuberculosis in clinical specimens. The test consists of a target-amplified nucleic acid probe for the in vitro detection of MTBC rRNA in smear-positive and -negative concentrated sediments prepared from respiratory

samples such as sputum and bronchial and tracheal aspirates. Although MTD is not yet FDA approved for nonrespiratory samples, investigators have shown that, with specific modifications, it may also detect M. tuberculosis in nonrespiratory specimens (52, 154).

The MTD is a two-part test in which amplification and detection occur in a single tube. It detects rRNA which is present at a level of approximately 2,000 copies per cell. This is advantageous over tests that target sequences present in only a single copy or in very low copy numbers (98). As few as one mycobacterium cell equivalent can be detected using this system (66). Initially, nucleic acids are released from mycobacterial cells by sonication. Subsequently, heat is applied to denature the nucleic acids and disrupt the secondary structure of rRNA. Then, using a constant temperature (42°C), transcription-mediated amplification of a specific 16S rRNA target by transcription of DNA intermediates results in multiple copies of the mycobacterial RNA final product, also known as an amplicon. MTBC-specific sequences are then detected in the RNA amplicon by a hybridization protection assay using a chemiluminescent DNA probe. This probe is complementary to the M. tuberculosis-specific sequences. When stable RNA-DNA hybrids are formed between the probe and the specific sequences, hybrids are selected and measured in a luminometer.

The AMTDT-1, the first version of the MTD, was evaluated extensively against culture methods and AFB smears with respiratory specimens. The AMTDT-2, the current version of the MTD, has an enhanced protocol

TABLE 5 Genotypic characteristics of the MTBC members[a]

Strain	mtp40	oxyR/ 285G	oxyR/ 285A	pncA/ 169C	pncA/ 169G	RD1	RD4	RD7	RD8	RD9	RD10
M. tuberculosis	+[b]	+	−	+	−	+	+	+	+	+	+
M. bovis	−	−	+	−	+	+	−	−	−	−	−
M. bovis BCG	−	−	+	−	+	−	−	−	−	−	−
M. africanum	V	+	−	+	−	+	+	+	+	−	+
M. canettii	+	+	−	+	−	ND	ND	ND	ND	ND	ND
M. tuberculosis subsp. caprae	−	−	+	+	−	ND	ND	ND	ND	ND	ND
M. microti	−	+	−	+	−	+	+	−	−	−	−

[a] Data from references 4, 45, 54, 148, 149, and 161.
[b] Not present in some strains; V, variable; ND, not determined; RD, locus numbering as to reference 54.

which includes (i) the use of a larger quantity of pretreated specimen (450 to 500 μl instead of the original 45 to 50 μl) (12); (ii) a reduction in the incubation time of the amplification reaction (60 to 30 min); and (iii) elimination of the termination reaction. AMTDT-2 has been reported as more sensitive than AMTDT-1 when applied to smear-negative specimens. On the other hand, AMTDT-2 is more susceptible than AMTDT-1 to inhibitory substances in the amplification reaction. To decrease the number of false-negative results due to inhibitory substances, an internal control for the evaluation of amplification inhibitors in clinical samples should be included in each test run (52). The turnaround time with AMTDT-2 has been shortened to 3.5 h, compared to AMTDT-1, which took 5 h to perform (52). The sensitivity and specificity of the AMTDT-2 are comparable to or better than those of AMTDT-1 (52). A potential problem with AMTDT-2 was recently reported when the test gave a discrepant positive result for a patient infected with M. celatum (138).

AMPLICOR M. tuberculosis PCR Test

The AMPLICOR M. tuberculosis PCR test (MTB) (Roche Diagnostic Systems, Branchburg, N.J.) is the first commercially available PCR test kit for detection of MTBC in clinical specimens and consists of three steps: specimen preparation, amplification, and detection.

Specimens are prepared by adding 100 μl of concentrated digested decontaminated specimen to 0.5 ml of wash buffer and centrifuging at 12,500 $\times$ g for 10 min. The supernatant is aspirated, and lysis reagent is added to the sediment. After vortexing, the suspension is incubated at 60°C to lyse the mycobacterial cells. The lysed material is subsequently neutralized by the addition of a neutralization reagent. AMPLICOR MTB amplifies a 584-bp region of the 16S rRNA gene sequence. Incorporation of dUTP instead of dTTP prevents carrier contamination in the amplification reaction, and the use of uracil-N-glycosylase (Amp Erase) enzymatically cleaves any contaminating amplicons from previous reactions. Amp Erase is inactivated during thermal cycling. Subsequently, 50 μl of neutralized specimen is added to 50 μl of master mix. Specimens and controls are then loaded into a thermal cycler for amplification. Detection is accomplished by hybridization of the amplified product to a DNA probe specific for MTB. A hybridized duplex is detected by using an avidin-horseradish peroxidase conjugate-tetramethyl benzidine substrate system. The reaction is stopped by addition of dilute hydrosulfuric acid. A result is considered positive if the absorbance at 450 nm is >0.35 (98).

The test requires approximately 6.5 to 8 h for completion. A total of 92 specimens can be analyzed during a single test run (39, 87). The sensitivity of the AMPLICOR MTB has been reported to be 66.7% (39) to 85% (87), with 99 to 100% specificity (39, 87). The sensitivity of specimens containing ≤100 CFU of M. tuberculosis per ml has been reported to be 69%, compared to 98% sensitivity in samples containing more than 1,000 CFU/ml (87).

Piersimoni et al. have compared the sensitivities, specificities, and positive and negative predictive values of the AMTDT and the AMPLICOR assays (98). The authors agree that both nucleic acid amplification methods were found to be rapid and specific for the detection of MTBC in respiratory specimens; however, the AMTDT was 100% sensitive compared to AMPLICOR at 99% in 33 smear-positive samples and the sensitivity of the AMTDT and the AMPLICOR was 87.5 and 66.7%, respectively, in 281 smear-negative samples (98).

MYCOBACTERIAL STRAIN TYPING

Molecular Typing Methods for M. tuberculosis Complex Strains

Historically, unusual drug susceptibility patterns and phage typing have been used for epidemiological studies of tuberculosis, but they have significant limitations (57, 121). Most strains are still susceptible to all antituberculous drugs and have identical drug susceptibility patterns. Moreover, strains isolated from patients in a single outbreak may present different drug resistance profiles due to resistance acquired during treatment. Phage studies also yielded limited results because of the scarcity of phage types and the presence of a predominant phage type in most areas. In tuberculosis, it is critical that the epidemiological tools be discriminating, accurate, and stable since epidemiological investigations may cover several years.

In 1990, the description of the repetitive insertion sequence IS6110 marked a major advance in the molecular epidemiology of tuberculosis (137). Since then, additional sequences of interest for M. tuberculosis fingerprinting have been described (100), some through deliberate searches in the genome sequence of the M. tuberculosis type strain H37Rv (49, 131). M. tuberculosis DNA fingerprinting has proven to be a powerful epidemiological tool (146).

IS6110 RFLP

The RFLP technique using the IS6110 repetitive sequence as a probe is considered the "gold standard" for typing MTBC strains. IS6110 is a 1,355-bp repetitive insertion sequence which presents variability in both the copy number, from 0 to about 25 in MTBC strains, and chromosomal positions. Although a mobile element, IS6110 is stable enough to ensure reliable epidemiological studies. Examination of RFLP patterns of strains isolated from patients with sequential positive cultures allowed the estimation of a 3- to 4-year half-life of IS6110 RFLP (42). In other words, RFLP patterns of 50% of M. tuberculosis strains may display one band shift within a 3- to 4-year period. Changes in the drug resistance profile do not alter a strain's fingerprint (26).

A standardized protocol has been proposed for IS6110 RFLP comparison (143). It involves the growth of M. tuberculosis, extraction of genomic DNA, restriction endonuclease digestion using PvuII, Southern blotting, and probing for IS6110. Standardization of the procedure facilitates interlaboratory comparability of patterns. However, comparison of profiles requires sophisticated software for image analysis and the availability of well-trained users (114).

Spoligotyping

The spoligotyping method (which stands for "spacer oligotyping") is based on the polymorphism of the direct repeat (DR) locus. This region, present in all MTBC strains in a unique locus, contains multiple, well-conserved 36-bp repeats interspersed with nonrepetitive short spacer sequences of 34 to 41 bp. The order of spacers is well conserved in all isolates, apart from a few duplications of spacers. Strains vary in the numbers of 36-bp repeated elements and in the presence or absence of some spacers. The strains are tested by hybridizing their PCR-amplified

DR regions to a membrane which consists of an array of 43 covalently bound oligonucleotides representing the polymorphic spacers identified in the M. *tuberculosis* H37Rv DR sequence (spacers 1 to 19, 22 to 32, and 37 to 43) and in the sequence of M. *bovis* BCG (spacers 20 to 21 and 33 to 36). Because MTBC isolates differ in the presence of the interspersed spacers, strains can be differentiated by their hybridization patterns (or spoligotypes). Spoligotypes appear highly stable, suggesting that isolates with different spoligotypes are rarely clonally related (48, 124).

Although polymorphic, the M. *tuberculosis* spoligotypes are characterized by the absence of spacers 33 to 36 whereas M. *bovis* spoligotypes usually lack spacers 39 to 43 and M. *africanum* spoligotypes lack spacers 8, 9, and 39 (Table 4) (68, 90, 150). Moreover, M. *microti* as well as M. *canettii* and M. *tuberculosis* subsp. *caprae,* two recently described new taxa in the M. *tuberculosis* complex, display very characteristic spoligotypes (4, 148, 149). Spoligotyping hence represents a useful method for the confirmation of specific identifications within MTBC. Moreover, spoligotyping allows the identification of prevalent genotypes, especially the Beijing genotype, frequently encountered in the Beijing area, other regions of Asia, the former USSR, and other geographical areas (146). In the United States, the largest known epidemic due to drug-resistant strains was due to the so-called "W" strain, an evolutionary branch of the Beijing family (1, 9).

The discriminative power of spoligotyping is less than that of IS6110 RFLP as indicated by the comparison of methods for typing of MTBC strains (79). Spoligotyping, however, is more discriminating than the reference method for strains with no or few copies of IS6110. Spoligotyping represents the method of choice for M. *bovis* strains and has been recommended for M. *tuberculosis* as a first-line test that may cost-effectively contribute to defining clusters to be further analyzed by complementary typing methods (107).

PCR Methods Targeting IS6110

Haas et al. (59) developed a rapid, highly sensitive and specific method for typing strains of M. *tuberculosis* based on IS6110 RFLP by PCR. The key feature of this method, termed mixed-linker PCR, is the ability to amplify multiple restriction fragments containing IS6110 sequences and variable sequences adjacent to the restriction site. The method shows 100% reproducibility and a differentiation level close to that of IS6110 RFLP (79). As expected, the method is not accurate for strains with few IS6110 copies. A similar, less complex method (ligation-mediated PCR) has also been found more discriminatory than spoligotyping for clinical M. *tuberculosis* strains with more than five IS6110 copies (14, 101).

PCR Methods Targeting Loci Other Than IS6110

Genetic loci containing a variable number of tandem repeats (VNTR) have been identified in the M. *tuberculosis* genome (49, 131). VNTR are a source of allelic polymorphism which can be analyzed by amplification of each locus and estimation of the size of the PCR products. Results can be conveniently coded in a simple numerical format, corresponding to the number of repeated units in each locus. VNTR typing was shown to be highly reproducible and stable (49, 79, 84). One VNTR method is based on 12 loci of a type of VNTR sequences called mycobacterial interspersed repetitive units (MIRUs). The 12 MIRU-VNTR loci present two to eight alleles which correspond to a potential of over 16 million different combinations. The

method yielded a discrimination power close to that of IS6110 RFLP typing and accurately clustered epidemiologically related strains (84).

Whole-Genome Fingerprinting Methods

Two newly developed methods show promising results for M. *tuberculosis* strain typing. Their feasibility and application in clinical laboratories will be eased with increasing use of sophisticated technologies that are at present restricted to some laboratories.

The detection of small-scale genomic deletions of more than 350 bp has been proposed as a suitable genotyping system for epidemiological studies. It relies on the use of a high-density oligonucleotide microarray harboring 20 probe pairs targeted to every open reading frame and intergenic region of M. *tuberculosis* H37Rv, thus totaling 111,488 probe pairs after the exclusion of noninformative probes from rRNA, tRNA, and highly repetitive PE and PPE genes. Hybridized DNA is detected with a confocal laser scanner. Based on a small-scale evaluation, the pattern of deletions detected was identical in epidemiologically related clones but differed between different clones, suggesting that the system is suitable for epidemiological studies (72).

The fluorescent amplified fragment length polymorphism analysis detects base substitutions within the whole genome. It follows the amplified fragment length polymorphism patented protocol and consists of restriction of genomic DNA, ligation to linkers, and selective amplification using a primer partly complementary to the restriction site (65). The first evaluation of the technique showed concordance with IS6110 RFLP for strains with multiple IS6110 copies. The technique was able to differentiate among epidemiologically unrelated strains with a single copy of IS6110 (56).

Feasibility and Technical Demands of M. tuberculosis Fingerprinting Methods

RFLP needs approximately 2 μg of high quality DNA and hence has to be performed with large quantities of cells. A subculture of the isolate or heavy growth on the original slant and a long turnaround time are required. The technical steps are both labor-intensive and lengthy. Moreover, sophisticated computer image analysis software is required for fingerprinting interpretation in large-scale analysis. The reference method, IS6110 RFLP, is offered by regional laboratories in the United States through a program funded by CDC. PCR-based methods require small amounts of genomic DNA (approximately 10 ng) and do not rely on growing cultures or even viable cells. These methods have the potential to be applied directly to strongly smear-positive specimens (59, 68), providing the opportunity for real-time epidemiology. However, technical pitfalls should not be underestimated, especially those due to the presence of PCR inhibitors and the use of multiplex PCR, and large-scale evaluation should be available before considering applications to specimens in clinical laboratories. RFLP- or PCR-based methods which rely on band matching for interpretation of the fingerprints may require reexamination of the DNAs from suspected similar isolates to be analyzed at the same time. By contrast, the digital format of the MIRU-VNTR technique is unambiguous and portable and allows easy storage in archives and easy interlaboratory comparisons. High-density oligonucleotide microarrays should be commercially available to be used for clinical laboratory purposes eventually.

Molecular Typing Methods for Slow-Growing NTM

Typing methods have to be applied to isolates belonging to the same species. The precise species identification of such isolates is thus a prerequisite for molecular typing. Assignment of the isolate(s) to the "complex" level (especially MAC) cannot be considered an accurate characterization. For mycobacteria, relevant typing methods either use specific molecular markers in RFLP methods or apply to the whole genome, e.g., pulsed-field gel electrophoresis (PFGE). The presence of repeated sequences (usually insertional elements such as IS6110) may greatly facilitate molecular studies of a given species, insofar as these molecular markers provide polymorphic and stable patterns.

In the absence of such repetitive sequences, PFGE remains the most useful typing technique because it can be applied in the absence of knowledge of the specific content of a species genome. However, PFGE is a fastidious technique which requires an actively growing culture and several days for completion. Standardization may be hampered by cell clumping and difficulties in controlling cell lysis resulting in different DNA yields from strain to strain, even from batch to batch of the same strain. Moreover, because of DNA degradation, some strains or species are untypeable by PFGE (94, 155).

By contrast, RFLP analyis is easier to perform and does not require living cells, although a consistent amount is needed. Standardization of DNA quantities can be readily performed by adjusting DNA solutions, whereas evaluation of DNA quantities in agarose cubes in the PFGE method is difficult. These difficulties may result in uneven patterns (light and overloaded lanes) since agarose cubes may release various DNA amounts.

In both techniques (RFLP analysis and PFGE), the degree of strain discrimination varies from species to species and may vary within a species from type to type. A comprehensive review of the various methods used for molecular epidemiology studies of the slowly growing mycobacterial species has been published (46).

M. avium Typing Methods

The first strain-typing method for M. avium was serotyping, based on a seroagglutination procedure originally developed by Schaefer (115). The serological specificity of serovar antigens is conferred by oligosaccharide residues of the C-mycoside glycopeptidolipids (15). Combined use of serotyping and species-specific DNA probes has shown that serovars 1 through 6 and 8 through 11 are M. avium while serovars 7, 12 through 17, 19, 20, and 25 are M. intracellulare (113). Multilocus enzyme electrophoresis (MEE) provides a wider range of polymorphism than serotyping (166).

These two phenotypic methods are of limited epidemiological value and have generally been replaced by genomic methods utilizing PFGE or RFLP analysis with the repetitive elements IS1245 or IS1311. Both of these molecular techniques have demonstrated a high degree of discrimination among M. avium strains. Using a standardized IS1245 RFLP typing method (147), M. avium isolates from humans show highly polymorphic patterns with a median number of 16 to 20 bands (58, 95). A PCR method based on amplification of sequences located between the homologous sequences IS1245 and IS1311 has been developed for a rapid strain typing of M. avium, with a level of discrimination similar to that IS1245 RFLP (97). The wide genetic variability of clinical strains using IS1245 is similarly shown by PFGE, with highly discriminant patterns (5, 58, 85, 95).

Isolates recovered from single patients exhibited stable IS1245 RFLP or PFGE patterns over months or even years (5, 85, 95).

Strains from birds share a characteristic IS1245 two-band pattern (7, 13, 58). This two-band pattern has seldom been found in humans, indicating that birds represent an unusual source of M. avium infection in human immunodeficiency virus-infected or uninfected patients (7, 95, 106).

M. kansasii Typing Methods

In M. kansasii, molecular markers show an intraspecific polymorphism which allows the definition of five subspecies (2, 94). The clustering of strains is identical regardless of the molecular marker used, indicating a robust subspecies delineation. The subspecies are characterized by distinct hsp65 alleles, which can be easily displayed by PRA analysis, and distinct major polymorphic tandem repeat (MPTR) RFLP patterns. (MPTR is a repetitive element shared with M. tuberculosis and M. gordonae.) All strains within each subspecies present a single hsp65 PRA pattern (defined with the restriction enzymes HaeIII and BstEII) and a single MPTR pattern. Either method can be used for subspecies recognition, although PRA is much easier to perform. Additional molecular markers aid in the recognition of subgroups within each subspecies. A repeat sequence, IS1652 (108), is found exclusively in subspecies II and III. IS1652 RFLP patterns of subspecies II are polymorphic whereas strains of subspecies III contain a single IS1652 copy in the same genome locus. Although polymorphic, IS1652 RFLP patterns do not present a high degree of discrimination and unrelated strains may have the same pattern. The degree of discrimination by PFGE is low for each subspecies, suggesting that the genotypic divergence between strains among each subspecies is low. An analysis of M. kansasii isolates from the United States showed that all strains belonged to subspecies I; approximately 50% of isolates had the same PFGE pattern identified in clinical and water isolates in France. These results confirm the predominance and the marked clonality of subspecies I (94; Y. Zhang, L. Mann, R. W. Wilson, B. A. Brown-Elliott, V. Vincent, and R. J. Wallace, Jr., Abstr. 101st Gen. Meet. Am. Soc. Microbiol. 2001, abstr. U-14, p. 700–701, 2001).

Typing Methods for Other NTM Slow-Growing Species

For the other slow-growing species, information on the degree of polymorphism displayed by the different techniques is limited. Additional epidemiological investigations are needed.

Molecular epidemiology of M. intracellulare can rely only on PFGE since the M. avium insertion sequences IS1245 and IS1311 are absent from all strains of M. intracellulare (58). Polymorphic PFGE patterns have been obtained for epidemiologically unrelated strains (85, 119).

IS1395, a specific insertion sequence, has been described in M. xenopi. All M. xenopi strains have the element in 3 to 18 copies. Despite this high copy number, the element provides a limited polymorphism and unrelated strains were shown to share several bands in IS1395 RFLP patterns. Comparable results were obtained with PFGE, suggesting high homogeneity of the M. xenopi genome (96).

Although rarely clinically significant, M. gordonae is a common laboratory contaminant and is frequently the cause of pseudo-outbreaks related to endoscopy, tap water, ice machines, or refrigerated fountains (155). Several molecular markers have been described in M. gordonae, including the polymorphic GC-rich sequence (PGRS) and MPTR repetitive elements, also present in MTBC and in M. kansasii, and two insertion sequences, IS1511 and IS1512, which display a high polymorphism (93a). PFGE has also been applied to M. gordonae (82).

The molecular epidemiology of M. celatum clearly differentiates M. celatum type 1 from M. celatum type 2 (93). A specific insertion sequence, IS1407, has been detected in M. celatum type 1 in three or four copies in identical genomic positions. The element is absent from M. celatum type 2. However, M. celatum type 2 strains display polymorphic PFGE patterns whereas strains of M. celatum type 1 present a single homogeneous pattern regardless of the enzyme used to generate the genomic restriction fragments. Further studies are needed to confirm the high homogeneity of M. celatum type 1 and to ascertain the polymorphism within M. celatum type 2.

A limited polymorphism was demonstrated within M. haemophilum with either a repetitive element in an RFLP study (76) or PFGE (167). Random amplification of polymorphic DNA (RAPD) typing also showed some polymorphism in M. malmoense (73). Several techniques, including amplified fragment length polymorphism and RFLP using IS2404, an insertion sequence specific to M. ulcerans (130), showed six types within M. ulcerans which correlated with the geographical origins of the strains (33).

Molecular Methods for Rapidly Growing Mycobacteria

Pulsed-Field Gel Electrophoresis
PFGE is the most widely used technique for typing RGM. Unrelated strains of RGM species are highly heterogeneous, and repeat isolates from the same strain are genetically indistinguishable. PFGE standards (134) have never been validated for RGM. Differences of two or three bands with a restriction enzyme may occur in strains from patients in outbreaks due to RGM, and generally comparable differences are produced with other restriction enzymes (61, 157). Different plasmid mobilities are one cause of the differences of one or two bands in some isolates, and PFGE provides a sensitive means of screening RGM strains for plasmids (61).

M. fortuitum
The first clinical epidemiological use of PFGE in mycobacterial strains was described by Burns et al. (20) in a nosocomial outbreak of respiratory tract colonization with M. fortuitum. Hector et al. (61) have shown that unrelated strains of M. fortuitum were highly diverse by PFGE analysis.

M. chelonae, M. abscessus, and M. immunogenum
Random and outbreak strains of M. chelonae, M. abscessus, and the recently described M. immunogenum have also been studied by PFGE (157). Although the technique is useful and random strains are highly diverse, DNA is spontaneously lysed or digested from approximately 60% of strains of M. abscessus and hence cannot be analyzed by PFGE. So far, the use of different extraction methods and attempts to inactivate a possible endonuclease have been unsuccessful (155). In the first study of M. chelonae and M. abscessus using PFGE, Wallace et al. evaluated a total of 92 patient and environmental isolates that included 12 noso-

comial outbreaks (some isolates identified as M. abscessus were later shown to be M. immunogenum) (157). Broken DNA was a problem in five outbreaks involving M. abscessus, and thus these outbreaks could not be assessed by this technique.

RAPD PCR
Guidelines for the use of RAPD PCR with RGM have been published (168). RAPD PCR is especially useful with M. abscessus since almost 60% of the strains of this species cannot be compared by PFGE (152, 168).

Using RAPD PCR, Zhang et al. (168) confirmed several previous observations concerning nosocomial outbreaks of M. abscessus. Moreover, their analysis of a surgical wound outbreak following cardiac surgery confirmed the presence of M. abscessus in the hospital water supply and in infected patients (168). RAPD PCR helps to identify laboratory contamination of samples. Lai et al. traced the origin of a laboratory pseudo-outbreak of M. abscessus to in-house prepared distilled water (81).

Multilocus Enzyme Electrophoresis
The MEE technique has been used to identify and evaluate isolates of MAC (47, 166), M. chelonae, M. abscessus, M. fortuitum, and M. smegmatis in a study of sternal wound RGM isolates (159). MEE was also used along with PFGE in the evaluation of the isolates of M. abscessus from the postinjection abscess outbreak (51), previously described by Wallace et al. (157).

Some applications of MEE include subtyping of mycobacteria for epidemiological studies and analysis of the genetic relatedness among mycobacterial strains to determine their classification by species clusters. MEE may also help define new species of mycobacteria among strains that do not cluster into recognized groups (166). Furthermore, MEE can be used to type strains regardless of their plasmid content and may provide strain differentiation that may not be evident by restriction enzyme analysis. Comparison of this technique with other typing systems such as PFGE has not been done, and specific guidelines for defining isolates as the same or different by MEE have not been published.

IMMUNODIAGNOSTIC TESTS FOR TUBERCULOSIS
A variety of immunodiagnostic tests for tuberculosis based on the recognition of specific host responses to the infecting organism have been described. Historically, the first immunodiagnostic test was the tuberculin skin test. The shortcomings of this test include the inability to distinguish active disease from past sensitization and unknown predictive values (122). ESAT-6, a T-cell antigen expressed in M. tuberculosis but absent in M. bovis BCG, may represent an alternative to purified protein derivative for delayed-type hypersensitivity tests (145). Various in vitro tests of cell-mediated immune responses to mycobacterial antigens have been described, but they are expensive and technically demanding and provide no more diagnostic information than the tuberculin skin test does at this time.

Much effort has been devoted to the development of serological tests for tuberculosis, but no test has found widespread clinical use (41). The specificity of serological tests with crude antigen preparations is too low for clinical application. Specificity can be increased by using purified antigens, but since not all patients respond to the same antigens, the increased specificity often results in decreased sensitivity (31, 41, 64). Sensitivity and specificity increase if enzyme-linked immunosorbent assay results obtained with a set of purified antigens are combined. The antigens tested in serological assays include the 38-kDa antigen (31, 41, 64, 169), lipoarabinomannan (112), antigen 60 (36), the antigen 85 complex (142), and glycolipids including phenolic glycolipid Tb1, 2,3-diacyltrehalose and lipooligosaccharide (118). Most patients with tuberculosis produce antibody to glycolipids and 38-kDa and 85 complex antigens, and most healthy controls do not. The use of a combination of purified glycolipid antigens resulted in a better specificity and sensitivity. However, a small proportion of tuberculous patients still have low levels or an absence of antibodies against any of these antigens. Lipoarabinomannan, an antigenic lipopolysaccharide of mycobacteria, is found in healthy controls, and the sensitivity and specificity of tests using this antigen are determined largely by the choice of cutoff titer. A test is commercially available (DynaGen, Cambridge, Mass.). Antigen 60 is a complex mixture of proteins, polysaccharides, and lipids obtained from BCG. These antigens are shared by different mycobacterial species. Semipurified antigen 60 is used in a commercially available serodiagnostic test for tuberculosis (Anda Biologicals, Strasbourg, France). A comparative study of antigen 60 and the three glycolipid antigens mentioned above (phenolic glycolipid Tb1, 2,3-diacyltrehalose, and lipooligosaccharide) showed that only 36% of the patients with tuberculosis had a positive response in the antigen 60 test whereas 84% showed a response to the three glycolipids (117).

A number of antigen capture assays based on enzyme-linked immunosorbent assay, radioimmunoassay, or agglutination of antibody-coated latex particles have been described (40). The results reported for some assays have been promising for CSF, but experience with sputum and other specimen types is limited. The sensitivities of immunoassays for detection of mycobacterial antigen in CSF ranged from 65.8 to 100% and the specificities ranged from 95 to 100% in six major studies (40). The use of antigen tests cannot be recommended at this time.

QUALITY ASSURANCE

General

Much of the information in this section was obtained from several recent publications (3, 6, 63, 75, 88, 89). The reader should consult these publications for more information and access to the primary literature. In addition to the specific recommendations listed here, standard components of laboratory quality assurance, such as personnel competency, procedure manuals, proficiency testing, and quality control of media, tests, and reagents, should be in place (see chapter 2).

The Public Health Service introduced the "Levels of Service" concept for mycobacteriology laboratories in 1967. In this scheme, laboratories determine the level of service which best fits the needs of the patient population they serve, the experience of their personnel, their laboratory facilities, and the number of specimens they receive. The concept of levels of service is supported by the CDC and the American Thoracic Society (ATS) (60, 80). The College of American Pathologists (CAP) proposed extents of service for participation in mycobacterial interlaboratory comparison surveys. ATS levels I, II, and III correlate with CAP extents 2, 3, and 4, respectively. ATS makes no

provision for laboratories in which no mycobacterial procedures are performed (CAP extent 1). Five types of mycobacteriology laboratories have been defined by the Clinical Laboratory Improvement Amendments (CLIA). These are modified from the extents described by CAP, but the definitions are awaiting consensus and thus may be modified in the future (165). All specimens submitted for mycobacterial examination should have cultures as well as smears performed. The ATS and the CDC recommend that laboratories examine a minimum of 10 to 15 AFB smears per week to maintain proficiency in performance and interpretation and that they process and culture 20 specimens per week to maintain proficiency in culture and the identification of M. tuberculosis. Recently, the Association of State and Territorial Public Health Laboratory Directors (ASTPHLD) proposed that only two levels of service be designated: (i) specimen collection, specimen transport, and (optional) microscopy of at least 20 smears per week; and (ii) complete mycobacteriology service from microscopy to complete species identification and drug susceptibility testing (158).

Personnel working in the clinical mycobacteriology laboratory must have proper training and certification in the specific functions that they perform. All laboratories performing mycobacteriology testing must be enrolled in a proficiency program which monitors a laboratory's performance by using external samples which are sent for testing. These programs must follow the specifications outlined in CLIA.

Multiple test parameters are monitored by adherence to the quality assurance guidelines described in the recent NCCLS standard document (89). Acceptable results derived from testing quality control reference strains do not guarantee accurate results with all clinical isolates. If atypical or inconsistent results are seen with clinical isolates, the test should be repeated in an attempt to ensure accuracy. Each laboratory should put its own policies into effect regarding the verification of atypical test results.

Quality control (QC) is vital for monitoring a laboratory's effectiveness in detecting and isolating mycobacteria. The CLIA and accreditation programs represent the minimum acceptable standards of practice (165), and laboratories performing mycobacterial testing should follow QC recommendations in the scientific literature and in ad hoc publications (6, 63, 89).

The laboratory must maintain a collection of well-characterized mycobacteria that are used for QC of test systems. These control organisms may be obtained from the American Type Culture Collection and proficiency testing programs. Frequently used stock cultures can be maintained on L-J slants or in 7H9 broth at 37°C or room temperature if subcultured monthly. Cultures on L-J slants may be held for up to 1 year if stored at 4°C. Such maintenance is not recommended for strains with drug resistance. Freezing of organisms suspended in skim milk or broth medium and storage at −20 to −70°C is the best option for long-term maintenance of stock cultures.

Routine QC tests are recommended with new lots of media used with commercial systems (63). Laboratories that prepare their own media must also document the performance characteristics of each new lot.

Ideally, positive control slides should be prepared from a concentrated sputum sample obtained from a patient with active tuberculosis. In practice, many laboratories use suspensions of stock cultures or seeded negative sputa as positive controls for acid-fast staining procedures. The *Clinical*

Microbiology Procedures Handbook (63) describes a method for preparing control slides. Control slides are also commercially available. An increase in the percentage of smear-positive but culture-negative specimens of > 2% that cannot be attributed to a response to mycobacterial therapy or the presence of AFB in the negative controls suggests that water or reagents used in the staining or the digestion procedures are contaminated with environmental mycobacteria (75). M. *gordonae* and M. *terrae* complex are most often involved. A procedure for detection of AFB in working solutions and reagents is described in the ASTPHLD/ CDC document (6). AFB may also be carried over from one slide to another in the oil used with the immersion lens. Oil should be removed from the lens after a positive slide is examined. The sensitivity of the AFB smear is directly related to the relative centrifugal force (RCF) (g force) attained during centrifugation. Thus, laboratories should calculate the RCF of their centrifuge and periodically monitor and document that they are reaching sufficient RCF by checking the revolutions per minute with a tachometer (75).

Laboratories should monitor and document contamination rates (percentage of specimens producing contaminating growth on culture media) for decontaminated specimens. Contamination rates of 3 to 5% are generally considered acceptable. Rates below 3% may indicate that the decontamination procedure is too harsh and that the procedure needs to be modified to minimize the lethal effect on mycobacteria. Contamination rates above 5% often indicate a too weak decontamination procedure which could compromise mycobacterial cultures due to overgrowth of contaminants (see chapter 36). It should be emphasized that the widespread use of liquid culture media (radiometric or not) increases the generation of aerosols; as a consequence, the risk of contamination between samples also increases. Laboratories that handle large numbers of isolates of MAC, M. *abscessus*, or specimens from patients with cystic fibrosis will probably have much higher contamination rates due to the high incidence of colonization of the sputum with gram-negative bacteria, especially *Pseudomonas aeruginosa.*

The processes involved in culturing mycobacteria are naturally prone to errors because of the multiple steps involved in processing cultures, the viability of mycobacteria for long periods in the laboratory environment, and the large number of mycobacteria present in some specimens (19). False-positive cultures may result from mislabeling, specimen switching during handling, specimen carryover (including proficiency testing specimens), contaminated reagents, or cross-contamination between culture tubes or vials (19, 30, 44, 120). Inclusion of a "positive control" (e.g., a suspension of M. *tuberculosis*) in the processing of patient specimens is discouraged due to the risk of cross-contamination. Cross-contamination of culture vials in the BACTEC radiometric system (sometimes skipping several vials) due to inadequately sterilized sample needles has been documented (10, 144). Standardized laboratory procedures that minimize the potential for errors leading to false-positive cultures should be followed, and mechanisms should be in place to rapidly recognize their occurrence. Transfers or inoculation of cultures must be accomplished by using individual transfer pipettes, single-delivery diluent tubes, or disposable labware. The order in which specimens are processed and the media are inoculated should be recorded. A negative control specimen following processing of patient specimens with the same digestion or decontamination solutions can be used for detecting possible specimen contamination of the solutions (6). Alternatively, the processing solutions may be planted directly. Laboratories should prospectively track positivity rates and establish a threshold which, when exceeded, will prompt an investigation (120). The significance of an isolate may be determined by reviewing the order in which specimens were handled for all manipulations (e.g., initial processing, liquid media readings, subculturing), the direct-smear results, the time to positivity, and the clinical history. Cross-contamination in the BACTEC or other automated systems is probably rare if the manufacturer's recommendations for operation and maintenance are closely followed.

Since the introduction of molecular fingerprinting of M. *tuberculosis* strains, false-positive cultures have been demonstrated to occur more frequently than previously assumed, from 1 to more than 10% (44, 102, 120, 144). The deleterious impact of these undesirable events may be minimized if the evidence of false positivity is established in a timely manner and a rapid molecular method of fingerprinting is available. It has been suggested that single positive cultures of M. *tuberculosis* strains grown from AFB smear-negative specimens should be analyzed by a PCR-derived typing technique to rule out laboratory contamination (102). Strains with identical fingerprints isolated within a 1-week period from different patients should be considered probably false positive (120).

The CDC and others have recommended that AFB smear results be available and positive results be reported within 24 h of specimen receipt (6, 135). The time required for identification and susceptibility testing of M. *tuberculosis* should average 14 to 21 days and 15 to 30 days from time of specimen receipt, respectively (6, 27).

Molecular Microbiology Methods

Nucleic acid amplification (NAA)-based assays require several levels of controls (e.g., to detect amplification inhibition as well as contamination between specimens) in addition to positive and negative controls (88). When used as approved by the FDA, NAA tests for M. *tuberculosis* diagnosis do not replace any previously recommended tests (29). Laboratories that test patient specimens by using research or "home-brew" methods or commercially available NAA assays for nonapproved or off-label indications and report their results must validate the assays and establish their performance characteristics prior to diagnostic use. Available information is often insufficient to guide test interpretation. Approved guidelines for molecular diagnostic methods in clinical microbiology are available from the NCCLS; in these documents, the development, validation, quality assurance, and routine use of NAA assays are addressed in detail (88). However, basing the identification of M. *tuberculosis* on a sole positive home-brew PCR result is not recommended because the results of these assays vary considerably (6, 28).

Potential probes and/or primers must be selected for sensitivity by using multiple clinical and reference strains of the target organism. Additionally, specificity must be evaluated by testing for cross-hybridization with other organisms which may be present in patient samples (88).

Several types of validation tests are used to evaluate the presence of target nucleic acid in the sample and to determine that it was isolated in a manner in which inhibitors or contaminants which might interfere with detection of the target have not been introduced. Testing to assess amplification should include positive and negative controls and controls for detection of the presence of inhibitors, such as an endogenous nucleic acid. Other quality control measures include those referring to assays of restriction enzymes, reagents, inspection of equipment, and laboratory design (i.e., separate areas for processing, amplification, and detection steps) (88).

EVALUATION, INTERPRETATION, AND REPORTING OF RESULTS

Adequate funding and focused training are critical in maintaining state-of-the-art mycobacteriology laboratories (11, 88, 139, 164). Laboratories play a pivotal role in the diagnosis and control of tuberculosis, and every effort should be made to implement sensitive and rapid methods for the detection, identification, and susceptibility testing of MTBC as well as other mycobacterial species. Specifically, these include (i) the use of fluorochrome stain for mycobacteria in smears, (ii) a broth-based or microcolony method for culture, (iii) the use of DNA probes or chromatographic analysis for identification, and (iv) direct susceptibility testing of smear-positive specimen concentrates by broth or agar methods.

The 24-h turnaround time for AFB smear results presents a challenge to most laboratories. The daily processing of specimens required to meet this goal adds considerable expense to the laboratory budget. Turnaround time goals for AFB smear results should be established for each institution after consultation with infection control practitioners and infectious-disease specialists.

NAA assays offer the promise of same-day detection and identification of M. tuberculosis. Implementation of this new technology presents several new challenges. Although the performance characteristics of many of these assays are quite good for smear-positive respiratory specimens, limited information exists on the use of these tests for diagnosis of paucibacillary pulmonary or extrapulmonary disease. The new technology will supplement rather than replace culture. Culture will still be required to obtain organisms for susceptibility testing and detect mycobacteria other than M. tuberculosis.

The significance of the isolation of NTM may be difficult to assess since many species are opportunistic pathogens, and the reader is referred to the criteria suggested by the ATS for this evaluation (3). In addition to these criteria, accurate identification of NTM will prevent rarely encountered pathogens from being mistaken for nonpathogenic species.

Thus, accurate and timely reporting of the results of AFB microscopy, culture, identification, and drug susceptibility tests is essential to the effective management of individual patients and to the appropriate implementation of public health and infection control measures.

REFERENCES

1. **Agerton, T. B., S. E. Valway, R. J. Blinkhorn, K. L. Shilkret, R. Reves, W. W. Schluter, B. Gore, C. J. Pozsik, B. B. Plikaytis, C. Woodley, and I. M. Onorato.** 1999. Spread of strain W, a highly drug-resistant strain of Mycobacterium tuberculosis, across the United States. Clin. Infect. Dis. **29:**85–92.

2. **Alcaide, F., I. Richter, C. Bernasconi, B. Springer, C. Hagenau, R. Schulze-Röbbecke, E. Tortoli, R. Martin, E. C. Böttger, and A. Telenti.** 1997. Heterogeneity and clonality among isolates of Mycobacterium kansasii: implications for epidemiological and pathogenicity studies J. Clin. Microbiol. **35:**1959–1964.

3. **American Thoracic Society.** 1997. Diagnosis and treatment of disease caused by nontuberculous mycobacteria. Am. J. Respir. Crit. Care Med. **156**(Suppl.)**:**S1–S25.

4. **Aranaz, A., E. Liebana, E. Gomez-Mampaso, J. C. Galan, D. Cousins, A. Ortega, J. Blazquez, F. Baquero, A. Mateos, G. Suarez, and L. Dominguez.** 1999. Mycobacterium tuberculosis subsp. caprae subsp. nov.: a taxonomic study of a new member of the Mycobacterium tuberculosis complex isolated from goats in Spain. Int. J. Syst. Bacteriol. **49:**1263–1273.

5. **Arbeit, R. D., A. Slutsky, T. W. Barber, J. N. Maslow, S. Niemczyk, J. O. I. Falkinham, G. T. O'Connor, and C. F. von Reyn.** 1993. Genetic diversity among strains of Mycobacterium avium causing monoclonal and polyclonal bacteremia in patients with AIDS. J. Infect. Dis. **167:**1384–1390.

6. **Association of State and Territorial Public Health Laboratory Directors and U.S. Department of Health and Human Services, P.H.S., Centers for Disease Control and Prevention.** 1995. Mycobacterium tuberculosis: Assessing Your Laboratory. Association of State and Territorial Public Health Laboratory Directors and Centers for Disease Control and Prevention, Atlanta, Ga.

7. **Bauer, J., A. B. Andersen, D. Askgaard, S. B. Giese, and B. Larsen.** 1999. Typing of clinical Mycobacterium avium complex strain cultures during a two-year period in Denmark by using IS1245. J. Clin. Microbiol. **37:**600–605.

8. **Bercovier, H., O. Kafri, and S. Sela.** 1986. Mycobacteria possess a surprisingly small number of ribosomal RNA genes in relation to the size of their genome. Biochem. Biophys. Res. Commun. **136:**1136–1141.

9. **Bifani, P. J., B. B. Plikaytis, V. Kapur, K. Stockbauer, X. Pan, M. L. Lutfey, S. L. Moghazeh, W. Eisner, T. M. Daniel, M. H. Kaplan, J. T. Crawford, J. M. Musser, and B. N. Krciswirth.** 1996. Origin and interstate spread of a New York City multidrug-resistant Mycobacterium tuberculosis clone family. JAMA **275:**452–457.

10. **Bignardi, G. E., S. P. Barrett, R. Hinkins, P. A. Jenkins, and M. P. Rebec.** 1994. False-positive Mycobacterium avium-intracellulare cultures with the Bactec 460 TB system. J. Hosp. Infect. **26:**203–210.

11. **Bird, B. R., M. M. Denniston, R. E. Huebner, and R. C. Good.** 1996. Changing practices in mycobacteriology: a follow-up survey of state and territorial public health laboratories. J. Clin. Microbiol. **34:**554–559.

12. **Bodmer, T., E. Möckl, K. Mühlemann, and L. Matter.** 1996. Improved performance of Gen-Probe Amplified Mycobacterium Tuberculosis Direct Test when 500 instead of 50 microliters of decontaminated sediment is used. J. Clin. Microbiol. **34:**222–223.

13. **Bono, M., T. Jemmi, C. Bernasconi, D. Burki, A. Telenti, and T. Bodmer.** 1995. Genotypic characterization of Mycobacterium avium strains recovered from animals and their comparison to human strains. Appl. Environ. Microbiol. **61:**371–373.

14. **Bonora, S., M. C. Gutierrez, G. Di Perri, F. Brunello, B. Allegranzi, M. Ligozzi, R. Fontana, E. Concia, and V. Vincent.** 1999. Comparative evaluation of ligation-mediated PCR and spoligotyping as screening methods for genotyping of Mycobacterium tuberculosis strains. J. Clin. Microbiol. **37:**3118–3123.

15. **Brennan, P. J.** 1989. Structure of mycobacteria: recent developments in defining cell wall carbohydrates and proteins. Rev. Infect. Dis. **11**(Suppl.)**:**S420–S430.

16. **Brosch, R., S. V. Gordon, K. Eiglmeier, T. Garnier, F. Tekaia, E. Yeraman, and S. T. Cole.** 2000. Genomics, biology, and evolution of the Mycobacterium tuberculosis

complex, p. 19–36. *In* G. F. Hatfull and W. R. Jacobs (ed.), *Molecular Genetics of Mycobacteria.* ASM Press, Washington, D.C.

17. **Brown, B. A., B. Springer, V. A. Steingrube, R. W. Wilson, G. E. Pfyffer, M. J. Garcia, M. C. Menendez, B. Rodriguez-Salgado, K. C. M Jost, Jr., S. H. Chiu, G. O. Onyi, E. C. Böttger, and R. J. Wallace, Jr.** 1999. *Mycobacterium wolinskyi* sp. nov. and *Mycobacterium goodii* sp. nov., two new rapidly growing species related to *Mycobacterium smegmatis* and associated with human wound infections: a cooperative study from the International Working Group on Mycobacterial Taxonomy. *Int. J. Syst. Bacteriol.* **49:**1493–1511.

18. **Brunello, F., M. Ligozzi, E. Cristelli, S. Bonora, E. Tortoli, and R. Fontana.** 2001. Identification of 54 mycobacterial species by PCR-restriction fragment length polymorphism analysis of the *hsp65* gene. *J. Clin. Microbiol.* **39:**2799–2806.

19. **Burman, W. J., B. L. Stone, R. R. Reves, M. L. Wilson, Z. Yang, H. El-Hajj, J. H. Bates, and M. D. Cave.** 1997. The incidence of false-positive cultures for *Mycobacterium tuberculosis. Am. J. Respir. Crit. Care Med.* **155:**321–326.

20. **Burns, D. N., R. J. J. Wallace, M. E. Schultz, Y. Zhang, S. Q. Zubairi, Y. Pang, C. L. Gibert, B. A. Brown, E. S. Noel, and F. M. Gordin.** 1991. Nosocomial outbreak of respiratory tract colonization with M. *fortuitum:* demonstration of the usefulness of pulsed-field gel electrophoresis in an epidemiologic investigation. *Am. Rev. Respir. Dis.* **144:**1153–1159.

21. **Butler, W. R., M. M. Floyd, V. A. Silcox, G. Cage, E. Desmond, P. S. Duffey, L. S. Guthertz, W. M. Gross, K. C. Jost, L. S. Ramos, L. Thibert, and N. G. Warren.** 1999. *Mycolic Acid Standards for HPLC Identification of Mycobacteria.* Centers for Disease Control and Prevention, U.S. Department of Health and Human Services, Atlanta, Ga.

22. **Butler, W. R., M. M. Floyd, V. A. Silcox, G. Cage, E. Desmond, P. S. Duffey, L. S. Guthertz, W. M. Gross, K. C. Jost, L. S. Ramos, L. Thibert, and N. G. Warren.** 1996. *Standardized Method for HPLC Identification of Mycobacteria.* Centers for Disease Control and Prevention, U.S. Department of Health and Human Services, Atlanta, Ga.

23. **Butler, W. R., K. C. Jost, and J. O. Kilburn.** 1991. Identification of mycobacteria by high-performance liquid chromatography. *J. Clin. Microbiol.* **29:**2468–2472.

24. **Butler, W. R., S. P. O'Connor, M. A. Yakrus, and W. M. Gross.** 1994. Cross-reactivity of genetic probe for detection of *Mycobacterium tuberculosis* with newly described species *Mycobacterium celatum. J. Clin. Microbiol.* **32:**536–538.

25. **Butler, W. R., L. Thibert, and J. O. Kilburn.** 1992. Identification of *Mycobacterium avium* complex strains and some similar species by high-performance liquid chromatography. *J. Clin. Microbiol.* **30:**2698–2704.

26. **Cave, M. D., K. D. Eisenach, G. Templeton, M. Salfinger, G. Mazurek, J. H. Bates, and J. T. Crawford.** 1994. Stability of DNA fingerprint pattern produced with IS6110 in strains of *Mycobacterium tuberculosis. J. Clin. Microbiol.* **32:**262–266.

27. **Centers for Disease Control.** 1992. National MDR-TB Task Force, National Action Plan to combat multi-drug resistant tuberculosis. *Morb. Mortal. Wkly. Rep.* **41:**1–71.

28. **Centers for Disease Control.** 1993. Diagnosis of tuberculosis by nucleic acid amplification methods applied to clinical specimens. *Morb. Mortal. Wkly. Rep.* **42:**686.

29. **Centers for Disease Control.** 1996. Nucleic acid amplification tests for tuberculosis. *Morb. Mortal. Wkly. Rep.* **45:**950–952.

30. **Centers for Disease Control and Prevention.** 1997. Multiple misdiagnoses of tuberculosis resulting from laboratory error—Wisconsin, 1996. *Morb. Mortal. Wkly. Rep.* **46:**797–801.

31. **Chan, S. L., Z. Reggiardo, T. M. Daniel, D. J. Girling, and D. A. Mitchison.** 1990. Serodiagnosis of tuberculosis using an ELISA with antigen 5 and a hemagglutination assay with glycolipid antigens. Results in patients with newly diagnosed pulmonary tuberculosis ranging in extent of disease from minimal to extensive. *Am. Rev. Respir. Dis.* **142:**385–389.

32. **Chapin-Robertson, K., S. Dahlberg, S. Waycott, J. Corrales, C. Kontnick, and S. C. Edberg.** 1993. Detection and identification of *Mycobacterium* directly from BACTEC bottles by using a DNA-rRNA probe. *Diagn. Microbiol. Infect. Dis.* **17:**203–207.

33. **Chemlal, K., G. Huys, P. A. Fonteyne, V. Vincent, A. G. Lopez, L. Rigouts, J. Swings, W. M. Meyers, and F. Portaels.** 2001. Evaluation of PCR-restriction profile analysis, IS2404 restriction fragment length polymorphism and amplified fragment length polymorphism fingerprinting for identification and typing of *Mycobacterium ulcerans* and M. *marinum. J. Clin. Microbiol.* **39:**3272–3278.

34. **Chun, J., L. L. Blackall, S. O. Kang, Y. C. Hah, and M. Goodfellow.** 1997. A proposal to reclassify *Nocardia pinensis* Blackall et al. as *Skermania piniformis* gen. nov., comb. nov. *Int. J. Syst. Bacteriol.* **47:**127–131.

35. **Clark-Curtiss, J. E., and G. P. Walsh.** 1989. Conservation of genomic sequences among isolates of *Mycobacterium leprae. J. Bacteriol.* **171:**4844–4851.

36. **Cocito, C. G.** 1991. Properties of the mycobacterial antigen complex A60 and its applications to the diagnosis and prognosis of tuberculosis. *Chest* **100:**1687–1693.

37. **Cole, S. T., R. Brosch, J. Parkhill, T. Garnier, C. Churcher, D. Harris, S. V. Gordon, K. Eiglmeier, S. Gas, C. E. Barry III, F. Tekaia, K. Badcock, D. Basham, D. Brown, T. Chillingworth, R. Connor, R. Davies, K. Devlin, T. Feltwell, S. Gentles, N. Hamlin, S. Holroyd, T. Hornsby, K. Jagels, A. Krogh, J. McLean, S. Moule, L. Murphy, K. Oliver, J. Osborne, M. A. Quail, M. A. Rajandream, J. Rogers, S. Rutter, K. Seeger, J. Skelton, R. Squares, S. Squares, J. E. Sulston, K. Taylor, S. Whitehead, and B. G. Barrell.** 1998. Deciphering the biology of *Mycobacterium tuberculosis* from the complete genome sequence. *Nature* **393:**537–544.

38. **Cole, S. T., K. Eiglmeier, J. Parkhill, K. D. James, N. R. Thomson, P. R. Wheeler, N. Honore, T. Garnier, C. Churcher, D. Harris, K. Mungall, D. Basham, D. Brown, T. Chillingworth, R. Connor, R. M. Davies, K. Devlin, S. Duthoy, T. Feltwell, A. Fraser, N. Hamlin, S. Holroyd, T. Hornsby, K. Jagels, C. Lacroix, J. Maclean, S. Moule, L. Murphy, K. Oliver, M. A. Quail, M. A. Rajandream, K. M. Rutherford, S. Rutter, K. Seeger, S. Simon, M. Simmonds, J. Skelton, R. Squares, S. Squares, K. Stevens, K. Taylor, S. Whitehead, J. R. Woodward, and B. G. Barrell.** 2001. Massive gene decay in the leprosy bacillus. *Nature* **409:**1007–1011.

39. **d'Amato, R. F., A. A. Wallman, L. H. Hochstein, P. M. Colaninno, M. Scardamaglia, E. Ardila, M. Ghouri, K. Kim, R. C. Patel, and A. Miller.** 1995. Rapid diagnosis of pulmonary tuberculosis by using Roche AMPLICOR *Mycobacterium tuberculosis* PCR test. *J. Clin. Microbiol.* **33:**1832–1834.

40. **Daniel, T. M.** 1989. Rapid diagnosis of tuberculosis: laboratory techniques applicable in developing countries. *Rev. Infect. Dis.* **11**(Suppl.)**:**S471–S478.

41. **Daniel, T. M., and S. M. Debanne.** 1987. The serodiagnosis of tuberculosis and other mycobacterial diseases by

enzyme-linked immunosorbent assay. *Am. Rev. Respir. Dis.* **135**:1137–1151.

42. de Boer, A. S., M. W. Borgdorff, P. E. de Haas, N. J. Nagelkerke, J. D. van Embden, and D. van Soolingen. 1999. Analysis of rate of change of IS*6110* RFLP patterns of *Mycobacterium tuberculosis* based on serial patient isolates. *J. Infect. Dis.* **180**:1238–1244.

43. Devallois, A., K. S. Goh, and N. Rastogi. 1997. Rapid identification of mycobacteria to species level by PCR-restriction fragment length polymorphism analysis of the *hsp65* gene and proposition of an algorithm to differentiate 34 mycobacterial species. *J. Clin. Microbiol.* **35**:2969–2973.

44. Dunlap, N. E., R. H. Harris, W. H. Benjamin, Jr., J. W. Harden, and D. Hafner. 1995. Laboratory contamination of *Mycobacterium tuberculosis* cultures. *Am. J. Respir. Crit. Care Med.* **152**:1702–1704.

45. Espinosa de los Monteros, L. E., J. C. Galan, M. Gutierrez, S. Samper, J. F. Garcia Marin, C. Martin, L. Dominguez, L. de Rafael, F. Baquero, E. Gomez-Mampaso, and J. Blazquez. 1998. Allele-specific PCR method based on *pncA* and *oxyR* sequences for distinguishing *Mycobacterium bovis* from *Mycobacterium tuberculosis*: intraspecific *M. bovis pncA* sequence polymorphism. *J. Clin. Microbiol.* **36**:239–242.

46. Falkinham, J. O., III. 1999. Molecular epidemiology: other mycobacteria, p. 136–160. *In* C. Ratledge and J. Dale (ed.), *Mycobacteria. Molecular Biology and Virulence.* Blackwell Science, Oxford, United Kingdom.

47. Feizabadi, M. M., I. D. Robertson, D. V. Cousins, D. J. Dawson, and D. J. Hampson. 1997. Use of multilocus enzyme electrophoresis to examine genetic relationships amongst isolates of *Mycobacterium intracellulare* and related species. *Microbiology* **143**:1461–1469.

48. Filliol, I., C. Sola, and N. Rastogi. 2000. Detection of a previously unamplified spacer within the DR locus of *Mycobacterium tuberculosis*: epidemiological implications. *J. Clin. Microbiol.* **38**:1231–1234.

49. Frothingham, R., and W. A. Meeker-O'Connell. 1998. Genetic diversity in the *Mycobacterium tuberculosis* complex based on variable numbers of tandem DNA repeats. *Microbiology* **144**:1189–1196.

50. Frothingham, R., and K. H. Wilson. 1993. Sequence-based differentiation of strains in the *Mycobacterium avium* complex. *J. Bacteriol.* **175**:2818–2825.

51. Galil, K., L. A. Miller, M. A. Yakrus, R. J. Wallace, Jr., D. G. Mosley, B. England, G. Huitt, M. M. McNeil, and B. A. Perkins. 1999. Abscesses due to *Mycobacterium abscessus* linked to injection of unapproved alternative medication. *Emerg. Infect. Dis.* **5**:681–687.

52. Gamboa, F., G. Fernandez, E. Padilla, J. M. Manterola, J. Lonca, P. J. Cardona, L. Matas, and V. Ausina. 1998. Comparative evaluation of initial and new versions of the Gen-Probe Amplified *Mycobacterium Tuberculosis* Direct Test for direct detection of *Mycobacterium tuberculosis* in respiratory and nonrespiratory specimens. *J. Clin. Microbiol.* **36**:684–689.

53. Glickman, S. E., J. O. Kilburn, W. R. Butler, and L. S. Ramos. 1994. Rapid identification of mycolic acid patterns of mycobacteria by high-performance liquid chromatography using pattern recognition software and a *Mycobacterium* library. *J. Clin. Microbiol.* **32**:740–745.

54. Gordon, S. V., R. Brosch, A. Billault, T. Garnier, K. Eiglmeier, and S. T. Cole. 1999. Identification of variable regions in the genomes of tubercle bacilli using bacterial artificial chromosome arrays. *Mol. Microbiol.* **32**:643–655.

55. Goto, M., S. Oka, K. Okuzumi, S. Kimura, and K. Shimada. 1991. Evaluation of acridinium-ester-labeled DNA probes for identification of *Mycobacterium tuberculosis* and *Mycobacterium avium-Mycobacterium intracellulare* complex in culture *J. Clin. Microbiol.* **29**:2473–2476.

56. Goulding, J. N., J. Stanley, N. Saunders, and C. Arnold. 2000. Genome-sequence-based fluorescent amplified-fragment length polymorphism analysis of *Mycobacterium tuberculosis*. *J. Clin. Microbiol.* **38**:1121–1126.

57. Gruft, H., R. Johnson, R. Claflin, and A. Loder. 1984. Phage-typing and drug-resistance patterns as tools in mycobacterial epidemiology. *Am. Rev. Respir. Dis.* **130**:96–97.

58. Guerrero, C., C. Bernasconi, D. Bürki, T. Bodmer, and A. Telenti. 1994. IS*1245*: a novel insertion element from *Mycobacterium avium* is a specific marker for analysis of strain relatedness. *J. Clin. Microbiol.* **33**:304–307.

59. Haas, W. H., W. R. Butler, C. L. Woodley, and J. T. Crawford. 1993. Mixed-linker polymerase chain reaction: a new method for rapid fingerprinting of isolates of the *Mycobacterium tuberculosis* complex. *J. Clin. Microbiol.* **31**:1293–1298.

60. Hawkins, J. E., R. C. Good, G. P. Kubica, P. R. J. Gangadharam, H. M. Gruft, K. D. Stottmeier, H. M. Sommers, and L. G. Wayne. 1983. Levels of laboratory services for mycobacterial diseases: official statement of the American Thoracic Society. *Am. Rev. Respir. Dis.* **128**:213.

61. Hector, J. S. R., Y. Pang, G. H. Mazurek, Y. Zhang, B. A. Brown, and R. J. Wallace, Jr. 1992. Large restriction fragment patterns of genomic *Mycobacterium fortuitum* DNA as strain-specific markers and their use in epidemiologic investigation of four nosocomial outbreaks. *J. Clin. Microbiol.* **30**:1250–1255.

62. Imaeda, T. 1985. Deoxyribonucleic acid relatedness among selected strains of *Mycobacterium tuberculosis*, *Mycobacterium bovis*, *Mycobacterium bovis* BCG, *Mycobacterium microti*, and *Mycobacterium africanum*. *Int. J. Syst. Bacteriol.* **35**:147–150.

63. Isenberg, H. D. 1993. *Clinical Microbiology Procedures Handbook*, vol. 1. American Society for Microbiology, Washington D.C.

64. Jackett, P. S., G. H. Bothamley, H. V. Batra, A. Mistry, D. B. Young, and J. Ivanyi. 1988. Specificity of antibodies to immunodominant mycobacterial antigens in pulmonary tuberculosis. *J. Clin. Microbiol.* **26**:2313–2318.

65. Janssen, P., R. Coopman, G. Huys, J. Swings, M. Bleeker, P. Vos, M. Zabeau, and K. Kersters. 1996. Evaluation of the DNA fingerprinting method AFLP as a new tool in bacterial taxonomy. *Microbiology* **142**:1881–1893.

66. Jonas, V., M. J. Alden, J. I. Curry, K. Kamisango, C. A. Knott, R. Lankford, J. M. Wolfe, and D. F. Moore. 1993. Detection and identification of *Mycobacterium tuberculosis* directly from sputum sediments by amplification of rRNA. *J. Clin. Microbiol.* **31**:2410–2416.

67. Jost, K. C. J., D. F. Dunbar, S. S. Barth, V. L. Headley, and L. B. Elliott. 1995. Identification of *Mycobacterium tuberculosis* and M. *avium* complex directly from smear-positive sputum specimens and BACTEC 12B cultures by high-performance liquid chromatography with fluorescence detection and computer-driven pattern recognition models. *J. Clin. Microbiol.* **33**:1270–1277.

68. Kamerbeek, J., L. Schouls, A. Kolk, M. van Agterveld, D. van Soolingen, S. Kuijper, A. Bunschoten, H. Molhuizen, R. Shaw, M. Goyal, and J. van Embden. 1997. Simultaneous detection and strain differentiation of *Mycobacterium tuberculosis* for diagnosis and epidemiology. *J. Clin. Microbiol.* **35**:907–914.

69. Kaminski, D. A., and D. J. Hardy. 1995. Selective utilization of DNA probes for identification of *Mycobacterium* species on the basis of cord formation in primary BACTEC 12B cultures. *J. Clin. Microbiol.* **33**:1548–1550.

70. **Kapur, V., L. L. Li, M. R. Hamrick, B. B. Plikaytis, T. M. Shinnick, A. Telenti, W. R. Jacobs, A. Banerjee, S. T. Cole, K. Y. Yuen, J. E. Clarridge, B. N. Kreiswirth, and J. M. Musser.** 1995. Rapid species assignment and unambiguous identification of mutations associated with antimicrobial resistance in *Mycobacterium tuberculosis* by automated DNA sequencing. *Arch. Pathol. Lab. Med.* **119:**131–138.

71. **Kasai, H., T. Ezaki, and S. Harayama.** 2000. Differentiation of phylogenetically related slowly growing mycobacteria by their *gyrB* sequences. *J. Clin. Microbiol.* **38:**301–308.

72. **Kato-Maeda, M., J. T. Rhee, T. R. Gingeras, H. Salamon, J. Drenkow, N. Smittipat, and P. M. Small.** 2001. Comparing genomes within the species *Mycobacterium tuberculosis*. *Genome Res.* **11:**547–554.

73. **Kauppinen, J., R. Mäntyjärvi, and M.-L. Katila.** 1994. Random amplified polymorphic DNA genotyping of *Mycobacterium malmoense*. *J. Clin. Microbiol.* **32:**1827–1829.

74. **Kellogg, J. A., D. A. Bankert, G. S. Withers, W. Sweimler, T. E. Kiehn, and G. E. Pfyffer.** 2001. Application of the Sherlock Mycobacteria Identification System using high-performance liquid chromatography in a clinical laboratory. *J. Clin. Microbiol.* **39:**964–970.

75. **Kent, P. T., and G. P. Kubica.** 1985. *Public Health Mycobacteriology: a Guide for the Level III Laboratory.* U.S. Department of Health and Human Services, Centers for Disease Control, Atlanta, Ga.

76. **Kikuchi, K., E. M. Bernard, T. E. Kiehn, D. Armstrong, and L. W. Riley.** 1994. Restriction fragment length polymorphism analysis of clinical isolates of *Mycobacterium haemophilum*. *J. Clin. Microbiol.* **32:**1763–1767.

77. **Kim, B. J., S. H. Lee, M. A. Lyu, S. J. Kim, G. H. Bai, G. T. Chae, E. C. Kim, C. Y. Cha, and Y. H. Kook.** 1999. Identification of mycobacterial species by comparative sequence analysis of the RNA polymerase gene (*rpoB*). *J. Clin. Microbiol.* **37:**1714–1720.

78. **Kirschner, R. A., B. Springer, U. Vogel, A. Meier, A. Wrede, M. Kieckenbeck, F. C. Bange, and E. C. Böttger.** 1993. Genotypic identification of mycobacteria by nucleic acid sequence determination: report of a 2-year experience in a clinical laboratory. *J. Clin. Microbiol.* **31:**2882–2889.

79. **Kremer, K., D. van Soolingen, R. Frothingham, W. H. Haas, P. W. Hermans, C. Martin, P. Palittapongarnpim, B. B. Plikaytis, L. W. Riley, M. A. Yakrus, J. M. Musser, and J. D. van Embden.** 1999. Comparison of methods based on different molecular epidemiological markers for typing of *Mycobacterium tuberculosis* complex strains: interlaboratory study of discriminatory power and reproducibility. *J. Clin. Microbiol.* **37:**2607–2618.

80. **Kubica, G. P., W. M. Gross, J. E. Hawkins, H. M. Sommers, A. L. Vestal, and L. G. Wayne.** 1975. Laboratory services for mycobacterial diseases. *Am. Rev. Respir. Dis.* **112:**773–787.

81. **Lai, K. K., B. A. Brown, J. A. Westerling, S. A. Fontecchio, Y. Zhang, and R. J. Wallace, Jr.** 1998. Long-term laboratory contamination by *Mycobacterium abscessus* resulting in two pseudo-outbreaks: recognition with use of random amplified polymorphic DNA (RAPD) polymerase chain reaction. *Clin. Infect. Dis.* **27:**169–175.

82. **Lalande, V., F. Barbut, A. Varnerot, M. Febvre, D. Nesa, S. Wadel, V. Vincent, and J. C. Petit.** 2001. Pseudo-outbreak of *Mycobacterium gordonae* associated with water from refrigerated fountains. *J. Hosp. Infect.* **48:**76–79.

83. **Lebrun, L., F. Espinasse, J. D. Poveda, and V. Vincent-Lévy-Frébault.** 1992. Evaluation of nonradioactive DNA probes for identification of mycobacteria. *J. Clin. Microbiol.* **30:**2476–2478.

84. **Mazars, E., S. Lesjean, A. L. Banuls, M. Gilbert, V. Vincent, B. Gicquel, M. Tibayrenc, C. Locht, and P. Supply.** 2001. High-resolution minisatellite-based typing as a portable approach to global analysis of *Mycobacterium tuberculosis* molecular epidemiology. *Proc. Natl. Acad. Sci. USA* **98:**1901–1906.

85. **Mazurek, G. H., S. Hartman, Y. Zhang, B. A. Brown, J. S. R. Hector, D. T. Murphy, and R. J. J. Wallace.** 1993. Large DNA selection fragment polymorphisms in the *Mycobacterium avium-M. intracellulare* complex: a potential epidemiological tool. *J. Clin. Microbiol.* **31:**390–394.

86. **Miller, N., S. Infante, and T. Cleary.** 2000. Evaluation of the LiPA MYCOBACTERIA assay for identification of mycobacterial species from BACTEC 12B bottles. *J. Clin. Microbiol.* **38:**1915–1919.

87. **Moore, D. F., J. I. Curry, C. A. Knott, and V. Jonas.** 1996. Amplification of rRNA for assessment of treatment response of pulmonary tuberculosis patients during antimicrobial therapy. *J. Clin. Microbiol.* **34:**1745–1749.

88. **National Committee for Clinical Laboratory Standards.** 1994. *Specifications for Molecular Microbiology Methods for Infectious Diseases.* NCCLS, Villanova, Pa.

89. **National Committee for Clinical Laboratory Standards.** 2000. *Susceptibility Testing of Mycobacteria, Nocardia, and Other Aerobic Actinomycetes: Tentative Standard.* NCCLS, Wayne, Pa.

90. **Niemann, S., E. Richter, and S. Rüsch-Gerdes.** 2000. Differentiation among members of the *Mycobacterium tuberculosis* complex by molecular and biochemical features: evidence for two pyrazinamide-susceptible subtypes of M. *bovis. J. Clin. Microbiol.* **38:**152–157.

91. **Park, H., H. Jang, C. Kim, B. Chung, C. L. Chang, S. K. Park, and S. Song.** 2000. Detection and identification of mycobacteria by amplification of the internal transcribed spacer regions with genus- and species-specific PCR primers. *J. Clin. Microbiol.* **38:**4080–4085.

92. **Parra, C. A., L. P. Londono, P. Del Portillo, and M. E. Patarroyo.** 1991. Isolation, characterization, and molecular cloning of a specific *Mycobacterium tuberculosis* antigen gene: identification of a species-specific sequence. *Infect. Immun.* **59:**3411–3417.

93. **Picardeau, M., T. J. Bull, G. Prod'hom, A. L. Pozniak, D. C. Shanson, and V. Vincent.** 1997. Comparison of a new insertion element, IS*1407*, with established molecular markers for the characterization of *Mycobacterium celatum*. *Int. J. Syst. Bacteriol.* **47:**640–644.

93a. **Picardeau, M., T. J. Bull, and V. Vincent.** 1997. Identification and characterization of ES-like elements in *Mycobacterium gordonae*. *FEMS Microbiol. Lett.* **154:**95–102.

94. **Picardeau, M., G. Prod'hom, L. Raskine, M. P. LePennec, and V. Vincent.** 1997. Genotypic characterization of five subspecies of *Mycobacterium kansasii*. *J. Clin. Microbiol.* **35:**25–32.

95. **Picardeau, M., A. Varnerot, T. Lecompte, F. Brel, T. May, and V. Vincent.** 1997. Use of different molecular typing techniques for bacteriological follow-up in a clinical trial with AIDS patients with *Mycobacterium avium* bacteremia. *J. Clin. Microbiol.* **35:**2503–2510.

96. **Picardeau, M., A. Varnerot, J. Rauzier, B. Gicquel, and V. Vincent.** 1996. *Mycobacterium xenopi* IS*1395*, a novel insertion sequence expanding the IS256 family. *Microbiology* **142:**2453–2461.

97. **Picardeau, M., and V. Vincent.** 1996. Typing of *Mycobacterium avium* isolates by PCR. *J. Clin. Microbiol.* **34:**389–392.

98. **Piersimoni, C., A. Callegaro, D. Nista, S. Bornigia, F. De Conti, G. Santini, and G. De Sio.** 1997. Comparative evaluation of two commercial amplification assays for di-

rect detection of *Mycobacterium tuberculosis* complex in respiratory specimens. *J. Clin. Microbiol.* **35:**193–196.

99. **Plikaytis, B. B., B. D. Plikaytis, M. A. Yakrus, W. R. Butler, C. L. Woodley, V. A. Silcox, and T. M. Shinnick.** 1992. Differentiation of slowly growing *Mycobacterium* species, including *Mycobacterium tuberculosis*, by gene amplification and restriction fragment length polymorphism analysis. *J. Clin. Microbiol.* **30:**1815–1822.

100. **Poulet, S., and S. T. Cole.** 1995. Characterization of the highly abundant polymorphic GC-rich-repetitive sequence (PGRS) present in *Mycobacterium tuberculosis*. *Arch. Microbiol.* **163:**87–95.

101. **Prod'hom, G., C. Guilhot, M. C. Gutierrez, A. Varnerot, B. Gicquel, and V. Vincent.** 1997. Rapid discrimination of *Mycobacterium tuberculosis* complex strains by ligation-mediated PCR fingerprint analysis *J. Clin. Microbiol.* **35:**3331–3334.

102. **Ramos, M., H. Soini, G. C. Roscanni, M. Jaques, M. C. Villares, and J. M. Musser.** 1999. Extensive cross-contamination of specimens with *Mycobacterium tuberculosis* in a reference laboratory. *J. Clin. Microbiol.* **37:**916–919.

103. **Reisner, B. S., A. M. Gatson, and G. L. Woods.** 1994. Use of Gen-Probe AccuProbes to identify *Mycobacterium avium* complex, *Mycobacterium tuberculosis* complex, *Mycobacterium kansasii*, and *Mycobacterium gordonae* directly from BACTEC TB broth cultures. *J. Clin. Microbiol.* **32:**2995–2998.

104. **Richter, E., S. Niemann, S. Rüsch-Gerdes, and S. Hoffner.** 1999. Identification of *Mycobacterium kansasii* by using a DNA probe (AccuProbe) and molecular techniques. *J. Clin. Microbiol.* **37:**964–970.

105. **Ringuet, H., C. Akoua-Koffi, S. Honore, A. Varnerot, V. Vincent, P. Berche, J. L. Gaillard, and C. Pierre-Audigier.** 1999. *hsp65* sequencing for identification of rapidly growing mycobacteria. *J. Clin. Microbiol.* **37:**852–857.

106. **Ritacco, V., K. Kremer, T. van der Laan, J. E. M. Pijnenburg, P. E. W. de Haas, and D. van Soolingen.** 1998. Use of IS*901* and IS*1245* in RFLP typing of *Mycobacterium avium* complex: relatedness among serovar reference strains, human and animal isolates. *Int. J. Tuberc. Lung Dis.* **2:**242–251.

107. **Roring, S., D. Brittain, A. E. Bunschoten, M. S. Hughes, R. A. Skuce, J. D. van Embden, and S. D. Neill.** 1998. Spacer oligotyping of *Mycobacterium bovis* isolates compared to typing by restriction fragment length polymorphism using PGRS, DR and IS*6110* probes. *Vet. Microbiol.* **61:**111–120.

108. **Ross, B. C., K. Jackson, M. Yang, A. Sievers, and B. Dwyer.** 1992. Identification of a genetically distinct subspecies of *Mycobacterium kansasii*. *J. Clin. Microbiol.* **30:**2930–2933.

109. **Roth, A., M. Fischer, M. E. Hamid, S. Michalke, W. Ludwig, and H. Mauch.** 1998. Differentiation of phylogenetically related slowly growing mycobacteria based on 16S–23S rRNA gene internal transcribed spacer sequences. *J. Clin. Microbiol.* **36:**139–147.

110. **Roth, A., U. Reischl, N. Schönfeld, L. Naumann, S. Emler, M. Fischer, H. Mauch, R. Loddenkemper, and R. M. Kroppenstedt.** 2000. *Mycobacterium heckeshornense* sp. nov., a new pathogenic slowly growing mycobacterium sp. causing cavitary lung disease in an immunocompetent patient *J. Clin. Microbiol.* **38:**4102–4107.

111. **Runyon, E. H.** 1970. Identification of mycobacterial pathogens using colony characteristics. *Am. J. Clin. Pathol.* **54:**578–586.

112. **Sada, E., P. J. Brennan, T. Herrera, and M. Torres.** 1990. Evaluation of lipoarabinomannan for the serolog-

ical diagnosis of tuberculosis. *J. Clin. Microbiol.* **28:**2587–2590.

113. **Saito, H., H. Tomioka, K. Sato, H. Tasaka, and D. J. Dawson.** 1990. Identification of various serovar strains of *Mycobacterium avium* complex by using DNA probes specific for *Mycobacterium avium* and *Mycobacterium intracellulare*. *J. Clin. Microbiol.* **28:**1694–1697.

114. **Salamon, H., M. R. Segal, A. Ponce de Leon, and P. M. Small.** 1998. Accommodating error analysis in comparison and clustering of molecular fingerprints. *Emerg. Infect. Dis.* **4:**159–168.

115. **Schaefer, W. B.** 1979. Serological identification of atypical mycobacteria, p. 323–344. *In* T. Bergan and J. R. Norris (ed.), *Methods in Microbiology*. Academic Press, Ltd., London, United Kingdom.

116. **Shinnick, T. M.** 1987. The 65-kilodalton antigen of *Mycobacterium tuberculosis*. *J. Bacteriol.* **169:**1080–1088.

117. **Simonney, N., J. M. Molina, M. Molimard, E. Oksenhendler, and P. H. Lagrange.** 1996. Comparison of A60 and three glycolipid antigens in an ELISA test for tuberculosis. *Clin. Microbiol. Infect.* **2:**214–222.

118. **Simonney, N., J. M. Molina, M. Molimard, E. Oksenhendler, and P. H. Lagrange.** 1997. Circulating immune complexes in human tuberculosis sera: demonstration of specific antibodies against *Mycobacterium tuberculosis* glycolipid (DAT, PGLTb1, LOS) antigens in isolated circulating immune complexes. *Eur. J. Clin. Investig.* **27:**128–134.

119. **Slutsky, A. M., R. D. Arbeit, T. W. Barber, J. Rich, C. F. von Reyn, W. Pieciak, M. A. Barlow, and J. N. Maslow.** 1994. Polyclonal infections due to *Mycobacterium avium* complex in patients with AIDS detected by pulsed-field gel electrophoresis of sequential clinical isolates. *J. Clin. Microbiol.* **32:**1773–1778.

120. **Small, P. M., N. B. McClenny, S. P. Singh, G. K. Schoolnik, L. S. Tompkins, and P. A. Mickelsen.** 1993. Molecular strain typing of *Mycobacterium tuberculosis* to confirm cross-contamination in the mycobacteriology laboratory and modification of procedures to minimize occurrence of false-positive cultures. *J. Clin. Microbiol.* **31:**1677–1682.

121. **Snider, D. E., W. D. Jones, and R. C. Good.** 1984. The usefulness of phage typing *Mycobacterium tuberculosis* isolates. *Am. Rev. Respir. Dis.* **130:**1095–1099.

122. **Snider, D. E., Jr.** 1982. The tuberculin skin test. *Am. Rev. Respir. Dis.* **125:**108–118.

123. **Soini, H., E. C. Böttger, and M. K. Viljanen.** 1994. Identification of mycobacteria by PCR-based sequence determination of the 32-kilodalton protein gene. *J. Clin. Microbiol.* **32:**2944–2947.

124. **Soini, H., X. Pan, A. Amin, E. A. Graviss, A. Siddiqui, and J. M. Musser.** 2000. Characterization of *Mycobacterium tuberculosis* isolates from patients in Houston, Texas, by spoligotyping. *J. Clin. Microbiol.* **38:**669–676.

125. **Somoskovi, A., J. E. Hotaling, M. Fitzgerald, V. Jonas, D. Stasik, L. M. Parsons, and M. Salfinger.** 2000. False-positive results for *Mycobacterium celatum* with the AccuProbe *Mycobacterium tuberculosis* complex assay. *J. Clin. Microbiol.* **38:**2743–2745.

126. **Springer, B., L. Stockman, K. Teschner, G. D. Roberts, and E. C. Böttger.** 1996. Two-laboratory collaborative study on identification of mycobacteria: molecular versus phenotypic methods. *J. Clin. Microbiol.* **34:**296–303.

127. **Sreevatsan, S., X. Pan, K. E. Stockbauer, N. D. Connell, B. N. Kreiswirth, T. S. Whittam, and J. M. Musser.** 1997. Restricted structural gene polymorphism in the *Mycobacterium tuberculosis* complex indicates evolutionarily recent global dissemination. *Proc. Natl. Acad. Sci. USA* **94:**9869–9874.

128. **Stahl, D. A., and J. W. Urbance.** 1990. The division between fast- and slow-growing species corresponds to natural relationships among the mycobacteria. *J. Bacteriol.* **172:**116–124.

129. **Steingrube, V. A., J. L. Gibson, B. A. Brown, Y. Zhang, R. W. Wilson, M. Rajagopalan, and R. J. Wallace, Jr.** 1995. PCR amplification and restriction endonuclease analysis of a 65-kilodalton heat shock protein gene sequence for taxonomic separation of rapidly growing mycobacteria. *J. Clin. Microbiol.* **33:**149–153.

130. **Stinear, T., B. C. Ross, J. K. Davies, L. Marino, R. M. Robins-Browne, F. Oppedisano, A. Sievers, and P. D. Johnson.** 1999. Identification and characterization of IS2404 and IS2606: two distinct repeated sequences for detection of *Mycobacterium ulcerans* by PCR. *J. Clin. Microbiol.* **37:**1018–1023.

131. **Supply, P., E. Mazars, S. Lesjean, V. Vincent, B. Gicquel, and C. Locht.** 2000. Variable human minisatellite-like regions in the *Mycobacterium tuberculosis* genome. *Mol. Microbiol.* **36:**762–771.

132. **Takewaki, S. I., K. Okuzumi, I. Manabe, M. Tanimura, K. Miyamura, K. I. Nakahara, Y. Yazaki, A. Ohkubo, and R. Nagai.** 1994. Nucleotide sequence comparison of the mycobacterial dnaJ gene and PCR-restriction fragment length polymorphism analysis for identification of mycobacterial species. *Int. J. Syst. Bacteriol.* **44:**159–166.

133. **Telenti, A., F. Marchesi, M. Balz, F. Bally, E. C. Böttger, and T. Bodmer.** 1993. Rapid identification of mycobacteria to the species level by polymerase chain reaction and restriction enzyme analysis. *J. Clin. Microbiol.* **31:**175–178.

134. **Tenover, F. C., R. D. Arbeit, R. V. Goering, P. A. Mickelsen, B. E. Murray, D. H. Persing, and B. Swaminathan.** 1995. Interpreting chromosomal DNA restriction patterns produced by pulsed field gel electrophoresis: criteria for bacterial strain typing. *J. Clin. Microbiol.* **33:**2233–2239.

135. **Tenover, F. C., J. T. Crawford, R. E. Huebner, L. J. Geiter, C. R. Horsburgh, Jr., and R. C. Good.** 1993. The resurgence of tuberculosis: is your laboratory ready? *J. Clin. Microbiol.* **31:**767–770.

136. **Thibert, L., and S. Lapierre.** 1993. Routine application of high-performance liquid chromatography for identification of mycobacteria. *J. Clin. Microbiol.* **31:**1759–1763.

137. **Thierry, D., M. D. Cave, K. D. Eisenach, J. T. Crawford, J. H. Bates, B. Gicquel, and J. L. Guesdon.** 1990. IS6110, an IS-like element of *Mycobacterium tuberculosis* complex. *Nucleic Acids Res.* **18:**188.

138. **Tjhie, J. H., A. F. van Belle, M. Dessens-Kroon, and D. van Soolingen.** 2001. Misidentification and diagnostic delay caused by a false-positive amplified *Mycobacterium tuberculosis* direct test in an immunocompetent patient with a *Mycobacterium celatum* infection. *J. Clin. Microbiol.* **39:**2311–2312.

139. **Tokars, J. I., J. R. Rudnick, K. Kroc, L. Manangan, G. Pugliese, R. E. Huebner, J. Chan, and W. R. Jarvis.** 1996. U.S. hospital mycobacteriology laboratories: status and comparison with state public health department laboratories. *J. Clin. Microbiol.* **34:**680–685.

140. **Tortoli, E., A. Nanetti, C. Piersimoni, P. Cichero, C. Farina, G. Mucignat, C. Scarparo, L. Bartolini, R. Valentini, D. Nista, G. Gesu, C. P. Tosi, M. Crovatto, and G. Brusarosco.** 2001. Performance assessment of new multiplex probe assay for identification of mycobacteria. *J. Clin. Microbiol.* **39:**1079–1084.

141. **Tortoli, E., M. T. Simonetti, and F. Lavinia.** 1996. Evaluation of reformulated chemiluminescent DNA probe (AccuProbe) for culture identification of *Mycobacterium kansasii*. *J. Clin. Microbiol.* **34:**2838–2840.

142. **Turneer, M., J. P. Van Vooren, J. De Bruyn, E. Serruys, P. Dierckx, and J. C. Yernault.** 1988. Humoral immune response in human tuberculosis: immunoglobulins G, A, and M directed against the purified P32 protein antigen of *Mycobacterium bovis* bacillus Calmette-Guerin. *J. Clin. Microbiol.* **26:**1714–1719.

143. **van Embden, J. D., M. D. Cave, J. T. Crawford, J. W. Dale, K. D. Eisenach, B. Gicquel, P. Hermans, C. Martin, R. McAdam, T. M. Shinnick, and P. M. Small.** 1993. Strain identification of *Mycobacterium tuberculosis* by DNA fingerprinting: recommendations for a standardized methodology. *J. Clin. Microbiol.* **31:**406–409.

144. **Vannier, A. M., J. J. Tarrand, and P. R. Murray.** 1988. Mycobacterial cross contamination during radiometric culturing. *J. Clin. Microbiol.* **26:**1867–1868.

145. **van Pinxteren, L. A., P. Ravn, E. M. Agger, J. Pollock, and P. Andersen.** 2000. Diagnosis of tuberculosis based on the two specific antigens ESAT-6 and CFP10. *Clin. Diagn. Lab. Immunol.* **7:**155–160.

146. **van Soolingen, D.** 2001. Molecular epidemiology of tuberculosis and other mycobacterial infections: main methodologies and achievements. *J. Intern. Med.* **249:** 1–26.

147. **van Soolingen, D., J. Bauer, V. Ritacco, S. C. Leao, I. Pavlik, V. Vincent, N. Rastogi, A. Gori, T. Bodmer, C. Garzelli, and M. J. Garcia.** 1998. IS1245 restriction fragment length polymorphism typing of *Mycobacterium avium* isolates: proposal for standardization. *J. Clin. Microbiol.* **36:**3051–3054.

148. **van Soolingen, D., T. Hoogenboezem, P. E. de Haas, P. W. Hermans, M. A. Koedam, K. S. Teppema, P. J. Brennan, G. S. Besra, F. Portaels, J. Top, L. M. Schouls, and J. D. van Embden.** 1997. A novel pathogenic taxon of the *Mycobacterium tuberculosis* complex, Canetti: characterization of an exceptional isolate from Africa. *Int. J. Syst. Bacteriol.* **47:**1236–1245.

149. **van Soolingen, D., A. G. van der Zanden, P. E. de Haas, G. T. Noordhoek, A. Kiers, N. A. Foudraine, F. Portaels, A. H. Kolk, K. Kremer, and J. D. van Embden.** 1998. Diagnosis of *Mycobacterium microti* infections among humans by using novel genetic markers. *J. Clin. Microbiol.* **36:**1840–1845.

150. **Viana-Niero, C., C. Gutierrez, C. Sola, I. Filliol, F. Boulahbal, V. Vincent, and N. Rastogi.** 2001. Genetic diversity of *Mycobacterium africanum* clinical isolates based on IS6110-restriction fragment length polymorphism analysis, spoligotyping, and variable number of tandem DNA repeats. *J. Clin. Microbiol.* **39:**57–65.

151. **Viljanen, M. K., L. Olkkonen, and M. L. Katila.** 1993. Conventional identification characteristics, mycolate and fatty acid composition, and clinical significance of MAIX AccuProbe-positive isolates of *Mycobacterium avium* complex. *J. Clin. Microbiol.* **31:**1376–1378.

152. **Villanueva, A., R. Villanueva, B. A. Vargas, F. Ruiz, S. Aguero, Y. Zhang, B. A. Brown, and R. J. Wallace, Jr.** 1997. Report on an outbreak of postinjection abscesses due to *Mycobacterium abscessus*, including management with surgery and clarithromycin therapy and comparison of strains by random amplified polymorphic DNA polymerase chain reaction. *Clin. Infect. Dis.* **24:**1147–1153.

153. **Vincent Lévy-Frébault, V., and F. Portaels.** 1992. Proposed minimal standards for the genus *Mycobacterium* and for description of new slowly growing *Mycobacterium* species. *Int. J. Syst. Bacteriol.* **42:**315–323.

154. **Vlaspolder, F., P. Singer, and C. Roggeveen.** 1995. Diagnostic value of an amplification method (GenProbe) compared with that of culture for diagnosis of tuberculosis. *J. Clin. Microbiol.* **33:**2699–2703.

155. **Wallace, R. J., Jr., B. A. Brown, and D. E. Griffith.** 1998. Nosocomial outbreaks/pseudo-outbreaks caused by nontuberculous mycobacteria. *Annu. Rev. Microbiol.* **52:** 453–490.

156. **Wallace, R. J., Jr., V. A. Silcox, M. Tsukamura, B. A. Brown, J. O. Kilburn, W. R. Butler, and G. Onyi.** 1993. Clinical significance, biochemical features, and susceptibility patterns of sporadic isolates of the *Mycobacterium chelonae*-like organism. *J. Clin. Microbiol.* **31:**3231–3239.

157. **Wallace, R. J., Jr., Y. Zhang, B. A. Brown, V. Fraser, G. H. Mazurek, and S. Maloney.** 1993. DNA large restriction fragment patterns of sporadic and epidemic nosocomial strains of *Mycobacterium chelonae* and *Mycobacterium abscessus. J. Clin. Microbiol.* **31:**2697–2701.

158. **Warren, N. G., and J. R. Cordts.** 1996. Clinical mycobacteriology. Activities and recommendations by the Association of State and Territorial Public Health Laboratory Directors. *Clin. Lab. Med.* **16:**731–743.

159. **Wasem, C. F., C. M. McCarthy, and L. W. Murray.** 1991. Multilocus enzyme electrophoresis analysis of the *Mycobacterium avium* complex and other mycobacteria. *J. Clin. Microbiol.* **29:**264–271.

160. **Wayne, L. G., R. C. Good, E. C. Böttger, R. Butler, M. Dorsch, T. Ezaki, W. Gross, V. Jonas, J. Kilburn, P. Kirschner, M. I. Krichevsky, M. Ridell, T. M. Shinnick, B. Springer, E. Stackebrandt, I. Tarnok, Z. Tarnok, H. Tasaka, V. Vincent, N. G. Warren, C. A. Knott, and R. Johnson.** 1996. Semantide- and chemotaxonomy-based analyses of some problematic phenotypic clusters of slowly growing mycobacteria, a cooperative study of the International Working Group on Mycobacterial Taxonomy. *Int. J. Syst. Bacteriol.* **46:** 280–297.

161. **Weil, A., B. B. Plikaytis, W. R. Butler, C. L. Woodley, and T. M. Shinnick.** 1996. The *mtp40* gene is not present in all strains of *Mycobacterium tuberculosis. J. Clin. Microbiol.* **34:**2309–2311.

162. **Williams, D. L., T. P. Gillis, and F. Portaels.** 1990. Geographically distinct isolates of *Mycobacterium leprae* exhibit no genotypic diversity by restriction fragment-length polymorphism analysis. *Mol. Microbiol.* **4:**1653–1659.

163. **Wilson, R. W., V. A. Steingrube, E. C. Böttger, B. Springer, B. A. Brown-Elliott, V. Vincent, J. K. C. Jost, Y. Zhang, M. J. Garcia, S. H. Chiu, G. Onyi, H. Rossmore, D. R. Nash, and R. J. Wallace, Jr.** 2001. *Mycobacterium immunogenum* sp. nov., a novel species related to *Mycobacterium abscessus* and associated with clinical disease, pseudo-outbreaks and contaminated metalworking fluids: an international cooperative study on mycobacterial taxonomy. *Int. J. Syst. Evol. Microbiol.* **51:**1751–1764.

164. **Woods, G. L., T. A. Long, and F. G. Witebsky.** 1996. Mycobacterial testing in clinical laboratories that participate in the College of American Pathologists Mycobacteriology Surveys. Changes in practices based on responses to 1992, 1993, and 1995 questionnaires. *Arch. Pathol. Lab. Med.* **120:**429–435.

165. **Woods, G. L., and J. C. Ridderhof.** 1996. Quality assurance in the mycobacteriology laboratory. *Clin. Lab. Med.* **16:**657–675.

166. **Yakrus, M. A., M. W. Reeves, and S. B. Hunter.** 1992. Characterization of isolates of *Mycobacterium avium* serotypes 4 and 8 from patients with AIDS by multilocus enzyme electrophoresis. *J. Clin. Microbiol.* **30:**1474–1478.

167. **Yakrus, M. A., and W. L. Straus.** 1994. DNA polymorphisms detected in *Mycobacterium haemophilum* by pulsed field gel electrophoresis. *J. Clin. Microbiol.* **32:**1083–1084.

168. **Zhang, Y., M. Rajagopalan, B. A. Brown, and R. J. Wallace, Jr.** 1997. Randomly amplified polymorphic DNA PCR for comparison of *Mycobacterium abscessus* strains from nosocomial outbreaks. *J. Clin. Microbiol.* **35:**3132–3139.

169. **Zhou, A. T., W. L. Ma, P. Y. Zhang, and R. A. Cole.** 1996. Detection of pulmonary and extrapulmonary tuberculosis patients with the 38-kilodalton antigen from *Mycobacterium tuberculosis* in a rapid membrane-based assay. *Clin. Diagn. Lab. Immunol.* **3:**337–341.

170. **Zolg, J. W., and S. Philippi-Schulz.** 1994. The superoxide dismutase gene, a target for detection and identification of mycobacteria by PCR. *J. Clin. Microbiol.* **32:** 2801–2812.

Neisseria and Moraxella catarrhalis*

WILLIAM M. JANDA AND JOAN S. KNAPP

38

TAXONOMY OF THE GENUS *NEISSERIA* AND THE COCCAL *MORAXELLA* SPECIES

Since the publication of *Bergey's Manual of Systematic Bacteriology* in 1984, the taxonomy of *Neisseria* species and *Moraxella* (*Branhamella*) *catarrhalis* has undergone substantial revision. At that time, the *Neisseriaceae* included four genera: *Neisseria*, *Moraxella*, *Kingella*, and *Acinetobacter*. The genus *Neisseria* consisted of 11 species that were considered "true neisseriae" and three animal species ("*N. caviae*," "*N. ovis*," and "*N. cuniculi*") that were *species incertae sedis*. The application of molecular techniques to these and related organisms has resulted in several taxonomic modifications to the family (27). In the forthcoming edition of *Bergey's Manual*, the family *Neisseriaceae* is classified in the β-subgroup of the *Proteobacteria*, which includes the "true neisseriae," *Kingella*, *Eikenella*, *Simmonsiella*, *Alysiella*, the former Centers for Disease Control and Prevention (CDC) groups M-5 and M-6, and EF-4. CDC groups M-5 and M-6 have been reclassified as *N. weaveri* and *N. elongata* subsp. *nitroreducens*, respectively (5, 39) (see chapters 39 and 49 for related species). At the same time, several proposals were made regarding the familial taxonomic position of the diplococcal species *Branhamella catarrhalis* and the rod-shaped moraxellae (e.g., family *Moraxellaceae* and family *Branhamaceae*). Molecular taxonomic methods suggest that members of the family *Moraxellaceae*, including *Moraxella* (*Branhamella*) *catarrhalis*, constitute part of a monophyletic taxon forming a distinct line of descent within the γ-subgroup of the *Proteobacteria*. *M. catarrhalis* (and the coccal moraxellae, *M. cuniculi* and *M. caviae*) form a distinct cluster within this genus; other clusters include the rod-shaped *Moraxella* spp. and the former "false neisseria" *M. ovis* (73). The family *Moraxellaceae* also includes *Acinetobacter* and *Psychrobacter* species (see chapter 49). Despite the familiarity of the name "*Branhamella catarrhalis*" to many clinical microbiologists, *Moraxella catarrhalis* has been accepted as the new name for this organism. Because of morphologic and biochemical similarities, *M. catarrhalis* and the "coccal moraxellae" are discussed in this chapter along with the *Neisseria* spp. The rod-shaped *Moraxella* species are considered with the nonfermentative gram-negative bacilli in chapter 49.

CHARACTERISTICS OF THE GENUS *NEISSERIA* AND THE COCCAL *MORAXELLA* SPECIES

Members of the genus *Neisseria* are coccal or rod-shaped gram-negative organisms that frequently occur in pairs or short chains. Diplococcal species have adjacent sides that are flattened, giving them a "coffee bean" appearance. Currently, *Neisseria* species (except for the three *N. elongata* subspecies and *N. weaveri*) are the only true coccal members of the family *Neisseriaceae*. *N. elongata* subspecies and *N. weaveri* are medium to large, plump rods that sometimes occur in pairs or short chains (5, 39). All species in the genus *Neisseria* inhabit mucous membrane surfaces of warm-blooded hosts. These organisms are aerobic and nonmotile and do not form spores; most species grow optimally at 35 to 37°C. The growth of *Neisseria* species is stimulated by CO_2 and humidity; some *N. gonorrhoeae* isolates have an obligate requirement for CO_2 not only for initial isolation but also for subsequent subculture. Atmospheric CO_2 shortens the lag phase by being assimilated for nucleic acid and protein biosynthesis. *Neisseria* species produce acid from carbohydrates oxidatively. All species in the genus are oxidase positive and, except for *N. elongata* subspecies *elongata* and *nitroreducens*, are catalase positive. In contrast, *Kingella* spp. are oxidase positive but catalase negative (see chapter 39).

While most *Neisseria* species are not exacting in their nutritional requirements for growth, the pathogenic species, and *N. gonorrhoeae* in particular, are more nutritionally demanding. *N. gonorrhoeae* does not grow in the absence of the amino acid cysteine and a usable energy source (i.e., glucose, pyruvate, or lactate). Some strains display requirements for amino acids, pyrimidines, and purines as a result of defective or altered biosynthetic pathways. Demonstration of these growth requirements forms the basis for a strain-typing method for gonococcal isolates called auxotyping (see below). The neisseriae are aerobic but do grow under anaerobic conditions if low concentrations of an alternative electron acceptor (e.g., nitrites) are present (54).

* This chapter contains information presented in chapter 38 by Joan S. Knapp and Emily H. Koumans in the seventh edition of this Manual.

The coccal moraxellae from animals are asaccharolytic and are variably hemolytic on media containing sheep, horse, rabbit, or human blood; they may produce a caramel-colored pigment. All coccal *Moraxella* spp. also produce butyrate esterase, the presence of which is used in clinical laboratories for rapid identification of *M. catarrhalis*.

CLINICAL SIGNIFICANCE

Members of the genus *Neisseria* that are found in humans include *N. gonorrhoeae*, *N. meningitidis*, *N. lactamica*, *N. sicca*, *N. subflava* (biovars subflava, flava, and perflava), *N. mucosa*, *N. flavescens*, *N. cinerea*, *N. polysaccharea*, and *N. elongata* subspecies *elongata*, *glycolytica*, and *nitroreducens*. *N. gonorrhoeae* subspecies *kochii* (*N. kochii*), a subspecies endemic in the Sudan but rarely isolated in other geographic areas, is both phenotypically and genetically related to *N. gonorrhoeae* and *N. meningitidis* (64). Among animal species, *N. canis* and *N. weaveri* are found as part of the normal respiratory tract flora of dogs, *N. denitrificans* is present in the respiratory tract of guinea pigs, and *N. macacae*, *N. dentiae*, and *N. iguanae* comprise part of the oral flora in rheseus monkeys, cows, and iguanid lizards, respectively. Most human *Neisseria* species are normal inhabitants of the upper respiratory tract and are not considered pathogens, although on occasion these organisms are isolated from infectious processes, particularly in the settings of underlying disease and immunosuppression. *N. gonorrhoeae* is always considered a pathogen, regardless of the site of isolation. *N. meningitidis* causes significant and often severe disease but may also colonize the human nasopharynx without causing disease. *M. catarrhalis* is the only coccal member of the genus *Moraxella* that is found in humans. *M. caviae* and *M. cuniculi* are found in the respiratory tracts of guinea pigs and rabbits, respectively.

N. gonorrhoeae is the causative agent of gonorrhea. In the United States, the incidence of gonorrhea increased during the 1960s and early 1970s, with the highest incidence—over 460 cases per 100,000 population—occurring in 1975. Since the mid-1980s and into the 1990s, the incidence of gonorrhea steadily declined. The decline in incidence continued through 1997, increased slightly in 1998 (from 122.0 to 131.6 cases/100,000), and then plateaued. In 1994, reported cases of *Chlamydia trachomatis* infection exceeded reported cases of gonococcal infection for the first time (29). The incidence of gonorrhea remains high among sexually active teenagers and young adults, with the highest attack rates found among 15- to 24-year-old males and females (87). Disproportionately high rates of gonococcal infection are also found among urban-dwelling African Americans, particularly females ages 15 to 19 years. Maintenance and transmission of gonorrhea are related to a social subset of "core transmitters" who have unprotected intercourse with multiple partners and either are asymptomatic or choose to ignore symptoms (86). Both social (i.e., low socioeconomic status, urban residence, lack of education, limited access to health care, unmarried status, minority race/ethnicity, male homosexuality, prostitution, histories of other sexually transmitted diseases) and behavioral (i.e., unprotected intercourse, multiple partners, other high-risk partners, drug use) risk factors have been identified for targeting by outreach/intervention and sexually transmitted disease control programs. In the United States, gonococcal infection has increasingly become a disease of the poor and disenfranchised and epidemiologic associations have been noted between gonorrhea, the use of crack cocaine and intravenous drugs, and the exchange of sex for money and drugs (87).

The risk of acquiring gonorrhea is multifactorial and is related to the number and sites of exposure. For heterosexual males, the risk of acquiring urethral infection from an infected female is about 20% for a single exposure and up to 80% for four exposures (44, 87). Due to anatomical considerations, the risk of infection for the female genital tract from a single exposure to an infected male is probably much higher. Transmission of rectal infection is also quite efficient, and recent studies among homosexual/bisexual men have demonstrated that urethral infection following fellatio with an infected partner may account for as much as 26% of urethral infections diagnosed in this population (59). Among women, use of hormonal contraceptive methods is associated with an increased risk of gonococcal infection, while barrier methods such as condoms and diaphragms used with spermicidal foams and gels exert a protective effect against infection (44).

In males, *N. gonorrhoeae* causes an acute urethritis with dysuria and urethral discharge (44, 87). The incubation period between organism acquisition and onset of symptoms averages 2 to 7 days (range, 1 to 14 days). After infection, 95 to 99% of men experience a urethral discharge that may be purulent, cloudy, or mucoid; the consistency of the discharge at presentation is affected by the length of time that the infection has been incubating and whether the patient has recently urinated. About 2.5% of men with gonorrhea presenting to sexually transmitted disease clinics are truly asymptomatic, and it is estimated that the prevalence of asymptomatic urogenital gonorrhea in men in the general population may be as high as 5%. If left untreated, most cases of gonorrhea in men resolve spontaneously, but in fewer than 10% of cases, ascending infection may result in gonococcal epididymitis, epididymo-orchitis, prostatitis, periurethral abscess, or urethral stricture.

In females, the primary gonococcal infection is present in the endocervix, with concomitant urethral infection occurring in 70 to 90% of persons. After an incubation period of 8 to 10 days, patients may present with cervicovaginal discharge, abnormal or intermenstrual bleeding, and abdominal or pelvic pain; the presence of pain suggests the presence of upper genital tract disease (44, 87). Gonococcal infection of the vaginal squamous epithelium of postpubertal women is uncommon, and in women with hysterectomies, the urethra is the most common primary site of infection. Symptoms of uncomplicated endocervical infection often resemble those of other conditions, such as cystitis or vaginal infections, and the symptoms of gonococcal endocervicitis are clouded by frequent coinfection with *Chlamydia trachomatis*, *Trichomonas vaginalis*, and/or *Candida albicans*. Between 20 and 75% of women present with a mucopurulent endocervical discharge. Infection of the Bartholin's and Skene's glands is seen in about one-third of women with genital tract infection. Endocervical gonorrhea may also complicate pregnancy and is a recognized cofactor for spontaneous abortion, chorioamnionitis, premature rupture of membranes, and premature delivery (87). Infants born to women with genital tract infection are at risk for developing gonococcal conjunctivitis ("ophthalmia neonatorum") or pharyngeal gonococcal infection.

Ascending gonococcal infection may occur in 10 to 20% of infected women and can result in acute pelvic inflammatory disease (PID) that may manifest as salpingitis (infection of the fallopian tubes), endometritis, and/or tubo-ovarian abscess, all of which can lead to scarring, ectopic pregnancies, sterility, and chronic pelvic pain (44, 87). Symptoms of gonococcal PID include bilateral lower abdominal pain, abnormal cervical discharge and bleeding, pain on motion, fever, and peripheral leukocytosis. PID caused by *N. gonorrhoeae* generally occurs early, rather than late, in infection and often during or shortly after the onset of menstruation. Women with salpingitis may also develop Fitz-Hugh–Curtis syndrome, which is a perihepatitis characterized by direct extension of the organisms from the fallopian tubes to the liver and peritoneum, resulting in right upper quadrant pain and adhesions between the liver and the anterior abdominal wall. In pregnant women, gonococcal infection is associated with increased risk of complications, including premature labor, premature rupture of the fetal membranes, spontaneous abortion, and infant morbidity.

N. gonorrhoeae may also cause pharyngeal and anorectal infections. Oropharyngeal gonococcal infection is seen in homosexual and bisexual men and heterosexual women who acquire the infection by engaging in orogenital sexual contact with an infected partner. Pharyngeal gonorrhea is also seen occasionally in heterosexual men as a result of performing cunnilingus with an infected partner. Over 90% of oropharyngeal gonococcal infections are asymptomatic and are diagnosed by culture of the organism from the throat (44, 87). Anorectal gonococcal infection is seen in homosexual/bisexual males who engage in unprotected anal intercourse. Women may also acquire rectal infections by this route, but most rectal infections in women are due to perianal contamination with infected cervicovaginal secretions. Rectal gonococcal infections are often asymptomatic, although some individuals experience acute proctitis with anorectal pain and itching, a mucopurulent discharge, bleeding, tenesmus, and constipation 5 to 7 days following infection (78). Anoscopic examination of the anal canal usually reveals an edematous and erythematous rectal mucosa and a purulent discharge associated with the anal crypts.

In a small percentage (approximately 0.5 to 3%) of infected individuals, gonococci invade the bloodstream, resulting in disseminated gonococcal infection (DGI) (44, 87). Disseminated disease may develop following infection at genital or extragenital sites, and repeated bouts of DGI have been observed in individuals with certain complement deficiencies (i.e., C7, C8, or C9) (33). DGI is characterized by low-grade fever, chills, hemorrhagic skin lesions, tenosynovitis, migratory polyarthralgias, and frank arthritis. Women have a greater risk of developing DGI during menstruation and during the second and third trimesters of pregnancy than at other times. The skin lesions are generally painful and appear as a papule that evolves into a necrotic pustule on an erythematous base. Very few lesions may be present, and most are found on the extremities. Cultures of skin lesions and synovial fluids from patients with DGI may be negative, suggesting that immune processes may contribute to the pathogenesis of DGI. In 30 to 40% of cases, organisms from the bloodstream may localize in one or more joints to cause a purulent and destructive gonococcal arthritis. Joint involvement is usually asymmetric and most commonly involves the knee, elbow, wrist, fingers, or ankle joints. Infected synovial fluid frequently contains 50,000 to 200,000 cells/mm^3, with 90% being polymorphonuclear leukocytes (PMNs).

Rare complications of DGI include endocarditis and meningitis (44, 87). Gonococcal endocarditis may develop in about 1 to 2% of patients with disseminated infection,

usually involves the aortic valve, and follows a rapid and destructive course. Pericarditis, pericardial effusions, and adult respiratory distress syndrome have also been reported in association with gonococcal bacteremia (87). Gonococcal meningitis is a rare complication of disseminated infection; it has features typical of meningitides caused by other organisms. Studies of isolates recovered from patients with DGI have shown that more invasive strains have unusual characteristics, including unique nutritional requirements (e.g., requirements for arginine, hypoxanthine, and uracil for growth [AHU strains]), defined PorIA serovar classification, resistance to the bactericidal action of normal human serum, and exquisite susceptibility to penicillin (56). With the decline in the prevalence of the AHU/PorIA auxotype/serovar in recent years, increasing numbers of disseminated infections have been associated with other auxotype/serovar classes, as has been noted in Australia (90). DGI may also present atypically in patients with underlying diseases, including human immunodeficiency virus infection and systemic lupus erythematosus (46).

Ocular gonococcal infections, once seen primarily among neonates who acquired the organism during passage through an infected birth canal ("ophthalmia neonatorum"), have been reported among adults who become infected via genital secretions (87). Laboratory personnel working with cultures may also become accidentally infected if care is not taken to protect the eyes (61). Infection of the eye results in periorbital cellulitis, a profuse purulent discharge, conjunctival injection, eyelid edema and erythema, and epithelial and stromal keratitis. Inadequate treatment of eye infections can lead to ulcerative keratitis, corneal perforation, and blindness. It should be noted that *N. cinerea* may also cause neonatal conjunctival infections, which are often initially misdiagnosed as gonococcal infections. Hence, it is important to identify gram-negative, oxidase-positive isolates with confirmatory tests before reporting conjunctival infections as gonococcal infections (31).

Cases of gonococcal infection in children during the newborn period are the result of ocular contamination during vaginal delivery. Transmission of gonorrhea from adults to children by fomites (e.g., shared towels) was proposed as a mode of transmission in older children. However, it is now recognized that gonococcal infections, including conjunctivitis and other sexually transmitted diseases in children beyond the immediate neonatal period, are indicators of sexual abuse (3). Gonococcal infections in children resemble those in adults, with some notable differences. *N. gonorrhoeae* causes a vaginitis, rather than a cervicitis, in prepubertal girls. The epithelium of the prepubertal vagina is composed of columnar epithelial cells, which are the cell types that *N. gonorrhoeae* preferentially infects. With the onset of puberty, these cells are replaced by a stratified squamous epithelium that is not susceptible to gonococcal infection. Female children with genital gonococcal infection generally present with a vaginal discharge. Urethral infection in male children, if present, resembles that seen in adults. Pharyngeal and rectal gonococcal infections, as in adults, are usually asymptomatic in children.

N. meningitidis causes a disease spectrum ranging from occult sepsis with rapid recovery to fulminant overwhelming fatal disease (6). The major virulence factor of disease-associated meningococci is the polysaccharide capsule. Thirteen meningococcal capsular polysaccharide serogroups (A, B, C, D, H, I, K, L, X, Y, Z, W135, and 29E) have been recognized, and most infections are caused by organisms belonging to serogroups A, B, C, Y, and W135. Meningococci cause epidemic and endemic meningitis, and serogroups A, B, and C are responsible for 90% of cases globally. Humans are the only natural host for *N. meningitidis*, and the organism is spread from person to person via the respiratory route. Meningococci also may be asymptomatically carried in the oropharynx and nasopharynx. Carriage rates range from about 8% up to 20%, with older children and young adults having higher rates than young children, and carriage may be transient, intermittent, or persistent (2). Carriage strains may be encapsulated (groupable) or nonencapsulated (nongroupable). Infection may result in the formation of serogroup-specific antibodies and broadly cross-reactive antibodies against several other outer membrane antigens. Individuals who are colonized with nongroupable strains also develop high titers of antibody against groupable strains, probably due to shared antigenic determinants. This response does not eliminate the carriage state, but it may protect the host from overt disease.

In some individuals, the meningococcal strain established in the upper respiratory tract enters the bloodstream and initiates systemic disease. Invasive meningococcal disease occurs in those who are newly infected with a strain against which bactericidal meningococcal serogroup-specific antibodies are lacking (6). Concurrent viral or mycoplasmal respiratory tract infection also facilitates systemic invasion by the organism. The risk of meningococcal disease is also higher among those with complement or properdin component deficiencies (e.g., C5, C6, C7, C8, and C9) (37). Other underlying conditions, such as hepatic failure, systemic lupus erythematosus, multiple myeloma, and asplenia, may also predispose to serious meningococcal disease (6).

The clinical spectrum of meningococcal disease includes meningoencephalitis, meningitis with or without meningococcemia, meningococcemia without meningitis, and bacteremia without septic complications (6). The onset of acute meningococcal meningitis is sudden, with fever and chills, myalgias, and arthralgias. Classic signs of meningitis, such as confusion, headache, fever, and nuchal rigidity, are seen only in about half of the patients, and vomiting may also be a part of the clinical presentation, particularly in children. Meningococcemia and widespread dissemination of the organism are heralded by the development of a rash, which is seen in about 50 to 60% of patients. This rash begins as a pink, maculopapular eruption and then becomes petechial. Initially these petechiae appear on the mucous membranes (e.g., the conjunctivae), and then they spread to the trunk and the lower extremities. Fulminant, rapidly progressive disease may result in the formation of additional cutaneous lesions that progress to form purpuric or ecchymotic areas of hemorrhage and necrosis. These lesions are indicators of systemic coagulopathies that are triggered by the release of various cytokines in response to meningococcal infection. About 10% of patients with meningococcemia develop purpura fulminans, resulting in extensive tissue destruction secondary to coagulopathy; aggressive monitoring of coagulation parameters and replacement of coagulation factors may benefit these patients. Diffuse neurologic and myocardial involvement are also seen more frequently in patients with meningococcal meningitis. Fulminant meningococcal shock may dominate the clinical picture of meningococcal meningitis and acute meningococcal sepsis (6, 96). The patient becomes unresponsive, with absence of superficial and deep tendon reflexes and a depressed sensorium. Due to peripheral vasoconstriction, gangrenous changes in the extremities may be noted and death may supervene as a result of disseminated intravascular coagulation. Autopsies reveal terminal myocarditis, with microthrombi and thromboses observed in many organs. The classic finding of acute hemorrhagic necrosis of the adrenal glands represents the anatomic hallmark of the Waterhouse-Friderichsen syndrome (95, 96). Meningitis with sepsis may have a mortality rate of up to 30%.

N. meningitidis may also cause acute or chronic bloodstream infection (meningococcemia) without meningitis (6). Patients present with a fever, headache, malaise, and peripheral leukocytosis, and meningococci are recovered from blood cultures. By that time, the patient is usually clinically well, and no therapy or a short course of therapy is administered. Patients with chronic meningococcemia are usually symptomatic, with a presentation similar to the gonococcal arthritis-dermatitis syndrome. Individuals with underlying deficiencies in properdin and other late complement components, other hypocomplementeric states (e.g., systemic lupus erythematosus), or human immunodeficiency virus infection are also at risk for serious meningococcal disease (36).

N. meningitidis also causes infections that result from hematogenous dissemination of the organism, including osteomyelitis, arthritis, cellulitis, pericarditis, endophthalmitis, and spontaneous bacterial peritonitis (6). Meningococcal pneumonia presents as a community-acquired pneumonia that is clinically similar to other acute bacterial pneumonias and occurs primarily in older persons with preexisting illnesses (99). Fulminant bacteremic supraglottitis has also been reported in association with serogroup B, C, and Y meningococcal infections (84). Meningococcal conjunctivitis has been described in adults, children, and neonates and may develop as a complication of systemic infection with *N. meningitidis* or as a primary infection (6). Complications of meningococcal infection limited to the eye include corneal ulcers, keratitis, subconjunctival hemorrhage, and iritis. *N. meningitidis* may also be isolated from the male urethra, the female genital tract, and the anal canal. In these sites, it may cause infections that are clinically indistinguishable from gonococcal infections (i.e., acute purulent urethritis, cervicitis, salpingitis, and proctitis). Orogenital, anogenital, and oroanal sexual practices are believed to be responsible for the presence of meningococci in these anogenital sites (24).

M. catarrhalis is found in the upper respiratory tracts of 1.5 to 5.4% of healthy adults and is more common in the respiratory tracts of healthy children (50.8%) and elderly adults (26.5%) (97). Infections of the respiratory tract and adjacent anatomic areas account for the majority of clinical conditions involving *M. catarrhalis*, including otitis media, sinusitis, bronchitis, and pneumonia (50). Otitis media and sinusitis caused by *M. catarrhalis* are seen mostly in children, while pneumonia is uncommon in the pediatric age group. Lower respiratory tract infections due to *M. catarrhalis* occur predominantly in elderly and immunocompromised patients, particularly individuals with chronic obstructive pulmonary disease, bronchiectasis, congestive heart failure, and predisposition to aspiration (50). Patients present with increasing production of purulent sputum and mild respiratory distress; pneumonic involvement is heralded by the appearance of low-grade fever, dyspnea, and production of increasing amounts of purulent sputum. *M. catarrhalis* bacteremia has been reported in association with infections of the respiratory tract and may occur secondary to otitis media, sinusitis, or pneumonia in immunocompromised patients (1).

M. *catarrhalis* has also been isolated from patients with primary bacteremia, endocarditis, meningitis, eye infections, urogenital tract infections, wound infections, septic arthritis, nosocomial respiratory tract infections, and continuous ambulatory peritoneal dialysis-associated peritonitis (50). Endocarditis has been reported in healthy individuals without prior valvular disease, in immunosuppressed patients with various underlying diseases (e.g., leukemia, lymphoma, immunoglobulin deficiency states, and AIDS), and following invasive procedures, such as balloon angioplasty (89). Rare cases of M. *catarrhalis* meningitis and ventriculitis have also occurred following surgical procedures involving the head and neck or from infected ventriculoperitoneal shunts or external ventricular drains (80). Ophthalmia neonatorum caused by M. *catarrhalis* results either from acquisition of the organism at birth from the mother's colonized genital tract or from respiratory tract secretions of the child's caretakers. Recovery of this organism from the male or female genital tract occurs rarely. Nosocomially acquired pneumonia due to M. *catarrhalis* has also been documented in both hospital respiratory units and pediatric intensive care units (50).

NEISSERIA GONORRHOEAE

Specimen Collection

Details of specimen collection are given in chapter 20.

The collection of appropriate specimens for diagnosis of gonococcal infection is dependent on the gender and sexual practices of the patient and on the clinical presentation. In all cases, specimens from genital sites (male urethra, female endocervix) should be collected. If the patient has a history of orogenital or anogenital sexual contacts, collection of oropharyngeal or anal canal specimens is also appropriate. In suspected cases of disseminated gonococcal infection, blood cultures and specimens from genital and extragenital sites should be obtained. Appropriate sites for culture are summarized in Table 1.

Specimens should be collected with Dacron or rayon swabs; calcium alginate may be toxic to gonococci (60). Cotton swabs may also be used; however, some brands of cotton contain fatty acids that may be inhibitory for gonococci. Therefore, calcium alginate and cotton swabs should be used only if the specimens are inoculated directly onto growth media or are transported in nonnutritive swab transport media. Some acceptable transport medium formulations contain charcoal to inactivate toxic materials present in the swab material or in the specimen itself. Instruments used to aid in the collection of specimens (e.g., vaginal specula) should be lubricated with warm water or saline because various water- and oil-based lubricants may also inhibit organism growth.

The role of the clinical microbiology laboratory in diagnosing gonococcal infections in children is crucial and involves the proper handling of appropriately collected specimens and the accurate identification of isolated organisms. Specimens from prepubertal females should be obtained from the vagina or urethra, the oropharynx, and the rectum and inoculated onto media as described below. Vaginal specimens are collected by swabbing the vaginal wall for 10 to 15 s to absorb any secretions; if the hymen is intact, the specimen is collected from the vaginal orifice. Specimens for diagnosis of rectal, urethral, and oropharyngeal gonococcal infections in children are collected as for adults.

Specimen Transport

Maximal recovery of gonococci is obtained when specimens are plated directly onto growth medium after collection.

TABLE 1 Body sites or specimens and culture media for the isolation of *N. gonorrhoeae*, *N. meningitidis*, and *M. catarrhalis*

Species	Syndrome	Gender[a]	Site(s) or specimen(s)	Media
N. gonorrhoeae	Uncomplicated	Female	Endocervix (Bartholin's gland), rectum,[b] urethra, pharynx[b]	Selective
		Male		
		Heterosexual	Urethra	Selective
		Homosexual, bisexual	Urethra, rectum,[b] pharynx[b]	Selective
	PID	Female	Endocervix, endometrium,[c] fallopian tubes	Selective, nonselective
	DGI		Endocervix (female), urethra (male), skin lesions	Selective, nonselective
			Joint fluid	Nonselective, selective
			Blood	Blood culture medium
	Ophthalmia		Conjunctiva	Nonselective
N. meningitidis	Meningitis		CSF, skin lesions	Nonselective
			Blood	Blood culture medium
			Nasopharynx	Selective, nonselective
M. catarrhalis	Pneumonia		Sputum (or more invasively obtained respiratory specimen)	Nonselective
	Otitis media		Tympanocentesis[d]	Nonselective
	Sinus		Sinus biopsy specimen or aspirate[d]	Nonselective

[a] Specified only if samples from different sites of males and females are cultured.
[b] If there is a history of oral-genital or anal-genital exposure.
[c] If a laparoscopic examination is performed.
[d] Not routinely performed.

However, this technique might not always be possible or practical, particularly in busy clinics or hospital emergency rooms. For these situations, various transport systems are available.

Nonnutritive Swab Transport Systems

Stuart's or Amies buffered semisolid transport media are used for transport of swab specimens for *N. gonorrhoeae*. Transport systems inoculated with specimens that may contain *N. gonorrhoeae* should be maintained at room temperature, since exposure to extremes in temperature (e.g., refrigeration) will compromise successful recovery. Some swab transport systems use sponges soaked with transport medium, while others use a semisolid medium with or without activated charcoal. Recent studies with newer swab collection devices (Copan Transystems; Copan Diagnostics, Inc., Corona, Calif. [now marketed as BBL Culture-Swab Plus; BD Biosciences, Sparks, Md.]) suggest that semisolid Amies transport medium with or without charcoal may preserve the viability of gonococci for as long as 48 h, although the viability of many gonococcal isolates may decrease noticeably after 24 h, and that these systems are superior to devices that use medium-soaked sponges (34, 68, 93). To prevent loss of organism viability, swab specimens submitted in transport medium should be inoculated onto growth medium within 6 h after collection.

Culture Medium Transport Systems

Transport of specimens already inoculated onto culture media presents several advantages over swab transport systems. Commercially available systems include JEMBEC plates containing various selective media (Remel, Inc., Lenexa, Kans.), the Gono-Pak (BD Biosciences), and the InTray GC system (BioMed Diagnostics, Inc., San Jose, Calif.) (8). While the Gono-Pak and JEMBEC products require refrigerated storage prior to use, the sealed InTray system permits storage of the medium at room temperature for up to 1 year. Media are inoculated with the specimen from a swab and placed in an impermeable plastic bag with a bicarbonate-citric acid pellet. Contact of the pellet with moisture via evaporation from the medium during incubation or by crushing an ampoule of water adjacent to the pellet generates a CO_2-enriched environment within the bag. Organisms remain viable in the CO_2-enriched environment during transport to a reference laboratory, but incubation for 18 to 24 h at 35°C prior to transport allows some initial outgrowth of the organisms and enhances survival.

Direct Examination of Clinical Specimens

In clinical settings, gonococcal urethritis in adult males is often diagnosed by the observation of gram-negative diplococci within or closely associated with PMNs on a smear prepared from the urethral discharge (Fig. 1). When properly performed, the Gram stain has a sensitivity of 90 to 95% and a specificity of 95 to 100% for diagnosing genital gonorrhea in symptomatic men (44, 87). In females, Gram stains of endocervical specimens collected under direct visualization of the cervix (i.e., with a speculum in place) may also be very helpful in diagnosis (see "Specimen Collection" above). Gram-stained smears of such specimens have a sensitivity of 50 to 70%, depending on the adequacy of the specimen and the patient population. An endocervical smear showing gram-negative intracellular diplococci, particularly from a woman with other signs and symptoms of gonococcal infection, is highly predictive. In asymptom-

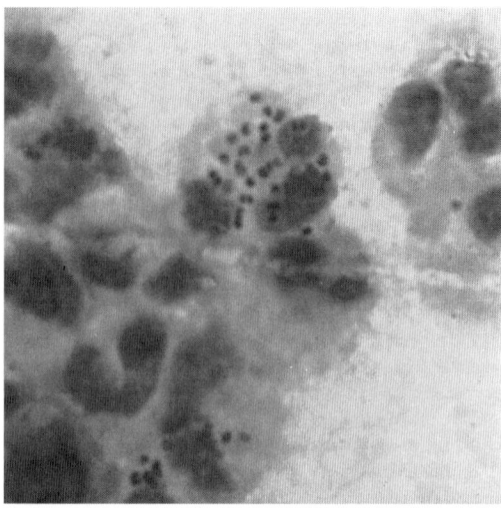

FIGURE 1 Gram stain of male urethral exudate. Some PMNs contain many diplococci; others contain none. Magnification, ×1,500.

atic women, however, the predictive value of the Gram stain is much lower. In patients with symptomatic proctitis, smears collected under direct visualization through an anoscope may provide a diagnosis in 70 to 80% of such patients, as opposed to blind collection, where Gram-stained smears have a sensitivity of only 40 to 60% (Fig. 2) (87). Because of the presence of other gram-negative coccobacilli and bipolar-staining bacilli in rectal and endocervical specimens contaminated with vaginal secretions, care must be taken not to overinterpret smears obtained from these sites. Gram-stained smears have no value in the diagnosis of pharyngeal gonococcal infection. Gram-stained smears should not be relied on for the diagnosis of gonorrhea but should be used adjunctively along with more specific tests.

Smears for Gram stain should always be prepared from urethral and endocervical sites and should be collected with

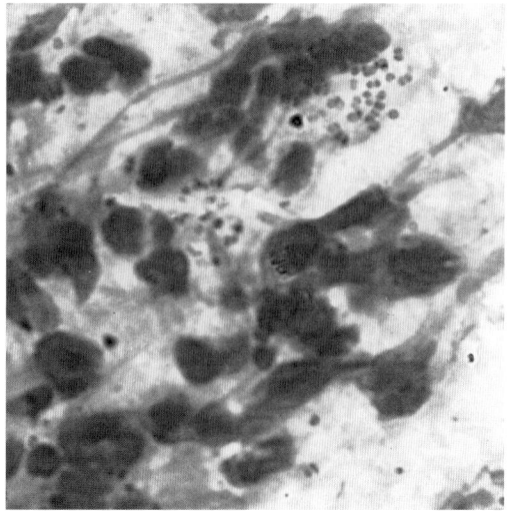

FIGURE 2 Gram stain of mucopurulent rectal exudate showing many diplococci inside PMNs. Magnification, ×1,500.

a different swab from that collected for culture. The swab is rolled gently over the surface of a glass slide in one direction only in order to minimize distortion and breakage of PMNs and preserve the characteristic appearance of the microorganisms. Gram-stained smears from men usually show moderate to many PMNs with two or more gram-negative intracellular diplococci (Fig. 1). Smears from men with early symptoms may show stringy proteinaceous material with few to moderate PMNs and predominantly extracellular diplococci. Smears prepared from specimens submitted in transport media may be more difficult to interpret due to distortion of the PMNs or to interfering substances (e.g., charcoal). Smears from normally sterile or minimally contaminated sites (e.g., joint fluid or skin lesions) should also be prepared.

Culture and Isolation Procedures

Various selective media allow recovery of *N. gonorrhoeae* from body sites harboring an endogenous bacterial flora. A variety of enriched selective media for culture of *N. gonorrhoeae* are available and include modified Thayer-Martin (MTM) medium, Martin-Lewis (ML) medium, GC-Lect medium (BD Biosciences), and New York City (NYC) medium. MTM, ML, and GC-Lect media are chocolate agar-based media that are supplemented with growth factors for fastidious microorganisms, whereas NYC medium is a clear peptone-corn starch agar-based medium containing yeast dialysate, citrated horse plasma, and lysed horse erythrocytes. These media contain antimicrobial agents that inhibit other microorganisms and allow the selective recovery of *N. gonorrhoeae*, *N. meningitidis*, and *N. lactamica* (Table 2). Vancomycin and colistin, antimicrobials present in all four formulations, inhibit gram-positive and gram-negative bacteria (including saprophytic *Neisseria* species), respectively. Trimethoprim is added to inhibit the swarming of *Proteus* spp. present in rectal and, occasionally, in cervicovaginal specimens. Nystatin, amphotericin B, or anisomycin is added to inhibit yeasts and molds. NYC medium also supports the growth of genital mycoplasmas and ureaplasmas. Media are commercially available in either petri dishes or JEMBEC plates. Formulas for these media are provided in chapter 27.

Commercially available selective media vary in their ability to support the growth of pathogenic *Neisseria* species and to inhibit the growth of nonpathogenic neisseriae and other contaminants (101). Failure of these various selective media to support gonococcal growth may also be due to the susceptibility of some *N. gonorrhoeae* strains to vancomycin. These strains account for a variable percentage of isolates depending on the geographic area (101).

Media for isolation of the pathogenic *Neisseria* should be at room temperature before inoculation and should not be excessively dry or moist. Specimens collected on swabs are firmly rolled in a Z pattern on the selective medium and cross-streaked with a bacteriologic loop. If a nonselective chocolate agar medium is also inoculated, these plates are streaked for isolation. The plates are incubated in a CO_2 incubator or a candle extinction jar at 35 to 37°C. The CO_2 level of the incubator should be 3 to 7%; higher CO_2 concentrations may actually inhibit the growth of some strains. The atmosphere should be moist, and, with candle jars, moisture evaporating from the medium during incubation is usually sufficient for organism growth. CO_2 incubators that are not equipped with humidifiers may be kept moist by placing a pan of water on the lower shelf. If candle jars are used, the candles should be made of white wax or bees' wax; scented or colored candles release volatile products during extinction, which may inhibit organism growth. Plates are inspected at 24, 48, and 72 h before a final report of "no growth" is issued. Suspect colonies are subcultured to chocolate agar, incubated, and used as inoculum for identification procedures.

Presumptive Identification

Colony Morphology

Gonococci produce several colony types in culture that are related to the piliation of organisms in the colony. Typical colonies tend to be small (about 0.5 mm in diameter), glistening, and raised. With subculture of individual piliated colonies, the culture can be maintained in this colonial type. With nonselective subculture (i.e., a "sweep" of growth), the other colony types become more evident, with all colonies eventually becoming the nonpiliated varieties. These colonies are larger (about 1 mm in diameter) and flatter and do not have the characteristic high profile and glistening highlights of piliated colony types. Cultures containing predominantly large-colony types often do not form smooth suspensions, because the colonies become gummy from autolysis and release of cellular DNA. The presence of multiple colony types on a subculture from a primary plate may give the appearance of a mixed culture. Careful scrutiny and subculture with the use of a dissecting microscope (magnification, ×10) enable one to become familiar with these colony types. Colony type variation is always observed with fresh isolates of *N. gonorrhoeae*. Atypical gonococci (i.e., those with multiple nutritional requirements such as the AHU-requiring or proline-arginine-uracil [PAU]-requiring strains) also produce various colony types, but these develop more slowly and require the use of a

TABLE 2 Antimicrobial agents in selective media for the pathogenic *Neisseria*

Antimicrobial agent	Amt of antimicrobial agent (µg/ml of medium) in:			
	MTM medium	ML medium	NYC medium	GC-Lect medium
Vancomycin	3	4	2	2
Lincomycin				1
Colistin	7.5	7.5	5.5	7.5
Nystatin	12.5			
Anisomycin		20		
Amphotericin B			1.2	1.5
Trimethoprim	5	5	5	5

dissecting microscope for detection and colony type characterization. Some *N. gonorrhoeae* strains grow on commercially available sheep blood agar, although growth takes longer and is not as luxuriant as on chocolate agar. However, other strains do not grow on sheep blood agar at all.

Gram Stain and Oxidase Test

Smears prepared from suspicious colonies should be examined with the Gram stain. The Gram stain of organisms from colonial growth should show uniform, characteristic gram-negative diplococci. Some of the organisms may appear as tetrads, particularly on smears prepared from young colonies. Organisms on smears prepared from older cultures may appear swollen and display a wide variation in counterstaining intensity, while smears prepared from partially autolyzed colonies may be uninterpretable. If it is necessary to perform a Gram stain from an older culture, individual colonies or growth should be selected from the margin of confluent growth to minimize the amount of lysed material in the smear. Examination by Gram stain is essential for presumptive identification because other organisms occasionally grow on selective media, particularly when oropharyngeal specimens are cultured (discussed below).

Oxidase test results are obtained with the tetramethyl derivative of the oxidase reagent (*N,N,N,N*-tetramethyl-1,4-phenylenediamine, 1% aqueous solution). A drop of this reagent is placed on a piece of filter paper, and a portion of the colonial growth is rubbed onto the reagent with a platinum loop, a cotton swab, or a wooden applicator stick. Alternatively, a loopful of growth is rubbed onto a cotton/Dacron swab which has been dipped in the oxidase solution. With fresh cultures, a dark purple color will appear on the filter paper within 10 s. Excellent results are obtained with the oxidase reagents that are packaged in crushable glass ampoules (e.g., BACTIDROP Oxidase; Remel Inc.).

Superoxol Test

Superoxol (30% hydrogen peroxide) is another helpful test for the rapid presumptive identification of *N. gonorrhoeae* (81). *N. gonorrhoeae* strains produce immediate, very brisk bubbling when some of the colony material is emulsified

with the reagent on a glass slide. Both *N. meningitidis* and *N. lactamica*, the other species that grow on selective media, generally produce weak, delayed bubbling, although some isolates of *N. meningitidis* and *M. catarrhalis* may also produce immediate, brisk bubbling similar to that produced by the gonococcus in this test. Isolates of oxidase-positive, gram-negative diplococci that are recovered from urogenital sites and that grow on selective media may be presumptively identified as *N. gonorrhoeae*. The superoxol test provides an additional presumptive test for identifying these isolates. Confirmatory identification tests are recommended for all isolates and are required for identification of isolates from extragenital sites (i.e., throat, rectum, blood, joint fluid, and cerebrospinal fluid [CSF]).

Differentiation of Other Organisms on Selective Media

Presumptive and confirmatory identification of *N. gonorrhoeae* species depends on the ability to differentiate these organisms from others that may also grow on selective media. These organisms include *Kingella denitrificans*, *M. catarrhalis*, other *Moraxella* species, *Acinetobacter* species, and *Capnocytophaga* species. *K. denitrificans* grows on MTM medium and produces colony types that resemble those of *N. gonorrhoeae*. The catalase test is useful in presumptively identifying gonococci and differentiating them from *K. denitrificans*. Gonococci produce vigorous bubbling when growth from the plate is immersed in 3% hydrogen peroxide (H_2O_2) or in superoxol; *K. denitrificans* produces a negative catalase reaction. *M. catarrhalis* and other *Moraxella* species, like gonococci, are oxidase positive and catalase positive. These organisms can be differentiated from *Neisseria* by the penicillin disk test (15). The organism is subcultured to a Trypticase-soy blood agar plate and streaked out to obtain confluent growth. A penicillin susceptibility disk (10 U of penicillin) is then placed on the inoculum. After overnight incubation in CO_2, a Gram stain is prepared from growth at the edge of the zone of inhibition. *Neisseria* species and *M. catarrhalis* retain their diplococcal morphology, although the cells may appear swollen (Fig. 3). Coccobacillary *Moraxella* species and *K. denitrificans* form long filaments or spindle-shaped cells under the influence of subinhibitory

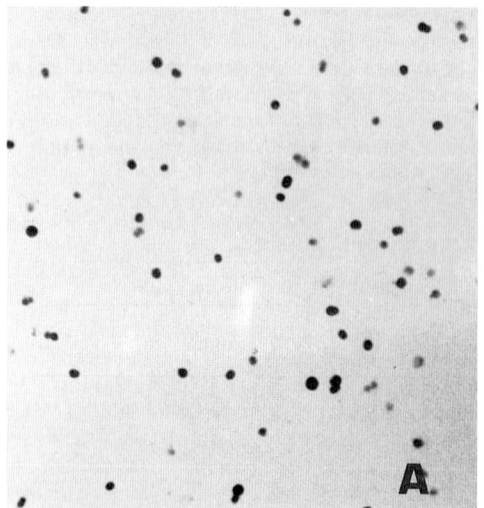
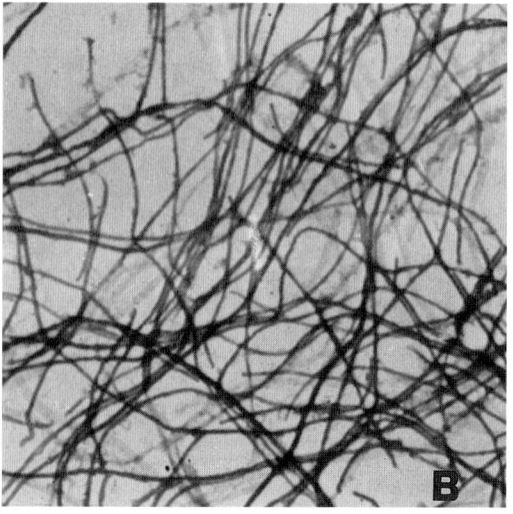

FIGURE 3 Cocci (A) and bacilli (B) exposed to subinhibitory concentrations of penicillin. Some cocci are swollen but still coccoid; bacilli form long strings. Magnification, ×1,000.

concentrations of penicillin. *Acinetobacter* spp. can exhibit diplococcal morphology and form filaments under the influence of penicillin, but these organisms are oxidase negative. *Capnocytophaga* species appear as pale-staining, gram-negative, slightly curved, fusiform bacteria and are both oxidase negative and catalase negative. On prolonged incubation (i.e., longer than 48 h) these organisms tend to spread due to gliding motility and may impede the recovery of gonococci from oropharyngeal specimens.

Confirmatory Identification Tests for *Neisseria* Species

Confirmatory tests for *N. gonorrhoeae*, *N. meningitidis*, and other *Neisseria* species include carbohydrate acidification tests, chromogenic enzyme substrate tests, immunologic tests (e.g., fluorescent antibody, staphylococcal coagglutination, and other tests), multitest identification systems, and DNA probe tests. Carbohydrate acidification tests and the multitest identification systems can be used to identify *N. gonorrhoeae*, *N. meningitidis*, and the other *Neisseria* species. Chromogenic substrate identification procedures are limited to identifying isolates that are able to grow on selective media (i.e., *N. gonorrhoeae*, *N. meningitidis*, *N. lactamica*, and some strains of *M. catarrhalis*). Fluorescent-antibody tests, coagglutination, other immunologic tests, and the DNA probe culture confirmation test are available for identification of *N. gonorrhoeae* only. The newer nucleic acid hybridization and nucleic acid amplification procedures are approved for direct detection of *N. gonorrhoeae* in genital tract and urine specimens only.

Acid Production from Carbohydrates

Conventional CTA Carbohydrates

The traditional technique for the identification of *Neisseria* species employs cystine-tryptic digest semisolid agar-base (CTA) medium containing 1% carbohydrate and a phenol red pH indicator. The usual test battery includes CTA-glucose, CTA-maltose, CTA-sucrose, and CTA-lactose, plus a carbohydrate-free CTA control. The lactose structural analogue *o*-nitrophenyl-β-D-galactopyranoside (ONPG) may be substituted for the lactose tube, and the addition of fructose to the test battery is helpful for identifying the various *N. subflava* biovars. Some commercial CTA formulations are supplemented with ascitic fluid to support the growth of more fastidious organisms. CTA media are inoculated with a dense suspension of the organism to be identified from a pure 18- to 24-h culture on chocolate agar. Either the inoculum is prepared in 0.5 ml of saline and divided among the tubes, or each tube is individually inoculated with a loopful of the organism. The inoculum is restricted to the top 0.5 in. of the agar-deep tubes. The tubes are incubated in a non-CO_2 incubator at 35°C with the caps tightened firmly. With a heavy inoculum, many isolates produce a detectable change in the color of the phenol red indicator within 24 h. If the inoculum is heavy enough, some strains change the indicator within 4 h. However, some fastidious gonococcal strains may require 24 to 72 h to produce sufficient acid to change the indicator. Because CTA medium containing 1% carbohydrate is used primarily for the detection of acid by fermentative organisms, the small amounts of acid produced oxidatively by some strains of *Neisseria* species may not be detected. In addition, this method may be problematic for differentiating *N. gonorrhoeae* and *N. cinerea*. Consequently, it is no longer favored for the detection of acid

production from carbohydrates. Table 3 shows the carbohydrate acidification profiles and other useful tests for the identification of *Neisseria* spp. recovered from humans.

Rapid Carbohydrate Test

The rapid carbohydrate test is a non-growth-dependent method for the detection of acid production from carbohydrates by *Neisseria* species. Small volumes (0.10 ml) of balanced salts solution (0.04 g of K_2HPO_4 per liter, 0.01 g of KH_2PO_4 per liter, 0.80 g of KCl per liter [pH 7.0]) with phenol red (0.5 ml of a 1% aqueous solution) indicator are dispensed in nonsterile tubes to which single drops of 20% filter-sterilized aqueous carbohydrates are added. A dense suspension of the organism is prepared in balanced salts solution, and 1 drop of this suspension is added to each of the carbohydrate-containing tubes. Tubes are incubated for 4 h at 35°C in a non-CO_2 incubator or a water bath. This method is economical, the reagents are easy to prepare and inoculate, and the results are clear-cut. The key to this technique is the use of reagent-grade carbohydrates. Maltose obtained from some bacteriologic media companies may produce positive or equivocal results for *N. gonorrhoeae* in the rapid carbohydrate test, presumably owing to the presence of contaminant glucose. Inocula for this procedure may be obtained from the primary culture if sufficient colonies are present and if the growth is less than 24 h old. Since growth does not occur in the test medium, small numbers of contaminants that may be present do not interfere with the 4-h result. However, incubation cannot be continued overnight. The RIM-*Neisseria* Test (Rapid Identification Method-Neisseria; Remel, Inc.) is a commercially available modification of the rapid acid production test, and evaluations have reported good agreement with conventional methods, although this test may not provide adequate differentiation between *N. gonorrhoeae* and *N. cinerea* (28, 30).

Chromogenic Enzyme Substrate Tests

The enzymatic identification systems use specific biochemical substrates that, after hydrolysis by bacterial enzymes, yield a colored end product that is detected immediately or after the addition of a diazo dye-coupling reagent. These tests are restricted to species that are able to grow on selective media: *N. gonorrhoeae*, *N. meningitidis*, and *N. lactamica*. Because some strains of *M. catarrhalis* grow on selective media, these systems also provide a presumptive identification of this organism. Chromogenic substrate identification tests should not be used to identify suspected gonococci or meningococci recovered on blood and/or chocolate agar without prior subculture of the isolate to selective media. The enzymatic activities that are detected in these systems include β-galactosidase, γ-glutamylaminopeptidase, and prolyl-hydroxyprolyl aminopeptidase. β-Galactosidase and γ-glutamylaminopeptidase are specific for *N. lactamica* and *N. meningitidis*, respectively. The absence of these activities and the presence of prolyl-hydroxyprolyl aminopeptidase identifies an organism as *N. gonorrhoeae*. Some *N. meningitidis* strains produce both γ-glutamylaminopeptidase and prolyl-hydroxyprolyl aminopeptidase. *M. catarrhalis* lacks all three of these enzymatic activities. The Gonochek II (EY Labs, San Mateo, Calif.) is a commercial system that detects all three enzyme activities in a single tube (28). The BactiCard *Neisseria* (Remel, Inc.) includes substrates for the three enzymes, as well as an indoxyl butyrate substrate for the identification of *M. catarrhalis* (see below) (W. M. Janda and M. Montero, *Abstr. 95th*

TABLE 3 Characteristics of *Neisseria* and related species of human origin[a]

Species	Colony morphology on chocolate agar	Growth on:			Acid from:					Reduction of NO₃	Polysaccharide from SUC	Tributyrin hydrolysis
		MTM, ML and NYC media	Chocolate or blood agar (22°C)	Nutrient agar (35°C)	GLU	MAL	LAC	SUC	FRU			
N. gonorrhoeae[b]	Beige to gray-brown, translucent, smooth, 0.5–1 mm in diameter	+	0	0	+	0	0	0	0	0	0	0
N. meningitidis	Beige to gray-brown, translucent, smooth, 1–3 mm in diameter	+	0	V	+	+	0	0	0	0	0	0
N. lactamica	Beige to gray-brown, translucent, smooth, 1–2 mm in diameter	+	V	+	+	+	+	0	0	0	0	0
N. cinerea[c]	Beige to gray-brown to yellowish, translucent, smooth, 1–2 mm in diameter	V	0	+	0	0	0	0	0	0	0	0
N. polysaccharea	Beige to gray-brown to yellow, translucent, smooth, 1–2 mm in diameter	V	+	+	+	+	0	V	0	0	+	0
N. subflava[d]	Greenish yellow, opaque, 1–3 mm in diameter, smooth to rough, sometimes adherent	V	+	+	+	+	0	V	V	0	V	0
N. sicca	White, opaque, 1–3 mm in diameter, adherent, wrinkled with age	0	+	+	+	+	0	+	+	0	+	0
N. mucosa	Greenish yellow, opaque, 1–3 mm in diameter	0	+	+	+	+	0	+	+	+	+	0
N. flavescens	Yellow, opaque, 1–2 mm in diameter	0	+	+	0	0	0	0	0	0	+	0
N. elongata[e]	Gray-brown, translucent, smooth, 1–2 mm in diameter, glistening, dry, claylike consistency	0	+	+	0	0	0	0	0	0	0	0
M. catarrhalis	Pinkish-brown, opaque, 1–3 mm in diameter, dry, "hockey puck" consistency	V	+	+	0	0	0	0	0	+	0	+
K. denitrificans	Beige to gray-brown, translucent, smooth, 1–2 mm in diameter	+	NT	+	+	0	0	0	0	+	0	0

[a] Symbols and abbreviations: +, strains typically positive but genetic mutants may be negative; V, strain dependent; NT, not tested; GLU, glucose; MAL, maltose; LAC, lactose; SUC, sucrose; FRU, fructose.
[b] *N. kochii* is considered to be a subspecies of *N. gonorrhoeae*; isolates of *N. kochii* exhibit characteristics of both *N. gonorrhoeae* and *N. meningitidis*, but are identified as *N. gonorrhoeae* by tests routinely used for the identification of *Neisseria* spp.
[c] Some strains grow on selective media.
[d] Includes biovars subflava, flava, and perflava. *N. subflava* bv. perflava strains produce acid from sucrose and fructose and produce polysaccharide from sucrose; *N. subflava* bv. flava strains produce acid from fructose; *N. subflava* bv. subflava strains do not produce polysaccharide.
[e] Rod-shaped organism. The catalase test is weakly positive or negative compared with those of other *Neisseria* spp. (catalase positive). Results in the table are for *N. elongata* subsp. *elongata*. Strains of *N. elongata* subsp. *glycolytica* may produce a weak acid reaction from D-glucose, are catalase positive, and do not reduce nitrate but do reduce nitrite. Strains of *N. elongata* subsp. *nitroreducens* (formerly CDC group M-6) may produce a weak acid reaction with D-glucose, are catalase negative, and reduce both nitrate and nitrite.

Gen. Meet. Am. Soc. Microbiol. 1995, abstr. C-303, p. 53, 1995). It should be noted that the interpretive guidelines for these tests do not allow for the fact that some nongonococcal neisseria isolates may be isolated on gonococcal selective media. Most of these species give a positive prolyl-hydroxyprolyl aminopeptidase reaction and may be misidentified as *N. gonorrhoeae* if additional tests are not performed.

Immunologic Methods for Culture Confirmation

Direct Fluorescent Monoclonal Antibody Test

The currently available direct fluorescent-antibody (DFA) culture confirmation procedure uses monoclonal antibodies that recognize epitopes on the PorI (protein I) principal outer membrane protein of *N. gonorrhoeae*. The DFA test (*Neisseria gonorrhoeae* Culture Confirmation Test; Wampole Laboratories, Cranberry, N.J.) is performed by preparing a smear on a DFA slide, overlaying the smear with the DFA reagent, and incubating the smear for 15 min. After rinsing and mounting, the slide is examined under a fluorescence microscope. Gonococci appear as apple-green fluorescent diplococci. The Wampole kit is the same product that was developed and marketed by Syva in 1986. At that time, the DFA reagent was highly sensitive and specific; however, at present, many strains of *N. gonorrhoeae* fail to stain with this reagent (49, 51). Serotyping and pulsed-field gel electrophoresis (PFGE) data indicate that β-lactamase-producing and non-β-lactamase-producing strains that are negative with the DFA reagent belong to a variety of serovars (9, 49). The anti-PorI monoclonal antibody cocktail used in the original product has not been modified since its initial marketing, and package insert claims of 99.6% sensitivity and 100% specificity are no longer valid. Isolates that fail to stain with the DFA reagent must be identified by another method. This caveat limits the real advantages of the DFA procedure, which included its rapidity, the ability to test colonies directly from primary cultures, and the small amount of growth required for test performance. The DFA test is not intended for direct detection and identification of organisms on smears from patient specimens.

Coagglutination Tests

Two coagglutination tests for the identification of *N. gonorrhoeae* are currently available: the Phadebact Monoclonal GC Test (Boule Diagnostics AB, Huddinge, Sweden) and the GonoGen I (New Horizons Diagnostics, Columbia, Md.). The Phadebact Monoclonal GC test uses monoclonal antibodies that detect heat-stable epitopes on the PorI outer membrane protein. Unlike the GC OMNI test previously marketed by Boule Diagnostics, the Monoclonal GC test contains one reagent that reacts with serogroup WI *N. gonorrhoeae* strains and a second reagent that reacts with serogroup WII/WIII strains. Because a negative control reagent is not included, gonococcal isolates react with either the WI or the WII/WIII reagent, depending on the PorI epitopes expressed by an individual isolate. A suspension (McFarland standard no. 0.5) prepared in buffered saline (pH 7.2 to 7.4) is boiled and mixed with test and control reagents on a cardboard slide. Agglutination within 1 min indicates a positive test. Freshly subcultured serogroup WI (ATCC 19424) and serogroup WII/III (ATCC 23051) strains are recommended for quality control but are not provided with the kit. The GonoGen I coagglutination test also uses staphylococcal cells coated with anti-PorI

monoclonal antibodies (65). This test kit contains test and control coagglutination reagents, with positive and negative gonococcal test control suspensions included. GonoGen I also uses a boiled organism suspension (McFarland no. 3) for testing. Agglutination with the test but not the control reagent constitutes a positive test. Careful attention to procedural details is necessary to prevent false-positive and false-negative results with either test. Some gonococci do not react with these reagents, and cross-reactions with other *Neisseria* species (i.e., *N. meingitidis*, *N. lactamica*, and *N. cinerea*) and *K. denitrificans* have been reported (28, 30, 49, 51).

GonoGen II

GonoGen II (New Horizons Diagnostics) uses anti-Por monoclonal antibodies conjugated to colloidal gold as the detection reagent. Colonies from agar medium are suspended in a lysing solution, and 1 drop of the antibody reagent is added. After 5 min, 2 drops of the suspension are passed through a membrane filter that retains antigen-antibody complexes. Concentration of the complex on the filter turns the filter red, identifying the organism as *N. gonorrhoeae*. Nongonococcal isolates result in the filter remaining white or pale pink. Some *N. gonorrhoeae* strains do not react with the conjugate and are not identified, and false-positive reactions have been noted with some *N. meningitidis* and *N. lactamica* strains (49, 51).

Multitest Identification Systems

Kit systems are available that identify *Neisseria* spp., *Haemophilus* spp., and other fastidious gram-negative organisms. These systems are the RapID NH (*Neisseria-Haemophilus*) (Remel, Inc.), the Vitek NHI (*Neisseria-Haemophilus* Identification) card (bioMérieux, Inc., Hazelwood, Mo.), the *Haemophilus-Neisseria* identification (HNID) panel (Dade/American Microscan, Sacramento, Calif.), and the API NH (bioMérieux, Inc., La Balme-les-Grottes, France) (7, 30, 47, 48). These kits use modified conventional tests and chromogenic substrates to provide identification within 2 to 4 h. The NHI card identifies the pathogenic *Neisseria* spp., *N. lactamica*, and *N. cinerea*, but *M. catarrhalis* cannot be differentiated from other *Moraxella* spp. (48). *N. cinerea* is not included in the database of the MicroScan HNID panel, resulting in misidentifications as *N. gonorrhoeae* or *M. catarrhalis*, and some *N. meningitidis* strains do not produce clear-cut reactions with key tests (47). RapID NH includes tests that enable the reliable identification of the pathogenic *Neisseria* spp., *N. cinerea*, and *M. catarrhalis*. The API NH identifies gonococci, meningococci, *N. lactamica*, and *M. catarrhalis* within 2 h; other *Neisseria* species required additional tests for correct species identification (7).

DNA Probe Test for Culture Confirmation

The Accuprobe *Neisseria gonorrhoeae* Culture Confirmation Test (Gen Probe, San Diego, Calif.) identifies *N. gonorrhoeae* by the detection of species-specific rRNA sequences. Organisms from growth on agar medium are lysed and mixed with a chemiluminescent acridinium ester-labeled single-stranded DNA probe that is complementary to gonococcal rRNA. DNA probe/rRNA hybrids are selected by a chemical process, and the presence of the probe in hybrids is detected by hydrolysis of the acridinium ester, with the consequent release of light energy. This energy is detected by a chemiluminometer and reported as relative light units. The Accuprobe test is more sensitive and specific than biochemical or immunologic culture confirmation tests and is particularly useful for confirming problem isolates (49).

Direct Probe and Amplified Probe Detection

Probe and nucleic acid amplification tests (NAATs) permit the direct detection of *N. gonorrhoeae* in clinical specimens. These tests have gained popularity because they permit the concurrent detection of *C. trachomatis*. They do not appreciably increase the number of cases of gonorrhea detected over the numbers detected with a proficient specimen transport and culture system. An advantage of these tests is that specimens may be transported and stored for several days before being tested in the laboratory; they do not require viable organisms. Thus, these tests may be used to detect *N. gonorrhoeae* in specimens from geographic areas distant from a laboratory and where facilities cannot maintain viable organisms. NAATs also permit the detection of *N. gonorrhoeae* in urine, thus avoiding the necessity for performing endocervical examinations or obtaining intraurethral swab specimens.

A major disadvantage associated with the use of nonculture nucleic acid probe tests or NAATs is that the results must be interpreted with care in the context of a clinical diagnosis. For example, since gonococcal DNA may still be present in specimens for up to 3 weeks after successful treatment of an infection, amplification tests should not be used to assess response to therapy. Results of NAATs may be used only to make a presumptive diagnosis of a gonococcal infection and are inadmissible evidence in medicolegal cases in the United States at this time. Other countries are less restrictive. An additional disadvantage is that isolates are not available for ongoing surveillance or for antimicrobial susceptibility testing if questions of treatment efficacy arise.

Nucleic Acid Hybridization (DNA Probe) Tests

Two nucleic acid probe assays, the Gen-Probe PACE 2 and PACE 2C assays (Gen-Probe Inc.) and the Hybrid Capture II assay (Digene Corp., Gaithersburg, Md.), are approved by the Food and Drug Administration (FDA) for detecting *N. gonorrhoeae*. In the Gen-Probe tests, an acridinium ester-labeled DNA probe for a specific sequence of *Chlamydia trachomatis* or *N. gonorrhoeae* rRNA is allowed to hybridize with any complementary rRNA in the specimen (52). An acridinium ester hybridization protection assay detects any DNA-RNA hybrids which are adsorbed to magnetic particles. The acridinium ester label is hydrolyzed from any unhybridized acridinium ester-labeled DNA probe. Chemiluminescence generated by the acridinium ester-DNA-rRNA hybrids is then detected with a luminometer that gives a numerical readout (52). The PACE 2C test detects both *N. gonorrhoeae* and *C. trachomatis* in a single test. If a positive result is obtained in this test, separate tests for the individual organisms must be performed. A probe competition assay may also be used to augment the specificity of the test. An unlabeled probe is incubated with the initially positive specimen; the unlabeled probe competitively inhibits binding of the labeled probe. A prescribed reduction in the signal obtained for the assay performed with and without the unlabeled probe verifies the initial positive test result.

The Digene assay uses RNA hybridization probes which are specific for both genomic DNA and cryptic plasmid DNA sequences of *C. trachomatis* and *N. gonorrhoeae* (66). In this test, RNA-DNA hybrids are "captured" in the wells of microtiter plates by hybrid-specific antibodies. The hybrids are detected with alkaline phosphatase-labeled anti–RNA-DNA hybrid antibodies, and the signal is amplified by using a chemiluminescent substrate detected by a luminometer. The Digene test kit has no supplemental tests to allow verification of the initial test result.

Nucleic Acid Amplification Tests

NAATs are designed to amplify *N. gonorrhoeae*-specific nucleic acid sequences; positive results may be obtained from as little as a single copy of the target DNA or RNA. Like other nonculture tests, NAATs do not require viable organisms (22). NAATs from three manufacturers are currently FDA cleared for the detection of *N. gonorrhoeae*: the Abbott LCx (Abbott Laboratories Inc., Abbott Park, Ill.), the Roche AMPLICOR (Roche Diagnostics, Indianapolis, Ind.), and the Becton Dickinson BDProbeTec (BD Biosciences) tests. The Abbott LCx test detects a 48-bp sequence in the *opa* genes in *N. gonorrhoeae*, which may be present in up to 11 copies per bacterial cell. The Roche AMPLICOR PCR test for *N. gonorrhoeae* detects a 201-bp sequence in the cytosine methyltransferase gene. The BDProbeTec ET detects a DNA sequence in the multicopy pilin gene-inverting protein homologue.

Most NAATs have been cleared by the FDA to detect *N. gonorrhoeae* in endocervical swabs from women, urethral swabs from men, and urine from men and women. Although not cleared by the FDA for this purpose, NAATs have been evaluated for detection of *N. gonorrhoeae* in self-collected vaginal specimens from women (43). NAATs are not FDA cleared or recommended for the detection of *N. gonorrhoeae* in either rectal or pharyngeal specimens.

The ability to detect *N. gonorrhoeae* in urine, thus avoiding the necessity to obtain an endocervical specimen or an intraurethral swab from men, is an important advantage of NAATs over tests which require "invasive" endocervical and intraurethral specimens. It should be noted, however, that some specimens contain inhibitors which may result in false-negative results in NAATs. Some NAATs may exhibit reduced sensitivity when used to screen for *N. gonorrhoeae* in urine from women and in swab specimens or urine from men (23, 62). It should also be noted that some NAATs for *N. gonorrhoeae* have reacted with isolates of nongonococcal *Neisseria* species including *N. cinerea*, *N. lactamica*, and *N. subflava* (35, 62). Supplemental procedures to enhance NAAT specificities are not packaged with commercial NAATs. Reproducibility problems have been identified with the Abbott Laboratories LCx assay that would not be detected by the quality control procedures provided by the manufacturer (41); the authors provide procedures for detecting and preventing problems (41).

Typing Systems

Phenotypic and genotypic typing systems are used to differentiate between strains of *N. gonorrhoeae*. The specific characteristics chosen depend on the question(s) being asked. Antimicrobial resistance is frequently the subject of investigation or surveillance. Susceptibilities are determined to a panel of agents including penicillin, tetracycline, spectinomycin, an extended-spectrum cephalosporin (ceftriaxone or cefixime), a fluoroquinolone (ciprofloxacin or ofloxacin), and a macrolide (erythromycin or azithromycin), and results are interpreted by NCCLS-recommended methods (67). Strains are usually described by their pattern of penicillin-tetracycline susceptibilities (penicillin-tetracycline resistance phenotype) (75). Penicillin-tetracycline resistance phenotypes include penicillin resistant (PenR), tetracycline resistant (TetR), chromosomally mediated resistance to penicillin and tetracycline (CMRNG), β-lactamase positive (PPNG), plasmid-mediated resistance to tetracycline (TRNG), strains with plasmid-mediated resistance to both penicillin and tetracycline (PP/TR), and isolates susceptible to both penicillin and tetracycline (Susc.) (75). PPNG and TRNG isolates may exhibit chromosomally mediated resistance to tetracycline (PPNG, TetR) and penicillin (TRNG, PenR), respectively. Intermediate resistance or resistance to other antimicrobial agents is appended to the penicillin-tetracycline resistance phenotype. For example, a PPNG isolate exhibiting resistance to ciprofloxacin (CipR) would be designated PPNG, CipR.

Phenotypic characterization also includes the determination of nutritional requirements for growth on a chemically defined medium (auxotyping) and serotyping with a panel of 12 monoclonal antibodies in coagglutination tests to define serovars (53, 82). Strains have been classified with a dual auxotype-serovar system, which provides greater discrimination among strains than is possible with either typing system alone (82). Auxotyping involves determination of the requirement of strains for individual metabolites for growth on a chemically defined medium. For example, if a strain fails to grow on a medium from which arginine has been omitted, the strain is recorded as arginine requiring. Thus, strains with single or multiple growth requirements may be identified. Serotyping is performed with a panel of monoclonal antibody coagglutination reagents; monoclonal antibodies are directed against epitopes on the PorI (protein I) molecule in the gonococcal outer membrane (82). Strains are divided into two major serogroups, IA and IB, on the basis of the protein I species expressed by the strain; further subdivision into serovars is made according to patterns of reaction with a panel of six protein IA- and protein IB-specific antibody reagents. Typing systems are not used for the identification of isolates as *N. gonorrhoeae*. Rather, they are used to compare isolates for molecular epidemiologic investigations, which may range from studies of the dynamics of gonococcal strains in communities and the geographic spread of antimicrobial-resistant strains to comparisons between strains for medicolegal investigations (82).

Gonococcal isolates may also be characterized by additional characteristics related to antimicrobial resistance. At least six different β-lactamase plasmids have been described in the gonococcus; these, as well as two conjugative plasmids (one possessing a *Tet*M determinant), have also been used to study the distribution of gonococcal strains (82). Strains possessing the *Tet*M determinant may, with PCR-based tests, be assigned to one of two types: American or Dutch (45). Mutations in the *gyr*A and *par*C genes in strains exhibiting decreased susceptibilities to fluoroquinolones may also be characterized (26).

In addition, molecular typing methods which characterize either specific genes or the whole chromosome have been used more recently to differentiate among gonococcal isolates. With older methods, such as PFGE and restriction endonuclease analysis, the whole chromosome is digested with restriction enzymes into fragments which are then separated in polyacrylamide gels (74, 100). Restriction endonuclease typing permitted differentiation among isolates belonging to the same serovar; however, restriction patterns are very complex and are often difficult to interpret (74). The PFGE method is tedious to perform, with restriction taking as long as 48 h and resulting in large fragments

which are difficult to separate on conventional gels. Thus, fragments which appear to be similar may, in fact, be different.

Recently developed typing methods involve amplification and restriction of individual genes or the whole chromosome (69, 70, 86, 94). Characterization of individual genes has included the Lip typing system, which permits the grouping of gonococcal isolates based on the number and sequence of pentamer amino acid repeats and their sequence within the *lip* gene (94). In contrast, Opa typing is based on identification of the restriction patterns of a family of 11 distinct and highly variable *opa* genes to give an *opa* type (69). One possible disadvantage of the Opa typing system is that types may evolve very rapidly, resulting in every isolate having a different type unless it is from a sexual partner or a short chain of sexual partners (69). A system to type the variable regions of the *porIB* gene using oligonucleotide probes has been developed (92). This system can detect differences in *porIB* among isolates belonging to the same serovar; however, this method requires the use of different hybridization conditions for individual probes.

In addition, two typing methods which characterize the entire chromosome are based on amplification fragment length polymorphism (AFLP). These methods use different restriction enzymes to digest the DNA (70, 86). The fluoresent AFLP has the same discriminatory power as the Opa typing system but is probably more stable than the latter system; the two AFLP typing systems have not been compared (70).

Antimicrobial Susceptibility

Antimicrobial resistance is now widespread among strains of *N. gonorrhoeae* and occurs as both chromosomally mediated resistance to a variety of agents and plasmid-mediated resistance to penicillins (penicillinase [β-lactamase]-producing) and to tetracycline (tetracycline-resistant *N. gonorrhoeae*) (75). Owing to the increased frequency of penicillin- and tetracycline-resistant strains of *N. gonorrhoeae* (Fig. 4), CDC has recommended that selected extended-spectrum cephalosporins and newer fluoroquinolones be used as primary therapy against uncomplicated gonococcal infections (18). Although tetracycline is no longer recommended for the treatment of gonorrhea, dual therapy including doxycycline or azithromycin is recommended for the empiric treatment of concurrent chlamydial infections. Although CDC no longer recommends test-of-cure cultures, if symptoms persist after treatment with one of the recommended therapies, patients should be reevaluated for *N. gonorrhoeae* infection by culture and the susceptibilities of any resulting gonococcal isolate should be determined (18). Although clinically significant resistance to extended-spectrum cephalosporins has not been confirmed, failure of infections to respond to treatment with CDC-recommended doses of fluoroquinolones (MIC of ciprofloxacin, ≥1.0 μg/ml; MIC of ofloxacin, ≥2.0 μg/ml) has been documented extensively (55). Strains with clinically significant resistance to fluoroquinolones are now widespread in the Far East and account for approximately 10% of isolates in Honolulu, Hawaii; they have been isolated from a number of cities in the United States (18–20, 55). In 1986, CDC implemented the Gonococcal Isolate Surveillance Project in 24 to 26 sentinel sites in the United States to monitor changes in antimicrobial susceptibilities in *N. gonorrhoeae* on a monthly basis. The susceptibilities of gonococcal isolates to penicillin, tetracycline, spectinomycin, ceftriax-

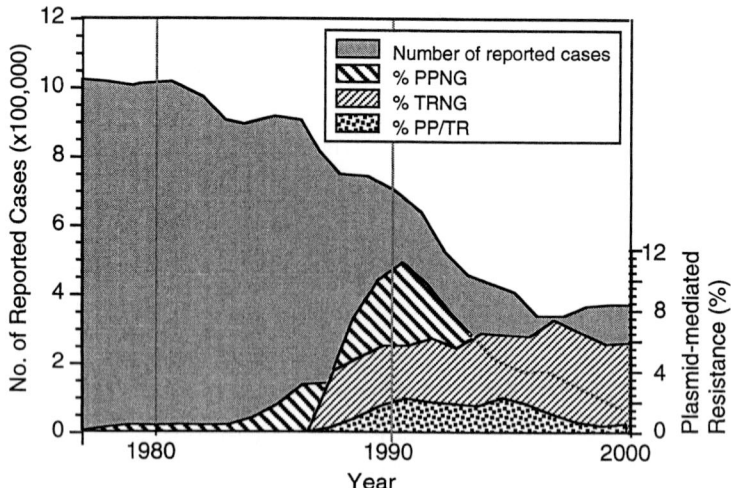

FIGURE 4 Percentage of cases of gonorrhea and frequency of gonorrhea caused by strains of *N. gonorrhoeae* with plasmid-mediated resistance to penicillin (PPNG), tetracycline (TRNG), and both penicillin and tetracycline (PP/TR) in the United States, 1978 to 2000, compared with the total number of reported cases. The number of infections with strains with plasmid-mediated resistance to penicillin is based on a combination of passive surveillance of strains with plasmid-mediated resistance to penicillin (1978 to 1987) and data provided by active surveillance in the Gonococcal Isolate Surveillance Project. Data for *N. gonorrhoeae* strains with plasmid-mediated resistance to tetracycline and to both penicillin and tetracycline are provided by the Gonococcal Isolates Surveillance Project (20, 21).

one, cefixime, ciprofloxacin, and azithromycin are measured, and the results are published annually (18, 19). These data are used when CDC revises the treatment recommendations for gonorrhea. It should also be noted that the prevalence of antimicrobial resistance in *N. gonorrhoeae* varies geographically within the United States and that it is necessary to conduct testing at the local level to obtain the most accurate assessment of resistance prevalence with which to assess appropriate treatment recommendations.

The susceptibilities of gonococcal isolates are determined by an agar dilution method, either on antibiotic-containing media or with the E test, or by a disk diffusion method recommended by the NCCLS (67). β-Lactamase production may be determined by a highly sensitive nitrocefin test. Ideally, susceptibilities to penicillin, tetracycline, spectinomycin, an extended-spectrum cephalosporin, a fluoroquinolone, and azithromycin should be determined for surveillance purposes. At a minimum, susceptibilities to the agents routinely used to treat gonorrhea should be determined; in clinical settings where PID is treated, susceptibility to antigonococcal agents (cefoxitin or cefotetan) recommended for the treatment of PID should be tested (16). Resistance to both penicillin and tetracycline may serve as an indicator of decreased susceptibility to extended-spectrum cephalosporins (98). Determination of spectinomycin susceptibilities is recommended if this agent is used as an alternative therapy for uncomplicated gonococcal infections.

Currently, azithromycin is not recommended for the routine treatment of uncomplicated gonococcal infections (16). This agent may be recommended for the treatment of gonorrhea in geographic areas where fluoroquinolone-resistant isolates are prevalent and if spectinomycin is not available (18–20). If azithromycin is used to treat gonorrhea, it is important that the FDA-cleared dose of 2 g of

azithromycin be used rather than the 1-g dose currently recommended for the primary treatment of chlamydial infections (16). Failure of infections to respond to therapy with 1 g of azithromycin and 2 g of azithromycin has been observed with gonococcal isolates for which the azithromycin MICs are 0.125 to 0.25 and ≤0.5 μg/ml, respectively (42, 91). Gonococcal isolates with azithromycin MICs of ≥1.0 μg/ml have been identified in a number of cities in the United States including an outbreak in Kansas City, Mo. (18, 19).

Because fluoroquinolone-resistant gonococcal isolates are prevalent in Hawaii and are being isolated more frequently in other cities in the United States and because resistance to extended-spectrum cephalosporins may emerge, it is important to determine the susceptibilities of gonococcal isolates from patients whose symptoms persist after treatment. Isolates that exhibit resistance or decreased susceptibility to the treatment agent should be submitted to a reference laboratory for confirmation. If possible, laboratories should implement a routine surveillance program to monitor the susceptibilities of gonococcal isolates in order to detect changes that may indicate the emergence of clinically significant resistance to therapeutic agents that may compromise treatment outcomes.

Evaluation, Interpretation, and Reporting of Results

The level of testing and the format for reporting of laboratory results should be directed by the sociodemographic characteristics (e.g., age and gender) of the patient clientele served and a working knowledge of the incidence and prevalence of clinically significant disease caused by *Neisseria* species, e.g., gonorrhea, in that population. When specimens are collected from patients at high risk for gonorrhea and there are no sociologic or medicolegal implications of a diagnosis of gonorrhea, a presumptive identification of *N. gonorrhoeae* may be sufficient if the diagnosis is intended to facilitate prompt and effective treatment of infections. However, when specimens are collected to confirm a clinical diagnosis in patients, e.g., women and children at low risk for gonorrhea, special concerns apply to laboratory processing and retention of specimens because of the medicolegal consequences that may ensue if an organism is identified as *N. gonorrhoeae*. Laboratorians and clinicians must know the patient population that they serve and decide to what levels of specificity identifications of *Neisseria* and related species must be made.

Special protocols should be developed for processing specimens from alleged victims of sexual abuse and assault. Suspect gonococci isolated from children must be confirmed by at least two different methods that involve different principles because certain social and medicolegal issues are raised following the release of test results (3). These tests may include carbohydrate utilization tests, immunologic methods (e.g., monoclonal antibody fluorescence tests or coagglutination tests), enzymatic procedures (e.g., chromogenic detection of specific enzyme activities), and the DNA probe culture confirmation test (see below). Of these, tests which detect acid production from glucose and the DNA probe culture confirmation test provide the least equivocal results for medicolegal purposes. Nongonococcal isolates may cross-react in gonococcal coagglutination tests and gonococcal isolates may not react in the monoclonal antibody fluorescence test (49). Nongonococcal isolates also give positive prolylhydroxyprolyl aminopeptidase reactions in enzyme substrate tests (e.g., GonoChek II and the BactiCard-Neisseria), as do gonococcal isolates. Communication between the clinician and the laboratory is essential to ensure that specimens of potential medicolegal importance are processed according to these criteria. In too many instances, because a specimen has not been clearly marked as being from a child, an organism has been identified by only one confirmatory test and discarded according to a routine protocol.

In general, with the exception of high-risk patients for whom presumptive identifications may suffice, similar principles apply to the identification of all gram-negative, oxidase-positive diplococci. Many tests are available for the confirmation of the identities of gram-negative, oxidase-positive diplococcal isolates from clinical specimens. Although many tests for the identification of *Neisseria* and related species are marketed as confirmatory tests, most do not provide sufficient information to accurately identify an isolate to the species level without the performance of additional tests. As noted earlier in the chapter, several species may give identical reactions in some tests; e.g., maltose-negative *N. meningitidis* and *K. denitrificans* may give reactions identical to those of *N. gonorrhoeae* in some acid production tests. In addition, problems have been identified with most tests for the identification of *N. gonorrhoeae* and related species, e.g., false-negative acid production reactions from glucose with *N. gonorrhoeae* or false-positive reactions from glucose with *N. cinerea*.

Culture confirmation tests are preferred for the identification of *Neisseria* and related species because they require the isolation of an organism which can be examined by multiple tests if the results of the primary tests are equivocal. In general, multitest systems provide the most comprehensive information about several biochemical characteristics that may, in some cases, allow the identification of an isolate. These tests are most useful if identification to the species level is required and may help characterize isolates in rare instances when hydrid organisms are isolated. Rapid

identification tests, including serologic and nucleic acid probe or amplification tests, that provide a "yes-no" answer, i.e., an isolate either is or is not *N. gonorrhoeae*, may be adequate if it is necessary only to eliminate *N. gonorrhoeae* as the causative agent; these tests are of limited usefulness when identification to the species level is required.

Because of the serious social and medicolegal consequences of misdiagnosing gonorrhea or misidentifying strains of *N. gonorrhoeae*, three levels of diagnosis are recommended for reporting diagnoses of gonorrhea. These levels are "suggestive," which is defined on the basis of clinical findings, "presumptive," and "definitive," with the last two levels including the results of laboratory diagnostic tests. A suggestive diagnosis is defined by the presence of (i) a mucopurulent endocervical or urethral exudate on physical examination and (ii) sexual exposure to a person infected with *N. gonorrhoeae*. A presumptive diagnosis of gonorrhea is made on the basis of two of the following three criteria: (i) typical gram-negative intracellular diplococci on microscopic examination of a smear of urethral exudate (men) or endocervical secretions (women); (ii) growth of *N. gonorrhoeae* from the urethra (men) or endocervix (women) on culture medium and demonstration of typical colonial morphology, positive oxidase reaction, and typical gram-negative morphology; and/or (iii) detection of *N. gonorrhoeae* by nonculture laboratory tests (e.g., antigen detection, nucleic acid probe tests, or NAATs). A definitive diagnosis requires (i) isolation of *N. gonorrhoeae* from sites of exposure (e.g., urethra, endocervix, throat, or rectum) by culture (usually on a selective medium) and demonstration of typical colonial morphology, positive oxidase reaction, and typical gram-negative morphology and (ii) confirmation of isolates by biochemical, enzymatic, serologic, or nucleic acid tests, e.g., carbohydrate utilization, rapid enzyme substrate tests, serologic methods such as coagglutination or fluorescent-antibody tests, or the DNA probe culture confirmation test.

For reporting purposes, the laboratory should perform species-level identification and confirmation with appropriate tests in order to report a definitive result of "*N. gonorrhoeae* confirmed" for the clinician unless otherwise requested. If an organism suspected to be *N. gonorrhoeae* is tested by rapid tests but not by additional confirmatory tests that compensate for problems associated with the primary test and is reported as "presumptive *N. gonorrhoeae*," it is important that a clinician receiving this report understands that additional tests may be required to confirm this identification. Ideally, to avoid confusion, an organism should be reported only as "gram-negative, oxidase-positive diplococcus isolated" unless it has been identified to the species level with sufficient tests to ensure the accuracy of the identification.

NEISSERIA MENINGITIDIS

Specimen Collection and Transport

Specimens helpful in the diagnosis of meningococcal disease include CSF, blood, aspirates, biopsy specimens, and nasopharyngeal and oropharyngeal swabs (Table 1). Occasionally, meningococci are sought in sputum and transtracheal aspirates. Genital, rectal, and oropharyngeal isolates of *N. meningitidis* may be recovered using the collection and inoculation procedures described for *N. gonorrhoeae*. Incubation conditions for inoculated media are the same as those described for *N. gonorrhoeae*. Meningococci grow well on all selective media for the pathogenic neisseriae, and vancomycin-susceptible strains have not been described. Recovery of both gonococci and meningococci from blood cultures may be adversely affected by the anticoagulant sodium polyanethol sulfonate that is present in blood culture media. This effect may be neutralized by addition of sterile gelatin (1% final concentration) to the media or by processing the blood specimen by lysis-centrifugation (i.e., Isolator; Wampole Laboratories).

Laboratory Safety

N. meningitidis is classified as a biosafety level 2 organism, which means that a biological safety cabinet must be used for the manipulation of specimens that have a substantial risk for the generation of aerosols (e.g., centrifuging, grinding, and blending). Recent reports of laboratory-acquired meningococcal infections suggest, however, that manipulation of cultures, rather than patient specimens, increases the risk of infection for microbiology laboratory technologists and technicians (17, 21). Such manipulations may include the preparation of heavy organism suspensions for inoculation into identification systems (which often use suspensions corresponding to no. 3 or 4 McFarland standards) and for serogrouping of isolates by slide agglutination. Use of a biological safety cabinet when manipulating cultures for these purposes would ensure protection of the laboratorian from aerosolized organisms. Alternative measures for protection from droplet aerosols, such as the use of splash guards and masks, are currently being assessed. Education and adherence to established laboratory safety precautions should minimize the risk of meningococcal infection for workers in the clinical microbiology laboratory. Laboratory policies should also be developed for situations that may require the administration of chemoprophylaxis to employees who are exposed to meningococci. Laboratories may also consider offering the quadrivalent meningococcal vaccine (which includes serogroups A, C, Y, and W135) to microbiology laboratory staff. Vaccination would decrease, but not eliminate, the potential risk of laboratory-acquired infections.

Direct Examination of Clinical Specimens

A rapid presumptive diagnosis of meningococcal meningitis can be made by direct examination of CSF using the Gram stain. If sufficient CSF (i.e., more than 1 to 2 ml) is received, the specimen should be centrifuged to obtain a pellet of material for examination and culture. Cytocentrifugation of CSF specimens enhances the detection of small numbers of organisms and increases the sensitivity of the Gram stain in comparison with conventionally centrifuged or uncentrifuged specimens. On Gram-stained smears prepared from clinical specimens, meningococci appear as gram-negative diplococci both inside and outside of PMNs. Organisms may display considerable size variation and tend to resist decolorization. Heavily encapsulated strains may have a distinct pink halo around the cells. Because the presence of inflammatory cells has prognostic value (e.g., with fulminant, rapidly fatal disease, many organisms and few inflammatory cells are present), the Gram stain report to the physician should include quantitation of both organisms and PMNs.

Direct tests for detection of meningococcal capsular polysaccharides in CSF, serum, and urine are also available (58). These direct antigen tests use antibody-sensitized latex agglutination or coagglutination to detect capsular antigens of meningococcal serogroups A, B, C, Y, and

W135. The serogroup B reagent also detects the cross-reacting Escherichia coli K1 antigen. These reagents are available from several vendors (BD Biosciences for latex tests; Boule Diagnostics AB for coagglutination tests). A negative test does not rule out meningitis caused by any of the organisms that commonly occur. In addition, false-positive latex agglutination tests may also occur, particularly with urine specimens, resulting in unnecessary treatment and prolonged hospitalization. These tests should always be performed in conjunction with a cytocentrifuged Gram stain and culture on enriched agar media. Due to the enhanced sensitivity of the Gram stain provided by specimen cytocentrifugation and the problems with the specificity of the antigen detection assays, most laboratories in the United States no longer perform these tests routinely.

A recent modification of the manual latex agglutination test involves performance of these assays in the presence of an ultrasonic standing wave. Antibody-coated latex particles suspended in the wave are subjected to physical forces that increase particle-to-particle contact, and enhanced agglutination occurs in the presence of antigen, resulting in increased sensitivity. Ultrasound-enhanced latex agglutination for the detection of meningococcal serogroups A, B, C, Y, and W135 has demonstrated increased sensitivity with CSF specimens without any loss in specificity and has also been used to enhance the detection of meningococcal polysaccharides in serum and to quantitate blood antigen concentrations (40, 85).

Culture and Isolation Procedures

For recovery of N. meningitidis, CSF specimens should be cultured on nonselective chocolate agar and sheep blood agar. Specimens that may harbor other organisms (e.g., oropharyngeal and nasopharyngeal swab specimens) should be inoculated onto both selective (e.g., MTM, ML, NYC, or GC-Lect agar) and nonselective media. Plates are incubated in 5 to 7% CO_2 at 35°C (CO_2 incubator or candle extinction jar) and inspected after 24, 48, and 72 h before a final report of "no growth" is issued. Suspicious colonies are subcultured to blood and chocolate agar for further identification.

Identification

Colony Morphology

Colonies of N. meningitidis are larger than gonococcal colonies, usually attaining a diameter of about 1 mm or more after 18 to 24 h of incubation. The colonies are low and convex, with a smooth, moist entire edge and a glistening surface. On sheep blood agar, colonies are usually gray, and heavily encapsulated strains may be mucoid. The medium beneath and adjacent to the colonies may exhibit a gray-green cast, particularly in areas of confluent growth. Young cultures have a smooth consistency, while older cultures become gummy due to autolysis.

Identification Procedures

N. meningitidis is identified by acid production tests or by chromogenic enzyme substrate tests. Identification procedures for meningococci (and gonococci as well) produce the best results when fresh 18- to 24-h subcultures on chocolate or blood agar are used in carbohydrate acidification tests. N. meningitidis acidifies glucose and maltose but not sucrose, fructose, or lactose (Table 3). In acid production tests, the acidic reaction in the maltose tube may be stronger than that in the glucose tube because maltose is degraded by the organism to two glucose molecules, which are then metabolized. Isolates recovered on selective media can be identified by chromogenic enzyme substrate tests as well. *N. meningitidis* strains produce γ-glutamylaminopeptidase, and some strains also produce prolyl-hydroxyprolyl aminopeptidase. Glucose-negative, maltose-negative, and asaccharolytic *N. meningitidis* strains may also be isolated from time to time. If such biochemically aberrant strains are recovered, chromogenic substrate confirmatory tests or serogrouping of the isolates should be performed.

Serogrouping and Typing

Slide agglutination is the most commonly used technique for serogrouping meningococci. A dense suspension of the organism is prepared in 0.5 to 1.0 ml of phosphate-buffered saline (pH 7.2) from a 12- to 18-h subculture on Trypticase soy blood agar. One drop of this suspension is mixed with 1 drop of meningococcal antisera on a sectored slide, and the slide is rotated for 2 to 4 min. Groupable strains generally agglutinate strongly within this time. Although isolates from systemic infections usually agglutinate rapidly, those from carriers may fail to agglutinate (nongroupable strains) or may autoagglutinate in the phosphate-buffered saline. Use of younger cultures from blood agar (6 to 8 h) or use of a serum-enriched medium, such as Trypticase soy agar containing 10% decomplemented horse serum, may resolve these problems. Antisera for the major meningococcal serogroups are available from BD Biosciences. Some of these nongroupable strains may actually be *N. polysaccharea*; testing for production of polysaccharide from sucrose will help identify this species (see below) (13).

In addition to serogroup determinations, *N. meningitidis* isolates may be serotyped and serosubtyped on the basis of their outer membrane protein and lipooligosaccharide antigens (95). These techniques are used mainly for investigations of epidemics and sporadic outbreaks of disease and are not amenable for use in routine clinical microbiology laboratories. In addition to these serologic techniques, several molecular techniques have been applied to investigations of meningococcal disease and to the epidemiology of *N. meningitidis* strains. These techniques include multilocus enzyme electrophoresis; restriction enzyme fragment length polymorphism analysis; rRNA probe technology (ribotyping); PCR amplicon restriction endonuclease analysis of the chromosomal *dhps* (dihydropteroatesynthase), *pilA-pilB*, and *porA* genes of *N. meningitidis*; and PFGE (71, 95, 96) (see chapters 12 and 17).

Antimicrobial Susceptibility

Despite the occasional recovery of *N. meningitidis* strains with decreased susceptibility to penicillin, penicillin G remains the drug of choice for treatment of meningococcal meningitis (6). Chloramphenicol is an alternative in penicillin-allergic patients. The broad-spectrum cephalosporins (i.e., cefotaxime, ceftriaxone, ceftizoxime, and ceftazidime) reach levels in CSF that may be several hundredfold the MIC for the infecting isolate and are also recommended treatment options. Patients with meningococcal disease also require intensive supportive care and monitoring for detection of complications and disease progression (96). Other biological agents (e.g., antiendotoxin and anticytokine monoclonal antibodies) may also play important roles as adjunctive therapies in the management of meningococcal septic shock.

As in the gonococcus, the antimicrobial susceptibility of *N. meningitidis* strains is also evolving (79). Historically,

penicillin-susceptible strains of *N. meningitidis* have penicillin MICs of ≤0.06 µg/ml, and this has been the case in the United States for many decades. Rare β-lactamase-producing meningococcal isolates have been encountered sporadically since 1983 in Canada, South Africa, and Spain; these isolates have penicillin MICs of >256 µg/ml. Since 1987, β-lactamase-negative *N. meningitidis* strains with penicillin MICs of >0.06 µg/ml have been isolated in Europe, South Africa, and the United States (79). These strains are variously referred to as being relatively resistant to penicillin, moderately susceptible to penicillin, and having diminished susceptibility to penicillin. In Spain, the prevalence of these strains has increased from 0.4% in 1985 to 67% in 1994, and in the United Kingdom, about 9% of strains show decreased susceptibility to penicillin. In 1997, 3 of 90 isolates accumulated at the CDC from 121 cases of reported meningococcal disease were moderately susceptible to penicillin, with penicillin MICs of 0.12 µg/ml (79). Strains with decreased susceptibility to penicillin have penicillin MICs ranging from 0.10 to 1.0 µg/ml, and resistant strains are defined as having penicillin MICs of ≥2 µg/ml. Most of the reported relatively resistant meningococci have belonged to either serogroup B or C. Diminished susceptibility to penicillin is apparently due to decreased binding of penicillin by altered meningococcal cell wall penicillin-binding proteins (PBP2 and PBP3). In the case of the PBP2 proteins, decreased binding of penicillin to the altered binding protein results from a mutation in the nucleotide sequence of the PBP2 gene, *penA*. Similar low-affinity forms of PBP2 are found in penicillin-resistant strains of other *Neisseria* species, including *N. lactamica*, *N. flavescens*, *N. polysaccharea*, and *N. gonorrhoeae* (14). The altered PBP2 found in these *N. meningitidis* strains apparently arose from recombinational events that resulted in the replacement of sequences in the native meningococcal *penA* gene with corresponding genetic material from the commensal *Neisseria* species.

The clinical significance of diminished penicillin susceptibility in *N. meningitidis* is unclear at present. Although both treatment failures and higher rates of complications have been observed in patients infected with relatively resistant strains, the administration of higher doses of penicillin has been clinically effective. Broad-spectrum cephalosporins, such as ceftriaxone and cefotaxime, are active against both susceptible and moderately susceptible *N. meningitidis* strains, but the MICs of some agents (e.g., cefuroxime, aztreonam, and imipenem) may be significantly higher than those for susceptible strains (72).

N. meningitidis strains have also demonstrated resistance to other antimicrobial agents. High-level chloramphenicol resistance has been reported in isolates from France and Vietnam. Fear of the spread of chloramphenicol resistance is justified since the drug is a mainstay of therapy for meningitis in sub-Saharan Africa. High-level resistance to sulfonamides, including trimethoprim-sulfamethoxazole, is widespread and is found commonly among epidemic serogroup A *N. meningitidis* strains. Rifampin resistance has also emerged, even during the administration of rifampin prophylaxis, and is due to alterations in cell membrane permeability or to mutations in the *rpoB* gene coding for the β-subunit of the meningococcal RNA polymerase. In 2000, an *N. meningitidis* strain with decreased susceptibility to ciprofloxacin (MIC, 0.25 µg/ml) was isolated from a patient with invasive meningococcal disease in Australia (83). Susceptible strains have ciprofloxacin MICs of ≤0.03 µg/ml. PCR amplification and sequencing of the *gyrA* gene of this isolate revealed a 3-nucleotide difference from wild type, ciprofloxacin-susceptible strains. Finally, some *N. meningitidis* strains have also acquired the *tet*M tetracycline resistance determinant.

Antimicrobial susceptibility testing of *N. meningitidis* isolates is difficult, and MIC determinations are the methods of choice. Accepted standards and susceptibility breakpoints for *N. meningitidis* are not available, and evaluations of disk diffusion methods using penicillin, oxacillin, ampicillin, and rifampin disks have produced disappointing results (10). Currently, the NCCLS recommends either broth microdilution or agar dilution MIC testing of *N. meningitidis* by using cation-supplemented Mueller-Hinton broth with 2 to 5% laked horse blood or Mueller-Hinton agar with 5% (vol/vol) sheep blood, respectively (67) (see chapter 71). For optimal growth of some *N. meningitidis* strains, this medium may require supplementation with IsoVitaleX (1%) (BD Biosciences) or GCHI enrichment (Remel, Inc.). The E test may also prove valuable in determining the antimicrobial susceptibility of individual meningococcal isolates. Since most clinical microbiology laboratories are not equipped to perform agar dilution tests, isolates from patients who are not responding to appropriate antimicrobial chemotherapy and any presumptively penicillin-resistant isolates should be tested for β-lactamase production with the chromogenic cephalosporin test (Cefinase nitrocefin disks; BD Biosciences) and forwarded to a reference laboratory for agar dilution susceptibility testing.

Evaluation, Interpretation, and Reporting of Results

Meningococci are isolated most frequently from the oro- or nasopharynges of asymptomatic carriers along with other organisms of the normal flora (6). Controversy exists about whether *N. meningitidis* isolated from throat cultures should be reported, since reporting implies that the organism is behaving as a pathogen at that anatomic site and requires treatment. Meningococci recovered from oropharyngeal cultures primarily represent carriage strains. Meningococcal carriage may be transient, intermittent, or chronic, and carriage alone is not predictive of the development of life-threatening disease (95). Invasive meningococcal disease generally occurs in susceptible individuals who become newly infected with a virulent strain as recently as 24 to 48 h prior to the development of symptoms (6, 96). While chemoprophylaxis with either rifampin, ciprofloxacin, or ceftriaxone is recommended for close contacts of individuals with severe disease, treatment of asymptomatic individuals who are meningococcal carriers is not recommended. In addition, unless selective medium is employed, colonies of *N. meningitidis* may not be noticed among the other members of the resident flora. Strains of *N. meningitidis* recovered from CSF, blood, and other normally sterile sites should be identified and reported. Isolates from sputum cultures must be interpreted with regard to clinical presentation and in consultation with clinicians caring for the patient, since the presence of meningococci in sputum may represent oropharyngeal contamination and not the cause of a pneumonic process. Because meningococci may be isolated from anogenital sites infected by gonococci, for medicolegal purposes, it is necessary to identify neisserial isolates from these sites to the species level by using confirmatory tests (24).

OTHER *NEISSERIA* SPECIES

Neisseria lactamica

N. lactamica resembles *N. meningitidis* in colony morphology and was initially thought to be a lactose-positive variant of *N. meningitidis*. This species is resident in the throat and is found more frequently in children than in adults (38). *N. lactamica* grows on selective media and produces acid from glucose, maltose, and lactose (Table 3). ONPG is also hydrolyzed and can be used as a substitute for lactose in the test battery. Some strains of this organism have been reported to cause false-positive reactions with some commercial coagglutination tests (49).

Neisseria cinerea

N. cinerea is part of the commensal flora of the upper respiratory tract and has been isolated from other sites, including the cervix, rectum, conjunctivae, blood, and CSF (31, 32, 57). *N. cinerea* grows on both blood and chocolate agar. On chocolate agar after 24 h of incubation, colonies of *N. cinerea* resemble the large-colony types of *N. gonorrhoeae*, are about 1 mm in diameter, and are smooth with entire edges. The organism does not produce acid from carbohydrates in either CTA-based media or the rapid acid production test (Table 3). Weak positive reactions with glucose after overnight incubation have been reported with some identification systems, and its positive prolyl-hydroxyprolyl aminopeptidase reaction may also result in misidentifications of *N. cinerea* as *N. gonorrhoeae* (32; Janda and Montero, *Abstr. 95th Gen. Meet. Am. Soc. Microbiol. 1995*). Most *N. cinerea* isolates, however, do not grow well on MTM medium or other selective media, which precludes testing of this organism on chromogenic substrate tests such as the BactiCard-Neisseria (Remel, Inc.). *N. cinerea* can be differentiated from the asaccharolytic species *N. flavescens* by its inability to produce polysaccharide from sucrose (see below) and the lack of a discernible yellow pigment. This species can also be separated from *M. catarrhalis*, another asaccharolytic species, by its negative nitrate reduction, DNase, and tributyrin hydrolysis reactions (Table 3).

A helpful test for differentiating *N. cinerea* from *N. gonorrhoeae* is the colistin susceptibility test. A suspension of the organism (MacFarland no. 5 turbidity standard) is prepared in broth and is swabbed onto a chocolate or blood agar plate as for a disk diffusion susceptibility test. A 10-µg colistin disk is placed on the inoculum, and the plate is incubated in CO_2 for 18 to 24 h. *N. cinerea* is colistin susceptible and produces a zone that is larger than or equal to 10 mm around the disk. Generally, *N. gonorrhoeae* grows up to the edge of the disk.

Neisseria flavescens

N. flavescens is found in the respiratory tract and is rarely associated with infectious processes. This organism grows as smooth, yellowish colonies on both blood and chocolate agar and grows on nutrient agar at 35°C. Most strains also grow at room temperature on chocolate or blood agar. This organism is able to synthesize iodine-positive polysaccharides from sucrose (see below) and can be differentiated from *M. catarrhalis* by its inability to reduce nitrate and its negative DNase and tributyrin hydrolysis reactions.

Neisseria subflava Biovars, *Neisseria mucosa*, and *Neisseria sicca*

N. subflava, *N. mucosa*, and *N. sicca* form part of the normal human upper respiratory tract flora and are occasional isolates from infectious processes, including endocarditis, bacteremia, meningitis, empyema, pericarditis, and pneumonia. Identification of the "nonpathogenic" *Neisseria* species is not generally necessary unless the organism is determined to be clinically significant or is isolated from a systemic site (e.g., blood or CSF) or in pure culture. Identification is based on colony morphology, growth on simple nutrient media, inability to grow on selective media, acid production from carbohydrates, reduction of nitrate and nitrite, and synthesis of a starch-like, iodine-staining polysaccharide from sucrose. Nitrate reduction and nitrite reduction are determined in medium (Trypticase soy or heart infusion broth) containing 0.1% (wt/vol) KNO_3 and 0.01% (wt/vol) KNO_2, respectively. Polysaccharide synthesis is determined by inoculating the organism onto brain heart infusion agar containing 1% sucrose. Medium lacking sucrose is inoculated as a negative control. After incubation at 35°C for 48 h, the plates are flooded with Gram's or Lugol's iodine (1:4 dilution). A positive test is indicated by the development of a deep blue color in and around the colonies synthesizing the polysaccharide. Good results may also be obtained by adding regular Gram's iodine (1 or 2 drops) to the sucrose-containing tube in the rapid carbohydrate degradation technique after 4 h of incubation. If the test is positive, a deep blue color appears in the tube. This is compared with the tan color seen in the other carbohydrate tubes (e.g., the maltose tube) after addition of Gram's iodine.

Strains of *N. subflava* can be subdivided into three biovars (biovars subflava, flava, and perflava) on the basis of acid production from fructose and sucrose and synthesis of iodine-positive polysaccharide from sucrose (Table 3). All three biovars reduce nitrite but not nitrate. *N. mucosa* has a carbohydrate utilization pattern similar to *N. subflava* bv. perflava and also produces the iodine-positive polysaccharide, but *N. mucosa* is able to reduce both nitrate and nitrite to N_2 gas. All of these organisms also display various degrees of yellow pigmentation. The *N. sicca* strains are biochemically identical to *N. subflava* bv. perflava, but they characteristically form dry (desiccated), adherent, leathery colonies on agar media that cannot be emulsified readily.

Neisseria polysaccharea

N. polysaccharea is found in the human oropharynx. This organism is an oxidase-positive, catalase-positive, gram-negative diplococcus that forms smooth yellow colonies (77). In the orginal description of this organism, the ability to grow on selective media (e.g., MTM agar) was a key characteristic. Subsequent studies indicate, however, that growth on selective media for the pathogenic *Neisseria* species is a variable characteristic of *N. polysaccharea* because of the colistin susceptibility of some strains (4). The organisms are resistant to vancomycin. After 24 h of growth, *N. polysaccharea* forms colonies about 2 mm in diameter on chocolate or blood agar. Acid is produced from glucose and maltose but not from fructose or lactose. Acid production from sucrose is variable and appears to depend on the types of media used to determine this characteristic. *N. polysaccharea* possesses an amylosucrase that synthesizes an acidic extracellular polysaccharide from sucrose. Production of various amounts of the material by different strains may explain the variable nature of the sucrose reaction. Nitrate is not reduced, whereas nitrite frequently is reduced. *N. polysaccharea* can be differentiated from *N. meningitidis* by polysaccharide synthesis and the γ-glutamylaminopeptidase tests. *N. polysaccharea* produces iodine-positive polysaccharide

from sucrose and is γ-glutamylaminopeptidase negative, whereas *N. meningitidis* does not produce iodine-positive polysaccharide from sucrose and is γ-glutamylaminopeptidase positive. Like *N. gonorrhoeae*, *N. lactamica*, and some *N. meningitidis* strains, *N. polysaccharea* is L-hydroxyprolylaminopeptidase positive (4). The organism requires cysteine for growth and does not grow on nutrient agar or on chocolate agar at 22°C.

Neisseria elongata Subspecies

N. elongata subspecies *elongata*, *glycolytica*, and *nitroreducens* are rod-shaped members of the genus *Neisseria*. The first two subspecies were recognized in the last edition of *Bergey's Manual of Systematic Bacteriology* as *Neisseria* species, whereas the last subspecies, formerly known as CDC group M-6, was recently reclassified in the genus. All subspecies are members of the human upper respiratory tract flora, and all have been isolated from infectious processes. These subspecies can be differentiated on the basis of catalase reactivity, acid production from glucose, and reduction of nitrate (Table 3).

Neisseria gonorrhoeae Subspecies kochii ("Neisseria kochii")

In 1986, seven isolates of an unusual *Neisseria* species were recovered from conjunctival cultures of children in two rural villages in Egypt (64). These isolates grew on chocolate agar and MTM medium and produced large, smooth colonies resembling meningococci. Like *N. gonorrhoeae*, these isolates required the amino acid cysteine for growth. The isolates were oxidase positive, produced acid from glucose only, and were γ-glutamylaminopeptidase negative. They did not react with fluorescent gonococcal monoclonal antibody reagents and failed to react with monoclonal coagglutination reagents used for serovar determinations for *N. gonorrhoeae*. These strains also had different surface proteins from the gonococcal strains to which they were compared. Plasmid analysis showed significant homology to plasmids commonly found in gonococcal strains. DNA homology experiments showed similarity to both *N. gonorrhoeae* and *N. meningitidis*; on this basis, the workers felt that these isolates did not represent a new species but, rather, a subspecies of *N. gonorrhoeae*. Since these isolates would probably be identified as *N. gonorrhoeae* in a clinical laboratory and since their site of isolation and their carbohydrate utilization pattern were similar to those associated with gonococci, these isolates have been named *N. gonorrhoeae* subsp. *kochii* or "*N. kochii*" (64).

Nonhuman Neisseria Species

On occasion, the clinical microbiology laboratory may recover *Neisseria* and *Moraxella* species of animal origin from human infections, such as bite wounds from animals. Isolates may include *N. canis*, *N. weaveri*, *N. denitrificans*, *N. macacae*, and the coccal moraxellae, *M. caviae* and *M. cuniculi*. All of these organisms exhibit typical gram-negative diplococcal morphology except for *N. weaveri*, which is a gram-negative rod. Like *M. catarrhalis*, the coccal moraxellae isolated from animals are asaccharolytic and hydrolyze tributyrin (Table 4).

MORAXELLA CATARRHALIS

Specimen Collection and Transport

For the diagnosis of otitis media and sinusitis, the specimens of choice are tympanocentesis fluid and sinus aspirates,

TABLE 4 Characteristics of *Neisseria* species and the coccal *Moraxella* species of animal origin[a]

Species	Cell morphology	Acid from:				Reduction of:		Polysaccharide from sucrose	Tributyrin hydrolysis
		Glucose	Maltose	Sucrose	Lactose	NO₃	NO₂		
N. canis	Diplococcus	0	0	0	0	+	0	0	0
N. macacae	Diplococcus	+	+	+	+	0	+	+	0
N. weaveri	Rod	0	0	0	0	0	+	NT	NT
N. iguanae	Diplococcus	V	0	0	NT	+	V	+	NT
M. caviae	Diplococcus	0	0	0	0	+	+	NT	+
M. cuniculi	Diplococcus	0	0	0	0	0	0	NT	+

[a] +, positive reaction; 0, negative reaction; V, variable reaction; NT, not tested.

respectively. However, these specimens are rarely submitted due to the difficulty of collection and the attendant discomfort to the patient. In patients with respiratory tract infections, M. catarrhalis may be recovered from expectorated sputum specimens. First morning, coughed sputum specimens are collected and sent to the laboratory as quickly as possible.

Direct Examination

Gram-stained smears of sputum from patients with M. catarrhalis lower respiratory tract infections (i.e., pneumonia or bronchitis) usually show numerous PMNs, mucus, and large numbers of extracellular gram-negtive diplococci measuring about 0.5 to 1.5 μm in diameter. A similar Gram stain appearance is seen on smears made from middle ear fluid and sinus aspirates.

Isolation and Identification

M. catarrhalis grows well on both blood and chocolate agars, and some strains also grow well on MTM and other selective media. Colonies are generally gray to white, opaque, and smooth and measure about 1 to 3 mm after 24 h of incubation. Characteristically, the colonies may be nudged across the plate intact with a bacteriological loop like a "hockey puck." Gram-stained smears from colonies show uniform gram-negative diplococci measuring 0.5 to 1.5 μm in diameter. M. catarrhalis is strongly oxidase positive and catalase positive. The organism does not produce acid from glucose or other carbohydrates and may actually turn peptone-based identification media alkaline. Most strains reduce nitrate and nitrite and produce DNase (Table 3). DNase activity is detected by heavily spot-inoculating on an area the size of a dime a plate of DNase test medium containing toluidine blue. After overnight incubation, hydrolysis of the DNA is detected by a change from blue to pink in the color of the medium around and under the inoculum. Staphylococcus aureus and S. epidermidis are also inoculated onto the plate as positive and negative DNase test controls, respectively.

M. catarrhalis may also be distinguished from Neisseria species by its ability to hydrolyze ester-linked butyrate groups (butyrate esterase) (88). This enzyme activity is detected with a substrate called tributyrin. A very rapid (2.5-min) and reliable indoxyl-butyrate hydrolysis spot test has also been described and is commercially available (Remel Inc.; Carr-Scarbourough, Stone Mountain, Ga.) (25). This test is also included on the BactiCard-Neisseria along with the three other chromogenic substrates for Neisseria identification (Janda and Montero, Abstr. 95th Gen. Meet. Am. Soc. Microbiol. 1995). The RapID NH system also contains a fatty acid ester hydrolysis test to assist in the

identification of M. catarrhalis. Indoxyl acetate, which is used for the identification of Campylobacter species, can also be used as a substrate for the esterase enzyme of M. catarrhalis (88). In addition, most clinically significant M. catarrhalis strains produce an inducible, cell-associated β-lactamase. Because of its inducible nature, rapid acidometric β-lactamase tests (i.e., those that rely on conversion of hydrolysis of penicillin to penicilloic acid) may yield false-negative results. The best results are obtained with the chromogenic cephalosporin (nitrocefin) test.

Typing Methods

With the recognition of M. catarrhalis as a primary pathogen in certain clinical settings and the knowledge that nosocomial infections have been documented, methods for strain typing have been investigated. These methods include enzymatic biotyping, polyacrylamide gel electrophoresis of whole-cell proteins, immunoblotting, PFGE, and restriction fragment length polymorphism endonuclease analysis (63). These methods have been applied to investigations of outbreaks of respiratory tract disease in critical-care units. Two DNA typing methods, probe-generated restriction fragment length polymorphism analysis and single-adaptor modified fragment polymorphism analysis, were recently used to demonstrate the existence of two subgroups within M. catarrhalis that may actually represent separate subspecies (11).

Antimicrobial Susceptibility

At present, most clinical isolates of M. catarrhalis produce β-lactamase enzymes. Two types of enzymes, BRO-1 (or Ravisio-type) and BRO-2 (or 1908-type), have been identified and can be differentiated by isoelectric focusing (12, 76). Strains that produce BRO-1 enzymes account for more than 90% of the β-lactamase-producing M. catarrhalis organisms isolated from clinical specimens, while BRO-2-producing strains account for the remaining isolates. M. catarrhalis strains that possess the BRO-1-type enzyme possess significantly greater enzymatic activity than do isolates that produce the BRO-2 enzyme. The latter strains may also have penicillin and ampicillin MICs that fall in the susceptible range when tested by microbroth dilution methods. Patients who have been infected with BRO-2 β-lactamase-producing M. catarrhalis strains have also responded clinically to ampicillin and penicillin. M. catarrhalis strains should be tested for β-lactamase production, preferably with the chromogenic cephalosporin test (Cefinase nitrocefin disks; BD Biosciences). NCCLS-approved performance standards for susceptibility testing of M. catarrhalis are not available.

Isolates of M. *catarrhalis* are generally susceptible to amoxicillin-clavulanate, expanded-spectrum and broad-spectrum cephalosporins (i.e., cefuroxime, cefotaxime, ceftriaxone, cefpodoxime, ceftibuten, and the oral agents cefixime and cefaclor), macrolides (i.e., azithromycin, clarithromycin, erythromycin), tetracyclines, and rifampin. While most isolates are susceptible to the fluoroquinolones, resistance to these agents has emerged in isolates recovered from patients who were receiving long-term therapy with such agents. Rare strains of M. *catarrhalis* may be resistant to tetracyclines, macrolides, or trimethoprim-sulfamethoxazole.

Evaluation, Interpretation, and Reporting of Results

The pathogenesis of M. *catarrhalis* sinusitis and otitis media involves contiguous spread of the organisms from a colonizing focus in the respiratory tract (50). However, isolation of M. *catarrhalis* from the upper respiratory tract (i.e., a throat culture) of children with otitis media or sinusitis does not provide evidence that the isolate is the cause of these infections. Rates of upper respiratory tract colonization by M. *catarrhalis* in children vary widely and are influenced by many factors (both environmental and genetic). The presence of the organism in the oropharynx or nasopharynx is not necessarily predictive of infection in contiguous anatomic sites. Isolates from sinus aspirates and middle ear specimens obtained by tympanocentesis should be identified and reported. Similarly, little is known about the pathogenesis of lower respiratory tract infection in adults with chronic lung diseases. Examination of Gram-stained smears of sputum specimens from patients with exacerbations of bronchitis and pneumonia due to M. *catarrhalis* usually reveals an abundance of leukocytes, the presence of many gram-negative diplococci as the exclusive or predominant bacterial morphotype, and the presence of intracellular gram-negative diplococci. Such specimens may yield M. *catarrhalis* in virtually pure culture, and the organism should be identified and reported. M. *catarrhalis* should also be identified and reported when recovered from normally sterile body fluids (e.g., blood).

REFERENCES

1. **Abuhammour, W. M., N. M. Abdel-Haq, B. I. Asmar, and A. S. Dajani.** 1999. *Moraxella catarrhalis* bacteremia: a 10-year experience. *South. Med. J.* **92:**1071–1074.
2. **Ala'Aldeen, D. A. A., K. R. Neal, K. Ait-Tahar, J. S. Nguyen-Van-Tam, A. English, T. J. Falla, P. M. Hawkey, and R. C. Slack.** 2000. Dynamics of meningococcal long-term carriage among university students and their implications for mass vaccination. *J. Clin. Microbiol.* **38:**2311–2316.
3. **American Academy of Pediatrics Committee on Child Abuse and Neglect.** 1998. Gonorrhea in prepubertal children. *Pediatrics* **101:**134–135.
4. **Anand, C. M., F. Ashton, H. Shaw, and R. Gordon.** 1991. Variability in growth of *Neisseria polysaccharea* on colistin-containing selective media for *Neisseria* spp. *J. Clin. Microbiol.* **29:**2434–2437.
5. **Andersen B. M., A. G. Steigerwalt, S. P. O'Connor, D. G. Hollis, R. S. Weyant, R. E. Weaver, and D. J. Brenner.** 1993. *Neisseria weaveri* sp. nov., formerly CDC group M-5, a gram-negative bacterium associated with dog bite wounds. *J. Clin. Microbiol.* **31:**2456–2466.
6. **Apicella, M. A.** 2000. *Neisseria meningitidis*, p. 2228–2241. *In* G. L. Mandell, J. E. Bennett, and R. Dolin (ed.), *Mandell, Douglas, and Bennett's Principles and Practice of Infectious Diseases*, 5th ed. Churchill-Livingstone, Inc., Philadelphia, Pa.
7. **Barbe, G., M. Babolet, J. M. Boeufgras, D. Monget, and J. Freney.** 1994. Evaluation of API NH, a new 2-hour system for identification of *Neisseria* and *Haemophilus* species and *Moraxella catarrhalis* in a routine clinical laboratory. *J. Clin. Microbiol.* **32:**187–189.
8. **Beverly, A., J. R. Bailey-Griffin, and J. R. Schwebke.** 2000. InTray GC medium versus modified Thayer-Martin agar plates for diagnosis of gonorrhea from endocervical specimens. *J. Clin. Microbiol.* **38:**3825–3826.
9. **Billings, S. D., D. Fuller, A. M. LeMonte, T. E. Davis, and A. L. Hartstein.** 1997. Characterization of DFA-negative, probe-positive *Neisseria gonorrhoeae* by pulsed field electrophoresis. *Diagn. Microbiol. Infect. Dis.* **29:**281–283.
10. **Block, C., Y. Davidson, and N. Keller.** 1998. Unreliability of disc diffusion test for screening for reduced penicillin susceptibility in *Neisseria meningitidis*. *J. Clin. Microbiol.* **36:**3103–3104.
11. **Bootsma, H. J., H. G. van der Heide, S. van de Pas, L. M. Schouls, and L. M. Mooi.** 2000. Analysis of *Moraxella catarrhalis* by DNA typing: evidence for a distinct subpopulation associated with virulence traits. *J. Infect. Dis.* **181:**1376–1387.
12. **Bootsma, H. J., H. van Dijk, J. Verhoef, A. Fleer, and F. R. Mooi.** 1996. Molecular characterization of the BRO beta-lactamase of *Moraxella (Branhamella) catarrhalis*. *Antimicrob. Agents Chemother.* **40:**966–972.
13. **Boquete, M. T., C. Marcos, and J. A. Saez-Nieto.** 1986. Characterization of *Neisseria polysaccharea* sp. nov. (Riou, 1983) in previously identified noncapsulated strains of *Neisseria meningitidis*. *J. Clin. Microbiol.* **23:**973–975.
14. **Bowler, L. D., Q.-Y. Zhang, J.-Y. Riou, and B. G. Spratt.** 1994. Interspecies recombination between the *penA* genes of *Neisseria meningitidis* and commensal *Neisseria* species during the emergence of penicillin resistance in *N. meningitidis*: natural events and laboratory simulation. *J. Bacteriol.* **176:**333–337.
15. **Catlin, B. W.** 1975. Cellular elongation under the influence of antibacterial agents: way to differentiate coccobacilli from cocci. *J. Clin. Microbiol.* **1:**102–105.
16. **Centers for Disease Control and Prevention.** 1998. 1998 sexually transmitted diseases treatment guidelines. *Morb. Mortal. Wkly. Rep.* **47:**59–63.
17. **Centers for Disease Control and Prevention.** 1999. *Biosafety in Microbiological and Biomedical Laboratories*, 4th ed. U.S. Department of Health and Human Services, Atlanta, Ga.
18. **Centers for Disease Control and Prevention.** 2000. Fluoroquinolone-resistance in *Neisseria gonorrhoeae*, Hawaii, 1999, and decreased susceptibility to azithromycin in *N. gonorrhoeae*, Missouri, 1999. *Morb. Mortal. Wkly. Rep.* **49:**833.
19. **Centers for Disease Control and Prevention.** 2000. *Gonococcal Isolate Surveillance Project.* [Online.] Centers for Disease Control and Prevention, Atlanta, Ga. http://www.cdc.gov/ncidod/dastlr/gcdir/Resist/gisp.html.
20. **Centers for Disease Control and Prevention.** 2000. *2000 Sexually Transmitted Disease Surveillance. Gonococcal Isolate Surveillance Project (GISP) Supplement.* [Online.] Centers for Disease Control and Prevention, Atlanta, Ga. http://www.cdc.gov/nchstp/dstd/Stats_Trends/Stats_and_Trends.htm.
21. **Centers for Disease Control and Prevention.** 2002. Laboratory-acquired meningococcal disease—United States, 2000. *Morb. Mortal. Wkly. Rep.* **71:**141–144.
22. **Chernesky, M. A.** 1999. Nucleic acid tests for the diagnosis of sexually transmitted diseases. *FEMS Immunol. Med. Microbiol.* **24:**437–446.

23. Crotchfelt, K. A., L. E. Welsh, D. DeBonville, M. Rosenstraus, and T. C. Quinn. 1997. Detection of *Neisseria gonorrhoeae* and *Chlamydia trachomatis* in genitourinary specimens from men and women by a coamplification PCR assay. *J. Clin. Microbiol.* **35:**1536–1540.

24. D'Antuono, A., F. Andalo, and C. Varotti. 1999. Acute urethritis due to *Neisseria meningitidis*. *Sex. Transm. Dis.* **75:**362.

25. Dealler, S. F., M. Abbott, M. J. Croughan, and P. M. Hawkey. 1989. Identification of *Branhamella catarrhalis* in 2.5 min with an indoxyl butyrate strip test. *J. Clin. Microbiol.* **27:**1390–1391.

26. Deguchi, T., M. Yasuda, M. Nakano, S. Ozeki, T. Ezaki, I. Saito, and Y. Kawada. 1996. Quinolone-resistant *Neisseria gonorrhoeae*: correlations of alterations in the GyrA subunit of DNA gyrase and the ParC subunit of topoisomerase IV with antimicrobial susceptibility profiles. *Antimicrob. Agents Chemother.* **40:**1020–1023.

27. Dewhirst, F. E., B. J. Paster, and B. L. Bright. 1989. *Chromobacterium, Eikenella, Kingella, Neisseria, Simonsiella,* and *Vitreoscilla* species comprise a major branch of the β-subgroup of the *Protobacteria* by 16S ribosomal nucleic acid sequence comparison: transfer of *Eikenella* and *Simonsiella* to the Family *Neisseriaceae* (emend.). *Int. J. Syst. Bacteriol.* **39:**258–266.

28. Dillon, J. R., M. Carballo, and M. Pauze. 1988. Evaluation of eight methods for identification of pathogenic *Neisseria* species: *Neisseria*-Kwik, RIM-N, Gonobio Test, Gonochek II, GonoGen, Phadebact GC OMNI test, and Syva MicroTrak test. *J. Clin. Microbiol.* **26:**493–497.

29. Division of STD Prevention. 1995. *Sexually Transmitted Diseases Surveillance, 1994.* U.S. Department of Health and Human Services, Public Health Service, Atlanta, Ga.

30. Dolter, J., L. Bryant, and J. M. Janda. 1990. Evaluation of five rapid systems for the identification of *Neisseria gonorrhoeae*. *Diagn. Microbiol. Infect. Dis.* **13:**265–267.

31. Dolter, J., J. Wong, and J. M. Janda. 1998. Association of *Neisseria cinerea* with ocular infections in paediatric patients. *J. Infect.* **36:**49–52.

32. Dossett, J. H., P. C. Applebaum, J. S. Knapp, and P. S. Totten. 1985. Proctitis associated with *Neisseria cinerea* misidentified as *Neisseria gonorrhoeae* in a child. *J. Clin. Microbiol.* **21:**575–577.

33. Ellison, R. T., III, J. G. Curd, P. F. Kohler, L. B. Reller, and F. N. Judson. 1987. Underlying complement deficiency in patients with disseminated gonococcal infection. *Sex. Transm. Dis.* **14:**201–204.

34. Farhat, S. E., M Thibault, and R. Devlin. 2001. Efficacy of a swab transport system in maintaining viability of *Neisseria gonorrhoeae* and *Streptococcus pneumoniae*. *J. Clin. Microbiol.* **39:**2958–2960.

35. Farrell, D. J. 1999. Evaluation of AMPLICOR *Neisseria gonorrhoeae* PCR using cppB nested PCR and 16S rRNA PCR. *J. Clin. Microbiol.* **37:**386–390.

36. Feliciano, R., W. Swedler, and J. Varga. 1999. Infection with uncommon subgroup Y *Neisseria meningitidis* in patients with systemic lupus erythematosus. *Clin. Exp. Rheumatol.* **17:**737–740.

37. Fijen, C. A. P., E. J. Kuijper, H. G. Tija, M. R. Daha, and J. Dankert. 1994. Complement deficiency predisposes for meningitis due to non-groupable meningococci and *Neisseria*-related bacteria. *Clin. Infect. Dis.* **18:**780–784.

38. Gold, R., I. Goldschneider, M. L. Lepow, T. F. Draper, and M. Randolph. 1978. Carriage of *Neisseria meningitidis* and *Neisseria lactamica* in infants and children. *J. Infect. Dis.* **137:**112–121.

39. Grant, P. E., D. J. Brenner, A. G. Steigerwalt, D. G. Hollis, and R. E. Weaver. 1990. *Neisseria elongata* subsp. *nitroreducens* subsp. nov., formerly CDC group M-6, a

gram-negative bacterium associated with endocarditis. *J. Clin. Microbiol.* **28:**2591–2596.

40. Gray, S. J., M. A. Sobanski, E. B. Kaczmarski, M. Guiver, W. J. Marsh, R. Borrow, R. A. Barnes, and W. T. Coakley. 1999. Ultrasound-enhanced latex immunoagglutination and PCR as complementary methods for non-culture-based confirmation of meningococcal disease. *J. Clin. Microbiol.* **37:**1797–1801.

41. Gronowski, A. M., S. Copper, D. Baorto, and P. R. Murray. 2000. Reproducibility problems with the Abbott laboratories LCx assay for *Chlamydia trachomatis* and *Neisseria gonorrhoeae*. *J. Clin. Microbiol.* **38:**2416–2418.

42. Handsfield, H. H., Z. A. Dalu, D. H. Martin, J. M. Douglas, Jr., J. M. McCarty, D. Schlossberg, and the Azithromycin Gonorrhea Study Group. 1994. Multicenter trial of single-dose azithromycin vs. ceftriaxone in the treatment of uncomplicated gonorrhea. *Sex. Transm. Dis.* **21:**107–111.

43. Hook, E. W., III, S. F. Ching, J. Stephens, K. F. Hardy, K. R. Smith, and H. H. Lee. 1997. Diagnosis of *Neisseria gonorrhoeae* infections in women by using the ligase chain reaction on patient-obtained vaginal swabs. *J. Clin. Microbiol.* **35:**2129–2132.

44. Hook, E. W., and H. H. Handsfield. 1999. Gonococcal infections in the adult, p. 451–466. *In* K. K. Holmes, P.-A. Mardh, P. F. Sparling, S. M. Lemon, W. E. Stamm, P. Piot, and J. Wasserheit (ed.), *Sexually Transmitted Diseases*, 3rd ed. McGraw-Hill Book Co., New York, N.Y.

45. Ison, C. A., N. Tekki, and M. J. Gill. 1993. Detection of the tetM determinant in *Neisseria gonorrhoeae*. *Sex. Transm. Dis.* **20:**329–333.

46. Jacoby, H. M., and B. J. Mady. 1995. Acute gonococcal sepsis in an HIV-infected woman. *Sex. Transm. Dis.* **22:**380–382.

47. Janda, W. M., J. J. Bradna, and P. Ruther. 1989. Identification of *Neisseria* spp., *Haemophilus* spp., and other fastidious gram-negative bacteria with the MicroScan *Haemophilus-Neisseria* identification panel. *J. Clin. Microbiol.* **27:**869–873.

48. Janda, W. M., P. J. Malloy, and P. C. Schreckenberger. 1987. Clinical evaluation of the Vitek *Neisseria-Haemophilus* identification card. *J. Clin. Microbiol.* **25:**37–41.

49. Janda, W. M., L. M. Wilcoski, K. L. Mandel, P. Ruther, and J. M. Stevens. 1993. Comparison of monoclonal antibody-based methods and a ribosomal ribonucleic acid probe test for *Neisseria gonorrhoeae* culture confirmation. *Eur. J. Clin. Microbiol. Infect. Dis.* **12:**177–184.

50. Karalus, R., and A. Campagnari. 2000. *Moraxella catarrhalis*: a review of an important human mucosal pathogen. *Microbes Infect.* **2:**547–559.

51. Kellogg, J. A., and L. K. Orwig. 1995. Comparison of GonoGen, GonoGen II, and MicroTrak direct fluorescent antibody test with carbohydrate fermentation for confirmation of culture isolates of *Neisseria gonorrhoeae*. *J. Clin. Microbiol.* **33:**474–476.

52. Kluytmans, J. A., H. G. Niesters, J. W. Mouton, W. G. Quint, J. A. Ijpelaar, J. H. VanRijsoort-Vos, L. Habbema, E. Stolz, M. F. Michel, and J. H. Wagenvoort. 1991. Performance of a nonisotopic DNA probe for detection of *Chlamydia trachomatis* in urogenital specimens. *J. Clin. Microbiol.* **29:**2685–2689.

53. Knapp, J. S. 1988. Historical perspectives and identification of *Neisseria* and related species. *Clin. Microbiol. Rev.* **1:**415–431.

54. Knapp, J. S., and V. L. Clark. 1984. Anaerobic growth of *Neisseria gonorrhoeae* coupled to nitrite reduction. *Infect. Immun.* **46:**176–181.

55. **Knapp, J. S., K. K. Fox, D. L. Trees, and W. L. Whittington.** 1997. Fluoroquinolone resistance in *Neisseria gonorrhoeae*. *Emerg. Infect. Dis.* **24:**142–148.

56. **Knapp, J. S., and K. K. Holmes.** 1975. Disseminated gonococcal infections caused by *Neisseria gonorrhoeae* with unique nutritional requirements. *J. Infect. Dis.* **132:**204–208.

57. **Knapp, J. S., P. A. Totten, M. H. Mulks, and B. H. Minshew.** 1984. Characterization of *Neisseria cinerea*, a non-pathogenic species isolated on Martin-Lewis medium selective for pathogenic *Neisseria* spp. *J. Clin. Microbiol.* **19:**63–67.

58. **Kurzynski, T. A., J. L. Kimball, and M. B. Polyak.** 1985. Evaluation of the Phadebact and Bactigen for detection of *Neisseria meningitidis* in cerebrospinal fluid. *J. Clin. Microbiol.* **21:**989–990.

59. **Lafferty, W., J. P. Hughes, and H. H. Handsfield.** 1997. Sexually transmitted diseases among men who have sex with men: Acquisition of gonorrhea and non-gonococcal urethritis by fellatio and implications for STD/HIV prevention. *Sex. Transm. Dis.* **24:**272–278.

60. **Lauer, B. A., and H. B. Masters.** 1988. Toxic effects of calcium alginate swabs on *Neisseria gonorrhoeae*. *J. Clin. Microbiol.* **26:**54–56.

61. **Malhotra, R., Q. N. Karim, and J. F. Acheson.** 1998. Hospital-acquired gonococcal conjunctivitis. *J. Infect.* **37:**305–312.

62. **Martin, D. H., C. Cammarata, B. Van der Pol, R. B. Jones, T. C. Quinn, C. A. Gaydos, K. Crotchfelt, J. Schachter, J. Moncada, D. Jungkind, B. Turner, and C. Peyton.** 2000. Multicenter evaluation of AMPLICOR and automated COBAS AMPLICOR CT/NG tests for *Neisseria gonorrhoeae*. *J. Clin. Microbiol.* **38:**3544–3549.

63. **Martinez, G., K. Ahmed, C. H. Zheng, K. Watanabe, K. Oishi, and T. Nagatake.** 1999. DNA restriction patterns produced by pulsed-field gel electrophoresis in *Moraxella catarrhalis* isolated from different geographical areas. *Epidemiol. Infect.* **122:**417–422.

64. **Mazloum, H., P. A. Totten, G. F. Brooks, C. R. Dawson, S. Falkow, J. S. Knapp, J. M. Koomey, C. J. Lammel, D. Peters, J. Schachter, W. S. Tang, and N. A. Vedros.** 1986. An unusual *Neisseria* isolated from conjunctival cultures in rural Egypt. *J. Infect. Dis.* **154:**212–224.

65. **Minshew, B. H., J. L. Beardsley, and J. S. Knapp.** 1985. Evaluation of GonoGen coagglutination test for serodiagnosis of *Neisseria gonorrhoeae*: identification of problem isolates by auxotyping, serotyping, and with a fluorescent antibody reagent. *Diagn. Microbiol. Infect. Dis.* **3:**41–46.

66. **Modarress, K. J., A. P. Cullen, W. J. S. Jaffurs, G. L. Troutman, N. Mousavi, R. A. Hubbard, S. Henderson, and A. T. Lorincz.** 1999. Detection of *Chlamydia trachomatis* and *Neisseria gonorrhoeae* in swab specimens by the Hybrid Capture II and PACE 2 nucleic acid probe tests. *Sex. Transm. Dis.* **26:**303–308.

67. **National Committee for Clinical Laboratory Standards.** 2001. *Methods for Dilution Antimicrobial Susceptibility Tests for Bacteria That Grow Aerobically.* Approved standard M7-A5. National Committee for Clinical Laboratory Standards, Wayne, Pa.

68. **Olsen, C. C., J. R. Schwebke, W. H. Benjamin, Jr., A. Beverly, and B. Waites.** 1999. Comparison of direct inoculation and Copan transport systems for isolation of *Neisseria gonorrhoeae* from endocervical specimens. *J. Clin. Microbiol.* **37:**3583–3585.

69. **O'Rourke, M., C. A. Ison, A. M. Renton, and B. G. Spratt.** 1995. Opa-typing: a high-resolution tool for studying the epidemiology of gonorrhoea. *Mol. Microbiol.* **17:**865–875.

70. **Palmer, H. M., and C. Arnold.** 2001. Genotyping *Neisseria gonorrhoeae* using fluorescent amplified fragment length polymorphism analysis. *J. Clin. Microbiol.* **39:**2325–2329.

71. **Peixuan, Z., H. Xujing, and X. Li.** 1995. Typing *Neisseria meningitidis* by analysis of restriction fragment length polymorphisms in the gene encoding the class 1 outer membrane protein: application to assessment of epidemics through the last four decades in China. *J. Clin. Microbiol.* **33:**458–462.

72. **Perez-Trallero, E., J. M. Garcia-Arenzana, I. Ayestaran, and J. Munoz-Baroja.** 1989. Comparative activity in vitro of 16 antimicrobial agents against penicillin-susceptible meningococci and meningococci with diminished susceptibility to penicillin. *Antimicrob. Agents Chemother.* **33:**1622–1623.

73. **Pettersson, B., A. Kodjo, M. Ronaghi, M. Uhlen, and T. Tonjum.** 1998. Phylogeny of the family *Moraxellaceae* by 16S rDNA sequence analysis, with special emphasis on differentiation of *Moraxella* species. *Int. J. Syst. Evol. Microbiol.* **48:**75–89.

74. **Poh, C. L., G. K. Loh, and J. W. Tapsall.** 1995. Resolution of clonal subgroups among *Neisseria gonorrhoeae* IB-2 and IB-6 serovars by pulsed-field gel electrophoresis. *Genitourin. Med.* **71:**145–149.

75. **Rice, R. J., and J. S. Knapp.** 1994. Comparative in vitro activities of penicillin G, amoxicillin-clavulanic acid, selected cephalosporins and quinolone antimicrobial agents against representative resistance phenotypes of *Neisseria gonorrhoeae*. *Antimicrob. Agents Chemother.* **38:**155–158.

76. **Richter, S. S., P. L. Winokur, A. B. Brueggemann, H. K. Huynh, R. R. Rhomberg, E. M. Wingert, and G. V. Doern.** 2000. Molecular characterization of the beta-lactamases from clinical isolates of *Moraxella* (*Branhamella*) *catarrhalis* obtained from 24 U.S. medical centers during 1994-1995 and 1997-1998. *Antimicrob. Agents Chemother.* **44:**444–446.

77. **Riou, J.-Y., and M. Guibourdenche.** 1987. *Neisseria polysaccharea* sp. nov. *Int. J. Syst. Bacteriol.* **37:**163–165.

78. **Rompalo, A. M.** 1999. Diagnosis and treatment of sexually acquired proctitis and proctocolitis: an update. *Clin. Infect. Dis.* **28**(Suppl.)**:**S84–S90.

79. **Rosenstein, N. E., S. A. Stocker, T. Popovic, F. C. Tenover, and B. A. Perkins.** 2000. Antimicrobial resistance of *Neisseria meningitidis* in the U.S., 1997. *Clin. Infect. Dis.* **30:**212–213.

80. **Rotta, A. T., B. I. Asmar, N. Ballal, and A. Canady.** 1995. *Moraxella catarrhalis* ventriculitis in a child with hydrocephalus and an external ventricular drain. *Pediatr. Infect. Dis. J.* **14:**397–398.

81. **Saginur, R., B. Clecner, J. Portnoy, and J. Mendelson.** 1982. Superoxol (catalase) test for identification of *Neisseria gonorrhoeae*. *J. Clin. Microbiol.* **15:**475–477.

82. **Sarafian, S. K., and J. S. Knapp.** 1989. Molecular epidemiology of gonorrhea. *Clin. Microbiol. Rev.* **2:**S49–S55.

83. **Schultz, T. R., J. W. Tapsall, P. A. White, and P. J. Newton.** 2000. An invasive isolate of *Neisseria meningitidis* showing decreased susceptibility to quinolones. *Antimicrob. Agents Chemother.* **45:**909–911.

84. **Schwam, E., and J. Cox.** 1999. Fulminant meningococcal supraglottitis: an emerging infectious syndrome. *Emerg. Infect. Dis.* **5:**464–467.

85. **Sobanski, M. A., R. A. Barnes, S. J. Gray, A. D. Carr, E. B. Kaczmarski, A. O'Rourke, K. Murphy, M. Cafferkey, R. W. Ellis, K. Pidcock, P. Hawtin, and W. T. Coakley.** 2000. Measurement of serum antigen concentration by ultrasound-enhanced immunoassay and correlation with clinical outcome in meningococcal disease. *Eur. J. Clin. Microbiol. Infect. Dis.* **19:**260–266.

86. **Spaargaren, J., J. Stoof, H. Fennema, R. Coutinho, and P. Savelkoul.** 2001. Amplified fragment length polymorphism fingerprinting for identification of a core group of *Neisseria gonorrhoeae* transmitters in the population attending a clinic for treatment of sexually transmitted diseases in Amsterdam, the Netherlands. *J. Clin. Microbiol.* **39:**2335–2337.

87. **Sparling, P. F., and H. H. Handsfield.** 2000. *Neisseria gonorrhoeae*, p. 2242–2258. *In* G. L. Mandell, J. E. Bennett, and R. Dolin (ed.), *Mandell, Douglas, and Bennett's Principles and Practice of Infectious Diseases*, 5th ed. Churchill Livingstone, Inc., Philadelphia, Pa.

88. **Speeleveld, E., J.-M. Fosspre, B. Gordts, and H. W. Landuyt.** 1994. Comparison of three rapid methods, tributyrine, 4-methylumbelliferyl butyrate, and indoxyl acetate, for rapid identification of *Moraxella catarrhalis. J. Clin. Microbiol.* **32:**1362–1363.

89. **Stefanou, J., A. V. Agelopoulou, N. V. Sipsas, M. Smilakou, and A. Avlami.** 2000. *Moraxella catarrhalis* endocarditis: case report and review of the literature. *Scand. J. Infect. Dis.* **32:**217–218.

90. **Tapsall, J. W., E. A. Phillips, T. R. Schultz, B. Way, and K. Withnall.** 1992. Strain characteristics and antibiotic susceptibility of *Neisseria gonorrhoeae* causing disseminated gonococcal infections in Australia. *Int. J. STD AIDS* **3:**273–277.

91. **Tapsall, J. W., T. R. Shultz, E. A. Limnios, B. Donovan, G. Lum, and B. P. Mulhall.** 1998. Failure of azithromycin therapy in gonorrhea and discorrelation with laboratory test parameters. *Sex. Transm. Dis.* **25:**505–508.

92. **Thompson, D. K., C. D. Deal, C. A. Ison, J. M. Zenilman, and M. C. Bash.** 2000. A typing system for *Neisseria gonorrhoeae* based on biotinylated oligonucleotide probes to PIB gene variable regions. *J. Infect. Dis.* **181:**1652–1660.

93. **Thompson, D. S., and S. A. French.** 1999. Comparison of commercial Amies transport systems with in-house Amies medium for recovery of *Neisseria gonorrhoeae. J. Clin. Microbiol.* **37:**3020–3021.

94. **Trees, D. L., A. J. Schultz, and J. S. Knapp.** 2000. Use of the neisserial lipoprotein (Lip) for subtyping *Neisseria gonorrhoeae. J. Clin. Microbiol.* **38:**2914–2916.

95. **Tzeng, Y.-L., and D. S. Stephens.** 2000. Epidemiology and pathogenesis of *Neisseria meningitidis.* Microbes Infect. **2:**687–700.

96. **van Deuren, M., P. Brandtzaeg, and J. W. M. van der Mer.** 2000. Update on meningococcal disease with emphasis on pathogenesis and clinical management. *Clin. Microbiol. Rev.* **13:**144–166.

97. **Vaneechoutte, M., G. Verschraegen, G. Claeys, B. Weise, and A. M. Van den Abeele.** 1990. Respiratory tract carrier rates of *Moraxella (Branhamella) catarrhalis* in adults and children and interpretation of isolation of *M. catarrhalis* from sputum. *J. Clin. Microbiol.* **28:**2674–2680.

98. **Whittington, W. L., and J. S. Knapp.** 1988. Trends in antimicrobial resistance in *Neisseria gonorrhoeae* in the United States. *Sex. Transm. Dis.* **15:**202–210.

99. **Winstead, J. M., D. S. McKinsey, S. Tasker, M. A. DeGroote, and L. M. Baddour.** 2000. Meningococcal pneumonia: characterization and review of cases seen over the past 25 years. *Clin. Infect. Dis.* **30:**87–94.

100. **Xia, M., M. C. Roberts, W. L. Whittington, K. K. Holmes, J. S. Knapp, J. A. Dillon, and R. Wi.** 1996. *Neisseria gonorrhoeae* with decreased susceptibility to ciprofloxacin: pulsed-field gel electrophoresis typing of strains from North America, Hawaii, and the Philippines. *Antimicrob. Agents Chemother.* **40:**2439–2440.

101. **Young, H., and A. Moyes.** 1996. An evaluation of pre-poured selective media for the isolation of *Neisseria gonorrhoeae. J. Med. Microbiol.* **44:**253–260.

Actinobacillus, Capnocytophaga, Eikenella, Kingella, Pasteurella, and Other Fastidious or Rarely Encountered Gram-Negative Rods*

ALEXANDER VON GRAEVENITZ, REINHARD ZBINDEN, AND REINIER MUTTERS

39

The bacterial genera covered in this chapter, i.e., *Actinobacillus*, *Pasteurella* (and related organisms), *Capnocytophaga*, *Dysgonomonas*, *Kingella*, *Eikenella*, *Simonsiella*, Group EF-4a, *Cardiobacterium*, *Suttonella*, *Chromobacterium*, and *Streptobacillus*, are taxonomically diverse but have certain traits in common that justify their discussion as a group. With a very few exceptions, they are facultatively anaerobic gram-negative rods but do not belong to the other facultatively anaerobic families of *Enterobacteriaceae*, *Vibrionaceae*, or *Aeromonadaceae*. Except for *Chromobacterium*, they do not possess flagella but may show surface translocation phenomena such as gliding or twitching (60). They are nutritionally fastidious; i.e., in the routine laboratory they need, with the exception of *Chromobacterium*, blood or chocolate agar or supplemented liquid media for growth, and most of them cannot grow on enteric media. Variable characteristics are failure to decolorize fully in the Gram stain, requirement for or stimulation by a 5 to 10% CO_2 atmosphere, and limited viability on solid media. Most species are susceptible to many antimicrobials but are resistant to vancomycin (although a small zone may form around a 30-μg vancomycin disk on blood agar); some are also resistant to colistin and thus will grow on Thayer-Martin or Martin-Lewis agar (e.g., *Kingella denitrificans* and *Capnocytophaga* spp.). Again, with the exception of *Chromobacterium*, these bacteria have a predilection for the oral cavity of animals and/or humans.

The low viability of many of them makes the use of transport media mandatory. Identification may present numerous difficulties because of similar biochemical characteristics, particularly between species of the genera *Actinobacillus* and *Pasteurella* (37, 81), which may call for molecular methods (47, 134). Automated or miniaturized diagnostic systems may not contain all species in their databases and/or may not yield correct diagnoses (19, 33, 46, 79). In some instances, the use of enzyme panels (e.g., APIZYM) may be helpful (37, 38, 59). Tubed identification media, e.g., triple sugar iron or Kligler agar, may not support growth. Gas formation, if present, is scant and may not be seen in such media (45). Traditional media used to check

acid formation from carbohydrates or reduction of nitrate or nitrite must be rich in peptones (serum should not be used since it may split maltose); better yet would be the use of cystine Trypticase agar with 1% carbohydrate and a large inoculum, e.g., cell paste or colonies on an agar block. Oxidase must be tested from colonies on blood-containing media with the tetramethyl-*p*-phenylenediamine dihydrochloride reagent (55). Catalase should be checked, if possible, in a liquid medium in order to avoid false-positive reactions due to transfer from blood agar and false-negative ones due to weak gas production. Indole formation may take 2 days and may be noticeable on xylene extraction only.

Susceptibility testing requires dilution systems because of slow growth and possible requirement for CO_2 (2, 67, 73, 82, 88). There are no NCCLS data for breakpoints and critical disk zones.

The genera *Haemophilus*, *Actinobacillus*, *Cardiobacterium*, *Eikenella*, and *Kingella* have often been lumped together by clinicians as "HACEK" bacteria because they occur in the human oral cavity and are able to cause a particular type of endocarditis characterized by a long duration of symptoms (2 weeks to 6 months) until the diagnosis is made, large vegetations, a tendency to embolization, and slow growth in blood cultures (in modern systems, up to 6 days) (29). Native and prosthetic valves may be affected. Prognosis is good with appropriate therapy, i.e., ampicillin alone or combined with an aminoglycoside.

ACTINOBACILLUS

The genus *Actinobacillus*, as well as the genera *Pasteurella* and *Haemophilus*, belongs to the family *Pasteurellaceae* (32). It consists of facultatively anaerobic, nonmotile, fastidious gram-negative rods which are coccoid to small (0.6 to 1.4 by 0.3 to 0.5 μm) on routine solid media and longer in serum broth and on media containing sugars. They show a tendency toward bipolar staining. Arrangement is single, in pairs, and in short chains.

Many species have been isolated only from animals so far (121) and are not discussed here. Of those isolated from animals and humans, only *A. lignieresii* (primary habitat in the oral cavity of sheep and cattle), *A. equuli* and *A. suis* (in the oral cavity of horses and pigs), and the primarily human

* This chapter contains information presented in chapter 42 by Barry Holmes, M. John Pickett, and Dannie G. Hollis in the seventh edition of this Manual.

species *A. ureae* (formerly *Pasteurella ureae*) and *A. hominis* belong to the genus *Actinobacillus* sensu stricto. The most conspicuous human species, *A. actinomycetemcomitans*, however, is, by DNA homology and 16S rRNA sequencing, more closely related to *Haemophilus aphrophilus* and *H. parahaemophilus* than to the other actinobacilli (97) and therefore has uncertain taxonomic status. It is a normal inhabitant of the human oral cavity but does not belong to the normal flora of animals (104).

Growth of actinobacilli requires enriched media but not necessarily hemin and is improved by a 5 to 10% CO_2 atmosphere. Colonies of the non-*A. actinomycetemcomitans* species are 2 mm in diameter after 24 h of growth at 37°C, are smooth or rough, and adhere to the agar surface. Smooth colonies are dome shaped and have a bluish hue when viewed by transmitted light. *A. actinomycetemcomitans* colonies initially show a central opaque dot which, on further incubation, develops into a star-like configuration like "crossed cigars" (Fig. 1). In serum broth, growth occurs in granules adherent to the side and bottom of the tube. Viability is limited (114).

Biochemical reactions are listed in Table 1; they include differential features with respect to *H. aphrophilus*. Separation of *A. hominis* from *A. equuli* may be difficult for strains of *A. hominis* that resemble those of *A. equuli* in being mannose positive (47). The composition of the main cellular fatty acids is similar in the entire genus ($C_{16:0}$, $C_{16:1\omega7c}$, $C_{14:0}$) and resembles that of *Haemophilus* (132). The guanine-plus-cytosine (G+C) content of the DNA is 40 to 43 mol%.

A. lignieresii causes actinobacillosis, a granulomatous disease in cattle and sheep in which, similar to actinomycosis, sulfur granules are formed in tissues (113). A very few human tissue infections have originated from cattle or sheep bite wounds or contact (102).

A. equuli and *A. suis* cause a variety of diseases in horses and pigs (9, 113). Human infections are mostly due to horse and pig bites or contact (9, 41, 111). Both species have also been isolated from human infections of the upper respiratory tract (114, 132).

A. hominis and *A. ureae* have been isolated most often as commensals or from infections of the human respiratory tract, *A. hominis* also, although rarely, from blood (47, 137) and *A. ureae* from blood, spinal fluid, and peritoneal dialysate (15, 96, 130, 134) in patients with various underlying diseases (47, 96).

A. actinomycetemcomitans is subdivided into five serotypes based on surface polysaccharides, which can be identified by multiplex PCR (126). Serotypes a to c are the most frequent ones. Serotype b is associated with periodontitis and β-lactamase production, bacteremia, and endocarditis; and serotype c is associated with extraoral infections but also with periodontal health (99). Known virulence factors are leukotoxin, which is not confined to one serotype (99) and is toxic to polymorphonuclear leukocytes and monocytes (97), and collagenase (107). Diseases caused by *A. actinomycetemcomitans* are mostly endocarditis (HACEK type), soft tissue infections, and periodontitis (29, 68); other organ systems are rarely affected (68). The organism may occur in combination with *Actinomyces* spp., particularly in soft tissue infections, where it can also be present in sulfur granules (6, 145). Selective media containing various compounds inhibitory for gram-positive organisms have been devised (5, 62), as have PCRs targeting the leukotoxin gene or specific sequences of the 16S rRNA gene (43, 48). Typing is classically done by serology but particular clones and transmission are more effectively traced by molecular techniques (129).

Susceptibility studies are extant for a few isolates of *A. ureae* and *A. hominis* which were susceptible to many antibiotics including penicillin (15, 47, 130). *A. actinomycetemcomitans* is mostly susceptible to cephalosporins, tetracycline, and fluoroquinolones; resistance to penicillin, amikacin, and macrolides is not uncommon (68, 73, 88, 142).

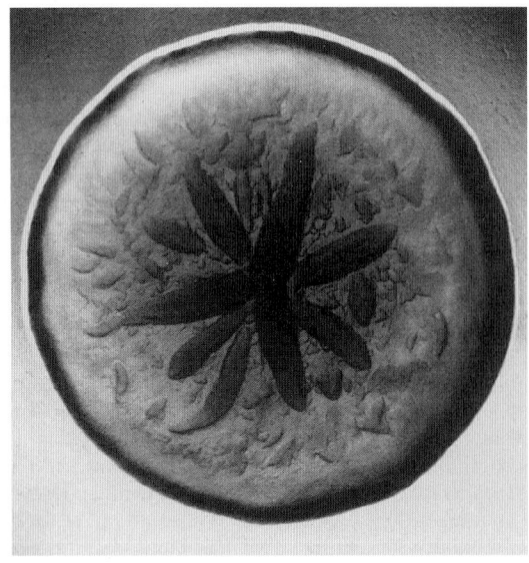
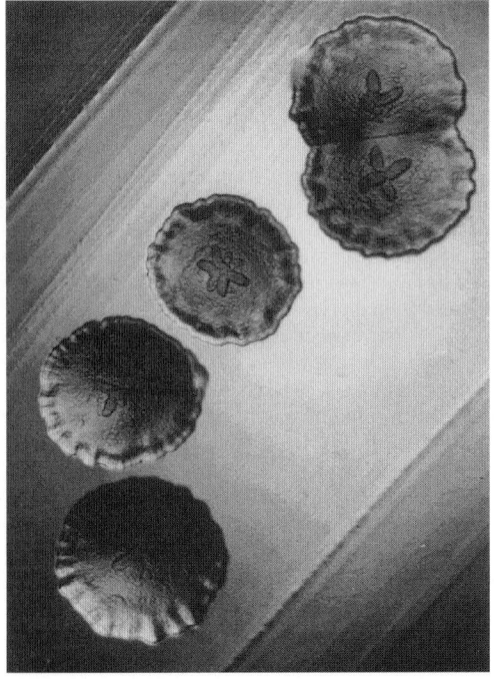

FIGURE 1 Star-shaped colonies of *Actinobacillus actinomycetemcomitans*.

TABLE 1 Biochemical reactions of *Actinobacillus* and *Haemophilus aphrophilus*[a,b]

Test	A. actinomycetemcomitans	A. equuli	A. hominis	A. lignieresii	A. suis[c]	A. ureae	H. aphrophilus
Catalase	+	v	+	v	v	+/w/−	−
Oxidase	−/w	+	+	+	+	+	v
Ornithine decarboxylase	−	−	−	−	−	−	−
Esculin hydrolysis	−	−	−	−	+	−	−
Urease	−	+	+	+	+	+	−
ONPG	−	+	+	+	+	−	+
Growth on MacConkey agar	−	v	+	v	v	−	v
Gas from glucose	v	−	−	−	−	−	+
Acid from:							
Xylose	v	+	+	+	+	−	−
Mannitol	v	+	+	+	v	+	−
Lactose	−	+	+	v	+	−	(+)
Sucrose	−	+	+	+	+	+	+
Maltose	+	+	+	+	+	+	+
Melibiose	−	+	+	−	+	−	ND
Trehalose	−	+	+	−	+	−	(+)

[a] Data from references 45, 47, 102, 114, and 132.
[b] +, ≥90% of strains positive; (+), ≥90% of strains positive after >48 h; −, ≥90% of strains negative; ONPG, *o*-nitrophenyl-β-D-galactopyranoside; ND, no data available; v, variable; w, weak; /, or. All species are indole negative and reduce nitrate to nitrite.
[c] Beta-hemolytic on sheep blood agar.

PASTEURELLA AND RELATED ORGANISMS

Like *Actinobacillus*, the genus *Pasteurella* belongs to the family *Pasteurellaceae*. Taxa that are, on the basis of DNA-DNA hybridization studies, more closely related to other genera (e.g., *Actinobacillus*) (94, 121), have been marked *[P.]* (7). Both groups occur in animals, and most of them also occur in humans.

Pasteurellae are coccoid to small, nonmotile, facultatively anaerobic gram-negative rods that occur singly, in pairs, or in short chains. The related species generally have a more pronounced rod-like morphology. *Pasteurella* spp. sensu stricto are nutritionally more fastidious than the related species, which may be able to grow on MacConkey agar. All pasteurellae are hemin and CO_2 independent, but a few strains require factor V (72). Colonies are 1 to 2 mm in diameter after 24 h of growth on blood agar at 37°C.

Biochemical reactions of species isolated from humans are given in Table 2. Beta-hemolysis is observed only in the former *[P.] haemolytica* complex, which occurs in animals and has recently been subdivided into the genus *Mannheimia* (trehalose-negative strains) (7) and *[P.] trehalosi* (trehalose-positive strains) (121). All species have an identical cellular fatty acid composition, with $C_{16:1\omega7c}$, $C_{16:0}$, and $C_{14:0}$ as the main components. In this regard, they are indistinguishable from members of the genera *Actinobacillus* and *Haemophilus* (132). There is also no single phenotypic feature that distinguishes the genus *Actinobacillus* from the genus *Pasteurella*. The G+C content of *Pasteurella* is between 37.7 and 45.9 mol% (94).

Pasteurellae are widespread in healthy and diseased wild and domestic animals. Their habitats are the nasopharynx and the gingiva. *Pasteurella* species sensu stricto which have

TABLE 2 Biochemical reactions of *Pasteurella* spp. and related species[a,b]

Reaction	P. canis	P. dagmatis	P. gallinarum	P. multocida	P. stomatis	[P.] aerogenes	[P.] bettyae	[P.] caballi	[P.] pneumotropica	Bisgaard taxon 16	"SP" group
Catalase	+	+	+	+	+	+	−	−	+	+	+
Oxidase	+	+	+	+	+	+	v	+	+	+	+
Indole	+	+	−	+	+	−	+	−	+	+	+
Urease	−	+	−	−	−	+	−	−	+	−	−
Ornithine decarboxylase	+	−	v	+	−	v	−	+	+	−	−
Growth on MacConkey agar	−	−	v	−	−	+	v	−	v	v	ND
Gas from glucose	−	v	−	−	−	+	+	+	−	−	+
Acid from:											
Lactose	−	−	−	−	−	v	−	+	−	−	+
Sucrose	+	+	+	+	+	+	−	+	+	+	+
Xylose	−	−	v	v	−	v	−	+	+	−	−
Maltose	−	+	+	−	−	+	−	+	+	+	+
Mannitol	−	−	−	+	−	−	−	+	−	−	−

[a] Data from references 16, 45, 115, and 132.
[b] +, ≥90% of strains positive; −, ≥90% of strains negative; ND, no data available; v, variable; w, weak. All species reduce nitrate to nitrite and are negative for arginine dihydrolase and esculin hydrolysis.

so far been isolated only from animals include *P. anatis* (from ducks), *P. avium* (from chickens and calves), *P. langaa* (from chickens), *P. lymphangitidis* (from cattle), *P. mairi* (from pigs), *P. testudinis* (from tortoises), *P. trehalosi* (from lambs), and *P. volantium* (from fowl) (94, 95, 121).

P. multocida, the species most frequently isolated from humans, also occurs in many animal species including dogs and cats. Its three subspecies, *multocida*, *septica*, and *gallicida*, can be separated on the basis of sorbitol and dulcitol fermentation (+/− in subsp. *multocida*, −/− in subsp. *septica*, and −/+ in the mostly avian subsp. *gallicida*; weakly sorbitol-positive strains of subsp. *multocida* can be recognized by a negative α-glucosidase test and a specific PCR profile [49]). On the basis of 16S rRNA gene sequencing, it has been speculated that subsp. *septica* may be a separate species (76). A 145-kDa cytotoxin is essential for causing atrophic rhinitis in pigs and can be detected by enzyme-linked immunosorbent assay or PCR (80), but there is so far little evidence that it plays a role in human infections (63). Other species isolated from humans are *P. canis* (associated with dogs), *P. stomatis*, and *P. dagmatis* (both associated with dogs and cats).

In an analysis of 159 strains of *Pasteurella* sensu stricto isolated from humans, approximately 60% were *P. multocida* subsp. *multocida*, 18% were *P. canis*, 13% were *P. multocida* subsp. *septica*, 5% were *P. stomatis*, and 3%, *P. dagmatis*. Over 90% of infections are wound infections or abscesses following bites, scratches, or licking of skin lesions (63). Infected cat bite wounds contain pasteurellae significantly more often than infected dog bite wounds do (127). Systemic disease is also well known, comprising septicemia, meningitis, endocarditis, arthritis, pneumonia with lung abscess, osteomyelitis, and peritonitis (40, 77, 85, 131). Patients with immune defects are at higher risk (131). Colonization of the bronchial tree in patients with underlying pulmonary disease is not uncommon (131).

P. gallinarum occurs primarily in poultry and has been isolated from the blood in humans (3, 8). The species diagnosis was subsequently put in doubt (46). A more recent case of neonatal meningitis, however, seems to be due to this species without doubt (1).

Media containing vancomycin, clindamycin, and/or amikacin have been used for selection of pasteurellae (10), and species-specific PCR assays have been used as well, albeit largely in veterinary research (65). Two species may even be encountered in one sample (143). Typing of *P. multocida* has traditionally been done by serological means. There are five capsular serogroups and 16 serotypes; human strains belong mostly to serogroup A (128). New typing techniques rely on molecular methods (17, 128). Recently the genome of the avian *P. multocida* strain Pm 70, 2,257,487 bp in length, has been sequenced (90).

Of undetermined taxonomic status but outside the genus *Pasteurella* and occasionally found in human specimens are [*P.*] *caballi*, found primarily in horses (115) and isolated from horse bites in humans (42); [*P.*] *bettyae*, formerly called HB-5, of uncertain natural habitat, isolated from human genitourinary tract infections (11, 18) and from blood of patients with peripartum bacteremia (117); [*P.*] *aerogenes*, found primarily in pigs, isolated from pig bites in humans (39, 81); [*P.*] *pneumotropica*, found primarily in rodents but also in dogs and cats, isolated from local and systemic infections in humans (27, 44); *Mannheimia* (formerly *P.*) *haemolytica*, found primarily in many domestic animals (the identification of a human strain from a patient with endocarditis [141] was subsequently put in doubt [79]);

the "SP" group, found primarily in guinea pigs, isolated from human blood and feces (45); and "Bisgaard taxon 16," found primarily in dogs and cats (16) and isolated from dog bites (37).

Pasteurellae are generally susceptible to β-lactam antibiotics, including penicillin, macrolides, tetracycline, and quinolones, and are resistant to clindamycin and amikacin; other aminoglycosides are only moderately active (51, 131). A few β-lactamase-positive strains of *P. multocida* (84) and *P. bettyae* (18) have been reported; they were susceptible to the combination of a β-lactam with clavulanic acid. *P. bettyae* may also be tetracycline resistant (18).

CAPNOCYTOPHAGA

The genus *Capnocytophaga* includes bacteria formerly called DF-1 and DF-2 and has been placed in the emended family *Flavobacteriaceae* (14). At present, it consists of seven species of facultatively anaerobic, fastidious gram-negative rods. Fusiform shapes, 2.5 to 7.5 by 0.4 to 0.6 μm, predominate, while curved filaments and coccoid and spindle forms may also be observed. Primary isolation of most strains requires 5 to 10% CO_2 and rich media; growth differences have even been observed on various Columbia blood agar bases (35). Colonies reach 2 to 3 mm in diameter after 2 to 4 days at 37°C, are convex or flat, are often slightly yellow when scraped off the agar surface, have regular edges or may show spreading, have sliding motility, and show adherence to the agar surface.

Biochemical test results are listed in Table 3. The G+C content is between 34 and 40 mol% (14). The cellular fatty acids are fairly uniform within the genus; (iC$_{15:0}$, ≥60%; i-3-OH C$_{17:0}$, ≥4%) (132). Species differentiation is also possible by use of (noncommercial) DNA probes and other molecular techniques (26). There may be cross-reactions between *C. ochracea* and *Legionella* spp. in latex agglutination tests (23).

The oxidase- and catalase-negative species *C. ochracea* (formerly DF-1), *C. gingivalis*, *C. sputigena*, *C. haemolytica* (beta-hemolytic), and *C. granulosa* (growing aerobically) are normal inhabitants of the human oral cavity, while the oxidase- and catalase-positive species *C. canimorsus* (formerly DF-2) and *C. cynodegmi* occur primarily in the oral cavities of dogs and cats (20). *C. granulosa* and *C. haemolytica* have also been isolated from human supragingival dental plaque (140); *C. ochracea*, *C. gingivalis*, and *C. sputigena* are associated with periodontitis (58). *C. ochracea* and the other oxidase-negative species may cause septicemia and other infections (endocarditis, endometritis, osteomyelitis, abscesses, peritonitis, and keratitis) in immunocompromised (mostly neutropenic) patients (54, 70, 100) as well as in immunocompetent ones (34, 36, 98, 116). Unfortunately, many published isolates have not been identified to species.

C. canimorsus is associated mainly with dog and cat bites or contact. Most patients with septicemia have been splenectomized or were alcoholics and had a poor prognosis. In fulminant cases, the organisms could be seen in direct blood smears (83). Other infections reported are meningitis, endocarditis, arthritis, and eye infections (71, 83). *C. cynodegmi* has been isolated from dog bite wounds and from eye infections (20, 91).

For isolation of *Capnocytophaga* spp., the use of enriched media is important; for specimens that are likely to yield mixed cultures, various selective media (24) and PCR (58) have been used.

TABLE 3 Biochemical reactions of *Capnocytophaga* spp., *Dysgonomonas* and related species, *Chromobacterium*, and *Streptobacillus*[a,b]

Reaction	C. ochracea	C. sputigena	C. gingivalis	C. granulosa	C. haemolytica	C. canimorsus	C. cynodegmi	D. capnocyto-phagoides	D. gadei	DF-3-like	Chromo-bacterium violaceum	S. moniliformis
Catalase	−	−	−	−	−	+	+	−	+	−	+	−
Oxidase	−	−	−	−	−	+	+	−	+	−	v	−
Indole	−	−	−	−	−	−	−	v	+	+	v	−
Arginine dihydrolase	−	−	−	ND	ND	+	+	−	−	−	+	+
Nitrate to nitrite	−	v	−	−	+	−	v	−	−	−	+	−
Esculin hydrolysis	+	+	−	−	+	v	+	v	+	+	+	v
Gelatinase	−	v	−	ND	ND	−	−	−	−	v	−	−
Starch hydrolysis	+	−	−	ND	ND	ND	ND	ND	+	ND	v	ND
ONPG	+	+	−	+	+	+	+	+	+	+	−	−
Acid from:												
Glucose	+	+	+	+	+	+	+	+	+	+	+[c]	+
Lactose	v	v	−	+	+	+	+	+	+	+	−	−
Sucrose	+	+	+	+	+	−	+	+	+	−	v	−
Xylose	−	−	−	−	−	−	−	+	+	−	−	−
Melibiose	−	−	−	−	−	+	−	+	+	ND	ND	ND
Main cellular fatty acids	i-15:0, 3OH-17:0	i-15:0, 3OH-17:0	i-15:0, 3OH-17:0	i-15:0, 3OH-17:0	i-15:0, 3OH-17:0	i-15:0, 3OH-17:0	i-15:0, 3OH-17:0	ai-15:0, i14:0, 15:0, i3OH-16:0	ai15:0, 16:0, i14:0	ai15:0, i15:0, 16:0, 18:2, i-3OH-17:0	16:1ω7c, 16:0, 18:1ω7c	16:0, 18:1, 18:2, 18:0

[a] Data from references 13, 20, 28, 61, and 132.
[b] +, ≥90% of strains positive; −, ≥90% of strains negative; ND, no data available; ONPG, *o*-nitrophenyl-β-D-galactopyranoside; v, variable. All species are negative for urease.
[c] Some strains form small amounts of gas.

Capnocytophaga spp. are usually susceptible to many antibiotics including narrow-, extended-, and broad-spectrum β-lactams, macrolides, tetracycline, clindamycin (surprisingly), and quinolones but resistant to aminoglycosides (67, 112). β-Lactamase-positive strains have occasionally been found (54, 67, 112); they were susceptible to β-lactam drug combinations with β-lactamase inhibitors.

DYSGONOMONAS AND DF-3-LIKE BACTERIA

Dysgonomonas, a recently outlined genus without family assignment, is closer to *Bacteroides forsythus* and *B. distasonis* than to *Capnocytophaga* (61). The G+C content is 38 mol%. Two species are recognized at present: *D. capnocytophagoides* (formerly CDC group DF-3) and *D. gadei* (61); group DF-3-like bacteria (28) have not been investigated taxonomically. All of these bacteria, however, resemble *Capnocytophaga* in their requirement for enriched media, facultative anaerobiosis, lack of flagella, and slow growth. Microscopically, they are coccoid to small gram-negative rods. Colonies have a strawberry-like odor and are neither adherent nor spreading.

The two species show few biochemical differences; the notable differences are in catalase production (Table 3) and in certain enzymatic (APIZYM) reactions (61). The differential characterization includes aerobically growing isolates of *Leptotrichia buccalis*, which have a different cellular fatty acid profile (mainly $C_{16:0}$ and c11/t9/t6 $C_{18:1}$) and produce only lactic acid from glucose whereas *Dysgonomonas* spp. produce propionic and succinic acid (13).

While only one human isolate of *D. gadei* (from a gallbladder) has been reported so far (61), numerous *D. capnocytophagoides* strains have been isolated, mostly from stools of immunocompromised patients (89). Selective media based on their natural antimicrobial resistance, e.g., those used for *Campylobacter jejuni* (56), have been used for this purpose. Diarrhea was reported in approximately half of these patients. One blood isolate was found to be identical by ribotyping to that from the stool of the same patient (56).

In contrast to oxidase-negative *Capnocytophaga* spp., *Dysgonomonas capnocytophagoides* strains are usually resistant to β-lactam antibiotics, aminoglycosides, macrolides, and quinolones but susceptible to tetracycline, imipenem, rifampin, and co-trimoxazole (56, 89).

KINGELLA

The genus *Kingella* belongs, with *Suttonella*, *Eikenella*, *Simonsiella*, *Alysiella*, the EF-4 bacteria, and *Neisseria*, in the emended family *Neisseriaceae* (110). It consists of three species; *K. kingae*, *K. denitrificans*, and *K. oralis*. They are facultatively anaerobic, nutritionally fastidious, short (2 to 3 by 0.4 μm) gram-negative rods with square ends, lying in pairs or chains, and they tend to decolorize unevenly on Gram stain. They do not possess flagella but may show twitching motility. Colonies develop to 1 to 2 mm in diameter in 48 h. One type is smooth with a central papilla; another shows pitting of the medium and spreading edges. A CO_2 atmosphere is not required, but its presence enhances growth. Viability on culture media is low. *K. kingae* shows a small but distinct zone of beta-hemolysis. The G+C contents are 47 mol% for *K. kingae*, 54 to 57 mol% for *K. denitrificans*, and 56 to 58 mol% for *K. oralis* (110).

Biochemical test results are listed in Table 4. Differentiation from the rod-shaped neisseriae, *N. elongata* and *N. weaveri*, is important (Table 5).

K. kingae may colonize the upper respiratory tract of humans, particularly of children (119, 138). The natural

TABLE 4 Biochemical reactions of selected members of the *Neisseriaceae*[a,b]

Reaction	*Cardiobacterium hominis*	*Suttonella indologenes*	*Kingella kingae*	*Kingella denitrificans*	*Kingella oralis*	*Eikenella corrodens*	EF-4a	EF-4b	*Simonsiella muelleri*
Catalase	−	v	−	−	−	−	+	+	−
Oxidase	+	+	+	+	+	+	+	+	+
Indole	+	+	−	−	−	−	−	−	−
Arginine dihydrolase	−	−	−	−	−	−	v	−	−
Nitrate to nitrite	−	−	−	+/G	−	+	+/G	+	v
Esculin hydrolysis	−	−	−	−	−	−	−	−	−
Ornithine decarboxylase	−	−	−	−	−	+	−	−	−
Growth on MacConkey agar	−	−	−	−	−	−	v	v	−
Alkaline phosphatase[c]	−	+	+	−	+	−	−	−	−
Acid (no gas) from:									
Glucose	+	+	+	+	+[w]	−	+	+	+
Lactose	−	−	−	−	−	−	−	−	−
Sucrose	+	+	−	−	−	−	−	−	−
Xylose	−	−	−	−	−	−	−	−	−
Maltose	+	+	+	−	−	−	−	−	+
Mannitol	+	−	−	−	−	−	−	−	−
Special features			Beta-hemolytic			LD v	Yellowish or no pigment	Yellowish or no pigment	
Main cellular fatty acids	18:1ω7c, 16:0,14:0	16:0, 18:1ω7c, 16:1ω7c, 14:0	14:0, 16:1ω7c, 16:0, 12:0	16:0, 14:0, 18:2, 18:1ω9c, 12:0	ND	16:0, 18:1ω7c, 16:1ω7c	16:0, 16:1ω7c, 18:1ω7c	16:0, 16:1ω7c, 18:1ω7c	16:1ω7c, 12:0, 14:0

[a] Data from references 31, 59, 74, and 132.
[b] +, ≥90% of strains positive; −, ≥90% of strains negative; G, gas; LD, lysine decarboxylase; v, variable; w, weak. All species are negative for urease.
[c] APIZYM system.

TABLE 5 Differentiation between *Kingella* and rod-shaped *Neisseria* species[a,b]

Feature	Kingella kingae	Kingella dentrificans	Kingella oralis	Neisseria elongata subsp. glycolytica	Neisseria elongata subsp. nitroreducens	Neisseria weaveri
Catalase	−	−	−	+	−	+
Nitrate to nitrite	−	+	−	−	+	−
Nitrate to gas	−	+	−	−	−	−
Alkaline phosphatase[c]	+	−	+	−	−	ND
Glucose acid	+	+	+[w]	+[W]	v	−
Maltose acid	+	−	−	−	−	−
Beta-hemolysis	+	−	−	−	−	−
Main cellular fatty acids	14:0, 16:1ω7c, 16:0	16:0, 14:0, 18:2, 18:1ω9c	ND	16:0, 16:1ω7c, 18:1ω7c	16:0, 16:1ω7c, 18:1ω7c	16:0, 16:1ω7c, 18:1ω7c

[a] Data from references 22, 30, 110, and 132.
[b] +, ≥90% of strains positive; −, ≥90% of strains negative; ND, no data available; v, variable; w, weak.
[c] APIZYM system.

habitat of *K. denitrificans* is unknown. *K. oralis* occurs in the human oral cavity (22, 30).

K. kingae infections show a predilection for infants and children, preferentially causing bone and joint infections (138). In adults, HACEK-type endocarditis is particularly conspicuous (29) but septicemia, keratitis, diskitis, and central nervous system infections (25, 122) have also been described. Ribotyping and pulsed-field gel electrophoresis have shown that person-to-person transmission does occur (119). *K. denitrificans* has been reported as an agent of endocarditis and of granulomatous disease in patients with AIDS (92). *K. oralis* may be associated with periodontitis (22).

Recovery of kingellae may be difficult. For isolates from areas of the body harboring normal flora, selective media containing clindamycin (30) or vancomycin (119) may be used. The use of blood culture media, e.g., BacT/Alert (64), and eubacterial PCR (123) significantly improves the rate of isolation from body fluids.

Kingellae are generally susceptible to β-lactam antibiotics, macrolides, tetracycline, co-trimoxazole, and quinolones (73, 139). β-Lactamase-positive strains have been observed (92, 122) but were susceptible to β-lactam drug combinations with clavulanic acid.

EIKENELLA

The genus *Eikenella* belongs to the emended family *Neisseriaceae* (110). So far, one species, *E. corrodens*, has been recognized, but DNA-DNA hybridization, cellular carbohydrates, and the occurrence of aberrant strains with positive catalase reactions (ca. 8%) suggest that there could be more than one genomospecies (69). The G+C content is 56 to 58 mol% (110).

Eikenellae are slender, straight, 0.3 to 0.4 by 1.5 to 4 μm, nonflagellated, facultatively anaerobic gram-negative rods. Twitching motility may be observed on some media. *E. corrodens* requires hemin for aerobic growth and consequently grows poorly or not at all aerobically on identification media such as triple sugar iron or Kligler's agar. The presence of 5 to 10% CO_2 may enhance growth but is not required if heme is present (50). Colonies are 1 to 2 mm in diameter after 48 h at 37°C, show clear centers often surrounded by spreading growth, and may pit the agar. They

smell of hypochlorite and assume a slightly yellow hue after several days.

Biochemical reactions are recorded in Table 4. Of diagnostic importance are the failure of these organisms to form acid from carbohydrates and the presence of ornithine decarboxylase and nitratase. Lysine decarboxylase may also be present.

The habitat of *E. corrodens* is the oral cavity of humans and some mammals (53, 69) and probably other gastrointestinal sites. Isolates are often found mixed with members of the oropharyngeal flora (124). In dental plaque, *E. corrodens* can be detected by PCR (48). Clindamycin has been used in selective media (118).

E. corrodens is an agent of oral (perhaps also periodontal), pleuropulmonary, abdominal, joint, bone, and wound infections (101). The wound infections may be caused by animal or human bites (124, 127). Endocarditis follows the HACEK pattern (29). The organism is generally susceptible to β-lactam antibiotics, tetracycline, and quinolones (52, 73, 124) but β-lactamase-positive strains have been reported (101, 124).

SIMONSIELLA

The genus *Simonsiella* belongs to the emended family *Neisseriaceae* (110). Its members are strictly aerobic gram-negative, crescent-shaped rods. They are arranged in multicellular filaments (10 to 50 by 2 to 8 μm), which are segmented into groups of mostly eight cells, resulting in a caterpillar-like appearance (Fig. 2). The long axis of each cell is perpendicular to the long axis of the filament, representing the width of the latter. Gliding motility and incomplete decolorization with Gram stain are usually observed. Simonsiellae are nutritionally fastidious, growing well on blood agar but not on enteric media. An optimal medium for microscopic recognition is BSTSY agar, which contains bovine serum, glucose, tryptic soy broth, and yeast extract (75). Colonies are 1 to 2 mm in diameter after 24 h at 37°C and produce a pale yellow pigment.

Three species which can be separated by biochemical tests (74) have been described. Their natural habitat is the oral cavity (except for teeth): *S. crassa* in sheep, *S. steedae* in dogs and cats, and *S. muelleri* in humans (74).

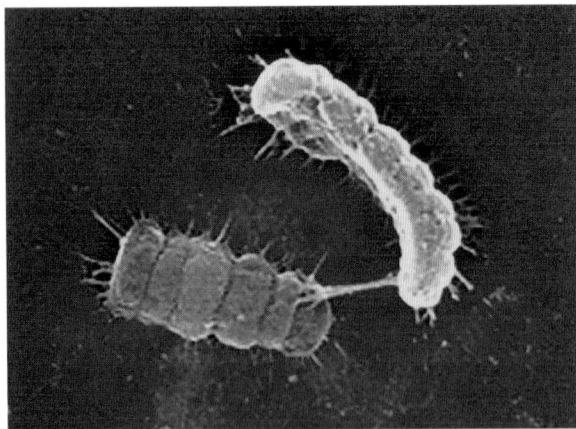

FIGURE 2 Scanning electron micrograph of a *Simonsiella* sp. with two multicellular filaments, giving the appearance of caterpillars. (Courtesy of L. Corboz, Zürich, Switzerland.)

S. muelleri is beta-hemolytic and has a G+C content of 40.3 to 41.8 mol%. The long axis of the cells measures 2.1 to 3.5 μm, and the short axis measures 0.5 to 0.9 μm. The organism has not been associated with human disease (21, 133).

One strain recovered from gastric aspirate of a newborn was tested for antimicrobial susceptibility and was susceptible to β-lactam antibiotics, tetracycline, and gentamicin but resistant to clindamycin (133).

GROUP EF-4a

Groups EF-4a and EF-4b belong to the emended family *Neisseriaceae* (110). EF-4a consists of nonmotile, coccoid to short, facultatively anaerobic gram-negative rods with a G+C content of 49.3 to 50.9 mol% (110); group EF-4a members differ from group EF-4b members in certain biochemical reactions and in the electrophoretic patterns of whole-cell proteins and lipopolysaccharides (57). EF-4a is fermentative and arginine dihydrolase positive (Table 4), and EF-4b is oxidative and arginine negative (see chapter 49). EF-4a reduces nitrate with or without gas formation (132), while EF-4b always reduces nitrate without gas formation. Colonies are slightly yellow or nonpigmented and may smell of popcorn. Cellular fatty acids of both groups are mainly $C_{16:0}$, $C_{16:1\omega7c}$, and $C_{18:1\omega7c}$ (132). Both groups are part of the normal oral flora of dogs, cats, and rodents, in which they may cause pulmonary infection (57). Human infections with EF-4a are associated with cat or dog bite or contact (82, 108, 127).

EF-4a organisms are susceptible to many antimicrobials but are variable in their susceptibility to penicillin and narrow-spectrum cephalosporins and resistant to clindamycin and trimethoprim. The latter has been used in a selective medium (108). Of note is the difference in the MIC of methicillin: $\geq$64 μg/ml for EF-4a strains but $\leq$32 μg/ml for EF-4b strains (4).

CARDIOBACTERIUM

The genus *Cardiobacterium*, which belongs to the family *Cardiobacteriaceae* (31), consists of one species, *C. hominis*, a nonmotile, facultatively anaerobic, fastidious gram-negative rod, 1 to 3 by 0.5 to 0.75 μm, occurring singly or in pairs, short chains, or rosettes, showing bulbous ends, and often staining irregularly. Pleomorphism disappears when yeast extract is present in the medium. Growth requires a capnophilic atmosphere. Colonies attain a diameter of 1 mm after 2 days at 37°C, are circular and opaque, and often pit the agar (132). The G+C content is 59 to 60 mol% (31).

Biochemical test results are recorded in Table 4. The positive indole reaction (which is sometimes weak) may initially suggest *Pasteurella* or *Suttonella*; the differential identification must include tests for catalase, mannitol fermentation, and possibly alkaline phosphatase. Also, cellular fatty acids of *Suttonella* and *Cardiobacterium* differ only quantitatively (Table 4), $C_{16:1\omega7c}$ being present only in very small amounts (<5%) in *C. hominis* (the same is true for $C_{18:1\omega7c}$ in *Pasteurella*) (132).

The normal habitat of *C. hominis* is the human upper respiratory tract and possibly also the genitourinary and gastrointestinal tracts (120). Human disease is confined largely to endocarditis typical of HACEK organisms (29, 86, 135); occasionally, *C. hominis* is isolated from other samples (105). Growth in blood culture media is typically slow. Culture-negative cases have been reported in which the diagnosis was made by eubacterial PCR followed by sequencing, or by serologic testing (93, 144).

The organism is susceptible to many antimicrobials except clindamycin (135), but β-lactamase-producing strains have been reported (86).

SUTTONELLA

The genus *Suttonella* belongs to the family *Cardiobacteriaceae* (31) and contains one species, *S. indologenes* (formerly *Kingella indologenes*), a plump, irregularly staining, nonmotile, fastidious, facultatively anaerobic gram-negative rod whose colonies may show spreading and/or pitting (132). The G+C content is 49 mol% (31). Characteristics differentiating *Suttonella* from morphologically and biochemically similar gram-negative rods are listed in Table 4. The organism, whose natural habitat is unknown, has only rarely been isolated from human sources, e.g., from diseased eyes (125, 132) and from blood cultures in patients with endocarditis (66). Its susceptibility resembles that of *C. hominis* (66).

CHROMOBACTERIUM

The genus *Chromobacterium*, which is the closest neighbor to the *Neisseriaceae* rRNA cluster (110), contains one species, *C. violaceum*, a facultatively anaerobic, gram-negative, straight rod, 0.8 to 1.2 by 2.5 to 6.0 μm, motile by one polar and one to four lateral flagella. It is less fastidious than most of the other bacteria described in this chapter (Table 3). Colonies are 1 to 2 mm in diameter after 24 h of growth at 30 to 35°C, round, and smooth; they smell of cyanide; and they may be beta-hemolytic. Most colonies produce a violet pigment called violacein, which is ethanol but not water soluble. Entirely nonpigmented strains exist as well and are frequently indole positive (132). The G+C content is 65 to 68 mol% (110).

Biochemical test results are listed in Table 3. Identification is easy if violacein is produced. Nonpigmented strains may be confused with *Aeromonas* spp., but, unlike aeromonads, are lysine, maltose, and mannitol negative. The principal cellular fatty acids do not differentiate between the two genera (see chapter 45).

The organism inhabits soil and water and is often found in semitropical and tropical climates (South Africa, Southeast Asia, Australia, and the southeastern United States). Infections in humans are rare. The portal of entry is usually a skin lesion leading to a wound infection, but oral intake may also occur. Septicemia may develop, is significantly associated with neutrophil dysfunction, and has a high case-fatality rate (78, 87, 106).

C. violaceum is generally resistant to narrow-, extended-, and broad-spectrum β-lactam antibiotics; shows variable susceptibility to aminoglycosides; and is susceptible to ciprofloxacin, co-trimoxazole, tetracycline, and imipenem (78, 87, 106).

STREPTOBACILLUS

The genus *Streptobacillus* consists of one species, *S. moniliformis*, which has a closer relationship to the *Mycoplasmatales* than to other bacteria as regards G+C content (24 to 26 mol%), lack of quinones, and serologic test results (136). There is a high degree of phenotypic and genotypic conformity between strains (132, 136).

S. moniliformis is a facultatively anaerobic, nonmotile, fastidious gram-negative rod of 1 to 5 by 0.3 to 0.5 μm. Some organisms, which become more numerous as the culture ages, develop into long filaments (100 to 150 μm) containing granules, bulbs (often in series) and bands (Fig. 3); coccal forms may also be observed. Older cultures tend to become gram variable.

Eubacterial and L-phase colonies occur, occasionally together in one culture. The former are 1 to 3 mm in diameter after 48 h, are round and smooth, and develop optimally in 48 to 72 h on blood agar in 10% CO_2 at 35 to 37°C. L-phase colonies develop better on clear, serum-supplemented media and give the characteristic "fried-egg" appearance with irregular outlines and coarse granular lipid globules. In liquid media, growth occurs mainly in the form of "puff balls" at the bottom. The organism does not grow on enteric media and even dies quickly on other media unless subcultured frequently. It is also inhibited by sodium polyanethol sulfonate present in blood culture media (136). Eubacterial PCR followed by sequencing has been used in a culture-negative case (12).

S. moniliformis is relatively inert biochemically (Table 3). Sugars are acidified weakly and in a delayed fashion

(132). The identification may be confirmed by use of the APIZYM system (38) or by cellular fatty acid analysis (Table 3). Serologic testing is unreliable (12).

S. moniliformis occurs naturally in the nasopharynx of wild and laboratory rats. Human infections result either from bites of rodents (rats, mice, squirrels, weasels, gerbils, and even cats or dogs that prey on them) or from consumption of contaminated food or water. The former infection is called rat-bite fever, and the latter is called Haverhill fever. The incubation period is usually 2 to 10 days. Characteristic are irregular fever with headaches, chills, myalgias, and arthralgias followed in a few days by a maculopapular rash on the extremities and sometimes polyarthritis (12). Complications such as endocarditis (109), myocarditis, pericarditis, meningitis, pneumonia, amnionitis, and abscesses may develop (103). Approximately half of the cases occur in children younger than 12 years (12).

S. moniliformis is susceptible to a wide range of antimicrobials, particularly penicillin and doxycycline, which are recommended for treatment (38, 109).

EVALUATION, INTERPRETATION, AND REPORTING OF RESULTS

Various species discussed in this chapter belong to the normal flora of humans, particularly the flora of the oral cavity, and their identification and reporting when isolated from normal flora do not seem justified. When found in other samples such as wounds, blood, or body fluids, their recognition is important since they often occur in mixed culture (e.g., in animal bites). Identification to species would be required for reasons of pathogenicity and epidemiology, since some species, e.g., *C. canimorsus*, may cause life-threatening disease. While identification is possible for larger laboratories, it may be challenging for smaller ones, which may not have the necessary material or personnel resources. However, analysis of colony and microscopic morphology, together with some simple biochemical tests such as oxidase, catalase, indole, nitratase, urease, ornithine decarboxylase, and growth on MacConkey agar, should go a long way toward making a species identification. Since disk susceptibility systems are not yet available for this group, a correct identification may also help in predicting susceptibility, as shown in some sections of this chapter. MIC testing is indicated for organisms whose resistance to certain antimicrobials has been previously reported in the literature.

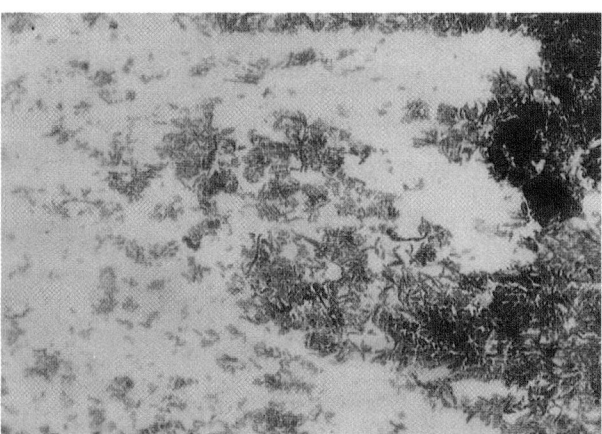

FIGURE 3 Microscopic morphology of *Streptobacillus moniliformis* grown on sheep blood agar (109).

REFERENCES

1. **Ahmed, K., P. P. Sein, M. Shahnawaz, and A. A. Hoosen.** 2002. *Pasteurella gallinarum* neonatal meningitis. *Clin. Microbiol. Infect.* **8:**55–57.
2. **Alcala, L., F. Garcia-Garrote, E. Cercenado, T. Pelaez, G. Ramos, and E. Bouza.** 1998. Comparison of broth microdilution method using *Haemophilus* test medium and agar dilution method for susceptibility testing of *Eikenella corrodens. J. Clin. Microbiol.* **36:**2386–2388.
3. **Al Fadel Saleh, M., M. S. Al-Madan, H. H. Erwa, I. Defonseka, S. Z. Sohel, and S. K. Sanyal.** 1995. First case of human infection caused by *Pasteurella gallinarum* causing infective endocarditis in an adolescent 10 years after surgical correction for truncus arteriosus. *Pediatrics* **95:**944–948.
4. **Allen, J. W., and T. L. Hanner.** 1997. Differentiation of EF-4 biovars by analysis of methicillin resistance. *Lab. Anim. Sci.* **47:**194–196.

5. **Alsina, M., E. Olle, and J. Frias.** 2001. Improved, low-cost selective culture medium for *Actinobacillus actinomycetemcomitans. J. Clin. Microbiol.* **39:**509–513.

6. **Amrikachi, M., B. Krishnan, C. J. Finch, and I. Shahab.** 2000. *Actinomyces* and *Actinobacillus actinomycetemcomitans-Actinomyces*-associated lymphadenopathy mimicking lymphoma. *Arch. Pathol. Lab. Med.* **124:**1502–1505.

7. **Angen, O., R. Mutters, D. A. Caugant, J. E. Olsen, and M. Bisgaard.** 1999. Taxonomic relationships of the *[Pasteurella] haemolytica* complex as evaluated by DNA-DNA hybridizations and 16S rRNA sequencing with proposal of *Mannheimia haemolytica* gen. nov., comb. nov., *Mannheimia granulomatis* comb. nov., *Mannheimia glucosida* sp. nov., *Mannheimia ruminalis* sp. nov. and *Mannheimia varigena* sp. nov. *Int. J. Syst. Bacteriol.* **49:**67–86.

8. **Arashima, Y., K. Kato, R. Kakuta, T. Fukui, K. Kumasaka, T. Tsuchiya, and K. Kawano.** 1999. First case of *Pasteurella gallinarum* isolation from blood of a patient with symptoms of acute gastroenteritis in Japan. *Clin. Infect. Dis.* **29:**698–699.

9. **Ashhurst-Smith, C., R. Norton, W. Thoreau, and M. M. Peel.** 1998. *Actinobacillus equuli* septicemia: an unusual zoonotic infection. *J. Clin. Microbiol.* **36:**2789–2790.

10. **Avril, J.-L., P.-Y. Donnio, and P. Pouedras.** 1990. Selective medium for *Pasteurella multocida* and its use to detect oropharyngeal carriage in pig breeders. *J. Clin. Microbiol.* **28:**1438–1440.

11. **Baddour, L. M., M. S. Gelfand, R. E. Weaver, T. C. Woods, M. Altwegg, L. W. Mayer, R. A. Kelley, and D. J. Brenner.** 1989. CDC group HB-5 as a cause of genitourinary infections in adults. *J. Clin. Microbiol.* **27:**801–805.

12. **Berger, C., M. Altwegg, A. Meyer, and D. Nadal.** 2001. Broad range polymerase chain reaction for diagnosis of rat-bite fever caused by *Streptobacillus moniliformis. Pediatr. Infect. Dis. J.* **20:**1181–1182.

13. **Bernard, K., C. Cooper, S. Tessier, and E. P. Ewan.** 1991. Use of chemotaxonomy as an aid to differentiate among *Capnocytophaga* species, CDC group DF-3, and aerotolerant strains of *Leptotrichia buccalis. J. Clin. Microbiol.* **29:**2263–2265.

14. **Bernardet, J.-F., P. Segers, M. Vancanneyt, F. Berthe, K. Kersters, and P. Vandamme.** 1996. Cutting a gordian knot: emended classification and description of the genus *Flavobacterium*, emended description of the family *Flavobacteriaceae*, and proposal of *Flavobacterium hydatis* nom. nov. (Basonym, *Cytophaga aquatilis* Strohl and Tait 1978). *Int. J. Syst. Bacteriol.* **46:**128–148.

15. **Bia, F., R. Marier, W. F. Collins, Jr, and A. von Graevenitz.** 1978. Meningitis and bacteremia caused by *Pasteurella ureae. Scand. J. Infect. Dis.* **10:**251–253.

16. **Bisgaard, M., and R. Mutters.** 1986. Characterization of some previously unclassified "*Pasteurella*" spp. obtained from the oral cavity of dogs and cats and description of a new species tentatively classified with the family *Pasteurellaceae* Pohl 1981 and provisionally called taxon 16. *Acta Pathol. Microbiol. Immunol. Scand. Sect. B* **94:**177–184.

17. **Boerlin, P., H. H. Siegrist, A. P. Burnens, P. Kuhnert, P. Mendez, G. Pretat, R. Lienhard, and J. Nicolet.** 2000. Molecular identification and epidemiological tracing of *Pasteurella multocida* meningitis in a baby. *J. Clin. Microbiol.* **38:**1235–1237.

18. **Bogaerts, J., J. Verhaegen, W. M. Tello, S. Allen, L. Verbist, E. Van Dyck, and P. Piot.** 1990. Characterization, in vitro susceptibility, and clinical significance of CDC group HB-5 from Rwanda. *J. Clin. Microbiol.* **28:**2196–2199.

19. **Brands, U., and W. Mannheim.** 1996. Use of two commercial rapid test kits for the identification of *Haemophilus*

20. **Brenner, D. J., D. G. Hollis, G. R. Fanning, and R. E. Weaver.** 1989. *Capnocytophaga canimorsus* sp. nov. (formerly CDC Group DF-2), a cause of septicemia following dog bite, and C. *cynodegmi* sp. nov., a cause of localized wound infection following dog bite. *J. Clin. Microbiol.* **27:**231–235.

21. **Carandina, G., M. Bacchelli, A. Virgili, and R. Strumia.** 1984. *Simonsiella* filaments isolated from erosive lesions of the human oral cavity. *J. Clin. Microbiol.* **19:**931–933.

22. **Chen, C.** 1996. Distribution of a newly described species, *Kingella oralis*, in the human oral cavity. *Oral Microbiol. Immunol.* **11:**425–427.

23. **Chen, S., L. Hichs, M. Yuen, D. Mitchell, and G. L. Gilbert.** 1994. Serological cross-reaction between *Legionella* spp. and *Capnocytophaga ochracea* by using latex agglutination test. *J. Clin. Microbiol.* **32:**3054–3055.

24. **Ciantar, M., D. A. Spratt, H. N. Newman, and M. Wilson.** 2000. Assessment of five culture media for the growth and isolation of *Capnocytophaga* spp. *Clin. Microbiol. Infect.* **7:**158–160.

25. **Claesson, B., E. Falsen, and B. Kjellman.** 1985. *Kingella kingae* infections: a review and a presentation of data from 10 Swedish cases. *Scand. J. Infect. Dis.* **17:**233–243.

26. **Conrads, G., R. Mutters, I. Seyfarth, and K. Pelz.** 1997. DNA-probes for the differentiation of *Capnocytophaga* species. *Mol. Cell. Probes* **11:**323–328.

27. **Cuadrado-Gomez, L. M., J. A. Arranz-Caso, J. Cuadros-Gonzales, and F. Albarran-Hernandez.** 1995. *Pasteurella pneumotropica* pneumonia in a patient with AIDS. *Clin. Infect. Dis.* **21:**445–446.

28. **Daneshvar, M. I., D. G. Hollis, and C. W. Moss.** 1991. Chemical characterization of clinical isolates which are similar to CDC Group DF-3 bacteria. *J. Clin. Microbiol.* **29:**2351–2353.

29. **Das, M., A. D. Badley, F. R. Cockerill, J. M. Steckelberg, and W. R. Wilson.** 1997. Infective endocarditis caused by HACEK microorganisms. *Annu. Rev. Med.* **48:**25–33.

30. **Dewhirst, F. E., C.-K. C. Chen, B. J. Paster, and J. J. Zambon.** 1993. Phylogeny of species in the family *Neisseriaceae* isolated from human dental plaque and description of *Kingella oralis* sp. nov. *Int. J. Syst. Bacteriol.* **43:**490–499. (Erratum, **44:**376, 1994.)

31. **Dewhirst, F. E., B. J. Paster, S. La Fontaine, and J. I. Rood.** 1990. Transfer of *Kingella indologenes* (Snell and Lapage 1976) to the genus *Suttonella* gen. nov. as *Suttonella indologenes* comb. nov.; transfer of *Bacteroides nodosus* (Beveridge 1941) to the genus *Dichelobacter* gen. nov. as *Dichelobacter nodosus* comb. nov., and assignment of the genera *Cardiobacterium*, *Dichelobacter*, and *Suttonella* to *Cardiobacteriaceae* fam. nov. in the gamma division of *Proteobacteria* on the basis of 16S rRNA sequence comparisons. *Int. J. Syst. Bacteriol.* **40:**426–433.

32. **Dewhirst, F. E., B. J. Paster, I. Olsen, and G. J. Fraser.** 1993. Phylogeny of the *Pasteurellaceae* as determined by comparison of 16S ribosomal ribonucleic acid sequences. *Zentbl. Bakteriol.* **279:**35–44.

33. **Dogan, B., S. Asikainen, and H. Jousimies-Somer.** 1999. Evaluation of two commercial kits and arbitrarily primed PCR for identification and differentiation of *Actinobacillus actinomycetemcomitans*, *Haemophilus aphrophilus*, and *Haemophilus paraphrophilus. J. Clin. Microbiol.* **37:**742–747.

34. **Duong, M., J. F. Besancenot, C. Neuwirth, M. Buisson, P. Chavanet, and H. Portier.** 1996. Vertebral osteomyelitis due to *Capnocytophaga* species in immunocompetent patients: report of two cases and review. *Clin. Infect. Dis.* **22:**1099–1101.

35. Dusch, H., R. Zbinden, and A. von Graevenitz. 1995. Growth differences of *Capnocytophaga canimorsus* strains and some other fastidious organisms on various Columbia-based blood agar media. *Zentbl. Bakteriol.* **282:**362–366.

36. Ebinger, M., T. Nichterlein, U. K. Schumacher, B. Manncke, D. Schmidt, and I. Böhn. 2000. Isolation of *Capnocytophaga granulosa* from an abscess in an immunocompetent adolescent. *Clin. Infect. Dis.* **30:**606–607.

37. Eckert, F., A. Stenzel, R. Mutters, W. Frederiksen, and W. Mannheim. 1991. Some unusual members of the family *Pasteurellaceae* isolated from human sources—phenotypic features and genomic relationships. *Zentbl. Bakteriol.* **275:**143–155.

38. Edwards, R., and R. G. Finch. 1986. Characterisation and antibiotic susceptibilities of *Streptobacillus moniliformis*. *J. Med. Microbiol.* **21:**39–42.

39. Ejlertsen, T., B. Gahrn-Hansen, P. Sogaard, O. Heltberg, and W. Frederiksen. 1996. *Pasteurella aerogenes* isolated from ulcers or wounds in humans with occupational exposure to pigs: a report of 7 Danish cases. *Scand. J. Infect. Dis.* **28:**567–570.

40. Elsaghier, A. A. F., C. C. Kibbler, and J. M. T. Hamilton-Miller. 1998. *Pasteurella multocida* as an infectious cause of endocarditis. *Clin. Infect. Dis.* **27:**410.

41. Escande, F., A. Bailly, S. Bone, and J. Lemozy. 1996. *Actinobacillus suis* infection after a pig bite. *Lancet* **348:**888.

42. Escande, F., E. Vallée, and F. Aubart. 1997. *Pasteurella caballi* infection following a horse bite. *Zentbl. Bakteriol.* **285:**440–444.

43. Flemming, T. F., S. Rüdiger, U. Hofmann, H. Schmidt, B. Plaschke, A. Strätz, B. Klaiber, and H. Karch. 1995. Identification of *Actinobacillus actinomycetemcomitans* in subgingival plaque by PCR. *J. Clin. Microbiol.* **33:**3102–3105.

44. Frebourg, N. B., G. Berthelot, R. Hocq, A. Chibani, and J.-F. Lemeland. 2002. Septicemia due to *Pasteurella pneumotropica*: 16S rRNA sequencing for diagnosis confirmation. *J. Clin. Microbiol.* **40:**687–689.

45. Frederiksen, W. 1981. Gas producing species within *Pasteurella* and *Actinobacillus*, p. 185–196. *In* M. Kilian, W. Frederiksen, and E. L. Biberstein (ed.), Haemophilus, Pasteurella, *and* Actinobacillus. Academic Press, Ltd., London, United Kingdom.

46. Frederiksen, W., and B. Tonning. 2001. Possible misidentification of *Haemophilus aphrophilus* as *Pasteurella gallinarum*. *Clin. Infect. Dis.* **32:**987–989.

47. Friis-Moller, A., J. J. Christensen, V. Fussing, A. Hesselbjerg, J. Christiansen, and B. Bruun. 2001. Clinical significance and taxonomy of *Actinobacillus hominis*. *J. Clin. Microbiol.* **39:**930–935.

48. Furcht, C., K. Eschrich, and K. Merte. 1996. Detection of *Eikenella corrodens* and *Actinobacillus actinomycetemcomitans* by use of the polymerase chain reaction (PCR) in vitro and in subgingival plaque. *J. Clin. Periodontol.* **23:**891–897.

49. Gerardo, S. H., D. M. Citron, M. C. Claros, H. T. Fernandez, and E. J. C. Goldstein. 2001. *Pasteurella multocida* subsp. *multocida* and *P. multocida* subsp. *septica* differentiation by PCR fingerprinting and α-glucosidase activity. *J. Clin. Microbiol.* **39:**2558–2564.

50. Goldstein, E. J. C., E. O. Agyare, and R. Silletti. 1981. Comparative growth of *Eikenella corrodens* on 15 media in three atmospheres of incubation. *J. Clin. Microbiol.* **13:**951–953.

51. Goldstein, E. J. C., D. M. Citron, C. V. Merriam, Y. Warren, and K. Tyrrell. 2000. Comparative in vitro activities of GAR-936 against aerobic and anaerobic animal and human bite wound pathogens. *Antimicrob. Agents Chemother.* **44:**2747–2751.

52. Goldstein, E. J. C., D. M. Citron, A. E. Vagvolgyi, and M. E. Gombert. 1986. Susceptibility of *Eikenella corrodens* to newer and older quinolones. *Antimicrob. Agents Chemother.* **30:**172–173.

53. Goldstein, E. J. C., L. A. Tarenzi, E. O. Agyare, and J. R. Berger. 1983. Prevalence of *Eikenella corrodens* in dental plaque. *J. Clin. Microbiol.* **17:**636–639.

54. Gomez-Garces, J.-L., J.-I. Alos, J. Sanchez, and R. Cogollos. 1994. Bacteremia by multidrug-resistant *Capnocytophaga sputigena*. *J. Clin. Microbiol.* **32:**1067–1069.

55. Grehn, M., and F. Müller. 1989. The oxidase reaction of *Pasteurella multocida* strains cultured on Mueller-Hinton medium. *J. Microbiol. Methods* **9:**333–336.

56. Grob, R., R. Zbinden, C. Ruef, M. Hackenthal, I. Diesterweg, M. Altwegg, and A. von Graevenitz. 1999. Septicemia caused by dysgonic fermenter 3 in a severely immunocompromised patient and isolation of the same microorganism from a stool specimen. *J. Clin. Microbiol.* **37:**1617–1618.

57. Hanner, T. L., J. W. Allen, A. Robertson-Byers, and S. L. Hurley. 1991. Characterization of eugonic fermenters group EF-4 by polyacrylamide gel electrophoresis and protein immunoblot analysis. *Am. J. Vet. Res.* **52:**1065–1068.

58. Hayashi, F., M. Okada, X. Zhong, and K. Miura. 2001. PCR detection of *Capnocytophaga* species in dental plaque samples from children aged 2 to 12 years. *Microbiol. Immunol.* **45:**17–22.

59. Heiske, A., and R. Mutters. 1994. Differentiation of selected members of the family *Neisseriaceae* (*Alysiella, Eikenella, Kingella, Simonsiella* and CDC Groups EF-4 and M-5) by carbohydrate fingerprints and selected phenotypic features. *Zentbl. Bakteriol.* **281:**67–79.

60. Henrichsen, J. 1972. Bacterial surface translocation: a survey and a classification. *Bacteriol. Rev.* **36:**478–503.

61. Hofstad, T., I. Olsen, E. R. Eribe, E. Falsen, M. D. Collins, and P. A. Lawson. 2000. *Dysgonomonas* gen. nov. to accommodate *Dysgonomonas gadei* sp. nov., an organism isolated from a human gall bladder, and *Dysgonomonas capnocytophagoides* (formerly CDC group DF-3). *Int. J. Syst. Evol. Microbiol.* **50:**2189–2195.

62. Holm, A., P. Rabe, S. Kalfas, and S. Edwardsson. 1987. Improved selective culture media for *Actinobacillus actinomycetemcomitans* and *Haemophilus aphrophilus*. *J. Clin. Microbiol.* **25:**1985–1988.

63. Holst, E., J. Rollof, L. Larsson, and J. P. Nielsen. 1992. Characterization and distribution of *Pasteurella* species recovered from infected humans. *J. Clin. Microbiol.* **30:**2984–2987.

64. Host, B., H. Schumacher, J. Prag, and M. Arpi. 2000. Isolation of *Kingella kingae* from synovial fluids using four commercial blood culture bottles. *Eur. J. Clin. Microbiol. Infect. Dis.* **19:**608–611.

65. Hunt, M. L., B. Adler, and K. M. Townsend. 2000. The molecular biology of *Pasteurella multocida*. *Vet. Microbiol.* **72:**3–25.

66. Jenny, D. B., P. W. Letendre, and G. Iverson. 1987. Endocarditis caused by *Kingella indologenes*. *Rev. Infect. Dis.* **9:**787–789.

67. Jolivet-Gougeon, A., A. Buffet, C. Dupuy, J.-L. Sixou, M. Bonnaure-Mallet, S. David, and M. Cormier. 2000. In vitro susceptibility of *Capnocytophaga* isolates to β-lactam antibiotics and β-lactamase inhibitors. *Antimicrob. Agents Chemother.* **44:**3186–3188.

68. Kaplan, A. H., D. J. Weber, E. Z. Oddone, and J. R. Perfect. 1989. Infection due to *Actinobacillus actinomycetemcomitans*: 15 cases and review. *Rev. Infect. Dis.* **11:**46–63.

69. **Kasten, R., R. Mutters, and W. Mannheim.** 1998. Catalase-positive *Eikenella corrodens* and *Eikenella*-like isolates of human and canine origin. *Zentbl. Bakteriol.* **288:**319–329.

70. **Kim, J. O., J. Ginsberg, K. L. McGowan.** 1996. *Capnocytophaga* meningitis in a cancer patient. *Pediatr. Infect. Dis. J.* **15:**636–637.

71. **Kooter, A. J., A. Derks, and W. L. E. Vasmel.** 1999. Rapidly progressive tricuspid valve endocarditis caused by *Capnocytophaga canimorsus* infection in an immunocompetent host. *Clin. Microbiol. Infect.* **5:**173–175.

72. **Krause, T., H. U. Bertschinger, L. Corboz, and R. Mutters.** 1987. V-factor dependent strains of *Pasteurella multocida* subsp. *multocida.* *Zentbl. Bakteriol.* **266:**255–260.

73. **Kugler, K. C., D. J. Biedenbach, and R. N. Jones.** 1999. Determination of the antimicrobial activity of 29 clinically important compounds tested against fastidious HACEK group organisms. *Diagn. Microbiol. Infect. Dis.* **34:**73–76.

74. **Kuhn, D. A., and D. A. Gregory.** 1978. Emendation of *Simonsiella muelleri* Schmid and description of *Simonsiella steedae* sp. nov., with designations of the respective proposed neotype and holotype strains. *Curr. Microbiol.* **1:**11–14.

75. **Kuhn, D. A., D. A. Gregory, G. E. Buchanan, Jr., M. D. Nyby, and K. R. Daly.** 1978. Isolation, characterization, and numerical taxonomy of *Simonsiella* strains from the oral cavities of cats, dogs, sheep and humans. *Arch. Microbiol.* **118:**235–241.

76. **Kuhnert, P., P. Boerlin, S. Emler, M. Krawinkler, and J. Frey.** 2000. Phylogenetic analysis of *Pasteurella multocida* subspecies and molecular identification of feline *P. multocida* subsp. *septica* by 16S rRNA gene sequencing. *Int. J. Med. Microbiol.* **290:**599–604.

77. **Kumar, A., H. R. Devlin, and H. Vellend.** 1990. *Pasteurella multocida* meningitis in an adult: case report and review. *Rev. Infect. Dis.* **12:**440–448.

78. **Lee, J., J. S. Kim, C. H. Nahm, J. W. Choi, J. Kim, S. H. Pai, K. H. Moon, K. Lee, and Y. Chong.** 1999. Two cases of *Chromobacterium violaceum* infection after injury in a subtropical region. *J. Clin. Microbiol.* **37:**2068–2070.

79. **Lester, A., J. O. Jarlov, H. Westh, and W. Frederiksen.** 1992. *Pasteurella haemolytica* diagnosis questioned. *J. Infect.* **25:**334–335.

80. **Lichtensteiger, C. A., S. M. Steenbergen, R. M. Lee, D. D. Polson, and E. R. Vimr.** 1996. Direct PCR analysis for toxigenic *Pasteurella multocida.* *J. Clin. Microbiol.* **34:**3035–3039.

81. **Lindberg, J., W. Frederiksen, B. Gahrn-Hansen, and B. Bruun.** 1998. Problems of identification in clinical microbiology exemplified by pig bite wound infections. *Zentbl. Bakteriol.* **288:**491–499.

82. **Lion, C., P. de Monchy, M. Weber, M. C. Conroy, F. Mory, and J. C. Burdin.** 1992. Sensibilité aux antibiotiques de quarante-quatre souches de bactéries du groupe EF4: étude des concentrations minimales inhibitrices par dilution en gélose. *Pathol. Biol.* **40:**471–478.

83. **Lion, C., F. Escande, and J. C. Burdin.** 1996. *Capnocytophaga canimorsus* infections in human: review of the literature and cases report. *Eur. J. Epidemiol.* **12:**521–533.

84. **Lion, C., A. Lozniewski, V. Rosner, and M. Weber.** 1999. Lung abscess due to β-lactamase-producing *Pasteurella multocida.* *Clin. Infect. Dis.* **29:**1345–1346.

85. **London, R. D., and E. J. Bottone.** 1991. *Pasteurella multocida:* zoonotic cause of peritonitis in a patient undergoing peritoneal dialysis. *Am. J. Med.* **91:**202–204.

86. **Lu, P.-L., P.-R. Hsueh, C.-C. Hung, L.-J. Teng, T.-N. Jang, and K.-T. Luh.** 2000. Infective endocarditis complicated with progressive heart failure due to β-lactamase-producing *Cardiobacterium hominis.* *J. Clin. Microbiol.* **38:**2015–2017.

87. **Macher, A. M., Th. B. Casale, and A. S. Fauci.** 1982. Chronic granulomatous disease of childhood and *Chromobacterium violaceum* infections in the Southeastern United States. *Ann. Intern. Med.* **97:**51–55.

88. **Madinier, I. M., T. B. Fosse, C. Hitzig, Y. Charbit, and L. R. Hannoun.** 1999. Resistance profile survey of 50 periodontal strains of *Actinobacillus actinomycetemcomitans.* *J. Periodontol.* **70:**888–892.

89. **Martinez-Sanchez, L., F. J. Vasallo, F. Garcia-Garrote, L. Alcala, M. Rodriguez-Créixems, and E. Bouza.** 1998. Clinical isolation of a DF-3 microorganism and review of the literature. *Clin. Microbiol. Infect.* **4:**344–346.

90. **May, B. J., Q. Zhang, L. L. Li, M. L. Paustian, T. S. Whittam, and V. Kapur.** 2001. Complete genomic sequence of *Pasteurella multocida,* Pm70. *Proc. Natl. Acad. Sci. USA* **98:**3460–3465.

91. **McNabb, A., and D. Colby.** 1990. *Capnocytophaga cynodegmi* isolated from a corneal ulcer. *Clin. Microbiol. Newsl.* **12:**126–127.

92. **Minamoto, G. Y., and E. M. Sordillo.** 1992. *Kingella denitrificans* as a cause of granulomatous disease in a patient with AIDS. *Clin. Infect. Dis.* **15:**1052–1053.

93. **Mueller, N. J., V. Kaplan, R. Zbinden, and M. Altwegg.** 1999. Diagnosis of *Cardiobacterium hominis* endocarditis by broad-range PCR from arterio-embolic tissue. *Infection* **27:**278–279.

94. **Mutters, R., P. Ihm, S. Pohl, W. Frederiksen, and W. Mannheim.** 1985. Reclassification of the genus *Pasteurella* Trevisan 1887 on the basis of deoxyribonucleic acid homology, with proposals for the new species *Pasteurella dagmatis, Pasteurella canis, Pasteurella stomatis, Pasteurella anatis,* and *Pasteurella langaa.* *Int. J. Syst. Bacteriol.* **35:**309–322.

95. **Mutters, R., K. Piechulla, K.-H. Hinz, and W. Mannheim.** 1985. *Pasteurella avium* (Hinz and Kunjara 1977) comb. nov. and *Pasteurella volantium* sp. nov. *Int. J. Syst. Bacteriol.* **35:**5–9.

96. **Noble, R. C., B. J. Marek, and S. B. Overman.** 1987. Spontaneous bacterial peritonitis caused by *Pasteurella ureae.* *J. Clin. Microbiol.* **25:**442–444.

97. **Olsen, J., H. N. Shah, and S. E. Gharbia.** 1999. Taxonomy and biochemical characteristics of *Actinobacillus actinomycetemcomitans* and *Porphyromonas gingivalis.* *Periodontology* **20:**14–52.

98. **Paerregaard, A., and E. Gutschik.** 1987. *Capnocytophaga* bacteremia complicating premature delivery by Cesarean section. *Eur. J. Clin. Microbiol.* **6:**580–581.

99. **Paju, S., P. Carlson, H. Jousimies-Somer, and S. Asikainen.** 2000. Heterogeneity of *Actinobacillus actinomycetemcomitans* strains in various human infections and relationships between serotype, genotype, and antimicrobial susceptibility. *J. Clin. Microbiol.* **38:**79–84.

100. **Parenti, D. M., and D. R. Snydman.** 1985. *Capnocytophaga* species: infections in nonimmunocompromised and immunocompromised hosts. *J. Infect. Dis.* **151:**140–147.

101. **Paul, K., and S. S. Patel.** 2001. *Eikenella corrodens* infections in children and adolescents: case reports and review of the literature. *Clin. Infect. Dis.* **33:**54–61.

102. **Peel, M. M., K. A. Hornidge, M. Luppino, A. M. Stacpoole, and R. E. Weaver.** 1991. *Actinobacillus* spp. and related bacteria in infected wounds of humans bitten by horses and sheep. *J. Clin. Microbiol.* **29:**2535–2538.

103. **Pins, M. R., J. M. Holden, J. M. Yang, S. Madoff, and M. J. Ferraro.** 1996. Isolation of presumptive *Streptobacillus moniliformis* from abscesses associated with the female genital tract. *Clin. Infect. Dis.* **22:**471–476.

104. **Pulverer, G., and H. Schütt-Gerowitt.** 1998. *Actinobacillus actinomycetemcomitans* in the human oral microflora. *Zentbl. Bakteriol.* **288:**87–92.

105. **Rechtman, D. J., and J. P. Nadler.** 1991. Abdominal abscess due to *Cardiobacterium hominis* and *Clostridium bifermentans. Rev. Infect. Dis.* **13:**418–419.

106. **Roberts, S. A., A. J. Morris, N. McIvor, and R. Ellis-Pegler.** 1997. *Chromobacterium violaceum* infection of the deep neck tissues in a traveler to Thailand. *Clin. Infect. Dis.* **25:**334–335.

107. **Robertson, P. B., M. Lantz, P. T. Marucha, K. S. Kornman, C. L. Trummel, and S. C. Holt.** 1982. Collagenolytic activity associated with *Bacteroides* species and *Actinobacillus actinomycetemcomitans. J. Periodontal Res.* **17:**275–283.

108. **Roebuck, J. D., and J. T. Morris.** 1999. Chronic otitis media due to EF-4 bacteria. *Clin. Infect. Dis.* **29:**1343–1344.

109. **Rordorf, T., C. Züger, R. Zbinden, A. von Graevenitz, and M. Pirovino.** 2000. *Streptobacillus moniliformis* endocarditis in an HIV-positive patient. *Infection* **28:**393–394.

110. **Rossau, R., G. Vandenbussche, S. Thielemans, P. Segers, H. Grosch, E. Göthe, W. Mannheim, and J. de Ley.** 1989. Ribosomal ribonucleic acid cistron similarities and deoxyribonucleic acid homologies of *Neisseria, Kingella, Eikenella, Simonsiella, Alysiella,* and Centers for Disease Control groups EF-4 and M-5 in the emended family *Neisseriaceae. Int. J. Syst. Bacteriol.* **39:**185–198.

111. **Ruddy, A., J. Hughes, and P. Bourbeau.** 1986. *Actinobacillus suis:* finger isolate following horse bite. *Clin. Microbiol. Newsl.* **24:**187–188.

112. **Rummens, J.-L., B. Gordts, and H. W. van Landuyt.** 1986. In vitro susceptibility of *Capnocytophaga* species to 29 antimicrobial agents. *Antimicrob. Agents Chemother.* **30:**739–742.

113. **Rycroft, A. N., and L. H. Garside.** 2000. *Actinobacillus* species and their role in animal disease. *Vet. J.* **159:**18–36.

114. **Sakazaki, R., E. Yoshizaki, K. Tamura, and S. Kuramochi.** 1984. Increased frequency of isolation of *Pasteurella* and *Actinobacillus* species and related organisms. *Eur. J. Clin. Microbiol. Infect. Dis.* **3:**244–248.

115. **Schlater, L. K., D. J. Brenner, A. G. Steigerwalt, C. W. Moss, M. A. Lambert, and R. A. Packer.** 1989. *Pasteurella caballi,* a new species from equine clinical specimens. *J. Clin. Microbiol.* **27:**2169–2174.

116. **Seger, R., J. Kloeti, A. von Graevenitz, J. Wüst, J. Briner, U. Willi, and H. Siegrist.** 1982. Cervical abscess due to *Capnocytophaga ochracea. Pediatr. Infect. Dis. J.* **1:**170–173.

117. **Shapiro, D. S., P. E. Brooks, D. M. Coffey, and K. F. Browne.** 1996. Peripartum bacteremia with CDC group HB-5 (*Pasteurella bettyae*). *Clin. Infect. Dis.* **22:**1125–1126.

118. **Slee, A. M., and J. M. Tanzer.** 1978. Selective medium for isolation of *Eikenella corrodens* from periodontal lesions. *J. Clin. Microbiol.* **8:**459–462.

119. **Slonim, A., E. S. Walker, E. Mishori, N. Porat, R. Dagan, and P. Yagupsky.** 1998. Person-to-person transmission of *Kingella kingae* among day care center attendees. *J. Infect. Dis.* **178:**1843–1846.

120. **Slotnick, I. J.** 1968. *Cardiobacterium hominis* in genitourinary specimens. *J. Bacteriol.* **95:**1175.

121. **Sneath, P. H. A., and M. Stevens.** 1990. *Actinobacillus rossii* sp. nov., *Actinobacillus seminis* sp. nov., nom. rev., *Pasteurella bettii* sp. nov., *Pasteurella lymphangitidis* sp. nov., *Pasteurella mairi* sp. nov., and *Pasteurella trehalosi* sp. nov. *Int. J. Syst. Bacteriol.* **40:**148–153.

122. **Sordillo, E. M., M. Rendel, R. Sood, J. Belinfanti, O. Murray, and D. Brook.** 1993. Septicemia due to

123. **Stähelin, J., D. Goldenberger, H. E. Gnehm, and M. Altwegg.** 1998. Polymerase chain reaction diagnosis of *Kingella kingae* arthritis in a young child. *Clin. Infect. Dis.* **27:**1328–1329.

β-lactamase-positive *Kingella kingae. Clin. Infect. Dis.* **17:**818–819.

124. **Stoloff, A. L., and M. L. Gillies.** 1986. Infections with *Eikenella corrodens* in a general hospital: a report of 33 cases. *Rev. Infect. Dis.* **8:**50–53.

125. **Sutton, R. G. A., M. F. O'Keeffe, M. A. Bundock, J. Jeboult, and M. P. Tester.** 1972. Isolation of a new *Moraxella* from corneal abscess. *J. Med. Microbiol.* **5:**148–150.

126. **Suzuki, N., Y. Nakano, Y. Yoshida, D. Ikeda, and T. Koga.** 2001. Identification of *Actinobacillus actinomycetemcomitans* serotypes by multiplex PCR. *J. Clin. Microbiol.* **39:**2002–2005.

127. **Talan, D. A., D. M. Citron, F. M. Abrahamian, G. J. Moran, and E. J. C. Goldstein.** 1999. Bacteriologic analysis of infected dog and cat bites. *N. Engl. J. Med.* **340:**85–92.

128. **Townsend, K. M., J. D. Boyce, J. Y. Chung, A. J. Frost, and B. Adler.** 2001. Genetic organization of *Pasteurella multocida cap* loci and development of a multiplex capsular PCR typing system. *J. Clin. Microbiol.* **39:**924–929.

129. **van Steenbergen, T. J. M., C. J. Bosch-Tijhof, A. J. van Winkelhoff, R. Gmür, and J. de Graaff.** 1994. Comparison of six typing methods for *Actinobacillus actinomycetemcomitans. J. Clin. Microbiol.* **32:**2769–2774.

130. **Verhaegen, J., H. Verbraeken, A. Cabuy, J. Vandeven, and J. Vandepitte.** 1988. *Actinobacillus* (formerly *Pasteurella*) *ureae* meningitis and bacteraemia: report of a case and review of the literature. *J. Infect.* **17:**249–253.

131. **Weber, D. J., J. S. Wolfson, M. N. Swartz, and D. C. Hooper.** 1984. *Pasteurella multocida* infections. Report of 34 cases and review of the literature. *Medicine* **63:**133–154.

132. **Weyant, R. S., C. W. Moss, R. E. Weaver, D. G. Hollis, J. G. Jordan, E. C. Cook, and M. I. Daneshvar.** 1996. *Identification of Unusual Pathogenic Gram-Negative Aerobic and Facultatively Anaerobic Bacteria,* 2nd ed. The Williams & Wilkins Co., Baltimore, Md.

133. **Whitehouse, R. L. S., H. Jackson, M. C. Jackson, and M. M. Ramji.** 1987. Isolation of *Simonsiella* sp. from a neonate. *J. Clin. Microbiol.* **25:**522–525.

134. **Whitelaw, A. C., I. M. Shankland, and B. G. Elisha.** 2002. Use of 16S rRNA sequencing for identification of *Actinobacillus ureae* isolated from a cerebrospinal fluid sample. *J. Clin. Microbiol.* **40:**666–668.

135. **Wormser, G. P., and E. J. Bottone.** 1983. *Cardiobacterium hominis:* review of microbiologic and clinical features. *Rev. Infect. Dis.* **5:**680–691.

136. **Wullenweber, M.** 1994. *Streptobacillus moniliformis*—a zoonotic pathogen. Taxonomic considerations, host species, diagnosis, therapy, geographical distribution. *Lab. Anim.* **29:**1–15.

137. **Wüst, J., J. Gubler, W. Mannheim, and A. von Graevenitz.** 1991. *Actinobacillus hominis* as a causative agent of septicemia in hepatic failure. *Eur. J. Clin. Microbiol. Infect. Dis.* **10:**693–694.

138. **Yagupsky, P., and R. Dagan.** 1997. *Kingella kingae:* an emerging cause of invasive infections in young children. *Clin. Infect. Dis.* **24:**860–866.

139. **Yagupsky, P., O. Katz, and N. Peled.** 2001. Antibiotic susceptibility of *Kingella kingae* isolates from respiratory carriers and patients with invasive infections. *J. Antimicrob. Chemother.* **47:**191–193.

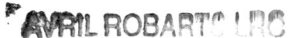

140. **Yamamoto, T., S. Kajiura, Y. Hirai, and T. Watanabe.** 1994. *Capnocytophaga haemolytica* sp. nov. and *Capnocytophaga granulosa* sp. nov., from human dental plaque. *Int. J. Syst. Bacteriol.* **44:**324–329.

141. **Yaneza, A. L., H. Jivan, P. Kumari, and M. S. Togoo.** 1991. *Pasteurella haemolytica* endocarditis. *J. Infect.* **23:** 65–67.

142. **Yogev, R., D. Shulman, S. T. Shulman, and W. G. Glogowski.** 1986. In vitro activity of antibiotics alone and in combination against *Actinobacillus actinomycetemcomitans. Antimicrob. Agents Chemother.* **29:**179–181.

143. **Zbinden, R., P. Sommerhalder, and U. von Wartburg.** 1988. Co-isolation of *Pasteurella dagmatis* and *Pasteurella multocida* from cat-bite wounds. *Eur. J. Clin. Microbiol. Infect. Dis.* **7:**203–204.

144. **Zbinden, R., A. Hany, R. Lüthy, D. Conen, and I. Heinzer.** 1998. Antibody response in six HACEK endocarditis cases under therapy. *APMIS* **106:**547–552.

145. **Zijlstra, E. E., G. R. Swart, F. J. M. Godfroy, and J. E. Degener.** 1992. Pericarditis, peumonia and brain abscess due to a combined *Actinomyces-Actinobacillus actinomycetemcomitans* infection. *J. Infect.* **25:**83–87.

Haemophilus

MOGENS KILIAN

40

TAXONOMY AND DESCRIPTION OF THE GENUS

Members of the genus *Haemophilus* are gram-negative, non-acid-fast, nonmotile, and non-spore-forming rods that may range from small coccobacilli to filamentous rods. They are obligate parasites that, with a few misclassified exceptions (e.g., *Haemophilus ducreyi*), are exclusively adapted to human mucosal membranes of the respiratory tract. Most species of animal origin originally included in the genus *Haemophilus* have been transferred to the genus *Pasteurella* or the genus *Actinobacillus*, which together with the genus *Haemophilus* and a few newly described genera of bacteria from animals constitute the family *Pasteurellaceae* (60).

The *Haemophilus* species associated with humans are *H. influenzae*, *H. aegyptius*, *H. haemolyticus*, *H. parainfluenzae*, *H. parahaemolyticus*, *H. ducreyi*, *H. aphrophilus*, *H. paraphrophilus*, *H. segnis*, and the poorly defined species *H. paraphrohaemolyticus*.

All *Haemophilus* species are facultatively anaerobic. The genus name refers to the fact that in vitro growth requires accessory growth factors contained in blood: X factor (hemin; "X" for unknown) and V factor (NAD; "V" for vitamin). *H. influenzae* requires both of these compounds, whereas most other species require only one of them (Table 1). Strains of a few species grow better in a humid atmosphere with added 5 to 10% CO_2. The optimal temperature is about 33 to 37°C (see below).

Haemophilus species ferment a characteristic range of carbohydrates; end products from the fermentation of glucose are succinic, lactic, and acetic acids. Strains of some species (e.g., *H. aphrophilus*) produce gas in fermentation media. Only the misplaced *H. ducreyi* is negative by traditional fermentation tests. All *Haemophilus* strains reduce nitrate and produce alkaline phosphatase (36). The G+C content of DNA of *Haemophilus* species ranges from 37 to 44 mol% (36). Predominant cell wall fatty acids are *n*-tetradecanoate (14:0), 3-hydroxy-tetradecanoate (3-OH-14:0), hexadecanoate (16:1), and *n*-hexadecanoate (16:0) (37).

Separate subpopulations of *H. influenzae* express polysaccharide capsules, of which six different serotypes, termed serotypes a through f, have been described.

By traditional taxonomic criteria, it is unjustified to maintain the recognition of *H. influenzae* and *H. aegyptius*

as separate species (13). However, one formal obstacle to combining the two is that the name *H. aegyptius* has priority over *H. influenzae*. Moreover, population genetic analyses reveal that they do constitute distinct populations of bacteria, and clinical experience indicates that they have distinct pathogenic potentials. This is also true for the so-called *H. influenzae* biogroup aegyptius (10; M. Kilian, K. Poulsen, and H. Lomholt, unpublished data). Likewise, some taxonomic studies have questioned the validity of *H. paraphrophilus* as a species separate from *H. aphrophilus*, despite differences in their growth factor requirements and other chemotaxonomic characteristics (15, 37).

According to nucleic acid hybridization studies and 16S rRNA sequence homologies, the species *H. ducreyi* does not belong in the genus *Haemophilus*, although it does appear to be a valid member of the family *Pasteurellaceae* (14, 22).

CLINICAL SIGNIFICANCE

Carriage

Haemophilus bacteria constitute approximately 10% of the normal bacterial flora of the healthy upper respiratory tract. The predominant species is *H. parainfluenzae*, which accounts for three-fourths of the *Haemophilus* flora both in the oral cavity and in the pharynx but is absent from the nasal cavity. Nonencapsulated *H. influenzae* strains, predominantly of biotypes II or III, are present in the pharynges of most healthy children (80%) but normally constitute less than 2% of the total bacterial flora (38, 39).

Nasopharyngeal colonization by *H. influenzae* is a dynamic phenomenon characterized by constant turnover of a mixture of clones, with a mean duration of carriage of 1.4 months (39, 70). During local infection a single clone of *H. influenzae* usually dominates the bacterial flora in the pharynx and nasal cavity. With increasing age of the individual, carriage of *H. influenzae* in the upper respiratory tract becomes less frequent (39, 54). In populations without vaccination, the rate of *H. influenzae* serotype b carriage by healthy individuals is below 1% during the first 6 months of life but averages 3 to 5% throughout the rest of childhood, although it may be considerably higher in selected populations (54, 84). Carriage in vaccinated children is becoming rare as a result of the antibodies induced by the conjugate vaccine (78). Carriage in healthy individuals of *H. aegyptius*

TABLE 1 Principal differential characteristics of *Haemophilus* species

Species	Factor requirement X[a]	V	Hemolysis	Glucose	Sucrose	Lactose	Mannose	Xylose	Presence of catalase	β-Galactosidase (ONPG[b] test)	H₂S production	CO₂ enhances growth
H. influenzae[c]	+	+	−	+	−	−	−	+[d]	+	−	−	−
H. aegyptius[c]	+	+	−	+	−	−	−	−	+	−	−	−
H. haemolyticus	+	+	+	+	−	−	−	+[d]	+	−	+	−
H. ducreyi	+	−	−[e]	−	−	−	−	−	−	−	−	−
H. parainfluenzae	−	+	−	+	+	−	+	−	D[f]	D	+	−
H. parahaemolyticus	−	+	+	+	+	−	−	−	+	−	+	−
H. segnis	−	+	−	w[g]	w	−	−	−	D	−	−	−
H. paraphrophilus[h]	−	+	−	+	+	+	+	D	−	+	+	+
H. aphrophilus[h]	w	−	−	+	+	+	+	−	−	+	+	+

a As determined by the porphyrin test.
b ONPG, *o*-nitrophenyl-β-D-galactopyranoside.
c For further characteristics, see Table 2.
d More than 90% of isolates are positive.
e Detection requires special media; see text.
f D, differences encountered.
g w, weak fermentation reaction.
h For further characteristics, see Table 3.

and *H. influenzae* biogroup aegyptius has not been demonstrated.

The species *H. parainfluenzae*, *H. aphrophilus*, *H. paraphrophilus*, and *H. segnis*, but not *H. influenzae*, are part of the normal oral microflora. The species *H. aphrophilus*, *H. paraphrophilus*, and *H. segnis* occur predominantly on tooth surfaces in the biofilm known as dental plaque. *H. haemolyticus* may be encountered primarily in gingival crevices, but its clinical relevance is unknown. Human saliva contains a mean number of more than 10⁷ haemophili per ml (38). Symptomless cervical carriage of the venereal pathogen *H. ducreyi* may occur (83).

Spread of the *Haemophilus* species that colonize the upper respiratory tract typically occurs by respiratory droplets, and spread of *H. ducreyi* is by sexual intercourse.

Disease

H. influenzae

Until the implementation of vaccination in many countries, *H. influenzae* was one of the three leading causes of bacterial meningitis worldwide. Most of these cases were in young children, with a peak incidence of infection at 6 to 7 months of age. Virtually all were caused by serotype b, and the majority belonged to biotype I. Both characteristics make them distinct from commensal strains. Strains with the same characteristics were also major etiologic agents of acute epiglottitis (obstructive laryngitis) associated with septicemia. The annual number of invasive *H. influenzae* serotype b infections in the United States is now below 100, all of which occur in unvaccinated or incompletely vaccinated children (1, 16). However, *H. influenzae* type b remains a leading cause of meningitis among unvaccinated children. It is estimated that at least 3 million cases of serious disease and 400,000 to 700,000 deaths occur in young children per year worldwide (63). Occasional cases of invasive infection caused by nonencapsulated strains or strains possessing a capsule, primarily of serotype f, occur, mostly in patients with significant underlying disease, such as malignancy, chronic obstructive pulmonary disease, alcoholism, and human immunodeficiency virus (HIV) infection. In children, underlying diseases are less common (26% of cases), and pneumonia and meningitis are equally represented (86). Strains carrying capsules of serotypes a, d, and e are occasionally isolated from patients with infections as well as from the healthy respiratory tract, whereas serotype c strains are rare (36, 88).

Invasion of the bloodstream by encapsulated strains of *H. influenzae* may also result in septic arthritis, osteomyelitis, cellulitis, and pericarditis (73, 84). Primary *H. influenzae* pneumonia is being recognized with increasing frequency in both children and adults and is sometimes complicated by bacteremia (44, 57). Most isolates from patients with pneumonia are non-type b strains. A recent literature review revealed that *H. influenzae* accounted for 7% of identified etiologic agents of childhood community-acquired pneumonia in North America and Europe and accounted for 21% of such agents in Africa and South America (57). Pneumonia was the predominant clinical syndrome in patients with *H. influenzae* serotype f disease (86).

Nonencapsulated *H. influenzae* strains (often collectively referred to by the misnomer "nontypeable"), indistinguishable from the *H. influenzae* strains found in the healthy respiratory tract (predominantly biotypes II and III), are frequent causes of infections in children. Nonencapsulated *H. influenzae* usually occurs at sites contiguous with the upper respiratory tract but typically is not a cause of bacteremia. Nonencapsulated *H. influenzae* is, after *Streptococcus pneumoniae*, the second most frequent cause of otitis media, the most common cause of purulent bacterial conjunctivitis, and an important cause of sinusitis and chronic or acute exacerbations of lower respiratory tract infections in patients with and without cystic fibrosis (26, 84). *H. influenzae* otitis media is usually associated with significantly increased proportions (>50% of the total bacterial flora) of the same clone in the nasopharynx (43). *H. influenzae* occasionally causes obstetric and neonatal infections, and in some countries these are predominantly due to biotype IV strains that constitute a distinct genospecies (69). Both *H. influenzae* and *H. parainfluenzae* have been implicated in urinary tract infections and peritonitis (2, 69, 90).

H. aegyptius

H. aegyptius (Koch-Weeks bacillus) is associated with an acute purulent and contagious form of conjunctivitis ("pink eye") that occurs in seasonal endemics, especially in hot climates (66).

H. influenzae Biogroup Aegyptius

Bacteria that share many of the properties of *H. aegyptius* cause a fulminant pediatric disease known as Brazilian purpuric fever (BPF), manifested by high fever, hemorrhagic skin lesions, septicemia, vascular collapse, hypotensive shock, and death, usually within 48 h of onset. It is characteristically preceded by purulent conjunctivitis that has resolved before the onset of fever. Since its initial recognition in 1984, several outbreaks of the disease have occurred in the neighboring states of São Paulo, Paraná, and Mato Grosso in Brazil (10). Although invasive, these bacteria are nonencapsulated and have been designated *H. influenzae* biogroup aegyptius (10), a term sometimes erroneously also applied to strains of *H. aegyptius*. Cases clinically similar to BPF were observed in Australia, but these were caused by strains distinct from BPF isolates (10).

H. ducreyi

H. ducreyi causes the venereal disease soft chancre or chancroid. The genital lesion begins as a tender papule that becomes pustular and that is then ulcerated over the course of 2 days. Lesions may merge to form larger ulcers that may be accompanied by unilateral inguinal lymphadenitis (bubo formation). *H. ducreyi* infection is an important cause of genital ulcers in Asia, Africa, and Latin America but is a less important cause of such ulcers in North America and most parts of Europe. Morbidity figures from the United States show an annual incidence of approximately 1,000 to 5,000 cases, concentrated primarily in major Eastern cities and in the South. However, PCR detection of *H. ducreyi* suggests that the prevalence of chancroid is underreported (61, 83). The disease has received renewed attention because it facilitates the transmission of HIV in populations in which it is endemic. Extragenital lesions may occur but are rare (40, 67, 83).

Other Species

H. parahaemolyticus may have previously unrecognized pathogenic properties, as it is often isolated from patients with pharyngitis in whom no other bacterial pathogen is detected, from patients with lower respiratory tract infections, and from patients with local abscesses in the oral

cavity (77; M. Kilian and K. Poulsen, unpublished data). Some of the oral *Haemophilus* species (*H. parainfluenzae, H. aphrophilus, H. paraphrophilus,* and *H. segnis*) are occasionally implicated in subacute endocarditis, brain abscesses, sinusitis, arthritis, osteomyelitis, and wound and postoperative infections (2, 21), which are often the result of a temporary bacteremic condition following dental treatments that result in a break of the oral mucosal barrier. Reported cases of meningitis ascribed to *H. parainfluenzae* can probably be explained by misidentification of *H. influenzae* isolates, as described below.

COLLECTION, TRANSPORT, AND STORAGE

Specimens of patient blood and cerebrospinal fluid (CSF) are obtained and processed as described in chapters 6 and 20. Prompt transport of these samples to the laboratory is mandatory to ensure the fastest possible diagnosis and survival of microorganisms in the sample. Additional specimens from which *Haemophilus* organisms may be isolated include aspirated synovial fluid, pericardial fluid, pleural fluid, pus, nasopharyngeal or throat swabs, purulent discharge from infected eyes, urine, and occasionally, vaginal swabs. It is important that samples taken from the respiratory tract remain representative of the infecting flora by avoidance of contamination with commensals as far as possible. Thus, throat swabs must be collected from the pharynx and not from the surface of the tongue or other sites in front of the palatinal arches. Likewise, for sampling of the lower respiratory tract, any method that bypasses the upper respiratory tract (e.g., bronchial washing) is preferred. Because most children carry *H. influenzae* in the upper respiratory tract, its mere detection is of limited value for establishment of the etiology of otitis media (25), although in most cases of purulent otitis media the etiologic agent will dominate the nasopharyngeal microflora (43).

Samples must be transported to the laboratory in a suitable transport medium or should be spread directly onto an appropriate agar medium whenever possible (especially conjunctival specimens). The viability of most *Haemophilus* organisms is readily lost as a result of drying out, and most *Haemophilus* organisms, particularly the more fastidious species such as *H. aegyptius*, do not survive for more than a few days in clinical samples.

Genital specimens for *H. ducreyi* culture should be collected from the base and the undermined margins of the chancroid lesion with a saline- or broth-moistened swab. Cultivation may be supplemented by aspiration of pus from infected bubonic lymph nodes, but isolation of *H. ducreyi* from pus is usually less successful than isolation from ulcer material (24, 83). Direct plating on selective media is preferable as it results in the highest levels of recovery. The use of transport media is a viable alternative only if a reliable source of refrigeration is available, as the viability of *H. ducreyi* in various transport media is completely lost within 1 day at room temperature. The best results were obtained by using thioglycolate-hemin-based transport media containing various combinations of selenium dioxide, albumin, and glutamine (20). After storage at 4°C for up to 4 days, 71% of samples from patients clinically diagnosed with chancroid yielded growth of *H. ducreyi*.

Haemophilus isolates may be stored for many years at room temperature after lyophilization in skim milk or at −135°C on dry cotton swabs heavily inoculated with bacteria from an agar culture transferred to a sterile empty vial. An alternative method of storage is freezing below −60°C of 24-h broth cultures or suspensions of freshly grown cells in broth medium containing 10% glycerol. Biweekly transfers on agar media can also maintain most strains. However, strains of *H. aegyptius* and *H. ducreyi* will rapidly die out.

DIRECT EXAMINATION

Microscopic Examination

CSF

A film of CSF previously concentrated by centrifugation at 10,000 × *g* or by filtration is stained by Gram's method or with methylene blue. Cytocentrifugation of CSF significantly increases the sensitivity of the Gram stain (76). Care should be exercised in destaining since the coccobacillary form of *H. influenzae* may morphologically resemble pneumococci. However, in CSF the organism may be relatively pleomorphic, with coccoid, coccobacillary, short rod, long rod, and filamentous forms. The bacteria may be few in number but are usually detected along with granulocytes by careful examination. Approximately 85% of patients with culture-proven *H. influenzae* meningitis yield positive Gram-stained smears of CSF (29).

Capsules present on bacteria in CSF can be demonstrated by several techniques, provided that a sufficient number of bacteria is present. The simplest method is by demonstration of the capsular swelling reaction (Quellung reaction). A drop of CSF is mixed on a slide with a drop of an antiserum against each of the capsular serotypes (Becton Dickinson Diagnostic Systems, Sparks, Md.). When mixed with the relevant antiserum, the capsule will appear swollen and sharply delineated by phase-contrast microscopy when it is compared with a control smear without added antiserum. Immunofluorescence staining achieved by the addition of a secondary layer of fluorescein-conjugated anti-rabbit immunoglobulins (DAKO, Carpinteria, Calif.) provides another excellent means of identifying and serotyping encapsulated strains of *H. influenzae* in clinical samples. It is important to include controls that rule out direct binding of the fluorescence-labeled secondary antibodies to the bacteria.

Respiratory Tract Specimens

The presence of small, pleomorphic Gram-negative rods in areas of the sample that contain polymorphonuclear leukocytes and no squamous epithelial cells strongly suggests that a *Haemophilus* species is etiologically involved, but the final diagnosis must be established by cultivation. Due to their small size and staining reaction, *Haemophilus* bacteria may easily be missed in Gram-stained smears of sputa. Direct microscopy is also an important tool in cases in which fluid is collected by bronchoalveolar lavage or transthoracic needle aspiration. An immunoperoxidase-conjugated monoclonal antibody (monoclonal antibody 8BD9) directed against outer membrane protein P6 has been successfully used for the detection of *H. influenzae* in sputa from patients with cystic fibrosis (51).

Other Specimens

Due to the fastidious nature of *H. aegyptius*, microscopic examination of Gram-stained smears of conjunctival scrapings, particularly from patients with seasonal conjunctivitis, is a useful supplement to cultivation. *H. aegyptius* organisms appear as long, slender gram-negative rods.

There is some doubt about the value of direct examination of Gram-stained smears or dark-field microscopy as an aid in the diagnosis of chancroid. Most genital ulcers have a polymicrobial flora, and the arrangements of *H. ducreyi* cells as long chains or "schools of fish," previously considered typical, appear to be more characteristic of smears prepared from cells grown in vitro (3, 83). The sensitivity of Gram staining does not exceed 50% (83). The development of assays for the direct detection of *H. ducreyi* in smears by immunofluorescence has been hindered, in part, by the poor specificities of polyclonal antisera. Monoclonal antibodies against various surface epitopes on *H. ducreyi* have been developed and used in field studies. Many show satisfactory specificities and sensitivities compared with the results of culture techniques (83), but none appear to be commercially available.

Antigen Detection

Various immunochemical techniques for detection of capsular antigen of serotype b in CSF and other body fluids have been developed, but with the rarity of this serotype and the limited sensitivity that these tests offer over microscopy of Gram-stained smears, they are now of limited clinical value (48).

CULTURE

Media

Attempts to isolate *Haemophilus* species must take into account the particular growth requirements of this group of bacteria (Table 1). The two growth factors hemin (X factor) and NAD (V factor) are contained in blood cells, but only X factor is directly available in conventional blood agar. To release V factor, the blood cells must be broken up by brief heating as, for example, in chocolate agar and Levinthal's medium. In addition to liberating V factor, heat treatment inactivates V factor-destroying enzymes (NADase) present in blood. The heat treatment is obtained by adding the blood (5% sheep, bovine, or horse blood) to the medium base when its temperature is reduced to approximately 80°C immediately after autoclaving. A comparison of six medium bases showed that a medium consisting of GC agar base plus 5% chocolatized sheep blood and 1% yeast autolysate promoted the best growth of *H. influenzae*, *H. parainfluenzae*, and most other species that may be isolated from humans, excluding *H. ducreyi* (71).

For *H. aegyptius*, which is particularly fastidious, chocolate agar supplemented with 1% growth factor supplements (IsoVitaleX [Becton Dickinson Diagnostic Systems], Vitox [Oxoid, Basingstoke, United Kingdom], or cofactors-vitamins-amino acids [CVA; Gibco Diagnostics, Grand Island, N.Y.]) provides a good medium for isolation, although primary growth from clinical samples is never luxuriant (19, 87).

Growth on conventional blood agar may be achieved by adding a source of V factor, traditionally done by cross-streaking the inoculated plate with a staphylococcus or enterococcus strain. These organisms excrete V factor and allow detection of *Haemophilus* organisms, which grow as satellite colonies (Fig. 1). Alternatively, V factor may be supplied by applying a filter paper disk or a strip saturated with V factor (Rosco A/S, Taastrup, Denmark) to the surface of the medium.

Due to the relatively slow growth and small size of *Haemophilus* colonies, their presence in cultures from sites

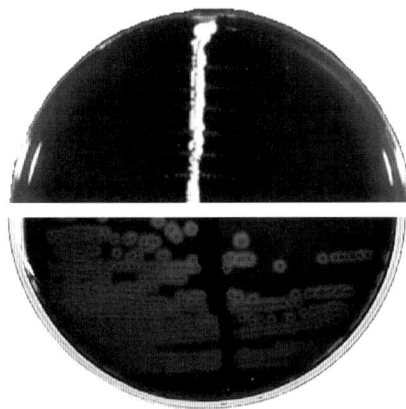

FIGURE 1 Growth of *Haemophilus* isolates on horse blood agar around a streak of *S. aureus*. The upper half shows the typical satellite growth characteristic of most *Haemophilus* species. The lower part shows the characteristic lack of satellite growth of a strain of *H. parahaemolyticus*, despite its requirement for V factor. Note that the colonies of *H. parahaemolyticus* resemble those of pyogenic streptococci on blood agar.

with a mixed flora may easily be overlooked. When necessary, this problem may be solved by including selective agents or a special incubation procedure. This is particularly important for attempts to detect *H. ducreyi*. GC-HgS, which consists of GC agar (GIBCO Laboratories) supplemented with 3 mg of vancomycin per liter, 1% hemoglobin, 5% fetal bovine serum, 1% IsoVitaleX (Becton Dickinson Diagnostic Systems), or some other comparable enrichment, has a high sensitivity for isolation of *H. ducreyi* from clinical specimens, as does Mueller-Hinton agar (BBL) supplemented with 5% chocolatized horse blood, 1% IsoVitaleX, and 3 mg of vancomycin per liter (MH-HB) (19). Strains of *H. ducreyi* that are inhibited by 3 mg of vancomycin per liter have been reported (33). However, this observation needs to be confirmed in other laboratories. It is generally accepted that a combination of two media (e.g., GC-HgS and MH-HB) is optimal for the isolation of *H. ducreyi*, possibly because of differences in nutritional requirements between strains (83), but the sensitivity for *H. ducreyi* is never 100% (19, 24, 83). Some lots of fetal calf serum inhibit the growth of *H. ducreyi*. Fetal calf serum can be replaced by either activated charcoal or bovine albumin, but not by newborn calf serum (82).

The problem of overgrowth of *H. influenzae* by *Pseudomonas aeruginosa* in cultures of sputa from patients with cystic fibrosis has been solved with some success by anaerobic incubation of inoculated chocolate agar plates containing 300 mg of bacitracin per liter. Detection of *Haemophilus* bacteria in cultures of specimens from the upper respiratory tract is also considerably improved by use of the latter medium (39). However, to be able to evaluate the relative proportion of haemophili in the microflora, a nonselective medium must be included.

Lower respiratory tract secretions and aspirates or swabs of pus from localized infections should be inoculated both on 5% blood agar cross-inoculated with a feeder strain and on chocolate agar.

Cultures of all *Haemophilus* organisms except *H. ducreyi* should be incubated at 35 to 37°C; cultures of *H. ducreyi* grow significantly better at 33°C. A moist atmosphere supplemented with 5 to 10% CO_2 is preferred by most strains

and is mandatory for the isolation of *H. ducreyi* and many strains of *H. aphrophilus* and *H. paraphrophilus*. Given optimal conditions, most *Haemophilus* species grow to colonies of at least 1 to 2 mm in diameter after incubation for 18 to 24 h. Fresh isolates of *H. aegyptius* and *H. ducreyi* require incubation for 3 to 4 days.

Modern commercial blood culture systems show excellent recovery of *Haemophilus* species from blood samples. However, the same systems will fail to recover *Haemophilus* species from normally sterile body fluids like pleural fluids, joint fluids, ascitic fluid, or dialysates unless blood (e.g., human blood [1:8; vol/vol]) or X- and V-factor enrichments are added (28, 64). Cultivation of spinal fluid or subcultivation from blood cultures should be performed on both chocolate agar and blood agar.

Appearance of Growth

With the exception of *H. aphrophilus* and *H. ducreyi*, all *Haemophilus* species that may be isolated from humans require V factor. Therefore, on blood agar these species will grow as satellite colonies around the staphylococcus streak. The two hemolytic species *H. parahaemolyticus* and *H. haemolyticus* usually do not show satellite growth or the phenomenon is less pronounced because of the release of V factor from lysed blood cells. Colonies of *H. parahaemolyticus* are surrounded by strong beta-hemolytic zones that resemble those induced by pyogenic streptococci (Fig. 1).

H. influenzae colonies on chocolate agar are grayish, semiopaque, smooth, and flat convex and reach a diameter of 1 to 2 mm after incubation for 24 h. In dense areas of the plate, encapsulated strains tend to grow confluently, in contrast to colonies of nonencapsulated strains, which remain separate. On clear agar media such as Levinthal's agar, colonies of encapsulated strains show a bright iridescence (red, blue, green, and yellow) when light is obliquely transmitted from behind. The phenomenon is most clearly detected in young (10- to 18-h) cultures and will gradually disappear during prolonged incubation. In some strains with capsules of serotypes other than type b, iridescence is not always clear-cut. Nonencapsulated strains examined in the same way show a more uniform bluish green color. Strains from patients with meningitis and epiglottitis virtually always produce indole, as do many nonencapsulated isolates (e.g., biovar II isolates). Release of indole gives the growth on agar media a characteristic pungent smell similar to that of *Escherichia coli*. Otherwise, *Haemophilus* strains emit a "mouse nest" smell.

Colonies of *H. parainfluenzae* may be up to 2 mm in diameter after incubation for 24 h and appear either smooth or rough and wrinkled. Most colonies are flat, grayish, and semiopaque. *H. aphrophilus* and *H. paraphrophilus* grow as rough, raised colonies that rarely attain a diameter exceeding 1 mm. When incubated in air without extra CO_2, these species will grow, if at all, as colonies of various sizes; the growth mimics that of a mixed culture. Fresh isolates of *H. aegyptius* and *H. segnis* grow as small (diameter, <1 mm) smooth colonies. Colonies of *H. ducreyi* are smooth and semitranslucently gray and attain a diameter of 0.1 to 0.5 mm on enriched chocolate agar after incubation for 3 days. They are characteristically cohesive and can be pushed intact across the surface of the agar.

Microscopy of Cultures

Gram-stained smears of *Haemophilus* isolates show small gram-negative rods with various degrees of polymorphism. The most extensive polymorphism, which may include long filamentous forms, is observed with the X-factor-independent species. *H. ducreyi* often appears as parallel rows of small rods in chains (with a "school of fish," "rail-road track," or "fingerprint" appearance).

IDENTIFICATION

X- and V-Factor Requirement

The satellite phenomenon, which may be detected in primary blood agar plate cultures, provides a convenient means for a tentative genus identification of all of the V-factor-requiring species that are regularly isolated from humans. However, other bacteria, such as occasional strains of *Pasteurella multocida*, some animal-pathogenic *Actinobacillus* and *Pasteurella* species (58), and some streptococci may also show satellite growth, although it is not always due to a V-factor requirement.

A small 5.25-kb plasmid that is normally present in *H. ducreyi* has been found to confer independence of V factor in occasional isolates of *H. parainfluenzae* (46, 92). How widespread such V-factor-independent strains of *H. parainfluenzae* are is not known.

A prerequisite for detection of the satellite phenomenon is an agar medium that lacks V factor. Since ordinary blood agar contains various amounts of free V factor, depending on the method of preparation and the length of storage, it is sometimes difficult to achieve convincing satellite growth on this medium. The special problem associated with hemolytic strains has already been mentioned. In case of doubtful reactions, far better results are obtained on a blood agar medium to which the blood (5 to 10%) is added before autoclaving. Since NAD is heat labile, this medium is completely devoid of V factor but otherwise satisfies all growth requirements of *Haemophilus* species, including X factor.

Determination of a requirement for X-factor is done in some laboratories by demonstrating growth around an X-factor-containing paper disk (Becton Dickinson Diagnostic Systems) on an agar medium or by comparing the growth on medium with blood and that on medium without blood. However, even when particular care is being exercised to avoid carrying over X factor with the inoculum, this method will result in erroneous results in up to 20% of cases (M. Kilian, unpublished observations). If the identity is not confirmed by biochemical tests, *H. influenzae* strains are often misidentified as *H. parainfluenzae* and occasionally vice versa. This undoubtedly explains some of the reported cases of meningitis ascribed to *H. parainfluenzae*. The porphyrin test (35) provides a more accurate and rapid means of determining the X-factor requirement.

Porphyrin Test

The porphyrin test is based on the observation (7) that hemin-independent *Haemophilus* strains excrete porphobilinogen and porphyrins, both of which are intermediates in the hemin biosynthetic pathway (Fig. 2), when supplied with δ-aminolevulinic acid. X-factor-requiring strains do not excrete these compounds because of a lack of enzymes involved in the biosynthesis of heme.

The substrate consists of 2 mM δ-aminolevulinic acid hydrochloride (Sigma Chemical Co., St. Louis, Mo.) and 0.8 mM $MgSO_4$ in 0.1 M phosphate buffer at pH 6.9. It is distributed in 0.5-ml quantities in small glass tubes and may be stored for several months in a refrigerator. Sterility is not required. The substrate is inoculated by suspending a heavy

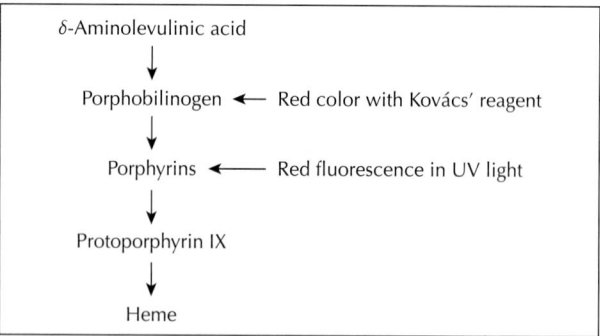

FIGURE 2 Principal steps of the heme biosynthetic pathway and methods for detection of intermediate compounds.

loopful of bacteria from an agar plate culture. After incubation for 4 h at 37°C, the mixture is exposed to UV light (wavelength, approximately 360 nm), preferably in a dark room. A red fluorescence from the bacterial cells or from the fluid indicates the presence of porphyrins; i.e., growth of the strain is not dependent on X factor. In cases of doubtful reactions, tubes may be reincubated for up to 24 h. An alternative way is to add 0.5 ml of Kovács' reagent (p-dimethylaminobenzaldehyde, 5 g; amyl alcohol, 75 ml; concentrated HCl, 25 ml), shake the mixture vigorously, and allow the phases to separate. A red color in the lower water phase is indicative of porphobilinogen. When this method of reading is used, it is advisable to include an inoculated tube without δ-aminolevulinic acid as a negative control. Kovács' reagent also gives a red color reaction with indole, which, however, will be present in the upper alcohol phase. Still, indole-positive strains of *H. influenzae* may erroneously be identified as X-factor independent in the absence of an appropriate control. Another disadvantage of this method of reading is that further incubation of samples with doubtful reactions is not possible.

Hemolysis

Hemolysis is detected on blood agar plates that are used for demonstration of V-factor requirement. For most species the use of horse, sheep, or bovine blood results in identical results, but only *H. parahaemolyticus* shows large hemolytic zones resembling those produced by *Streptococcus agalactiae*. Demonstration of the hemolytic activity of *H. ducreyi* requires specialized media. Reproducible results have been obtained with bilayer horse blood agar plates consisting of GC agar base, 1% X factor-V factor supplement, and 5% horse blood. All strains examined were less hemolytic on sheep blood agar (81).

Biochemical Tests, General

Table 1 shows the key reactions for further differentiation of the *Haemophilus* species. Tests for fermentation of glucose, sucrose, and lactose are important for species identification. They are performed in 1% solutions of the respective carbohydrates in phenol red broth base (Becton Dickinson Diagnostic Systems) supplemented with X and V factors (10 mg/liter each; Sigma Chemical Co.) after autoclaving (36). Reactions are usually clear-cut after 24 h of incubation, but some species such as *H. segnis* and *H. aegyptius* show weak reactions.

Hydrogen sulfide production is demonstrated by placing a lead test paper strip (BDH, Gallard-Schlesinger, New

York, N.Y.) in the lid of an inoculated chocolate agar plate. Distinct blackening of the strip after 2 days of incubation is indicative of hydrogen sulfide production (36).

The ability to reduce nitrate, which is a characteristic of all *Haemophilus* species, can be demonstrated after 5 days of growth in Levinthal's broth with 0.1% (wt/vol) potassium nitrate. Strains of *H. aphrophilus* and *H. paraphrophilus* may, however, reduce nitrate beyond nitrite, which may result in a negative reaction for nitrite (36).

H. influenzae and *H. parainfluenzae* may be subdivided into eight biotypes or biovars each (23, 36) on the basis of three biochemical reactions that are also important in the differentiation between some of the species: indole production, urease, and ornithine decarboxylase activities (Table 2). Biotypes of *H. influenzae* show a relationship to the source of isolation (30, 36, 59): while respiratory tract, middle ear, and eye infections are usually caused by biotype II and III strains, biotype IV has been associated with genital infections (69, 90). There is also correlation between the biotypes and the capsular serotypes of *H. influenzae* strains (36), in agreement with the fact that the serotypes constitute separate evolutionary lineages, in contrast to serotypes of *S. pneumoniae* (55, 56). The vast majority of serotype a, b, and f strains belong to biotype I; serotype c strains are usually biotype II; and strains with serotype d or e capsules are biotype IV. Subtyping on the basis of outer membrane proteins, lipopolysaccharides, or

TABLE 2 Differential tests for *H. influenzae*, *H. parainfluenzae*, *H. aegyptius*, *H. parahaemolyticus*, and *H. segnis* and for biotyping of *H. influenzae* and *H. parainfluenzae*

Species and biotype	Indole	Urease	Ornithine decarboxylase
H. influenzae			
Biotype I	+	+	+
Biotype II	+	+	−
Biotype III	−	+	−
Biotype IV	−	+	+
Biotype V	+	−	+
Biotype VI	−	−	+
Biotype VII	+	−	−
Biotype VIII	−	−	−
H. aegyptius[a]	−	+	−
H. influenzae biogroup aegyptius[a]	−	+	−
H. parainfluenzae			
Biotype I	−	−	+
Biotype II	−	+	+
Biotype III	−	+	−
Biotype IV	+	+	+
Biotype V	−	−	−
Biotype VI	+	−	+
Biotype VII	+	+	−
Biotype VIII	+	−	−
H. parahaemolyticus	−	+	−
H. segnis	−	−	−

[a] For differentiation of *H. aegyptius*, *H. influenzae* biotype III, and *H. influenzae* biogroup aegyptius, see text for further information.

isoenzymes has also been done. However, for epidemiological purposes, typing by DNA-based techniques (DNA fingerprinting, ribotyping, pulsed-field gel electrophoresis, multilocus sequence typing, multilocus enzyme electrophoresis [MLEE], etc.) is preferred because of their superior discriminatory powers (31, 42, 55, 74).

Direct Enzyme Tests for Biotyping

The three biochemical reactions used in the identification and biotyping of *H. influenzae* and *H. parainfluenzae* may be performed as rapid tests (36). An additional advantage of these tests is that growth is not required. All three test media (0.3- to 0.5-ml quantities) are inoculated with a heavy loopful of bacteria from an agar culture, and the results are read after incubation for 4 h. (The test for ornithine decarboxylase may in some cases require additional incubation for 18 to 20 h.)

Indole Test
The substrate for the indole test is 1% L-tryptophan in 0.05 M phosphate buffer at pH 6.8. After inoculation and incubation for 4 h, 1 volume of Kovács' reagent is added and the mixture is shaken. A red color in the upper alcohol phase indicates the presence of indole.

Urease Test
The substrate for the urease test is 0.1 g of KH_2PO_4, 0.1 g of K_2HPO_4, 0.5 g of NaCl, and 0.5 ml of 1:500 phenol red in 100 ml of distilled water. The pH is adjusted to 7.0 with NaOH, and 10.4 ml of a 20% (wt/vol) aqueous solution of urea is added (for 1:500 phenol red, dissolve 0.2 g of phenol red in NaOH and add distilled water to 100 ml). The development of a red color within 4 h after inoculation indicates urease activity.

Ornithine Decarboxylase Test
The substrate for the ornithine decarboxylase test is the medium used regularly for other bacteria (see chapter 27). For *Haemophilus* organisms the substrate is inoculated with a heavy loopful of bacteria from an agar plate culture. The development of a purple color within 4 to 24 h indicates ornithine decarboxylase activity.

Alternative Methods

Several commercial kits are available for identification of *Haemophilus* species once the V-factor requirement has been determined, e.g., API NH (bioMérieux Inc., Hazelwood, Mo.), Vitek NHI Card V1308 (bioMérieux), the Haemophilus ID Test kit (Remel, Lenexa, Kans.), the RIM-H system (Austin Biological Laboratories, Austin, Tex.), and RapidID NF (Innovative Diagnostics, Norcross, Ga.) (62, 68). However, most of these kits do not provide sufficient information to accurately identify an isolate to the species level without additional tests. Therefore, it is advisable that more unusual findings be confirmed by traditional tests.

DNA-Based Identification

If the technology is available, isolates of most *Haemophilus* species and related genera may easily be identified by determining a partial 16S rRNA gene sequence and comparing it with the sequences of type strains available in databases accessible on the Internet (e.g., at http://www.ncbi.nlm.nih.gov/BLAST/). Because of their close similarities the technique will not differentiate between *H.*

influenzae, *H. aegyptius*, and *H. influenzae* biogroup aegyptius or between *H. aphrophilus* and *H. paraphrophilus*.

A DNA probe based on specific 16S rRNA sequences for identification of cultures of *H. influenzae* is commercially available under the name Accuprobe (Gen-Probe Inc., San Diego, Calif.), which has been demonstrated to have a high sensitivity and a high specificity compared to the results of conventional identification methods (18). A highly sensitive and specific PCR-based noncommercial system for simultaneous detection of *H. influenzae*, *Neisseria meningitidis*, and *S. pneumoniae* in clinical samples of CSF, plasma, serum, and whole blood has been described (17).

A noncommercial multiplex PCR assay that allows simultaneous detection of the major etiologic agents of genital ulcer disease, *H. ducreyi*, *Treponema pallidum*, and herpes simplex virus types 1 and 2, has a sensitivity for detection of 1 to 10 *H. ducreyi* organisms and is thus greatly superior to cultivation (61). It has proved valuable in clinical settings in the United States and Africa (8, 49, 53, 80), where the resolved sensitivity ranged from 95 to 98.4% and the resolved specificity seems to be greater than 99%. Compared with this technique, the sensitivity of *H. ducreyi* culture with selective media varied from 44 to 75%. DNA probes do not have the sensitivity needed to detect *H. ducreyi* in clinical specimens but have been used to confirm the identification of *H. ducreyi* isolates (8).

A PCR-based method that allows differentiation of *H. aphrophilus*, *H. paraphrophilus*, and *Actinobacillus actinomycetemcomitans* has been described. Strains of all three species yielded a distinct pattern of restriction enzyme fragments of PCR-amplified 16S rRNA genes (72).

Particular Identification Problems

The differentiation of *H. influenzae*, *H. aegyptius*, and *H. influenzae* biogroup aegyptius by standard laboratory techniques is impossible at present. The three taxa form distinct clusters by phylogenetic analysis based on multiple genetic and phenotypic traits including the electrophoretic mobilities of selected housekeeping enzymes (as determined by MLEE) (Kilian et al., unpublished data). Both *H. aegyptius* and *H. influenzae* biogroup aegyptius have the same key biochemical characteristics as *H. influenzae* biotype III (Table 2). Since the latter does not possess the invasive potential of BPF strains or the ability to cause serious endemic conjunctivitis like *H. aegyptius* strains do, it is important to develop means for exact identification. *H. aegyptius* lacks the ability to ferment xylose, in contrast to the vast majority of *H. influenzae* strains (10, 47). Additional characteristics that may be of use in the separation of *H. aegyptius* from *H. influenzae* are its poorer in vitro growth, its more slender and rodlike shape, its ability to agglutinate human erythrocytes as a result of more stable pilus expression, and its susceptibility to the now unavailable troleandomycin (47). However, none of these characteristics will unequivocally differentiate *H. aegyptius* from *H. influenzae*, and it is not yet clear how isolates of *H. influenzae* biogroup aegyptius behave in these tests. It has been reported that the distinct outer membrane protein profiles of *H. aegyptius* and *H. influenzae* biotype III may be used as adjuncts to differentiate the two species, but the validity of this for the identification of fresh isolates is not clear, as a certain outer membrane protein pattern was used to define *H. aegyptius* (12).

Strains of *H. influenzae* biogroup aegyptius share the inability to ferment xylose and the slender rod morphology of *H. aegyptius*. Isolates from the initial outbreak of BPF

belonged to the so-called BPF clone, which was defined by five features: (i) a 24-MDa plasmid with a specific profile after restriction endonuclease digestion, (ii) a characteristic whole-bacteria protein profile, (iii) a specific MLEE pattern, (iv) one of two characteristic rRNA hybridization patterns, and (v) a positive reaction in a sandwich enzyme immunoassay with BPF case strain-specific monoclonal antibodies. However, it is now clear that not all BPF isolates carry the 24-MDa plasmid (79) and, furthermore, that several distinct clones have been implicated in subsequent outbreaks. To what extent these isolates share the five characteristics of the original clone is yet unknown. The same is true for the characteristic pilin epitope described by Weyant et al. (91).

Isolates of *H. ducreyi* may be presumptively identified by their adherent colony characteristics, their appearance in Gram-stained smears, and positive oxidase and negative catalase reactions. Confirmation can be achieved by demonstrating a negative porphyrin test result, the inability to ferment carbohydrates, and a positive reaction for nitrate reduction. However, commercial identification systems fail to reveal the ability to reduce nitrate, and a positive oxidase reaction is only obtained with tetramethyl-*p*-phenylenediamine (36, 52).

H. aphrophilus and *A. actinomycetemcomitans* are not easily distinguished from certain *Pasteurella* species, which potentially may explain two recent reports of the isolation of *Pasteurella gallinarum* from human cases of endocarditis and bacteremia (27). Criteria for the identification of such bacteria may be found elsewhere (60) (see also chapter 39).

Biochemical reactions that are valuable in separating *H. aphrophilus* and *H. paraphrophilus* from the closely related *A. actinomycetemcomitans* and other bacteria that resemble these species are provided in Table 3.

CAPSULAR TYPING

Separation of the six serotypes of *H. influenzae* is based on structurally distinct capsular polysaccharides. Until vaccination against *H. influenzae* type b was introduced, identification of serotype b strains was of particular practical significance as invasive pathogenicity was almost exclusively associated with that serotype. There is no doubt that the exclusive focus on serotype b in many laboratories has resulted in an underestimation of infections caused by other serotypes, as mentioned above.

Evaluation of cases of apparent vaccine failure necessitates definitive serotyping. Furthermore, the decline of *H. influenzae* serotype b carriage raised concerns about an increase in the rates of *H. influenzae* carriage and disease caused by other serotypes and by nonencapsulated strains. Recently reported results of a study of Alaskan residents aged 10 years and older suggest such an increase (from 0.5 to 1.1 per 100,000 population per year) (65). It is therefore advisable that laboratories that are unable to perform appropriate serotyping of isolates refer these isolates to reference laboratories such as the Centers for Disease Control and Prevention (Atlanta, Ga.).

Capsular serotyping may be carried out by slide agglutination, coagglutination with staphylococci or latex particles coated with type-specific antibodies, a capsular swelling test, and immunofluorescence microscopy.

Bacterial suspensions used for serologic typing of isolates must be prepared from a young (12- to 18-h) agar culture, since the capsular structure tends to deteriorate in older cultures. A smooth suspension of bacteria is made in normal saline containing formalin (0.5%; vol/vol) and must be of sufficient density to permit the antigen-antibody reaction to proceed to completion within 1 min. In a strong positive slide agglutination reaction, all bacteria are agglutinated and the fluid between the clusters is clear.

As polyclonal antisera contain various proportions of antibodies to somatic antigens, agglutination may occur as a result of reaction with somatic antigens. Therefore, serotyping with antisera should be performed only for cultures in which the texture of colonies or their ability to show iridescence (see above) suggests capsule formation, and only strong reactions occurring within 1 min should be taken as a positive reaction. Antisera for serotyping of encapsulated *H. influenzae* isolates are available from Becton Dickinson Diagnostic Systems and from some state laboratories. A coagglutination test for detection of serotype b is available under the product name Phadebact (Boule Diagnostics AB, Huddinge, Sweden).

For screening of nasopharyngeal swab cultures for the presence of encapsulated strains, Levinthal's agar containing antiserum is a valuable and sensitive tool (50). However, the method is too expensive for general use.

Antigenic similarities to the six capsular polysaccharides of *H. influenzae* have been found in a number of unrelated bacteria. However, these cross-reactions should not create practical problems for laboratory diagnosis. Bacteria possessing antigens cross-reactive with the type b capsule include *S. pneumoniae* serotypes 6, 15a, 29, and 35a, *E. coli* K100, *Staphylococcus aureus*, *Staphylococcus epidermidis*, *Streptococcus pyogenes*, *Enterococcus faecalis*, *Bacillus alvei*, and *Bacillus pumilus* (4, 9).

While traditional serotyping is liable to occasional misinterpretations, the capsule serotype of an isolate may be unequivocally determined by detection of serotype-specific gene sequences. The most attractive method is PCR capsular genotyping, which is easier to perform than probe analysis as there is no need for lengthy DNA extractions, Southern blotting, and hybridization. This PCR methodology may also be used to detect deletion mutants and the amplification pattern of the *capB* locus (31), which differentiates two distinct evolutionary divisions (divisions I and II) of *H. influenzae* type b with different pathogenic potentials (55). Three-primer sets for amplification of serotype-specific gene sequences are shown in Table 4.

ANTIBIOTIC SUSCEPTIBILITY

Wild-type strains of the *Haemophilus* species are susceptible to ampicillin, to cephalosporins, and to chloramphenicol, sulfonamides, tetracycline, and the macrolide-azalide-ketolide group of antimicrobials. However, mainly because of the spread of conjugative plasmids, a large proportion of clinical isolates are resistant to ampicillin and most other β-lactam antibiotics, chloramphenicol, and the tetracyclines (6, 11, 32, 75). Resistance to β-lactams is in most cases a result of TEM-1- and ROB-1-type β-lactamase production. The likelihood that an *H. influenzae* isolate will be resistant to ampicillin due to β-lactamase production is 5 to 30% in most countries, but in certain areas it may exceed 60%. There have also been β-lactamase-negative strains for which ampicillin MICs were slightly increased (>4.0 mg/liter) (5). Those strains are referred to as β-lactamase-negative, ampicillin-resistant (BLNAR) strains. Their diminished susceptibilities to β-lactam antibiotics, including some of the cephalosporins, are due to mutations in genes encoding the penicillin-binding proteins (85). In a recent

TABLE 3 Differential tests for *H. aphrophilus*, *H. paraphrophilus*, and some related species

Species	X factor required	V factor required	Indole	Urease	Ornithine decarboxylase	Lysine decarboxylase	Glucose	Sucrose	Lactose	Mannitol	Nitrate reduction	Presence of catalase
H. aphrophilus	+[a]	-	-	-	-	-	+	+	+	-	+	-
H. paraphrophilus	-	+	-	-	-	-	+	+	+	-	+	-
A. actinomycetemcomitans	-	-	-	-	-	-	+	-	-	D[b]	+	+
Eikenella corrodens	-	-	-	-	+	+	-	-	-	-	+	-
Cardiobacterium hominis	-	-	+	-	-	-	+	+	-	+	-	-
Suttonella indologenes	-	-	+	-	-	-	+	+	-	-	-	-
H. haemoglobinophilus	+	-	+	-	-	-	+	+	-	+	+	+

a The requirement for hemin is often lost upon subcultivation, and the porphyrin test is weakly positive.
b D, differences encountered.

TABLE 4 Serotype-specific three-primer sets for demonstration of capsular serotype-specific genes in *H. influenzae*[a]

Primer name	Primer sequences
a_1	CTA CTC ATT GCA GCA TTT GC
a_2	GAA TAT GAC CTG ATC TTC TG
a_3	AGT GGA CTA TTC CTG TTA CAC
b_1	GCG AAA GTG AAC TCT TAT CTC TC
b_2	GCT TAC GCT TCT ATC TCG GTG AA
b_3	ACC ATG AGA AAG TGT TAG CG
c_1	TCT GTG TAG ATG ATG GTT CA
c_2	CAG AGG CAA GCT ATT AGT GA
c_3	TGG CAG CGT AAA TAT CCT AA
d_1	TGA TGA CCG ATA CAA CCT GT
d_2	TCC ACT CTT CAA ACC ATT CT
d_3	CTC TTC TTA GTG CTG AAT TA
e_1	GGT AAC GAA TGT AGT GGT AG
e_2	GCT TTA CTG TAT AAG TCT AG
e_3	CAG CTA TGA ACA AGA TAA CG
f_1	GCT ACT ATC AAG TCC AAA TC
f_2	CGC AAT TAT GGA AGA AAG CT
f_3	AAT GCT GGA GTA TCT GGT TC

[a] The data are from reference 31.

Spanish survey, 9.3% of 1,730 isolates (~12% of β-lactamase-negative isolates) from patients with community-acquired respiratory tract infections had the BLNAR phenotype (45). The clinical relevance of BLNAR strains is unclear since there are few data to support or refute the assumption that infections with such strains will fail to respond to therapy with ampicillin or other β-lactams.

In the same survey, the rate of macrolide nonsusceptibility was about 1% for azithromycin and 10% for clarithromycin, and in most cases these were categorized as intermediate resistance. Ciprofloxacin resistance is still rare (the rate in Spain is 0.1%) (45).

Considerable geographical and temporal differences in the antimicrobial susceptibilities of *H. ducreyi* isolates have been recorded. There is very little information concerning chromosomally mediated resistance in *H. ducreyi*. However, most clinical isolates contain plasmids, which may encode resistance, either separately or in combination, to sulfonamides, aminoglycosides, tetracyclines, chloramphenicol, and β-lactam antibiotics. It is not unusual for a single isolate to contain multiple resistance plasmids. Both TEM-1 and ROB-1 β-lactamases have been identified in isolates from Thailand (83). Most clinical isolates of *H. ducreyi* worldwide are susceptible to erythromycin, which is the drug recommended as the primary treatment by the World Health Organization and by the Centers for Disease Control and Prevention. However, strains for which the erythromycin MIC is 4 mg/liter have been isolated in Thailand and Singapore (83). Alternative recommended drugs are azithromycin, ciprofloxacin, ceftriaxone, amoxicillin plus clavulanic acid, spectinomycin, and trimethoprim-sulfamethoxazole. The prevalence and spectrum of antimicrobial resistance make it important that clinical isolates of *H. ducreyi* be routinely monitored for resistance.

Comprehensive and up-to-date in vitro susceptibility data for other *Haemophilus* species are not available. However, there are indications that the prevalence of resistance in these species is higher than that in *H. influenzae*. Both β-lactamase-mediated and non-β-lactamase-mediated resistance to ampicillin have been observed in *H. parainfluenzae* (34, 89). A PCR-based screening of nasopharyngeal haemophili of a group of individuals in the United Kingdom revealed that 59% carried plasmids encoding β-lactamase. Of these, 83% were in *H. parainfluenzae* and 17% were in *H. influenzae* (41). Transmissible resistance to chloramphenicol and aminoglycosides has been described in *H. parainfluenzae*, *H. parahaemolyticus*, and *H. paraphrophilus* (37).

EVALUATION, INTERPRETATION, AND REPORTING

Detection of *Haemophilus* species by culture is uncomplicated and reliable, provided that the correct media and incubation procedures are being applied. Only for *H. ducreyi* do isolation procedures show suboptimal sensitivities. Once they become commercially available, PCR methods will become important in the diagnosis of *H. ducreyi* infections.

Interpretation of laboratory findings is also, in most cases, uncomplicated. Isolation of *Haemophilus* species from sites other than the upper respiratory tract and from normally sterile sites is almost always clinically significant. The mere detection of *H. influenzae* in a sample from the nasopharynx is of no clinical significance. However, a strong predominance in the flora suggests an impaired balance that may be associated with sinusitis, otitis media, or some other local infection in the area. It is therefore important that findings be interpreted on this basis and that they be reported in semiquantitative terms. It is also unavoidable that sputum samples are contaminated with haemophili during passage through the pharynx and oral cavity. The sample must be evaluated by microscopy prior to culture to make sure that small gram-negative rods in the sample are associated with inflammatory cells and not with squamous epithelial cells from the upper respiratory tract. Even in samples that bypass the upper respiratory tract, a mixture of bacteria often renders the interpretation difficult.

Detection of *H. ducreyi* in samples from genital ulcers or in inguinal lymph node aspirates is always clinically relevant and should be followed by proper antibacterial therapy.

With the virtual elimination of *H. influenzae* serotype b disease, the demands on the clinical microbiology laboratory in this area have changed dramatically. Methods specifically designed to detect antigens of *H. influenzae* type b are of less importance, and more emphasis should be placed on other serotypes. In this context, it is important to realize that observations made for one human population do not necessarily apply to other populations. Population genetic analyses of *H. influenzae* isolates suggest that clones of *H. influenzae* may be strictly adapted to humans with a particular genetic background and do not spread freely among human populations (56). As there is significant coupling of gene loci (linkage disequilibrium) in the *H. influenzae* population, such differences may include antibiotic resistance markers as well as virulence traits.

REFERENCES

1. **Adams, W. G., K. A. Deaver, S. L. Cochi, B. D. Plikaytis, E. R. Zell, C. V. Broome, and J. D. Wenger.** 1996. Decline in childhood *Haemophilus influenzae* type b (Hib) disease in the vaccine era. *JAMA* **269:**221–226.

2. **Albritton, W. L.** 1982. Infections due to *Haemophilus* species other than *H. influenzae*. *Annu. Rev. Microbiol.* **36:**199–216.

3. **Albritton, W. L.** 1989. Biology of *Haemophilus ducreyi*. *Microbiol. Rev.* **53:**377–389.

4. **Argaman, M., T.-Y. Liu, and J. B. Robbins.** 1974. Polyribitol phosphate: an antigen of four gram-positive bacteria cross-reactive with the capsular polysaccharide of *Haemophilus influenzae*, type b. *J. Immunol.* **112:**649–655.

5. **Barry, A. L., P. C. Fuchs, and S. D. Brown.** 2001. Identification of β-lactamase-negative, ampicillin-resistant strains of *Haemophilus influenzae* with four methods and eight media. *Antimicrob. Agents Chemother.* **45:** 1585–1588.

6. **Barry, A. L., P. C. Fuchs, and M. A. Pfaller.** 1993. Susceptibilities of beta-lactamase-producing and -nonproducing ampicillin-resistant strains of *Haemphilus influenzae* to ceftibuten, cefaclor, cefuroxime, cefixime, cefotaxime, and amoxicillin-clavulanic acid. *Antimicrob. Agents Chemother.* **37:**14–18.

7. **Biberstein, E. L., P. D. Mini, and M. G. Gills.** 1963. Action of *Haemophilus* cultures on δ-aminolevulinic acid. *J. Bacteriol.* **86:**814–819.

8. **Black, C. M., and S. A. Morse.** 2000. The use of molecular techniques for the diagnosis and epidemiologic study of sexually transmitted infections. *Curr. Infect. Dis.* **2:**31–43.

9. **Bradshaw, M. W., R. Schneerson, J. C. Parke, and J. B. Robbins.** 1971. Bacterial antigens cross-reactive with the capsular polysaccharide of *Haemophilus influenzae* type b. *Lancet* **6:**1095–1096.

10. **Brenner, D. J., L. W. Mayer, G. M. Carlone, L. H. Harrison, W. F. Bibb, M. C. C. Brandileone, F. O. Sottnek, K. Irino, M. W. Reeves, J. M. Swenson, K. A. Birkness, R. S. Weyant, S. F. Berkley, T. C. Woods, A. G. Steigerwalt, P. A. D. Grimont, R. M. McKinney, D. W. Fleming, L. L. Gheesling, R. C. Cooksey, R. J. Akko, C. V. Broome, and The Brazilian Purpuric Fever Study Group.** 1988. Biochemical, genetic, and epidemiologic characterization of *Haemophilus influenzae* biogroup aegyptius *(Haemophilus aegyptius)* strains associated with Brazilian purpuric fever. *J. Clin. Microbiol.* **26:**1524–1534.

11. **Campos, J., S. Garcia-Tornel, J. M. Gairi, and I. Fabregues.** 1986. Multiply resistant *Haemophilus influenzae* type b causing meningitis: comparative clinical and laboratory study. *J. Pediatr.* **108:**897–902.

12. **Carlone, G. M., F. O. Sottnek, and B. D. Plikaytis.** 1985. Comparison of outer membrane protein and biochemical profiles of *Haemophilus aegyptius* and *Haemophilus influenzae* biotype III. *J. Clin. Microbiol.* **22:**708–713.

13. **Casin, I., F. Grimont, and P. A. Grimont.** 1986. Deoxyribonucleic acid relatedness between *Haemophilus aegyptius* and *Haemophilus influenzae*. *Ann. Inst. Pasteur Microbiol.* **137B:**155–163.

14. **Casin, I., F. Grimont, P. A. D. Grimont, and M.-J. Sanson-Le-Pors.** 1985. Lack of deoxyribonucleic acid relatedness between *Haemophilus ducreyi* and other *Haemophilus* species. *Int. J. Syst. Bacteriol.* **35:**22–25.

15. **Caugant, D. A., R. K. Selander, and I. Olsen.** 1990. Differentiation between *Actinobacillus (Haemophilus) actinomycetemcomitans, Haemophilus aphrophilus* and *Haemophilus paraphrophilus* by multilocus enzyme electrophoresis. *J. Gen. Microbiol.* **136:**2135–2141.

16. **Centers for Disease Control and Prevention.** 1999. Impact of vaccines universally recommended for children—United States, 1900–1998. *Morb. Mortal. Wkly. Rep.* **48:** 243–248.

17. **Corless, C. E., M. Guiver, R. Borrow, V. Edwards-Jones, A. J. Fox, and E. B. Kaczmarski.** 2001. Simultaneous detection of *Neisseria meningitidis, Haemophilus influenzae*, and *Streptococcus penumoniae* in suspected cases of meningitis and septicemia using real-time PCR. *J. Clin. Microbiol.* **39:**1553–1558.

18. **Daly, J. A., N. L. Clifton, K. C. Seskin, and W. M. Goosh III.** 1991. Use of rapid, nonradioactive DNA probes in culture confirmation tests to detect *Streptococcus agalactiae, Haemophilus influenzae*, and *Enterococcus* spp. from pediatric patients with significant infections. *J. Clin. Microbiol.* **29:**80–82.

19. **Dangor, Y., S. D. Miller, H. J. Koornhof, and R. C. Ballard.** 1992. A simple medium for the primary isolation of *Haemophilus ducreyi*. *Eur. J. Microbiol. Infect. Dis.* **11:** 930–934.

20. **Dangor, Y., F. Radebe, and R. C. Ballard.** 1993. Transport media for *Haemophilus ducreyi*. *Sex. Transm. Dis.* **20:**5–9.

21. **Darras-Joly, C., O. Lortholary, J.-L. Mainardi, J. Etienne, L. Guillevin, J. Acar, and the *Haemophilus* Endocarditis Study Group.** 1997. *Haemophilus* endocarditis: report of 42 cases in adults and review. *Clin. Infect. Dis.* **24:**1087–1094.

22. **Dewhirst, F. E., B. J. Paster, I. Olsen, and G. J. Frasen.** 1992. Phylogeny of 54 representative strains of species in the family *Pasteurellaceae* as determined by comparison of 16S rRNA sequences. *J. Bacteriol.* **174:**2002–2013.

23. **Doern, G. V., and K. C. Chapin.** 1987. Determination of biotypes of *Haemophilus influenzae* and *Haemophilus parainfluenzae*. A comparison of methods and a description of a new biotype (VIII) of *H. parainfluenzae*. *Diagn. Microbiol. Infect. Dis.* **7:**269–272.

24. **Dylewski, J., H. Nisanze, G. Maitha, and A. Ronald.** 1986. Laboratory diagnosis of *Haemophilus ducreyi*: sensitivity of culture media. *Diagn. Microbiol. Infect. Dis.* **4:**241–245.

25. **Faden, H., J. Stanievich, L. Brodsky, J. Bernstein, and P. L. Ogra.** 1990. Changes in nasopharyngeal flora during otitis media of childhood. *Pediatr. Infect. Dis. J.* **9:**623–626.

26. **Foxwell, A. R., J. M. Kyd, and A. W. Cripps.** 1998. Nontypeable *Haemophilus influenzae*: pathogenesis and prevention. *Microbiol. Mol. Biol. Rev.* **62:**294–308.

27. **Frederiksen, W., and B. Tønning.** 2001. Possible misidentification of *Haemophilus aphrophilus* as *Pasteurella gallinarum*. *Clin. Infect. Dis.* **32:**987–988.

28. **Fuller, D. D., T. E. Davis, P. C. Kibsey, L. Rosmus, L. W. Ayers, M. Ott, M. A. Saubolle, and D. L. Sewell.** 1994. Comparison of BACTEC Plus 26 and 27 media with and without fastidious organism supplement with conventional methods for culture of sterile body fluids. *J. Clin. Microbiol.* **32:**1488–1491.

29. **Greenlee, J. L.** 1990. Approach to diagnosis of meningitis. Cerebrospinal fluid evaluation. *Infect. Dis. Clin. N. Am.* **4:**583–597.

30. **Harper, J. J., and M. H. Tilse.** 1991. Biotypes of *Haemophilus influenzae* that are associated with noninvasive infections. *J. Clin. Microbiol.* **29:**2539–2542.

31. **Herbert, M. A., D. Crook, and E. R. Moxon.** 1998. Molecular methods for *Haemophilus influenzae*, p. 243–263. *In* N. Woodford and A. P. Johnson (ed.), *Molecular Bacteriology. Protocols and Clinical Applications*. Humana Press Inc., Totowa. N.J.

32. **Jacobs, M. R., S. Bajaksouzian, A. Zilles, G. Lin, G. A. Pankuch, and P. C. Appelbaum.** 1999. Susceptibilities of *Streptococcus pneumoniae* and *Haemophilus influenzae* to 10 oral antimicrobial agents based on pharmacodynamic parameters: 1997 U.S. surveillance study. *Antimicrob. Agents Chemother.* **43:**1901–1908.

33. Jones, C., T. Rosen, J. Clarridge, and S. Collins. 1990. Chancroid: results from an outbreak in Houston, Texas. *South. Med. J.* **83:**1384–1389.

34. Kauffman, C. A., A. G. Bergman, and C. S. Hertz. 1979. Antimicrobial resistance of *Haemophilus* species in patients with chronic bronchitis. *Am. Rev. Respir. Dis.* **120:**1382–1385.

35. Kilian, M. 1974. A rapid method for the differentiation of *Haemophilus* strains. The porphyrin test. *Acta Pathol. Microbiol. Scand. Sect. B* **82:**835–842.

36. Kilian, M. 1976. A taxonomic study of the genus *Haemophilus* with the proposal of a new species. *J. Gen. Microbiol.* **93:**9–62.

37. Kilian, M. *Haemophilus* Winslow, Broadhurst, Buchanan, Krumwiede, Rogers and Smith 1917, 561. *In* G. M. Garrity et al. (ed.), *Bergey's Manual of Systematic Bacteriology*, in press. Springer Verlag Inc., New York, N.Y.

38. Kilian, M., and C. R. Schiøtt. 1975. Haemophili and related bacteria in the human oral cavity. *Arch. Oral. Biol.* **20:**791–796.

39. Kuklinska, D., and M. Kilian. 1984. Relative proportions of *Haemophilus* species in the throat of healthy children and adults. *Eur. J. Clin. Microbiol.* **3:**249–252.

40. Lagergård, T. 1995. *Haemophilus ducreyi*: pathogenesis and protective immunity. *Trends Microbiol.* **3:**87–91.

41. Leaves, N. I., I. Dimopoulou, I. Hayes, S. Kerridge, T. Falla, O. Secka, R. A. Adegbola, M. P. Slack, T. E. Peto, and D. W. Crook. 2000. Epidemiological studies of large resistance plasmids in *Haemophilus*. *J. Antimicrob. Chemother.* **45:**599–604.

42. Leaves, N. I., and J. Z. Jordens. 1994. Development of a ribotyping scheme for *Haemophilus influenzae* type b. *Eur. J. Clin. Microbiol. Infect. Dis.* **13:**1038–1045.

43. Long, S. S., F. M. Henretig, M. J. Teter, and K. L. McGowan. 1983. Nasopharyngeal flora and acute otitis media. *Infect. Immun.* **41:**987–991.

44. Macfarlane, J., W. Holmes, P. Gard, R. Macfarlane, D. Rose, V. Weston, M. Leinonen, P. Saikku, and S. Myint. 2001. Prospective study of the incidence, aetiology and outcome of adult lower respiratory tract illness in the community. *Thorax* **56:**109–114.

45. Marco, F., J. García-de-Lomas, C. García-Rey, E. Bouza, L. Aguilar, C. Fernández-Mazarrasa, and The Spanish Surveillance Group for Respiratory Pathogens. 2001. Antimicrobial susceptibilities of 1,730 *Haemophilus influenzae* respiratory tract isolates in Spain in 1998–1999. *Antimicrob. Agents Chemother.* **45:**3226–3228.

46. Martin, P. R., R. J. Shea, and M. H. Mulks. 2001. Identification of a plasmid-encoded gene from *Haemophilus ducreyi* which confers NAD independence. *J. Bacteriol.* **183:**1168–1174.

47. Mazloum, H. A., M. Kilian, Z. M. Mohamed, and M. D. Said. 1982. Differentiation of *Haemophilus aegyptius* and *Haemophilus influenzae*. *Acta Pathol. Microbiol. Immunol. Scand. Sect. B* **90:**109–112.

48. Mein, J., and G. Lum. 1999. CSF bacterial antigen detection tests offer no advantage over Gram's strain in the diagnosis of bacterial meningitis. *Pathology* **31:**67–69.

49. Mertz, K. J., J. B. Weiss, R. M. Webb, W. C. Levine, J. S. Lewis, K. A. Orle, P. A. Totten, J. Overbaugh, S. A. Morse, M. M. Currier, M. Fishbein, and M. E. St Louis. 1998. An investigation of genital ulcers in Jackson, Mississippi, with use of a multiplex polymerase chain reaction assay: high prevalence of chancroid and human immunodeficiency virus infection. *J. Infect. Dis.* **178:**1060–1066.

50. Michaels, R. H., F. E. Stonebraker, and J. B. Robbins. 1975. Use of antiserum agar for detection of *Haemophilus influenzae* type b in the pharynx. *Pediatr. Res.* **9:**513–516.

51. Möller, L. V. M, G. J. Ruijs, H. G. M. Heijerman, J. Dankert, and L. van Alphen. 1992. *Haemophilus influenzae* is frequently detected with monoclonal antibody 8BD9 in sputum samples from patients with cystic fibrosis. *J. Clin. Microbiol.* **30:**2495–2497.

52. Morse, S. A. 1989. Chancroid and *Haemophilus ducreyi*. *Clin. Microbiol. Rev.* **2:**137–157.

53. Morse, S. A., D. L. Trees, Y. Htun, F. Radebe, K. A. Orle, Y. Dangor, C. M. Beck-Sague, S. Schmid, G. Fehler, J. B. Weiss, and R. C. Ballard. 1997. Comparison of clinical diagnosis and standard laboratory and molecular methods for the diagnosis of genital ulcer disease in Lesotho: association with human immunodeficiency virus infection. *J. Infect. Dis.* **175:**583–589.

54. Moxon, E. R. 1985. The carrier state: *Haemophilus influenzae*. *J. Antimicrob. Chemother.* **18**(Suppl. A):17–24.

55. Musser, J. M., D. M. Granoff, P. E. Pattison, and R. K. Selander. 1985. A population genetic framework for the study of invasive diseases caused by serotype b strains of *Haemophilus influenzae*. *Proc. Natl. Acad. Sci. USA* **82:**5078–5082.

56. Musser, J. M., J. S. Kroll, D. M. Granoff, E. R. Moxon, B. R. Brodeur, J. Campos, H. Dabernat, W. Frederiksen, J. Hamel, G. Hammond, E. A. Høiby, K. E. Jonsdottir, M. Kabeer, I. Kallings, W. N. Khan, M. Kilian, K. Knowles, H. J. Koornhof, B. Law, K. I. Li, J. Montgomery, P. E. Pattison, J.-C. Piffaretti, A. K. Takala, M. L. Thong, R. A. Wall, J. I. Ward, and R. K. Selander. 1990. Global genetic structure and molecular epidemiology of encapsulated *Haemophilus influenzae*. *Rev. Infect. Dis.* **12:**75–111.

57. Nascimento-Carvalho, C. M. 2001. Etiology of childhood community acquired pneumonia and its implications for vaccination. *Braz. J. Infect. Dis.* **5:**87–97.

58. Niven, D. F., and T. O'Reilly. 1990. Significance of V-factor dependency in the taxonomy of *Haemophilus* species and related organisms. *Int. J. Syst. Bacteriol.* **40:**1–4.

59. Oberhofer, T. R., and A. E. Back. 1979. Biotypes of *Haemophilus* encountered in clinical laboratories. *J. Clin. Microbiol.* **10:**168–174.

60. Olsen, I., F. E. Dewhirst, B. J. Paster, and H.-J. Busse. Family *Pasteurellaceae* POHL 1981, 382. *In* G. M. Garrity et al. (ed.), *Bergey's Manual of Systematic Bacteriology*, in press. Springer Verlag Inc., New York, N.Y.

61. Orle, K. A., C. A. Gates, D. H. Martin, B. A. Body, and J. B. Weiss. 1996. Simultaneous PCR detection of *Haemophilus ducreyi*, *Treponema pallidum*, and herpes simplex virus types 1 and 2 from genital ulcers. *J. Clin. Microbiol.* **34:**49–54.

62. Palladino, S., B. J. Leahy, and T. L. Newall. 1990. Comparison of the RIM-H rapid identification kit with conventional tests for the identification of *Haemophilus* spp. *J. Clin. Microbiol.* **28:**1862–1863.

63. Peltola, H. 2000. Worldwide *Haemophilus influenzae* type b disease at the beginning of the 21st century: global analysis of the disease burden 25 years after the use of the polysaccharide vaccine and a decade after the advent of conjugates. *Clin. Microbiol. Rev.* **13:**302–317.

64. Pennekamp, A., R. Zbinden, and A. von Graevenitz. 1996. Detection of *Haemophilus influenzae* and *Haemophilus parainfleunzae* from body fluids in blood culture bottles. *J. Microbiol. Methods* **25:**303–307.

65. Perdue, D. G., L. R. Bulkow, B. G. Gellin, M. Davidson, K. M. Petersen, R. J. Singleton, and A. J. Parkinson. 2000. Invasive *Haemophilus influenzae* disease in Alaskan residents aged 10 years and older before and after infant vaccination programs. *JAMA* **283:**3089–3094.

66. **Pittman, M., and D. J. Davis.** 1950. Identification of the Koch-Weeks bacillus (*Hemophilus aegyptius*). *J. Bacteriol.* **59:**413–426.

67. **Plummer, F. A., L. J. D'Costa, H. Nisanze, J. Dylewski, P. Karasira, and A. R. Ronald.** 1983. Epidemiology of *Haemophilus ducreyi* in Nairobi, Kenya. *Lancet* **ii:**1293–1295.

68. **Quentin, R., I. Dubarry, C. Martin, B. Catteier, and A. Goudeau.** 1992. Evaluation of four commercial methods for identification and biotyping of genital and neonatal strains of *Haemophilus* species. *Eur. J. Clin Microbiol. Infect. Dis.* **11:**546–549.

69. **Quentin, R., R. Ruimy, A. Rosenau, J. M. Musser, and R. Christen.** 1996. Genetic identification of cryptic genospecies of *Haemophilus* causing urogenital and neonatal infections by PCR using specific primers targeting genes coding for 16S rRNA. *J. Clin. Microbiol.* **34:**1380–1385.

70. **Raymond, J., L. Armand-Lefevre, F. Moulin, H. Dabernat, A. Commeau, D. Gendrel, and P. Berche.** 2001. Nasopharyngeal colonization by *Haemophilus influenzae* in children living in an orphanage. *Pediatr. Infect. Dis. J.* **20:**779–784.

71. **Rennie, R., T. Gordon, Y. Yaschuk, P. Tomlin, P. Kibsey, and W. Albritton.** 1992. Laboratory and clinical evaluations of media for the primary isolation of *Haemophilus* species. *J. Clin. Microbiol.* **30:**1917–1921.

72. **Riggio, M. P., and A. Lennon.** 1997. Rapid identification of *Actinobacillus actinomycetemcomitans*, *Haemophilus aphrophilus*, and *Haemophilus paraphrophilus* by restriction enzyme analysis of PCR-amplified 16S rRNA genes. *J. Clin. Microbiol.* **35:**1630–1632.

73. **Saez-Llorens, X., J. Velarde, and C. Canton.** 1994. Pediatric osteomyelitis in Panama. *Clin. Infect. Dis.* **19:**323–324.

74. **Saito, M., A. Umeda, and S.-I. Yoshida.** 1999. Subtyping of *Haemophilus influenzae* strains by pulsed-field gel electrophoresis. *J. Clin. Microbiol.* **37:**2142–2147.

75. **Scriver, S. R., S. L. Walmsley, C. L. Kau, D. J. Hoban, J. Brunton, A. McGeer, T. C. Moore, E. Witwicki, Canadian *Haemophilus* Study Group, and D. E. Low.** 1994. Determination of antimicrobial susceptibilities of Canadian isolates of *Haemophilus influenzae* and characterization of their beta-lactamases. *Antimicrob. Agents Chemother.* **38:**1678–1680.

76. **Shanholtzer, C. J., P. J. Schaper, and L. R. Peterson.** 1982. Concentrated Gram-stained smears prepared with a cytospin centrifuge. *J. Clin. Microbiol.* **16:**1052–1056.

77. **Sims, W.** 1970. Oral haemophili. *J. Med. Microbiol.* **3:**615–625.

78. **Takala, A. K., J. Eskola, M. Leinonen, H. Käyhty, A. Nissinen, E. Pekkanen, and P. H. Mäkelä.** 1991. Reduction of oropharyngeal carriage of *Haemophilus influenzae* type b (Hib) in children immunized with an Hib conjugate vaccine. *J. Infect. Dis.* **164:**982–986.

79. **Tondella, M. L., F. D. Quinn, and B. A. Perkins.** 1995. Brazilian purpuric fever caused by *Haemophilus influenzae* biogroup aegyptius strains lacking the 3031 plasmid. *J. Infect. Dis.* **171:**209–212.

80. **Totten, P. A., J. M. Kuypers, C.-Y. Chen, M. J. Alfa, L. M. Parsons, S. M. Dutro, S. A. Morse, and N. B. Kiviat.** 2000. Etiology of genital ulcer disease in Dakar, Senegal, and comparison of PCR and serologic assays for detection of *Haemophilus ducreyi*. *J. Clin. Microbiol.* **38:**268–273.

81. **Totten, P. A., D. V. Norn, and W. E. Stamm.** 1995. Characterization of the hemolytic activity of *Haemophilus ducreyi*. *Infect. Immun.* **63:**4409–4416.

82. **Totten, P. A., and W. E. Stamm.** 1994. Clear broth and plate media for culture of *Haemophilus ducreyi*. *J. Clin. Microbiol.* **32:**2019–2023.

83. **Trees, D. L., and S. A. Morse.** 1995. Chancroid and *Haemophilus ducreyi*: an update. *Clin. Microbiol. Rev.* **8:**357–375.

84. **Turk, D. C.** 1984. The pathogenicity of *Haemophilus influenzae*. *J. Med. Microbiol.* **18:**1–16.

85. **Ubukata, K., Y. Shibasaki, K. Yamamoto, N. Chiba, K. Hasegawa, Y. Takeuchi, K. Sunakawa, M. Inoue, and M. Konno.** 2001. Association of amino acid substitutions in penicillin-binding protein 3 with β-lactam resistance in β-lactamase-negative ampicillin-resistant *Haemophilus influenzae*. *Antimicrob. Agents Chemother.* **45:**1693–1699.

86. **Urwin, G., J. A. Krohn, K. Deaver-Robinson, J. D. Wenger, M. M. Farley, and the *Haemophilus influenzae* Study Group.** 1996. Invasive disease due to *Haemophilus influenzae* serotype f: clinical and epidemiological characteristics in the *H. influenzae* serotype b vaccine era. *Clin. Infect. Dis.* **22:**1077–1078.

87. **Vastine, D. W., C. R. Dawson, I. Hoshiwara, C. Yoneda, T. Daghfous, and M. Messadi.** 1974. Comparison of media for the isolation of *Haemophilus* species from cases of seasonal conjunctivitis associated with severe endemic trachoma. *Appl. Microbiol.* **28:**688–690.

88. **Waggoner-Fountain, L. A., J. O. Hendley, E. J. Cody, A. A. Perriello, and L. G. Donowitz.** 1995. The emergence of *Haemophilus influenzae* types e and f as significant pathogens. *Clin. Infect. Dis.* **21:**1322–1324.

89. **Walker, C. N., and P. W. Smith.** 1980. Ampicillin resistance in *Haemophilus parainfluenzae*. *Am. J. Clin. Pathol.* **74:**229–232.

90. **Wallace, R. J., C. J. Baker, F. J. Quinones, D. G. Hollis, R. E. Weaver, and K. Wiss.** 1983. Nontypable *Haemophilus influenzae* (biotype 4) as a neonatal, maternal and genital pathogen. *Rev. Infect. Dis.* **5:**123–135.

91. **Weyant, R. S., W. F. Bibb, D. O. Stephens, B. P. Holloway, W. F. Moo-Penn, K. A. Birkness, L. O. Helsel, and L. W. Mayer.** 1990. Purification and characterization of a pilin specific for Brazilian purpuric fever-associated *Haemophilus influenzae* biogroup aegyptius (*H. aegyptius*) strains. *J. Clin. Microbiol.* **28:**756–763.

92. **Windsor, H. M., R. C. Gromkova, and H. J. Koornhof.** 1991. Plasmid-mediated NAD independence in *Haemophilus parainfluenzae*. *J. Gen. Microbiol.* **137:**2415–2421.

Enterobacteriaceae: Introduction and Identification

J. J. FARMER III

41

In the fifth edition of this Manual in 1991, Farmer and Kelly commented that it was becoming more difficult to cover the family *Enterobacteriaceae* in a single chapter. The family includes the plague bacillus *Yersinia pestis;* the typhoid bacillus *Salmonella* serotype Typhi (*Salmonella typhi*); four genera with species that often cause diarrhea and other intestinal infections; seven species that frequently cause nosocomial infections; many other organisms that occasionally cause human or animal infections; dozens of species that occasionally occur in human clinical specimens; and many other species that do not occur in human clinical specimens but can be confused with those that do. In the sixth edition, the material on *Enterobacteriaceae* was divided among three chapters: an introduction to the family that described the overall plan for isolation and identification; a chapter that covered *Salmonella, Shigella, Escherichia coli,* and *Yersinia,* the enteric pathogens; and a chapter that covered the remaining genera and species in the family. In the seventh edition a fourth chapter was added that covered *Klebsiella, Enterobacter, Citrobacter,* and *Serratia.* In the eighth edition there are also four chapters. However, *Yersinia* now has its own chapter, chapter 43; and *Klebsiella, Enterobacter, Citrobacter,* and *Serratia,* along with *Plesiomonas* (see this chapter) and all the remaining genera of *Enterobacteriaceae,* are in chapter 44.

Because of space limitations, many topics in the present chapter are discussed briefly and only a few primary literature citations are given. Several books, reviews, and chapters are recommended for more detailed information (1, 7, 8, 17, 25, 30, 33, 39, 44).

NOMENCLATURE AND CLASSIFICATION

The nomenclature and classification of the genera, species, subspecies, biogroups, and serotypes of *Enterobacteriaceae* have always been topics for hot debate and differing opinions (7, 8, 17, 24–27, 30, 39, 44). Until recently, genera and species were defined by biochemical and antigenic analysis. Newer techniques, such as nucleic acid hybridization and nucleic acid sequencing, that measure evolutionary distance (see chapters 17 and 19) have made it possible to determine the evolutionary relationships of organisms in the family (7–9, 14, 30, 39). The use of DNA-DNA hybridization has led to the discovery of many new species and

has resulted in the proposed reclassification of some of the older ones (7, 8, 30).

This chapter includes the different names and classifications that clinical microbiologists are likely to encounter in the scientific literature and in material accompanying commercial products. The nomenclature and classification given in Tables 1 to 3 are a compromise based on all available evidence; they include most of the genera, species, subspecies, biogroups, and unnamed Enteric Groups included in the family. If two names are widely used for the same organism, both are mentioned in this chapter with one in parentheses. Most of the "nonclinical" organisms in the family are also included, because there is a possibility that they will be isolated from a human clinical specimen some day (7, 8, 30).

Most of the newly described organisms in Tables 1 and 2 are only very rarely found in clinical specimens (30); most clinically significant isolates belong to 20 to 25 species that have been well known for many years (25). This is illustrated by the lists of genera that most often cause bacteremia (Table 4), nosocomial infections (Table 5), and infections of the gastrointestinal tract (Tables 6 and 7). The internet site of J. P. Euzéby (www.bacterio.cict.fr) gives nomenclature, classifications, original literature citations, and other information for all of the genera and species in the family *Enterobacteriaceae* and its relatives.

New Species That Occur in
Human Clinical Specimens

Several new "clinical" species have been described since the seventh edition was published in 1999. These include *Citrobacter gillenii* (11), originally known as *Citrobacter* species 10; *Citrobacter murliniae* (11), originally known as *Citrobacter* species 11; *Enterobacter cowanii* (38); *Klebsiella granulomatis* (14); *Proteus hauseri* (49); and Enteric Group 137 (59).

It is becoming more and more difficult to keep Table 1 current. For example, *Klebsiella granulomatis* (*Calymmatobacterium granulomatis*) does not grow on most bacteriological media and lacks a type strain that can be grown and described. Another problem has been the unavailability of certain strains (43). Hopefully, all the newly described species of *Enterobacteriaceae* will eventually be characterized, studied, and added.

TABLE 1 Biochemical reactions of the named species, biogroups, and Enteric Groups of the family *Enterobacteriaceae*[a,d]

Organism	Indole production	Methyl red	Voges-Proskauer	Citrate (Simmons)	Hydrogen sulfide (TSI)	Urea hydrolysis	Phenylalanine deaminase	Lysine decarboxylase	Arginine dihydrolase	Ornithine decarboxylase	Motility (36°C)	Gelatin hydrolysis (22°C)	Growth in KCN	Malonate utilization	D-Glucose, acid	D-Glucose, gas	Lactose fermentation	Sucrose fermentation	D-Mannitol fermentation	Dulcitol fermentation	Salicin fermentation	Adonitol fermentation	myo-Inositol fermentation	D-Sorbitol fermentation	L-Arabinose fermentation	Raffinose fermentation	L-Rhamnose fermentation	Maltose fermentation	D-Xylose fermentation	Trehalose fermentation	Cellobiose fermentation	alpha-Methyl-D-glucoside fermentation	Erythritol fermentation	Esculin hydrolysis	Melibiose fermentation	D-Arabitol fermentation	Glycerol fermentation	Mucate fermentation	Tartrate, Jordan's	Acetate utilization	Lipase (corn oil)	DNase at 25°C	Nitrate → Nitrite	Oxidase, Kovacs	ONPG test	Yellow pigment	D-Mannose fermentation
Budvicia																																															
B. aquatica*[b]	0	93	0	0	80	33	0	0	0	0	27	0	0	0	100	53	87	0	60	0	0	0	0	0	80	0	100	0	93	0	0	0	0	0	0	27	0	20	27	0	0	0	100	0	93	0	0
Buttiauxella																																															
B. agrestis	0	100	0	100	0	0	0	0	0	100	100	0	80	60	100	100	100	0	100	0	100	0	0	0	100	100	100	100	100	100	100	0	0	100	100	0	60	100	60	0	0	0	100	0	100	0	100
B. brennerae	0	100	0	99	0	0	0	0	0	33	100	0	100	100	100	100	67	0	100	0	100	0	0	0	100	100	33	100	100	100	99	40	0	100	100	67	67	67	0	0	0	0	100	0	100	0	100
B. ferragutiae	0	100	0	95	0	0	0	0	0	80	60	5	40	100	100	100	60	0	100	0	100	0	0	0	100	100	100	100	100	100	100	2	0	100	100	80	60	80	40	0	0	0	100	0	100	0	100
B. gaviniae	0	100	0	100	0	0	0	0	20	80	80	0	60	100	100	40	60	0	100	0	100	0	0	0	100	0	100	60	100	100	100	75	0	100	0	0	0	80	93	0	0	0	100	0	100	0	100
B. izardi	33	100	0	33	0	0	0	0	0	100	100	60	67	100	100	100	100	0	100	0	100	0	0	0	100	33	100	100	100	100	100	33	0	100	67	0	33	100	67	33	0	0	100	0	100	0	100
B. noackiae*	0	100	0	33	0	0	100	0	0	0	0	0	0	0	100	100	100	0	100	0	100	0	0	0	100	100	100	100	100	100	100	0	0	100	100	0	100	100	0	0	0	0	100	0	100	0	100
B. warmboldiae	0	100	0	33	0	0	100	0	0	0	100	0	33	100	100	100	100	0	100	0	100	0	0	0	100	100	100	100	100	100	100	0	0	100	67	0	0	0	0	0	0	0	100	0	100	0	100
Cedecea																																															
C. davisae*	0	100	50	95	0	0	0	0	50	95	95	0	86	91	100	70	19	100	100	0	99	0	0	0	0	10	0	100	100	100	100	5	0	45	0	0	0	0	0	44	91	0	100	0	90	0	100
C. lapagei*	0	40	80	99	0	0	0	0	80	0	80	0	100	99	100	100	60	0	100	0	100	0	0	0	0	0	0	100	0	100	100	0	0	100	0	0	0	0	0	75	100	0	100	0	99	0	100
C. neteri*	0	100	50	95	0	0	0	0	100	100	100	0	65	100	100	100	35	100	100	0	100	0	0	0	0	0	100	100	100	100	100	0	0	100	0	0	65	100	93	86	100	0	100	0	97	0	100
Cedecea species 3*	0	100	50	100	0	0	0	0	50	0	100	0	100	100	100	100	0	50	100	0	100	0	0	100	0	0	100	100	100	100	100	50	0	100	67	0	67	100	0	50	100	50	100	0	100	0	100
Cedecea species 5*	0	100	100	100	0	0	0	0	50	0	100	0	100	100	100	100	0	100	100	0	100	0	67	100	0	0	100	100	100	100	100	50	0	100	33	0	100	100	0	50	50	0	100	0	100	0	100
Citrobacter																																															
C. freundii*	33	100	0	78	78	44	0	0	67	0	89	0	89	11	89	78	78	89	100	11	0	0	0	100	100	44	100	100	89	100	44	11	0	0	100	0	100	100	100	44	0	0	100	0	89	0	100
C. diversus (koseri)*	99	100	0	99	0	75	0	0	80	99	95	0	0	95	98	98	50	40	99	40	15	99	0	99	99	0	99	100	100	100	99	40	0	1	0	98	99	95	90	75	0	0	100	0	99	0	100
C. amalonaticus*	100	100	0	95	5	85	0	0	85	95	95	0	93	1	97	97	35	9	100	1	30	0	0	100	99	5	100	100	99	100	100	2	0	5	0	0	60	96	96	86	0	0	100	0	97	0	100
C. farmeri*	100	100	0	10	5	59	0	0	50	100	95	0	95	5	96	75	15	100	100	2	9	0	5	100	99	100	100	100	100	100	100	75	0	5	100	0	65	100	100	80	0	0	100	0	100	0	100
C. youngae*	15	100	0	75	65	80	0	0	67	5	95	0	95	5	96	93	25	20	100	85	10	0	5	100	100	10	100	100	100	100	45	0	0	5	10	0	90	100	93	65	0	0	100	0	90	0	100
C. braakii*	33	100	0	87	60	47	0	0	67	93	95	0	100	5	100	75	80	7	100	33	0	0	0	100	100	7	100	100	100	100	73	33	0	0	80	0	87	100	100	53	0	0	100	0	80	0	100
C. werkmanii*	0	100	0	100	100	100	0	0	100	0	100	0	100	100	100	100	17	0	100	100	0	0	0	100	100	0	100	100	100	100	0	0	0	0	100	0	0	100	100	0	0	0	100	0	100	0	100
C. sedlakii*	83	100	0	83	0	100	0	0	100	100	100	0	0	100	100	100	100	0	100	0	17	0	0	100	100	0	100	100	100	100	0	0	0	17	100	0	83	100	100	83	0	0	100	0	100	0	100
C. rodentium*	0	100	0	0	67	100	0	0	33	0	0	0	100	100	100	0	0	0	100	100	0	0	0	100	100	0	100	100	100	100	0	0	0	0	67	0	0	67	100	0	0	0	100	0	67	0	100
C. gillenii*	0	100	0	33	67	0	0	0	33	67	67	0	100	100	100	33	67	33	100	33	0	0	0	100	100	33	100	100	100	100	67	0	0	0	67	0	67	67	100	0	0	0	100	0	67	0	100
C. murliniae*	100	100	0	100	67	67	0	0	67	0	100	0	100	100	100	100	67	33	100	33	33	0	0	100	100	33	100	100	100	100	100	0	0	0	33	0	100	100	100	33	0	0	100	0	100	0	100
Edwardsiella																																															
E. tarda*	99	100	0	1	100	0	0	100	0	100	98	0	0	0	100	100	0	0	0	0	0	0	0	0	0	0	0	100	0	0	0	0	0	0	0	0	30	0	0	0	0	0	100	0	0	0	100
E. tarda biogroup 1*	100	100	0	0	0	0	0	100	0	100	100	0	0	0	100	50	0	0	0	0	0	0	0	0	9	0	0	100	0	0	0	0	0	0	0	0	65	0	25	0	0	0	100	0	0	0	100
E. hoshinae*	50	50	0	0	0	0	0	95	0	95	100	0	0	100	100	35	0	100	100	0	50	0	0	0	13	0	100	100	0	0	9	9	0	0	0	0	100	0	0	0	0	0	100	0	0	0	100
E. ictaluri	0	0	0	0	0	0	0	100	0	65	0	0	0	0	100	50	0	0	0	0	0	0	0	0	0	0	0	100	0	0	0	0	0	0	0	0	100	0	0	0	0	0	100	0	0	0	100
Enterobacter																																															
E. aerogenes*	0	5	98	95	0	2	0	98	0	98	97	0	98	95	100	100	95	100	100	5	100	98	95	100	100	96	99	99	89	100	100	95	0	98	99	0	98	90	95	50	0	0	100	0	100	0	95
E. cloacae*	5	5	100	100	0	65	0	0	97	96	95	0	98	75	100	97	93	97	100	15	75	25	15	95	100	97	92	100	99	100	99	85	0	30	90	15	98	75	30	75	0	0	99	0	99	0	100
E. agglomerans group*	20	50	70	50	0	20	20	0	0	0	85	2	35	65	98	20	40	75	99	15	65	7	15	30	100	30	85	89	93	97	55	7	0	60	50	50	30	40	25	30	0	0	85	0	90	75	98
E. gergoviae*	0	5	100	99	0	93	0	90	0	100	85	0	96	100	98	98	55	98	99	5	9	0	0	0	99	97	97	100	97	99	99	55	0	97	97	0	30	2	93	30	0	0	100	0	97	75	100
E. sakazakii*	11	5	100	99	0	1	50	0	94	91	96	0	98	18	98	98	99	100	100	0	92	0	75	1	100	99	100	100	100	100	73	96	0	100	100	0	87	2	96	96	0	98	100	0	100	98	100
E. taylorae* (cancerogenus)	0	7	100	70	0	1	0	0	99	55	97	0	98	91	100	100	10	0	100	0	0	0	0	9	100	0	100	99	100	100	73	1	0	90	0	15	0	75	1	35	0	0	100	0	91	0	100
E. amnigenus biogroup 1*	0	5	100	100	0	1	0	0	9	55	92	0	100	91	100	70	35	100	100	0	91	0	0	9	100	100	100	100	100	100	100	55	0	100	0	0	35	35	9	35	0	0	100	0	100	0	100
E. amnigenus biogroup 2*	0	65	100	100	0	0	0	0	35	100	100	0	100	100	100	35	75	0	100	0	100	0	0	100	100	70	100	97	100	100	95	55	0	100	100	11	0	100	9	0	0	0	100	0	91	0	100
E. asburiae*	0	100	2	100	0	60	0	21	95	95	0	0	97	3	95	50	75	100	100	0	100	0	0	100	100	30	5	97	97	100	95	95	0	95	0	0	11	21	30	87	0	0	100	0	100	0	100

(*Enterobacter* continued on next page)

(Continued)

TABLE 1 Biochemical reactions of the named species, biogroups, and Enteric Groups of the family *Enterobacteriaceae*[a,d]   (*Continued*)

Organism	Indole production	Methyl red	Voges-Proskauer	Citrate (Simmons)	Hydrogen sulfide (TSI)	Urea hydrolysis	Phenylalanine deaminase	Lysine decarboxylase	Arginine dihydrolase	Ornithine decarboxylase	Motility (36°C)	Gelatin hydrolysis (22°C)	Growth in KCN	Malonate utilization	D-Glucose, acid	D-Glucose, gas	Lactose fermentation	Sucrose fermentation	D-Mannitol fermentation	Dulcitol fermentation	Salicin fermentation	Adonitol fermentation	myo-Inositol fermentation	D-Sorbitol fermentation	L-Arabinose fermentation	Raffinose fermentation	L-Rhamnose fermentation	Maltose fermentation	D-Xylose fermentation	Trehalose fermentation	Cellobiose fermentation	alpha-Methyl-D-glucoside fermentation	Erythritol fermentation	Esculin hydrolysis	Melibiose fermentation	D-Arabitol fermentation	Glycerol fermentation	Mucate fermentation	Tartrate, Jordan's	Acetate utilization	Lipase (corn oil)	DNase at 25°C	Nitrate → Nitrite	Oxidase, Kovacs	ONPG test	Yellow pigment	D-Mannose fermentation
Enterobacter (*continued*)																																															
*E. hormaechei**	0	57	100	96	0	87	4	0	78	91	52	0	100	100	100	83	9	100	100	87	44	0	0	0	100	0	100	100	96	100	100	83	0	0	0	0	4	96	13	74	0	0	0	0	95	0	0
*E. intermedium**	0	20	100	65	0	0	0	0	0	89	89	0	100	100	100	100	100	65	100	100	100	0	0	100	100	100	100	100	100	100	100	0	0	100	100	0	100	100	0	0	0	0	100	0	100	0	100
E. cancerogenus	0	0	100	100	0	0	0	0	100	100	0	0	100	100	100	100	65	100	100	0	100	0	0	0	100	100	100	100	100	100	100	100	0	100	100	0	0	100	100	33	0	0	100	0	100	0	100
E. dissolvens	0	0	100	100	0	100	0	0	100	100	0	0	100	100	100	100	0	100	100	0	100	0	0	0	100	100	100	100	100	100	100	100	0	100	100	0	0	100	0	100	0	0	100	0	100	0	100
E. nimipressuralis	0	100	0	0	100	0	0	0	0	0	0	0	100	100	100	100	0	100	100	0	100	0	0	100	100	100	100	100	100	100	100	100	0	100	100	0	0	100	0	0	0	0	100	0	100	0	100
E. pyrinus	0	29	86	0	0	86	0	100	100	100	43	0	0	86	100	100	14	0	100	0	0	100	100	100	100	100	100	100	100	100	100	0	0	100	14	100	14	0	86	14	0	0	100	0	100	0	100
Escherichia																																															
*E. coli**	98	99	0	1	1	1	0	90	17	65	95	0	3	0	100	95	95	50	98	60	40	5	1	94	99	50	80	95	95	98	2	0	0	35	75	5	75	95	95	90	0	0	100	0	95	0	98
E. coli, inactive*	80	95	0	1	1	1	0	40	3	20	5	0	1	0	100	5	25	15	93	40	10	3	1	75	85	15	65	80	70	90	2	0	0	5	40	5	65	30	85	40	0	0	98	0	45	0	97
*E. fergusonii**	98	100	0	17	0	0	0	95	5	100	93	0	94	0	100	95	0	0	98	60	65	98	0	0	100	0	92	96	96	96	96	0	0	46	0	100	20	97	96	96	0	0	100	0	83	0	100
*E. hermannii**	99	100	0	1	0	0	0	6	6	0	0	0	15	35	100	97	45	45	100	19	40	0	0	0	100	40	97	100	100	96	97	0	0	40	0	0	8	78	2	78	0	0	100	0	98	98	100
*E. vulneris**	0	100	0	0	0	0	0	85	30	0	100	0	0	85	100	97	15	8	100	0	30	0	0	1	100	99	93	100	100	100	100	25	0	20	100	0	25	50	50	30	0	0	100	0	100	50	100
E. blattae	0	100	0	50	0	0	0	100	0	100	0	0	0	100	100	100	0	0	100	0	0	0	100	100	100	0	100	100	100	75	0	0	0	100	14	0	100	0	50	0	0	0	100	0	100	0	100
Shigella																																															
S. dysenteriae (Group A)*	45	99	0	0	0	0	0	0	2	0	0	0	0	0	100	0	5	1	0	5	0	0	0	30	45	30	30	15	4	90	0	0	0	0	55	1	10	0	75	0	0	0	99	0	30	0	100
S. flexneri (Group B)*	50	100	0	0	0	0	0	0	5	0	0	0	0	0	100	3	1	1	95	1	0	0	0	29	60	40	5	30	2	65	0	0	0	0	15	0	10	0	30	8	0	0	99	0	1	0	100
S. boydii (Group C)*	25	100	0	0	0	0	0	0	18	2	0	0	0	0	100	0	1	0	97	5	0	0	0	43	94	1	1	20	11	85	0	0	0	0	25	8	50	10	50	0	0	0	100	0	10	0	100
S. sonnei (Group D)*	0	100	0	0	0	0	0	0	2	98	0	0	0	0	100	0	2	1	99	0	0	0	0	2	95	3	75	90	2	100	5	0	0	0	0	0	15	10	90	0	0	0	100	0	90	0	100
Ewingella																																															
*E. americana**	0	84	95	95	0	0	0	0	6	0	60	0	5	0	100	98	70	0	100	0	80	0	0	0	0	0	23	16	13	99	10	0	0	50	0	99	24	35	35	10	0	0	97	0	85	0	99
Hafnia																																															
*H. alvei**	0	40	85	10	0	4	0	100	6	98	85	0	95	50	100	98	5	10	99	0	13	0	0	0	95	2	97	98	98	95	15	0	0	7	0	0	95	70	70	15	0	0	99	0	90	0	100
H. alvei biogroup 1	0	85	70	0	0	0	0	100	0	45	0	0	100	45	100	70	0	0	55	0	55	0	0	0	0	0	0	100	70	70	0	0	0	0	0	0	0	30	30	0	0	0	100	0	30	0	100
Klebsiella																																															
*K. pneumoniae**	0	10	98	98	0	95	0	98	0	0	0	0	98	93	100	97	98	99	99	30	99	90	95	99	99	99	99	98	99	99	98	90	2	99	99	98	97	90	95	75	0	0	99	0	99	0	99
*K. oxytoca**	99	20	95	95	0	90	1	99	0	0	0	0	97	98	100	97	100	100	99	55	100	100	98	99	99	100	100	100	99	100	100	100	0	100	100	98	99	93	98	93	0	0	100	0	100	1	100
*K. ornithinolytica**	100	96	70	100	0	100	0	100	0	100	0	0	100	100	100	100	100	100	100	10	100	100	95	100	98	100	100	100	100	100	100	100	0	100	100	100	100	96	100	95	0	0	100	0	100	0	100
*K. planticola**	20	98	98	100	0	98	0	100	0	0	0	0	100	100	100	100	100	100	100	15	100	97	100	92	100	100	100	100	100	100	100	100	0	80	97	100	100	100	100	62	0	0	100	0	100	1	100
*K. ozaenae**	0	98	0	30	0	10	0	40	6	3	0	0	88	3	100	50	30	20	100	2	97	100	100	65	90	90	55	95	95	98	92	70	0	30	100	95	65	25	50	0	0	0	80	0	80	0	100
*K. rhinoscleromatis**	0	100	0	0	0	0	0	0	0	0	0	0	80	95	100	0	0	75	100	0	98	100	95	100	100	100	96	95	100	100	100	100	0	100	100	100	50	100	50	20	0	0	100	0	0	0	100
K. terrigena	0	60	100	40	0	0	0	100	0	20	0	0	100	100	100	80	100	100	100	20	100	100	80	100	100	100	100	100	100	100	100	100	0	100	100	100	100	100	100	20	0	0	100	0	100	0	100
Kluyvera																																															
*K. ascorbata**	92	100	0	96	0	0	0	97	0	100	98	0	92	96	100	93	98	98	100	25	100	0	0	40	100	98	100	100	99	100	100	98	0	99	99	0	40	90	35	50	0	0	100	0	100	0	100
*K. cryocrescens**	90	100	0	80	0	0	0	23	0	98	90	0	86	86	100	95	95	81	100	0	100	0	0	45	100	100	100	100	91	100	100	95	0	100	100	0	5	81	19	86	0	0	100	0	100	0	100
*K. georgiana**	100	100	0	100	0	0	0	100	0	100	0	0	83	50	100	17	83	100	100	33	100	0	0	0	100	83	100	100	100	100	100	100	0	100	100	0	33	83	50	83	0	0	100	0	100	0	100
Leclercia																																															
*L. adecarboxylata**	100	100	0	0	0	0	0	0	0	0	79	0	97	93	100	97	93	66	100	86	100	93	0	0	100	66	100	100	100	100	100	0	0	100	100	96	3	93	83	28	0	0	100	0	100	37	100
Leminorella																																															
*L. grimontii**	0	100	0	100	100	0	0	0	0	0	0	0	0	0	100	33	0	0	0	0	0	0	0	0	100	0	0	83	0	0	0	0	0	0	0	0	17	100	100	0	0	0	100	0	0	0	0
*L. richardii**	0	0	0	100	100	0	0	0	0	0	0	0	0	0	100	0	0	0	0	0	0	0	0	0	100	0	0	0	0	0	0	0	0	0	0	0	0	50	100	0	0	0	100	0	0	0	0

(*Continued*)

TABLE 1 (Continued)

Organism	Indole production	Methyl red	Voges-Proskauer	Citrate (Simmons)	Hydrogen sulfide (TSI)	Urea hydrolysis	Phenylalanine deaminase	Lysine decarboxylase	Arginine dihydrolase	Ornithine decarboxylase	Motility (36°C)	Gelatin hydrolysis (22°C)	Growth in KCN	Malonate utilization	D-Glucose, acid	D-Glucose, gas	Lactose fermentation	Sucrose fermentation	D-Mannitol fermentation	Dulcitol fermentation	Salicin fermentation	Adonitol fermentation	myo-Inositol fermentation	D-Sorbitol fermentation	L-Arabinose fermentation	Raffinose fermentation	L-Rhamnose fermentation	Maltose fermentation	D-Xylose fermentation	Trehalose fermentation	Cellobiose fermentation	alpha-Methyl-D-glucoside fermentation	Erythritol fermentation	Esculin hydrolysis	Melibiose fermentation	D-Arabitol fermentation	Glycerol fermentation	Mucate fermentation	Tartrate, Jordan's	Acetate utilization	Lipase (corn oil)	DNase at 25°C	Nitrate → Nitrite	Oxidase, Kovacs	ONPG test	Yellow pigment	D-Mannose fermentation
Moellerella																																															
M. wisconsensis*	0	100	0	80	0	0	0	0	0	0	0	0	70	0	100	100	100	100	60	0	0	100	0	0	100	100	0	30	0	0	0	0	0	0	100	75	10	0	30	10	0	0	90	0	90	0	100
Morganella																																															
M. morganii ss morganii*	95	95	0	0	20	95	95	1	0	95	95	0	98	1	99	90	1	0	0	0	0	0	0	0	0	0	0	0	0	0	0	0	0	0	0	0	5	0	95	0	0	0	90	0	10	0	98
M. morganii biogroup 1*	100	95	0	0	15	100	100	100	0	80	0	0	90	5	100	93	0	0	0	0	0	0	0	0	0	0	0	0	0	0	0	0	0	0	0	0	100	7	100	0	0	0	90	0	20	0	100
M. morganii ss sibonii*	50	86	0	0	7	100	93	29	0	64	79	0	79	0	100	86	0	7	0	0	0	0	0	0	0	0	0	0	0	100	0	0	0	0	0	0	7	7	100	0	0	0	100	0	0	0	100
Obesumbacterium																																															
O. proteus biogroup 2	0	15	0	0	0	0	0	100	0	0	0	0	0	0	100	0	0	0	0	0	0	0	0	0	0	0	0	50	15	85	0	0	0	0	0	0	0	0	15	0	0	0	100	0	0	0	85
Pragia																																															
P. fontium	0	100	0	89	89	0	0	0	0	0	100	0	0	0	100	0	0	0	0	0	78	0	0	0	0	0	0	0	0	0	0	0	0	78	0	0	0	0	0	0	0	0	100	0	0	0	0
Pantoea																																															
P. dispersa	0	82	64	100	0	0	9	0	0	0	100	0	82	9	100	0	0	1	100	0	0	0	0	0	100	0	91	82	100	100	55	0	0	0	0	0	27	0	9	100	0	0	91	0	91	27	0
Photorhabdus																																															
P. luminescens (25°C)	50	0	0	50	0	25	0	0	0	0	100	50	0	0	75	0	0	0	0	0	0	0	0	0	0	0	0	25	0	0	0	0	0	0	0	0	0	0	50	0	92	50	0	0	0	50	100
P. asymbiotica*	0	0	0	20	0	60	0	0	0	0	100	80	20	0	100	0	0	0	0	0	0	0	0	0	0	0	0	0	0	0	0	0	0	0	0	0	0	0	60	20	80	60	0	0	0	60	100
Plesiomonas																																															
P. shigelloides*	100	90	0	0	0	0	3	98	98	99	95	0	1	0	100	0	80	0	0	0	0	0	95	0	0	0	0	95	0	100	0	0	0	0	70	0	35	0	50	8	0	0	100	99	90	0	10
Proteus																																															
P. mirabilis*	2	97	50	65	98	98	98	0	0	99	94	90	97	2	100	96	2	15	0	0	0	0	0	0	0	1	1	0	98	0	1	0	0	0	0	0	70	0	87	20	92	50	95	0	5	0	0
P. vulgaris*	98	95	0	15	95	95	99	0	0	0	95	91	99	0	100	85	2	97	0	0	50	5	0	0	0	1	5	97	98	98	0	60	0	50	0	0	60	0	80	25	80	50	100	0	10	0	0
P. penneri*	0	100	0	0	30	100	99	0	0	1	85	50	99	0	100	45	1	15	2	0	0	0	0	0	0	1	0	100	100	55	0	80	0	0	0	0	55	0	85	5	45	40	90	0	1	0	0
P. myxofaciens	0	100	100	50	0	100	100	0	0	0	46	100	100	0	100	100	0	100	0	0	0	0	0	0	0	0	0	100	0	100	0	100	0	0	0	0	100	0	100	0	100	50	100	0	0	0	0
Providencia																																															
P. rettgeri*	99	93	0	95	0	98	98	0	0	0	94	0	97	2	100	10	5	15	100	0	50	100	90	1	0	5	70	2	10	0	3	5	75	35	5	100	70	90	95	60	0	0	100	0	5	0	0
P. stuartii*	98	100	0	93	0	30	98	0	0	0	85	0	99	2	100	0	2	50	10	0	2	5	95	1	0	7	0	1	7	98	5	0	1	0	0	0	60	0	80	75	80	10	100	0	10	0	0
P. alcalifaciens*	99	99	0	98	0	0	98	0	0	1	96	0	99	0	100	85	1	15	1	0	1	98	0	0	0	1	1	1	1	2	0	0	1	0	0	0	50	0	90	25	45	40	100	0	1	0	0
P. rustigianii*	98	65	0	15	0	0	99	0	0	0	30	0	99	1	100	35	0	35	2	0	0	0	0	0	0	0	0	0	0	2	0	0	0	0	0	0	5	0	50	5	5	0	100	0	0	0	0
P. heimbachae	0	85	0	50	0	0	100	0	0	0	46	0	8	0	100	0	0	0	0	0	0	92	46	0	0	0	100	54	8	0	0	0	0	0	0	92	100	0	69	0	100	0	100	0	0	0	100
Rahnella																																															
R. aquatilis*	0	88	94	94	0	0	95	0	0	0	6	0	0	0	100	98	100	100	100	88	100	0	0	94	100	94	94	94	94	100	100	0	0	100	100	0	13	30	6	6	0	0	100	0	100	0	100
Salmonella																																															
Group I^c strains*																																															
Most serotypes*	1	100	0	95	95	1	0	98	70	97	95	0	0	0	100	96	1	1	100	96	0	0	35	95	99	2	95	97	97	99	5	5	0	5	95	0	5	90	90	90	0	2	100	0	2	0	100
Serotype Typhi*	0	100	0	0	97	0	0	98	3	0	97	0	0	0	100	0	1	0	100	0	0	0	0	99	2	0	0	97	82	100	0	0	0	0	0	0	20	100	100	1	0	0	100	0	0	0	100
Serotype Choleraesuis*	0	100	0	25	50	0	0	95	55	100	95	0	0	0	100	95	0	0	98	5	0	0	0	90	100	1	100	95	100	30	0	0	1	0	45	1	20	0	85	0	0	0	98	0	0	0	95
Serotype Paratyphi A*	0	100	0	0	10	0	0	15	15	95	95	0	0	0	100	99	0	0	100	90	0	0	0	95	80	0	95	95	95	100	5	0	0	0	95	0	10	0	0	1	0	10	100	0	0	0	100
Serotype Gallinarum*	0	90	0	0	90	0	0	90	10	1	0	0	0	0	100	0	0	0	100	90	0	0	5	100	100	10	10	90	70	90	5	0	0	0	90	0	0	50	50	0	0	0	100	0	0	0	100
Serotype Pullorum*	2	90	0	0	90	0	0	100	10	95	0	0	0	0	100	90	0	1	100	90	0	0	5	100	100	1	100	100	90	90	5	1	0	0	96	0	25	0	50	95	0	2	100	0	15	0	95
Group II strains*	1	100	0	100	99	0	0	99	70	100	98	0	0	95	100	99	1	1	100	0	0	0	5	100	99	1	99	100	100	99	1	1	0	15	8	0	25	90	50	95	0	2	100	0	15	0	95
Group IIIa strains*	1	100	0	99	99	0	0	99	70	99	99	0	0	0	100	99	15	5	100	1	0	0	0	99	99	1	99	98	100	99	1	1	0	1	95	0	10	90	20	75	0	2	100	0	92	0	95
Group IIIb strains*	2	100	0	98	100	0	0	99	70	100	98	0	0	100	100	100	85	5	100	1	0	0	0	100	99	1	98	98	100	99	50	1	0	10	70	0	0	65	65	70	0	2	100	0	94	0	100
Group IV strains*	0	100	0	98	0	0	0	94	94	100	99	0	95	0	100	100	0	0	100	0	60	0	0	100	0	0	88	100	100	100	0	0	0	95	0	0	0	88	0	89	0	0	100	0	94	0	95
Group V strains*	0	100	0	94	0	0	0	67	0	100	100	0	100	0	100	94	0	0	100	94	0	0	0	0	100	0	100	100	100	100	0	0	0	0	94	0	33	89	100	89	0	0	100	0	94	0	95
Group VI strains*	0	100	0	89	100	0	0	100	67	100	100	0	100	22	100	94	22	0	100	67	0	0	0	0	94	0	100	100	100	100	0	0	0	0	89	0	0	100	0	0	0	0	100	0	44	0	100

(Continued)

TABLE 1 Biochemical reactions of the named species, biogroups, and Enteric Groups of the family *Enterobacteriaceae*[a,d] *(Continued)*

Organism	Indole production	Methyl red	Voges-Proskauer	Citrate (Simmons)	Hydrogen sulfide (TSI)	Urea hydrolysis	Phenylalanine deaminase	Lysine decarboxylase	Arginine dihydrolase	Ornithine decarboxylase	Motility (36°C)	Gelatin hydrolysis (22°C)	Growth in KCN	Malonate utilization	D-Glucose, acid	D-Glucose, gas	Lactose fermentation	Sucrose fermentation	D-Mannitol fermentation	Dulcitol fermentation	Salicin fermentation	Adonitol fermentation	myo-Inositol fermentation	D-Sorbitol fermentation	L-Arabinose fermentation	Raffinose fermentation	L-Rhamnose fermentation	Maltose fermentation	D-Xylose fermentation	Trehalose fermentation	Cellobiose fermentation	alpha-Methyl-D-glucoside fermentation	Erythritol fermentation	Esculin hydrolysis	Melibiose fermentation	D-Arabitol fermentation	Glycerol fermentation	Mucate fermentation	Tartrate, Jordan's	Acetate utilization	Lipase (corn oil)	DNase at 25°C	Nitrate → Nitrite	Oxidase, Kovacs	ONPG test	Yellow pigment	D-Mannose fermentation
Serratia																																															
*S. marcescens**	1	20	98	98	0	15	0	99	0	99	97	90	95	3	100	55	2	99	99	0	95	40	75	99	0	2	0	96	7	99	5	0	1	95	0	0	95	0	75	50	98	98	98	0	95	0	
S. marcescens biogroup 1*	0	100	60	30	0	15	0	55	4	65	17	30	70	0	100	0	4	100	96	0	92	30	30	100	0	0	0	70	7	99	4	0	0	96	0	0	92	5	50	4	75	98	83	0	75	0	99
S. liquefaciens group*	1	93	60	90	0	3	0	55	0	95	95	90	70	2	100	75	10	98	100	0	97	5	60	95	98	85	15	98	100	100	5	5	0	97	75	0	95	0	75	40	85	85	100	0	93	0	100
*S. rubidaea**	60	20	100	95	0	2	0	0	0	0	85	90	25	94	100	30	70	99	100	0	98	99	20	1	100	99	1	99	99	100	94	1	0	94	99	85	20	5	70	80	35	99	100	0	100	0	100
S. odorifera biogroup 1*	50	60	100	95	0	5	0	100	0	100	100	94	0	0	100	0	97	0	100	0	98	55	100	100	100	7	95	100	100	100	88	0	7	40	96	0	50	0	100	65	65	100	100	0	70	0	100
S. odorifera biogroup 2*	50	60	100	97	0	5	0	94	0	100	100	60	19	0	100	13	80	100	97	0	45	55	50	65	100	94	94	100	94	100	88	0	0	81	93	0	50	5	55	55	65	100	100	0	70	0	100
*S. plymuthica**	0	94	80	75	0	0	0	0	0	0	50	60	30	0	100	40	15	100	100	0	94	0	50	0	100	7	35	94	94	100	88	0	0	100	0	0	0	0	17	40	77	100	100	0	80	0	100
*S. ficaria**	75	75	75	100	0	0	0	0	0	0	100	100	0	0	100	0	0	100	100	0	100	0	0	0	100	100	0	100	40	100	6	70	0	100	93	100	88	0	100	80	20	100	92	8	100	0	100
S. entomophila	0	20	100	100	0	0	0	0	0	0	100	100	100	0	100	15	0	100	100	0	100	0	55	0	100	70	100	100	40	100	0	8	0	100	0	60	0	0	58	15	0	100	100	0	100	0	100
*"Serratia" fonticola**	0	100	9	91	0	13	0	100	0	97	91	0	70	88	100	79	97	21	100	91	100	100	30	100	100	100	76	97	85	100	6	91	0	100	98	100	88	0	58	0	0	0	100	0	100	0	100
Tatumella																																															
*T. ptyseos**	0	0	5	2	0	0	90	0	0	0	0	0	0	0	100	0	0	98	0	0	55	0	0	0	0	11	0	0	9	93	0	0	0	0	25	0	7	0	0	0	0	0	98	0	0	0	100
Trabulsiella																																															
*T. guamensis**	40	100	0	88	100	0	0	100	50	100	100	0	100	0	100	100	0	0	100	0	13	0	0	100	100	0	100	100	100	100	100	0	0	40	0	0	0	100	50	88	0	0	100	0	100	0	100
Xenorhabdus																																															
X. nematophilus (25°C)	40	0	0	0	0	0	0	0	0	0	0	80	0	0	80	0	0	0	0	0	0	0	0	0	0	0	0	0	0	0	0	0	0	0	0	0	0	0	60	0	0	20	20	0	0	60	80
Yersinia																																															
*Y. enterocolitica**	50	97	2	0	0	75	0	0	0	95	2	0	2	0	100	5	5	95	98	0	20	0	30	99	98	5	1	75	70	98	75	0	0	25	1	40	90	0	85	15	55	5	98	0	95	0	100
*Y. frederiksenii**	100	100	5	15	0	70	0	0	0	95	5	0	0	0	100	40	40	100	100	0	92	0	20	100	100	30	99	100	100	100	96	0	0	85	0	100	85	5	55	15	55	0	100	0	100	0	100
*Y. intermedia**	30	100	5	5	0	80	0	0	0	100	5	0	10	5	100	18	35	100	100	0	100	0	15	100	100	45	100	100	100	100	100	77	0	100	80	45	60	6	88	18	12	0	94	0	90	0	100
*Y. kristensenii**	0	92	0	0	0	77	0	0	0	92	5	0	0	0	100	23	8	0	100	0	15	0	15	100	77	0	0	100	85	100	25	0	0	0	0	45	70	8	40	8	0	0	100	0	70	0	100
*Y. rohdei**	0	62	0	0	0	62	0	0	0	25	5	0	0	0	100	0	0	0	100	0	0	0	0	60	100	62	0	100	38	100	0	0	0	50	50	0	38	0	100	8	0	0	88	0	50	0	100
Y. aldovae	0	80	0	0	0	60	0	0	0	40	0	0	0	0	100	0	0	20	80	0	0	0	60	100	100	0	0	100	100	100	100	0	0	0	0	0	20	0	100	0	0	0	100	0	20	0	100
*Y. bercovieri**	0	80	0	0	0	60	0	0	0	80	0	0	0	0	100	0	20	100	100	0	20	0	0	100	100	0	0	60	60	100	100	0	0	20	0	0	50	0	100	0	0	0	100	0	80	0	100
*Y. mollaretii**	0	80	0	0	0	20	0	0	0	80	0	0	0	0	100	0	40	100	100	0	20	0	0	100	100	0	1	80	60	100	100	0	0	50	0	0	50	0	100	0	0	0	100	0	20	0	100
*Y. pestis**	0	80	0	0	0	5	0	0	0	0	0	0	0	0	100	0	0	0	97	0	70	0	0	50	50	15	70	95	100	100	0	0	0	50	20	0	50	0	50	0	0	0	85	0	50	0	100
*Y. pseudotuberculosis**	0	100	0	0	0	95	0	0	5	0	0	0	0	0	100	0	0	0	100	0	25	0	50	0	50	5	5	95	100	100	5	0	0	67	70	0	30	0	50	0	0	0	95	0	70	0	100
*"Yersinia" ruckeri**	0	97	10	0	0	0	0	50	5	100	91	30	15	0	100	5	0	0	100	0	0	0	0	0	5	0	0	95	0	95	0	0	0	0	0	0	30	0	30	25	0	0	75	0	50	0	100
Yokenella (Koserella)																																															
*Y. regensburgei**	0	100	0	92	0	0	0	100	8	100	100	0	92	0	100	100	0	100	100	0	8	0	0	0	100	25	100	100	100	100	100	0	0	67	92	0	0	0	0	25	0	0	100	0	100	0	100
Enteric Group 58*	0	100	0	85	0	70	0	100	0	85	100	100	100	85	100	85	30	100	100	85	100	0	0	100	100	0	100	100	100	100	100	55	0	0	0	0	30	0	60	45	0	0	100	0	100	0	100
Enteric Group 59*	10	100	0	100	0	30	30	0	60	0	100	100	80	90	100	100	80	100	100	0	100	0	0	0	100	0	100	100	100	100	100	10	0	85	0	10	70	60	50	50	0	0	100	0	100	25	100
Enteric Group 60*	0	100	0	0	50	50	0	0	0	100	75	0	0	0	100	0	0	50	50	0	0	100	0	0	25	75	75	0	0	100	100	0	0	100	25	0	0	65	75	0	0	0	100	0	90	0	100
Enteric Group 63	0	100	0	0	0	0	100	100	0	100	65	100	100	100	100	100	0	100	100	0	100	0	0	100	100	0	100	100	100	100	100	65	0	100	0	100	0	0	50	0	0	0	100	0	70	0	100
Enteric Group 64	0	100	0	50	0	0	0	0	50	0	100	100	100	100	100	50	100	100	100	0	50	0	100	100	100	100	100	100	100	100	100	0	0	50	0	0	100	100	50	0	0	0	100	0	50	0	100
Enteric Group 68*	0	100	50	0	0	0	0	50	0	0	0	100	100	100	100	100	100	25	100	0	100	0	0	100	100	100	100	100	100	100	100	100	0	100	100	0	50	0	0	25	0	100	100	0	0	0	100
Enteric Group 69	0	0	100	100	0	0	0	100	100	100	100	100	100	100	100	100	100	100	100	0	100	100	0	100	100	100	100	100	100	100	100	0	0	100	100	0	0	0	0	25	0	0	100	0	100	0	100
Enteric Group 137*	100	100	0	0	0	70	0	0	20	0	91	100	100	100	100	100	100	100	100	0	100	0	0	100	100	100	100	100	100	100	100	80	0	100	100	0	100	0	100	100	0	0	100	0	100	0	100

[a] Each number is the percentage of positive reactions after 2 days of incubation at 36°C (unless a different temperature is indicated). The vast majority of these positive reactions occur within 24 h. Reactions that become positive after 2 days are not considered. Abbreviations: TSI, triple sugar iron agar; ONPG, o-nitrophenyl-β-D-galactopyranoside.

[b] An "*" indicates that the organism occurs in human clinical specimens.

[c] The Roman numerals refer to the seven *Salmonella* subgroups that are biochemically and genetically distinct.

[d] Revision: December 2001.

TABLE 2 Some new and unusual genera and species that have been classified[a] in the family *Enterobacteriaceae* and which do not normally occur[b] in human clinical specimens

Unculturable or extremely fastidious organisms whose
 classification as *Enterobacteriaceae* has been based mainly
 on 16S rRNA sequencing data
  Genus *Aranicola*
    A. proteolyticus
  Genus *Arsenophonus*
    A. nasoniae
    "*A. tiatominarum*"
  Genus *Buchnera*
    B. aphidicola
  Genus *Calymmatobacterium*
    C. granulomatis (*Klebsiella granulomatis*)

Genera associated with, or pathogenic for, plants
  Genus *Brenneria*, 6 species
  Genus *Erwinia*, 28 species, 5 subspecies
  Genus *Pectobacterium*, 6 species, 5 subspecies

Other organisms:
  Genus *Pantoea*, 7 species, 2 subspecies
  Genus "*Phlomobacter*," 1 species
  Genus *Xenorhabdus*, 4 species

  [a] The table includes some organisms whose eventual classification may be as "relatives" of *Enterobacteriaceae*. For more information about these organisms, refer to the internet site of J. P. Euzéby (www.bacterio.cict.fr).
  [b] There have been clinical isolates for a few of the organisms.

Organisms That Do Not Occur in Human Clinical Specimens

New or unusual *Enterobacteriaceae* that do not occur in human clinical specimens are listed in Table 2, and more

TABLE 4 Distribution of *Enterobacteriaceae* and other organisms in patients with bacteremia[a]

Organism	No. of cases
Family *Enterobacteriaceae*	
Escherichia coli	1,751
Klebsiella species	765
Enterobacter species	399
Serratia species	136
Proteus mirabilis	122
Salmonella, all serotypes	93
Citrobacter species	76
Enterobacter agglomerans complex	44
Morganela morganii	26
Other organisms (for comparison)	
Staphyloccus aureus	2,151
Coagulase-negative staphylococci	1,256
Enterococcus species	794
Streptococcus pneumoniae	475
Pseudomonas aeruginosa	451
Beta-hemolytic streptococci	307
Acinetobacter species	206
Viridans group streptococci	154
Stenotrophomonas maltophilia	69
Haemophilus species	27
Corynebacterium species	20

  [a] Adapted from reference (20), which included nosocomial and community-acquired bloodstream infections in 48 institutions in Canada, the United States, and Latin America. Bacteremia is not a reportable disease in the United States. Also see reference 23 for data covering a 3-year period and over 10,000 bloodstream infections in the United States.

TABLE 3 Vernacular names and use of the term "complex"[a] suggested for reporting isolates that are difficult to identify completely[b]

Vernacular name	Organisms included, definition, and comment
Citrobacter freundii complex	In addition to *Citrobacter freundii*, this term includes *C. braakii*, *C. gilenii*, *C. murliniae*, *C. werkmanii*, and *C. youngae*, which are difficult to differentiate (9, 11).
Enterobacter agglomerans complex	This term includes over 60 named organisms: the species of *Brenneria*, *Erwinia*, *Pectobacterium*, *Pantoea*, and a dozen additional "*Enterobacter agglomerans* DNA-DNA hybridization groups"[c]; and perhaps also *Enterobacter cowanii*.
Enterobacter cloacae complex	*Enterobacter cloacae* is made up of at least five DNA-DNA hybridization groups (8). The definition of the complex could be expanded to also include *Enterobacter amnigenus*, *Enterobacter intermedium*, and *Enterobacter kobei*, which are difficult to differentiate.
Klebsiella pneumoniae complex	In addition to *K. pneumoniae*, the term includes the closely related species (subspecies) *K. ozaenae* and *K. rhinoscleromatis* and two less closely related species, *K. planticola* and *K. terrigena*, which are difficult to differentiate.
Kluyvera-Buttiauxella complex	This complex includes two genera with almost a dozen species (Table 1).
Proteus vulgaris complex	*Proteus vulgaris* is made up of at least four DNA-DNA hybridization groups. The definition of the complex could be expanded to include the closely related species *P. penneri* and *P. hauseri*, which can often be differentiated.
Rahnella aquatilis complex	*Rahnella aquatilis* is made up of at least three DNA-DNA hybridization groups.
Serratia liquefaciens complex	The term includes *S. liquefaciens* and two closely related species, *S. grimesii* and *S. proteamaculans* (with its two subspecies *proteamaculans* and *quinovora*), which are difficult to differentiate.
Yersinia enterocolitica complex	In addition to *Y. enterocolitica*, the term includes the closely related species *Y. aldovae*, *Y. bercovieri*, *Y. frederiksenii*, *Y. intermedia*, *Y. kristensenii*, and *Y. mollaretti*, which are difficult to differentiate (4).

  [a] The word "group" is an alternative term for "complex"; e.g., the *Enterobacter agglomerans* group.
  [b] An alternative approach would be to report only the genus name (e.g., "*Citrobacter* species" or "*Kluyvera* species"). However, the terms in this table have a narrower definition.
  [c] Some of the "*Enterobacter agglomerans* DNA-DNA hybridization groups" can rarely occur in human clinical specimens.

TABLE 5 Important causes of nosocomial infections in the United States[a]

Organism	No. (%) of isolates in:				All infections
	Urinary tract infection	Wound or surgical site	Pneumonia	Blood	
Enterobacteriaceae					
Escherichia coli	20,218 (25.1)	3,600 (9.2)	1,607 (5.2)	1,511 (5.2)	27,871 (13.7)
Enterobacter, all species	4,232 (5.2)	2,850 (7.3)	3,257 (10.6)	1,316 (4.5)	12,757 (6.2)
Klebsiella pneumoniae	5,544 (6.9)	1,250 (3.2)	2,230 (7.2)	1,280 (4.4)	11,015 (5.4)
Proteus mirabilis	4,077 (5.1)	1,246 (3.2)	779 (2.5)	197 (0.7)	4,662 (2.3)
Citrobacter, all species	1,553 (1.9)	598 (1.5)	418 (1.4)	174 (0.6)	2,912 (1.4)
Serratia marcescens	688 (0.9)	548 (1.4)	1,112 (3.6)	351 (1.2)	3,010 (1.5)
Other organisms for comparison					
Enterococci	12,595 (15.6)	4,998 (12.8)	607 (2.0)	2,594 (9.0)	22,033 (10.8)
Pseudomonas aeruginosa	9,309 (11.5)	3,169 (8.1)	5,162 (16.8)	1,095 (3.8)	20,307 (9.9)
Staphyloccus aureus	1,569 (2.1)	7,371 (18.8)	5,352 (17.4)	4,625 (16.0)	23,187 (11.4)
Coagulase-negative staphylococci	3,035 (3.8)	5,147 (13.1)	637 (2.1)	8,481 (29.3)	20,465 (10.0)
Candida albicans	5,933 (7.4)	984 (2.5)	1,419 (4.6)	1,380 (4.8)	10,706 (5.2)
Streptococcus, all species	1,265 (1.6)	1,303 (3.3)	1,050 (3.4)	1,053 (3.6)	4,998 (2.4)
Candida, other species	1,763 (2.2)	229 (0.6)	245 (0.8)	879 (3.0)	3,370 (1.7)

[a] Based on nosocomial infection surveillance of over 200,000 cases for the United States, 1986 to 1989 (56) and 1990 to 1996 (unpublished data). Because of changes in hospital practices and in the national surveillance system, future updates of these data may not be possible. See references 20 and 23 for more recent but less comprehensive data.

information and literature citations can be found at the internet site previously cited. Many of these are not included in Table 1.

The Expanding Number of *Enterobacteriaceae* Species

How many species of *Enterobacteriaceae* are there? There are probably many hundreds, if not thousands. This is becoming more apparent as methods such as DNA-DNA hybridization and 16S rRNA sequencing are being used to study strains isolated from human clinical specimens, plants, animals, and the environment. One example is the recent study by Müller et al. (48), who found six new species of *Buttiauxella* and two new species of *Kluyvera* in a large collection of strains isolated from snails. Similarly, additional DNA-DNA hybridization subgroups, which are probably new species (sometimes called genomospecies), have been found in systematic studies of *Enterobacter cloacae* (7), *Proteus vulgaris* (49), *Rahnella aquatilis* (10), and *Citrobacter* (9, 11). Most of the *Enterobacteriaceae* that clinical microbiologists encounter every day belong to just a few of the many species described (25). However, the expanding number of *Enterobacteriaceae* species is becoming a serious problem for reference laboratories and for commercial identification systems, whose identification methods are becoming inadequate for complete and accurate identification. When a commercial identification system gives an unusual organism for a final identification, there are several possibilities to consider: the identification is correct, just unusual; the identification is incorrect; another aerobic or anaerobic organism is present and the biochemical profile is the result of the metabolic activities of the mixture; or a handling or coding error was made somewhere along the way. Before a final report of an unusual organism is issued, it is advisable to do as much checking as possible. This could include repeating the biochemical tests in the same commercial system after confirming the absence of a contaminating aerobic or anaerobic organism, testing the isolate in another commercial identification system, and comparing the strain's antibiogram with known patterns

reported for this organism. If these steps do not resolve the problem, the state health department can be contacted for advice, and the culture will often be accepted for further study. Different commercial systems often give different identifications for the same strain. The "gold standard" for identification is DNA-DNA hybridization (16S rRNA sequencing is a less accurate but more readily available alternative), but a reference laboratory's identification based on phenotypic characteristics is the final step in most cases.

Changes in Classification

Contrary to popular opinion, there is no designated international body that considers all proposed changes in classification and then issues an "official classification." For many years there has been a Subcommittee on *Enterobacteriaceae* of the International Committee on Systematic Bacteriology, whose responsibility is the nomenclature and classification of *Enterobacteriaceae*. This Subcommittee can make recommendations on matters of classification but has done so sparingly in the past. Even if this Subcommittee studies a specific "proposed reclassification," it can only make a recommendation, which can then be accepted or rejected by the scientific community. It should be emphasized that changes in classification are decided by usage, not by a judicial decision or action (see chapter 19 for further discussion). Sometimes two classifications are widely used, and both can be "correct." Classifications are correct if they conform to all the rules in the *Bacteriological Code (International Code of Nomenclature of Bacteria)*. However, classifications can be useful or not useful and can be frequently used in the literature or rarely used.

Proposed Changes in Classification Incorporated in Table 1

Since the sixth edition (1995) of this Manual, many "alternative classifications" have been proposed in the literature. Some of these appear to be totally justified and have been incorporated in Table 1. However, others have not been fully discussed or widely accepted by the scientific community (21). Table 1 gives the nomenclature and clas-

TABLE 6 *Salmonella* isolates in the United States for 1968 to 1998[a]

Rank	Serotype	No. of isolates: 1968–1998	No. of isolates: 1998
1	Typhimurium	301,548	8,796
2	Enteritidis	145,405	5,906
3	Heidelberg	82,442	1,900
4	Newport	60,983	2,272
5	Infantis	32,392	591
6	Agona	27,414	989
7	Saintpaul	21,646	476
8	Hadar	20,715	544
9	Montevideo	19,928	824
10	Thompson	17,858	564
11	Javiana	16,662	1,170
12	Oranienburg	16,339	691
13	Typhi	16,333	382
14	Munchen	14,495	645
15	Derby	10,680	172
16	Branderup	10,452	500
17	Blockley	9,734	60
18	Anatum	7,983	138
19	Panama	7,026	117
20	Java	6,865	250
	Subgroups 3A and 3B	985	62
	Paratyphi A		85
	Paratyphi B		189
	Paratyphi C		0
	Choleraesuis		23
	Choleraesuis variety Kunzendorf		13
	Total *Salmonella* isolates	1,056,511	33,781

[a] Data are from the Centers for Disease Control and Prevention (15). A free paper copy of this *Salmonella* atlas (15) can be obtained by contacting Richard Bishop (rbishop1@cdc.gov), Centers for Disease Control and Prevention, Mail Stop C09, 1600 Clifton Rd., Atlanta, GA 30333. A free copy of the annual *Salmonella* surveillance reports can be obtained from Centers for Disease Control and Prevention, Foodborne and Diarrheal Diseases Branch, Mail Stop A38, 1600 Clifton Rd., Atlanta, GA 30333. Recent surveillance reports can also be viewed on the internet at http://www.cdc.gov/ncidod/dbmd/phlisdata/salmonella.htm. (Note: These are very large documents, so it is essential to download individual parts for viewing.)

sification used by the reference laboratories at the Foodborne and Diarrheal Diseases Laboratory Section, Centers for Disease Control and Prevention. It may differ from other nomenclatures and classifications.

In the seventh edition, the genus *Plesiomonas* was classified in the family *Vibrionaceae* with *Aeromonas* and both

TABLE 7 *Shigella* isolates in the United States for 2000[a]

Rank	Serotype	Isolates
1	*Shigella sonnei* (serogroup D)	10,134
2	*Shigella flexneri* (serogroup B)	1,732
3	*Shigella boydii* (serogroup C)	174
4	*Shigella dysenteriae* (serogroup A)	56
	Not completely typed	636
	Total *Shigella* isolates	12,732

[a] Data are from the Centers for Disease Control and Prevention (16). A free copy of recent *Shigella* surveillance reports can be obtained from Centers for Disease Control and Prevention, Foodborne and Diarrheal Diseases Branch, Mail Stop A38, 1600 Clifton Rd., Atlanta, GA 30333. Recent surveillance reports can also be viewed on the internet at http://www.cdc.gov/ncidod/dbmd/phlisdata/shigella.htm. (Note: These are very large documents, so it is essential to download individual parts for viewing.)

genera were covered in chapter 32. Because *Plesiomonas* is closer to *Enterobacteriaceae* than to *Vibrionaceae* based on 16S rRNA sequencing and because it contains the enterobacterial common antigen, it has been included in the *Enterobacteriaceae* (Table 1) for the present edition. However, *Plesiomonas* is oxidase positive, a characteristic not shared with other species of *Enterobacteriaceae*, and is a distant relative of *Escherichia coli*, the type species of the type genus of *Enterobacteriaceae*. Thus, the classification of *Plesiomonas* in the family *Enterobacteriaceae* might best be viewed as tentative.

In Table 1, the organism originally classified (5, 31) as *Xenorhabdus luminescens* DNA hybridization group 5 is now classified as *Photorhabdus asymbiotica* (34). It has caused rare cases of bacteremia and wound infection in the United States (31) and Australia (50).

The names *Citrobacter diversus* and *Citrobacter koseri* have both been used in the literature for some time, but the name *Citrobacter diversus* has been used much more frequently. Many workers recognized the phenotypic similarity of these two organisms and thought that they might be the same. The species have different type strains, and so considering them to be the same will always be a subjective matter. They can be considered "subjective synonyms" but not "objective synonyms" (which must have the same type strain). The name *Citrobacter diversus* became the correct name for this organism on 1 January 1980, when the *Approved Lists of Bacterial Names* was issued, because under the laws of priority it was the older name. However, in 1993 the Judicial Commission of the International Committee on Systematic Bacteriology issued an Opinion (40) that the name *Citrobacter koseri* should be conserved over the name *Citrobacter diversus*, even though the name *Citrobacter diversus* was the older name, was on the *Approved Lists of Bacterial Names*, was the correct name under the rules of the *Bacteriological Code*, and was the name used most frequently in the literature. This "opinion" needs much more discussion by the scientific community, which is beyond the scope of this chapter; therefore, both names are included in Table 1.

Phenotypic and 16S rRNA sequencing data indicate that *Kluyvera cochleae* is almost identical to *Enterobacter intermedium*. All evidence indicates that it is a junior subjective synonym, and thus an illegitimate name, which is why it is not included in Table 1.

Other Proposed Changes in Nomenclature and Classification

Proposed Classification of Three *Klebsiella* Species in *Raoultella*

In 2001, Drancourt et al. (21) proposed that *Klebsiella planticola*, *K. ornithinolytica*, and *K. terrigena* be classified in a new genus, *Raoultella*, as *R. planticola*, *R. ornithinolytica*, and *R. terrigena*. These three species are extremely similar to *Klebsiella pneumoniae* in their phenotypic properties, making differentiation very difficult (30). This alternative classification needs further evaluation.

Enterobacter agglomerans Group—*Pantoea*

Enterobacter agglomerans—*Pantoea* complex is a confusing subject, and writers continue to make errors in the definition and circumscription (boundaries) of *Pantoea agglomerans*. In 1972, Ewing and Fife redefined the name *Enterobacter agglomerans* to include a wide variety of organisms known under many different names. These investigators also defined 11 different biogroups to recognize the phenotypic diversity of the many strains included in *Enterobacter agglomerans*. This name has become useful for clinical microbiologists, and it has been used extensively in the literature. Systematic analysis by Brenner and coworkers using DNA-DNA hybridization indicated that *Enterobacter agglomerans* is very heterogeneous, with at least 14 DNA hybridization groups (7). For this reason, the names "*Enterobacter agglomerans* complex" and "*Enterobacter agglomerans* group" (30) have been used to better indicate the heterogeneity of this "species" (Tables 2 and 3). However, it has been very difficult to find simple tests to differentiate and identify all of the DNA hybridization groups (30). For this reason, workers have been reluctant to subdivide the *Enterobacter agglomerans* group until a definitive classification could be proposed (30). Gavini et al. (35) took the first step toward more logical classification for this complex group by proposing that the group of six strains defined by Brenner et al. as "DNA hybridization group 13 of *Enterobacter agglomerans*" be classified in a new genus, *Pantoea*. They also defined a new species in the genus, *Pantoea dispersa* (35), that corresponded to *Enterobacter agglomerans* DNA hybridization group 3 of Brenner (7).

However, this new classification has caused some problems. Some authors have broadened the original definition of Gavini et al. for *Pantoea agglomerans*. Since DNA-DNA hybridization is not routinely done and since simple tests are not available to definitively identify strains to the level of DNA hybridization group, it seems prudent to retain the vernacular name "*Enterobacter agglomerans* complex" as a convenient name for clinical microbiologists for routine identification (Table 3). This term is defined biochemically in Table 1, and it should be emphasized that it is used merely for convenience and because the name *Enterobacter agglomerans* is well understood and widely used in the literature. Eventually, this term will be replaced with a better classification. When definitive testing in a reference laboratory (usually including DNA hybridization) is done, more precise names can be used in reporting. Examples could include *Pantoea agglomerans* (DNA hybridization group 13), *Pantoea dispersa* (DNA hybridization group 3), *Enterobacter agglomerans* DNA hybridization group 1, etc. Table 3 gives the vernacular name *Enterobacter agglomerans* complex, a term that may prove useful for reporting isolates in most microbiology laboratories since few can do DNA-DNA hybridization.

Enterobacter taylorae-*Enterobacter cancerogenus*

Enterobacter taylorae and *Enterobacter cancerogenus* may be two names for the same organism (36). However, they have different type strains; therefore, they are not "objective synonyms" under the rules of the *Bacteriological Code*. Until the identity of these two organisms is confirmed by other laboratories, both names will be used (Table 1).

Nomenclature, Classification, and Reporting of the Genus *Salmonella*

After much study and discussion, there is now good agreement on much of the nomenclature and classification of the genus *Salmonella* (25, 32, 47, 51, 53). However, there are still several problem areas where different names and classifications are being used. These include the names *Salmonella choleraesuis* versus *Salmonella enterica* (24); the use of the terms "serotype" (12, 47) versus "serovar" (51, 52) (both terms are often abbreviated as "ser."); the best way to write the names of the serotypes (serovars); the use of names versus antigenic formulas for some of the serotypes; and the argument whether some well-known serotype names should be eliminated and combined with other serotypes (12, 47, 51, 52).

Historical Species Concept in the Genus *Salmonella*

Until the 1970s, the species concept in the genus *Salmonella* was based on epidemiology, host range, biochemical reactions, and antigenic structure (the O antigen, phases 1 and 2 of the H antigen, and the Vi antigen, if present), and strains that differed in one or all of these properties were given distinct names. Names such as *Salmonella typhi*, *Salmonella cholerae-suis* (originally some names such as this one were written with a hyphen, which was eventually dropped), *Salmonella paratyphi* A, *Salmonella paratyphi* A var. *durazzo*, *Salmonella typhimurium*, *Salmonella typhimurium* var. *copenhagen*, *Salmonella enteritidis*, and *Salmonella newport* began to appear, and the list rapidly expanded to include hundreds of names. Some workers believed that these names really represented biological species, but others thought they were antigenic and biochemical varieties with an uncertain evolutionary relationship. However, there was universal agreement that the names were an extremely useful way to communicate about the particular serotypes and the disease they caused. Most authors wrote the serotype names in italics as a species in the genus *Salmonella*, for example, *Salmonella typhimurium* (25, 32). Several recent proposals to the Judicial Commission, International Committee on Systematic Bacteriology, have requested that important serotype names be preserved (24, 26, 27).

Basis for the Current Classification of the Genus *Salmonella*

In 1973, Crosa et al. (18) used DNA-DNA hybridization to show that *Salmonella* strains could be grouped into five main evolutionary groups. Two (possibly three) additional groups are now known (6, 51, 53). The vast majority of strains that cause human infections occur in DNA hybridization group 1 (I). Strains isolated from animals and the environment clustered into the four other groups, designated DNA groups 2 (II), 3a (IIIa), 3b (IIIb), and 4 (IV). Over the years, different authors have used different terms to refer to these evolutionary groups: DNA-DNA hybridization groups (18, 32), multilocus enzyme electrophoresis clusters (6, 53), subgenera, species (see the *Approved Lists of Bacterial Names* and www.bacterio.cict.fr), and subspecies (47, 51, 52).

A Single Species of *Salmonella*, *Salmonella choleraesuis*

Crosa et al. (18) showed that all five groups of *Salmonella* are very highly related. With the operational species definition usually used in DNA hybridization, these five groups could be considered to belong to the same species. Under the rules of the *Bacteriological Code*, the name of this species has to be *Salmonella choleraesuis*. However, this species name can cause confusion, since *Salmonella choleraesuis* would have two totally different meanings, one as a species and one as a serotype.

A Single Species of *Salmonella, Salmonella enterica*

There has been support for making an exception to the rules of the *Bacteriological Code* and using a name that would not cause confusion. There was a formal proposal to coin a new name, *Salmonella enterica* (24), that would replace the name *Salmonella choleraesuis* as the species name to represent most of the serotypes of *Salmonella*. The main advantage of this proposal is that it would reduce confusion by using a new name that has never been used as a serotype name. However, the proposal to replace the name *Salmonella choleraesuis* with *Salmonella enterica* was denied by the Judicial Commission of the International Committee on Systematic Bacteriology. Thus, the same *Salmonella choleraesuis* remains the correct name. *Salmonella enterica* is currently an "illegitimate name." A second proposal to the Judicial Commission is now pending and, if approved, would change the status of *Salmonella enterica* from "without standing in nomenclature, thus illegitimate" to "with standing in nomenclature, and legitimate." The name *Salmonella enterica* is being used by the World Health Organization's International Center for *Salmonella* (51) and by some of the World Health Organization's National Centers for *Salmonella*, including the one in the United States (12). The name is also being used widely in the literature.

Different Nomenclatures for Serotype Names

Another point of disagreement concerns the method of writing serotype names. For almost 100 years, serotype names have been written as species (the "serotype as species" nomenclature), and this method is still widely used. An example of this nomenclature: "*Salmonella enteritidis* is one of the most common serotypes in the United States and in many European countries."

Recently, the World Health Organization's International Center for *Salmonella*, a laboratory at the Institut Pasteur, Paris, France, introduced a different nomenclature in which the serotype name is capitalized and not written in italics. In this nomenclature, the name *Salmonella enteritidis* in the previous paragraph would be written in one of the following ways: "*Salmonella* serovar Enteritidis," "*Salmonella* ser. Enteritidis," or "*Salmonella* Enteritidis." The nomenclature described by McWhorter-Murlin and Hickman-Brenner (47) is similar, but they recommend using the term "serotype" instead of "serovar" (17). The main advantage of these nomenclatures is that they do not artificially treat the serotypes as species. The main disadvantage is that they create a new nomenclature, which differs from one that has been widely accepted and used for over 70 years. There have been literally hundreds of thousands of uses of the "serotype as species" nomenclature in the literature. The International *Salmonella* Center's nomenclature is being used (often with modifications) by some of the National Centers for *Salmonella*, including the one in the United States (12, 47). However, other National Centers for *Salmonella*, such as the one in England, continue to use the "serotype as species" nomenclature (for examples, see publications from the World Health Organization's National Center for *Salmonella* in England and epidemiological tabulations in the English epidemiological bulletin, *CDR Reports* [see www:phls.co.uk; then click on "New Electronic CDR Weekly"]). Since *Salmonella* names are being written differently by different authors and different National Centers for *Salmonella*, it is not surprising that the literature is beginning to reflect this confusion. Recent examples of the way "serotype Typhimurium" is being written include *Salmonella* serotype Typhimurium, *Salmonella* ser. Typhimurium, *Salmonella typhimurium*, *Salmonella* Typhimurium, *Salmonella* typhimurium, *Salmonella* serovar Typhimurium, and *Salmonella* serovar typhimurium. When the above variations are combined with the four species/subspecies possibilities, i.e., *Salmonella choleraesuis*, *Salmonella choleraesuis* subspecies *choleraesuis*, *Salmonella enterica*, and *Salmonella enterica* subspecies *enterica*, the number of possible variations is multiplied considerably. One example of the almost endless possibilities is *Salmonella enterica* subspecies *enterica* serovar Typhimurium.

Simple Laboratory Reports for *Salmonella* Isolates

Most clinical microbiology laboratories will identify *Salmonella* isolates with a commercial identification system and then with *Salmonella* "grouping antisera," to identify the O antigen group. These two methods usually give definitive results, and a simple report can be issued such as "*Salmonella* serogroup B", avoiding the complex problems described above. A reference laboratory can do definitive serotyping and biochemical testing and can determine the complete serotype. A report such as "*Salmonella* serotype Typhimurium" can be issued. This simple wording concentrates on the actual laboratory results and avoids the subgenus/species/subspecies concept. Abbreviating "serotype" and "serovar" as "ser." would be a further simplification and would avoid the disagreement over these two terms.

Nomenclature for Shiga Toxins/Verotoxins Produced by *E. coli* and *Shigella*

In a similar vein to the problems described for *Salmonella*, several different names are being used in the literature for the cytotoxins produced by *E. coli* and *Shigella*. This topic is critical because of the importance of *E. coli* O157 and other strains that produce these toxins (see chapter 42). Several different commercial assays for these toxins are being marketed; therefore, it is essential to read the package insert carefully to determine exactly which toxin(s) the kit is detecting and to word laboratory reports accordingly.

For almost 100 years, it has been known that *Shigella dysenteriae* serogroup O1 produces a potent cytotoxin known as Shiga toxin. More recently, it has been shown that certain strains of *E. coli* that cause intestinal infections produced a similar toxin, which was first detected because it was cytotoxic for Vero cells in tissue culture. A number of recent studies have defined these proteins from *Shigella dysenteriae* O1 and *E. coli*, and there is agreement that they comprise a family of toxins. They are being referred to in the literature as Shiga toxin (ST), Shiga-like toxins (SLT), and verotoxins (VT); and at least five different toxins are involved (13). The *E. coli* (EC) strains that produce these toxins are often referred to as "STEC" and "VTEC". Recently, Calderwood et al. (13) summarized the data available and proposed a new nomenclature for the toxins and for their corresponding genes. They recommended that strains of *E. coli* that produce these toxins be called "Shiga toxin-producing" *E. coli*, which would replace the previous term, "Shiga-like toxin producing." They also recommended that the new toxin name be cross-referenced with the corresponding verotoxin name. With this nomenclature, a laboratory report for a stool culture might be worded, "positive for *E. coli* O157:H7, which produces Shiga toxins Stx1 (VT1) and Stx2 (VT2)." Hopefully the differences between those using the two different nomenclatures will be resolved, resulting in a single nomenclature.

Proposed Reclassification of *Calymmatobacterium granulomatis* as *Klebsiella granulomatis*

Calymmatobacterium granulomatis is an organism that has received little attention in industrialized countries. In the seventh edition of this Manual, *Calymmatobacterium* was mentioned only twice (p. 25 and 50). It was listed as an aerobic bacterium that can be found in the genital area, and under the topic "Specimen Management" it was mentioned under the diseases granuloma inguinale or ulcerative donovanosis, with the notes "mostly a tropical disease" and "culture is nonproductive." *C. granulomatis* has been described as a highly pleomorphic gram-negative rod that does not grow on laboratory media. Diagnosis of granuloma inguinale has been based on showing the presence of "Donovan bodies" in Giemsa-stained smears of mononuclear cells or histiocytes from the patient's genital ulcers.

It had been assumed for almost a century that *Calymmatobacterium granulomatis* has no relationship to the "easy-to-culture" organisms of the family Enterobacteriaceae. Carter et al. (14) recently proposed that *Calymmatobacterium granulomatis* be reclassified in the genus *Klebsiella* as *Klebsiella granulomatis*. This proposal was based both on nucleotide sequence relatedness and on disease similarity. Granuloma inguinale is a disease similar to rhinoscleroma, also a tropical disease (nose infection) caused by *Klebsiella rhinoscleromatis*. While this alternative classification is being evaluated and tested, it would be helpful to write both scientific names, with writer's preference listed first: "*Calymmatobacterium granulomatis (Klebsiella granulomatis)*" or "*Klebsiella granulomatis (Calymmatobacterium granulomatis).*"

"Unculturable *Enterobacteriaceae*" as Possible Causes of Human Diseases of Unknown Etiology

That *Calymmatobacterium granulomatis* is probably an unculturable species of *Klebsiella* is a stunning finding. This suggests that other diseases of unknown etiology may be caused by unculturable Enterobacteriaceae. It is possible that strains of Enterobacteriaceae have evolved in a host-parasite relationship in such a way that they become unculturable or difficult to culture. Examples of this host adaptation have already been demonstrated in insects. The unculturable Enterobacteriaceae species *Buchnera aphidicola* and the slow-growing species *Arsenophonus nasoniae* are well-documented examples from insect pathology. Unculturable Enterobacteriaceae should be looked for in diseases of unknown etiology including Crohn's disease, ulcerative colitis, tropical sprue, "Brainerd diarrhea" (see www.cdc.gov/ncidod/dpd/parasites/diarrhea/brainerd_diarrhea.htm), and ankylosing spondylitis.

DESCRIPTION OF THE FAMILY *ENTEROBACTERIACEAE*

Most genera and species in the family Enterobacteriaceae share the following properties: they are gram negative and rod shaped; do not form spores; are motile by peritrichous flagella or nonmotile; grow on peptone or meat extract media without the addition of sodium chloride or other supplements; grow well on MacConkey agar; grow both aerobically and anaerobically; are active biochemically; ferment (rather than oxidize) D-glucose and other sugars, often with gas production; are catalase positive and oxidase negative; reduce nitrate to nitrite; contain the enterobacterial common antigen; and have a 39 to 59% guanine-plus-cytosine (G + C) content of DNA (1, 8, 28, 30).

Host-adapted species that are unculturable, difficult to culture, or slow growing appear to have evolved in some genera (Table 2). When techniques that measure evolutionary distance are used, genera and species in the family should also be more closely related to *Escherichia coli*, the type species of the type genus of the family, than they are to organisms in other families. Tables 1 to 3 expand on this definition and give most of the exceptions.

NATURAL HABITATS

Enterobacteriaceae are widely distributed on plants and in soil, water, and the intestines of humans and animals (1, 33). Some species occupy very limited ecological niches. *Salmonella typhi* causes typhoid fever and is found only in humans (37). In contrast, strains of *Klebsiella pneumoniae* are distributed widely in the environment and contribute to biochemical and geochemical processes (44). However, strains of *K. pneumoniae* also cause human infections, ranging from asymptomatic colonization of the intestinal, urinary, and respiratory tracts to fatal pneumonia, septicemia, and meningitis.

CLINICAL SIGNIFICANCE

Strains of *Enterobacteriaceae* are associated with abscesses, pneumonia, meningitis, septicemia, and infections of wounds, the urinary tract, and the intestine. They are a major component of the normal intestinal flora of humans but are relatively uncommon as normal flora of other body sites. Several species of *Enterobacteriaceae* are very important causes of nosocomial infections (Table 5). *Enterobacteriaceae* may account for 80% of clinically significant isolates of gram-negative bacilli and 50% of clinically significant bacteria in clinical microbiology laboratories. They account for nearly 50% of septicemia cases (Table 4), more than 70% of urinary tract infections, and a significant percentage of intestinal infections.

Human Extraintestinal Infections

Except for the species of *Shigella*, which rarely cause infections outside the gastrointestinal tract, many species of *Enterobacteriaceae* commonly cause extraintestinal infections. However, a small number of species, i.e., *E. coli*, *Klebsiella pneumoniae*, *K. oxytoca*, *Proteus mirabilis*, *Enterobacter aerogenes*, the *Enterobacter cloacae* complex, and *Serratia marcescens*, account for most of these infections (Tables 4 and 5). Urinary tract infections, primarily cystitis, are the most common (56), followed by respiratory, wound, bloodstream, and central nervous system infections. Many of these infections, especially sepsis and meningitis, are life-threatening and are often hospital acquired. Because of the severity of these infections, prompt isolation, identification, and susceptibility testing of *Enterobacteriaceae* isolates are essential.

Human Intestinal Infections

Several organisms in the family *Enterobacteriaceae* are also important causes (Tables 6 and 7) of intestinal infections of humans and animals worldwide. Although other species in the family have been associated with diarrhea (58) or even implicated as causes of diarrhea, only organisms in four genera, *Escherichia* (22, 29, 42, 60), *Salmonella* (18, 32, 37, 51), *Shigella* (25), and *Yersinia* (3, 41, 54), have been clearly documented as enteric pathogens. These four genera are discussed in chapters 42 and 43. Other *Enterobacteriaceae* such as *Citrobacter*, *Edwardsiella*, *Hafnia*, *Morganella*, *Proteus*, *Klebsiella*, *Enterobacter*, and *Serratia*, have an "association with diarrhea" and occasionally have been implicated (1, 58). Strains that produce biologically active compounds (these are often overstated as being "enterotoxin-producing strains") of these *Enterobacteriaceae* have been isolated from people with diarrhea (58), but the etiological role of these strains is uncertain. Some laboratories issue reports for stool cultures such as, "*Klebsiella pneumoniae* isolated in essentially pure culture (10 of 10 colonies tested); please consult the laboratory to discuss possible significance," to reflect this drastic change in the stool flora. There is no evidence that strains of these other genera are important causes of diarrhea.

In contrast, the evidence for the etiological role of *Plesiomonas shigelloides* (see chapter 44) in diarrhea is somewhat stronger. A safe generalization would be that "certain strains of *P. shigelloides* may cause diarrhea in certain people under certain conditions, but it is probably not an intrinsic pathogen." For an intrinsic pathogen, most strains would cause diarrhea in most people, under most conditions.

SPECIMEN COLLECTION, TRANSPORT, AND PROCESSING

Extraintestinal Specimens

Enterobacteriaceae are recovered from infections at many different body sites, and normal practices (see chapters 6 and 20) for collecting blood, respiratory, wound, urine, and other specimens should be followed.

Intestinal Specimens

Stool cultures are usually submitted to the laboratory with a request to isolate and identify the cause of a possible intestinal infection, usually manifested as diarrhea. The groups of *Enterobacteriaceae* usually associated with diarrhea in the United States are *Salmonella* (15), *Shigella* (16), and certain pathogenic strains of *E. coli* and *Yersinia enterocolitica*.

Stool specimens require special attention to both collection and transportation and should be obtained early in the course of illness, when the causative agent is likely to be present in the largest numbers on primary plates. At this stage, the use of enrichment broths should be unnecessary. If rapid processing (within 2 h of collection) is not possible, a small portion of feces or a swab coated with feces should be placed in transport medium, such as Stuart, Amies, Cary-Blair, or buffered glycerol saline. Cary-Blair is probably the best overall transport medium for diarrheal stools. More information about the isolation, identification, typing, and virulence testing of isolates of *Salmonella*, *Shigella*, *E. coli*, and *Y. enterocolitica* is given in chapters 42 and 43.

Microscopic Examination

Stool specimens should be examined visually for the presence of blood or mucus, but microscopic examination should not be done routinely because of its lack of specificity (55). Although identification by fluorescent-antibody staining is theoretically possible for all enteric pathogens, it has been of limited success because the method is difficult and there are many serological cross-reactions among the species of *Enterobacteriaceae* (25). This technique has been limited to detection of *Salmonella* strains (primarily by the food industry) and certain serogroups of *E. coli* and to outbreak investigations.

ISOLATION

Extraintestinal Specimens

Most strains of *Enterobacteriaceae* grow readily on the plating media commonly used in clinical microbiology laboratories (see chapter 20). MacConkey agar, generally interchangeable with eosin methylene blue agar, is usually used, because it allows a preliminary grouping of enteric and other gram-negative bacteria. The most common isolates of *Enterobacteriaceae* have a characteristic appearance on blood agar and MacConkey agar that is useful for preliminary identification (Table 8). Broth enrichment can increase the isolation rate if small numbers of *Enterobacteriaceae* are present, but this step is not normally required.

Intestinal Specimens

Media that should be used routinely for intestinal specimens include a nonselective medium such as blood agar, a differential medium of low to moderate selectivity such as MacConkey agar, and a more selective differential medium such as xylose-lysine-deoxycholate (XLD) agar or Hektoen

TABLE 8 Colonial appearance of the most common *Enterobacteriaceae* on MacConkey agar and sheep blood agar[a]

Genus or species	Appearance and typical colony diameter on:	
	MacConkey agar	Sheep blood agar[b]
Salmonella and *Shigella*	Colorless, flat, 2–3 mm	Smooth, 2–3 mm
Yersinia enterocolitica	Colorless, less than 1 mm	Smooth, less than 1 mm
Escherichia coli (lactose positive)	Red, usually surrounded by precipitated bile, 2–3 mm	Smooth, 2–3 mm
Escherichia coli (lactose negative)	Colorless, 2–3 mm	Smooth, 2–3 mm
Klebsiella pneumoniae	Pink, mucoid, 3–4 mm	Mucoid, 3–4 mm
Enterobacter	Pink, not as mucoid as *Klebsiella*, 2–4 mm	Smooth, 3–4 mm
Proteus vulgaris and *Proteus mirabilis*	Colorless, flat, often swarming slightly, 2–3 mm	Swarming in waves to cover plate
Other *Proteus*, *Providencia*, and *Morganella* species	Colorless, flat, no swarming, 2–3 mm	Flat, 2–3 mm, no swarming

[a] Most strains appear this way, but there are exceptions.
[b] Unlike *Vibrionaceae*, most strains of *Enterobacteriaceae* are nonhemolytic. However, a few strains of *E. coli*, and occasionally other organisms, are strongly hemolytic.

enteric agar. A broth enrichment such as selenite (or GN or tetrathionate) can be included, particularly if the specimen is not optimal. A highly selective medium such as brilliant green agar or bismuth sulfite agar can also be included for isolating strains of *Salmonella*. A special plate, such as sorbitol-MacConkey agar (or one of its modifications), can be added to enhance the isolation of Shiga toxin-producing strains of *E. coli* O157:H7. This medium should be used if the stool is frankly bloody or if the patient has a diagnosis of hemolytic-uremic syndrome, and it can be used for all fecal specimens if resources permit (see chapter 42). When *Y. enterocolitica* is suspected, a selective-differential medium, such as CIN (cefsulodin-irgasan-novobiocin) agar (also called *Yersinia* selective agar), can be added (see chapter 43). A complete stool culture procedure should also include media for isolation of *Campylobacter* and possibly *Vibrio* strains in areas where cholera and other *Vibrio* infections are common.

IDENTIFICATION

There are many different approaches to identifying strains of *Enterobacteriaceae* (30).

Conventional Biochemical Tests in Tubes

Tube testing was once used by all clinical microbiology laboratories, and it is still widely used in reference and public health laboratories (25, 30). Although some laboratories prepare their own media from commercial dehydrated powders, most of the common media are also available commercially in glass tubes that are ready to inoculate. Growth from a single colony is inoculated into each tube, and the tests are read at 24 h and usually also at 48 h. In many reference laboratories, most tests are often kept for 7 days to detect delayed reactions. Unfortunately, the media and tests are not completely standardized, and few laboratories use exactly the same formulations or procedures. Even with these variables, this approach usually results in correct identifications of the common species of *Enterobacteriaceae*. Table 1 gives the results for *Enterobacteriaceae* in

47 tests (for the media and methods used to generate the data in this table, see references 25, 28, and 30).

Computer Analysis To Assist in Identification

Two microcomputer programs have been developed in the Enteric Reference Laboratories to assist with the identification of *Enterobacteriaceae* cultures. "George" and "Strain matcher" were described in the 1985 review of the family (30). A detailed description and information for obtaining them are available from the author, and hopefully the programs will eventually be available via the Internet.

Screening Tests, Using All Information Available

Over the years, our Enteric Reference Laboratories have found that many genera, species, and serotypes can be tentatively identified with a minimum number of screening tests (Table 9). More precise identification can be made by using a complete set of tests or commercial identification systems. Because of the limited availability of certain reagents (bacteriophage O1, *Yersinia* sera, etc.), these screening tests may be more useful in a reference or research laboratory. Another problem will be government regulations for testing human clinical specimens.

Example 1. A blood isolate has the following properties: colonies on MacConkey agar are 2 to 3 mm in diameter, are bright red and nonmucoid, and have precipitated bile around them; it is indole positive and 4-methylumbelliferyl-β-D-glucuronidase (MUG) positive; it grows at 44.5°C; and it is antibiotic resistant. These results are completely compatible with *Escherichia coli*.

Example 2. An isolate from the feces of a diarrhea patient has the following properties: colonies on MacConkey agar are 2 to 3 mm in diameter and colorless; colonies on XLD agar are 2 to 3 mm and black; the isolate agglutinates in *Salmonella* polyvalent O serum and in O-group B serum; the MUCAP test (hydrolysis of 4-methylumbelliferyl caprylate; Biolife, Milan, Italy) and lysis by bacterio-

TABLE 9 Screening tests for genera and species of *Enterobacteriaceae* often isolated from human clinical specimens[a]

Organism (genus, species, or serotype)	Test or property[b]
Salmonella	Lactose⁻, sucrose⁻, H_2S^+, O1 phage⁺[c], MUCAP⁺[d], agglutinates in polyvalent serum,[b] typical colonies on media selective/differential for *Salmonella* (brilliant green agar, SS agar, Rambach agar, etc.), lysed by the *Salmonella*-specific bacteriophage,[c] often antibiotic resistant
Salmonella typhi	H_2S^+ (trace amount only), agglutinates in group D serum
Shigella	Nonmotile, lysine⁻, gas⁻, agglutinates in polyvalent serum, biochemically inactive, often antibiotic resistant, PhoE⁺[d] molecular test
Shigella dysenteriae	Agglutinates in group A serum, D-mannitol⁻
Shigella dysenteriae O1 . . .	Catalase⁻, agglutinates in O1 serum, Shiga toxin⁺
Shigella flexneri	Agglutinates in group B serum, D-mannitol⁺
Shigella boydii	Agglutinates in group C serum, D-mannitol⁺
Shigella sonnei	Agglutinates in group D serum, D-mannitol⁺, ornithine decarboxylase⁺, lactose⁺ (delayed), colony variation from smooth to rough
Escherichia coli	Extremely variable biochemically, indole⁺, MUG⁺, grows at 44.5°C, sometimes antibiotic resistant, PhoE⁺ molecular test[d]
Escherichia coli O157:H7 .	Colorless colonies on sorbitol-MacConkey agar, MUG⁻, D-sorbitol⁻ (or delayed), agglutinates in O157 serum and H7 serum
Yersinia	Grows on CIN agar, often more active biochemically at 25 than 36°C (motile at 25°C, nonmotile at 36°C), urea⁺
Yersinia enterocolitica, pathogenic serotypes . .	CR-MOX⁺, pyrazinamidase⁻, salicin⁻, esculin⁻, agglutinate in O typing sera: 3; 4,32; 5,27; 8; 9; 13a,13b; 18; 20; or 21
Yersinia enterocolitica O3 (a pathogenic serotype)	D-Xylose⁻, agglutinates in O3 serum, tiny colonies at 24 h on plating media
Yersinia enterocolitica, nonpathogenic serotypes	CR-MOX⁻, pyrazinamidase⁺, salicin⁺, esculin⁺, do not agglutinate in typing O sera: 3; 4,32; 5,27; 8; O9; 13a,13b; 18; 20; or 21
Citrobacter	Citrate⁺, lysine decarboxylase⁻, often grows on CIN agar, strong characteristic odor
Hafnia	Lysed by *Hafnia*-specific bacteriophage,[c] often more active biochemically at 25 than 36°C
Klebsiella	Mucoid colonies, encapsulated cells, nonmotile, lysine⁺, very active biochemically, ferments most sugars, VP⁺, malonate⁺, resistant to carbenicillin and ampicillin
Enterobacter	Variable biochemically, citrate⁺, VP⁺, resistant to cephalothin
Serratia	DNase⁺, gelatinase⁺, lipase⁺, resistant to colistin and cephalothin
Serratia marcescens	L-arabinose⁻
Serratia, other species . . .	L-arabinose⁺
Proteus-Providencia-Morganella	Phenylalanine⁺, tyrosine hydrolysis⁺, often urea⁺, resistant to colistin
Proteus	Swarms on blood agar, pungent odor, H_2S^+, gelatin⁺, lipase⁺
Proteus mirabilis	Urea⁺, indole⁻, ornithine⁺, maltose⁻
Proteus vulgaris	Urea⁺, indole⁺, ornithine⁻, maltose⁺
Providencia	No swarming, H_2S^-, ornithine⁻, gelatin⁻, lipase⁻
Morganella	Very inactive biochemically, no swarming, citrate⁻, H_2S^-, ornithine⁺, gelatin⁻, lipase⁻, urea⁺
Plesiomonas shigelloides . . .	Oxidase⁺, lysine⁺, arginine⁺, ornithine⁺, *myo*-inositol⁺

[a] This table gives only the general properties of the genera, species, and serogroups, so there will be exceptions. See Table 1 and chapters 42 to 44 for more details and more precise data. The properties listed for a genus or group of genera generally apply to each of its species, and the properties listed for a species generally apply to each of its serotypes.

[b] Biochemical test results are given as percentages in Table 1. The serological tests refer to slide agglutination in group or individual antisera (O1, O3, etc.) for *Salmonella*, *Shigella*, *Yersinia*, and *E. coli*.

[c] These are two bacteriophage tests useful for identification.

[d] Abbreviations: CIN, cefsulodin-irgasan-novobiocin agar (a plating medium selective for *Yersinia*); CR-MOX, Congo red, magnesium oxalate agar (a differential medium useful for distinguishing pathogenic from nonpathogenic strains of *Yersinia*); MUCAP, 4-methylumbelliferyl caprylate (a genus-specific test for *Salmonella*); MUG, 4-methylumbelliferyl-β-D-glucuronidase; ONPG, o-nitrophenyl-β-D-galactopyranoside; PhoE, a test done by PCR that is sensitive and specific for *E. coli/Shigella* (see the text and reference 57); VP, Voges-Proskauer.

phage O1 are positive; and it is antibiotic resistant. All these results are compatible with *Salmonella* serogroup B.

"Kits" for Identification

A kit is defined as a panel of miniaturized or standardized tests that are available commercially. The approach for using kits is similar to the conventional tube method, with the main differences being in the miniaturization, number of tests available, suspending medium, and method of reading and interpreting results (sometimes by machine). Kits are now used by most American laboratories; they are discussed in chapter 14. Kits usually give the correct identification for the most common species of *Enterobacteriaceae*, but they may not be as accurate for some of the new species. It is important to check the instruction manual to determine which organisms are included in the database and the number of strains that were used to define each organism. The main problem with kit-based identification is that the tests used (usually about 20 tests) are becoming inadequate to differentiate all of the current species of *Enterobacteriaceae* given in Tables 1 to 3. This is also becoming a problem with conventional tube tests, even when the 47 tests listed in Table 1 are used. Unusual identifications or "no identification" obtained with a kit could be verified by other methods or approaches, but referral to a reference laboratory may be the best alternative. Other methods might include a different kit (which will have similar limitations) or more expensive research techniques such as molecular tests or 16S rRNA sequencing.

Molecular Methods of Identification

Molecular methods have proved useful for identification to the level of family, genus, species, serotype, clone, and strain and for differentiating pathogenic from nonpathogenic strains (see chapter 17). For example, a PCR test for the *phoE* gene appears to be a sensitive and specific test for determining if a strain belongs to the *Escherichia-Shigella* group (57). However, few if any of these molecular methods are commercially available. In the United States, commercial tests must also be approved by the Food and Drug Administration if they are used on human clinical specimens. These problems have greatly restricted the use of molecular methods in clinical microbiology laboratories. However, they have proved extremely useful in a research setting. In the United States, to conform with the CLIA regulations (Clinical Laboratory Improvement Amend-

ments of 1988, also called CLIA '88), it is necessary to report these research results with a disclaimer unless all the CLIA requirements have been met.

Problem Strains

Most strains of *Enterobacteriaceae* grow rapidly on plating media and on media used for biochemical identification, but occasionally a slow-growing or fastidious strain is encountered. Some strains grow poorly on blood agar but much better on chocolate agar incubated in a candle jar. This characteristic suggests a possible nutritional requirement or a mutation involving respiration. There are slow-growing strains of *E. coli*, *K. pneumoniae*, and *Serratia marcescens*, and typical biochemical reactions of these strains usually require extended incubation. Another type of problem organism is sometimes isolated from patients who are being treated with antimicrobial agents. Li et al. described such "pleiotropic" (having multiple phenotypic expression) mutants of *S. marcescens* (46) and *Salmonella* after exposure to gentamicin. These strains react atypically in many of the standard biochemical tests and are difficult to identify. A different type of pleiotropic mutant induced by chemical exposure was reported by Lannigan and Hussian (45). A *Salmonella* strain lost the ability to produce hydrogen sulfide, reduce nitrate to nitrite, and produce gas from glucose because of chlorate resistance acquired after exposure to Dakin's solution (a solution that contains chlorate and is found in hospitals). Some atypical and slow-growing strains become more typical and grow better when they are transferred several times. Laboratories occasionally isolate strains that grow rapidly but have a biochemical reaction profile that does not fit any of the described species, biogroups, or Enteric Groups of

TABLE 10 Intrinsic antimicrobial resistance in some common *Enterobacteriaceae*

Genus or species	Most strains are resistant to:
Buttiauxella species	Cephalothin
Cedecea species	Polymyxins, ampicillin, cephalothin
Citrobacter amalonaticus	Ampicillin
Citrobacter freundii	Cephalothin
Citrobacter diversus (*C. koseri*)	Cephalothin, carbenicillin
Edwardsiella tarda	Colistin
Enterobacter cloacae	Cephalothin
Enterobacter aerogenes	Cephalothin
Many other *Enterobacter* species	Cephalothin
Escherichia hermannii	Ampicillin, carbenicillin
Ewingella americana	Cephalothin
Hafnia alvei	Cephalothin
Klebsiella pneumoniae	Ampicillin, carbenicillin
Kluyvera ascorbata	Ampicillin
Kluyvera cryocrescens	Ampicillin
Proteus mirabilis	Polymyxins, tetracycline, nitrofurantoin
Proteus vulgaris	Polymyxins, ampicillin, nitrofurantoin, tetracycline
Morganella morganii	Polymyxins, ampicillin, cephalothin
Providencia rettgeri	Polymyxins, cephalothin, nitrofurantoin, tetracycline
Other *Providencia*[a] species	Polymyxins, nitrofurantoin
Serratia marcescens[b]	Polymyxins, cephalothin, nitrofurantoin
Serratia fonticola	Ampicillin, carbenicillin, cephalothin
Other *Serratia* species	Polymyxins,[c] cephalothin

[a] Most strains of *Providencia stuartii* are also resistant to cephalothin and tetracycline.

[b] *Serratia marcescens* can also be resistant to ampicillin, carbenicillin, streptomycin, and tetracycline.

[c] Most *Serratia* species are resistance to polymyxins, but some strains have unusual zones of inhibition, 10 to 12 mm or larger, even though they are resistant when tested by other methods.

Enterobacteriaceae. At present, this type of culture can only be reported as "unidentified". It may be an atypical strain of one of the organisms listed in Tables 1 to 3, or it may belong to a new species that has not been described (30, 59). Additional testing at a state, national, or international reference laboratory can often answer this question and has in the past led to the discovery of new causes of human infections (7–11, 30, 48, 59).

ANTIBIOTIC SUSCEPTIBILITY

Several methods are available for testing the antibiotic susceptibility of *Enterobacteriaceae*, but the most popular are disk diffusion (2) and broth dilution (see chapters 15 and 69 to 75). In addition, the reader should consult a current textbook or review of infectious diseases for a description of antibiotic usage in clinical practice.

When antibiotics were first introduced, there was only slight resistance among the species of *Enterobacteriaceae*. Today, antibiotic resistance is much more common among strains isolated from humans and animals. Resistance patterns vary depending on the organism and its origin.

Intrinsic Resistance

Intrinsic resistance is a genetic property of most strains of a species and evolved long before the clinical use of antibiotics. This evolution can best be shown by studying strains isolated and stored before the antibiotic era or by studying a large collection of strains from a wide variety of sources that presumably have had less exposure to antibiotics. For example, essentially all strains of *Serratia marcescens* have intrinsic resistance to penicillin G, colistin, and cephalothin. Table 10 lists some species of *Enterobacteriaceae* and their intrinsic resistance patterns.

The Antibiogram as a Marker in Epidemiological Studies

Antibiotic susceptibility testing is usually done on isolates that are clinically significant and provides an "antibiogram" that is useful for comparing isolates in epidemiologic studies. When the selective ecological pressure of antibiotics is changed, the resistance patterns of epidemic (or endemic) strains may also change. These changes have been documented in outbreaks that have lasted for several months or longer. Even with these limitations in stability, the antibiogram is probably the most useful and practical laboratory marker for comparing strains and can be extremely helpful in recognizing and analyzing infection problems.

Use of Antibiograms for Identification

The antibiogram of a culture can be compared with those of known isolates (Table 10) to provide a different approach to identification. When the antibiogram and identification are incompatible (for example, a strain of *Klebsiella* that is susceptible to ampicillin and carbenicillin, or a culture of *Enterobacter* that is susceptible to cephalothin), the culture should be streaked and checked for purity. In addition, both the identification and the antibiogram may have to be repeated.

Some of the material in this chapter was taken from or adapted from publications by authors from the Centers for Disease Control and Prevention, including other chapters and reviews of the family. I thank these authors for allowing me to use this material with a minimum of editing and rewriting. Thanks also to Robert Gaynes, Hospital Infections Program, Centers for Disease Control and Prevention, for providing the unpublished data in Table 5 for 1992 to 1996, and special thanks to the many people who did biochemical testing of the cultures tabulated in Table 1.

REFERENCES

1. **Balows, A., H. G. Trüper, M. Dworkin, W. Harder, and K.-H. Schleifer (ed.).** 1992. *The Prokaryotes*, 2nd ed., vol. 3, p. 2673–2937. Springer-Verlag KG, Berlin, Germany.
2. **Bauer, A. W., W. M. M. Kirby, J. C. Sherris, and M. Turck.** 1966. Antibiotic susceptibility testing by a standardized single disk method. *Am. J. Clin. Pathol.* **45:**493–496.
3. **Bercovier, H., D. J. Brenner, J. Ursing, A. G. Steigerwalt, G. R. Fanning, J. M. Alonso, G. A. Carter, and H. H. Mollaret.** 1980. Characterization of *Yersinia enterocolitica sensu stricto. Curr. Microbiol.* **4:**201–206.
4. **Bercovier, H., J. Ursing, D. J. Brenner, A. G. Steigerwalt, G. R. Fanning, G. P. Carter, and H. H. Mollaret.** 1980. *Yersinia kristensenii*: a new species of *Enterobacteriaceae* composed of sucrose-negative strains (formerly called *Yersinia enterocolitica* or *Yersinia enterocolitica*-like). *Curr. Microbiol.* **4:**219–224.
5. **Boemare, N. E., R. J. Akhurst, and R. G. Mourant.** 1993. DNA relatedness between *Xenorhabdus* spp. (*Enterobacteriaceae*), symbiotic bacteria of entomopathogenic nematodes, and a proposal to transfer *Xenorhabdus luminescens* to a new genus, *Photorhabdus* gen. nov. *Int. J. Syst. Bacteriol.* **43:**249–255.
6. **Boyd, E. F., F.-S. Wang, T. S. Whittam, and R. K. Selander.** 1996. Molecular genetic relationships of the salmonellae. *Appl. Environ. Microbiol.* **62:**804–808.
7. **Brenner, D. J.** 1992. Additional genera of *Enterobacteriaceae*, p. 2922–2937. *In* A. Balows, H. G. Trüper, M. Dworkin, W. Harder, and K.-H. Schleifer (ed.), *The Prokaryotes*, 2nd ed. Springer-Verlag KG, Berlin, Germany.
8. **Brenner, D. J.** 1992. Introduction to the family *Enterobacteriaceae*, p. 2673–2695. *In* A. Balows, H. G. Trüper, M. Dworkin, W. Harder, and K.-H. Schleifer (ed.), *The Prokaryotes*, 2nd ed. Springer-Verlag KG, Berlin, Germany.
9. **Brenner, D. J., P. A. D. Grimont, A. G. Steigerwalt, G. R. Fanning, E. Ageron, and C. F. Riddle.** 1993. Classification of citrobacteria by DNA hybridization: designation of *Citrobacter farmeri* sp. nov., *Citrobacter youngae* sp. nov., *Citrobacter braakii* sp. nov., *Citrobacter werkmanii* sp. nov., *Citrobacter sedlakii* sp. nov., and three unnamed *Citrobacter* genomospecies. *Int. J. Syst. Bacteriol.* **43:**645–658.
10. **Brenner, D. J., H. E. Müller, A. G. Steigerwalt, A. M. Whitney, C. M. O'Hara, and P. Kämpfer.** 1998. Two new *Rahnella* genomospecies that cannot be phenotypically differentiated from *Rahnella aquatilis. Int. J. Syst. Bacteriol.* **48:**141–149.
11. **Brenner, D. J., C. M. O'Hara, P. A. D. Grimont, J. M. Janda, E. Falsen, E. Aldova, E. Ageron, J. Schindler, S. L. Abbott, and A. G. Steigerwalt.** 1999. Biochemical identification of *Citrobacter* species defined by DNA hybridization and description of *Citrobacter gillenii* sp. nov. (formerly *Citrobacter* genomospecies 10) and *Citrobacter murliniae* sp. nov. (formerly *Citrobacter* genomospecies 11). *J. Clin. Microbiol.* **37:**2619–2624.
12. **Brenner, F. W., R. G. Villar, F. J. Angulo, R. Tauxe, and B. Swaminathan.** 2000. *Salmonella* nomenclature. *J. Clin. Microbiol.* **38:**2465–2467.
13. **Calderwood, S. B., D. W. K. Acheson, G. T. Keusch, T. J. Barrett, P. M. Griffin, N. A. Strockbine, B. Swaminathan, J. B. Kaper, M. M. Levine, B. S. Kaplan, H. Karch, A. D. O'Brien, T. G. Obrig, Y. Takeda, P. I. Tarr, and I. K. Wachsmuth.** 1996. Proposed new nomenclature for SLT (VT) family. *ASM News* **62:**118–119.

14. Carter, J. S., F. J. Bowden, I. Bastian, G. M. Myers, K. S. Sriprakash, and D. J. Kemp. 1999. Phylogenetic evidence for reclassification of *Calymmatobacterium granulomatis* as *Klebsiella granulomatis* comb. nov. *Int. J. Syst. Bacteriol.* **49:**1695–1700.

15. Centers for Disease Control and Prevention. 2001. *An Atlas of Salmonella in the United States*. Centers for Disease Control and Prevention, Atlanta, Ga.

16. Centers for Disease Control and Prevention. 2001. Shigella *Surveillance: Annual Summary, 2000*. Centers for Disease Control and Prevention, Atlanta, Ga.

17. Collier, L., A. Balows, and M. Sussman (ed.). 1998. *Topley and Wilson's Microbiology and Microbial Infections*, 9th ed., vol. 2 and 3. Edward Arnold, London, England.

18. Crosa, J. H., D. J. Brenner, W. H. Ewing, and S. Falkow. 1973. Molecular relationships among the salmonelleae. *J. Bacteriol.* **115:**307–315.

19. Dickey, R. S., and C. H. Zumoff. 1988. Emended description of *Enterobacter cancerogenus* comb. nov. (formerly *Erwinia cancerogena*). *Int. J. Syst. Bacteriol.* **38:**371–374.

20. Diekema, D. J., M. A. Pfaller, R. N. Jones, G. V. Doern, P. L. Winokur, A. C. Gales, H. S. Sader, K. Kugler, and M. Beach. 1999. Survey of bloodstream infections due to gram-negative bacilli: frequency of occurrence and antimicrobial susceptibility of isolates collected in the United States, Canada, and Latin America for the SENTRY antimicrobial surveillance program, 1997. *Clin. Infect. Dis.* **29:**595–607.

21. Drancourt, M., C. Bollet, A. Carta, and P. Rousselier. 2001. Phylogenetic analysis of *Klebsiella* species delineate *Klebsiella* and *Raoultella* gen. nov. with description of *Raoultella ornithinolytica* comb. nov., *Raoultella terrigena* comb. nov. and *Raoultella planticola* comb. nov. *Int. J. Syst. Evol. Microbiol.* **51:**925–932.

22. DuPont, H. L., S. B. Formal, R. B. Hornick, M. J. Snyder, J. P. Libonati, D. G. Sheahan, E. H. LaBrec, and J. P. Kalas. 1971. Pathogenesis of *Escherichia coli* diarrhea. *N. Engl. J. Med.* **285:**1–9.

23. Edmond, M. B., S. E. Wallace, D. K. McClish, M. A. Pfaller, R. N. Jones, and R. P. Wenzel. 1999. Nosocomial bloodstream infections in United States hospitals: a three-year analysis. *Clin. Infect. Dis.* **29:**239–244.

24. Euzeby, J. P. 1999. Revised *Salmonella* nomenclature: designation of *Salmonella enterica* (ex Kauffmann and Edwards) Le Minor and Popoff 1987 sp. nov., nom. rev. as the neotype species of the genus *Salmonella* Lignieres 1900 (Approved Lists 1980), rejection of the name *Salmonella choleraesuis* (Smith 1894) Weldin 1927 (Approved Lists 1980), and conservation of the name *Salmonella typhi* (Schroeter 1886) Warren and Scott 1930 (Approved Lists 1980). Request for an opinion. *J. Syst. Bacteriol.* **49:**927–930.

25. Ewing, W. H. 1986. *Edwards and Ewing's Identification of Enterobacteriaceae*, 4th ed. Elsevier Science Publishing Co., New York, N.Y.

26. Ezaki, T., M. Amano, Y. Kawamura and E. Yabuuchi. 2000. Proposal of *Salmonella paratyphi* sp. nov., nom. rev. and request for an opinion to conserve the epithet *paratyphi* in the binary combination *Salmonella paratyphi* as *nomen epitheton conservandum*. *Int. J. Syst. Evol. Microbiol.* **50:**941–944.

27. Ezaki, T., Y. Kawamura and E. Yabuuchi. 2000. Recognition of the nomenclatural standing of *Salmonella typhi* (Approved Lists 1980), *Salmonella enteritidis* (Approved Lists 1980) and *Salmonella typhimurium* (Approved Lists 1980), and conservation of the specific epithets *enteritidis* and *typhimurium*. Request for an opinion. *Int. J. Syst. Evol. Microbiol.* **50:**945–947.

28. Farmer, J. J., III, M. A. Asbury, F. W. Hickman, D. J. Brenner, and The *Enterobacteriaceae* Study Group. 1980. *Enterobacter sakazakii*: a new species of "*Enterobacteriaceae*" isolated from clinical specimens. *Int. J. Syst. Bacteriol.* **30:**569–584.

29. Farmer, J. J., III, and B. R. Davis. 1985. H7 antiserum-sorbitol fermentation medium: a single tube screening medium for detecting *Escherichia coli* O157:H7 associated with hemorrhagic colitis. *J. Clin. Microbiol.* **22:**620–625. (*Note:* This paper has a misprint in the formula for MacConkey sorbitol agar. The paper says to use 22.2 g of MacConkey agar base; the correct amount is 40 g, which is given in the instructions on the bottle.)

30. Farmer, J. J., III, B. R. Davis, F. W. Hickman-Brenner, A. McWhorter, G. P. Huntley-Carter, M. A. Asbury, C. Riddle, H. G. Wathen, C. Elias, G. R. Fanning, A. G. Steigerwalt, C. M. O'Hara, G. K. Morris, P. B. Smith, and D. J. Brenner. 1985. Biochemical identification of new species and biogroups of *Enterobacteriaceae* isolated from clinical specimens. *J. Clin. Microbiol.* **21:**46–76.

31. Farmer, J. J., III, J. H. Jorgensen, P. A. D. Grimont, R. J. Akhurst, G. O. Poinar, Jr., E. Ageron, G. V. Pierce, J. A. Smith, G. P. Carter, K. L. Wilson, and F. W. Hickman-Brenner. 1989. *Xenorhabdus luminescens* (DNA hybridization group 5) from human clinical specimens. *J. Clin. Microbiol.* **27:**1594–1600.

32. Farmer, J. J., III, A. C. McWhorter, D. J. Brenner, and G. K. Morris. 1984. The *Salmonella-Arizona* group of *Enterobacteriaceae*: nomenclature, classification and reporting. *Clin. Microbiol. Newsl.* **6:**63–66.

33. Farmer, J. J., III, J. G. Wells, P. M. Griffin, and I. K. Wachsmuth. 1987. *Enterobacteriaceae* infections, p. 233–296. *In* B. B. Wentworth (ed.), *Diagnostic Procedures for Bacterial Infections*, 7th ed. American Public Health Association, Washington, D.C.

34. Fischer-Le Saux, M., V. Viallard, B. Brunel, P. Normand, and N. Boemare. 1999. Polyphasic classification of the genus *Photorhabdus* and proposal of new taxa: *P. luminescens* subsp. *luminescens* subsp. nov., *P. luminescens* subsp. *akhurstii* subsp. nov., *P. luminescens* subsp. *laumondii* subsp. nov., *P. temperata* sp. nov., and *P. asymbiotica* sp. nov. *Int. J. Syst. Bacteriol.* **49:**1645–1656.

35. Gavini, F., J. Mergaert, A. Beji, C. Mielcarek, D. Izard, K. Kersters, and J. De Ley. 1989. Transfer of *Enterobacter agglomerans* (Beijerinck 1888) Ewing and Fife 1972 to *Pantoea* gen. nov. as *Pantoea agglomerans* comb. nov. and description of *Pantoea dispersa* sp. nov. *Int. J. Syst. Bacteriol.* **39:**337–345.

36. Grimont, P. A. D., and E. Ageron. 1989. *Enterobacter cancerogenus* (Urosevic, 1966) Dickey and Zumoff 1988, a senior subjective synonym of *Enterobacter taylorae* Farmer et al. (1985). *Res. Microbiol.* **140:**459–465.

37. Hickman, F. W., and J. J. Farmer III. 1978. *Salmonella typhi*: identification, antibiograms, serology, and bacteriophage typing. *Am. J. Med. Technol.* **44:**1149–1159.

38. Inoue, K., K. Sugiyama, Y. Kosako, R. Sakazaki, and S. Yamai. 2000. *Enterobacter cowanii* sp. nov., a new species of the family *Enterobacteriaceae*. *Curr. Microbiol.* **41:**417–420.

39. Janda, J. M., and S. L. Abbott. 1998. *The Enterobacteria*. Lippincott-Raven, Philadelphia, Pa.

40. Judicial Commission of the International Committee on Systematic Bacteriology. 1993. Rejection of the name *Citrobacter diversus* Werkman and Gillen. *Int. J. Syst. Bacteriol.* **43:**392.

41. Kandolo, K., and G. Wauters. 1985. Pyrazinamidase activity in *Yersinia enterocolitica* and related organisms. *J. Clin. Microbiol.* **21:**980–982.

42. **Karmali, M. A.** 1989. Infection by verocytotoxin-producing *Escherichia coli. Clin. Microbiol. Rev.* **2:**15–38.

43. **Kosako, Y., K. Tamura, R. Sakazaki, and K. Miki.** 1996. *Enterobacter kobei* sp. nov., a new species of *Enterobacteriaceae* resembling *Enterobacter cloacae. Curr. Microbiol.* **33:** 261–265.

44. **Krieg, N. R., and J. G. Holt (ed.).** 1984. *Bergey's Manual of Systematic Bacteriology,* vol. 1, p. 408–516. The Williams & Wilkins Co., Baltimore, Md.

45. **Lannigan, R., and Z. Hussian.** 1993. Wound isolate of *Salmonella typhimurium* that became chlorate resistant after exposure to Dakin's solution: concomitant loss of hydrogen sulfide production, gas production, and nitrate reduction. *J. Clin. Microbiol.* **31:**2497–2498.

46. **Li, K., J. J. Farmer III, and A. Coppola.** 1974. A novel type of resistant bacteria induced by gentamicin. *Trans. N. Y. Acad. Sci.* **36:**369–396.

47. **McWhorter-Murlin, A. C., and F. W. Hickman-Brenner.** 1994. *Identification and Serotyping of* Salmonella *and an Update of the Kauffmann-White Scheme; Appendix A, Kauffmann-White Scheme, Alphabetical List of* Salmonella *Serotypes* (updated 1994); *Appendix B, Kauffmann-White Scheme, List of* Salmonella *Serotypes by O Group* (updated 1994). Foodborne and Diarrheal Diseases Laboratory Section, Centers for Disease Control and Prevention, Atlanta, Ga.

48. **Müller, H. E., D. J. Brenner, G. R. Fanning, P. A. D. Grimont, and P. Kämpfer.** 1996. Emended description of *Buttiauxella agrestis* with recognition of six new species of *Buttiauxella* and two new species of *Kluyvera: Buttiauxella ferragutiae* sp. nov., *Buttiauxella gaginiae* sp. nov., *Buttiauxella brennerae* sp. nov., *Buttiauxella izardii* sp. nov., *Buttiauxella noackiae* sp. nov., *Buttiauxella warmboldiae* sp. nov., *Kluyvera cochleae* sp. nov., and *Kluyvera georgiana* sp. nov. *Int. J. Syst. Bacteriol.* **46:**50–63.

49. **O'Hara, C. M., F. W. Brenner, A. G. Steigerwalt, B. C. Hill, B. Holmes, P. A. D. Grimont, P. M. Hawkey, J. L. Penner, J. M. Miller, and D. J. Brenner.** 2000. Classification of *Proteus vulgaris* biogroup 3 with recognition of *Proteus hauseri* sp. non., nom. rev. and unnamed *Proteus* genomospecies 4, 5 and 6. *Int. J. Syst. Evol. Microbiol.* **50:**1869–1875.

50. **Peel, M. M., D. A. Alfredson, J. G. Gerrard, J. M. Davis, J. M. Robson, R. J. McDougall, B. L. Scullie, and R. J. Akhurst.** 1999. Isolation, identification, and molecular characterization of strains of *Photorhabdus luminescens* from infected humans in Australia. *J. Clin. Microbiol.* **37:**3647–3653.

51. **Popoff, M. Y.** 2001. *Antigenic Formulas of the* Salmonella *Serovars,* 8th ed. WHO Collaborating Centre for Reference and Research on *Salmonella,* Institut Pasteur, Paris, France.

52. **Popoff, M. Y.** 2001. *Guidelines for the Preparation of* Salmonella *Antisera.* WHO Collaborating Centre for Reference and Research on *Salmonella,* Institut Pasteur, Paris, France.

53. **Reeves, M. W., G. M. Evins, A. A. Heiba, B. D. Plikaytis, and J. J. Farmer III.** 1989. Clonal nature of *Salmonella typhi* and its genetic relatedness to other salmonellae as shown by multilocus enzyme electrophoresis, and proposal of *Salmonella bongori* comb. nov. *J. Clin. Microbiol.* **27:** 313–320.

54. **Riley, G., and S. Toma.** 1989. Detection of pathogenic *Yersinia enterocolitica* by using Congo red-magnesium oxalate agar medium. *J. Clin. Microbiol.* **27:**213–214.

55. **Savola, K. L., E. J. Baron, L. S. Tompkins, and D. J. Passaro.** 2001. Fecal leukocyte stain has diagnostic value for outpatients but not inpatients. *J. Clin. Microbiol.* **39:** 266–269.

56. **Schaberg, D. R.** 1991. Major trends in the microbial etiology of nosocomial infections. *Ann. Intern. Med.* **91**(Suppl. 3B)**:**72S–75S.

57. **Sprierings, G., C. Ockhuijsen, H. Hofstra, and J. Tommassen.** 1993. Polymerase chain reaction for the specific detection of *Escherichia coli/Shigella. Res. Microbiol.* **144:** 557–564.

58. **Wadstrom, T., A. Aust-Kettis, D. Habte, J. Holmgren, G. Meeuwisse, R. Mollby, and O. Soderlind.** 1976. Enterotoxin-producing bacteria and parasites in stool of Ethiopian children with diarrhoeal disease. *Arch. Dis. Child.* **51:**865–870.

59. **Warren, J. R., J. J. Farmer III, F. E. Dewhirst, K. Birkhead, T. Zembower, L. R. Peterson, L. Sims, and M. Bhattacharya.** 2000. Outbreak of nosocomial infections due to extended-spectrum β-lactamase-producing strains of Enteric Group 137, a new member of the family *Enterobacteriaceae* closely related to *Citrobacter farmeri* and *Citrobacter amalonaticus. J. Clin. Microbiol.* **38:**3946–3952.

60. **Wells, J. G., B. R. Davis, I. K. Wachsmuth, L. W. Riley, R. S. Remis, R. Sokolow, and G. K. Morris.** 1983. Laboratory investigation of hemorrhagic colitis outbreaks associated with a rare *Escherichia coli* serotype. *J. Clin. Microbiol.* **18:**512–520.

Escherichia, Shigella, and Salmonella

CHERYL A. BOPP, FRANCES W. BRENNER, PATRICIA I. FIELDS,
JOY G. WELLS, AND NANCY A. STROCKBINE

42

TAXONOMY

Escherichia, *Shigella*, and *Salmonella* are classified in the family *Enterobacteriaceae*, which is addressed in chapter 41 of this Manual (42). Species in these three genera are gram-negative rods that grow well on MacConkey agar. When these organisms are motile, the motility is by peritrichous flagella; however, all strains of *Shigella* and some strains of *Escherichia* and *Salmonella* are nonmotile. All ferment D-glucose; *Escherichia* and *Salmonella* strains usually produce gas. *Shigella* is phenotypically similar to *Escherichia coli* and, with the exception of *Shigella boydii* serotype 13, would be considered the same species by DNA-DNA hybridization analysis (17).

NATURAL HABITATS

Escherichia, *Shigella*, and *Salmonella* are isolated most frequently from the intestines of humans and animals. Because *E. coli* is ubiquitous in human and animal feces, the presence of this species in water is considered to be an indicator of fecal contamination. Some species or serotypes are isolated only from humans (e.g., *Salmonella* serotype Typhi and *Shigella dysenteriae* serotype 1), while others (e.g., *Salmonella* serotypes Gallinarum and Marina) are strongly associated with certain animal hosts. These genera can be isolated from fecally contaminated foods or water but probably do not occur as free-living organisms in the environment. *Salmonella* strains can, however, survive for long periods, perhaps years, in the environment (61).

COLLECTION, TRANSPORT, AND STORAGE OF FECAL SPECIMENS

Information on the collection, transport, and storage of specimens from extraintestinal sites is provided in chapter 20.

Fecal specimens can include whole stools, swabs prepared from whole stools, or rectal swabs with visible fecal staining. Ideally, stool specimens should be examined as soon as they are received in the laboratory. If whole-stool specimens are not processed immediately, they should be either refrigerated or frozen at −70°C as soon as possible after collection. All fecal specimens that cannot be examined within 1 to 2 h and all rectal swabs should be immediately placed in transport medium and refrigerated. The swab should be completely covered by the transport medium to keep it sufficiently moist for optimal recovery of the organisms. If specimens in transport medium are not examined within 3 days, they should be frozen immediately, preferably at −70°C.

Many of the commercially available transport media (e.g., Cary-Blair, Stuart's, and Amies transport media) are satisfactory for these organisms. Although acceptable for the transport of *E. coli*, *Salmonella*, and *Shigella*, buffered glycerol saline should not be used for specimens that must also be tested for *Campylobacter* and *Vibrio*.

ESCHERICHIA

Description of the Genus

The genus *Escherichia* is composed of motile or nonmotile bacteria that conform to the definitions of the family *Enterobacteriaceae* (42). There are five species in this genus: *Escherichia blattae*, *E. coli*, *E. fergusonii*, *E. hermannii*, and *E. vulneris*. The type species is *E. coli*. Biochemical reactions typical of each *Escherichia* species are listed in chapter 41.

Clinical Significance

Of the five *Escherichia* species, *E. coli* is the species usually isolated from human specimens. It is part of the bowel flora of healthy individuals; however, certain strains may cause extraintestinal and intestinal infections in immunocompromised as well as healthy individuals. Urinary tract infections, bacteremia, meningitis, and diarrheal disease are the most frequent clinical syndromes and are caused primarily by a limited number of pathogenic clones of *E. coli*. *E. hermannii* and *E. vulneris* are most often obtained from wound infections but have also been isolated from infections at other body sites, while *E. fergusonii* is most frequently identified from human feces (9). *E. blattae*, which is a commensal organism of cockroaches, is not recovered from human specimens.

Diarrheagenic *E. coli*

There are at least four categories of recognized diarrheagenic *E. coli*: Shiga toxin-producing *E. coli* (STEC) (also referred to as enterohemorrhagic *E. coli* [EHEC]), enterotoxigenic *E. coli* (ETEC), enteropathogenic *E. coli* (EPEC), and enteroinvasive *E. coli* (EIEC) (Table 1) (79). The clinical significance of several other groups of putative diarrheagenic *E. coli,* including enteroaggregative *E. coli* (EaggEC), is unclear.

STEC: O157 and Other STEC Serogroups

We refer to the STEC category of diarrheagenic *E. coli* according to the toxins that these organisms produce, e.g., STEC rather than EHEC, because the essential genetic features that define organisms capable of causing hemorrhagic colitis and hemolytic-uremic syndrome (HUS) are not clear. *E. coli* serotypes O157:H7 and O157:nonmotile (NM) (O157 STEC) produce one or more Shiga toxins, also called verocytotoxins, and are the most frequently identified diarrheagenic *E. coli* serotypes in North America and Europe. Each year an estimated 73,000 cases of illness and 60 deaths are caused by O157 STEC in the United States (74).

E. coli O157:H7 and other STEC serotypes cause illness that can present as mild nonbloody diarrhea, severe bloody diarrhea (hemorrhagic colitis), and HUS (47). Additional symptoms of *E. coli* O157:H7 infection include abdominal cramps and lack of a high fever. Of patients with O157 STEC diarrhea, approximately 8% develop HUS, a condition characterized by microangiopathic hemolytic anemia, thrombocytopenia, and acute renal failure.

O157 STEC is thought to cause at least 80% of cases of HUS in North America and is recognized as a common cause of bloody diarrhea in developed countries (47). In the United States, the rates of isolation of O157 STEC from fecal specimens exceed the rates of isolation of other common enteric pathogens, particularly *Shigella,* in some geographic areas and some age groups (101). Many U.S. clin-

ical laboratories do not routinely culture stools for O157 STEC; as a result, many illnesses are not detected (15, 29).

O157 STEC colonizes dairy and beef cattle; not surprisingly, ground beef has caused more O157 STEC outbreaks than any other vehicle of transmission (47). Other known vehicles of transmission include raw milk, sausage, roast beef, unchlorinated municipal water, apple cider, raw vegetables, and sprouts (alfalfa and radish). O157 STEC spreads easily from person to person because the infectious dose is low; outbreaks associated with person-to-person spread have occurred in schools, long-term care institutions, families, and day care facilities (8).

More than 150 non-O157 STEC serotypes have been isolated from persons with diarrhea or HUS (http://www.microbionet.com.au/frames/feature/vtec/brief01.html). In some countries, non-O157 STEC strains, particularly *E. coli* serotypes O111:NM and O26:H11, are more commonly isolated than O157 STEC, although most outbreaks and cases of HUS are attributed to O157 STEC (Table 1) (25, 47, 49, 54, 73, 78, 85, 86, 107). In the United States, *E. coli* O157:H7 is the most frequently isolated STEC but increasingly non-O157 STEC are identified as causes of outbreaks and sporadic illness (26, 72, 107). At the Centers for Disease Control and Prevention (CDC) *E. coli* Reference Laboratory, 72% of all non-O157 STEC isolates received between 1983 and 2000 belonged to eight serogroups (O26, O111, O103, O121, O45, O145, O165, and O113) (N. A. Strockbine, unpublished data). Because most laboratory methods for the detection of O157 STEC do not detect non-O157 STEC, the numbers of documented infections with serotypes other than O157:H7 or O157:NM are probably underestimated.

ETEC

ETEC, which produces heat-labile *E. coli* enterotoxin (LT), heat-stable *E. coli* enterotoxin (ST), or both LT and ST, is an important cause of diarrhea in developing countries, particularly among young children (79). ETEC also is a frequent cause of traveler's diarrhea. Ten U.S. outbreaks were reported to the Centers for Disease Control and Prevention (CDC) from 1995 to 2001, while only 15 outbreaks occurred during the preceding 25 years (37; C. A. Bopp, unpublished data). ETEC is infrequently identified in the United States, but this is attributable, at least in part, to the fact that few laboratories are capable of identifying this pathogen. ETEC strains, particularly those associated with outbreaks, tend to cluster in a few serotypes (Table 1).

The most prominent symptoms of ETEC illness are diarrhea and abdominal cramps, sometimes accompanied by nausea and headache but usually with little vomiting or fever (37). Although ETEC is usually associated with relatively mild watery diarrhea, illness in recent ETEC outbreaks has been notable for its prolonged duration.

EPEC

In the past, EPEC strains were defined as certain *E. coli* serotypes that were epidemiologically associated with infantile diarrhea but did not produce enterotoxins or Shiga toxins and were not invasive. The traditional EPEC serotypes are listed in Table 1; typically these serotypes show a distinct pattern of localized adherence to HeLa and HEp-2 cells. These serotypes usually also demonstrate actin aggregation in the fluorescent actin stain test, which correlates with the attaching-and-effacing lesion in vivo (79). Because of the lack of simple diagnostic methods for EPEC, few laboratories attempt to identify these organisms.

TABLE 1 Frequently encountered serotypes of diarrheagenic *E. coli*[a]

ETEC	EPEC	EIEC	STEC	
O6:NM	**O55:NM**	O28:NM	O1:NM	**O111:H8**
O6:H16	**O55:H6**	O29:NM	O2:H6	**O113:H21**
O8:H9	O55:H7	O112:NM	O2:H7	**O118:H2**
O15:H11	O86:NM	O124:NM	O5:NM	O118:H12
O20:NM	O86:H34	O124:H7	O9:NM	O118:H16
O25:NM	**O111:NM**	**O124:H30**	O14:NM	**O121:H19**
O25:H42	**O111:H2**	O136:NM	O22:H5	O128:NM
O27:NM	O111:H12	**O143:NM**	O22:H8	O128:H2
O27:H7	O111:H21	O144:NM	O26:NM	O128:H45
O27:H20	**O114:NM**	O152:NM	**O26:H11**	O137:H41
O49:NM	**O114:H2**	**O164:NM**	O45:H2	**O145:NM**
O63:H12	O119:H6	O167:NM	O48:H21	O153:H2
O78:H11	**O125:H21**	ONT:NM	O50:H7	O153:H25
O78:H12	O126:NM		O55:H7	**O157:NM**
O128:H7	O126:H27		O79:H7	**O157:H7**
O148:H28	**O127:NM**		O83:H1	O163:H19
O153:H45	**O127:H6**		O91:NM	O165:NM
O159:NM	O127:H9		O91:H10	O165:H25
O159:H4	O127:H21		O91:H21	O172:NM
O159:H20	**O128:H2**		O103:H2	Orough:H9
O167:H5	0128:H12		O104:NM	ONT:NM
O169:H41	O142:H6		**O104:H21**	
	O157:H45		**O111:NM**	
			O111:H2	

[a] Outbreak-associated serotypes are shown in bold type. NM, nonmotile; NT, not typeable; Orough, O antigen rough and serotype not determined.

The incidence of EPEC-associated nursery outbreaks has declined in developed countries since the 1960s, but in the past 20 years there have been several outbreaks in day care centers and nurseries in the United States (79). EPEC infections are rare in developed countries but are a recognized cause of infantile diarrhea in the developing world.

The symptoms of severe, prolonged, and nonbloody diarrhea, vomiting, and fever in infants or young toddlers are characteristic of EPEC illness (79). Infection with EPEC has been associated with chronic diarrhea; sequelae may include malabsorption, malnutrition, weight loss, and growth retardation.

EIEC

EIEC strains invade cells of the colon and produce a generally watery but occasionally bloody diarrhea by a pathogenic mechanism similar to that of *Shigella*. EIEC is very rare in the United States and is less common than ETEC or EPEC in the developing world (79). EIEC strains, like ETEC and EPEC strains, are associated with only a few characteristic serotypes (Table 1). Three large outbreaks of diarrhea caused by EIEC have been reported in the United States (79).

Putative Diarrheagenic *E. coli*

EAggEC, which exhibits a specific pattern of aggregative adherence to HEp-2 cells in culture, has been associated with diarrhea in children in Chile, persistent diarrhea in children in Mexico and Kenya, and bloody diarrhea in children in India (79). These organisms may also have a role in chronic diarrhea among human immunodeficiency virus-infected patients (88). EAggEC was isolated from children with diarrhea during an outbreak in Japan (53).

Diffusely adherent *E. coli* (DAEC) strains, which exhibit a diffuse pattern of adherence to HEp-2 cells, have been implicated as causes of diarrhea in some studies but not others (79). Little is known about their associated clinical syndrome, epidemiology, and pathogenic mechanisms. In a retrospective case-control study, the majority of children infected with DAEC strains had watery diarrhea without blood or fecal leukocytes (87). In one study, DAEC infections were significantly associated with diarrhea in children 1 to 5 years of age but were not associated with illness in infants (64).

Cytotoxic necrotizing factor (CNF)-producing *E. coli* strains produce a toxin that induces morphological alterations (multinucleation) and death in tissue cultures (24). Two forms have been described: CNF1 and CNF2. CNF1-producing strains were originally detected in infants with enteritis and were later detected in humans with extraintestinal infections (13, 23). Most CNF1-producing strains are also hemolytic, although the toxin is distinct from hemolysin (23). CNF2-producing strains have been isolated from animals with diarrhea (38, 83, 103). The role of these strains in human diarrheal disease has not been definitively determined (79).

Cytolethal distending toxin (CLDT)-producing *E. coli* strains produce a heat-labile factor that induces cytotonic and cytotoxic changes in Chinese hamster ovary cells similar to those caused by LT (55). This factor does not affect Y-1 cells. The results of one study in Bangladesh suggested that CLDT-producing *E. coli* strains are not associated with diarrhea, but other studies are needed to establish their status as etiologic agents (4).

Isolation Procedures

Isolation procedures for extraintestinal infections are covered in chapter 20.

Isolation Procedures for STEC

All stools submitted for culture of bacterial enteric pathogens should also be examined for O157 STEC (5, 48, 108). Culture for non-O157 STEC is indicated for patients with HUS, bloody diarrhea, or a history of bloody diarrhea (48, 108) and should be considered for other patients with diarrhea. Criteria that have been proposed for screening stools for non-O157 STEC include severity of illness, age, and epidemiologic or exposure information (57, 96).

Because there is no selective isolation medium for non-O157 STEC, testing for Shiga toxin in the stool is the best option for the laboratory to detect these organisms. Commercial enzyme-linked immunosorbent assays are a sensitive means of detecting Shiga toxin (40, 70). Isolation and serotyping of STEC from fecal specimens that are positive by EIA should always be attempted because serotype information is important for public health purposes and may also help in clinical decisions.

Enrichment

Although broth enrichment is widely used for the recovery of O157 STEC from foods, there is little evidence that it enhances isolation from human fecal specimens. However, immunomagnetic separation, a technique shown to increase the rate of isolation of O157 STEC from food specimens, has been adapted to culture of stools. Immunomagnetic separation enhances the detection of O157 STEC from patients with HUS, patients presenting a long time after the onset of illness, asymptomatic carriers, or specimens that have been stored or transported improperly (32, 36, 56). IMS beads for O157, O111, and O26 are available commercially (Table 2), or laboratories may produce beads with other O-specific antibodies (85).

Plating Media

Because O157 STEC strains ferment lactose, they are impossible to differentiate from other lactose-fermenting organisms on lactose-containing media. Most O157 STEC strains do not ferment the carbohydrate D-sorbitol overnight, in contrast to the approximately 80% of other *E. coli* strains that ferment sorbitol rapidly. Thus, sorbitol-containing MacConkey agar (SMAC) is used for isolation of O157 STEC. Sorbitol-nonfermenting colonies are suspect (71). In some areas of central Europe, sorbitol-fermenting O157 STEC strains are commonly isolated from patients with HUS (12); these organisms are very rare in North America (W. M. Johnson, personal communication; N. A. Strockbine, unpublished data).

Cefixime-tellurite SMAC is mostly used for culture of animal and food specimens because of its selectivity, but it also is used for culture of human specimens (32, 121). It has been reported that a few O157:NM strains fail to grow on cefixime-tellurite SMAC (56).

Commercial Rapid Diagnostic Methods

A number of commercial immunoassays are now available for testing for Shiga toxin or O157 lipopolysaccharide and other O antigens in stools, enrichment broths of stool specimens, colony sweeps, or individual colonies (Table 2). Isolation of STEC from fecal specimens that are positive by one of these rapid diagnostic methods is important for

TABLE 2 Partial listing of commercial suppliers of reagents for detection of STEC[a]

Antisera for tube agglutination
    Difco Laboratories (Division of Becton Dickinson and Co., Sparks, Md.)
        O157 and H7 antisera
    SA Scientific, San Antonio, Tex.
        O157 and H7 antisera
    Denka Seiken Co., Ltd., Tokyo, Japan
        O157, H7, O145, O128, O111, O103, O91, O26, and other *E. coli* O antisera
Latex slide agglutination reagents
    Denka Seiken Co., Ltd., Tokyo, Japan
        O157, O111, and O26 reagents
    Murex Biotech Ltd., Dartford, United Kingdom
        O157 and H7 reagents
    Oxoid Inc., Ogdensburg, N.Y.
        O157, O145, O128, O111, O103, O91, O26 reagents
    ProLab Diagnostics, Inc., Ontario, Canada
        O157 and H7 reagents
    Remel, Lenexa, Kans.
        O157 and H7 reagents
Immunomagnetic beads
    Dynal Biotech Inc., Lake Success, N.Y.
        Anti-O157 labeled beads
    Denka Seiken Co., Ltd., Tokyo, Japan
        Anti-O157, anti-O111, and anti-O26 labeled beads
O157 Immunoassays
    Meridian Diagnostics Inc., Cincinnati, Ohio
        For testing stool specimens or enrichment broths for O157 antigen
    Denka Seiken Co., Ltd., Tokyo, Japan
        For testing colony sweeps or individual colonies for O157, O111, or O26 antigens
Shiga toxin immunoassays
    Meridian Diagnostics Inc., Cincinnati, Ohio
        For testing stool specimens, enrichment broths, colony sweeps, or individual colonies for Shiga toxin
    Alexon-Trend, Ramsey, Minn.
        For testing stool specimens or enrichment broths for Shiga toxin
    Denka Seiken Co., Ltd., Tokyo, Japan
        For testing colony sweeps or individual colonies for Shiga toxin
    Oxoid Inc., Ogdensburg, N.Y.
        For testing individual colonies for Shiga toxin

[a] Not intended to be a comprehensive listing. The U.S. Food and Drug Administration has not approved all of these reagents for use with clinical specimens. This table does not include reagents or tests specifically intended for examination of food, water, or environmental specimens. The online version of the Bacteriological Analytical Manual lists many tests for food specimens (www.fda.gov). Inclusion does not constitute endorsement by CDC.

public health purposes. Determination of the subtype of O157 STEC and the serotype of a non-O157 STEC isolate is valuable for outbreak investigations and surveillance purposes (see "Subtyping" and "Identification" below).

Screening Procedures for STEC Strains

For the isolation of O157 STEC from SMAC, colorless (nonfermenting) colonies are tested with O157 antiserum or latex reagent (Table 2) (104). If the O157 latex reagent is used, it is important to test positive colonies with the latex control reagent to rule out nonspecific reactions. The

manufacturers of these kits recommend that strains reacting with both the antigen-specific and control latex reagents be heated and retested. However, in a study that followed this procedure, none of the nonspecifically reacting strains were subsequently identified as O157 STEC (14).

The MUG reaction (4-methylumbelliferyl-beta-D-glucuronide for detection of beta-glucuronidase activity), used in conjunction with sorbitol fermentation and O157 antiserum, is helpful for screening for these strains from human specimens (98). MUG-positive, urease-positive O157 STEC strains have been isolated in the United States but are still rare (50) (Strockbine, unpublished).

For the recovery of STEC from stool specimens which test positive for Shiga toxin, either SMAC or MacConkey agar should be inoculated. It is advantageous to use SMAC because O157 STEC can be quickly and easily identified. If sorbitol-nonfermenting colonies are negative with O157 latex, then sorbitol-fermenting colonies (because most non-O157 STEC strains ferment sorbitol) and a representative sample of sorbitol-nonfermenting colonies may be selected for Shiga toxin testing. Latex reagents and antisera for detecting certain non-O157 STEC serotypes are now available (Table 2) and could also be used to test colonies from Shiga toxin-positive specimens or to serogroup Shiga toxin-positive isolates.

Virtually all O157 STEC and 60 to 80% of non-O157 STEC produce a characteristic *E. coli* hemolysin, referred to as enterohemolysin (Ehly), which is distinct from the alpha-hemolysin produced by other *E. coli* strains (11). A special medium, washed sheep blood agar supplemented with calcium (WSBA-Ca), is used as a differential medium for the detection of enterohemolytic activity (11). Ehly-producing colonies can be differentiated from alpha-hemolysin-producing colonies on WSBA-Ca because the latter are visible after 3 to 4 h of incubation. After 3 to 4 h, colonies are marked for the appearance of alpha-hemolysin and the plates are examined again after 18 to 24 h. Incorporation of mitomycin C into the WSBA-Ca enhances the appearance of the Ehly hemolysis and increases the proportion of non-O157 STEC strains that exhibit this activity (109). Because many non-O157 STEC strains do not demonstrate the enterohemolytic phenotype and because enterohemolytic nontoxigenic strains have been reported, additional screening methods should be used in conjunction with WSBA-Ca medium (10, 97).

Presumptive STEC isolates should be sent to a reference laboratory or a public health laboratory for further characterization.

Isolation Methods for ETEC, EPEC, EIEC, and the Putative Diarrheagenic *E. coli*

Methods for the identification of ETEC, EPEC, EIEC, and the putative diarrheagenic *E. coli* are generally available only in reference or research settings. Public health and reference laboratories usually examine specimens for these pathogens only when an outbreak has occurred and specimens are negative for routine bacterial pathogens. ETEC should be considered a possible etiologic agent of watery diarrhea for which no pathogen has been identified (37). EPEC should be considered a possible pathogen in outbreaks of severe nonbloody diarrhea in infants or young toddlers, particularly in nursery or day care settings. EIEC should be considered a possible etiologic agent in outbreaks of diarrhea, bloody or nonbloody, when other routine bacterial agents have been ruled out.

Fecal specimens should be plated on a differential medium of low selectivity (e.g., MAC). Between 5 and 20 colonies, mostly lactose fermenting but with a representative sample of nonfermenting colonies, should be selected and inoculated onto a nonselective agar slant. These colonies are then screened for virulence-associated characteristics appropriate to the pathogen being sought (see "Virulence Testing" below). Arrangements to send *E. coli* isolates from well-characterized outbreaks to CDC for testing can be made through local and state health departments.

Screening Procedures for ETEC, EPEC, and EIEC Strains

ETEC or EPEC strains cannot be distinguished from other *E. coli* strains by biochemical screening techniques. Many EIEC strains are nonmotile and fail to decarboxylate lysine; however, some EIEC strains are motile or lysine positive.

Use of commercial antisera to the classical EPEC somatic (O) and capsular (K) antigens yields many false-positive results. Further testing with H (flagellar) antisera would reduce the number of false-positive reports. However, this type of testing is not practical for the average clinical microbiology laboratory.

Identification

Biochemical Identification

Biochemical identification of presumptive O157 STEC isolates is necessary because other species may cross-react with O157 antiserum or latex reagents, including *Salmonella* O group N, *Yersinia enterocolitica* serotype O9, *Citrobacter freundii*, and *E. hermannii*. Special biochemical tests (cellobiose fermentation, growth in the presence of KCN) may be necessary to differentiate *E. hermannii* from *E. coli*, but because *E. hermannii* is rarely detected in stool specimens, use of these tests is not cost-effective for most laboratories.

Serotyping

The serologic classification of *E. coli* is generally based on the O antigen (somatic) and the H antigen (flagellar) (9). The O and H antigens of *E. coli* are stable and reliable strain characteristics, and although 175 O antigens and 53 H antigens are currently recognized, the actual number of serotype combinations associated with diarrheal disease is limited (Table 1). Determination of the O and H serotypes of *E. coli* strains implicated in diarrheal disease is particularly useful in epidemiologic investigations (Table 1). Even though antisera for the tube agglutination test are available from several manufacturers, most laboratories do not attempt complete *E. coli* serotyping because it is costly. For well-characterized outbreaks with no identified etiologic agent, arrangements may be made through state health departments to send *E. coli* isolates to CDC for virulence testing and serotyping.

Serologic Confirmation of O157 STEC

Confirmation of *E. coli* O157:H7 requires identification of the H7 flagellar antigen. H7-specific antisera and latex reagents are commercially available (Table 2), but detection of the H7 flagellar antigen often requires multiple passages (104). Isolates that are nonmotile or negative for the H7 antigen should be tested for the production of Shiga toxins or the presence of Shiga toxin gene sequences.

Approximately 85% of O157 isolates from humans received by CDC are serotype O157:H7, 12% are nonmotile, and 3% are H types other than H7 (Strockbine, unpublished). *E. coli* O157:NM strains frequently produce Shiga

toxin and are otherwise very similar to O157:H7, but no O157 strain from human illness with an H type other than H7 has been found to produce Shiga toxin (Strockbine, unpublished) (44, 113).

Virulence Testing

STEC (primarily non-O157 STEC), ETEC, EPEC, EIEC, and EAggEC (and other putative diarrheagenic *E. coli* strains) are identified by detection of their respective virulence-associated factors (characteristic toxins, adherence, or invasiveness). Techniques for virulence testing include bioassays (e.g., cell culture or in vivo testing), immunologic methods (e.g., immunoblotting or EIA), or the detection of gene sequences by DNA-based methods (e.g., PCR or colony blot hybridization). The laboratory's capability for performing the different types of assays will guide its selection of appropriate tests.

Most methods involve the screening of isolated colonies. If PCR techniques are used, a sweep of confluent growth from a MAC plate may be screened. If the PCR assay is positive, isolated colonies may then be picked and screened individually. This approach has worked well for some laboratories (J. Besser-Wiek, D. Boxrud, J. Bender, M. Sullivan, L. Carroll, and F. Leano, *Abstr. 96th Gen. Meet. Am. Soc. Microbiol. 1996*, abstr. C364, 1996; J. G. Wells, unpublished data).

STEC

Two distinct Shiga toxins, Stx1 and Stx2, also referred to as verocytotoxins, have been described. In addition, there are several variant forms of Stx2, including Stx2c, Stx2d, Stx2e, and Stx2f, which in one study were more frequently identified from asymptomatic carriers than from HUS patients (45). All of these toxins are similar to the Shiga toxin expressed by *S. dysenteriae* serotype 1, and the Stx1 toxins produced by O157 STEC and other STEC serotypes are virtually identical. STEC may produce either Stx1 or Stx2 or both toxins. The production of Stx or the genes encoding Stx can be detected by a variety of biological, immunologic, or nucleic acid-based assays (Table 2) (79). Protocols for several of these tests (e.g., cell culture, DNA probing, and PCR) are available (82, 102).

Many STEC strains possess other virulence-associated characteristics including the production of intimin, a 60-MDa EHEC plasmid that also plays a role in cell adherence, and Ehly production, which was discussed above (see "Screening Procedures for STEC Strains") (79).

ETEC

The enterotoxins produced by ETEC, ST and LT, have been purified and sequenced and may be detected by a variety of biological, immunologic, and nucleic acid-based assays (79). Two structurally distinct STs have been identified. Strains that produce ST only or ST in combination with LT have caused most ETEC outbreaks in the United States (37).

At least two commercial immunoassays are available for the identification of ETEC strains from culture supernatants. The ST EIA kit (Denka Seiken Co., Ltd.) is a competitive EIA for the detection of ST only (99, 105). A reversed passive latex agglutination assay (VET-RPLA; Oxoid, Ogdensburg, N.Y.) detects both cholera toxin and LT, which are highly related antigenically. The effectiveness of the VET-RPLA may be optimized by use of a culture medium designed for LT production, such as Biken's medium, rather than the medium recommended by the manufacturer (120).

EPEC

Laboratory identification of EPEC involves the identification of virulence-associated characteristics, particularly patterns of adherence to certain cells, by various methods including tissue culture, immunoassay, and DNA-based assays. No commercial kits are available for the detection of attachment-related virulence factors (e.g., intimin and the EPEC adherence factor [EAF], which is plasmid mediated) (79). An EIA has been described for the detection of EAF-positive *E. coli*, but the specific antibody is not commercially available.

To diagnose EPEC illness, a laboratory may find it convenient to set up an assay using either oligonucleotide probes or PCR primers that detect *eae* (intimin gene) or the EAF plasmid. Alternately, a laboratory with tissue culture facilities may set up cell culture adherence assays for the localized adherence pattern typically expressed by EPEC.

EIEC

EIEC can be identified by various in vivo assays, immunoassays, and nucleic acid-based assays for invasiveness, but no commercial kits or reagents are available. Cell culture invasion assays or DNA-based assays for the *ipaC* or *ipaH* invasion-related factors are, for the most part, practical only in research settings (79, 100). Plasmid DNA electrophoresis may be used to detect the large (120- to 140-MDa) plasmid associated with invasiveness, but this plasmid is easily lost when the isolate is subcultured. Because of shared invasiveness-related characteristics, these assays also detect *Shigella* strains.

Subtyping

Several methods of subtyping have been used for *E. coli* O157:H7 isolates. In particular, pulsed-field gel electrophoresis (PFGE) methods are useful (79). A national molecular subtyping network, PulseNet, was established in 1996 by CDC to facilitate the subtyping of bacterial foodborne pathogens, including *E. coli* O157:H7, *Shigella*, nontyphoidal *Salmonella* serotypes, and *Listeria monocytogenes* (110). Successful detection of outbreaks by this network of state and local public health laboratories is dependent on submission of isolates by clinical laboratories for confirmation and subtyping. Determination of the serotype and the antimicrobial susceptibility pattern is usually adequate for defining outbreak strains of ETEC, EPEC, and EIEC. Plasmid typing or PFGE methods may also be helpful for distinguishing between background isolates and outbreak strains, but neither method has been widely used for these *E. coli* groups.

Serodiagnostic Tests

At present, serodiagnostic tests for diarrheagenic *E. coli* are valuable only for seroepidemiology surveys and are not useful for the diagnosis of sporadic infections. Assays that measure antibody response to lipopolysaccharide have been used to detect STEC infection in culture-negative HUS patients (79).

Antimicrobial Susceptibilities

STEC

Antimicrobial therapy for O157 STEC diarrhea or HUS has not been demonstrated to be efficacious and safe (47). Consequently, the antimicrobial susceptibility pattern is usually determined only for epidemiologic studies. Until recently, *E. coli* O157:H7 isolates were almost uniformly sensitive to antimicrobial agents. However, since the early 1990s, O157 and other STEC strains have demonstrated slowly increasing levels of resistance to certain antibiotics, particularly streptomycin, sulfonamides, and tetracycline (101) (www.cdc.gov/narms/).

ETEC, EPEC, EIEC, and Other Diarrheagenic *E. coli* Strains

Treatment with an appropriate antibiotic can reduce the severity and duration of symptoms of ETEC infection (79). Antimicrobial resistance, particularly to tetracycline, is common among ETEC strains isolated from outbreaks in the United States (37). Antibiotic treatment may be helpful for diarrhea caused by EPEC (79). Most EPEC strains associated with outbreaks are resistant to multiple antimicrobial agents (39). Little information about the efficacy of antimicrobial treatment or the prevalence of resistance is available for EIEC or other putative diarrheagenic *E. coli* strains (e.g., EAggEC), but determination of the antimicrobial susceptibility pattern may be helpful in establishing whether isolates are associated with an outbreak.

Interpretation and Reporting of Results

STEC

A presumptive diagnosis of an O157 STEC (isolate positive for O157 antigen) or a non-O157 STEC (isolate positive for Shiga toxin) infection should be reported to the clinician as soon as the laboratory obtains this result. It would be advisable to indicate on the report that non-O157 STEC strains cause diarrhea and HUS. Clusters and outbreaks of STEC should be reported to public health authorities. Presumptive STEC isolates should be confirmed by demonstration of the O157 and H7 antigens or assay for Shiga toxin and should be identified biochemically as *E. coli*. STEC isolates should be forwarded to a local or state public health laboratory for serotyping and/or molecular subtyping.

ETEC, EPEC, and EIEC

Generally, the ETEC, EPEC, and EIEC classes of diarrheagenic *E. coli* are identified only during outbreak investigations. A laboratorian reporting these results, which usually will be a retrospective diagnosis obtained by a reference laboratory, should provide an explanation of the clinical significance of these organisms and should perhaps refer the clinician to the reference laboratory for further information. All suspected outbreaks should be reported to public health authorities.

SHIGELLA

Description of the Genus

The genus *Shigella* is composed of nonmotile bacteria that conform to the definition of the family *Enterobacteriaceae* (42). There are four subgroups of *Shigella* that historically have been treated as species: subgroup A as *Shigella dysenteriae*, subgroup B as *Shigella flexneri*, subgroup C as *Shigella boydii*, and subgroup D as *Shigella sonnei*. From a genetic standpoint, the four species of *Shigella* and *E. coli* represent a single genomospecies, with >75% nucleotide similarity by DNA-DNA reassociation studies (18, 19). Using a genetic definition for species, the four species of *Shigella* would be regarded as serologically defined anaerogenic biotypes of *E. coli*. The current nomenclature of *Shigella* is maintained largely for medical purposes because of the useful association of the genus epithet with the distinctive disease (shigellosis) caused by these organisms. The type species is S. dysenteriae. Shigella does not form gas from fermentable carbohydrates, with the exception of certain strains of S. flexneri serotype 6, S. boydii serotype 13, and S. boydii serotype 14. Compared with Escherichia, Shigella strains are less active in their use of carbohydrates. S. sonnei strains ferment lactose on extended incubation, but other species generally do not use this substrate in conventional medium.

Clinical Significance

Members of the genus Shigella have been recognized since the late 19th century as causative agents of bacillary dysentery (1). Shigella causes bloody diarrhea (dysentery) and nonbloody diarrhea. Shigellosis often begins with watery diarrhea accompanied by fever and abdominal cramps but may progress to classic dysentery with scant stools containing blood, mucus, and pus. Ulcerations, which are restricted to the large intestine and rectum, typically do not penetrate beyond the lamina propria. Bloodstream infections can occur but are rare. All four subgroups of Shigella are capable of causing dysentery, but S. dysenteriae serotype 1 has been associated with a particularly severe form of illness thought to be related to its production of Shiga toxin. Infection can also be asymptomatic, particularly infection with S. sonnei strains. Although these organisms are very important as causes of gastrointestinal infections, they rarely cause other types of infections. Complications of shigellosis include HUS, which is associated with S. dysenteriae 1 infection, and Reiter chronic arthritis syndrome, which is associated with S. flexneri infection (1). The identification of Shigella species is important for both clinical and epidemiologic purposes.

Humans and other large primates are the only natural reservoirs of Shigella bacteria. Most transmission is by person-to-person spread, but infection is also caused by ingestion of contaminated food or water. Shigellosis is most common in situations in which hygiene is limited (e.g., child care centers and other institutional settings). In populations without running water and indoor plumbing, shigellosis can become an endemic problem. Sexual transmission of Shigella among men who have sex with men also occurs.

In the United States, an estimated 450,000 cases of shigellosis occur each year, with 70 deaths (74). Up to 20% of all U.S. cases of shigellosis are related to international travel. Most infections in the United States and other developed countries are caused by S. sonnei; S. flexneri is the second most common serogroup.

In the developing world, the most prevalent Shigella species are S. flexneri and S. dysenteriae 1, with the latter being the most frequent cause of epidemic dysentery. Since 1979, a prolonged S. dysenteriae 1 epidemic has affected southern Africa, and major epidemics have also occurred in other parts of Africa, in Asia, and in Central America. Infection with S. dysenteriae 1 is associated with high rates of morbidity and mortality in developing countries, particularly when antimicrobial resistance or its misdiagnosis as amoebiasis makes appropriate treatment problematic.

Isolation Procedures

Enrichment and Plating Media

There is no reliably effective enrichment medium for all Shigella isolates, but gram-negative (GN) broth and Selenite broth are frequently used. For the optimal isolation of Shigella, two different selective media should be used: a general-purpose plating medium of low selectivity (e.g.,

MAC) and a more selective agar medium (e.g., xylose lysine desoxycholate agar [XLD]). Desoxycholate citrate agar (DCA) and Hektoen Enteric agar (HE) are suitable alternatives to XLD as media with moderate to high selectivities. Salmonella-shigella agar (SS) should be used with caution because it inhibits the growth of some strains of S. dysenteriae 1.

Screening Procedures

Shigella strains appear as lactose- or xylose-nonfermenting colonies on the isolation media described above. S. dysenteriae 1 colonies may be smaller on all of these media, and these strains generally grow best on media with low selectivities (e.g., MAC). S. dysenteriae 1 colonies on XLD agar are frequently very tiny, unlike other Shigella species.

Suspect colonies may be screened biochemically or serologically on Kligler iron agar (KIA) or triple sugar iron agar (TSI). Shigella species characteristically produce an alkaline slant and an acid butt (K/A) but do not produce gas or H_2S. A few strains of S. flexneri 6 and a very few strains of S. boydii produce gas in KIA or TSI. The motility, urea, and lysine decarboxylase tests (all are negative for Shigella) can be used to further screen isolates before doing serologic testing (Table 3). Isolates that react appropriately with the screening biochemicals should then be identified with a complete set of biochemical tests, with automated systems or self-contained commercial kits being satisfactory, and should be tested with grouping antisera. Confirmation requires both biochemical and serologic identification, and laboratories that do not perform both types of tests should send Shigella isolates to a reference laboratory.

Identification

Biochemical

Because the somatic antigens of most serotypes of Shigella are either identical or related to those of E. coli, suspicious cultures that are serologically negative should be tested further biochemically (42). Shigella and inactive E. coli (anaerogenic or lactose nonfermenting) are frequently difficult to distinguish by routine biochemical tests; Table 3 lists certain useful reactions. The biochemical reactions of Shigella are given in Table 4. Although S. dysenteriae and S.

TABLE 3 Differentiation of E. coli and Shigella

Test	Reaction of the following species[a]:		
	Shigella	Inactive E. coli[b]	E. coli
Lysine decarboxylase	−	d	+
Motility	−	−	+
Gas from glucose	−	−	+
Acetate utilization	−	d	+
Christiansen's citrate[c]	−	d	d
Mucate	−	d	+
Lactose	−	d	+

[a] Abbreviations: +, 90% or more positive within 1 or 2 days; −, no reaction (90% or more) in 7 days; d, different reactions [+, (+), −]. Adapted from reference 42.
[b] Nonmotile, anaerogenic biotypes sometimes referred to as Alkalescens-Dispar bioserotypes.
[c] Christiansen's citrate medium tests for citrate utilization in the presence of organic nitrogen. The more commonly used citrate utilization test, Simmons citrate, is not useful for discriminating between E. coli and Shigella (see chapter 41).

TABLE 4 Antigenic scheme and biochemical reactions of *Shigella* serotypes[a]

Subgroup, serotype [antigenic formula]	No. of strains examined (reference)	Indol	Arginine	Ornithine	Lactose	Sucrose	D-mannitol	Dulcitol	D-Sorbitol	Raffinose	D-Xylose	Glycerol	β-Galactosidase (ONPG)[b]
Subgroup A (*S. dysenteriae*)													
1	122 (41)	0	13 (7)	0 (0)	0 (8)	0 (11)	0 (0)	0 (0)	0 (0)	0 (0)	0 (0)	0 (100)	100 (0)
2	224 (41)	100	0 (0)	0 (0)	0 (0)	<1 (0)	0 (0)	0 (0)	9 (59)	0 (0)	0 (0)	8 (88)	2 (0)
3	159 (41)	0	2 (94)	0 (0)	0 (0)	0 (0)	0 (0)	0 (0)	77 (23)	0 (0)	0 (0)	5 (95)	25 (0)
4	31 (41)	0	0 (0)	0 (0)	0 (0)	0 (0)	0 (0)	0 (0)	7 (87)	0 (0)	0 (0)	23 (77)	70 (0)
5	29 (41)	0	20 (73)	0 (0)	0 (0)	0 (0)	0 (0)	90 (10)	97 (3)	0 (0)	0 (0)	84 (16)	0 (0)
6	17 (41)	0	0 (94)	0 (0)	0 (0)	0 (0)	0 (0)	0 (0)	94 (0)	0 (0)	0 (0)	0 (38)	71 (0)
7	39 (41)	100	0 (50)	0 (0)	0 (0)	0 (0)	0 (0)	0 (0)	0 (0)	0 (0)	0 (0)	0 (0)	85 (0)
8	25 (41)	100	0 (95)	0 (0)	0 (0)	0 (0)	0 (0)	0 (0)	0 (0)	0 (0)	76 (20)	80 (20)	50 (0)
9	7 (41)	0	29 (43)	0 (0)	0 (0)	0 (0)	0 (0)	0 (0)	14 (0)	0 (0)	0 (0)	57 (43)	0 (0)
10	3 (41)	0	0 (100)	0 (0)	0 (0)	0 (0)	0 (0)	0 (0)	100 (0)	0 (0)	100 (0)	0 (0)	0 (0)
11	19 (119)	0	0 (0)	0 (0)	0 (0)	0 (0)	0 (0)	0 (0)	0 (21)	0 (0)	0 (84)	58 (95)	63 (84)
12	13 (119)	0	0 (0)	0 (0)	0 (0)	0 (0)	0 (0)	0 (0)	0 (77)	0 (0)	0 (69)	54 (92)	54 (69)
13	19 (119)	0	58 (84)	0 (0)	0 (0)	0 (0)	0 (0)	0 (0)	79 (100)	0 (0)	0 (0)	0 (100)	0 (0)
14	8 (6)	0	0 (0)	0 (0)	0 (0)	0 (0)	0 (0)	0 (0)	NT[c]	0 (0)	0 (0)	0 (100)	0 (0)
15	10 (6)	0	0 (0)	0 (0)	0 (0)	0 (0)	0 (0)	0 (0)	NT	0 (0)	0 (0)	0 (100)	0 (0)
Subgroup B (*S. flexneri*)													
1a [I:4]	76 (CDC)	83	0 (0)	0 (0)	0 (0)	0 (11)	100 (0)	0 (0)	0 (0)	54 (32)	0 (0)	0 (0)	0 (0)
1b [I:4,6]	52 (CDC)	33	4 (6)	0 (0)	0 (0)	0 (60)	100 (0)	0 (0)	0 (0)	81 (19)	0 (0)	0 (5)	0 (0)
2a [II:3,4]	159 (CDC)	73	0 (0)	0 (0)	0 (0)	0 (9)	100 (0)	0 (0)	3 (2)	20 (28)	0 (0)	0 (0)	0 (0)
2b [II:7,8]	40 (CDC)	78	0 (0)	0 (0)	0 (0)	11 (32)	0	0 (0)	68 (0)	69 (6)	0 (0)	0 (0)	0 (0)
3a [III:(3,4),6,7,8]	120 (CDC)	83	0 (0)	0 (0)	0 (0)	8 (52)	91 (1)	0 (0)	85 (6)	65 (6)	0 (0)	0 (0)	0 (2)
3b [III:(3,4),6]	9 (CDC)	64	0 (5)	0 (5)	0 (0)	0 (33)	100 (0)	0 (0)	22 (11)	63 (37)	0 (13)	0 (0)	0 (11)
4a [IV:3,4]	479 (41)	74	0 (0)	0 (0)	0 (0)	1 (19)	76 (1)	0 (0)	37 (12)	38 (0)	10 (4)	0 (5)	NT
4b [IV:6]	148 (41)	70	0 (0)	0 (0)	0 (0)	0 (44)	99 (0)	0 (0)	4 (0)	77 (16)	0 (0)	0 (0)	NT
4c [IV:7,8]	212 (91)	0	0 (0)	0 (0)	0 (0)	0 (0)	100 (0)	0 (0)	0 (0)	41 (60)	0 (0)	0 (0)	NT
5a [V:(3,4)]	25 (CDC)	31	0 (7)	0 (0)	0 (4)	0 (25)	96 (0)	0 (0)	0 (8)	56 (12)	4 (0)	0 (4)	0 (8)
5b [V:7,8]	4 (CDC)	95	0 (0)	0 (0)	0 (0)	0 (30)	98 (0)	0 (0)	100 (0)	47 (25)	0 (0)	0 (0)	NT
6 [VI:4], bioserotype Boyd 88	483 (41)	0	52 (12)	0 (0)	0 (0)	0 (0)	100 (0)	4 (75)	17 (74)	0 (0)	0 (3)	59 (29)	NT

(Continued on next page)

TABLE 4 Antigenic scheme and biochemical reactions of *Shigella* serotypes[a] *(Continued)*

Subgroup, serotype [antigenic formula]	No. of strains examined (reference)	Indol	Arginine	Ornithine	Lactose	Sucrose	D-mannitol	Dulcitol	D-Sorbitol	Raffinose	D-Xylose	Glycerol	β-Galactosidase (ONPG)[b]
6 [VI:4], bioserotype Manchester	100 (41)	0	5 (5)	0 (0)	0 (0)	0 (0)	100 (0)	29 (57)	45 (46)	0 (0)	2 (73)	67 (33)	NT
6 [VI:4], bioserotype Newcastle	7 (41)	0	0 (75)	0 (0)	0 (0)	0 (0)	0 (0)	0 (100)	0 (80)	0 (0)	0 (0)	50 (50)	NT
X [:7,8]	4 (CDC)	75	0 (0)	0 (0)	0 (0)	0 (75)	100 (0)	0 (0)	50 (0)	100 (0)	0 (0)	0 (0)	0 (0)
Y [:3,4]	23 (CDC)	30	4 (13)	0 (13)	0 (0)	0 (26)	96 (0)	0 (5)	16 (0)	30 (26)	0 (0)	0 (10)	5 (5)
Subgroup C (S. boydii)													
1	109 (41)	0	2 (73)	0 (0)	0 (0)	0 (0)	100 (0)	1 (0)	40 (60)	0 (0)	13 (85)	0 (96)	8 (0)
2	121 (41)	0	48 (38)	0 (0)	0 (0)	0 (0)	100 (0)	1 (0)	11 (41)	0 (0)	0 (0)	80 (20)	3 (0)
3	25 (41)	0	50 (25)	0 (0)	0 (0)	0 (0)	100 (0)	55 (20)	95 (5)	0 (0)	18 (68)	58 (33)	22 (0)
4	100 (41)	0	27 (57)	0 (0)	0 (0)	1 (1)	99 (0)	0 (28)	10 (63)	0 (0)	0 (0)	75 (25)	0 (0)
5	58 (41)	100	0 (0)	0 (0)	0 (0)	0 (0)	100 (0)	0 (0)	28 (72)	0 (0)	4 (94)	9 (52)	0 (0)
6	7 (41)	0	0 (0)	0 (0)	0 (0)	0 (0)	71 (14)	43 (57)	86 (14)	0 (0)	0 (100)	33 (67)	0 (0)
7	48 (41)	100	8 (17)	0 (0)	0 (0)	0 (0)	100 (0)	0 (0)	90 (6)	0 (0)	98 (0)	0 (100)	50 (0)
8	17 (41)	0	13 (53)	0 (0)	0 (0)	0 (0)	100 (0)	0 (0)	58 (42)	0 (0)	29 (65)	10 (90)	50 (0)
9	15 (41)	100	0 (0)	0 (0)	0 (0)	0 (0)	93 (0)	0 (0)	87 (13)	0 (0)	0 (0)	0 (60)	75 (0)
10	91 (41)	0	62 (29)	0 (0)	0 (0)	0 (0)	93 (0)	97 (3)	56 (6)	0 (0)	4 (79)	65 (30)	24 (0)
11	61 (41)	100	0 (0)	0 (0)	0 (0)	0 (0)	100 (0)	0 (41)	32 (26)	0 (0)	61 (40)	0 (90)	0 (0)
12	14 (41)	0	0 (0)	100 (0)	0 (0)	0 (0)	100 (0)	0 (7)	0 (7)	0 (0)	0 (0)	14 (0)	0 (0)
13	10 (41)	100	0 (11)	1 (0)	0 (0)	0 (0)	100 (0)	0 (0)	100 (0)	0 (0)	0 (0)	0 (43)	0 (0)
14	17 (41)	0	7 (93)	0 (0)	0 (0)	0 (0)	45 (0)	0 (0)	60 (40)	0 (0)	7 (93)	0 (100)	0 (0)
15	11 (41)	100	0 (0)	0 (0)	0 (18)	0 (0)	91 (0)	0 (0)	91 (9)	0 (0)	0 (0)	0 (78)	33 (0)
16	4 (118)	100	0 (0)	0 (0)	0 (0)	0 (0)	100 (0)	0 (0)	100 (0)	0 (0)	100 (0)	33 (100)	0 (0)
17	7 (118)	100	0 (0)	0 (0)	0 (0)	0 (0)	100 (0)	0 (0)	100 (0)	0 (0)	100 (0)	0 (100)	20 (0)
18	31 (118)	0	6 (25)	0 (0)	0 (0)	0 (0)	100 (0)	0 (0)	75 (0)	0 (0)	18 (85)	19 (100)	18 (52)
19	36 (CDC)	0	42 (44)	0 (0)	0 (0)	0 (0)	100 (0)	0 (0)	49 (47)	0 (0)	33 (67)	28 (72)	6 (33)
Subgroup D													
S. sonnei	640 (41)	0	1 (5)	99 (0)	2 (88)	<1 (85)	99 (0)	0 (1)	1 (1)	3 (82)	1 (0)	13 (33)	95 (0)

[a] Values without parentheses are percentages of isolates tested with positive test results within 1 or 2 days of incubation at 35 to 37°C. Values in parentheses are percentages of isolates tested with a delayed positive test result, e.g., decarboxylase tests positive on day 3 or 4 and other tests positive after 3 to 7 days of incubation at 35 to 37°C. Data were compiled from findings published by Ewing (41), Wathen-Grady et al. (118, 119), Ansaruzzaman et al. (6), and Pryamukhina and Khomenko (91) and from unpublished findings from the reference laboratory at CDC, 1972 to 2002.
[b] β-Galactosidase activity determined with the substrate *o*-nitrophenyl-β-D-galactopyranoside.
[c] NT, not tested.

sonnei are biochemically distinct, *S. flexneri* and *S. boydii* are often biochemically indistinguishable, so that serologic grouping is essential.

Serotyping

Serologic testing is essential for the identification of *Shigella*. Three of the four subgroups, A (*S. dysenteriae*), B (*S. flexneri*), and C (*S. boydii*), are made up of a number of serotypes. Subgroup A has 15 serotypes; subgroup B has 8 serotypes (with serotypes 1 to 5 being subdivided into 11 subserotypes); and subgroup C has 19 serotypes. Subgroup D (*S. sonnei*) is made up of a single serotype and is the most common subgroup in the United States, followed by subgroup B (*S. flexneri*). Subgroups A and C are rare. Several provisional *Shigella* serotypes have also been described, which are held sub judice until findings from the characterization of representative isolates show them to be unique. Antisera for the identification of provisional serotypes are typically available only at reference laboratories. The currently recognized serotypes of *Shigella* and their biochemical profiles are shown in Table 4.

Serologic identification is typically performed by slide agglutination with polyvalent somatic (O) antigen-grouping sera followed, in some cases, by testing with monovalent antisera for specific serotype identification. Monovalent antiserum to *S. dysenteriae* 1 is required to identify this serotype and is not widely available. Because of the potentially serious nature of illness associated with this serotype, isolates that agglutinate in subgroup A reagent should be sent immediately to a reference laboratory for further serotyping.

Biochemically typical *Shigella* isolates that agglutinate poorly or that do not agglutinate at all should be suspended in saline and heated in a water bath at 100°C for 15 to 30 min. After cooling, the antigen suspension is tested in normal saline to determine if it is rough (agglutinates spontaneously). If the heated and cooled suspension is not rough, it may then be retested for agglutination in antisera.

Subtyping

A variety of methods have been used to subtype *Shigella*, including colicin typing (particularly for *S. sonnei*), plasmid profiling, restriction fragment length polymorphism analysis, PFGE, and ribotyping (3, 16, 43, 46, 67, 106). For an overview of the epidemiologic use of typing methods, see chapter 12.

Serodiagnostic Tests

Several serodiagnostic assays based on different antigens possessed by *Shigella* have been described (N. Strockbine, S. Fernandez, B. Mahon, E. Oaks, W. Picking, and E. Mintz, *Abstr. 97th Gen. Meet. Am. Soc. Microbiol. 1997,* abstr. V-20, 1997) (66, 117). These assays are practical only in research settings for seroepidemiology surveys and are not currently used for the diagnosis of infection in individual patients.

Antimicrobial Susceptibilities

Shigella infections are often treated with antimicrobial agents. Because of the widespread antimicrobial resistance among *Shigella* strains, all isolates should undergo susceptibility testing (www.cdc.gov/narms/). Reporting of susceptibility results to the clinician is particularly important for *S. dysenteriae* 1 isolates. Infections caused by these strains are often acquired during international travel to areas where most strains are multidrug resistant (112). In certain areas

of Africa and Asia, *S. dysenteriae* 1 strains are resistant to all locally available antimicrobial agents, including nalidixic acid, but are still susceptible to the fluoroquinolones (95).

Interpretation and Reporting of Results

A preliminary report of suspected *Shigella* infection may be issued if biochemical or serologic screening tests are positive. If serotyping results are available, these should also be reported, particularly if the isolate is *S. dysenteriae* 1. All *Shigella* isolates should be tested for antimicrobial susceptibility. Before a final report is issued, isolates should be confirmed by both serologic and biochemical methods. Isolates, particularly those from individuals with dysentery-like illness, that are biochemically identified as *Shigella* but that are serologically negative may be new serotypes of *Shigella* and should be sent to a reference laboratory for further characterization. Isolates from sites other than the gastrointestinal tract that resemble *Shigella* should be carefully scrutinized for gas production and other differentiating characteristics (Table 3). These isolates should be sent to a reference laboratory for confirmation because they are more likely to be anaerogenic *E. coli*, certain strains of which may cross-react with *Shigella* antiserum.

SALMONELLA

Description of the Genus

The genus *Salmonella* is composed of motile bacteria that conform to the definition of the family *Enterobacteriaceae* (42). Two species are currently recognized in the genus *Salmonella*, *Salmonella enterica* and *Salmonella bongori* (formerly subspecies V) (92). *Salmonella enterica* has been subdivided into six subspecies: (*S. enterica* subsp. *enterica*, designated subspecies I; *S. enterica* subsp. *salamae*, subspecies II; *S. enterica* subsp. *arizonae*, subspecies IIIa; *S. enterica* subsp. *diarizonae*, subspecies IIIb; *S. enterica* subsp. *houtenae*, subspecies IV; and *S. enterica* subsp. *indica*, subspecies VI). The type species is *S. enterica* subsp. *enterica*. See the Nomenclature section (below) and chapter 41 for a discussion of these six subspecies and *S. bongori*.

Subspecies I strains are usually isolated from humans and warm-blooded animals. Subspecies II, IIIa, IIIb, IV, and VI strains and *S. bongori* are usually isolated from cold-blooded animals and the environment (rarely from humans). The biochemical tests useful for identification of *Salmonella* and for subspecies differentiation are given in Tables 5 and 6, respectively.

Nomenclature for *Salmonella* and Distribution of Serotypes

The World Health Organization (WHO) Collaborating Centre for Reference and Research on *Salmonella*, which is located at the Pasteur Institute in Paris, France, designates serotypes (serovars) belonging to *S. enterica* subsp. *enterica* (subspecies I) with a name which is related to the geographical place where the serotype was first isolated (90). The serotype name is written in roman (not italicized) letters, and the first letter is a capital letter (for example, *Salmonella* serotype [ser.] Typhimurium or *Salmonella* Typhimurium). Serotypes belonging to other subspecies are designated by their antigenic formulae following the subspecies name (for example, *S. enterica* subsp. *salamae* ser. 50:z:e,n,x or *Salmonella* serotype II 50:z:e,n,x). The National *Salmonella* Reference Laboratory at CDC uses this nomenclature, with the minor deviation of using the term "serotype" instead of

TABLE 5 Biochemical tests useful in differentiating *Salmonella* from other members of the family *Enterobacteriaceae* and identifying *Salmonella* serotypes Typhi and Paratyphi A[a]

Test	Nontyphoidal *Salmonella* subsp. I reaction	*Salmonella* serotype Typhi reaction	*Salmonella* serotype Paratyphi A reaction
TSI	K/Ag	K/A	K/Ag
H₂S (TSI)	+	+[weak]	− or +[weak]
Indole	−	−	−
Methyl red	+	+	+
Voges-Proskauer	−	−	−
Citrate (Simmons)	+	−	−
Urea	−	−	−
Lysine decarboxylase	+	+	−
Arginine dihydrolase	+	d	(+)
Ornithine decarboxylase	+	−	+
Motility	+	+	+
Mucate	+	−	−
Malonate	−	−	−
L(+)-Tartrate (*d*-tartrate[b])	+	+	−
Growth in KCN	−	−	−
Glucose	Ag	A	Ag
Lactose	−	−	−
Sucrose	−	−	−
Salicin	−	−	−
Dulcitol	Ag	−	Ag[2 days]
Inositol	d	−	−
Sorbitol	Ag	A	Ag
ONPG[c]	−	−	−
Galacturonate	−	−	−

[a] Reactions after incubation at 37°C. K, alkaline slant; A, acid; g, gas; +, 90% or more positive within 1 or 2 days; (+), positive reaction after 3 or more days; −, no reaction (90% or more) in 7 days; d, different reactions [+, (+), −]. Adapted from reference 42. See Table 4 for reactions of the other subspecies.
[b] Sodium potassium tartrate (42).
[c] ONPG, *o*-nitrophenyl-β-D-galactopyranoside for detection of β-galactosidase activity.

TABLE 6 Biochemical reactions useful for differentiating *Salmonella* species and subspecies[a]

Test	Species or subspecies (no. of strains tested)						
	S. enterica						*S. bongori* (formerly V) (16)
	I (650)	II (146)	IIIa (120)	IIIb (155)	IV (120)	VI (9)	
Dulcitol	+	+	−	−	−	d[b]	+
Lactose	−	−	−[c]	+[d]	−	d[e]	−
ONPG	−	−[f]	+	+	−	d[g]	+
Salicin	−	−	−	−	+[h]	−	−
Sorbitol	+	+	+	+	+	−	+
Galacturonate	−	+	−	+	+	+	+
Malonate	−	+	+	+	−	−	−
Mucate	+	+	+	−[i]	−	+	+
Growth in KCN	−	−	−	−	+	−	+
Gelatin (strip)	−	+	+	+	+	+	−
L(+)-Tartrate (*d*-tartrate[j])	+	−	−	−	−	−	−

[a] Reactions after incubation at 37°C. +, 90% or more positive within 1 or 2 days; (+), positive reaction after 3 or more days; −, no reaction (90% or more) in 7 days; d, different reactions [+, (+), −]. Adapted from reference 42.
[b] A total of 67% were positive.
[c] A total of 15% were positive.
[d] A total of 85% were positive.
[e] A total of 22% were positive.
[f] A total of 15% were positive.
[g] A total of 44% were positive.
[h] A total of 60% were positive.
[i] A total of 30% were positive.
[j] Sodium potassium tartrate (42).

"serovar," and strongly encourages its use because it communicates the appropriate taxonomic relationship of the more than 2,500 antigenically distinct members of these two species (22).

Currently, there are 2,501 *Salmonella* serotypes (90). Most of these serotypes, including *Salmonella* serotype Typhi, belong to subspecies I (1,478 recognized serotypes) and are found in O groups A, B, C$_1$, C$_2$, D, and E. The two most commonly isolated serotypes in the United States are *Salmonella* serotypes Typhimurium and Enteritidis (31). Serotypes belonging to subspecies II (498 serotypes), IIIa (94 serotypes), IIIb (327 serotypes), IV (71 serotypes), VI (12 serotypes), and *S. bongori* (21 serotypes) are found primarily in O groups O11 (F) through O67 (the higher O groups) (60, 62, 63, 92). The genus "*Arizona*" was incorporated into the genus *Salmonella* as subspecies IIIa, containing the monophasic strains, and subspecies IIIb, containing the diphasic strains (94).

Clinical Significance

Strains of nontyphoidal *Salmonella* usually cause an intestinal infection (accompanied by diarrhea, fever, and abdominal cramps) that often lasts 1 week or longer (52, 77). Less commonly, nontyphoidal *Salmonella* can cause localized infections (e.g., osteomyelitis or urinary tract infection) or bacteremia, especially in immunocompromised persons. Persons of all ages are affected; the incidence is highest in infants. *Salmonella* is ubiquitous in animal populations, and human illness is usually linked to foods of animal origin. Salmonellosis also is transmitted by direct contact with animals, by nonanimal foods, by water, and occasionally by human contact. Each year, an estimated 1.4 million cases of illness and 600 deaths are caused by nontyphoidal salmonellosis in the United States (74).

Typhoid fever is a serious bloodstream infection that is common in the developing world. However, it is rare in the United States, where an estimated 800 cases with fewer than five deaths occur each year; >70% of U.S. cases are related to foreign travel (2, 74, 75). Typhoid fever typically presents with a sustained debilitating high fever and headache, without diarrhea. Illness is milder in young children (nonspecific fever) (75, 77). Humans are the only reservoir and may be healthy carriers. Typhoid fever typically has a low infectious dose (<10^3) and a long, highly variable incubation period (1 to 6 weeks). It is transmitted through person-to-person contact or fecally contaminated food and water. A syndrome similar to typhoid fever is caused by "paratyphoidal" strains of *Salmonella*: *Salmonella* serotypes Paratyphi A, Paratyphi B, and Paratyphi C. These serotypes are rare in the United States.

Disease caused by *Salmonella* serotype Enteritidis in the United States is part of an expanding global pandemic. The proportion of reported *Salmonella* isolates in the United States that were *Salmonella* serotype Enteritidis increased from 5% in 1976 to a peak of 26% in 1994 (30). From 1993 to 2000, state and territorial health departments reported 409 *Salmonella* serotype Enteritidis outbreaks to CDC. In these outbreaks, the dominant location was a commercial venue (e.g., restaurants, delicatessens, and cafeterias). Eighty percent of identified vehicles were foods containing raw or lightly cooked shell eggs. The WHO Collaborating Center for Enteric Phage Typing developed a phage-typing system that is used internationally to monitor *Salmonella* serotype Enteritidis phage types (51). Although phage type 8 is currently the most common type among isolates from outbreaks in the United States, *Salmonella* serotype Enter-

itidis phage type 4 infections were first identified in California and other western states during 1993 and 1994 and have spread rapidly to other regions of the United States (84).

A strain of *Salmonella* serotype Typhimurium phage type DT104 resistant to ampicillin, chloramphenicol, streptomycin, sulfonamides, and tetracycline (ACSSuT) has emerged in the United Kingdom and the United States as the predominant strain of this serotype; it comprised 28% of *Salmonella* serotype Typhimurium isolates in 2000 (28). In 1996, the first outbreak of pentadrug-resistant DT104 infection in the United States was reported (27), and outbreaks have occurred each year since.

Isolation Procedures

Enrichment

Maximal recovery of *Salmonella* from fecal specimens is obtained by using an enrichment broth, although isolation from acutely ill persons is usually possible by direct plating of specimens. Enrichment broths for *Salmonella* are usually highly selective and inhibit certain serotypes of *Salmonella*, particularly *Salmonella* serotype Typhi. The three selective enrichment media most widely used to isolate *Salmonella* from fecal specimens are tetrathionate broth, tetrathionate broth with brilliant green, and Selenite broth (SEL). SEL may also be used for the recovery of *Salmonella* serotype Typhi and *Shigella*, although its value as enrichment for the latter has not been clearly established. Specimens that might contain organisms inhibited by selective enrichment broths should be plated directly or cultured in a nonselective enrichment broth (e.g., GN broth).

A number of commercial rapid diagnostic tests are available for the testing of foods, but to our knowledge, none has been evaluated in the literature for use with fecal specimens.

Plating Media

Many differential plating media, varying from slightly selective to highly selective, are available for the isolation of *Salmonella* from fecal specimens. Media of low selectivity include MAC and eosin methylene blue. Media of intermediate selectivity include XLD, DCA, SS, and HE. Highly selective media include bismuth sulfite agar, the preferred medium for the isolation of *Salmonella* serotype Typhi, and brilliant green agar. Bismuth sulfite, XLD, and HE all have H$_2$S indicator systems, which are helpful for the detection of lactose-positive *Salmonella* strains. Most laboratories today use HE or XLD because these media may also be used for the isolation of *Shigella*.

In the developing world, typhoid fever is frequently diagnosed solely on clinical grounds, but isolation of the causative organism is necessary for a definitive diagnosis. *Salmonella* serotype Typhi is more frequently isolated from blood cultures than from fecal specimens. Blood cultures are positive for 80% of typhoid patients during the first week of fever but show decreasing positive results thereafter.

Screening Procedures

A latex agglutination kit has been described for screening for *Salmonella* from SEL enrichment broth (Wellcolex Color *Salmonella*; Murex Diagnostics, Inc., Norcross, Ga.) (76). This kit can also be used to screen individual colonies from primary plates.

Suspect colonies may be inoculated onto a screening medium such as KIA or TSI. On KIA or TSI, most *Salmo-*

nella strains produce a K/AG+ reaction, indicating that glucose is fermented with gas and H_2S production. On these media, *Salmonella* serotype Typhi isolates are characteristically K/A but do not produce gas, and only a small amount of H_2S is visible at the site of the stab and in the stab line. Lysine iron agar is also a useful screening medium because most *Salmonella* isolates, even those that ferment lactose, decarboxylate lysine and produce H_2S. Alternately, isolates may be identified by a battery of biochemical tests or by slide agglutination with antisera for *Salmonella* O groups A, B, C_1, C_2, D, and E. Isolates suspected of being *Salmonella* serotype Typhi should be tested serologically with *Salmonella* Vi and O group D antisera (see the discussion below).

If the biochemical reactions for a particular isolate are not characteristic but *Salmonella* antigens are found, the cultures should be plated on MAC or eosin methylene blue to obtain a pure culture, tested with a complete set of biochemical tests, or forwarded to a reference laboratory.

Identification

Clinical laboratories may issue a preliminary report of *Salmonella* when an isolate is positive either with O group antisera or by biochemical identification methods. An isolate is confirmed as *Salmonella* when the O serogroup has been determined and biochemical identification has been completed. The methods described below for serotyping are intended primarily for reference laboratories.

Biochemical Identification

Suspect colonies from one of the differential plating media mentioned above can be identified biochemically as *Salmonella* spp. with traditional media in tubes or commercial biochemical systems. Methods of biochemical identification and specific commercial manual and automated identification systems are covered in chapter 14. The species and subspecies of *Salmonella* can be identified biochemically, as indicated in Tables 5 and 6. Table 5 records biochemical reactions that are helpful for identifying nontyphoidal *Salmonella* subspecies I and distinguishing *Salmonella* serotypes Typhi and Paratyphi A from nontyphoidal *Salmonella* strains. Table 6 lists the biochemical reactions that are useful for differentiating *Salmonella* species and subspecies.

Serotyping

Salmonella spp. are serotyped according to their O (somatic) antigens, Vi (capsular) antigen, and H (flagellar) antigens (20, 21). Serotype can be expressed as a name or as the antigenic formula. The antigenic formulae of *Salmonella* serotypes are listed in the Kauffmann-White scheme and are expressed as follows: O antigen(s), Vi (when present):H antigen(s) (phase 1):H antigen(s) (phase 2, when present). For example, the antigenic formula for *Salmonella* serotype Typhimurium is 4,5,12:i:1,2. Updating of the Kauffmann-White scheme is the responsibility of the WHO Collaborating Centre for Reference and Research on *Salmonella*. The Kauffmann-White scheme is updated annually with a listing of new serotypes (90), and the latest revision of the complete scheme is published every 5 years (89).

Determination of O Antigens

O (heat-stable somatic) antigens are identified by first testing the isolate in O grouping antisera, which react with one or multiple antigens in each group, and then in the appropriate O single-factor antisera, which react with individual antigens (20). The approach most commonly used for determining O antigens is to initially test the isolates by slide agglutination in antisera against O groups A to E because approximately 95% of *Salmonella* isolates belong to one of these O groups. If no agglutination occurs in antisera for these O groups, the isolate is tested in pools containing the remaining *Salmonella* O antisera, O11 through O67.

Detection of the Vi Antigen and Identification of *Salmonella* Serotype Typhi (9,12,[Vi]:d:_)

The Vi antigen, a heat-labile capsular polysaccharide, is useful for the identification of *Salmonella* serotype Typhi. It is also occasionally detected in *Salmonella* serotype Dublin, *Salmonella* serotype Paratyphi C, and some *Citrobacter* strains. Vi antigen is identified by slide agglutination with a specific antiserum.

If *Salmonella* serotype Typhi is suspected, the culture is first tested live (unheated) in O group D antiserum (which contains antibodies to O antigens 9 and 12) and Vi antiserum on a slide. The Vi capsular polysaccharide can mask the O antigens, blocking their reactivity with the O grouping antiserum. If only the Vi antiserum is positive, the bacterial suspension is heated in boiling water for 15 min to remove the capsule, cooled, and tested again in the same antisera. After heating, *Salmonella* serotype Typhi isolates are negative in the Vi antiserum but positive in the O group D antiserum. Expression of the Vi antigen by *Salmonella* serotype Typhi is variable but tends to occur more frequently in freshly isolated cultures than in cultures that have been subcultured. If the strain is typical for *Salmonella* serotype Typhi on TSI or KIA (see "Screening Procedures" above), is urease negative, and reacts in O group D or Vi antisera, a presumptive report is made. The identity of the isolate is confirmed by biochemical testing (Tables 5 and 6) and determination of the H (flagellar) antigen (see below) before a final report is issued. *Salmonella* serotype Typhi strains typically express only one flagellar antigen, Hd.

Determination of H Antigens

H (flagellar) antigens are typically determined by tube agglutination tests using broth cultures. Isolates are initially tested with H typing antisera, which recognize individual or multiple antigens, and then with H single-factor antisera, which recognize individual antigens. Most *Salmonella* serotypes are either monophasic (express one type of H antigen) or diphasic (express two different types of H antigen). Typically, individual cells of a diphasic serotype express antigen(s) from only one phase at a time; however, both phases may be detected in the whole culture.

In cultures that have a mixture of cells in different phases, it is possible to detect both phases of a diphasic strain in a single assay. When only one phase is detected (either phase 1 or phase 2), the strain should be inoculated into a semisolid medium to which sterile antiserum of the detected phase has aseptically been added. Growth of the strain in this semisolid agar immobilizes cells expressing the detected antigen(s) and allows the growth of bacteria expressing the antigen(s) in the other phase. After phase reversal, the strain is tested in appropriate H typing and single-factor antisera to complete the serotyping. A strain must be actively motile to ensure the good development of H antigens, and sometimes it must be passed through one or more tall tubes of semisolid agar before H antigens can be detected. When a *Salmonella* strain is nonmotile, it is identified biochemically (Tables 5 and 6) and by the O antigens that it expresses.

Identification Problems

Several potential problems may prevent accurate serotype determination. The strain may express the Vi capsular antigen, which can block the binding of antibodies against the O antigens. The strain may be rough, i.e., fails to make complete O antigens. Rough strains have a tendency to cross-agglutinate in different antisera. The strain may be mucoid and will not agglutinate in antisera. When O antigens are not recognized, a strain is confirmed as a *Salmonella* species by its H antigens and a set of biochemical tests (Tables 5 and 6).

Many laboratories are likely to overlook *Salmonella* serotype Paratyphi A because they do not screen with O group A antiserum or because it is H₂S negative, lysine negative, and citrate negative (Table 5). *Salmonella* serotype Paratyphi B and *Salmonella* serotype Java can be confused because they have an identical antigenic formula (4,5,12:b:1,2), but they can be distinguished biochemically. *Salmonella* serotype Java is tartrate positive, while *Salmonella* serotype Paratyphi B is tartrate negative. Disease caused by *Salmonella* serotype Paratyphi B is usually typhoid-like and rare in the United States, while *Salmonella* serotype Java infection is usually typical nontyphoidal salmonellosis. The WHO Collaborating Centre for Reference and Research on *Salmonella* has combined these two serotypes and refers to *Salmonella* serotype Java as *Salmonella* serotype Paratyphi B, variety L(+)tartrate positive. Similarly, *Salmonella* serotype Choleraesuis and *Salmonella* serotype Paratyphi C have the same antigenic formula (6,7:c:1,5) but are differentiated biochemically. *Salmonella* serotype Paratyphi C may express the Vi antigen.

Citrobacter and *E. coli* strains may possess O, H, or Vi antigens that are related to those of *Salmonella*; biochemical identification may be necessary to confirm that an isolate is *Salmonella* (see Table 5 in this chapter and Table 1 in chapter 27).

Subtyping

Subtyping methods other than serotyping are frequently used for common serotypes (e.g., Typhimurium, Enteritidis, and Typhi). Various phenotypic methods (e.g., phage typing, antimicrobial susceptibility pattern determination, and biotyping) and genotyping methods (e.g., plasmid fingerprinting, PFGE, IS200 profiling, and random amplified polymorphic DNA analysis) have been developed for subtyping within serotypes of *Salmonella* (65, 80, 81, 114). PFGE is the current method of choice for the subtyping of most *Salmonella* serotypes and is the basis for PulseNet.

Serodiagnostic Tests

The Widal test is commonly used for serodiagnosis of *Salmonella* enteric fever; it measures agglutinating antibodies to the O and H antigens of *Salmonella* serotype Typhi (68). It is often used when isolation of *Salmonella* serotype Typhi is not feasible but produces false-negative and false-positive reactions and does not provide a definitive diagnosis of individual cases of infection (33, 58). Other serodiagnostic techniques are used for the detection of antibodies to other antigens (e.g., outer membrane proteins, lipopolysaccharide, flagellin protein, and Vi antigen) (34). Vi assays may be helpful, particularly when specimens for culture are unobtainable or are unlikely to be positive, such as retrospective epidemiologic investigations in which chronic carriers are being sought (68).

Antimicrobial Susceptibilities

Antimicrobial therapy is not recommended for uncomplicated *Salmonella* gastroenteritis, and routine susceptibility testing of fecal isolates is not warranted for treatment purposes. However, determination of antimicrobial resistance patterns is often valuable for surveillance purposes and may be performed periodically to monitor the development and spread of antimicrobial resistance among *Salmonella* isolates.

In contrast to uncomplicated salmonellosis, treatment with the appropriate antimicrobial agent can be crucial for patients with invasive *Salmonella* and typhoidal infections, and the susceptibilities of these isolates should be reported as soon as possible (59). The untreated case mortality rate for typhoid fever is >10%; when patients with typhoid fever are treated with appropriate antibiotics, the rate should be <1%.

CDC performed antimicrobial susceptibility testing of selected *Salmonella* isolates at 5-year intervals from 1979 to 1995. These investigations found an increasing prevalence of isolates resistant to at least one antimicrobial agent, from 16% during 1979 to 1980 to 29% during 1989 to 1990 (59, 69, 93). In 2000, 26% of nontyphoidal *Salmonella* isolates were resistant to one or more antimicrobials (28). Resistance to at least one antimicrobial agent among *Salmonella* serotype Typhi infections has increased from 24% in 1999 to 28% in 2000 (28) (http://www.cdc.gov/narms/annuals.htm). Recent reports from abroad have also noted an increasing level of resistance to one or more antimicrobial agents in *Salmonella* isolates, particularly in *Salmonella* serotype Typhi strains (2, 7, 35, 111, 115, 116). In particular, reduced susceptibility to ciprofloxicin among *Salmonella* serotype Typhi isolates and increasing numbers of treatment failures are of concern (115).

Among *Salmonella* serotype Typhimurium isolates submitted to CDC through the National Antimicrobial Resistance Monitoring System, the prevalence of the ACSSuT resistance pattern was 28% in both 1999 (102 of 362 strains) and 2000 (84 of 303 strains) (28). The emergence of a multiply resistant clone of *Salmonella* serotype Newport has also been noted (28), but so far it seems to be a significant problem only in the United States.

Interpretation and Reporting of Results

A preliminary report can be issued as soon as a presumptive identification of *Salmonella* is obtained. In most situations, a presumptive identification would be based on biochemical findings obtained either by traditional or commercial systems or by a serologic reaction in *Salmonella* O grouping antisera. A confirmed identification requires both biochemical and serologic identification methods. Because the National *Salmonella* Surveillance System depends on the receipt of serotype information for *Salmonella* strains isolated in the United States for the tracking of outbreaks of infection, laboratories should follow the procedures recommended by their state health departments for submitting isolates for further characterization, including complete serotyping. The susceptibilities of typhoidal *Salmonella* strains and strains from normally sterile sites should be tested, and the strains should be forwarded to a reference or public health laboratory for complete biochemical and serologic characterization.

REFERENCES

1. **Acheson, D. W. K., and G. T. Keusch.** 1995. *Shigella* and enteroinvasive *Escherichia coli*, p. 763–784. *In* M. J. Blaser, J. I. Ravdin, H. B. Greenberg, and R. L. Guerrant (ed.), *Infections of the Gastrointestinal Tract.* Raven Press, New York, N.Y.

2. **Ackers, M. L., N. D. Puhr, R. V. Tauxe, and E. D. Mintz.** 2000. Laboratory-based surveillance of *Salmonella* serotype Typhi infections in the United States: antimicrobial resistance on the rise. JAMA **283:**2668–2673.

3. **Albert, M. J., K. V. Singh, B. E. Murray, and J. Erlich.** 1990. Molecular epidemiology of *Shigella* infection in Central Australia. *Epidemiol. Infect.* **105:**51–57.

4. **Albert, M. J., S. M. Faruque, A. S. Faruque, K. A. Bettelheim, P. K. Neogi, N. A. Bhuiyan, and J. B. Kaper.** 1996. Controlled study of cytolethal distending toxin-producing *Escherichia coli* infections in Bangladeshi children. *J. Clin. Microbiol.* **34:**717–719.

5. **American Gastroenterological Association.** 1995. Consensus Conference Statement. *Escherichia coli* O157:H7 infections—an emerging national health crisis, July 11–13, 1994. *Gastroenterology* **108:**1923–1934.

6. **Ansaruzzaman, M., A. K. M. G. Kibriya, A. Rahman, P. K. B. Neogi, A. S. G. Faruque, B. Rowe, and M. J. Albert.** 1995. Detection of provisional serovars of *Shigella dysenteriae* and designation as *S. dysenteriae* serotypes 14 and 15. *J. Clin. Microbiol.* **33:**1423–1425.

7. **Aysev, A. D., H. Guriz, and B. Erdem.** 2001. Drug resistance of *Salmonella* strains isolated from community infections in Ankara, Turkey, 1993-99. *Scand. J. Infect. Dis.* **33:**420–422.

8. **Belongia, E. A., M. T. Osterholm, J. T. Soler, D. A. Ammend, J. E. Braun, and K. L. MacDonald.** 1993. Transmission of *Escherichia coli* O157:H7 infection in Minnesota child day-care facilities. JAMA **269:**883–888.

9. **Bettelheim, K. A.** 1992. The genus *Escherichia*, p. 2696–2736. *In* A. Balows, H. G. Trüper, M. Dworkin, W. Harder, and K.-H. Schleifer (ed.), *The Prokaryotes,* 2nd ed. Springer-Verlag KG, Berlin, Germany.

10. **Bettelheim, K. A.** 1995. Identification of enterohaemorrhagic *Escherichia coli* by means of their production of enterohaemolysin. *J. Appl. Bacteriol.* **79:**178–180.

11. **Beutin, L., M. A. Montenegro, I. Orskov, F. Orskov, J. Proada, S. Zimmerman, and R. Stephan.** 1989. Close association of verocytotoxin (Shiga-like toxin) production with enterohemolysin production in strains of *Escherichia coli*. *J. Clin. Microbiol.* **27:**2559–2564.

12. **Bitzan, M., K. Ludwig, M. Klemt, H. Konig, J. Buren, and D. E. Muller-Wiefel.** 1993. The role of *Escherichia coli* O157 infections in the classical (enteropathic) haemolytic uraemic syndrome: results of a Central European multicentre study. *Epidemiol. Infect.* **110:**183–196.

13. **Blanco, J. E., J. Blanco, M. Blanco, M. P. Alonso, and W. H. Jansen.** 1994. Serotypes of CNF1-producing *Escherichia coli* strains that cause extra intestinal infections in humans. *Eur. J. Epidemiol.* **10:**707–711.

14. **Borczyk, A. A., N. Harnett, M. Lombos, and H. Lior.** 1990. False-positive identification of *Escherichia coli* O157 by commercial latex agglutination tests. *Lancet* **336:**946–947.

15. **Boyce, T. G., A. G. Pemberton, J. G. Wells, and P. M. Griffin.** 1995. Screening for *Escherichia coli* O157:H7: a nationwide survey of clinical laboratories. *J. Clin. Microbiol.* **33:**3275–3277.

16. **Bratoeva, M. P., J. F. Jopn, and N. L. Barg.** 1992. Molecular epidemiology of trimethoprim-resistant *Shigella boydii* serotype 2 strains from Bulgaria. *J. Clin. Microbiol.* **30:**1428–1431.

17. **Brenner, D. J.** 1992. Introduction to the family *Enterobacteriaceae*, p. 2673–2695. *In* A. Balows, H. G. Trüper, M. Dworkin, W. Harder, and K.-H. Schleifer (ed.), *The Prokaryotes,* 2nd ed. Springer-Verlag KG, Berlin, Germany.

18. **Brenner, D. J., G. R. Fanning, F. J. Skerman, and S. Falkow.** 1972. Polynucleotide sequence divergence among strains of *Escherichia coli* and closely related organisms. *J. Bacteriol.* **109:**933–965.

19. **Brenner, D. J., G. R. Fanning, G. V. Miklos, and A. G. Steigerwalt.** 1973. Polynucleotide sequence relatedness among *Shigella* species. *Int. J. Syst. Bacteriol.* **23:**1–7.

20. **Brenner, F. W., and A. C. McWhorter-Murlin.** 1998. *Identification and Serotyping of* Salmonella. Centers for Disease Control and Prevention, Atlanta, Ga.

21. **Brenner, F. W.** 1998. *Modified Kauffmann-White Scheme.* Centers for Disease Control and Prevention, Atlanta, Ga.

22. **Brenner, F. W., R. G. Villar, F. J. Angulo, R. Tauxe, and B. Swaminathan.** 2000. *Salmonella* nomenclature. *J. Clin. Microbiol.* **38:**2465–2467.

23. **Caprioli, A., V. Falbo, F. M. Ruggeri, L. Baldassarri, R. Bisicchia, G. Ippolito, E. Romoli, and G. Donelli.** 1987. Cytotoxic necrotizing factor production by hemolytic strains of *Escherichia coli* causing extra intestinal infections. *J. Clin. Microbiol.* **25:**146–149.

24. **Caprioli, A., V. Falbo, L. G. Roda, F. M. Ruggeri, and C. Zona.** 1983. Partial purification and characterization of an *Escherichia coli* toxic factor that induces morphological cell alterations. *Infect. Immun.* **39:**1300–1306.

25. **Caprioli, A., and A. E. Tozzi.** 1998. Epidemiology of Shiga toxin-producing *Escherichia coli* infections in continental Europe, p. 38–48. *In* J. B. Kaper and A. D. O'Brien (ed.), Escherichia coli *O157:H7 and Other Shiga Toxin-Producing* E. coli *Strains.* ASM Press, Washington, D.C.

26. **Centers for Disease Control and Prevention.** 2000. *Escherichia coli* O111:H8 outbreak among teenage campers—Texas, 1999. *Morb. Mortal. Wkly. Rep.* **49:**321–324.

27. **Centers for Disease Control and Prevention.** 1997. Multidrug-resistant *Salmonella* serotype Typhimurium—United States, 1996. *Morb. Mortal. Wkly. Rep.* **46:**308–310.

28. **Centers for Disease Control and Prevention.** 2000. *NARMS 2000 Annual Report.* Centers for Disease Control and Prevention, Atlanta, Ga.

29. **Centers for Disease Control and Prevention.** 2001. Preliminary FoodNet data on the incidence of foodborne illnesses—selected sites, United States, 2000. *Morb. Mortal. Wkly. Rep.* **50:**241–246.

30. **Centers for Disease Control and Prevention.** 1997. *Salmonella Surveillance, 1996.* Centers for Disease Control and Prevention, Atlanta, Ga.

31. **Centers for Disease Control and Prevention.** 2001. *Salmonella Surveillance: Annual Summary, 2000.* Centers for Disease Control and Prevention, Atlanta, Ga.

32. **Chapman, P. A., and C. A. Siddons.** 1996. A comparison of immunomagnetic separation and direct culture for the isolation of verocytotoxin-producing *Escherichia coli* O157 from cases of bloody diarrhoea, non-bloody diarrhoea and asymptomatic contacts. *J. Med. Microbiol.* **44:**267–271.

33. **Chart, H., J. S. Cheesbrough, and D. J. Waghorn.** 2000. The serodiagnosis of infection with *Salmonella typhi*. *J. Clin. Pathol.* **53:**851–853.

34. **Chart, H., L. R. Ward, and B. Rowe.** 1998. An immunoblotting procedure comprising O = 9,12 and H = d antigens as an alternative to the Widal agglutination assay. *J. Clin. Pathol.* **51:**854–856.

35. **Cruchaga, S., A. Echeita, A. Aladuena, J. Garcia-Pena, N. Frias, and M. A. Usera.** 2001. Antimicrobial resistance in salmonellae from humans, food and animals in Spain in 1998. *J. Antimicrob. Chemother.* **47:**315–321.

36. **Cubbon, M. D., J. E. Coia, M. F. Hanson, and F. M. Thomson-Carter.** 1996. A comparison of immunomagnetic separation, direct culture and polymerase chain reaction for the detection of verocytotoxin-producing *Escherichia coli* O157 in human faeces. *J. Med. Microbiol.* **44:** 219–222.

37. **Dalton, C. B., E. D. Mintz, J. G. Wells, C. A. Bopp, and R. V. Tauxe.** 1999. Outbreaks of enterotoxigenic *Escherichia coli* infection in American adults: a clinical and epidemiologic profile. *Epidemiol. Infect.* **123:**9–16.

38. **De Rycke, J., J. F. Guillot, and R. Boivin.** 1997. Cytotoxins in nonenterotoxigenic strains of *Escherichia coli* isolated from feces of diarrheic calves. *Vet. Microbiol.* **15:** 137–150.

39. **Donnenberg, M. S.** 1995. Enteropathogenic *Escherichia coli,* p. 709–726. *In* M. J. Blaser, P. D. Smith, J. I. Ravdin, H. B. Greenberg, and R. L. Guerrant (ed.), *Infections of the Gastrointestinal Tract.* Raven Press, New York, N.Y.

40. **Dylla, B. L., E. A. Vetter, J. G. Hughes, and F. R. Cockerill III.** 1995. Evaluation of an immunoassay for direct detection of *Escherichia coli* O157 in stool specimens. *J. Clin. Microbiol.* **33:**222–224.

41. **Ewing, W. H.** 1971. *Biochemical Reactions of* Shigella. Center for Disease Control, Atlanta, Ga.

42. **Ewing, W. H.** 1986. *Edwards and Ewing's Identification of Enterobacteriaceae,* 4th ed. Elsevier Science Publishing Co. Inc., New York, N.Y.

43. **Faruque, S. M., K. Haider, M. M. Rahman, A. R. M. A. Alim, Q. S. Ahmad, M. J. Albert, and R. B. Sack.** 1992. Differentiation of *Shigella flexneri* strains by rRNA gene restriction patterns. *J. Clin. Microbiol.* **30:**2996–2999.

44. **Fields, P. I., K. Blom, H. J. Hughes, L. O. Helsel, P. Feng, and B. Swaminathan.** 1997. Molecular characterization of the gene encoding H antigen in *Escherichia coli* and development of a PCR-restriction fragment length polymorphism test for identification of *E. coli* O157:H7 and O157:NM. *J. Clin. Microbiol.* **35:**1066–1070.

45. **Friedrich, A. W., M. Bielaszewska, W. L. Zhang, M. Pulz, T. Kuczius, A. Ammon, and H. Karch.** 2002. *Escherichia coli* harboring Shiga toxin 2 gene variants: frequency and association with clinical symptoms. *J. Infect. Dis.* **185:**74–84.

46. **Gebre-Yohannes, A., and B. S. Drasar.** 1990. Plasmid profiles of *Shigella dysenteriae* type 1 isolates from Ethiopia with special reference to R-plasmids. *J. Med. Microbiol.* **33:**101–106.

47. **Griffin, P. M., P. S. Mead, and S. Sivapalasingam.** 2002. *Escherichia coli* O157:H7 and other enterohemorrhagic *Escherichia coli,* p. 627–642. *In* M. J. Blaser, J. I. Ravdin, H. B. Greenberg, and R. L. Guerrant (ed.), *Infections of the Gastrointestinal Tract,* 2nd ed. Lippincott Williams & Wilkins, New York, N.Y.

48. **Guerrant, R. L., T. Van Gilder, T. S. Steiner, N. M. Thielman, L. Slutsker, R. V. Tauxe, T. Hennessy, P. M. Griffin, H. DuPont, R. B. Sack, P. Tarr, M. Neill, I. Nachamkin, L. B. Reller, M. T. Osterholm, M. L. Bennish, and L. K. Pickering.** 2001. Practice guidelines for the management of infectious diarrhea. *Clin. Infect. Dis.* **32:**331–351.

49. **Hashimoto, H., K. Mizukoshi, M. Nishi, T. Kawakita, S. Hasui, Y. Kato, Y. Ueno, R. Takeya, N. Okuda, and T. Takeda.** 1999. Epidemic of gastrointestinal tract infection including hemorrhagic colitis attributable to Shiga toxin 1-producing *Escherichia coli* O118:H2 at a junior high school in Japan. *Pediatrics* **103:**141.

50. **Hayes, P. S., K. Blom, P. Feng, J. Lewis, N. A. Strockbine, and B. Swaminathan.** 1995. Isolation and characterization of a β-glucuronidase-producing strain of *Esche-*

richia coli O157:H7 in the United States. *J. Clin. Microbiol.* **33:**3347–3348.

51. **Hickman-Brenner, F. W., A. D. Stubbs, and J. J. Farmer III.** 1991. Phage typing of *Salmonella enteritidis* in the United States. *J. Clin. Microbiol.* **29:**2817–2823.

52. **Hohmann, E. L.** 2001. Nontyphoidal salmonellosis. *Clin. Infect. Dis.* **32:**263–269.

53. **Itoh, Y., I. Nagano, M. Kunishima, and T. Ezaki.** 1997. Laboratory investigation of enteroaggregative *Escherichia coli* O untypable:H10 associated with a massive outbreak of gastrointestinal illness. *J. Clin. Microbiol.* **35:**2546–2550.

54. **Johnson, R. P., R. C. Clarke, J. B. Wilson, S. C. Read, K. Rahn, S. A. Renwick, K. Sandhu, D. Alves, M. A. Karmali, H. Lior, S. A. McEwen, J. S. Spika, and C. L. Gyles.** 1996. Growing concerns and recent outbreaks involving non-O157:H7 serotypes of verotoxigenic *Escherichia coli. J. Food Prot.* **59:**1112–1122.

55. **Johnson, W. M., and H. Lior.** 1988. A new heat-labile cytolethal distending toxin (CLDT) produced by *Escherichia coli* isolates from clinical material. *Microb. Pathog.* **4:**103–113.

56. **Karch, H., C. Janetzki-Mittman, S. Aleksic, and M. Datz.** 1996. Isolation of enterohemorrhagic *Escherichia coli* O157 strains from patients with hemolytic-uremic syndrome by using immunomagnetic separation, DNA-based methods, and direct culture. *J. Clin. Microbiol.* **34:**516–519.

57. **Karch, H., M. Bielaszewska, M. Bitzan, and H. Schmidt.** 1999. Epidemiology and diagnosis of Shiga toxin-producing *Escherichia coli* infections. *Diagn. Microbiol. Infect. Dis.* **34:** 229–243.

58. **Koeleman, J. G., D. F. Regensburg, F. van Katwijk, and D. M. MacLaren.** 1992. Retrospective study to determine the diagnostic value of the Widal test in a non-endemic country. *Eur. J. Clin. Microbiol. Infect. Dis.* **11:**167–170.

59. **Lee, L. A., N. D. Puhr, E. K. Mahoney, N. H. Bean, and R. V. Tauxe.** 1994. Increase in antimicrobial-resistant *Salmonella* infections in the United States, 1989–1990. *J. Infect. Dis.* **170:**128–134.

60. **Le Minor, L., G. Chamoiseau, E. Barbe, C. Charie-Marsaines, and L. Egron.** 1969. Dix nouveau serotypes de *Salmonella* isoles au Tchad. *Ann. Inst. Pasteur* (Paris) **116:** 775–780.

61. **Le Minor, L.** 1992. The genus *Salmonella,* p. 2760–2774. *In* A. Balows, H. G. Truper, M. Dworkin, W. Harder, and K.-H. Schleifer (ed.), *The Prokaryotes,* 2nd ed. Springer-Verlag KG, Berlin, Germany.

62. **Le Minor, L., M. Y. Popoff, B. Laurent, and D. Herman.** 1986. Individualization d'une septieme sous-espece de *Salmonella: S. choleraesuis* subsp. *Indica* subsp. nov. *Ann. Inst. Pasteur/Microbiol.* **137B:**211–217.

63. **Le Minor, L., M. Veron, and M. Y. Popoff.** 1982. Taxonomie des *Salmonella. Ann. Inst. Pasteur/Microbiol.* **133B:**223–243.

64. **Levine, M. M., C. Ferreccio, V. Prado, M. Cayazzo, P. Abrego, J. Martinez, L. Maggi, M. M. Baldini, W. Martin, D. Maneval, B. Kay, L. Guers, H. Lior, S. S. Wasserman, and J. P. Nataro.** 1993. Epidemiologic studies of *Escherichia coli* diarrheal infections in a low socioeconomic level peri-urban community in Santiago, Chile. *Am. J. Epidemiol.* **138:**849–869.

65. **Lin, A. W., M. A. Usera, T. J. Barrett, and R. A. Goldsby.** 1996. Application of random amplified polymorphic DNA analysis to differentiate strains of *Salmonella enteritidis. J. Clin. Microbiol.* **34:**870–876.

66. **Lindberg, A. A., P. D. Cam, N. Chan, L. K. Phu, D. D. Trach, G. Lindberg, K. Karlsson, A. Karnell, and E. Ekwall.** 1991. Shigellosis in Vietnam: seroepidemiologic

studies with use of lipopolysaccharide antigens in enzyme immunoassays. *Rev. Infect. Dis.* **13**(Suppl. 4)**:**S213–S237.

67. **Litwin, C. M., A. L. Storm, S. Chipowsky, and K. J. Ryan.** 1991. Molecular epidemiology of *Shigella* infections: plasmid profiles, serotype correlation, and restriction endonuclease analysis. *J. Clin. Microbiol.* **29:**104–108.

68. **Losonsky, G. A., and M. M. Levine.** 1997. Immunologic methods for diagnosis of infections caused by diarrheagenic members of the families *Enterobacteriaceae* and *Vibrionaceae*, p. 484–497. *In* N. R. Rose, E. C. de Macario, J. D. Folds, H. C. Lane, and R. M. Nakamura (ed.), *Manual of Clinical Laboratory Immunology*, 5th ed. ASM Press, Washington, D.C.

69. **MacDonald, K. L., M. L. Cohen, N. T. Hargrett-Bean, J. G. Wells, N. D. Puhr, S. F. Collin, and P. A. Blake.** 1987. Changes in antimicrobial resistance of *Salmonella* isolated from humans in the United States. *JAMA* **258:** 1496–1499.

70. **Mackenzie, A. M., P. Lebel, E. Orrbine, P. C. Rowe, L. Hyde, F. Chan, W. Johnson, P. N. McLaine, and The SYNSORB Pk Study Investigators.** 1998. Sensitivities and specificities of Premier *E. coli* O157 and Premier EHEC enzyme immunoassays for diagnosis of infection with verotoxin (Shiga-like toxin)-producing *Escherichia coli. J. Clin. Microbiol.* **36:**1608–1611.

71. **March, S. B., and S. Ratnam.** 1986. Sorbitol-MacConkey medium for detection of *Escherichia coli* O157:H7 associated with hemorrhagic colitis. *J. Clin. Microbiol.* **23:**869–872.

72. **McCarthy, T. A., N. L. Barrett, J. L. Hadler, B. Salsbury, R. T. Howard, D. W. Dingman, C. D. Brinkman, W. F. Bibb, and M. L. Cartter.** 2001. Hemolytic-uremic syndrome and *Escherichia coli* O121 at a lake in Connecticut, 1999. *Pediatrics* **108**(4)**:**E59.

73. **McMaster, C., E. A. Roch, G. A. Willshaw, A. Doherty, W. Kinnear, and T. Cheasty.** 2001. Verocytotoxin-producing *Escherichia coli* serotype O26:H11 outbreak in an Irish creche. *Eur. J. Clin. Microbiol. Infect. Dis.* **20:** 430–432.

74. **Mead, P. S., L. Slutsker, V. Dietz, L. F. McCaig, J. S. Bresee, C. Shapiro, P. M. Griffin, and R. V. Tauxe.** 1999. Food-related illness and death in the United States. *Emerg. Infect. Dis.* **5:**607–625.

75. **Mermin, J. H., J. M. Townes, M. Gerber, N. Dolan, E. D. Mintz, and R. V. Tauxe.** 1998. Typhoid fever in the United States, 1985–1994: changing risks of international travel and increasing antimicrobial resistance. *Arch. Intern. Med.* **158:**633–638.

76. **Metzler, J., and I. Nachamkin.** 1988. Evaluation of a latex agglutination test for the detection of *Salmonella* and *Shigella* spp. by using broth enrichment. *J. Clin. Microbiol.* **26:**2501–2504.

77. **Miller, S. I., E. L. Hohmann, and D. A. Pegues.** 1995. *Salmonella* (including *Salmonella* Typhi), p. 2013–2033. *In* G. L. Mandell, J. E. Bennett, and R. Dolin (ed.), *Principles and Practice of Infectious Diseases.* Churchill Livingstone, Inc., New York, N.Y.

78. **Morabito, S., H. Karch, P. Mariani-Kurkdjian, H. Schmidt, F. Minelli, E. Bingen, and A. Caprioli.** 1998. Enteroaggregative, Shiga toxin-producing *Escherichia coli* O111:H2 associated with an outbreak of hemolytic-uremic syndrome. *J. Clin. Microbiol.* **36:**840–842.

79. **Nataro, J. P., and J. B. Kaper.** 1998. Diarrheagenic *Escherichia coli. Clin. Microbiol. Rev.* **11:**142–201.

80. **Navaro, F., T. Llovet, M. A. Echeita, P. Coll, A. Aladueña, M. A. Usera, and G. Prats.** 1996. Molecular typing of *Salmonella enterica* serovar Typhi. *J. Clin. Microbiol.* **34:**2831–2834.

81. **Olsen, J. E., M. N. Skov, O. Angen, E. J. Threlfall, and M. Bisgaard.** 1997. Genomic relationships between selected phage types of *Salmonella enterica* subsp. *enterica* serotype *typhimurium* defined by ribotyping, IS200 typing, and PFGE. *Microbiology* **43:**1471–1479.

82. **Olsvik, O., and N. A. Strockbine.** 1993. PCR detection of heat-stable, heat-labile, and Shiga-like toxin genes in *Escherichia coli*, p. 271–276. *In* D. H. Persing, T. F. Smith, F. C. Tenover, and T. J. White (ed.), *Diagnostic Molecular Microbiology: Principles and Applications.* American Society for Microbiology, Washington, D.C.

83. **Oswald, E., J. DeRycke, J. F. Guillot, and R. Boivin.** 1989. Cytotoxic effect of multinucleation in HeLa cell cultures associated with the presence of Vir plasmid in *Escherichia coli* strains. *FEMS Microbiol. Lett.* **58:**95–100.

84. **Passaro, D. J., R. Reporter, L. Mascola, L. Kilman, G. B. Malcolm, H. Rolka, S. S. Werner, and D. J. Vugia.** 1996. Epidemic *Salmonella enteritidis* infection in Los Angeles County, California. The predominance of phage type 4. *West. J. Med.* **63:**126–130.

85. **Paton, A. W., R. M. Ratcliff, R. M. Doyles, J. Seymour-Murray, D. Davos, J. A. Lanser, and J. C. Paton.** 1996. Molecular microbiological investigation of an outbreak of hemolytic-uremic syndrome caused by dry fermented sausage contaminated with Shiga-like toxin-producing *Escherichia coli. J. Clin. Microbiol.* **34:**1622–1627.

86. **Paton, A. W., M. C. Woodrow, R. M. Doyle, J. A. Lanser, and J. C. Paton.** 1999. Molecular characterization of a Shiga toxigenic *Escherichia coli* O113:H21 strain lacking *eae* responsible for a cluster of cases of hemolytic-uremic syndrome. *J. Clin. Microbiol.* **37:**3357–3361.

87. **Poitrineau, P., C. Forestier, M. Meyer, C. Jallat, C. Rich, G. Malpuech, and C. De Champs.** 1995. Retrospective case-control study of diffusely adhering *Escherichia coli* and clinical features in children with diarrhea. *J. Clin. Microbiol.* **33:**1961–1962.

88. **Polotsky, Y., J. P. Nataro, D. Kotler, T. J. Barrett, and J. M. Orenstein.** 1997. HEp-2 cell adherence patterns, serotyping, and DNA analysis of *Escherichia coli* isolates from eight patients with AIDS and chronic diarrhea. *J. Clin. Microbiol.* **35:**1952–1958.

89. **Popoff, M. Y.** 2001. *Antigenic Formulas of the* Salmonella *Serovars*, 8th ed. WHO Collaborating Centre for Reference and Research on Salmonella, Pasteur Institute, Paris, France.

90. **Popoff, M. Y., J. Bockemuhl, F. W. Brenner, and L. L. Gheesling.** 2001. Supplement 2000 (no. 44) to the Kauffmann-White scheme. *Res. Microbiol.* **152:**907–909.

91. **Pryamukhina, N. S., and N. A. Khomenko.** 1988. Suggestion to supplement *Shigella flexneri* classification scheme with the subserovar *Shigella flexneri* 4c: phenotypic characteristics of strains. *J. Clin. Microbiol.* **26:**1147–1149.

92. **Reeves, M. W., G. M. Evins, A. A. Heiba, B. D. Plikaytis, and J. J. Farmer III.** 1989. Clonal nature of *Salmonella typhi* and its genetic relatedness to other salmonellae as shown by multilocus enzyme electrophoresis and proposal of *Salmonella bongori* comb. nov. *J. Clin. Microbiol.* **27:** 313–320.

93. **Riley, L. W., M. L. Cohen, J. E. Seals, M. J. Blaser, K. A. Birkness, N. T. Hargrett, S. M. Martin, and R. A. Feldman.** 1984. Importance of host factors in human salmonellosis caused by multiresistant strains of *Salmonella. J. Infect. Dis.* **149:**878–883.

94. **Rohde, R.** 1979. Serological integration of all known *Arizona* species into the Kauffmann-White schema. *Zentbl. Bakteriol. Parasitenkd. Infektionskr. Hyg. I Abt. Orig. Reihe A* **243:**148–176.

95. **Sack, R. B., M. Rahman, M. Yunus, and E. H. Khan.** 1997. Antimicrobial resistance in organisms causing diarrheal disease. *Clin. Infect. Dis.* **24**(Suppl. 1):S102–S105.

96. **Scheutz, F., L. Beutin, and H. R. Smith.** 2001. Clinical detection of verocytotoxin-producing *E. coli* (VTEC), p. 25–56. *In* G. Duffy, P. Garvey, and D. A. McDowell (ed.), *Verocytotoxigenic E. coli.* Food & Nutrition Press, Inc., Trumbull, Conn.

97. **Schmidt, H., and H. Karch.** 1996. Enterohemolytic phenotypes and genotypes of Shiga toxin-producing *Escherichia coli* O111 strains from patients with diarrhea and hemolytic-uremic syndrome. *J. Clin. Microbiol.* **34**:2364–2367.

98. **Scotland, S. M., T. Cheasty, A. Thomas, and B. Rowe.** 1991. Beta-glucuronidase activity of Vero cytotoxin-producing strains of *Escherichia coli*, including serogroup O157, isolated in the United Kingdom. *Lett. Appl. Microbiol.* **13**:42–44.

99. **Scotland, S. M., G. A. Willshaw, B. Said, H. R. Smith, and B. Rowe.** 1989. Identification of *Escherichia coli* that produce heat-stable enterotoxin STA by a commercially available enzyme-linked immunoassay and comparison of the assay with infant mouse and DNA probe tests. *J. Clin. Microbiol.* **27**:1697–1699.

100. **Sethabutr, O., P. Echeverria, C. W. Hoge, L. Bodhidatta, and C. Pitarangsi.** 1994. Detection of *Shigella* and enteroinvasive *Escherichia coli* by PCR in the stools of patients with dysentery in Thailand. *J. Diarrhoeal Dis. Res.* **12**:265–269.

101. **Slutsker, L., A. A. Ries, K. D. Greene, J. G. Wells, L. Hutwagner, and P. M. Griffin.** 1997. *Escherichia coli* O157:H7 diarrhea in the United States: clinical and epidemiologic features. *Ann. Intern. Med.* **126**:505–513.

102. **Smith, H. R., and S. M. Scotland.** 1993. Isolation and identification methods for *Escherichia coli* O157 and other Vero cytotoxin producing strains. *J. Clin. Pathol.* **46**:10–17.

103. **Smith, H. W.** 1974. A search for transmissible pathogenic characters in invasive strains of *Escherichia coli*: the discovery of a plasmid-controlled toxin and a plasmid-controlled lethal character closely associated, or identical, with colicine V. *J. Gen. Microbiol.* **83**:95–111.

104. **Sowers, E. G., J. G. Wells, and N. A. Strockbine.** 1996. Evaluation of commercial latex reagents for identification of O157 and H7 antigens of *Escherichia coli. J. Clin. Microbiol.* **34**:1286–1289.

105. **Stavric, S., B. Buchanan, and J. Speirs.** 1992. Comparison of a competitive enzyme immunoassay kit and the infant mouse assay for detecting *Escherichia coli* heat-stable enterotoxin. *Lett. Appl. Microbiol.* **14**:47–50.

106. **Strockbine, N. A., J. Parsonnet, K. Greene, J. A. Kiehlbauch, and I. K Wachsmuth.** 1991. Molecular epidemiologic techniques in analysis of epidemic and endemic *Shigella dysenteriae* type 1 strains. *J. Infect. Dis.* **163**:406–409.

107. **Strockbine, N. A., J. G. Wells, C. A. Bopp, and T. J. Barrett.** 1998. Overview of detection and subtyping methods, p. 331–356. *In* J. B. Kaper and A. D. O'Brien (ed.), *Escherichia coli O157:H7 and Other Shiga Toxin-Producing E. coli strains.* ASM Press, Washington, D.C.

108. **Subcommittee of the PHLS Advisory Committee on Gastrointestinal Infections.** 2000. Guidelines for the control of infection with Vero cytotoxin producing *Escherichia coli* (VTEC). *Commun. Dis. Public Health* **3**:14–23.

109. **Sugiyama, K., K. Inoue, and R. Sakazaki.** 2001. Mitomycin-supplemented washed blood agar for the isolation of Shiga toxin-producing *Escherichia coli* other than O157:H7. *Lett. Appl. Microbiol.* **33**:193–195.

110. **Swaminathan, B., T. J. Barrett, S. B. Hunter, and R. V. Tauxe.** 2001. PulseNet: the molecular subtyping network for foodborne bacterial disease surveillance, United States. *Emerg. Infect. Dis.* **7**:382–389.

111. **Szych, J., A. Cieslik, J. Paciorek, and S. Kaluzewski.** 2001. Antibiotic resistance in *Salmonella enterica* subsp. enterica strains isolated in Poland from 1998 to 1999. *Int. J. Antimicrob. Agents* **18**:37–42.

112. **Tauxe, R. V., N. D. Puhr, J. G. Wells, N. Hargrett-Bean, and P. A. Blake.** 1990. Antimicrobial resistance of *Shigella* isolates in the USA: the importance of international travelers. *J. Infect. Dis.* **162**:1107–1111.

113. **Thomas, A., H. Chart, T. Cheasty, H. R. Smith, J. A. Frost, and B. Rowe.** 1993. Vero cytotoxin-producing *Escherichia coli*, particularly serogroup O157, associated with human infections in the United Kingdom: 1989–91. *Epidemiol. Infect.* **110**:591–600.

114. **Threlfall, E. J., and J. A. Frost.** 1990. The identification, typing, and fingerprinting of *Salmonella*: laboratory aspects and epidemiological applications. *J. Appl. Bacteriol.* **68**:5–16.

115. **Threlfall, E. J., and L. R. Ward.** 2001. Decreased susceptibility to ciprofloxacin in *Salmonella enterica* serotype Typhi, United Kingdom. *Emerg. Infect. Dis.* **7**:448–450.

116. **Van Looveren, M., M. L. Chasseur-Libotte, C. Godard, C. Lammens, M. Wijdooghe, L. Peeters, and H. Goossens.** 2001. Antimicrobial susceptibility of nontyphoidal *Salmonella* isolated from humans in Belgium. *Acta Clin. Belg.* **56**:180–186.

117. **Verbrugh, H. A., D. R. Mekkes, R. P. Verkoyen, and J. E. Landbeer.** 1987. Widal type serology using live antigen for diagnosis of *Shigella flexneri* dysentery. *Eur. J. Clin. Microbiol. Infect. Dis.* **5**:540–542.

118. **Wathen-Grady, H. G., B. R. Davis, and G. K. Marris.** 1985. Addition of three new serotypes of *Shigella boydii* to the *Shigella* schema. *J. Clin. Microbiol.* **21**:129–132.

119. **Wathen-Grady, H. G., L. E. Britt, N. A. Strockbine, and I. K. Wachsmuth.** 1990. Characterization of *Shigella dysenteriae* serotypes 11, 12, and 13. *J. Clin. Microbiol.* **28**:2580–2584.

120. **Yam, W. C., M. L. Lung, and M. H. Ng.** 1992. Evaluation and optimization of a latex agglutination assay for detection of cholera toxin and Escherichia coli heat-labile toxin. *J. Clin. Microbiol.* **30**:2518–2520.

121. **Zadik, P. M., P. A. Chapman, and C. A. Siddons.** 1993. Use of tellurite for the selection of verocytotoxigenic *Escherichia coli* O157. *J. Med. Microbiol.* **39**:155–158.

Yersinia*

JOCHEN BOCKEMÜHL AND JANE D. WONG

43

TAXONOMY

In 1944, Van Loghem proposed the transfer of *Pasteurella pestis* and *Pasteurella pseudotuberculosis* to his newly defined genus *Yersinia*, named after Alexandre Yersin, who had first isolated the plague bacillus in 1894. In 1964, Frederiksen further included *Pasteurella* X (syn. *Bacterium enterocoliticum*) which previously had been described by Schleifstein and Coleman.

Following intensive taxonomic studies in the 1980s, the genus *Yersinia* at present includes 10 established species: *Yersinia pestis*, *Y. pseudotuberculosis*, *Y. enterocolitica*, *Y. frederiksenii*, *Y. intermedia*, *Y. kristensenii*, *Y. bercovieri*, *Y. mollaretii*, *Y. rohdei*, and *Y. aldovae*. The taxonomic status of "*Y.*" *ruckeri*, a fish pathogen, is still uncertain. *Y. pestis*, *Y. pseudotuberculosis*, and certain strains of *Y. enterocolitica* are of pathogenic importance for humans and certain warm-blooded animals, whereas the other species are of environmental origin and, according to present knowledge, may at best act as opportunists. However, they are frequently isolated from clinical materials and therefore must be identified to the species level.

Members of the genus *Yersinia* exhibit 10 to 32% relatedness to other members of the family *Enterobacteriaceae* by DNA-DNA hybridization. The DNA G+C content of the genus is in the range of 46.0 to 48.5 mol%. Based on DNA-DNA hybridization, *Y. enterocolitica* exhibits 43 to 64% relatedness to *Y. pestis* and *Y. pseudotuberculosis* (20). The genetic difference between *Y. pestis* and *Y. pseudotuberculosis*, on the other hand, is on the subspecies level and would taxonomically justify the inclusion of both into one species (1, 3).

DESCRIPTION OF THE GENUS

Members of the genus *Yersinia* are non-spore-forming, gram-negative, rod-shaped or coccoid cells 0.5 to 0.8 μm in width and 1 to 3 μm in length. Except for *Y. pestis*, which is nonmotile, the other species are motile at 22 to 30°C but not at 37°C; motile cells are peritrichously flagellated (36). Yersiniae grow under aerobic and anaerobic culture condi-

tions between 0 and 45°C, with an optimum at 25 to 28°C, on nonselective and certain selective media. Only *Y. pestis* has special nutritional requirements for L-valine, L-methionine, L-phenylalanine, and glycine or L-threonine. These requirements limit its survival outside the mammalian or flea host.

Glucose is fermentatively utilized, with the formation of acid; gas and hydrogen sulfide are not produced. There is no growth in the presence of KCN. Phenylalanine and tryptophan are not deaminated, gelatin is not liquified, lysine is not decarboxylated, and arginine is not dehydrolyzed. Nitrate is reduced to nitrite, catalase is produced, but oxidase is absent. Acetoin is produced at 25 to 28°C (not at 37°C) by most strains of *Y. enterocolitica*, *Y. frederiksenii*, *Y. intermedia*, and *Y. aldovae* but not by the remaining *Yersinia* species. With the exception of *Y. pestis*, urease is produced at 25 to 28°C. Ornithine is decarboxylated by all the species but *Y. pestis* and *Y. pseudotuberculosis* (Table 1).

Virulence Factors of Pathogenic *Yersinia*

Y. pestis, *Y. pseudotuberculosis*, and the pathogenic bioserotypes of *Y. enterocolitica* have the same basic virulence mechanisms, although their routes of invasion as well as the clinical symptoms that they cause are different. A majority of the genes involved in pathogenicity are located on virulence plasmids, although some are chromosomally determined. Virulence factors and their genes have been used for both phenotypic and genotypic detection of pathogenic strains in clinical specimens. Furthermore, they have proved useful for the differentiation of pathogenic and nonpathogenic strains, especially of *Y. enterocolitica*, in which both occur naturally. The major virulence genes of *Yersinia* and their gene products are listed in Table 2.

The three pathogenic species share a 70- to 75-kb plasmid carrying a number of genes which are especially important for *Y. enterocolitica* and *Y. pseudotuberculosis*. They encode a number of proteins (*Yersinia* outer proteins [Yops]) with antiphagocytic properties, which are secreted and translocated by a type III secretion system (13, 45). Loss of the plasmid results in decreased pathogenicity and an inability to cause disseminated disease.

In addition, *Y. pestis* contains two plasmids absent from *Y. enterocolitica* and *Y. pseudotuberculosis*. The 9.5-kb plasmid encodes plasminogen activator (Pla) and the bacteriocin pesticin (Pst). The 110-kb plasmid encodes murine

* This chapter contains information presented in chapter 30 by Stojanka Aleksic and Jochen Bockemühl in the seventh edition of this Manual.

TABLE 1 Biochemical differentiation of Yersinia species after incubation at 25°C for 48 h[a]

Yersinia species	Reaction[b]										
	Motility	Urease	Voges-Proskauer	Indole	Citrate (Simmons)	Ornithine	Sucrose	Rhamnose	Cellobiose	Melibiose	Sorbose
Y. pestis	−	−	−	−	−	−	−	−	−	d	−
Y. pseudotuberculosis	+	+	−	−	−	−	−	+	−	+	−
Y. enterocolitica	+	+	+	d	−	+	+	−	+	−	d
Y. intermedia	+	+	+	+	+	+	+	+	+	+	+
Y. frederiksenii	+	+	+	+	d	+	+	+	+	−	+
Y. kristensenii	+	+	−	d	−	+	−	−	+	−	+
Y. aldovae	+	+	+	−	d	+	−	+	−	−	−
Y. rohdei[c]	+	d[d]	−	−	+	+	+	−	+	d	+
Y. mollaretii[e]	+	+	−	−	−	+	+	−	+	−	+
Y. bercovieri[e]	+	+	−	−	−	+	+	−	+	−	−

[a] Modified from references 2 and 36 and from our own unpublished data.
[b] +, ≥90% of strains positive; d, 11 to 89% of strains positive; −, ≥90% of strains negative.
[c] For Y. rohdei biotype 1, melibiose positive and raffinose positive; for Y. rohdei biotype 2, melibiose negative and raffinose negative.
[d] Delayed, positive after 7 days.
[e] For fucose (acid production), Y. mollaretii is negative and Y. bercovieri is positive.

toxin (Ymt) and the structural gene for the fraction 1 (F1) protein capsule. Recently, Hinnebusch et al. (34) have shown that the 70-kb plasmid that is required to produce disease in mammals is not required for Y. pestis to infect and block the proventriculus of the flea. Those investigators suggest that the 110-kb plasmid may contain genes important for producing disease in both the mammal and the flea, while the 9.5-kb and the 70-kb plasmids are required to produce disease only in the mammal.

Chromosomally encoded virulence factors of Y. enterocolitica and Y. pseudotuberculosis include Inv (invasin) and Ail (attachment-invasion locus); both of these are adhesins and support translocation of the organisms across the epithelial barrier via the phagocytic M cells. The high-pathogenicity island, present in Y. pestis, Y. pseudotuberculosis, and strains of biogroup 1B of Y. enterocolitica, harbors the genes for a siderophore named yersiniabactin which provides iron to the bacterial cells and increases pathogenicity (54). In Y. pestis, an important gene locus termed hsm (pgm) carries the genes for a hemin storage system (Hms) which is essential for the blockage of the flea proventriculus (34, 35). The role of a thermostable enterotoxin produced by pathogenic strains of Y. enterocolitica is still under discussion, although a clinical association has been suggested (17).

NATURAL HABITATS

Y. pestis

Rodents are the natural reservoir of the plague bacteria. Transmission in these populations occurs mainly via their fleas but occasionally also by direct contact and cannibalism. Each mammalian species tends to support its own flea species, and at least 80 species are involved in transmitting Y. pestis (33, 52). The Oriental rat flea, Xenopsylla cheopis, is considered the classic and most effective vector of plague. Oropsylla montana, the flea of ground squirrels (Spermophilus lateralis and Spermophilus beecheyi), is an important vector in California. The flea of the prairie dogs (Cynomys spp.), Oropsylla hirsuta, is important in New Mexico, as are the fleas of rock squirrels (Spermophilus variegatus), Oropsylla montana, and Hoplopsyllus anomalus. Arizona and Colorado, too, harbor endemic vector populations.

Transmission of plague from a flea to a mammal depends on blockage of the flea proventriculus (part of the foregut) by a mass of Y. pestis cells. Blockage is dependent upon synthesis of proteins encoded by the hms locus on the chromosome, which is induced at 26 to 30°C. "Blocked fleas" cannot pump blood into their stomachs and will repeatedly bite the host mammal in a futile attempt to feed; their life spans are reduced due to starvation. Blockage of the proventriculus in fleas thus supports transmission of the organisms to the mammalian host (35). A flea ingests 0.03 to 0.5 μl of blood (33) during a blood meal. This small amount of blood must contain large amounts of plague bacteria for blockage to occur. Thus, to maintain a natural transmission cycle in nature, the mammalian host must have a high level of bacteremia.

More than 200 mammalian species have been reported to be naturally infected with Y. pestis; however, rodents are of principal importance. Highly susceptible hosts include various species of mice, rats, voles, gerbils, ground squirrels, rabbits, and prairie dogs. If such susceptible populations migrate into areas occupied by infected species, this may be followed by dramatic increases in mortality and decimation of the invaders. Their fleas then search for new hosts, including humans, and transmit the disease. Such epizootic outbreaks have occurred in the past and were the cause of many of the large classical epidemics. Today, plague is more or less confined to endemic foci in Africa, the Americas, and Asia, where local epidemics or increased incidences may occur. In the United States, domestic cats repeatedly have been infected, and this mode of infection has caused 23 of the 297 human cases (7.7%) from 1977 to 1998 (24). Five of these cases (22%) presented as primary pneumonic plague; this is significant from a public health perspective, since unrecognized primary pneumonic plague poses a significant threat of spreading rapidly through a population.

Cats are likely to be exposed by ingesting Y. pestis-infected rodents rather than by flea bites. The cat flea, Ctenocephalides felis, is a very poor plague vector (51). Humans who contract plague from cats are either scratched or bitten or have inhaled respiratory secretions directly from cats. Veterinarians, in particular those in Arizona, California, Colorado, and New Mexico, should be aware of

TABLE 2 Virulence genes of pathogenic *Yersinia* with emphasis on their diagnostic use

Yersinia species	Gene(s)	Genetic location	Gene product	Function	Expression	Diagnostic use (reference[s])
Y. pestis	*caf1*	Plasmid, 110 kb	F1 capsular protein	Antiphagocytic	37°C	Fluorescent staining with FITC[a] conjugate, serology tests; PCR, detection of pathogenic strains (10, 50, 53, 55)
Y. pestis	*ymt*	Plasmid, 110 kb	Murine toxin protein	Phospholipase D; erythrocyte lysis in flea proventriculus	30°C	
Y. pestis	*pla*	Plasmid, 9.5 kb	Plasminogen activator (outer surface protease)	Fibrinolysis	37°C	PCR, detection of pathogenic strains (34, 50)
				Coagulase	28°C	
Y. pestis	*hms*	Chromosome	Hemin storage protein	Iron or hemin binding, flea blockage	26 to 30°C	Congo red or hemin binding (39, 63)
Y. pestis	*psaA*	Chromosome	pH 6 antigen	Fimbrial structural component	37°C (low pH)	
Y. enterocolitica, Y. pseudotuberculosis, Y. pestis	HPI[b] (*ybt*)	Chromosome	Yersiniabactin (siderophore)	Iron uptake	37°C	Pesticin sensitivity; siderophore production; Congo red phenotype (51)
Y. enterocolitica, Y. pseudotuberculosis	*invA*	Chromosome	Invasin	Adhesin	26°C (pH 8); 37°C (low pH)	PCR, detection of pathogenic strains (48)
Y. enterocolitica, Y. pseudotuberculosis	*ail*	Chromosome	Attachment-invasion-locus protein (Ail)	Adhesin	37°C	PCR, detection of pathogenic strains (22, 40)
Y. enterocolitica	*yst*	Chromosome	Heat-stable enterotoxin	Enterotoxin	26°C	Colony blot, detection of *Y. enterocolitica* (19), species specific
Y. enterocolitica, Y. pseudotuberculosis, Y. pestis	*virF*	Plasmid, 70 kb	VirF protein	Transcriptional activator for expression of Yops	37°C	PCR, detection of pathogenic strains (21, 71)
Y. enterocolitica, Y. pseudotuberculosis	*yadA*	Plasmid, 70 kb	Membrane protein with lollipop-shaped surface projection	Adhesion to cells and extracellular matrix proteins	37°C	Autoagglutination test; PCR, detection of pathogenic strains (42, 43, 44)
Y. enterocolitica, Y. pseudotuberculosis, Y. pestis	*yop* genes	Plasmid, 70 kb	Yops, secreted and translocated by type III secretion apparatus	Antiphagocytic	37°C	Detection of class-specific serum antibodies against YopB, YopD, YopE, YopH, YopM, and LcrV in yersiniosis (30, 60)
Y. enterocolitica, Y. pseudotuberculosis, Y. pestis	*ysc* (*lcr*)	Plasmid, 70 kb	Proteins of type III secretion apparatus	Effectors of Yop secretion	37°C	

[a] FITC, fluorescein isothiocyanate.
[b] HPI, high-pathogenicity island.

this risk to their patients, their patients' owners, and themselves.

Plague Pandemics

Plague is one of the oldest recorded infectious diseases. A recent study on the population genetic structure of *Y. pestis* suggests that the plague bacterium emerged 1,500 to 20,000 years ago as a clone that evolved from *Y. pseudotuberculosis* and that first caused outbreaks in Africa (1).

More than 150 epidemics, most of them associated with three main pandemics, have been reported. It has been hypothesized that the first (A.D. 541 to 544), second (A.D. 1330 to 1480), and third (A.D. 1885) pandemics were caused by three different but genetically constant biotypes of *Y. pestis*, i.e., biotypes Antiqua, Medievalis, and Orientalis, respectively (18). These historically and epidemiologically combined data were recently substantiated by Achtmann et al. (1) who developed a phylogenetic tree based on the chromosomal locations of the insertion element IS100. Those investigators showed that strains of biotype Antiqua continue to be isolated in central and east Africa, the supposed origin of the first pandemic wave; that biotype Medievalis continues to be isolated in Kurdistan, where the second pandemic wave passed through; and that biotype Orientalis is still isolated in most of the countries to which isolates were imported as a result of marine shipping at the end of the 19th century.

Between 1985 and 1999, 23 countries reported a total of 29,020 cases of plague to the World Health Organization, showing an increasing trend of morbidity with an average fatality rate of about 11% (70). Major epidemics and outbreaks in Tanzania (1991), Zaire (1992 to 1993), Peru (1993 to 1994), India (1994), and Madagascar (1995) with fatality rates of 4.6 to 22.3% have demonstrated that plague is far from being eradicated.

Enteropathogenic and Nonpathogenic *Yersinia* Species

Y. enterocolitica and *Y. pseudotuberculosis* are distributed worldwide but occur mainly in the moderate and subtropical climatic areas of the Americas; Europe; north, central, and east Asia; South Africa; and Australia. On the other hand, they are rare or lacking in the tropical regions of Africa and Southeast Asia.

Y. pseudotuberculosis is found in numerous wild and domestic mammals as well as birds. Outbreaks occur mainly in captive rodent populations (animals involved in fur farming and experimental animals), zoo animals, poultry farms (turkeys, ducks, and pigeons), and pet-bird breeding facilities. The disease may vary from acute septicemia to a subacute or chronic course with fever, weakness, diarrhea, respiratory disorders, and paralysis. In wild, domestic, and pet animals, sporadic cases of pseudotuberculosis or asymptomatic infections prevail. The main reservoirs of *Y. pseudotuberculosis* are rodents (mice and rats), lagomorphs (hares and rabbits), and wild birds. The organisms survive for prolonged periods in soil and river water (23).

Y. enterocolitica has a wide distribution and can be found in humans; in all warm-blooded wild, domestic, and pet animals; and occasionally, in or on reptiles, fish, and shellfish. The organisms are also isolated from food, soil, and surface water. Pigs are important reservoirs for human-pathogenic serogroups O:3 and O:9; the organisms especially colonize pigs' tonsils. Only certain serogroups are obligatory pathogens for animals; these include O:1,2a,3 (biotype 3) and O:2a,2b,3 (biotype 5) for chinchillas, hares,

rabbits, cattle, sheep, and goats. These serogroups occasionally have also caused disease in humans. The remaining serotypes, including the human pathogens, frequently colonize animals but do not cause disease.

Whereas the nonpathogenic serotypes of *Y. enterocolitica* biotype 1A (Table 3) apparently are able to propagate independently in the environment, this is less likely for the pathogenic serotypes; however, pathogenic serotypes may survive for prolonged periods outside their hosts. Thus, contaminated surface water, soil, and vegetation may become sources for infections of humans and animals.

Y. frederiksenii, *Y. kristensenii*, *Y. intermedia*, *Y. rohdei*, *Y. aldovae*, *Y. mollaretii*, and *Y. bercovieri* are primarily environmental organisms but occasionally colonize warm- and cold-blooded hosts in a transient manner. *Y. mollaretii*, *Y. intermedia*, *Y. bercovieri*, and *Y. kristensenii* seem to be especially adapted to the aquatic environment. "*Y.*" *ruckeri* is a fish pathogen which causes red mouth disease.

CLINICAL SIGNIFICANCE

Y. pestis (Plague)

The clinical course of plague in animals and humans is similar. Following infection by a flea or animal bite or via otherwise injured skin or mucous membrane, the organisms must disseminate rapidly. This might be supported by the *pla* gene product, a cell surface protease which activates plasminogen and thus promotes fibrinolysis at the site of infection. It has been hypothesized that this protease further interferes with the alternative pathway of complement activation, followed by reduced chemoattraction of polymorphonuclear neutrophils (59). Thus, abscess formation and localization of the infection are inhibited, and the organisms may be spread and transported to the nearest lymph node. Once they are ingested by macrophages, the *Y. pestis* organisms survive and proliferate to high numbers due to their production of antiphagocytic and toxic outer proteins (Yops) and the capsular F1 protein.

An intense inflammatory response produces the characteristic swelling or "bubo" which gives bubonic plague its name. Depending on the immunity of the host, bacteria leaking into the bloodstream may cause a secondary septicemia and be transported to various organs. This stage of the disease, septicemic plague, may be followed by menin-

TABLE 3 Biotypes of *Y. enterocolitica*[a] after incubation at 25°C for 48 h

Test	Reaction[b] for biotype:					
	1A	1B	2	3	4	5
Lipase (Tween esterase)	+	+	−	−	−	−
Esculin	+	−	−	−	−	−
Salicin	+	−	−	−	−	−
Indole	+	+	(+)	−	−	−
Xylose	+	+	+	+	−	d
Trehalose	+	+	+	+	+	−
NO$_3$ → NO$_2$	+	+	+	+	+	−
DNase	−	−	−	−	+	+
Pyrazinamidase[c]	+	−	−	−	−	−

[a] Modified from reference 67 with permission of the publisher S. Karger AG, Basel, Switzerland.
[b] +, ≥90% of strains positive; d, 11 to 89% of strains positive; −, ≥90% of strains negative; (+), weakly positive reaction.
[c] According to Kandolo and Wauters (41).

gitis or pneumonia when the organisms parasitize the alveolar macrophages. Patients suffering from pneumonic plague can transmit Y. pestis via aerosols to other persons. The resulting form of primary pneumonia is usually followed by a very acute course, since Y. pestis acquired from another human already expresses all the virulence factors required for the disease. Patients with plague often develop necrotic lesions in the peripheral blood vessels, giving the skin a blackish coloration which, in the past, led to the name "black death" (58). Human plague can thus be classified into three general syndromes, i.e., bubonic plague, primary and secondary septicemic plague, and primary and secondary pneumonic plague (15, 51).

Highly susceptible animal species usually develop acute to subacute septicemic plague with necrosis or necrotic nodules in the lymph nodes, liver, and spleen; they succumb to the infection within approximately 6 days. Cats typically develop acute febrile illness, followed by bacteremia, pneumonia, and buboes. They die within 6 to 20 days (26); the histopathology is similar to that described for human plague (66). More resistant animal species experience bubonic plague characterized by lymphadenopathy with purulent focal necrosis.

Plague induces a long-lasting immunity, which, however, is not absolute (6). Two types of vaccine have been developed; one is derived from an attenuated, Hsm (Pgm)-deficient strain (live vaccine [Institut Pasteur, Paris, France]). Madagascar, China, Russia, and Kazakhstan still manufacture a live attenuated vaccine. The other consists of a formalin-inactivated whole-cell preparation from a virulent strain of Y. pestis (47). The United States no longer manufactures this vaccine, but Australia, Great Britain, and India still do. Although controlled field trials are lacking, the latter proved to have a certain effectiveness in soldiers exposed to virulent plague bacteria during the Vietnam War (47). The protection is variable and particularly low against the pneumonic form. Vaccination is therefore limited to certain conditions such as staff working with virulent Y. pestis cultures or military personnel operating in areas where the infection is endemic.

Y. pestis belongs to the group of microorganisms that might be misused as a biological weapon. The most threatening form would be the application of aerosolized plague bacteria. It has been estimated that, in a worst-case scenario, 50 kg of aerosolized Y. pestis released over a city of 5 million inhabitants could cause pneumonic plague in up to 150,000 persons, 36,000 of whom would die. The agents would remain viable as an aerosol for 1 h for a distance of up to 10 km (38). If Y. pestis was used as a biological weapon, the epidemiology would differ substantially from that of naturally occurring infection, in that the release of the organism for this purpose would primarily cause the pneumonic form of the disease (38).

Y. enterocolitica, Y. pseudotuberculosis, and Nonpathogenic Species

Infections due to Y. enterocolitica and Y. pseudotuberculosis may be acquired by ingestion of contaminated food or water or, rarely, by direct person-to-person transmission, e.g., in kindergartens, schools, or hospitals. Y. enterocolitica is a common cause of human infection, whereas Y. pseudotuberculosis is primarily an animal pathogen. The incubation period varies between 4 and 7 days in Y. enterocolitica and is unknown for Y. pseudotuberculosis (6).

Both species have an affinity for the lymphoid tissue and penetrate into the ileal mucosa via the M cells of Peyer's patches. From the basolateral site they invade the intestinal epithelial cells. However, more important is the successful elimination of the phagocytes, which they effect with the aid of secreted outer proteins (Yops) in a three-step interaction (57). The first step is the paralysis of the phagocytic machinery by injecting a set of effector proteins by use of a type III secretion system. These proteins inhibit several eukaryotic signal transduction pathways and thus effectively counteract internalization of the bacteria. The second step includes the suppression of tumor necrosis factor alpha production in macrophages, impeding the recognition of bacterial lipopolysaccharide and suppressing the immune response. The third step finally leads to induction of apoptosis and cell death in macrophages. Thus, pathogenic yersiniae may spread and penetrate into the lymph nodes, where they multiply. The inflammatory response causes pain in the lower abdominal region, which is a typical symptom and which may be mistaken for appendicitis.

Intestinal yersiniosis may present in three clinical forms: enteritis, terminal ileitis or mesenteric lymphadenitis causing "pseudoappendicitis," and septicemia (4). Watery, sometimes bloody stools are characteristic of Y. enterocolitica infection but are rarely caused by Y. pseudotuberculosis. Bloody diarrhea is observed mainly in adults and less frequently in children; and it is often accompanied by fever, vomiting, and, typically, abdominal pain. Terminal ileitis, mesenteric lymphadenitis, and pseudoappendicitis may also be produced by Y. enterocolitica; but these are the characteristic symptoms in Y. pseudotuberculosis infection that are especially common in children older than 5 years and adolescents. Whereas adults usually overcome intestinal yersiniosis within 1 to 2 weeks, disease in children may last for up to 4 weeks (4).

Septicemia is a rare event that occurs in adults, mostly in association with severe underlying disease. The clinical course may include focal abscesses in the liver and spleen, pneumonia, septic arthritis, meningitis, endocarditis, osteomyelitis, and development of a mycotic aneurysm (4). Although rare, an asymptomatic bacteremia may occur in healthy children. A special case is septicemia in patients who have iron overload due to hemolytic anemia (thalassemia, sickle cell disease, or aplastic anemia) or who are undergoing therapeutic application of iron compounds. Siderophore (yersiniabactin)-producing strains of Y. enterocolitica serogroups O:8, O:13a,13b, and O:20 have been isolated from patients with hemolytic anemia, whereas the non-siderophore-producing strains of serogroups O:3, O:5,27, and O:9 are associated with iron compound treatment (11, 31).

Yersinia is one of a few organisms associated with transfusion-related septicemia because of its ability to multiply at 4°C. Since the mid-1970s, septicemia caused by transfusion of contaminated blood and blood products has been noted worldwide (4, 7). Amazingly, in all reported cases, only non-siderophore-producing serogroups O:3, O:9, O:5,27, and O:1,2a,3 have been recovered from blood specimens. Serogroup O:8 has not been isolated; it was shown that O:8 more readily loses serum resistance at 4°C than the other pathogenic serogroups do (5).

Following intestinal infection by both Y. enterocolitica and Y. pseudotuberculosis, immunologically mediated extraintestinal disease develops in some patients, particularly those who display histocompatibility antigen HLA-B27. These sequelae primarily include reactive arthritis and, rarely, myocarditis, glomerulonephritis, thyroiditis, and erythema nodosum. They usually have a favorable prognosis, but they may last for years. In patients who develop reactive arthritis, antigens of the causative agents, such as the lipopolysaccharides and the *Yersinia* heat shock protein, but not living *Yersinia* or their DNA, have been shown to persist for years in the inflamed joints, where they consecutively trigger a local T- and B-cell response (27). Furthermore, it has been reported that certain *Yersinia* antigens show similarities to host antigens of the joints and to thyroid epithelial cells, causing antibodies to bacterial surface structures to cross-react with the host tissue (64). Concomitantly, elevated concentrations of *Yersinia*-specific immunoglobulin A (IgA) antibodies in serum have regularly been demonstrated, suggesting that the triggering organisms are not efficiently eliminated but persist, probably in the intestinal mucosa or the mesenteric lymph nodes (16, 27). It appears likely that microbial debris from the intestinal region is transported by blood circulation into the joints since structures of *Yersinia* cells have been demonstrated in peripheral blood phagocytes from arthritis patients for up to 4 years (27). Interestingly, postinfective sequelae have mainly been reported from Europe in association with Y. enterocolitica serogroup O:3 and O:9 infections, but they are rare in the United States (4).

Y. kristensenii, Y. intermedia, Y. mollaretii, Y. bercovieri, Y. frederiksenii, and Y. rohdei are frequently isolated from clinical materials. A specific pathogenic potential has not been established for these organisms, although a novel heat-stable enterotoxin (YbST) has recently been described in two strains of Y. bercovieri (62). The role of these *Yersinia* species in opportunistic infections of immunocompromised hosts has yet to be elucidated.

COLLECTION, TRANSPORT, AND STORAGE OF SPECIMENS

Safety Procedures

Local and state health authorities must be immediately notified of suspected and presumptive cases of plague. Furthermore, plague is notifiable to the World Health Organization according to the International Health Regulations. Standard bacteriological practices of biosafety level 2 are usually sufficient for clinical laboratories handling Y. pestis, but special precautions must be used if aerosols are produced or deceased animals are handled. Such activities, as well as procedures with cultures of Y. pestis, can be performed in a biological safety cabinet with biosafety level 3 practices (9) (see chapters 3 and 9).

If Y. pestis was not expected but is discovered in the course of examination, the activities must be stopped. The isolate should be preserved for further identification and susceptibility testing in a biological safety cabinet, and all remaining culture materials should be destroyed by autoclaving. The laboratory bench and equipment used for handling of the material must be disinfected. Laboratory personnel must be informed of possible clinical symptoms and are obligated to immediately report any signs of disease. If infection cannot be ruled out, prophylaxis with orally administered doxycycline or ciprofloxacin may be considered.

Specimen Collection and Transport

In humans, Y. pestis can be isolated from blood (see chapters 6 and 20), by bubo aspiration (obtained by injection of 1 ml of sterile saline and immediate aspiration), from spu-

tum, from throat swabs or throat washings, from skin swabs or scrapings, and from cerebrospinal fluid in patients with meningitis. At autopsy, blood and tissue specimens from the buboes, liver, spleen, and lungs should be collected.

In areas of endemicity, rodent carcasses are tested for surveillance purposes. Sick cats that may have been exposed to the plague bacterium should be tested as well. Living or dead animals should be treated with an insecticide before specimens are collected; fleas are collected for bacteriological examination. Blood from the heart and tissue specimens from the lymph nodes, liver, spleen, and other organs are collected; bone marrow and brain tissue are appropriate specimens from decaying cadavers. Y. pestis may even be isolated 1 to 2 months postmortem if the material is inoculated into mice, rats, or guinea pigs. Cary-Blair or Stuart's medium is a suitable transport medium for swabs.

Isolation of Y. enterocolitica and Y. pseudotuberculosis is attempted from stool specimens in patients with intestinal disease; from blood in patients with septicemia; and from lymph nodes, intestinal tissue, or pus if abdominal surgery or a biopsy has been performed. Feces, mesenteric and pharyngeal lymphatic tissue, abscess material, or nodules in the liver and spleen are collected from animals. Examination of food and water may be useful for epidemiological reasons; local public health authorities should assist with such studies.

In the late stage of the disease (2 or more weeks after onset), if antibiotics have been administered or if appropriate material cannot be recovered for culture, serum specimens should be taken for detection of specific antibodies against the three pathogenic *Yersinia* species. For transport and storage of suspected clinical specimens or cultures of *Yersinia* species, the general principles described in chapter 20 are applicable.

DIRECT DETECTION AND ISOLATION PROCEDURES

Y. pestis

Microscopy after Giemsa, Wright, Wayson, or methylene blue staining (see chapter 27) may be helpful; a typical appearance after staining is supportive but not confirmatory. Y. pestis organisms present in clinical material commonly display bipolarity and resemble safety pins due to retention of stain by the cytoplasm (Fig. 1); this morphology is not displayed by Gram staining or in cultured organisms.

Direct microscopic detection of the capsular F1 antigen in clinical specimens can be attempted by use of a fluorescent-antibody stain. The fluorescent-antibody reagent is not commercially available, but testing can be performed at state health department laboratories, as well as some city and county laboratories. Contact your state health department laboratory for instructions.

The capsular F1 antigen is expressed mainly at 37°C. Samples that have been refrigerated for more than 30 h, cells from cultures incubated below 35°C, or extracts from fleas will be negative (51). A positive fluorescent F1 antigen test result may be taken as confirmatory evidence of Y. pestis infection.

PCR (50) with primers derived from the *pla* (plasminogen activator protein) and *caf1* (capsular F1 antigen) genes, which are harbored by two different Y. pestis virulence plasmids, is a rapid and sensitive method for the presumptive diagnosis of plague in clinical specimens or fleas. However, the method has not yet been sufficiently validated and

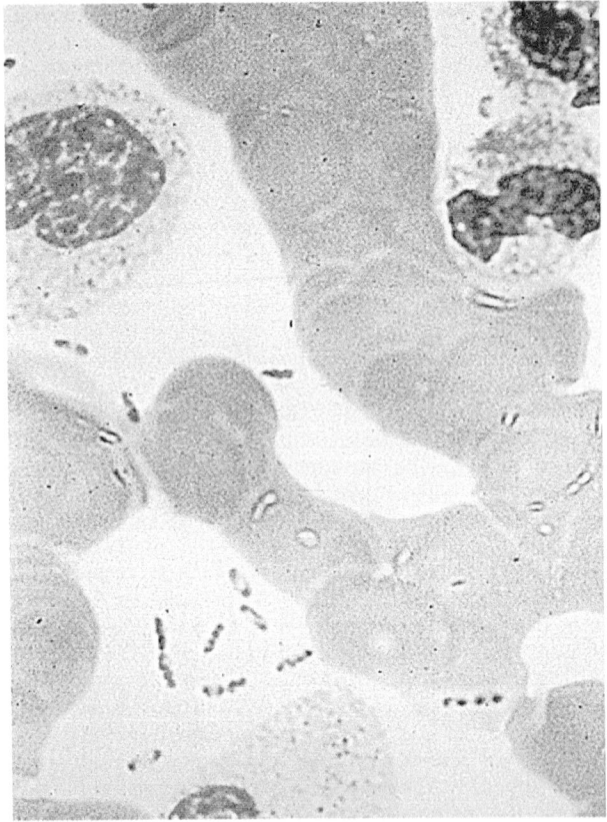

FIGURE 1 Wayson stain of *Y. pestis* in blood (courtesy of CDC).

showed a lower sensitivity compared to those of culture and an enzyme-linked immunosorbent assay (ELISA) for the capsular F1 antigen in a field trial in Madagascar (53).

Animal testing can be used if heavily contaminated specimens must be examined. Fleas are usually examined by this method. The samples are homogenized in sterile saline, of which 0.1 to 0.2 ml is subcutaneously or intraperitoneally inoculated into mice, rats, or guinea pigs. If virulent *Y. pestis* organisms are present, the animals die within 2 to 6 days and the organisms can be isolated from the blood, liver, and spleen. Again, safety considerations restrict the use of this procedure to specialized laboratories.

Isolation of the organisms in culture is the most certain etiological proof of *Y. pestis* infection. Nonselective media, such as 5% blood agar or brain heart infusion (BHI) agar, can be used for sterile materials such as blood, bubo aspirates, or biopsy specimens. Selective media such as MacConkey agar and cefsulodin-irgasan-novobiocin (CIN) agar with a reduced cefsulodin content (4 μg/ml), which is commercially available, are suitable for contaminated specimens such as sputum and swabs (throat, skin, and organs). Enrichment cultures of sterile specimens should be made in BHI broth. Blood specimens may be enriched in commercial blood culture media. For contaminated materials, MacConkey broth can be used. As a specific selective enrichment medium, CIN broth with 4 μg of cefsulodin per ml may be used. Fluid and plate cultures are incubated at 35°C for 7 days before they are reported as negative.

On all solid media, *Y. pestis* grows as pinpoint colonies after a 24-h incubation at 35°C. The morphology becomes more typical after 48 h, when the organisms are nonhemolytic on blood agar, smooth or mucoid on BHI agar, and lactose negative on MacConkey agar. Larger colonies have irregular edges, demonstrating a hammered-metal appearance under a dissecting microscope. Upon further growth, the centers of the colonies are raised and older colonies often assume a fried-egg configuration (Fig. 2) (12).

Y. enterocolitica, Y. pseudotuberculosis, and Other *Yersinia* Species

Certain chromosomal and plasmid-located virulence genes, such as *invA, ail, yst, yadA,* and *virF,* have been used for the detection of pathogenic *Y. enterocolitica* and *Y. pseudotuberculosis* by PCR and DNA colony blot hybridization (Table 2). These methods, however, are not required in the routine laboratory because isolation of *Y. enterocolitica* and *Y. pseudotuberculosis* usually is not problematic. For patients with chronic infections, however, yersiniae may be difficult to isolate from specimens obtained during surgery, such as organ tissues and lymph nodes. For such situations, in situ

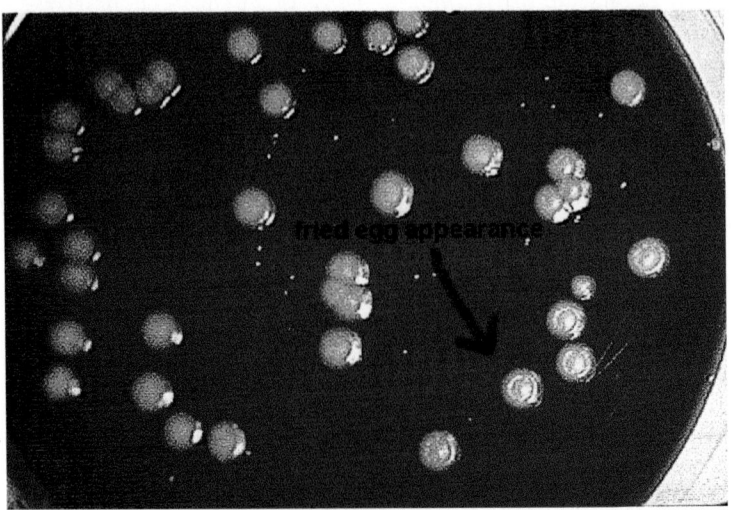

FIGURE 2 Typical fried-egg-shaped colonies of *Y. pestis* on sheep blood agar (courtesy of CDC).

indirect immunofluorescence, an rRNA-targeted PCR, and a fluorescent in situ hybridization method have been recommended (37, 65). Such tests, however, are available only in specialized laboratories.

Enrichment of stool specimens is usually not necessary for patients with diarrhea but is advised for patients with terminal ileitis or postinfectious arthritis without diarrhea, when the number of excreted organisms is low. As a simple and efficient isolation method, cold enrichment in 0.15 M phosphate-buffered saline (pH 7.4) can be used. The cultures are kept at 4°C for up to 21 days with weekly subcultures. However, this method also propagates the nonpathogenic *Yersinia* species, which may overgrow the pathogens or render their identification difficult. Except for cold-enrichment procedures, cultures for intestinal *Yersinia* species should preferably be incubated at 25 to 30°C, which yields better growth than incubation at 35°C. Both species grow well on all nonselective or moderately selective media used for the isolation of members of the family *Enterobacteriaceae*. CIN agar is the best selective agar. This medium is commercially available with different cefsulodin concentrations (4 to 15 µg/ml). We suggest use of the lower concentration, which produces better growth of *Y. enterocolitica* and *Y. pseudotuberculosis* and which also allows the isolation of *Y. pestis* and *Aeromonas* species. Suspected colonies of *Y. enterocolitica* (and *Aeromonas*) are approximately 2 mm in diameter after 48 h at 25 to 30°C. *Y. enterocolitica* is recognized by its red center surrounded by a translucent zone ("bulls-eye"), which is lacking in *Y. pseudotuberculosis*. MacConkey and salmonella-shigella agars may also be used for the isolation of enteropathogenic yersiniae. The organisms grow as lactose-negative, pinpoint or flat colonies 1 mm in diameter after 24 h at 25 to 30°C, depending on the selectivity of the media.

IDENTIFICATION

Yersiniae are metabolically more active at 25 to 30°C than at 35°C. Therefore, incubation at lower temperatures is strongly advised for most biochemical tests and should be used for the reactions listed in Tables 1 and 3. Biochemical reactions for yersiniae at 35°C are shown in Table 1 of chapter 41.

Yersinia spp. are included in the databases of most commercial identification systems, such as Microscan, Vitek, API, Biolog, and BBL Crystal ID (68). In the experience of the California State Department of Health Services, in 60% of human plague cases it was the identification of an organism as *Y. pestis* by one of these systems that first led to a diagnosis of human plague. However, not all differential tests for *Yersinia* spp. summarized in Table 1 are included in these identification systems, which are, furthermore, based on results obtained at 35°C. Slow growth of field strains, especially of *Y. pestis*, in artificial media and a low level of biochemical activity at 35°C may lead to wrong or doubtful identifications, especially in the hands of inexperienced laboratory workers (8, 38, 46, 49). Although most isolates may be correctly identified to the genus level, it is strongly advised to forward suspected *Yersinia* strains to a reference laboratory whenever the laboratory diagnosis does not agree with the clinical picture, when the material from which it had been isolated is unusual, or when the growth appearance in culture is atypical. This is especially true for *Y. pestis*, for which conventional bacteriology is still needed for correct laboratory diagnosis (68).

Y. pestis is identified by the biochemical reactions summarized in Table 1, in conjunction with Table 1 in chapter 41. After 2 to 5 days of incubation at 25 to 30°C, the organisms are nonmotile, ferment glucose without production of gas, and hydrolyze esculin but do not decarboxylate ornithine or hydrolyze urea. In fluid media, they show a stalactitic growth, which sediments after slight shaking. If *Y. pestis* is suspected, notify your state health department laboratory immediately for instructions on forwarding the isolate for further testing.

Y. enterocolitica, *Y. pseudotuberculosis*, and the non-pathogenic *Yersinia* species are characterized by anaerogenic fermentation of glucose and other carbohydrates, urease production, motility below 30°C but not at 35°C, and a lack of phenylalanine deaminase and lysine decarboxylase. However, *Y. enterocolitica* strains produce small gas bubbles of about 2 mm in diameter if they are tested in glucose broth with a Durham tube. Differentiation of the species within the genus *Yersinia* is performed by the tests summarized in Table 1. For further differentiation of related genera, refer to Table 1 in chapter 41.

Strains of *Y. enterocolitica* should be further characterized by their biotypes since strains of biotype 1A are mostly nonpathogenic (Table 3). Positive reactions with salicin and esculin are indicative of this biotype. On the other hand, pathogenic serotypes of *Y. enterocolitica* are associated with biotypes 1B, 2, 3, 4, and 5 (Table 3), which may be helpful if agglutinating sera are not available.

The presence of the 70-kb virulence plasmid and expression of YadA in strains of *Y. enterocolitica* and *Y. pseudotuberculosis* can reliably be determined by the autoagglutination test (43). When the test is positive, parallel cultures in tubes containing methyl red–Voges-Proskauer medium (Bacto MR-VP medium; Difco Laboratories, Becton Dickinson Microbiological Systems, Sparks, Md.) at room temperature and at 37°C show clearing of the medium, with sticky growth agglutinating at the bottom of the tube after 24 to 48 h at 37°C, in contrast to a uniform turbidity at room temperature. Virulence plasmid-negative strains, on the other hand, grow with uniform turbidity at both temperatures (Fig. 3).

The virulence plasmid is easily lost after subculture at 35°C. Virulent strains grown on nutrient agar at 25 to 30°C frequently dissociate into small (plasmid-positive) and large (plasmid-negative) colonies. Less common phenotypic tests for recognizing virulent organisms are the uptake of Congo red at temperatures below 30°C (63) and calcium dependency at 37°C on magnesium oxalate agar (32).

Serotyping of isolates of *Y. enterocolitica* and *Y. pseudotuberculosis* is appropriate for epidemiologic and diagnostic reasons. Enteropathogenic strains of *Y. enterocolitica* fall into a narrow scope of serogroups which are associated with distinct biotypes. Pathogenic serogroups O:8, O:4,32, O:13a,13b, O:18, O:20, and O:21 are found nearly exclusively in the United States; they all belong to biotype 1B (American strains). Worldwide, serogroups O:3 (biotype 4), O:5,27 (biotypes 2 and 3), and O:9 (biotypes 2 and 3) prevail; the first two mentioned are increasingly identified in the United States. Serogroups O:1,2a,3 (biotype 3) and O:2a,2b,3 (biotype 5) are pathogenic for animals and humans but are rarely isolated from patients.

SEROLOGICAL TESTS

The use of paired serum samples taken during the acute and convalescent phases of the disease or at 1- to 2-week

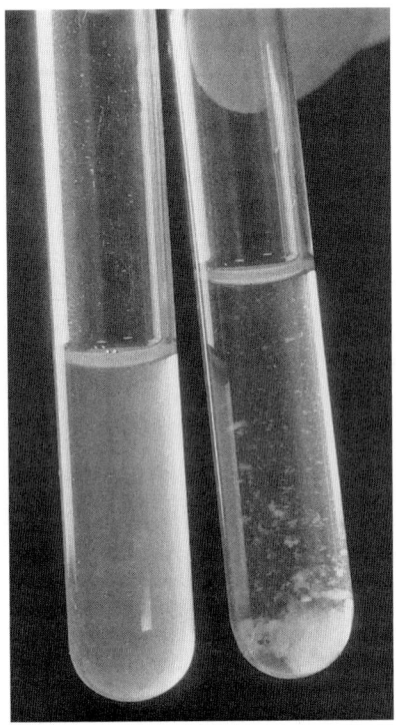

FIGURE 3 Autoagglutination test in MR-VP medium (Difco) after 24 h of incubation at 37°C and slight shaking. Left, virulence plasmid-negative strain of *Y. enterocolitica* O:6,30 (biotype 1A); right, virulence plasmid-positive strain of *Y. enterocolitica* O:3 (biotype 4).

intervals is preferable for serological tests. For the detection of *Y. pestis*, the capsular F1 antigen is the target antigen. The antibody response can be tested by a passive hemagglutination assay or ELISA. A titer of ≥1:10 for antibody directed against the capsular F1 antigen in a validated test system is presumptive, and a fourfold rise or fall of the antibody titer is confirmatory of recent infection in persons who have not previously been infected or vaccinated; these tests are available at the Centers for Disease Control and Prevention (CDC) (51).

Antibodies directed against pathogenic serogroups O:3, O:9, O:5,27, and O:8 of *Y. enterocolitica* can be detected by tube or microtiter agglutination with heated (1 h at 100°C) (O antigens) and formalin-killed (OH antigens) whole-cell preparations in parallel. Agglutination tests for *Y. pseudotuberculosis* are performed with formalin-killed cells (OH antigens). O-antigen titers of ≥1:40 and OH-antigen titers of ≥1:160 or a fourfold rise of the titers in paired serum specimens may be considered confirmatory. It is important to know that *Y. enterocolitica* O:9 and *Brucella* species cross-react with identical titers. Whole-cell antigens absorbed to microtiter wells can be used for separate detection of IgG and IgA antibodies by indirect enzyme immunoassay (28). When performed under standardized conditions, the tests described above are reliable for the diagnosis of intestinal infections (terminal ileitis, lymphadenitis, and pseudoappendicitis). The tests are performed in specialized laboratories; test kits are not commercially available.

Reactive arthritis and other immunologically mediated extraintestinal diseases seem to be especially associated with the formation of IgA antibodies (60). Yops have proved to be very useful for their detection, especially YopD and LcrV (V antigen), but also YopB, YopE, YopH, and YopM. Their isolation from calcium-deficient culture supernatants and subsequent purification by sodium dodecyl sulfate-polyacrylamide gel electrophoresis have been described by Heesemann and coworkers (30). The mixture of purified Yops is immobilized to microtiter wells and tested by indirect ELISA or electroblotted onto nitrocellulose membranes and tested by immunoblotting (Western blotting) analysis. The IgG and IgA classes of antibodies can be tested for separately. The method is highly specific and sufficiently sensitive, and it detects both *Y. enterocolitica* and *Y. pseudotuberculosis* infections. Lipopolysaccharide-mediated cross-reaction with *Brucella* does not occur. In immunoblotting analysis, anti-Yop IgG may persist for years, whereas IgA antibodies usually disappear within months after elimination of the organisms; their prolonged presence suggests persistent *Yersinia* infection (16). Test kits are commercially available (Genzyme Virotech GmbH, Rüsselsheim, Germany; Mikrogen GmbH, Martinsried, Germany [the test kit from the latter uses recombinant Yops]).

TREATMENT AND ANTIBIOTIC SUSCEPTIBILITIES

Early treatment of plague with antibiotics is mandatory in view of the high mortality, which is over 50% in untreated patients (6, 51). Streptomycin and gentamicin given parenterally are the antibiotics of choice (6, 38, 51). Most treated patients recover rapidly and become afebrile within 3 days. Alternatively, doxycycline, ciprofloxacin, or chloramphenicol may be given intravenously (6, 38, 51). Other antibiotics such as sulfonamides, trimethoprim-sulfamethoxazole, or ampicillin appear to be less effective (6). In a mass-casualty setting following a bioterrorist attack or for postexposure prophylaxis, oral doxycycline and ciprofloxacin have been recommended as preferred choices (38). In view of the high rate of mortality from untreated plague, especially pneumonic plague, these antibiotics were also recommended for children and pregnant women (38).

Whereas antibiotic resistance in *Y. pestis* has never been a recognized problem, multidrug resistance mediated by a transferable plasmid has been identified in one isolate from a patient in Madagascar (25). The strain was resistant to ampicillin, chloramphenicol, kanamycin, streptomycin, spectinomycin, sulfonamides, tetracycline, and minocycline. However, a recent study with strains recovered over a 21-year period has shown that, in vitro, *Y. pestis* has remained highly susceptible not only to drugs traditionally used for the treatment of plague but also to newer antibiotic agents, such as broad-spectrum cephalosporins and quinolones. The investigators noted in vitro resistance only to rifampin and imipenem (69).

Intestinal infections with *Y. enterocolitica* and *Y. pseudotuberculosis* are mostly self-limited and need no specific antibiotic treatment. In immunocompromised patients, enteritis may be treated prophylactically. Oral doxycycline or trimethoprim-sulfamethoxazole has been recommended for such patients as well as for patients with complicated gastrointestinal or focal extraintestinal infections in general (14).

In contrast to *Y. pseudotuberculosis*, *Y. enterocolitica* serogroups O:3 and O:9 produce two chromosomally determined β-lactamases (types A and B, respectively), which are variably expressed (61). These account for resistance to ampicillin, cephalothin, and carbenicillin. *Y. enterocolitica* O:8 is susceptible to ampicillin but is variably resistant to carbenicillin and cephalothin. O:8 strains, like most biotype 1B strains, predominantly produce a type A β-lactamase (61). In vitro antibacterial activity does not necessarily reflect in vivo efficacy. Clinically, administration of broad-spectrum cephalosporins, often in combination with aminoglycosides, has resulted in successful outcomes for most patients with extraintestinal infections, including septicemia (4). Fluoroquinolones (ciprofloxacin) and expanded spectrum cephalosporins, such as cefotaxime and ceftriaxone, may be regarded as the most active antimicrobial agents for the treatment of *Y. enterocolitica* O:3 infections (56).

The usefulness of antibiotic treatment in patients with reactive arthritis and other immunopathological disorders is still under discussion. Although persistence of the organisms in the intestines or mesenteric lymph nodes may be assumed, prospective and retrospective studies so far have not yielded solid evidence in favor of antibiotic therapy.

INTERPRETATION AND REPORTING OF RESULTS

Clinically, plague should be suspected if the patient has recently returned from or lives in an area where plague is endemic, reports a history of contact with rodents or house cats or has flea bites, and presents with a severe febrile disease. The presence of painful swelling of inguinal, axillary, or cervical lymph nodes, septicemia, pneumonia, or meningitis is indicative. Detection of typical morphology in Wayson- or methylene blue-stained smears of clinical material is supportive for plague, and the diagnosis is confirmed by isolation of the organisms and identification by biochemical reactions and detection of specific virulence factors. At the earliest suspicion of plague, be it on clinical or bacteriological grounds, the case must immediately be reported to local and state health administrations, and further diagnostic steps should be performed by or in close collaboration with the CDC. If cases of plague, especially of pneumonic plague, occur in persons who have no known risk factors and who live in locations where enzootic infection is not known and where prior rodent deaths have not been observed, bioterrorist action should be taken into consideration (38).

Enteropathogenic *Y. enterocolitica* and *Y. pseudotuberculosis* must be taken into consideration in patients with enteritis of unknown origin, in patients complaining of persistent abdominal pain (terminal ileitis, lymphadenitis, or pseudoappendicitis), and in patients with arthritis following intestinal illness. Detection of *Y. pseudotuberculosis* or pathogenic serogroups of *Y. enterocolitica* in stool specimens is confirmatory if no other enteropathogenic organisms are isolated. However, in patients with terminal ileitis and mesenteric lymphadenitis, as well as in those with reactive arthritis, isolation of the organisms from stool specimens is rare. Septicemic yersiniosis is not associated with specific clinical features; isolation of either *Yersinia* strain from blood cultures is confirmatory.

Determination of antibodies directed against the prevailing serogroups of *Y. pseudotuberculosis* and pathogenic *Y. enterocolitica* by a quantitative agglutination test (Widal reaction) or enzyme immunoassay or evidence of antibodies against Yops by ELISA or immunoblotting is diagnostic for intestinal infections as well as extraintestinal complications (reactive arthritis and other conditions).

Isolates of *Y. enterocolitica* should be tested according to their biotypes and serogroups, since all pathogenic strains are associated with defined bioserogroups. Detection of the 70-kb virulence plasmid by either genotypic (PCR or DNA colony blot hybridization) or phenotypic (e.g., autoagglutination test) methods should be reported. Isolates of *Y. enterocolitica* biotype 1A generally lack the virulence markers of classical invasive *Yersinia* strains and therefore are considered nonpathogenic. However, a novel mechanism of invading tissue culture cells has recently been identified in a number of such strains, and this mechanism may contribute to diarrhea (29). Until more facts are available, biotype 1A strains might tentatively be regarded as causative if they are isolated in large numbers from a patient with diarrhea, if no other enteropathogens are isolated, and if they disappear from the intestines after cessation of the symptoms.

Y. frederiksenii, *Y. kristensenii*, *Y. intermedia*, *Y. mollaretii*, *Y. bercovieri*, *Y. rohdei*, and *Y. aldovae* have no established pathogenic potential in immunocompetent patients. Their detection in stool specimens should be reported as "nonpathogenic yersiniae isolated."

We are grateful to May Chu, Centers for Disease Control and Prevention, Atlanta, Ga., and Jürgen Heesemann, Max von Pettenkofer-Institut, University of Munich, Munich, Germany, for helpful discussions and advice.

REFERENCES

1. **Achtmann, M., K. Zurth, G. Morelli, G. Torrea, A. Guiyoule, and E. Carniel.** 1999. *Yersinia pestis*, the cause of plague, is a recently emerged clone of *Yersinia pseudotuberculosis*. *Proc. Natl. Acad. Sci. USA* **96:**14043–14048.
2. **Aleksic, S., A. G. Steigerwalt, J. Bockemühl, G. P. Huntley-Carter, and D. J. Brenner.** 1987. *Yersinia rohdei* sp. nov. isolated from human and dog feces and surface water. *Int. J. Syst. Bacteriol.* **37:**327–332.
3. **Bercovier, H., H. H. Mollaret, J. M. Alonso, J. Brault, G. R. Fanning, A. G. Steigerwalt, and D. J. Brenner.** 1980. Intra- and interspecies relatedness of *Yersinia pestis* by DNA hybridization and its relationship to *Yersinia pseudotuberculosis*. *Curr. Microbiol.* **4:**225–229.
4. **Bottone, E. J.** 1997. *Yersinia enterocolitica*: the charisma continues. *Clin. Microbiol. Rev.* **10:**257–276.
5. **Buchholz, D. H., J. P. AuBuchon, E. L. Snyder, R. Kandler, S. Edberg, V. Piscitelli, C. Pickard, and P. Napychank.** 1992. Removal of *Yersinia enterocolitica* from AS-1 red cells. *Transfusion* **32:**667–672.
6. **Butler, T.** 1994. *Yersinia* infections: centennial of the discovery of the plague bacillus. *Clin. Infect. Dis.* **19:**655–661.
7. **Centers for Disease Control and Prevention.** 1997. Red blood cell transfusions contaminated with *Yersinia enterocolitica*—United States, 1991–1996, and initiation of a national study of detecting bacteria-associated transfusion reactions. *Morb. Mortal. Wkly. Rep.* **46:**553–555.
8. **Centers for Disease Control and Prevention.** 1997. Fatal human plague—Arizona and Colorado, 1996. *Morb. Mortal. Wkly. Rep.* **46:**617–620.
9. **Centers for Disease Control and Prevention and National Institutes of Health.** 1999. *Biosafety in Microbiological and Biomedical Laboratories*, 4th ed. U.S. Government Printing Office, Washington, D.C.
10. **Chanteau, S., L. Rabarijaona, T. O'Brien, L. Rahalison, J. Hager, P. Boisier, J. Burans, and M. Rasolomaharo.** 1998. F1 antigenaemia in bubonic plague patients, a

marker of gravity and efficacy of therapy. *Trans. R. Soc. Trop. Med. Hyg.* **92:**572–573.

11. **Chin, H. Y., D. M. Flynn, A. V. Hoffrand, and D. Politis.** 1986. Infection with *Yersinia enterocolitica* in patients with iron overload. *Br. Med. J.* **292:**97.

12. **Chu, M. C.** 2000. *Laboratory Manual of Plague Diagnostic Tests.* U.S. Government Printing Office, Washington, D.C.

13. **Cornelis, G. R., A. Boland, A. P. Boyd, C. Geuijen, M. Iriarte, C. Neyt, M. P. Sory, and I. Stanier.** 1998. The virulence plasmid of *Yersinia*, an antihost genome. *Microbiol. Mol. Biol. Rev.* **62:**1315–1352.

14. **Cover, T. L., and R. C. Aber.** 1989. *Yersinia enterocolitica.* *N. Engl. J. Med.* **321:**16–24.

15. **Crook, L. D., and B. Tempest.** 1992. Plague, a clinical review of 27 cases. *Arch. Intern. Med.* **152:**1253–1256.

16. **De Koning, J., J. Heesemann, J. A. A. Hoogkamp-Korstanje, J. J. M. Festen, P. M. Houtman, and P. L. M. Van Oijen.** 1989. *Yersinia* in intestinal biopsy specimens from patients with seronegative spondylarthropathy: correlation with specific serum IgA antibodies. *J. Infect. Dis.* **159:**109–112.

17. **Delor, I., and G. R. Cornelis.** 1992. Role of *Yersinia enterocolitica* Yst toxin in experimental infection of young rabbits. *Infect. Immun.* **60:**4269–4277.

18. **Devignat, R.** 1951. Variétés de l'espèce *Pasteurella pestis.* Nouvelle hypothèse. *Bull. W. H. O.* **4:**247–263.

19. **Durisin, M. D., A. Ibrahim, and M. W. Griffith.** 1998. Detection of pathogenic *Yersinia enterocolitica* using a digoxigenin labelled probe targeting the *yst* gene. *J. Appl. Microbiol.* **84:**285–292.

20. **Ewing, W. H.** 1986. Identification of *Enterobacteriaceae*, 4th ed. Elsevier, New York, N.Y.

21. **Feng, P. S., P. Keasler, and W. E. Hill.** 1992. Direct identification of *Yersinia enterocolitica* in blood by polymerase chain reaction. *Transfusion* **32:**850–854.

22. **Fenwick, S. G., and A. Murray.** 1991. Detection of pathogenic *Yersinia enterocolitica* by the polymerase chain reaction. *Lancet* **337:**496–497.

23. **Fukushima, H., M. Gomyoda, K. Shiozawa, S. Kaneko, and M. Tsubokura.** 1988. *Yersinia pseudotuberculosis* infection contracted through water contaminated by a wild animal. *J. Clin. Microbiol.* **26:**584–585.

24. **Gage, K. L., D. T. Dennis, K. A. Orloski, P. Ettestad, T. L. Brown, P. J. Reynolds, W. J. Pape, C. L. Fritz, L. G. Carter, and J. D. Stein.** 2000. Cases of cat-associated human plague in the western US, 1977–1998. *Clin. Infect. Dis.* **30:**893–900.

25. **Galimand, M., A. Guiyoule, G. Gerbaud, B. Rasoamanana, S. Chanteau, E. Carniel, and P. Courvalin.** 1997. Multidrug resistance in *Yersinia pestis* mediated by a transferable plasmid. *N. Engl. J. Med.* **337:**677–680.

26. **Gasper, P. W., A. M. Barnes, T. J. Quan, J. P. Benziger, L. G. Carter, M. L. Beard, and G. O. Maupin.** 1993. Plague (*Yersinia pestis*) in cats: description of experimentally induced disease. *J. Med. Entomol.* **30:**20–26.

27. **Granfors, K., R. Merilahti-Palo, R. Luukkainen, T. Möttönen, R. Lahesmaa, P. Probst, E. Märker-Hermann, and P. Toivanen.** 1998. Persistence of *Yersinia* antigens in peripheral blood cells from patients with *Yersinia enterocolitica* O:3 infection with or without reactive arthritis. *Arthritis Rheum.* **41:**855–862.

28. **Granfors, K., M. K. Viljanen, and A. Toivanen.** 1981. Measurement of immunoglobulin M, immunoglobulin G, and immunoglobulin A antibodies against Y. *enterocolitica* by enzyme-linked immunosorbent assay. Comparison of lipopolysaccharide and whole bacterium as antigen. *J. Clin. Microbiol.* **14:**6–14.

29. **Grant, T., V. Bennet-Wood, and R. M. Robins-Browne.** 1998. Identification of virulence-associated characters in clinical isolates of *Yersinia enterocolitica* lacking classical virulence markers. *Infect. Immun.* **66:**1113–1120.

30. **Heesemann, J., U. Gross, N. Schmidt, and R. Laufs.** 1986. Immunochemical analysis of plasmid-encoded proteins released by enteropathogenic *Yersinia* sp. grown in calcium-deficient media. *Infect. Immun.* **54:**561–567.

31. **Heesemann, J., K. Hantke, T. Vocke, E. Saken, A. Rakin, I. Stojiljkovic, and R. Berner.** 1993. Virulence of *Yersinia enterocolitica* is closely associated with siderophore production, expression of an iron-repressible outer membrane polypeptide of 65,000 Da and pesticin sensitivity. *Mol. Microbiol.* **8:**397–408.

32. **Higuchi, K., and J. I. Smith.** 1961. Studies on the nutrition and physiology of *Pasteurella pestis*. VI. A differential plating medium for the estimation of mutation rate to avirulence. *J. Bacteriol.* **81:**605–608.

33. **Hinnebusch, B. J.** 1997. Bubonic plague: a molecular genetic case history of the emergence of an infectious disease. *J. Mol. Med.* **75:**645–652.

34. **Hinnebusch, B. J., E. R. Fischer, and T. G. Schwan.** 1998. Evaluation of the role of the *Yersinia pestis* plasminogen activator and other plasmid-encoded factors in temperature-dependent blockage of the flea. *J. Infect. Dis.* **178:**1406–1415.

35. **Hinnebusch, B. J., R. D. Perry, and T. G. Schwan.** 1996. Role of the *Yersinia pestis* hemin storage (*hms*) locus in the transmission of plague to fleas. *Science* **273:**367–370.

36. **Holt, J. G., N. R. Krieg, P. H. A. Sneath, J. T. Staley, and S. T. Williams (ed.).** 1994. *Bergey's Manual of Determinative Bacteriology*, 9th ed. The Williams & Wilkins Co., Baltimore, Md.

37. **Hoogkamp-Korstanje, J. A., J. de Koning, and J. Heesemann.** 1988. Persistence of *Yersinia enterocolitica* in man. *Infection* **16:**81–85.

38. **Inglesby, T. V., D. T. Dennis, D. A. Henderson, J. G. Bartlett, M. S. Ascher, E. Eitzen, A. D. Fine, A. M. Friedlander, J. Hauer, J. F. Koerner, M. Layton, J. McDade, M. T. Osterholm, T. O'Toole, G. Parker, T. M. Pearl, P. K. Russel, M. Schoch-Spana, and K. Tonat.** 2000. Plague as a biological weapon. Medical and public health management. *JAMA* **283:**2281–2290.

39. **Jackson, S., and T. W. Burrows.** 1956. The pigmentation of *Pasteurella pestis* on a defined medium containing haemin. *Br. J. Exp. Pathol.* **37:**570–576.

40. **Jourdan, A. D., S. C. Johnson, and I. V. Wesley.** 2000. Development of a fluorogenic 5′ nuclease PCR assay for detection of the *ail* gene of pathogenic *Yersinia.* *Appl. Environ. Microbiol.* **66:**3750–3755.

41. **Kandolo, K., and G. Wauters.** 1985. Pyrazinamidase activity in *Yersinia enterocolitica* and related organisms. *J. Clin. Microbiol.* **21:**980–982.

42. **Kapperud, G., K. Dommarsness, M. Skurnik, and E. Hornes.** 1990. A synthetic oligonucleotide probe based on the *yopA* gene for detection and enumeration of virulent *Yersinia enterocolitica.* *Appl. Environ. Microbiol.* **56:**17–23.

43. **Laird, W. J., and D. C. Cavanaugh.** 1980. Correlation of autoagglutination and virulence of yersiniae. *J. Clin. Microbiol.* **11:**430–432.

44. **Lantz, P. G., R. Knutsson, Y. Blixt, W. A. Al-Soud, E. Borch, and P. Radström.** 1998. Detection of pathogenic *Yersinia enterocolitica* in enrichment media and pork by a multiplex PCR: a study of sample preparation and PCR-inhibitory components. *Int. J. Food Microbiol.* **45:**93–105.

45. **Lee, V. T., and O. Schneewind.** 1999. Type III secretion machines and the pathogenesis of enteric infections caused by *Yersinia* and *Salmonella. Immunol. Rev.* **168:**241–255.

46. Linde, H. J., H. Neubauer, H. Meyer, S. Aleksic, and N. Lehn. 1999. Identification of *Yersinia* species by the Vitek GNI card. *J. Clin. Microbiol.* **37:**211–214.

47. Meyer, K. F. 1970. Effectiveness of live or killed plague vaccines in man. *Bull. W. H. O.* **42:**653–666.

48. Nakajima, H., M. Inoue, T. Mori, K. I. Itoh, E. Arakawa, and H. Watanabe. 1992. Detection and identification of *Yersinia pseudotuberculosis* and pathogenic *Yersinia enterocolitica* by an improved polymerase chain reaction. *J. Clin. Microbiol.* **30:**2484–2486.

49. Neubauer, H., T. Sauer, H. Becker, S. Aleksic, and H. Meyer. 1998. Comparison of systems for identification and differentiation of species within the genus *Yersinia*. *J. Clin. Microbiol.* **36:**3366–3368.

50. Norkina, O. V., A. N. Kulichenko, A. L. Gintsburg, I. V. Tuchkov, Y. A. Popov, M. U. Aksenov, and I. G. Drosdov. 1994. Development of a diagnostic test for *Yersinia pestis* by the polymerase chain reaction. *J. Appl. Bacteriol.* **76:**240–245.

51. Perry, R. D., and J. D. Fetherston. 1997. *Yersinia pestis*— etiologic agent of plague. *Clin. Microbiol. Rev.* **10:**35–66.

52. Pollitzer, R. 1954. *Plague. World Health Organization Monograph Series 22.* World Health Organization, Geneva, Switzerland.

53. Rahalison, L., E. Vololonirina, M. Ratsitorahina, and S. Chanteau. 2000. Diagnosis of bubonic plague by PCR in Madagascar under field conditions. *J. Clin. Microbiol.* **38:**260–263.

54. Rakin, A., C. Nölting, S. Schubert, and J. Heesemann. 1999. Common and specific characteristics of the high-pathogenicity island of *Yersinia enterocolitica*. *Infect. Immun.* **67:**5265–5274.

55. Rasoamanana, B., F. Leroy, P. Boisier, M. Rasolomaharo, P. Buchy, E. Carniel, and S. Chanteau. 1997. Field evaluation of an immunoglobulin G anti-F1 enzyme-linked immunosorbent assay for serodiagnosis of human plague in Madagascar. *Clin. Diagn. Lab. Immunol.* **4:**587–591.

56. Rastawicki, W., R. Gierczynski, M. Jagielski, S. Kulazewski, and J. Jeljaszewicz. 2000. Susceptibility of Polish clinical strains of *Yersinia enterocolitica* serotype O:3 to antibiotics. *Int. J. Antimicrob. Agents* **13:**297–300.

57. Ruckdeschel, K. 2000. *Yersinia* species disrupt immune responses to subdue the host. *ASM News* **66:**470–477.

58. Salyers, A. A., and D. D. Whitt. 1994. *Yersinia* infections, p. 213–228. *In* A. A. Salyers and D. D. Whitt (ed.), *Bacterial Pathogenesis.* American Society for Microbiology, Washington, D.C.

59. Sodeinde, O. A., Y. V. B. K. Subrahmanyam, K. Stark, T. Quan, Y. Bao, and J. D. Goguen. 1992. A surface protease and the invasive character of plague. *Science* **258:**1004–1007.

60. Ståhlberg, T. H., J. Heesemann, K. Granfors, and A. Toivanen. 1989. Immunoblot analysis of IgM, IgG, and IgA responses to plasmid encoded released proteins of *Yersinia enterocolitica* in patients with or without yersinia triggered reactive arthritis. *Ann. Rheum. Dis.* **48:**577–581.

61. Stock, I., P. Heisig, and B. Wiedemann. 2000. Beta-lactamase expression in *Yersinia enterocolitica* biovars 1A, 1B, and 3. *J. Med. Microbiol.* **49:**403–408.

62. Sulakvelidze, A., A. Kreger, A. Joseph, R. M. Robins-Browne, A. Fasano, G. Wauters, N. Harnett, L. DeTolla, and J. G. Morris. 1999. Production of enterotoxin by *Yersinia bercovieri*, a recently identified *Yersinia enterocolitica*-like species. *Infect. Immun.* **67:**968–971.

63. Surgalla, M. J., and E. D. Beesley. 1969. Congo red-agar plating medium for detecting pigmentation in *Pasteurella pestis*. *Appl. Microbiol.* **18:**834–837.

64. Toivanen, P., and A. Toivanen. 1994. Does *Yersinia* induce autoimmunity? *Int. Arch. Allergy Immunol.* **104:**107–111.

65. Trebesius, K., D. Harmsen, A. Rakin, J. Schmelz, and J. Heesemann. 1998. Development of rRNA-targeted PCR and in situ hybridization with fluorescently labelled oligonucleotides for detection of *Yersinia* species. *J. Clin. Microbiol.* **36:**2557–2564.

66. Watson, R. P., T. W. Blanchard, M. G. Mense, and P. W. Gasper. 2001. Histopathology of experimental plague in cats. *Vet. Pathol.* **38:**165–172.

67. Wauters, G., K. Kandolo, and M. Janssens. 1987. Revised biogrouping scheme of *Yersinia enterocolitica*. *Contrib. Microbiol. Immunol.* **9:**14–21.

68. Wilmoth, B. A., M. C. Chu, and T. J. Quan. 1996. Identification of *Yersinia pestis* by BBL crystal enteric/nonfermenter identification system. *J. Clin. Microbiol.* **34:**2829–2830.

69. Wong, J. D., J. R. Barash, R. F. Sandfort, and J. M. Janda. 2000. Susceptibilities of *Yersinia pestis* strains to 12 antimicrobial agents. *Antimicrob. Agents Chemother.* **44:**1995–1996.

70. World Health Organization. 2000. Human plague in 1998 and 1999. *Wkly. Epidemiol. Rec.* **75:**338–344.

71. Wren, B. W., and S. Tabaqchali. 1990. Detection of pathogenic *Yersinia enterocolitica* by the polymerase chain reaction. *Lancet* **336:**693.

Klebsiella, Enterobacter, Citrobacter, Serratia, Plesiomonas, and Other Enterobacteriaceae

SHARON L. ABBOTT

44

TAXONOMY

Recent taxonomic changes among genera of the family *Enterobacteriaceae* included in this chapter are covered in Tables 1 and 2. Inclusion of *Plesiomonas shigelloides* within the family is a reflection of the taxonomic upheavals occurring throughout the bacterial community. Phylogenic studies involving both 16S and 5S rRNA sequencing have shown that *Plesiomonas* clearly clusters with the genus *Proteus* within the family *Enterobacteriaceae* (86, 87, 111). Since members of the *Enterobacteriaceae* have been oxidase negative by definition (38), the characteristics of the family will need to be redefined to accommodate the inclusion of the genus *Plesiomonas* in the next edition of *Bergey's Manual*. For the present, however, the interrelationship between *Proteus vulgaris* (87) and *Plesiomonas* demonstrated by rRNA sequencing warrants its inclusion in this chapter.

After the creation of nine new *Citrobacter* species from the heterogeneous *C. freundii* complex and the renaming of *C. diversus* as *C. koseri* and *C. amalonaticus* biogroup 1 as *C. farmeri*, *Citrobacter* has remained relatively stable. With the recent proposal of the species epithets *C. gillenii* and *C. murliniae* for strains previously known as *Citrobacter* genomospecies 10 and 11, respectively (23), all members within this genus are now named. This may change, however, since 16S rRNA sequencing has established that a newly recognized opportunistic pathogen, enteric group 137, has >99% similarity to *C. amalonaticus* and *C. farmeri* (124). The genus *Enterobacter* has one new proposed species. Strains belonging to NIH group 42 (Tokyo, Japan) which had previously clustered within the *Enterobacter agglomerans* complex were named *Enterobacter cowanii* by Inoue et al. (62). The *E. agglomerans* complex itself was placed in the genus *Pantoea* as *P. agglomerans* in 1989 by Gavini et al. (46). Since this change has had ample time to be accepted and is currently in use in the literature, the epithet *agglomerans* is included in *Pantoea* in this chapter. Despite the genus change, this species remains heterogeneous at the DNA level, containing as many as 18 different hybridization groups (20). *E. cloacae* is also a heterogeneous species containing at least five DNA groups (51). Biochemical identification of strains within both of these species is complicated by this heterogeneity. *Klebsiella* has undergone perhaps the most tumultuous changes, with the proposed

removal of three species, *K. ornithinolytica*, *K. terrigena*, and *K. planticola*, to the newly created genus *Raoultella* (34). This proposal is based on 16S rDNA and *rpoB* gene sequencing and carbon assimilation studies. A proposal has also been made to transfer the nonculturable bacterium *Calymmatobacterium granulomatis*, the causative agent of donovanosis (genital ulceration), to the genus *Klebsiella* (26, 74) (Table 2). This change is supported by 16S rDNA and *phoE* (phosphatase porin) gene sequencing data plus the fact that *K. (C.) granulomatis* causes ulcerative lesions similar to those produced by *K. ozaenae* and *K. rhinoscleromatis*. No recent changes have occurred within the genus *Serratia*.

In addition to the inclusion of *Plesiomonas*, this chapter has been expanded to cover other genera of the *Enterobacteriaceae* including *Proteus*, *Providencia*, *Morganella*, and *Hafnia* (Table 1). Few taxonomic changes have occurred within these genera, with the exception of the addition of *Proteus hauseri* (formerly genomospecies 3 of *P. vulgaris*) by O'Hara et al. (99). Three other *Proteus* genomospecies, designated 4, 5, and 6, also previously within *P. vulgaris*, remain unnamed (99). In this edition of the Manual, miscellaneous genera within the *Enterobacteriaceae* have been moved to this chapter and are listed in Table 2. *Edwardsiella* currently includes three species, *E. tarda*, a clinically significant species in humans, *E. ictaluri*, an important fish pathogen, and *E. hoshinae*. With the exception of *E. tarda* and *K. (C.) granulomatis*, the genera in the first column of Table 2 are primarily opportunistic pathogens. Numbered genomospecies designations within a genus are given when they are composed of a single strain or too few organisms to be named or if they cannot be separated from other members of their genus by available phenotypic tests. The genera listed in the last two columns of Table 2 are not isolated from human clinical specimens or are isolated but may not be significant, and most of them will be unfamiliar to clinical microbiologists. A number of these taxa cannot be grown on laboratory media, so they are unlikely to be confused with or necessitate separation from the genera seen in humans. References have been included for organisms that are isolated only from nonhuman sources, and they will not be discussed further.

TABLE 1 Nomenclature, isolation source, and significance of selected genera of the family *Enterobacteriaceae*[a]

Current (previous) designation	Clinical data			Environmental data
	Frequency	Source	Significance	
Citrobacter				
C. amalonaticus	++	**Feces,** blood, wound, UT, RT	2	Unknown, one isolate from an animal
C. braakii	+++	**Feces,** UT, RT, wound	2	Similar to *C. freundii*; some species have unknown reservoir
C. farmeri (C. amalonaticus biogroup 1)	++	**Feces,** UT, wound	2	Unknown
C. freundii	++++	All sites, feces most common	1	Water, soil, fish, animals, food
C. koseri (C. diversus)	+++	All sites, **CSF**		Unknown
C. rodentium			1	Pathogenic for mice
C. sedlakii	−			Same as for *C. braakii*
C. werkmanii	+	Feces, blood, CSF	2	Same as for *C. braakii*
C. youngae	++	**Feces,** wound	3	Same as for *C. braakii*
C. gillenii (Citrobacter DNA group 10)	++++	**Feces,** UT, blood, CSF	2	Food
C. murliniae (Citrobacter DNA group 11)	+	Feces	3	Same as for *C. braakii*
Enterobacter				
E. aerogenes	++++	All sites	1	Water soil sewage, animals, dairy products
E. amnigenus biogroup 1	−			Plants
E. amnigenus biogroup 2	−			Water
E. asburiae	++	**UT,** RT, feces, wound, blood	2	Water
E. cancerogenus (E. taylorae)	++	**Wound,** RT, feces	2	Animals, water
E. cloacae	++++	All sites	1	Water, soil, sewage, meat
E. cowanii (P. agglomerans/ Japanese NIH group 42)	Unk	UT, RT, blood, wound	3	Unknown
E. dissolvens (Erwinia)	−			Diseased corn stalks
E. gergoviae	++	RT, UT, blood	2	Water, cosmetics
E. hormaechei	+	RT, wound, blood	2	Unknown, one isolation from a frog
E. intermedium	+	Wound, blood, bile, feces	2	Water, soil
E. kobei	Unk	Unk	Unk	Food
E. nimipressuralis (Erwinia)	−			Diseased elms
E. pyrinus (Erwinia)	−			Diseased pear trees
E. sakazakii	++	RT, wound, CSF	1	Unknown
Hafnia alvei	++	**Feces,** blood, RT	2	Ubiquitous
Klebsiella				
K. pneumoniae	++++	All sites, RT/UT most common	1	Ubiquitous, including foods and water
K. pneumoniae subsp. ozaenae	++	**Nasal discharge,** RT, UT, blood	2	Unknown
K. pneumoniae subsp. rhinoscleromatis	++	Nasal discharge	1	Unknown
K. oxytoca	++++	All sites	1	Ubiquitous, including foods and water
Morganella				
M. morganii subsp. morganii	++	All sites	1	Unknown, isolations from mammalian and reptile gastrointestinal tract
M. morganii subsp. sibonii	++	Same	1	Same as above
Pantoea agglomerans (Enterobacter)	+++	All sites	2	Plants
Plesiomonas shigelloides	+++	**Feces,** blood	1	Aquatic habitats and animals

(Continued on next page)

TABLE 1 Nomenclature, isolation source, and significance of selected genera of the family *Enterobacteriaceae*[a]   (Continued)

Current (previous) designation	Clinical data			Environmental data
	Frequency	Source	Significance	
Proteus				
P. hauseri (*P. vulgaris* genomospecies 3)	+	Unk	Unk	Unknown, probably similar to *P. mirabilis*
P. mirabilis	++++	**UT,** blood, CSF	1	Animals, birds, fresh- and saltwater fish, foods
P. myxofaciens	−			Gypsy moth
P. penneri	++	**UT,** blood, wound, feces, eye	1	Probably similar to *P. mirabilis*
P. vulgaris	+++	**UT,** wound, stool, RT	1	Probably similar to *P. mirabilis*
Providencia				
P. alcalifaciens	+++	All sites, UT/feces common	1	Mammals, water
P. heimbachae	+	Feces	3	Penguins
P. rettgeri	+++	All sites, UT common	1	Same as for *P. alcalifaciens*, insects
P. rustigianii	+	Feces	3	Unknown
P. stuartii	+++	All sites, UT common	1	Mammals
Raoultella				
R. ornithinolytica (*Klebsiella*)	+	Wound, UT, blood	2	Food
R. planticola (*Klebsiella*)	Unk		3	Plants, water
R. terrigena (*Klebsiella*)	Unk		3	Soil, water
Serratia				
S. entomophila	−			New Zealand grass grub, water
S. ficaria	+	RT, wound	3	Fig wasps, figs, plants
S. fonticola	+	**Wound,** RT	3	Water, birds
S. liquefaciens group (*S. liquefaciens* sensu stricto, *S. proteamaculans*, *S. grimesii*)	+++	RT, wound	2	Plants, insects, mammals, birds, dairy products
S. marcescens	++++	All sites, RT common	1	Water, soil, plants, vegetables, animals, insects
S. marcescens biogroup 1	+	**UT,** RT	2	Unknown
S. odorifera biogroup 1	+	RT, wound, feces, blood, UT	2	Plants
S. odorifera biogroup 2		Same as biogroup 1		Same as biogroup 1
S. plymuthia	+	RT	3	Water, plants, small mammals
S. rubidaea	+	RT, wound, blood, UT, feces	2	Water plants

[a] Abbreviations and symbols: ++++, frequent; +++, occasional; ++, rare; +, very rare; −, not yet isolated from humans; CSF, cerebrospinal fluid; RT, respiratory tract; Unk, unknown; UT, urinary tract; 1, major pathogenic species of humans; 2, proven cause of disease in rare instances; 3, isolated from humans, significance unknown. Bold denotes the most common source. Data are from references 21, 23, 34, 46, 50, 51, 52, 62, 64, 79, 85, 92, 99, 100, 101, and 115.

DESCRIPTION OF GENERA

Members belonging to the family *Enterobacteriaceae* are gram-negative facultative anaerobic rods or coccobacilli ranging from 0.3 to 1.0 μm wide and 0.6 to 6.0 μm long. Of the organisms in Tables 1 and 2 isolated from human specimens, all *Klebsiella*, *Leminorella*, *Moellerella*, *Tatumella*, and *Enterobacter asburiae* strains are nonmotile, although any strain of any genus may be nonmotile. Prototrophic strains grow readily on ordinary media. Among these genera, auxotrophic strains from clinical specimens are rare. However, cysteine-requiring urinary isolates of *K. pneumoniae*, which grow as pinpoint colonies on routine media, do occur. If encountered, these strains require supplementation of biochemical media or commercial identification systems with 0.63 mM cysteine for accurate identification. While some strains of *S. plymuthica* may not grow at 37°C, most other members of these genera grow well between 25 and 37°C. Essentially only *Klebsiella* and *Raoultella* (*Klebsiella*) spp. are encapsulated, but strains from all genera may grow as mucoid or rough colonies. Five genera produce

pigment. Some strains of *S. marcescens* and most *S. rubidaea* and *S. plymuthica* strains produce a red pigment, prodigiosin, which may appear throughout the entire colony or as only a red center or margin. Most strains of *E. sakazakii* and some strains of *P. agglomerans*, *Leclercia adecarboxylata*, and *Photorhabdus* spp. form yellow-pigmented colonies, which range from bright to pale yellow. Weak pigment producers may be detected only by observing growth placed on a swab or filter paper. The yellow pigment may be enhanced by incubation at 25°C. *Photorhabdus luminescens* cultures are luminescent, giving a visible glow in a darkroom after 5 min. *S. odorifera*, as indicated by its name, and some *Cedecea* spp. strains produce a pungent (potato-like) odor due to the production of alkyl-methoxypyrazines (50). Species of *Proteus* and *Providencia* oxidatively deaminate α-amino acids, producing pyruvic acids. L-Phenylalanine deamination yields a green color when ferric chloride is added; however, deamination of *dl*-tryptophan produces the deep reddish brown pigment often seen in media inoculated with these organisms without the addition of ferric chloride

TABLE 2 Other members of the family *Enterobacteriaceae*[a]

Human pathogens or opportunists	Primarily environmental strains[b]	Nonhuman isolates
Edwardsiella tarda	*Budvicia aquatica*[c] (7, 19)	*Arsenophonus nasoniae*[e] (47, 125)
Ewingella americana	*Buttiauxella noackiae*[d] (91)	*Brenneria* species[f] (57)
Klebsiella (Calymmatobacterium) granulomatis	*Edwardsiella hoshinae*[c,d] (55)	*Buchnera aphidicola*[e] (93)
Cedecea davisae	*Trabulsiella guamensis*[c] (88)	*Buttiauxella* species[c,e] (91)
Cedecea lapagei	*Pragia fontium*[c] (6)	*Edwardsiella ictaluri*[d] (58)
Cedecea neteri		*Kluyvera cochleae*[d] (91)
Cedecea genomospecies 3		*Obesumbacterium proteus*[c] (64)
Cedecea genomospecies 5		*Pantoea* species[c,f] (57, 73)
Kluyvera ascorbata		*Pectobacterium* species[f] (117)
Kluyvera cryocrescens		*Photorhabdus* species[e] (42)
Kluyvera georgiana		*Sodalis glossinidius*[e] (31)
Leclercia adecarboxylata		*Wigglesworthia glossinidia*[e] (2)
Leminorella grimontii		*Xenorhabdus* species[e] (17)
Leminorella richardii		
Leminorella genomospecies 3		
Moellerella wisconsensis		
Photorhabdus luminescens		
Rahnella aquatilis		
Rahnella genomospecies 2 (22)		
Rahnella genomospecies 3		
Tatumella ptyseos		
Yokenella regenburgei		

[a] References are given in parentheses. Genomospecies listed cannot be biochemically separated from other species within their genus and/or only a single strain exists.
[b] Rare human isolates of no, or questionable, significance.
[c] Environmental isolates.
[d] Fish, marine, animal, or bird isolates.
[e] Insect isolate or pathogens.
[f] Plant isolate or phytopathogens.

(107). *Proteus* species also produce swarmer cells that are elongated forms created when cells fail to septate or divide. These cells, which are profusely covered with flagella, act in concert to produce swarming motility on solid media (14).

Plesiomonas shigelloides organisms are also gram-negative facultative anaerobes growing as straight rods of similar size to the other *Enterobacteriaceae*. However, unlike other *Enterobacteriaceae*, *P. shigelloides* strains are oxidase positive, do not produce gas from glucose (other *Enterobacteriaceae* are variable), and are susceptible to O/129 vibriostatic agent (2,4-diamino-6,7-diisopropylpteridine). Both *P. shigelloides* and enterobacteria grow at similar salt concentrations (0 to 5%) and pH ranges (4.0 to 8.0).

NATURAL HABITAT AND CLINICAL SIGNIFICANCE

The *Enterobacteriaceae* are widespread throughout the environment (Tables 1 and 2). The citrobacteria are primarily inhabitants of the intestinal tract; thus, their presence in the environment may reflect fecal excretion by humans and animals. The natural habitat of some *Citrobacter* species is unknown.

Many species of the genera listed in Table 1 are commonly recognized nosocomial pathogens. The most currently available National Nosocomial Infections Surveillance System (109) data rank *Enterobacter* species and *K. pneumoniae* between the fifth and seventh most common agents of nosocomial urinary tract, bloodstream, cardiovascular, and ear, nose, and throat infections (109). They rank third and fourth, respectively, as a cause of hospital-acquired pneumonia. Although less prevalent than other etiologic agents, *Klebsiella* and *Enterobacter* cause significant infections. For instance, in one study, when found intraoperatively, *Klebsiella* and *Enterobacter* species had a 68 and 100% probability, respectively, of causing a wound infection; the probability rates for *Escherichia coli* or *Staphylococcus aureus*, which were isolated three times more often during surgery, were only 31 and 55%, respectively (121). While *K. pneumoniae* and *E. cloacae* cause sepsis four to five times less often than gram-positive organisms, they are twice as likely to cause patient mortality (123). Species of both of these genera were among the most commonly involved in relapse or reinfection in one study on recurrent bacteremia (126). Additionally, Wendt et al. (125) found that of eight patients with a positive blood specimen for klebsiellae that showed multiple colony morphologies upon plating, two actually had more than one strain of *Klebsiella* present, as ascertained by pulsed-field gel electrophoresis (PFGE). Both *Klebsiella* and *Enterobacter* are frequent causes of urinary tract infections (UTIs). Surveillance studies in 1997 found that 7 and 5% of UTIs in Europe were caused by *Klebsiella* and *Enterobacter* spp., respectively (43), and that 12 and 4% of UTIs in North America were caused by *Klebsiella* and *Enterobacter* spp., respectively (71). *Klebsiella* is carried in the nasopharynx and the bowel; however, feces is probably the most significant source of patient infections (90). Approximately one-third of patients carry *Klebsiella* in their stools, but rates may increase as much as threefold during hospitalization and antimicrobial usage in adults. Fecal carriage rates for children may be as high as 90 to 100%, even in the absence of antimicrobial therapy. *K. rhinoscleromatis* and *K. ozaenae* cause granulomatous infections termed rhinoscleroma and atrophic rhinitis, respectively. Both are chronic diseases of the upper respiratory tract; although atrophic rhinitis is restricted to the nose, rhinoscleroma may spread to the trachea and larynx (64). Both diseases occur most frequently in tropical areas of the world; transmission is thought to be from person to person, although prolonged contact with persons producing airborne nasal secretions is required. *Klebsiella* (*C.*) *granulomatis* causes chronic genital ulcers and is also predominantly seen in tropical countries (56). It is believed that *K.* (*C.*). *granulomatis* is sexually transmitted and that the only known reservoir is humans.

Strains proposed as *Raoultella* (*Klebsiella*) *planticola* and *Raoultella* (*Klebsiella*) *terrigena*, which are difficult to distinguish from *Klebsiella pneumoniae* without special tests, are generally believed to be environmental strains. This has been disputed by recent studies in Europe that have found that 3.5 to 19% of clinical strains of *Klebsiella* are actually *R. planticola* and that these strains have pathogenicity features similar to those found in *K. pneumoniae* (106). However, in the United States, a survey of 436 *Klebsiella* strains isolated from newborns found only one isolate which could be identified as *R. planticola*, indicating that its prevalence may differ geographically (128). Nosocomial *Enterobacter* colonization and infection are frequently associated with contaminated medical devices and instrumentation; however, *Enterobacter* species are commonly consumed in food, and an endogenous source should also be considered (64). A number of *Enterobacter* species were previously members of the genus *Erwinia* and are isolated from plants or trees (Table 1), where they may cause disease. The clinical microbiologist must be aware of these species as potential transients or commensals within clinical specimens. *Citrobacter* species and *S. marcescens* constitute 1 to 2% of nosocomial bloodstream, cardiovascular, and ear, nose, and throat infections (109). *S. marcescens* causes 4% of hospital-acquired pneumonias, ranking as the seventh most common agent in this category (109). Nosocomial *Citrobacter* spp. are now most commonly isolated from pneumonia and ear, nose, and throat infections (109) and from the urinary tract, where they are generally present in pure culture (60 to 75%) and are clinically significant (60 to 65%) (41, 82). In Europe and North America, *Citrobacter* spp. accounted for 2 to 3% of UTIs in 1997 (43, 71). Sepsis involving *Citrobacter* is often polymicrobic (64). Mortality rates as high as 48 to 50% have been reported; death is more often associated with polymicrobic than monomicrobic infections. *C. koseri* sepsis arising from endogenous sources typically originates from the genitourinary tract, while *C. freundii* bacteremia or septicemia arises from the urinary tract, gallbladder, or gastrointestinal tract (35). *Citrobacter* meningitis is almost exclusively associated with *C. koseri* and involves children younger than 2 months, with the highest onset rates noted in neonates with a mean age of 7 days (64). An exceedingly large number (>75%) of these infants develop brain abscesses, and those who survive are generally afflicted with neurological defects. The most prominent risk factor is prior colonization; during outbreaks, colonization rates of 27% have been noted, in contrast to the normal rate of <1% (81, 129). Person-to-person spread from hospital personnel and, less often, from mother to offspring is the most likely source; sampling of inanimate or environmental reservoirs in hospitals usually fails to yield *Citrobacter*. *Citrobacter* species previously belonging to the *C. freundii* complex, including the two newly named species, *C. gillenii* and *C. murliniae*, are found in clinical, animal, food, and environmental specimens (21,

23). It is unclear what role many of these species may play in human infections; for some, the numbers of strains available are insufficient to determine clinical significance in humans or to establish a reservoir for infections. *C. rodentium* is the cause of murine colonic hyperplasia (85). This disease is self-limiting in adult mice but causes significant morbidity and mortality in infant mice when outbreaks occur in mouse colonies (85). Although *Serratia* spp. are seldom a cause of primary infection, they are notorious nosocomial pathogens and colonizers. The predominant mode of transmission is from person to person, but various medical apparatuses, intravenous fluids, and other solutions have often been implicated as well (64). Patients with indwelling catheters, particularly those with UTIs, serve as a primary reservoir for transmission via hospital personnel. In children, the gastrointestinal tract is a common source of infections. Outbreaks transmitted by hand are often insidious and may occur over a long period, subsiding and then peaking a number of times before recognition and infection control efforts can contain them. Pigment production in *S. marcescens* appears to be a marker that the strain is environmental in origin and of low virulence (11). Specific O and K types are associated with strains involved with human colonization and infection (10, 11). These strains tend to be able to adhere to host cells based on the presence of hemagglutinins. Further studies are required to determine whether adherence, which precedes colonization and infection, may be due to the polysaccharide or whether the polysaccharide is merely associated with other adherence factors. Most other species of *Serratia* have also been isolated from humans, where they, too, are usually transiently present or cause opportunistic infections. *S. ficaria* is isolated predominantly from figs or fig wasps (64). Only *S. entomophila* has yet to be isolated from humans; it causes amber disease in the New Zealand grass grub (64).

Proteus, *Providencia*, and *Morganella* are widespread in the environment and are normal inhabitants of the gut. *Proteus* spp. ranked as the fourth and fifth leading cause of UTIs in Europe and North America, respectively, in 1997 (43, 71). While *Proteus* spp., especially *P. mirabilis*, are common causes of uncomplicated UTIs, they frequently affect the upper urinary tract as well, causing renal scarring and kidney stone formation (89). Ammonia and CO_2 produced in urine by the urease of *Proteus* lowers the pH, causing precipitation of soluble ions and the formation of stones, composed of struvite or apatite crystals, within the urinary tract. These crystals, which can be visualized within urine agar (filter-sterilized human urine solidified with agar) that has been inoculated with *Proteus*, are composed of magnesium ammonium phosphate or calcium phosphate (89). Since *P. mirabilis*, *P. penneri*, *Morganella*, and *P. alcalifaciens* have been isolated with greater frequency from diarrheal stools than from normal stools, it has been speculated that they may cause diarrhea. However, of these agents, only *P. alcalifaciens* plays a potential role in gastroenteritis. Studies by several groups have shown that *P. alcalifaciens* is invasive in HEp-2 cell assays (4, 69) and elicits diarrhea in the RITARD (reversible intestinal-tie adult rabbit diarrhea) model (4). However, some strains isolated in pure culture or in large numbers from diarrheal stools have failed to invade cell lines. The inability of these noninvasive strains to penetrate epithelial cells may be explained by the fact that they appear unable to adhere to cell lines, a prerequisite to invasion (75).

Hafnia alvei has also been linked to gastrointestinal disease. *Hafnia*, isolated in pure culture from the diarrheal stool of a 9-month-old child, was found to produce fluid in a RITARD model (3). A 1994 study of tourists returning to Finland found that 5% of patients with diarrhea had *Hafnia* in their stool while >300 asymptomatic individuals were negative for *Hafnia* (110). To date, putative virulence characteristics have not been demonstrated in hafniae. Isolates originally identified as *H. alvei* prototypical diarrheal strains, thought to possess the *eae* gene (attaching-effacing), thus giving further credence to the role of *Hafnia* in diarrhea (5), were eventually found to be *Escherichia* spp. (66). Extraintestinal infections caused by *H. alvei* are unusual but can occur in immunocompetent individuals as well as those with underlying diseases, although the latter group is more likely to be affected (108). These infections are often community acquired and are believed to arise from the gastrointestinal tract. *Hafnia* appears to have a predilection for the biliary tree and may produce abscesses at the site of infection (108).

In humans, *Plesiomonas shigelloides* is primarily associated with diarrheal disease. Infections occur most frequently in individuals who live in or travel to tropical countries; a history of seafood consumption is common. A retrospective study of *Plesiomonas* infection undertaken in Hong Kong found an infection rate of 5.9% over a 4-year period, with increasing numbers of isolations during 3 of the 4 years of the study (130). Most infections are self-limiting; however, hospitalization may be required for severe infections and/or in those with underlying conditions. Symptoms associated with *Plesiomonas* diarrhea vary, and patients may present with either a secretory or a dysenteric type of disease. In the study by Wong et al. (130), 73% of patients had watery diarrhea and 25% had bloody diarrhea. Abdominal pain is commonly reported and may be severe; dehydration and fever are also present in one-third to one-half of the patients (63, 68). Patients may also report chronic diarrhea for 2 weeks or longer. Association of *P. shigelloides* with diarrheal disease has been hampered by the inability to demonstrate putative virulence factors and the lack of an animal model. However, *Plesiomonas* has recently been observed both in membrane-bound vacuoles and free within the cytosol of cultured human colon cells examined by transmission electron microscopy (120). A beta-hemolysin described previously (65) and now shown to be calcium and iron dependent (12) probably plays a role in the infectious process by releasing *P. shigelloides* from intracellular vacuoles. The dysenteric form of diarrhea seen in some patients may be explained by the organism's ability to invade and multiply within human gastrointestinal cells. Association of *Plesiomonas* with secretory diarrheal infections is more tenuous, although cholera-like, heat-stable, and heat-labile toxins (63) have been described. The lipopolysaccharide of *Plesiomonas* may also play a role in the infectious process. Sequencing data have shown that the O17 antigen, belonging to the most common serogroup of *Plesiomonas*, and the form 1 antigen of *S. sonnei* have almost identical gene regions (28). Sepsis caused by *Plesiomonas* is rare but has been documented (63). Although plesiomonads have an aquatic reservoir, wound infections associated with water contact similar to those found with *Aeromonas* species are not encountered. *Edwardsiella tarda* is yet another aquatic organism and is an infrequent cause of gastroenteritis in humans, with most infections occurring after contact with fish or turtles. The low carriage rate of this organism, except in tropical areas of the world, and the ability to produce a cell-associated hemolysin and invade HEp-2 cells are indicators that *E. tarda* is a diarrheal agent (68). Serious wound

infections, including myonecrosis, have been reported in immunocompetent individuals who had aquatic exposure (116). Systemic infections usually occur in patients with liver disease or iron overload conditions.

Except for *E. tarda*, the other *Enterobacteriaceae* listed in the left-hand column of Table 2 cause opportunistic infections and are not frequently encountered in the clinical laboratory (64). Some, like *Cedecea* spp. (53), *Leminorella* spp. (60), *Moellerella* (59), and *Tatumella* (61), are rarely isolated from nonhuman sources, making it difficult to determine reservoirs for these organisms (64). Strains of *Ewingella* (54), *Leclercia* (118), and *Kluyvera* spp. (39) have been found in a variety of foods, water, or animals (snails and slugs) and are probably, like many *Enterobacteriaceae*, ubiquitous in the environment (64). Other genera that have been isolated from human specimens have more specific natural habitats. These include *Rahnella* (64), all of whose initially described isolates were recovered from water and which probably serves as the reservoir for human infections, or *Yokenella* (78) and *Photorhabdus luminescens* (17, 40), which are common in insects and have caused infections resulting from insect bites (64).

ISOLATION

For the most part, the clinically relevant strains covered in this chapter are not difficult to isolate from sterile body sites. Cockerill et al. (30) did find, however, that during culturing of blood, both *E. cloacae* and *S. marcescens* grew significantly better in aerobic culture than in nonvented or anaerobic culture; no difference was noted for other major species of the genera in this chapter. *S. marcescens* was recovered significantly more often from the Isolator system than by Septi-Chek (67 and 38 isolations, respectively; $P = 0.006$). Isolation from nonsterile body or environmental sites may require specialized media.

CHROMagar Orientation (CHROMagar Co., Paris, France) is a medium that was developed to isolate and differentiate gram-negative, gram-positive, and yeast urinary tract pathogens (114). Presumptive identification of organisms is based on the colony color produced by the enzymatic action of the organism on chromogenic substrates in the medium. A comparison of this medium with the standard media used for urine culture, 5% sheep blood and MacConkey agars, yielded identical results in a test of 900 urine samples (114). Of 190 positive specimens in this study, *P. mirabilis*, *P. vulgaris*, and *Morganella* were all correctly identified directly from the plate by their colony color, although a spot indole was required to separate *Morganella* and *P. mirabilis*. In this study, colony colors for *Klebsiella*, *Citrobacter*, and *Enterobacter* were too similar to be identified from the CHROMagar without additional selected biochemical tests. CHROMagar prevents swarming of *Proteus*, allowing easier detection of multiple pathogens, and antimicrobial susceptibility tests can be performed directly without the need for subculturing. Ohkusu (102) expanded the usage of CHROMagar Orientation to cover isolation of pathogenic organisms from wound, stool, and a variety of other specimens in addition to urine. Using colony color on CHROMagar in combination with indole, lysine, and ornithine decarboxylase tests and serologic testing, 466 of 472 isolates (98.7%) were correctly identified, including 15 species of *Klebsiella*, *Citrobacter*, *Enterobacter*, *Proteus*, *Morganella*, and *Providencia*.

E. tarda, which is a lactose-negative, H_2S-positive organism, is indistinguishable from *Salmonella* on enteric plating media (opaque or opaque with black centers). A positive indole reaction and lack of agglutination in specific *Salmonella* antisera differentiate *E. tarda* strains from *Salmonella*.

Plesiomonas is also easily isolated, growing on blood agar (BA) as a 2- to 3-mm, opaque, convex colony or as a non-lactose-, non-sucrose-fermenting colony on enteric plating media. It does not grow on thiosulfate-citrate-bile salts-sucrose medium, but it does grow well on, and can be isolated from, cefsulodin-Irgasan-novobiocin (CIN) medium. Because it does not ferment mannitol, the colonies are opaque but do not have a pink center on CIN medium. It must be separated from other oxidase-positive organisms (*Pseudomonas* and *Aeromonas*) that can also grow on this medium, although *Aeromonas* should have a pink center with an opaque apron. Inositol fermentation and a positive reaction in Moeller's lysine, arginine, and ornithine tests differentiate *Plesiomonas* from other organisms.

Other *Enterobacteriaceae* that are involved in opportunistic infections and that may be present in a variety of specimen types generally grow well on commonly used laboratory media (64). Some genera are lactose or sucrose fermenters and give the appearance of normal flora on enteric plating media, while others may produce H_2S and appear *Salmonella*-like. *Rahnella*, *Ewingella*, and especially *Tatumella* may require 48 h for growth. *Tatumella* also grows poorly on Mueller-Hinton agar, and a broth dilution method may be required for susceptibility testing. Strains of *Tatumella* do not survive well at room temperature and should be stored at −70°C. K. (C.) granulomatis, as with many of the organisms in the third column of Table 2, does not grow on conventional laboratory media. Since K. (C.) granulomatis does not stain well with Gram reagents, the Giemsa- or Wright-stained impression smear of lesions showing Donovan bodies has been the method most commonly used to detect this organism. However, Donovan bodies, which are pleomorphic bipolar-staining bodies shaped like a closed safety pin, are not always present and therefore are not reliable for diagnosis. Recently, growth in HEp-2 monolayers has been achieved (27). Primers to the *phoE* and *scrA* (sucrose regulon) genes have been used to identify and separate K. (C.) granulomatis from *Klebsiella* species. *Klebsiella* species are positive for both genes, while K. (C.) granulomatis possesses only the *phoE* gene (26).

IDENTIFICATION

The biochemical tests most useful for separating species within each genus are described in Tables 3 through 13. Full biochemical profiles for each species can be found in chapter 41. Correct identification to species level is increasingly important in recognizing strains that are of high risk for carrying extended-spectrum β-lactamases, cephalosporinases, or carbapenemases (83). Identification problems arising from the use of commercial systems vary with each genus. *Serratia* spp. are generally easily identified by commercial systems, except for the *S. liquefaciens* group; separation of members within this group requires carbon assimilation tests (64). These tests can be performed using a combination of API 50CH, API 50AO, and API 50AA (carbohydrate, organic acid, and amino acid panels, respectively; bioMérieux, Hazelwood, Mo.) strips (50). *Citrobacter* identification is hampered because few systems include newer species in their databases. Automated systems appear to fare worse than manual systems, with <90% accuracy in identifying members previously within the *C. freundii* complex (64). Many strains require supplemental conventional biochemical tests, especially for differentiation of *C. koseri* from *C. amalonaticus*. Most of the commonly employed commercial systems have difficulties in identifying *C. amalonaticus*, with 6 to 41% of strains tested giving an incorrect identification (64). A PYR (L-pyroglutamic acid to detect pyrrolidonyl peptidase) test may be useful for separating biochemically atypical strains of *Citrobacter* (positive) from *Salmonella* (negative) (15). Of the *Klebsiella* spp., *K. ozaenae* and *K. rhinoscleromatis* do the poorest in commercial systems, probably as a result of slow growth. These species can be difficult to separate using conventional biochemicals as well. R. (*Klebsiella*) planticola and R. (*Klebsiella*) terrigena cannot be readily separated from *Klebsiella* without temperature growth or carbon assimilation tests, which are not readily available in most clinical laboratories. Members of the genus *Enterobacter* appear to confound commercial systems more often than do other genera in the *Enterobacteriaceae*, probably because of the heterogeneity of several of the species. Six commonly employed systems failed to identify one or more of several species (E. cloacae, E. aerogenes, P. agglomerans, and E. sakazakii) with ≥90% accuracy a total of 14 times (64). H. alvei, which biochemically most closely resembles members of the genus *Enterobacter* and

TABLE 3 Separation of members of the genus *Citrobacter*[a]

Species	Indole	ODC	Malonate	Acid[b] from:			
				Sucrose	Dulcitol	Melibiose	Adonitol
C. amalonaticus	+	+	−	−	−	−	−
C. braakii	V	+	−	−	V	V	−
C. farmeri	+	+	−	+	−	+	−
C. freundii (sensu stricto)	V	−	−	+	−	+	−
C. koseri	+	+	+	V	V	−	+
C. rodentium	−	+	+	−	−	−	−
C. sedlakii	V	+	+	−	+	+	−
C. werkmanii	−	−	+	−	−	−	−
C. youngae	V	−	−	V	+	−	−
C. gillenii	−	−	+	V	−	V	−
C. murliniae	+	−	−	V	+	V	−

[a] Abbreviations and symbols: ODC, ornithine decarboxylase; +, ≥85%; V, 15 to 85%; −, ≤15%.
[b] Fermentation reactions in commercial identification systems should be similar to reactions in conventional fermentation broths (1% carbohydrate in broth with indicator).

TABLE 4 Differentiation of *Pantoea agglomerans* and members of the genus *Enterobacter*[a]

| Species | LDC | ADH | ODC | VP | Acid[b] from: | | | | | | | Yellow pigment |
					Sucrose	Adonitol	Sorbitol	Rhamnose	α-Methyl glucoside	Esculin	Melibiose	
Human species												
E. aerogenes	+	−	+	+	+	+	+	+	+	+	+	−
P. agglomerans	−	−	−	V	V	V	−	V	V	−	V	V	V
E. amnigenus biogroup 1	−	−	V	+	+	−	−	+	V	+	+	−
E. asburiae	−	V	+	−	+	−	+	−	+	+	−	−
E. cancerogenus	−	+	+	+	−	−	−	+	−	+	−	−
E. cloacae	−	+	+	+	+	V	+	+	V	V	+	−
E. cowanii[c]	−	−	−	+	+	−	+	+	−	+	+	V
E. gergoviae	+	−	+	+	+	−	−	+	−	+	+	−
E. hormaechei	−	V	+	+	+	−	−	+	V	−	−	−
E. intermedium	−	−	V	+	V	−	+	+	+	+	+	−
E. kobei	−	+	+	−	+	−	+	+	+	V	+	−
E. sakazakii	−	+	+	+	+	−	−	+	+	+	+	+
Environmental species												
E. amnigenus biogroup II	−	V	+	+	−	−	+	+	+	+	+	−
E. dissolvens	−	+	+	+	+	−	+	+	+	+	+	−
E. nimipressuralis	−	−	+	+	−	−	+	+	+	+	+	−
E. pyrinus[d]	+	−	+	V	+	−	−	+	−	+	V	−

[a] Abbreviations and symbols: LDC, lysine decarboxylase; ADH, arginine dihyrolase; ODC, ornithine decarboxylase; VP, Voges-Proskauer; +, ≥90%; V, 11 to 89%; −, ≤10%.

[b] See Table 3, footnote b.

[c] Separated from *P. agglomerans* by a negative malonate reaction and fermentation of sorbitol (62).

[d] Separated from *E. gergoviae* by positive reactions in potassium cyanide broth and *myo*-inositol.

Yokenella regensburgei (Table 11), is usually correctly identified in commercial systems. Two members of the genus *Proteus* can be rapidly identified with minimal testing. Gram-negative and oxidase-negative organisms that swarm on BA and appear flat with tapered edges on MacConkey agar may be reported as *Proteus*. *Proteus* spp. that are spot indole negative and ampicillin susceptible may be reported as *P. mirabilis* (13, 104). *P. penneri*, which is a rare clinical isolate, also fits the above description but can be separated from *P. mirabilis* by its negative reactions in ornithine decarboxylase and maltose. Spot indole-positive, ampicillin-resistant strains are reported as *P. vulgaris* (13). *P. hauseri*, previously a subgroup of *P. vulgaris*, can be differentiated from *P. vulgaris* by a negative salicin or esculin

reaction (98). Although it occurs in clinical specimens, *P. hauseri* is infrequently seen in the laboratory (67). If an organism does not fit any one of the above qualifications, it must be fully identified by commercial or conventional biochemical methods (13). Most commercially available systems satisfactorily identify *Proteus*, with reports varying between 95 to 100% accuracy for different systems. *Providencia*, however, is not identified to the same level of accuracy in commercial systems, and the rates vary from 79 to 100% (98). When *Providencia* spp. are misidentified, they are usually called *Morganella* or *Proteus*. Urea-positive *P. stuartii* may be misidentified as *P. rettgeri*, or the system may require additional tests for identification. *P. heimbachae* is not included in commercial system databases (98). M.

TABLE 5 Separation of some members of the genera *Klebsiella* and *Raoultella*[a]

| Species | Indole | ODC | VP | Malonate | ONPG | Growth at: | | Acid[b] from D-melezitose |
						10°C	44°C	
R. ornithinolytica	+	+	V	+	+	+	NA	NA
K. oxytoca	+	−	+	+	+	−	+	−
K. ozaenae	−	−	−	−	V	NA	NA	NA
K. pneumoniae	−	−	+	+	+	−	+	−
R. planticola	V	−	+	+	+	+	−	−
R. terrigena	−	V	+	+	+	+	−	+
K. rhinoscleromatis	−	−	−	+	−	NA	NA	NA

[a] Abbreviations and symbols: ODC, ornithine decarboxylase; VP, Voges-Proskauer; ONPG, *o*-nitrophenyl-β-D-galactopyranoside; NA, not available; +, ≥90%; V, 11 to 89%; −, ≤10%.

[b] See Table 3, footnote b.

TABLE 6 Biochemical characterization of members of the genus *Serratia*[a]

Species	LDC	ODC	Mal	Acid[b] from:							Red pigment	Odor
				Arabinose	L-Rhamnose	D-Xylose	Sucrose	Adonitol	D-Sorbitol	Cellobiose		
S. entomophila[c]	−	−	−	−	−	V	+	−	−	−	−	−
S. ficaria	−	−	V	+	V	+	+	−	+	+	−	V
S. fonticola	+	+	V	+	V	V	V	+	+	−	−	−
S. liquefaciens group	+	+	−	+	V	+	+	−	+	−	−	−
S. marcescens	+	+	−	−	−	−	+	V	+	−	V	−
S. marcescens biogroup 1	V	V	−	−	−	−	+	V	+	−	NA	−
S. odorifera biogroup 1	+	+	−	+	+	+	+	V	+	+	−	+
S. odorifera biogroup 2	+	−	−	+	+	+	−	V	+	+	−	+
S. plymuthica[d]	−	−	−	+	−	+	+	−	V	V	+	−
S. rubidaea	V	−	+	+	−	+	+	+	−	+	+	−

[a] Abbreviations and symbols: LDC, lysine decarboxylase; ODC, ornithine decarboxylase; Mal, malonate; +, ≥90%; V, 11 to 89%; −, ≤10%; NA, information not available.
[b] See Table 3, footnote *b*.
[c] Growth at 37°C but biochemical characterization optimal at 30°C.
[d] May fail to grow at 37°C.

morganii subsp. *morganii* is identified 100% of the time in commercial systems according to most studies, although 2-h identification methods misidentify it about 66% of the time. *M. morganii* subsp. *sibonii* is not included in most databases and may be separated from subsp. *morganii* only by a positive reaction in trehalose.

The two agents of gastroenteritis, *Plesiomonas* (Table 13) and *E. tarda* (Table 12), are easily separated from both other enteric pathogens and normal flora, and their identification presents no difficulty in either conventional or commercial systems. Sequencing data have shown that the somatic antigen that occurs in the most common serogroup

of *Plesiomonas* (serogroup 17) and the form 1 antigen of *S. sonnei* have almost identical gene regions (28). Thus, if *Shigella* serotyping is performed on strains of *Plesiomonas*, as sometimes happens, cross-reactions may occur.

Reactions to identify other enterobacteria isolated from clinical specimens are listed in Tables 8 through 12. The organisms are grouped with the genera with which they would most probably be confused and from which they must be differentiated. Many of the agents in these tables are included in commercial system databases. Unfortunately, the number of strains available to use in challenge studies is very limited; therefore, the ability of these systems to ac-

TABLE 7 Separation of members of the genera *Proteus*, *Providencia*, and *Morganella*[a]

Organism	Indole	H₂S	Urea	ODC	Acid[b] from:				
					Maltose	D-Adonitol	D-Arabitol	Trehalose	myo-Inositol
Proteus									
P. hauseri	+	V	+	−	+	−	−	+	−
P. mirabilis	−	+	+	+	−	−	−	+	−
P. penneri	−	V	+	−	+	−	−	V	−
P. vulgaris[c]	+	+	+	−	+	−	−	V	−
Providencia									
P. alcalifaciens	+	−	−	−	−	+	−	−	−
P. heimbachae	−	−	−	−	V	+	+	−	V
P. rettgeri	+	−	+	−	−	+	+	−	+
P. rustigianii	+	−	−	−	−	−	−	−	−
P. stuartii	+	−	V	−	−	−	−	+	+
Morganella									
M. morganii subsp. *morganii*	+	−[d]	+	+[e]	−	−	−	−	−
M. morganii subsp. *sibonii*	V	−[d]	+	+[e]	−	−	−	+	−

[a] Abbreviations and symbols: H₂S, hydrogen sulfide; ODC, ornithine decarboxylase; +, ≥90%; V, 11 to 89%; −, ≤10%.
[b] See Table 3, footnote *b*.
[c] *P. vulgaris* genomospecies 4, 5, and 6 cannot be differentiated phenotypically.
[d] Some members of some biogroups are H₂S positive.
[e] Some members of some biogroups are ornithine decarboxylase negative.

TABLE 8 Separation of *Cedecea* from selected *Enterobacter* species (VP, ADH, and ODC variable or positive)[a]

Organism	Acid[b] from:					
	D-Sorbitol	Raffinose	L-Rhamnose	Melibiose	D-Arabitol	Sucrose
C. davisae	−	−	−	−	+	+
C. lapagei	−	−	−	−	+	−
E. cloacae	+	+	+	+	V	+
E. sakazakii	−	+	+	+	−	+
E. cancerogenus	−	−	+	−	−	−

[a] Abbreviations and symbols: VP, Voges-Proskauer; ADH, arginine dihydrolase; ODC, ornithine decarboxylase; +, ≥90%; V, 11 to 89%; −, ≤10%.
[b] See Table 3, footnote *b*.

curately identify these organisms is really unknown. *Ewingella* and *Tatumella* are poor growers and are biochemically inactive. *Kluyvera* can be identified only to genus level by these systems; species determination requires an ascorbate test, Irgasan susceptibility, and/or gas-liquid chromatography profiles (64). *Photorhabdus luminescens* is not included in commercial databases.

The use of molecular methods (see chapter 17) to determine the presence and/or identity of bacteria directly from clinical specimens or from isolates is increasingly reported but not universally available. These methods offer a great advantage when bacteria are difficult or impossible to culture, such as *K. (C.) granulomatis*, or in diseases such as keratitis, where cultures are negative 40 to 60% of the time (76). Testing specimens with universal primers based on conserved regions of the bacterial chromosome can determine within 1 h if a patient has a bacterial infection (16). Normally sterile clinical specimens found negative by these assays would not then require culturing, saving considerably on laboratory resources. However, numerous problems remain to be worked out with these methods of bacterial identification. For ribosomal DNA sequencing, these include, but are not limited to, DNA extraction protocols, ambiguous profiles arising from testing mixed cultures, the presence of too few species in the databases, and percent similarity cutoff guidelines for identification at the species or genus level (33).

The ability to trace the spread or involvement of nosocomial pathogens in outbreaks caused by the *Enterobacteriaceae* has become a major responsibility and problem for the laboratory. Biotyping using commercially available identification systems is seldom suitably discriminating unless an unusual marker or profile is present. Biotyping schemes using carbon assimilation tests have been developed, particularly for *Serratia* (50), but may be difficult to perform. Typing all genera for which traditional typing methods are

TABLE 9 Differentiation of *Kluyvera* from commonly seen indole-positive, VP-negative organisms[a]

Organism	Citrate	Urea	LDC	KCN
Kluyvera	+	−	+	+
C. koseri	+	V	−	−
Morganella	−	+	−	+
Providencia	+	+/−	−	+
E. coli	−	−	+	−

[a] Abbreviations and symbols: VP, Voges-Proskauer; LDC, lysine decarboxylase; KCN, potassium cyanide; +, ≥90%; V, 11 to 89%; −, ≤10%. *Leclercia* and *E. tarda* are also indole positive and VP negative and can be found in Tables 10 and 12, respectively.

available (serotyping, bacteriocins, and bacteriophages) would necessitate multiple sets of reagents, which are not readily available and/or are economically prohibitive. Molecular techniques including plasmid analysis, ribotyping, PFGE, and various PCR methods all appear satisfactorily discriminatory, with some working better for a specific genus or species than others (see chapter 17). The variety of PCR techniques is proliferating at an astonishing pace, especially repetitive-element PCR methods for the *Enterobacteriaceae*. Care in the performance and interpretation of these assays is critical since many PCR techniques have not been standardized (36, 49). For now, since a single method applicable to most strains is preferable, at least economically, PFGE still remains the most universally accepted standardized technique for epidemiological studies. The disadvantage of a long turnaround time (usually 4 days) has been partially overcome by a rapid PFGE protocol that is suitable for most enteric bacteria as well as other common clinical strains (45).

ANTIMICROBIAL SUSCEPTIBILITY

Resistance among members of the *Enterobacteriaceae* is increasing at a slow but inexorable pace (9), especially in organisms known to harbor extended-spectrum β-lactamases (ESBL), cephalosporinases, and carbapenemases (Table 14) (for resistance mechanisms, see chapters 68, 74, and 75). In one 9-year study of nosocomial isolates, as the number of intrinsically β-lactamase-susceptible organisms such as *E. coli* and *Proteus* decreased, the number of intrinsically β-lactamase-resistant species, notably *Enterobacter* and *Klebsiella* species, increased (97). While ESBLs are most prevalent in *K. pneumoniae*, they have been reported in almost all clinically significant members of the *Enterobacteriaceae* (70, 72, 83, 97). Ambler class C chromosomally mediated carbapenemases are seen in *E. cloacae* and *S. marcescens*, while the Ambler class B carbapenemase IMP-1, originally found in *S. marcescens*, has recently been found in *K. pneumoniae* (77). Because IMP-1 may be located on a plasmid, it poses a greater risk for intra- and inter-hospital spread than do cephalosporinases that are only chromosomally encoded. In Japan, 4.4% of >3,000 *S. marcescens* isolates tested were IMP-1 producers (8). Resistance to amikacin and fluoroquinolones in the same strains was also noted. Ambler class C plasmid-mediated cephalosporinases have emerged in *K. pneumoniae* in various regions of the world, including the United States, while the chromosomally mediated AmpC cephalosporinases are found in *Citrobacter* spp., *Morganella*, *Providencia*, *P. vulgaris*, and *C. koseri* (83).

TABLE 10 Separation of LDC-, ODC-, and ADH-negative unusual *Enterobacteriaceae* found in clinical specimens[a]

Organism	Motility	Gas from glucose	KCN	VP	Acid[b] from:		
					Sucrose	Arabinose	Trehalose
Ewingella	V	−	−	+	−	−	+
Leclercia	V	+	+	−	V	+	+
Moellerella	−	−	V	−	+	−	−
Rahnella	−	+	−	+	+	+	+
Tatumella	−	−	−	−	+	−	+
Photorhabdus luminescens	+	−	−	−	−	−	−

[a] Abbreviations and symbols: LDC, lysine decarboxylase; ODC, ornithine decarboxylase; ADH, arginine dihydrolase; KCN, potassium cyanide; VP, Voges-Proskauer; +, ≥90%; V, 11 to 89%; −, ≤10%. *Budvicia* is also LDC, ODC, and ADH negative and can be found in Table 12.
[b] See Table 3, footnote b.

Several reports have indicated that *Enterobacter* species are the primary reservoir for ESBLs (96, 123). Neuwirth et al. (96) reported plasmid transmission of a TEM-24 ESBL from *E. aerogenes* to strains of *K. pneumoniae*, *P. vulgaris*, *P. mirabilis*, and *S. marcescens* in their institution. Transfer occurred in vivo to any organism present in a patient site that was also colonized with the ESBL-producing *E. aerogenes*.

The spread of ESBL-producing strains can be controlled, without restricting antimicrobial usage, by using barrier precautions and cohorting patients after discharge from the intensive care unit (84), since transmission occurs primarily on the hands of hospital staff (105). However, Patterson and Yu (105) recommend a three-pronged effort to control ESBL-producing organisms that includes enhancing surveillance and control within the intensive care unit, increasing laboratory capability in the detection of ESBLs, and limiting the empirical use of antibiotics. While the selective pressure for antimicrobial resistance in the presence of widespread unremitting antimicrobial use is hard to deny, drug resistance has been found in bacteria isolated from wild rodents that have not had exposure to antibiotics (48). A total of 126 isolates of *H. alvei*, *Serratia* spp., *Enterobacter* spp., *Cedecea* spp., and *Providencia* spp. resistant to multiple antibiotics including cefuroxime were isolated from 108 wild rodents. The origin and persistence of resistance in this wild population are unknown but indicate that selective processes in addition to antimicrobial usage are involved in the maintenance of resistance genes. Furthermore, restriction of specific antimicrobials may reduce resistance in one or several species but select for resistance in others, substituting one problem for another (80).

Apart from its use for infection control, the cost-effectiveness of laboratory testing for ESBLs has been questioned since ESBL detection is unlikely to affect patient outcome (37). Studies to determine the outcomes of serious infections caused by organisms considered cephalosporin "sus-

ceptible" or "intermediate" in vitro found that 54% of patients who were treated with a cephalosporin experienced therapy failure (104). These patients either succumbed to their infections or required a change in therapy to achieve a cure. UTIs caused by ESBL-producing organisms can be successfully treated with cephalosporins, eliminating the need to test urine isolates for ESBL production for therapeutic consideration; however, testing may be required for infection control efforts to prevent horizontal transfer of these strains (104).

Since NCCLS ESBL detection methods are recommended only for *Klebsiella* and *E. coli* (94, 95), guidelines suggested for testing ESBL-producing strains of *Enterobacter* have evolved to include using cefpirome or, preferably, cefepime disks placed 20 mm apart from the amoxicillin-clavulanic acid disk (122). Using this method, Tzelepi et al. (122) were able to detect ESBLs in 28 of 31 *Enterobacter* isolates (90%), while other methods detected only 6.4 to 61.3% of the ESBL strains, indicating that the incidence of ESBLs may be underestimated in strains of *Enterobacter* with derepressed β-lactamases. Strains of *P. vulgaris* may present difficulties in susceptibility testing when agar methods are employed. Agar dilution, E-test, or disk diffusion assays may give falsely susceptible results, as indicated by broth dilution MICs that may be as much as 10 dilutions higher than those seen with agar dilution. This phenomenon may be due to the presence of an inducible class A β-lactamase, CumA, which appears to be suppressed when cultures are grown on agar (103).

Other resistances noted worldwide among the *Enterobacteriaceae* include imipenem resistance, which typically emerges during therapy to treat ceftazidime- and aminoglycoside-resistant strains and appears reversible with cessation of therapy (1, 18). An unusual plasmid-borne AmpC β-lactamase with cefoxitin susceptibility has been reported in *Klebsiella* (113). Ciprofloxacin resistance, influenced by antibiotic usage and the clonal spread between patients of strains containing ESBLs, has been found in strains of *K. pneumoniae* and *K. oxytoca*, with rates as high as 7.2 and 3.4%, respectively (24). Cefepime resistance in *Enterobacter* spp. and *K. oxytoca* strains has been reported recently (112). In a Belgian study, 7 and 2% of *E. aerogenes* strains were reported to be resistant to cefepime and imipenem, respectively (32). All strains resistant to imipenem were resistant to cefepime, although the reverse was not true. Additionally, of 249 strains tested, 76% were resistant to both ceftazidime and ciprofloxacin and 46% had ESBLs present; 90% of strains remained aminoglycoside susceptible.

TABLE 11 Separation of *Yokenella* from *Hafnia*[a]

Organism	VP	Citrate	Acid[b] from:	
			Melibiose	Glycerol
Yokenella	−	+	+	−
Hafnia alvei	+	−	−	+

[a] Abbreviations and symbols: VP, Voges-Proskauer; +, ≥90%; V, 11 to 89%; −, ≤10%.
[b] See Table 3, footnote b.

TABLE 12 Separation of H$_2$S-positive members of the *Enterobacteriaceae*[a]

Organism	LDC	ODC	Urea	Acid[b] from arabinose	Citrate	KCN	ONPG
Leminorella spp.	−	−	−	+	V[c]	−	−
Edwardsiella tarda	+	+	−	−	−	−	−
Budvicia aquatilis[d]	−	−	V	V	−	−	+
Pragia fontium[d]	−	−	−	−	V	−	−
Trabulsiella guamensis[d]	+	+	−	+	V	+	+
Salmonella subgroup 1	+	+	−	+	+	−	−
Citrobacter	−	V	V	+	V	+	+
Proteus	−	V	+	−	V	+	−

[a] Abbreviations and symbols: H$_2$S, hydrogen sulfide; LDC, lysine decarboxylase; ODC, ornithine decarboxylase; KCN, potassium cyanide; ONPG, *o*-nitrophenol-β-D-galactopyranoside; +, ≥90%; V, 11 to 89%; −, ≤10%.
[b] See Table 3, footnote *b*.
[c] *L. grimontii* is positive; *L. richardii* is negative.
[d] Found in clinical specimens but of questionable or no significance.

TABLE 13 Differentiation of *P. shigelloides* from other clinically significant members of the *Vibrionaceae* and the *Aeromonadaceae*[a]

Organism	LDC	ODC	ADH	Gas from glucose	Acid[b] from: Sucrose	Acid[b] from: Inositol	Growth in: TCBS	Growth in: 0% NaCl	O/129 susceptibility
Plesiomonas	+	+	+	−	−	+	−	+	+
Aeromonas spp.	V	−[c]	+	V	V	−	−	+	−
Vibrio spp.[d]	+	+	−	−	V	−	+	V	+

[a] Abbreviations and symbols: LDC, lysine decarboxylase; ODC, ornithine decarboxylase; ADH, arginine dihydrolase; TCBS, thiosulfate-citrate-bile salts-sucrose; O/129, 2,4-diamino-6,7-diisopropylpteridine.
[b] See Table 3, footnote *b*.
[c] Only *A. veronii* biotype veronii is positive.
[d] *V. hollisae* is LDC, ODC, and ADH negative; only *V. fluvialis* and *V. furnissii* are ADH positive; *V. furnissii* produces gas; *V. cincinnatiensis* ferments inositol; *V. cholerae* and *V. mimicus* grow in 0% NaCl.

TABLE 14 ESBLs, cephalosporinases, and carbapenemases of the *Enterobacteriaceae*[a]

Ambler class	Bush class	Enzyme class	Substrate	Clavulanic acid	Organism(s)	Location
Serine β-lactamase						
A	2b	Restricted-spectrum β-lactamase	Aminopenicillins, carboxypenicillins	S	*K. pneumoniae* Several other genera	Plasmid Chromosome
A	2be	Extended-spectrum β-lactamase	Extended-spectrum β-lactams	S	*Klebsiella* spp., *S. marcescens*, *Enterobacter* spp., *Proteus* spp., *C. freundii*, *M. morganii*	Plasmid
A	2f	Carbapenemase	Carbapenems, aztreonam	S	*Enterobacter* spp., *S. marcescens*	Chromosome
A	2e	Cefuroximases	Cephalosporins	S	*Proteus* spp., *C. koseri*	Chromosome
C	1	Cephalosporinase	Extended-spectrum β-lactams, cephamycins, aztreonam	R	*K. pneumoniae*, several other genera	Plasmid
C	1	Cephalosporinase	Extended-spectrum β-lactams, aztreonam	R	*Enterobacter* spp., *C. freundii*, *S. marcescens*, *Proteus* spp., *M. morganii*	Chromosome
Metallo-β-lactamase						
B	3	Carbapenemase	Oxyamino-cephalosporins, aztreonam	R	*K. pneumoniae* *S. marcescens*	Plasmid Chromosome

[a] Abbreviations: S, susceptible; R, resistant. Data from references 25 and 97.

Strains of *P. mirabilis* are resistant to nitrofurantoin but susceptible to trimethoprim-sulfamethoxazole, ampicillin, amoxicillin, piperacillin, cephalosporins, aminoglycosides, and imipenem. Although most strains are susceptible to ciprofloxacin, resistance occurs with unrestricted use of the drug (98). *P. penneri* and *P. vulgaris* have a similar resistance profile to *Morganella*, although *P. penneri* is more resistant to penicillin than is *P. vulgaris*. All three organisms are susceptible to broad-spectrum cephalosporins, cefoxitin, cefepime, aztreonam, aminoglycosides, and imipenem. They are resistant to piperacillin, amoxicillin, ampicillin, cefoperazone, cefuroxime, and cefazolin. Some automated systems may not be able to detect resistance to broad- and expanded-spectrum cephalosporins in *Morganella* and indole-positive *Proteus* (98). Three- and six-hour automated tests may not involve sufficiently long incubations to detect resistant bacteria and may result in false reports of susceptibility of *Morganella* and *Providencia* (98). *Providencia rettgeri* and *P. stuartii* are resistant to gentamicin and tobramycin but susceptible to amikacin. Urine isolates are susceptible to broad- and expanded-spectrum cephalosporins, ciprofloxacin, amoxicillin-clavulanic acid, imipenem, and trimethoprim-sulfamethoxazole. *Providencia heimbachae*, although infrequently seen in humans, is resistant to tetracycline, most cephalosporins, gentamicin, and amikacin. Human isolates of *E. tarda* are susceptible to cephalosporins, aminoglycosides, imipenem, ciprofloxacin, aztreonam, and antibiotic–β-lactamase inhibitor combination agents (29). Isolates from fish and fishponds may be more resistant because of the use of antibiotics prophylactically in fish farming. Almost all strains of *E. tarda* produce β-lactamases, even though they are susceptible to β-lactams. *P. shigelloides* is resistant to ampicillin, carbenicillin, piperacillin, and ticarcillin and is variably resistant to most aminoglycosides and tetracycline (63). Cephalosporins, quinolones, carbapenems, and trimethoprim-sulfamethoxazole show good activity against *P. shigelloides*.

Freney et al. (44) performed susceptibility tests on 120 isolates of uncommonly isolated species of *Klebsiella*, *Enterobacter*, and *Serratia* and found their susceptibilities to be similar to those of conventional species within each genus. Because they are infrequently seen in clinical laboratories, resistance profiles of many of the other *Enterobacteriaceae* are found only in individual case reports. Susceptibilities vary from isolate to isolate even within a genus, so that no empirical guidelines are available for therapy prior to susceptibility testing of the suspected strain.

EVALUATION, INTERPRETATION, AND REPORTING OF RESULTS

When any of the species included in this chapter are identified with a high level of accuracy (>90% probability) by a commercial system, the identification is probably reliable. However, when organisms are isolated from a source in which they may be considered significant, such as blood or cerebrospinal fluid and the identification has a probability of <90%, the isolate should be identified by conventional methods or sent to a reference laboratory that uses these techniques. In the interim, the isolate may be reported to the physician with a presumptive identification. For strains seen more commonly, the antimicrobial susceptibility profile may be a helpful adjunct for deciding if identifications with lower probabilities are reliable. Rare species that are identified with low probabilities should always be sent to a reference labo-

ratory, accompanied by a brief history. Colony appearance on MacConkey and BA plates, spot oxidase and indole reactions, and ampicillin susceptibility or resistance are sufficient for reporting *Proteus mirabilis* and *Proteus vulgaris* (13). At the very least, susceptibility testing of strains of *Klebsiella* that appear to contain ESBLs should be performed by the methods in NCCLS documents (119) M100-S9 (94) or M100-S10 (95). Any strain of the *Enterobacteriaceae* that has been shown to have an ESBL or AmpC cephalosporinase should be reported as resistant to all penicillins, expanded-spectrum cephalosporins, and aztreonam (105).

REFERENCES

1. **Ahmad, M., C. Urban, N. Mariano, P. A. Bradford, E. Calcagni, S. J. Projan, K. Bush, and J. J. Rahal.** 1999. Clinical characteristics and molecular epidemiology associated with imipenem-resistant *Klebsiella pneumoniae*. *Clin. Infect. Dis.* **29:**352–355.
2. **Aksoy, S.** 1995. *Wigglesworthia* gen. nov. and *Wigglesworthia glossinidia* sp. nov., taxa consisting of the mycetocyte-associated, primary endosymbionts of tsetse flies. *Int. J. Syst. Bacteriol.* **45:**848–851.
3. **Albert, M. J., K. Alam, M. M. Islam, J. Montanaro, A. S. Rhaman, K. Haider, M. A. Hossain, A. K. Kibriyan, and S. Tzipori.** 1991. *Hafnia alvei*, a probable cause of diarrhea in humans. *Infect. Immun.* **59:**1507–1513.
4. **Albert, M. J., M. Ansaruzzaman, N. A. Bhuiyan, P. K. B. Neogi, and A. S. G. Faruque.** 1995. Characteristics of invasion of HEp-2 cells by *Providencia alcalifaciens*. *J. Med. Microbiol.* **42:**186–190.
5. **Albert, M. J., S. M. Faruque, M. Ansaruzzaman, M. M. Islam, K. Haider, K. Alam, I. Kabir, and R. Robins-Browne.** 1992. Sharing of virulence-associated properties at the phenotypic and genetic levels between enteropathogenic *Escherichia coli* and *Hafnia alvei*. *J. Med. Microbiol.* **37:**310–314.
6. **Aldova, E., O. Hausner, D. J. Brenner, D. Kocmoud, J. Schindler, B. Potuznikova, and P. Petras.** 1988. *Pragia fontium* gen. nov., sp. nov. of the family *Enterobacteriaceae*, isolated from water. *Int. J. Syst. Bacteriol.* **38:**183–189.
7. **Aldova, E., O. Hausner, and M. Gabrhelova.** 1984. *Budvicia*—a new genus of *Enterobacteriaceae*. Data on phenotypic characters. *J. Hyg. Epidemiol. Microbiol. Immunol.* **28:**234–237.
8. **Arakawa, Y., Y. Ike, M. Nagasawa, N. Shibata, Y. Doi, K. Shibayama, T. Yagi, and T. Kurata.** 2000. Trends in antimicrobial-drug resistance in Japan. *Emerg. Infect. Dis.* **6:**572–575.
9. **ASCP Susceptibility Group.** 1997. United States geographic bacteria susceptibility patterns. *Diagn. Microbiol. Infect. Dis.* **35:**143–151.
10. **Aucken, H. M., and T. L. Pitt.** 1998. Different O and K serotype distributions among clinical and environmental strains of *Serratia marcescens*. *J. Med. Microbiol.* **47:**1097–1104.
11. **Aucken, H. M., and T. L. Pitt.** 1998. Antibiotic resistance and putative virulence factors of *Serratia marcescens* with respect to O and K serotypes. *J. Med. Microbiol.* **47:**1105–1113.
12. **Baratela, K. C., H. O. Saridakis, L. C. J. Gaziri, and J. S. Pelayo.** 2001. Effects of medium composition, calcium, iron and oxygen in haemolysin production by *Plesiomonas shigelloides* isolated from water. *J. Appl. Microbiol.* **90:**482–487.
13. **Baron, E. J.** 2001. Rapid identification of bacteria and yeast: summary of a National Committee for Clinical

Laboratory standards proposed guidelines. *Clin. Infect. Dis.* **33:**220–225.

14. **Belas, R.** 1992. The swarming phenomenon of *Proteus mirabilis. ASM News* **58:**15–22.

15. **Bennett, A. R., S. MacPhee, R. Betts, and D. Post.** 1999. Use of pyrrolidonyl peptidase to distinguish *Citrobacter* from *Salmonella. Lett. Appl. Microbiol.* **28:**175–178.

16. **Bergeron, M. G.** 2000. Genetic tools for the simultaneous identification of bacterial species and their antibiotic resistance genes: impact on clinical practice. *Int. J. Antimicrob. Agents* **16:**1–3.

17. **Boemare, N. E., R. J. Akhurst, and R. G. Mourant.** 1993. DNA relatedness between *Xenorhabdus* spp. (*Enterobacteriaceae*), symbiotic bacteria of entomopathogenic nematodes, and a proposal to transfer *Xenorhabdus luminescens* to a new genus, *Photorhabdus* gen. nov. *Int. J. Syst. Bacteriol.* **43:**249–255.

18. **Bornet, C., A. Davin-Regli, C. Bosi, J.-M. Pages, and C. Bollet.** 2000. Imipenem resistance of *Enterobacter aerogenes* mediated by outer membrane permeability. *J. Clin. Microbiol.* **38:**1048–1052.

19. **Bouvet, O. M. M., P. A. D. Grimont, C. Richard, E. Aldova, O. Hausner, and M. Gabrhelova.** 1985. *Budvicia aquatica* gen. nov.: a hydrogen sulfide-producing member of the *Enterobacteriaceae. Int. J. Syst. Bacteriol.* **35:**60–64.

20. **Brenner, D. J., G. R. Fanning, J. K. L. Knutson, A. G. Steigerwalt, and M. I. Krichevsky.** 1984. Attempts to classify Herbicola group-*Enterobacter agglomerans* strains by deoxyribonucleic acid hybridization and phenotypic tests. *Int. J. Syst. Bacteriol.* **34:**45–55.

21. **Brenner, D. J., P. A. D. Grimont, A. G. Steigerwalt, G. R. Fanning, E. Ageron, and C. F. Riddle.** 1993. Classification of citrobacteria by DNA hybridization: designation of *Citrobacter farmeri* sp. nov., *Citrobacter youngae* sp. nov., *Citrobacter braakii* sp. nov., *Citrobacter werkmanii* sp. nov., *Citrobacter sedlakii* sp. nov., and three unnamed *Citrobacter* genomospecies. *Int. J. Syst. Bacteriol.* **43:**645–658.

22. **Brenner, D. J., H. E. Muller, A. G. Steigerwalt, A. M. Whitney, C. M. O'Hara, and P. Kampfer.** 1998. Two new *Rahnella* genomospecies that cannot be phenotypically differentiated from *Rahnella aquatilis. Int. J. Syst. Bacteriol.* **48:**141–149.

23. **Brenner, D. J., C. M. O'Hara, P. A. D. Grimont, J. M. Janda, E. Falsen, E. Aldova, E. Ageron, J. Schindler, S. L. Abbott, and A. G. Steigerwalt.** 1999. Biochemical identification of *Citrobacter* species defined by DNA hybridization and description of *Citrobacter gillenii* sp. nov. (formerly *Citrobacter* genomospecies 10) and *Citrobacter murliniae* sp. nov. (formerly *Citrobacter* genomospecies 11). *J. Clin. Microbiol.* **37:**2619–2624.

24. **Brisse, S., D. Milatovic, A. C. Fluit, J. Verhoef, and F.-J. Schmitz.** 2000. Epidemiology of quinolone resistance of *Klebsiella pneumoniae* and *Klebsiella oxytoca* in Europe. *Eur. J. Clin. Microbiol. Infect. Dis.* **19:**64–68.

25. **Bush, K., G. A. Jacoby, and A. A. Medeiros.** 1995. A functional classification scheme for β-lactamases and its correlation with molecular structure. *Antimicrob. Agents Chemother.* **39:**1211–1233.

26. **Carter, J. S., F. J. Bowden, I. Bastain, G. M. Myers, K. S. Sriprakash, and D. J. Kemp.** 1999. Phylogenetic evidence for reclassification of *Calymmatobacterium granulomatis* as *Klebsiella granulomatis* comb. nov. *Int. J. Syst. Bacteriol.* **49:**1695–1700.

27. **Carter, J., S. Hutton, K. S. Sriprakash, D. J. Kemp, G. Lum, J. Savage, and F. J. Bowden.** 1997. Culture of the causative organism of donovanosis (*Calymmatobacterium*

28. **Chida, T., N. Okamura, K. Ohtani, Y. Yoshida, E. Arakawa, and H. Watanbe.** 2000. The complete DNA sequence of the O antigen gene region of *Plesiomonas shigelloides* serotype O17 which is identical to *Shigella sonnei* form I antigen. *Microbiol. Immunol.* **44:**161–172.

29. **Clark, R. B., P. D. Lister, and J. M. Janda.** 1991. In vitro susceptibilities of *Edwardsiella tarda* to 22 antibiotics and antibiotic-β-lactamase-inhibitor agents. *Diagn. Microbiol. Infect. Dis.* **14:**173–175.

30. **Cockerill, F. R., III, J. G. Hughes, E. A. Vetter, R. A. Mueller, A. L. Weaver, D. M. Ilstrup, J. E. Rosenblatt, and W. R. Wilson.** 1997. Analysis of 281,797 consecutive blood cultures performed over an eight-year period: trends in microorganism isolated and the value of anaerobic culture of blood. *Clin. Infect. Dis.* **24:**403–418.

31. **Dale, C., and I. Maudlin.** 1999. *Sodalis* gen. nov. and *Sodalis glossinidius* sp. nov., a microaerophilic secondary endosymbiont of the tsetse fly *Glossina morsitans morsitans. Int. J. Syst. Bacteriol.* **49:**267–275.

32. **De Gheldre, Y., M. J. Struelens, Y. Glupczynski, P. De Mol, N. Maes, C. Nonhoff, H. Chetoui, C. Sion, O. Ronveaux, M. Vaneechoutte, and Le Groupement pour le Dépistage, l'Etude et la Prévention des Infections Hospitalières (GDEPIH-GOSPIZ).** 2001. National epidemiologic surveys of *Enterobacter aerogenes* in Belgian hospitals from 1996 to 1998. *J. Clin. Microbiol.* **39:**889–896.

33. **Drancourt, M., C. Bollet, A. Carlioz, R. Martelin, J.-P. Gayral, and D. Raoult.** 2000. 16S ribosomal DNA sequence analysis of a large collection of environmental and clinical unidentifiable bacterial isolates. *J. Clin. Microbiol.* **38:**3623–3630.

34. **Drancourt, M., C. Bollet, A. Carta, and P. Rousselier.** 2001. Phylogenetic analyses of *Klebsiella* species delineate *Klebsiella* and *Raoultella* gen. nov., with description of *Raoultella ornithinolytica* comb. nov., *Raoultella terrigena* comb. nov. and *Raoultella planticola* comb. nov. *Int. J. Syst. Evol. Bacteriol.* **51:**925–932.

35. **Drelichman, V., and J. D. Band.** 1985. Bacteremias due to *Citrobacter diversus* and *Citrobacter freundii. Arch. Intern. Med.* **145:**1808–1810.

36. **Ehrlich, G. D.** 1991. Caveats of PCR. *Clin. Microbiol. Newsl.* **13:**149–151.

37. **Emery, C. L., and L. A. Weymouth.** 1997. Detection and clinical significance of extended-spectrum β-lactamases in a tertiary-care medical center. *J. Clin. Microbiol.* **35:**2061–2067.

38. **Farmer, J. J., III.** 1984. Other genera of the family *Enterobacteriaceae*, p. 506–516. *In* N. R. Krieg and J. G. Holt. (ed.), *Bergey's Manual of Systematic Bacteriology*, vol. 1. The Williams & Wilkins Co., Baltimore, Md.

39. **Farmer, J. J., III, G. R. Fanning, G. P. Huntley-Carter, B. Holmes, F. W. Hickman, C. Richard, and D. J. Brenner.** 1981. *Kluyvera*, a new (redefined) genus in the family *Enterobacteriaceae*: identification of *Kluyvera ascorbata* sp. nov. and *Kluyvera cryocrescens* sp. nov. in clinical specimens. *J. Clin. Microbiol.* **13:**919–933.

40. **Farmer, J. J., III, J. H. Jorgeson, P. A. D. Grimont, R. J. Akhurst, G. O. Poinar, E. Ageron, G. V. Pierce, and J. A. Smith.** 1989. *Xenorhabdus luminescens* (DNA hybridization group 5) from human clinical specimens. *J. Clin. Microbiol.* **27:**1594–1600.

41. **Fields, B. N., M. M. Uwaydah, L. J. Kunz, and M. N. Swarz.** 1967. The so-called "paracolon" bacteria. *Am. J. Med.* **42:**89–106.

42. **Fischer-LeSaux, M., V. Viallard, B. Brunel, P. Normand, and N. Boemare.** 1999. Polyphasic classification of

the genus *Photorhabdus* and proposal of new taxa: *P. luminescens* subsp. *luminescens* subsp. nov., *P. luminescens* subsp. *akhurstii* subsp. nov., *P. luminescens* subsp. *laumondii* subsp. nov., *P. temperata* sp. nov., and *P. asymbiotica* sp. nov. *Int. J. Syst. Bacteriol.* **49:**1645–1656.

43. **Fluit, A. C., M. E. Jones, F.-J. Schmitz, J. Acar, R. Gupta, and J. Verhoef.** 2000. Antimicrobial resistance among urinary tract infection (UTI) isolates in Europe: results from the SENTRY antimicrobial surveillance program 1997. *Antonie Leeuwenhoek* **77:**147–152.

44. **Freney, J., M. O. Husson, F. Gavini, S. Madier, A. Martra, D. Izard, H. Leclerc, and J. Fleurette.** 1988. Susceptibilities to antibiotics and antiseptics of new species of the family *Enterobacteriaceae*. *Antimicrob. Agents Chemother.* **32:**873–876.

45. **Gautom, R. K.** 1997. Rapid pulsed-field gel electrophoresis protocol for typing of *Escherichia coli* O157:H7 and other gram-negative organisms in 1 day. *J. Clin. Microbiol.* **35:**2977–2980.

46. **Gavini, E., J. Mergaert, A. Beji, C. Mielcarek, D. Izard, K. Kersters, and J. De Ley.** 1989. Transfer of *Enterobacter agglomerans* (Beijerinck 1988) Ewing and Fife 1972 to *Pantoea* gen. nov. as *Pantoea agglomerans* comb. nov. and description of *Pantoea dispersa* sp. nov. *Int. J. Syst. Bacteriol.* **39:**337–345.

47. **Gherna, R. L., J. H. Werren, W. Weisburg, R. Cote, C. R. Woese, L. Mandelco, and D. J. Brenner.** 1991. *Arsenophonas nasoniae* gen. nov., sp. nov., the causative agent of the son-killer trait in the parasitic wasp *Nasonia vitripennis*. *Int. J. Syst. Bacteriol.* **41:**563–565.

48. **Gilliver, M. A., M. Bennett, M. Begon, S. M. Hazel, and C. A. Hart.** 1999. Antibiotic resistance found in wild rodents. *Nature* **401:**233–234.

49. **Goering, R. V.** 1998. The molecular epidemiology of nosocomial infection, p. 131–147. *In* S. Specter, M. Bendinella, and H. Friedman (ed.), *Rapid Detection of Infectious Agents.* Plenum Press, New York, N.Y.

50. **Grimont, F., and P. A. D. Grimont.** 1981. The genus *Serratia*, p. 2822–2848. *In* M. P. Starr, H. Stolp, H. G. Trüper, and H. G. Schlegel (ed.), *The Prokaryotes: a Handbook on Habitats, Isolation, and Identification of Bacteria.* Springer-Verlag KG, Berlin, Germany.

51. **Grimont, F., and P. A. D. Grimont.** 1991. The genus *Enterobacter*, p. 2797–2815. *In* A. Balows, H. G. Trüper, M. Dworkin, W. Harder, and K.-H. Schleifer (ed.), *The Prokaryotes: a Handbook on Habitats, Isolation, and Identification of Bacteria*, 2nd ed. Springer-Verlag KG, Berlin, Germany.

52. **Grimont, F., P. A. D. Grimont, and C. Richard.** 1991. The genus *Klebsiella*, p. 2775–2796. *In* M. P. Starr, H. Stolp, H. G. Trüper, A. Balows, and H. G. Schlegel (ed.), *The Prokaryotes: a Handbook on the Biology of Bacteria: Ecophysiology, Isolation, Identification, Applications*, 2nd ed. Springer-Verlag KG, Berlin, Germany.

53. **Grimont, P. A. D., F. Grimont, J. J. Farmer III, and M. A. Asbury.** 1981. *Cedecea davisae* gen. nov., sp. nov., new *Enterobacteriaceae* from clinical specimens. *Int. J. Syst. Bacteriol.* **31:**317–326.

54. **Grimont, P. A. D., J. J. Farmer III, F. Grimont, M. A. Asbury, D. J. Brenner, and C. Deval.** 1983. *Ewingella americana* gen. nov., sp. nov., a new *Enterobacteriaceae* isolated from clinical specimens. *Ann. Microbiol. (Inst. Pasteur)* **134A:**39–52.

55. **Grimont, P. A. D., F. Grimont, C. Richard, and R. Sakazaki.** 1980. *Edwardsiella hoshinae*, a new species of *Enterobacteriaceae. Curr. Microbiol.* **4:**347–351.

56. **Hart, C. A., and S. K. Rao.** 1999. Donovanosis. *J. Med. Microbiol.* **48:**707–709.

57. **Hauben, L., E. R. B. Moore, L. Vauterin, M. Steenackers, J. Maegaert, L. Verdonck, and J. Swings.** 1999. Phylogenetic position of phytopathogens within the *Enterobacteriaceae. Syst. Appl. Microbiol.* **21:**384–397.

58. **Hawke, J. P., A. C. McWhorter, A. G. Steigerwalt, and D. J. Brenner.** 1981. *Edwardsiella ictaluri* sp. nov., the causative agent of enteric septicemia of catfish. *Int. J. Syst. Bacteriol.* **31:**396–400.

59. **Hickman-Brenner, F. W., G. P. Huntley-Carter, Y. Saitoh, A. G. Steigerwalt, J. J. Farmer III, and D. J. Brenner.** 1984. *Moellerella wisconsensis*, a new genus and species of *Enterobacteriaceae* found in human stool specimens. *J. Clin. Microbiol.* **19:**460–463.

60. **Hickman-Brenner, F. W., M. P. Vohra, G. P. Huntley-Carter, G. R. Fanning, V. A. Lowery III, D. J. Brenner, and J. J. Farmer III.** 1985. *Leminorella*, a new genus of *Enterobacteriaceae*: identification of *Leminorella grimontii* sp. nov. and *Leminorella richardii* sp. nov. found in clinical specimens. *J. Clin. Microbiol.* **21:**234–239.

61. **Hollis, D. G., F. W. Hickman G. R. Fanning, J. J. Farmer III, R. E. Weaver, and D. J. Brenner.** 1981. *Tatumella ptyseos* gen. nov., sp. nov., a member of the family *Enterobacteriaceae* found in clinical specimens. *J. Clin. Microbiol.* **14:**79–88.

62. **Inoue, K., K. Sugiyama, Y. Kosako, R. Sakazaki, and S. Yamai.** 2000. *Enterobacter cowanii* sp. nov., a new species of the family *Enterobacteriaceae. Curr. Microbiol.* **41:**417–420.

63. **Janda, J. M.** 2001. *Aeromonas* and *Plesiomonas*, p. 1237–1270. *In* M. Sussman (ed.), *Molecular Medical Microbiology.* Academic Press, Ltd., London, United Kingdom.

64. **Janda, J. M., and S. L. Abbott.** 1998. *The Enterobacteria.* Lippincott-Raven, Philadelphia, Pa.

65. **Janda, J. M., and S. L. Abbott.** 1993. Expression of hemolytic activity in *Plesiomonas shigelloides. J. Clin. Microbiol.* **31:**1206–1208.

66. **Janda, J. M., S. L. Abbott, and M. J. Albert.** 1999. Prototypal diarrheagenic strains of *Hafnia alvei* are actually members of the genus *Escherichia. J. Clin. Microbiol.* **37:**2399–2401.

67. **Janda, J. M., S. L. Abbott, S. Khashe, and W. Probert.** 2001. Biochemical identification and characterization of DNA groups within the *Proteus vulgaris* complex. *J. Clin. Microbiol.* **39:**1231–1234.

68. **Janda, J. M., S. L. Abbott, and J. G. Morris.** 1995. *Aeromonas, Plesiomonas* and *Edwardsiella*, p. 905–917. *In* M. J. Blaser, P. D. Smith, J. I. Ravdin, H. B. Greenberg, and R. L. Guerrant (ed.), *Infections of the Gastrointestinal Tract.* Raven Press, New York, N.Y.

69. **Janda, J. M., S. L. Abbott, D. Woodward, and S. Khashe.** 1998. Invasion of HEp-2 and other eukaryotic cell lines by *Providenciae*: further evidence supporting the role of *Providencia alcalifaciens* in bacterial gastroenteritis. *Curr. Microbiol.* **37:**159–165.

70. **Jones, R. N., S. G. Jenkins, D. J. Hoban, M. A. Pfaller, and R. Ramphal.** 2000. In vitro efficacy of six cephalosporins tested against *Enterobacteriaceae* isolated at 38 North American medical centres participating in the SENTRY antimicrobial surveillance program, 1997–1998. *Int. J. Antimicrob. Agents* **15:**111–118.

71. **Jones, R. N., K. C. Kugler, M. A. Pfaller, P. L. Winokur, and the SENTRY Surveillance Group, North America.** 1999. Characteristics of pathogens causing urinary tract infections in hospitals in North America: results from the SENTRY antimicrobial surveillance program, 1997. *Diagn. Microbiol. Infect. Dis.* **35:**55–63.

72. **Jones, R. N., and M. Pfaller.** 1998. Bacterial resistance: a worldwide problem. *Diagn. Microbiol. Infect. Dis.* **31:**379–388.

73. **Kageyama, B., M. Nakae, S. Yagi, and T. Sonoyama.** 1992. *Pantoea punctata* sp. nov., *Pantoea citrea* sp. nov., and *Pantoea terrea* sp. nov. isolated from fruit and soil samples. *Int. J. Syst. Bacteriol.* **42:**203–210.

74. **Kharsany, A. B. M., A. A. Hoosens, P. Kiepela, P. Kirby, and A. W. Sturm.** 1999. Phylogenetic analysis of *Calymmatobacterium granulomatis* based on rRNA gene sequences. *J. Med. Microbiol.* **48:**841–847.

75. **Khashe, S., D. J. Scales, S. L. Abbott, and J. M. Janda.** 2001. Non-invasive *Providencia alcalifaciens* strains fail to attach to HEp-2 cells. *Curr. Microbiol.* **43:**414–417.

76. **Knox, C. M., V. Cevellos, and D. Dean.** 1998. 16S ribosomal DNA typing for identification of pathogens in patients with bacterial keratits. *J. Clin. Microbiol.* **36:** 3492–3496.

77. **Koh, T. H., G. S. Babini, N. Woodford, L.-H. Sng, L. M. C. Hall, and D. M. Livermore.** 1999. Carbapenem-hydrolysing IMP-1 β-lactamase in *Klebsiella pneumoniae* from Singapore. *Lancet* **353:**2162.

78. **Kosako, Y., R. Sakazaki, and E. Yoshizaki.** 1984. *Yokenella regensburgei* gen. nov., sp. nov.: a new genus and species in the family *Enterobacteriaceae*. *Jpn. J. Med. Sci. Biol.* **37:**117–124.

79. **Kosako, Y., K. Tamura, R. Sakazaki, and K. Miki.** 1996. *Enterobacter kobei* sp. nov., a new species of the family *Enterobacteriaceae* resembling *Enterobacter cloacae*. *Curr. Microbiol.* **33:**261–265.

80. **Landman, D., M. Chocklingam, and J. M. Quale.** 1999. Reduction in the incidence of methicillin-resistant *Staphylococcus aureus* and ceftazidime-resistant *Klebsiella pneumoniae* following changes in a hospital antibiotic formulary. *Clin. Infect. Dis.* **28:**1062–1066.

81. **Lin, F.-Y. C., W. F. Devoe, C. Morrison, J. Libonati, P. Powers, R. J. Gross, B. Rowe, E. Israel, and J. G. Morris.** 1987. Outbreak of neonatal *Citrobacter diversus* meningitis in a suburban hospital. *Pediatr. Infect. Dis. J.* **6:**50–55.

82. **Lipsky, B. A., E. W. Hook III, A. A. Smith, and J. J. Plorde.** 1980. *Citrobacter* infections in humans: experience at the Seattle Veterans Administration Medical Center and a review of the literature. *Rev. Infect. Dis.* **2:**746–760.

83. **Livermore, D. M.** 1995. β-Lactamases in laboratory and clinical resistance. *Clin. Microbiol. Rev.* **8:**557–584.

84. **Lucet, J.-C., D. Decre, A. Fichelle, M.-L. Joly-Guillou, M. Pernet, C. Deblangy, M.-J. Kosmann, and B. Regnier.** 1999. Control of a prolonged outbreak of extended-spectrum β-lactamase-producing *Enterobacteriaceae* in a university hospital. *Clin. Infect. Dis.* **29:**1411–1418.

85. **Luperchio, S. A., J. V. Newman, C. A. Dangler, M. D. Schrenzel, D. J. Brenner, A. G. Steigerwalt, and D. B. Schauer.** 2000. *Citrobacter rodentium*, the causative agent of transmissable murine colonic hyperplasia, exhibits clonality: synonymy of *C. rodentium* and mouse-pathogenic *Escherichia coli*. *J. Clin. Microbiol.* **38:**4343–4350.

86. **MacDonell, M. T., and R. R. Colwell.** 1985. Phylogeny of the *Vibrionaceae*, and recommendation for two new genera, *Listonella* and *Shewanella*. *Syst. Appl. Microbiol.* **6:**171–182.

87. **Martinez-Murcia, A. J., S. Beniloch, and M. D. Collins.** 1992. Phylogenetic interrelationships of members of the genera *Aeromonas* and *Plesiomonas* as determined by 16S ribosomal DNA sequencing: lack of congruence with results of DNA-DNA hybridizations. *Int. J. Syst. Bacteriol.* **42:**412–421.

88. **McWhorter, A. C., R. L. Haddock, F. A. Nocon, A. G. Steigerwalt, D. J. Brenner, S. Aleksic, J. Bockmuhl, and J. J. Farmer III.** 1991. *Trabulsiella guamensis*, a new genus and species of the family *Enterobacteriaceae* that resembles *Salmonella* subgroups 4 and 5. *J. Clin. Microbiol.* **29:**1480–1485.

89. **Mobley, H. L.** 2000. Virulence of the two primary uropathogens. *ASM News* **66:**403–410.

90. **Montgomerie, J. Z.** 1979. Epidemiology of *Klebsiella* and hospital-associated infections. *Rev. Infect. Dis.* **1:**736–753.

91. **Muller, H. E., D. J. Brenner, G. R. Fanning, P. A. D. Grimont, and P. Kampfer.** 1996. Emended description of *Buttiauxella agrestis* with recognition of six new species of *Buttiauxella* and two new species of *Kluyvera: Buttiauxella ferragutiae* sp. nov., *Buttiauxella gaviniae* sp. nov., *Buttiauxella brennerae* sp. nov., *Buttiauxella izarddii* sp. nov., *Buttiauxella noackiae* sp. nov., *Buttiauxella warmboldiae* sp. nov., *Kluyvera cochleae* sp. nov., and *Kluyvera georgiana* sp. nov. *Int. J. Syst. Bacteriol.* **46:**50–63.

92. **Muller, H. E., C. M. O'Hara, G. R. Fanning, F. W. Hickman-Brenner, J. M. Swenson, and D. J. Brenner.** 1986. *Providencia heimbachae*, a new species of *Enterobacteriaceae* isolated from animals. *Int. J. Syst. Bacteriol.* **36:**252–256.

93. **Munson, M. A., P. Baumann, and M. G. Kinsey.** 1991. *Buchnera* gen. nov. and *Buchnera aphidicola* sp. nov., a taxon consisting of the mycetocyte-associated, primary endosymbionts of aphids. *Int. J. Syst. Bacteriol.* **41:**566–568.

94. **National Committee for Clinical Laboratory Standards.** 1999. *Performance Standards for Antimicrobial Susceptibility Testing. Ninth Informational Supplement, M100-S9.* National Committee for Clinical Laboratory Standards, Wayne, Pa.

95. **National Committee for Clinical Laboratory Standards.** 2000. *Performance Standards for Antimicrobial Susceptibility Testing. Tenth Informational Supplement, M100-S10.* National Committee for Clinical Laboratory Standards, Wayne, Pa.

96. **Neuwirth, C., E. Siebor, A. Pechinot, J.-M. Duez, M. Pruneaux, F. Garel, A. Kazmierczak, and R. Labia.** 2001. Evidence of in vivo transfer of a plasmid encoding the extended-spectrum β-lactamase TEM-24 and other resistance factors among different members of the family *Enterobacteriaceae*. *J. Clin. Microbiol.* **39:**1985–1988.

97. **Nordmann, P.** 1998. Trends in β-lactam resistance among *Enterobacteriaceae*. *Clin. Infect. Dis.* **27**(Suppl. 1): S100–S106.

98. **O'Hara, C. M., F. W. Brenner, and J. M. Miller.** 2000. Classification, identification, and clinical significance of *Proteus, Providencia*, and *Morganella*. *Clin. Microbiol. Rev.* **13:**534–546.

99. **O'Hara, C. M., F. W. Brenner, A. G. Steigerwalt, B. C. Hill, B. Holmes, P. A. D. Grimont, P. M. Hawkey, J. L. Penner, J. M. Miller, and D. J. Brenner.** 2000. Classification of *Proteus vulgaris* biogroup 3 with recognition of *Proteus hauseri* sp. nov., nom. rev. and unnamed *Proteus* genomospecies 4, 5, and 6. *Int. J. Syst. Evol. Microbiol.* **50:**1869–1875.

100. **O'Hara, C. M., A. G. Steigerwalt, D. Green, M. Mc-Dowell, B. C. Hill, D. J. Brenner, and J. M. Miller.** 1999. Isolation of *Providencia heimbachae* from human feces. *J. Clin. Microbiol.* **37:**3048–3050.

101. **O'Hara, C. M., A. G. Steigerwalt, B. C. Hill, J. J. Farmer III, G. R. Fanning, and D. J. Brenner.** 1989. *Enterobacter hormaechei*, a new species of the family *Enterobacteriaceae* formerly known as enteric group 75. *J. Clin. Microbiol.* **27:**2046–2049.

102. **Ohkusu, K.** 2000. Cost-effective and rapid presumptive identification of gram-negative bacilli in routine urine, pus, and stool cultures: evaluation of the use of CHROMagar orientation medium in conjunction with simple biochemical tests. *J. Clin. Microbiol.* **38:**4586–4592.

103. Ohno, A., Y. Ishii, L. Ma, and K. Yamaguchi. 2000. Problems related to determination of MICs of oximino-type expanded-spectrum cephems for *Proteus vulgaris*. *J. Clin. Microbiol.* **38:**677–681.

104. Paterson, D. L., W.-C. Ko, A. Von Gottberg, J. M. Casellas, L. Mulazimoglu, K. P. Klugman, R. A. Bonomo, L. B. Rice, J. G. McCormack, and V. L. Yu. 2001. Outcome of cephalosporin treatment for serious infections due to apparently susceptible organisms producing extended-spectrum β-lactamases: implications for the clinical microbiology laboratory. *J. Clin. Microbiol.* **39:**2206–2212.

105. Paterson, D. L., and V. L. Yu. 1999. Editorial response: extended-spectrum β-lactamases: a call for improved detection and control. *Clin. Infect. Dis.* **29:**1419–1422.

106. Podschun, R., A. Fischer, and U. Ullman. 2000. Expression of putative virulence factors by clinical isolates of *Klebsiella planticola*. *J. Med. Microbiol.* **49:**115–119.

107. Polster, M., and M. Svobodova. 1964. Production of reddish-brown pigment from *dl*-tryptophan by enterobacteria of the *Proteus-Providencia* group. *Experientia* **20:**637–638.

108. Ramos, A., and D. Damaso. 2000. Extraintestinal infection due to *Hafnia alvei*. *Eur. J. Microbiol. Infect. Dis.* **19:**708–710.

109. Richards, M. J., J. R. Edwards, D. H. Culver, and R. P. Gaynes. 1999. Nosocomial infections in medical intensive care units in the United States. *Crit. Care Med.* **27:**887–892.

110. Ridell, J., A. Siitonen, L. Paulin, L. Mattila, H. Korkeala, and M. J. Albert. 1994. *Hafnia alvei* in stool specimens from patients with diarrhea and healthy controls. *J. Clin. Microbiol.* **32:**2335–2337.

111. Ruimy, R., V. Breittmayer, P. Elbaze, B. Lafay, O. Boussemart, M. Gauthier, and R. Christen. 1994. Phylogenetic analysis and assessment of the genera *Vibrio*, *Photobacterium*, *Aeromonas*, and *Plesiomonas* deduced from small-subunit rRNA sequences. *Int. J. Syst. Bacteriol.* **44:**416–426.

112. Sabella, C., M. Touhy, G. Hall, A. C. Gales, M. E. Erwin, and R. N. Jones. 2000. Emergence of cefepime-resistance in *Klebsiella oxytoca* clinical isolate due to alteration in the outer membrane permeability. *Clin. Microbiol. Newsl.* **22:**37–39.

113. Sahly, H., V. Boehme, R. Podschun, A. Bauernfeind, U. R. Folsch, and U. Ullmann. 1999. Infection and chronic colonization of intensive care unit patient's respiratory tract by a *Klebsiella pneumoniae* strain producing a novel AmpC β-lactamase different from that known. *Clin. Infect. Dis.* **26:**1338–1339.

114. Samra, Z., M. Heifetz, J. Talmor, E. Bain, and J. Bahar. 1998. Evaluation of use of a new chromogenic agar in detection of urinary tract pathogens. *J. Clin. Microbiol.* **36:**990–994.

115. Schonheyder, H. C., K. T. Jensen, and W. Frederiksen. 1994. Taxonomic notes: synonymy of *Enterobacter cancerogenus* (Urosevic 1966) Dickey and Zumoff 1988 and *Enterobacter taylorae* Farmer et al. 1985 and resolution of an ambiguity in the biochemical profile. *Int. J. Syst. Bacteriol.* **44:**586–587.

116. Slaven, E. M., F. A. Lopez, S. M. Hart, and C. V. Sanders. 2001. Myonecrosis caused by *Edwardsiella tarda*: a case report and case series of extraintestinal *E. tarda* infections. *Clin. Infect Dis.* **32:**1430–1433.

117. Sproer, C., U. Mendrock, J. Swiderski, E. Lang, and E. Stackebrandt. 1999. The phylogenetic position of *Serratia*, *Buttiauxella* and some other genera of the family Enterobacteriaceae. *Int. J. Syst. Bacteriol.* **49:**1433–1438.

118. Tamura, K., R. Sakazaki, Y. Kosako, and E. Yoshizaki. 1986. *Leclercia adecarboxylata* gen. nov., comb. nov., formerly known as *Escherichia adecarboxylata*. *Curr. Microbiol.* **13:**179–184.

119. Tenover, F. C., M. J. Mohammed, T. S. Gorton, and Z. F. Dembek. 1999. Detection and reporting of organisms producing extended-spectrum β-lactamases: survey of laboratories in Connecticut. *J. Clin. Microbiol.* **37:**4065–4070.

120. Theodoropoulos, C., T. H. Wong, M. O'Brien, and D. Stenzel. 2001. *Plesiomonas shigelloides* enters polarized human intestinal Caco-2 cells in an in vitro model system. *Infect. Immun.* **69:**2260–2269.

121. Twum-Danso, K., C. Grant, S. A. Al-Suleiman, S. Abdel-Khader, M. S. Al-Awami, H. Al-Breiki, S. Taha, A.-A. Ashoor, and L. Wosornu. 1992. Microbiology of postoperative wound infection: a prospective study of 1770 wounds. *J. Hosp. Infect.* **21:**29–37.

122. Tzelepi, E., P. Giakkoupi, D. Sofianou, V. Loukova, A. Kemeroglou, and A. Tsarkis. 2000. Detection of extended-spectrum β-lactamases in clinical isolates of *Enterobacter cloacae* and *Enterobacter aerogenes*. *J. Clin. Microbiol.* **38:**542–546.

123. Vallis, J., C. León, and F. Alvarez-Lerma. 1997. Nosocomial bacteremia in critically ill patients: a multi-center study evaluating epidemiology and prognosis. *Clin. Infect. Dis.* **24:**387–395.

124. Warren, J. R., J. J. Farmer III, F. E. Dewhirst, K. Birkhead, T. Zembower, L. R. Peterson, L. Sims, and M. Bhattacharya. 2000. Outbreak of nosocomial infections due to extended-spectrum β-lactamase-producing strains of Enteric Group 137, a new member of the family Enterobacteriaceae closely related to *Citrobacter farmeri* and *Citrobacter amalonaticus*. *J. Clin. Microbiol.* **38:**3946–3952.

125. Wendt, C., S. A. Messer, R. J. Hollis, M. A. Pfaller, and L. A. Herwaldt. 1998. Epidemiology of polyclonal gram-negative bacteremia. *Diagn. Microbiol. Infect. Dis.* **32:**9–13.

126. Wendt, C., S. A. Messer, R. J. Hollis, M. A. Pfaller, R. P. Wenzel, and L. A. Herwaldt. 1999. Recurrent gram-negative bacteremia: incidence and clinical patterns. *Clin. Infect. Dis.* **28:**611–617.

127. Werren, J. H., S. W. Skinner, and A. M. Huger. 1986. Male-killing bacteria in a parasitic wasp. *Science* **231:**990–992.

128. Westbrook, G. L., C. M. O'Hara, S. B. Roman, and J. M. Miller. 2000. Incidence and identification of *Klebsiella planticola* in clinical isolates with emphasis on newborns. *J. Clin. Microbiol.* **38:**1495–1497.

129. Williams, W. W., J. Mariano, M. Spurrier, H. D. Donnell, Jr., R. L. Breckenridge, Jr., R. L. Anderson, I. K. Wachsmuth, C. Thornsberry, D. R. Graham, D. W. Thibeault, and J. R. Allen. 1984. Nosocomial meningitis due to *Citrobacter diversus* in neonates: new aspects of epidemiology. *J. Infect. Dis.* **150:**229–235.

130. Wong, T. Y., H. Y. Tsui, M. K. So, J. Y. Lai, C. W. S. Tse, and T. K. Ng. 2000. *Plesiomonas shigelloides* infection in Hong Kong: retrospective study of 167 laboratory-confirmed cases. *Hong Kong Med. J.* **6:**375–380.

Aeromonas*

SHARON L. ABBOTT

45

TAXONOMY

Aeromonas is the only genus within the family *Aeromonadaceae*, established in 1986 by Colwell et al. (5), which is pathogenic for humans. Because of frequent reclassifications and constant amended or extended descriptions, *Aeromonas* taxonomy remains confusing to microbiologists not working with these organisms on a daily basis. Table 1 contains a concise list of the currently recognized species. DNA hybridization group numbers, which no longer serve a meaningful purpose, and synonymous species designations for *Aeromonas veronii* bv. sobria (*A. ichthiosmia*) and *A. trota* (*A. enteropelogenes*) (4) are not included for simplicity. *Aeromonas* group 501 (DNA hybridization group 13), which is made up of *A. schubertii*-like organisms, and *Aeromonas* sp. DNA hybridization group 11 (17), which is made up of *A. eucrenophila/A. encheleia*-like organisms, are also not addressed in the table. These groups contain few strains, their taxonomic status has yet to be resolved and is still highly debated, and most importantly, neither group has been shown to be significant in human or animal disease. All other *Aeromonas* species listed in Table 1, with the exception of *A. salmonicida* subsp. *pectinolytica*, which has been found only in heavily polluted waters in Argentina (19), were published in the previous edition of this Manual.

Finally, because of its clinical significance, it bears repeating that clinical strains referred to as "*A. sobria*" are, in fact, *A. veronii* bv. sobria and should be reported as such. It usually is not necessary to definitively separate members of the *A. hydrophila* complex (*A. hydrophila*, *A. bestiarum*, and *A. salmonicida*) or the *A. caviae* complex (*A. caviae*, *A. media*, and *A. eucrenophila*), especially when they are isolated from feces (see "Interpretation and Reporting of Results" below).

DESCRIPTION OF THE GENUS

Members of the genus *Aeromonas* are gram-negative facultative anaerobes that are straight rods or coccoid cells ranging from 1.0 to 3.5 μm long and 0.3 to 1.0 μm wide.

They possess polar, monotrichous flagella, but young cultures grown on solid media may be peritrichous. Fish strains of *A. salmonicida* are nonmotile, but members of any species may be nonmotile. Aeromonads are defined as oxidase- and catalase-positive organisms that reduce nitrate to nitrite and ferment D-glucose and a variety of other carbohydrates and alcoholic sugars to acid or acid with gas. Human (mesophilic) strains grow between 10 and 42°C, but occasional isolates may be more active in some biochemical assays at 22 to 25°C. Psychrophilic strains from fish and the environment (*A. popoffii* and *A. salmonicida*) seldom grow above 37°C and preferentially grow at 22 to 25°C. In brain heart infusion broth at 28°C, growth occurs between pH 4.5 and 9.0 and at salt concentrations between 0 and 4%. Aeromonads are prolific producers of extracellular enzymes, including hemolysins, proteases, chitinase, chondroitinase, amylase, DNase, esterases, peptidases, and arylamidases. In general, aeromonads are resistant to O/129 vibriostatic agent (2,4-diamino-6,7-diisopropylpteridine), but rare strains have been reported as susceptible. Primary cellular fatty acids produced include hexadecanoic acid (16:0) and two unsaturated acids, hexadecenoic acid (16:1) and octadecenoic acid (18:1). The guanine-plus-cytosine content of their DNA ranges from 57 to 64%.

NATURAL HABITATS

Aeromonads are inhabitants of aquatic ecosystems worldwide. These include groundwater and drinking water at treatment plants and in distribution systems and reservoirs as well as clean or polluted lakes and rivers. *Aeromonas* may also be found in marine environments but only in brackish water or water with a low saline content. A viable but nonculturable state has been described for *Aeromonas* in low-nutrient-containing habitats such as chlorinated drinking water or chemically polluted waters. Most *Aeromonas* species, particularly those associated with human infections, are found in a wide variety of fresh produce, meat (beef, poultry, pork), and dairy products (raw milk, ice cream) (13). *A. veronii* bv. sobria is a symbiont in the gut of medicinal leeches, where it may grow as a pure culture (9). In fisheries, psychrophilic strains of *Aeromonas* cause severe infections resulting in considerable economic loss. Infections in frogs, pigs, cattle, birds, and marine animals have also been reported (13).

* This chapter contains information presented in chapter 32 by Martin Altwegg in the seventh edition of this Manual.

TABLE 1 Members of the genus *Aeromonas*[a]

Organism	Human isolation (extraintestinal/fecal)	Human pathogen (extraintestinal/fecal)	Frequency in humans	Pathogenic for animals, fish, reptiles
A. hydrophila complex				
A. hydrophila	Both	Both	Common	Yes
A. bestiarum	No/yes	—/no	One case	Yes
A. salmonicida	No/yes	Neither	Rare	
subsp. salmonicida				Yes
subsp. achromogenes				Yes
subsp. masoucida				Yes
subsp. smithia				Yes
subsp. pectinolytica				No
A. caviae complex				
A. caviae	Both	Both	Common	Yes
A. media	No/yes	—/yes	Rare	No
A. eucrenophila	Yes/yes	No/—	Very rare	No
A. veronii bv. sobria	Both	Both	Common	Yes
A. veronii bv. veronii	Both	Both	Rare	No
A. jandaei	Both	Yes/unknown	Rare	No
A. trota	Both	Neither	Rare	No
A. schubertii	Yes/no	Yes/—	Rare	No
A. encheleia	Yes/no	No/—	One case	No
A. allosaccharophila	No/yes	—/no	Rare	Yes
A. sobria	Neither	—	—	No
A. popoffii	Neither	—	—	No

[a] Abbreviations and symbols: bv., biovar; —, not applicable.

CLINICAL SIGNIFICANCE

Aeromonas gastroenteritis ranges from an acute watery diarrhea (most common form) to dysenteric illness to chronic illness. Stools from acute watery diarrhea are loose (take the shape of their container), and erythrocytes and fecal leukocytes are absent. Accompanying symptoms include abdominal pain (60 to 70%), fever and vomiting (20 to 40%), and nausea (40%) (13). Infections are usually self-limiting, but children may require hospitalization due to dehydration. *A. caviae* is the most common species associated with these infections. Albert et al. (2), in a recent comprehensive study done in Bangladesh, found that the presence of loose stools was associated with *Aeromonas* strains possessing an *alt* gene encoding a heat-labile cytotonic enterotoxin. Patients with more severe disease and watery diarrhea had strains that possessed both the *alt* gene and a second gene, *ast*, which encodes a heat-stable cytotonic enterotoxin. A total of seven different *Aeromonas* species were associated with diarrhea in this study.

A. veronii bv. sobria strains may be associated with rare cholera-like disease characterized by abdominal pain (60%) and fever and nausea (20%) (13). In dysenteric diarrhea resembling shigellosis, patients suffer from severe abdominal pain and have bloody stools containing mucus and polymorphonuclear leukocytes. About 10 to 15% of patients with either cholera-like or dysenteric diarrhea are coinfected with another enteric pathogen(s).

Complications from *Aeromonas* diarrheal disease include hemolytic uremic syndrome (3) or kidney disease requiring kidney transplantation (7). These more severe infections are usually associated with *A. hydrophila* or *A. veronii* bv. sobria. Also, nonresolvable, intermittent diarrhea can occur months after the initial infection and may persist for months or several years.

Aeromonas can also be isolated from a wide variety of extraintestinal sites, although blood and wounds are by far the most common sources. *Aeromonas* septicemia occurs rarely in immunocompetent hosts, and most cases are associated with patients with liver disease and hematological malignancies. Fatality rates range from 30 to 50% in these infections. Wound infections are usually preceded by traumatic injury that occurs in contact with water. These infections range from relatively uncomplicated cases of cellulitis to myonecrotic infections with a poor prognosis. Surveys indicate that only 17 to 52% of *Aeromonas* wound infections are monomicrobic (13). The predominant *Aeromonas* species isolated from wound infections is *A. hydrophila*. Use of medicinal leeches postoperatively to enhance blood flow to surgical sites has resulted in wound infection rates of 20%, primarily with *A. veronii* bv. sobria (9). Other extraintestinal infections from which aeromonads have been isolated include ocular, respiratory, and urinary tract infections; meningitis; osteomyelitis; cholecystitis; endocarditis; and peritonitis (12). The exact involvement of *Aeromonas* in some of these infections is arguable but is more credible if the organism is present in pure culture.

COLLECTION, TRANSPORT, AND STORAGE OF SPECIMENS

Aeromonads survive well in specimens; any of the widely used transport media are acceptable for transport, including buffered glycerol in saline (chapter 20). Feces are always preferable to rectal swabs for isolation of enteric pathogens, and stools should be collected in the acute phase of disease.

ISOLATION PROCEDURES

Aeromonads generally grow well on a variety of enteric differential and selective agars, although sucrose- and/or lactose-fermenting strains usually resemble nonpathogens on these media. Blood agar (BA) with 20 μg of ampicillin per ml (ABA) is useful for isolating all *Aeromonas* species except *A. trota*, which is susceptible to ampicillin. Since most clinically relevant species are beta-hemolytic, including an increasing number of *A. caviae* strains, beta-hemolytic colonies on BA should be screened with oxidase and a spot indole, if available. Any colonies positive for both tests should be characterized further. Modified cefsulodin-Irgasan-novobiocin (CIN) (4 μg of cefsulodin per ml versus 15 μg/ml in unmodified CIN) is also an excellent isolation medium for aeromonads. On this medium, *Aeromonas* colonies will have a pink center with an uneven, clear apron and will be indistinguishable from *Yersinia enterocolitica* morphologically. We incubate CIN at 25°C to enhance the recovery of *Yersinia*, but we are still able to recover *Aeromonas* within 24 h at this temperature. For optimal isolation, use of both ABA and modified CIN is recommended (15). A xylose-galactosidase medium (XGM), containing novobiocin, bile salts, xylose, and two galactopyranosides, has been evaluated in Europe for the isolation of *Aeromonas*, *Salmonella*, *Shigella*, and *Yersinia* spp. (8). *Aeromonas* species, which form green colonies, were isolated more frequently from XGM agar (36%) than from any other medium except CIN (43%), but XGM had fewer false positives (11% for XGM versus 60% for CIN). Thiosulfate-citrate-bile salts-sucrose (TCBS) medium is usually inhibitory to aeromonads. Enrichment in alkaline peptone water enhances recovery of *Aeromonas* from populations that generally would be expected to shed low numbers of organisms (carriers, convalescent-phase patients, and those with subclinical infections). For patients with acute diarrhea, enrichment is probably unnecessary (20).

IDENTIFICATION

Aeromonas spp. are most easily confused in the laboratory with other oxidase-positive fermenters, i.e., *Vibrio* and *Plesiomonas* spp. *Plesiomonas* is easily differentiated from *Aeromonas* by positive reactions in Moeller's lysine, ornithine, and arginine tests and by fermentation of *m*-inositol. Vibrios may be more difficult to distinguish from aero-

monads, which is particularly true for *Vibrio fluvialis* and *A. caviae*. Resistance to O/129 vibriostatic agent and the inability to grow in salt concentrations of ≥6% usually indicate the genus *Aeromonas*. *Vibrio cholerae* O139, a cholera toxin-positive, non-salt-requiring, O/129 vibriostatic agent-resistant vibrio, is a major exception to this rule. However, the decarboxylase pattern (positive for lysine and ornithine, negative for arginine), production of gas from glucose, and fermentation of salicin will separate this organism from aeromonads. Biochemical tests useful for separating *Aeromonas* species believed to cause disease in humans are given in Table 2. Members of the *A. hydrophila* complex (*A. hydrophila*, *A. bestiarum*, and *A. salmonicida*) may be separated by fermentation reactions at 24 h (35°C) for salicin (95, 0, and 100%, respectively) and D-sorbitol (0, 0, and 67%, respectively) and gluconate oxidation (68, 0, and 0%, respectively) (1). *A. caviae* complex members (*A. caviae*, *A. media*, and *A. eucrenophila*) are separated by citrate utilization (100, 82, and 0%, respectively) and glycerol (73, 91, and 0%, respectively) and D-mannose (27, 100, and 100%, respectively) fermentation (1).

Because isolates do not survive well at room or refrigerator temperature in the laboratory for long periods (>1 month), even in media deep freezing at −70°C is recommended for their storage.

SEROLOGIC RESPONSE

Most serologic assays that have been used to detect antibodies to *Aeromonas* (tube agglutination, immunoblot, and enzyme-linked immunoassay) have low sensitivity and specificity and are not considered reliable. An immunoglobulin A (IgA) (fecal antibody) response to *Aeromonas* somatic lipopolysaccharides and exotoxins has been reported (6). Crivelli et al. (6) found secretory IgA to *Aeromonas* in 10 of 13 stools from patients when the stool was extracted with Jacalin, a lectin with high affinity for human IgA.

ANTIBIOTIC SUSCEPTIBILITIES

Although they in part reflect previously known data, two recent articles on *Aeromonas* antimicrobial susceptibilities (14, 18) are notable. Both studies included only strains well characterized to the species level and expand susceptibility

TABLE 2 Biochemical tests to separate *Aeromonas* species involved in human disease[a]

Species	Test result									
	VP	LDC	ADH	ODC	Gas (glucose)	Acid from:			Esculin hydrolysis	Cephalothin[b]
						Arabinose	Sucrose	Mannitol		
A. caviae	−	−	+	−	−	A	A	A	+	R
A. hydrophila	+	+	+	−	+	V	A	A	+	R
A. jandaei	+	+	+	−	+	−	−	A	−	R
A. schubertii	V	V	+	−	−	−	−	−	−	S
A. trota[c]	−	+	+	−	V	−	V	A	−	R
A. veronii bv. sobria	+	+	+	−	+	−	A	A	−	S
A. veronii bv. veronii	+	+	−	+	+	−	A	A	+	S

[a] Abbreviations and symbols: VP, Voges-Proskauer; LDC, lysine decarboxylase; ADH, arginine dihydrolase; ODC, ornithine decarboxylase; +, ≥90% of strains positive; V, 11 to 89% of strains positive; −, ≤10% of strains positive; A, acid; S, susceptible; R, resistant. Data taken from reference 1.
[b] Tested by NCCLS standard methods (chapters 69 and 70).
[c] *A. trota* is ampicillin susceptible; other species are usually resistant.

information on aeromonads isolated less frequently from clinical specimens. A general antimicrobial susceptibility profile for *Aeromonas* derived from both of these investigations as well as other studies (11, 16) is given in Table 3. Ciprofloxacin, commonly used to treat gram-negative infections, remains active against all species of *Aeromonas*, with little or no resistance reported in studies in the United States and Europe (14, 18). Two to three percent of *A. caviae*, *A. hydrophila*, and *A. veronii* bv. sobria strains in Asia have been reported to be ciprofloxacin resistant (16). Data from Ko et al. (16) in Taiwan indicate that susceptibilities may differ from one geographic area to another, suggesting that antimicrobial susceptibility testing of local isolates is necessary. *Aeromonas* species express three chromosomal β-lactam-induced β-lactamases, including a group 1 molecular class C cephalosporinase, a group 2d molecular class D penicillinase, and a group 3 molecular class B metallo-β-lactamase (carbapenemase) (21). The presence of these β-lactamases in *Aeromonas*, in particular the carbapenemase, may not be detected by conventional susceptibility methods. Rossolini et al. (21) noted that conventional susceptibility test methods underestimated resistance to carbapenems. The MICs for truly carbapenem-susceptible strains were below the susceptible breakpoint even when a large inoculum was tested, while the MICs for strains possessing carbapenemase activity were much higher only when a large inoculum was used. It may be necessary for strains of species known to potentially carry carbapenemases (*A. hydrophila*, *A. veronii* bv. sobria, *A. veronii* bv. veronii, and *A. jandaei*) to be tested with the higher inoculum if imipenem or meropenem therapy is being considered. CphA, one of several enzymes responsible for resistance to carbapenems, hydrolyzes nitrocefin poorly or not at all, indicating that the nitrocefin test is not reliable for detecting carbapenemases (10, 21).

TABLE 3 *Aeromonas* species susceptibilities

Susceptibility[a]	Antibiotic agent
Resistant	Ampicillin (except *A. trota* [100% susceptible])
Variable	Ticarcillin or piperacillin (except *A. veronii* bv. veronii [100% resistant], *A. trota* [100% susceptible])
	Cephalothin
	Cefazolin
	Cefoxitin (except *A. veronii* bv. veronii 100% susceptible)
	Cefuroxime
	Ceftriaxone
	Cefotaxime
	Cefepime
Susceptible	Ciprofloxacin
	Gentamicin
	Amikacin
	Tobramycin (*A. veronii* bv. veronii [42% resistant])
	Imipenem (*A. jandaei* [65% resistant], *A. veronii* bv. veronii [67% resistant])
	Trimethoprim-sulfamethoxazole

[a] Resistant or susceptible, ≥90% of all isolates resistant or susceptible; variable, 10 to 90% of isolates susceptible.

INTERPRETATION AND REPORTING OF RESULTS

Regardless of the site of isolation (intestinal or extraintestinal), aeromonads should at least be identified either as belonging to the *A. hydrophila* or *A. caviae* complex or as *A. veronii* bv. sobria and not "*A. sobria*." For routine isolates recovered from uncomplicated cases of gastroenteritis, this level of identification is probably sufficient. Although there is strong evidence that some aeromonads are gastrointestinal pathogens, there is no convincing evidence, at present, that all fecal isolates of *Aeromonas* are involved in diarrheal disease. Thus, the significance of the recovery of aeromonads from stool specimens should be interpreted cautiously and must rely on both laboratory information and clinical interpretation. Because of this, the relative quantity of *Aeromonas* recovered on enteric media (few colonies, moderate growth, predominant organism) should be reported in conjunction with the *Aeromonas* complex or species identification. For complicated cases of diarrhea, i.e., prolonged bloody diarrhea in pediatric patients or chronic gastroenteritis of >1-month duration or in cancer patients with positive fecal cultures in which *Aeromonas* tends to disseminate, a definite identification to species level is warranted. In several instances, bloody diarrhea due to *Aeromonas* in adults was in fact masking underlying malignancies of the bowel.

For extraintestinal isolates (from blood or wounds), the same general rules should apply to species identification of aeromonads. Although it is clear that both the in vitro and the in vivo pathogenic potentials of *Aeromonas* species and strains vary considerably, for the present time, there are no universal markers or indicators available that dictate when isolates should be definitively identified to the species level. Thus, for extraintestinal isolates, identification of aeromonads beyond complexes to a definitive species should be reserved for strains exhibiting unusual resistance patterns, associated with nosocomial outbreaks, or for publication purposes in the description of traditional species associated with new disease processes or newly described species isolated from new anatomic sites.

REFERENCES

1. **Abbott, S. L., W. K. W. Cheung, S. Kroske-Bystrom, T. Malekzadeh, and J. M. Janda.** 1992. Identification of *Aeromonas* strains to the genospecies level in the clinical laboratory. *J. Clin. Microbiol.* **30:**1262–1266.
2. **Albert, M. J., M. Ansaruzzaman, K. A. Talukder, A. K. Chopra, I. Kuhn, M. Rahman, A. S. G. Faruque, M. Sirajul Islam, R. B. Sack, and R. Mollby.** 2000. Prevalence of enterotoxin genes in *Aeromonas* spp. isolated from children with diarrhea, healthy controls, and the environment. *J. Clin. Microbiol.* **38:**3785–3790.
3. **Bogdanovic, R., M. Cobeljic, V. Markovic, V. Nikolic, M. Ognjanovic, L. Sarjanovic, and D. Makic.** 1991. Haemolytic-uremic syndrome associated with *Aeromonas hydrophila* enterocolitis. *Pediatr. Nephrol.* **5:**293–295.
4. **Collins, M. D., A. J. Martinez-Murcia, and J. Cai.** 1994. *Aeromonas enteropelogenes* and *Aeromonas ichthiosmia* are identical to *Aeromonas trota* and *Aeromonas veronii*, respectively, as revealed by small-subunit rRNA sequence analysis. *Int. J. Syst. Bacteriol.* **43:**855–856.
5. **Colwell, R. R., M. R. MacDonell, and J. DeLey.** 1986. Proposal to recognize the family *Aeromonadaceae* fam. nov. *Int. J. Syst. Bacteriol.* **36:**473–477.
6. **Crivelli, C., A. Demarta, and R. Peduzzi.** 2001. Intestinal secretory immunoglobulin A (sIgA) response to *Aeromo-*

nas exoproteins in patients with naturally acquired *Aeromonas* diarrhea. *FEMS Immunol. Med. Microbiol.* **30:**31–35.

7. **Filler, G., J. H. H. Ehrich, E. Strauch, and L. Beutin.** 2000. Acute renal failure in an infant associated with cytotoxic *Aeromonas sobria* isolated from patient's stool and from aquarium water as suspected source of infection. *J. Clin. Microbiol.* **38:**469–470.

8. **Garcia-Arguayo, J. M., P. Ubedo, and M. Gobernado.** 1999. Evaluation of xylose-galactosidase medium, a new plate for the isolation of *Salmonella, Shigella, Yersinia* and *Aeromonas* species. *Eur. J. Clin. Microbiol. Infect. Dis.* **18:**77–78.

9. **Graf, J.** 1999. Symbiosis of *Aeromonas veronii* biovar sobria and *Hirudo medicinalis*, the medicinal leech: a novel model for digestive tract associations. *Infect. Immun.* **67:**1–7.

10. **Hayes, M. V., C. J. Thomson, and S. G. B. Amyes.** 1996. The "hidden" carbapenemase of *Aeromonas hydrophila*. *J. Antimicrob. Chemother.* **37:**33–44.

11. **Janda, J. M.** 2001. *Aeromonas* and *Plesiomonas*, p. 1237–1270. *In* M. Sussman (ed.), *Molecular Medical Microbiology*, vol. 2. Academic Press, London, United Kingdom.

12. **Janda, J. M., and S. L. Abbott.** 1998. Evolving concepts regarding the genus *Aeromonas*: an expanding panorama of species, disease presentations, and unanswered questions. *Clin. Infect. Dis.* **27:**332–344.

13. **Janda, J. M., S. L. Abbott, and J. G. Morris.** 1995. *Aeromonas, Plesiomonas* and *Edwardsiella*, p. 905–917. *In* M. J. Blaser, P. D. Smith, J. I. Ravdin, H. B. Greenberg, and R. L. Guerrant (ed.), *Infections of the Gastrointestinal Tract*. Raven Press, Ltd., New York, N.Y.

14. **Kampfer, P., C. Christmann, J. Swings, and G. Huys.** 1999. In vitro susceptibilities of *Aeromonas* genomic species to 69 antimicrobial agents. *Syst. Appl. Microbiol.* **22:**662–669.

15. **Kelly, M. T., E. M. D. Stroh, and J. Jessop.** 1988. Comparison of blood agar, ampicillin blood agar, MacConkey-ampicillin-Tween agar, and modified cefsulodin-irgasan-novobiocin agar for isolation of *Aeromonas* spp. from stool specimens. *J. Clin. Microbiol.* **26:**1738–1740.

16. **Ko, W. C., K. W. Yu, C. Y. Liu, C. T. Huang, H. S. Leu, and Y. C. Chuang.** 1996. Increasing antibiotic resistance in clinical isolates of *Aeromonas* strains in Taiwan. *Antimicrob. Agents Chemother.* **40:**1260–1262.

17. **Martinez-Murcia, A. J.** 1999. Phylogenetic positions of *Aeromonas encheleia, Aeromonas popoffii, Aeromonas* DNA hybridization group 11 and *Aeromonas* group 501. *Int. J. Syst. Bacteriol.* **49:**1403–1408.

18. **Overman, T. L., and J. M. Janda.** 1999. Antimicrobial susceptibility patterns of *Aeromonas jandaei, A. schubertii, A. trota,* and *A. veronii* biotype veronii. *J. Clin. Microbiol.* **37:**706–708.

19. **Pavan, M. E., S. L. Abbott, J. Zorzopulos, and J. M. Janda.** 2000. *Aeromonas salmonicida* subsp. *pectinolytica* subsp. nov., a new pectinase-positive subspecies isolated from a heavily polluted river. *Int. J. Syst. Evol. Microbiol.* **50:**1119–1124.

20. **Robinson, J., J. Beaman, L. Wagener, and V. Burke.** 1986. Comparison of direct plating with the use of enrichment culture for isolation of *Aeromonas* spp. from faeces. *J. Med. Microbiol.* **22:**315–317.

21. **Rossolini, G. M., T. Walsh, and G. Amicosante.** 1996. The *Aeromonas* metallo-β-lactamases: genetics, enzymology, and contribution to drug resistance. *Microb. Drug Resist.* **2:**245–251.

Vibrio

J. J. FARMER III, J. MICHAEL JANDA, AND KAREN BIRKHEAD

46

TAXONOMY

The genus *Vibrio* is classified in the family *Vibrionaceae*, and it is the type genus for the family (23). Since several different classifications are being used for the *Vibrio* species, commonly used synonyms are listed. Many new *Vibrio* species have been described since publication of the previous edition of this Manual (23), but only *Vibrio vulnificus* biogroup 3 (9) occurs in human clinical specimens.

DESCRIPTION OF THE GENUS

Most *Vibrio* species have the following properties (22, 23): they occur as small straight, slightly curved, curved, or comma-shaped gram-negative rods 0.5 to 0.8 μm in width and 1.4 to 2.6 μm in length; they are motile with monotrichous or multitrichous polar flagella when grown in liquid media; some species produce numerous lateral flagella when grown on solid media; they do not require vitamins or amino acids; the growth of all *Vibrio* species is stimulated by Na$^+$, and Na$^+$ is an absolute requirement for most species; they are facultative anaerobes and oxidase positive; they ferment D-glucose, producing acid but rarely gas; they reduce nitrate to nitrite; and they grow on thiosulfate-citrate-bile salts-sucrose (TCBS) medium (Tables 1 to 6).

NATURAL HABITATS

Vibrio species are primarily aquatic, and the species distribution is usually dependent on the temperature, Na$^+$ concentration, nutrient content of the water, and plants and animals present (23, 57). *Vibrio* species are very common in marine and estuarine environments and on the surfaces and in the intestinal tracts of marine animals. In marine and estuarine environments, vibrios are commonly isolated from sediment, the water column, plankton, and shellfish. Seafood often found to harbor *Vibrio* species (24, 26, 41) include bivalve shellfish (oysters, clams, mussels), crabs, shrimp, and prawns. Vibrios have also been recovered from brackish lakes within the continental United States, and nonhalophilic vibrios have even been isolated from freshwater sources. A number of vibrios have been reported to exist in the natural environment (e.g., the ocean) in a dormant state; these are referred to as "viable but nonculturable" (VNC). According to this hypothesis, vibrios are alive but cannot be cultured when plated onto common plating media. This VNC state is not universally accepted (6), and if it is true, its role in *Vibrio* ecology and pathogenicity is unclear.

CLINICAL SIGNIFICANCE

Twelve *Vibrio* species occur in human clinical specimens (Table 2), and all except *V. furnissii* are apparently pathogenic for humans (20, 22, 23, 24). Vibrios usually cause either diarrhea or extraintestinal infections, but some, such as *V. cholerae*, can cause both. *V. cholerae* and *V. parahaemolyticus* are well-documented causes of diarrhea. More recently, *V. fluvialis* (39), *V. hollisae* (30, 46), and *V. mimicus* (21) have also been implicated, but they are less common. *V. furnissii* (19), *V. metschnikovii* (17), and *V. vulnificus* (20) have been isolated from the feces of patients with diarrhea (particularly those who have eaten raw oysters), and their etiological role is unproven but deserves systematic investigation (23). Investigators have overstated the etiological role of the last three *Vibrio* species, as is often the case with *Aeromonas* and *Plesiomonas*.

Vibrios are often isolated from blood, wounds of arms and legs, infected eyes and ears, and the gallbladder; but they are rarely reported from patients with meningitis, pneumonia, and infection of the reproductive organs or urinary tract (22).

V. cholerae

V. cholerae is the most important species in the genus *Vibrio*. It has caused many epidemics of cholera and millions of deaths (3, 8, 10, 37, 45, 52, 57). It is now divided into three major subgroups: *V. cholerae* O1, *V. cholerae* O139, and *V. cholerae* non-O1.

V. cholerae O1

V. cholerae serogroup O1 is the organism responsible for seven pandemics (52) of cholera (1816–1817, 1829, 1852, 1863, 1881, 1889, and 1961 to the present). In patients with severe cholera or "cholera gravis" there is massive diarrhea, with large volumes of "rice water stool" (clear fluid with flecks of mucus) passed painlessly. The amount of fluid passed can be a liter or more per hour. In 4 to 6 days this would amount to over twice the body weight. There is usually vomiting and little desire to eat. If left untreated,

706

TABLE 1 Properties of the genus *Vibrio* and differentiation from three other phenotypically similar oxidase-positive genera and from *Enterobacteriaceae*

Test or property	Reaction or property of[a]:				
	Vibrio	*Photobacterium*	*Aeromonas*	*Plesiomonas*	*Enterobacteriaceae*
Associated with diarrhea and extraintestinal infections in humans	+	−	+	+	+
Enterobacterial common antigen (eca)	−	−	−	+	+
Oxidase reaction	+	+	+	+	−
Na$^+$ is required for growth or stimulates growth	+	+	−	−	−
Sensitive to the vibriostatic compound O-129[b]	+	+	−	+	−
Lipase production	+	V	+	−	V
D-Mannitol fermentation	+	−	+	−	+
Guanine + cytosine content of DNA (mol%)	38–51	40–44	57–63	51	38–60
Sheathed polar flagellum	+	−	−	−	−
Peritrichous flagella when grown on solid media	V	−	−	−	V
Accumulates poly-β-hydroxybutyrate but does not utilize β-hydroxybutyrate	−	+	NA	NA	NA

[a] Symbols and abbreviations: +, most species and strains are positive; −, most species and strains are negative; V, species-to-species variation; NA, data not available.

[b] Done on Trypticase soy agar with O-129 disks (Oxoid), 150 μg per disk, as described by Farmer and Hickman-Brenner (22).

the patient becomes prostrate with symptoms of severe dehydration, electrolyte imbalance, painful muscle cramps, watery eyes, loss of skin elasticity, and anuria (absence of urine excretion). Death can occur very quickly after the onset of symptoms because of the severe dehydration. This is the terrifying disease that caused such fear in the 19th and early 20th century when the word "cholera" was mentioned. Interestingly, there is a correlation between human blood types and susceptibility to *V. cholerae* infection.

In areas where cholera is endemic, many individuals will have either a mild diarrhea or only asymptomatic colonization of the intestine. This pattern of mild disease has been much more common in the seventh cholera pandemic caused by the eltor biogroup of *V. cholerae*.

Treatment for the most severe cases of cholera is intravenous therapy with large volumes of a balanced salts solution which restores water and electrolyte balance and prevents acidosis. Cases with mild or moderate illness are often treated with oral electrolyte solutions. Tetracycline therapy reduces the period of excretion but is not a substitute for rehydration. Antibiotic resistance is becoming more common in *V. cholerae*, particularly strains circulating in the developing world (34, 57).

The pathogenesis of diarrhea due to *V. cholerae* O1 is well understood. A large number of organisms (10^8 organisms in some human volunteer experiments) are ingested, and some cells survive the acid pH of the stomach and pass into the small intestine. There they multiply and produce cholera toxin, which results in the massive fluid loss.

Originally it was thought that *V. cholerae* O1 did not occur in aquatic environments unless they had been contaminated with feces from patients with cholera. However, recent indigenous cases of *V. cholerae* O1 infection in the United States and Australia (57), along with ecological studies in areas where cholera is endemic, have suggested there may also be a free-living state.

V. cholerae O139

V. cholerae serogroup O139 (synonym: *V. cholerae* O139 Bengal) is a relatively new organism that causes epidemic cholera (3). It emerged in October 1992 in Madras,

India, and by 1994 had spread to many Asian countries and had been imported into industrialized countries. The symptoms in this outbreak were typical of cholera, but the organism did not react in *V. cholerae* O1 antisera or in O2-138 antisera. Thus, it was named *V. cholerae* O139, and reagents for its detection have been produced commercially (29). Unlike *V. cholerae* O1, strains of O139 produce a capsule (58), as do some strains of *V. cholerae* non-O1 (45). It has been speculated that the emergence of this strain is the beginning of the eighth cholera pandemic.

V. cholerae Non-O1

V. cholerae non-O1 strains (synonyms: "nag vibrios"; "non-agglutinating vibrios"; "non-cholera vibrios"; *V. cholerae* "non-O1, non-O139"; and *V. cholerae* non-O1,139) do not agglutinate in O1 or O139 antisera but are otherwise typical strains of *V. cholerae* in their biochemical reactions. They usually do not produce cholera toxin (18, 45, 52, 57) but can produce other toxins (32). They can cause a severe cholera-like disease, but they are usually isolated from patients with mild diarrhea, extraintestinal infections, seafood, and the environment. *V. cholerae* non-O1 strains have also caused septicemia in patients with cirrhosis or other underlying diseases (45). Strains have also been isolated from ears, wounds, the respiratory tract, and urine (22, 45).

V. mimicus

V. mimicus was first described in 1981 by Davis et al. (21), and most isolates were from patients with diarrhea, which usually occurred after the consumption of uncooked seafood, particularly raw oysters. *V. mimicus* is similar to *V. cholerae* non-O1 in most of its clinical, epidemiological, and ecological aspects.

V. parahaemolyticus

V. parahaemolyticus was not documented as a cause of acute gastroenteritis until 1950. It causes gastroenteritis with nausea, vomiting, abdominal cramps, low-grade fever, and chills. The diarrhea is usually watery but can sometimes be bloody. The disease is usually mild and self-limiting but can

TABLE 2 Key differential tests[a] for six groups of the 12 *Vibrio* species that occur in clinical specimens

Test	Group 1		Group 2,	Group 3,	Group 4,	Group 5			Group 6			
	V. cholerae	*V. mimicus*	*V. metschnikovii*	*V. cincinnatiensis*	*V. hollisae*	*V. damsela*	*V. fluvialis*	*V. furnissii*	*V. alginolyticus*	*V. parahaemolyticus*	*V. vulnificus*	*V. harveyi*
Growth in nutrient broth with:												
No NaCl added	+	+	−	−	−	−	−	−	−	−	−	−
1% NaCl added	+	+	+	+	+	+	+	+	+	+	+	+
Oxidase production	+	+	−	+	+	+	+	+	+	+	+	+
Nitrate reduction to nitrite	+	+	−	+	+	+	+	+	+	+	+	+
myo-Inositol fermentation			V	+								
Arginine dihydrolase					−	+	+	+	−	−	−	−
Lysine decarboxylase					−				+	+	+	+
Ornithine decarboxylase					−							

Reactions of the species in[b]:

[a] The key differential reactions that define the six groups are as follows: *V. cholerae* and *V. mimicus* do not require NaCl for growth; *V. metschnikovii* is negative for oxidase production and nitrate reduction to nitrite; *V. cincinnatiensis* ferments *myo*-inositol; *V. hollisae* is negative for arginine dihydrolase, lysine decarboxylase, and ornithine decarboxylase (i.e., is triple decarboxylase negative); the three species in group 5 are arginine positive; and the four species in group 6 are arginine negative and lysine positive.

[b] All data except those for oxidase production and nitrate reduction are for reactions that occur within 2 days at 35 to 37°C; oxidase production and nitrate reduction reactions are done only at day 1. Symbols: +, most strains positive (generally, about 90 to 100% of strains are positive); −, most strains negative (generally, about 0 to 10% of strains are positive); V, strain-to-strain variation (generally, about 25 to 75% of strains are positive). See Table 3 for the exact percentages.

TABLE 3 Biochemical test results and other properties of the 12 *Vibrio* species that occur in human clinical specimens

Test[a]	% Positive for[b]:											
	V. cholerae	*V. mimicus*	*V. metschnikovii*	*V. cincinnatiensis*	*V. hollisae*	*V. damsela*	*V. fluvialis*	*V. furnissii*	*V. alginolyticus*	*V. parahaemolyticus*	*V. vulnificus* biogroup 1	*V. harveyi*
Indole production (HIB, 1% NaCl)*	99	98	20	8	97	0	13	11	85	98	97	100
Methyl red (1% NaCl)	99	99	96	93	0	100	96	100	75	80	80	100
Voges-Proskauer (1% NaCl; Barritt)*	75	9	96	0	0	95	0	0	95	0	0	50
Citrate (Simmons)	97	99	75	21	0	0	93	100	1	3	75	0
H$_2$S on TSI	0	0	0	0	0	0	0	0	0	0	0	0
Urea hydrolysis	0	1	0	0	0	0	0	0	0	15	1	0
Phenylalanine deaminase	0	0	0	0	0	0	0	0	1	1	35	NG
Arginine (Moeller's; 1% NaCl)*	0	0	60	0	0	95	93	100	0	0	0	0
Lysine (Moeller's; 1% NaCl)*	99	100	35	57	0	50	0	0	99	100	99	100
Ornithine (Moeller's; 1% NaCl)*	99	99	0	0	0	0	0	0	50	95	55	0
Motility (36°C)	99	98	74	86	0	25	70	89	99	99	99	0
Gelatin hydrolysis (1% NaCl, 22°C)	90	65	65	0	0	6	85	86	90	95	75	0
KCN test (percent that grow)	10	2	0	0	0	5	65	89	15	20	1	0
Malonate utilization	1	0	0	0	0	0	0	11	0	0	0	0
D-Glucose, acid production*	100	100	100	100	100	100	100	100	100	100	100	50
D-Glucose, gas production*	0	0	0	0	0	10	0	100	0	0	0	0
Acid production from:												
D-Adonitol	0	0	0	0	0	0	0	0	1	0	0	0
L-Arabinose*	0	1	0	100	97	0	93	100	1	80	0	0
D-Arabitol*	0	0	0	0	0	0	65	89	0	0	0	0
Cellobiose*	8	0	9	100	0	0	30	11	3	5	99	50
Dulcitol	0	0	0	0	0	0	0	0	0	3	0	0
Erythritol	0	0	0	0	0	0	0	0	0	0	0	0
D-Galactose	90	82	45	100	100	90	96	100	20	92	96	0
Glycerol	30	13	100	100	0	0	7	55	80	50	1	0
myo-Inositol	0	0	40	100	0	0	0	0	0	0	0	0
Lactose*	7	21	50	0	0	0	3	0	0	1	85	0
Maltose*	99	99	100	100	0	100	100	100	100	99	100	100
D-Mannitol*	99	99	96	100	0	0	97	100	100	100	45	50
D-Mannose	78	99	100	100	100	100	100	100	99	100	98	50
Melibiose	1	0	0	7	0	0	3	11	1	1	40	0

(Continued on next page)

TABLE 3 Biochemical test results and other properties of the 12 *Vibrio* species that occur in human clinical specimens (*Continued*)

Test[a]	% Positive for:[b]											
	V. cholerae	*V. mimicus*	*V. metschnikovii*	*V. cincinnatiensis*	*V. hollisae*	*V. damsela*	*V. fluvialis*	*V. furnissii*	*V. alginolyticus*	*V. parahaemolyticus*	*V. vulnificus* biogroup 1	*V. harveyi*
α-Methyl-D-glucoside	0	0	25	57	0	5	0	0	1	0	0	0
Raffinose	0	0	0	0	0	0	0	11	0	0	0	0
L-Rhamnose	0	0	0	0	0	0	0	45	0	1	0	0
Salicin*	1	0	9	100	0	0	0	0	4	1	95	0
D-Sorbitol	1	0	45	0	0	0	3	0	1	1	0	0
Sucrose*	100	0	100	100	0	5	100	100	99	1	15	50
Trehalose	99	94	100	100	0	86	100	100	100	99	100	50
D-Xylose	0	0	0	43	0	0	0	0	0	0	0	0
Mucate-acid production	1	0	0	0	0	0	0	0	0	0	0	0
Tartrate (Jordan)	75	12	35	0	65	0	35	22	95	93	84	50
Esculin hydrolysis	0	0	60	0	0	0	8	0	3	1	40	0
Acetate utilization	92	78	25	14	0	0	70	65	0	1	7	0
Nitrate reduced to nitrite*	99	100	0	100	100	100	100	100	100	100	100	100
Oxidase*	100	100	0	100	100	95	100	100	100	100	100	100
DNase (25°C)	93	55	50	79	0	75	90	100	95	92	50	100
Lipase*	92	17	100	36	0	0	40	89	85	90	92	0
ONPG test*	94	90	50	86	0	0	65	35	0	5	75	0
Yellow pigment at 25°C	0	0	0	0	0	0	0	0	0	0	0	0
Tyrosine clearing	13	30	5	0	3	0	0	45	70	77	75	0
Growth in nutrient broth with:												
0% NaCl*	100	100	0	0	0	0	0	0	0	0	0	0
1% NaCl*	100	100	100	100	99	100	99	99	99	100	99	100
6% NaCl*	53	49	78	100	83	95	96	100	100	99	65	100
8% NaCl*	1	0	44	62	0	0	71	78	94	80	0	0
10% NaCl*	0	0	4	0	0	0	4	0	69	2	0	0
12% NaCl*	0	0	0	0	0	0	0	0	17	1	0	0
Swarming (marine agar, 25°C)[c]	−	−	−	+	−	−	−	−	+	+	−	+
String test	100	100	100	80	100	80	100	100	91	64	100	100
O-129, zone of inhibition[d]	99	95	90	25	40	90	31	0	19	20	98	100
Polymyxin B (% with any zone of inhibition)	22	88	100	92	100	85	100	89	63	54	3	100

[a] Symbols and abbreviations: *, the test is recommended as part of the routine set for *Vibrio* identification; 1% NaCl, 1% NaCl has been added to the standard media to enhance growth; HIB, heart infusion broth; Barritt, the Barritt reagent for the Voges Proskauer test contains α-naphthol for greater sensitivity; TSI, triple sugar iron agar; ONPG, *o*-nitrophenyl-β-D-galactopyranoside; a positive string test indicates that cells are lysed when they are suspended in a 0.5% sodium deoxycholate solution. For more details about media and methods, see reference 22. The approximate number of strains studied for each organism can be found in Table 6.

[b] The numbers indicate the percentage of strains that are positive after 48 h of incubation at 36°C (unless other conditions are indicated). Most of the positive reactions occur during the first 24 h. NG, no growth, which means that the organism does not grow, probably because the NaCl concentration is too low.

[c] Symbols: +, most strains positive (generally about 90 to 100% of strains are positive); −, most strains negative (generally, about 0 to 10% of strains are positive).

[d] The content of the disk was 150 μg.

TABLE 4 Growth of *Vibrio* species on TCBS agar

Organism	% of strains with the following colony appearance on TCBS agar:		Growth and plating efficiency
	Green	Yellow	
V. cholerae	0	100	Good
V. mimicus	100	0	Good
V. parahaemolyticus	99	1	Good
V. alginolyticus	0	100	Good
V. fluvialis	0	100	Good
V. furnissii	0	100	Good
V. hollisae	100	0	Very poor
V. harveyi	0	100	Good
V. damselae	95	5	Reduced at 36°C
V. metschnikovii	0	100	May be reduced
V. cincinnatiensis	0	100	Very poor
V. vulnificus	90[a]	10[a]	Good
"Marine vibrios"	Variable	Variable	Variable
Aeromonas and *Enterobacteriaceae*	No growth	No growth	Most strains are totally inhibited

[a] The original report describing this species gave the proportion of strains positive for sucrose fermentation as 3%. At the *Vibrio* Laboratory of the Centers for Disease Control and Prevention, about 15% of the strains have been sucrose positive. The 10% value in the table represents a composite value.

be fatal (the fatality rate was 7% in the first outbreak). Rehydration is usually the only treatment needed, but in some severe cases the patient will require hospital admission. Antimicrobial therapy may be beneficial.

Foodborne outbreaks and sporadic cases occur worldwide and are usually associated with the consumption of raw or contaminated seafood. In Japan, *V. parahaemolyticus* is an extremely important diarrheal agent, causing 50 to 70% of the cases of foodborne enteritis, almost always associated with the consumption of raw fish or shellfish. Cross-contamination after the food is cooked is another important mechanism of spread. Outbreaks are not common in the United States. Recently, a pandemic clone of serotype O3:K6 has emerged (49). Strains of this serotype also caused an unusually high proportion of *V. parahaemolyticus* foodborne disease outbreaks in Taiwan (from 1996 to

TABLE 5 Differentiation of the three *V. vulnificus* biogroups[a]

Test	Result for biogroup[b]:		
	1	2	3
Ornithine decarboxylase	55	−	+
Indole production	+	−	+
D-Mannitol fermentation	45	−	−
D-Sorbitol fermentation	−	+	−
Citrate (Simmons)	(+)	+	−
Salicin fermentation	+	+	−
Cellobiose fermentation	+	+	−
Lactose fermentation	(+)	+	−
ONPG[c] test	(+)	+	−

[a] The first three tests are important for differentiating biogroup 2 from biogroups 1 and 3. The remaining tests are important for differentiating biogroup 3 from biogroups 1 and 2. Adapted from Bisharat et al. (9).
[b] Symbols: +, most (90% or greater) strains positive; (+), many strains (75 to 89.9%) positive; −, most strains negative (10% or less are positive). Numbers give the actual percentage of strains that are positive.
[c] ONPG, *o*-nitrophenyl-β-D-galactopyranoside.

1999), suggesting something unusual in the organism's ecology, epidemiology, or virulence (15).

V. vulnificus

V. vulnificus (synonyms: "L+ *Vibrio*", "Lac+ *Vibrio*", and *Beneckea vulnifica*) has been recognized as a distinct species of *Vibrio* since 1976. It has primarily been associated with two disease syndromes: primary septicemia and wound infection (11). Primary septicemia is a very serious infection in patients with preexisting liver disease and has a fatality rate of about 50%. In most cases the disease begins several days after the patient has eaten raw oysters. Cultures of blood and skin lesions are usually positive. *V. vulnificus* also causes severe wound infections, usually after trauma and exposure to marine animals or the marine environment (11), where it is commonly isolated.

V. vulnificus Biogroups 2 and 3

Little information has been published about the recently described vibrios *V. vulnificus* biogroups 2 and 3. *V. vulnificus* biogroup 2 was originally isolated from diseased eels, but in 1995 Amaro and Biosca (5) isolated it from a human wound infection. *V. vulnificus* biogroup 3 was described in 1999 by Bisharat et al. (9), who isolated it from patients with wound infections and bacteremia. Cases have been limited to Israel and were acquired from exposure to live fish (tilapia) grown in aquaculture.

V. fluvialis

V. fluvialis (synonyms: "Group F *Vibrios*" and "Group EF6") was first named in 1981 and appears to cause sporadic cases of diarrhea worldwide (39). It was also implicated in a large outbreak of diarrhea in Bangladesh (33).

V. furnissii

V. furnissii (synonyms: "*V. fluvialis* biovar II", "*V. fluvialis* aerogenic", and "*V. fluvialis* gas+") was described as a separate *Vibrio* species in 1983 (13). It is apparently rare in human clinical specimens, and stool is the most common

TABLE 6 Use of antibiotic susceptibility patterns as an aid in identifying the 12 *Vibrio* species that occur in human clinical specimens

Antibiotic	% Strains susceptible[a]:											
	V. cholerae (480)[b]	*V. mimicus* (75)	*V. metschnikovii* (22)	*V. cincinnatiensis* (14)	*V. hollisae* (34)	*V. damsela* (21)	*V. fluvialis* (25)	*V. furnissii* (9)	*V. alginolyticus* (69)	*V. parahaemolyticus* (144)	*V. vulnificus* biogroup 1 (130)	*V. harveyi* (2)
Penicillin G (10 U, 12–21 mm)[c]	2	3	9	0	97	0	0	0	0	0	2	0
Ampicillin (10 μg, 12–13 mm)	87	97	31	36	100	52	32	11	0	12	99	0
Carbenicillin (100 μg, 18–22 mm)	64	8	27	7	100	14	16	0	0	1	54	0
Cephalothin (30 μg, 15–17 mm)	98	100	100	100	100	76	40	0	32	17	65	100
Colistin (10 μg, 9–10 mm)	4	61	91	93	100	76	100	100	25	11	2	0
Tetracycline (30 μg, 15–18 mm)	98	100	73	93	97	86	88	89	94	98	99	100
Sulfadiazine (250 μg, 13–16 mm)	26	17	5	36	56	71	36	11	16	3	28	50
Chloramphenicol (30 μg, 13–17 mm)	99	100	100	100	100	10	88	100	100	100	100	100
Streptomycin (10 μg, 12–14 mm)	60	61	32	86	100	24	84	100	54	17	42	50
Kanamycin (30 μg, 14–17 mm)	92	89	14	79	100	43	88	100	62	37	53	100
Gentamicin (10 μg, 13–14 mm)	98	99	100	100	100	100	100	100	100	97	100	100
Nalidixic acid (30 μg, 14–18 mm)	99	99	100	100	100	100	100	100	97	99	99	100

[a] Studied at the *Vibrio* Laboratory of the Centers for Disease Control and Prevention and done on Mueller-Hinton agar (with no added NaCl) at 35 to 37°C.

[b] The number of strains studied for each organism is given in parentheses.

[c] The first number in parentheses is the disk content. The next two numbers give the zone size range for the intermediate category. For example, 12–21 mm means that strains of intermediate susceptibility have zones that are 12 to 21 mm in diameter, resistant strains have zones that are 6 to 11 mm in diameter, and susceptible strains have zones that are 22 mm in diameter or larger. The breakpoints listed are the ones established for members of the family *Enterobacteriaceae* in the early 1970s for each antibiotic and have been used in the *Vibrio* Laboratory of the Centers for Disease Control and Prevention for almost 30 years for taxonomic studies. They may differ from the current breakpoints given for antibiotics used for the treatment of human infections. Thus, these data should only be used as an aid in identifying isolates.

source. *V. furnissii* has a clear association with diarrhea but an unproven etiological role (22, 23), although its role has been suggested (19). Microbiologists should be alert in detecting this organism and should look for evidence both for and against its etiological role in individual cases of diarrhea. Lee et al. (39) showed that *V. furnissii* is widespread in the aquatic environment and is more common in estuaries.

V. hollisae

V. hollisae (synonyms: "group EF13" and "Enteric Group 42") was named a new halophilic *Vibrio* species in 1982 (30) and apparently causes sporadic cases of diarrhea (1, 46). The thermostable direct hemolysin (*tdh*) gene of *V. parahaemolyticus* occurs in essentially all strains of *V. hollisae* and may have been acquired by horizontal transfer in the distant past (48).

V. damsela

V. damsela (synonyms: *V. damselae*, *Photobacterium damsela*, *P. damsela* subsp. *damsela*, *P. damselae*, *P. damselae* subsp. *damselae*, *Listonella damsela*, and *L. damselae*) was described in 1981 by Love et al. (43), who isolated it from wound infections of damselfish off the California coast and from human wound infections. Its etiological role as a cause of serious human infections was strengthened by additional reports of wound infections, with or without bacteremia (25, 46, 56). Isolates have also been recovered from marine fish, sewage, oysters, and a wound on a raccoon (23).

V. alginolyticus

V. alginolyticus is very common in the marine environment (22, 34) and has been isolated from infections of soft tissues, wounds, the ears, and, occasionally, the eyes. There is a clear association of *V. alginolyticus* with infections at these sites, but its etiological role has often been assumed rather than definitively shown in many of the reported cases. However, most investigators list *V. alginolyticus* as a pathogenic *Vibrio* species, particularly of wound and ear infections.

V. metschnikovii

V. metschnikovii has frequently been isolated from fresh, brackish, and marine waters (38). However, in 1981 Jean-Jacques et al. (35) reported that it caused peritonitis and bacteremia in a patient with an inflamed gallbladder. Subsequently, *V. metschnikovii* has been isolated from additional patients with bacteremia (28). It has also been isolated from the urine of two patients (22), a foot ulcer (22), and from five children with diarrhea (17). However, its etiological role as a cause of diarrhea is unproven.

V. cincinnatiensis

V. cincinnatiensis was first reported by Brayton et al. (12) from a patient with bacteremia and meningitis. Subsequent isolates have been from feces (intestine), the ear, a foot or leg wound, animals, and water (22).

V. harveyi (V. carchariae)

In 1984 Grimes et al. (27) described *V. carchariae* as a urease-positive halophilic vibrio isolated from a brown shark (*Carcharhinus plumbeus*) that had died in captivity in a large aquarium. In 1989 Pavia et al. (50) described an isolate of *V. carchariae* from a human wound infection following a shark bite. Subsequently, it was shown that *V. carchariae* is almost identical to *V. harveyi* in phenotype (23, 51), and the type strains of the two species are 88% related

by DNA-DNA hybridization (51). The two organisms also have identical or almost identical 16S rRNA sequences. The evidence seems conclusive that the two species are (subjective) synonyms. *V. harveyi* is the older name; thus, it has priority (23, 51).

COLLECTION, TRANSPORT, AND STORAGE OF SPECIMENS

Extraintestinal specimens are collected and processed without special attention to *Vibrio* species. The collection, processing, and isolation of *Vibrio* species from extraintestinal specimens (e.g., blood and wounds) does not typically present a problem in the clinical laboratory because most *Vibrio* strains are found as the only pathogen. In addition, most pathogenic vibrios grow well on common plating media such as MacConkey agar and blood agar designed for the isolation of gram-negative bacilli.

Stool specimens (14, 23) should be collected early, preferably within the first 24 h of illness and before the patient has received any antimicrobial agents. If feces are unavailable, rectal swabs may also be used (14). Purgatives may increase the yield if small numbers of vibrios are present. (*Laboratory Methods for the Diagnosis of Epidemic Dysentery and Cholera* [14] is available without charge by contacting the Foodborne and Diarrheal Diseases Laboratory Section, Centers for Disease Control and Prevention, Mailstop C03, 1600 Clifton Rd. N.E., Atlanta, GA 30333, Attention: Mrs. Cheryl Bopp. Fax: (404) 639-3333. E-mail: cab4@cdc.gov.)

Stool or rectal swab specimens should be inoculated on isolation plates with minimal delay. The viability of *Vibrio* species is well maintained at the alkaline pH of rice water stool, but the viability of *Vibrio* species in formed stools is unpredictable. Vibrios are very susceptible to desiccation. If there will be a delay in the plating of a culture (especially when it must be transported by courier), rectal swabs or fecal material should be placed in the semisolid transport medium of Cary and Blair, which maintains the viability of *Vibrio* in culture for up to 4 weeks. Buffered glycerol-saline, often used in enteric bacteriology, is an unsatisfactory transport medium even for short periods. Tellurite-taurocholate-peptone medium or alkaline peptone water can be used for "enrichment transport" in areas where specimens are collected in the field and can be plated within 12 to 24 h. In the absence of available suitable transport media, strips of blotting paper may be soaked in liquid stool and inserted into airtight plastic bags.

Direct examination of stool material is not recommended for general purposes. However, stools may be examined by dark-field microscopy for the characteristic size, shape, and darting motility of vibrios, especially after brief incubation in broth. Direct microscopic identification of *V. cholerae* O1 in feces by "O1 serum immobilization" is described in a subsequent section.

ISOLATION PROCEDURES

In many laboratories both extraintestinal and stool specimens will be processed with no special media or methods specific for vibrios, but special efforts will be appropriate in areas where vibrios are encountered more frequently (14). One recent study (44) in Gulf Coast states of the United States surveyed the laboratory practices of more than 100 centers and found that only 20% of the sites routinely cultured stools specifically for *Vibrio* species. Since the routine culture for vibrios even in areas of high prevalence is not common, it is important that physicians alert the laboratory of the possibility of *Vibrio* infections by relaying relevant information in the clinical history for the patient. Such information should include whether the patient has consumed seafood; has a history of marine, marine-associated (e.g., shellfish), or brackish water penetrating injuries (40); has recently participated in aquatic activities (swimming, bathing, diving); or has hobbies such as keeping of aquaria. In all instances, it is extremely helpful if the specimen is accompanied by a note such as "*Vibrio* species are suspected," "the patient ate raw oysters in New Orleans," or "the patient's foot was cut while wading in brackish water."

Several commercial companies produce media and reagents useful in vibrio work (BD Biosciences, Sparks, Md. [http.www.bd.com/microbiology]; Denka Seiken Co. Ltd., Tokyo, Japan [http://www.science net.com.au/ds2broch1.htm]; New Horizons Diagnostics Corp., Columbia Md. [www.nhdiag. com]; Oxoid Inc., Ogdensburg, N.Y. [www.oxoid.ca; Oxoid distributes Denka Seiken products]; and Remel, Lenexa, Kans. [www.remelinc.com]). There are several good general media (22, 23) for the isolation of *Vibrio* species. Marine agar (BD Biosciences) is a nonselective medium, and essentially all *Vibrio* strains will grow on it. Alkaline peptone water is probably the most useful liquid enrichment medium. Specimens are enriched at 36°C in alkaline peptone water and are then subcultured after 8 h and again at 16 to 24 h. TCBS agar is commercially available (BD Biosciences, Oxoid) and is extremely useful for isolating *V. cholerae* and *V. parahaemolyticus* from stool specimens. It is also probably the most widely used medium for isolating *Vibrio* strains from human clinical specimens and the environment (Table 4). Its main advantage is that it increases a laboratory worker's awareness of suspect *Vibrio* colonies, and in some laboratories, its use will result in the detection of *Vibrio* isolates that otherwise would be missed.

Cultures of *Vibrio* grow well on blood agar where they may be beta-hemolytic (*V. cholerae* non-O1 and some *V. cholerae* O1 strains of the eltor biotype), alpha-hemolytic (*V. vulnificus* and many others), or nonhemolytic (7). *Vibrio* strains usually grow on MacConkey agar (sometimes with a reduced plating efficiency) and will appear as colorless (lactose-negative) colonies. *Vibrio* cultures often do not grow well on more selective plating media for enteric organisms.

Oxidase testing can be done on colonies from blood agar and on lactose-negative colonies from selective media. However, lactose-positive colonies from selective media can give a false-negative oxidase reaction. Oxidase screening of colonies appears to be a cost-efficient method for detecting *Vibrio* isolates from cultures of stool and extraintestinal specimens. Its main advantage is that it avoids the expense of adding a plate of TCBS agar. Individual colonies can be tested for oxidase production, or the reagent can be added to an area of growth on the plate.

DIRECT DETECTION OF *V. CHOLERAE* O1 IN FECES

In rice water stools from patients with cholera, *V. cholerae* O1 is usually present in very high numbers, often 10^6 to 10^8 organisms per ml of stool, and can be recovered essentially as a pure culture (36). Thus, there is enough *V. cholerae* O1 antigen present to agglutinate particles (latex or *Staphylococcus aureus* cells) coated with antibodies to the O1 antigen (16, 36).

A second method for direct detection is the microscopic immobilization test, which detects the rapid loss of motility of *V. cholerae* O1 cells in the presence of O1 antiserum (52), as observed with a microscope.

Antibodies to *V. cholerae* O139 could also be included in both of these assays. These direct methods seem most appropriate in the hands of experienced personnel in geographic areas where cholera is common or in areas where laboratory facilities are scarce or unavailable.

IDENTIFICATION

Only 12 *Vibrio* species occur in human clinical specimens, and their identification is not difficult (22, 23). However, strains of *Vibrio* are rare compared to *Enterobacteriaceae*, so laboratory personnel may not be as familiar with them. Clinical laboratories will typically identify *Vibrio* strains with the commercial identification system that they use to identify gram-negative organisms. State health departments and reference laboratories typically use conventional biochemical tests to identify vibrios.

The first generation of commercial identification systems had problems identifying vibrios. One product originally used distilled water as the suspending medium, which caused the rapid lysis of halophilic *Vibrio* cultures and gave aberrant results. Saline was later substituted as the suspending medium to eliminate this problem.

Literature from commercial companies should be consulted for a list of the *Vibrio* species included in the product's database, published evaluations of the product, and the formula of the kit's suspending medium and tests to determine if the Na^+ content is sufficient. There needs to be a comprehensive evaluation of commercial products for their ability to identify clinical and environmental *Vibrio* species. One of the most common errors of commercial systems is that they misidentify cultures of *Aeromonas* as *V. fluvialis* or *V. furnissii* and vice versa (2). This is not surprising since these three organisms are phenotypically similar. There is a good check on a commercial system's identification of a culture as one of the halophilic vibrio species: determine its oxidase reaction (Tables 1 and 2), growth in nutrient broth with 1% NaCl and without NaCl (Tables 1 and 2), and growth on TCBS agar (Table 4). Disagreements in any of these key properties warn of a possible misidentification.

The first and most important step in identifying a *Vibrio* strain is to suspect that it is a member of the genus (Tables 1 to 4). For *Vibrio* identification by standard tube tests, NaCl should be added to several biochemical test media (Table 3) because the commercial formulas do not include NaCl. Otherwise, halophilic *Vibrio* species will not grow or will grow poorly and give negative reactions in tests that should be positive. Fortunately, commercial media for most of the biochemical tests are formulated to contain 0.5 to 1.0% NaCl.

Identification of environmental and seafood isolates can be extremely difficult because over 60 species of *Vibrio*, *Photobacterium*, and their relatives must be considered (22, 23). 16S rRNA sequencing may prove a good alternative to phenotypic methods for identifying this complex group of organisms.

Research tests have been described for many of the *Vibrio* species (23, 34, 57), but for a number of technical and regulatory reasons (23) these seem more appropriate for reference and research laboratories. These include 16S rRNA sequencing, DNA-based diagnostic tests, pulsed-field gel electrophoresis for strain typing, and detection of toxins and virulence factors (14, 23, 34, 57).

IDENTIFYING THE INDIVIDUAL VIBRIO SPECIES

The most common Vibrio species isolated from human clinical specimens are V. cholerae (O1, O139, non-O1), V. parahaemolyticus, V. alginolyticus, V. vulnificus, V. fluvialis, and V. mimicus (22, 23, 31).

In countries where cholera is common, there is no need to do a large number of biochemical tests to confirm a culture as V. cholerae. Agglutination in V. cholerae O1 or O139 antiserum is usually sufficient. However, complete biochemical testing (Tables 2 and 3) should be done in countries where cholera is rare. In industrial countries, identification to the species level will typically come first, and cultures identified as V. cholerae should be immediately tested in O1 and O139 antisera.

Phenotypically, V. cholerae O139 is almost identical to V. cholerae O1 eltor, and it is identified by its agglutination in O139 antiserum. Another possible differential characteristic is susceptibility to the compound O-129. V. cholerae O139 strains are usually O-129 resistant, whereas most O1 isolates (except in Bangladesh and surrounding regions) are O-129 sensitive (3).

Strains that are identified as V. cholerae but that do not agglutinate in O1 or O139 antiserum are identified as V. cholerae non-O1. Further serotyping would yield a more precise identification such as V. cholerae O13, but complete serotyping is done by only a few reference laboratories. The test for Na$^+$ requirement differentiates V. cholerae from the halophilic Vibrio species (Table 2), and sucrose fermentation differentiates V. cholerae from its very close relative V. mimicus (Table 3).

Strains of V. parahaemolyticus are usually typical in their biochemical reactions (Tables 2 and 3), but in the late 1970s (22, 34) urea-positive strains emerged and were very common. V. alginolyticus is biochemically similar to V. parahaemolyticus; but it usually swarms, is Voges-Proskauer positive, and grows in higher concentrations of NaCl (Table 3). It is often misidentified as V. parahaemolyticus and vice versa.

V. vulnificus strains grow well on blood agar and TCBS agar. Most strains are sucrose negative and green on TCBS agar, but occasional strains (Table 4) are sucrose positive and produce yellow colonies. V. vulnificus is unique among Vibrio species because it ferments lactose, salicin, and cellobiose and is ONPG$^+$ (o-nitrophenyl-β-D-galactopyranoside positive) (Table 3). It has no zone of inhibition or a small zone of inhibition around colistin, but it has large zones of inhibition around ampicillin and carbenicillin (Table 6). V. vulnificus biogroups 2 and 3 are difficult to identify without doing a complete set of biochemical tests (Table 3), but eventually, they should be included in commercial identification systems. Table 5 gives the differential reactions.

V. fluvialis and V. furnissii are often confused with Aeromonas (2) since members of all three taxa are usually arginine dihydrolase positive and biochemically similar. In contrast to strains of Aeromonas, V. fluvialis, and V. furnissii are slightly halophilic and will grow in nutrient broth only if NaCl is added (Table 3). Phenotypically, V. furnissii is

almost identical to V. fluvialis, and gas production is the key differential test (Table 3).

V. hollisae strains are fastidious. They grow on blood agar but not on MacConkey or TCBS agar (Table 4). Strains are halophilic, triple decarboxylase negative, and poorly motile and have a characteristic fermentation pattern (Tables 2 and 3). V. hollisae strains also have a unique antibiogram (30), with very large zones of inhibition around all antibiotics, including penicillin (Table 6).

V. damsela has a unique biochemical profile (Tables 2 and 3) and resistance pattern (Table 6), which make identification easy.

V. metschnikovii is unique among the pathogenic Vibrio species because it is oxidase negative and does not reduce nitrate to nitrite (Tables 2 and 3).

V. cincinnatiensis ferments myo-inositol (Table 3), which should make it easy to identify.

V. harveyi is biochemically distinct (Table 3) and is resistant to ampicillin, carbenicillin, and colistin (Table 6), which can be helpful in identification.

COMMERCIAL PRODUCTS FOR DETECTING CHOLERA TOXIN AND THE THERMOSTABLE DIRECT HEMOLYSIN OF V. PARAHAEMOLYTICUS

Until recently the detection of cholera toxin was limited to a few reference laboratories because the methodology was complex. However, there is a now a commercially available kit (Oxoid) that determines cholera toxin production by pure cultures. Because of antigenic cross-reactions, the assay also detects the heat-labile enterotoxin (LT) of Escherichia coli strains. The assay is based on reverse passive latex agglutination (antibody-coated latex particles) in 96-well plates (4).

About 96% of the V. parahaemolyticus strains from patients with well-documented gastroenteritis are Kanagawa positive, but only about 1% of the strains isolated from the environment are positive. Most pathogenic strains of V. parahaemolyticus produce a toxin named thermostable direct hemolysin (TDH), also known as the Kanagawa toxin. This toxin is coded by the genes tdh1 and tdh2x, and it has been detected in a number of vibrios including V. cholerae non-O1, V. mimicus, and V. hollisae (48). The toxin was originally detected by the hemolysis of red blood cells on Wagatsuma agar (Kanagawa reaction), a difficult procedure with technical limitations. Now, a commercially available kit (Oxoid) detects this toxin by reverse passive latex agglutination in 96-well plates. This test is easier to standardize and read than the Kanagawa reaction but is limited to reference laboratories. Kanagawa-negative strains of V. parahaemolyticus can apparently cause gastroenteritis by producing a second toxin named TDH-related toxin (TRH) and encoded by the trh gene. Although tdh and trh share 70% sequence homology, they are different genes. There are no commercial products for the detection of TRH.

SEROTYPING AND SERODIAGNOSIS

Serotyping schemes are available for several of the Vibrio species (53–55, 57), but complete serotyping is done in only a few specialized reference laboratories. However, clinical laboratories should maintain V. cholerae O1 and O139 antisera (BD Biosciences, New Horizons, Oxoid) so that these two important pathogens can be identified completely and reported immediately.

Serodiagnosis of cholera can be established with a high degree of certainty by titration of acute- and convalescent-phase sera in agglutination, vibriocidal, or antitoxin tests (42). The reagents are not commercially available, so this technique will normally be limited to a few reference laboratories.

ANTIMICROBIAL SUSCEPTIBILITY TESTING

The *Vibrio* species important in clinical microbiology usually grow well on Mueller-Hinton agar and broth, but some of the environmental marine vibrios grow poorly (22, 23) because of their requirement for larger amounts of Na$^+$. Antibiotic resistance is rare in *Vibrio* compared with *Enterobacteriaceae* (20, 22, 23, 34, 57). Table 6 summarizes the results for over 1,000 isolates studied in a reference laboratory. In most cases resistance is probably intrinsic to the species rather than acquired through plasmid transfer or antibiotic exposure. The main exception is that strains of *V. cholerae* apparently become resistant through exposure to antibiotics (20, 57). In cholera outbreaks, resistance can be acquired by the acquisition of R factors.

Unlike the *Enterobacteriaceae*, there are few interpretive standards for vibrios. However, in 1998 the National Committee for Clinical Laboratory Standards (NCCLS) published interpretive standards for *V. cholerae* for ampicillin, tetracycline, trimethoprim-sulfamethoxazole, chloramphenicol, and sulfonamides (47). Because *Vibrio* species grow rapidly and are similar to *Enterobacteriaceae* in many ways, a first approximation might be to use the interpretive standards for the *Enterobacteriaceae* for other antibiotics and all *Vibrio* species. This approach was adopted almost 30 years ago and is described in Table 6. In defense of this position, a limited number of strains of the *Enterobacteriaceae* were used in studies to set interpretive standards for the entire family, and most of the new species of *Enterobacteriaceae* have not been studied. Presumably, additional NCCLS standards will be developed to cover additional antibiotics and the other *Vibrio* species.

Resistance patterns can be helpful in differentiating species that are phenotypically similar. *V. hollisae* has very large zones of inhibition around most antibiotics (30), and its antibiogram is unique among the *Vibrio* species (Table 6). Resistance to polymyxin antibiotics (polymyxin B and colistin) can be useful in detecting an isolate of the eltor biogroup of *V. cholerae* or *V. vulnificus*, because most other *Vibrio* species are susceptible to this antibiotic (Table 6). Patterns of resistance to colistin, ampicillin, and carbenicillin can also be useful for differentiation (23).

INTERPRETATION AND REPORTING OF RESULTS

The isolation of *V. cholerae* O1 or O139 should be reported immediately to the attending physician because of the severe dehydration that cholera can produce. The case should also be reported to public health authorities, and the isolate should be submitted for confirmation and toxin testing. If no other potential pathogens are present, cultures of the other *Vibrio* species that are known to cause diarrhea will often be clinically significant. However, raw oysters are often the implicated food, and they may contain many different possible pathogens and many *Vibrio* species. A few colonies of a *Vibrio* species on a plate of TCBS medium would probably not be significant, whereas a pure culture in high numbers probably would. This is particularly true for *V. parahaemolyticus*; there is a danger of confusing nonpathogenic strains passing through the intestine for actual infection. Most strains isolated from oysters and from the marine environment do not have the genes associated with human pathogenicity; thus, toxin testing would be necessary to confirm the suspected etiological role. In the experience of one of us (J.M.J.), most isolates of *V. parahaemolyticus* from human feces contain pathogenicity genes. If strains do not have the pathogenicity genes, their presence probably represents transient passage through the intestine rather than infection.

The same warning should be emphasized for *Vibrio* isolates from other specimens such as wounds and ears. Isolation of vibrios could represent infection, transient colonization, or merely the vibrio flora always present in seawater or brackish water.

Vibrio strains from blood or spinal fluid are always significant. Blood or wound specimens that are culture positive for *V. vulnificus* (and perhaps *V. damsela*) should also be reported immediately because of the life-threatening nature of infections with these organisms. The clinical significance of *Vibrio* strains in many other specimens will be more difficult to determine, and since physicians are not familiar with many *Vibrio* species, it would be helpful to provide a telephone consultation when a *Vibrio* is identified.

REFERENCES

1. **Abbott, S. L., and J. M. Janda.** 1994. Severe gastroenteritis associated with *Vibrio hollisae* infection: report of two cases and review. *Clin. Infect. Dis.* **18:**310–312.
2. **Abbott, S. L., L. S. Seli, M. Catino, Jr., M. A. Hartley, and J. M. Janda.** 1998. Misidentification of unusual *Aeromonas* species as members of the genus *Vibrio*: a continuing problem. *J. Clin. Microbiol.* **36:**1103–1104.
3. **Albert, M. J.** 1994. *Vibrio cholerae* O139 Bengal. *J. Clin. Microbiol.* **32:**2345–2349.
4. **Almeida, M. J., F. W. Hickman-Brenner, E. G. Sowers, N. D. Puhr, J. J. Farmer III, and I. K. Wachsmuth.** 1990. Comparison of a latex agglutination assay and an enzyme-linked immunosorbent assay for detecting cholera toxin. *J. Clin. Microbiol.* **28:**128–130.
5. **Amaro, C., and E. G. Biosca.** 1996. *Vibrio vulnificus* biotype 2, pathogenic for eels, is also an opportunistic pathogen for humans. *Appl. Environ. Microbiol.* **62:**1454–1457.
6. **Barer, M. R.** 1997. Viable but not-culturable and dormant bacteria: time to resolve an oxymoron and a misnomer? *J. Med. Microbiol.* **46:**629–631.
7. **Barrett, T. J., and P. A. Blake.** 1981. Epidemiological usefulness of changes in hemolytic activity of *Vibrio cholerae* El Tor during the seventh pandemic. *J. Clin. Microbiol.* **13:**126–129.
8. **Bennish, M. L.** 1994. Cholera: pathophysiology, clinical features, and treatment, p. 229–255. *In* I. K. Wachsmuth, P. A. Blake, and O. Olsvik (ed.), Vibrio cholerae *and* Cholera: Molecular to Global Perspectives. ASM Press, Washington, D.C.
9. **Bisharat, N., V. Agmon, R. Finkelstein, R. Raz, G. Ben-Dror, L. Lerner, S. Soboh, R. Colodner, D. N. Cameron, D. L. Wykstra, D. L. Swerdlow, J. J. Farmer III, and the Israel Vibrio Study Group.** 1999. Clinical, epidemiological, and microbiological features of Vibrio

vulnificus biogroup 3 causing outbreaks of wound infection and bacteraemia in Israel. *Lancet* **354:**1421–1424.

10. **Blake, P. A.** 1994. Historical perspectives on pandemic cholera, p. 293–295. *In* I. K. Wachsmuth, P. A. Blake, and O. Olsvik (ed.), *Vibrio cholerae and Cholera: Molecular to Global Perspectives.* ASM Press, Washington, D.C.

11. **Blake, P. A., M. H. Merson, R. E. Weaver, D. G. Hollis, and P. C. Heublein.** 1979. Disease caused by a marine *Vibrio*: clinical characteristics and epidemiology. *N. Engl. J. Med.* **300:**1–5.

12. **Brayton, P. R., R. B. Bode, R. R. Colwell, M. T. Mac-Donell, H. L. Hall, D. J. Grimes, P. A. West, and T. N. Bryant.** 1986. *Vibrio cincinnatiensis* sp. nov., a new human pathogen. *J. Clin. Microbiol.* **23:**104–108.

13. **Brenner, D. J., F. W. Hickman-Brenner, J. V. Lee, A. G. Steigerwalt, G. R. Fanning, D. G. Hollis, J. J. Farmer III, R. E. Weaver, and R. J. Seidler.** 1983. *Vibrio furnissii* (formerly aerogenic biogroup of *Vibrio fluvialis*), a new species isolated from human feces and the environment. *J. Clin. Microbiol.* **18:**816–824.

14. **Centers for Disease Control and Prevention.** 1999. *Laboratory Methods for the Diagnosis of Epidemic Dysentery and Cholera.* Centers for Disease Control and Prevention, Atlanta, Ga.

15. **Chiou, C.-S., S.-Y. Hsu, S.-I. Chiu, T.-K. Wang, and C.-S. Chao.** 2000. *Vibrio parahaemolyticus* serovar O3:K6 as cause of unusually high incidence of food-borne disease outbreaks in Taiwan from 1996 to 1999. *J. Clin. Microbiol.* **38:**4621–4625.

16. **Colwell, R. R., J. A. K. Hasan, A. Huq, L. Loomis, R. J. Siebeling, M. Torres, S. Galvez, S. Islam, M. Tamplin, and D. Bernstein.** 1992. Development and evaluation of a rapid, simple, sensitive monoclonal antibody-based coagglutination test for direct detection of *Vibrio cholerae* O1. *FEMS Immunol. Med. Microbiol.* **8:**293–298.

17. **Dalsgaard, A., A. Alarcon, C. F. Lanata, T. Jensen, H. J. Hansen, F. Delgado, A. I. Gil, M. E. Penny, and D. Taylor.** 1996. Clinical manifestations and molecular epidemiology of five cases of diarrhoea in children associated with *Vibrio metschnikovii* in Arequipa, Peru. *J. Med. Microbiol.* **45:**494–500.

18. **Dalsgaard, A., M. J. Albert, D. N. Taylor, T. Shimada, R. Meza, O. Serichantalergs, and P. Echeverria.** 1995. Characterization of *Vibrio cholerae* non-O1 serogroups obtained from an outbreak of diarrhea in Lima, Peru. *J. Clin. Microbiol.* **33:**2715–2722.

19. **Dalsgaard, A., P. Glerup, L. L. Hoybye, A. M. Paarup, R. Meza, M. Bernal, T. Shimada, and D. N. Taylor.** 1997. *Vibrio furnissii* isolated from humans in Peru: a possible human pathogen? *Epidemiol. Infect.* **119:**143–149.

20. **Daniels, N. A., M. C. Evans, and P. M. Griffin.** 2000. Noncholera vibrios, p. 137–147. *In* W. M. Scheld, W. A. Craig, and J. M. Hughes (ed.), *Emerging Infections 4.* ASM Press, Washington, D.C.

21. **Davis, B. R., G. R. Fanning, J. M. Madden, A. G. Steigerwalt, H. B. Bradford, Jr., H. L. Smith, Jr., and D. J. Brenner.** 1981. Characterization of biochemically atypical *Vibrio cholerae* strains and designation of a new pathogenic species, *Vibrio mimicus. J. Clin. Microbiol.* **14:**631–639.

22. **Farmer, J. J., III, and F. W. Hickman-Brenner.** 1992. *Vibrio* and *Photobacterium*, p. 2952–3011. *In* A. Balows, H. G. Trüper, M. Dworkin, W. Harder, and K. H. Schleifer (ed.), *The Prokaryotes*, 2nd ed. Springer-Verlag, Berlin, Germany.

23. **Farmer, J. J., III, J. M. Janda, F. W. Hickman-Brenner, D. N. Cameron, and K. M. Birkhead.** Genus *Vibrio. In* G. M. Garrity (ed.), *Bergey's Manual of Systematic Bacteriology*, 2nd ed., in press. Springer-Verlag, New York, N.Y.

24. **Feldhusen, F.** 2000. The role of seafood in bacterial food-borne diseases. *Microbes Infect.* **2:**1651–1660.

25. **Fraser, S. L., B. K. Purcell, B. Delgado, Jr., A. E. Baker, and A. C. Whelen.** 1997. Rapidly fatal infection due to *Photobacterium (Vibrio) damsela. Clin. Infect. Dis.* **25:**935–936.

26. **Greenlees, K. J., J. Machado, T. Bell, and S. F. Sundlof.** 1998. Food borne microbial pathogens of cultured aquatic species. *Vet. Clin. N. Am. Food Anim. Pract.* **14:**101–112.

27. **Grimes, D. J., J. Stemmler, H. Hada, E. B. May, D. Maneval, F. M. Hetrick, R. T. Jones, M. Stoskopf, and R. R. Colwell.** 1984. *Vibrio* species associated with mortality of sharks held in captivity. *Microb. Ecol.* **10:**271–282.

28. **Hardardittir, H., K. Vikenes, A. Digranes, J. Lassen, and A. Halstensen.** 1994. Mixed bacteremia with *Vibrio metschnikovii* in an 83-year-old female patient. *Scand. J. Infect. Dis.* **26:**493–494.

29. **Hasan, J. A. K., A. Huq, G. B. Nair, S. Garg, A. K. Mukhopadhyay, L. Loomis, D. Bernstein, and R. R. Colwell.** 1995. Development and testing of monoclonal antibody-based rapid immunodiagnostic kits for direct detection of *V. cholerae* O139 synonym Bengal. *J. Clin. Microbiol.* **33:**2935–2939.

30. **Hickman-Brenner, F. W., J. J. Farmer III, D. G. Hollis, G. R. Fanning, A. G. Steigerwalt, R. E. Weaver, and D. J. Brenner.** 1982. Identification of *Vibrio hollisae* sp. nov. from patients with diarrhea. *J. Clin. Microbiol.* **15:**395–401.

31. **Hlady, W. G., and K. C. Klontz.** 1996. The epidemiology of *Vibrio* infections in Florida, 1981–1993. *J. Infect. Dis.* **173:**1176–1183.

32. **Honda, T., M. Arita, T. Takeda, M. Yoh, and T. Miwatani.** 1985. Non-O1 *Vibrio cholerae* produces two newly identified toxins related to *Vibrio parahaemolyticus* hemolysin and *Escherichia coli* heat-stable enterotoxin. *Lancet* **ii:**163–164.

33. **Huq, M. I., A. K. M. J. Alam, D. J. Brenner, and G. K. Morris.** 1980. Isolation of *Vibrio*-like group, EF-6, from patients with diarrhea. *J. Clin. Microbiol.* **11:**621–624.

34. **Janda, J. M.** 1998. *Vibrio*, *Aeromonas* and *Plesiomonas*, p. 1065–1089. *In* L. Collier (ed.), *Topley & Wilson's Microbiology & Microbial Infections*, 9th ed. Oxford University Press, New York, N.Y.

35. **Jean-Jacques, W., K. R. Rajashekaraiah, J. J. Farmer III, F. W. Hickman, J. G. Morris, and C. A. Kallick.** 1981. *Vibrio metschnikovii* bacteremia in a patient with cholecystitis. *J. Clin. Microbiol.* **14:**711–712.

36. **Jesudason, M. V., C. P. Thangavelu, and M. K. Lalitha.** 1984. Rapid screening of fecal samples for *Vibrio cholerae* by a coagglutination technique. *J. Clin. Microbiol.* **19:**712–713.

37. **Kaper, J. B., J. G. Morris, Jr., and M. M. Levine.** 1995. Cholera. *Clin. Microbiol. Rev.* **8:**48–86.

38. **Lee, J. V., T. J. Donovan, and A. L. Furniss.** 1978. Characterization, taxonomy, and emended description of *Vibrio metschnikovii. Int. J. Syst. Bacteriol.* **28:**99–111.

39. **Lee, J. V., P. Shread, L. Furniss, and T. N. Bryant.** 1981. Taxonomy and description of *Vibrio fluvialis* sp. nov. (synonym group F vibrios, group EF-6). *J. Appl. Bacteriol.* **50:**73–94.

40. **Lehane, L., and G. T. Rawlin.** 2000. Topically acquired bacterial zoonoses from fish: a review. *Med. J. Aust.* **173:**256–259.

41. **Lipp, E. K., and J. B. Rose.** 1997. The role of seafood in foodborne diseases in the United States of America. *Rev. Sci. Tech.* **16:**620–640.

42. **Losonsky, G. A., and M. M. Levine.** 1997. Immunologic methods for diagnosis of infections caused by diarrhea-

genic members of the families *Enterobacteriaceae* and *Vibrionaceae*, p. 484–497. *In* N. R. Rose, E. C. de Macario, J. D. Folds, H. C. Lane, and R. M. Nakamura (ed.), *Manual of Clinical Laboratory Immunology*, 5th ed. ASM Press, Washington, D.C.

43. **Love, M. D., D. Teebken-Fisher, J. E. Hose, J. J. Farmer III, F. W. Hickman-Brenner, and G. R. Fanning.** 1981. *Vibrio damsela*, a marine bacterium, causes skin ulcers on the damselfish *Chromis punctipinnis*. *Science* **214:**1139–1140.

44. **Marano, N. N., N. A. Daniels, A. N. Easton, A. Mc-Shan, B. Ray, J. G. Wells, P. M. Griffin, and F. J. Angulo.** 2000. A survey of stool culturing practices for *Vibrio* species at clinical laboratories in Gulf Coast states. *J. Clin. Microbiol.* **38:**2267–2270.

45. **Morris, J. G., Jr.** 1994. Non-O group 1 *Vibrio cholerae* strains not associated with epidemic disease, p. 103–115. *In* I. K. Wachsmuth, P. A. Blake, and O. Olsvik (ed.), Vibrio cholerae *and Cholera: Molecular to Global Perspectives.* ASM Press, Washington, D.C.

46. **Morris, J. G., Jr., R. Wilson, D. G. Hollis, R. E. Weaver, H. G. Miller, C. O. Tacket, F. W. Hickman, and P. A. Blake.** 1982. Illness caused by *Vibrio damsela* and *Vibrio hollisae*. *Lancet* **i:**1294–1297.

47. **National Committee for Clinical Laboratory Standards.** 1998. *Performance Standards for Antimicrobial Susceptibility Testing.* Eighth informational supplement. NCCLS document M100-S8. National Committee for Clinical Laboratory Standards, Wayne, Pa.

48. **Nishibuchi, M., J. M. Janda, and T. Ezaki.** 1996. The thermostable direct hemolysin gene (*tdh*) of *Vibrio hollisae* is dissimilar in prevalence to and phylogenetically distant from the *tdh* genes of other vibrios: implications in the horizontal transfer of the *tdh* gene. *Microbiol. Immunol.* **40:**59–65.

49. **Okuda, J., M. Ishibashi, E. Hayakawa, T. Nishino, Y. Takeda, A. K. Mukhopadhyay, S. Garg, S. K. Bhatta-charya, G. B. Nair, and M. Nishibuchi.** 1997. Emergence of a unique O3:K6 clone of *Vibrio parahaemolyticus* in Calcutta, India, and isolation of strains from the same clonal group from Southeast Asian travelers arriving in Japan. *J. Clin. Microbiol.* **35:**3150–3155.

50. **Pavia, A. T., J. A. Bryan, K. L. Maher, T. R. Hester, Jr., and J. J. Farmer III.** 1989. *Vibrio carchariae* infection after a shark bite. *Ann. Intern. Med.* **111:**85–86.

51. **Pedersen, K., L. Verdonck, B. Austin, D. A. Austin, A. R. Blanch, P. A. D. Grimont, J. Jofre, S. Koblavi, J. L. Larsen, T. Tiainen, M. Vigneulle, and J. Swings.** 1998. Taxonomic evidence that *Vibrio carchariae* Grimes *et al.* 1985 is a junior synonym of *Vibrio harveyi* (Johnson and Shunk 1936) Baumann *et al.* 1981. *Int. J. Syst. Bacteriol.* **48:**749–758.

52. **Pollitzer, R.** 1959. *Cholera.* World Health Organization, Geneva, Switzerland.

53. **Shimada, T., E. Arakawa, K. Itoh, T. Okitsu, A. Matsushima, Y. Asai, S. Yamai, T. Nakazato, G. B. Nair, M. J. Albert, and Y. Takeda.** 1994. Extended serotyping scheme for *Vibrio cholerae*. *Curr. Microbiol.* **28:**175–178.

54. **Shimada, T., Y. Kosako, K. Inoue, M. Ohtomo, S. Matsushita, S. Yamada, and Y. Kudoh.** 1991. *Vibrio fluvialis* and *Vibrio furnissii* serotyping scheme for international use. *Curr. Microbiol.* **22:**335–337.

55. **Shimada, T., and R. Sakazaki.** 1984. On the serology of *Vibrio vulnificus*. *Jpn. J. Med. Sci. Biol.* **37:**241–246.

56. **Shin, J. H., M. G. Shin, S. P. Suh, D. W. Ryang, J. S. Rew, and F. S. Nolte.** 1996. Primary *Vibrio damsela* septicemia. *Clin. Infect. Dis.* **22:**856–857.

57. **Wachsmuth, I. K., P. A. Blake, and O. Olsvik (ed.).** 1994. Vibrio cholerae *and Cholera: Molecular to Global Perspectives.* ASM Press, Washington, D.C.

58. **Weintraub, A., G. Widmalm, P.-E. Jansson, M. Jansson, K. Hultenby, and M. J. Albert.** 1994. *Vibrio cholerae* O139 Bengal possesses a capsular polysaccharide which confers increased virulence. *Microb. Pathol.* **16:**235–241.

Pseudomonas

DEANNA L. KISKA AND PETER H. GILLIGAN

47

TAXONOMY

The original classification of the genus *Pseudomonas* into five rRNA homology groups (73) has undergone extensive revision, resulting in the reclassification of many *Pseudomonas* species into separate genera. These genera include *Burkholderia, Stenotrophomonas, Comamonas, Shewanella, Ralstonia, Methylobacterium, Sphingomonas, Acidovorax,* and *Brevundimonas* (47). The genus *Pseudomonas* (sensu stricto) comprises rRNA homology group 1 and includes the type species, *Pseudomonas aeruginosa,* as well as the species listed in Table 1. Many species of "pseudomonads" remain in the genus, although recent phylogenetic studies based on 16S rRNA sequences warrant their transfer to new or existing genera (3, 47). A revised description of the genus *Pseudomonas* (sensu stricto) is anticipated in the near future and would limit the species to those corresponding to rRNA homology group I (3). The genus *Pseudomonas* can be distinguished from related genera on the basis of cellular fatty acid composition. Characteristic fatty acids include $C_{16:0}$, $C_{16:1cis9}$, and $C_{18:1cis11}$ (92). Also, members of *Pseudomonas* (sensu stricto) can be identified by the presence of the outer membrane lipoprotein I (*oprI*) gene as detected by PCR and/or Southern blot analysis (22, 88).

P. *stutzeri*, P. *putida*, and P. *fluorescens* demonstrate considerable heterogeneity at the intraspecies level. P. *stutzeri* can be divided into eight genomovars based on 16S rRNA gene sequence analysis and DNA hybridization studies (85, 86). Genomovar 6 is sufficiently different from the type strain that it has been given species status as P. *balearica* (8). Phylogenetic analyses utilizing internally transcribed spacer sequences have demonstrated that genomovar 7 forms a distinct phylogenetic branch and should receive a new species designation (36). This is consistent with previous studies of phenotypic (85) and genotypic (8) characteristics.

Five biovars of P. *fluorescens* (I to V) and two biovars of P. *putida* (A and B) are recognized in *Bergey's Manual,* 9th ed. (41). Two additional biovars of these species have been reported, P. *fluorescens* biovar VI and P. *putida* biovar C (6). Sequence analysis of the DNA gyrase B subunit gene (*gyrB*) and 16S rRNA restriction fragment length polymorphism (RFLP) analysis have demonstrated a close relationship between P. *putida* biovar B and P. *fluorescens* biovar VI (54, 99). This is consistent with the similar phenotypic charac-

teristics exhibited by these two strains. Reclassification of P. *putida* biovar B strains is likely, based on these findings (99). P. *putida* biovar C does not show a close relationship to any *Pseudomonas* (sensu stricto) species by 16S rRNA RFLP analysis and so may represent a new genus (54).

Two new species of *Pseudomonas* have been recovered from clinical specimens, P. *veronii* and P. *monteilii*. P. *veronii* is most closely related to P. *fluorescens* biovars II and V and P. *monteilii* is most closely related to P. *putida* biovar A by DNA hybridization studies (24, 25).

GENERAL DESCRIPTION

Pseudomonas spp. are aerobic, non-spore-forming, gram-negative rods which are straight or slightly curved (41). They are 1.5 to 5 μm in length and 0.5 to 1.0 μm in width and possess a strictly respiratory metabolism with oxygen as the terminal electron acceptor. Some isolates can grow under anaerobic conditions by using nitrate or arginine as terminal electron acceptors. *Pseudomonas* spp. are motile due to the presence of one or more polar flagella. Clinical isolates are oxidase positive (with the exception of P. *luteola* and P. *oryzihabitans*) and catalase positive and grow on MacConkey agar, appearing as lactose nonfermenters. Most species degrade glucose oxidatively and convert nitrate to either nitrite or nitrogen gas. Certain species have distinctive colony morphologies or pigmentation, as described below. They are nutritionally quite versatile, with different species being able to utilize a variety of simple and complex carbohydrates, alcohols, and amino acids as carbon sources. Certain species can multiply at 4°C, but most are mesophilic, with optimal growth temperatures between 30 and 37°C.

NATURAL HABITATS

Pseudomonas spp. have a worldwide distribution with a predilection for moist environments (41). They are found in water and soil and on plants, including fruits and vegetables. Some *Pseudomonas* species are well recognized as phytopathogens, and many species were first described in that context. Because of their ability to survive in aqueous environments, these organisms, particularly P. *aeruginosa,* have become problematic in the hospital environment. P. *aeruginosa* has been found in a variety of aqueous solutions

719

TABLE 1 Characteristics of *Pseudomonas* spp. found in clinical specimens[a]

Test	P. aeruginosa (n = 201)	P. fluorescens (n = 155)	P. putida (n = 16)	P. veronii (n = 8)	P. monteilii (n = 10)	P. stutzeri (n = 28)	P. mendocina (n = 4)	P. pseudoalcaligenes (n = 34)	P. alcaligenes (n = 26)	P. luteola (n = 34)	P. oryzihabitans (n = 36)
Oxidase	99	97	100	100	100	100	100	100	96	0	0
Growth:											
MacConkey	100	100	100	ND[d]	ND	100	100	100	96	100	100
Cetrimide	94	89	81 (6)	ND	90	4	75 (25)	56 (18)	15	0	25 (28)
6.0% NaCl	65	43	100	ND	0	80 (16)	100	62 (6)	41	74	62
42°C	100	0	0	0	0	69	100	94	0	94	33
Nitrate reduction	98	19	0	100	0	100	100	100	54	62	6
Gas from nitrate	93	3	0	100	0	100	100	0	0	0	0
Pyoverdin	65	96	93	100	100	0	0	0	0	0	0
Arginine dihydrolase	100	97	100	100	100	0[e]	100	78	12	100	14
Lysine decarboxylase	0	0	0	ND	0	0	0	0	0	0	7
Ornithine decarboxylase	0	0	0	ND	0	0	0	0	0	0	3
Indole	0	0	0	ND	0	0	0	0	0	0	0
Litmus milk[b]	89 pep	95 pep	62 k	ND	ND	57 k	25 (75) k	38 k	46 k	44 k	57 k
Hydrolysis:											
Urea	48 (9)	21 (31)	31 (44)	25	50	33 (22)	50	3 (6)	0	26 (38)	77
Gelatin[f]	82	100	0	13	0	0	0	0	0	61	17
Acetamide	100	6 (12)	0	0	0	0	0	ND	ND	ND	ND
Esculin	0	0	0	ND	0	0	0	0	0	100	0
Starch	0	0	0	ND	0	100	0	0	0	0	0
Acid from[c]:											
Glucose	97	100	100	100	100	96 (4)	100	9	0	100	100
Fructose	ND	ND	ND	100	100	ND	ND	79 (21)	0	ND	ND
Xylose	90	100	100	100	0	93 (7)	75 (25)	18 (12)	0	100	100
Lactose	<1	24	25 (13)	ND	0	0	0	0	0	3 (24)	14 (22)
Sucrose	0	48	0	100	0	0	0	0	0	12	25
Maltose	<1	2	31	ND	0	100	0	0	0	100	97
Mannitol	70	53	25	100	0	89 (4)	0	0	0	76 (18)	100
Simmons citrate	95	93	94 (6)	ND	100	82 (14)	100	26 (9)	57 (8)	100	97
No. of flagella	1	>1	>1	1	ND	1	1	1	1	>1	1

[a] Results are given as percentage of positive strains; percentages in parentheses represent strains with delayed reactions. Data are from references 24, 25, 41, and 98.
[b] Type of reaction on litmus milk; pep, peptonization; k, alkaline.
[c] Oxidative-fermentative basal medium with 1% carbohydrate.
[d] ND, no data.
[e] *P. stutzeri*-like organisms (formerly CDC group 3b) are arginine dihydrolase positive.
[f] Results are for a 7-day incubation.

including disinfectants, ointments, soaps, irrigation fluids, eye drops, and dialysis fluids and equipment (69). *P. aeruginosa* is frequently found in the aerators and traps of sinks; in baby, whirlpool, and hydrotherapy baths; in respiratory therapy equipment; and on showerheads. It is also found on the surface of many types of raw fruits and vegetables; therefore, profoundly immunosuppressed individuals should not consume these foods because subsequent gastrointestinal colonization by *P. aeruginosa* may lead to bacteremia. In addition to its nosocomial sources, *P. aeruginosa* may be found in swimming pools, hot tubs, contact lens solutions, cosmetics, artificial fingernails, illicit injectable drugs, and the inner soles of sneakers (12, 26, 27, 40, 52, 75). All have been sources of infection.

P. aeruginosa is found infrequently as part of the microbial flora of healthy individuals. In these persons, the gastrointestinal tract is the most frequent site of colonization but other moist body sites may become colonized, including the throat, nasal mucosa, and moist skin surfaces such as the axillae and perineum. Rates of colonization increase in hospitalized patients, particularly in those who have been hospitalized for extended periods and/or have received broad-spectrum antimicrobial therapy or chemotherapy. The colonization sites in these patients are similar to those in healthy persons but also include the lower respiratory tract, especially in intubated patients (65, 75).

The distribution of other *Pseudomonas* spp. in the environment is similar to that of *P. aeruginosa*. Contamination of aqueous solutions such as distilled water, soaps, disinfectants, and injectable medicines with these organisms has led to pseudoinfections, most commonly pseudobacteremia, as well as true bacteremia and other infections (16, 48, 57, 91). *P. veronii* was first recovered from mineral water springs (25).

P. pseudoalcaligenes has a highly unusual habitat. It has been found in concentrations of $>10^8$ organisms/ml in metalworking fluid, a mixture of water and petroleum products. Metalworkers are exposed to aerosols containing 10^5 organisms/m^3 with no apparent ill effects (64).

CLINICAL SIGNIFICANCE

P. aeruginosa

P. aeruginosa is the most important human pathogen in the genus *Pseudomonas* with respect both to the numbers and types of infections caused and to their associated morbidity and mortality (75). The spectrum of disease caused by this agent ranges from superficial skin infections to fulminant sepsis.

Probably the most superficial infection associated with this organism is folliculitis, acquired in swimming pools, water slides, whirlpools, and hot tubs or by using contaminated sponges (12, 60). Superficial infections of the ear canal due to *P. aeruginosa* frequently develop in those involved in aquatic sports, such as competitive swimmers. This condition is aptly named "swimmer's ear." It should not be confused with a much more severe ear infection called malignant otitis externa. In this infection, seen primarily in diabetics and the elderly, *P. aeruginosa* can invade the underlying tissues, damaging cranial nerves and causing a temporal bone and basilar skull osteomyelitis. Meningitis may result (87). Successful treatment of this infection requires surgical debridement and antimicrobial therapy.

P. aeruginosa infection of the eyes usually follows minor trauma to the cornea. These infections are frequently asso-

ciated with contact lens use. Contaminated contact lens solution and the use of tap water during lens care have been implicated as sources of infection (40). *P. aeruginosa* infection of the eye can cause corneal ulcers, which may progress to loss of ocular function if not promptly treated.

P. aeruginosa is a common cause of osteomyelitis of the calcaneus in children. A puncture wound, usually caused by a nail penetrating a sneaker, occurs within the month preceding the development of this infection. The inner pad of the sneaker is the source of *P. aeruginosa* (26).

P. aeruginosa is a cause of community-acquired pneumonia (CAP) in a small number of patients. These individuals tend to be middle-aged, frequently have a history of smoking, and have been exposed to aerosolized water from sources such as home whirlpools or humidifying devices. Because this is an unusual cause of CAP, patients rarely receive appropriate empiric antimicrobial therapy and mortality is quite high (33%). Because 92% of the patients reported in the literature were bacteremic, it is likely that only the most severely ill are described and that mortality with *P. aeruginosa* CAP is actually lower (37).

Bacteremia and septic shock due to *P. aeruginosa* continue to be major problems in hospitalized patients with underlying malignancies, cardiopulmonary disease, renal failure, or diabetes (11). In cancer patients, it is responsible for between 5 and 31% of culture-proven cases of bacteremia (63). Mortality due to *P. aeruginosa* bacteremia in that patient population varies widely, from as low as 5% to as high as 50% in patients with polymicrobial bacteremia (63). In a recent study of patients who have received bone marrow transplants for a variety of malignancies or immunodeficiency disorders, *P. aeruginosa* was responsible for only 3% of bacteremic episodes but the mortality in this patient population was 40% (18). In two different surveys of North American hospitals, it was the third most common gram-negative bacillus recovered from blood (23, 96) after *Escherichia coli* and *Klebsiella pneumoniae*. Bacteremia due to *P. aeruginosa* in intravenous drug users is usually associated with bacterial endocarditis, a result of injecting contaminated drugs. Replacement of the infected valve is usually necessary (52). These individuals may also develop osteomyelitis of a variety of bones.

P. aeruginosa is the leading cause of nosocomial respiratory tract infection. Patients receiving ventilatory assistance have a 20-fold-higher likelihood of developing nosocomial pneumonia, with *P. aeruginosa* being the most frequently identified etiologic agent. In this patient population, mortality is 40 to 50% (65, 75). *P. aeruginosa* also causes nosocomial urinary tract infections, wound infections, and peritonitis in patients on chronic ambulatory peritoneal dialysis (2, 9). Wound infections due to *P. aeruginosa* are particularly troublesome in burn patients. Although the incidence of such infections has declined in these patients, the high rate of sepsis following these wound infections is responsible for significant mortality rates (70).

An unusual "mucoid" phenotype of *P. aeruginosa* chronically infects approximately 70 to 80% of adolescents and adults with cystic fibrosis (CF) (31). Once infected, CF patients rarely, if ever, clear this organism. Overproduction of alginate, a polysaccharide polymer, is responsible for the wet, "mucoid" appearance typical of colonies of the mucoid phenotype. The events which surround the establishment of the mucoid phenotype in the lungs of CF patients are not well understood despite being the focus of intense study (34). It is speculated that following infection with a nonmucoid isolate, emergence of the mucoid phenotype is due to random mutation in the gene cluster that controls alginate synthesis. Growth of mucoid *P. aeruginosa* as "microcolonies," which are small clusters of organisms surrounded by large amounts of alginate, is central to the development of chronic infection in the airway of CF patients (19). This form of growth is believed to inhibit phagocytosis, increase antibiotic resistance, and induce a significant immune response in the lungs of CF patients via the action of neutrophil-derived elastase. High levels of elastase damage the lungs and have a cumulative, deleterious effect on pulmonary function over a period of years or even decades, eventually resulting in death (34). Bacteremia is rare, probably due to the high level of circulating antibodies to various *P. aeruginosa* virulence factors in these patients (51). Mucoid *P. aeruginosa* occasionally is seen causing pulmonary infections in individuals with other chronic lung diseases or urinary tract infections secondary to indwelling catheters (66, 78).

Other *Pseudomonas* Species

Pseudomonas species other than *P. aeruginosa* infrequently cause infection. Because of their low virulence, infections due to these species are often iatrogenic and are associated with the administration of contaminated solutions, medicines, and blood products or the presence of indwelling catheters (33, 57, 59, 61, 79, 90).

P. fluorescens and *P. putida* have the ability to grow at 4°C, and *P. fluorescens* can be isolated from the skin of a small proportion of blood donors (90), resulting in occasional transfusion-associated septicemia in the recipient. *P. putida* and *P. fluorescens* have been reported as agents of catheter-related bacteremia in cancer patients (1, 42). Both *P. fluorescens* and *P. stutzeri* have been implicated in outbreaks of pseudobacteremia (48, 91).

P. stutzeri is an unusual cause of human infection. It has been reported to cause bacteremia in immunosuppressed persons (76), meningitis in a human immunodeficiency virus-infected individual (84), pneumonia in alcoholics (16), and osteomyelitis (81). Iatrogenic infections due to *P. stutzeri* include endophthalmitis following cataract surgery (45) and bacteremia in hemodialysis patients as a result of contaminated dialysis fluid (33). *P. stutzeri* has also been recovered from wounds, the respiratory tract of intubated patients, and the urinary tract, although its pathogenic role in those settings is unclear (71).

P. oryzihabitans increasingly is being recognized as a cause of bacteremia in immunocompromised patients with central venous access devices. As with *P. aeruginosa*, synthetic bath sponges can be a source of bacteremia with this organism in patients with Hickman catheters (61). Because of the organism's low virulence, patients bacteremic with this organism can be successfully treated with parenteral antimicrobials and do not require removal of their foreign bodies (59). This organism has also been reported to cause peritonitis in patients undergoing chronic ambulatory peritoneal dialysis. Cellulitis, abscesses, wound infections, and meningitis following neurosurgical procedures have also been reported (57).

P. luteola is a rare cause of infections in humans. There have been case reports of a variety of different infections including cellulitis, osteomyelitis, peritonitis, endocarditis, and meningitis in patient following a neurosurgical procedure. Bacteremia is the most frequently reported infection with this organism (79, 80).

Other *Pseudomonas* species are found even less frequently in human infection. *P. alcaligenes* was the cause of

catheter-related endocarditis in a bone marrow transplant recipient (62). *P. mendocina* has been isolated from two cases of endocarditis (5, 46). *P. veronii* has been reported to be associated with an intestinal inflammatory pseudotumor (17). *P. monteilii* has been isolated from stool, bile, placenta, bronchial aspirates, pleural fluid, and urine, but its clinical significance is unknown (24).

COLLECTION, TRANSPORT, AND STORAGE

Pseudomonas spp. can survive in a variety of hostile environments and at temperatures found in clinical settings. Therefore, standard collection, transport, and storage techniques as outlined in chapters 6 and 20 are sufficient to ensure recovery of these organisms from clinical specimens.

DIRECT EXAMINATION

Pseudomonas spp. have similar Gram stain morphologies and are not easily distinguished from other glucose-nonfermenting gram-negative bacilli. Mucoid *P. aeruginosa* can be seen as microcolonies in the sputum of CF patients, appearing as clusters of thin gram-negative rods surrounded by more darkly staining amorphous gram-negative material. Several PCR amplification methods have been described for the direct detection of *P. aeruginosa* in clinical specimens, particularly from CF patients. Although PCR, in some cases, was demonstrated to be more sensitive than culture, the clinical relevance of this finding requires further investigation (20, 21, 93). A fluorescent in situ hybridization method has been described for the direct detection of *P. aeruginosa* and other common pathogens in CF patients (39). The sensitivity of fluorescent in situ hybridization was lower than that of culture but it provided a rapid (4-h), specific diagnosis of the pathogen(s) present in respiratory samples. Because of the rapid growth and ease of identification of *P. aeruginosa* and the need to perform susceptibility testing on clinically significant isolates, molecular methods for detecting *P. aeruginosa* currently have little practical value. Serologic diagnosis of pseudomonad infections is not used in clinical settings.

CULTURE AND ISOLATION

Pseudomonas spp. grow well on standard laboratory media such as tryptic soy agar with 5% sheep blood or chocolate agar. Such media can be used to recover the organisms from clinical specimens, such as cerebrospinal fluid, joint fluid, or peritoneal dialysis fluid, where a mixed flora is not anticipated. All members of the genus *Pseudomonas* grow in broth blood culture systems, and so special blood culture techniques are not required. Isolation of these organisms from specimens containing a mixed flora is facilitated by the use of selective media. MacConkey agar is a useful selective medium for the isolation of most *Pseudomonas* spp., including mucoid strains of *P. aeruginosa* from CF patients. Selective agents such as cetrimide, acetamide, nitrofurantoin, and 9-chloro-9-[4-(diethylamino)phenyl]-9,10-dihydro-10-phenylacridine hydrochloride (C390) may be used to isolate *P. aeruginosa* from clinical and environmental samples (14, 38, 53, 55).

IDENTIFICATION

Fluorescent Group

P. aeruginosa, P. fluorescens, P. putida, P. veronii, and P. monteilii

Members of the fluorescent pseudomonad group produce pyoverdin, a water-soluble yellow-green or yellow-brown pigment which fluoresces under short-wavelength UV light. Most *P. aeruginosa* isolates are easily recognized on primary isolation media on the basis of characteristic colonial morphology, production of diffusible pigments, and a grape-like or corn taco-like odor. Colonies are usually spreading and flat, and have serrated edges and a metallic sheen which is often associated with autolysis of the colonies (100). Other colonial variants exist, including smooth, coliform, gelatinous, dwarf, and mucoid forms. Mucoid colonial variants are particularly prevalent in respiratory tract specimens from CF patients (31). *P. aeruginosa* produces a number of water-soluble pigments. When pyoverdin combines with the blue, water-soluble, phenazine pigment, pyocyanin, the bright green color characteristic of *P. aeruginosa* is created. This organism may also produce one of two other water-soluble pigments: pyorubrin (red) or pyomelanin (brown to brown-black). *P. aeruginosa* can be confidently identified on the basis of a positive oxidase test, a triple sugar iron agar reaction of alkaline over no change, growth at 42°C, and production of bright blue to blue-green, red, or brown diffusible pigments on Mueller-Hinton or other non-dye-containing agars. Occasional *P. aeruginosa* strains produce only pyoverdin, which would not differentiate them from other fluorescent pseudomonads. The ability of *P. aeruginosa* to grow at 42°C distinguishes it from these other species (Table 1). Nonpigmented *P. aeruginosa* strains may also occur; frequently they are highly mucoid strains recovered from the respiratory secretions of CF patients. In practice, the finding of a highly mucoid, glucose-nonfermenting, gram-negative rod in respiratory specimens from CF patients is sufficient to identify the organism as *P. aeruginosa*. However, when a nonpigmented isolate is recovered in a clinical setting other than this, key biochemical characteristics include growth at 42°C, hydrolysis of acetamide, and reduction of nitrates to nitrogen gas. Additional characteristics include resistance to the combination of C390 and phenanthroline, the presence of the exotoxin A gene (~95% of strains), and the presence of $C_{19:0\ cyc11-12}$ fatty acid (14, 92, 95).

P. fluorescens and *P. putida* do not possess a distinctive colony morphology or odor. Their inability to reduce nitrates to nitrogen gas and their ability to produce acid from xylose distinguish these two species from the other fluorescent pseudomonads. In most clinical settings, there is little need to differentiate between these organisms since they are of low virulence and usually not clinically significant. However, because of the well-known association between *P. fluorescens* and contaminated blood products, accurate identification may be important for isolates from patients who recently received blood products and developed bacteremia. *P. fluorescens* can be differentiated from *P. putida* based on its ability to grow at 4°C and ability to hydrolyze gelatin; *P. putida* can do neither. A significant number of *P. fluorescens* isolates may require 4 to 7 days of incubation for accurate detection of gelatin hydrolysis. According to the package insert for API 20NE (bioMérieux Vitek, Hazelwood, Mo.), only 39% of *P. fluorescens* isolates demonstrate gelatin hydrolysis in the 24- to 48-h incubation time for this system.

P. monteilii can be distinguished from the other members of the fluorescent group by the inability to reduce nitrates to nitrogen gas and inability to produce acid from xylose. *P. veronii* can be distinguished by the ability to reduce nitrates to nitrogen gas and the inability to hydrolyze acetamide or grow at 42°C.

Other fluorescent pseudomonads are rarely encountered in clinical specimens. Many of these isolates are negative for arginine dihydrolase activity. Identification as "*Pseudomonas* species not *aeruginosa*" and susceptibility testing of the isolates, when appropriate, is sufficient in most circumstances. When necessary, these isolates can be referred to reference laboratories, where more extensive biochemical batteries and cell wall fatty acid analysis can be used to establish a definitive identification. PCR amplification of 16S rDNA followed by RFLP analysis has been used to successfully identify and characterize members of the fluorescent pseudomonad group (54).

Nonfluorescent Group

P. stutzeri and *P. mendocina*

Most *P. stutzeri* isolates are easily recognized on primary isolation media by their distinctive dry, wrinkled colony morphology, which is similar to the morphology of *Burkholderia pseudomallei*. *P. stutzeri* can be distinguished from the latter species by its lack of arginine dihydrolase activity and inability to produce acid from lactose. *P. stutzeri* colonies can pit or adhere to the agar and are buff to brown. The adherence can make removal of colonies from agar medium difficult. Because of the difficulty in making suspensions of specific turbidity, commercial susceptibility systems may not work well with this organism. Not all isolates of *P. stutzeri* produce wrinkled colonies; such strains can be distinguished from other pseudomonads by their ability to hydrolyze starch, which is a unique reaction for this species.

P. mendocina colonies are smooth, nonwrinkled, and flat, producing a brownish yellow pigment. Key biochemical characteristics of this species include the ability to reduce nitrates to nitrogen gas, arginine dihydrolase activity, and inability to hydrolyze acetamide or starch.

P. alcaligenes and *P. pseudoalcaligenes*

These organisms are encountered rarely in clinical and environmental samples (62). They do not have a distinctive colony morphology, nor do they produce pigments. Compared to other pseudomonads, they are biochemically inert. Characteristics that distinguish them from other biochemically inert gram-negative rods are a positive oxidase reaction, motility due to a polar flagellum, and growth on MacConkey agar. *P. alcaligenes* is distinguished from *P. pseudoalcaligenes* by its inability to oxidize sugars and lack of growth at 42°C; *P. pseudoalcaligenes* weakly oxidizes fructose. Isolates of these organisms are difficult to identify, and many laboratories, especially those using commercial systems, may appropriately call these isolates "*Pseudomonas* sp. not *aeruginosa*." If the clinical situation dictates a definitive identification, assistance from reference laboratories should be sought.

P. luteola and *P. oryzihabitans*

P. luteola and *P. oryzihabitans* can be distinguished from other pseudomonads by their negative oxidase reaction and production of an intracellular, nondiffusible yellow pigment. Both organisms typically exhibit rough, wrinkled, adherent colonies or, more rarely, smooth colonies. *P. luteola* can be differentiated from *P. oryzihabitans* on the basis of its ability to hydrolyze *o*-nitrophenyl-β-D-galactopyranoside (ONPG) and esculin.

Use of Commercial Systems for Identification of *Pseudomonas* spp.

Many laboratories use commercial systems rather than conventional biochemical tests to identify *Pseudomonas* spp. Commercial systems developed for the identification of glucose-nonfermenting gram-negative rods include the Vitek gram-negative identification (GNI) card and API 20NE (bioMérieux Vitek), N/F and RapID NF Plus (Remel, Inc., Lenexa, Kans.), MicroScan W/A Neg Combo panels (Dade Behring MicroScan, Inc., Deerfield, Ill.), and Crystal E/NF (BD Diagnostic Systems, Sparks, Md.). It may take 4 to 48 h to obtain an identification with these systems depending on whether the system identifies the organism on the basis of preformed enzymes (rapid) or substrate utilization. The accuracy of these commercial systems for identifying pigmented *P. aeruginosa* ranges from 70 to 100% but, on average, is greater than 90% (4, 30, 50, 82, 83). However, the use of an expensive commercial system for identification of *P. aeruginosa* is unwarranted when a few simple tests will suffice. When the commercial systems are challenged with nonpigmented, atypical *P. aeruginosa* strains, many of the systems perform inadequately (49). The most accurate system in this regard appears to be RapID NF Plus, which does not rely on pigment production as a key characteristic for identification (49).

Although the *Pseudomonas* spp. listed in Table 1 are in most of the commercial system databases, published evaluations of these systems often include very few, if any, *Pseudomonas* spp. other than *P. aeruginosa* (30, 82, 83). However, certain statements can be made concerning the value of commercial systems for identifying some *Pseudomonas* spp. RapID NF Plus and API 20NE appear to accurately identify *P. fluorescens* and *P. putida*, although the former system does not distinguish *P. fluorescens* from *P. putida* (4, 50). Differentiating these organisms may be clinically relevant if a patient develops bacteremia with a blood transfusion as a potential source. These systems also appear to perform well with *P. stutzeri* (4, 50). However, if other *Pseudomonas* spp. are encountered or if other commercial systems are used, identification should be confirmed by alternative methods if clinically indicated.

TYPING SYSTEMS

Because of its importance as a cause of nosocomial outbreaks and its role in CF lung disease, there has been great interest in developing typing systems to study the clonal relationship among isolates of *P. aeruginosa*. Conventional typing methods such as serotyping, antibiograms, phage typing, bacteriocin typing, and biotyping are not sufficiently discriminatory to be used for strain typing (43). Molecular methods have replaced these methods and are now the "gold standard" for epidemiologic studies. Ribotyping, pulsed field gel electrophoresis, and a variety of PCR-based techniques have been used to type *P. aeruginosa*. Ribotyping is the least discriminatory of these methods (35, 77). In most circumstances, PCR-based techniques, such as random amplified polymorphic DNA analysis and enterobacterial repetitive intergenic consensus PCR, are suffi-

ciently discriminatory to be useful in studying the molecular epidemiology of *P. aeruginosa* (56, 77). In addition, these techniques are much more rapid and less labor-intensive than pulsed-field gel electrophoresis.

ANTIMICROBIAL SUSCEPTIBILITY

International monitoring of antimicrobial susceptibility in the industrialized world is now available for *P. aeruginosa*. Since monitoring is typically hospital based, data for *P. aeruginosa* are skewed toward isolates causing nosocomial infections. In North America, susceptibility of >75% was typically seen with antipseudomonal penicillins (piperacillin and piperacillin-tazobactam), the aminoglycosides (tobramycin and amikacin), ciprofloxacin, cefepime, ceftazidime, meropenem, and imipenem. Susceptibilities to the monobactam aztreonam and the fluoroquinolone levofloxacin were in the 50 to 80% range. Antimicrobial resistance among *P. aeruginosa* isolates was more pronounced in Latin America and to a lesser degree in Europe, resulting in susceptibility rates as much as 25% lower for all classes of antimicrobials compared to isolates recovered in North America (28). In a European survey, approximately 80% of *P. aeruginosa* isolates were susceptible to gentamicin and tobramycin, with amikacin showing greater activity at 92% (89). The organism is uniformly resistant to antistaphylococcal penicillins, ampicillin, amoxicillin-clavulanic acid, ampicillin-sulbactam, tetracyclines, macrolides, rifampin, chloramphenicol, trimethoprim-sulfamethoxazole, narrow- and extended-spectrum cephalosporins, and oral broad-spectrum cephalosporins (cefixime and cefpodoxime).

Nosocomially acquired *P. aeruginosa* isolates tend to be more resistant to antimicrobials than do community-acquired strains, frequently displaying resistance to multiple classes of antimicrobials. Development of resistance may occur during antimicrobial therapy and is particularly well documented during monotherapy. It has become increasingly clear that resistance development in *P. aeruginosa* is multifactorial, with mutations in genes encoding porins, efflux pumps, penicillin-binding proteins, and chromosomal β-lactamase all contributing to resistance to β-lactams, carbapenems, aminoglycosides, and fluoroquinolones (58, 72, 97). In addition, *P. aeruginosa* strains may contain extended-spectrum β-lactamases as well as metallo-β-lactamases, which can degrade imipenem. Genes encoding these enzymes can be either chromosomal or located on plasmids or integrons (44, 58, 74).

As the numbers of multidrug-resistant *P. aeruginosa* isolates including those resistant to all β-lactams, carbapenems, aminoglycosides, and fluoroquinolones become increasingly larger (28, 58), the search for antimicrobial agents with alternative mechanisms of action has intensified. This has resulted in the revisiting of the use of colistin and polymyxin B, once believed to be too toxic, as therapeutic agents for *P. aeruginosa*. Currently there are no recommended breakpoints for susceptibility testing of either agent. Results of a recent study suggest that disk diffusion testing of colistin and polymyxin B shows relatively poor correlation with MIC determinations and that only MIC testing should be done. Using this method, all *P. aeruginosa* isolates tested were found to be sensitive to ≤2 μg/ml (29). The use of synergistic combinations of drugs may also be considered. It has been shown that both aminoglycosides and fluoroquinolones may be synergistic when tested in combination with β-lactams and/or carbapenems

(72, 97). Synergy testing is best done in research or reference laboratory settings.

Because isolates of *P. aeruginosa* may be susceptible only to imipenem, it is important that susceptibility tests showing false resistance to imipenem be avoided. It is well known that imipenem can be unstable in both frozen and dried susceptibility panels. At least one pseudo-outbreak, originally thought to be due to imipenem-resistant *P. aeruginosa*, has been reported (15). Increases in imipenem MICs with quality control strains should be investigated thoroughly, especially if a concurrent increase in the recovery of imipenem-resistant clinical isolates is seen.

Recent studies (13) of different approaches to susceptibility testing of *P. aeruginosa* isolates recovered from respiratory secretions of CF patients have shown that both disk diffusion and E test (AB BioDisk North America Inc., Piscataway, N.J.) have good correlaton with microbroth dilution MIC determinations and that microbroth MICs have excellent correlation with agar dilution MIC determinations. Currently, there are no data on the accuracy of commercial susceptibility systems for *P. aeruginosa* recovered from CF patients. Another challenging issue when performing susceptibility testing on *P. aeruginosa* isolates from CF patients is the frequent presence of multiple colony morphotypes. Although frequently clonally related (10), these individual morphotypes may have significantly different antibiograms. Testing individual morphotypes is labor-intensive and expensive. Studies done to compare the testing of individual morphotypes with mixtures of those morphotypes have shown that mixed-morphotype testing does not detect resistance as accurately as individual-morphotype testing (67).

In the final stages of chronic CF lung infection, *P. aeruginosa* may be resistant to all available antimicrobials. In these patients, high-dose aerosolized tobramycin may be of value. It should be noted that with this treatment strategy, the achievable tobramycin airway concentration is in the range of 100 to 200 μg/ml (32). Laboratories in institutions caring for large numbers of CF patients should be able to determine whether isolates resistant to tobramycin by standard methods are susceptible at these higher levels. Such testing should be done by MIC determination. It is not known whether the tobramycin E test is accurate at determining susceptibility at this high drug concentration.

INTERPRETATION OF RESULTS

P. aeruginosa is considered a true pathogen when isolated from any sterile site. Recovery of this organism from sites which harbor an indigenous microflora is significant when associated with a typical clinical syndrome, such as folliculitis or otitis externa. Colonization of the upper airways and endotracheal tubes can occur in intubated patients and must be distinguished from true infection in this setting (7) because patients with pneumonia have a high mortality rate and require aggressive antimicrobial therapy. Gram stains of secretions obtained by endotracheal suction which reveal large quantities of gram-negative rods and polymorphonuclear leukocytes support the diagnosis of nosocomial pneumonia (7). The absence of gram-negative rods and the presence of squamous epithelial cells indicate that the specimen is not useful for determining if the patient has pneumonia and should be rejected (68).

The presence of *P. aeruginosa*, especially isolates with a mucoid phenotype, in the respiratory tracts of young children may indicate that the individual has CF. Testing for the presence of sweat chloride should then be initiated. In cultures from patients with cystic fibrosis, the different colonial morphotypes of *P. aeruginosa* (smooth, rough, and mucoid) should be reported. The presence of mucoid colonies suggests chronic infection in these patients.

The recovery of multiple *P. aeruginosa* isolates in a nosocomial setting with the same unusual antibiogram or phenotypic characteristic(s) should alert laboratory/infection control personnel to the possibility of a nosocomial outbreak.

Although other pseudomonads are isolated infrequently from clinical specimens, they have been associated with infections, particularly bacteremia. Recovery of these organisms from blood, sterile fluids, or blood unit bags should be considered significant until proven otherwise. Limited studies have shown that 75% of these isolates are clinically significant (96). Hospital infection control should be notified if an unusual pseudomonad is found in more than one patient, since contaminated hospital equipment or injectables may be involved (9, 79, 90). In these situations, consideration should be given to sending the isolates to a reference laboratory for definitive identification. The clinical significance of these organisms in specimens from contaminated sites is often unclear. Although rare, these organisms may cause wound infections, cellulitis, abscesses, and pneumonia. In these instances, the specimen Gram stain, the predominance of the organism in culture, and the absence of more common pathogens should be used to guide judgment as to whether the organism is significant.

REFERENCES

1. **Anaissie, E., V. Fainstein, P. Miller, K. Hassamali, S. Pitlik, G. P. Bodey, and K. Rolston.** 1987. *Pseudomonas putida:* newly recognized pathogen in patients with cancer. *Am. J. Med.* **82:**1191–1194.
2. **Anonymous.** 1997. National Nosocomial Surveillance (NNIS) report, data summary from October 1986–April 1997, issued May 1997. A report from NNIS System. *Am. J. Infect. Control* **25:**477–487.
3. **Anzai, Y., H. Kim, J.-Y. Park, H. Wakabayashi, and H. Oyaizu.** 2000. Phylogenetic affiliation of the pseudomonads based on 16S rRNA sequence. *Int. J. Syst. Evol. Microbiol.* **50:**1563–1589.
4. **Appelbaum, P. C., and D. J. Leathers.** 1984. Evaluation of the Rapid NFT system for identification of gram-negative, nonfermenting rods. *J. Clin. Microbiol.* **20:**730–734.
5. **Aragone, M. R., D. M. Maurizi, and L. O. Clara.** 1992. *Pseudomonas mendocina,* an environmental bacterium isolated from a patient with human infective endocarditis. *J. Clin. Microbiol.* **30:**1583–1584.
6. **Barrett, E. L., R. E. Solanes, J. S. Tang, and N. J. Palleroni.** 1986. *Pseudomonas fluorescens* biovar V: its resolution into distinct component groups and the relationship of these groups to other *P. fluorescens* biovars, to *P. putida,* and to psychrotropic pseudomonads associated with food spoilage. *J. Gen. Microbiol.* **132:**2709–2721.
7. **Baselski, V.** 1993. Microbiologic diagnosis of ventilator-associated pneumonia. *Infect. Dis. Clin. North Am.* **7:**331–357.
8. **Bennasar, A., R. Rossello-Mora, J. Lalucat, and E. R. B. Moore.** 1996. 16S rRNA gene sequence analysis relative to genomovars of *Pseudomonas stutzeri* and proposal of *Pseudomonas balearica* sp. nov. *Int. J. Syst. Bacteriol.* **46:**200–205.
9. **Bernardini, J., B. Piraino, and M. Sorkin.** 1987. Analysis of continuous ambulatory peritoneal dialysis-related

Pseudomonas aeruginosa infections. *Am. J. Med.* **83:**829–832.

10. **Bingen, E., E. Denamur, B. Picard, P. Goullet, N. Lambert-Zechovsky, P. Foucaud, J. Navarro, and J. Elion.** 1992. Molecular epidemiological analysis of *Pseudomonas aeruginosa* strains causing failure of antibiotic therapy in cystic fibrosis patients. *Eur. J. Clin. Microbiol. Infect. Dis.* **11:**432–437.

11. **Boffi El Amari, E., E. Chamot, R. Auckenthaler, J. C. Pechere, and C. Van Delden.** 2001. Influence of previous exposure to antibiotic therapy on the susceptibility pattern of *Pseudomonas aeruginosa* bacteremic isolates. *Clin. Infect. Dis.* **33:**1859–1864.

12. **Bottone, E. J., and A. A. Perez II.** 1993. *Pseudomonas aeruginosa* folliculitis acquired through use of a contaminated loofah sponge: an unrecognized potential public health problem. *J. Clin. Microbiol.* **31:**480–483.

13. **Burns, J. L., L. Saiman, S. Whittier, D. Larone, J. Krzewinski, Z. Liu, S. A. Marshall, and R. N. Jones.** 2000. Comparison of agar diffusion methodologies for antimicrobial susceptibility testing of *Pseudomonas aeruginosa* isolates from cystic fibrosis patients. *J. Clin. Microbiol.* **38:**1818–1822.

14. **Campbell, M. E., S. W. Farmer, and D. P. Speert.** 1988. New selective medium for *Pseudomonas aeruginosa* with phenanthroline and 9-chloro-9-[4-(diethylamino)phenyl]-9,10-dihydro-10-phenylacridine hydrochloride (C-390). *J. Clin. Microbiol.* **26:**1910–1912.

15. **Carmeli, Y., K. Eichelberger, D. Soja, J. Dakos, L. Venkataraman, P. DeGirolami, and M. Samore.** 1998. Failure of quality control measures to prevent reporting of false resistance to imipenem, resulting in a pseudo-outbreak of imipenem-resistant *Pseudomonas aeruginosa.* *J. Clin. Microbiol.* **36:**595–597.

16. **Carratala, J., A. Salazar, J. Mascaro, and M. Santin.** 1992. Community-acquired pneumonia due to *Pseudomonas stutzeri.* *Clin. Infect. Dis.* **14:**792.

17. **Cheuk, W., P. C. Y. Woo, K. Y. Yuen, P. H. Yu, and J. K. C. Chan.** 2000. Intestinal inflammatory pseudotumour with regional lymph node involvement: identification of a new bacterium as the aetiological agent. *J. Pathol.* **192:**289–292.

18. **Collins, B. A., H. L. Leather, J. R. Wingard, and R. Ramphal.** 2001. Evolution, incidence, and susceptibility of bacterial bloodstream isolates from 519 bone marrow transplant patients. *Clin. Infect. Dis.* **33:**947–953.

19. **Costerton, J. W., P. S. Stewart, and E. P. Greenberg.** 1999. Bacterial biofilms: a common cause of persistent infections. *Science* **284:**1318–1322.

20. **da Silva Filho, L. V., J. E. Levi, C. N. Oda Bento, S. R. da Silva Ramos, and T. Rozov.** 1999. PCR identification of *Pseudomonas aeruginosa* and direct detection in clinical samples from cystic fibrosis patients. *J. Med. Microbiol.* **48:**357–361.

21. **De Vos, D., A. Lim, Jr., J.-P. Pirnay, M. Struelens, C. Vandenvelde, L. Duinslaeger, A. Vanderkelen, and P. Cornelis.** 1997. Direct detection and identification of *Pseudomonas aeruginosa* in clinical samples such as skin biopsy specimens and expectorations by multiplex PCR based on two outer membrane lipoprotein genes, *oprI* and *oprL. J. Clin. Microbiol.* **35:**1295–1299.

22. **De Vos, D., A. Lim, P. De Vos, A. Sarniguet, K. Kersters, and P. Cornelis.** 1993. Detection of the outer membrane lipoprotein I and its gene in flourescent and non-fluorescent pseudomonads: its implication for taxonomy and diagnosis. *J. Gen. Microbiol.* **139:**2215–2223.

23. **Diekema, D. J., M. A. Pfaller, R. N. Jones, G. V. Doern, P. L. Winokur, A. C. Gales, H. S. Sader, K. Kugler, M. Beach, and the SENTRY Participants Group (Ameri-**

cas). 1999. Survey of blood stream infections due to gram-negative bacilli: frequency of occurrence and antimicrobial susceptibility of isolates collected in the United States, Canada, and Latin America for the SENTRY antimicrobial surveillance program, 1997. *Clin. Infect. Dis.* **29:**595–607.

24. **Elomari, M., L. Coroler, S. Verhille, D. Izard, and H. Leclerc.** 1997. *Pseudomonas monteilii* sp. nov. isolated from clinical specimens. *Int. J. Syst. Bacteriol.* **47:**846–852.

25. **Elomari, M., L. Coroler, B. Hoste, M. Gillis, D. Izard, and H. Leclerc.** 1996. DNA relatedness among pseudomonas strains isolated from natural mineral waters and proposal of *Pseudomonas veronii* sp. nov. *Int. J. Syst. Bacteriol.* **46:**1138–1144.

26. **Fisher, M. C., J. F. Goldsmith, and P. H. Gilligan.** 1985. Sneakers as a source of *Pseudomonas aeruginosa* in children with osteomyelitis following puncture wounds. *J. Pediatr.* **106:**607–609.

27. **Foca, M., K. Jacob, S. Whittier, P. D. Latta, S. Factor, D. Rubenstein, and L. Saiman.** 2000. Endemic *Pseudomonas aeruginosa* infection in a neonatal intensive care unit. *N. Engl. J. Med.* **343:**695–700.

28. **Gales, A. C., R. N. Jones, J. Turnidge, R. Rennie, and R. Ramphal.** 2001. Characterization of *Pseudomonas aeruginosa* isolates: occurrence rates, antimicrobial susceptibility patterns, and molecular typing in the global SENTRY Antimicrobial Surveillance Program, 1997–1999. *Clin. Infect. Dis.* **32**(Suppl. 2):S146–S155.

29. **Gales, A. C., A. O. Reis, and R. N. Jones.** 2001. Contemporary assessment of antimicrobial susceptibility testing methods for polymyxin B and colistin: review of available interpretative criteria and quality control guidelines. *J. Clin. Microbiol.* **39:**183–190.

30. **Geiss, H. K., and M. Geiss.** 1992. Evaluation of a new commercial system for the identifcation of Enterobacteriaceae and non-fermentative bacteria. *Eur. J. Clin. Microbiol. Infect. Dis.* **11:**610–616.

31. **Gilligan, P. H.** 1991. Microbiology of airway disease in patients with cystic fibrosis. *Clin. Microbiol. Rev.* **4:**35–51.

32. **Gilligan, P. H.** 1996. Report on the consensus document for microbiology and infectious diseases in cystic fibrosis. *Clin. Microbiol. Newsl.* **18:**83–87.

33. **Goetz, A., V. L. Yu, J. E. Hanchett, and J. D. Rihs.** 1983. *Pseudomonas stutzeri* bacteremia associated with hemodialysis. *Arch. Intern. Med.* **143:**1909–1912.

34. **Govan, J. R. W., and V. Deretic.** 1996. Microbial pathogenesis in cystic fibrosis: mucoid *Pseudomonas aeruginosa* and *Burkholderia cepacia. Microbiol. Rev.* **60:**539–574.

35. **Grundman, H., C. Schneider, D. Hartung, F. D. Daschner, and T. L. Pitt.** 1995. Discriminatory power of three DNA-based typing techniques for *Pseudomonas aeruginosa. J. Clin. Microbiol.* **33:**528–534.

36. **Guasp, C., E. R. B. Moore, J. Lalucat, and A. Bennasar.** 2000. Utility of internally transcribed 16S–23S rDNA spacer regions for the definition of *Pseudomonas stutzeri* genomovars and other *Pseudomonas* species. *Int. J. Syst. Evol. Microbiol.* **50:**1629–1639.

37. **Hatchette, T. F., R. Gupta, and T. J. Marrie.** 2000. *Pseudomonas aeruginosa* community-acquired pneumonia in previously healthy adults: case report and review of literature. *Clin. Infect. Dis.* **31:**1349–1356.

38. **Hedberg, M.** 1969. Acetamide agar medium selective for *Pseudomonas aeruginosa. Appl. Microbiol.* **17:**481.

39. **Hogardt, M., K. Trebesius, A. M. Geiger, M. Hornef, J. Rosenecker, and J. Heesemann.** 2000. Specific and rapid detection by fluorescent in situ hybridization of bacteria in clinical samples obtained from cystic fibrosis patients. *J. Clin. Microbiol.* **38:**818–825.

40. Holland, S. P., J. S. Pulido, T. K. Shires, and J. W. Costerton. 1993. *Pseudomonas aeruginosa* ocular infections, p. 159–176. *In* R. B. Fick, Jr. (ed.), Pseudomonas aeruginosa: *the Opportunist*. CRC Press, Inc., Boca Raton, Fla.

41. Holt, J. G., N. R. Kreig, P. H. A. Sneath, J. T. Staley, and S. T. Williams. 1994. *Bergey's Manual of Systematic Bacteriology*, 9th ed., p. 93–94, 151–168. The Williams & Wilkins Co., Baltimore, Md.

42. Hsueh, P.-R., L.-J. Teng, H.-J. Pan, Y.-C. Chen, C.-C. C. Sun, S.-W. Ho, and K.-T. Luh. 1998. Outbreak of *Pseudomonas fluorescens* bacteremia among oncology patients. *J. Clin. Microbiol.* **36**:2914–2917.

43. International *Pseudomonas aeruginosa* Typing Study Group. 1994. A multicenter comparison of methods for typing strains of *Pseudomonas aeruginosa* predominantly from patients with cystic fibrosis. *J. Infect. Dis.* **169**:134–142.

44. Iyobe, S., H. Kusadokoro, J. Ozaki, N. Matsumura, S. Minami, S. Haruta, T. Sawai, and K. O'Hara. 2000. Amino acid substitutions in a variant of imp-1 metallo-β-lactamase. *Antimicrob. Agents Chemother.* **44**:2023–2027.

45. Jiraskova, N., and P. Rozsival. 1998. Delayed-onset *Pseudomonas stutzeri* endophthalmitis after uncomplicated cataract surgery. *J. Cataract Refract. Surg.* **24**:866–867.

46. Johansen, H. K., K. Kjeldsen, and N. Hoiby. 2001. *Pseudomonas mendocina* as a cause of chronic infective endocarditis in a patient with situs inversus. *Clin. Microbiol. Infect.* **7**:650–652.

47. Kersters, K., W. Ludwig, M. Vancanneyt, P. DeVos, M. Gillis, and K.-H. Schleifer. 1996. Recent changes in the classification of the pseudomonads: an overview. *Syst. Appl. Microbiol.* **19**:465–477.

48. Keys, T. F., L. J. Melton III, M. D. Maker, and D. M. Ilstrup. 1983. A suspected hospital outbreak of pseudobacteremia due to *Pseudomonas stutzeri*. *J. Infect. Dis.* **147**:489–493.

49. Kiska, D. L., A. Kerr, M. C. Jones, J. A. Caracciolo, B. Eskridge, M. Jordan, S. Miller, D. Hughes, N. King, and P. H. Gilligan. 1996. Accuracy of four commercial systems for identification of *Burkholderia cepacia* and other gram-negative nonfermenting bacilli recovered from patients with cystic fibrosis. *J. Clin. Microbiol.* **34**:886–891.

50. Kitch, T. T., M. R. Jacobs, and P. C. Appelbaum. 1992. Evaluation of the 4-hour RapID NF Plus method for identification of 345 gram-negative nonfermentative rods. *J. Clin. Microbiol.* **30**:1267–1270.

51. Klinger, J. D., D. C. Straus, C. B. Hilton, and J. A. Bass. 1978. Antibodies to proteases and exotoxin A of *Pseudomonas aeruginosa* in patients with cystic fibrosis: demonstration by radioimmunoassay. *J. Infect. Dis.* **138**:49–58.

52. Komshian, S. V., O. C. Tablan, W. Palutke, and M. P. Reyes 1990. Characteristics of left-sided endocarditis due to *Pseudomonas aeruginosa* in the Detroit Medical Center. *Rev. Infect. Dis.* **12**:693–702.

53. Krueger, C. L., and W. Sheikh. 1987. A new selective medium for isolating *Pseudomonas* spp. from water. *Appl. Environ. Microbiol.* **53**:895–897.

54. Laguerre, G., L. Rigottier-Gois, and P. Lamanceau. 1994. Fluorescent *Pseudomonas* species categorized by using polymerase chain reaction (PCR)/restriction fragment analysis of 16S rDNA. *Mol. Ecol.* **3**:479–487.

55. Lambre, D. W., and P. Stewart. 1972. Evaluation of Pseudosel agar as an aid in the identification of *Pseudomonas aeruginosa*. *Appl. Microbiol.* **23**:377–381.

56. Lau, Y. J., P. Y. F. Liu, B. S. Hu, J. M. Shyr, Z. Y. Shi, W. S. Tsai, Y. H. Lin, and C. Y. Tseng. 1995. DNA fingerprinting of *Pseudomonas aeruginosa* serotype 011 by enterobacterial repetitive intergenic consensus-polymerase chain reaction and pulsed-field gel electrophoresis. *J. Hosp. Infect.* **31**:61–66.

57. Lin, R.-D., P.-R. Hsueh, J.-C. Chang, L.-J. Teng, S.-C. Chang, S.-W. Ho, W.-C. Hsieh, and K.-T. Luh. 1996. *Flavimonas oryzihabitans* bacteremia: clinical features and microbiological characteristics of isolates. *Clin. Infect. Dis.* **24**:867–873.

58. Livermore, D. M. 2002. Mulitple mechanisms of antimicrobial resistance in *Pseudomonas aeruginosa*: our worst nightmare? *Clin. Infect. Dis.* **34**:634–640.

59. Lucas, K. G., T. E. Kiehn, K. A. Sobeck, D. Armstrong, and A. E. Brown. 1994. Sepsis caused by *Flavimonas oryzihabitans*. *Medicine* **73**:209–214.

60. Maniatis, A. N., C. Karkavitsas, N. A. Maniatis, E. Tsiftsakis, V. Genimata, and N. J. Legakis. 1995. *Pseudomonas aeruginosa* folliculitis due to non-0:11 serogroups: acquisition through use of contaminated synthetic sponges. *Clin. Infect. Dis.* **21**:437–439.

61. Marín, M., M. D. G. de Viedma, P. Martin-Rabadán, M. Rodríguez-Créxmes, and E. Bouza. 2000. Infection of Hickman catheter by *Pseudomonas* (formerly *Flavimonas*) *oryzihabitans* traced to a synthetic bath sponge. *J. Clin. Microbiol.* **38**:4577–4579.

62. Martino, P., A. Micozzi, M. Venditti, G. Gentile, C. Girmenia, R. Raccah, S. Santilli, N. Alessandri, and F. Mandelli. 1990. Catheter-related right-sided endocarditis in bone marrow transplant recipients. *Rev. Infect. Dis.* **12**:250–257.

63. Maschmeyer, G., and I. Braveny. 2000. Review of the incidence of prognosis of *Pseudomonas aeruginosa* infections in cancer patients in the 1990s. *Eur. J. Clin. Microbiol. Infect. Dis.* **19**:915–925.

64. Mattsby-Baltzer, I., L. Edebo, B. Järvholm, B. Lavenius, and T. Soderstrom. 1990. Subclass distribution of IgG and IgA antibody response to *Pseudomonas pseudoalcaligenes* in humans exposed to metal-working fluid. *J. Allergy Clin. Immunol.* **6**:231–238.

65. Mayhall, C. G. 1997. Nosocomial pneumonia: diagnosis and prevention. *Infect. Dis. Clin. North Am.* **11**:427–457.

66. McAvoy, M. J., V. Newton, A. Paull, J. Morgan, P. Gacesa, and N. J. Russell. 1989. Isolation of mucoid *Pseudomonas aeruginosa* from non-CF patients and characterization of the structure of secreted alginate. *J. Med. Microbiol.* **28**:1831–1839.

67. Morlin, G. L., D. L. Hedges, A. L. Smith, and J. L. Burns. 1994. Accuracy and cost of antibiotic susceptibility testing of mixed morphotypes of *Pseudomonas aeruginosa*. *J. Clin. Microbiol.* **32**:1027–1030.

68. Morris, A. J., D. C. Tanner, and L. B. Reller. 1993. Rejection criteria for endotracheal aspirates from adults. *J. Clin. Microbiol.* **31**:1027–1029.

69. Morrison, A. J., Jr., and R. P. Wenzel. 1984. Epidemiology of infections due to *Pseudomonas aeruginosa*. *Rev. Infect. Dis.* **6**(Suppl. 3):S627–S642.

70. Mousa, H. A. 1997. Aerobic, anaerobic and fungal burn wound infections. *J. Hosp. Infect.* **37**:317–323.

71. Noble, R. C., and S. B. Overman. 1994. *Pseudomonas stutzeri* infection. A review of hospital isolates and a review of the literature. *Diagn. Microbiol. Infect. Dis.* **19**:51–56.

72. Pai, H., J.-W. Kim, J. Kim, J. H. Lee, K. W. Choe, and N. Gotoh. 2001. Carbapenem resistance mechanisms in *Pseudomonas aeruginosa* clinical isolates. *Antimicrob. Agents Chemother.* **45**:480–484.

73. Palleroni, N. J., R. Kunisawa, R. Contopoulou, and M. Doudoroff. 1973. Nucleic acid homologies in the genus *Pseudomonas*. *Int. J. Syst. Bacteriol.* **23**:333–339.

74. Philippon, L. N., T. Naas, A.-T. Bouthors, V. Barakett, and P. Nordmann. 1997. OXA-18, a class D clavulanic acid inhibited extended-spectrum β-lactamase from *Pseudomonas aeruginosa*. *Antimicrob. Agents Chemother.* **41**:2188–2195.

75. **Pollack, M.** 2000. *Pseudomonas aeruginosa*, p. 1980–2003. *In* G. L. Mandell, J. E. Bennett, and R. Dolin (ed.), *Principles and Practice of Infectious Diseases*, 5th ed. Churchill Livingstone, Inc., New York, N.Y.

76. **Potvliege, C., J. Jonckheer, C. Lenclud, and W. Hansen.** 1987. *Pseudomonas stutzeri* pneumonia and septicemia in a patient with multiple myeloma. *J. Clin. Microbiol.* **25:**458–459.

77. **Pujana, I., L. Gallego, M. J. Canduela, and R. Cisterna.** 2000. Specific and rapid identification of multiple-antibiotic resistant *Pseudomonas aeruginosa* clones isolated in an intensive care unit. *Diagn. Microbiol. Infect. Dis.* **36:**65–68.

78. **Pujana, I., L. Gallego, G. Martin, F. Lopez, J. Canduela, and R. Cisterna.** 1999. Epidemiological analysis of sequential *Pseudomonas aeruginosa* isolates from chronic bronchiectasis patients without cystic fibrosis. *J. Clin. Microbiol.* **37:**2071–2073.

79. **Rahav, G., A. Simhon, Y. Mattan, A. E. Moses, and T. Sacks.** 1995. Infections with *Chryseomonas luteola* (CDC group Ve-1) and *Flavimonas oryzihabitans* (CDC group Ve-2). *Medicine* **74:**83–88.

80. **Rastogi, S., and S. J. Sperber.** 1998. Facial cellulites and *Pseudomonas luteola* bacteremia in an otherwise healthy patient. *Diagn. Microbiol. Infect. Dis.* **32:**303–305.

81. **Reisler, R. B., and H. Blumberg.** 1999. Community-acquired *Pseudomonas stutzeri* vertebral osteomyelitis in a previously healthy patient: case report and review. *Clin. Infect. Dis.* **29:**667–669.

82. **Rhoads, S., L. Marinelli, C. A. Imperatrice, and I. Nachamkin.** 1995. Comparison of the MicroScan Walkaway system and Vitek system for identification of gram-negative bacteria. *J. Clin. Microbiol.* **33:**3044–3046.

83. **Robinson, A., Y. S. McCarter, and J. Tetreault.** 1995. Comparison of Crystal enteric/nonfermenter system, API 20E system, and Vitek Automicrobic system for identification of gram-negative bacilli. *J. Clin. Microbiol.* **33:**364–370.

84. **Roig, P., A. Orti, and V. Navarro.** 1996. Meningitis due to *Pseudomonas stutzeri* in a patient infected with human immunodeficiency virus. *Clin. Infect. Dis.* **22:**587–588.

85. **Rossello, R., E. Garcia-Valdes, J. Lalucat, and J. Ursing.** 1991. Genotypic and phenotypic diversity of *Pseudomonas stutzeri*. *Syst. Appl. Microbiol.* **14:**150–157.

86. **Rossello-Mora, R. A., J. Lalucat, K. N. Timmis, and E. R. B. Moore.** 1996. Strain JM300 represents a new genomovar within *Pseudomonas stutzeri*. *Syst. Appl. Microbiol.* **19:**596–599.

87. **Rubin, J., and V. L. Yu.** 1990. Malignant external otitis: insights into pathogenesis, clinical manifestations, diagnosis, and therapy. *Am. J. Med.* **85:**391–398.

88. **Saint-Onge, A., F. Romeyer, P. Lebel, L. Masson, and R. Brousseau.** 1992. Specificity of the *Pseudomonas aeruginosa* PAO1 lipoprotein I gene as a DNA probe and PCR target region within the Pseudomonadaceae. *J. Gen. Microbiol.* **138:**733–741.

89. **Schmitz, F.-J., J. Verhoef, A. C. Fluit, and the SENTRY Participants Group.** 1999. Prevalence of aminoglycoside resistance in 20 European university hospitals participating in the European SENTRY antimicrobial surveillance programme. *Eur. J. Clin. Microbiol. Infect. Dis.* **18:**414–421.

90. **Scott, J. F., E. Boulton, J. R. W. Govan, R. S. Miles, D. B. L. McClelland, and C. V. Prowse.** 1988. A fatal transfusion reaction associated with blood contaminated with *Pseudomonas fluorescens*. *Vox Sang.* **54:**201–204.

91. **Simor, A. E., J. Ricci, A. Lau, R. M. Bannatyne, and L. Ford-Jones.** 1985. Pseudobacteremia due to *Pseudomonas fluorescens*. *Pediatr. Infect. Dis.* **4:**508–512.

92. **Stead, D. E.** 1992. Grouping of plant-pathogenic and some other *Pseudomonas* spp. by using cellular fatty acid profiles. *Int. J. Syst. Bacteriol.* **42:**281–295.

93. **van Belkum, A., N. H. M. Renders, S. Smith, S. E. Overbeck, and H. A. Verbrugh.** 2000. Comparison of conventional and molecular methods for the detection of bacterial pathogens in sputum samples from cystic fibrosis patients. *FEMS Immunol. Med. Microbiol.* **27:**51–57.

94. **Vancanneyt, M., U. Torck, D. Dewettinck, M. Vaerewijck, and K. Kersters.** 1996. Grouping of pseudomonads by SDS-PAGE of whole-cell proteins. *Syst. Appl. Microbiol.* **19:**493–500.

95. **Vasil, M. L., C. Chamberlain, and C. C. R. Grant.** 1986. Molecular studies of *Pseudomonas* exotoxin A gene. *Infect. Immun.* **52:**538–548.

96. **Weinstein, M. P., M. L. Towns, S. M. Quartey, S. Mirrett, L. G. Reimer, G. Parmigiani, and B. Reller.** 1997. The clinical significance of positive blood cultures in the 1990s: a prospective comprehensive evaluation of the microbiology, epidemiology, and outcome of bacteremia and fungemia in adults. *Clin. Infect. Dis.* **24:**584–602.

97. **Westbrock-Wadman, S., D. R. Sherman, M. J. Hickey, S. N. Coulter, Y. Q. Zhu, P. Warrener, L. Y. Nguyen, R. M. Shawar, K. R. Folger, and C. K. Stover.** 1999. Characterization of a *Pseudomonas aeruginosa* efflux pump contributing to aminoglycoside impermeability. *Antimicrob. Agents Chemother.* **43:**2975–2983.

98. **Weyant, R. S., C. W. Moss, R. E. Weaver, D. G. Hollis, J. G. Jordan, E. C. Cook, and M. I. Daneshvar.** 1995. *Identification of Unusual Pathogenic Gram-Negative Aerobic and Facultatively Anaerobic Bacteria*, p. 318–319, 340–341, 470–503. The Williams & Wilkins Co., Baltimore, Md.

99. **Yamamoto, S., and S. Harayama.** 1998. Phylogenetic relationships of *Pseudomonas putida* strains deduced from the nucleotide sequences of *gyrB*, *rpoD*, and 16S rRNA genes. *Int. J. Syst. Bacteriol.* **48:**813–819.

100. **Zierdt, C. H.** 1971. Autolytic nature of iridescent lysis in *Pseudomonas aeruginosa*. *Antonie Leeuwenhoek* **37:**319–337.

Burkholderia, Stenotrophomonas, Ralstonia, Brevundimonas, Comamonas, Delftia, Pandoraea, and Acidovorax

PETER H. GILLIGAN, GARY LUM,
PETER A. R. VANDAMME, AND SUSAN WHITTIER

48

TAXONOMY

The genus *Pseudomonas* was described more than 100 years ago, and its classification and description have been revised thoroughly on several occasions (97). In 1973, its taxonomic heterogeneity was revealed by the work of Palleroni et al., who delineated five major species clusters (referred to as rRNA homology groups) among the pseudomonads (130). The phylogenetic distance between each of these rRNA homology groups was more correctly interpreted by the inclusion of representatives of a wide variety of *Proteobacteria* in DNA-rRNA hybridization experiments (57) that led to the gradual dissection of the genus over the following decades (97). The name *Pseudomonas* was confined to rRNA homology group I organisms because they comprised the type species, *Pseudomonas aeruginosa* (see chapter 47).

The nomenclatural rearrangements of the genus *Pseudomonas* entailed the creation of several new genera (Table 1). Some of these encompassed complete rRNA homology groups (e.g., rRNA homology group IV species were reclassified in the genus *Brevundimonas*), whereas others encompassed only partial groups. rRNA group II pseudomonads were reclassified into the genera *Burkholderia* and *Ralstonia* (196, 197). More recently, the novel genus *Pandoraea* was shown to represent a third subgroup in the same phylogenetic lineage (34). The rRNA group II pseudomonads form a remarkable group of primary and opportunistic human, animal, and plant pathogens, as well as environmental species with a considerable potential for biological control, remediation, and plant growth promotion. During the past decade, the interest in several peculiar characteristics of these organisms led to the discovery and description of a multitude of novel species. The genus *Burkholderia* now contains more than 20 validly named species, most of which have been isolated from soil and water samples. Some other novel *Burkholderia*-like species were found to represent a distinct phylogenetic lineage with a position intermediate between that of the genera *Burkholderia* and *Ralstonia* and were classified in the novel genus *Pandoraea* (34).

Although several *Burkholderia* species have been isolated from human clinical samples, only a few, notably *Burkholderia cepacia*, *B. mallei*, and *B. pseudomallei*, are generally recognized as human or animal pathogens. Recent taxonomic studies by 16S rDNA sequence analysis, DNA-DNA hybridization experiments, whole-cell protein and fatty acid analyses, and biochemical characterization revealed that *B. cepacia*-like bacteria belonged to at least nine distinct genomic species (genomovars), referred to collectively as the *B. cepacia* complex (171). *B. cepacia* complex species have a high degree of 16S rDNA sequence similarity (98 to 99%) and moderate levels of whole-genome DNA-DNA hybridization (30 to 50%) (171, 172). Following identification of distinguishing phenotypic characteristics, the names *B. multivorans* and *B. stabilis* have been proposed for genomovars II and IV, respectively (171, 172). Genomovar V was identified as *B. vietnamiensis*, an organism that until recently was isolated primarily from the rice rhizosphere (69). In the absence of differential biochemical tests to separate genomovar III from genomovar I (*B. cepacia*), the former remained unnamed.

Continued international collaborative studies in the context of the International *B. cepacia* Working Group (http://go.to/cepacia) revealed an even more complex picture of the underestimated biodiversity of these bacteria, and recently, three additional *B. cepacia* complex genomovars have been identified. *B. cepacia* genomovar VI (38) could be differentiated biochemically from all *B. cepacia* complex genomovars except *B. multivorans* and therefore remained unnamed. In contrast, *B. cepacia* genomovars VII and VIII could be differentiated from other *B. cepacia* complex bacteria and were formally proposed as *B. ambifaria* (39) and *B. anthina* (170), respectively. In addition, *B. pyrrocinia*, another soil organism, has the same high 16S rDNA sequence similarity and moderate DNA-DNA hybridization levels as *B. cepacia* complex genomovars and should be considered a ninth member of the *B. cepacia* complex (170).

Apart from the *B. cepacia* complex species, *B. mallei*, and *B. pseudomallei*, the genus *Burkholderia* now comprises 15 validly described species; most of these organisms are not associated with human disease and are not discussed further here. Organisms associated with human infections include *B. fungorum*, *B. gladioli* (including strains previously classified as *B. cocovenenans* [36]), and *B. thailandensis* (19, 37, 195).

In the genus *Ralstonia*, the number of species has increased drastically during the past few years. The genus was established in 1995 to accommodate species previously

TABLE 1 Current classification of selected *Pseudomonas* rRNA homology group II to V organisms which have been recovered from humans

Pseudomonas rRNA homology group	Former species designation	Current species designation
II	*Pseudomonas cepacia*	*Burkholderia cepacia* complex
		genomovar I: *B. cepacia*
		genomovar II: *B. multivorans*
		genomovar III (unnamed species)
		genomovar IV: *B. stabilis*
		genomovar V: *B. vietnamiensis*
		genomovar VI (unnamed species)
		genomovar VII: *B. ambifaria*
		genomovar VIII: *B. anthina*
		genomovar IX: *B. pyrrocinia*
	Pseudomonas gladioli	*Burkholderia gladioli*
	Pseudomonas cocovenenans	*Burkholderia gladioli*
	Pseudomonas mallei	*Burkholderia mallei*
	Pseudomonas pseudomallei	*Burkholderia pseudomallei*
		Burkholderia thailandensis
	Pseudomonas (Burkholderia) pickettii	*Ralstonia pickettii*
	Pseudomonas pickettii biovar 3/'thomasii'	*Ralstonia mannitolilytica*
III	*Pseudomonas (Comamonas) acidovorans*	*Delftia acidovorans*
	Pseudomonas testosteroni	*Comamonas testosteroni*
	Pseudomonas delafieldii	*Acidovorax delafieldii*
	Pseudomonas facilis	*Acidovorax facilis*
IV	*Pseudomonas diminuta*	*Brevundimonas diminuta*
	Pseudomonas vesicularis	*Brevundimonas vesicularis*
V	*Pseudomonas (Xanthomonas) maltophilia*	*Stenotrophomonas maltophilia*
		Stenotrophomonas africana

known as *Alcaligenes eutrophus*, *Pseudomonas solanacearum*, and *Pseudomonas pickettii* (197). Since then, several additional species isolated from environmental or human clinical sources, or both, have been delineated using integrated phenotypic and genotypic taxonomic studies. Human pathogens include *R. pickettii* (144), *R. paucula* (previously known as Centers for Disease Control group IVc-2) (169), *R. gilardii* (35), and *R. mannitolilytica* (previously known as *R. pickettii* biovar 3/'thomasii') (52).

The genus *Pandoraea* was created to accommodate various isolates tentatively identified as *B. cepacia*, *R. pickettii*, or *R. paucula*. Five distinct species, *P. apista* (the type species), *P. pulmonicola*, *P. pnomenusa*, *P. sputorum*, and *P. norimbergensis*, were distinguished by sodium dodecyl sulfate-polyacrylamide gel electrophoresis of whole-cell proteins, amplified fragment length polymorphism fingerprinting, DNA-DNA hybridization, and 16S rDNA sequence analysis. In addition, four strains, each representing a distinct novel *Pandoraea* species, presently remain unnamed (34, 50).

Organisms in the *Pseudomonas* rRNA homology group III are now classified in a new family, the *Comamonadaceae*, which includes the genera *Comamonas*, *Delftia*, and *Acidovorax* (184, 189). The genus *Comamonas* was originally created in 1985 and included a single species, *C. terrigena*. Two years later, *Pseudomonas acidovorans* and *Pseudomonas testosteroni* were reclassified as members of the genus *Comamonas* (166). More recently, *C. acidovorans* was reclassified as *Delftia acidovorans* (184).

Originally, *Acidovorax facilis* was classified as *Hydrogenomonas facilis* based on its ability to oxidize hydrogen (147). Poly-β-hydroxybutyrate metabolism studies resulted in the transfer of this species to the genus *Pseudomonas*, along with a new species called *P. delafieldii* (51). DNA-rRNA hybridization studies led to the proposal of a new genus, *Acidovorax*, which includes three species, *A. facilis*, *A. delafieldii*, and *A. temperans*, all members of homology group III (190).

Brevundimonas diminuta and *B. vesicularis* were originally classified as members of *Pseudomonas* rRNA homology group IV (11). Phenotypically, this categorization seemed appropriate. However, based on DNA-rRNA hybridization studies, 16S rRNA cataloging, and 16S rRNA sequencing, the reclassification as *Brevundimonas* constituting homology group IV was proposed (149).

The genomic classification of *Stenotrophomonas maltophilia* has been a circuitous one. In 1961, the organism was designated *Pseudomonas maltophilia* based on flagellar characteristics (85). *P. maltophilia* belonged to *Pseudomonas* rRNA homology group V, and therefore in 1983, its transfer to the genus *Xanthomonas* was proposed (164). This proposal was based on genotypic and phenotypic characteristics including DNA-rRNA hybridizations, cellular fatty acid composition, and growth parameters. However, many differences were also noted, including flagellum number, nitrate reduction, fimbriation, and plant pathogenicity. Therefore, the genus designation of *Stenotrophomonas*, consisting of the species *S. maltophilia* and *S. africana*, has been established (58, 129).

GENERAL DESCRIPTION

Burkholderia, Ralstonia, Brevundimonas, Comamonas, Delftia, Pandoraea, and *Acidovorax* spp. are aerobic, non-spore-forming, gram-negative rods which are straight or slightly curved. They are 1 to 5 μm in length and 0.5 to 1.0 μm in width (83). *Stenotrophomonas* spp. are straight bacilli and tend to be slightly smaller (0.7 to 1.8 μm in length and 0.4 to 0.7 μm in width) (83). With the exception of *B. mallei*, these organisms are motile due to the presence of one or more polar flagella (128). These bacteria are catalase positive, and most, with the exception of *Stenotrophomonas*, are oxidase positive. All grow on MacConkey agar, except for certain strains of *B. vesicularis*, and appear as nonfermenters. The majority of species degrade glucose oxidatively, and most degrade nitrate to either nitrite or nitrogen gas. Certain species have distinctive colony morphologies or pigmentation. They are nutritionally quite versatile, with different species being able to utilize a variety of simple and complex carbohydrates, alcohols, and amino acids as carbon sources. Certain species can multiply at 4°C, but most are mesophilic, with optimal growth temperatures of between 30 and 37°C (128). For some genera, growth at higher temperatures (i.e., 42°C) can be useful for species identification.

NATURAL HABITATS

Burkholderia, Stenotrophomonas, Ralstonia, Brevundimonas, Comamonas, Delftia, Pandoraea, and *Acidovorax* spp. are environmental organisms found in water, soil, and on plants including fruits and vegetables. They have a worldwide distribution. Members of these genera are widely recognized as phytopathogens, and many species were first described in that context. Because of their ability to survive in aqueous environments, these organisms have become particularly problematic in the hospital environment.

The natural distribution of *Burkholderia cepacia* complex is being intensively studied because of interest in its use as a biologic control agent in bioremediation of soils contaminated with toxic wastes and because of its pathogenicity in patients with cystic fibrosis (73). Studies have shown that, unlike *P. aeruginosa*, *B. cepacia* complex is infrequently recovered from environmental sites such as sinks, swimming pools, showers, and salad bars (73, 118). However, it is frequently recovered from soil and environmental water samples (9, 62, 104), provided that appropriate growth conditions are used to inhibit the growth of vast numbers of other environmental bacteria. Studies of a variety of foodstuffs and bottled water have shown that *B. cepacia* is likely to be found in unpasteurized dairy products (15, 117). At-risk patients should avoid consumption of these products.

B. pseudomallei and *B. thailandensis* are found primarily in tropical and subtropical areas. They are particularly prevalent environmentally in the rice-growing regions of northern Thailand because of high concentrations of the organism in rice paddy surface water (103). Both species can be recovered from rice paddies in southern and central Vietnam (132). Reports have suggested that *B. pseudomallei* may also occur with some degree of frequency on the Indian subcontinent but goes unrecognized (48).

Because of the increasing frequency of nosocomial infections due to *S. maltophilia*, its presence in hospital environments is being more closely examined. Like *P. aeruginosa*, *S. maltophilia* is ubiquitous in aqueous environments and can be readily cultured from water sources in homes and hospitals (54).

CLINICAL SIGNIFICANCE

Burkholderia spp.

The genus *Burkholderia* contains two organisms frequently encountered as human pathogens, *B. pseudomallei* and *B. cepacia* complex.

B. pseudomallei is the causative organism of the disease melioidosis. The organism is acquired either by inhalation or by contact of cut or abraded skin with contaminated soil or water (47, 103). Risk factors include alcoholism, diabetes mellitus, renal failure, and penetrating wounds (42, 44). The clinical presentation of melioidosis is sufficiently variable to make diagnosis difficult in areas where the infection is not endemic. In areas where it is endemic, a high clinical index of suspicion during the monsoonal season and the availability of a microbiology laboratory proficent in isolating the microorganism make the diagnosis only slightly less difficult. The illness can manifest as an acute, subacute, or chronic process, with death occurring in some cases. However, serosurveillance indicates that the majority of those infected remain asymptomatic (93, 103). Because of the potential of *B. pseudomallei* as a bioterrorism agent, its isolation from patients who do not give a history of travel to a disease-endemic area should be immediately reported to local or state public health authorities. For further details, see chapter 10 or www.bt.cdc.gov.

While pneumonia is the most common presentation, the detection of *B. pseudomallei* in the blood of patients with signs of septicemia substantially increases the risk of mortality. Mortality in patients with fulminant sepsis is high, approaching 90% in patients with high-grade bacteremia, as evidenced by the presence of >100 CFU/ml of blood or blood culture showing growth in the first 24 h of incubation (167). Genitourinary infections are well described (44), and, given the number of prostatic infections detected, all patients with melioidosis should have their abdomens imaged, for example, by computed tomography (44). Neurological melioidosis exists, but rather than presenting as a meningitis, it is more consistent with a brain stem encephalitis associated with peripheral weakness or flaccid paralysis (43, 44, 193). Brain abscess due to *B. pseudomallei* has also been reported (102).

Chronic infections with this organism can mimic those with *Mycobacterium tuberculosis*. Like *M. tuberculosis*, *B. pseudomallei* can survive within phagocytes (89), produce nodular lesions visible on chest radiography, and cause granulomatous lesions in a variety of tissues. The disease may lie quiescent for many years, only to reactivate, a more common finding than reinfection (42, 56, 89). Based on molecular genotyping studies, relapse following appropriate antimicrobial therapy has been observed in as many as 15% of patients (56).

Melioidosis is most prevalent in Southeast Asia and Northern Australia but occurs in tropical and subtropical regions throughout the world. Because so much of the combat in the Vietnam war occurred in the rice-growing regions, concern exists that a significant number of veterans of that conflict may be latently infected with this organism, reactivation may become increasingly common as that population ages (100). As travel to Southeast Asia has become more frequent for individuals living in industrialized countries, reports of infection in travelers returning to Europe and the United States are becoming more common (48), including infections in patients with cystic fibrosis (CF) (148, 178). This organism should be considered in the differential diagnosis of any individual with a fever of unknown origin or a tuberculosis-like disease who has a history of travel to a region with endemic infection, even if the travel preceded the illness by decades (48, 100).

B. cepacia is well recognized as a nosocomial pathogen, causing infections associated with contaminated equipment, medications, mouthwash, and disinfectants including povidone-iodine and benzalkonium chloride (158). These infections include bacteremia, particularly in patients with indwelling catheters, urinary tract infection, septic arthritis, peritonitis, and respiratory tract infection (127, 134). Nosocomial outbreaks of B. cepacia respiratory tract infections in ventilated patients have been attributed to contamination of nebulizers or medication such as albuterol given by nebulizers (133, 142). Because B. cepacia appears to be of low virulence in patients who do not have CF or chronic granulomatous disease (CGD), morbidity and mortality associated with these infections are low. B. cepacia pseudobacteremia due to contaminated disinfectants has been described (41, 127). Isolation of B. cepacia from the blood of multiple patients over a short period should be investigated for possible pseudobacteremia.

B. cepacia complex is an important pathogen in two patient populations with genetic diseases, CF and CGD patients (67, 108, 191). In CGD patients, B. cepacia is the second most common cause of bacteremia and third leading cause of pneumonia. It is the second leading cause of death, responsible for the demise of 20% of this patient population (191).

In the United States, approximately 3% of CF patients are infected with this organism. The rates of infection are higher in adults with CF (6 to 7%), and infection rates as high as 20 to 30% have been reported in some CF centers (46, 90). CF patients chronically infected with B. cepacia complex have decreased survival compared to those not infected with this complex (107). Approximately 20% of CF patients who become infected with B. cepacia develop the "cepacia syndrome" (67). These patients frequently have mild lung disease prior to B. cepacia infection but experience rapid decline in lung function, frequent bacteremia (an unusual occurrence in CF patients), and death due to lung failure. Autopsy results reveal multiple lung abscesses containing B. cepacia, a pathologic finding similar to that seen in fulminant B. pseudomallei disease (67). Recent studies have shown that strains of B. cepacia complex are invasive in a number of different cell culture models (95). Autopsies from patients with cepacia syndrome are also consistent with invasion of the respiratory epithelium (146). The virulence factors responsible for the invasive phenotype have not been identified.

Molecular typing techniques have played an important role in our understanding of the epidemiology of B. cepacia in CF patients. A clone of this bacterium which has a highly unusual adhesin called cable pilin (71) was shown to have been spread from a CF center in Canada to other Canadian centers as well as centers in England and Scotland and then on to CF centers in continental Europe (153, 162). Studies suggest that transmission occurs primarily via close personal contact, with kissing being implicated as one

transmission mode (72). Nosocomial spread from CF patients to non-CF patients has also been documented in the intensive care unit ICU setting (82). Because of the retrospective nature of that study, the mode of transmission could not be determined.

The recent advances in our understanding of the complexity of the taxonomy of B. cepacia have clinical implications. Although nine genomovars are now recognized in the B. cepacia complex, over 85% of the isolates recovered from CF patients belong to two genomovars, B. cepacia genomovar III (50%) and the species B. multivorans (38%) (genomovar II) (110). The highly transmissible, cable pilin-positive clone that has been spread intercontinentally among CF patients is a genomovar III clone. Subclassifying members of the B. cepacia complex appears to be of particular importance in lung transplantation in CF patients. Because of their profound immunosuppression, CF patients who have received lung transplants are particularly vulnerable to infection with B. cepacia. Studies have shown that CF patients who are infected with B. cepacia prior to transplantation have a poorer outcome than do CF transplant recipients infected with other organisms pretransplantation (30). Many transplant centers refuse to consider B. cepacia complex-infected patients for transplantation because of concerns about potentially poor outcomes. A recent study has shown that this poor outcome is found primarily in patients infected with B. cepacia genomovar III. These genomovar III strains were all cable pilin gene negative and genotypically unique, suggesting that other virulence factors are important in the lung pathology seen in these patients (5).

B. gladioli has also been isolated from both the CF and the CGD patients (13, 75, 91, 145). This organism was first recognized in CF patients due to its ability to grow on a selective medium used to isolate B. cepacia (32). Reports have implicated this organism as the cause of pulmonary exacerbation and multiple abscesses in CF patients (13, 75, 91), but there has been some controversy about whether these strains were actually misidentified strains of B. cepacia complex (108, 151). B. gladioli has also been recovered from the blood and tissue of other immunocompromised patients (75).

B. mallei is the etiologic agent of glanders, a disease of livestock, particularly horses, mules, and donkeys. Both B. mallei and B. pseudomallei have been identified as potential agents of bioterrorism. The only human case of B. mallei in the past 50 years in the United States was recently laboratory acquired (26).

Stenotrophomonas

The significance of S. maltophilia in cultures is not always clear and must be interpreted in conjunction with patient information. Stenotrophomonas is recognized as a significant nosocomial pathogen and can be associated with substantial morbidity and mortality (53). Risk factors for colonization and infection include mechanical ventilation (158), broad-spectrum antibiotic prophylaxis (158), chemotherapeutic regimens (10, 114, 119), the use of central venous catheters (119), and neutropenia (158, 176). Infections caused by S. maltophilia are numerous and include bacteremia (119, 158), meningitis (70, 123), urinary tract infection (176), mastoiditis (158), epididymitis (158), conjunctivitis (135), endocarditis (76), continuous ambulatory peritoneal dialysis-associated peritonitis (165), bursitis (53), keratitis (159), endophthalmitis (92), cholangitis (131), and a wide range of mucocutaneous and soft tissue infections that may mimic disseminated fungal infections (175). Septicemia can be accompanied by ecthyma gangrenosa, a type of skin lesion more commonly associated with *Pseudomonas aeruginosa* and *Vibrio* spp. (17, 175). Mortality is significantly associated with malignancy, neutropenia, immunosuppressive therapy, and the overall severity of disease (63). Pneumonia is uncommon, and isolation from the respiratory tract is usually indicative of colonization (87). The role of *Stenotrophomonas* as an emerging pathogen, rather than just a colonizer (179), in patients with CF is under consideration. While the literature is sparse, there is some evidence which suggests a progressive decline in pulmonary function in patients chronically colonized with $>10^5$ to 10^6 CFU/ml (94). In the United States, the data from the 1999 Cystic Fibrosis Foundation registry reported that this organism was isolated from 6.4% of CF patients (46). Microbiology data gleaned from CF clinical trials demonstrated a prevalence of 10.2% (23). As microbiology laboratories become more proficient at the isolation and accurate identification of organisms isolated from CF patients, the role of *Stenotrophomonas* may become clearer. A new species of *Stenotrophomonas*, *S. africana*, was proposed in 1997 (58). This organism was isolated from the spinal fluid of a human immunodeficiency virus-positive Rwandan refugee with primary meningoencephalitis. 16S rRNA gene sequence analysis demonstrated significant homology to *S. maltophilia*.

Other Genera

In general, *Acidovorax*, *Brevundimonas*, *Comamonas*, *Delftia*, *Pandoraea*, and *Ralstonia* spp. are infrequently isolated from clinical specimens. *Acidovorax* spp. have been isolated from a variety of clinical sources; however, their role as a true pathogen has not been established (190).

Isolated incidents of *B. vesicularis* bacteremias have been reported in a hemodialysis patient, an open-heart surgery patient, a patient with sickle cell anemia, and an immunosuppressed individual (66, 125, 139, 173). It has been isolated from peritoneal dialysis fluid, an oral abscess, and a scalp wound (24, 99). It has also been recognized in cervical specimens because of its ability to produce bright orange colonies on Thayer-Martin agar (126). *B. diminuta* has been associated with a limited number of bacteremias (99).

Although typically regarded as nonpathogenic (166), *D. acidovorans* strains have been recovered from a variety of environmental sites, including dental water units (160), and clinical sites; they have been linked to certain disease states. *D. acidovorans* has also been reported to cause infection. It has been identified as the etiologic agent of bacteremia (25, 59), intravenous drug use-associated endocarditis (84), indwelling central venous catheter-associated bacteremia (25), ocular infections (20), and acute suppurative otitis (143).

One report described 10 adult cases of *C. testosteroni* infections, with the most common site of isolation being the peritoneal cavity (12). The majority of these infections were polymicrobic.

There is little information currently about the role of *Pandoraea* spp. in human infections. The organism has been isolated in episodes of bacteremia and from the respiratory tree of patients with cystic fibrosis. Like *B. gladioli* and *B. cepacia*, it has also been isolated from the lungs of a CGD patient (50).

R. pickettii has been recovered from a variety of clinical specimens (144) and is an infrequent cause of bacteremia (64, 101), meningitis (60), endocarditis (74), and osteomy-

elitis (185). It has been identified in several nosocomial outbreaks due to contamination of intravenous products (61), "sterile" water (113), saline (31), chlorhexidine solutions (185), respiratory therapy solutions (115), and intravenous catheters (141). It has also been associated with pseudobacteremias (177) and asymptomatic colonization (115). *R. pickettii* may be recovered from the respiratory tract of CF patients. Because of biochemical similarities, *R. pickettii* may be confused with members of the *B. cepacia* complex. *R. pickettii* does not appear to cause pulmonary-disease exacerbations in CF patients.

Little clinical information exists about three newly recognized species of *Ralstonia*, *R. gilardii*, *R. paucula*, and *R. mannitolilytica*. *R. gilardii* has been recovered from cerebrospinal fluid (35), while *R. mannitolilytica* has been recovered from blood, nosocomial meningitis, and sputum specimens from CF patients (52). Cases of *R. paucula* bacteremia, peritonitis, and tenosynovitis have all been reported, with most cases occurring in patients with underlying immunodeficiencies (169).

COLLECTION, TRANSPORT, AND STORAGE

The genera described in this chapter are all organisms that can survive in a variety of hostile environments and at temperatures found in clinical settings. Therefore, standard collection, transport, and storage techniques as outlined in chapters 6 and 20 are sufficient to ensure the recovery of these organisms from clinical specimens.

DIRECT EXAMINATION

The genera have similar morphologies and are not easily distinguished from each other on the basis of Gram stain, with the exception of *B. pseudomallei*. Direct Gram stain of *B. pseudomallei*-positive specimens often reveals small gramnegative bacilli demonstrating bipolar staining, making the cells resemble "safety pins" (Fig. 1) (103). It is not uncommon for the presumptive laboratory diagnosis to be made on the examination of the initial Gram-stained smear.

Because septicemia with *B. pseudomallei* is frequently fatal, several rapid direct-detection methods have been developed in research laboratories, including urinary antigen detection using latex agglutination (LA) and enzyme immunoassay (EIA), direct fluorescent-antibody (DFA) stains, and PCR (55, 77, 154, 180). The EIA for detection of urinary antigen is more sensitive than LA, with an overall sensitivity of 71% in patients with melioidosis compared with an LA sensitivity of 62% (with concentrated urine) or only 17.5% (with unconcentrated urine). The EIA has an even higher sensitivity (84%) for samples from septicemic patients. Cross-reactions with other urinary tract pathogens including *Klebsiella pneumoniae* and *Escherichia coli* have been reported with EIA but not LA; therefore, EIA results must be interpreted cautiously (55, 154).

Antibodies raised against heat-killed whole cells of *B. pseudomallei* have been used to prepare a reagent for DFA staining. When this DFA reagent was used to stain clinical specimens from patients with suspected melioidosis, it showed a sensitivity of 73%, similar to that of other bacterial DFA stains. The reagent (not available commercially) apparently does not cross-react with other organisms, although the number of isolates tested for cross-reaction was small (180).

Reports on the use of PCR for the direct detection of *B. pseudomallei* in clinical specimens indicate that the cur-

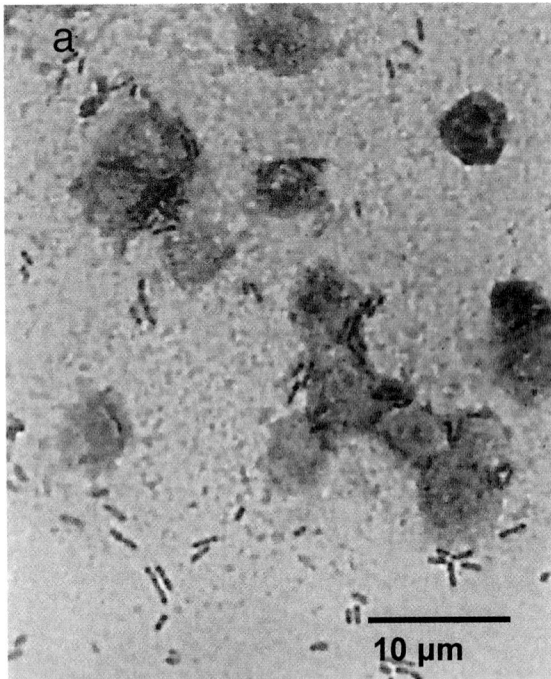

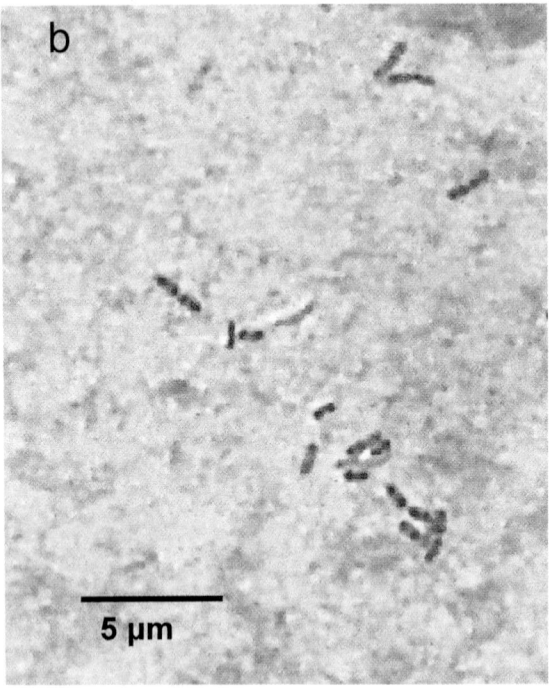

FIGURE 1 (a) Gram stain of *B. pseudomallei* in a blood culture; (b) Gram stain of *B. pseudomallei* from a colony on blood agar.

organisms, with particular emphasis on the identification of members of the *B. cepacia* complex. Molecular amplification kits for detection or identification of these organisms are not commercially available.

CULTURE AND ISOLATION

Organisms have been recovered from a variety of clinical specimens. They grow well on standard laboratory media such as 5% sheep blood or chocolate agar. Such media can be used to recover the organisms from clinical specimens, such as cerebrospinal fluid, joint fluid, or peritoneal dialysis fluid, where a mixed flora is not anticipated. All members of these genera which have been reported to be recovered from blood, including *B. pseudomallei* (167), grow in broth blood culture systems within the standard 5-day incubation period, so that special blood culture techniques such as lysis-centrifugation or extended incubation periods are not required.

The use of selective media facilitates the isolation of these organisms from specimens with mixed flora. With the exception of *B. vesicularis*, MacConkey agar is a useful selective medium for the isolation of most species of these genera.

Burkholderia species grow on MacConkey agar (Fig. 2a), but the use of specific selective media with the ability to inhibit *P. aeruginosa* is preferred for the isolation of *B. cepacia* and *B. pseudomallei*. Three media, PC (for "*Pseudomonas cepacia*") (68), OFPBL (for "oxidative-fermentative base, polymyxin b, bacitracin, lactose") (183), and BCSA (for "*B. cepacia* selective agar") (80) agars, are useful for the recovery of *B. cepacia* from respiratory secretions of CF patients. All three media contain antimicrobials that inhibit the growth of most *P. aeruginosa* strains. A multicenter comparison of these three media showed that BCSA was superior, being both more sensitive (more *B. cepacia* isolates were recovered) and specific (fewer other types of organisms grew) than PC or OFPBL agar (80). These studies provide strong evidence that BCSA is the medium of choice for the recovery of *B. cepacia* from respiratory tract specimens from CF patients.

Ashdown medium is effective for the isolation of *B. pseudomallei*; crystal violet and gentamicin act as selective agents. It has been shown to be superior to MacConkey agar or MacConkey agar supplemented with colistin for the recovery of *B. pseudomallei* from clinical specimens containing mixed bacterial flora, such as throat, rectal, and sputum specimens (7, 194). An enrichment broth consisting of Ashdown medium supplemented with 50 mg of colistin per liter allowed the recovery of 25% more *B. pseudomallei* isolates compared with direct plating of clinical specimens on Ashdown agar (182).

For the recovery of *B. pseudomallei* from rectal and throat swabs, selective broth should be inoculated at the bedside and selective media should be inoculated in the laboratory. During the monsoonal season, specimens such as sputum, urine, and wound swabs should be inoculated onto Ashdown's agar (7, 182, 193). Broths should be incubated at 35 to 37°C for up to 7 days and then subcultured onto Ashdown's agar for incubation at 35 to 37°C for another 7 days. Subculture from broth should be done earlier if a pellicle at the liquid-air interface is observed or if the broth changes from a deep purple to a deep pink due to a change in pH affecting the neutral red indicator.

rently used primer sets and assay conditions are sensitive but lack specificity, resulting in positive predictive values of only 70% (77). PCR primer sets have been described for detection of members of the *B. cepacia* complex, *B. gladioli*, and *S. maltophilia* (14, 109, 112, 187, 188). PCR detection of these organisms directly in clinical specimens has remained an infrequently used research tool. Rather, PCR has been used as a tool to identify clinical isolates of these

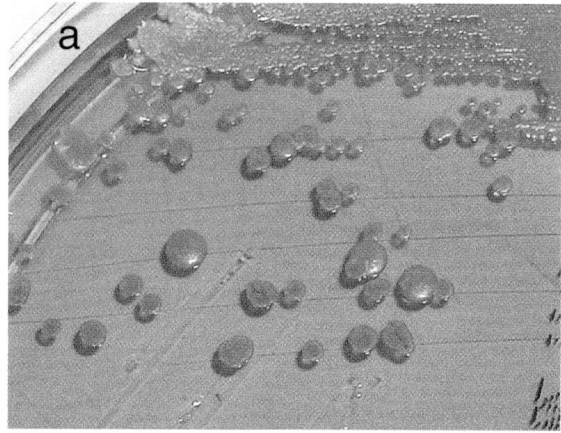

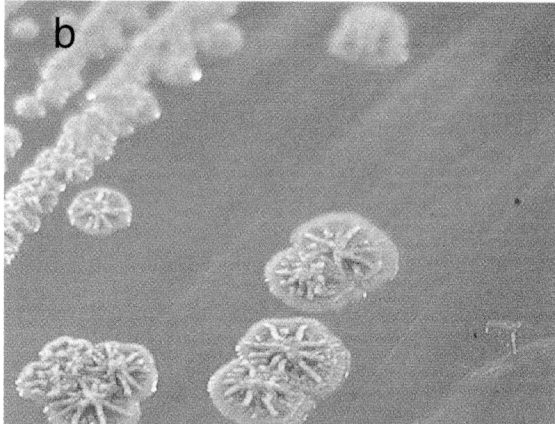

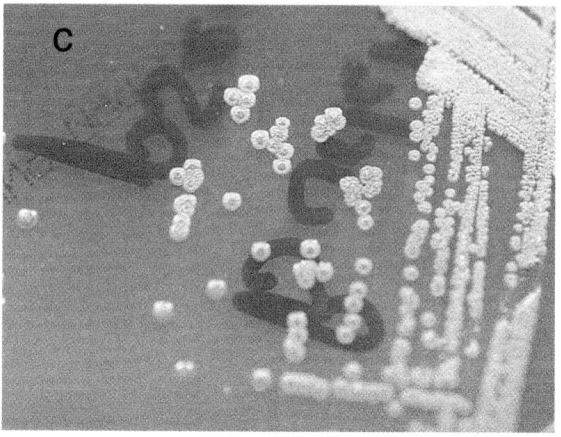

FIGURE 2 (a) B. pseudomallei colonies on MacConkey agar; (b) B. pseudomallei colonies on blood agar; (c) B. pseudomallei colonies on Ashdown medium agar.

IDENTIFICATION

Burkholderia spp.

Burkholderia spp. can be recovered on most aerobically incubated primary isolation media used in the clinical laboratory to isolate enteric gram-negative bacilli. Some Burkholderia species have distinctive growth characteristics. Growth of B. pseudomallei in the first 1 to 2 days often reveals small smooth colonies, which gradually change after a few days to dry wrinkled colonies similar to Pseudomonas

stutzeri (Fig. 2b). On Ashdown agar, the colonies take on a deep pink color due to the absorption of the neutral red (Fig. 2c) (181). B. pseudomallei also often produces a distinctive earthy odor which is very pronounced on opening a petri dish growing the microorganism or even opening an incubator door when a positive plate is present. While B. pseudomallei is not strictly a biosafety level 3 microorganism, precautions should be taken to avoid "sniffing" plates, during centrifugation, and when large-volume enrichment broths are being handled. All cultures suspected of containing B. pseudomallei should be handled in a biological safety cabinet (8).

B. cepacia, especially when recovered from the respiratory tracts of CF patients, may require 3 days of incubation before colonies are seen on selective media. On MacConkey agar, these colonies may be punctate and tenacious, while on blood agar or selective medium such as BCSA, PC, or OFPBL, the colonies are smooth and slightly raised; occasional isolates are mucoid. On MacConkey agar, colonies of B. cepacia frequently become dark pink to red due to oxidation of lactose after extended incubation (4 to 7 days). Most clinical isolates are nonpigmented, but on iron-containing media such as a TSI slant, many strains produce a bright yellow pigment. B. cepacia has a characteristic dirt-like odor.

B. mallei is the most easily identified member of this genus because it is nonmotile (Table 2). Other characteristics helpful in identifying B. mallei are its reduction of nitrate to nitrite, arginine dihydrolase activity, and oxidation of glucose. It fails to oxidize sucrose or maltose (186).

If B. pseudomallei is suspected, all efforts should be made to confirm or exclude the identification. Key identifying features include a positive oxidase reaction, production of gas from nitrate, multitrichous polar flagella, and arginine dihydrolase and gelatinase activities (Table 2) (186). Cellular fatty acid profiles may be useful for differentiating B. pseudomallei from other genera but are not especially useful when differentiating between environmental (B. thailandensis) and human pathogenic strains of B. pseudomallei (136) or other species of pathogenic Burkholderia species including B. mallei, B. cepacia, and B. gladioli (186).

B. pseudomallei needs to be differentiated from P. stutzeri and B. cepacia in clinical specimens. P. stutzeri appears very similar to B. pseudomallei after a few days of incubation. Both B. pseudomallei and B. cepacia have been isolated from at-risk patients with CF (67, 148, 178). A misidentification can have seriously adverse consequences. While B. pseudomallei produces gas from nitrate and is arginine dihydrolase positive, most B. cepacia complex isolates are negative for both. P. stutzeri is negative for arginine dihydrolase, O-F glucose, and gelatin hydrolysis. P. stutzeri also has only one flagellum, while B. pseudomallei has more than one (186).

There have been reports linking virulence or lack of virulence in B. pseudomallei with the ability to assimilate arabinose. Environmental strains tend to be arabinose assimilators, while those that do not assimilate arabinose are almost always found as clinical isolates. There is debate over the validity of a proposed new name for the environmental strain Burkholderia thailandensis sp. nov., with differences of opinion over the degree of genetic relatedness between the classical and environmental strains as well as the proposed specific names (3, 18, 19, 27, 138).

Early reliance was placed on commercially available strip biochemical systems like the API 20NE (bioMérieux, Hazelwood, Mo.) (49) and even the API 20E. Recent

TABLE 2 Characteristics of *B. mallei*, *B. pseudomallei*, and *B. thailandensis*[a]

Test	B. mallei	B. pseudomallei	B. thailandensis
Oxidase	v	+	+
Growth:			
MacConkey	+	+	+
42°C	−	+	+
Nitrate reduction	+	+	+
Gas from nitrate	−	+	+
Arginine dihydrolase	+	+	+
Lysine decarboxylase	−	−	−
Ornithine decarboxylase	−	−	−
Hydrolysis:			
Urea	v	v	v
Citrate	−	v	v
Gelatin	−	v	v
Esculin	−	v	v
Acid from:			
Glucose	+	+	+
Xylose	v	+	+
Lactose	v	+	+
Sucrose	−	v	v
Maltose	−	+	+
Mannitol	−	+	+
Arabinose	ND[b]	−	+
Motility	0	100%+	100%+
No. of flagella	0	≥2	≥2

[a] Data from references 19 and 186. +, >90% positive; −, >90% negative; v, variable.

[b] ND, not determined.

studies using the Microbact 24E strip (MedVet, Adelaide, Australia) show that this system more accurately identifies *B. pseudomallei* than does the API 20NE system (86). Experience with automated systems such as the Vitek-1 (T. R. Olma, G. Lum, and D. Mitchell, *Proc. Aust. Soc. Antimicrob. Annu. Sci. Meet.*, abstr. 0063, 2000) (bioMérieux, Durham, N.C.) and MicroScan WalkAway (Dade International Inc., West Sacramento, Calif.) indicate that they reliably identify *B. pseudomallei*. Limited, preliminary studies (Olma et al., *Proc. Aust. Soc. Antimicrob. Annu. Sci. Meet.*) indicate that Vitek-2 (bioMérieux) may also reliably identify *B. pseudomallei*, but further studies to confirm these findings are needed.

Recent taxonomic advances have demonstrated that *B. cepacia* is a complex of at least nine closely related genomic species (or genomovars) collectively referred to as the *B. cepacia* complex. Commercial bacterial identification systems are not able to distinguish among members of the *B. cepacia* complex and often fail to separate *B. cepacia* com-

plex from closely related species or genera such as *B. gladioli*, *R. pickettii*, *R. mannitolilytica*, and *Pandoraea* spp. (81, 98, 151, 174). In most clinical situations, this would be considered of minimal importance. However, for a CF patient, accuracy as close to 100% as possible is essential because CF patients infected with *B. cepacia* often become medical and social outcasts due to concern about spread of the organism to other individuals with CF (73). They also are excluded from lung transplantation in many centers (5). When *B. cepacia*, *B. gladioli*, or *R. pickettii* is identified in a CF patient by a commercial system, the identity of the isolate should be confirmed by conventional biochemical testing (81) and, if necessary, CFA analysis or molecular techniques. To aid clinical microbiologists in the United States, the U.S. Cystic Fibrosis Foundation has established a *B. cepacia* Reference Laboratory, which uses a combination of phenotypic and genotypic methods (described below) to confirm the identity of suspected *B. cepacia* isolates (109). For further information concerning the *B. cepacia* Reference Laboratory, contact the U.S. Cystic Fibrosis Center at www.cff.org.

An extensive biochemical analysis of *B. cepacia* complex and phenotypically similar species has recently been reported for genomovars I to VII (Table 3) (81). *B. multivorans* and *B. stabilis* could reliably be separated from the other members of the *B. cepacia* complex by phenotypic methods. *B. multivorans*, *B. stabilis*, and *B. cepacia* genomovar VI all fail to oxidize sucrose. *B. stabilis* is ornithine decarboxylase positive, while *B. multivorans* and *B. cepacia* genomovar VI isolates are negative. Differentiation of *B. multivorans* and *B. cepacia* genomovar VI can be challenging, since the only commonly used biochemical test that differentiates the two, lysine decarboxylase, is positive in only 53% of *B. multivorans* strains (81). Phenotypic characterization of *B. anthina* (genomovar VIII) and *B. pyrrocinia* (genomovar IX) is currently quite limited, although a small number of strains examined using the API Rapid NE (bioMérieux Vitek Inc., Durham, N.C.) were correctly identified as belonging to the *B. cepacia* complex. Two characteristics are particularly helpful to differentiate *B. anthina* from most other *B. cepacia* complex isolates. On BCSA agar, the isolates turned the medium alkaline (pink color production), which is most unusual for organisms capable of utilizing sucrose. In addition, the colony color and morphology would be best described as "creamy" whereas most other *B. cepacia* complex isolates are typically grey and either moist or dry (depending on the genomovar) (170).

Phenotypic differentiation of isolates of *B. cepacia* complex from isolates of *R. pickettii* and *B. gladioli* can be difficult (Table 3). Most isolates of the *B. cepacia* complex oxidize either sucrose, adonitol, or both, while *R. pickettii* fails to oxidize either. Most but not all strains of the *B. cepacia* complex are lysine decarboxylase positive, while *R. pickettii* is negative. CFA analysis may be helpful in distinguishing between these two organisms as well (197). *B. gladioli* isolates are unable to oxidize lactose, maltose, and sucrose and usually can be differentiated from *B. cepacia* on the basis of these phenotypic characteristics. However, some *B. cepacia* genomovar III isolates that have been recovered from CF patients fail to acidify sugars (81). They can be differentiated from *B. gladioli* and *Pandoraea* on the basis of a positive lysine decarboxylase test; the other organisms are negative. *B. cepacia* complex and *B. gladioli* have the same CFA profile, so that this identification approach for separating these two organisms has no value

TABLE 3 Characteristics of *B. cepacia* complex and phenotypically similar organisms[a]

| Test | % of strains positive | | | | | | | | | |
| | B. cepacia complex | | | | | | | B. gladioli | Pandoraea species | R. pickettii |
	Genomovar I	Genomovar II	Genomovar III	Genomovar IV	Genomovar V	Genomovar VI	Genomovar VII			
Oxidase[b]	100	100	100	100	100	100	100	0	67	100
Growth:										
MacConkey	83	96	84	93	83	100	100	96	100	50
BCSA	100	100	100	100	100	100	100	18	100	100
42°C	43	100	84	0	100	100	22	4	89	83
Pigment yellow	78	2	3	0	0	0	0	44	0	0
Pigment brown	4	2	14	0	0	0	6	33	0	0
Lysine decarboxylase	100	53	99	100	100	0	100	0	0	0
Ornithine decarboxylase	30	0	71	100	0	0	0	0	0	0
Acid from[c]:										
Glucose	100	100	95 (96)	100	100	100	100	100	11 (89)	100
Maltose	39 (70)	98 (99)	78 (86)	93	97 (100)	100	100	0	0	92
Lactose	61 (91)	100	79 (88)	93	97 (100)	100	100	0	0	92
Xylose	87 (100)	98 (99)	88 (92)	44 (78)	75 (86)	100	100	96	0	83 (92)
Sucrose	87 (91)	0	88 (91)	0	94 (97)	0	94	0	0	0
Adonitol	70 (78)	91 (92)	79 (87)	78 (96)	0	100	100	93 (96)	0	0
PNPG or ONPG[d]	100	98	99	0	100	100	100	100	0	0
Nitrate to nitrite reduction[e]	4	94	31	4	47	100	67	33	11	17
Gelatin liquefaction[e]	74	2	55	93	0	0	94	70	0	33
Esculin hydrolysis[e]	56	2	33	0	0	0	56	11	0	0

[a] The number of strains positively identified as being of a particular genomovar or species are as follows: for genomovar I, 23; for genomovar II (*B. multivorans*), 109; for genomovar III, 139; for genomovar IV (*B. stabilis*), 27; for genomovar V (*B. vietnamiensis*), 36; for genomovar VI, 9; for genomovar VII (*B. ambifaria*), 18; for *B. gladioli*, 27; for *Pandoraea* species, 9; and for *R. pickettii*, 12. Data from reference 81.

[b] In tests using the Pathotech cytochrome oxidase strip, the slow, weak reaction occurred in 10 to 30 s and the fast, strong reaction occurred in less than 10 s. Only *R. pickettii* displayed a fast, strong reaction.

[c] Oxidation test results were recorded after 3 days of incubation (data in parentheses were recorded after 7 days of incubation).

[d] PNPG, *P*-nitrophenyl-β-D-glucoside; ONPG, *O*-nitrophenyl-β-D-galactopyranoside.

[e] Results presented are from the API 20 NE strip test.

(120, 161). Conventional biochemical tests may need as long as 7 days of incubation before becoming positive for the *B. cepacia* complex and related organisms.

Recently, several molecular diagnostic approaches have been described for the specific identification of *B. cepacia* complex bacteria and their separation from biochemically similar species. However, while these novel methods were being developed, the knowledge of the taxonomic complexity of these bacteria continued to increase. The novel taxonomic insights (38, 39) explained why some strains remained difficult or impossible to identify (81) but also immediately challenged the validity of the newly developed assays.

Sequence polymorphisms of 16S and 23S rRNA genes have been used to develop PCR tests to identify the first five *B. cepacia* complex genomovars (14, 109) These assays could identify *B. multivorans* and *B. vietnamiensis* but failed to distinguish among *B. cepacia* genomovars I and III and *B. stabilis*. A single PCR test has been developed for the identification of the last three genomovars as a group. Subsequently, additional PCR tests were described to separate *B. cepacia* genomovar III from *B. stabilis*, but neither species could be distinguished from *B. cepacia* genomovar I (188). Primer pairs for the rapid identification of all *Burkholderia* and *Ralstonia* isolates have also been described (109).

Restriction fragment length polymorphism analysis of the 16S rRNA genes using six different restriction enzymes has further refined PCR identification of the *B. cepacia* complex (150). Restriction analysis using *Dde*I yielded different patterns for (i) *B. multivorans*, (ii) *B. vietnamiensis*, and (iii) *B. cepacia* genomovars I and III and *B. stabilis* as a group. Restriction analysis using *Cfo*I, however, allowed the separation of *B. stabilis* from *B. cepacia* genomovars I and III. Using the same two restriction enzymes, *B. cepacia* genomovar VI could be identified at the genomovar level; *B. ambifaria* (genomovar VII) could not be differentiated from *B. cepacia* genomovars I and III (62).

Another molecular approach to differentiating the *B. cepacia* complex was to develop assays based on polymorphisms present in the *recA* gene (112). PCR primer pairs were designed for the specific identification of *B. cepacia* genomovar I, *B. multivorans*, *B. stabilis*, and *B. vietnamiensis*. Two different primer pairs were required to detect all *B. cepacia* genomovar III isolates examined. In a subsequent study (39), a primer pair for the specific detection of *B. ambifaria* (genomovar VII) was described as well. In addition to this "direct" PCR approach, an alternative strategy based on restriction fragment length polymorphism analysis of PCR-amplified *recA* genes was proposed. The primers used for the initial amplification of the *recA* gene were chosen to specifically detect *B. cepacia* complex bacteria. This assay can therefore be used for the rapid identification of *B. cepacia* complex bacteria at the group level.

Two additional genomic approaches, amplified fragment length polymorphism fingerprinting (40) and automated ribotyping (21), proved useful for the differentiation of *B. cepacia* complex bacteria. However, both methods are expensive and require a considerable database before isolates can reliably be identified. This renders them impractical for use in a routine diagnostic laboratory. Whole-cell protein electrophoresis was also described as a useful method to separate *B. cepacia* genomovars (171) but subsequent studies revealed a poor discriminatory power between *B. cepacia* genomovars I and III and *B. ambifaria* (39, 40). In addition, cellular fatty acid methyl ester analysis is very useful for identification of *Burkholderia* strains at the genus level but proved unreliable for identification of individual *B. cepacia* complex genomovars or for their separation from closely related species (33, 171).

Ralstonia

Of the *Ralstonia* species, *R. pickettii* is the most frequently isolated from clinical specimens (144). *R. pickettii* grows slowly on primary isolation media and may require ≥72 h of incubation before colonies are visible. The newly classified *R. mannitolilytica* can be distinguished from other *Ralstonia* species by its acidification of D-arabitol and mannitol and by its inability to reduce nitrate (Table 4) (52). Both *R. gilardii* and *R. paucula* are biochemically inert, being unable to acidify carbohydrates. *R. paucula* is urease positive, while *R. gilardii* is urease negative. *R. gilardii* has a characteristic cellular fatty acid profile that allows it to be differentiated from other *Ralstonia* species (35, 52).

Pandoraea

Overall, the biochemical profile of *Pandoraea* strains is similar to that of *Burkholderia* and *Ralstonia* species that may be isolated from clinical specimens (34, 50, 81). The lack of saccharolytic activity is indicative of *Pandoraea* but is also seen with selected *Ralstonia* species as well. This requires *Pandoraea* strains to be differentiated from *Burkholderia* and *Ralstonia* strains by their specific *Dde*I 16S rDNA restriction profile (81). A quantitative comparison of the whole-cell fatty acid profiles of these three genera allows the differentiation of *Pandoraea* strains from the others (35, 50). However, using the commercially available Microbial Identification System database (Microbial ID, Inc., Newark, Del.), these organisms are mostly identified with low identification scores as *Burkholderia* or *Ralstonia* species (35, 81) due to a lack of discriminatory fatty acids.

Stenotrophomonas maltophilia

Key features for identifying *S. maltophilia* include a negative oxidase reaction, oxidation of glucose and maltose with a more intense reaction with the latter, positive reactions for DNase and lysine decarboxylase, and a tuft of polar flagella (Table 5) (186). Detection of extracellular DNase activity by *S. maltophilia* is a key to differentiating this species from most other glucose-oxidizing, gram-negative bacilli. It can be detected on tube or plate DNase medium with a methyl green indicator. DNase-positive organisms produce a zone of clearing around the colonies on this medium (see chapter 27). Care must be taken when interpreting the DNase reaction, since one report documented the misidentification of *S. maltophilia* as *B. cepacia* partially based on false-negative DNase reactions that were finalized within 48 h of incubation rather than 72 h (22). Selected isolates of *Flavobacterium* and *Shewanella* spp. may also be DNase positive (see chapter 49). On sheep blood agar, colonies appear rough and lavender-green and have an ammonia odor. *S. maltophilia* has a characteristic cellular fatty acid profile with large amounts (>30%) of 13-methyl tetradecanoic acid ($C_{15:0\ iso}$) and lesser amounts (>10%) of 12-methyl tetradecanoic acid ($C_{15:0\ anteiso}$) and *cis*-9-hexadecenoic acid ($C_{16:1\ cis9}$) (186).

Acidovorax, Brevundimonas, Delftia, and Comamonas

Characteristics of *Acidovorax*, *Brevundimonas*, *Delftia*, and *Comamonas* are given in Table 5.

TABLE 4 Characteristics of *Ralstonia* spp.[a]

Tests	R. pickettii	R. paucula	R. gilardii	R. mannitolilytica
Catalase	+	+	+	+
Oxidase	+	+	−	+
Growth at 42°C	v	v	+	+
Colistin resistance	+	−	ND[b]	+
Nitrate reduction	+	−	−	−
Hydrolysis:				
Tween 80	+	+	ND	+
Urease	+	+	−	+
Acid from:				
L-Arabinose	+	−	−	+
D-Arabitol	−	−	ND	+
Glucose	+	−	ND	+
Inositol	−	−	ND	−
Lactose	v	−	ND	+
Maltose	v	−	ND	+
Mannitol	−	−	ND	+
Sucrose	−	−	ND	−
Xylose	+	−	−	+
Motility	+	+	+	+
Flagella	1 polar	Peritrichous	1 polar	1 polar

[a] Data from reference 52; +, >90% positive; −, >90% negative; v, variable.
[b] ND, not determined.

Acidovorax species, rarely encountered in clinical and environmental samples, are straight to slightly curved gram-negative bacilli which occur either singly or in short chains. They are oxidase positive and nonpigmented and have a single polar flagellum. Urease activity varies among strains (186, 190).

B. diminuta and *B. vesicularis*, infrequently encountered in clinical and environmental samples, have growth requirements for specific vitamins, including pantothenate, biotin, and cyanocobalamin. An additional growth requirement for *B. diminuta* is cysteine. Most strains of *B. diminuta* grow on MacConkey agar, while only approximately 25% of *B. vesicularis* strains do so. On primary isolation media, *B. diminuta* colonies are chalk white while many strains of *B. vesicularis* are characterized by an orange intracellular pigment. These organisms are oxidase positive, have a single polar flagellum, and weakly oxidize glucose (*B. vesicularis* more so than *B. diminuta*), and the vast majority fail to reduce nitrate to nitrite. The most reliable method for differentiating these two species is the test for esculin hydrolysis. Almost all strains of *B. vesicularis* (88%) are reported to hydrolyze this substrate, while *B. diminuta* strains rarely do (5%) (Table 5) (186).

Comamonas spp. are straight to slightly curved gram-negative bacilli which occur singly or in pairs. The organisms are catalase and oxidase positive and have a single tuft of polar flagella. All *Comamonas* species reduce nitrate to nitrite. Phenotypic differentation of *C. terrigenia* from *C. testosteroni* is difficult, and as a result isolates are typically reported as *Comamonas* spp. (Table 5).

D. acidovorans is phenotypically similar to *Comamonas*. Key characteristics of the species are oxidization of fructose and mannitol. One-quarter of the strains produce a fluorescent pigment, while approximately half of the strains may produce a soluble yellow to tan one (186, 189).

TYPING SYSTEMS

Several molecular methods are available to assess strain relatedness in nosocomial outbreak investigations. These methods have proven to be much more discriminatory and reproducible than phenotypically based systems (16, 31, 140, 168). Pulsed-field gel electrophoresis and ribotyping are the most accurate, albeit technically challenging, typing methods. They have been used to study outbreaks and more global epidemiologic questions for *B. cepacia* (5, 82, 133, 162), *B. pseudomallei* (106), *R. pickettii* (31), and *S. maltophilia* (16, 168). The restriction endonucleases *XbaI* and *SpeI*, frequently used for chromosomal digestion in pulsed-field gel electrophoresis, typically yield 20 to 30 fragments for analysis. This is not surprising since *B. cepacia* strains have as many as four chromosomes and a very large genome size (5 to 9 Mb) (105).

Typing methods have not been reported for *Brevundimonas*, *Delftia*, *Comamonas*, or *Acidovorax* spp.

SEROLOGIC TESTS

Of the organisms discussed in this chapter, serologic tests have been used clinically only to diagnose *B. pseudomallei*

TABLE 5 Characteristics of *Acidovorax*, *Brevundimonas*, *Delftia*, *Comamonas*, and *Stenotrophomonas* spp. found in clinical specimens[a]

Test	Acidovorax delafieldii (n = 2)	A. facilis (n = 2)	A. temperans (n = 2)	Brevundimonas diminuta (n = 68)	B. vesicularis (n = 94)	Delftia acidovorans (n = 69)	Comamonas spp. (n = 28)	Stenotrophomonas maltophilia (n = 228)
Oxidase	100	100	100	100	98	100	100	0
Growth:								
MacConkey	100	0	100	100	43	100	100	100
Cetrimide	0	0	0	0	0	4	0	2
6.0% NaCl	0	0	0	21	23	6	0	22
42°C	50	0	100	38	19	29	68	48
Nitrate reduction	100	100	100	3	5	99	96	39
Gas from nitrate	0	0	100	0	0	0	0	0
Pigment	Yellow, soluble	None	Yellow, soluble	Brown-tan, soluble	52% yellow-orange, insoluble[d]	26% fluorescent, 44% yellow-tan; soluble	27% yellow-brown, soluble	Brown-tan, soluble
Arginine dihydrolase	100	100	0	0	0	0	0	0
Lysine decarboxylase	0	0	0	0	0	0	0	93
Ornithine decarboxylase	0	0	0	0	0	0	0	0
Indole	0	0	0	0	0	0	0	0
Hemolysis	0	0	0	0	0	0	0	1
Hydrolysis:								
Urea	100	100	50	13	2	0	7	3
Citrate	100	0	0	1	1	94	47	34
Gelatin	0	100	0	68	25	11	0	93
Esculin	0	0	0	5	88	0	0	39
Acid from:								
Glucose[b]	100	100	100	21	87	0	0	85
Xylose	85	100	0	0	27	0	0	35
Lactose	0	0	0	0	0	0	0	60
Sucrose	0	0	0	0	0	0	0	63
Maltose	0	0	0	0	94	0	0	100
Mannitol	50	100	50	0	0	100	0	0
H$_2$S[c]	100	100	100	34	49	57	0	95
Motility	100	100	100	100	100	100	100	100
No. of flagella	1–2	1–2	1–2	1–2	1–2	>2	>2	>2

[a] Data from reference 186. Results are the percentage of strains positive.
[b] Oxidative-fermentation basal medium with 1% carbohydrate.
[c] Lead acetate paper.
[d] Pigment observed on Thayer-Martin agar.

infections. The indirect hemagglutination assay, although not available commercially, is the most widely used test in regions of endemic infection (45). It is done using a prepared antigen from strains of *B. pseudomallei* sensitized to sheep cells and includes unsensitized cells as a control. This assay can be adapted to a microtiter plate test system. Because of high antibody background levels in healthy individuals (2), cross-reactions with other organisms including *B. cepacia* (2), and the rapid onset of septicemic disease, the indirect hemagglutination assay is of limited clinical value. Interpretation in areas of endemic infection is difficult, and all results must be viewed in a clinical context. IHA titers may rise to high levels in culture-negative individuals, but a particular titer cutoff that indicates disease has not been established. In regions of endemic infection, single titers are reported without any interpretation (2, 4). The need for acute- and convalescent-phase titers to aid in interpretation is paramount when attempting to establish serologically the diagnosis of subacute or chronic *B. pseudomallei* infection (124).

ANTIMICROBIAL SUSCEPTIBILITY

Specific interpretive criteria are not available for susceptibility testing of *Burkholderia*, *Pandoraea*, *Stenotrophomonas*, *Acidovorax*, *Brevundimonas*, *Delftia*, *Comamonas*, and *Ralstonia* spp. Those which are established for *Pseudomonas* are typically applied in accordance with NCCLS recommendations. MIC microbroth dilution tests or E tests are likely to yield the most reliable susceptibility results for this group of organisms. The disk diffusion method is not recommended (121, 122).

Like those for other nonfermenters, in vitro results for *B. pseudomallei* are not always consistent with in vivo outcomes. Many agents have antimicrobial activity in vitro, including ceftazidime, cefoperazone, amoxicillin-clavulanic acid, ampicillin-sulbactam, chloramphenicol, and doxycycline. Both trimethoprim-sulfamethoxazole (TMP-SMX) and the fluoroquinoles are used clinically, although in vitro susceptibility results are variable (28, 29, 88, 96, 155, 163, 192). E tests have proved satisfactory for determining in vitro resistance or susceptibility, especially for TMP-SMX (88) as opposed to disk diffusion techniques, which have been disappointing (111, 157) and which should probably be avoided.

Current trends in the management of melioidosis involve acutely ill patients receiving ceftazidime and TMP-SMX, with TMP-SMX continuing as eradication therapy for a number of months after hospital discharge (156). In patients requiring intensive care, a carbapenem, TMP-SMX, and granulocyte colony-stimulating factor are being used in some centers (44, 88, 152).

B. cepacia is one of the most antimicrobially resistant organisms encountered in the clinical laboratory. The organism is usually susceptible only to piperacillin, cefoperazone, ceftazidime, chloramphenicol, and TMP-SMX. Susceptibility to imipenem and meropenem is variable (137). Strains recovered from CF patients who have received repeated antimicrobial courses are frequently resistant to all known antimicrobial agents (67). The value of synergy testing of these isolates is controversial. Both double and triple synergy tests have been reported, with triple combinations showing greater activity than either double combinations or single agents. Antagonism with both double and triple combinations was also frequently observed. There have been no studies correlating in vitro synergy results

with patient response to the recommended therapy (1, 116).

Because of the potential role of *B. mallei* as a bioterrorism agent, studies have been recently done to determine the activity of a variety of agents against this organism. *B. mallei* had a similar susceptibility profile to that of *B. pseudomallei*, except that *B. mallei* is susceptible to the aminoglycosides while *B. pseudomallei* is resistant. Besides the aminoglycosides, *B. mallei* is susceptible to ceftazidime, imipenem, piperacillin, ciprofloxacin, and doxycycline. Resistance to most penicillins, cephalosporins, ofloxacin, rifampin, and chloramphenicol is common (78, 96). The E test gave consistently lower MICs than did broth dilution (78).

S. maltophilia is intrinsically resistant to many classes of antibiotics. Resistance develops quickly, and the slow growth and increased mutation rate often result in discordance between in vitro susceptibility results and clinical outcome (65). Resistance to β-lactam agents is mediated by the production of at least two β-lactamases, one of which is zinc dependent and resistant to β-lactamase inhibitors and breaks down imipenem. Aminoglycoside and quinolone resistance is the result of mutations in the outer membrane proteins. TMP-SMX is the drug of choice and continues to be active against most strains of *S. maltophilia*. It is often used in combination with minocycline or ticarcillin-clavulanic acid for treatment of serious infections.

The issue of susceptibility testing of *S. maltophilia* remains challenging and is being addressed by an NCCLS subcommittee. Although difficulties have been reported with all methods, the microbroth dilution, the E test (198), or the agar dilution method is preferred over disk susceptibility because of interpretation inconsistencies associated with disk susceptibility testing (6). However, trailing end points and colonies or hazes of growth within the zone of inhibition plague even the NCCLS-recommended methods. Many U.S. laboratories comment on the effectiveness of TMP-SMX and will test additional antibiotics such as minocycline, ceftazidime, ticarcillin-clavulanate and ciprofloxacin upon request only.

In general, *C. testosteroni* is susceptible to extended- and broad-spectrum cephalosporins, carbapenems, quinolones, and TMP-SMX (12). *D. acidovorans* is frequently resistant to the aminoglycosides.

REFERENCES

1. **Aaron, S. D., W. Ferris, D. A. Henry, D. P. Speert, and N. E. MacDonald.** 2000. Multiple combination bactericidal antibiotic testing for patients with cystic fibrosis infected with *Burkholderia cepacia*. *Am. J. Respir. Crit. Care Med.* **161:**1206–1212.
2. **Alexander, A. D., D. L. Huxsoll, A. R. Warner, Jr., V. Shepler, and A. Dorsey.** 1970. Serological diagnosis of human melioidosis with indirect hemagglutination and complement fixation tests. *Appl. Microbiol.* **20:**825.
3. **Anuntagool, N., P. Intachote, V. Wuthiekanun, N. J. White, and S. Sirisinha.** 1998. Lipopolysaccharide from nonvirulent Ara⁺ *Burkholderia pseudomallei* isolates is immunologically indistinguishable from lipopolysaccharide from virulent Ara⁻ clinical isolates. *Clin. Diagn. Lab. Immunol.* **5:**225–229.
4. **Anuntagool, N., P. Rugdech, and S. Sirisinha.** 1993. Identification of specific antigens of *Pseudomonas pseudomallei* and evaluation of their efficacies for diagnosis of melioidosis. *J. Clin. Microbiol.* **31:**1232–1236.
5. **Aris, R. M., J. C. Routh, J. J. LiPuma, D. G. Heath, and P. H. Gilligan.** 2001. Lung transplantation for cystic fi-

brosis patients with *Burkholderia cepacia* complex: survival linked to genomovar type. *Am. J. Respir. Crit. Care Med.* 164:2102–2106.

6. Arpi, M., M. A. Victor, I. Mortenson, A. Gottschau, and B. Bruun. 1996. In vitro susceptibility of 124 *Xanthomonas maltophilia* isolates: comparison of the agar dilution method with the E test and two agar diffusion methods. *APMIS* 104:108–114.

7. Ashdown, L. R. 1979. An improved screening technique for isolation of *Pseudomonas pseudomallei* from clinical specimens. *Pathology* 11:293–297.

8. Ashdown, L. R. 1992. Melioidosis and safety in the clinical laboratory. *J. Hosp. Infect.* 21:301–306.

9. Balandreau, J., V. Viallard, B. Cournoyer, T. Coenye, S. Laevens, and P. Vandamme. 2001. *Burkholderia cepacia* genomovar III is a common plant-associated bacterium. *Appl. Environ. Microbiol.* 67:982–985.

10. Balaz, M., A. Demitrovicova, S. Spanik, L. Drgona, I. Krupova, S. Grausova, K. Kralovicova, J. Trupl, A. Kunova, and V. Krcmery. 1996. Etiology of bacteremia in patients with various malignancies: is there an association between certain antineoplastic drugs and microorganisms? *Bratislavske Lekarske Listy* 97:675–679.

11. Ballard, R. W., M. Doudoroff, and R. Y. Stanier. 1968. Taxonomy of the aerobic pseudomonads: *Pseudomonas diminuta* and *Pseudomonas vesicularis*. *J. Gen. Microbiol.* 53:349–361.

12. Barbaro, D. J., and P. A. Mackowiak. 1987. *Pseudomonas testosteroni* infections: eighteen recent cases and review of the literature. *Rev. Infect. Dis.* 9:124–129.

13. Barker, P. M., R. E. Wood, and P. H. Gilligan. 1997. Lung infection with *Burkholderia gladioli* in a child with cystic fibrosis: acute clinical and spirometric deterioration. *Pediatr. Pulmonol.* 24:123–125.

14. Bauernfeind, A., I. Schneider, R. Jungwirth, and C. Roller. 1999. Discrimination of *Burkholderia multivorans* and *Burkholderia vietnamiensis* from *Burkholderia cepacia* genomovars I, III and IV by PCR. *J. Clin. Microbiol.* 37:1335–1339.

15. Berriatura, E., I. Ziluaga, C. Miguel-Virto, P. Uribarren, R. Juste, S. Laevens, P. Vandamme, and J. R. W. Govan. 2001. Outbreak of subclinical mastitis in a flock of dairy sheep associated with *Burkholderia cepacia* complex infection. *J. Clin. Microbiol.* 39:990–994.

16. Bingen, E. D., K. Denamur, and J. Elion. 1994. Use of ribotyping in epidemiological surveillance of nosocomial outbreaks. *Clin. Microbiol. Rev.* 7:311–327.

17. Bottone, E. J., M. Reitano, J. M. Janda, K. Troy, and J. Cuttner. 1986. *Pseudomonas maltophilia* exoenzyme activity as a correlate in pathogenesis of ecthyma gangrenosum. *J. Clin. Microbiol.* 24:995–997.

18. Brett, P. J., D. Deshazer, and D. E. Woods. 1997. Characterization of *Burkholderia pseudomallei* and *Burkholderia pseudomallei*-like strains. *Epidemiol. Infect.* 118:137–148.

19. Brett, P. J., D. DeShazer, and D. E. Woods. 1998. *Burkholderia thailandensis* sp. nov., a *Burkholderia pseudomallei*-like species. *Int. J. Syst. Bacteriol.* 48:317–320.

20. Brinser, J. H., and E. Torczynski. 1977. Unusual *Pseudomonas* corneal ulcers. *Am. J. Ophthalmol.* 84:462–466.

21. Brisse, S., C. M. Verduin, D. Milatovic, A. Fluit, J. Verhoef, S. Laevens, P. Vandamme, B. Tummler, H. A. Verbrugh, and A. van Belkum. 2000. Distinguishing species of the *Burkholderia cepacia* complex and *Burkholderia gladioli* by automated ribotyping. *J. Clin. Microbiol.* 38:1876–1884.

22. Burdge, D. R., M. A. Noble, M. E. Campbell, V. L. Krelland, and D. P. Speert. 1995. *Xanthomonas maltophilia* misidentified as *Pseudomonas cepacia* in cultures of sputum

from patients with cystic fibrosis: a diagnostic pitfall with major clinical implications. *Clin. Infect. Dis.* 20:445–448.

23. Burns, J. L., J. Emerson, J. R. Stapp, D. L. Yim, J. Krzewinski, L. Louden, B. W. Ramsey, and C. R. Clausen. 1998. Microbiology of sputum from patients at cystic fibrosis centers in the United States. *Clin. Infect. Dis.* 27:158–163.

24. Calegari, L., K. Gezuele, E. Torres, and C. Carmona. 1996. Botryomycosis caused by *Pseudomonas vesicularis*. *Int. J. Dermatol.* 35:817–818.

25. Castagnola, E., L. Tasso, M. Conte, M. Nantron, A. Barretta, and R. Giacchino. 1994. Central venous catheter-related infection due to *Comamonas acidovorans* in a child with non-Hodgkin's lymphoma. *Clin. Infect. Dis.* 19:559–560.

26. Centers for Disease Control and Prevention. 2000. Laboratory-acquired human glanders—Maryland. *Morb. Mortal. Wkly. Rep.* 49:532–535.

27. Chaiyaroj, S. C., K. Kotrnon, S. Koonpaew, N. Anantagool, N. J. White, and S. Sirisinha. 1999. Differences in genomic macrorestriction patterns of arabinose-positive (*Burkholderia thailandensis*) and arabinose-negative *Burkholderia pseudomallei*. *Microbiol. Immunol.* 43:625–630.

28. Chaowagul, W. 2000. Recent advances in the treatment of severe melioidosis. *Acta Trop.* 74:133–137.

29. Chaowagul, W., A. J. Simpson, Y. Suputtamongkol, M. D. Smith, B. J. Angus, and N. J. White. 1999. A comparison of chloramphenicol, trimethoprim-sulfamethoxazole, and doxycycline with doxycycline alone as maintenance therapy for melioidosis. *Clin. Infect. Dis.* 29:375–380.

30. Chaparro, C., J. Maurer, C. Gutierrez, M. Krajden, C. Chan, T. Winton, S. Keshavjee, M. Scavuzzo, E. Tullis, M. Hutcheon, and S. Kesten. 2001. Infection with *Burkholderia cepacia* in cystic fibrosis; outcome following lung transplantation. *Am. J. Respir. Crit. Care Med.* 163:43–48.

31. Chetoui, H., P. Melin, M. J. Struelens, E. Delhalle, M. Mutro Nigo, R. De Ryck, and P. De Mol. 1997. Comparison of biotyping, ribotyping, and pulsed field gel electrophoresis for investigation of a common-source outbreak of *Burkholderia pickettii* bacteremia. *J. Clin. Microbiol.* 35:1398–1403.

32. Christenson, J. C., D. F. Welch, G. Mukwaya, M. J. Muszynski, R. E. Weaver, and D. J. Brenner. 1989. Recovery of *Pseudomonas gladioli* from respiratory tract specimens of patients with cystic fibrosis. *J. Clin. Microbiol.* 27:270–273.

33. Clode, F. E., A. Louise, L. Metherel, and T. L. Pitt. 1999. Nosocomial acquisition of *Burkholderia gladioli* in patients with cystic fibrosis. *Am. J. Respir. Crit. Care Med.* 160:374–375.

34. Coenye, T., E. Falsen, B. Hoste, M. Ohlén, J. Goris, J. R. W. Govan, M. Gillis, and P. Vandamme. 2000. Description of *Pandoraea* gen. nov. with *Pandoraea apista* sp. nov., *Pandoraea pulmonicola* sp. nov., *Pandoraea pnomenusa* sp. nov., *Pandoraea sputorum* sp. nov., and *Pandoraea norimbergensis* comb. nov. *Int. J. Syst. Evol. Microbiol.* 50:887–899.

35. Coenye, T., E. Falsen, M. Vancanneyt, B. Hoste, J. R. W. Govan, K. Kersters, and P. Vandamme. 1999. Classification of some *Alcaligenes faecalis*-like isolates from the environment and human clinical samples as *Ralstonia gilardii* sp. nov. *Int. J. Syst. Bacterial.* 49:405–413.

36. Coenye, T., B. Holmes, K. Kersters, J. R. W. Govan, and P. Vandamme. 1999. *Burkholderia cocovenenans* (van Damme et al. 1960) Gillis et al. 1995 and *Burkholderia vandii* Urakami et al. 1994 are junior subjective synonyms of *Burkholderia gladioli* (Severini 1913) Yabuuchi et al.

1993 and *Burkholderia plantarii* (Azegami et al. 1987) Urakami et al. 1994, respectively. *Int. J. Syst. Bacteriol.* **49:**37–42.

37. **Coenye, T., S. Laevens, A. Willems, M. Ohlén, W. Hannant, J. R. W. Govan, M. Gillis, E. Falsen, and P. Vandamme.** 2001. *Burkholderia fungorum* sp. nov. and *Burkholderia caledonica* sp. nov., two new species isolated from the environment, animals and human clinical samples. *Int. J. Syst. Evol. Microbiol.* **51:**1099–1107.

38. **Coenye, T., J. J. LiPuma, D. Henry, B. Hoste, K. Vandemeulebroucke, M. Gillis, D. P. Speert, and P. Vandamme.** 2001. *Burkholderia cepacia* genomovar VI, a new member of the *Burkholderia cepacia* complex isolated from cystic fibrosis patients. *Int. J. Syst. Evol. Microbiol.* **51:** 271–279.

39. **Coenye, T., E. Mahenthiralingam, D. Henry, J. J. LiPuma, S. Laevens, M. Gills, D. P. Speert, and P. Vandamme.** 2001. *Burkholderia ambifaria* sp. nov., a novel member of the *Burkholderia cepacia* complex including biocontrol and cystic fibrosis-related isolates. *Int. J. Syst. Evol. Microbiol.* **51:**1481–1490.

40. **Coenye, T., L. M. Schouls, J. R. W. Govan, K. Kersters, and P. Vandamme.** 1999. Identification of *Burkholderia* species and genomovars from cystic fibrosis patients by AFLP fingerprinting. *Int. J. Syst. Bacteriol.* **49:**1657–1666.

41. **Craven, D. E., B. Moody, M. G. Connolly, N. R. Kollisch, K. D. Stottmeier, and W. R. McCabe.** 1981. Pseudobacteremia caused by povidone-iodine solution contaminated with *Pseudomonas cepacia*. *N. Engl. J. Med.* **305:**621–623.

42. **Currie, B. J., D. A. Fisher, N. M. Anstey, and S. P. Jacups.** 2000. Melioidosis: acute and chronic disease, relapse and re-activation. *Trans. R. Soc. Trop. Med. Hyg.* **94:**301–304.

43. **Currie, B. J., D. A. Fisher, D. M. Howard, and J. N. Burrow.** 2000. Neurological melioidosis. *Acta Trop.* **74:** 145–151.

44. **Currie, B. J., D. A. Fisher, D. M. Howard, J. N. Burrow, D. Lo, S. Selva-Nayagam, N. M. Anstey, S. E. Huffam, P. L. Snelling, P. J. Marks, D. P. Stephens, G. D. Lum, S. P. Jacups, and V. L. Krause.** 2000. Endemic melioidosis in tropical northern Australia: a 10-year prospective study and review of the literature. *Clin. Infect. Dis.* **31:** 981–986.

45. **Cuzzubbo, A. J., V. Chenthamarakshan, J. Vadivelu, S. D. Puthucheary, D. Rowland, and P. L. Devine.** 2000. Evaluation of a new commercially available immunoglobulin M and immunoglobulin G immunochromatographic test for diagnosis of melioidosis infection. *J. Clin. Microbiol.* **38:**1670–1671.

46. **Cystic Fibrosis Foundation.** 2000. *Patient Registry 1999 Annual Data Report.* Cystic Fibrosis Foundation, Bethesda, Md.

47. **Dance, D. A. B.** 1991. Melioidosis: the tip of the iceberg? *Clin. Microbiol. Rev.* **4:**52–60.

48. **Dance, D. A. B., M. D. Smith, H. M. Aucken, and T. L. Pitt.** 1999. Imported melioidosis in England and Wales. *Lancet* **353:**208.

49. **Dance, D. A. B., V. Wuthiekanun, P. Naigowit, and N. J. White.** 1989. Identification of *Pseudomonas pseudomallei* in clinical practice: use of simple screening tests and API 20NE *J. Clin. Pathol.* **42:**645–648.

50. **Daneshvar, M. I., D. G. Hollis, A. G. Steigerwalt, A. M. Whitney, L. Spangler, M. P. Douglas, J. G. Jordan, J. P. MacGregor, B. C. Hill, F. C. Tenover, D. J. Brenner, and R. S. Weyant.** 2001. Assignment of CDC Weak Oxidizer Group 2 (WO-2) to the genus *Pandoraea* and characterization of three new Pandoraea genomospecies. *J. Clin. Microbiol.* **39:**1819–1826.

51. **Davis, D. H., R. Y. Stanier, M. Doudoroff, and M. Mandel.** 1970. Taxonomic studies on some gram negative polarly flagellated "hydrogen bacteria" and related species. *Arch. Mikrobiol.* **70:**1–13.

52. **De Baere, T., S. Steyaert, G. Wauters, P. Des Vos, J. Goris, T. Coenye, T. Suyama, G. Verschraegen, and M. Vaneechoutte.** 2001. Classification of *Ralstonia pickettii* biovar 3/"thomasii" strains (Pickett 1994) and of new isolates related to nosocomial recurrent meningitis as *Ralstonia mannitolytica* sp. nov." *Int. J. Syst. Evol. Microbiol.* **51:**547–558.

53. **Denton, M., and K. Kerr.** 1998. Microbiological and clinical aspects of infection associated with *Stenotrophomonas maltophilia*. *Clin. Microbiol. Rev.* **11:**57–80.

54. **Denton, M., N. J. Todd, K. G. Kerr, P. M. Hawkey, and J. M. Littlewood.** 1998. Molecular epidemiology of *Stenotrophomonas maltophilia* isolated from clinical specimens from patients with cystic fibrosis and associated environmental samples. *J. Clin. Microbiol.* **36:**1953–1958.

55. **Desakorn, V., M. D. Smith, V. Wuthiekanun, D. A. Dance, H. Aucken, P. Suntharasamai, A. Rajchanuwong, and N. J. White.** 1994. Detection of *Pseudomonas pseudomallei* antigen in urine for the diagnosis of melioidosis. *Am. J. Trop. Med. Hyg.* **51:**627–633.

56. **Desmarchelier, P. M., D. A. Dance, W. Chaowagul, Y. Suputtamongkol, N. J. White, and T. L. Pitt.** 1993. Relationships among *Pseudomonas pseudomallei* isolates from patients with recurrent melioidosis. *J. Clin. Microbiol.* **31:**1592–1596.

57. **De Vos, P., and J. De Ley.** 1983. Intra- and intergeneric similarities of *Pseudomonas* and *Xanthomonas* ribosomal ribonucleic acid cistrons. *Int. J. Syst. Bacteriol.* **33:**487–509.

58. **Drancourt, M., C. Bollet, and D. Raoult.** 1997. *Stenotrophomonas africana* sp. nov., an opportunistic pathogen in Africa. *Int. J. Syst. Bacteriol.* **47:**160–163.

59. **Ender, T. E., D. P. Dooley, and R. H. Moore.** 1996. Vascular catheter-related *Comamonas acidovorans* bacteremia managed with preservation of the catheter. *Pediatr. Infect. Dis. J.* **15:**918–920.

60. **Fass, R. J., and J. Barnishan.** 1976. Acute meningitis due to a *Pseudomonas*-like group Va-1 bacillus. *Ann. Intern. Med.* **84:**51–52.

61. **Fernandez, C., I. Wilhelm, E. Andradas, C. Gaspar, J. Gomez, J. Romera, J. Mariano, O. Corral, M. Rubio, J. Elviro, and J. Fereres.** 1996. Nosocomial outbreak of *Burkholderia pickettii* infection due to a manufactured intravenous product used in three hospitals. *Clin. Infect. Dis.* **22:**1092–1095.

62. **Fiore, A., S. Laevens, A. Bevivino, C. Dalmastri, S. Tabacchioni, P. Vandamme, and L. Chiarini.** 2001. *Burkholderia cepacia* complex: distribution of genomovars among isolates from the maize rhizosphere in Italy. *Environ. Microbiol.* **3:**137–143.

63. **Fujita, J., I. Yamadori, G. Xu, S. Hojo, K. Negayama, H. Miyawaki, Y. Yamaji, and J. Takahara.** 1996. Clinical features of *Stenotrophomonas maltophilia* in immunocompromised patients. *Respir. Med.* **90:**35–38.

64. **Fujita, S., T. Yoshida, and F. Matsubara.** 1981. *Pseudomonas pickettii* bacteremia. *J. Clin. Microbiol.* **13:**781–782.

65. **Garrison, M. W., D. E. Anderson, D. M. Campbell, K. C. Carroll, C. L. Malone, and J. D. Anderson.** 1996. *Stenotrophomonas maltophilia*: emergence of multidrug resistant strains during therapy and in an in vitro pharmodynamic chamber model. *Antimicrob. Agents Chemother.* **40:**2859–2864.

66. **Gilad, J., A. Borer, N. Peled, K. Riesenberg, S. Tager, A. Appelbaum, and F. Schlaeffer.** 2000. Hospital-acquired *Brevundimonas vesicularis* septicemia following open-heart

surgery: case report and literature review. *Scand. J. Infect. Dis.* **32**:90–91.

67. **Gilligan, P. H.** 1991. Microbiology of airway disease in patients with cystic fibrosis. *Clin. Microbiol. Rev.* **4**:35–51.

68. **Gilligan, P. H., P. A. Gage, L. M. Bradshaw, D. V. Schidlow, and B. T. DeCicco.** 1985. Isolation medium for the recovery of *Pseudomonas cepacia* from respiratory secretions of patients with cystic fibrosis. *J. Clin. Microbiol.* **22**:5–8.

69. **Gillis, M., T. Van Van, R. Bardin, M. Goor, P. Hebbar, A. Willems, P. Segers, K. Kersters, T. Heulin, and M. P. Fernandez.** 1995. Polyphasic taxonomy in the genus *Burkholderia* leading to an emended description of the genus and proposition of *Burkholderia vietnamiensis* sp. nov. for N₂-fixing isolates from rice in Vietnam. *Int. J. Syst. Bacteriol.* **45**:274–289.

70. **Girijaratnakumari, T., A. Raja, R. Ramani, B. Antony, and P. G. Shivananda.** 1993. Meningitis due to *Xanthomonas maltophilia. J. Postgrad. Med.* **39**:153–155.

71. **Goldstein, R., L. Sun, R.-Z. Jiang, U. Sajjan, J. F. Forstner, and C. Campanelli.** 1995. Structurally variant classes of pilus appendage fibers coexpressed from *Burkholderia (Pseudomonas) cepacia. J. Bacteriol.* **177**:1039–1052.

72. **Govan, J. R. W., P. H. Brown, J. Maddison, C. J. Doherty, J. W. Nelson, M. Dodd, A. P. Greening, and A. K. Webb.** 1993. Evidence for transmission of *Pseudomonas cepacia* by social contact in cystic fibrosis. *Lancet* **342**:15–19.

73. **Govan, J. R. W., J. E. Hughes, and P. VanDamme.** 1996. *Burkholderia cepacia*: medical, taxonomic and ecological issues. *J. Med. Microbiol.* **45**:395–407.

74. **Graber, C. D., L. Jervey, W. E. Ostrander A. H. Sally, and R. E. Weaver.** 1968. Endocarditis due to a lanthanic, unclassified gram-negative bacterium (group IVd). *Am. J. Clin. Pathol.* **49**:220–223.

75. **Graves, M., T. Robin, A. M. Chipman, J. Wong. S. Khashe, and J. M. Janda.** 1997. Four additional cases of *Burkholderia gladioli* infection with microbiological correlates and review. *Clin. Infect. Dis.* **25**:838–842.

76. **Gutierrez, R. F., M. M. Masia, J. Cortes, V. Ortez de la Tabla, V. Mainar, and A. Vilar.** 1996. Endocarditis caused by *Stenotrophomonas maltophilia*: case report and review. *Clin. Infect. Dis.* **23**:1261–1265.

77. **Haase, A., M. Brennan, S. Barrett, Y. Wood, S. Huffam, D. O'Brien, and B. Currie.** 1998. Evaluation of PCR for diagnosis of melioidosis. *J. Clin. Microbiol.* **36**:1039–1041.

78. **Heine, H. S., M. J. England, D. M. Waag, and W. R. Byrne.** 2001. In vitro antibiotic susceptibilities of *Burkholderia mallei* (causative agent of glanders) determined by broth microdilution and E-test. *Antimicrob. Agents Chemother.* **45**:2119–2121.

79. **Henry, D. A., M. E. Campbell, J. J. LiPuma, and D. P. Speert.** 1997. Identification of *Burkholderia cepacia* isolates from patients with cystic fibrosis and use of a simple selective medium. *J. Clin. Microbiol.* **35**:614–619.

80. **Henry, D., M. Campbell, C. McGimpsey, A. Clarke, L. Louden, J. L. Burns, M. H. Roe, P. Vandamme, and D. Speert.** 1999. Comparison of isolation media for recovery of *Burkholderia cepacia* complex from respiratory secretions of patients with cystic fibrosis. *J. Clin. Microbiol.* **37**:1004–1007.

81. **Henry, D. A., E. Mahenthiralingam, P. Vandamme, T. Coenye, and D. P. Speert.** 2001. Phenotypic methods for determining genomovar status of the *Burkholderia cepacia* complex. *J. Clin. Microbiol.* **39**:1073–1078.

82. **Holmes, A., R. Nolan, R. Taylor, R. Finley, M. Riley, R. Jiang, S. Steinbach, and R. Goldstein.** 1999. An epidemic of *Burkholderia cepacia* transmitted between patients with and without cystic fibrosis. *J. Infect. Dis.* **179**:1197–1205.

83. **Holt, J., G. N. R. Krieg, P. H. A. Sneath, J. T. Staley, and S. T. Williams.** 1994. *Bergey's Manual of Determinative Bacteriology*, 9th ed. The Williams & Wilkins Co., Philadelphia, Pa.

84. **Horowitz, H., S. Gilroy, S. Feinstein, and G. Gilardi.** 1990. Endocarditis associated with *Comamonas acidovorans. J. Clin. Microbiol.* **28**:143–145.

85. **Hugh, R., and E. Ryschenkow.** 1961. *Pseudomonas maltophilia*, an *Alcaligenes*-like organism. *J. Gen. Microbiol.* **26**:123–132.

86. **Inglis, T. J., D. Chiang, G. S. Lee, and L. Chor-Kiang.** 1998. Potential misidentification of *Burkholderia pseudomallei* by API 20NE. *Pathology* **30**:62–64.

87. **Irifune, K., T. Ishida, K. Shimoguchi, J. Ohtake, T. Tanaka, N. Morikawa, M. Kaku, H. Koga, S. Kohno, and K. Hara.** 1994. Pneumonia caused by *Stenotrophomonas maltophilia* with a mucoid phenotype. *J. Clin. Microbiol.* **32**:2856–2857.

88. **Jenney, A. W., G. Lum, D. A. Fisher, and B. J. Currie.** 2001. Antibiotic susceptibility of *Burkholderia pseudomallei* from tropical northern Australia and implications for therapy of melioidosis. *Int. J. Antimicrob. Agents* **17**:109–113.

89. **Jones, A. L., T. J. Beveridge, and D. E. Woods.** 1996. Intracellular survival of *Burkholderia pseudomallei. Infect. Immun.* **64**:782–790.

90. **Jones, A. M., M. E. Todd, and A. K. Webb.** 2001. *Burkholderia cepacia*: current clinical issues, environmental controversies and ethical dilemmas. *Eur. Respir. J.* **17**:295–301.

91. **Jones, A. M., T. N. Stanbridge B. J. Isalaka, M. E. Dodd, and A. K. Webb.** 2001. *Burkholderia gladioli*: recurrent abscesses in patient with cystic fibrosis. *J. Infect.* **42**:69–71.

92. **Kaiser, G. M., P. C. Tso, R. Morris, and D. McCurdy.** 1997. *Xanthomonas maltophilia* endophthalmitis after cataract extraction. *Am. J. Ophthal.* **123**:410–411.

93. **Kanaphun, P., N. Thirawattanasuk, Y. Suputtamongkol, P. Naigowit, D. A. B. Dance, M. D. Smith, and N. J. White.** 1993. Serology and carriage of *Pseudomonas pseudomallei*: a prospective study in 1000 hospitalized children in northeast Thailand. *J. Infect. Dis.* **167**:230–233.

94. **Karpati, F., A. S. Malmborg, H. Alfredsson, L. Hjelte, and B. Strandvik.** 1994. Bacterial colonization with *Xanthomonas maltophilia*—a retrospective study in a cystic fibrosis patient population. *Infection* **22**:258–263.

95. **Keig, P. M., E. Ingham, and K. G. Kerr.** 2001. Invasion of human type II pneumocytes by *Burkholderia cepacia. Microb. Pathog.* **30**:167–170.

96. **Kenny, D. J., P. Russell, D. Rogers, S. M. Eley, and R. W. Titball.** 1999. In vitro susceptibilities of *Burkholderia mallei* in comparison to those of other pathogenic *Burkholderia* spp. *Antimicrob. Agents Chemother.* **43**:2773–2775.

97. **Kersters, K., W. Ludwig, M. Vancanneyt, P. De Vos, M. Gillis, and K. H. Schleifer.** 1996. Recent changes in the classification of the pseudomonads: an overview. *Syst. Appl. Microbiol.* **19**:465–477.

98. **Kiska, D. L., A. Kerr, M. C. Jones, J. A. Caracciolo, B. Eskridge, M. Jordan, S. Miller, D. Hughes, N. King, and P. Gilligan.** 1996. Accuracy of four commercial systems for identification of *Burkholderia cepacia* and other gram-negative nonfermenting bacilli recovered from patients with cystic fibrosis. *J. Clin. Microbiol.* **34**:886–891.

99. **Koneman, E. W., S. D. Allen, W. M. Janda, P. C. Schreckenberger, and W. C. Winn, Jr. (ed.).** 1997. The nonfermentative gram negative bacilli, p. 253–320. *In Color Atlas and Textbook of Diagnostic Microbiology*, 5th ed. Lippincott Williams & Wilkins Co., Philadelphia, Pa.

100. **Koponen, M. A., D. Zlock, D. L. Palmer, and T. L. Merlin.** 1991. Melioidosis. Forgotten, but not gone! *Arch. Intern. Med.* **151**:605–608.

101. **Lacey, S., and S. V. Want.** 1991. *Pseudomonas pickettii* infections in a pediatric oncology unit. *J. Hosp. Infect.* **17**:45–51.

102. **Lath, R., and V. Rajshekhar.** 1998. Brain abscess as the presenting feature of melioidosis. *Br. J. Neurosurg.* **12**: 170–172.

103. **Leelarasamee, A., and S. Bovornkitti.** 1989. Melioidosis: review and update. *Rev. Infect. Dis.* **11**:413–425.

104. **Leff, L. G., R. M. Kernan, J. V. McArthur, and L. J. Shimkets.** 1995. Identification of aquatic *Burkholderia* (*Pseudomonas*) *cepacia* by hybridization with species-specific rRNA gene probes. *Appl. Environ. Microbiol.* **61**:1634–1636.

105. **Lessie, T. G., W. Hendrickson, B. D. Manning, and R. Devereux.** 1996. Genomic complexity and plasticity of *Burkholderia cepacia. FEMS Microbiol. Lett.* **144**:117–128.

106. **Lew, A. E., and P. M. Desmarchelier.** 1993. Molecular typing of *Pseudomonas pseudomallei*: restriction fragment length polymorphisms of rRNA genes. *J. Clin. Microbiol.* **31**:533–539.

107. **Liou, T. G, F. R. Adler, S. C. FitzSimmons, B. C. Cahill, J. R. Hibbs, and Bruce C. Marshall.** 2001. Predictive 5-year survivorship model for cystic fibrosis. *Am. J. Epidemiol.* **153**:345–352.

108. **LiPuma, J. J.** 1998. *Burkholderia cepacia*: management issues and new insights. *Clin. Chest Med.* **19**:473–486.

109. **LiPuma, J. J., B. J. Dulaney, J. D. McMenamin, P. W. Whitby, T. L. Stull, T. Coenye, and P. Vandamme.** 1999. Development of rRNA-based PCR assays for identification of *Burkholderia cepacia* complex isolates recovered from cystic fibrosis patients. *J. Clin. Microbiol.* **37**: 3167–3170.

110. **LiPuma, J. J., L. Spilker, H. Gill, P. W. Campbell III, L. Liu, and E. Mahenthiralingam.** 2001. Disproportionate distribution of *Burkholderia cepacia* complex species and transmissibility marker in cystic fibrosis. *Am. J. Respir. Crit. Care Med.* **163**:92–96.

111. **Lumbiganon, P., U. Tattawasatra, P. Chetchotisakd, S. Wongratanacheewin, and B. Thinkhamrop.** 2000. Comparison between the antimicrobial susceptibility of *Burkholderia pseudomallei* to trimethoprim-sulfamethoxazole by standard disk diffusion method and by minimal inhibitory concentration determination. *J. Med. Assoc. Thai.* **83**:856–860.

112. **Mahenthiralingam, E., J. Bischof, S. K. Byrne, C. Radomski, J. E. Davies, Y. Av-Gay, and P. Vandamme.** 2000. DNA-based diagnostic approaches for the identification of *Burkholderia cepacia* complex, *Burkholderia vietnamiensis, Burkholderia multivorans, Burkholderia stabilis,* and *Burkholderia cepacia* genomovars I and III. *J. Clin. Microbiol.* **38**:3165–3173.

113. **Maki, D. G, B. S. Klein, R. D. McCormick, C. J. Alvarado, M. A. Zilz, S. M. Stolz, C. A. Hassemer, J. Gould, and A. R. Liegel.** 1991. Nosocomial *Pseudomonas pickettii* bacteremias traced to narcotic tampering: a case for selective drug screening of health care personnel. *JAMA* **265**:981–986.

114. **Martino, R., C. Martinez, R. Pericas, R. Salazar, C. Sola, S. Brunet, A. Sureda and A. Domingo-Albos.** 1996. Bacteremia due to glucose non-fermenting gram-negative bacilli in patients with hematological neoplasias and solid tumors. *Eur. J. Clin. Microbiol. Infect. Dis.* **15**:610–615.

115. **McNeil, M. M., S. L. Solomon, R. L. Anderson, B. J. Davis, R. F. Spengler, R. E. Reisberg, C. Thornsberry, and W. J. Martone.** 1985. Nosocomial *Pseudomonas pic-*

116. **Moore, J. E., M. Crowe, A. Shaw, J. McCaughan, A. O. B. Redmond, and J. S. Elborn.** 2001. Antibiotic resistance in *Burkholderia cepacia* at two regional cystic fibrosis centres in Northern Ireland: is there a need for synergy testing? *J. Antimicrob. Chemother.* **48**:315–329.

117. **Moore, J. E., B. McIlhatton, A. Shaw, P. G. Murphy, and J. S. Elborn.** 2001. Occurrence of *Burkholderia cepacia* in foods and waters: clinical implications for patients with cystic fibrosis. *J. Food Prot.* **64**:1076–1078.

118. **Mortensen, J. E., M. C. Fisher, and J. J. LiPuma.** 1995. Recovery of *Pseudomaonas cepacia* and other *Pseudomonas* species from the environment. *Infect. Control Hosp. Epidemiol.* **16**:30–32.

119. **Muder, R. R., A. P. Harris, S. Muller, M. Edmond, J. W. Chow, K. Papadakis, M. W. Wagener, G. P. Bodey, and J. M. Steckelberg.** 1996. Bacteremia due to *Stenotrophomonas maltophilia*: a prospective multicenter study of 91 episodes. *Clin. Infect. Dis.* **22**:508–512.

120. **Mukwaya, G. M., and D. F. Welch.** 1989. Subgrouping of *Pseudomonas cepacia* by cellular fatty acid composition. *J. Clin. Microbiol.* **27**:2640–2646.

121. **National Committee for Clinical Laboratory Standards.** 2000. *Methods for Dilution Antimicrobial Susceptibility Tests for Bacteria That Grow Aerobically. Approved Standard M7-A5.* NCCLS, Wayne, Pa.

122. **National Committee for Clinical Laboratory Standards.** 2002. *Performance Standards for Antimicrobial Susceptibility Testing. Twelfth Informational Supplement. Approved Standard M100-S12.* NCCLS, Wayne, Pa.

123. **Nguyen, M. H., and R. R. Muder.** 1994. Meningitis due to *Xanthomonas maltophilia*: case report and review. *Clin. Infect. Dis.* **19**:325–326.

124. **Norzah, A., M. Y. Rohani, P. T. Chang, and A. G. M. Kamel.** 1996. Indirect hemagglutination antibodies against *Burkholderia pseudomallei* in normal blood donors and suspected cases of melioidosis in Malaysia. *S.E. Asian J. Trop. Med. Public Health* **27**:263–266.

125. **Oberhelman, R. A., J. R. Humbert, and F. W. Santorelli.** 1994. *Pseudomonas vesicularis* causing bacteremia in a child with sickle cell anemia. *South. Med. J.* **87**:821–822.

126. **Otto, L. A., B. S. Deboo, E. L. Capers, and M. J. Pickett.** 1978. *Pseudomonas vesicularis* from cervical specimens. *J. Clin. Microbiol.* **7**:341–345.

127. **Pallent, L. J., W. B. Hugo, D. J. W. Grant, and A. Davies.** 1983. *Pseudomonas cepacia* as contaminant and infective agent. *J. Hosp. Infect.* **4**:9–13.

128. **Palleroni, N. J.** 1984. Genus I. *Pseudomonas* Migula 1894, 237^{AL}, p. 141–199. *In* N. R. Krieg and J. G. Holt (ed.), *Bergey's Manual of Systematic Bacteriology*, vol. 1. The Williams & Wilkins Co., Baltimore, Md.

129. **Palleroni, N. J., and J. F. Bradbury.** 1993. *Stenotrophomonas*, a new bacterial genus for *Xanthomonas maltophilia* (Hugh 1980) Swings et al. *Int. J. Syst. Bacteriol.* **43**:606–609.

130. **Palleroni, N. J., R. Kunisawa, R. Contopoulo, and M. Doudoroff.** 1973. Nucleic acid homologies in the genus *Pseudomonas. Int. J. Syst. Bacteriol.* **23**:333–339.

131. **Papadakis, K. A., S. E. Vartivarian, M. E. Vassilaki, and E. J. Anaissie.** 1995. *Stenotrophomonas maltophilia*: an unusual cause of biliary sepsis. *Clin. Infect. Dis.* **21**:1032–1034.

132. **Parry, C. M., V. Wethiekanum, N. T. T. Hoa, T. S. Diep, L. T. T. Thao, P. V. Loc, B. A. Wills, J. Wain, T. T. Hien, N. J. White, and J. J. Farrar.** 1999. Melioidosis in southern Vietnam: clinical surveillance and

environmental sampling. *Clin. Infect. Dis.* **29**:1323–1326.

133. **Pegues, C. F., D. F. Pegues, D. S. Ford, P. L. Hibberd, L. A. Carson, C. M. Raine, and D. C. Hooper.** 1996. *Burkholderia cepacia* respiratory acquisition: epidemiology and molecular characterization of a large nosocomial outbreak. *Epidemiol. Infect.* **116**:309–317.

134. **Pegues, D. A., L. A. Carson, R. L. Anderson, M. J. Norgard, T. A. Agent, W. R. Jarvis, and C. H. Woernle.** 1993. Outbreak of *Pseudomonas cepacia* bacteremia in oncology patients. *Clin. Infect. Dis.* **16**:407–411.

135. **Penland, R. L., and K. R. Wilhelmus.** 1996. *Stenotrophomonas* ocular infections. *Arch. Ophthalmol.* **114**:433–436.

136. **Phung, L. V., T. B. Tran, H. Hotta, E. Yabuuchi, and I. Yano** 1995. Cellular lipid and fatty acid compositions of *Burkholderia pseudomallei* strains isolated from human and environment in Viet Nam. *Microbiol. Immunol.* **39**:105–116.

137. **Pitkin, D. H., W. Sheikh, and H. L. Nadler.** 1997. Comparative in vitro activity of meropenem versus other extended-spectrum antimicrobials against randomly chosen and selected resistant clinical isolates tested in 26 North American centers. *Clin. Infect. Dis.* **24**(Suppl. 2):S238–S248.

138. **Pitt, T. L., S. Trakulsomboon, and D. A. Dance.** 2000. Molecular phylogeny of *Burkholderia pseudomallei*. *Acta Trop.* **74**:181–185.

139. **Planes, M., A. Ramirez, F. Fernandez, J. A. Capdivila, and C. Tolosa.** 1992. *Pseudomonas vesicularis* bacteremia. *Infection* **20**:367–368.

140. **Rabkin C. S., W. R. Jarvis, R. L. Anderson, J. Govan, J. Kliger, J. LiPuma, W. Jarvis, W. J. Martone, H. Monteil, C. Richard, S. Shigeta, A. Sosa, T. Stull, J. Swenson, and D. Woods.** 1989. *Pseudomonas cepacia* typing systems: collaborative study to assess their potential in epidemiologic investigations. *Rev. Infect. Dis.* **11**:600–607.

141. **Raveh, D., A. Simhon, Z. Gimmon, T. Sacks, and M. Shapiro.** 1993. Infections caused by *Pseudomonas pickettii* in association with permanent indwelling intravenous devices: four cases and a review. *Clin. Infect. Dis.* **17**:877–880.

142. **Reboli, A. C., R. Koshinski, K. Arias, K. Marks-Austin, D. Stiertz, and T. L. Stull.** 1996. An outbreak of *Burkholderia cepacia* lower respiratory tract infection associated with contaminated albuterol nebulization solution. *Infect. Control Hosp. Epidemiol.* **17**:741–743.

143. **Reina, J., I. Llompart, and P. Alomar.** 1991. Acute suppurative otitis caused by *Comamonas acidovorans*. *Clin. Microbiol. Newsl.* **13**:38–39.

144. **Riley, P. S., and R. E. Weaver.** 1975. Recognition of *Pseudomonas pickettii* in the clinical laboratory: biochemical characterization of 62 strains. *J. Clin. Microbiol.* **1**:61–64.

145. **Ross, J. P., S. M. Holland, V. J. Gill, E. S. DeCarlo, and J. I. Gallin.** 1995. Severe *Burkholderia (Pseudomonas) gladioli* infection in chronic granulomatous disease: report of two successfully treated cases. *Clin. Infect. Dis.* **21**:1291–1293.

146. **Sajjan, U., M. Corey, A. Humar, E. Tullis, E. Cutz, C. Ackerley, and J. Fostner.** 2001. Immunolocalisation of *Burkholderia cepacia* in the lungs of cystic fibrosis patients. *J. Med. Microbiol.* **50**:535–546.

147. **Schatz, A., and C. Bovell, Jr.** 1952. Growth and hydrogenase activity of a new bacterium, *Hydrogenomonas facilis*. *J. Bacteriol.* **63**:87–98.

148. **Schülin, T., and I. Steinmetz.** 2001. Chronic melioidosis in a patient with cystic fibrosis. *J. Clin. Microbiol.* **39**:1676–1677.

149. **Segers, P., M. Vancanneyt, B. Pot, U. Torck, B. Hoste, D. Dewettinck, E. Falsen, K. Kersters, and P. De Vos.** 1994. Classification of *Pseudomonas diminuta* Leifson and Hugh 1954 and *Pseudomonas vesicularis* Busing, Doll, and Freytag 1953 in *Brevundimonas* gen. nov. as *Brevundimonas diminuta* comb. nov. and *Brevundimonas vesicularis* comb. nov., respectively. *Int. J. Syst. Bacteriol.* **44**:499–510.

150. **Segonds, C., T. Heulin, N. Marty, and G. Chabanon.** 1999. Differentiation of *Burkholderia* species by PCR-restriction fragment length polymorphism analysis of the 16S rRNA gene and application to cystic fibrosis isolates. *J. Clin. Microbiol.* **37**:2201–2208.

151. **Shelly, D. B., T. Spilker, E. J. Gracely, T. Coenye, P. Vandamme, and J. J. LiPuma.** 2000. Utility of commercial systems for identification of *Burkholderia cepacia* complex from cystic fibrosis sputum culture. *J. Clin. Microbiol.* **38**:3112–3115.

152. **Simpson, A. J., Y. Suputtamongkol, M. D. Smith, B. J. Angus, A. Rajanuwong, V. Wuthiekanun, P. A. Howe, A. L. Walsh, W. Chaowagul, and N. J. White.** 1999. Comparison of imipenem and ceftazidime as therapy for severe melioidosis. *Clin. Infect. Dis.* **29**:381–387.

153. **Smith, D. L., L. B. Gumery, E. G. Smith, D. E. Stableforth, M. E. Kaufmann, and T. L. Pitt.** 1993. Epidemic of *Pseudomonas cepacia* in an adult cystic fibrosis unit: evidence of person-to-person transmission. *J. Clin. Microbiol.* **31**:3017–3022.

154. **Smith, M. D., V. Wuthiekanun, A. L. Walsh, N. Teerawattanasook, V. Desakorn, Y. Suputtamongkol, T. L. Pitt, and N. J. White.** 1995. Latex agglutination for rapid detection of *Pseudomonas pseudomallei* antigen in urine of patients with melioidosis. *J. Clin. Pathol.* **48**:174–176.

155. **Smith, M. D., V. Wuthiekanun, A. L. Walsh, and N. J. White.** 1994. Susceptibility of *Pseudomonas pseudomallei* to some newer beta-lactam antibiotics and antibiotic combinations using time-kill studies. *J. Antimicrob. Chemother.* **33**:145–149.

156. **Sookpranee, M., P. Boonma, W. Susaengrat, K. Bhuripanyo, and S. Punyagupta.** 1992. Multicenter prospective randomized trial comparing ceftazidime plus co-trimoxazole with chloramphenicol plus doxycycline and co-trimoxazole for treatment of severe melioidosis. *Antimicrob. Agents Chemother.* **36**:158–162.

157. **Sookpranee, T., M. Sookpranee, M. A. Mellencamp, and L. C. Preheim.** 1991. *Pseudomonas pseudomallei*, a common pathogen in Thailand that is resistant to the bactericidal effects of many antibiotics. *Antimicrob. Agents Chemother.* **35**:484–489.

158. **Spencer, R. C.** 1995. The emergence of epidemic, multiple-antibiotic resistant *Stenotrophomonas maltophilia* and *Burkholderia cepacia*. *J. Hosp. Infect.* **30**(Suppl.):453–464.

159. **Spraul, C. W., G. E. Lang, and G. K. Lang.** 1996. *Xanthomonas maltophilia* keratitis associated with contact lenses. *CLAO J.* **22**:158.

160. **Stampi, S., F. Zanetti, A. Bergamaschi, and G. De Luca.** 1999. *Comamonas acidovorans* contamination of dental water units. *Lett. Appl. Microbiol.* **29**:52–55.

161. **Stead, D. E.** 1992. Grouping of plant-pathogenic and some other *Pseudomonas* spp. by using cellular fatty acid profiles. *Int. J. Syst. Bacteriol.* **42**:281–285.

162. **Sun, L., R.-Z. Jiang, S. Steinbach, A. Holmes, C. Campanelli, J. Forstner, U. Sajjan, Y. Tan, M. Riley, and R. Goldstein.** 1995. The emergence of a highly transmissi-

ble lineage of cbl⁺ *Pseudomonas* (*Burkholderia*) *cepacia* causing CF centre epidemics in North America and Britain. *Nat. Med.* **1:**661–666.

163. **Suputtamongkol, Y., A. Rajchanuwong, W. Chaowagul, D. A. Dance, M. D. Smith, V. Wuthiekanun, A. L. Walsh, S. Pukrittayakamee, and N. J. White.** 1994. Ceftazidime vs. amoxicillin/clavulanate in the treatment of severe melioidosis. *Clin. Infect. Dis.* **19:** 846–853.

164. **Swing, J., P. de Vos, M. van den Mooter, and J. de Ley.** 1983. Transfer of *Pseudomonas maltophilia* Hugh 1981 to the genus *Xanthomonas* as *Xanthomonas maltophilia* (Hugh 1981) comb. nov. *Int. J. Syst. Bacteriol.* **33:**409–413.

165. **Szeto, C. C., P. K. Li, C. B. Leung, A. W. Yu, S. F. Lui, and K. N. Lai.** 1997. *Xanthomonas maltophilia* peritonitis in uremic patients receiving continuous ambulatory peritoneal dialysis. *Am. J. Kidney Dis.* **29:**91–95.

166. **Tamaoka, J., D. M. Ha, and K. Komagata.** 1987. Reclassification of *Pseudomonas acidovorans* den Dooren de Jong 1926 and *Pseudomonas testosteroni* Marcus and Talalay 1956 as *Comamonas acidovorans* comb. nov. and *Comamonas testosteroni* comb. nov., with an emended description of the genus *Comamonas*. *Int. J. Syst. Bacteriol.* **37:**52–59.

167. **Tiangitayakorn, C., S. Songsivilai, N. Piyasangthong, and T. Dharakul.** 1997. Speed of detection of *Burkholderia pseudomallei* in blood cultures and its correlation with clinical outcome. *Am J. Trop. Med.* **57:**96–99.

168. **Van Couwenberghe, C., and S. Cohen.** 1994. Analysis of epidemic and endemic isolates of *Xanthomonas maltophilia* by contour clamped homogeneous electric field gel electrophoresis. *Infect. Control Hosp. Epidemiol.* **15:**691–696.

169. **Vandamme, P., J. Goris, T. Coenye, B. Hoste, D. Janssens, K. Kersters, P. De Vos, and E. Falsen.** 1999. Assignment of Centers for Disease Control group IVc-2 to the genus *Ralstonia* as *Ralstonia paucula* sp. nov. *Int. J. Syst. Bacteriol.* **49:**663–669.

170. **Vandamme, P., D. Henry, T. Coenye, S. Nzula, M. Vancanneyt, J. J. LiPuma, D. P. Speert, J. R. W. Govan, and E. Mahenthiralingam.** 2002. *Burkholderia anthina* sp. nov. and *Burkholderia pyrrocinia*, two additional *Burkholderia cepacia* complex bacteria, may confound results of new molecular diagnostic tools. *FEMS Immunol. Med. Microbiol.* **33:**143–149.

171. **Vandamme, P., B. Holmes, M. Vancanneyt, T. Coenye, B. Hoste, R. Coopman, H. Revets, S. Lauwers, M. Gillis, K. Kersters, and J. R. W. Govan.** 1997. Occurrence of multiple genomovars of *Burkholderia cepacia* in cystic fibrosis patients and proposal of *Burkholderia multivorans* sp. nov. *Int. J. Syst. Bacteriol.* **47:**1188–1200.

172. **Vandamme, P., E. Mahenthiralingam, B. Holmes, T. Coenye, B. Hoste, P. De Vos, D. Henry, and D. P. Speert.** 2000. Identification and population structure of *Burkholderia stabilis* sp. nov. (formerly *Burkholderia cepacia* genomovar IV). *J. Clin. Microbiol.* **38:**1042–1047.

173. **Vanholder, R., E. Vanhaecke, and S. Ringoir.** 1992. *Pseudomonas* septicemia due to deficient disinfectant mixing during reuse. *Int. J. Artif. Organs* **15:**19–24.

174. **van Pelt, C., C. M. Verduin, W. H. F. Goessens, M. C. Vos, B. Tümmler, C. Segonds, F. Reubsaet, H. Verbrugh, and A. van Belkum.** 1999. Identification of *Burkholderia* spp. in the clinical microbiology laboratory: comparison of conventional and molecular methods. *J. Clin. Microbiol.* **37:**2158–2164.

175. **Vartivarian, S. E., K. A. Papadakis, J. A. Palacios, J. T. Manning, and E. J. Anaissie.** 1994. Mucocutaneous and soft tissue infections caused by *Xanthomonas maltophilia*. A new spectrum. *Ann. Intern. Med.* **121:**969–973.

176. **Vartivarian, S. E., K. A. Papadakis, and E. J. Anaissie.** 1996. *Stenotrophomonas maltophilia* urinary tract infection. A disease that is usually severe and complicated. *Arch. Intern. Med.* **156:**433–435.

177. **Verschraegen, G., G. Claeys, G. Meeus, and M. Delanghe.** 1985. *Pseudomonas pickettii* as a cause of pseudobacteremia. *J. Clin. Microbiol.* **21:**278–279.

178. **Visca, P., G. Cazzola, A. Petrucca, and C. Braggion.** 2001. Travel-associated *Burkholderia pseudomallei* infection (melioidosis) in a patient with cystic fibrosis: a case report. *Clin. Infect. Dis.* **32:**15–16.

179. **Vu-Thien, H., D. Moissenet, M. Valcin, C. Dulot, G. Tournier, and A. Garbarg-Chenon.** 1996. Molecular epidemiology of *Burkholderia cepacia*, *Stenotrophomonas maltophilia* and *Alcaligenes xylosoxidans* in a cystic fibrosis center. *Eur. J. Clin. Microbiol. Infect. Dis.* **15:**876–879.

180. **Walsh, A. L., M. D. Smith, V. Wuthiekanun, Y. Suputtamongkol, V. Desakorn, W. Chaowagul, and N. J. White.** 1994. Immunofluorescence microscopy for the rapid diagnosis of melioidosis. *J. Clin. Pathol.* **47:**377–379.

181. **Walsh, A. L., and V. Wuthiekanun.** 1996. The laboratory diagnosis of melioidosis. *Br. J. Biomed. Sci.* **53:**249–253.

182. **Walsh, A. L., V. Wuthiekanun, M. D. Smith, Y. Suputtamongkol, and N. J. White.** 1995. Selective broths for the isolation of *Pseudomonas pseudomallei* from clinical samples. *Trans. R. Soc. Trop. Med. Hyg.* **89:**124.

183. **Welch, D. F., M. J. Muszynski, C. H. Pai, M. J. Marcon, M. M. Hribar, P. H. Gilligan, J. M. Matsen, P. A. Ahlin, B. C. Hilman, and S. A. Chartrand.** 1987. Selective and differential medium for recovery of *Pseudomonas cepacia* from the respiratory tracts of patients with cystic fibrosis. *J. Clin. Microbiol.* **25:**1730–1734.

184. **Wen, A., M. Fegan, C. Hayward, S. Chakraborty, and L. I. Sly.** 1999. Phylogenetic relationships among members of the *Comamonadaceae*, and description of *Delftia acidovorans* (den Dooren de Jong 1926 and Tamaoka *et al.* 1987) gen. nov., comb. nov. *Int. J. Syst. Bacteriol.* **49:** 567–576.

185. **Wertheim, W. A., and D. M. Markovitz.** 1992. Osteomyelitis and intervertebral discitis caused by *Pseudomonas pickettii*. *J. Clin. Microbiol.* **30:**2506–2508.

186. **Weyant, R. S., C. W. Moss, R. E. Weaver, D. G. Hollis, J. G. Jordan, E. C. Cook, and M. I. Daneshvar.** 1996. *Identification of Unusual Pathogenic Gram-Negative Aerobic and Facultatively Anaerobic Bacteria*, 2nd ed. The Williams & Wilkins Co., Baltimore, Md.

187. **Whitby, P. W., K. B. Carter, J. L. Burns, J. A. Royall, J. J. LiPuma, and T. L. Stull.** 2000. Identification and detection of *Stenotrophomonas maltophilia* by rRNA-directed PCR. *J. Clin. Microbiol.* **38:**4305–4309.

188. **Whitby, P., K. B. Carter, K. L. Hatter, J. J. LiPuma, and T. L. Stull.** 2000. Identification of members of the *Burkholderia cepacia* complex by species-specific PCR. *J. Clin. Microbiol.* **38:**2962–2965.

189. **Willems, A., J. DeLay, M. Gillis, and K. Kersters.** 1991. *Comamonadaceae*, a new family encompassing the acidovorans rRNA complex, including *Variovorax paradoxus* gen. nov., comb nov., for *Alcaligenes paradoxus* (Davis 1969). *Int. J. Syst. Bacteriol.* **41:**445–450.

190. **Willems, A., E. Falsen, B. Pot, B. Hoste, P. Vandamme, M. Gillis, K. Kersters, and J. De Ley.** 1990. *Acidovorax*, a new genus for *Pseudomonas facilis*, *Pseudomonas delafieldii*, E. Falsen (EF) group 13, EF group 16 and several clinical isolates with the species *Acidovorax* comb. nov., *Acidovorax delafieldii* comb. nov., and *Acidovorax temperans* sp. nov. *Int. J. Syst. Bacteriol.* **40:**384–398.

191. Winkelstein, J. A., M. C. Marino, R. B. Johnston, Jr., J. Boyle, J. Curnutte, J. I. Gallin, H. L. Malech, S. M. Holland, H. Ochs, P. Quie, R. H. Buckley, C. B. Foster, S. J. Chanock, and H. Dickler. 2000. Chronic granulomatous disease. *Medicine* **79:**155–159.

192. Winton, M. D., E. D. Everett, and S. A. Dolan. 1988. Activities of five new fluoroquinolones against *Pseudomonas pseudomalleii. Antimicrob. Agents Chemother.* **32:** 928–929.

193. Woods, M. L., Jr., B. J. Currie, D. M. Howard, A. Tierney, A. Watson, N. M. Anstey, J. Philpott, V. Asche, and K. Withnall. 1992. Neurological melioidosis: seven cases from the Northern Territory of Australia. *Clin. Infect. Dis.* **15:**163–169.

194. Wuthiekanun, V., D. A. Dance, Y. Wattanagoon, Y. Supputtamongkol, W. Chaowagul, and N. J. White. 1990. The use of selective media for the isolation of *Pseudomonas pseudomallei* in clinical practice. *J. Med. Microbiol.* **33:**121–126.

195. Yabuuchi, E., Y. Kawamura, T. Ezaki, M. Ikedo, S. Dejsirilert, N. Fujiwara, T. Naka, and K. Kobayashi. 2000. *Burkholderia uboniae* sp. nov., L-arabinose assimilating but different from *Burkholderia thailandensis* and *Burkholderia vietnamiensis. Microbiol. Immunol.* **44:**307–317.

196. Yabuuchi, E., Y. Kosako, H. Oyaizu, I. Yano, H. Hotta, Y. Hashimoto, T. Ezaki, and M. Arakawa. 1992. Proposal of *Burkholderia* gen. nov; and transfer of seven species of the *Pseudomonas* homology group II to the new genus, with the type species *Burkholderia cepacia* (Palleroni and Holmes 1981) comb. nov. *Microbiol. Immunol.* **36:**1251–1275.

197. Yabuuchi, E., Y. Kosako, I. Yano, H. Hotta, and Y. Nishiuchi. 1995. Transfer of two *Burkholderia* and an *Alcaligenes* species to *Ralstonia* gen. nov.: proposal of *Ralstonia pickettii* (Ralston, Palleroni and Doudoroff 1973) comb. nov., *Ralstonia solanacearum* (Smith 1896) comb. nov. and *Ralstonia eutropha* (Davis 1969) comb. nov. *Microbiol. Immunol.* **39:**897–904.

198. Yao, J. D., M. Louie, L. Louie, J. Goodfellow, and A. E. Simor. 1995. Comparison of E test and agar dilution for antimicrobial susceptibility testing of *Stenotrophomonas maltophilia. J. Clin. Microbiol.* **33:**1428–1430.

Acinetobacter, Achromobacter, Chryseobacterium, Moraxella, and Other Nonfermentative Gram-Negative Rods*

PAUL C. SCHRECKENBERGER, MARYAM I. DANESHVAR,
ROBBIN S. WEYANT, AND DANNIE G. HOLLIS

49

The organisms covered in this chapter belong to a group of taxonomically diverse nonfermentative gram-negative bacilli. They all share the common phenotypic features of failing to acidify the butt of Kligler or triple sugar iron agar or of oxidative-fermentative media and grow significantly better under aerobic than under anaerobic conditions; many strains fail to grow anaerobically. The organisms covered in this chapter are either nonmotile or motile, often with peritrichous flagella; oxidase and growth on MacConkey agar are variable and, with the exception of *Neisseria elongata* subsp. *elongata* and *nitroreducens*, they are catalase positive.

Methods used to grow and identify the members of this group are those used for *Pseudomonas* spp. (see chapter 47). Initial incubation should be at 35 to 37°C, although many pink-pigmented strains grow better at ≤30°C and may be detected only on plates left at room temperature after the initial readings are taken. In such cases, all identification tests should be carried out at that temperature. In fact, some of the commercial kits, such as the API20 NE, are designed to be incubated at 30°C. Growth on certain selective primary media (e.g., MacConkey or salmonella-shigella agar) is variable; there can be significant lot-to-lot variations in the media. Nonfermenters that grow on MacConkey agar generally form colorless colonies.

Although certain nonfermenting bacilli (NFBs) are on occasion frank pathogens, e.g., *Pseudomonas aeruginosa*, *Burkholderia pseudomallei*, and *Chryseobacterium meningosepticum*, NFBs are generally considered to be of low virulence and often occur in mixed cultures, making it difficult to determine when to work up cultures and when to perform susceptibility studies. Decisions regarding the significance of NFBs in a clinical specimen must take into account the clinical condition of the patient and the source of the specimen submitted for culture. In general, the recovery of an NFB in pure culture from a normally sterile site warrants identification and susceptibility testing whereas predominant growth of an NFB from a nonsterile specimen, such as a culture of an endotracheal specimen from a patient with no clinical signs or symptoms of pneumonia, would not be

worked up further. Because many NFBs exhibit multiple antibiotic resistance, patients taking antibiotics often become colonized with NFBs. NFB species isolated in mixed cultures can usually be reported by descriptive identification, e.g., "growth of *P. aeruginosa* and two varieties of nonfermenting gram-negative bacilli not further identified." The Gram stain made from the clinical material should be used to guide the laboratory decision on how far to work up the specimen.

Decisions about performing susceptibility testing are complicated by the fact that there are no National Committee for Clinical Laboratory Standards (NCCLS) interpretive guidelines for disk diffusion testing of the organisms included in this chapter except for *Acinetobacter* species. Furthermore, results obtained with certain organisms (e.g., *Chryseobacterium* species) by disk diffusion and E-test methods do not correlate with results obtained by conventional MIC methods (See "*Chryseobacterium*" below). In general, laboratories should try to avoid performing susceptibility testing on the organisms included in this chapter. When clinical necessity dictates that susceptibility testing be performed, an overnight MIC method is recommended.

When laboratory identification of this group of organisms is deemed necessary, a simplified approach is recommended whereby unknown isolates are initially characterized and placed into one of eight groups based on microscopic morphology, oxidase reaction, motility, acidification of carbohydrates, requirement of NaCl for growth, indole production, and production of pink-pigmented colonies (Fig. 1). Further characterization is made on the basis of the biochemical reactions given in Tables 1 through 8. Additional differential tests can be found in other publications (120, 174, 212). Carbon assimilation is determined in mineral basal medium as described in chapter 27. In our experience, indole production is best demonstrated by inoculation of heart infusion broth and incubation at 35 to 37°C followed by extraction with xylene and addition of Ehrlich's reagent. The oxidase test is performed using N,N,N,N-tetramethyl-p-phenylenediamine dihydrochloride (0.5%). Motility is easily determined by using a wet mount preparation of a young colony from a blood agar plate. For some strains, motility can best be demonstrated after incubation of cultures at room temperature.

Traditional diagnostic systems, e.g., those based on oxidative-fermentative media, aerobic low-peptone media, or

* This chapter contains information presented in chapter 35 by Paul C. Schreckenberger and Alexander von Graevenitz in the seventh edition of this Manual.

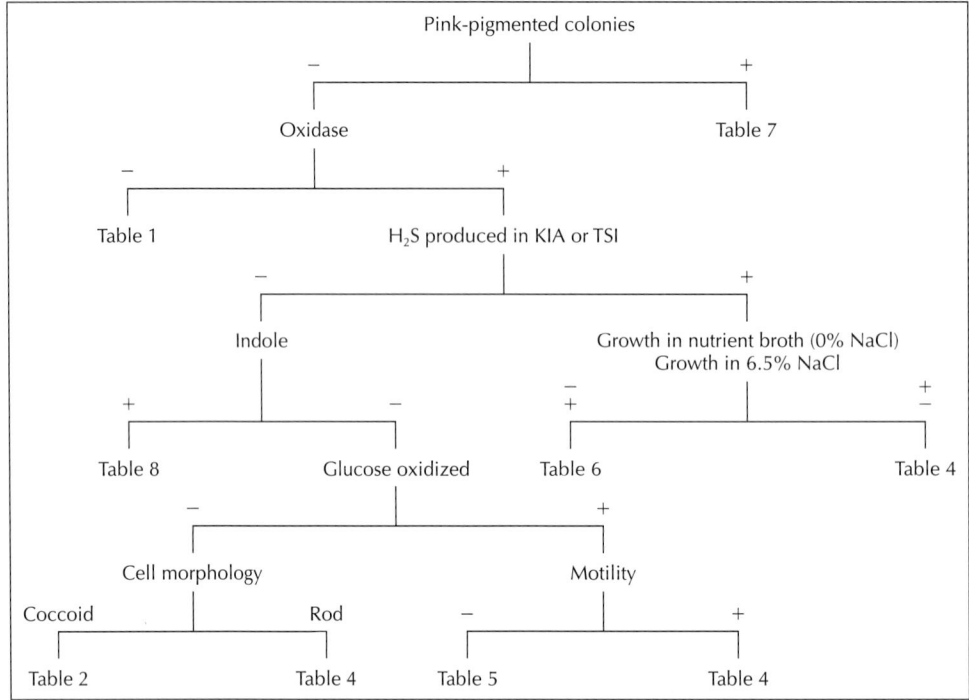

FIGURE 1 Identification of miscellaneous gram-negative nonfermenters. KIA, Kligler iron agar; TSI, triple sugar iron agar.

buffered single substrates, have now been replaced in many laboratories by commercial kits. The ability of commercial kits to identify this group of nonfermenters is variable and often results in an identification to the genus or group level only, necessitating the use of supplemental biochemical testing for species identification (12, 105, 117, 124, 144, 186). If such kits are used, the laboratory must be familiar with the extent of the database; organisms not included will be unidentified or identified incorrectly. Because assimilation test results often depend on the basal medium used, most of those results are not included in the tables presented here. Identification of nonfermenters by automated fatty acid analysis has also been attempted (202). In view of the difficulties inherent in this approach (145), it is recommended that fatty acid profiles be used only in conjunction with traditional or commercial diagnostic systems. The fatty acid profiles for the most common species of nonfermenting bacilli have been published by Weyant et al. (212) and are included in the tables presented here. In recent years, it has become possible to use 16S rRNA gene sequence information to identify unusual gram-negative nonfermenters in reference laboratories (68). The impact of this technology will probably be reflected in future editions of this Manual.

OXIDASE-NEGATIVE GROUP
See Table 1.

Acinetobacter spp.

General Description
The genus *Acinetobacter* consists of strictly aerobic, gram-negative coccobacillary rods that are oxidase negative, non-

motile, usually nitrate negative, and nonfermentative. Individual cells are 1 to 1.5 by 1.5 to 2.5 μm in size, sometimes difficult to decolorize, and frequently arranged in pairs. Clinical microbiologists should be alert to the fact that *Acinetobacter* species may initially appear as gram-positive cocci in direct smears prepared from positive blood culture bottles (B. J. Harrington, Letter, *Clin. Microbiol. Newsl.* **19:**191, 1997). In the stationary growth phase and on nonselective agars, coccobacillary forms predominate, while early growth in fluid media and growth on plates containing cell wall-active antimicrobial agents yield mostly rods. Colonies are smooth, opaque, and slightly smaller than those of members of the family *Enterobacteriaceae*. Many strains grow on MacConkey agar as either colorless or slightly pinkish colonies. Some strains are fastidious, showing punctate colonies on blood agar, and fail to grow in nutrient broth (212). Certain glucose-oxidizing acinetobacters may also cause a unique brown discoloration of heart infusion agar with tyrosine or blood agar into which glucose is incorporated (179, 212). We have also observed this phenomenon on MacConkey and Mueller-Hinton agars with a clinical isolate of *A. baumannii*. Differential and selective media have been described for isolation of *Acinetobacter* spp. from contaminated specimens (86, 100).

Taxonomy
The genus was originally placed within the family *Neisseriaceae* but has since been moved to the family *Moraxellaceae* (169). Studies based on DNA-DNA hybridization have resulted in the description of 25 DNA homology groups (also called genomospecies) within the genus *Acinetobacter* (19, 21, 60, 97, 140, 141, 190). While only 10 species have been named (19, 140, 141), differential bio-

chemical and growth tests have been published for at least 19 species (19, 21, 61, 140, 141). However, the authors feel that the majority of the genomospecies cannot be separated reliably by phenotypic tests. Most published reactions are based on five or fewer isolates. Genomospecies 1, 2, 3, and 13 of Tjernberg and Ursing (190) may be difficult to separate in the clinical laboratory and have been referred to as the *Acinetobacter calcoaceticus-Acinetobacter baumannii* complex (61). Because of problems in the clinical laboratory in separating the DNA groups by phenotypic tests, we have chosen to separate the *Acinetobacter* species in Table 1 into two groups, saccharolytic and asaccharolytic. Most glucose-oxidizing nonhemolytic clinical strains are *A. baumannii*, most glucose-negative nonhemolytic ones are *Acinetobacter lwoffii*, and most hemolytic ones are *Acinetobacter haemolyticus*. A transformation assay has been described that can be used for genus level identification of *Acinetobacter* (106).

Natural Habitat and Clinical Significance

Acinetobacter species are widely distributed in nature and in the hospital environment, are the second most commonly isolated nonfermenters in human specimens (*P. aeruginosa* being the first), are able to survive on moist and dry surfaces (62), and may be present in foodstuffs (88) and on healthy human skin (175). *Acinetobacter* spp. are generally considered to be nonpathogenic to healthy individuals but may cause infections in debilitated individuals. The species most frequently isolated from humans is *A. baumannii* (with 19 biotypes identified by assimilation tests [20] and 34 serovars [191]), followed by *A. lwoffii*, *A. haemolyticus*, *Acinetobacter johnsonii*, genomospecies 3 (with 26 serovars [191]), and genomospecies 6 (22, 109, 175, 190). *Acinetobacter ursingii* causes bloodstream infections in hospitalized patients (140), and rare cases of infection caused by *Acinetobacter junii*, particularly in pediatric patients, have been reported (11, 110, 158). A case of community-acquired *Acinetobacter radioresistens* bacteremia in a human immunodeficiency virus-positive patient has also been reported (205).

The ability of this microorganism to acquire antimicrobial multiresistance and its high capacity for survival on most environmental surfaces has led to an increased concern regarding hospital-acquired infections. Corbella et al. have shown that the digestive tract of intensive care unit patients is an important epidemiologic reservoir for multiresistant *A. baumannii* infections in hospital outbreaks, and they suggest that a fecal surveillance program might be considered for early implementation of patient isolation precautions in an outbreak setting (39). Hospital-acquired infections are most likely to involve the respiratory tract (most often related to endotracheal tubes or tracheostomies), urinary tract, and wounds (including catheter sites) and may progress to septicemia (9, 11, 36, 56, 176, 203, 213). Sporadic cases of continuous ambulatory peritoneal dialysis peritonitis, endocarditis, meningitis, osteomyelitis, arthritis, and corneal perforation have also been reported (9, 103, 158). There are an increasing number of reports of *Acinetobacter* species as agents of nosocomial pneumonia, particularly ventilator-associated pneumonia in patients confined to hospital intensive care units (9). Risk factors are antibiotic treatment and/or surgery, instrumentation, mechanical ventilation, and stay in intensive care units; clinical isolates, however, are more often colonizers than infecting agents (9, 36, 213). Hospital outbreaks have been investigated by various typing methods (11, 67, 119, 126). Community-acquired *Acinetobacter* pneumonias have also

been reported in which a fatal outcome was strongly associated with inappropriate initial antibiotic therapy (2).

Antibiotic Susceptibility

Cephalothin is ineffective against *Acinetobacter* spp., while trimethoprim-sulfamethoxazole, imipenem, imipenem-cilastatin, ampicillin-sulbactam, ticarcillin-clavulanate, piperacillin-tazobactam, amoxicillin-clavulanate, doxycycline, and quinolones are effective against most strains (9, 36, 59, 101, 103, 204), but susceptibility testing is required for each clinically significant strain. Multiply resistant strains including carbapenem-resistant *Acinetobacter* species have been reported in nosocomial outbreaks (18, 131, 214). Although the carbapenems are still the most active antimicrobials against *Acinetobacter* species, nearly 11% of the nosocomial isolates have been reported resistant to this drug group (59).

CDC Group EO-5

CDC eugonic oxidizer group 5 (EO-5) (M. I. Daneshvar, D. G. Hollis, C. W. Moss, J. G. Jordan, J. P. MacGregor, and R. S. Weyant, *Abstr. 98th Gen. Meet. Am. Soc. Microbiol. 1998*, abstr. C-204, p. 165, 1998) consists of glucose-oxidizing gram-negative rods that have a biochemical profile similar to *A. baumannii*. They are nonmotile and oxidase negative, but unlike *Acinetobacter* species, they fail to grow on MacConkey agar. Some strains produce a yellow soluble pigment. Cellular fatty acid analysis is also useful in differentiating EO-5 strains from *Acinetobacter*. Other characteristics are given in Table 1. Isolates have been recovered from blood, peritoneal fluid, transtracheal aspirate, gallbladder, and an arm wound (Daneshvar et al., *Abstr. 98th Gen. Meet. Am. Soc. Microbiol. 1998*). Antibiotic susceptibility data are not available.

CDC Group NO-1

CDC nonoxidizer group 1 (NO-1) bacteria (71) are oxidase negative, asaccharolytic, nonmotile, coccoid to medium-sized gram-negative rods that form small colonies on sheep blood agar (SBA). Other differential features are shown in Table 1. Nitrate, but not nitrite, is reduced; however, since approximately 6% of asaccharolytic *Acinetobacter* spp. reduce nitrate, the definitive differential test between the two groups is the transformation assay (106, 212), which is negative with group NO-1. Cellular fatty acid profiles are also useful in making this differentiation. Most strains have been isolated from human wounds resulting from dog or cat bites (108). They are susceptible to antibiotics used for infections by gram-negative organisms, including aminoglycosides, β-lactam antibiotics, tetracyclines, quinolones, and sulfonamides (71).

Bordetella spp.

The *Bordetella* species are discussed in detail in chapter 50. There are six *Bordetella* spp. that are nonfastidious and grow on ordinary culture media (i.e., sheep blood and MacConkey agars) and biochemically resemble either *Acinetobacter* spp. or *Alcaligenes* spp. This is the reason these organisms are included in this chapter. Three species (*B. holmesii*, *B. parapertussis*, and *B. trematum*) are oxidase negative and are included in Table 1, and three species are oxidase positive (*B. avium*, *B. bronchiseptica*, and *B. hinzii*) and are included in Table 3. *B. holmesii* (formerly CDC group NO-2) is nitrate negative (differentiating it from NO-1 strains) and produces a brown soluble pigment on heart infusion-tyrosine agar. Other differential tests are given in Table 1.

TABLE 1 Oxidase-negative group[a]

| Test | Acinetobacter species[b] | | CDC group EO-5 (10) | CDC group NO-1 (22) | Bordetella holmesii (13) | Bordetella parapertussis (12) | Bordetella trematum (1) | Pseudomonas oryzihabitans[c] (36) | Pseudomonas luteola[c] (34) | Massilia timonae[d] (1) |
	Asaccharolytic (270)	Saccharolytic (77)								
Motility; flagella	0	0	0	0	0	0	100; pe	100; p. 1–2	100; p. >2	100; p. 1
Acid from:[e]										
D-Glucose	0	95 (5)	100	0[f]	0	0	0	100	100	0
D-Xylose	<1	98	100	0	0	0	0	100	100	0
D-Mannitol	0	0	0	0	0	0	0	100	76 (18)	0
Lactose	0	62 (13)	0	0	0	0	0	14 (22)	3 (24)	0
Sucrose	0	0	0	0	0	0	0	25	12	0
Maltose	0	17 (37)	0	0	0	0	0	97 (3)	100	0
Catalase	>99	100	100	100	38	100	100	94	100	100
Growth on:										
MacConkey	74 (4)	96	10w	5 (15)	77 (23)	100	100	100	100	100
Salmonella-shigella	9 (2)	10 (2)	0	0	0	0	100	22	68	ND
Cetrimide	<1	2	0	0	0	0	0	25 (28)	0	ND
Simmons citrate	30 (3)	63 (3)	0	0	0	67 (8)	100w	97	100	0
Urea, Christensen's	8 (18)	22 (24)	(10w)	5w	0	100	0	77	26 (38)	0
Nitrate reduction	6	8	0	100	0	0	0[i]	6	62	0
H₂S (lead acetate paper)	51	38	50	5, 45w	62	17	100	97	12	ND
Gelatin hydrolysis[g]	2	6	0	0	0	0	0	17	61	100

Characteristic										
Pigment:										
Insoluble	0	0	0	0	0	0	0	100 yel	97 yel	100 st
Soluble	12 yel-tan	22 br-yel-tan	20 yel	0	100 br	100 br	0	0	0	0
Growth at:										
25°C	98	100	90	20	67	60	100	100	100	100
35°C	98	100	90	100	100	100	100	100	100	100
42°C	48	72	0	15	0	18	0	33	94	ND
Esculin hydrolysis	0	0	0	0	0	0	0	0	100	100
Lysine decarboxylase	0	10	0	0	0	ND	0	7	0	ND
Arginine dihydrolase	9, 6w	19	0	0	0	ND	0	14	100	100
Ornithine decarboxylase	0	5	0	0	0	ND	0	3	0	ND
Nutrient broth, 0% NaCl	86 (1)	99	90	10 (5)	46 (15)	92	100	100	100	100
Nutrient broth, 6% NaCl	19	13	0	0	0	0	100	62	74 (3)	0
Major CFAs[h]	16:0[i], 16:1ω7c, 18:1ω9c	16:0[i], 16:1ω7c, 18:1ω9c	16:0, 18:1ω7c	16:0, 16:1ω7c, 18:1ω7c	16:0, 17:0cyc	16:0, 17:0cyc	16:0, 17:0cyc	16:0, 16:1ω7c, 18:1ω7c	16:0, 16:1ω7c, 18:1ω7c	16:0, 16:1ω7c

[a] Unless otherwise indicated, data are from the CDC Special Bacteriology Reference Laboratory (212). All taxa were negative (<10% positive) for gas from nitrate, nitrite reduction, indole production, acid in triple sugar iron slant or butt, and H_2S in triple sugar iron. Numbers in parentheses after the organisms indicate the number of strains. Numbers indicate the percentage of strains. Numbers indicate the percentage positive at 2 days of incubation; parentheses indicate a delayed reaction (3 to 7 days of incubation); w, weak reaction; pe, peritrichous; p, polar; br, brown; yel, yellow; st, straw color; ND, not determined or not available.

[b] A total of 25 *Acinetobacter* genomospecies have been described. See the text.

[c] Included in the table only; the description is covered in chapter 47.

[d] Data from reference 121.

[e] Oxidative-fermentative basal medium with 1% carbohydrate.

[f] Usually does not grow in oxidative-fermentative medium.

[g] 14 days of incubation.

[h] CFA, cellular fatty acid. The number before the colon indicates the number of carbons; the number after the colon is the number of double bonds; ω, the position of the double bond counting from the hydrocarbon end of the carbon chain; c, cis isomer; cyc, a cyclopropane ring structure.

[i] Cannot distinguish most *Acinetobacter* species by CFA (109).

[j] Nitrate reduction reported variable by other authors (see chapter 50).

B. bronchiseptica is rapid urease positive and must be differentiated from *Ralstonia paucula* (see Table 3) and *Oligella ureolytica* (see Table 2).

Massilia timonae

M. timonae is an actively motile (one polar flagellum), strictly aerobic gram-negative rod that is oxidase negative, catalase positive, and asaccharolytic. Additional phenotypic characteristics are given in Table 1. Colonies appear pale yellow, are distinctively tenacious on agar media, and have a tendency to form flocs and films in liquid medium (121). Isolates have been recovered from a surgical wound and the blood of a patient with common variable immunodeficiency (121, 182). *M. timonae* is susceptible to most antibiotics, with resistance reported to ampicillin, cephalothin, and aztreonam (121, 182).

OXIDASE-POSITIVE, INDOLE-NEGATIVE, ASACCHAROLYTIC COCCOID-SHAPED NONFERMENTERS

See Table 2.

Moraxella spp. and Psychrobacter phenylpyruvicus

The classification of species belonging to the family *Moraxellaceae* is still evolving and has been reviewed by Pettersson et al. (150). Members of the genus *Moraxella* are oxidase-positive, nonmotile, asaccharolytic coccobacilli that are often plump, occur predominantly in pairs and sometimes in short chains, and have a tendency to resist decolorization (43).

Moraxellae are parasitic on human skin and mucous membranes. *Moraxella osloensis*, *Moraxella nonliquefaciens*, and *M. lincolnii* are part of the normal flora of the human respiratory tract, while most *M. canis* strains have been found in the upper respiratory tracts of dogs and cats. These and other moraxellae are rare agents of infections (conjunctivitis, keratitis, meningitis, septicemia, endocarditis, arthritis, and otolaryngologic infections) (64, 104, 177, 200). The most frequently isolated species is *M. nonliquefaciens*, which forms smooth, translucent to semiopaque colonies 0.1 to 0.5 mm in diameter after 24 h and 1 mm in diameter after 48 h of growth on SBA plates. Occasionally, these colonies spread and pit the agar. The colonial morphologies of *M. lincolnii* (197), *M. osloensis*, and *Psychrobacter phenylpyruvicus* (formerly *Moraxella phenylpyruvica*) are similar, but pitting is rare. On the other hand, pitting is common in *Moraxella lacunata*, whose colonies are smaller and form dark haloes on chocolate agar. Colonies of *Moraxella atlantae* are small (usually 0.5 mm in diameter) and show pitting and spreading (23). Most *Moraxella canis* colonies resemble those of the *Enterobacteriaceae* (large, smooth colonies) and may produce a brown pigment when grown on starch-containing Mueller-Hinton agar (99). Some strains may also produce very slimy colonies resembling colonies of *Klebsiella pneumoniae* (99). Microscopically, *M. canis* resembles *Moraxella catarrhalis*, which is discussed in chapter 38. Animal species include *M. bovis* (isolated from healthy cattle and other animals, including horses), *M. boevrei* and *M. caprae* (goats), *M. caviae* (guinea pigs), *M. cuniculi* (rabbits), and *M. ovis* (sheep).

Biochemical reactions for the human isolates are listed in Table 2. Most laboratories do not determine the species of moraxellae because of the similarity in pathogenic significance of the species and because many strains are somewhat fastidious and biochemical reactions are often negative or equivocal. *M. atlantae*, *M. lacunata*, and *M. nonliquefaciens* are similar in many of their features. Growth of *M. atlantae* is stimulated by bile salts and sodium desoxycholate, while growth of *M. lacunata* and *M. nonliquefaciens* is not. Only *M. lacunata* liquefies gelatin, while both *M. lacunata* and *M. nonliquefaciens* reduce nitrate to nitrite (23, 152). Separation of *M. lacunata* and nonspreading *M. nonliquefaciens* may prove difficult, because gelatin hydrolysis (with any method) and liquefaction of Loeffler slants may take more than 1 week. In some instances, fatty acid analysis may help determine the species (212); in other cases, quantitative transformation of a high-level streptomycin resistance marker can be used (107). The differential diagnosis of *P. phenylpyruvicus* and *Brucella* spp. is of great practical importance and requires microscopy (*Brucella* are tiny coccobacilli) and tests for acidification of xylose and glucose (153, 154). *P. phenylpyruvicus* is asaccharolytic, whereas *Brucella* spp. utilize xylose and usually glucose when a sufficiently sensitive method for detecting the acidification of glucose is employed (153). Microbiologists should be aware that *Brucella* species that are unwittingly inoculated into certain commercial identification systems may be misidentified as *P. phenylpyruvicus* or *Haemophilus influenzae* (5, 6, 148). The tributyrin test may be positive for several *Moraxella* spp. and therefore cannot be used to separate them from *M. catarrhalis* (149). Likewise, γ-glutamyl aminopeptidase occurs not only in *M. canis* but also in some strains of other moraxellae (99).

Most *Moraxella* strains are susceptible to penicillin and its derivatives, cephalosporins, tetracyclines, quinolones, and aminoglycosides (52, 167, 183). Production of β-lactamase has been only rarely reported in *Moraxella* species other than *M. catarrhalis* (104, 167).

Oligella spp.

The genus *Oligella* consists of two species: *O. urethralis* (formerly *Moraxella urethralis* and CDC group M-4) and *O. ureolytica* (formerly CDC group IVe) (168). *O. urethralis* is nonmotile, while most strains of *O. ureolytica* are motile by peritrichous flagella. Biochemical features that help differentiate *Oligella* spp. from *Moraxella* spp. are listed in Table 2. *O. urethralis* is similar to *Moraxella* spp. in that isolates are coccobacillary, oxidase positive, and nonmotile. Colonies are smaller than those of *M. osloensis* and are opaque to whitish. *O. urethralis* and *M. osloensis* have additional biochemical similarities, e.g., accumulation of poly-β-hydroxybutyric acid and failure to hydrolyze urea, but they can be differentiated on the basis of nitrite reduction and alkalinization of formate, itaconate, proline, and threonine (all positive in *O. urethralis* and negative in *M. osloensis*) (155). Cellular fatty acid analysis can also be used to differentiate these two species (212).

Colonies of *O. ureolytica* are slow growing on blood agar, producing pinpoint colonies after 24 h but large colonies after 3 days of incubation. Colonies are white, opaque, entire, and nonhemolytic. *O. ureolytica* strains are both phenylalanine deaminase and rapid urease positive, with the urease reaction often turning positive within minutes after inoculation. In this regard, *O. ureolytica* is similar to *Bordetella bronchiseptica* and *Ralstonia paucula*, from which it must be differentiated. Cellular fatty acid analysis is useful since the CFA profiles are different for each of these species (212).

Both *Oligella* spp. have been isolated chiefly from the human urinary tract, and both have been reported to cause urosepsis (159, 166). A case of septic arthritis due to *O. urethralis* has also been reported (132). *O. urethralis* is generally susceptible to most antibiotics, including penicillin, while *O. ureolytica* exhibits variable susceptibility patterns (52).

OXIDASE-POSITIVE, INDOLE-NEGATIVE, ASACCHAROLYTIC, ROD-SHAPED NONFERMENTERS

See Table 3.

Alcaligenes faecalis and Asaccharolytic *Achromobacter* spp.

Members of the genera *Alcaligenes* and *Achromobacter* are rods (0.5 by 1 to 0.5 by 2.6 μm) with peritrichous flagella. Both phylogenetically and biochemically, they are closely related to members of the genus *Bordetella* (see chapter 50). They occur mainly in the environment and show limited action on carbohydrates. Colonies are nonpigmented and similar in size to those of *Acinetobacter* spp. Medically important species are divided into the asaccharolytic species (Table 3), including *Alcaligenes faecalis*, *Achromobacter piechaudii* (216), and *Achromobacter xylosoxidans* subsp. *denitrificans* (216), and the saccharolytic species (see Table 4) *Achromobacter xylosoxidans* subsp. *xylosoxidans* (216) as well as the unnamed *Achromobacter* groups B, E, and F (73, 74). The asaccharolytic species are rarely observed as human pathogens (16, 116, 206). *A. faecalis* is the most frequently isolated species and characteristically produces colonies with a thin spreading irregular edge. Some strains (previously named "*Alcaligenes odorans*") produce a characteristic fruity odor (sometimes described as the odor of green apples) and cause a greenish discoloration of blood agar medium. A key biochemical feature of this species is its ability to reduce nitrite but not nitrate. It is often found in mixed cultures, particularly in samples of diabetic ulcers of the feet and lower extremities, and its clinical significance is difficult to determine. *A. piechaudii* has been recovered from blood, recurrent ear discharge, nose, pharynx, and soil (111, 116, 147). In one instance the blood isolate was associated with an infected Hickman catheter in a patient with hematological malignancy (111). *A. faecalis* and *A. piechaudii* have been reported to be resistant to ampicillin, aztreonam, and gentamicin and to be of variable susceptibility to other antimicrobials (16, 111). The clinical significance of *A. xylosoxidans* subsp. *denitrificans* remains to be elucidated; however, an organism that is biochemically similar, known as *Alcaligenes*-like group 1, has been recovered from blood, urine, knee joint, brain abscess, and bronchial washings, suggesting that it may have greater potential to cause human infection. It can be differentiated from *A. xylosoxidans* subsp. *denitrificans* by cellular fatty acid composition, failure to grow on salmonella-shigella agar, failure to alkalinize tartrate and acetamide, and a positive urease reaction (Table 3) (212).

Myroides spp.

Vancanneyt et al. (195) determined that the organism formerly classified as *Flavobacterium odoratum* consisted of a heterogenous group that comprised two distinct species, for which they proposed the names *Myroides odoratus* and *Myroides odoratimimus*. Cells of both species are gram-negative rods 0.5 μm in diameter and 1 to 2 μm long. Various colony types may occur, but most colonies are yellow pig-

mented and form effuse, spreading colonies that may be confused with the colony morphology of a *Bacillus* species. A characteristic fruity odor (similar to the odor of *A. faecalis*) is produced by most strains. *Myroides* organisms grow on most media including MacConkey agar. Growth occurs at 18 to 37°C but not at 42°C. They are asaccharolytic but are oxidase, catalase, urease, and gelatinase positive. Indole is not produced, and nitrite (but not nitrate) is reduced (Table 3). There are no routine phenotypic tests for differentiating the two *Myroides* species, their differences being confined to assimilation tests and cellular fatty acids ($C_{13:0}$ and $C_{15:0}$) (195). Organisms identified as *M. odoratus* have been found mostly in urine but also in wound, sputum, blood, and ear specimens (82, 218). Clinical infection with *Myroides* spp. is exceedingly rare; however, cases of rapidly progressive necrotizing fasciitis and bacteremia (94) and recurrent cellulitis with bacteremia (3) have been reported. Most strains are resistant to penicillins, cephalosporins, aminoglycosides, aztreonam, and carbapenems (82).

Neisseria weaveri and *Neisseria elongata*

Although assigned to the genus *Neisseria*, the rod-shaped bacteria *Neisseria weaveri* and *Neisseria elongata* morphologically resemble nonfermenting gram-negative bacilli and therefore are listed in Table 3 to help in the differentiation of these phenotypically similar bacteria. The *Neisseria* species are covered in detail in chapter 38.

Ralstonia spp.

Ralstonia paucula is the name given to the organism formerly designated CDC group IVc-2 (198). It is a short to medium-sized gram-negative rod that is asaccharolytic and motile by peritrichous flagella. Cells may stain irregularly. It is rapid urease positive and can be differentiated from the phenotypically similar organisms, *B. bronchiseptica* and *O. ureolytica*, by a usually negative nitrate reduction test and its cellular fatty acid composition (Table 3).

Ralstonia gilardii is the new designation for an *Alcaligenes faecalis*-like organism that has been isolated from human clinical sources and the environment (37). *R. gilardii* can be differentiated from *A. faecalis* by the absence of nitrite reduction, failure to utilize acetamide, the presence of polar rather than peritrichous flagella, and cellular fatty acid composition (Table 3). The *Ralstonia* species are discussed in more detail in chapter 48.

Gilardi Rod Group 1

Gilardi rod group 1 consists of oval to medium-length asaccharolytic gram-negative rods that resemble *N. weaveri* in many respects except that Gilardi rod group 1 isolates do not reduce nitrite and are strongly phenylalanine deaminase positive, producing a dark green slant after addition of FeCl₃ (10%), while *N. weaveri*, when positive, produces a weak to moderate reaction (Table 3). Isolates of Gilardi rod group 1 have been recovered from a variety of human sources including leg, arm, and foot wounds, an oral lesion, urine, and blood; however, their pathogenic potential has yet to be determined (137). They are susceptible to many antimicrobial agents including various penicillins, cephalothin, and chloramphenicol (137).

TABLE 2 Oxidase-positive, indole-negative, asaccharolytic, coccoid nonfermenters[a]

Test	Moraxella atlantae[b] (73)	Moraxella canis (1)	Moraxella catarrhalis (74)	Moraxella lacunata[b] (66)	Moraxella lincolnii (1)	Moraxella nonliquefaciens[b] (243)	Moraxella osloensis (163)	Oligella ureolytica (37)	Oligella urethralis (22)	Psychrobacter phenylpyruvicus (50)	Asaccharolytic Psychrobacter immobilis (5)
Motility; flagella	0	0	0	0	0	0	0	100[c]; pe	0	0	0
Growth on MacConkey	80 (20)	100	5	2	0	8 (2)	70	62 (27)	96	80 (6)	40
Simmons citrate	0	0	0	0	0	0	0	14 (16)	46	0	20
Urea, Christensen's	0	0	68	0	0	0	0	97	0	100	(20)
Nitrate reduction	0	100	92	98	0	95	24	100	0	68	40 (20)
Gas from nitrate	0	0	0	0	0	0	0	60	0	0	0
Nitrite reduction	3	ND	86	0	0[d]	0	0	100	100	0	ND
H$_2$S (lead acetate paper)	61	100	73	34	0	83	74	38	9	47	20 (20)
Gelatin hydrolysis[e]	0	0	0	42	0	0	0	0	0	0	0
Growth at:											
25°C	51	100	85	33	100	93	96	67	50	85	100
35°C	99	100	97	73	100	88	98	88	100	100	40
42°C	46	100w	23	0	0	15	51	18	59	29	20
Phenylalanine deaminase	0	ND	ND	17	ND	ND	14	100[i]	100	97	ND
Penicillin sensitivity[f]	100	ND	ND	95	ND	99	92	ND	100	73	ND
Loeffler slant digestion	ND	ND	ND	100	ND	0	0	ND	ND	ND	ND

Characteristic										
Sodium acetate alkalinization	ND	43	84	ND	100	0	0	0	ND	ND	ND
Nutrient broth, 0% NaCl	100	53	96	19 (3)	98	22	0	5	47	100	0
Nutrient broth, 6% NaCl	60	19	59	15 (5)	12	0	0	2	ND	100w	0
DNase[g]	ND	0	0	0	0	0	0	0	100	100	0
Major CFAs[h]	16:1ω7c, 17:1ω8c, 18:1ω9c	16:0, 16:1ω7c, 18:1ω9c, 18:2	16:0, 18:1ω7c	16:0, 18:1ω7c	16:1ω7c, 18:1ω9c	16:0, 16:1ω7c, 18:1ω9c	16:0, 16:1ω7c, 18:1ω9c	16:0, 16:1ω7c, 16:0a1c, 17:1ω8c, 18:0, 18:1ω9c, 18:2, 18:0alc[i]	16:1ω7c, 17:1ω8c, 18:1ω9c	18:1ω9c	16:0, 18:0, 18:1ω9c, 18:2

[a] Unless otherwise indicated, data are from the CDC Special Bacteriology Reference Laboratory (212). All taxa were positive (≥90%) for catalase. All were negative (<10% positive) for acid from D-glucose, D-xylose, D-mannitol, lactose, sucrose, and maltose; growth on SS and cetrimide agars, esculin hydrolysis, acid production in triple sugar iron agar, and H_2S production in triple sugar iron agar. Numbers indicate the percentage positive at 2 days of incubation; parentheses indicate a delayed reaction (3 to 7 days incubation); w, weak reaction; pe, peritrichous; ND, not determined or not available. Numbers in parentheses after the organisms indicate the number of strains.

[b] Usually does not grow in oxidative-fermentative medium.

[c] Motility may be delayed or difficult to demonstrate.

[d] Nitrite-positive strains have been described (197).

[e] 14 days of incubation.

[f] Based on results obtained by streaking a blood agar plate with growth from an 18- to 36-h culture and then placing a 10-U penicillin disk on the streaked area. A positive reaction is indicated by the appearance of a zone of inhibition.

[g] Data from reference 99.

[h] The number before the colon indicates the number of carbons; the number after the colon is the number of double bonds; ω, the position of the double bond counting from the hydrocarbon end of the carbon chain; c, cis isomer; alc, alcohol.

[i] Two profiles exist. Most strains of M. lacunata II differ from M. lacunata I by lower amounts of 17:1ω 8c, 16:1ω7c, and 18:1ω9c, higher levels of 18:0 (16% vs 3%), and higher levels of 16:0 alc and 18:0 alc. However, there is some overlap in the relative amounts of these acids in some strains of both groups which prohibit their differentiation solely on the basis of CFA data (212).

[j] Data from P. Schreckenberger.

TABLE 3 Oxidase-positive, indole-negative, asaccharolytic, rod-shaped nonfermenters[a]

Test	Achromobacter xylosoxidans subsp. denitrificans (4)	Achromobacter piechaudii (5)	Alcaligenes faecalis (49)	CDC Alcaligenes-like group 1 (8)	Bordetella avium (3)[c]	Bordetella bronchiseptica (85)	Bordetella hinzii (2)
Motility; flagella	100; pe	100; pe	100; pe	100; pe	100; pe	100; pe	100; pe
Acid from D-glucose	0	0	0	0	0	0	0
Catalase	100	100	98	100	100	100	100
Growth on:							
MacConkey	100	100	100	100	100	100	100
Salmonella-shigella	100	100	100	13	100	99	100
Centrimide	25 (25)	80 (20)	59	0	0	0	0
Simmons citrate	100	100	100	100	33w	98 (1)	100
Urea, Christensen's	0	0	2	75	0	99	0
Nitrate reduction	100	100	0	100	0	92	0
Gas from nitrate	100	0	0	100	0	0	0
Nitrite reduction	ND	0	100	100	0	ND	0
H_2S (lead acetate paper)	25W	100[e]	8	13	67	74	50
Gelatin hydrolysis[f]	0	0	22	0	0	0	0
Pigment:							
Insoluble	0	0	0	0	0	0	0
Soluble	25 yel	0	22 yel	0	33 yel	0	0
Growth at:							
25°C	100	100	100	100	100	99	100
35°C	100	100	100	100	100	100	100
42°C	25w	60	18	50	100	78	100
Alkalinization of:							
Acetamide	33 (33)	0	83	0	0	0	0
Serine	33 (33)	40 (40)	39	(75)	(50w)	30 (61)	50
Tartrate	75 (25)	80 (20)	6	0	0	5	0
Arginine dihydrolase	0	0	0	(33)	0	0	50 (50)
Nutrient broth, 0% NaCl	100	100	100	100	100	100	100
Nutrient broth, 6% NaCl	25	100[g]	98 (2)	13	67	82 (5)	100
Major CFAs[h]	16:0, 16:1ω7c, 17:0cyc	16:0, 16:1ω7c, 17:0cyc	3-OH-14:0, 16:0, 16:1ω7c, 17:0cyc	16:0, 16:1ω7c, 17:0cyc, 18:1ω7c	16:0, 17:0cyc	16:0, 16:1ω7c, 17:0cyc	16:0, 17:0cyc

   [a] Unless otherwise indicated, data are from the CDC Special Bacteriology Reference Laboratory (212). All taxa were negative (<10% positive) for acid production from D-xylose, D-mannitol, lactose, sucrose, and maltose; acid in triple sugar iron agar, H_2S production in triple sugar iron agar, esculin hydrolysis, lysine decarboxylase and ornithine decarboxylase activity. Numbers in parentheses after the organisms indicate the number of strains. Numbers indicate the percentage positive at 2 days of incubation; parentheses indicate a delayed reaction (3 to 7 days of incubation); w, weak reaction; pe, peritrichous; p, polar; ND, not determined or not available; yel, yellow; amb, amber.

   [b] The *Myroides* genus consists of two phenotypically similar species: M. *odoratus* and M. *odoratimimus*. The type strain of M. *odoratus* did not grow on MacConkey agar; in contrast, the type strain of M. *odoratimimus* grew heavily. *Ralstonia paucula* was formerly CDC group IVc-2.

   [c] All from avian sources.

OXIDASE-POSITIVE, INDOLE-NEGATIVE, SACCHAROLYTIC, MOTILE, ROD-SHAPED NONFERMENTERS

See Table 4.

Achromobacter xylosoxidans subsp. xylosoxidans

Achromobacter xylosoxidans subsp. *xylosoxidans* is a relatively frequent agent of infection in immunocompromised patients, causing both local and systemic infections in nosocomial settings (33, 48, 211). A. *xylosoxidans* subsp. *xylosoxidans* has also been found to colonize the respiratory tract of intubated children and patients with cystic fibrosis, leading to exacerbation of pulmonary symptoms (49). Methods for epidemiologic typing of A. *xylosoxidans* subsp. *xylosoxidans* have been described (33, 123). Susceptibilities are unpredictable, requiring testing of individual isolates. Strains are frequently resistant to aminoglycosides, ampicillin, narrow- and extended-spectrum cephalosporins, chloramphenicol, and flluoroquinolones but are usually susceptible to antipseudomonal broad-spectrum cephalosporins, piperacillin, ticarcillin-clavulanic acid, imipenem, and trimethoprim-sulfamethoxazole (15, 183, 206). Panresistance has been reported in at least one clinically significant infection (211).

Ochrobactrum spp. and Achromobacter Groups B, E, and F

Ochrobactrum anthropi (81) is the name given to the urease-positive *Achromobacter* species formerly designated CDC group Vd (biotypes 1 and 2) and *Achromobacter* groups A, C, and D of Holmes et al. (80). Subsequent studies have shown, however, that biogroup C and some strains belonging to biogroup A constitute a homogeneous DNA-DNA hybridization group separate from O. *anthropi*, which has been given the new species designation of *Ochrobactrum intermedium* (201). Both *Ochrobactrum* species are closely

Myroides species[b] (74)	Neisseria weaveri (132)	Neisseria elongata subsp. elongata (15)	Neisseria elongata subsp. glycolytica (2)	Neisseria elongata subsp. nitroreducens (26)	Ralstonia paucula[b] (36)	Ralstonia gilardii[d] (8)	Gilardi rod group 1 (15)
0	0	0	0	0	100; pe	100; 1-2P	0
0	0	0	0[i]	23	0	0	0
100	100	0	100	0	100	100	100
91 (5)	27 (18)	13 (53)	50 (50)	19 (35)	94 (6)	ND	93
30 (11)	0	0	0	0	3 (6)	ND	80
0	0	0	0	0	0 (3)	0	0
0	0	0	0	0	100	0	0
100	0	0	0	0	100	0	0
0	0	0	0	100	11	0	0
0	0	0	ND	0	0	0	0
83	100	92	50	100	ND	0	0
16	86	67	100	100	51	ND	87
96	0	0	0	0	0	0	0
85 yel	0	0	0	0	0	0	60 amb
0	24 yel	13 yel	50 yel	15 yel	22 yel	0	0
100	94	67	100	62	94	ND	100
100	100	100	100	100	100	100	100
31	41	27	0	23	86	100	80
(2w)	2	0	0	0	ND	0	0
5, 2w	0	0	0	0	ND	100	0
(2w)	0	0	0	0	100	0	0
(9)	0	ND	ND	0	ND	0	0
100	85	100	100	88	100	100	100
20 (5)	18	0	0	4	11	0	7 (13)
i15:0	16:0, 16:1ω7c, 18:1ω7c	16:0, 16:1ω7c, 18:1ω7c	16:0, 16:1ω7c, 18:1ω7c	16:0, 16:1ω7c, 18:1ω7c	16:0, 16:1ω7c, 17:0cyc, 18:1ω7c	16:0, 16:1ω7c	14:0, 16:0, 18:1ω7c, 19:0cyc

[d] Data from reference 37.

[e] H$_2$S triple sugar iron (butt), the line of the stab became dark in 3 to 7 days with three strains.

[f] 14 days of incubation.

[g] Light growth at 48 h, heavier at 7 days.

[h] The number before the colon indicates the number of carbons; the number after the colon is the number of double bonds; ω, the position of the double bond counting from the hydrocarbon end of the carbon chain; c, cis isomer; i, iso; 3-OH, a hydroxyl group at the 3 (β) position from the carboxyl end; cyc, a cyclopropane ring structure.

[i] Acid production may be detected in rapid sugar test base.

related to Brucella spp., with Ochrobactrum intermedium occupying a phylogenetic position intermediate between O. anthropi and Brucella (201). The two species have identical phenotypic properties. They appear as medium-length rods with peritrichous flagella, but individual cells may have a single flagellum only. Colonies on SBA resemble those of the Enterobacteriaceae, except that those of Ochrobactrum are smaller. Colonies measure about 1 mm in diameter and appear circular, low convex, smooth, shining, and entire.

O. anthropi has been isolated from various environmental and human sources, predominantly from patients with catheter-related bacteremias (35, 81, 113, 170) and rarely with other infections (129), including one case of meningitis (30). Pulsed-field gel electrophoresis and PCR genome fingerprinting based on repetitive chromosomal sequences have both been used successfully for epidemiologic typing of outbreak strains (199). O. anthropi strains are usually resistant to β-lactams, such as broad-spectrum penicillins, broad-spectrum cephalosporins, aztreonam, and amoxicillin-clavulanate, but are usually susceptible to aminoglycosides, fluoroquinolones, imipenem, tetracycline, and trimethoprim-sulfamethoxazole (14, 35, 113, 170).

There are no currently available biochemical tests that separate O. intermedium from O. anthropi; however, it has been suggested that colistin (polymyxin E) and polymyxin B resistance can be used to separate O. intermedium (resistant) from O. anthropi (susceptible) (201). One case of pyogenic liver infection due to O. intermedium has been reported (134); however, because of the close phenotypic similarity between O. anthropi and O. intermedium, it is possible that certain infections thought to be caused by O. anthropi were actually caused by O. intermedium.

Achromobacter groups B and E constitute biotypes of a single new species that has yet to be named (73, 74, 76). Achromobacter group F is genetically distinct from groups

TABLE 4 Oxidase-positive, indole-negative, saccharolytic, motile, rod-shaped nonfermenters[a]

Test	Achromobacter xylosoxidans subsp. xylosoxidans (135)	"Achromobacter" group B[b] (3)	"Achromobacter" group E[b] (2)	"Achromobacter" group F[b] (2)	Rhizobium radiobacter (66)	Agrobacterium yellow group (3)	Ochrobactrum species[c] (14)
Motility, flagella	100; pe	100; p, L	100; p, L	100	100; pe	100; p, 1–2[e]	100; pe
Acid from:							
D-Glucose	78	100	100	100	94 (6)	33 (67)	93 (7)
D-Xylose	99	100	100	100	97 (3)	67 (33)	100
D-Mannitol	0	(67)	0	100	94 (6)	0	43 (14)
Lactose	0	(33)	(100)[f]	ND	79 (21)	(100)	0
Sucrose	0	(100)	(100)	100	95 (5)	(100)	50
Maltose	0	33 (67)	100	100	97 (3)	100	64
Catalase	98	100	100	ND	98	100	100
Growth on:							
MacConkey	100	100	100	0	100	(33)	100
Salmonella-shigella	98	100	100	ND	20 (5)	0	100
Cetrimide	95 (1)	0	50 (50)	ND	0	0	100
Simmons citrate	95	100	100	0	97 (3)	0	64
Urea, Christensen's	0	100	100	100	88 (9)	(33)	100
Nitrate reduction	100	100	(100)[i]	100	83	0	86
Gas from nitrate	60	100	100	0	5	0	43
Nitrite reduction	ND	100[h]	100[h]	0	38	0	ND
TSI slant, acid	0	0	0	0	0	0	0
TSI butt, acid	0	0	0	0	0	0	0
H$_2$S (TSI butt)	0	0	(50)	ND	11 (3)	0	43
H$_2$S (lead acetate paper)	0	(100)	100	ND	100	100	100
Gelatin hydrolysis[i]	0	0	0	ND	2	0	0
Pigment:							
Insoluble	0	0	0	ND	0	100 yel	0
Soluble	5 br	67 yel	50 tan	ND	21 yel	0	21 yel
Growth at:							
25°C	98	100	100	ND	100	100	100
35°C	100	100	100	ND	100	100	100
42°C	84	100	100	ND	32	0	64
Esculin hydrolysis	0	100	100	100	100	67 (33)	29 (7)
Lysine decarboxylase	0	0	0	ND	0	0	0
Arginine dihydrolase	13	100	100	0	8	0	71
Ornithine decarboxylase	0	0	0	ND	0	0	0
Nutrient broth, 0% NaCl	100	100	100	ND	100	67 (33)	100
Nutrient broth, 6% NaCl	69	100	100	ND	18	0	60
3-Ketolactonate	ND	0	0	ND	100	100	0
ONPG	0[l]	100[m]	100[m]	0[m]	100[l]	ND	0[l]
Major CFAs[j]	16:0, 16:1ω7c, 17:0cyc	18:1ω7c	18:1ω7c	ND	16:0, 16:1ω7c, 19:0cyc	16:0, 18:1ω7c	18:0, 18:1ω7c, 19:0cyc

[a] Unless otherwise indicated, data are from CDC Special Bacteriology Reference Laboratory (212). Numbers indicate the percentage positive at 2 days incubation; parentheses indicate a delayed reaction (3 to 7 days of incubation); w, weak reaction; ND, not determined or not available; pe, peritrichous; p, polar; L, lateral; br, brown; yel, yellow; pk, pink; TSI, triple sugar iron. Numbers in parentheses after the organisms indicate the number of strains.

[b] The following tests are useful in distinguishing among "Achromobacter" groups B, E, and F: L-rhamnose, D-sorbitol, and cellobiose: B (+, +, +); E (+, −, +), and F (−, ND, +) (73).

[c] Colistin resistance has been suggested to differentiate O. intermedium (colistin resistant) from O. anthropi (colistin sensitive) (201).

[d] Glycerol and rhamnose oxidation are absent in S. paucimobilis and present in S. parapaucimobilis.

[e] Motility may be difficult to demonstrate.

[f] Acid production was detected only after 21 days of incubation.

B and E (73, 74). *Achromobacter* group B has been isolated from patients with septicemia (75, 102). Isolates of *Achromobacter* groups E and F have also been recovered from blood (73, 74). Susceptibility to chloramphenicol, ciprofloxacin, gentamicin, imipenem, tobramycin, and trimethoprim-sulfamethoxazole has been reported for isolates of *Achromobacter* group B recovered from blood (75, 102).

OFBA-1 (6)	CDC Group Ic (34)	CDC Group O-1 (62)	CDC Group O-2 (66)	CDC Group O-3 (13)	Herbaspirillum species 3 (1)	Sphingomonas paucimobilis[d] (1)	Sphingomonas parapaucimobilis[d] (2)	Pseudomonas-like group 2 (11)	Shewanella putrefaciens (24)
100; p, 1–2	100; p, 1–2	100; p. 1–2[e]	100; p. 1–2 or p, L[e]	100; p. 1–2[e]	100; >2p	100; p. 1–2	100; p. 1–2	100; p. >2	100; p. 1–2
100	97	69 (31)	73 (11)	100	100	100w	(100)	100	17 (33)
100	0	0	2	100	100	100	100	100	0
67 (33)	0	0	2	0	100	0	0	100	0
67 (33)	0	0	2	0	100w	100	50 (50)	100	0
67 (33)	0	0	64 (36)	100	0	100	100	0	96 (4)
67 (33)	100	0	71 (27)	100	0	100	50 (50)	0	92 (8)
100	97	98	91	23, 62w	100	100	100	100	100
100	100	6 (40)	5 (5)	(38)	ND	0	0	100	100
100	100	0	0	0	ND	0	0	0	(8)
100	94	0	0	0	100	0	0	0	4
33 (33)	41 (15)	0	0	0	100	0	0[g]	100	4 (4)
33 (17)	18 (15)	2	12	0	100	0	0	91 (9)	4 (8)
100	100	0	15	8	0	0	0	18	100
100	0	0	0	0	0	0	0	0	0
ND	0	0	ND	0	ND	ND	ND	ND	ND
100	0	0	18	0	0	0	100w	0	0
33 (67)	0	0	20	0	0	0	0	0	0
0	3	0	0	0	0	0	0	0	96
50	100	93	91	15	100	0	100	89	100
50	0	25	38	0	0	0	0	0	65
0	9w pk	100 yel	100 yel	0	0	100 yel	100 yel	0	0
0	32 tan-br	0	0	0	0	0	0	0	71 br
100	100	90	89	92	100	100	100	80	100
100	100	100	100	100	100	100	100	100	96
100	97	24	31	40	100	100w	0	20	38
0	0	93 (2)	64	92 (8)	0	100	100	0	0
0	0	0	0	0	ND	ND	ND	0	0
100	100	0	22	0	ND	ND	ND	30	0
0	0	0	6	0	ND	ND	ND	0	100
100	100	34	92	100	100	100	100	100	100
75	91	0	22	0	0	0	50	0	43
ND	ND	ND	ND	ND	ND	0	0	ND	ND
ND	ND	ND	ND	ND	ND	100[l]	ND	ND	ND
16:0, 19:0cyc	ND	16:0, 18:1ω7c	ND[k]	16:0, 16:1ω7c, 18:1ω7c	16:0, 16:1ω7c, 18:1ω7c	16:0, 18:1ω7c	16:0, 17:1ω6c, 18:1ω7c	16:0, 16:1ω7c, 18:1ω7c	i-15:0, 16:1ω7c, 17:1ω8c

[g] Reported to be positive by Yabuuchi et al. (217).

[h] When tested at 48 h of incubation, nitrite reduction may be observed only in media containing <0.01% nitrite.

[i] 14 days of incubation.

[j] The number before the colon indicates the number of carbons; the number after the colon is the number of double bonds; ω, the position of the double bond counting from the hydrocarbon end of the carbon chain; c, *cis* isomer; cyc, a cyclopropane ring structure; i, *iso*; ND, not determined.

[k] Fatty acid profile analysis, performed on six strains in our laboratory, indicates that this group is heterogeneous.

[l] Data from P. Schreckenberger.

[m] Data from reference 80.

Rhizobium (Agrobacterium) radiobacter

The former genus *Agrobacterium* contained several species of plant pathogens occurring worldwide in soils. Four distinct species of *Agrobacterium* were recognized: *Agrobacterium radiobacter* (formerly *A. tumefaciens* and CDC group Vd-3), *Agrobacterium rhizogenes* (subsequently transferred to the genus *Sphingomonas* as *S. rosa*), *Agrobacterium vitis*, and *Agrobacterium rubi* (173). The separation of the phenotypically indistinguishable species *A. tumefaciens* and *A. radiobacter* was based on the presence of a plant tumor-inducing plasmid in *A. tumefaciens* but not in *A. radiobacter*. Genetic studies showed that the two species were the same, and a proposal was made to reject the name *A. tumefaciens* and to designate *A. radiobacter* as the type species for the genus *Agrobacterium* (173). Recently, Young et al. (219) proposed an emended description of the genus *Rhizobium* to include all species of *Agrobacterium*. Following this proposal, the new combinations are *Rhizobium radiobacter*, *Rhizobium rhizogenes*, *Rhizobium rubi*, and *Rhizobium vitis* (219). Cells are 0.6 to 1.0 by 1.5 to 3.0 μm long and occur singly and in pairs. Colonies of *R. radiobacter* grow optimally at 25 to 28°C but also grow at 35°C. They appear circular, convex, smooth, and nonpigmented to light beige on SBA, with a diameter of 2 mm at 48 h. Colonies may appear wet looking and become extremely mucoid and pink on MacConkey agar with prolonged incubation (Fig. 2).

R. *radiobacter* has been most frequently isolated from blood, followed by peritoneal dialysate, urine, and ascitic fluid (50, 96). The majority of cases have occurred in patients with transcutaneous catheters or implanted biomedical prostheses, and effective treatment often requires removal of the device (51). *R. radiobacter* septicemia has also been reported in hospitalized patients with advanced human immunodeficiency virus disease (130). One case of endophthalmitis caused by an *R. radiobacter*-like (3-ketolactonate-negative) organism has also been reported (133). Most strains are susceptible to broad-spectrum cephalosporins, carbapenems, tetracyclines, and gentamicin but not to tobramycin (50, 206). Testing of individual isolates is recommended for clinically significant cases.

Agrobacterium Yellow Group

Organisms in the *Agrobacterium* yellow group are represented by slender, medium to long gram-negative rods that produce a yellow insoluble growth pigment and most closely resemble *Sphingomonas paucimobilis* and CDC group O-1 and O-2 organisms. Growth on MacConkey agar is variable, motility occurs via a single polar flagellum, oxidase and catalase are positive, and glucose, xylose, lactose, sucrose, and maltose, but not mannitol, are oxidized. Only a positive 3-ketolactonate reaction differentiates this organism from *S. paucimobilis* (Table 4). The organism has been isolated from blood and peritoneal fluid (187, 212).

OFBA-1

OFBA-1 is an unclassified, medium to long, gram-negative, motile rod with one or two polar flagella; it has the unusual property of producing acid in OF base medium without carbohydrate, hence the acronym OFBA, for "OF base acid." The organism most closely resembles *P. aeruginosa* biochemically due to beta-hemolysis, growth at 42°C, presence of arginine dihydrolase, nitrate reduction to gas, and utilization of most carbohydrates (209, 212). Unlike *P. aeruginosa*, it is negative for pyocyanin and pyoverdin production and acetamide hydrolysis. Isolates have been recovered from blood, leg ulcer, abdominal wound, bronchial wash, and a catheter tunnel infection in a patient on continuous ambulatory peritoneal dialysis (209, 212).

CDC Group Ic

Members of CDC group Ic are gram-negative, slender, short to long, motile rods with one to two polar flagella. The organisms grow well on MacConkey, salmonella-shigella, and usually cetrimide agars; oxidize glucose and maltose; reduce nitrate to nitrite without gas; produce H_2S on lead acetate paper (usually strong); are arginine dihydrolase positive, urease and citrate variable, and esculin and gelatin hydrolysis negative; and grow well at 25, 35, and usually 42°C. Other characteristics are listed in Table 4. Most isolates have come from human sources including urine, sputum, blood, and other sites (212). Antibiotic susceptibility data are not available.

CDC Groups O-1, O-2, and O-3

CDC groups O-1, O-2, and O-3 are phenotypically similar, motile, and usually oxidase positive, gram-negative rods. Groups O-1 and O-2 are yellow pigmented and most closely resemble *Agrobacterium* yellow group and *Sphingomonas* species. These organisms grow poorly or not at all on MacConkey agar, usually hydrolyze esculin, but are otherwise inactive. All are motile, although motility may be difficult to demonstrate. O-1 appear as uniformly short gram-negative rods, O-2 appear as slightly pleomorphic rods with some cells appearing thin in the central portion with thickened ends, and O-3 cells appear as thin, medium to slightly long curved rods with tapered ends (sickle-like) (42, 212). O-3 is the only group in which yellow growth pigment is not produced and the only group of predominantly curved rods. Most isolates of O-3 grow well on CAMPY CVA (campylobacter agar with cefoperazone, vancomycin, and amphotericin B) plates under microaerophilic conditions, hence creating the potential for misidentification of O-3 organisms as *Campylobacter* (42). Organisms of all three O groups have been isolated from a variety of clinical sources. One case of group O1-associated pneumonia complicated by bronchopulmonary fistula and bacteremia has been reported (160). Antibiotic susceptibility data have been reported only for group O-3. All isolates tested were susceptible to the aminoglycosides, trimethoprim-sulfamethoxazole, and imipenem. Resistance was noted to most β-lactams, and variable susceptibility was noted for chloramphenicol, tetracycline, ciprofloxacin, and amoxicillin-clavulanate (42).

Sphingomonas spp.

On the basis of its 16S rRNA sequence and the presence of unique sphingoglycolipid and ubiquinone types, a new genus, *Sphingomonas*, was created for the organism formerly known as *Pseudomonas paucimobilis* and CDC group IIk-1 (217). Since the original proposal, numerous novel species originating from various environments have been added to the genus *Sphingomonas*.

Members of this genus are known to be decomposers of aromatic compounds and, as such, are expected to be used for bioremediation of the environment. It is now known that members of the genus *Sphingomonas* can be divided into four phylogenetic groups, each representing a different genus. Consequently, three new genera, *Sphingobium*, *Novosphingobium*, and *Sphingopyxis*, in addition to the genus *Sphingomonas* have been created to accommodate the four phylogenetic groups (188). The emended genus *Sphingomonas* contains at least 12 species, of which only *S. paucimobilis*, designated the type species, and *S. parapaucimobilis* are thought to be important clinically.

S. *paucimobilis* is characterized by medium to long motile rods with a polar flagellum. However, few cells are actively motile in broth culture, thus making motility a difficult characteristic to demonstrate. Motility occurs at 18 to 22°C but not at 37°C. The oxidase reaction is weakly positive, although occasional strains may be oxidase negative. Colonies are slow growing on blood agar medium, with only

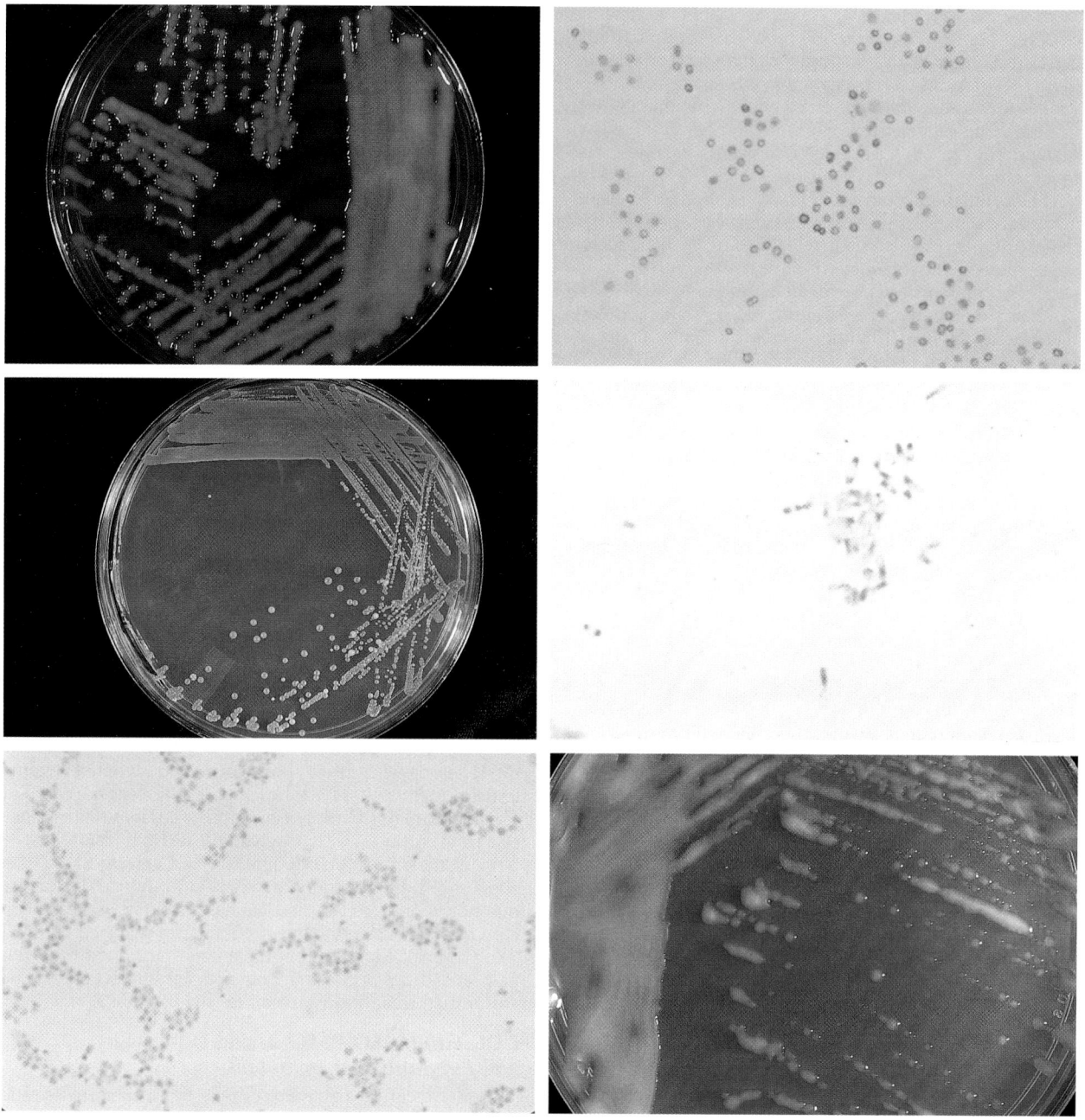

FIGURE 2 (top left)   *Rhizobium radiobacter* on MacConkey agar after 48 h of incubation.

FIGURE 3 (top right)   Gram stain of EO-2 showing the characteristic donut shaped morphology.

FIGURE 4 (middle left)   *Methylobacterium* on Sabouraud dextrose agar, showing coral-pigmented colonies.

FIGURE 5 (middle right)   Gram stain of *Methylobacterium*, showing pleomorphic gram-negative rods with vacuoles.

FIGURE 6 (bottom left)   Gram stain of *Roseomonas*, showing gram-negative coccoid rods.

FIGURE 7 (bottom right)   *Roseomonas* on Sabouraud dextrose agar, showing pink mucoid colonies.

small colonies appearing after 24 h of incubation. Older colonies demonstrate a deep yellow (mustard color) pigment. Growth occurs at 37°C but not at 42°C, with optimum growth occurring at 30°C. Isolates are strongly esculin hydrolysis positive and produce a zone of growth inhibition around a vancomycin disk (30 μg) placed on a blood agar plate inoculated with a pure culture isolate (unpublished data). *S. paucimobilis* is widely distributed in the environment, including water, and has been isolated from a variety of clinical specimens, including blood, cerebrospinal fluid, peritoneal fluid, urine, wounds, vagina, and cervix, and from the hospital environment (77, 92, 136, 161). Most strains are susceptible to tetracycline, chloramphenicol, trimethoprim-sulfamethoxazole, and aminoglycosides; their susceptibility to other antimicrobial agents including fluoroquinolones varies (52, 92, 161).

The cellular and colonial characteristics of S. parapaucimobilis are similar to those of S. paucimobilis. It is differentiated from S. paucimobilis by blackening of lead acetate paper suspended over Kligler iron agar, ability to grow and alkalinize Simmons' citrate medium, and a negative extracellular deoxyribonuclease reaction (217). Clinical isolates have been obtained from the sputum, urine, and vagina (217). Antibiotic susceptibility data are not available.

Pseudomonas-Like Group 2

The organisms in Pseudomonas-like group 2 were previously included in a heterogeneous group of organisms designated CDC group IVd (45). Strains are oxidase positive and motile with polar tufts of flagella and are urea, O-nitrophenyl-β-D-galactopyranoside (ONPG), and phenylalanine deaminase positive (45). Isolates are similar to Burkholderia gladioli but do not oxidize dulcitol or inositol. Other characteristics are given in Table 4. Colonies tend to stick to the agar. Human clinical isolates have been obtained from the respiratory tract, blood, spinal fluid, feces, urine, and dialysate (118).

Herbaspirillum Species 3

Herbaspirillum is a gram-negative, generally curved, and sometimes helical bacillus. Individual cells are 0.6 to 0.7 μm wide and 1.5 to 5.0 μm long and have one to three or more flagella on one or both poles (4). A group of clinical isolates previously described as EF-1 has been shown by molecular hybridization to belong to the genus Herbaspirillum and is designated as a new unnamed species, Herbaspirillum species 3 (4). The organism is oxidase and urease positive; catalase is weak or variable. Other reactions are given in Table 4. Isolates have been recovered from the respiratory tract, feces, urine, ears, eyes, and wound sites (4). Antibiotic susceptibility data are not available.

OXIDASE-POSITIVE, INDOLE-NEGATIVE, SACCHAROLYTIC, NONMOTILE, COCCOID OR ROD-SHAPED NONFERMENTERS

See Table 5.

Sphingobacterium and Pedobacter

Sphingobacterium spp. are oxidase-positive, indole-negative gram-negative rods that form yellow-pigmented colonies. They have no flagella but may exhibit sliding motility. They are nonproteolytic and produce acid from carbohydrates. The currently described species of Sphingobacterium are Sphingobacterium multivorum (formerly Flavobacterium multivorum, CDC group IIk-2), Sphingobacterium spiritivorum (includes species formerly designated Flavobacterium spiritivorum, Flavobacterium yabuuchiae, and CDC group IIk-3), Sphingobacterium mizutaii, Sphingobacterium thalpophilum, Sphingobacterium faecium, Sphingobacterium antarcticum, and unnamed species Sphingobacterium genomospecies 1 and 2 (189, 215). The former Sphingobacterium species Sphingobacterium heparinum and Sphingobacterium piscium have been

placed in a new genus Pedobacter as Pedobacter heparinus and Pedobacter piscium (184). The genus Pedobacter contains several species of heparinase-producing bacteria found in soil, activated sludge, or fish but not from human sources. Steyn and colleagues have shown that all these organisms constitute a separate rRNA branch in the rRNA superfamily V for which they have proposed a new family called the Sphingobacteriaceae (184).

S. multivorum and S. spiritivorum are the two species that have been most frequently recovered from human clinical specimens. They can be distinguished from the similar organism Sphingomonas paucimobilis (formerly IIk-1) by lack of motility, urease production, and resistance to polymyxin B (S. paucimobilis is usually motile, urease negative, and usually susceptible to polymyxin B). S. multivorum has been isolated from various clinical specimens but has only rarely been associated with serious infections (peritonitis and sepsis) (58, 79, 157). Blood and urine have been the most common sources for the isolation of S. spiritivorum (78). S. mizutaii has been isolated from blood, cerebrospinal fluid, and wound specimens and can be differentiated from S. multivorum by its failure to grow on MacConkey agar and usual lack of urease (212). S. thalpophilum has been recovered from wounds, blood, eyes, abscesses, and abdominal incisions (212). A positive nitrate test and growth at 42°C differentiates S. thalpophilum from other Sphingobacterium species. Sphingobacterium species are generally resistant to aminoglycosides and polymyxin B while susceptible in vitro to the quinolones and trimethoprim-sulfamethoxazole. Susceptibility to β-lactam antibiotics is variable, requiring testing of individual isolates (183).

CDC Group EF-4b

EF-4b, along with EF-4a, was originally designated eugonic fermenter group 4 (EF-4); however, EF-4b does not ferment glucose, does not hydrolyze arginine, and does not produce gas from nitrate, which separates it from the glucose-fermenting strains now designated CDC group EF-4a (see chapter 39). EF-4b strains are coccoid to short rods that are nonmotile and oxidase and catalase positive. Colonies on culture plates are nonpigmented and are reported to smell like popcorn. Most isolates have been recovered from human infections following dog and cat bites (212). The antibiotic susceptibility resembles that of EF-4a.

CDC Groups EO-2, EO-3, and EO-4 and Psychrobacter immobilis

The classification of groups EO-2, EO-3, and EO-4 and saccharolytic Psychrobacter immobilis strains is incomplete. All are strongly oxidase-positive, nonmotile, saccharolytic coccobacilli and grow, sometimes poorly, on MacConkey agar. In contrast to the EO (eugonic oxidizer) groups, P. immobilis grows best at 20°C and only occasionally at 37°C. EO-3 and many EO-4 strains have a yellow, nondiffusible pigment that is not observed with either EO-2 or P. immobilis. Microscopically, EO-2 is characterized by distinctive "O-shaped" cells (Fig. 3) upon Gram stain examination due to the presence of vacuolated or peripherally stained cells, and P. immobilis is characterized by paired, coccoid organisms. P. immobilis is divided into saccharolytic and asaccharolytic strains. Saccharolytic P. immobilis strains (Table 5) share all of the characteristics of the asaccharolytic strains (Table 2) except that glucose, xylose, and lactose, but not sucrose and maltose, are oxidized. Asaccharolytic strains are phenotypically similar to P. phenylpyruvicus. The diagnosis of P. immobilis can be confirmed by transformation studies,

TABLE 5 Oxidase-positive, indole-negative, saccharolytic, nonmotile, coccoid or rod-shaped nonfermenters[a]

Test	Sphingobacterium mizutaii (6)	Sphingobacterium multivorum (22)	Sphingobacterium spiritivorum (13)	Sphingobacterium thalpophilum (10)	CDC group EF-4b (34)	CDC group EO-2 (11)	CDC group EO-3 (7)	CDC group EO-4[a] (8)	Psychrobacter immobilis (saccharolytic strains) (7)
Acid from:									
D-Glucose	67 (33)	100	100	100	70 (26)	91 (9)	100	100	57 (43)
D-Xylose	(100)	100	92 (8)	100	0	91 (9)	100	100	57 (43)
D-Mannitol	0	0	100	0	0	0	57 (43)	0	0
Lactose	100	100	92 (8)	100	0	45 (55)	71 (29)	0	57 (43)
Sucrose	50 (50)	100	100	100	0	0	0	0	0
Maltose	50 (50)	100	92 (8)	100	0	(9)	14 (14)	0	0
Catalase	100	100	100	100	100	82	100	100	100
Growth on MacConkey	0	100	(46)	100	65 (6)	64 (18)	100	87 (13)	40
Simmons citrate	0	0	0	0	14 (6)	64 (36)	29 (71)	87	20
Urea, Christensen's	0	95	62 (38)	90 (10)	0	36 (55)	14 (86)	62 (38)	(43)
Nitrate reduction	0	0	0	100	97	100	0	0	86
Gas from nitrate	0	0	0	0	0	18	0	0	0
Nitrite reduction	100[b]	0	0	0	71	0[c]	0[c]	0	0[c]
TSI slant, acid	17	55 (5)	0	100	0	0	0	0	0
TSI butt, acid	17	5 (76)	0	10 (70)	6	0	0	0	0
H2S (lead acetate paper)[d]	100	86 (5)	56	100	88	64 (9)	100	100	43 (14)
Gelatin hydrolysis	0	0	15	40	9	0	0	0	0
Pigment:									
Insoluble	33 yel[e]	57 light yel	54 pale yel	50 pale yel	50 yel	0	100 yel	75 yel	0
Soluble	0	0	0	0	0	55 yel	0	0	0
Growth at:									
25°C	100	100	100	100	88	73	100	100	100
35°C	100	100	100	100	100	100	100	100	57
42°C	0	0	9	100	69	36	14	0	0
Esculin hydrolysis	100	100	100	100	0	0	0	0	0
Arginine dihydrolase	25	0	25	0	0	ND	ND	14	29
Nutrient broth, 0% NaCl	100	100	100	100	0	64	71	87	43 (57)
Nutrient broth, 6% NaCl	0	25	0	10		36	43	13	100
Major CFAs[f]	i-15:0, i-2-OH-15:0, 16:1ω7c	i-15:0, i-2-OH-15:0, 16:1ω7c	i-15:0, i-2-OH-15:0	15:0, 16:1ω7c	16:0, 16:1ω7c, 18:1ω7c	16:0, 18:1ω7c	18:1ω7c	18:1ω7c	16:1ω7c, 18:1ω9c

[a] Data are from the CDC Special Bacteriology Reference Laboratory (212). All taxa were negative (≤10% positive) for motility, growth on salmonella-shigella and cetrimide agars, production of H2S in triple sugar iron (TSI), lysine decarboxylase, and ornithine decarboxylase activity. Numbers indicate the percentage positive at 2 days of incubation; parentheses indicate a delayed reaction (3 to 7 days of incubation); w, weak reaction; ND, not determined or not available; yel, yellow. CDC group EO-4 was described previously. (Weyant et al., Abstr. 99th Gen. Meet. Am. Soc. Microbiol. 1999). Numbers in parentheses after the organisms indicate the number of strains.

[b] A partial reduction may be observed with 0.1% nitrite. A full reduction is observed with 0.01% nitrite.

[c] 14 days of incubation.

[d] 14 days of incubation.

[e] Pigment production may be enhanced by room temperature incubation.

[f] The number before the colon indicates the number of carbons; the number after the colon is the number of double bonds; ω, the position of the double bond counting from the hydrocarbon end of the carbon chain; c, cis isomer; i, iso; 2-OH, a hydroxyl group at the 2 (β) position from the carboxyl end.

TABLE 6 Halophilic nonfermenters[a]

Test	*Alishewanella fetalis*[b] (1)	*Halomonas venusta*[c] (15)	*Shewanella algae* (26)	CDC halophilic nonfermenter group 1[a] (6)
Motility; flagella	0	100; pe	100; p, 1–2	100; pe
Acid from or assimilation of:				
D-Glucose	0	100	0	17 (83)
D-Xylose	0	0	0	0
D-Mannitol	0	80	0	33 (67)
Lactose	0	0	0	0
Sucrose	0	80	0	67 (33)
Maltose	0	100	0	67 (33)
Growth on:				
MacConkey	100	100	100	100
Salmonella-shigella	100	ND	92 (4)	83
Cetrimide	ND	ND	8	17
Citrate	0	100	8	100
Urea, Christensen's	0	100	42	(100)
Nitrate reduction	100	100	100	33
Gas from nitrate	ND	ND	0	0
Nitrite reduction	100	ND	ND	ND
H$_2$S (TSI butt)	0	ND	100	0
H$_2$S (lead acetate paper)	ND	ND	100	100
Gelatin hydrolysis[d]	100	0	100	0
Pigment:				
Insoluble	ND	ND	0	17 pk, 17 yel
Soluble	ND	ND	0	67 tan-amb
Growth at 42°C	100	ND	23	17
Esculin hydrolysis	100	100	0	0
Lysine decarboxylase	ND	0	0	0
Arginine dihydrolase	0	0	0	0
Ornithine decarboxylase	ND	0	0	0
Nutrient broth, 0% NaCl	ND	ND	0	0
Nutrient broth, 6% NaCl	100	100	100	100
Major CFAs[e]	16:1ω7c, 17:1ω8c	16:0, 18:1ω9c	i-15:0, 16:1ω7c, 17:1ω8c	16:0, 18:1ω7c

[a] Unless otherwise indicated, data are from the CDC Special Bacteriology Reference Laboratory (212). All taxa were positive (>90%) for catalase, oxidase, and growth at 25 and 35°C. All were negative for indole production and acid production in triple sugar iron (TSI) agar. Numbers indicate the percentage positive at 2 days of incubation; parentheses indicate a delayed reaction (3 to 7 days of incubation); w, weak reaction; ND, not determined; pe, peritrichous; p, polar; amb, amber; pk, pink; yel, yellow. Unless otherwise noted, carbohydrate results represent acid production. CDC halophilic nonfermenter group 1 results are based on unpublished data from the CDC Special Bacteriology Reference Laboratory. Numbers in parentheses after the organisms indicate the number of strains.
[b] Data from reference 55. Carbohydrate results are from assimilation tests.
[c] Data from reference 207. Carbohydrate results are from assimilation tests.
[d] 7 to 14 days of incubation.
[e] The number before the colon indicates the number of carbons; the number after the colon is the number of double bonds; ω, the position of the double bond counting from the hydrocarbon end of the carbon chain; c, cis isomer; i, iso.

cellular fatty acid profile, and optimal growth temperatures of <35°C (138, 212). Many strains of *P. immobilis* have an odor resembling phenylethyl alcohol agar (roses) and are resistant to penicillin but susceptible to most other antibiotics (63, 127). All four groups have been recovered from clinical specimens. EO-2 has been isolated from various human wound infections and shows a high level of homology to *Paracoccus* species (R. S. Weyant, A. G. Steigerwalt, A. M. Whitney, M. I. Daneshvar, J. G. Jordan, L. W. Mayer, S. Rassouli, W. Barchet, C. Munro, L. Shuttleworth, and K. Bernard, Abstr. 2nd Int. Conf. Emerg. Infect. Dis., p. 103, 2000). EO-3 has been reported to cause peritonitis in a patient on continuous peritoneal dialysis (40). EO-4 has been recovered from blood, urine, and a nasal sinus, but the clinical significance of these isolates is unknown (R. S. Weyant, M. I. Daneshvar, J. G. Jordan, J. P. MacGregor, and D. G. Hollis, Abstr. 99th Gen. Meet. Am. Soc. Microbiol. 1999, abstr. C-196, p. 144, 1999). One

case of ocular infection and one case of infant meningitis have been reported to be caused by *P. immobilis* (63, 127).

HALOPHILIC NONFERMENTERS

See Table 6. Organisms included in Table 6 require NaCl for growth and thus are referred to as halophilic nonfermenters. While most studies report growth in 6% NaCl, our experience is that the organisms also grow in 6.5% NaCl, which is commonly available in clinical microbiology laboratories.

Shewanella and *Alishewanella*

The organism formerly called *Pseudomonas putrefaciens*, *Alteromonas putrefaciens*, *Achromobacter putrefaciens*, and CDC group Ib has now been placed in the genus *Shewanella* (128). Colonies on SBA are convex, circular, smooth, and occasionally mucoid; produce a brown to tan soluble pigment; and cause green discoloration of the medium. Cells are long, short, or filamentous. Motility is due to a single polar flagellum. Ornithine decarboxylase, nitrate reductase, and DNase are always produced, and with few exceptions, hydrogen sulfide (H_2S) is produced in Kligler's and triple sugar iron agars (shewanellae are the only nonfermenters that produce H_2S in these media). The Centers for Disease Control and Prevention (CDC) recognizes two biotypes based on the requirement of NaCl for growth, oxidation of sucrose and maltose, and the ability to grow on salmonella-shigella agar (212). Owen et al. (146) have shown that organisms identified as *Shewanella putrefaciens* comprise at least four clearly separated genomic groups (I to IV). Based on the taxonomic proposals of Nozue et al. (142) and Simidu et al. (181), strains belonging to Owen's genomic group IV (synonymous with CDC biotype 2) should be identified as *Shewanella alga* (corrected to *S. algae* [192]). Khashe and Janda (114) have reported that *S. algae* is the predominant human clinical isolate (77%), while *S. putrefaciens* (CDC biotype 1) represents the majority of nonhuman isolates (89%). *S. algae* requires NaCl for growth and is therefore placed in Table 6 with the halophilic nonfermenters. *S. putrefaciens* is nonhalophilic and is included with saccharolytic, rod-shaped nonfermenters in Table 4. Although infrequent isolates in the clinical laboratory, *S. putrefaciens* and *S. algae* have been recovered from a wide variety of clinical specimens and are associated with a broad range of human infections including cellulitis, otitis media, ocular infection, abscesses, osteomyelitis, peritonitis, and septicemia (25, 28, 32, 41, 85, 98, 115). Many of these infections were probably caused by *S. algae*. Shewanellae are generally susceptible to most antimicrobial agents effective against gram-negative rods except penicillin and cephalothin (52, 206). Recent investigations have noted that the mean MICs of penicillin, ampicillin, and tetracycline for *S. algae* were higher than the corresponding MICs for *S. putrefaciens* (54, 114).

Alishewanella fetalis is a halophilic gram-negative rod that grows at temperatures between 25 and 42°C, with optimum growth at 37°C. NaCl is required for growth. It can withstand NaCl concentrations up to 8% but does not grow at 10% NaCl, which helps differentiate this species from *S. algae*, which can grow in 10% NaCl (55). Also, unlike *S. algae*, it is esculin hydrolysis positive. It is oxidase and catalase positive and asaccharolytic. It does not produce H_2S in the butt of triple sugar iron and Kligler iron agar. Other reactions are given in Table 6. It has been isolated from a human fetus at autopsy; however, its association with clinical infection is unknown (55).

Halomonas venusta and CDC Halophilic Nonfermenter Group 1

Halomonas venusta was originally described as *Alcaligenes venustus* (7) but later transferred to the new genus *Deleya*, as *Deleya venusta*, by Bauman (8). In 1996, Dobson and Franzmann proposed combining the genus *Deleya* into a more broadly defined genus, *Halomonas* (47). Von Graevenitz et al. were the first to report a human infection caused by *H. venusta* in a wound that originated from a fish bite. It was reported to be susceptible to most antibiotics (207).

CDC halophilic nonfermenter group 1 consists of six phenotypically similar isolates received by CDC between 1971 and 1998 that are similar to *H. venusta* except for esculin hydrolysis and CFA composition. Five of these are from human blood cultures, and the sixth is from a hip wound culture (unpublished data from CDC).

PINK-PIGMENTED NONFERMENTERS
See Table 7.

Methylobacterium spp.
Members of the genus *Methylobacterium* are pink-pigmented bacteria that are able to utilize methanol as a sole source of carbon and energy, although this characteristic may be lost on subculture. They occur mostly on vegetation but may also be found in the hospital environment. Nine named species (*Methylobacterium extorquens*, *Methylobacterium organophilum*, *Methylobacterium rhodinum*, *Methylobacterium rhodesianum*, *Methylobacterium zatmanii*, *Methylobacterium aminovorans*, *Methylobacterium radiotolerans*, *Methylobacterium mesophilicum*, and *Methylobacterium fujisawaense*) and additional unassigned biovars are recognized on the basis of carbon assimilation type, electrophoretic type, and DNA-DNA homology grouping (65, 66, 193). *Methylobacterium mesophilicum* (formerly *Pseudomonas mesophilica*, *Pseudomonas extorquens*, and *Vibrio extorquens*) and *Methylobacterium zatmanii* have been the two most commonly reported species isolated in clinical samples. Methylobacteria are oxidase positive and motile by one polar or lateral flagellum, although motility is often difficult to demonstrate. Isolates are slow growing on ordinary media, producing 1-mm-diameter colonies in 4 to 5 days on SBA, modified Thayer-Martin, Sabouraud, buffered charcoal-yeast extract, and Middlebrook 7H11 agars, with best growth occurring on Sabouraud agar and usually no growth occurring on MacConkey agar. Optimum growth occurs from 25 to 30°C. Colonies are dry and appear pink or coral in incandescent light (Fig. 4). Under UV light, *Methylobacterium* species appear dark due to absorption of UV light (165). On Gram stain, the cells appear as large, vacuolated, pleomorphic rods that stain poorly and may resist decolorization (Fig. 5). Oxidation of sugars (xylose and sometimes glucose) is weak; urea and starch are hydrolyzed.

Methylobacterium species have been reported to cause septicemia, continuous ambulatory peritoneal dialysis-related peritonitis, skin ulcers, synovitis, and other infections, often in immunocompromised patients, as well as pseudoinfections (53, 87, 112, 125, 171). Tap water has been implicated as a possible agent of transmission in hospital environments, and methods for monitoring water systems for methylobacteria have been described (163). Active drugs include aminoglycosides and trimethoprim-sulfamethoxazole, whereas β-lactam drugs show variable patterns (27). They are best tested for susceptibility by agar or broth dilution at 30°C for 48 h (27).

Roseomonas spp.
Members of the genus *Roseomonas* (165) are also pink pigmented but differ in morphologic and biochemical characteristics from *Methylobacterium* spp. (Table 7). They are nonvacuolated and rather plump and coccoid, and they form mostly pairs and short chains (Fig. 6). They grow on SBA, modified Thayer-Martin, and usually MacConkey agars at 37°C, but best growth is observed on Sabouraud agar. Colonies are mucoid and runny (Fig. 7). They are separated from *Methylobacterium* by their inability to oxidize methanol and assimilate acetamide and by their lack of absorption of long-wave UV light (165). All strains are weakly oxidase positive (often after 30 s) or oxidase negative, catalase positive, and urease positive. The genus includes three named (*Roseomonas gilardii*, *Roseomonas cervicalis*, and *Roseomonas fauriae*) and three unnamed genomospecies. Clinical isolates have been recovered from

TABLE 7 Pink-pigmented nonfermenters[a]

Test	Methylobacterium species[b] (90)	Roseomonas cervicalis (7)	Roseomonas gilardii (21)	Roseomonas genomospecies 4 (3)	Roseomonas genomospecies 5 (3)	Roseomonas genomospecies 6 (1)	Roseomonas fauriae (5)
Motility; flagella	100; p. 1	100; p. 1–2	33; p. 1–2[c]	67; p. 1–2[d]	0	100; p. 1–2	100; p. 1–2
Acid from:							
D-Glucose	40	0	(43)	0	0	0	20
D-Xylose	94	43	19 (57)	100	67	0	80 (20)
D-Mannitol	2	0	14 (38)	0	0	0	0
Oxidase	96	100	52	100	100	100	100
Growth on:							
MacConkey	15	100	43 (52)	100	67 (33)	100w	60 (40)
Salmonella-shigella	0	0	0	0	0	0	20
Simmons citrate	2 (3)	86 (14)	100	0	33	(100)	60 (20)
Urea, Christensen's	29 (26)	86 (14)	71 (29)	67 (33)	100	100	100
Nitrate reduction	25	0	5	100	0	100	100
Gas from nitrate	0	0	0	0	0	0	20
H₂S (lead acetate paper)	47	100	100	100	100	100	100
Growth at 42°C	12	100	67	100	67	100	100
Esculin hydrolysis	0	0	0	0	0	0	100
Nutrient broth, 0% NaCl	93	100	100	100	100	100	100
Nutrient broth, 6% NaCl	0	0	24	33	0	0	20
Major CFAs[e]	18:1ω7c	16:0, 18:1ω7c	16:0, 18:1ω7c, 19:0cyc, 2-OH-19:0cyc	16:0, 18:1ω7c	16:0, 3-OH-16:0, 18:1ω7c	3-OH-14:0, 16:1ω7c, 18:1ω7c	16:1ω7c, 18:1ω7c

[a] Unless otherwise indicated, data are from the CDC Special Bacteriology Reference Laboratory (212). Numbers indicate the percentage positive at 2 days of incubation; parentheses indicate a delayed reaction (3 to 7 days of incubation); w, weak reaction; p, polar; pk, pink. All taxa were positive (≥90%) for catalase and growth at 25 and 35°C. All were negative for acid from lactose, sucrose, and maltose; growth on cetrimide agar, indole production, gelatin hydrolysis, acid in triple sugar iron agar, and H₂S production in triple sugar iron agar. Numbers in parentheses after the organisms indicate the number of strains.

[b] At least nine species and additional biovars have been described (see the text).

[c] Motility was more easily demonstrated in oxidative-fermentative medium than in motility medium. Motile strains demonstrated either one or two polar flagella or detached flagella.

[d] Motile strains demonstrated one or two flagella.

[e] The number before the colon indicates the number of carbons; the number after the colon is the number of double bonds; ω, the position of the double bond counting from the hydrocarbon end of the carbon chain; c, cis isomer; i, iso; OH, a hydroxyl group at the 2(α) or 3(β) position from the carboxyl end; cyc, a cyclopropane ring structure.

blood, wounds, exudates, abscesses, genitourinary sites, chronic ambulatory peritoneal dialysis fluid, and bone (13, 122, 139, 164, 165, 172, 185; L. Alcala, F. J. Vasallo, E. Cercenado, F. Garcia-Garrote, M. Rodriguez-Creixems, and E. Bouza, Letter, *J. Clin. Microbiol.* 35:2712, 1997). In a review of the laboratory, clinical, and epidemiologic data on 35 patients from whom *Roseomonas* was isolated, Struthers et al. reported that *Roseomonas* spp. appear to have a low pathogenic potential for humans but that some species, particularly *R. gilardii*, may be significant pathogens in persons with underlying medical complications (185). *Roseomonas* species are susceptible to aminoglycosides, tetracycline, and imipenem (165); however, in catheter-related infections, eradication of the organism has proven difficult unless the infected catheter is removed (164; Alcala et al., letter).

OXIDASE-POSITIVE, INDOLE-POSITIVE, NONMOTILE OR MOTILE, YELLOW-PIGMENTED NONFERMENTERS
See Table 8.

Family *Flavobacteriaceae* and CDC Groups IIc, IIe, IIg, IIh, and IIi
The taxonomy of organisms belonging to the genus *Flavobacterium* and other closely aligned genera has undergone extensive revision, resulting in an emended description of the family *Flavobacteriaceae* and an emended classification and description of the genus *Flavobacterium* (10, 195, 196). These changes are summarized below.

1. *Flavobacterium balustinum, Flavobacterium gleum, Flavobacterium indologenes, Flavobacterium indoltheticum, Flavobacterium meningosepticum,* and *Flavobacterium scophthalmum* have been moved to a new genus, *Chryseobacterium,* with *Chryseobacterium gleum* as the type species (196).

2. *Flavobacterium breve* represents a distinct genetic taxon and has been reclassified as *Empedobacter brevis* (196).

3. *Flavobacterium odoratum* has been placed in a new genus, *Myroides,* as *Myroides odoratus/odoratimimus* (195) (see above).

4. The emended genus of *Flavobacterium* contains the following species: *Flavobacterium acidificum, Flavobacterium acidurans, Flavobacterium aquatile, Flavobacterium branchiophilum, Flavobacterium columnare, Flavobacterium flevense, Flavobacterium frigidarium, Flavobacterium gillisiae, Flavobacterium hibernum, Flavobacterium hydatis, Flavobacterium johnsoniae, Flavobacterium oceanosedimentum, Flavobacterium pectinovorum, Flavobacterium psychrophilum, Flavobacterium resinovorum, Flavobacterium saccharophilum, Flavobacterium succinicans, Flavobacterium tegetincola, Flavobacterium thermophilum,* and *Flavobacterium xanthum* (10). These remaining species of *Flavobacterium* are all indole negative and are not found in human clinical specimens.

5. *Weeksella zoohelcum* has been reclassified as *Bergeyella zoohelcum* (196). *Weeksella virosa* remains the type species and only species in the genus *Weeksella.*

Chryseobacterium, Empedobacter, and Unnamed CDC Groups
The natural habitats of *Chryseobacterium, Empedobacter,* and the unnamed CDC groups are soil, plants, foodstuffs, and water sources, including those in hospitals. Species in these genera are oxidase positive, indole positive, and nonmotile. The indole reaction is often weak and difficult to

demonstrate; therefore, the more sensitive Ehrlich method should be used. Pigment formation with these organisms is variable. Colonies of *Chryseobacterium meningosepticum* are smooth and fairly large (1 to 2 mm in diameter after 24 h) but show only weak (if any) production of yellow pigment. In contrast, colonies of *Chryseobacterium indologenes* are deep yellow due to the production of the water-insoluble pigment, flexirubin (151). Colonies of *Empedobacter brevis* are pale yellow. Microscopically, cells of *C. meningosepticum, C. indologenes,* and groups IIe, IIh, and IIi are thinner in their central than their peripheral portions and include filamentous forms; IIh cells are significantly smaller than those of other species. It should be emphasized that test results (e.g., DNase, indole, urea, and starch hydrolysis) in this group are dependent on the choice of medium, reagents, and length of incubation (151). *C. indologenes, Chryseobacterium gleum,* and CDC group IIb are tabulated individually in Table 8. Group IIb is genetically heterogeneous and includes strains of *C. indologenes, C. gleum,* and probably additional genomospecies. Additional DNA-DNA hybridization studies are required to resolve this issue. Phenotypic separation between *C. indologenes* and *C. gleum* has been difficult; however, acid production from xylose and growth at 41°C are consistently positive in DNA groups clustering around the type strain of *C. gleum* (194).

C. indologenes is the most frequent human isolate, although it rarely has clinical significance (206). It has been documented to cause bacteremia in hospitalized patients with severe underlying disease, although the mortality is relatively low even among patients who were given antibiotics without activity against *C. indologenes* (90). Nosocomial infections due to *C. indologenes* have been linked to the use of indwelling devices during hospital stay (91, 93, 143). *C. meningosepticum* is the species most often associated with significant disease in humans, causing neonatal meningitis and nosocomial miniepidemics (17, 34, 180) verifiable by ribotyping (38) and random amplified polymorphic DNA fingerprinting (34) and, rarely, adult pneumonia and septicemia (17, 178, 206). A case of respiratory colonization and infection following aerosolized polymyxin B treatment has also been described (26).

E. brevis and the unnamed CDC groups IIc, IIe, IIg, IIh, and IIi are rarely recovered from clinical material, and little is known about their involvement in clinical disease. One case of meningitis caused by CDC group IIe has been reported (210), and the phenotypic characteristics of several clinical isolates of CDC groups IIc and IIg have also been recently described (70, 72).

The appropriate choice of effective antimicrobial agents for treatment of chryseobacterial infections is difficult. *Chryseobacterium* spp. are inherently resistant to many antimicrobial agents commonly used to treat infections caused by gram-negative bacteria (aminoglycosides, β-lactam antibiotics, tetracyclines, and chloramphenicol) but are often susceptible to agents generally used for treating infections caused by gram-positive bacteria (rifampin, clindamycin, erythromycin, sparfloxacin, trimethoprim-sulfamethoxazole, and vancomycin) (52, 183, 206). While early investigators recommended vancomycin for treating serious infection with *C. meningosepticum* (69, 156), recent studies have shown greater in vitro activity of minocycline, rifampin, trimethoprim-sulfamethoxazole, and quinolones (17, 57, 183). Among the quinolones, sparfloxacin and levofloxacin are more active than ciprofloxacin and ofloxacin (183). Di Pentima et al. (46) have provided evidence to suggest that the combination of intravenous vancomycin

TABLE 8 Oxidase-positive, indole-positive, nonmotile or motile nonfermenters[a]

Test	Chryseobacterium meningosepticum (149)	Chryseobacterium gleum (type strain)	Chryseobacterium indologenes (type strain)	CDC group IIb[b] (155)	CDC group IIc (20)	CDC group IIe (30)	CDC group IIg (12)	CDC group IIh (21)	CDC group IIi (23)	Empedobacter brevis (7)	Weeksella virosa (87)	Bergeyella zoohelcum (4)	Balneatrix alpica (1)
Motility, flagella	0	−	−	0	0	0	0	0	0	0	0	0	100; p, 1–2
Acid from:													
D-Glucose	95 (4)	(+)	(+)	92 (6)	100	83 (17)	0	85 (15)	91 (9)	85 (15)	0	0	100
D-Xylose	2 (1)	(+)	−	30 (1)	0	0	0	5	87 (13)	0	0	0	0
D-Mannitol	91 (8)	−	−[b]	10	0	0	0	0	0	0	0	0	(100)
Lactose	42 (15)	−	−	0	0	0	0	0	91 (9)	0	0	0	0
Sucrose	0	−	−	13 (1)	100	0	0	0	91 (9)	0	0	0	0
Maltose	93 (7)	(+)	(+)	92 (6)	100	97 (3)	0	95	91 (9)	85 (15)	0	0	100
Starch	0	−	(+)	100	ND	ND	ND	ND	ND	75	ND	ND	(100)
Trehalose	100	(+)	(+)	100	ND	ND	ND	ND	ND	0	ND	ND	0
ONPG	100	ND	−	57	ND	ND	ND	ND	ND	0	ND	ND	ND
Catalase	100	+	+	99	100	100	92	100	100	100	98	100	100
Oxidase	99	+	+	96	100	100	100	100	100	100	100	100	100
Growth on MacConkey	89 (3)	+	(+)[b]	54 (9)	0	3	100	0	0	100	(10)	2	0
Citrate	9 (3)	+[b]	+	2 (1)	0	0	0	0	14 (18)	0	0	0	100
Urea, Christensen's	3 (5)	(+)	−[b]	14 (28)	0	0	0	0	0	0	0	100	0
Nitrate reduction	0	+	−	22	90	ND	0	ND	ND	0[c]	0	0	100
Nitrite reduction	50[c]	+	−	20	90	ND	100	ND	ND	0	0	0	0
TSI slant, acid	0	−	−	1	60 (20)	0	0	0	0	0	0	0	0
TSI butt, acid	(3)	−	−	5 (5)	10 (70)	0	0	5	0	0	0	0	0

	1	2	3	4	5	6	7	8	9	10	11	12	13
H₂S (lead acetate paper)	98	+	+	99	100	87	50	100	70	100	95	59	100
Gelatin hydrolysis[d]	91	+	+	78	20	3	0	7	0	100	100	98	0
Yellow insoluble pigment	0	+	+	99	0	7w	0	0	22	85w	0	0	0
Growth at: 25°C	100	+	+	100	100	90	100	100	100	100	58	30	100
35°C	100	+	+	100	100	100	100	100	100	100	100	95	100
42°C	45	+	–	42	5	0	90	5	36	0	70	10	100
Esculin hydrolysis	99	+	+	70	100	0	0	100	96	0	0	0	0
Lysine decarboxylase	0[c]	ND	ND	12	0	0	ND	0	0	0	0	0	0
Arginine dihydrolase	33[c]	ND	ND	24	(20)	0	ND	0	0	0	0	100	0
Nutrient broth, 0% NaCl	100	+	+	100	100	97	100	86	100	100	99	15	100
Nutrient broth, 6% NaCl	7	–	–	0	10	3	0	5	9	0	7	0	0
CFAs[e]	i-15:0, i-2-OH-15:0, i-3-OH-17:0	i-15:0, i-2-OH-15:0, i-17:1ω8c	i-15:0, i-2-OH-15:0, i-17:1ω8c	i-15:0, i-2-OH-15:0, i-17:1ω8c	i-15:0, i-2-OH-15:0, i-3-OH-17:0, i-17:1ω8c	i-15:0, a-15:0, i-2-OH-15:0, i-17:1ω8c	3-OH-14:0, 16:0, 16:1ω7c, 18:1ω7c	i-15:0, a-15:0	i-15:0, i-2-OH-15:0, i-3-OH-17:0	i-15:0, 16:1ω7c	i-15:0, i-2-OH-15:0	i-15:0	16:0, 16:1ω7c, 18:1ω7c

[a] Unless otherwise indicated, data are from the CDC Special Bacteriology Reference Laboratory (212). All taxa were negative (<10% positive) for growth on salmonella-shigella agar, H₂S production in triple sugar iron (TSI), and ornithine decarboxylase activity. Numbers indicate the percentage positive at 2 days of incubation; parentheses indicate a delayed reaction (3 to 7 days of incubation); w, weak reaction; ND, not determined or not available; p, polar. Numbers in parentheses after the organisms indicate the number of strains.

[b] The original description of C. gleum lists the type strain as citrate negative. In the original description of C. indologenes, 30% of strains (4 of 13) oxidized mannitol, 46% of strains (6 of 13) grew on MacConkey agar, and 38% of strains (5 of 13) reduced nitrate to gas. CDC group IIb includes C. indologenes and C. gleum (212).

[c] Fewer than five strains tested.

[d] 7 to 14 days of incubation.

[e] The number before the colon indicates the number of carbons; the number after the colon is the number of double bonds; ω, the position of the double bond counting from the hydrocarbon end of the carbon chain; c, cis isomer; i, iso; a, anteiso; OH, a hydroxyl group at the 2(α) or 3(β) position from the carboxyl end; cyc, a cyclopropane ring structure.

and rifampin is an appropriate regimen for initial empirical therapy of *C. meningosepticum* meningitis in newborns. *C. indologenes* is reported to be uniformly resistant to cephalothin, cefotaxime, ceftriaxone, aztreonam, aminoglycosides, erythromycin, clindamycin, vancomycin, and teicoplanin, while susceptibility to piperacillin, cefoperazone, ceftazidime, imipenem, quinolones, minocycline, and trimethoprim-sulfamethoxazole is variable, requiring testing of individual isolates (90, 93, 183, 208). Further complicating the choice of appropriate antimicrobial therapy is the fact that MIC breakpoints for resistance and susceptibility of chryseobacteria have not been established by the National Committee for Clinical Laboratory Standards (NCCLS) and the results of disk diffusion testing have been shown to be unreliable in predicting antimicrobial susceptibility to *Chryseobacterium* species (1, 31, 57, 208). The E test has been shown to be a possible alternative to the standard agar dilution method for testing cefotaxime, ceftazidime, amikacin, minocycline, ofloxacin, and ciprofloxacin but not piperacillin (89). Definitive therapy for clinically significant isolates should be guided by individual susceptibility patterns determined by an MIC method.

Weeksella and Bergeyella

Vandamme et al. (196) have shown that *Weeksella virosa* (formerly CDC group IIf) (83) and *Weeksella zoohelcum* (formerly CDC group IIj) (84) represent separate genetic taxa and thus have proposed the reclassification of one of these species, *Weeksella zoohelcum*, as *Bergeyella zoohelcum*. These organisms are 0.6 to 2 to 3 μm long, with parallel sides and rounded ends. Both species are oxidase positive and indole positive, fail to grow on MacConkey agar, and are nonpigmented and nonsaccharolytic. Both species have the unusual feature of being susceptible to penicillin, a feature that allows them to be easily differentiated from the related genera of *Chryseobacterium* and *Sphingobacterium*. *W. virosa* colonies are mucoid and adherent to the agar, and they develop tan to brown pigmentation; *B. zoohelcum* colonies are sticky and tan to yellow. *W. virosa* is urease negative and polymyxin B susceptible; *B. zoohelcum* is rapid urease positive and polymyxin B resistant. *W. virosa* occurs mainly in urine and vaginal samples (83, 162), whereas, *B. zoohelcum* is isolated mainly from wounds caused by animal (mostly dog) bites (84; J. Reina and N. Borrell, Letter, *Clin. Infect. Dis.* 14:1162–1163, 1992). Meningitis or septicemia due to *B. zoohelcum* has occurred in patients either bitten by a dog (24, 135) or with continuous contact with cats (F. Noell, M. F. Gorce, C. Garde, and C. Bîzet, Letter, *Lancet* ii:332, 1989). Both organisms are susceptible to most antibiotics; however, at present no specific antibiotic treatment is recommended, and so antibiotic susceptibility testing should be performed on significant clinical isolates.

Balneatrix

The genus *Balneatrix* contains a single species, *Balneatrix alpica* (44), that was first isolated in 1987 during an outbreak of pneumonia and meningitis among persons who attended a hot (37°C)-spring spa in Southern France (29, 44, 95). Isolates from eight patients were recovered from blood, cerebrospinal fluid, and sputum, and one was recovered from water. The bacterium is described as a gram-negative, straight or curved rod that is motile by a single polar flagellum, and strictly aerobic. Growth occurs at 20 to 46°C, producing colonies that are 2 to 3 mm in diameter, convex, and smooth. The center of the colonies is pale yellow after 2 to 3 days and pale brown after 4 days. Growth occurs on chocolate and tryptic soy agars but not on MacConkey agar. It is oxidase positive and nonfermentative but oxidizes glucose, mannose, fructose, maltose, sorbitol, mannitol, glycerol, and inositol. Indole is produced, and nitrate is reduced to nitrite (Table 8). Gelatin is weakly hydrolyzed, and lecithinase is positive. It is similar to *C. meningosepticum* but can be differentiated by its positive motility and nitrate and negative ONPG reactions. *B. alpica* is reported to be susceptible to penicillin G and all other β-lactam antibiotics and to all aminoglycosides, chloramphenicol, tetracycline, erythromycin, sulfonamides, trimethoprim, ofloxacin, and nalidixic acid. It is resistant to clindamycin and vancomycin (29).

REFERENCES

1. Aber, R. C., C. Wennersten, and R. C. Moellering, Jr. 1978. Antimicrobial susceptibility of flavobacteria. *Antimicrob. Agents Chemother.* **14**:483–487.
2. Anstey, N. M., B. J. Currie, and K. M. Withnall. 1992. Community-acquired *Acinetobacter* pneumonia in the northern territory of Australia. *Clin. Infect. Dis.* **14**:83–91.
3. Bachman, K. H., D. L. Sewell, and L. J. Strausbaugh. 1996. Recurrent cellulitis and bacteremia caused by *Flavobacterium odoratum*. *J. Clin. Microbiol.* **22**:1112–1113.
4. Baldani, J. I., B. Pot, G. Kirchhof, E. Falsen, V. L. D. Baldani, F. L. Olivares, B. Hoste, K. Kersters, A. Hartmann, M. Gillis, and J. Dobereiner. 1996. Emended description of *Herbaspirillum*; inclusion of [*Pseudomonas*] *rubrisubalbicans*, a mild plant pathogen, as *Herbaspirillum rubrisubalbicans* comb. nov.; and classification of a group of clinical isolates (EF Group 1) as *Herbaspirillum* species 3. *Int. J. Syst. Bacteriol.* **46**:802–810.
5. Barham, W. B., P. Church, J. E. Brown, and S. Paparello. 1993. Misidentification of *Brucella* species with use of rapid bacterial identification systems. *Clin. Infect. Dis.* **17**:1068–1069.
6. Batchelor, B. I., R. J. Brindle, G. F. Gilks, and J. B. Selkon. 1992. Biochemical misidentification of *Brucella melitensis* and subsequent laboratory-acquired infections. *J. Hosp. Infect.* **22**:159–162.
7. Baumann, L., P. Baumann, M. Mandel, and R. D. Allen. 1972. Taxonomy of aerobic marine eubacteria. *J. Bacteriol.* **110**:402–429.
8. Baumann, L., R. D. Bowditch, and P. Baumann. 1983. Description of *Deleya* gen. nov. created to accommodate the marine species *Alcaligenes aestus*, *A. pacificus*, *A. cupidus*, *A. venustus*, and *Pseudomonas marina*. *Int. J. Syst. Bacteriol.* **33**:793–802.
9. Bergogne-Berezin, E., and K. J. Towner. 1996. *Acinetobacter* spp. as nosocomial pathogens: microbiological, clinical, and epidemiological features. *Clin. Microbiol. Rev.* **9**:148–165.
10. Bernardet, J.-F., P. Segers, M. Vancanneyt, F. Berthe, K. Kersters, and P. Vandamme. 1996. Cutting a Gordian knot: emended classification and description of the genus *Flavobacterium*, emended description of the family *Flavobacteriaceae*, and proposal of *Flavobacterium hydatis*, nom. nov. (basonym, *Cytophaga aquatilis* Strohl and Tait 1978). *Int. J. Syst. Bacteriol.* **46**:128–148.
11. Bernards, A. T., A. J. de Beaufort, L. Dijkshoorn, and C. P. A. van Boven. 1997. Outbreak of septicaemia in neonates caused by *Acinetobacter junii* investigated by amplified ribosomal DNA restriction analysis (ARDRA) and four typing methods. *J. Hosp. Infect.* **35**:129–140.
12. Bernards, A. T., J. van der Toorn, C. P. A. van Boven, and L. Dijkshoorn. 1996. Evaluation of the ability of a commercial system to identify *Acinetobacter* genomic species. *Eur. J. Clin. Microbiol. Infect. Dis.* **15**:303–308.

13. **Bibashi, E., D. Sofianou, K. Kontopoulou, E. Mitsopoulos, and E. Kokolina.** 2000. Peritonitis due to *Roseomonas fauriae* in a patient undergoing continuous ambulatory peritoneal dialysis. *J. Clin. Microbiol.* **38:**456–457.

14. **Bizet, C., and J. Bizet.** 1995. Sensibilité comparée de *Ochrobactrum anthropi, Agrobacterium tumefaciens, Alcaligenes faecalis, Alcaligenes denitrificans* subsp. *denitrificans, Alcaligenes denitrificans* subsp. *xylosidans et Bordetella bronchiseptica* vis-à-vis de 35 antibiotiques dont 17 β-lactamines. *Pathol. Biol.* **43:**258–263.

15. **Bizet, C., F. Tekaia, and A. Philippon.** 1993. In-vitro susceptibility of *Alcaligenes faecalis* compared with those of other *Alcaligenes* spp. to antimicrobial agents including seven β-lactams. *J. Antimicrob. Chemother.* **32:**907–910.

16. **Bizet, J., and C. Bizet.** 1997. Strains of *Alcaligenes faecalis* from clinical material. *J. Infect.* **35:**167–169.

17. **Bloch, K. C., R. Nadarajah, and R. Jacobs.** 1997. *Chryseobacterium meningosepticum:* an emerging pathogen among immunocompromised adults. *Medicine* **76:**30–40.

18. **Bou, G., G. Cervero, M. A. Dominguez, C. Quereda, and J. Martinez-Beltran.** 2000. PCR-based DNA fingerprinting (REP-PCR, AP-PCR) and pulsed-field gel electrophoresis characterization of a nosocomial outbreak caused by imipenem- and meropenem-resistant *Acinetobacter baumannii. Clin. Microbiol. Infect.* **6:**635–643.

19. **Bouvet, P. J. M., and P. A. D. Grimont.** 1986. Taxonomy of the genus *Acinetobacter* with the recognition of *Acinetobacter baumannii* sp. nov., *Acinetobacter haemolyticus* sp. nov., *Acinetobacter johnsonii* sp. nov., and *Acinetobacter junii* sp. nov. and emended descriptions of *Acinetobacter calcoaceticus* and *Acinetobacter lwoffii. Int. J. Syst. Bacteriol.* **36:**228–240.

20. **Bouvet, P. J. M., and P. A. D. Grimont.** 1987. Identification and biotyping of clinical isolates of *Acinetobacter. Ann. Inst. Pasteur Microbiol.* **138:**569–578.

21. **Bouvet, P. J. M., and S. Jeanjean.** 1989. Delineation of new proteolytic genomic species in the genus *Acinetobacter. Res. Microbiol.* **140:**291–299.

22. **Bouvet, P. J. M., S. Jeanjean, J. F. Vieu, and L. Dijkshoorn.** 1990. Species, biotype, and bacteriophage type determinations compared with cell envelope protein profiles for typing *Acinetobacter* strains. *J. Clin. Microbiol.* **28:**170–176.

23. **Bovre, K., J. E. Fuglesang, N. Hagen, E. Jantzen, and L. O. Froholm.** 1976. *Moraxella atlantae* sp. nov. and its distinction from *Moraxella phenylpyrouvica. Int. J. Syst. Bacteriol.* **26:**511–521.

24. **Bracis, R., K. Seibers, and R. M. Julien.** 1979. Meningitis caused by Group IIj following a dog bite. *West. J. Med.* **131:**438–440.

25. **Brink, A. J., A. van Straten, and A. J. van Rensburg.** 1995. *Shewanella (Pseudomonas) putrefaciens* bacteremia. *Clin. Infect. Dis.* **20:**1327–1332.

26. **Brown, R. B., D. Phillips, M. J. Barker, R. Pieczarka, M. Sands, and D. Teres.** 1989. Outbreak of nosocomial *Flavobacterium meningosepticum* respiratory infections associated with use of aerosolized polymyxin B. *Am. J. Infect. Control* **17:**121–125.

27. **Brown, W. J., R. L. Sautter, and A. E. Crist, Jr.** 1992. Susceptibility testing of clinical isolates of *Methylobacterium* species. *Antimicrob. Agents Chemother.* **36:**1635–1638.

28. **Butt, A. A., J. Figueroa, and D. H. Martin.** 1997. Ocular infection caused by three unusual marine organisms. *Clin. Infect. Dis.* **24:**740.

29. **Casalta, J. P., Y. Peloux, D. Raoult, P. Brunet, and H. Gallais.** 1989. Pneumonia and meningitis caused by a new nonfermentative unknown gram-negative bacterium. *J. Clin. Microbiol.* **27:**1446–1448.

30. **Centers for Disease Control and Prevention.** 1996. *Ochrobactrum anthropi* meningitis associated with cadaveric pericardial tissue processed with a contaminated solution—Utah, 1994. *Morb. Mortal. Wkly. Rep.* **45:**671–673.

31. **Chang, J.-C., P.-R. Hsueh, J.-J. Wu, S.-W. Ho, W.-C. Hsieh, and K.-T. Luh.** 1997. Antimicrobial susceptibility of flavobacteria as determined by agar dilution and disk diffusion methods. *Antimicrob. Agents Chemother.* **41:**1301–1306.

32. **Chen, Y.-S., Y.-C. Liu, M.-Y. Yen, J.-H. Wang, J.-H. Wang, S.-R. Wann, and D.-L. Cheng.** 1997. Skin and soft-tissue manifestations of *Shewanella putrefaciens* infection. *Clin. Infect. Dis.* **25:**225–229.

33. **Cheron, M., E. Abachin, E. Guerot, M. El-Bez, and M. Simonet.** 1994. Investigation of hospital-acquired infections due to *Alcaligenes denitrificans* subsp. *xylosoxidans* by DNA restriction fragment length polymorphism. *J. Clin. Microbiol.* **32:**1023–1026.

34. **Chiu, C.-H., M. Waddingdon, W.-S. Hsieh, D. Greenberg, P. C. Schreckenberger, and A. M. Carnahan.** 2000. Atypical *Chryseobacterium meningosepticum* and meningitis and sepsis in newborns and the immunocompromised, Taiwan. *Emerg. Infect. Dis.* **6:**481–486.

35. **Cieslak, T. J., M. L. Robb, C. J. Drabick, and G. W. Fischer.** 1992. Catheter-associated sepsis caused by *Ochrobactrum anthropi:* report of a case and review of related nonfermentative bacteria. *Clin. Infect. Dis.* **14:**902–907.

36. **Cisneros, J. M., M. J. Reyes, J. Pachon, B. Becerril, F. J. Caballero, J. L. Garcia-Garmendia, C. Ortiz, and A. R. Cobacho.** 1996. Bacteremia due to *Acinetobacter baumannii:* epidemiology, clinical findings, and prognostic features. *Clin. Infect. Dis.* **22:**1026–1032.

37. **Coenye, T., E. Falsen, M. Vancanneyt, B. Hoste, J. R. W. Govan, K. Kersters, and P. Vandamme.** 1999. Classification of *Alcaligenes faecalis*-like isolates from the environment and human clinical samples as *Ralstonia gilardii* sp. nov. *Int. J. Syst. Bacteriol.* **49:**405–413.

38. **Colding, H., J. Bangsborg, N.-E. Fiehn, T. Bennekov, and B. Bruun.** 1994. Ribotyping for differentiating *Flavobacterium meningosepticum* isolates from clinical and environmental sources. *J. Clin. Microbiol.* **32:**501–505.

39. **Corbella, X., M. Pujol, J. Ayats, M. Sendra, C. Ardanuy, M. A. Dominguez, J. Linares, J. Ariza, and F. Gudiol.** 1996. Relevance of digestive tract colonization in the epidemiology of nosocomial infections due to multiresistant *Acinetobacter baumannii. Clin. Infect. Dis.* **23:**329–334.

40. **Daley, D., S. Neville, and K. Kociuba.** 1997. Peritonitis associated with a CDC group EO-3 organism. *J. Clin. Microbiol.* **35:**3338–3339.

41. **Dan, M., R. Gutman, and A. Biro.** 1992. Peritonitis caused by *Pseudomonas putrefaciens* in patients undergoing continuous ambulatory peritoneal dialysis. *Clin. Infect. Dis.* **14:**359–360.

42. **Daneshvar, M. I., B. Hill, D. G. Hollis, C. W. Moss, J. G. Jordan, J. P. MacGregor, F. Tenover, and R. S. Weyant.** 1998. CDC group O-3: phenotypic characteristics, fatty acid composition, isoprenoid quinone content, and in vitro antimicrobic susceptibilities of an unusual gram-negative bacterium isolated from clinical specimens. *J. Clin. Microbiol.* **36:**1674–1678.

43. **Das, K., S. Shah, and M. H. Levi.** 1997. Misleading Gram stain from a patient with *Moraxella (Branhamella) catarrhalis* bacteremia. *Clin. Microbiol. Newsl.* **19:**85–88.

44. **Dauga, C., M. Gillis, P. Vandamme, E. Ageron, F. Grimont, K. Kersters, C. de Mahenge, Y. Peloux, and P. A. D. Grimont.** 1993. *Balneatrix alpica* gen. nov., sp.

nov., a bacterium associated with pneumonia and meningitis in a spa therapy centre. *Res. Microbiol.* **144:**35–46.

45. **Dees, S. B., D. G. Hollis, R. E. Weaver, and C. W. Moss.** 1983. Cellular fatty acid composition of *Pseudomonas marginata* and closely associated bacteria. *J. Clin. Microbiol.* **18:**1073–1078.

46. **Di Pentima, M. C., E. O. Mason, Jr., and S. L. Kaplan.** 1998. In vitro antibiotic synergy against *Flavobacterium meningosepticum*: implications for therapeutic options. *Clin. Infect. Dis.* **26:**1169–1176.

47. **Dobson, S. J., and P. D. Franzmann.** 1996. Unification of the genera *Deleya* (Baumann et al. 1983), *Halomonas* (Vreeland et al. 1980), and *Halovibrio* (Fendrich 1988) and the species *Paracoccus halodenitrificans* (Robinson and Gibbons 1952) into a single genus, *Halomonas*, and placement of the genus *Zymobacter* in the family *Halomonadaceae. Int. J. Syst. Bacteriol.* **46:**550–558.

48. **Duggan, J. M., S. J. Goldstein, C. E. Chenoweth, C. A. Kauffman, and S. F. Bradley.** 1996. *Achromobacter xylosoxidans* bacteremia: report of four cases and review of the literature. *Clin. Infect. Dis.* **23:**569–576.

49. **Dunne, W. M., Jr., and S. Maisch.** 1995. Epidemiological investigation of infections due to *Alcaligenes* species in children and patients with cystic fibrosis: use of repetitive-element-sequence polymerase chain reaction. *Clin. Infect. Dis.* **20:**836–841.

50. **Dunne, W. M., Jr., J. Tillman, and J. C. Murray.** 1993. Recovery of a strain of *Agrobacterium radiobacter* with a mucoid phenotype from an immunocompromised child with bacteremia. *J. Clin. Microbiol.* **31:**2541–2543.

51. **Edmond, M. B., S. A. Riddler, C. M. Baxter, B. M. Wicklund, and A. W. Pasculle.** 1993. *Agrobacterium radiobacter*: a recently recognized opportunistic pathogen. *Clin. Infect. Dis.* **16:**388–391.

52. **Fass, R. J., and J. Barnishan.** 1980. In vitro susceptibility of nonfermentative gram-negative bacilli other than *Pseudomonas aeruginosa* to 32 antimicrobial agents. *Rev. Infect. Dis.* **2:**841–853.

53. **Flournoy, D. J., R. L. Petrone, and D. W. Voth.** 1992. A pseudo-outbreak of *Methylobacterium mesophilica* isolated from patients undergoing bronchoscopy. *Eur. J. Clin. Microbiol. Infect. Dis.* **11:**240–243.

54. **Fonnesbech Vogel, B., K. Jørgensen, H. Christensen, J. E. Olsen, and L. Gram.** 1997. Differentiation of *Shewanella putrefaciens* and *Shewanella alga* on the basis of whole-cell protein profiles, ribotyping, phenotypic characterization, and 16S rRNA gene sequence analysis. *Appl. Environ. Microbiol.* **63:**2189–2199.

55. **Fonnesbech Vogel, B., K. Venkateswaran, H. Christensen, E. Falsen, G. Christiansen, and L. Gram.** 2000. Polyphasic taxonomic approach in the description of *Alishewanella fetalis* gen. nov., sp. nov., isolated from a human foetus. *Int. J. Syst. Evol. Microbiol.* **50:**1133–1142.

56. **Forster, D. H., and F. D. Daschner.** 1998. *Acinetobacter* species as nosocomial pathogens. *Eur. J. Clin. Microbiol. Infect. Dis.* **17:**73–77.

57. **Fraser, S. L., and J. H. Jorgensen.** 1997. Reappraisal of the antimicrobial susceptibilities of *Chryseobacterium* and *Flavobacterium* species and methods for reliable susceptibility testing. *Antimicrob. Agents Chemother.* **41:**2738–2741.

58. **Freney, J., W. Hansen, C. Ploton, H. Meugnier, S. Madier, N. Bornstein, and J. Fleurette.** 1987. Septicemia caused by *Sphingobacterium multivorum. J. Clin. Microbiol.* **25:**1126–1128.

59. **Gales, A. C., R. N. Jones, K. R. Forward, J. Linares, H. S. Sader, and J. Verhoef.** 2001. Emerging importance of multidrug-resistant *Acinetobacter* species and *Stenotrophomonas maltophilia* as pathogens in seriously ill patients: geographic patterns, epidemiological features, and trends in the SENTRY antimicrobial surveillance program (1997–1999). *Clin. Infect. Dis.* **32**(Suppl. 2):104–113.

60. **Gerner-Smidt, P., and I. Tjernberg.** 1993. *Acinetobacter* in Denmark. II. Molecular studies of the *Acinetobacter calcoaceticus-Acinetobacter baumannii* complex. *APMIS* **101:**826–832.

61. **Gerner-Smidt, P., I. Tjernberg, and J. Ursing.** 1991. Reliability of phenotypic tests for identification of *Acinetobacter* species. *J. Clin. Microbiol.* **29:**277–282.

62. **Getchell-White, S. I., L. G. Donowitz, and D. H. M. Gröschel.** 1989. The inanimate environment of an intensive care unit as a potential source of nosocomial bacteria: evidence for long survival of *Acinetobacter calcoaceticus. Infect. Control Hosp. Epidemiol.* **10:**402–407.

63. **Gini, G. A.** 1990. Ocular infection caused by *Psychrobacter immobilis* acquired in the hospital. *J. Clin. Microbiol.* **28:**400–401.

64. **Graham, D. R., J. D. Band, C. Thornsberry, D. G. Hollis, and R. E. Weaver.** 1990. Infections caused by *Moraxella, Moraxella urethralis, Moraxella*-like groups M-5 and M-6, and *Kingella kingae* in the United States, 1953–1980. *Rev. Infect. Dis.* **12:**423–431.

65. **Green, P. N., and I. J. Bousfield.** 1983. Emendation of *Methylobacterium* Patt, Cole, and Hanson 1976; *Methylobacterium rhodinum* (Heumann 1962) comb. nov. corrig.; *Methylobacterium radiotolerans* (Ito and Iizuka 1971) comb. nov. corrig.; and *Methylobacterium mesophilicum* (Austin and Goodfellow 1979) comb. nov. *Int. J. Syst. Bacteriol.* **33:**875–877.

66. **Green, P. N., I. J. Bousfield, and D. Hood.** 1988. Three new *Methylobacterium* species: M. *rhodesianum* sp. nov., M. *zatmanii* sp. nov., and M. *fujisawaense* sp. nov. *Int. J. Syst. Bacteriol.* **38:**124–127.

67. **Grundmann, H. J., K. J. Towner, L. Dijkshoorn, P. Gerner-Smidt, M. Maher, H. Seifert, and M. Vaneechoutte.** 1997. Multicenter study using standardized protocols and reagents for evaluation of reproducibility of PCR-based fingerprinting of *Acinetobacter* spp. *J. Clin. Microbiol.* **35:**3071–3077.

68. **Harmsen, D., C. Singer, J. Rothgänger, T. Tønjum, G. Sybren de Hoog, H. Shah, J. Albert, and M. Frosch.** 2001. Diagnostics of *Neisseriaceae* and *Moraxellaceae* by ribosomal DNA sequencing: ribosomal differentiation of medical microorganisms. *J. Clin. Microbiol.* **39:**936–942.

69. **Hawley, H. B., and D. W. Gump.** 1973. Vancomycin therapy of bacterial meningitis. *Am. J. Dis. Child.* **126:**261–264.

70. **Hollis, D. G., M. I. Daneshvar, C. W. Moss, and C. N. Baker.** 1995. Phenotypic characteristics, fatty acid composition, and isoprenoid quinone content of CDC group IIg bacteria. *J. Clin. Microbiol.* **33:**762–764.

71. **Hollis, D. G., C. W. Moss, M. I. Daneshvar, L. Meadows, J. Jordan, and B. Hill.** 1993. Characterization of Centers for Disease Control group NO-1, a fastidious, nonoxidative, gram-negative organism associated with dog and cat bites. *J. Clin. Microbiol.* **31:**746–748.

72. **Hollis, D. G., C. W. Moss, M. I. Daneshvar, and P. L. Wallace-Shewmaker.** 1996. CDC group IIc: phenotypic characteristics, fatty acid composition, and isoprenoid quinone content. *J. Clin. Microbiol.* **34:**2322–2324.

73. **Holmes, B., M. Costas, A. C. Wood, and K. Kersters.** 1990. Numerical analysis of electrophoretic protein patterns of "Achromobacter" group B, E and F strains from human blood. *J. Appl. Bacteriol.* **68:**495–504.

74. **Holmes, B., M. Costas, A. C. Wood, R. J. Owen, and D. D. Morgan.** 1990. Differentiation of *Achromobacter*-like strains from human blood by DNA restriction endo-

nuclease digest and ribosomal RNA gene probe patterns. *Epidemiol. Infect.* **105:**541–551.

75. Holmes, B., R. Lewis, and A. Trevett. 1992. Septicaemia due to *Achromobacter* group B: a report of two cases. *Med. Microbiol. Lett.* **1:**177–184.

76. Holmes, B., C. W. Moss, and M. I. Daneshvar. 1993. Cellular fatty acid compositions of "*Achromobacter* groups B and E." *J. Clin. Microbiol.* **31:**1007–1008.

77. Holmes, B., R. J. Owen, A. Evans, H. Malnick, and W. R. Willcox. 1977. *Pseudomonas paucimobilis*, a new species isolated from human clinical specimens, the hospital environment, and other sources. *Int. J. Syst. Bacteriol.* **27:**133–146.

78. Holmes, B., R. J. Owen, and D. G. Hollis. 1982. *Flavobacterium spiritivorum*, a new species isolated from human clinical specimens. *Int. J. Syst. Bacteriol.* **32:**157–165.

79. Holmes, B., R. J. Owen, and R. E. Weaver. 1981. *Flavobacterium multivorum*, a new species isolated from human clinical specimens and previously known as group IIK, biotype 2. *Int. J. Syst. Bacteriol.* **31:**21–34.

80. Holmes, B., C. A. Pinning, and C. A. Dawson. 1986. A probability matrix for the identification of Gram-negative, aerobic, non-fermentative bacteria that grow on nutrient agar. *J. Gen. Microbiol.* **132:**1827–1842.

81. Holmes, B., M. Popoff, M. Kiredjian, and K. Kersters. 1988. *Ochrobactrum anthropi* gen. nov., sp. nov. from human clinical specimens and previously known as group Vd. *Int. J. Syst. Bacteriol.* **38:**406–416.

82. Holmes, B., J. J. S. Snell, and S. P. Lapage. 1979. *Flavobacterium odoratum*: a species resistant to a wide range of antimicrobial agents. *J. Clin. Pathol.* **32:**73–77.

83. Holmes, B., A. G. Steigerwalt, R. E. Weaver, and D. J. Brenner. 1986. *Weeksella virosa* gen. nov., sp. nov. (formerly Group IIf), found in human clinical specimens. *Syst. Appl. Microbiol.* **8:**185–190.

84. Holmes, B., A. G. Steigerwalt, R. E. Weaver, and D. J. Brenner. 1986. *Weeksella zoohelcum* sp. nov. (formerly Group IIj), from human clinical specimens. *Syst. Appl. Microbiol.* **8:**191–196.

85. Holt, H. M., P. Sogaard, and B. Gahrn-Hansen. 1997. Ear infections with *Shewanella alga*: a bacteriologic, clinical and epidemiologic study of 67 cases. *Clin. Microbiol. Infect.* **3:**329–334.

86. Holton, J. 1983. A note on the preparation and use of a selective and differential medium for the isolation of the *Acinetobacter* spp. from clinical sources. *J. Appl. Bacteriol.* **66:**24–26.

87. Hornei, B., E. Luneberg, H. Schmidt-Rotte, M. Maab, K. Weber, F. Heits, M. Frosch, and W. Solbach. 1999. Systemic infection of an immunocompromised patient with *Methylobacterium zatmanii*. *J. Clin. Microbiol.* **37:**248–250.

88. Houang, E. T. S., Y. W. Chu, C. M. Leung, K. Y. Chu, J. Berlau, K. C. Ng, and A. F. B. Cheng. 2001. Epidemiology and infection control implications of *Acinetobacter* spp. in Hong Kong. *J. Clin. Microbiol.* **39:**228–234.

89. Hsueh, P.-R., J.-C. Chang, L.-J. Teng, P.-C. Yang, S.-W. Ho, W.-C. Hsieh, and K.-T. Luh. 1997. Comparison of Etest and agar dilution method for antimicrobial susceptibility testing of *Flavobacterium* isolates. *J. Clin. Microbiol.* **35:**1021–1023.

90. Hsueh, P.-R., T.-R. Hsiue, J.-J. Wu, L.-J. Teng, S.-W. Ho, W.-C. Hsieh, and K.-T. Luh. 1996. *Flavobacterium indologenes* bacteremia: clinical and microbiological characteristics. *Clin. Infect. Dis.* **23:**550–555.

91. Hsueh, P.-R., L.-J. Teng, S.-W. Ho, W.-C. Hsieh, and K.-T. Luh. 1996. Clinical and microbiological characteristics of *Flavobacterium indologenes* infections associated with indwelling devices. *J. Clin. Microbiol.* **34:**1908–1913.

92. Hsueh, P.-R., L.-J. Teng, P.-C. Yang, Y.-C. Chen, H.-J. Pan, S.-W. Ho, and K.-T. Luh. 1998. Nosocomial infections caused by *Sphingomonas paucimobilis*: clinical features and microbiological characteristics. *Clin. Infect. Dis.* **26:**676–681.

93. Hsueh, P.-R., L.-J. Teng, P.-C. Yang, S.-W. Ho, W.-C. Hsieh, and K.-T. Luh. 1997. Increasing incidence of nosocomial *Chryseobacterium indologenes* infections in Taiwan. *Eur. J. Clin. Microbiol. Infect. Dis.* **16:**568–574.

94. Hsueh, P.-R., J.-J. Wu, T.-R. Hsiue, and W.-C. Hsieh. 1995. Bacteremic necrotizing fasciitis due to *Flavobacterium odoratum*. *Clin. Infect. Dis.* **21:**1337–1338.

95. Hubert, B., A. de Mahenge, F. Grimont, C. Richard, Y. Peloux, C. de Mahenge, J. Fleurette, and P. A. D. Grimont. 1991. An outbreak of pneumonia and meningitis caused by a previously undescribed gram-negative bacterium in a hot spring spa. *Epidemiol. Infect.* **107:**373–381.

96. Hulse, M., S. Johnson, and P. Ferrieri. 1993. *Agrobacterium* infections in humans: experience at one hospital and review. *Clin. Infect. Dis.* **16:**112–117.

97. Ibrahim, A., P. Gerner-Smidt, and W. Liesack. 1997. Phylogenetic relationship of the twenty-one DNA groups of the genus *Acinetobacter* as revealed by 16S ribosomal DNA sequence analysis. *Int. J. Syst. Bacteriol.* **47:**837–841.

98. Iwata, M., K. Tateda, T. Matsumoto, N. Furuya, S. Mizuiri, and K. Yamaguchi. 1999. Primary *Shewanella alga* septicemia in a patient on hemodialysis. *J. Clin. Microbiol.* **37:**2104–2105.

99. Jannes, G., M. Vaneechoutte, M. Lannoo, M. Gillis, M. Vancanneyt, P. Vandamme, G. Verschraegen, H. van Heuverswyn, and R. Rossau. 1993. Polyphasic taxonomy leading to the proposal of *Moraxella canis* sp. nov. for *Moraxella catarrhalis*-like strains. *Int. J. Syst. Bacteriol.* **43:**438–449.

100. Jawad, A., P. M. Hawkey, J. Heritage, and A. M. Snelling. 1994. Description of Leeds *Acinetobacter* medium, a new selective and differential medium for isolation of clinically important *Acinetobacter* spp., and comparison with Herellea agar and Holton's agar. *J. Clin. Microbiol.* **32:**2353–2358.

101. Jellison, T. K., P. S. McKinnon, and M. J. Rybak. 2001. Epidemiology, resistance, and outcomes of *Acinetobacter baumannii* bacteremia treated with imipenem-cilastatin or ampicillin-sulbactam. *Pharmacotherapy* **21:**142–148.

102. Jenks, P. J., and E. J. Shaw. 1997. Recurrent septicaemia due to "*Achromobacter* Group B." *J. Infect.* **34:**143–145.

103. Jiménez-Mejias, M. E., J. Pachón, B. Becerril, J. Palomino-Nicás, A. Rodriguez-Cobacho, and M. Revuelta. 1997. Treatment of multidrug-resistant *Acinetobacter baumannii* meningitis with ampicillin/sulbactam. *Clin. Infect. Dis.* **24:**932–935.

104. Johnson, D. W., G. Lum, G. Nimmo, and C. M. Hawley. 1995. *Moraxella nonliquefaciens* septic arthritis in a patient undergoing hemodialysis. *Clin. Infect. Dis.* **21:**1039–1040.

105. Joyanes, P., M. Del Carmen Conejo, L. Martínez-Martínez, and E. J. Perea. 2001. Evaluation of the Vitek 2 system for the identification and susceptibility testing of three species of nonfermenting gram-negative rods frequently isolated from clinical specimens. *J. Clin. Microbiol.* **39:**3247–3253.

106. Juni, E. 1972. Interspecies transformation of *Acinetobacter*: genetic evidence for a ubiquitous genus. *J. Bacteriol.* **112:**917–931.

107. Juni, E., G. A. Heym, M. J. Maurer, and M. L. Miller. 1987. Combined genetic transformation and nutritional

assay for identification of *Moraxella nonliquefaciens*. *J. Clin. Microbiol.* **25**:1691–1694.

108. **Kaiser, R. M., R. L. Garman, M. G. Bruce, R. S. Weyant, and D. A. Ashford.** 2002. Clinical significance and epidemiology of NO-1, an unusual bacterium associated with dog and cat bites. *Emerg. Infect. Dis.* **8**:171–174.

109. **Kämpfer, P.** 1993. Grouping of *Acinetobacter* genomic species by cellular fatty acid composition. *Med. Microbiol. Lett.* **2**:394–400.

110. **Kappstein, I., H. Grundmann, T. Hauer, and C. Niemeyer.** 2000. Aerators as a reservoir of *Acinetobacter junii*: an outbreak of bacteraemia in paediatric oncology patients. *J. Hosp. Infect.* **44**:27–30.

111. **Kay, S. E., R. A. Clark, K. L. White, and M. M. Peel.** 2001. Recurrent *Achromobacter piechaudii* bacteremia in a patient with hematological malignancy. *J. Clin. Microbiol.* **39**:808–810.

112. **Kaye, K. M., A. Macone, and P. H. Kazanjian.** 1992. Catheter infection caused by *Methylobacterium* in immunocompromised hosts: report of three cases and review of the literature. *Clin. Infect. Dis.* **14**:1010–1014.

113. **Kern, W. V., M. Oethinger, A. Kaufhold, E. Rozdzinski, and R. Marre.** 1993. *Ochrobactrum anthropi* bacteremia: report of four cases and short review. *Infection* **21**:306–310.

114. **Khashe, S., and J. M. Janda.** 1998. Biochemical and pathogenic properties of *Shewanella alga* and *Shewanella putrefaciens*. *J. Clin. Microbiol.* **36**:783–787.

115. **Kim, J. H., R. A. Cooper, K. E. Welty-Wolf, L. J. Harrell, P. Zwadyk, and M. E. Klotman.** 1989. *Pseudomonas putrefaciens* bacteremia. *Rev. Infect. Dis.* **11**:97–104.

116. **Kiredjian, M., B. Holmes, K. Kersters, I. Guilvout, and J. de Ley.** 1986. *Alcaligenes piechaudii*, a new species from human clinical specimens and the environment. *Int. J. Syst. Bacteriol.* **36**:282–287.

117. **Kiska, D. L., A. Kerr, M. C. Jones, J. A. Caracciolo, B. Eskridge, M. Jordan, S. Miller, D. Hughes, N. King, and P. H. Gilligan.** 1996. Accuracy of four commercial systems for identification of *Burkholderia cepacia* and other gram-negative nonfermenting bacilli recovered from patients with cystic fibrosis. *J. Clin. Microbiol.* **34**:886–891.

118. **Knuth, B. D., M. R. Owen, and R. Latorraca.** 1969. Occurrence of an unclassified organism group IVd. *Am. J. Med. Technol.* **35**:227–232.

119. **Koeleman J. G. M., J. Stoof, D. J. Biesmans, P. H. M. Savelkoul, and C. M. J. E. Vandenbroucke-Grauls.** 1998. Comparison of amplified ribosomal DNA restriction analysis, random amplified polymorphic DNA analysis, and amplified fragment length polymorphism fingerprinting for identification of *Acinetobacter* genomic species and typing of *Acinetobacter baumannii*. *J. Clin. Microbiol.* **36**:2522–2529.

120. **Koneman, E. W., S. D. Allen, W. M. Janda, P. C. Schreckenberger, and W. C. Winn, Jr.** 1997. *Color Atlas and Textbook of Diagnostic Microbiology*, 5th ed. p. 253–320. The J. B. Lippincott Co., Philadelphia, Pa.

121. **La Scola, B., R. J. Birtles, M.-N. Mallet, and D. Raoult.** 1998. *Massilia timonae* gen. nov., sp. nov., isolated from blood of an immunocompromised patient with cerebellar lesions. *J. Clin. Microbiol.* **36**:2847–2852.

122. **Lewis, L., F. Stock, D. Williams, S. Weir, and V. J. Gill.** 1997. Infections with *Roseomonas gilardii* and review of characteristics used for biochemical identification and molecular typing. *Am. J. Clin. Pathol.* **108**:210–216.

123. **Lin, Y.-H., P. Y.-F. Liu, Z.-Y. Shi, Y.-J. Lau, and B.-S. Hu.** 1997. Comparison of polymerase chain reaction and pulsed-field gel electrophoresis for the epidemiological typing of *Alcaligenes xylosoxidans* subsp. *xylosoxidans* in a burn unit. *Diagn. Microbiol. Infect. Dis.* **28**:173–178.

124. **Ling, T. K. W., P. C. Tam, Z. K. Liu, and A. F. B. Cheng.** 2001. Evaluation of Vitek 2 rapid identification and susceptibility testing system against gram-negative clinical isolates. *J. Clin. Microbiol.* **39**:2964–2966.

125. **Liu, J.-W., J.-J. Wu, H.-M. Chen, A.-H. Huang, W.-C. Ko, and Y.-C. Chuang.** 1997. *Methylobacterium mesophilicum* synovitis in an alcoholic. *Clin. Infect. Dis.* **24**:1008–1009.

126. **Liu, P. Y.-F., and W.-L. Wu.** 1997. Use of different PCR-based DNA fingerprinting techniques and pulsed-field gel electrophoresis to investigate the epidemiology of *Acinetobacter calcoaceticus-Acinetobacter baumannii* complex. *Diagn. Microbiol. Infect. Dis.* **28**:19–28.

127. **Lloyd-Puryear, M., D. Wallace, T. Baldwin, and D. G. Hollis.** 1991. Meningitis caused by *Psychrobacter immobilis* in an infant. *J. Clin. Microbiol.* **29**:2041–2042.

128. **MacDonell, M. T., and R. R. Colwell.** 1985. Phylogeny of the *Vibrionaceae*, and recommendation for two new genera, *Listonella* and *Shewanella*. *Syst. Appl. Microbiol.* **6**:171–182.

129. **Mahmood, M. S., A. R. Sarwari, M. A. Khan, Z. Sophie, E. Khan, and S. Sami.** 2000. Infective endocarditis and septic embolization with *Ochrobactrum anthropi*: case report and review of literature. *J. Infect.* **40**:287–290.

130. **Manfredi, R., A. Nanetti, M. Ferri, A. Mastroianni, O. V. Coronado, and F. Chiodo.** 1999. Emerging gram-negative pathogens in the immunocompromised host: *Agrobacterium radiobacter* septicemia during HIV disease. *Microbiologica* **22**:375–382.

131. **Manikal, V. M., D. Landman, G. Saurina, E. Oydna, H. Lal, and J. Quale.** 2000. Endemic carbapenem-resistant *Acinetobacter* species in Brooklyn, New York: citywide prevalence, interinstitutional spread, and relation to antibiotic usage. *Clin. Infect. Dis.* **31**:101–106.

132. **Mesnard, R., J. M. Sire, P. Y. Donnio, J. Y. Riou, and J. L. Avril.** 1992. Septic arthritis due to *Oligella urethralis*. *Eur. J. Clin. Microbiol. Infect. Dis.* **11**:195–196.

133. **Miller, J. M., C. Novy, and M. Hiott.** 1996. Case of bacterial endophthalmitis caused by an *Agrobacterium radiobacter*-like organism. *J. Clin. Microbiol.* **34**:3212–3213.

134. **Moller, L. V. M., J. P. Arends, H. J. M. Harmsen, A. Talens, P. Terpstra, and M. J. H. Slooff.** 1999. *Ochrobactrum intermedium* infection after liver transplantation. *J. Clin. Microbiol.* **37**:241–244.

135. **Montejo, M., K. Aguirrebengoa, J. Ugalde, L. Lopez, J. A. S. Nieto, and J. L. Hernández.** 2001. *Bergeyella zoohelcum* bacteremia after a dog bite. *Clin. Infect. Dis.* **33**:1608–1609.

136. **Morrison, A. J., and J. A. Shulman.** 1986. Community-acquired bloodstream infection caused by *Pseudomonas paucimobilis*: case report and review of literature. *J. Clin. Microbiol.* **24**:853–855.

137. **Moss, C. W., M. I. Daneshvar, and D. G. Hollis.** 1993. Biochemical characteristics and fatty acid composition of Gilardi rod group 1 bacteria. *J. Clin. Microbiol.* **31**:689–691.

138. **Moss, C. W., P. L. Wallace, D. G. Hollis, and R. E. Weaver.** 1988. Cultural and chemical characterization of CDC groups EO-2, M-5, and M-6, *Moraxella* (*Moraxella*) species, *Oligella urethralis*, *Acinetobacter* species, and *Psychrobacter immobilis*. *J. Clin. Microbiol.* **26**:484–492.

139. **Nahass, R. G., R. Wisneski, D. J. Herman, E. Hirsh, and K. Goldblatt.** 1995. Vertebral osteomyelitis due to *Roseomonas* species: case report and review of the evaluation of vertebral osteomyelitis. *Clin. Infect. Dis.* **21**:1474–1476.

140. Nemec, A., T. De Baere, I. Tjernberg, M. Vaneechoutte, T. J. K. van der Reijden, and L. Dijkshoorn. 2001. *Acinetobacter ursingii* sp. nov. and *Acinetobacter schindleri* sp. nov., isolated from human clinical specimens. *Int. J. Syst. Evol. Microbiol.* **51:**1891–1899.

141. Nishimura, Y., T. Ino, and H. Hzuka. 1988. *Acinetobacter radioresistens* sp. nov. isolated from cotton and soil. *Int. J. Syst. Bacteriol.* **38:**209–211.

142. Nozue, H., T. Hayashi, Y. Hashimoto, T. Ezaki, K. Hamasaki, K. Ohwada, and Y. Terawaki. 1992. Isolation and characterization of *Shewanella alga* from human clinical specimens and emendation of the description of *S. alga* Simidu et al., 1990, 335. *Int. J. Syst. Bacteriol.* **42:**628–634.

143. Nulens, E., B. Bussels, A. Bols, B. Gordts, and H. W. Van Landuyt. 2001. Recurrent bacteremia by *Chryseobacterium indologenes* in an oncology patient with a totally implanted intravascular device. *Clin. Microbiol. Infect.* **7:**391–393.

144. O'Hara, C. M., G. L. Westbrook, and J. M. Miller. 1997. Evaluation of Vitek GNI+ and Becton Dickinson Microbiology Systems Crystal E/NF identification systems for identification of members of the family *Enterobacteriaceae* and other gram-negative, glucose-fermenting and non-glucose-fermenting bacilli. *J. Clin. Microbiol.* **35:**3269–3273.

145. Osterhout, G. J., V. H. Shull, and J. D. Dick. 1991. Identification of clinical isolates of gram-negative nonfermentative bacteria by an automated cellular fatty acid identification system. *J. Clin. Microbiol.* **29:**1822–1830.

146. Owen, R. J., R. M. Legros, and S. P. Lapage. 1978. Base composition, size and sequence similarities of genome deoxyribonucleic acids from clinical isolates of *Pseudomonas putrefaciens. J. Gen. Microbiol.* **104:**127–138.

147. Peel, M. M., A. J. Hibberd, B. M. King, and H. G. Williamson. 1988. *Alcaligenes piechaudii* from chronic ear discharge. *J. Clin. Microbiol.* **26:**1580–1581.

148. Peiris, V., S. Fraser, M. Fairhurst, D. Weston, and E. Kaczmarski. 1992. Laboratory diagnosis of brucella infection: some pitfalls. *Lancet* **339:**1415–1416.

149. Perez, J. L., A. Pulido, F. Pantozzi, and R. Martin. 1990. Butyrate esterase (tributyrin) spot test, a simple method for immediate identification of *Moraxella (Branhamella) catarrhalis. J. Clin. Microbiol.* **28:**2347–2348.

150. Pettersson, B., A. Kodjo, M. Ronaghi, M. Uhlen, and T. Tonjum. 1998. Phylogeny of the family *Moraxellaceae* by 16S rRNA sequence analysis, with special emphasis on differentiation of *Moraxella* species. *Int. J. Syst. Bacteriol.* **48:**75–89.

151. Pickett, M. J. 1989. Methods for identification of flavobacteria. *J. Clin. Microbiol.* **27:**2309–2315.

152. Pickett, M. J. 1994. Moraxellae: differential features for identification of *Moraxella atlantae, M. lacunata,* and *M. nonliquefaciens. Med. Microbiol. Lett.* **3:**397–400.

153. Pickett, M. J. 1994. Identification of *Brucella* species with a procedure for detecting acidification of glucose. *Clin. Infect. Dis.* **19:**976.

154. Pickett, M. J., and E. L. Nelson. 1955. Speciation within the genus *Brucella.* IV. Fermentation of carbohydrates. *J. Bacteriol.* **69:**333–336

155. Pickett, M. J., A. von Graevenitz, G. E. Pfyffer, V. Pünter, and M. Altwegg. 1996. Phenotypic features distinguishing *Oligella urethralis* from *Moraxella osloensis. Med. Microbiol. Lett.* **5:**265–270.

156. Plotkin, S. A., and J. C. McKitrick. 1966. Nosocomial meningitis of the newborn caused by a flavobacterium. *JAMA* **198:**194–196.

157. Potvliege, C., C. Dejaegher-Bauduin, W. Hansen, M. Dratwa, F. Collart, C. Tielemans, and E. Youras-

sowsky. 1984. *Flavobacterium multivorum* septicemia in a hemodialyzed patient. *J. Clin. Microbiol.* **19:**568–569.

158. Prashanth, K., M. P. M. Ranga, V. A. Rao, and R. Kanungo. 2000. Corneal perforation due to *Acinetobacter junii:* a case report. *Diagn. Microbiol. Infect. Dis.* **37:**215–217.

159. Pugliese, A., B. Pacris, P. E. Schoch, and B. A. Cunha. 1993. *Oligella urethralis* urosepsis. *Clin. Infect. Dis.* **17:**1069–1070.

160. Purcell, B. K., and D. P. Dooley. 1999. Centers for Disease Control and Prevention Group O1 bacterium-associated pneumonia complicated by bronchopulmonary fistula and bacteremia. *Clin. Infect. Dis.* **29:**945–946.

161. Reina, J., A. Bassa, I. Llompart, D. Portela, and N. Borrell. 1991. Infections with *Pseudomonas paucimobilis:* report of four cases and review. *Rev. Infect. Dis.* **13:**1072–1076.

162. Reina, J., J. Gil, F. Salva, J. Gomez, and P. Alomar. 1990. Microbiological characteristics of *Weeksella virosa* (formerly CDC Group IIf) isolated from the human genitourinary tract. *J. Clin. Microbiol.* **28:**2357–2359.

163. Rice, E. W., D. J. Reasoner, C. H. Johnson, and L. A. DeMaria. 2000. Monitoring for methylobacteria in water systems. *J. Clin. Microbiol.* **38:**4296–4297.

164. Richardson, J. D. 1997. Failure to clear a *Roseomonas* line infection with antibiotic therapy. *Clin. Infect. Dis.* **25:**155.

165. Rihs, J. D., D. J. Brenner, R. E. Weaver, A. G. Steigerwalt, D. G. Hollis, and V. L. Yu. 1993. *Roseomonas,* a new genus associated with bacteremia and other human infections. *J. Clin. Microbiol.* **31:**3275–3283.

166. Rockhill, R. C., and L. I. Lutwick. 1978. Group IVe-like gram-negative bacillemia in a patient with obstructive uropathy. *J. Clin. Microbiol.* **8:**108–109.

167. Rosenthal, S. L., L. F. Freundlich, G. L. Gilardi, and F. Y. Clodomar. 1978. In vitro antibiotic sensitivity of *Moraxella* species. *Chemotherapy* **24:**360–363.

168. Rossau, R., K. Kersters, E. Falsen, E. Jantzen, P. Segers, A. Union, L. Nehls, and J. de Ley. 1987. *Oligella,* a new genus including *Oligella urethralis* comb. nov. (formerly *Moraxella urethralis*) and *Oligella ureolytica* sp. nov. (formerly CDC group IVe): relationship to *Taylorella equigenitalis* and related taxa. *Int. J. Syst. Bacteriol.* **37:**198–210.

169. Rossau, R., A. Van Landschoot, M. Gillis, and J. de Ley. 1991. Taxonomy of *Moraxellaceae* fam. nov., a new bacterial family to accommodate the genera *Moraxella, Acinetobacter,* and *Psychrobacter* and related organisms. *Int. J. Syst. Bacteriol.* **41:**310–319.

170. Saavedra, J., C. Garrido, D. Folgueira, M. J. Torres, and J. T. Ramos. 1999. *Ochrobactrum anthropi* bacteremia associated with a catheter in an immunocompromised child and review of the pediatric literature. *Pediatr. Infect. Dis. J.* **18:**658–660.

171. Sanders, J. W., J. W. Martin, M. Hooke, and J. Hooke. 2000. *Methylobacterium mesophilicum* infection: case report and literature review of an unusual opportunistic pathogen. *Clin. Infect. Dis.* **30:**936–938.

172. Sandoe, J. A. T., H. Malnick, and K. W. Loudon. 1997. A case of peritonitis caused by *Roseomonas gilardii* in a patient undergoing continuous ambulatory peritoneal dialysis. *J. Clin. Microbiol.* **35:**2150–2152.

173. Sawada, H., H. Ieki, H. Oyaizu, and S. Matsumoto. 1993. Proposal for rejection of *Agrobacterium tumefaciens* and revised descriptions for the genus *Agrobacterium* and for *Agrobacterium radiobacter* and *Agrobacterium rhizogenes. Int. J. Syst. Bacteriol.* **43:**694–702.

174. **Schreckenberger, P. C.** 2000. *Practical Approach to the Identification of Glucose Non-Fermenting Gram-Negative Bacilli,* 2nd ed. University of Illinois College of Medicine at Chicago, Chicago, Ill.

175. **Seifert, H., L. Dijkshoorn, P. Gerner-Smidt, N. Pelzer, I. Tjernberg, and M. Vaneechoutte.** 1997. Distribution of *Acinetobacter* species on human skin: comparison of phenotypic and genotypic identification methods. *J. Clin. Microbiol.* **35:**2819–2825.

176. **Seifert, H., A. Strate, and G. Pulverer.** 1995. Nosocomial bacteremia due to *Acinetobacter baumannii:* clinical features, epidemiology and predictors of mortality. *Medicine* (Baltimore) **74:**340–349.

177. **Shah, S. S., A. Ruth, and S. E. Coffin.** 2000. Infection due to *Moraxella osloensis:* case report and review of the literature. *Clin. Infect. Dis.* **30:**179–181.

178. **Sheridan, R. I., C. M. Ryan, M. S. Pasternack, J. M. Weber, and R. G. Tompkins.** 1993. Flavobacterial sepsis in massively burned pediatric patients. *Clin. Infect. Dis.* **17:**185–187.

179. **Siau, H., K.-Y. Yuen, P.-L. Ho, W. K. Luk, S. S. Y. Wong, P. C. Y. Woo, R. A. Lee, and W.-T. Hui.** 1998. Identification of acinetobacters on blood agar in presence of D-glucose by unique browning effect. *J. Clin. Microbiol.* **36:**1404–1407.

180. **Siegman-Igra, Y., D. Schwartz, G. Soferman, and N. Konforti.** 1987. *Flavobacterium* group IIb bacteremia: report of a case and review of *Flavobacterium* infections. *Med. Microbiol. Immunol.* **176:**103–111.

181. **Simidu, U., K. Kita-Tsukamoto, T. Yasumoto, and M. Yotsu.** 1990. Taxonomy of four marine bacterial strains that produce tetrodotoxin. *Int. J. Syst. Bacteriol.* **40:**331–336.

182. **Sintchenko, V., P. Jelfs, A. Sharma, L. Hicks, and G. L. Gilbert.** 2000. *Massilia timonae:* an unusual bacterium causing wound infection following surgery. *Clin. Microbiol. Newsl.* **22:**149–151.

183. **Spangler, S. K., M. A. Visalli, M. R. Jacobs, and P. C. Appelbaum.** 1996. Susceptibilities of non-*Pseudomonas aeruginosa* gram-negative nonfermentative rods to ciprofloxacin, ofloxacin, levofloxacin, D-ofloxacin, sparfloxacin, ceftazidime, piperacillin, piperacillin-tazobactam, trimethoprim-sulfamethoxazole, and imipenem. *Antimicrob. Agents Chemother.* **40:**772–775.

184. **Steyn, P. L., P. Segers, M. Vancanneyt, P. Sandra, K. Kersters, and J. J. Joubert.** 1998. Classification of heparinolytic bacteria into a new genus, *Pedobacter,* comprising four species: *Pedobacter heparinus* comb. nov., *Pedobacter piscium* comb. nov., *Pedobacter africanus* sp. nov., and *Pedobacter saltans* sp. nov. Proposal of the family *Sphingobacteriaceae* fam. nov. *Int. J. Syst. Bacteriol.* **48:**165–177.

185. **Struthers, M., J. Wong, and J. M. Janda.** 1996. An initial appraisal of the clinical significance of *Roseomonas* species associated with human infections. *Clin. Infect. Dis.* **23:**729–733.

186. **Sung, L. L., D. I. Yang, C. C. Hung, and H. T. Ho.** 2000. Evaluation of autoSCAN-W/A and the Vitek GNI+ AutoMicrobic system for identification of non-glucose-fermenting gram-negative bacilli. *J. Clin. Microbiol.* **38:**1127–1130.

187. **Swann, R. A., S. J. Foulkes, B. Holmes, J. B. Young, R. G. Mitchell, and S. T. Reeders.** 1985. "*Agrobacterium* yellow group" and *Pseudomonas paucimobilis* causing peritonitis in patients receiving continuous ambulatory peritoneal dialysis. *J. Clin. Pathol.* **38:**1293–1299.

188. **Takeuchi, M., K. Hamana, and A. Hiraishi.** 2001. Proposal of the genus *Sphingomonas sensu stricto* and three new genera, *Sphingobium, Novosphingobium* and *Sphingo-*

pyxis, on the basis of phylogenetic and chemotaxonomic analyses. *Int. J. Syst. Evol. Microbiol.* **51:**1405–1417.

189. **Takeuchi, M., and A. Yokota.** 1992. Proposals of *Sphingobacterium faecium* sp. nov., *Sphingobacterium piscium* sp. nov., *Sphingobacterium heparinum* comb. nov., *Sphingobacterium thalpophilum* comb. nov. and two genospecies of the genus *Sphingobacterium,* and synonymy of *Flavobacterium yabuuchiae* and *Sphingobacterium spiritivorum. J. Gen. Appl. Microbiol.* **38:**465–482.

190. **Tjernberg, I., and J. Ursing.** 1989. Clinical strains of *Acinetobacter* classified by DNA-DNA hybridization. *APMIS* **97:**595–605.

191. **Traub, W. H., and B. Leonhard.** 1994. Serotyping of *Acinetobacter baumannii* and genospecies 3: an update. *Med. Microbiol. Lett.* **3:**120–127.

192. **Trüper, H. G., and L. De Clari.** 1997. Taxonomic note: necessary correction of specific epithets formed as substantives (Nouns) "in apposition." *Int. J. Syst. Bacteriol.* **47:**908–909.

193. **Urakami, T., H. Araki, K.-I. Suzuki, and K. Komagata.** 1993. Further studies of the genus *Methylobacterium* and description of *Methylobacterium aminovorans* sp. nov. *Int. J. Syst. Bacteriol.* **43:**504–513.

194. **Ursing, J., and B. Bruun.** 1991. Genotypic heterogeneity of *Flavobacterium* group IIb and *Flavobacterium breve,* demonstrated by DNA-DNA hybridization. *APMIS* **99:**780–786.

195. **Vancanneyt, M., P. Segers, U. Torck, B. Hoste, J.-F. Bernardet, P. Vandamme, and K. Kersters.** 1996. Reclassification of *Flavobacterium odoratum* (Stutzer 1929) strains to a new genus, *Myroides,* as *Myroides odoratus* comb. nov. and *Myroides odoratimimus* sp. nov. *Int. J. Syst. Bacteriol.* **46:**926–932.

196. **Vandamme, P., J.-F. Bernardet, P. Segers, K. Kersters, and B. Holmes.** 1994. New perspectives in the classification of the flavobacteria: description of *Chryseobacterium* gen. nov., *Bergeyella* gen. nov., and *Empedobacter* nom. rev. *Int. J. Syst. Bacteriol.* **44:**827–831.

197. **Vandamme, P., M. Gillis, M. Vancanneyt, B. Hoste, K. Kerster, and E. Falsen.** 1993. *Moraxella lincolnii* sp. nov., isolated from the human respiratory tract, and reevaluation of the taxonomic position of *Moraxella osloensis. Int. J. Syst. Bacteriol.* **43:**474–481.

198. **Vandamme, P., J. Goris, T. Coenye, B. Hoste, D. Janssens, K. Kersters, P. De Vos, and E. Falsen.** 1999. Assignment of Centers for Disease Control group IV c-2 to the genus *Ralstonia* as *Ralstonia paucula* sp. nov. *Int. J. Syst. Bacteriol.* **49:**663–669.

199. **van Dijck, P., M. Delmee, H. Ezzedine, A. Deplano, and M. J. Struelens.** 1995. Evaluation of pulsed-field gel electrophoresis and rep-PCR for the epidemiological analysis of *Ochrobactrum anthropi* strains. *Eur. J. Clin. Microbiol. Infect. Dis.* **14:**1099–1102.

200. **Vaneechoutte, M., G. Claeys, S. Steyaert, T. De Baere, R. Peleman, and G. Verschraegen.** 2000. Isolation of *Moraxella canis* from an ulcerated metastatic lymph node. *J. Clin. Microbiol.* **38:**3870–3871.

201. **Velasco, J., C. Romero, I. Lopez-Goni, J. Leiva, R. Diaz, and I. Moriyon.** 1998. Evaluation of the relatedness of *Brucella* spp. and *Ochrobactrum anthropi* and description of *Ochrobactrum intermedium* sp. nov., a new species with a closer relationship to *Brucella* spp. *Int. J. Syst. Bacteriol.* **48:**759–768.

202. **Veys, A., W. Callewaert, E. Waelkens, and K. van den Abbeele.** 1989. Application of gas-liquid chromatography to the routine identification of nonfermenting gram-negative bacteria in clinical specimens. *J. Clin. Microbiol.* **27:**1538–1542.

203. **Villers, D., E. Espaze, M. Coste-Burel, F. Giauffret, E. Ninin, F. Nicolas, and H. Richet.** 1998. Nosocomial *Acinetobacter baumannii* infections: microbiological and clinical epidemiology. *Ann. Intern. Med.* **129:**182–189.

204. **Visalli, M. A., M. R. Jacobs, T. D. Moore, F. A. Renzi, and P. C. Appelbaum.** 1997. Activities of β-lactams against *Acinetobacter* genospecies as determined by agar dilution and E-test MIC methods. *Antimicrob. Agents Chemother.* **41:**767–770.

205. **Visca, P., A. Petrucca, P. De Mori, A. Festa, E. Boumis, A. Antinori, and N. Petrosillo.** 2001. Community-acquired *Acinetobacter radioresistens* bacteremia in an HIV-positive patient. *Emerg. Infect. Dis.* **7:**1032–1035.

206. **von Graevenitz, A.** 1985. Ecology, clinical significance, and antimicrobial susceptibility of infrequently encountered glucose-nonfermenting gram-negative rods, p. 181–232. *In* G. L. Gilardi (ed.), *Nonfermentative Gram-Negative Rods: Laboratory Identification and Clinical Aspects.* Marcel Dekker, Inc., New York, N.Y.

207. **von Graevenitz, A., J. Bowman, C. Del Notaro, and M. Ritzler.** 2000. Human infection with *Halomonas venusta* following fish bite. *J. Clin. Microbiol.* **38:**3123–3124.

208. **von Graevenitz, A., and M. Grehn.** 1977. Susceptibility studies on *Flavobacterium* II-b. *FEMS Microbiol. Lett.* **2:**289–292.

209. **von Graevenitz, A., G. E. Pfyffer, M. J. Pickett, R. E. Weaver, and J. Wüst.** 1993. Isolation of an unclassified non-fermentative gram-negative rod from a patient on continuous ambulatory peritoneal dialysis. *Eur. J. Clin. Microbiol. Infect. Dis.* **12:**568–570.

210. **Watson, K. C., and I. Muscat.** 1983. Meningitis caused by a *Flavobacterium*-like organism (CDC IIe strain). *J. Infect.* **7:**278–279.

211. **Weitkamp, J.-H., Y.-W. Tang, D. W. Haas, N. K. Midha, and J. E. Crowe, Jr.** 2000. Recurrent *Achromobacter xylosoxidans* bacteremia associated with persistent lymph node infection in a patient with hyperimmunoglobulin M syndrome. *Clin Infect. Dis.* **31:**1183–1187.

212. **Weyant, R. S., C. W. Moss, R. E. Weaver, D. G. Hollis, J. G. Jordan, E. C. Cook, and M. I. Daneshvar.** 1996. *Identification of Unusual Pathogenic Gram-Negative Aerobic and Facultatively Anaerobic Bacteria,* 2nd ed. The Williams & Wilkins Co., Baltimore, Md.

213. **Wisplinghoff, H., M. B. Edmond, M. A. Pfaller, R. N. Jones, R. P. Wenzel, and H. Seifert.** 2000. Nosocomial bloodstream infections caused by *Acinetobacter* species in United States hospitals: clinical features, molecular epidemiology, and antimicrobial susceptibility. *Clin. Infect. Dis.* **31:**690–697.

214. **Wood, C. A., and A. C. Reboli.** 1993. Infections caused by imipenem-resistant *Acinetobacter calcoaceticus* biotype *anitratus. J. Infect. Dis.* **168:**1602–1603.

215. **Yabuuchi, E., T. Kaneko, I. Yano, C. W. Moss, and N. Miyoshi.** 1983. *Sphingobacterium* gen. nov., *Sphingobacterium spiritivorum* comb. nov., *Sphingobacterium multivorum* com. nov., *Sphingobacterium mizutae* sp. nov., and *Flavobacterium indologenes* sp. nov.: glucose-nonfermenting gram-negative rods in CDC groups IIk-2 and IIb. *Int. J. Syst. Bacteriol.* **33:**580–598.

216. **Yabuuchi, E., Y. Kawamura, Y. Kosako, and T. Ezaki.** 1998. Emendation of genus *Achromobacter* and *Achromobacter xylosoxidans* (Yabuuchi and Yano) and proposal of *Achromobacter ruhlandii* (Packer and Vishniac) comb. nov., *Achromobacter piechaudii* (Kiredjian et al.) comb. nov., and *Achromobacter xylosoxidans* subsp. *denitrificans* (Rüger and Tan) comb. nov. *Microbiol. Immunol.* **42:**429–438.

217. **Yabuuchi, E., I. Yano, H. Oyaizu, Y. Hashimoto, T. Ezaki, and H. Yamamoto.** 1990. Proposals of *Sphingomonas paucimobilis* gen. nov. and comb. nov., *Sphingomonas parapaucimobilis* sp. nov., *Sphingomonas yanoikuyae* sp. nov., *Sphingomonas adhaesiva* sp. nov., *Sphingomonas capsulata* comb. nov., and two genospecies of the genus *Sphingomonas. Microbiol. Immunol.* **34:**99–119.

218. **Yağci, A., N. Çerikçioğlu, M. E. Kaufmann, H. Malnick, G. Söyletir, F. Babacan, and T. L. Pitt.** 2000. Molecular typing of *Myroides odoratimimus (Flavobacterium odoratum)* urinary tract infections in a Turkish hospital. *Eur. J. Clin. Microbiol. Infect. Dis.* **19:**731–732.

219. **Young, J. M., L. D. Kuykendall, E. Martinez-Romero, A. Kerr, and H. Sawada.** 2001. A revision of *Rhizobium* Frank 1889, with an emended description of the genus, and the inclusion of all species of *Agrobacterium* Conn 1942 and *Allorhizobium undicola* de Lajundie *et al.* 1998 as new combinations: *Rhizobium radiobacter, R. rhizogenes, R. rubi, R. undicola* and *R. vitis. Int. J. Syst. Evol. Microbiol.* **51:**89–103.

*Bordetella**

MIKE J. LOEFFELHOLZ

50

TAXONOMY

The genus *Bordetella* is named for J. Bordet, who, with O. Gengou, described the bacterium in 1906 (6). The type species, *B. pertussis*, was originally called *Haemophilus pertussis* by Bordet and Gengou. In addition to *B. pertussis*, the genus consists of *B. bronchiseptica* (24), *B. parapertussis* (20), *B. avium* (52), *B. hinzii* (87), *B. holmesii* (93), and *B. trematum* (86). Phylogenetic analysis based on 16S rRNA gene sequencing has demonstrated that *B. pertussis, B. parapertussis, B. bronchiseptica*, and *B. holmesii* are very closely related (49). In spite of considerable genetic relatedness among some *Bordetella* species, current literature still refers to seven distinct species.

DESCRIPTION OF THE GENUS

Bordetella organisms are small gram-negative coccobacilli. Some species are motile. They are strictly aerobic, with optimal growth at 35 to 37°C. All species oxidize amino acids, but none ferment carbohydrates. While all species have relatively simple nutritional requirements, fastidiousness varies depending on the degree of sensitivity to toxic substances and metabolites found in common laboratory media. *B. pertussis* is the most fastidious species and is inhibited by constituents present in many media, including fatty acids, metal ions, sulfides, and peroxides. Isolation of *B. pertussis* requires media containing protective substances such as charcoal, blood, or starch. The other *Bordetella* species are less fastidious and will grow on routine agars containing blood and on MacConkey agar. Growth rates of *Bordetella* species are generally inversely related to fastidiousness; *B. pertussis* grows slowly, while *B. avium* and *B. bronchiseptica* grow rapidly. Table 1 lists some of the common characteristics used to differentiate *Bordetella* species.

B. pertussis produces a number of virulence factors that are responsible for pathogenesis. These virulence factors include toxins (pertussis toxin, adenylate cyclase toxin, and tracheal cytotoxin) and components that mediate adherence to ciliated epithelial cells of the respiratory tract (pertussis toxin [PT], fimbriae, filamentous hemagglutinin

[FHA], and pertactin). Other virulence factors include dermonecrosis (heat-labile) toxin, lipopolysaccharide (endotoxin), and tracheal colonization factor. For a review of virulence factors, see reference 51. *Bordetella* species other than *B. pertussis* also express virulence factors. *B. parapertussis* and *B. bronchiseptica* produce pertactin and FHA (7, 12). Promoter and structural genes for PT are present in both *B. parapertussis* and *B. bronchiseptica* but are not expressed (2).

NATURAL HABITATS

B. pertussis produces disease only in humans, who also serve as the sole reservoir. *B. parapertussis*, once thought to be strictly a human pathogen, is also found in sheep (13). Genotypic strain analysis showed that human and ovine *B. parapertussis* strains are distinct (90). *B. pertussis* has historically been considered a strict respiratory pathogen, causing localized infection of the ciliated epithelium of the bronchial tree. However, its detection in alveolar macrophages (8) and isolation from blood (48) indicate the potential for invasive infection. *B. bronchiseptica* is a respiratory tract pathogen of a variety of animals, including dogs, swine, cats, and rabbits (27). *B. avium* is found in birds and causes coryza in turkeys (52). *B. hinzii* colonizes the respiratory tracts of poultry but has not been associated with disease in poultry (87). On rare occasions *B. bronchiseptica* and *B. hinzii* cause disease in humans (11, 95). *B. avium* is strictly a veterinary pathogen; to date, no infections have been reported in humans, although *B. avium*-like organisms have been isolated from human specimens (16). *B. holmesii* and *B. trematum* are infrequently associated with both respiratory and nonrespiratory infections in humans (83, 85, 93). *B. holmesii* has recently been linked to pertussis-like symptoms (97).

CLINICAL SIGNIFICANCE

The incubation period of pertussis is usually 7 to 10 days, with a range of approximately 4 to 21 days (9). The symptoms that develop following the incubation period can be classified as either typical (classical) or atypical. Classical pertussis consists of a catarrhal stage lasting 1 to 2 weeks, a paroxysmal stage lasting 1 to 6 weeks (as long as 10 weeks), and a convalescent stage lasting 2 to 4 weeks (as long as

---

* This chapter contains information presented in chapter 40 by Jörg E. Hoppe in the seventh edition of this Manual.

TABLE 1 Differential characteristics of *Bordetella* spp.[a]

Characteristic	B. pertussis	B. parapertussis	B. bronchiseptica	B. avium	B. hinzii	B. holmesii	B. trematum
Catalase	+	+	+	+	+	+[b]	+
Oxidase	+	−	+	+	+	−	−
Nitrate reduction	−	−	+	−	−	−	V
Urease production	−	+ (24 h)	+ (4 h)	−	V	−	−
Motility	−	−	+	+	+	−	+
Growth on:							
Blood agar	−	+	+	+	+	+	+
MacConkey agar	−	V (delayed)	+	+	+	+ (delayed)	+

[a] Modified from references 11, 86, 93, and earlier editions of this Manual. Responses: +, activity or growth present; −, not present; V, variable.
[b] Some strains may exhibit a weak reaction.

several months). Patient symptoms during the catarrhal stage are nonspecific and include rhinorrhea, sneezing, low-grade fever, and occasional mild cough. Pertussis is frequently unsuspected during this period. The paroxysmal stage of pertussis is characterized by the presence of one or more of the pathognomonic signs of pertussis: episodes of paroxysmal cough, whoop, and posttussive vomiting. The severity of respiratory symptoms gradually decreases during the convalescent stage. Atypical symptoms in older children and adults consist of a prolonged, nondescript cough. The differential diagnosis of atypical pertussis includes bronchitis and upper respiratory tract infections caused by adenovirus, parainfluenza virus, respiratory syncytial virus, *Chlamydophila* (formerly *Chlamydia*) *pneumoniae*, and *Mycoplasma pneumoniae* (30, 31). Infants with pertussis may present with choking and apnea, while cough may be absent. Infants are more likely than other age groups to suffer from severe disease and complications, including cyanosis and pneumonia, and to die (5). Adults experience more complications from pertussis than adolescents (15).

B. pertussis is responsible for the vast majority of pertussis cases and causes more severe respiratory symptoms than other *Bordetella* species associated with pertussis syndrome. Worldwide, *B. pertussis* causes an estimated 50 million cases of pertussis and 350,000 deaths, primarily among children in countries lacking organized vaccination programs (51). *B. pertussis* is transmitted from person to person via respiratory droplets and is highly contagious, infecting 80 to 90% of susceptible contacts. Since *B. pertussis* is spread by respiratory droplets, relatively close contact (within several feet) is required for transmission; transmission over long distances via aerosols does not occur. A carrier state is not generally recognized for *B. pertussis*. Sensitive nonculture tests such as PCR can detect organisms in asymptomatic immune persons (36), but this is more likely to represent a transient colonization or infection rather than a prolonged carrier state. The disease is endemic, with epidemics consistently occurring every 3 to 5 years (9). The number of reported pertussis cases in the United States has increased steadily since the 1980s, in spite of continued high levels of vaccination coverage. Explanations offered for the increased incidence include heightened awareness and reporting of disease (particularly the atypical presentation, and disease in older persons), and the use of more sensitive laboratory diagnostic tests.

Immunity to pertussis following natural infection or vaccination wanes after 5 to 12 years. As a result, *B. pertussis* is a significant cause of respiratory disease in older children and adults (5, 11, 29, 72, 96), who, in countries with vaccination programs, have replaced young children as

the primary reservoir of *B. pertussis*. Serologic evidence indicates that as much as 12 to 32% of chronic cough illness in adults is due to *B. pertussis* (10, 66, 72, 96). However, in two studies in which culture was performed, *B. pertussis* was not isolated from any seropositive subjects (66, 96). Therefore, the public health significance of this high seroprevalence is unclear.

Vaccines have dramatically reduced the public health impact of pertussis. The initial heat-killed, whole-cell vaccines have been largely replaced by multicomponent acellular vaccines, which are associated with fewer side effects (73). The efficacy of whole-cell and acellular vaccines is estimated to be between 60 and 90% (9). Currently available pertussis vaccines are formulated for children younger than 7 years. However, the recognition of the importance of *B. pertussis* as a cause of respiratory disease in adolescents and adults has stimulated recent evaluations of the immunogenicity and safety of acellular pertussis vaccines in older persons (80, 85).

B. parapertussis causes a pertussis syndrome similar to but usually less severe than that caused by *B. pertussis* (37, 63). While *B. parapertussis* may be quite prominent in isolated outbreaks (58), overall it accounts for fewer than 5% of all pertussis cases (22, 88). Symptomatic *B. parapertussis* infections more commonly present as a nonspecific cough illness or bronchitis. *B. bronchiseptica* (18, 95) and, more recently, *B. holmesii* (97) have been implicated as infrequent causes of pertussis syndrome and other respiratory illnesses. Most reported cases of *B. bronchiseptica* respiratory disease have been associated either with underlying conditions such as immunosuppression or with exposure to animals.

COLLECTION, TRANSPORT, AND STORAGE OF SPECIMENS

Excellent summaries of specimen collection and handling for optimal detection of *B. pertussis* are available (71), including several earlier editions of this Manual. Preferred specimens for laboratory diagnosis of pertussis are nasopharyngeal (NP) aspirates and posterior NP swabs. When properly collected, these specimens contain the ciliated respiratory epithelial cells for which *B. pertussis* exhibits tropism. NP aspirates yield more positive culture results than do NP swabs (32). Aspirates offer additional advantages over swabs; there is usually sufficient specimen for multiple analyses (important when verifying new test procedures), and the specimen collection technique may be preferred by clinicians and parents of young patients (32). Throat swabs are inferior specimens for culture; they do not sample the ciliated epithelium, and they contain large numbers of members of the normal flora, which can result in over-growth of isolation media. In one study, significantly fewer infections were detected by culture using throat swabs compared to NP swabs (62). However, recent data suggest that throat swabs may be suitable for PCR diagnosis of *B. pertussis* infection (22).

To obtain an NP aspirate, a narrow catheter or infant feeding tube is inserted through the nostril to the posterior nasopharynx. A mucous trap and hand-operated vacuum pump are connected to the other end, and suction is applied while the tube is in place and while slowly withdrawing it back through the nostril. Any secretions remaining in the tube should be flushed into the trap by aspirating *Bordetella* transport medium or phosphate-buffered saline. Additionally, the catheter tip can be cut off and placed into suitable transport medium for shipping. Swab specimens are collected by inserting a small swab on a flexible (usually aluminum wire) shaft through the nostril. The placement of the swab is important. Figure 1 depicts the correct positioning of the patient's head and placement of the swab. The swab should then be rotated for several seconds before being withdrawn. It is generally recommended that two NP swab specimens be collected, one through each nostril. This provides separate swabs if multiple laboratory tests are to be performed. Specimens are then either directly plated or placed in a suitable medium for transport.

Several transport media are readily available for NP specimens. Regan-Lowe (RL) transport medium contains half-strength charcoal agar and horse blood, with cephalexin added to suppress growth of the normal NP flora. Substitution of 2.5 μg of methicillin per ml or 0.625 μg of oxacillin per ml for cephalexin reportedly allows the growth of *B. holmesii* (64). Other appropriate transport media include 1% acid-hydrolyzed casein (Casamino Acids; Becton Dickinson, Sparks, Md.) and Amies medium with charcoal. These two media provide less than 24 h of stability, limiting their use to on-site laboratories or requiring overnight shipping. Unlike Casamino Acids and Amies medium, RL transport medium also functions as an enrichment medium for *B. pertussis*. Preincubation of specimens in RL transport medium is controversial. Preincubation at 36°C may enhance the recovery of *B. pertussis* due to multiplication of

organisms. Some recommend against preincubation due to overgrowth of cephalexin-resistant members of the flora (9). Transport at 4°C provides better recovery of *B. pertussis* than does transport at room temperature (34, 69) but adds additional costs due to packaging and weight.

Swab material should be calcium alginate or Dacron if culture isolation is to be performed (45). Cotton contains inhibitors that will decrease isolation rates of *B. pertussis* (45). Dacron is recommended if PCR testing is performed, since calcium alginate can inhibit PCR (91). The inhibitory effect of calcium alginate on PCR amplification may depend in part on the specimen extraction procedure. Crude proteinase K extracts were completely inhibitory to PCR (91).

Because of the lability of *B. pertussis* outside of its normal host environment, proper handling and shipping conditions are critical for optimal culture sensitivity. For culture testing, direct plating of NP specimens onto agar plates provides optimal sensitivity (44). However, this requires clinician participation and training and is not practical for off-site reference and public health laboratories.

For direct fluorescent-antibody (DFA) testing, the specimen collection kit should contain a glass slide, on which a smear is prepared from an NP swab immediately after collection. The slide is allowed to air dry and is then transported to the laboratory. Alternatively, smears can be prepared at the laboratory from liquid transport medium containing an NP swab or from NP aspirates.

For PCR testing, swabs can be transported dry (59), in transport medium, or in saline. Transport in liquid medium provides a specimen from which multiple aliquots can be tested, whereas processing a dry swab for PCR testing leaves no unextracted specimen material available for repeat analysis if required.

DIRECT DETECTION

DFA Testing

The direct detection of *B. pertussis* in NP secretions by using fluorochrome-conjugated antibody provides the most rapid and simple diagnosis of pertussis. Commercially available antibodies are polyclonal (Becton Dickinson) or monoclonal, recognizing a lipooligosaccharide epitope (Accu-Mab; Altachem Pharma, Edmonton, Alberta, Canada) (1). The monoclonal antibodies are available as a dual-fluorochrome reagent for the detection of both *B. pertussis* and *B. parapertussis* in a single smear. A head-to-head comparison of the polyclonal and monoclonal reagents showed that they had similar sensitivity (84). Factors to consider when choosing an antibody source include cost and performance in the laboratory's own hands.

Regardless of the antibody used, the direct detection of *B. pertussis* using DFA lacks both sensitivity and specificity. Compared to culture, DFA sensitivity in several published studies ranged from 30 to 71% (21, 25, 33, 59). DFA-positive, culture-negative specimens are not unusual. When DFA was compared to an expanded "gold standard" (e.g., two positive nonculture tests or a clinical diagnosis), its sensitivity ranged from half that of culture (33) to threefold greater than that of culture (59). The large range in DFA performance reflects variation in the sensitivities of both the DFA procedure and the culture procedures against which it is compared. The specificity of DFA is highly variable, due to the cross-reactivity of immunological reagents and the subjectivity of fluorescence interpretation.

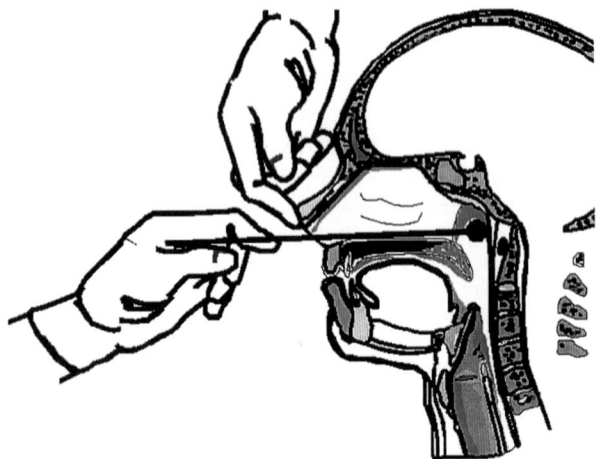

FIGURE 1 Correct positioning of patient's head and placement of the swab for collection of NP specimens reprinted from reference 9. (Courtesy of Kris Bisgard, Centers for Disease Control and Prevention.)

In a study conducted by Loeffelholz et al., several specimens positive only by DFA were considered to be true positives because of strong clinical or epidemiological evidence of infection (59). Other studies have shown extremely poor DFA specificity (21, 33). Notwithstanding the variable performance, DFA testing can provide valuable information when appropriate quality assurance and quality control measures are implemented to maximize specificity. DFA testing should be performed only as an adjunct to culture or PCR, and the results should be considered presumptive.

Antibody for DFA testing must be appropriately titrated before use. To control for staining specificity, control slides should contain separate smears of *B. pertussis* and *B. parapertussis*. Smears should contain 10 to 100 organisms per oil immersion field. Suspensions of control organisms can be prepared in phosphate-buffered saline with a turbidity equivalent to a McFarland no. 1 standard. Stained smears are examined under a fluorescent microscope for the presence or absence and degree of fluorescence. Slides are viewed initially at a magnification of ×400. Any fluorescence is examined at ×1,000 magnification to confirm morphology. *Bordetella* organisms appear as small coccobacillary rods with pronounced peripheral apple green fluorescence and dark centers. Fluorescence must be intense, and other staining characteristics and morphology must be ignored.

Nucleic Acid Detection

In many laboratories, nucleic acid detection methods such as PCR have replaced DFA as the routine nonculture test method or have even become the primary diagnostic test. The Centers for Disease Control and Prevention recommends that PCR be used as a presumptive assay in conjunction with culture (9). Depending on batching, PCR can provide a rapid result, which is important for patient management and control of outbreaks. PCR has consistently been shown to be more sensitive than DFA or culture, in some cases, dramatically more (22, 26, 28, 35, 36, 59, 88, 92). The range in PCR performance compared to culture is due in part to variation in the sensitivity of culture. PCR tests themselves vary in sensitivity, depending on the nucleic acid extraction method, the amount of specimen amplified, the amplification conditions and efficiency, and the DNA detection format.

The lack of a standardized or Food and Drug Administration-cleared, commercially available PCR test for *B. pertussis* and the lack of a widely available quality assurance program to assess interlaboratory performance are significant shortcomings of PCR. As a result, extensive method validation on the part of the laboratory is required before the test is offered for diagnostic use. The laboratory must develop and implement quality control and an ongoing quality assurance program. Consensus recommendations for the diagnosis of *B. pertussis* infections by PCR have been proposed (65). These recommendations focus heavily on quality assurance and control and on verification of assay performance (clinical sensitivity and specificity, analytical specificity). Strict adherence to quality assurance practices is necessary to avoid false-positive PCR results due to contamination of reaction mixtures with previously amplified DNA. These practices include separation of pre- and post-PCR work areas, unidirectional workflow, and incorporation of reagents or procedures that modify the PCR product and prevent it from serving as a template in subsequent reactions. Positive and negative controls must be able to monitor the entire PCR assay procedure. While there are no established guidelines about the number of negative controls to include in each run, some laboratories routinely include a negative control for approximately every five specimens.

Chromosomal regions targeted by PCR include the pertussis toxin promoter region (28, 46, 78), a region upstream of the porin gene (23, 57), repetitive insertion sequences IS*481* of *B. pertussis* (26, 35, 89) and IS*1001* of *B. parapertussis* (89), the adenylate cyclase gene (17), and a region upstream of the flagellin gene (47). A set of primers targeted to the toxin promoter was shown not to detect *B. parapertussis* or *B. bronchiseptica* (28, 46). However, in one study, these primers did amplify and detect a single *B. bronchiseptica* isolate tested (C. Thompson, M. Loeffelholz, L. Holcomb, K. Long, and M. Gilchrist, *Abstr. 97th Gen. Meet. Am. Soc. Microbiol.*, abstr. C24, 1997). A PCR assay designed to detect and differentiate *B. pertussis*, *B. parapertussis*, and *B. bronchiseptica* targeted conserved toxin promoter sequences that bracketed a variable region (78). All three species yielded a PCR product that was differentiated by restriction enzyme analysis. Primers targeting the IS*481* repetitive insertion sequence of *B. pertussis* were originally reported to cross-react weakly with *B. bronchiseptica* (26). PCR assays utilizing the same upstream primer and a different downstream primer did not cross-react with *B. bronchiseptica* (35, 59). More recently, primers targeting IS*481* have been shown to detect *B. holmesii* (60). Sequence analysis of IS*481* PCR products from *B. pertussis* and *B. holmesii* isolates showed nearly 100% homology (77). PCR assays targeting a region upstream of the porin gene generated product from *B. pertussis*, *B. parapertussis*, and *B. bronchiseptica* that was distinguishable in agarose gels (57) or by hybridization to species-specific probes (23). Nested PCR assays for the detection of *Bordetella* have been described (22, 79). While these assays were reported to be sensitive and specific, nested PCR is inherently more susceptible to contamination than is unnested PCR. It is my opinion that when PCR conditions are properly optimized, nesting of PCR is not required for the accurate, sensitive diagnosis of most infectious diseases, including pertussis.

Presumably because of its greater sensitivity and ability to detect dead organisms, PCR remains positive longer during the course of disease than does culture (88, 92) and is more likely to remain positive following antibiotic therapy (19, 92). Longitudinal analysis of erythromycin-treated infants showed that after 4 days of treatment, 56 and 89% of NP swab specimens were positive by culture and PCR, respectively (19), whereas after 7 days of treatment, no specimens were positive by culture but 56% were still positive by PCR. The higher sensitivity of PCR is also marked among persons with mild or atypical symptoms (82) and among older persons (88, 92).

ISOLATION

Culture provides the most specific diagnosis of pertussis and produces isolates for genotypic analysis and antimicrobial susceptibility testing. The sensitivity of culture varies greatly, depending on patient factors (including prior antibiotic therapy, duration of symptoms, age, and vaccination status), specimen transport conditions, the type and quality of media used, and other conditions. While PCR testing is also affected by these factors, culture is affected to a greater degree due to its requirement for viable organisms. The highest isolation rates are achieved when specimens are inoculated onto media immediately after collection from the patient. Since this is often not possible, transport media are available that, with various degrees of success, maintain the viability of *B. pertussis*. These media are described earlier in this chapter.

Several media have been described for the isolation of *B. pertussis*. Traditional media consist of bases such as potato infusion (Bordet-Gengou [BG] medium) or charcoal (RL medium) supplemented with glycerol, peptones, and horse or sheep blood. An antimicrobial agent is added to reduce the growth of the normal flora. Cephalexin is the agent of choice, yet growth of resistant members of the NP flora is still quite common (71). RL medium provides better isolation of *B. pertussis* than does BG medium (69, 71). The shelf life of media ranges from 5 days for BG medium to 4 to 8 weeks for RL medium (75).

Plates are incubated in ambient air at 35 to 36°C and examined daily for suspicious colonies. In one study, *B. pertussis* colony development was more rapid in ambient air than in air containing 5 to 10% carbon dioxide (43). The humidity must be sufficient to prevent the desiccation of agar plates during the long incubation period. While most *B. pertussis* colonies become visible after 3 to 4 days of incubation (*B. parapertussis* becomes visible after 2 to 3 days), an incubation time of 7 days has historically been recommended. In one study, 12 days of incubation recovered more isolates than did 7 days of incubation (50).

IDENTIFICATION

Phenotypic

On RL agar, young *B. pertussis* colonies are round, domed, mercury-silver colored, and shiny. *B. parapertussis* colonies are similar but are grayer and less domed. On BG agar, *B. pertussis* and *B. parapertussis* produce zones of hemolysis.

Colonies with the above characteristics are Gram stained. *Bordetella* organisms appear as gram-negative coccobacilli or short rods. Suspensions of colonies are prepared in phosphate-buffered saline, applied to slides, and identified with specific antisera. Both *B. pertussis* and *B. parapertussis* controls should be included. For identification with fluorescent antibodies, colony suspensions should be dilute (as described earlier in this chapter) to avoid dulling of fluorescence. Fluorescence is interpreted as described earlier in this chapter. For identification by slide agglutination, a suspension heavier than that used for fluorescent staining (equivalent to a MacFarland no. 3 standard) is prepared. Repeatedly forcing the suspension through a pipette—a procedure that may generate aerosols—will break up clumps. Colonies grown on antibiotic-free RL agar produce more homogenous suspensions for easier interpretation of agglutination. In addition to identification using specific antisera, *Bordetella* species can be identified using biochemical tests based on differential phenotypic characteristics (Table 1). Oxidase-positive, nonfermentative gram-negative rods, particularly *Oligella ureolytica* and CDC group IVc-2, can be misidentified as *B. bronchiseptica*. *B. bronchiseptica* differs from CDC group IVc-2 by having a positive nitrate reduction test and from *O. ureolytica* by having a negative nitrite reduction test and by showing penicillin susceptibility.

Commercially obtained strains (American Type Culture Collection, Manassas, Va.) or clinical isolates can serve as controls for quality control of media and reagents. Fresh clinical isolates are preferred, to avoid laboratory adaptation of strains. Clinical isolates should be frozen as soon as possible at −70°C in glycerol. Once plated, cultures lose viability quickly and must be replaced regularly.

Biosafety level 2 practices are recommended when working with *Bordetella*. Routine manipulations of specimens and isolates can be conducted on open bench tops.

Genotypic Strain Typing

Pulsed-field gel electrophoresis (PFGE) methods for the identification of *B. pertussis* strains have been described previously (9, 68). PFGE has been proven to be valuable in tracking outbreak transmission patterns (9, 67). It has also been used to identify *B. parapertussis* (74) and *B. bronchiseptica* isolates (4). The rare-cutting restriction enzyme XbaI is used in most PFGE procedures for typing *B. pertussis*, *B. parapertussis*, and *B. bronchiseptica* (4, 9, 74). Other genotypic methods used to discriminate *Bordetella* isolates include restriction enzyme analysis (81), arbitrarily primed PCR (randomly amplified polymorphic DNA) (98), PCR targeting a specific repetitive element (67), and ribotyping (76). Comparative analysis of PFGE and PCR-based typing methods for discrimination of *B. pertussis* isolates showed PFGE to be more discriminatory (67). Standardized approaches to genotypic analysis of *B. pertussis* isolates have focused on PFGE (9, 68).

SEROLOGIC TESTS

Serologic methods used to detect antibody responses to *B. pertussis* include enzyme-linked immunosorbent assay (ELISA), agglutination, complement fixation, immunoblotting, indirect hemagglutination, and toxin neutralization (71). ELISAs are available from a number of manufacturers on several continents. The immunoblot format is also commercially available (MarBlot; Trinity Biotech, Wicklow, Ireland). Serologic tests are still not widely used, particularly in the United States. This is due to the lack of a Food and Drug Administration-cleared test, the lack of standardized interpretive criteria, and the need for paired sera for the most specific diagnosis. Because of ease of use and sensitivity, ELISAs in microwell plate format have become the method of choice. ELISAs have been used to measure immunoglobulin A (IgA), IgG, and IgM levels to PT, FHA, pertactin, and fimbriae. Generally, IgG and IgA responses to PT or FHA are considered reliable indicators of *Bordetella* infection. At least 90% of infected persons develop IgG to PT and FHA (71). An IgG response to PT is specific for *B. pertussis*, since no other *Bordetella* species expresses PT. FHA is expressed by *B. pertussis* and *B. parapertussis*. However, other bacteria including *Haemophilus influenzae* possess epitopes that cross-react with FHA. An evaluation of several commercial ELISAs showed that the results lacked concordance (54). Clinical sensitivity and assay reproducibility were among the other assay parameters evaluated.

Comparative analyses of serologic testing, culture, DFA, and PCR have generally shown serologic testing to be the most sensitive method for diagnosis of *B. pertussis* infections (28, 33, 88). In one study, PCR was positive in only 21% of patients with positive serology (either high IgG or IgA concentrations in a single specimen or significant increases in antibody concentrations in paired specimens) (88).

The most specific serodiagnosis of pertussis is the demonstration of seroconversion or a fourfold rise in the concentration of IgG against PT. However, this diagnostic approach is often hampered by the lack of true acute-phase specimens (related to the nonspecific symptoms in the early stages of disease) and the lack of convalescent-phase specimens due to the lack of patient follow-up. Alternative strategies for serodiagnosis have been evaluated but may suffer from poor specificity. These strategies vary, depending on the age and vaccination status of the patient. For the serologic diagnosis of pertussis in unvaccinated children, demonstration of increases in the concentrations of IgG or IgA to PT or FHA is a suitable approach, although young infants may not produce IgA (88). Testing of single specimens collected early in the disease (1 to 3 weeks after onset of cough) showed a low sensitivity (94). Serodiagnosis of pertussis in vaccinated children is more problematic due to rapid increases in antibody concentration and the ensuing difficulty in detecting significant rises in titer. In this population, high IgA or IgG titers in a single specimen may distinguish responses to vaccination from responses to infection. IgA is rarely detected in uninfected vaccinees (71). IgA-specific ELISAs and immunoblot assays are available. Serodiagnosis of pertussis in adolescents and adults is often based on high antibody titers in a single specimen, since increases in antibody concentrations are infrequently detected (71). Regardless of the patient population, the results of serologic testing from a single specimen should receive considerable scrutiny. The specificity of this approach depends on the particular assay and cutoff used (14).

ANTIMICROBIAL SUSCEPTIBILITY

Erythromycin and the newer macrolides, including azithromycin and clarithromycin, are the drugs of choice for treatment and prophylaxis of pertussis (3, 70). Two erythromycin-resistant strains of *B. pertussis* have been described (53, 56), but resistance does not appear to be spreading. An acceptable alternative for individuals intolerant of macrolides is trimethoprim-sulfamethoxazole (TMP-SMX) (40). Among the fluoroquinolones, ciprofloxacin, levofloxacin, and gemifloxacin showed the highest activities against *B. pertussis* (42, 70).

While antibiotics are generally less active against *B. parapertussis* than against *B. pertussis* (55), *B. parapertussis* is susceptible to macrolides, fluoroquinolones, and TMP-SMX (39, 70). *B. bronchiseptica* and other *Bordetella* species generally have antimicrobial susceptibility profiles similar to those of other nonfermentative gram-negative bacilli.

Antibiotic susceptibility testing of *B. pertussis* is not standardized. Methods include the E-test (AB Biodisk, Solna, Sweden), agar dilution, and disk diffusion (38, 41, 53). Agar dilution has been performed with Mueller-Hinton agar supplemented with 5% horse blood (41), as well as BG agar containing 20% horse blood (38). RL agar without cephalexin is commonly used for the disk diffusion and E-test methods (38, 56). In most studies, agar dilution has served as the reference method. It is recommended that strains determined to be nonsusceptible by disk diffusion also be tested by agar dilution (9). Studies have demonstrated good agreement among diffusion tests and agar dilution for determining erythromycin resistance in *B. pertussis* (38, 53). Less agreement was observed among TMP-SMX MICs (38).

EVALUATION AND INTERPRETATION OF RESULTS

The diagnosis of pertussis can be challenging, given the frequent atypical presentation and the shortcomings of laboratory tests. Indeed, no single laboratory test can be considered a gold standard. While culture is virtually 100% specific, its sensitivity is often low due to poorly collected specimens, long specimen transport time, and patient factors such as duration of symptoms and prior antibiotic treatment.

Nucleic acid amplification methods such as PCR generally offer greater sensitivity compared to culture. PCR has frequently been shown to provide the specific diagnosis of pertussis when culture is negative. In many laboratories, PCR performed daily or several times per week has replaced DFA as the primary rapid test for *B. pertussis*. The major shortcomings of nucleic acid amplification methods are the potential for false-positive results due to contamination, the lack of standardization among assays, and the interpretation of a positive result for *B. pertussis* DNA in the absence of a positive culture. While the combination of a positive PCR result and a negative culture result for the same patient usually reflects the greater sensitivity of PCR, there are situations when a positive PCR result alone may not have clinical or public health relevance. Therefore, positive PCR results must be interpreted in conjunction with patient symptoms, treatment status, and epidemiological factors. Culture, serology, and, to a greater extent, PCR have shown that asymptomatic *B. pertussis* infections occur (36, 61). In one study, 92% of preschool-aged children with positive PCR results remained free of symptoms (36). During pertussis outbreaks, laboratories may be pressured to test specimens from asymptomatic "contacts" of cases. In fact, while these individuals may share a day care center or school classroom with a patient, they often do not meet the criteria for exposure to *B. pertussis*. Positive laboratory results (usually by the sensitive PCR test) for these asymptomatic persons confound treatment and outbreak response decisions. Given the general belief that a long-lasting carrier state for pertussis does not exist, PCR-positive asymptomatic persons are unlikely to contribute significantly, if at all, to the spread of pertussis.

Serology has the potential to contribute substantially to the diagnosis of pertussis, when standardized tests and interpretive criteria that reliably diagnose recent infections in vaccinated populations are available. Interpretive criteria for a single serum specimen will have more clinical utility than those that require paired sera. For the optimal use and interpretation of serology and other tests for pertussis, the laboratory must have information on the patient's symptoms, antibiotic treatment, exposure to other ill persons, vaccination status, and age and on the level of disease activity in the community.

REFERENCES

1. **Archambault, D., P. Rondeau, P. Martin, and B. R. Brodeur.** 1991. Characterization and comparative bactericidal activity of monoclonal antibodies to *Bordetella pertussis* lipooligosaccharide A. *J. Gen. Microbiol.* **137:**905–911.
2. **Arico, B., and R. Rappuoli.** 1987. *Bordetella parapertussis* and *Bordetella bronchiseptica* contain transcriptionally silent pertussis toxin genes. *J. Bacteriol.* **169:**2847–2853.
3. **Bass, J. W.** 1986. Erythromycin for treatment and prevention of pertussis. *Pediatr. Infect. Dis. J.* **5:**154–157.
4. **Binns, S. H., A. J. Speakman, S. Dawson, M. Bennett, R. M. Gaskell, and C. A. Hart.** 1998. The use of pulsed-field gel electrophoresis to examine the epidemiology of *Bordetella bronchiseptica* isolated from cats and other species. *Epidemiol. Infect.* **120:**201–208.

5. **Black, S.** 1997. Epidemiology of pertussis. *Pediatr. Infect. Dis. J.* **16:**S85–S89.

6. **Bordet, J., and O. Gengou.** 1906. Le microbe de la coqueluche. *Ann. Inst. Pasteur* **20:**731–741.

7. **Boursaux-Eude, C., and N. Guiso.** 2000. Polymorphism of repeated regions of pertactin in *Bordetella pertussis, Bordetella parapertussis,* and *Bordetella bronchiseptica. Infect. Immun.* **68:**4815–4817.

8. **Bromberg, K., G. Tannis, and P. Steiner.** 1991. Detection of *Bordetella pertussis* associated with the alveolar macrophages of children with human immunodeficiency virus infection. *Infect. Immun.* **59:**4715–4719.

9. **Centers for Disease Control and Prevention.** 2000. *Guidelines for the Control of Pertussis Outbreaks.* Centers for Disease Control and Prevention, Atlanta, Ga.

10. **Cherry, J. D.** 1999. Epidemiological, clinical, and laboratory aspects of pertussis in adults. *Clin. Infect. Dis.* **28:** S112–S117.

11. **Cookson, B. T., P. Vandamme, L. C. Carlson, A. M. Larson, J. V. Sheffield, K. Kersters, and D. H. Spach.** 1994. Bacteremia caused by a novel *Bordetella* species, "*B. hinzii.*" *J. Clin. Microbiol.* **32:**2569–2571.

12. **Cotter, P. A., M. H. Yuk, S. Mattoo, B. J. Akerley, J. Boschwitz, D. A. Relman, and J. F. Miller.** 1998. Filamentous haemagglutinin of *Bordetella bronchiseptica* is required for efficient establishment of tracheal colonization. *Infect. Immun.* **66:**5921–5929.

13. **Cullinane, L. C., M. R. Alley, R. B. Marshall, and B. W. Manktelow.** 1987. *Bordetella parapertussis* from lambs. *N. Z. Vet. J.* **35:**175.

14. **De Melker, H. E., F. G. A. Versteegh, M. A. E. Conyn-van Spaendonck, L. H. Elvers, G. A. M. Berbers, A. van der Zee, and J. F. P. Schellekens.** 2000. Specificity and sensitivity of high levels of immunoglobulin G antibodies against pertussis toxin in a single serum sample for diagnosis of infection with *Bordetella pertussis. J. Clin. Microbiol.* **38:**800–806.

15. **De Serres, G., R. Shadmani, B. Duval, N. Boulianne, P. Dery, M. Douville-Fradet, L. Rochette, and S. A. Halperin.** 2000. Morbidity of pertussis in adolescents and adults. *J. Infect. Dis.* **182:**174–179.

16. **Dorittke, C., P. Vandamme, K.-H. Hinz, E. M. Schemken-Birk, and C.-H. Wirsing von König.** 1995. Isolation of a *Bordetella avium*-like organism from a human specimen. *Eur. J. Clin. Microbiol. Infect. Dis.* **14:**451–454.

17. **Douglas, E., J. G. Coote, R. Parton, and W. McPheat.** 1993. Identification of *Bordetella pertussis* in nasopharyngeal swabs by PCR amplification of a region of the adenylate cyclase gene. *J. Med. Microbiol.* **38:**140–144.

18. **Dworkin, M. S., P. S. Sullivan, S. E. Buskin, R. D. Harrington, J. Olliffe, R. D. MacArthur, and C. E. Lopez.** 1999. *Bordetella bronchiseptica* infection in human immunodeficiency virus-infected patients. *Clin. Infect. Dis.* **28:**1095–1099.

19. **Edelman, K., S. Nikkari, O. Ruuskanen, Q. He, M. Viljanen, and J. Mertsola.** 1996. Detection of *Bordetella pertussis* by polymerase chain reaction and culture in the nasopharynx of erythromycin-treated infants with pertussis. *Pediatr. Infect. Dis. J.* **15:**54–57.

20. **Eldering, G., and P. Kendrick.** 1938. *Bacillus para-pertussis:* a species resembling both *Bacillus pertussis* and *Bacillus bronchisepticus* but identical with neither. *J. Bacteriol.* **35:** 561–572.

21. **Ewanowich, C. A., L. W. L. Chui, M. G. Paranchych, M. S. Peppler, R. G. Marusyk, and W. L. Albritton.** 1993. Major outbreak of pertussis in northern Alberta, Canada: analysis of discrepant direct fluorescent-antibody and culture results by using polymerase chain reaction methodology. *J. Clin. Microbiol.* **31:**1715–1725.

22. **Farrell, D. J., G. Daggard, and T. K. S. Mukkur.** 1999. Nested duplex PCR to detect *Bordetella pertussis* and *Bordetella parapertussis* and its application in diagnosis of pertussis in nonmetropolitan southeast Queensland, Australia. *J. Clin. Microbiol.* **37:**606–610.

23. **Farrell, D. J., M. McKeon, G. Daggard, M. J. Loeffelholz, C. J. Thompson, and T. K. S. Mukkur.** 2000. Rapid-cycle PCR method to detect *Bordetella pertussis* that fulfills all consensus recommendations for use of PCR in diagnosis of pertussis. *J. Clin. Microbiol.* **38:**4499–4502.

24. **Ferry, N. S.** 1912. *Bacillus bronchisepticus (bronchicanis):* the cause of distemper in dogs and a similar disease in other animals. *Vet. J.* **68:**376–391.

25. **Gilligan, P. H., and M. C. Fisher.** 1984. Importance of culture in laboratory diagnosis of *Bordetella pertussis* infections. *J. Clin. Microbiol.* **20:**891–893.

26. **Glare, E. M., J. C. Paton, R. R. Premier, A. J. Lawrence, and I. T. Nisbet.** 1990. Analysis of a repetitive DNA sequence from *Bordetella pertussis* and its application to the diagnosis of pertussis using the polymerase chain reaction. *J. Clin. Microbiol.* **28:**1982–1987.

27. **Goodnow, R. A.** 1980. Biology of *Bordetella bronchiseptica. Microbiol. Rev.* **44:**722–738.

28. **Grimprel, E., P. Begue, I. Anjak, F. Betsou, and N. Guiso.** 1993. Comparison of polymerase chain reaction, culture, and western immunoblot serology for diagnosis of *Bordetella pertussis* infection. *J. Clin. Microbiol.* **31:**2745–2750.

29. **Guris, D., P. M. Strebel, B. Bardenheier, M. Brennan, R. Tachdjian, E. Finch, M. Wharton, and J. R. Livengood.** 1999. Changing epidemiology of pertussis in the United States: increasing incidence among adolescents and adults, 1990–1996. *Clin. Infect. Dis.* **28:**1230–1237.

30. **Hagiwara, K., K. Ouchi, N. Tashiro, M. Azuma, and K. Kobayashi.** 1999. An epidemic of a pertussis-like illness caused by *Chlamydia pneumoniae. Pediatr. Infect. Dis. J.* **18:**271–275.

31. **Hallander, H. O., J. Gnarpe, H. Gnarpe, and P. Olin.** 1999. *Bordetella pertussis, Bordetella parapertussis, Mycoplasma pneumoniae, Chlamydia pneumoniae* and persistent cough in children. *Scand. J. Infect. Dis.* **31:**281–286.

32. **Hallander, H. O., E. Reizenstein, B. Renemar, G. Rasmuson, L. Mardin, and P. Olin.** 1993. Comparison of nasopharyngeal aspirates with swabs for culture of *Bordetella pertussis. J. Clin. Microbiol.* **31:**50–52.

33. **Halperin, S. A., R. Bortolussi, and A. J. Wort.** 1989. Evaluation of culture, immunofluorescence, and serology for the diagnosis of pertussis. *J. Clin. Microbiol.* **27:**752–757.

34. **Halperin, S. A., A. Kasina, and M. Swift.** 1992. Prolonged survival of *Bordetella pertussis* in a simple buffer after nasopharyngeal secretion aspiration. *Can. J. Microbiol.* **38:**1210–1213.

35. **He, Q., J. Mertsola, H. Soini, M. Skurnik, O. Ruuskanen, and M. K. Viljanen.** 1993. Comparison of polymerase chain reaction with culture and enzyme immunoassay for diagnosis of pertussis. *J. Clin. Microbiol.* **31:**642–645.

36. **He, Q., G. Schmidt-Schlapfer, M. Just, H. C. Matter, S. Nikkari, M. K. Viljanen, and J. Mertsola.** 1996. Impact of polymerase chain reaction on clinical pertussis research: Finnish and Swiss experiences. *J. Infect. Dis.* **174:**1288–1295.

37. **Heininger, U., K. Stehr, S. Schmitt-Grohe, C. Lorenz, R. Rost, P. D. Christenson, M. Uberall, and J. D. Cherry.** 1994. Clinical characteristics of illness caused by *Bordetella parapertussis* compared with illness caused by *Bordetella pertussis. Pediatr. Infect. Dis. J.* **13:**306–309.

38. Hill, B. C., C. N. Baker, and F. C. Tenover. 2000. A simplified method for testing *Bordetella pertussis* for resistance to erythromycin and other antimicrobial agents. *J. Clin. Microbiol.* **38**:1151–1155.

39. Hoppe, J. E., and A. Eichhorn. 1989. Activity of new macrolides against *Bordetella pertussis* and *Bordetella parapertussis. Eur. J. Clin. Microbiol. Infect. Dis.* **8**:653–654.

40. Hoppe, J. E., U. Halm, H. J. Hagedorn, and A. Kraminer-Hagedorn. 1989. Comparison of erythromycin ethylsuccinate and co-trimoxazole for treatment of pertussis. *Infection* **17**:227–231.

41. Hoppe, J. E., and T. Paulus. 1998. Comparison of three media for agar dilution susceptibility testing of *Bordetella pertussis* using six isolates. *Eur. J. Clin. Microbiol. Infect. Dis.* **17**:391–393.

42. Hoppe, J. E., E. Rahimi-Galougahi, and G. Seibert. 1996. In vitro susceptibilities of *Bordetella pertussis* and *Bordetella parapertussis* to four fluoroquinolones (levofloxacin, d-ofloxacin, ofloxacin, and ciprofloxacin), cefpirome, and meropenem. *Antimicrob. Agents Chemother.* **40**:807–808.

43. Hoppe, J. E., and M. Schlagenhauf. 1989. Comparison of three kinds of blood and two incubation atmospheres for cultivation of *Bordetella pertussis* on charcoal agar. *J. Clin. Microbiol.* **27**:2115–2117.

44. Hoppe, J. E., and J. Schwaderer. 1989. Direct plating versus use of transport medium for detection of *Bordetella* species from nasopharyngeal swabs. *Eur. J. Clin. Microbiol. Infect. Dis.* **8**:264–265.

45. Hoppe, J. E., and A. Weiss. 1987. Recovery of *Bordetella pertussis* from four kinds of swabs. *Eur. J. Clin. Microbiol.* **6**:203–205.

46. Houard, S., C. Hackel, A. Herzog, and A. Bollen. 1989. Specific identification of *Bordetella pertussis* by the polymerase chain reaction. *Res. Microbiol.* **140**:477–487.

47. Hozbor, D., F. Fouque, and N. Guiso. 1999. Detection of *Bordetella bronchiseptica* by the polymerase chain reaction. *Res. Microbiol.* **150**:333–341.

48. Janda, W. M., E. Santos, J. Stevens, D. Celig, L. Terrile, and P. C. Schreckenberger. 1994. Unexpected isolation of *Bordetella pertussis* from a blood culture. *J. Clin. Microbiol.* **32**:2851–2853.

49. Kattar, M. M., J. F. Chavez, A. P. Limaye, S. L. Rassoulian-Barrett, S. L. Yarfitz, L. C. Carlson, Y. Houze, S. Swanzy, B. L. Wood, and B. T. Cookson. 2000. Application of 16S rRNA gene sequencing to identify *Bordetella hinzii* as the causative agent of fatal septicemia. *J. Clin. Microbiol.* **38**:789–794.

50. Katzko, G., M. Hofmeister, and D. Church. 1996. Extended incubation of culture plates improves recovery of *Bordetella* spp. *J. Clin. Microbiol.* **34**:1563–1564.

51. Kerr, J. R., and R. C. Matthews. 2000. *Bordetella pertussis* infection: pathogenesis, diagnosis, management, and the role of protective immunity. *Eur. J. Clin. Microbiol. Infect. Dis.* **19**:77–88.

52. Kersters, K., K.-H. Hinz, A. Hertle, P. Segers, A. Lievens, O. Siegmann, and J. De Ley. 1984. *Bordetella avium*, sp. nov., isolated from the respiratory tracts of turkeys and other birds. *Int. J. Syst. Bacteriol.* **34**:56–70.

53. Korgenski, E. K., and J. A. Daly. 1997. Surveillance and detection of erythromycin resistance in *Bordetella pertussis* isolates recovered from a pediatric population in the Intermountain West region of the United States. *J. Clin. Microbiol.* **35**:2989–2991.

54. Kosters, K., M. Riffelmann, B. Dohrn, and C. H. von Konig. 2000. Comparison of five commercial enzyme-linked immunosorbent assays for detection of antibodies to *Bordetella pertussis. Clin. Diagn. Lab. Immunol.* **7**:422–426.

55. Kurzynski, T. A., D. M. Boehm, J. A. Rott-Petri, R. F. Schell, and P. E. Allison. 1988. Antimicrobial suscepti-

bilities of *Bordetella* species isolated in a multicenter pertussis surveillance project. *Antimicrob. Agents Chemother.* **32**:137–140.

56. Lewis, K., M. A. Saubolle, F. C. Tenover, M. F. Rudinsky, S. D. Barbour, and J. D. Cherry. 1995. Pertussis caused by an erythromycin-resistant strain of *Bordetella pertussis. Pediatr. Infect. Dis. J.* **14**:388–391.

57. Li, Z., D. L. Jansen, T. M. Finn, S. A. Halperin, A. Kasina, S. P. O'Connor, T. Aoyama, C. R. Manclark, and M. J. Brennan. 1994. Identification of *Bordetella pertussis* infection by shared-primer PCR. *J. Clin. Microbiol.* **32**:783–789.

58. Linnemann, C. C., and E. B. Perry. 1977. *Bordetella parapertussis.* Recent experience and a review of the literature. *Am. J. Dis. Child.* **131**:560–563.

59. Loeffelholz, M. J., C. J. Thompson, K. S. Long, and M. J. R. Gilchrist. 1999. Comparison of PCR, culture, and direct fluorescent-antibody testing for detection of *Bordetella pertussis. J. Clin. Microbiol.* **37**:2872–2876.

60. Loeffelholz, M. J., C. J. Thompson, K. S. Long, and M. J. R. Gilchrist. 2000. Detection of *Bordetella holmesii* using *Bordetella pertussis* IS481 PCR assay. *J. Clin. Microbiol.* **38**:467.

61. Long, S. S., C. J. Welkon, and J. L. Clark. 1990. Widespread silent transmission of pertussis in families: antibody correlates of infection and symptomatology. *J. Infect. Dis.* **161**:480–486.

62. Marcon, M. J., A. C. Hamoudi, H. J. Cannon, and M. M. Hribar. 1987. Comparison of throat and nasopharyngeal swab specimens for culture diagnosis of *Bordetella pertussis* infection. *J. Clin. Microbiol.* **25**:1109–1110.

63. Mastrantonio, P., P. Stefanelli, M. Giuliano, Y. Herrera Rojas, M. Ciofi degli Atti, A. Anemona, and A. E. Tozzi. 1998. *Bordetella parapertussis* infection in children: epidemiology, clinical symptoms, and molecular characteristics of isolates. *J. Clin. Microbiol.* **36**:999–1002.

64. Mazengia, E., E. A. Silva, J. A. Peppe, R. Timperi, and H. George. 2000. Recovery of *Bordetella holmesii* from patients with pertussis-like symptoms: use of pulsed-field gel electrophoresis to characterize circulating strains. *J. Clin. Microbiol.* **38**:2330–2333.

65. Meade, B. D., and A. Bollen. 1994. Recommendations for the use of the polymerase chain reaction in the diagnosis of *Bordetella pertussis* infections. *J. Med. Microbiol.* **41**:51–55.

66. Mink, C. M., J. D. Cherry, P. Christenson, K. Lewis, E. Pineda, D. Shlian, J. A. Dawson, and D. A. Blumber. 1992. A search for *Bordetella pertussis* infection in university students. *Clin. Infect. Dis.* **14**:464–471.

67. Moissenet, D., M. Valcin, V. Marchand, E. Grimprel, P. Begue, A. Garbarg-Chenon, and H. Vu-Thien. 1996. Comparative DNA analysis of *Bordetella pertussis* clinical isolates by pulsed-field gel electrophoresis, randomly amplified polymorphism DNA, and ERIC polymerase chain reaction. *FEMS Microbiol. Lett.* **143**:127–132.

68. Mooi, F. R., H. Hallander, C. H. Wirsing von Konig, B. Hoet, and N. Guiso. 2000. Epidemiological typing of *Bordetella pertussis* isolates: recommendations for a standard methodology. *Eur. J. Clin. Microbiol. Infect. Dis.* **19**:174–181.

69. Morrill, W. E., J. M. Barbaree, B. S. Fields, G. N. Sanden, and W. T. Martin. 1988. Effects of transport temperature and medium on recovery of *Bordetella pertussis* from nasopharyngeal swabs. *J. Clin. Microbiol.* **26**:1814–1817.

70. Mortensen, J. E., and G. L. Rodgers. 2000. In vitro activity of gemifloxacin and other antimicrobial agents against isolates of *Bordetella pertussis* and *Bordetella parapertussis. J. Antimicrob. Chemother.* **45**:47–49.

71. **Müller, F.-M. C., J. E. Hoppe, and C.-H. Wirsing von König.** 1997. Laboratory diagnosis of pertussis: state of the art in 1997. *J. Clin. Microbiol.* **35:**2435–2443.

72. **Nennig, M. E., H. R. Shinefield, K. M. Edwards, S. B. Black, and B. H. Fireman.** 1996. Prevalence and incidence of adult pertussis in an urban population. *JAMA* **275:**1672–1674.

73. **Pichichero, M. E., M. A. Deloria, M. B. Rennels, E. L. Anderson, K. M. Edwards, M. D. Decker, J. A. Englund, M. C. Steinhoff, A. Deforest, and B. D. Meade.** 1997. A safety and immunogenicity comparison of 12 acellular pertussis vaccines and one whole-cell pertussis vaccine given as a fourth dose in 15- to 20-month-old children. *Pediatrics* **100:**772–788.

74. **Porter, J. F., K. Connor, and W. Donachie.** 1996. Differentiation between human and ovine isolates of *Bordetella parapertussis* using pulsed-field gel electrophoresis. *FEMS Microbiol. Lett.* **135:**131–135.

75. **Regan, J., and F. Lowe.** 1977. Enrichment medium for the isolation of *Bordetella*. *J. Clin. Microbiol.* **6:**303–309.

76. **Register, K. B., A. Boisvert, and M. R. Ackermann.** 1997. Use of ribotyping to distinguish *Bordetella bronchiseptica* isolates. *Int. J. Syst. Bacteriol.* **47:**678–683.

77. **Reischl, U., N. Lehn, G. N. Sanden, and M. J. Loeffelholz.** 2001. Real-time PCR assay targeting IS*481* of *Bordetella pertussis* and molecular basis for detecting *Bordetella holmesii*. *J. Clin. Microbiol.* **39:**1963–1966.

78. **Reizenstein, E., B. Johansson, L. Mardin, J. Abens, R. Möllby, and H. O. Hallander.** 1993. Diagnostic evaluation of polymerase chain reaction discriminative for *Bordetella pertussis*, *B. parapertussis*, and *B. bronchiseptica*. *Diagn. Microbiol. Infect. Dis.* **17:**185–191.

79. **Reizenstein, E., L. Lindberg, R. Möllby, and H. O. Hallander.** 1996. Validation of nested *Bordetella* PCR in pertussis vaccine trial. *J. Clin. Microbiol.* **34:**810–815.

80. **Rothstein, E. P., E. L. Anderson, M. D. Decker, G. A. Poland, K. S. Reisinger, M. M. Blatter, R. M. Jacobson, C. A. Mink, D. Gennevois, A. E. Izu, F. Sinangil, and A. G. Langenberg.** 1999. An acellular pertussis vaccine in healthy adults: safety and immunogenicity. *Vaccine* **17:**2999–3006.

81. **Sacco, R. E., K. B. Register, and G. E. Nordholm.** 2000. Restriction endonuclease analysis discriminates *Bordetella bronchiseptica* isolates. *J. Clin. Microbiol.* **38:**4387–4393.

82. **Schlapfer, G., H. P. Senn, R. Berger, and M. Just.** 1993. Use of the polymerase chain reaction to detect *Bordetella pertussis* in patients with mild or atypical symptoms of infection. *Eur. J. Clin. Microbiol. Infect. Dis.* **12:**459–463.

83. **Tang, Y. W., M. K. Hopkins, C. P. Kolbert, P. A. Hartley, P. J. Severance, and D. H. Persing.** 1998. *Bordetella holmesii*-like organisms associated with septicemia, endocarditis, and respiratory failure. *Clin. Infect. Dis.* **26:**389–392.

84. **Tilley, P. A., M. V. Kanchana, I. Knight, J. Blondeau, N. Antonishyn, and H. Deneer.** 2000. Detection of *Bordetella pertussis* in a clinical laboratory by culture, polymerase chain reaction, and direct fluorescent antibody; accuracy, and cost. *Diagn. Microbiol. Infect. Dis.* **37:**17–23.

85. **Tran Minh, N. N., Q. He, K. Edelman, A. Putto-Laurila, H. Arvilommi, M. K. Viljanen, and J. Mertsola.** 2000. Immune responses to pertussis antigens eight years after booster immunization with acellular vaccines in adults. *Vaccine* **18:**1971–1974.

86. **Vandamme, P., M. Heyndrickx, M. Vancanneyt, B. Hoste, P. De Vos, E. Falsen, K. Kersters, and K.-H. Hinz.** 1996. *Bordetella trematum* sp. nov., isolated from wounds and ear infections in humans, and reassessment of *Alcaligenes denitrificans* Rüger and Tan 1983. *Int. J. Syst. Bacteriol.* **46:**849–858.

87. **Vandamme, P., J. Hommez, M. Vancanneyt, M. Monsieurs, B. Hoste, B. Cookson, C.-H. Wirsing von König, K. Kersters, and P. J. Blackall.** 1995. *Bordetella hinzii* sp. nov., isolated from poultry and humans. *Int. J. Syst. Bacteriol.* **45:**37–45.

88. **van der Zee, A., C. Agterberg, M. Peeters, F. Mooi, and J. Schellekens.** 1996. A clinical validation of *Bordetella pertussis* and *Bordetella parapertussis* polymerase chain reaction: comparison with culture and serology using samples from patients with suspected whooping cough from a highly immunized population. *J. Infect. Dis.* **174:**89–96.

89. **van der Zee, A., C. Agterberg, M. Peeters, J. Schellekens, and F. R. Mooi.** 1993. Polymerase chain reaction assay for pertussis: simultaneous detection and discrimination of *Bordetella pertussis* and *Bordetella parapertussis*. *J. Clin. Microbiol.* **31:**2134–2140.

90. **van der Zee, A., H. Groenendijk, M. Peeters, and F. R. Mooi.** 1996. The differentiation of *Bordetella parapertussis* and *Bordetella bronchiseptica* from humans and animals as determined by DNA polymorphism mediated by two different insertion sequence elements suggests their phylogenetic relationship. *Int. J. Syst. Bacteriol.* **46:**640–647.

91. **Wadowsky, R. M., S. Laus, T. Libert, S. J. States, and G. D. Ehrlich.** 1994. Inhibition of PCR-based assay for *Bordetella pertussis* by using calcium alginate fiber and aluminum shaft components of a nasopharyngeal swab. *J. Clin. Microbiol.* **32:**1054–1057.

92. **Wadowsky, R. M., R. H. Michaels, T. Libert, L. A. Kingsley, and G. D. Ehrlich.** 1996. Multiplex PCR-based assay for detection of *Bordetella pertussis* in nasopharyngeal swab specimens. *J. Clin. Microbiol.* **34:**2645–2649.

93. **Weyant, R. S., D. G. Hollis, R. E. Weaver, M. F. M. Amin, A. G. Steigerwalt, S. P. O'Connor, A. M. Whitney, M. I. Daneshvar, C. W. Moss, and D. J. Brenner.** 1995. *Bordetella holmesii* sp. nov., a new gram-negative species associated with septicemia. *J. Clin. Microbiol.* **33:**1–7.

94. **Wirsing von König, C.-H., D. Gounis, S. Laukamp, H. Bogaerts, and H. J. Schmitt.** 1999. Evaluation of a single-sample serological technique for diagnosing pertussis in unvaccinated children. *Eur. J. Clin. Microbiol. Infect. Dis.* **18:**341–345.

95. **Woolfrey, B. F., and J. A. Moody.** 1991. Human infections associated with *Bordetella bronchiseptica*. *Clin. Microbiol. Rev.* **4:**243–255.

96. **Wright, S. W., K. M. Edwards, M. D. Decker, and M. H. Zeldin.** 1995. Pertussis infection in adults with persistent cough. *JAMA* **273:**1044–1046.

97. **Yih, W. K., E. A. Silva, J. Ida, N. Harrington, S. M. Lett, and H. George.** 1999. *Bordetella holmesii*-like organisms isolated from Massachusetts patients with pertussis-like symptoms. *Emerg. Infect. Dis.* **5:**441–443.

98. **Yuk, M. H., U. Heininger, G. Martinez de Tejada, and J. F. Miller.** 1998. Human but not ovine isolates of *Bordetella parapertussis* are highly clonal as determined by PCR-based RAPD fingerprinting. *Infection* **26:**270–273.

Francisella and *Brucella**

MAY C. CHU AND ROBBIN S. WEYANT

51

Francisella and *Brucella* are small, nonmotile, gram-negative coccobacilli. The genera are composed of zoonotic agents pathogenic for humans and animals. These genera have been linked because of their similarities in appearance, clinical symptoms, the enzootic nature of the agents, and serologic cross-reactivity by agglutination tests (9, 79, 145). Evidence based on the divergent DNA relatedness index, biochemical characteristics, and genome sequences has led to the recognition that *Francisella* and *Brucella* are distinct. *Brucella* belongs to the α-proteobacteria, which are in the same class as the *Rickettsia*, *Ehrlichia*, and *Bartonella*, while *Francisella* belongs to the γ-proteobacteria, which taxonomically are closer to the enteric bacteria, *Legionella*, *Pseudomonas*, and *Pasteurella*. Presumptive differentiation and identification of *Francisella* and *Brucella* are possible by oxidase, urea hydrolysis, cysteine auxotrophy, and cellular fatty acids (Table 1). *Francisella* and *Brucella* remain linked by their reputation as being the causes of two of the more frequent laboratory-acquired infections (40) and are considered to be potential bioterrorism agents (53).

Francisella tularensis and the members of the genus *Brucella* are considered Select Biological Agents of Human Disease, and the transfer of these organisms, in whole or in part, is regulated by U.S. Federal Code 42 CFR Part 72.6 (40). Laboratories that work with, send, or receive these organisms must be registered with the Centers for Disease Control and Prevention (CDC) unless they are used for CLIA-regulated diagnostic work. Further information on this process is available from the CDC Office of Health and Safety at http://www.cdc.gov/od/ohs/lrsat.

FRANCISELLA

Taxonomy

Tularemia is the disease caused by infection with members of the *Francisella* genus. It is an enzoosis affecting a wide range of animals and humans. It was described in detail in the first part of the 20th century (52, 63, 83). The etiologic agent was isolated in 1910 by McCoy and Chapin from a ground squirrel die-off in Tulare County in Calif. (83).

Francis, for whom the genus is named, recognized and confirmed that a number of diverse and widespread epidemiologically distinct clinical entities were really one disease and proposed the name "tularemia" to describe the disease in humans (52). Two other members from North America have been added to the *Francisellaceae*: *F. novicida*, now reclassified as *F. tularensis* subsp. *novicida*, was recovered in 1951 from water and *F. philomiragia* was isolated in 1969 from muskrats and the surrounding water environment (62). These two latter species are infrequently isolated and are not often implicated in clinical disease. The genus members have been separated into two pathogenic groups: one that causes serious illness in humans and is often lethal for animals, and one that is considered of lesser virulence for humans and animals (66). The pathogenic members of this genus exist as intracellular parasites; therefore, the duration of antibiotic therapy may have to be extended in order to eliminate the infection. All genus members are susceptible to aminoglycosides and tetracyclines. It is the widespread epizootic nature of tularemia, its potential to cause severe and fatal disease in humans, its reputation as a laboratory hazard, and its potential use as a biological warfare agent that has given tularemia its notoriety. *F. tularensis* has been developed as a biological weapon, and projections about its impact, if used as a weapon in an urban setting, depict a scenario devastating to public health services and of huge economic burden (39).

The species of *Francisella* share morphological characteristics, similar biochemical activities, a high degree of DNA relatedness (49, 50, 62), and a unique cellular fatty acid profile (41, 62). There are two recognized species, *F. tularensis* and *F. philomiragia* (62, 115). Subspecies designation continues to be in transition as new information about host relationships, geographic origin, virulence, and phenotypic, biochemical, and genetic features are revealed. Four subspecies (subsp.) or biovars of *F. tularensis* are listed in the most recent edition of *Bergey's Manual* (115): *F. tularensis* subsp. *tularensis* (type A), *F. tularensis* subsp. *holarctica* (type B, formerly known as *F. tularensis* subsp. *palaearctica*), *F. tularensis* subsp. *mediaasiatica* (1, 93, 109), and *F. tularensis* subsp. *novicida*. The members of this genus have been associated with the natural outdoors environment, small mammals, and arthropods. *Wolbachia persica* isolated from *Argas persicus* ticks and two tick endosymbionts, from *Dermacentor andersoni* and from *Ornithodoros moubata*, share

* This chapter contains information presented in chapters 41 and 44 by Daniel S. Shapiro and Jane D. Wong in the seventh edition of this Manual.

TABLE 1 Presumptive differentiation of *Francisella* and *Brucella* from similar gram-negative genera[a]

Test	F. tularensis	Brucella spp.[b]	Bartonella spp.[b]	Acinetobacter sp.	Psychrobacter phenylpyruvicus[c]	Oligella sp.	Bordetella bronchiseptica	Haemophilus influenzae
Oxidase	−	+	−	−	+	+	+	v
Urea hydrolysis	−	+	−	v	+	+	+	v
Gram stain morphology	Tiny ccb	Tiny ccb	Thin rod	Broad ccb	Broad ccb	Tiny ccb	Thin rod	Small ccb
Specimen source	Ulcer, wound, blood, aspirates	Blood, bone marrow	Blood, bone marrow, lymph node	v	v	Urinary tract	v	v
X or V factor requirement	−	−	−[d]	−	−	−	−	+
Cysteine enhancement	+	−	−	−	−	−	−	−
Motility	−	−	−	−	−	v	+	−
Major CFA[e]	10:0; 14:0; 16:0; 18:1ω9c; 3-OH-18:0	16:0; 18:1ω7c; 18:0; 19:0cyc[11-12]	16:0; 17:0; 18:1ω7c	16:1ω7c; 16:0; 18:1ω9c	16:1ω7c; 16:0; 18:2; 18:1ω9c	16:0; 18:1ω7c	16:1ω7c; 16:0; 17:0cyc	14:0; 16:1ω7c; 16:0

[a] +, greater than or equal to 90% positive; −, less than or equal to 10% positive; v, variable (11 to 89% positive); ccb, coccobacilli.
[b] Does not include *B. bacilliformis*, which is the only motile species.
[c] Formerly *Moraxella phenylpyruvica*.
[d] Although not strictly required, hemin (X factor) enhances growth and biochemical activity for many strains.
[e] The acids listed represent at least 10% of the total CFA composition. The number before the colon indicates the number of carbons; the number after the colon is the number of double bonds; ω indicates the position of the double bond counting from the hydrocarbon end of the carbon chain; OH indicates a hydroxy group at the 2(α)- or 3(β)-position from the carboxyl end; c indicates *cis* isomer.

16S rRNA sequence similarity with *Francisellaceae* (50, 115).

Description of the Genus

The genus *Francisella* comprises tiny gram-negative coccobacilli that can be distinguished from other families by several features (Table 1). Members of the genus take up Gram's counterstain (safranin) poorly; are strict aerobes, weakly catalase positive, nonmotile, and non-spore forming; and react with a limited number of carbohydrates (Table 2). Only a few sugars (glucose, maltose, sucrose, and glycerol) are utilized by most of the members of the genus. Acid is produced without gas. Unique fatty acids are associated with the genus (Table 1) (62, 115). For most species, in vitro growth is enhanced by sulfhydryl supplementation. The organisms in the genus have ≥98% 16S rRNA sequence similarity (50). Single plasmids of various sizes have been associated with individual isolates of *F. tularensis* subsp. *holarctica*, *F. tularensis* subsp. *novicida* (115), and, recently, two strains of *F. philomiragia* (M. Chu, unpublished observation).

Description of the Species

The two *Francisella* species are quite homogeneous, with only a few key differences serving to differentiate them (Table 2). *F. philomiragia* is more biochemically reactive than *F. tularensis*; it also differs by its ability to ferment maltose and is oxidase positive using Kovac's reagent. Subspecies differentiation is less distinctive; single biochemical differences in glycerol fermentation and glucose utilization are used to define the biovars. *F. tularensis* subsp. *tularensis*, designated type A, is the most virulent of all the subspecies, with a 50% lethal dose of ≤10 cells for laboratory mice and rabbits (41, 66). *F. tularensis* subsp. *tularensis* and *F. tularensis* subsp. *mediaasiatica* have the greatest similarity in that they utilize glycerol (1), possess citrulline ureidase activity (77, 109), and, along with *F. tularensis* subsp. *novicida*, have the same 16S rRNA signature nucleotide sequence (50, 109). *F. tularensis* subsp. *mediaasiatica* differs from *F. tularensis* subsp. *tularensis* by its inability to utilize glucose and its comparatively lower virulence (1). Type B organisms (*F. tularensis* subsp. *holarctica*) may be differentiated by their inability to utilize glycerol, an absence of citrulline ureidase activity, and the presence of a unique 16S rRNA signature sequence. *F. tularensis* subsp. *holoarctica* is of intermediate virulence, with a 50% lethal dose of ≤1,000 cells for laboratory animals (41, 66). *F. tularensis* subsp. *novicida* can be distinguished from the other subspecies by its ability to grow independently of cysteine supplementation and by its comparatively larger vegetative cell size. *F. tularensis* subsp. *novicida* is considered to be of low virulence like *F. tularensis* subsp. *mediasiaactica* and *F. philomiragia* but otherwise shares genetic characteristics of *F. tularensis* subsp. *tularensis* (62, 109, 115).

Natural Habitats

Global Distribution

Francisellaceae are distributed widely within the northern hemisphere (holarctic region) in a variety of natural habitats, from the Arctic Circle south to about latitude 20°N (63). Regions south of this latitude, Australia, and Central and South America appear to be untouched by tularemia (63). Tularemia is associated with a wide range of habitats and hosts, with over 100 species of wild animals, birds, and arthropod vectors being involved (63, 67, 93). Habitats

where the Lagomorpha (*Sylvilagus* [rabbits], *Lepus* [hares], and *Oryctolagus* [Old World hares]) and the Rodentia (water voles, muskrat, lemmings, voles, and beavers) thrive are important in maintaining tularemia-enzootic foci (11, 63, 87, 94). Biting arthropod vectors, primarily tabanid flies (*Chrysops* and *Tabanus*), ticks (*Dermacentor*, *Ixodes*, and *Amblyomma*), and mosquitoes (*Culicidae* in Europe and Russia), are implicated in the mechanical transmission of tularemia. By their presence in the natural environment, infections with *Francisella* are usually acquired in association with outdoor activities; via contact with contaminated air, water, soil, or vegetation; by handling ill or dead animals; and from infective insect bites (3, 48, 87, 104, 122, 146).

Distribution in North America

F. tularensis subsp. *tularensis* was thought to occur only in North America, where it has been most closely associated with infection in lagomorphs and humans. Recently it was found that the distribution of *F. tularensis* subsp. *tularensis* appears not to be limited to North America; it has been isolated from mites and fleas in Europe but has not been associated with human infection there (60). In contrast, infection with *F. tularensis* subsp. *holarctica* is less virulent; it has a much wider distribution, in both the Old World and New World, and is associated with a greater variety of animals, primarily hares and rodents, and with contaminated environmental source outbreaks. *F. tularensis* subsp. *mediaasiatica* is found in circumscribed geographical regions in Kazakhstan and Turkmenistan and has been isolated from hares and ticks but not from humans (1). *F. tularensis* subsp. *novicida* has been described primarily in North America (35, 62). Of the 15 known isolates of *F. philomiragia*, 1 was recovered from Switzerland and the rest were recovered in North America (112, 135).

Since the 1940s, when several thousand cases annually were sometimes reported, the incidence of reported tularemia cases in the United States has steadily declined to about 100 to 200 cases each year. All states except Hawaii have reported cases. From 1995 to 1999, tularemia was removed as a nationally notifiable disease, but it was reinstated in 2000 because of concerns about its potential use as a bioterrorism agent (33). Despite its removal from nationally notifiable disease status between 1995 and 1999, the number of cases reported annually to CDC did not differ substantially from previous years. A total of 1,367 human cases were reported to CDC between 1990 and 2000 (Fig. 1) (33). Most cases occur in south-central and western states. The epidemiology of tularemia in the United States has not changed significantly in the past several decades. It remains a rural disease, and most patients acquire tularemia from tick or deerfly bites or by contact with infected animals, particularly rabbits. Cultures of isolates recovered in the United States from 1996 to 2001 consist of equal proportions of type A and type B genotypes, and these overwhelmingly predominate; isolations of *F. tularensis* subsp. *novicida* and *F. philomiragia* are rare.

Clinical Significance

F. tularensis subsp. *tularensis* and *F. tularensis* subsp. *holarctica*

Tularemia has been known historically by a number of synonyms such as plague-like disease, rabbit fever, deerfly fever, market men's disease, glandular type of tick fever, conjunctivitis tularensis, Ohara's or Yao-byo disease, and

TABLE 2 *Francisella* spp. characteristics

Characteristics	*F. tularensis* subspecies				*F. philomiragia*[c]
	tularensis[a]	*holarctica*[b]	*mediaasiatica*	*novicida*[c]	
Gram stain (culture)	Faintly staining, pleomorphic, single, rarely chained, gram-negative coccobacilli	As for subsp. *tularensis*	As for subsp. *tularensis*	As for subsp. *tularensis*	As for subsp. *tularensis*
Cell size (μm)	0.2 by 0.2–0.7	0.2 by 0.2–0.7	0.2 by 0.2–0.7	0.7 by 1.7	0.7 by 1.7
Growth on:					
Standard agar[d]	−	−	−	+	+
Chocolate agar, 48 h	2–4 mm, raised, gray, smooth, moist, butyrous entire colonies, usually no agar discoloration	As for subsp. *tularensis*	As for subsp. *tularensis*	As for subsp. *tularensis* but 5 mm in diam	>5-mm, white, smooth, mucoid, entire colonies; no agar discoloration
Cysteine heart blood agar, 48 h	2-mm, pearl-white to ivory color with green tint and prominent opalescent sheen; smooth, butyrous, and green-yellow discoloration of agar medium	As for subsp. *tularensis*	Not tested	5-mm colonies with features the same as type A and type B	Colonies are >5 mm, creamy white-grey, mucoid, and smooth with a purple-tinted opalescent sheen
Requires cystine/cysteine	+	+	+	−	−
Catalase	Weakly +	Weakly +	Weakly +	Weakly +	Weakly +
Oxidase (Kovacs)	−	−	−	−	+
Acid from:					
Glucose[e]	+	+	−	+	+
Maltose	+	+	−	V[i]	+
Sucrose	−	−	+	+	V
Glycerol	+	−	+	+	+
Relative virulence (mice)	High	Intermediate	Low	Low	Low
DNA typing					
16S rRNA probe[f]	Type A	Type B	Type A	Type A	Type A
PCR primers[g]	Species specific	Species specific	Species specific	Species specific	Does not react
VNTR and IS probe[h]	Strain specific	Strain specific	Strain specific	Strain specific	Strain specific

[a] Type A, predominantly found in North America and associated with a severe form of disease in humans and rabbits.

[b] Type B, found throughout the Northern Hemisphere and associated with a less severe form of disease in humans; associated with humans and rodents (muskrats, field mice, beaver, voles, and water rats).

[c] Associated with low virulence and infrequently isolated.

[d] Standard bacteriological media: blood, Trypticase soy, and brain heart infusion.

[e] Delayed or variable reaction. *F. tularensis* subsp. *mediaasiatica* does not ferment glucose (1).

[f] Probes that define type A and type B sequences (49).

[g] PCR primers: Tul-4, T-cell epitope (75); FopA and p43,000 antigen (115).

[h] VNTR, variable number of tandem repeats: allelic variation, subspecies and strain specific (47). IS, insertion element PCR (type B specific) or Southern hybridization pattern (subspecies and strain specific).

[i] Variable or slow reaction.

water rat trappers' disease. These synonyms attest to the variety of clinical presentations, the infectious agent's ubiquitous presence in nature, and the way in which the infection may be acquired by humans.

The clinical spectrum depends on the mode of transmission, the virulence of the infecting strain, the degree of systemic involvement, the immune status of the host, and timely diagnosis and treatment. Tularemia can be misdiag-

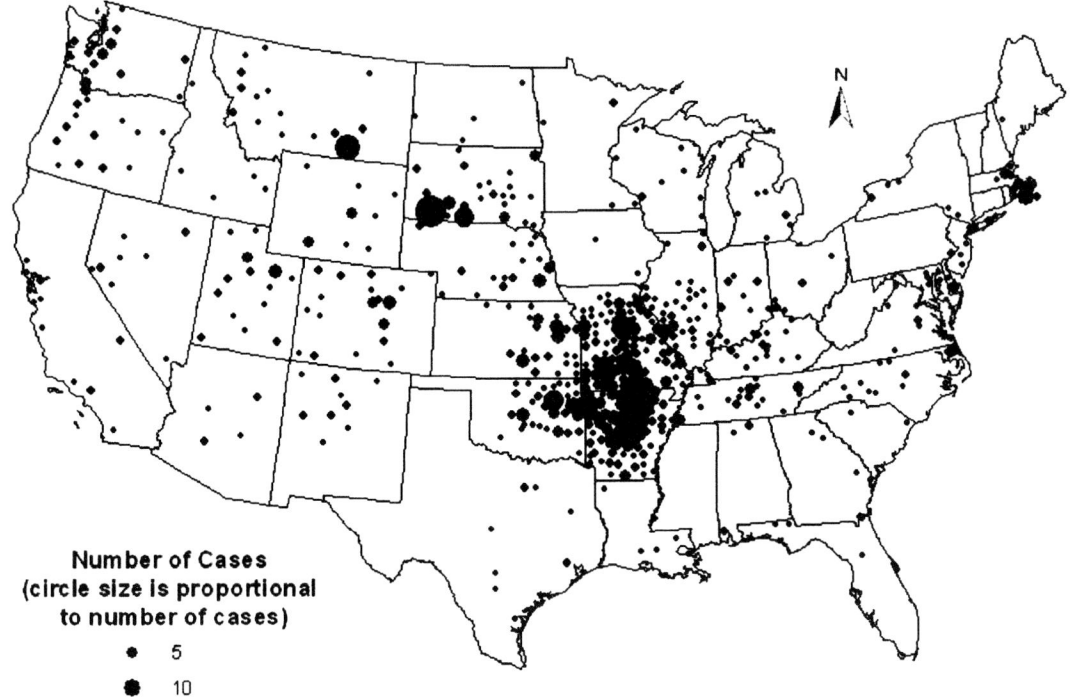

**Number of Cases
(circle size is proportional
to number of cases)**

• 5

● 10

FIGURE 1 Distribution of tularemia cases in the United States, 1990–2000. Numbers are based on 1,347 cases reporting county of residence in the lower continental United States. Alaska reported 10 cases in 4 counties from 1990 to 2000.

nosed early in infection since its symptoms are not unique: sudden onset of chills, fever, headache, and generalized malaise characterize each onset of illness. The differential diagnosis includes a wide range of infectious diseases, such as cat-scratch fever, syphilis, mycobacterial infections, anthrax, brucellosis, legionellosis, and plague. The incubation period averages 3 to 5 days, but onset occurs in as little as 2 days or up to 14 days after infection. Without treatment, nonspecific symptoms usually persist for several weeks to months, with sweats, chills, progressive weakness, and weight loss being characteristic. Prior to the advent of antibiotics, the overall mortality from infections with the more severe type A strains was in the range of 5 to 15%; however, fatality rates as high as 30 to 60% have been reported for untreated typhoidal and pneumonic forms of the disease. In the United States, untreated type B strain infections were rarely fatal; the fatality rate for all forms in recent years has been less than 2% (39).

Patients may present with any one or more of the classically described forms of tularemia: ulceroglandular, glandular, oculoglandular, pharyngeal, typhoidal, and pneumonic. The most common form is ulceroglandular disease (45 to 80% of the reported cases), indicating that the portal of entry is via infective insect bite (ticks, flies, and mosquitoes) or other inoculation through the skin barrier usually associated with handling contaminated materials (skinning infected animals). Pharyngeal lymphadenopathy suggests a portal of entry via ingestion of contaminated water or food, as was the case with the recent food- and waterborne outbreak in Kosovo (104). Typhoidal tularemia is the most difficult form to recognize because there is no identified portal of entry and because localization signs are absent. Any of the initial forms of tularemia may be complicated by

bacteremic spread, leading to various secondary tularemic symptoms such as pneumonia, sepsis, or meningitis.

F. tularensis subsp. *novicida*

Until 1989, a single 1951 Utah water isolate was defined as *F. tularensis* subsp. *novicida* and no human infection had been linked with it. During a subsequent study of 16 unusual human bacterial isolates, 14 were identified as *F. philomiragia* and 2 were identified as *F. tularensis* subsp. *novicida* (62). The two latter isolates, along with two from Texas (35), are the only ones causing human cases described in the literature. Fever, chills, cough, shortness of breath, and chest pain were the common symptoms described. All cases were identified after the isolates, recovered from blood and from granulomatous tissue, were characterized. Two patients manifested skin lesions, one had cervical lymphadenopathy, and one had a debilitating illness. A human isolate was recovered from a cervical lymph node of a patient in Utah in 2000 (Chu, unpublished).

F. philomiragia

F. philomiragia appears to be mostly an opportunistic agent, infecting patients with a previous underlying condition that renders them more susceptible. A total of 15 cases were described between 1974 and 1997. All but one involved a host with an impaired physical barrier to infection (near-drowning) or impaired immunologic defenses (chronic granulomatous disease or myeloproliferative disease) (112, 135). The U.S. patients were from nine different states, and one patient was from Switzerland (112, 135). In most cases *F. philomiragia* was isolated from normally sterile sites: blood, bone marrow, cerebrospinal fluid, pericardial fluid. The drowning and water exposure cases were associated with saltwater, in contrast to *F. tularensis* infections, which are associated with freshwater sources.

Unusual Occurrences of Tularemia

There is an increasing awareness of unusual occurrences of tularemia in animals and humans. Tularemia in domestic pets (138) may increase the risk to family members and veterinarians (10). Recently, the risk from wild-caught prairie dogs has been noted (74). Tularemia has been described in captive-monkey colonies (42, 91, 98, 99, 134). Rare cases of tularemia have been associated with postprosthetic replacement surgery (36), underlying debilitating conditions posttransplantation (90), a shunt infection (97), underlying human immunodeficiency virus infection (57), and chronic granulomatous disease (76). Pneumonic tularemia cases have been associated with lawn mowing or other activities that could have aerosolized infectious particles (48, 80, 82, 92, 122). Recent occurrence of pneumonic cases associated with lawn-mowing or brush-cutting activities in Martha's Vineyard, Mass., in 2000 and 2001 serve to underscore the gaps in our understanding of the transmission dynamics of tularemia (48).

Handling, Transport, and Storage of Specimens

Laboratory Safety

Working with live *F. tularensis* can be hazardous. *F. tularensis* has a long and notorious history of infecting laboratory personnel who were working with infectious materials (27, 40, 67, 95). This was especially so before laminar-flow cabinets, vaccination, and appropriate antibiotic therapy became available. Clinical specimens should be handled under biosafety level 2 conditions with universal precautions and transferred to biosafety level 3 as soon as *F. tularensis* is suspected (40). Hundreds of laboratory-acquired infections have been documented, including infections in the pioneer scientists who first investigated the natural history of the disease; they acquired infections by handling infected animals, removing arthropods from carcasses, and working with live cultures (67). The greatest risk of laboratory-acquired tularemia is by aerosol inhalation while working with infected materials and cultures. The infectiousness of the organisms is high, and they should be handled by trained and, preferably, vaccinated personnel.

Transport and Storage of Specimens

Specimens should be stored chilled in appropriate medium until processed in the laboratory. Freezing of tissues is recommended but not swab specimens because of lysis of live bacteria upon thawing. Although *F. tularensis* may survive for long periods in the environment, successful laboratory recovery is not high, and so efforts should be made to maintain the integrity of the isolates and avoid delay in transporting the specimens to the laboratory for testing. Ectoparasites may be stored intact in 2% NaCl, transported to the laboratory for identification, and then processed for evidence of *F. tularensis*. Clinical specimens should be placed in Amies agar with charcoal, a commercial transport system designed for anaerobic and aerobic pathogens (BD, Franklin Lakes, N.J.). *F. tularensis* should remain viable for 7 days at ambient room temperature when stored in Amies medium (68). Stuart medium, designed for transporting gonococcal specimens, and saline were inadequate in keeping *F. tularensis* viable during transport (68). For PCR, specimens should be collected in guanidine isothio-cyanate-containing buffer, which should preserve *F. tularensis* DNA for up to 1 month (68).

Direct Examination

The *F. tularensis* subspecies cannot be clearly differentiated from each other by microscopy. Cultures and fresh clinical specimens (ulcer or wound swabs, touch-prep fresh tissues, or aspirates) but not thick blood or environmental samples can be directly examined. Under microscopic examination of gram-stained specimens or culture, *Francisella* cells (single, pleomorphic) are so tiny and faintly staining that they can be easily missed. Thus, direct Gram staining is usually of no diagnostic value. To improve visualization, direct fluorescent-antibody (DFA) staining, using a labeled hyperimmune rabbit polyclonal antibody prepared by immunizations with *F. tularensis* subsp. *tularensis* cells (CDC, Ft. Collins, Colo.), will presumptively identify *F. tularensis* subsp. *tularensis* and *F. tularensis* subsp. *holarctica*. This DFA reagent does not react with *F. tularensis* subsp. *novicida* or *F. philomiragia*. DFA reagents prepared by other laboratories may have cross-reactivity with *F. philomiragia* (115) and *Legionella* (108). Immunohistochemical (IHC) staining, using a monoclonal antibody directed against the lipopolysaccharide, has been successfully used to visualize *F. tularensis* in formalin-fixed tissues in both intra- and extracellular sites (59).

Molecular Detection

The presence of *F. tularensis* in specimens taken from ulcers, wounds, tissues, and the environment (animal feces and urine, water, hay infusion, mud, and ectoparasites) may be determined by detection of *F. tularensis* lipopolysaccharide antigen using a rapid hand-held assay (12, 58), or by an antigen capture enzyme-linked immunosorbent assay (cELISA) (12, 58, 86). DNA detection by PCR has been widely applied directed at unique target regions (51, 61, 68, 75, 114). The detection limit of the handheld assay has been estimated to be 10^6 bacteria/ml, while the limit is 10^3 bacteria/ml for cELISA and 10^2 bacteria/ml for PCR (58). These are specialized tests and are not widely available, although PCR technologies have become more commonly used for screening purposes.

Culture and Isolation

Procedures for Recovery and Isolation

F. tularensis is not readily recovered by culture and is not easily identified even when it is cultured. The pathogenic *F. tularensis* bacteria are fastidious, requiring supplementation with sulfhydryl compounds (cysteine, cystine, thiosulfate, or IsoVitaleX) to grow on artificial medium. *F. tularensis* grows well on chocolate agar (CA), buffered charcoal yeast extract (BCYE) agar, and Thayer-Martin (TM) agar; in thioglycolate broth and in general bacteriological media (tryptic soy broth and Mueller-Hinton broth) supplemented with 1 to 2% IsoVitaleX; and on cysteine heart blood agar supplemented with 9% chocolatized sheep blood (CHAB). The organisms grow slowly (60-min generation time); therefore, robust growth is obtained by prolonged incubation (48 h or longer) or by plating on highly nutritive media such as CHAB. *F. tularensis* cultures should be incubated at 35 to 37°C aerobically and observed daily for 10 to 14 days; CO_2 does not impede its growth. Incorporation of antibiotics in the medium (penicillin, 100,000 U/ml; polymyxin B sulfate, 100,000 U/ml; and cycloheximide, 0.1 mg/ml) suppresses growth of the normal flora and prevents it from overwhelming the *F. tularensis* organisms (41). Complex protein or nutritionally enriched specimens such as blood or tissue provide an intrinsic source of sulfhydryl compounds that permit *F. tularensis* growth. Upon subculture, the fastidiousness of *F. tularensis* becomes evident as the exogenous compounds are depleted, leading to the loss of its viability unless the subculture is propagated on cysteine-supplemented media. If a subculture fails to grow successfully on agar, inoculation of laboratory mice with a suspension of the original specimen or inoculated medium may assist in reviving the culture.

Specimens should be taken based on clinical presentation and before administration of antibiotics. Fresh clinical material, likely to contain high concentrations of *F. tularensis* organisms, such as ulcers, wounds, and lymphoid tissue (liver, spleen, affected lymph node), are inoculated directly on an agar plate using the sample-laden swab or bacteriological loop. Larger inocula are necessary for the recovery of *F. tularensis* from specimens that contain a lower concentration of the organisms: blood, aspirates of pharyngeal washes, bronchial washes, pleural fluid, urine, and environmental samples (41, 67, 125, 127). A total of 3 to 10 ml of whole blood should be inoculated into blood culture bottles (41, 112). Environmental specimens, impinged air samples, and collected water are concentrated through a 0.22- or 0.45-μm-pore-size nitrocellulose filter, and the filter-trapped organisms are released by vigorous agitation of the filter in less than 5 ml of sterile buffer (41). The inoculum should be spread on as many agar plates as necessary at a seeding volume of 0.5 ml/agar plate. A portion of the inoculum (0.1 ml) may be injected subcutaneously into mice for enhanced recovery. Preserved, formalin-fixed tissues should be examined by IHC staining (59).

Identification

Presumptive and Confirmatory Identification
An exposure history consistent with risks known to be associated with tularemia, suggestive clinical symptoms, and the presence of poorly staining, tiny gram-negative coccobacilli should raise the suspicion of tularemia (Fig. 2). A positive test result with any one of (i) DFA (Fig. 3), (ii) IHC staining (Fig. 4), (iii) slide agglutination test, (iv) PCR, or (v) single antibody titer by serologic test provides a presumptive diagnosis. Confirmation of infection would include the identification of a culture as *F. tularensis* and/or a fourfold titer difference in acute- and convalescent-phase serum samples, with one of the paired samples having a positive titer. The slide agglutination test presumptively identifies a suspect culture by mixing polyclonal rabbit anti-*F. tularensis* antibody with safranin-stained cells. Biochemical reactions are supportive of identification but are not reliable for confirmation, since *Francisella* spp. are not very reactive. Fatty acid profiles may also be used to presumptively identify the organism as belonging to the *Francisella* genus (41, 62). There is no specific bacteriophage lysis test for *F. tularensis*.

Bacteriological Growth
Colony morphology of *F. tularensis* is most distinctive when it is grown on CHAB. On CA, *F. tularensis* colonies have an entire edge; they are gray, smooth, raised, and moist with a butyrous consistency. *F. tularensis* subsp. *novicida* grows more robustly than the other subspecies and is cysteine independent (Table 2). Colonies of *F. philomiragia* on CA are >5 mm in size with an entire edge; they are white,

smooth, raised, mucoid, and cysteine independent. On CHAB, *F. tularensis* exhibits a prominent and unique opalescent sheen due to its production of H$_2$S; this iridescent sheen is less prominent in *F. philomiragia* than in *F. tularensis* and is absent in cultures of other gram-negative organisms such as *Yersinia*, *Brucella*, *Haemophilus*, and *Pasteurella* spp.

Molecular Typing of Species and Subspecies
F. tularensis and *F. philomiragia* may be differentiated by protein profiling, 16S rRNA sequencing (50, 109, 115), various types of PCR approaches (61, 69, 101), and insertion element (IS) typing (Table 2). When the genomic sequences of both the prototypic type A strain, Schu 4 (100), and type B, live vaccine strain, are completely determined, additional target areas may be identified for more precise typing and for study of strain pathogenesis.

Using 16S rRNA sequences, genus, species, and subspecies strains can be determined (50). PCR is more sensitive than recovery by culture (83% compared to 62%) (68). A variety of PCR methods have been used to type isolates by genus, by species, or by individual isolates or small groups (61, 69, 101). Rapid PCR methods using the *Taqman* 5' nuclease assay have a detection limit of less than 100 CFU under controlled laboratory conditions (61). IS typing (M. Chu, submitted for publication) and multilocus variable-number tandem repeat analysis using three to six allelic markers have been successful in typing biovars and strains (47, 69). PCR methods for clinical laboratory use as a rapid detection approach during bioterrorism situations are undergoing evaluation and validation by the Rapid Response Advanced Technology Laboratory at CDC.

Serologic Testing
Serologic testing is the most common method by which *F. tularensis* infections are diagnosed (126). Serum, plasma from citrated or heparinized blood, and filter paper-extracted serum proteins (137) can be used in serologic assays. Antibodies may be detected as early as 1 week after onset (about 2 weeks after infection). By 2 weeks after onset, antibody may be detected in 89 to 95.4% of samples (15, 123, 126). Antibodies can persist for more than 10 years (15, 133). Immunoglobulin M (IgM), IgA, and IgG antibodies appear simultaneously (126, 131). IgM antibody can last for many years; therefore, its presence does not indicate early or recent infection (15, 126). Agglutination, by the tube agglutination (TA) or microagglutination (MA) method, is the standard serologic test for determining the presence of antibody to tularemia (23, 126). A single specimen with a TA titer of ≥1:160 or an MA titer of ≥1:128 can be interpreted as a presumptive positive result when there are compatible symptoms of tularemia and an absence of a history of vaccination or previous exposure. Confirmatory serodiagnosis requires a fourfold titer difference between acute- and convalescent-phase specimens taken at least 14 days apart, with one of the pair of serum specimens showing a positive titer by TA or MA. The formalin-killed whole-cell agglutination antigen (BBL Microbiology Systems, Cockeysville, Md.) may have low-level cross-reactivity primarily with *Brucella* antibodies, but the level of reactivity is typically ≤1:20 and does not interfere with the interpretation of a positive result (9, 13, 79). ELISA formats that identify immunoglobulin classes (13, 14, 123, 131) and antigen detection (58, 86, 125) have been adopted for use in parts of Europe where tularemia is endemic. Cellular (14, 131) and recombinant (133) antigens used for ELISAs are

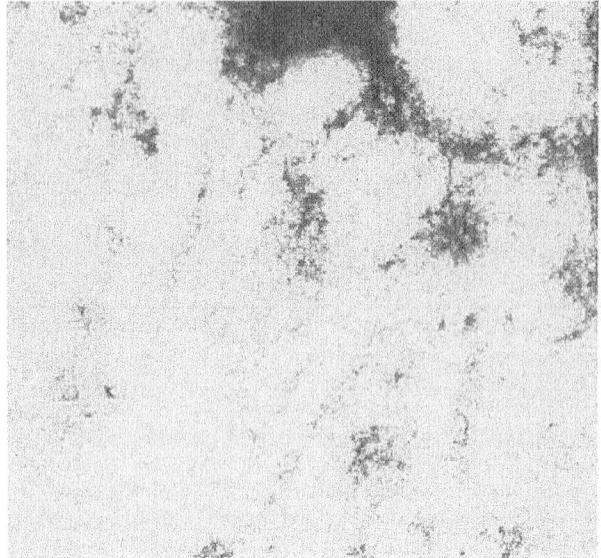

FIGURE 2 *Francisella tularensis* Gram stain. Cells are tiny (0.2 by 0.2 to 0.7 μm) and stain poorly with safranin. Magnification, ×630.

more sensitive and specific than agglutination, but their use in enzootic serosurveillance is limited by host specificity. Antigenic difference between the type A and type B biovars has not been demonstrated (88). The serologic tests thus react with anti-type A and anti-type B antibodies and usually do not react with anti-*F. tularensis* subsp. *novicida* and anti-*F. philomiragia* antibodies.

F. tularensis organisms are intracellular bacteria and are capable of eliciting both humoral and cell-mediated immunity (126). The latter response has been known to remain strong 25 years after infection (43). A skin test was previously used to measure specific tularemia reactivity to intradermally injected extracts (25). Host T cells retain proliferative responses to unique *F. tularensis* membrane proteins, with a concomitant increase in gamma interferon- and interleukin-2 levels (43, 120, 121). Tests for measuring cell-mediated immune responses are specialized and are not routinely used for diagnosis of tularemia.

Antimicrobial Susceptibilities of *F. tularensis* and Prevention and Control of Disease in Humans

Antimicrobial Susceptibility Test Methods

Antimicrobial susceptibility testing of *F. tularensis* is not usually performed in clinical microbiology laboratories because of safety concerns associated with working with these organisms (27, 95). Mueller-Hinton medium supplemented with 2% IsoVitaleX or CHAB must be used because of the fastidiousness of the pathogenic *F. tularensis* organisms. Susceptibility to the antibiotics recommended for treatment and prophylaxis, i.e., chloramphenicol, ciprofloxacin, gentamicin, streptomycin, and tetracycline, should be tested against the *F. tularensis* isolate. No known naturally occurring strains resistant to the drugs recommended for treatment exist. The nature of penicillin resistance has not been defined. Standardized methods have been published for susceptibility testing using broth, agar dilution (7), disk diffusion (110), and E test (65, 70). No breakpoint standards have been set since there are no known naturally drug-resistant strains except for erythromycin resistance in *F. tularensis* subsp. *holarctica* strains of northern Europe (93).

Treatment

F. tularensis infections are treatable with narrow-spectrum antibiotics, and drug resistance, with the exception of erythromycin resistance, in wild-type isolates is not known.

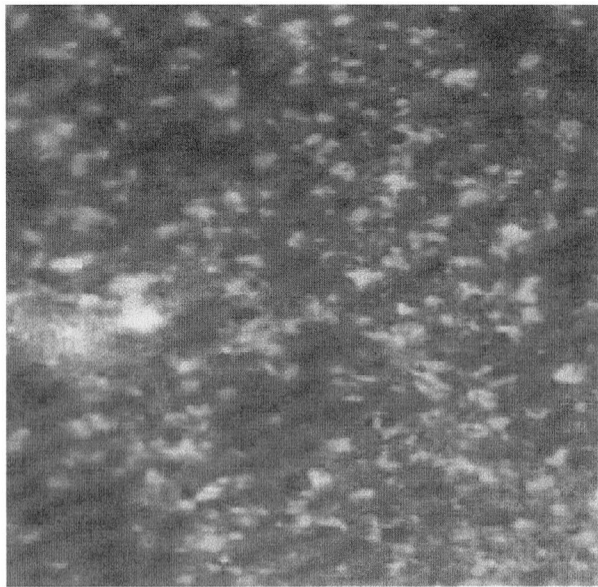

FIGURE 3 DFA staining of *Francisella tularensis* in liver tissue. Magnification, ×400.

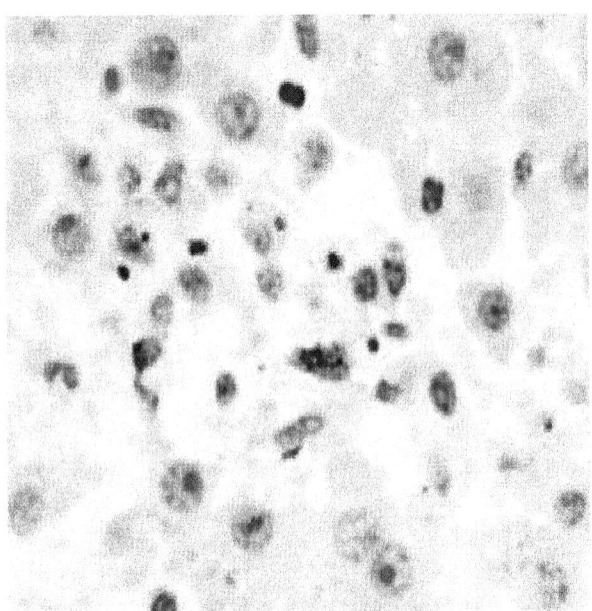

FIGURE 4 IHC staining of *Francisella tularensis* (red) in liver tissue (blue) using mouse monoclonal antibody against *F. tularensis* LPS and gold-labeled anti-mouse secondary antibody. Magnification, ×1,000.

Appropriate and early treatment is effective. Streptomycin is the drug of choice. It is given to adults in a dosage of 0.5 to 1.0 g intramuscularly every 12 h for 7 to 10 days (39). Gentamicin is an alternative drug, which can be given at 3 to 5 mg/kg/day intramuscularly in equal divided doses at 8-h intervals for 10 days. Doxycycline or chloramphenicol may be used in combination with an aminoglycoside or used alone in less severe cases. Treatment with bacteriostatic agents, doxycycline, or chloramphenicol alone may result in treatment failures or relapses. An extended dosage schedule of 14 to 21 days may be necessary to prevent relapses. Ciprofloxacin has been used successfully to treat a limited number of patients (70, 110, 124); these clinical results, coupled with its low effective MIC, suggest that ciprofloxacin may become a useful addition to the armamentarium of drugs recommended for treating tularemia. All *Francisella* isolates examined to date are β-lactamase positive, and so penicillins and cephalosporins are not effective and should not be used to treat tularemia.

Prevention and Control

F. tularensis is a well-entrenched enzootic agent and is unlikely to be eliminated even from limited natural foci. *F. tularensis* can survive for long periods in a cold, moist environment (11, 66, 94). Avoidance of infective exposure is the principal means of preventing tularemia. The public should be educated about the risks for acquiring the disease in tularemia-endemic regions and warned especially not to handle dead or ill animals, particularly rabbits, hares, and water rodents. Gloves and protective clothing should be worn when skinning or preparing such animals for food. People should be advised to thoroughly cook these animals before eating them. Repellents should be used to avoid arthropod bites, and ticks should be removed promptly. Chlorinated municipal water is safe from tularemia, but untreated water can be a ready source of infection; outbreaks have followed drinking the water from contaminated wells or streams and even from eating freshwater crustaceans (3, 104).

Isolation of patients is not necessary, since person-to-person spread does not occur; therefore, treatment of close contacts of tularemia patients is not recommended (39). Universal precautions to avoid direct contact with contaminated secretions are advised. Laboratory personnel are at high risk of acquiring typhoidal or pulmonary tularemia via inhalation. When handling specimens from patients suspected of having tularemia, laboratory personnel should work in a class II biosafety cabinet, and all work should be moved to biosafety level 3 conditions once an isolate is confirmed as *F. tularensis*. Persons who have a recognized high-risk exposure (e.g., spill, aerosol spray, or puncture of skin) to *F. tularensis* should be given oral antibiotic prophylaxis. If the exposure is considered to be of low risk (e.g., handling culture in the biosafety cabinet, preparing and making slides), these persons should be placed on fever watch for 10 days and treated if they develop symptoms. Vaccination may be advised for persons who are working with live cultures or those who are at risk because of occupational duties. A live attenuated vaccine has been used to immunize millions of persons living in northern European countries and Russia. A variant of this vaccine, LVS, has been used in the United States since 1959 for immunization of personnel who are at risk of laboratory infection. The vaccine is administered as a single dose of 0.06 ml by scarification. Antibodies develop within 3 weeks and may persist at reduced levels for months or years. Human volunteer studies demonstrated only partial protection against aerosol challenges after vaccination. A review of vaccination records at the U.S. Army microbiological laboratories from 1960 to 1969 revealed a total of 11 cases of laboratory-acquired tularemia (1 case per 1,000 at-risk employee-years) (27) in vaccinated personnel. However, LVS vaccinees were thought to have had milder symptoms than the unvaccinated persons. The greatest protection of vaccination was against typhoidal and pneumonic forms; it was less effective against the ulceroglandular form of tularemia. This vaccine is administered under investigational use in the United States (U.S. Army Medical Research and Development Command, Ft. Detrick, Frederick, Md.). It is currently under Food and Drug Administration review, and its availability in the future is undetermined.

BRUCELLA

Taxonomy

The genus *Brucella* consists of small, nonmotile, gram-negative coccobacilli that are pathogenic for humans and animals. The first human cases of brucellosis were described in 1861 by J. A. Marston, a physician with the British army stationed at Malta (78). The causative agent of brucellosis was first cultivated in 1886 by Sir David Bruce from spleen tissues of victims of Malta fever (24). Bruce assigned the name *Micrococcus melitensis* to these isolates. In 1895, B. Bang, a Danish veterinarian, isolated an organism, which he designated *Bacillus abortus*, from cases of bovine abortion (8). In 1918, Alice Evans, an American bacteriologist who would later become the first female President of the American Society for Microbiology, demonstrated a high level of similarity between these organisms (45). Shortly thereafter, Meyer and Shaw proposed the new genus *Brucella*, to include both the agents of Malta fever and Bang's disease as *B. melitensis* and *B. abortus*, respectively (84). In 1929, Huddleston proposed a third species, *B. suis*, to include strains originally isolated by Traum in 1914 from aborted swine (64, 129). Two additional species were identified in the 1950s: *B. ovis*, an agent of reproductive disease in sheep, and *B. neotomae*, isolated from the desert wood rat in Utah (26, 119). Neither of these species have been associated with human disease. In 1966, Carmichael and Bruner described a sixth *Brucella* species, *B. canis*, which is a causative agent of canine abortion (29). Over the past 10 years, multiple studies have described phenotypically unique *Brucella* strains isolated from marine mammals. Two additional species names, "*B. maris*" and "*B. delphini*," have been suggested to represent these isolates (46, 85).

The 16S rRNA gene sequence-based phylogenetic tree illustrated in Fig. 5 shows the taxonomic location of the genus *Brucella*. This genus, *Ochrobactrum*, and *Mycoplana* form the family *Brucellaceae*. *Mycoplana* species are soil organisms that have not been associated with human disease, and *Ochrobactrum anthropi* is a soil organism and opportunistic human pathogen. The close phylogenetic relationship between the members of the family *Brucellaceae* suggests that they may have evolved from a common free-living soil organism. According to the taxonomic outline presented in the second edition of *Bergey's Manual of Systematic Bacteriology*, the *Brucellaceae* are part of the proposed order "*Rhizobiales*," which is in the proposed class "*Alphaproteobacteria*" of the phylum *Proteobacteria* and domain *Bacteria* (55). Other members of the "*rhizobiales*" as-

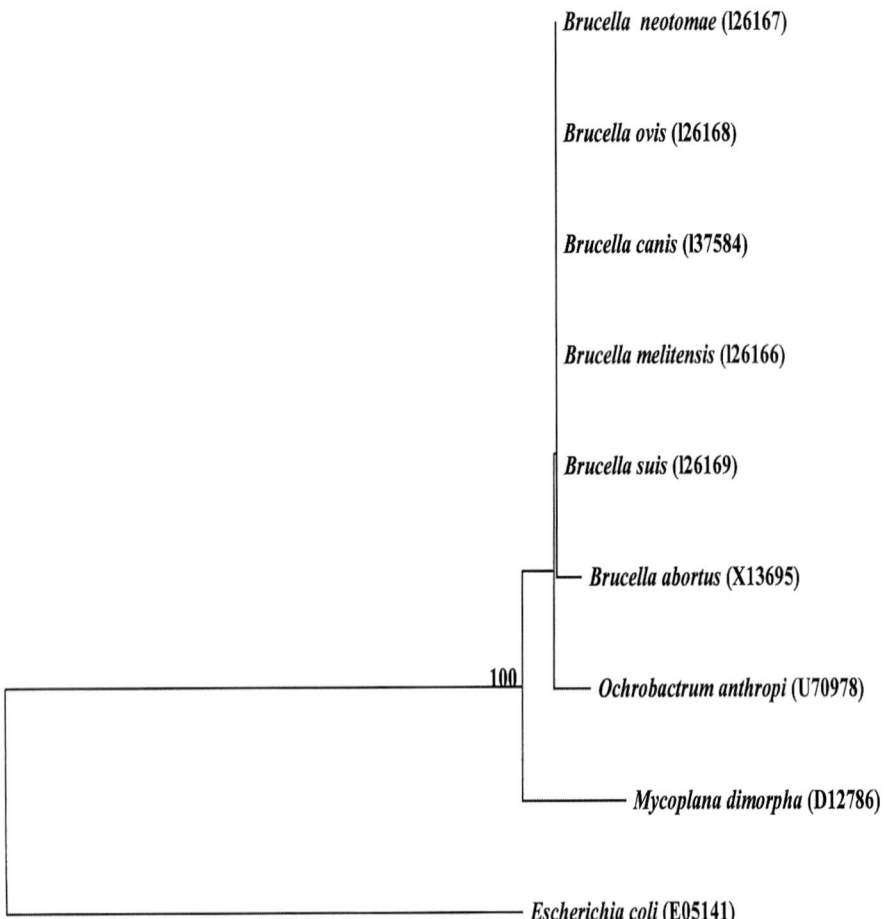

FIGURE 5 Phylogeny tree based on representative 16S rRNA gene sequences of the validly published *Brucella* species and other taxa in the family *Brucellaceae*. GenBank sequence accession numbers are given in parentheses.

sociated with human disease include *Bartonella* (family *Bartonellaceae*), *Afipia* (proposed family "*Bradyrhyzobiaceae*"), and *Methylobacterium* and *Roseomonas* (proposed family "*Methylobacteriaceae*").

The taxonomy of the genus *Brucella* suffers from a dichotomy between the morphologic and molecular definitions of species. There are six historically recognized and validly published species: *B. melitensis*, *B. abortus*, *B. suis*, *B. canis*, *B. ovis*, and *B. neotomae*. Three of these species contain multiple biovars; three for *B. melitensis*, seven for *B. abortus*, and five for *B. suis*. These species and biovars are defined by their host specificity, tolerance to fuchsin and thionin, CO_2 requirement, rate of urease activity, agglutination in monospecific adsorbed rabbit antiserum, and susceptibility to *Brucella* Tbilisi phage (136). However, DNA relatedness and multilocus enzyme electrophoresis studies indicate that all these organisms, along with the recent marine mammal-derived strains, represent a single species (54, 130). Recent molecular taxonomic studies show that although a high overall level of relatedness exists, the historically recognized species can be differentiated by restriction polymorphisms of major outer membrane genes, insertion sequences, and whole-chromosomal preparations

(132). This chapter follows the guidelines of the International Committee on Systematic Bacteriology subcommittee on the taxonomy of *Brucella* and retains the historical taxonomy (38).

Description of the Genus

Brucellae are gram-negative cocci, bacilli, or short rods, 0.5 to 0.7 μm in diameter and 0.6 to 1.5 μm in length. In Gram-stained preparations of pure cultures they are arranged singly and, less frequently, in pairs, short chains, or small groups (Fig. 6A). Bipolar staining is usually not observed. They are nonmotile and do not produce flagella. Their metabolism is aerobic, with oxygen or nitrate acting as the terminal electron acceptor via a cytochrome-based electron transport system. Strains are positive for nitrate reductase, oxidase, and catalase, although weak reactions may be observed with some strains in the last two tests. Strains are negative for indole production, gelatin liquefaction, and hemolysis. The methyl red and Voges-Proskauer tests are negative. Enhanced CO_2 may be required for growth of some strains, especially on primary isolation. Growth occurs between 20 and 40°C, with an optimum growth temperature of 37°C. The optimum growth pH

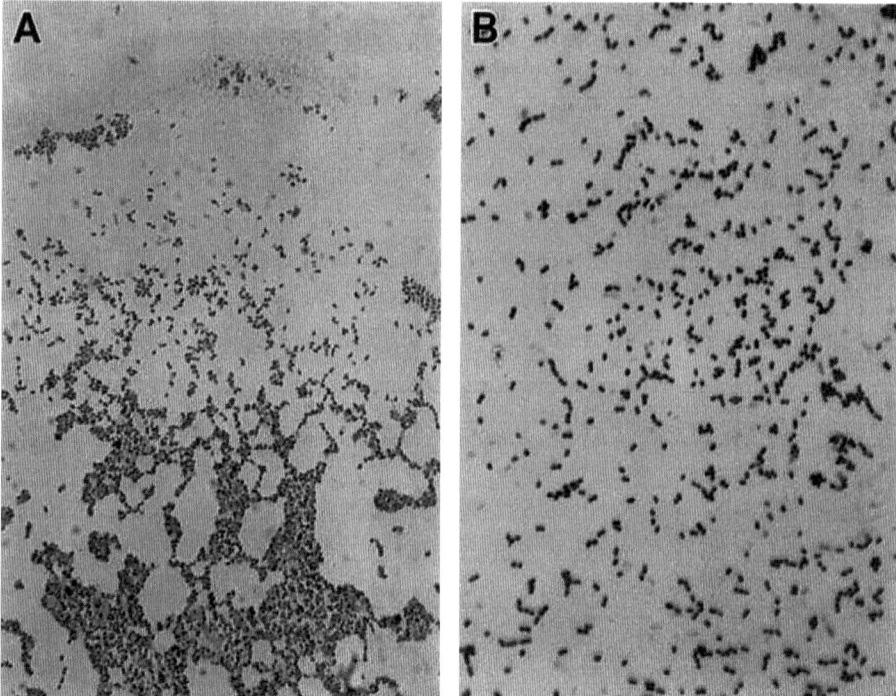

FIGURE 6 Gram stains of *Brucella abortus* (A) and *Acinetobacter* species (B). Magnification, ×750.

ranges from 6.6 to 7.4. Most strains require complex growth media containing several amino acids, thiamine, nicotinamide and magnesium ions; some strains may be induced to grow on minimal media containing an ammonium salt as the sole nitrogen source. Growth is improved by serum or blood, but hemin (X factor) and NAD (V factor) are not essential. When grown on blood agar at optimal temperature and atmosphere, colonies are usually 0.5 to 1.0 mm in diameter, raised, and convex, with an entire edge and a smooth shiny surface. *B. canis* and *B. ovis* characteristically produce nonsmooth colonies. Nonsmooth variants of the other species also occur. The G+C content of the DNA is 55 to 58 mol%. The DNA of most strains is divided into two replicons (71). Brucellae are intracellular parasites, transmissible to a wide range of animal species including humans (37).

Natural Habitats

Brucellae exist as naturally occurring parasites in a wide variety of animal species. Four *Brucella* species, *B. abortus*, *B. melitensis*, *B. suis*, and *B. canis*, cause brucellosis when transmitted to humans. *B. abortus* occurs primarily in cattle but has also been isolated from horses, buffalo, camels, yaks, and American bison. *B. melitensis* is most commonly isolated from goats and sheep but has also been isolated from alpacas and camels. In recent years *B. melitensis* has become established in cattle in Brazil, Colombia, and Israel (145). The primary hosts for *B. suis* are swine (biovars 1 to 3) and reindeer and caribou (biovar 4). *B. canis* is usually isolated from kennel-bred dogs but also has been found in coyotes and foxes. The brucellae that are nonpathogenic for humans include *B. ovis*, *B. neotomae*, and the marine mammal strains. *B. ovis* has been isolated from sheep, and *B. neotomae* has been isolated from a desert wood rat. The marine

mammal strains have been isolated from porpoises, dolphins, and seals (21). *Brucella* species are associated with chronic lifelong infections in animals, where organisms localize within the reproductive system and cause abortion and sterility. Significant numbers of organisms are shed through the milk, urine, and products of birth (145).

Clinical Significance

Brucellosis is a zoonosis of worldwide importance, particularly in developing countries. This disease is highly endemic in the Mediterranean basin, the Middle East, western Asia, Africa, and Latin America. According to the World Health Organization, the annual incidence of reported cases in areas of endemic infection varies from less than 1 to 78 per 100,000, with serologic evidence of exposure found in as much as 20% of the population (139). Mainly due to an aggressive program to eradicate infected bovines, the annual incidence of brucellosis in the United States has been reduced to less than 0.5 case per 100,000 (32). The epidemiology of brucellosis in the United States has changed over the past 20 years. Occupations traditionally associated with increased risk include farmers, veterinarians, abattoir workers, and laboratory personnel. However, effective control measures in the cattle industry and an increase in the ingestion of unpasteurized goat milk products imported from countries with endemic infection have shifted brucellosis from a predominantly occupational to a predominantly food-borne disease, especially in California and Texas (34).

Brucellosis is usually transmitted to humans by direct contact through abraded skin or mucosal surfaces, consumption of contaminated food products, or inhalation. Agricultural workers, veterinarians, and others in occupations that involve handling of animals or uncooked animal tissues are at higher risk for direct inoculation. Individuals who ingest unpasteurized dairy products, especially from areas of endemic infection, are at significant risk for foodborne brucellosis (145). Brucellosis continues to be one of the most common laboratory-acquired infections. Practices associated with transmission in the laboratory include unprotected handling of specimens, sniffing of plates, mouth pipetting, and exposure of the eyes, nose, or mouth to infectious aerosols (40). Brucellosis may also be potentially transmitted in association with biowarfare, bioterrorism, or biocriminal activities. B. suis was one of the agents included in the U.S. offensive biological weapons research program, prior to its termination in 1969 (53). In areas of hyperendemic infection, such as Saudi Arabia, brucellosis is associated with a high incidence of spontaneous abortion in pregnant women (72).

Brucellae are facultative intracellular pathogens. After transmission to the host, they are able to resist intracellular killing by neutrophils and are released into the blood. Once liberated into the bloodstream, they may infect a variety of organs but are most often localized in the reticuloendothelial system, where they reside within phagocytic cells. Granulomas or abscesses most often develop in the bone marrow, liver, spleen, lymph nodes, or lungs. Other sites of infection may include subcutaneous tissue, testes, epididymis, ovary, gallbladder, kidneys, and brain. Meningitis and endocarditis are commonly reported complications (89). Factors associated with the intracellular survival of brucellae are not well understood. The production of respiratory burst inhibitors, including GMP, AMP, and Cu-Zn superoxide dismutase, is well documented, and more recent studies suggest that Brucella cells are able to retard phagosomal maturation by disrupting normal intracellular trafficking (4, 18, 28). The upcoming availability of the B. melitensis and B. suis genomic sequences promises to uncover other potential virulence mechanisms (16).

Brucellosis is a systemic disease that may involve any of the major organ systems. The clinical manifestations of this disease are therefore highly variable. Symptoms most commonly described include relapsing fever, chills, night sweats, headache, body aches, anorexia, and malaise. In addition, localized foci of infection may occur in the liver, reticuloendothelial system, bones and joints, genitourinary tract, central nervous system, eyes, skin, lungs, and heart (endocarditis) (145). The incubation period is generally 10 to 14 days postexposure but may range from 5 to more than 35 days, and the onset of symptoms may be acute or insidious (89, 145).

The ability of brucellae to cause deep-seated infections results in various long-term sequelae including chronic brucellosis, treatment relapse, and delayed convalescence. Chronic brucellosis is generally defined as persistence of the infection for more than 1 year. This condition may occur in untreated patients or as a result of treatment relapse. The symptoms usually associated with chronic brucellosis include fever, weight loss, and malaise. The treatment of brucellosis involves long-term antibiotic therapy, and relapses may occur if therapy is discontinued prematurely or if the organisms are in a particularly deep focus of infection. These relapses usually occur within 3 to 6 months of the discontinuation of therapy. Delayed convalescence is a condition associated with nonspecific complaints of ill health and fatigue after apparently successful treatment. This condition may be differentiated from "true" chronic brucellosis by serologic testing. Chronic brucellosis is characterized by high titers of IgG antibodies in the serum,

whereas delayed convalescence is associated with negligible titers (143, 145).

Collection, Handling, Storage, and Transport of Specimens

Optimal specimens for the diagnosis of brucellosis in humans include blood and bone marrow for culture and serum for serologic testing. Brucellae may also be recovered from spleen, liver, or abscess specimens. For optimal results, multiple blood cultures should be drawn during febrile episodes (89). The general collection, handling, storage, and transport guidelines for these specimens given in this manual (see chapter 20) are applicable here. If possible, specimens for culture should be collected prior to the initiation of antibiotic therapy. Specimens that cannot be processed within 1 h of collection should be refrigerated. Acute-phase serum specimens should be collected as soon as possible after the onset of symptoms, and convalescent-phase specimens should be collected 14 to 21 days thereafter. Serum specimens should be shipped and stored frozen. If freezing is not possible, serum specimens can be preserved by adding 10 μl of a 1% merthiolate solution per ml of serum. Blood specimens may also be collected for PCR analysis. The method of collection should complement the ensuing molecular protocol. For example, the protocol of Matar et al., which includes Ficoll-Hypaque purification of mononuclear cells followed by a DNA purification step, recommends collection of whole blood in EDTA tubes (81). Conversely, the method of Queipo-Ortuno et al., which uses an osmotic erythrocyte lysis approach to purify peripheral lymphocytes, recommends the collection of whole blood in sodium citrate tubes and storage at $-20°C$ (102). Specimens from patients with suspected brucellosis should be labeled appropriately so that laboratory exposures to this agent can be minimized.

Direct Examination of Specimens

Direct microscopic examination of blood or bone marrow is not sufficiently sensitive to be useful in the diagnosis of brucellosis. There is no laboratory protocol for DFA staining. However, in recent years, new direct-detection methods using molecular approaches, particularly numerous rapid assay formats, have been described (6, 81, 103, 107). Although none of these methods has yet achieved broad acceptance in the clinical microbiology community, laboratories that serve areas of endemic infection would be well advised to investigate these molecular approaches.

Culture and Isolation

Blood and bone marrow are the specimens from which brucellae are most often isolated in cases of human disease. Bone marrow has been reported to be superior to blood when nonautomated blood culture systems are utilized (56). However, the improvement in sensitivity and time of detection demonstrated by current automated blood culture technology suggests that a reexamination of this issue is in order. The optimal procedure for processing bone marrow is by lysing 0.5 to 1.5 ml of bone marrow cells in pediatric Isolator tubes (pediatric Isolator tubes do not require centrifugation) and then inoculating the entire tube contents onto agar plates. If this is not available, the material should be inoculated into a blood culture system. Depending on the volume available, pediatric bottles should be considered. If brucellosis is suspected and there is insufficient material to inoculate both aerobic and anaerobic components, the aerobic component should be used. Brucellae grow in the aerobic component of essentially all semiautomated and automated blood culture systems, although differences exist in the time of detection and sensitivity depending upon the system used.

Biphasic bottles (Castenada bottles) containing tryptose broth, brain heart infusion broth, or brucella broth with 2.5% agar slants containing the same basal medium have been the historical method of choice for culturing brucellae from blood (31, 89). These bottles are inoculated with blood to a final concentration of 10% (vol/vol) and incubated under 10% CO_2 tension for up to 6 weeks at 35 to 37°C. At 3-day intervals the bottles are tilted to allow the inoculated broth to wash over the agar slant and then returned to the upright position. Growth, as indicated by turbidity in the broth or formation of colonies on the agar surface, is monitored visually on a daily basis. Hemoline performance biphasic medium (bioMérieux, Marcy l'Etoile, France), an updated version of the Castenada bottle, has been recently introduced. Various studies have reported times to detection ranging from less than 6 days to more than 27 days for biphasic bottles (56, 105, 111).

Lysis centrifugation is a method which involves osmotic lysis of erythrocytes followed by concentration of bacteria by centrifugation and direct plating of the concentrate onto culture media (17). This system is available commercially as the Isolator Microbial Tube (Wampole Laboratories, Cranbury, N.J.). This method significantly improves the sensitivity and time to detection of brucellae in blood compared with Castenada bottles (46). Compared with early versions of automated blood culture systems, such as BACTEC 460 and BACTEC NR, the lysis centrifugation approach produced shorter times to detection but in some cases the automated systems produced higher sensitivity rates (73).

Recent studies with the newer continuous-monitoring systems indicate that the BACTEC 9000 series is able to achieve times to detection that are comparable to those of lysis centrifugation (>95% positive within 7 days incubation) without sacrificing sensitivity (140). Published studies assessing the ability of the BacT/Alert system to rapidly detect brucellae in blood all suffer from a small sample size and have given widely variable results. Casas et al. in 1994 reported that 1 of 11 positive cultures from five brucellosis patients was detected within 7 days by the BacT/Alert system (30). However, Solomon and Jackson in 1992 and Roiz et al. in 1998 both reported 100% detection within 1 week for one and five patients, respectively, with BacT/Alert (106, 117). Although continuous monitoring systems represent a significant improvement in time of detection over biphasic bottles, holding blood culture bottles from suspected brucellosis patients for 21 days remains a prudent approach. For more information regarding the detection of brucellae in blood cultures, the reader should consult the excellent 1999 review by Yagupsky (141).

Although brucellae have a lower growth rate than most bacteria studied in the clinical laboratory, these organisms are not nutritionally fastidious. Growth is obtained on most commonly used media including Trypticase soy (with and without 5% sheep blood), brucella, brain heart infusion, heart infusion, and chocolate agars. Selective media such as Thayer-Martin and Martin-Lewis agars also support the growth of most *Brucella* strains. Growth on MacConkey agar is variable and has been observed on approximately 50% of the strains studied at CDC (136).

Identification

Rapid preliminary identification of *Brucella* not only is important from a diagnostic perspective, but also has significant public health and laboratory safety implications. Fortunately, commonly detected characteristics, such as cellular and colonial morphology, are very useful for preliminary identification. Brucellae are gram-negative coccobacilli that are smaller than other gram-negative organisms usually encountered in the clinical laboratory. A Gram-stained preparation of a *B. abortus* strain is shown in Fig. 6A. Note the size difference between the *Brucella* cells and the cells of the *Acinetobacter* strain shown in Fig. 6B. When grown on agar plates streaked for isolation, *Brucella* strains usually appear as undifferentiated growth in the primary streaked area, with no discrete colonies observed in other quadrants until much later in the incubation of the culture. When they are observed, *Brucella* colonies rarely grow to a maximum diameter of greater than 1 mm.

The phenotypic differentiation of *Brucella* and *Francisella* from other similar clinically encountered organisms is given in Table 1. A positive urease test is characteristic of the genus *Brucella*. *B. suis* and some *B. melitensis* strains produce a rapid reaction that can be observed within 5 min of inoculation on a Christensen's urea slant. The other *Brucella* species usually produce a positive reaction after overnight incubation. Other urease-positive species that may be confused with *Brucella* include *Psychrobacter phenylpyruvicus*, *Oligella ureolytica*, *Bordetella bronchiseptica*, and some *Haemophilus influenzae* biogroups. Characteristics useful in differentiating between these species include X- and V-factor requirement, motility, and, in the case of *O. ureolytica*, specimen source. Organisms that are phenotypically similar to *F. tularensis* include *Bartonella* and *Acinetobacter* species. Cysteine enhancement is useful in differentiating among these species. Cellular fatty acid (CFA) profiles are also very useful in differentiating *Francisella* and *Brucella* from other similar taxa, and a commercially available system has been developed for CFA analysis (Sherlock; Microbial Identification System [MIDI] Inc.; www.midi-inc.com). The *Brucella* CFA profile is characterized by significant amounts (≥10% of total CFA composition) of capric, myristic, palmitic, oleic, and β-hydroxystearic acids, and the *Francisella* profile is characterized by significant amounts of palmitic, *cis*-vaccenic, stearic, and lactobacillic acids (136).

Identification and biotype designation of *Brucella* isolates are achieved by the tests given in Table 3. Detailed descriptions of these and other reference methods may be found in the monographs by Alton et al. (2) and Young (142). Many of these tests require specialized reagents and should be performed in a biological safety cabinet. For these reasons, species identification and biotyping of these organisms are performed primarily in reference laboratories. A growth requirement for elevated CO_2 levels is observed in some strains of *B. abortus*. This requirement is sometimes lost by multiple passages in the laboratory. The CO_2 requirement test is performed by streaking two plates of general-use media (Trypticase soy agar with or without 5% sheep blood or heart infusion agar with or without 5% rabbit blood) and then incubating one plate in ambient air and the other plate in 5% CO_2. Plates are examined at daily intervals, and the growth on the plates is compared. The H_2S test is performed by inoculating a slant of brucella or heart infusion agar with fresh growth of the test organism. After inoculation, a lead acetate paper strip (Fisher Scien-

TABLE 3 Phenotypic identification of *Brucella* species and biovars associated with human infections[a]

Species	Biovar	CO₂ required	H₂S production[b]	Urease[c] <5 min	Urease[c] >5 min	Thionin 1:25 ×10³	Thionin 1:50 ×10³	Thionin 1:100 ×10³	Basic fuchsin 1:50 ×10³	Basic fuchsin 1:100 ×10³	Aggl. monospecific serum[d] B. abortus	Aggl. monospecific serum[d] B. melitensis	Acriflavin	Lysis by phage Tb[d,e] RTD	Lysis by phage Tb[d,e] RTD ×10⁴
B. melitensis	1	−	−	v	+	−	+	+	+	+	−	+	−	−	−
	2	−	−	v	+	−	+	+	+	+	+	+	−	−	−
	3	−	+	v	+	−	+	+	+	+	+	+	−	−	−
B. abortus	1	v	+	−	+	−	−	+	+	+	+	−	−	+	+
	2	+	+	−	+[f]	−	−	+	+	+	+	−	−	+	+
	3	v	+	−	+	−	+	+	+	+	+	−	−	+	+
	4	v	+	−	+	−	−	+	+	+	−	+	−	+	+
	5	−	−	−	+	+	+	+	+	+	−	+	−	+	+
	6	−	v	−	+	−	+	+	+	+	+	−	−	+	+
	7[g]	v	+	−	+	−	+	+	+	+	+	+	−	+	+
B. suis	1	−	+	+[h]		+	+	+	−[i]	−	+	−	−	−	+
	2	−	−	+[h]		−	+	+	+	+	+	−	−	−	+
	3	−	−	+[h]		+	+	+	+	+	+	−	−	−	+
	4	−	−	+[h]		+	+	+	+	+	+	+	−	−	+
	5	−	−	+[h]		+	+	+	−	−	−	+	−	−	+
B. canis		−	−	+[h]		+	+	+	−[i]	v	−	−	+[j]	−	−

[a] Reactions based on those obtained in the SBRL, CDC; those given in *Laboratory Techniques in Brucellosis*, 2nd ed., World Health Organization, Geneva, Switzerland, 1975.

[b] Heart infusion agar with lead acetate paper.

[c] Warm urea slant inoculated heavily.

[d] Agglutination and phage procedures given in *Laboratory Techniques in Brucellosis*, 2nd ed.

[e] Tbilisi, a *Brucella* phage originally isolated in the former USSR, has been designated as the reference phage.

[f] Rare strains are urease negative.

[g] Formerly *B. abortus* biovar 9; biovars 7 and 8 were deleted by the International Committee on Bacterial Taxonomy, Subcommittee on Taxonomy of *Brucella* (reference 6 in the *Brucella abortus* description).

[h] Usually immediate or instant reaction.

[i] Some strains studied in SBRL, CDC, grew at this concentration.

[j] *B. canis* forms a stringy mass or "gel" of increased viscosity when suspended in phenolized saline and agglutinates in specific antiserum.

tific, Hanover Park, Ill.; no. 14-862) is suspended above the slant so that the paper and the medium do not come in contact. The tube is incubated at 35°C and examined daily for 6 days. A positive reaction is indicated by the development of a dark gray or black color on the strip. At the CDC Special Bacteriology Reference Laboratory, the urease test for *Brucella* identification is performed on commercially available Christensen's urea slants (136). The slant is inoculated with a freshly grown culture, incubated at room temperature for 5 min, and examined for the development of a pronounced pink color. If no color change is noted, the slant is incubated at 35°C and examined the next day. *B. suis* strains typically produce a positive reaction within 5 min, whereas the other *Brucella* species usually require a longer incubation time.

Tolerance to the dyes thionin and basic fuchsin is determined by examining the growth on agar plates containing 1:25,000, 1:50,000, and 1:100,000 dilutions of dye. The dilutions are made by adding 0.8, 0.4, or 0.2 ml of 1% stock solutions to 20 ml of heart infusion agar that has cooled to 50°C prior to pouring. The inoculum is prepared by suspending a loopful of bacterial growth from a freshly grown culture into 1 ml of physiological saline. A sterile cotton swab is immersed into the bacterial suspension and used to inoculate the dye plates and one control plate containing no dye. A single streak is made across each of the dye plates and, lastly, a control plate containing no dye. The plates are inverted and incubated at 35°C for up to 4 days (if increased CO_2 is required, the plates may be incubated in a 5% CO_2 incubator or a candle jar) and examined for growth on a daily basis.

The acriflavin and gel formation tests are useful in differentiating *B. canis* from other *Brucella* species. The acriflavin reagent is made at a concentration of 1 mg/ml in distilled water. The test is performed by placing a drop of reagent on a slide and mixing it with fresh growth of the test organism. Agglutination of the organisms is indicative of a positive test. The gel formation test is performed by making a heavy suspension of a fresh culture in a small volume (<100 μl) of phenolized saline (0.5% phenol in buffered saline) in a 13- by 100-mm screw-cap test tube. The tube is allowed to stand at room temperature for 30 min and then is observed for gel formation. Gel formation can be determined by inserting a bacteriological loop in the suspension and looking for the formation of a short, mucoid string as the loop is withdrawn. Another technique for observing gel formation is tilting the tube and comparing the viscosity of the test suspension with that of buffered saline in a control tube. If no reaction is observed at 30 min, the tube may be incubated at room temperature overnight and observed the next day. *B. canis* strains are characteristically positive for these tests, whereas the other *Brucella* species are usually negative.

Lysis by phage Tbilisi is particularly useful in differentiating *B. melitensis* from *B. abortus* and *B. suis*. This reagent is commercially available from the American Type Culture Collection (ATCC 23448-B1). The routine test dose (RTD) is determined by testing 10-fold Trypticase soy or heart infusion broth dilutions of stock phage suspension against a control *B. abortus* strain such as ATCC 23448. The highest dilution at which a complete plaque is observed is the RTD. The test is performed by suspending cells from a fresh culture to a final concentration of approximately 10^9 cells per ml and then inoculating a Trypticase soy or heart infusion agar plate with a sterile cotton swab to produce a uniform inoculum on the surface of the plate.

After allowing the inoculum to dry, 10-μl volumes of the RTD and RTD $\times$ 10^4 are applied to the plate and allowed to adsorb into the medium. The plates are then inverted, incubated at 35°C, and read on a daily basis for 2 days. CO_2-requiring isolates should be incubated in a 5% CO_2 incubator or a candle jar.

The technical complexity and biohazard risk associated with traditional methods for *Brucella* species identification make this a prime area for molecular approaches. Although the high level of DNA homology among the species and biovars of this organism has been a confounding factor, a few molecular identification techniques have been described. Probably the best-established molecular method for identification of *Brucella* is the AMOS PCR assay, originally developed by the U.S. Department of Agriculture in 1994 (19). This assay, which takes advantage of species-specific locations of the insertion element IS711, has been used to differentiate among three biovars of *B. abortus*, all biovars of *B. melitensis* and *B. ovis*, and biovar 1 of *B. suis*. The AMOS assay has been modified to differentiate the *B. abortus* vaccine strains RB-51 and S19 from wild-type strains and has been adapted to LightCycler real-time detection technology (20, 103). Although this assay identifies the biovars most commonly encountered in the U.S. agricultural sector, it does not identify *B. canis* and many of the *B. suis* biovars. More recently Tcherneva et al. have used random amplified polymorphic DNA with 10-base primers (128) and Sifuentes-Rincon et al. have used restriction analysis of the *omp2* locus after PCR amplification to differentiate strains of the six *Brucella* species (113).

Serologic Testing

Serologic testing is a valuable adjunct to culture-based and molecular methods for the laboratory diagnosis of brucellosis. Demonstration of a specific antibody response can provide useful diagnostic information, and the characterization of the response (predominantly IgM versus IgG) assists in differentiating acute infection from recurrent disease (116). Various serologic assays have been described, including the serum agglutination test (SAT), the Rose Bengal test, the Coombs anti-human globulin test, the complement fixation test, ELISA, and the rapid dipstick test (5, 116, 118). The SAT is the most widely used test in the United States (145). This test can be used in a tube or microplate agglutination format and can be modified to differentiate IgG from IgM titers by pretreatment of specimens with 2-mercaptoethanol. The standard SAT method uses killed whole-cell *B. abortus* antigen and detects antibodies against *B. abortus*, *B. suis*, and *B. melitensis* but not *B. canis*. For paired specimens, a fourfold rise in SAT titer between the acute- and convalescent-phase sample is indicative of brucellosis. For single specimens, an SAT titer of ≥160 is suggestive of brucellosis. Cross-reactions may be observed with antibodies directed against *Francisella tularensis*, *Vibrio cholerae*, or *Yersinia enterocolitica* (145). The rapid dipstick assay, a relatively simple screening procedure for *Brucella*-specific IgM, shows promise as a field test in areas without direct access to a reference laboratory (116).

Antimicrobial Susceptibility and Therapy

Successful treatment of brucellosis requires long-term combination antibiotic therapy. The World Health Organization-recommended regimen is doxycycline (200 mg/day) in combination with rifampin (600 to 900 mg/day, orally) for 6 weeks (139). The combination of doxycycline and streptomycin is also effective. In children younger than 8 years, the combination of trimethoprim-sulfamethoxazole with an aminoglycoside has resulted in successful treatment without the side effects of tetracyclines in this age group (145).

In vitro susceptibility testing of *Brucella* isolates is not recommended. For many agents, including β-lactams and quinolones, high levels of in vitro activity do not correlate with clinical efficacy (144). In the majority of cases, the lack of well-established interpretive standards and the increased biohazard risk associated with manipulating these organisms far outweigh any benefit obtained through in vitro susceptibility testing.

Control and Prevention of Brucellosis

Human brucellosis in the United States has gradually decreased from approximately 300 cases per year in the 1970s to approximately 100 cases per year in the late 1990s. The control of this disease in domestic herds has played a major role in the reduction of human cases. Control in cattle has been achieved by serologic surveillance, vaccination (*B. abortus* strain 19), and elimination of reactor cattle (22). In recent years, the strain 19 vaccine has been replaced by the rough *B. abortus* strain RB51 (96). The RB51 vaccine has many advantages over the strain 19 vaccine. RB51 has a lower level of virulence for humans than strain 19, and vaccination with RB51 does not interfere with serologic screening for infection with wild-type strains. A useful marker for identification of RB51 in the laboratory is resistance to rifampin, which is not commonly observed in wild-type strains.

As the epidemiology of brucellosis has evolved in the United States, with a substantial increase in the proportion of food-borne infections and a recognition of *Brucella* as a potential agent of bioterrorism, new and exciting research opportunities have arisen. There is a great need for assays to rapidly and reliably detect brucellae in food and in the environment. The recent advances in *Brucella* genomics should play a significant role in this area.

REFERENCES

1. **Aikimbaev, M. A.** 1996. Taxonomy of genus *Francisella*. *Rep. Acad. Sci. Kaz. SSR Ser. Biol.* **5:**42–44.
2. **Alton, G. G., L. M. Jones, R. D. Angus, and J. M. Verger.** 1988. *Techniques for the Brucellosis Laboratory*, p. 44. Institut National de la Recherche Agronomique, Paris, France.
3. **Anda, P., J. S. del Pozo, J. M. D. Garcia, R. Escudero, F. J. G. Peña, M. C. L. Velasco, R. E. Sellek, M. R. J. Chillarón, L. P. S. Serrano, and J. F. M. Navarro.** 2001. Waterborne outbreak of tularemia associated with crayfish fishing. *Emerg. Infect. Dis.* **7:**575–582.
4. **Arenas, G. B, A. S. Staskevich, A. Aballay, and L. S. Mayorga.** 2000. Intracellular trafficking of *Brucella abortus* in J774 macrophages. *Infect. Immun.* **68:**4255–4263.
5. **Ariza, J., T. Pellicer, R. Pallares, and F. Gudiol.** 1992. Specific antibody profile in human brucellosis. *Clin. Infect. Dis.* **14:**131–140.
6. **Baily, G. G., J. B. Krahn, B. S. Drasar, and N. G. Stoker.** 1992. Detection of *Brucella melitensis* and *Brucella abortus* by DNA amplification. *J. Trop. Med. Hyg.* **95:**271–275.
7. **Baker, C. N., D. G. Hollis, and C. Thornsberry.** 1985. Antimicrobial susceptibility testing of *Francisella tularensis* with a modified Mueller-Hinton broth. *J. Clin. Microbiol.* **22:**212–215.
8. **Bang, B.** 1897. The etiology of epizootic abortion. *J. Comp. Pathol. Ther.* **10:**125–149.
9. **Behan, K. A., and G. C. Klein.** 1982. Reduction of *Brucella* species and *Francisella tularensis* cross-reacting agglutinins by dithiothreitol. *J. Clin. Microbiol.* **16:**756–757.
10. **Behr, M.** 2000. Laboratory-acquired lymphadenopathy in a veterinary pathologist. *Lab. Anim.* **29:**23–25.
11. **Bell, J. F., and S. J. Stewart.** 1975. Chronic shedding tularemia nephritis in rodents: possible relation to occurrence of *Francisella tularensis* in lotic waters. *J. Wildl. Dis.* **11:**421–436.
12. **Berdal, B. P., R. Mehl, N. K. Meidell, A. M. Lorentzen-Styr, and O. Scheel.** 1996. Field investigations of tularemia in Norway. *FEMS Immunol. Med. Microbiol.* **13:**191–195.
13. **Bevanger L., J. A. Maeland, and A. I. Naess.** 1988. Agglutinins and antibodies to *Francisella tularensis* outer membrane antigens in the early diagnosis of disease during an outbreak of tularemia. *J. Clin. Microbiol.* **26:**433–437.
14. **Bevanger, L., J. A. Maeland, and A. I. Naess.** 1989. Competitive enzyme immunoassay for antibodies to a 43,000-molecular-weight *Francisella tularensis* outer membrane protein for the diagnosis of tularemia. *J. Clin. Microbiol.* **27:**922–926.
15. **Bevanger, L., J. A. Maeland, and A. I. Kvam.** 1994. Comparative analysis of antibodies to *Francisella tularensis* antigens during the acute phase of tularemia and eight years later. *Clin. Diagn. Lab. Immunol.* **1:**238–240.
16. **Boschiroli, M. L., V. Foulongne, and D. O'Callaghan.** 2001. Brucellosis: a worldwide zoonosis. *Curr. Opin. Microbiol.* **4:**58–64.
17. **Braun, W., and J. Kelsh.** 1954. Improved method for cultivation of *Brucella* from the blood. *Proc. Soc. Exp. Biol. Med.* **85:**154–155.
18. **Bricker, B. J., L. B. Tabatabai, B. A. Judge, B. L. Deyoe, and J. E. Mayfield.** 1990. Cloning, expression, and occurrence of the *Brucella* Cu-Zn superoxide dismutase. *Infect. Immun.* **58:**2935–2939.
19. **Bricker, B. J., and S. M. Halling.** 1994. Differentiation of *Brucella abortus* biovars 1, 2, and 4, *Brucella melitensis*, *Brucella ovis*, and *Brucella suis* biovar 1 by PCR. *J. Clin. Microbiol.* **32:**2660–2666.
20. **Bricker, B. J., and S. M. Halling.** 1995. Enhancement of the *Brucella* AMOS PCR assay for differentiation of *Brucella abortus* vaccine strains S19 and RB51. *J. Clin. Microbiol.* **33:**1640–1642.
21. **Bricker, B. J., D. R. Ewalt, A. P. MacMillan, G. Foster, and S. Brew.** 2000. Molecular characterization of *Brucella* strains isolated from marine mammals. *J. Clin. Microbiol.* **38:**1258–1262.
22. **Brown, G. M.** 1977. The history of the brucellosis eradication program in the United States. *Ann. Sclavo* **19:**18–34.
23. **Brown, S. L., F. T. McKinney, G. C. Klein, and W. L. Jones.** 1980. Evaluation of a safranin-O-stained antigen microagglutination test for *Francisella tularensis* antibodies. *J. Clin. Microbiol.* **11:**146–148.
24. **Bruce, D.** 1887. Note on the discovery of a microorganism in Malta Fever. *Practitioner* **36:**161–170.
25. **Buchanan, T. M., G. F. Brooks, and P. S. Brachman.** 1971. The tularemia skin test—325 skin tests in 210 persons: serologic correlation and review of the literature. *Ann. Intern. Med.* **74:**336–343.
26. **Buddle, M. B.** 1956. Studies on *Brucella ovis* (n. sp.), a cause of genital disease of sheep in New Zealand and Australia, *J. Hyg. Camb.* **54:**351–364.
27. **Burke, D. S.** 1977. Immunization against tularemia: analysis of the effectiveness of live *Francisella tularensis* vaccine in prevention of laboratory-acquired tularemia. *J. Infect. Dis.* **135:**55–60.

28. **Canning, P. C., J. A. Roth, and B. L. Dayoe.** 1986. Release of 5'-guanosine monophosphate and adenine by *Brucella abortus* and their role in the intracellular survival of the bacteria. *J. Infect. Dis.* **154:**464–470.

29. **Carmichael, L. E., and D. W. Bruner.** 1968. Characteristics of a newly recognized species of *Brucella* responsible for infectious canine abortions. *Cornell Vet.* **48:**579–592.

30. **Casas, J., Y. Partal, J. Llosa, J. Leiva, J. M. Navarro, and M. de la Rosa.** 1994. Deteccion de *Brucella* por un sistema automatico de hemocultivos: Bact/Alert. *Enferm. Infec. Microbiol. Clin.* **12:**497–500.

31. **Castenada, M. R.** 1947. A practical method for routine blood cultures in brucellosis. *Proc. Soc. Exp. Biol. Med.* **64:**114–115.

32. **Centers for Disease Control and Prevention.** 1997. Summary of notifiable diseases, United States, 1996. *Morb. Mortal. Wkly. Rep.* **45:**26.

33. **Centers for Disease Control and Prevention.** 2002. Tularemia—United States, 1990–2000. *Morbid. Mort. Wkly. Rep.* **51:**182–184.

34. **Chomel, B. B., E. E. DeBess, D. M. Mangiamele, K. F. Reilly, T. B. Farver, R. K. Sun, and L. R. Barrett.** 1994. Changing trends in the epidemiology of human brucellosis in California from 1973 to 1992: a shift toward food-borne transmission. *J. Infect. Dis.* **170:**1216–1223.

35. **Clarridge, J. E., III, T. J. Raich, A. Sjöstedt, G. Sandström, R. O. Darouiche, R. M. Shawar, P. R. Georghiou, C. Osting, and L. Vo.** 1996. Characterization of two unusual clinically significant *Francisella* strains. *J. Clin. Microbiol.* **34:**1995–2000.

36. **Cooper, C. L., P. Van Caeseele, J. Canvir, and L. E. Nicoll.** 1999. Chronic prosthetic device infection with *Francisella tularensis. Clin. Infect. Dis.* **29:**1589–1591.

37. **Corbel, M. J., and W. J. Brinley-Morgan.** 1984. Genus *Brucella*, p. 377–388. *In* N. R. Krieg and J. G. Holt (ed.), *Bergey's Manual of Systematic Bacteriology*, vol. 1. The Williams & Wilkins Co., Baltimore, Md.

38. **Corbel, M. J.** 1988. International committee on systematic bacteriology subcommittee on the taxonomy of *Brucella. Int. J. Syst. Bacteriol.* **38:**450–452.

39. **Dennis, D. T., T. V. Inglesby, D. A. Henderson, J. G. Bartlett, M. S. Ascher, E. Eitzen, A. D. Fine, A. M. Friedlander, J. Hauer, M. Layton, S. R. Lillibridge, J. E. McDade, M. T. Osterholm, T. O'Toole, G. Parker, T. M. Perl, P. K. Russell, and K. Tonat.** 2001. Tularemia as a biological weapon: medical and public health management. *JAMA* **285:**2763–2773.

40. **Department of Health and Human Services, Public Health Service.** 1999. *Biosafety in Microbiological and Biomedical Laboratories*, 3rd ed. HHS publication (CDC) 93-8395. Department of Health and Human Services, Washington, D.C.

41. **Eigelsbach, H. T., and V. G. McGann.** 1984. Genus *Francisella* Dorofe'ev 1947, p. 394–399. *In* N. R. Krieg and J. G. Holt (ed.), *Bergey's Manual of Systematic Bacteriology*, vol. 1. The Williams & Wilkins Co., Baltimore, Md.

42. **Emmons, R. W., J. D. Woodie, M. S. Taylor, and G. S. Nygaard.** 1970. Tularemia in a pet squirrel monkey (*Saimiri sciureus*). *Lab. Anim. Care* **30:**1149–1153.

43. **Ericsson, M., G. Sandström, A. Sjöstedt, and A. Tarnvik.** 1994. Persistence of cell-mediated immunity and decline of humoral immunity to the intracellular bacterium *Francisella tularensis. J. Infect. Dis.* **170:**110–114.

44. **Etemadi, H., A. Raissadat, M. J. Pickett, Y. Zafari, and P. Vahedifar.** 1984. Isolation of *Brucella* spp. from clinical specimens. *J. Clin. Microbiol.* **64:**115.

45. **Evans, A. C.** 1918. Further studies on *Bacterium abortus* and related bacteria. II. A comparison of *Bacterium abortus*

with *Bacterium bronchosepticus* and with the organism which causes Malta fever. *J. Infect. Dis.* **22:**580–593.

46. **Ewalt, D. R., J. B. Payeur, B. M. Martin, D. R. Cummins, and W. G. Miller.** 1994. Characteristics of a *Brucella* species from a bottlenose dolphin (*Tursiops truncatus*). *J. Vet. Diagn. Investig.* **6:**448–452.

47. **Farlow, J., K. L. Smith, J. Wong, M. Abrams, M. Lytle, and P. Keim.** 2001. *Francisella tularensis* strain typing using multiple-locus variable-number tandem repeat analysis. *J. Clin. Microbiol.* **39:**3186–3192.

48. **Feldman, K. A., R. Enscore, S. Lathrop, B. Matyas, M. McGuill, M. Schriefer, D. Stiles-Enos, D. Dennis, and E. Hayes.** 2001. Outbreak of primary pneumonic tularemia on Martha's Vineyard. *N. Engl. J. Med.* **345:**1601–1606.

49. **Forsman, M., G. Sandström, and B. Jaurin.** 1990. Identification of *Francisella* species and discrimination of type A and type B strains of *F. tularensis* by 16S rRNA analysis. *Appl. Environ. Microbiol.* **56:**949–955.

50. **Forsman, M., G. Sandström, and A. Sjöstedt.** 1994. Analysis of 16S ribosomal DNA sequences of *Francisella* strains and utilization for determination of the phylogeny of the genus and for identification of strains by PCR. *Int. J. Syst. Bacteriol.* **44:**38–46.

51. **Forsman, M., A. Nyrén, A. Sjöstedt, L. Sjökvist, and G. Sandström.** 1995. Identification of *Francisella tularensis* in natural water samples by PCR. *FEMS Microbiol. Ecol.* **16:**83–92.

52. **Francis, E.** 1921. The occurrence of tularemia in nature as a disease of man. *Public Health Rep.* **36:**1731–1738.

53. **Franz, E. R., P. B. Jahrling, A. M. Friedlander, D. J. McClain, D. L. Hoover, W. R. Bryne, J. A. Pavlin, G. W. Christopher, and E. M. Eitzen.** 1997. Clinical recognition and management of patients exposed to biological warfare agents. *JAMA* **278:**399–411.

54. **Gandara, B., A. Lopez Merino, M. A. Rogel, and E. Martinez-Romero.** 2001. Limited genetic diversity of *Brucella* spp. *J. Clin. Microbiol.* **39:**235–240.

55. **Garrity, G. M., and J. G. Holt.** 2001. Taxonomic outline of the *Archaea* and *Bacteria*, p. 155–166. *In* D. R. Boone and R. C. Castenholz (ed.), *Bergey's Manual of Systematic Bacteriology*, 2nd ed., vol. 1. Springer-Verlag, New York, N.Y.

56. **Gotuzzo, E., C. Carrillo, J. Guerra, and L. Llosa.** 1986. An evaluation of diagnostic methods for brucellosis—the value of bone marrow culture. *J. Infect. Dis.* **153:**122–125.

57. **Gries, D. M., and M. P. Fairchok.** 1996. Typhoidal tularemia in a human immunodeficiency virus-infected adolescent. *Pediatr. Infect. Dis. J.* **15:**838–840.

58. **Grunow, R., W. Splettstoesser, S. McDonald, C. Otterbein, T. O'Brien, C. Morgan, J. Aldrich, E. Hofer, E. Finke, and H. Meyer.** 2000. Detection of *Francisella tularensis* in biological specimens using a capture enzyme-linked immunosorbent assay, and immunochromatographic handheld assay, and a PCR. *Clin. Diagn. Lab. Immunol.* **7:**86–90.

59. **Guarner, J., P. R. Breer, J. C. Bartlett, M. C. Chu, W. J. Shleh, and S. R. Zaki.** 1999. Immunohistochemical detection of *Francisella tularensis* in formalin-fixed paraffin-embedded tissue. *Appl. Immunohistochem. Mol. Morphol.* **7:**122–126.

60. **Guryčová, D.** 1998. First isolation of *Francisella tularensis* subsp. *tularensis* in Europe. *Eur. J. Epidemiol.* **14:**707–802.

61. **Higgins, J. A., Z. Hubalek, J. Halouzka, K. L. Elkins, A. Sjostedt, M. Shipley, and M. S. Ibrahim.** 2000. Detection of *Francisella tularensis* in infected mammals and vectors using a probe-based polymerase chain reaction. *Am. J. Trop. Med. Hyg.* **62:**310–318.

62. **Hollis, D. G., R. E. Weaver, A. G. Steigerwalt, J. D. Wenger, C. W. Moss, and D. J. Brenner.** 1989. *Francisella*

philomiragia comb. nov. (formerly *Yersinia philomiragia*) and *Francisella tularensis* biogroup novicida (formerly *Francisella novicida*) associated with human disease. *J. Clin. Microbiol.* **27**:1601–1608.

63. **Hopla, C. E., and A. K. Hopla.** 1994. Tularemia, p. 113–126. *In* G. W. Beran and J. H. Steele (ed.), *Handbook of Zoonoses*, 2nd ed. CRC Press, Inc., Boca Raton, Fla.

64. **Huddleston, I. F.** 1929. Differentiation of the species of the genus *Brucella*. *Am. J. Public Health* **21**:491–498.

65. **Ikäheimo, I., H. Syrjälä, J. Karhukorpi, R. Schildt, and M. Koskela.** 2000. *In vitro* antibiotic susceptibility of *Francisella tularensis* isolated from humans and animals. *J. Antimicrob. Chemother.* **46**:287–290.

66. **Jellison, W. L., C. R. Owen, J. F. Bell, and G. M. Kohls.** 1961. Tularemia and animal populations: ecology and epizootiology. *Wildl. Dis.* **17**:1–15.

67. **Jellison, W. L.** 1974. *Tularemia in North America, 1930–1974.* University of Montana, Missoula.

68. **Johansson, A., L. Gerglund, U. Eriksson, I. Göransson, R. Wollin, M. Forsman, A. Tärnvik, and A. Sjöstedt.** 2000. Comparative analysis of PCR versus culture for diagnosis of ulceroglandular tularemia. *J. Clin. Microbiol.* **38**:22–26.

69. **Johansson, A., A. Ibrahim, I. Göransson, U. Eriksson, D. Guryŏvá, J. E. Clarridge III, and A. Sjöstedt.** 2000. Evaluation of PCR-based methods for discrimination of *Francisella* species and subspecies and development of a specific PCR that distinguishes the two major subspecies of *Francisella tularensis*. *J. Clin. Microbiol.* **38**:4180–4185.

70. **Johansson, A., L. Berglund, L. Gothefors, A. Sjöstedt, and A. Tärnvik.** 2000. Ciprofloxacin for treatment of tularemia in children. *Pediatr. Infect. Dis. J.* **19**:449–453.

71. **Jumas-Bilak, E., S. Michaux-Charachon, G. Bourg, D. O'Callaghan, and M. Ramuz.** 1998. Differences in chromosome number and genome rearrangements in the genus *Brucella*. *Mol. Microbiol.* **27**:99–106.

72. **Khan, M. Y., M. W. Mah, and Z. A. Memish.** 2001. Brucellosis in pregnant women. *Clin. Infect. Dis.* **32**:1172–1177.

73. **Kolman, S., M. C. Maayan, G. Gotesman, L. A. Rozenzajn, B. Wolach, and R. Lang.** 1991. Comparison of the BACTEC and lysis concentration methods for recovery of *Brucella* species from clinical specimens. *Eur. J. Clin. Microbiol. Infect. Dis.* **10**:647–648.

74. **La Regina, M. L., J. Longro, and M. Wallace.** 1986. *Francisella tularensis* infection in captive, wild caught prairie dogs. *Lab. Anim. Sci.* **4**:178–180.

75. **Long, G. W., J. J. Oprandy, R. B. Narayanan, A. H. Fortier, K. R. Porter, and C. A. Nacy.** 1993. Detection of *Francisella tularensis* in blood by polymerase chain reaction. *J. Clin. Microbiol.* **31**:152–154.

76. **Maranan, M. C., D. Schiff, D. C. Johnson, C. Abrahams, M. Wylam, and S. I. Gerber.** 1997. Pneumonic tularemia in a patient with chronic granulomatous disease. *Clin. Infect. Dis.* **25**:630–633.

77. **Marchette, N. J., and P. S. Nicholes.** 1961. Virulence and citrulline ureidase activity of *Pasteurella tularensis*. *J. Bacteriol.* **82**:26–32.

78. **Marsten, J. A.** 1861. Report on fever (Malta). *Great Br. Army Med. Dept. Rep.* **3**:520–521.

79. **Massachusetts Medical Society.** 1985. Case records of the Massachusetts General Hospital (case 27-1985). *N. Engl. J. Med.* **313**:36–42.

80. **Massachusetts Medical Society.** 2000. Case records of the Massachusetts General Hospital (case 14-2000). *N. Engl. J. Med.* **342**:1430–1437.

81. **Matar, G., I. A. Khneisser, and A. M. Abdelmoor.** 1996. Rapid laboratory comfirmation of human brucellosis by PCR analysis of a target sequence on the 31-kilodalton *Brucella* antigen DNA. *J. Clin. Microbiol.* **34**:477–478.

82. **McCarthy, V. P., and M. D. Murphy.** 1990. Lawnmower tularemia. *Pediatr. Infect. Dis. J.* **9**:298–300.

83. **McCoy, G. W., and C. W. Chapin.** 1912. *Bacterium tularense* the cause of a plague-like disease of rodents. *U.S. Public Health Hosp. Bull.* **53**:17–23.

84. **Meyer, K. F., and E. B. Shaw.** 1920. A comparison of the morphologic, culture and biochemical characteristics of *B. abortus* and *B. melitensis*: studies on the genus *Brucella* nov. gen. I. *J. Infect. Dis.* **27**:173–184.

85. **Miller, W. G., L. G. Adams, T. A. Ficht, N. F. Cheville, J. P. Payeur, D. R. Harley, C. House, and S. H. Ridgway.** 1999. *Brucella*-induced abortions and infection in bottlenose dolphins (*Tursiops truncatus*). *J. Zoo Wildl. Med.* **30**:100–110.

86. **Mörner, T., G. Sandström, and R. Matsson.** 1988. Comparison of serum and lung extracts for surveys of wild animals for antibodies to *Francisella tularensis* biovar *palaearctica*. *J. Wildl. Dis.* **24**:10–14.

87. **Mörner, T., G. Sandström, R. Matsson, and P. Nilsson.** 1988. Infections with *Francisella tularensis* biovar *palaearctica* in hares (*Lepus tumidus, Lepus europaeus*) from Sweden. *J. Wildl. Dis.* **24**:422–433.

88. **Mörner, T., R. Matsson, M. Forsman, K. E. Johansson, and G. Sandström.** 1993. Identification and classification of different isolates of *Francisella tularensis*. *J. Vet. Med.* **40**:613–620.

89. **Moyer, N. P., and W. J. Hausler, Jr.** 1992. The genus *Brucella*, p. 2384–2400. *In* A. Balows, H. G. Trüper, M. Dworkin, W. Harder, and K.-H. Schleifer (ed.), *The Prokaryotes*, vol. III. Springer-Verlag, New York, N.Y.

90. **Naughton, M., R. Brown, D. Adkins, and J. DiPersio.** 1999. Tularemia—an unusual cause of a solitary pulmonary nodule in the post-transplant setting. *Bone Marrow Transplant.* **24**:197–199.

91. **Nayar, G. P. S., G. J. Crawshaw, and J. L. Neufeld.** 1979. Tularemia in a group of nonhuman primates. *J. Am. Vet. Med. Assoc.* **175**:962–963.

92. **Ohara, S., T. Sato, and M. Homma.** 1994. Serological studies on *Francisella tularensis*, *Francisella novicida*, *Yersinia philomiragia*, and *Brucella abortus*. *Int. J. Syst. Bacteriol.* **24**:191–196.

93. **Olsufjev, N. G., and I. S. Mescheryakova.** 1982. Infraspecific taxonomy of tularemia agent *Francisella tularensis* McCoy et Chapin. *J. Hyg. Epidemiol. Microbiol. Immunol.* **3**:291–299.

94. **Olsufjev, N. G., K. N. Shlygina, and E. V. Ananova.** 1984. Persistence of *Francisella tularensis* McCoy et Chapin tularemia agent in the organism of highly sensitive rodents after oral infection. *J. Hyg. Epidemiol. Microbiol. Immunol.* **4**:441–454.

95. **Overholt, E. I., W. D. Tigertt, P. J. Kadull, M. K. Ward, N. D. Charkes, R. M. Rene, T. E. Salzman, and M. Stephens.** 1961. An analysis of forty-two cases of laboratory-acquired tularemia. *Am. J. Med.* **30**:785–806.

96. **Palmer, M. V., J. F. Cheville, and A. E. Jensen.** 1996. Experimental infection of pregnant cattle with the vaccine candidate *Brucella abortus* strain RB51: pathologic, bacteriologic, and serologic findings. *Vet. Pathol.* **33**:682–691.

97. **Pittman, T., D. Williams, and A. D. Friedman.** 1996. A shunt infection caused by *Francisella tularensis*. *Pediatr. Neurosurg.* **24**:50–51.

98. **Posthaus, H., M. Welle, T. Mörner, J. Nicolet, and P. Kuhnert.** 1998. Tularemia in a common marmoset (*Callithrix jacchus*) diagnosed by 16S rRNA sequencing. *Vet. Microbiol.* **61**:145–150.

99. Preiksaitis, J. K., G. J. Crawshaw, G. S. P. Nayar, and H. G. Stiver. 1979. Human tularemia at an urban zoo. *Can. Med. Assoc. J.* **121:**1097–1099.

100. Prior, R. G., L. Klasson, P. Larsson, K. Williams, L. Lindler, A. Sjöstedt, T. Svensson, I. Tamas, B. W. Wren, P. C. F. Oyston, S. G. E. Andersson, and R. W. Titball. 2001. Preliminary analysis and annotation of the partial genome sequence of *Francisella tularensis* strain Schu 4. *J. Appl. Microbiol.* **91:**614–620.

101. Puente-Redondo, V. A. de la, N. García del Blanco, C. B. Gutiérrez-Martin, F. J. García-Peña, and E. F. Rodríguez Ferri. 2000. Comparison of different PCR approaches for typing of *Francisella tularensis* strains. *J. Clin. Microbiol.* **38:**1016–1022.

102. Queipo-Ortuno, M. I., P. Morata, P. Ocon, P. Manchado, and J. D. Colmenero. 1997. Rapid diagnosis of human brucellosis by peripheral-blood PCR assay. *J. Clin. Microbiol.* **35:**2927–2930.

103. Redklar, R., S. Rose, B. Bricker, and V. delVecchio. 2001. Real-time detection of *Brucella abortus*, *Brucella melitensis*, and *Brucella suis*. *Mol. Cell. Probes* **15:**43–52.

104. Reintjes, R., I. Dedushaj, A. Gjini, T. R. Jorgensen, B. Cotter, A. Lieftucht, F. D'Ancona, D. T. Dennis, M. A. Kosoy, G. Mulliqi-Osmani, R. Grunow, A. Kalaveshi, L. Gashi, and I. Humolli. 2002. Tularemia outbreak investigation in Kosovo: case control and environmental studies. *Emerg. Infect. Dis.* **8:**69–73.

105. Rodriguez-Torrez, A., J. Fermoso, and R. Landinez. 1983. Brucellosis. *Medicine* **48:**3126–3136. (In Spanish.)

106. Roiz, M. P., F. G. Peralta, R. Valle, and R. Arjona. 1998. Microbiological diagnosis of brucellosis. *J. Clin. Microbiol.* **36:**1819.

107. Romero, C., C. Gamazo, M. Pardo, and I. Lopez-Goni. 1995. Specific detection of *Brucella* DNA by PCR. *J. Clin. Microbiol.* **33:**615–617.

108. Roy, T. M., D. Fleming, and W. H. Anderson. 1989. Tularemic pneumonia mimicking Legionnaires' disease with false-positive direct fluorescent antibody stains for *Legionella*. *South. Med. J.* **82:**1429–1431.

109. Sandström, G., A. Sjöstedt, M. Forsman, N. V. Pavlovich, and B. N. Mishankin. 1992. Characterization and classification of strains of *Francisella tularensis* isolated in the Central Asian focus of the Soviet Union, and in Japan. *J. Clin. Microbiol.* **30:**172–175.

110. Scheel, O., T. Hoel, T. Sandvik, and B. P. Berdal. 1993. Susceptibility pattern of Scandinavian *Francisella tularensis* isolates with regard to oral and parental antimicrobial agents. *Acta Pathol. Microbiol. Immunol. Scand.* **101:**33–36.

111. Serrano, M. L., J. Llosa, C. Castells, J. Mendoza, J. M. Navarro, and M. de la Rosa. 1987. Detection radiometrica de bacteriemias por *Brucella*. *Enferm. Infec. Microbiol. Clin.* **5:**139–142.

112. Sicherer, S. H., E. J., Asturias, J. A. Winkelstein, J. D. Dick, and R. E. Willoughby. 1997. *Francisella philomiragia* sepsis in chronic granulomatous disease. *Pediatr. Infect. Dis. J.* **16:**420–422.

113. Sifuentes-Rincon, A. M., A. Revol, and H. A. Barrera-Saldana. 1997. Detection and differentiation of the six *Brucella* species by polymerase chain reaction. *Mol. Med.* **3:**734–739.

114. Sjöstedt, A., U. Eriksson, L. Berglund, and A. Tärnvik. 1997. Detection of *Francisella tularensis* in ulcers of patients with tularemia by PCR. *J. Clin. Microbiol.* **35:**1045–1048.

115. Sjöstedt, A. *Francisella*. *In* D. J. Brenner, N. R. Krieg, J. T. Staley, and G. M. Garrity (ed.), *Bergey's Manual of Systematic Bacteriology*, 2nd ed., vol. 2. *The Proteobacteria*, in press. Springer-Verlag, New York, N.Y.

116. Smits, H. L., M. A. Basahi, R. Diaz, T. Marrodan, J. T. Douglas, A. Rocha, J. Veerman, M. M. Zheludkov, O. W. M. Witte, J. de Jong, G. G. Gussenhoven, M. G. A. Goris, and M. A. W. G. van der Hoorn. 1999. Development and evaluation of a rapid dipstick assay for serodiagnosis of acute human brucellosis. *J. Clin. Microbiol.* **37:**4179–4182.

117. Solomon, J. M., and D. Jackson. 1992. Rapid diagnosis of *Brucella melitensis* in blood: some operational characteristics of the BACT/ALERT. *J. Clin. Microbiol.* **30:**222–224.

118. Spink, W. W., N. B. McCullough, L. M. Hutchings, and C. K. Mingle. 1954. A standardized antigen and agglutination technique for human brucellosis. *Am. J. Clin. Pathol.* **24:**466–468.

119. Stoenner, H. G., and D. B. Lackman. 1957. A new species of *Brucella* isolated from the desert woodrat *Neotoma lepida*. *Am. J. Vet. Res.* **18:**947–951.

120. Surcel, H. M., J. Ilonen, K. Poikonen, and E. Herva. 1989. *Francisella tularensis*-specific T-cell clones are human leukocyte antigen class II restricted, secrete interleukin-2 and gamma interferon, and induce immunoglobulin production. *Infect. Immun.* **57:**2906–2908.

121. Surcel, H. M., M. Sarvas, I. M. Helander, and E. Herva. 1989. Membrane proteins of *Francisella tularensis* LVS differ in ability to induce proliferation of lymphocytes from tularemia-vaccinated individuals. *Microb. Pathog.* **7:**411–419.

122. Syrjälä, H. P., V. Kujala, V. Myllyla, and A. Salminen. 1985. Airborne transmission of tularemia in farmers. *Scand. J. Infect. Dis.* **17:**371–375.

123. Syrjälä, H., P. Koskela, T. Ripatti, A. Salminen, and E. Heva. 1986. Agglutination and ELISA methods in the diagnosis of tularemia in different clinical forms and severities of the disease. *J. Infect. Dis.* **153:**142–145.

124. Syrjälä, H., R. Schildt, and S. Räisäinen. 1991. In vitro susceptibility of *Francisella tularensis* to fluoroquinolones and treatment of tularemia with norfloxacin and ciprofloxacin. *Eur. J. Clin. Microbiol. Infect. Dis.* **10:**68–70.

125. Tärnvik, A., S. Löfgren, L. Öhlund, and G. Sandström. 1987. Detection of antigen in urine of a patient with tularemia. *Eur. J. Clin. Microbiol.* **6:**318–319.

126. Tärnvik, A. 1989. Nature of protective immunity to *Francisella tularensis*. *Rev. Infect. Dis.* **11:**440–451.

127. Tärnvik, A., C. Henning, E. Falsen, and G. Sandström. 1989. Isolation of *Francisella tularensis* biovar *palaearctica* from human blood. *Eur. J. Clin. Microbiol. Infect. Dis.* **8:**146–150.

128. Tcherneva, E., N. Rijpens, B. Jersek, and L. M. Herman. 2000. Differentiation of *Brucella* species by random amplified polymorphic DNA analysis. *J. Appl. Microbiol.* **88:**69–80.

129. Traum, J. 1914. *Report of the Chief of the Bureau of Animal Industry*, p. 30. U.S. Department of Agriculture, Washington, D.C.

130. Verger, J. M., F. Grimont, P. A. D. Grimont, and M. Grayon. 1985. *Brucella*, a monospecific genus as shown by deoxyribonucleic acid hybridization. *Int. J. Syst. Bacteriol.* **35:**292–295.

131. Viljanen, M. K., T. Nurmi, and A. Salminen. 1983. Enzyme-linked immunosorbent assay (ELISA) with bacterial sonicate antigen for IgM, IgA, and IgG antibodies to *Francisella tularensis*: comparison with bacterial agglutination test and ELISA with lipopolysaccharide antigen. *J. Infect. Dis.* **148:**715–720.

132. Vizcaino, N., A. Cloeckaert, J. M. Verger, M. Grayon, and L. Fernandez-Lago. 2000. DNA polymorphism in the genus *Brucella*. *Microb. Infect.* **2:**1089–1100.

133. **Waag, D. M., K. T. McKee, Jr., G. Sandström, L. L. K. Pratt, C. R. Bolt, M. J. England, G. O. Nelson, and J. C. Williams.** 1995. Cell-mediated and humoral immune responses after vaccination of human volunteers with the live vaccine strain of *Francisella tularensis*. *Clin. Diagn. Lab. Immunol.* **2:**143–148.

134. **Waggie, K. S., P. A. Day-Lollini, P. A. Marphy-Hackley, J. R. Blum, and G. W. Morrow.** 1997. Diagnostic exercise: illness, cutaneous hemorrhage, and death in two squirrel monkeys (*Saimiri sciureus*). *Lab. Anim. Sci.* **47:**647–649.

135. **Wenger, J. D., D. G. Hollis, R. E. Weaver, C. N. Baker, G. R. Brown, D. J. Brenner, and C. V. Broome.** 1989. Infection caused by *Francisella philomiragia* (formerly *Yersinia philomiragia*): a newly recognized human pathogen. *Ann. Intern. Med.* **110:**888–892.

136. **Weyant, R. S., C. W. Moss, R. E. Weaver, D. G. Hollis, J. G. Jordan, E. C. Cook, and M. I. Daneshvar.** 1996. *Identification of Unusual Pathogenic Gram-Negative Aerobic and Facultatively Anaerobic Bacteria*, 2nd ed. The Williams & Wilkins Co., Baltimore, Md.

137. **Wolff, K. L., and B. W. Hudson.** 1974. Paper-strip blood-sampling technique for the detection of antibody to the plague organism *Yersinia pestis*. *Appl. Microbiol.* **28:**323–325.

138. **Woods, J. P., M. A. Crystal, R. J. Morton, and R. J. Panciera.** 1998. Tularemia in two cats. *J. Am. Vet. Med. Assoc.* **212:**81–83.

139. **World Health Organization.** 1997. *Brucellosis*. Fact sheet N173. www.who.int/inf-fs/en/fact173.html. [Online.] World Health Organization, Geneva, Switzerland.

140. **Yagupsky, P., N. Peled, J. Press, O. Abramson, and M. Abu-Rashid.** 1997. Comparison of BACTEC 9240 Peds Plus medium and Isolator 1.5 Microbial Tube for detection of *Brucella melitensis* from blood cultures. *J. Clin. Microbiol.* **35:**1382–1384.

141. **Yagupsky, P.** 1999. Detection of brucellae in blood cultures. *J. Clin. Microbiol.* **37:**3437–3442.

142. **Young, E. J.** 1989. Treatment of brucellosis in humans, p. 127–141. *In* E. J. Young and M. J. Corbel (ed.), *Brucellosis: Clinical and Laboratory Aspects*. CRC Press, Inc., Boca Raton, Fla.

143. **Young, E. J.** 1991. Serologic diagnosis of human brucellosis: analysis of 214 cases by agglutination tests and review of the literature. *Rev. Infect. Dis.* **13:**359–372.

144. **Young, E. J.** 1999. *Brucella* species, p. 71–89. *In* V. L. Yu, T. C. Merigan, Jr., and S. L. Barriere (ed.), *Antimicrobial Therapy and Vaccines*. The Williams & Wilkins Co., Baltimore, Md.

145. **Young, E. J.** 2000. *Brucella* species, p. 2386–2393. *In* G. L. Mandell, J. E. Bennett, and R. Dolin (ed.), *Mandell, Douglas, and Bennett's Principles and Practice of Infectious Diseases*, vol. 2. Churchill Livingstone, Inc., Philadelphia, Pa.

146. **Young, L. S., D. S. Bicknell, B. G. Archer, J. M. Clinton, L. J. Leavens, J. C. Feeley, and P. S. Brachman.** 1969. Tularemia epidemic: Vermont. 1968: forty-seven cases linked to contact with muskrats. *N. Engl. J. Med.* **280:**1253–1260.

Legionella*

JANET E. STOUT, JOHN D. RIHS, AND VICTOR L. YU

52

A dramatic outbreak of pneumonia after the American Legion Convention in Philadelphia, Pa., in 1976 precipitated one of the most extensive epidemiologic investigations in the history of medicine. The outcome of the investigation was the identification of a previously unknown agent of disease. The newly discovered bacterium was assigned to the family Legionellaceae, the genus Legionella (for "legion"), and the species pneumophila (for "lung loving") (19). There are now more than 40 named species, of which approximately half have been implicated in human disease (Table 1); the remainder have been isolated from environmental sources, usually water. There are more than 60 serogroups among the numerous species (10); however, most cases of legionellosis are caused by Legionella pneumophila serogroups 1, 4, and 6 (98). Other than L. pneumophila, the species most commonly associated with illness are L. micdadei, L. longbeachae, L. dumoffii, and L. bozemanii (23, 46).

TAXONOMY

A single genus and species (Legionella pneumophila) was originally proposed for the family Legionellaceae (19). Subsequent isolation of Legionella-like bacteria and analysis of DNA relatedness resulted in a proposal to divide the family into three separate genera: Legionella, Tatlockia, and Fluoribacter (56). However, further analysis by DNA-DNA hybridization, guanine-plus-cytosine content, and 16S rRNA-encoding (rDNA) sequencing analysis supports the delineation of the phylogeny within the Legionellaceae family as one monophyletic family belonging to the gamma subdivision of the Proteobacteria (55, 68). This family now includes 45 species and over 60 serogroups (2), some of which have been isolated from cocultivation with amoebae and termed "Legionella-like amoebal pathogens" (1, 108). One such organism, Sarcobium lyticum, has been transferred to the genus Legionella as Legionella lytica comb. nov. (68).

DESCRIPTION OF THE GENUS

Legionella species are small (0.3 to 0.9 μm wide and approximately 2 μm long); faintly staining gram-negative rods with polar flagella (except L. oakridgensis). They generally appear as small coccobacilli in infected tissue or secretions, whereas long filamentous forms (up to 20 μm long) can be seen when they are grown in culture media. Legionellaceae are obligately aerobic slow-growing nonfermentative bacteria. They are distinguished from other saccharolytic bacteria by their requirement for L-cysteine and iron salts for primary isolation on solid media and by their unique cellular fatty acids and ubiquinones. Gas-liquid chromatography demonstrates unusually large amounts of cellular branched-chain fatty acids and respiratory ubiquinones with 10 or more isoprene units (162). Differences among species have also been assessed by phenotypic (166) and chemotaxonomic tests. Phenotypic tests include composition of lipopolysaccharide (132), electrophoretic protein profiles (85), monoclonal antibodies (20), fatty acid composition (32), and cellular carbohydrates (54). Genotypic tests include random amplified polymorphic DNA profiles (6, 90), heteroduplex analysis of 5S rRNA gene sequences (114), and computer-assisted matching of tDNA intergenic length polymorphism patterns (58).

NATURAL HABITATS

Legionella organisms are readily found in natural aquatic bodies, and some species have been recovered from soil (134). The organisms can survive under a wide range of conditions, including temperatures of 0 to 63°C, pH of 5.0 to 8.5, and dissolved oxygen concentrations of 0.2 to 15 ppm in water (52). Temperature is a critical determinant for Legionella proliferation. Colonization of hot-water tanks is more likely if the tank temperatures are 40 to 50°C (104 to 122°F) (117, 159). Legionella and other microorganisms become attached to surfaces in an aquatic environment, forming a biofilm. Legionella attaches to and colonizes various materials found in water systems including plastics, rubber, and wood (124, 169). Organic sediments, scale, and inorganic precipitates provide Legionella with a surface for attachment and a protective barrier (169). Interestingly, the growth of other environmental organisms is stimulated by organic sediment, which in turn leads to the formation of by-products that stimulate the growth of Legionella (140).

---

* This chapter contains information presented in chapter 37 by Washington C. Winn, Jr., in the seventh edition of this Manual.

TABLE 1 Biochemical and phenotypic differentiation of *Legionella* species implicated in infections[a,b]

Species	Browning on tyrosine-supplemented agar	Gelatinase production	Hippurate hydrolysis	Oxidase	β-Lactamase production	Autofluorescence (365-nm UV light)	Flagella
L. pneumophila	+	+	+	±	+	−	+
L. micdadei	−	−	−	+	−	−	+
L. bozemanii	+	+	−	±	±	+(BW)	+
L. dumoffii	+	+	−	−	+	+(BW)	+
L. longbeachae	+	+	−	+	±	−	+
L. jordanis	+	+	−	+	+	−	+
L. feeleii	+	−	±	−	−	−	+
L. gormanii	+	+	−	−	+	+(BW)	+
L. wadsworthii	−	+	−	−	+	+(YG)	+
L. hackeliae	+	+	−	+	+	−	+
L. maceachernii	±	±	−	+	−	−	+
L. oakridgensis	+	+	−	−	+(W)	−	−
L. birminghamensis	±	+	−	±	+	+(YG)	+
L. cherrii	+	+	−	−	+	+(BW)	+
L. sainthelensi	+	+	−	+	+	−	+
L. cincinnatiensis	+	+	−	−	+	−	+
L. tucsonensis	−	+	−	−	+	+(BW)	+
L. anisa	+	+	−	+	+	+(BW)	+
L. lansingensis	−	−	−	+	−	−	+
L. parisiensis	+	+	−	+	+	+(BW)	+

[a] Data from references 68, 156, and 164.
[b] Symbols: +, positive; −, negative; ±, variable reaction; W, weak reaction; BW, blue-white autofluorescence; YG, yellow-green autofluorescence.

Commensal bacteria such as *Empedobacter brevis* (*Flavobacterium breve*), *Pseudomonas*, *Alcaligenes*, and *Acinetobacter* and blue-green algae (*Cyanobacterium* spp.) can stimulate the growth of *Legionella* in the aquatic environment (140, 148, 161). *L. pneumophila* can also infect and multiply within soil-dwelling and aquatic species of amoebae (*Hartmanella*, *Acanthamoeba*, and *Naegleria*) and ciliated protozoa (*Tetrahymena*), including amoebae isolated from hot-water tanks (49, 50). When the protozoan host ruptures, large numbers of motile *Legionella* organisms are freed (12). It has been suggested that *Legionella* could be transmitted to humans via inhalation of amoebic vesicles (8, 127); however, there has been no clinical evidence to support this popular theory. Amoebic cysts may also contribute to its survival under unfavorable environmental conditions such as elevated chlorine levels.

Legionella bacteria are relatively chlorine tolerant (81). This enables the organisms to survive the water treatment process and pass into water distribution systems. Studies have shown that *Legionella* organisms are present in all segments of community water supplies, including water treatment facilities (29, 133, 160). The aquatic environment of *Legionella* also includes man-made habitats such as cooling towers, evaporative condensers, whirlpool spas, decorative fountains, and potable-water distribution systems (89). Water distribution systems colonized with *Legionella* are now recognized as the primary source of nosocomial infections and a significant source of sporadic community-acquired cases (14, 89, 141, 142). In fact, the water distribution systems of hospitals have been the source of the majority of nosocomial cases reported to the Centers for Disease Control and Prevention, (CDC) (22, 23). The British Communicable Disease Surveillance Centre reported that 19 of 20 hospital outbreaks of Legionnaires' disease in the United Kingdom from 1980 to 1992 were attributed to hospital potable-water distribution systems (74). Acquisition of Legionnaires' disease has been linked to contamination of water supplies in residences, rehabilitation centers, nursing homes, and industrial buildings (139).

CLINICAL SIGNIFICANCE

The spectrum of illness due to *Legionella* spp. ranges from a mild, self-limited illness (Pontiac fever) to a disseminated and often fatal disease. Pontiac fever is characterized by the onset of an acute, self-limiting flu-like illness without pneumonia. The syndrome derives its name from an outbreak of the disease in Pontiac, Mich., in 1968 (59, 154). The incubation period is short (24 to 48 h), and the attack rate is generally high (≥90%). Complete recovery occurs within 1 week without antibiotic therapy. Pontiac fever has been attributed to exposure to several *Legionella* species, including *L. pneumophila* serogroups 1, 6, and 7; *L. micdadei*; *L. feeleii*; and *L. anisa* (44, 93, 147). Diagnosis has typically been made by showing specific seroconversion.

In studies from Europe and North America, *Legionella* is a cause of 2 to 15% of all sporadic community-acquired pneumonias requiring hospitalization (107). *L. pneumophila* is among the top three or four microbial etiologies of community-acquired pneumonia (45). Patients with community-acquired Legionnaires' disease are more likely to have severe community-acquired pneumonia, as defined by greater degrees of abnormality of vital signs, more extensive infiltrates on chest radiograph, and admission to intensive care units (30, 45, 122, 149, 153). Coinfections with other pulmonary pathogens have been documented in rare anecdotal reports, i.e., with *Streptococcus pneumoniae*, *Chlamydophila pneumoniae*, *Haemophilus* species, and *Mycobacterium tuberculosis* (37).

Both community-acquired and nosocomial cases of legionellosis are now being seen in children (17, 60, 119). Most pediatric patients with Legionnaires' disease have been immunosuppressed. The incidence of Legionnaires' disease in AIDS patients is low (15); however, the clinical manifestations are more severe (98). Extrapulmonary infections involving *Legionella* do occur rarely and involve the heart, sinuses, skin and soft tissue, peritoneum, kidney, pancreas, liver, and bowel (91).

Cigarette smoking, chronic lung disease, and immuno-suppression (especially by corticosteroids) have been consistently implicated as risk factors (24, 125). Surgery is a major predisposing factor in nosocomial infection, with transplant recipients at the highest risk (71, 80).

Legionnaires' disease is not transmitted directly from person to person. Water containing the bacterium accesses the respiratory tract by inhalation of aerosols or aspiration. Aerosol-generating systems that have been linked to disease transmission include cooling towers, respiratory therapy equipment, mist machines, and whirlpools (18, 94). Aspiration has been underappreciated as a mode of transmission (16, 97, 152, 168, 170). Nasogastric tubes have been implicated in several studies of nosocomial legionellosis; microaspiration of contaminated water was the presumed mode of transmission (16, 97, 152).

After *Legionella* enters the upper respiratory tract, the organism is cleared by cilia on respiratory epithelial cells and the normal pulmonary immune system. Impaired mucociliary clearance followed by aspiration may increase the risk of infection. Virulent *Legionella* strains are flagellated and adhere to human respiratory epithelial cells via pili (135). It is well established that *Legionella* replicates within alveolar macrophages (69). Alveolar epithelial cells also provide an alternate site for replication, which may contribute to the severity of pneumonia in patients with Legionnaires' disease. A number of *Legionella* virulence factors have been described, including a pore-forming toxin, type IV pili, flagella, and type II and IV secretion systems (28, 96, 128, 144). A number of these virulence factors are regulated by genes including *dot* (defective for organelle trafficking), *mip* (macrophage infectivity potentiator), and *icm* (intracellular multiplication) (144).

Nosocomial Legionnaires' disease is relatively common among hospitals in the U.S. National Nosocomial Infections Surveillance System (51). A high proportion (42%) of hospitals with transplantation programs have reported cases. Of these hospitals, 77% had diagnostic tests for *Legionella* available within the hospital. The incidence of nosocomial *Legionella* pneumonia is therefore directly correlated to three factors: (i) the availability of specialized diagnostic tests readily available in-house (especially sputum culture and urinary antigen), (ii) the presence of *Legionella* in the hospital water supply, and (iii) the presence of susceptible hosts.

Legionnaires' disease can be prevented by eradication of the bacterium from its reservoir. Recent data suggest that active environmental surveillance and disinfection can significantly reduce nosocomial legionellosis (C. Squier, S. Krystofiak, J. McMahon, M. M. Wagener, and J. E. Stout, *Abstr. Annu. Meet. Assoc. Pract. Infect. Control*, session 2403, ref. no. 149, 2001). An extensive review of the various approaches to controlling *Legionella* in water systems has been published elsewhere (88). Thermal eradication and copper-silver ionization are commonly used methods (138).

COLLECTION, TRANSPORT, AND STORAGE OF SPECIMENS

Specimens submitted for culture should be collected by the usual methods and delivered to the laboratory as promptly

as possible (see chapter 20). If a delay in culturing is expected, samples should be refrigerated (164), since *Legionella* remains viable for at least a week in refrigerated clinical specimens and even longer in frozen specimens. As per standard laboratory practice in the United States, samples should be processed in a biological safety cabinet. Standard laboratory safety precautions are adequate for handling specimens for the diagnosis of *Legionella* infections. There are no reported laboratory-acquired cases of Legionnaires' disease.

Specimens for culture of *Legionella* species should be obtained prior to initiation of antimicrobial therapy. All sputum specimens submitted for *Legionella* culture should be cultured regardless of the presence of squamous epithelial cells (70).

Patients with severe Legionnaires' disease are often bacteremic. Bacteremia tends to occur late in the progression of the disease and usually portends death (123). *Legionella* has been recovered from blind subculture of blood culture bottles (25, 123); however, these are rare occurrences since the organism does not multiply in blood culture media (D. M. Cirillo, E. J. Baron, and G. Marchiaro, *Abstr. 99th Gen. Meet. Am. Soc. Microbiol. 1999*, abstr. C-255, p. 189, 1999). One study used blood culture bottles supplemented with cysteine and iron to recover *Legionella*, but these are not commercially available (123).

Serum for detection of antibodies to *L. pneumophila* should be collected during the acute and convalescent phases of illness; convalescent-phase samples should be collected approximately 6 to 12 weeks after onset of symptoms. However, the maximum rise in antibody titer may not occur until between 12 and 24 weeks after illness (R. M. Vickers, Y. C. Yee, J. D. Rihs, M. M. Wagener, and V. L. Yu., *Abstr. 94th Gen. Meet. Am. Soc. Microbiol. 1994*, abstr. C-17, p. 493, 1994).

Urine specimens for the detection of *L. pneumophila* serogroup 1 antigen should be collected as clean-catch samples in standard sterile containers and assayed within 24 h of collection. Antigen excretion is unaffected by therapy and can remain positive for several weeks (126).

DIRECT DETECTION OF *LEGIONELLA*

Legionella is not easily visualized by Gram stain of respiratory specimens; therefore, alternative staining methods are necessary. Carbol fuchsin (without heating and acid-alcohol decolorizing) and crystal violet with or without Lugol's iodine (the half-Gram stain) have been suggested as alternative methods (167). Silver stains, including the Dieterle and Warthin-Starry stains, allow visualization of *Legionella* in paraffin-fixed tissues. *Legionella micdadei* can stain weakly acid fast in tissue with the Kinyoun and Fite stains and in smears with the modified Ziehl-Neelsen stain from tissue or sputum specimens (65). The acid fastness is rarely seen in *L. micdadei* grown from culture.

Legionella in respiratory secretions is more often visualized by immunofluorescence microscopy, also known as the direct fluorescent-antibody stain (DFA). The sensitivity of the DFA stain is much lower than for culture (range, 25 to 75%), which has resulted in the suggestion that this test should not be performed routinely (Table 2) (37). DFA may be performed if the direct culture of the specimen is overgrown by competing members of the microflora. At this point, the specimen undergoes acid pretreatment and DFA staining (see "Isolation Procedures" below). We have found the monoclonal antibody DFA reagent (MONOFLUO;

TABLE 2 Diagnostic testing modalities for Legionnaires' disease[a]

Test	Sensitivity (%)	Specificity (%)	Cost/test ($)	Advantages	Disadvantages
Culture	80	100	9	Most sensitive method; inexpensive; all species detected; no special equipment; isolate available for typing	May take 3–4 days for result; affected by therapy; sputum may be difficult to obtain or not available; bacterial overgrowth
DFA	33–70	96–99	16	Same-day results (1–2 h); not affected by therapy	Experienced personnel required; UV microscope required; no isolate available; limited species and serogroups detected
PCR	64–100	88–100	50	Same-day results (2–3 h); not affected by therapy; detects multiple species	Experienced personnel and dedicated space required; expensive; no isolate available
Urinary antigen (EIA)	70–80	99	16	Same-day results (2–3 h); not affected by therapy; urine easily obtained	Only *L. pneumophila* serogroup 1 detected; no isolate available
Urinary antigen immunochromatographic	80	97–100	16	Same-day results (15 min); not affected by therapy; little training necessary	Only *L. pneumophila* serogroup 1 detected; no isolate available
Serology (seroconversion)	40–75	96–99	21	Helpful in outbreak investigations	Acute and convalescent-phase sera required; no isolate available

[a] Data from references 9, 76, and 163.

Bio-Rad Laboratories, Redmond, Wash.) to be superior to polyclonal reagents for detecting *L. pneumophila* in respiratory specimens because background fluorescence is reduced and cross-reactivity with non-*Legionella* bacteria has not occurred in our experience (see Fig. 2G). Polyclonal reagents are available from a variety of suppliers (SciMedx, Corp., Denville, N.J.; Monoclonal Technologies, Atlanta, Ga.; Meridian Diagnostics, Inc., Cincinnati, Ohio; Zeus Technologies, Raritan, N.J.). Cross-reactions with other bacterial species have been reported with both the polyclonal reagents (*Bacteroides fragilis*, *Pseudomonas* spp., *Stenotrophomonas maltophilia*) and the monoclonal reagent (*Bacillus cereus*) (43, 53, 126). Strong cross-reactivity of polyclonal anti-*Legionella* antiserum was also demonstrated for isolates of *Bordetella pertussis* (109). However, if one uses the monoclonal reagent for screening and interprets both the staining intensity and the cell morphology, a misidentification is unlikely.

In many hospitals, cases of Legionnaires' disease due to *L. pneumophila* serogroup 1 are often diagnosed by the urinary antigen test rather than by DFA or culture (79). In fact, reports from the CDC and others indicate that the introduction of the urinary antigen test into some hospital laboratories has resulted in the detection of unrecognized endemic nosocomial outbreaks of Legionnaires' disease (79, 86). The urinary antigen test has several advantages over culture. For many patients with Legionnaires' disease, obtaining an adequate sputum specimen is difficult if not impossible. The test format is an enzyme immunoassay (EIA) which is available commercially from two U.S. suppliers (Wampole Laboratories, a division of Carter-Wallace Inc., Cranbury, N.J.; and Bartels, Issaquah, Wash.). The Biotest urine antigen test is also an EIA (Biotest AG, Dreieich, Germany). This test is not currently available in the United States. Both the Binax (Binax, Portland, Maine) and Biotest assays are capable of detecting Legion-

naires' disease due to non-serogroup 1 *L. pneumophila* and other species (11). However, the sensitivity and specificity of these tests for detecting other serogroups and species are currently unknown.

False-positive results have been reported with the urine EIAs. The package insert of the Bartels kit indicates that a false-positive result can occur in a small percentage of urine specimens from patients with bacteremia due to *Streptococcus pneumoniae*. False-positive results have also been reported for the Binax EIA (31) but were due to nonspecific protein binding. Therefore, the sensitivity and specificity of the urinary antigen test have been reported to be 80 to 99% and 99%, respectively (Table 2) (37). Sensitivity has been improved by concentration of urine samples, and specificity has been improved by boiling the samples (34). The results of the urinary antigen test can be available within hours, whereas culture results require 3 to 5 days (75). The disadvantage of the urinary antigen test is that it is specific only for *L. pneumophila* serogroup 1. This limitation has not been considered a major disadvantage of the test because the vast majority of cases of Legionnaires' disease cases are caused by this species and serogroup (172).

Although the antibody used in the urinary antigen test has specificity for *L. pneumophila* serogroup 1, there have been reports of cross-reactivity with other serogroups of *L. pneumophila* (11, 27). The antigen can be detected in a patient's urine even after antibiotic treatment has been initiated. In our experience, most patients will remain positive for *Legionella* urinary antigen for weeks (and even months on rare occasions). In our laboratory, the urinary antigen test became negative for the majority of 66 culture-confirmed cases of Legionnaires' disease due to *L. pneumophila* serogroup 1 within 60 days. The sensitivity and specificity of the urine antigen test were approximately 85 and 100%, respectively, without concentration or boiling of the samples (Vickers et al., *Abstr. 94th Gen. Meet. Am. Soc.*

Microbiol. 1994). The sensitivity was only 85% because the test was negative for several patients who had small numbers (<10 CFU) of *L. pneumophila* serogroup 1 isolated from their sputum.

A rapid urinary antigen test, the Binax NOW *Legionella* urinary antigen test, is commercially available that yields a result in less than 15 min. It is an immunochromatographic membrane (ICT) assay that is performed using a swab that has been dipped in urine and inserted into the card-type test device. The reaction is read as presence or absence of a visually detectable pink to purple line that results from the antigen-antibody reaction. The ICT assay is comparable to the EIA, with a sensitivity of 80% and specificity of 97 to 100% (Table 2) (33, 137). This format of the urinary antigen test seems to be less prone to false-positive reactions.

Although PCR-based assays for detection of *Legionella* in clinical samples are highly specific, they are not more sensitive than culture (76, 101). The primary advantage of this technique is the ability to detect *Legionella* rapidly and to detect species other than *L. pneumophila*. DNA amplification by PCR of *Legionella* has been reported from patients with pneumonia by using throat swab specimens, bronchoalveolar lavage fluid, urine, and serum (3, 13, 73, 76, 95, 120, 121). Depending on the study, the sensitivity and specificity have been reported to be 64 to 100% and 88 to 100%, respectively (Table 2). Primer sequences of the macrophage infectivity potentiator (*mip*) gene of *L. pneumophila* and 16S and 5S rRNA genes have been used in PCR assays. A PCR kit (EnviroAmp; Perkin-Elmer Cetus, Norwalk, Conn.) had been used successfully to detect *Legionella* in both clinical and environmental samples (101), but it is no longer commercially available (100). PCR assays hold the promise of a rapid and specific diagnosis. A rapid (2- to 3-h) real-time PCR assay was recently reported to be able to detect the most clinically relevant *Legionella* species, and it successfully detected *L. pneumophila* in bronchoalveolar lavage fluid specimens that were also culture positive (121).

Given that clinical experience has not yet shown PCR to be more sensitive than culture (64), the CDC does not recommend the routine use of genetic probes or PCR for detection of *Legionella* in clinical samples (26).

ISOLATION PROCEDURES

Culture remains the most sensitive method for the diagnosis of Legionnaires' disease. The reported sensitivity and specificity for culture are 80 to 90% and 100%, respectively (Table 2) (37). In addition to respiratory tract specimens, *Legionella* has been detected in blood, pleural, pericardial, and peritoneal fluids, as well as prosthetic valves and sternal wounds (91, 112).

Legionella species are primary pathogens of the lower respiratory tract. Appropriate (and optimal) respiratory specimens for culture include expectorated sputum, tracheal aspirate, bronchoscopy specimens, pleural fluid, and lung tissue. Respiratory specimens that are difficult or impossible to obtain more than once, such as lung tissue, pleural fluid, and bronchoscopy samples, should be routinely cultured for *Legionella*, regardless of whether the test was ordered (Fig. 1). Even the isolation of a single colony confirms the diagnosis of Legionnaires' disease.

Legionellae are fastidious slow-growing bacteria. The likelihood of isolating *Legionella* from clinical specimens is greatest when there is little or no competition from other

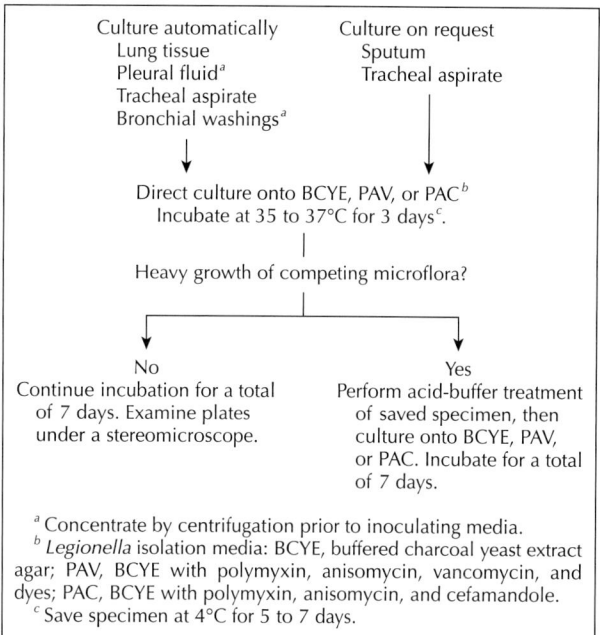

FIGURE 1 Procedure for processing clinical samples for *Legionella* culture (136). Reprinted with permission from HC Information Resources, Fallbrook, Calif.

organisms. The culture work-up for samples likely to have competing members of the flora, such as sputum sample, should always include selective media. Culture of sputum and tracheal suction specimens for *Legionella* should be performed only when specifically requested, since isolation of *Legionella* from this type of sample is difficult and requires the use of both selective media and pretreatment techniques to optimize recovery.

Expectorated sputum and bronchoscopy specimens can give similar yields with the use of selective media and acid pretreatment (40). The fact that bronchoscopy specimens sometimes give the first clue to an outbreak of legionellosis is probably because, in most hospitals, culture for *Legionella* is more likely to be ordered for bronchoscopy specimens (106).

Sputum, tracheal suction, and bronchoscopy samples can be plated with a sterile swab directly onto media and then streaked. If the sample contains areas of purulence or blood, these areas should be selected and cultured. Pleural fluid, if present in adequate volume (>1 ml), should be centrifuged at a minimum of 1,500 × g for 15 min. After centrifugation, the supernatant is removed, leaving approximately 0.5 ml. The sediment is resuspended before being plated. Bronchoscopy samples, if very dilute, can also be concentrated by centrifugation. Lung tissue samples are first homogenized using a small amount of sterile nutrient broth and then cultured. Figure 1 depicts an algorithm for the processing of clinical specimens for the culture of *Legionella* spp. (136).

Legionella does not grow on standard microbiological media due to its fastidious growth requirements. Microbiologists should be aware that *Legionella* has been isolated on chocolate II agar (60); however, the use of chocolate agar for *Legionella* culture is not recommended. A charcoal yeast extract agar was specifically formulated to grow *Legionella* (47, 48). Buffered charcoal yeast extract (BCYE) agar (47),

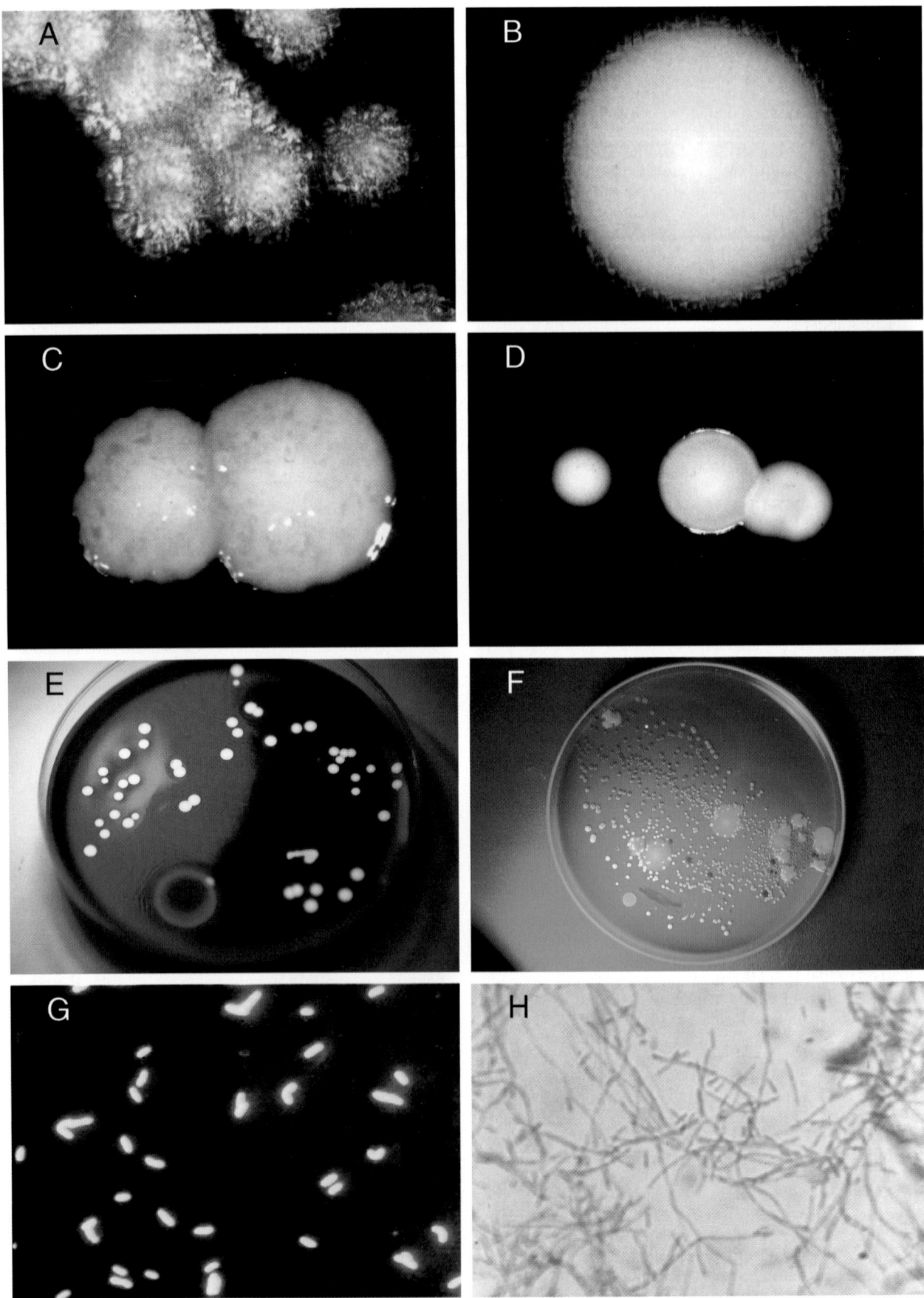

buffered with ACES [*N*-(2-acetamido)-2-aminoethane sulfonic acid] (10 mg/ml) (113) and supplemented with α-ketoglutarate (1 mg/ml), L-cysteine (400 μg/ml), and ferric pyrophosphate (250 μg/ml) (pH 6.9), is the primary medium for isolation of *Legionella* by culture. Both α-ketoglutarate and activated charcoal stimulate *Legionella* growth by decreasing the production of toxic peroxides; α-ketoglutarate does so indirectly by inhibiting cysteine oxidation (115), and charcoal does so directly by promoting the decomposition of peroxides (66). Yeast extract, L-cysteine, and ferric pyrophosphate supply vitamins, minerals, and other specific nutrients essential for growth, while the ACES buffer maintains a critical pH of 6.85 to 6.95. The addition of albumin counteracts the inhibitory effects of starch and may improve the recovery of *L. micdadei*, *L. bozemanii*, and *L. anisa* in culture (105).

The standard medium for isolation of *Legionella* from contaminated clinical specimens (PAV) is BCYE supplemented with polymyxin (80 U/ml), anisomycin (40 μg/ml), vancomycin (1 μg/ml), and dyes (bromocresol purple, 10 μg/ml; bromothymol blue, 10 μg/ml); the antimicrobial agents prevent the overgrowth of *Legionella* by competing organisms, while the dyes impart a distinctive color to the *Legionella* organisms (36, 84, 113, 157). The presence of the dyes makes the identification of *L. micdadei* and *L. maceachernii* easier. Their colonies appear blue due to uptake of the bromothymol blue dye, whereas *L. pneumophila* appears apple green (157). For maximal sensitivity, we recommend the simultaneous use of three media: BCYE; BCYE with polymyxin (80 U/ml), anisomycin (40 μg/ml), and cefamandole (4 μg/ml) (PAC); and BCYE with polymyxin, anisomycin, vancomycin, and dyes (PAV) (antimicrobial concentrations cited above). We have found that if yeast overgrowth occurs despite the presence of anisomycin in the selective media, addition of fluconazole (80 μg/ml) can aid in the recovery of *Legionella* from such samples (87).

All three media (BCYE, PAV, and PAC) are commercially available. Most commercial media have passed an internal quality assurance test before being shipped; however, we recommend that each laboratory perform its own quality control check for adequate growth. Not all commercial media have been shown to pass such a simple quality control check (84).

It is also important to note that not all *Legionella* species grow equally well in the presence of antimicrobial agents (84). For example, *L. micdadei* does not grow in the presence of cefamandole. One study showed that 11 *Legionella* spp. that grew on PAV failed to grow on PAC (84). Some species, like *L. feeleii*, do not grow well on either selective medium. In one instance, we isolated *L. feeleii* only from the BCYE plate after acid pretreatment of the specimen. This illustrates the need for the use of multiple selective media and BCYE for optimal recovery of *Legionella* species.

Even with the use of selective media, some cultures may be overgrown by competing members of the flora. This usually occurs with specimens from hospitalized patients or nursing-home residents who are colonized with highly re-sistant nosocomial bacteria. Recovery of legionellae from these samples may be enhanced by the use of an acid pretreatment (21). Acid pretreatment is performed by diluting the sample 1:5 with a KCl-HCl buffer (pH 2.2). The sample is briefly vortexed to obtain a homogeneous mixture and incubated at room temperature for 4 min. It is then immediately cultured onto selective and nonselective BCYE media. This procedure may be done at the time of initial processing, or the sample may be refrigerated and retrieved later if the direct culture reveals bacterial overgrowth. We refrigerate all respiratory specimens for 1 week by placing them in separate bins marked by the days of the week. This practice has proven invaluable when a patient's urine sample is positive for *Legionella* urinary antigen but the physician ordered only routine work-up of the sputum sample. On such occasions, we have been able to go back to the refrigerated specimen and isolate *Legionella*. Specimens may also be heat pretreated to 60°C for 3 min to reduce the number of members of the competing flora (164).

If there is a pleural effusion, thoracentesis should be performed and the fluid should be evaluated by DFA, culture, and the *Legionella* antigen test used for urine (110).

Blood cultures may also be performed, but blood should not be considered the specimen of choice. If blood cultures for *Legionella* are ordered, the samples should be processed using lysis-centrifugation and plated directly onto BCYE. Conventional and automated blood-culturing systems do not support the growth of *Legionella*. However, viable organisms may be recovered from the bottles if blind subcultures are made onto BCYE. To increase the chance of recovery, 0.5 ml of the blood-broth mixture should be transferred and spread over the entire area of several plates.

The culture plates are incubated in humidified room air at 35 to 37°C and observed daily for 7 days. The use of CO_2 is not necessary for the growth of *Legionellaceae*. The slow-growing colonies of *Legionella* can usually be detected 24 h earlier if the plates are examined under a stereoscopic microscope. Very young colonies demonstrate a characteristic speckled green, blue, or pinkish purple iridescence (Fig. 2A). This iridescence can be seen easily through the dissecting stereo microscope if a light source is directed toward the plates at a slight angle. Colonies mature in 3 or 4 days, are 3 to 4 mm in diameter, entire, and convex, and have a frosted-glass internal appearance (Fig. 2B). Aging colonies lose most of their iridescence and develop grayish white centers. Colonies of non-*L. pneumophila* species can be mucoid and protuberant in appearance with irregular edges (Fig. 2C and D). The plates should also be examined using a long-wavelength (365-nm) UV lamp. Certain species of *Legionella* (*L. bozemanii*, *L. dumoffii*, *L. cherrii*, *L. gormanii*, *L. tucsonensis*, *L. anisa*, and *L. parisiensis*) autofluoresce blue-white under UV light (Fig. 2E). *L. rubrilucens* and *L. erythra* demonstrate a red autofluorescence (Fig. 2F), and *L. wadsworthii* and *L. birminghamensis* demonstrate a yellow-green autofluorescence (Table 1).

Colonies demonstrating characteristic morphology should first be Gram stained. Those that reveal thin gram-

FIGURE 2 (A and B) *Legionella* species may appear as characteristic ground-glass colonies with iridescent edges, which is typical of *L. pneumophila*. (C and D) Non-*pneumophila* species may appear as mucoid protuberant colonies (C) or raised greyish white colonies (D). (E and F) The colonies of certain species of *Legionella* autofluoresce either blue-white (E) or red (F) under long-wavelength UV light. (G) Immunofluorescent staining of either respiratory specimens or culture isolates should reveal short coccobacilli that stain a bright (3 to 4+) apple green. (H) Gram stain morphology of *L. pneumophila* shows thin, faintly staining gram-negative bacilli.

negative rods can be further tested to determine if L-cysteine is essential for growth. This can be done simply by subculturing the isolate in parallel to BCYE agar and 5% sheep blood agar. A BCYE medium without cysteine is also available for this purpose. Isolates found to grow only on BCYE, with typical colony morphology and staining characteristics, can be presumptively identified as *Legionella* (Fig. 3). Further testing, such as DFA, should be performed to identify the organism as definitively belonging to the family *Legionellaceae*.

If *Legionella* has been isolated from a clinical specimen, the isolate should be subcultured and frozen at −20 or −70°C. Epidemiologic investigations are often initiated well after the patient has been discharged. The growth from one BCYE plate should be suspended into 1.0 ml of brucella broth containing 15% glycerol, vortexed, and frozen.

Hospital-acquired Legionnaires' disease occurs after exposure to *Legionella* in the water distribution system. Epidemiologic investigations of these cases include environmental cultures. Selective media are also used for the isolation of *Legionella* from environmental specimens; however, the formulations are slightly different from those used for clinical culture. For potable-water samples, either swab or water samples, we found the use of BCYE agar and DGVP to yield optimal results (145). DGVP contains the dyes bromocresol purple and bromothymol blue, glycine, vancomycin, and polymyxin B. If a water sample is collected, a minimum of 200 ml should be collected (after the swab sample) and 100 ml is filter concentrated using a 47-mm, 0.2-μm-pore-size polycarbonate filter. Water samples from a cooling tower should also be plated on *Legionella* selective media that contains an antifungal agent such as cycloheximide. Most environmental specimens should undergo acid pretreatment prior to inoculation of selective media.

IDENTIFICATION

Although *Legionellaceae* share a number of phenotypic characteristics (Table 1), these characteristics are of limited value in species identification (68). The usual basis for identification includes culture characteristics (requirement for cysteine), nonfermentative metabolism, and serotyping (by slide agglutination or DFA staining). Combinations of these traits have been used with variable degrees of accuracy in distinguishing among the numerous *Legionella* species (156, 158). The identification algorithm used in our laboratory is depicted in Fig. 3.

Specific antibody reactions, as detected by indirect immunofluorescence, direct immunofluorescence, crossed immunoelectrophoresis (5), slide agglutination (165), and immunodiffusion (111), can also be used for identification of *Legionella* species.

The availability and quality of reagents for identification of *Legionella* spp. by DFA staining or slide agglutination have substantially improved, so that a diagnosis of infection due to *L. pneumophila* can be made with great confidence. A latex agglutination test is now available that allows the identification of *L. pneumophila* serogroup 1 or serogroups 2 to 14 and detection of seven other *Legionella* species (Oxoid Ltd., Basingstoke, England). DFA staining reagents (see also "Direct Detection" above) are available as monoclonal and polyclonal, monovalent and polyvalent reagents. One reagent is a polyclonal-polyvalent reagent capable of reacting with 22 species and 31 serogroups of *Legionella* (Remel, Lenexa, Kans.).

There is considerable potential for misidentification at the serotype level due to significant cross-reactivity among the various serogroups of *L. pneumophila* (166). For example, an isolate of *L. pneumophila* serogroup 6 shows some degree of staining with polyclonal reagents for serogroups 3 and 6. We have also seen a clinical isolate identified as *L. pneumophila* serogroup 12 that stained with DFA reagents to *L. pneumophila* serogroups 1 and 6. The blue-white-fluorescing species also show some cross-reactivity with the monovalent-polyclonal reagents. Isolates of *L. anisa* show cross-reactivity with the reagent for *L. bozemanii*, making it difficult to differentiate between these species (55, 67, 68, 166). While differences in staining patterns can be discerned with experience, clinical isolates that react with multiple reagents should be sent to CDC for confirmation.

Both phenotypic and genotypic differences among strains of *L. pneumophila* have been used in epidemiologic investigations to link patient isolates to an environmental reservoir (7, 151). These methods include serotyping (151), monoclonal antibody subtyping (92), isoenzyme analysis (131), protein and carbohydrate profiling (54), plasmid analysis (62), restriction fragment length polymorphism of rRNA (ribotyping) or chromosomal DNA (4, 151), amplified fragment length polymorphism (150), repetitive-element PCR (57), restriction endonuclease analysis of whole-cell DNA with or without pulsed-field gel electrophoresis (PFGE) (62, 83, 130), arbitrarily primed PCR (72, 83, 118, 151), and 16S-23S spacer analysis (151).

For epidemiologic investigations, a combination of phenotypic and genotypic methods may be necessary for maximal discrimination. Studies have shown that there may be limited genetic heterogeneity among subtypes of *L. pneumophila* (35, 82, 143). Therefore, the results of molecular subtyping must be interpreted with caution. It has been recommended that both a phenotypic method (monoclonal subtyping) and a genotypic method (PFGE) be used for optimal comparison of epidemiologically linked clinical and environmental isolates of *L. pneumophila* (35).

Among the currently available techniques for molecular subtyping of *Legionella* isolates, either PFGE or arbitrarily primed PCR is commonly used (83, 118, 129).

SEROLOGICAL TESTS

Indirect fluorescent-antibody (IFA) and enzyme-linked immunosorbent assays have been the most commonly used methods for *L. pneumophila* serological testing. The CDC recommends that only IFA results for *L. pneumophila* serogroup 1 be used for diagnostic purposes due to insufficient information on the sensitivity and specificity of tests for other serogroups and species (26, 37). Diagnosis is based on a fourfold rise in antibody titer to ≥1:128; therefore, both acute- and convalescent-phase sera are required. Anywhere from 4 to 24 weeks is often required to detect an antibody response, the use of both immunoglobulin M (IgM) and IgG assays gives maximal sensitivity, and 25 to 40% of patients may have elevated titers in the first week of disease (Vickers et al., *Abstr. 94th Gen. Meet. Am. Soc. Microbiol. 1994*). Some patients never demonstrate a fourfold increase in titer (102, 104). In addition, the reported sensitivity and specificity are approximately 75 and 96%, respectively (Table 2) (37). Serological testing is useful in epidemiologic studies but less helpful to the clinician in making an immediate diagnosis of Legionnaires' disease for an individual patient. On the other hand, if the seroprevalence of *L. pneumophila* antibody titers within the community is known

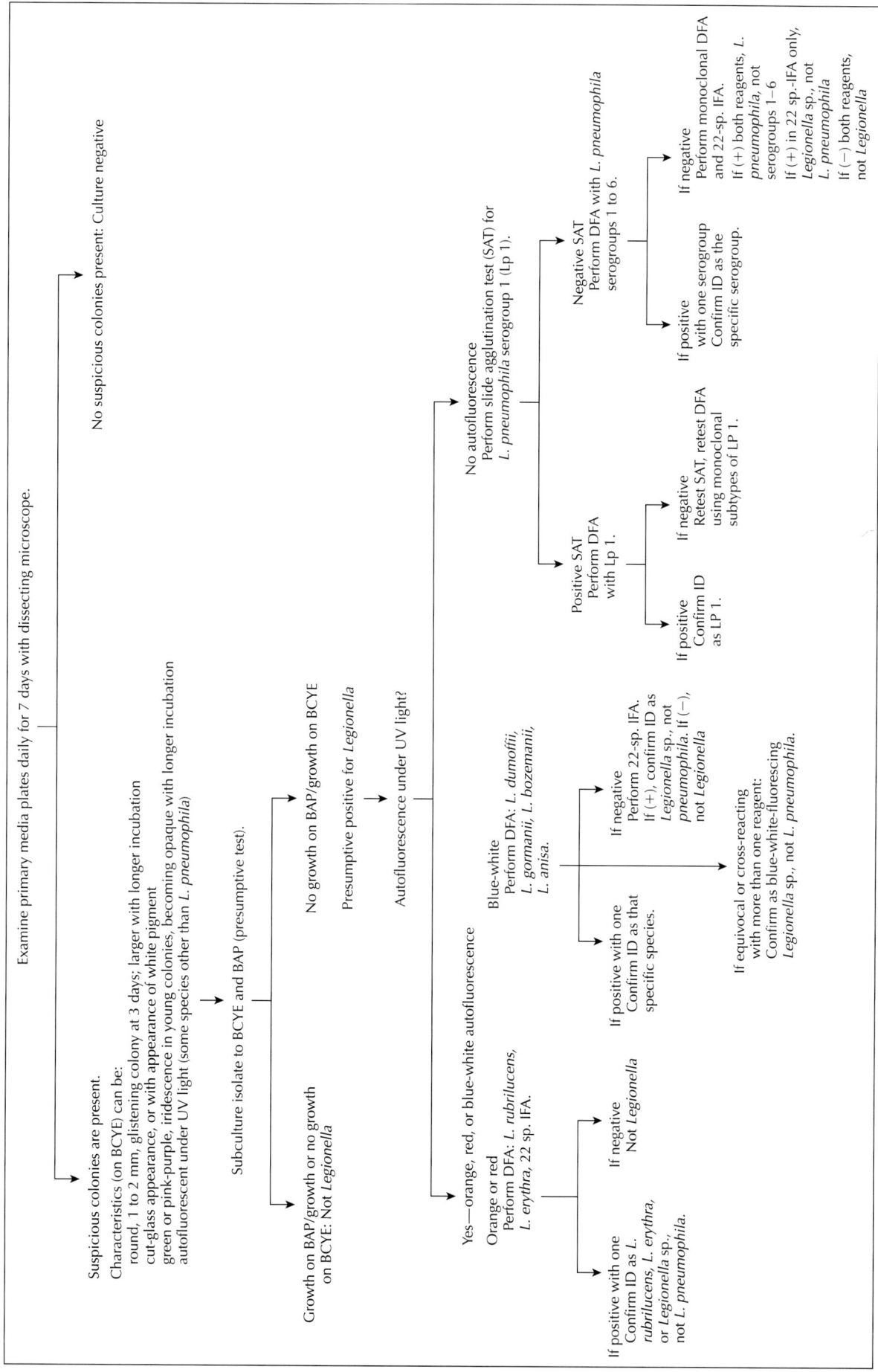

FIGURE 3 *Legionella* identification chart.

to be low, a single elevated titer (1:256) may possibly indicate the presence of acute disease. However, in one study, acute-phase antibody titers of ≥256 failed to discriminate between definitive cases of Legionnaires' disease and nondefinitive cases (116). Also, a single elevated titer does not confirm a case of Legionnaires' disease because IFA titers of ≥1:256 have been found in 1 to 16% of healthy adults (26), and the positive predictive value of a convalescent-phase titer is unacceptably low (116). False-positive results can rarely occur as a result of cross-reaction with antibody to other gram-negative organisms (43). Taken together, these facts show that the utility of serological testing as a diagnostic tool is limited.

L. pneumophila IgG/IgM enzyme-linked immunosorbent assay kits are commercially available (Carter Wallace-Wampole, Cranbury, N.J., and Virion-Serion, Würzburg, Germany). IFA reagents are also available commercially (SciMedx, Zeus Technologies, and Trinity Biotech, Bray, Colo.).

ANTIMICROBIAL SUSCEPTIBILITIES

Legionella species are facultative intracellular pathogens. As such, they can avoid the effects of antimicrobial agents that cannot penetrate host cell membranes. For example, agents that cannot penetrate macrophages, such as penicillins and cephalosporins, demonstrate activity in MIC assays but are clinically ineffective (38). In vitro antibiotic susceptibility studies have been problematic due to a lack of standardized methods, variable susceptibility results depending on the type of medium used, and poor correlation to clinical observations. Three methods are generally used for susceptibility testing: extracellular testing in broth or agar, intracellular testing in tissue culture, and studies using infected guinea pigs (38).

Resistance to antimicrobial therapy has been suspected due to persistent recovery of *Legionella* from respiratory cultures despite macrolide therapy (77, 146). However, it could not be demonstrated. For example, when MICs for isolates recovered from specimens taken early and late in the course of therapy were compared, no difference was observed (146).

Erythromycin, rifampin, tetracycline, fluoroquinolones and newer macrolide/azalide antimicrobial agents are considered to be effective agents in the treatment of Legionnaires' disease (171). In vitro and in vivo results have shown the following agents to be highly active: azithromycin, clarithromycin, ciprofloxacin, pefloxacin, levofloxacin, moxifloxacin, fleroxacin, trovafloxacin, minocycline, doxycycline, and the ketolides (38, 41, 42; K. Sens, S. Mietzner, A. Sagnimeni, J. E. Stout, and V. L. Yu, *Program Abstr. 40th Intersci. Conf. Antimicrobiol. Agents Chemother.*, abstr. 2159, 2000). Synergy in vitro has also been shown for trimethoprim-sulfamethoxazole, erythromycin, rifampin, and macrolide-quinolone combinations (99, 103). Variable results (including antagonism) have been reported for quinolones plus rifampin (63, 103). *Legionella* species that lack β-lactamase presumably may be susceptible to β-lactam agents, but clinical experience indicates a high likelihood of failure. However, as intravenous formulations of the newer macrolides have become available, the newer quinolones and macrolides have displaced erythromycin as the drug of choice (39, 155).

EVALUATION, INTERPRETATION, AND REPORTING OF RESULTS

Unlike most other respiratory pathogens, *Legionella* does not colonize the respiratory tract. Even a single colony isolated from a culture confirms the diagnosis of Legionnaires' disease.

Immunofluorescent staining (DFA) results are reported as positive or negative. Both the intensity of the staining and the morphology of the organism should be noted. On a scale of 1 to 4, a strong positive is 3–4+ fluorescence intensity. Also to be noted is the number of fluorescent cells per well of the slide. If the monoclonal immunofluorescent antibody is used for screening respiratory specimens, even the presence of a few appropriately staining cells is considered a positive result.

The urinary antigen test is also reported as positive or negative based on the ratio-to-negative of the EIA or the presence/absence of even a faint pink to purple line on the card (ICT). A positive value for the EIA is ≥3.0; however, some data suggest that values between 2.5 and 3.0 may also be positive (61). If the ratio-to-negative is in this range, we report the result as "suspicious" and request another specimen.

Serological test results are presumptive only if results are available for only a single specimen. A fourfold rise to ≥128 between the acute- and convalescent-phase titers is required for a definitive diagnosis based on serological testing (26).

REFERENCES

1. **Adeleke, A., J. Pruckler, R. Benson, T. Rowbotham, M. Halablab, and B. Fields.** 1996. *Legionella*-like amebal pathogens—phylogenetic status and possible role in respiratory diseases. *Emerg. Infect. Dis.* **2:**225–230.
2. **Adeleke, A. A., B. S. Fields, R. F. Benson, M. I. Daneshvar, J. M. Pruckler, R. M. Ratcliff, T. G. Harrison, R. S. Weyant, R. J. Birtles, D. Raoult, and M. A. Halablab.** 2001. *Legionella drozanskii* sp. nov., *Legionella rowbothamii* sp. nov. and *Legionella fallonii* sp. nov.: three unusual new *Legionella* species. *Int. J. Syst. Evol. Microbiol.* **51:**1151–1160.
3. **Ballard, A. L., N. K. Fry, L. Chan, S. B. Surman, J. V. Lee, T. G. Harrison, and K. J. Towner.** 2000. Detection of *Legionella pneumophila* using a real-time PCR hybridization assay. *J. Clin. Microbiol.* **38:**4215–4218.
4. **Bangsborg, J. M., P. Gerner-Smidt, H. Colding, N. E. Fiehn, B. Bruun, and N. Hoiby.** 1995. Restriction fragment length polymorphism of rRNA genes for molecular typing of members of the family *Legionellaceae. J. Clin. Microbiol.* **33:**402–406.
5. **Bangsborg, J. M., G. Shand, E. Pearlman, and N. Hoiby.** 1991. Cross-reactive *Legionella* antigens and the antibody response during infection. *APMIS* **99:**854–865.
6. **Bansal, N. S., and F. McDonell.** 1997. Identification and DNA fingerprinting of *Legionella* strains by randomly amplified polymorphic DNA analysis. *J. Clin. Microbiol.* **35:** 2310–2314.
7. **Barbaree, J. M.** 1993. Selecting a subtyping technique for use in investigations of legionellosis epidemics, p. 169–172. *In* J. M. Barbaree, R. F. Brieman, and A. P. Dufour (ed.), Legionella: *Current Status and Emerging Perspectives.* American Society for Microbiology, Washington, D.C.
8. **Barker, J., and M. R. W. Brown.** 1994. Trojan horses of the microbial world: protozoa and the survival of bacterial pathogens in the environment. *Microbiology* **140:**1253–1259.

9. **Barthe, C., J. R. Joly, D. Ramsay, M. Boissinot, and N. Benhamou.** 1988. Common epitope on the lipopolysaccharide of *Legionella pneumophila* recognized by monoclonal antibody. *J. Clin. Microbiol.* **26:**1016–1023.

10. **Benson, R. F., and B. S. Fields.** 1998. Classification of the genus *Legionella. Semin. Respir. Infect.* **13:**90–99.

11. **Benson, R. F., P. W. Tang, and B. S. Fields.** 2000. Evaluation of the Binax and Biotest urinary antigen kits for detection of Legionnaires' disease due to multiple serogroups and species of *Legionella. J. Clin. Microbiol.* **38:** 2763–2765.

12. **Berk, S., R. Ting, G. Turner, and R. Ashburn.** 1999. Production of respirable vesicles containing live *Legionella pneumophila* cells by two *Acanthamoeba* spp. *Appl. Environ. Microbiol.* **64:**279–286.

13. **Bernander, S., H.-S. Hanson, B. Johansson, and L. V. von Stedingk.** 1997. A nested polymerase chain reaction for detection of *Legionella pneumophila* in clinical specimens. *Clin. Microbiol. Infect.* **3:**95–101.

14. **Best, M., V. L. Yu, J. Stout, A. Goetz, R. R. Muder, and F. Taylor.** 1983. *Legionellaceae* in the hospital water supply—epidemiological link with disease and evaluation of a method of control of nosocomial Legionnaires' disease and Pittsburgh pneumonia. *Lancet* **ii:**307–310.

15. **Blatt, S. P., M. J. Dolan, C. W. Hendrix, and G. P. Melcher.** 1994. Legionnaires' disease in HIV-infected patients: eight cases and review. *Clin. Infect. Dis.* **18:**227–232.

16. **Blatt, S. P., M. D. Parkinson, E. Pace, P. Hoffman, D. Dolan, P. Lauderdale, R. A. Zajac, and S. P. Melcher.** 1993. Nosocomial Legionnaires' disease: aspiration as a primary mode of transmission. *Am. J. Med.* **95:**16–22.

17. **Brady, M.** 1989. Nosocomial Legionnaires' disease in a children's hospital. *J. Pediatr.* **115:**46–50.

18. **Breiman, R. F.** 1993. Modes of transmission in epidemic and nonepidemic *Legionella* infection: directions for further study, p. 30–35. *In* J. M. Barbaree, R. M. Breiman, and A. P. Dufour (ed.), Legionella: *Current Status and Emerging Perspectives.* American Society for Microbiology, Washington, D.C.

19. **Brenner, D. J., A. G. Steigerwalt, and J. E. McDade.** 1979. Classification of the Legionnaires' disease bacterium: *Legionella pneumophila,* genus novum, species nova, of the family *Legionellaceae. Ann. Intern. Med* **90:**656–658.

20. **Brindle, R. J., T. N. Bryant, and P. W. Draper.** 1989. Taxonomic investigation of *Legionella pneumophila* using monoclonal antibodies. *J. Clin. Microbiol.* **27:**536–539.

21. **Buesching, W. J., R. A. Brust, and L. W. Ayers.** 1983. Enhanced primary isolation of *Legionella pneumophila* from clinical specimens by low-pH treatment. *J. Clin. Microbiol.* **17:**1153–1155.

22. **Butler, J. C., B. S. Fields, and R. F. Breiman.** 1997. Issues in the control of nosocomial legionellosis. *Infect. Dis. Clin. Pract.* **7:**117–118.

23. **Butler, J. C., B. S. Fields, and R. F. Breiman.** 1997. Prevention and control of legionellosis. *Infect. Dis. Clin. Pract.* **6:**458–464.

24. **Carratala, J., F. Gudiol, R. Pallares, R. Verdaguer, J. Ariza, and F. Manresa.** 1994. Risk factors for nosocomial *Legionella pneumophila* pneumonia. *Am. J. Respir. Crit. Care. Med.* **149:**625–629.

25. **Carter, D. M.** 1993. Blood culture detection of *Legionella* in a transplant patient. *Clin. Microbiol. Newsl.* **15:**151–152.

26. **Centers for Disease Control and Prevention.** 1997. Guidelines for prevention of nosocomial pneumonia. *Morb. Mortal. Wkly. Rep.* **46:**31–34.

27. **Chang, F. Y., S. L. Jacobs, S. M. Colodny, J. E. Stout, and V. L. Yu.** 1996. Nosocomial Legionnaires' disease caused by *Legionella pneumophila* serogroup 5: laboratory and epidemiological implications. *J. Infect. Dis.* **174:** 1116–1119.

28. **Cianciotto, N. P., J. K. Stamos, and D. W. Kamp.** 1995. Infectivity of *Legionella pneumophila mip* mutant for alveolar epithelial cells. *Curr. Microbiol.* **30:**247–250.

29. **Colbourne, J. S., and P. J. Dennis.** 1989. The ecology and survival of *Legionella pneumophila. Thames Water Authority J. Inst. Water Environ. Manage.* **3:**345–350.

30. **Cunha, B. A.** 1998. Clinical features of Legionnaires' disease. *Semin. Respir. Infect.* **13:**116–127.

31. **Deforges, L., P. Legrand, J. Tankovic, C. Brun-Buisson, P. Lang, and C. J. Soussy.** 1999. Case of false-positive results of the urinary antigen test for *Legionella pneumophila. Clin. Infect. Dis.* **29:**953–954.

32. **Diogo, A., A. Verissimo, M. F. Nobre, and M. S. daCosta.** 1999. Usefulness of fatty acid composition for differentiation of *Legionella* species. *J. Clin. Microbiol.* **37:** 2248–2254.

33. **Dominguez, J., N. Gali, L. Matas, P. Pedroso, A. Hernandez, and E. Padilla.** 1999. Evaluation of a rapid immunochromatographic assay for the detection of *Legionella* antigen in urine samples. *Eur. J. Clin. Microbiol. Infect. Dis.* **18:**896–898.

34. **Dominguez, J. A., J. M. Manterola, R. Blavia, N. Sopena, F. J. Belda, E. Padilla, M. Gimenez, M. Sabria, J. Morera, and V. Ausina.** 1996. Detection of *Legionella pneumophila* serogroup 1 antigen in nonconcentrated urine and urine concentrated by selective ultrafiltration. *J. Clin. Microbiol.* **34:**2334–2336.

35. **Drenning, S. D., J. E. Stout, J. R. Joly, and V. L. Yu.** 2001. Unexpected similarity of pulsed-field gel electrophoresis patterns of unrelated clinical isolates of *Legionella pneumophila,* serogroup 1. *J. Infect. Dis.* **183:**628–632.

36. **Edelstein, P. H.** 1981. Improved semiselective medium for isolation of *Legionella pneumophila* from contaminated clinical and environmental specimens. *J. Clin. Microbiol.* **14:** 298–303.

37. **Edelstein, P. H.** 1993. Legionnaires' disease. *Clin. Infect. Dis.* **16:**741–749.

38. **Edelstein, P. H.** 1995. Antimicrobial chemotherapy for Legionnaires' disease: a review. *Clin. Infect. Dis.* **21**(Suppl. 3):S265–S276.

39. **Edelstein, P. H.** 1998. Antimicrobial chemotherapy for Legionnaires' disease: time for a change. *Ann. Intern. Med.* **129:**328–330.

40. **Edelstein, P. H.** 2000. Detection of selected fastidious bacteria. *Clin. Infect. Dis.* **31:**846.

41. **Edelstein, P. H., M. A. C. Edelstein, K. H. Lehr, and J. Ren.** 1996. In-vitro activity of levofloxacin against clinical isolates of *Legionella* spp., its pharmacokinetics in guinea pigs, and use in experimental *Legionella pneumophila* pneumonia. *J. Antimicrob. Chemother.* **37:**117–126.

42. **Edelstein, P. H., M. A. C. Edelstein, J. Ren, R. Polzer, and R. P. Gladue.** 1996. Activity of trovafloxacin (CP-99, 219) against *Legionella* isolates: in vitro activity, intracellular accumulation and killing in macrophages, and pharmacokinetics and treatment of guinea pigs with *L. pneumophila* pneumonia. *Antimicrob. Agents Chemother.* **40:** 314–331.

43. **Edelstein, P. H., R. M. McKinney, R. D. Meyer, M. A. Edelstein, C. J. Krause, and S. M. Finegold.** 1980. Immunologic diagnosis of Legionnaires' disease: cross-reactions with anaerobic and microaerophilic organisms and infections caused by them. *J. Infect. Dis.* **141:**652–655.

44. **Fallon, R. J., and T. J. Rowbotham.** 1990. Microbiological investigations into an outbreak of Pontiac fever due to *Legionella micdadei* associated with use of a whirlpool spa. *J. Clin. Pathol.* **43:**479–483.

45. **Fang, G. D., M. Fine, J. Orloff, D. Arisumi, V. L. Yu, W. Kapoor, T. Grayston, S. P. Wang, R. Kohler, R. Muder, Y. C. Ying, J. D. Rihs, and R. M. Vickers.** 1990. New and emerging etiologies for community-acquired pneumonia with implications for therapy: a prospective multicenter study of 359 cases. *Medicine* **69:**307–316.

46. **Fang, G. D., V. L. Yu, and R. M. Vickers.** 1989. Disease due to *Legionellaceae* (other than *Legionella pneumophila*): historical, microbiological, clinical and epidemiological review. *Medicine* **68:**116–139.

47. **Feeley, J. C., R. J. Gibson, and G. W. Gorman.** 1979. Charcoal yeast extract agar: primary isolation medium for *Legionella pneumophila*. *J. Clin. Microbiol.* **10:**437–441.

48. **Feeley, J. C., G. W. Gorman, R. E. Weaver, D. C. Mackel, and H. W. Smith.** 1978. Primary isolation media for Legionnaires' disease bacterium. *J. Clin. Microbiol.* **8:**320–325.

49. **Fields, B. S.** 1993. *Legionella* and protozoa: interaction of a pathogen and its natural host, p. 129–136. *In* J. M. Barbaree, R. F. Breiman, and A. P. Dufour (ed.), Legionella: *Current Status and Emerging Perspectives.* American Society for Microbiology, Washington, D.C.

50. **Fields, B. S.** 1996. The molecular ecology of legionellae. *Trends Microbiol.* **4:**286–290.

51. **Fiore, A. E., J. C. Butler, T. G. Emori, and R. P. Gaynes.** 1999. A survey of methods to detect nosocomial legionellosis among participants in the National Nosocomial Infectious Surveillance System. *Infect. Control Hosp. Epidemiol.* **20:**412–416.

52. **Fliermans, C. B.** 1984. Philosophical ecology: *Legionella* in historical perspective, p. 285–289. *In* C. Thornsberry, A. Balows, and J. C. Feeley (ed.), Legionella—*Proceedings of the 2nd International Symposium.* American Society for Microbiology, Washington, D.C.

53. **Flournoy, D. J., K. A. Belobraydic, S. L. Silberg, C. H. Lawrence, and P. J. Guthrie.** 1988. False positive *Legionella pneumophila* direct immunofluorescent monoclonal antibody test caused by *Bacillus cereus* spores. *Diagn. Microbiol. Infect. Dis.* **9:**123–125.

54. **Fox, A., P. Y. Lau, A. Brown, S. L. Morgan, Z. I. Zhu, M. Lema, and M. D. Walla.** 1984. Capillary gas chromatographic analysis of carbohydrates of *Legionella pneumophila* and other members of the family *Legionellaceae*. *J. Clin. Microbiol.* **19:**326–332.

55. **Fry, N. K., S. Warwick, N. A. Saunders, and T. M. Embley.** 1991. The use of 16S ribosomal RNA analysis to investigate the phylogeny of the family *Legionellaceae*. *J. Gen. Microbiol.* **137:**1215–1222.

56. **Garrity, G. M., A. Brown, and R. M. Vickers.** 1980. *Tatlockia* and *Fluoribacter:* two new genera of organisms resembling *Legionella pneumophila*. *Int. J. Syst. Bacteriol.* **30:**609–614.

57. **Georghiou, P. R., A. M. Doggett, M. A. Kielhofner, J. E. Stout, D. A. Watson, J. R. Lupski, and R. J. Hamill.** 1994. Molecular fingerprinting of *Legionella* species by repetitive element PCR. *J. Clin. Microbiol.* **32:**2989–2994.

58. **Gheldre, Y. D., N. Maes, F. Lo Presti, J. Etienne, and M. Struelens.** 2001. Rapid identification of clinically relevant *Legionella* spp. by analysis of transfer DNA intergenic spacer length polymorphism. *J. Clin. Microbiol.* **39:**162–169.

59. **Glick, T. H., M. B. Gregg, B. Berman, G. Mallison, W. W. Rhodes, Jr., and I. Kassanoff.** 1978. Pontiac fever. An epidemic of unknown etiology in a health department. I. Clinical and epidemiologic aspects. *Am. J. Epidemiol.* **107:**149–160.

60. **Green, M., E. R. Wald, K. Dashefsky, K. Barbadora, and R. M. Wadowsky.** 1996. Field inversion gel electrophoretic analysis of *Legionella pneumophila* strains associated with nosocomial legionellosis in children. *J. Clin. Microbiol.* **34:**175–176.

61. **Hackman, B. A., J. F. Plouffe, R. F. Benson, B. S. Fields, and R. F. Breiman.** 1996. Comparison of Binax Legionella urinary antigen EIA kit with Binax RIA urinary antigen kit to detect *Legionella pneumophila*, serogroup 1 antigen. *J. Clin. Microbiol.* **34:**1579–1580.

62. **Harrison, T. G., N. A. Saunders, A. Haththotuwa, G. Hallas, R. J. Birtles, and A. G. Taylor.** 1990. Phenotypic variation amongst genotypically homogeneous *Legionella pneumophila* serogroup 1 isolates: implications for the investigation of outbreaks of Legionnaires' disease. *Epidemiol. Infect.* **104:**171–180.

63. **Havlichek, D., L. Saravolatz, and D. Pohlod.** 1987. Effect of quinolones and other antimicrobial agents on cell-associated *Legionella pneumophila* Antimicrob. Agents Chemother. **31:**1529–1534.

64. **Hayden, M. K., J. R. Uhl, X. Qian, M. K. Hopkins, M. C. Aubry, A. H. Limper, R. V. Lloyd, and F. R. Cockerill.** 2000. Direct detection of *Legionella* species from bronchoalveolar lavage and open lung biopsy specimens: comparison of LightCycler PCR, in situ hybridization, direct fluorescence antigen detection, and culture. *J. Clin. Microbiol.* **39:**2618–2626.

65. **Hilton, E., R. A. Freedman, F. Cintron, H. D. Isenberg, and C. Singer.** 1986. Acid-fast bacilli in sputum: a case of *Legionella micdadei* pneumonia. *J. Clin. Microbiol.* **24:**1102–1103.

66. **Hoffman, P. S., L. Pine, and S. Bell.** 1983. Production of superoxide and hydrogen peroxide in medium used to culture *L. pneumophila:* catalytic decomposition by charcoal. *Appl. Environ. Microbiol.* **45:**784–791.

67. **Hookey, J. V., R. J. Birtles, and N. A. Saunders.** 1995. Intergenic 16S rRNA gene (rDNA)-23S rDNA sequence length polymorphism in members of the family *Legionellaceae*. *J. Clin. Microbiol.* **33:**2377–2381.

68. **Hookey, J. V., N. A. Saunders, N. K. Fry, R. J. Birtles, and T. G. Harrison.** 1996. Phylogeny of *Legionellaceae* based on small-subunit ribosomal DNA sequences and proposal of *Legionella lytica* comb. nov. for *Legionella*-like amoebal pathogens. *Int. J. Syst. Bacteriol.* **46:**526–531.

69. **Horwitz, M. A.** 1993. Toward an understanding of host and bacterial molecules mediating *L. pneumophila* pathogenesis, p. 55–62. *In* J. M. Barbaree, R. F. Breiman, and A. P. Dufour (ed.), Legionella: *Current Status and Emerging Perspectives.* American Society for Microbiology, Washington, D.C.

70. **Ingram, J. G., and J. Plouffe.** 1994. Danger of sputum purulence screens in culture of *Legionella* species. *J. Clin. Microbiol.* **32:**209–210.

71. **Johnson, J. T., V. L. Yu, M. Best, R. M. Vickers, A. Goetz, R. Wagner, H. Wicker, and A. Woo.** 1985. Nosocomial legionellosis uncovered in surgical patients with head and neck cancer: implications for epidemiologic reservoir and mode of transmission. *Lancet* **ii:**298–300.

72. **Jonas, D., W. M. Heinz-Georg, P. Matthes, D. Hartung, B. Jahn, F. D. Daschner, and B. Jansen.** 2000. Comparative evaluation of three different genotyping methods for investigation of nosocomial outbreaks of Legionnaires' disease in hospitals. *J. Clin. Microbiol.* **38:**2284–2291.

73. **Jonas, D., A. Rosenbaum, S. Weyrich, and S. Bhakdi.** 1995. Enzyme-linked immunoassay for detection of PCR-amplified DNA of legionellae in bronchoalveolar fluid. *J. Clin. Microbiol.* **33:**1247–1252.

74. **Joseph, C. A., J. M. Watson, T. G. Harrison, and C. L. R. Bartlett.** 1994. Nosocomial Legionnaires' disease in England and Wales. *Epidemiol. Infect.* **112:**329–345.

75. **Kazandjian, D., R. Chiew, and G. L. Gilbert.** 1997. Rapid diagnosis of *Legionella pneumophila* serogroup 1 infection

with the Binax enzyme immunoassay urinary antigen test. *J. Clin. Microbiol.* **35:**954–956.

76. **Kessler, H. H., F. F. Reinthaler, A. Pschaid, K. Pierer, B. Kleinhappl, E. Eber, and E. Marth.** 1993. Rapid detection of *Legionella* species in bronchoalveolar lavage fluids with the EnviroAmp Legionella PCR amplification and detection kit. *J. Clin. Microbiol.* **31:**3325–3328.

77. **Ko, Y.-Y., C.-H. Chen, C.-L. Lai, and R.-P. Perng.** 1996. Recurrent infection of *Legionella* pneumonia: a case report. *Chin. Med. J.* **57:**365–369.

78. **Kool, J. L., D. Bergmire-Sweat, J. C. Butler, E. W. Brown, D. J. Peabody, D. S. Massi, J. C. Carpenter, J. M. Pruckler, R. F. Benson, and B. S. Fields.** 1999. Hospital characteristics associated with colonization of water systems by *Legionella* and risk of nosocomial Legionnaires' disease: a cohort study of 15 hospitals. *Infect. Control Hosp. Epidemiol.* **20:**798–805.

79. **Kool, J. L., A. E. Fiore, C. M. Kioski, E. W. Brown, R. F. Benson, J. M. Pruckler, C. Glasby, J. C. Butler, G. D. Cage, J. C. Carpenter, R. M. Mandel, B. England, and R. F. Breiman.** 1998. More than ten years of unrecognized nosocomial transmission of Legionnaires' disease among transplant patients. *Infect. Control Hosp. Epidemiol.* **19:**898–904.

80. **Korvick, J., and V. L. Yu.** 1987. Legionnaires' disease: an emerging surgical problem. *Ann. Thorac. Surg.* **43:**341–347.

81. **Kuchta, J. M., S. J. States, J. E. McGlaughlin, J. H. Overmeyer, R. M. Wadowsky, A. M. McNamara, R. S. Wolford, and R. B. Yee.** 1985. Enhanced chlorine resistance of tap water-adapted *Legionella pneumophila* as compared with agar medium-passage strains. *J. Appl. Microbiol.* **50:**21–26.

82. **Lawrence, C., M. Reyrolle, S. Dubrou, F. Forey, B. Decludt, C. Goulvestre, P. Matsiota-Bernard, J. Etienne, and C. Nauciel.** 1999. Single clonal origin of a high proportion of *Legionella pneumophila* serogroup 1 isolates from patients and the environment in the area of Paris, France, over a 10-year period. *J. Clin. Microbiol.* **37:**2652–2655.

83. **Lawrence, C., E. Ronco, S. Dubrou, R. Leclero, C. Nauciel, and P. Matsiota-Bernard.** 1999. Molecular typing of *L. pneumophila* serogroup one isolates from patients and the nosocomial environment by arbitrarily primed PCR and pulsed-field gel electrophoresis. *J. Med. Microbiol.* **48:**327–333.

84. **Lee, T. C., R. M. Vickers, V. L. Yu, and M. M. Wagener.** 1993. Growth of 28 *Legionella* species on selective culture media: a comparative study. *J. Clin. Microbiol.* **31:**2761–2768.

85. **Lema, M., and A. Brown.** 1983. Electrophoretic characterization of soluble protein extracts of *Legionella pneumophila* and other members of the family *Legionellaceae*. *J. Clin. Microbiol.* **17:**1132–1140.

86. **Lepine, L. A., D. B. Jernigan, J. C. Butler, J. M. Pruckler, R. F. Benson, F. Kim, J. L. Hadler, M. L. Cartter, and B. S. Fields.** 1998. A recurrent outbreak of nosocomial Legionnaire's disease detected by urinary antigen testing: evidence for long-term colonization of a hospital plumbing system. *Infect. Control Hosp. Epidemiol.* **19:**905–910.

87. **Lin, A., J. E. Stout, J. D. Rihs, R. M. Vickers, and V. L. Yu.** 1999. Improved *Legionella* selective media by the addition of fluconazole: results of *in vitro* testing and clinical evaluation. *Diagn. Microbiol. Infect. Dis.* **34:**173–175.

88. **Lin, Y. E., J. E. Stout, and V. L. Yu.** 1998. Disinfection of water distribution systems for *Legionella*. *Semin. Respir. Infect.* **13:**147–159.

89. **Lin, Y. E., R. D. Vidic, J. E. Stout, and V. L. Yu.** 1998. *Legionella* in water distribution systems. *J. Am. Water Works Assoc.* **90:**112–121.

90. **Lo Presti, F., S. Riffard, F. Vandenesch, and J. Etienne.** 1998. Identification of *Legionella* species by random amplified polymorphic DNA profiles. *J. Clin. Microbiol.* **36:**3193–3197.

91. **Lowry, P. W., and L. S. Tompkins.** 1993. Nosocomial legionellosis: a review of pulmonary and extrapulmonary syndromes. *Am. J. Infect. Control* **21:**21–27.

92. **Luck, P. C., R. J. Birtles, and J. H. Helbig.** 1995. Correlation of MAb subgroups with genotype in closely related *Legionella pneumophila* serogroup 1 strains from a cooling tower. *J. Med. Microbiol.* **43:**50–54.

93. **Luttichau, H. R., C. Vinther, S. A. Uldum, J. Moller, M. Faber, and J. S. Jensen.** 1998. An outbreak of Pontiac fever among children following use of a whirlpool. *Clin. Infect. Dis.* **26:**1374–1378.

94. **Mahoney, F. J., C. W. Hoge, T. A. Farley, J. M. Barbaree, R. F. Breiman, R. Benson, and L. M. McFarland.** 1992. Community-wide outbreak of Legionnaires' disease associated with a grocery store mist machine. *J. Infect. Dis.* **165:**736–739.

95. **Maiwald, M., M. Schill, C. Stockinger, J. H. Helbig, P. C. Luck, W. Witzleb, and H. G. Sonntag.** 1995. Detection of *Legionella* DNA in human and guinea pig urine samples by the polymerase chain reaction. *Eur. J. Clin. Microbiol. Infect. Dis.* **14:**25–33.

96. **Marra, A., and H. A. Shuman.** 1992. Genetics of *Legionella pneumophila* virulence. *Annu. Rev. Genet.* **26:**51–69.

97. **Marrie, T. J., D. Haldane, and S. Macdonald.** 1991. Control of endemic nosocomial Legionnaires' disease by using sterile potable water for high risk patients. *Epidemiol. Infect.* **107:**591–605.

98. **Marston, B. J., H. B. Lipman, and R. F. Breiman.** 1994. Surveillance for Legionnaires' disease. Risk factors for morbidity and mortality. *Arch. Intern. Med.* **154:**2417–2422.

99. **Martin, S. J., S. L. Pendland, C. Chen, P. Schreckenberger, and L. H. Danziger.** 1996. In vitro synergy testing of macrolide-quinolone combinations against 41 clinical isolates of *Legionella*. *Antimicrob. Agents Chemother.* **40:**1419–1421.

100. **Martin, W. T., B. S. Fields, and L. C. Hutwagoner.** 1993. Comparison of culture and polymerase chain reaction to detect legionellae in environmental samples, p. 175. *In* J. M. Barbaree, R. F. Breiman, and A. P. Dufour (ed.), Legionella: *Current Status and Emerging Perspectives.* American Society for Microbiology, Washington, D.C.

101. **Matsiota-Bernard, P., E. Pitsouni, N. Legakis, and C. Nauciel.** 1994. Evaluation of commercial amplification kit for detection of *Legionella pneumophila* in clinical samples. *J. Clin. Microbiol.* **32:**1503–1505.

102. **McWhinney, P. H., P. L. Ragunathan, and T. J. Rowbotham.** 2000. Failure to produce detectable antibodies to *Legionella pneumophila* by an immunocompetent adult. *J. Infect. Dis.* **41:**91–92.

103. **Moffie, B. G., and R. P. Mouton.** 1988. Sensitivity and resistance of *Legionella pneumophila* to some antibiotics and combination of antibiotics. *J. Antimicrob. Chemother.* **22:**457–462.

104. **Monforte, R., R. Estruch, J. Vidal, R. Cervera, and A. Urbano-Marquez.** 1988. Delayed seroconversion in Legionnaires' disease. *Lancet* **ii:**513.

105. **Morrill, W. E., J. M. Barbaree, B. S. Fields, G. N. Sanden, and W. T. Martin.** 1990. Increased recovery of *Legionella micdadei* and *Legionella bozemanii* on buffered charcoal yeast extract agar supplemented with albumin. *J. Clin. Microbiol.* **28:**616–618.

106. **Muder, R. R., J. E. Stout, and V. L. Yu.** 2000. Nosocomial *Legionella micdadei* infection in transplant pa-

tients: fortune favors the prepared mind. *Am. J. Med.* **108:**346–348.

107. **Muder, R. R., V. L. Yu, and G. D. Fang.** 1989. Community-acquired Legionnaires' disease. *Semin. Respir. Infect.* **4:**32–39.

108. **Newsome, A. L., T. M. Scott, R. F. Benson, and B. S. Fields.** 1998. Isolation of an amoeba naturally harboring a distinctive *Legionella* species. *Appl. Environ. Microbiol.* **64:**1688–1693.

109. **Ng, V., L. Weir, M. K. York, and W. K. Hadley.** 1992. *Bordetella pertussis* versus non-*L. pneumophila Legionella* spp.: a continuing diagnostic challenge. *J. Clin. Microbiol.* **30:**3300–3301.

110. **Oliverio, M. J., M. A. Fisher, R. M. Vickers, V. L. Yu, and A. Menon.** 1991. Diagnosis of Legionnaires' disease by radioimmunoassay of *Legionella* antigen in pleural fluid. *J. Clin. Microbiol.* **29:**2893–2894.

111. **Orrison, L. H., W. F. Bibb, W. B. Cherry, and L. Thacker.** 1983. Determination of antigenic relationships among legionellae and non-legionellae by direct fluorescent-antibody and immunodiffusion tests. *J. Clin. Microbiol.* **17:**332–337.

112. **Pasculle, A. W.** 2000. Update on *Legionella*. *Clin. Microbiol. Newsl.* **22:**97–101.

113. **Pasculle, A. W., J. C. Feeley, R. J. Gibson, L. G. Cordes, R. L. Myerowitz, C. M. Patton, G. W. Gorman, C. L. Carmack, J. W. Ezzell, and J. N. Dowling.** 1980. Pittsburgh pneumonia agent: direct isolation from human lung tissue. *J. Infect. Dis.* **141:**727–732.

114. **Pinar, A., S. Ahkee, R. D. Miller, J. A. Rameriez, and J. T. Summersgill.** 1997. Use of heteroduplex analysis to classify legionellae on the basis of 5S rRNA gene sequences. *J. Clin. Microbiol.* **35:**1609–1611.

115. **Pine, L., P. S. Hoffman, G. B. Malcolm, R. F. Benson, and M. J. Franzus.** 1986. Role of keto acids and reduced oxygen-scavenging enzymes in the growth of *Legionella* species. *J. Clin. Microbiol.* **23:**33–42.

116. **Plouffe, J. F., T. M. File, and R. F. Breiman.** 1995. Reevaluation of the definition of Legionnaires' disease: use of the urinary antigen assay. *Clin. Infect. Dis.* **20:**1286–1291.

117. **Plouffe, J. F., L. R. Webster, and B. Hackman.** 1983. Relationship between colonization of hospital buildings with *Legionella pneumophila* and hot water temperatures. *Appl. Environ. Microbiol.* **46:**769–770.

118. **Pruckler, J. M., L. A. Mermel, and R. F. Benson.** 1995. Comparison of *Legionella pneumophila* isolates by arbitrarily primed PCR and pulsed-field gel electrophoresis: Analysis from seven epidemic investigations. *J. Clin. Microbiol.* **33:**2872–2875.

119. **Quaresima, T., and M. Castellani Pastoris.** 1992. Infezioni da *Legionella* sp. nel bambino. *Riv. Ital. Pediatr.* **18:**125–136.

120. **Ramirez, J. A., S. Ahkee, A. Tolentino, R. D. Miller, and J. T. Summersgill.** 1996. Diagnosis of *Legionella pneumophila*, *Mycoplasma pneumoniae*, or *Chlamydia pneumoniae* lower respiratory infection using the polymerase chain reaction on a single throat swab specimen. *Diagn. Microbiol. Infect. Dis.* **24:**7–14.

121. **Rantakokko-Jalava, K., and J. Jalava.** 2001. Development of conventional and real-time PCR assays for detection of *Legionella* DNA in respiratory specimens. *J. Clin. Microbiol.* **39:**2904–2910.

122. **Rello, J., E. Quintana, V. Ausina, A. Net, and G. Prats.** 1993. A three year study of severe community-acquired pneumonia with emphasis on outcome. *Chest* **103:**232–235.

123. **Rihs, J. D., V. L. Yu, J. J. Zuravleff, A. Goetz, and R. R. Muder.** 1985. Isolation of *Legionella pneumophila*

124. **Rogers, J., A. B. Dowsett, P. J. Dennis, J. V. Lee, and C. W. Keevil.** 1994. Influence of temperature and plumbing material selection on biofilm formation and growth of *Legionella pneumophila* in a model potable water system containing complex microbial flora. *Appl. Environ. Microbiol.* **60:**1585–1592.

125. **Roig, J., X. Aguilar, J. Ruiz, C. Domingo, E. Mesalles, J. Manterola, and J. Morera.** 1991. Comparative study of *Legionella pneumophila* and other nosocomial-acquired pneumonias. *Chest* **99:**344–350.

126. **Roig, J., C. Domingo, and J. Morera.** 1994. Legionnaires' disease. *Chest* **105:**1817–1825.

127. **Rowbotham, T. J.** 1986. Current views on the relationships between amoebae legionellae, and man. *Isr. J. Med. Sci.* **22:**678–689.

128. **Roy, C. R., K. Beger, and R. R. Isbert.** 1998. *Legionella pneumophila* DotA protein is required for early phagosome decisions that occur within minutes of bacterial uptake. *Mol. Microbiol.* **28:**663–674.

129. **Saunders, N. A., T. G. Harrison, A. Haththotuwa, N. Kachwalla, and A. G. Taylor.** 1990. A method for typing strains of *Legionella pneumophila* serogroup one by analysis of restriction fragment length polymorphisms. *J. Med. Microbiol.* **31:**45–55.

130. **Schoonmaker, D., T. Heimberger, and G. Birkhead.** 1992. Comparison of ribotyping and restriction enzyme analysis using pulsed-field gel electrophoresis for distinguishing *Legionella pneumophila* isolates obtained during a nosocomial outbreak. *J. Clin. Microbiol.* **30:**1491–1498.

131. **Selander, R. K., R. M. McKinney, T. S. Whittam, W. F. Bibb, D. J. Brenner, F. S. Nolte, and P. E. Pattison.** 1985. Genetic structure of populations of *Legionella pneumophila*. *J. Bacteriol.* **163:**1021–1037.

132. **Sonesson, A., E. Jantzen, K. Bryn, T. Tangen, J. Eng, and U. Zahringer.** 1994. Composition of 2,3-dihydroxy fatty acid-containing lipopolysaccharides from *Legionella israelensis*, *Legionella maceachernii*, and *Legionella micdadei*. *Microbiology* **140:**1261–1271.

133. **States, S. J., L. Conley, J. M. Kuchta, B. M. Oleck, M. J. Lipovich, R. S. Wolford, R. M. Wadowsky, A. M. McNamara, J. L. Sykora, and G. Keleti.** 1987. Survival and multiplication of *Legionella pneumophila* in municipal drinking water systems. *Appl. Environ. Microbiol.* **53:**979–986.

134. **Steele, T. W., C. Y. Moore, and N. Sangster.** 1990. Distribution of *Legionella longbeachae* serogroup 1 and other legionellae in potting soil in Australia. *Appl. Environ. Microbiol.* **56:**2984–2988.

135. **Stone, B. J., and Y. A. Kwaik.** 1998. Expression of multiple pili by *Legionella pneumophila*: identification and characterization of a type IV pilin gene and its role in adherence to mammalian and protozoan cells. *Infect. Immun.* **66:**1768–1775.

136. **Stout, J. E.** 1999. *Culture Methodology for* Legionella *Species.* [Online.] HC Information Resources, Inc., Fallbrook, Calif. http://www.hcinfo.com.

137. **Stout, J. E.** 2000. Laboratory diagnosis of Legionnaires' disease: the expanding role of the *Legionella* urinary antigen test. *Clin. Microbiol. Newsl.* **22:**62–64.

138. **Stout, J. E., Y. S. E. Lin, A. M. Goetz, and R. R. Muder.** 1998. Controlling *Legionella* in hospital water systems: experience with the superheat-and-flush method and copper-silver ionization. *Infect. Control Hosp. Epidemiol.* **19:**911–914.

139. **Stout, J. E., and V. L. Yu.** 1997. Current concepts: legionellosis. *N. Engl. J. Med.* **337:**682–687.

from blood with the BACTEC system: a prospective study yielding positive results. *J. Clin. Microbiol.* **22:**422–424.

140. **Stout, J. E., V. L. Yu, and M. Best.** 1985. Ecology of *Legionella pneumophila* within water distribution systems. *Appl. Environ. Microbiol.* **49:**221–228.

141. **Stout, J. E., V. L. Yu, P. Muraca, J. Joly, N. Troup, and L. S. Tompkins.** 1992. Potable water as the cause of sporadic cases of community-acquired Legionnaires' disease. *N. Engl. J. Med.* **326:**151–154.

142. **Straus, W. L., J. F. Plouffe, T. M. File, Jr., H. B. Lipman, B. H. Hackman, S. J. Salstrom, R. F. Benson, and R. F. Breiman.** 1996. Risk factors for domestic acquisition of Legionnaires' disease. *Arch. Intern. Med.* **156:**1685–1692.

143. **Struelens, M. J., N. Maes, F. Rost, A. Deplano, F. Jacobs, C. Liesnard, N. Bornstein, F. Grimont, S. Lauwers, and M. P. McIntyre.** 1992. Genotypic and phenotypic methods for the investigation of a hospital-acquired *Legionella pneumophila* outbreak and efficacy of control measures. *J. Infect. Dis.* **166:**22–30.

144. **Swanson, M. S., and B. K. Hammer.** 2000. *Legionella pneumophila* pathogenesis: a fateful journey from amoebae to macrophages. *Annu. Rev. Microbiol.* **54:**567–613.

145. **Ta, A. C., J. E. Stout, V. L. Yu, and M. M. Wagener.** 1995. Comparison of culture methods for monitoring *Legionella* species in hospital potable water systems and recommendations for standardization of such methods. *J. Clin. Microbiol.* **33:**2118–2123.

146. **Tan, J. S., T. M. File, Jr., L. P. DiPersio, R. Hamor, L. D. Saravolatz, and J. E. Stout.** 2001. Persistently positive culture results in a patient with community-acquired pneumonia due to *Legionella pneumophila.* *Clin. Infect. Dis.* **32:**1562–1566.

147. **Thomas, D. L., L. M. Mundy, and P. C. Tucker.** 1993. Hot tub legionellosis: Legionnaires' disease and pontiac fever after a point-source exposure to *Legionella pneumophila.* *Arch. Intern. Med.* **153:**2597–2599.

148. **Tison, D. L., D. H. Pope, W. B. Cherry, and C. B. Fliermans.** 1980. Growth of *Legionella pneumophila* in association with blue-green algae (cyanobacteria). *Appl. Environ. Microbiol.* **39:**456–459.

149. **Torres, A., J. Sera-Batlles, A. Ferrer, P. Jimenez, R. Celis, E. Cobo, and R. Rodriguez-Roisin.** 1991. Severe community-acquired pneumonia. Epidemiology and prognostic factors. *Am. Rev. Respir. Dis.* **144:**312–318.

150. **Valsangiacomo, C., F. Baggi, V. Gaia, T. Balmelli, R. Peduzzi, and J. C. Piffaretti.** 1995. Use of amplified fragment length polymorphisms in molecular typing of *Legionella pneumophila* and application to epidemiological studies. *J. Clin. Microbiol.* **33:**1716–1719.

151. **van Belkum, A., H. Mass, H. Verbrugh, and N. van Leeuwen.** 1996. Serotyping, ribotyping, PCR-mediated ribosomal 16S-23S spacer analysis, and arbitrarily primed PCR for epidemiological studies on *Legionella pneumophila.* *Res. Microbiol.* **147:**405–413.

152. **Venezia, R. A., M. D. Agresta, E. M. Hanley, K. Urquhart, and D. Schoonmaker.** 1994. Nosocomial legionellosis associated with aspiration of nasogastric feedings diluted in tap water. *Infect. Cont. Hosp. Epidemiol.* **15:**529–533.

153. **Vergis, E. N., E. Abbas, and V. L. Yu.** 2000. *Legionella* as a cause of severe pneumonia. *Semin. Respir. Infect.* **4:**295–304.

154. **Vergis, E. N., and V. L. Yu.** 1998. Legionellosis, p. 2235–2246. *In* A. P. Fishman, J. A. Elias, J. A. Fishman, M. A. Grippi, L. R. Kaiser, and R. N. Senior (ed.), *Fishman's Pulmonary Diseases and Disorders.* McGraw-Hill, New York, N.Y.

155. **Vergis, E. N., and V. L. Yu.** 1998. Macrolides are ideal for empiric therapy of community-acquired pneumonia in the immunocompetent host. *Semin. Respir. Infect.* **12:** 327–328.

156. **Vesey, G., P. J. Dennis, J. Lee, and A. A. West.** 1988. Further development of simple tests to differentiate the *Legionella.* *J. Appl. Bacteriol.* **65:**339–345.

157. **Vickers, R. M., A. Brown, and G. M. Garrity.** 1981. Dye-containing buffered charcoal yeast extract medium for the differentiation of members of the family *Legionellaceae.* *J. Clin. Microbiol.* **13:**380–382.

158. **Vickers, R. M., and V. L. Yu.** 1984. Clinical laboratory differentiation of *Legionellaceae* family members with pigment production and fluorescence on media supplemented with aromatic substrates. *J. Clin. Microbiol.* **19:**583–587.

159. **Vickers, R. M., V. L. Yu, S. S. Hanna, P. Muraca, W. Diven, N. Carmen, and F. B. Taylor.** 1987. Determinants of *Legionella pneumophila* contamination of water distribution systems: 15 hospital prospective study. *Infect. Control* **8:**357–363.

160. **Voss, L., K. S. Button, R. C. Lorenz, and O. H. Tuovinen.** 1986. *Legionella* contamination of a preoperational treatment plant. *J. Am. Water Works Assoc.* **78:**70–75.

161. **Wadowsky, R. M., and R. B. Yee.** 1985. Effect of non-*Legionellaceae* bacteria on the multiplication of *Legionella pneumophila* in potable water. *Appl. Environ. Microbiol.* **49:**1206–1210.

162. **Waite, R.** 1988. Confirmation of identity of legionellae by whole cell fatty-acid and isoprenoid quinone profiles, p. 69–101. *In* T. G. Harrison and A. G. Taylor (ed.), *A Laboratory Manual for* Legionella. John Wiley & Sons, Inc., Chichester, United Kingdom.

163. **Waterer, G. W., V. S. Baselski, and R. G. Wunderink.** 2001. *Legionella* and community-acquired pneumonia: a review of current diagnostic tests from a clinician's viewpoint. *Am. J. Med.* **110:**41–48.

164. **Wilkinson, H. W.** 1988. *Hospital Laboratory Diagnosis of* Legionella *Infections.* Centers for Disease Control, Atlanta, Ga.

165. **Wilkinson, H. W., and B. J. Fikes.** 1980. Slide agglutination tests for serogrouping *Legionella pneumophila* and atypical *Legionella*-like organisms. *J. Clin. Microbiol.* **11:**99–101.

166. **Wilkinson, I. J., N. Sangster, R. M. Ratcliff, P. A. Mugg, D. E. Davos, and J. A. Lanser.** 1990. Problems associated with identification of *Legionella* species from the environment and isolation of six possible new species. *Appl. Environ. Microbiol.* **56:**796–802.

167. **Winn, W. C., Jr., and A. W. Pasculle.** 1982. Laboratory diagnosis of infections caused by *Legionella* species. *Clin. Lab. Med.* **2:**343–369.

168. **Wright, J. B., M. A. Athar, T. M. van Olm, J. S. Wootliff, and J. S. Costerton.** 1989. Atypical legionellosis: isolation of *Legionella pneumophila* serogroup 1 from a patient with aspiration pneumonia. *J. Hosp. Infect.* **13:**187–190.

169. **Wright, J. B., I. Ruseska, M. Athar, S. Corbett, and J. W. Costerton.** 1989. *Legionella pneumophila* grows adherent to surfaces in vitro and in situ. *Infect. Control Hosp. Epidemiol.* **10:**408–415.

170. **Yu, V. L.** 1993. Could aspiration be the major mode of transmission for *Legionella? Am. J. Med.* **95:**13–15.

171. **Yu, V. L.** 1993. *Legionella* infections, p. 141–146. *In* H. D. Neu, L. S. Young, and S. H. Zinner (ed.), *The New Macrolides, Azalides, and Streptogramins.* Marcel Dekker, Inc., New York, N.Y.

172. **Yu, V. L., J. Plouffe, M. Castellani-Pastoris, J. E. Stout, M. Schousboe, A. Widmer, J. Summersgill, T. File, C. Heath, D. Paterson, and A. Chereshky.** 2002. Distribution of *Legionella* species and serogroups isolated by culture in patients with sporadic community-acquired legionellosis: an international collaborative survey. *J. Infect. Dis.* **186:**127–128.

Bartonella and *Afipia*

DAVID F. WELCH AND LEONARD N. SLATER

53

TAXONOMY

The genus *Bartonella* is named for A. L. Barton, who described the intraerythrocytic bacterium, *Bartonella bacilliformis*, in 1909. The genus *Afipia* is named for the Armed Forces Institute of Pathology, Washington, D.C., where *Afipia felis* was first described as an agent of cat scratch disease. *Bartonella* and *Afipia* are members of the class *Alphaproteobacteria* (57), order *Rhizobiales*. *Bartonella* is the only genus of the family *Bartonellaceae*. *Afipia* is one of seven genera belonging to the family *Bradyrhizobiaceae*. The species formerly within *Rochalimaea* and *Grahamella* are now in the genus *Bartonella* (6, 9), and in addition there are several newly recognized species: *B. koehlerae* (24), *B. alsatica* (31), *B. tribocorum* (32), *B. birtlesii* (21), *B. schoenbuchii* (20), "*B. weissii*" (7), and "*B. washoensis*" (7). *B. vinsonii* is now divided into the three subspecies *vinsonii*, *berkhoffii*, and *arupensis* (42, 72). Closely related to *Bartonella*, based on 16S rRNA similarity, are *Brucella* and *Agrobacterium*. Phylogenetic data place *Bartonella* and *Afipia* in the same order with *Methylobacterium* and *Roseomonas*, examples of other related genera that may also be encountered in clinical specimens. The *Rickettsiaceae* (*Rickettsia* and *Ehrlichia*), which originally contained *Rochalimaea*, are more distantly related (9).

DESCRIPTION OF THE GENERA

The genus *Bartonella* is currently composed of 16 validated and 2 provisionally described species and 3 subspecies (Table 1). The type species of the genus is *B. bacilliformis*. *Bartonella* spp. are small (0.6- by 1.0-µm) gram-negative rods that are often slightly curved. They are oxidase negative, aerobic, and highly fastidious. They do not produce acid from carbohydrates. All members of the genus can be cultured on enriched (blood-containing) bacteriologic culture medium in the presence of air or 5% CO_2. For this and the other medically important species, the optimal temperature varies from 25–30°C (*B. bacilliformis*) to 35–37°C (*B. henselae*, *B. quintana*, and *B. elizabethae*). *B. clarridgeiae*, *B. grahamii*, and *B. vinsonii* subspp. *berkhoffii* and *arupensis* are potentially pathogenic, and they are variable with respect to optimal growth temperatures. Some members of the genus are motile. *B. bacilliformis* and *B. clarridgeiae* have flagella. Electron microscopy of *B. henselae* and *B. quintana*

does not reveal flagella, but these species typically display twitching motility in wet mounts due to the presence of pili. The pili are also associated with marked cytoadherence and may mediate specific interaction with host endothelial cells and erythrocytes, leading to epi- or intracellular localization.

The genus *Afipia* consists of *A. felis* (type species of the genus), *A. broomeae*, *A. clevelandensis*, and several unnamed *Afipia* genospecies (8). They differ from *Bartonella* spp. in that they are urease and oxidase positive. Most *Afipia* strains produce acid from D-xylose. Their generation time is usually shorter and they are less fastidious nutritionally than *Bartonella* spp. *A. felis* is also a facultatively intracellular pathogen. The optimal temperature for growth is 30°C.

NATURAL HABITATS

Limited to the Andes mountain region of South America, *B. bacilliformis* had received little attention outside its zone of endemicity in recent years until related bacteria of the genus formerly named *Rochalimaea* were found to be pathogens in patients with AIDS (67, 68, 74). Its strictly regional occurrence is due to the limited distribution of its sandfly (*Lutzomyia verrucarum*) vector. *B. quintana* is globally distributed. Outbreaks of trench fever (also known as Volhynia fever, Meuse fever, His-Werner disease, shinbone fever, shank fever, and quintan or 5-day fever) have been focal and widely separated, often associated with conditions of poor sanitation and personal hygiene which may predispose to exposure to *Pediculus humanus*, the only known vector of *B. quintana*. Nonhuman vertebrate reservoirs have not been identified for *B. bacilliformis* or *B. quintana*. The species derived from the genus *Grahamella* (*B. grahamii*, *B. talpae*, *B. peromysci*, *B. taylorii*, and *B. doshiae*) occur almost exclusively in nonhuman vertebrate reservoirs. These and the newer species *B. tribocorum*, *B. alsatica*, *B. birtlesii* and *B. schoenbuchii* are species specific with respect to erythrocytic parasitism of rodents, birds, fish, or other animals. In addition, coinfection by different *Bartonella* species or with the agents *Borrelia burgdorferi* and *Babesia microti* may occur frequently in naturally infected mice and cats (33).

B. henselae is globally endemic; serologic studies indicate that infection of domestic cats is worldwide, with the prev-

TABLE 1 Members of the genus *Bartonella*

Known to be pathogenic in humans	Unlikely to be transmitted to humans
B. bacilliformis	B. vinsonii subsp. vinsonii
B. henselae	B. taylorii
B. quintana	B. doshiae
B. elizabethae	B. tribocorum
B. clarridgeiae	B. alsatica
B. vinsonii subsp. berkhoffii	B. birtlesii
B. vinsonii subsp. arupensis	B. koehlerae
B. grahamii	B. peromysci
	B. schoenbuchii
	B. talpae
	"B. weissii"
	"B. washoensis"

alence of antibodies in cats being higher in warm, humid climates where cat fleas are abundant (13, 37, 76). Rates of bacteremia in cats can vary, even between geographically close locales, but generally tend to be higher among feral animals in any given locale. *B. henselae* bacteremia has been documented in healthy domestic cats which have been specifically associated with bacillary angiomatosis (BA) or typical cat scratch disease (CSD) in their human contacts. Transmission of *B. henselae* to humans has been linked to cats in numerous studies. The major arthropod vector of *B. henselae* is the cat flea, *Ctenocephalides felis* (14). Ticks are also occasionally involved (49). Fleas appear to serve primarily as vectors for cat-to-cat transmission; their contribution to human infection is not yet defined. *B. clarridgeiae* and *B. koehlerae* are recognized as agents of asymptomatic infection of cats (15, 28, 30). *B. clarridgeiae*, like *A. felis*, appears occasionally to be transmitted to humans (41). However, much less is known about their full geographic distribution or potential vectors. *A. felis* is apparently not a common zoonotic agent among cats or dogs. Although dogs have been linked epidemiologically to CSD, one study failed to implicate them in the epidemiology of CSD (22). Like *B. clarridgeiae*, the other identified *Bartonella* species appear to infect mainly birds, reptiles, and nonhuman mammals. Ticks may well be vectors of their transmission (12), and humans may become rare incidental hosts of infection. Recent evidence suggests that hospital water supplies may be a reservoir of *Afipia* spp. (44).

CLINICAL SIGNIFICANCE

Oroya Fever and Verruga Peruana: *B. bacilliformis*

The suspected link between Oroya fever and verruga peruana was confirmed tragically in 1885 by Daniel Carrión, a medical student who had himself injected with material from a verruga and subsequently died of Oroya fever. The eponym "Carrión's disease" has since denoted the full spectrum of *B. bacilliformis* infection. Acute *B. bacilliformis* infection results in bacteremic illness (Oroya fever), often with severe extravascular hemolysis, anemia, and an increased susceptibility to opportunistic infection. Descriptions from the late 19th and early 20th centuries suggest that without antimicrobial therapy, there could be a high fatality rate among persons lacking endemic exposure. Newer data suggest that even in areas where the infection is not endemic, the majority of *B. bacilliformis* infections

may be asymptomatic or mild (43). The late-stage (within months) manifestation known as verruga peruana is characterized by nodular skin lesions with a variety of shapes and hues; mucosal and internal lesions can also occur (62). Histologically, the infection is associated with neovascular proliferation, and bacteria are evident in the affected tissue. Such lesions may develop at one site while receding at another, persist for months to years, and eventually become fibrotic with involution. At this stage, the prognosis of these patients is good.

Bacteremic Illness, Endocarditis: Primarily *B. quintana* and *B. henselae*

In recent years, *B. quintana* bacteremic infection (trench fever) outside of patients with human immunodeficiency virus (HIV) infection has been identified sporadically, mainly in homeless persons in North America and Europe (35). Trench fever is characterized by a spectrum of self-limited clinical patterns. In the shortest form, a single bout of fever lasts 4 to 5 days. In the more typical periodic form, there are three to five, sometimes up to eight, febrile paroxysms, each lasting about 5 days. The continuous form is manifested by 2 to 6 weeks of uninterrrupted fever. Afebrile infection is the least common form.

B. quintana or *B. henselae* bacteremia in HIV-infected persons develops insidiously, involving recurring fevers, sometimes headache, and hepatomegaly, but other localizing symptoms are often lacking. By way of contrast, *B. henselae* bacteremia in persons not infected with HIV more often presents with abrupt onset of fever which persists or becomes relapsing. *B. henselae* bacteremia can evolve into long-term asymptomatic persistence. *Bartonella* spp. may well represent important pathogens in "culture-negative" endocarditis and should be added to the list of fastidious gram-negative bacteria which have been similarly implicated, i.e., the HACEK group, consisting of *Haemophilus*, *Actinobacillus*, *Cardiobacterium*, *Eikenella*, and *Kingella*.

Bacillary Angiomatosis and Peliosis: *B. quintana* and *B. henselae*

Bacillary angiomatosis (BA, also referred to as epithelioid angiomatosis or bacillary epithelioid angiomatosis) is a disorder of neovascular proliferation that was originally described as involving skin and regional lymph nodes of HIV-infected persons (16, 40, 70). It has since been demonstrated to be able to involve a variety of internal organs including the liver, spleen, bone, brain, lungs, and bowel and to occur in other immunocompromised as well as immunocompetent hosts. In bacillary peliosis, which involves the liver and/or the spleen in HIV-infected persons and other immunosuppressed persons, the affected tissues contain numerous blood-filled, partially endothelial cell-lined cystic structures (47). Clumps of bacilli may be identified by Warthin-Starry staining. Either species can cause cutaneous lesions, but subcutaneous and osseous lesions are more often associated with *B. quintana* and hepatosplenic lesions are associated only with *B. henselae* (38).

Cat Scratch Disease: *B. henselae*, *B. clarridgeiae*, and *Afipia felis*

The various manifestations comprising CSD have been recognized over the past 100 years, but "la maladie des griffes du chat" was not defined as a syndrome until 1950 (19). CSD then remained an infection in search of an agent for more than 40 years. Hence, most cases have been identified by clinical and pathologic criteria, supplemented by reactions to unstandardized skin test antigens in some cases. It is reasonable to ascribe the majority of CSD cases to *B. henselae* based on the numerous lines of evidence developed in recent years. However, it remains likely that occasional CSD cases are caused by other agents, such as *A. felis* (1, 8) or *B. clarridgeiae* (41). Other *Afipia* spp. have been isolated from only skeletal and/or pleuropulmonary sites of one patient each and not in the setting of CSD; their roles as pathogens remain speculative.

CSD is the most commonly recognized manifestation of human infection with *Bartonella*. In the United States, the number of CSD cases is estimated to approach 25,000 annually (34). In typical CSD (about 89% of cases), a cutaneous papule or pustule develops at a site of inoculation (usually a scratch or bite) within a week after contact with an animal (most commonly a kitten). Regional lymphadenopathy develops in 1 to 7 weeks. About one-third of patients have fever, and about one-sixth develop lymph node suppuration. Histopathologic examination of nodes reveals a mixture of inflammatory reactions including granulomata and stellate necrosis.

Atypical CSD (about 11%) includes Parinaud's oculoglandular syndrome (self-limited granulomatous conjunctivitis and ipsilateral, usually preauricular, lymphadenitis) and various other presentations (51), including self-limited granulomatous hepatitis and splenitis, retinitis, and encephalitis. In recent years, serologic testing has suggested that some cases of mononucleosis-like syndromes and fevers of undetermined origin may be ascribed to atypical CSD (36, 52). The importance of accurate history regarding animal exposure cannot be overemphasized when evaluating a patient with findings consistent with one of these syndromes. Fortunately, in most CSD cases, whether typical or atypical, spontaneous resolution occurs in weeks to months. Beyond Parinaud's oculoglandular syndrome, other ophthalmologic manifestations of *B. henselae* infection have been recognized (17). Neuroretinitis manifests as sudden loss of visual acuity. The most common retinal manifestation results in a macular exudate (macular star formation). Like other manifestations of CSD, ocular complications are usually self-limited. They warrant antimicrobial therapy, however, because of association with bacteremia and vision loss.

HIV-Associated Neurologic Syndromes

B. henselae and *B. quintana* have been implicated in a small proportion of cases of HIV-associated brain lesions, meningoencephalitis, encephalopathy, or neuropsychiatric disease which cannot be ascribed to other causes. Intracerebral BA was first recognized in 1990 (69). *B. henselae* has also been identified by immunofluorescence staining and by PCR amplification postmortem in the brains of AIDS patients with dementia and with an elevated ratio of cerebrospinal fluid to serum *B. henselae*-reactive antibody (58). A small fraction of cases of HIV-associated dementia or neuropsychological decline may result from *Bartonella* infections and therefore may be potentially treatable with antibiotics.

COLLECTION, TRANSPORT, AND STORAGE OF SPECIMENS

The specimen source of most isolates of *Bartonella* and *Afipia* spp. is blood or tissue. Approaches typically used for recovery of other pathogens from such sites are generally suitable (see chapters 6 and 20), although the fastidious nature of these organisms requires that precautions be taken to minimize the interval from collection to processing. If storage of specimens prior to culture is necessary, they should be kept frozen at −20°C or below. A controlled study of the effects of blood collection and handling methods has shown that blood specimens which were collected from *B. henselae*-infected cats into both EDTA and Isolator (Wampole, Cranbury, N.J.) blood lysis tubes yielded a good recovery and that blood collected into tubes containing EDTA can be plated after 26 days at −65°C with no loss of sensitivity (10). *Bartonella* spp. are broadly susceptible to antimicrobial agents in vitro, so specimens should be collected prior to antimicrobial therapy, especially with the tetracyclines and macrolides. *B. henselae* is also inhibited by concentrations of sodium polyanethol sulfonate (SPS) that are found in blood culture media. Addition of agents that neutralize SPS toxicity (e.g., gelatin) or use of resin-containing media (primarily to lyse erythrocytes) is another precaution that should be taken if blood is cultured in commercially designed blood culture systems. Lytic blood culture systems (e.g., Isolator) combine the protective effect of free hemoglobin against SPS toxicity with the release of intracellular organisms.

Collection of tissue from affected lymph nodes by fine-needle aspiration (FNA) is a less invasive alternative to biopsy. While many investigators have found FNA samples to be insufficient for DNA amplification of infectious agents, Avidor et al. (2) have developed an accurate PCR method for diagnosis of CSD from FNA specimens. A further advantage is the ability to use glass microscope slides for collecting FNA (or primary-lesion) specimens, which may also be stored and shipped at room temperature. DNA is extracted from the specimen spotted on a slide and then purified with a QIAmp Blood Kit (Qiagen; Hilden, Germany, and Valencia, Calif.) followed by PCR.

ISOLATION PROCEDURES

Direct Examination

Although stained blood films have been used to detect intraerythrocytic *B. bacilliformis* in patients with Oroya fever, the magnitude of bacteremia associated with the other species is usually too low for this technique to be practical. Means of direct examination that may prove useful include Warthin-Starry silver staining of fixed tissue sections (Fig. 1) and detection of organisms in tissue by using an immunocytochemical labeling technique (60); however, reagents for immunocytochemical labeling are not widely available. Bacilli may be demonstrable by Warthin-Starry staining during the early stages of lymphadenopathy in CSD but typically not during the later granulomatous stage of inflammation. Successful staining of organisms in tissue by the Warthin-Starry method also depends on careful attention to details of the procedure (see chapter 27). Critical steps include those of washing glassware in potassium dichromate-sulfuric acid solution, making the developer from solutions heated separately at 54 to 56°C (and maintained at this temperature after they are mixed) for 30 min, and then using the developer as soon as it is mixed.

Direct detection of *Bartonella* spp. is also possibly by amplification of DNA from tissue, pus, or skin lesions. A gene fragment specific for either citrate synthase or a heat shock protein of *B. henselae* is demonstrable by PCR in the

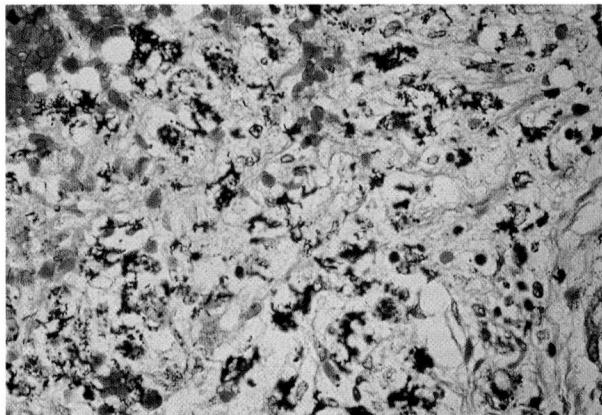

FIGURE 1 Warthin-Starry silver stain of a liver tissue section containing clusters of *B. henselae*. Magnification, ×530.

majority of patients with CSD (1, 66). Species-specific restriction fragment length polymorphism with a 16S rRNA fragment has been successfully applied with various clinical specimens (53). Amplification of rRNA with universal primers followed by direct nucleotide sequence analysis of the amplification product or hybridization with a specific probe is another, more sensitive but more laborious approach. These tests are performed by a few reference laboratories or academic centers.

Culture

Since the majority of isolates require more than 7 days of incubation before they can be detected, routine bacterial culture protocols usually do not allow *Bartonella* spp. to be detected. Attempts to isolate *Bartonella* spp. may be driven by the clinical picture, but throughout the spectrum of manifestations, many symptoms are not distinctive enough to guide the diagnosis and thus to inform the laboratory that special cultures are needed. If clinically directed culturing is relied on to detect *Bartonella* spp., it is indicated in the settings of atypical CSD (cultures are not recommended for diagnosis of most cases of CSD); fever of unknown origin with history of cat exposure; fever, lymphadenitis, or encephalitis of unknown origin in the immunocompromised patient; and BA-peliosis. Culture protocols designed to yield other slowly growing organisms (for example, *Histoplasma capsulatum* or *Mycobacterium avium* complex on noninhibitory media) can also result in the recovery of *Bartonella* spp.

A. felis and *Bartonella* spp. also have been isolated (from lymph node biopsy samples or aspirates) by using various cell lines. HeLa cell or primary cell cultures of human monocytes support the growth of *A. felis*, and *B. henselae* and *B. quintana* grow in endothelial cell cultures. In both systems, elongated pleomorphic organisms become visible in Gimenez-stained (see chapter 27) preparations 72 h after inoculation of the cell cultures. In some instances, coculture with a eukaryotic cell line may be a more sensitive isolation method than agar techniques. LaScola and Raoult (45) found that subculture of blood culture broth into shell vials yielded significantly more isolates of *B. henselae* or *B. quintana* than did a standard bacteriologic method. A defined cell-free medium has also been described which permits the recovery of both *Afipia* and *Bartonella* spp. (75). In general, any protocol designed to recover *Bartonella* spp.

would also be adequate for recovery of *Afipia* spp. because the latter is less fastidious.

Blood

Cultures of samples from patients with infective endocarditis due to *Bartonella* spp. are rarely positive, but the organism can be recovered from blood of patients with other bacteremic conditions. Direct plating (Isolator) or broth-based systems can be adapted for detection of *Bartonella* spp. Isolator-processed blood should be plated on enriched (chocolate- or blood-containing) medium incubated at 35 to 37°C under conditions of 5 to 10% CO_2 and >40% humidity. The optimal handling of blood for recovery of *Bartonella* spp. probably involves the use of the Isolator in conjunction with freshly prepared rabbit blood (5 to 7%) heart-infusion agar plates. For optimal growth, the medium should be as freshly prepared as possible. Plates can be sealed with Parafilm or Shrink Seal after the first 24 h of incubation to preserve the moisture content of the medium. Such plates usually can be incubated for up to 30 days without undergoing noticeable deterioration. Considering that the length of time required for detection of *Bartonella* spp. allows other slowly growing pathogens including *Mycobacterium tuberculosis* to grow on the same plates, appropriate safety precautions should be taken with positive cultures.

Alternative approaches to use of the Isolator include the use of a broth-based or biphasic culture system. Improved growth has been obtained in brucella broth supplemented with hemin (250 g/ml) and peptic digest of blood (8% Fildes reagent), but this technique has been applied primarily to propagation rather than primary isolation (65). Similarly, isolates can be propagated on buffered charcoal yeast extract medium, but this is not recommended for primary isolation of *Bartonella* spp. whereas it may be a practical approach for recovery of *Afipia* spp. *B. henselae* has been isolated in the biphasic Septi-Chek system (Roche Diagnostics, Nutley, N.J.) after prolonged incubation in excess of 40 days. Evidence of growth, if any, in the broth phase is given by the presence of a pellicle or adherent film on the glass surface. Biphasic media reportedly serve to isolate *A. felis* (26), but experience to date is so limited that methods of choice, with the possible exception of the tissue culture protocol of Birkness et al. (5), cannot be stated with certainty.

Bartonella spp. usually grow best on solid or semisolid media. In broth, they often do not produce turbidity or convert enough oxidizable substrate to CO_2 for CO_2 detection-based blood culture systems to indicate growth. However, several isolates have been initially detected using BACTEC and resin-containing media combined with acridine orange staining at the termination of a 7-day incubation period, with recovery subsequently achieved by subculture to solid media.

Tissue

B. henselae and *B. quintana* have been isolated from liver, spleen, lymph node, and skin after homogenization either by direct plating or by cocultivation with an endothelial cell line (38). While the cocultivation method may be more successful in recovering organisms from specimens such as tissue, it is not practical for most microbiology laboratories. Freshly prepared heart infusion agar containing 5 or 10% defibrinated rabbit or horse blood supports better growth of most strains than do other media such as chocolate or 5% sheep blood, although the last two have been used successfully. Other necessary conditions include a humid atmosphere and incubation at 35 to 37°C for 3 to 4 weeks. *B. bacilliformis* and *Afipia* spp. have a lower (25 to 30°C) optimal temperature for growth. Selective culture techniques have not been developed, and so recovery of isolates from certain specimens such as skin may be impossible if indigenous or contaminating flora members are present. The medium (modified RPMI 1640) described by Wong et al. (75) may also be useful for recovery of *B. henselae* from both tissue and blood.

IDENTIFICATION

Bartonella spp.

Colonies of *Bartonella* spp. are of two morphologic types: (i) irregular, raised, whitish, rough ("cauliflower," "molar tooth," or "verrucous"), and dry in appearance or (ii) smaller, circular, tan, and moist in appearance, tending to pit and adhere to the agar. Both types are usually present in the same culture (Fig. 2). The degree of colonial heterogeneity varies by species and by strain, with *B. henselae* typically being characterized by a greater proportion of rough colonies than *B. quintana*, which may even appear as uniformly smooth in primary cultures. Repeated subcultures of *B. henselae* tend to have increasing proportions of smooth colonies. Cultures of *B. henselae* on blood agar produce an odor similar to the caramel odor (diacetyl) produced by the "*Streptococcus milleri*" group. The Gram stain of a colony reveals small, faintly staining, gram-negative, slightly curved rods resembling *Campylobacter, Helicobacter,* or *Haemophilus*. Cells, especially those of *B. henselae*, are very autoadherent, as can be demonstrated by attempting to scrape colonies off a culture plate with a loop. In a wet mount, there is twitching motility of cells. These features, plus a lengthy (>7-day) incubation before the appearance of colonies and negative catalase and oxidase reactions, are sufficient for presumptive identification of *B. henselae* or *B. quintana*. Additional methods may be employed to confirm the identity of isolates, or isolates may be referred to a laboratory experienced with *Bartonella* spp. for confirmatory identification. Although not widely available, a reliable method is immunofluorescence with antisera monospecific for the individual species of *Bartonella* (46). Characteriza-

tion using conventional tests may also produce results that identify the *Bartonella* spp. and distinguish them from *A. felis* (Table 2).

Motility

Isolates most likely to be encountered, i.e., *B. henselae* or *B. quintana*, do not possess flagella but do produce a twitching motion when suspended in saline and examined microscopically under a coverslip. This motility is presumably related to adherence, with both features being mediated by fine fimbriae (pili) that are visible under the electron microscope in negative-stained preparations.

Cellular Fatty Acid Composition

Determination of cellular fatty acid composition by gas-liquid chromatography is outlined in chapter 14. Fatty acid methyl esters are prepared from cells harvested after 7 days of incubation at 35°C in 5% CO_2 on plates containing 5% rabbit blood heart infusion agar. Other media may not provide comparable results. This approach is useful in identifying and distinguishing *Bartonella* spp. in that they have relatively simple gas-liquid chromatography profiles consisting mainly of $C_{18:1}$, $C_{18:0}$, and $C_{16:0}$ acids. *B. elizabethae* contains a greater amount of $C_{17:0}$ than the other species. An unusual branched-chain fatty acid (11-methyloctadec-12-enoic acid) is found in *Afipia* spp. (8) but not in *Bartonella* spp.

Identification Kits

Although none of the various commercially available identification systems contain *Bartonella* spp. in their databases, the RapID ANA II, Rapid ID 32 A, and MicroScan rapid anaerobe systems have been used as aids to identification. With the MicroScan rapid anaerobe panel and careful adjustment of inoculum size, it is possible to distinguish *B. henselae* and *B. quintana* based on biotype codes derived from the reactions in this panel (73). If the inoculum size used in performing the MicroScan tests is equivalent to a McFarland no. 3 standard, the biotype codes usually obtained are 10077640 (*B. henselae*), 10073640 (*B. quintana*), and 10077240 (*B. bacilliformis*). Difficulty in separating *B. quintana* from *B. henselae* occurs when inocula heavier than McFarland no. 3 are used in these panels. In other systems, such as API, the biochemical reactivity of *B. quintana* and *B. henselae* has been enhanced by addition of 100 μg of hemin per ml to test media (23).

Afipia Species

Afipia spp. can be identified based on conventional phenotypic tests. Because they exhibit weaker growth at 35 than 30°C, incubations should be carried out at the latter temperature. Colonies develop at 72 h on blood agar or on buffered charcoal yeast extract agar. They are greyish white, glistening, convex, and opaque. Delayed, weak growth of *A. clevelandensis* may occur on MacConkey agar. Biochemical characteristics useful in differentiation among the *Afipia* and *Bartonella* spp. are shown in Table 2.

Species and Strain Identification by Molecular Techniques

Several molecular techniques for comparing isolates and a few for distinguishing species of *Bartonella* have been described. One of the original methods was that of Matar et al. (54), a PCR-based restriction fragment length polymorphism method for subtyping of isolates of *B. henselae*. Vari-

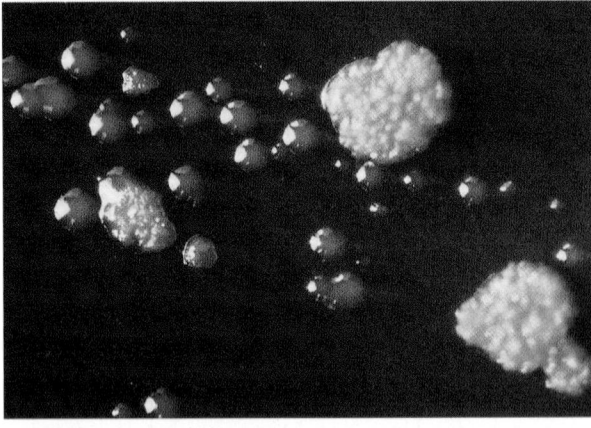

FIGURE 2 *B. henselae* after 7 days of incubation on chocolate agar, showing heterogeneity of colonies. Magnification, ×21.

TABLE 2 Differential characteristics of selected *Bartonella* species and *A. felis*[a]

Characteristic	B. bacilliformis	B. quintana	B. henselae	B. elizabethae	B. clarridgeiae	B. grahamii	B. vinsonii subsp. vinsonii	B. vinsonii subsp. berkhoffii	B. vinsonii subsp. arupensis	A. felis
Optimal growth temp (°C)	25–30	35–37	35–37	35–37	35–37	35–37	35–37	35–37	35–37	25–30
Growth in nutrient broth	−	v	−	−	−	−	−	−	−	+
Growth on heart infusion agar with X factor	−	v	−	+	−	−	v	−	+	+
Hemolysis	−	−	−	w	−	−	−	−	−	−
Growth in <10 days	+	+	v	+	+	+	+	+	+	+
Oxidase	−	v	v	−	−	−	v	−	−	+
Catalase	+	−	v	−	−	−	v	v	−	+
Nitrate reduction	−	−	−	−	−	−	−	−	−	+
Indole	−	−	−	−	−	−	−	−	−	−
Urease	−	−	−	−	−	−	−	−	−	+
Glucose oxidation or fermentation	−	−	−	−	−	−	−	−	−	−
Voges-Proskauer	−	−	−	−	−	+	−	NA	NA	NA
p-Nitrophenyl-β-D-galactopyranosidase	−	−	−	−	−	−	−	−	−	NA
p-Nitrophenyl-α-D-galactopyranosidase	−		−	−		−	−	−	−	NA
bis-p-Nitrophenylphosphatase	+	v	+	+	NA	NA	+	+	+	NA
p-Nitrophenyl-N-acetyl-β-D-glucosaminidase	−	−	−	−	−	−	−	−	−	NA
p-Nitrophenyl-α-D-glucopyranosidase	−	−	−	−	−	−	−	−	−	NA
p-Nitrophenyl-β-D-glucopyranosidase	−	−	−	−	−	−	−	−	−	NA
p-Nitrophenylphosphatase	NA	−	−	−	NA	NA	−	−	−	NA
p-Nitrophenyl-α-L-fucopyranosidase	−	−	−	−	−	−	−	−	−	NA
p-Nitrophenyl-α-D-mannopyranosidase	−	−	−	−	−	−	−	−	−	NA
L-Leucine-β-naphthylamidase	+	+	+	+	NA	+	+	+	+	NA
DL-Methionine-β-naphthylamidase	+	+	+	+	NA	NA	+	+	w	NA
L-Lysine-β-naphthylamidase (alkaline)	+	+	+	+	NA	NA	+	+	+	NA
L-Lysine-β-naphthylamidase (acidic)	+	−	+	w	NA	NA	−	+	−	NA
Glycylglycine-β-naphthylamidase	+	+	+	+	NA	NA	+	+	+	NA
Glycine-β-naphthylamidase	+	+	+	+	+	NA	+	+	+	NA
L-Proline-β-naphthylamidase	+	+	+	+	+	v	v	+	−	NA
L-Arginine-β-naphthylamidase	+	+	+	+	+	NA	+	+	+	NA
L-Pyrrolindonyl-β-naphthylamidase	−	−	−	−	NA	NA	−	−	−	NA
L-Tryptophan-β-naphthylamidase	+	+	+	+	NA	NA	+	+	+	NA
3-Indoxylphosphatase	+	−	−	−	+	−	+	+	+	NA
Flagella	+	+	+	−	+	−	−	−	−	+
Twitching motility	−	−	+	−	−	−	−	−	−	
Major cellular fatty acids (CFA) constituting >80% of total CFA	C18:1ω7C, C16:0, C16:1ω7C	C18:1ω7C, C16:0, C18:0	C18:1ω7C, C18:0, C16:0	C18:1ω7C, C17:0, C16:0	C18:1ω7C, C16:0, C18:0	NA	C18:1ω7C, C18:0, C16:0, C17:0	C18:1ω7C, C18:0, C16:0	C18:1ω7C, C18:0, C16:0, C17:0	C18:1ω7C, C19:0CYC, CBR19:1

[a] +, positive; −, negative; w, weakly positive; v, strains vary; NA, data not available.

ants of *B. henselae* have also been found among bacteremic isolates from cats (and their owners) by using enterobacterial repetitive intergenic consensus PCR (39) and sodium dodecyl sulfate-polyacrylamide gel electrophoresis (63). Newer approaches that can be used to identify the pathogenic species of *Bartonella* include the PCR genomic fingerprinting technique of Handley and Regnery (29). A selective amplification of restriction endonuclease-cleaved fragments results in a series of amplicons that are resolved by polyacrylamide gel electrophoresis.

SEROLOGIC TESTS

Serologic testing is becoming a mainstay of diagnosis, particularly for CSD and central nervous system infection. Since culturing of *Bartonella* spp. is difficult and time-consuming, such alternative means of identifying the infectious agents are important. However, serologic cross-reactions can occur, most notably with *Coxiella burnetii* and *Chlamydia* spp. and between *Bartonella* spp. Human antibody responses to *Bartonella* species have been measured by a variety of techniques. Tests for *B. henselae* and, in some cases, other *Bartonella* spp. are performed by the Centers for Disease Control and Prevention, and many state and commercial reference laboratories. Kits are available in Europe, but not in the United States.

B. bacilliformis

Enzyme immunoassay (EIA) utilizing a complex antigen preparation to reduce cross-reactions may be the most sensitive test for detecting immunoglobulin G (IgG) antibodies among endemically exposed persons. An IgG immunoblot assay using a simple sonic lysate antigen has a reported 94% sensitivity for chronic infection but only 70% sensitivity for acute infection; these sensitivities come at the expense of optimal specificity (50). An IgG immunofluorescence assay has reported sensitivities for acute disease and the convalescent phase of 82 and 93%, respectively, but substantial cross-reaction with other *Bartonella* species occurs (11). IgM antibodies can be detected by immunofluorescence in samples from persons with active Oroya fever as well as some persons without blood smear evidence of acute bacteremic infection.

B. quintana and B. henselae

Prior to the discovery of *B. henselae* and development of assays for it, EIA and radioimmunoprecipitation were comparable and both were deemed superior to hemagglutination or immunofluorescence assays in sensitivity. When the same EIA was used, all patients in a small series of persons with acute primary or relapsed trench fever had measurable, although often low, levels of anti-*B. quintana* antibodies. Since the consolidation and expansion of the *Bartonella* genus, (human) IgG antibody responses to the major *Bartonella* human pathogens have been found to be substantially cross-reactive, raising some doubts about the utility of these earlier tests.

Modern serologic studies continue to be evaluated (4, 48, 56, 77). Most studies to date have been flawed by the absence of definitive proof of infection with a particular agent by which to calibrate the serologic response, mainly because of the extremely difficult nature of culture recovery. As diagnostic techniques utilizing DNA amplification for definitive diagnosis of infection have become more widely used, definitive comparitors for serologic findings have become available.

The performance of the immunofluorescent-antibody (IFA) test varies in different studies. The method involving Vero cell-cocultured bacteria as antigen, employed by the Centers for Disease Control and Prevention, has both high sensitivity and specificity for detecting anti-*B. henselae* IgG, ranging from 84 to 95% and from 94 to 98%, respectively. However, this method does not measure IgM antibodies and has a high *B. quintana* IgG cross-reaction when using antigen from contemporary isolates (18, 61, 76). Results of IFA tests have been less satisfactory in studies performed in Europe, with findings typically of lower sensitivity and specificity (5, 25, 59, 64, 77). It is possible that in Europe, a higher seroprevalence of IgG antibodies cross-reactive with *B. henselae* due to exposure to non-*henselae Bartonella* species may result in inferior performance of the IFA test compared with that in the United States. In addition, IFA tests in general suffer from interobserver variation and are not suitable for automation or for screening large numbers of specimens.

Recently, an EIA using partially purified proteins of presumed outer membrane origin as antigen has been evaluated in a large study of definitively proven CSD cases, in which all patients met stringent clinical criteria and had culture and/or PCR evidence of *B. henselae* infection. Even applying very stringent criteria for positive results, resulting in a specificity of >98%, this study determined the EIA sensitivity to be 75% for anti-*B. henselae* IgG alone, 48% for IgM alone, and 85% overall when positive IgG and/or IgM results were accepted as diagnostic (27).

Despite cross-reaction, the differential magnitude of antibody reactions to *B. quintana* and *B. henselae* in serologic tests may allow us to infer which may be culpable in a particular infection. This would be especially important when they cause overlapping syndromes, such as fever with bacteremia or BA, but less so in CSD where *B. quintana* is not implicated. Since the skin test antigen for CSD is not commercially available or standardized and since it carries the potential risk of transmitting infection, serologic testing should replace skin testing in aiding the diagnosis of CSD.

Afipia felis

There are limited, if any, roles for serologic testing to diagnose *Afipia* infections. In studies of CSD patients, no higher levels of antibodies to *A. felis* were found than among controls, while most CSD patients had evidence of elevated anti-*Bartonella* antibodies by the IFA test and of anti-*Bartonella* IgM by EIA compared to controls (71).

ANTIMICROBIAL SUSCEPTIBILITY

Antimicrobial susceptibility testing can be performed by incorporation of antimicrobial agents into either blood or chocolate agar or into *Haemophilus* test medium by using a broth microdilution technique. However, in vitro susceptibility of *B. henselae* and *B. quintana* may not predict an in vivo response to therapy. Testing of isolates is problematic for strains displaying the most fastidious growth characteristics. The E test (AB Biodisk, Solna, Sweden) can also be used to assess susceptibility. Generally, isolates are susceptible in vitro to most antibacterial agents tested, including β-lactams, tetracyclines, macrolides, aminoglycosides, fluoroquinolones, rifampin, chloramphenicol, and co-trimoxazole, but resistant to nalidixic acid. In vitro resistance to penicillin, ampicillin, tetracycline, and vancomycin has been noted. *B. quintana* is similar to *B. henselae* in its in vitro susceptibility pattern, except for resistance to aminoglycosides.

The routine use of rifabutin, clarithromycin, and azithromycin for the prevention of *M. avium* complex infections in persons with advanced HIV disease has reduced the incidence of *Bartonella* infections in that population. There have been anecdotal reports of the utility of various agents in the treatment of CSD. However, only azithromycin has been demonstrated to accelerate the resolution of the lymphadenopathy of typical CSD in a placebo-controlled double-blind study (3). While the value of antibiotic therapy of CSD remains subject to debate, azithromycin should be considered the agent of choice if antimicrobial administration is contemplated. For BA and peliosis, bacteremia, endocarditis, and other manifestations of either *B. quintana* or *B. hensaelae* infection, erythromycin or doxycycline is the agent of choice based on the efficacy, low cost, and ease of administration of these drugs. Despite in vitro findings suggesting susceptibility, treatment with a variety of β-lactams appears largely ineffective. Responses to trimethoprim-sulfamethoxazole and fluoroquinolones in other manifestations of *Bartonella* infections have been inconsistent. The standard treatment for *B. bacilliformis* infection is oral chloramphenicol.

Afipia spp. are more resistant than *Bartonella* spp. In axenic medium, *A. felis* displays susceptibility to imipenem, aminoglycosides, and rifampin when using either the broth or the agar dilution technique. When grown in HeLa cells, *A. felis* is susceptible to amikacin and tobramycin but appears resistant to other compounds (55). It is generally nonsusceptible to penicillins, cephalosporins, and quinolones. Documented cases of infection due to *Afipia* are too few to draw conclusions about in vivo correlation.

EVALUATION, INTERPRETATION, AND REPORTING OF RESULTS

Serologic data provide the most cost-effective support for the diagnosis of typical CSD, within the limitations of the tests that are currently available. An optimized PCR assay would be expected to approach 100% sensitivity. Atypical CSD and other manifestations of *Bartonella* infection are usually best approached by serology combined with culture or PCR. Serologic tests with antigens more specific than whole cell may also play a role in corroborating these entities. PCR amplification may enable the identification of *B. henselae* in clinical material such as cerebrospinal fluid or brain tissue in the absence of positive cultures. While the value of culturing for *Bartonella* spp. is limited in certain cases by practicality issues of fresh-medium availability, length of incubation, and unknown efficiency, the use of cultures in conjunction with serology is justified in selected cases. In addition to blood, *B. henselae* and *B. quintana* have been cultured from a variety of tissue sources, albeit infrequently.

REFERENCES

1. **Avidor, B., Y. Kletter, S. Abulafia, Y. Golan, M. Ephros, and M. Giladi.** 1997. Molecular diagnosis of cat scratch disease: a two-step approach. *J. Clin. Microbiol.* **35**:1924–1930.
2. **Avidor, B., M. Varon, S. Marmor, B. Lifschitz-Mercer, Y. Kletter, M. Ephros, and M. Giladi.** 2001. DNA amplification for the diagnosis of cat scratch disease. *Am. J. Clin. Pathol.* **15**:900–909.
3. **Bass, J. W., B. C. Freitas, A. D. Freitas, C. L. Sisler, D. S. Chan, J. M. Vincent, D. A. Person, J. R. Claybaugh, R. R. Wittler, M. E. Weisse, R. L. Regnery, and L. N. Slater.** 1998. Prospective randomized double-blind placebo-controlled evaluation of azithromycin for treatment of cat scratch disease. *Pediatr. Infect. Dis. J.* **17**:447–452.
4. **Bergmans, A. M., M. F. Peeters, J. F. Schellekens, M. C. Vos, L. J. Sabbe, J. M. Ossewaarde, H. Verbakel, H. J. Hooft, and L. M. Schouls.** 1997. Pitfalls and fallacies of cat scratch disease serology: evaluation of *Bartonella henselae*-based indirect fluorescence assay and enzyme-linked immunoassay. *J. Clin. Microbiol.* **35**:1931–1937.
5. **Birkness, K. A., V. G. George, E. H. White, D. S. Stephens, and F. D. Quinn.** 1992. Intracellular growth of *Afipia felis*, a putative etiologic agent of cat scratch disease. *Infect. Immun.* **60**:2280–2287.
6. **Birtles, R. J., T. G. Harrison, N. A. Saunders, and D. H. Molyneux.** 1995. Proposals to unify the genera *Grahamella* and *Bartonella*, with descriptions of *Bartonella talpae* comb. nov., *Bartonella peromysci* sp. nov., *Bartonella taylorii* sp. nov., and *Bartonella doshiae* sp. nov. *Int. J. Syst. Bacteriol.* **45**:1–8.
7. **Breitschwerdt, E. B., and D. L. Kordick.** 2000. Bartonella infection in animals: carriership, reservoir potential, pathogenicity, and zoonotic potential for human infection. *Clin. Microbiol. Rev.* **13**:428–438.
8. **Brenner, D. J., D. G. Hollis, C. W. Moss, C. K. English, G. S. Hall, V. Judy, J. Radosevic, K. A. Birkness, W. F. Bibb, F. D. Quinn, B. Swaminathan, R. E. Weaver, M. W. Reeves, S. P. O'Connor, P. S. Hayes, F. C. Tenover, A. G. Steigerwalt, B. A. Perkins, M. I. Daneshvar, B. C. Hill, J. A. Washington, T. C. Woods, S. B. Hunter, T. L. Hadfield, G. W. Ajelio, A. F. Kaufman, D. J. Wear, and J. D. Wenger.** 1991. Proposal of *Afipia* gen. nov., with *Afipia felis* sp. nov. (formerly the cat scratch disease bacillus), *Afipia clevelandensis* sp. nov. (formerly the Cleveland Clinic Foundation strain), *Afipia broomeae* sp. nov., and three unnamed genospecies. *J. Clin. Microbiol.* **29**:2450–2460.
9. **Brenner, D. J., S. P. O'Connor, H. H. Winkler, and A. G. Steigerwalt.** 1993. Proposals to unify the genera *Bartonella* and *Rochalimaea*, with descriptions of *Bartonella quintana* comb nov., *Bartonella vinsonii* comb nov., *Bartonella henselae* comb. nov., and *Bartonella elizabethae* comb nov, and to remove the family *Bartonellaceae* from the order *Rickettsiales*. *Int. J. Syst. Bacteriol.* **43**:777–786.
10. **Brenner, S. A., J. A. Rooney, P. Manzewitsch, and R. L. Regnery.** 1997. Isolation of *Bartonella* (*Rochalimaea*) *henselae*—effects of methods of blood collection and handling. *J. Clin. Microbiol.* **35**:544–547.
11. **Chamberlin, J., L. Laughlin, S. Gordon, S. Romero, N. Solórzano, and R. L. Regnery.** 2000. Serodiagnosis of *Bartonella bacilliformis* infection by indirect fluorescence antibody assay: test development and application to a population in an area of bartonellosis endemicity. *J. Clin. Microbiol.* **38**:4269–4271.
12. **Chang, C. C., B. B. Chomel, R. W. Kasten, V. Romano, and N. Tietze.** 2001. Molecular evidence of *Bartonella* spp. in questing adult *Ixodes pacificus* ticks in California. *J. Clin. Microbiol.* **39**:1221–1226.
13. **Chomel, B. B., R. C. Abbott, R. W. Kasten, K. A. Floyd-Hawkins, P. H. Kass, C. A. Glaser, N. Pedersen, and J. E. Koehler.** 1995. *Bartonella henselae* prevalence in domestic cats in California: risk factors and association between bacteremia and antibody titers. *J. Clin. Microbiol.* **33**:2445–2450.
14. **Chomel, B. B., R. W. Kasten, K. Floyd-Hawkins, B. Chi, K. Yamamoto, J. Roberts-Wilson, A. N. Gurfield,**

R. C. Abbott, N. C. Pederson, and J. E. Koehler. 1996. Experimental transmission of *Bartonella henselae* by the cat flea. *J. Clin. Microbiol.* **34**:1952–1956.

15. Clarridge, J. E., III, T. J. Raich, D. Pirwani, B. Simon, L. Tsai, M. C. Rodriguez-Barradas, R. Regnery, A. Zollo, D. C. Jones, and C. Rambo. 1995. Strategy to detect and identify *Bartonella* species in a routine clinical laboratory yields *Bartonella henselae* from human immunodeficiency virus-infected patient and unique *Bartonella* strain from his cat. *J. Clin. Microbiol.* **33**:2107–2113.

16. Cockerell, C. J., G. F. Webster, M. A. Whitlow, and A. E. Friedman-Kien. 1987. Epithelioid angiomatosis: a distinct vascular disorder in patients with the acquired immunodeficiency syndrome or AIDS-related complex. *Lancet* **ii**:6544–6546.

17. Cunningham, E. T., and J. E. Koehler. 2000. Ocular bartonellosis. *Am. J. Ophthalmol.* **130**:340–349.

18. Dalton, M. J., L. E. Robinson, J. Cooper, R. L. Regnery, J. G. Olson, and J. E. Childs. 1995. Use of *Bartonella* antigens for the serologic diagnosis of cat-scratch disease at a national referral center. *Arch. Intern. Med.* **155**:1670–1676.

19. Debré, R., M. Lamy, M. L. Jammet, L. Costil, and P. Mozziconacci. 1950. La maladie des griffes de chat. *Semin. Hop. Paris* **26**:1895–1904.

20. Dehio, C., C. Lanz, R. Pohl, P. Behrens, D. Bermond, Y. Piemont, K. Pelz, and A. Sander. 2001. *Bartonella schoenbuchii* sp. nov., isolated from the blood of wild roe deer. *Int. J. Syst. Evol. Microbiol.* **51**:1557–1565.

21. Delphine, B., R. Heller, F. Barrat, D. Gilles, G. Delacour, C. Dehio, A. Alliot, H. Monteil, B. Chomel, H.-J. Boulouis, and Y. Piemont. 2000. *Bartonella birtlesii* isolated from small mammals (*Apodemus* spp.). *Int. J. Syst. Evol. Microbiol.* **50**:1973–1979.

22. Demers, D. M., J. W. Bass, J. M. Vincent, D. A. Person, D. K. Noyes, C. M. Staege, C. P. Samlaska, N. H. Lockwood, R. L. Regnery, and B. E. Anderson. 1995. Cat-scratch disease in Hawaii: etiology and seroepidemiology. *J. Pediatr.* **127**:23–26.

23. Drancourt, M., and D. Raoult. 1993. Proposed tests for the routine identification of *Rochalimaea* species. *Eur. J. Clin. Microbiol.* **4**:112–114.

24. Droz, S., B. Chi, E. Horn, A. G. Steigerwalt, A. M. Whitney, and D. J. Brenner. 1999. *Bartonella koehlerae* sp. nov., isolated from cats. *J. Clin. Microbiol.* **37**:1117–1122.

25. Dupon, M., A.-M. Savin de Larclause, P. Brouqui, M. Drancourt, D. Raoult, A. De Mascare, and J.-Y. Lacut. 1996. Evaluation of serological response to *Bartonella henselae*, *Bartonella quintana*, and *Afipia felis* antigens in 64 patients with suspected cat scratch disease. *Scand. J. Infect. Dis.* **28**:361–366.

26. English, C. K., D. J. Wear, A. M. Margileth, C. R. Lissner, and G. P. Walsh. 1988. Cat-scratch disease. Isolation and culture of the bacterial agent. *JAMA* **269**:1347–1354.

27. Giladi, M., Y. Kletter, B. Avidor, E. Metzkor-Cotter, M. Varon, Y. Golan, M. Weinberg, I. Riklis, M. Ephros, and L. Slater. 2001. Enzyme immunoassay for the diagnosis of cat scratch disease defined by polymerase chain reaction. *Clin. Infect. Dis.* **33**:1852–1858.

28. Gurfield, A. N., H.-J. Boulouis, B. B. Chomel, R. Heller, R. W. Kasten, K. Yamamoto, and Y. Piemont. 1997. Coinfection with *Bartonelle clarridgeiae* and *Bartonella henselae* and with different *Bartonella henselae* strains in domestic cats. *J. Clin. Microbiol.* **35**:2120–2123.

29. Handley, S. A., and R. L. Regnery. 2000. Differentiation of pathogenic *Bartonella* species by infrequent restriction site PCR. *J. Clin. Microbiol.* **38**:3010–3015.

30. Heller, R., M. Artois, V. Xemar, D. De Briel, G. Hervè, B. Jaulhac, H. Monteil, and Y. Piemont. 1997. Prevalence of *Bartonella henselae* and *Bartonella clarridgeiae* in stray cats. *J. Clin. Microbiol.* **35**:1327–1331.

31. Heller, R., M. Kubina, P. Mariet, P. Riegel, G. Delacour, C. Dehio, F. Lamarque, R. Kasten, H. J. Boulouis, H. Monteil, B. Chomel, and Y. Piemont. 1999. *Bartonella alsatica* sp. nov., a new *Bartonella* species isolated from the blood of wild rabbits. *Int. J. Syst. Bacteriol.* **49**:283–288.

32. Heller, R., P. Riegel, Y. Hansmann, G. Delacour, D. Bermond, C. Dehio, F. Lamarque, H. Monteil, B. Chomel, and Y. Piemont. 1998. *Bartonella tribocorum* sp. nov., a new *Bartonella* species isolated from the blood of wild rats. *Int. J. Syst. Bacteriol.* **48**:1333–1339.

33. Hofmeister, E. K., C. P. Kolbert, A. S. Abdulkarim, J. M. H. Magera, M. Hopkins, J. R. Uhl, A. Ambayaye, S. R. Telford, F. R. Cockerill, and D. H. Persing. 1998. Cosegregation of a novel *Bartonella* species with *Borrelia burgdorferi* and *Babesia microti* in *Peromyscus leucopus*. *J. Infect. Dis.* **177**:409–416.

34. Jackson, L. A., B. A. Perkins, and J. D. Wenger. 1993. Cat scratch disease in the United States: an analysis of three national databases. *Am. J. Public Health* **83**:1707–1711.

35. Jackson, L. A., and D. H. Spach. 1996. Emergence of *Bartonella quintana* infection among homeless persons. *Emerg. Infect. Dis.* **2**:141–144.

36. Jacobs, R. F., and G. E. Schultze. 1998. *Bartonella henselae* as a cause of prolonged fever of unknown origin in children. *Clin. Infect. Dis.* **26**:80–84.

37. Jameson, P., C. Greene, R. Regnery, M. Dryden, A. Marks, J. Brown, J. Cooper, B. Glaus, and R. Greene. 1995. Prevalence of *Bartonella henselae* antibodies in pet cats throughout regions of North America. *J. Infect. Dis.* **172**:1145–1149.

38. Koehler, J. E., F. D. Quinn, T. G. Berger, P. E. LeBoit, and J. W. Tappero. 1992. Isolation of *Rochalimaea* species from cutaneous osseous lesions of bacillary angiomatosis. *N. Engl. J. Med.* **327**:1625–1632.

39. Koehler, J. E., M. A. Sanchez, C. S. Garrido, M. J. Whitfield, F. M. Chen, T. G. Berger, M. C. Rodriguez-Barradas, P. E. LeBoit, and J. W. Tappero. 1997. Molecular epidemiology of *Bartonella* infections in patients with bacillary angiomatosis-peliosis. *N. Engl. J. Med.* **337**:1876–1883.

40. Koehler, J. E., and J. W. Tappero. 1993. Bacillary angiomatosis and bacillary peliosis in patients infected with human immunodeficiency virus. *Clin. Infect. Dis.* **17**:612–624.

41. Kordick, D. L., E. J. Hilyard, T. L. Hadfield, K. H. Wilson, A. G. Steigerwalt, D. J. Brenner, and E. B. Breitschwerdt. 1997. *Bartonella clarridgeiae*, a newly recognized zoonotic pathogen causing inoculation papules, fever and lymphadenopathy (cat scratch disease). *J. Clin. Microbiol.* **35**:1813–1818.

42. Kordick, D. L., B. Swaminathan, C. E. Greene, K. H. Wilson, A. M. Whitney, O. C. Steve, D. G. Hollis, G. M. Matar, A. G. Steigerwalt, G. B. Malcolm, P. S. Hayes, T. L. Hadfield, E. B. Breitschwerdt, and D. J. Brenner. 1996. *Bartonella vinsonii* subsp. *berkhoffii* subsp. nov., isolated from dogs; *Bartonella vinsonii* subsp. *vinsonii*; and emended description of *Bartonella vinsonii*. *Int. J. Syst. Bacteriol.* **46**:704–709.

43. Kosek, M., R. Lavarello, R. H. Gilman, J. Delgado, C. Maguiña, M. Verástegui, A. G. Lescano, V. Mallqui, J. C. Kosek, S. Recavarren, and L. Cabrera. 2000. Natural history of infection with *B. bacilliformis* in a nonendemic population. *J. Infect. Dis.* **182**:865–872.

44. **La Scola, B., and D. Raoult.** 1999. *Afipia felis* in hospital water supply in association with free-living amoebae. *Lancet* **353:**1330.

45. **La Scola, B., and D. Raoult.** 1999. Culture of *Bartonella quintana* and *Bartonella henselae* from human samples: a 5-year experience (1993 to 1998). *J. Clin. Microbiol.* **37:** 1899–1905.

46. **Liang, Z., and D. Raoult.** 2000. Differentiation of *Bartonella* species by a microimmunofluorescence assay, sodium dodecyl sulfate-polyacrylamide gel electrophoresis, and western immunoblotting. *Clin. Diagn. Lab. Immunol.* **7:**617–624.

47. **Liston, T. E., and J. E. Koehler.** 1996. Granulomatous hepatitis and necrotizing splenitis due to *Bartonella henselae* in a patient with cancer: case report and review of hepatosplenic manifestations of *Bartonella* infection. *Clin. Infect. Dis.* **22:**951–957.

48. **Litwin, C. M., T. B. Martins, and H. R. Hill.** 1997. Immunologic response to *Bartonella henselae* as determined by enzyme immunoassay and Western blot analysis. *Am. J. Clin. Pathol.* **108:**202–209.

49. **Lucey, D., M. J. Dolan, C. W. Moss, M. Garcia, D. G. Hollis, S. Wegner, G. Morgan, R. Almeida, D. Leong, K. S. Greisen, D. F. Welch, and L. N. Slater.** 1992. Relapsing illness due to *Rochalimaea henselae* in normal hosts: implication for therapy and new epidemiologic associations. *Clin. Infect. Dis.* **14:**683–688.

50. **Mallqui, V., E. C. Speelmon, M. Verástegui, C. Maguiña-Vargas, P. Pinell-Salles, R. Lavarello, J. Delgado, M. Kosek, S. Romero, Y. Arana, and R. H. Gilman.** 2000. Sonicated diagnostic immunoblot for bartonellosis. *Clin. Diagn. Lab. Immunol.* **7:**1–5.

51. **Margileth, A. M., D. J. Wear, and C. K. English.** 1987. Systemic cat scratch disease: report of 23 patients with prolonged or recurrent severe bacterial infection. *J. Infect. Dis.* **155:**390–402.

52. **Massei, F., F. Messina, M. Massimetti, P. Macchia, and G. Maggiore.** 2000. Pseudoinfectious mononucleosis: a presentation of *Bartonella henselae* infection. *Arch. Dis. Child.* **83:**443–444.

53. **Matar, G. M., J. E. Koehler, G. Malcolm, M. A. Lambert-Fair, J. Tappero, S. B. Hunter, and B. Swaminathan.** 1999. Identification of *Bartonella* species directly in clinical specimens by PCR-restriction fragment length polymorphism analysis of a 16S rRNA gene fragment. *J. Clin. Microbiol.* **37:**4045–4047.

54. **Matar, G. M., B. Swaminathan, S. B. Hunter, L. N. Slater, and D. F. Welch.** 1993. Polymerase chain reaction-based restriction fragment length polymorphism analysis of a fragment of the ribosomal operon from *Rochalimaea* species for subtyping. *J. Clin. Microbiol.* **31:**1730–1734.

55. **Maurin, M., H. Lepocher, D. Mallet, and D. Raoult.** 1993. Antibiotic susceptibilities of *Afipia felis* in axenic medium and in cells. *Antimicrob. Agents Chemother.* **37:** 1410–1413.

56. **Not, T., M. Canciani, E. Buratii, G. Dal Molin, A. Tommasini, C. Trevisiol, and A. Ventura.** 1999. Serologic response to *Bartonella henselae* in patients with cat scratch disease and in sick and healthy children. *Acta Paediatr.* **88:**284–289.

57. **O'Connor, S. P., M. Dorsch, A. G. Steigerwalt, D. J. Brenner, and E. Stackebrandt.** 1991. 16S rRNA sequences of *Bartonella bacilliformis* and cat scratch disease bacillus reveal phylogenetic relationships with the alpha-2 subgroup of the class *Proteobacteria*. *J. Clin. Microbiol.* **29:**2144–2150.

58. **Patnaik, M., W. A. Schwartzman, and J. B. Peter.** 1995. *Bartonella henselae:* detection in brain tissue of patients with AIDS-associated neurological disease. *J. Investig. Med.* **43:**368A.

59. **Rath, P. M., G. von Recklinghausen, and R. Ansorg.** 1997. Seroprevalence of immunoglobulin G antibodies to *Bartonella henselae* in cat owners. *Eur. J. Clin. Microbiol. Infect. Dis.* **16:**326–327.

60. **Reed, J., D. J. Brigati, S. D. Flynn, N. S. McNutt, K. W. Min, D. F. Welch, and L. N. Slater.** 1992. Immunocytochemical identification of *Rochalimaea henselae* in bacillary (epithelioid) angiomatosis, parenchymal bacillary peliosis, and persistent fever with bacteremia. *Am. J. Surg. Pathol.* **16:**650–657.

61. **Regnery, R. L., J. G. Olson, B. A. Perkins, and W. Bibb.** 1992. Serological response to "*Rochalimeae henselae*" antigen in suspected cat-scratch disease. *Lancet* **339:**1443–1445.

62. **Ricketts, W. E.** 1949. Clinical manifestations of Carrion's disease. *Arch. Intern. Med.* **84:**751–781.

63. **Sander, A., C. Buhler, K. Pelz, E. Voncramm, and W. Bredt.** 1997. Detection and identification of two *Bartonella henselae* variants in domestic cats in Germany. *J. Clin. Microbiol.* **35:**584–587.

64. **Sander, A., M. Posselt, K. Oberle, and W. Bredt.** 1998. Seroprevalence of antibodies to *Bartonella henselae* in patients with cat scratch disease and in healthy controls: evaluation and comparison of two commercial serological tests. *Clin. Diagn. Lab. Immunol.* **5:**486–490.

65. **Schwartzman, W. A., C. A. Nesbit, and E. J. Baron.** 1993. Development and evaluation of a blood-free medium for determining growth curves and optimizing growth of *Rochalimaea henselae*. *J. Clin. Microbiol.* **31:** 1882–1885.

66. **Scott, M. A., T. L. McCurley, C. L. Vnencak-Jones, C. Hager, J. A. McCoy, B. Anderson, R. D. Collins, and K. M. Edwards.** 1996. Cat scratch disease—detection of *Bartonella henselae* DNA in archival biopsies from patients with clinically, serologically, and histologically defined disease. *Am. J. Pathol.* **149:**2161–2167.

67. **Slater, L. N., D. F. Welch, D. Hensel, and D. W. Coody.** 1990. A newly recognized fastidious Gram-negative pathogen as a cause of fever and bacteremia. *N. Engl. J. Med.* **323:**1587–1593.

68. **Slater, L. N., D. F. Welch, and K. W. Min.** 1992. *Rochalimaea henselae* causes bacillary angiomatosis and peliosis hepatitis. *Arch. Intern. Med.* **152:**602–606.

69. **Spach, D. H., L. A. Panther, D. R. Thorning, J. E. Dunn, J. J. Plorde, and R. A. Miller.** 1992. Intracerebral bacillary angiomatosis in a patient infected with the human immunodeficiency virus. *Ann. Intern. Med.* **116:**740–742.

70. **Stoler, M. H., T. A. Bonfiglio, R. T. Steigbigel, and M. Pereira.** 1983. An atypical subcutaneous infection associated with acquired immune deficiency syndrome. *Am. J. Clin. Pathol.* **80:**714–718.

71. **Szelc-Kelly, C. M., S. Goral, G. I. Perez-Perez, B. A. Perkins, R. L. Regnery, and K. M. Edwards.** 1995. Serologic responses to *Bartonella* and *Afipia* antigens in patients with cat scratch disease. *Pediatrics* **96:**1137–1142.

72. **Welch, D. F., K. C. Carroll, E. K. Hofmeister, D. H. Persing, D. Robison, A. G. Steigerwalt, and D. J. Brenner.** 1999. Isolation of a new subspecies, *Bartonella vinsonii* subsp. *arupensis*, from a cattle rancher: identity with isolates found in conjunction with *Borrelia burgdorferi* and *Babesia microti* among naturally infected mice. *J. Clin. Microbiol.* **37:**2598–2601.

73. **Welch, D. F., D. M. Hensel, D. A. Pickett, V. H. San Joaquin, A. Robinson, and L. N. Slater.** 1993. Bacteremia in a child due to *Rochalimaea henselae:* a practical identification of isolates in the clinical laboratory. *J. Clin. Microbiol.* **31:**2381–2386.

74. **Welch, D. F., D. A. Pickett, L. N. Slater, A. G. Steigerwalt, and D. J. Brenner.** 1992. *Rochalimaea henselae* sp. nov., a cause of septicemia, bacillary angiomatosis, and parenchymal bacillary peliosis. *J. Clin. Microbiol.* **30:**275–280.

75. **Wong, M. T., D. C. Thornton, R. C. Kennedy, and M. J. Dolan.** 1995. A chemically defined liquid medium that supports primary isolation of *Rochalimaea (Bartonella) henselae* from blood and tissue specimens. *J. Clin. Microbiol.* **33:**742–744.

76. **Zangwill, K. M., D. H. Hamilton, B. A. Perkins, R. L. Regnery, B. D. Plikaytis, J. L. Hadler, M. L. Cartter, and J. D. Wenger.** 1993. Cat scratch disease in Connecticut. Epidemiology, risk factors, and evaluation of a new diagnostic test. *N. Engl. J. Med.* **329:**8–13.

77. **Zbinden, R., N. Michael, M. Sekulovski, A. von Graevenitz, and D. Nadal.** 1997. Evaluation of commercial slides for detection of immunoglobulin G against *Bartonella henselae* by indirect immunofluorescence. *Eur. J. Clin. Microbiol. Infect. Dis.* **16:**648–652.

Clostridium*

STEPHEN D. ALLEN, CHRISTOPHER L. EMERY,
AND DAVID M. LYERLY

54

TAXONOMY

Historically, the genus *Clostridium* has long contained obligately anaerobic (or aerotolerant) endospore-forming rods that do not form spores in the presence of air, are usually gram positive (at least in early stages of growth), and do not carry out a dissimilatory sulfate reduction (31, 39). Probably as a result of this simple definition, as Collins et al. suggested, the genus has become one of the largest and most diverse genera of bacteria and "is clearly in need of revision" (39). Although significant genetic diversity within the genus has long been known (82), studies using 16S rRNA gene sequences determined by PCR direct sequencing and the construction of phylogenetic trees revealed that the genus *Clostridium* is extremely heterogeneous and could be divided into several phylogenetic clusters. The type species, *Clostridium butyricum*, and most of the medically important *Clostridium* species were placed in cluster 1, which was equivalent to rRNA group I of Johnson and Francis (82). In 1994, Collins et al. named five new genera of spore-forming rods: *Caloramator*, *Filifactor*, *Moorella*, *Oxobacter*, and *Oxalophagus* (39). They also proposed 11 new species combinations. None of these new generic and species designations was of medical significance. Since the seventh edition of this Manual was published, relatively few nomenclature changes within the genus *Clostridium* have had medical significance. However, the name *C. putrificum* was rejected while *C. botulinum* and *C. sporogenes* were conserved, although strains of *C. putrificum*, *C. botulinum*, and *C. sporogenes* were known to be genetically related at the species level. This decision was made to avoid the confusion that could have resulted from renaming all strains of this group as a single species (i.e., *C. botulinum*) (86). On the basis of DNA-DNA hybridization similarities and other data, *C. hylemonae* and *C. hiranonis* were the names proposed for two new species of human intestinal bacteria with bile acid 7α-dehydroxylating activity (92, 93). The resulting 7α-dehydroxylation of cholic and chenodeoxycholic acids, yielding deoxycholic and lithocholic acids, respectively, has long been postulated to be a risk factor for the development of colorectal cancer (76, 136). Currently, more than 150 species of *Clostridium* are validly published. Fortunately for the clinical microbiologist, the number of species commonly encountered as agents of infection in properly collected clinical specimens from humans is relatively small (Table 1).

DESCRIPTION OF THE GENUS

While it is clear that the anaerobic spore-forming rods are phylogenetically diverse and that much progress has been made toward full rRNA sequencing of many species, their taxonomic classification still has not been resolved (39, 157). For this reason, the description of the genus that follows remains similar to that which was used in the seventh edition of this text. The vegetative cells of most species are rod shaped and straight or curved, but cells vary from short coccoid rods to long filamentous forms. The rod-shaped cells may be rounded, tapered, or blunt ended. Cells may occur singly, in pairs, or in chains of various lengths. In certain species (e.g., *C. cocleatum* and *C. spiroforme*), many rods may be joined to form tight coils or spiral configurations (30). Most species stain gram positive during the early stage of growth; however, some, such as *C. ramosum* and *C. clostridioforme*, almost always appear gram negative after overnight culture. Several species (e.g., *C. tetani*) appear gram negative by the time spores have formed. All but a few species are motile by means of peritrichous flagella. Nonmotile species isolated from clinical specimens include *C. perfringens*, *C. ramosum*, and *C. innocuum*. The spores of clostridia are ovoid to spherical and distend the vegetative cells. Certain species, e.g., *C. perfringens*, produce spores only under special culture conditions. Although the majority of *Clostridium* species are obligate anaerobes, there is considerable species variation with respect to oxygen toxicity; some species (e.g., *C. haemolyticum* and *C. novyi* type B) are strict obligate anaerobes and will not grow when exposed to even trace amounts of oxygen. A few aerotolerant species (*C. tertium*, *C. carnis*, *C. histolyticum*, and occasional strains of *C. perfringens*) show scant growth on solid media incubated in a 5 to 10% CO_2 incubator in air or in a candle jar.

Aerotolerant clostridia may be confused with certain facultatively anaerobic *Bacillus* species. However, members of the genus *Clostridium* usually form spores only under

* This chapter contains information presented in chapter 46 by Stephen D. Allen, Christopher L. Emery, and Jean A. Siders in the seventh edition of this Manual.

TABLE 1 *Clostridium* species most frequently encountered in clinical specimens at Indiana University Hospital Anaerobe Laboratory, 1989 through 2001[a]

Species	Isolates	
	No.	% of total
C. perfringens	515	20
C. clostridioforme	421	16
C. innocuum	380	15
C. ramosum	357	14
C. difficile	287	11
C. butyricum	113	4
C. cadaveris	99	4
C. bifermentans	53	2
C. sporogenes	49	2
C. glycolicum	44	2
C. septicum	42	2
C. tertium	39	2
C. sordellii	30	1
C. subterminale	27	1
C. paraputrificum	23	1
C. symbiosum	24	1
C. baratii	15	1
Other recognized species[b]	37	1

[a] S. D. Allen and J. A. Siders, unpublished data. The total of 2,555 isolates does not include 270 isolates (10% of 2,825 isolates) that did not belong to a recognized species. All of the isolates were from properly collected specimens and did not include fecal samples for *C. difficile* testing.

[b] Includes one to six isolates of each of the following: *C. beijerinckii, C. botulinum, C. carnis, C. celatum, C. coccoides, C. cochlearium, C. ghoni, C. hastiforme, C. histolyticum, C. indolis, C. limosum, C. malenominatum, C. novyi, C. putrefaciens, C. putrificum,* and *C. sphenoides.*

anaerobic conditions and almost never produce catalase. Also, aerotolerant clostridia show much better growth (i.e., they form larger colonies) under anaerobic conditions than in air, unlike *Bacillus* species.

Catalase is rarely produced, and then the reaction is only weakly positive. In addition, clostridia lack a cytochrome system and thus react negatively in the cytochrome oxidase test. Clostridia are usually fermentative or proteolytic or both, but some are asaccharolytic and nonproteolytic. Many clostridia produce a range of short-chain fatty acids (e.g., acetate and butyrate) when grown in peptone-yeast extract-glucose or chopped-meat–carbohydrate medium, and many produce a variety of other fermentation products (e.g., acetone, butanol, and other alcohols).

NATURAL HABITATS

Although *Clostridium* species are ubiquitous in nature, their principal habitats are the soil and the intestinal tracts of many animals, including humans (151). The species most frequently isolated from soil are *C. subterminale, C. sordellii, C. sporogenes, C. indolis, C. bifermentans, C. mangenotii,* and *C. perfringens* (149). Others regularly found in soil samples, but somewhat less frequently, are *C. botulinum* and *C. tetani* (150). The widespread occurrence of *C. perfringens,* including its spores, in soil samples almost guarantees the frequent presence of this organism on surfaces exposed to dust contamination, including many food items (151). However, the average daily intake of *C. perfringens* on foods consumed by humans is probably small (e.g., $<5 \times 10^2$ organisms per day) (151).

Clostridia were recovered frequently from the feces of infants studied during the first week of life (159). However, breast-fed infants 1 month of age were less likely to be colonized by clostridia than formula-fed infants were. As reviewed elsewhere (159), the feces of infants 6 to 20 months old tend to contain about the same numbers of *C. perfringens* (essentially all toxin type A) as adults (e.g., $\sim 10^3$ to 10^8 CFU per g). The feces of infants commonly contain *C. difficile,* but it is seen less frequently ($\leq 3\%$) in healthy adults (58). Several additional *Clostridium* species such as *C. innocuum, C. ramosum, C. paraputrificum, C. sporogenes, C. tertium, C. bifermentans,* and *C. butyricum* reside in the lower intestinal tracts of humans as part of the normal flora. With certain notable exceptions, most species occur as harmless saprophytes.

Diseases caused by clostridia from an external source (e.g., food-borne botulism, tetanus, and myonecrosis) are well-known historically and are clinically important. Outbreaks of hospital-acquired diarrhea may be caused by a single strain of *C. difficile* in geographically separated hospitals (89, 140). Endogenous infections involving other clostridia that are a part of the host's own microflora are more common than exogenous infections, however. As is true for other endogenous infections involving anaerobes (endocarditis, brain abscess, aspiration pneumonia, intra-abdominal abscess, etc.), the development of clostridial disease is usually associated with special circumstances. Common predisposing factors include trauma, operative procedures, vascular stasis, obstruction, treatment of cancer patients with immunosuppressive agents or chemotherapeutic agents, prior treatment with antimicrobial agents (as in pseudomembranous colitis), and underlying illness such as leukemia, carcinoma, or diabetes mellitus (108). Under the right conditions, clostridia can invade and multiply in essentially any tissue of the body.

CLINICAL SIGNIFICANCE

Tissue Infections Due to *C. perfringens*

C. perfringens is the species most commonly isolated from human clinical specimens, excluding feces. It is encountered in a wide variety of clinical settings ranging from simple contamination of wounds to traumatic or nontraumatic myonecrosis, clostridial cellulitis, intra-abdominal sepsis, gangrenous cholecystitis, postabortion infection with devastating septicemia, intravascular hemolysis, bacteremia in various clinical settings, aspiration pneumonia, necrotizing pneumonia, thoracic empyema, subdural empyema, and brain abscess (63).

Clostridial myonecrosis (gas gangrene) involves a breakdown of muscle tissue related to the action of potent extracellular protein toxins, particularly the alpha-toxin (a phospholipase C) and theta-toxin (a thiol-activated cytolysin) (27, 28). It is a rapidly progressive, life-threatening condition with liquefactive necrosis of muscle, gas (primarily insoluble hydrogen and nitrogen) formation, and associated systemic manifestations (e.g., hypotension, renal failure, and hemolysis) (64). Blood cultures are positive in about 15% of patients (163). Although *C. perfringens* type A is the species most commonly involved in gas gangrene, *C. septicum, C. novyi* B, *C. histolyticum, C. bifermentans,* and *C. sordellii* are other potential causes. *C. fallax, C. sporogenes,* and *C. tertium* have been encountered in patients with myonecrosis, but their clinical importance in this condition is less clear.

In addition to the habitats mentioned above, *C. perfringens* has also been isolated from the vaginal vaults or cervices of approximately 1 to 9% of healthy pregnant and nonpregnant women (41). Gas gangrene of the uterus, now rare in the United States, occurred most frequently as a consequence of illegal or self-induced abortions. It has also followed spontaneous abortion, vaginal delivery, cesarean section, amniocentesis, and uterine tumors in nonpregnant women (64).

Various gas-producing bacteria may form gas in tissue without causing myonecrosis; those that do so most frequently, particularly after laceration-type wounds involving soft tissue other than muscle, are the clostridia, especially *C. perfringens* (64). Crepitant cellulitis caused by clostridia, also called anaerobic cellulitis, characteristically involves subcutaneous tissues or retroperitoneal tissues and can progress to fulminant systemic disease (108). In contrast to clostridial myonecrosis, the muscle is usually not involved to a significant extent and remains viable. The outlook for patients who have clostridial infections confined to subcutaneous tissues is usually not as ominous as that for patients with myonecrosis, provided that the correct diagnosis and treatment are initiated early in the course of illness. Pertinent findings in crepitant cellulitis include abundant gas in the tissue, often more than in myonecrosis; tissue swelling without much discoloration of the overlying skin; minimal pain; and a thin, sweet-smelling or sometimes foul-smelling exudate that may contain numerous polymorphonuclear leukocytes and bacteria (108). On occasion, however, polymorphonuclear leukocytes are absent because of the activity of the leukolytic toxins of the clostridia. The presence of boxcar-shaped, gram-variable rods and no leukocytes in a Gram-stained preparation of infected tissue should lead one to suspect clostridial infection. These infections are frequently polymicrobial.

Clostridium species are commonly encountered in a variety of polymicrobial infections involving the abdomen, including peritonitis, intra-abdominal abscesses, and septicemia in patients with obstructive or perforating lesions of the terminal ileum or large bowel (63). *C. perfringens* and *C. septicum* have been documented in patients with overwhelming sepsis and gangrenous necrosis of the small intestine or large bowel.

C. perfringens produces a variety of biologically active proteins, or toxins, that play an important role in pathogenicity (73, 109). On the basis of mouse lethality assays and specific neutralization of four toxins produced in culture fluids, five toxin types of *C. perfringens* have been identified (types A through E) (72) (Table 2). Clostridia of all five types that produce lethal toxins produce phospholipase C, or alpha-toxin, which plays a major role in the pathogenesis of myonecrosis caused by *C. perfringens* (27, 28). Alpha-toxin has several additional properties. It produces the opaque zone of lecithin hydrolysis products that surrounds colonies of *C. perfringens* growing on egg yolk agar plates. It gives rise to an outer zone of partial hemolysis that encircles a smaller zone of complete hemolysis produced by theta-toxin (a heat-labile, oxygen-labile hemolysin easily detected around colonies of *C. perfringens* growing on sheep blood agar). Alpha-toxin is also active against the membranes of muscle cells, leukocytes, and platelets, and it has necrotizing activity that leads to the death of a variety of host cells and tissues. These effects are probably related to its interaction with eukaryotic cell membranes and hydrolysis of sphingomyelin and phosphatidylcholine, resulting in lysis of the affected cells (164). In addition to

producing alpha-toxin, type B strains of *C. perfringens* produce lethal beta- and epsilon-toxins, type D strains produce lethal epsilon-toxin, and type E strains uniquely produce an iota-toxin as well as alpha-toxin (Table 2).

A variety of apparently less important bioactive proteins, or minor toxins, which may or may not serve as virulence factors, are produced by *C. perfringens* (138). These include lambda-toxin (a protease), kappa-toxin (a collagenase), mu-toxin (a hyaluronidase), a neuraminidase, and a DNase (151).

C. perfringens and Food Poisoning

For many years, *C. perfringens* has been one of the most common bacterial causes of food-borne illness in the United States (130, 146). Almost all U.S. outbreaks and cases of *C. perfringens* food-borne gastroenteritis appear to be due to type A strains. In *C. perfringens* type A food-borne disease, the food vehicle is almost always an improperly cooked meat or a meat product, such as gravy, that has cooled slowly after cooking or may have been inadequately reheated. Spores surviving the initial cooking germinate, and vegetative cells proliferate during slow cooling or insufficient reheating. *C. perfringens* type A food-borne illness should be suspected when there is an outbreak of diarrhea with crampy abdominal pain within about 7 to 15 h after the consumption of a suspected food (146). However, the incubation period may range up to 30 h. Most patients are afebrile; nausea and vomiting occur in less than one-third of patients, and the stools are frequently foamy and foul smelling. Illness results from the ingestion of food with about 10^8 or more viable vegetative cells, which, in the alkaline environment of the small intestine, undergo sporulation, producing an enterotoxin in the process (146). The enterotoxin, a single polypeptide with a molecular weight of about 35,000, accumulates within *C. perfringens* cells when they sporulate and is released into the intestine when the sporulating cells undergo lysis and release their spores (97). After it is released into the small intestine, the enterotoxin apparently binds to receptors on the surface of intestinal epithelial cells and causes cytotoxic damage to cell membranes and permeability alterations leading to diarrhea and cramping abdominal symptoms (97). Animal model studies have revealed that *C. perfringens* enterotoxin causes significant histopathological damage to the small intestine, including necrosis of villus cells (147). In humans, the illness is usually mild, and most patients recover within 2 to 3 days after onset. The diagnosis is problematic, and the disease undoubtedly is underdiagnosed. Laboratory confirmation has traditionally been performed by culture from epidemiologically implicated food of at least 10^5 organisms per g and by the demonstration, using a quantitative spore selection technique, of median spore counts of at least 10^6 *C. perfringens* spores per g of feces collected within 24 h after the onset of illness (146). Assays that have been used to detect the enterotoxin include Vero cell toxin neutralization, Western immunoblotting (98), reverse passive latex agglutination (Oxoid USA, Columbia, Md.), and commercial enzyme-linked immunosorbent assay (ELISA) kits (TechLab, Blacksburg, Va.). Although PCR assays and digoxigenin-labeled probe assays (to detect all or part of the *C. perfringens* enterotoxin gene) (98) can indicate the potential of a *C. perfringens* isolate to produce enterotoxin in vitro without a requirement for sporulation, gene probe assays do not indicate whether an isolate can sporulate and produce enterotoxin within the intestinal tract of a patient (73). Laboratory testing for *C. perfringens* food-borne illness

TABLE 2 Distribution of major toxins among types of *C. perfringens*

Toxin type	Occurrence and country where originally found	Alpha-toxin		Beta-toxin		Epsilon-toxin		Iota-toxin	
		Presence or absence	Characteristics	Presence or absence	Characteristics	Presence or absence	Characteristics	Presence or absence	Characteristics
A[a]	Gas gangrene of humans and animals Intestinal flora of humans and animals Putrefactive processes in soil, etc. (United States) Food poisoning (United Kingdom)	+	Lethal, lecithinase, hemolytic, necrotizing	−	Lethal, necrotizing	−	Lethal, permease	−	Lethal, dermonecrotic, ADP ribosylating
B	Lamb dysentery Enterotoxemia of foals (United Kingdom) Enterotoxemia of sheep and goats (Iran)	+		+		+		−	
C	Enterotoxemia of sheep (struck) (United Kingdom) Enteritis necroticans of humans (pig-bel) (Papua New Guinea)	+		+		−		−	
D	Enterotoxemia of sheep, lambs, goats, cattle, possibly humans (Australia)	+		−		+		−	
E	Sheep and cattle, pathogenicity doubted (United Kingdom)	+		−		−		+	

[a] Also called phospholipase C.

is a public health laboratory function that should be performed concomitantly with provision of epidemiologic support. Ideally, isolates of the same serotype can be cultured from epidemiologically incriminated food and ill persons but not from control subjects. Unfortunately, the experience with serotyping of *C. perfringens* at the Centers for Disease Control and Prevention (CDC) has not been highly successful (73).

Enteritis Necroticans (Pig-Bel, Necrotizing Enteritis, and Necrotizing Enterocolitis [NEC])

Caused by beta-toxin-producing strains of *C. perfringens* type C, enteritis necroticans is a life-threatening infectious disease characterized by ischemic necrosis of the small bowel (5). Recognized in Papua New Guinea during the 1960s, where it then was the most frequent cause of death in children, it has been associated with pig feasts and occurs both sporadically and in outbreaks (127). "Pig-bel" is the pidgin English name used in the highlands of Papua New Guinea to describe this condition. The clinical features

usually begin within hours to 1 week after a large amount of meat has been eaten and include abdominal pain and tenderness, distention, and vomiting, sometimes with bloody diarrhea. The patient may become febrile and hypotensive, with signs of septicemia and intestinal obstruction, and may die within 24 h of onset. The pathologic spectrum of the disease includes an acute, patchy, hemorrhagic, necrotizing process involving the jejunum. In severe cases, there may be gas gangrene of the entire small bowel with involvement of the proximal large bowel as well (5). Evidence implicating the beta-toxin produced by type C strains of *C. perfringens* in the etiology of pig-bel includes the success of immunization against the toxin which resulted in a decreased incidence of the disease in New Guinea (107). Among the factors likely to be involved in the pathogenesis of enteritis necroticans are (i) overeating (i.e., pork and other meats), which might distend the bowel and cause partial obstruction; (ii) poor nutrition, which leads to low levels of production of the pancreatic proteases (particularly trypsin, which ordinarily destroys beta-toxin);

(iii) a diet rich in trypsin inhibitors (e.g., sweet potatoes, peanuts, and soy beans); and (iv) trypsin inhibitors produced by *Ascaris lumbricoides*. Enteritis necroticans occurs in other developing countries of the world (127). It has also been recognized in the United States, the United Kingdom, and other developed nations, especially involving adults who are malnourished or who have chronic illnesses (e.g., diabetes or alcoholic liver disease) (49, 67, 134). The surgical and medical treatment of enteritis necroticans is beyond the scope of this chapter but has been addressed elsewhere (127). There is concern that enteritis necroticans is more common than appreciated and is probably underreported (108).

NEC is a serious gastrointestinal disease that affects low-birth-weight (premature) infants who are hospitalized in neonatal intensive care units (103). As reviewed by Kliegman et al., the etiology and pathogenesis of this condition remain speculative in spite of more than 1,000 publications on NEC over the last 4 decades (96). In the United States, NEC affects an estimated 2,000 to 4,000 infants each year and is a significant cause of morbidity and mortality (e.g., 20 to 35%) in neonatal intensive care units (96, 103). Pathologically, there are many similarities between NEC and pig-bel, including the patterns of necrosis and inflammation that occur in these conditions (95). An interesting finding in both diseases is the presence of abnormal intestinal gas cysts or pneumatosis intestinalis. The source of the gas, which contains hydrogen, methane, and carbon dioxide, is probably the fermentative activities of intestinal bacteria (96). Similar disease caused by *C. perfringens* has been reported for neonatal piglets (94) and in experimental animal studies (168). Epidemiologic data (e.g., outbreaks of the disease) also support an important role for *C. perfringens* or perhaps other gas-producing microorganisms (e.g., certain other clostridia or *Klebsiella* spp.) in the pathogenesis of NEC (95, 103).

CDAD, AAD, and Colitis

C. difficile, the major cause of antibiotic-associated diarrhea (AAD) and pseudomembranous colitis, is also the most frequently identified cause of hospital-acquired diarrhea (84). The organism has been isolated from diverse natural habitats, including soil, hay, sand, dung from various large mammals (cows, donkeys, and horses), and the feces of dogs, cats, rodents, and humans (111). *C. difficile* is carried asymptomatically as part of the gastrointestinal flora of as many as half of all healthy neonates during the first year of life; the carriage rate decreases to the adult carrier rate of 3% or less in children older than 2 years (109). Rates of carriage of *C. difficile* in asymptomatic adult populations have varied from 1.9% in Sweden to 15.4% of young adults in Japan (13, 128). As reviewed by Gerding et al., hospitalized patients frequently become colonized with this organism (60). McFarland et al. reported that 21% of 399 patients with negative cultures on admission to a hospital with a high prevalence of *C. difficile*-associated disease (CDAD) acquired *C. difficile* during hospitalization (120). Of these patients, 63% remained asymptomatic while 37% developed diarrhea. Antimicrobial agents of all classes and several anticancer chemotherapeutic agents have been implicated in the development of CDAD or pseudomembranous colitis (84). The most commonly reported agents have been ampicillin, amoxicillin, clindamycin, and various cephalosporins; the carbapenems, quinolones, macrolides (e.g., clarithromycin and azithromycin), aminoglycosides, and tetracyclines appear to carry lower risks (60, 62, 169).

C. difficile is susceptible to the antimicrobial agents that lead to the onset of CDAD. Most strains, for example, are susceptible to penicillin, erythromycin, tetracycline, chloramphenicol, clindamycin, metronidazole, vancomycin, and cotrimoxazole (37, 46). Metronidazole and vancomycin, which are used to treat the disease, are active against all strains tested to date. In some instances, particular strains were resistant to chloramphenicol, rifampin, erythromycin, clindamycin, and tetracycline, resulting in outbreaks of CDAD.

In CDAD, the primary initating event involves the disruption of the protective intestinal flora during treatment with antibiotics and antineoplastic agents. As the level of antibiotic drops to below inhibitory concentrations, nosocomial pathogens such as *C. difficile* are able to enter the intestine and begin to grow. Toxigenic as well as nontoxigenic isolates are capable of forming spores and existing in the hospital environment. As a result, either type can infect the colon and utilize the nutrients that are available because of the lack of competition by the normal flora. Only the toxigenic isolates, however, are associated with disease, and in fact, the nontoxigenic isolates may be protective through competitive exclusion (21). Whether the organism attaches to the colonic wall is not clear, but it is more likely that the organism grows throughout the lumen of the colon. Toxigenic strains produce and release toxins A and B as the cells grow and lyse. The onset of the disease is due to the action of toxins A and B, both of which are glucosyltransferases that monoglucosylate factor Rho (and other low-molecular-mass G proteins), which is involved in the control of the cytoskeletal system (1). This activity, along with the inflammatory response, results in the histopathological events leading to *C. difficile*-associated diarrhea and colitis.

C. difficile produces at least three potential virulence factors: a 308-kDa enterotoxin (toxin A) that induces a positive fluid response in the rabbit ligated ileal loop model, a 270-kDa cytotoxin (toxin B) that induces cytopathic effects in numerous tissue culture cell lines (123), and a substance that inhibits bowel motility (87). Toxin A also produces cytopathic effects in cell cultures but is less potent than toxin B in most cell culture lines (123). Both toxins interfere with the actin cytoskeletons of intestinal epithelial cells, thereby rendering the cells nonfunctional. As reviewed elsewhere, the mechanism through which toxins A and B disrupt the cytoskeleton involves modification of Rho family proteins by UDP-glucose-dependent glycosylation (123).

Until recently, all toxigenic isolates of *C. difficile* were believed to produce both toxin A and toxin B. In the early 1990s, an isolate that produced only toxin B was described, and characterization studies suggested that the isolate carried a truncated *toxA* gene (23, 110, 165). Furthermore, biological activity assays indicated that toxin B from this particular isolate was more toxic than toxin B from typical A$^+$/B$^+$ isolates. At the time, however, the clinical significance of this "atypical" isolate was not known. In the late 1990s, reports of atypical A$^-$/B$^+$ isolates and their association with clinical disease began to appear (2, 4, 112). It appears now that like A$^+$/B$^+$ isolates, atypical A$^-$/B$^+$ isolates may be associated with a wide range of clinical findings ranging from asymptomatic carriage to fatal pseudomembranous colitis. There also is increasing evidence that atypical isolates may be associated with outbreaks in hospitals (2, 4). This is of particular concern since these isolates will be missed in facilities which base their diagnosis solely on the use of toxin A-specific tests. The incidence of A$^-$/B$^+$ isolates in CDAD is not known, and additional epidemiological studies are needed for this purpose. In the United States and Canada, A$^-$/B$^+$ isolates have been identified in more than eight distinct geographical locations. In England, it has been estimated that about 5% of CDAD is due to these atypical isolates (25). Recent evidence suggests that the incidence may be quite high in some institutions (M. S. Burday, R. Sood, and W. Alpaugh, *Abstr. 101st Gen. Meet. Am. Soc. Microbiol.*, abstr. C-188, 2001). Atypical A$^-$/B$^+$ isolates have been associated with fatal pseudomembranous colitis (2, 4, 85).

A characteristic feature of A$^-$/B$^+$ isolates is the deletion of a large region of about 1.7 kb within the portion of the *toxA* gene encoding the repeating region (i.e., the binding portion of the toxin) (88, 124). Located within the repeating region are epitopes recognized by the monoclonal antibody used in many toxin A-specific ELISAs. Because this portion of the toxin is deleted, A$^-$/B$^+$ isolates are not detected in toxin A-specific ELISAs. In addition to the deletion in *toxA*, the active site of the toxin B gene is modified in A$^-$/B$^+$ isolates, resulting in a toxin B that more closely resembles the lethal toxin of *C. sordellii* (166).

Reports suggest that *C. perfringens* is a less frequently identified cause of AAD (22). Enterotoxin-producing *C. perfringens* type A has been isolated from AAD patients who are negative for *C. difficile* and who have no other apparent causes of the disease. Coinfection with *C. difficile* and enterotoxigenic *C. perfringens* type A has been reported for AAD patients. The incidence of *C. perfringens*-associated AAD has been estimated at 5 to 20%, but additional epidemiological studies are needed to more accurately determine the role of this organism in AAD (29). Some *C. perfringens* isolates from AAD were shown to carry *cpe* on a plasmid, whereas isolates associated with food poisoning carried the gene on the chromosome (154).

C. difficile is an important cause of enteric infections in the elderly and in nursing home residents (148). *C. difficile* is a problem not only when antibiotics are used, but also for patients with bowel stasis, those who have had bowel surgery, and those with no known risk factors, although this form of the disease is less common than that associated with antibiotic use. Clinical symptoms range from mild diarrhea to toxic megacolon (84). In the most severe form, the disease may include bowel perforation and death, although these events are unlikely to occur in appropriately treated patients.

C. septicum and Bacteremia

C. septicum is isolated only rarely from the feces of healthy individuals and is not recovered often from cultures of blood from otherwise healthy individuals. Increasingly, the isolation of this swarming organism (Fig. 1) from anaerobic blood cultures has been associated with other underlying disease processes, often serious neoplastic disease. The portal of entry for *C. septicum* into the bloodstream is believed to be the ileocecal region of the bowel. Whether *C. septicum* is part of the indigenous microflora of this site, at least in low concentrations, has not been established. *C. septicum* has, however, been found in the lumens of 10 to 68% of normal appendices and in none of 30 nonlumen appendiceal tissue samples from gangrenous or perforated appendices (19, 58).

C. septicum bacteremia is associated with malignancies, especially leukemia and lymphoma or carcinoma of the large bowel. As many as 70 to 85% of patients whose blood cultures are positive for this organism have some underlying malignancy (20, 91). While the nature of this association between *C. septicum* and underlying malignancy remains to be determined, it has not been shown to involve 7α-dehydroxylation of bile acids (77, 93). Another clinically important association has been observed between *C. septicum* bacteremia, neutropenia, and enterocolitis involving the terminal ileum or cecum (90, 104). The neutropenia has been related both to chemotherapy for leukemia or other neoplastic diseases and to cyclic neutropenia and drug-induced agranulocytosis.

Not all patients with *C. septicum* bacteremia have malignancy or neutropenic enterocolitis. Patients with diabetes mellitus, severe atherosclerotic cardiovascular disease, or gas gangrene may also develop *C. septicum* bacteremia (101). The clinical importance of recognizing *C. septicum* bacteremia and starting appropriate treatment without delay cannot be overemphasized. Patients with this condition are usually acutely and gravely ill, frequently have high temperatures, and often show metastatic spread of myonecrosis to distant anatomic sites. Mortality rates are significant (68% or greater). Although appropriate antibiotic therapy with β-lactam antibiotics and aggressive surgical intervention early in the course of the illness have both been recommended to aid in avoiding a devastating outcome (101, 102), some survivors have received antibiotics and supportive care alone (83).

C. botulinum and Botulism

C. botulinum, the cause of a rare but life-threatening foodborne illness, is widely distributed in soil and aquatic habitats throughout the world. Microorganisms designated *C. botulinum*, along with unique strains of *C. butyricum*, *C. baratii*, and *C. argentinense*, can produce the most lethal poison known, namely, botulinum neurotoxin (BoNT) (70). There are seven antigenic toxin types of BoNT (A through G), determined by serologic toxin neutralization tests, and they serve as useful clinical and epidemiologic markers. Toxin types A, B, and E of *C. botulinum* are the principal causes of botulism in humans. Strains of *C. butyricum* (15, 52, 142), which produce type E neurotoxin, and strains of *C. baratii* (68, 118), which produce type F neurotoxin, have been implicated rarely in human botulism. *C. argentinense*, which produces type G neurotoxin (162), has been isolated from soil in Argentina and from autopsy materials from five individuals who died suddenly, but *C. argentinense* has not been clearly implicated in botulism (70). *C. botulinum* types C and D are associated primarily with botulism in birds and mammals (151). Type C can be subdivided into two toxin types, C1 and C2; C1 is a neurotoxin, and C2 causes vascular permeability and has enterotoxic activity (151).

Each BoNT is synthesized during growth of the organism as a single inactive protein (~150 kDa) that is released during lysis of the bacterial cells (109). Activation of the molecule requires proteolytic cleavage into two disulfide-linked polypeptide chains, a 50-kDa light chain and a 100-kDa heavy chain (143). BoNT production in type C and D *C. botulinum* is mediated by bacteriophages and can be lost by curing the organisms of their prophages (71). In contrast to those for all of the other toxin types of *C. botulinum*, the genes for type G BoNT are carried on a plasmid (170). The genes encoding the BoNT complexes for toxin types A, B, E, and F are assumed to be located on chromosomal DNA (81).

There are four naturally occurring categories of botulism: (i) classical food-borne botulism, an intoxication

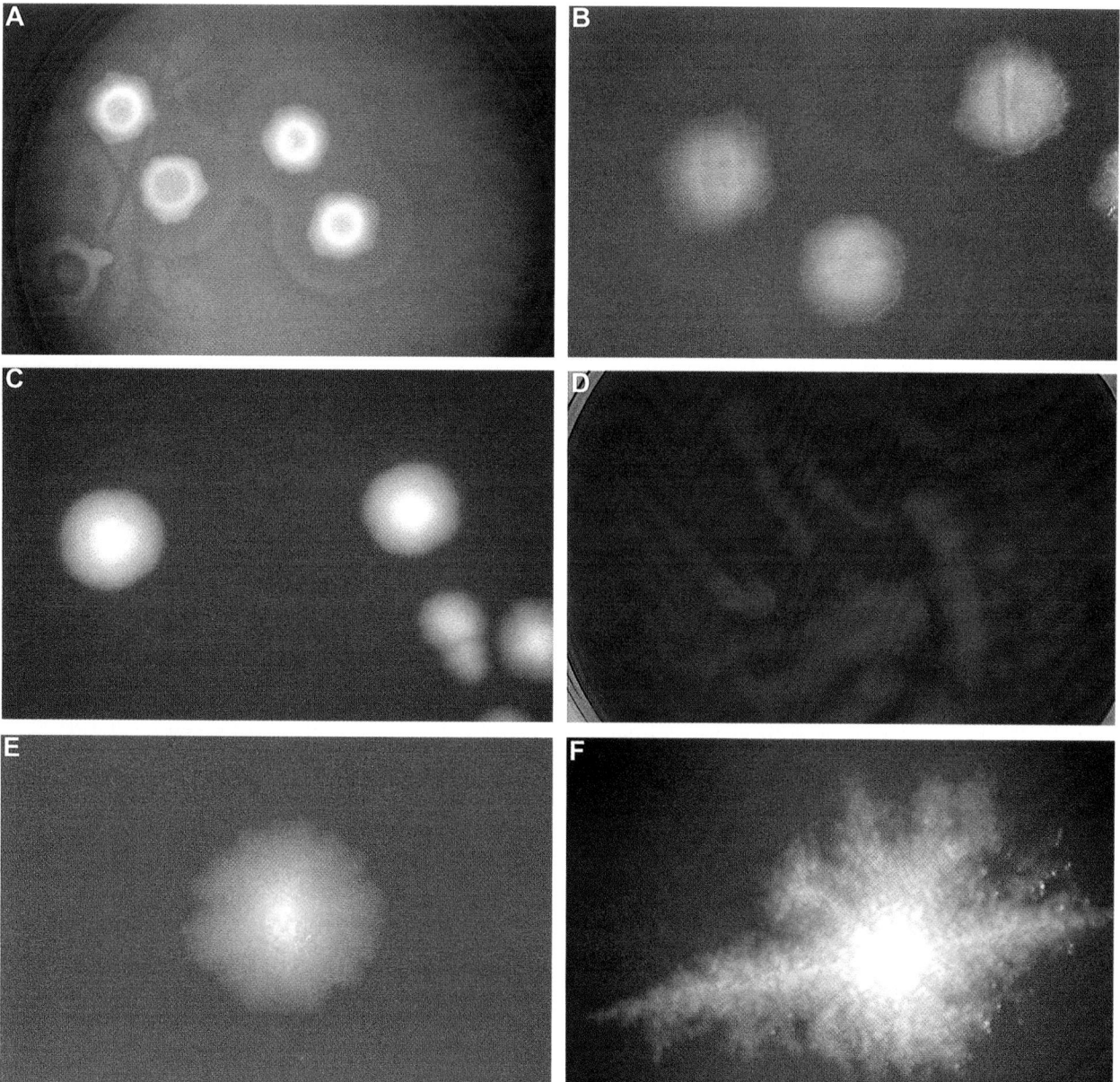

FIGURE 1 Colony characteristics typical of selected common and/or clinically important *Clostridium* species on CDC Anaerobe Blood Agar (prepared with sheep blood; see text for more information). (A) *C. perfringens* colonies surrounded by double zone of hemolysis. There is an inner narrow zone of complete hemolysis due to theta-toxin and an outer, wider zone of partial hemolysis due to the alpha-toxin. (B) Dissecting microscope close-up view (magnification, ×7 to ×15) of the same *C. perfringens* colonies shown in panel A. The 3- to 5-mm-diameter colonies are slightly raised, relatively flat, and semitranslucent with irregular margins. (C) *C. ramosum*: dissecting microscope view showing ~2-mm, nonhemolytic semitranslucent colonies with opaque centers and entire to slightly irregular margins. (D) *C. septicum*: swarming, flat, translucent, markedly irregular surface growth with hemolysis beneath the surface growth. The darkness of the medium is related to the incubation conditions (low oxidation-reduction potential). (E) *C. innocuum*: 3 to 4 mm, convex, grey-white, semitranslucent with internal flecking; nonhemolytic, but some strains may be hemolytic. (F) *C. difficile*: ~3 to 5 mm, nonhemolytic, grey-white, with birefringent, crystalline internal structure and irregular, rhizoid margins.

caused by the ingestion of preformed botulinal toxin in contaminated food; (ii) wound botulism, which results from elaboration of botulinal toxin in vivo after growth of *C. botulinum* in an infected wound; (iii) infant botulism, in which botulinal toxin is elaborated in vivo in the intestinal tract of an infant colonized with *C. botulinum*; and (iv) botulism due to intestinal colonization in children and adults (70).

Aerosolized Botulinum Toxin as a Bioweapon

There now is a fifth category of botulism: inhalational botulism, which results from aerosolization of botulinum toxin. This form has been demonstrated experimentally in monkeys and accidentally in three veterinary personnel in Germany who were exposed to reaerosolized BoNT from rabbits and guinea pigs with aerosolized type A botulinum on their fur (12). As reviewed by Arnon et al. (12), terrorists have already attempted to use aerosolized botulinum toxin as a bioweapon in Japan but were not successful. After Operation Desert Storm ended in 1991, Iraq admitted to having produced 19,000 liters of concentrated botulinum toxin and to having loaded more than half of it into specially designed military weapons (e.g., missiles). According to Arnon et al., 19,000 liters of concentrated botulinum toxin is more than enough to kill the entire human population by inhalation (12).

Regardless of the category of botulism, the toxin enters the bloodstream from the site where it was produced or absorbed (e.g., gut, wound, or lung) and then is carried through the bloodstream to peripheral nerve endings, particularly the neuromuscular junctions of motor neurons, where it binds irreversibly to the presynaptic membranes. A portion of the toxin molecule probably penetrates the plasma membrane by receptor-mediated endocytosis and is internalized into the nerve cell. The neurotoxin molecule acts within the nerve terminal at the neuromuscular junction to prevent the release of acetylcholine (143). The characteristic clinical hallmark of botulism is an acute flaccid paralysis, which begins with bilateral cranial nerve impairment involving muscles of the face, head, and pharynx and then descends symmetrically to involve muscles of the thorax and extremities. In naturally occurring food-borne botulism, gastrointestinal symptoms (e.g., abdominal cramps, nausea, vomiting, or diarrhea) occurring probably secondarily in response to other bacterial metabolites present in the food may precede the neurological signs of descending flaccid paralysis. Gastrointestinal symptoms or signs are not likely to be seen if purified botulinum toxin is released in aerosols or ingested in foods or liquids. Death may result from respiratory failure caused by paralysis of the tongue or muscles of the pharynx that occlude the upper airway or from paralysis of the diaphragm and intercostal muscles. Patients diagnosed with food-borne or wound botulism should immediately receive trivalent (type ABE) antitoxin and intensive respiratory care. Botulinum toxin, as a weapon in bioterrorism, is covered further in chapter 10.

C. botulinum and Infant Botulism

In the United States, infant botulism (a reportable disease) is the most frequently recognized form of botulism. Although it has been documented in at least 13 other countries, it is rare outside the United States (70). Of the 1,678 cases reported in the United States between 1976 and 1999, about 45% were in California (33, 34). Across the United States, the geographical distribution of toxin types in infant botulism cases has paralleled the distribution of *C. botuli-*

num toxin types in soil sampled from different locations (150). Type A has been the most frequent BoNT type in cases of infant botulism in states west of the Mississippi River, whereas type B cases have predominated east of the Mississippi (10). Interestingly, one infant from Hawaii had both type A and B strains of *C. botulinum* (69). Two other cases were caused by a strain(s) of *C. botulinum* that produced toxins requiring both type B and F antitoxins for neutralization (69). In another interesting case, type F infant botulism was caused by an organism that most closely resembled *C. baratii* in its cultural and biochemical characteristics (68). Type E botulism, caused by toxigenic strains of *C. butyricum*, was confirmed in two infants from Italy (70). Although most infected infants are 3 weeks to 6 months old, the age range is 6 to 363 days (9). Preformed toxin has not been detected in any food or liquid ingested by these infants. To date, the only clearly defined risk factors have been breast-feeding and exposure to honey, which is a potential source of spores. The CDC has recommended that honey not be fed to infants less than 1 year old (156). Another concern, although not proven, is that spores have also been found in a limited number of samples of corn syrup, which is often given to infants for treatment of decreased frequency of bowel movements (156). Whatever the sources, the ingested spores of *C. botulinum* germinate within the intestinal tract, and the vegetative cells multiply and produce the neurotoxin, which is then absorbed into the bloodstream. Decreased frequency of bowel movements, which may also be a sign of decreased intestinal motility, may be an additional risk factor for infant botulism (156). The first sign of illness is invariably constipation, which is often overlooked. Infants who are ultimately hospitalized usually develop lethargy and mild weakness with feeding difficulties, pooled oral secretions, and an altered cry. They eventually become floppy, lose head control, and may go on to develop ophthalmoplegia, ptosis, flaccid facial expression, dysphagia, other signs of cranial nerve deficits, and generalized muscular weakness. Respiratory insufficiency necessitating respiratory therapy also may occur, as in other forms of botulism (10). There is a spectrum of clinical features in infant botulism, ranging from mild illness not requiring hospitalization to sudden death, which accounts for a small percentage of cases of sudden infant death syndrome (11).

C. tetani and Tetanus

Tetanus, the strictly toxigenic disease caused by *C. tetani*, is often associated with puncture wounds that do not appear to be serious infections, particularly in animals. The organism and its spores can be isolated from a variety of sources, including soil and the intestinal contents of numerous animal species. A potent neurotoxin, tetanospasmin, is elaborated at the site of apparent minor trauma and rapidly binds to neural tissue, provoking a characteristic paralysis and spasms (see below). Tetanus is largely a disease of nonimmunized animals and humans, since an effective toxoid has been in use for many years.

Tetanus is an extremely dramatic illness. Spasticity is characteristic of tetanus, whereas flaccid paralysis is characteristic of botulism (42), because tetanospasmin acts within the central nervous system, and the activity of BoNT is confined to the peripheral nervous system. Tetanospasmin is synthesized as a single, inactive polypeptide chain (150 kDa). Upon lysis of *C. tetani*, the toxin is cleaved by an intrinsic protease to produce a dichain, consisting of a heavy chain (100 kDa) and a light chain (50 kDa) linked by a disulfide bond (143). The heavy chain is the part of the molecule that binds to neuronal cells. The light chain, a zinc endopeptidase, binds to protein components of the neuroexocytotic apparatus and inhibits the exocytosis of the neurotransmitter (γ-aminobutyric acid in this case) at synapses within the central nervous system (143). Thus, inhibitory impulses to the motor neurons are blocked; uninhibited firing of motor nerve transmissions continues, resulting in prolonged muscle spasms of both flexor and extensor muscles that can persist for weeks. In the United States, tetanus is reported most frequently in California, Michigan, Texas, and Florida and other areas of the rural South (80). While most cases involve persons aged $\geq$60 years, injection of drugs (i.e., "skin popping") has recently become an important risk factor in younger persons (80). It would be unusual for the clinical laboratory to be requested to isolate *C. tetani* from a wound, since tetanus usually presents few diagnostic problems for the clinician.

OTHER CLOSTRIDIAL DISEASES

Clostridium spp. and Bacteremia

At Indiana University and Riley Hospitals (Clarian Health Partners, Indianapolis, Ind.), where anaerobic blood cultures remain as a standard part of a high-volume blood culture system, approximately 9% of all blood cultures during the years 1996 through 2001 yielded clinically significant bacteria. During this period, clostridia accounted for about 1% of the significant isolates (S. D. Allen and J. A. Siders, unpublished data). The species encountered most frequently in positive blood cultures was *C. perfringens*, which usually represents 20 to $\geq$50% of the *Clostridium* bloodstream isolates per year. Other *Clostridium* species found less frequently in positive blood cultures include *C. innocuum*, *C. septicum*, *C. ramosum*, *C. clostridioforme*, *C. difficile*, *C. bifermentans*, *C. sordellii*, *C. tertium*, *C. paraputrificum*, *C. cadaveris*, and *C. sporogenes* (26). Underlying conditions commonly associated with clostridial bacteremia have included chronic alcoholism, sepsis following intra-abdominal surgery, necrosis of the small intestine and large bowel, genitourinary tract disorders (including septic abortions), cardiovascular disease, pulmonary diseases, underlying malignancy, diabetes, and decubitus ulcers (26, 63). Bacteremia involving *C. perfringens* and certain other clostridia is not always associated with a serious underlying illness (63). Isolates are sometimes of doubtful significance or may even represent contaminants. Clostridia of the intestinal flora deposited transiently in the perianal area could be spread to a venipuncture site; alternatively, blood culture isolates could reflect transient bacteremia of no clinical significance.

Although as many as 7 to 8% of all cases of infective endocarditis may have been caused by anaerobes during the early 1970s, clostridia were relatively uncommon (18). Reports during the 1990s suggest that clostridial endocarditis is becoming more prevalent than it was during the 1970s (38). *Clostridium* species encountered in infective endocarditis have included *C. perfringens*, *C. septicum*, *C. sordellii*, *C. bifermentans*, *C. histolyticum*, *C. clostridioforme*, *C. sporogenes*, and *C. innocuum* (40, 45, 137).

Additional Clostridial Species of Interest

In the spring of 2000, *C. novyi* was implicated in a large outbreak of illness among injecting-drug users (IDUs) in England, Wales, Scotland, and Ireland, suggesting soil or fecal contamination of drugs or other materials that were in common to these individuals (35). *C. novyi* is a fastidious, strict obligate anaerobe that has been reported only occasionally in recent years for patients with clinical illness. It is probably underreported because of its demanding growth requirements and its tendency to lose viability unless anaerobic conditions are optimal. A number of these IDU patients, including one from England who had necrotizing fasciitis, had *C. novyi* as the only pathogen (129). The relatively large number of cases and the severity of illnesses associated with this outbreak are noteworthy. IDUs are at high risk for tetanus (80) and probably for other clostridial diseases as well. Although it is rare, the subcutaneous injection of Mexican black tar heroin has been associated with wound botulism in Hispanic IDUs (36, 47).

Numerous other clostridial species are occasionally associated with disease. Species such as *C. sordellii*, *C. histolyticum*, *C. bifermentans*, *C. fallax*, *C. sporogenes*, and *C. tertium* have all been associated with histotoxic clostridial disease (see the discussion of *C. perfringens* above) (55, 151). *C. sordellii* has also been cited as producing a cytotoxin similar to that of *C. difficile* (see the discussion of *C. difficile* above) (65).

COLLECTION, TRANSPORT, AND STORAGE OF CLINICAL SPECIMENS

As with other anaerobic bacteria, the proper selection, collection, and transport of clinical specimens are extremely important for the laboratory diagnosis of clostridial infections. For recommended collection and transport procedures in general, refer to chapter 20. Several tissue specimens should be taken from the active site of infections when gas gangrene is suspected, because clostridia are often not distributed uniformly in pathological lesions. In addition to standard aspirates and tissues, selected clostridial illnesses require special specimens.

Specimens for Confirmation of *C. perfringens* Food-Borne Illness

For a laboratory confirmation of *C. perfringens* food-borne illness, most clinical laboratories need to use the services of a reference laboratory (e.g., local or state public health laboratory; see chapter 13).

Specimens To Aid in Diagnosis of Enteritis Necroticans (*C. perfringens* Type C)

Important considerations in the diagnosis of intestinal illness caused by *C. perfringens* type C include examination of the patient's medical history and clinical findings, direct gross and microscopic examination of pathologic specimens, bacteriologic workup of appropriate specimens, and assays for toxins (or toxin genes) in pathologic materials or bacteriologic cultures (e.g., supernatants of broth cultures). Thus, if enteritis necroticans is suspected, the specimens to collect include three blood cultures collected from three different venipuncture sites, stool (at least 25 g, or 25 ml if liquid), and lumen contents, or tissue from the involved bowel (e.g., surgical specimen or autopsy material). Specimens should be transported in tightly sealed leakproof containers for the following: direct Gram stain, culture, isolation, identification, and typing of *C. perfringens*. Although at this writing no immunologic procedures or molecular assays are commercially available for detection of the beta-toxin or the beta-toxin gene of *C. perfringens* type

C, PCR assays for genotyping *C. perfringens* are being used in certain research or referral laboratories to aid in diagnosis (121, 152, 153). Accordingly, DNA can be extracted for this purpose from formalin-fixed intestinal tissue or culture and amplified by PCR using primers specific for the *cpa* and *cpb* genes of *C. perfringens* type C.

Specimens for *C. difficile* Culture and Toxin Assay

A single, freshly passed fecal specimen (ideally 10 to 20 ml of watery stool; minimum of 5.0 ml or 5 g) is the preferred specimen for *C. difficile* culture and toxin assay (59). To lessen the chance of obtaining positive culture results from patients merely colonized with the organism, only liquid or unformed stool specimens should be processed. An exception could be made for epidemiologic surveys to determine the degree of *C. difficile* carriage in a population. Swab specimens are inadequate for the toxin assay because the volume of sample obtained is too small, although swabs have been used successfully to detect carriers during epidemiologic investigations (119). Other appropriate specimens include lumen contents and surgical or autopsy samples of the large bowel. Specimens should be transported in tightly sealed, leakproof plastic or glass containers without transport medium. For optimal recovery, stool specimens should be cultured within 2 h of collection; although spores will survive in refrigerated stool for several days, there will probably be a large decrease in the number of viable vegetative cells of *C. difficile* in refrigerated specimens. Stools may be placed in an anaerobic environment (anaerobic transport vial or swab) if culture must be performed after storage. Adequate recovery of *C. difficile* may be expected from stools stored at 5°C for up to 2 days. Specimens for toxin assay may be stored at 5°C for up to 3 days and should be frozen at −70°C if a longer delay before performance of the assay is anticipated. Freezing at −20°C results in a dramatic loss of cytotoxin activity (132).

Specimens for Suspected Neutropenic Enterocolitis Involving *C. septicum*

The specimens of choice for suspected neutropenic enterocolitis involving *C. septicum* are three blood cultures collected from three different venipuncture sites, stool (at least 25 g, or 25 ml if liquid), and lumen contents or tissue from the involved ileocecal area collected at surgery or autopsy and transported in tightly sealed leakproof containers. In addition, a biopsy sample of muscle (or an aspirate of fluid from the involved area, taken with a needle and syringe) should be collected if the patient is also suspected of having myonecrosis or another form of progressive infection.

Specimens for *C. botulinum* Culture and Toxin Assay

Most hospital laboratories are not properly equipped to process specimens from patients suspected of having botulism. Attending physicians should notify their State Health Department or the CDC (24-h/7-day emergency service) immediately when there is a suspected case of botulism and before collecting any specimens so that appropriate action can be taken to establish the diagnosis, initiate treatment, and investigate the potential outbreak. Some State Health Department Laboratories also provide diagnostic laboratory services for botulism. The appropriate CDC telephone numbers for the Foodborne and Diarrheal Diseases Branch follow: days, (404) 639-2206 (Monday to Friday, 8:30 a.m. to 4:30 p.m. Eastern Time); nights and weekends, (404) 639-2888.

The diagnosis of botulism can be confirmed by the laboratory demonstration of BoNT in serum, feces, gastric contents, or vomitus or by the recovery of *C. botulinum* from the feces of the patient, since the organism has been isolated only rarely from asymptomatic individuals during food-borne outbreaks (33, 71). Ideally, 15 to 20 ml of serum (not whole blood), 25 to 50 g of stool, and the suspect food(s) should be collected. Specimens from patients with suspected wound botulism include serum, feces, tissue, exudate, or swab samples from the wound. When infant botulism is suspected, serum (2 ml) and as much stool as possible should be collected. In most instances, the diagnosis of infant botulism has been confirmed by the detection of the toxin or *C. botulinum* or both in feces. Toxin has been detected in serum only infrequently in infants with this diagnosis. During a bioterrorist attack, serum, gastric aspirates, feces, and environmental or nasal swabs could be useful for detecting aerosolized botulinum toxin that has been inhaled (12, 167). All specimens should be refrigerated until they can be transported to the laboratory for testing (12).

DIRECT EXAMINATION

Gas gangrene is an extremely urgent situation, requiring a rapid clinical diagnosis. The direct examination of a Gram-stained smear of the wound may be useful for establishing the diagnosis. Characteristic findings are the absence of inflammatory cells and other cellular outlines and the presence of clostridia in smears prepared from the central areas of the lesion. In contrast, nonclostridial anaerobic cellulitis may involve anaerobic cocci, facultatively anaerobic cocci, *Bacteroides* spp., *Fusobacterium* spp., and/or other microbial species. Cell outlines of striated muscle cells and granulocytes remain intact in the latter condition (114).

Special note should be made of gram-positive rods with or without spores, because sporulation in tissue is not common for the two species most frequently encountered in wound and abscess materials, *C. perfringens* and *C. ramosum*. *C. perfringens* usually appears as large, relatively short, fat, gram-positive rods in tissue smears; the cells of *C. ramosum* are more slender and longer (99). *C. perfringens* may or may not be encapsulated in smears from wounds; capsules usually are present in smears of endometrial specimens from postabortion *C. perfringens* infections. Special spore stains offer no advantage over Gram stains for the demonstration of spores.

Examination with a phase microscope may be helpful if the spores are close to maturity. If spores are present, their shapes (spherical or oval) and positions (terminal, subterminal, or central) in the cells should be noted. An excellent medium for the demonstration of spores is a chopped-meat agar slant. The culture should be incubated anaerobically at 5 to 7°C below the optimum temperature for growth of clostridia. For most species, 30°C is satisfactory, but 37°C is better for inducing sporulation of *C. perfringens*. If spores are not visible, their presence may be deduced by subjecting a suspension of the isolate to heat (80°C) or ethanol treatment (described below).

A monograph and color atlas containing 230 examples of Gram-stained smear preparations (along with a CD-ROM version), including many photomicrographs of various *Clostridium* species, other anaerobes, and numerous other microorganisms in clinical specimens, was published recently (114). Other publications containing representative Gram stain preparations plus other illustrations related to the diagnosis of anaerobic infections are also available (54, 99, 163).

CULTURE AND ISOLATION OF CLOSTRIDIA OTHER THAN *C. DIFFICILE*

A summary of useful procedures for culture and isolation of clostridia is provided below. For more detailed information on the topic, the *Clinical Microbiology Procedures Handbook* for anaerobic bacteriology (79), the manual by Summanen et al. (163), and the text by Koneman et al. (99) provide detailed procedures. Clostridia usually produce good growth on commercially available CDC anaerobe blood agar and phenylethyl alcohol blood agar (PEA) after 1 to 2 days of incubation. Brucella 5% sheep blood agar, Columbia agar, or brain heart infusion agar supplemented with yeast extract, vitamin K, and hemin may also be used as the nonselective blood agar medium; colony characteristics vary on these different media. A few species, such as *C. perfringens*, form colonies after overnight incubation. When clostridia are suspected in wound or abscess specimens (e.g., from gas gangrene), it is recommended that egg yolk agar (modified McClung-Toabe formula) be inoculated in addition to blood agar and PEA (44).

After incubation, the blood agar and PEA cultures should be examined under a dissecting microscope, with note being made of the hemolysis pattern, colony structure, and any evidence of swarming or motile colonies. Egg yolk agar should be examined for evidence of lecithinase or lipase production. Lecithinase activity is indicated by the development of an insoluble, opaque, whitish precipitate within the agar. An iridescent sheen or oil on water appearance (pearly layer) on the surface growth indicates lipase activity. Proteolysis, the third reaction that can be seen on egg yolk agar, is indicated by a zone of translucent clearing in the medium around the colonies. In addition to the modified McClung-Toabe egg yolk agar formulation, the same reactions can be visualized on the hemin-supplemented egg yolk agar formulation recommended by Summanen et al. (163) or on Lombard-Dowell egg yolk agar (99).

Isolation of additional strains in the presence of swarming *Proteus* species or *C. septicum* may require short incubation times (18 to 24 h), subculture onto PEA, or use of anaerobe blood agar with ≥4% agar (stiff blood agar) (44). When isolated colonies can be picked, they should be subcultured to chopped-meat medium, and the culture should be incubated overnight and used for the inoculation of differential media. In addition, chopped-meat–carbohydrate broth (78) should be inoculated for gas-liquid chromatography.

Spore Selection Techniques

Heat (80°C) or ethanol procedures (100) are commonly used in public health laboratories for the selective isolation of *C. botulinum* and *C. perfringens* from feces and foods (33, 73). These techniques can aid in the isolation of *C. difficile* from feces and are less costly than cycloserine-cefoxitin-fructose agar (CCFA) medium (115). They can also save time in isolation of clostridia from other kinds of specimens containing a mixture of microorganisms (e.g., wounds and abscesses) (99). Ethanol may be more effective than heat if the specimen contains relatively heat-sensitive clostridia (e.g., *C. botulinum* type E and some strains of *C. perfringens* involved in food-borne outbreaks) (100). Heat treatment

may be more effective than alcohol if homogenization is incomplete and the specimen contains particulate matter that is not penetrated adequately by the alcohol. For any spore selection technique, an untreated control subculture should be prepared.

Alcohol Treatment

To a 1-ml sample of a fecal suspension, homogenate of a wound or exudate, etc., in a sterile screw-cap tube, an equal volume of absolute (or 95%) ethanol is added (100). The specimen is gently mixed at room temperature (22 to 25°C for 1 h). An Ames aliquot mixer (Miles Laboratories, Inc., Elkhart, Ind.) is a convenient way to provide continuous mixing. The treated material is subcultured and used to inoculate chopped-meat–glucose (or chopped-meat–glucose–starch) medium, anaerobe blood agar, or egg yolk agar. The culture is incubated and inspected for growth.

Heat Treatment

For heat treatment (44), a tube of chopped-meat–glucose–starch medium is preheated in an 80°C water bath for 5 min and 1 ml of sample suspension is added. The culture is heated for 10 min and the tube is removed and cooled in cold water. The treated sample suspension is subcultured into an unheated tube of chopped-meat–glucose–starch medium and onto an anaerobe blood agar and egg yolk agar plate. The cultures are incubated anaerobically and examined for growth.

Tests (Including Culture) for Diagnosis of *C. difficile* Disease

Controversy exists about which of the multiple methods for the detection of *C. difficile* and its toxins (Table 3) is optimal. Toxin detection and neutralization by a tissue culture cytotoxin assay are often considered the "gold standard" when new detection methods are evaluated. Toxigenic culture, although it requires 3 or 4 days, tests *C. difficile* isolates for toxin production and has higher sensitivity and equivalent specificity compared to the cytotoxicity assay (84, 133, 158). In studies designed to evaluate the diagnostic utility of detection methods, a confirmed diagnosis of *C. difficile*-associated diarrhea on the basis of both clinical and laboratory criteria probably represents the ultimate gold standard.

Direct stool cytotoxin neutralization assays have not detected toxin in as many as 15 to 38% of patients with confirmed CDAD (48, 158). Unfortunately, some patients without positive direct stool cytotoxin assay results have progressed to pseudomembranous colitis and death (48, 106).

It is important to note that culture alone (without subsequent testing of all *C. difficile* isolates for toxin production) leads to lower specificity and misdiagnosis of CDAD when high background rates of asymptomatic *C. difficile* carriage exist. This situation has led some investigators to conclude that cytotoxicity assays are more specific than culture and that culture should not be used as a means of detecting *C. difficile* in patients with CDAD (66). However, for properly performed toxigenic culture, this conclusion does not hold.

To perform a toxigenic culture, a stool specimen or fecal swab should be inoculated directly onto CCFA (containing 500 μg of cycloserine per ml) with horse blood (115). Commercially available CCFA with the recommended horse blood formulation (Remel, Lenexa, Kans.) has performed satisfactorily in our laboratory. The culture should

TABLE 3 Methods and tests for the detection of *C. difficile* and its toxins

Method	Entity detected	Advantages	Limitations	Available tests and sources
Toxigenic culture	Organism	Most sensitive, specific	Efficiency varies from lab to lab; use of stereomicroscope recommended	CCFA with horse blood preferred; 500 μg of cycloserine and prereduction of medium increase the isolation rate of *C. difficile* (Remel, Lenexa, Kans.)
Latex agglutination	Glutamate dehydrogenase	Rapid, simple	Not extremely sensitive; does not distinguish between toxigenic and nontoxigenic strains of *C. difficile*	CDT (Becton Dickinson Microbiology Systems, Sparks, Md.) Meritec *C. difficile* (Meridian Diagnostics, Inc., Cincinnati, Ohio)
Membrane EIA	Glutamate dehydrogenase	Rapid, simple	More sensitive than latex agglutination; does not distinguish between toxigenic and nontoxigenic strains of *C. difficile*	ImmunoCard *C. difficile* (Meridian Diagnostics, Inc., Cincinnati, Ohio) Triage *C. difficile* panel (Biosite Diagnostics, Inc., San Diego, Calif.)
Tissue culture	Toxin B	Sensitive, specific	Most assays require 24–48 h to complete; toxin B can be inactivated, resulting in false-negative results	*C. difficile* Toxin/Antitoxin (TechLab, Inc., Blacksburg, Va.) *C. difficile* Tox-B Test (Wampole Laboratories, Cranberry, N.J., and TechLab Inc., Blacksburg, Va.) *C. difficile* Toxititer (Bartels, Inc., Issaguah, Wash.) Cytoxi (Advanced Clinical Diagnostics, Toledo, Ohio)
EIA	Toxin A	Rapid, simple, specific	Some kits have higher sensitivity than others; some kits may yield indeterminant readings Does not detect atypical A−/B+ isolates that cause disease	CD-Tox (Porton, Cambridge, England) Premier (Meridian Diagnostics, Inc., Cincinnati, Ohio) Prospect II *C. difficile* toxin A microplate (Alexon-Trend, Sunnyvale, Calif.) *C. difficile* Tox-A Test (Wampole Laboratories, Cranberry, N.J., and TechLab, Inc., Blacksburg, Va.) Toxin A EIA (Bartels, Inc., Issaguah, Wash.) Toxin CD Test (Becton Dickinson Microbiology Systems, Sparks, Md.) VIDAS-CDA (bioMérieux Vitek, Hazelwood, Mo.) Triage *C. difficile* panel (Biosite Diagnostics, Inc., San Diego, Calif.) *C. difficile* toxin A microplate assay (Remel, Lenexa, Kans.)
Membrane EIA	Toxin A	Rapid	Not as sensitive as microwell EIAs	ImmunoCard Toxin A test (Meridian Diagnostics, Inc., Cincinnati, Ohio) *C. difficile* Toxin A (Oxoid, Inc., Ogdensburg, N.Y.) Triage *C. difficile* Panel (Biosite Diagnostics, Inc., San Diego, Calif.)
OIA[a] (optical measurement)	Toxin A	Rapid, simple	Less sensitive than EIA	CdTOX A OIA (ThermoBiostar, Boulder, Colo.)
EIA	Toxins A and B	Rapid, simple, specific	Some kits have higher sensitivity than others; some kits may yield indeterminant readings	*C. difficile* TOX A/B II (Wampole Laboratories, Cranberry, N.J., and TechLab, Inc., Blacksburg, Va.) Cd Toxin A+B (Rohm Pharma, Darmstadt, Germany) Premier A+B (Meridian Diagnostics, Inc., Cincinnati, Ohio)

[a] OIA, optical immunoassay.

be incubated anaerobically at 35 to 37°C for 18 to 24 h before observation. Following incubation, the plates should be examined by using a dissecting microscope to select colonies of *C. difficile* for toxin analysis (99, 115, 133). Colonies of *C. difficile* are yellowish to white, circular to irregular, and flat, with a rhizoid or erose edge and a ground-glass appearance. The colonies have a distinctive odor like *p*-cresol (or horse manure). In addition, *C. difficile* colonies on CCFA can fluoresce chartreuse under UV light (163). Four to six characteristic colonies should be subcultured to chopped-meat–carbohydrate or brain heart infusion broth and incubated anaerobically at 35 to 37°C for 24 h. The isolates are tested for in vitro toxin production by performing a cytotoxin assay on filtered 24-h broths. Because *C. difficile* recovery rates vary significantly when media from different manufacturers are used (115), the importance of appropriate quality control of commercially prepared CCFA cannot be overemphasized.

In addition to the use of CCFA medium, *C. difficile* from fecal samples can be isolated by using the alcohol or heat shock spore selection technique. After 18 to 24 h of incubation, colonies from treated samples are nonhemolytic, 2 to 4 mm in diameter, creamy yellow to grey-white, and irregular; have a coarsely mottled to mosaic internal structure and a matte or dull surface; and are slightly raised when viewed under a dissecting microscope (Fig. 1). The odor remains distinctive. Gram staining of *C. difficile* reveals gram-positive to gram-variable rods that are thin, even sided, and 0.5 μm wide by 3 to 5 μm long. If spores are present, they are subterminal. As described above (for CCFA), isolates obtained by a spore selection technique should also be tested for in vitro toxin production.

Presumptive identification of *C. difficile* can be made by demonstrating typical colonies, Gram stain morphology, and characteristic odor. Definitive identification depends on demonstration of the unique pattern of short-chain fatty acid metabolic products by gas-liquid chromatography (see Table 5) and by biochemical characterization of isolates (78, 99, 163).

Commercially available cytotoxin B neutralization assays, including the *Clostridium difficile* TOX-B test (TechLab) and the Bartels cytotoxicity assay (Bartels, Inc., Issaquah, Wash.), are available (6). Toxin neutralization assays are highly specific because parallel tests of a patient's stool sample are run with specific antisera, which neutralizes any toxin-mediated cytotoxic effect. No standards or National Committee for Clinical Laboratory Standards (NCCLS) guidelines exist for performing the cytotoxin neutralization assay (66). An accurate cytotoxin neutralization assay result, and hence an accurate comparison to other detection methods such as toxigenic culture, depends on multiple factors including specimen centrifugation, cell line, and the subjective interpretation of cytopathic effect (144). Submitting two additional stool specimens from patients suspected of having CDAD increases toxin detection by only 10% (14). Because of the lower sensitivity of the cytotoxin neutralization assays, toxigenic culture should remain an option for the diagnostic evaluation of some patients with CDAD (48, 84, 133, 158).

Most of the multiple enzyme immunoassays (EIAs) for detection of toxin A and/or toxin B in stool are microwell formats, but several membrane-based EIAs are available. Despite extensive testing, relatively few studies have compared EIAs to toxigenic culture for patients with confirmed CDAD. Instead, most studies have compared these tests to tissue culture assay. In general, the relative sensitivity and

specificity values for the various tests vary considerably, depending upon the laboratory and the method to which the test is compared. A review of the literature which summarized comparative studies for eight commercial EIA kits reported that the sensitivity and specificity ranged from 34 to 100% and 88 to 100%, respectively (66). The membrane-based EIAs offer a shorter turnaround time than many of the microwell formats, although that of the microwell EIAs from Meridian Diagnostics, Inc., and TechLab, Inc./Wampole Laboratories can be shortened considerably by utilizing a shaking incubation step. The microwell formats offer increased sensitivity and specificity over the membrane-based EIAs (50). A primary consideration when choosing a test is the fact that atypical A⁻/B⁺ isolates from CDAD patients will be negative in the toxin A-specific tests. Interest in tests that detect both toxin A and toxin B has increased (85, 105) because there have been instances in which outbreaks due to A⁻/B⁺ isolates have gone undetected due to the use of a toxin A-specific EIA (2, 4). A primary limitation of the tests that detect glutamate dehydrogenase is the fact that this enzyme is produced by both toxigenic and nontoxigenic isolates. For this reason, the predictive positive value is low for these tests. Their greatest utility probably lies in their use as a negative screen to aid in ruling out CDAD and as a rapid screen in outbreak situations. Commercially available tests for CDAD are summarized in Table 3 and described in more detail elsewhere (6). Performance data for the EIAs are summarized in Table 4.

PCR amplification methods have been used to differentiate between toxigenic and nontoxigenic strains of *C. difficile*, to detect the presence of *C. difficile* in specimens, and to detect fragments of the toxin A and toxin B gene sequences (8, 88, 124). While this research is of considerable interest, there are no simple-to-use commercial kits and equipment for molecular applications related to *C. difficile* (6). Although PCR amplification procedures can detect the genes for toxins A and B, these methods do not detect either toxin in a clinical specimen.

A single-step assay which combines *C. difficile* toxin gene detection and molecular typing has been developed (141). In addition, a number of other molecular, as well as phenotypic, typing methods have been used to study the epidemiology of nosocomial infections involving *C. difficile* (24, 89, 126). However, there are no strain-specific control measures, and most hospital microbiology laboratories do not attempt to type *C. difficile* (17).

Laboratory Investigation of *C. perfringens* Food-Borne Illness

Methods for the enumeration of *C. perfringens* organisms in foods and *C. perfringens* spores in feces with egg yolk-free tryptose-sulfite-cycloserine agar are described in detail by Hauschild (74). Also see chapter 13. Although methods for the detection of *C. perfringens* enterotoxin in feces have been described previously, these assays are still considered experimental and are generally not used in clinical laboratories, except in research settings (113, 146, 152).

IDENTIFICATION OF CLOSTRIDIA OTHER THAN *C. DIFFICILE*

A number of strategies are available for the phenotypic characterization and identification of clostridia (44, 78, 99, 163). One of the traditional methods has included the use of prereduced anaerobically sterilized (PRAS) media for the determination of fermentation profiles and other characteristics (78). Although the CDC conventional media described by Dowell and Hawkins (44) provide an excellent system for characterizing clostridia and can be used, Table 5 is based on results obtained with PRAS media, and a few of the reactions differ. Thus, if CDC conventional media are used, the CDC publications on anaerobic bacteriology should be consulted (44). The cultures are incubated for 24 to 72 h at 35 to 37°C; overnight incubation is often sufficient for most clostridia because they grow rapidly. Gram stains of the chopped-meat culture are examined to determine the presence, positions, and shapes of the spores. If spores are not found, a tube of chopped-meat medium is inoculated, heated at 70°C for 10 min, and incubated. Growth in this heated tube usually indicates the presence of spores, although none may be apparent microscopically. Alternatively, an alcohol spore selection technique may be helpful for clostridia with heat-sensitive spores (100).

The short-chain acid-metabolic products from chopped-meat–carbohydrate broth culture are determined by gas-liquid chromatography (78, 99, 163). The results will not be identical if peptone-yeast extract-glucose is used (44, 78). In addition, analyses of cellular fatty acids are practical, accurate, and sensitive methods for characterization of isolates that simplify the identification of clostridia (Table 5) (7). The identification of *Clostridium* species can be made without the analyses of either metabolic products or cellular

fatty acids, but such identification usually involves more time. Table 5 includes most of the *Clostridium* species commonly isolated from clinical specimens. Additional information can be found elsewhere (30, 43, 73, 78, 99, 151, 163). In the current era of managed competition and ever-increasing budget tightening, there has been increasing interest in finding less costly alternatives to conventional identification procedures.

A number of commercial kits have been marketed for the rapid identification of anaerobes; these are described in considerable detail in the *Manual of Commercial Methods in Clinical Microbiology* (6). In general, Gram reaction, cellular morphology, colony characteristics, and aerotolerance of isolates should always be determined in conjunction with use of these packaged microsystems. When kits are used to identify the clostridia, results are incorrect relatively frequently (6, 16). Intended for use with the Vitek system for automated identification of medically important anaerobic and microaerophilic bacteria of human origin, the Vitek Anaerobe Identification card (ANI; bioMérieux Vitek, Hazelwood, Mo.) is a plastic card containing 30 small wells, 28 of which contain substrates for biochemical tests (6). This system identified only 64% of 44 *Clostridium* isolates (in general) correctly but gave correct identifications for eight of eight *C. perfringens* isolates (145). The AN-Ident (bioMérieux Vitek), one of the first commercially available 4-h packaged kits to be marketed with a database for identification of anaerobes, has recently been discontinued (D. Pincus, personal communication, 2002). In the late 1980s, a system for anaerobe identification now called the "rapid ID 32 A" (bioMérieux Vitek) was introduced in Europe. As summarized elsewhere, this product has been the subject of a number of studies with widely differing results (6). According to one of the more recent evaluations, the rapid ID 32 A had problems in identifying clostridia other than *C. perfringens* or *C. ramosum* (122). The rapid ID 32 A was introduced to the U.S. market relatively recently.

In a comparison against Virginia Polytechnic Institute conventional methods, 74% of the 130 strains of *Clostridium* species tested (overall) were identified correctly to the species level by the RapID-ANA II (Innovative Diagnostic Systems, Inc., Atlanta, Ga.) without the need for additional tests (116). Two of the more common clostridia encountered clinically, *C. perfringens* and *C. ramosum*, were accurately identified by using the RapID-ANA II, but identifications were less likely to be correct for other common species (e.g., *C. difficile*, *C. innocuum*, and *C. clostridioforme*) (116). Similarly, the BBL Crystal anaerobe identification system (Becton Dickinson, Cockeysville, Md.) correctly identified 76 of 103 *Clostridium* isolates but did not identify any strains of *C. innocuum*, *C. sporogenes*, or *C. tetani* that were tested; in addition, some strains of *C. septicum* and *C. difficile* required retesting to achieve correct identifications (32). Commercial kits are not without significant costs, especially if clostridia other than *C. perfringens* are to be identified (16). In addition to the need to determine Gram reaction, cellular morphology, colony characteristics, and aerotolerance of isolates when using the kits, other useful supplemental tests for the clostridia include tests for lipase and lecithinase on egg yolk agar, the reduction of nitrate, a test for gelatin hydrolysis, and metabolic product analysis using gas-liquid chromatography (6).

TABLE 4 Summary of performance data compiled for immunodiagnostic products marketed for the detection of *C. difficile*

Test	Sensitivity (%)	Specificity (%)
Alexon-Trend Prospect II CD Toxin A	82–85	98–100[d,h]
Bartel Toxin A, Prima	87	98[i]
bioMérieux VIDAS Toxin A II	65–85	99–100[d,i]
Biosite Triage *C. difficile* Panel (antigen or toxin A)	68–100	83–90[i,j]
Meridian ImmunoCard Toxin A	65–92	95–100[c,e,g]
Meridian Premier Cytoclone CD Toxin A/B	77–83	99–100[d,i]
Meridian Toxin A	87–94	97–99[e,h]
Meridian Premier Toxins A and B	84–95	97–99[f]
TechLab/Wampole CD Tox A/B	80–94	99–100[a,b,d,f,h,i]

[a] R. Aldeen, M. Bingham, A. Aiderzada, J. Kucera, M. Bale, and K. Carroll, *Abstr. 98th Gen. Meet. Am. Soc. Microbiol.*, abstr. C-181, p. 161, 1998.

[b] S. D. Allen, G. G. Korba, and J. A. Siders, *Anaerobe 2000 Int. Congr. Confed. Anaerobe Soc.*, abstr. VIII-P1, p. 167, 2000.

[c] F. Barbut, M. Mace, V. Lalande, P. Tilleux, and J.-C. Petit, *Abstr. 97th Gen. Meet. Am. Soc. Microbiol.*, abstr. C-261, p. 166, 1997.

[d] M. Campion, A. T. Evangelista, and J. Mortensen, *Abstr. 99th Gen. Meet. Am. Soc. Microbiol.*, abstr. C-2, p. 105, 1999.

[e] C. Gleaves, R. J. Dworkin, L. Olson, and M. Campbell, *Abstr. 97th Gen. Meet. Am. Soc. Microbiol.*, abstr. C-266, p. 167, 1997.

[f] C. Gleaves, R. Aldeen, K. Schwarz, M. Campbell, and K. Carroll, *Abstr. 100th Gen. Meet. Am. Soc. Microbiol.*, abstr. C-252, p. 188, 2000.

[g] S. Riddell, P. Gilligan, and L. McMillon, *Abstr. 97th Gen. Meet. Am. Soc. Microbiol.*, abstr. C-254, p. 165, 1997.

[h] M. R. Smith, T. P. Ferguson, S. K. Zimmerman, J. A. Kee, L. Neville, and K. C. Chapin, *Abstr. 100th Gen. Meet. Am. Soc. Microbiol.*, abstr. C-246, p. 187, 2000.

[i] D. Turgeon, J. Quick, L. Carlson, P. Miller, B. Ulness, A. Cent, T. Novicki, M. Coyle, A. Limaye, and T. Fritsche, *Abstr. 100th Gen. Meet. Am. Soc. Microbiol.*, abstr. C-247, p. 187, 2000.

[j] References 60 and 97.

Presumptive Identification of Commonly Encountered Clostridia

Simplified flowcharts for presumptive identification of anaerobes by using minimal resources were devised by Baron and Citron (16). Somewhat different approaches and schemata for relatively low-cost presumptive identification of anaerobes have been described elsewhere (99, 163). The first 12 species listed in Table 1 represent approximately 95% of all the *Clostridium* organisms isolated at the Indiana University Medical Center Anaerobe Laboratory. Some key characteristics that aid in the presumptive identification of these most common species, without the use of gas-liquid chromatography, commercial packaged kits, or other costly resources, are listed below. Based on their ability to hydrolyze gelatin, these 12 species can be divided into two groups: proteolytic (gelatin hydrolysis positive) and nonproteolytic (gelatin hydrolysis negative).

Proteolytic Group

- *C. perfringens*: double zone of hemolysis, boxcar-shaped rods, spores rare, lecithinase positive. *C. baratii* mimics these characteristics but does not hydrolyze gelatin.
- *C. difficile*: creamy-yellow to grey-white, irregular coarse mottled to mosaic internal structure, matte or dull surface; subterminal to free spores or spores infrequent; gelatin hydrolysis can be slow for half of the strains; mannitol positive.
- *C. cadaveris*: white-grey, entire to slightly irregular, raised to slightly convex; oval terminal spores, spot indole positive, DNase positive.
- *C. sporogenes*: medusa-head colonies, possible swarmer; subterminal and many free spores, lipase positive.
- *C. bifermentans*: grey-white, irregular, scalloped edge; many free spores often chaining, urease negative, indole and lecithinase positive. *C. sordellii* is similar but is urease positive.
- *C. septicum*: swarms, subterminal spores often "citron" forms, DNase positive, sucrose negative.

Nonproteolytic Group

- *C. clostridioforme*: colonies resemble *Bacteroides fragilis* but usually have a slightly irregular edge, gram negative, football shaped; spores are rare.
- *C. innocuum*: grey-white to brilliant greenish, coarsely mottled to mosaic internal structure; terminal spores may be difficult to find, nonmotile, mannitol positive, lactose and maltose negative.
- *C. ramosum*: colonies resemble *B. fragilis* but usually have a slight irregular edge; gram-variable, palisading, slender rods, nonmotile, mannitol positive.
- *C. butyricum*: very large irregular, mottled to mosaic internal structure, subterminal spores, ferments many carbohydrates.
- *C. tertium*: aerotolerant, terminal spores from anaerobically incubated media only.
- *C. glycolicum*: grey-white, entire to scalloped edge, convex; subterminal and free spores, DNase positive.

(Colonies of some of the more common and/or clinically important species are shown in Fig. 1.)

Toxin tests are necessary for the identification of a few species (44, 73, 151). *C. sporogenes* cannot be differentiated with certainty from the proteolytic group I strains of *C.*

botulinum unless toxin tests are used. A few strains of group III *C. botulinum* produce lecithinase as well as lipase and are difficult to distinguish from *C. novyi* type A except by toxin tests or by the use of a *C. novyi* fluorescent-antibody conjugate (151). To test for toxin, the following procedure is used. Two tubes of chopped-meat–glucose medium are inoculated. One tube is incubated at 37°C overnight, and the other is incubated at 37°C for 3 days. If no toxin is found in the overnight culture, the 3-day culture is tested. The culture is centrifuged, and 1.2-ml volumes of the supernatant are placed in several tubes. Appropriate antiserum (0.3 ml) is added per tube for the various species suspected. The well-mixed suspensions are allowed to stand for 30 min at room temperature or at 37°C, and then 0.5-ml portions of control supernatant (without antiserum) and antiserum mixtures are injected intraperitoneally into each of two mice. The mice are observed for 3 days, and any deaths are recorded. Only specific sera for laboratory testing should be used for toxin identification; therapeutic sera are often unsatisfactory because they may contain antibodies to toxins of species other than those listed on the label. An excellent source of diagnostic clostridial antisera is TechLab. As a supplement to the methods described above, the various types of *C. botulinum* can be presumptively identified on the basis of differences in their cellular fatty acid profiles (Table 5) (7, 61).

SUSCEPTIBILITY TO ANTIMICROBIAL AGENTS

Surgical measures are especially important in the treatment of gas gangrene and a number of other *Clostridium*-mediated diseases (108). Despite concerns of increasing penicillin resistance among *C. perfringens* isolates (117) and poor outcomes in animals treated experimentally with this antibiotic alone, penicillin G (10×10^6 to 24×10^6 U per day) is still considered the drug of choice for gas gangrene in some texts (108). β-Lactamase has not been demonstrated in *C. perfringens*. Resistance to penicillin in *C. perfringens* may involve a decreased affinity of penicillin-binding protein 1 (75), but its practical significance remains unclear. At Indiana University Hospital, penicillin (at ≤8 μg/ml) was active in vitro against 100% of the 57 *C. perfringens* strains tested. Nonetheless, in a mouse model of gas gangrene, outcomes were better for mice treated with clindamycin, metronidazole, rifampin, chloramphenicol, or tetracycline alone, or with clindamycin plus penicillin, than they were for animals that received penicillin G alone (160, 161). Also in these studies, the combination of metronidazole with penicillin G was antagonistic. Thus, for treatment of gas gangrene, it seems wise to select an alternative to penicillin alone, such as the combination of clindamycin plus penicillin G (108). However, as a note of caution, in vitro susceptibility testing has revealed resistance to clindamycin in *C. perfringens* (9% of strains in our laboratory were resistant to ≤4 μg of clindamycin per ml). Imipenem, which is active in vitro against 100% of *Clostridium* species that we have tested (99), is considered a prudent alternative (108).

Resistance to penicillin is especially common in *C. ramosum*, *C. clostridioforme*, and *C. butyricum* (53, 139); these species produce β-lactamases that are induced by β-lactam antibiotics (75). *C. tertium* is also resistant to β-lactam antibiotics and is a bit unusual among the clostridia in that it also is resistant to both metronidazole and clindamycin (63, 155).

TABLE 5 Differential characteristics of commonly encountered clostridia[a]

Species	Spores	Egg yolk agar LEC	Egg yolk agar LIP	Growth on aerobic blood agar	Gelatin hydrolysis	Milk digestion	Indole production	Carbohydrate fermentation Glucose	Maltose	Lactose	Sucrose	Salicin	Mannitol
C. bifermentans	OS	+	−	−	+	+	+	+	w/−	−	−	−	−
C. botulinum[c]													
Group Ic[d]	OS	−	+	−	+	+	−	+	−/w	−	−	−	−
Group IIc[d]	OS	−/+	+	−	+	+	−/+	+	V	−	−	−	−
Group IIIc[d]	OS	−	+	−	+	−	−	+	+/w	−	+/w	−	−
C. butyricum	OS	−	−	−	−	−	−	+	+	+	+	+	−/+
C. cadaveris	OT	−	−	−	+	+	+	+	−	−	−	−	−
C. chauvoei[e]	OS	−	−	−	+	−	−	+	+/w	+/w	+/w	−	−
C. clostridioforme	OS	−	−	−	−	−	−/+	+	+/w	+/−	−	+/−	−
C. difficile	OS	−	−	−	+	−	−	+	−	−	−	−/w	+/−
C. histolyticum	OS	−	−	V	+	+	−	−	−	−	−	−	−
C. innocuum[f]	OT	−	−	−	−	−	−	+	−	−	+	+	+
C. limosum	OS	+	−	−	+	+	−	−	−	−	−	−	−
C. novyi A	OS	+	+	−	+	−	−	+	V	−	−	−/+	−
C. novyi B	OS	+	−	−	+	+	+/−	+	V	−	−	−	−
C. paraputrificum	OT	−	−	−	−	−	−	+	+	+	+	+	−
C. perfringens[f]	OS	+	−	−	+	+	−	+	+	+	+	−	−
C. ramosum[f]	R/OT	−	−	−	−	−	−	+	+	+	+	+	+/−
C. septicum	OS	−	−	−	+	+	−	+	+	+	−	V	−
C. sordellii	OS	+	−	−	+	+	+	+	w/+	−	−	−	−
C. sphenoides	RS/T	−	−	−	−	−	−	+	+	w/+	w/−	w/+w	w/+
C. sporogenes	OS	−	+	−	+	+	−	+	−/w	−	−	−	−
C. subterminale	OS	−/+	−	−	+	+	−	−	−	−	−	−	−
C. tertium	OT	−	−	+	−	−	−	+	+	+	+	+	+/w
C. tetani	RT	−	−	−	+	+/−	V	−	−	−	−	−	−

[a] Based on the use of PRAS media as described by Holdeman et al. (78). Key: +, positive reaction; −, negative reaction; V, variable reaction; w, weak reaction; /, either/or; O, oval; R, round; S, subterminal; T, terminal; LEC, lecithinase production; LIP, lipase production. Fermentation products: A, acetate; B, butyrate; F, formate; IB, isobutyrate; IC, isocaproate; IV, isovalerate; P, propionate; V, valerate. Parentheses indicate that it may or may not be present. Capital letters indicate major peaks; lowercase letters indicate minor peaks. PYG, peptone-yeast extract-glucose medium. CMC, chopped-meat–carbohydrate medium.

[b] Major fatty acid methyl esters are listed. Data derived from the Moore database version 3.9, September 1995, Sherlock, Microbial Identification System, MIDI, Inc., Newark, DE 19713.

Although clindamycin is still active against many species of commonly encountered anaerobic bacteria in the United States, a number of clostridial species are frequently resistant to it. Resistance to this antibiotic has been documented for some strains of C. perfringens (as noted above), C. ramosum, C. difficile, C. tertium, C. subterminale, C. butyricum, C. sporogenes, and C. innocuum (63, 99).

Chloramphenicol, piperacillin, metronidazole, imipenem, and combinations of β-lactam drugs with β-lactam inhibitors (e.g., ampicillin-sulbactam) are active against nearly all of the clostridia, with only a few exceptions (63, 99). The clostridia have shown variable resistance to the cephalosporins and tetracyclines, and they are usually resistant to the aminoglycosides. Many clostridia other than C. perfringens (particularly C. ramosum, C. clostridioforme, and C. innocuum) are resistant to cefoxitin, cefotaxime, ceftazidime, ceftizoxime, cefoperazone, and other broad-spectrum β-lactam drugs (3, 53, 99, 139).

Most strains of C. innocuum are only moderately susceptible to vancomycin (3). It has been suggested that C. innocuum is intrinsically resistant to this compound (125). In general, most of the currently available quinolone agents have only low or intermediate activity against anaerobes and have not been recommended for treatment of mixed infections involving anaerobes, including those involving the clostridia.

Severe C. difficile-associated intestinal disease is usually treated with oral vancomycin or metronidazole, although most strains of C. difficile are susceptible to a number of antimicrobial agents in vitro (including penicillins, tetracycline, and quinolones). For patients unable to tolerate oral antibiotics but requiring therapy, parenteral vancomycin or metronidazole has been recommended (57). Antibiotic therapy often results in relapse of disease, so discontinuation of the offending agent or change to an agent less likely to cause diarrhea should be considered the primary intervention of choice (57). A current concern about the use of vancomycin is the potential emergence of vancomycin-resistant enterococci (56, 135).

EVALUATION, INTERPRETATION, AND REPORTING OF RESULTS

As a note of caution, the isolation of a Clostridium species from a clinical specimen may or may not be significant clinically, and culture results should be interpreted in relation to the patient's clinical findings (151). Clostridia (e.g., C. perfringens) of the patient's own intestinal microflora may be present on the skin and thus can contaminate blood samples or other specimens that are collected and transported to the laboratory. In addition, most clostridia currently encountered in wounds, exudates, blood, and other normally sterile body fluids are opportunistic and unlikely to cause progressive histotoxic disease unless conditions are suitable in a compromised host. As discussed earlier in this

Principal metabolic products on PYG or CMC	Other	Cellular fatty acids[b]
A, (p), (ib), (b), (iv), (ic)	Urease negative	16:0, 18:1*cis* 9, 19cyc9, 10/:1
A, (p), ib, B, IV, (v), (ic)		14:0, 16:0, 18:1*cis* 9, 18:1*cis* 9dma
A, P, B, (v)		14:0, 16:0, 18:1*cis* 9
A, B		14:0, 16:0, 18:1*cis* 9
A, B		16:0, 18:1*cis* 9
A, (p), B (from PY = A, p, ib, v, iv)		14:0, 16:0, 18:1*cis* 9
A, B		14:0, 16:0, 18:1*cis* 9
A	Spores seldom observed: usually gram negative	16:0, 18:1*cis* 11dma
A, (p), ib, B, iv, (v), ic		16:0, 16:0dma, 18:1*cis* 9, 19cyc 9, 10/:1
A	Aerotolerant	14:0, 16:0, 18:1*cis* 9, 18:1*cis* 9dma
A, V		16:0, 18:1*cis* 9
A		12:0, 18:1*cis* 9, 18:1*cis* 9dma
A, P, B		14:0, 18:1*cis* 9, 18:1*cis* 9dma
A, P, B		14:0, 15:0, 16:0, 18:1*cis* 9
A, B		16:0, 18:1*cis* 9, 18:1*cis* 9dma
A, (p), B	Spores seldom observed; double zone of hemolysis	12:0, 14:0
A	Spores seldom observed; frequently gram negative	16:0, 16:0dma, 18:1*cis*
A, (p), B	Spreading colony	14:0, 16:0, 18:1*cis* 9
A, (p), (ib), (iv), (ic)	Usually urease positive	18:1*cis* 9, 19cyc 9, 10:1
A	Usually gram negative	16:0, 18:1*cis* 11dma
A, (p), ib, B, iv, (v), (ic)		14:0, 16:0, 18:1*cis* 9
A, (p), ib, B, IV, (ic)		16:0, 18:1*cis* 9, 18:1*cis* 9dma
A, B	Aerotolerant	14:0, 16:0, 18:1*cis* 9
A, p, B		14:0, 18:1*cis* 9, 18:1*cis* 9dma

[c] Group I contains proteolytic strains (A, B, and F), group II contains types C and D, and group III contains saccharolytic strains (B, E, and F).
[d] Toxin neutralization test required for identification.
[e] Pathogenic for herbivores.
[f] C. innocuum, C. perfringens, and C. ramosum are nonmotile and pathogenic for herbivores.

chapter, one of the important exceptions to this generalization is *C. septicum*, which rarely is encountered in blood cultures except from patients who have underlying malignancy or neutropenic sepsis (101, 102). *C. septicum* sepsis is an infectious disease emergency that requires prompt and clear communication between the laboratory and the clinician to institute early treatments with antimicrobial agents and surgical measures to improve outcomes (131). Several other clostridia (e.g., *C. bifermentans, C. sporogenes, C. innocuum, C. cadaveris, C. subterminale,* and *C. tertium*) that lack pathogenic properties (i.e., do not produce toxins and are nonpathogenic for animals) are occasionally isolated from clinical specimens (151). Still others (e.g., *C. carnis, C. fallax,* and *C. limosum*) have been isolated so infrequently from properly collected clinical specimens and studied so little that their clinical significance is especially hard to interpret (151).

The accurate and timely reporting of preliminary results (e.g., findings from direct microscopic examinations of clinical specimens), as well as early culture results after 24 and 48 h of incubation, can be extremely valuable to the physician (99, 163). The colony characteristics and microscopic features of some clostridia (e.g., *C. perfringens, C. sordellii,* and *C. sporogenes*) can be so distinctive that preliminary or presumptive reports can be made even before aerotolerance studies are completed (99). Nonetheless, final identification reports based on accurate, definitive identifications are needed to better define the role of clostridia in diseases, to aid the clinician in selecting optimal treatments, for public health purposes (e.g., hospital-acquired CDAD), and for academic purposes (99).

A number of *C. difficile* toxin EIAs provide same-day test results and acceptable specificities but slightly lower sensitivities than those of toxigenic culture or cytotoxicity assays (6). EIAs should not be relied upon as the sole laboratory test for *C. difficile* toxin. An EIA which detects both toxin A and toxin B may be optimal since atypical A⁻/B⁺ isolates have been associated with patients who have a clinical history consistent with CDAD. Reliable and timely results can be provided by culturing for the organism and performing a rapid EIA directly on the stool. If *C. difficile* is isolated but the toxin assay performed directly on feces is negative, *C. difficile* could be tested for toxin if warranted clinically.

The decision about which of the various test strategies available for the detection of *C. difficile* and its toxins should be chosen for an individual laboratory is the responsibility of the laboratory director. The Society for Hospital Epidemiology of America Position Paper provides an excellent review of the advantages and disadvantages of the different diagnostic procedures (60). For smaller laboratories without anaerobic chambers, incubation of the recommended formulation of prereduced CCFA in anaerobic jars, bags, and pouches provides acceptable recovery (51). As described above, quality control of media and use of a stereomicroscope are essential for accurate isolation and identification of *C. difficile*. EIAs can be performed on isolates to detect toxin production and provide same-day results. Commercially available cytotoxin neutralization assays may provide a low-cost alternative to the more expensive EIAs, but they have a longer turnaround time and require experienced personnel for interpretation. Screening tests for glutamate dehydrogenase produced by *C. difficile* may allow rapid preliminary identification in nosocomial outbreaks and epidemiological investigations.

We thank Jean A. Siders for her many significant contributions to this chapter and Deborah Blue-Hnidy for her helpful editorial suggestions.

REFERENCES

1. **Aktories, K., and I. Just.** 1995. Monoglucosylation of low-molecular-mass GTP-binding Rho proteins by clostridial cytotoxins. *Trends Cell Biol.* **5:**441–443.
2. **al-Barrak, A., J. Embil, B. Dyck, K. Olekson, D. Nicoll, M. Alfa, and A. Kabani.** 1999. An outbreak of toxin A negative, toxin B positive *Clostridium difficile*-associated diarrhea in a Canadian tertiary-care hospital. *Can. Commun. Dis. Rep.* **25:**65–69.
3. **Alexander, C. J., D. M. Citron, J. S. Brazier, and E. J. Goldstein.** 1995. Identification and antimicrobial resistance patterns of clinical isolates of *Clostridium clostridioforme, Clostridium innocuum,* and *Clostridium ramosum* compared with those of clinical isolates of *Clostridium perfringens. J. Clin. Microbiol.* **33:**3209–3215.
4. **Alfa, M. J., A. Kabani, D. Lyerly, S. Moncrief, L. M. Neville, A. Al-Barrak, G. K. Harding, B. Dyck, K. Olekson, and J. M. Embil.** 2000. Characterization of a toxin A-negative, toxin B-positive strain of *Clostridium difficile* responsible for a nosocomial outbreak of *Clostridium difficile*-associated diarrhea. *J. Clin. Microbiol.* **38:**2706–2714.
5. **Allen, S. D.** 1997. Pig-bel and other necrotizing disorders of the gut involving *Clostridium perfringens,* p. 717–724. *In* D. H. Connor, F. W. Chandler, D. A. Schwartz, H. J. Manz, and E. E. Lack (ed.), *Pathology of Infectious Diseases.* Appleton & Lange, Norwalk, Conn.
6. **Allen, S. D., C. L. Emery, and J. A. Siders.** 2002. Anaerobic bacteriology, p. 50–81. *In* A. L. Truant (ed.), *Manual of Commercial Methods in Clinical Microbiology.* ASM Press, Washington, D.C.
7. **Allen, S. D., J. A. Siders, M. J. Riddell, J. A. Fill, and W. S. Wegener.** 1995. Cellular fatty acid analysis in the differentiation of *Clostridium* in the clinical microbiology laboratory. *Clin. Infect. Dis.* **20:**S198–S201.
8. **Alonso, R., C. Munoz, S. Gros, D. Garcia de Viedma, T. Pelaez, and E. Bouza.** 1999. Rapid detection of toxigenic *Clostridium difficile* from stool samples by a nested PCR of toxin B gene. *J. Hosp. Infect.* **41:**145–149.
9. **Arnon, S. S.** 1997. Human tetanus and human botulism, p. 95–115. *In* J. I. Rood, B. A. McClane, J. G. Songer, and R. W. Titball (ed.), *The Clostridia: Molecular Biology and Pathogenesis.* Academic Press, New York, N.Y.
10. **Arnon, S. S.** 1989. Infant botulism, p. 601–609. *In* S. M. Finegold and W. L. George (ed.), *Anaerobic Infections in Humans.* Academic Press, New York, N.Y.
11. **Arnon, S. S., K. Damus, and J. Chin.** 1981. Infant botulism: epidemiology and relation to sudden infant death syndrome. *Epidemiol. Rev.* **3:**45–66.
12. **Arnon, S. S., R. Schechter, T. V. Inglesby, D. A. Henderson, J. G. Bartlett, M. S. Ascher, E. Eitzen, A. D. Fine, J. Hauer, M. Layton, S. Lillibridge, M. T. Oster-

holm, T. O'Toole, G. Parker, T. M. Perl, P. K. Russell, D. L. Swerdlow, and K. Tonat.** 2001. Botulinum toxin as a biological weapon: medical and public health management. *JAMA* **285:**1059–1070.
13. **Aronsson, B., R. Mollby, and C. E. Nord.** 1985. Antimicrobial agents and *Clostridium difficile* in acute enteric disease: epidemiological data from Sweden, 1980–1982. *J. Infect. Dis.* **151:**476–481.
14. **Aronsson, B., R. Mollby, and C. E. Nord.** 1984. Diagnosis and epidemiology of *Clostridium difficile* enterocolitis in Sweden. *J. Antimicrob. Chemother.* **14:**85–95.
15. **Aureli, P., L. Fenicia, B. Pasolini, M. Gianfranceschi, L. M. McCroskey, and C. L. Hatheway.** 1986. Two cases of type E infant botulism caused by neurotoxigenic *Clostridium butyricum* in Italy. *J. Infect. Dis.* **154:**207–211.
16. **Baron, E. J., and D. M. Citron.** 1997. Anaerobic identification flowchart using minimal laboratory resources. *Clin. Infect. Dis.* **25:**S143–S146.
17. **Bartlett, J. G.** 2002. Clinical practice. Antibiotic-associated diarrhea. *N. Engl. J. Med.* **346:**334–339.
18. **Bayer, A. S., and W. M. Scheld.** 2000. Endocarditis and intravascular infections, p. 857–902. *In* G. L. Mandell, J. E. Bennett, and R. Dolin (ed.), *Mandell, Douglas, and Bennett's Principles and Practice of Infectious Diseases,* 5th ed. Churchill Livingstone, Philadelphia, Pa.
19. **Bennion, R. S., E. J. Baron, J. E. Thompson, Jr., J. Downes, P. Summanen, D. A. Talan, and S. M. Finegold.** 1990. The bacteriology of gangrenous and perforated appendicitis—revisited. *Ann. Surg.* **211:**165–171.
20. **Bodey, G. P., S. Rodriguez, V. Fainstein, and L. S. Elting.** 1991. Clostridial bacteremia in cancer patients. A 12-year experience. *Cancer* **67:**1928–1942.
21. **Borriello, S. P., and F. E. Barclay.** 1986. An in-vitro model of colonisation resistance to *Clostridium difficile* infection. *J. Med. Microbiol.* **21:**299–309.
22. **Borriello, S. P., F. E. Barclay, A. R. Welch, M. F. Stringer, G. N. Watson, R. K. Williams, D. V. Seal, and K. Sullens.** 1985. Epidemiology of diarrhoea caused by enterotoxigenic *Clostridium perfringens. J. Med. Microbiol.* **20:**363–372.
23. **Borriello, S. P., B. W. Wren, S. Hyde, S. V. Seddon, P. Sibbons, M. M. Krishna, S. Tabaqchali, S. Manek, and A. B. Price.** 1992. Molecular, immunological, and biological characterization of a toxin A-negative, toxin B-positive strain of *Clostridium difficile. Infect. Immun.* **60:**4192–4199.
24. **Brazier, J. S.** 2001. Typing of *Clostridium difficile. Clin. Microbiol. Infect.* **7:**428–431.
25. **Brazier, J. S., S. L. Stubbs, and B. I. Duerden.** 1999. Prevalence of toxin A negative/B positive *Clostridium difficile* strains. *J. Hosp. Infect.* **42:**248–249.
26. **Brook, I.** 1989. Anaerobic bacterial bacteremia: 12-year experience in two military hospitals. *J. Infect. Dis.* **160:**1071–1075.
27. **Bryant, A. E., R. Y. Chen, Y. Nagata, Y. Wang, C. H. Lee, S. Finegold, P. H. Guth, and D. L. Stevens.** 2000. Clostridial gas gangrene. I. Cellular and molecular mechanisms of microvascular dysfunction induced by exotoxins of *Clostridium perfringens. J. Infect. Dis.* **182:**799–807.
28. **Bryant, A. E., R. Y. Chen, Y. Nagata, Y. Wang, C. H. Lee, S. Finegold, P. H. Guth, and D. L. Stevens.** 2000. Clostridial gas gangrene. II. Phospholipase C-induced activation of platelet gpIIbIIIa mediates vascular occlusion and myonecrosis in *Clostridium perfringens* gas gangrene. *J. Infect. Dis.* **182:**808–815.
29. **Carman, R. J.** 1997. *Clostridium perfringens* in spontaneous and antibiotic-associated diarrhoea of man and other animals. *Rev. Med. Microbiol.* **8:**S43–S45.

30. **Cato, E. P., W. L. George, and S. M. Finegold.** 1986. Genus *Clostridium* Prazmowski 1880, 23^AL^, p. 1141–1200. *In* P. H. A. Sneath, N. S. Mair, M. E. Sharpe, and G. H. Holt (ed.), *Bergey's Manual of Systematic Bacteriology*, vol. 2. Williams & Wilkins, Baltimore, Md.

31. **Cato, E. P., and E. Stackebrandt.** 1989. Taxonomy and phylogeny, p. 1–26. *In* N. P. Minton and D. J. Clark (ed.), *Clostridia*. Plenum Press, New York, N.Y.

32. **Cavallaro, J. J., L. S. Wiggs, and J. M. Miller.** 1997. Evaluation of the BBL Crystal Anaerobe identification system. *J. Clin. Microbiol.* **35:**3186–3191.

33. **Centers for Disease Control and Prevention.** 1998. *Botulism in the United States 1899–1996: Handbook for Epidemiologists, Clinicians, and Laboratory Workers.* Centers for Disease Control and Prevention, Atlanta, Ga.

34. **Centers for Disease Control and Prevention.** 2001. Summary of notifiable diseases, United States, 1999. *Morb. Mortal. Wkly. Rep.* **48:**1–104.

35. **Centers for Disease Control and Prevention.** 2000. Update: *Clostridium novyi* and unexplained illness among injecting-drug users—Scotland, Ireland, and England, April–June 2000. *Morb. Mortal. Wkly. Rep.* **49:**543–545.

36. **Centers for Disease Control and Prevention.** 1995. Wound botulism—California, 1995. *Morb. Mortal. Wkly. Rep.* **44:**889–892.

37. **Clabots, C. R., C. J. Shanholtzer, L. R. Peterson, and D. N. Gerding.** 1987. In vitro activity of efrotomycin, ciprofloxacin, and six other antimicrobials against *Clostridium difficile. Diagn. Microbiol. Infect. Dis.* **6:**49–52.

38. **Cohen, C. A., L. M. Almeder, A. Israni, and J. N. Maslow.** 1998. *Clostridium septicum* endocarditis complicated by aortic-ring abscess and aortitis. *Clin. Infect. Dis.* **26:**495–496.

39. **Collins, M. D., P. A. Lawson, A. Willems, J. J. Cordoba, J. Fernandez-Garayzabal, P. Garcia, J. Cai, H. Hippe, and J. A. Farrow.** 1994. The phylogeny of the genus *Clostridium*: proposal of five new genera and eleven new species combinations. *Int. J. Syst. Bacteriol.* **44:**812–826.

40. **Cutrona, A. F., C. Watanakunakorn, C. R. Schaub, and A. Jagetia.** 1995. *Clostridium innocuum* endocarditis. *Clin. Infect. Dis.* **21:**1306–1307.

41. **Decker, W. H., and W. Hall.** 1966. Treatment of abortions infected with *Clostridium welchii. Am. J. Obstet. Gynecol.* **95:**395–399.

42. **Dowell, V. R., Jr.** 1984. Botulism and tetanus: selected epidemiologic and microbiologic aspects. *Rev. Infect. Dis.* **6:**S202–S207.

43. **Dowell, V. R., Jr., and S. D. Allen.** 1981. Anaerobic bacterial infections, p. 171–213. *In* A. Balows and W. J. Hausler (ed.), *Diagnostic Procedures for Bacterial, Mycotic, and Parasitic Infections*, 6th ed. American Public Health Association, Washington, D.C.

44. **Dowell, V. R., Jr., and T. M. Hawkins.** 1981. *Laboratory Methods in Anaerobic Bacteriology*. CDC Laboratory Manual, HHS publication no. (CDC) 81-8272. Government Printing Office, Washington, D.C.

45. **Durmaz, B., H. E. Agel, E. Sonmez, R. Turkoz, and E. Aydin.** 2000. Infective endocarditis due to *Clostridium histolyticum. Clin. Microbiol. Infect.* **6:**561–563.

46. **Dzink, J., and J. G. Bartlett.** 1980. In vitro susceptibility of *Clostridium difficile* isolates from patients with antibiotic-associated diarrhea or colitis. *Antimicrob. Agents Chemother.* **17:**695–698.

47. **Elston, H. R., M. Wang, and L. K. Loo.** 1991. Arm abscesses caused by *Clostridium botulinum. J. Clin. Microbiol.* **29:**2678–2679.

48. **Fang, F. C., D. N. Gerding, and L. R. Peterson.** 1996. Diagnosis of *Clostridium difficile* colitis. *Ann. Intern. Med.* **125:**515.

49. **Farrant, J. M., Z. Traill, C. Conlon, B. Warren, N. Mortensen, F. V. Gleeson, and D. P. Jewell.** 1996. Pigbel-like syndrome in a vegetarian in Oxford. *Gut* **39:**336–337.

50. **Fedorko, D. P., H. D. Engler, E. M. O'Shaughnessy, E. C. Williams, C. J. Reichelderfer, and W. I. Smith, Jr.** 1999. Evaluation of two rapid assays for detection of *Clostridium difficile* toxin A in stool specimens. *J. Clin. Microbiol.* **37:**3044–3047.

51. **Fekety, R., and the American College of Gastroenterology Practice Parameters Committee.** 1997. Guidelines for the diagnosis and management of *Clostridium difficile*-associated diarrhea and colitis. *Am. J. Gastroenterol.* **92:**739–750.

52. **Fenicia, L., G. Franciosa, M. Pourshaban, and P. Aureli.** 1999. Intestinal toxemia botulism in two young people, caused by *Clostridium butyricum* type E. *Clin. Infect. Dis.* **29:**1381–1387.

53. **Finegold, S. M.** 1989. Therapy of anaerobic infections, p. 793–818. *In* S. M. Finegold and W. L. George (ed.), *Anaerobic Infections in Humans*. Academic Press, Inc., New York, N.Y.

54. **Finegold, S. M., E. J. Baron, and H. M. Wexler.** 1992. *A Clinical Guide to Anaerobic Infections*. Star Publishing Company, Belmont, Calif.

55. **Finegold, S. M., and W. L. George (ed.).** 1989. *Anaerobic Infections in Humans*. Academic Press, New York, N.Y.

56. **Garbutt, J. M., B. Littenberg, B. A. Evanoff, D. Sahm, and L. M. Mundy.** 1999. Enteric carriage of vancomycin-resistant *Enterococcus faecium* in patients tested for *Clostridium difficile. Infect. Control Hosp. Epidemiol.* **20:**664–670.

57. **George, W. L.** 1989. Antimicrobial agent-associated diarrhea and colitis, p. 661–678. *In* S. M. Finegold and W. L. George (ed.), *Anaerobic Infections in Humans*. Academic Press, Inc., New York, N.Y.

58. **George, W. L., and S. M. Finegold.** 1985. Clostridia in the human gastrointestinal flora, p. 1–37. *In* S. P. Borriello (ed.), *Clostridia in Gastrointestinal Disease*. CRC Press, Inc., Boca Raton, Fla.

59. **Gerding, D. N., and J. S. Brazier.** 1993. Optimal methods for identifying *Clostridium difficile* infections. *Clin. Infect. Dis.* **16:**S439–S442.

60. **Gerding, D. N., S. Johnson, L. R. Peterson, M. E. Mulligan, and J. Silva, Jr.** 1995. *Clostridium difficile*-associated diarrhea and colitis. *Infect. Control Hosp. Epidemiol.* **16:**459–477.

61. **Ghanem, F. M., A. C. Ridpath, W. E. Moore, and L. V. Moore.** 1991. Identification of *Clostridium botulinum, Clostridium argentinense*, and related organisms by cellular fatty acid analysis. *J. Clin. Microbiol.* **29:**1114–1124.

62. **Gorbach, S. L.** 1999. Antibiotics and *Clostridium difficile. N. Engl. J. Med.* **341:**1689–1691.

63. **Gorbach, S. L.** 1998. *Clostridium perfringens* and other clostridia, p. 1925–1933. *In* S. L. Gorbach, J. G. Bartlett, and N. R. Blacklow (ed.), *Infectious Diseases*, 2nd ed. W. B. Saunders Company, Philadelphia, Pa.

64. **Gorbach, S. L.** 1998. Gas gangrene and other clostridial skin and soft tissue infections, p. 915–922. *In* S. L. Gorbach, J. G. Bartlett, and N. R. Blacklow (ed.), *Infectious Diseases*, 2nd ed. W. B. Saunders Company, Philadelphia, Pa.

65. **Green, G. A., V. Schue, R. Girardot, and H. Monteil.** 1996. Characterisation of an enterotoxin-negative, cytotoxin-positive strain of *Clostridium sordellii. J. Med. Microbiol.* **44:**60–64.

66. **Gröschel, D. H.** 1996. *Clostridium difficile* infection. *Crit. Rev. Clin. Lab. Sci.* **33:**203–245.

67. **Gui, L., C. Subramony, J. Fratkin, and M. D. Hughson.** 2002. Fatal enteritis necroticans (pigbel) in a diabetic adult. *Mod. Pathol.* **15:**66–70.

68. **Hall, J. D., L. M. McCroskey, B. J. Pincomb, and C. L. Hatheway.** 1985. Isolation of an organism resembling *Clostridium baratii* which produces type F botulinal toxin from an infant with botulism. *J. Clin. Microbiol.* **21:**654–655.

69. **Hatheway, C. L.** 1988. Botulism, p. 111–133. *In* A. Balows, W. J. Hausler, Jr., M. Ohashi, and A. Turano (ed.), *Laboratory Diagnosis of Infectious Diseases: Principles and Practice,* vol. 1. Springer, New York, N.Y.

70. **Hatheway, C. L.** 1998. *Clostridium botulinum,* p. 1919–1925. *In* S. L. Gorbach, J. G. Bartlett, and N. R. Blacklow (ed.), *Infectious Diseases,* 2nd ed. W. B. Saunders Company, Philadelphia, Pa.

71. **Hatheway, C. L.** 1993. *Clostridium botulinum* and other clostridia that produce botulinum neurotoxin, p. 3–20. *In* A. H. W. Hauschild and K. L. Dodds (ed.), *Clostridium botulinum: Ecology and Control in Foods.* Marcel Dekker, Inc., New York, N.Y.

72. **Hatheway, C. L.** 1990. Toxigenic clostridia. *Clin. Microbiol. Rev.* **3:**66–98.

73. **Hatheway, C. L., and E. A. Johnson.** 1998. *Clostridium:* the spore-bearing anaerobes, p. 731–782. *In* L. Collier, A. Balows, and B. Duerden (ed.), *Systematic Bacteriology,* 9th ed., vol. 2. Edward Arnold Publisher, New York, N.Y.

74. **Hauschild, A. H.** 1975. Criteria and procedures for implicating *Clostridium perfringens* in food-borne outbreaks. *Can. J. Public Health* **66:**388–392.

75. **Hecht, D. W., M. H. Malamy, and F. P. Tally.** 1989. Mechanisms of resistance and resistance transfer in anaerobic bacteria, p. 755–769. *In* S. M. Finegold and W. L. George (ed.), *Anaerobic Infections in Humans.* Academic Press, Inc. New York, N.Y.

76. **Hill, M. J.** 1988. Gut flora and cancer in humans and laboratory animals, p. 461–502. *In* I. R. Rowland (ed.), *Role of the Gut Flora in Toxicity and Cancer.* Academic Press, Inc., New York, N.Y.

77. **Hill, M. J., B. S. Drasar, R. E. Williams, T. W. Meade, A. G. Cox, J. E. Simpson, and B. C. Morson.** 1975. Faecal bile-acids and clostridia in patients with cancer of the large bowel. *Lancet* **i:**535–539.

78. **Holdeman, L. V., E. P. Cato, and W. E. C. Moore (ed.).** 1977. *Anaerobe Laboratory Manual,* 4th ed. Virginia Polytechnic Institute and State University, Blacksburg.

79. **Isenberg, H. D. (ed.).** 1992. *Clinical Microbiology Procedures Handbook,* vol. 1. American Society for Microbiology, Washington, D.C.

80. **Izurieta, H. S., R. W. Sutter, P. M. Strebel, B. Bardenheier, D. R. Prevots, M. Wharton, and S. C. Hadler.** 1997. Tetanus surveillance—United States, 1991–1994. *CDC Surveill. Summ.* **46**(no. SS-2)**:**15–25.

81. **Johnson, E. A., and M. Bradshaw.** 2001. *Clostridium botulinum* and its neurotoxins: a metabolic and cellular perspective. *Toxicon* **39:**1703–1722.

82. **Johnson, J. L., and B. S. Francis.** 1975. Taxonomy of the clostridia: ribosomal ribonucleic acid homologies among the species. *J. Gen. Microbiol.* **88:**229–244.

83. **Johnson, S., M. R. Driks, R. K. Tweten, J. Ballard, D. L. Stevens, D. J. Anderson, and E. N. Janoff.** 1994. Clinical courses of seven survivors of *Clostridium septicum* infection and their immunologic responses to alpha toxin. *Clin. Infect. Dis.* **19:**761–764.

84. **Johnson, S., and D. N. Gerding.** 1998. *Clostridium difficile*-associated diarrhea. *Clin. Infect. Dis.* **26:**1027–1034. (Quiz, 1035–1036.)

85. **Johnson, S., S. A. Kent, K. J. O'Leary, M. M. Merrigan, S. P. Sambol, L. R. Peterson, and D. N. Gerding.** 2001. Fatal pseudomembranous colitis associated with a variant *Clostridium difficile* strain not detected by toxin A immunoassay. *Ann. Intern. Med.* **135:**434–438.

86. **Judicial Commission of the International Committee on Systematic Bacteriology.** 1999. Rejection of *Clostridium putrificum* and conservation of *Clostridium botulinum* and *Clostridium sporogenes*—Opinion 69. *Int. J. Syst. Bacteriol.* **49**(Part 1)**:**339.

87. **Justus, P. G., J. L. Martin, D. A. Goldberg, N. S. Taylor, J. G. Bartlett, R. W. Alexander, and J. R. Mathias.** 1982. Myoelectric effects of *Clostridium difficile:* motility-altering factors distinct from its cytotoxin and enterotoxin in rabbits. *Gastroenterology* **83:**836–843.

88. **Kato, H., N. Kato, S. Katow, T. Maegawa, S. Nakamura, and D. M. Lyerly.** 1999. Deletions in the repeating sequences of the toxin A gene of toxin A-negative, toxin B-positive *Clostridium difficile* strains. *FEMS Microbiol. Lett.* **175:**197–203.

89. **Kato, H., N. Kato, K. Watanabe, T. Yamamoto, K. Suzuki, S. Ishigo, S. Kunihiro, I. Nakamura, G. E. Killgore, and S. Nakamura.** 2001. Analysis of *Clostridium difficile* isolates from nosocomial outbreaks at three hospitals in diverse areas of Japan. *J. Clin. Microbiol.* **39:**1391–1395.

90. **King, A., A. Rampling, D. G. Wright, and R. E. Warren.** 1984. Neutropenic enterocolitis due to *Clostridium septicum* infection. *J. Clin. Pathol.* **37:**335–343.

91. **Kirchner, J. T.** 1991. *Clostridium septicum* infection. Beware of associated cancer. *Postgrad. Med.* **90:**157–160.

92. **Kitahara, M., F. Takamine, T. Imamura, and Y. Benno.** 2000. Assignment of *Eubacterium* sp. VPI 12708 and related strains with high bile acid 7alpha-dehydroxylating activity to *Clostridium scindens* and proposal of *Clostridium hylemonae* sp. nov., isolated from human faeces. *Int. J. Syst. Evol. Microbiol.* **50:**971–978.

93. **Kitahara, M., F. Takamine, T. Imamura, and Y. Benno.** 2001. *Clostridium hiranonis* sp. nov., a human intestinal bacterium with bile acid 7alpha-dehydroxylating activity. *Int. J. Syst. Evol. Microbiol.* **51:**39–44.

94. **Kliegman, R. M.** 1979. Neonatal necrotizing enterocolitis: implications for an infectious disease. *Pediatr. Clin. N. Am.* **26:**327–344.

95. **Kliegman, R. M., and A. A. Fanaroff.** 1984. Necrotizing enterocolitis. *N. Engl. J. Med.* **310:**1093–1103.

96. **Kliegman, R. M., W. A. Walker, and R. H. Yolken.** 1993. Necrotizing enterocolitis: research agenda for a disease of unknown etiology and pathogenesis. *Pediatr. Res.* **34:**701–708.

97. **Kokai-Kun, J. F., and B. A. McClane.** 1997. The *Clostridium perfringens* enterotoxin, p. 325–357. *In* J. I. Rood, B. A. McClane, J. G. Songer, and R. W. Titball (ed.), *The Clostridia: Molecular Biology and Pathogenesis.* Academic Press, New York, N.Y.

98. **Kokai-Kun, J. F., J. G. Songer, J. R. Czeczulin, F. Chen, and B. A. McClane.** 1994. Comparison of Western immunoblots and gene detection assays for identification of potentially enterotoxigenic isolates of *Clostridium perfringens. J. Clin. Microbiol.* **32:**2533–2539.

99. **Koneman, E. W., S. D. Allen, W. M. Janda, P. C. Schreckenberger, and W. C. Winn, Jr.** 1997. *Color Atlas and Textbook of Diagnostic Microbiology,* 5th ed. Lippincott-Raven Publishers, Philadelphia, Pa.

100. **Koransky, J. R., S. D. Allen, and V. R. Dowell, Jr.** 1978. Use of ethanol for selective isolation of sporeforming microorganisms. *Appl. Environ. Microbiol.* **35:**762–765.

101. **Koransky, J. R., M. D. Stargel, and V. R. Dowell, Jr.** 1979. *Clostridium septicum* bacteremia. Its clinical significance. *Am. J. Med.* **66:**63–66.

102. **Kornbluth, A. A., J. B. Danzig, and L. H. Bernstein.** 1989. *Clostridium septicum* infection and associated malignancy. Report of 2 cases and review of the literature. *Medicine (Baltimore)* **68:**30–37.

103. **Kosloske, A. M.** 1994. Epidemiology of necrotizing enterocolitis. *Acta Paediatr. Suppl.* **396:**2–7.

104. **Kudsk, K. A.** 1992. Occult gastrointestinal malignancies producing metastatic *Clostridium septicum* infections in diabetic patients. *Surgery* **112:**765–770.

105. **Kuijper, E. J., J. de Weerdt, H. Kato, N. Kato, A. P. van Dam, E. R. van der Vorm, J. Weel, C. van Rheenen, and J. Dankert.** 2001. Nosocomial outbreak of *Clostridium difficile*-associated diarrhoea due to a clindamycin-resistant enterotoxin A-negative strain. *Eur. J. Clin. Microbiol. Infect. Dis.* **20:**528–534.

106. **Lashner, B. A., J. Todorczuk, D. F. Sahm, and S. B. Hanauer.** 1986. *Clostridium difficile* culture-positive toxin-negative diarrhea. *Am. J. Gastroenterol.* **81:**940–943.

107. **Lawrence, G. W., D. Lehmann, G. Anian, C. A. Coakley, G. Saleu, M. J. Barker, and M. W. Davis.** 1990. Impact of active immunisation against enteritis necroticans in Papua New Guinea. *Lancet* **336:**1165–1167.

108. **Lorber, B.** 2000. Gas gangrene and other clostridium-associated diseases, p. 2549–2561. *In* G. L. Mandell, J. E. Bennett, and R. Dolin (ed.), *Mandell, Douglas and Bennett's Principles and Practice of Infectious Diseases*, 4th ed., vol. 2. Churchill Livingstone, Philadelphia, Pa.

109. **Lyerly, D. M., and S. D. Allen.** 1997. The clostridia, p. 559–623. *In* A. M. Emmerson, P. Hawkey, and S. Gillespie (ed.), *Principles and Practice of Clinical Bacteriology.* John Wiley & Sons, New York, N.Y.

110. **Lyerly, D. M., L. A. Barroso, T. D. Wilkins, C. Depitre, and G. Corthier.** 1992. Characterization of a toxin A-negative, toxin B-positive strain of *Clostridium difficile.* *Infect. Immun.* **60:**4633–4639.

111. **Lyerly, D. M., H. C. Krivan, and T. D. Wilkins.** 1988. *Clostridium difficile*: its disease and toxins. *Clin. Microbiol. Rev.* **1:**1–18.

112. **Lyerly, D. M., L. M. Neville, D. T. Evans, J. Fill, S. Allen, W. Greene, R. Sautter, P. Hnatuck, D. J. Torpey, and R. Schwalbe.** 1998. Multicenter evaluation of the *Clostridium difficile* TOX A/B TEST. *J. Clin. Microbiol.* **36:**184–190.

113. **Mahony, D. E., E. Gilliatt, S. Dawson, E. Stockdale, and S. H. Lee.** 1989. Vero cell assay for rapid detection of *Clostridium perfringens* enterotoxin. *Appl. Environ. Microbiol.* **55:**2141–2143.

114. **Marler, L. M., J. A. Siders, and S. D. Allen.** 2001. *Direct Smear Atlas: a Monograph of Gram-Stained Preparations of Clinical Specimens.* Lippincott Williams & Wilkins, Philadelphia, Pa.

115. **Marler, L. M., J. A. Siders, L. C. Wolters, Y. Pettigrew, B. L. Skitt, and S. D. Allen.** 1992. Comparison of five cultural procedures for isolation of *Clostridium difficile* from stools. *J. Clin. Microbiol.* **30:**514–516.

116. **Marler, L. M., J. A. Siders, L. C. Wolters, Y. Pettigrew, B. L. Skitt, and S. D. Allen.** 1991. Evaluation of the new RapID-ANA II system for the identification of clinical anaerobic isolates. *J. Clin. Microbiol.* **29:**874–878.

117. **Marrie, T. J., E. V. Haldane, C. A. Swantee, et al.** 1981. Susceptibility of anaerobic bacteria to nine antimicrobial agents and demonstration of decreased susceptibility of *Clostridium perfringens* to penicillin. *Antimicrob. Agents Chemother.* **19:**51–55.

118. **McCroskey, L. M., C. L. Hatheway, B. A. Woodruff, J. A. Greenberg, and P. Jurgenson.** 1991. Type F botulism due to neurotoxigenic *Clostridium baratii* from an unknown source in an adult. *J. Clin. Microbiol.* **29:**2618–2620.

119. **McFarland, L. V., M. B. Coyle, W. H. Kremer, and W. E. Stamm.** 1987. Rectal swab cultures for *Clostridium difficile* surveillance studies. *J. Clin. Microbiol.* **25:**2241–2242.

120. **McFarland, L. V., M. E. Mulligan, R. Y. Kwok, and W. E. Stamm.** 1989. Nosocomial acquisition of *Clostridium difficile* infection. *N. Engl. J. Med.* **320:**204–210.

121. **Meer, R. R., and J. G. Songer.** 1997. Multiplex polymerase chain reaction assay for genotyping *Clostridium perfringens.* *Am. J. Vet. Res.* **58:**702–705.

122. **Moll, W. M., J. Ungerechts, G. Marklein, and K. P. Schaal.** 1996. Comparison of BBL Crystal ANR ID Kit and API rapid ID 32 A for identification of anaerobic bacteria. *Zentralbl. Bakteriol.* **284:**329–347.

123. **Moncrief, J. S., D. M. Lyerly, and T. D. Wilkins.** 1997. Molecular biology of the *Clostridium difficile* toxins, p. 369–392. *In* J. I. Rood, B. A. McClane, J. G. Songer, and R. W. Titball (ed.), *The Clostridia: Molecular Biology and Pathogenesis.* Academic Press, New York, N.Y.

124. **Moncrief, J. S., L. Zheng, L. M. Neville, and D. M. Lyerly.** 2000. Genetic characterization of toxin A-negative, toxin B-positive *Clostridium difficile* isolates by PCR. *J. Clin. Microbiol.* **38:**3072–3075.

125. **Mory, F., A. Lozniewski, V. David, J. P. Carlier, L. Dubreuil, and R. Leclercq.** 1998. Low-level vancomycin resistance in *Clostridium innocuum.* *J. Clin. Microbiol.* **36:**1767–1768.

126. **Mulligan, M. E., L. R. Peterson, R. Y. Kwok, C. R. Clabots, and D. N. Gerding.** 1988. Immunoblots and plasmid fingerprints compared with serotyping and polyacrylamide gel electrophoresis for typing *Clostridium difficile.* *J. Clin. Microbiol.* **26:**41–46.

127. **Murrell, T. G. C.** 1989. Enteritis necroticans, p. 639–659. *In* S. M. Finegold and W. L. George (ed.), *Anaerobic Infections in Humans.* Academic Press, San Diego, Calif.

128. **Nakamura, S., M. Mikawa, S. Nakashio, M. Takabatake, I. Okado, K. Yamakawa, T. Serikawa, S. Okumura, and S. Nishida.** 1981. Isolation of *Clostridium difficile* from the feces and the antibody in sera of young and elderly adults. *Microbiol. Immunol.* **25:**345–351.

129. **Noone, M., M. Tabaqchali, and J. B. Spillane.** 2002. *Clostridium novyi* causing necrotising fasciitis in an injecting drug user. *J. Clin. Pathol.* **55:**141–142.

130. **Olsen, S. J., L. C. MacKinnon, J. S. Goulding, N. H. Bean, and L. Slutsker.** 2000. Surveillance for foodborne-disease outbreaks—United States, 1993–1997. *Morb. Mortal. Wkly. Rep. CDC Surveill. Summ.* **49:**1–62.

131. **Pelletier, J. P., J. A. Plumbley, E. A. Rouse, and S. J. Cina.** 2000. The role of *Clostridium septicum* in paraneoplastic sepsis. *Arch. Pathol. Lab. Med.* **124:**353–356.

132. **Peterson, L. R., and P. J. Kelly.** 1993. The role of the clinical microbiology laboratory in the management of *Clostridium difficile*-associated diarrhea. *Infect. Dis. Clin. N. Am.* **7:**277–293.

133. **Peterson, L. R., P. J. Kelly, and H. A. Nordbrock.** 1996. Role of culture and toxin detection in laboratory testing for diagnosis of *Clostridium difficile*-associated diarrhea. *Eur. J. Clin. Microbiol. Infect. Dis.* **15:**330–336.

134. **Petrillo, T. M., C. M. Beck-Sague, J. G. Songer, C. Abramowsky, J. D. Fortenberry, L. Meacham, A. G. Dean, H. Lee, D. M. Bueschel, and S. R. Nesheim.** 2000. Enteritis necroticans (pigbel) in a diabetic child. *N. Engl. J. Med.* **342:**1250–1253.

135. **Poduval, R. D., R. P. Kamath, M. Corpuz, E. P. Norkus, and C. S. Pitchumoni.** 2000. *Clostridium difficile* and vancomycin-resistant enterococcus: the new nosocomial alliance. *Am. J. Gastroenterol.* **95:**3513–3515.

136. **Reddy, B. S.** 1981. Dietary fat and its relationship to large bowel cancer. *Cancer Res.* **41:**3700–3705.

137. **Ridgway, E. J., and E. D. Grech.** 1993. Clostridial endocarditis: report of a case caused by *Clostridium septicum* and review of the literature. *J. Infect.* **26:**309–313.

138. **Rood, J. I., B. A. McClane, J. G. Songer, and R. W. Titball (ed.).** 1997. *The Clostridia: Molecular Biology and Pathogenesis.* Academic Press, New York, N.Y.

139. **Rosenblatt, J. E.** 1989. Susceptibility testing of anaerobic bacteria. *Clin. Lab. Med.* **9:**239–254.

140. **Samore, M. H.** 1999. Epidemiology of nosocomial *Clostridium difficile* diarrhoea. *J. Hosp. Infect.* **43**(Suppl.): S183–S190.

141. **Saulnier, P., E. Chachaty, F. Hilali, and A. Andremont.** 1997. Single-step polymerase chain reaction for combined gene detection and epidemiological typing in three bacterial models. *FEMS Microbiol. Lett.* **150:**311–316.

142. **Schechter, R., and S. S. Arnon.** 1999. Commentary: where Marco Polo meets Meckel: type E botulism from *Clostridium butyricum*. *Clin. Infect. Dis.* **29:**1388–1393.

143. **Schiavo, G., and C. Montecucco.** 1997. The structure and mode of action of botulinum and tetanus toxins, p. 295–322. *In* J. I. Rood, B. A. McClane, J. G. Songer, and R. W. Titball (ed.), *The Clostridia: Molecular Biology and Pathogenesis.* Academic Press, New York, N.Y.

144. **Schleupner, M. A., D. C. Garner, K. M. Sosnowski, C. J. Schleupner, L. J. Barrett, E. Silva, D. Hirsch, and R. L. Guerrant.** 1995. Concurrence of *Clostridium difficile* toxin A enzyme-linked immunosorbent assay, fecal lactoferrin assay, and clinical criteria with *C. difficile* cytotoxin titer in two patient cohorts. *J. Clin. Microbiol.* **33:**1755–1759.

145. **Schreckenberger, P. C., D. M. Celig, and W. M. Janda.** 1988. Clinical evaluation of the Vitek ANI card for identification of anaerobic bacteria. *J. Clin. Microbiol.* **26:**225–230.

146. **Shandera, W. X., C. O. Tacket, and P. A. Blake.** 1983. Food poisoning due to *Clostridium perfringens* in the United States. *J. Infect. Dis.* **147:**167–170.

147. **Sherman, S., E. Klein, and B. A. McClane.** 1994. *Clostridium perfringens* type A enterotoxin induces tissue damage and fluid accumulation in rabbit ileum. *J. Diarrhoeal Dis. Res.* **12:**200–207.

148. **Simor, A. E., S. L. Yake, and K. Tsimidis.** 1993. Infection due to *Clostridium difficile* among elderly residents of a long-term-care facility. *Clin. Infect. Dis.* **17:**672–678.

149. **Smith, L. D.** 1975. Common mesophilic anaerobes, including *Clostridium botulinum* and *Clostridium tetani*, in 21 soil specimens. *Appl. Microbiol.* **29:**590–594.

150. **Smith, L. D.** 1978. The occurrence of *Clostridium botulinum* and *Clostridium tetani* in the soil of the United States. *Health Lab. Sci.* **15:**74–80.

151. **Smith, L. D. S., and B. L. Williams.** 1984. *The Pathogenic Anaerobic Bacteria,* 3rd ed. Charles C. Thomas, Springfield, Ill.

152. **Songer, J. G.** 1997. Molecular and immunological methods for the diagnosis of clostridial diseases, p. 491–503. *In* J. I. Rood, B. A. McClane, J. G. Songer, and R. W. Titball (ed.), *The Clostridia: Molecular Biology and Pathogenesis.* Academic Press, New York, N.Y.

153. **Songer, J. G., and R. R. Meer.** 1996. Genotyping of *Clostridium perfringens* by polymerase chain reaction is a useful adjunct to diagnosis of clostridial enteric disease in animals. *Anaerobe* **2:**197–203.

154. **Sparks, S. G., R. J. Carman, M. R. Sarker, and B. A. McClane.** 2001. Genotyping of enterotoxigenic *Clostridium perfringens* fecal isolates associated with antibiotic-associated diarrhea and food poisoning in North America. *J. Clin. Microbiol.* **39:**883–888.

155. **Speirs, G., R. E. Warren, and A. Rampling.** 1988. *Clostridium tertium* septicemia in patients with neutropenia. *J. Infect. Dis.* **158:**1336–1340.

156. **Spika, J. S., N. Shaffer, N. Hargrett-Bean, S. Collin, K. L. MacDonald, and P. A. Blake.** 1989. Risk factors for infant botulism in the United States. *Am. J. Dis. Child.* **143:**828–832. (Erratum, **144:**60, 1990.)

157. **Stackebrandt, E., and F. A. Rainey.** 1997. Phylogenetic relationships, p. 3–19. *In* J. I. Rood, B. A. McClane, J. G. Songer, and R. W. Titball (ed.), *The Clostridia: Molecular Biology and Pathogenesis.* Academic Press, New York, N.Y.

158. **Staneck, J. L., L. S. Weckbach, S. D. Allen, J. A. Siders, P. H. Gilligan, G. Coppitt, J. A. Kraft, and D. H. Willis.** 1996. Multicenter evaluation of four methods for *Clostridium difficile* detection: ImmunoCard C. difficile, cytotoxin assay, culture, and latex agglutination. *J. Clin. Microbiol.* **34:**2718–2721.

159. **Stark, P. L., and A. Lee.** 1982. The microbial ecology of the large bowel of breast-fed and formula-fed infants during the first year of life. *J. Med. Microbiol.* **15:**189–203.

160. **Stevens, D. L., B. M. Laine, and J. E. Mitten.** 1987. Comparison of single and combination antimicrobial agents for prevention of experimental gas gangrene caused by *Clostridium perfringens*. *Antimicrob. Agents Chemother.* **31:**312–316.

161. **Stevens, D. L., K. A. Maier, B. M. Laine, et. al.** 1987. Comparison of clindamycin, rifampin, tetracycline, metronidazole, and penicillin for efficacy in prevention of experimental gas gangrene due to *Clostridium perfringens*. *J. Infect. Dis.* **155:**220.

162. **Suen, J. C., C. L. Hatheway, A. G. Steigerwalt, and D. J. Brenner.** 1988. *Clostridium argentinense*, sp. nov.: a genetically homogenous group composed of all strains of *Clostridium botulinum* toxin type G and some nontoxigenic strains previously identified as *Clostridium subterminale* or *Clostridium hastiforme*. *Int. J. Syst. Bacteriol.* **38:** 375–381.

163. **Summanen, P., E. J. Baron, D. M. Citron, C. A. Strong, H. M. Wexler, and S. M. Finegold.** 2002. *Wadsworth Anaerobic Bacteriology Manual,* 6th ed. Star Publishing, Belmont, Calif.

164. **Titball, R. W.** 1993. Bacterial phospholipases C. *Microbiol. Rev.* **57:**347–366.

165. **Torres, J. F.** 1991. Purification and characterisation of toxin B from a strain of *Clostridium difficile* that does not produce toxin A. *J. Med. Microbiol.* **35:**40–44.

166. **von Eichel-Streiber, C., I. Zec-Pirnat, M. Grabnar, and M. Rupnik.** 1999. A nonsense mutation abrogates production of a functional enterotoxin A in *Clostridium difficile* toxinotype VIII strains of serogroups F and X. *FEMS Microbiol. Lett.* **178:**163–168.

167. **Woodruff, B. A., P. M. Griffin, L. M. McCroskey, J. F. Smart, R. B. Wainwright, R. G. Bryant, L. C. Hutwagner, and C. L. Hatheway.** 1992. Clinical and laboratory comparison of botulism from toxin types A, B, and E in the United States, 1975–1988. *J. Infect. Dis.* **166:**1281–1286.

168. **Yale, C. E., and E. Balish.** 1992. The relative lethality of intestinal bacteria for gnotobiotic rats with experimental intestinal strangulation. *J. Med.* **23:**265–277.

169. **Yip, C., M. Loeb, S. Salama, L. Moss, and J. Olde.** 2001. Quinolone use as a risk factor for nosocomial *Clostridium difficile*-associated diarrhea. *Infect. Control Hosp. Epidemiol.* **22:**572–575.

170. **Zhou, Y., H. Sugiyama, H. Nakano, and E. A. Johnson.** 1995. The genes for the *Clostridium botulinum* type G toxin complex are on a plasmid. *Infect. Immun.* **63:**2087–2091.

Peptostreptococcus, Propionibacterium, Lactobacillus, Actinomyces, and Other Non-Spore-Forming Anaerobic Gram-Positive Bacteria*

BERNARD J. MONCLA AND SHARON L. HILLIER

55

The anaerobic gram-positive cocci and non-spore-forming rods constitute a genetically and phenotypically diverse group of bacteria. These organisms are, for the most part, components of the normal flora of the skin, vagina, or mucosal surfaces of humans and animals. Like many other anaerobes, they can be opportunistic pathogens when they gain access to normally sterile body sites. Hence, infections caused by this group of organisms are usually considered to be of endogenous origin. The recovery of these organisms from clinical infections is summarized in Table 1. They are most likely found in mixed infections together with anaerobic gram-negative rods or facultatively anaerobic organisms.

Gram-positive anaerobic bacteria may be separated on the basis of their mol percent G+C contents of their DNA into two major subdivisions, which appear to represent separate phylogenetic lines. The subdivision with low (<50%) G+C contents represents a more ancient line and includes the genera *Mogibacterium* (98), *Lactobacillus* (103), *Clostridium* and *Bulleidia* (31), *Eubacterium* (23), *Holdemania* (152), *Catenibacterium* (69), *Atopobium* (26), and *Peptostreptococcus* and *Peptococcus* (36, 37). The subdivision with high (>50%) G+C contents includes the genera *Bifidobacterium* (126), *Actinomyces* (79), *Arcanobacterium* (107), *Propionibacterium* (32), *Mobiluncus* (79), *Slackia* (147), *Cryptobacterium* (97), *Collinsella* (70), *Actinobaculum* (80), and *Eggerthella* (72).

These genera fall into discrete units on the basis of the amino acid contents of the cell wall, the major end products of glucose fermentation, and the mol percent G+C contents; however, considerable work remains before this group of organisms is fully understood (32).

Anaerobic gram-positive cocci and non-spore-forming rods are often undetected or unrecognized by many clinical laboratories since many of them require extended anaerobic incubation with selective or complex media for growth. Specimens from oral or pelvic abscesses are often negative for most anaerobes after 48 h of incubation, and extended anaerobic incubation is required to accurately detect the etiologic agents of these infections.

After recovery and isolation, these microorganisms are difficult to identify accurately. Most of the commercial rapid identification systems that identify many of the fast-growing anaerobic gram-negative rods correctly are inadequate for identification of the organisms discussed in this chapter. However, correct identification at least to the genus level may provide useful information for the clinician. For example, recovery of a *Lactobacillus* species from the blood is suggestive of a genital or rectal source of the infection, whereas recovery of a *Propionibacterium* species may suggest a skin source.

ANAEROBIC GRAM-POSITIVE COCCI

Description of the Genera

The genera *Peptostreptococcus, Anaerococcus, Gallicola, Finegoldia, Micromonas, Schleiferella (Peptoniphilus),* and *Peptococcus* include gram-positive obligately anaerobic non-spore-forming sometimes elongated cocci. Cells may occur in pairs, tetrads, irregular masses, or chains. These species are chemoorganotrophs that metabolize peptones and amino acids to acetic acid and often produce isobutyric, butyric, isovaleric, or isocaproic acid. Obligately anaerobic cocci belonging to the genus *Streptococcus* produce lactic acid as the major product of glucose metabolism.

Taxonomy

A considerable body of evidence indicated that the *Peptostreptococcus* genus was in need of taxonomic revision (35). Because of differences within the species with respect to carbohydrate fermentation, glutamate dehydrogenase, metabolic end products, peptidoglycan structure, and 16S rRNA sequence data, it has recently been proposed that the genus be reclassified into at least five new genera (Table 2) (35, 96, 115). Ezaki et al. (35) proposed *Anaerococcus, Peptoniphilus,* and *Gallicola* to accommodate many of the *Peptostreptococcus* species (Table 2). Another group proposed the new genus *Schleiferella* to accommodate several of the *Peptostreptococcus* species (115). Both *Peptoniphilus* and *Schleiferella* are pending synonyms; however, by taxonomic rules, *Schleiferella* has priority and will likely take precedence.

The genus *Peptococcus* currently includes only one species, *Peptococcus niger.*

* This chapter contains information presented in chapter 47 by Arne C. Rodloff, Sharon L. Hillier, and Bernard J. Moncla in the seventh edition of this Manual.

TABLE 1 Recovery of anaerobic gram-positive rods and cocci from various specimen types[a]

Site	% of patients yielding isolates of:				
	Anaerobic gram-positive cocci	Actinomyces	Eubacterium	Lactobacillus[b]	Propionibacterium
Appendix	23	11	34	21	6
Kidney abscess	83	0	17	0	17
Bladder abscess	100	0	50	0	0
Periurethral abscess	71	0	0	0	0
Bartholin gland abscess	42	0	8	4	0
Penile abscess	86	0	0	0	0
Scrotal or testicular abscess	48	5	5	0	0
Periapical abscess	68	14	9	23	0
Orofacial infection	33	0	13	33	0
Penile wound	66	0	0	0	0
Periodontal pockets[c]	60	75	43	NA[d]	15
Breast abscess	51	0	2	0	27
Peritonsillar abscess	36	0	0	2	10
Blood	11	0	2	0.2	36
Nostril (normal)	16	0	0	0	75
Vagina	87	7	3	14	22

[a] Data from references 5, 12, 13, 14, 15, 39, 55, and 154.
[b] Obligately anaerobic strains only.
[c] B. J. Moncla, unpublished data from University of Washington Periodontal Clinic, 1984 through 1989.
[d] NA, no attempts were made to recover *Lactobacillus* spp. in these studies.

The genus *Streptococcus* currently includes two strictly anaerobic species, *Streptococcus hansenii* and *Streptococcus pleomorphus*. *Streptococcus parvulus* has been transferred to the genus *Atopobium* as *Atopobium parvulum* (26). The obligately anaerobic *Streptococcus* species are rarely found in clinical specimens, and their taxonomic position remains unclear. Analyses of the 16S rRNA, DNA base composition, and peptidoglycan type suggest that *S. hansenii* is related to *Clostridium coccoides* (153) and *Clostridium amniovalericum*, whereas *S. pleomorphus* appears to be closely

TABLE 2 Proposed and validated revisions to the genus *Peptostreptococcus*

Basonym	Current or proposed nomenclature
P. anaerobius	Unchanged
P. asaccharolyticus . . .	*Peptoniphilus asaccharolyticus, Schleiferella asaccharolytica*
P. barnesae	*Gallicola barnesae*
P. harei	*Peptoniphilus harei, Schleiferella harei*
P. heliotrinireducens . .	*Slackia heliotrinireducens*
P. hydrogenalis	*Anaerococcus hydrogenalis*
P. indolicus	*Peptoniphilus indolicus, Schleiferella indolica*
P. ivorii	*Peptoniphilus ivorii*
P. lacrimalis	*Peptoniphilus lacrimalis, Schleiferella lacrimalis*
P. lactolyticus	*Anaerococcus lactolyticus*
P. magnus	*Finegoldia magna*
P. micros	*Micromonas micros*
P. octavius	*Anaerococcus octavius*
P. prevotii	*Anaerococcus prevotii*
P. productus	Unchanged
P. tetradius	*Anaerococcus tetradius*
P. vaginalis	*Anaerococcus vaginalis*
Peptococcus niger	Unchanged

related to *Clostridium innocuum* (84). *A. parvulum*, which can be recovered from the gingival crevice, is more closely related to *Actinomyces* species (26, 68).

Anaerobic gram-positive cocci of other genera, including *Ruminococcus* and *Coprococcus*, can be isolated from the rumens of animals and the stomachs and bowels of humans. However, their isolation from clinical specimens is exceedingly rare (94).

Natural Habitat

The anaerobic gram-positive cocci are widely distributed as members of the normal flora in humans and animals. They can be recovered routinely from the skin, oropharynx, upper respiratory tract, gut, and urogenital tract (99); in particular, they are recovered from the vaginas of 90% of pregnant women, with *Anaerococcus prevotii, Anaerococcus tetradius, Finegoldia magna*, and *Peptoniphilus asaccharolyticus* being the most common species recovered (55). Likewise, these organisms can be recovered from 60% of periodontal pocket specimens but are relatively uncommon in saliva. *P. niger* is present in the vaginas of 20 to 30% of pregnant women but has been only infrequently recovered from clinical specimens (55).

Clinical Significance

The role of "anaerobic streptococci" in human infections has been recognized since the early 1900s. One report (55) listed a wide variety of species recovered from the endometria of women with postpartum fever, including *F. magna* (41%), *A. tetradius* (26%), *Schleiferella asaccharolytica* (20%), *Peptostreptococcus anaerobius* (19%), *A. prevotii* (15%), and, less frequently, *P. niger* (4%). These organisms are also frequently recovered from tubo-ovarian abscesses, the fallopian tubes, or endometria of women with pelvic inflammatory disease, septic abortions, and patients with amnionitis and infection of the placental membranes (chorioamnionitis) (56). In patients with pelvic inflammatory disease, these organisms are often part of a mixed infection in association with *Prevotella* and *Porphyromonas* species or facultatively anaerobic bacteria such as *Escherichia coli* (56).

Anaerobic gram-positive cocci are isolated from patients with a wide variety of head and neck infections, including periodontitis, chronic otitis media, chronic sinusitis, purulent nasopharyngitis, and brain abscess (12, 15, 16, 17). The source of anaerobic cocci in brain abscess is related to the presence of these bacteria in otitis and sinusitis and their subsequent spread into the central nervous system. Anaerobic gram-positive cocci present in the gingiva can also spread hematogenously following dental manipulations or extractions to cause endocarditis or brain abscess (50). Aspiration from the oral cavity may cause pulmonary disease such as pneumonitis, lung abscess, empyema, or necrotizing pneumonia. Again, these infections are usually polymicrobic.

Spillage of fecal contents into the peritoneum following appendicitis, diverticulitis, surgery, penetrating trauma, or cancer can lead to intra-abdominal mixed infections involving anaerobic gram-positive cocci, *Bacteroides* species, *Clostridium* species, and facultatively anaerobic bacteria such as members of the family *Enterobacteriaceae* and enterococci. Intestinal perforation or cancer may also lead to liver abscess, which involves obligate anaerobes in at least half of all cases (6). In one study, *Peptostreptococcus* species were isolated in one of four specimens from patients with perforated appendicitis and peritonitis (5).

Bacteremia due to anaerobic gram-positive cocci most commonly follows obstetric or gynecologic infections, including postpartum endometritis and amnionitis. Over a 6-year period in Turku, Finland, *Peptostreptococcus* species were recovered from 7 of 57 patients who developed clinically significant bacteremias (122), although none of these infections was lethal. An additional 24 patients developed clinically insignificant bacteremia, and 3 of the cases were due to *Peptostreptococcus* species. Thus, the recovery of anaerobic gram-positive cocci from the blood is not as frequently associated with fatal infection as is bacteremia due to *Bacteroides* species, but *Peptostreptococcus* spp. should not be routinely interpreted as clinically insignificant. The most common isolates include *F. magna*, *S. asaccharolytica*, and *P. anaerobius* (13, 15). Infection of bone, joints, and grafts may also occur, with *F. magna* being of major importance in these processes (8).

P. niger has been associated with sheep foot rot (111), but its role in human infections is unclear.

Collection and Transport of Specimens

The appropriate specimen collection and transport methods for obligately anaerobic gram-positive rods and cocci are similar to those for other anaerobes (chapter 20). In general, aspirates or biopsy specimens are considered the optimal samples for culture of obligate anaerobic bacteria. Such specimens are less likely to be contaminated with microorganisms of the normal flora and are also less likely to be exposed to the detrimental effects of oxygen and desiccation. Appropriate samples should be transported to the laboratory within 30 min. Swab specimens should be accepted only after consultation. In all cases, it is imperative to use an anaerobic transport system, since anaerobic cocci are quickly rendered nonviable when exposed to O_2. Anaerobic transport media that have been evaluated for use with anaerobic cocci include the B-D Port-a-Cul anaerobic transport tube (Becton Dickinson Microbiology Products, Cockeysville, Md.) and the Anaerobic Transport Tube

(Anaerobe Systems, Morgan Hill, Calif.). It has been demonstrated that *Peptostreptococcus* species have 100% viability after 24 h at room temperature in the Port-a-Cul anaerobic transport tube. A modified Stuart transport medium has also been reported to provide adequate protection for *F. magna* and *P. anaerobius* for up to 48 h (11, 109, 140). Finally, an Amies medium without charcoal (Venturi Transystem; Copan Diagnostics, Corona, Calif.) was shown to be equivalent to the Port-a-Cul anaerobic transport tube in protecting *P. anaerobius* and other anaerobes (62). However, studies have demonstrated that survival decreases rapidly after 24 h (109). These data suggest that rapid transportation to the laboratory is essential irrespective of the transport system chosen if preservation of *Peptostreptococcus* species is desired. It should be noted that *P. anaerobius* is susceptible to sodium polyanethol sulfonate (Liquoid), and this characteristic has even been used for identification purposes (151). However, this also suggests that blood culture systems containing Liquoid as an additive are inadequate for the recovery of this species.

The optimal temperature for transport is somewhat controversial. A report by Tvede and Hoiby (140) indicates that transportation at either 4 or 22°C does not influence the survival of anaerobic bacteria; however, our experience suggests better recovery when the specimens are held at 18 to 22°C.

Direct Examination

Although direct examination of clinical specimens with a Gram stain is always desirable, little specific information about the presence of anaerobic cocci can be determined since facultatively anaerobic and obligately anaerobic cocci cannot be distinguished. Moreover, anaerobic cocci may display a rod shape, and, finally, cocci with a cell wall structure typical of gram-negative organisms (*Megasphaera*) may appear as a gram-positive organism on initial microscopic examination.

Isolation Procedures

The anaerobic cocci grow well on most nonselective plating media suitable for anaerobic isolation. Brucella, Columbia, or Schaedler agar base supplemented with 5% sheep blood, vitamin K, and hemin generally yield good growth within 48 to 72 h. One report has suggested that Centers for Disease Control and Prevention (CDC) agar base gives better recovery of *A. tetradius*, *P. anaerobius*, and *S. asaccharolytica* than brucella blood agar (128).

There is no single selective medium for growing anaerobic gram-positive cocci. The addition of nalidixic acid and Tween 80 (94) or oxolinic acid (110) may enhance the recovery of gram-positive anaerobes in mixed infections. Columbia CNA agar supplemented with glutathione and lead acetate can be used as a differential medium for *Micromonas micros*. Unlike other cocci, *M. micros* rapidly utilizes the reduced form of glutathione to form hydrogen sulfide, which reacts with lead acetate to form a black precipitate under the colony in the medium (139).

Acceptable broth media include peptone-yeast extract-glucose, chopped meat-glucose, and thioglycolate supplemented with hemin, vitamin K, and rabbit serum (5%). Supplementation with Tween 80 (final concentration, 0.02%) may stimulate growth in broth media. Most laboratories no longer inoculate broth enrichment media for isolation of anaerobes.

For recovery of anaerobic gram-positive cocci from blood, anaerobic tryptic or Trypticase soy broth incubated for a minimum of 5 days has been used by many laboratories. By comparison, aerobic blood culture bottles never yield anaerobic gram-positive cocci from the blood, and short-term incubation of anaerobic blood culture bottles similarly fails to detect these organisms.

Identification Procedures

Anaerobic gram-positive cocci do not always stain as gram-positive cocci. For instance, P. productus and Peptostreptococcus anaerobius may be elongated and resemble gram-positive coccobacilli. Any of the gram-positive cocci may, with age, rapidly lose their positivity by Gram staining. To add to the confusion, anaerobic gram-negative cocci, including Veillonella and Megasphaera spp., appear at times to be gram-positive organisms. Preparation of Gram stains from a variety of media, both broth and solid, and examination of subcultures at different ages may help in assessing the correct cellular morphology and Gram stain reaction. Gram-positive cocci that resemble rods while on agar medium will assume a more coccoid appearance when grown in broth. Vancomycin susceptibility testing as well as the KOH and antibiotic disk tests or a test with L-alanine-4-nitroanilide (LANA) as a substrate for alanine aminopeptidase (see below) are useful for establishing that a microorganism is gram positive in instances in which gram-variable or gram-negative staining is observed (7). Accurate Gram staining of organisms in this group requires fixing and staining under anaerobic conditions, i.e., in an anaerobic chamber (67).

Assignment of an anaerobic gram-positive coccus to a specific genus can be somewhat difficult if gas chromatography is not available. Any identification of anaerobic gram-positive cocci that is made without the aid of chromatographic analysis of metabolic fatty acids must be considered presumptive. Even though the rapid identification systems can readily identify many species of anaerobic gram-positive cocci, the accuracy of the identification is directly related to the knowledge and experience of the individual reading the test (2, 19, 73). For example, the reported accuracy of the RapID-ANA II system for members of the genus Peptostreptococcus ranges from 15% for A. prevotii to 100% for M. micros (22, 87). The Rapid ID32A kit (bioMerieux Vitek, Inc., Hazelwood, Mo.) correctly identified only 1 of 12 A. prevotii isolates in one study (100). The authors noted that A. prevotii is heterogeneous according to preformed enzyme profiles and that further taxonomic clarification may be required. Thus, the difficulty in correctly identifying these organisms may be due in part to our lack of understanding of the true taxonomic status of some anaerobic gram-positive cocci. Tables 3 and 4 can be used to distinguish the genera and species of anaerobic gram-positive cocci. By contrast, S. asaccharolytica is identified by most commercial systems.

The three species of anaerobic gram-positive cocci most commonly seen in clinical specimens are F. magna, P. anaerobius, and S. asaccharolytica. Colonies of F. magna are minute to 0.5 mm in diameter, raised, dull, smooth, and nonhemolytic. The cells are 0.7 to 1.2 μm in diameter and appear in a tightly packed arrangement. M. micros colonies are minute to 1 mm in diameter, convex, and dull. The cells are smaller than those of F. magna, being 0.3 to 0.7 μm in diameter. However, strain variability under different growth conditions makes differentiation of these two species on the basis of cellular morphology subjective. While most colonies of M. micros are smooth, a rough variant from periodontitis patients has also been described (142). The

colonies of P. anaerobius are usually somewhat larger (1 mm in diameter) and nonhemolytic, while the individual cells are smaller (0.5 to 0.6 μm in diameter) than those of F. magna. Very young cultures of P. anaerobius may have elongated cells in chains. The colonies of P. anaerobius may have a pungently sweet odor. S. asaccharolytica colonies are minute to 2 mm in diameter and may have a slightly yellow pigment on blood agar. The individual cells are 0.5 to 1.5 μm in diameter and are arranged in pairs, tetrads, or irregular clumps. Anaerococcus vaginalis, Anaerococcus lacrimalis, and Anaerococcus lactolyticus appear as short chains or in masses.

P. niger is rarely recovered from clinical specimens, although it is likely that this isolate has gone unnoticed within mixed anaerobic cultures from clinical specimens. On initial isolation, colonies are black to olive green. The pigment may not be visible to the naked eye but is evident under a dissecting microscope. It fades quickly upon exposure to oxygen. After subculture or in older cultures, the colony can take on a mustard yellow pigment. Colonies are convex and circular with a shiny, smooth appearance. They are weakly catalase positive. P. niger strains are indole, urease, and coagulase negative; nitrate is not reduced; and esculin and starch are not hydrolyzed. Hydrogen sulfide (in sulfide-indole-motility medium) and ammonia are produced. The only definitive means of differentiating Peptococcus from other anaerobic gram-positive cocci is by analyzing G+C content ratios or by genetic sequencing. This is obviously not practical, and the Peptococcus must be presumptively identified on the basis of pigment production and the catalase reaction.

Procedures for Determination of Gram Stain Characteristics Using KOH Solubility, Antibiotic Sensitivity Disk Test, and LANA Test

KOH Solubility Test

The KOH solubility test procedure is used to aid in the determination of Gram stain reactions. Place 2 drops of a 3% KOH solution on a microscope slide. A 2-mm loopful of bacterial growth from an appropriate medium is stirred into the solution with a circular motion. The reaction is considered positive if increased viscosity or stringiness is observed within the first 30 s (suggesting a gram-positive organism).

Antibiotic Sensitivity

Antibiotic disks may be helpful in differentiating gram-positive and gram-negative organisms. Vancomycin (5 μg/disk), colistin (10 μg/disk), and erythromycin (60 μg/disk) (Oxoid Inc., Nepean, Ontario, Canada) are placed onto the surface of an inoculated blood agar plate and incubated for 24 to 48 h. Most gram-positive organisms are vancomycin and erythromycin susceptible (zone sizes, ≥10 mm) and colistin resistant. These results cannot be used for treatment decisions.

LANA Test

The LANA test uses LANA as a substrate for an aminopeptidase and may be useful in the differentiation of gram-positive and gram-negative isolates. The test is available commercially from Hardy Diagnostics, Santa Maria, Calif. (www.hardydiagnostics.com) as Lanagram. The test is relatively simple, as described by the manufacturer. One Lanagram tablet is placed in a small test tube with 2 or 3 drops of distilled or deionized water to which sufficient bacteria

TABLE 3 Differential characteristics of *Anaerococcus*, *Gallicola*, *Micromonas*, *Finegoldia*, *Schleiferella* (*Peptoniphilus*), *Peptostreptococcus*, and *Peptococcus* spp.[a]

Species (no. of strains examined)	Terminal VFA	Production of:				Carbohydrate fermentation reaction					Production of saccharolytic and proteolytic enzymes										
		Indole	Urease	ALP	ADH	Glucose	Lactose	Raffinose	Ribose	Mannose	αGAL	βGAL	αGLU	βGUR	ArgA	ProA	PheA	LeuA	PyrA	TyrA	HisA
F. magna (116)	A	−	−	d	d	−/w	−	−	−	−	−	−	−	−	+	+	+	+	+	−/w	−/w
M. micros (31)	A	−	−	+	−	−	−	−	−	−	−	−	−	−	+	+	+	+	+	+	+
S. heliotrinireducens (6)	A	−	−	−	+	−	−	−	−	−	−	−	−	−	d	+	+	+	−	w	w
P. productus (1)	A	−	−	−	−	+	+	+	d	d	+	−	+	−	−	−	−	−	−	−	−
G. barnesae	A (B)	w	−	−	−	+	−	−	−	−	−	−	−	−	−	−	−	−	−	−	−
S. asaccharolytica (52)	B	d	−	−	−	−	−	−	−	−	−	−	−	−	+	−	−	d	−	d	w
S. indolicus (6)	B	+	−	+	−	−	−	−	−	−	−	−	−	−	+	−	+	+	−	w	+
S. harei (13)	B	d	−	−	−	−	−	−	−	−	−	−	−	−	+	−	−	−/w	−	w	+
S. lacrimalis (1)	B	−	−	−	−	−	−	−	−	−	−	−	−	−	+	−	+	+	+	d	+
"trisimilis" group (4)[b]	B	+	−	d	−	+	w	−/w	−/w	+	−	d	−	−	−	−	−	−	−	−	−
A. hydrogenalis (14)	B	+	d	−/w	−	+	+	+	+	+	+	−	d	−	−	−	−	−	+	−	−
A. prevotii (type strain)	B	−	+	−	−	−	−	+	+	+	−	−	+	+	+	−	−	−	−	w	+
A. tetradius (type strain)	B	−	+	−	−	−	−	−	−	+	−	−	+	+	+	−	w	+	w	w	w
prevotii/tetradius group (34)	B	−	d	−	−	d	d	d	d	d	d	d	+	+	+	−	d	d	d	d	d
A. lactolyticus (1)	B	−	+	−	−	+	+	−	−	+	−	+	−	−	+	−	−	−	−	−	−
A. vaginalis (29)	B	d	−	−/w	+	+	−	−	−	d	−	−	−/w	−	+	−	−	+	−	−	+
"β-GAL" group (24)[b]	B	−	−	w	d	+	+	−	+	+	−	w/+	−/w	−	+	−	−	+	w	−	−
P. ivorii (4)	IV	−	−	−	−	−	−	−	−	−	−	−	−	−	+	+	−	−	−	−	−
P. anaerobius (63)	IC (IV)	−	−	−	−	+	−	−	−	w	−	+	−	−	−	+	−	−	−	−	−
A. octavius (6)	C	−	−	−	−	+	−	−	+	+	−	−	−	−	−	+	−	−	w	−	−
P. niger (1)	C	−	−	−	−	−	−	−	−	−	−	−	−	−	−	−	−	−	−	−	−

[a] Data from references 5, 34, 57, 82, 95, and 135. Abbreviations and symbols: VFA, volatile fatty acids; A, acetate; B, butyrate; IV, isovalerate; IC, isocarborate; C, n-caproate; ALP, alkaline phosphatase; ADH, arginine dihydrolase; αGAL, α-galactosidase; βGAL and βGAL, β-galactosidase; αGLU, α-glucosidase; βGUR, β-glucoronidase; ArgA, arginine arylamidase (AMD); PheA, phenylalanine AMD; LeuA, leucine AMD; PyrA, pyroglutamyl AMD; HisA, histidine AMD; −, >90% negative; w, weakly positive; +, >90% positive; d, different reactions.
[b] Undescribed strains that cluster in whole-cell composition as assessed by pyrolysis mass spectrometry.

TABLE 4 Biochemical characteristics of the anaerobic streptococci and *A. parvulum*[a]

Characteristic	*S. hansenii*	*S. pleomorphus*	*A. parvulum*
Aerotolerance	−	−	−
Acid from:			
Cellobiose	−	−	+
Fructose	−	+	+
Galactose	+	−	+
Inulin	−	NT	+
Lactose	+	−	+
Maltose	+	−	+
Mannose	−	d	+
Salicin	−	−	+
Sucrose	−	−	+
Raffinose	+	NT	−
Production of H_2S[b]	+	w	−
Esculin hydrolysis	d	NT	+

[a] Adapted from references 68 and 131 with permission of Williams & Wilkins, Baltimore, Md. Abbreviations and symbols: +, positive; −, negative; w, weak; d, differs among strains; NT, not tested. All species produced lactic acid from carbohydrate fermentation and fail to ferment mannitol, sorbitol, and starch.
[b] Determined in sulfide-indole-motility medium.

are added to result in a milky suspension (usually two to three well-isolated colonies), and the mixtures incubated at 35°C for 5 to 30 min. A positive reaction results in a yellow color, indicating that the isolate is gram negative. Recommended controls include *E. coli* ATCC 25922 (positive control) and *Bacillus subtilis* ATCC 6633 (negative control). False-negative reactions may occur if medium-derived dye is carried over, resulting in the masking of yellow pigment; therefore, a saline control should be included. Isolates with a yellow pigment may give a false-positive reaction, which is apparent immediately upon the addition of the bacteria, and for isolates with a yellow pigment a true-positive result would be observed as a deepening of the yellow color.

Antimicrobial Susceptibility

Most *Peptostreptococcus* isolates (96%) are susceptible to β-lactam antibiotics (Table 5). However, MICs as high as 64 μg/ml have been reported for ticarcillin and cefotaxime. Clindamycin and metronidazole are slightly less active: 84 and 88% of isolates, respectively, are susceptible. However, there is evidence of inducible macrolide-lincosamide resistance, with *S. asaccharolytica* being the most resistant to erythromycin (117). Some strains that are clindamycin susceptible and erythromycin resistant have inducible clindamycin resistance. While most quinolones have limited activities against *Peptostreptococcus* species, trovafloxacin was an exception (Table 5). Ciprofloxacin was less active (1).

Evaluation, Interpretation, and Reporting of Results

The significance of finding anaerobic gram-positive cocci in clinical specimens depends on the specimen and the likelihood that it was contaminated by the bacterial flora of the skin or mucous membranes. Hence, interpretation of the

TABLE 5 Antimicrobial susceptibilities of anaerobic gram-positive cocci and *P. niger*[a]

Antimicrobial agent	Breakpoint (mg/liter)	No. of strains tested	MIC (mg/liter) for anaerobic gram-positive cocci[b]			*P. niger*		
			50%	90%	Range	No. of strains tested	MIC_{50} (mg/liter)	MIC range (mg/liter)
Penicillin G	2	60	0.2	8	≤0.06–128	4	0.1	0.1–0.5
Ampicillin	2	98	2	32	≤0.06–128	4	0.1	≤0.06–2
Piperacillin	128	35	0.5	8	≤0.06–32	4	0.2	≤0.06–0.5
Mezlocillin	128	35	0.5	16	≤0.06–128	4	0.2	0.2–1
Cefuroxime	16	35	0.5	16	≤0.06–≥256	4	0.2	≤0.06–1
Cefpodoxime	ND	63	1	32	≤0.12–264	0	ND	ND
Cefixime	ND	63	8	≥64	0.5–≥64	0	ND	ND
Cefoxitin	64	123	1	8	≤0.06–64	4	0.5	0.2–4
Cefoperazone	64	60	0.5	4	≤0.06–64	4	0.2	≤0.06–8
Cefotaxime	64	35	2	8	≤0.06–16	4	1	≤0.06–2
Imipenem	16	60	1	16	≤0.06–≥256	4	1	0.5–8
Clindamycin	4	88	2	16	≤0.06–128	0	ND	ND
Erythromycin	4	33	4	>32	0.03–>32			
Lincomycin	4	35	4	≥256	≤0.06–≥256	4	8	0.5–32
Ofloxacin	4	83	2	16	≤0.06–≥32	0	ND	ND
Norfloxacin	4	39	4	32	≤0.06–128	4	1	0.5–8
Ciprofloxacin	4	139	2	4	≤0.06–32	0	ND	ND
Trovafloxacin	8	14	0.06	0.5	0.015–0.5	NA	NA	NA
Tinidazole	32	35	2	32	≤0.06–≥256	4	1	1–16
Metronidazole	32	147	2	64	≤0.06–≥256	4	1	0.5–8
Tetracycline	16	35	2	16	≤0.06–32	4	1	0.2–8
Doxycycline		63	4	16	≤0.06–32	0	NA	NA

[a] Includes data compiled from references 1, 47, 48, 85, 111, 149, and 150. Abbreviations: 50% (MIC_{50}) and 90%, MICs at which 50 and 90% of strains, respectively, are inhibited. NA, not applicable; ND, no data available.
[b] Includes *P. anaerobius*, *S. asaccharolytica*, and *M. micros*.

culture result is dependent on the nature and quality of the specimen submitted to the laboratory. When anaerobic cocci are the only isolates in a clinical specimen, one should still keep in mind that they most often occur in mixed infections. This might have implications in selecting an appropriate antimicrobial therapy.

ANAEROBIC NON-SPORE-FORMING GRAM-POSITIVE RODS

Description of the Genera
Members of the anaerobic non-spore-forming gram-positive rods are gram-positive asporogenous rods, obligately anaerobic or facultatively anaerobic, motile or nonmotile, chemoorganotrophic, and saccharolytic or asaccharolytic.

Taxonomy
The group of anaerobic non-spore-forming gram-positive rods has undergone significant taxonomic changes over the past several years (Table 6) and now includes the traditional genera *Propionibacterium*, *Eubacterium*, *Bifidobacterium*, *Lactobacillus*, *Actinomyces*, and *Mobiluncus*, as well as, as of recently, *Bulleidia* (31), *Collinsella* (70), *Eggerthella* (72), *Mogibacterium* (98), *Atopobium* (26), *Catenibacterium* (69), *Cryptobacterium* (97), *Slackia* (147), *Actinobaculum* (80), and *Holdemania* (152). *Arcanobacterium* and *Actinobaculum* represent genera whose members have traditionally been included in this group of microorganisms, and

indeed, studies show a very close relationship and intermixing among these bacteria; however, *Arcanobacterium* is discussed in detail in chapter 34 with the corynebacteria. These genera are taxonomically quite diverse but share many phenotypic characteristics. Since in the past bacterial taxonomy has relied heavily on descriptive aspects of these organisms, which resulted in the grouping of genera into families that were probably not appropriate genetically, numerous additional revisions are to be expected.

Several species of *Actinomyces* beyond those listed in the previous edition of this Manual have been described more recently: *Actinomyces bowdenii* (108), *A. radicidentis* (24), *A. urogenitalis* (101), *A. canis* (60), *A. catuli* (61), and *A. funkei* (81). Studies of 16S rRNA sequences have delineated many of these new genera and species, resulting in several taxonomic changes. The former *A. pyogenes* and *A. bernardiae* have been transferred to the genus *Arcanobacterium* as *Arcanobacterium pyogenes* and *Arcanobacterium bernardiae*, respectively (42, 107). The former *A. humiferus* is now *Cellulomonas humilata* (25), and *A. suis* has been reclassified as *Actinobaculum suis*, a genus that also includes *A. schaalii* (80). Studies of 16S rRNA sequence data for *Actinomyces*, *Mobiluncus*, *Rothia*, and *Arcanobacterium* indicate that these genera are phylogenetically intermixed with *Actinomyces* species and that the genus *Actinomyces* clearly represents at least several different distinct genera (78, 79, 80, 107, 124, 125); see chapters 34 and 35 for a complete discussion of the actinomycetes that grow aerobically.

TABLE 6 Taxonomic revisions within the anaerobic gram-positive rods

Current nomenclature	Newly described	Basonym or synonym
Actinobaculum schaalii	Yes	
Actinobaculum suis		*Actinomyces suis*
Arcanobacterium bernardiae		*Actinomyces bernardiae*
Actinomyces bowdenii	Yes	
Actinomyces canis	Yes	
Actinomyces catuli	Yes	
Actinomyces funkei	Yes	
Cellulomonas humilata		*Actinomyces humiferus*
Actinomyces pyogenes		*Arcanobacterium pyogenes*
Actinomyces radicidentis	Yes	
Actinomyces urogenitalis	Yes	
Atopobium minutum		*Lactobacillus minutum*
Atopobium parvulum		*Streptococcus parvulum*
Atopobium rimae		*Lactobacillus rimae*, *Lactobacillus* D02
Atopobium vaginae	Yes	
Bulleidia extructa	Yes	
Catenibacterium mitsuokai	Yes	
Collinsella intestinalis	Yes	
Collinsella stercoris	Yes	
Cryptobacterium curtum	Yes	
Collinsella aerofaciens		*Eubacterium aerofaciens*
Slackia exigua		*Eubacterium exiguum* (*Eubacterium* D-6 group)
Atopobium fossor		*Eubacterium fossor*
Eggerthella lenta		*Eubacterium lentum*
Eggerthella minutum		*Eubacterium tardum*
Mogibacterium timidum		*Eubacterium timidum*
Fusobacterium sulci		*Eubacterium sulci*
Holdemania filiformis	Yes	
Lactobacillus uli	Yes	
Mogibacterium pumilum	Yes	
Mogibacterium vescum	Yes	

Addenda to the *Lactobacillus* species include *Lactobacillus uli* (103). At least 34 *Lactobacillus* species are currently recognized and at least 19 other distinct groups of unnamed species are known, but only a few are encountered in the clinical laboratory.

While recovery of these anaerobic rods from vaginal specimens had been reported earlier, this group of microorganisms was not recognized formally and was not given the name *Mobiluncus* until 1984 (133). The genus *Mobiluncus* is composed of obligately anaerobic, gram-variable or gram-negative, curved, non-spore-forming rods with tapered ends. The rods occur singly or in pairs and may have a gull-wing appearance. They are motile by multiple subpolar flagella. Even though single organisms stain gram negative to gram variable, they possess a multilayered gram-positive type of cell wall lacking the lipopolysaccharide 2-keto-3-deoxyoctulonic acid and hydroxylated fatty acids typically found in the cell walls of gram-negative organisms (20). These organisms are susceptible to vancomycin and resistant to colistin, which is consistent with the susceptibility patterns of other gram-positive organisms (38). 16S rRNA sequencing has demonstrated that the genus *Mobiluncus* is closely related to the genus *Actinomyces* (79).

Historically, the genus *Eubacterium* has been a repository for species of anaerobic gram-positive bacteria whose taxonomic position was not well understood. *Eubacterium aerofaciens* has been transferred to the genus *Collinsella* as *Collinsella aerofaciens* (71). Two distinct groups of *Eubacterium* species are known; those which utilize carbohydrates are better understood, while those which fail to attack sugar have been more problematic. Microorganisms within the latter group, which are generally unreactive in conventional phenotypic tests, had been grouped together in the genus *Eubacterium*. Several new genera have been described to accommodate these isolates. *Eubacterium lentum* is now in the genus *Eggerthella* as *Eggerthella lenta* (72). Other new genera are *Catenibacterium* (69), *Bulleidia* (31), *Mogibacterium* (98), and *Holdemania* (152). *Eubacterium exiguum* (formerly *Eubacterium* group D6 [112]) has been reclassified as *Slackia exigua* (147), and *Eubacterium timidum* has been changed to *Mogibacterium timidum* (98). *Eggerthella minutum* and *Eubacterium tardum* are synonymous, and *E. minutum* has priority (146). New combinations may seem remarkable to the practicing clinical microbiologist. For example, 16S rRNA studies have demonstrated that *Fusobacterium sulci* is most closely related to *Eubacterium* and has resulted in the new combination of *Eubacterium sulci* (65). However, this organism is phenotypically most like a *Fusobacterium*. Many workers believe there are still many undescribed taxa among the *Eubacterium* spp. (69, 71, 97, 152). A brief description of these newly described genera is given below.

Cryptobacterium

The *Eubacterium*-like genus *Cryptobacterium* consists of one species, and the description is based on two isolates from human periodontal pockets (97). The sole species of this genus, *Cryptobacterium curtum*, is inert in most conventional biochemical tests and is therefore phenotypically similar to the *Eubacterium* group; however, genetic studies suggest that the genus represents a distinct lineage from *Eubacterium* (97). These organisms are strictly anaerobic, very short gram-positive rods that are nonmotile and non-spore forming. Other characteristics are given in Tables 7, 8, and 9.

Mogibacterium

The organisms in the genus *Mogibacterium* are strictly anaerobic, short gram-positive rods that are nonmotile and non-spore forming and that grow poorly in broth media. A distinguishing characteristic is the production of phenyl acetate as the sole metabolic product in peptone-yeast extract-glucose medium. For other characteristics, see Table 7. The three species of this genus are M. *pumilum*, M. *vesicum*, and M. *timidum* (formerly *E. timidum*), which can be differentiated only by DNA relatedness studies and 16S rRNA sequencing. They have been isolated from human periodontal infections (98).

Bulleidia

The species in the genus *Bulleidia*, *B. extructa*, is a strictly anaerobic, short gram-positive rod that is nonmotile and non-spore forming and that grows poorly in broth media but that is stimulated by the addition of 0.5% Tween 80 along with a fermentable carbohydrate, glucose, or maltose (31). *B. extructa* does not produce H_2S or hydrolyze esculin but does hydrolyze arginine. The sole species can be differentiated from *Erysipelothrix rhusiopathiae* (which grows in air and in 20% bile and which produces H_2S) and *Holdemania*, which hydrolyzes esculin but not arginine (152). *B. extructa* has been isolated from human periodontal pockets and dentoalveolar infections.

Collinsella

The genus *Collinsella*, which consists of three species (Table 9), was created to accommodate species which had previously been classified as *Eubacterium*. The most important species is *C. aerofaciens*, which is one of the dominant species in human feces (70, 71, 93).

Atopobium

The genus *Atopobium* was proposed to accommodate several species from the genera *Lactobacillus* and *Streptococcus* (*Lactobacillus minutus*, *Lactobacillus rimae*, and *S. parvulus*) and the recently described species *Atopobium vaginae* (26, 68). Phylogenetically they are associated with the actinomycete branch of the gram-positive rod-shaped organisms and may often be confused phenotypically with lactic acid bacteria (68). They have been isolated from a wide range of human infections and from healthy individuals.

Slackia

The genus *slackia* was proposed to accommodate species with low G+C contents, formerly *Eubacterium exiguum* (earlier, the *Eubacterium* S group) and *Peptostreptococcus heliotrinireducens* (147). *Slackia* species resemble *Eggerthella lenta* (formerly *Eubacterium lentum*) in that they are generally unreactive in most biochemical tests. Phylogenetic studies indicate that the genus is most closely related to *Atopobium* and *Eggerthella* (147).

Eggerthella

The genus *Eggerthella* has resulted from the reclassification of one species, *Eubacterium lentum*, since genetically it shares few characteristics with the type strain of *Eubacterium* (147).

Holdemania

Holdemania filiformis is a *Eubacterium*-like organism which is a member of the *Clostridium* subphylum of the gram-posi-

TABLE 7 Differentiation of genera of anaerobic gram positive rods[a]

Genus	Primary characteristic	Fatty acid production[b]	Cell characteristics	Mol % G+C content[g]
Propionibacterium	Propionic acid major end product	A, P, (iv), (s), (1)[c]	Cells 0.5–0.8 by 1.5 µm, morphology; may vary considerably including diphtheroidal or club shaped with one end round and the other end tapered or coccoid, bifid, or branched	59–67 (T_m)
Mogibacterium	Phenylacetic acid	Traces of acetic, succinic, or lactic acid	Cells 0.2–0.3 by 1.0–1.5 µm, occurring singly as short chains or clumps; differentiation of species is by 16S rRNA sequence or DNA homology	45–46 (HPLC)
Mobiluncus	Major succinic and lactic acids with acetic acid	S, L, A	Curved rods, motile	49–52 (T_m)
Lactobacillus	Lactic acid primary or sole metabolic product	L, (s), (a)	Slender cells may be long or short, often with boxy ends; may appear slightly bent or as coryneform rods	35–53 (T_m)
Atopobium	Lactic acid primary or sole metabolic product	L	Cells elongated gram-positive cocci occurring in singles, pairs, or short chains	G+C, 44 (T_m)
Bifidobacterium	Major acetic acid greater than lactic acid	A, L[d]	Rods with or without one bifurcated end; ends may appear club-like	C, 57–64 (T_m)
Bulleidia	Acetic and lactic acids with a smaller amount of succinic	A, L, trace s	Rods occur 0.5 by 0.8–2.0 µm as singles or pairs aligned side by side	38 (HPLC)
Holdemania	Acetic and lactic acids with a smaller amount of succinic acid	A, L, (s)	Short to long rods in pairs and short chains; growth in prereduced anaerobically sterilized medium stimulated by 0.2% Tween 80	38 (HPLC)
Collinsella	Lactic, acetic, and fumaric acids with hydrogen gas	H_2, L, A, F, E abundant	Cells 0.3–0.4 by 1.3–2.0 µm occurring in chains of 2–20, producing abundant ethanol	60–65 (HPLC)
Eggerthella	Acetic, lactic, and succinic acids with hydrogen gas	H_2, a, l, s	Cells 0.2–4 by 0.2–2.0 µm	62 (T_m)
Eubacterium[h]	Major acetic, butyric, and fumaric acids	A, B, F[e]		30–40 (T_m)
Catenibacterium	Acetic, lactic, and butyric acids	A, L, B, iv	Cells 0.4–2.0 µm occurring in tangled chains	36–39 (HPLC)
Actinobaculum	Acetic acid solely or with traces of formic acid	A	Cells straight to slightly curved	50–57 (T_m)
Cryptobacterium	Acetic acid or no end products	None	Very short rods (0.4 by 0.8–1.0 µm) as singles or in masses	50–51 (HPLC)
Slackia	Acetic acid or no end products	A or none	Cells are short bacilli to cocci (0.5–1.0 µm) as singles or clumps; growth stimulated by the addition of 0.5% arginine	60–64 (HPLC)
Actinomyces	Succinic acid in the presence of CO_2 and lactic acid with small amounts of acetic and formic acids	S, L, a[f]	Straight or slightly curved rods 0.2–1.0 µm; considerable variation, with true branching with or without clubs; may occur as singles or pairs with diphtheroidal arrangement or may be pleomorphic	55–68 (T_m)

[a] Data compiled from references 29, 31, 57, 69, 72, 80, 92, 97, 124, 127, 131, 147, and 152.

[b] Volatile fatty acids; A, acetic acid; S, succinic acid; B, butyric acid; E, ethanol; F, formic acid; L, lactic acid; P, propionic acid; IV, isovaleric acid; parentheses indicate variable production or, if produced, usually present only in trace amounts; lowercase letters represent products usually produced in small amounts. Determined in peptone-yeast extract-glucose broth cultures.

[c] Under anaerobic conditions, *P. propionicum* ferments glucose to CO_2, acetic acid, propionic acid, and small amounts of lactic and succinic acids. In air, glucose is converted to CO_2 and acetic acid.

[d] Acetic and lactic acids are produced in a molar ratio of 3:2.

[e] Metabolic products formed by *Eubacterium* species vary (see Table 9).

[f] Production of succinic acid is stimulated by growth in enriched CO_2.

[g] Moles percent G+C content determinations were by melting point analysis (T_m) or high-pressure liquid chromatography (HPLC).

[h] See Tables 9 to 11.

TABLE 8 Characteristics of *Actinomyces* and *Actinobaculum* spp.[a]

Characteristic	A. suis	A. schaalii	A. bowdenii	A. canis	A. catuli	A. denticolens	A. europaeus	A. funkei	A. georgiae	A. gerencseriae	A. graevenitzii	A. howellii
Catalase		−	+	+	d	−	−	−	−	−	−	+
Nitrate reduction	−	−	+	−	+	+	−	+	−	−	−	−
Gelatin hydrolysis	−	−	−	−	−				d	−	−	−
H₂S production		−							d			
Esculin hydrolysis		−	+	−	+	+	d	−	+	+	−	−
Pink pigment on blood agar							−	−	−	−	+	
CAMP reaction		w					−	+	−	−	−	
Method[b]		+	+	+	+		+			+	+	+
Isolated from animals	+		+	+		+						+
Fatty acids[c]		A, S					S			L, S, f	L, S	
Urease	+	−	−				−	−	−	−	−	−
Acid from:												
Esculin	−	−		−			−		−		−	
Glucose	−	+	+	+	+		+		+	+	+	
Glycerol						d			d	−		
Glycogen		−		+	−		d		+	−		
Mannitol		−	−	−		d	−	−	−	+[e]	−	
meso-Inositol						+		−	d	−		
Raffinose	−			v		+	−	−	−	+	−	
Sucrose	−	d	+	d	+		d		+	+	+	
Trehalose	+	v	+	−		−		−	+	+	d	
Xylose	+	−	−	+	−	−	−	+	+	+	−	
Beta-hemolysis on sheep blood agar			−		−		d		−	d		
Mol % G+C DNA content[d]	55 (T_m)	57 (HPLC)				66–68 (HPLC)	61–63 (HPLC)		65–69 (T_m)	70–71 (T_m)	62 (Unk)	

[a] Adapted from references 27, 29, 41, 43, 60, 61, 66, 80, 81, 89, 106, 124, 129, 131, and 157. Abbreviations and symbols for biochemical reactions: +, most strains positive; −, most strains negative; d, variable results reported; −/w, most isolates are negative or a weak reaction is observed; +/w, most strains are positive or a weak reaction is observed.

[b] Positivity for sugar utilization and enzyme activities were obtained with the following API bioMerieux rapid systems: API ZYM, API Coryne, API50CH, Rapid ID32A, and Rapid ID32 Strep.

tive bacteria and is phylogenetically associated with *Erysipelothrix* (152).

Catenibacterium

Catenibacterium is another *Eubacterium*-like genus that is taxonomically a member of the *Clostridium* subphylum of the gram-positive bacteria and is phylogenetically associated with *Lactobacillus catenaformis* and *Lactobacillus vitulinus* (69). The six strains evaluated for the original report were all isolated from the feces of highlanders in Papua New Guinea.

Actinobaculum

The recently described genus *Actinobaculum* includes the reclassified species *Actinomyces suis* as *Actinobaculum suis* and a new human-derived species, *Actinobaculum schaalii* (80).

Natural Habitat

The natural habitats of *Actinomyces* and *Atopobium* spp. appear to be the mucosal surfaces of humans and animals. The *Actinomyces* spp. *A. bovis*, *A. bowdenii*, *A. denticolens*, *A. howellii*, *A. hordeovulneris*, *A. hyovaginalis*, *A. slackii*, *A. catuli*, and *A. suis* have not been isolated from humans.

Many of the more recently described taxa have been isolated from the oral cavities of humans, infected periodontal pockets, and dentoalveolar infections (*Bulleidia*, *Mogibacterium*, *Cryptobacterium*) or from feces (*Collinsella*, *Catenibacterium*, *Holdemania*). *Eubacterium* species have been isolated from humans, animals, and various sources in nature.

Bifidobacterium species are found in the intestines of humans and animals and in sewage. *Eubacterium* species are also found in the intestines and in the oral cavities (periodontia) of humans and other animals and in various plant products.

Propionibacterium species can be isolated from skin and the moist epithelium of the conjunctiva, oral cavity, and large intestine.

Although most isolates of *Lactobacillus* species are facultative anaerobes, approximately 20% of the human isolates are obligately anaerobic. *Lactobacillus* species are found in the mouth (in both saliva and plaque), the intestinal tract, the vaginas of humans and other mammals, and a variety of food products.

The natural habitat of *Mobiluncus* spp. is the reproductive tract and rectum of humans and other primates. *Mobiluncus* species have been found in 50 to 65% of vaginal specimens from women with bacterial vaginosis (59). How-

A. hyovaginalis	*A. israelii*	*A. meyeri*	*A. naeslundii* I	*A. naeslundii* II	*A. neuii* subsp. *anitratus*	*A. neuii* subsp. *neuii*	*A. viscosus*	*A. odontolyticus*	*A. radicidentis*	*A. radingae*	*A. turicensis*	*A. urogenitalis*	*P. propionicum*
−	−	−	−/d	+/d	+	+	+	−	+	−	−	−	−
+	d	−	d	+	−	+	+	+	d	−	−	+	+
−	−	−	−	−	−	−	−	−	w	−	−	−	d
	+	−	+	+	−	−	+	+					d
+	+	−	+	+	+	−	+	d	w/+	+	−	+	−
	−	−	−	−	−	−	−	+	+	−	−	+	−
	−	+	−	+	+	+	−	−	−	+	−	−	
+										+	+	+	+
+													
−	−	d	+	+	−	−	+	−	d	−			
	−	−	+	+	−	−	−	d	d				
	+	+	+	+	+	+	+	+	+	+	+		
	−	d	d		+	+	−	d			+		d
	−	d	−	d	d	d	−	d		−	−	−	
	+	−	−	+	−	−	−	−	+	d	−	d	d
d	+	−	+	+	−	−	−	−		d	+		d
−	+	−	+	+	+	+	−	−		d	−	+	+
	+	+	+	+	+	+	+	+	+	+	+	+	
−	+	−	+	+	+	+	−	−	+	d	−	+	+
+	+	+	d	+	+	+	d	d	−	+	+	+	+
−	−	−	−			−	−		−/w	−/w		+
63 (Unk)	57–67 (T_m)	64–67 (T_m)	66 (T_m)	66 (T_m)	55 (T_m)	55 (T_m)	62–68 (T_m)	62 (T_m)		60 (HPLC)	58 (HPLC)	61 (T_m)	63–65 (T_m)

[c] Volatile fatty acids; A, acetic acid; S, succinic acid; F, formic; L, lactic acid; lowercase letters represent products usually produced in small amounts. Determined in peptone-yeast extract-glucose broth cultures.

[d] Mole percent G+C content determinations were by melting point analysis (T_m) or high-pressure liquid chromatography (HPLC); Unk, method used for determination unknown.

[e] The type strain was positive, while six of six field isolates were negative (123).

ever, they are recovered from fewer than 10% of specimens from women with normal, *Lactobacillus*-predominant flora. They may be recovered together with other bacteria associated with bacterial vaginosis from the vaginas of children with no history of sexual abuse. *Mobiluncus* spp. have been cultured from rectal swabs from women with bacterial vaginosis and from rectal and urethral specimens from the male sex partners of women with bacterial vaginosis.

Clinical Significance

Information on the occurrence of anaerobic gram-positive rods in clinical materials is difficult to obtain. Both methodologic and taxonomic problems contribute to our inability to obtain such data. However, results from individual laboratories specializing in anaerobes indicate that the prevalence of these anaerobes in various infections is much greater than is reflected by their isolation frequencies in many other clinical laboratories. For example, Finegold (39) determined that *Actinomyces* spp. were isolated in his laboratory from 14% of the infections involving anaerobes, while other workers reported a much lower incidence.

Actinomycosis is the most frequently encountered disease entity involving *Actinomyces* spp. The incidence of actinomycosis in the United States is difficult to determine, since this disease is not reportable. While there are few recent reports on this subject, Slack and Gerencser (129) concluded that "actinomycosis occurs throughout the world and is neither a rare nor a common disease." Actinomycosis is observed twice as frequently in men as in women, and the anatomical distribution is about 60% cervicofacial, 15% thoracic, 20% abdominal, and 5% other types. Clinically, actinomycosis other than the cervicofacial type is often misdiagnosed as a malignant tumor (136).

Actinomycosis is characterized as a chronic granulomatous lesion that becomes suppurative and that forms abscesses and draining sinuses (118). A purulent actinomycotic discharge, usually containing macroscopic sulfur granules that appear as whitish, yellow, or brown granular bodies, may be present. *Actinomyces israelii* is the most common cause of actinomycosis in humans, but some of the other *Actinomyces* spp. (i.e., *A. naeslundii*, *A. meyeri*, *A. odontolyticus*, *A. gerencseriae*, and *A. viscosus*), as well as *Propionibacterium propionicum*, may also be etiologic agents. These infections are usually polymicrobic. Frequently, *Fusobacterium* spp., *Eikenella corrodens*, *Capnocytophaga* spp., *Actinobacillus actinomycetemcomitans*, black-pigmented *Prevotella* spp., *Porphyromonas asaccharolytica*, *Porphyromonas gingivalis*, and streptococci are also found in various com-

TABLE 9 Characteristics of nonsaccharolytic species of *Eubacterium*[a]

Species	Cellular characteristics	Colony morphology	Fatty acid production[b]	Utilization of pyruvate	Nitrate reduction	Gelatin hydrolysis	Esculin hydrolysis	Hydrogen production
E. brachy	Short or coccoidal, chaining, 0.4–0.8 by 0.1–3.0 μm in PY[c]	Circular, entire, low convex, occasionally rough	ib, iv, ic, (a), (f), (l), (s), (hc)	−, +	−	−	−	+
E. combesii	Singles, pairs, short chains, and palisade arrangements; motile; 0.6–0.8 by 3.0–10 μm in PYG[d]	Circular, entire to irregular convex, semiopaque, whitish yellow, shiny, smooth	A, B, iv, l, ib, (p), (f)	+		+	d	+
E. infirmum	Short rods (0.5 by 2.0 μm); cells occur as singles	Colonies are approximately 1 mm, circular, convex, and translucent	a, B					
E. minutum	Short rods (0.5 by 1.0–1.5 μm), in singles, pairs, and clumps	Colonies on brain heart infusion-blood agar are 0.3 by 0.5 mm, circular, convex, entire, translucent	B or b	−	−	−	−	
E. nodatum	Branched, filamentous, or club-shaped cells; nonmotile; 0.5–0.9 by 2.0–12 μm in PY	Molar tooth, heaped, or raspberry; 0.5–1.0 mm in diameter	(a), (s)	+	−	−	−	−
E. saphenum[e]	Short rods	After 7 days, colonies are 0.3 by 0.5 mm, circular, convex, and translucent	a, b	−	−	−	−	
E. yurii	Straight rods with slightly rounded edges, form unique three-dimensional brushlike aggregates	Colonies spread on blood agar, measuring about 10 mm in 48 h; pale yellow pigment may be evident	B, A, p			−	−	

[a] Data compiled from references 23, 53, 58, 113, and 141. Abbreviations and symbols for biochemical reactions: +, most strains positive; −, most strains negative; w, reaction weak; d, reaction variable.

[b] ic, isocaproate; iv, isovalerate; ib, isobutyrate; a, acetate; b, butyrate; l, lactate; s, succinate; f, formate; p, propionate; v, valerate; paa, phenylacetate; hc, hydrocinnamate. Capital letters represent 1 meq of product per 100 ml of culture; lowercase letters represent <1 meq of product per 100 ml of culture; products in parentheses are not produced uniformly.

[c] PY, peptone-yeast extract.

[d] PYG, peptone-yeast extract-glucose.

[e] Resembles *E. nodatum* except for a lack of production of ammonia from arginine.

binations. It is believed that these associated microorganisms contribute significantly to the pathogenesis of actinomycosis (129, 130). *Actinobaculum schaalii* was isolated from a human blood culture (80).

The *Actinomyces* species *A. israelii*, *A. naeslundii*, *A. viscosus*, *A. odontolyticus*, *A. meyeri*, *A. turicensis*, *A. radingae*, and *A. neuii* are causative agents in various diseases in humans and must be considered opportunistic pathogens (126). All except *A. neuii*, *A. turicensis*, *A. radicidentis*, and *A. meyeri* are found in large numbers in saliva and subgingival plaques. *A. israelii*, *A. gerencseriae*, *A. odontolyticus*, *A.*

georgiae, and *A. naeslundii* have been studied extensively and are believed to play significant roles in dental caries and periodontal disease (9). *Actinomyces* species may also be involved in pelvic inflammatory disease associated with intrauterine contraceptive devices (40, 138, 158) and pyogenic liver abscess (90). Evans (33) estimated that between 1.6 and 11.6% of intrauterine device users have *A. israelii* infection.

In a 7-year study of 294 *Actinomyces*-like isolates which were not easily identifiable, DNA probes were used to identify three recently described species (*A. radingae*, *A.*

turicensis, and A. europaeus) (121). Of these, 128 isolates belonged to the three species. In a small number of cases, one of these Actinomyces species was the sole isolate. About 90% were A. turicensis, while only 3 and 6% were A. radingae and A. europaeus, respectively. A. radingae occurred in skin-related infections, and A. europaeus occurred in urinary tract infections. Similar results were also reported by G. Funke (personal communication cited in reference 121). More isolates came from women than from men, and most (the only exception being A. turicensis) were obtained from genital tract infections (143). In laboratories which can recognize A. neuii, A. radingae, and A. turicensis, they are among the most common Actinomyces isolates (44). It should also be noted that A. neuii infections do not usually present as typical Actinomyces infections, that is, with discharge of sulfur granules (44).

Propionibacteria have been recovered from mixed infections of the skin (16, 135). The role of Propionibacterium acnes in acne vulgaris is widely accepted (18). Induction of proinflammatory cytokines (144) with or without specific cell-mediated immunity (74) by Propionibacterium antigens may play a role in the pathogenesis. Often, propionibacterial infections have been linked to surgical procedures or foreign bodies (64). Propionibacterium acnes is the predominant member of the anaerobic flora from conjunctival cultures of adults and children and has been reported to cause uveitis and endophthalmitis (64). P. acnes, Propionibacterium aridium, and Propionibacterium granulosum are also pathogenic in infections of bone, joints, and the central nervous system (64) and may cause endocarditis, especially after prosthetic valve implantation (49). P. acnes has also been associated with the SAPHO syndrome (synovitis, acne pustulosis, hyperostosis, and osteomyelitis) (77). Thus, although Propionibacterium species often originate from the normal flora, they can act as primary pathogens and should not be immediately dismissed as contaminants. However, in a recent study, recovery of Propionibacterium species from the blood accounted for only 5% of clinically significant bacteremias and 50% of clinically insignificant bacteremias, suggesting that this group of microorganisms is a more frequent cause of insignificant anaerobic bacteremias (122). Finally, the ability of Propionibacterium spp. to modulate the immune response to unrelated antigens has been well documented (114, 120).

Propionibacterium propionicum is a recognized agent of lacrimal canaliculitis and produces abscesses in animals when injected (10).

Eubacterium species and Eubacterium-like organisms are not frequently reported from clinical specimens, probably because of the difficulty in recognizing them. Eubacterium species are usually isolated in mixed culture from abscesses and wounds and very rarely from blood cultures. E. lentum is the species most frequently observed. Several species have been associated with periodontal disease: Eubacterium nodatum, M. timidum, Eubacterium brachy, and Slackia (91, 92, 145). A study by Hill et al. (53) suggests that these species are involved in numerous infections at other sites such as the head and neck, thorax, bones, skin, and pelvis.

We do not have sufficient information to understand the role of many of the newly described genera and species in various disease processes. Catenibacterium and Holdemania have been isolated from feces and not from infected sites. A number of species (Mogibacterium, Bulleidia, and Cryptobacterium) have been isolated from infected periodontal pockets, but their role in periodontal disease is not defined. Atopobium species (A. rimae, A. parvulum, and A. minu-

tum) occur in periodontally diseased sites and dental and pelvic abscesses (26).

Bifidobacterium species are infrequently encountered in clinical materials. Bifidobacterium dentium (formerly Actinomyces eriksonii and later Bifidobacterium eriksonii) appears to be the only Bifidobacterium species with pathogenic potential. It has been isolated from dental caries (91) and from various clinical materials such as genital and lower respiratory tract specimens (16). Bifidobacterium longum and Bifidobacterium breve are found only rarely in human clinical materials. Recent reports claim that administration of B. breve to preterm infants improved weight gain and reduced abnormal abdominal signs (75).

Most Lactobacillus species recovered from clinical specimens are microaerophilic, but obligately anaerobic isolates can also be recovered. They are rarely pathogenic and might even be beneficial in the treatment of bacterial vaginosis (105) and diarrhea (104, 116, 156). However, lactobacilli have been reported to cause endocarditis, neonatal meningitis, chorioamnionitis, pleuropulmonary infections, and bacteremia (3, 28, 30, 83). In addition, lactobacilli may play a role in dental caries (91, 119). Identification of anaerobic lactobacilli to the species level is extremely difficult and, given the low levels of pathogenicity of the organisms, is rarely indicated. The difficulty in identifying lactobacilli can lead to confusion about the probable source of some infections due to Lactobacillus species. For example, a case of peritonitis associated with a vancomycin-resistant Lactobacillus rhamnosus isolate in a continuous peritoneal dialysis patient was initially identified as being due to Lactobacillus acidophilus (76), although the latter species is susceptible to vancomycin (52). Superinfection due to Lactobacillus spp. may be possible only in an immunocompromised host, and identification of this organism to the species level is often inaccurate because of the poor reproducibilities of current commercial methods.

The pathogenic potential of Mobiluncus spp. is not well understood. It is unclear whether the rare isolation of Mobiluncus spp. from clinical specimens is due to the inability of many laboratories to isolate and identify this fastidious microorganism or to its low level of pathogenicity. While Mobiluncus spp. are present in the vaginas of many women with bacterial vaginosis, their role in the etiology of this syndrome is not known. However, bacterial vaginosis in pregnant women is associated with premature rupture of membranes and preterm birth (88). The pathogenic potential of Mobiluncus spp. has been supported by its isolation from breast abscesses, umbilical discharge, and blood cultures (46, 134). Mobiluncus spp. can also be recovered from the endometrial aspirates of women with pelvic inflammatory disease and from the chorioamnion of the placenta from preterm deliveries (54). While they have been recovered in pure cultures from some sterile-site specimens, they are most often found in association with other anaerobes (134).

Collection and Transport of Specimens

This group includes microorganisms that are anaerobic, aerotolerant, or facultatively anaerobic. Therefore, samples should be treated as anaerobic and handled as outlined above for anaerobic cocci (also see chapter 20).

Direct Examination

Direct microscopic examination of clinical materials is an excellent presumptive method for detection of anaerobic gram-positive rods and should be used whenever possible.

In pathology laboratories, specimens are sectioned, stained with Brown-Brenn stain, and examined for sulfur granules, which are considered diagnostic for actinomycosis (Fig. 1).

A variety of clinical samples are suitable for examination for the presence of sulfur granules: surgically removed tissues, tissues recovered at autopsy, bronchial washings, body fluids, purulent exudates, intrauterine devices, Papanicolaou smears, and gauze from draining wounds. Sulfur granules are irregular in shape and size (ranging from 0.1 to 5 mm), hard, and usually yellowish. They may be large enough to be seen with the unaided eye; granules from patients with oral actinomycosis sometimes resemble popcorn husks. If sulfur granules are observed, one granule should be removed with an inoculating needle, loop, or sterile forceps; placed in a drop of water on a microscope slide; and then gently crushed with a second slide. A wet mount should be examined under low power (×100). The granules have distinctly irregular edges. Upon reduction of the light intensity, the peripheries of the granules give the appearance of numerous club-shaped masses of filaments radiating from the granule, which is usually difficult to distinguish. The clubs should become very distinct at higher magnification (×1,000). They should be refractile, and their appearance has been described as hyaline. Having made these initial observations, one must confirm the presence of filaments. The coverslip is removed, and the specimen is dried, heat fixed, and Gram stained. Gram-positive branched and unbranched filaments should be easily discernible.

However, it is usually necessary to fix, section, and stain tissue specimens to demonstrate sulfur granules; therefore, these specimens should be referred to the pathology laboratory. Other organisms that may produce granules with clubs are *Nocardia*, *Streptomyces*, and *Staphylococcus* species (botryomycosis). The presence of *Staphylococcus* species can be ruled out by morphology and the Gram stain reaction. To distinguish *Actinomyces* from *Nocardia* isolates, granules should be stained for acid fastness with the modified acid-fast stain (see chapters 27 and 35) (129).

Routine culture of vaginal specimens for isolation of *Mobiluncus* spp. are costly and not clinically useful. The acceptable alternative is identification of curved rod morphotypes on Gram-stained vaginal smears (102).

Isolation Procedures

Clinicians should indicate clearly which specimens are to be cultured for the presence of non-spore-forming anaerobic gram-positive rods, particularly *Actinomyces* spp., since additional steps are required for proper setup and since the incubation period should be extended. Routinely used anaerobic plate media, anaerobic blood culture media, enriched thioglycolate medium, and chopped meat-glucose medium will support the growth of these microorganisms.

The usual procedures for anaerobes should be followed. Many of these organisms require a high moisture content for optimal growth, and so fresh medium should be used. Laboratories unable to prepare their own media may wish to consider the use of commercially prepared, prereduced, anaerobically sterilized blood agar, available from Anaerobe Systems. These media have an extended shelf life of up to 6 months and yield results comparable to those obtained with fresh media (86).

Sulfur granules, if present, should be placed in a sterile petri dish and rinsed with thioglycolate broth. They should then be transferred with a sterile Pasteur pipette to a sterile tube or preferably a Ten Broeck grinder (available from various sources) with approximately 0.5 ml of thioglycolate broth. The granules should be crushed with the tip of a sterile glass rod and immediately inoculated on anaerobic blood agar and phenylethylalcohol blood agar plates (1 drop of inoculum each). Plates should be streaked to achieve well-isolated colonies. Thioglycolate broth medium should be inoculated with 2 drops of inoculum near the bottom of the tube; the screw caps should be left loose to allow exchange of gases. Solid media should be incubated in an anaerobic jar or anaerobic chamber at 35 to 37°C. All cultures should be examined for growth after 48 h and then reincubated for 5 to 7 days. It may be necessary to hold the plates for as long as 2 to 4 weeks. Plate media incubated in anaerobic glove boxes should be protected from desiccation.

Actinomyces species may grow on many common bacteriological media; however, isolation from specimens rich in microflora may be particularly troublesome. Cultures of genital swabs or intrauterine devices may present a considerable problem, since the number of organisms may be quite large and many different species are present. Traynor et al. (138) described a method in which swabs are soaked in 5 ml of thioglycolate broth, samples are diluted 10-fold in the same medium (10^{-1} to 10^{-4} dilutions), and dilutions are plated on Columbia blood agar with and without 2.5 mg of metronidazole per liter (138). Although this method would not inhibit many organisms such as streptococci and lactobacilli, it appears to give results comparable to the visual results obtained by using fluorescent antibodies in a direct microscopic examination for actinomycetes (138). A selective medium for bifidobacteria has been described (4).

Identification Procedures

Traditionally, inclusion in a group of microorganisms was based primarily on morphologic and biochemical criteria. Although considerable progress has been made in understanding the taxonomy of anaerobic non-spore-forming gram-positive rods, reliable, accessible, and consistent tests for identification of many of these species are still not available. At least part of the problem stems from the difficulty in obtaining a uniform inoculum. Identification is

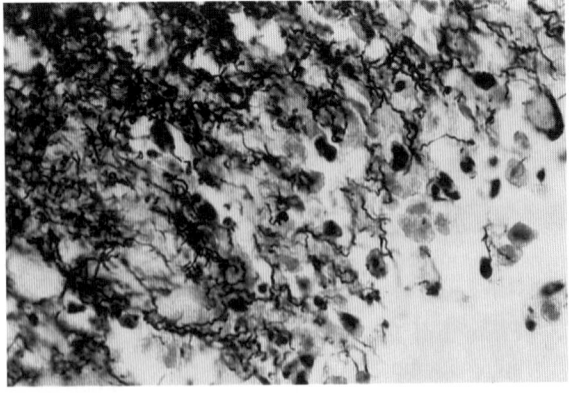

FIGURE 1 Microscopic morphology of *Actinomyces* species in a sulfur granule taken from an oral soft tissue section stained with the Brown-Brenn modification of the Gram stain. Note the characteristic appearance of the club-shaped filaments and the numerous polymorphonuclear leukocytes. Magnification, ×100. (Courtesy of Dolphine Oda, Department of Oral Biology, University of Washington, Seattle.)

TABLE 10 Characteristics of *Eubacterium*-like organisms[a]

Characteristic	*Eggerthella lentum*	*Collinsella aerofaciens*	*Collinsella stercoris*	*Collinsella intestinalis*	*Slackia exigua*	*Slackia heliotrinireducens*	*Catenibacterium mitsuokai*	*Holdemania filiformis*	*Bulleidia extructa*	*Cryptobacterium curtum*
Mol % G+C content[b]	61 (T_m)				60–64 (HPLC)	61 (HPLC)	36–39 (HPLC)	38 (HPLC)	38 (Unk)	50–51 (Unk)
Metabolic products[c]	a, l, s	A, f, l, trace s			None	a	A, L, B, l	a, l, trace s	a, l, (ts)	None
H_2 production	–[d]	+						w		–
Catalase	–				–	–	–	–	–	–
Gelatin hydrolysis	–	–			–		–			–
Esculin hydrolysis	–	+, –			–	–	–	+	–	–
Nitrate reduction	+				–	–	–	–	–	–
Starch hydrolysis		–					+			–
Ammonia from arginine					+	+		–		+
Arginine hydrolysis					+	+		–	+	+
Acid production from:										
Esculin		d	–	–	–					–
Cellobiose		d	+	+	–		+			–
Glucose		–, +	+	+	–			+		
Lactose		+	+	–	–	–	+	w		–
Maltose		+	+	–	–	–	+	w	+	
Raffinose		d	–	–			–	–		
Rhamnose		d	–	+	–		–	–		
Ribose		d	–	–						
Sucrose		d	d	–	–	–	+	+		
Trehalose		d	–	–			–	–		
Xylose	–	–	+	+				–	+	
N-Acetyl-glucosaminidase		–	+	+						–
β-Galactosidase		d	+	–						–
Rapid ID 32A code	2000 0000 00				2000 0337 00	2000 0237 05		0500 0041 20	2000 0120 00	

[a] Data compiled from references 31, 53, 57, 69, 70, 92, 97, 112, and 147. Abbreviations and symbols for biochemical reactions: +, most strains positive; –, most strains negative; d, variable results reported; –/w, most isolates are negative or a weak reaction is observed; +/w, most isolates are positive or a weak reaction is observed.

[b] Mole percent G+C content determinations were by melting point analysis (T_m) or high-pressure liquid chromatography (HPLC); Unk, method used for determination unknown.

[c] Volatile fatty acids; A, acetic acid; S, succinic acid; B, butyric acid; E, ethanol; F, formic; L, lactic acid; P, propionic acid; IV, isovaleric acid; parentheses indicate variable production or, if produced, usually present only in trace amounts; lowercase letters represent products usually produced in small amounts. Determined in peptone-yeast extract-glucose broth cultures.

[d] Hydrogen gas production, as determined in reference 57.

further complicated by the fact that the techniques used in the more recent descriptions of species, which use commercial systems such as API rapid test systems, are different from the techniques described in the older literature, in which characteristics were determined by using growth characteristics, gas-liquid chromatographic analysis of metabolic products, and the mole percent G+C content of the organism's DNA. The mole percent G+C contents for this group of organisms range from 30 to 55%, demonstrating that this is a heterogeneous group. This is supported by the fact that the metabolic end products fall into four groups: (i) butyric acid plus other short-chain fatty acids and alcohols (*Eubacterium*, *Catenibacterium*); (ii) a combination of lactic, acetic, succinic, and formic acids with or without H_2 (*Actinomyces*, *Eggerthella*, *Collinsella*, *Holdemania*); (iii) a single (acetic) or no detectable acids (*Cryptobacterium*, *Actinobaculum*, *Slackia*); and (iv) phenylacetic acid with traces of acetic, succinic, or lactic acid (*Mogibacterium*). Although analysis of cellular fatty acids is used for identification in other areas of clinical microbiology, a database of a useful size for this group of microorganisms that would make the technique useful is not yet available. The use of DNA probe technologies is of considerable utility in clearly identifying, categorizing, and determining the species of new isolates, but the use of such technologies is not practical in the clinical microbiology setting. However, our knowledge and expertise in using DNA probes are rapidly expanding and should eventually allow the use of such technologies.

Colony and cell morphologies are a means of presumptively separating anaerobic gram-positive rods into genera; however, these characteristics can be both variable and diverse. For example, *Actinomyces* species on blood agar yield numerous colony types, ranging from smooth to molar tooth-like. Moreover, the colony appearances and micromorphologies of *Actinomyces* and *Propionibacterium* species may vary with different culture media and the ages and conditions of the culture. (Excellent photographs and drawings may be found in references 57, 127, and 131.) Some species of *Actinomyces* may appear coccoid, and *Eubacterium sulci* stains gram negative (65). It has been reported that a reliable Gram stain requires preparation, fixation, and staining under anaerobic conditions, which is not practical in clinical laboratories (67).

The key for the presumptive genus identification of anaerobic gram-positive rods is depicted in Table 7. As shown, gas chromatography of metabolic products is probably the most important tool in identifying gram-positive anaerobes. Some other genera may be eliminated from consideration by relatively simple means. The presence of bacterial endospores indicates *Bacillus* or *Clostridium* species. Some organisms appear more rod-like or diphtheroidal on solid medium than in broth culture. *Streptococcus mutans*, *Streptococcus intermedius*, *Gemella morbillorum*, and others form elongated cells on solid media more rapidly than in broth culture and may on initial inspection be mistaken for rods. *Nocardia*, *Rothia*, *Corynebacterium*, *Erysipelothrix*, and *Listeria* species may be ruled out by testing for aerobic growth. The observation of rods with clubs or bifurcated ends should suggest a species of *Bifidobacterium*, but this morphology may also be observed in other genera. Non-partial-acid-fast branched filaments are good indicators of *Actinomyces* species.

All *Actinomyces* species except *A. meyeri* are facultatively anaerobic; *A. meyeri* is strictly anaerobic or, very rarely, microaerophilic. It may be difficult to obtain isolates in pure culture; therefore, several subcultures are recommended to ensure purity before biochemical tests are carried out.

Differentiation of several *Actinomyces* species may be difficult. *A. naeslundii* and *A. viscosus* are very similar phenotypically, but *A. viscosus* is catalase positive (30% H_2O_2). *A. israelii* and *P. propionicum* both produce acetic and lactic acids as end products of carbohydrate metabolism; however, *P. propionicum* produces propionic acid, whereas *A. israelii* produces succinic acid. Differential characteristics for species of *Actinomyces* spp. and *P. propionicum* are summarized in Tables 7 and 8. Phenotypically, *A. israelii* and other *Actinomyces* species are very similar to *E. nodatum*, but the production of butyric acid by some *Eubacterium* species is a differential characteristic (53, 57). Some *Actinomyces* spp. actually require CO_2 before they can produce succinate.

Eubacterium spp. and the *Eubacterium*-like species (Tables 9, 10, and 11) are easily confused with each other and other anaerobic gram-positive rods; however, gas-liquid chromatographic analysis of metabolic end products is very useful for differentiation (53, 57, 92) (Tables 9 and 10). Cells may be either uniform or pleomorphic on Gram stain, and growth is obligately anaerobic.

Moore and Moore (93) reported three phenotypic groups of *E. aerofaciens*, based on sugar utilization patterns. Recently, Kageyama et al. (71) reported a fourth group and further noted that their 181 isolates of the newly named *C. aerofaciens* could be subdivided into 16 subgroups.

The key characteristic (Table 12) of *Bifidobacterium* spp. is the production of acetate and lactate at a molar ratio of 2:3, which distinguishes these organisms from other lactic acid- and acetic acid-producing gram-positive anaerobic rods. Some strains are able to grow in ambient air with CO_2.

Lactobacillus spp. can usually be identified on the basis of long, parallel-sided, thin gram-positive rods (compared to the morphologies of *Bacillus* spp.) on Gram stain; a negative catalase test; and a major lactic acid peak from glucose by gas chromatography.

Two species of *Mobiluncus* are recognized: *Mobiluncus curtisii* and *Mobiluncus mulieris*. They are oxidase, catalase, and indole negative and do not produced H_2S. Both species of *Mobiluncus* are positive for proline aminopeptidase and α-D-glucosidase and negative for phosphatases and β-D-glucosidase. They are weakly saccharolytic and produce succinic and acetic acids during fermentation with or without lactic acid. Growth is not stimulated by formate and fumarate. The strains are motile by multiple subterminal flagella. The colonies are colorless, translucent, smooth, and convex and may have a watery appearance, especially on very moist or fresh media. Colonies have a maximum diameter of 2 to 3 mm after 5 days of uninterrupted anaerobic incubation. They may be less than 1 mm in diameter after 2 days of incubation. Although cells of both species are curved and slightly pointed rods, *M. curtisii* can be differentiated from *M. mulieris* most easily by its length and its gram-variable rather than gram-negative staining (Table 13). Gas chromatographic analysis of peptone yeast broth supplemented with starch and 2% serum is of some use in distinguishing the two species. *M. curtisii* produces a major succinate peak and a minor acetate peak, while *M. mulieris* generally produces major succinate and acetate peaks with or without a minor lactate peak.

For identification of *Atopobium* spp., see Table 14.

Several commercial systems for the identification of anaerobic bacteria have been evaluated for gram-positive

TABLE 11 Flowchart for identification of selected *Eubacterium* spp.[a]

I. Butyric acid produced
    A. Caproic acid produced: *E. alactolyticum*
    B. Caproic acid not produced, acid from glucose
        1. Indole produced: *E. saburreum*
        2. Indole not produced
            a. Nitrate reduced
                i. Esculin hydrolyzed: *E. multiforme*
                  aa. Glycogen acid: *E. budayi*
                  bb. Glycogen not acid, maltose not acid, motile, phospholipase C not produced: *E. multiforme*
                  cc. Glycogen not acid, major acetic acid maltose acid, phospholipase C not produced: *E. nitrogenes*
                ii. Esculin not hydrolyzed: *E. monoforme*
            b. Nitrate not reduced
                i. Major lactic acid from glucose
                  aa. H_2S produced: *E. rectale*
                  bb. H_2S not produced: *E. cylindroides*
                 ii. No major lactic acid from glucose
                  aa. Acid from glucose and esculin hydrolyzed: *E. limosum*
                  bb. No acid from glucose or maltose, gelatin hydrolyzed: *E. combesii*
                  cc. Weak acid from glucose and maltose, gelatin not hydrolyzed: *E. nodatum*
II. Butyric acid not produced
    A. Acid from glucose
        1. Indole produced: *E. tenue*
        2. Indole not produced
            a. Major lactic acid from glucose: *C. aerofaciens* (see *Collinsella*)
            b. No lactic acid from glucose: *E. contortum*
    B. No acid from glucose: *E. lentum, E. brachy, E. timidum, E. yurii*

[a] Modified from references 57 and 92 with permission of Williams & Wilkins, Baltimore, Md.

TABLE 12 Characteristics of *Bifidobacterium* spp.[a]

Species	Arabinose	Cellobiose	Fermentation of glycogen	Melezitose	Sucrose	Occurrence in human material			
						Clinical	Mouth	Feces	Vagina
B. adolescentis	v	+	+	−	+			+	
B. bifidum	−	−	−	−	−	+		+	+
B. breve	−	+	+	v	+	+		+	+
B. catenulatum	v	+	v	−	+			+	+
B. dentium	+	+	+	+	+	+	+	+	+
B. globosum	+	v	+	−	+			+	
B. infantis	−	−[+]	−	−	+			+	+
B. longum	+	−[+]	−	+[w]	+	+		+	

[a] Acid production in peptone yeast extract glucose broth; +, pH below 5.5, or positive; w, pH 5.5 to 5.9 or weak; −, pH above 5.9 or negative; v, variable; superscript, reaction of some strains of a species. Fermentation patterns of *Bifidobacterium* species overlap considerably; DNA-DNA hybridization is required for the definitive identification of some species. All *Bifidobacterium* species produce acid from glucose.

TABLE 13 Characteristics of *Mobiluncus* spp.[a]

Characteristic	M. mulieris	M. curtisii	M. curtisii group SLH-29
Length (μm)	2.9	1.7	1.3–1.7
Gram reaction	−	d	−
Hippurate hydrolysis	−	+	d (27)
α-D-Galactosidase	−	+	d (7)
Arginine dihydrolase	−	+	+
Proline aminopeptidase	+	+	+
α-D-Glucosidase	+	+	+
β-D-Glucosidase	−	−	−

[a] Adapted from references 127 and 133. Abbreviations and symbols: d, variable; −, negative; +, positive. Values in parentheses are the percentage of isolates positive.

TABLE 14 Characteristics for differentiation of *Atopobium* species[a]

Species	Acid phosphatase	Arginine dihydrolase	Leucine arylamidase	Glycine arylamidase	β-Galactosidase
A. vaginae	+	+	+	+	−
A. minutum	−	+	−	−	−
A. parvulum	+	−	+	+	+
A. rimae	+	−	−	−	−

[a] Adapted from reference 68 with permission of the International Union of Microbiological Societies. *Atopobium* species are facultatively anaerobic, with lactic acid being the major acid produced and with cells occurring as elliptical cocci or being rod shaped. Symbols: −, negative; +, positive.

rods. While the number of isolates evaluated in each study is relatively small, the overall accuracies of these systems are low and vary depending on the species (21, 63). More recent reports suggest that molecular methods like PCR-restriction fragment length polymorphism analysis may be helpful in permitting a definitive identification of anaerobic gram-positive rods (9, 51, 155).

As with aerobic gram-positive organisms, analysis of cellular fatty acids may aid in the identification of anaerobic bacteria (45). However, this technique does not lend itself to nonspecialist laboratories.

Antimicrobial Susceptibility

New information on the antimicrobial susceptibilities of anaerobic gram-positive rods is sparse compared with the information available for other anaerobic species. Many reports fail to give results for specific species, opting instead to combine data for the group (47, 48). Recent advances in taxonomy should allow us to better understand antibiotic sensitivities and resistance within this group. Although data are limited, quinolones have limited activity against *A. odontolyticus* and *A. israelii* (48). It is generally accepted that the anaerobic gram-positive non-spore-forming rods are susceptible to penicillin G, carbenicillin, and chloramphenicol (148, 149). Other antimicrobial agents, particularly metronidazole, have been reported to have various efficiencies. Clindamycin, erythromycin, and tetracycline were active against 94, 88, and 60% of isolates tested, respectively (137, 148, 149). *M. curtisii* is uniformly resistant to metronidazole, but it is doubtful whether this fact has clinical significance (132). Women with bacterial vaginosis who are treated with oral or intravaginal metronidazole rarely have persistent *M. curtisii* immediately after therapy.

Eradication of some of these organisms from the sites of infection may be difficult, particularly in actinomycotic or actinomycosis-like infections, since blood supplies to the infected site(s) may be inadequate, multiple abscesses may be present, and surrounding tissue with granulation may impede the penetration of antimicrobial agents. Therefore, in these cases surgical intervention and prolonged therapy are usually recommended (39, 118). Current recommended antibiotic regimens call for intravenous antibiotics for 4 to 6 weeks, followed by oral administration for 6 to 12 months.

Evaluation, Interpretation, and Reporting of Results

As with the anaerobic gram-positive cocci, interpretation of culture results may require additional clinical information about how the specimen was obtained. Direct observation of sulfur granules is the most sensitive method for diagnosis of actinomycosis. Specimens yielding anaerobic gram-positive rods will often yield two or three other organisms as well; therefore, one should not automatically dismiss mixed cultures as contaminated. *P. acnes* has been implicated as the etiologic agent of prosthetic device infection. These organisms, which can form biofilms on devices, can cause infiltration of inflammatory cells into the infected site. Evaluating the clinical specimens for inflammatory cells may help guide interpretation of cultures yielding these organisms. On the other hand, since these microorganisms are members of the endogenous flora of the skin, oral cavity, genital tract, and gut, contamination by the normal flora during specimen acquisition can occur, but inflammatory cells are rarely present in the specimen. Therefore, communication with the physician submitting the specimen for culture is essential.

REFERENCES

1. **Aldridge, K. E., D. Ashcroft, and K. A. Bowman.** 1997. Comparative in vitro activities of trovafloxacin (CP 99,219) and other antimicrobials against clinically significant anaerobes. *Antimicrob. Agents Chemother.* **41:**484–487.
2. **Appelbaum, P. C., C. S. Kaufmann, and J. W. Depenbusch.** 1985. Accuracy and reproducibility of a four-hour method for anaerobe identification. *J. Clin. Microbiol.* **21:**894–898.
3. **Bayer, A. S., A. W. Chow, D. Betts, and L. B. Guze.** 1978. Lactobacillemia—report of nine cases. Important clinical and therapeutic considerations. *Am. J. Med.* **64:**808–813.
4. **Beeruns, H.** 1990. Selective medium for *Bifidobacterium.* *Lett. Appl. Microbiol* **11:**155–157.
5. **Bennion, R. S., J. E. Thompson, E. J. Baron, and S. M. Finegold.** 1990. Gangrenous and perforated appendicitis with peritonitis: treatment and bacteriology. *Clin. Ther.* **12:**31–44.
6. **Bjornson, H. S.** 1989. Biliary tract and hepatic infections, p. 333–347. *In* S. M. Finegold and W. L. George (ed.), *Anaerobic Infections in Humans.* Academic Press, Inc., San Diego, Calif.
7. **Bourgault, S. A. M., and F. Lamotte.** 1988. Evaluation of the KOH test and the antibiotic disk test in routine clinical anaerobic bacteriology. *J. Clin. Microbiol.* **26:**2144–2146.
8. **Bourgault, A. M., J. E. Rosenblatt, and R. H. Fitzgerald.** 1980. *Peptococcus magnus:* a significant human pathogen. *Ann. Intern. Med.* **93:**244–248.
9. **Brailsford, S. R., R. B. Tregaskis, H. S. Leftwich, and D. Beighton.** 1999. The predominant *Actinomyces* spp. isolated from infected dentin of active root caries lesions. *J. Dent. Res.* **78:**1525–1534.
10. **Brazier, J. S., and V. Hall.** 1993. *Propionibacterium propionicum* and infections of the lacrimal apparatus. *Clin. Infect. Dis.* **17:**892–893.

11. **Brook, I.** 1987. Comparison of two transport systems for recovery of aerobic and anaerobic bacteria from abscesses. *J. Clin. Microbiol.* **24:**2020–2022.

12. **Brook, I.** 1988. Aerobic and anaerobic bacteriology of purulent nasopharyngitis in children. *J. Clin. Microbiol.* **26:**592–594.

13. **Brook, I.** 1988. Anaerobic bacteria in suppurative genitourinary infections. *J. Urol.* **141:**889–893.

14. **Brook, I.** 1988. Microbiology of non-puerperal breast abscesses. *J. Infect. Dis.* **157:**377–379.

15. **Brook, I.** 1988. Recovery of anaerobic bacteria from clinical specimens in 12 years at two military hospitals. *J. Clin. Microbiol.* **26:**1181–1188.

16. **Brook, I., and E. H. Frazier.** 1993. Significant recovery of nonsporulating anaerobic rods from clinical specimens. *Clin. Infect. Dis.* **16:**476–480.

17. **Brook, I., R. B. Kiehlich, and S. Grimm.** 1981. Bacteriology of acute periapical abscess in children. *J. Endodontol.* **7:**378–380.

18. **Brown, S. K., and A. R. Shalita.** 1998. Acne vulgaris. *Lancet* **351:**1871–1876.

19. **Burlage, R. S., and P. D. Ellner.** 1985. Comparison of the PRAS II, AN-Ident, and RapID ANA systems for identification of anaerobic bacteria. *J. Clin. Microbiol.* **22:**32–35.

20. **Carlone, G. M., M. L. Thomas, R. J. Arko, G. O. Guerrant, C. W. Moss, J. M. Swenson, and S. A. Morse.** 1986. Cell wall characteristics of *Mobiluncus* species. *Int. J. Syst. Bacteriol.* **36:**288–296.

21. **Cavallaro, J. J., L. S. Wiggs, and J. M. Miller.** 1997. Evaluation of the BBL Crystal anaerobe identification system. *J. Clin. Microbiol.* **35:**3186–3191.

22. **Celig, D. M., and P. C. Schreckenberger.** 1991. Clinical evaluation of the RapID ANA II panel for identification of anaerobic bacteria. *J. Clin. Microbiol.* **29:**457–462.

23. **Cheeseman, S. L., S. J. Hiom, A. J. Weightman, and W. G. Wade.** 1996. Phylogeny of oral asaccharolytic *Eubacterium* species determined by 16S ribosomal DNA sequence comparison and proposal of *Eubacterium infirmum* sp. nov. and *Eubacterium tardum* sp. nov. *Int. J. Syst. Bacteriol.* **46:**957–959.

24. **Collins, M. D., L. Hoyles, G. Kalfas, G. Sundquist, T. Monsen, N. Nikolaitchouk, and E. Falsen.** 2000. Characterization of *Actinomyces* isolates from infected root canals of teeth: description of *Actinomyces radicidentis* sp. nov. *J. Clin. Microbiol.* **38:**3399–3403.

25. **Collins, M. D., and C. Pascual.** 2000. Reclassification of *Actinomyces humiferus* (Gledhill and Casida) as *Cellulomonas humilata* nom. corrig., comb. nov. *Int. J. Syst. Evol. Microbiol.* **50:**661–663.

26. **Collins, M. D., and S. Wallbanks.** 1992. Comparative sequence analysis of 16S rRNA genes of *Lactobacillus minutus*, *Lactobacillus rimae* and *Streptococcus parvulus*: proposal for creation of a new genus, *Atopobium*. *FEMS Microbiol. Lett.* **95:**235–240.

27. **Collins, M. S., S. Stubbs, J. Hommez, and L. A. Devriese.** 1993. Molecular taxonomic studies of *Actinomyces*-like bacteria isolated from purulent lesions in pigs and description of *Actinomyces hyovaginalis* sp. nov. *Int. J. Syst. Bacteriol.* **43:**471–473.

28. **Cox, S. M., L. E. Phillips, L. J. Mercer, C. E. Stager, S. Waller, and S. Faro.** 1986. Lactobacillemia of amniotic fluid origin. *Obstet. Gynecol.* **68:**134–135.

29. **Cummins, C. S., and J. S. Johnson.** 1986. Genus I. *Propionibacterium* Orla Jensen 1909, 337[AL], p. 1346–1363. *In* P. H. A. Sneath, N. S. Mair, M. E. Sharpe, and J. G. Holt (ed.), *Bergey's Manual of Systematic Bacteriology*, vol. 2. The Williams & Wilkins Co., Baltimore, Md.

30. **Davis, A. J., P. A. James, and P. M. Hawkey.** 1986. *Lactobacillus* endocarditis. *J. Infect.* **12:**169–174.

31. **Downes, J., B. Olsvik, S. J. Hiom, S. A. Spratt, S. L. Cheeseman, I. Olsen, A. J. Weightman, and W. G. Wade.** 2000. *Bulleidia extructa* gen. nov. sp. nov., isolated from the oral cavity. *Int. J. Syst. Evol. Microbiol.* **50:**979–983.

32. **Embly, T. M., and E. Stackebrandt.** 1994. The molecular phylogeny and systematics of the actinomycetes. *Annu. Rev. Microbiol.* **48:**257–289.

33. **Evans, D. T. P.** 1993. *Actinomyces israelii* in the female genital tract: a review. *Genitourin. Med.* **69:**54–59.

34. **Ezaki, T., S. L. Liu, Y. Hashimoto, and E. Yabuchi.** 1990. *Peptostreptococcus hydrogenalis* sp. nov. from human fecal and vaginal flora. *Int. J. Syst. Bacteriol.* **40:**305–306.

35. **Ezaki, T., Y. Kawamura, N. Li, Z. Li, L. Shao, and S. Shu.** 2001. Proposal of the genera *Anaerococcus* gen. nov., *Peptoniphilus* gen. nov. and *Gallicola* gen. nov. for members of the genus *Peptostreptococcus*. *Int. J. Syst. Evol. Microbiol.* **51:**1521–1528.

36. **Ezaki, T., N. Yamamoto, K. Ninomiya, S. Suzuki, and E. Yabuuchi.** 1983. Transfer of *Peptococcus indolicus*, *Peptococcus asaccharolyticus*, *Peptococcus prevotii*, and *Peptococcus magnus* to the genus *Peptostreptococcus* and proposal of *Peptostreptococcus tetradius* sp. nov. *Int. J. Syst. Bacteriol.* **33:**683–698.

37. **Ezaki, T., and E. Yabuuchi.** 1986. Transfer of *Peptococcus heliotrinireducens* Corrig. to the genus *Peptostreptococcus*: *Peptostreptococcus heliotrinireducens* 1983 comb. nov. *Int. J. Syst. Bacteriol.* **36:**107–108.

38. **Fenollar, F., and D. Raoult.** 2000. Comparison of a commercial disk test with vancomycin and colimycin susceptibility testing for identification of bacteria with abnormal Gram staining reactions. *Eur. J. Microbiol. Infect. Dis.* **19:**33–38.

39. **Finegold, S. M.** 1989. General aspects of anaerobic infection, p. 135–153. *In* S. M. Finegold and W. L. George (ed.), *Anaerobic Infections in Humans*. Academic Press, Inc., San Diego, Calif.

40. **Fiorino, A.-S.** 1996. Intrauterine contraceptive device-associated actinomycotic abscess and *Actinomyces* detection on cervical smear. *Obstet. Gynecol.* **87:**142–149.

41. **Funke, G., N. Alvarez, C. Pascual, E. Falsen, E. Akervall, L. Sabbe, L. Schouls, N. Weiss, and M. D. Collins.** 1997. *Actinomyces europaeus* sp. nov., isolated from human clinical specimens. *Int. J. Syst. Bacteriol.* **47:**687–692.

42. **Funke, G., C. P. Ramos, J. F. Fernandez-Garayzabal, N. Weiss, and M. D. Collins.** 1995. Description of a human-derived Centers for Disease Control coryneform group 2 bacteria as *Actinomyces bernardiae* sp. nov. *Int. J. Syst. Bacteriol.* **45:**57–60.

43. **Funke, G., S. Stubbs, A. von Graevenitz, and M. D. Collins.** 1994. Assignment of human-derived CDC group 1 coryneform bacteria and CDC group 1-like bacteria to the genus *Actinomyces* as *Actinomyces neuii* subsp. *neuii* sp. nov. subsp. nov., and *Actinomyces neuii* subsp. *anitratus* subsp. nov. *Int. J. Syst. Bacteriol.* **44:**167–171.

44. **Funke, G. N., and A. von Graevenitz.** 1995. Infections due to *Actinomyces neuii* (former "CDC coryneform group 1" bacteria). *Infection* **23:**73–75.

45. **Funke, G. N., A. von Graevenitz, J. E. Clarridge III, and K. A. Bernard.** 1997. Clinical microbiology of coryneform bacteria. *Clin. Microbiol. Rev.* **10:**125–159.

46. **Glupczynski, Y., M. Labbe, F. Crockaert, F. Pepersack, P. Van Der Auwera, and E. Yourassowsky.** 1984. Isolation of *Mobiluncus* in four cases of extragenital infections in adult women. *Eur. J. Clin. Microbiol.* **3:**433–435.

47. **Goldstein, E. J. C., and D. M. Citron.** 1991. Susceptibility of anaerobic bacteria isolated from intra-abdominal infections to ofloxacin and interaction of ofloxacin with

metronidazole. *Antimicrob. Agents Chemother.* **35:**2447–2449.

48. **Goldstein, E. J. C., D. M. Citron, C. V Merriam, K. Tyrrell, and Y. Warren.** 1991. Activities of gemifloxacin (SB 265805, LB20304) compared to those of other oral antimicrobial agents against unusual anaerobes. *Antimicrob. Agents Chemother.* **43:**2726–2730.

49. **Gunthard, H., A. Hany, M. Turina, and J. Wüst.** 1994. *Propionibacterium acnes* as a cause of aggressive aortic valve endocarditis and importance of tissue grinding: case report and review. *J. Clin. Microbiol.* **32:**3043–3045.

50. **Hall, G., A. Heimdahl, and C. E. Nord.** 1998. Comparison of E test and agar dilution methods for determining antibiotic susceptibilities of anaerobic bacteria and viridans streptococci isolated from blood. *Anaerobe* **4:**29–33.

51. **Hall, V., G. L. O'Neill, J. T. Magee, and B. I. Duerden.** 1999. Development of amplified 16S ribosomal DNA restriction analysis for identification of *Actinomyces* species and comparison with pyrolysis-mass spectrometry and conventional biochemical tests. *J. Clin. Microbiol.* **37:**2255–2261.

52. **Hamilton-Miller, J. M. T., and S. Shah.** 1998. Vancomycin susceptibility as an aid to the identification of lactobacilli. *Lett. Appl. Microbiol.* **26:**153–154.

53. **Hill, G. B., O. M. Ayers, and A. P. Kohan.** 1987. Characterization and sites of infection of *Eubacterium nodatum*, *Eubacterium timidum*, *Eubacterium brachy*, and other asaccharolytic eubacteria. *J. Clin. Microbiol.* **25:**1540–1545.

54. **Hillier, S. L., M. A. Krohn, N. B. Kiviat, D. H. Watts, and D. A. Eschenbach.** 1991. Microbiologic causes and neonatal outcomes associated with chorioamnion infection. *Am. J. Obstet. Gynecol.* **165:**955–961.

55. **Hillier, S. L., M. A. Krohn, L. K. Rabe, S. J. Klebanoff, and D. A. Eschenbach.** 1993. Normal vaginal flora, H_2O_2-producing lactobacilli and bacterial vaginosis in pregnant women. *Clin. Infect. Dis.* **16**(Suppl. 4):S273–S281.

56. **Hillier, S. L., D. H. Watts, M. F. Lee, and D. A. Eschenbach.** 1990. Etiology and treatment of post cesarean section endometritis after cephalosporin prophylaxis. *J. Reprod. Med.* **35:**322–328.

57. **Holdeman, L. V., E. P. Cato, and W. E. C. Moore (ed.).** 1977. *Anaerobe Laboratory Manual*, 4th ed. Virginia Polytechnic Institute and State University, Blacksburg.

58. **Holdeman, L. V., E. P. Cato, J. A. Burmeister, and W. E. C. Moore.** 1980. Descriptions of *Eubacterium timidum* sp. nov., *Eubacterium brachy* sp. nov., and *Eubacterium nodatum* sp. nov. isolated from human periodontitis. *Int. J. Syst. Bacteriol.* **30:**163–169.

59. **Holst, E., B. Wathne, B. Hovelius, and P.-A. Mardh.** 1987. Bacterial vaginosis: microbiological and clinical findings. *Eur. J. Clin. Microbiol.* **6:**536–541.

60. **Hoyles, L., E. Falsen, G. Foster, C. Pascual, C. Greko, and M. D. Collins.** 2000. *Actinomyces canis* sp. nov., isolated from dogs. *Int. J. Syst. Evol. Microbiol.* **50:**1547–1551.

61. **Hoyles, L., E. Falsen, C. Pascual, B. Sjoden, G. Foster, D. Henderson, and M. D. Collins.** 2001. *Actinomyces catuli* sp. nov., from dogs. *Int. J. Syst. Evol. Microbiol.* **51:**679–682.

62. **Hudspeth, M. K., D. M. Citron, and E. J. C. Goldstein.** 1997. Evaluation of a novel specimen transport system (Venturi Transystem) for anaerobic bacteria. *Clin. Infect. Dis.* **25:**132–133.

63. **Hudspeth, M. K., S. H. Gerardo, D. M. Citron, and E. J. C. Goldstein.** 1998. Evaluation of the RapID CB Plus system for the identification of *Corynebacterium* species and other gram-positive rods. *J. Clin. Microbiol.* **36:**543–547.

64. **Jakab, E., R. Zbinden, J. Gubler, C. Ruef, A. von Graevenitz, and M. Krause.** 1998. Severe infections caused by *Propionibacterium acnes*: an underestimated pathogen in late postoperative infections. *Yale J. Biol. Med.* **69:**477–482.

65. **Jalava, J., and E. Eerola.** 1999. Phylogenetic analysis of *Fusobacterium alocis* and *Fusobacterium sulci* based on 16S rRNA gene sequences: proposal of *Filifactor alocis* (Cato, Moore and Moore) comb. nov. and *Eubacterium sulci* (Cato, Moore and Moore) comb. nov. *Int. J. Syst. Evol. Microbiol.* **49:**1375–1379.

66. **Johnson, J. L., L. V. H. Moore, B. Kaneko, and W. E. C. Moore.** 1990. *Actinomyces georgiae* sp. nov., *Actinomyces gerencseriae* sp. nov., designation of two genospecies of *Actinomyces naeslundii*, and inclusion of *A. naeslundii* serotypes II and III and *Actinomyces viscosus* serotype II in *A. naeslundii* genospecies 2. *Int. J. Syst. Bacteriol.* **40:**273–286.

67. **Johnson, M. J., E. Thatcher, and M. E. Cox.** 1995. Techniques for controlling variability in Gram staining of obligate anaerobes. *J. Clin. Microbiol.* **33:**755–758.

68. **Jovita, M. R., M. D. Collins, B. Sjoden, and E. Falsen.** 1999. Characterization of a novel *Atopobium* isolate from the human vagina: description of *Atopobium vaginae* sp. nov. *Int. J. Syst. Evol. Microbiol.* **49:**1573–1576.

69. **Kageyama, A., and Y. Benno.** 2000. *Catenibacterium mitsuokai* gen. nov., a gram-positive anaerobic bacterium isolated from human faeces. *Int. J. Syst. Evol. Microbiol.* **50:**1595–1599.

70. **Kageyama, A., and Y. Benno.** 2000. Emendation of genus *Collinsella* and proposal of *Collinsella stercoris* sp. nov. and *Collinsella intestinalis* sp. nov. *Int. J. Syst. Evol. Microbiol.* **50:**1767–1774.

71. **Kageyama, A., Y. Yoshimi, and T. Nakase.** 1999. Phylogenetic and phenotypic evidence for the transfer of *Eubacterium aerofaciens* to the genus *Collinsella* as *Collinsella aerofaciens* gen. nov., comb. nov. *Int. J. Syst. Evol. Microbiol.* **49:**557–565.

72. **Kageyama, A., Y. Yoshimi, and T. Nakase.** 1999. Phylogenetic evidence for the transfer of *Eubacterium lentum* to the genus *Eggerthella* as *Eggerthella lenta* gen. nov., comb. nov. *Int. J. Syst. Evol. Microbiol.* **49:**1725–1732.

73. **Karachewski, N. O., E. L. Busch, and C. L. Wells.** 1985. Comparison of PRAS II, RapID ANA, and API 20A systems for identification of anaerobic bacteria. *J. Clin. Microbiol.* **21:**122–126.

74. **Karvonen, S. L., L. Rasanen, W. J. Cunliffe, K. T. Holland, J. Karvonen, and T. Reunala.** 1994. Delayed hypersensitivity to *Propionibacterium acnes* in patients with severe nodular acne and acne fulminans. *Dermatology* **189:**344–349.

75. **Kitajima, H., Y. Sumida, R. Tanaka, N. Yuki, H. Takayama, and M. Fujimura.** 1997. Early administration of *Bifidobacterium breve* to preterm infants: randomized controlled trial. *Arch. Dis. Child. Fetal Neonatal Med.* **76:**F101–F107.

76. **Klein, G., E. Zill, R. Schindler, and J. Louwers.** 1998. Peritonitis associated with vancomycin-resistant *Lactobacillus rhamnosus* in a continuous ambulatory peritoneal dialysis patient: organism identification, antibiotic therapy, and case report. *J. Clin. Microbiol.* **36:**1781–1783.

77. **Kotilainen, P., R. Merilahti-Palo, O. P. Lehtonen, I. Manner, I. Helander, T. Mottonen, and E. Rintala.** 1996. *Propionibacterium acnes* isolated from sternal osteitis in a patient with SAPHO syndrome. *J. Rheumatol.* **23:**1302–1304.

78. **Kronvall, G., M. Lanner-Sjöberg, L. V. von Stedingk, H. Hanson, B. Pettersson, and E. Falsen.** 1997. Whole cell protein and partial 16S rRNA gene sequence analysis

suggest the existence of a second *Rothia* species. *Clin. Microbiol. Infect.* **4:**225–263.

79. **Lassnig, C., M. Dorsch, J. Wolters, E. Schaber, G. Stöffler, and E. Stackebrandt.** 1989. Phylogenetic evidence for the relationship between the genera *Mobiluncus* and *Actinomyces. FEMS Microbiol. Lett.* **65:**17–22.

80. **Lawson, P. A., E. Falsen, E. Akervall, P. Vandamme, and M. D. Collins.** 1997. Characterization of some *Actinomyces*-like isolates from human clinical specimens: reclassification of *Actinomyces suis* (Soltys and Spratling) as *Actinobaculum suis* comb. nov. and description of *Actinobaculum schaalii* sp. nov. *Int. J. Syst. Bacteriol.* **47:**899–903.

81. **Lawson, P. A., N. Nikolaitchouk, E. Falsen, K. Westling, and M. D. Collins.** 2001. *Actinomyces funkei* sp. nov., isolated from human clinical specimens. *Int. J. Syst. Evol. Microbiol.* **51:**853–855.

82. **Li, N., Y. Hashimoto, S. Adnan, H. Miura, H. Yamamoto, and T. Ezaki.** 1992. Three new species of the genus *Peptostreptococcus* isolated from humans: *Peptostreptococcus vaginalis* sp. nov., *Peptostreptococcus lacrimalis* sp. nov., and *Peptostreptococcus lactolyticus* sp. nov. *Int. J. Syst. Bacteriol.* **42:**602–605.

83. **Lorenz, R. P., P. C. Appelbaum, R. M. Ward, and J. J. Botti.** 1982. Chorioamnionitis and possible neonatal infection associated with *Lactobacillus* species. *J. Clin. Microbiol.* **16:**558–561.

84. **Ludwig, W., R. Weizenegger, R. Kilpper-Bälz, and K. H. Schleifer.** 1988. Phylogenetic relationships of anaerobic streptococci. *Int. J. Syst. Bacteriol.* **38:**15–18.

85. **Madinger, N. E., J. A. McGregor, P. J. McKinney, S. T. Dembeck, C. S. Haskell, and Z. Johnson.** 1993. Comparative antibiotic susceptibilities of anaerobes associated with infection of the female reproductive tract. *Clin. Infect. Dis.* **16**(Suppl. 4):S349–S352.

86. **Mangels, J. I., and B. P. Douglas.** 1989. Comparison of four commercial brucella agar media for growth of anaerobic organisms. *J. Clin. Microbiol.* **27:**2268–2271.

87. **Marler, L. M., J. A. Siders, L. C. Wolters, Y. Pettigrew, B. L. Skitt, and S. D. Allen.** 1991. Evaluation of the new RapID-ANA II system for the identification of clinical anaerobic isolates. *J. Clin. Microbiol.* **29:**874–878.

88. **McGregor, J. A., J. I. French, W. Jones, K. Milligan, P. J. McKinney. E. Patterson, and R. Parker.** 1994. Bacterial vaginosis is associated with prematurity and vaginal fluid mucinase and sialidase: results of a controlled trial of topical clindamycin cream. *Am. J. Obstet. Gynecol.* **170:**1048–1060.

89. **Miller, P. H. L. S. Wiggs, and M. Miller.** 1995. Evaluation of RapID ANA II systems for identification of *Actinomyces* species from clinical specimens. *J. Clin. Microbiol.* **33:**329–330.

90. **Miyamoto, M. I., and F. C. Fang.** 1993. Pyogenic liver abscess involving *Actinomyces*: case report and review. *Clin. Infect. Dis.* **16:**303–309.

91. **Moore, L. V. H., W. E. C. Moore, E. P. Cato, R. M. Smibert, J. A. Burmeister, and A. M. Best.** 1987. Bacteriology of human gingivitis. *J. Dent. Res.* **6:**989–995.

92. **Moore, W. E. C., and L. V. H. Moore.** 1986. Genus *Eubacterium* Prevot 1938, 294[AL], p. 1353–1373. *In* P. H. A. Sneath, N. S. Mair, M. E. Sharpe, and J. G. Holt (ed.), *Bergey's Manual of Systematic Bacteriology*, vol. 2. The Williams & Wilkins Co., Baltimore, Md.

93. **Moore, W. E. C., and L. V. H. Moore.** 1974. Human fecal flora: the normal flora of 20 Japanese-Hawaiians. *Appl. Microbiol.* **27:**961–979.

94. **Murdoch, D. A.** 1998. Gram-positive anaerobic cocci. *Clin. Microbiol. Rev.* **11:**81–120.

95. **Murdoch, D. A., M. D. Collins, A. Willems, J. M. Hardie, K. A. Young, and T. J. Magee.** 1997. Description of three new species of the genus *Peptostreptococcus* from human clinical specimens: *Peptostreptococcus harei* sp. nov., *Peptostreptococcus ivorii* sp. nov., and *Peptostreptococcus octavius* sp. nov. *Int. J. Syst. Bacteriol.* **47:**781–787.

96. **Murdoch, D. A., H. N. Shah, S. E. Gharbia, and D. Rajendram.** 2000. Proposal to restrict the genus *Peptostreptococcus* (Kluyver & van Niel 1936) to *Peptostreptococcus anaerobius. Anaerobe* **6:**257–260.

97. **Nakazawa, F., S. E. Poco, T. Ikeda, M. Sako, S. Kalfas, G. Sundqvist, and E. Hoshino.** 1999. *Cryptobacterium curtum* gen. nov., sp. nov., a new genus of gram-positive anaerobic rod isolated from human oral cavities. *Int. J. Syst. Evol. Microbiol.* **49:**1193–1200.

98. **Nakazawa, F., M. Sato, S. E. Poco, Jr., T. Hashimura, T. Ikeda, S. Kalfas, G. Sundquist, and E. Hoshino.** 2000. Description of *Mogibacterium pumilum* gen. nov., sp. nov., and *Mogibacterium vescum* gen. nov., sp. nov., and reclassification of *Eubacterium timidum* (Holdeman et al. 1980) as *Mogibacterium timidum* gen. nov., comb. nov. *Int. J. Syst. Evol. Microbiol.* **50:**679–688.

99. **Neut, C., V. Lesieur, C. Romond, and H. Beerens.** 1985. Analysis of gram-positive anaerobic cocci in oral, fecal and vaginal flora. *Eur. J. Clin. Microbiol.* **4:**435–437.

100. **Ng, J., L.-K. Ng, A. W. Chow, and J. R. Dillon.** 1994. Identification of five *Peptostreptococcus* species isolated predominantly from the female genital tract by using the rapid ID32A system. *J. Clin. Microbiol.* **32:**1302–1307.

101. **Nikolaitchouk, N., L. Hoyles, E. Falsen, J. M. Grainger, and M. D. Collins.** 2000. *Actinomyces* isolates from samples from the human urogenital tract: description of *Actinomyces urogenitalis* sp. nov. *Int. J. Syst. Evol. Microbiol.* **50:**1649–1654.

102. **Nugent, T., M. Krohn, and S. L. Hillier.** 1991. Reliability of diagnosing bacterial vaginosis is improved by a standardized method of Gram stain interpretation. *J. Clin. Microbiol.* **29:**297–301.

103. **Olsen, I., J. L. Johnson, L. V. Moore, and W. E. Moore.** 1991. *Lactobacillus uli* sp. nov. and *Lactobacillus rimae* sp. nov. from the human gingival crevice and emended descriptions of *Lactobacillus minutus* and *Streptococcus parvulus. Int. J. Syst. Bacteriol.* **41:**261–266.

104. **Pant, A. R., S. M. Graham, S. J. Allen, S. Harikul, A. Sabcharoen, L. Cuevas, and C. A. Hart.** 1996. *Lactobacillus* GG and acute diarrhea in young children in the tropics. *J. Trop. Pediatr.* **42:**162–165.

105. **Parent, D., M. Bossens, D. Bayot, C. Kirkpatrick, F. Graf, F. E. Wilkinson, and R. R. Kaiser.** 1996. Therapy of bacterial vaginosis using exogenously-applied *Lactobacilli acidophili* and a low dose of estriol: a placebo-controlled multicentric clinical trial. *Arzneimittelforschung* **46:**68–73.

106. **Pascual Ramos, C., E. Falsen, N. Alvarez, E. Äkervall, B. Sjäden, and M. D. Collins.** 1997. *Actinomyces graevenitzii* sp. nov., isolated from human clinical specimens. *Int. J. Syst. Bacteriol.* **47:**885–888.

107. **Pascual Ramos, C., G. Foster, and M. D. Collins.** 1997. Phylogenetic analysis of the genus *Actinomyces* based on 16S rRNA gene sequences: description of *Arcanobacterium phocae* sp. nov., *Arcanobacterium bernardiae* comb. nov., and *Arcanobacterium pyogenes* comb. nov. *Int. J. Syst. Bacteriol.* **47:**46–53.

108. **Pascual Ramos, C., G. Foster, E. Falsen, K. Bergstrom, C. Greko, and M. D. Collins.** 1999. *Actinomyces bowdenii* sp. nov., isolated from canine and feline clinical specimens. *Int. J. Syst. Evol. Microbiol.* **49:**1873–1877.

109. **Perry, J. L.** 1997. Assessment of swab transport systems for aerobic and anaerobic organism recovery. *J. Clin. Microbiol.* **35:**1269–1271.

110. **Petts, D. N., W. Champion, and G. Raymond.** 1988. Oxolinic acid as a selective agent for the isolation of nonsporing anaerobes from clinical material. *Lett. Appl. Microbiol.* **6:**65–67.

111. **Piriz, S., R. Cuenca, J. Valle, and S. Vadillo.** 1992. Susceptibilities of anaerobic bacteria isolated from animals with ovine foot rot to 28 antimicrobial agents. *Antimicrob. Agents Chemother.* **36:**198–201.

112. **Poco, S. E., T. Ikeda, M. Sato, T. Sato, and E. Hoshino.** 1996. *Eubacterium exiguum* sp. nov., isolated from human oral lesions. *Int. J. Syst. Bacteriol.* **46:**1120–1124.

113. **Poco, S. E., F. Nakazawa, M. Sato, and E. Hoshino.** 1996. *Eubacterium minutum* sp. nov., isolated from human periodontal pockets. *Int. J. Syst. Bacteriol.* **46:**31–34.

114. **Pulverer G., J. Beuth, W. Roszkowski, H. Burrichter, K. Roszkowski, A. Yassin, H. L. Ko, and J. Jeljaszewicz.** 1990. Bacteria of human physiological microflora liberate immunomodulating peptides. *Zentbl. Bakteriol. Parasitenkd. Infektkrankh. Hyg. Abt. 1 Orig.* **272:**467–476.

115. **Rajendram, D., H. N. Shah, S. E. Gharbia, and D. A. Murdoch.** 2001. Reclassification of *Peptostreptococcus asaccharolyticus* (Distaso 1912) Ezaki, Yamamoto, Ninomiya, Suzuki and Yabuuchi 1983 as *Schleiferella asaccharolytica* comb. nov., *Peptostreptococcus indolicus* (Christiansen 1934) Ezaki, Yamamoto, Ninomiya, Suzuki and Yabuuchi 1983 as *Schleiferella indolica* comb. nov., *Peptostreptococcus lacrimalis* Li, Hashimoto, Adnan, Miura, Yamamoto and Ezaki 1992 as *Schleiferella lacrimalis* comb. nov. and *Peptostreptococcus harei* (Murdoch, Collins, Willems, Hardie, Young and Magee 1997) as *Schleiferella harei* comb. nov. *Anaerobe* **7:**93–101.

116. **Raza, S., S. M. Graham, S. J. Allen, S. Sultana, L. Cuevas, and C. A. Hart.** 1995. *Lactobacillus* GG promotes recovery from acute nonbloody diarrhea in Pakistan. *Pediatr. Infect. Dis.* **14:**107–111.

117. **Reig, M., A. Moreno, and F. Baquero.** 1992. Resistance of *Peptostreptococcus* spp. to macrolides and lincosamides: inducible and constitutive phenotypes. *Antimicrob. Agents Chemother.* **36:**662–664.

118. **Reiner, S. L., J. M. Harrelson, S. E. Miller, G. B. Hill, and H. A. Gallis.** 1987. Primary actinomycosis of an extremity: a case report and review. *Rev. Infect. Dis.* **9:**581–589.

119. **Roeters, F. J., J. S. van der Hoeven, R. C. Burgersdijk, and M. J. Schaeken.** 1995. Lactobacilli, mutant streptococci and dental caries: a longitudinal study in 2-year-old children up to the age of 5 years. *Caries Res.* **29:**272–279.

120. **Roszkowski, W., K. Roszkowski, H. L. Ko, J. Beuth, and J. Jeljaszewicz.** 1990. Immunomodulation by propionibacteria. *Zentbl. Bakteriol. Parasitenkd. Infektkrankh. Hyg. Abt. 1 Orig.* **274:**289–298.

121. **Sabbe, L. J. M., D. Van De Merwe, L. Schouls, A. Bergmans, M. Vaneechoutte, and P. Vandamme.** 1999. Clinical spectrum of infections due to the newly described *Actinomyces* species *A. turicensis, A. radingae,* and *A. europaeus. J. Clin. Microbiol.* **37:**8–13.

122. **Salonen, J. H., E. Erola, and O. Meurman.** 1998. Clinical significance and outcome of anaerobic bacteremia. *Clin. Infect. Dis.* **26:**1413–1417.

123. **Sarkonen, N., E. Könönen, P. Summanen, M. Könönen, and H. Jousimies-Somer.** 2001. Phenotypic identification of *Actinomyces* and related species isolated from human sources. *J. Clin. Microbiol.* **39:**3955–3961.

124. **Schaal, K. P.** 1986. Genus *Actinomyces* Harz 1877, 133[AL], p. 1383–1418. *In* P. H. A. Sneath, N. S. Mair, M. E. Sharpe, and J. G. Holt (ed.), *Bergey's Manual of Systematic Bacteriology,* vol. 2. The Williams & Wilkins Co., Baltimore, Md.

125. **Schaal, K. P.** 1992. The genera *Actinomyces, Arcanobacterium* and *Rothia,* vol. I, p. 850–905. *In* A. Balows, H. G. Truper, M. Dworkin, W. Harder, and K. H. Schleifer (ed.), *The Prokaryotes,* 2nd ed. *A Handbook on the Biology of Bacteria: Ecophysiology, Isolation, Identification, Applications.* Springer-Verlag, New York, N.Y.

126. **Schaal, K. P., and H. J. Lee.** 1992. Actinomycete infections in humans: a review. *Gene* **115:**201–211.

127. **Schwebke, J. R., S. A. Lukehart, M. C. Roberts, and S. L. Hillier.** 1991. Identification of two new antigenic subgroups within the genus *Mobiluncus. J. Clin. Microbiol.* **29:**2204–2208.

128. **Sheppard, A., C. Cammarata, and D. H. Martin.** 1990. Comparison of different medium bases for the semiquantitative isolation of anaerobes from vaginal secretions. *J. Clin. Microbiol.* **28:**455–457.

129. **Slack, J. M., and M. A. Gerencser.** 1975. Actinomyces, Filamentous Bacteria: Biology and Pathogenicity. Burgess Publishing Co., Minneapolis, Minn.

130. **Smego, R. A., Jr., and G. Foglia.** 1998. Actinomycosis. *Clin. Infect. Dis.* **26:**1155–1163.

131. **Sneath, P. H. A., N. S. Mair, M. E. Sharpe, and J. G. Holt (ed.).** 1986. *Bergey's Manual of Systematic Bacteriology,* vol. 2. The Williams & Wilkins Co., Baltimore, Md.

132. **Spiegel, C. A.** 1987. Susceptibility of *Mobiluncus* species to 23 antimicrobial agents and 15 other compounds. *Antimicrob. Agents Chemother.* **31:**249–252.

133. **Spiegel, C. A., and M. Roberts.** 1984. *Mobiluncus* gen. nov., *Mobiluncus curtisii* subsp. *curtisii* sp. nov., *Mobiluncus curtisii* subsp. *holmesii* subsp. nov., and *Mobiluncus mulieris* sp. nov., curved rods from the human vagina. *Int. J. Syst. Bacteriol.* **34:**177–184.

134. **Sturm, A. W.** 1989. *Mobiluncus* species and other anaerobic bacteria in nonpuerperal breast abscess. *Eur. J. Clin. Microbiol.* **8:**789–792.

135. **Summanen, P., E. J. Baron, D. M. Citron, C. A. Strong, H. M. Wexler, and S. M. Finegold.** 1993. *Wadsworth Anaerobic Bacteriology Manual,* 5th ed. Star Publishing, Belmont, Calif.

136. **Sumoza, D., I. Raad, and E. Douglas.** 2000. Differentiating thoracic actinomycosis from lung cancer. *Infect. Med.* **17:**695–698.

137. **Sutter, V. L., and S. M. Finegold.** 1976. Susceptibility of anaerobic bacteria to 23 antimicrobial agents. *Antimicrob. Agents Chemother.* **10:**736–752.

138. **Traynor, R. M., D. Pavatt, H. L. D. Duguid, and I. D. Duncan.** 1981. Isolation of actinomycetes from cervical specimens. *J. Clin. Pathol.* **34:**914–916.

139. **Turng, B. F., J. M. Guthmiller, G. E. Minah, and W. A. Falkler, Jr.** 1996. Development and evaluation of a selective and differential medium for the primary isolation of *Peptostreptococcus micros. Oral Microbiol. Immunol.* **11:**356–361.

140. **Tvede, M., and N. Hoiby.** 1992. Experimental studies of survival of anaerobic bacteria at 4°C and 22°C in two different transport systems. *APMIS* **100:**1048–1052.

141. **Uematsu, H., F. Nakazawa, T. Ikeda, and E. Hoshino.** 1993. *Eubacterium saphenus* sp. nov., isolated from human periodontal pockets. *Int. J. Syst. Bacteriol.* **43:**302–304.

142. **van Dalen, P. J., T. J. M. van Steenbergen, M. M. Cowan, H. J. Busscher, and J. de Graaff.** 1993. Description of two morphotypes of *Peptostreptococcus micros. Int. J. Syst. Bacteriol.* **43:**787–798.

143. **Vandamme, P., E. Falsen, V. Vancanneyt, M. Van Esbroeck, D. Van de Merwe, A. Bergmans, L. Schouls, and L. Sabbe.** 1998. Characterization of *Actinomyces*

turicensis and *Actinomyces radingae* strains from human clinical samples. *Int. J. Syst. Evol. Microbiol.* **48:**505–510.

144. **Vowels, B. R., S. Yang, and J. J. Leyden.** 1995. Induction of proinflammatory cytokines by a soluble factor of *Propionibacterium acnes*: implications for chronic inflammatory acne. *Infect. Immun.* **63:**3158–3165.

145. **Wade, W. G.** 1996. The role of *Eubacterium* species in periodontal disease and other oral infections. *Microb. Ecol. Health Dis.* **9:**367–370.

146. **Wade, W. G., H. Downs, M. A. Munson, and A. J. Wightman.** 1999. *Eubacterium minutum* is an earlier synonym of *Eubacterium tardum* and has priority. *Int. J. Syst. Evol. Microbiol.* **49:**1939–1941.

147. **Wade, W. G., J. Downes, D. Dymock, S. J. Hiom, A. J. Weightman, F. E. Dewhirst, B. J. Paster, J. Tzellas, and B. Coleman.** 1999. The family *Coriobacteriaceae*: reclassification of *Eubacterium exiguum* (Poco et al. 1996) and *Peptostreptococcus heliotrinireducens* (Lanigan 1976) as *Slackia exigua* gen. nov., comb. nov. and *Slackia heliotrinireducens* gen. nov., and *Eubacterium lentum* (prevot 1938) as *Eggerthella lenta* gen. nov., comb. nov. *Int. J. Syst. Evol. Microbiol.* **49:**595–600.

148. **Wexler, H. M., and S. M. Finegold.** 1988. In vitro activity of cefotetan compared with that of other antimicrobial agents against anaerobic bacteria. *Antimicrob. Agents Chemother.* **32:**601–604.

149. **Wexler, H. M., and S. M. Finegold.** 1988. In vitro activity of cefoperazone plus sulbactam compared with that of other antimicrobial agents against anaerobic bacteria. *Antimicrob. Agents Chemother.* **32:**403–406.

150. **Whiting, J. L., N. Cheng, and A. W. Chow.** 1987. Interactions of ciprofloxacin with clindamycin, metronidazole, cefoxitin, cefotaxime, and mezlocillin against gram-positive and gram-negative anaerobic bacteria. *Antimicrob. Agents Chemother.* **31:**1379–1382.

151. **Wideman, P. A., V. L. Vargo, D. Citronbaum, and S. M. Finegold.** 1976. Evaluation of the sodium polyanethol sulfonate disk test for the identification of *Peptostreptococcus anaerobius*. *J. Clin. Microbiol.* **4:**330–333.

152. **Willems, A., W. E. C. Moore, N. Weiss, and M. D. Collins.** 1997. Phenotyptic and phylogenetic characterization of some *Eubacterium*-like isolates containing a novel type B wall murein from human feces: description of *Holdemania filiformis* gen. nov., sp. nov. *Int. J. Syst. Bacteriol.* **47:**1201–1204.

153. **Willems, A., and M. D. Collins.** 1995. Phylogenetic analysis of *Ruminococcus flavefaciens*, the type species of the genus *Ruminococcus*, does not support the reclassification of *Streptococcus hansenii* and *Peptostreptococcus productus* as ruminococci. *Int. J. Syst. Bacteriol.* **45:**572–575.

154. **Williams, B. L., G. F. McCann, and F. D. Schoenknecht.** 1983. Bacteriology of dental abscesses of endodontic origin. *J. Clin. Microbiol.* **18:**770–774.

155. **Wilson, K. H., R. B. Blitchington, and R. C. Green.** 1990. Amplification of bacterial 16S ribosomal DNA with polymerase chain reaction. *J. Clin. Microbiol.* **28:** 1942–1946.

156. **Witsell, D. L., C. G. Garrett, W. G. Yarbrough, S. P. Dorrestein, A. F. Drake, and M. C. Weissler.** 1995. Effect of *Lactobacillus acidophilus* on antibiotic-associated gastrointestinal morbidity: a prospective randomized trial. *J. Otolaryngol.* **24:**230–233.

157. **Wüst, J., N. Weiss, G. Funke, and M. D. Collins.** 1995. Assignment of *Actinomyces pyogenes*-like (CDC coryneform group E) bacteria to the genus *Actinomyces* as *Actinomyces radingae* sp. nov. and *Actinomyces turicensis* sp. nov. *Lett. Appl. Microbiol.* **20:**76–81.

158. **Yoonessi, M., K. Crickard, I. S. Cellino, S. K. Satchidanand, and W. Fett.** 1985. Association of *Actinomyces* and intrauterine contraceptive devices. *J. Reprod. Med.* **30:**48–52.

Bacteroides, Porphyromonas, Prevotella, Fusobacterium, and Other Anaerobic Gram-Negative Bacteria

HANNELE R. JOUSIMIES-SOMER,* PAULA H. SUMMANEN,
HANNAH WEXLER, SYDNEY M. FINEGOLD,
SAHEER E. GHARBIA, AND HAROUN N. SHAH

56

TAXONOMY

The anaerobic gram-negative bacteria are part of the normal flora of the mouth, upper respiratory tract, intestinal tract, and urogenital tract of humans and animals. Anaerobic spirochetes are covered in chapter 61, and *Campylobacter* spp. other than *Campylobacter rectus*, *Campylobacter curvus*, *Campylobacter gracilis*, and *Campylobacter showae* are discussed in chapter 57. The initial differentiation of these genera is based on cellular morphology, motility, flagellar arrangement, and an analysis of metabolic end products by gas-liquid chromatography (GLC) (Table 1) (33, 35, 45, 84). Species definition is based on biochemical characteristics, nucleic acid base composition, and homology (see chapter 19). *Acidaminococcus*, *Megasphaera*, and *Veillonella* are the genera of anaerobic, gram-negative cocci (Table 1). In the majority of clinical specimens, only organisms of the genera *Bacteroides*, *Porphyromonas*, *Prevotella*, *Fusobacterium*, *Campylobacter*, *Sutterella*, *Bilophila*, and *Veillonella* are encountered.

Bacteroides spp., *Porphyromonas* spp., *Prevotella* spp., *Fusobacterium* spp., *Campylobacter* spp., *Sutterella* sp., and *Bilophila* sp. may be presumptively characterized on the basis of colony and cellular morphology, pigment production, fluorescence under long-wave UV light, atmospheric growth characteristics, sensitivity to special-potency antibiotic disks, and certain rapidly determined biochemical characteristics. A definitive species-level identification requires a battery of biochemical tests, cellular fatty acid profiling, and occasionally, molecular methods (see chapter 17). Definitive identification is not feasible for all anaerobic isolates because of financial constraints and is not ordinarily important for clinical purposes. Generally, for clinical purposes (especially for the initiation of empiric therapy), it is sufficient to know the broad groupings of isolates and their usual pattern of susceptibility to antimicrobial agents. However, all laboratories performing anaerobic cultures should be able to isolate different anaerobes, store them, and forward them to a reference laboratory for further testing if clinically indicated.

The taxonomy of anaerobic bacteria, especially that of the gram-negative rods, has been in a state of great change in recent years (45, 47). The methods used for taxonomic studies have mainly been based on nucleic acid analyses such as DNA-DNA hybridization and 16S rRNA gene (rDNA) sequencing. The latter classification approach, based on phylogenetic relatedness, does not necessarily correlate with phenotypic characteristics, such as Gram-staining properties, morphology, atmospheric growth requirements, and sporulation, concepts that were earlier considered cornerstones in the classification of anaerobes (40). In fact, several species currently included in anaerobic gram-negative rods and all gram-negative cocci (*Butyrivibrio* spp., *Catonella morbi*, *Dialister pneumosintes*, *Fusobacterium* spp., *Leptotrichia* spp., *Johnsonella ignava*, *Tissierella* spp., *Mitsuokella multiacida*, *Selenomonas* spp., *Centipeda periodontii*, *Acidaminococcus fermentans*, *Megasphaera elsdenii*, and *Veillonella* spp.) cluster within the *Clostridium* subphylum of the gram-positive bacteria (15, 41, 45, 47). Recently, *Fusobacterium alocis* was reclassified as *Filifactor alocis* and *Fusobacterium sulci* was reclassified as *Eubacterium sulci* (38) and therefore placed in lineages of gram-positive bacteria.

The genus *Bacteroides* includes bile-resistant species that were formerly described as the "*Bacteroides fragilis*" group (including *Bacteroides eggerthii*) (84). However, the *B. fragilis* group organisms *Bacteroides distasonis* and *Bacteroides merdae* are related to *Tannerella forsythensis* (formerly *Bacteroides forsythus*) and cluster close to *Porphyromonas* on the basis of 16S rDNA sequencing (77). Similarly, *Bacteroides splanchnicus* falls far outside the group and probably represents a new genus (77). On the other hand, *Prevotella heparinolytica* and *Prevotella zoogleoformans* cluster among the *B. fragilis* group, although they are sensitive to bile (77). Inclusion of these species warrants redefinition of the *B. fragilis* group. *B. forsythus* was recently renamed *T. forsythensis* (82). The taxonomic positions of other species still included in the genus *Bacteroides* remain uncertain, but all of these will ultimately be transferred to other genera. The genera *Prevotella* (pigmented or nonpigmented, saccharolytic organisms) and *Porphyromonas* (pigmented or nonpigmented, asaccharolytic or weakly saccharolytic organisms) were previously included in the genus *Bacteroides*. *Porphyromonas catoniae* is the only nonpigmented taxon in the genus *Porphyromonas* (96). Several new species have recently been included in these genera (41, 44, 45, 47). Animal strains of *Porphyromonas gingivalis* have been renamed *Porphyromonas gulae* (30). 16S rRNA sequencing

---

* Deceased.

TABLE 1 Differentiation of genera of gram-negative anaerobic bacteria

Characteristic	Genus
Gram-negative bacilli	
Rod-shaped cells or coccobacilli	
I. Nonmotile or peritrichous flagella	
A. Produce butyric acid (without isobutyric and isovaleric acids). .	*Fusobacterium*
B. Produce major lactic acid	*Leptotrichia*
C. Produce acetic acid and hydrogen sulfide; reduce sulfate.	*Desulfovibrio* (*piger*)
D. Not as above (A, B, or C)	*Anaerorhabdus*
	Bacteroides
	Bilophila
	Campylobacter (*gracilis*)
	Catonella
	Dialister
	Dichelobacter
	Fibrobacter
	Johnsonella
	Megamonas
	Mitsuokella
	Porphyromonas
	Prevotella
	Rikenella
	Ruminobacter
	Sebaldella
	Sutterella
	Tannerella
	Tissierella
II. Polar flagella, motile	
A. Fermentative	
1. Produce butyric acid	*Butyrivibrio*
2. Produce succinic acid	
a. Spiral-shaped cells.	*Succinivibrio*
b. Ovoid cells.	*Succinimonas*
3. Produce propionic and acetic acids	*Anaerovibrio*
B. Nonfermentative	
1. Produce succinic acid from fumarate	*Campylobacter*
2. Produce hydrogen sulfide; reduce sulfate.	*Desulfovibrio*
III. Tufts of flagella on concave side of curved cells; fermentative	*Selenomonas*
	Centipeda
IV. Bipolar tufts of flagella	*Anaerobiospirillum*
Gram-negative cocci	
Spherical or kidney bean-shaped cells	
I. Produce propionic and acetic acids.	*Veillonella*
II. Produce butyric and acetic acids.	*Acidaminococcus*
III. Produce isobutyric, butyric, isovaleric, valeric, and caproic acids.	*Megasphaera*

results have identified two closely related pigmented, bile-resistant, saccharolytic, gram-negative "species" conforming to a new genus (80). The asaccharolytic, formate- and fumarate-requiring gram-negative rods *Bacteroides ureolyticus*, *C. gracilis* (formerly *B. gracilis*), *C. curvus*, *C. rectus*, and *Sutterella wadsworthensis* are microaerophiles. *Campylobacter hominis* is a newly described anaerobic campylobacter from the human gastrointestinal tract (54). *Wolinella succinogenes*, isolated from the bovine rumen, is the only species remaining in the genus *Wolinella*. The taxonomic position of *B. ureolyticus* has remained uncertain; additional studies are required to determine whether these organisms should be transferred to the genus *Campylobacter* or if they represent a new genus. Sulfate-reducing *Desulfomonas pigra* was recently renamed *Desulfovibrio piger* and the genus *Desulfomonas* was suppressed (57).

The anaerobic, gram-negative cocci are identified presumptively on the basis of colonial and cellular morphologies, fluorescence under long-wave UV light, sensitivities to special-potency antibiotic disks, and some rapidly determined biochemical characteristics. A definite identification relies on carbohydrate fermentation test results and fatty acid profiles of metabolic end products determined by GLC.

For recent taxonomic changes see references 38, 41, 44, and 45.

DESCRIPTION OF THE GROUP

The anaerobic gram-negative bacteria are differentiated from the facultatively anaerobic bacteria by their inability to grow in the presence of oxygen and their susceptibility to metronidazole. Metronidazole resistance among anaerobes is extremely rare if proper anaerobic testing conditions are used; any unusual finding in this setting should trigger further testing. Some of the species included here are indeed microaerophiles and are often resistant to metronidazole; the appropriate atmospheric requirements should be determined for all isolates.

NATURAL HABITATS AND CLINICAL SIGNIFICANCE

Gram-negative anaerobic rods are the anaerobes most commonly encountered in clinical infections; they are found in more than half of the specimens yielding anaerobes (23, 24, 26, 45). Among the anaerobes encountered in clinical specimens, members of the bile-resistant B. fragilis group are the most commonly encountered and are more virulent and resistant to antimicrobial agents than most other anaerobes. B. fragilis and Bacteroides thetaiotaomicron are of the greatest clinical significance. They are recovered from most intra-abdominal infections and may occur in infections at other sites. Members of the B. fragilis group are major constituents of the normal colonic flora and are also found in smaller numbers in the female genital tract but are not common in the mouth or upper respiratory tract (24). B. fragilis strains producing a potent zinc-dependent metalloprotease or enterotoxin with a variety of pathological effects on intestinal mucosal cells have recently been identified (75). Enterotoxin-producing B. fragilis strains have been isolated from the intestinal tracts of young farm animals and small children with diarrhea and in cases of extra-abdominal infections including bacteremia, but they have also been isolated from fecal samples from healthy children and adults and from vaginal samples from pregnant women (49, 55, 76). Further epidemiological surveys are necessary to clarify the clinical significance of enterotoxin-producing B. fragilis findings in different populations. To date, three types of enterotoxins that have different virulences and geographical distributions have been characterized. B. splanchnicus is frequently isolated from patients with intra-abdominal infections.

The pigmented anaerobic gram-negative rods are composed of saccharolytic and asaccharolytic species of the genera Prevotella and Porphyromonas and a group of organisms probably representing a new genus and species (for an update, see references 41, 43, 44, and 80). Several species of these genera are found in human clinical specimens. Prevotella corporis, Prevotella denticola, Prevotella intermedia, Prevotella loescheii, Prevotella melaninogenica, Prevotella nigrescens, Prevotella pallens, Prevotella tannerae, Porphyromonas endodontalis, and P. gingivalis are found in the human oral cavity. Likewise, the nonpigmented species P. catoniae and nonpigmented variants of P. endodontalis are mainly encountered in the oral cavity (53, 90). Some are important pathogens in oral, dental, and bite infections and may produce infections of the head, neck, and lower respiratory tract. P. gingivalis is the putative key pathogen in aggressive forms of adult periodontitis and, together with P. endodontalis, is often involved in root canal infections and complications of these infections such as odontogenic sinusitis. Some of the above-named pigmented organisms plus Porphyromonas asaccharolytica are also prevalent in the urogenital and intestinal tracts and are important in infections arising from these sources. In addition to the P. endodontalis-like organisms and the pigmented bile-resistant organisms mentioned above, P. gingivalis has also been isolated from extraoral sources, especially from patients

with appendicitis (27, 66, 80, 94). Porphyromonas spp. of animal origin have been encountered in humans with animal bite infections (13, 27, 37, 91). Strains phenotypically similar to but genotypically different from Porphyromonas levii have been isolated from various types of human clinical infections including pleuropulmonary infections, skin and soft tissue infections, and bacterial vaginosis (46).

The bile-sensitive, nonpigmented, saccharolytic Prevotella strains recovered from human samples presently include 12 species. They are found in the same settings as the pigmented gram-negative rods (27). Prevotella bivia and Prevotella disiens are found in female patients with genital tract infections and less frequently in patients with oral infections; these strains are often resistant to the β-lactam antibiotics, including penicillin, aminopenicillins, and cephalosporins. Prevotella oris and Prevotella buccae are found in a variety of oral, pleuropulmonary (14), and other infections. The P. oralis group, which is relatively infrequently encountered in samples from humans, is now represented by P. oralis, P. veroralis, P. buccalis, and P. oulorum. The clinical significance of Prevotella enoeca from oral samples is poorly defined (72).

P. zoogleoformans (indole negative) is rarely isolated from human clinical specimens, whereas P. heparinolytica (indole positive) is often found in the oral cavity and in association with oral infections. Prevotella dentalis is a common isolate from infected root canals and from periodontal pockets. We have also encountered this organism in mandibular and gum abscesses and in sialadenitis (89). M. multiacida, a nonmotile gram-negative anaerobic rod, sometimes isolated from the intestinal tract, is not related to P. dentalis but is most closely related to Selenomonas species, which in turn seem to belong to cluster IX of the Clostridium subphylum of the gram-positive bacteria (15). The nonpigmented, saccharolytic organism Megamonas hypermegas has not, to our knowledge, been isolated from human clinical specimens.

The nonpigmented, asaccharolytic, or weakly fermentative species Anaerorhabdus furcosus, Bacteroides capillosus, Bacteroides coagulans, D. pneumosintes, Bacteroides putredinis, Desulfovibrio spp., and Tissierella praeacuta inhabit the intestinal tract and have occasionally been recovered from miscellaneous infections (40). T. forsythensis (Bacteroides forsythus), a fusiform gram-negative rod, is a putative pathogen recovered from subgingival sites in patients with periodontitis and is often isolated together with C. rectus and Fusobacterium nucleatum. Bacteroides tectus and phenotypically similar Bacteroides pyogenes are often associated with canine or feline oral flora and are prevalent in infections in humans who have sustained animal bites (2, 27, 29, 37). Bilophila wadsworthia, a bile-resistant organism, is present in small numbers in the bowel flora of healthy persons, yet it is the third most common anaerobe recovered from gangrenous or perforated appendixes and is a common constituent of the microbiota in other intra-abdominal infections. It has also been isolated from various other clinical specimens including blood, brain abscess, liver abscess, pericardial fluid, joint fluid, and pleural fluid as well as from human feces and vaginal and oral secretions (4, 6, 27, 48). B. wadsworthia is easily overlooked in cultures owing to its fastidious growth.

Members of the formate-fumarate-requiring B. ureolyticus-Campylobacter group including B. ureolyticus, C. gracilis, C. curvus, C. rectus, and S. wadsworthensis have been isolated from various types of infections. B. ureolyticus has been recovered from pulmonary, head and neck, intra-abdominal, urogenital, bone, and soft tissue infections. *C. gracilis* has been recognized as an important pathogen in serious visceral or head and neck infections and, in general, in infections above the diaphragm, and *S. wadsworthensis* is an important pathogen in infections below the diaphragm, especially abdominal infections (68, 95). *Campylobacter* spp. are primarily oral isolates found in patients with oral infections and periodontitis; *C. rectus* has been implicated as a putative pathogen at sites of active periodontal break-down (21, 92).

Fusobacterium nucleatum is the *Fusobacterium* sp. most commonly encountered in clinical infections (9, 45). This organism is found in the mouth and in the genital, gastro-intestinal, and upper respiratory tracts. It is often involved in the same types of infections as the pigmented *Prevotella* spp. and *Porphyromonas* spp. *F. nucleatum* may be found as the sole infecting agent in pleuropulmonary infections (14). *Fusobacterium necrophorum* is a very virulent anaerobe that may cause severe infection, usually in children or young adults, originating from pharyngotonsillitis, some-times in association with infectious mononucleosis (64). It was the most common anaerobe isolated from peritonsillar abscesses in young adults (42). In addition to peritonsillar abscesses, local complications include neck space infections and jugular vein septic thrombophlebitis. There may also be pleural effusion with empyema and multiple metastatic abscesses (most frequently in the lungs, pleural space, liver, and large joints) related to bacteremia (postanginal sepsis syndrome or Lemierre's disease) (64, 74). *F. necrophorum* is now encountered in serious infections much less often than it was in the era before antimicrobial agents, but this makes it more treacherous, because many clinicians may not be familiar with the syndrome. *F. necrophorum* has been sep-arated into two subspecies; *F. necrophorum* subsp. *necropho-rum* contains lipase-positive, hemagglutinin-producing bio-var A, and *F. necrophorum* subsp. *funduliforme* contains lipase-negative, non-hemagglutinin-producing biovar B. *Fusobacterium mortiferum* and *Fusobacterium varium* are mainly encountered in patients with intra-abdominal in-fections. *Fusobacterium russii* has been implicated in animal-bite infections (27), and *Fusobacterium ulcerans* is found in tropical ulcer. *Fusobacterium prausnitzii*, which is not a real fusobacterium but, rather, is related to some *Eubacterium* spp. and *Clostridium* spp., is one of the major components of fecal anaerobic flora, but little is known about its patho-genic potential.

Capnocytophaga spp. of human origin are often isolated only in anaerobic culture, and they are common in the oral cavity. *Leptotrichia buccalis* is a common mouth organism and may be found in the vagina and intestinal tract. Isola-tion of *Capnocytophaga* spp. or *Leptotrichia* spp. from blood cultures is often linked to patients (primarily adolescents) with hematological malignancies and is a direct clue to the presence of oral mucosal lesions in the patient (3, 8, 27). *Leptotrichia sanguinegens* has been isolated from cultures of blood from pregnant and elderly women and neonates (33).

Selenomonas sputigena, *Selenomonas artemidis*, *Selenomo-nas dianae*, *Selenomonas flueggei*, *Selenomonas infelix*, and *Selenomonas noxia* are all oral organisms, as is *Centipeda periodontii*, which closely resembles and phylogenetically clusters with *Selenomonas* in the *Clostridium* subphylum of the gram-positive bacteria (15, 92); these organisms are found in subgingival sites in patients with periodontitis (73, 92).

The motile organisms *Succinivibrio dextrinosolvens*, *Bu-tyrivibrio fibrisolvens*, and *Desulfovibrio* spp. including the nonmotile species *D. piger* (*D. pigra*) are found as members of the normal colonic flora but may occasionally be encoun-tered in patients with clinical infections, such as appendi-citis (4, 40). *Desulfovibrio* has been recovered in a culture of blood from an immunocompromised patient and from a pyogenic liver abscess in another patient (67, 93). The sites of normal carriage of *Anaerobiospirillum succiniciproducens* and *Anaerobiospirillum thomasii* in humans are unknown, but *Anaerobiospirillum* species are common in the fecal flora of cats and dogs (59). Strains of *Anaerobiospirillum* have been isolated from cultures of blood from compromised patients and from fecal specimens of patients with diarrhea (59, 60). In the latter case, a zoonotic role for *Anaerobiospirillum* spp. has been proposed.

Acidaminococcus fermentans, *Megasphaera elsdenii*, and *Veillonella parvula* are part of the normal human fecal flora, and *V. parvula*, as well as *V. atypica* and *V. dispar*, is part of the normal oral flora. Anaerobic gram-negative cocci are seldom pathogenic. *Veillonella* spp. are isolated more fre-quently from clinical specimens than are *Megasphaera* sp. or *Acidaminococcus* sp. *Veillonella* spp. have been encountered in patients with oral, bite-wound, head and neck, and miscellaneous soft tissue infections (45).

COLLECTION, TRANSPORT, AND STORAGE OF SPECIMENS

General guidelines for collection, transport, and storage of specimens are discussed in chapters 6 and 20. Sites normally harboring a rich indigenous flora, such as the intestinal tract or vagina, should not be sampled and cultured for anaerobes except under special circumstances and by using special methods (e.g., quantitative study of upper small bowel flora in patients with the blind loop syndrome). Lower respiratory tract specimens and endometrial samples are especially difficult to obtain without contaminating the sample with indigenous flora. Double-lumen-catheter bron-chial brushings and bronchoalveolar lavage fluid trans-ported immediately to the laboratory under anaerobic con-ditions and cultured quantitatively, as well as pleural fluid, represent good respiratory tract specimens. An endometrial suction curette (Pipelle; Unimar, Wilton, Conn.) biopsy provides a good sample from the endometrium (28). In-structions for collection of specimens from different body sites and by various methods are given in more detail elsewhere (25, 28, 36, 45).

Ulcers should be carefully debrided, and proper samples should be collected from the base or progressive edge, where bacteria actively multiply, rather than from unremoved crust or surface pus, which are often contaminated by other bacteria not reflecting the true infecting flora.

Pus, when present, is best aspirated into a syringe through a needle and injected into an anaerobic transport vial containing an oxidation-reduction indicator. Syringes used for aspiration should not be used as transporters be-cause of the potential danger of needlestick injuries or accidental expulsion and because oxygen diffuses through plastic syringes. Pieces of infected tissue obtained by exci-sion or biopsy are always preferable to pus, which is, in turn, preferable to a specimen obtained with a swab. Swabs are prone to drying and may carry a volume of sample too small to be cultured on several media or quantitatively. Tissue samples are best transported in loosely capped containers sealed in anaerobic gas-impermeable bags. For small tissue and biopsy specimens and for subgingival and root canal samples, a semisolid anaerobic transport medium in which the specimen can be submerged may be used. The dental specimens can be collected with a curette or with the use of paper points after careful removal of supragingival plaque (45). The material from currettes or the paper points are transported in a transport medium, such as VMGA III (Viability Medium, Göteborg, anaerobically prepared and sterilized), containing glass beads to facilitate dispersion of aggregates in plaque (16). In the case of failed peri-implants, the whole fixture is placed in VMGA III (45).

The conditions and time of transport should not affect the viability or relative proportions of bacteria present in the specimen if appropriate transport systems are used (7). Fast transport is important when Gram stain and culture results are needed early for guidance of therapy. Specimens should not be refrigerated, as oxygen diffuses better at lower temperatures. More detailed information on transport systems and anaerobic techniques can be found elsewhere (25, 36, 45).

DIRECT DETECTION

The following methods of direct examination may be useful for the detection of gram-negative, non-spore-forming anaerobic bacteria: macroscopic examination, Gram stain, dark-field or phase-contrast microscopy, and GLC.

The gross appearance (purulence, necrotic tissue), fluorescence of the sample under long-wave (366-nm) UV light, and the odor of the specimen can give the laboratory valuable clues to the presence of anaerobes. A fetid or putrid odor due to volatile short-chain fatty acids and amines is always associated with the presence of anaerobes in the sample. Black, necrotic tissue and/or red fluorescence of the sample may be indicative of the presence of pigmented gram-negative rods.

Molecular methods, such as nucleic acid probe hybridization, PCR amplification, and direct demonstration of nucleic acid sequences by 16S rDNA sequencing, are not yet standardized or produced for commercial distribution for the direct demonstration of medically important anaerobes from clinical specimens. However, a number of oral microbiology laboratories and commercial concerns have sets of probes designed for the identification of indicator bacteria of periodontal disease (17, 88) and nonoral gram-negative rods (79). In due time, molecular methods undoubtedly will offer a potential option when accurate identification and rapid diagnosis are indicated in laboratories supplied with the appropriate equipment, competence, and funding (see chapter 17).

Of the conventional methods, the Gram stain is by far the simplest and the most likely to yield significant information. Gram-stained smears should be prepared from all specimens accepted for anaerobic culture. The morphotypes and relative quantities of both the host and the bacterial cells present in the preparation will give clues to the presence of particular bacterial species and suggest the need for special selective media. Furthermore, the Gram stain information also provides quality control for specimen transport and isolation efficiency (28). It is recommended that direct smears be fixed in methanol for 30 s to preserve the host and bacterial cell morphologies (61). Standard Gram stain procedures and reagents are used, except that 0.5% basic fuchsin, which enhances the staining of gram-negative anaerobes, is substituted for safranin as the counterstain (45). In thick films from exudates and bloody fluids, recognition of organisms may be facilitated by staining with acridine orange. Dark-field and phase-contrast microscopy may be helpful in the detection of small, poorly staining organisms (*D. pneumosintes*), for the direct observation of motility (*Campylobacter* spp.), for the notation of spores (*Clostridium* spp.), and for the recognition of morphotypes not cultivable on ordinary media (spirochetes).

Direct gas chromatographic analysis of specimens other than blood does not add relevant information to what is obtainable from Gram-stained smears.

ISOLATION PROCEDURES AND MEDIA

The use of selective media along with nonselective media will increase the yield and save time in terms of recognition and isolation of colonies. Fresh or prereduced media (commercially available from Anaerobe Systems, Morgan Hill, Calif.) are recommended, as both considerably increase the isolation efficiency (62, 78). Nonselective media made from different basal media differ in their abilities to support the growth of certain groups of anaerobes; brucella base is superior to Trypticase soy (CDC base agar) and Schaedler base for isolation of gram-negative rods, but CDC base better supports the growth of anaerobic gram-positive cocci. Brain heart infusion base is superior to Trypticase soy in isolation efficiency for *Eubacterium* species but is inferior for pigmented gram-negative rods from subgingival and other samples (73, 86). Fastidious anaerobe agar (Lab M, Bury, England) produces luxuriant growth of fusobacteria and some formate-fumarate-requiring species and can be used as a base medium with or without selective agents. In academic centers performing large-scale anaerobic bacteriology, it would be ideal to use two different basal media to maximize isolation efficiency (28).

Isolation methods have been published elsewhere (10, 45, 81). The minimum medium setup includes (i) a nonselective, enriched, brucella base sheep blood agar plate supplemented with vitamin K₁ and hemin (BAP); (ii) a kanamycin-vancomycin laked sheep blood agar (KVLB) for the selection of *Bacteroides* and *Prevotella* spp. KVLB allows growth and rapid pigmentation of most *Prevotella* spp., but the concentration of vancomycin (7.5 µg/ml) will inhibit most *Porphyromonas* spp.; for the isolation of *Porphyromonas* spp., KVLB medium with a reduced vancomycin concentration (2 µg/ml) may be prepared; and (iii) a *Bacteroides* bile-esculin agar plate (BBE) for specimens from areas below the diaphragm for the selection and presumptive identification of the *B. fragilis* group and *Bilophila* sp. BBE and KVLB are also available as biplates. When indicated, a phenylethyl alcohol-sheep blood agar plate, used to prevent overgrowth by aerobic gram-negative rods and swarming of some clostridia, may be inoculated. When fusobacteria are clinically suspected as the cause of infection, *Fusobacterium* neomycin-vancomycin agar or *Fusobacterium* selective agar may be used (45). Also, a selective medium for culturing *Anaerobiospirillum* spp. from fecal specimens has been described (60). After inoculation, the anaerobic plates should immediately be placed in an anaerobic environment, such as an anaerobic bag, jar, or chamber. After incubation for 48 h at 36°C, the plates are examined. In routine clinical microbiology, a total incubation period of at least 7 days for primary plates is recommended. In our experience with shorter incubation times, some anaerobic species, such as *Porphyromonas* spp., may not be detected.

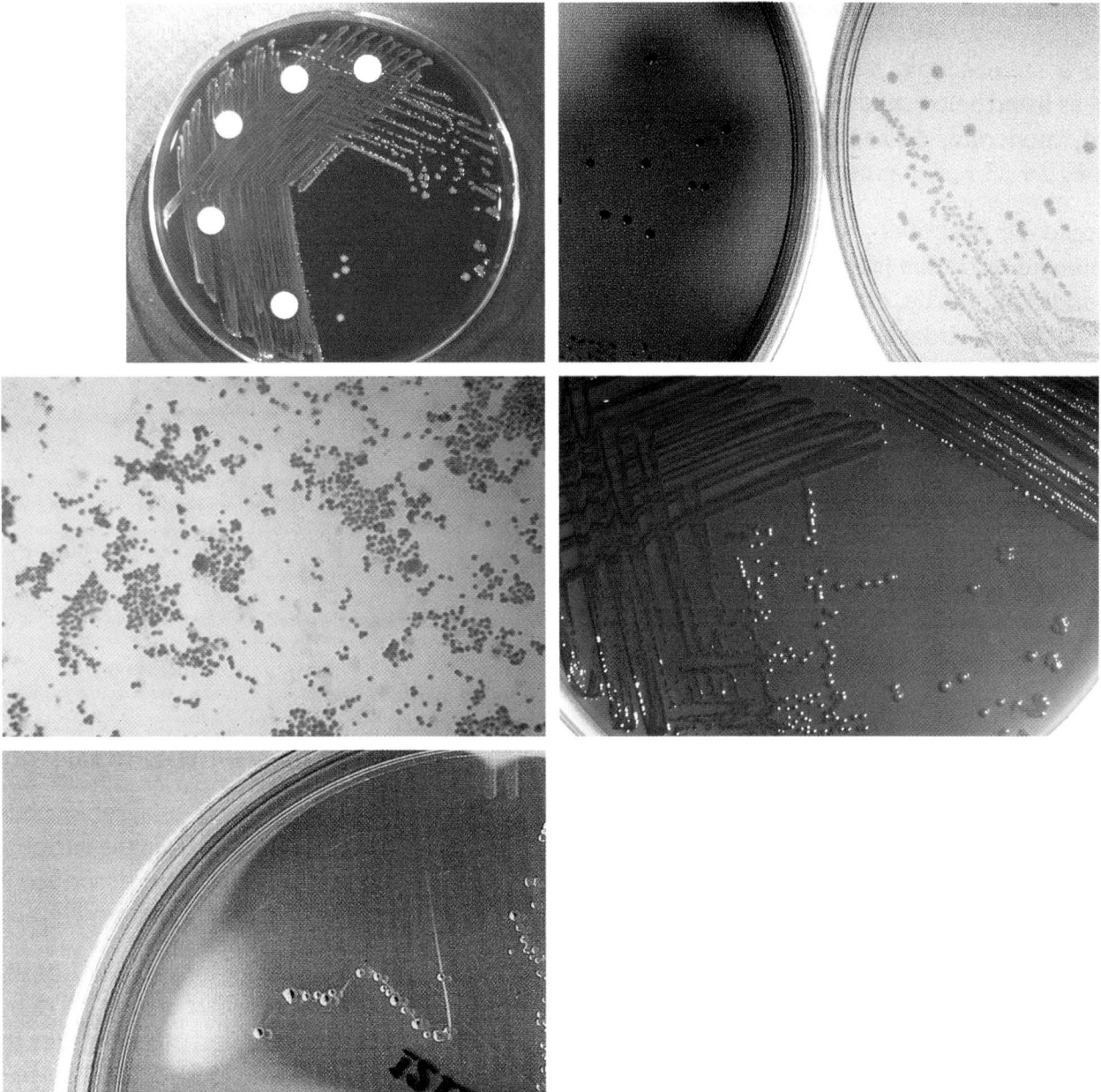

FIGURE 1 (top left)   Placement of special-potency antibiotic disks. A blank disk for indole testing may be added (usually after growth has occurred).

FIGURE 2 (top right)   Colonies of *Bacteroides fragilis* (left) and *Bacteroides vulgatus* (right) on BBE. Note the blackening of the agar and colonies due to esculin hydrolysis and bile precipitation.

FIGURE 3 (middle left)   Coccobacillary cells of *Prevotella melaninogenica*.

FIGURE 4 (middle right)   Pigmented colonies of *Porphyromonas* sp.

FIGURE 5 (bottom)   Colony morphology of *Bilophila wadsworthia* on BBE. Note the black centers.

IDENTIFICATION

Different colony types are subcultured to (i) a brucella BAP to which special-potency antibiotic disks (colistin, 10 μg; kanamycin, 1,000 μg; and vancomycin, 5 μg) are added (a nitrate disk may also be added) (Fig. 1); (ii) a chocolate agar plate that is incubated in 5 to 10% CO_2; and (iii) blood agar, which is incubated in air (for aerotolerance testing; a blood agar plate is optional, but it is useful for differentiation of *Haemophilus*, capnophilic organisms, and β-hemolysis of microaerophilic streptococci). A laked rabbit blood agar plate (LRBA) for the rapid demonstration of pigment production (laked rabbit blood agar is the most reliable and effective medium) (44) and an egg yolk agar plate (EYA) for the demonstration of lipase and proteolytic activities may also be inoculated at this point. The primary plates are reincubated along with the purity and test plates.

Preliminary Examination of Isolates

The characteristics that are noted from BAP include detailed Gram stain and colony morphology, pigment, fluorescence (long-wave UV light) (the results of last two tests are also recorded from an LRBA), hemolysis, and greening or pitting of the agar. Furthermore, the spot indole reaction (*para*-dimethylaminocinnamaldehyde reagent), the nitrate reduction test, tests for sensitivities to special-potency antibiotic disks, catalase (15% H_2O_2; preferably, colonies from EYAs are tested), and motility tests from a broth culture or plate (hanging drop or wet mount) are done with colonies from BAPs. Motile isolates are studied further as indicated in Table 1; most often, these will be *Campylobacter* spp. Another approach is the use of Lombard-Dowell Presumpto plates (Presumpto I, II, and III plates; available from Remel Laboratories and Anaerobe Systems [as monoplates on request]) developed at the Centers for Disease Control and Prevention; these may give additional important information for the presumptive identification of the anaerobic gram-negative rods (22). Good growth is necessary for the proper interpretation of test results on this medium.

The primary plates are reinspected after 4 or more days to detect slow growers, new morphotypes, or late pigmenters. In oral microbiology laboratories, two rapid in situ tests have been used. The rapid differentiation of lactose-fermenting species from lactose-nonfermenting species is determined by applying 4-methylumbelliferyl-D-galactoside reagent (catalog no. M-1633; Sigma Chemical Co., St. Louis, Mo.) to the colonies and screening for fluorescent (lactose-positive) colonies under long-wave UV light (1). The carboxy-L-arginine-7-amino-4-methylcoumarin amide HCl (CAAM) test demonstrates the trypsin-like activities of suspected colonies of *P. gingivalis*; the colonies are treated with the CAAM reagent (catalog no. C-9396; Sigma) and screened for blue-white fluorescence under long-wave UV light (87).

Presumptive Identification of Species

Most of the clinically significant gram-negative rods can be placed into broad groups with relatively few tests, and some can be presumptively identified with ease (Table 2). The special-potency antibiotic disk pattern can be used to separate the gram-negative rods into several groups. A zone size equal to or greater than 10 mm is considered to indicate a sensitive isolate (45).

Most of the *Bacteroides* and *Prevotella* spp. are resistant to vancomycin and kanamycin and are variable in sensitivity to colistin; *Porphyromonas* spp. are generally sensitive to vancomycin and resistant to colistin. The *B. fragilis* group can be identified presumptively by their special-potency antibiotic disk pattern (resistant to the antibiotics in all three disks) and by growth equal to or greater than the control growth in 20% bile, as determined by a tube test, by a bile disk test (45), or on BBE (Fig. 2). Coccobacillary organisms that fluoresce red or produce black colonies are in the pigmented *Prevotella* spp.-*Porphyromonas* spp. group (Fig. 3 and 4).

Fusobacterium spp., *B. ureolyticus*, *Campylobacter* spp., *Bilophila* sp., *Sutterella* sp., and *Leptotrichia* spp. are resistant to vancomycin but sensitive to both colistin and kanamycin. *B. ureolyticus*, *Campylobacter*, *Bilophila*, and *Sutterella* colonies are usually much smaller and more translucent than those of fusobacteria; *Leptotrichia* colonies are large and gray and have a convoluted ("brain surface") texture. Furthermore, the most commonly encountered fusobacteria, *F. nucleatum* and *F. necrophorum*, are indole positive and nitrate negative. On microscopic inspection, fusobacteria are usually bigger than the other bacteria with the same identification disk profile, excluding the large tapered cells of *Leptotrichia*. An anaerobic, gram-negative, catalase-negative rod that requires formate and fumarate for growth in broth culture or that pits agar may be presumptively identified as *B. ureolyticus* or a *Campylobacter* sp.; *B. ureolyticus* is urease positive (Table 2, footnote *d*). To document the formate-fumarate requirement, inoculate one tube of peptone yeast (or thioglycolate) broth medium containing the additive (0.3%) and one tube not containing the additive (control) (Table 2, footnote *b*). Compare the intensity of growth. A strongly catalase-positive, bile-resistant, often urease-positive gram-negative rod can be presumptively identified as *Bilophila* sp. (Fig. 5). Microaerophilic and catalase- and urease-negative but bile-resistant organisms growing in *Campylobacter* atmosphere (2 to 6% oxygen) are probably *S. wadsworthensis*.

Desulfovibrio piger (*Desulfomonas pigra*) (nonmotile), other *Desulfovibrio* spp. (motile), and the capnophilic, often yellow-pigmented *Capnocytophaga* spp. are resistant to vancomycin and colistin but sensitive to kanamycin. *Desulfovibrio* cells are curved or spiral; *Capnocytophaga* cells resemble fusobacteria with tapered ends. *Selenomonas* spp. may have the same special-potency disk patterns as *Desulfovibrio* and *Capnocytophaga* spp., but we have also encountered strains that are sensitive to colistin. *Selenomonas* cells are curved and motile, as are those of *C. periodontii*, a closely related species that forms swarming colonies.

Most organisms not fitting the above-described groupings are *Bacteroides* spp. or *Prevotella* spp. but occasionally are representatives of the other genera listed in Table 1.

Gram-negative cocci are sensitive to colistin and usually to kanamycin but are resistant to vancomycin. Small, gram-negative cocci that reduce nitrate or nitrite and that grow as small grayish white, translucent colonies that may fluoresce red under UV light can be presumptively identified as *Veillonella* spp.

Rapid Identification

Whenever possible, simple tests should be used for the rapid and, to the extent that they permit, definitive identification of anaerobes (5). These include tests for colony and microscopic morphologies; the spot indole, catalase, lipase, and lecithinase tests; the nitrate disk test; the bile disk test; growth stimulation tests; and tests for sensitivities to special-potency antibiotic disks. Furthermore, rapid tests based on the presence of preformed enzymes produce clinically meaningful results in a timely fashion (see "Other Approaches to Identification"). Tables 2 to 8 incorporate the results of these tests; they can be used for the rapid identification of many commonly encountered anaerobic gram-negative rods and cocci.

Identification of the most commonly encountered bile-resistant members of the *B. fragilis* group is based on the special-potency disk profile and the results of a few tests that can be performed rapidly, including the catalase, indole, esculin, and α-fucosidase tests (Table 3, footnote *b*). On these grounds the members of this group can be reported as *B. fragilis* group, most closely related to *B. fragilis*, or other organisms in this group according to the reactions obtained (Tables 2 and 3). Further tests are performed when indicated. *Porphyromonas* spp. are easily identified even to the species level with the aid of the special-potency disk profile and the results of a few tests including the indole, catalase, lipase, and some rapid enzyme tests (see Tables 2 and 6) (44, 94). An indole- and lipase-positive coccobacillus that forms black-pigmented colonies or that fluoresces red may be identified as *P. intermedia/P. nigrescens* group; *Prevotella pallens* resembles these two species but has lighter pigment and is lipase negative (50, 51). We have also encountered a few *P. asaccharolytica* strains that are lipase positive. A rapid enzyme test for α-glucosidase (with Rosco Diagnostic Tablets [Taastrup, Denmark] or the WEE-Tabs system [Key Scientific Products, Round Rock, Tex.]) is helpful; *P. intermedia/P. nigrescens* and *P. pallens* are positive, and *P. asaccharolytica* is negative. Furthermore, *P. asaccharolytica* is generally sensitive to the special-potency vancomycin disk. Any indole-negative strains must be identified further by other biochemical tests. A lipase-positive, indole-negative, pigmented gram-negative rod could be either *P. loescheii* or Virginia Polytechnic Institute "*Prevotella* DIC-20" genospecies (97).

B. ureolyticus, *C. gracilis*, other "anaerobic" *Campylobacter* spp., and *Sutterella* sp. are thin gram-negative rods with rounded ends that produce the *Fusobacterium* disk pattern. The colonies are small and translucent or transparent and may produce greening of the agar. Three colony morphotypes exist: smooth and convex, pitting (Fig. 6), and spreading. All colony types can occur in the same culture. These organisms are asaccharolytic and nitrate or nitrate reducing, and they require supplementation of broth media with formate and fumarate for growth (Table 2, footnote *b*). *C. rectus*, *C. curvus*, *C. concisus*, and *C. showae* are motile and oxidase positive; unlike the first three, *C. showae* is catalase positive. *C. gracilis* is nonmotile and urease negative and, thus, is differentiated from urease-positive *B. ureolyticus* (Table 2, footnotes *d* and *e*). *Bilophila* sp., which phenotypically resembles *B. ureolyticus*, is distinguished from the above-mentioned species by its resistance to bile and its strong catalase reaction. *Sutterella* sp. is also resistant to bile but is urease and catalase negative, whereas *Bilophila* is catalase positive and usually urease positive (95).

F. nucleatum is a thin rod with tapering ends (Fig. 7) and is indole positive. The needle-shaped morphology is shared with the microaerophilic, indole-negative *Capnocytophaga* spp. and *Leptotrichia* spp., as discussed above. *F. nucleatum* fluoresces chartreuse under UV light and often produces greening of the agar after exposure to air. At least three different colony morphotypes of *F. nucleatum* exist (20, 31). Due to considerable phenotypic and genotypic heterogeneity and uncertainty of valid criteria for the separation of the *F. nucleatum* subspecies, it is hard to judge whether the reported colonial morphologies consistently coincide with the subspecies designations. *F. nucleatum* subsp. *nucleatum* colonies may be small, grayish white, and smooth; *F. nucleatum* subsp. *fusiforme* colonies may also be small (<0.5 to 1 mm), granular, and irregular (bread crumb shaped) (Fig. 8); and *F. nucleatum* subsp. *polymorphum* colonies often are large, speckled, smooth, translucent, and butyrous. *F. necrophorum* subsp. *necrophorum* is lipase positive and usually bile sensitive. It is a pleomorphic long rod with round ends and

often has bizarre forms. It produces indole, fluoresces chartreuse, produces greening of the agar, and often demonstrates beta-hemolysis around the grayish to yellow dull, umbonate colonies (Fig. 9). Lipase-negative strains require further biochemical testing. *F. mortiferum* is indole negative and extremely pleomorphic; it has filaments containing swollen areas with large, round bodies and exhibiting irregular staining (Fig. 10). *F. necrophorum* may have a similar morphology but usually has fewer round bodies. A bile-resistant fusobacterium isolated from BBE may be identified as *F. mortiferum* or *F. varium*; *F. mortiferum* is positive for *o*-nitrophenyl-β-D-galactopyranoside (Table 3, footnote *b*), whereas *F. varium* is negative.

Small, gram-negative cocci that fluoresce red under UV light and that reduce nitrate or nitrite are probably *Veillonella* spp. *Megasphaera* cells are large (>1.5 μm). *Megasphaera* and *Acidaminococcus* colonies do not fluoresce.

Definitive Identification

A definitive identification of an anaerobic isolate should be obtained for all isolates from blood, spinal fluid, and organs or body cavities; when the patient is gravely ill and not responding to treatment; and when a prolonged and expensive treatment is indicated. Definitive identification is also indicated in unusual case presentations, when a nosocomial infection is suspected, and in some teaching-hospital settings.

The definitive identification of most species requires certain additional biochemical tests, metabolic end product analysis, and/or cell wall fatty acid profiling by GLC (45). Even in good research or reference laboratories, a percentage of strains will not be identified definitively. If such strains are isolated from blood or closed-space infections, molecular methods such as 16S rRNA sequencing may prove helpful if it is available or provided by a referral laboratory. Curved rods that are not *Campylobacter* spp. should be checked for motility and identified as set out in Table 1. Organisms with small, translucent, spreading colonies that are not *B. ureolyticus*-like should also be checked for motility. Very large fusiform rods that are isolated from the mouth or urogenital tract and that have one pointed end, one blunt end, and gray, relatively large, sometimes spreading, convoluted colonies (often growing on neomycin-vancomycin agar on primary isolation) are suggestive of *Leptotrichia* spp. The characteristic GLC pattern shows major amounts of lactic acid. The results in Tables 3 to 8 are based on reactions in prereduced, anaerobically sterilized (PRAS) liquid media (34, 45). A shortened and simplified scheme (arabinose, trehalose, rhamnose, and xylan tests) for the identification of the *B. fragilis* group with commercial PRAS biochemicals and the addition of bromthymol blue at 24 h postincubation has been described (12). **Do not interpret the results from other systems with the tables given here.** Gas chromatographic analysis may be performed on broth that shows good growth of the organism (34, 45). Each lot of uninoculated broth must be assayed in parallel with samples to determine the background amounts of acetic and succinic acids, and if chopped-meat broth is used, an uninoculated broth is assayed for lactic acid. Fermentation end products vary depending on the substrate available to the organism. Use of substrates other than those on which the results in the identification tables are based may lead to misinterpretation of the GLC pattern and misidentification of the organism. For instance, saccharolytic organisms produce larger amounts of isoacids in the absence of a fermentable

TABLE 2 Group identification of anaerobic gram-negative rods[a]

Species	Vancomycin (5 μg)	Kanamycin (1,000 μg)	Colistin (10 μg)	Growth in 20% bile	Catalase	Indole
B. fragilis group	R	R	R	+	V	V
Other Bacteroides spp.	R	R	V	−[+]	−[+]	V
Pigmented species	V	R	V	−	−[+]	V
Porphyromonas spp.	S	R	R	−	V	+[−]
Prevotella spp.	R	R[S]	V	−	−	V
P. intermedia-P. nigrescens-P. pallens	R	R[S]	S	−	−	+
P. loescheii	R	R	V	−	−	−
Other Prevotella sp.	R	R	V	−	−[+]	−[+]
Campylobacter spp./B. ureolyticus	R	S	S	−	−[+]	−
B. ureolyticus	R	S	S	−	−	−
Campylobacter spp.[g]	R	S	S	−	−	−
C. gracilis	R	S	S	−	−	−
Sutterella sp.	R	S	S	+	−	−
Bilophila sp.[h]	R	S	S	+	+	−
Desulfovibrio piger[i]	R	S	R	V	V	−
Desulfovibrio spp.[i]	R	S	R	V	V	−
Fusobacterium spp.	R	S	S	V	−	V
F. nucleatum	R	S	S	−	−	+
F. necrophorum	R	S	S	−[+]	−	+
F. varium/F. mortiferum	R	S	S	+	−	V
Capnocytophaga spp.	R	S	R	−	−	−
Leptotrichia spp.	R	S	S	+[−]	−	−
Selenomonas spp.	R	S	R	−	−	−
Veillonella spp.	R	S	S	−	V	−

[a] R, resistant; S, susceptible; R[S], most strains resistant, some strains susceptible; V, variable; +, positive reaction for majority of strains; −, negative reaction; +[−], most strains positive; −[+], most strains negative, some strains positive.

[b] Compare the growth of the organism in an unsupplemented thioglycolate broth with growth in a broth supplemented with formate and fumarate additive: dissolve 3 g of sodium formate, 3 g of fumaric acid, and 20 pellets of sodium hydroxide in 50 ml of distilled water; adjust the pH to 7; and filter sterilize. Add 0.5 ml of additive to 10 ml of culture broth (34, 45).

[c] Use the spot nitrate disk test (45).

[d] Make a heavy suspension of the organism in 0.5 ml of sterile urea broth (Difco Laboratories, Detroit, Mich.) or in sterile water and insert a urea tablet (Rosco Diagnostic Tablets [Rosco] or WEE-Tabs [Key Scientific Products]). Incubate the tubes aerobically for up to 24 h. A bright pink or red is positive; this color usually appears within 15 to 30 min.

carbohydrate, and a fermentable carbohydrate is required for the detection of lactic acid.

Colonies of the B. fragilis group on brucella BAP are 2 to 3 mm in diameter, circular, entire, convex, and gray to white. The cells may be uniform, bipolarly stained, or pleomorphic (some may contain vacuoles) (Fig. 11); this difference is medium and age dependent. The presence of ovoid cells suggests B. ovatus. Good growth in or stimulation by 20% bile (2% oxgall) is characteristic of the B. fragilis group; the exception to this rule is the poor growth of B. uniformis in bile. Some organisms not belonging to the B. fragilis group (non-B. fragilis group) are bile resistant.

TABLE 3 Characteristics of B. fragilis group and B. splanchnicus[a]

Species	Growth on BBE	Indole	Catalase	Esculin hydrolysis	α-Fucosidase[b]
B. caccae[d]	+	−	−[+]	+	+
B. distasonis[e]	+	−	+[−]	+	−
B. fragilis[d]	+	−	+	+	+
B. merdae[e]	+	−	−[+]	+	−
B. vulgatus	+	−	−[+]	−[+]	+
B. eggerthii	+	+	−	+	−
B. ovatus	+	+	+[−]	+	+[−]
B. stercoris	+	+	−	+[−]	V
B. thetaiotaomicron	+	+	+	+	+
B. uniformis	W[+]	+	−[+]	+	+[−]
B. splanchnicus	+	+	−	+	+

[a] +, Positive reaction for the majority of strains; −, negative reaction; V, variable reaction; W, weak reaction; +[−], most strains positive; −[+], most strains negative, some strains positive; −[w], most strains negative, some strains weakly positive. For sugars: +, pH < 5.5; W, pH 5.5 to 5.8; −, pH > 5.8.

[b] Make a heavy suspension (heavier than a McFarland no. 2 standard) of the organism in 0.25 ml of sterile saline. Insert a tablet of substrate (Rosco Diagnostic Tablets or WEE-Tabs). Incubate for 4 h (or overnight). Yellow color, positive; colorless, negative.

Lipase	Pigment	Red fluorescence	Growth stimulated by formate-fumarate[b]	Nitrate reduction[c]	Urease[d]	Motility[e]	Pitting of agar[f]	Slender cells with pointed ends
−		−						
−								
V	+	+[-]						
−[+]	+[-]	+[-]						
V	+	+						
+[-]	+	+						
V	+	+						
−[+]	−	−						
−			+	+	V	V	V	
−			+	+	+	−	V	
−			+	+	−	+[-]	V	
−			+	+	−	−	V	
−			+	+	−	−	V	
−			−	+	+[-]	−	−	
−			−	−[+]	−[+]	−	−	
−			−	V	−[+]	+	−	
V								V
−				−				+
+[-]				−				−
−								−
−				+				

[e] Check motility with a young broth culture supplemented with formate and fumarate.
[f] Formate and fumarate should be added to broth media for this group of organisms.
[g] C. rectus, C. curvus, and C. showae.
[h] Growth stimulated by 1% pyruvate (final concentration).
[i] Desulfoviridin positive. Inoculate a tube of liquid medium supplemented with 1% pyruvate and 0.25% magnesium sulfate. Incubate until the turbidity indicates good growth. Centrifuge the tube to obtain a pellet. Pipette a heavy drop of the pellet onto a slide. Add a drop of 2 N NaOH to the pellet, and immediately observe under long-wave (366 nm) UV light. Positive, red fluorescence; negative, no fluorescence.

These include B. splanchnicus, B. tectus, B. pyogenes, M. multiacida, Bilophila sp., a newly described pigmented gram-negative rod (80), and some fusobacteria. Not all of these, however, grow on BBE. Morphologic characteristics, special-potency identification disks, and some biochemical reactions differentiate these species. Most of the B. fragilis group organisms blacken the BBE (esculin hydrolyzed), although B. vulgatus may not hydrolyze esculin. Table 3 is a key for the differentiation of members of the bile-resistant B. fragilis group.

Members of the non-B. fragilis group, nonpigmented anaerobic gram-negative rods, form three major subgroups:

Arabinose	Cellobiose	Rhamnose	Salicin	Sucrose	Trehalose	Xylose	Xylan	Fatty acids from PYG[c]
+	+[-]	+[-]	−[+]	+	+	+	−	A, p, S, (iv)
−[+]	+	V	+	+	+	+	−	A, p, S, (pa, ib, iv, l)
−	+[-]	−	−	+	−	+	−	A, p, S, pa, (ib, iv, l)
−[+]	V	+	+	+	+	+	−	A, p, S, (ib, iv)
+	−	+	−	+	−	+	−[+]	A, p, S
+	−[+]	+[-]	−	−	−	+	+	A, p, S, (ib, iv, l)
+	+	+	+	+	+	+	+	A, p, S, pa, (ib, iv, l)
−[+]	−[+]	+	−[+]	+	−	+	V	A, p, S, (ib, iv)
+	+[-]	+	−[+]	+	+	+	−	A, p, S, pa, (ib, iv, l)
+	+	−[+]	+[-]	+	−[w]	+	V	a, p, l, S, (ib, iv)
+	−	−	−	−	−	−	−	A, P, S, ib, b, iv, (l)

Fermentation of:

[c] Capital letters indicate major metabolic products from peptone-yeast-glucose (PYG), lowercase letters indicate minor products, and parentheses indicate a variable reaction for the following fatty acids: A, acetic; P, propionic; IB, isobutyric; B, butyric; IV, isovaleric; V, valeric; L, lactic; S, succinic; PA, phenylacetic. Note that isoacids are primarily from carbohydrate-free media (e.g., peptone-yeast extract) in the case of saccharolytic organisms.
[d] B. caccae is L-arabinose positive with Rosco Diagnostic Tablets; B. fragilis is negative.
[e] B. merdae is β-glucuronidase-positive with Rosco Diagnostic Tablets; B. distasonis is negative.

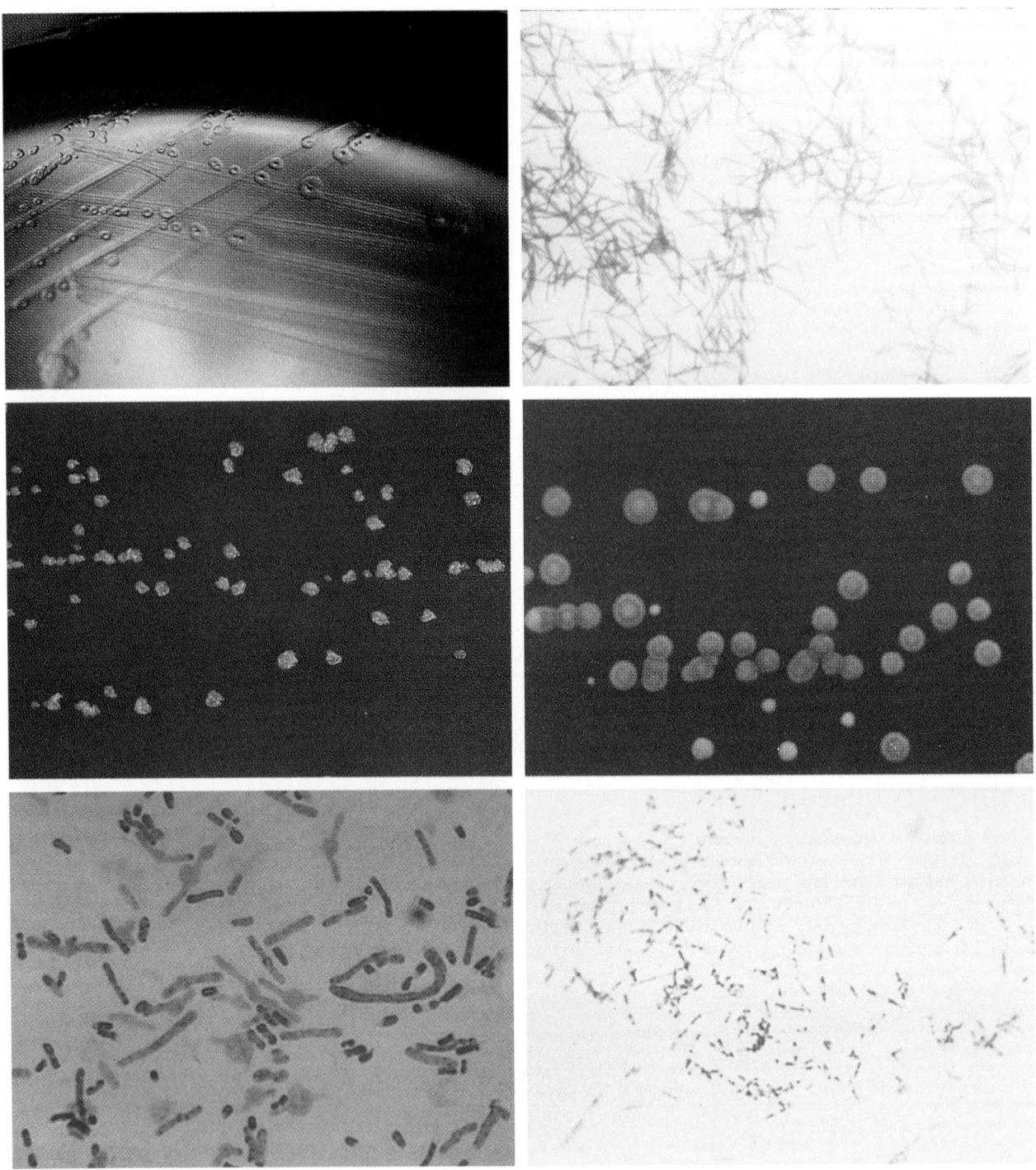

FIGURE 6 (top left)   Pitting colonies of *Bacteroides ureolyticus*.

FIGURE 7 (top right)   Cells of *Fusobacterium nucleatum*. Note the slender shape with pointed ends.

FIGURE 8 (middle left)   Bread crumb-shaped colonies of *Fusobacterium nucleatum*. Note the greening of the agar.

FIGURE 9 (middle right)   Umbonate colonies of *Fusobacterium necrophorum*.

FIGURE 10 (bottom left)   Microscopic morphology of *Fusobacterium mortiferum*. There is marked pleomorphism and irregularity of staining. Note the filaments with swellings along their course.

FIGURE 11 (bottom right)   Pleomorphic, irregularly staining cells of *Bacteroides fragilis*.

(i) saccharolytic, (ii) saccharolytic and proteolytic, and (iii) asaccharolytic. Tables 4 and 5 list the more commonly encountered or clinically important species in this group.

The saccharolytic organisms fall into two categories, i.e., pentose fermenters and nonfermenters (arabinose and xylose are usually tested). Pentose fermentation may be difficult to demonstrate owing to suboptimal growth in the test medium; therefore, a screening test for the presence of the preformed enzyme β-xylosidase is recommended (for the procedure see Table 3, footnote b). P. oris and P. buccae are pentose fermenters (Table 4). They are phenotypically very similar but can be differentiated by the α-fucosidase and N-acetyl-β-glucosaminidase tests (Table 3, footnote b) (19); furthermore, P. buccae is usually sensitive to the special-potency colistin disk, whereas P. oris is not. P. zoogleoformans and P. heparinolytica may also ferment pentoses. Both produce viscous material in broth cultures, and on solid media the colonies often adhere to the agar. The positive indole reaction of P. heparinolytica differentiates these two species. The indole production is sometimes very difficult to demonstrate and should be tested from a pure culture on an EYA and/or from an old (>5-day-old) culture because it tends to be a weak reaction. Other pentose fermenters include bile-resistant M. multiacida and B. splanchnicus and bile-sensitive P. dentalis. Unlike most Prevotella and Bacteroides species, M. multiacida is both nitrate and inositol positive. P. dentalis forms characteristic, "water-drop," viscous colonies on blood agar. A positive N-acetyl-β-glucosaminidase reaction differentiates it from P. buccae, and a negative α-fucosidase reaction differentiates it from P. oris. The far better growth of P. dentalis on CDC blood agar than on brucella blood agar is an additional feature to facilitate the identification of the species.

Salicin, cellobiose, xylan, and sucrose are the key sugars in the differentiation of P. oralis, P. buccalis, P. veroralis, P. oulorum, and P. enoeca (Table 4). Furthermore, P. oulorum produces catalase and is lipase positive (71). Certain strains of the saccharolytic pigmented Prevotella spp. require more than 21 days to develop pigment, and these strains (especially P. loescheii) closely resemble P. veroralis. Darker, more opaque colonies and salicin and cellobiose reactions may aid in differentiation of the strains. It has been reported that P. loescheii, P. tannerae, "Prevotella sp. strain DIC-20," and some strains of P. melaninogenica, P. denticola, P. enoeca, and P. veroralis cannot be differentiated by conventional biochemical tests; cellular fatty acid analysis was the only reliable method for the separation of these species (70, 72, 97).

P. bivia and P. disiens are both saccharolytic and strongly proteolytic (Table 4). Gelatin and milk are usually digested within 2 to 3 days (milk digestion may take longer). Differentiation is based on lactose fermentation; P. bivia is lactose positive, and P. disiens is lactose negative. Furthermore, P. bivia is both N-acetyl-β-glucosaminidase and α-fucosidase positive, but P. disiens is negative for both. Under long-wave UV light, P. bivia and P. disiens colonies may fluoresce light orange to pink (coral), and P. disiens also may produce a brown pigment on LRBA that makes differentiation from the phenotypically similar P. corporis difficult. P. bivia and P. enoeca share the same phenotypic characteristics, but P. enoeca is gelatin negative; it is usually isolated from oral or oral-associated sources, whereas P. bivia is more often found in nonoral samples.

Asaccharolytic, nonpigmented Anaerorhabdus spp., Bacteroides spp., and Tissierella spp. are infrequently isolated from clinical specimens (Table 5). B. capillosus coagulates

milk, and may grow better with Tween 80-supplemented media. D. pneumosintes is a very tiny rod best seen by darkfield examination (it almost resembles Veillonella spp. by Gram staining) and forms minute colonies that may require magnification to be seen. T. forsythensis (B. forsythus) is a fusiform rod that exhibits a wide variety of enzyme activities including trypsin-like activity and N-acetyl-β-glucosaminidase, α-fucosidase, and β-glucuronidase activities. However, its growth is minimal in broth media, and it requires N-acetylmuramic acid; therefore, it is often seen as satellite colonies around colonies of other organisms, especially fusobacteria. Desulfovibrio spp. are sulfate-reducing bacteria and can be confirmed by the desulfoviridin test (Table 2, footnote i). The species are motile (except for recently included D. piger) and produce copious amounts of H_2S.

The pigmented Prevotella spp. and Porphyromonas spp. (Table 6) vary greatly in the degree and rapidity of pigment production, depending primarily on the type of blood and the composition of the base medium used in the agar. A period of 2 to 21 days may be required even on LRBA to detect pigmentation, which ranges from buff to tan to black. The identities of strains not showing pigmentation within 21 days must be established by other biochemical tests to avoid confusion with the P. oralis group of organisms. The pigmented Prevotella and Porphyromonas spp. fluoresce pink, orange, or brick red under UV light. Fluorescence is best demonstrated in young cultures; in older cultures, especially on laked blood agar, the fluorescence is more or less masked depending on the intensity of pigment production (44).

The indole-positive species P. intermedia and P. nigrescens produce dark pigment; the pigment produced by P. pallens is lighter. The use of oligonucleotide probes or determination of arbitrarily primed PCR and enzyme electrophoretic mobility profiles are needed for species differentiation (51, 66). The unusual special-potency antibiotic disk pattern (sensitivity to vancomycin), in addition to asaccharolytic properties, separates most Porphyromonas spp. from the other pigment producers. P. asaccharolytica, P. endodontalis, and P. gingivalis are all asaccharolytic and phenotypically very similar. The key differential tests include tests for phenylacetic acid production, trypsin-like activity, and N-acetyl-β-glucosaminidase and α-fucosidase activities (Table 6). Unlike most Porphyromonas spp., P. catoniae, P. levii, and P. levii-like organisms (frequently isolated from human clinical specimens) are indole negative and weakly saccharolytic; the latter characteristic is also shared with the animal strains of Porphyromonas macacae. Most of the Porphyromonas spp. of animal origin are differentiated from the human strains by a positive catalase reaction; Porphyromonas crevioricanis, however, is catalase negative (44).

Table 7 characterizes the more commonly isolated fusobacteria. The conversion of threonine and lactate to propionic acid is important in the differentiation of these species. Bizarre pleomorphic rods with very large round bodies are suggestive of F. mortiferum (Fig. 10). This organism may grow on BBE and turn the agar black. F. ulcerans, isolated from tropical ulcer, closely resembles F. mortiferum but is esculin negative. F. periodonticum, an oral isolate, is indole positive and bile sensitive and converts threonine but not lactate to propionate. Contrary to earlier reports, we have failed to demonstrate glucose, fructose, or galactose fermentation by the type strain; this bacterium is indistinguishable from F. nucleatum. Fusobacterium russii is indole

TABLE 4 Characteristics of nonpigmented saccharolytic *Prevotella* spp. and other genera[a]

Subgroup and species	Growth in 20% bile	Indole	Esculin hydrolysis	α-Fucosidase[b]	ONPG[c] (β-galactosidase)[b]	N-Acetyl-β-glucosaminidase[b]	β-Xylosidase[b]
Pentose fermenters							
M. *multiacida*	+	−	+	+	+	+	+
P. *buccae*	−	−	+	−	+	−	+
P. *dentalis*	−	−	V	−	+	+	V
P. *heparinolytica*[e]	−	+	+	+	+	+	+
P. *oris*	−	−	+	+	+	+	+
P. *zoogleoformans*[e]	−	−	+	+	+	+	+
Not pentose fermenters							
P. *buccalis*	−	−	+	+	+	+	−
P. *enoeca*	−	−	V	+	+	+	−
P. *oralis*	−	−	+	+	+	+	−[f]
P. *oulorum*[g]	−	−	+	−	+	+	−
P. *veroralis*	−	−	+	+	+	+	−
Proteolytic							
P. *bivia*	−	−	−	+	+	+	−
P. *disiens*	−	−	−	−	−	−	−
Capnocytophaga spp.	−	−	+[−]				
Leptotrichia buccalis	+[−]	−	+				
Leptotrichia sanguinegens		−	+				
Selenomonas sp.	−	−	V				

[a] See Table 3, footnote *a*.
[b] See Table 3, footnote *b*.
[c] ONPG, *o*-nitrophenyl-β-D-galactopyranoside.
[d] See Table 3, footnote *c*.

negative and does not convert lactate or threonine to propionate.

Veillonella spp. are nonfermentative and produce acetic and propionic acids (Table 8). A. *fermentans* produces acetic and butyric acids. M. *elsdenii* ferments glucose and produces multiple fatty acids, including caproic acid.

Other Approaches to Identification

Several microsystems for the identification of anaerobes are currently available. The API 20A system (bioMérieux Vitek, Hazelwood, Mo.) and the Minitek system (Becton Dickinson MicroSystems, Cockeysville, Md.) are microtube biochemical systems that produce results in 24 to 48 h and have computerized databases. The API 20A and Minitek systems are best suited for identification of saccharolytic, fast-growing organisms such as members of the B. *fragilis* group and many clostridia. Most asaccharolytic organisms cannot be identified by these systems, and some fastidious organisms (e.g., some *Prevotella* spp.) fail to grow in them. Even for many saccharolytic organisms, supplemental tests, including GLC, are often required for definitive identification. The color reactions in both of these systems are not always clear-cut, as shades of brown or no color (API 20A system) and yellow-orange (Minitek system) can make interpretation of the test results difficult.

The rapid (2- to 4-h) identification systems based on detection of preformed (constitutive) enzymes by use of chromogenic or fluorogenic substrates, or a combination of both, include the RapID ANA II system (Innovative Diagnostic Systems, Inc., Norcross, Ga.), the Rapid ID 32A system (bioMérieux, Marcy l'Etoile, France), the ANI Card, AN-IDent, and API ZYM systems (bioMérieux Vitek), the MicroScan system (Dade Behring MicroScan,

Inc., Sacramento, Calif.), and the BBL Crystal Anaerobe (ANR) Identification (ID) system (Becton Dickinson Diagnostic Systems, Franklin Lakes, N.J.), as mentioned in chapter 14. The overall performance of these systems has varied from moderate to good; 53 to 100% of the isolates are identified to the species level (11, 18, 39, 56, 65, 83). The Crystal Anaerobe (ANR) Identification (ID) system was reported to identify 91% of the B. *fragilis* group and all of the *Prevotella* and *Porphyromonas* strains tested to the species level; 53% of the non-B. *fragilis* group *Bacteroides* spp. were identified correctly (11). The Rapid ID 32A system was found to be 78.4 to 90.6% accurate for the B. *fragilis* group (39, 56); a supplemental test for catalase activity increased the accuracy to 94.6% (39). The Rapid ID 32A system identified 95.5% of the fusobacteria correctly (56); however, poor discrimination between F. *nucleatum* and F. *necrophorum* has been noted (18). Similarly, the Rapid ID 32A system accurately assigned *Prevotella* and *Porphyromonas* species to the genus level, but it less accurately differentiated between the species (18). The RapID ANA II system identified 62% of the gram-negative rods correctly (65). Use of the rapid identification systems is indicated when an identification is not achieved by using the tests described in "Rapid Identification" but before more time-consuming tests, such as fermentation tests and GLC, are used. These systems are also suited for the identification of slowly growing fastidious gram-negative rods and cocci, since no growth in the test medium is required. When using rapid identification systems, all the information available on the organism should be considered. The performance of all these systems is, of course, affected by the source and nature of the isolates; the accuracy can be further increased by certain simple supplemental tests and

Fermentation of:								Fatty acids from PYG[d]
Arabinose	Cellobiose	Glucose	Lactose	Salicin	Sucrose	Xylose	Xylan	
+	+	+	+	+	+	+		A, L, S
+	+	+	+	+	+	+		A, S, (p, ib, b, iv)
+	+	+	+	−	W	V		A, S
+	+	+	+	+	+	+		A, p, S, (iv)
+⁻	+	+	+	+	+	+		A, S, (p, ib, iv)
V	+	+	+	V	+	V		A, P, S, (ib, iv)
−	+	+	+	−	+	−	−	a, iv, S
−	−	+	+	−	−	−		a, S
−	+	+	+	+	+	−	−	A, S, (l)
−	−	+	+	−	+	−	−	A, S
−	+	+	+	−	+	−	+	a, S
−	−	+	+	−	−	−		A, iv, S, (ib)
−	−	+	−	−	−	−		A, S, (p, ib, iv)
−	−⁺	+	V	−	+	−		A, S
−⁺	+⁻	+	+⁻	+⁻	+	−		L, (a, s)
−	+	+	−	+	−	−		L, (a)
−	−	+⁻	V	−	+⁻	−		A, P

ᵉ Produces viscous sediment in broth and colonies usually adhere to agar.
ᶠ Positive with 4-methylumbelliferyl substrates (58).
ᵍ Catalase and lipase positive.

by GLC. The API ZYM system, which allows the detection of 19 preformed enzymes in 4 h, does not have a database; only data compiled from different publications is available, but it is a useful supplement for identification of clinically encountered anaerobic bacteria, especially the *Porphyromonas* spp. (Table 6) (19, 32, 94).

Individually available tablets containing single, dual, or triple enzyme substrates (Rosco Diagnostic Tablets [Rosco]; WEE-Tabs [Key Scientific Products]) are much cheaper than commercial kits; they can be applied in a number of situations and allow flexibility in tailoring the set to best suit special needs (19, 37). The use of 4-methylumbelliferone derivatives of many substrates (Sigma) permits rapid and inexpensive spot tests based on fluorescence (58, 63, 69, 79). It should be noted, however, that reactions obtained by fluorogenic and the different chromogenic test applications may not completely agree, owing to divergent substrate concentrations, affinities, and buffering conditions in the different systems. Therefore, it is important to name the system used for identification when reporting enzyme reactions, particularly in publications.

A recently developed method for identification of anaerobes is based on analysis of whole-cell fatty acids by capillary column GLC (45). An extensive database (MIDI, Inc., Newark, Del.) for anaerobes has been compiled, largely by the Virginia Polytechnic Institute Anaerobe Laboratory, and it is updated frequently. An option for creating a cumulative database is also available. Nucleic acid probes are not yet commercially available for the identification of clinically important anaerobes. Determination of arbitrarily primed PCR profiles may be useful in differentiation of certain species such as *P. intermedia* and *P. nigrescens* (51, 66).

Matrix-assisted laser desorption ionization–time of flight mass spectrometry (MALDI-TOF-MS) is a versatile and emerging technology in the field of biomedical sciences. The addition of an organic matrix to biomolecules results in a rapid cocrystallization in a spatial array on a sample plate. Each sample is analyzed by exposure to a fixed, pulsed laser beam that liberates and ionizes a portion of the sample. The ions, which are generated within nanoseconds, travel through a "flight" tube to a detector where differences in mass-to-ionic charge ratios result in separation of the ions. The results from multiple laser pulses are collected electronically in spectral channels and are converted from a time value into a mass value and displayed as a spectrum. In practice, minimal sample preparation from a single colony is required (85). The mass spectral profiles produced are stable and reproducible and can be stored in a database and used for subsequent matching of the patterns of different species and strains. At the generic level, representative members of *Bacteroides*, *Prevotella*, and *Porphyromonas* may be readily distinguished by comparison of their mass spectral profiles over the range of 500 to 3,000 Da (Fig. 12). Various genera are being examined, and the results will show whether MALDI-TOF-MS will be applicable as a new tool for identification of microorganisms in diagnostic and research laboratories.

Identification of unusual isolates by 16S rRNA sequencing is gradually being adopted by reference laboratories and is also commercially available (see chapter 17).

A commercially available computer software program (The Anaerobe Educator; Anaerobe Systems, Morgan Hill, Calif.) allows interactive self-learning about identification of the most commonly occurring clinically important anaerobes based on phenotypic characteristics.

TABLE 5 Characteristics of nonpigmented weakly saccharolytic or nonsaccharolytic gram-negative bacilli[a]

Species	Growth in 20% bile	Glucose	Catalase	Indole	Nitrate	Motility
Anaerorhabdus furcosus	+⁻	W	−	−	−	−
Bilophila wadsworthia[g]	+	−	+	−	+	−
Bacteroides capillosus	−⁺	W⁻ʰ	−	−	−	−
B. coagulans	+	−	−	+	−	−
B. putredinis	+⁻	−	+⁻	+	−	−
B. pyogenes[f]	+	W	−	−	−	−
B. tectus[f]	+	W	−	−	−	−
B. ureolyticus	−	−	−⁺	−	+	−
Campylobacter spp.	−	−	−	−	+	+⁻
C. gracilis	−	−	−	−	+	−
Desulfovibrio piger[g]	V	−	V	−	−⁺	−
Desulfovibrio spp.[g]	V	−	V	−	V	+
Dialister pneumosintes	−	−	−	−	−	−
Sutterella wadsworthensis	+	−	−	−	+	−
Tannerella forsythensis	−	−	−	−	−	−
Tissierella praeacuta	+	−	−	−	V	+

[a] See Table 3, footnote *a*.
[b] F/F, formate-fumarate. See Table 2, footnote *b*.
[c] See Table 2, footnote *i*.
[d] See Table 2, footnote *d*.

TABLE 6 Characteristics of pigmented *Porphyromonas* spp. and *Prevotella* spp.[a]

Species and origin	Indole	Lipase	Catalase	Esculin hydrolysis	α-Fucosidase[b]	α-Galactosidase[b]	β-Galactosidase[b]
Porphyromonas, asaccharolytic or weakly saccharolytic							
Human origin							
P. asaccharolytica	+	−	−				
P. catoniae[d]	−	−	−	−	+	−⁺	+
P. endodontalis	+	−	−	−	−	−	−ᶠ
P. gingivalis[e]	+	−	−	−	−	−	−
P. levii-like[e,g]	−	−	−	−	−	−	+
Animal origin[g]							
P. canoris	+	−	+	−	−	−	+
P. cangingivalis	+	−	+	−	−	−	−
P. cansulci	+	−	+ʷ	−	−	−	−
P. circumdentaria	+	−	+	−	−	−	−
P. crevioricanis	+	NA	−	−	−	NA	NA
P. gingivicanis	+	NA	+	−	−	NA	NA
P. gulae	+	−	+	−	−	−	−ᶠ
P. macacae	+	+	+	−	−	+	−ᶠ
Prevotella, saccharolytic							
P. corporis	−	−	−	−	−	−	−
P. denticola	−	−	−	+⁻	+	+	+
P. intermedia	+	+⁻	−	−	+	−	−
P. loescheii	−	V	−	+⁻	+	+	+
P. melaninogenica	−	−	−	−⁺	+	+	+
P. nigrescens[h]	+	+⁻	−	−	+	−	−
P. pallens	+	−	−	−	+	−	−
P. tannerae	−	−	−	−	+	−	+

[a] See Table 3, footnote *a*. +ʷ, most strains positive; some strains weakly positive.
[b] Reaction by the API ZYM system or with Rosco Diagnostic Tablets (see Table 3, footnote *b*). Reactivity in these systems is not always identical (see footnote *f*).
[c] See Table 3, footnote *c*.
[d] Nonpigmented.

F/F required[b]	Desulfoviridin[c]	Urease[d]	Esculin hydrolysis	Gelatin hydrolysis	Fatty acids from PYG[e]
−	−	−	+	−[w]	a, l, (s)
−	w[−]	+[−]	−	−	A, (s)
−	−	−	+	−[w]	a, s, (p, l)
−	−	−	−	+	a, (p, l, s)
−	−	−	−	+	a, P, ib, b, IV, S, (l), pa
−	−	−	+	+	a, P, ib, b, IV, S, (l)
−	−	−	+	+	A, p, iv, S, pa
+	−	+	−	−	A, S
+	−	−	−	−	a, S
+	−	−	−	−	a, S
−	+	−[+]	−	−	A
−	+	−[+]	−	−	A
−	−	−	−	−[w]	a, (l, s)
+	−	−	−	−	a, S
−	−	−	+	+	A, S, pa
−	−	−	−	+	A, p, ib, B, IV, s, (l)

[e] See Table 3, footnote c.

[f] Animal origin; also isolated from bite infections in humans. Quantitative differences between some cellular fatty acids may help in differentiation of these species (29).

[g] Bilophila sp. is colistin sensitive; Desulfovibrio spp. are colistin resistant.

[h] w[−], most strains weakly positive, some strains negative.

N-Acetyl-β-glucosaminidase[b]	Chymotrypsin	Trypsin	Fermentation of:				Fatty acids from PYG[c]
			Glucose	Cellobiose	Lactose	Sucrose	
			−	−	−	−	
+	−[+]	+[−]	W	−	W	−	a, P, iv, l, S
−	−	−	−	−	−	−	A, P, ib, B, IV, s
+	+	−	−	−	−	−	A, P, ib, B, IV, s, pa
+	−	+	W	−	W	−	A, P, ib, B, IV, s
+	−	+	−	−	−	−	A, P, ib, b, IV, s
−	−	+	−	−	−	−	A, p, ib, B, IV
−	−	−	−	−	−	−	A, P, ib, B, IV, S, pa
−	−	−	−	−	−	−	A, P, ib, b, IV, s, pa
−	−	NA	−	−	−	−	A, p, ib, B, IV, s
−	−	NA	−	−	−	−	
+	+	−	−	−	−	−	A, P, ib, B, IV, s, pa
+	+	+	W	−	W	−	A, P, ib, B, IV, s, pa
−	−	+[−]	+	−	−	−	A, ib, iv, S, (b)
+	−	−	+	−[+]	+	+	A, S, (ib, iv, l)
−	−	−	+	−	−	+[−]	A, iv, S, (p, ib)
+	−	−	+	+	+	+	a, S, (l)
+	−	−	+	−[+]	+	+	A, S, (ib, iv, l)
−	−	−	+	−	−	+[−]	A, iv, S, (p, ib)
−	−	−	+	−	−	+	A, S, (p, ib)
+	−	−	+	−	+	V	A, iv, S, (ib)

[e] P. gingivalis does not show fluorescence; P. levii-like may show weak or no fluorescence.

[f] Negative by the API ZYM system; positive by the Rosco o-nitrophenyl-β-D-galactopyranoside test.

[g] May be isolated from bite infections; NA, information not available.

[h] P. intermedia shares the same characteristics. Differentiation based on enzyme electrophoresis, oligonucleotide probe analysis, or arbitrarily primed PCR (66).

TABLE 7 Characteristics of *Fusobacterium* species[a]

Species	Distinctive cellular morphology	Indole	Growth on BBE or 20% bile	Lipase	ONPG[b]	Glucose	Fructose	Lactose	Mannose	Lactate converted to propionate	Threonine converted to propionate	Fatty acids from PYG[c]
F. gonidiaformans	Gonidial forms	+	−	−	−	−	−	−	−	−	+	A, p, B, (l, s)
F. mortiferum	Bizarre; round bodies	−	+	−	+	$+^w$	$+^w$	+	$+^w$	−	+	a, p, B, (v, l, s)
F. naviforme	Boat shape	+	−	−	−	w^-	−	−	−	+	−	a, B, L, (p, s)
F. necrophorum[d]	Large, pleomorphic	+	$-^+$	$+^-$	−	$-^w$	$-^w$	−	−	+	+	A, p, B, (l, s)
F. nucleatum[e]	Slender, pointed ends	+	−	−	−	$-^w$	$-^w$	−	−	−	+	A, p, B, (l, s)
F. russii	Large, rounded ends	−	−	$-^+$	−	−	−	−	−	−	−	a, B, L
F. varium	Large, rounded ends	$+^-$	+	+	−	w^+	w^+	−	$+^w$	−	+	a, p, B, L, (s)
F. ulcerans[f]	Large, rounded ends	−	+	−	−	+	w^-	−	$+^-$	−	+	a, p, B, l, (s)

[a] See Table 3, footnote a. $+^w$, most strains positive, some strains weakly positive; w^-, most strains weakly positive, some strains negative; w^+, most strains weakly positive, some strains positive.
[b] ONPG, o-Nitrophenyl-β-D-galactopyranoside. See Table 3, footnote b.
[c] See Table 3, footnote c.
[d] Lipase-positive strains, *F. necrophorum* subsp. *necrophorum*; lipase-negative strains, *F. necrophorum* subsp. *funduliforme*.
[e] *F. periodonticum* shares the same characteristics and probably is *F. nucleatum*.
[f] Nitrate positive.

SEROLOGICAL TESTS

Serological procedures are not practical for the identification of anaerobic bacteria from colonies. Furthermore, no standardized tests are available for the detection of antibodies or antigens in clinical specimens that would be useful for this group of organisms.

ANTIBIOTIC SUSCEPTIBILITIES

Susceptibility testing of anaerobes is discussed in chapter 72. The susceptibility patterns obtained in the Wadsworth Anaerobic Bacteriology Laboratory for the most commonly encountered gram-negative rods of clinical significance and for *Veillonella* spp. are noted in Table 9. Resistance is increasingly common among anaerobic gram-negative rods. This is particularly true for the members of the *B. fragilis* group, which are not uncommonly resistant to expanded- and broad-spectrum cephalosporins (including β-lactamase-resistant drugs such as cefoxitin) and clindamycin. Strains of the *B. fragilis* group with resistance to imipenem and metronidazole are also encountered. The previously reported resistance to several antimicrobial agents in the group containing both *C. gracilis* and *S. wadsworthensis* was found to be partly due to a technical artifact (lack of formate-fumarate additive in susceptibility testing media). The true resistance seems to be confined to *Sutterella*; *Sutterella* spp. are more resistant to antimicrobial agents such as metronidazole and some β-lactam drugs than *C. gracilis* (68, 95).

β-Lactamase production (nitrocefin test positivity) is common among the species of the *B. fragilis* group and *B. wadsworthia*; almost all strains are β-lactamase positive. Approximately 30 to 50% of *Prevotella* spp. are also β-lactamase producers, and even higher proportions of β-lactamase producers have been reported among certain species when several isolates per sample were tested (41, 52). An increasing number of β-lactamase-positive *F. nucleatum* strains have been encountered. Occasional strains of *C. gracilis*, *B. coagulans*, *B. splanchnicus*, *D. piger* (*D. pigra*), *F. mortiferum*, *F. varium*, *Megamonas hypermegas*, *M. multiacida*, and *Porphyromonas* spp. may produce β-lactamase. Animal-derived *Porphyromonas* spp. are more often β-lactamase producers than those derived from humans (44). *Leptotrichia* spp. as well as *Capnocytophaga* spp. are sometimes β-lactamase producers and are resistant to aminoglycosides and vancomycin; *Leptotrichia* spp. are resistant to erythromycin as well (8, 27). Furthermore, erythromycin and the newer extended-spectrum macrolides commonly used for the treatment of upper respiratory tract infections, such as tonsillitis, otitis media, and maxillary sinusitis, are not active against fusobacteria.

TABLE 8 Characteristics of gram-negative cocci[a]

Species	Nitrate reduction	Catalase	Fatty acids from PYG[b]
Veillonella spp.	+	V	A, p
Acidaminococcus fermentans	−	−	A, B
Megasphaera elsdenii	−	−	a, ib, b, iv, v, C

[a] +, positive reaction for most strains; −, negative reaction for most strains; V, variable reaction.
[b] See Table 3, footnote c.

TABLE 9 Activities of various drugs against anaerobic gram-negative bacteria (Wadsworth agar dilution procedure)[a]

Drug	NCCLS breakpoint (μg/ml)			% Susceptible[b]								
	Susceptible	Intermediate	Resistant	B. fragilis	B. fragilis group[c]	Prevotella spp.	Porphyromonas spp.	Fusobacterium spp.	C. gracilis[d]	Sutterella spp.[d]	Bilophila sp.[e]	Veillonella spp.
Cefotaxime	16	32	≥64	50–69	<50	>95	>95	85–95			70–84	
Cefotetan	16	32	≥64	85–95	50–69			85–95			>95	
Cefoxitin	16	32	≥64	>95	85–95	>95	>95	>95	>95	>95	>95	>95
Ceftizoxime	32	64	≥128	85–95	85–95	>95	>95	>85–95	>95	85–95	>95	>95
Ceftriaxone	16	32	≥64	70–84	<50	85–95	>95	>85–95	>95	>95		>95
Chloramphenicol	8	16	≥32	>95	>95	>95	>95	>95	>95	>95	>95	>95
Clindamycin	2	4	≥8	85–95	70–84	>95	>95	70–95	>95	50–69	85–95	>95
Imipenem[f]	4	8	≥16	>95	>95	>95	>95	>95	>95	>95	>95	>95
Meropenem	4	8	≥16	>95	>95	>95	>95	>95	>95	>95	>95	>95
Metronidazole	8	16	≥32	>95	>95	>95	>95	>95	>95	70–84	>95	>95
Penicillin G[g]	0.5	1	≥2	<50	<50	<50	85–95	70–95			<50	70–90
Amoxicillin-clavulanate	4/2	8/4	≥16/8	>95	85–95	>95	>95	85–95	>95	>95	>95	
Piperacillin	32	64	≥128	>95	85–95	>95	>95	85–95	>95	85–95	>95	
Piperacillin-tazobactam	32/4	64/4	≥128/4	>95	>95	>95	>95	>95	>95	85–95	>95	
Ticarcillin	32	64	≥128			>95	>95		>95		>95	
Ticarcillin-clavulanate	32/2	64/2	≥128/2	>95	>95	>95	>95	85–95	>95	>95	>95	>95
Trovafloxacin	2	4	≥8	85–95	70–95	50–95	>95	70–95	>95	85–95	>95	>95

[a] NCCLS approved method M11-A5; data are from the Wadsworth Anaerobic Bacteriology Laboratory.
[b] According to the NCCLS-approved breakpoints (approved method M11-A5), using the intermediate category as susceptible.
[c] Includes the species B. fragilis.
[d] The use of formate-fumarate additive is recommended (Table 3, footnote b).
[e] Addition of 1% pyruvate to the test medium is recommended.
[f] Biapenem exhibits similar activity.
[g] Strains producing β-lactamase should be considered resistant.

OMZ311P.Int0001_lc_comb_, 9344Bfragilis0005, July 13 b0001
%Int.   100% = 1925 mV 885 mV 787 mV

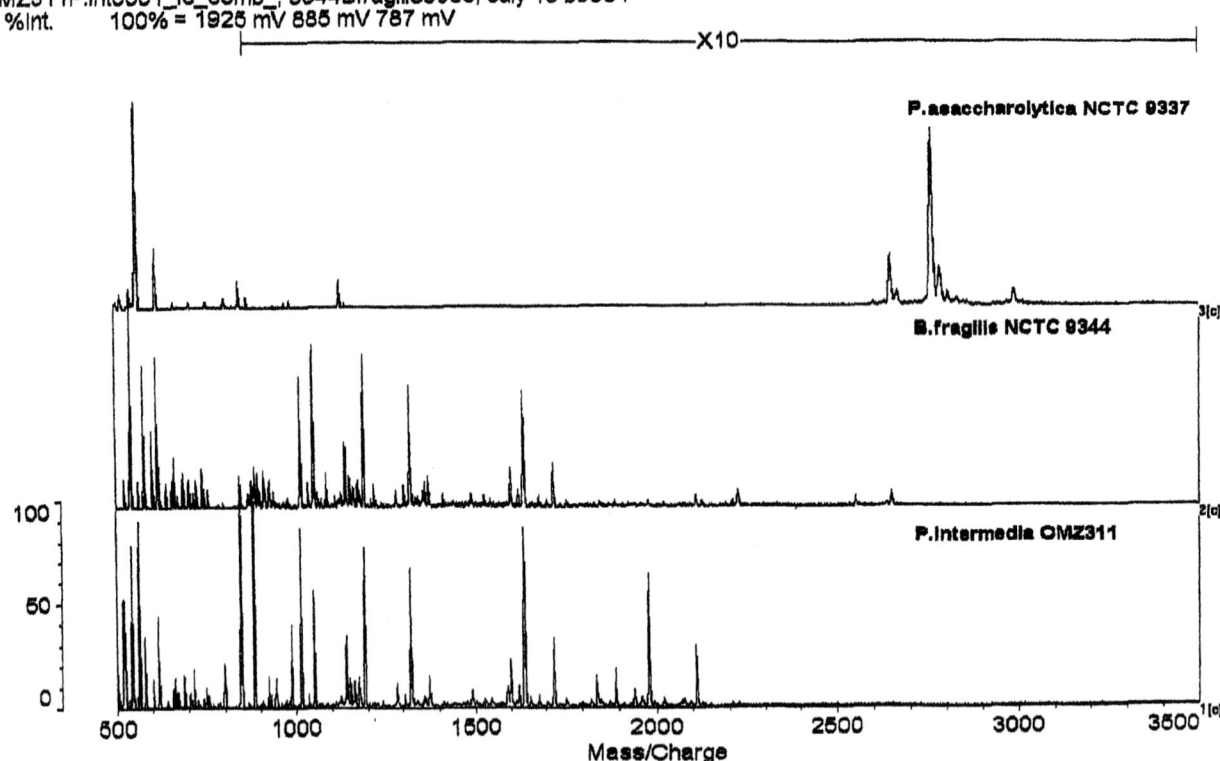

FIGURE 12 Comparison of the mass spectral profiles of representative species of *Bacteroides*, *Prevotella*, and *Porphyromonas* spp. showing the vast differences in mass ions over the range of 500 to 3,000 Da.

Mechanisms of resistance other than β-lactamase (including high-level metalloenzyme production) include changes in penicillin-binding proteins and in outer membrane porin channels. Plasmids conferring resistance are also encountered.

EVALUATION, INTERPRETATION, AND REPORTING OF RESULTS

Because anaerobic bacteriology is time-consuming, several interim reports are desirable. The initial report can give Gram stain results. Bacterial and host cell morphologies and the relative quantities seen in the smear give a good overall impression of the specimen quality, the nature of the polymicrobial infection, and even morphologies suggestive of certain anaerobes. Furthermore, Gram stain results can guide the laboratory in choosing media for the optimal recovery of the predicted organisms. At 24 h, preliminary information on the aerobic and facultatively anaerobic flora is available, and at 48 h, more definite information on the nonanaerobes and preliminary but clinically useful information on the anaerobes can be given (28).

Interpretation of results of a mixed culture containing multiple isolates is difficult. In general, bacterial isolates that are most predominant, empirically most virulent, and most resistant to antimicrobials should be given the most attention. Rough quantitation of the different isolates recovered, together with Gram stain results (provided that the specimen was properly taken and transported), is helpful. The bacteria present in pure culture or in large numbers

are probably of major importance, as are organisms recovered again on a repeat culture and organisms isolated from normally sterile sites. The nature of the bacteria found can also give clues to their importance in the infectious process. Certain taxa, including the *B. fragilis* group, *Fusobacterium* spp., and some *Prevotella* spp., are much more important clinically in terms of the frequency of occurrence, the severity of the infection produced, and antimicrobial resistance.

Microbiologists must be willing to consult with the clinician on interpretation of the relevance of the findings. The laboratory should provide the clinician with a gradual introduction to new taxonomy by reporting both the new and old names in parallel for at least 1 to 2 years. Reports must be readily available for phone or direct contact. Statements of specimen quality and possible limitations of methods used serve as the most important feedback to the clinician. Dialogue between the clinician and the microbiologist should be frequent.

REFERENCES

1. **Alcoforado, G. A., T. L. McKay, and J. Slots.** 1987. Rapid method for detection of lactose fermenting oral microorganisms. *Oral Microbiol. Immunol.* 2:35–38.
2. **Alexander, C. J., D. M. Citron, S. Hunt Gerardo, M. C. Claros, D. Talan, and E. J. C. Goldstein.** 1997. Characterization of saccharolytic *Bacteroides* and *Prevotella* isolates from infected dog and cat bite wounds in humans. *J. Clin Microbiol.* 35:406–411.

3. Baquero, F., J. Fernández, F. Dionda, A. Erice, J. Pérez de Oteiza, J. A. Reguera, and M. Reig. 1990. Capnophilic and anaerobic bacteremia in neutropenic patients: an oral source. *Rev. Infect. Dis.* **2**(Suppl. 12):S157–S160.

4. Baron, E. J., R. Bennion, J. Thompson, C. Strong, P. Summanen, M. McTeague, and S. M. Finegold. 1992. A microbial comparison between acute and complicated appendicitis. *Clin. Infect. Dis.* **14:**227–231.

5. Baron, E. J., and D. M. Citron. 1997. Anaerobic identification flowchart using minimal laboratory resources. *Clin. Infect. Dis.* **25:**S143–S146.

6. Baron, E. J., M. Curren, G. Henderson, H. Jousimies-Somer, K. Lee, K. Lechowitz, C. A. Strong, P. Summanen, K. Tuner, and S. M. Finegold. 1992. *Bilophila wadsworthia* isolates from clinical specimens. *J. Clin. Microbiol.* **30:**1882–1884.

7. Baron, E. J., C. A. Strong, M. McTeague, M.-L. Vaisanen, and S. M. Finegold. 1995. Survival of anaerobes in original specimens transported by overnight mail services. *Clin. Infect. Dis.* **20:**S174–S177.

8. Beebe, J. L., and E. W. Koneman. 1995. Recovery of uncommon bacteria from blood: association with neoplastic disease. *Clin. Microbiol. Rev.* **8:**336–356.

9. Bolstad, A. I., H. B. Jensen, and V. Bakken. 1996. Taxonomy, biology, and periodontal aspects of *Fusobacterium nucleatum*. *Clin. Microbiol. Rev.* **9:**55–71.

10. Byrd, L. 1992. Examination of primary culture plates for anaerobic bacteria, p. 2.4.1–2.4.6. *In* H. D. Isenberg (ed.), *Clinical Microbiology Procedures Handbook*. American Society for Microbiology, Washington, D.C.

11. Cavallaro, J. J., L. S. Wiggs, and J. M. Miller. 1997. Evaluation of the BBL crystal anaerobe identification system. *J. Clin. Microbiol.* **35:**3186–3191.

12. Citron, D. M., E. J. Baron, S. M. Finegold, and E. J. C. Goldstein. 1990. Short prereduced anaerobically sterilized (PRAS) biochemical scheme for identification of clinical isolates of bile-resistant *Bacteroides* species. *J. Clin. Microbiol.* **28:**2220–2223.

13. Citron, D. M., S. Hunt Gerardo, M.-C. Claros, F. Abrahamian, D. Talan, and E. J. C. Goldstein. 1996. Incidence and characterization of *Porphyromonas* species isolated from infected dog and cat bite wounds in humans by biochemical and PCR fingerprinting. *Clin. Infect. Dis.* **23**(Suppl.1):S78–S82.

14. Civen, R., H. Jousimies-Somer, M. Marina, L. Borenstein, H. Shah, and S. M. Finegold. 1995. A retrospective review of cases of anaerobic empyema and update of bacteriology. *Clin. Infect. Dis.* **20**(Suppl. 2):S224–S229.

15. Collins, M. D, P. A. Lawson, and A. Willems. 1994. The phylogeny of the genus *Clostridium*: proposal of five new genera and eleven new species combinations. *Int. J. Syst. Bacteriol.* **44:**812–826.

16. Dahlen, G., P. Pipattanagovit, B. Rosling, and Å. J. R. Möller. 1993. A comparison of two transport media for saliva and subgingival samples. *Oral Microbiol. Immunol.* **8:**375–382.

17. Dix, K., S. M. Watanabe, S. McArdle, D. I. Lee, C. Randolph, B. Moncla, and D. E. Schwartz. 1990. Species-specific oligonucleotide probes for the identification of periodontal bacteria. *J. Clin. Microbiol.* **28:**319–323.

18. Downes, J., J. Hardie, and I. Phillips. 1999. Evaluation of the Rapid ID 32A system for identification of anaerobic gram-negative bacilli, excluding the *Bacteroides fragilis* group. *Clin. Microbiol. Infect.* **5:**319–326.

19. Durmaz, B., H. R. Jousimies-Somer, and S. M. Finegold. 1995. Enzymatic profiles of *Prevotella*, *Porphyromonas*, and *Bacteroides* species obtained with the API ZYM system and Rosco diagnostic tablets. *Clin. Infect. Dis.* **20**(Suppl. 2):S192–S194.

20. Dzink, J. L., M. T. Sheenan, and S. S. Socransky. 1990. Proposal of three subspecies of *Fusobacterium nucleatum* Knorr 1922: *Fusobacterium nucleatum* subsp. *nucleatum* subsp. nov.; *Fusobacterium nucleatum* subsp. *polymorphum* subsp. nov., nov. rev., comb. nov.; *Fusobacterium nucleatum* subsp. *vincentii* subsp. nov., nov. rev., comb. nov. *Int. J. Syst. Bacteriol.* **40:**74–78.

21. Dzink, J. L., S. S. Socransky, and A. D. Haffajee. 1988. The predominant cultivable microbiota of active and inactive lesions of destructive periodontal diseases. *J. Clin. Periodontol.* **15:**316–323.

22. Engelkirk, P. G., J. Duben-Engelkirk, and V. R. Dowell, Jr. 1992. *Principles and Practice of Clinical Anaerobic Bacteriology*. Star Publishing Company, Belmont, Calif.

23. Finegold, S. M. 1995. Anaerobic infections in humans: an overview. *Anaerobe* **1:**3–9.

24. Finegold, S. M. 1995. Overview of clinically important anaerobes. *Clin. Infect. Dis.* **20:**S205–S207.

25. Finegold, S. M., E. J. Baron, and H. M. Wexler. 1991. *A Clinical Guide to Anaerobic Infections*. Star Publishing Company, Belmont, Calif.

26. Finegold, S. M., and W. L. George (ed.). 1989. *Anaerobic Infections in Humans*. Academic Press, Inc., San Diego, Calif.

27. Finegold, S. M., and H. Jousimies-Somer. 1997. Recently described anaerobic bacteria: medical aspects. *Clin. Infect. Dis.* **25**(Suppl. 2):S88–S93.

28. Finegold, S. M., H. R. Jousimies-Somer, and H. M. Wexler. 1993. Current perspectives on anaerobic infections: diagnostic approaches. *Infect. Dis. Clin. N. Am.* **7:**257–275.

29. Forsblom, B., D. N. Love, and H. R. Jousimies-Somer. 1997. Characterization of anaerobic, gram-negative, non-pigmented saccharolytic rods from subgingival sites of dogs. *Clin. Infect. Dis.* **25**(Suppl. 2):S100–S106.

30. Fournier, D., C. Mouton, P. Lapierre, T. Kato, K. Okuda, and C. Ménard. 2001. *Porphyromonas gulae* sp. nov., an anaerobic gram-negative coccobacillus from the gingival sulcus of various animal hosts. *Int. J. Syst. Evol. Microbiol.* **51:**1179–1189.

31. Gharbia, S. E., and H. N. Shah. 1992. *Fusobacterium nucleatum* subsp. *fusiforme* subsp. nov. and *Fusobacterium nucleatum* subsp. *animalis* subsp. nov. as additional subspecies within *Fusobacterium nucleatum*. *Int. J. Syst. Bacteriol.* **42:**296–298.

32. Gruner, E., A. Graevenitz, and M. Altwegg. 1992. The API ZYM system: tabulated review from 1977 to date. *J. Microbiol. Methods* **16:**101–118.

33. Hanff, P. A., J.-A. Rosol-Donoghue, C. A. Spiegel, K. H. Wilson, and L. H. Moore. 1995. *Leptotrichia sanguinegens* sp. nov., a new agent of postpartum and neonatal bacteremia. *Clin. Infect. Dis.* **20**(Suppl. 2):S237–S239.

34. Holdeman, L. V., E. P. Cato, and W. E. C. Moore (ed.). 1977. *Anaerobic Laboratory Manual*, 4th ed. Virginia Polytechnic Institute and State University, Blacksburg.

35. Holdeman, L. V., R. W. Kelley, and W. E. C. Moore. 1984. Anaerobic gram-negative straight, curved and helical rods. Family 1. *Bacteroidaceae* Pribram 1933, 10^AL, p. 602–662. *In* N. R. Krieg and J. G. Holt (ed.), *Bergey's Manual of Systematic Bacteriology*, vol. 1. The Williams & Wilkins Co., Baltimore, Md.

36. Holden, J. 1992. Collection and transport of clinical specimens for anaerobic culture, p. 2.2.1–2.2.7. *In* H. D. Isenberg (ed.), *Clinical Microbiology Procedures Handbook*. American Society for Microbiology, Washington, D.C.

37. Hudspeth, M. K., S. Hunt Gerardo, D. M. Citron, and E. J. C. Goldstein. 1997. Growth characteristics and a novel method for identification (the WEE-TAB system) of

Porphyromonas species isolated from infected dog and cat bite wounds in humans. *J. Clin. Microbiol.* **35:**2450–2453.

38. **Jalava, J., and E. Eerola.** 1999. Phylogenetic analysis of *Fusobacterium alocis* and *Fusobacterium sulci* based on 16S rRNA gene sequences: proposal of *Filifactor alocis* (Cato, Moore and Moore) comb. nov. and *Eubacterium sulci* (Cato, Moore and Moore) comb. nov. *Int. J. Syst. Bacteriol.* **49:**1375–1379.

39. **Jenkins, S. A., D. B. Drucker, M. G. Keaney, and L. A. Ganguli.** 1991. Evaluation of the RAPID ID 32A system for the identification of *Bacteroides fragilis* and related organisms. *J. Appl. Bacteriol.* **71:**360–365.

40. **Johnson, C. C., and S. M. Finegold.** 1987. Uncommonly encountered, motile, anaerobic gram-negative bacilli associated with infection. *Rev. Infect. Dis.* **9:**1150–1162.

41. **Jousimies-Somer, H.** 1997. Recently described clinically important anaerobic bacteria: taxonomic aspects and update. *Clin. Infect. Dis.* **25**(Suppl. 2)**:**S78–S87.

42. **Jousimies-Somer, H., S. Savolainen, A. Mäkitie, and J. Ylikoski.** 1993. Bacteriologic findings in peritonsillar abscesses in young adults. *Clin. Infect. Dis.* **16**(Suppl. 4)**:** 292–298.

43. **Jousimies-Somer, H., and P. Summanen.** 1997. Microbiology terminology update: clinically significant anaerobic gram-positive and gram-negative bacteria (excluding spirochetes). *Clin. Infect. Dis.* **25:**11–14.

44. **Jousimies-Somer, H. R.** 1995. Update on the taxonomy and the clinical and laboratory characteristics of pigmented anaerobic gram-negative rods. *Clin. Infect. Dis.* **20**(Suppl. 2)**:**S187–S191.

45. **Jousimies-Somer, H. R., P. H. Summanen, D. M. Citron, E. J. Baron, H. M. Wexler, and S. M. Finegold.** 2002. *Wadsworth Anaerobic Bacteriology Manual*, 6th ed. Star Publishing Company, Belmont, Calif.

46. **Jousimies-Somer, H. R., P. Summanen, and S. M. Finegold.** 1995. *Bacteroides levii*-like organisms isolated from clinical specimens. *Clin. Infect. Dis.* **20**(Suppl. 2)**:**S208–S209.

47. **Jousimies-Somer, H. R., P. H. Summanen, and S. M. Finegold.** 1999. *Bacteroides, Porphyromonas, Prevotella, Fusobacterium*, and other anaerobic gram-negative rods and cocci, p. 690–711. *In* P. R. Murray, E. J. Baron, M. A. Pfaller, F. C. Tenover, and R. H. Yolken. (ed.), *Manual of Clinical Microbiology*, 7th ed. ASM Press, Washington, D.C.

48. **Kasten, M. J., J. E. Rosenblatt, and D. R. Gustafson.** 1992. *Bilophila wadsworthia* bacteremia in two patients with hepatic abscess. *J. Clin. Microbiol.* **30:**2502–2503.

49. **Kato, N. H., H. Kato, K. Watanabe, and K. Ueno.** 1996. Association of enterotoxigenic *Bacteroides fragilis* with bacteremia. *Clin. Infect. Dis.* **23:**S83–S86.

50. **Könönen, E., E. Eerola, E. V. G. Frandsen, J. Jalava, J. Mättö, S. Salmenlinna, and H. R. Jousimies-Somer.** 1998. Phylogenetic characterization and proposal of a new pigmented species to the genus *Prevotella: Prevotella pallens* sp. nov. *Int. J. Syst. Bacteriol.* **48:**47–51.

51. **Könönen, E., J. Mättö, M.-L. Väisänen-Tunkelrott, E. V. G. Frandsen, I. Helander, S. M. Finegold, and H. R. Jousimies-Somer.** 1998. Biochemical and genetic characterization of a *Prevotella intermedia/Prevotella nigrescens*-like organism. *Int. J. Syst. Bacteriol.* **48:**39–46.

52. **Könönen, E., S. Nyfors, J. Mättö, S. Asikainen, and H. R. Jousimies-Somer.** 1997. β-lactamase production among oral pigmented *Prevotella* species in young children. *Clin. Infect. Dis.* **25**(Suppl. 2)**:**S272–S274.

53. **Könönen, E., M.-L. Väisänen, S. M. Finegold, R. Heine, and H. Jousimies-Somer.** 1996. Cellular fatty acid analysis of *Porphyromonas catoniae*—a frequent colonizer of the oral cavity in children. *Anaerobe* **2:**329–335.

54. **Lawson, A. J., S. L. W. On, J. M. J. Logan, and J. Stanley.** 2001. *Campylobacter hominis* sp. nov., from the human gastrointestinal tract. *Int. J. Syst. Evol. Microbiol.* **51:**651–660.

55. **Leszczynski, P., A. van Belkum, H. Pituch, H. Verbrugh, and F. Meisel-Mikolajczyk.** 1997. Vaginal carriage of enterotoxigenic *Bacteroides fragilis* in pregnant women. *J. Clin. Microbiol.* **35:**2899–2903.

56. **Looney, W. J., A. J. Gallusser, and H. K. Modde.** 1990. Evaluation of the ATB 32 A system for identification of anaerobic bacteria isolated from clinical specimens. *J. Clin. Microbiol.* **28:**1519–1524.

57. **Loubinoux, J., F. M. A. Valente, I. A. C. Pereira, A. Costa, P. A. D. Grimont, and A. E. Le Faou.** 2002. Reclassification of the only species of the genus *Desulfomonas, Desulfomonas pigra*, as *Desulfovibrio piger* comb. nov. *Int. J. Syst. Evol. Microbiol.* **52:**1305–1308.

58. **Maiden, M. F. J., A. Tanner, and P. J. Macuch.** 1996. Rapid characterization of periodontal bacterial isolates by using fluorogenic substrate tests. *J. Clin. Microbiol.* **34:** 376–384.

59. **Malnick, H.** 1997. *Anaerobiospirillum thomasii* sp. nov., an anaerobic spiral bacterium isolated from the feces of cats and dogs and from diarrheal feces of humans, and emendation of the genus *Anaerobiospirillum. Int. J. Syst. Bacteriol.* **47:**381–384.

60. **Malnick, H., K. Williams, J. Phil-Ebosie, and A. S. Levy.** 1990. Description of a medium for isolating *Anaerobiospirillum* spp., a possible cause for zoonotic disease, from diarrheal feces and blood of humans and use of the medium in a survey of human, canine, and feline feces. *J. Clin. Microbiol.* **28:**1380–1384.

61. **Mangels, J. I., M. Cox, and L. H. Lindberg.** 1984. Methanol fixation: an alternative to heat fixation of smears before staining. *Diagn. Microbiol. Infect. Dis.* **2:**129–137.

62. **Mangels, J. I., and B. P. Douglas.** 1989. Comparison of four commercial brucella agar media for growth of anaerobic organisms. *J. Clin. Microbiol.* **27:**2268–2271.

63. **Mangels, J. I., I. Edvalson, and M. Cox.** 1993. Rapid presumptive identification of *Bacteroides fragilis* group organisms with use of 4-methylumbelliferone-derivative substrates. *Clin. Infect. Dis.* **16**(Suppl. 4)**:**S319–S321.

64. **Mann, K. A.** 1994. Lemierre's syndrome following infectious mononucleosis. *Clin. Microbiol. Newsl.* **16:**158–159.

65. **Marler, L. M., J. A. Siders, L. C. Wolters, Y. Pettigrew, B. L. Skitt, and S. D. Allen.** 1991. Evaluation of the new RapID-ANA II system for the identification of clinical anaerobic isolates. *J. Clin. Microbiol.* **29:**874–878.

66. **Mättö J., S. Asikainen, M.-L. Väisänen, M. Saarela, P. Summanen, S. M. Finegold, and H. R. Jousimies-Somer.** 1997. *Porphyromonas gingivalis, Prevotella intermedia* and *Prevotella nigrescens* in extraoral and some odontogenic infections. *Clin. Infect. Dis.* **25**(Suppl. 2)**:**S194–S198.

67. **McDougall, R., J. Robson, D. Paterson, and W. Tee.** 1997. Bacteremia caused by a recently described novel *Desulfovibrio* species. *J. Clin. Microbiol.* **35:**1805–1808.

68. **Molitoris, E., H. M. Wexler, and S. M. Finegold.** 1997. Sources and antimicrobial susceptibilities of *Campylobacter gracilis* and *Sutterella wadsworthensis. Clin. Infect. Dis.* **25**(Suppl. 2)**:**S264–S265.

69. **Moncla, B. J., P. Braham, L. K. Rabe, and S. L. Hillier.** 1991. Rapid presumptive identification of black-pigmented gram-negative anaerobic bacteria by using 4-methylumbelliferone derivatives. *J. Clin. Microbiol.* **29:** 1955–1958.

70. **Moore, L. V. H., D. M. Bourne, and W. E. C. Moore.** 1994. Comparative distribution and taxonomic value of cellular fatty acids in thirty-three genera of anaerobic gram-negative bacilli. *Int. J. Syst. Bacteriol.* **44:**338–347.

71. **Moore, L. V. H., E. P. Cato, and W. E. C. Moore.** 1991. *Anaerobe Laboratory Manual Update: a Supplement to the VPI Anaerobe Laboratory Manual*, 4th ed. Virginia Polytechnic Institute and State University, Blacksburg.

72. **Moore, L. V. H., J. L. Johnson, and W. E. C. Moore.** 1994. Description of *Prevotella tannerae* sp. nov. and *Prevotella enoeca* sp. nov. from human gingival crevice and emendation of the description of *Prevotella zoogleoformans*. *Int. J. Syst. Bacteriol.* **44:**599–602.

73. **Moore, W. E. C.** 1987. Microbiology of periodontal disease. *J. Periodont. Res.* **22:**335–341.

74. **Moreno, S., J. G. Altozano, B. Pinilla, J. C. Lopez, B. de Quiros, A. Ortega, and E. Bouza.** 1989. Lemierre's disease: postanginal bacteremia and pulmonary involvement caused by *Fusobacterium necrophorum*. *Rev. Infect. Dis.* **11:**319–324.

75. **Obiso, R. J., D. M. Lyerly, R. L. Van Tassell, and T. D. Wilkins.** 1995. Proteolytic activity of the *Bacteroides fragilis* enterotoxin causes fluid secretion and intestinal damage in vivo. *Infect. Immun.* **63:**3820–3826.

76. **Pantosti, A., M. Malpeli, M. Wilks, M. G. Menozzi, and B. D'Ambrosio.** 1997. Detection of enterotoxigenic *Bacteroides fragilis* by PCR. *J. Clin. Microbiol.* **35:**2482–2486.

77. **Paster, B. J., F. E. Dewhirst, I. Olsen, and G. J. Fraser.** 1994. Phylogeny of *Bacteroides*, *Prevotella*, and *Porphyromonas* spp. and related bacteria. *J. Bacteriol.* **176:**725–732.

78. **Peterson, L. R.** 1997. Effect of media on transport and recovery of anaerobic bacteria. *Clin. Infect. Dis.* **25**(Suppl. 2)**:**S134–S136.

79. **Rabe, L. K., D. Sheiness, and S. L. Hillier.** 1995. Comparison of the use of oligonucleotide probes, 4-methylumbelliferyl derivatives, and conventional methods for identifying *Prevotella bivia*. *Clin. Infect. Dis.* **20**(Suppl. 2)**:**S195–S197.

80. **Rautio, M., H. Saxén, M. Lönnroth, M.-L. Väisänen, R. Nikku, and H. R. Jousimies-Somer.** 1997. Characteristics of an unusual anaerobic pigmented gram-negative rod isolated from normal and inflamed appendices. *Clin. Infect. Dis.* **25**(Suppl. 2)**:**S107–S110.

81. **Reischelderfer, C., and J. I. Mangels.** 1992. Culture media for anaerobes, p. 2.3.1–2.3.8. *In* H. D. Isenberg (ed.), *Clinical Microbiology Procedures Handbook*. American Society for Microbiology, Washington, D.C.

82. **Sakamoto, M., M. Suzuki, M. Umeda, I. Ishikawa, and Y. Benno.** 2002. Reclassification of *Bacteroides forsythus* (Tanner et al. 1986) as *Tannerella forsythensis* corrig. gen. nov., comb. nov. *Int. J. Syst. Evol. Microbiol.* **52:**841–849.

83. **Schreckenberger, P. C., D. M. Celig, and W. M. Janda.** 1988. Clinical evaluation of the Vitek ANI card for identification of anaerobic bacteria. *J. Clin. Microbiol.* **26:**225–230.

84. **Shah, H. N., and M. D. Collins.** 1989. Proposal to restrict the genus *Bacteroides* (Castellani and Chalmers) to *Bacteroides fragilis* and closely related species. *Int. J. Syst. Bacteriol.* **39:**85–87.

85. **Shah, H. N., C. J. Keys, S. E. Gharbia, K. Ralphson, F. Trundle, I. Brookhouse, and M. A. Claydon.** 2000. The application of matrix-assisted laser desorption/ionisation time of flight mass spectrometry to profile the surface of intact bacterial cells. *Microb. Ecol. Health Dis.* **12:**241–246.

86. **Sheppard, A., C. Cammarata, and D. H. Martin.** 1990. Comparison of different bases for the semiquantitative isolation of anaerobes from vaginal secretions. *J. Clin. Microbiol.* **28:**455–457.

87. **Slots, J.** 1987. Detection of colonies of *Bacteroides gingivalis* by a rapid fluorescence assay for trypsin-like activity. *Oral Microbiol. Immunol.* **2:**139–141.

88. **Socransky, S. S., S. Smith, L. Martin, B. J. Paster, F. E. Dewhirst, and A. E. Levin.** 1994. "Checkerboard" DNA-DNA hybridization. *BioTechniques* **17:**788–793.

89. **Summanen, P. H., P. J. Hancher, M. J. Flynn, and J. Slots.** 1996. Obstructive sialadenitis secondary to parotic sialolithiasis: a case report. *Anaerobe* **2:**81–84.

90. **Suzuki, K., T. Ikeda, H. Nakamura, and F. Yoshimura.** 1997. Isolation and characterization of a nonpigmented variant of *Porphyromonas endodontalis*. *Oral Microbiol. Immunol.* **12:**155–161.

91. **Talan, D. A., D. M. Citron, F. M. Abrahamian, G. J. Moran, E. J. Goldstein, for the Emergency Medicine Animal Bite Study Group.** 1999. Bacteriologic analysis of infected dog and cat bites. *N. Engl. J. Med.* **340:**85–92.

92. **Tanner, A., M. F. J. Maiden, B. J. Paster, and F. E. Dewhirst.** 1994. The impact of 16S ribosomal RNA-based phylogeny on the taxonomy of oral bacteria. *Periodontology 2000* **5:**26–51.

93. **Tee, W., M. Dyall-Smith, W. Woods, and D. Eisen.** 1996. Probable new species of *Desulfovibrio* isolated from a pyogenic liver abscess. *J. Clin. Microbiol.* **34:**1760–1764.

94. **Väisänen, M.-L., M. Kiviranta, P. Summanen, S. M. Finegold, and H. R. Jousimies-Somer.** 1997. *Porphyromonas endodontalis*-like organisms isolated from extraoral sources. *Clin. Infect. Dis.* **23**(Suppl. 2)**:**S191–S193.

95. **Wexler, H. M., D. Reeves, P. H. Summanen, E. Molitoris, M. McTeague, J. Duncan, K. Wilson, and S. M. Finegold.** 1996. *Sutterella wadsworthensis* gen. nov., sp. nov., bile-resistant microaerophilic *Campylobacter gracilis*-like clinical isolates. *Int. J. Syst. Bacteriol.* **46:**252–258.

96. **Willems, A., and M. D. Collins.** 1995. Reclassification of *Oribaculum catoniae* (Moore and Moore 1994) as *Porphyromonas catoniae* comb. nov. and emendation of the genus *Porphyromonas*. *Int. J. Syst. Bacteriol.* **45:**578–581.

97. **Wu, C.-C., J. L. Johnson, W. E. C. Moore, and L. V. H. Moore.** 1992. Emended descriptions of *Prevotella denticola*, *Prevotella loescheii*, *Prevotella veroralis*, and *Prevotella melaninogenica*. *Int. J. Syst. Bacteriol.* **42:**536–541.

Campylobacter and *Arcobacter*

IRVING NACHAMKIN

57

TAXONOMY

Three closely related genera, *Campylobacter*, *Arcobacter*, and the newly added genus *Sulfurospirillum*, are included in the family *Campylobacteraceae* (100, 141). The family *Campylobacteraceae* includes 16 species in the genus *Campylobacter*, 4 species in the genus *Arcobacter*, and 5 species in the genus *Sulfurospirillum*. Several new species have recently been proposed, including *Campylobacter hominis*, which is isolated from healthy human feces and which is closely related to *C. gracilis* and *C. sputorum* (76), and *C. lanienae*, which is isolated from healthy human feces and which is closely related to *C. hyointestinalis* (80). *Bacteroides ureolyticus* is somewhat related to *Campylobacter*; however, comparison of its 16S rRNA sequence with that of *Campylobacter* and phenotypic tests suggest major differences (100). Some isolates previously thought to be *C. gracilis* have now been renamed *Sutterella wadsworthensis* and are more related to *Alcaligenes* and *Bordetella* (155).

Campylobacters are curved, S-shaped, or spiral rods that are 0.2 to 0.9 μm wide and 0.5 to 5 μm long. Some species such as *C. hominis* form straight rods. *Campylobacter* species are gram-negative, non-spore-forming rods that may form spherical or coccoid bodies in old cultures or cultures exposed to air for prolonged periods. Organisms are usually motile by means of a single polar unsheathed flagellum at one or both ends, but they may lack flagella. The species are generally microaerobic with a respiratory type of metabolism; however, some strains grow aerobically or anaerobically. An atmosphere containing increased hydrogen may be required by some species for microaerobic growth (143).

Arcobacters are gram-negative, slightly curved, curved, S-shaped, or helical non-spore-forming rods that are 0.2 to 0.9 μm wide and 1 to 3 μm long. The organisms are motile with a single polar unsheathed flagellum. Arcobacters grow at 15, 25, and 30°C but have variable growth at 37 and 42°C. Organisms are microaerobic and do not require increased hydrogen for growth. Arcobacters may grow aerobically at 30°C and anaerobically at 35 to 37°C. Most strains are nonhemolytic. *Arcobacter skirrowii* may be alpha-hemolytic. Most *Arcobacter* strains are susceptible to nalidixic acid but variable to cephalothin (145).

Originally classified as free-living *Campylobacter* species, *Sulfurospirillum* spp. are slender, curved, gram-negative rods that are 0.1 to 0.5 μm wide and 1 to 3 μm long. All of the species are sulfur reducers and exhibit variable metabolic activities. *Sulfurospirillum deleyianum* is the type species of the genus. These species have no known pathogenicity for humans or animals, are environmental organisms isolated from water sediments, and will not be discussed in this chapter (141).

NATURAL HABITATS

Campylobacter species are primarily zoonotic, with a variety of animals implicated as reservoirs for infection (Table 1). In addition to food animals such as poultry, cattle, sheep, and pigs, *Campylobacter* species may be present in domestic pets. Humans appear to be the only recognized reservoirs for the periodontal pathogens.

CLINICAL SIGNIFICANCE

C. jejuni and *C. coli*

C. jejuni subsp. *jejuni* (referred to as *C. jejuni* throughout this chapter) and *C. coli* have been recognized since the late 1970s as agents of gastrointestinal infection. Many clinical and epidemiologic investigations have established *C. jejuni* as one of the most common causes of sporadic bacterial enteritis in the United States. Studies by the Centers for Disease Control and Prevention suggest that 2.4 million cases occur annually in the United States, an incidence of infection similar to that in the United Kingdom and other developed nations (35). *C. jejuni* continues to be the most common enteric pathogen isolated from patients with diarrhea, as suggested by the Foodborne Diseases Active Surveillance Network, FoodNet (20). *Campylobacter* infections are usually sporadic, occurring in the summer months and early fall, and usually follow ingestion of improperly handled or cooked food, primarily poultry products. The incidence of infection follows a bimodal age distribution, with the highest incidence in infants and young children, followed by a second peak in young adults 20 to 40 years old. Outbreaks usually occur in the spring and fall months, and in recent years, most outbreaks have been associated with contaminated food or water. Milk-borne outbreaks, while common in the 1980s and early 1990s, have not been reported since 1992 (35).

TABLE 1 Reservoirs for *Campylobacter* and *Arcobacter* species[a]

Reservoir	Species
Humans	*C. jejuni, C. sputorum* bv. sputorum, *C. concisus, C. curvus, C. rectus, C. showae, C. gracilis*
Cattle	*C. jejuni, C. fetus* subsp. *fetus* or *C. fetus* subsp. *venerealis, C. hyointestinalis, C. sputorum* bv. paraureolyticus and faecalis, *A. butzleri, A. cryaerophilus, A. skirrowii*
Sheep	*C. fetus, C. sputorum* bv. faecalis, *A. cryaerophilus, A. skirrowii*
Pigs	*C. coli, C. hyointestinalis, C. mucosalis, A. butzleri, A. cryaerophilus, A. skirrowii*
Birds	*C. jejuni, C. coli, C. lari*
Domestic pets	*C. jejuni, C. lari, C. upsaliensis, C. hyointestinalis, C. helveticus*

[a] The information in this table is from references 94, 122, and 142.

The incidence of campylobacter infection in developing countries such as Mexico and Thailand is much higher than that in the United States (99). In developing countries, *Campylobacter* is frequently isolated from individuals who may or may not have diarrheal disease. Most symptomatic infections occur in infancy and early childhood, and the incidence decreases with age. Travelers to developing countries are at risk for developing *Campylobacter* infection, with isolation rates of 0 to 39% reported in different studies (99).

C. jejuni and *C. coli* are the most common *Campylobacter* species associated with diarrheal illness and are clinically indistinguishable. Most laboratories do not routinely distinguish these organisms. Approximately 5 to 10% of cases reported as being due to *C. jejuni* in the United States are probably due to *C. coli*, but this percentage may be higher in other parts of the world (99).

A spectrum of illness is seen during *C. jejuni* or *C. coli* infection, and patients may be asymptomatic to severely ill. Symptoms and signs usually include fever, abdominal cramping, and diarrhea (with or without blood or fecal white blood cells) that lasts several days to more than 1 week. Symptomatic infections are usually self-limited, but relapses may occur in 5 to 10% of untreated patients (11). *Campylobacter* infection may mimic acute appendicitis and result in unnecessary surgery. Extraintestinal infections have been reported following *Campylobacter* enteritis and include bacteremia, hepatitis, cholecystitis, pancreatitis, abortion and neonatal sepsis, hemolytic uremic syndrome, nephritis, prostatitis, urinary tract infection, peritonitis, myocarditis, and focal infections including meningitis, septic arthritis, and abscess formation (123). Bacteremia has been reported to occur at a rate of 1.5 per 1,000 intestinal infections, with the highest rate occurring in the elderly (124). Persistent diarrheal illness and bacteremia may occur in immunocompromised hosts such as in patients with human immunodeficiency virus infection (109) and may be difficult to treat. Deaths attributable to *C. jejuni* infection are uncommon but do occur (35).

Guillain-Barré syndrome (GBS) and reactive arthritis are both late-onset complications of *Campylobacter* infection. *C. jejuni* infection is now the most recognized infection preceding the development of GBS, an acute paralytic disease of the peripheral nervous system. Certain Penner heat-stable (HS) serotypes such as HS:19 (67) and HS:41 (38) appear to be overrepresented in some GBS cases; other, more common serotypes are frequently reported as well (95). Certain serotypes of *C. jejuni* express ganglioside-like structures in the core region of the lipooligosaccharide. The pathogenesis of *Campylobacter*-induced GBS likely involves host immune responses to these ganglioside-like epitopes and, in the susceptible host, mediates damage in the peripheral nerve, where ganglioside targets are highly enriched (51).

Reactive arthritis sometimes follows campylobacter infection, with the onset of pain and joint swelling occurring days to weeks after the diarrhea and lasting from a few weeks to nearly a year. Reiter's syndrome may also occur in some patients (123). The pathogenesis of campylobacter infection and joint involvement is unknown, but HLA B27 positivity is strongly associated with the condition (123).

Little is known about the pathogenesis of campylobacter enteric infection. The infective dose of *Campylobacter* is not clearly defined, but as few as 1,000 organisms may be capable of causing illness (10). The signs and symptoms of infection suggest an invasive mechanism of disease. In vitro and in vivo studies suggest that *Campylobacter* first colonizes the intestinal mucous layer mediated by motility and then invades and/or translocates through the epithelial surface to the underlying tissue, where other putative virulence factors are then elaborated (65, 148). *C. jejuni* express a cytolethal distending toxin; however, the role of the toxin in pathogenesis is not understood (70, 111). *Campylobacter* spp. do not produce a classic cholera-like enterotoxin (153).

Campylobacter Species Other Than *C. jejuni* and *C. coli*

C. fetus subsp. *fetus* is primarily associated with bacteremia and extraintestinal infections in patients with underlying diseases, which may lead to a poor outcome in some patients (11). *C. fetus* subsp. *fetus* is also associated with septic abortions, septic arthritis, abscesses, meningitis, endocarditis, mycotic aneurysm, thrombophlebitis, peritonitis, and salpingitis (11). Although gastroenteritis does occur with this species, the incidence is probably underestimated because the organism does not grow well at 42°C and is usually susceptible to cephalothin, an antimicrobial agent used in some common selective media for stool culture (24). *C. fetus* subsp. *venerealis* causes bovine venereal campylobacteriosis and is a cause of infertility; it has rarely been isolated from human infections (137). *C. fetus* subsp. *fetus* produces a surface protein capsule composed of a high-molecular-weight surface array protein that is essential for the virulence of the organism. This high-molecular-weight protein confers resistance to serum-mediated killing and phagocytosis and may explain why *C. fetus* subsp. *fetus* is able to cause systemic infection (137).

C. upsaliensis is a thermotolerant species that appears to be an important cause of diarrhea and bacteremia in humans and that is also associated with canine and feline gastroenteritis (42, 77). *C. upsaliensis* is susceptible to many antimicrobial agents present in *C. jejuni*-selective media;

thus, it is usually not isolated on routine primary isolation media. *C. lari* is a thermophilic species first isolated from gulls of the genus *Larus* and from other avian species, dogs, cats, and chickens. *C. lari* has been infrequently reported from humans with bacteremia and gastrointestinal and urinary tract infections. A waterborne outbreak of infection that occurred in 1985 affected over 100 individuals (129).

Other *Campylobacter* species have been isolated from clinical specimens of patients with a variety of diseases, but their pathogenic roles have not been determined. *C. jejuni* subsp. *doylei* is a nitrate-negative subspecies of *C. jejuni* rarely recovered from patients with upper gastrointestinal tract infections and gastroenteritis (42, 127). *C. hyointestinalis* has been occasionally associated with proctitis and diarrhea in human infection (25). *C. concisus* is associated primarily with periodontal disease but has also been isolated from patients with bacteremia, foot ulcer, and upper and lower gastrointestinal tract infections (59, 144). The role of *C. concisus* as a cause of diarrheal disease is not established, and several studies suggest that the organism is not pathogenic (30, 147). *C. sputorum* biovars have been associated with lung, axillary, scrotal, and groin abscesses (88). *C. sputorum* bv. paraureolyticus, formerly referred to as catalase-negative, urease-positive campylobacter, has been isolated from patients with diarrhea, but the significance of this finding is unknown (101). *C. mucosalis* was isolated from two children with enteritis (34). *C. helveticus* (126) has been recovered from domestic cats and dogs and has not been reported from human sources. *C. rectus* is primarily isolated from patients with active periodontal infections but has also been isolated from a patient with pulmonary infection (115, 125). *C. curvus* is also isolated from patients with periodontal infections, but its role in gastrointestinal infections is unknown (30). *C. showae* has been isolated from the human gingival crevice (31). *C. gracilis* has been isolated from patients with appendicitis and peritonitis, bacteremia, soft tissue abscesses, and pulmonary infections (89). A more extensive review on the clinical significance of non-*C. jejuni* or *C. coli* species was recently published (72).

Arcobacter

Arcobacters are aerotolerant, *Campylobacter*-like organisms frequently isolated from bovine and porcine products of abortion and feces of animals with enteritis (154). Two of the five *Arcobacter* species have been associated with human infection. *A. butzleri* has been isolated from patients with bacteremia, endocarditis, peritonitis, and diarrhea (64, 132, 145). *A. cryaerophilus* has previously been characterized into two DNA-related groups, groups 1A and 1B (64). *A. cryaerophilus* group 1B has been isolated from patients with bacteremia and diarrhea (53, 64, 145). Group 1A has been isolated from animal sources (64). *A. nitrofigilis* is a nitrogen-fixing bacterium found on the roots of a small marsh plant in Nova Scotia, Canada, and is not associated with human disease (86).

COLLECTION, TRANSPORT, AND STORAGE OF SPECIMENS

Fecal Samples

Fecal specimens are the preferred sample for isolating *Campylobacter* species from patients with gastrointestinal infections; however, rectal swabs are acceptable for culture. For hospitalized patients, the "3-day" rule (rejection of specimens collected >72 h after admission) should be used as a criterion for the acceptability of routine culture requests (45, 50). For routine purposes, testing of a single stool sample has high sensitivity for detection of common enteric pathogens, but testing of two samples may be desirable, depending upon the clinical circumstances, such as a >2-h delay in transport of the first sample that could affect recovery (140). A transport medium should be used when a delay of more than 2 h is anticipated and for transport of rectal swabs. Several types of transport media that are useful for *Campylobacter* have been described, including alkaline peptone water with thioglycolate and cystine (151), modified Stuart medium (2), and Cary-Blair medium (19). Transport media such as commercial Stuart medium and buffered glycerol saline do not appear to perform well (151). Cary-Blair medium containing reduced agar (1.6 g/liter) appears to be the most suitable as a single transport medium for *Campylobacter* as well as other enteric pathogens (151). Specimens received in Cary-Blair medium should be stored at 4°C if processing is not performed immediately. Use of Cary-Blair medium supplemented with laked sheep blood may be useful for prolonged storage of stool samples and recovery of *C. jejuni* (152).

Blood

Campylobacter species, primarily *C. fetus*, *C. jejuni*, and *C. upsaliensis*, have been isolated from blood; however, in only a few studies have optimal conditions for isolating *Campylobacter* from blood culture systems been evaluated. Both the BACTEC system (aerobic bottles) and the Septi-Chek system appear to support the growth of the common *Campylobacter* species (63, 71, 150). Other systems, such as anaerobic broth or lysis-centrifugation, may not be as sensitive (63).

DIRECT EXAMINATION

Campylobacters are not easily visualized with the safranin counterstain commonly used in the Gram stain procedure; carbol fuchsin or 0.1% aqueous basic fuchsin should be used as the counterstain for smears of stools or pure cultures (105, 117). Because of their characteristic microscopic morphology, campylobacters may be detected with the reagents mentioned above by direct Gram stain examination of stools obtained from patients with acute enteritis at a sensitivity ranging from 66 to 94% and at a specificity above 95% (105, 117). Phase-contrast microscopy and dark-field microscopy have been used to directly detect motile campylobacters in fresh stool samples; however, the sensitivities of these approaches have not been studied widely, and in the author's experience, these approaches require significant microscopic expertise (61, 104).

Fecal white blood cells may be present during *Campylobacter* infection and have been reported in as few as 25% to as many as 80% of patients with culture-proven cases (32, 40). Some authors suggest that a test for the presence of leukocytes in stools be used to direct culture to improve the cost-effectiveness of diagnosis (44). While the likelihood of *Campylobacter* or other enteroinvasive pathogens may be higher in the presence of fecal leukocytes, the absence of fecal leukocytes does not rule out disease (140). Thus, routine examination of stool samples for fecal leukocytes is not recommended as a test for predicting bacterial infection or for selective culturing for *Campylobacter* or other stool pathogens (45).

ISOLATION PROCEDURES

Most *Campylobacter* species require a microaerobic atmosphere containing approximately 5% O_2, 10% CO_2, and 85% N_2 for optimal recovery. Several manufacturers produce microaerobic gas generator packs that are suitable for routine use. A tri-gas incubator (136) or evacuation and replacement of an anaerobic jar with the approximate gas mixture may also be used for routine cultures (91). The concentration of oxygen generated in candle jars is suboptimal for the isolation of *Campylobacter* and should not be used for routine laboratory isolation procedures (81). Some species of *Campylobacter*, such as *C. sputorum*, *C. concisus*, *C. mucosalis*, *C. curvus*, *C. rectus*, and *C. hyointestinalis*, require hydrogen for primary isolation and growth. These species may not be recovered under conventional microaerobic conditions since the amount of hydrogen generated in properly used commercial gas generator packs is <2% (92). A gas mixture of 10% CO_2, 6% H_2, and balanced N_2 used in an evacuation-replacement jar is sufficient for isolating hydrogen-requiring species (92).

A number of selective media are recommended for the isolation of *C. jejuni* and *C. coli*. These include blood-free media, such as charcoal cefoperazone deoxycholate agar (CCDA; Oxoid Inc. North America, Nepean, Ontario, Canada) (56) and charcoal-based selective medium (CSM; Oxoid Inc.) (62), and blood-containing media, such as Campy-CVA medium (L. B. Reller, S. Mirrett, and L. G. Reimer, Abstr. 83rd Annu. Meet. Am. Soc. Microbiol. 1983, abstr. C-274, p. 357, 1983) and Skirrow medium (121). A charcoal-based medium containing cefoperazone, amphotericin, and teicoplanin (CAT medium) is a selective medium for the primary isolation of *C. upsaliensis* (6). Two recent studies, however, did not isolate *C. upsaliensis* from any stool samples with this medium (30, 49). *C. upsaliensis* may occasionally be recovered on some other selective media. *C. upsaliensis* isolates are recovered by using a filtration method, and some strains may grow better in a hydrogen-enriched atmosphere (42, 72).

To achieve the highest yield of campylobacters from stool samples, a combination of media, including either CCDA or CSM as one of the media, appears to be the optimal method (28, 46) and may increase the recovery of campylobacters by as much as 10 to 15% over the use of a single medium. If only a single medium can be used because of budgetary constraints, our laboratory has had very good experience with the Campy-CVA formulation, but a charcoal-based medium such as CCDA works just as well. CCDA was found to be the most sensitive for detecting *C. jejuni* and *C. coli* when it was compared with Skirrow medium, CAT agar, and the filtration technique of Engberg et al. (30).

Most of these selective media have one or more antimicrobial agents, mainly cefoperazone, as the primary inhibitors of enteric bacterial flora. The antimicrobial agents, such as cephalothin, colistin, and polymyxin B, present in some selective medium formulations are inhibitory to some strains of *C. jejuni* and *C. coli* (41, 98) and are inhibitory to *C. fetus* subsp. *fetus*. *C. jejuni* subsp. *doylei*, *C. upsaliensis*, and *A. butzleri* generally will not grow on cephalothin-containing media. When choosing selective media for the primary isolation of *Campylobacter* from fecal samples, laboratories should use cefoperazone-containing media and discontinue using cephalothin-containing formulations.

If *Campylobacter* infection is suspected at the time that blood specimens are drawn, broth media should be subcul-

tured after 24 to 48 h to a nonselective blood agar medium and the plates should be incubated under microaerobic conditions at 37°C. This procedure will allow for the isolation of thermophilic and nonthermophilic species. Similarly, blood drawn in Isolator (Wampole Laboratories, Cranbury, N.J.) tubes for bacterial culture should be inoculated on a nonselective blood agar plate incubated under microaerobic conditions at 37°C if *Campylobacter* infection is suspected. If a curved, gram-negative rod is observed upon Gram stain examination of a positive blood culture bottle, an aliquot should be cultured on a nonselective blood agar plate and incubated under microaerobic conditions at 37°C. An alternative staining method, such as acridine orange staining, may also be useful for detecting campylobacters in blood culture bottles if the Gram stain results are negative.

Optimal conditions for the recovery of *Arcobacter* from clinical specimens have not been determined. *Arcobacter* species were first isolated on semisolid media designed to isolate *Leptospira* species (145, 154). *Arcobacter* species are aerotolerant and have been recovered on certain selective media, such as Campy-CVA (5), incubated under microaerobic conditions at 37°C and on nonselective media used with the filtration method. Several other media have been reported to recover *Arcobacter* species but have not been studied in clinical settings (5, 22, 145; A. Borczyk, S. D. Rosa, and H. Lior, Abstr. 91st Annu. Meet. Am. Soc. Microbiol. 1991, abstr. C-267, p. 386, 1991).

Enrichment Cultures

A number of enrichment broths have been formulated to enhance the recovery of *Campylobacter* from stool samples, such as Preston enrichment (13), Campy-thio (12), *Campylobacter* enrichment broth (85), and other formulations (1, 21, 66, 119). Enrichment cultures may be beneficial in instances in which low numbers of organisms may be expected due to delayed transport to the laboratory or after the acute stage of disease, when the concentration of organisms may be low, such as in the investigation of GBS following acute *Campylobacter* infection (15, 93, 131). The clinical effectiveness and the cost-effectiveness of using enrichment cultures as part of the routine stool culture setup have not been studied adequately.

Filtration

Filtration should be used as a complement to direct culture to selective plating media and not as a replacement. Various investigators have cultured stools using a filtration method with a nonselective medium to isolate antibiotic-susceptible *C. jejuni* and *C. coli* as well as other *Campylobacter* species (30, 41, 42) and *Arcobacter* species (64) susceptible to antibiotics present in most selective media. The method is based on the principle that campylobacters can pass through membrane filters (pore sizes, 0.45 to 0.65 μm) with relative ease (because of their motility), while other stool flora are retained during the short processing time. Cellulose acetate membrane filters with a 0.65-μm pore size are recommended for routine use (J. G. Wells, N. D. Puhr, C. M. Patton, M. A. Nicholson, M. A. Lambert, and R. Jerris, Abstr. Annu. 89th Meet. Am. Soc. Microbiol. 1989, abstr. C231, p. 432, 1989). The filtration technique is performed by placing a sterile 0.65-μm-pore-size cellulose acetate filter onto the surface of an agar medium such as antibiotic-free CCDA, CSM, or blood-containing medium. Ten to 15 drops of fecal suspension are placed on the filter, and the plate is incubated at 37°C for

1 h. The filter is then removed and the plate is incubated at 37°C under microaerobic conditions, preferably with an atmosphere containing increased hydrogen (for the hydrogen-requiring species). Stool samples containing ~10^5 CFU of campylobacter per ml will be detected by this method, and thus, the filtration method is not as sensitive as primary culture with selective media (42).

Species within the genera *Campylobacter* and *Arcobacter* have different optimal temperatures for growth. The choice of incubation temperature for routine stool cultures is therefore critical in determining the spectrum of species that will be isolated. By convention, most laboratories use 42°C as the primary incubation temperature for *Campylobacter*. This temperature allows growth of *C. jejuni* and *C. coli* on selective media. *C. upsaliensis* also grows well at 42°C but usually is not recovered on selective media. *C. fetus* grows poorly at this temperature and generally will not be recovered. *Arcobacter* species are not thermophilic and generally cannot be recovered at 42°C.

In contrast, most *Campylobacter* and *Arcobacter* species grow well at 37°C. Selective media, such as Skirrow medium, were devised for use at 42°C and have poor selective properties at 37°C, whereas CCDA and CSM show good selective properties at 37°C (28). Plates should be incubated for 72 h before the results are reported as negative. Engberg et al. (30) also found that incubation of CCDA for 5 to 6 days increased the yield of *C. jejuni* and *C. coli* compared with that after 2 days of incubation.

Because of the expense of including several types of media and filtration in the initial workup for campylobacters, a practical approach is to use a single medium, such as Campy-CVA or CCDA (or equivalent) incubated at 42°C, for the isolation of thermophilic campylobacters in the workup of acute bacterial gastroenteritis. If the primary culture workup is unrevealing and, based on clinical consultation, additional testing is required, additional stool samples should be plated on multiple selective media (e.g., CCDA or CVA), processed by the filtration method, and incubated at 37°C under microaerobic conditions.

IDENTIFICATION

Depending on the medium used, *Campylobacter* colonies may have different appearances. In general, *Campylobacter* spp. produce gray, flat, irregular, and spreading colonies, particularly on freshly prepared media; spreading along the streak line is commonly seen. As the moisture content decreases, colonies may form round, convex, and glistening colonies, with little spreading observed. Hemolysis on blood agar is not observed. *Arcobacter* spp. are morphologically similar to *Campylobacter* spp. (141, 145).

For initial analysis, a Gram stain examination of the colony should be performed along with an oxidase test. Oxidase-positive colonies exhibiting a characteristic Gram stain appearance (e.g., gram-negative, curved to S-shaped rods) on selective media incubated at 42°C under microaerobic conditions can be reliably reported as *Campylobacter* spp. until other biochemical tests are performed (Table 2). The Gram stain appearance of *Arcobacter* colonies may differ from that of typical *Campylobacter* colonies. *A. butzleri* is only slightly curved, and *A. cryaerophilus* tends to be much more helical in appearance. Commercial systems for identification of *Campylobacter* species have not been found to be more accurate than conventional tests (57). Unfortunately, *Campylobacter* species are difficult to differentiate from *Arcobacter* species on the basis of pheno-

typic tests. However, an aerotolerant species (i.e., a species that grows under aerobic conditions) that grows on Mac-Conkey agar (under microaerobic conditions) could be presumptively identified as *Arcobacter* sp. The failure to grow on MacConkey agar, however, does not rule out an *Arcobacter* species.

For species other than *C. jejuni*, phenotypic characterization becomes more problematic. With the increasing prevalence of fluoroquinolone-resistant species, use of the disk identification assays, a mainstay for many years, is no longer useful in most circumstances. Because many of the species of *Campylobacter* and *Arcobacter* are difficult to identify, however, molecular methods have been developed to differentiate a number of species.

The most common species, *C. jejuni* is relatively easy to identify phenotypically; however, hippurate-negative strains may be more difficult to identify. Except for hippuricase activity, which *C. coli* lacks, both *C. coli* and *C. jejuni* are similar biochemically. As such, molecular methods are needed to accurately identify *C. coli*. *C. jejuni*, *C. coli*, other *Campylobacter* species, and *Arcobacter* species have been reported to be reliably differentiated based on polymorphism in the *ceuE* gene (39), a GTPase gene (146), the 16S rRNA gene (48, 75, 78, 84), the 23S rRNA gene (9, 33, 55), and the *glyA* gene (4) by PCR and/or PCR-restriction fragment length polymorphism analysis.

Several phenotypic tests have been described for identifying *Campylobacter* spp. The most routinely useful tests for initial identification include growth temperature studies (e.g., growth at 25, 37, and 42°C), catalase production, hippurate hydrolysis, indoxyl acetate hydrolysis, nitrate reduction, production of H_2S, and antibiotic sensitivity determined by the disk method (8). The methods for the routinely useful tests have been published elsewhere (8, 58, 91).

Hydrolysis of sodium hippurate is the major test for distinguishing between *C. jejuni* (and also *C. jejuni* subsp. *doylei*) and other *Campylobacter* species. Strains that are isolated on selective media that grow at 42°C, are oxidase positive, show characteristic microscopic morphology, and give a positive result for hippurate hydrolysis should be reported as *C. jejuni* subsp. *jejuni*; and for routine clinical purposes, no other tests need to be performed. Methods for this test are described elsewhere (82, 114). Commercially available disk methods for rapid hippurate hydrolysis testing compare favorably with the tube method (18). A large inoculum (i.e., a full loop) should be used for this test. Occasional strains of *C. jejuni* may be hippurate hydrolysis negative (90, 139). Gas-liquid chromatography for detecting benzoic acid (liberated from the hydrolysis of sodium hippurate) is the most sensitive assay for hippurate hydrolysis (90) and can be used for more definitive determination. Molecular detection of the *hipO* (hippuricase) gene by PCR may be useful for identifying phenotypically negative isolates (47).

Inhibition (susceptibility) or resistance of *Campylobacter* spp. to nalidixic acid and cephalothin has routinely been used as an aid for species identification. Tests can be performed by standard disk diffusion techniques with any nonselective medium that supports the growth of the *Campylobacter* strain; 30-μg nalidixic acid and 30-μg cephalothin disks should be incubated at 37°C for nonthermophilic campylobacters and at 42°C for thermophilic strains for 1 to 2 days. Any zone of inhibition indicates susceptibility. Some variability does exist with this test, and even with *C. jejuni* and *C. coli*, many strains may not give the expected

TABLE 2 Phenotypic properties of *Campylobacter* and *Arcobacter* species[a]

Organism	Catalase	Nitrate reduction	H₂ required	Urease	H₂S (TSI)	Hippurate hydrolysis	Indoxyl acetate hydrolysis	Growth at: 25°C	42°C	Growth in or on: 3.5% NaCl	1% Glycine	MacConkey agar	Susceptibility to: Nalidixic acid	Cephalothin
C. jejuni	+	+	−	−	−	+	+	−	+	−	+	−	V	R
C. jejuni subsp. doylei	V	−	−	−	−	V	+	−	−	V	+	−	S	S
C. coli	+	+	−	−	V	−	+	−	+	−	+	V	V	R
C. fetus subsp. fetus	+	+	−	−	−	−	−	+	V	−	+	V	V	S
C. fetus subsp. venerealis	V	+	−	−	−	−	−	+	−	−	−	V	V	S
C. lari	+	+	−	V	−	−	−	−	+	−	+	−	R	R
C. upsaliensis	−	+	−	−	−	−	+	−	V	−	+	V	S	V
C. hyointestinalis subsp. hyointestinalis	+	+	V	−	+	−	−	V	+	−	+	V	R	V
C. hyointestinalis subsp. lawsonii	+	+	V	+	+[b]	−	−	−	+	−	V	V	R	S
C. lanienae	+	+	ND	ND	−	−	−	−	+	−	−	ND	R	R
C. sputorum bv. sputorum[b]	−	+	+	−	+	−	−	−	+	−	+	+	S	S
C. sputorum bv. faecalis	+	+	+	+	+	−	−	−	+	−		+	R	S
C. sputorum bv. paraureolyticus	−	+	+	+	+	−	−	ND	ND	V	+	ND	R	V
C. helveticus	−	+	−	−	−	−	+	−	+	−	V	−	S	S
C. hominis	−	V	+[c]	ND	−	−	−	−	−	−	−	−	V	ND
C. mucosalis	−	−	+	−	+	−	−	−	+	−	V	V	V	S
C. concisus	−	V	+	−	+	−	−	−	V	−	V	+	V	S
C. curvus	−	+	+	−	−	−	V	−	V	−	+	V	R	S
C. rectus	V	+	+	−	V	V	+	−	V	−	−	−	V	S
C. showae	+	V	+	−	−	−	V	−	V	−	V	+	S	S
C. gracilis[c]	V	V	ND	−	−	−	V	−	V	−	+	V	V	R
A. cryaerophilus	V	+	−	−	−	−	+	+	−	V	V	V	V	R
A. butzleri	V	+	−	−	−	−	+	+	+	−	V	V	V	S
A. nitrofigilis	+	+	−	+	−	−	+	+	−	+	−	−	S	S
A. skirrowii	+	+	−	−	−	−	+	+	+	−	−	−	S	R
B. ureolyticus	V	+	+	+	−	−	−	−	V	+	+	V	S	S

[a] +, positive reaction; −, negative reaction; TSI, triple sugar iron; W, weak reaction; V, variable reaction; ND, not determined; S, susceptible; R, resistant. Adapted from references 31, 64, 76, 80, 112, 126, 141, 143, and 145.
[b] Strains of C. sputorum and C. hyointestinalis subsp. lawsonii normally produce large amounts of H₂S in triple sugar iron agar (76).
[c] Anaerobic growth only.

results. Occasional strains of *C. jejuni* and *C. coli* may be cephalothin susceptible. Resistance to nalidixic acid in *C. jejuni* or *C. coli* strains has been increasing in many parts of the world, with rates of resistance reported to be as high as 80% (29). Since there is cross-resistance between the fluoroquinolones and nalidixic acid, the finding of nalidixic acid resistance does not exclude the identification of *C. jejuni* or *C. coli*. As such, disk identification tests are no longer appropriate for the initial characterization of *Campylobacter* isolates from stool cultures. Hippurate hydrolysis-positive strains should be reported as *C. jejuni*, regardless of the results obtained by the nalidixic acid disk technique. Detection of a nalidixic acid-resistant strain of *C. jejuni* should also alert the laboratory and suggest to the physician that the strain may be resistant to fluoroquinolones, and further susceptibility testing may be warranted if antimicrobial therapy with this class of drugs is used.

Indoxyl acetate hydrolysis (83, 87, 112) is useful for differentiating some thermophilic *Campylobacter* species (Table 2). The disk method is rapid (5 to 30 min) and easy to perform. Disks are prepared by making a 20% solution of indoxyl acetate in acetone and adding 25 μl to a blank paper disk (0.6 cm). The disk is dried at room temperature and stored at 4°C in a brown tube with desiccant. Disks are also available from commercial sources. A large loopful of growth from a plate is placed on the disk, and a drop of sterile distilled water is added. Hydrolysis of indoxyl acetate is indicated by the appearance of a dark blue or blue-green color. Weakly positive strains show a pale blue color in 10 to 30 min. No color change is indicative of a negative reaction.

Additional tests can be performed to aid in the identification of *Campylobacter* spp. (Table 2). To obtain consistent and reproducible results, a standardized suspension and inoculum should be used for phenotypic tests. For growth temperature and oxygen tolerance studies, a suspension of the organism in heart infusion broth or tryptic soy broth at a turbidity of a McFarland no. 1 turbidity standard should be used. A fiber-tipped swab dipped in the broth suspension should be used to make a single streak across the plate (Mueller-Hinton agar with 5% sheep blood is a suitable medium), and the plates should be incubated at the desired temperature and/or under the desired atmospheric conditions (8, 91).

The H₂S reaction on triple sugar iron medium works best if the medium is freshly prepared. The nitrate reduction test is performed with nitrate broth medium (91) as described by Barrett et al. (8). Nitrate medium is inoculated with 0.1 ml of bacterial suspension. Strains that do not grow in nitrate broth medium can be inoculated into semisolid Mueller-Hinton broth with 0.3% agar and 0.2% potassium nitrate by stabbing the agar several times with bacterial growth from an agar plate. Development of a red reaction after addition of appropriate reagents indicates reduction of nitrate (73).

Nonculture Methods

A number of commercial systems have been developed as an aid to identifying *Campylobacter* spp. to the genus level. Two immunologic assays that use isolated colonies (ID Campy [Integrated Diagnostics, Baltimore, Md.] and Campyslide [BBL Microbiology Systems, Cockeysville, Md.]) (52, 96) can identify *C. jejuni* and *C. coli* but cannot differentiate the two. At the time of evaluation, the ID Campy (formerly Meritec Campy jcl; Meridian Diagnostics, Cincinnati, Ohio) assay could not reliably identify *C. lari*

(96). A DNA probe (Accuprobe; Gen-Probe Inc., San Diego, Calif.) directed against *Campylobacter* rRNA sequences identifies *C. jejuni C. jejuni* subsp. *doylei*, *C. coli*, and *C. lari* and was 100% sensitive for all isolates tested (113, 135); however, the probe also hybridized with 2 of 17 *C. hyointestinalis* strains (113). Thus, these methods may be useful for confirming *Campylobacter* if other tests are not conclusive.

A commercially available system for the detection of *Campylobacter* antigen in stool samples is now available (ProSpecT *Campylobacter*; Alexon-Trend, Inc., Ramsey, Minn.). When compared with culture, this immunoassay had a sensitivity and a specificity of 89 and 99%, respectively, in a study conducted by Hindiyeh and colleagues (49) in the Salt Lake City, Utah, region. The enzyme immunoassay was found to cross-react with *C. upsaliensis*; however, *C. upsaliensis* was not isolated from any patients in that study. Tolcin et al. (138) found the assay to be highly sensitive (96%) and specific (98.2%) compared with culture in an analysis of 50 frozen culture-positive stool samples. In an analysis of 30 culture-positive stool samples by Endtz and colleagues (26), the assay had a sensitivity of 80% and antigen was detected in the same positive samples stored for up to 8 to 9 days at 4°C. Several investigators have evaluated PCR for directly detecting *Campylobacter* in stool samples (74, 78, 102, 103, 128, 149). The major obstacle in the development of a PCR assay for stools for the clinical laboratory is the lack of a simple and practical DNA extraction procedure for stools that eliminates PCR inhibitors.

Epidemiologic Typing Systems

Many typing systems have been devised to study the epidemiology of *Campylobacter* infections, and they vary in complexity and ability to discriminate between strains. These methods include serotyping, biotyping, bacteriocin sensitivity testing, detection of preformed enzymes, auxotyping, lectin binding, phage typing, multilocus enzyme electrophoresis, and molecular methods such as restriction endonuclease analysis, ribotyping, and PCR (97, 106). The most frequently used system is serotyping. Two major serotyping schemes are used worldwide and detect heat-labile (HL) (79) and HS (108) antigens. The HL serotyping scheme originally described by Lior et al. (79) can detect over 100 serotypes of *C. jejuni*, *C. coli*, and *C. lari*. Uncharacterized bacterial surface antigens and, in some serotypes, flagellar antigens are the serodeterminants for this serotyping system (3). The HS serotyping scheme of Penner and Hennessy (108) detects 60 types of *C. jejuni* and *C. coli* (106). Initially thought to detect lipopolysaccharide antigenic determinants, the HS system was recently shown to detect a *Campylobacter* capsular polysaccharide (60). Serotyping is performed only in a few reference laboratories because of the time and expense needed to maintain quality antisera. A combination of serotyping and molecular methods should be used for studying the epidemiology of campylobacter infections (97).

SEROLOGIC TESTS

Serum immunoglobulin (IgG), IgM, and IgA levels rise in response to infection, but IgA appears in serum and feces during the first few weeks of infection and then the level falls rapidly (11). Serum antibody assays vary in both sensitivity and specificity for detecting campylobacter infections, and test performance appears to be population dependent. Patients with campylobacter infection may have false-positive legionella antibody test results (14). Serologic testing appears to be useful for epidemiologic investigations and is not recommended for routine diagnosis.

ANTIMICROBIAL SUSCEPTIBILITY

C. jejuni and *C. coli* have variable susceptibilities to a variety of antimicrobial agents, including macrolides, fluoroquinolones, aminoglycosides, chloramphenicol, nitrofurantoin, and tetracycline (11). Most isolates are not susceptible to cephalosporins and penicillins (11). Azithromycin and erythromycin are the drugs of choice for treating *C. jejuni* gastrointestinal infections, and for infections caused by susceptible organisms, ciprofloxacin or norfloxacin may also be used (37). Early therapy of *Campylobacter* infection with erythromycin or ciprofloxacin is effective in eliminating the organism from stools and may also reduce the duration of symptoms associated with infection (23, 40, 110, 116).

C. jejuni is generally susceptible to erythromycin, with resistance rates of less than 5% (107, 118). Rates of erythromycin resistance in *C. coli* vary considerably, with up to 80% of strains showing resistance in some studies (54, 69, 107, 130). Although ciprofloxacin has been effective in treating *Campylobacter* infections, the emergence of ciprofloxacin resistance during therapy has been reported (17, 40, 110, 133, 157). Several in vitro studies now show significant rates of resistance to fluoroquinolones (16, 27, 29, 36, 43, 120, 156), and thus, the effectiveness of this class of drugs may be diminished. *C. jejuni* and *C. coli* may also produce a β-lactamase that appears to be active against amoxicillin, ampicillin, and ticarcillin; this enzyme has been reported to be inhibited by clavulanic acid but not by sulbactam or tazobactam (68).

Parenteral therapy is used to treat systemic *C. fetus* infections; drugs used include erythromycin, ampicillin, aminoglycosides, and chloramphenicol, depending upon the type of infection (11). *C. gracilis* is generally susceptible to a variety of antimicrobial agents, including amoxicillin-clavulanate, cefoxitin, ceftriaxone, clindamycin, metronidazole, and piperacillin-tazobactam (89).

Susceptibility tests for *Campylobacter* are not standardized; consequently, the literature contains some variability in the susceptibility data reported. Recommendations for the agar dilution method include the use of Mueller-Hinton agar supplemented with 5% horse or sheep blood and incubated for 16 to 18 h under microaerobic conditions (134). The E-test (PDM Epsilometer; AB Biodisk, Solna, Sweden) with Mueller-Hinton agar with 5% sheep blood has been found to compare favorably with agar dilution methods (7, 54).

INTERPRETATION AND REPORTING OF RESULTS

Campylobacter species, including the common thermophilic species *C. jejuni* and *C. coli*, should be sought in all diarrheic stools submitted to the laboratory for routine culture. Except for epidemiologic purposes, cultures of formed stools should not be performed. Isolation of *Campylobacter* from a patient with acute diarrhea is usually significant since the carrier rate in developed countries is quite low; however, in developing countries, the significance of isolation might be more difficult to interpret, especially in the presence of

other enteric pathogens. In acute infection, there is usually a high number of organisms in the stool; however, the quantity of organisms is neither related to the severity of infection nor indicative of a carrier state. Other species, such as *C. fetus* subsp. *fetus* and *C. upsaliensis*, may be important causes of diarrhea and are not isolated on routine selective media. Special methods including alternative incubation techniques would be required, as described in this chapter. Oxidase-positive, curved gram-negative rods that are hippurate hydrolysis positive should be reported as *C. jejuni* without further workup. The importance of identifying other species will depend upon the clinical circumstance, but identification tests should always be performed on isolates from blood or other sterile sites since this could influence antimicrobial therapy decisions. Given that fluoroquinolone resistance is present in a significant proportion of *C. jejuni* isolates, susceptibility testing is suggested for isolates from patients who are receiving or being considered for therapy of gastroenteritis. Susceptibility testing should be performed on all systemic isolates.

REFERENCES

1. **Agulla, A., F. J. Merino, P. A. Villasante, J. V. Saz, A. Diaz, and A. C. Velasco.** 1987. Evaluation of four enrichment media for isolation of *Campylobacter jejuni*. *J. Clin. Microbiol.* **25:**174–175.
2. **Aho, M., M. Kauppi, and J. Hirn.** 1988. The stability of small number of campylobacteria in four different transport media. *Acta Vet. Scand.* **29:**437–442.
3. **Alm, R. A., P. Guerry, M. E. Power, H. Lior, and T. J. Trust.** 1991. Analysis of the role of flagella in the heat-labile Lior serotyping scheme of thermophilic campylobacters by mutant allele exchange. *J. Clin. Microbiol.* **29:**2438–2445.
4. **Al Rashid, S. T., I. Dakuna, H. Louie, D. Ng, P. Vandamme, W. Johnson, and V. L. Chan.** 2000. Identification of *Campylobacter jejuni, C. coli, C. lari, C. upsaliensis, Arcobacter butzleri,* and *A. butzleri*-like species based on the *glyA* gene. *J. Clin. Microbiol.* **38:**1488–1494.
5. **Anderson, K. F., J. A. Kiehlbauch, D. C. Anderson, H. M. McClure, and I. K. Wachsmuth.** 1993. *Arcobacter (Campylobacter) butzleri* associated diarrheal illness in a nonhuman primate. *Infect. Immun.* **61:**2220–2223.
6. **Aspinall, S. T., D. R. A. Wareing, P. G. Hayward, and D. N. Hutchinson.** 1996. A comparison of a new campylobacter selective medium (CAT) with membrane filtration for the isolation of thermophilic campylobacters including *Campylobacter upsaliensis*. *J. Appl. Bacteriol.* **80:**645–650.
7. **Baker, C. N.** 1992. The E-test and *Campylobacter jejuni*. *Diagn. Microbiol. Infect. Dis.* **15:**469–472.
8. **Barrett, T. J., C. M. Patton, and G. K. Morris.** 1988. Differentiation of *Campylobacter* species using phenotypic characterization. *Lab. Med.* **19:**96–102.
9. **Bastyns, K., D. Cartuyvels, S. Chapelle, P. Vandamme, H. Goossens, and R. De Wachter.** 1995. A variable 23S rDNA region is a useful discriminating target for genus-specific and species-specific PCR amplification in *Arcobacter* species. *Syst. Appl. Microbiol.* **18:**353–356.
10. **Black, R. E., M. M. Levine, M. L. Clements, T. P. Hughs, and M. J. Blaser.** 1988. Experimental *Campylobacter jejuni* infections in humans. *J. Infect. Dis.* **157:**472–480.
11. **Blaser, M. J.** 2000. *Campylobacter jejuni* and related species, p. 2276–2285. *In* G. L. Mandell, J. E. Bennett, and R. Dolin (ed.), *Principles and Practice of Infectious Diseases*. Churchill Livingstone, Philadelphia, Pa.

12. Blaser, M. J., I. D. Berkowitz, F. M. LaForce, J. Craven, L. B. Reller, and W. L. Wang. 1979. Campylobacter enteritis: clinical and epidemiologic features. *Ann. Intern. Med.* **91:**179–185.

13. Bolton, F. J., and L. Robertson. 1982. A selective medium for isolating *Campylobacter jejuni/coli*. *J. Clin. Pathol.* **35:**462–467.

14. Boswell, T. C. J., and G. Kudesia. 1992. Serological cross-reactions between *Legionella pneumophila* and *Campylobacter* in the indirect fluorescent antibody test. *Epidemiol. Infect.* **109:**291–295.

15. Bowen-Jones, J. 1989. Infection and cross-infection in a paediatric gastro-enteritis unit. *Curationis* **12:**30–33.

16. Bowler, I. C. J. W., M. Connor, M. P. A. Lessing, and D. Day. 1996. Quinolone resistance and *Campylobacter* species. *J. Antimicrob. Chemother.* **38:**315.

17. Burnens, A. P., M. Heitz, I. Brodard, and J. Nicolet. 1996. Sequential development of resistance to fluoroquinolones and erythromycin in an isolate of *Campylobacter jejuni*. *Zentbl. Bakteriol. Parasitenkd. Infektkrankh. Hyg. Abt. 1 Orig.* **283:**314–321.

18. Cacho, J. B., P. M. Aguirre, A. Hernanz, and A. C. Velasco. 1989. Evaluation of a disk method for detection of hippurate hydrolysis by *Campylobacter* spp. *J. Clin. Microbiol.* **27:**359–360.

19. Cary, S. G., and E. B. Blair. 1964. New transport medium for shipment of clinical specimens. I. Fecal specimens. *J. Bacteriol.* **88:**96–98.

20. Centers for Disease Control and Prevention. 2001. Preliminary FoodNet data on the incidence of foodborne illnesses—selected sites, United States, 2000. *Morb. Mortal. Wkly. Rep.* **50:**241–246.

21. Chan, F. T. H., and A. M. R. Mackenzie. 1984. Advantage of using enrichment-culture techniques to isolate *Campylobacter jejuni* from stools. *J. Infect. Dis.* **149:**481–482.

22. de Boer, E., J. J. H. C. Tilburg, D. L. Woodward, H. Lior, and W. M. Johnson. 1996. A selective medium for the isolation of *Arcobacter* from meats. *Lett. Appl. Microbiol.* **23:**64–66.

23. Dryden, M. S., R. J. E. Gabb, and S. K. Wright. 1996. Empirical treatment of severe acute community-acquired gastroenteritis with ciprofloxacin. *Clin. Infect. Dis.* **22:**1019–1025.

24. Edmonds, P., C. M. Patton, T. J. Barrett, G. K. Morris, A. G. Steigerwalt, and D. J. Brenner. 1985. Biochemical and genetic characteristics of atypical *Campylobacter fetus* subsp. *fetus* isolated from humans in the United States. *J. Clin. Microbiol.* **21:**936–940.

25. Edmonds, P., C. M. Patton, P. M. Griffin, T. J. Barrett, G. P. Schmid, C. N. Baker, M. A. Lambert, and D. J. Brenner. 1987. *Campylobacter hyointestinalis* associated with human gastrointestinal disease in the United States. *J. Clin. Microbiol.* **25:**685–691.

26. Endtz, H. P., C. W. Ang, N. Van Den Braak, A. Luijendijk, B. C. Jacobs, P. de Man, J. M. van Duin, A. van Belkum, and H. A. Verbrugh. 2000. Evaluation of a new commercial immunoassay for rapid detection of *Campylobacter jejuni* in stool samples. *Eur. J. Clin. Microbiol. Infect. Dis.* **19:**794–797.

27. Endtz, H. P., G. J. Ruijs, B. van Klingeren, W. H. Jansen, T. van der Reyden, and R. P. Mouton. 1991. Quinolone resistance in campylobacter isolated from man and poultry following the introduction of fluoroquinolones in veterinary medicine. *J. Antimicrob. Chemother.* **27:**199–208.

28. Endtz, H. P., G. J. Ruijs, A. H. Zwinderman, T. van der Reijden, M. Biever, and R. P. Mouton. 1991. Comparison of six media, including a semisolid agar, for the isolation of various *Campylobacter* species from stool specimens. *J. Clin. Microbiol.* **29:**1007–1010.

29. Engberg, J., F. M. Aarestrup, D. E. Taylor, P. Gerner-Smidt, and I. Nachamkin. 2001. Quinolone and macrolide resistance in *Campylobacter jejuni* and *C. coli*: resistance mechanisms and trends in human isolates. *Emerg. Infect. Dis.* **7:**24–34.

30. Engberg, J., S. L. W. On, C. S. Harrington, and P. Gerner-Smidt. 2000. Prevalence of *Campylobacter*, *Arcobacter*, *Helicobacter*, and *Sutterella* spp. in human fecal samples as estimated by a reevaluation of isolation methods for *Campylobacter*. *J. Clin. Microbiol.* **38:**286–291.

31. Etoh, Y., F. E. Dewhirst, B. J. Paster, A. Yamamoto, and N. Goto. 1993. *Campylobacter showae* sp. nov., isolated from the human oral cavity. *Int. J. Syst. Bacteriol.* **43:**631–639.

32. Fan, K., A. J. Morris, and L. B. Reller. 1993. Application of rejection criteria for stool cultures for bacterial enteric pathogens. *J. Clin. Microbiol.* **31:**2233–2235.

33. Fermer, C., and E. O. Engvall. 1999. Specific PCR identification and differentiation of the thermophilic campylobacters, *Campylobacter jejuni*, *C. coli*, *C. lari*, and *C. upsaliensis*. *J. Clin. Microbiol.* **37:**3370–3373.

34. Figura, N., P. Guglielmetti, A. Zanchi, N. Partini, D. Armellini, P. F. Bayeli, M. Bugnoli, and S. Verdiani. 1993. Two cases of *Campylobacter mucosalis* enteritis in children. *J. Clin. Microbiol.* **31:**727–728.

35. Friedman, C. R., J. Neimann, H. C. Wegener, and R. V. Tauxe. 2000. Epidemiology of *Campylobacter jejuni* infections in the United States and other industrialized nations, p. 121–138. *In* I. Nachamkin and M. J. Blaser (ed.), *Campylobacter*, 2nd ed. ASM Press, Washington, D.C.

36. Gaunt, P. N., and L. J. V. Piddock. 1996. Ciprofloxacin resistant *Campylobacter* spp. in humans: an epidemiological and laboratory study. *J. Antimicrob. Chemother.* **37:**747–757.

37. Gilbert, D. N., R. C. Moellering, Jr., and M. A. Sande. 2000. *The Sanford Guide to Antimicrobial Therapy*. Antimicrobial Therapy, Inc., Hyde Park, Vt.

38. Goddard, E. A., A. J. Lastovica, and A. C. Argent. 1997. *Campylobacter* O:41 isolation in Guillain-Barré syndrome. *Arch. Dis. Child.* **76:**526–528.

39. Gonzalez, I., K. A. Grant, P. T. Richardson, S. F. Park, and M. D. Collins. 1997. Specific identification of the enteropathogens *Campylobacter jejuni* and *Campylobacter coli* by using a PCR test based on the *ceuE* gene encoding a putative virulence determinant. *J. Clin. Microbiol.* **35:**759–763.

40. Goodman, L. J., G. M. Trenholme, R. L. Kaplan, J. Segreti, D. Hines, R. Petrak, J. A. Nelson, K. W. Mayer, W. Landau, and G. W. Parkhurst. 1990. Empiric antimicrobial therapy of domestically acquired acute diarrhea in urban adults. *Arch. Intern. Med.* **150:**541–546.

41. Goossens, H., M. De Boeck, H. Coignau, L. Vlaes, C. Van den Borre, and J.-P. Butzler. 1986. Modified selective medium for isolation of *Campylobacter* spp. from feces: comparison with Preston medium, a blood-free medium, and a filtration system. *J. Clin. Microbiol.* **24:**840–843.

42. Goossens, H., L. Vlaes, M. De Boeck, B. Pot, K. Kersters, J. Levy, P. de Mol, J. P. Butzler, and P. Vandamme. 1990. Is "*Campylobacter upsaliensis*" an unrecognised cause of human diarrhoea? *Lancet* **335:**584–586.

43. Grandien, M., G. Sterner, M. Kalin, and L. Engardt. 1990. Management of pregnant women with diarrhoea at term and of healthy carriers of infectious agents in stools at delivery. *Scand. J. Infect. Dis. Suppl.* **71:**9–18.

44. Guerrant, R. L., and D. A. Bobak. 1991. Bacterial and protozoal gastroenteritis. *N. Engl. J. Med.* **325:**327–340.

45. Guerrant, R. L., T. Van Gilder, T. S. Steiner, N. M. Thielman, L. Slutsker, R. V. Tauxe, T. Hennessy, P. M.

Griffin, H. L. DuPont, R. B. Sack, P. I. Tarr, M. Neill, I. Nachamkin, L. B. Reller, M. T. Osterholm, M. L. Bennish, and L. K. Pickering. 2001. Practice guidelines for managing infectious diarrhea. *Clin. Infect. Dis.* **32:** 331–351.

46. **Gun-Monro, J., R. P. Rennie, J. H. Thornley, H. L. Richardson, D. Hodge, and J. Lynch.** 1987. Laboratory and clinical evaluation of isolation media for *Campylobacter jejuni. J. Clin. Microbiol.* **25:**2274–2277.

47. **Hani, E., and V. L. Chan.** 1995. Expression and characterization of *Campylobacter jejuni* benzoylglycine amidohydrolase (hippuricase) gene in *Escherichia coli. J. Bacteriol.* **177:**2396–2402.

48. **Harmon, K. M., and I. V. Wesley.** 1996. Identification of *Arcobacter* isolates by PCR. *Lett. Appl. Microbiol.* **23:**241–244.

49. **Hindiyeh, M., S. Jense, S. Hohmann, H. Benett, C. Edwards, W. Aldeen, A. Croft, J. Daly, S. Mottice, and K. C. Carroll.** 2000. Rapid detection of *Campylobacter jejuni* in stool specimens by an enzyme immunoassay and surveillance for *Campylobacter upsaliensis* in the greater Salt Lake City area. *J. Clin. Microbiol.* **38:**3076–3079.

50. **Hines, J., and I. Nachamkin.** 1996. Effective use of the clinical microbiology laboratory for diagnosing diarrheal diseases. *Clin. Infect. Dis.* **23:**1292–1301.

51. **Ho, T. W., G. M. McKhann, and J. W. Griffin.** 1998. Human autoimmune neuropathies. *Annu. Rev. Neurosci.* **21:**187–226.

52. **Hodinka, R. L., and P. H. Gilligan.** 1988. Evaluation of the Campyslide agglutination test for confirmatory identification of selected *Campylobacter* species. *J. Clin. Microbiol.* **26:**47–49.

53. **Hsueh, P.-R., L.-J. Teng, P.-C. Yang, S.-K. Wang, S.-C. Chang, S.-W. Ho, W.-C. Hsieh, and K.-T. Luh.** 1997. Bacteremia caused by *Arcobacter cryaerophilus* 1B. *J. Clin. Microbiol.* **35:**489–491.

54. **Huang, M. B., C. N. Baker, S. Banerjee, and F. C. Tenover.** 1992. Accuracy of the E test for determining antimicrobial susceptibilities of staphylococci, enterococci, *Campylobacter jejuni*, and gram-negative bacteria resistant to antimicrobial agents. *J. Clin. Microbiol.* **30:** 3243–3248.

55. **Hurtado, A., and R. J. Owen.** 1997. A molecular scheme based on 23S rRNA gene polymorphisms for rapid identification of *Campylobacter* and *Arcobacter* species. *J. Clin. Microbiol.* **35:**2401–2404.

56. **Hutchinson, D. N., and F. J. Bolton.** 1984. Improved blood free selective medium for the isolation of *Campylobacter jejuni* from faecal specimens. *J. Clin. Pathol.* **37:** 956–957.

57. **Huysmans, M. B., J. D. Turnidge, and J. H. Williams.** 1995. Evaluation of API Campy in comparison with conventional methods for identification of thermophilic campylobacters. *J. Clin. Microbiol.* **33:**3345–3346.

58. **Isenberg, H. (ed. in chief).** 1992. *Clinical Microbiology Procedures Handbook.* American Society for Microbiology, Washington, D.C.

59. **Johnson, C. C., and S. M. Finegold.** 1987. Uncommonly encountered motile, anaerobic gram-negative bacilli associated with infection. *Rev. Infect. Dis.* **9:**1150–1162.

60. **Karlyshev, A. V., D. Linton, N. A. Gregson, A. J. Lastovica, and B. W. Wren.** 2000. Genetic and biochemical evidence of a *Campylobacter jejuni* capsular polysaccharide that accounts for Penner serotype specificity. *Mol. Microbiol.* **35:**529–541.

61. **Karmali, M. A., and P. C. Fleming.** 1979. Campylobacter enteritis in children. *J. Pediatr.* **94:**527–533.

62. **Karmali, M. A., A. E. Simor, M. Roscoe, P. C. Flemming, S. S. Smith, and J. Lane.** 1986. Evaluation of a blood-free, charcoal-based, selective medium for the isolation of *Campylobacter* organisms from feces. *J. Clin. Microbiol.* **23:**456–459.

63. **Kasten, M. J., F. Allerberger, and J. P. Anhalt.** 1991. *Campylobacter* bacteremia: clinical experience with three different blood culture systems at Mayo Clinic 1984–1990. *Infection* **19:**88–90.

64. **Kiehlbauch, J. A., D. J. Brenner, M. A. Nicholson, C. N. Baker, C. M. Patton, A. G. Steigerwalt, and I. K. Wachsmuth.** 1991. *Campylobacter butzleri* sp. nov. isolated from humans and animals with diarrheal illness. *J. Clin. Microbiol.* **29:**376–385.

65. **Konkel, M. E., L. A. Joens, and P. F. Mixter.** 2000. Molecular characterization of *Campylobacter jejuni* virulence determinants, p. 217–240. *In* I. Nachamkin and M. J. Blaser (ed.), *Campylobacter*, 2nd ed. ASM Press, Washington, D.C.

66. **Korhonen, L. K., and P. J. Martikainen.** 1990. Comparison of some enrichment broths and growth media for the isolation of thermophilic campylobacters from surface water samples. *J. Appl. Bacteriol.* **68:**593–599.

67. **Kuroki, S., T. Saida, M. Nukina, T. Haruta, M. Yoshioka, Y. Kobayashi, and H. Nakanishi.** 1993. *Campylobacter jejuni* strains from patients with Guillain-Barré syndrome belong mostly to Penner serogroup 19 and contain β-N-acetylglucosamine residues. *Ann. Neurol.* **33:** 243–247.

68. **Lachance, N., C. Gaudreau, F. Lamothe, and L. A. Larivière.** 1991. Role of the β-lactamase of *Campylobacter jejuni* in resistance to β-lactam agents. *Antimicrob. Agents Chemother.* **35:**813–818.

69. **Lachance, N., C. Gaudreau, F. Lamothe, and F. Turgeion.** 1993. Susceptibilities of β-lactamase-positive and -negative strains of *Campylobacter coli* to β-lactam agents. *Antimicrob. Agents Chemother.* **37:**1174–1176.

70. **Lara-Tejero, M., and J. E. Galan.** 2001. CdtA, CdtB, and CdtC form a tripartite complex that is required for cytolethal distending toxin activity. *Infect. Immun.* **69:**4358–4365.

71. **Lastovica, A. J., E. Le Roux, and J. L. Penner.** 1989. "*Campylobacter upsaliensis*" isolated from blood cultures of pediatric patients. *J. Clin. Microbiol.* **27:**657–659.

72. **Lastovica, A. J., and M. B. Skirrow.** 2000. Clinical significance of *Campylobacter* and related species other than *Campylobacter jejuni*, p. 89–121. *In* I. Nachamkin and M. J. Blaser (ed.), *Campylobacter*, 2nd ed. ASM Press, Washington, D.C.

73. **Lauderdale, T.-L., K. C. Chapin, and P. R. Murray.** 1999. Reagents, p. 1665–1673. *In* P. R. Murray, E. J. Baron, M. A. Pfaller, F. C. Tenover, and R. H. Yolken (ed.), *Manual of Clinical Microbiology*, 7th ed. ASM Press, Washington, D.C.

74. **Lawson, A. J., D. Linton, J. Stanley, and R. J. Owen.** 1997. Polymerase chain reaction and speciation of *Campylobacter upsaliensis* and *C. helveticus* in human faeces and comparison with culture techniques. *J. Appl. Microbiol.* **83:**375–380.

75. **Lawson, A. J., J. M. J. Logan, G. L. O'Neill, M. Desai, and J. Stanley.** 1999. Large-scale survey of *Campylobacter* species in human gastroenteritis by PCR and PCR–enzyme-linked immunosorbent assay. *J. Clin. Microbiol.* **37:** 3860–3864.

76. **Lawson, A. J., S. L. W. On, J. M. J. Logan, and J. Stanley.** 2001. *Campylobacter hominis* sp. nov., from the human gastrointestinal tract. *Int. J. Syst. Evol. Microbiol.* **51:**651–660.

77. **Lindblom, G.-B., E. Sjogren, J. Hansson-Westerberg, and B. Kaijser.** 1995. *Campylobacter upsaliensis*, *C. sputo-*

rum sputorum and *C. concisus* as common causes of diarrhea in Swedish children. *Scand. J. Infect. Dis.* **27:**187–188.

78. **Linton, D., A. J. Lawson, R. J. Owen, and J. Stanley.** 1997. PCR detection, identification to species level, and fingerprinting of *Campylobacter jejuni* and *Campylobacter coli* direct from diarrheic samples. *J. Clin. Microbiol.* **35:** 2568–2572.

79. **Lior, H., D. L. Woodward, J. A. Edgar, L. J. Laroche, and P. Gill.** 1982. Serotyping of *Campylobacter jejuni* by slide agglutination based on heat-labile antigenic factors. *J. Clin. Microbiol.* **15:**761–768.

80. **Logan, J. M. J., A. Burnens, D. Linton, A. J. Lawson, and J. Stanley.** 2000. *Campylobacter lanienae* sp. nov., a new species isolated from workers in an abattoir. *Int. J. Syst. Evol. Microbiol.* **50:**865–872.

81. **Luechtefeld, N. W., L. B. Reller, M. J. Blaser, and W.-L. L. Wang.** 1982. Comparison of atmospheres of incubation for primary isolation of *Campylobacter fetus* subsp. *jejuni* from animal specimens: 5% oxygen versus candle jar. *J. Clin. Microbiol.* **15:**53–57.

82. **MacFaddin, J. F.** 2000. Hippurate hydrolysis test, p. 188–204. *In* J. F. MacFaddin (ed.), *Biochemical Tests for Identification of Medical Bacteria.* Lippincott Williams & Wilkins, Philadelphia, Pa.

83. **MacFaddin, J. F.** 2000. Indoxyl substrate hydrolysis tests, p. 233–238. *In* J. F. MacFaddin (ed.), *Biochemical Tests for Identification of Medical Bacteria.* Lippincott Williams & Wilkins, Philadelphia, Pa.

84. **Marshall, S. M., P. L. Melito, D. L. Woodward, W. M. Johnson, F. G. Rodgers, and M. R. Mulvey.** 1999. Rapid identification of *Campylobacter, Arcobacter,* and *Helicobacter* isolates by PCR-restriction fragment length polymorphism analysis of the 16S rRNA gene. *J. Clin. Microbiol.* **37:**4158–4160.

85. **Martin, W. T., C. M. Patton, G. K. Morris, M. E. Potter, and N. D. Puhr.** 1983. Selective enrichment broth for isolation of *Campylobacter jejuni. J. Clin. Microbiol.* **17:** 853–855.

86. **McClung, C. R., D. G. Patriquin, and R. E. Davis.** 1983. *Campylobacter nitrofigilis* sp. nov., a nitrogen-fixing bacterium associated with roots of *Spartina alterniflora* Loisel. *Int. J. Syst. Bacteriol.* **33:**605–612.

87. **Mills, C. K., and R. L. Cherna.** 1987. Indoxyl acetate hydrolysis. *J. Clin. Microbiol.* **25:**1560–1561.

88. **Mishu, B., C. M. Patton, and R. V. Tauxe.** 1992. Clinical and epidemiological features of non-jejuni, non-coli *Campylobacter* species, p. 31–41. *In* I. Nachamkin, M. J. Blaser, and L. S. Tompkins (ed.), Campylobacter jejuni: *Current Status and Future Trends.* American Society for Microbiology, Washington, D.C.

89. **Molitoris, E., H. M. Wexler, and S. M. Finegold.** 1997. Sources and antimicrobial susceptibilities of *Campylobacter gracilis* and *Sutterella wadsworthensis. Clin. Infect. Dis.* **25S:** S264–S265.

90. **Morris, G. K., M. R. El Sherbeeny, C. M. Patton, H. Kodaka, G. L. Lombard, P. Edmonds, D. G. Hollis, and D. J. Brenner.** 1985. Comparison of four hippurate hydrolysis methods for identification of thermophilic *Campylobacter* spp. *J. Clin. Microbiol.* **22:**714–718.

91. **Morris, G. K., and C. M. Patton.** 1985. *Campylobacter,* p. 302–308. *In* E. H. Lennette, A. Balows, W. J. Hausler, Jr., and H. J. Shadomy (ed.), *Manual of Clinical Microbiology,* 4th ed. American Society for Microbiology, Washington, D.C.

92. **Nachamkin, I.** 1995. *Campylobacter* and *Arcobacter,* p. 483–491. *In* P. R. Murray, E. J. Baron, M. A. Pfaller, F. C. Tenover, and R. H. Yolken (ed.), *Manual of Clinical Microbiology,* 6th ed. ASM Press, Washington, D.C.

93. **Nachamkin, I.** 1997. Microbiologic approaches for studying *Campylobacter* in patients with Guillain-Barré syndrome. *J. Infect. Dis.* **176**(Suppl. 2)**:**S106–S114.

94. **Nachamkin, I.** 2001. *Campylobacter jejuni,* p. 179–192. *In* M. P. Doyle, L. R. Beuchat, and T. J. Montville (ed.), *Food Microbiology: Fundamentals and Frontiers,* 2nd ed. ASM Press, Washington, D.C.

95. **Nachamkin, I., B. M. Allos, and T. W. Ho.** 1998. *Campylobacter* and Guillain-Barré syndrome. *Clin. Microbiol. Rev.* **11:**555–567.

96. **Nachamkin, I., and S. Barbagallo.** 1990. Culture confirmation of *Campylobacter* spp. by latex agglutination. *J. Clin. Microbiol.* **28:**817–818.

97. **Newell, D. G., J. A. Frost, B. Duim, J. A. Wagenaar, R. H. Madden, J. van der Plas, and S. L. W. On.** 2000. New developments in the subtyping of *Campylobacter* species, p. 27–44. *In* I. Nachamkin and M. J. Blaser (ed.), *Campylobacter,* 2nd ed. ASM Press, Washington, D.C.

98. **Ng, L. K., D. E. Taylor, and M. E. Stiles.** 1988. Characterization of freshly isolated *Campylobacter coli* strains and suitability of selective media for their growth. *J. Clin. Microbiol.* **26:**518–523.

99. **Oberhelman, R. A., and D. N. Taylor.** 2000. *Campylobacter* infections in developing countries, p. 139–153. *In* I. Nachamkin and M. J. Blaser (ed.), *Campylobacter,* 2nd ed. ASM Press, Washington, D.C.

100. **On, S. L. W.** 2001. Taxonomy of *Campylobacter, Arcobacter, Helicobacter* and related bacteria: current status, future prospects and immediate concerns. *J. Appl. Microbiol.* **90:**1S–15S.

101. **On, S. L. W., H. I. Atabay, J. E. L. Corry, C. S. Harrington, and P. Vandamme.** 1998. Emended description of *Campylobacter sputorum* and revision of its infrasubspecific (biovar) divisions, including C. *sputorum* biovar *paraureolyticus,* a urease-producing variant from cattle and humans. *Int. J. Syst. Bacteriol.* **48:**195–206.

102. **Oyofo, B. A., Z. S. Mohran, S. El-Etr, M. O. Wasfy, and L. F. Peruski.** 1996. Detection of enterotoxigenic *Escherichia coli, Shigella,* and *Campylobacter* spp. by multiplex PCR assay. *J. Diarrh. Dis. Res.* **14:**207–210.

103. **Oyofo, B. A., S. A. Thornton, D. H. Burr, T. J. Trust, O. R. Pavlovskis, and P. Guerry.** 1992. Specific detection of *Campylobacter jejuni* and *Campylobacter coli* by using polymerase chain reaction. *J. Clin. Microbiol.* **30:** 2613–2619.

104. **Paisley, J. W., S. Mirrett, B. A. Lauer, M. Roe, and L. B. Reller.** 1982. Dark-field microscopy of human feces for presumptive diagnosis of *Campylobacter fetus* subsp. *jejuni* enteritis. *J. Clin. Microbiol.* **15:**61–63.

105. **Park, C. H., D. L. Hixon, A. S. Polhemus, C. B. Ferguson, S. L. Hall, C. C. Risheim, and C. B. Cook.** 1983. A rapid diagnosis of campylobacter enteritis by direct smear examination. *Am. J. Clin. Pathol.* **80:**388–390.

106. **Patton, C. M., and I. K. Wachsmuth.** 1992. Typing schemes: are current methods useful?, p. 110–128. *In* I. Nachamkin, M. J. Blaser, and L. S. Tompkins (ed.), Campylobacter jejuni: *Current Status and Future Trends.* American Society for Microbiology, Washington, D.C.

107. **Pazzaglia, G., R. B. Sack, E. Salazar, A. Yi, E. Chea, R. Leon-Barua, C. E. Guerrero, and J. Palomino.** 1991. High frequency of coinfecting enteropathogens in *Aeromonas*-associated diarrhea of hospitalized Peruvian infants. *J. Clin. Microbiol.* **29:**1151–1156.

108. **Penner, J. L., and J. N. Hennessy.** 1980. Passive hemagglutination technique for serotyping *Campylobacter fetus* subsp. *jejuni* on the basis of soluble heat-stable antigens. *J. Clin. Microbiol.* **12:**732–737.

109. **Perlman, D. M., N. M. Ampel, R. B. Schifman, D. L. Cohn, C. M. Patton, M. L. Aguirre, W.-L. L. Wang, and M. J. Blaser.** 1988. Persistent *Campylobacter jejuni* infections in patients infected with human immunodeficiency virus (HIV). *Ann. Intern. Med.* **108:**540–546.

110. **Petruccelli, B. P., G. S. Murphy, J. L. Sanchez, S. Walz, R. DeFraites, J. Gelnett, R. L. Haberberger, P. Echeverria, and D. N. Taylor.** 1992. Treatment of traveler's diarrhea with ciprofloxacin and loperamide. *J. Infect. Dis.* **165:**557–560.

111. **Pickett, C. L.** 2000. *Campylobacter* toxins and their role in pathogenesis, p. 179–190. *In* I. Nachamkin and M. J. Blaser (ed.), *Campylobacter*, 2nd ed. ASM Press, Washington, D.C.

112. **Popovic-Uroic, T., C. M. Patton, M. A. Nicholson, and J. A. Kiehlbauch.** 1990. Evaluation of the indoxyl acetate hydrolysis test for rapid differentiation of *Campylobacter*, *Helicobacter*, and *Wolinella* species. *J. Clin. Microbiol.* **28:**2335–2339.

113. **Popovic-Uroic, T., C. M. Patton, I. K. Wachsmuth, and P. Roeder.** 1991. Evaluation of an oligonucleotide probe for identification of *Campylobacter* species. *Lab. Med.* **22:**533–539.

114. **Pratt-Ripplin, K., and M. Pezzlo.** 1992. Identification of commonly isolated aerobic gram-positive bacteria, p. 1.20.21–1.20.22. *In* H. Isenberg (ed. in chief), *Clinical Microbiology Procedures Handbook.* American Society for Microbiology, Washington, D.C.

115. **Rams, T. E., D. Feik, and J. Slots.** 1993. *Campylobacter rectus* in human periodontitis. *Oral Microbiol. Immunol.* **8:**230–235.

116. **Salazar-Lindo, E., R. B. Sack, E. Chea-Woo, B. A. Kay, I. Piscoya, and R. Y. Leon-Barua.** 1986. Early treatment with erythromycin of *Campylobacter jejuni*-associated dysentery in children. *J. Pediatr.* **109:**3555–3560.

117. **Sazie, E. S. M., and A. E. Titus.** 1982. Rapid diagnosis of *Campylobacter* enteritis. *Ann. Intern. Med.* **96:**62–63.

118. **Sjögren, E., B. Kaijser, and M. Werner.** 1992. Antimicrobial susceptibilities of *Campylobacter jejuni* and *Campylobacter coli* isolated in Sweden: a 10-year follow-up report. *Antimicrob. Agents Chemother.* **36:**2847–2849.

119. **Sjögren, E., G.-B. Lindblom, and B. Kaijser.** 1987. Comparison of different procedures, transport media, and enrichment media for isolation of *Campylobacter* species from healthy laying hens and humans with diarrhea. *J. Clin. Microbiol.* **25:**1966–1968.

120. **Sjogren, E., G. B. Lindblom, and B. Kaijser.** 1997. Norfloxacin resistance in *Campylobacter jejuni* and *Campylobacter coli* isolates from Swedish patients. *J. Antimicrob. Chemother.* **40:**257–261.

121. **Skirrow, M. B.** 1977. *Campylobacter* enteritis: a "new" disease. *Br. Med. J.* **ii:**9–11.

122. **Skirrow, M. B.** 1994. Diseases due to *Campylobacter*, *Helicobacter* and related bacteria. *J. Comp. Pathol.* **111:**113–149.

123. **Skirrow, M. B., and M. J. Blaser.** 2000. Clinical aspects of *Campylobacter* infection, p. 69–88. *In* I. Nachamkin and M. J. Blaser (ed.), *Campylobacter*, 2nd ed. ASM Press, Washington, D.C.

124. **Skirrow, M. B., D. M. Jones, E. Sutcliffe, and J. Benjamin.** 1993. *Campylobacter* bacteremia in England and Wales, 1981–1991. *Epidemiol. Infect.* **110:**567–573.

125. **Spiegel, C. A., and G. Telford.** 1984. Isolation of *Wolinella recta* and *Actinomyces viscosus* from an actinomycotic chest wall mass. *J. Clin. Microbiol.* **20:**1187–1189.

126. **Stanley, J., A. P. Burnens, D. Linton, S. L. W. On, M. Costas, and R. J. Owen.** 1992. *Campylobacter helveticus* sp. nov., a new thermophilic species from domestic animals: characterization, and cloning of a species-specific DNA probe. *J. Gen. Microbiol.* **138:**2293–2303.

127. **Steele, T. W., and R. J. Owen.** 1988. *Campylobacter jejuni* subspecies *doylei* (subsp. nov.), a subspecies of nitrate-negative campylobacters isolated from human clinical specimens. *Int. J. Syst. Bacteriol.* **38:**316–318.

128. **Takeshi, K., T. Ikeda, A. Kubo, Y. Fujinaga, S. Makino, K. Oguma, E. Isogai, S. Yoshida, H. Sunagawa, T. Ohyama, and H. Kimura.** 1997. Direct detection by PCR of *Escherichia coli* O157 and enteropathogens in patients with bloody diarrhea. *Microbiol. Immunol.* **41:**819–822.

129. **Tauxe, R. V., C. M. Patton, P. Edmonds, T. J. Barrett, D. J. Brenner, and P. A. Blake.** 1985. Illness associated with *Campylobacter laridis*, a newly recognized *Campylobacter* species. *J. Clin. Microbiol.* **21:**222–225.

130. **Taylor, D. N., M. J. Blaser, P. Echeverria, C. Pitarangsi, L. Bodhidatta, and W.-L. L. Wang.** 1987. Erythromycin resistant *Campylobacter* infections in Thailand. *Antimicrob. Agents Chemother.* **31:**438–442.

131. **Taylor, D. N., P. Echeverria, C. Pitarangsi, J. Seriwatana, L. Bodhidatta, and M. J. Blaser.** 1988. Influence of strain characteristics and immunity on the epidemiology of *Campylobacter* infections in Thailand. *J. Clin. Microbiol.* **26:**863–868.

132. **Taylor, D. N., J. H. Kiehlbauch, W. Tee, C. Pitarangsi, and P. Echeverria.** 1991. Isolation of group 2 aerotolerant *Campylobacter* species from Thai children with diarrhea. *J. Infect. Dis.* **163:**1062–1067.

133. **Tee, W., A. Mijch, E. Wright, and A. Yung.** 1995. Emergence of multidrug resistance in *Campylobacter jejuni* isolates from three patients infected with human immunodeficiency virus. *Clin. Infect. Dis.* **21:**634–638.

134. **Tenover, F. C., C. N. Baker, C. L. Fennell, and C. A. Ryan.** 1992. Antimicrobial resistance in *Campylobacter* species, p. 66–73. *In* I. Nachamkin, M. J. Blaser, and L. S. Tompkins (ed.), Campylobacter jejuni: *Current Status and Future Trends.* American Society for Microbiology, Washington, D.C.

135. **Tenover, F. C., L. Carlson, S. Barbagallo, and I. Nachamkin.** 1990. DNA probe culture confirmation assay for identification of thermophilic *Campylobacter* species. *J. Clin. Microbiol.* **28:**1284–1287.

136. **Thompson, J. S., D. S. Hodge, D. E. Smith, and Y. A. Yong.** 1990. Use of tri-gas incubator for routine culture of *Campylobacter* species from fecal specimens. *J. Clin. Microbiol.* **28:**2802–2803.

137. **Thompson, S. A., and M. J. Blaser.** 2000. Pathogenesis of *Campylobacter fetus* infections, p. 321–347. *In* I. Nachamkin and M. J. Blaser (ed.), *Campylobacter*, 2nd ed. ASM Press, Washington, D.C.

138. **Tolcin, R., M. M. LaSalvia, B. A. Kirkley, E. A. Vetter, F. Cockerill, and G. W. Procop.** 2000. Evaluation of the Alexon-Trend ProSpecT *Campylobacter* Microplate Assay. *J. Clin. Microbiol.* **38:**3853–3855.

139. **Totten, P. A., C. M. Patton, F. C. Tenover, T. J. Barrett, W. E. Stamm, A. G. Steigerwalt, J. Y. Lin, K. K. Holmes, and D. J. Brenner.** 1987. Prevalence and characterization of hippurate-negative *Campylobacter jejuni* in King County, Washington. *J. Clin. Microbiol.* **25:**1747–1752.

140. **Valenstein, P., M. Pfaller, and M. Yungbluth.** 1996. The use and abuse of routine stool microbiology: a College of American Pathologists Q-Probes study of 601 institutions. *Arch. Pathol. Lab. Med.* **120:**206–211.

141. **Vandamme, P.** 2000. Taxonomy of the family *Campylobacteraceae*, p. 3–26. *In* I. Nachamkin and M. J. Blaser

(ed.), *Campylobacter*, 2nd ed. ASM Press, Washington, D.C.

142. **Vandamme, P., M. I. Daneshvar, F. E. Dewhirst, B. J. Paster, K. Kersters, H. Goossens, and C. W. Moss.** 1995. Chemotaxonomic analyses of *Bacteroides gracilis* and *Bacteroides ureolyticus* and reclassification of *B. gracilis* as *Campylobacter gracilis* comb. nov. *Int. J. Syst. Bacteriol.* **45:**145–152.

143. **Vandamme, P., and J. De Ley.** 1991. Proposal for a new family, *Campylobacteraceae. Int. J. Syst. Bacteriol.* **41:** 451–455.

144. **Vandamme, P., E. Falsen, B. Pot, B. Hoste, K. Kersters, and J. De Ley.** 1989. Identification of EF group 22 campylobacters from gastroenteritis cases as *Campylobacter concisus. J. Clin. Microbiol.* **27:**1775–1781.

145. **Vandamme, P., M. Vancanneyt, B. Pot, L. Mels, B. Hoste, D. Dewettinck, L. Vlaes, C. Van Den Borre, R. Higgins, J. Hommez, K. Kersters, J.-P. Butzler, and H. Goossens.** 1992. Polyphasic taxonomic study of the emended genus *Arcobacter* with *Arcobacter butzleri* comb. nov. and *Arcobacter skirrowii* sp. nov., an aerotolerant bacterium isolated from veterinary specimens. *Int. J. Syst. Bacteriol.* **42:**344–356.

146. **van Doorn, L. J., A. V. Van Haperen, A. Burnens, M. Huysmans, P. Vandamme, B. A. J. Giesendorf, M. J. Blaser, and W. G. V. Quint.** 1999. Rapid identification of thermotolerant *Campylobacter jejuni*, *Campylobacter coli*, *Campylobacter lari*, and *Campylobacter upsaliensis* from various geographic regions by a GTPase-based PCR-reverse hybridization assay. *J. Clin. Microbiol.* **37:**1790–1796.

147. **Van Etterijck, R., J. Breynaert, H. Revets, T. Devreker, Y. Vandenplas, P. Vandamme, and S. Lauwers.** 1996. Isolation of *Campylobacter concisus* from feces of children with and without diarrhea. *J. Clin. Microbiol.* **34:**2304–2306.

148. **van Vliet, A. H. M., and J. M. Ketley.** 2001. Pathogenesis of enteric *Campylobacter* infection. *J. Appl. Microbiol.* **90:**45S–56S.

149. **Waegel, A., and I. Nachamkin.** 1996. Detection and molecular typing of *Campylobacter jejuni* in fecal samples by polymerase chain reaction. *Mol. Cell. Probes* **10:**75–80.

150. **Wang, W.-L. L., and M. J. Blaser.** 1986. Detection of pathogenic *Campylobacter* species in blood culture systems. *J. Clin. Microbiol.* **23:**709–714.

151. **Wang, W.-L. L., L. B. Reller, B. Smallwood, N. W. Luechtefeld, and M. J. Blaser.** 1983. Evaluation of transport media for *Campylobacter jejuni* in human fecal specimens. *J. Clin. Microbiol.* **18:**803–807.

152. **Wasfy, M., B. Oyofo, A. Elgindy, and A. Churilla.** 1995. Comparison of preservation media for storage of stool samples. *J. Clin. Microbiol.* **33:**2176–2178.

153. **Wassenaar, T. M.** 1997. Toxin production by *Campylobacter* spp. *Clin. Microbiol. Rev.* **10:**466–476.

154. **Wesley, I. V.** 1994. *Arcobacter* infections, p. 181–190. *In* G. W. Beran (ed.), *CRC Handbook of Zoonosis.* CRC Press, Inc., Boca Raton, Fla.

155. **Wexler, H. M., D. Reeves, P. H. Summanen, E. Molitoris, M. McTeague, J. Duncan, K. H. Wilson, and S. M. Finegold.** 1996. *Sutterella wadsworthensis* gen. nov., sp. nov., bile-resistant microaerophilic *Campylobacter gracilis*-like clinical isolates. *Int. J. Syst. Bacteriol.* **46:**252–258.

156. **Wistrom, J., M. Jertborn, E. Ekwall, K. Norlin, B. Soderquist, A. Stromberg, R. Lundholm, H. Hogevik, L. Lagergren, G. Englund, and S. R. Norrby.** 1992. Empiric treatment of acute diarrheal disease with norfloxacin. *Ann. Intern. Med.* **117:**202–208.

157. **Wretlind, B., A. Stromberg, L. Ostlund, E. Sjogren, and B. Kaijser.** 1992. Rapid emergence of quinolone resistance in *Campylobacter jejuni* in patients treated with norfloxacin. *Scand. J. Infect. Dis.* **24:**685–686.

Helicobacter

JAMES VERSALOVIC AND JAMES G. FOX

58

TAXONOMY

Gastric spiral-shaped bacteria have been observed in animals and humans for more than 100 years. The first recorded observations of gastric spiral-shaped bacteria in animals were made by Rappin in 1881 and Bizzozero in 1893. In 1896, Salomon noted spiral bacteria in the stomachs of dogs, cats, and Norway rats (128). In 1982, *Campylobacter pyloridis* (later known as *Helicobacter pylori*) was successfully cultured from stomach biopsy specimens of human patients with gastritis (152). Subsequently other spiral gram-negative bacteria have been observed and isolated from the gastrointestinal tracts of mammals such as cats, dogs, ferrets, and rodents (33).

Initially, many spiral gram-negative bacteria isolated from the mammalian gastrointestinal tract were grouped as campylobacters. This classification was based on similar microscopic and ultrastructural morphologies, common microaerobic growth requirements, and similar ecologic niches (Table 1). However, partial sequencing of 16S rRNA genes provided evidence that *Campylobacter pylori* belonged in a different genus (124). The genus *Helicobacter* was formally distinguished from other gram-negative curved rods (e.g., *Campylobacter*) following extensive analysis of enzymatic activities, fatty acid profiles, growth characteristics, nucleic acid hybridization profiles, and 16S rRNA sequence analysis (39, 101, 111, 145). Recent sequencing of the *Campylobacter jejuni* and *H. pylori* (1, 141) genomes has emphasized differences between *Campylobacter* and *Helicobacter* organisms.

DESCRIPTION OF THE GENUS

The genus *Helicobacter* comprises 20 species formally validated by international rules of nomenclature (20, 101), with at least 7 species awaiting validation or representing candidate species. The genus includes spiral or curved bacilli ranging from 0.3 to 1.0 μm in width and 1.5 to 10.0 μm in length. Helicobacters are gram-negative, non-spore-forming rods that may form spheroid or coccoid bodies with prolonged culture. These bacteria are motile and usually possess multiple bipolar sheathed flagella (Table 1). *H. pylori* isolates, in contrast to other *Helicobacter* species, have multiple monopolar sheathed flagella. Several helicobacters (e.g., *Helicobacter pullorum* and *Helicobacter canadensis*) have

unsheathed flagella like the campylobacters. The animal gastric helicobacters, *Helicobacter bizzozeronii*, *Helicobacter felis*, and *Helicobacter salomonis*, as well as the human-animal gastric pathogen "*Helicobacter heilmannii*" (formerly *Gastrospirillum hominis*), have distinctive tightly spiraled morphologies under light and transmission electron microscopy (Fig. 1C). *H. pylori* can be induced in liquid culture to assume the morphology of "*H. heilmannii*," so these distinctions may not be absolute in vivo (24).

These organisms are microaerobic and possess respiratory metabolic capabilities. Successful cultivation of helicobacters requires a humid atmosphere maintained at 37°C with reduced levels of oxygen (5 to 10%) and increased levels of carbon dioxide (5 to 12%). Atmospheric hydrogen (as much as 5 to 10%) either is required or stimulates the growth of these organisms. Most *Helicobacter* species grow poorly, if at all, in routine aerobic atmospheres. Several helicobacters, including *H. felis* (70), *Helicobacter hepaticus* (31), and *Helicobacter rodentium* (130), can grow both anaerobically and microaerobically.

Several biochemical and genetic criteria distinguish this genus, although significant intragenus variation exists with respect to each trait (Table 1). All helicobacters are oxidase positive and appear to be relatively inert with respect to carbohydrate pathways by conventional methods. Nuclear magnetic resonance spectroscopy (51) and genomic (76) studies have revealed the existence of carbohydrate catabolic pathways in *H. pylori* (51). Comparative genomic analysis of *H. pylori* supports the presence of important catabolic pathways such as the pentose phosphate shunt, Entner-Doudoroff pathway, glycolysis, and an altered noncylic version of the Krebs reaction sequence (76). Members of the genus *Helicobacter* have G+C contents ranging from 30 to 48 mol% (33), similar to those of the campylobacters.

NATURAL HABITATS

Helicobacter species have been isolated from the gastrointestinal and hepatobiliary tracts of mammals and birds (Table 1). In this chapter, we refer to gastric (stomach) and enterohepatic (intestine and liver/bile) helicobacters in order to distinguish these organisms according to their preferred niche(s) in the gastrointestinal tract. Gastric helicobacters possess several unifying features including phylogenetic clustering, urease activity, and the ability to form

TABLE 1 Habitats and phenotypic characteristics of *Helicobacter* species[a]

Helicobacter taxon	Source(s)	Primary site	Catalase production	Nitrate reduction	Alkaline phosphatase	Urease	Indoxyl acetate hydrolysis	γ-Glutamyl transferase	Growth At 42°C	Growth With 1% glycine	Resistance to[b] Nalidixic acid	Resistance to[b] Cephalothin	Flagella
Human													
H. bizzozeronii[c]	Human, cat, dog, primate	Stomach	+	+	+	+	+	+	+	−	R	S	Bipolar
H. canis	Human, cat, dog	Intestine	−	−	+	−	+	+	+	−	S	I	Bipolar
H. canadensis	Human	Intestine	+	±	−	−	+	−	+	+	R	R	Mono/Bipolar
H. cinaedi	Human, hamster, macaque	Intestine	+	+	−	−	−	−	−	+	S	I	Bipolar
H. fennelliae	Human	Intestine	+	−	+	−	+	−	−	+	S	S	Bipolar
H. pullorum	Human, chicken	Intestine	+	+	−	−	−	ND[d]	+	−	R	S	Monopolar
H. pylori	Human, macaque, cat	Stomach	+	−	+	+	−	+	+	−	R	S	Monopolar
Helicobacter sp. strain flexispira taxon 8[e]	Human, dog, sheep, mouse	Intestine	±	−	−	+	−	+	+	−	R	R	Bipolar
H. winghamensis	Human	Intestine	−	−	−	−	+	ND	−	+	R	R	Bipolar
Nonhuman													
H. acinonychis	Cheetah	Stomach	+	−	+	+	−	+	−	−	R	S	Bipolar
H. bilis	Mouse, dog, rat	Intestine	+	+	−	+	−	+	+	+	R	R	Bipolar
H. cholecystus	Hamster	Liver	+	+	+	−	−	−	+	+	I	R	Monopolar
H. felis	Cat, dog	Stomach	+	+	+	+	−	−	+	−	R	S	Bipolar
H. hepaticus	Mouse	Intestine	+	+	−	+	+	−	−	+	R	R	Bipolar
H. mesocricetorum	Hamster	Intestine	+	+	+	−	ND	+	+	−	S	R	Bipolar
H. muridarum	Mouse, rat	Intestine	+	−	+	+	+	+	−	−	R	R	Bipolar
H. mustelae	Ferret, mink	Stomach	+	+	+	+	+	+	+	−	S	R	Peritrichous
H. pametensis	Birds, swine	Intestine	+	+	+	−	−	−	+	+	S	S	Bipolar
H. rodentium	Mouse	Intestine	+	+	−	−	−	−	+	+	R	R	Bipolar
H. salomonis	Dog	Stomach	+	+	+	+	+	+	−	ND	R	S	Bipolar
H. trogontum	Rat	Intestine	+	+	−	+	−	+	+	ND	R	R	Bipolar

[a] Data are from references 20, 29, 31, 32, 33, 46, 58, 86, 111, 130, 135, 136, 145, and 149. All *Helicobacter* species are oxidase positive and lack the ability to oxidize or ferment carbohydrates in routine reactions.

[b] Resistance is determined by disk diffusion. Isolates are incubated for several days at 37°C on blood-containing medium containing 30-μg antibiotic disks. Microaerobic conditions are typically used, and exact incubation times vary among organisms. Resistance (R) is defined as the complete absence of an inhibition zone, whereas intermediate (I; zones usually <15 mm) and susceptible (S; zones usually >20 mm in diameter) isolates have visible inhibition zones of various sizes.

[c] Probably the same as "*H. heilmannii*." "*H. heilmannii*" (formerly *Gastrospirillum hominis*) has the same phenotype as listed here for *H. bizzozeronii*. Only a single "*H. heilmannii*" strain has been isolated by culture (3), and so it is not included in Table 1.

[d] ND, not determined.

[e] Formerly regarded as "*Flexispira rappini*," now has been subgrouped into 10 taxa (20).

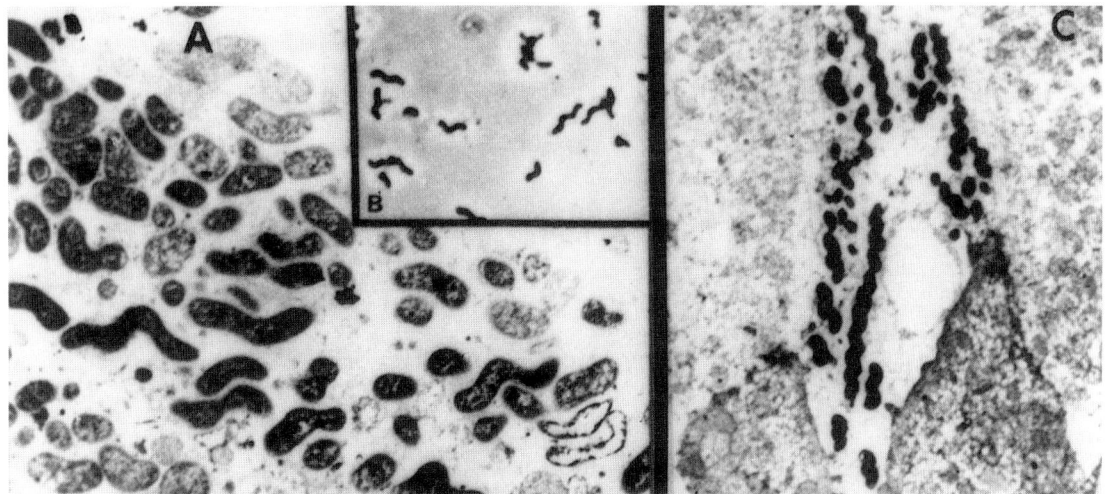

FIGURE 1 Microscopic morphology of *H. pylori* and "*H. heilmannii.*" (A) Transmission electron micrograph of a gastric biopsy specimen from an *H. pylori*-infected individual. (B) Phase-contrast micrograph of *H. pylori*. (C) Transmission electron micrograph of bacteria resembling "*H. heilmannii*" in the gastric pits of an infected cat. Adapted from reference 33 with permission.

discrete colonies on plated media (149). Gastric helicobacters primarily inhabit the stomach either within or beneath the mucous gel layer adjacent to the epithelium and rarely invade the bloodstream (in contrast to enterohepatic helicobacters). *H. pylori* colonizes the cardia, corpus, and antrum (distal portion) of the human stomach. These organisms may also be found transiently in areas of gastric metaplasia of the proximal small intestine (duodenum), saliva, gastric juice (vomitus), and feces.

Evidence suggests that fecal-oral and oral-oral modes of interhuman transmission are likely to represent routes of dissemination of *H. pylori*. Oral-oral transmission is supported by the frequent presence of *H. pylori* in the oral cavities of infected individuals (25, 106). *H. pylori* has been isolated frequently from dental plaque (120), saliva (109), and vomitus (109). Crowded living conditions and the lack of hot running water have been associated with an increased likelihood of *H. pylori* infection (80, 87). Although *Helicobacter* organisms have never been cultured from environmental sources, molecular (56) and immunologic (52) methods have been used to detect *Helicobacter* DNA in municipal water supplies and groundwater samples. These findings raise the possibility of fecal-oral transmission via contaminated municipal water sources. Epidemiologic analyses of intrafamilial *H. pylori* infection support the occurrence of direct person-to-person spread as a primary mode of transmission (90, 151, 153), occurring chiefly in early childhood. Evidence supports the notion that children serve as the primary source of infection in families (25).

H. pylori naturally infects other mammals such as cats (28) and nonhuman primates (45) and has caused experimental infections of laboratory mice (77). The presence of *H. pylori* in secretions and feces of naturally infected cats (34) and sheep (21) has raised the possibility of zoonotic transmission of gastric helicobacters to humans. "*Helicobacter heilmannii*" also resides in the human stomach (53, 54). Like *H. pylori*, "*H. heilmannii*"-like organisms (33, 71, 121), *H. bizzozeronii* (46), *H. felis* (70, 111), and "*H. suis*" (19) have been isolated from the stomachs of cats, dogs, nonhuman primates, and swine. An exception, urease-negative

Helicobacter cinaedi, has been detected by PCR amplification of DNA from gastric biopsy specimens of human patients with gastritis (113).

In contrast to the gastric helicobacters, enterohepatic helicobacters inhabit the intestinal (small intestine, colon, and rectum) and hepatobiliary tracts of mammals and birds. In humans, enterohepatic helicobacters (*H. canadensis*, *Helicobacter canis*, *H. cinaedi*, *Helicobacter fennelliae*, *H. pullorum*, and *Helicobacter winghamensis*) have been isolated from rectal swabs and feces (10, 86, 135, 136).

CLINICAL SIGNIFICANCE

Gastric Helicobacters

H. pylori has been associated with peptic ulcer disease and cancers of the human gastrointestinal tract. Warren and Marshall (152) first proposed the association of *H. pylori* with peptic ulcer disease and gastric cancer. In February 1994, the National Institutes of Health Consensus Development Conference concluded that *H. pylori* infection represents the major cause of peptic ulcer disease and stated that all patients with confirmed peptic ulcer disease associated with *H. pylori* infection should receive antimicrobial treatment (94). In June 1994, the International Agency for Research on Cancer Working Group of the World Health Organization identified *H. pylori* as a group I, or definite, human carcinogen. Approximately 50% of the world's population is estimated to be infected with *H. pylori*. Seroprevalence of *H. pylori* generally increases with age, ranging from 5–27% in early childhood to levels exceeding 70% in adults older than 50 years (78). Seroprevalence studies demonstrate an acquisition rate of 3 to 4% in selected populations per decade (131).

Persons infected with *H. pylori* may develop acute gastritis (abdominal pain, nausea, and vomiting) within 2 weeks following infection. *H. pylori* establishes a chronic infection in the majority of infected individuals, represented by chronic gastritis of different types. Prominent mucosal inflammation in chronic active gastritis is often evident in the antrum (antral predominant gastritis), predisposing to hyperacidity and duodenal ulcer disease. In contrast, multifocal atrophic pangastritis or atrophic corpus-predominant gastritis results from long-standing infection and is characterized by glandular atrophy, intestinal metaplasia, and sparse inflammatory cells. Many patients infected with *H. pylori* have recurrent abdominal symptoms (nonulcer dyspepsia) without ulcer disease (81). Inflammation of the duodenum (duodenitis) often occurs in patients with *H. pylori* infection, and duodenal ulcers develop in as many as 16% of infected individuals. *H. pylori* infection has been associated with the majority of duodenal and gastric ulcers (2). In patients with long-standing *H. pylori* infection, persistent inflammation can lead to multifocal atrophic gastritis. Multifocal atrophic gastritis is a recognized precursor state for gastric ulcer disease and gastric adenocarcinoma (47). *H. pylori* infection represents an independent risk factor for the development of atrophic gastritis (61), gastric ulcer disease (137), gastric adenocarcinomas (99, 107), and gastric mucosa-associated lymphoid tissue (MALT) lymphomas (108, 156).

"*H. heilmannii*" (formerly *Gastrospirillum hominis*) has been observed in human gastric biopsy specimens (53, 54, 133) and cultured from human stomach tissue (3). The species name has not been formally recognized since there is significant nucleic acid sequence variation among various human isolates, resulting in the designation of multiple genotypes 1 and 2 among other clones (18). Infection with "*H. heilmannii*" has been associated with mild to moderate gastritis in cats and dogs (100), peptic ulcer disease in swine (121) and gastritis, peptic ulcer disease, and gastric MALT lymphomas in humans (53, 54, 92, 142). "*H. heilmannii*" is relatively uncommon, being present in less than 1% of human esophagogastroduodenal (EGD) endoscopy specimens, in contrast to *H. pylori*, which was present in 59% of such specimens (54). *Helicobacter* species have been observed and isolated from the stomach tissue of other mammals including cats, dogs, ferrets, rodents, and nonhuman primates (Table 1).

Enterohepatic Helicobacters

Multiple species including *H. cinaedi* and *H. fennelliae* have been implicated as causes of human gastroenteritis, particularly in immunocompromised individuals (41, 68, 122). More recently, cases of human gastroenteritis have been associated with infection by *H. canadensis* (29), *H. canis* (136), *H. pullorum* (33, 135), and *H. winghamensis* (86). "*Helicobacter* sp. strain flexispira" organisms have been divided into 10 taxonomic taxa (20). "*Helicobacter* sp. strain flexispira taxon 8" includes clinically relevant isolates that have been implicated in cases of human gastroenteritis (4, 125) and bacteremia (20). In contrast to *H. pylori*, *H. cinaedi* was identified from the blood of multiple patients with febrile bacteremia and was associated with a multifocal cellulitis or monoarticular arthritis in a subset of infected individuals (9, 63). *H. cinaedi* (previously identified as *Helicobacter* sp. strain Mainz) (146) was cultured from the blood and joint fluid of a human immunodeficiency virus type 1 (HIV-1)-infected male with septic arthritis and recurrent fevers (58). *H. fennelliae* has occasionally been isolated from human blood (96) and was associated with septic shock in a non-HIV-1-infected individual (55). Presumably, these bacteremia-associated helicobacters invaded the bloodstream via colonization of the human lower gastrointestinal tract.

Enterohepatic *Helicobacter* species have been detected in the human hepatobiliary tract. *H. bilis* and *H. pullorum* were detected in bile specimens from Chilean patients with chronic cholecystitis (30). *Helicobacter* spp. were identified in liver specimens of patients with primary sclerosing cholangitis (98), cholangiocarcinoma (97), and hepatocellular carcinoma (5, 97) by genus-specific PCR amplification and partial DNA sequencing. Additionally, serum antibodies to *H. hepaticus* and *H. pylori* antigens were detected in human patients with chronic liver disease, specifically primary sclerosing cholangitis (98). Possible cross-reactivities with other *Helicobacter* antigens could not be excluded. The pathogenetic significance of PCR amplification and serologic findings are not clear since organisms have not been cultured from the human hepatobiliary tract.

Several enterohepatic helicobacters have not been isolated to date from human specimens, even though they cause significant diseases in other mammals (Table 1). In addition to the intestine, enterohepatic helicobacters colonize and cause inflammation in the mammalian hepatobiliary tract. For example, the isolation of *H. cinaedi* from the colon and liver of a 2-year-old rhesus monkey (32) implicates this organism as a possible etiologic agent of chronic hepatitis in nonhuman primates. *H. hepaticus* infection was associated with multifocal necrotic hepatitis in several strains of barrier-maintained mice and was implicated in the development of hepatic adenomas and hepatocellular carcinomas in A/JCr mice and more recently in $B_6C_3F_1$ mice (31, 35).

COLLECTION, TRANSPORT, AND STORAGE OF SPECIMENS

Blood Specimens

Given that *H. pylori* specifically adheres to the gastric mucosal epithelium and causes superficial gastric infections, it has rarely been isolated from human blood. In contrast, enterohepatic helicobacters translocate across the intestinal barrier and cause invasive infections. If bacteremia is suspected, peripheral venous blood should be collected as recommended by the manufacturer in commercially available aerobic and anaerobic blood culture bottles. The Isolator system (Wampole Laboratories, Cranbury, N.J.) can be used as an alternative collection system but is not essential. Culture conditions are described below.

Feces

Gastric helicobacters, *H. pylori* and "*H. heilmannii*," are rarely isolated from human fecal specimens. By contrast, enterohepatic helicobacters, like campylobacters, can be cultivated routinely by modified stool culture. These organisms are probably underisolated due to primary efforts directed at isolation of thermophilic campylobacters (e.g., *C. jejuni*). Fresh stool specimens should be submitted in a sterile container and processed as a routine specimen. Enterohepatic helicobacters rapidly lose viability, and it is important to transfer to plated media in a rapid time frame (preferably within 4 h of collection).

Gastric Biopsy Specimens

Human gastric biopsy specimens are necessary for direct tissue diagnosis of *H. pylori* or "*H. heilmannii*" by the rapid urease test or histopathologic testing. Furthermore, the proper collection, storage, and transport of gastric biopsy specimens are important for bacteriologic culture of *H.*

pylori. Culture of *H. pylori* may be necessary for antimicrobial suscepitiby testing, diagnostic confirmation, or epidemiologic studies. Importantly, "*H. heilmannii*" has been rarely cultured from human tissue (3). Since *H. pylori* rapidly loses viability at room temperature, biopsy specimens that must be maintained at ambient temperature should be plated within 2 h. *H. pylori* is sensitive to desiccation and ambient atmosphere, and so appropriate transport media should be used (114). Recommended transport media include brucella broth (Remel, Lenexa, Kans.) with 20% glycerol, cysteine-Albimi broth with 20% glycerol, or Stuart's transport medium (44, 114). The authors recommend brucella broth with 20% glycerol since the broth is available commercially and eliminates the need to weigh out and mix reagents. A single biopsy sample can be immersed with the aid of sterile forceps into 1 ml of storage or transport medium.

In contrast to Stuart's transport medium, glycerol-containing media may serve as both transport and storage media for gastric biopsy specimens (44). Storage time, temperature, and medium are important variables. Isolates from 81% of biopsy specimens stored at 4°C in glycerol-containing media for 1 week remained viable, whereas isolates from only 19% of biopsy specimens stored at 4°C for 2 weeks were cultivable (44). In contrast, 100% of biopsy specimens stored at $-20°C$ in glycerol-containing media for 4 weeks remained culturable for *H. pylori*. Only cysteine-Albimi medium with 20% glycerol was evaluated for long-term storage, and 14 of 16 gastric biopsy specimens stored for at least 5 years at $-70°C$ yielded *H. pylori* (44). For prolonged transport (exceeding 4 days) of cultures by air mail, chocolate agar slants preincubated in a microaerobic atmosphere proved to be a better transport medium for the recovery of *H. pylori* than did chocolate agar plates in Campy Pouches (BBL Microbiology Systems, Cockeysville, Md.) (157).

DIRECT EXAMINATION AND DETECTION

Antigen Detection

Direct fecal antigen detection of *H. pylori* has been approved by the Food and Drug Administration for diagnosis and follow-up testing. Meridian Bioscience (Cincinnati, Ohio) has developed a commercial kit (Premier Platinum HpSA) for the rapid, noninvasive detection of *H. pylori* antigens by enzyme immunoassay. *H. pylori* antigens from fresh human fecal specimens are detected by polyclonal antibodies adsorbed to microwells. The sensitivities and specificities of fecal antigen detection were approximately 89 and 94 to 95%, respectively, in multiple studies (75, 91). Direct fecal antigen testing may be a cost-effective approach for diagnostic screening based on its accuracy in the setting of low to intermediate pretest probability of infection (144). Antigen detection may be useful in cases in which the urea breath test (described below) is difficult to perform (e.g., in pediatric patients) or antibody results are less reliable (e.g., in HIV-1-infected individuals).

Biopsy and Histologic Testing

In patients with chronic gastritis or suspected peptic ulcer disease, *H. pylori* infection may be diagnosed by direct detection of organisms in tissue collected by EGD endoscopy. In cases of duodenal ulcer disease, biopsy samples are obtained from the gastric antrum or corpus. Adequate sampling is the primary issue affecting the sensitivity of histo-

logic testing since *H. pylori* infection may be patchy. At least two biopsy specimens (from the antrum and corpus) should be obtained. Following fixation in formalin, routine hematoxylin-and-eosin staining and special stains are used for histopathologic testing and organism detection, respectively. Various special stains, including Giemsa and the modified Steiner silver stain, may be useful for visualizing *H. pylori* adjacent to the gastric mucosa (118). Fluorescence in situ hybridization with species-specific 16S rDNA probes (Creatogen GmBH, Augsburg, Germany) represents a sophisticated approach to the detection of *H. pylori* (126) and "*H. heilmannii*" (142) in human gastric biopsy specimens. *H. pylori* and "*H. heilmannii*" can be distinguished by organism morphology in gastric biopsy specimens (Fig. 1).

DNA Amplification

Since rapid urease testing and histologic examination yield excellent sensitivities and specificities for the diagnosis of *H. pylori* infection, PCR amplification of gastric biopsy specimens may not be cost-effective as a primary diagnostic strategy. "Home brew" PCR and RT-PCR (22) methods which specifically detect *H. pylori* in gastric biopsy specimens have been developed and include different target genes such as 23S rDNA (74), *glmM* (73), and *vacA* (148). Comparisons of different target sequences in gastric biopsy specimens yielded different positive and negative predictive values (73). Maeda et al. reported a PCR assay based on 23S rDNA target sequences that yielded specific amplification of *H. pylori* from gastric biopsy specimens and contained the macrolide resistance-determining region (74). Identification of macrolide resistance mutations (described below) by restriction digestion of PCR amplicons (112) or real-time detection (13) may be useful for follow-up testing. A recent study has indicated that biopsy specimens submitted for rapid urease testing may be used for molecular resistance studies by PCR-based mutational analysis after storage at room temperature for up to 8 weeks (112). PCR detection may preclude the need for subsequent EGD endoscopies for invasive testing and follow-up macrolide susceptibility testing. Species-specific PCR assays have been developed for other helicobacters such as *H. pullorum* (29) and *H. hepaticus* (123). No PCR-based tests are commercially available.

Smear Evaluation

Imprint cytology specimens do not require overnight formalin fixation and provide a rapid adjunct to histopathologic examination of antral biopsy specimens. After biopsy specimens are collected with forceps, imprints are made by pressing a needle against the tissue on a glass slide or by simply rubbing the tissue over the slide. Cytology specimens may be prepared immediately following biopsy by staining the imprints with a rapid Giemsa or Gram stain, and *H. pylori* or "*H. heilmannii*" organisms may be directly visualized. Such an approach has been demonstrated to match or outperform conventional histologic testing in multiple studies (16, 89, 110). When imprint smears were used, 30 of 32 biopsy specimens with positive *H. pylori* cultures yielded visible organisms with the Gram stain (110). The Gram stain may be modified by counterstaining with carbol fuchsin (0.5% [wt/vol]) for easier visualization. "*H. heilmannii*" organisms were diagnosed in 11 of 100 patients with dyspepsia by imprint cytology, and imprint cytology may be more sensitive than histologic testing for detection of this organism (16). Direct fecal smears, like fecal cultures, lack utility for the diagnosis of *H. pylori*.

Urease Testing

H. pylori produces large amounts of extracellular urease, which can be detected within hours following placement of gastric biopsy tissue in a urea-containing medium (50, 79). Urease catalyzes the hydrolysis of urea into ammonia and carbamate. The net effect of ammonia production is increased local pH. Biopsy samples are placed in an agar gel or on a paper strip containing a pH indicator. If organisms are present in sufficient numbers in the antral biopsy sample, a color change will occur as a result of urea breakdown and ammonia production by *H. pylori* urease (119, 158). Commercial rapid urease tests include the agar gel-based tests (e.g., CLOtest [Kimberly-Clark, Neenah, Wis.] and Hp*fast* [GI Supply, Camp Hill, Pa.]) or paper strip tests (e.g., PyloriTek [Horizons International Corp., Ponce, P.R.]). The sensitivity of detection depends on the organism load in the mucosal biopsy specimen and the number of biopsy specimens collected but generally approaches or exceeds 90%. At least one fresh biopsy specimen from the gastric angle or antrum should be submitted for rapid urease testing, and biopsy specimens should be stored at 4°C prior to testing. The sensitivity of rapid urease testing is maximized if specimens are obtained from the gastric angle (155) and if multiple specimens are obtained (83). Rapid urease tests enable convenient detection of *H. pylori* infection within 3 h in most cases, although the agar gel-based tests (e.g., CLOtest and Hp*fast*) usually require 24 h of incubation for maximal sensitivity. Immunologic rapid urease testing, although not yet commercially available, combines antigenic and enzyme activity-based detection of *H. pylori* urease in gastric biopsy specimens, thus improving the sensitivity and specificity (129). Agar gel-based rapid urease tests are cost-effective and widely used approaches for the screening of biopsy tissue for *H. pylori* infection.

Noninvasive urease testing by sampling human breath specimens has enabled the direct detection of *H. pylori* infection without endoscopy (65, 132). In 1996 and 1997, the Food and Drug Administration approved both ^{13}C- and ^{14}C-based urea breath tests (UBT), respectively, for the diagnosis of *H. pylori*. In the UBT (72), a solution containing isotopically labeled urea is consumed by the patient. Isotopically labeled carbon dioxide formed by *H. pylori* urease activity in the stomach is absorbed into the bloodstream and exhaled in the breath sample collected 30 min after ingestion of labeled urea. The ^{13}C-labeled carbon dioxide must be detected by gas isotope ratio mass spectrometry, whereas the ^{14}C-labeled carbon dioxide may be analyzed by scintillation particle counting. Infrared spectroscopy (88) and the laser-assisted ratio analyzer based on laser optogalvanic spectroscopy (11) have been used as alternatives to isotope ratio mass spectrometry for the detection of ^{13}C-labeled carbon dioxide (88). The UBT has excellent sensitivity and specificity, both exceeding 95% for the initial diagnosis of active infection in untreated patients (7, 78) and for treatment follow-up at 6 weeks after therapy (65, 132). Detection of postingestion labeled carbon in blood, the ^{13}C urea blood test, yielded a sensitivity of 89% and a specificity of 96% in a recent U.S. multicenter study (12). The ^{13}C urea blood test, Ez-HBT, is available commercially from Metabolic Solutions (Nashua, N.H.).

CULTURE AND ISOLATION PROCEDURES

Gastric Helicobacters

Unlike campylobacters, *H. pylori* is usually diagnosed by noncluture methods such as histologic, serologic, or urease testing. However, the increasing prevalence of nitroimidazole and macrolide resistance (104) has revitalized efforts to culture organisms from patients with recurrent dyspepsia or ulcer disease for antimicrobial susceptibility testing. *H. pylori* may be routinely isolated by culture from human gastric biopsy samples.

Consistent isolation of *H. pylori* from gastric biopsy specimens requires processing by homogenization or vortexing prior to plating (114). *H. pylori* organisms, like most helicobacters, are microaerobes, requiring reduced oxygen concentrations and elevated levels of carbon dioxide. Helicobacters typically grow best in freshly prepared, moist media incubated in a warm (37°C) atmosphere with carbon dioxide (5 to 10%), nitrogen (80 to 90%), and oxygen (5 to 10%). Humid atmospheres enriched in hydrogen content (5 to 8%) improve the yield of *H. pylori*. Primary isolation of *H. pylori* from gastric biopsy specimens requires 5 to 7 days in a microaerobic atmosphere created by a variable-atmosphere incubator, partially evacuated anaerobic jars with defined gas mixtures, or commercial gas-generating sachets (CampyPak Plus [BD Diagnostic Systems, Sparks, Md.], Anaeropack-Campylo [Remel, Lenexa, Kans.], and others). A dedicated CO_2 incubator (10 to 12% CO_2) is useful for subculturing *H. pylori* but is not recommended for primary isolation.

Nonselective media enriched with blood or serum are recommended for the cultivation of *H. pylori* from gastric biopsy specimens for a minimum period of 5 days. Such a strategy maximizes the sensitivity of culture. Various agar media including brain heart infusion agar, brucella agar, Columbia agar, or Skirrow's agar supplemented with horse blood, horse serum, or sheep blood have been used to cultivate *H. pylori* (49). We recommend commercially available brucella agar plates with 5% horse blood (Remel) or brain heart infusion agar supplemented with 7% horse blood as the preferred media. One study documented the superiority of brain heart infusion agar supplemented with 7% fresh whole defibrinated horse blood (96% recovery) versus commercial Trypticase soy agar with 5% sheep blood (78% recovery) and Columbia blood agar with cyclodextrin (32% recovery) for the isolation of *H. pylori* (42). In the report on culturing of "*H. heilmannii*" from human gastric biopsy samples (3), specimens were cultivated for up to 7 days on nonselective media containing 7% lysed horse blood (Statens Seruminstitut, Copenhagen, Denmark) in an atmosphere of 5% oxygen and 10% carbon dioxide.

Enterohepatic Helicobacters

Selective enriched media and a microaerobic atmosphere are essential for the cultivation of helicobacters from feces or rectal swabs. *H. canadensis*, *H. canis*, *H. cinaedi*, *H. fennelliae*, *H. pullorum*, "*Helicobacter* sp. strain flexispira taxon 8," and *H. winghamensis* have been isolated from humans with gastroenteritis. Fresh stool specimens should be plated directly onto selective media and incubated for a minimum of 3 days (3 to 7 days) at 37°C in a microaerobic atmosphere. The authors recommend selective CVA medium (Columbia agar base with 5% sheep blood and cefoperazone, vancomycin, and amphotericin B [Remel]) and a defined microaerobic atmosphere in partially evacuated anaerobic jars (5 to 10% carbon dioxide, 5 to 10% hydrogen, 5 to 10% oxygen) for the successful isolation of most enterohepatic helicobacters from human feces (146). Commercial gas-generating sachets (e.g., CampyPak Plus) have been used to isolate enterohepatic helicobacters, but because of increased atmospheric hydrogen requirements, the amount of hydrogen may be inadequate in such systems. Alternatively, *H. winghamensis* was isolated from human stool on nonselective Mueller-Hinton agar supplemented with 10% sheep blood in a defined microaerobic atmosphere as described above (86).

Blood culture isolates have been detected in aerobic and anaerobic bottles (usually aerobic bottles only) by using routine media with prolonged incubation (minimum 6 days) in automated instruments such as the BACTEC (Becton Dickinson, Franklin Lakes, N.J.) (9) or the BacT/Alert (Organon Teknika, Durham, N.C.) (103) systems. Enterohepatic helicobacters in blood cultures may require special stains for organisms such as *H. cinaedi*. The authors of a multicenter study which included 22 *H. cinaedi* blood isolates noted that these thin, gull-shaped organisms were generally not visible on Gram staining and required acridine orange staining, dark-field microscopy, or Giemsa staining for visualization (63). A modified Gram stain with carbol fuchsin (0.5% [wt/vol]) as the counterstain is recommended for detection. Instrument-positive blood cultures should be stained with acridine orange if Gram stains are negative.

Nonselective, blood-enriched media are preferred for the isolation of helicobacters from primary blood culture media and sterile body fluids. *H. cinaedi* isolates from positive blood cultures have been cultivated in 2 to 3 days at 37°C on nonselective blood media (e.g., brucella or Columbia agar base with 5% horse or sheep blood) in a microaerobic atmosphere (e.g., CampyPak Plus or partially evacuated jars with defined microaerobic atmospheres as described above). Supplementation of atmospheric hydrogen (5 to 10%) permitted the successful culture of *H. cinaedi* under microaerobic conditions (146). Supplementation of atmospheric hydrogen is done by the addition of gas-generating sachets to closed containers or, ideally, by direct supplementation with gas tanks containing 5 to 10% hydrogen. The only documented examples of *Helicobacter* cultivation from nonblood sterile body fluids include the isolation of *H. cinaedi* in nonselective Trypticase soy broth (103) and *Helicobacter* sp. strain Mainz (reclassified as *H. cinaedi*) (146) from joint fluid on nonselective blood agar (58) at 37°C.

IDENTIFICATION

Helicobacters yield various colony phenotypes on blood agar, ranging from discrete, gray, and translucent colonies of *H. pylori* and gastric helicobacters to various swarming phenotypes of intestinal helicobacters. Enterohepatic helicobacters yield a swarming phenotype with a thin film (e.g., *H. cinaedi* and *H. fennelliae*) or a thick, mucoid film similar to campylobacters (e.g., *H. pullorum* and *H. canadensis*). Helicobacters have a characteristic morphology by light microscopy that resembles that of other gram-negative spiral or curved bacteria (Fig. 1; Table 1). These organisms usually appear faint on conventional Gram staining and may require counterstaining with carbol fuchsin (0.5% [wt/vol]) for enhanced visualization. Most *Helicobacter* isolates are motile if observed by phase-contrast microscopy. Helicobacters are routinely tested for cytochrome oxidase, catalase, and urease activities (Table 1) (84). All helicobacters are oxidase positive. Most *Helicobacter* species, including *H. pylori*, are catalase positive (Table 1).

Gastric Helicobacters

The morphology of helicobacters observed in gastric biopsy specimens may differ markedly from that observed in a Gram-stained preparation of cultured organisms. For example, *H. pylori* usually appears as a curved or straight rod in culture whereas stained tissue biopsy specimens usually reveal a helical or more strikingly curved appearance. "*H. heilmannii*" (probably identical to *H. bizzozeronii* [Table 1]) is usually distinguished from *H. pylori* by its larger size and more pronounced helical morphology in gastric biopsy specimens (Fig. 1) (54). *H. felis* has also been found in human gastric biopsy specimens (36, 69) and cannot be distinguished from "*H. heilmannii*" or *H. bizzozeronii* by light microscopy.

H. pylori infection is presumptively diagnosed by microscopic morphology (Gram stain or biopsy) and the presence of catalase, oxidase, and urease activities. *C. jejuni*, a urease-negative relative of *H. pylori*, has been identified in a gastric biopsy specimen from a patient with a gastric ulcer (127). This report highlights the need to perform biopsy-based rapid urease testing or the UBT on patients who are refractory to therapy and have spiral or curved gram-negative bacteria visible in gastric biopsy specimens. The rapid urease, indoxyl acetate hydrolysis, and hippurate hydrolysis tests distinguish *H. pylori* and *C. jejuni* (see chapter 57) (102, 117). Commercial tests for urease (Christensen's urea agar slant [Remel or BBL Microbiology Systems]), indoxyl acetate (Remel), and hippurate hydrolysis (Remel) are available and are convenient for the rapid identification of cultured specimens. In a study of 400 clinical isolates, all *H. pylori* isolates were positive for cytochrome oxidase, catalase, and urease activities (Table 1) (82). In contrast to *C. jejuni*, *H. pylori* is urease positive and lacks the ability to hydrolyze hippurate or indoxyl acetate.

Enterohepatic Helicobacters

The enterohepatic helicobacters possess several distinguishing biochemical characteristics. Most intestinal helicobacters isolated from humans, such as *H. canadensis*, *H. cinaedi*, *H. fennelliae*, and *H. pullorum*, lack urease activity. Distinguishing catalase-positive, urease-negative helicobacters from the enteric campylobacters (e.g., *C. jejuni*) may be especially challenging. Unlike *C. jejuni* and *Campylobacter coli*, *H. cinaedi* and *H. fennelliae* do not survive at 42°C and *H. cinaedi* does not hydrolyze indoxyl acetate (Table 1) (117). Indoxyl acetate hydrolysis distinguishes *C. jejuni* and *C. coli* from *H. pullorum* (Table 1). *H. pullorum* is distinguished from *Campylobacter lari* only by its resistance to nalidixic acid. A nalidixic acid-resistant *C. lari* isolate would require species-specific PCR of 16S rRNA target sequences (135) for differentiation from *H. pullorum*. *H. canadensis* was initially characterized as a separate cluster of *H. pullorum*-like isolates capable of hydrolyzing indoxyl acetate and resistant to nalidixic acid (29). Unlike other helicobacters, *H. canis* is catalase and urease negative. To distinguish *H. canis* from catalase-negative campylobacters, the nitrate reduction and indoxyl acetate hydrolysis tests may be useful (Table 1).

SEROLOGIC TESTS

Serologic testing represents a primary screening method for the diagnosis of *H. pylori* infection. Pooled *H. pylori* antigens consisting of high-molecular-weight surface-associated proteins, acid extracts, or whole-cell lysates (sonicates) are used in most serologic assays. Various cytosolic and cell surface-associated proteins represent immunodominant antigens recognized by serum antibodies from infected individuals (64). Infection with *H. pylori* results in a vigorous local and systemic humoral response to multiple antigens (64, 140). In contrast to serum immunoglobulin M (IgM), serum IgA and IgG levels persist for months or years and correlate with active infection in untreated individuals (8, 93, 115). Only a minority of individuals did not show evidence of systemic seroconversion following infection (83). Anti-*H. pylori* serum IgG levels are more consistently elevated than are serum IgA levels. Consequently, serum IgG immunoassays yield greater sensitivities and specificities than do serum IgA assays in comparative studies (67).

Commercial enzyme-linked immunosorbent assays (ELISAs) detecting anti-*H. pylori* serum IgG are the serologic tests of choice (67) for the primary screening of patients with uncomplicated infections. Such recommended ELISA-based tests include HM-CAP (Enteric Products, Westbury, N.Y.), *H. pylori* IgG ELISA (Wampole Laboratories), and Premier (Meridian Bioscience) assays. Overall, the medians of the sensitivity and specificity for all commercially available *H. pylori* serology kits were 92 and 83%, respectively (67). Performance varied significantly between commercial serologic kits, with the top performers exceeding 90% in sensitivity and specificity and the bottom performers failing to reach 90% in sensitivity or 80% in specificity (67). Anti-*H. pylori* serologic assays from various commercial sources have highly variable sensitivities (57 to 100%) and specificities (31 to 100%) (67). Importantly, positive (95 to 100%) and negative (84 to 89%) predictive values for serologic tests were comparable to those of histologic tests, rapid urease tests, and UBT (14). ELISA serologic testing had the lowest cost per correct diagnosis, but the overall accuracy was lower than that of stool antigen testing or UBT (144). Patients infected with "*H. heilmannii*" were usually negative by anti-*H. pylori* IgG assays (54). Serum IgA immunoassays may be used as second-line tests for assessing equivocal or possibly false-negative anti-*H. pylori* serum IgG results. The key advantage of serum IgA studies is that follow-up testing may be performed with the same serum sample. In one study (59), more than 7% of samples with a negative serum IgG test result were found to possess detectable anti-*H. pylori* serum IgA and to be associated with symptoms consistent with *H. pylori* infection. With sensitivities of 39 to 82%, serum IgA assays lack the requisite sensitivity to serve as primary screening tests but may be useful in cases when infection is strongly suspected and the serum IgG result is negative or equivocal.

Although serum IgG assays remain the tests of choice for screening patient sera, whole-blood immunoassays are being used with increasing frequency in physicians' offices and point-of-care testing protocols. Qualitative point-of-care immunoassays produce rapid results (4 to 10 min) with heparinized whole blood or capillary blood specimens. Rapid whole-blood immunoassays have lower sensitivities (usually 80 to 90%) and comparable specificities compared to laboratory-based serum enzyme immunoassays (23, 139). Concerns regarding interoffice variability with point-of-care whole-blood assays have been raised. Whole-blood card-based immunoassays represent acceptable approaches for diagnostic screening in the outpatient setting, assuming that negative results are confirmed by laboratory ELISA-based serum IgG testing, fecal antigen testing, or UBT.

Sustained immunoglobulin responses to multiple antigens of *H. cinaedi* and *H. fennelliae* have been documented (27). Little is known about the nature of the immunoglobulin class and subclass responses following infection by *H. cinaedi* and *H. fennelliae*. No commercial serologic assays have been developed to monitor infection with *H. cinaedi* or other enterohepatic helicobacters.

ANTIBIOTIC SUSCEPTIBILITIES

Multidrug regimens are required to attain successful cure rates (exceeding 90%) for *H. pylori* infection (57). Either a nitroimidazole (e.g., metronidazole) or a macrolide (e.g., clarithromycin) must be included as part of the multidrug regimen to attain high cure rates. Antacid medications such as proton pump inhibitors (e.g., omeprazole) or H_2 antagonists (e.g., ranitidine) are usually added to reduce acid output and accelerate ulcer healing. Successful treatment regimens include metronidazole-omeprazole-clarithromycin for 7 to 14 days, triple-agent metronidazole-based therapy (tetracycline-metronidazole-bismuth) for 14 days, or triple-agent clarithromycin-based therapy (tetracycline or amoxicillin-clarithromycin-bismuth) for 14 days. The prevalence of *H. pylori* strains resistant to either metronidazole or clarithromycin has been increasing in various geographic regions (85, 105, 143). Infections with *H. pylori* strains resistant to clarithromycin or metronidazole have been associated with a greater incidence of treatment failures than have infections with susceptible strains (6, 143). Alternative approaches such as rifabutin-based salvage therapies may be required for treatment of patients failing standard triple therapy because of the presence of resistant *H. pylori* (116).

Various susceptibility testing methods such as broth microdilution, disk diffusion, the E test, and agar dilution have been used to assess antimicrobial resistance in *H. pylori* (17, 43, 48). The National Committee for Clinical Laboratory Standards (NCCLS) recommends an agar dilution standard for *H. pylori* susceptibility testing (95). Mueller-Hinton agar base with 5% aged sheep blood and incubation for 72 h at 35°C were selected by NCCLS for susceptibility testing by agar dilution (see chapter 71). *H. pylori* resistance in vitro to clarithromycin is clinically relevant, and an MIC breakpoint of 1 µg/ml is recommended by NCCLS (95). Point mutations in the 23S rRNA gene confer stable macrolide resistance (150), and either of two predominant mutations (15) may be detected by PCR amplification and restriction enzyme digestion (112, 138, 150). Alternatively, reverse hybridization following PCR amplification has demonstrated improved detection of mutations in mixed *H. pylori* populations in gastric biopsy specimens (147). In contrast to clarithromycin, in vitro susceptibility testing for metronidazole has not been standardized, although elevated MICs (>8 µg/ml) have been correlated with treatment failures (6). Multiple null mutations in the NADPH nitroreductase gene (*rdxA*) represent the primary molecular bases for metronidazole resistance in *H. pylori* (38, 60, 66), leading to the inability of cells to reduce and activate nitroimidazole compounds intracellularly.

Eradication of "*H. heilmannii*" by antimicrobial therapy resulted in the resolution of gastritis and peptic ulcer disease (37, 53, 54). Since "*H. heilmannii*" has been rarely cultured (3), antibiotic susceptibility testing has been described only for multiple isolates from a single patient (3). "*H. heilmannii*" isolates were susceptible to amoxicillin, ciprofloxacin, erythromycin, and tetracycline and resistant to nalidixic acid and metronidazole (3). "*H. heilmannii*" infections have been successfully treated with bismuth alone and combination therapies that included amoxicillin, metronidazole, and omeprazole (3, 53, 54).

Bacteremias due to intestinal helicobacters require drug combinations in prolonged intravenous-treatment regimens, often including aminoglycosides. "*Helicobacter* sp. strain flexispira taxon 8" bacteremias required multiagent regimens including aminoglycosides such as amikacin (134) or gentamicin (154) for clearance of infections. Effective therapy for *H. cinaedi* infection has included ciprofloxacin, gentamicin, or tetracycline for at least 2 to 3 weeks (9, 63, 103). In vitro susceptibility testing of *H. cinaedi* (26, 62, 63) appears to be meaningful, and in vitro resistance has been correlated with treatment failures in patients medicated with erythromycin (9) or ciprofloxacin (63). Relatively limited therapeutic experience is available for *H. fennelliae* infections. Gentamicin (96) and ampicillin-sulbactam (55) have been used successfully to treat bacteremia caused by *H. fennelliae*. Neither in vitro susceptibility testing data nor treatment recommendations have been reported for cases of gastroenteritis caused by *H. canis* or *H. pullorum*. NCCLS recommendations are not available for antimicrobial susceptibility testing of organisms other than *H. pylori*.

INTERPRETATION AND REPORTING OF RESULTS

For the diagnosis of *H. pylori* infection, the patient's clinical status dictates whether noninvasive or invasive approaches are used (91). Asymptomatic individuals at risk (40) should be screened by ELISA-based IgG serologic testing, fecal antigen detection, or UBT. Negative rapid whole-blood immunoassays, if performed at the point of care, should be confirmed by laboratory-based serum IgG immunoassays, fecal antigen detection, or UBT. If serum IgG results are equivocal and arranging a separate stool or breath collection is problematic for the patient, the same serum specimen could be used to determine serum IgA levels. Either fecal antigen testing or UBT is recommended as the method of choice to confirm *H. pylori* infection in symptomatic patients with nonulcer dyspepsia lacking "alarm" features. As early as 6 weeks following therapy, direct-detection methods such as fecal antigen testing or UBT can establish whether successful eradication or treatment failure has occurred.

Patients with "alarm" features (40) such as old age, weight loss, or gastrointestinal bleeding should undergo EGD endoscopy. Rapid urease testing of gastric biopsy specimens can be used to assess the *H. pylori* infection status. If results are positive, they can be reported as "positive and consistent with *H. pylori* infection." Histologic tests of gastric biopsy specimens should be interpreted by the histopathologist. Routine hematoxylin and eosin staining indicates the nature of the gastritis or the presence of gastric adenocarcinoma or gastric MALT lymphoma. *H. pylori* organisms may be visible on Gram staining of impression smears or special stains such as Giemsa or modified Steiner stain. "*H. heilmannii*" infection must be diagnosed by bacterial morphology in gastric biopsy specimens, since this organism is rarely cultured.

To perform antimicrobial susceptibility testing, bacteriologic culture of *H. pylori* from gastric biopsy specimens is recommended. Successful culture of *H. pylori* from biopsy specimens may be reported if organisms have the typical gram-negative morphology and cytochrome oxidase, catalase, and urease activities. Primary biopsy cultures should be incubated for at least 7 days before a negative report is made. Susceptibility testing should be performed by the NCCLS reference method (95) or a substantially equivalent method. Molecular resistance testing (mutation detection) may be used as an alternative to detect the presence of discrete mutations conferring macrolide resistance (112).

Enterohepatic helicobacters such as *H. cinaedi* and *H. fennelliae* must be isolated by microbiologic culture of blood or feces for a definitive diagnosis. If the Gram stain is negative, microscopic morphology may be assessed by a modified Gram stain, Giemsa stain, acridine orange stain, or dark-field microscopy. Appropriate biochemical tests must be performed (Table 1). Human enterohepatic helicobacters are typically urease negative and may be easily confused with campylobacters. Even with supplemental tests, the distinctions can be difficult without genotypic tests such as species-specific PCR amplification or DNA sequencing.

REFERENCES

1. **Alm, R. A., L. S. Ling, D. T. Moir, B. L. King, E. D. Brown, P. C. Doig, D. R. Smith, B. Noonan, B. C. Guild, B. L. deJonge, G. Carmel, P. J. Tummino, A. Caruso, M. Uria-Nickelsen, D. M. Mills, C. Ives, R. Gibson, D. Merberg, S. D. Mills, Q. Jiang, D. E. Taylor, G. F. Vovis, and T. J. Trust.** 1999. Genomic-sequence comparison of two unrelated isolates of the human gastric pathogen *Helicobacter pylori*. *Nature* **397:**176–180.
2. **Anand, B. S., and D. Y. Graham.** 1999. Ulcer and gastritis. *Endoscopy* **31:**215–225.
3. **Andersen, L. P., K. Boye, J. Blom, S. Holck, A. Norgaard, and L. Elsborg.** 1999. Characterization of a culturable "*Gastrospirillum hominis*" (*Helicobacter heilmannii*) strain isolated from human gastric mucosa. *J. Clin. Microbiol.* **37:**1069–1076.
4. **Archer, J. R., S. Romero, A. E. Ritchie, M. E. Hamacher, B. M. Steiner, J. H. Bryner, and R. F. Schell.** 1988. Characterization of an unclassified microaerophilic bacterium associated with gastroenteritis. *J. Clin. Microbiol.* **26:**101–105.
5. **Avenaud, P., A. Marais, L. Monteiro, B. Le Bail, S. P. Bioulac, C. Balabaud, and F. Megraud.** 2000. Detection of *Helicobacter* species in the liver of patients with and without primary liver carcinoma. *Cancer* **89:**1431–1439.
6. **Bazzoli, F., D. Berretti, L. De Luca, G. Nicolini, P. Pozzato, S. Fossi, and M. Zagari.** 1999. What can be learnt from the new data about antibiotic resistance? Are there any practical clinical consequences of *Helicobacter pylori* antibiotic resistance? *Eur. J. Gastroenterol. Hepatol.* **11**(Suppl. 2)**:**S39–S42.
7. **Bazzoli, F., M. Zagari, S. Fossi, P. Pozzato, L. Ricciardiello, C. Mwangemi, A. Roda, and E. Roda.** 1997. Urea breath tests for the detection of *Helicobacter pylori* infection. *Helicobacter* **2**(Suppl. 1)**:**S34–S37.
8. **Blecker, U., S. Lanciers, B. Hauser, D. I. Mehta, and Y. Vandenplas.** 1995. Serology as a valid screening test for *Helicobacter pylori* infection in asymptomatic subjects. *Arch. Pathol. Lab. Med.* **119:**30–32.
9. **Burman, W. J., D. L. Cohn, R. R. Reves, and M. L. Wilson.** 1995. Multifocal cellulitis and monoarticular arthritis as manifestations of *Helicobacter cinaedi* bacteremia. *Clin. Infect. Dis.* **20:**564–570.
10. **Burnens, A. P., J. Stanley, U. B. Schaad, and J. Nicolet.** 1993. Novel *Campylobacter*-like organism resembling *Helicobacter fennelliae* isolated from a boy with gastroenteritis and from dogs. *J. Clin. Microbiol.* **31:**1916–1917.

11. **Cave, D. R., S. V. Zanten, E. Carter, E. F. Halpern, S. Klein, C. Prather, M. Stolte, and L. Laine.** 1999. A multicentre evaluation of the laser assisted ratio analyser (LARA): a novel device for measurement of $^{13}CO_2$ in the ^{13}C-urea breath test for the detection of *Helicobacter pylori* infection. *Aliment. Pharmacol. Ther.* **13:**747–752.

12. **Chey, W. D., U. Murthy, P. Toskes, S. Carpenter, and L. Laine.** 1999. The ^{13}C-urea blood test accurately detects active *Helicobacter pylori* infection: a United States, multicenter trial. *Am. J. Gastroenterol.* **94:**1522–1524.

13. **Chisholm, S. A., R. J. Owen, E. L. Teare, and S. Saverymuttu.** 2001. PCR-based diagnosis of *Helicobacter pylori* infection and real-time determination of clarithromycin resistance directly from human gastric biopsy samples. *J. Clin. Microbiol.* **39:**1217–1220.

14. **Cutler, A. F., S. Havstad, C. K. Ma, M. J. Blaser, G. I. Perez-Perez, and T. T. Schubert.** 1995. Accuracy of invasive and noninvasive tests to diagnose *Helicobacter pylori* infection. *Gastroenterology* **109:**136–141.

15. **Debets-Ossenkopp, Y. J., M. Sparrius, J. G. Kusters, J. J. Kolkman, and C. M. Vandenbroucke-Grauls.** 1996. Mechanism of clarithromycin resistance in clinical isolates of *Helicobacter pylori*. *FEMS Microbiol. Lett.* **142:**37–42.

16. **Debongnie, J. C., J. Mairesse, M. Donnay, and X. Dekoninck.** 1994. Touch cytology. A quick, simple, sensitive screening test in the diagnosis of infections of the gastrointestinal mucosa. *Arch. Pathol. Lab Med.* **118:**1115–1118.

17. **DeCross, A. J., B. J. Marshall, R. W. McCallum, S. R. Hoffman, L. J. Barrett, and R. L. Guerrant.** 1993. Metronidazole susceptibility testing for *Helicobacter pylori*: comparison of disk, broth, and agar dilution methods and their clinical relevance. *J. Clin. Microbiol.* **31:**1971–1974.

18. **De Groote, D., R. Ducatelle, and F. Haesebrouck.** 2000. Helicobacters of possible zoonotic origin: a review. *Acta Gastroenterol. Belg.* **63:**380–387.

19. **De Groote, D., L. J. van Doorn, R. Ducatelle, A. Verschuuren, F. Haesebrouck, W. G. Quint, K. Jalava, and P. Vandamme.** 1999. 'Candidatus Helicobacter suis', a gastric *Helicobacter* from pigs, and its phylogenetic relatedness to other gastrospirilla. *Int. J. Syst. Bacteriol.* **49:**1769–1777.

20. **Dewhirst, F. E., J. G. Fox, E. N. Mendes, B. J. Paster, C. E. Gates, C. A. Kirkbride, and K. A. Eaton.** 2000. 'Flexispira rappini' strains represent at least 10 *Helicobacter* taxa. *Int. J. Syst. Evol. Microbiol.* **50:**1781–1787.

21. **Dore, M. P., A. R. Sepulveda, H. El Zimaity, Y. Yamaoka, M. S. Osato, K. Mototsugu, A. M. Nieddu, G. Realdi, and D. Y. Graham.** 2001. Isolation of *Helicobacter pylori* from sheep—implications for transmission to humans. *Am. J. Gastroenterol.* **96:**1396–1401.

22. **Engstrand, L., A. M. Nguyen, D. Y. Graham, and F. A. El Zaatari.** 1992. Reverse transcription and polymerase chain reaction amplification of rRNA for detection of *Helicobacter* species. *J. Clin. Microbiol.* **30:**2295–2301.

23. **Faigel, D. O., N. Magaret, C. Corless, D. A. Lieberman, and M. B. Fennerty.** 2000. Evaluation of rapid antibody tests for the diagnosis of *Helicobacter pylori* infection. *Am. J. Gastroenterol.* **95:**72–77.

24. **Fawcett, P. T., K. M. Gibney, and K. M. Vinette.** 1999. *Helicobacter pylori* can be induced to assume the morphology of *Helicobacter heilmannii*. *J. Clin. Microbiol.* **37:**1045–1048.

25. **Feldman, R. A.** 2001. Epidemiologic observations and open questions about disease and infection caused by *Helicobacter pylori*, p. 29–51. *In* M. Achtman and S. Suerbaum (ed.), Helicobacter pylori: *Molecular and Cellular Biology.* Horizon Scientific Press. Wymondham, United Kingdom.

26. **Flores, B. M., C. L. Fennell, K. K. Holmes, and W. E. Stamm.** 1985. In vitro susceptibilities of *Campylobacter*-like organisms to twenty antimicrobial agents. *Antimicrob. Agents Chemother.* **28:**188–191.

27. **Flores, B. M., C. L. Fennell, and W. E. Stamm.** 1989. Characterization of *Campylobacter cinaedi* and C. *fennelliae* antigens and analysis of the human immune response. *J. Infect. Dis.* **159:**635–640.

28. **Fox, J. G., M. Batchelder, R. Marini, L. Yan, L. Handt, X. Li, B. Shames, A. Hayward, J. Campbell, and J. C. Murphy.** 1995. *Helicobacter pylori*-induced gastritis in the domestic cat. *Infect. Immun.* **63:**2674–2681.

29. **Fox, J. G., C. C. Chien, F. E. Dewhirst, B. J. Paster, Z. Shen, P. L. Melito, D. L. Woodward, and F. G. Rodgers.** 2000. *Helicobacter canadensis* sp. nov. isolated from humans with diarrhea as an example of an emerging pathogen. *J. Clin. Microbiol.* **38:**2546–2549.

30. **Fox, J. G., F. E. Dewhirst, Z. Shen, Y. Feng, N. S. Taylor, B. J. Paster, R. L. Ericson, C. N. Lau, P. Correa, J. C. Araya, and I. Roa.** 1998. Hepatic *Helicobacter* species identified in bile and gallbladder tissue from Chileans with chronic cholecystitis. *Gastroenterology* **114:**755–763.

31. **Fox, J. G., F. E. Dewhirst, J. G. Tully, B. J. Paster, L. Yan, N. S. Taylor, M. J. Collins, Jr., P. L. Gorelick, and J. M. Ward.** 1994. *Helicobacter hepaticus* sp. nov., a microaerophilic bacterium isolated from livers and intestinal mucosal scrapings from mice. *J. Clin. Microbiol.* **32:**1238–1245.

32. **Fox, J. G., L. Handt, B. J. Sheppard, S. Xu, F. E. Dewhirst, S. Motzel, and H. Klein.** 2001. Isolation of *Helicobacter cinaedi* from the colon, liver, and mesenteric lymph node of a rhesus monkey with chronic colitis and hepatitis. *J. Clin. Microbiol.* **39:**1580–1585.

33. **Fox, J. G., and A. Lee.** 1997. The role of *Helicobacter* species in newly recognized gastrointestinal tract diseases of animals. *Lab. Anim. Sci.* **47:**222–255.

34. **Fox, J. G., S. Perkins, L. Yan, Z. Shen, L. Attardo, and J. Pappo.** 1996. Local immune response in *Helicobacter pylori*-infected cats and identification of H. *pylori* in saliva, gastric fluid and faeces. *Immunology* **88:**400–406.

35. **Fox, J. G., L. Yan, B. Shames, J. Campbell, J. C. Murphy, and X. Li.** 1996. Persistent hepatitis and enterocolitis in germfree mice infected with *Helicobacter hepaticus*. *Infect. Immun.* **64:**3673–3681.

36. **Germani, Y., C. Dauga, P. Duval, M. Huerre, M. Levy, G. Pialoux, P. Sansonetti, and P. A. Grimont.** 1997. Strategy for the detection of *Helicobacter* species by amplification of 16S rRNA genes and identification of H. *felis* in a human gastric biopsy. *Res. Microbiol.* **148:**315–326.

37. **Goddard, A. F., R. P. Logan, J. C. Atherton, D. Jenkins, and R. C. Spiller.** 1997. Healing of duodenal ulcer after eradication of *Helicobacter heilmannii*. *Lancet* **349:**1815–1816.

38. **Goodwin, A., D. Kersulyte, G. Sisson, S. J. Veldhuyzen van Zanten, D. E. Berg, and P. S. Hoffman.** 1998. Metronidazole resistance in *Helicobacter pylori* is due to null mutations in a gene (*rdxA*) that encodes an oxygen-insensitive NADPH nitroreductase. *Mol. Microbiol.* **28:**383–393.

39. **Goodwin, C. S., T. Armstrong, T. Chilvers, M. Peters, M. D. Collins, L. Sly, W. McConnell, and W. E. S. Harper.** 1989. Transfer of *Campylobacter pylori* and *Campylobacter mustelae* to *Helicobacter* gen. nov. as *Helicobacter pylori* comb. nov. and *Helicobacter mustelae* comb. nov., respectively. *Int. J. System. Bacteriol.* **39:**397–405.

40. **Graham, D. Y., and L. Rabeneck.** 1996. Patients, payers, and paradigm shifts: what to do about *Helicobacter pylori*. *Am. J. Gastroenterol.* **91:**188–190.

41. **Grayson, M. L., W. Tee, and B. Dwyer.** 1989. Gastroenteritis associated with *Campylobacter cinaedi*. *Med. J. Aust.* **150:**214–215.

42. **Hachem, C. Y., J. E. Clarridge, D. G. Evans, and D. Y. Graham.** 1995. Comparison of agar based media for primary isolation of *Helicobacter pylori. J. Clin. Pathol.* **48:** 714–716.

43. **Hachem, C. Y., J. E. Clarridge, R. Reddy, R. Flamm, D. G. Evans, S. K. Tanaka, and D. Y. Graham.** 1996. Antimicrobial susceptibility testing of *Helicobacter pylori.* Comparison of E-test, broth microdilution, and disk diffusion for ampicillin, clarithromycin, and metronidazole. *Diagn. Microbiol. Infect. Dis.* **24:**37–41.

44. **Han, S. W., R. Flamm, C. Y. Hachem, H. Y. Kim, J. E. Clarridge, D. G. Evans, J. Beyer, J. Drnec, and D. Y. Graham.** 1995. Transport and storage of *Helicobacter pylori* from gastric mucosal biopsies and clinical isolates. *Eur. J. Clin. Microbiol. Infect. Dis.* **14:**349–352.

45. **Handt, L. K., J. G. Fox, L. L. Yan, Z. Shen, W. J. Pouch, D. Ngai, S. L. Motzel, T. E. Nolan, and H. J. Klein.** 1997. Diagnosis of *Helicobacter pylori* infection in a colony of rhesus monkeys (*Macaca mulatta*). *J. Clin. Microbiol.* **35:**165–168.

46. **Hanninen, M. L., I. Happonen, S. Saari, and K. Jalava.** 1996. Culture and characteristics of *Helicobacter bizzozeronii*, a new canine gastric *Helicobacter* sp. *Int. J. Syst. Bacteriol.* **46:**160–166.

47. **Hansson, L. E., O. Nyren, A. W. Hsing, R. Bergstrom, S. Josefsson, W. H. Chow, J. F. Fraumeni, Jr., and H. O. Adami.** 1996. The risk of stomach cancer in patients with gastric or duodenal ulcer disease. *N. Engl. J. Med.* **335:** 242–249.

48. **Hardy, D. J., C. W. Hanson, D. M. Hensey, J. M. Beyer, and P. B. Fernandes.** 1988. Susceptibility of *Campylobacter pylori* to macrolides and fluoroquinolones. *J. Antimicrob. Chemother.* **22:**631–636.

49. **Hazell, S. L.** 1993. *Helicobacter pylori*, p. 273–283. *In* C. S. Goodwin and B. W. Worsley (ed.), Helicobacter pylori: *Biology and Clinical Practice.* CRC Press, Inc., Boca Raton, Fla.

50. **Hazell, S. L., T. J. Borody, A. Gal, and A. Lee.** 1987. *Campylobacter pyloridis* gastritis. I. Detection of urease as a marker of bacterial colonization and gastritis. *Am. J. Gastroenterol.* **82:**292–296.

51. **Hazell, S. L., and G. L. Mendz.** 1997. How *Helicobacter pylori* works: an overview of the metabolism of *Helicobacter pylori. Helicobacter* **2:**1–12.

52. **Hegarty, J. P., M. T. Dowd, and K. H. Baker.** 1999. Occurrence of *Helicobacter pylori* in surface water in the United States. *J. Appl. Microbiol.* **87:**697–701.

53. **Heilmann, K. L., and F. Borchard.** 1991. Gastritis due to spiral shaped bacteria other than *Helicobacter pylori*: clinical, histological, and ultrastructural findings. *Gut* **32:**137–140.

54. **Hilzenrat, N., E. Lamoureux, I. Weintrub, E. Alpert, M. Lichter, and L. Alpert.** 1995. *Helicobacter heilmannii*-like spiral bacteria in gastric mucosal biopsies. Prevalence and clinical significance. *Arch. Pathol. Lab. Med.* **119:**1149–1153.

55. **Hsueh, P. R., L. J. Teng, C. C. Hung, Y. C. Chen, P. C. Yang, S. W. Ho, and K. T. Luh.** 1999. Septic shock due to *Helicobacter fennelliae* in a non-human immunodeficiency virus-infected heterosexual patient. *J. Clin. Microbiol.* **37:**2084–2086.

56. **Hulten, K., S. W. Han, H. Enroth, P. D. Klein, A. R. Opekun, R. H. Gilman, D. G. Evans, L. Engstrand, D. Y. Graham, and F. A. El Zaatari.** 1996. *Helicobacter pylori* in the drinking water in Peru. *Gastroenterology* **110:** 1031–1035.

57. **Hunt, R. H.** 1997. Peptic ulcer disease: defining the treatment strategies in the era of *Helicobacter pylori. Am. J. Gastroenterol.* **92:**36S–40S.

58. **Husmann, M., C. Gries, P. Jehnichen, T. Woelfel, G. Gerken, W. Ludwig, and S. Bhakdi.** 1994. *Helicobacter* sp. strain Mainz isolated from an AIDS patient with septic arthritis: case report and nonradioactive analysis of 16S rRNA sequence. *J. Clin. Microbiol.* **32:**3037–3039.

59. **Jaskowski, T. D., T. B. Martins, H. R. Hill, and C. M. Litwin.** 1997. Immunoglobulin A antibodies to *Helicobacter pylori. J. Clin. Microbiol.* **35:**2999–3000.

60. **Jenks, P. J., R. L. Ferrero, and A. Labigne.** 1999. The role of the rdxA gene in the evolution of metronidazole resistance in *Helicobacter pylori. J. Antimicrob. Chemother.* **43:**753–758.

61. **Kawaguchi, H., K. Haruma, K. Komoto, M. Yoshihara, K. Sumii, and G. Kajiyama.** 1996. *Helicobacter pylori* infection is the major risk factor for atrophic gastritis. *Am. J. Gastroenterol.* **91:**959–962.

62. **Kiehlbauch, J. A., D. J. Brenner, D. N. Cameron, A. G. Steigerwalt, J. M. Makowski, C. N. Baker, C. M. Patton, and I. K. Wachsmuth.** 1995. Genotypic and phenotypic characterization of *Helicobacter cinaedi* and *Helicobacter fennelliae* strains isolated from humans and animals. *J. Clin. Microbiol.* **33:**2940–2947.

63. **Kiehlbauch, J. A., R. V. Tauxe, C. N. Baker, and I. K. Wachsmuth.** 1994. *Helicobacter cinaedi*-associated bacteremia and cellulitis in immunocompromised patients. *Ann. Intern. Med.* **121:**90–93.

64. **Kimmel, B., A. Bosserhoff, R. Frank, R. Gross, W. Goebel, and D. Beier.** 2000. Identification of immunodominant antigens from *Helicobacter pylori* and evaluation of their reactivities with sera from patients with different gastroduodenal pathologies. *Infect. Immun.* **68:**915–920.

65. **Klein, P. D., H. M. Malaty, R. F. Martin, K. S. Graham, R. M. Genta, and D. Y. Graham.** 1996. Noninvasive detection of *Helicobacter pylori* infection in clinical practice: the 13C urea breath test. *Am. J. Gastroenterol.* **91:** 690–694.

66. **Kwon, D. H., J. A. Pena, M. S. Osato, J. G. Fox, D. Y. Graham, and J. Versalovic.** 2000. Frameshift mutations in rdxA and metronidazole resistance in North American *Helicobacter pylori* isolates. *J. Antimicrob. Chemother.* **46:** 793–796.

67. **Laheij, R. J., H. Straatman, J. B. Jansen, and A. L. Verbeek.** 1998. Evaluation of commercially available *Helicobacter pylori* serology kits: a review. *J. Clin. Microbiol.* **36:**2803–2809.

68. **Laughon, B. E., A. A. Vernon, D. A. Druckman, R. Fox, T. C. Quinn, B. F. Polk, and J. G. Bartlett.** 1988. Recovery of *Campylobacter* species from homosexual men. *J. Infect. Dis.* **158:**464–467.

69. **Lavelle, J. P., S. Landas, F. A. Mitros, and J. L. Conklin.** 1994. Acute gastritis associated with spiral organisms from cats. *Dig. Dis. Sci.* **39:**744–750.

70. **Lee, A., S. L. Hazell, J. O'Rourke, and S. Kouprach.** 1988. Isolation of a spiral-shaped bacterium from the cat stomach. *Infect. Immun.* **56:**2843–2850.

71. **Lee, A., and J. O'Rourke.** 1993. Gastric bacteria other than *Helicobacter pylori. Gastroenterol. Clin. North Am.* **22:**21–42.

72. **Logan, R. P. H.** 1993. Breath tests to detect *Helicobacter pylori*, p. 307–326. *In* C. S. Goodwin and B. W. Worsley (ed.), Helicobacter pylori: *Biology and Clinical Practice.* CRC Press, Inc., Boca Raton, Fla.

73. **Lu, J. J., C. L. Perng, R. Y. Shyu, C. H. Chen, Q. Lou, S. K. Chong, and C. H. Lee.** 1999. Comparison of five PCR methods for detection of *Helicobacter pylori* DNA in gastric tissues. *J. Clin. Microbiol.* **37:**772–774.

74. **Maeda, S., H. Yoshida, K. Ogura, F. Kanai, Y. Shiratori, and M. Omata.** 1998. *Helicobacter pylori* specific nested PCR

assay for the detection of 23S rRNA mutations associated with clarithromycin resistance. *Gut* **43:**317–321.

75. **Makristathis, A., E. Pasching, K. Schutze, M. Wimmer, M. L. Rotter, and A. M. Hirschl.** 1998. Detection of *Helicobacter pylori* in stool specimens by PCR and antigen enzyme immunoassay. *J. Clin. Microbiol.* **36:**2772–2774.

76. **Marais, A., G. L. Mendz, S. L. Hazell, and F. Megraud.** 1999. Metabolism and genetics of *Helicobacter pylori:* the genome era. *Microbiol. Mol. Biol. Rev.* **63:**642–674.

77. **Marchetti, M., B. Arico, D. Burroni, N. Figura, R. Rappuoli, and P. Ghiara.** 1995. Development of a mouse model of *Helicobacter pylori* infection that mimics human disease. *Science* **267:**1655–1658.

78. **Marshall, B. J.** 1994. *Helicobacter pylori. Am. J. Gastroenterol.* **89:**S116–S128.

79. **Marshall, B. J., J. R. Warren, G. J. Francis, S. R. Langton, C. S. Goodwin, and E. D. Blincow.** 1987. Rapid urease test in the management of *Campylobacter pyloridis*-associated gastritis. *Am. J. Gastroenterol.* **82:**200–210.

80. **McCallion, W. A., L. J. Murray, A. G. Bailie, A. M. Dalzell, D. P. O'Reilly, and K. B. Bamford.** 1996. *Helicobacter pylori* infection in children: relation with current household living conditions. *Gut* **39:**18–21.

81. **McCarthy, C., S. Patchett, R. M. Collins, S. Beattie, C. Keane, and C. O'Morain.** 1995. Long-term prospective study of *Helicobacter pylori* in nonulcer dyspepsia. *Dig. Dis. Sci.* **40:**114–119.

82. **McNulty, C. A., and J. C. Dent.** 1987. Rapid identification of *Campylobacter pylori* (*C. pyloridis*) by preformed enzymes. *J. Clin. Microbiol.* **25:**1683–1686.

83. **Megraud, F.** 1996. Advantages and disadvantages of current diagnostic tests for the detection of *Helicobacter pylori. Scand. J. Gastroenterol. Suppl.* **215:**57–62.

84. **Megraud, F., F. Bonnet, M. Garnier, and H. Lamouliatte.** 1985. Characterization of "*Campylobacter pyloridis*" by culture, enzymatic profile, and protein content. *J. Clin. Microbiol.* **22:**1007–1010.

85. **Megraud, F., N. Lehn, T. Lind, E. Bayerdorffer, C. O'Morain, R. Spiller, P. Unge, S. V. van Zanten, M. Wrangstadh, and C. F. Burman.** 1999. Antimicrobial susceptibility testing of *Helicobacter pylori* in a large multicenter trial: the MACH 2 study. *Antimicrob. Agents Chemother.* **43:**2747–2752.

86. **Melito, P. L., C. Munro, P. R. Chipman, D. L. Woodward, T. F. Booth, and F. G. Rodgers.** 2001. *Helicobacter winghamensis* sp. nov., a novel *Helicobacter* sp. isolated from patients with gastroenteritis. *J. Clin. Microbiol.* **39:**2412–2417.

87. **Mendall, M. A., P. M. Goggin, N. Molineaux, J. Levy, T. Toosy, D. Strachan, and T. C. Northfield.** 1992. Childhood living conditions and *Helicobacter pylori* seropositivity in adult life. *Lancet* **339:**896–897.

88. **Mion, F., R. Ecochard, J. Guitton, and T. Ponchon.** 2001. [^{13}C]O2 breath tests: comparison of isotope ratio mass spectrometry and non-dispersive infrared spectrometry results. *Gastroenterol. Clin. Biol.* **25:**375–379.

89. **Misra, S. P., M. Dwivedi, V. Misra, and S. C. Gupta.** 1993. Imprint cytology—a cheap, rapid and effective method for diagnosing *Helicobacter pylori. Postgrad. Med. J.* **69:**291–295.

90. **Mitchell, H. M., T. Bohane, R. A. Hawkes, and A. Lee.** 1993. *Helicobacter pylori* infection within families. *Zentralbl. Bakteriol.* **280:**128–136.

91. **Monteiro, L., A. de Mascarel, A. M. Sarrasqueta, B. Bergey, C. Barberis, P. Talby, D. Roux, L. Shouler, D. Goldfain, H. Lamouliatte, and F. Megraud.** 2001. Diagnosis of *Helicobacter pylori* infection: noninvasive methods compared to invasive methods and evaluation of two new tests. *Am. J. Gastroenterol.* **96:**353–358.

92. **Morgner, A., N. Lehn, L. P. Andersen, C. Thiede, M. Bennedsen, K. Trebesius, B. Neubauer, A. Neubauer, M. Stolte, and E. Bayerdorffer.** 2000. *Helicobacter heilmannii*-associated primary gastric low-grade MALT lymphoma: complete remission after curing the infection. *Gastroenterology* **118:**821–828.

93. **Morris, A. J., M. R. Ali, G. I. Nicholson, G. I. Perez-Perez, and M. J. Blaser.** 1991. Long-term follow-up of voluntary ingestion of *Helicobacter pylori. Ann. Intern. Med.* **114:**662–663.

94. **National Institutes of Health.** 1994. NIH Consensus Conference. *Helicobacter pylori* in peptic ulcer disease. NIH Consensus Development Panel on *Helicobacter pylori* in Peptic Ulcer Disease. *JAMA* **272:**65–69.

95. **NCCLS.** 2002. *Performance Standards for Antimicrobial Susceptibility Testing: Twelfth Informational Supplement.* M100-S12. NCCLS, Wayne, Pa.

96. **Ng, V. L., W. K. Hadley, C. L. Fennell, B. M. Flores, and W. E. Stamm.** 1987. Successive bacteremias with "*Campylobacter cinaedi*" and "*Campylobacter fennelliae*" in a bisexual male. *J. Clin. Microbiol.* **25:**2008–2009.

97. **Nilsson, H. O., R. Mulchandani, K. G. Tranberg, and T. Wadstrom.** 2001. *Helicobacter* species identified in liver from patients with cholangiocarcinoma and hepatocellular carcinoma. *Gastroenterology* **120:**323–324.

98. **Nilsson, H. O., J. Taneera, M. Castedal, E. Glatz, R. Olsson, and T. Wadstrom.** 2000. Identification of *Helicobacter pylori* and other *Helicobacter* species by PCR, hybridization, and partial DNA sequencing in human liver samples from patients with primary sclerosing cholangitis or primary biliary cirrhosis. *J. Clin. Microbiol.* **38:**1072–1076.

99. **Nomura, A., G. N. Stemmermann, P. H. Chyou, I. Kato, G. I. Perez-Perez, and M. J. Blaser.** 1991. *Helicobacter pylori* infection and gastric carcinoma among Japanese Americans in Hawaii. *N. Engl. J. Med.* **325:**1132–1136.

100. **Norris, C. R., S. L. Marks, K. A. Eaton, S. Z. Torabian, R. J. Munn, and J. V. Solnick.** 1999. Healthy cats are commonly colonized with "*Helicobacter heilmannii*" that is associated with minimal gastritis. *J. Clin. Microbiol.* **37:**189–194.

101. **On, S. L.** 2001. Taxonomy of *Campylobacter, Arcobacter, Helicobacter* and related bacteria: current status, future prospects and immediate concerns. *J. Appl. Microbiol.* **90:**1S–15S.

102. **On, S. L., and B. Holmes.** 1992. Assessment of enzyme detection tests useful in identification of campylobacteria. *J. Clin. Microbiol.* **30:**746–749.

103. **Orlicek, S. L., D. F. Welch, and T. L. Kuhls.** 1993. Septicemia and meningitis caused by *Helicobacter cinaedi* in a neonate. *J. Clin. Microbiol.* **31:**569–571.

104. **Osato, M. S., R. Reddy, S. G. Reddy, R. L. Penland, and D. Y. Graham.** 2001. Comparison of the Etest and the NCCLS-approved agar dilution method to detect metronidazole and clarithromycin resistant *Helicobacter pylori. Int. J. Antimicrob. Agents* **17:**39–44.

105. **Osato, M. S., R. Reddy, S. G. Reddy, R. L. Penland, H. M. Malaty, and D. Y. Graham.** 2001. Pattern of primary resistance of *Helicobacter pylori* to metronidazole or clarithromycin in the United States. *Arch. Intern. Med.* **161:**1217–1220.

106. **Oshowo, A., D. Gillam, A. Botha, M. Tunio, J. Holton, P. Boulos, and M. Hobsley.** 1998. *Helicobacter pylori:* the mouth, stomach, and gut axis. *Ann. Periodontol.* **3:**276–280.

107. **Parsonnet, J., G. D. Friedman, D. P. Vandersteen, Y. Chang, J. H. Vogelman, N. Orentreich, and R. K.**

Sibley. 1991. *Helicobacter pylori* infection and the risk of gastric carcinoma. *N. Engl. J. Med.* **325:**1127–1131.

108. Parsonnet, J., S. Hansen, L. Rodriguez, A. B. Gelb, R. A. Warnke, E. Jellum, N. Orentreich, J. H. Vogelman, and G. D. Friedman. 1994. *Helicobacter pylori* infection and gastric lymphoma. *N. Engl. J. Med.* **330:** 1267–1271.

109. Parsonnet, J., H. Shmuely, and T. Haggerty. 1999. Fecal and oral shedding of *Helicobacter pylori* from healthy infected adults. *JAMA* **282:**2240–2245.

110. Parsonnet, J., K. Welch, C. Compton, R. Strauss, T. Wang, P. Kelsey, and M. J. Ferraro. 1988. Simple microbiologic detection of *Campylobacter pylori*. *J. Clin. Microbiol.* **26:**948–949.

111. Paster, B. J., A. Lee, J. G. Fox, F. E. Dewhirst, L. A. Tordoff, G. J. Fraser, J. L. O'Rourke, N. S. Taylor, and R. Ferrero. 1991. Phylogeny of *Helicobacter felis* sp. nov., *Helicobacter mustelae*, and related bacteria. *Int. J. Syst. Bacteriol.* **41:**31–38.

112. Pena, J. A., J. G. Fox, M. J. Ferraro, and J. Versalovic. 2001. Molecular resistance testing of *Helicobacter pylori* in gastric biopsies. *Arch. Pathol. Lab Med.* **125:**493–497.

113. Pena, J. A., K. McNeil, J. G. Fox, and J. Versalovic. 2002. Molecular evidence of *Helicobacter cinaedi* organisms in human gastric biopsy specimens. *J. Clin. Microbiol.* **40:**1511–1513.

114. Perez-Perez, G. I. 2000. Accurate diagnosis of *Helicobacter pylori*. Culture, including transport. *Gastroenterol. Clin. North Am.* **29:**879–884.

115. Perez-Perez, G. I., B. M. Dworkin, J. E. Chodos, and M. J. Blaser. 1988. *Campylobacter pylori* antibodies in humans. *Ann. Intern. Med.* **109:**11–17.

116. Perri, F., V. Festa, R. Clemente, M. R. Villani, M. Quitadamo, N. Caruso, M. L. Bergoli, and A. Andriulli. 2001. Randomized study of two "rescue" therapies for *Helicobacter pylori*-infected patients after failure of standard triple therapies. *Am. J. Gastroenterol.* **96:**58–62.

117. Popovic-Uroic, T., C. M. Patton, M. A. Nicholson, and J. A. Kiehlbauch. 1990. Evaluation of the indoxyl acetate hydrolysis test for rapid differentiation of *Campylobacter*, *Helicobacter*, and *Wolinella* species. *J. Clin. Microbiol.* **28:**2335–2339.

118. Powers, C. N. 1998. Diagnosis of infectious diseases: a cytopathologist's perspective. *Clin. Microbiol. Rev.* **11:** 341–365.

119. Puetz, T., N. Vakil, S. Phadnis, B. Dunn, and J. Robinson. 1997. The Pyloritek test and the CLO test: accuracy and incremental cost analysis. *Am. J. Gastroenterol.* **92:**254–257.

120. Pytko-Polonczyk, J., S. J. Konturek, E. Karczewska, W. Bielanski, and A. Kaczmarczyk-Stachowska. 1996. Oral cavity as permanent reservoir of *Helicobacter pylori* and potential source of reinfection. *J. Physiol. Pharmacol.* **47:**121–129.

121. Queiroz, D. M., G. A. Rocha, E. N. Mendes, S. B. De Moura, A. M. De Oliveira, and D. Miranda. 1996. Association between *Helicobacter* and gastric ulcer disease of the pars esophagea in swine. *Gastroenterology* **111:**19–27.

122. Quinn, T. C., S. E. Goodell, C. Fennell, S. P. Wang, M. D. Schuffler, K. K. Holmes, and W. E. Stamm. 1984. Infections with *Campylobacter jejuni* and *Campylobacter*-like organisms in homosexual men. *Ann. Intern. Med.* **101:**187–192.

123. Riley, L. K., C. L. Franklin, R. R. Hook, Jr., and C. Besch-Williford. 1996. Identification of murine helicobacters by PCR and restriction enzyme analyses. *J. Clin. Microbiol.* **34:**942–946.

124. Romaniuk, P. J., B. Zoltowska, T. J. Trust, D. J. Lane, G. J. Olsen, N. R. Pace, and D. A. Stahl. 1987. *Campylobacter pylori*, the spiral bacterium associated with human gastritis, is not a true *Campylobacter* sp. *J. Bacteriol.* **169:**2137–2141.

125. Romero, S., J. R. Archer, M. E. Hamacher, S. M. Bologna, and R. F. Schell. 1988. Case report of an unclassified microaerophilic bacterium associated with gastroenteritis. *J. Clin. Microbiol.* **26:**142–143.

126. Russmann, H., V. A. Kempf, S. Koletzko, J. Heesemann, and I. B. Autenrieth. 2001. Comparison of fluorescent in situ hybridization and conventional culturing for detection of *Helicobacter pylori* in gastric biopsy specimens. *J. Clin. Microbiol.* **39:**304–308.

127. Sahay, P., A. P. West, D. Birkenhead, and P. M. Hawkey. 1995. *Campylobacter jejuni* in the stomach. *J. Med. Microbiol.* **43:**75–77.

128. Salomon, H. 1898. Uber das Spirillum des Saugetiermagens und sein Verhalten zu den Belegzellen. *Zentbl. Bakeriol. Parasitenkd. Infektionskr. Hyg. Abt 1* **19:**422–441.

129. Sato, T., M. A. Fujino, Y. Kojima, F. Kitahara, A. Morozumi, K. Nagata, M. Nakamura, and H. Hosaka. 2000. Evaluation of immunological rapid urease testing for detection of *Helicobacter pylori*. *Eur. J. Clin. Microbiol. Infect. Dis.* **19:**438–442.

130. Shen, Z., J. G. Fox, F. E. Dewhirst, B. J. Paster, C. J. Foltz, L. Yan, B. Shames, and L. Perry. 1997. *Helicobacter rodentium* sp. nov., a urease-negative *Helicobacter* species isolated from laboratory mice. *Int. J. Syst. Bacteriol.* **47:**627–634.

131. Sipponen, P., T. U. Kosunen, I. M. Samloff, O. P. Heinonen, and M. Siurala. 1996. Rate of *Helicobacter pylori* acquisition among Finnish adults: a fifteen year follow-up. *Scand. J. Gastroenterol.* **31:**229–232.

132. Slomianski, A., T. Schubert, and A. F. Cutler. 1995. [^{13}C]urea breath test to confirm eradication of *Helicobacter pylori*. *Am. J. Gastroenterol.* **90:**224–226.

133. Solnick, J. V., J. O'Rourke, A. Lee, B. J. Paster, F. E. Dewhirst, and L. S. Tompkins. 1993. An uncultured gastric spiral organism is a newly identified *Helicobacter* in humans. *J. Infect. Dis.* **168:**379–385.

134. Sorlin, P., P. Vandamme, J. Nortier, B. Hoste, C. Rossi, S. Pavlof, and M. J. Struelens. 1999. Recurrent "*Flexispira rappini*" bacteremia in an adult patient undergoing hemodialysis: case report. *J. Clin. Microbiol.* **37:** 1319–1323.

135. Stanley, J., D. Linton, A. P. Burnens, F. E. Dewhirst, S. L. On, A. Porter, R. J. Owen, and M. Costas. 1994. *Helicobacter pullorum* sp. nov.-genotype and phenotype of a new species isolated from poultry and from human patients with gastroenteritis. *Microbiology* **140:**3441–3449.

136. Stanley, J., D. Linton, A. P. Burnens, F. E. Dewhirst, R. J. Owen, A. Porter, S. L. On, and M. Costas. 1993. *Helicobacter canis* sp. nov., a new species from dogs: an integrated study of phenotype and genotype. *J. Gen. Microbiol.* **139:**2495–2504.

137. Sung, J. J., S. C. Chung, T. K. Ling, M. Y. Yung, V. K. Leung, E. K. Ng, M. K. Li, A. F. Cheng, and A. K. Li. 1995. Antibacterial treatment of gastric ulcers associated with *Helicobacter pylori*. *N. Engl. J. Med.* **332:**139–142.

138. Szczebara, F., L. Dhaenens, P. Vincent, and M. O. Husson. 1997. Evaluation of rapid molecular methods for detection of clarithromycin resistance in *Helicobacter pylori*. *Eur. J. Clin. Microbiol. Infect. Dis.* **16:**162–164.

139. The European *Helicobacter pylori* Study Group. 1997. Current European concepts in the management of *Helicobacter pylori* infection. The Maastricht Consensus Report. *Gut* **41:**8–13.

140. **Tinnert, A., A. Mattsson, I. Bolin, J. Dalenback, A. Hamlet, and A. M. Svennerholm.** 1997. Local and systemic immune responses in humans against *Helicobacter pylori* antigens from homologous and heterologous strains. *Microb. Pathog.* **23:**285–296.

141. **Tomb, J. F., O. White, A. R. Kerlavage, R. A. Clayton, G. G. Sutton, R. D. Fleischmann, K. A. Ketchum, H. P. Klenk, S. Gill, B. A. Dougherty, K. Nelson, J. Quackenbush, L. Zhou, E. F. Kirkness, S. Peterson, B. Loftus, D. Richardson, R. Dodson, H. G. Khalak, A. Glodek, K. McKenney, L. M. Fitzegerald, N. Lee, M. D. Adams, E. K. Hickey, D. E. Berg, J. D. Gocayne, T. R. Utterback, J. D. Peterson, J. M. Kelley, M. D. Cotton, J. M. Weidman, C. Fujii, C. Bowman, L. Watthey, E. Wallin, W. S. Hayes, M. Borodovsky, P. D. Karp, H. O. Smith, C. M. Fraser, and J. C. Venter.** 1997. The complete genome sequence of the gastric pathogen *Helicobacter pylori*. *Nature* **388:**539–547.

142. **Trebesius, K., K. Adler, M. Vieth, M. Stolte, and R. Haas.** 2001. Specific detection and prevalence of *Helicobacter heilmannii*-like organisms in the human gastric mucosa by fluorescent in situ hybridization and partial 16S ribosomal DNA sequencing. *J. Clin. Microbiol.* **39:**1510–1516.

143. **Vakil, N., B. Hahn, and D. McSorley.** 1998. Clarithromycin-resistant *Helicobacter pylori* in patients with duodenal ulcer in the United States. *Am. J. Gastroenterol.* **93:**1432–1435.

144. **Vakil, N., D. Rhew, A. Soll, and J. J. Ofman.** 2000. The cost-effectiveness of diagnostic testing strategies for *Helicobacter pylori*. *Am. J. Gastroenterol.* **95:**1691–1698.

145. **Vandamme, P., E. Falsen, R. Rossau, B. Hoste, P. Segers, R. Tytgat, and J. De Ley.** 1991. Revision of *Campylobacter*, *Helicobacter*, and *Wolinella* taxonomy: emendation of generic descriptions and proposal of *Arcobacter* gen. nov. *Int. J. Syst. Bacteriol.* **41:**88–103.

146. **Vandamme, P., C. S. Harrington, K. Jalava, and S. L. On.** 2000. Misidentifying helicobacters: the *Helicobacter cinaedi* example. *J. Clin. Microbiol.* **38:**2261–2266.

147. **van Doorn, L. J., Y. J. Debets-Ossenkopp, A. Marais, R. Sanna, F. Megraud, J. G. Kusters, and W. G. Quint.** 1999. Rapid detection, by PCR and reverse hybridization, of mutations in the *Helicobacter pylori* 23S rRNA gene, associated with macrolide resistance. *Antimicrob. Agents Chemother.* **43:**1779–1782.

148. **van Doorn, L. J., C. Figueiredo, R. Sanna, A. Plaisier, P. Schneeberger, W. de Boer, and W. Quint.** 1998. Clinical relevance of the *cagA*, *vacA*, and *iceA* status of *Helicobacter pylori*. *Gastroenterology* **115:**58–66.

149. **Versalovic, J., and J. G. Fox.** 2001. Taxonomy and phylogeny of *Helicobacter*, p. 15–28. *In* M. Achtman and S. Suerbaum (ed.), Helicobacter pylori: *Molecular and Cellular Biology*. Horizon Scientific Press, Wymondham, United Kingdom.

150. **Versalovic, J., D. Shortridge, K. Kibler, M. V. Griffy, J. Beyer, R. K. Flamm, S. K. Tanaka, D. Y. Graham, and M. F. Go.** 1996. Mutations in 23S rRNA are associated with clarithromycin resistance in *Helicobacter pylori*. *Antimicrob. Agents Chemother.* **40:**477–480.

151. **Vincent, P., F. Gottrand, P. Pernes, M. O. Husson, M. Lecomte-Houcke, D. Turck, and H. Leclerc.** 1994. High prevalence of *Helicobacter pylori* infection in cohabiting children. Epidemiology of a cluster, with special emphasis on molecular typing. *Gut* **35:**313–316.

152. **Warren, J. R., and B. J. Marshall.** 1983. Unidentified curved bacilli on gastric epithelium in active chronic gastritis. *Lancet* **i:**1273–1275.

153. **Webb, P. M., T. Knight, S. Greaves, A. Wilson, D. G. Newell, J. Elder, and D. Forman.** 1994. Relation between infection with *Helicobacter pylori* and living conditions in childhood: evidence for person to person transmission in early life. *Br. Med. J.* **308:**750–753.

154. **Weir, S., B. Cuccherini, A. M. Whitney, M. L. Ray, J. P. MacGregor, A. Steigerwalt, M. I. Daneshvar, R. Weyant, B. Wray, J. Steele, W. Strober, and V. J. Gill.** 1999. Recurrent bacteremia caused by a *"Flexispira"*-like organism in a patient with X-linked (Bruton's) agammaglobulinemia. *J. Clin. Microbiol.* **37:**2439–2445.

155. **Woo, J. S., H. M. el Zimaity, R. M. Genta, M. M. Yousfi, and D. Y. Graham.** 1996. The best gastric site for obtaining a positive rapid urease test. *Helicobacter* **1:**256–259.

156. **Wotherspoon, A. C., C. Ortiz-Hidalgo, M. R. Falzon, and P. G. Isaacson.** 1991. *Helicobacter pylori*-associated gastritis and primary B-cell gastric lymphoma. *Lancet* **338:**1175–1176.

157. **Xia, H. X., C. T. Keane, J. Chen, J. Zhang, E. J. Walsh, A. P. Moran, J. S. Hua, F. Megraud, and C. A. O'Morain.** 1994. Transportation of *Helicobacter pylori* cultures by optimal systems. *J. Clin. Microbiol.* **32:**3075–3077.

158. **Yousfi, M. M., H. M. el Zimaity, R. A. Cole, R. M. Genta, and D. Y. Graham.** 1997. Comparison of agar gel (CLOtest) or reagent strip (PyloriTek) rapid urease tests for detection of *Helicobacter pylori* infection. *Am. J. Gastroenterol.* **92:**997–999.

Leptospira and *Leptonema**

PAUL N. LEVETT

59

TAXONOMY

Serologic Classification

The genus *Leptospira* is comprised of spiral-shaped bacteria with hooked ends (33). This genus and the genus *Leptonema* make up the family *Leptospiraceae* within the order *Spirochaetales* and class "*Spirochaetes*" of the recently proposed phylum *Spirochaetes* (25). The genus was formerly divided into two species, *Leptospira interrogans*, comprising all pathogenic strains, and *Leptospira biflexa*, containing the saprophytic strains isolated from the environment (23, 33). *L. biflexa* and *L. interrogans* were differentiated by a number of biochemical tests (33).

Both *L. interrogans* sensu lato and *L. biflexa* sensu lato are divided into serovars defined by agglutination after cross-absorption with homologous antigen (16, 33, 35). Serovars are considered distinct if more than 10% of the homologous titer remains in at least one of the two antisera on repeated testing (32). Over 60 serovars of *L. biflexa* sensu lato and more than 200 serovars of *L. interrogans* sensu lato are recognized. Serovars that are antigenically related have traditionally been grouped into serogroups (35). Serogroups have no taxonomic standing, but the concept has proved useful for epidemiological understanding, particularly when the serological results from the microscopic agglutination test (MAT) are being interpreted. The serogroups of *L. interrogans* sensu lato and some common serovars are shown in Table 1.

Genotypic Classification

The phenotypic classification of leptospires has been replaced by a genotypic one, in which 12 named species and 5 unnamed genomospecies include all serovars of *Leptospira* spp. (10, 47, 49, 71). DNA hybridization studies have also confirmed the taxonomic status of the monospecific genus *Leptonema* (10, 48). The genetically defined species of *Leptospira* do not correspond to the previous two species (*L. interrogans* sensu lato and *L. biflexa* sensu lato), and both pathogenic and nonpathogenic serovars occur within some species (36). Neither serogroup nor serovar reliably predicts

the true species of *Leptospira*. Moreover, genetic heterogeneity within serovars occurs (10, 24), resulting in strains of some serovars being classified in multiple species (Table 2). In addition, the phenotypic characteristics formerly used to differentiate *L. interrogans* sensu lato from *L. biflexa* sensu lato do not differentiate the genetically defined species (10, 71).

The reclassification of leptospires on genotypic grounds is taxonomically correct and provides a strong foundation for future classifications. However, the molecular classification is problematic for clinical microbiologists, because it is incompatible with the system of serogroups with which clinicians and epidemiologists are familiar. Clinical laboratories will have to retain the serological classification of pathogenic leptospires until simpler DNA-based identification methods are developed and validated (36). In addition, the retention of *L. interrogans* and *L. biflexa* as specific names in the genomic classification allows for nomenclatural confusion. In this chapter, specific names refer to the genetically defined species, including *L. interrogans* sensu stricto and *L. biflexa* sensu stricto.

DESCRIPTION OF THE FAMILY

Leptospires are tightly coiled spirochetes, usually 0.1 μm by 6 to 20 μm. The helical conformation is right-handed, while the amplitude is approximately 0.1 to 0.15 μm and the wavelength is approximately 0.5 μm (22). The cells have pointed ends, either or both of which are usually bent into a distinctive hook (Fig. 1). Two axial filaments (periplasmic flagella), with polar insertions, are located in the periplasmic space. Leptospires exhibit two distinct forms of movement, either translational (rapid back and forth movements) or rotational (spinning rapidly about the long axis of the cell) (26). Morphologically, all leptospires are indistinguishable.

Leptospires are obligate aerobes with an optimum growth temperature of 28 to 30°C. The optimum pH for growth is 7.2 to 7.6. They produce both catalase and oxidase. They grow in simple media enriched with vitamins (vitamins B_2 and B_{12} are growth factors), long-chain fatty acids, and ammonium salts (33).

Leptonema illini, the sole member of the genus *Leptonema*, is morphologically similar to leptospires but is distinguished by a higher guanine-plus-cytosine ratio

---

* This chapter contains information presented in chapter 52 by Robbin S. Weyant, Sandra L. Bragg, and Arnold F. Kaufmann in the seventh edition of this Manual.

TABLE 1 Serogroups and some serovars of *L. interrogans* sensu lato

Serogroup	Serovar(s)
Icterohaemorrhagiae	icterohaemorrhagiae
	copenhageni
	lai
Hebdomadis	hebdomadis
	jules
	kremastos
Autumnalis	autumnalis
	fortbragg
	bim
Pyrogenes.	pyrogenes
Bataviae.	bataviae
Grippotyphosa	grippotyphosa
	canalzonae
	ratnapura
Canicola	canicola
Australis	australis
	bratislava
	lora
Pomona.	pomona
Javanica.	javanica
Sejroe	sejroe
	saxkoebing
	hardjo
Panama	panama
	mangus
Cynopteri	cynopteri
Djasiman	djasiman
Sarmin	sarmin
Mini	mini
	georgia
Tarassovi	tarassovi
Ballum.	ballum
	arborea
Celledoni.	celledoni
Louisiana	louisiana
	lanka
Ranarum	ranarum
Manhao.	manhao
Shermani	shermani
Hurstbridge	hurstbridge

TABLE 2 Leptospiral serovars found in multiple species[a]

Serovar	Species
bataviae	*L. interrogans, L. santarosai*
bulgarica	*L. interrogans, L. kirschneri*
grippotyphosa	*L. kirschneri, L. interrogans*
hardjo	*L. borgpetersenii, L. interrogans,*
	L. meyeri
icterohaemorrhagiae.	*L. interrogans, L. inadai*
kremastos	*L. interrogans, L. santarosai*
mwogolo.	*L. kirschneri, L. interrogans*
paidjan.	*L. kirschneri, L. interrogans*
pomona	*L. interrogans, L. noguchii*
pyrogenes	*L. interrogans, L. santarosai*
szwajizak.	*L. interrogans, L. santarosai*
valbuzzi	*L. interrogans, L. kirschneri*

[a] Based on data reported by Brenner et al. (10) and by Feresu et al. (24).

(54.2%). The organism has been isolated on only a handful of occasions and is not considered a human pathogen (22).

NATURAL HABITAT

Leptospires are ubiquitous, either free-living in water or associated with renal infection of animals. Leptospirosis is presumed to be the most widespread zoonosis in the world (69). The source of infection in humans is usually either direct or indirect contact with the urine of an infected animal. The incidence is very much higher in warm-climate countries than in temperate regions, due mainly to longer survival of leptospires in the environment in warm, humid conditions. The disease is seasonal, with peak incidence occurring in summer or fall in temperate regions, where temperature is the limiting factor in survival of leptospires, and during rainy seasons in warm-climate regions, where rapid desiccation would otherwise prevent survival. Water-borne transmission has been documented; point contamination of water supplies has resulted in several outbreaks of leptospirosis (36).

Animals, including humans, can be divided into maintenance hosts or accidental (incidental) hosts. A maintenance host is defined as a species in which infection is endemic, usually transferred from animal to animal by direct contact. Infection is usually acquired at an early age, and the prevalence of chronic excretion in the urine increases with the age of the animal. Other animals (such as humans) may become infected by indirect contact with the maintenance host. Animals may be maintenance hosts of some serovars but incidental hosts of others, infection with which may cause severe or fatal disease. The most important maintenance hosts are small mammals, which may transfer infection to domestic farm animals, dogs, and humans. Different rodent species may be reservoirs of distinct serovars, but rats are generally maintenance hosts for serovars of the serogroup Icterohaemorrhagiae and mice are generally maintenance hosts for serogroup Ballum serovars. Domestic animals are also maintenance hosts: dairy cattle may harbor serovars hardjo and pomona; pigs may harbor pomona, tarassovi, or bratislava; and dogs may harbor canicola. Distinct variations in maintenance hosts and the serovars they carry occur throughout the world, and these associations may change over time. Knowledge of the prevalent serovars and their maintenance hosts is essential in understanding the epidemiology of the disease.

CLINICAL SIGNIFICANCE

Human infections may be acquired through occupational, recreational, or avocational exposures. Occupation is a significant risk factor for humans. Direct contact with infected animals accounts for most infections in farmers, veterinarians, abattoir workers, rodent control workers, and people in other occupations which require contact with animals, while indirect contact is important for sewer workers, miners, soldiers, septic tank cleaners, fish farmers, rice field workers, and sugar cane cutters. Livestock farming is a major occupational risk factor throughout the world. The highest risk is associated with dairy farming and is associated with serovar hardjo and in particular with milking of dairy cattle. There is a significant risk associated with recreational exposures occurring in water sports.

The usual portal of entry is through abrasions or cuts in the skin or via the conjunctiva. The great majority of infections are either subclinical or of very mild severity, and

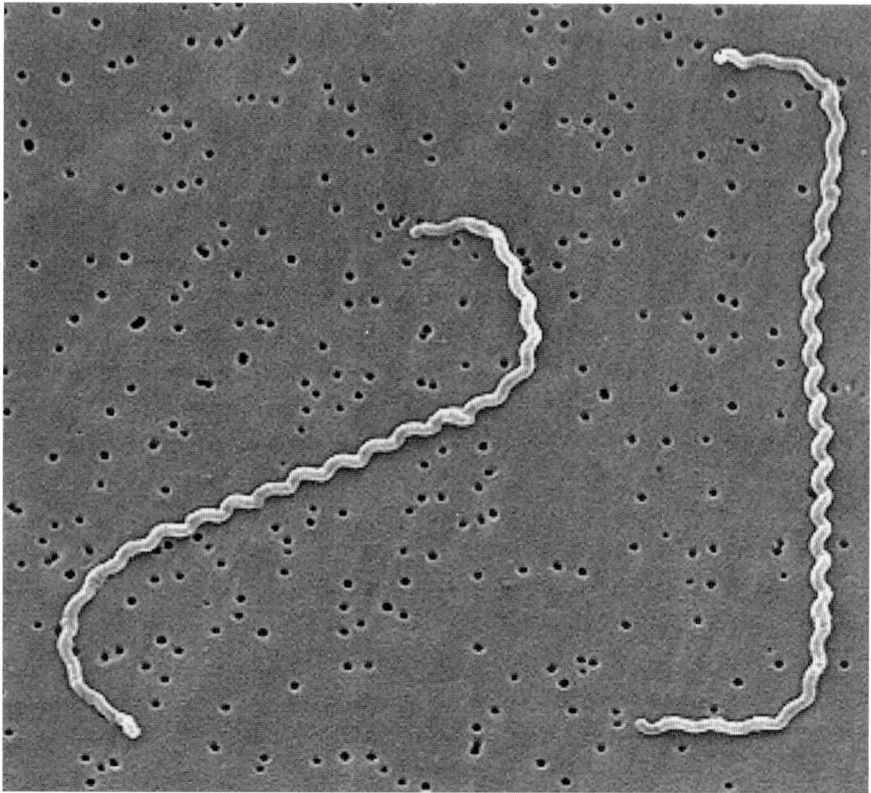

FIGURE 1   Scanning electron micrograph of leptospiral cells bound to a 0.2-μm-pore-size filter. Magnification, approximately ×3,500.

the patients will probably not seek or be brought to medical attention. The clinical presentation of leptospirosis is biphasic, with a septicemic phase lasting about a week, followed by the immune phase, characterized by antibody production and excretion of leptospires in the urine. Most of the complications of leptospirosis are associated with localization of leptospires within the tissues during the immune phase and thus occur during the second week of the illness.

The overwhelming majority of the recognized cases present with a febrile illness of sudden onset, the symptoms of which include chills, headache, myalgia, abdominal pain, and conjunctival suffusion. Aseptic meningitis may be found in ≤25% of all leptospirosis cases. Between 5 and 10% of all patients with leptospirosis have the icteric form of the disease (Weil's disease), in which the clinical course is often very rapidly progressive. In addition to jaundice, patients with icteric leptospirosis may develop acute renal failure, pulmonary hemorrhage, and cardiac arrhythmias. Severe cases often present late in the course of the disease, and this contributes to the high mortality rate, which ranges between 5 and 15%.

COLLECTION, TRANSPORT, AND STORAGE OF SPECIMENS

Leptospires can be isolated from blood, cerebrospinal fluid (CSF), and peritoneal dialysate fluids during the first 10 days of illness. These specimens should be collected before antibiotic therapy is initiated and while the patient is febrile. Under optimal conditions, 1 or 2 drops of blood are

inoculated directly into culture medium at the bedside. There are no transport media available, but blood can be collected and shipped at ambient temperature in tubes containing heparin, oxalate, or citrate (22). Survival of leptospires in commercial blood culture media for several days has been reported (46).

Urine can be cultured after the first week of illness. Specimens should be collected aseptically into sterile containers without preservatives and must be processed within a short time of collection; best results are obtained when the delay is less than 1 h.

ISOLATION PROCEDURES

Microscopic Demonstration

Leptospires in clinical material may be visualized by dark-field microscopy (×100 magnification) or by immunofluorescence or light microscopy after appropriate staining. Dark-field microscopic examination of body fluids such as blood, urine, CSF, or dialysate fluid is insensitive and lacks specificity (4, 66, 68). Approximately 10^4 leptospires/ml is necessary for one cell per field to be visible by dark-field microscopy (64). Direct dark-field microscopy of blood is also subject to misinterpretation of fibrin or protein threads, which may demonstrate Brownian motion (22, 64, 68). Leptospires in tissues were first visualized by silver staining (56), and the Warthin-Starry stain is widely used for histologic examination. More recently, immunohistochemical methods have been applied (65, 73, 74). Immunohistochemical staining can be performed at the Centers for

Disease Control and Prevention, Atlanta, Ga. (contact Sherif Zaki at szaki@cdc.gov).

Molecular Diagnosis

Several primer pairs for PCR detection of leptospires have been described, some based on specific gene targets such as 16S or 23S ribosomal genes or repetitive elements, while others have been constructed from genomic libraries (36). However, few have been shown to amplify leptospiral DNA from either human or veterinary clinical material, and only two methods have been subjected to extensive clinical evaluation (11, 43). Both methods were found to be more sensitive than culture, but one approach targeted a 331-bp fragment of the 16S RNA gene of both pathogenic and nonpathogenic leptospires (42), whereas the other approach requires the use of two primer pairs for detection of all pathogenic serovars (27, 28). By use of these two approaches, leptospiral DNA has been amplified from serum, urine, aqueous humor, CSF, and tissues obtained at autopsy.

A limitation of PCR-based diagnosis of leptospirosis is the inability of most PCR assays to identify the infecting serovar. While this is not significant for individual patient management, the identity of the serovar has both epidemiological and public health value.

Isolation of Leptospires

Leptospiremia occurs during the first stage of the disease, beginning before the onset of symptoms and usually finishing by the end of the first week of the acute illness (41). Therefore, blood cultures should be taken as soon as possible after the patient's presentation. One or 2 drops of blood (approximately 50 μl) are inoculated into 10 ml of semisolid oleic acid-albumin medium (19, 34), such as Ellinghausen-McCullough-Johnson-Harris (EMJH) medium (Difco Laboratories, Sparks, Md.) or PLM-5 (Intergen Co., Purchase, N.Y.), containing 0.1% agar and 200 μg of 5-fluorouracil per ml, at the patient's bedside. Care should be taken to avoid overinoculation of the medium, as blood contains inhibitors of leptospiral growth. For the greatest recovery rate, multiple cultures should be performed, but this is rarely possible. Inoculation of media with further 10-fold dilutions of blood samples may increase recovery (59). Survival of leptospires in commercial blood culture media for up to a week has been reported (46).

Other samples that may be cultured during the first week of illness include CSF and peritoneal dialysate. Urine cultures may yield growth from the beginning of the second week of symptomatic illness. Survival of leptospires in voided human urine is limited, so urine should be processed immediately, by neutralization of pH with sodium bicarbonate followed by centrifugation. After centrifugation in 15-ml tubes for 30 min at 1,500 × g, the sediment is resuspended in phosphate-buffered saline and inoculated into semisolid medium containing 5-fluorouracil as described above.

Cultures are incubated in sealed bottles at 28 to 30°C and examined weekly by dark-field microscopy for up to 13 weeks before being discarded. Growth often develops in a discrete band, several millimeters below the surface of the medium, known as a Dinger's ring. Cultures that show growth of other bacteria may be passed through a 0.2- or 0.45-μm pore-size filter before subculture into fresh medium.

Identification

Isolated leptospires are identified either by serological methods or, more recently, by molecular techniques. Traditional methods relied on cross-agglutinin absorption (16). The number of laboratories that can perform these identification methods is very small. The use of panels of monoclonal antibodies allows laboratories that can perform the MAT to identify isolates with relative rapidity (61). Monoclonal antibodies are available from the World Health Organization/Office International des Épizooties (WHO/OIE) Leptospirosis Reference Laboratory at the Royal Tropical Institute, Amsterdam, The Netherlands.

Because of the difficulties associated with serological identification of leptospiral isolates, there has been great interest in molecular methods for identification and subtyping (31, 61). Methods employed have included digestion of chromosomal DNA by restriction endonucleases, analysis of restriction fragment length polymorphisms, ribotyping, pulsed-field gel electrophoresis, and a number of PCR-based approaches (36).

SEROLOGICAL TESTS

Most cases of leptospirosis are diagnosed by serology. Antibodies are detectable in the blood approximately 5 to 7 days after the onset of symptoms. The definitive serologic investigation in leptospirosis remains the MAT, in which patients' sera are reacted with live or killed antigen suspensions of leptospiral serovars. After incubation, the serum-antigen mixtures are examined microscopically for agglutination and the titers are determined. The MAT is a complex test to control, perform, and interpret (63), the use of which is limited to regional or national reference laboratories. Protocols for performing the MAT have been described in detail elsewhere (2, 20, 59). The range of antigens used should include serovars representative of all serogroups (20, 63) and all locally common serovars (62). Titers of antibody to local isolates are often higher than titers of antibody to laboratory stock strains of serovars within the same serogroup. It is customary to include also one of the serovars of the nonpathogenic species *L. biflexa* (30, 60). The wide range of antigens is used in order to detect infections with uncommon, or previously undetected, serovars.

The test is read by dark-field microscopy. The end point is the highest dilution of serum in which 50% agglutination occurs. Because of the difficulty in detecting the titer at which 50% of the leptospires are agglutinated, the end point is determined by the presence of approximately 50% free, unagglutinated leptospires, by comparison with the control suspension (20). Considerable effort is required to reduce the subjective effect of observer variation, even within laboratories.

Interpretation of the MAT is complicated by the high degree of cross-reaction that occurs between different serogroups, especially in acute-phase samples. Paradoxical reactions, in which the highest titers detected are of antibody to a serogroup unrelated to the infecting one, are also common (36). The broad cross-reactivity in the acute phase, followed by relative serogroup specificity in convalescent-phase samples, results from the detection in the MAT of both immunoglobulin M (IgM) and IgG antibodies and the presence of several common antigens among leptospires (1, 13, 39).

Paired sera are required to confirm a diagnosis with certainty. A fourfold or greater rise in titer between paired sera confirms the diagnosis, regardless of the interval between samples. The interval between the first and second samples depends very much on the delay between the onset of symptoms and presentation of the patient. If symptoms typical of leptospirosis are present, an interval of 3 to 5 days may be adequate to detect rising titers. However, if the patient presents earlier in the course of the disease, or if the date of onset is not known precisely, then an interval of 10 to 14 days between samples is more appropriate. Less often, seroconversion does not occur with such rapidity, and a longer interval between samples (or repeated sampling) is necessary. MAT serology is insensitive, particularly in early-acute-phase specimens (5, 9, 14). Moreover, patients with fulminant leptospirosis may die before seroconversion occurs (11, 14, 50).

A presumptive diagnosis can be made by detection of a single elevated titer in association with an acute febrile illness. The magnitude of such a titer is dependent upon the background level of exposure in the population, and hence the seroprevalence. In the current Centers for Disease Control and Prevention case definition, a titer of ≥200 in a patient with a clinically compatible illness is used to indicate a probable case (12).

Titers following acute infection may be extremely high (≥25,600) and may take months, or even years, to fall to low levels (4, 8, 40, 51). Thus, in a high-incidence population, a low cutoff titer for presumptive diagnosis is inappropriate and will generate many false-positive diagnoses. In areas of endemicity, a single titer of ≥800 in symptomatic patients is generally indicative of leptospirosis (21), but titers as high as ≥1,600 have been recommended (2). Rarely, seroconversion may be delayed for many weeks after recovery, and longer serological follow-up will be necessary to confirm the diagnosis.

Formolized antigens have been used in the MAT in order to overcome some of the difficulties associated with the use of live antigens. Titers obtained with these antigens are somewhat lower, and more cross-reactions are detected (20, 45). Agglutination of formolized antigens is qualitatively different from that seen with live antigens (2). However, for laboratories without the staff or expertise to maintain live antigens, formolized and lyophilized antigens may represent a good alternative. These antigens are not available commercially but may be obtained from WHO Collaborating Centers.

The MAT is the most appropriate test to employ in epidemiological serosurveys, since it can be applied to sera from any animal species and because the range of antigens utilized can be expanded or decreased as required. It is usual to use a titer of ≥100 as evidence of past exposure (20). Contrary to a widely held belief, the MAT is a serogroup-specific assay. However, conclusions about infecting serovars cannot be drawn without isolates; at best, the MAT data can give a general impression of which serogroups are present within a population.

Because of the complexity of the MAT, rapid screening tests for leptospiral antibodies in acute infection have been developed. Several assays are available commercially. An indirect hemagglutination assay (IHA) (58) was shown to have a sensitivity of 92% and a specificity of 95% compared with the MAT (57). Recent estimates of sensitivity of the IHA (Focus Technologies, Cypress, Calif.) in populations in which leptospirosis is endemic have varied, due partly to differences in case ascertainment and study design (17, 38, 72). IgM antibodies become detectable during the first week of illness, allowing the diagnosis to be confirmed and treat-

ment to be initiated while it is likely to be most effective. IgM detection has repeatedly been shown to be more sensitive than the MAT when the first specimen is taken early in the acute phase of the illness (14, 50, 67). IgM dipstick assays (manufactured by PanBioINDX, Baltimore, Md., and Organon Teknika, Boxtel, The Netherlands) have been shown to be as sensitive as a microtiter plate IgM enzyme-linked immunosorbent assay (29, 37). Other rapid assays described recently include a latex agglutination assay (55) and a lateral-flow assay (54), both available outside the United States from Organon Teknika BV, Boxtel, The Netherlands. A microcapsule agglutination test using a synthetic polymer microcapsule in place of red blood cells (7, 53) was more sensitive than either the MAT or an IgM enzyme-linked immunosorbent assay with early-acute-phase samples (6) but failed to detect infections caused by some serovars (6, 52).

ANTIBIOTIC SUSCEPTIBILITIES

Leptospires are susceptible to many antimicrobial agents, including β-lactams, macrolides, tetracyclines, fluoroquinolones, and streptomycin (3, 22). Resistance to other aminoglycosides and to vancomycin has been reported (22). Problems in the determination of susceptibility include the long incubation time required (18), the use of media containing serum (44, 70), and the difficulty in quantifying growth accurately. These constraints have limited the development of rapid, standardized methods for susceptibility testing. Penicillin and doxycycline are both effective for treatment of leptospirosis and remain the drugs of choice (36).

EVALUATION, INTERPRETATION, AND REPORTING OF RESULTS

A diagnosis of leptospirosis can be made by isolation of the organism or amplification of leptospiral DNA from blood, urine, or other specimens; by demonstration of leptospires in tissues by immunohistochemical staining; or by detection of a fourfold or greater rise in titers between acute- and convalescent-phase serum samples tested by the same method at the same time. In populations and/or regions in which leptospirosis is not endemic, MAT titers of ≥200 in a single specimen obtained after the onset of symptoms are suggestive but not diagnostic of acute or recent leptospirosis. A titer of ≥800 in the presence of compatible symptoms is strong evidence of recent or current leptospirosis (20). Delayed seroconversions are common. Assays that detect IgM antibodies give presumptive evidence of recent exposure to leptospirosis but require confirmation, since IgM titers are persistent (15). Cross-reactive antibodies, sometimes with significant seroconversion, are associated with syphilis, relapsing fever, Lyme disease, and legionellosis. Negative test results in the presence of compatible symptoms do not rule out the diagnosis of leptospirosis, and further samples should be examined. The isolation of leptospires, the demonstration of leptospiral DNA by molecular methods, or the detection of leptospires in tissues by immunohistochemistry confirms the diagnosis and differentiates between current infection and past exposure, which may not be clearly differentiated by serology.

Despite recent advances in molecular detection and characterization of leptospires and in the development of rapid serologic tests, there are still few laboratories throughout the world with the appropriate capabilities for *Lepto-spira* diagnostics. WHO Collaborating Centers for Lepto-spirosis are located in Atlanta, Ga.; Amsterdam, The Netherlands; Hereford, United Kingdom; Paris, France; and Brisbane, Australia. Additional information regarding lep-tospirosis and diagnostic centers of expertise is available at the International Leptospirosis Society (ILS) website (http://www.med.monash.edu.au/microbiology/staff/adler/ilspage.htm) and through the ILS list server located there.

REFERENCES

1. **Adler, B., and S. Faine.** 1978. The antibodies involved in the human immune response to leptospiral infection. *J. Med. Microbiol.* **11:**387–400.
2. **Alexander, A. D.** 1986. Serological diagnosis of leptospi-rosis, p. 435–439. *In* N. R. Rose, H. Friedman, and J. L. Fahey (ed.), *Manual of Clinical Laboratory Immunology,* 3rd ed. American Society for Microbiology, Washington, D.C.
3. **Alexander, A. D., and P. L. Rule.** 1986. Penicillins, cephalosporins, and tetracyclines in treatment of hamsters with fatal leptospirosis. *Antimicrob. Agents Chemother.* **30:**835–839.
4. **Alston, J. M., and J. C. Broom.** 1958. *Leptospirosis in Man and Animals.* E. & S. Livingstone, Edinburgh, Scotland.
5. **Appassakij, H., K. Silpapojakul, R. Wansit, and J. Woodtayakorn.** 1995. Evaluation of the immunofluores-cent antibody test for the diagnosis of human leptospirosis. *Am. J. Trop. Med. Hyg.* **52:**340–343.
6. **Arimitsu, Y., E. Kmety, Y. Ananyina, G. Baranton, I. R. Ferguson, L. Smythe, and W. J. Terpstra.** 1994. Evalua-tion of the one-point microcapsule agglutination test for diagnosis of leptospirosis. *Bull. W. H. O.* **72:**395–399.
7. **Arimitsu, Y., S. Kobayashi, K. Akama, and T. Matuhasi.** 1982. Development of a simple serological method for diagnosing leptospirosis: a microcapsule agglutination test. *J. Clin. Microbiol.* **15:**835–841.
8. **Blackmore, D. K., L. M. Schollum, and K. M. Moriarty.** 1984. The magnitude and duration of titres of leptospiral agglutinins in human sera. *N. Z. Med. J.* **97:**83–86.
9. **Brandão, A. P., E. D. Camargo, E. D. da Silva, M. V. Silva, and R. V. Abrão.** 1998. Macroscopic agglutination test for rapid diagnosis of human leptospirosis. *J. Clin. Microbiol.* **36:**3138–3142.
10. **Brenner, D. J., A. F. Kaufmann, K. R. Sulzer, A. G. Steigerwalt, F. C. Rogers, and R. S. Weyant.** 1999. Further determination of DNA relatedness between sero-groups and serovars in the family *Leptospiraceae* with a proposal for *Leptospira alexanderi* sp. nov. and four new *Leptospira* genomospecies. *Int. J. Syst. Bacteriol.* **49:**839–858.
11. **Brown, P. D., C. Gravekamp, D. G. Carrington, H. Van de Kemp, R. A. Hartskeerl, C. N. Edwards, C. O. R. Everard, W. J. Terpstra, and P. N. Levett.** 1995. Evalu-ation of the polymerase chain reaction for early diagnosis of leptospirosis. *J. Med. Microbiol.* **43:**110–114.
12. **Centers for Disease Control and Prevention.** 1997. Case definitions for infectious conditions under public health surveillance. *Morb. Mortal. Wkly. Rep.* **46** (RR-10):49.
13. **Chapman, A. J., B. Adler, and S. Faine.** 1987. Genus-specific antigens in *Leptospira* revealed by immunoblotting. *Zentbl. Bakteriol.* **264:**279–283.
14. **Cumberland, P. C., C. O. R. Everard, and P. N. Levett.** 1999. Assessment of the efficacy of the IgM enzyme-linked immunosorbent assay (ELISA) and microscopic agglutina-tion test (MAT) in the diagnosis of acute leptospirosis. *Am. J. Trop. Med. Hyg.* **61:**731–734.
15. **Cumberland, P. C., C. O. R. Everard, J. G. Wheeler, and P. N. Levett.** 2001. Persistence of anti-leptospiral IgM,

16. **Dikken, H., and E. Kmety.** 1978. Serological typing methods of leptospires. *Methods Microbiol.* **11:**259–307.
17. **Effler, P. V., H. Y. Domen, S. L. Bragg, T. Aye, and D. M. Sasaki.** 2000. Evaluation of the indirect hemagglu-tination assay for diagnosis of acute leptospirosis in Ha-waii. *J. Clin. Microbiol.* **38:**1081–1084.
18. **Ellinghausen, H. C.** 1983. Growth, cultural characteris-tics, and antibacterial sensitivity of *Leptospira interrogans* serovar *hardjo. Cornell Vet.* **73:**225–239.
19. **Ellinghausen, H. C., and W. G. McCullough.** 1965. Nutrition of *Leptospira pomona* and growth of 13 other serotypes: fractionation of oleic albumin complex and a medium of bovine albumin and polysorbate 80. *Am. J. Vet. Res.* **26:**45–51.
20. **Faine, S.** 1982. *Guidelines for the Control of Leptospirosis.* World Health Organization, Geneva, Switzerland.
21. **Faine, S.** 1988. Leptospirosis, p. 344–352. *In* A. Balows, W. J. Hausler, M. Ohashi, and A. Turano (ed.), *Laboratory Diagnosis of Infectious Diseases. Principles and Practice,* vol. 1. Springer-Verlag, New York, N.Y.
22. **Faine, S., B. Adler, C. Bolin, and P. Perolat.** 1999. *Leptospira* and *Leptospirosis,* 2nd ed. MedSci, Melbourne, Australia.
23. **Faine, S., and N. D. Stallman.** 1982. Amended descrip-tions of the genus *Leptospira* Noguchi 1917 and the species *L. interrogans* (Stimson 1907) Wenyon 1926 and *L. biflexa* (Wolbach and Binger 1914) Noguchi 1918. *Int. J. Syst. Bacteriol.* **32:**461–463.
24. **Feresu, S. B., C. A. Bolin, H. van de Kemp, and H. Korver.** 1999. Identification of a serogroup Bataviae *Lep-tospira* strain isolated from an ox in Zimbabwe. *Zentbl. Bakteriol.* **289:**19–29.
25. **Garrity, G. M., and J. G. Holt.** 2001. The road map to the Manual, p. 119–166. *In* D. R. Boone, R. W. Castenholz, and G. M. Garrity (ed.), *Bergey's Manual of Systematic Bacteriology,* 2nd ed., vol. 1. Springer-Verlag, New York, N.Y.
26. **Goldstein, S. F., and N. W. Charon.** 1988. Motility of the spirochete *Leptospira. Cell Motility Cytoskeleton* **9:**101–110.
27. **Gravekamp, C., H. van de Kemp, D. Carrington, G. J. J. M. van Eys, C. O. R. Everard, and W. J. Terpstra.** 1991. Detection of leptospiral DNA by PCR in serum from patients with *copenhageni* infections, p. 151–164. *In* Y. Kobayashi (ed.), *Leptospirosis. Proceedings of the Leptospirosis Research Conference 1990.* University of To-kyo Press, Tokyo, Japan.
28. **Gravekamp, C., H. van de Kemp, M. Franzen, D. Car-rington, G. J. Schoone, G. J. J. M. van Eys, C. O. R. Everard, R. A. Hartskeerl, and W. J. Terpstra.** 1993. Detection of seven species of pathogenic leptospires by PCR using two sets of primers. *J. Gen. Microbiol.* **139:**1691–1700.
29. **Gussenhoven, G. C., M. A. W. G. van der Hoorn, M. G. A. Goris, W. J. Terpstra, R. A. Hartskeerl, B. W. Mol, C. W. van Ingen, and H. L. Smits.** 1997. LEPTO dipstick, a dipstick assay for detection of *Leptospira*-specific immunoglobulin M antibodies in human sera. *J. Clin. Microbiol.* **35:**92–97.
30. **Hergt, R.** 1976. Meaning of serotype Patoc (biflexa com-plex) for the diagnosis of leptospirosis by microscopic agglutination test. *Zentbl. Bakteriol.* **235:**506–511.
31. **Herrmann, J. L.** 1993. Genomic techniques for identifi-cation of *Leptospira* strains. *Pathol. Biol.* **41:**943–950.

32. **International Committee on Systematic Bacteriology Subcommittee on the Taxonomy of *Leptospira*.** 1987. Minutes of the meeting, 5 and 6 September 1986, Manchester, England. *Int. J. Syst. Bacteriol.* **37:**472–473.

33. **Johnson, R. C., and S. Faine.** 1984. *Leptospira*, p. 62–67. In N. R. Krieg and J. G. Holt (ed.), *Bergey's Manual of Systematic Bacteriology*, vol. 1. Williams & Wilkins, Baltimore, Md.

34. **Johnson, R. C., and V. G. Harris.** 1967. Differentiation of pathogenic and saprophytic leptospires. 1. Growth at low temperatures. *J. Bacteriol.* **94:**27–31.

35. **Kmety, E., and H. Dikken.** 1993. Classification of the species *Leptospira interrogans* and history of its serovars. University Press Groningen, Groningen, The Netherlands.

36. **Levett, P. N.** 2001. Leptospirosis. *Clin. Microbiol. Rev.* **14:**296–326.

37. **Levett, P. N., S. L. Branch, C. U. Whittington, C. N. Edwards, and H. Paxton.** 2001. Two methods for rapid serological diagnosis of acute leptospirosis. *Clin. Diagn. Lab. Immunol.* **8:**349–351.

38. **Levett, P. N., and C. U. Whittington.** 1998. Evaluation of the indirect hemagglutination assay for diagnosis of acute leptospirosis. *J. Clin. Microbiol.* **36:**11–14.

39. **Lin, M., O. Surujballi, K. Nielsen, S. Nadin-Davis, and G. Randall.** 1997. Identification of a 35-kilodalton serovar-cross-reactive flagellar protein, FlaB, from *Leptospira interrogans* by N-terminal sequencing, gene cloning, and sequence analysis. *Infect. Immun.* **65:**4355–4359.

40. **Lupidi, R., M. Cinco, D. Balanzin, E. Delprete, and P. E. Varaldo.** 1991. Serological follow-up of patients in a localized outbreak of leptospirosis. *J. Clin. Microbiol.* **29:**805–809.

41. **McCrumb, F. R., J. L. Stockard, C. R. Robinson, L. H. Turner, D. G. Levis, C. W. Maisey, M. F. Kelleher, C. A. Gleiser, and J. E. Smadel.** 1957. Leptospirosis in Malaya. I. Sporadic cases among military and civilian personnel. *Am. J. Trop. Med. Hyg.* **6:**238–256.

42. **Merien, F., P. Amouriaux, P. Pérolat, G. Baranton, and I. Saint Girons.** 1992. Polymerase chain reaction for detection of *Leptospira* spp. in clinical samples. *J. Clin. Microbiol.* **30:**2219–2224.

43. **Merien, F., G. Baranton, and P. Pérolat.** 1995. Comparison of polymerase chain reaction with microagglutination test and culture for diagnosis of leptospirosis. *J. Infect. Dis.* **172:**281–285.

44. **Oie, S., K. Hironaga, A. Koshiro, H. Konishi, and Z. Yoshii.** 1983. In vitro susceptibilities of five *Leptospira* strains to 16 antimicrobial agents. *Antimicrob. Agents Chemother.* **24:**905–908.

45. **Palmer, M. F., S. A. Waitkins, and S. W. Wanyangu.** 1987. A comparison of live and formalised leptospiral microscopic agglutination test. *Zentbl. Bakteriol.* **265:**151–159.

46. **Palmer, M. F., and W. J. Zochowski.** 2000. Survival of leptospires in commercial blood culture systems revisited. *J. Clin. Pathol.* **53:**713–714.

47. **Pérolat, P., R. J. Chappel, B. Adler, G. Baranton, D. M. Bulach, M. L. Billinghurst, M. Letocart, F. Merien, and M. S. Serrano.** 1998. *Leptospira fainei* sp. nov., isolated from pigs in Australia. *Int. J. Syst. Bacteriol.* **48:**851–858.

48. **Ramadass, P., B. D. W. Jarvis, R. J. Corner, M. Cinco, and R. B. Marshall.** 1990. DNA relatedness among strains of *Leptospira biflexa*. *Int. J. Syst. Bacteriol.* **40:**231–235.

49. **Ramadass, P., B. D. W. Jarvis, R. J. Corner, D. Penny, and R. B. Marshall.** 1992. Genetic characterization of pathogenic *Leptospira* species by DNA hybridization. *Int. J. Syst. Bacteriol.* **42:**215–219.

50. **Ribeiro, M. A., C. S. N. Assis, and E. C. Romero.** 1994. Serodiagnosis of human leptospirosis employing immunodominant antigen. *Serodiagn. Immunother. Infect. Dis.* **6:**140–144.

51. **Romero, E. C., C. R. Caly, and P. H. Yasuda.** 1998. The persistence of leptospiral agglutinin titers in human sera diagnosed by the microscopic agglutination test. *Rev. Inst. Med. Trop. Sao Paulo* **40:**183–184.

52. **Sehgal, S. C., P. Vijayachari, and V. Subramaniam.** 1997. Evaluation of leptospira micro capsule agglutination test (MCAT) for serodiagnosis of leptospirosis. *Indian J. Med. Res.* **106:**504–507.

53. **Seki, M., T. Sato, Y. Aritmitsu, T. Matuhasi, and S. Kobayashi.** 1987. One-point method for serological diagnosis of leptospirosis: a microcapsule agglutination test. *Epidemiol. Infect.* **99:**399–405.

54. **Smits, H. L., C. K. Eapen, S. Sugathan, M. Kuriakose, M. H. Gasem, C. Yersin, D. Sasaki, B. Pujianto, M. Vestering, T. H. Abdoel, and G. C. Gussenhoven.** 2001. Lateral-flow assay for rapid serodiagnosis of human leptospirosis. *Clin. Diagn. Lab. Immunol.* **8:**166–169.

55. **Smits, H. L., M. A. van Der Hoorn, M. G. Goris, G. C. Gussenhoven, C. Yersin, D. M. Sasaki, W. J. Terpstra, and R. A. Hartskeerl.** 2000. Simple latex agglutination assay for rapid serodiagnosis of human leptospirosis. *J. Clin. Microbiol.* **38:**1272–1275.

56. **Stimson, A. M.** 1907. Note on an organism found in yellow-fever tissue. *Public Health Rep.* **22:**541.

57. **Sulzer, C. R., J. W. Glosser, F. Rogers, W. L. Jones, and M. Frix.** 1975. Evaluation of an indirect hemagglutination test for the diagnosis of human leptospirosis. *J. Clin. Microbiol.* **2:**218–221.

58. **Sulzer, C. R., and W. L. Jones.** 1973. Evaluation of a hemagglutination test for human leptospirosis. *Appl. Microbiol.* **26:**655–657.

59. **Sulzer, C. R., and W. L. Jones.** 1978. *Leptospirosis: Methods in Laboratory Diagnosis*. U.S. Department of Health, Education and Welfare, Atlanta, Ga.

60. **Tan, D. S. K., and Q. B. Welch.** 1974. Evaluation of *Leptospira biflexa* antigens for screening human sera by the microscopic agglutination (MA) test in comparison with the sensitized-erythrocyte-lysis (SEL) test. *Southeast Asian J. Trop. Med. Public Health* **5:**12–16.

61. **Terpstra, W. J.** 1992. Typing leptospira from the perspective of a reference laboratory. *Acta Leiden.* **60:**79–87.

62. **Torten, M.** 1979. Leptospirosis, p. 363–420. In H. E. Stoenner, M. Torten, and W. Kaplan (ed.), *CRC Handbook Series in Zoonoses. Section A: Bacterial, Rickettsial and Mycotic Diseases*, vol. I. CRC Press, Boca Raton, Fla.

63. **Turner, L. H.** 1968. Leptospirosis. II. Serology. *Trans. R. Soc. Trop. Med. Hyg.* **62:**880–889.

64. **Turner, L. H.** 1970. Leptospirosis. III. Maintenance, isolation and demonstration of leptospires. *Trans. R. Soc. Trop. Med. Hyg.* **64:**623–646.

65. **Uip, D. E., V. Amato Neto, and M. S. Duarte.** 1992. Diagnóstico precoce da leptospirose por demonstração de antígenos através de exame imuno-histoquímino em músculo da panturrilha. *Rev. Inst. Med. Trop. Sao Paulo* **34:**375–381.

66. **Vijayachari, P., A. P. Sugunan, T. Umapathi, and S. C. Sehgal.** 2001. Evaluation of darkground microscopy as a rapid diagnostic procedure in leptospirosis. *Indian J. Med. Res.* **114:**54–58.

67. **Winslow, W. E., D. J. Merry, M. L. Pirc, and P. L. Devine.** 1997. Evaluation of a commercial enzyme-linked immunosorbent assay for detection of immunoglobulin M antibody in diagnosis of human leptospiral infection. *J. Clin. Microbiol.* **35:**1938–1942.

68. **Wolff, J. W.** 1954. The laboratory diagnosis of leptospirosis. C. C. Thomas, Springfield, Ill.
69. **World Health Organization.** 1999. Leptospirosis worldwide, 1999. *Wkly. Epidemiol. Rec.* **74:**237–242.
70. **Wylie, J. A. H., and E. Vincent.** 1947. The sensitivity of organisms of the genus *Leptospira* to penicillin and streptomycin. *J. Pathol. Bacteriol.* **59:**247–254.
71. **Yasuda, P. H., A. G. Steigerwalt, K. R. Sulzer, A. F. Kaufmann, F. Rogers, and D. J. Brenner.** 1987. Deoxyribonucleic acid relatedness between serogroups and serovars in the family *Leptospiraceae* with proposals for seven new *Leptospira* species. *Int. J. Syst. Bacteriol.* **37:**407–415.
72. **Yersin, C., P. Bovet, H. L. Smits, and P. Perolat.** 1999. Field evaluation of a one-step dipstick assay for the diagnosis of human leptospirosis in the Seychelles. *Trop. Med. Int. Health* **4:**38–45.
73. **Zaki, S. R., W.-J. Shieh, and the Epidemic Working Group.** 1996. Leptospirosis associated with outbreak of acute febrile illness and pulmonary haemorrhage, Nicaragua, 1995. *Lancet* **347:**535.
74. **Zaki, S. R., and R. A. Spiegel.** 1998. Leptospirosis, p. 73–92. *In* A. M. Nelson and C. R. Horsburgh (ed.), *Pathology of Emerging Infections 2.* American Society for Microbiology, Washington, D.C.

*Borrelia**

BETTINA WILSKE AND MARTIN E. SCHRIEFER

60

TAXONOMY

Bacteria of the genus *Borrelia* belong to the order *Spirochaetales,* which encompasses the families *Spirochaetaceae* and *Leptospiraceae* (114). *Borrelia* and *Treponema* are the two genera of the family *Spirochaetaceae* that cause human disease. The type species of the genus *Borrelia* is *Borrelia anserina,* which causes borreliosis in birds. On the basis of 16S rRNA sequence analyses, spirochetes form a distinct entity (division D) within the eubacterial kingdom. They are neither gram-positive nor gram-negative organisms. In the case of the spirochetes, the morphological criteria agree with the phylogenetic relationship, a rare trait in other bacterial groups.

DESCRIPTION OF THE GENUS

Common Characteristics

Borreliae are similar in length (8 to 30 μm) but wider (0.2 to 0.5 μm) than the two other human-pathogenic spirochetes, the treponemes and the leptospires (Fig. 1) (10). They are highly motile organisms with corkscrew and oscillating motilities (corresponding to the helical and the flat-wave forms of the organisms, respectively). In contrast to the exoflagella of other bacteria, the flagella of borreliae, as well as those from all other spirochetes, are endoflagella. The endoflagella (7 to 20 per terminus) are localized beneath the outer membrane and insert subterminally at both ends of the protoplasmic cylinder (63). The protoplasmic cylinder consists of a peptidoglycan layer and an inner membrane which encloses the internal components of the cell. In contrast to the treponemes, microtubules have not been detected in borreliae and their flagella are unsheathed (10). If cultivable, borreliae grow slowly under microaerophilic (7) or anaerobic (81) conditions. They require *N*-acetylglucosamine and long-chain saturated and unsaturated fatty acids and produce lactic acid through glucose fermentation (52).

The Genome

The genome of the borreliae is composed of a linear chromosome, which is unusual among bacteria, and both linear and circular plasmids. First described for *B. burgdorferi* and subsequently for several relapsing fever borreliae and *B. anserina,* the linear chromosome of borreliae is rather small, with a size of approximately 1,000 kb. Also atypical of most bacteria, borreliae have a low G+C content of approximately 30 mol%.

The complete nucleotide sequences of the chromosome and 11 plasmids have been published for the type strain *B. burgdorferi* B31 (35). A total of 59% of the chromosomal open reading frames (ORFs) have homologs in other bacterial species; in contrast, homologs have been identified for only one-third of the plasmid ORFs. The genome encodes a basic set of proteins for DNA replication, transcription, and energy metabolism but, interestingly, does not encode proteins for most cellular biosynthetic pathways. The low metabolic capacity and the identification of homologs for 16 different membrane transporters indicate that *B. burgdorferi* acquires many essential components from its environment. Of some surprise is the tremendous number (>100) of genes that encode lipoproteins, suggesting an essential role of these molecules in the life cycle of the spirochete.

Linear plasmids were first observed in *B. hermsii* (73) and were subsequently found in *B. burgdorferi* (9). The linear plasmids of *B. hermsii* contain genes encoding outer membrane lipoproteins, called variable major proteins (VMPs). These genes are silent except when they are translocated to an expression site immediately adjacent to one of the linear plasmid telomeres. This mechanism of antigenic variation closely resembles that of the African trypanosome, the causative agent of sleeping sickness. Antigenic variation due to recombination of VMP-like sequence cassettes has also been described for *B. burgdorferi.* These genes are called *vls* genes, and besides highly variable regions, they also have highly conserved sequences which encode immunogenic epitopes (64, 117). The latter finding may be of utility in the development of improved serodiagnostic tests (64).

The human-pathogenic species of *B. burgdorferi* contain a large linear plasmid of 50 to 57 kb. This plasmid encodes two major outer surface proteins, OspA and OspB, which

---

* This chapter contains information presented in chapter 53 by Tom G. Schwan, Willy Burgdorfer, and Patricia A. Rosa in the seventh edition of this Manual.

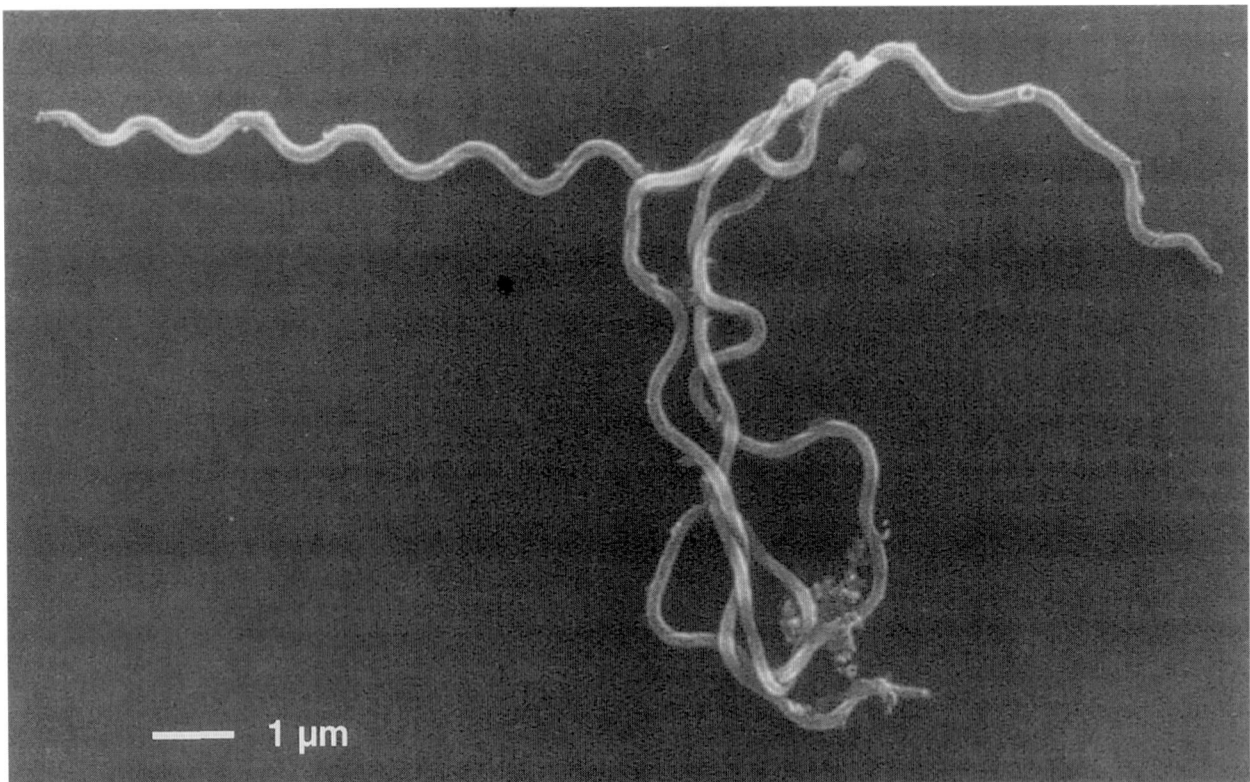

FIGURE 1   *B. burgdorferi* seen by scanning electron microscopy (provided by Gerhard Wanner, Munich, Germany).

are tandemly arrayed in one operon (14, 44). The first gene detected on a circular plasmid was the gene encoding OspC, another major outer surface protein of *B. burgdorferi* (36, 68, 86, 110). Sequence analysis of the *ospC* genes from different strains suggested that gene exchange might play a role in the diversity of Lyme disease borreliae (49, 65).

Species Diversity

Classification of *B. burgdorferi* has been studied in more detail than that of the other species of the genus *Borrelia*. Shortly after detection of the causative agent of Lyme borreliosis by Burgdorfer et al. in the early 1980s (18) it was named *B. burgdorferi* (54). Recent examination of the genotypic and phenotypic characteristics of numerous strains from different geographic and biologic sources indicated that more than one species of *Borrelia* were causative agents of Lyme borreliosis (11, 67, 111). Studies published since 1992 have divided *B. burgdorferi* sensu lato into three human-pathogenic species: *B. burgdorferi* sensu stricto, *B. afzelii*, and *B. garinii* (6, 19). Seven other species of *B. burgdorferi* sensu lato have recently been described (Table 1) (100), and of these, only *B. valaisiana* appears to have human-pathogenic potential (83). Other, uncharacterized species of *B. burgdorferi* sensu lato may play a role in Lyme borreliosis (99). In North America, *B. burgdorferi* sensu stricto is the only human-pathogenic species, whereas all three species have been isolated from humans in Europe. There is a strong prevalence of *B. afzelii* among human skin isolates from Europe, whereas isolates from cerebrospinal fluid (CSF) are most commonly *B. garinii* (Table 2) (19, 31, 109). Recently, more extended studies (using *ospA* PCR)

have shown that the strains causing Lyme arthritis are also heterogeneous (Table 2) (30, 98) and not primarily limited to *B. burgdorferi* sensu stricto, as previously assumed. The classification of other borreliae has not been studied in the same detail as *B. burgdorferi* sensu lato.

A scheme for species identification based on vector specificity was initially proposed for relapsing fever borreliae (i.e., *B. turicatae*, *B. parkeri*, and *B. hermsii* are transmitted by the ticks *Ornithodoros turicata*, *Ornithodoros parkeri*, and *Ornithodoros hermsi*, respectively). Because of the extreme dependence of these ticks on their hosts, the entire life cycle is often completed within the nesting confines of a single host and humans are rarely exposed to the vector-tick. Despite these restrictive relationships, the DNA-DNA similarity between relapsing fever species is greater than 70%. This value, a maximal level proposed for species discrimination, has prompted suggestions that these spirochetes may represent a single species. The species status of other cultivable borreliae, such as *B. anserina*, *B. crocidurae*, *B. recurrentis*, and *B. coriaceae*, has been supported by findings of greater DNA-DNA dissimilarity (23, 52).

NATURAL HABITATS

The life cycle of the borreliae is dependent on ecosystems that support a habitat suitable for competent arthropod vectors and vertebrate reservoir hosts. The ecological components that maintain *Borrelia* species in nature are quite diverse and are spread throughout the world (Table 1).

TABLE 1 Characteristics of arthropod-borne borreliae[a]

Borrelia spp.	Arthropod vector	Animal reservoir	Geographic distribution	Disease
B. recurrentis	Pediculus humanus humanus	Humans	Worldwide	Louse-borne (epidemic) relapsing fever
B. duttonii	O. moubata	Humans	Central, eastern, and southern Africa	Tick-borne (endemic) relapsing fever
B. hispanica	O. erraticus	Rodents	Spain, Portugal, Morocco, Algeria, Tunisia	Hispano-African tick-borne relapsing fever
B. crocidurae, B. merionesi, B. microti, B. dipodilli	O. erraticus	Rodents	Morocco, Libya, Egypt, Turkey, Senegal, Kenya	North African tick-borne relapsing fever
B. persica	O. tholozani	Rodents	Western China, Kashmir, Iraq, Egypt, former USSR, India	Asiatic-African tick-borne relapsing fever
B. caucasica	O. verrucosus	Rodents	Caucasus to Iraq	Caucasian tick-borne relapsing fever
B. hermsii	O. hermsi	Rodents	Western United States	American tick-borne relapsing fever
B. turicatae	O. turicata	Rodents	Southwestern United States	American tick-borne relapsing fever
B. parkeri	O. parkeri	Rodents	Western United States	American tick-borne relapsing fever
B. mazzottii	O. talajae	Rodents	Southern United States, Mexico, Central and South America	American tick-borne relapsing fever
B. venezuelensis	O. rudis (syn. O. venezulensis)	Rodents	Central and South America	American tick-borne relapsing fever
B. burgdorferi	Ixodes scapularis	Rodents	Eastern and midwestern United States	Lyme borreliosis
	I. pacificus	Rodents	Western United States	Lyme borreliosis
	I. ricinus	Rodents	Europe	Lyme borreliosis
B. garinii	I. ricinus, I. persulcatus	Rodents	Europe, Asia	Lyme borreliosis
	I. uriae	Seabirds	Bipolar	?
B. afzelii	I. ricinus, I. persulcatus	Rodents	Europe, Asia	Lyme borreliosis
B. japonica	I. ovatus	Rodents	Japan	?
B. andersonii	I. dentatus	Rabbits	United States	?
B. bissetii	I. scapularis, I. pacificus	Rodents	United States	?
B. tanukii	I. tanukii, I. ovatus	Rodents	Japan	?
B. turdae	I. turdus	?	Japan	?
B. valaisiana	I. ricinus	?	Europe, Asia	?
B. lusitaniae	I. ricinus	?	Europe, North Africa	?
B. lonestarii	Amblyoma americanum	?	United States	One reported human case (48)
B. miyamotoi	I. persulcatus	Rodents	Japan	?
B. theileri	Rhipicephalus spp. Boophilus spp.	Cattle, horses, sheep	South Africa, Australia, North America, Europe	Bovine borreliosis
B. coriaceae	O. coriaceus	Deer?	Western United States	Epizootic bovine abortion?
B. anserina	Argas spp.	Fowl	Worldwide	Avian borreliosis

[a] Borreliae are grouped into three groups: relapsing fever borreliae, B. burgdorferi sensu lato, and others. The table is modified from reference 89.

Relapsing Fever Borreliae

Most relapsing fever borreliae are transmitted by soft ticks of the genus *Ornithodoros* (Fig. 2a). The exception is *B. recurrentis*, which is vectored by the body louse (*Pediculus humanus humanus*). Infection in this human-specific ectoparasite is limited to the hemolymph, and spirochetes are not passed transovarially to louse progeny. Thus, humans serve as the sole reservoir of *B. recurrentis*. *B. duttonii* is vectored by the soft tick *Ornithodoros moubata* and, as is the case for *B. recurrentis*, humans serve as the only known reservoir. Notably, these human-adapted borreliae are very closely related genetically (23). The remaining relapsing fever *Borrelia* species are transmitted by ticks of other *Ornithodoros* species and have wild animal reservoirs, mostly rodents (Table 1). The soft ticks feed rapidly, within 10 to 45 min, and mostly at night. All developmental stages of these ticks prefer to feed on a single species of mammal, and humans are rare and circumstantial hosts.

TABLE 2 Distribution of species of B. burgdorferi sensu lato as well as of OspA types in European isolates from ticks, CSF, skin, and synovial fluid specimens[a]

Species	OspA type	% Distribution			
		Ticks ($n = 90$)	CSF ($n = 43$)	Skin ($n = 68$)	Synovial fluid[b] ($n = 20$)
B. burgdorferi sensu stricto	1	20	19	6	33
B. afzelii	2	9	12	84	29
B. garinii[c]	3–7	71	69	10	38

[a] The data presented in this table are from previous reports (30, 98, 105).

[b] Identification of organisms from synovial fluid samples as B. burgdorferi sensu lato is based on the results of ospA PCR. Too few isolates could be recovered by culture to estimate the species distribution.

[c] Tick and CSF isolates differ in the percentage of OspA types 4 and 6. OspA type 6 is found in 53% of the tick isolates but only 23% of the CSF isolates. In contrast, OspA type 4 was found in 28% of the CSF isolates but was not isolated from ticks.

B. burgdorferi sensu lato

The Lyme disease borreliae of B. burgdorferi sensu lato are transmitted by hard ticks (genus Ixodes) (Fig. 2b). In contrast to Ornithodoros, Ixodes species feed on three different hosts, depending on the developmental stage of the tick (93). The larvae and nymphs feed primarily on small rodents, whereas adult ticks feed on a variety of mammals (deer, raccoons, domestic and wild carnivores, larger domestic animals, and birds). The feeding period of Ixodes species ticks is rather long (several days to over a week) and contributes to their geographic dispersal along with the movement of the host. Birds, particularly migratory seabirds, can transport the ticks (Ixodes uriae) over very long distances and thus distribute borreliae (especially B. garinii) worldwide (70). There appears to be an association between certain B. burgdorferi sensu lato species and certain vertebrate hosts, e.g., B. afzelii and small rodents and B. garinii and birds, possibly due to different serum sensitivities of the borreliae (45, 60). In unfed ticks, B. burgdorferi sensu lato lives in the midgut. During the blood meal on humans or mice, molecular changes (e.g., a switch from OspA to OspC expression) are induced in the borreliae that lead to their migration to the salivary glands (34, 91). This migration process takes >36 h in Ixodes scapularis (24). In Ixodes

ricinus, however, spirochete migration within the tick and transmission to the mammalian host have been observed with ticks feeding for as few as 17 h (56). Therefore, differences may exist between the transmission times for different species of ticks and/or borreliae.

CLINICAL SIGNIFICANCE

Relapsing Fever

Relapsing fever is an infectious disease with an acute onset of clinical signs and symptoms including high fever, shaking chills, severe headache, nausea, myalgias, and severe malaise. Initial physical findings often are conjunctival effusion, petechiae, and diffuse abdominal tenderness. Fever attacks of 3 to 7 days are interspersed with afebrile periods of days to weeks. More detailed descriptions of louse-borne relapsing fever (17) and tick-borne relapsing fever in North America (29) and a general overview have been published elsewhere (94).

Louse-borne relapsing fever is, in general, more severe than tick-borne relapsing fever, but the number of febrile attacks is often fewer. In tick-borne relapsing fever, up to 13 febrile attacks have been reported, and a rash is more often

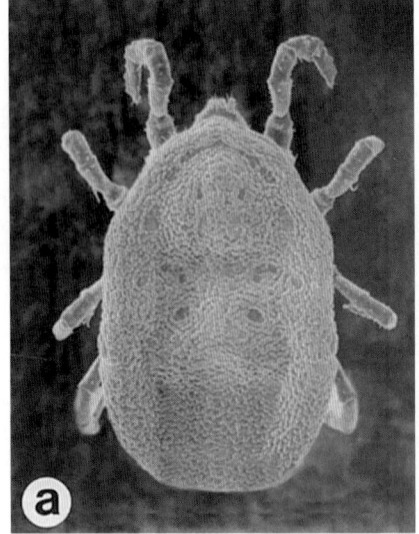
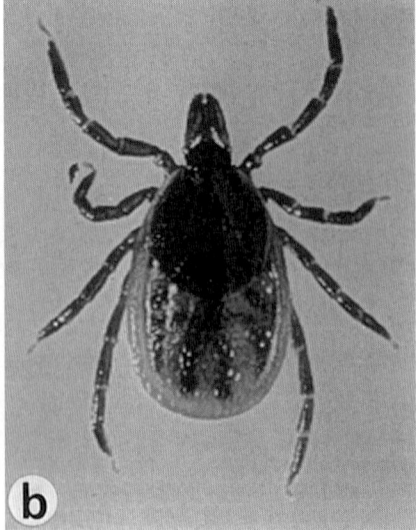

FIGURE 2 Two genera of ticks are vectors for relapsing fever and Lyme borreliosis: Ornithodoros (a) and Ixodes (b).

reported in tick-borne relapsing fever than in louse-borne relapsing fever (28 versus 8%). Splenomegaly, hepatomegaly, and jaundice are observed in 77, 66, and 36% of patients with louse-borne relapsing fever, respectively, whereas these signs are reported in only 41, 17, and 7% of patients with tick-borne relapsing fever, respectively. In louse-borne relapsing fever, 34% of the patients have respiratory symptoms and 30% have central nervous system involvement, but only 16% of the patients with tick-borne relapsing fever present with respiratory symptoms and only 9% present with central nervous system involvement (55, 94). Complications leading to death (mortality rates of up to 40% among patients with louse-borne relapsing fever) are acute heart and hepatic failure, cerebral hemorrhage, and other compromises (poor nutrition and coinfection with other diseases) common in many areas of endemicity. During pregnancy, relapsing fever (especially that caused by *B. recurrentis*) may also lead to congenital infection and fetal death.

Lyme Borreliosis

Lyme borreliosis can be defined by early localized, early disseminated, and late-stage manifestations similar to the three stages of syphilis (95). The natural course of untreated *B. burgdorferi* infections varies considerably, and clinical manifestations can occur alone or in various combinations (71, 95, 102). In the majority of cases the infection is self-limiting, but in rare cases, *B. burgdorferi* may persist, even after antibiotic treatment (79).

Erythema migrans (EM) at the site of the infectious tick bite is the most common manifestation of early (stage I) Lyme borreliosis and occurs in 60 to 90% of patients. The center of the expanding annular lesion often fades to produce a bull's-eye appearance. However, the extension, color intensity, and duration of EM vary considerably; and alternate rash etiologies must be ruled out. General symptoms such as fever, myalgia, headache, and, rarely, meningismus may accompany the primary EM lesion. In untreated patients, EM typically resolves within 3 to 4 weeks.

In some patients, hematogenous dissemination of spirochetes to other organs and tissues occurs within days to weeks of infection. During this early stage (stage II), patients often feel quite ill and may present with fatigue, headache, fever, malaise, arthralgia, and myalgia. Multiple (secondary) areas of erythema are common among patients in the United States but are uncommon in Europe. Neurologic structures, including the meninges, brain, spinal cord, peripheral nerves, and nerve roots, are also potential sites of disseminated, early infection. Fifteen to 20% of untreated patients in the United States develop neurologic involvement, most commonly facial nerve palsy (unilateral or bilateral), meningitis, and radiculoneuropathy. CSF findings in cases of Lyme meningitis almost always include a mononuclear pleocytosis (10 to 1,000 cells/μl), elevated protein concentrations, and normal glucose levels. Meningitis or even facial palsy without meningismus is more common among children than adults. Severe encephalitis is occasionally observed in stage II. Borrelial lymphocytoma, a reddish to livid swelling of the skin in typical locations such as the earlobe, mamilla, or scrotum, is manifested among some patients in Europe. Bannwarth's syndrome, first described in Germany in 1944, is the most common neurologic manifestation of early, disseminated Lyme borreliosis in Europe. The syndrome is characterized initially by intense, migratory, or focal radicular pain, particularly at night, and by cranial nerve palsy. Pareses of the extremities

and the trunk are less frequent. Further clinical manifestations of stage II may include Lyme carditis, dysrhythmia with atrioventricular conduction blocks, and ophthalmoborreliosis.

Lyme arthritis and acrodermatitis chronica atrophicans (ACA), which occur months to years after the initial infection, are the most common manifestations of late (stage III) disease. Lyme arthritis can take a monoarticular or oligoarticular, intermittent, or, less frequently, chronic course. Patients with ACA initially develop an infiltrative stage, followed by alterations characteristic of the atrophic stage: creased skin with livid discolorations and plastic protrusion of vessels. ACA is observed almost exclusively in Europe, a finding highly correlated with *B. afzelii* infections. Chronic neuroborreliosis is a very rare manifestation of late (stage III) disease. Parapareses and tetrapareses are its most common symptoms. Examination of the CSF reveals a marked elevation of the protein concentration, with a low to moderate increase in the number of cells in the CSF. The detection of intrathecally produced specific antibodies is regarded as the best marker of neuroborreliosis and the most relevant criterion for its discrimination from multiple sclerosis.

Early manifestations of Lyme borreliosis are observed most frequently in the spring, summer, and autumn time frame, coinciding with tick activity. Late manifestations do not show a seasonal pattern.

COLLECTION, TRANSPORT, AND STORAGE OF SPECIMENS

The specimen types used for laboratory confirmation of borreliosis are presented in Table 3.

Blood and Serum

For relapsing fever, blood is the specimen of choice. During febrile attacks, large numbers of borreliae may easily be detected by dark-field or bright-field microscopy of a wet-mount blood sample or a stained blood smear, respectively (see "Detection and Isolation Procedures," "Microscopy"). At this time, the level of spirochetemia may reach 10^6 to 10^8 cells ml^{-1} (51). Blood from acutely ill patients is also the best source for culture confirmation (22, 23, 75). However, the spirochetemia diminishes with each successive relapse, and visualization or culture isolation of borreliae is often unsuccessful during afebrile periods. In contrast to relapsing fever, spirochetemia in Lyme borreliosis patients is below the level of microscopic confirmation. Even under special conditions (three specimens of 3 ml of plasma cultured in 70 ml of medium for 12 weeks), in which specimens positive by culture have been derived from up to 50% of patients with EM (115), attempts to confirm Lyme borreliosis by culture of blood samples are of low diagnostic priority (39).

Serum is suitable for detection of indirect (antibody) evidence of exposure to borreliae. Specific antibody detection tests are the tests that are the most widely used for laboratory confirmation of Lyme borreliosis and have recently been applied to confirmation of relapsing fever cases as well (see "Serologic Diagnosis").

Cerebrospinal Fluid

In suspected neuroborreliosis patients, CSF (along with a serum sample drawn at the same time) should be obtained for determination of cell counts-cell differentials, protein

TABLE 3 Specimen types used for diagnosis of Lyme borreliosis

Clinical manifestation	Specimens for:	
	Direct pathogen detection (culture, PCR)	Antibody detection
Stage I (early or localized; days through weeks after tick bite), EM	Skin biopsy	Serum
Stage II (early or disseminated; weeks through months after tick bite)		
Multiple areas of erythema	Skin biopsy	Serum
Borrelial lymphocytoma	Skin biopsy	Serum
Lyme carditis	Endomyocardial biopsy specimen	Serum
Neuroborreliosis	CSF	Paired serum-CSF[a]
Stage III (late/persistent; months through years after tick bite)		
Arthritis	Synovial fluid, biopsy specimen	Serum
Acrodermatitis chronica atrophicans	Skin biopsy specimen	Serum
Chronic neuroborreliosis	CSF	Paired serum-CSF[a]

[a] Paired serum and CSF specimens are obtained on the same day for CSF antibody/serum antibody index determination.

contents, and intrathecal immunoglobulin (immunoglobulin M [IgM] and IgG) synthesis. Laboratory confirmation of neuroborreliosis is most readily achieved by demonstration of borrelia-specific, intrathecal antibody production (see "Serologic Diagnosis," "Detection of Intrathecally Produced Antibodies"). CSF can also be used for culture or PCR; however, the detection rates by these approaches are only about 20% (31).

Synovial Fluid or Synovial Biopsy Specimen

Investigation of synovial fluid or, preferably, a synovial biopsy specimen, by PCR is indicated in patients in whom Lyme arthritis is suspected (69). Culture is usually negative, with few exceptions. Due to the high protein permeability of the synovium, synovial fluid and serum display roughly equivalent antibody titers. Thus, significant indices for intra-articular antibody synthesis cannot be demonstrated, and it is absolutely sufficient to monitor antibody in serum.

Skin Biopsy Specimens

Skin biopsy specimens are the best sources for isolation of *B. burgdorferi*, and spirochetes can be isolated from most untreated patients with early and late dermatoborreliosis (EM and ACA, respectively) (Table 4). In patients with EM, the rate of success of culture is highest (up to 86%) with biopsy specimens taken close (4 mm inside) to the expanding border of the lesion (13). Without treatment, *B. burgdorferi* can persist for long periods of time in the skin, as shown by isolation of the organism from a 10-year-old acrodermatitis lesion (4). Biopsy specimens (taken after thorough disinfection of the skin) should be sent in a small amount of sterile saline as soon as possible to the microbiological laboratory.

Other Materials

If available, other biopsy materials from the heart, brain, and eye can be investigated for detection of borreliae. For example, *B. burgdorferi* has been isolated from an iris biopsy specimen of a patient with iridocyclitis and panuveitis (78).

Ticks are often tested for borreliae as part of epidemiologic studies to assess the risk to human populations in a given geographic area. Although specialized laboratories offer diagnostic services for individual ticks, detection of spirochetes within ticks by PCR or other methods has not been shown to provide clinically useful information.

General Remarks for Collection and Transport

For culture, collection and preparation of specimens under sterile conditions are of utmost importance. Body fluids should be transported without any additives, and biopsy specimens should be placed in a small quantity of sterile saline or suitable culture medium (see "Culture Isolation"). Samples should reach the laboratory as quickly as possible (within 2 to 4 h). Before specimens are collected and transported, the laboratory should be contacted so that details related to methodology can be agreed upon. If postal transport is unavoidable, overnight delivery is recommended.

DETECTION AND ISOLATION PROCEDURES

Evidence of borrelia in clinical samples can be determined by direct methods such as microscopy, culture, and nucleic acid detection and by indirect methods such as the detection of antibody responses. Critical evaluation of the patient's pretest history and presentation is necessary in order to select the most useful test approach and to optimize its performance.

Microscopy

Direct microscopic visualization of borrelia in clinical samples is only applicable to cases of relapsing fever. During

TABLE 4 Sensitivity of methods for direct pathogen detection in Lyme borreliosis

Specimen	Sensitivity
Skin (EM lesion, acrodermatitis)..........................	50–70% when using culture or PCR
CSF (neuroborreliosis, stage II)..........................	10–30% when using culture or PCR
Synovial fluid[a] (Lyme arthritis)..........................	50–70% when using PCR (culture is only extremely seldom positive)

[a] Higher sensitivity of direct pathogen detection from synovial biopsy specimens.

acute phases, the level of spirochetemia often reaches 10^6 to 10^8 cells ml^{-1} and motile spirochetes can be visualized by dark-field microscopy from wet preparations made from a drop of blood. This simple confirmatory test is often overlooked because of the increasingly common use of automated differential blood counts. Spirochetes can also be visualized by stained (e.g., Giemsa) thin or thick blood films (Fig. 3). Detection of low-level spirochetemias may be assisted by a microhematocrit concentration technique (38). The hematocrit capillary is filled 75% with citrated blood and is centrifuged for 2 min. The region containing the buffy coat is than examined directly under a microscope at ×400 to ×1,000 magnification (89). Failure to observe spirochetes does not rule out disease, and other diagnostic methods (see "Culture Isolation" and "Animal Inoculation") may be considered. In Lyme borreliosis patients, spirochete numbers in blood or other tissues are below the level of microscopic detection, and microscopy is best applied to the monitoring of borrelial growth in cultured tissues or fluids.

Culture Isolation

Many Lyme and relapsing fever borreliae are successfully cultured in artificial media. However, for diagnostic purposes, culturing is a slow, time-consuming method characterized by modest sensitivity, especially with patient body fluids (Table 4). For these reasons culture attempts are most often limited to research applications and are performed by reference laboratories (e.g., the National Reference Center for Borreliae in Germany and the Centers for Disease Control and Prevention [CDC] in the United States).

Several media such as modified Kelly medium (e.g., Barbour-Stoenner-Kelly II medium [BSK II] and BSKH) or modified Kelly medium Preac-Mursic (MKP) (7, 74, 81) are capable of supporting the growth of borreliae. A commercial preparation of BSKH is available from Sigma Chemical Co., St. Louis, Mo. Optimum growth (the generation time of *B. burgdorferi* is about 7 to 20 h) in these media is obtained at 30 to 33°C under microaerophilic conditions. Positive cultures of EM lesion and synovial biopsy specimens or fluid samples (blood and CSF) may be obtained in

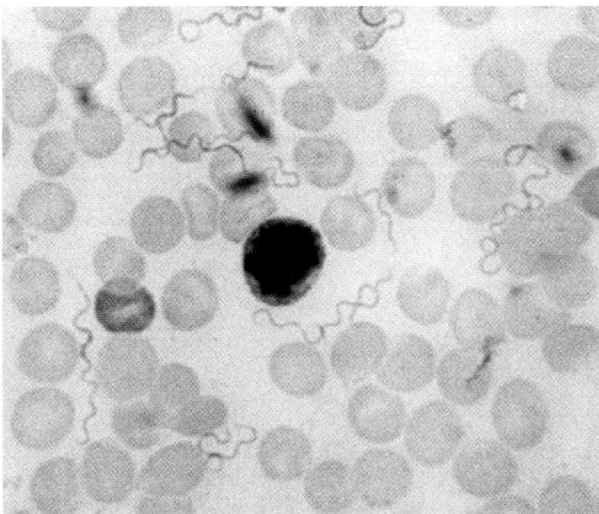

FIGURE 3 *B. hermsii* in a thin smear of rodent blood. Giemsa stain. Magnification, ×1,000.

as few as 4 days; but most isolates require several weeks of incubation, and negative cultures should be monitored for at least 6 weeks.

Antigen Detection

Enzyme-linked immunosorbent assay and immunoblotting have been used for the detection of borrelial antigen in body fluids including CSF and urine (21, 47). However, the validity of antigen detection methods is controversial, and their use is no longer recommended (59).

Nucleic Acid Detection Methods

Nucleic acid amplification techniques (NATs) for borreliae have been most widely used for phylogenetic analysis and investigation of pathogenic mechanisms and zoonotic disease. In addition, standardized methods of DNA extraction and amplification have yet to be validated in multicenter clinical diagnostic studies. Therefore, NATs for the diagnosis of Lyme borreliosis should be restricted to experienced and specialized laboratories with the ability to verify amplicons by use of specific hybridization probes, sequencing, or equivalent methods. For patients with suspected exposure outside of North America, it is imperative that the targets selected for NATs are sensitive for all human-pathogenic species, and species identification from the amplification products is preferable (113).

Under circumstances in which antibody detection and culture isolation fail to provide case confirmation, NATs can serve as separate adjuncts to clinical diagnosis. A variety of chromosomal and plasmid targets for NATs have been developed (for a review, see reference 88). For PCR, an analytical sensitivity of approximately 10 to 20 borreliae per test sample has been demonstrated. Test sensitivities for both NATs and culture are greater with tissue specimens than with body fluids. Only NAT with synovial fluid seems to be more sensitive than culture. Nocton et al. (69) reported a sensitivity of 96% and Bradley et al. (15) reported a sensitivity of 86% (six of seven specimens) for NATs with synovial fluid from American patients with Lyme arthritis. Depending on the method used, European investigators have found NAT sensitivities ranging between 50 and 70% (30, 82, 98). With skin biopsy and CSF specimens, NATs demonstrated diagnostic sensitivities of approximately 60 and 20%, respectively (16, 31). A prospective study of PCR and culture detection of *B. burgdorferi* in EM biopsy specimens from Slovenian patients showed that they had comparable sensitivities (36% for culture with MKP, 24% for culture with BSKII, 25% for PCR, 54% for at least one positive test, and 6% for all three tests positive) (72).

PCR amplification of *B. burgdorferi* sequences from urine has been described (82, 88) but remains very controversial, and doubts persist, especially regarding the specificity of the method. Although *Borrelia*-specific DNA was demonstrated in over 70% of skin biopsy specimens from patients with florid EM, parallel testing of urine samples gave uniformly negative results (16). NATs are therefore not recommended as primary diagnostic tools with urine samples.

Animal Inoculation

Animal inoculation as a diagnostic tool for relapsing fever is indicated if the borreliae are not cultivable in artificial media, in the case of fever-free intervals, or during later relapses in which the numbers of borrellae in the blood are rather low. Animal inoculation can also be used for purification of contaminated cultures. Mice, rats, and hamsters have been used for in vivo culture of relapsing fever borreliae. Animal inoculation is not a useful diagnostic approach for Lyme borreliosis.

IDENTIFICATION

Molecular Techniques

The classical approach for examining relationships among closely related taxa, recommended by the Ad Hoc Committee on Reconciliation of Approaches to Bacterial Systematics, is DNA-DNA reassociation analysis (101). This is the currently used reference method for species delineation within *B. burgdorferi* sensu lato (6). Relapsing fever borrelia have been typed on the basis of DNA-DNA reassociation analysis and flagellin gene analysis (23, 52). A number of additional molecular-genetic methods, including pulsed-field gel electrophoresis of large restriction fragments (12) and PCR and sequence analysis or restriction fragment length polymorphism (RFLP) analysis of the 16S rRNA and 16S ribosomal DNA and of the 5S-23S intergenic spacer region (62, 76), have also been described for species differentiation (summarized in reference 100). RFLP analysis of the 5S-23S intergenic spacer region is the method the most often used to determine and compare *B. burgdorferi* sensu lato species. Analysis of certain protein-encoding genes, especially of the *ospA* gene, has also been used for *B. burgdorferi* sensu lato species identifications (31, 109). Some approaches also enable subspecies characterization (e.g., *ospA* and *ospC* gene analysis) (104). However, in most cases, diagnosis and effective management of individual patients are independent of species determinations beyond the Lyme and relapsing fever groups.

Immunological Techniques

A species-specific monoclonal antibody which binds selectively to the flagellin of *B. hermsii* can be used to identify this species in cultures of isolates or infected tissues (90). Antibody responses to GlpQ, an antigen expressed by relapsing fever species but not Lyme borreliosis species, have been used to discriminate the two infections (75, 92). For *B. burgdorferi* sensu lato, serotyping is the most common phenotyping method. Using monoclonal antibodies, a serotyping system has been established and confirmed by sequence analysis of OspA. Eight different serotypes have been described for Europe (104, 109). Phenotypic analysis of OspC revealed 15 different serotypes (105). Some monoclonal antibodies are species specific: H3TS for *B. burgdorferi* sensu stricto (11, 109), 117.3 and L32 14G7 for *B. afzelii* (19, 104), and D6 and L18 A14 for *B. garinii* (6, 104).

SEROLOGIC DIAGNOSIS

Borrelia Antigens and Human Humoral Immune Response

Immunologically relevant antigens of *B. burgdorferi* are encoded on both its plasmids and its chromosome. More than 100 different plasmid-encoded lipoproteins have been identified (35). Analysis of the humoral immune response in patients with Lyme borreliosis with regard to the immunodominant protein antigens of *B. burgdorgeri* (Fig. 4b) reveals specific, stage-dependent characteristics that are also diagnostically relevant.

The early antibody response is largely IgM and is mainly directed against the outer membrane-associated protein

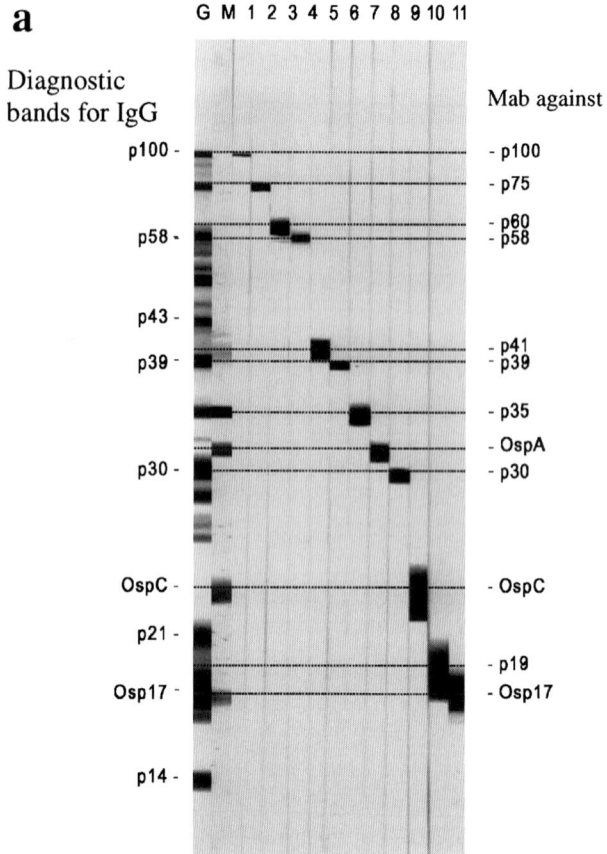

a

G M 1 2 3 4 5 6 7 8 9 10 11

Diagnostic bands for IgG

Mab against

p100 - — - p100
— - p75
— - p60
p58 - — - p58
p43 - —
— - p41
p39 - — - p39
— - p35
— - OspA
p30 - — - p30
OspC - — - OspC
p21 - —
— - p19
Osp17 - — - Osp17
p14 - —

FIGURE 4 Immunoblotting. (a) Identification of diagnostic bands with monoclonal antibodies (Mab). Lanes: G, IgG antibody; M, IgM antibody; 1 to 10, sera from European patients. (b) Immunoblots for patients with early (neuroborreliosis stage II) and late (acrodermatitis) disease. Lanes: +, reference serum (IgG); lanes 1 to 7, sera from European patients. Note that the antigen used is *B. afzelii* strain PKo. (Fig. 4a and b are modified from Fig. 1 and 5, respectively, of reference 43).

OspC, p35, and the flagellum subunits p37 (FlaA) and p41 (FlaB) (1, 3, 32, 43, 106) (Fig. 4b). The level of IgM antibody to most spirochetal antigens peaks within the first weeks of infection. However, persistence of this immunoglobulin class in patients with Lyme borreliosis is directly related to disease duration and/or dissemination prior to treatment, and IgM antibodies against OspC and flagellum subunits p37 (FlaA) and p41 (FlaB) are often detected many months after effective treatment and cure (1). Therefore, IgM reactivity should not be taken as a sole marker of early or active disease. The IgG response increases and broadens slowly over the first weeks of disease. Among the reactive antigens to which there is an early IgG response are p37 (FlaA), p41 (FlaB), and OspC (1). During early disseminated (stage II) disease, IgG levels increase and reactivity against p39 (BmpA) and p58 often appears (Fig. 4b). The late-stage immune response (stage III) is characterized by IgG antibodies to a wide variety of antigens (8, 28, 43). Using *B. burgdorferi* sensu stricto strain B31 as the antigen for immunoblotting, Dressler et al. (28) found that the immunorelevant and best discriminatory antigens for IgG antibodies among North American patients were p18, p21 (OspC), p28, p30, p37 (FlaA), p41 (FlaB), p45, p58,

b Neuroborreliosis Stage II

Acrodermatitis

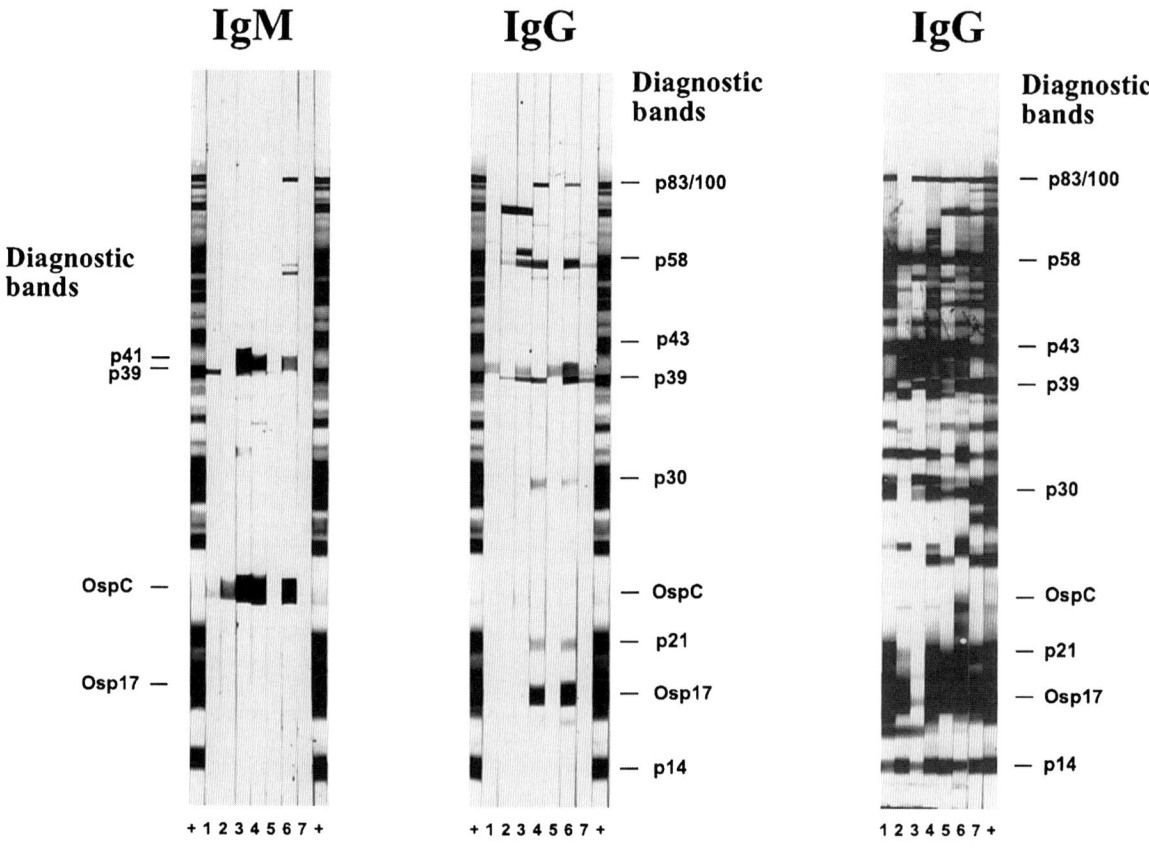

IgM

IgG

IgG

FIGURE 4 (Continued)

p66, and p93. Approximately 80% of the serum specimens from European patients with late disease (arthritis and ACA) reacted with p14, Osp17, p21 (not OspC), p30, p39, p43, p58, and p83/100 (homologue of p93) of *B. afzelii* strain PKo. Interestingly, IgG antibodies against OspC were detected in only 20% of these patients (Fig. 4b) (43). The frequency of IgG reactivity to OspC in American patients with late disease is higher (48%) than that in similar European patients. However, also in American patients, IgG immune responses to other antigens, such as p58 (93%) and p93 (88%), are higher than OspC immune responses (28). Spirochetal expression of OspC is presumably downregulated in many patients with chronic disease, especially in Europe. Nonetheless, detection of anti-OspC is a valuable diagnostic correlate in patients with early neuroborreliosis. OspC derived from *B. garinii* showed the best sensitivity among European patients (43).

Although the outer membrane protein OspA is abundantly expressed in culture by most strains, it is downregulated at the time of initial infection in the mammalian host. This explains why antibodies against OspA are rarely observed in patients with early disease. Among American patients with late disease, 42% (28) were reactive to OspA, whereas only 5 to 7% of European patients were reactive to OspA (43, 106). Notably, OspA antibodies are quite common in a special group of patients from the United States

who suffer from therapy-refractory forms of Lyme arthritis (3).

Recently, Zhang et al. (117) detected an antigen (VlsE) of *B. burgdorferi* that contains highly variable and highly conserved regions. Initial studies suggest that antibody elicited to a specific, constant-region epitope may be a sensitive and specific marker of exposure in Lyme borreliosis patients (64).

Immunofluorescence Assay

For the immunofluorescence assay (IFA), whole borreliae fixed on glass slides are used as the antigen. IFA has been used for the serodiagnosis of Lyme borreliosis as well as of relapsing fever. Serodiagnosis of relapsing fever, however, is challenged by variable expression of the major membrane proteins. The specificity of IFA for the serodiagnosis of Lyme borreliosis may be improved by adsorption of sera with *Treponema phagedenis* sonicate (IFA-ABS) (113). For the IgM test, pretreatment of the sera with anti-IgG immune serum is recommended to avoid false-positive test results due to rheumatoid factor as well as false-negative results due to high IgG antibody levels. As in all antibody detection assays, it is important to verify the expression of OspC within cultures used as the antigen source. Although IFA is relatively easy to perform, it is not easy to standardize, and evaluation of test results requires expertise not always available in the routine laboratory. In general, antibody titers ≥1:64 are regarded as positive in the IFA-ABS, and antibody titers ≥1:256 are regarded as positive in the unadsorbed IFA. Sera from patients with syphilis are often positive in the unadsorbed IFA and are only rarely positive in the IFA-ABS (113).

Enzyme Immunoassay

Different modifications of the enzyme immunoassay (EIA) have been used for the diagnosis of Lyme borreliosis. In the indirect EIA, antigen is coated onto the plates, followed by incubation with the patient's serum, enzyme-labeled anti-IgM or anti-IgG immune serum, and the EIA substrate. Capture IgM EIAs (μ-capture EIAs) have been specifically designed to avoid false-positive reactivity due to rheumatoid factor (42). False-positive reactivity due to rheumatoid factor can be also overcome by pretreatment of the sera with anti-IgG (106). EIA has the advantages of objective measurement, quantification, and high throughput. Many different antigen preparations have been used, including whole-cell sonicates (85), isolated flagella (40), detergent extracts (106), recombinant antigens (57, 61, 106), and synthetic peptides (64). Use of crude antigen preparations, such as whole-cell sonicates, often results in unacceptable specificity. New-generation tests, which use enriched, specific, or recombinant antigens, are under evaluation. New-generation tests with an octyl β-D-glucopyranoside (OGP)-detergent extract and Reiter treponeme absorbent, isolated flagella, and the C6 peptide of VlsE are available from Dade Behring (Marburg, Germany), Dakopatts (Copenhagen, Denmark), and Immunetics (Cambridge, Mass.), respectively.

Immunoblotting

Western immunoblotting enables assessment of the humoral immune response to individual protein antigens as resolved by sodium dodecyl sulfate-polyacrylamide gel electrophoresis (SDS-PAGE). Western immunoblotting is regarded as a supplementary assay (in the United States) or a confirmatory assay (in Europe). This implies that it should be used only when a screening assay is reactive (equivocal or positive). Antigen preparations for Western immunoblotting include whole-cell lysates or recombinant antigen mixtures that are transferred after SDS-PAGE to blot membranes.

The advantage of immunoblotting with whole-cell lysate is that antibodies against a large number (~50) of antigens can be detected. Herein also lies a significant challenge to the diagnostic laboratorian: discerning reactivity between specific and nonspecific or cross-reactive antigens that may not be clearly resolved from each other. Thus, reliable identification of the immunoreactive bands is imperative. This is best accomplished through the use of monoclonal antibodies (Fig. 4a) (5, 113). Immunoblotting for Lyme borreliosis is considered technically complex, and in order to realize its maximal performance and utility, standardization and careful quality control must be used.

Numerous immunoblotting tests which use antigens of various strains or genospecies of B. burgdorferi sensu lato are commercially available. Recommendations for interpretation of the Borrelia immunoblot have been published by the Association of State and Territorial Public Health Laboratory Directors (ASTPHLD) and CDC as well as by the German Society for Hygiene and Microbiology (DGHM) (5, 113).

In the United States, immunoblot interpretation rules have been recommended which refer to the detection of antibody against whole-cell antigens of specific B. burgdorferi sensu stricto strains (strains 2591, low-passage strain 297, and low-passage strain B31) (5, 28, 32). The IgM immunoblot is interpreted as positive if two or more bands for the following proteins are reactive: OspC, the 39-kDa protein (BmpA), and the 41-kDa protein (FlaB). The IgG immunoblot is interpreted as positive if five or more bands for the following proteins are reactive: proteins of 18, 21 (OspC), 28, 30, 39 (BmpA), 41 (FlaB), 45, 58, 66, and 93 kDa. If the immunoblot is used within the first 4 weeks of disease onset (during early disease or stage I or II of disease) both IgM and IgG immunoblotting should be performed. A positive IgM immunoblot alone is not recommended for use in determination of infection in persons with illness for >1 month because the likelihood of a false-positive test result for current infection is high in these individuals.

Interpretation of the antibody response among European patients is complicated by the risk of infection with B. burgdorferi sensu stricto, B. garinii, or B. afzelii. In addition, immunoblotting studies have shown that the immune response of European patients compared with that of American patients is restricted to a narrower spectrum of Borrelia proteins (27). Interpretive rules defined in a species- and strain-specific manner have been determined (43) and independently corroborated (58). B. afzelii strain PKo is preferred to strains PBi (B. garinii) and PKa2 (B. burgdorferi sensu stricto) because the first strain, even though it has the same sensitivity as the last two strains, permits a two-band criterion for the IgG test (the sample must be positive for at least two bands among the bands for p14, Osp17, p21, OspC, p30, p39 [BmpA], p43, p58, and p83/100 [Fig. 4b]), whereas the last two strains have only a single-band criterion (for B. garinii PBi, the sample must be positive for at least one band among the bands for p17, p21, OspC, p30, p39 [BmpA], and p83/100; for B. burgdorferi sensu stricto PKa2, the sample must be positive for at least one band among the bands for p17a, p21, OspC, p56, p58, and p83/100) (113). According to the general Deutsches Institut für Normung (DIN) recommendations for immunoblotting tests (DIN 58967, part 40), at least a two-band criterion should be used for interpretation of a positive IgG immunoblotting result. For IgM immunoblotting, a detectable immune response is restricted to only a few bands. Therefore, the IgM blot is regarded as positive if there is strong reactivity to OspC (113).

For commercial immunoblotting tests the user should verify that all relevant antigens are present and that interpretation rules have been established for defined patient and control populations. Every assay must include positive and negative controls. It must also be ensured that the positive control is capable of detecting all diagnostically relevant bands. If necessary, more than one control must be included. Furthermore, a cutoff control with borderline reactivity must be included in the analysis of samples from every patient group. In blot evaluations, a scored band must have an intensity equal to or greater than that for the cutoff control. Commercial Western immunoblotting test kits, licensed by the Food and Drug Administration (FDA), are available from five different manufacturers. Current listings of 510K, FDA-approved serodiagnostics assays for Lyme disease can be found at http://www.accessdata.fda.gov/scripts/cdrh/cfdocs/cfPMN/pmn.cfm under product code LSR.

Differences in the reactivities of sera with different strains may play a role in the sensitivity of the immunoblotting assay (43). Many of the technical complexities of whole-cell lysate immunoblotting may be alleviated by the use of recombinant antigens. Antibody responses to a number of recombinant antigens, their peptide fragments, or chimeras of multiple peptides have been assessed as diagnostic markers of infection (37, 106, 107). Recombinant blots with Osp17, OspC, p39 (BmpA), truncated p41 (FlaB), p58, and p83/100 have been demonstrated to have sensitivity for the detection of Lyme borreliosis, with the exception of the earliest stage of disease (EM), comparable to that of the whole-cell immunoblotting assay (107). Recombinant blots containing these antigens (except p58) are commercially available (Mikrogen, Munich, Germany). These and other studies suggest that the recombinant antigen-based assays are much easier to standardize and perform.

Two-Step Approach in Serodiagnosis

A two-step approach is recommended by ASTPHLD and CDC (in the United States) (5, 53), for the serodiagnosis of Lyme borreliosis: "All serum specimens submitted for Lyme disease testing should be evaluated in a two-step process, in which the first step is a sensitive serological test, such as an enzyme immunoassay (EIA) or immunofluorescence assay (IFA). All specimens found to be positive or equivocal by a sensitive EIA or IFA should be tested by a standardized Western blot procedure. Specimens found to be negative should not be tested further" (5). This procedure is also recommended in the *Quality Standards for Microbiological Diagnosis of Infectious Diseases* for Lyme borreliosis published by the German expert group on the diagnosis of Lyme borreliosis of DGHM (Fig. 5) (113). The concept of a two-step approach, which aims at increasing the predictive value of a positive test result with each step, requires that the tests be performed in succession (50, 113). Simultaneous performance of the screening and confirmatory assays will reduce the test specificity of the entire procedure.

Detection of Intrathecally Produced Antibodies

Detection of the intrathecal *Borrelia*-specific immune response is one of the most valuable diagnostic tools for the diagnosis of neuroborreliosis. Methods that take into account the potential dysfunction of the blood-CSF barrier, a common finding in neuroborreliosis, are required for accurate assessment of intrathecal antibody production. Since the permeability of the blood-CSF barrier may change rapidly in patients with inflammatory diseases like acute neuroborreliosis, CSF and serum must be obtained at the same time. Long-used procedures for detection of specific intrathecal antibody production in the diagnosis of neurosyphilis have been modified for the diagnosis of neuroborreliosis (41, 96, 112). The most frequently used method is the determination of the CSF antibody/serum antibody index (the specific antibody index [AI]).

This method requires measurement of the specific antibodies in the blood and in the CSF by means of a calibrated standard curve and determination of a quotient from the

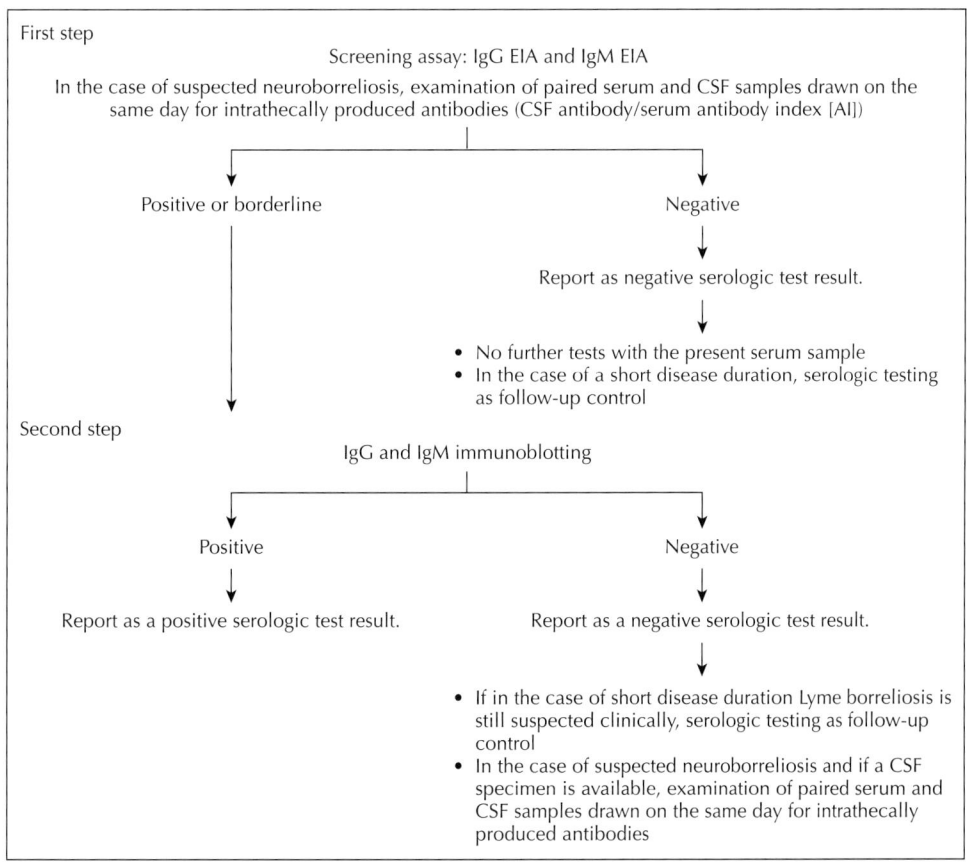

FIGURE 5 Two-step approach for serodiagnosis.

antibody units and the IgG concentrations in CSF and serum:

$$AI = \frac{\text{EIA units in CSF} \times \text{total IgG concentration in serum}}{\text{EIA units in serum} \times \text{total IgG concentration in CSF}}$$

For the determination of AI, EIAs, that allow quantitative measurement are suitable (112). The total IgG concentrations in serum and CSF are determined nephelometrically.

Alternatively, both serum and CSF can be used for EIA after adjustment so that they contain identical concentrations of total IgG (e.g., 1 mg/dl). If this does not lead to optical densities within the linear range of the standard curve, higher or lower concentrations of total IgG will have to be used in a new assay.

When CSF and serum are diluted so that they contain identical concentrations of total IgG (e.g., 1 mg of IgG/dl), the index is calculated by a simplified formula:

$$AI = \frac{\text{EIA units in CSF}}{\text{EIA units in serum}}$$

By calculating the AI, CSF and serum are compared with regard to the portion of pathogen-specific IgG antibodies in the total IgG content. An AI of ≥ 2.0 is considered significantly elevated (66, 113). Lower indices are also considered significant by some investigators. However, there is a higher risk of false-positive results due to the technical imprecision of measurement of immunoglobulin levels and antibody titers. False-positive AI results are also likely with neurosyphilis patients when their samples are tested against whole-cell or flagellar sonicates in an EIA. If neither clinical findings nor a serodiagnosis of syphilis sheds light on the matter, EIAs with *T. phagedenis* adsorption (Dade-Behring, Marburg, Germany) can be helpful for differential diagnosis.

Other suitable methods for determination of intrathecal antibody production are the μ- or γ-capture EIA (Dakopatts, Copenhagen, Denmark) (41) and IgG-matched immunoblotting (112). IgG-matched immunoblotting allows comparison of the spectrum of antibodies (against various *Borrelia* proteins) in serum and CSF and thus permits one to draw conclusions as to the specificity of the intrathecal antibody response.

For patients with neuroborreliosis, the intrathecal antibody production increases over time. Antibody was detected in 80 to 90% of patients between 8 and 41 days after the onset of disease and in up to 100% of patients after 41 days after onset (41). However, in cases of short duration, the intrathecal immune response may be absent, especially in children. Cases have also been reported in which only the IgM antibody test performed with CSF showed a positive result and no specific antibodies were detected in serum samples taken at the same time (20).

Vaccination and Its Impact on Serology

In the United States, a vaccine against Lyme borreliosis has been licensed for use in humans. The vaccine (Lymerix) is a lipidated recombinant of OspA derived from a *B. burgdorferi* sensu stricto strain and requires three doses at 0, 1, and 12 months. The efficacy of the vaccine in protecting against definite disease was 49% after two doses and 76% after three doses (97).

The first indication that OspA immunization protected animals from challenge was reported in 1990 (33, 87). The mechanism by which OspA antibodies protect vaccinated individuals appears to take place largely within the midgut of the blood-feeding tick (25). Antibody raised against another surface-associated protein, OspC, has also been shown to protect animals against challenge with homologous *B. burgdorferi* species (80). Currently, both OspA and OspC vaccines are being developed by industry for use in Europe.

In general, most currently available EIAs do not differentiate between immune responses due to vaccination and those due to natural infection. For this purpose new tests which detect non-vaccine-induced immune responses in vaccine recipients must be developed. Such EIAs can be designed by using strain variants that lack the respective vaccine protein (OspA-less and OspC-less variants) or by use of recombinant antigen- or peptide-based tests. The confounding Western immunoblotting reactivity to antigens other than p31 often observed among OspA vaccine recipients is due to fragments of OspA (or cross-reactive OspB) that migrate independently of the intact molecule during SDS-PAGE. Despite these issues and concerns, the experienced Lyme borreliosis laboratorian is often able to distinguish OspA vaccination from early infection using the standard two-test paradigm (2).

ANTIBIOTIC SUSCEPTIBILITY

The antimicrobial susceptibility of *Borrelia* species has been studied intensively in vitro (52, 77). As for other slowly growing bacteria, standard methods for determination of the minimal bactericidal concentration have not been established. However, despite the different methods used, there is general agreement on the in vitro susceptibilities of the borreliae to antimicrobials, as follows: *B. burgdorferi* sensu lato is sensitive to macrolides, tetracyclines, semisynthetic penicillins, and the expanded- and broad-spectrum cephalosporins; is moderately sensitive to penicillin G and chloramphenicol; and is resistant to trimethoprim, sulfomethoxazole, rifampin, the aminoglycosides, and the quinolones (52). The susceptibilities of the relapsing fever borreliae (*B. hermsii* and *B. turicatae*) to the antibiotics penicillin G, amoxicillin, ceftriaxone, erythromycin, azithromycin, doxycycline, and tetracycline were investigated, and no significant difference from those of the Lyme disease borreliae was found (52). Recently, several newer antimicrobial agents were tested against *B. burgdorferi* sensu lato, resulting in high sensitivities for everninomycin and meropenem (26) and streptogramin and mezlocillin (46).

In vivo studies have been conducted with experimentally infected gerbils (77) and hamsters (52). Good in vivo activity was achieved with amoxicillin, cefotaxime, ceftriaxone, tetracycline, doxycycline, and azithromycin in the studies with gerbils and hamsters; but penicillin G required high doses for in vivo activity.

Recommendations for Antibiotic Therapy

All clinical manifestations of *B. burgdorferi* infection must be treated with antibiotics. The antibiotic, dosage, duration, and route of application depend on the clinical picture and the stage of the disease (103, 116).

In case of a solitary EM lesion, oral treatment with doxycycline, amoxicillin, or cefuroxime for 2 weeks is recommended. Disseminated infections require parenteral treatment with cephalosporins (ceftriaxone, one dose of 2 g/day intravenously [i.v.], or cefotaxime, three doses of 2 g/day i.v.) or parenteral high-dose treatment with penicillin G (four doses of 3 g/day i.v.). In patients with acrodermatitis, the same antibiotics and daily doses used to treat EM are recommended. In patients with Lyme arthritis, oral treatment with doycycline may be tried first, but in case of a poor therapeutic response, the patient should be treated i.v. with cephalosporins or penicillin G. Cephalosporins or penicillin G administered i.v. are also recommended for the treatment of tertiary neuroborreliosis. All patients with late manifestations should be treated for 3 to 4 weeks.

Interpretation and Reporting of Results

General Aspects
Clinical criteria (case history, clinical findings) are decisive factors in the diagnosis and ordering of microbiological laboratory tests. Although laboratory test results may confirm a clinical suspicion, the predictive value of these findings is directly related to the pretest probability. It should be kept in mind that the lower the probability of the clinical diagnosis is, the lower the predictive value of a positive test result will be. For the differential diagnosis of arthritis, a negative serologic test result has a high negative predictive value for Lyme arthritis since nearly all cases are seropositive. Whether or not a detected immune response corresponds with the patient's presentation is a question that can be answered only by the clinician, e.g., by use of clinical case definitions applicable to the various manifestations of Lyme borreliosis. Therefore, the microbiological report should not contain any therapy recommendations.

Serologic Report
The serologic report should contain the following points:

1. Recording of individual test results. Results of the screening assay are reported as positive, borderline or equivocal, or negative. The immunoblotting assay results are reported as positive or negative. In case of a positive result, the reactive diagnostic bands should also be reported (113). However, caution against overinterpretation of minimally reactive blots must be emphasized (e.g., IgG reactivity against p41 is expected in approximately 50% of healthy adults in the United States and Europe and is therefore excluded from the European criteria for the IgG immunoblotting assay).

2. An assessment of the final result of the two-step approach regarding its immunodiagnostic significance (e.g., whether specific antibodies have been detected or not).

3. An assessment of serologic findings as to the stage of the immune response, as far as test results allow pertinent statements to this effect (see below).

4. Recommendations for further reasonable diagnostic methods (PCR, culture) or for a serologic follow-up, if indicated.

Patterns of Serologic Results in Various Stages of Lyme Borreliosis
Antibody tests performed in the early stage of Lyme borreliosis may show a negative or a borderline result (Table 5), often due to insufficient time for the full evolution of the immune response. In some cases seroconversion occurs even after the initiation of antibiotic treatment (108). Thus, in the presence of a positive clinical correlation, a repeat serology may be warranted up to 6 weeks after the onset of disease. During the early stage of Lyme borreliosis, detection of IgM is consistent with an active infection. On the other hand, an IgM assay may be negative during early disease, most likely due to insufficient time for the evolu-

tion of a complete antibody response or, in the face of a robust IgG response, due to an anamnestic response to reinfection. Usually, only a few bands are detected by immunoblotting in patients with early disease (IgG and IgM) (Fig. 4b).

In late disease a positive test for IgG antibodies is mandatory for serologic confirmation. In many cases, IgM antibodies are often absent. In principle, an IgM test is not useful for establishment of the diagnosis of late disease. The sole detection of IgM (without the detection of IgG) even rules out the diagnosis of late Lyme disease manifestations. A false-positive result for IgM due to a polyclonal immune response in the context of herpesvirus infections or autoimmune diseases and rheumatoid disorders must also be considered. In many cases the origin of such IgM findings remains unclear. IgM antibodies may also be detected differentially in patients with late disease, according to the test method used. For example, positive IgM EIA or IgM immunoblotting assay results were demonstrated in 20 to 40% of patients with late disease, whereas positive results were detected in only 5% of these patients by the IgM immunofluorescence test (106). The IgG immunoblotting assay usually shows a broad band pattern (Fig. 4b). However, positive findings for IgG with a broad band pattern in the immunoblot are compatible not only with active Lyme disease but also with past, spontaneously resolved, or sufficiently treated infections. Such patterns of results are often found in members of high-risk groups with frequent exposures to ticks (for example, forest workers), who do not show any clinical manifestations.

In patients with neuroborreliosis, apart from the serum findings, the detection of pathogen-specific, intrathecally produced antibodies, i.e., an elevated AI, is of utmost importance for the diagnosis. In most cases, determination of the IgG AI will be sufficient. Neuroborreliosis in children is a notable exception to the rule because in those patients only the IgM AI may be positive, particularly in patients in whom the disease duration has been short. Also common to the latter circumstances are positive CSF findings preceding positive serum findings. Therefore, examination of paired serum and CSF specimens is mandatory in each case. Since a positive AI may be detectable as long as years after treatment and cure, repeated testing is not suitable for monitoring of the success of therapy. Diagnosis of chronic neuroborreliosis is based on demonstration of a positive AI. Detection of antibodies against *B. burgdorferi* in serum alone is not sufficient, and direct detection of the pathogen by culture or NATs is unsuccessful.

Influence of Antimicrobial Therapy on Serodiagnosis
Clinicians are often tempted to order repeated posttreatment serologic tests in an effort to correlate cure and

TABLE 5 Sensitivity of antibody detection methods in the diagnosis of Lyme disease

Stage	Sensitivity	Remarks
I	20–50	Predominance of IgM
II	70–90	Presence of IgM and IgG; in cases of long disease duration, predominance of IgG
III	Nearly 100[a]	Usually solely IgG

[a] Negative only for patients with a very short duration of symptoms.

decreasing antibody titers. However, IgG antibodies against *B. burgdorferi* persist for a long time even after successful therapy. Significant changes in titer can be expected only several months after the end of therapy; in patients with late manifestations, even years may elapse. Moreover, a decrease in the antibody titer does not rule out persistence of the pathogen. Hence, there is practically no indication for serologic follow-up aimed at an assessment of the success of the therapy. Treatment success therefore must always be assessed according to clinical criteria.

Direct Detection of the Pathogen (Culture and NATs)

The indication for the direct detection of the pathogen by means of PCR or culture is restricted to specific cases. Table 4 gives an overview of the success rates to be expected. Detection of the pathogen by culture is the best evidence for an infection with *B. burgdorferi*. Contaminations are rather uncommon. In contrast, PCR, due to its higher contamination rate, is likely to yield more false-positive results. As in other infectious diseases, the medical report should specify the species found, e.g., *B. afzelii*, not just *B. burgdorferi* sensu lato. Sequence analysis of amplicons increases the diagnostic validity because detection of sequences of genes (e.g., the *ospA* gene) that differ from those of laboratory control strains excludes contamination. It must always be borne in mind that, as with serologic results, direct detection of the pathogen must be evaluated in the context of the clinical picture. Upon medical assessment of the results, the serologic findings must always be taken into account. An improbable finding for Lyme arthritis would be a positive PCR result with a synovial biopsy specimen and a negative serology result. In the case of a positive serology result, however, a positive NAT result will support the diagnosis of Lyme borreliosis. Moreover, positive PCR and/or culture results are important diagnostic criteria in the case of clinically equivocal or atypical skin manifestations. A negative PCR result does not rule out a diagnosis of Lyme disease. The transport of tissues under less than optimum conditions or the presence of inhibitory substances in the sample may result in negative findings. If inhibitory substances have been detected (the detection procedure is described in reference 84), these findings must be stated in the report. Direct detection of the pathogen is not suitable for the monitoring of treatment success because of the high likelihood of false-negative results. However, cultivation of *B. burgdorferi* after therapy is evidence of treatment failure.

Sources of Error in Serodiagnosis

False results, both negative and positive, can result from the test itself or the nature of the immune response. Seronegative results within the first days of disease are common. In Europe, differences between the test antigen and the species causing infection may also contribute to seronegative findings. In addition, deficiencies in diagnostic antigen expression will compromise the sensitivities of tests. Of utmost importance, however, are the diagnostic gaps (seronegativity) in the early stage of disease. The high levels of background reactivity of many first-generation, whole-cell-based assays often result in lower specificities and therefore the frequent occurrence of false-positive results. Cross-reactivity with treponemes can largely be avoided by use of the Reiter treponeme adsorbent, although syphilis serology should be performed in cases in which treponeme exposure cannot be ruled out. Continued test development and evaluation promise to provide second-

and third-generation assays with improved performances in terms of their sensitivities and specificities. Nonetheless, critical assessment of the patient's pretest risk factors, clinical history, and presentation will provide the best direction for laboratory test use and minimize false test outcomes for current and future diagnostic tests.

REFERENCES

1. Aguero-Rosenfeld, M. E., J. Nowakowski, S. Bittker, D. Cooper, R. B. Nadelman, and G. P. Wormser. 1996. Evolution of the serologic response to *Borrelia burgdorferi* in treated patients with culture-confirmed erythema migrans. *J. Clin. Microbiol.* **34:**1–9.

2. Aguero-Rosenfeld, M. E., J. Roberge, C. A. Carbonaro, J. Nowakowski, R. B. Nadelman, and G. P. Wormser. 1999. Effects of OspA vaccination on Lyme disease serologic testing. *J. Clin. Microbiol.* **37:**3718–3721.

3. Akin, E., G. L. McHugh, R. A. Flavell, E. Fikrig, and A. C. Steere. 1999. The immunoglobulin (IgG) antibody response to OspA and OspB correlates with severe and prolonged Lyme arthritis and the IgG response to P35 correlates with mild and brief arthritis. *Infect. Immun.* **67:**173–181.

4. Åsbrink, E., and A. Hovmark. 1988. Early and late cutaneous manifestations in Ixodes-borne borreliosis (erythema migrans borreliosis, Lyme borreliosis). *Ann. N. Y. Acad. Sci.* **539:**4–15.

5. Association of State and Territorial Public Health Laboratory Directors and the Centers for Disease Control and Prevention. 1995. Recommendations, p. 1–5. In *Proceedings of the Second National Conference on the Serologic Diagnosis of Lyme Disease.* Association of State and Territorial Public Health Laboratory Directors, Washington, D.C.

6. Baranton, G., D. Postic, I. Saint Girons, P. Boerlin, J.-C. Piffaretti, M. Assous, and P. A. D. Grimont. 1992. Delineation of *Borrelia burgdorferi* sensu stricto, *Borrelia garinii* sp. nov., and group VS461 associated with Lyme borreliosis. *Int. J. Syst. Bacteriol.* **42:**378–383.

7. Barbour, A. G. 1984. Isolation and cultivation of Lyme disease spirochetes. *Yale J. Biol. Med.* **57:**521–525.

8. Barbour, A. G., W. Burgdorfer, E. Grunwaldt, and A. C. Steere. 1983. Antibodies of patients with Lyme disease to components of the *Ixodes dammini* spirochete. *J. Clin. Investig.* **72:**504–515.

9. Barbour, A. G., and C. F. Garon. 1987. Linear plasmids of the bacterium *Borrelia burgdorferi* have covalently closed ends. *Science* **237:**409–411.

10. Barbour, A. G., and S. F. Hayes. 1986. Biology of *Borrelia* species. *Microbiol. Rev.* **50:**381–400.

11. Barbour, A. G., R. A. Heiland, and T. R. Howe. 1985. Heterogeneity of major proteins in Lyme disease borreliae: a molecular analysis of North American and European isolates. *J. Infect. Dis.* **152:**478–484.

12. Belfaiza, J., D. Postic, E. Bellenger, G. Baranton, and I. S. Girons. 1993. Genomic fingerprinting of *Borrelia burgdorferi* sensu lato by pulsed-field gel electrophoresis. *J. Clin. Microbiol.* **31:**2873–2877.

13. Berger, B. W., R. C. Johnson, C. Kodner, and L. Coleman. 1992. Cultivation of *Borrelia burgdorferi* from erythema migrans lesions and perilesional skin. *J. Clin. Microbiol.* **30:**359–361.

14. Bergström, S., V. G. Bundoc, and A. G. Barbour. 1989. Molecular analysis of linear plasmid-encoded major surface proteins, OspA and OspB, of the Lyme disease spirochete *Borrelia burgdorferi*. *Mol. Microbiol.* **3:**479–486.

15. **Bradley, J. F., R. C. Johnson, and J. L. Goodman.** 1994. The persistence of spirochetal nucleic acids in active Lyme arthritis. *Ann. Intern. Med.* **120:**487–489.

16. **Brettschneider, S., H. Bruckbauer, N. Klugbauer, and H. Hofmann.** 1998. Diagnostic value of PCR for detection of *Borrelia burgdorferi* in skin biopsy and urine samples from patients with skin borreliosis. *J. Clin. Microbiol.* **36:**2658–2665.

17. **Bryceson, A. D. E., E. H. O. Parry, P. L. Perine, D. A. Warrell, D. Vukotich, and C. S. Leithead.** 1970. Louse-borne relapsing fever. A clinical and laboratory study of 62 cases in Ethiopia and a reconsideration of the literature. *Q. J. Med.* **39:**129–170.

18. **Burgdorfer, W., A. G. Barbour, S. F. Hayes, J. L. Benach, E. Grunwaldt, and J. P. Davis.** 1982. Lyme disease—a tick-borne spirochetosis? *Science* **216:**1317–1319.

19. **Canica, M. M., F. Nato, L. Du Merle, J. C. Mazie, G. Baranton, and D. Postic.** 1993. Monoclonal antibodies for identification of *Borrelia afzelii* sp. nov. associated with late cutaneous manifestations of Lyme borreliosis. *Scand. J. Infect. Dis.* **25:**441–448.

20. **Christen, H.-J., F. Hanefeld, H. Eiffert, and R. Thomssen.** 1993. Epidemiology and clinical manifestations of Lyme borreliosis in childhood. A prospective multicentre study with special regard to neuroborreliosis. *Acta Paediatr. Suppl.* **386:**1–75.

21. **Coyle, P. K., S. E. Schutzer, A. L. Belman, L. B. Krupp, and Z. Dheng.** 1992. Cerebrospinal fluid immunologic parameters in neurologic Lyme disease, p. 31–44. *In* S. E. Schutzer (ed.), *Lyme Disease: Molecular and Immunologic Approaches.* Cold Spring Harbor Laboratory Press, Cold Spring Harbor, N.Y.

22. **Cutler, S. J., D. Fekade, K. Hussein, K. A. Knox, A. Melka, K. Cann, A. R. Emilianus, D. A. Warrell, and D. J. M. Wright.** 1994. Successful in-vitro cultivation of *Borrelia recurrentis. Lancet* **343:**242.

23. **Cutler, S. J., J. Moss, M. Fukunaga, D. J. M. Wright, D. Fekade, and D. Warrell.** 1997. *Borrelia recurrentis* characterization and comparison with relapsing-fever, Lyme-associated, and other *Borrelia* spp. *Int. J. Syst. Bacteriol.* **47:**958–968.

24. **De Silva, A. M., and E. Fikrig.** 1995. Growth and migration of *Borrelia burgdorferi* in *Ixodes* ticks during blood feeding. *Am. J. Trop. Med. Hyg.* **53:**397–404.

25. **De Silva, A. M., S. R. Telford III, L. R. Brunet, S. W. Barthold, and E. Fikrig.** 1996. *Borrelia burgdorferi* OspA is an arthropod-specific transmission-blocking Lyme disease vaccine. *J. Exp. Med.* **183:**271–275.

26. **Dever, L. L., C. V. Torigian, and A. G. Barbour.** 1999. In vitro activities of the everninomicin SCH 27899 and other newer antimicrobial agents against *Borrelia burgdorferi. Antimicrob. Agents Chemother.* **43:**1773–1775.

27. **Dressler, F., R. Ackermann, and A. C. Steere.** 1994. Antibody responses to the three genomic groups of *Borrelia burgdorferi* in European Lyme borreliosis. *J. Infect. Dis.* **169:**313–318.

28. **Dressler, F., J. A. Whalen, B. N. Reinhardt, and A. C. Steere.** 1993. Western blotting in the serodiagnosis of Lyme disease. *J. Infect. Dis.* **167:**392–400.

29. **Dworkin, M. S., D. E. Anderson, Jr., T. G. Schwan, P. C. Shoemaker, S. N. Banerjee, B. O. Kassen, and W. Burgdorfer.** 1998. Tick-borne relapsing fever in the northwestern United States and southwestern Canada. *Clin. Infect. Dis.* **26:**122–131.

30. **Eiffert, H., A. Karsten, R. Thomssen, and H.-J. Christen.** 1998. Characterization of *Borrelia burgdorferi* strains in Lyme arthritis. *Scand. J. Infect. Dis.* **30:**265–268.

31. **Eiffert, H., A. Ohlenbusch, H.-J. Christen, R. Thomssen, A. Spielman, and F.-R. Matuschka.** 1995. Nondif-ferentiation between Lyme disease spirochetes from vector ticks and human cerebrospinal fluids. *J. Infect. Dis.* **171:**476–479.

32. **Engström, S. M., E. Shoop, and R. C. Johnson.** 1995. Immunoblot interpretation criteria for serodiagnosis of early Lyme disease. *J. Clin. Microbiol.* **33:**419–427.

33. **Fikrig, E., S. W. Barthold, F. S. Kantor, and R. A. Flavell.** 1990. Protection of mice against the Lyme disease agent by immunizing with recombinant OspA. *Science* **250:**553–556.

34. **Fingerle, V., G. Liegl, U. Munderloh, and B. Wilske.** 1998. Expression of outer surface proteins A and C of *Borrelia burgdorferi* in *Ixodes ricinus* ticks removed from humans. *Med. Microbiol. Immunol.* **187:**121–126.

35. **Fraser, C. M., S. Casjens, W. M. Huang, G. G. Sutton, R. Clayton, R. Lathigra, O. White, K. A. Ketchum, R. Dodson, E. K. Hickey, M. Gwinn, B. Dougherty, J.-F. Tomb, R. D. Fleischmann, D. Richardson, J. Peterson, A. R. Kerlavage, J. Quackenbush, S. Salzberg, M. Hanson, R. van Vugt, N. Palmer, M. D. Adams, J. Gocayne, J. Weidman, T. Utterback, L. Watthey, L. McDonald, P. Artiach, C. Bowman, S. Garland, C. Fujii, M. D. Cotton, K. Horst, K. Roberts, B. Hatch, H. O. Smith, and J. C. Venter.** 1997. Genomic sequence of a Lyme disease spirochaete, *Borrelia burgdorferi. Nature* **390:**580–586.

36. **Fuchs, R., S. Jauris, F. Lottspeich, V. Preac-Mursic, B. Wilske, and E. Soutschek.** 1992. Molecular analysis and expression of a Borrelia burgdorferi gene encoding a 22 kDa protein (pC) in Escherichia coli. *Mol. Microbiol.* **6:**503–509.

37. **Gilmore, R. D., Jr., R. L. Murphree, A. M. James, S. A. Sullivan, and B. J. B. Johnson.** 1999. The *Borrelia burgdorferi* 37-kilodalton immunoblot band (P37) used in serodiagnosis of early Lyme disease is the *flaA* gene product. *J. Clin. Microbiol.* **37:**548–552.

38. **Goldsmid, J. M., and K. Mahomed.** 1972. The use of the microhematocrit technic for the recovery of *Borrelia duttonii* from the blood. *Am. J. Clin. Pathol.* **58:**165–169.

39. **Goodman, J. L., J. F. Bradley, A. E. Ross, P. Goellner, A. Lagus, B. Vitale, B. W. Berger, S. Luger, and R. C. Johnson.** 1995. Bloodstream invasion in early Lyme disease: results from a prospective, controlled, blinded study using the polymerase chain reaction. *Am. J. Med.* **99:**6–12.

40. **Hansen, K., P. Hindersson, and N. S. Pedersen.** 1988. Measurement of antibodies to the *Borrelia burgdorferi* flagellum improves serodiagnosis in Lyme disease. *J. Clin. Microbiol.* **26:**338–346.

41. **Hansen, K., and A.-M. Lebech.** 1991. Lyme neuroborreliosis: a new sensitive diagnostic assay for intrathecal synthesis of *Borrelia burgdorferi*-specific immunoglobulin G, A, and M. *Ann. Neurol.* **30:**197–205.

42. **Hansen, K., K. Pii, and A.-M. Lebech.** 1991. Improved immunoglobulin M serodiagnosis in Lyme borreliosis by using a μ-capture enzyme-linked immunosorbent assay with biotinylated *Borrelia burgdorferi* flagella. *J. Clin. Microbiol.* **29:**166–173.

43. **Hauser, U., G. Lehnert, R. Lobentanzer, and B. Wilske.** 1997. Interpretation criteria for standardized Western blots for three European species of *Borrelia burgdorferi* sensu lato. *J. Clin. Microbiol.* **35:**1433–1444.

44. **Howe, T. R., L. W. Mayer, and A. G. Barbour.** 1985. A single recombinant plasmid expressing two major outer surface proteins of the Lyme disease spirochete. *Science* **227:**645–646.

45. **Humair, P.-F., and L. Gern.** 2000. The wild hidden face of Lyme borreliosis in Europe. *Microb. Infect.* **2:**915–922.

46. **Hunfeld, K.-P., J. Weigand, T. A. Wichelhaus, E. Kekoukh, P. Kraiczy, and V. Brade.** 2001. In vitro activity

of mezlocillin, meropenem, aztreonam, vancomycin, teicoplanin, rebostamycin and fusidic acid against *Borrelia burgdorferi*. *Int. J. Antimicrob. Agents* **17:**203–208.

47. **Hyde, F. W., R. C. Johnson, T. J. White, and C. E. Shelburne.** 1989. Detection of antigens in urine of mice and humans infected with *Borrelia burgdorferi*, etiologic agent of Lyme disease. *J. Clin. Microbiol.* **27:**58–61.

48. **James, A. M., D. Liveris, G. P. Wormser, I. Schwartz, M. A. Montecalvo, and B. J. B. Johnson.** 2001. *Borrelia lonestarii* infection after a bite by an *Amblyoma americanum* tick. *J. Infect. Dis.* **183:**1810–1814.

49. **Jauris-Heipke, S., G. Liegl, V. Preac-Mursic, D. Roessler, E. Schwab, E. Soutschek, G. Will, and B. Wilske.** 1995. Molecular analysis of genes encoding outer surface protein C (OspC) of *Borrelia burgdorferi* sensu lato: relationship to *ospA* genotype and evidence of lateral gene exchange of *ospC*. *J. Clin. Microbiol.* **33:**1860–1866.

50. **Johnson, B. J. B., K. E. Robbins, R. E. Balley, B.-L. Cao, S. L. Sviat, R. B. Craven, L. W. Mayer, and D. T. Dennis.** 1996. Serodiagnosis of Lyme disease: accuracy of a two-step approach using a flagella-based ELISA and immunoblotting. *J. Infect. Dis.* **174:**346–353.

51. **Johnson, R. C.** 1998. Borreliosis, p. 955–967. *In* L. H. Collier and W. W. Topley (ed.), *Topley & Wilson's Microbiology and Microbiol Infections*, 9th ed. Arnold, London, United Kingdom.

52. **Johnson, R. C.** 1998. Borrelia, p. 1277–1286. *In* L. H. Collier and W. W. Topley (ed.), *Topley & Wilson's Microbiology and Microbiol Infections*, 9th ed. Arnold, London, United Kingdom.

53. **Johnson, R. C., and B. J. B. Johnson.** 1997. Lyme disease: serodiagnosis of *Borrelia burgdorferi* sensu lato infection, p. 526–533. *In* R. R. Noel, E. Conway de Macario, J. D. Folds, H. C. Lane, and R. M. Nakamura (ed.), *Manual of Clinical Laboratory Immunology*, 5th ed. ASM Press, Washington, D.C.

54. **Johnson, R. C., G. P. Schmid, F. W. Hyde, A. G. Steigerwald, and D. J. Brenner.** 1984. *Borrelia burgdorferi* sp. nov.: etiologic agent of Lyme disease. *Int. J. Syst. Bacteriol.* **34:**496–497.

55. **Johnson, W. D., Jr.** 1995. *Borrelia* species (relapsing fever), p. 2141–2143. *In* G. L. Mandell, J. E. Bennett, and R. Dolin (ed.), *Mandell, Douglas and Bennett's Principles and Practice of Infectious Diseases*, 4th ed. Churchill Livingstone, New York, N.Y.

56. **Kahl, O., C. Janetzki-Mittmann, J. S. Gray, R. Jonas, J. Stein, and R. de Boer.** 1998. Risk of infection with *Borrelia burgdorferi* sensu lato for a host in relation to the duration of nymphal *Ixodes ricinus* feeding and the method of tick removal. *Zentbl. Bakteriol.* **287:**41–52.

57. **Kaiser, R., and S. Rauer.** 1999. Advantage of recombinant borrelial proteins for serodiganosis of neuroborreliosis. *J. Med. Microbiol.* **48:**5–10.

58. **Kaiser, R., and S. Rauer.** 1999. Serodiagnosis of neuroborreliosis: comparison of reliability of three confirmatory assays. *Infection* **27:**177–181.

59. **Klempner, M. S., C. H. Schmid, L. Hu, A. C. Steere, G. Johnson, B. McCloud, R. Noring, and A. Weinstein.** 2001. Intralaboratory reliability of serologic and urine testing for Lyme disease. *Am. J. Med.* **110:**217–219.

60. **Kurtenbach, K., H.-S. Sewell, N. H. Ogden, S. E. Randolph, and P. A. Nuttall.** 1998. Serum complement sensitivity as a key factor in Lyme disease ecology. *Infect. Immun.* **66:**1248–1251.

61. **Lawrenz, M. B., J. M. Hardham, R. T. Owens, J. Nowakowski, A. C. Steere, G. P. Wormser, and S. J. Norris.** 1999. Human antibody responses to VlsE antigenic variation protein of *Borrelia burgdorferi*. *J. Clin. Microbiol.* **37:**3997–4004.

62. **Le Fleche, A., D. Postic, K. Girardet, O. Peter, and G. Baranton.** 1997. Characterization of *Borrelia lusitaniae* sp. nov. by 16S ribosomal DNA sequence analysis. *Int. J. Syst. Bacteriol.* **47:**921–925.

63. **Li, C., M. A. Motaleb, M. Sal, S. F. Goldstein, and N. W. Charon.** 2000. Spirochete periplasmic flagella and motility. *J. Mol. Microbiol. Biotechnol.* **2:**345–354.

64. **Liang, F. T., E. Aberer, M. Cinco, L. Gern, C. M. Hu, Y. N. Lobet, M. Ruscio, P. E. Voet, V. E. Weynants, and M. T. Philipp.** 2000. Antigenic conservation of an immunodominant invariable region of the VlsE lipoprotein among European pathogenic genospecies of *Borrelia burgdorferi* s.l. *J. Infect. Dis.* **182:**1455–1462.

65. **Livey, I., C. P. Gibbs, R. Schuster, and F. Dorner.** 1995. Evidence for lateral transfer and recombination in OspC variation in Lyme disease *Borrelia*. *Mol. Microbiol.* **18:**257–269.

66. **Luft, B. J., C. R. Steinman, H. C. Neimark, B. Muralidhar, T. Rush, M. Finkel, M. Kunkel, and R. J. Dattwyler.** 1992. Invasion of the central nervous system by Borrelia burgdorferi in acute disseminated infection. *JAMA* **267:**1364–1367.

67. **Marconi, R. T., and C. F. Garon.** 1992. Phylogenetic analysis of the genus *Borrelia*: a comparison of North American and European isolates of *Borrelia burgdorferi*. *J. Bacteriol.* **174:**241–244.

68. **Marconi, R. T., D. S. Samuels, and C. F. Garon.** 1993. Transcriptional analyses and mapping of the *ospC* gene in Lyme disease spirochetes. *J. Bacteriol.* **175:**926–932.

69. **Nocton, J. J., F. Dressler, B. J. Rutledge, P. N. Rys, D. H. Persing, and A. C. Steere.** 1994. Detection of *Borrelia burgdorferi* DNA by polymerase chain reaction in synovial fluid from patients with Lyme arthritis. *N. Engl. J. Med.* **330:**229–234.

70. **Olsen, B., D. C. Duffy, T. G. T. Jaenson, Å. Gylfe, J. Bonnedahl, and S. Bergström.** 1995. Transhemispheric exchange of Lyme disease spirochetes by seabirds. *J. Clin. Microbiol.* **33:**3270–3274.

71. **Pfister, H.-W., B. Wilske, and K. Weber.** 1994. Lyme borreliosis: basic science and clinical aspects. *Lancet* **343:**1013–1016.

72. **Picken, M. M., R. N. Picken, D. Han, Y. Cheng, E. Ruzic-Sabljic, J. Cimperman, V. Maraspin, S. Lotric-Furlan, and F. Strle.** 1997. A two year prospective study to compare culture and polymerase chain reaction amplification for the detection and diagnosis of Lyme borreliosis. *Mol. Pathol.* **50:**186–193.

73. **Plasterk, R. H. A., M. I. Simon, and A. G. Barbour.** 1985. Transposition of structural genes to an expression sequence on a linear plasmid causes antigenic variation in the bacterium *Borrelia hermsii*. *Nature* **318:**257–263.

74. **Pollack, R. J., S. R. Telford III, and A. Spielman.** 1993. Standardization of medium for culturing Lyme disease spirochetes. *J. Clin. Microbiol.* **31:**1251–1255.

75. **Porcella, S. F., S. J. Raffel, M. E. Schrumpf, M. E. Schriefer, D. T. Dennis, and T. G. Schwan.** 2000. Serodiagnosis of louse-borne relapsing fever with glycerophosphodiester phosphodiesterease (GlpQ) from *Borrelia recurrentis*. *J. Clin. Microbiol.* **38:**3561–3571.

76. **Postic, D., M. V. Assous, P. A. D. Grimont, and G. Baranton.** 1994. Diversity of *Borrelia burgdorferi* sensu lato evidenced by restriction fragment length polymorphism of *rrf* (5S)-*rrl* (23S) intergenic spacer amplicons. *Int. J. Syst. Bacteriol.* **44:**743–752.

77. **Preac-Mursic, V.** 1993. Antibiotic susceptibility of *Borrelia burgdorferi* in vitro and in vivo, p. 301–311. *In* K. Weber and W. Burgdorfer (ed.), *Aspects of Lyme Borreliosis*. Springer, Berlin, Germany.

78. Preac-Mursic, V., H.-W. Pfister, H. Spiegel, R. Burk, B. Wilske, S. Reinhardt, and R. Boehmer. 1993. First isolation of *Borrelia burgdorferi* from an iris biopsy. *J. Clin. Neurol. Ophthalmol.* **13:**155–161.

79. Preac-Mursic, V., K. Weber, H.-W. Pfister, B. Wilske, B. Gross, A. Baumann, and J. Prokop. 1989. Survival of *Borrelia burgdorferi* in antibiotically treated patients with Lyme borreliosis. *Infection* **17:**355–359.

80. Preac-Mursic, V., B. Wilske, E. Patsouris, S. Jauris, G. Will, E. Soutschek, S. Reinhardt, G. Lehnert, U. Klockmann, and P. Mehraein. 1992. Active immunization with pC protein of *Borrelia burgdorferi* protects gerbils against *Borrelia burgdorferi* infection. *Infection* **20:**342–349.

81. Preac-Mursic, V., B. Wilske, and S. Reinhardt. 1991. Culture of *Borrelia burgdorferi* on six solid media. *Eur. J. Microbiol. Infect. Dis.* **10:**1076–1079.

82. Priem, S., M. G. Rittig, T. Kamradt, G. R. Burmester, and A. Krause. 1997. An optimized PCR leads to rapid and highly sensitive detection of *Borrelia burgdorferi* in patients with Lyme borreliosis. *J. Clin. Microbiol.* **35:**685–690.

83. Rijpkema, S. G. T., D. J. Tazelaar, M. J. C. H. Molkenboer, G. T. Noordhoek, G. Plantinga, L. M. Schouls, and J. F. P. Schellekens. 1997. Detection of *Borrelia afzelii*, *Borrelia burgdorferi* sensu stricto, *Borrelia garinii* and group VS116 by PCR in skin biopsies of patients with erythema migrans and acrodermatitis chronica atrophicans. *Clin. Microbiol. Infect.* **3:**109–116.

84. Roth, A., H. Mauch, and U. B. Göbel. 1997. *MIQ1, Nucleic Acid Amplification Techniques*, 2nd ed. *Qualitätsstandards in der Mikrobiologisch-Infektiologischen Diagnostik.* H. Mauch and S. Lütticken (ed.). Urban & Fischer Verlag, Munich, Germany.

85. Russell, H., J. S. Sampson, G. P. Schmid, H. W. Wilkinson, and B. Plikaytis. 1984. Enzyme-linked immunosorbent assay and indirect immunofluorescence assay for Lyme disease. *J. Infect. Dis.* **149:**465–470.

86. Sadziene, A., B. Wilske, M. S. Ferdows, and A. G. Barbour. 1993. The cryptic *ospC* gene of *Borrelia burgdorferi* B31 is located on a circular plasmid. *Infect. Immun.* **61:**2192–2195.

87. Schaible, U. E., M. D. Kramer, K. Eichmann, M. Modolell, C. Museteanu, and M. M. Simon. 1990. Monoclonal antibodies specific for the outer surface protein (OspA) prevent Lyme borreliosis in severe combined immunodeficiency (scid) mice. *Proc. Natl. Acad. Sci. USA* **87:**3768–3772.

88. Schmidt, B. L. 1997. PCR in laboratory diagnosis of human *Borrelia burgdorferi* infections. *Clin. Microbiol. Rev.* **10:**185–201.

89. Schwan, T. G., W. Burgdorfer, and P. A. Rosa. 1999. Borrelia, p. 746–758. *In* P. R. Murray, E. J. Baron, M. A. Pfaller, F. C. Tenover, and R. H. Yolken (ed.), *Manual of Clinical Microbiology*, 8th ed. ASM Press, Washington, D.C.

90. Schwan, T. G., K. L. Gage, R. H. Karstens, M. E. Schrumpf, S. F. Hayes, and A. G. Barbour. 1992. Identification of the tick-borne relapsing fever spirochete *Borrelia hermsii* by using a species-specific monoclonal antibody. *J. Clin. Microbiol.* **30:**790–795.

91. Schwan, T. G., J. Piesman, W. T. Golde, M. C. Dolan, and P. A. Rosa. 1995. Induction of an outer surface protein on *Borrelia burgdorferi* during tick feeding. *Proc. Natl. Acad. Sci. USA* **92:**2909–2913.

92. Schwan, T. G., M. E. Schrumpf, B. J. Hinnebusch, D. E. Anderson, Jr., and M. E. Konkel. 1996. GlpQ: an antigen for serological discrimination between relapsing fever and Lyme borreliosis. *J. Clin. Microbiol.* **34:**2483–2492.

93. Sonenshine, D. E. 1991. *Biology of Ticks*, p. 1–447. Oxford University Press, New York, N.Y.

94. Southern, P. M., and J. P. Sanford. 1969. Relapsing fever: a clinical and microbiological review. *Medicine* **48:**129–149.

95. Steere, A. C. 1989. Medical progress—Lyme disease. *N. Engl. J. Med.* **321:**586–596.

96. Steere, A. C., V. P. Berardi, K. E. Weeks, E. L. Logigian, and R. Ackermann. 1990. Evaluation of the intrathecal antibody response to *Borrelia burgdorferi* as a diagnostic test for Lyme neuroborreliosis. *J. Infect. Dis.* **161:**1203–1209.

97. Steere, A. C., V. K. Sikand, F. Meurice, D. L. Parenti, E. Fikrig, R. T. Schoen, J. Nowakowski, C. H. Schmid, S. Laukamp, C. Buscarino, D. S. Krause, and The Lyme Disease Vaccine Study Group. 1998. Vaccination against Lyme disease with recombinant *Borrelia burgdorferi* outer-surface lipoprotein A with adjuvant. *N. Engl. J. Med.* **339:**209–215.

98. Vasiliu, V., P. Herzer, D. Rössler, G. Lehnert, and B. Wilske. 1998. Heterogeneity of *Borrelia burgdorferi* sensu lato demonstrated by an *ospA*-type-specific PCR in synovial fluid from patients with Lyme arthritis. *Med. Microbiol. Immunol.* **187:**97–102.

99. Wang, G., A. P. van Dam, and J. Dankert. 1999. Phenotypic and genetic characterization of a novel *Borrelia burgdorferi* sensu lato isolate from a patient with Lyme borreliosis. *J. Clin. Microbiol.* **37:**3025–3028.

100. Wang, G., A. P. van Dam, I. Schwartz, and J. Dankert. 1999. Molecular typing of *Borrelia burgdorferi* sensu lato taxonomic, epidemiological, and clinical implications. *Clin. Microbiol. Rev.* **12:**633–653.

101. Wayne, L. G., D. J. Brenner, R. R. Colwell, P. A. D. Grimont, O. Kandler, M. I. Krichevsky, I. H. Moore, W. E. C. Moore, R. G. E. Murray, E. Stackebrandt, M. P. Starr, and H. G. Trüper. 1987. Report of the Ad Hoc Committee on Reconciliation of Approaches to Bacterial Systematics. *Int. J. Syst. Bacteriol.* **37:**463–464.

102. Weber, K., and W. Burgdorfer. 1993. *Aspects of Lyme Borreliosis*. Springer, Berlin, Germany.

103. Weber, K., and H.-W. Pfister. 1994. Clinical management of Lyme borreliosis. *Lancet* **343:**1017–1020.

104. Wilske, B., U. Busch, H. Eiffert, V. Fingerle, H.-W. Pfister, D. Rössler, and V. Preac-Mursic. 1996. Diversity of OspA and OspC among cerebrospinal fluid isolates of *Borrelia burgdorferi* sensu lato from patients with neuroborreliosis in Germany. *Med. Microbiol. Immunol.* **184:**195–201.

105. Wilske, B., U. Busch, V. Fingerle, S. Jauris-Heipke, V. Preac-Mursic, D. Rössler, and G. Will. 1996. Immunological and molecular variability of OspA and OspC. Implications for *Borrelia* vaccine development. *Infection* **24:**208–212.

106. Wilske, B., V. Fingerle, P. Herzer, A. Hofmann, G. Lehnert, H. Peters, H.-W. Pfister, V. Preac-Mursic, E. Soutschek, and K. Weber. 1993. Recombinant immunoblot in the serodiagnosis of Lyme borreliosis. *Med. Microbiol. Immunol.* **182:**255–270.

107. Wilske, B., C. Habermann, V. Fingerle, B. Hillenbrand, S. Jauris-Heipke, G. Lehnert, I. Pradel, D. Rössler, and U. Schulte-Spechtel. 1999. An improved recombinant IgG immunoblot for serodiagnosis of Lyme borreliosis. *Med. Microbiol. Immunol.* **188:**139–144.

108. Wilske, B., and V. Preac-Mursic. 1993. Microbiological diagnosis of Lyme borreliosis, p. 267–300. *In* K. Weber and W. Burgdorfer (ed.), *Aspects of Lyme Borreliosis*. Springer, Berlin, Germany.

109. Wilske, B., V. Preac-Mursic, U. B. Göbel, B. Graf, S. Jauris-Heipke, E. Soutschek, E. Schwab, and G. Zumstein. 1993. An OspA serotyping system for *Borrelia burgdorferi* based on reactivity with monoclonal antibod-

ies and OspA sequence analysis. *J. Clin. Microbiol.* **31:** 340–350.

110. **Wilske, B., V. Preac-Mursic, S. Jauris, A. Hofmann, I. Pradel, E. Soutschek, E. Schwab, G. Will, and G. Wanner.** 1993. Immunological and molecular polymorphisms of OspC, an immunodominant major outer surface protein of *Borrelia burgdorferi. Infect. Immun.* **61:**2182–2191.

111. **Wilske, B., V. Preac-Mursic, G. Schierz, R. Kühbeck, A. G. Barbour, and M. Kramer.** 1988. Antigenic variability of *Borrelia burgdorferi. Ann. N. Y. Acad. Sci.* **539:**126–143.

112. **Wilske, B., G. Schierz, V. Preac-Mursic, K. von Busch, R. Kühbeck, H. W. Pfister, and K. Einhäupl.** 1986. Intrathecal production of specific antibodies against *Borrelia burgdorferi* in patients with lymphocytic meningoradiculitis (Bannwarth's syndrome). *J. Infect. Dis.* **153:** 304–314.

113. **Wilske, B., L. Zöller, V. Brade, M. Eiffert, U. B. Göbel, G. Stanek, and H. W. Pfister.** 2000. *MIQ 12, Lyme-Borreliose. Qualitätsstandards in der Mikrobiologisch-Infektiologischen Diagnostik.* H. Mauch and S. Lütticken (ed.). Urban & Fischer Verlag, Munich, Germany. (English version: http://alpha1.mpk.med.uni-muenchen.de/bak/nrz-borrelia/miq-lyme/index.html or http://www.dghm.org/red/index.html?cname=MIQ.)

114. **Woese, C.** 1987. Bacterial evolution. *Microbiol. Rev.* **51:**221–271.

115. **Wormser, G. P., S. Bittker, D. Cooper, J. Nowakowski, R. B. Nadelman, and C. Pavia.** 2000. Comparison of the yields of blood cultures using serum or plasma from patients with early Lyme disease. *J. Clin. Microbiol.* **38:**1648–1650.

116. **Wormser, G. P., R. B. Nadelman, R. J. Dattwyler, D. T. Dennis, E. D. Shapiro, A. C. Steere, T. J. Rush, D. W. Rahn, P. K. Coyle, D. H. Persing, D. Fish, and B. J. Luft.** 2000. Practice guidelines for the treatment of Lyme disease. *Clin. Infect. Dis.* **31**(Suppl. 1):S1–S14.

117. **Zhang, J.-R., J. M. Hardham, A. G. Barbour, and S. J. Norris.** 1997. Antigenic variation in Lyme disease borreliae by promiscuous recombination of VMP-like sequence cassettes. *Cell* **89:**275–285.

Treponema and Other Human Host-Associated Spirochetes

STEVEN J. NORRIS, VICTORIA POPE, ROBERT E. JOHNSON, AND SANDRA A. LARSEN

61

GENERAL TAXONOMY

The genus *Treponema* (order *Spirochaetales*, family *Spirochaetaceae*) includes four invasive human pathogens (Table 1), a large number of oral spirochetes found in the gingival crevices, and a few commensal skin organisms. In 1984, the nomenclature was restructured so that the species *Treponema pallidum* now includes three of the human pathogens: *T. pallidum* subsp. *pallidum* (venereal syphilis), *T. pallidum* subsp. *endemicum* (endemic syphilis), and *T. pallidum* subsp. *pertenue* (yaws) (109). *T. carateum* (pinta) remains a separate species due to the lack of genetic information. The pathogenic treponemes in this group are very closely related, to the extent that they are distinguished primarily by their patterns of pathogenesis in humans and experimentally infected animals. They are morphologically indistinguishable and, where examined, have >95% DNA homology by hybridization (26), a high degree of sequence identity of known genes (77–79), nearly identical protein profiles (see reference 82 for a review), and shared reactivity with monoclonal antibodies (75). Recent data indicate that there may be some subspecies differences, as well as differences between *T. pallidum* and *T. paraluiscuniculi*, a rabbit pathogen, in the flanking-region sequences of the 15.5-kDa lipoprotein gene (12). In addition, differences in the *tpr* and *arp* genes have been used for the molecular subtyping of *T. pallidum* strains (13, 14, 90); this approach is useful in epidemiologic studies (113). According to structure, host dependence, protein content, and DNA sequence similarities (12), *T. paraluiscuniculi* appears to be closely related to the human pathogens; however, it causes venereal spirochetosis of rabbits and is not known to cause human disease. *Brachyspira aalborgi* and *Brachyspira* (formerly *Serpulina*) *pilosicoli* are recently described intestinal spirochetes found in humans and other animals and are phylogenetically distinct from the other human host-associated spirochetes. Because of the distinctive nature of invasive treponemal pathogens, oral spirochetes, and intestinal spirochetes, these three groups are discussed separately below.

In contrast to the close relationship among the human pathogens, *T. pallidum* subsp. *pallidum* has <5% DNA homology to other spirochetes such as *T. phagedenis*, *T. refringens*, and *Brachyspira* (formerly *Serpulina*) *hyodysenteriae* (26). However, rRNA sequence similarities indicate an evolutionary relationship between the members of the genus *Treponema* (85). The sequence of the 1.13×10^6-bp *T. pallidum* subsp. *pallidum* Nichols genome was published in 1998 (30), and sequencing of the 2.8×10^6-bp genome of the oral spirochete *Treponema denticola* is nearing completion (http://www.tigr.org). The resulting information will be of value in characterizing the similarities and differences of these organisms.

SPIROCHETES ASSOCIATED WITH HUMAN TREPONEMATOSES

Description

T. pallidum subsp. *pallidum* (*T. pallidum*) and related human pathogens are spirochetes ~0.18 μm in diameter and ranging in length from 6 to 20 μm (Fig. 1). These organisms are coiled into regular helices (6 to 14 per cell) with a wavelength of 1.1 μm and an amplitude of ~0.3 μm. The ends are pointed and lack the hook shape characteristic of some commensal human spirochetes. Suspensions of *T. pallidum* are best visualized by dark-field microscopy, although the bacterium can also be seen by phase-contrast microscopy. Unstained organisms are not visible by standard bright-field microscopy because of the small cell diameter. Fresh preparations of the organism exhibit rapid rotation about the axis (the characteristic corkscrew motility) due to the action of flagella inserted in both ends and extending down the cell body within the periplasmic space (Fig. 1). Flexing and reversal of rotation can occur also, but translational motion is not observed unless *T. pallidum* is in a viscous medium. The human treponemal pathogens (Table 1) cannot be distinguished at either the light or electron microscopy level.

T. pallidum subsp. *pallidum* and the other pathogenic treponemes are extremely fastidious organisms that die readily on desiccation or exposure to atmospheric levels of oxygen, and they have not yet been cultured continuously in vitro. Although limited multiplication of *T. pallidum* subsp. *pallidum* has been obtained in a complex tissue culture system (18, 81), this procedure is limited to the research laboratory setting. Direct culture of *T. pallidum* from clinical specimens has not been accomplished.

TABLE 1 Characteristics of the human treponematoses[a]

Organism	Disease	Distribution	Predominant age of onset	Transmission	Congenital infection
T. pallidum subsp. pallidum	Venereal syphilis	Worldwide	Adolescents, adults	Sexual contact	Yes
T. pallidum subsp. pertenue	Yaws (frambesia, pian)	Tropical areas, Africa, South America, Caribbean, Indonesia	Children	Skin contact	No
T. pallidum subsp. endemicum	Endemic syphilis (bejel, dichuchwa)	Arid areas, Africa, Middle East	Children to adults	Mucous membrane	Rarely
T. carateum	Pinta (carate, cute)	Semiarid warm areas, Central and South America	Children, adolescents	Skin contact	No

[a] Data from references 23, 24, 87, 88, and 119.

Natural Habitat

The *T. pallidum* subspecies and *T. carateum* are obligate parasites of humans and are not known to have any animal or environmental reservoirs. Venereal syphilis has a worldwide distribution, with the incidence varying widely according to geographic location and socioeconomic group

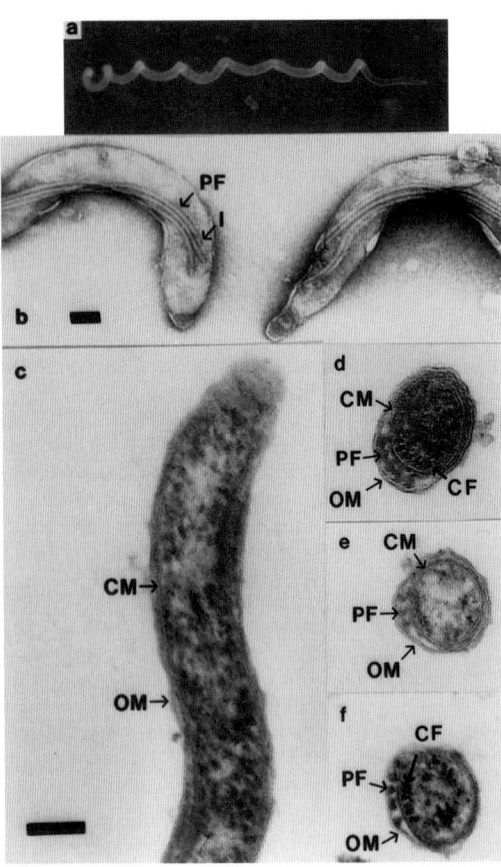

FIGURE 1 Morphology of *T. pallidum*. (a) Scanning electron micrograph showing spiral shape. (b) Negatively stained view of the tips of two organisms. Note the insertion points (I) of periplasmic flagella (PF) near the ends. (c to f) Electron micrographs of ultrathin sections, showing the outer membrane (OM), the cytoplasmic membrane (CM), periplasmic flagella (PF), and the location of the cytoplasmic filaments (CF). Bars, 0.1 μm. (Reprinted from reference 80a with permission of Kluwer.)

(Table 1). Endemic syphilis is restricted to desert and temperate regions of North Africa and the Middle East. Yaws occurs most commonly in tropical or desert regions of Africa, South America, and Indonesia. Pinta is found primarily in tropical areas of Central and South America.

Clinical Significance

Syphilis is still a common sexually transmitted disease in many areas of the world, despite the availability of effective therapy. In 1999, the World Health Organization estimated that the worldwide annual incidence of sexually acquired syphilis was 12 million cases (121). In the United States, 31,575 cases were reported in 2000, including 5,979 cases of primary and secondary syphilis and 529 cases of congenital syphilis in infants younger than 1 year. The reported incidence in the United States has decreased dramatically from the 135,043 total reported cases at the peak of a syphilis epidemic in 1990 (21). The national rate of reported primary and secondary syphilis cases has dropped below the year 2000 target of 4 per 100,000 (Fig. 2). Syphilis disproportionately affects African Americans living in poverty in the United States; overall, the rate of primary and secondary cases is 21-fold greater in non-Hispanic blacks than in non-Hispanic whites. Over 50% of the reported primary and secondary syphilis cases are localized in 21 counties and one city. This concentration of incident syphilis provides an opportunity to focus intensive control activities. In 1999, the U.S. Centers for Disease Control and Prevention (CDC), in collaboration with other federal partners, launched a National Plan To Eliminate Syphilis in the United States, using a combination of improved surveillance, strengthened community involvement, rapid outbreak response, expanded clinical and laboratory services, and enhanced health promotion (http://www.cdc.gov/stopsyphilis/Plan.pdf). Syphilis elimination is defined as the absence of sustained transmission (i.e., no transmission after 90 days of the report of an imported index case). The overall goal is to reduce the number of primary and secondary syphilis cases to ≤1,000 per year and to increase the proportion of syphilis-free counties to >90% by 2005. An attempt to extend eradication efforts worldwide would present additional challenges (100).

Transmission of *T. pallidum* infection occurs through direct contact with active lesions. The transmission of *T. pallidum* subsp. *pallidum* infection, the cause of venereal syphilis, usually occurs consequent to contact with lesions of an infected individual during sexual intercourse. Transplacental infection of the fetus also occurs in infected pregnant women.

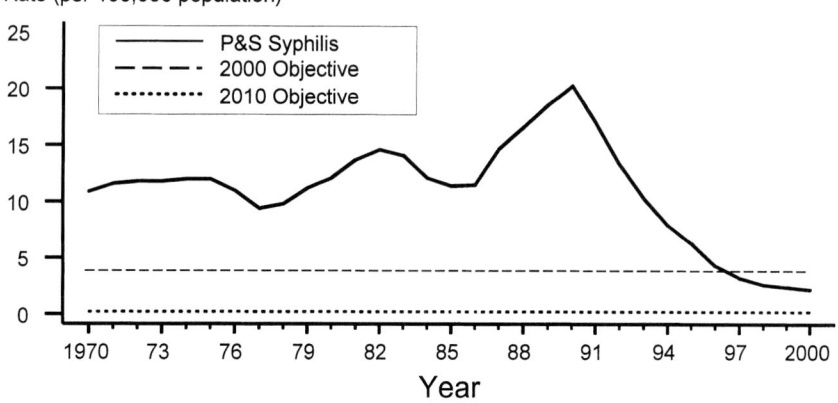

FIGURE 2 Rates of reported primary and secondary syphilis cases per 100,000 population in the United States, 1970 to 2000. The objectives of ≤4 cases per 100,000 for the year 2000 and 0.2 case per 100,000 in 2010 are indicated. Source: CDC.

Venereal syphilis exhibits a wide variety of clinical manifestations (Table 2). The natural history of venereal syphilis is divided into early and late syphilis. Early syphilis is defined by the Centers for Disease Control and Prevention (CDC) as the first year of infection, the interval during which an individual was potentially infectious. Transmission is rare in cases of longer than 1 year's duration, defined as late syphilis.

Early syphilis is itself subdivided into primary, secondary, and early latent stages. The primary stage is characterized by the appearance of one or more 0.3- to 2.0-cm indurated lesions which typically are painless and usually become encrusted or ulcerated. These lesions, called chancres, occur at the point of organism entry after a 10- to 90-day incubation period and contain large numbers of *T. pallidum* organisms. Chancres are generally located in the anogenital region, and in women they may be present on the vagina or cervix and hence may not be readily observed. The lesions may also occur on the lips, oral mucosa, fingers, or other areas of contact. Secondary syphilis is a disseminated infection characterized by protean dermatologic manifestations that are not localized to the site of organism entry and may be accompanied by fever and malaise. Typically, multiple lesions are observed and may be either macular or papular in appearance. Additional dermatologic manifestations include patchy hair loss and rashes, which vary in appearance from macular to papular. So-called "nickel and dime" macular lesions on the palms of the hands, soles of the feet, and other locations are a common presentation. Raised lesions called condylomata lata may occur in moist intertriginous areas, and erosions called mucous patches may appear on mucosa, such as in the mouth. Neurologic symptoms and signs and, less commonly, disease manifestations involving other organ systems may also occur during secondary stage syphilis. Although dissemination of *T. pallidum* occurs early in infection, these secondary-syphilis manifestations, which reflect dissemination, do not appear until 6 weeks to 6 months after infection. Primary and secondary syphilis manifestations may overlap, but each resolves spontaneously within a few weeks of onset.

Numerous treponemes are often present in the ulcers of primary syphilis and the moist intertriginous and mucosal lesions of secondary syphilis. Transmission occurs as a consequence of contact with these primary- and secondary-stage lesions. Nonvenereal transmission is rare. Individuals with venereal syphilis are no longer infectious after healing of secondary syphilis lesions. However, relapses of secondary syphilis can occur in about 25% of untreated patients. Such relapses are uncommon after the first year of infection (33).

Latent syphilis consists of the intervals between or following episodes of primary and secondary syphilis when the infected individual demonstrates no clinical manifestations of disease. In the CDC definition, early latent syphilis consists of intervals of latency occurring within the first year of infection. Late latent syphilis is defined as asymptomatic syphilis occurring more than 12 months after the appearance of the primary chancre. About 60 to 85% of persons with untreated late latent syphilis will remain in the latent stage for life. Two-thirds of the syphilis cases reported in the United States are diagnosed during latent infection and are identified primarily through a combination of serologic reactivity, patient history, and case tracing.

Tertiary (late) syphilis consists of the disease manifestations of syphilis that may occur after extended periods (usually years to decades) of late latent syphilis. Longitudinal observations of untreated syphilis patients at the beginning of the 20th century indicated that approximately one-third remain latently infected for life, one-third undergo "biological cure" (i.e., lose serologic reactivity), and the remaining one-third develop late syphilis (33). The manifestations of late syphilis consist of several characteristic conditions of the central nervous system, disease of the aortic valve and thoracic aorta, and a chronic inflammatory condition called a gumma, which usually involves the skin or bone but may occur in any organ (119). The cardiovascular and gummatous forms of syphilis are now rarely encountered, presumably because of effective therapy of early syphilis and antimicrobial therapy administered for other infections.

Recent studies have shown that viable *T. pallidum* is present in the cerebrospinal fluid (CSF) of patients with the primary and secondary stages of syphilis, indicating that central nervous system infection occurs very early in the course of disease (58). Neurologic manifestations, including syphilitic meningitis, may occur as early as 3 months postinfection; thus, neurosyphilis should not be considered solely

TABLE 2 Common manifestations of treponematoses

Venereal syphilis (*T. pallidum* subsp. *pallidum*)
  Primary (local): 10–90 days postinfection (average, 21 days)
    Chancre (single or multiple, skin or mucous membranes)
    Regional lymphadenopathy
  Secondary (disseminated): 6 wk–6 mo postinfection
    Multiple secondary lesions (skin or mucous membranes)
    Generalized lymphadenopathy, fever, malaise
    Condylomata lata
    Alopecia
    Asymptomatic or symptomatic CNS[a] involvement
      (meningovascular syphilis)
  Latent (early, ≤1 yr duration; late, >1 yr duration)
    Reactive serologic tests for syphilis
    Asymptomatic
  Tertiary (late, chronic): months to years postinfection
    Gummatous (monocytic infiltrates, tissue destruction, any
      organ)
    Cardiovascular (aortic aneurysm)
    Late forms of neurosyphilis (paresis, tabes dorsalis, optic
      atrophy)
  Congenital
    Early (onset, <2 years): fulminant, disseminated infection,
      mucocutaneous lesions, osteochondritis, anemia,
      hepatosplenomegaly, CNS involvement
    Late (persistence, >2 years): interstitial keratitis, bone and
      tooth deformities, eighth-nerve deafness, neurosyphilis,
      other tertiary manifestations

Yaws (*T. pallidum* subsp. *pertenue*)
  Early: onset 9–90 days postinfection (average, 21 days)
    Primary lesion (mother yaw): papular, nontender, often
      pruritic, crusted or ulcerated
    Disseminated lesions (daughter yaws): often resemble
      primary lesion, or varied appearance
    Malaise, fever, lymphadenopathy
    Osteitis, periostitis, other bone and joint manifestations
  Latent: positive serologic tests, no other signs of infection
  Late: 10% of patients
    Destructive lesions of bone and cartilage (e.g., ulcerative
      rhinopharyngitis)
    Hyperkeratotic skin lesions

Endemic syphilis (*T. pallidum* subsp. *endemicum*)
  Early
    Primary lesion not usually detected
    Secondary: multiple oropharyngeal, cutaneous lesions
    Generalized lymphadenopathy
    Periostitis
  Latent: positive serologic tests, no other signs of infection
  Late: destructive skin, bone, and cartilage lesions

Pinta (*T. carateum*): restricted to skin
  Early
    Initial lesion: hyperkeratotic, pigmented papule or plaque
    Disseminated skin lesions (pintids)
    Regional lymphadenopathy
  Late: pigmentary changes in skin (hyper- and
    hypopigmentation)

_____
[a] CNS, central nervous system.

a late manifestation of the disease (42). Numerous case reports indicate that human immunodeficiency virus (HIV) infection may result in an increased severity of early syphilis and a poor response to therapy (98), although the results of prospective therapy trials suggest that HIV infection does not markedly affect the natural history of syphilis in most instances of coinfection (98, 101).

Congenital syphilis results from the transmission of *T. pallidum* across the placenta during pregnancy (31). Early congenital syphilis tends to occur when the mother has early syphilis during the course of pregnancy and may result in stillbirth or fulminant infection of the newborn (Table 2). Late manifestations of congenital syphilis are the outcome of chronic, untreated infection and can result in multiple stigmata (Table 2) that are often not obvious until the second decade of life.

Yaws, endemic syphilis, and pinta were common infections in areas of endemic infection prior to the World Health Organization's eradication program that began in 1948; in the early 1950s, it was estimated that 200 million people were exposed to yaws during their lifetimes (87). Nowadays, areas where the diseases are endemic are more restricted, but decreased surveillance has led to a recrudescence of infection in many areas (63). Transmission of endemic treponematoses occurs through direct contact with early lesions or with contaminated fingers or drinking or eating utensils. Yaws and endemic syphilis commonly are transmitted among children (2 to 15 years of age), whereas pinta usually has a later onset (ages 15 to 30 years). Many of the manifestations of yaws and endemic syphilis are similar to those of veneral syphilis (Table 2); the lesions of pinta appear to be restricted to the skin. Congenital transmission of the endemic treponematoses is rare.

Detection and Identification of *T. pallidum* in Tissue and Tissue Exudates

General Principles

Treponemes are not readily detectable with common laboratory stains but can be visualized using dark-field microscopy, the direct fluorescent-antibody–*T. pallidum* (DFA-TP) test, or immunohistochemistry (IHC) methods (37). Currently, dark-field microscopy and DFA-TP tests are commonly used to detect *T. pallidum* in primary- or secondary-lesion exudates, while a modification of the DFA-TP for tissue (DFAT-TP) (52) and IHC are used for tissue sections. Because of the technical challenges of dark-field microscopy, DFA-TP is recommended for all but the most experienced laboratories. Similarly, silver-staining techniques (114) commonly used in the past for histologic staining of treponemes are both problematic and nonspecific and should be replaced by the more reliable immunologic procedures. PCR has been introduced as a method for detecting *T. pallidum* infection (as described subsequently) but is not widely available at present.

Specimen Collection

Specimens collected from the epidermal and mucosal lesions of primary, secondary, and early congenital syphilis are most useful, because the lesions tend to contain high concentrations of treponemes. Active lesions prior to the healing stages serve as the best source of organisms. The site should be cleansed and gently abraded with sterile gauze and saline until a serous exudate appears. A specimen for dark-field microscopy is collected on a glass slide and covered with a coverslip; a specimen for DFA-TP examination

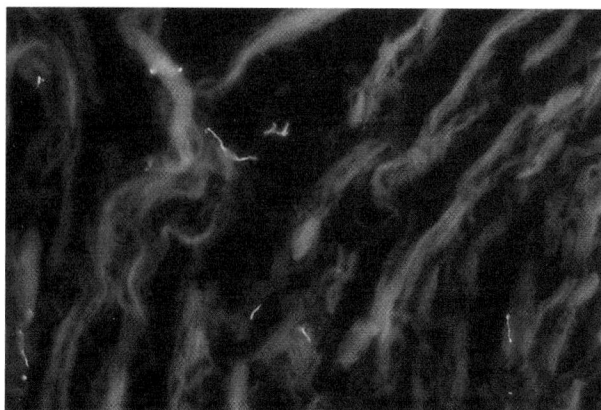

FIGURE 3 DFAT-TP of an umbilical cord section from an infant with congenital syphilis.

of serous fluids is collected on a slide and then air dried. The specimen should consist of serous fluid free of erythrocytes, other organisms, and tissue debris. Tissue specimens for DFAT-TP or IHC should be from formalin-fixed, paraffin-embedded sections cut 2 μm thick.

Detection Methods

When dark-field microscopy is used, the potential presence of morphologically similar, nonpathogenic spirochetes within and near the genitalia requires that *T. pallidum* be viewed in its "living state" to observe its characteristic morphology and motility. Furthermore, it is difficult or impossible to differentiate *T. pallidum* from other parasitic spirochetes of the gastrointestinal tract by using dark-field microscopy; therefore, samples from oral or rectal lesions should be examined by the DFA-TP test, because the conjugates used are specific for pathogenic strains of *Treponema*. Exudates should be examined as soon as possible (ideally within 20 min) to ensure retention of motility. *T. pallidum* is very sensitive to exposure to oxygen, heat, nonphysiologic pH, and desiccation.

Samples for DFA-TP are air dried onto slides and therefore do not require cell viability or immediate examination. Either labeled polyclonal anti-*T. pallidum* antibody (ViroStat, Portland, Maine) or labeled monoclonal antibody (CDC, Atlanta, Ga.) can be used. Samples for DFA-TP can also be sent to the Syphilis Diagnostic Immunology Section of the CDC for testing.

Tissue sections can be stained using either the IHC stain (Dako, Carpinteria, Calif.) (37) or the DFAT-TP test (52), since both use the *T. pallidum*-specific antibodies for detection. Either monoclonal antibody, which is directed against the 37-kDa flagellar protein, or Reiter-absorbed polyclonal antibody can be used; the absorbed polyclonal antibody is used most commonly. Any tissue can be examined, but most frequently paraffin-embedded sections are made from specimens collected from the skin, brain, gastrointestinal tract, placenta, or umbilical cord (Fig. 3). Often DFAT-TP or IHC is used to diagnose late-stage or congenital syphilis, although organism concentrations tend to be low during late adult syphilis, in congenital syphilis, and in resolving lesions of early syphilis (108). IHC may offer an advantage for use with tissue since a fluorescence microscope is not needed and the hematoxylin counterstain permits the examination of tissue structure simultaneously with the observation of treponemes (37).

The oldest and most definitive method for detection of *T. pallidum* infection is rabbit infectivity testing (RIT) (118). This technique probably offers the most sensitive method of detecting infectious treponemes (60) and is used as the "gold standard" for measuring the sensitivities of detection methods such as the PCR (36, 105). However, use of RIT is limited to research settings.

The newest technique for direct detection of *T. pallidum* is PCR (36, 56, 89, 105). PCR as a tool for detecting *T. pallidum* is used by only a few laboratories and is considered an experimental procedure for syphilis diagnosis. However, the PCR test is available at CDC for specimens from patients with suspected neurosyphilis (i.e., reactive serum serology, abnormal CSF or neurologic findings, and a history of syphilis) or patients with genital ulcer disease. The test also appears useful in detecting congenital syphilis, with sensitivity equivalent to RIT for amniotic fluid samples (10, 41, 73).

The optimal sample source for PCR is controversial (80). For example, one study found whole blood and lesion material, both exudate and tissue, to be satisfactory samples for PCR, whereas the appropriateness of serum and CSF as sample sources for PCR is still under consideration (80, 120). Purification of DNA from the sample is important in terms of sensitivity and reproducibility, due to the presence of components in tissue and serum that may inhibit PCR amplification. Contamination of the samples collected for PCR with extraneous DNA from other specimens can be a major problem and may account for some of the variable results noted by some researchers. Also, storage and transport of the sample prior to testing may seriously affect the results (120).

Serologic Tests

General Principles

Humoral antibodies produced in response to *T. pallidum* infection become detectable in the primary stage, increase in concentration during the secondary stage, and decline during latent infection. Antibody detection tests supplement the direct organism detection methods used for the diagnosis of primary and secondary syphilis and are the only practical methods of diagnosis during latent and late syphilis.

Available serologic tests for syphilis are subdivided into nontreponemal and treponemal assays (Table 3). Nontreponemal tests detect so-called reaginic antibodies that react with lipoidal particles containing the phospholipid cardiolipin. They are commonly used for screening and have the advantage of being widely available, inexpensive, convenient to perform on large numbers of specimens, and useful for determining the efficacy of treatment. Limitations of the nontreponemal serologic tests include their lack of sensitivity in early primary syphilis cases and in late syphilis and the possibilities of a prozone reaction or of false-positive results. Treponemal tests use *T. pallidum* subsp. *pallidum* or its derivatives (e.g., recombinant proteins) as the antigen and detect anti-*T. pallidum* antibodies. In the United States, treponemal tests have been used primarily to verify reactivity in the nontreponemal tests. The treponemal tests also may be used to confirm a clinical impression of late syphilis in which the nontreponemal test is nonreactive. Unfortunately, treponemal tests are technically more difficult and costly to perform than nontreponemal tests and cannot be used to monitor treatment or reinfection. For 85% of persons who are successfully treated,

TABLE 3 Sensitivity and specificity of serologic tests for syphilis

Test	Sensitivity (%)[a]				Specificity (nonsyphilis) (%)[a]
	Primary	Secondary	Latent	Late	
Nontreponemal tests					
VDRL	78 (74–87)	100	95 (88–100)	71 (37–94)	98 (96–99)
RPR card	86 (77–100)	100	98 (95–100)	73	98 (93–99)
USR	80 (72–88)	100	95 (88–100)		99
TRUST	85 (77–86)	100	98 (95–100)		99 (98–99)
Treponemal tests					
FTA-ABS	84 (70–100)	100	100	96	97 (94–100)
FTA-ABS DS	80 (69–90)	100	100		98 (97–100)
TP-PA	88 (86–100)	100	100		96 (95–100)
IgG EIA	—————————— 97 (97–100) ——————————		[b]		99 (98–100)

[a] Ranges in CDC studies are given in parentheses.
[b] Not broken down by stage of syphilis.

treponemal test results remain reactive for years, if not for life.

Specimen Collection

Universal safety precautions should be observed when collecting, preparing, and examining specimens (52). Serum is the specimen of choice for both nontreponemal and treponemal tests. However, the rapid plasma reagin (RPR) card test and toluidine red unheated serum test (TRUST) may also be performed with plasma samples. The technician must check the product insert to be sure that the plasma sample has not been stored for longer than the recommended storage time and that the blood was collected in the specified anticoagulant. Plasma cannot be used in the VDRL test, since the sample must be heated before testing; in addition, plasma cannot be used in the treponemal tests for syphilis. The Venereal Disease Research Laboratory (VDRL) test is the only nontreponemal test that can be used for testing CSF. The CSF is not heated before the test is performed. The fluorescent treponemal antibody-absorption (FTA-ABS) test can be used with CSF specimens to rule out syphilis, but the test may be reactive in persons who do not have neurosyphilis (46).

When screening for congenital syphilis, CDC recommends testing of the mother's serum rather than cord blood. Recent studies compared the reactivity of the mother's serum, cord blood, and infant's serum and found that the maternal sample is the best indicator of infection, followed by neonatal serum; cord blood is the least reactive (15). Infant's serum is the specimen of choice for the immunoglobulin M (IgM)-specific tests.

Nontreponemal Tests

All available nontreponemal tests are based on an antigen composed of an alcoholic solution containing measured amounts of cardiolipin, cholesterol, and sufficient purified lecithin to produce standard reactivity (53). The nontreponemal (reagin) tests measure IgM and IgG antibodies to lipoidal material released from damaged host cells as well as antibodies to lipoprotein-like material and possibly cardiolipin released from the treponemes (4, 62). The antilipoidal antibodies can be produced not only as a consequence of treponemal infections but also during autoimmune diseases, pregnancy, nontreponemal diseases of an acute and chronic nature in which tissue damage occurs, and other conditions (Table 4).

The standard nontreponemal tests use flocculation of lipoidal particles to indicate reactivity. The test antigen is mixed with the patient's serum on a solid matrix and rotated for a specified number of minutes before the results are read. The lipid particles are too small to be visualized without magnification unless a colored reagent (e.g., carbon particles) is added. Likewise, the antigen-antibody complex that occurs with serum from individuals with syphilis remains suspended, and flocculation rather than agglutination or precipitation occurs. The VDRL and unheated serum reagin (USR) tests are flocculation tests requiring microscopic examination, whereas reactions in the RPR test and TRUST, because of the addition of colored particles, can be read without magnification. All of the nontreponemal tests have approximately the same sensitivity and specificity (Table 3).

TABLE 4 Causes of false-positive reactions in serologic tests for syphilis[a]

Disease or condition	Type of test affected	
	Nontreponemal test	Treponemal test
Autoimmune disease	Yes	Yes
Malaria	Yes	No
Recent immunizations	Yes	No
Dermatologic diseases	Yes	Yes
Cardiovascular disease	Yes	Yes
Tuberculosis	Yes	No
Leprosy	Yes	Yes
Intravenous drug abuse	Yes	No
Viral infections	Yes	No
Febrile illness	Yes	Yes
Pregnancy	Yes	No
HIV	Yes	No
Other sexually transmitted diseases	Yes	No
Age	No	Yes
Multiple blood transfusions	Yes	No
Lyme disease	No	Yes
Endemic treponematoses	Yes	Yes
Transient unknown causes	Yes	Yes
Technical errors	Yes	Yes

[a] Data from references 6, 44, 53, and 59.

Any of these nontreponemal tests can be performed as quantitative tests by preparing serial twofold dilutions of the patient's serum to reach an end-point titer. Qualitative nontreponemal tests are used to screen for syphilis. Quantitative nontreponemal tests establish a baseline of reactivity from which change can be measured following treatment. The baseline serum sample should be drawn on the day that treatment is begun, and the same test that is used in the initial testing should be used to monitor treatment (28, 29, 107). Treatment success is defined by a decrease in titer of at least fourfold within a time interval that varies with stage of infection (10). Conversely, a fourfold increase in titer suggests treatment failure or reinfection.

Qualitative test results for the microscopic tests (the VDRL test and USR test) are reported as reactive, weakly reactive, or nonreactive. Qualitative test results for the macroscopic tests (the RPR card test and TRUST) are reported as reactive (regardless of the size of the flocculant) or nonreactive. Quantitative results may be reported as the reciprocal of the dilution, for example, 4 dils, a titer of 4, or R4 rather than a 1:4 dilution. The end point reported is the last dilution giving a fully reactive, not weakly reactive, result. In direct comparisons, the microscopic VDRL and USR tests often exhibit lower titers than the macroscopic nontreponemal tests, underscoring the need to consistently use the same test in monitoring the treatment efficacy in each patient.

Prozone reactions occur in 1 to 2% of patients with secondary syphilis. Any undiluted serum sample exhibiting a weakly reactive, atypical, or, on rare occasions, "rough negative" reaction should be diluted as in the quantitative assay. In samples exhibiting a prozone effect, the reactivity increases and then decreases as the end-point titer is approached.

In some low-risk populations, false-positive reactions may outnumber true-positive reactions. Nontreponemal test results must be interpreted according to the stage of syphilis suspected and the population being tested and should be confirmed using a treponemal test. When the nontreponemal tests are used as a screening test in a low-risk population, all reactive results should be confirmed with a treponemal test. Approximately 20% of those with early primary syphilis have nonreactive nontreponemal test results on the initial visit (Table 3). In secondary syphilis, nearly all patients have end-point titers of ≥1:8 in nontreponemal tests. For patients with atypical lesions and/or nontreponemal-test titers <1:8, the nontreponemal tests should be repeated and a confirmatory treponemal test should be performed. Even without treatment, the nontreponemal test may be weakly reactive or even nonreactive in the late stages of syphilis.

In congenital syphilis, a paradigm commonly used in the past was that the infant was infected with *T. pallidum* if the infant's nontreponemal test titer at delivery was higher than the mother's titer. However, a lower titer in the infant's serum than in the mother's serum does not rule out congenital syphilis. Examination of serum sample pairs from mothers and infants with congenital syphilis indicated that only 22% of the infants had a titer higher than that of the mother (112).

In any form of syphilis, patients should be monitored to ensure that treatment is effective, i.e., that signs and symptoms have resolved and that the titer of the quantitative nontreponemal test has declined fourfold, which indicates cure (28, 29, 107). A rise in titer following treatment establishes treatment failure or reinfection. For most pa-

tients treated in early syphilis, the titers decline until little or no reaction is detected after 3 years (28, 52, 53, 99). Patients who are treated in the latent or late stage or patients who have had multiple episodes of syphilis may show a more gradual decline in titer (27, 98). A low titer persists in approximately 50% of these patients after 2 years (27). As far as can be determined, this persistent seropositivity does not signify treatment failure or reinfection, and these patients are likely to remain serofast even if they are retreated (27). Recent studies indicate that HIV infection may delay the decline in antibody titer detected by nontreponemal tests for syphilis in patients with primary or secondary syphilis (98). The prognostic significance of this finding is unknown, since these patients did not experience clinical treatment failure during the 1-year posttreatment observation period. A delayed decline in antibody titer was not associated with detection of *T. pallidum* in CSF, and enhanced therapy did not appear to prevent the delay (98).

Treponemal Tests
The greatest value of the treponemal tests is in distinguishing true- and false-positive nontreponemal test results and in establishing the diagnosis of late latent or late syphilis. Problems may arise when these tests are used as screening procedures, because about 1% of the general population gives false-positive results and treponemal tests generally remain reactive for life following adequate treatment for syphilis. However, a reactive treponemal test result on a sample that is also reactive in a nontreponemal test is highly specific for treponemal infection.

If used appropriately as confirmatory tests, the treponemal tests have few limitations; their greatest limitation is cost. They vary in their sensitivity for the detection of early primary syphilis and the late stages of syphilis (Table 3). Treponemal test results should be obtained if late or late latent syphilis is suspected and the nontreponemal test results are nonreactive. The laboratory should be informed that late syphilis is suspected; otherwise, according to laboratory policy, a treponemal test may not be performed when the nontreponemal test result is nonreactive. Treponemal tests are 100% reactive in secondary and latent syphilis. Again, these findings should be interpreted in the light of treatment history.

Although false-positive treponemal test results are often transient and their cause is unknown, a definite association has been made between false-positive FTA-ABS test results and the diagnosis of systemic, discoid, and drug-induced varieties of lupus erythematosus (53). Patients with systemic lupus erythematosus can give false-positive FTA-ABS test results that exhibit an "atypical beading" fluorescence pattern. Patients whose serum specimens give this type of reaction should be screened for autoimmune disease, including a test for serum anti-DNA antibodies. Other possible causes of false-positive reactions are listed in Table 4. In these instances, the treponemal agglutination test, Western blot, or absorption with Reiter treponeme may be the only means of differentiating between syphilis and a false-positive reaction. If both the FTA-ABS and *Treponema pallidum* particle agglutination (TP-PA) tests are reactive, the sample is most probably (~95%) from a person who has or has had syphilis (94). However, the final decision rests with clinical judgment.

FTA-ABS Tests
The FTA-ABS test is an indirect fluorescent-antibody technique (52). Reagents for this test are available from

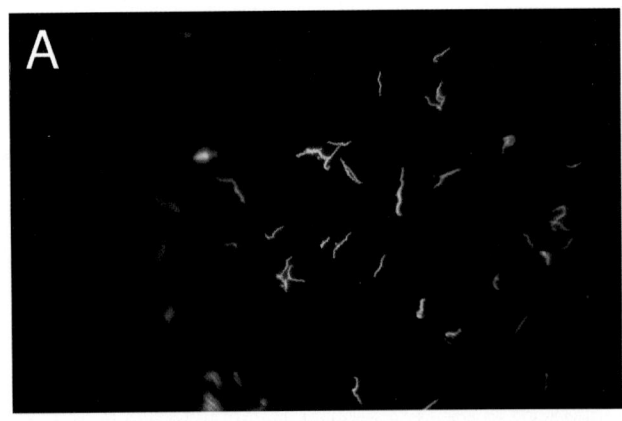

FIGURE 4 FTA-ABS DS test. (A) Counterstain with FITC-labeled anti-*T. pallidum* conjugate, demonstrating the location of *T. pallidum* cells within the microscopic field. (B) Reactive result obtained with tetramethylrhodamine isothiocyanate-labeled anti-human IgG, indicating the presence of anti-*T. pallidum* antibodies in the patient's serum.

several manufacturers, including Zeus Scientific, Inc. (Raritan, N.J.), SciMedx Corp. (Denville, N.J.), Lee Laboratories (Grayson, Ga.), and Hemagen Diagnostics, Inc. (Columbia, Md.). In this procedure, the antigen used is *T. pallidum* subsp. *pallidum* Nichols. A 1:5 dilution of the patient's serum sample in sorbent (an extract from cultures of the nonpathogenic Reiter treponeme) is layered on a microscope slide to which *T. pallidum* spirochetes have been fixed. Fluorescein isothiocyanate (FITC)-labeled anti-human immunoglobulin is added and binds with any patient anti-*T. pallidum* antibodies, resulting in spirochetes that are visible when examined by fluorescence microscopy.

A modification of the standard FTA-ABS test is the FTA-ABS double-staining (DS) test (Fig. 4). The FTA-ABS DS technique uses a tetramethylrhodamine isothiocyanate-labeled anti-human IgG (Fig. 4B) and a counterstain with FITC-labeled anti-*T. pallidum* conjugate (Fig. 4A). The counterstain was developed for use with microscopes with incident illumination to eliminate the need to locate the treponemes by dark-field microscopy when the patient's serum does not contain antibodies to *T. pallidum*. Counterstaining the organism ensures that the nonreactive result is due to the absence of antibodies and not to the absence of treponemes on the slide.

Results of both FTA-ABS tests are reported as reactive, reactive minimal, or nonreactive or as the observance of atypical fluorescence. Specimens initially read as 1+ (reactive minimal) should always be retested. If the results are again read as 1+, they should be reported as such with the statement that "in the absence of historical or clinical evidence of treponemal infection, this test result should be considered equivocal." A second specimen should be obtained 1 to 2 weeks after the initial specimen and submitted to the laboratory for serologic testing. Atypical staining patterns such as beaded fluorescence should be reported to alert the physician to possible autoimmune disease.

Sources of errors are numerous with the FTA-ABS tests, because they are multicomponent tests and each component must be matched with the other ones. Conjugates must be properly titrated, and controls for reactive, reactive minimal, and nonreactive samples and for nonspecific staining and sorbent must be included. The reactive control must be diluted properly to produce the reactive minimal control (1+). Slides must be evaluated to ensure that the

antigen is adhering. In addition, the microscope must be in proper operating condition with the appropriate filters in place (see chapter 18, Table 4). Finally, experience is an important factor in the consistent interpretation of FTA-ABS tests.

TP-PA Test

The TP-PA test (Fujirebio America, Fairfield, N.J.) (3, 19, 91) has replaced the microhemagglutination assay for antibodies to *Treponema pallidum* (MHA-TP). Instead of erythrocytes, the test uses gelatin particles sensitized with *T. pallidum* subsp. *pallidum* antigens. There is no separate absorption step; therefore, the test is simpler to set up and requires less preparation time. The serum sample is diluted in the microtiter plate. Sensitized gelatin particles are added to the 1:20 serum dilution, making a final serum dilution of 1:40. Anti-*T. pallidum* antibodies in the serum react with the sensitized particles, forming a mat of agglutinated particles in the microtiter plate. Unsensitized particles are included as a control for nonspecific reactivity.

Results are reported as reactive, nonreactive, or inconclusive. Reactive results are reported for a range of agglutination patterns, from a smooth mat of agglutinated particles surrounded by a smaller red circle of unagglutinated particles with agglutination outside the circle (1+), to a smooth mat of agglutinated particles covering the entire bottom of the well (4+). Nonreactive results are reported when a definite compact button, with or without a very small hole in its center, forms in the center of the well. A button of unagglutinated particles having a small hole in the center is initially read as "±," and the test should be repeated. If the same pattern is again observed, then the report should be "nonreactive." Because the TP-PA uses gelatin particles rather than sheep erythrocytes, which were the antigen carrier in the MHA-TP, nonspecific agglutination of the unsensitized particles rarely, if ever, occurs. The sources of error with the TP-PA are usually associated with the use of dusty or improper plates, pipetting errors, or vibrations in the laboratory.

Newer Serologic Tests for Syphilis

Several tests using the enzyme immunoassay (EIA) format have been developed for the diagnosis of syphilis (45, 52, 54, 74, 86, 106, 123). The Captia Syphilis-G test (Trinity

Biotech, Dublin, Ireland; BioRad, Richmond, Calif.; and Wampole Laboratories, Princeton, N.J.) and the Trep-Chek test (Phoenix Bio-Tech Corp., Mississauga, Ontario, Canada) are designed as confirmatory tests for syphilis. Initial evaluations of these EIAs have found that they have sensitivities and specificities similar to those of the other treponemal tests (54, 74, 91, 123) (Table 3). Nine EIAs using either *T. pallidum* sonicates or recombinant antigens were compared in the analysis of primary syphilis specimens that were nonreactive in the MHA-TP test (106); this study revealed that several EIAs had sensitivities similar to that of the IgM FTA-ABS test.

The Captia Syphilis-G test has also been cleared by the U.S. Food and Drug Administration as a screening test for syphilis. Laboratories using this test to screen should confirm a reactive Syphilis-G test result by repeating the test and by also performing an RPR test. If the RPR test is nonreactive, a second treponemal test should be performed to rule out the possibility of a false-positive EIA. Laboratorians and clinicians should remember that use of a treponemal test such as the Syphilis-G test as a screening procedure will detect old treated cases as well as active untreated cases of syphilis. The Syphilis-M test (Trinity Biotech, BioRad, and Wampole Laboratories) is based on the use of anti-human IgM antibody to capture IgM in the patient's serum, followed by the use of a purified *T. pallidum* antigen to detect IgM antibodies in the patient's serum directed toward *T. pallidum* (45). This test is most useful in the diagnosis of congenital syphilis. One study found that the IgM capture EIA was more sensitive than the FTA-ABS 19S IgM test in detecting probable cases of congenital syphilis (112); however, another study found the test to be equal in sensitivity to the IgM Western blot for the detection of neonatal congenital syphilis but less sensitive than the Western blot for the detection of delayed-onset congenital syphilis (7). The usefulness of the Syphilis-M test in adult onset syphilis has not been determined fully.

Another test format being increasingly used is Western blot analysis for *T. pallidum* (9, 32, 52, 61). This test is performed as an experimental test in the Syphilis Diagnostic Immunology Activity Laboratory at CDC. The test uses IgG conjugate and appears to be at least as sensitive and specific as the FTA-ABS tests, and efforts have been made to standardize the procedure (9, 32). To date, many investigators agree that the detection of antibodies to the immunodeterminants with molecular masses of 15.5, 17, 44.5, and 47 kDa appears to be diagnostic for acquired syphilis (82). Western blot analysis for *T. pallidum* has value as a diagnostic test for congenital syphilis when an IgM-specific conjugate is used (7, 22, 55, 105). The IgM Western blot analysis for congenital syphilis appears to have a greater specificity and sensitivity than does the IgM EIA.

Tests utilizing recombinant *T. pallidum* antigens are currently under evaluation. These include a rapid test utilizing 47-, 17-, and 15.5-kDa recombinant proteins (25, 122), an EIA (104), and a Western blot format recombinant assay (103). It is anticipated that serologic assays involving recombinant antigens will become more widely used in the future, given the difficulties in preparing *T. pallidum* antigen preparations from infected rabbit tissue.

Interpretation and Reporting of Results

The following is a brief discussion of the parameters involved in the diagnosis of syphilis and other treponematoses. Procedures for the direct detection of *T. pallidum* and

the serologic diagnosis of syphilis are described in detail in *A Manual of Tests for Syphilis* (52).

Diagnostic Criteria for Venereal Syphilis

For the laboratory diagnosis of syphilis, each stage has a particular testing requirement (Table 5) (11). Because *T. pallidum* cannot be cultured readily (18, 81), other laboratory methods to identify infection have been developed. The current tests for syphilis fall into three categories: direct microscopic examination, used to detect *T. pallidum* in lesion exudates or tissue specimens; nontreponemal tests, used to detect anticardiolipin antibodies; and treponemal tests, used to detect antitreponemal antibodies. In the United States, the traditional testing scheme is direct microscopic examination of lesion exudates followed by a nontreponemal test which, if reactive, is confirmed with a treponemal test (Fig. 5). In recent years, use of enzyme immunoassays has led to screening with a treponemal test followed by an RPR or other nontreponemal test. This approach may eliminate many false-positive reactions due to nonspecific nontreponemal test reactivity (Table 4); however, as the rates of syphilis decline, an increasing proportion of individuals who test reactive to treponemal tests will be persons with previously treated cases of syphilis or with falsely reactive treponemal test results. In addition, the low sensitivity of nontreponemal tests in detecting long-duration infection is an important disadvantage to their use as confirmatory tests. Therefore, the use of modified serologic screening procedures for syphilis requires careful consideration of the sensitivity and specificity of both the screening and confirmatory steps.

During the primary stage of syphilis, dark-field microscopy and the DFA-TP test (52) are the methods of choice for definitive diagnosis. If the chancre is starting to heal or the patient has used either topical or systemic antibiotics, the number of treponemes may be too small to be detected or they may become nonmotile or degraded. Humoral antibodies, as detected by the current serologic tests for syphilis, usually appear 1 to 4 weeks after the chancre(s) has formed. Thus, a reactive serologic test result may be expected if the chancre is healing. More generally, conversion to reactivity of a serologic test for syphilis or a rise in nontreponemal test titer over 1 to 2 weeks supports a diagnosis of syphilis even if a dark-field or DFA microscopic examination is negative.

By the secondary stage of syphilis, the organism has invaded every organ of the body and virtually all body fluids. At this stage, generally all serologic tests for syphilis are reactive and treponemes may be found in lesions prior to the healing stage. Although *T. pallidum* can be detected in the CSF of a substantial minority of patients with secondary syphilis, routine CSF examination is not considered necessary at this stage in the absence of neurologic symptoms or signs. A relationship between detection of treponemes in the CSF of patients with early syphilis, the development of late neurosyphilis, and the potential for reducing any such increased risk of developing neurosyphilis through enhanced therapy has not been established (72). Nontreponemal and treponemal serologic tests are consistently reactive in the early latent stage, but the patient is asymptomatic. Nontreponemal tests may become nonreactive in late latent syphilis. Routine CSF examination for the detection of neurosyphilis is probably indicated for the patient with coexistent latent syphilis and HIV infection (98), whereas the need for lumbar puncture in

TABLE 5 Criteria for diagnosis of syphilis[a]

Early syphilis
  Primary
    Confirmed (requires 1 *and* 2)
      1. One or more chancres (ulcers)
      2. Direct microscopic identification of *T. pallidum* in clinical specimens (dark field or DFA-TP)
    Probable (requires 1 *and* either 2 or 3)
      1. A clinically compatible case with one or more chancres
      2. Reactive nontreponemal or treponemal test and no previous history of syphilis
      3. For persons with a history of syphilis, a fourfold increase in titer on a quantitative nontreponemal test when results of past tests are compared with the most recent test results
  Secondary
    Confirmed
      Direct microscopic identification of *T. pallidum* in clinical specimens (dark field or DFA-TP)
    Probable (requires 1 *and* either 2 or 3)
      1. Skin or mucous membrane lesions typical of secondary syphilis
        a. Macular, papular, follicular, papulosquamous, or pustular
        b. Condylomata lata (anogenital region or mouth)
        c. Mucous patches (oropharynx or cervix)
      2. Reactive nontreponemal test titer of ≥1:4 and no previous history of syphilis
      3. For persons with a history of syphilis, a fourfold increase in the most recent nontreponemal test titer when compared with previous test results
  Early latent
    Probable (requires 1 *and* either 2 or 3 *and* either 4, 5, or 6)
      1. Absence of signs and symptoms of syphilis
      2. No past diagnosis of syphilis and reactive nontreponemal and treponemal test results
      3. A past history of syphilis therapy and a current nontreponemal test titer demonstrating fourfold or greater increase from the last nontreponemal test titer (obtained ≥1 yr ago)
      4. A history of symptoms consistent with primary or secondary syphilis during the previous 12 mo
      5. A history of sexual exposure to a partner who had confirmed or probable early syphilis (documented independently as duration of <1 yr)
      6. Documented seroconversion or fourfold or greater increase in titer of a nontreponemal test during the previous 12 mo
  Late latent
    Probable (requires 1 *and* either 2 or 3 *and* 4)
      1. Absence of signs and symptoms
      2. No past diagnosis of syphilis and reactive nontreponemal and treponemal test results
      3. A past history of syphilis therapy and a current nontreponemal test titer demonstrating fourfold or greater increase from the last nontreponemal test titer (obtained >1 yr ago)
      4. No evidence of having acquired the disease within the preceding 12 months

Latent of unknown duration
  Probable (requires 1 *and* either 2 or 3 *and* 4)
    1. Absence of signs and symptoms
    2. No past diagnosis of syphilis and reactive nontreponemal and treponemal test results
    3. A past history of syphilis therapy and a current nontreponemal test titer demonstrating fourfold or greater increase from the last nontreponemal test titer
    4. Patient does not meet the criteria for early latent syphilis, is aged 13–35 yr, and has a nontreponemal titer of >1:32

Late syphilis
  Benign (gummatous) and cardiovascular
    Confirmed (requires 1 *and* 2)
      1. Clinically compatible case
      2. Observation by direct microscopic examination of treponemes in tissue sections by DFAT-TP or detection by other methods (e.g., PCR)
    Probable (requires 1, 2, *and* 3)
      1. Clinically compatible case
      2. A reactive treponemal test
      3. No known history of treatment for syphilis
  Neurosyphilis
    Confirmed (requires 1, 2, *and* either 3 or 4)
      1. Clinical signs consistent with neurosyphilis
      2. A reactive serum treponemal test
      3. A reactive VDRL-CSF on a spinal fluid sample
      4. Identification of *T. pallidum* in CSF or tissue by microscopic examination or equivalent methods
    Probable (requires 1, 2, *and* 3)
      1. Clinical signs consistent with neurosyphilis
      2. A reactive serum treponemal test
      3. Elevated CSF protein or leukocyte count in the absence of other known causes

Neonatal congenital syphilis
  Confirmed (requires 1 *and* 2)
    1. Clinically compatible case
    2. Demonstration of *T. pallidum* by direct microscopic examination of specimens from lesions, placenta, umbilical cord, nasal discharge, or autopsy material
  Probable (requires 1, 2, *and* 3)
    1. Infant born to a mother who had untreated or inadequately[b] treated syphilis at delivery, regardless of findings in the infant
    2. An infant with a reactive treponemal test result
    3. One of the following additional criteria:
      a. Clinical sign or symptom of congenital syphilis on physical examination
      b. Abnormal CSF finding without other cause
      c. Reactive VDRL-CSF test result
      d. Reactive IgM antibody test specific for syphilis
  Syphilitic stillbirth (requires 1 *and* 2)
    1. A fetal death that occurs after a 20-wk gestation or in which the fetus weighs >500 g
    2. Mother had untreated or inadequately[b] treated syphilis at delivery

[a] Adapted from reference 11.
[b] Nonpenicillin therapy or penicillin given less than 30 days before delivery.

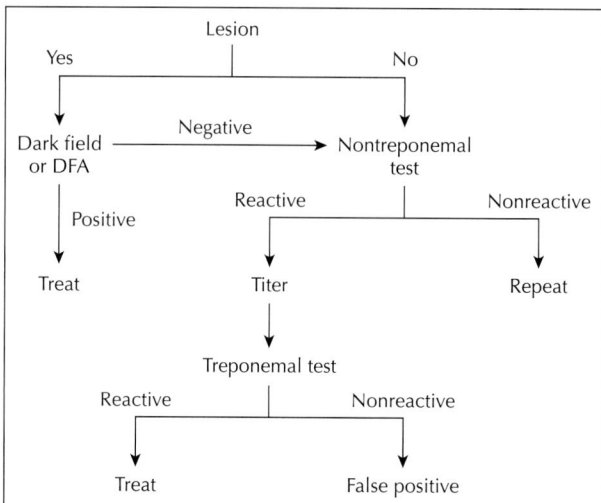

FIGURE 5 Routine screening scheme for early syphilis in the United States.

patients with latent syphilis but without HIV infection is controversial (10).

Neurologic forms of syphilis (e.g., syphilitic meningitis) may develop early as well as late in the course of syphilis (58, 98); therefore, neurosyphilis is classified by itself and is no longer restricted to the late stages of syphilis. The diagnosis of neurosyphilis is based on a combination of clinical and laboratory test criteria (Table 5). Neurosyphilis may take many forms, and manifestations consistent with neurosyphilis may not always be present (42). CSF examination, including the VDRL-CSF slide test and total protein and leukocyte counts, should be performed with CSF fluid of patients who fulfill any of the following criteria: neurologic or ophthalmic symptoms and signs consistent with neurosyphilis, evidence of active tertiary syphilis, treatment failure, or HIV infection with late latent syphilis or syphilis of unknown duration (10). CSF abnormalities include lymphocytosis (>4 cells/mm^3), elevated protein levels, and VDRL-CSF reactivity (57).

The VDRL-CSF test is highly specific (99.8%) for neurosyphilis, but its sensitivity is only about 50%. A nonreactive result does not rule out neurosyphilis, but a reactive result is diagnostic. An FTA-ABS test can also be performed on CSF. This test has 100% sensitivity and 94% specificity for neurosyphilis. A nonreactive FTA-ABS CSF result can therefore help rule out a diagnosis of neurosyphilis.

Late or tertiary syphilis is a chronic, progressive disease, and symptoms may not be evident until 10 to 20 years after the initial infection. Although rare, earlier onset of late or tertiary syphilis has been reported for individuals coinfected with HIV (48). Approximately 71% of patients with late-stage syphilis have reactive nontreponemal tests; however, treponemal tests are almost always reactive and may constitute the only laboratory confirmation of diagnosis (Table 5). Gummatous syphilis consists of granuloma-like lesions (gummas) containing lymphocytes and macrophages but few if any detectable spirochetes. Diagnosis of cardiovascular syphilis is made on the basis of findings that indicate aortic insufficiency or thoracic aortic aneurysm, reactive treponemal test results, and no known history of treatment of syphilis. Late forms of neurosyphilis include paresis (in-

fection of the brain parenchyma, resulting in behavioral changes including psychoses), tabes dorsalis (ataxia, paresthesias, and other manifestations resulting from posterior spinal cord and dorsal root ganglia degeneration), and optic atrophy (119).

The choice and interpretation of tests for the diagnosis of syphilis are the same for HIV-infected and uninfected patients, but additional considerations apply to HIV-infected individuals (34, 47, 72, 98). The titers of nontreponemal serologic test results may be higher in patients coinfected with HIV than in those without coexistent HIV infection, or the number of primary chancres may be increased (92). Also, patients with advanced HIV immunodeficiency may become falsely seronegative for syphilis (35, 40).

Diagnostic Criteria for Congenital Syphilis

A primary stage does not occur in congenital syphilis, because the organisms enter the fetal circulation directly (124). Treponemes or the effects thereof are detectable in almost every tissue of the infant. Currently, the diagnosis of neonatal congenital syphilis depends on a combination of results from physical, radiographic, serologic, and direct microscopic examinations (Table 5). Clinical signs of early congenital syphilis include hepatosplenomegaly, cutaneous lesions, osteochondritis, and snuffles (nasal discharge containing large numbers of *T. pallidum*) (49, 119). Roughly half of live-born neonates with congenital syphilis have normal physical findings at the time of birth. If the infant is not treated, other stigmata that may develop later in life include tooth and bone malformations, deafness, blindness, and learning disabilities (Table 2).

Definitive diagnosis is based on the identification of spirochetes in tissues, lesion exudates, or secretions by dark-field examination, DFA-TP, PCR, or other means (Table 5). The standard serologic tests for syphilis, which detect reactive IgG as well as other isotypes, may reflect antibodies passively transferred from the mother to the infant rather than IgM antibodies produced by an infected fetus during gestation. IgM-specific treponemal antibody tests are available and may be useful in the diagnosis of congenital syphilis (see "Serologic Tests" above). In syphilitic stillbirths, detection of the treponemes in the tissues is definitive for the diagnosis of congenital syphilis (93).

Diagnostic Criteria for Other Treponematoses

Serologic tests for syphilis are uniformly reactive with yaws, pinta, and nonvenereal endemic syphilis (bejel) (5, 76). Therefore, the patient history, the clinical appearance and anatomic locations of the lesions, the mode of transmission, and the age of the individual are the only criteria that can be used to diagnose these infections as separate entities (5) (Table 1). PCR may be useful in distinguishing these infections in a research setting (12).

Yaws, pinta, and nonvenereal syphilis are often contracted during childhood, but the nontreponemal test titers in affected individuals may remain reactive in adulthood, presenting a dilemma in the diagnosis of subsequent cases of venereal syphilis. Adults from geographic regions in which endemic treponematoses were virtually eliminated by mass campaigns in the 1950s and 1960s would be expected to have nontreponemal test titers of <1:8 (1). Therefore, any titer of ≥1:8 for adults from these regions is probably indicative of venereal syphilis. Likewise, titers of ≥1:8 for children indicate a possible resurgence of yaws in the populations of these areas (88).

Recently, methods utilizing PCR and DNA amplification techniques have begun to be able to distinguish between the various subspecies of *T. pallidum* and *T. carateum*, as well as various strains of *T. pallidum* subsp. *pallidum* (12, 90). These techniques are being used in some research laboratories to help determine the epidemiology of syphilis outbreaks (113).

Treatment and Antimicrobial Susceptibilities

CDC has published recommendations for the treatment of syphilis (10) based, in part, on detailed reviews of the literature (2, 97). Routine antimicrobial susceptibility testing of *T. pallidum* is not practical due to the lack of a suitable in vitro culture system, although a number of methods have been applied to the determination of antibiotic sensitivity in the research laboratory (81). *T. pallidum* strains appear to be uniformly susceptible to penicillin and other β-lactams. Penicillin regimens have been the mainstay of syphilis therapy since their introduction in the 1940s. Because treatment with benzathine penicillin as recommended for early syphilis yields low levels of penicillin in the central nervous system, the current recommendations include multiple doses of penicillin G for the treatment of neurosyphilis. Ceftriaxone, amoxicillin, and ampicillin are active against *T. pallidum* in vitro and also appear to be effective in the treatment of early syphilis. Ceftriaxone has a long half-life in serum and reaches high levels in the central nervous system. However, multiple doses are required, and there is a 3 to 7% risk of adverse reactions in penicillin-allergic individuals; in addition, the data on efficacy in patients are limited. Therefore, the use of ceftriaxone as an alternative therapy for syphilis is recommended only when better-established regimens are contraindicated.

Tetracycline has long been the second-line drug recommended for treatment of syphilis in patients allergic to penicillin. However, the in vitro activity of tetracycline against *T. pallidum* is markedly lower than the activity of penicillin and, in limited comparative trials, treatment failure appears to be more common with tetracycline. Doxycycline has been considered equivalent to tetracycline in recent treatment recommendations. Azithromycin shows promise as an effective treatment against syphilis and other sexually transmitted bacterial infections. This antibiotic is concentrated within cells; the resulting prolonged half-life offers the potential for reduced dosing, but a standard treatment regimen has not as yet been established. In vitro studies indicate that quinolone compounds have low antimicrobial activity against *T. pallidum* (81).

OTHER HUMAN HOST-ASSOCIATED SPIROCHETES

In addition to *T. pallidum* and related pathogens, a number of anaerobic treponemes and other spirochetes are parasites of humans. These include groups of spirochetes found in the oral cavity (particularly the gingival crevices), in sebaceous secretions in the genital region, and in the colon and rectum (Table 6). In general, these spirochetes are considered commensal organisms. However, there is evidence that spirochetes are involved in gingivitis and periodontal disease and that overgrowth of intestinal spirochetes may correlate with the occurrence of diarrhea or other bowel disorders.

TABLE 6 Other human host-associated spirochetes

Type	Habitat	Species
Oral spirochetes	Dental plaque in gingival crevices	*Treponema denticola* *Treponema socranskii* *Treponema vincentii* *Treponema pectinovorum* *Treponema skoliodontum* *Treponema maltophilum* *Treponema medium* *Treponema amylovorum* *Treponema parvum*
Skin-associated spirochetes	Sebaceous secretions in genital region	*Treponema phagedenis* *Treponema refringens* *Treponema minutum*
Intestinal spirochetes	Colon, rectum, feces	*Brachyspira pilosicoli* *Brachyspira aalborgi*

Oral Spirochetes

A variety of spirochetes inhabit supragingival and subgingival plaques in humans; only a small proportion of these have been cultured in vitro and characterized (16, 20, 84). Those that have been cultivated and identified to the species level are within the genus *Treponema* (Table 6). They are spiral-shaped organisms ranging from 0.15 to 0.30 μm in diameter and from 5 to 16 μm long (with lengths being variable within each species). Although the species differ from one another slightly in terms of cell diameter and helical configuration, it is generally not possible to identify them on morphologic grounds; genotypic characteristics and biochemical parameters such as growth requirements, carbohydrate fermentation, and enzymatic activities are used to identify species (109).

The oral spirochetes listed in Table 6 are difficult to isolate from healthy gingiva. However, they increase in both prevalence and number of organisms present in patients with gingivitis or periodontal disease, an inflammation of gum tissue that frequently precedes bone resorption and subsequent tooth loss. Treponemes are detected in the subgingival plaque of 88 to 97% of patients with periodontal disease (69). *T. socranskii* is the most common isolate in patients without periodontal disease, followed by *T. denticola* and *T. pectinovorum*. These organisms are isolated from a greater proportion of patients with periodontal disease than patients without the disease (69, 110, 111). Recent studies utilizing PCR amplification of 16S rRNA gene sequences have revealed that oral spirochetes are a heterogeneous group, consisting of up to 60 different species and as yet uncultured "phylotypes" (20, 84); as many as 23 phylotypes of treponemes have been identified in the lesions of individual periodontitis patients (16). All of the oral spirochetes clearly fall under the genus *Treponema* (85). Up to 415 cultured and uncultured bacterial species have been identified in human subgingival plaque (84), but treponemes represent one of the most prevalent groups (70, 71). Although it is difficult to establish a causal relationship in polymicrobial infections such as periodontitis, oral spirochetes are almost certainly involved in its etiology.

The term "pathogen-related oral spirochetes" has been used to describe a subset of oral spirochetes that have invasive properties and react with monoclonal antibodies against the *T. pallidum* flagellar protein FlaA (96); however, recent studies (17, 95) indicate that cultivated pathogen-related oral spirochete isolates represent a heterogeneous group with rRNA sequence similarities to *T. vincentii* or *T. medium*. This finding does not preclude the possibility that the heterogeneous group of oral *Treponema* species may include a subset of as yet uncharacterized organisms with particularly invasive or pathogenic properties.

The isolation and characterization of oral spirochetes require special media and strict anaerobic conditions (67, 68, 109–111) and are restricted primarily to research laboratories. At present, there is insufficient evidence linking particular oral spirochetes to pathologic conditions to warrant their detection and identification for diagnostic purposes.

Nonpathogenic Spirochetes of the Genital Region

T. phagedenis, *T. refringens*, and *T. minutum* are treponemal species that inhabit the smegma (sebaceous secretions and desquamated epithelial cells) found beneath the prepuce and in other epithelial folds of the genital region. *T. phagedenis* and *T. refringens* are 0.20 to 0.25 μm in diameter, whereas *T. minutum* tends to be smaller (0.15 to 0.20 μm). Although *T. phagedenis* and *T. refringens* have ≤5% homology to *T. pallidum* by DNA-DNA hybridization (26), comparison of 16S rRNA sequences indicates that they are related to the pathogenic treponemes. These harmless members of the normal flora could potentially be misidentified as *T. pallidum* in dark-field microscopy preparations from skin sites. Careful cleansing of the site as described in the "Specimen Collection" section under "Detection and Identification of *T. pallidum* in Tissue and Tissue Exudates" (above) obviates this possibility. Also, the DFA-TP test (52) is specific for pathogenic treponemes and can be used with specimens potentially contaminated with other organisms. The skin-associated treponemes may be collected with sterile moistened swabs and placed in anaerobic transport medium or directly in selective medium containing rifampin (2 μg/ml) and polymyxin (800 μg/ml). They are readily cultured in peptone-yeast extract-glucose medium or in thioglycolate medium with 10% heat-inactivated rabbit serum under anaerobic conditions at 37°C (67). Growth is usually observed within 1 to 2 weeks.

Intestinal Spirochetes

The presence of spirochetes in the colon, rectum, and feces of humans has been recognized for more than 100 years (102). Since the description of "human intestinal spirochetosis" in 1967 (39), there has been a resurgence in interest in the possible involvement of intestinal spirochetes in diarrhea and other gastrointestinal diseases (38), as well as in the apparently high prevalence of these organisms in homosexual males and HIV-infected individuals (102).

Morphologically, most human intestinal spirochetes are relatively short (3 to 6 μm long on average) and are 0.2 to 0.4 μm in diameter with one to two helices per cell. Longer cells may also be present. They have pointed ends and four to six periplasmic flagella attached subterminally in a single row at each end of the cell. The human intestinal spirochetes identified thus far fall into two species: *Brachyspira* (formerly *Serpulina*) *pilosicoli* and *Brachyspira aalborgi*. *B. pilosicoli* was initially named *Serpulina pilosicoli* (116, 117); however, this and other *Serpulina* species (e.g. *B. hyodysenteriae*, a cause of swine dysentery) were reclassified recently as *Brachyspira* based on phenotypic characteristics, rRNA sequence analysis, and DNA hybridization studies (83). *B.*

pilosicoli has a broad range of natural hosts, including swine, mice, rats, dogs, and chickens. *B. aalborgi* (43) is genetically and phenotypically distinct from *B. pilosicoli* (50, 116) and thus far has been identified only in humans.

B. pilosicoli and *B. aalborgi* are obligate anaerobes but grow in a variety of media containing blood. Until recently, *B. aalborgi* had been cultured on only one occasion (resulting in the type strain), leading to the conclusion that it was rare relative to *B. pilosicoli*. However, recent PCR analyses of human colonic biopsy specimens indicate that *B. aalborgi* is a common cause of human intestinal spirochetosis (51, 64, 65). In two series of histologically diagnosed cases of intestinal spirochetosis from Australia, Norway, and the United States, *B. aalborgi* sequences were detected in 62.5 and 82.5% of the cases whereas *B. pilosicoli* sequences were detected in only 0 and 14.3% (64, 65). In 2000, Kraaz et al. (51) isolated a second strain of *B. aalborgi* by using a selective medium consisting of tryptose soy agar with 10% bovine blood, 400 μg of spectinomycin per ml, and 5 μg of polymyxin per ml. They found that a selective medium commonly used for the culture of intestinal spirochetes inhibited the growth of this strain, presumably due to the inclusion of vancomycin and colistin.

When observed in association with rectal or colonic tissue, these organisms are typically attached by the tip to the apical surface of the columnar epithelial cells. Although the spirochetes can form a dense layer visible by light microscopy (using hematoxylin-and-eosin- or silver-staining techniques), signs of tissue damage or inflammation are usually absent.

A clear association between intestinal spirochetes and disease has not been established (102). Spirochetes can be present in healthy individuals as well as those with diarrhea or other gastrointestinal symptoms. In the early 1900s, several studies examined the presence of spirochetes in human stool specimens by light microscopy. In those studies, involving more than 100 patients, the proportion of subjects with spirochetes ranged from 3.3 to 61%. Recent examinations of rectal biopsy specimens from heterosexual patients by light and electron microscopy or culture have indicated the presence of spirochetes in 1.9 to 6.9% of subjects, and helical organisms were also associated with normal and inflamed appendixes. Higher proportions of homosexual males have been reported to have intestinal spirochetes. At present, there is no clear evidence for an association between intestinal spirochetosis and HIV infection.

B. pilosicoli was isolated from routine anaerobic cultures of blood from seven critically ill patients, including those with stroke, ethylene glycol intoxication, severe arteriopathy, peritonitis, and myeloma (115). The clinical significance and cause-and-effect relationship of *B. pilosicoli* bacteremia and life-threatening illness remain to be determined.

Colonic or rectal biopsy samples can serve as a source of material for culture, histologic examination for spirochetes, or PCR; fresh stool specimens or rectal swabs may also be examined by dark-field microscopy for the presence of spirochetes (102). Positive samples can be cultured under anaerobic conditions at 37°C in the presence of 5 to 10% CO_2 by being streaked onto Trypticase soy agar medium with 5 to 10% defibrinated horse or calf blood and 400 μg of spectinomycin per ml (with or without 5 μg of polymyxin B per ml) to inhibit the growth of other bacteria. After 5 to 14 days of incubation, growth appears as a thin film or as discrete, pinpoint colonies. Longer culture intervals may be required for *B. aalborgi*. Weak beta-hemolysis is typically observed. In the isolation of *Brachyspira* from anaerobic blood cultures, automated detection was not obtained uniformly and required a minimum of 5.6 to 14.9 days (depending on the strain); however, the organisms could be subcultured and observed by dark-field microscopy (8, 115). An alternative method of detection is PCR, using rRNA and/or NADH oxidase *(nox)* gene sequences as targets (51, 64); this approach can also be adapted for use with fixed, paraffin-embedded tissue specimens (64) or with human feces (66).

No commercial kits or serologic procedures for detection of human intestinal spirochetosis are available, and no data on antimicrobial susceptibility or treatment have been reported. Clearly, more information is needed to establish the potential medical importance of these organisms.

REFERENCES

1. **Antal, G. M., and G. Causse.** 1985. The control of endemic treponematoses. *Rev. Infect. Dis.* **7**(Suppl. 2): S220–S226.
2. **Augenbraun, M. H., and R. Rolfs.** 1999. Treatment of syphilis, 1998: nonpregnant adults. *Clin. Infect. Dis.* **28**(Suppl. 1):S21–S28.
3. **Backhouse, J. L., and S. I. Neseroff.** 2001. *Treponema pallidum* Western blot: comparison with the FTA-ABS test as a confirmatory test for syphilis. *Diagn. Microbiol. Infect. Dis.* **39**:9–14.
4. **Belisle, J. T., M. E. Brandt, J. D. Radolf, and M. V. Norgard.** 1994. Fatty acids of *Treponema pallidum* and *Borrelia burgdorferi* lipoproteins. *J. Bacteriol.* **176**:2151–2157.
5. **Benenson, A. S.** 1990. Pinta, p. 323–324; Nonvenereal endemic syphilis, p. 425–426; and Yaws, p. 483–486. *In* A. S. Benenson (ed.), *Control of Communicable Diseases in Man,* 15th ed. American Public Health Association, Washington, D.C.
6. **Birnbaum, N. R., R. H. Goldschmidt, and W. O. Buffett.** 1999. Resolving the common clinical dilemmas of syphilis. *Am. Fam. Physician* **59**:2233–2240.
7. **Bromberg, K., S. Rawstron, and G. Tannis.** 1993. Diagnosis of congenital syphilis by combining *Treponema pallidum*-specific IgM detection with immunofluorescent antigen detection for *T. pallidum. J. Infect. Dis.* **168**:238–242.
8. **Brooke, C. J., K. R. Margawani, A. K. Pearson, T. V. Riley, I. D. Robertson, and D. J. Hampson.** 2000. Evaluation of blood culture systems for detection of the intestinal spirochaete *Brachyspira (Serpulina) pilosicoli* in human blood. *J. Med. Microbiol.* **49**:1031–1036.
9. **Byrne, R. E., S. Laske, M. Bell, D. Larson, J. Phillips, and J. Todd.** 1992. Evaluation of a *Treponema pallidum* Western immunoblot assay as a confirmatory test for syphilis. *J. Clin. Microbiol.* **30**:115–122.
10. **Centers for Disease Control and Prevention.** 1998. 1998 Sexually transmitted diseases treatment guidelines. *Morb. Mortal. Wkly. Rep.* **47**(RR-1):28–49.
11. **Centers for Disease Control and Prevention.** 1997. Conditions under public health surveillance. *Morb. Mortal. Wkly. Rep.* **46**:34–37.
12. **Centurion-Lara, A., C. Castro, R. Castillo, J. M. Shaffer, W. C. Van Voorhis, and S. A. Lukehart.** 1998. The flanking region sequences of the 15-kDa lipoprotein gene differentiate pathogenic treponemes. *J. Infect. Dis.* **177**:1036–1040.
13. **Centurion-Lara, A., C. Godornes, C. Castro, W. C. Van Voorhis, and S. A. Lukehart.** 2000. The *tprK* gene is heterogeneous among *Treponema pallidum* strains and has multiple alleles. *Infect. Immun.* **68**:824–831.
14. **Centurion-Lara, A., E. S. Sun, L. K. Barrett, C. Castro, S. A. Lukehart, and W. C. Van Voorhis.** 2000. Multiple alleles of *Treponema pallidum* repeat gene D in *Treponema pallidum* isolates. *J. Bacteriol.* **182**:2332–2335.
15. **Chhabra, R. S., L. P. Brion, M. Castro, L. Freundlich, and J. H. Glaser.** 1993. Comparison of maternal sera, cord blood and neonatal sera for detection of presumptive congenital syphilis: relationship with maternal treatment. *Pediatrics* **91**:88–91.
16. **Choi, B. K., B. J. Paster, F. E. Dewhirst, and U. B. Göbel.** 1994. Diversity of cultivable and uncultivable oral spirochetes from a patient with severe destructive periodontitis. *Infect. Immun.* **62**:1889–1895.
17. **Choi, B. K., C. Wyss, and U. B. Gobel.** 1996. Phylogenetic analysis of pathogen-related oral spirochetes. *J. Clin. Microbiol.* **34**:1922–1925.
18. **Cox, D. L.** 1994. Culture of *Treponema pallidum. Methods Enzymol.* **236**:390–405.
19. **Deguchi, M., H. Hosotsubo, N. Yamashita, T. Ohmine, and S. Asari.** 1994. Evaluation of gelatin particle agglutination method for detection of *Treponema pallidum* antibody. *J. Jpn. Assoc. Infect. Dis.* **68**:1271–1277.
20. **Dewhirst, F. E., M. A. Tamer, R. E. Ericson, C. N. Lau, V. A. Levanos, S. K. Boches, J. L. Galvin, and B. J. Paster.** 2000. The diversity of periodontal spirochetes by 16S rRNA analysis. *Oral Microbiol. Immunol.* **15**:196–202.
21. **Division of STD Prevention.** 2001. *Sexually Transmitted Disease Surveillance, 2000.* Centers for Disease Control and Prevention, Atlanta, Ga.
22. **Dobson, S. R. M., L. H. Taber, and R. E. Baughn.** 1988. Recognition of *Treponema pallidum* antigens by IgM and IgG antibodies in congenitally infected newborns and their mothers. *J. Infect. Dis.* **157**:903–910.
23. **Engelkens, H. J. H., J. Judanarso, A. P. Oranje, V. D. Vuzevski, P. L. A. Niemel, J. J. van der Sluis, and E. Stolz.** 1991. Endemic treponematoses. I. Yaws. *Int. J. Dermatol.* **30**:77–83.
24. **Engelkens, H. J. H., P. L. A. Niemel, J. J. van der Sluis, A. Meheus, and E. Stolz.** 1991. Endemic treponematoses. II. Pinta and endemic syphilis. *Int. J. Dermatol.* **30**:231–238.
25. **Fears, M. B., and V. Pope.** 2001. Syphilis Fast latex agglutination test, a rapid confirmatory test. *Clin. Diagn. Lab. Immunol.* **8**:841–842.
26. **Fieldsteel, A. H.** 1983. Genetics, p. 39–54. *In* R. F. Schell and D. M. Musher (ed.), *Pathogenesis and Immunology of Treponemal Infection.* Marcel Dekker, Inc., New York, N.Y.
27. **Fiumara, N. J.** 1979. Serologic responses to treatment of 128 patients with late latent syphilis. *Sex. Transm. Dis.* **6**:243–246.
28. **Fiumara, N. J.** 1978. Treatment of early latent syphilis of less than one year's duration. *Sex. Transm. Dis.* **5**:85–88.
29. **Fiumara, N. J.** 1980. Treatment of primary and secondary syphilis: serological response. *JAMA* **243**:2500–2502.
30. **Fraser, C. M., S. J. Norris, G. M. Weinstock, et al.** 1998. Complete genome sequence of *Treponema pallidum,* the syphilis spirochete. *Science* **281**:375–388.
31. **Genc, M., and W. J. Ledger.** 2000. Syphilis in pregnancy. *Sex. Transm. Infect.* **76**:73–79.
32. **George, R. W., V. Pope, and S. A. Larsen.** 1991. Use of the Western blot for the diagnosis of syphilis. *Clin. Immunol. Newsl.* **8**:124–128.
33. **Gjestland, T.** 1955. The Oslo study of untreated syphilis: an epidemiologic investigation of the natural course of syphilis infection based upon a re-study of the Boeck-Bruusgaard material. *Acta Dermatovenereol.* **35**:1–368.
34. **Gourevitch, M. N., P. A. Selwyn, D. Davenny, D. Buono, E. E. Schoenbaum, R. S. Klein, and F. H. Friedland.** 1993. Effects of HIV infection on the serologic

manifestation and response to treatment of syphilis in intravenous drug users. *Ann. Intern. Med.* **118:**350–355.

35. **Gregory, N., M. Sanchez, and M. R. Buchness.** 1990. The spectrum of syphilis in patients with human immunodeficiency virus infection. *J. Am. Acad. Dermatol.* **22:** 1061–1067.

36. **Grimprel, E., P. J. Sanchez, G. D. Wendel, J. M. Burstain, G. H. McCracken, Jr., J. D. Radolf, and M. V. Norgard.** 1991. Use of polymerase chain reaction and rabbit infectivity testing to detect *Treponema pallidum* in amniotic fluid, fetal and neonatal sera, and cerebrospinal fluid. *J. Clin. Microbiol.* **29:**1711–1718.

37. **Guarner, J., K. Southwick, P. Greer, J. Bartlett, M. Fears, A. Santander, S. Blanco, V. Pope, W. Levine, and S. Zaki.** 2000. Testing umbilical cords for funisitis due to *Treponema pallidum* infection, Bolivia. *Emerg. Infect. Dis.* **6:**487–492.

38. **Hampson, D. J., and T. B. Stanton (ed.).** 1996. *Intestinal Spirochetes in Domestic Animals and Humans.* CAB International, Wallingford, England.

39. **Harland, W. A., and F. D. Lee.** 1967. Intestinal spirochaetosis. *Br. Med. J.* **3:**718–719.

40. **Hicks, C. B., P. M. Benson, G. P. Lupton, and E. C. Tramont.** 1987. Seronegative secondary syphilis in a patient infected with the human immunodeficiency virus (HIV) with Kaposi sarcoma. *Ann. Intern. Med.* **107:**492–495.

41. **Hollier, L. M., T. W. Harstad, P. J. Sanchez, D. M. Twickler, and G. D. Wendel, Jr.** 2001. Fetal syphilis: clinical and laboratory characteristics. *Obstet. Gynecol.* **97:**947–953.

42. **Hook, E. W., III, and C. M. Marra.** 1992. Acquired syphilis in adults. *N. Engl. J. Med.* **326:**1060–1069.

43. **Hovind-Hougen, K., A. Birch-Andersen, R. Henrik-Nielsen, M. Orholm, J. O. Pedersen, P. S. Teglbjaerg, and E. H. Thaysen.** 1982. Intestinal spirochetosis: morphological characterization and cultivation of the spirochete *Brachyspira aalborgi* gen. nov., sp. nov. *J. Clin. Microbiol.* **16:**1127–1136.

44. **Hunter, E. F., H. Russell, C. E. Farshy, J. S. Sampson, and S. A. Larsen.** 1986. Evaluation of sera from patients with Lyme disease in the fluorescent treponemal antibody-absorption tests for syphilis. *Sex. Transm. Dis.* **13:**232–236.

45. **Ijsselmuiden, O. E., J. J. van der Sluis, A. Mulder, E. Stolz, K. P. Bolton, and R. V. W. van Eijk.** 1989. An IgM capture enzyme-linked immunosorbent assay to detect IgM antibodies to treponemes in patients with syphilis. *Genitourin. Med.* **65:**79–83.

46. **Jaffe, H. W., S. A. Larsen, M. Peters, D. F. Jove, B. Lopez, and A. L. Schroeter.** 1978. Tests for treponemal antibody in CSF. *Arch. Intern. Med.* **138:**252–255.

47. **Janier, M., C. Chastang, E. Spindler, S. Strazzi, C. Rabian, A. Marcelli, and P. Morel.** 1999. A prospective study of the influence of HIV status on seroreversion of serologic tests for syphilis. *Dermatology* **198:**362–369.

48. **Johns, D. R., M. Tierney, and D. Felsenstein.** 1987. Alteration in the natural history of neurosyphilis by concurrent infection with the human immunodeficiency virus. *N. Engl. J. Med.* **316:**1569–1572.

49. **Kaufman, R. E., O. G. Jones, J. H. Blount, and P. J. Wiesner.** 1977. Questionnaire survey of reported early congenital syphilis, problems in diagnosis, prevention and treatment. *Sex. Transm. Dis.* **4:**135–139.

50. **Koopman, M. B. H., A. Käsbohrer, G. Beckmann, B. A. M. van der Zeijst, and J. G. K. Kusters.** 1993. Genetic similarity of intestinal spirochetes from humans and various animal species. *J. Clin. Microbiol.* **31:**711–716.

51. **Kraaz, W., B. Pettersson, U. Thunberg, L. Engstrand, and C. Fellstrom.** 2000. *Brachyspira aalborgi* infection diagnosed by culture and 16S ribosomal DNA sequencing using human colonic biopsy specimens. *J. Clin. Microbiol.* **38:**3555–3560.

52. **Larsen, S. A., V. Pope, R. E. Johnson, and E. J. Kennedy, Jr.** 1998. *A Manual of Tests for Syphilis*, 9th ed. American Public Health Association, Washington, D.C.

53. **Larsen, S. A., and B. M. Steiner.** 1995. Laboratory diagnosis and interpretation of tests for syphilis. *Clin. Microbiol. Rev.* **8:**1–21.

54. **Lefèvre, J. C., M. A. Bertrand, and R. Bauriaud.** 1990. Evaluation of the Captia enzyme immunoassays for detection of immunoglobulins G and M to *Treponema pallidum* in syphilis. *J. Clin. Microbiol.* **28:**1704–1707.

55. **Lewis, L. L., L. H. Taber, and R. E. Baughn.** 1990. Evaluation of immunoglobulin M Western blot analysis in the diagnosis of congenital syphilis. *J. Clin. Microbiol.* **28:**296–302.

56. **Liu, H., B. Rodes, C.-Y. Chen, and B. Steiner.** 2001. New tests for syphilis: rational design of a PCR method for detection of *Treponema pallidum* in clinical specimens using regions of the DNA polymerase I gene. *J. Clin. Microbiol.* **39:**1941–1946.

57. **Luger, A. F., B. L. Schmidt, and M. Kaulich.** 2000. Significance of laboratory findings for the diagnosis of neurosyphilis. *Int. J. STD AIDS* **11:**224–234.

58. **Lukehart, S. A., E. W. Hook III, S. A. Baker-Zander, A. C. Collier, C. W. Critchlow, and H. H. Handsfield.** 1988. Invasion of the central nervous system by *Treponema pallidum*: implications for diagnosis and treatment. *Ann. Intern. Med.* **109:**855–862.

59. **Magnarelli, L. A., J. N. Miller, J. F. Anderson, and G. R. Riviere.** 1990. Cross-reactivity of nonspecific treponemal antibody in serologic tests for Lyme disease. *J. Clin. Microbiol.* **28:**1276–1279.

60. **Magnuson, H. J., and H. Eagle.** 1948. The minimal infectious inoculum of *Spirochaeta pallida* (Nichols strain), and a consideration of its rate of multiplication in vivo. *Am. J. Syph.* **32:**1–18.

61. **Marangoni, A., V. Sambri, A. Olmo, A. D'Antuono, M. Negosanti, and R. Cevenini.** 1999. IgG western blot as a confirmatory test in early syphilis. *Zentbl. Bakteriol.* **289:** 125–133.

62. **Matthews, H. M., T. K. Yang, and H. M. Jenkin.** 1979. Unique lipid composition of *Treponema pallidum* (Nichols virulent strain). *Infect. Immun.* **24:**713–719.

63. **Meheus, A., and G. M. Antal.** 1992. The endemic treponematoses: not yet eradicated. *World Health Stat. Q.* **45:** 228–237.

64. **Mikosza, A. S., T. La, C. J. Brooke, C. F. Lindboe, P. B. Ward, R. G. Heine, J. G. Guccion, W. B. de Boer, and D. J. Hampson.** 1999. PCR amplification from fixed tissue indicates frequent involvement of *Brachyspira aalborgi* in human intestinal spirochetosis. *J. Clin. Microbiol.* **37:**2093–2098.

65. **Mikosza, A. S., T. La, W. B. de Boer, and D. J. Hampson.** 2001. Comparative prevalences of *Brachyspira aalborgi* and *Brachyspira (Serpulina) pilosicoli* as etiologic agents of histologically identified intestinal spirochetosis in Australia. *J. Clin. Microbiol.* **39:**347–350.

66. **Mikosza, A. S., T. La, K. R. Margawani, C. J. Brooke, and D. J. Hampson.** 2001. PCR detection of *Brachyspira aalborgi* and *Brachyspira pilosicoli* in human faeces. *FEMS Microbiol. Lett.* **197:**167–170.

67. **Miller, J. N., R. M. Smibert, and S. J. Norris.** 1992. The genus *Treponema*, p. 3537–3559. *In* A. Balows, H. G. Trüper, M. Dworkin, W. Harder, and K.-H. Schiefer (ed.), *The Prokaryotes. A Handbook on the Biology of Bacteria, Ecophysiology, Isolation, Identifications, and Applications*, 2nd ed. Springer-Verlag, Inc., New York, N.Y.

68. **Moore, L. V. H., W. E. C. Moore, E. P. Cato, R. M. Smibert, J. A. Burmeister, A. M. Best, and R. R. Ranney.** 1987. Bacteriology of human gingivitis. *J. Dent. Res.* **66:**989–995.

69. **Moore, W. E., and L. V. Moore.** 1994. The bacteria of periodontal diseases. *Periodontolology 2000* **5:**66–77.

70. **Moter, A., C. Hoenig, B. Choi, B. Riep, and U. Göbel.** 1998. Molecular epidemiology of oral treponemes associated with periodontal disease. *J. Clin. Microbiol.* **36:**1399–1403.

71. **Mullaly, B., B. Dace, C. Shelburne, L. Wolff, and W. Coulter.** 2000. Prevalence of periodontal pathogens in localized and generalized forms of early-onset periodontitis. *J. Periodontal Res.* **35:**232–241.

72. **Musher, D. M.** 1991. Syphilis, neurosyphilis, penicillin, and AIDS. *J. Infect. Dis.* **163:**1201–1206.

73. **Nathan, L., V. R. Bohman, P. J. Sanchez, N. K. Leos, D. M. Twickler, and J. Wendel.** 1997. In utero infection with *Treponema pallidum* in early pregnancy. *Prenatal Diagn.* **17:**119–123.

74. **Nayar, R., and J. M. Campos.** 1993. Evaluation of the DCL Syphilis-G enzyme immunoassay test kit for the serologic diagnosis of syphilis. *Am. J. Clin. Pathol.* **99:**282–285.

75. **Noordhoek, G. T., A. Cockayne, L. M. Schouls, R. H. Meloen, E. Stolz, and J. D. A. van Embden.** 1990. A new attempt to distinguish serologically the subspecies of *Treponema pallidum* causing syphilis and yaws. *J. Clin. Microbiol.* **28:**1600–1607.

76. **Noordhoek, G. T., H. J. H. Engelkens, J. Judanarso, J. van der Stek, G. N. M. Aelbers, J. J. van der Sluis, J. D. A. van Embden, and E. Stolz.** 1991. Yaws in West Sumatra, Indonesia: clinical manifestations, serological findings, and characterisation of new *Treponema* isolates by DNA probes. *Eur. J. Clin. Microbiol. Infect. Dis.* **10:**12–19.

77. **Noordhoek, G. T., P. W. M. Hermans, A. N. Paul, L. M. Schouls, J. J. van der Sluis, and J. D. A. van Embden.** 1989. *Treponema pallidum* subspecies *pallidum* (Nichols) and *Treponema pallidum* subspecies *pertenue* (CDC 2575) differ in at least one nucleotide: comparison of two homologous antigens. *Microb. Pathog.* **6:**29–42.

78. **Noordhoek, G. T., B. Wieles, J. J. van der Sluis, and J. D. A. van Embden.** 1990. Polymerase chain reaction and synthetic DNA probes—a means of distinguishing the causative agents of syphilis and yaws? *Infect. Immun.* **58:**2011–2013.

79. **Noordhoek, G. T., E. C. Wolters, M. E. J. De Jonge, and J. D. A. van Embden.** 1991. Detection by polymerase chain reaction of *Treponema pallidum* DNA in cerebrospinal fluid from neurosyphilis patients before and after antibiotic treatment. *J. Clin. Microbiol.* **29:**1976–1984.

80. **Norgard, M. V.** 1993. Clinical and diagnostic issues of acquired and congenital syphilis encompassed in the current syphilis epidemic. *Curr. Opin. Infect. Dis.* **6:**9–16.

80a.**Norris, S. J.** 1988. Syphilis, p. 1–31. *In* D. J. M. Wright (ed.), *Immunology of Sexually Transmitted Diseases.* MTP Press Ltd., Lancaster, England.

81. **Norris, S. J., D. L. Cox, and G. M. Weinstock.** 2001. Biology of *Treponema pallidum:* correlation of functional activities with genome sequence data. *J. Mol. Microbiol. Biotechnol.* **3:**37–62.

82. **Norris, S. J., and the *Treponema pallidum* Polypeptide Research Group.** 1993. Polypeptides of *Treponema pallidum:* progress toward understanding their structural, functional, and immunologic roles. *Microbiol. Rev.* **57:**750–779.

83. **Ochiai, S., Y. Adachi, and K. Mori.** 1997. Unification of the genera *Serpulina* and *Brachyspira,* and proposals of *Brachyspira hyodysenteriae* comb. nov., *Brachyspira innocens*

84. **Paster, B., S. Boches, J. Galvin, R. Ericson, C. Lau, V. Levanos, A. Sahasrabudhe, and F. Dewhirst.** 2001. Bacterial diversity in human subgingival plaque. *J. Bacteriol.* **183:**3770–3783.

85. **Paster, B., and F. Dewhirst.** 2000. Phylogenetic foundation of spirochetes. *J. Mol. Microbiol. Biotechnol.* **2:**341–344.

86. **Pedersen, N. S., O. Orum, and S. Mouritsen.** 1987. Enzyme-linked immunosorbent assay for detection of antibodies to venereal disease research laboratory (VDRL) antigen in syphilis. *J. Clin. Microbiol.* **25:**1711–1716.

87. **Perine, P. L., D. R. Hopkins, P. L. A. Niemel, R. K. St. John, G. Causse, and G. M. Antal.** 1984. *Handbook of Endemic Treponematoses: Yaws, Endemic Syphilis, and Pinta.* World Health Organization, Geneva, Switzerland.

88. **Perine, P. L., J. W. Nelson, J. O. Lewis, S. Liska, E. F. Hunter, S. A. Larsen, V. K. Agadzi, F. Kofi, J. A. K. Ofori, M. R. Tam, and M. A. Lovett.** 1985. New technologies for use in the surveillance and control of yaws. *Rev. Infect. Dis.* **7:**S295–S299.

89. **Pietravalle, M., F. Pimpinelli, A. Maini, E. Capoluongo, C. Felici, L. D'Auria, A. Di Carlo, and F. Ameglio.** 1999. Diagnostic relevance of polymerase chain reaction technology for *T. pallidum* in subjects with syphilis in different phases of infection. *Microbiologia* **22:**99–104.

90. **Pillay, A., H. Liu, C. Y. Chen, B. Holloway, W. Sturm, B. Steiner, and S. A. Morse.** 1998. Molecular subtyping of *Treponema pallidum* subspecies *pallidum. Sex. Transm. Dis.* **25:**408–414.

91. **Pope, V., M. B. Fears, W. E. Morrill, A. Castro, and S. E. Kikkert.** 2000. Comparison of the Serodia *Treponema pallidum* particle agglutination, Captia Syphilis-G, and Spiro Tek Reagin II tests with standard test techniques for diagnosis of syphilis. *J. Clin. Microbiol.* **38:**2543–2545.

92. **Rampalo, A. M., M. R. Joesoef, J. A. O'Donnell, M. Augenbraun, W. Brady, J. D. Radolf, R. Johnson, and R. T. Rolfs.** 2001. Clinical manifestations of early syphilis by HIV status and gender—results of the syphilis and HIV study. *Sex. Transm. Dis.* **28:**158–165.

93. **Rawstron, S. A., J. Vetrano, G. Tannis, and K. Bromberg.** 1997. Congenital syphilis: detection of *Treponema pallidum* in stillborns. *Clin. Infect. Dis.* **24:**24–27.

94. **Rein, M. F., G. W. Banks, L. C. Logan, S. A. Larsen, J. C. Feeley, D. S. Kellogg, and P. J. Wiesner.** 1980. Failure of the *Treponema pallidum* immobilization test to provide additional diagnostic information about contemporary problem sera. *Sex. Transm. Dis.* **7:**101–105.

95. **Riviere, G., K. Smith, S. Willis, and K. Riviere.** 1999. Phenotypic and genotypic heterogeneity among cultivable pathogen-related oral spirochetes and *Treponema vincentii. J. Clin. Microbiol.* **37:**3676–3680.

96. **Riviere, G. R., K. S. Weisz, D. F. Adams, and D. D. Thomas.** 1991. Pathogen-related oral spirochetes from dental plaque are invasive. *Infect. Immun.* **59:**3377–3380.

97. **Rolfs, R. T.** 1995. Treatment of syphilis, 1993. *Clin. Infect. Dis.* **20**(Suppl. 1):S23–S38.

98. **Rolfs, R. T., M. R. Joesoef, E. F. Hendershot, A. M. Rompalo, M. H. Augenbraun, M. Chiu, G. Bolan, S. C. Johnson, P. French, E. Steen, J. D. Radolf, S. Larsen, and The Syphilis and HIV Study Group.** 1997. A randomized trial of enhanced therapy for early syphilis in patients with and without human immunodeficiency virus infection. *N. Engl. J. Med.* **337:**307–314.

99. **Romanowski, B., R. Sutherland, F. H. Fick, D. Mooney, and E. J. Love.** 1991. Serologic response to treatment of infectious syphilis. *Ann. Intern. Med.* **114:**1005–1009.

100. **Rompalo, A.** 2001. Can syphilis be eradicated from the world? *Curr. Opin. Infect. Dis.* **14:**41–44.
101. **Rompalo, A. M., M. R. Joesoef, J. A. O'Donnell, M. Augenbraun, W. Brady, J. D. Radolf, R. Johnson, R. T. Rolfs, and the Syphilis and HIV Study Group.** 2001. Clinical manifestations of early syphilis by HIV status and gender: results of the Syphilis and HIV Study. *Sex. Transm. Dis.* **28:**158–165.
102. **Ruane, P. J., M. M. Nakata, J. F. Reinhardt, and W. L. George.** 1989. Spirochete-like organisms in the human gastrointestinal tract. *Rev. Infect. Dis.* **11:**184–196.
103. **Sambri, V., A. Marangoni, C. Eyer, C. Reichhuber, E. Soutschek, M. Negosanti, A. D'Antuono, and R. Cevenini.** 2001. Western immunoblotting with five *Treponema pallidum* recombinant antigens for serologic diagnosis of syphilis. *Clin. Diagn. Lab. Immunol.* **8:**534–539.
104. **Sambri, V., A. Marangoni, M. A. Simone, A. D'Antuono, M. Negosanti, and R. Cevenini.** 2001. Evaluation of recomWell Treponema, a novel recombinant antigen-based enzyme-linked immunosorbent assay for the diagnosis of syphilis. *Clin. Microbiol. Infect.* **7:**200–205.
105. **Sanchez, P. J., G. D. Wendel, Jr., E. Grimprel, M. Goldberg, M. Hall, O. Arencibia-Mireles, J. D. Radolf, and M. V. Norgard.** 1993. Evaluation of molecular methodologies and rabbit infectivity testing for the diagnosis of congenital syphilis and neonatal central nervous system invasion by *Treponema pallidum. J. Infect. Dis.* **167:**148–157.
106. **Schmidt, B. L., M. Edjlalipour, and A. Luger.** 2000. Comparative evaluation of nine different enzyme-linked immunosorbent assays for determination of antibodies against *Treponema pallidum* in patients with primary syphilis. *J. Clin. Microbiol.* **38:**1279–1282.
107. **Schroeter, A. L., J. B. Lucas, E. V. Price, and V. H. Falcone.** 1973. Treatment of early syphilis and reactivity of serologic tests. *JAMA* **221:**471–476.
108. **Schwartz, D. A., S. A. Larsen, R. J. Rice, M. Fears, and C. Beck-Sague.** 1995. Pathology of the umbilical cord in congenital syphilis. *Hum. Pathol.* **26:**784–791.
109. **Smibert, R. M.** 1984. Genus III: *Treponema* Schaudinn 1905, 1728[AL], p. 49–57. *In* N. R. Krieg and J. G. Holt (ed.), *Bergey's Manual of Systematic Bacteriology*, vol. 1. The Williams & Wilkins Co., Baltimore, Md.
110. **Smibert, R. M., and J. A. Burmeister.** 1983. *Treponema pectinovorum* sp. nov. isolated from humans with periodontitis. *Int. J. Syst. Bacteriol.* **33:**852–856.
111. **Smibert, R. M., J. L. Johnson, and R. R. Ranney.** 1984. *Treponema socranskii* sp. nov., *Treponema socranskii* subsp. *socranskii* subsp. nov., *Treponema socranskii* subsp. *buccale* subsp. nov., and *Treponema socranskii* subsp. *paredis* subsp.

112. nov. isolated from the human periodontia. *Int. J. Syst. Bacteriol.* **34:**457–462.
112. **Stoll, B. J., F. K. Lee, S. A. Larsen, E. Hale, D. Schwartz, R. J. Rice, R. Ashby, R. Holmes, and A. J. Nahmias.** 1993. Improved serodiagnosis of congenital syphilis with combined assay approach. *J. Infect. Dis.* **167:**1093–1099.
113. **Sutton, M. Y., H. Liu, B. Steiner, A. Pillay, T. Mickey, L. Finelli, S. Morse, L. E. Markowitz, and M. E. St. Louis.** 2001. Molecular subtyping of *Treponema pallidum* in an Arizona County with increasing syphilis morbidity: use of specimens from ulcers and blood. *J. Infect. Dis.* **183:**1601–1606.
114. **Swisher, B. L.** 1987. Modified Steiner procedure for microwave staining of spirochetes and nonfilamentous bacteria. *J. Histotechnol.* **10:**241–243.
115. **Trott, D. J., N. S. Jensen, I. Saint Girons, S. L. Oxberry, T. B. Stanton, D. Lindquist, and D. J. Hampson.** 1997. Identification and characterization of *Serpulina pilosicoli* isolates recovered from the blood of critically ill patients. *J. Clin. Microbiol.* **35:**482–485.
116. **Trott, D. J., T. B. Stanton, N. S. Jensen, G. E. Duhamel, J. L. Johnson, and D. J. Hampson.** 1996. *Serpulina pilosicoli* sp. nov., the agent of porcine intestinal spirochetosis. *Int. J. Syst. Bacteriol.* **46:**206–215.
117. **Trott, D. J., T. B. Stanton, N. S. Jensen, and D. J. Hampson.** 1996. Phenotypic characteristics of *Serpulina pilosicoli* the agent of intestinal spirochaetosis. *FEMS Microbiol. Lett.* **142:**209–214.
118. **Turner, T. B., and D. H. Hollander.** 1957. *Biology of the Treponematoses.* World Health Organization, Geneva, Switzerland.
119. **U.S. Public Health Service.** 1968. *Syphilis: a Synopsis.* U.S. Government Printing Office, Washington, D.C.
120. **Wicher, K., G. T. Noordhoek, F. Abbruscato, and V. Wicher.** 1992. Detection of *Treponema pallidum* in early syphilis by DNA amplification. *J. Clin. Microbiol.* **30:**497–500.
121. **World Health Organization.** 2001. *Global Prevalence and Incidence of Selected Curable Sexually Transmitted Diseases: Overview and Estimates.* WHO/HIV_AIDS/2001.02. World Health Organization, New York, N.Y.
122. **Young, H., A. Moyes, I. de Ste Croix, and A. McMillan.** 1998. A new recombinant antigen latex agglutination test (Syphilis Fast) for the rapid serological diagnosis of syphilis. *Int. J. STD AIDS* **9:**196–200.
123. **Young, H. A. M., A. McMillan, and J. Patterson.** 1992. Enzyme immunoassay for antitreponemal IgG: screening or confirmatory test? *J. Clin. Pathol.* **45:**37–41.
124. **Zenker, P. N., and S. M. Berman.** 1990. Congenital syphilis: reporting and reality. *Am. J. Public Health* **80:**271–272.

Mycoplasma and Ureaplasma

KEN B. WAITES, YASUKO RIKIHISA,
AND DAVID TAYLOR-ROBINSON

62

TAXONOMY AND NOMENCLATURE

Bacteria commonly referred to as mycoplasmas ("fungus-form") are included within the class Mollicutes ("soft skin"), which is composed of four orders, five families, eight genera, and at least 183 known species, as shown in Table 1. Table 2 lists 16 species isolated from humans, excluding occasional animal mycoplasmas that have been detected in humans from time to time, usually in immunosuppressed hosts, but which are generally considered transient colonizers. Mollicutes are eubacteria that have evolved from clostridial-like gram-positive cells by gene deletion. The availability of species-specific PCR technology is ameliorating difficulties of both culture and identification for fastidious mollicutes. Therefore, additional noncultivable, and thus presently unknown, species are likely to be discovered.

DESCRIPTION OF MOLLICUTES

Mollicutes are smaller than conventional bacteria, in cellular dimensions as well as genome size, making them the smallest free-living organisms known. Mycoplasmas associated with humans range from coccoid cells of about 0.2 to 0.3 μm in diameter, as in Ureaplasma spp. and Mycoplasma hominis (78), to tapered rods 1 to 2 μm long and 0.1 to 0.2 μm wide in the case of M. pneumoniae and M. penetrans (120). Mollicutes are contained by a trilayered cell membrane and do not possess a cell wall. The permanent lack of a cell wall barrier makes the mollicutes unique among prokaryotes and differentiates them from bacterial L forms, for which the lack of the cell wall is but a temporary reflection of environmental conditions. Lack of a cell wall also renders these organisms insensitive to the activity of β-lactam antimicrobials, prevents them from staining by Gram stain, and is largely responsible for their pleomorphic form. The extremely small genome (<600 kb in M. genitalium) and limited biosynthetic capabilities explain the parasitic or saprophytic existence of these organisms, their sensitivity to environmental conditions, and their fastidious growth requirements, which can complicate detection by culture. Mollicutes require enriched growth medium supplemented with nucleic acid precursors. Except for acholeplasmas, asteroleplasmas, and mesoplasmas, mollicutes require sterols in growth media, which is supplied by the addition of serum. Growth rates in culture medium vary

among individual species, with generation times of approximately 1 h for Ureaplasma spp., 6 h for M. pneumoniae, and 16 h for M. genitalium (50).

Typical mycoplasmal colonies vary from 15 to ≥300 μm in diameter. Colonies of some species, such as M. hominis, often exhibit a "fried-egg" appearance owing to the contrast in deeper growth in the center of the colony with more shallow growth at the periphery (Fig. 1), while others, such as M. pneumoniae, produce spherical colonies (Fig. 2). Whereas colonies of mycoplasmal species may be observed with the naked eye, those produced by ureaplasmas are typically 15 to 60 μm in diameter and require low-power microscopic magnification (Fig. 3).

Mycoplasmas of human origin can be classified according to whether they ferment glucose, utilize arginine, or hydrolyze urea (Table 2). Except for hydrolysis of urea, which is unique for ureaplasmas, these biochemical features are not sufficient for species distinction. Anaeroplasmas and asteroleplasmas, which occur in ruminants, are strictly anaerobic and oxygen sensitive, while most other mollicutes are facultative anaerobes.

Attachment of M. pneumoniae to host cells in the respiratory tracts of humans is a prerequisite for colonization and infection. Cytadherence, mediated by the P1 adhesin protein, is followed by induction of ciliostasis, chronic inflammation, and cytotoxicity mediated by hydrogen peroxide, which also acts as a hemolysin (8). M. pneumoniae stimulates B and T lymphocytes and induces the formation of autoantibodies which react with a variety of host tissues and the I antigen on erythrocytes, which is responsible for production of cold agglutinins. M. genitalium also possesses a terminal structure, the MgPa adhesin, which facilitates its attachment to epithelial cells. Factors involved with Ureaplasma and M. hominis attachment have not been well characterized, but ureaplasmas are known to produce immunoglobulin A (IgA) protease, which may be associated with disease production. Ureaplasmas also release ammonia through urealytic activity (108).

NATURAL HABITATS

Mollicutes are common in practically all mammalian species, as well as many other vertebrates in which they have been sought. Although most mollicutes have species-specific host-organism associations, some mycoplasmas and

TABLE 1 Classification and some distinguishing features of mycoplasmas (class *Mollicutes*)

Classification of class *Mollicutes*	Distinguishing features			
	Sterol required	Genome size (kbp)	Mol% G+C of DNA	Other
Order I: *Mycoplasmatales*				
Family I: *Mycoplasmataceae*				
Genus I: *Mycoplasma* (105 species)[a]	Yes	580–1,380	23–41	
Genus II: *Ureaplasma* (7 species)[b]	Yes	730–1,160	27–30	Urea metabolized
Order II: *Entomoplasmatales*				
Family I: *Entomoplasmataceae*				
Genus I: *Entomoplasma* (6 species)	Yes	790–1,140	27–29	
Genus II: *Mesoplasma* (12 species)	No	870–1,100	27–30	Requires 0.04% Tween 80
Family II: *Spiroplasmataceae*				
Genus I: *Spiroplasma* (34 species)	Yes	940–2,200	25–31	Helical structure
Order III: *Acholeplasmatales*[c]				
Family I: *Acholeplasmataceae*				
Genus I: *Acholeplasma* (14 species)	No	1,500–1,690	27–36	
Order IV: *Anaeroplasmatales*				
Family I: *Anaeroplasmataceae*				Obligate anaerobes
Genus I: *Anaeroplasma* (4 species)	Yes	ca. 1,600	29–33	
Genus II: *Asteroleplasma* (1 species)	No	ca. 1,600	40	

[a] Cell wall-less uncultivated parasitic bacteria that attach to the surface of erythrocytes and also occur free in the plasma, previously classified in the genera *Haemobartonella* and *Eperythrozoon*, are currently given candidatus status in the genus *Mycoplasma*. Their G+C content and sterol requirements are unknown.

[b] *U. urealyticum* and *U. parvum*, formerly considered biovars of *U. urealyticum*, are now classified as two separate species and are the only ureaplasmas of human origin.

[c] Phytoplasmas are uncultivable mollicutes of plants and insects genetically related to the *Acholeplasmatales* but have not been assigned individual genus and species designations.

acholeplasmas of animal origin occur in a wide variety of different animal hosts. Mollicutes can also be isolated from insects (entomoplasmas) and plants (spiroplasmas).

In humans, mycoplasmas and ureaplasmas are mucosally associated, residing predominantly in the respiratory and urogenital tracts and rarely penetrating the submucosa, except in cases of immunosuppression or instrumentation,

when they may invade the bloodstream and disseminate to many different organs and tissues throughout the body. Many mollicutes exist as commensals in the oropharynx (*M. salivarium*, *M. orale*, *M. buccale*, *M. faucium*, *M. lipophilum*, and *Acholeplasma laidlawii*) and have been associated with invasive disease only in very rare circumstances. *M. fermentans* has been detected by culture, and more

TABLE 2 Primary sites of colonization, metabolism, and pathogenicity of mollicutes of human origin

Species	Primary site of colonization		Metabolism of:		Pathogenicity
	Oropharynx	Genitourinary tract	Glucose	Arginine	
M. salivarium	+	−	−	+	−
M. orale	+	−	−	+	−
M. buccale	+	−	−	+	−
M. faucium	+	−	−	+	−
M. lipophilum	+	−	−	+	−
M. pneumoniae	+	−	+	−	+
M. hominis	+	+	−	+	+
M. genitalium	?+[a]	+	+	−	+
M. fermentans	+	+	+	+	+
M. primatum	−	+	−	+	−
M. spermatophilum	−	+	−	+	−
M. pirum	?	?	+	+	−
M. penetrans	−	+	+	+	?
Ureaplasma sp.[b]	+	+	−	−	+
A. laidlawii	+	−	+	−	−
A. oculi	?	?	+	−	−

[a] The organism has been found in the oropharynx, but whether that is a common or primary location is not known.

[b] Metabolizes urea.

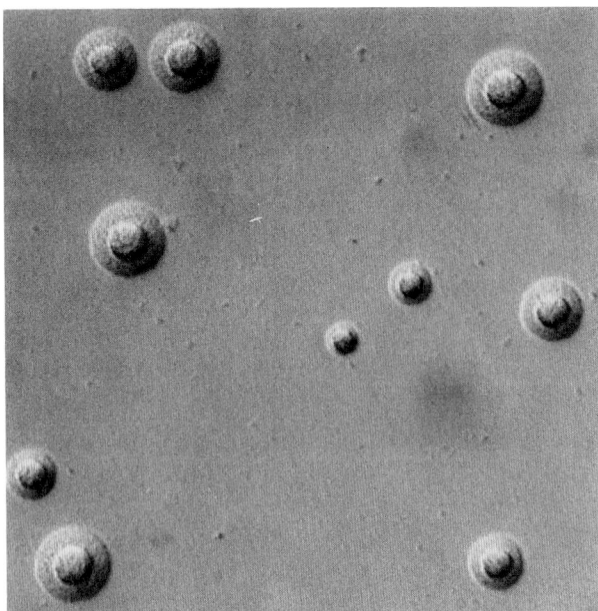

FIGURE 1 Fried-egg-type colonies of M. *hominis* up to 110 μm in diameter. Magnification, ×132.

recently by means of PCR assays, in various body sites, including the urogenital tract, throat, lower respiratory tract, and other body locations including joints (2–4, 82, 83), but its primary site of colonization and true disease potential are incompletely understood. Oral commensal mycoplasmas occasionally spread to the lower respiratory tract and can cause diagnostic confusion with M. *pneumoniae*.

Frequent occurrence of pathogenic species such as M. *hominis* and ureaplasmas in the lower urogenital tract in healthy men and women has so far precluded a complete understanding of their disease-producing capabilities. Organisms such as M. *hominis*, although most commonly

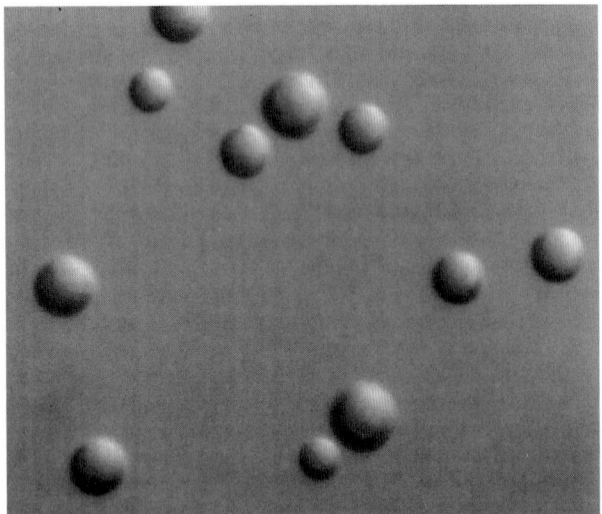

FIGURE 2 Spherical colonies of M. *pneumoniae* up to 100 μm in diameter. Magnification, ×98.

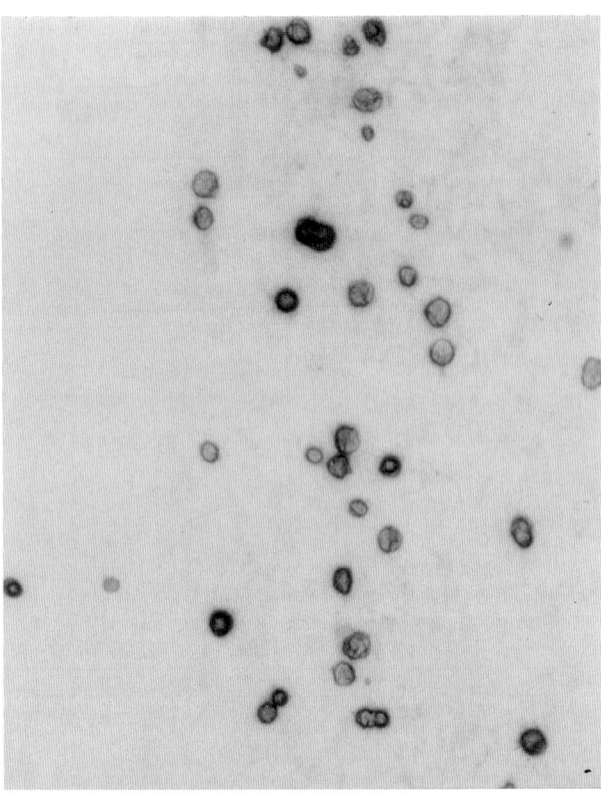

FIGURE 3 Granular brown urease-positive colonies *of Urea-plasma* species 15 to 60 μm in diameter from a vaginal specimen growing on A 8 agar. Magnification, ×100.

isolated from the urogenital tract, can also disseminate to other body sites, particularly if host defenses are impaired. M. *primatum*, M. *spermatophilum*, and A. *oculi* have been detected in the urogenital tract but are not associated with disease. Recent studies using PCR assays have demonstrated frequent occurrence of M. *genitalium* in the urogenital tract in men with urethritis (45, 46, 97, 107) and of M. *penetrans* in urine of homosexual males with human immunodeficiency virus (HIV)-associated disease (63, 117, 118). Although mycoplasmas are generally considered to be extracellular organisms, intracellular localization is now appreciated for M. *fermentans*, M. *penetrans*, M. *genitalium*, and M. *pneumoniae* (8, 25). Intracellular localization may be responsible for protecting the organism from antibodies and antibiotics, as well as contributing to disease chronicity and difficulty in cultivation. Variation in surface antigens of M. *hominis* and *Ureaplasma* spp. may be related to persistence of these organisms at invasive sites. In humans, mycoplasmas and ureaplasmas may be transmitted by direct contact between hosts, i.e., venereally through genital-genital or oral-genital contact; vertically from mother to offspring either at birth or in utero; by respiratory aerosols or fomites in the case of M. *pneumoniae*; or even by nosocomial acquisition through transplanted tissues.

CLINICAL SIGNIFICANCE

Respiratory Infections

M. *pneumoniae* was first identified and described in the early 1960s. It causes approximately 20% of all community-acquired pneumonias in the general population and up to 50% of pneumonias in certain confined groups (36, 73, 94). Although M. *pneumoniae* has long been associated with pneumonias in school-aged children, adolescents, and young adults, in recent years this organism has also been shown to occur endemically and occasionally epidemically in older persons, as well as children younger than 5 years (36, 47, 73, 94). The most typical clinical syndrome is tracheobronchitis, often accompanied by upper respiratory tract manifestations. Pneumonia develops in about one-third of persons who are infected. The incubation period is generally 2 to 3 weeks, and spread throughout households is common. The organism may persist in the respiratory tract for several months after initial infection and sometimes for years in hypogammaglobulinemic patients, possibly because the organism attaches strongly to and invades epithelial cells mediated by the P1 adhesin protein (36, 94, 102). Disease tends not to be seasonal, subclinical infections are common, and the disease is ordinarily mild. However, severe infections requiring hospitalization and even deaths are known to occur, especially in middle-aged and elderly persons (66).

Extrapulmonary complications including meningoencephalitis, ascending paralysis, transverse myelitis, pericarditis, hemolytic anemia, arthritis, and mucocutaneous lesions occur in some cases. Other nonspecific manifestations include nausea, vomiting, and diarrhea. An autoimmune response is thought to play a role in some extrapulmonary complications. However, M. *pneumoniae* has been isolated directly from cerebrospinal, pericardial, and synovial fluids, as well as other extrapulmonary sites, and additional evidence of direct invasion by this organism has been documented by the use of the PCR assay (94). Clinical manifestations are not sufficiently unusual to allow differentiation from infections caused by other common bacteria, particularly *Chlamydophila pneumoniae*. Recent data from animal models as well as clinical studies relying primarily on detection of organisms using the PCR assay have suggested a potential role of chronic infections with M. *pneumoniae* and C. *pneumoniae* as etiologic or exacerbating factors in bronchial asthma (67). Additional clinical studies are required to determine the ultimate significance of these preliminary findings.

M. *fermentans* has been recovered from the throats of children with pneumonia, in some of whom no other etiologic agent was identified, but the frequency of its occurrence in healthy children is not known (94). M. *fermentans* has been detected in adults with an acute influenza-like illness (62) and in bronchoalveolar lavage fluid, peripheral blood lymphocytes, and bone marrow from patients with AIDS and respiratory disease (2, 4). It is apparent that respiratory infection with M. *fermentans* is not necessarily linked with immunodeficiency, but the organism may also behave as an opportunistic respiratory pathogen.

Genitourinary Infections

Following puberty, *Ureaplasma* spp. and M. *hominis* can be isolated from the lower genital tract in many sexually active adults, with ureaplasmas being the more common organisms detected. Difficulty in accepting M. *hominis* and *Ureaplasma* spp. as causes of disease has arisen either because samples cannot be obtained easily from the affected site (for example, the fallopian tube) or because the organisms are recovered from asymptomatic individuals. Nevertheless, there is evidence that these species play etiologic roles in some genital tract diseases of both men and women. However,

the organisms reach the upper tract and cause disease only in a subpopulation of individuals who are colonized in the lower tract.

Results of human and animal inoculation studies and observations of immunocompromised patients support the notion that ureaplasmas are a cause of nonchlamydial, nongonococcal urethritis (NGU) in men, with further evidence supplied by therapeutic and serologic studies (91, 96, 98). Evidence that M. *hominis* causes NGU is lacking (91). M. *genitalium* has been detected by PCR technology significantly more often in urethral specimens from men with acute NGU than from those without urethritis (45, 49, 97, 107). Antibody responses have been detected in some men with acute disease, and this mycoplasma has also caused urethritis in nonhuman primates (94). M. *fermentans*, M. *penetrans*, and M. *pirum* were not detected in the urethras of men with urethritis by PCR assays, suggesting that these organisms are unlikely to play a pathogenic role in this condition (27). There is no evidence that M. *hominis* is a cause of the urethral syndrome in women, but ureaplasmas may be involved (88).

M. *hominis* and *Ureaplasma* spp. have not been detected by culture of prostatic biopsy samples from patients with chronic abacterial prostatitis (28), and M. *genitalium* has been found rarely by using a PCR assay (59). In contrast, ureaplasmas have been recovered from an epididymal aspirate from a patient suffering from nonchlamydial, nongonococcal acute epididymo-orchitis accompanied by a specific antibody response (48) and may be an infrequent cause of the disease. *Ureaplasma* spp. produce urease and induce crystallization of struvite and calcium phosphates in urine in vitro (43) and calculi in animal models (103). In addition, ureaplasmas have been found in urinary calculi of patients with infection-type stones more frequently than those with metabolism-type stones, suggesting a possible causal association (40). M. *hominis* has been isolated from the upper urinary tract only in patients with symptoms of acute pyelonephritis, often with an antibody response (106), and may cause about 5% of cases of such disease. Obstruction or instrumentation of the urinary tract may be predisposing factors. Ureaplasmas have not been associated in the same way.

Mollicutes do not cause vaginitis but are among various microorganisms that proliferate in patients with bacterial vaginosis (BV) and may contribute to the condition (101). BV may lead to pelvic inflammatory disease, and M. *hominis* has been isolated from the endometrium and fallopian tubes of about 10% of women with laparoscopy-diagnosed salpingitis accompanied by a specific antibody response (101). However, the significance of this mycoplasma is difficult to assess in an individual case when several microorganisms are present. *Ureaplasma* spp. have been isolated directly from affected fallopian tubes, but not alone. This, together with the negative results of serologic tests and of inoculating nonhuman primates as well as fallopian tube organ cultures (94), does not support a causal relationship for ureaplasmas in PID. M. *genitalium*, however, may play a role, as indicated by its significant association with cervicitis (65) and endometritis (22) by serologic data (70) and the results of non-human primate inoculation (94). In addition, there is serologic evidence that this mycoplasma causes some cases of tubal infertility in women (20). That ureaplasmas might cause infertility remains speculative (92, 93), as does the possibility that these organisms could affect sperm (41, 92).

Ureaplasmas have been isolated from internal organs of spontaneously aborted fetuses and from stillborn and premature infants more often than from induced abortions or normal full-term infants (100). The results of some serologic and therapeutic studies (41) have also supported a role for these organisms in fetal morbidity. BV is a possible confounding factor which must be considered in the association between ureaplasmas in the chorioamnion and low birth weight. Ureaplasmas at this site are directly associated with inflammation (32) and may invade the amniotic sac early in pregnancy in the presence of intact fetal membranes, causing persistent infection and adverse pregnancy outcome (15).

The notion that *M. hominis* organisms cause fever in some women after abortion or after normal delivery is based on their isolation from the blood of about 10% of such women but not from afebrile women who have had abortions or from healthy pregnant women (41, 93). In addition, antibody responses have been detected in about half of febrile aborting women but in only a few of those who remain afebrile (41, 93). Similar observations have been made for the isolation of *Ureaplasma* spp. (31). Case reports suggest that at least in some individuals, ureaplasmas alone may play a causal role in spontaneous abortion and premature birth (18).

Neonatal Infections

Colonization of infants by genital mycoplasmas may occur by ascension from the lower genital tract of the mother at the time of delivery or in utero earlier in gestation and may be transient and without sequelae. The rate of vertical transmission may be 18 to 55% among infants born to colonized mothers (18). *Ureaplasma* spp. and *M. hominis* may be isolated from neonates born to mothers with intact membranes and delivered by cesarean section, indicative of transplacental in utero transmission (18). Congenital pneumonia, bacteremia, progression to chronic lung disease of prematurity, and even death have occurred in very-low-birth-weight infants (<1,000 g) as a result of ureaplasmal infection of the lower respiratory tract (17). Both *M. hominis* and *Ureaplasma* spp. have been isolated from maternal and umbilical cord blood, as well as the blood of neonates. Both species can also invade the cerebrospinal fluid of neonates (111). Either mild, subclinical meningitis without sequelae or neurologic damage with permanent handicaps may ensue (111). Colonization of healthy full-term infants declines after 3 months of age, and fewer than 10% of older children and sexually inexperienced adults are colonized with genital mycoplasmas (18). While *M. fermentans* has been detected in pure culture from placenta and amniotic fluid in the presence of inflammation, no prospective studies to date have been performed to determine its occurrence and significance, if any, in neonates. Vertical transmission of *M. genitalium* from mother to neonate has been reported (64), but its significance in neonates is unknown.

Routine screening of neonates for genital mycoplasmas is not clinically justified based on the available evidence that many healthy neonates may be colonized without consequence. However, if there is clinical, radiological, or laboratory evidence of pneumonia, meningitis, or overall instability, particularly in preterm neonates in whom there are no obvious alternative etiologies, infection with *M. hominis* or *Ureaplasma* spp. should be considered.

Systemic Infections and Immunosuppressed Hosts

Extrapulmonary and extragenital mycoplasmal infections probably occur more often than is currently recognized. In many instances, these organisms are considered only after other likely etiologic agents have been excluded and/or there is no improvement following treatment with antimicrobials inactive against mycoplasmas. *M. hominis* is alone among pathogenic mycoplasmas of human origin which may occasionally be detected in routine bacteriologic cultures, so that there have been many instances of accidental discovery when mycoplasmas were not specifically sought. There is considerable evidence that mollicutes can cause invasive disease of the joints and respiratory tract with bacteremic dissemination in immunosuppressed persons, especially individuals with hypogammaglobulinemia (18, 39, 91, 94, 99, 102). Mycoplasmas are probably the most common etiologic agents of septic arthritis in the setting of congenital antibody deficiency states and should always be considered early when attempting to diagnose these conditions (18, 39, 91, 99, 102). In some patients, the arthritis responds to antibiotic therapy, whereas in others, disease and organisms persist for many months despite antimicrobial and anti-inflammatory treatment and gammaglobulin replacement. In some cases, arthritis has been associated with subcutaneous abscesses and chronic urethrocystitis (99). *M. hominis* bacteremia has been demonstrated after renal transplantation, trauma, and genitourinary manipulations. *M. hominis* has also been found in wound infections, brain abscesses, and osteomyelitis lesions (69). Numerous mycoplasmal species, including *M. fermentans*, *U. urealyticum*, and *M. salivarium*, have been detected by culture and/or PCR in synovial fluid of persons with rheumatoid arthritis, although the precise contribution of these organisms to this disease condition is still uncertain (82, 93). The significance of *M. fermentans* (53, 119), *M. penetrans* (63, 116–118), and other mycoplasmas in persons infected with HIV, with or without AIDS, has received a great deal of attention. However, the notion that *M. fermentans* is important in disease progression lacks firm support (4). *M. hominis* has been isolated on numerous occasions from sternal wounds in recipients of heart or lung transplants (94).

COLLECTION, TRANSPORT, AND STORAGE OF SPECIMENS

Specimen Type and Collection

Body fluids appropriate for mycoplasmal culture include blood, synovial fluid, amniotic fluid, cerebrospinal fluid, urine, prostatic secretions, semen, wound aspirates, sputum, pleural fluid, bronchoalveolar lavage fluid, and other tracheobronchial secretions, depending on the clinical condition and organisms of interest. Swabs from the nasopharynx, cervix and/or vagina, wounds, and urethra are also acceptable. Tissue from biopsy or autopsy, including placenta, endometrium, bone chips, and urinary calculi, can also be cultured. When swabs are used, care must be taken to sample the desired site vigorously to obtain as many cells as possible since mycoplasmas are cell associated. If determination of the localization of mycoplasmas in the genitourinary tract is desired, urine specimens can be obtained at various stages during urination or after prostatic massage. Care should be taken to avoid collection of specimens that are contaminated by lubricants or antiseptics commonly used in gynecologic practice. Calcium alginate, Dacron, or polyester swabs with aluminum or plastic shafts are preferred. Wooden-shaft cotton swabs should be avoided because of potential inhibitory effects. Swabs should always be removed from specimens before transportation to the laboratory.

Mycoplasmas can be successfully isolated from blood by inoculating blood, free of anticoagulant, into liquid mycoplasmal growth media at the bedside at a 1:10 ratio, using as much blood as possible (at least 10 ml in adults). Mycoplasmas are inhibited by sodium polyanethol sulfonate, the anticoagulant used in most commercial blood culture media, but the inhibitory effect can be overcome by addition of gelatin (1% wt/vol) (74). Use of commercial blood culture media with or without automated blood culture instruments is not recommended for detection of mycoplasmas. Continuously monitored, nonradiometric, automated blood culture systems have been evaluated for their ability to detect the growth of *M. hominis*. Thus far, none has been shown to flag bottles containing the organism, even when additional metabolic substrate and gelatin are added. The organism may survive in these media for several days, however (110).

Transport and Storage

Mycoplasmas are extremely sensitive to adverse environmental conditions, particularly drying and heat. Specimens should be inoculated at the bedside whenever possible, using appropriate transport and/or culture media. Specific mycoplasma media such as SP-4 or Shepard's 10 B broths (84, 109) or 2 SP (10% heat-inactivated fetal calf serum with 0.2 M sucrose in 0.02 M phosphate buffer [pH 7.2]) are acceptable transport media and can also be used for sample preparation for PCR assays. Other media available commercially for transport and storage of specimens are Stuart's medium, Trypticase soy broth with 0.5% bovine serum albumin, and Mycotrans (Irvine Scientific, Irvine, Calif.). A3B broth (Remel, Inc., Lenexa, Kans.) is available as a transport medium, whereas Remel arginine broth, 10 B, and SP-4 transport broths also serve as growth media. Liquid specimens do not require special transport media if cultures can be inoculated within 1 h, provided that the specimens are protected from evaporation. Tissues can be placed in a sterile container which can be tightly closed and delivered to the laboratory immediately. Otherwise, tissue specimens should be placed in transport media if a >1-h delay in culture inoculation is anticipated. Specimens should be refrigerated if immediate transportation to the laboratory is not possible. If specimens must be shipped and/or if the storage time is likely to exceed 24 h prior to processing, the specimen in transport medium should be frozen at $-70°C$ to prevent loss of viability and to minimize bacterial overgrowth if the specimen is from a nonsterile site. Mollicutes can be stored for long periods in appropriate growth or transport media at $-70°C$ or in liquid nitrogen (38). Frozen specimens can be shipped with dry ice to a reference laboratory if necessary. When specimens are to be examined, they should be thawed rapidly in a 37°C water bath.

NONCULTURAL DETECTION

Although culture is well adapted to species which can be isolated easily and rapidly from clinical specimens, such as *M. hominis* and *Ureaplasma* spp., it is not ideal for the detection of fastidious and/or extremely slowly growing organisms such as *M. genitalium* and, to a considerable degree, *M. pneumoniae*. Therefore, alternate means of detection should be used even if culture is attempted for these

organisms. The same types of specimens used for culture can also be used for noncultural detection of human mycoplasmas, but transportation conditions do not have to maintain organism viability. Several different methods for direct or amplified detection of mycoplasmas in clinical specimens have been described.

Antigen Detection Techniques

Rapid methods developed for antigenic detection of *M. pneumoniae* have included direct immunofluorescence, counterimmunoelectrophoresis, immunoblotting, and antigen capture enzyme immunoassay (EIA) (9, 40, 56, 93). The utility and general acceptance of these techniques have been reduced by low sensitivity and cross-reactivity with other mycoplasmas found in the respiratory tract. The use of optimum antibody mixtures can increase detection sensitivity within the range of 10^3 to 10^4 CFU/100 μl of specimen (9). Considering that the concentration of *M. pneumoniae* cells typically found in the sputum of infected patients is approximately 10^2 to 10^6 CFU/ml, antigen detection techniques are at the limit of sensitivity for detection and are not recommended for diagnostic purposes.

DNA Probes

DNA hybridization techniques for the diagnosis of *M. pneumoniae* infection were developed in the early 1980s (75). The 16S rRNA genes have been widely used as targets, as have probes consisting of rDNA. Because probes are relatively insensitive, the more recently available amplification techniques such as the PCR assay have largely supplanted them, and none is sold commercially in the United States.

PCR Amplification

PCR systems have been developed for all of the clinically important mycoplasma species that infect humans (9, 11, 24, 26, 34, 42, 45–47, 49, 51, 57, 58, 75, 80, 82, 89, 118). Targets include 16S rRNA genes and other repetitive sequences such as the insertion-like elements of *M. fermentans* (119), the P1 adhesin of *M. pneumoniae* (23), and the MgPa adhesin gene of *M. genitalium* (26, 49). Urease genes have been used for *Ureaplasma* spp. (11). For slowly growing organisms such as *M. pneumoniae*, and especially for extremely fastidious species for which optimum cultivation techniques are not established, such as *M. genitalium* and *M. fermentans*, the use of PCR assays may be the only practical means of detecting their presence in clinical material. The sensitivity of the PCR is very high, corresponding to a single organism when purified DNA is used. However, comparison of the PCR technique with culture and/or serology, in the case of *M. pneumoniae*, has yielded varied results, and large-scale experience with this procedure is still limited for any mollicute species. Positive PCR results for *M. pneumoniae* in culture-negative specimens from person without evidence of respiratory disease suggests inadequate specificity or persistence of the organism after infection or its existence in asymptomatic carriers. Quantitative studies may be useful in drawing conclusions. PCR is also a very good tool for identification of an unknown mycoplasma previously obtained by culture. It can be used for characterization of strains within a species, and for detection of a specific feature, such as the presence of an antibiotic resistance determinant. PCR technology appears to be less valuable for routine diagnostic purposes in the case of the more rapidly growing and easily cultivable organisms, such as *M. hominis* and *Ureaplasma* spp. Presently, PCR detection for mycoplasmas and most other microorganisms of clinical significance is still too expensive and complex to be carried out routinely in most clinical microbiology laboratories. Some drawbacks must still be corrected, such as the problem of contamination and the presence of inhibitors. Multiplex PCR tests, detecting several mycoplasmas or even combinations of mycoplasmas and other agents of community-acquired pneumonia, such as C. pneumoniae and Legionella pneumophila, may eventually prove useful for screening purposes (44). The possible development of commercial PCR kits in the future should bring about better standardization of the technique, and if available at a reasonable cost, PCR could become a major method for the diagnosis of mycoplasmal infections. Detailed information concerning PCR methods and controls has been provided (9, 75).

ISOLATION PROCEDURES

Growth Media and Inoculation
Growth of mycoplasmas pathogenic for humans requires the presence of serum, growth factors such as yeast extract, and a metabolic substrate. No single formulation is ideal for all pertinent species because of different properties, optimum pH, and substrate requirements. SP-4 broth and agar (pH 7.5) (109) are the best media overall and can be used for both M. pneumoniae and M. hominis, provided that arginine is added for the latter. Shepard's 10 B broth (pH 6.0) (84) can be used for M. hominis and Ureaplasma spp., with A 8 agar (85) as the corresponding solid medium. Refer to Appendix 1 for the compositions of these media. Penicillin G or a broad-spectrum semisynthetic penicillin (1,000 IU/ml) should be added to minimize bacterial overgrowth, especially for specimens from nonsterile sites. Addition of a pH indicator, such as phenol red, is important for detection of growth because mycoplasmas usually do not produce turbidity in broth culture owing to their small cell size.

Lack of commercially prepared media in the past has effectively prevented many laboratories, except those in institutions with especially high volumes or specific research interests in mycoplasmal diseases, from offering on-site mycoplasma detection. For self-prepared media, quality control is crucial for each of the main components. These controls must consist of the quantitative growth of mycoplasma strain(s) in two media that differ only in the component to be tested. New lots or batches of broth are considered satisfactory if the numbers of organisms that grow are within one 10-fold dilution of the reference batch. Agar plates should ideally support the growth of at least 90% of the colonies that are supported by the reference media. Sterility of commercially purchased medium components, such as horse serum, must be confirmed prior to their use. If a reference laboratory is to be used for mycoplasma testing, it is necessary to ask whether the medium used is self-prepared or purchased from a manufacturer and the type of quality control procedures performed should be verified. Quality control test organisms should include type strains and low-passage clinical isolates of the species of interest. When testing ureaplasmas, it is recommended to include at least one representative from the two biovar groups. Recommended choices include serotypes 3 and either 5, 7, or 8. Type strains of M. pneumoniae, M. hominis, and U. urealyticum designated by the American Type Culture Collection are available commercially for quality control testing. Testing inhibitory properties of media against the growth of various other organisms probably present in specimens from nonsterile sites may also be worthwhile to prevent the loss of mycoplasmas due to overgrowth of contaminating organisms.

Specimens should always be mixed well before being used to inoculate media, and fluids should be centrifuged ($600 \times g$ for 15 min) and the pellet inoculated. Urine can be filtered through a 0.45-μm-pore-size filter if bacterial contamination is suspected. Furthermore, it is wise to mince, not grind, tissues in broth prior to diluting. Serial dilution of specimens in broth to at least 10^{-3} with subculture of each dilution onto agar is an extremely important step in the cultivation process since it will help overcome possible interference by antibiotics, antibodies, and other inhibitors, including bacteria, that may be present in clinical specimens (93). Omission of this critical dilution step may be one reason why some laboratories have difficulty in recovering the organisms. Dilution also helps to overcome the problem of rapid decline in culture viability, which is particularly common with ureaplasmas, and it also provides information about the number of organisms present in the specimen. DNA fluorochrome stains such as Hoechst 33258 (ICN Biomedicals, Costa Mesa, Calif.) (Appendix 2) or acridine orange stain may be useful when applied to body fluids such as amniotic fluid after cytocentrifugation but are not specific for mycoplasmas. Positive and negative controls must always be included when these stains are used.

Incubation Conditions and Subcultures
Broths should be incubated at 37°C under atmospheric conditions. Agar plates yield the best growth if they are incubated in an atmosphere of room air supplemented with 5 to 10% CO_2 or in an anaerobic environment of 95% N_2 plus 5% CO_2. A candle jar or anaerobe jar with GasPak catalyst is adequate if dedicated incubators are not available. The relatively high growth rates of M. hominis and Ureaplasma spp. make identification of most positive cultures possible within 2 to 4 days, whereas M. pneumoniae usually requires 21 days or more. Several mycoplasmal species of human origin can produce similar biochemical reactions, and identification can be accomplished only by specific tests on organisms once isolated. All broths that have changed color should be subcultured into a fresh tube of the corresponding broth (0.1 ml into 0.9 ml) and onto agar (0.02 ml). Subcultures must be performed soon after the color change occurs, particularly if the organism belongs to Ureaplasma spp., because the culture can lose viability within a few hours. Subculture also increases the diagnostic yield since some strains may not grow sufficiently from the original specimen inoculated initially onto solid media. Blind subculture periodically during incubation may improve the yield of M. pneumoniae and other mycoplasmas since a color change may not always be evident, even if growth occurs. Cultures should be incubated for at least 7 days before being designated negative for genital mycoplasmas and 4 weeks for M. pneumoniae. The growth rate of M. fermentans is similar to that of M. pneumoniae. However, for M. fermentans, M. genitalium, and mycoplasmas of human origin other than M. pneumoniae, M. hominis, or Ureaplasma spp., cultivation conditions are not well established. Due to the advent of PCR assays for use in research and reference laboratories, the need to refine culture techniques for these slowly growing and fastidious organisms is less critical than previously.

Development of Colonies

Broth cultures for *Ureaplasma* spp. should be examined for color changes resulting from hydrolysis of urea twice daily for up to 7 days because of the steep death phase of this organism in culture. This is less critical for *Mycoplasma* spp., for which once-daily inspection of broth cultures is sufficient. Agar plates should be examined, using a stereomicroscope at ×20 to ×60 magnification, daily for *Ureaplasma* spp., at 1- to 3-day intervals for M. *hominis,* and every 3 to 5 days for M. *pneumoniae* and other slower-growing species. Mycoplasmal colonies must be distinguished from artifacts such as air bubbles, water or lipid droplets, or other debris, which can be confusing. *Ureaplasma* colonies (Fig. 3) can be identified on A 8 agar by urease production in the presence of $CaCl_2$ indicator contained in the medium. The larger M. *hominis* colonies are urease negative and often have the typical fried-egg appearance (Fig. 1). Other species, such as M. *pneumoniae* and M. *genitalium,* will produce much smaller spherical colonies, which may or may not demonstrate the fried-egg appearance (Fig. 2). Methylene blue stain applied directly to the agar plate is sometimes useful if there is uncertainty about whether mycoplasmal colonies are present. Mycoplasmal colonies stain blue with this reagent. M. *hominis* is the only pathogenic mycoplasma of humans cultivable on bacteriological media such as chocolate agar or blood agar, but the pinpoint translucent colonies are easily overlooked and routine bacterial cultures may be discarded sooner than the time needed for M. *hominis* colonies to develop, which may require 4 days or more in some cases. Occurrence of suspicious colonies warrants subculture to appropriate mycoplasma media.

Commercial Media and Culture Kits

In response to the growing desire of many independent or hospital-based clinical laboratories to offer mycoplasmal cultures on-site, numerous companies in the United States and Europe have developed various transport and growth media systems patterned after the original formulations developed by researchers in the field of mycoplasmology. A variety of kits for detection, quantitation, identification, and antimicrobial susceptibility testing of *Ureaplasma* spp. and M. *hominis* from urogenital specimens are available in several European countries but not in the United States. These products are sold by various international suppliers such as bioMérieux, Marcy l'Etoile, France, and International Microbio, Toulon Cedex, France. A more complete description of these commercial kits sold in Europe is provided in the *Manual of Commercial Methods in Clinical Microbiology* (116).

Mycoscreen GU (Irvine Scientific, Santa Ana, Calif.) is a broth-based culture system for screening clinical specimens for genital mycoplasmas. Vials showing evidence of growth as indicated by a color change must be subcultured to the Mycotrim GU Triphasic flask system, Mycotrim GU agar, or other solid medium for isolation and identification. A comparable system, Mycotrim RS, has been adapted for detection of M. *pneumoniae* in respiratory specimens. Remel, Inc., has developed several formulations of transport and growth media, including 10 B broth, A 7 agar, A 8 agar, SP-4 broth, and SP-4 agar.

Some kits and other commercial products and media have been evaluated to a limited degree by independent investigators (1, 12, 21, 72, 87, 115, 116, 121). Commercial products and kits may be of particular value if the need to detect mycoplasmas arises infrequently in laboratories which do not specialize in mycoplasma detection, but users should be aware of the potential limitations of existing products. Problems with some of the commercially prepared products have included contamination of serum with mycoplasmas of animal origin and inadequate quality control. If commercially prepared media are to be used, it is advisable that laboratories perform internal quality control tests.

IDENTIFICATION

Because of their cellular dimensions, mycoplasmas, like chlamydiae and rickettsiae, cannot be clearly visualized by routine light microscopy. Lack of a cell wall precludes visualization of mycoplasmas by Gram staining, but this procedure may prove useful to exclude contaminating bacteria. M. *hominis* occasionally appears as pinpoint colonies on bacteriologic media, and the lack of a Gram reaction by these colonies gives a clue to their possible mycoplasmal identity, warranting further, more specific evaluation and subculture to mycoplasmal media. Giemsa stains may be used, but the results can be difficult to interpret because of debris and artifacts in clinical specimens, which can be confused with mycoplasmas due to their small size. Even though the numerous large-colony mycoplasmal species which may be isolated from humans cannot be identified based on colonial morphology or a particular biochemical profile, the body site of origin and rate of growth, in conjunction with biochemical features, give some clues. Biochemical properties such as glucose, arginine, or urea hydrolysis are determined based on color changes in the absence of turbidity in the appropriate broth. Utilization of glucose by a mycoplasma in SP-4 broth will produce an acidic shift (red to yellow) whereas utilization of arginine will produce a change from red to deeper red in this broth in the presence of the phenol red pH indicator. Urea or arginine hydrolysis in 10 B broth causes an alkaline shift of orange to deep red. Thus, a slowly growing glycolytic organism grown from the respiratory tract that produces spherical colonies on SP-4 agar after approximately 5 to 20 days of incubation and that exhibits hemolytic activity and hemadsorption when colonies are overlaid with a 5% suspension of guinea pig erythrocytes (Appendix 3) is most likely to be M. *pneumoniae.* An alkaline color change which occurs after overnight incubation without turbidity in 10 B broth containing urea is almost certainly due to *Ureaplasma* spp., whereas a urogenital specimen that produces an alkaline reaction within 24 to 72 h in broth supplemented with arginine is likely to contain M. *hominis.* Examination of colony morphology is sufficient to identify *Ureaplasma* spp., and it is important to keep in mind that these organisms often coexist with M. *hominis* in urogenital specimens.

To identify an organism completely to species level, a number of different techniques are available, although they are more appropriately within the province of a reference laboratory than a hospital microbiology laboratory because of their complexity and the lack of commercial availability of the serologic test reagents required. Agar growth inhibition using filter paper disks impregnated with species-specific antisera applied to agar plates on which the unknown organism is inoculated is one method, but several antisera may be required to encompass multiple strains within a given species. Because of possible cross-reactions between related species, such as M. *pneumoniae* and M. *genitalium,* rigorous proof of the specificity of the method must be documented by testing multiple isolates of the same species as controls. Epi-immunofluorescence or immunoperoxidase techniques enable colonies on agar to be identified directly so that mixtures of different species can be readily discerned. Immunoblotting with monoclonal antibodies, metabolism inhibition tests, mycoplasmacidal tests, and PCR assays have also been used to identify mycoplasmas to the species level (18, 90, 96).

SEROLOGIC TESTS

M. pneumoniae Respiratory Disease

Historically, serology has been the most common laboratory means for diagnosis of M. pneumoniae respiratory tract infections. Although culture and, more recently, PCR are also used to detect the presence of M. pneumoniae in respiratory specimens, persistence of the organism for variable lengths of time following acute infection makes it difficult in some cases to assess the significance of a positive culture or assay without additional confirmatory tests such as seroconversion. M. pneumoniae has both lipid and protein antigens which elicit antibody responses in clinical infections that can be detected after about 1 week of illness, peaking at 3 to 6 weeks, and then gradually declining, allowing several different serological assays based on different antigens and technologies.

Complement fixation (CF), using the chloroform-methanol-extractable lipid antigen, has been the reference method for serologic testing for M. pneumoniae in the past (35, 54) and gives results that are comparable to those obtained with whole-organism antigen. Although CF measures mainly the early IgM response, it does not differentiate among antibody classes, which is desirable to differen-

tiate acute from remote infection. Therefore, seroconversion, defined as a fourfold change in titer, measured in paired sera collected 2 to 4 weeks apart and assayed simultaneously provides the greatest diagnostic accuracy with CF, particularly in adults older than 40 years in whom an IgM response may be minimal or absent, presumably because of reinfection (16). When IgM is present, the duration of detectability may be variable (86). Antibody production may also be delayed in some infections or may even be absent if the patient is immunosuppressed.

CF is far from being a "gold standard" for diagnosis. It suffers from low sensitivity and specificity because the glycolipid antigen mixture used is not specific for M. pneumoniae and may be found in other microorganisms, as well as human tissues and even plants. Cross-reactions with other organisms, most notably M. genitalium (61), are well recognized, and false-positive results due to cross-reactive autoantibodies induced by acute inflammation from other unrelated causes may occur. Confirmation of positive CF results by Western blotting can overcome the problem with cross-reactivity but adds further to the time and expense of testing (16, 54). In most clinical laboratories, CF has been replaced by alternative techniques with greater sensitivity and specificity, many of which have been developed and sold as commercial kits. Table 3 summarizes some of the most popular commercially available serologic assays used to detect M. pneumoniae infection in the United States.

An immunofluorescent-antibody (IFA) assay, direct and indirect hemagglutination using IgM capture, and other particle agglutination antibody assays have been developed to detect antibody to M. pneumoniae (5–7, 23, 33, 52, 60, 86). The IFA assay consists of M. pneumoniae antigen

TABLE 3 Major test kits for detection of serum antibodies to M. pneumoniae sold in the United States

Product name	Manufacturer or distributor	Antibodies measured	Assay format	No. of tests per kit	Specimen throughput	Assay time Start to finish	Assay time Hands on
M. pneumoniae Antibody (MP) Test System	Zeus Scientific, distributed by Wampole Laboratories	IgM and IgG separately	Indirect immunofluorescence	100	Each slide contains 10 wells	2.5 h	30 min
Chromalex Mycoplasma pneumoniae Antibody Latex Test System	Shared Systems, Inc.	All classes simultaneously	Latex particle agglutination	100	Each slide contains 8 wells	15–20 min	15–20 min
ETI-MP IgM or IgG	Savyon, manufactured for Diasorin	IgM and IgG separately	Enzyme immunoassay	192	Strips of 8 wells	2.5 h	15–20 min
ImmunoCard	Meridian Diagnostics	IgM only	Qualitative, membrane-based enzyme immunoassay	30	1 specimen per card	12 min	10 min
M. pneumoniae IgG/IgM Antibody Test System	Remel, Inc.	IgM and IgG simultaneously	Qualitative membrane-based enzyme-linked immunobinding membrane assay	10	1 specimen per card	10 min	2–3 min
Mycoplasma IgG and IgM ELISA Test System	Zeus Scientific, Inc.	IgM and IgG separately	Enzyme immunoassay	96	Strips of 8 wells	50 min	5–10 min
GenBio ImmunoWELL Mycoplasma pneumoniae IgM or IgG	GenBio, distributed by Remel, Inc.	IgM and IgG separately	Enzyme immunoassay	96	Strips of 8 wells	IgG 2.35 h, IgM 2.75 h	15–20 min

affixed to microscope slides and measures IgM and IgG separately. This assay is technically simple to perform but is subjective in its interpretation and requires a fluorescence microscope, and the presence of M. *pneumoniae*-specific IgG may interfere with IgM results (5). Microimmunofluorescence for IgM is more specific but less sensitive than CF, according to one study (86). Qualitative and semiquantitative particle agglutination assays using either latex beads or gelatin that detect IgM and IgG simultaneously can be technically easy to perform, but they do not offer any significant advantages over other methods such as EIAs.

EIAs were developed in the 1970s, and several test formats are marketed commercially by various companies. Assays may require the use of washed whole organisms, sonicated whole-cell antigen preparations, detergent-lysed organisms, or other formulations. Thus, not all of the assays can be considered equivalent. EIAs are more sensitive than CF or culture, have good specificity, and are less technically demanding. The need for acute- and convalescent-phase sera collected 2 to 4 weeks apart and tested simultaneously for both IgG and IgM to accurately detect acute M. *pneumoniae* infection using EIAs has remained the obvious limitation for prompt point-of-care diagnosis (5, 19, 35, 69, 104, 105). However, a qualitative membrane-based EIA specific for IgM, the ImmunoCard (Meridian Diagnostics, Cincinnati, Ohio), has been developed for rapidly detecting an acute M. *pneumoniae* infection using a single serum specimen (5, 8, 105). The ImmunoCard assay has the advantages of being technically much simpler and quicker (10 min) to perform than other types of assays. Its potential disadvantage is lack of sensitivity for detection of some M. *pneumoniae* infections in some adults in whom the IgM response may be minimal (105). The Remel EIA is another rapid point-of-care qualitative serologic assay that detects both IgM and IgG simultaneously This test has shown good sensitivity and specificity compared to other EIAs, IFAs, and CF tests (35, 104, 105). There remains a need for improved serologic reagents for detecting acute M. *pneumoniae* infection. Purified P1 adhesin protein as the antigenic basis of such tests may eventually prove useful. According to data provided by the manufacturer in the package insert for the Meridian ImmunoCard, the relative sensitivity was 82 to 94% and the specificity was 87 to 93% compared to microwell EIA for IgM to M. *pneumoniae* with discrepancies resolved by commercial immunofluorescence assay, latex particle agglutination, and CF testing. For the Remel IgG/IgM Antibody test, data from the manufacturer based on multiple studies indicate a relative sensitivity of 94.7% and specificity of 99.4% compared with commercial microtiter EIA and commercial IFAs.

Cold agglutinins, detected by agglutination of type O Rh-negative erythrocytes at 4 °C, occur in association with M. *pneumoniae* infection in about 50% of cases (16). Titers of 64 to 128 or a fourfold or greater rise in titer suggest a recent M. *pneumoniae* infection, but the test is nonspecific, and cold agglutinins may be induced by a wide variety of viral infections as well as noninfectious conditions such as collagen-vascular diseases. Due to these limitations, detection of cold agglutinins is not recommended for serologic diagnosis of M. *pneumoniae* infection.

Infections Due to Genital Mycoplasmas

The ubiquity of most genital mycoplasmas in humans makes interpretation of antibody titers difficult, and the mere existence of antibodies alone cannot be considered significant. However, when invasive extragenital disease occurs, elevation of antibody titers is often apparent. The unique susceptibility of hypogammaglobulinemic persons to invasive infections due to *Ureaplasma* spp. testifies to the importance of the humoral immune response for protection against disease due to this organism (18). Although it has been suggested that increases in the titers of type-specific antibodies against certain ureaplasmal serovars occur in women with pregnancy wastage and in infants with respiratory disease compared to control patients, more comparative data from well-characterized and carefully matched control populations are needed to fully appreciate the value of antibody determination in these settings (18). Patients with an intact humoral immune system and with invasive infection caused by M. *hominis* almost without exception seroconvert or have a significant rise in existing antibody titer (41, 100, 101, 106).

No single serologic test has proved satisfactory for identifying genital mycoplasma infections. Serologic tests for M. *hominis* and *Ureaplasma* spp., using the techniques of microimmunofluorescence, metabolism inhibition, and EIA, have been described (13, 14, 90, 96). Although not commercially available, a rapid and reproducible microimmunofluorescence assay for M. *genitalium* has also been developed (37) and shown to detect antibody responses in men with NGU (93) and women with salpingitis (70). CF has not been shown to be sufficiently sensitive or specific for use with genital mycoplasmal infections. No serologic tests for genital mycoplasmas have been standardized and made commercially available in the United States, and they cannot be recommended for routine diagnostic purposes at present.

ANTIBIOTIC SUSCEPTIBILITY TESTING

Methods Used

Several methods of susceptibility testing used for conventional bacteria have been employed for testing mycoplasmas. Agar dilution has been used extensively as a reference method (10, 55, 112). It has the advantages that there is a relatively stable end point over time, the inoculum size does not have a great effect, and it allows detection of mixed cultures readily. However, this technique is not practical for testing small numbers of strains or occasional isolates which may be encountered in diagnostic laboratories. Agar disk diffusion is not useful for testing mycoplasmas since there has been no correlation between inhibitory zones and MICs and the relatively slow growth of some of these organisms further limits this technology. Microbroth dilution to determine MICs is probably the most practical and widely used method. It is economical and allows several antimicrobials to be tested in the same microtiter plate, but it has numerous disadvantages in that preparation of antimicrobial dilutions is labor-intensive and the end point tends to shift over time. Limited comparisons of agar dilution with microbroth dilution indicated that the two methods provided similar results for erythromycin and tetracycline against ureaplasmas (112).

Studies using the E test (AB BIODISK, Solna, Sweden) agar gradient diffusion technique for detection of tetracycline resistance in M. *hominis* yielded results comparable to microbroth dilution (113). Additional comparative studies have also validated this method for the determination of in vitro susceptibilities of M. *hominis* to fluoroquinolones (114) and susceptibilities of ureaplasmas to various antimicrobials (29). The E test has the advantages of simplicity of agar-based testing, an end point which does not shift over time, not having a large inoculum effect, and easy adaptation for testing single isolates. The E test is most cost-effective if only a small number of drugs are of interest, such as screening for tetracycline resistance.

Irrespective of the method, there are no universally accepted standards for pH, media, incubation conditions, or duration of incubation for performing mycoplasmal or urea-plasmal susceptibility tests. No MIC breakpoints specific for these organisms are endorsed by any regulatory agency. Lack of specific guidelines for susceptibility testing methods and interpretation of results has led to diverse and often inconsistent susceptibility profiles for mollicutes, especially for the genital mycoplasmas. However, a new National Committee for Clinical Laboratory Standards (NCCLS) subcommittee has been formed to address these issues.

A control strain for which there are reproducible MICs, determined by the individual laboratory, of the drugs being tested must be included with each assay for validation purposes. This can be a commercially purchased type strain from the American Type Culture Collection or a well-studied clinical isolate for which there are reproducible MICs. An inoculum of 10^4 to 10^5 CFU/ml has been recommended as the optimum inoculum for broth-based testing (10, 115). Nonstandardized conditions at low pH (6.0) can affect MICs, especially those of macrolides, making them appear less active in vitro, but such conditions may be required for adequate growth of organisms such as *Ureaplasma* spp. (55).

Bactericidal activity can be tested directly from the wells in microbroth dilution MIC assays by removing the mixture of organisms and antibiotic, diluting it to subinhibitory concentrations in fresh medium, and observing for a color change as evidence of growth. Detailed descriptions of procedures for susceptibility testing techniques are available in reference texts (10, 115).

Although some reference laboratories have adopted MIC breakpoints for other bacteria for use in interpretation of MICs when testing mycoplasmas, this practice should be used with caution, and it may be preferable to report MICs and allow clinicians to draw their own conclusions about the suitability of a particular agent for use in the treatment of a specific infection. For most antimicrobial agents of potential use against mollicutes, MICs of ≤1 μg/ml should be considered likely to reflect effective treatment. Tetracycline-resistant *M. hominis* and *Ureaplasma* spp. can readily be distinguished by broth or agar-based methods since the MICs for resistant strains are generally ≥8 μg/ml whereas the MICs for susceptible strains are consistently ≤2 μg/ml, with no overlap between the two distinct populations (112, 113). Since susceptibility testing of mycoplasmas should be performed only in special circumstances, the most practical approach for laboratories which offer this service might be to test drugs on a case-by-case basis according to specific physician and patient needs, including only the agents being considered for actual treatment.

Commercial MIC kits for use with genital mycoplasmas have been available in Europe for several years. They consist of microwells containing dried antimicrobials, generally in two concentrations corresponding to the thresholds proposed for conventional bacteria to classify a strain as susceptible, intermediate, or resistant. Abele-Horn et al. (1) performed a comprehensive evaluation of the Mycofast "All In" (International Microbio) and Mycoplasma IST (bio-Mérieux) kits in comparison to standard methods and found that the results for tetracycline correlated better than

those for other agents, which showed wider differences, but they did not endorse either of these products for clinical purposes. Inoculum size can influence MICs, and direct inoculation with the clinical specimens without a defined inoculum or preculture, as is done with the Mycofast "All In, " the Mycoplasma IST, and the Mycofast Evolution 2 (International Microbio) kits, may contribute to error. Observations of gynecological specimens indicated that large numbers of mycoplasmas, exceeding 10^5 per ml, can cause MICs to be elevated twofold or more (1). Renaudin and Bébéar (76) evaluated the SIR Mycoplasma kit (Bio-Rad Laboratories, Hercules, Calif.) and reported that when a defined inoculum was used, this product gave results comparable to those obtained by established MIC determination. This product is adapted for use with *Ureaplasma* spp. and *M. hominis* after a primary culture, so that a standard inoculum can be incorporated into the test system. The Mycokit-ATB (PBS Orgenics, Courbevoie, France) also includes procedures for standardization of the inoculum prior to determination of antimicrobial susceptibilities. Experience with these products is still relatively limited, but from a practical standpoint, microbiology laboratories in European countries where these products are available may want to consider their use when antimicrobial susceptibility testing of genital mycoplasmas is desired for clinical purposes. If a product is to be used, those in which a known inoculum of organisms is utilized may yield the most accurate results.

Susceptibility Profiles and Antimicrobial Resistance

A great deal of conflicting information concerning the relative activities of various antimicrobial agents against mycoplasmas has arisen over the past several years. In addition to the lack of standardized techniques, small sample sizes in published reports, samples collected in a non-random manner without respect to drug exposure, vague end points subject to fluctuation, and changes in resistance over time have further confounded the issue. Information on in vitro susceptibilities is greatest for *M. pneumoniae*, *M. hominis*, and *Ureaplasma* spp., but in some recent studies the activities of numerous antimicrobials against *M. fermentans* and *M. genitalium* have been evaluated. Although incompletely studied, *M. genitalium* has susceptibilities generally similar to those of *M. pneumoniae* while *M. fermentans* has susceptibilities generally similar to those of *M. hominis*, with some exceptions. A comparison of the MICs of several antimicrobial agents tested against these mollicutes is shown in Table 4.

Susceptibility Testing and Treatment of Mycoplasmal Infections

Due to the lack of a cell wall, mollicutes are innately resistant to all β-lactams. Sulfonamides, trimethoprim, and rifampin are also inactive. Resistance to macrolides and lincosamides is variable according to species, with *M. hominis* being resistant to erythromycin but susceptible to clindamycin; for *Ureaplasma* spp. the reverse is true. Newer macrolides and azalides have shown in vitro activity comparable to erythromycin for *M. pneumoniae* and *Ureaplasma* spp.

M. pneumoniae has remained predictably susceptible to newer fluoroquinolones, tetracyclines, and macrolides, so that susceptibility testing is not indicated except for the in vitro evaluation of new and previously untested agents. Tetracycline resistance has been well documented in recent years in both *M. hominis* and *Ureaplasma* spp. to variable

TABLE 4 MIC ranges of various antimicrobials for M. *pneumoniae*, M. *hominis*, M. *fermentans*, M. *genitalium*, and *Ureaplasma* sp.[a]

Antimicrobial	MIC (µg/ml) of antimicrobial for:				
	M. *pneumoniae*	M. *hominis*	M. *genitalium*	M. *fermentans*	U. *urealyticum*
Tetracycline	0.63–0.25	0.2–2[b]	ND[c]	0.1–1	0.05–2[b]
Doxycycline	0.02–0.5	0.1–2[b]	≤0.01–0.3	0.05–1	0.02–1[b]
Erythromycin	≤0.004–0.06	32–>1,000	≤0.01	0.5–64	0.02–4
Roxithromycin	≤0.01	>16	0.01	32–64	0.1–2
Clarithromycin	≤0.004–0.125	16–>256	≤0.01	1–64	≤0.004–2
Azithromycin	≤0.004–0.01	4–64	≤0.01	≤0.003–0.05	0.5–4
Josamycin	≤0.01–0.02	0.05–2	0.01–0.02	0.1–0.5	0.5–4
Telithromycin	≤0.015	2–16	≤0.015	0.06–0.25	≤0.015–0.06
Clindamycin	≤0.008–2	≤0.008–2	0.2–1	0.01–0.25	0.2–64
Lincomycin	4–8	0.2–1	ND	ND	8–256
Pristinamycin	0.02–0.05	0.1–0.5	ND	ND	0.1–1
Chloramphenicol	2	4–25	ND	0.5–10	0.4–8
Gentamicin	4	2–16	ND	0.25–>500	0.1–13
Ciprofloxacin	0.5–2	0.1–4	2	0.02–>64	0.1–16
Ofloxacin	0.05–2	0.1–64	1–2	0.02–25	0.2–25
Levofloxacin	0.5–1	0.1–0.5	0.5–1	0.05	0.2–1
Sparfloxacin	≤0.008–0.5	<0.008–0.1	0.05–0.1	≤0.01–0.05	0.003–1
Gatifloxacin	0.031–0.125	0.016–0.063	ND	0.008–0.016	0.125–1
Moxifloxacin	0.06–0.12	0.06	0.03	≤0.015–0.06	0.12–0.5
Gemifloxacin	0.05–0.125	0.0025–0.01	0.05	0.001–0.01	0.063–0.5
Rifampin	ND	>1,000	ND	25–>50	>1,000
Quinupristin/dalfopristin	0.008–0.06	0.25–8	ND	ND	0.12–0.5
Nitrofurantoin	ND	6–500	ND	0.1–2.5	13–>1,000

[a] Data were compiled from multiple published studies in which different methods and often different antimicrobial concentrations were used.
[b] Tetracycline-susceptible strains only.
[c] ND, no data available.

degrees, mediated by the *tet*M transposon, which codes for a protein that binds to the ribosomes, protecting them from the actions of these drugs (77). The extent to which tetracycline resistance occurs in genital mycoplasmas varies geographically and according to prior antimicrobial exposure in different populations, but it may approach 40% for M. *hominis* in some groups. Other agents active at the bacterial ribosome such as streptogramins, ketolides, aminoglycosides, and chloramphenicol may show in vitro inhibitory activity against some mollicute species. Although data are very limited, oxazolidinones, which act at the 30S ribosome, appear less active against mycoplasmas than do other agents mentioned above.

Extragenital infections, often in immunocompromised hosts, may be caused by multidrug-resistant mycoplasmas, making guidance of chemotherapy by in vitro susceptibility tests important in this clinical setting. Eradication of infection under these circumstances can be extremely difficult, requiring prolonged therapy even when the organisms are susceptible to the expected agents. This difficulty highlights the facts that mollicutes are inhibited but not killed by most commonly used bacteriostatic antimicrobial agents in concentrations achievable in vivo and that a functioning immune system plays an integral part in their eradication. The need for bactericidal agents to treat systemic infections in immunocompromised hosts has led to considerable interest in the fluoroquinolones. New quinolones such as gemifloxacin, levofloxacin, moxifloxacin, gatifloxacin, and sparfloxacin tend to have greater in vitro activity than do older agents such as ciprofloxacin and ofloxacin. Treatment of mycoplasmal and ureaplasmal infections has been reviewed (95).

EVALUATION, INTERPRETATION, AND REPORTING OF RESULTS

Tests offered through diagnostic microbiology laboratories should focus on the species known to cause human disease and for which cultivation techniques are best defined. Unusual organisms, or those for which cultivation conditions are not established, may be detectable by PCR technology offered through a few specialized research or reference laboratories. Such organisms should be sought only after consultation with clinicians and personnel from the reference laboratory. Except for *Ureaplasma* spp., which can be identified by urease production and distinct colony morphology, until species identification can be confirmed, a preliminary report of "large-colony *Mycoplasma* species" is appropriate. In many instances, as in culturing specimens from the lower genital tract, this may be sufficient. Isolates from normally sterile sites and/or from immunosuppressed persons should be identified to species level if possible.

M. pneumoniae

Detection of M. *pneumoniae* in culture is time-consuming and not overly sensitive. However, isolation of the organism from respiratory tract specimens is clinically significant in most instances and should be correlated with the presence of clinical respiratory disease, since a small proportion of asymptomatic carriers may exist. Detection by PCR technology is becoming more widely available through reference laboratories, but a positive result must still be correlated with clinical events. The finding of a positive PCR result in the absence of seroconversion, positive culture, or clinical disease suggests inadequate specificity of the PCR assay used, persistence of the organism after the infection has resolved clinically, or the presence of an asymptomatic carrier state. Reliable serologic testing is critical for accurate diagnosis of *M. pneumoniae* respiratory disease, and EIA for detection of IgG and IgM antibody is the method of choice. EIA is widely available, is more sensitive than culture, and is comparable in sensitivity to PCR for detection of infection, provided that sufficient time has elapsed for the host to mount an immune response. A fourfold rise in antibody titer between acute- and convalescent-phase sera is considered diagnostic. In children, adolescents, and young adults, a single positive IgM result using appropriate immunoglobulin class-specific reagents may be considered diagnostic in most cases.

M. hominis

M. hominis can be detected in culture within a few days. It is occasionally discovered in routine bacteriologic media from appropriate clinical material, but this should not be relied on for detection. Its isolation in any quantity from normally sterile body fluids or tissues is significantly associated with disease, but quantitation of organisms present may be of value in other circumstances. When mycoplasmas are detected in nonsterile sites such as the female lower genital tract in numbers of $\geq 10^5$ organisms, they are most likely to be associated with BV.

Ureaplasma Species

Ureaplasma spp. can be detected in culture within 24 to 48 h. The characteristic colony morphology and urease production are sufficient for identification. Isolation in any quantity from normally sterile body fluids or tissues is significantly associated with disease. The presence of fewer than 10^4 organisms in the male urethra is unlikely to be significant (41).

Identification of specific biovars of *Ureaplasma*, which are now proposed for separation into two species, *U. urealyticum* and *U. parvum* (57, 58, 79, 81), is not practical or necessary for diagnostic purposes based on presently available information. Whether there is a difference in the pathogenicity among the ureaplasmal biovars has been the subject of several evaluations, but data reported thus far are inconclusive. This issue is now being investigated more extensively owing to the advent of PCR technology, which allows isolates to be classified more readily.

Hemotropic and Other Mycoplasmas

Optimum culture techniques for detecting species other than M. *pneumoniae*, M. *hominis*, and *Ureaplasma* spp. in clinical specimens are less well defined. However, detection of M. *genitalium* by a PCR assay without quantitation is likely to be significant.

Noncultivable cell wall-less parasitic bacteria that attach to the surface of erythrocytes and also occur free in the plasma, previously classified in the genera *Haemobartonella* and *Eperythrozoon*, are currently given the *Candidatus* status in the genus *Mycoplasma* based on 16S rRNA gene sequences (71), and the organisms infect a wide array of animal hosts, including primates. Species are named on the basis of the host animal species, e.g., "*Candidatus* Mycoplasma haemofelis" (cats), "*Candidatus* Mycoplasma haemomuris" (mice), "*Candidatus* Mycoplasma haemosuis" (pigs), "*Candidatus* Mycoplasma wenyonii" (cattle), "*Candidatus* Mycoplasma haemominutum" (cats), and "*Candidatus* Mycoplasma erythrodidelphis" (opossum). These hemotropic bacteria form a new

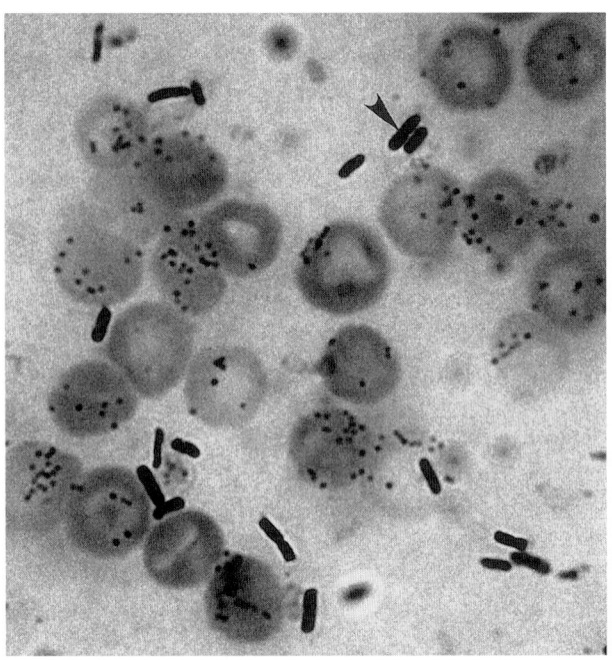

FIGURE 4 *H. muris* on erythrocytes of an infected mouse. *Escherichia coli* (arrowhead) was added to the mouse blood for size comparison. Giemsa stain; magnification, ×1,879. (Reproduced with permission from reference 76a.)

phylogenetic cluster within the so-called pneumoniae group of the genus *Mycoplasma*. Whether hemotropic mycoplasmas found in domestic and wild animals infect humans remains to be demonstrated. However, there has been an ultrastructural observation of *Haemobartonella*-like organisms infecting six AIDS patients in Brazil (30). Infections in animal hosts are typically asymptomatic or latent until the hosts are stressed, receive chemotherapy, or are splenectomized. Clinical signs of disease include anemia, fever, anorexia, lethargy, and icterus.

Infection is detected by examination of blood smears stained by Romanowsky methods. The organisms appear as pleomorphic cocci, 0.3 to 0.7 μm in diameter (Fig. 4). PCR assays and serologic tests have been developed for the detection of some species. All species that have been examined are inhibited by the tetracyclines but resistant to penicillins, cephalosporins, and other cell wall-active antibiotics.

APPENDIX 1
Medium Formulations for Cultivation of Mycoplasmas from Humans

A 8 agar

Purpose

A 8 is a differential agar medium useful for isolating genital mycoplasmas. Urea is included in this medium to enhance the differentiation of *Ureaplasma* spp. from non-urea-hydrolyzing mycoplasmas.

Ingredients and preparation

Mix the following ingredients in a flask in the order specified to prepare 1 liter. Adjust the pH to 5.5 with 2 N HCl. Autoclave for 15 min at 121°C. Cool in a 56°C water bath.

Base

825 ml of ultrapurified water

0.15 g of CaCl₂ dihydride (dissolve before adding other ingredients)

24 g of Trypticase soy broth (Becton Dickinson)

2 g of yeast extract (Difco)

1.7 g of putrescine dihydrochloride

0.2 g of DNA

10.5 g of Select Agar (Becton Dickinson)

Supplements: Prepare and filter sterilize (0.2-μm-pore-size filter) each supplement separately. Mix, add supplements to base agar, and adjust the pH to 6.0. Pour plates, and after 2 h invert them and keep them at room temperature overnight. Small petri plates (60 mm) that can be used for agar require 7.5 ml, whereas standard 100-mm plates require 10 ml. Place plates in sealed plastic bags, and refrigerate at 4°C. The plates will usually perform in a satisfactory manner for at least 4 weeks. Loss of inhibitory effect of antibiotics when plates older than 4 weeks are used may result in bacterial overgrowth and inability to detect mycoplasmas when culturing specimens from nonsterile sites.

200 ml horse serum (HyClone)

5 ml IsovitalX (Becton Dickinson)

10 ml 10% urea

1 ml GHL tripeptide solution (Calbiochem-Novabiochem)

5 ml 2% L-cysteine (prepare fresh on day of use)

1,000 IU of penicillin per ml to prevent bacterial overgrowth

10 B broth

Purpose
10 B is an enriched broth medium useful for cultivation of *Ureaplasma* spp. and *M. hominis.*

Ingredients and preparation
Mix the following ingredients in a flask in the order specified to prepare 1 liter. Adjust the pH to 5.5 with 2 N HCl. Autoclave for 15 min at 12°C, and cool before adding supplements.

Base

825 ml ultra-purified water

14 g of Mycoplasma broth base without crystal violet (Becton Dickinson)

2 g of arginine

0.2 g of DNA

1 ml of 1% phenol red (prepare fresh monthly)

Supplements: Prepare and filter sterilize (0.2-μm-pore-size filter) each supplement separately, and add supplements to base. Adjust the pH to 5.9 to 6.1. Dispense broth aseptically into sterile tubes, each containing 0.9 to 1.0 ml. 10 B broth will usually perform in a satisfactory manner for at least 4 weeks when stored at 4°C. Loss of inhibitory effect of antibiotics when broths older than 4 weeks are used may result in bacterial overgrowth and inability to detect mycoplasmas.

200 ml of horse serum (Hyclone)

100 ml of 25% yeast extract (Difco)

5 ml of IsoVitalX (Becton Dickinson)

4 ml of 10% urea

2.5 ml of 4% L-cysteine (prepare fresh on day of use)

Heat-inactivated fetal bovine serum can also be used instead of horse serum

SP-4 broth and agar

Purpose
SP-4 broth is an enriched growth medium used for the cultivation of many *Mycoplasma* species, including *M. pneumoniae.* Agar may

be added to SP-4 broth for preparation of solid medium, and glucose and/or arginine and urea may be added as metabolic substrates, depending on which mycoplasmas are being sought.

Ingredients and preparation
Mix the following ingredients in a flask in the order specified to prepare 1 liter. Autoclave for 15 min at 121°C, and cool before adding supplements. For agar, cool in a 56°C water bath.

Base

643 ml of ultrapurified water

3.5 g of Mycoplasma broth base without crystal violet (Becton Dickinson)

10 g of tryptone (Difco)

5.3 g of peptone (Difco)

2 g of arginine (only if medium is to be used to isolate *M. hominis*) (Sigma)

2 ml of 1% phenol red (prepare fresh monthly)

0.2 g of DNA

15 g of Noble Agar (only if preparing SP-4 agar) (Difco)

Supplements: Prepare and filter sterilize (0.2-μm-pore-size filter) each supplement separately, and add supplements to base. Adjust the pH to 7.4 to 7.6. If agar is added, pour plates, and after 2 h invert them; keep them at room temperature overnight. Small petri plates (60 mm) that can be used for agar require 7.5 ml, whereas standard 100-mm plates require 10 ml. The volume of broth required for individual cultures is dictated by the length of incubation required, e.g., 1.8 to 4.5 ml for *M. pneumoniae* and 0.9 to 1 ml for the genital mycoplasmas. Place plates in plastic bags, and refrigerate at 4°C. Plates usually perform in a satisfactory manner for at least 4 weeks. Loss of inhibitory effect of antibiotics when broths or agar plates older than 4 weeks are used may result in bacterial overgrowth and inability to detect mycoplasmas when culturing specimens from nonsterile sites

50 ml of 10× CMRL 1066 (Gibco)

35 ml of 25% yeast extract (Difco)

100 ml of 2% yeastolate (Difco)

170 ml of heat-inactivated (56°C for 30 min) fetal bovine serum (HyClone)

10 ml of 50% glucose

1,000 IU of penicillin per ml to prevent bacterial overgrowth

APPENDIX 2
Procedure for Hoechst Staining of Body Fluids To Detect Mycoplasmas

Background

Since mycoplasmas do not stain with the Gram stain owing to their lack of a cell wall, alternative means must be devised to observe them in human body fluids. A technique of DNA fluorochrome staining developed for screening cell cultures for *Mycoplasma* contamination can be adapted for observation of mycoplasmas in body fluids such as cerebrospinal fluid, amniotic fluid, and synovial fluid. This stain is thought to bind to the DNA helix by intercalation, thereby causing all prokaryotic organisms to fluoresce when stained with it.

Materials and reagents
Fluorochrome stain stock solution

5 mg of DNA Fluorochrome Hoechst 33258 (ICN Biomedicals, Costa Mesa, Calif.)

100 ml of citrate phosphate buffer

0.01 g of merthiolate

Mix thoroughly at 22 to 25°C with magnetic stirrer for 30 min. Wrap bottle in aluminum foil, and store in the dark at 2 to 8°C.

The stain is light and heat sensitive.

Fluorochrome stain working solution

> 5 μl of stock solution
> 4.995 ml of citrate phosphate buffer (final concentration, 0.05 μg/ml)

Mix thoroughly with a magnetic stirrer at room temperature for 30 min. Prepare fresh each day of use from stock solution.

Citrate phosphate buffer

> 16.188 g of Na_2HPO_4
> 9.03 g of citric acid monohydrate
> 1,000 ml of distilled water

Adjust the pH to 5.5, and filter sterilize.

Carnoy's fixative

> 1:3 solution of glacial acetic acid in methanol

Prepare fresh each day, and use within 4 h.

Mounting solution

> 100 ml of citrate phosphate buffer
> 50 ml of glycerol

Adjust the pH to 5.5, and store at 2 to 8°C.

Other materials

> Microscope slides and coverslips
> Pipettes
> Stock solution of M. hominis PG21

Equipment

> Fluorescence microscope

Procedure

1. Pipette a small volume of the specimen onto a microscope slide, and allow to air dry. Concentration of the clinical specimen by centrifugation, as well as cytocentrifuge preparations, is also acceptable. Prepare a positive control slide from the stock solution of M. hominis PG21 in the same manner. Sterile saline can be used as a negative control, if desired. Control slides can be prepared in advance and stored frozen at −70°C, if desired.
2. Fix slides by flooding them with Carnoy's fixative for 2 min.
3. Reapply fixative, and let stand for 5 min.
4. Reapply fixative, and let stand for 10 min.
5. Pour off fixative, and allow slides to air dry.
6. Apply working solution of DNA stain (usually 1:1,000 of stock stain) sufficient to immerse the slide. Stain for 10 min at room temperature in the dark.
7. Pour off stain.
8. Wash four times with a slow stream of deionized water.
9. Allow the slides to air dry.
10. Mount a coverslip onto each slide with 13 μl of mounting solution.
11. Examine the slides under ×1,000 magnification with oil immersion on a fluorescence microscope. Examine positive and negative controls first. A minimum of 10 fields should be scanned before designating specimens negative. Slides can be stored at 4°C in the dark for future reference.

Limitations

False-positive test results may be caused by microbiological contamination of the dye, high background, or damaging nuclear fragmentation of mammalian cells from the hosts in the specimen. Filtering the specimen to remove host cells may improve performance. The presence of extranuclear fluorescence is not specific for mycoplasmas and may represent prokaryotic DNA from other bacteria. A positive test should be compared with culture results for proper interpretation. Emission is best when observed using filter combinations that exclude light below 460 nm. Fluorescence is influenced by pH and the mounting medium, and so the instructions about materials and techniques described in this procedure should be followed exactly.

APPENDIX 3
Hemadsorption Test for Identification of M. pneumoniae

Background

The hemadsorption test procedure involves flooding colonies on agar with a dilute suspension of washed guinea pig erythrocytes, incubating, washing, and examining colonies microscopically for adherent erythrocytes. Hemadsorption is unique to M. pneumoniae and M. genitalium among mycoplasmas isolated from humans. Since M. genitalium is much more fastidious and very slow growing and has not been reliably isolated from humans using culture methods described for M. pneumoniae, a positive hemadsorption test provides a strong basis for identification of an organism as M. pneumoniae.

Materials and reagents

> Mycoplasma colonies <10 days old on SP-4 agar: unknown Mycoplasma colonies, M. pneumoniae colonies (positive control), M. hominis colonies (negative control)
> Guinea pig erythrocytes (Biowhittaker)
> Sterile phosphate-buffered saline (PBS) (pH 7.2)
> 15-ml conical centrifuge tubes
> Pipetting device and sterile disposable pipette tips

Procedure

1. Prepare a 10% working suspension of washed guinea pig erythrocytes by transferring 5 to 8 ml of the blood and an equal volume of sterile PBS (pH 7.2) aseptically into a 15-ml conical centrifuge tube.
2. Centrifuge at 900 × g for 5 min at room temperature. Discard the supernatant, and resuspend the cell pellet in 10 ml of PBS by gently pipetting up and down several times.
3. Centrifuge at 900 × g for 5 min at room temperature, and repeat the washing procedure.
4. Discard the supernatant, and measure the packed-cell volume. Add a volume of PBS equal to 9 times the packed-cell volume to yield a 10% suspension.
5. Store the suspension at 4°C, and use within 7 days. Do not use if there is evidence of hemolysis or bacterial contamination.
6. Use this stock solution to prepare a 0.5% working solution by combining 1 part 10% suspension to 19 parts sterile PBS.
7. Flood agar plates containing the unknown mycoplasma and positive and negative controls with the suspension of 0.5% guinea pig erythrocytes.
8. Cover the plates, and incubate at room temperature for 30 min.
9. Tilt the plates, and aspirate the cell suspension from the agar surface.
10. Flood the plate with PBS to wash the agar surface, rocking the plate back and forth.
11. Aspirate and discard the PBS.
12. Observe the plates macroscopically and microscopically under a stereomicroscope for absorption of erythrocytes to the surface of the colonies.
13. M. pneumoniae will hemadsorb, whereas M. hominis and other large-colony mycoplasmas that are cultivable on SP-4 agar in 4 to 20 days will not do so.

REFERENCES

1. **Abele-Horn, M., C. Blendinger, C. Becher, P. Emmerling, and G. Ruckdeschel.** 1996. Evaluation of commercial kits for quantitative identification and tests on antibiotic susceptibility of genital mycoplasmas. *Zentbl. Bakteriol.* **284:**540–549.

2. **Ainsworth, J. G., J. Clarke, R. Goldin, and D. Taylor-Robinson.** 2000. Disseminated *Mycoplasma fermentans* in AIDS patients: several case reports. *Int. J. STD AIDS* **11:**751–755.

3. **Ainsworth, J. G., S. Hourshid, J. Clarke, D. Mitchell, J. N. Weber, and D. Taylor-Robinson.** 1994. Detection of *Mycoplasma fermentans* in HIV-positive individuals undergoing bronchoscopy. *IOM Lett.* **3:**319–320.

4. **Ainsworth, J. G., S. Hourshid, P. J. Easterbrook, C. B., Gilroy, J. N. Weber, and D. Taylor-Robinson.** 2000. *Mycoplasma* species in rapid and slow HIV progressors. *Int. J. STD AIDS* **11:**76–79.

5. **Alexander, T. S., L. D. Gray, J. A. Kraft, D. S. Leland, M. T. Nikaido, and D. H. Willis.** 1996. Performance of Meridian ImmunoCard *Mycoplasma* test in a multicenter clinical trial. *J. Clin. Microbiol.* **34:**1180–1183.

6. **Aubert, G., B. Pozzzetto, O. G. Gaudin, J. Hafic, A. D. Mbida, and A. Ros.** 1992. Evaluation of five commercial tests: complement fixation, microparticle agglutination, indirect immunofluorescence, enzyme-linked immunosorbent assay and latex agglutination, in comparison to immunoblotting for *Mycoplasma pneumoniae* serology. *Ann. Biol. Chem.* **50:**593–597.

7. **Barker, C. E., M. Sillis, and T. G. Wreghitt.** 1990. Evaluation of Serodia Myco II particle agglutination test for detecting *Mycoplasma pneumoniae* antibody: comparison with μ-capture ELISA and indirect immunofluorescence. *J. Clin. Pathol.* **43:**163–165.

8. **Baseman, J. B., and J. G. Tully.** 1997. Mycoplasmas: sophisticated, reemerging, and burdened by their notoriety. *Emerg. Infect. Dis.* **3:**21–32.

9. **Bébéar, C., B. de Barbeyrac, C. M. Bébéar, H. Renaudin, and A. Allery.** 1997. New developments in diagnostic and treatment alternatives of mycoplasma infections in humans. *Wien. Klin. Wochenschr.* **15:**594–599.

10. **Bébéar, C., and J. A. Robertson.** 1996. Determination of minimal inhibitory concentration, p. 189–197. *In* J. G. Tully and S. Razin (ed.), *Molecular and Diagnostic Procedures in Mycoplasmology.* Academic Press, Inc., New York, N.Y.

11. **Blanchard, A., J. Hentschel, L. Duffy, K. Baldus, and G. H. Cassell.** 1993. Detection of *Ureaplasma urealyticum* by polymerase chain reaction in the urogenital tract of adults, in amniotic fluid and in the respiratory tract of newborns. *Clin. Infect. Dis.* **17**(Suppl. 1):S83–S89.

12. **Broitman, N. L., C. M. Floyd, C. A. Johnson, L. M. de la Maza, and E. Peterson.** 1992. Comparison of commercially available media for detection and isolation of *Ureaplasma urealyticum* and *Mycoplasma hominis.* *J. Clin. Microbiol.* **30:**1335–1337.

13. **Brown, M. B., G. H. Cassell, D. Taylor-Robinson, and M. C. Shepard.** 1983. Measurement of antibody to *Ureaplasma urealyticum* by an enzyme-linked immunosorbent assay and detection of antibody responses in patients with nongonococcal urethritis. *J. Clin. Microbiol.* **17:**288–295.

14. **Brown, M. B., G. H. Cassell, W. M. McCormack, and J. K. Davis.** 1987. Measurement of antibody to *Mycoplasma hominis* by an enzyme-linked immunosorbent assay and detection of antibody responses in women with postpartum fever. *Am. J. Obstet. Gynecol.* **156:**701–708.

15. **Cassell, G. H., R. O. Davis, K. B. Waites, M. B. Brown, P. A. Marriott, S. Stagno, and J. K. Davis.** 1983. Isolation of *Mycoplasma hominis* and *Ureaplasma urealyticum* from amniotic fluid at 16–20 weeks of gestation: potential effect on outcome of pregnancy. *Sex. Transm. Dis.* **10**(Suppl.):294–302.

16. **Cassell, G. H., G. Gambill, and L. Duffy.** 1996. ELISA in respiratory infections of humans, p. 123–136. *In* J. G. Tully and S. Razin (ed.), *Molecular and Diagnostic Procedures in Mycoplasmology.* Academic Press, Inc., New York, N.Y.

17. **Cassell, G. H., K. B. Waites, D. T. Crouse, P. T. Rudd, K. C. Canupp, S. Stagno, and G. R. Cutter.** 1988. Association of *Ureaplasma urealyticum* infection of the lower respiratory tract with chronic lung disease and death in very-low-birth-weight infants. *Lancet* **ii:**240–244.

18. **Cassell, G. H., K. B. Waites, and D. T. Crouse.** 2001. Mycoplasmal infections, p. 733–767. *In* J. S. Remington and J. O. Klein (ed.), *Infectious Diseases of the Fetus and Newborn Infant,* 5th ed. The W. B. Saunders Co., Inc., Philadelphia, Pa.

19. **Cimolai, N., and A. C. H. Cheong.** 1996. An assessment of a new diagnostic indirect enzyme immunoassay for the detection of anti-*Mycoplasma pneumoniae* IgM. *Clin. Microbiol. Infect. Dis.* **105:**205–209.

20. **Clausen, H. F., J. Fedder, M. Drasbek, P. K. Nielsen, B. Toft, H. J. Ingerslev, and G. Birkelund.** 2001. Serological investigation of *Mycoplasma genitalium* in infertile women. *Hum. Reprod.* **16:**1866–1874.

21. **Clegg, A., M. Passey, M. Yoannes, and A. Michael.** 1997. High rates of genital mycoplasma infections in the highlands of Papua New Guinea determined both by culture and a commercial detection kit. *J. Clin. Microbiol.* **35:** 197–200.

22. **Cohen, C. R., L. E. Manhart, E. A. Bukusi, S. Astete, R. C. Brunham, K. K. Holmes, S. K. Sinei, J. J. Bwayo, and P. A. Totten.** 2002. Association between *Mycoplasma genitalium* and acute endometritis. *Lancet* **359:**765–766.

23. **Coombs, R. R. A., G. Easter, P. Matejtschuk, and T. G. Wreghitt.** 1988. Red-cell IgM-antibody capture assay for the detection of *Mycoplasma pneumoniae*-specific IgM. *Epidemiol. Infect.* **100:**101–109.

24. **Cunliffe, N. A., S. Fergusson, F. Davidson, A. Lyon, and P. W. Ross.** 1996. Comparison of culture with the polymerase chain reaction for detection of *Ureaplasma urealyticum* in endotracheal aspirates of preterm infants. *J. Med. Microbiol.* **45:**27–30.

25. **Dallo, S. F., and J. B. Baseman.** 2000. Intracellular DNA replication and long-term survival of pathogenic mycoplasmas. *Microb. Pathog.* **29:**301–309.

26. **de Barbeyrac, B., C. Berner-Poggi, F. Febrer, H. Renaudin, M. Dupon, and C. Bébéar.** 1993. Detection of *Mycoplasma pneumoniae* and *Mycoplasma genitalium* in clinical samples by polymerase chain reaction. *Clin. Infect. Dis.* **17**(Suppl. 1):83–89.

27. **Deguchi T., C. B. Gilroy, and D. Taylor-Robinson.** 1996. Failure to detect *Mycoplasma fermentans*, *Mycoplasma penetrans*, or *Mycoplasma pirum* in the urethra of patients with acute nongonococcal urethritis. *Eur. J. Clin. Microbiol. Infect. Dis.* **15:**169–171.

28. **Doble, A., B. J. Thomas, P. M. Furr, M. M. Walker, J. R. W. Harris, R. O. Witherow, and D. Taylor-Robinson.** 1989. A search for infectious agents in chronic abacterial prostatitis using ultrasound guided biopsy. *Br. J. Urol.* **64:**297–301.

29. **Dosa, E., E. Nagy, W. Falk, I. Szoske, and U. Ballies.** 1999. Evaluation of the Etest for susceptibility testing of *Mycoplasma hominis* and *Ureaplasma urealyticum.* *J. Antimicrob. Chemother.* **43:**575–578.

30. **Duarte M. I., M. S. Oliveira, M. A. Shikanai-Yasuda, O. N. Mariano, C. F. Takakura, C. Pagliari, and C. E. Corbett.** 1992. *Haemobartonella*-like microorganism infection in AIDS patients: ultrastructural pathology. *J. Infect. Dis.* **165:**976–977.

31. **Eschenbach, D. A.** 1986. *Ureaplasma urealyticum* as a cause of post-partum fever. *Pediatr. Infect. Dis. J.* **5**(Suppl.):258–261.

32. Eschenbach, D. A. 1993. *Ureaplasma urealyticum* and premature birth. *Clin. Infect. Dis.* **17**(Suppl. 1):100–106.

33. Eschevarria, J. M., P. Leon, P. Balfagon, J. A. Lopez, and M. V. Fernandez. 1990. Diagnosis of *Mycoplasma pneumoniae* infection by microparticle agglutination and antibody capture enzyme-immunoassay. *Eur. J. Clin. Microbiol. Infect. Dis.* **9**:217–220.

34. Falguera, M., A. Nogues, A. Ruiz-Gonzalez, M. Garcia, and T. Puig. 1996. Detection of *Mycoplasma pneumoniae* by polymerase chain reaction in lung aspirates from patients with community-acquired pneumonia. *Chest* **110**: 972–976.

35. Fedorko, D. P., D. D. Emery, S. M. Franklin, and D. D. Congdon. 1995. Evaluation of a rapid enzyme immunoassay system for serologic diagnosis of *Mycoplasma pneumoniae* infection. *Diagn. Microbiol. Infect. Dis.* **23**:85–88.

36. Foy, H. M. 1993. Infections caused by *Mycoplasma pneumoniae* and possible carrier state in different populations of patients. *Clin. Infect. Dis.* **17**(Suppl. 1):37–46.

37. Furr, P. M., and D. Taylor-Robinson. 1984. Microimmunofluorescence technique for detection of antibody to *Mycoplasma genitalium*. *J. Clin. Pathol.* **37**:1072–1074.

38. Furr, P. M., and D. Taylor-Robinson. 1990. Long-term viability of stored mycoplasmas and ureaplasmas. *J. Med. Microbiol.* **31**:203–206.

39. Furr, P. M., D. Taylor-Robinson, and A. D. B. Webster. 1994. Mycoplasmas and ureaplasmas in patients with hypogammaglobulinaemia and their role in arthritis: microbiological observations over 20 years. *Ann. Rheum. Dis.* **53**:183–187.

40. Gerstenecker, B., and E. Jacobs. 1993. Development of a capture-ELISA for the specific detection of *Mycoplasma pneumoniae* in patient's material, p. 195–205. *In* I. Kahane and A. Adoni (ed.), *Rapid Diagnosis of Mycoplasmas*. Plenum Press, New York, N.Y.

41. Glatt, A. E., W. M. McCormack, and D. Taylor-Robinson. 1989. Genital mycoplasmas, p. 279–293. *In* K. K. Holmes, P-A. Mårdh, P. F. Sparling, P. J. Wiesner, W. Cates, S. M. Lemon, and W. E. Stamm (ed.), *Sexually Transmitted Diseases*, 2nd ed. McGraw Hill Book Co., New York, N.Y.

42. Grau, O., R. Kovacic, R. Griffais, V. Launay, and L. Montagnier. 1994. Development of PCR-based assays for the detection of two human mollicute species, *Mycoplasma penetrans* and M. *hominis*. *Mol. Cell. Probes* **8**:139–148.

43. Grenabo, L., H. Hedelin, and S. Pettersson. 1988. Urinary infection stones caused by *Ureaplasma urealyticum*: a review. *Scand. J. Infect. Dis.* **53**(Suppl.):46–49.

44. Gröndahl, B., W. Puppe, A. Hoppe, I. Kühne, J. A. I. Weidl, and H.-J. Schmitt. 1999. Rapid identification of nine microorganisms causing acute respiratory tract infections by single-tube multiplex reverse transcription PCR: feasibility study. *J. Clin. Microbiol.* **37**:1–7.

45. Horner, P., B. Thomas, C. B. Gilroy, M. Egger, and D. Taylor-Robinson. 2001. Role of *Mycoplasma genitalium* and *Ureaplasma urealyticum* in acute and chronic nongonococcal urethritis. *Clin. Infect. Dis.* **32**:995–1003.

46. Horner, P. J., C. B. Gilroy, B. J. Thomas, R. O. M. Naidoo, and D. Taylor-Robinson. 1993. Association of *Mycoplasma genitalium* with acute non-gonococcal urethritis. *Lancet* **342**:582–585.

47. Ieven, M., D. Ursi, H. Van Bever, W. Quint, H. G. M. Niesters, and H. Goosens. 1996. Detection of *Mycoplasma pneumoniae* by two polymerase chain reactions and role of M. *pneumoniae* in acute respiratory tract infections in pediatric patients. *J. Infect. Dis.* **173**:1445–1452.

48. Jalil, N., A. Doble, C. Gilchrist, and D. Taylor-Robinson. 1988. Infection of the epididymis by *Ureaplasma urealyticum*. *Genitourin. Med.* **64**:367–368.

49. Jensen, J. S., S. A. Uldum, J. Sondergard-Anderson, J. Vuust, and K. Lind. 1991. Polymerase chain reaction for detection of *Mycoplasma genitalium* in clinical samples. *J. Clin. Microbiol.* **29**:46–50.

50. Jensen, J. S., H. T. Hansen, and K. Lind. 1996. Isolation of *Mycoplasma genitalium* strains from the male urethra. *J. Clin. Microbiol.* **34**:286–291.

51. Kai, M. S., H. Kamiya, H. Yabe, I. Takakura, K. Shiozama, and A. Ozawa. 1993. Rapid detection of *Mycoplasma pneumoniae* in clinical samples by the polymerase chain reaction. *J. Med. Microbiol.* **38**:166–170.

52. Karppelin, M., K. Hakkarainen, M. Kleemola, and A. Miettinen. 1993. Comparison of three serological methods for diagnosing *Mycoplasma pneumoniae* infection. *J. Clin. Pathol.* **46**:1120–1123.

53. Katseni, V. L., C. B. Gilroy, B. K. Ryait, K. Ariyoshi, P. D. Bieniasz, J. N. Weber, and D. Taylor-Robinson. 1993. *Mycoplasma fermentans* in individuals seropositive and seronegative for HIV-1. *Lancet* **341**:271–273.

54. Kenny, G. E. 1992. Serodiagnosis, p. 505–512. *In* J. Maniloff, R. N. McElhaney, L. R. Finch, and J. B. Baseman (ed.), *Mycoplasmas: Molecular Biology and Pathogenesis*. American Society for Microbiology, Washington, D.C.

55. Kenny, G. E., and F. D. Cartwright. 1993. Effect of pH, inoculum size, and incubation time on the susceptibility of *Ureaplasma urealyticum* to erythromycin *in vitro*. *Clin. Infect. Dis.* **17**(Suppl. 1):215–218.

56. Kok, T.-W., G. Varkanis, B. P. Marmion, J. Martin, and A. Esterman. 1988. Laboratory diagnosis of *Mycoplasma pneumoniae* infection. I. Direct detection of antigen in respiratory exudates by enzyme immunoassay. *Epidemiol. Infect.* **101**:669–684.

57. Kong, F., G. James, Z. Ma, S. Gordon, W. Bin, and G. L. Gilbert. 1999. Phylogenetic analysis of *Ureaplasma urealyticum*—support for the establishment of a new species, *Ureaplasma parvum*. *Int. J. Syst. Bacteriol.* **4**:1879–1889.

58. Kong, F., Z. Ma, G. James, S. Gordon, and G. L. Gilbert. 2000. Species identification of *Ureaplasma parvum* and *Ureaplasma urealyticum* using PCR-based assays. *J. Clin. Microbiol.* **38**:1175–1179.

59. Krieger, J. N., D. E. Riley, M. C. Roberts, and R. E. Berger. 1996. Prokaryotic sequences in patients with chronic idiopathic prostatitis. *J. Clin. Microbiol.* **34**:3120–3128.

60. Lieberman, D., S. Horowitz, O. Horowitz, F. Schlaeffer, and A. Porath. 1995. Microparticle agglutination versus antibody capture enzyme immunoassay for diagnosis of community acquired *Mycoplasma pneumoniae* pneumonia. *Eur. J. Clin. Microbiol. Infect. Dis.* **14**:577–584.

61. Lind, K. 1982. Serological cross-reaction between *Mycoplasma genitalium* and M. *pneumoniae*. *Lancet* **ii**:1158–1159.

62. Lo, S. C., D. J. Wear, S. L. Green, P. G. Jones, and J. F. Legier. 1993. Adult respiratory distress syndrome with or without systemic disease associated with infections due to *Mycoplasma fermentans*. *Clin Infect. Dis.* **17**(Suppl. 1): 259–263.

63. Lo, S. C., M. M. Hayes, J. G. Tully, R. Y. Wang, H. Kotani, P. F. Pierce, D. L. Rose, and J. W. K. Shih. 1992. *Mycoplasma penetrans* sp. nov., from the urogenital tract of patients with AIDS. *Int. J. Syst. Bacteriol.* **42**:357–364.

64. Luki, N., P. Lebel, M. Boucher, B. Doray, J. Turgeon, and R. Brousseau. 1998. Comparison of polymerase chain reaction assay with culture for detection of genital mycoplasmas in perinatal infections. *Eur. J. Clin. Microbiol.* **17**:255–263.

65. Manhart, L. E., S. M. Dutro, K. K. Holmes, C. E. Stevens, C. W. Critchlow, D. A. Eschenbach, and P. A. Totten. 2001. *Mycoplasma genitalium* is associated with

mucopurulent cervicitis. *Int. J. STD AIDS* **12**(Suppl. 2): 69.

66. **Marston, B. J., J. F. Plouffe, T. M. File, B. A. Hackman, S.-J. Salstrom, H. B. Lipman, M. S. Kolczak, R. F. Breiman, and the Community Based Pneumonia Study Group.** 1997. Incidence of community-acquired pneumonia requiring hospitalization. *Arch. Intern. Med.* **157:**1709–1718.
67. **Martin, R. J., M. Kraft, H. W. Chu, E. A. Berns, and G. H. Cassell.** 2001. A link between chronic asthma and chronic infection. *J. Allergy Clin. Immunol.* **107:**595–601.
68. **Matas, L., J. Domínguez, F. De Ory, N. García, N. Gali, P. J. Cardona, A. Hernández, C. Rodrigo, and V. Ausina.** 1998. Evaluation of Meridian ImmunoCard mycoplasma test for the detection of *Mycoplasma pneumoniae*-specific IgM in pediatric patients. *Scand. J. Infect. Dis.* **30:**289–293.
69. **Meyer, R. D., and W. Clough.** 1993. Extragenital *Mycoplasma hominis* infections in adults: emphasis on immunosuppression. *Clin. Infect. Dis.* **17**(Suppl. 1):243–249.
70. **Møller, B. R., D. Taylor-Robinson, and P. M. Furr.** 1984. Serological evidence implicating *Mycoplasma genitalium* in pelvic inflammatory disease. *Lancet* **i:**1102–1103.
71. **Neimark, H., K.-E. Johansson, Y. Rikihisa, and J. Tully.** 2001. Proposal to transfer some members of the genera *Haemobartonella* and *Eperythrozoon* to the genus *Mycoplasma* with descriptions of 'Candidatus Mycoplasma hemofelis', 'Candidatus Mycoplasma hemomuris', 'Candidatus Mycoplasma hemosuis' and 'Candidatus Mycoplasma wenyonii'. *Int. J. Syst. Evol. Microbiol.* **51:**891–899.
72. **Phillips, L. E., K. H. Goodrich, R. M. Turner, and S. Faro.** 1986. Isolation of *Mycoplasma* species and *Ureaplasma urealyticum* from obstetrical and gynecological patients by using commercially available medium formulations. *J. Clin. Microbiol.* **24:**377–379.
73. **Porath, A., F. Schlaeffer, and D. Lieberman.** 1997. The epidemiology of community-acquired pneumonia among hospitalized adults. *J. Infect.* **34:**41–48.
74. **Pratt, B.** 1990. Automatic blood culture systems: detection of *Mycoplasma hominis* in SPS-containing media, p. 778–781. *In* G. Staneck, G. H. Cassell, J. G. Tully, and R. F. Whitcomb (ed.), *Recent Advances in Mycoplasmology*. Gustav Fischer Verlag, Stuttgart, Germany.
75. **Razin, S.** 1994. DNA probes and PCR in diagnosis of mycoplasma infections. *Mol. Cell. Probes* **8:**497–511.
76. **Renaudin, H., and C. Bébéar.** 1990. Evaluation des systemes *Mycoplasma* PLUS et SIR *Mycoplasma* pour la detection quantitative et l'etude de la sensibilite aux antibiotiques des mycoplasmes genitaux. *Pathol. Biol.* **38:**431–435.
76a. **Rikihisa, Y., M. Kawahara, B. Wen, G. Kociba, P. Fuerst, F. Kawamori, C. Suto, S. Shibata, and M. Futohashi.** 1997. Western immunoblot analysis of *Haemobartonella muris* and comparison of 16S rRNA gene sequences of *H. muris*, *H. felis*, and *Eperythrozoon suis*. *J. Clin Microbiol.* **35:**823–829.
77. **Roberts, M. C.** 1992. Antibiotic resistance, p. 513–523. *In* J. Maniloff, R. N. McElhaney, L. R. Finch, and J. B. Baseman (ed.), *Mycoplasmas: Molecular Biology and Pathogenesis.* American Society for Microbiology, Washington, D.C.
78. **Robertson, J. A., M. Alfa, and E. S. Boatman.** 1983. The morphology of the cells and colonies of *Mycoplasma hominis*. *Sex. Transm. Dis.* **10**(Suppl.):232–239.
79. **Robertson, J. A., L. A. Howard, C. L. Zinner, and G. W. Stemke.** 1994. Comparison of 16S-RNA genes within the T960 and parvo biovars of ureaplasmas isolated from humans. *Int. J. Syst. Bacteriol.* **44:**836–838.

80. **Robertson, J. A., A. Verkris, C. Bébéar, and G. W. Stemke.** 1993. Polymerase chain reaction using 16S-RNA gene sequences distinguishes the two biovars of *Ureaplasma urealyticum*. *J. Clin. Microbiol.* **31:**824–830.
81. **Robertson, J. A., G. W. Stemke, J. W. Davis, Jr., R. Harasawa, D. Thirkill, F. Kong, M. C. Shepard, and D. K. Ford.** 2002. Proposal of *Ureaplasma parvum* sp. nov. and emended description of *Urealasma urealyticum* (Shepard et al. 1974) Robertson et al. 2001. *Int. J. Syst. Evol. Microbiol.* **52:**587–597.
82. **Schaeverbeke, T., H. Renaudin, M. Clerc, L. Lequen, J. P. Vernhes, B. de Barbeyrac, B. Bannwarth, C. Bébéar, and J. Dehais.** 1997. Systematic detection of mycoplasmas by culture and polymerase chain reaction (PCR) procedures in 209 synovial fluid samples. *Br. J. Rheumatol.* **36:**310–314.
83. **Schaeverbeke, T., C. B. Gilroy, C. Bébéar, J. Dehais, and D. Taylor-Robinson.** 1996. *Mycoplasma fermentans* in joints of patients with rheumatoid arthritis and other joint diseases. *Lancet* **347:**1418.
84. **Shepard, M. C.** 1983. Culture media for ureaplasmas, p. 137–146. *In* S. Razin and J. G. Tully (ed.), *Methods in Mycoplasmology*, vol. 1, Academic Press, Inc., New York, N.Y.
85. **Shepard, M. C., and C. D. Lunceford.** 1978. Serological typing of *Ureaplasma urealyticum* isolates from urethritis patients by an agar growth inhibition method. *J. Clin. Microbiol.* **8:**566–574.
86. **Sillis, M.** 1990. The limitation of IgM assays in the serological diagnosis of *Mycoplasma pneumoniae* infection. *J. Med. Microbiol.* **33:**253–258.
87. **Sillis, M.** 1993. Genital mycoplasmas revisited—an evaluation of a new culture medium. *Br. J. Biomed. Sci.* **50:** 89–91.
88. **Stamm, W. E., K. Running, J. Hale, and K. K. Holmes.** 1983. Etiologic role of *Mycoplasma hominis* and *Ureaplasma urealyticum* in women with the acute urethral syndrome. *Sex. Transm. Dis.* **10**(Suppl.):318–322.
89. **Talkington, D. F., W. L. Thacker, D. W. Keller, and J. S. Jensen.** 1998. Diagnosis of *Mycoplasma pneumoniae* infection in autopsy and open-lung biopsy tissues by nested PCR. *J. Clin. Microbiol.* **36:**1151–1153.
90. **Taylor-Robinson, D.** 1983. Metabolism inhibition test, p. 411–417. *In* J. G. Tully and S. Razin (ed.), *Methods in Mycoplasmology*, vol. 1, Academic Press, Inc., New York, N.Y.
91. **Taylor-Robinson, D.** 1985. Mycoplasmal and mixed infections of the human male urogenital tract and their possible complications, p. 27–63. *In* S. Razin and M. F. Barile (ed.), *The Mycoplasmas*, vol. 4. Academic Press, Inc., New York, N.Y.
92. **Taylor-Robinson, D.** 1986. Evaluation of the role of *Ureaplasma urealyticum* in infertility. *Pediatr. Infect. Dis. J.* **5**(Suppl.):262–265.
93. **Taylor-Robinson, D.** 1989. Genital mycoplasma infections. *Clin. Lab. Med.* **9:**501–523.
94. **Taylor-Robinson, D.** 1996. Infections due to species of *Mycoplasma* and *Ureaplasma*: an update. *Clin. Infect. Dis.* **23:**671–684.
95. **Taylor-Robinson, D., and C. Bébéar.** 1997. Antibiotic susceptibilities of mycoplasmas and treatment of mycoplasmal infections. *J. Antimicrob. Chemother.* **40:**622–630.
96. **Taylor-Robinson, D., and G. W. Csonka.** 1981. Laboratory and clinical aspects of mycoplasmal infections of the human genitourinary tract. *Rec. Adv. Sex. Transm. Dis.* **2:**151–186.
97. **Taylor-Robinson, D., and P. J. Horner.** 2001. The role of *Mycoplasma genitalium* in non-gonococcal urethritis. *Sex. Transm. Infect.* **77:**229–231.

98. **Taylor-Robinson, D., P. M. Furr, and A. D. B. Webster.** 1985. *Ureaplasma urealyticum* causing persistent urethritis in a patient with hypogammaglobulinaemia. *Genitourin. Med.* **61:**404–408.

99. **Taylor-Robinson, D., P. M. Furr, and A. D. B. Webster.** 1986. *Ureaplasma urealyticum* in the immunocompromised host. *Pediatr. Infect. Dis. J.* **5**(Suppl.):236–238.

100. **Taylor-Robinson, D., and W. M. McCormack.** 1979. Mycoplasmas in human genitourinary infections, p. 307–366. *In* J. G. Tully and R. F. Whitcomb (ed.), *The Mycoplasmas*, vol. 2. Academic Press, Inc., New York, N.Y.

101. **Taylor-Robinson, D., and P. E. Munday.** 1988. Mycoplasmal infection of the female genital tract and its complications, p. 228–247. *In* M. J. Hare (ed.), *Genital Tract Infection in Women*. Churchill Livingstone, Edinburgh, United Kingdom.

102. **Taylor-Robinson, D., A. D. B. Webster, P. M. Furr, and G. L. Asherson.** 1980. Prolonged persistence of *Mycoplasma pneumoniae* in a patient with hypogammaglobulinaemia. *J. Infect.* **2:**171–175.

103. **Texier-Maugein, J., M. Clerc, A. Vekris, and C. Bébéar.** 1987. *Ureaplasma urealyticum*-induced bladder stones in rats and their prevention by flurofamide and doxycycline. *Isr. J. Med. Sci.* **23:**565–567.

104. **Thacker, W. L., and D. F. Talkington.** 1995. Comparison of two rapid commercial tests with complement fixation for serologic diagnosis of *Mycoplasma pneumoniae* infections. *J. Clin. Microbiol.* **33:**1212–1214.

105. **Thacker, W. L., and D. F. Talkington.** 2000. Analysis of complement fixation and commercial enzyme immunoassays for detection of antibodies to *Mycoplasma pneumoniae* in human serum. *Clin. Diagn. Lab. Immunol.* **7:**778–780.

106. **Thomsen, A. C.** 1978. Mycoplasmas in human pyelonephritis: demonstration of antibodies in serum and urine. *J. Clin. Microbiol.* **8:**197–202.

107. **Totten, P. A., M. A. Schwartz, K. E. Sjöström, G. E. Kenny, H. H. Handsfield, J. B. Weiss, and W. L. H. Whittington.** 2001. Association of *Mycoplasma genitalium* with nongonococcal urethritis in heterosexual men. *J. Infect. Dis.* **183:**269–276.

108. **Tryon, V. V., and J. B. Baseman.** 1992. Pathogenic determinants and mechanisms, p. 457–471. *In* J. Maniloff, R. N. McElhaney, L. R. Finch, and J. B. Baseman (ed.), *Mycoplasmas: Molecular Biology and Pathogenesis*. American Society for Microbiology, Washington, D.C.

109. **Tully, J. G., D. L. Rose, R. F. Whitcomb, and R. P. Wenzel.** 1979. Enhanced isolation of *Mycoplasma pneumoniae* from throat washings with a newly modified culture medium. *J. Infect. Dis.* **139:**478–482.

110. **Waites, K. B., and K. C. Canupp.** 2001. Evaluation of BacT/ALERT System for detection of *Mycoplasma hominis* in simulated blood cultures. *J. Clin. Microbiol.* **39:**4328–4331.

111. **Waites, K. B., P. T. Rudd, D. T. Crouse, K. C. Canupp, K. G. Nelson, C. Ramsey, and G. H. Cassell.** 1988. Chronic *Ureaplasma urealyticum* and *Mycoplasma hominis* infections of central nervous system in preterm infants. *Lancet* **i:**17–21.

112. **Waites, K. B., T. A. Figarola, T. Schmid, D. M. Crabb, L. B. Duffy, and J. W. Simecka.** 1991. Comparison of agar versus broth dilution techniques for determining antibiotic susceptibilities of *Ureaplasma urealyticum*. *Diagn. Microbiol. Infect. Dis.* **14:**265–271.

113. **Waites, K. B., D. M. Crabb, L. B. Duffy, and G. H. Cassell.** 1997. Evaluation of the Etest for detection of tetracycline resistance in *Mycoplasma hominis*. *Diagn. Microbiol. Infect. Dis.* **27:**117–122.

114. **Waites, K. B., K. C. Canupp, and G. E. Kenny.** 1999. In vitro susceptibilities of *Mycoplasma hominis* to six fluoroquinolones determined by Etest. *Antimicrob. Agents Chemother.* **43:**2571–2573.

115. **Waites, K. B., C. M. Bébéar, J. A. Robertson, D. F. Talkington, and G. E. Kenny.** 2001. *Cumitech 34, Laboratory Diagnosis of Mycoplasmal Infections.* Coordinating ed., F. S. Nolte. American Society for Microbiology, Washington, D.C.

116. **Waites, K. B., D. F. Talkington, and C. M. BéBéar.** 2002. Mycoplasmas, p. 201–224. *In* A. Truant (ed.), *Manual of Commercial Methods in Clinical Microbiology*. American Society for Microbiology, Washington, D.C.

117. **Wang, R. Y. H., J. W. K. Shih, T. Grandinetti, P. F. Pierce, M. M. Hayes, D. J. Wear, H. J. Alter, and S. C. Lo.** 1992. High frequency of antibodies to *Mycoplasma penetrans* in HIV-infected patients. *Lancet* **340:**1312–1316.

118. **Wang, R. Y. H., J. W. K. Shih, S. H. Weiss, T. Grandinetti, P. F. Pierce, M. Lange, H. J. Alter, D. J. Wear, C. L. Davies, R. K. Mayur, and S. C. Lo.** 1993. *Mycoplasma penetrans* infection in male homosexuals with AIDS: high seroprevalence and association with Kaposi's sarcoma. *Clin. Infect. Dis.* **17:**724–729.

119. **Wang, R. Y. H., W. S. Wu, M. S. Dawson, J. W. H. Shih, and S. C. Lo.** 1992. Selective detection of *Mycoplasma fermentans* by polymerase reaction and by using a nucleotide sequence within the insertion sequence-like element. *J. Clin. Microbiol.* **30:**245–248.

120. **Wilson, M. H., and A. M. Collier.** 1976. Ultrastructural study of *Mycoplasma pneumoniae* in organ culture. *J. Bacteriol.* **125:**332–339.

121. **Wood, J. C., R. M. Lu, E. M. Peterson, and L. M. de la Maza.** 1985. Evaluation of Mycotrim-GU for isolation of *Mycoplasma* species and *Ureaplasma urealyticum*. *J. Clin. Microbiol.* **22:**789–792.

Chlamydia and *Chlamydophila*[*]

JAMES B. MAHONY, BRIAN K. COOMBES, AND MAX A. CHERNESKY

63

Members of the *Chlamydiaceae* are highly evolved pathogens capable of infecting a wide range of warm- and cold-blooded animals and a variety of cell types ranging from soil protists such as *Acanthamoeba* to brain microglial cells. These bacteria are nonmotile, gram-negative, obligate intracellular organisms that possess a unique developmental cycle consisting of metabolically inactive infectious elementary bodies (EBs) and metabolically active but noninfectious reticulate bodies (RBs) (Fig. 1). This unique developmental cycle differentiates them from all other microorganisms (73) and is the basis for their taxonomic classification into a separate order, *Chlamydiales*. Chlamydiae replicate in the cytoplasm of host cells within an endosomal vacuole which appears under light microscopy as an intracellular inclusion. Chlamydiae are susceptible to many broad-spectrum antibiotics. Although they have the metabolic pathways to synthesize ATP, they are considered energy parasites since they use ATP produced by host cells for their own energy requirements. Under adverse environmental conditions such as glucose or amino acid starvation, elevated temperatures, or the presence of suboptimal antibiotic concentrations, chlamydiae revert to nonreplicating persistent bodies (PBs) (Fig. 1F), displaying an altered pattern of gene expression (68) that may contribute to their intracellular survival. The complete genome sequences of both *Chlamydia trachomatis* and *C. pneumoniae* have now been revealed (52, 101).

TAXONOMY

Historically, because of their unique developmental life cycle, all chlamydiae were placed into their own order, *Chlamydiales*, family *Chlamydiaceae*, within one genus, *Chlamydia* (73, 80), and four recognized species, *C. trachomatis*, *C. psittaci*, *C. pecorum*, and *C. pneumoniae*. However, recent analysis of 16S and 23S rRNA gene sequences has indicated that a new taxonomic classification may be warranted (32). It has been proposed that the order *Chlamydiales* be divided into four families as follows: (i) *Chlamydiaceae*, to contain two genera, *Chlamydia* (to in-

clude *C. trachomatis*, *C. muridarum*, and *C. suis*) and *Chlamydophila* (to include *C. pneumoniae*, *C. pecorum*, *C. psittaci*, *C. abortus*, *C. caviae*, and *C. felis*); (ii) *Simkaniaceae*, to include *Simkania negevensis*; (iii) *Parachlamydiaceae*, to include *Parachlamydia acanthamoeba* (strain BN9); and (iv) an unnamed family, to include *Waddlia* strain WSU 86-1044. *C. trachomatis* causes trachoma, conjunctivitis, lymphogranuloma venereum (LGV), genital tract diseases, pneumonia in infants and immunocompromised hosts, and reactive arthritis (Reiter's syndrome). It has been divided into three biovars, trachoma, LGV, and mouse pneumonitis (MoPn), and contains 18 recognized serovars. *C. trachomatis*-like organisms have been isolated from ferrets and swine; however, their relationship to the three known biovars is not known. *C. trachomatis* is sensitive to sulfonamides and produces a glycogen-like material within the inclusion that stains with iodine. *C. psittaci* strains infect many avian species and mammals, causing psittacosis, ornithosis, feline pneumonitis, and bovine abortion. Humans are infected secondarily from animals and develop pneumonia or systemic infection, including endocarditis. *C. psittaci* is resistant to the action of sulfonamides and produces inclusions that do not stain with iodine. *C. pneumoniae* causes a variety of respiratory tract infections (pharyngitis, sinusitis, bronchitis, and pneumonia) in humans and also infects a range of animals from koalas to snakes (39, 40). *C. pneumoniae* is a major cause of community-acquired pneumonia, and an increasing body of evidence has linked it to atherosclerosis and coronary artery disease. A fourth species, *C. pecorum*, has also been described, but its role as a pathogen is not clear and specialized reagents are required for its identification (35).

DESCRIPTION OF THE GENUS

Growth Cycle

The unique biphasic growth cycle is shared by all chlamydiae. EBs (diameter, ~0.3 μm) attach to a susceptible host cell via an unknown cellular receptor(s) and bacterial ligand(s). The binding process may also involve adhesive interactions between heparan sulfate-like molecules in *C. trachomatis* (117) and *C. pneumoniae* (116), which may function in adherence of the bacteria to the host cell surface. Chlamydial uptake is an invasive process since

---

[*] This chapter contains material presented in chapter 57 by Julius Schachter and Walter E. Stamm in the seventh edition of this Manual.

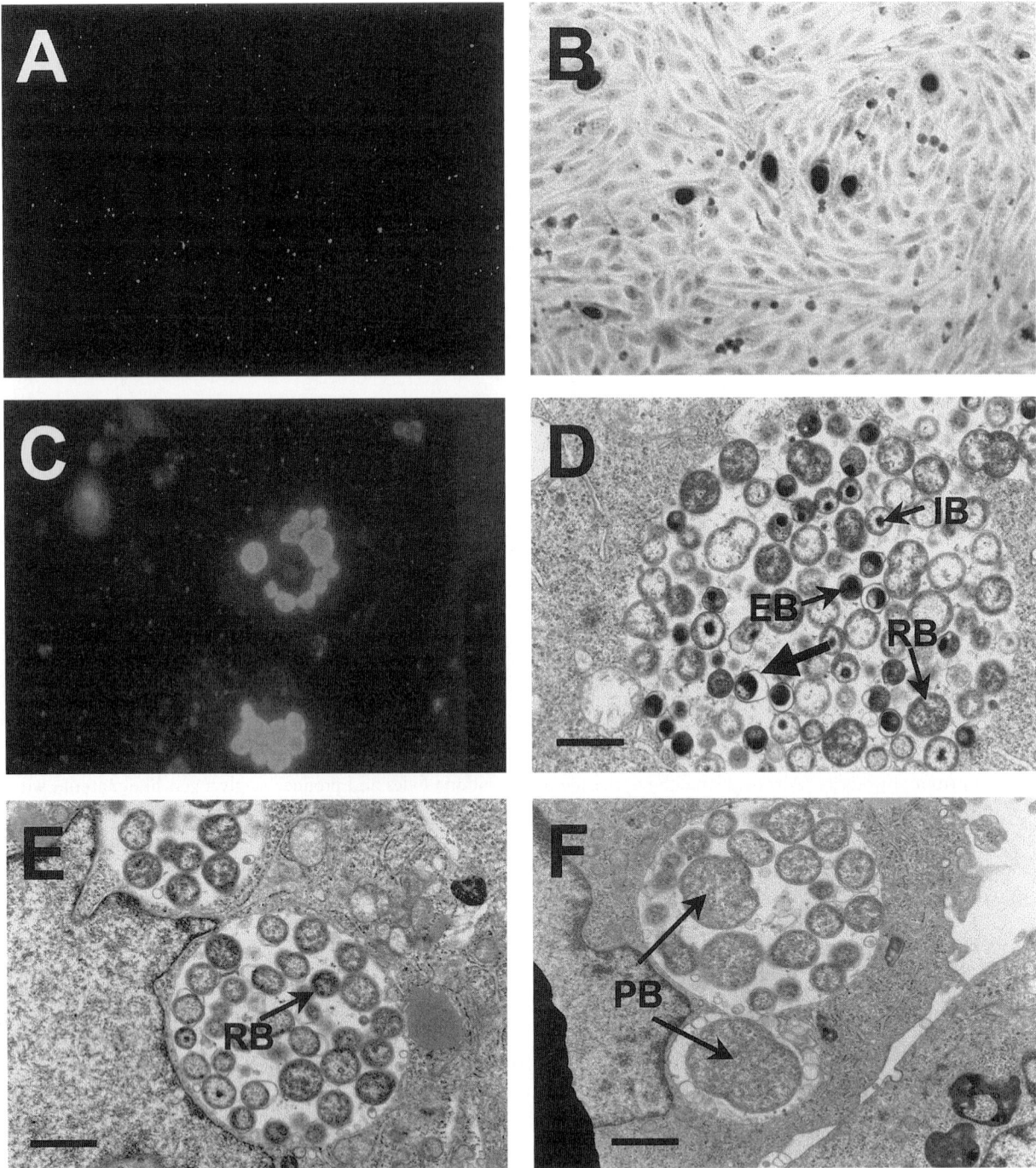

FIGURE 1 Identification of C. trachomatis and C. pneumoniae by a variety of staining techniques. (A) DFA staining of C. trachomatis EBs in a cervical smear, using a fluorescein-labeled monoclonal antibody directed at the MOMP. (B) Intracytoplasmic inclusions of C. trachomatis in cell culture stained with iodine. (C) Nonfusogenic inclusions of C. pneumoniae stained with a fluorescein-labeled monoclonal antibody directed to LPS. (D) Intracytoplasmic inclusion containing C. pneumoniae EBs, RBs, and intermediate bodies (IB) viewed by transmission electron microscopy. The large arrow indicates a loose outer membrane, occasionally seen for C. pneumoniae. Bar, 1 μm. (E) C. pneumoniae RBs grown in the absence of gamma interferon. (F) C. pneumoniae persistent bodies (PB) induced by growth in the presence of gamma interferon.

these bacteria infect nonphagocytic cells as well as phagocytes through a process that resembles receptor-mediated endocytosis. Chlamydiae remain bound inside a vacuole called an inclusion during the intracellular stage of their developmental cycle. The inclusion membrane is derived from the host cell plasma membrane during infection. Through an unknown process requiring bacterial protein synthesis, inclusions are stable, not maturing into late endosomes or fusing with lysosomes. Intracellular EBs reorganize into less condensed RBs (diameter, ~1 μm) that initiate RNA and DNA synthesis and divide by binary fission. Cultures of *C. trachomatis* appear to have a shortened developmental cycle (48 h) compared to *C. pneumoniae* (72 h) and require less time for propagation in vitro. The growth phase marked by binary fission of RBs lasts for 24 to 72 h after infection as assessed in cell culture models and is followed by asynchronous reorganization of RBs into EBs. The signals that control this process and the bacterial proteins required for morphological transformation are poorly understood but involve, in part, oxidation of cysteine-rich outer membrane proteins to create a rigid and osmotically stable EB that is adapted for extracellular survival. EBs are lytically released from host cells to initiate a new growth cycle in neighboring cells.

Antigenic Relationships

Chlamydiae contain both common antigens and species-specific antigens that play a role in pathogenesis and diagnosis of infection. The major common antigen is lipopolysaccharide (LPS), which contains a ketodeoxyoctanoic acid-reactive moiety (60). Type-specific antigens have also been characterized in *C. trachomatis* and *C. psittaci* that define specific biovars and/or serovars of these species. To date, type-specific antigens have not been characterized for *C. pneumoniae*, and so isolates of this species are serologically identical. DNA sequencing and monoclonal antibodies have been used to study the antigenic heterogeneity of the major outer membrane protein (MOMP), encoded by the *ompA* gene of *C. trachomatis*. These studies have identified four surface-exposed variable domains that allow serotyping of the organism using the microimmunofluorescence (MIF) test. In *C. pneumoniae*, OmpA appears to be located at a more conserved genetic locus yet is still a target for neutralizing immunoglobulins directed against conformational epitopes of this protein (114). The immunodominance of OmpA in *C. pneumoniae* has been questioned. It is possible that the variable regions in *C. pneumoniae* OmpA are not recognized by the human immune system, perhaps because they are masked by one or more of the large polymorphic outer membrane proteins as suggested by Christiansen et al. (23). A 60-kDa cysteine-rich outer membrane protein doublet (OmcB) is also an immunodominant species-specific antigen possessing genus-specific epitopes. Most sera from *Chlamydia*-infected patients contain antibodies against OmcB.

CLINICAL SIGNIFICANCE

C. trachomatis is the most common sexually transmitted bacterial agent. Serovars A, B, Ba, and C are associated with endemic trachoma, the most common preventable form of blindness, while serovars L1, L2, and L3 are associated with LGV. Serovars D through K are the major causes of nongonococcal urethritis and epididymitis in men and may induce Reiter's syndrome, proctitis, and conjunc-

tivitis in both men and women and cervicitis, urethritis, endometritis, salpingitis, and perihepatitis in women (89, 98). Salpingitis may lead to tubal scarring, infertility, and ectopic pregnancy. *C. trachomatis* in the cervix may be transmitted to a neonate during passage through an infected birth canal, resulting in neonatal pneumonia (5). Vaginal, pharyngeal, and enteric infections in neonates have also been recognized.

Infections with *C. trachomatis* have been associated with increased rates of transmission of human immunodeficiency virus (HIV) (110). Chlamydia-induced inflammation resulting in increased recruitment of CD4 lymphocytes into the genital tract (leading to an increased number of HIV targets) and increased HIV replication is thought to contribute to enhanced transmission. Between one-half and two-thirds of chlamydial infections in men and women may be asymptomatic and are not diagnosed and treated. In women ascending infection may include endometritis and salpingitis leading to pelvic inflammatory disease, ectopic pregnancy, or tubal factor infertility. Screening programs aimed at controlling chlamydial infections and preventing their consequences in high-risk women have been implemented in some jurisdictions with some success (45; H. H. Handsfield, Abstract and Commentary, JAMA **280**:1800–1801, 1998).

Psittacosis is a zoonosis usually contracted by humans following an exposure to an infected avian species. *C. psittaci* is ubiquitous among avian species, and infection usually involves the intestinal tract. The organism is shed in the feces and is readily spread by aerosols. *C. psittaci* is also common in domestic animals, and in some parts of the world these infections have important economic consequences because *C. psittaci* causes systemic and debilitating diseases, including abortions, in cattle. Human chlamydial infections resulting from exposure to infected domestic mammals occur but are relatively uncommon.

C. pneumoniae infections are very common worldwide (41). Seroepidemiologic studies suggest that infections are commonly acquired in later childhood, adolescence, and early adulthood, resulting in seroprevalences up to 70% by the fifth decade of life. Manifestations of infection include pharyngitis, bronchitis, mild pneumonia, and exacerbation of asthma (47). Within households, schools, and workplace environments, transmission is thought to occur via respiratory secretions. *C. pneumoniae* has been linked with atherosclerosis, coronary artery disease (115), and stroke. *C. pneumoniae* DNA and antigens have been detected in atheromas by a variety of techniques including PCR, in situ hybridization, and immunohistochemical staining, and the organism has been isolated from atheromatous tissue (49, 83). *C. pneumoniae* DNA has recently been detected in cerebrospinal fluid of multiple sclerosis patients and in postmortem brain tissues of Alzheimer's disease patients (2, 48, 97). An etiologic role in atherosclerosis is currently under intense scrutiny.

COLLECTION, TRANSPORT, AND STORAGE

Chlamydiae are relatively labile organisms, and viability can be maintained by keeping specimens cold and minimizing the time between specimen collection and processing in the laboratory. For successful culture of chlamydiae, swabs, scrapings, and small tissue samples should be forwarded to the laboratory in a special chlamydial transport medium such as 2SP (0.2 M sucrose-phosphate transport medium containing 10 μg of gentamicin/ml, 25 μg of vancomycin/ml, and 25 U of nystatin/ml) or SPG (75 g of sucrose, 0.52 g of KH_2PO_4, 1.22 g of Na_2HPO_4, 0.72 g of glutamic acid, and H_2O to 1 liter [pH 7.4 to 7.6]) supplemented with bovine serum, albumin, streptomycin, vancomycin, and nystatin (see chapter 27). Broad-spectrum antibiotics such as tetracyclines, macrolides, or penicillin cannot be used in the transport media since they have activity against chlamydiae. Aminoglycosides and fungicides are the mainstays and can be safely used. Chlamydial specimens should be refrigerated on receipt in the laboratory, and if they cannot be processed within 24 h after collection, they should be frozen at −70°C. C. psittaci strains are usually more stable, and some may persist in a contaminated environment for months without losing viability. The stability of C. pneumoniae has not been well studied, but these organisms have been extremely difficult to grow from clinical specimens, which may be due in part to reduced viability or their presence in tissue as nonreplicating PBs.

When specimens are collected for enzyme immunoassay (EIA), direct fluorescent-antibody (DFA), or nucleic acid amplification (NAA) procedures, the descriptions and procedural instructions given in the product's package insert should be followed. This includes the use of swabs or specific transport media specified by the manufacturers, since the use of other materials may impair the sensitivity and/or specificity of the test.

For cytological examination, impression smears of tissues or scrapings should be air dried and fixed with absolute methanol before staining for the DFA test.

C. trachomatis

For cytology, isolation in culture, or antigen detection methods, epithelial cell specimens should be collected by vigorous swabbing or scraping of the involved sites. Purulent discharges which lack infected epithelial cells are inappropriate and should be cleaned from the site before the sample is collected. Appropriate sites include the conjunctiva for trachoma-inclusion conjunctivitis and the male anterior urethra (several centimeters into the urethra) and the cervix (within the endocervical canal) for genital tract infection. Because C. trachomatis infects columnar or squamocolumnar cells, cervical specimens must be collected at the transitional zone or within the opening of the cervix. The organism also infects the female urethra, and recovery rates may be improved by collecting a specimen from the urethra as well as from the cervix and sending both to the laboratory. Vaginal swabs are inappropriate for these detection methods.

A variety of swab types can be used, but toxicity related to materials in swabs can be problematic. It is useful, therefore, to test swab types for toxicity in cell cultures or interference in nonculture assays when proprietary swabs are not provided by the manufacturer (65). As a general rule, swabs with wooden shafts should not be used. Cotton, Dacron, and calcium alginate swabs may all be used, although toxicity has been noted with specific lots of each. The cytobrush has also been used to collect endocervical specimens. It appears to collect more cells than swabs and has been associated in some investigators' experience with higher recovery rates of chlamydiae and higher rates of antigen detection by DFA (72). Regardless of whether a cytobrush or swab is used, clinicians and other health care providers must be trained to collect adequate specimens for chlamydial detection.

In women with salpingitis, samples may be collected by needle aspiration of the involved fallopian tube. Endometrial specimens have also yielded chlamydiae. In other clinical situations, the rectal mucosa, nasopharynx, and throat may be sampled. For infants with pneumonia, swabs may be collected from the posterior nasopharynx or the throat; however, nasopharyngeal or tracheobronchial aspirates collected by intubation are better specimens. For LGV strains, bubo pus, rectal or urethral swabbings, or biopsy samples should be collected.

First-void urine (FVU) specimens from men and women and vaginal swab specimens from women are excellent specimens for detection of C. trachomatis by NAA tests (17, 27, 44, 100, 103). FVU is the first 10 to 30 ml of urine, and specimens should be obtained at least 2 h after the last micturition. It is not necessary and may not be advantageous to obtain the first urine specimen passed in the morning. Subsequent processing of the urine specimen varies depending on the manufacturer's instructions. The urine sample is centrifuged, and the sediment is resuspended into the proprietary diluent for detection of nucleic acids.

C. psittaci

Appropriate specimens include sputum and blood. C. psittaci has been recovered in cell cultures from a variety of anatomic sites sampled by biopsy or at necropsy. Specimens for isolation are likely to be contaminated, and so the specimen should be collected into a medium that contains appropriate antibiotics to inhibit the growth of unwanted bacteria or fungi.

C. pneumoniae

Sputum (12, 106), bronchoalveolar lavage fluid (28), nasopharyngeal and throat swabs (9, 12, 36), ear and nasopharyngeal aspirates (10), gargled water (78), and tissues obtained at biopsy or autopsy (57) are suitable. Blood specimens, especially peripheral blood mononuclear cells (PBMC), appear to be excellent for C. pneumoniae nucleic acid detection (11, 94).

Nasopharyngeal specimens should be collected with swabs that have been pretested for cell culture toxicity and PCR inhibitors (13, 43). Transport media for culturing C. pneumoniae should also be tested for PCR inhibitors (9). Conditions for transportation of specimens for C. pneumoniae testing are similar to those stated above for C. trachomatis.

ISOLATION PROCEDURES

Biosafety Considerations

C. trachomatis is a biocontainment level 2 (BCL 2) agent and is not considered a particularly dangerous pathogen to handle in the laboratory. However, a number of laboratory-acquired infections, usually manifested as follicular conjunctivitis, have occurred. The LGV biovar is a more invasive organism, and severe cases of pneumonia or lymphadenitis have occurred when researchers were exposed to aerosols created by laboratory procedures such as sonication or centrifugation (6). C. psittaci (BCL 3) is considered a dangerous organism to handle in the laboratory. For many years it was a major cause of laboratory-acquired infections, usually resulting from exposure to aerosols. The stability of the organism in the environment is also a potential problem. This organism should therefore not be handled in laboratories without appropriate BCL 3 facilities. Laboratory infections with *C. pneumoniae* have also occurred, but these have generally been mild and have involved the upper respiratory tract.

Specimen Processing

General guidelines for processing specimens are listed below. Fresh samples are preferred, but frozen material (−70°C) is acceptable. Commercial tests should be used only for approved specimens (as listed in the product insert).

Ocular and Genital Tract Specimens

For ocular and genital tract sites, the laboratory usually receives swabs in transport medium containing antibiotics. Specimens to be assayed by commercial EIA, DFA, nucleic acid hybridization (NAH), or NAA should be handled as specified in the package insert. Homemade test protocols should be validated based on performance and consensus per guidelines of accrediting agencies.

Bubo Pus

To prepare bubo pus, the viscous material is ground and then suspended in nutrient broth or cell culture medium to at least 20% by weight. Even when the pus is not viscous, dilution is advisable. If the bubo is not fluctuant, sterile saline may be injected and aspirated for isolation attempts. The material should be tested for bacterial contaminants by plating on appropriate agar media and inoculating into cell cultures for isolation of chlamydiae.

Blood

Although chlamydiae have been isolated from clotted blood, whole blood may be inferior to fractionated blood. Blood clots should be ground and beef heart broth or cell culture medium (see chapter 27) should be added to make a 10% suspension. The suspension is inoculated directly into cell culture by using serial dilutions (from 1:2 to 1:10) since the concentrated material may be toxic to the cells. Peripheral blood mononuclear cells (PBMC) are purified by layering blood (diluted 1:2 with phosphate-buffered saline [usually 10 ml]) over 3 ml of Ficoll-Hypaque (Histopaque; Sigma, St. Louis, Mo.) and centrifuging for 10 min at 1,000 × g. PBMC are collected from the plasma/Ficoll-Hypaque interface by removing the top (plasma) layer and collecting 2 ml of the PBMC layer. Alternatively, mononuclear cells can be obtained with a CPT Vacutainer (BD Diagnostic Systems, Franklin Lakes, N.J.) as specified by the manufacturer.

Sputum or Throat Washings

To prepare an emulsion of sputum or throat washings, the sample is suspended in 2 to 10 times (depending on its consistency) its volume in cell culture medium; it is emulsified thoroughly by shaking with glass beads in a sterile, tightly stoppered container. Extracts should be centrifuged for 20 to 30 min at 100 × g to remove coarse material before the supernatant fluid is inoculated onto cell monolayers. Serial dilutions may be required if the inoculum is toxic to the cells.

Fecal Samples

Human rectal swabs for *C. trachomatis* and avian material for *C. psittaci* are suspended in cell culture medium containing penicillin and streptomycin. The suspension is shaken thoroughly and centrifuged at 300 × g for 10 min, and the supernatant fluid is removed. It may be further diluted (1:2 and 1:20) with culture medium before being inoculated into cell culture.

Tissue Samples

Frozen tissue is thawed, weighed, minced with sterile scissors, and ground with a mortar and pestle or homogenizer. A volume of cell culture medium required to make a 10 to 20% suspension is added, and the suspension is thoroughly mixed. For tissue specimens, serial dilutions (1:10 to 1:100) are often required for inoculation to prevent toxicity.

Isolation in Cell Culture

Historically, chlamydiae were grown in the yolk sacs of embryonated hen eggs. Most if not all chlamydiae appear to be able to grow in cell culture if the inoculum is centrifuged onto preformed cell monolayers. *C. psittaci* and LGV strains of *C. trachomatis* are capable of serial growth in cell culture without centrifugation. A number of different cell lines have been used to support the growth of chlamydiae. It appears that no single cell line is markedly superior to others, since successful isolation has been performed with monkey kidney, HeLa, HL, HEp-2, and McCoy cells, among others. McCoy, HEp-2, and HeLa cells are most commonly used for *C. trachomatis*. *C. pneumoniae* from clinical specimens is more difficult to grow. This organism grows poorly in McCoy and HeLa cells; HL cells and HEp-2 cells are more sensitive for its recovery (88).

Clinical specimens should be inoculated onto cycloheximide-treated monolayer cultures of McCoy cells (87) or other appropriate cells at 35 to 37°C. Detection involves centrifugation of the specimen onto the cell monolayer followed by incubation for 48 to 72 h and staining for intracytoplasmic inclusions. Fluorescein-conjugated fluorescent monoclonal antibody stains (Pathfinder; Kallestad, Chaska, Minn.) is the most sensitive method for detecting inclusions in cell culture and also allows earlier detection of inclusions. For *C. trachomatis* iodine staining can also be used but it is less sensitive. For *C. psittaci* and *C. pneumoniae*, inclusions can be demonstrated with group-specific fluorescent monoclonal antibodies or Giemsa stain (see chapter 27).

For the shell vial method, McCoy cells are plated onto 12-mm glass coverslips in 15-mm-diameter (1-dram [1 dram = 3.697 ml]) disposable glass vials. The cells (approximately 1×10^5 to 2×10^5) are selected to give a light, confluent monolayer after 24 to 48 h of incubation at 37°C in 5% CO_2. For optimal results, the cells should be used within 24 h after reaching confluency.

Clinical specimens are shaken with 5-mm glass beads to lyse the cells and release the chlamydiae before being used for inoculation. This procedure is safer and more convenient than sonication. For inoculation, the medium is removed from the cell monolayer and 0.1 to 1 ml of inoculum is added to the cells. The specimen is centrifuged onto the cell monolayer at approximately 3,000 × g at room temperature for 1 h. Shell vials are incubated at 35°C in 5% CO_2 for 2 h to allow uptake of chlamydiae, and then the medium is discarded and replaced with medium containing 1 μg of cycloheximide per ml. The cells are incubated at 35°C in 5% CO_2 for 48 to 72 h, and one coverslip is examined for inclusions by immunofluorescence, iodine staining, or Giemsa staining. The use of immunofluorescence can speed the process, since inclusions can clearly be seen (although they are smaller) at 24 h postinfection. Giemsa stain is more sensitive than iodine stain, but the microscopic evaluation is more difficult. Slide reading can be facilitated by examining the Giemsa-stained coverslip by dark-field microscopy.

If passage of positive material or blind passage of negative material is desired, the material should be passaged at 72 to 96 h postinoculation. The cell monolayer is disrupted by shaking with 5-mm glass beads on a Vortex mixer; the material is subjected to low-speed centrifugation (500 × g) for 10 min to remove cell debris, and the supernatant is reinoculated as described above. For symptomatic patients, the majority of specimens positive for C. trachomatis are identified in the first passage. For screening of asymptomatic patients, who often have a smaller bacterial burden at the infected site, a blind passage may be required to detect positive material.

For trachoma, inclusion conjunctivitis, and genital tract infections, culture is performed as described above. For LGV, the aspirated bubo pus must be diluted (10^{-1} and 10^{-2}) before inoculation. Second passages should always be made, because detritus from the inoculum may make it difficult to read the slides. For many C. psittaci isolation attempts, it may be convenient to lengthen the incubation period to 5 to 10 days before examining the coverslips for inclusions. These organisms do not require centrifugation for cell-to-cell infection. For C. pneumoniae, it may be necessary to repeat the centrifugation on days 3 and 5 and to perform up to five blind passages to improve recovery rates (79, 105).

Laboratories processing large numbers of specimens can use flat-bottom 48- or 96-well microtiter plates rather than shell vials. For this method, cells are plated either onto small glass coverslips in wells or, more commonly, directly into the plates. Processing and incubation are as described above, but microscopy is modified to use either long working objectives or inverted microscopes. This procedure offers considerable savings of reagents and time and may be useful when large numbers of patients are being screened. The microtiter technique may, however, be less sensitive than the shell vial technique for screening asymptomatic patients, who harbor fewer organisms, and a blind passage may be necessary to detect all positives.

Continuous quality control is important for maintaining a sensitive and specific culture system. To test the validity of specimen collection, periodic evaluation of slides by DFA permits evaluation of the cellular adequacy of the specimens being obtained. To test the adequacy of specimen transport, periodic transport of specimens with known numbers of chlamydia inclusion-forming units (IFU) can be used to assess loss of viability during transport. Daily inoculation of positive controls with a known number of IFU of chlamydiae is useful to determine the sensitivity of the cell culture system. Laboratories using the microtiter method should evaluate possible episodes of cross-contamination by reinoculation of any positive specimen occurring in wells adjacent to a high-titer positive specimen.

Yolk Sac Isolation

The yolk sac method is no longer used for evaluation of clinical specimens, but it is still used to prepare antigens for the microimmunofluorescence (micro-IF) test.

IDENTIFICATION

Most laboratories now use cell culture for isolation, and the basic procedure for identification of chlamydiae involves demonstration of intracytoplasmic inclusions by IF, iodine (Fig. 1B), or Giemsa staining procedures. Fluorescent-anti-body staining with group-specific antibody provides both morphological and immunological identification of chlamydiae and is therefore preferable to other staining methods, especially for use in less experienced laboratories.

C. trachomatis isolates can be serotyped by using serovar- or type-specific and subspecies-specific monoclonal antibodies. These antibodies can be used in several assay formats, but the most readily adaptable, sensitive, and specific method appears to be the microwell typing system, in which inclusions in microtiter wells are stained with pools of serovar-specific and subspecies-specific monoclonal antibodies (102). Typing of C. trachomatis isolates by genetic analysis involving restriction fragment length polymorphism analysis or sequencing of a single gene such as ompA provides useful genotyping information for strain clonality and relatedness studies (29, 34). Although serotyping and genotyping of chlamydial strains may be of use in epidemiological studies, it is of little clinical use unless medicolegal issues are involved.

In addition to typing C. trachomatis isolates with commercially available monoclonal antibodies, other methods of typing have been developed. These include the use of restriction endonuclease patterns of PCR-amplified DNA and direct sequencing of the variable domains in the ompA gene (8). These variable regions include the peptides responsible for species, serovar, and serogroup specificities. Variability in the amino acid sequence of the variable-region peptides may predict antigenic variants. Since these tests were first applied, more subtypes have been identified, and this process will probably continue, particularly if, as expected, these variants originate from immune selection. C. pneumoniae may be identified by use of commercially available group-specific monoclonal antibodies (Syva Microtrak Chlamydia Culture Confirmation Test, Trinity Biotech, Jamestown, N.Y.) or species-specific antibodies (RR2 or CF2; Washington Research Foundation, Seattle, Wash.). Differentiation of C. psittaci and C. pecorum is a research procedure, since there are no commercially available reagents for this purpose.

NONCULTURE DIAGNOSTIC TESTS

General Comments

The proliferation of new and more sensitive assays has led to a recognition that standardized approaches to evaluating their accuracy are needed. Initially, cell culture was thought to have a sensitivity close to 100% with very few false-positive results. Our thinking about this changed as antigen detection methods were developed, because a substantial number of antigen-positive and culture-negative specimens could be confirmed as containing organisms by DFA or by concurrence of multiple EIA results. This phenomenon probably reflected the presence in specimens of nonviable chlamydiae that died during transport and processing. Some package inserts that claimed 90% sensitivity for EIA were actually reflecting 90% compared to culture, which, in some laboratories, was 50 to 80% as defined using a combined reference standard for positivity. The expansion of the "gold standard" to include multiple nonculture tests to differentiate true-positive results from culture-negative results was helpful in evaluating the antigen detection methods (50). When NAA tests were introduced, the use of antigen detection methods proved inadequate because the NAA tests were far more sensitive. Therefore, it became necessary to use alternate nucleic acid targets to confirm some of the culture-negative and antigen-negative, nucleic acid-positive specimens (66, 67). In many evaluations, the NAA tests detected 20 to 30% more positive specimens than could be detected by the earlier technologies. The introduction of these tests also showed that there was considerably more variability in the sensitivity of culture from laboratory to laboratory than was true for the NAA tests.

The NAA tests are not a perfect gold standard, because none are consistently 100% sensitive on clinical specimens, probably due to the presence of inhibitors. The ideal gold standard for chlamydia diagnostics includes a sensitive NAA test together with a sensitive culture system to detect specimens that are negative in the NAA test due to the presence of inhibitors.

In comparisons of technologies, almost all studies have shown extra positive results with newer, more sensitive tests. This has led to the use of discrepant analysis to confirm whether these new positive results were true positives or false positives. A theoretical debate has ensued over this approach to diagnosis for cases when the arbitrating test was not used on all of the specimens that were negative in the comparative tests (42). From a practical point of view, discrepant analysis has been helpful, enabling an understanding of the sensitivity and specificity ranges of the various technologies. The few extra positive results found in the double-negative specimens generally had an insignificant effect on the percentages and did not justify the work and cost involved (M. Chernesky, J. Sellors, and J. Mahony, Letter, *Stat. Med.* **17:**1064–1065, 1998; J. Schachter, Letter, *J. Clin. Epidemiol.* **54:**210–215, 2001).

A further expansion of the gold standard has evolved as multiple specimens from each patient have been tested. Noninvasive specimens such as FVU (17) and vaginal (44, 113), vulvar (100), or introital swabs (103) often yield positive results in *C. trachomatis* NAA assays. Thus, discrepant analysis and multiple samples tested by more than one assay have enabled the gold standard to be defined as detection of an "infected patient" (18). Comparisons can now be made of the diagnostic abilities of particular tests performed on particular types of specimens. Only the NAA tests have been effective on noninvasive specimens, probably due to their greater sensitivity and a lack of sufficient antigens or viable organisms to be detected by EIA or culture.

Because of high costs and low throughput of current NAA tests, the concept of pooling urine samples (56) or swabs (53) has been evaluated. This appears to be an accurate and cost-beneficial maneuver when infection prevalence is low.

The principles discussed above are relevant for *C. trachomatis* infections. Specimens from individuals with other chlamydial infections may not easily yield organisms in cell cultures and have little or no antigen. The use of serologic testing for the diagnosis of *C. pneumoniae* has had variable success and questionable validity. Thus, NAA tests have been developed to detect *C. pneumoniae* nucleic acid sequences in either a single or nested PCR format (13). Other techniques for diagnosis of *C. pneumoniae* include immunocytochemistry and detection of circulating immune complexes (31). The sensitivity of these assays is unknown.

Direct Cytological Examination

Infections of the conjunctiva, urethra, or cervix can be diagnosed by demonstrating typical intracytoplasmic inclusions. For Giemsa staining, the smear is air dried, fixed with absolute methanol for at least 5 min, and dried again. It is then covered with the freshly prepared diluted Giemsa stain for at least 1 h. The slide is rapidly rinsed in 95% ethanol to remove excess dye and then dried and examined microscopically. The inclusions are basophilic and stain pinkish blue. Cytological testing to detect inclusions is particularly useful in diagnosing acute inclusion conjunctivitis of the newborn, in whom the sensitivity of this method exceeds 90%. Cytological testing is relatively insensitive in diagnosing adult conjunctival and genital tract infections.

Diagnostic tests involving monoclonal antibodies are based on detecting EBs in smears (Fig. 1A). The DFA test has approximately 75 to 85% sensitivity and 98 to 99% specificity compared with culture and lower sensitivity compared to NAA tests (16). The test requires a trained microscopist who can distinguish between fluorescing chlamydial particles and nonspecific fluorescence. Several DFA assays are commercially available, using monoclonal antibodies directed against MOMP (Syva Microtrak; Trinity Biotech) or LPS (Pathfinder; Kallestad). Monoclonal antibodies to the LPS will stain all chlamydiae, but the specimen may be more difficult to read because of uneven distribution of LPS on the chlamydial particle (25). The anti-MOMP monoclonal antibodies are prepared against *C. trachomatis;* therefore, they are species specific and will not stain *C. psittaci* or *C. pneumoniae*. The quality of fluorescence is better, because MOMP is evenly distributed on the chlamydial particle. The procedure offers rapid diagnosis, taking only 30 min to perform. A variation on the DFA procedure involves centrifugation of the transport medium being used for other tests (cell culture, NAA or EIA), preparation of a slide from the sediment, and staining with the fluorescent antibody reagents. This is often used as a confirmatory test for positives in other tests.

Enzyme Immunoassay

A number of EIAs are commercially available for detection of chlamydial antigens in clinical specimens (16, 24, 72). These products use either monoclonal or polyclonal antibodies to detect chlamydial LPS, which is more soluble than MOMP. These tests can theoretically detect all chlamydiae, but they have not been extensively evaluated for the diagnosis of infections with *C. psittaci* or *C. pneumoniae* and are not approved for this use. Most EIAs take several hours to perform and are suitable for batch processing.

The performance profiles of the commercially available *C. trachomatis* EIAs vary considerably, but increases in sensitivity using cultures as the reference standard have been achieved by using cycling enzymes to amplify the signal component in the IDEA PCE test (DAKO Ltd., Ely, United Kingdom) (22, 103, 104). Without confirmation, the tests have a specificity on the order of 97%. Therefore, they are not amenable to screening low-prevalence populations because of the low predictive value of a positive result in such groups. To address this problem, confirmatory tests have been developed. In one of the assays, all tests giving positive results are repeated in the presence of a monoclonal antibody directed against the group-specific epitope on the LPS. This results in blocking of the specific reactions but not of the false-positive results. The appropriate application of confirmatory tests increases the specificity to about 99.5% (71). Another approach to confirmation is to test a specimen by a second test based on a different principle, for example a DFA test based on MOMP detection to confirm an LPS-based EIA.

Several commercial point-of-care tests have been developed and have shown variable performance traits. They are usually performed within 30 min and facilitate immediate treatment of infected patients. Currently available point-of-care tests are 60 to 70% sensitive compared with NAA tests (21, 33, 55, 74, 84, 92) and specificity may also be less than 100%. These tests are not inexpensive and are not intended to be used in laboratory settings. If their performance can be improved and their costs can be decreased, they will offer the ability to test populations that are difficult to access and that almost inevitably fail to return for follow-up care, allowing for treatment of more cases (38).

Nucleic Acid Hybridization

Commercially available NAH tests for *C. trachomatis* in some parts of the world have been used as extensively as EIAs in laboratories handling large numbers of specimens on a daily basis. One commercially available probe test (PACE 2; Gen-Probe, San Diego, Calif.) utilizes DNA-RNA hybridization in an effort to increase sensitivity by detecting chlamydial RNA. Available data suggest that it is about as sensitive as the better antigen detection and cell culture methods and is relatively specific (24, 58). Another NAH test, Hybrid Capture II for *C. trachomatis* (Digene Corp., Gaithersburg, Md.), uses a signal amplification component to increase the sensitivity to approximately 90% of NAA assays (70, 91).

Nucleic Acid Amplification

Five nucleic acid amplification methods are currently licensed for detection of *C. trachomatis* in clinical specimens: PCR Amplicor (Roche Molecular Systems, Indianapolis, Ind.), ligase chain reaction LCx assay (Abbott Laboratories, Abbott Park, Ill.), transcription-mediated amplification AMP-CT and APTIMA Combo 2 (Gen-Probe), and strand displacement amplification ProbeTec (BD Diagnostic Systems). Only approved specimens as outlined in package inserts should be tested in these assays. At the time of writing, NAA test results for chlamydiae cannot be used for medicolegal purposes, since they are not legally admissible in U.S. courts. The principles behind these assays are described in chapter 17, which contains a thorough discussion of the methods. The PCR, ligase chain reaction, and strand displacement amplification assays amplify nucleotide sequences of the cryptic plasmid, which is present in multiple copies in each *C. trachomatis* EB. The transcription-mediated amplification reaction is directed against rRNA, which is also present in multiple copies. Theoretically, given the multiplicity of target sites for the amplification procedures being used, these techniques should be able to detect less than one EB. They can do so in purified suspensions of chlamydial particles; however, the actual sensitivity with clinical specimens is lower because of sampling variability and inhibition of the amplification reactions by factors in the specimens (4, 6, 19, 62). All the assays appear to be highly specific if problems with cross-contamination of reactions are avoided (76). Clinical evaluations of the amplification methods (4, 17, 27, 100) have demonstrated that they are more sensitive than culture and the other nonculture methods (microscopy, immunoassays, and NAH assays). The NAA assays are becoming the tests of choice for diagnosis of *C. trachomatis* infection in routine clinical laboratories. However, when organisms are needed for further study, isolation in cell culture will continue to be used.

Since no commercial NAA kits are available for *C. pneumoniae* at present, the value of using in-house-developed tests for diagnosis and the meaning of the presence of nucleic acid in a clinical specimen in relation to disease deserve attention. Several different formats including nested, nonnested, and enzyme time-released touchdown PCR targeting several different genes, namely, the *Pst*I fragment, *ompA*, 16S rRNA, and the 60-kDa cysteine-rich protein gene (*omcB*), have been described (9, 14, 37, 61, 77, 105, 106, 111). Current approaches to help interpret variable findings in clinical studies using PCR assays for *C. pneumoniae* have focused on standardizing the PCR protocols, including the choice of target genes, primers, PCR conditions, detection systems, and nucleic acid extraction techniques (1, 63). At the time of writing, companies are developing *C. pneumoniae* NAA tests, which may be submitted for Food and Drug Administration approval as a clinical test or provided as a research tool. Methods for quantitation of chlamydial nucleic acids are being developed and involve real-time PCR or nucleic acid sequence-based amplification of RNA (46, 96).

Serological Tests

Serological testing has been used for the diagnosis of acute and chronic *C. pneumoniae* infections, acute *C. psittaci* infections, and some acute and chronic *C. trachomatis* infections. The difficulty inherent in interpretation of the results of antibody studies for chlamydiae is that most studies lack appropriate control groups and reference standards of infection (20). The serological methods used are complement fixation (CF), IF, and EIA, using group- or species-specific antigens or a combination of these to measure immunoglobulin G (IgG), IgA, IgM, or total classes of antibodies to individual or multiple chlamydial serovars. The serological assay formats used are the MIF test (109), the whole-inclusion immunofluorescence test (85), EIA using EBs or RBs (81) or infected cells (69), and a recombinant enzyme-linked immunosorbent assay to LPS. Other tests include indirect hemagglutination, neutralization, precipitation, gel diffusion, enzyme-linked fluorescence or immunoperoxidase, and immunelectrophoresis. Several reports have described *C. pneumoniae* and *C. trachomatis* protein profiles with possible species- and group-specific immunoreactivities in Western blot analysis (7, 82), but interpretation is difficult. Most of the serological assays listed above employ in-house methods, although a few have been commercialized and are being used by clinical laboratories (MRL Diagnostics, Cypress, Calif.; Labsystems Oy, Helsinki, Finland; Sero-CP [Savyon Diagnostics, Kiryat Minrav, Ashdod, Israel]; and IPAzyme Chlamydia [Medac Diagnostics, Hamburg, Germany]).

Efforts are being made to link *C. pneumoniae* antibody titers and/or immunoglobulin types to differentiate acute from chronic and past infection (107). For *C. trachomatis* infections, IgM testing by microimmunofluorescence or EIA has been useful in identifying infants with pneumonia (64, 90) and total antibody determination by CF or whole-inclusion immunofluorescence has been useful in identifying patients with tubal factor infertility (26).

Complement Fixation Test

The classical CF serological test, once the stalwart test for diagnosis of chlamydial infection, is rarely performed today. It is based on antibody reactivity to the group-specific chlamydial LPS antigen and has been useful in the diagnosis of systemic chlamydial infections such as psittacosis and LGV. With this procedure, paired sera usually show at least a fourfold increase in antibody titer during an acute infection, although in some cases it may take 2 to 4 weeks to detect seroconversion. For patients with LGV, it is often difficult to demonstrate rising antibody titers in the CF test since patients usually present to physicians after the acute stage. In these cases, single sera that demonstrate titers greater than 64 have been supportive of the clinical diagnosis of LGV. Titers of 16 or greater are considered to provide significant evidence of previous exposure to chlamydiae. However, compared with culture, the CF test lacks sensitivity for the diagnosis of trachoma, inclusion conjunctivitis, or related genital infections caused by *C. trachomatis*. This test is also incapable of discriminating between chlamydial species, since it is based on the group-specific LPS antigen.

Microimmunofluorescence Test

The microimmunofluorescence test (micro-IF or MIF), developed by Wang (108), is the current method of choice for the serodiagnosis of acute chlamydial infection. It is a more sensitive technique for the measurement of antichlamydial antibodies and has the added advantage of being able to discriminate between chlamydial species and serovars of *C. trachomatis*. The MIF test allows quantitative determination of antibody reactivity to chlamydial EBs or single chlamydial antigens from various species on a glass slide solid support. It can be used for the diagnosis of psittacosis, LGV, ocular infection, and genital tract infection, providing that appropriately timed paired acute- and convalescent-phase sera are available. However, it is often difficult to demonstrate a rise in antibody titers due to the chronic and persistent nature of some chlamydial infections. This is particularly true among sexually active individuals attending sexually transmitted disease clinics, since these individuals are often chronically or repeatedly infected, making new seroconversions difficult to identify. In general, first attacks of chlamydial urethritis have been regularly associated with seroconversion. Individuals with systemic infections (epididymitis or salpingitis) usually have much higher antibody levels than do those with superficial infections, and women tend to have higher antibody levels than men.

MIF testing has also been useful in the diagnosis of respiratory *C. pneumoniae* infections and is the serological method of choice for the diagnosis of acute infections caused by this species. Only a single serovar for *C. pneumoniae* has been recognized using the MIF method, and cross-reactivity with other chlamydial species is negligible when the test is appropriately performed. Serum samples are generally screened for IgM and IgG antibody at a 1:8 dilution, and positive reactions are then tested at twofold dilutions to 1:1,024. The diagnostic criteria for acute infection with *C. pneumoniae* generally include paired sera demonstrating at least a fourfold rise in titer and single serum samples with IgM antibody titers of ≥16 and/or IgG titers of ≥512 (59), although it should be noted that there are no standardized criteria for serological positivity using the MIF technique. In general, while single serum samples may have a presumptive diagnostic value when evaluated in light of clinical symptoms, paired or serial sera allow determinations of antibody titer changes, thus offering a more precise serologic determination. It is questionable whether IgA antibody is a useful marker for either acute or chronic infection with *C. pneumoniae* since the production of antichlamydial IgA is inconsistent in different individuals.

MIF testing is useful in diagnosing *C. trachomatis* infection in neonates. High levels of IgM antibody are regularly associated with disease (90). IgG antibodies are less useful because infants present clinically when they still have a high level of maternal IgG. Since 6 to 9 months is required for maternal antichlamydial antibodies to disappear, infants older than 9 months may be tested for IgG. Infants with inclusion conjunctivitis or respiratory tract carriage of chlamydiae without pneumonia usually have very low levels of IgM antibodies. Thus, a single IgM titer of ≥32 may support the diagnosis of chlamydial pneumonia in these cases.

A simplified MIF method described by Wang et al. is recommended for testing infants (109). A limitation of this test is its use of only one antigen, which results in failure to detect 15 to 25% of infections. The MIF test is performed using chlamydiae grown in either yolk sacs or cell culture (108). Briefly, EBs suspended in yolk sacs are spotted on glass microscope slides and the spots are fixed with acetone and air dried. Serial dilutions of patient sera are reacted with clusters of antigen dots containing representative serovars or strains, and bound antibody is detected with fluorescein-conjugated anti-IgG or IgM antibody. The last dilution of serum showing uniform staining of EBs throughout the antigen dot is defined as the antibody titer.

Recombinant Immunoassays

Recombinant EIAs measure antibodies (IgG and/or IgM, depending on the test) reactive against single chlamydial antigens, usually LPS or MOMP. In contrast to the earlier CF tests for antichlamydial LPS antibodies, most commercially available recombinant immunoassays for antichlamydial LPS serological testing (Medac) use a chlamydia-specific recombinant fragment of the LPS, 3-deoxy-D-*manno*-2-octulopyranosonic acid, which reduces the cross-reactivity with antibodies directed against LPS from other gram-negative bacteria. Since heterogeneity in the humoral responses to chlamydia has been documented among individuals, it is possible that EIA tests based on single chlamydial antigens may show a significant proportion of false-negative results. New EIAs for the diagnosis of *C. pneumoniae* may benefit from efforts to identify major antigenic determinants in this species that are broadly immunodominant among infected individuals. Comparisons of these recombinant immunoassays with traditional CF tests and with the gold standard MIF test for the diagnosis of chlamydial infections have now been reported (3, 75, 93). A general finding from these comparisons is that the sensitivity and specificity of results obtained for serum antibodies to peptides or recombinant antigens are slightly lower than those of results obtained using whole EBs as the antigen. These results probably reflect the heterogeneous and variable humoral responses to some single chlamydial antigens among individuals in a population.

ANTIMICROBIAL SUSCEPTIBILITY TESTING

Only a few clinical isolates of *C. trachomatis* with antimicrobial resistance have been described (51, 59, 95). Drug resistance in *C. pneumoniae* has not yet been reported. Susceptibility testing has had little clinical utility to date, but concerns about antimicrobial resistance in chlamydiae persist and are based on the induction of antibiotic-resistant *C. trachomatis* in the laboratory by subinhibitory concentrations of antimicrobials (30, 54). Chlamydial species are susceptible to the tetracycline, macrolide, and fluoroquinolone classes of antibiotics. The most active of these include doxycycline, erythromycin, azithromycin, rifampin, ofloxacin, and clindamycin, which are used to treat chlamydial infections (112). Antimicrobial susceptibility testing in chlamydiae is typically performed in cell culture with increasing concentrations of antibiotic (15, 86). Drug efficacy is then determined by staining cells with fluorescently labeled antichlamydial antibodies and microscopically enumerating the intracellular chlamydial inclusions (99). Both the MIC (the lowest concentration of antibiotic producing no visible inclusions) and the MBC (the lowest concentration of antibiotic producing no viable bacterial progeny) can be measured by this method. However, antimicrobial susceptibility testing of chlamydiae is problematic due to the lack of standardized techniques and the variability introduced by the type of cell culture system used, different cell types, inoculum size, and the timing and duration of antibiotic application to the cell culture. Furthermore, it is unclear whether the end points measured by in vitro susceptibility testing (MIC and MBC) are relevant when applied to a naturally occurring infection, with dividing and nondividing bacteria which infect multiple cell types in vivo. Thus, the results of in vitro susceptibility testing may not predict the microbiological efficacy in vivo. For these reasons, susceptibility testing is not routinely performed by clinical laboratories.

INTERPRETATION AND REPORTING OF RESULTS

Chlamydiae are pathogenic microorganisms, and infections need to be reported and treated with appropriate antibiotics. Interpretation of serological results is particularly challenging. Antibody titers from a single serum sample are not recommended, especially for *C. pneumoniae*. If serological testing is to be performed for diagnostic purposes, paired sera should be tested in the same assay on the same day and a fourfold rise or fall in titer is diagnostic of a recent infection. For EIAs, the difference in optical density should be significant beyond the day-to-day variation in readings of the particular test. The presence of IgM above the test cutoff can also be interpreted as indicative of a recent infection if appropriate controls and rheumatoid factor elimination are used. Only experienced laboratories should perform serological testing. Reporting of serological results should include sufficient information about the test used and the reasons for the interpretations of the results.

C. trachomatis infections are ideally diagnosed by isolation or detection in clinical specimens. Although specimen adequacy will influence the success rate, from a practical point of view most laboratories would not evaluate specimens because of difficulties in acquiring subsequent specimens from patients with sexually transmitted diseases. For detection of chlamydial antigens, nucleic acids, or EBs in clinical specimens by DFA, EIA, NAH, or NAA, a positive test result indicates a current infection. For detection of EBs by DFA, the manufacturer's cutoff for positivity should be used or modified as the reader gains an increased level of confidence in reading positive and negative specimens. For commercially produced tests, the worker should follow the package insert carefully, testing only specimens approved for use in each test. Because false-positive results may arise with EIA and NAH, confirmatory tests should be performed on all positives. Properly performed NAA tests should have high specificity and do not usually require confirmation of positives. For EIA, NAH, or NAA, the use of a gray zone defined by the manufacturer's cutoff ± 20% can be used to identify low-positive specimens falling just below the cutoff. Specimens falling within the gray zone may be called indeterminate and should be confirmed where possible by a

second test. Specimens positive for *C. pneumoniae* DNA by an in-house PCR assay should be confirmed by probe hybridization. Reporting of positive results for chlamydiae should include the test result, the type of test used, and a clinical interpretation where appropriate.

REFERENCES

1. **Apfalter, P., F. Blasi, J. Boman, C. A. Gaydos, M. Kundi, M. Maass, A. Makristathis, A. Meijer, R. Nadrchal, K. Persson, M. Rotter, C. Y. W. Tong, G. Stanek, and A. Hirschl.** 2001. Multicenter comparison trial of DNA extraction methods and PCR assays for detection of *Chlamydia pneumoniae* in endarterectomy specimens. *J. Clin. Microbiol.* **39:**519–524.
2. **Balin, B. J., H. C. Gerard, E. J. Arking, et al.** 1998. Identification and localization of *Chlamydia pneumoniae* in the Alzheimer's brain. *Med. Microbiol. Immunol.* **187:**23–42.
3. **Bas, S., P. Muzzin, B. Ninet, J. E. Bornand, C. Scieux, and T. L. Vischer.** 2001. Chlamydial serology: comparative diagnostic value of immunoblotting, microimmunofluorescence tests, and immunoassays using different recombinant proteins as antigens. *J. Clin. Microbiol.* **39:**1369–1377.
4. **Bauwens, J. E., A. M. Clark, and W. E. Stamm.** 1993. Diagnosis of *Chlamydia trachomatis* endocervical infections by a commercial polymerase chain reaction assay. *J. Clin. Microbiol.* **31:**3023–3027.
5. **Beem, M. O., and E. M. Saxon.** 1977. Respiratory-tract colonization and a distinctive pneumonia syndrome in infants infected with *Chlamydia trachomatis*. *N. Engl. J. Med.* **296:**306–310.
6. **Berg, E., G. Anestad, H. Moi, G. Storvold, and K. Skaug.** 1997. False-negative results of a ligase chain reaction assay to detect *Chlamydia trachomatis* due to inhibitors in urine. *Eur. J. Clin. Microbiol. Infect. Dis.* **16:**727–731.
7. **Biendo, M., F. Eb, F. Lefebvre, and J. Orifila.** 1996. Limits of the immunofluorescence test and advantages of immunoblotting in the diagnosis of chlamydiosis. *Clin. Diagn. Lab. Immunol.* **3:**706–709.
8. **Black, C. M., J. A. Tharpe, and H. Russell.** 1992. Distinguishing *Chlamydia* species by restriction analysis of the major outer membrane protein gene. *Mol. Cell. Probes* **6:**395–400.
9. **Black, C. M., P. I. Fields, T. O. Messmer, and B. P. Berdal.** 1994. Detection of *Chlamydia pneumoniae* in clinical specimens by polymerase chain reaction using nested primers. *Eur. J. Clin. Microbiol. Infect. Dis.* **13:**752–756.
10. **Block, S. L., M. R. Hammerschlag, J. Hendrick, R. Tyler, A. Smith, P. Roblin, C. Gaydos, D. Pham, T. C. Quinn, R. Palmer, and J. McCarty.** 1997. *Chlamydia pneumoniae* in acute otitis media. *Pediatr. Infect. Dis. J.* **16:**858–862.
11. **Boman, J., S. Soderberg, J. Forsberg, L. S. Birgander, A. Allard, K. Persson, E. Jidell, U. Kumlin, P. Juto, A. Waldenstrom, and G. Wadell.** 1988. High prevalence of *Chlamydia pneumoniae* DNA in peripheral blood mononuclear cells in patients with cardiovascular disease and in middle-aged blood donors. *J. Infect. Dis.* **178:**274–277.
12. **Boman, J., A. Allard, K. Persson, M. Lundborg, P. Juto, and G. Wadell.** 1997. Rapid diagnosis of respiratory *Chlamydia pneumoniae* infection by nested touchdown polymerase chain reaction compared with culture and antigen detection by EIA. *J. Infect. Dis.* **175:**1523–1526.
13. **Boman, J., C. A. Gaydos, and T. C. Quinn.** 1999. Molecular diagnosis of *Chlamydia pneumoniae* infection. *J. Clin. Microbiol.* **37:**3791–3799.

14. Campbell, L. A., M. Perez Melgosa, D. J. Hamilton, C. C. Kuo, and J. T. Grayston. 1992. Detection of *Chlamydia pneumoniae* by polymerase chain reaction. *J. Clin. Microbiol.* **30:**434–439.

15. Cevenini, R., V. Sambri, and M. LaPlaca. 1986. Comparative *in vitro* activity of RU 28965 against *Chlamydia trachomatis*. *Eur. J. Clin. Microbiol.* **5:**598–600.

16. Chernesky, M. A., J. B. Mahony, S. Castriciano, M. Mores, I. O. Stewart, S. F. Landis, W. Seidelman, E. J. Sargeant, and C. Leman. 1986. Detection of *Chlamydia trachomatis* antigens by enzyme immunoassay and immunofluorescence in genital specimens from symptomatic and asymptomatic men and women. *J. Infect. Dis.* **154:**141–148.

17. Chernesky, M. A., D. Jang, H. Lee, J. D. Burczak, H. Hu, J. Sellors, S. J. Tomazic-Allen, and J. B. Mahony. 1994. Diagnosis of *Chlamydia trachomatis* infections in men and women by testing first void urine (FVU) with ligase chain reaction (LCR). *J. Clin. Microbiol.* **32:**2682–2685.

18. Chernesky, M. A., D. Jang, J. Sellors, K. Luinstra, S. Chong, S. Castriciano, and J. Mahony. 1997. Urinary inhibitors of polymerase chain reaction and ligase chain reaction and testing of multiple specimens may contribute to lower assay sensitivities for diagnosing *Chlamydia trachomatis* infection in women. *Mol. Cell. Probes* **11:**243–249.

19. Chernesky, M., S. Chong, D. Jang, K. Luinstra, M. Faught, and J. Mahony. 1998. Inhibition of amplification of *Chlamydia trachomatis* plasmid DNA by the ligase chain reaction associated with female urines. *Clin. Microbiol. Infect.* **4:**397–400.

20. Chernesky, M., K. Luinstra, J. Sellors, J. Schachter, J. Moncada, O. Caul, I. Paul, L. Mikaelian, B. Toye, J. Paavonen, and J. Mahony. 1998. Can serology diagnose upper genital tract *Chlamydia trachomatis* infection? *Sex. Transm. Dis.* **25:**14–19.

21. Chernesky, M., D. Jang, J. Krepel, J. Sellors, and J. Mahony. 1999. Impact of reference standard sensitivity on accuracy of rapid antigen detection assays and a leukocyte esterase dipstick for diagnosis of *Chlamydia trachomatis* infection in first-void urine specimens from men. *J. Clin. Microbiol.* **37:**2777–2780.

22. Chernesky, M., D. Jang, D. Copes, J. Patel, A. Petrich, K. Biers, A. Sproston, and J. Kapala. 2001. Comparison of a polymer conjugate-enhanced enzyme immunoassay to a ligase chain reaction for diagnosis of *Chlamydia trachomatis* in endocervical swabs. *J. Clin. Microbiol.* **39:**2306–2307.

23. Christiansen, G., A. S. Madsen, K. Knudsen, P. Mygind, and S. Birkelund. 1998. Stability of the outer membrane proteins of *Chlamydia pneumoniae*, p. 271–274. *In* R. S. Stephens, G. I. Byrne, G. Christiansen, I. N. Clarke, J. T. Grayston, R. G. Rank, G. L. Ridgeway, P. Saikku, J. Schachter, and W. E. Stamm (ed.), *Chlamydial Infections. Proceedings of the Ninth International Symposium on Human Chlamydial Infections*. International Chlamydia Symposium, Napa Valley, Calif.

24. Clarke, L. M., M. F. Sierra, B. J. Daidone, N. Lopez, J. M. Covino, and W. M. McCormack. 1993. Comparison of the Syva MicroTrak enzyme immunoassay and Gen-Probe PACE 2 with cell culture for diagnosis of cervical *Chlamydia trachomatis* infection in a high-prevalence female population. *J. Clin. Microbiol.* **31:**968–971.

25. Cles, L. D., K. Bruch, and W. E. Stamm. 1988. Staining characteristics of six commercially available monoclonal immunofluorescence reagents for direct diagnosis of *Chlamydia trachomatis* infections. *J. Clin. Microbiol.* **26:**1735–1737.

26. Conway, D., C. M. A. Glazener, E. O. Caul, J. Hodgson, M. G. R. Hull, S. K. R. Clarke, and G. M. Stirrat. 1984. Chlamydial serology in fertile and infertile women. *Lancet* **i:**191–193.

27. Crotchfelt, K., B. Pare, C. Gaydos, and T. Quinn. 1998. Detection of *Chlamydia trachomatis* by the Gen-Probe AMPLIFIED *Chlamydia trachomatis* assay (AMP CT) in urine specimens from men and women and endocervical specimens from women. *J. Clin. Microbiol.* **36:**391–394.

28. Dalhoff, K., and M. Maass. 1996. *Chlamydia pneumoniae* pneumonia in hospitalized patients. Clinical characteristics and diagnostic value of polymerase chain reaction detection in BAL. *Chest* **110:**351–356.

29. Dean, D., E. Oudens, G. Bolan, N. Padian, and J. Schachter. 1995. Major outer membrane protein variants of *Chlamydia trachomatis* are associated with severe upper genital tract infections and histopathology in San Francisco. *J. Infect. Dis.* **172:**1013–1022.

30. Dessus-Babus, S., C. M. Bebear, A. Charron, C. Bebear, and B. de Barbeyrac. 1998. Sequencing of gyrase and topoisomerase IV quinolone-resistance-determining regions of *Chlamydia trachomatis* and characterization of quinolone-resistant mutants obtained in vitro. *Antimicrob. Agents Chemother.* **42:**2474–2481.

31. Dowell, S., R. Peeling, J. Boman, G. Carlone, B. Fields, J. Guarner, M. Hammerschlag, L. Jackson, C. Kuo, M. Maass, T. Messmer, D. Talkington, M. Tondella, S. Zaki, P. Apfalter, C. Bandea, C. Black, L. Campbell, C. Cohen, C. Deal, I. W. Fong, C. Gaydos, J. T. Grayston, M. Leinonen, J. Mahony, S. O'Connor, J. M. Ossewaarde, J. Papp, K. Persson, P. Saikku, L. Schindler, A. Schuchat, V. Stevens, C. Taylor, C. Van Beneden, S. P. Wang, and E. Zell. 2001. Standardizing *Chlamydia pneumoniae* assays: recommendations from the Centers for Disease Control and Prevention (USA), and the Laboratory Centre for Disease Control (Canada). *Clin. Infect. Dis.* **33:**492–503.

32. Everett, K. D., R. M. Bush, and A. A. Andersen. 1999. Emended description of the order *Chlamydiales*, proposal of *Parachlamydiaceae* fam. nov. and *Simkaniaceae* fam. nov., each containing one monotypic genus, revised taxonomy of the family *Chlamydiaceae*, including a new genus and five new species and standards for the identification of organisms. *Int. J. Syst. Bacteriol.* **49:**415–440.

33. Ferris, D. G., W. H. Martin, D. M. Mathis, J. C. H. Steele, Jr., P. M. Fischer, and K. M. Styslinger. 1991. Noninvasive detection of *Chlamydia trachomatis* urethritis in men by a rapid enzyme immunoassay test. *J. Fam. Pract.* **33:**73–78.

34. Frost, E., S. Delandes, S. Veilleux, and D. Bourgaux-Ramoisy. 1991. Typing *Chlamydia trachomatis* by detection of restriction fragment length polymorphism in the gene encoding the major outer membrane protein. *J. Infect. Dis.* **172:**1013–1022.

35. Fukushi, H., and K. Hirai. 1992. Proposal of *Chlamydia pecorum* sp. nov. for *Chlamydia* strains derived from ruminants. *Int. J. Syst. Bacteriol.* **42:**306–308.

36. Garnett, P., O. Brogan, C. Lafong, and C. Fox. 1998. Comparison of throat swabs with sputum specimens for the detection of *Chlamydia pneumoniae* antigen by direct immunofluorescence. *J. Clin. Pathol.* **51:**309–311.

37. Gaydos, C. A., T. C. Quinn, and J. J. Eiden. 1992. Identification of *Chlamydia pneumoniae* by DNA amplification of the 16S rRNA gene. *J. Clin. Microbiol.* **30:**796–800.

38. Gift, T. L., M. S. Pate, E. W. Hook III, and W. J. Kassler. 1999. The rapid test paradox: when fewer cases detected lead to more cases treated. *Sex. Transm. Dis.* **26:**232–240.

39. Grayston, J. T., C. C. Kuo, L. A. Campbell, and S. P. Wang. 1989. *Chlamydia pneumoniae* strain TWAR. *Int. J. Syst. Bacteriol.* **39:**88–90.

40. Grayston, J. T. 1992. Infections caused by *Chlamydia pneumoniae* strain TWAR. *Clin. Infect. Dis.* **5:**757–761.

41. Grayston, J. T. 2000. Background and current knowledge of *Chlamydia pneumoniae* and atherosclerosis. *J. Infect. Dis.* **181**(Suppl. 3):S402–S410.

42. Hadgu, A. 1996. The discrepancy in discrepant analysis. *Lancet* **348:**592–593.

43. Hammerschlag, M. R. 1995. Diagnostic methods for intracellular pathogens. *Clin. Microbiol. Infect.* **1:**S3–S8.

44. Hook, E., K. Smith, C. Mullen, J. Stephens, L. Rinehardt, M. Pate, and H. Lee. 1997. Diagnosis of genitourinary *Chlamydia trachomatis* infections by using the ligase chain reaction on patient-obtained vaginal swabs. *J. Clin. Microbiol.* **35:**2133–2135.

45. Howell, M. R., T. C. Quinn, and C. A. Gaydos. 1998. Screening for *Chlamydia trachomatis* in asymptomatic women attending family planning clinics. A cost-effectiveness analysis of three strategies. *Ann. Intern. Med.* **128:**277–284.

46. Huang, J., F. J. DeGraves, D. Gao, P. Feng, T. Schlapp, and B. Kaltenboeck. 2001. Quantitative detection of *Chlamydia* spp. by fluorescent PCR in the LightCycler®. *BioTechniques* **30:**150–157.

47. Hyman, C. L., M. H. Augenbraun, P. M. Roblin, J. Schachter, and M. R. Hammerschlag. 1991. Asymptomatic respiratory tract infection with *Chlamydia pneumoniae* TWAR. *J. Clin. Microbiol.* **29:**2082–2083.

48. Ikejima, H., S. Haranaga, H. Takemura, T. Kamo, Y. Takahashi, H. Friedman, and Y. Yamamoto. 2001. PCR-based method for isolation and detection of *Chlamydia pneumoniae* DNA in cerebrospinal fluids. *Clin. Diagn. Lab. Immunol.* **8:**499–502.

49. Jackson, L. A., L. A. Campbell, R. A. Schmidt, C. Kuo, A. L. Cappuccio, M. J. Lee, and J. T. Grayston. 2000. Specificity of detection of *Chlamydia pneumoniae* in cardiovascular atheroma. *J. Infect. Dis.* **181**(Suppl. 3):S447–S448.

50. Jang, D., J. W. Sellors, J. B. Mahony, L. Pickard, and M. A. Chernesky. 1992. Effects of broadening the gold standard on the performance of a chemiluminometric immunoassay (Magic Lite) to detect *Chlamydia trachomatis* antigens in centrifuged first void urine and urethral swabs from men. *Sex. Transm. Dis. J.* **19:**315–319.

51. Jones, R. B., B. Van der Pol, D. H. Martin, and M. K. Shepard. 1990. Partial characterization of *Chlamydia trachomatis* isolates resistant to multiple antibiotics. *J. Infect. Dis.* **162:**1309–1315.

52. Kalman, S., W. P. Mitchell, R. Marathe, C. Lammel, J. Fan, R. W. Hyman, L. Olinger, J. Grimwood, R. W. Davis, and R. S. Stephens. 1999. Comparative genomes of *Chlamydia pneumoniae* and *C. trachomatis*. *Nat. Genet.* **21:**385.

53. Kapala, J., D. Copes, A. Sproston, J. Patel, D. Jang, A. Petrich, J. Mahony, K. Biers, and M. Chernesky. 2000. Pooling cervical swabs and testing by ligase chain reaction are accurate and cost-saving strategies for diagnosis of *Chlamydia trachomatis*. *J. Clin. Microbiol.* **38:**2480–2483.

54. Keshishyan, H., L. Hanna, and E. Jawefz. 1973. Emergence of rifampin-resistance in *Chlamydia trachomatis*. *Nature* **244:**173–174.

55. Kluytmans, J. A. J. W., W. H. F. Goessens, J. W. Mouton, J. H. Van Rijsoort-Vos, H. G. M. Niesters, W. G. V. Quint, L. Habbema, E. Stolz, and J. H. T. Wagenvoort. 1993. Evaluation of Clearview and Magic Lite tests, polymerase chain reaction, and cell culture for

56. Krepel, J., J. Patel, A. Sproston, F. Hopkins, D. Jang, J. Mahony, and M. Chernesky. 1999. The impact on accuracy and cost of ligase chain reaction testing by pooling urine specimens for the diagnosis of *Chlamydia trachomatis* infections. *Sex. Transm. Dis.* **26:**504–507.

57. Kuo, C. C., L. A. Jackson, L. A. Campbell, and J. T. Grayston. 1995. *Chlamydia pneumoniae* (TWAR). *Clin. Microbiol. Rev.* **8:**451–461.

58. Lauderdale, T. L., L. Landers, I. Thorneycroft, and K. Chapin. 1999. Comparison of the PACE 2 assay, two amplification assays, and Clearview enzyme immunoassay for detection of *Chlamydia trachomatis* in female endocervical and urine specimens. *J. Clin. Microbiol.* **37:**2223–2229.

59. Lefevre, J.-C., and J.-P. Lepargneur. 1998. Comparative *in vitro* susceptibility of a tetracycline-resistant *Chlamydia trachomatis* strain isolated in Toulouse (France). *Sex. Transm. Dis.* **25:**350–352.

60. Maaheimo, H., P. Kosma, L. Brade, H. Brade, and T. Peters. 2000. Mapping the binding of synthetic disaccharides representing epitopes of chlamydial lipopolysaccharide to antibodies with NMR. *Biochemistry* **39:**12778–12788.

61. Madico, G., T. C. Quinn, J. Boman, and C. A. Gaydos. 2000. Touchdown enzyme time release-PCR for detection and identification of *Chlamydia trachomatis*, *C. pneumoniae*, and *C. psittaci* using the 16S-23S spacer rRNA genes. *J. Clin. Microbiol.* **38:**1085–1093.

62. Mahony, J., S. Chong, D. Jang, K. Luinstra, M. Faught, D. Dalby, J. Sellors, and M. Chernesky. 1998. Urine specimens from pregnant and non-pregnant women inhibitory to amplification of *Chlamydia trachomatis* nucleic acid by PCR, ligase chain reaction, and transcription-mediated amplification: identification of urinary substances associated with inhibition and removal of inhibitory activity. *J. Clin. Microbiol.* **36:**3122–3126.

63. Mahony, J., S. Chong, B. K. Coombes, M. Smieja, and A. Petrich. 2000. Analytical sensitivity, reproducibility of results, and clinical performance of five PCR assays for detecting *Chlamydia pneumoniae* DNA in peripheral blood mononuclear cells. *J. Clin. Microbiol.* **38:**2622–2627.

64. Mahony, J. B., J. Schachter, and M. A. Chernesky. 1983. Detection of antichlamydial immunoglobulin G and M antibodies by enzyme-linked immunosorbent assay. *J. Clin. Microbiol.* **18:**270–275.

65. Mahony, J. B., and M. A. Chernesky. 1985. Effect of swab type and storage temperature on the isolation of *Chlamydia trachomatis* from clinical specimens. *J. Clin. Microbiol.* **22:**865–867.

66. Mahony, J. B., K. E. Luinstra, J. W. Sellors, D. Jang, and M. A. Chernesky. 1992. Confirmatory PCR testing for *Chlamydia trachomatis* in first void urine from asymptomatic and symptomatic men. *J. Clin. Microbiol.* **30:**2241–2245.

67. Mahony, J. B., K. E. Luinstra, J. W. Sellors, and M. A. Chernesky. 1993. Comparison of plasmid- and chromosome-based polymerase chain reaction assays for detecting *Chlamydia trachomatis* nucleic acids. *J. Clin. Microbiol.* **31:**1753–1758.

68. Mathews, S., C. George, C. Flegg, D. Stenzel, and P. Timms. 2001. Differential expression of ompA, ompB, pyk, nlpD and Cpn0585 genes between normal and interferon-γ treated cultures of *Chlamydia pneumoniae*. *Microb. Pathog.* **30:**337–345.

69. Mattila, A., A. Miettinen, P. K. Heinonen, K. Teisala, R. Punnonen, and J. Paavonen. 1993. Detection of serum antibodies to *Chlamydia trachomatis* in patients with chla-

mydial and nonchlamydial pelvic inflammatory disease by the IPAzyme chlamydia and enzyme immunoassay. *J. Clin. Microbiol.* **31:**998–1000.

70. **Modarress, K. J., A. P. Cullen, W. J. Jaffurs, G. L. Troutman, N. Mousavi, R. A. Hubbard, S. Henderson, and A. Lorincz.** 1999. Detection of *Chlamydia trachomatis* and *Neisseria gonorrhoeae* in swab specimens by the Hybrid Capture II and Pace 2 nucleic acid probe tests. *Sex. Transm. Dis.* **26:**303–308.

71. **Moncada, J., J. Schachter, G. Bolan, J. Engelman, L. Howard, I. Mushahwar, G. Ridgway, G. Mumtaz, W. Stamm, and A. Clark.** 1990. Confirmatory assay increases specificity of the Chlamydiazyme test for *Chlamydia trachomatis* infection of the cervix. *J. Clin. Microbiol.* **28:**1770–1773.

72. **Moncada, J., J. Schachter, G. Bolan, J. Nathan, M. A. Shafer, A. Clark, J. Schwebke, W. Stamm, T. Mroczkowski, Z. Seliborska, et al.** 1992. Evaluation of Syva's enzyme immunoassay for the detection of *Chlamydia trachomatis* in urogenital specimens. *Diagn. Microbiol. Infect. Dis.* **15:**663–668.

73. **Moulder, J. W.** 1984. Order *Chlamydiales* and family *Chlamydiaceae*, p. 729–739. *In* N. R. Krieg and J. G. Holt (ed.), *Bergey's Manual of Systematic Bacteriology*, vol. 1. The Williams & Wilkins Co., Baltimore, Md.

74. **Pate, M. S., P. B. Dixon, K. Hardy, M. Crosby, and E. W. Hook III.** 1998. Evaluation of the Biostar Chlamydia OIA assay with specimens from women attending a sexually transmitted disease clinic. *J. Clin. Microbiol.* **36:**2183–2186.

75. **Persson, K., and J. Boman.** 2000. Comparison of five serologic tests for diagnosis of acute infections by *Chlamydia pneumoniae*. *Clin. Diagn. Lab. Immunol.* **7:**739–744.

76. **Peterson, E., V. Darrow, J. Blanding, S. Aarnaes, and L. de la Maza.** 1997. Reproducibility problems with the AMPLICOR PCR *Chlamydia trachomatis* test. *J. Clin. Microbiol.* **35:**957–959.

77. **Petitjean, J., F. Vincent, M. Fretigny, A. Vabret, J. D. Poveda, J. Brun, and F. Freymuth.** 1998. Comparison of two serological methods and a polymerase chain reaction–enzyme immunoassay for the diagnosis of acute respiratory infections with *Chlamydia pneumoniae* in adults. *J. Med. Microbiol.* **47:**615–621.

78. **Prucki, P. M., C. Aspock, A. Makristathis, M. L. Rotter, H. Wank, B. Willinger, and A. M. Hirschi.** 1995. Polymerase chain reaction for detection of *Chlamydia pneumoniae* in gargled-water specimens of children. *Eur. J. Clin. Microbiol. Infect. Dis.* **14:**141–144.

79. **Pruckler, J. M., N. Masse, V. A. Stevens, L. Gang, Y. Yang, E. R. Zell, S. F. Dowell, and B. S. Fields.** 1999. Optimizing culture of *Chlamydia pneumoniae* by using multiple centrifugations. *J. Clin. Microbiol.* **37:**3399–3401.

80. **Pudjiatmoko, H., Y. Fukushi, Y. Ochiai, T. Yamaguchi, and K. Hirai.** 1997. Phylogenetic analysis of the genus *Chlamydia* based on 16S rRNA gene sequences. *Int. J. Syst. Bacteriol.* **47:**425–431.

81. **Puolakkainen, M., E. Vesterinen, E. Purola, P. Saikku, and J. Paavonen.** 1986. Persistence of chlamydial antibodies after pelvic inflammatory disease. *J. Clin. Microbiol.* **23:**924–928.

82. **Puolakkainen, M., C.-C. Kuo, A. Shor, S.-P. Wang, T. Grayston, and L. A. Campbell.** 1993. Serological response to *Chlamydia pneumoniae* in adults with coronary arterial fatty streaks and fibrolipid plaques. *J. Clin. Microbiol.* **31:**2212–2214.

83. **Ramirez, J. A., and The *Chlamydia pneumoniae*/Atherosclerosis Study Group.** 1996. Isolation of *Chlamydia pneumoniae* from the coronary artery of a patient with coronary atherosclerosis. *Ann. Intern. Med.* **125:**979–982.

84. **Reichart, C. A., C. A. Gaydos, W. E. Brady, T. C. Quinn, and E. W. Hook III.** 1990. Evaluation of Abbott Testpack® Chlamydia for detection of *Chlamydia trachomatis* in patients attending sexually transmitted diseases clinics. *Sex. Transm. Dis.* **17:**147–151.

85. **Richmond, S. J., and E. O. Caul.** 1975. Fluorescent antibody studies in chlamydial infections. *J. Clin. Microbiol.* **1:**345–352.

86. **Ridgeway, G. L., J. M. Owen, and J. D. Oriel.** 1976. A method for testing the susceptibility of *Chlamydia trachomatis* in a cell culture system. *J. Antimicrob. Chemother.* **2:**71–76.

87. **Ripa, K. T., and P. A. March.** 1977. Cultivation of *Chlamydia trachomatis* in cycloheximide-treated McCoy cells. *J. Clin. Microbiol.* **6:**328–331.

88. **Roblin, P. M., W. Dunornay, and M. R. Hammerschlag.** 1992. Use of Hep-2 cells for improved isolation and passage of *Chlamydia pneumoniae*. *J. Clin. Microbiol.* **30:**1968–1971.

89. **Schachter, J.** 1978. Chlamydial infections. *N. Engl. J. Med.* **298:**428, 490, 540.

90. **Schachter, J., M. Grossman, and P. M. Azimi.** 1982. Serology of *Chlamydia trachomatis* in infants. *J. Infect. Dis.* **146:**530–535.

91. **Schachter, J., E. Hook, W. McCormack, T. Quinn, M. Chernesky, S. Chong, J. Girdner, P. Dixon, L. DeMeo, E. Williams, A. Cullen, and A. Lorincz.** 1999. Ability of the Digene Hybrid Capture II test to identify *Chlamydia trachomatis* and *Neisseria gonorrhoeae* in cervical specimens. *J. Clin. Microbiol.* **37:**3668–3671.

92. **Schubiner, H. H., W. D. LeBar, S. Joseph, C. Taylor, and C. Jemal.** 1992. Evaluation of two rapid tests for the diagnosis of *Chlamydia trachomatis* genital infections. *Eur. J. Clin. Microbiol. Infect. Dis.* **11:**553–556.

93. **Schumacher, A., A. B. Lerkerod, I. Seljeflot, L. Sommervoll, I. Holme, J. E. Otterstad, and H. Arnesen.** 2001. *Chlamydia pneumoniae* serology: Importance of methodology in patients with coronary heart disease and healthy individuals. *J. Clin. Microbiol.* **39:**1859–1864.

94. **Smieja, M., S. Chong, M. Natarajan, A. Petrich, L. Rainen, and J. Mahony.** 2001. Circulating nucleic acids of *Chlamydia pneumoniae* and cytomegalovirus in patients undergoing coronary angiography. *J. Clin. Microbiol.* **39:**596–600.

95. **Somani, J., V. B. Bhullar, K. A. Workowski, C. E. Farshy, and C. M. Black.** 2000. Multiple drug-resistant *Chlamydia trachomatis* associated with clinical treatment failure. *J. Infect. Dis.* **181:**1421–1427.

96. **Song, X., B. K. Coombes, and J. B. Mahony.** 2000. Quantitation of *Chlamydia trachomatis* 16S rRNA using NASBA amplification and a bioluminescent microtiter plate assay. *Combin. Chem. High Throughput Screen.* **3:**303–313.

97. **Sriram, S., C. W. Stratton, Y. Song-yi, A. Tarp, L. Ding, J. D. Bannan, and W. M. Mitchell.** 1999. *Chlamydia pneumoniae* infection of the central nervous system in multiple sclerosis. *Ann. Neurol.* **46:**6–14.

98. **Stamm, W. E., L. A. Koutsky, J. K. Benedetti, J. L. Jourden, R. C. Brunham, and K. K. Holmes.** 1984. *Chlamydia trachomatis* urethral infections in men. Prevalence, risk factors, and clinical manifestations. *Ann. Intern. Med.* **100:**47–51.

99. **Stamm, W. E.** 2000. Potential for antimicrobial resistance in *Chlamydia pneumoniae*. *J. Infect. Dis.* **181**(Suppl. 3)**:**S456–S459.

100. **Stary, A., B. Najim, and H. H. Lee.** 1997. Vulval swabs as alternative specimens for ligase chain reaction detection of genital chlamydial infection in women. *J. Clin. Microbiol.* **35:**836–838.

101. **Stephens, R. S., S. Kalman, C. Lammel, J. Fan, R. Marathe, L. Aravind, W. Mitchell, L. Olinger, R. L. Tatusov, Q. Zhao, E. V. Koonin, and R. W. Davis.** 1998. Genome sequence of an obligate intracellular pathogen of humans: *Chlamydia trachomatis. Science* **282:** 754–759.

102. **Suchland, R. J., and W. E. Stamm.** 1991. Simplified microtiter cell culture method for rapid immunotyping of *Chlamydia trachomatis. J. Clin. Microbiol.* **29:**1333–1338.

103. **Tanaka, M., H. Nakayama, H. Yoshida, K. Takahashi, T. Nagafuji, T. Hagiwara, and J. Kumazawa.** 1998. Detection of *Chlamydia trachomatis* in vaginal specimens from female commercial sex workers using a new improved enzyme immunoassay. *Sex. Transm. Infect.* **74:** 435–438.

104. **Tanaka, M., H. Nakayama, K. Sagiyama, M. Haraoka, H. Yoshida, T. Hagiwara, K. Akazawa, and S. Naito.** 2000. Evaluation of a new amplified enzyme immunoassay (EIA) for the detection of *Chlamydia trachomatis* in male urine, female endocervical swab, and patient obtained vaginal swab specimens. *J. Clin. Pathol.* **53:**350–354.

105. **Tjhie, H. T. J., R. Roosendaal, J. M. M. Walboomers, J. J. H. Theunissen, R. R. M. Tjon Lim Sang, C. J. L. M. Meijer, D. M. MacLaren, and A. J. C. van den Brule.** 1993. Detection of *Chlamydia pneumoniae* using a general *Chlamydia* polymerase chain reaction with species differentiation after hybridization. *J. Microbiol. Methods* **18:**137–150.

106. **Tong, C. Y., and M. Sillis.** 1993. Detection of *Chlamydia pneumoniae* and *Chlamydia psittaci* in sputum samples by PCR. *J. Clin. Pathol.* **46:**313–317.

107. **Tuuminen, T., S. Varjo, H. Ingman, T. Weber, J. Oksi, and M. Viljanen.** 2000. The prevalence of *Chlamydia pneumoniae* and *Mycoplasma pneumoniae* immunoglobulin G and A antibodies in a healthy Finnish population as analyzed by quantitative enzyme immunoassays. *Clin. Diagn. Lab. Immunol.* **7:**734–738.

108. **Wang, S. P.** 1971. A micro-immunofluorescence method. Study of antibody response to TRIC organisms in mice, p. 273–318. *In* R. L. Nichols (ed.), *Trachoma and Related Disorders Caused by Chlamydial Agents.* Excerpta Medica, Amsterdam, The Netherlands.

109. **Wang, S. P., J. T. Grayston, E. R. Alexander, and K. K. Holmes.** 1975. Simplified microimmunofluorescence test with trachoma-lymphogranuloma venereum (*Chlamydia trachomatis*) antigens for use as a screening test for antibody. *J. Clin. Microbiol.* **1:**250–255.

110. **Wasserheit, J. N.** 1994. Effect of changes in human ecology and behavior on patterns of sexually transmitted diseases, including human immunodeficiency virus infection. *Proc. Natl. Acad. Sci. USA* **91:**2430–2435.

111. **Watson, M. W., P. R. Lambden, and I. N. Clarke.** 1991. Genetic diversity and identification of human infection by amplification of the chlamydial 60-kilodalton cysteine-rich outer membrane protein gene. *J. Clin. Microbiol.* **29:**1188–1193.

112. **Welsh, L. E., C. A. Gaydos, and T. C. Quinn.** 1992. In vitro activities of azithromycin, erythromycin and tetracycline against *Chlamydia trachomatis* and *Chlamydia pneumoniae. Antimicrob. Agents Chemother.* **36:**291–294.

113. **Wiesenfeld, H. C., R. P. Heine, A. Rideout, I. Macio, F. DiBiasi, and R. L. Sweet.** 1996. The vaginal introitus: a novel site for *Chlamydia trachomatis* testing in women. *Am. J. Obstet. Gynecol.* **174:**1542–1546.

114. **Wolf, K., E. Fischer, D. Mead, G. Zhong, R. Peeling, B. Whitmire, and H. D. Caldwell.** 2001. *Chlamydia pneumoniae* major outer membrane protein is a surface-exposed antigen that elicits antibodies primarily directed against conformation-dependent determinants. *Infect. Immun.* **69:**3082–3091.

115. **Wong, Y. K., K. D. Dawkins, and M. E. Ward.** 1999. Circulating *Chlamydia pneumoniae* DNA as a predictor of coronary artery disease. *J. Am. Coll. Cardiol.* **34:**1435–1439.

116. **Wuppermann, F. N., J. H. Hegemann, and C. A. Jantos.** 2001. Heparan sulfate-like glycosaminoglycan is a cellular receptor for *Chlamydia pneumoniae. J. Infect. Dis.* **184:**181–187.

117. **Zhang, J. P., and R. S. Stephens.** 1992. Mechanism of *C. trachomatis* attachment to eukaryotic cells. *Cell* **69:** 861–869.

Rickettsia

DAVID H. WALKER AND DONALD H. BOUYER

64

TAXONOMY

DNA sequence data of the 16S rRNA, 17-kDa lipoprotein, citrate synthase, rickettsial outer membrane proteins A (OmpA) and B (OmpB), and 120-kDa cytoplasmic antigenic protein genes have delineated the phylogeny of the genus *Rickettsia* (1, 2, 13, 49, 50, 53, 55) (Fig. 1). The typhus group and spotted fever group (SFG), defined originally by their distinctive lipopolysaccharide antigens, make up the genus along with other species such as *R. bellii*, *R. canadensis*, and the *Rickettsia* species isolated from ladybird beetles, which as currently characterized do not have phenotypes that fit so neatly into these groups (38, 51, 52, 59, 60) (Table 1). *Orientia* (formerly *Rickettsia*) *tsutsugamushi* diverges from the genus *Rickettsia* by approximately 10% in the 16S rRNA gene and differs greatly in its cell wall structure, containing completely unrelated proteins and lacking lipopolysaccharide and peptidoglycan (36, 57) (Table 1). There is no consensus about the criteria that define the placement of two strains of *Rickettsia* into separate species, a situation that is most apparent in the SFG. The SFG contains bacteria that are generally recognized as human pathogens (*R. rickettsii*, *R. akari*, *R. conorii*, *R. africae*, *R. sibirica*, *R. japonica*, *R. honei*, and *R. australis*), as well as a rapidly growing list of organisms identified only in arthropods. Most of these species of undetermined pathogenicity, including *R. montanensis*, *R. bellii*, *R. rhipicephali*, and *R. amblyommii*, are presumed to be nonpathogenic and are much more prevalent in U.S. ticks than is pathogenic *R. rickettsii*. In Europe, *R. slovaca* and *R. helvetica* have recently been proposed as human pathogens, but other rickettsiae (e.g., *R. massiliae*) have not been associated with disease (12, 35, 46). According to some opinions, the criteria that have been applied to the molecular phylogeny of other bacteria would define as few as four pathogenic *Rickettsia* species in the spotted fever group, namely, *R. akari*, *R. australis*, *R. felis*, and all the rest lumped together as one, whereas tradition, geographic distribution, and clinical manifestations would place even very closely related organisms such as *R. conorii*, *R. sibirica*, and *R. africae* in separate species (Fig. 1; Table 2). SFG isolates from Israel and the Astrakhan region of Russia appear to be minor genetic variations of *R. conorii*, which may also contain strain-specific conformational epitopes, especially in OmpA. Similarly, SFG isolates from *Hyalomma asiaticum*

ticks in Inner Mongolia and two patients in France appear to represent a strain of *R. sibirica* and SFG isolates from ticks in northeastern China are very closely related to *R. japonica* (14, 71).

DESCRIPTION OF THE GENERA AND NATURAL HABITATS

Species of *Rickettsia* are small (0.3 to 0.5 μm by 1 to 2 μm) obligately intracellular bacteria of the alpha subdivision of the *Proteobacteria*, with a gram-negative cell wall structure that contains lipopolysaccharide, peptidoglycan, a major 135-kDa S-layer protein (OmpB), a 17-kDa lipoprotein, and, for SFG rickettsiae, a surface-exposed protein (OmpA) containing a variable number of near-identical tandem repeat units (59). OmpA and OmpB encode proteins with a predicted β-autotransporter that appears to be posttranslationally removed in the mature cell wall proteins. *Rickettsia* spp. appear to be surrounded by an electron-lucent slime layer, reside free in the cytosol of their host cell, and are found in an arthropod host for at least a part of their life cycle, where they are maintained by transovarian transmission and/or cycles involving horizontal transmission to mammalian hosts (30) (Table 2).

Orientia tsutsugamushi (0.3 to 0.5 μm by 0.8 to 1.5 μm) has a major surface protein of 54 to 58 kDa as well as 110-, 80-, 46-, 43-, 39-, 35-, 28-, and 25-kDa surface proteins but lacks muramic acid, glucosamine, 2-keto-3-deoctulonic acid, and hydroxy fatty acids, suggesting the absence of lipopolysaccharide and peptidoglycan (57). Compared with *Rickettsia* spp., *Orientia* has a more plastic gram-negative cell wall with a thicker outer leaflet and thinner inner leaflet of the outer envelope; it does not have a slime layer. *Orientia* resides free in the cytosol and is maintained in nature by transovarian transmission in trombiculid chiggers, which transmit the infection to humans during feeding at the larval stage (Table 2).

CLINICAL SIGNIFICANCE

In addition to Rocky Mountain spotted fever, rickettsialpox, murine typhus, flying squirrel-associated *R. prowazekii* infection, and cat flea-transmitted *R. felis* infection, which are indigenous to the United States, there is a significant potential for imported cases of African tick bite fever,

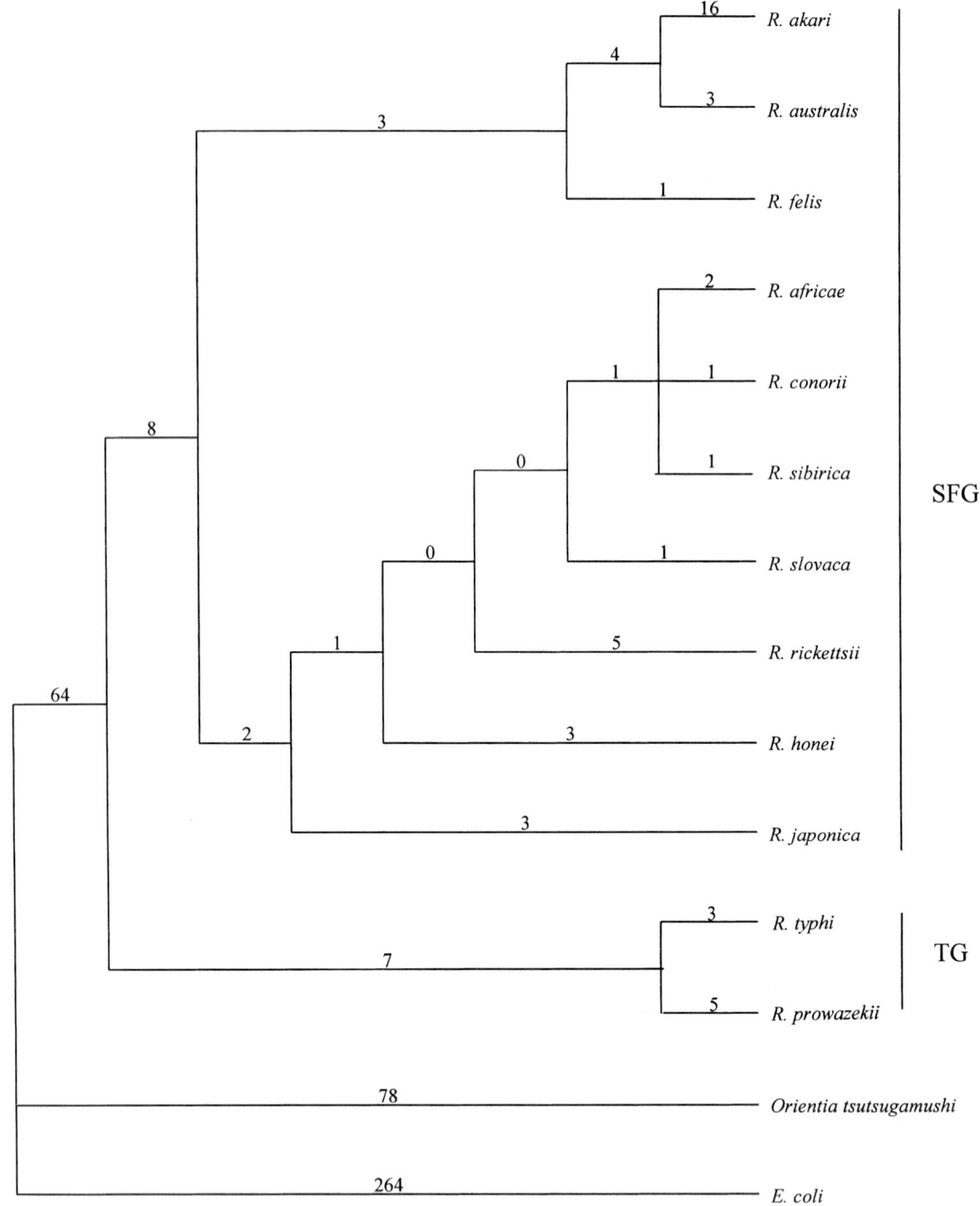

FIGURE 1 Phylogeny of known pathogenic rickettsiae as determined by unweighed maximum-parsimony analyses of 16S rRNA gene sequences prepared by PAUP 4.0 software with *Escherichia coli* as the outgroup. Numerical values on the branches represent the quantity of genetic divergence from the nearest node.

boutonneuse fever, murine typhus, scrub typhus, and even louse-borne typhus (9, 19–21, 34, 37, 42, 51, 63, 67, 69). Other rickettsioses such as North Asian tick typhus, Flinders Island spotted fever, Japanese spotted fever, and Queensland tick typhus, either because of their geographic distribution and infrequent travel exposure to them or because of their incidence, are unlikely to be imported. Rocky Mountain spotted fever, louse-borne typhus, and

scrub typhus are life-threatening illnesses even for young, previously healthy persons. Murine typhus, boutonneuse fever, and North Asian tick typhus can have a fatal outcome in patients who are elderly or have underlying diseases or other risk factors.

An average of 7 days after tick bite inoculation of rickettsiae, patients with Rocky Mountain spotted fever develop fever, severe headache, malaise, and myalgia, fre-

TABLE 1 Characteristics of *Rickettsia* spp. and *Orientia tsutsugamushi*[a]

Organisms	LPS[b]	PG[c]	OmpA	OmpB	17-kDa lipoprotein	56-kDa protein
SFG	S	+	+	+	+	0
Typhus group	T	+	0	+	+	0
R. canadensis	T	+	+	+	+	0
R. bellii	B	+	0	ND	+	0
O. tsutsugamushi	0	0	0	0	0	+

[a] +, present; 0, absent; ND, not determined.
[b] LPS, lipopolysaccharide; S, SFG lipopolysaccharide present; T, typhus group lipopolysaccharide present; B, *bellii* type lipopolysaccharide present.
[c] PG, peptidoglycan.

quently accompanied by nausea, vomiting, and abdominal pain and sometimes by cough (19, 20). Rash typically appears only after 3 to 5 days of illness. Rickettsiae infect the endothelial cells lining the blood vessels, frequently leading to increased vascular permeability and focal hemorrhages (17). In severe cases, rickettsial encephalitis with coma and seizures and noncardiogenic pulmonary edema are grave conditions that often presage death (62).

Rickettsialpox has been recognized mainly as an urban disease which manifests a disseminated vesicular rash and an eschar at the location of rickettsial inoculation by the feeding mite (21). Although it is clinically a typical spotted fever rickettsiosis, no fatalities have been recorded. The complete spectrum of clinical manifestations of *R. felis* infections has yet to be determined. This disease suffers from diagnostic neglect despite its widening recognized geographic distribution and the prevalence of cat flea exposure (43, 51, 52, 70).

Murine typhus causes rash in only slightly more than half of the infected patients, cough and chest radiographic infiltrates suggesting pneumonia in many patients, and severe illness with seizures, coma, and renal and respiratory failure necessitating intensive care unit admission in 10% of hospitalized patients (9).

Patients who have returned from Africa and develop fever, one or more eschars, and in some cases regional lymphadenopathy and a maculopapular or vesicular rash are very likely to be infected with *R. africae* (42).

COLLECTION, TRANSPORT, AND STORAGE OF SPECIMENS

Blood should be collected as early as possible in the course of illness. For the isolation of rickettsiae, blood should be obtained in a sterile heparin-containing vial before the administration of antimicrobial agents that are active

TABLE 2 Etiology, epidemiology, and ecology of rickettsial diseases

Organism	Disease	Geographic distribution	Typical mode of transmission to humans	Natural cycle
R. rickettsii	Rocky Mountain spotted fever	Western Hemisphere	Tick bite	Transovarian in ticks and rodent-tick cycles
R. akari	Rickettsialpox	United States, Ukraine, Croatia, Korea	Mite bite	Transovarian in mites and mite-mouse cycles
R. conorii	Boutonneuse fever	Southern Europe, Africa, Middle East	Tick bite	Transovarian in ticks
R. africae	African tick bite fever	Eastern and southern Africa, Caribbean	Tick bite	Transovarian in ticks
R. sibirica	North Asian tick typhus	Asia	Tick bite	Transovarian in ticks
R. japonica	Japanese spotted fever	Japan	Tick bite	Ticks
R. australis	Queensland tick typhus	Australia	Tick bite	Ticks
R. honei	Flinders Island spotted fever	Australia	Tick bite	Unknown
R. felis	Cat flea typhus	North and South America, Europe	Not known	Transovarian in cat fleas
R. prowazekii	Primary louse-borne typhus	Worldwide	Infected louse feces rubbed into broken skin or mucous membranes or inhaled as aerosol	Human-louse cycle; flying squirrel-flea and/or -louse cycle
R. prowazekii	Brill-Zinsser disease	Worldwide	Recrudescence years after primary attack of louse-borne typhus	
R. typhi	Murine typhus	Worldwide	Infected flea feces rubbed into broken skin or mucous membranes or as aerosol	Rat-flea cycle; opposum-flea cycle
O. tsutsugamushi	Scrub typhus	Japan, eastern Asia, northern Australia, west and southwest Pacific	Chigger bite	Transovarian in mites

against rickettsiae (20, 25, 28). Heparinized blood collected during the acute stage of spotted fever rickettsiosis is also useful for immunocytologic detection of circulating endothelial cells containing rickettsiae (25). For isolation and immunocytologic diagnosis, blood should be stored temporarily at 4°C and processed as promptly as possible. If inoculation of cell culture or animals must be delayed for more than 24 h, plasma, buffy coat, or whole blood should be frozen rapidly and stored at −70°C or in liquid nitrogen. EDTA- or sodium citrate-anticoagulated blood collected in the acute state has been used effectively for the diagnosis of murine typhus, epidemic typhus, Japanese spotted fever, scrub typhus, and, with lower sensitivity, Rocky Mountain spotted fever and African tick bite fever by PCR (15, 42, 51, 54, 56, 58, 69). If whole blood, plasma, or buffy coat cannot be processed for PCR within several days, it should be stored at −20°C or lower.

For serologic diagnosis, blood is collected as early in the course of disease as possible and a second sample is collected after 1 or 2 weeks; if a fourfold rise in the antibody titer has not occurred, a third sample is collected 3 or 4 weeks after onset. The serum may be stored for several days at 4°C but should be stored frozen at −20°C or lower for longer periods to avoid degradation of the antibodies. However, blood samples collected by finger stick on appropriate blotting paper in remote areas and sent by ordinary mail can be eluted for serologic diagnosis (11).

A 3-mm-diameter punch biopsy of a skin lesion, preferably a maculopapule containing a petechia or the margin of an eschar, should be collected as soon as possible (19, 32, 61). Although treatment should not be delayed, it is best to perform the biopsy prior to the completion of 24 h of treatment with a tetracycline or chloramphenicol. For immunohistologic detection of SFG or typhus group rickettsiae, the specimen can be snap-frozen for frozen sectioning or fixed in formaldehyde for the preparation of paraffin-embedded sections (17, 21, 32, 61–63, 65). The former approach yields an answer more rapidly, but freezing artifacts distorts the architecture of the tissue, whereas the latter is more convenient for shipping to a reference laboratory. Rickettsial DNA or infected endothelial cells can also be recovered from eschars for detection by PCR or cultivation of rickettsiae, respectively (26). Aseptically collected autopsy specimens, e.g., spleen and lung, are useful for rickettsial isolation; ideally they are inoculated fresh, or they are held for 24 h at 4°C or stored frozen at −70°C for longer periods if the specimen must be shipped to a public health or reference laboratory. Autopsy tissues can also be examined for the presence of rickettsiae by immunohistochemistry or PCR.

Body lice (*Pediculus humanus corporis*) removed from patients suspected of having epidemic typhus can be examined for the presence of rickettsiae. Body lice acquire rickettsiae and remain infected for life, thus providing a useful specimen for PCR diagnosis even after a prolonged period of shipping at ambient temperature and humidity, conditions that do not ensure survival of the lice (48).

ISOLATION PROCEDURES

Rickettsial isolation is performed in few laboratories. Cumbersome historic methods such as inoculation of adult male guinea pigs, mice, or the yolk sac of embryonated chicken eggs have been supplanted by cell culture methods, except for isolation of *O. tsutsugamushi* by intraperitoneal inoculation of mice (20, 25, 28, 69). Vero, L-929, HEL, and MRC5 cells have been used in antibiotic-free media to isolate rickettsiae. The best results reported have been achieved with heparin-anticoagulated plasma or buffy coat collected from patients suspected to have boutonneuse fever before administration of antirickettsial therapy.

Samples containing 0.5 ml of clinical triturated material mixed with 0.5 ml of tissue culture medium are inoculated as promptly as possible onto 3.7-ml shell vials with 12-mm round coverslips containing a confluent layer of cells and centrifuged at 700 × g for 1 h at room temperature to enhance the attachment and entry of rickettsiae into host cells (4, 25, 28). After removal of the inoculum, the shell vials are washed with phosphate-buffered saline and incubated with minimal essential medium containing 10% fetal calf serum in an atmosphere containing 5% CO_2 at 34°C. At 48 and 72 h, a coverslip is examined by Giemsa or Gimenez staining or by immunofluorescence with antibodies against SFG and typhus group rickettsiae. Detection of 4 or more organisms is interpreted as a positive result. In France, this method has yielded a diagnosis in 59% of samples from patients with boutonneuse fever who had neither been treated nor developed antibodies to *R. conorii* prior to collection of the sample (25). Rickettsiae were detected at 48 h of growth in 82% of the positive samples. Of course, universal precautions should be exercised, as is always appropriate for handling clinical specimens, and work should be performed in a laminar-flow biosafety hood with use of gloves and gown. Although the quantity of rickettsiae in the cell culture is relatively small, aerosol, internal, or contact exposure should be avoided as for mycobacteria, fungi, and viruses.

IDENTIFICATION OF RICKETTSIAL ISOLATES

Rickettsiae isolated in cell culture can be identified by indirect immunofluorescence with group-, species-, and strain-specific monoclonal antibodies in laboratories where they are available. In an increasing number of laboratories, rickettsial isolates are identified by molecular methods such as PCR amplification of genes that are genus specific (17-kDa protein, citrate synthase, or OmpB genes) or SFG specific (OmpA gene) followed by restriction fragment length polymorphism analysis (47). Determination of DNA sequences offers the opportunity to identify unique isolates that may represent novel strains or even species. *Orientia tsutsugamushi*, being more distantly related to *Rickettsia* spp., lacks the above cell wall genes but can be identified by PCR of the gene encoding the major immunodominant 56-kDa surface protein.

A well-established method for identifying the species of rickettsial isolates is microimmunofluorescence serotyping with mouse sera prepared precisely by intravenous inoculation with a substantial yet nonlethal dose of viable rickettsiae on days 0 and 7 and collection of the typing sera on day 10 (39). These antibodies react at high titer with conformational species-specific epitopes of OmpA and OmpB. Antibodies against group-specific lipopolysaccharide develop later in the murine immune response to *Rickettsia*. This rather cumbersome and expensive method requires propagation of large quantities of the isolate as well as the prototype strains that are desired to be compared for use as antigens for immunofluorescence titer determination as well as for development of the typing sera. Thus, biohazard containment facilities and procedures are necessary. Genetic analysis allows the evaluation of a larger portion of the genome and is currently favored.

DIRECT DETECTION IN CLINICAL SAMPLES BY IMMUNOLOGIC AND GENETIC METHODS

The diagnoses of Rocky Mountain spotted fever, boutonneuse fever, murine typhus, louse-borne typhus, and rickettsialpox have been established by immunohistochemical detection of rickettsiae in cutaneous biopsy specimens of rash and eschar lesions (17, 20, 21, 32, 61, 63, 65). Direct immunofluorescence staining with a fluorescein-conjugated polyclonal antiserum that is reactive with *R. rickettsii*, *R. conorii*, and *R. akari* has been applied successfully to frozen sections and formalin-fixed, paraffin-embedded sections of maculopapular rash lesions and eschars (Fig. 2, left). Unfortunately there is no commercial conjugate available for this purpose. Monoclonal antibodies that are specific for lipopolysaccharides of either SFG or typhus group rickettsiae have been used to detect rickettsiae by immunoperoxidase staining of formalin-fixed, paraffin-embedded tissues from patients with Rocky Mountain spotted fever, boutonneuse fever, rickettsialpox, murine typhus, and louse-borne typhus, as well as of tissues of animals experimentally infected with *R. australis*, *R. sibirica*, and *R. japonica* (63, 64) (Fig. 2, right). The sensitivity and specificity of immunohistochemical detection of *R. rickettsii* in cutaneous biopsy specimens are 70 and 100%, respectively (20, 61). Eschar biopsy specimens are sensitive specimens for the diagnosis of SFG rickettsioses that manifest that lesion and should be considered for diagnostic evaluation in patients suspected to have rickettsialpox, boutonneuse fever, or African tick bite fever.

Immunocytochemical detection of *R. conorii* in circulating endothelial cells has been accomplished by capture of the endothelial cells from blood samples by using magnetic beads coated with a monoclonal antibody to a human endothelial cell surface antigen followed by immunofluorescent staining of the intracellular rickettsiae (25). Over a 6-year period, this method achieved a sensitivity of 50% and a specificity of 94%. Rickettsiae were detected in 56% of untreated patients and 29% of patients receiving antirickettsial treatment. *O. tsutsugamushi* has recently been identified immunohistochemically in human endothelial cells, macrophages, and cardiac myocytes (33). In situ hybridization has not been reported for the detection of rickettsiae in tissue samples.

PCR has been applied to the amplification of *R. rickettsii*, *R. conorii*, *R. japonica*, *R. typhi*, *R. prowazekii*, *R. africae*, *R. felis*, *R. helvetica*, *R. slovaca*, and *O. tsutsugamushi* DNA, usually from peripheral blood, buffy coat, or plasma but occasionally from fresh, frozen, or paraffin-embedded tissue or arthropod vectors from patients (15, 35, 42, 46, 48, 51, 54, 56, 58, 69). For all pathogenic *Rickettsia* spp., the 17-kDa lipoprotein gene is the principal target, and the primers CATTACTTGGTTCTCAATTCGGT and GTTT-TATTAGTGGTTACGTAACC, which amplify a 231-bp DNA fragment, are used (51). The citrate synthase, 16S rRNA, and OmpA genes have also been amplified diagnostically, with the *Rickettsia* species being identified through either restriction fragment length polymorphism analysis using *Alu*I and *Xba*I or sequencing of the PCR product (51). For *O. tsutsugamushi*, the 56-kDa protein gene is the usual

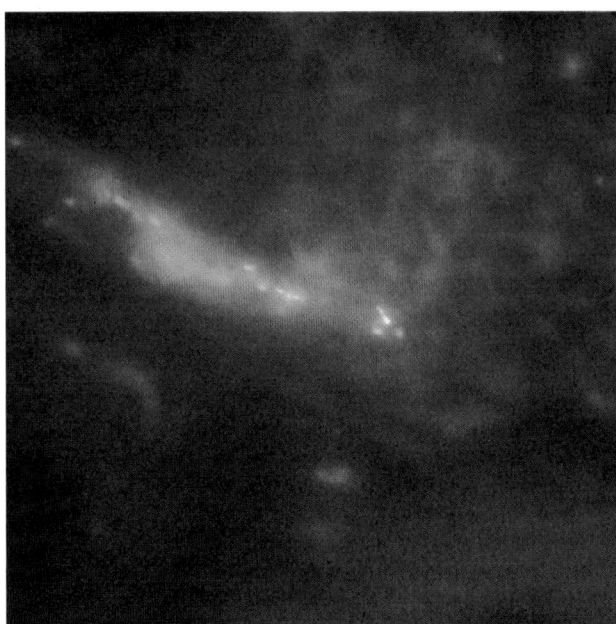
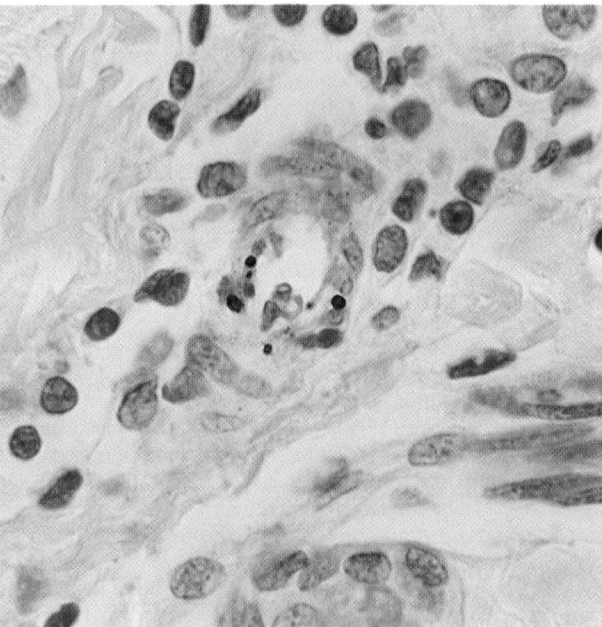

FIGURE 2 (Left) Direct immunofluorescence staining of skin biopsy specimens with anti-SFG *Rickettsia* antibodies facilitates rapid diagnosis. Rickettsiae are present in the vessel wall. (Right) Demonstration of rickettsial organisms in the microvasculature of the dermis in a patient with a history of Rocky Mountain spotted fever. Rickettsiae are seen in the vessel wall. An immunoperoxidase stain, using monoclonal antibodies directed against SFG lipopolysaccharide, was used. Magnification, ×800.

target of diagnostic PCR amplification for scrub typhus (56).

Molecular and immunohistochemical diagnostic testing, the most useful methods for establishing a diagnosis during the acute stage of illness when therapeutic decisions are critical, are, to the best of our knowledge, available in only a few reference laboratories, including ours. Individual cases for immunohistochemistry may be referred to the following laboratories after contacting the directors for consultation: David H. Walker, M.D., Department of Pathology, University of Texas Medical Branch, 301 University Blvd., Keiller Building, Room 1.116, Galveston, TX 77555-0609, telephone (409) 772-2682, fax (409) 772-2500, e-mail dwalker@utmb.edu; J. Stephen Dumler, M.D., Division of Medical Microbiology, Department of Pathology, The Johns Hopkins Medical Institutions, Meyer B1-193, 600 North Wolfe Street, Baltimore, MD 21287, telephone (410) 955-5077, fax (410) 614-8087, e-mail sdumler@jhmi.edu; and Sherif Zaki, M.D., Ph.D., Department of Pathology, Centers for Disease Control and Prevention, 1600 Clifton Road Mail Stop G32, CDC, Atlanta, GA 30333, telephone (404) 639-3133, e-mail sxz1@cdc.gov.

SEROLOGIC TESTS

In most clinical microbiology laboratories, assays for antibodies to rickettsiae are the only tests performed. This situation is unfortunate for the patient with a life-threatening, acutely incapacitating rickettsial disease because these assays are useful principally for serologic confirmation of the diagnosis in convalescence and usually do not provide information that is helpful in making critical therapeutic decisions during the acute illness. Patients who die of rickettsioses usually receive many antibiotics, none of which have antirickettsial activity owing in part to the lack of laboratory data providing clinical guidance for a rickettsial diagnosis. The earlier a diagnosis is established, the shorter the course of rickettsial illness after an appropriate antirickettsial antibiotic is administered.

Serologic assays for the diagnosis of rickettsial infections in contemporary use include the "gold standard" indirect immunofluorescence assay (IFA), indirect immunoperoxidase assay, latex agglutination, enzyme immunoassay (EIA), Proteus vulgaris OX-19 and OX-2 and Proteus mirabilis OX-K strain agglutination, line blot, and Western immunoblotting (7, 9, 10, 16, 18, 20–23, 40, 45, 61, 68, 69). Only a portion of these assays are available as commercial kits or as assays performed in reference laboratories for some, but not all, rickettsial diseases. Other serologic tests such as indirect hemagglutination, microagglutination, and complement fixation are no longer in general use.

The IFA contains all the rickettsial heat-labile protein antigens and the group-shared lipopolysaccharide antigen and thus provides group-reactive serologic test results. IFA reagents are available commercially for SFG and typhus group rickettsiae from Pan Bio, Inc. (Baltimore, Md.), Focus Technologies (Cypress, Calif.), and Bio-Mérieux (Marcy l'Etoile, France), and for O. tsutsugamushi from Pan Bio, Inc. In cases of Rocky Mountain spotted fever, IFA detects antibodies at a diagnostic titer of ≥64, usually in the second week of illness. Effective antirickettsial treatment must be initiated by day 5 of illness to avoid a potentially fatal outcome. Other rickettsioses prevalent in the United States and Europe allow more leeway except in patients with particular risk factors for severe disease. For boutonneuse fever, a diagnostic IFA titer of ≥40 occurs in

46% of patients between days 5 and 9 of illness, in 90% between 20 and 29 days, and in 100% thereafter (45). In murine typhus, diagnostic IFA titers are present in 50% of patients by the end of the first week of illness and in nearly all by 15 days after onset (9). In areas where particular rickettsial diseases are endemic, a higher diagnostic cutoff titer is required. For example, for the IFA diagnosis of scrub typhus in patients residing in these areas, an IFA titer to O. tsutsugamushi of ≥400 is 96% specific and 48% sensitive, with the sensitivity rising from 29% in the first week to 56% in the second week (7). Lowering the diagnostic cutoff titer to 100 raises the sensitivity only to 84% and reduces the specificity to 78%. These considerations are not as important when testing patients who have visited areas of endemic infection for only a short period. The stated cutoff titer may serve as a guide, but each laboratory performing the test should establish its own cutoff titers for the patient population and the microscope and reagents used and the laboratorian's judgement of the minimal positive signal.

Indirect immunoperoxidase assays for scrub typhus, murine typhus, boutonneuse fever, and presumably other rickettsioses yield results similar to IFA when the immunoglobulin G (IgG) diagnostic titer is set at 128 and that of IgM is set at 32 (22). Advantages include the use of a more generally available light microscope rather than a UV microscope and the production of a permanent slide result.

Latex agglutination test reagents are available commercially from Pan Bio, Inc., only for Rocky Mountain spotted fever in the United States. Latex beads coated with an extracted rickettsial protein-carbohydrate complex containing rickettsial lipopolysaccharide are agglutinated mainly by IgM antibodies, and there are reports of a sensitivity of 71 to 94% and a specificity of 96 to 99% (16). A diagnostic titer of 128 is often detected early in the second week of illness, by which time treatment should have already been started empirically.

EIAs have been developed in various formats including the use of antigens coated onto microtiter wells or immobilized on nitrocellulose or other sheets and have been employed in the commercial reference laboratory setting. Dot EIA kits are commercially available as Dip-S-Ticks from Pan Bio, Inc., for detecting antibodies against R. rickettsii, R. conorii, R. typhi, and O. tsutsugamushi (22, 68). There are at the time of this writing no publications in the peer-reviewed literature regarding the use of the dot EIA for the diagnosis of Rocky Mountain spotted fever. Compared with an IFA titer of ≥64 for the diagnosis of murine typhus, the dot EIA showed a sensitivity of 88% and specificity of 91% (22). The dot EIA for diagnosis of scrub typhus had sensitivities and specificities of only 80 and 77%, respectively, when compared with an IFA cutoff titer of 64, and 89 and 66%, respectively, at an IFA cutoff titer of 128 (68). These SFG and R. typhi kits detect cross-reactive antibodies, as demonstrated by clinical and epidemiologic data in an outbreak of African tick bite fever (6). The dot EIA of R. conorii antigen provided early diagnostic evidence of an SFG rickettsiosis. Subsequent analysis revealed poor specificity with a high rate of false-positive results. These assays make available diagnostic tools that do not require expensive, specialized equipment, but they suffer from apparent low specificity as well as all the limitations of serologic diagnosis that is made most often in the convalescent stage. The use of these tests for paired sera from populations with clinical (fever, headache, and rash) and epidemiologic (tick exposure) features consistent with rickettsiosis would most probably yield useful information.

The assays that have been most widely used for the diagnosis of rickettsial diseases are agglutination of the OX-19 and OX-2 strains of *P. vulgaris* for rickettsioses and the OX-K strain of *P. mirabilis* for *O. tsutsugamushi* infections. These assays have been largely discredited owing to their poor sensitivity and specificity (18, 61). They should be replaced by more accurate serologic methods such as IFA. There is great potential for the development of useful serodiagnostic tests involving recombinant rickettsial antigens. For example, the recombinant 56-kDa surface protein of *O. tsutsugamushi* has been demonstrated to be effective for the diagnosis of scrub typhus (24). However, there are situations in developing countries where the choice is between the *Proteus* agglutination tests and none at all for the detection of important public health problems such as outbreaks of louse-borne typhus. In fact, the evidence leading to the recent recognition of some emerging infectious diseases such as Japanese spotted fever and Flinders Island spotted fever included *Proteus* agglutinating antibodies.

The presence of shared antigens of OmpA, OmpB, and group-specific lipopolysaccharide impedes the establishment of a species-specific diagnosis by serologic methods. The criterion of a fourfold or greater difference in IFA titers between the two suspected agents distinguished infections by *R. prowazekii* and *R. typhi* in only 34% of cases and infections by *R. africae* and *R. conorii* in only 26% (27, 42). Western immunoblot detection of antibodies against OmpA or OmpB of only one *Rickettsia* species has also been proposed as a criterion for species-specific diagnosis. However, it was effective in distinguishing *R. prowazekii* and *R. typhi* infections or *R. africae* and *R. conorii* infections in only half of the cases (27, 42). Cross-absorption of sera prior to IFA or Western immunoblotting is more effective in establishing a species-specific diagnosis, but it is cumbersome and expensive. However, interpretation of these results requires careful evaluation of valid control experiments, the quality and quantity of each antigen preparation, and the potential for the occurrence of infection by an untested, even as yet unrecognized, agent. In the past, knowledge of the geographic origin of the case has sufficed to make a specific diagnosis. However, the increasing number and geographic overlap of rickettsioses challenge the old assumptions. If important clinical differences in severity and treatment are identified, this epidemiologic problem will become a pragmatic clinical issue.

ANTIMICROBIAL SUSCEPTIBILITY TESTING

Data supporting the use of doxycycline or another tetracycline antibiotic as the drug of choice for the treatment of infections caused by *Rickettsia* spp. and *O. tsutsugamushi* and the use of chloramphenicol as an alternative drug have been derived principally from empirical experience and retrospective case studies. In addition to historic studies of the activity of antimicrobial agents against these obligately intracellular bacteria in infected animals and embryonated eggs, studies of the effects of antimicrobial agents in cell culture have supported the consideration of alternative drugs such as fluoroquinolones, josamycin, and clarithromycin. Among the fluoroquinolones, levofloxacin has been shown to be particularly active in vitro as a bacteriostatic agent against SFG rickettsiae (29). Indeed several fluoroquinolones, josamycin, and azithromycin have been used successfully for the treatment of boutonneuse fever under certain circumstances but cannot be recommended for more pathogenic rickettsioses (3, 8, 31, 41, 44). Except for

cases of scrub typhus in Thailand which have not responded to doxycycline or chloramphenicol, for which azithromycin may be effective, there is little concern about the development of antimicrobial resistance in these rickettsiae (41, 66). Chloramphenicol has been used to treat Rocky Mountain spotted fever during pregnancy, and josamycin has been used for boutonneuse fever. Antimicrobial susceptibility studies of rickettsiae are not routinely performed.

INTERPRETATION AND REPORTING OF RESULTS

When reporting the results of an assay for antibodies in a single serum sample, the laboratorian seldom knows the duration of illness and whether the serum sample is from the acute or convalescent phase of infection. For sera that are nonreactive by dot EIA, by IFA at a dilution of 1:64, by indirect immunoperoxidase assay at a dilution of 1:128, by latex agglutination at a dilution of 1:64, or by Weil-Felix *Proteus* agglutination at a titer of 1:160, the laboratory report should state that no antibodies were detected at the particular cutoff dilution, which may differ in some laboratories and some patient populations, that negative results are expected in the acute stage of rickettsial illness, and that a second sample should be submitted to evaluate the possibility of seroconversion if no alternative diagnosis has been established. If paired acute- and convalescent-phase sera separated by an appropriate interval are available, they should be tested simultaneously. It is wise to test for all the rickettsial and ehrlichial agents to which the patient is likely to have been exposed in the United States. SFG rickettsiae, *Ehrlichia chaffeensis*, *Anaplasma phagocytophila*, and *R. typhi* are the likely agents unless travel to a scrub typhus-endemic area has occurred. If the paired sera are negative, the report should state that the results do not support the diagnosis of rickettsial infection but that occasionally antibody synthesis is delayed, particularly when early antirickettsial therapy was given. If a single serum sample contains an IFA antibody titer of ≥64, an IgM IFA titer of ≥1:32, an indirect immunoperoxidase antibody titer of ≥128, a latex agglutination titer of ≥64, or a Weil-Felix titer of ≥1:320, the laboratory report should state that antibodies reactive with the particular rickettsial antigen were detected at the measured titer, that the result provides supportive evidence for the diagnosis of the rickettsial disease, and that a convalescent-phase sample should be submitted to assess the possibility of seroconversion. If paired sera measured simultaneously show a fourfold or greater rise in titer, the report should state that the results strongly support the rickettsial diagnosis indicated by the tested antigen. If a significant titer was detected in the acute-phase sample but no rise or only a single doubling-dilution rise was measured, the report should state that an additional later sample should be tested to check for a fourfold rise or fall in titer. The possibility that recrudescent typhus could be distinguished from primary louse-borne typhus by the absence of IgM antibodies to *R. prowazekii* and of *Proteus* OX-19 agglutinating antibodies has been shown recently not to be the case (10). The manufacturers of the dot EIA have recommended the interpretation that strongly reactive samples (three or four dots) may indicate the presence of a specific antibody response and that weakly reactive samples (one or two dots) are infrequent but possible in normal populations. Retesting 2 to 3 weeks later would establish the diagnosis if three or four dots develop in the convalescent-phase serum sample and should always be performed.

Isolation of a rickettsia from blood or tissue may be interpreted as indicating an etiologic role. The level of identification of the isolate should be stated, whether it is identified only to a group containing particular organisms or to the species level.

Immunohistologic and immunocytologic diagnostic interpretation states the method, reactivity of the method (e.g., antibody reactive with SFG rickettsiae), and location of the antigen (e.g., in vascular endothelium and frequently adjacent vascular smooth muscle for *R. rickettsii*). Detection of three or more rickettsiae in vascular endothelium in biopsy specimens or four or more rickettsiae in captured circulating endothelial cells is diagnostic of rickettsial infection.

Interpretation of PCR results should state the target gene, the organisms that would be detected, and the presence or absence of a DNA product of a particular size. If a specific oligonucleotide probe or DNA sequencing confirmed the specificity of the identification, this result should be stated. For negative immunohistologic, immunocytologic, and PCR results, it should always be stated that the failure to detect the agent does not exclude the diagnosis, along with data regarding the sensitivity and specificity of the assay in the particular laboratory and the effects of antirickettsial treatment on the sensitivity.

Special efforts should be made to establish the diagnosis of fatal cases including rickettsial isolation, immunohistology, PCR, and serologic testing on samples collected at necropsy.

REFERENCES

1. **Anderson, B. E., G. A. McDonald, D. C. Jones, and R. L. Regnery.** 1990. A protective protein antigen of *Rickettsia rickettsii* has tandemly repeated, near-identical sequences. *Infect. Immun.* **58:**2760–2769.
2. **Anderson, B. E., R. L. Regnery, G. M. Carlone, T. Tzianabos, J. E. McDade, Z. Y. Fu, and W. J. Bellini.** 1987. Sequence analysis of the 17-kilodalton-antigen gene from *Rickettsia rickettsii*. *J. Bacteriol.* **169:**2385–2390.
3. **Bella, F., B. Font, S. Uriz, T. Munoz, E. Espejo, J. Traveria, J. A. Serrano, and F. Segura.** 1990. Randomized trial of doxycycline versus josamycin for Mediterranean spotted fever. *Antimicrob. Agents Chemother.* **34:**937–938.
4. **Birg, M. L., B. La Scola, V. Roux, P. Brouqui, and D. Raoult.** 1999. Isolation of *Rickettsia prowazekii* from blood by shell vial cell culture. *J. Clin. Microbiol.* **37:**3722–3724.
5. **Bouyer, D. H., J. Stenos, P. Crocquet-Valdes, C. G. Moron, V. L. Popov, J. E. Zavala-Velazquez, L. D. Foil, D. R. Stothard, A. F. Azad, and D. H. Walker.** 2001. *Rickettsia felis*: molecular characterization of a new member of the spotted fever group. *Int. J. Syst. Evol. Microbiol.* **51:**339–347.
6. **Broadhurst, L. E., D. J. Kelly, C.-T. Chan, B. L. Smoak, J. F. Brundage, J. B. McClain, and R. N. Miller.** 1998. Laboratory evaluation of a dot-blot enzyme immunoassay for serologic confirmation of illness due to *Rickettsia conorii*. *Am. J. Trop. Med. Hyg.* **58:**786–789.
7. **Brown, G. W., A. Shirai, C. Rogers, and M. G. Groves.** 1983. Diagnostic criteria for scrub typhus: probability values for immunofluorescent antibody and Proteus OXK agglutinin titers. *Am. J. Trop. Med. Hyg.* **32:**1101–1107.
8. **Cascio, A., C. Colomba, D. Di Rosa, L. Salsa, L. di Martino, and L. Titone.** 2001. Efficacy and safety of clarithromycin as treatment for Mediterranean spotted fever in children: a randomized controlled trial. *Clin. Infect. Dis.* **33:**409–411.
9. **Dumler, J., J. P. Taylor, and D. H. Walker.** 1991. Clinical and laboratory features of murine typhus in south Texas, 1980 through 1987. *JAMA* **266:**1365–1370.
10. **Eremeeva, M. E., N. M. Balayeva, and D. Raoult.** 1994. Serological response of patients suffering from primary and recrudescent typhus: comparison of complement fixation reaction, Weil-Felix test, microimmunofluorescence, and immunoblotting. *Clin. Diagn. Lab. Immunol.* **1:**318–324.
11. **Fenollar, F., and D. Raoult.** 1999. Diagnosis of rickettsial diseases using samples dried on blotting paper. *Clin. Diagn. Lab. Immunol.* **6:**483–488.
12. **Fournier, P. E., F. Grunnenberger, B. Jaulhac, G. Gastinger, and D. Raoult.** 2000. Evidence of *Rickettsia helvetica* infection in humans, eastern France. *Emerg. Infect. Dis.* **6:**389–392.
13. **Fournier, P. E., V. Roux, and D. Raoult.** 1998. Phylogenetic analysis of spotted fever group rickettsiae by study of the outer surface protein rOmpA. *Int. J. Syst. Bacteriol.* **48:**839–849.
14. **Fournier, P. E., H. Tissot-Dupont, H. Gallais, and D. R. Raoult.** 2000. *Rickettsia mongolotimonae*: a rare pathogen in France. *Emerg. Infect. Dis.* **6:**290–292.
15. **Furuya, Y., T. Katayama, Y. Yoshida, and I. Kaiho.** 1995. Specific amplification of *Rickettsia japonica* DNA from clinical specimens by PCR. *J. Clin. Microbiol.* **33:**487–489.
16. **Hechemy, K. E., R. L. Anacker, R. N. Philip, K. T. Kleeman, J. N. MacCormack, S. J. Sasowski, and E. E. Michaelson.** 1980. Detection of Rocky Mountain spotted fever antibodies by a latex agglutination test. *J. Clin. Microbiol.* **12:**144–150.
17. **Horney, L. F., and D. H. Walker.** 1988. Meningoencephalitis as a major manifestation of Rocky Mountain spotted fever. *South. Med. J.* **81:**915–918.
18. **Kaplan, J. E., and L. B. Schonberger.** 1986. The sensitivity of various serologic tests in the diagnosis of Rocky Mountain spotted fever. *Am. J. Trop. Med. Hyg.* **35:**840–844.
19. **Kaplowitz, L. G., J. J. Fischer, and P. F. Sparling.** 1981. Rocky Mountain spotted fever: a clinical dilemma. *Curr. Clin. Top. Infect. Dis.* **2:**89–108.
20. **Kaplowitz, L. G., J. V. Lange, J. J. Fischer, and D. H. Walker.** 1983. Correlation of rickettsial titers, circulating endotoxin, and clinical features in Rocky Mountain spotted fever. *Arch. Intern. Med.* **143:**1149–1151.
21. **Kass, E. M., W. K. Szaniawski, H. Levy, J. Leach, K. Srinivasan, and C. Rives.** 1994. Rickettsialpox in a New York City hospital, 1980 to 1989. *N. Engl. J. Med.* **331:**1612–1617.
22. **Kelly, D. J., C. T. Chan, H. Paxton, K. Thompson, R. Howard, and G. A. Dasch.** 1995. Comparative evaluation of a commercial enzyme immunoassay for the detection of human antibody to *Rickettsia typhi*. *Clin. Diagn. Lab. Immunol.* **2:**356–360.
23. **Kelly, D. J., P. W. Wong, E. Gan, and G. E. Lewis, Jr.** 1988. Comparative evaluation of the indirect immunoperoxidase test for the serodiagnosis of rickettsial disease. *Am. J. Trop. Med. Hyg.* **38:**400–406.
24. **Kim, I.-S., S.-Y. Seong, S.-G. Woo, M.-S. Choi, and W.-H. Chang.** 1993. High-level expression of a 56-kilodalton protein gene (*bor56*) of *Rickettsia tsutsugamushi* Boryong and its application to enzyme-linked immunosorbent assays. *J. Clin. Microbiol.* **31:**598–605.
25. **La Scola, B., and D. Raoult.** 1996. Diagnosis of Mediterranean spotted fever by cultivation of *Rickettsia conorii* from blood and skin samples using the centrifugation-shell vial technique and by detection of *R. conorii* in circulating

endothelial cells: a 6-year follow-up. *J. Clin. Microbiol.* **34:**2722–2727.

26. **La Scola, B., and D. Raoult.** 1997. Laboratory diagnosis of rickettsioses: current approaches to diagnosis of old and new rickettsial diseases. *J. Clin. Microbiol.* **35:**2715–2727.

27. **La Scola, B., L. Rydkina, J. B. Ndihokubwayo, S. Vene, and D. Raoult.** 2000. Serological differentiation of murine typhus and epidemic typhus using cross-adsorption and Western blotting. *Clin. Diagn. Lab. Immunol.* **7:**612–616.

28. **Marrero, M., and D. Raoult.** 1989. Centrifugation-shell vial technique for rapid detection of Mediterranean spotted fever rickettsia in blood culture. *Am. J. Trop. Med. Hyg.* **40:**197–199.

29. **Maurin, M., and D. Raoult.** 1997. Bacteriostatic and bactericidal activity of levofloxacin against *Rickettsia rickettsii, Rickettsia conorii,* 'Israeli spotted fever group rickettsia' and *Coxiella burnetii. J. Antimicrob. Chemother.* **39:**725–730.

30. **McDade, J. E., C. C. Shepard, M. A. Redus, V. F. Newhouse, and J. D. Smith.** 1980. Evidence of *Rickettsia prowazekii* infections in the United States. *Am J. Trop. Med. Hyg.* **29:**277–284.

31. **Meloni, G., and T. Meloni.** 1996. Azithromycin vs. doxycycline for Mediterranean spotted fever. *Pediatr. Infect. Dis. J.* **15:**1042–1044.

32. **Montenegro, M. R., S. Mansueto, B. C. Hegarty, and D. H. Walker.** 1983. The histology of "taches noires" of boutonneuse fever and demonstration of *Rickettsia conorii* in them by immunofluorescence. *Virchows Arch.* **400:**309–317.

33. **Moron, C. L., H. M. Feng, D. J. Wear, and D. H. Walker.** 2000. Identification of the target cells of *Orientia tsutsugamushi* in human cases of scrub typhus. *Mod. Pathol.* **14:**752–759.

34. **Niang, M., P. Brouqui, and D. Raoult.** 1999. Epidemic typhus imported from Algeria. *Emerg. Infect. Dis.* **5:**716–718.

35. **Nilsson, K., O. Lindquist, and C. Pahlson.** 1999. Association of *Rickettsia helvetica* with chronic perimyocarditis in sudden cardiac death. *Lancet* **354:**1169–1173.

36. **Oaks, E. V., R. M. Rice, D. J. Kelly, and C. K. Stover.** 1989. Antigenic and genetic relatedness of eight *Rickettsia tsutsugamushi* antigens. *Infect. Immun.* **57:**3116–3122.

37. **Parola, P., D. Vogelaers, C. Roure, F. Janbon, and D. Raoult.** 1998. Murine typhus in travelers returning from Indonesia. *Emerg. Infect. Dis.* **4:**677–680.

38. **Philip, R. N., E. A. Casper, R. L. Anacker, J. Cory, S. F. Hayes, W. Burgdorfer, and C. E. Yunker.** 1983. *Rickettsia bellii* sp. nov.: a tick-borne rickettsia, widely distributed in the United States, that is distinct from the spotted fever and typhus biogroups. *Int. J. Syst. Bacteriol.* **33:**94–106.

39. **Philip, R. N., E. A. Casper, W. Burgdorfer, R. K. Gerloff, L. E. Hughes, and E. J. Bell.** 1978. Serologic typing of rickettsiae of the spotted fever group by microimmunofluorescence. *J. Immunol.* **121:**1961–1968.

40. **Raoult, D., and G. A. Dasch.** 1989. Line blot and western blot immunoassays for diagnosis of Mediterranean spotted fever. *J. Clin. Microbiol.* **27:**2073–2079.

41. **Raoult, D., and M. Drancourt.** 1991. Antimicrobial therapy of rickettsial diseases. *Antimicrob. Agents Chemother.* **35:**2457–2462.

42. **Raoult, D., P.-E. Fournier, F. Fenollar, M. Jensenius, T. Prioe, J. J. De Pina, G. Caruso, N. Jones, H. Laferl, J. E. Rosenblatt, and T. J. Marrie.** 2001. *Rickettsia africae,* a tick-borne pathogen in travelers to sub-Saharan Africa. *N. Engl. J. Med.* **344:**1501–1510.

43. **Raoult, D., B. La Scola, M. Enea, P. E. Fournier, V. Foux, F. Fenollar, M. A. Galvao, and X. de Lamballerie.** 2001. A flea-associated rickettsia pathogenic for humans. *Emerg. Infect. Dis.* **7:**73–81.

44. **Raoult, D., and M. Maurin.** 1999. *Rickettsia* species, p. 568–574. *In* V. L. Yu, T. C. Merigan, Jr., and S. L. Barriere (ed.), *Antimicrobial Therapy and Vaccines.* The Williams & Wilkins Co., Baltimore, Md.

45. **Raoult, D., S. Rousseau, B. Toga, C. Tamalet, H. Gallais, P. De Micco, and P. Casanova.** 1984. Diagnostic sérologique de la fièvre boutonneuse méditerranéenne. *Pathol. Biol.* **32:**791–794.

46. **Raoult, D., V. Roux, W. Xu, and M. Maurin.** 1997. A new tick-transmitted disease due to *Rickettsia slovaca. Lancet* **350:**128–129.

47. **Regnery, R. L., C. L. Spruill, and B. D. Plikaytis.** 1991. Genotypic identification of rickettsiae and estimation of intraspecies sequence divergence for portions of two rickettsial genes. *J. Bacteriol.* **173:**1576–1589.

48. **Roux, V., and D. Raoult.** 1999. Body lice as tools for diagnosis and surveillance of reemerging diseases. *J. Clin. Microbiol.* **37:**596–599.

49. **Roux, V., and D. Raoult.** 2000. Phylogenetic analysis of members of the genus *Rickettsia* using the gene encoding the outer-membrane protein rOmpB *(ompB). Int. J. Syst. Evol. Microbiol.* **50:**1449–1455.

50. **Roux, V., E. Rydkina, M. Eremeeva, and D. Raoult.** 1997. Citrate synthase gene comparison, a new tool for phylogenetic analysis, and its application for the rickettsiae. *Int. J. Syst. Bacteriol.* **47:**252–261.

51. **Schriefer, M. E., J. B. Sacci, Jr., J. S. Dumler, M. G. Bullen, and A. F. Azad.** 1994. Identification of a novel rickettsial infection in a patient diagnosed with murine typhus. *J. Clin. Microbiol.* **32:**949–954.

52. **Schriefer, M. E., J. B. Sacci, Jr., J. A. Higgins, and A. F. Azad.** 1994. Murine typhus: updated roles of multiple urban components and a second typhus like rickettsia. *J. Med. Entomol.* **31:**681–685.

53. **Sekyova, Z., V. Roux, and D. Raoult.** 2001. Phylogeny of *Rickettsia* spp. inferred by comparing sequences of 'gene D' which encodes an intracytoplasmic protein. *Int. J. Syst. Evol. Microbiol.* **51:**1353–1360.

54. **Sexton, D. J., S. S. Kanj, K. Wilson, G. R. Corey, B. C. Hegarty, M. G. Levy, and E. B. Breitschwerdt.** 1994. The use of a polymerase chain reaction as a diagnostic test for Rocky Mountain spotted fever. *Am. J. Trop. Med. Hyg.* **50:**59–63.

55. **Stothard, D. R., and P. A. Fuerst.** 1995. Evolutionary analysis of the spotted fever and typhus groups of *Rickettsia* using 16S rRNA gene sequences. *Syst. Appl. Microbiol.* **18:**52–61.

56. **Sugita, Y., Y. Yamakawa, K. Takahashi, T. Nagatani, K. Okuda, and H. Nakajima.** 1993. A polymerase chain reaction system for rapid diagnosis of scrub typhus within six hours. *Am. J. Trop. Med. Hyg.* **49:**636–640.

57. **Tamura, A., N. Ohashi, H. Urakami, and S. Miyamura.** 1995. Classification of *Rickettsia tsutsugamushi* in a new genus, *Orientia* gen. nov., as *Orientia tsutsugamushi* comb. nov. *Int. J. Syst. Bacteriol.* **45:**589–591.

58. **Tzianabos, T., B. E. Anderson, and J. E. McDade.** 1989. Detection of *Rickettsia rickettsii* DNA in clinical specimens by using polymerase chain reaction technology. *J. Clin. Microbiol.* **27:**2866–2868.

59. **Vishwanath, S.** 1991. Antigenic relationships among the rickettsiae of the spotted fever and typhus groups. *FEMS Microbiol. Lett.* **81:**341–344.

60. **von der Schulenburg, J. H., M. Habig, J. J. Sloggett, K. M. Webberley, D. Bertrand, G. D. Hurst, and M. E. Majerus.** 2001. Incidence of male-killing *Rickettsia* spp. (alpha-proteobacteria) in the ten-spot ladybird beetle

Adalia decempunctata L. (Coleoptera: Coccinellidae). *Appl. Environ. Microbiol.* **67**:270–277.

61. **Walker, D. H., M. S. Burday, and J. D. Folds.** 1980. Laboratory diagnosis of Rocky Mountain spotted fever. *South. Med. J.* **73**:1443–1447.

62. **Walker, D. H., C. G. Crawford, and B. G. Cain.** 1980. Rickettsial infection of pulmonary microcirculation: the basis for interstitial pneumonitis in Rocky Mountain spotted fever. *Hum. Pathol.* **11**:263–272.

63. **Walker, D. H., H.-M. Feng, S. Ladner, A. N. Billings, S. R. Zaki, D. J. Wear, and B. Hightower.** 1997. Immunohistochemical diagnosis of typhus rickettsioses using an anti-lipopolysaccharide monoclonal antibody. *Mod. Pathol.* **10**:1038–1042.

64. **Walker, D. H., S. D. Hudnall, W. K. Szaniawski, and H. M. Feng.** 1999. Monoclonal antibody-based immunohistochemical diagnosis of rickettsialpox: the macrophage is the principal target. *Mod. Pathol.* **12**:529–533.

65. **Walker, D. H., F. M. Parks, T. G. Betz, J. P. Taylor, and J. W. Muehlberger.** 1989. Histopathology and immunohistologic demonstration of the distribution of *Rickettsia typhi* in fatal murine typhus. *Am. J. Clin. Pathol.* **91**:720–724.

66. **Watt, G., C. Chouriyagune, R. Ruangweerayud, P. Watcharapichat, D. Phulsuksombati, K. Jongsakul, P. Teja-Isavadharm, D. Bhodhidatta, K. D. Corcoran, G. A. Dasch, and D. Strickman.** 1996. Scrub typhus infections poorly responsive to antibiotics in northern Thailand. *Lancet* **348**:86–89.

67. **Watt, G., and D. Strickman.** 1994. Life-threatening scrub typhus in a traveler returning from Thailand. *Clin. Infect. Dis.* **18**:624–626.

68. **Weddle, J. R., T.-C. Chan, K. Thompson, H. Paxton, D. J. Kelly, G. Dasch, and D. Strickman.** 1995. Effectiveness of a dot-blot immunoassay of anti-*Rickettsia tsutsugamushi* antibodies for serologic analysis of scrub typhus. *Am. J. Trop. Med. Hyg.* **53**:43–46.

69. **Williams, W. J., S. Radulovic, G. A. Dasch, J. Lindstrom, D. J. Kelly, C. N. Oster, and D. H. Walker.** 1994. Identification of *Rickettsia conorii* infection by polymerase chain reaction in a soldier returning from Somalia. *Clin. Infect. Dis.* **19**:93–99.

70. **Zavala-Velazquez, J. E., J. A. Ruiz-Sosa, R. A. Sanchez-Elias, G. Becerra-Carmona, and D. H. Walker.** 2000. *Rickettsia felis* rickettsiosis in Yucatan. *Lancet* **356**:1079–1080.

71. **Zhang, J. Z., M. Y. Fan, Y. M. Wu, P. E. Fournier, V. Roux, and D. Raoult.** 2000. Genetic classification of "*Rickettsia heilongjiangii*" and "*Rickettsia hulinii*," two Chinese spotted fever group rickettsiae. *J. Clin. Microbiol.* **38**:3498–3501.

Ehrlichia, Anaplasma, Neorickettsia, and Aegyptianella

MARIA E. AGUERO-ROSENFELD AND J. STEPHEN DUMLER

65

TAXONOMY

Members of the genera *Ehrlichia* and *Anaplasma* have become important agents of human disease and have recently been successfully cultured in vitro. Together with a number of other pathogens in several genera, they are obligate intracellular bacteria currently placed in the order *Rickettsiales*. While most closely related to the genera *Rickettsia* and *Orientia*, organisms classically considered ehrlichiae could be divided into four major clades. The most recently proposed changes in taxonomic classification of this group of bacteria (Fig. 1) are extensive and largely based upon sequence analysis of 16S rRNA genes and *groESL* operons (35). The phylogenetic approach is further supported by serologic cross-reactions, comparisons among major immunodominant surface proteins, and the cellular tropisms of these bacteria (30, 57). Critical changes include assignment of all members of the tribes *Ehrlichieae* and *Wolbachieae* into the family *Anaplasmataceae* with elimination of the tribe structure of the family *Rickettsiaceae*. All tick-borne bacteria of *Anaplasmataceae* are now grouped within two closely related genera, *Ehrlichia* and *Anaplasma*. The former members of the *Ehrlichia phagocytophila* group that includes the species *Ehrlichia equi* and the human granulocytic ehrlichiosis (HGE) agent are merged into a single species within the genus *Anaplasma* as *A. phagocytophila*. Because of incorrect Latin usage, the name of this species was again changed to *Anaplasma phagocytophilum* (Notification List published in *Int. J. Syst. Bacteriol. Evol. Microbiol.* 52:5–6, 2002), now considered the valid designation. Reassigned into this genus are the former *Ehrlichia* species *E. platys* and *E. bovis*, now *A. platys* and *A. bovis*. *Cowdria ruminantium*, a ruminant pathogen closely related to *Ehrlichia canis*, is reassigned into the genus *Ehrlichia* as *E. ruminantium*, while the non-tick-transmitted species *Ehrlichia sennetsu* and *Ehrlichia risticii* are assigned into the genus *Neorickettsia*. Members of the *Wolbachia* genus are otherwise not reassigned. Thus, human pathogens are now present in the genera *Ehrlichia* (*Ehrlichia chaffeensis* and *Ehrlichia ewingii*), *Anaplasma* (*A. phagocytophilum*), and *Neorickettsia* (*Neorickettsia sennetsu*), and helminth infection by *Wolbachia* spp. may be a determinant of severity with human filariasis (96).

While *Ehrlichia* species infect predominantly leukocytes of humans and other mammals, *Anaplasma* species infect bone marrow-derived cells of all lineages in different animal hosts. *Neorickettsia* species infect predominantly mononuclear phagocytes and occasionally enterocytes in mammalian hosts. The genus *Aegyptianella* is currently listed as incerta sedis. *Wolbachia* spp. are endocytosymbionts of insects and helminths that are transmitted only by transovarial and transstadial (between stages of development) passage. For historical reasons and because of similarities among human pathogens in these genera, they will be referred to in this chapter as ehrlichiae and the diseases will be referred to as ehrlichioses.

DESCRIPTION OF THE GENERA

Kurloff first described intracellular inclusions resembling *Ehrlichia*-like organisms in mononuclear cells of guinea pigs in 1889 while working at Paul Ehrlich's laboratory (87). Theiler discovered and named the tick-borne intraerythrocytic bacterial pathogen of ruminants *Anaplasma marginale* in 1910. Moshkovsky proposed the genus name *Ehrlichia*, in honor of the earlier discovery in Ehrlich's laboratory, for the dog pathogen known as *Rickettsia canis*. *Ehrlichia* and *Anaplasma* spp. are obligate intracellular gram-negative bacteria that propagate and reside in cytoplasmic membrane-lined vacuoles in bone marrow-derived cells, including granulocytes, monocytes, erythrocytes, and platelets, and for *E. ruminantium*, also within endothelial cells (84, 98, 102). For the genera *Ehrlichia* and *Anaplasma*, organisms are transmitted by tick bite, whereas organisms in the genera *Wolbachia* and *Neorickettsia* are not. Individual small (0.2- to 0.4-μm) dense forms of bacterial cells resembling chlamydial elementary bodies have been described, as have larger forms (0.8 to 1.5 μm) resembling reticulate bodies (81). Both are capable of binary fission, and a developmental cycle has not been demonstrated. After a few days, the elementary bodies dividing in the phagosome form an initial pleomorphic inclusion that matures into a microscopic colony known as a morula. *N. sennetsu* grows as bacterial cells that may maintain their individual vacuolar membranes when they undergo binary fission, and thus an intracellular inclusion may not be identified by light microscopy. Cell lysis is a feature of the infectious process and leads to the release of cell-free bacteria that can infect other competent cells (16). Unlike *Rickettsia* spp., members of the genera *Ehrlichia* and *Anaplasma* do not show thickening of either leaflet of the outer membrane, and the outer mem-

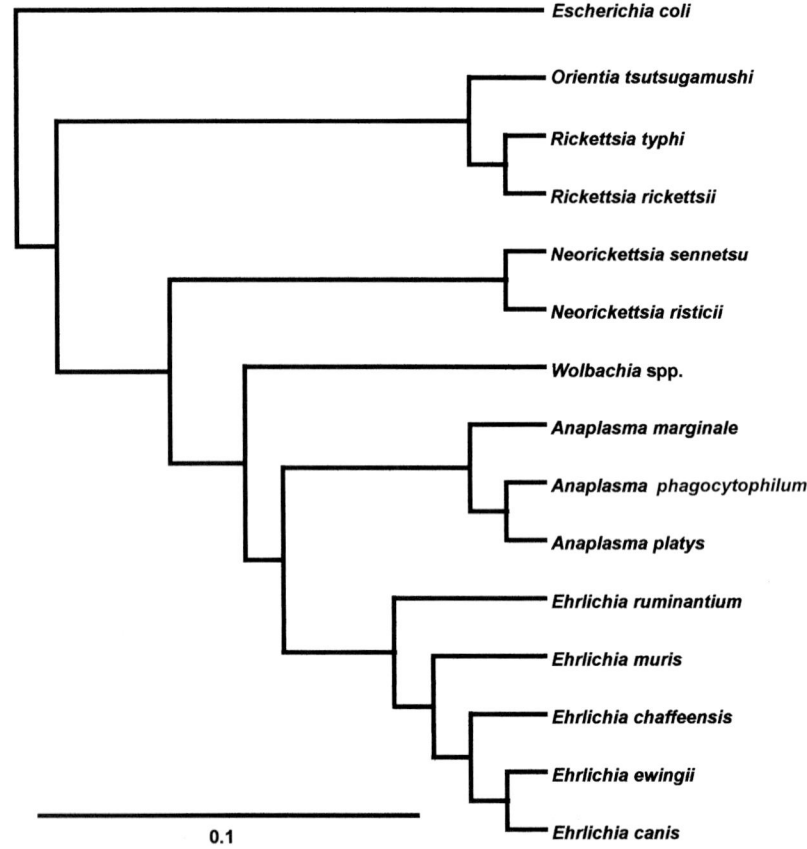

FIGURE 1 Neighbor-joining phylogenetic tree inferred from 16S rRNA gene sequences of selected *Ehrlichia*, *Anaplasma*, *Neorickettsia*, and *Wolbachia* spp. *Escherichia coli* is used as an outgroup. The bar represents the estimated number of substitutions per site.

brane appears to be more ruffled in *A. phagocytophilum* than in *N. sennetsu* or *E. chaffeensis* (84). By transmission electron microscopy, *Ehrlichia* and *Anaplasma* spp. do not appear to contain significant amounts of peptidoglycan. The genome size of *N. sennetsu* is approximately 800 kb, whereas those of *E. chaffeensis* and *A. phagocytophilum* are 1,200 and 1,500 kb, respectively. Host cell-free *Ehrlichia* and *Anaplasma* spp. metabolize L-glutamine but not glucose or glucose-6-phosphate, suggesting that they lack a conventional glycolytic pathway (103).

A. *marginale* and *Aegyptianella* spp. are tick-transmitted intraerythrocytic bacteria of ruminants and of birds, amphibians, or reptiles, respectively. These organisms reside in small membrane-bound inclusions (15) and are not known to be associated with human disease.

NATURAL HABITATS

Ehrlichia and *Anaplasma* spp. are zoonotic agents that are transmitted to animals and humans most frequently after a tick bite or possibly by ingestion of fish infested by *Neorickettsia*-infected flukes (Table 1). *Wolbachia* spp. are symbionts of a broad range of arthropods and helminths. Thus, most species have the potential for vertebrate and invertebrate life stages. The tick vectors for species known to infect humans include members of the *Ixodes persulcatus* group (including *I. scapularis*, *I. pacificus*, and *I. ricinus*) for *A. phagocytophilum* (63, 83, 97), *Amblyomma americanum*

(lone star tick) and perhaps *Dermacentor variabilis* (dog tick) for *E. chaffeensis*, *A. americanum* for *E. ewingii* (4, 5), and *Rhipicephalus sanguineus* (brown dog tick) for *E. canis* (88). Although poorly studied, transovarial transmission in ticks does not appear to occur, and thus, *Ehrlichia* and *Anaplasma* species depend upon high levels of bacteremia and in some cases persistent infection for enzootic maintenance (63, 88). Transstadial and interstadial transmission in ticks allows ehrlichiae to be acquired from blood meals on naturally infected animals by the immature stages of ticks (larvae and nymphs), which can transmit the ehrlichiae to other mammalian hosts after molting to the next stage (nymph or adult). Humans are only inadvertently infected and represent an end-stage host for ehrlichiae. Natural maintenance of tick-borne ehrlichiae depends upon the presence of appropriate tick vectors and mammalian hosts in the local environment.

Natural reservoirs that are known to exist for *E. chaffeensis* involve both white-tailed deer (*Odocoileus virginianus*) and domestic dogs and perhaps other animals that host *A. americanum* ticks (28, 62). The identities of the major reservoirs for *A. phagocytophilum* have been incompletely investigated, although small mammals, especially the white-footed mouse (*Peromyscus leucopus*) in the eastern United States and other small mammals such as chipmunks (*Tamias striatus*) and voles (*Clethrionomys gapperi*), are naturally infected and are frequent hosts of the immature stages of *I. scapularis* (97, 100). The role of white-

TABLE 1 Selected features of *Ehrlichia, Anaplasma, Neorickettsia,* and *Aegyptianella* species of human and veterinary interest

Organism name	Former denomination(s)	Vector	Disease[a]	Hosts developing disease	Infected cells	Reservoir hosts
Anaplasma phagocytophilum	Ehrlichia equi; Ehrlichia phagocytophila; HGE agent	Ixodes persulcatus group	EGE; Tick-borne fever; HGE	Horses; Ruminants; Humans, dogs	Granulocytes	Deer, sheep; White-footed mice
Anaplasma marginale, Anaplasma centrale, Anaplasma ovis		Several tick species	Ruminant anaplasmosis	Cattle (sheep, goats)	Erythrocytes	Ruminants; Wild cervids?
Anaplasma platys	Ehrlichia platys	Rhipicephalus sanguineus?; Amblyomma spp.?	Canine cyclic thrombocytopenia	Dogs	Platelets	Ruminants?
Anaplasma bovis	Ehrlichia bovis	Rhipicephalus appendiculatus; Amblyomma variegatum	Bovine ehrlichiosis	Cattle	Mononuclear leukocytes	Ruminants?; Rabbits?
Ehrlichia chaffeensis		Amblyomma americanum; Dermacentor variabilis	HME	Humans; Dogs	Mononuclear leukocytes	White-tailed deer; Domestic dogs; Others?
Ehrlichia ewingii		Amblyomma americanum	CGE; E. ewingii ehrlichiosis	Dogs; Humans	Granulocytes	Canids?
Ehrlichia canis		Rhipicephalus sanguineus	CME	Dogs	Mononuclear leukocytes	Canids
Ehrlichia ruminantium	Cowdria ruminantium	Amblyomma species	Cowdriosis (heartwater)	Domestic and wild ruminants	Granulocytes; Endothelial cells	Ruminants
Ehrlichia muris		Haemaphysalis flava	Not named	Laboratory mice	Mononuclear leukocytes	Not known
Neorickettsia sennetsu	Ehrlichia sennetsu	Unknown; Possibly acquired by ingestion?	Sennetsu fever	Humans	Mononuclear leukocytes	Fluke-infested fish
Neorickettsia risticii	Ehrlichia risticii	Ingestion of fluke-infested insects	Potomac horse fever	Horses	Mononuclear leukocytes	Juga sp. flukes
Neorickettsia helminthoeca		Ingestion of fluke-infested salmonid fish	Salmon poisoning disease	Dogs, bears	Mononuclear leukocytes	Fluke-infested fish
Aegyptianella spp. (genus and species incertae sedis)		Amblyomma spp.	Not known	Birds, amphibians, reptiles	Erythrocytes	Not known

[a] EGE, equine granulocytic ehrlichiosis; CGE, canine granulocytic ehrlichiosis; CME, canine monocytic ehrlichiosis.

footed mice as a reservoir of *A. phagocytophilum* in nature has recently been questioned, since immunity that develops after infection may render them temporarily host incompetent (61). Persistent or prolonged infection of animal reservoirs is essential for maintenance of zoonotic pathogens. Mice infected with *Borrelia burgdorferi* remain infected for many months, which is essential for continuous transmission to different stages of developing *I. scapularis* ticks (42). In Europe, red deer, sheep, cattle, and goats are persistently infected and serve as reservoirs of *A. phagocytophilum*. The reservoir for *N. sennetsu* is not known; however, epidemiological data suggest that consumption of raw fish was associated with sennetsu fever. Other species of *Neorickettsia* seem to have a complex transmission process involving trematode stages. *N. risticii*, the agent of Potomac horse fever, appears to be transmitted to horses by accidental ingestion of insects carrying *N. risticii*-infected cercariae (65). Similarly, *Neorickettsia helminthoeca* infects dogs through ingestion of trematode-infested fish.

Over 20 species of ticks have been identified in the transmission of *A. marginale* worldwide (60). Other modes of transmission, such as accidental inoculation of infected erythrocytes or blood-sucking insects, have also been reported for *A. marginale*. Tick vectors also appear to be important in the transmission of members of the genus *Aegyptianella* to birds and amphibians (54).

CLINICAL SIGNIFICANCE

Human Diseases

HME

The causative agent of human monocytotropic ehrlichiosis (HME) is *E. chaffeensis*, a monocytotropic ehrlichia that was first identified as a human pathogen in a patient with a severe febrile illness after tick bites in 1986 (67). More than 742 cases of HME have been identified by the Centers for Disease Control and Prevention between 1986 and 1997 (70); however, serologic data compiled at a major commercial laboratory that performs serologic testing for *E. chaffeensis* comprises more than 722 diagnostic serologic results between 1992 and 1995 alone, suggesting that HME occurs much more frequently than is reported (98). Passive and active case identification has revealed that clinically apparent HME occurs as frequently as or more frequently than Rocky Mountain spotted fever in Oklahoma, Georgia, Maryland, Tennessee, and North Carolina (90, 98). Most cases are identified in the south central and southeastern United States, but increasingly infections have been identified in the mid-Atlantic region as well. Prospective evaluation of individuals with high rates of tick exposure shows that approximately 75% of seroconversions with antibody to *E. chaffeensis* are subclinical (43).

The median incubation period for HME is 9 days, and two of every three patients are males; the median age is 44 years (43). Patients typically present with high fever (97%), headache (81%), malaise (84%), and myalgia (68%), usually without other specific physical findings. Manifestations of gastrointestinal involvement (nausea, vomiting, diarrhea), respiratory involvement (cough or pulmonary infiltrates), and joint pain are rare. Central nervous system involvement (stiff neck, confusion) and meningitis have been described (90). Rash is identified in only 36% of patients and is only infrequently petechial. In spite of the nonspecific clinical symptoms and signs, laboratory findings are abnormal for at least 86% of patients, including leukopenia (60 to 74%) with lymphopenia and neutropenia, thrombocytopenia (72%), and increased serum aspartate transaminase activities (86 to 88%). Severe complications include a toxic shock-like syndrome with multiorgan failure, meningoencephalitis, diffuse alveolar damage associated with adult respiratory distress syndrome, and fulminant infections in patients immunocompromised by human immunodeficiency virus, high-dose corticosteroids, or organ transplantation (6, 36, 41, 69, 75, 86). The case fatality rate of approximately 2 to 3% would be higher if effective antimicrobial therapy were not available.

HGE

The causative agent of HGE is *A. phagocytophilum*, causing an illness identical to that of the formerly named *E. equi* and *E. phagocytophila* in horses and ruminants, respectively (12, 66; D. Fish, M. Papero, C. Gingrich-Baker, and R. T. Coughlin, *Program Abstr. 13th Sesqui-Annu. Meet. Am. Soc. Rickettsiol.*, abstr. 75, 1997). HGE was first identified in 1990 in a patient from Wisconsin after tick bites in an area where *E. chaffeensis* and its tick vector do not exist (8). Although the most frequent mode of transmission is through the bite of an infected *Ixodes* tick, other modes of infection are likely to exist; perinatal transmission has been reported (51). Transmission by accidental inoculation of infected blood or by transfusion is probably rare but should also be considered.

As for HME, HGE is not a reportable illness in most states; thus, the true incidence and prevalence of the infection are unknown. However, prospective passive case collection in northwestern Wisconsin from 1990 through 1995 revealed a yearly incidence of 16 cases per 100,000 population, with peak rates identified as high as 58 cases per 100,000 in some counties in 1995 (10). From 1986 through 1997, 449 cases of HGE were reported by 30 state health departments in the United States (70). The highest annual incidences were in the Northeast and upper Midwest states. Infected patients were identified in many other states, as well as in several European countries (17, 26, 31, 80, 94, 98). In 1999, over 200 HGE cases were reported in the United States, doubling the number of HME cases reported that year. Two-thirds of those cases occurred in Connecticut and upstate New York (22). Subclinical infection is probably the norm, as nearly 14% of the population assessed in northwestern Wisconsin has antibodies indicative of prior infection (9). The tick vectors for HME and HGE coexist in the mid-Atlantic, southern New England states, and the southern Midwest. Thus, both diseases can occur in these areas (26).

HGE has a median incubation period of 5 to 11 days after *Ixodes* sp. tick bites and occurs in patients with a median age of 43 to 60 years (1, 10). Twice as many men have the illness as women (11). Patients present with high fever, myalgias, headache, and malaise, with gastrointestinal, respiratory, musculoskeletal, or central nervous system involvement in fewer patients. Rash is observed in less than 11% of patients. Leukopenia with lymphopenia, thrombocytopenia, and increased serum aspartate transaminase activities are present in most patients during early stages of the disease. The hematological abnormalities may normalize before antimicrobial treatment, and lymphocytosis with atypical lymphocytes has been observed after the first week of infection (11, 53). Severe complications of HGE include a septic shock-like illness with multiorgan failure, adult respiratory distress syndrome, and opportunistic infections

(10, 46, 53, 99); meningitis has not been documented with HGE. At least six deaths have been associated with HGE; at least three of those patients had opportunistic infections, including *Candida* esophagitis, *Cryptococcus* pneumonia, invasive pulmonary aspergillosis, and herpes esophagitis (10, 46, 99).

Sennetsu Ehrlichiosis
Named after the Japanese term for glandular fever, *N. sennetsu* was first isolated from patients with suspected infectious mononucleosis in 1953 (71). Rarely identified now, patients develop a self-limited febrile illness with chills, headache, malaise, sore throat, anorexia, and generalized lymphadenopathy. Cases were identified only in Japan and possibly Malaysia. Laboratory findings include early leukopenia and atypical lymphocytes in the peripheral blood during early convalescence. No fatalities or severe complications have been reported.

Other Human Ehrlichioses
In 1996, an *E. canis*-like agent was isolated from the blood of an asymptomatic man from Venezuela who had morulae in peripheral blood monocytes. Serological investigations of children with febrile illness and healthy adults exposed to dogs with canine ehrlichiosis in that geographic area showed two healthy individuals with antibodies reacting with the Venezuelan human ehrlichia agent, *E. chaffeensis*, *E. canis*, and *E. muris*. Comparison of the 16S rRNA gene of the Venezuelan human ehrlichia agent with those of two strains of *E. canis* showed 1 or 2 base differences (79).

The agent causing canine granulocytic ehrlichiosis, *E. ewingii*, was also recently implicated in human disease in four cases from Missouri. Three of the four patients were receiving immunosuppressive therapy and presented with clinical and routine laboratory findings indistinguishable from those of HME. Two of the four patients showed inclusions in peripheral granulocytes, and PCR of blood using 16S rRNA primers identified a sequence that matched that of *E. ewingii* (21). The infection may be more prevalent than previously suspected, since nearly 10% of blood samples submitted for PCR testing in one Midwest laboratory contained *E. ewingii* DNA.

While *Wolbachia* spp. are not known to be directly pathogenic for humans or animals, emerging experimental evidence indicates a potential role for the intracellular bacterial components ("symbionts") of such helminths as *Brugia malayi, Onchocerca volvulus,* and *Wuchereria bancrofti* as potentiators of the inflammatory reactions that are considered significant parts of the pathogenesis of the parasite infection (96).

Animal Diseases
Members of the genera *Ehrlichia, Anaplasma, Neorickettsia,* and *Aegyptianella* and related genera were known as veterinary pathogens long before they were recognized as human pathogens. Work in this area by dedicated veterinary microbiologists has contributed tremendously to the recognition and understanding of the diseases these pathogens cause in humans.

Canine Ehrlichiosis
Canine monocytic ehrlichiosis caused by *E. canis* was originally described in Algeria in 1935 and later in other areas of the world (84). It caused fatal disease in U.S. military dogs during the Vietnam conflict. This disease has acute,

subclinical, and chronic phases and presents with leukopenia, thrombocytopenia, and hypergammaglobulinemia.

E. ewingii causes canine granulocytic ehrlichiosis, which is usually milder in presentation than canine monocytic ehrlichiosis and is sometimes associated with polyarthritis (40). Unlike *E. canis, E. ewingii* has not yet been cultured in vitro. Canine granulocytic ehrlichiosis caused by *A. phagocytophilum* has also been reported (38, 91).

A. platys is a thrombocytotropic bacterium that causes mild cyclical fevers and thrombocytopenia in dogs; remittent clinical signs are associated with the presence of morulae in platelets of infected dogs, suggesting persistence (84).

Equine Ehrlichiosis
Potomac horse fever is a febrile gastrointestinal disease of horses caused by *N. risticii* organisms that infect monocytes (49). Potomac horse fever occurs in different geographic areas, including North America and Europe, and presents with depression, anorexia, lethargy, fever, colic, watery diarrhea, dehydration, leukopenia, and sometimes abortion. The transmission involves a complex aquatic ecosystem in which infected insects seem to be implicated (65).

Equine granulocytic ehrlichiosis caused by *A. phagocytophilum*, formerly *E. equi*, is a seasonal disease first described in 1969. Although it has been described as occurring mostly in the foothills of Northern California (64), it also occurs in other regions of the United States and Europe. It causes a self-limiting disease in horses similar to HGE in humans (12) and appears to be transmitted in California through the bite of infected *I. pacificus* ticks. Tick-borne fever of ruminants is caused by the granulocytotropic *A. phagocytophilum*, formerly *E. phagocytophila*, and is transmitted via the bite of infected *I. ricinus* ticks in Europe (44).

Anaplasmosis of Ruminants
A. marginale is the etiologic agent of bovine anaplasmosis, the most prevalent tick-borne disease of cattle worldwide. Mechanical transmission by biting flies and other insects may also occur. Organisms develop as an intraerythrocytic inclusion and can produce severe anemia, weight loss, abortion, and sometimes death. A feature of this infection is the persistent low-level bacteremia even after clinical recovery; therefore, infected animals become a reservoir of infection for transmission to other animals. This feature is shared with the related *A. phagocytophilum* infections of deer and *A. platys* infection of dogs. Antigenic variation has been postulated to play a role in the persistence of *A. marginale* infection and transmission (77). Successful cultivation of this agent has been achieved in a tick cell line, IDE8 (15), and transiently in erythrocyte cultures.

Aegyptianella Infection of Birds and Amphibians
Members of the genus *Aegyptianella* infect erythrocytes of different animal species throughout the world. The type species is *Aegyptianella pullorum* of birds. Other species, such as *A. bacterifera*, have been associated with infections in amphibians. *A. botuliformis*, which infects helmeted guineafowls in Africa, appears to be transmitted through the bite of infected *Amblyomma* species (54). The exact relationships of these species to the family *Anaplasmataceae* is not known.

Cowdriosis (Heartwater)
Ehrlichia (Cowdria) ruminantium is an intracellular bacterium that infects neutrophils and endothelial cells of cattle,

sheep, goats, and certain wildlife species (84). Cowdriosis is an acute disease that can cause mortality rates of up to 90% in susceptible ruminants. It occurs most frequently in sub-Saharan Africa and the islands of the Atlantic, Indian Ocean, and Caribbean Sea and is transmitted by *Amblyomma* tick vectors.

Neorickettsiosis of Canines

N. helminthoeca, the agent of salmon poisoning disease, infects mononuclear cells and is acquired by dogs after ingesting salmonid fish encysted with a fluke harboring the organism (84). Molecular and antigenic analyses have established a close relationship between *N. helminthoeca*, *N. risticii* (formerly *E. risticii*), and *N. sennetsu* (formerly *E. sennetsu*). Further similarities may exist in their modes of transmission.

COLLECTION, TRANSPORT, AND STORAGE OF SPECIMENS

EDTA- or acid-citrate-dextrose-anticoagulated blood or cerebrospinal fluid (CSF) and serum should be obtained for diagnosis or confirmation of HME or HGE. Currently, there are three methods for diagnosis during the acute phase of illness, when ehrlichiae are likely to be present in circulating peripheral blood or CSF leukocytes: PCR amplification of *Ehrlichia* or *Anaplasma* species nucleic acids; detection of morulae in the cytoplasm of infected leukocytes by use of nonspecific Romanowsky stains (e.g., Giemsa or Wright) or by use of specific immunocytologic or immunohistologic stains with *E. chaffeensis* or *A. phagocytophilum* antibodies; and culture of *Ehrlichia* or *Anaplasma* species from blood or CSF. EDTA-anticoagulated blood is the most useful specimen for most tests and should be obtained during the acute phase of illness (27, 32, 45).

Samples for PCR should be tested promptly, but if the blood is maintained at 4°C, it may still be possible to amplify nucleic acids several days to a week or more later. If delays beyond several days are anticipated, the blood should be frozen at −20°C until used. There is less experience with collection and storage of CSF for PCR, but it is expected that similar conditions will yield appropriate results. PCR using serum or plasma is far less sensitive than PCR using samples that contain infected leukocytes.

Peripheral blood buffy coat smears or cytocentrifuged preparations of CSF cells should be prepared within several hours of obtaining the samples, since leukocytes degenerate rapidly. Once prepared, air-dried blood smears and cytocentrifuged CSF preparations are stable at room temperature for months or years.

The culture conditions for *Ehrlichia* and *Anaplasma* species are still being optimized. Currently, the preferred specimen for culture is peripheral blood. Samples should be obtained by sterile venipuncture or lumbar puncture and submitted as soon as possible to the laboratory that will attempt culture. Usually, this will require overnight courier service, since culture is currently performed in only a few public health and research laboratories. Samples to be cultured should be maintained at approximately 4°C during shipping; it is important to avoid freezing, which is likely to reduce the content of viable ehrlichiae. EDTA-anticoagulated blood stored for up to 18 days at 4°C has also been successfully used to culture *A. phagocytophilum* in vitro (58). After cultivation, ehrlichia-infected cells may be stored in a frozen state at −80°C for several months or in liquid nitrogen for longer periods. Storage of infected cells is best accomplished when more than 50 to 90% of the host cells are infected and is achieved by suspension of at least 10^6 cells per ml in tissue culture medium that contains 10% dimethyl sulfoxide and at least 30% fetal bovine serum.

LABORATORY CONFIRMATION OF *E. CHAFFEENSIS*

Isolation Procedures

E. chaffeensis has been isolated from peripheral blood of more than 30 patients with HME, and an *E. canis*-like organism was isolated only once from an asymptomatic human (25, 27, 32, 76, 79, 90; G. M. Shore, S. M. Folk, D. C. Bartley, J. W. Sumner, and C. D. Paddock, *Program Abstr. 13th Sesqui-Annu. Meet. Am. Soc. Rickettsiol.*, abstr. 82, 1997). The cell most frequently used for primary isolation is the canine histiocytic cell line, DH82; however, *E. chaffeensis* has been successfully cultivated in other cells, including the human macrophage-like THP-1 cells, the fibroblast-like HEL-22 cells, Vero cells, and HL60 cells, a human promyelocytic cell line differentiated to the monocytic pathway, among others (14, 16, 25, 47). Isolation may be successful even when infected leukocytes are not observed on examination of peripheral blood (90). The usual format for isolation involves direct inoculation of leukocyte fractions or, less optimally, placement of whole blood into flasks with a confluent layer of adherent cells or into flasks that contain approximately 2×10^5 to 1×10^6 nonadherent cells per ml of tissue culture medium. Macrophage-like cells that are highly phagocytic may be adversely affected by the presence of numerous erythrocytes; thus, it is recommended that either (i) leukocytes be fractionated from erythrocytes by density gradient centrifugation (e.g., Ficoll-Paque), (ii) leukocytes be harvested after erythrocyte lysis (hypotonic lysis, NH_4Cl lysis, etc.), or (iii) cell confluency be reestablished after cultivation with erythrocyte-containing samples by addition of uninfected host cells. Since *E. chaffeensis* may be present in a very small proportion of peripheral blood leukocytes, it is usually advisable to inoculate cultures with as many peripheral blood leukocytes as possible. This may be difficult because of the leukopenia that often accompanies HME. A method using 2 to 3 ml of EDTA-anticoagulated blood, diluted in 2 volumes of sterile Hanks' balanced salt solution and then subjected to Histopaque (Sigma, St. Louis, Mo.) gradient separation of leukocytes, gave a high yield of isolation in a recent study of the use of culture to diagnose HME (90).

The blood mononuclear cells are resuspended in a 2-ml volume of tissue culture medium supplemented with 5% fetal bovine serum and allowed to interact with adherent host cells in a 25-cm^2 flask for 3 h; the interaction is usually enhanced by incubation with rocking at 37°C in 5% CO_2. The inoculum is removed if significant erythrocyte contamination is present, and the monolayer is replenished with 5 ml of fresh tissue culture medium. Since *Ehrlichia* species are bacteria, antibiotics in the medium must be avoided. The generation time of *E. chaffeensis* may be 8 h or more, and thus, cultures must be maintained to allow a slow logarithmic or stable growth phase to avoid having the host cells outgrow the ehrlichiae.

The presence of infected cells is determined by sampling the medium (DH82 cells and THP-1 cells) or by lightly scraping part of the monolayer. Aliquots of the culture are cytocentrifuged and then subjected to Romanowsky or immunofluorescent staining, and cells are examined for the presence of intracytoplasmic morulae or *E. chaffeensis* antigen (Fig. 2). Culture may require 1 month or more but has been achieved in as little as a few days (27, 32, 90; Shore et al., *13th Sesqui-Annu. Meet. Am. Soc. Rickettsiol.*). Confirmation of the infectious agent is currently best achieved by PCR amplification using species-specific primers (3).

Identification

Romanowsky and Immunohistologic Identification

Patients with suspected HME should have Romanowsky-stained (Giemsa or Wright stain) peripheral blood or buffy coat leukocytes examined for the presence of ehrlichial morulae. This method is very insensitive, identifying up to 29% (2 of 7) of culture-confirmed *E. chaffeensis*-infected patients (90). Ordinarily, *E. chaffeensis* is detected predominantly in monocytes, and its detection seems to correlate with severity of infection. When present, ehrlichial morulae are small (1- to 3-μm diameter), round-to-oval clusters of bacteria that stain basophilic to amphophilic with Romanowsky stains (see Fig. 4). These clusters are present in the cytoplasm and have a stippled appearance owing to individual bacteria within the vacuole.

Immunohistologic methods may be used to identify *E. chaffeensis* within human tissues, including bone marrow, liver, and spleen. An immunohistologic study of bone marrow, however, detected *E. chaffeensis* in only 40% of specimens obtained during the active infection (33). Most immunohistologic studies have been performed using polyclonal antibodies that react with other *Ehrlichia* species. A monoclonal antibody may specifically detect *E. chaffeensis* in human tissues (108). Unfortunately, commercial sources for direct immunohistologic detection of *E. chaffeensis* are not currently available.

PCR

The most widely used PCR method for amplification of *E. chaffeensis* nucleic acids from clinical samples uses the HE1/HE3 primer set (5, 39, 89). This primer pair amplifies a 389-bp fragment of the 16S rRNA gene sequences. The product may be detected by simple nucleic acid staining (e.g., ethidium bromide) after agarose gel electrophoresis or by Southern hybridization of the amplified products using an internal probe that is reported to increase analytical sensitivity. A clinical evaluation of *E. chaffeensis* PCR using the HE1/HE3 system showed a sensitivity of 79 to 100% compared with detection of *E. chaffeensis* or *E. canis* antibodies in convalescence; however, *E. chaffeensis* nucleic acids were frequently detected in patients who never developed antibodies, a finding of uncertain significance given the high degree of analytical specificity demonstrated with this system (5, 89). Similar results occur with a nested PCR that employs broad-range "*Ehrlichia* genus" primers in an initial step followed by PCR with the HE1/HE3 primer pair (89). Other targets for PCR that have not been evaluated for clinical sensitivity or specificity include the *groESL* operon; a variable-length PCR target of unknown significance that is present in *E. chaffeensis* (90, 93; Shore et al., *13th Sesqui-Annu. Meet. Am. Soc. Rickettsiol.*); the 120-kDa antigen gene that encodes an immunodominant antigen with tandemly repeated subunits that may vary among *E. chaffeensis* isolates; and the quinolinate synthase A gene, *nadA* (110, 111; Shore et al., *13th Sesqui-Annu. Meet. Am. Soc. Rickettsiol.*). PCR of whole blood using a nested PCR with broad-range 16S rRNA primers (8F and

1448R) followed by a second (nested) reaction with primers 15F and 208R yielded results similar to those of culture in a recent study (90).

Serologic Tests

The majority of cases of HME are diagnosed by retrospective serologic confirmation, and serology is the most sensitive method for diagnostic confirmation. The most widely used test is an indirect fluorescent-antibody (IFA) test that utilizes ehrlichia-infected cells fixed to glass slides. Ehrlichial antigens may be difficult to prepare and are available mostly through public health and research laboratories, although commercial production and distribution are now available. IFA serodiagnostic kits are currently available through Focus Technologies (Cypress, Calif.). and PanBio Inc. (Columbia, Md.). Immunoblot procedures are becoming increasingly popular because of the perception of increased specificity (18, 24, 104).

Currently, there is little standardization for any method of ehrlichial serology, and cutoff titers are dependent upon validation in individual laboratories that perform these assays. The algorithm for serologic testing by IFA test includes an initial screen at a dilution of 1:64 or 1:80 for antibodies to *E. chaffeensis*. Reactive samples are then titrated.

E. chaffeensis IFA

E. chaffeensis antibodies are detected by IFA test using *E. chaffeensis* Arkansas strain-infected DH82 canine macrophage-like cells. Sera are serially diluted starting at a dilution of 1:64. The presence of antibodies is detected after incubation with fluorescein isothiocyanate-conjugated anti-human immunoglobulins. A positive reaction is detected by the fluorescent demonstration of typical intracytoplasmic ehrlichial morula morphology. It is important to identify the appropriate proportion of infected cells as determined by use of a positive-control serum and the appropriate morphology for each antigen preparation to preclude false-positive interpretations. Prescreening for autoantibodies or routine removal of rheumatoid factors will lessen the risk of misinterpretation due to antibodies reactive with cellular components, including nuclear or cytoplasmic antigens. A fourfold increase or decrease in antibody titer, with a peak titer or a single convalescent-phase titer of ≥64, in a patient with a consistent clinical history supports the diagnosis of HME. Antibody titers may be detected in a small proportion of subjects without HME because of the presence of antigens that are highly conserved among bacterial species, including heat shock proteins (29, 104). Acute-phase sera should be obtained at the time of presentation with acute illness, and convalescent-phase sera are best obtained 3 to 6 weeks later (29).

The precise sensitivity and specificity of the IFA test for *E. chaffeensis* are not known but are assumed to be high because of a high degree of correlation of presence of *E. chaffeensis* antibodies and characteristic clinical findings (43). Although immunoglobulin M (IgM) testing is routinely performed, no evaluation of its sensitivity or specificity for the confirmation of HME has been published. Previously, the serologically cross-reactive *E. canis* was used as a surrogate antigen; however, this serodiagnostic assay has a lower sensitivity than that obtained with *E. chaffeensis*, and its use should be discouraged (5). The role of immunoblots in diagnosis is not well established; however, many patients with *E. chaffeensis* infection can be differentiated from patients with HGE by the demonstration of

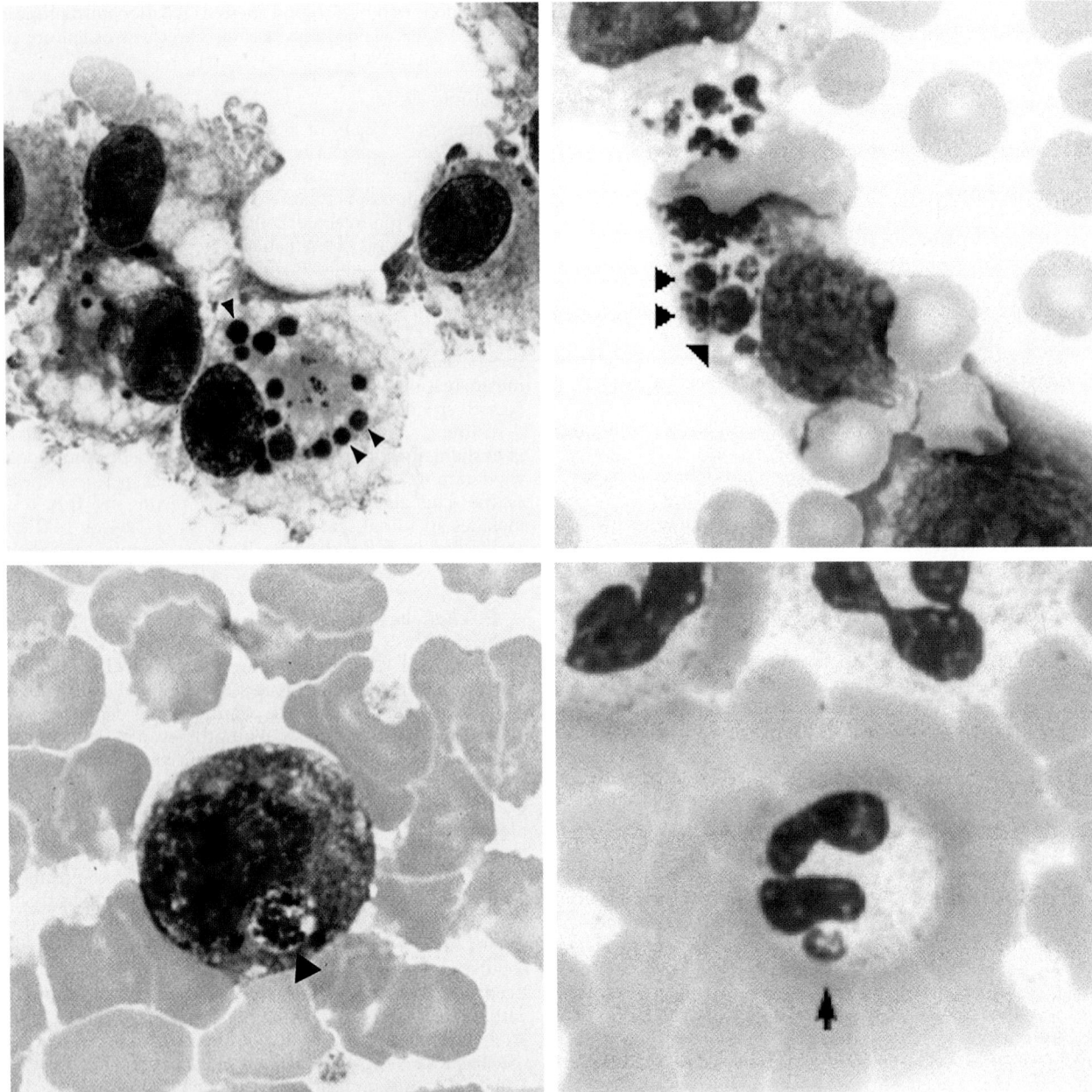

FIGURE 2 (top left)   *E. chaffeensis* cultured in the canine histiocyte cell line, DH82. Note the presence of basophilic, stippled, intracytoplasmic inclusions approximately 2 to 3 μm in diameter (arrowheads). The smaller intracytoplasmic granules may also be ehrlichial morulae (Romanowsky [Leukostat] stain; original magnification, ×1,000).

FIGURE 3 (top right)   *A. phagocytophilum* cultured in the human promyelocytic cell line HL60 from the blood of an infected patient. Note the presence of multiple basophilic, stippled, intracytoplasmic inclusions (arrowheads) in an HL60 cell (Wright stain; original magnification, ×915).

FIGURE 4 (bottom)   *E. chaffeensis* (A [left]) and *A. phagocytophilum* (B [right]) in peripheral blood leukocytes. Note that the *E. chaffeensis* morula (arrowhead) is present in a monocyte (A) and that the *A. phagocytophilum* morula (arrow) is present in a neutrophil (B) (Wright stain; original magnification, ×915).

antibodies reactive with one or more of the 22-, 28-, 29-, or 120-kDa antigens of *E. chaffeensis* (18, 24). A recombinant 120-kDa protein that has been applied in a dot blot method appears to offer a sensitive and specific serologic confirmation tool (109). Antibodies to *E. chaffeensis* have also been detected in patients diagnosed with Rocky Mountain spotted fever, Q fever, brucellosis, Lyme disease, and Epstein-Barr virus infections, suggesting that false-positive reactions do occur (29, 104). Antigenic diversity among isolates of *E. chaffeensis* is well described (25) but may not affect the detection of the polyclonal antibody response that is generated with human infection. Several reports have characterized patients with HME without antibody responses, even long after onset (39, 86, 90). However, in the few cases in which *E. chaffeensis* infection has been most clearly proven by cultivation of the agent, most patients who survived developed clear serologic reactions detected by IFA methods during convalescence (25, 27, 32, 90; Shore et al., *13th Sesqui-Annu. Meet. Am. Soc. Rickettsiol.*). Hypothetical reasons for false-negative results include infection by antigenically diverse strains (unproven) and abrogation of antibody response by early therapy (90).

LABORATORY CONFIRMATION OF HGE

Isolation Procedures

A. phagocytophilum has been successfully cultivated from human patients more often than has *E. chaffeensis, E. canis,* or *N. sennetsu* because of the larger number of organisms that are present in peripheral blood in many infected patients. More than 45 isolates have been cultured from infected patients at a single medical center. Isolation is best achieved in the human promyelocytic cell line HL60 (45) and has also been accomplished when ehrlichiae are not observed in peripheral blood smears. The optimal conditions for recovery of these bacteria have not been conclusively determined, but cultivation in HL60 cells has been achieved with or without the presence of granulocyte-differentiating chemicals (e.g., dimethyl sulfoxide or retinoic acid) (46, 48). Because erythrocytes do not adversely affect the HL60 cells, direct inoculation of EDTA-anticoagulated blood is effective. Fractionation of blood into leukocytes by preparation of buffy coat or by isolation of granulocyte fractions by density gradient centrifugation is also effective (85). Ordinarily, approximately 100 to 500 μl of EDTA-anticoagulated blood containing approximately 10^2 to 10^4 infected granulocytes is inoculated into a total of approximately 100-fold-more uninfected HL60 cells that are in the exponential growth phase and are subsequently maintained at a concentration between 2×10^5 and 1×10^6 cells per ml of tissue culture medium.

Cultures are examined every 2 to 3 days by Romanowsky staining of cytocentrifuged preparations of 20 to 50 μl of culture suspensions. Ehrlichial morulae appear as small aggregates of basophilic bacteria in the cytoplasm of the HL60 cells (Fig. 3). Since HL60 cells may contain a variety of cytoplasmic granules, immunocytology can be very helpful for the inexperienced laboratorian. Unfortunately, immunohistological reagents are currently not commercially available. Cultures usually require between 5 and 10 days of cultivation before morulae are clearly identified, but infected cells may be detected as early as 3 days postinoculation. The time to detection of organisms in culture correlates with the amount of bacteria present in blood at the time of culture inoculation (58). Definitive identification is

achieved by PCR amplification using species-specific primers (23, 45, 78) or by sequence analysis of 16S rRNA genes that have been amplified by universal eubacterial PCR (23). The exact length of incubation before cultures are considered negative is still unknown, but they should be kept for at least 14 days, with the cell density maintained at about 2×10^5/ml.

Identification

Romanowsky and Immunohistologic Identification

Examination of Romanowsky-stained (Giemsa or Wright stain) peripheral blood or buffy coat leukocytes for the presence of ehrlichial morulae is highly valuable in the diagnosis of HGE. Usually, 800 to 1,000 granulocytes are examined under $\times 500$ to $\times 1,000$ magnification for the presence of morulae (1, 10). Since most patients presenting with positive smears have less than 1% infected granulocytes and usually have leukopenia, buffy coat preparations will have a higher yield than peripheral smears. Infection rates as high as 40% of peripheral granulocytes have been described (8). As for HME, the presence of detectable infected granulocytes in peripheral blood seems to correlate with the severity of infection (1, 8, 10). The sensitivity of the buffy coat smear examination in the acute phase of HGE is approximately 60% (11). When present, ehrlichial morulae are small (1- to 3-μm diameter), round-to-oval clusters of bacteria that stain basophilic to amphophilic with Romanowsky stains (Fig. 4). These clusters are present in the cytoplasm of neutrophils or eosinophils and have a stippled appearance owing to individual bacteria within the vacuole.

Immunohistologic methods may also be used to identify *A. phagocytophilum* group ehrlichiae within human tissues, including bone marrow, liver, and spleen.

A. phagocytophilum PCR

Multiple PCR assays for detection of *A. phagocytophilum* nucleic acids have been published (23, 37, 45, 78, 89, 92). Most utilize regions of the 16S rRNA gene that are relatively specific as targets for amplification. Since the formerly named *E. phagocytophila, E. equi,* and the HGE agent differ by only two or three nucleic acids over the nearly 1,500-bp 16S rRNA gene, a specific PCR based on this gene cannot distinguish among them. The most frequently applied and evaluated method employs the primer set ge9f and ge10r, which amplifies a 919-bp fragment, most often used as a single-stage reaction, with or without a hybridization probe to enhance sensitivity (23, 37). A popular alternative is the use of nested PCR with an outer set of primers that anneal to and amplify eubacterial 16S rRNA genes, followed by an internal PCR with *A. phagocytophilum*-specific primers (13, 89). To date, only one clinical evaluation to assess sensitivity and specificity, comparing the assay to a serological standard, has been performed. The method employs modifications to enhance sensitivity, including a proofreading thermostable polymerase and alternative nucleic acid-binding dye detection (37). In the prospective evaluation, the PCR detected *A. phagocytophilum* nucleic acids in acute-phase blood from 6 of 7 patients who developed *A. phagocytophilum* antibodies in convalescence, and the PCR correctly classified 10 suspected patients without seroconversions, for an overall clinical sensitivity of 86% and specificity of 100%. In direct clinical application, the sensitivity of PCR for diagnosis has not been as rewarding, with a sensitivity of approximately 50%

in a study that included 23 cases, 8 culture confirmed and 15 not confirmed by culture (50). All eight culture-confirmed cases, however, tested positive by PCR using different PCR primer sets. At least one PCR-positive patient from whom *A. phagocytophilum* was isolated in cell culture never developed a detectable antibody response (1). PCR amplification of the *groESL* region using a nested reaction has also been useful for detecting ehrlichial DNA in blood during the acute phase. Primers HS1 and HS6 are used in the primary reaction, followed by primers HS43 and HS45. The size of the amplified product distinguishes *E. chaffeensis* from *A. phagocytophilum* (528 versus 480 bp, respectively) (92).

Serology of HGE

A. phagocytophilum IFA

A. phagocytophilum is a single species that now includes three previously distinct organisms, *E. phagocytophila*, *E. equi*, and the HGE agent (12, 23, 45). Thus, IFA serologic testing is performed with any of these antigens (30, 55, 101). Previously, most testing was done with neutrophils obtained from the blood of animals experimentally infected with *E. phagocytophila* or *E. equi* (8, 30, 66). Currently, the preferred method for testing human sera is the use of a human isolate propagated in the human HL60 promyelo-cyte cell line (2, 26, 45, 48, 55, 74, 82). It is now well demonstrated that antigenic diversity exists among *A. phagocytophilum* isolates, but it is unlikely that such diversity affects detection under clinical circumstances (7, 101, 113). Interpretation of immunofluorescent patterns is similar to that for *E. chaffeensis* and requires an experienced microscopist. IFA kits are currently available from Focus Technologies and PanBio Inc.

Sera should be screened at a single dilution (1:64 or 1:80), and the presence of antibodies is determined after incubation with fluorescein isothiocyanate-conjugated anti-human IgG and IgM. If specimens test reactive, they are serially diluted to determine the end point titer. A serologic confirmation of the diagnosis is achieved when a fourfold rise in titer is demonstrated in convalescence with a minimum titer of 80 or when a single antibody titer of ≥80 is demonstrated for a patient with clinical features typical of HGE (1, 10). Approximately 25 to 45% of infected patients will have antibodies at the time of presentation (1, 2, 10); however, up to 14% of the population in some regions of high endemicity possesses antibodies, rendering this early serologic information less useful (9). The typical response during the acute phase of infection is a rapid rise (within 2 weeks of onset) in antibody levels, reaching high titers (≥640) within the first month (2). In a treated cohort of patients whose diagnosis of HGE was confirmed by culture, the antibody titers declined gradually over the next few months and about half had detectable antibodies by IFA test 1 year after infection (2). However, many patients will have antibodies detectable for months to years after initial infection (11).

The sensitivity and specificity of the HGE serologic tests are both believed to be high because of good correlation between typical clinical cases and serologic reactions to *A. phagocytophilum* group antigens (1, 2, 10, 70). HGE serology had a sensitivity of 91.3% in a group of 24 culture-confirmed patients (2) and a median sensitivity of 95% among a group of 28 patients diagnosed by culture, PCR, or presence of morulae in blood smears (101). IgM testing appears to be a useful tool for identification of recent

infection, although the sensitivity may not be as high as that for IgG testing (101). An enzyme-linked immunosorbent assay (ELISA)-based method (82) and immunoblots have been described (7, 30, 55, 82, 104, 113), but their diagnostic utility is still being investigated. Immunoblots may be used to differentiate among *A. phagocytophilum* and *E. chaffeensis* infections by demonstration of a major *A. phagocytophilum* antigen of approximately 44 kDa in sera of HGE patients (30, 55, 104). Cross-reactivity between *E. chaffeensis* and *A. phagocytophilum* group has been observed in IFA tests. In those circumstances, testing with both antigens will often show higher titers with antigens of the homologous infecting agent (1, 100).

False-positive reactions have been observed for patients with other rickettsial infections, Q fever, and Epstein-Barr virus infections. Many patients with HGE develop antibodies that react with *B. burgdorferi* by ELISA and demonstrate diagnostic IgG or IgM immunoblots (107). Although some patients have been confirmed by culture to have concurrent infection with *A. phagocytophilum* and *B. burgdorferi*, the statistical probability that this mechanism accounts for most of these concurrent positive serologic results is very low (73, 104, 106). Another explanation is exposure to the various tick-borne agents at different times rather than from a single tick bite. The most frequent scenario is the presence of antibodies to the various agents in individuals living in areas of high endemicity (9, 68). Autoantibodies to platelets and other leukocyte components can cause false-positive IFA tests (105).

Other immunoassays employing recombinant p44 antigens have been developed and show promise as alternatives to IFA tests (95, 112). Antigens of 42 to 49 kDa are immunodominant in *A. phagocytophilum* infection and are encoded by a multigene family (72) similar to that of the major surface proteins (*msp* proteins) of *A. marginale* (77).

ANTIBIOTIC SUSCEPTIBILITIES

Routine antimicrobial susceptibility testing of *Ehrlichia* or *Anaplasma* species isolates is unnecessary. These bacteria are maintained enzootically by transmission among ticks and feral mammalian reservoir hosts (4, 62, 78, 97, 100). The level of exposure of such vertebrate and invertebrate hosts to antimicrobial selection factors is very low, and thus antimicrobial resistance is very unlikely. Most patients with either HME or HGE become afebrile and have clinical improvement within 48 h of therapy with a tetracycline antibiotic, including doxycycline, the drug of choice (10, 43). Retrospective analysis of patients with HME has shown a significant degree of efficacy for tetracyclines or chloramphenicol compared with other broad-spectrum antimicrobial agents (43). With in vitro studies, tetracycline antibiotics are uniformly bactericidal for *Ehrlichia* and *Anaplasma* species, whereas the MICs of chloramphenicol cannot be safely achieved in humans with HME or HGE (19, 52, 59). In contrast, the antibiotics most frequently used for patients who have had recent tick bites, amoxicillin and ceftriaxone, and broad-spectrum antibiotics that might be prescribed for undifferentiated fever such as other cephalosporins, aminoglycosides, and macrolides are not effective for inhibition of ehrlichial growth in vitro. The rifamycins (rifampin and rifabutin) can achieve effective inhibition or killing of *Ehrlichia* and *Anaplasma* species in vitro, and the fluoroquinolones (ofloxacin, levofloxacin, and trovafloxacin) have very low MICs for human isolates of *A. phagocytophilum* (52, 59). Rifampin has been successfully used to treat HGE during pregnancy and appears to be a useful alternative for patients who cannot receive tetracyclines (20).

Whereas persistent infections with *Ehrlichia* and *Anaplasma* species may occur frequently in naturally and experimentally infected animals even after treatment with tetracycline (44, 56), persistence of ehrlichiae in humans has rarely been documented (34, 86). Therapy is usually highly effective at eliminating ehrlichiae from the blood of infected humans.

INTERPRETATION AND REPORTING OF RESULTS

The current algorithm for identification and confirmation of infections by *Ehrlichia* and *Anaplasma* species requires a complete evaluation of the history, physical examination, and laboratory results that will suggest the diagnosis. Before specific tests for etiologic determination are attempted, a decision concerning therapy should be made, since delays may lead to increased morbidity and perhaps mortality. At the time of acute illness and prior to institution of antiehrlichial therapy, EDTA-anticoagulated blood should be obtained for PCR amplification of *E. chaffeensis* and *A. phagocytophilum* and considered for the possibility of in vitro cultivation. *A. phagocytophilum* has been cultured more frequently than *E. chaffeensis* during the acute phase and provides a definite proof of the infection. Since *A. phagocytophilum* remains viable under refrigeration conditions for several days, specimens could be transported to a remote laboratory that performs culture (58). A peripheral blood or buffy coat smear should be examined for the presence of morulae, which would confirm the presumptive diagnosis. Serum should be obtained and tested for antibodies to *E. chaffeensis* or *A. phagocytophilum*, with an aliquot saved for repeat testing when a convalescent-phase serum sample is obtained 2 to 4 weeks later.

The presence of intracytoplasmic inclusions within a leukocyte in peripheral blood might be due to the presence of overlying platelets, Döhle bodies, toxic granulations, nuclear fragments, Auer rods in blasts, other bacteria, yeasts, inorganic materials, or granules of normal large granular lymphocytes or granulocytes. If the typical morphology of an *Ehrlichia* or *Anaplasma* sp. morula is observed, an assessment as to the hematopoietic lineage and the percentage of cells that contain morulae should be made and reported. A report that identifies such structures should state only that structures consistent with *Ehrlichia* or *Anaplasma* species morulae are identified and that definitive identification relies upon other specific laboratory evaluations.

A positive PCR result should be reported as such, indicating the presence of *E. chaffeensis* or *A. phagocytophilum* DNA, and it should be made clear that a positive PCR is not equivalent to the culture of ehrlichiae from blood. Laboratories that use a broad-range PCR to identify *Ehrlichia* or *Anaplasma* sp. DNA in blood may also detect *E. ewingii* infection, which may mimic either HME or HGE (21). In addition, false-positive reactions can occur due to amplicon contamination. Careful techniques involving physical separation of PCR setup, amplification, and post-amplification analysis as well as biochemical inactivation protocols may be needed to avoid contamination. A negative PCR result does not exclude the possibility of HME, HGE, or ehrlichiosis due to *E. ewingii*. Possible explanations for a false-negative PCR result include (i) an exces-

sively long interval after the onset of clinical manifestations or tick bite until the blood sample was obtained, (ii) previous antimicrobial therapy, and (iii) the analytical and clinical sensitivities and specificities of the PCR assay used in the testing laboratory. Detection sensitivity limits should be stated as "xx copies/ml," "xx bacteria/ml," or "xx infected cells/ml," while clinical sensitivity data concerning the laboratory's clinical validation of the assay using samples from proven patients with and without the disease should be readily available.

IFA serologic test results should be reported as the titer of antibodies determined to be reactive with *E. chaffeensis* or *A. phagocytophilum*, including the positive cutoff values determined in the laboratory. An interpretation should indicate whether the titers determined are considered "significant" or "positive" on the basis of a fourfold increase or decrease or as single high-titered sera. Additionally, all interpretations should be made in the context of typical clinical and epidemiological information. It should be remembered that infections with *E. ewingii* would yield serologic patterns considered diagnostic of *E. chaffeensis* that are difficult to differentiate even with immunoblot methods. Immunoblot analyses should provide information about antibodies that react with specific antigens considered unique or diagnostic of infection with a single species of *Ehrlichia* or *Anaplasma*.

REFERENCES

1. **Aguero-Rosenfeld, M. E., H. W. Horowitz, G. P. Wormser, D. F. McKenna, J. Nowakowski, J. Munoz, and J. S. Dumler.** 1996. Human granulocytic ehrlichiosis (HGE): a case series from a single medical center in New York State. *Ann. Intern. Med.* **125:**904–908.

2. **Aguero-Rosenfeld, M. E., F. Kalantarpour, M. Baluch, H. W. Horowitz, D. F. McKenna, J. T. Raffalli, T.-C. Hsieh, J. Wu, J. S. Dumler, and G. P. Wormser.** 2000. Serology of culture-confirmed cases of human granulocytic ehrlichiosis. *J. Clin. Microbiol.* **38:**635–638.

3. **Anderson, B. E., J. E. Dawson, D. C. Jones, and K. H. Wilson.** 1991. *Ehrlichia chaffeensis*, a new species associated with human ehrlichiosis. *J. Clin. Microbiol.* **29:**2838–2842.

4. **Anderson, B. E., K. G. Sims, J. G. Olson, J. E. Childs, J. F. Piesman, C. M. Happ, G. O. Maupin, and B. J. B. Johnson.** 1993. *Amblyomma americanum*: a potential vector of human ehrlichiosis. *Am. J. Trop. Med. Hyg.* **49:**239–244.

5. **Anderson, B. E., J. W. Sumner, J. E. Dawson, T. Tzianabos, C. R. Greene, J. G. Olson, D. B. Fishbein, M. Olsen-Rasmussen, B. P. Hollowau, E. H. George, and A. F. Azad.** 1992. Detection of the etiologic agent of human ehrlichiosis by polymerase chain reaction. *J. Clin. Microbiol.* **30:**775–780.

6. **Antony, S. J., J. S. Dummer, and E. Hunter.** 1995. Human ehrlichiosis in a liver transplant recipient. *Transplantation* **60:**879–880.

7. **Asanovich, K. M., J. S. Bakken, J. E. Madigan, M. Aguero-Rosenfeld, G. P. Wormser, and J. S. Dumler.** 1997. Antigenic diversity of granulocytic *Ehrlichia* isolates from humans in Wisconsin and New York and a horse from California. *J. Infect. Dis.* **176:**1029–1034.

8. **Bakken, J. S., J. S. Dumler, S.-M. Chen, M. R. Eckman, L. L. Van Etta, and D. H. Walker.** 1994. Human granulocytic ehrlichiosis in the upper Midwest United States. A new species emerging? *JAMA* **272:**212–218.

9. **Bakken, J. S., P. Goellner, M. Van Etten, D. Z. Boyle, O. L. Swonger, S. Mattson, J. Krueth, R. L. Tilden, K.**

Asanovich, J. Walls, and J. S. Dumler. 1998. Seroprevalence of human granulocytic ehrlichiosis among permanent residents of northwestern Wisconsin. *Clin. Infect. Dis.* **27:**1491–1496.

10. Bakken, J. S., J. Krueth, C. Wilson-Nordskog, R. L. Tilden, K. Asanovich, and J. S. Dumler. 1996. Clinical and laboratory characteristics of human granulocytic ehrlichiosis. *JAMA* **275:**199–205.

11. Bakken, J. S., M. E. Aguero-Rosenfeld, R. L. Tilden, G. P. Wormser, H. W. Horowitz, J. T. Raffalli, M. Baluch, D. Riddell, J. J. Walls, and J. S. Dumler. 2001. Serial measurements of hematologic counts during the active phase of human granulocytic ehrlichiosis. *Clin. Infect. Dis.* **32:**862–870.

12. Barlough, J. E., J. E. Madigan, E. DeRock, J. S. Dumler, and J. S. Bakken. 1995. Protection against *Ehrlichia equi* is conferred by prior infection with the human granulocytotropic ehrlichia (HGE agent). *J. Clin. Microbiol.* **33:**3333–3334.

13. Barlough, J. E., J. E. Madigan, E. DeRock, and L. Bigornia. 1996. Nested polymerase chain reaction for detection of *Ehrlichia equi* genomic DNA in horses and ticks (*Ixodes pacificus*). *Vet. Parasitol.* **63:**319–329.

14. Barnewell, R. E., Y. Rikihisa, and E. H. Lee. 1997. *Ehrlichia chaffeensis* inclusions are early endosomes which selectively accumulate transferrin receptor. *Infect. Immun.* **65:**1455–1461.

15. Blouin, E. F., and K. M. Kocan. 1998. Morphology and development of *Anaplasma marginale* (Rickettsiales: Anaplasmataceae) in cultured *Ixodes scapularis* (Acari: Ixodidae) cells. *J. Med. Entomol.* **35:**788–797.

16. Brouqui, P., M. L. Birg, and D. Raoult. 1994. Cytopathic effect, plaque formation, and lysis of *Ehrlichia chaffeensis* grown on continuous cell lines. *Infect. Immun.* **62:**405–411.

17. Brouqui, P., J. S. Dumler, R. Lienhard, M. Brossard, and D. Raoult. 1995. Human granulocytic ehrlichiosis in Europe. *Lancet* **346:**782–783.

18. Brouqui, P., C. Lecam, J. Olson, and D. Raoult. 1994. Serologic diagnosis of human monocytic ehrlichiosis by immunoblot analysis. *Clin. Diagn. Lab. Immunol.* **1:**645–649.

19. Brouqui, P., and D. Raoult. 1992. In vitro antibiotic susceptibility of the newly recognized agent of ehrlichiosis in humans, *Ehrlichia chaffeensis. Antimicrob. Agents Chemother.* **36:**2799–2803.

20. Buitrago, M. I., J. W. IJdo, P. Rinaudo, H. Simon, J. Copel, J. Gadbaw, R. Heimer, E. Fikrig, and F. J. Bia. 1998. Human granulocytic ehrlichiosis during pregnancy treated successfully with rifampin. *Clin. Infect. Dis.* **27:**213–215.

21. Buller, R. S., M. Arens, S. P. Hmiel, C. D. Paddock, J. W. Sumner, Y. Rikihisa, A. Unver, M. Gaudreault-Keener, F. A. Manian, A. M. Liddell, N. Schmulewitz, and G. A. Storch. 1999. *Ehrlichia ewingii*, a newly recognized agent of human ehrlichiosis. *N. Engl. J. Med.* **341:**148–155.

22. Centers for Disease Control and Prevention. 2001. Summary of notifiable diseases, United States 1999. *Morb. Mortal. Wkly. Rep.* **48:**5.

23. Chen, S. M., J. S. Dumler, J. S. Bakken, and D. H. Walker. 1994. Identification of a granulocytotropic *Ehrlichia* species as the etiologic agent of human disease. *J. Clin. Microbiol.* **32:**589–595.

24. Chen, S. M., J. S. Dumler, H.-M. Feng, and D. H. Walker. 1994. Identification of the antigenic constituents of *Ehrlichia chaffeensis. Am. J. Trop. Med. Hyg.* **50:**52–58.

25. Chen, S. M., X. J. Yu, V. L. Popov, E. L. Westerman, F. G. Hamilton, and D. H. Walker. 1997. Genetic and antigenic diversity of *Ehrlichia chaffeensis*: comparative analysis of a novel human strain from Oklahoma and previously isolated strains. *J. Infect. Dis.* **175:**856–863.

26. Comer, J. A., W. L. Nicholson, J. G. Olson, and J. E. Childs. 1999. Serologic testing for human granulocytic ehrlichiosis at a National Referral Center. *J. Clin. Microbiol.* **37:**558–564.

27. Dawson, J. E., B. E. Anderson, D. B. Fishbein, J. L. Sanchez, C. S. Goldsmith, K. H. Wilson, and C. W. Duntley. 1991. Isolation and characterization of an *Ehrlichia* sp. from a patient diagnosed with human ehrlichiosis. *J. Clin. Microbiol.* **29:**2741–2745.

28. Dawson, J. E., and S. A. Ewing. 1992. Susceptibility of dogs to infection with *Ehrlichia chaffeensis*, the causative agent of human ehrlichiosis. *Am. J. Vet. Res.* **53:**1322–1327.

29. Dawson, J. E., D. B. Fishbein, T. R. Eng, M. A. Redus, and N. R. Greene. 1990. Diagnosis of human ehrlichiosis with the indirect fluorescent antibody test: kinetics and specificity. *J. Infect. Dis.* **162:**91–95.

30. Dumler, J. S., K. M. Asanovich, J. S. Bakken, P. Richter, R. Kimsey, and J. E. Madigan. 1995. Serologic cross-reaction among *Ehrlichia equi, Ehrlichia phagocytophila*, and human granulocytic ehrlichia. *J. Clin. Microbiol.* **33:**1098–1103.

31. Dumler, J. S., and J. S. Bakken. 1996. Human granulocytic ehrlichiosis in Wisconsin and Minnesota: a frequent infection with the potential for persistence. *J. Infect. Dis.* **173:**1027–1030.

32. Dumler, J. S., S. M. Chen, K. Asanovich, E. Trigiani, V. L. Popov, and D. H. Walker. 1995. Isolation and characterization of a new strain of *Ehrlichia chaffeensis* from a patient with nearly fatal monocytic ehrlichiosis. *J. Clin. Microbiol.* **33:**1704–1711.

33. Dumler, J. S., J. E. Dawson, and D. H. Walker. 1993. Human ehrlichiosis: hematopathology and immunohistologic detection of *Ehrlichia chaffeensis. Hum. Pathol.* **24:**391–396.

34. Dumler, J. S., W. L. Sutker, and D. H. Walker. 1993. Persistent infection with *Ehrlichia chaffeensis. Clin. Infect. Dis.* **17:**903–905.

35. Dumler, J. S., A. F. Barbet, C. P. J. Bekker, G. A. Dasch, G. H. Palmer, S. C. Ray, Y. Rikihisa, and F. R. Rurangirwa. 2001. Reorganization of genera in the families *Rickettsiaceae* and *Anaplasmataceae* in the order *Rickettsiales*: unification of some species of *Ehrlichia* with *Anaplasma, Cowdria* with *Ehrlichia*, and *Ehrlichia* with *Neorickettsia*, designation of six new species combinations and designation of *Ehrlichia equi* and "HGE agent" as subjective synonyms of *Ehrlichia phagocytophila. Int. J. Syst. Evol. Microbiol.* **51:**2145–2165.

36. Dunn, B. E., T. P. Monson, J. S. Dumler, C. C. Morris, A. B. Westbrook, J. L. Duncan, J. E. Dawson, K. G. Sims, and B. E. Anderson. 1992. Identification of *Ehrlichia chaffeensis* morulae in cerebrospinal fluid mononuclear cells. *J. Clin. Microbiol.* **30:**2207–2210.

37. Edelman, D. C., and J. S. Dumler. 1996. Evaluation of an improved PCR diagnostic assay for human granulocytic ehrlichiosis. *Mol. Diagnosis* **1:**41–49.

38. Egenvall, A., B. N. Bonnett, A. Gunnarsson, A. Hedhammar, M. Shoukri, S. Bornstein, and K. Artursson. 2000. Seroprevalence of granulocytic *Ehrlichia* spp. and *Borrelia burgdorferi* sensu lato in Swedish dogs 1991–94. *Scand. J. Infect. Dis.* **32:**19–25.

39. Everett, E. D., K. A. Evans, R. B. Henry, and G. McDonald. 1994. Human ehrlichiosis in adults after tick exposure: diagnosis using polymerase chain reaction. *Ann. Intern. Med.* **120:**730–735.

40. **Ewing, S. A., W. R. Roberson, R. G. Buckner, and C. S. Hayat.** 1971. A new strain of *Ehrlichia canis*. *J. Am. Vet. Med. Assoc.* **159:**1771–1774.

41. **Fichtenbaum, C. J., L. R. Peterson, and G. J. Weil.** 1993. Ehrlichiosis presenting as a life-threatening illness with features of the toxic shock syndrome. *Am. J. Med.* **95:** 351–357.

42. **Fish, D.** 1995. Environmental risk and prevention of Lyme disease. *Am. J. Med.* **98:**2S–8S.

43. **Fishbein, D. B., J. E. Dawson, and L. E. Robinson.** 1994. Human ehrlichiosis in the United States, 1985 to 1990. *Ann. Intern. Med.* **120:**736–743.

44. **Foggie, A.** 1951. Studies on the infectious agent of tick-borne fever in sheep. *J. Pathol. Bacteriol.* **63:**1–15.

45. **Goodman, J. L., C. Nelson, B. Vitale, J. S. Dumler, J. E. Madigan, T. J. Kurtti, and U. G. Munderloh.** 1996. Direct cultivation of the causative agent of human granulocytic ehrlichiosis. *N. Engl. J. Med.* **334:**209–215.

46. **Hardalo, C., V. Quagliarello, and J. S. Dumler.** 1995. Human granulocytic ehrlichiosis in Connecticut: report of a fatal case. *Clin. Infect. Dis.* **21:**910–914.

47. **Heimer, R., D. Tisdale, and J. E. Dawson.** 1998. A single tissue culture system for the propagation of the agents of the human ehrlichioses. *Am. J. Trop. Med. Hyg.* **58:**812–815.

48. **Heimer, R., A. Van Andel, G. P. Wormser, and M. L. Wilson.** 1997. Propagation of granulocytic *Ehrlichia* spp. from human and equine sources in HL-60 cells induced to differentiate into functional granulocytes. *J. Clin. Microbiol.* **35:**923–927.

49. **Holland, C. J., E. Weiss, W. Burgdorfer, A. I. Cole, and I. Kakoma.** 1985. *Ehrlichia risticii* sp. nov.: etiologic agent of equine monocytic ehrlichiosis (synonym, Potomac horse fever). *Int. J. Syst. Bacteriol.* **35:**524–526.

50. **Horowitz, H. W., M. E. Aguero-Rosenfeld, D. F. Mc-Kenna, D. Holmgren, T.-C. Hsieh, S. A. Varde, S. J. Dumler, J. M. Wu, I. Schwartz, Y. Rikihisa, and G. P. Wormser.** 1998. Clinical and laboratory spectrum of culture-proven granulocytic ehrlichiosis: comparison with culture-negative cases. *Clin. Infect. Dis.* **27:**1314–1317.

51. **Horowitz, H. W., E. Kilchevsky, S. Haber, M. Aguero-Rosenfeld, R. Kranwinkel, E. K. James, S. J. Wong, F. Chu, D. Liveris, and I. Schwartz.** 1998. Perinatal transmission of the agent of human granulocytic ehrlichiosis. *N. Engl. J. Med.* **339:**375–378.

52. **Horowitz, H. W., T.-C. Hsieh, M. E. Aguero-Rosenfeld, F. Kalantarpour, I. Chowdhury, G. P. Wormser, and J. Wu.** 2001. Antimicrobial susceptibility of *Ehrlichia phagocytophila*. *Antimicrob. Agents Chemother.* **45:**786–788.

53. **Hossain, D., M. E. Aguero-Rosenfeld, H. W. Horowitz, J. M. Wu, T.-C. Hsieh, N. Sachdeva, S. J. Peterson, J. S. Dumler, and G. P. Wormser.** 1999. Clinical and laboratory evolution of a culture-confirmed case of human granulocytic ehrlichiosis. *Connect. Med.* **63:**265–270.

54. **Huchzermeyer, F. W., I. G. Horak, J. F. Putterill, and R. A. Earle.** 1992. Description of *Aegyptianella botuliformis* n. sp. (*Rickettsiales: Anaplasmataceae*) from the helmeted guineafowl, *Numida meleagris*. *Onderstepoort J. Vet. Res.* **59:**97–101.

55. **IJdo, J. W., Y. Zhang, E. Hodzic, L. A. Magnarelli, M. L. Wilson, S. R. Telford III, S. W. Barthold, and E. Fikrig.** 1997. The early humoral response in human granulocytic ehrlichiosis. *J. Infect. Dis.* **176:**687–692.

56. **Iqbal, Z., and Y. Rikihisa.** 1994. Reisolation of *Ehrlichia canis* from blood and tissues of dogs after doxycycline treatment. *J. Clin. Microbiol.* **32:**1644–1649.

57. **Jongejan, F., L. A. Wassink, M. J. C. Thielemans, N. M. Perie, and G. Uilenberg.** 1989. Serotypes in *Cowdria ruminantium* and their relationship with *Ehrlichia phagocy-tophila* determined by immunofluorescence. *Vet. Microbiol.* **21:**31–40.

58. **Kalantarpour, F., I. Chowdhury, G. P. Wormser, and M. E. Aguero-Rosenfeld.** 2000. Survival of the human granulocytic (HGE) agent under refrigeration conditions. *J. Clin. Microbiol.* **38:**2398–2399.

59. **Klein, M. B., C. M. Nelson, and J. L. Goodman.** 1997. Antibiotic susceptibility of the newly cultivated agent of human granulocytic ehrlichiosis: promising activity of quinolones and rifamycins. *Antimicrob. Agents Chemother.* **41:**76–79.

60. **Kocan, K. M.** 1995. Targeting ticks for control of selected hemoparasitic diseases of cattle. *Vet. Parasitol.* **57:**121–151.

61. **Levin, M. L., and D. Fish.** 2000. Immunity reduces reservoir host competence of *Peromyscus leucopus* for *Ehrlichia phagocytophila*. *Infect. Immun.* **68:**1514–1518.

62. **Lockhart, J. M., W. R. Davidson, D. E. Stallknecht, J. E. Dawson, and E. W. Howerth.** 1997. Isolation of *Ehrlichia chaffeensis* from wild white-tailed deer (*Odocoileus virginianus*) confirms their role as natural reservoir hosts. *J. Clin. Microbiol.* **35:**1681–1686.

63. **MacLeod, J. R., and W. S. Gordon.** 1933. Studies in tick-borne fever of sheep. Transmission by the tick, *Ixodes ricinus*, with a description of the disease produced. *Parasitology* **25:**273–285.

64. **Madigan, J. E., and D. Gribble.** 1987. Equine ehrlichiosis in northern California: 49 cases (1968–1981). *J. Am. Vet. Med. Assoc.* **190:**445–448.

65. **Madigan, J. E., N. Pusterla, E. Johnson, J.-S. Chae, J. Berger Pusterla, E. DeRock, and S. P. Lawler.** 2000. Transmission of *Ehrlichia risticii*, the agent of Potomac horse fever, using naturally infected aquatic insects and helminth vectors: preliminary report. *Equine Vet. J.* **32:** 275–279.

66. **Madigan, J. E., P. J. Richter, R. B. Kimsey, J. E. Barlough, J. S. Bakken, and J. S. Dumler.** 1995. Transmission and passage in horses of the agent of human granulocytic ehrlichiosis. *J. Infect. Dis.* **172:**1141–1144.

67. **Maeda, K., N. Markowitz, R. C. Hawley, M. Ristic, D. Cox, and J. McDade.** 1987. Human infection with *Ehrlichia canis*, a leukocytic rickettsia. *N. Engl. J. Med.* **316:** 853–856.

68. **Magnarelli, L. A., J. S. Dumler, and J. F. Anderson.** 1995. Coexistence of antibodies to tick-borne pathogens of babesiosis, ehrlichiosis, and Lyme borreliosis in human sera. *J. Clin. Microbiol.* **33:**3054–3057.

69. **Marty, A. M., J. S. Dumler, G. Imes, H. P. Brusman, L. L. Smrkovski, and D. M. Frisman.** 1995. Ehrlichiosis mimicking thrombotic thrombocytopenic purpura. Case report and pathological correlation. *Hum. Pathol.* **26:**920–925.

70. **McQuiston, J. H., C. D. Paddock, R. C. Holman, and J. E. Childs.** 1999. The human ehrlichioses in the United States. *Emerg. Infect. Dis.* **5:**635–642.

71. **Misao, T., and Y. Kobayashi.** 1954. Studies on infectious mononucleosis. I. Isolation of etiologic agent from blood, bone marrow, and lymph node of a patient with infectious mononucleosis by using mice. *Tokyo Iji Shinshi* **71:**683–686.

72. **Murphy, C. I., J. R. Storey, J. Recchia, L. A. Doros-Richert, C. Gingrich-Baker, K. Munroe, J. S. Bakken, R. T. Coughlin, and G. A. Beltz.** 1998. Major antigenic proteins of the agent of human granulocytic ehrlichiosis are encoded by members of a multigene family. *Infect. Immun.* **66:**3711–3718.

73. **Nadelman, R. B., H. W. Horowitz, T.-C. Hsieh, J. M. Wu, M. Aguero-Rosenfeld, L. Schwartz, J. Nowakowski, S. Varde, and G. P. Wormser.** 1997. Simulta-

neous human granulocytic ehrlichiosis and Lyme borreliosis. *N. Engl. J. Med.* **337:**27–30.

74. Nicholson, W. L., J. A. Comer, J. W. Sumner, C. Gingrich-Baker, R. T. Coughlin, L. A. Magnarelli, J. G. Olson, and J. E. Childs. 1997. An indirect immunofluorescent assay using a cell culture-derived antigen for detection of antibodies to the agent of human granulocytic ehrlichiosis. *J. Clin. Microbiol.* **35:**1510–1516.

75. Paddock, C. D., D. P. Suchard, K. L. Grumbach, W. K. Hadley, R. L. Kerschmann, N. W. Abbey, J. E. Dawson, B. E. Anderson, K. G. Sims, J. S. Dumler, and B. G. Herndier. 1993. Fatal seronegative ehrlichiosis in a patient with HIV infection. *N. Engl. J. Med.* **329:**1164–1167.

76. Paddock, C. D., J. W. Sumner, G. M. Shore, D. C. Bartley, R. C. Elie, J. G. McQuade, C. R. Martin, C. S. Goldsmith, and J. E. Childs. 1997. Isolation and characterization of *Ehrlichia chaffeensis* strains from patients with fatal ehrlichiosis. *J. Clin. Microbiol.* **35:**2496–2502.

77. Palmer, G. H., W. C. Brown, and F. R. Rurangirwa. 2000. Antigenic variation in the persistence and transmission of the ehrlichia *Anaplasma marginale. Microb. Infect.* **2:**167–176.

78. Pancholi, P., C. P. Kolbert, P. D. Mitchell, K. D. Reed, J. S. Dumler, J. S. Bakken, S. R. Telford III, and D. H. Persing. 1995. *Ixodes dammini* as a potential vector of human granulocytic ehrlichiosis. *J. Infect. Dis.* **172:**1007–1012.

79. Perez, M., Y. Rikihisa, and B. Wen. 1996. *Ehrlichia canis*-like agent isolated from a man in Venezuela: antigenic and genetic characterization. *J. Clin. Microbiol.* **34:**2133–2139.

80. Petrovec, M., S. L. Furlan, T. A. Zupanc, F. Strle, P. Brouqui, V. Roux, and J. S. Dumler. 1997. Human disease in Europe caused by a granulocytic *Ehrlichia. J. Clin. Microbiol.* **35:**1556–1559.

81. Popov, V. L., S.-M. Chen, H.-M. Feng, and D. H. Walker. 1995. Ultrastructural variation of cultured *Ehrlichia chaffeensis. J. Med. Microbiol.* **43:**411–421.

82. Ravyn, M. D., J. L. Goodman, C. B. Kodner, D. K. Westad, L. A. Coleman, S. M. Engstrom, C. M. Nelson, and R. C. Johnson. 1998. Immunodiagnosis of human granulocytic ehrlichiosis by using culture-derived human isolates. *J. Clin. Microbiol.* **36:**1480–1488.

83. Richter, P. J., R. B. Kimsey, J. E. Madigan, et al. 1996. *Ixodes pacificus* as a vector of *Ehrlichia equi. J. Med. Entomol.* **33:**1–5.

84. Rikihisa, Y. 1991. The tribe *Ehrlichieae* and ehrlichial diseases. *Clin. Microbiol. Rev.* **4:**286–308.

85. Rikihisa, Y., N. Zhi, G. P. Wormser, B. Wen, H. W. Horowitz, and K. E. Hechemy. 1997. Ultrastructural and antigenic characterization of a granulocytic ehrlichiosis agent directly isolated and stably cultivated from a patient in New York State. *J. Infect. Dis.* **175:**210–213.

86. Roland, W. E., G. McDonald, C. W. Cauldwell, and E. D. Everett. 1995. Ehrlichiosis—a cause of prolonged fever. *Clin. Infect. Dis.* **20:**821–825.

87. Silverstein, A. M. 1998. On the naming of Rickettsia after Paul Ehrlich. *Bull. Hist. Med.* **72:**731–733.

88. Smith, R. D., D. M. Sells, E. H. Stephenson, M. Ristic, and D. L. Huxsoll. 1997. Development of *Ehrlichia canis*, causative agent of canine ehrlichiosis, in the tick *Rhipicephalus sanguineus* and its differentiation from a symbiotic rickettsia. *Am. J. Vet. Res.* **37:**119–126.

89. Standaert, S. M., J. E. Dawson, W. Schaffner, J. E. Childs, K. L. Biggie, J. Singleton, Jr., R. R. Gerhardt, M. L. Knight, and R. H. Hutcheson. 1995. Ehrlichiosis in a golf-oriented retirement community. *N. Engl. J. Med.* **333:**420–425.

90. Standaert, S. M., T. Yu, M. A. Scott, J. E. Childs, C. D. Paddock, W. L. Nicholson, J. Singleton, Jr., and M. J. Blaser. 2000. Primary isolation of *Ehrlichia chaffeensis* from patients with febrile illnesses: clinical and molecular characteristics. *J. Infect. Dis.* **181:**1082–1088.

91. Suksawat, J., B. C. Hegarty, and E. B. Breitschwerdt. 2000. Seroprevalence of *Ehrlichia canis, Ehrlichia equi*, and *Ehrlichia risticii* in sick dogs from North Carolina and Virginia. *J. Vet. Intern. Med.* **14:**50–55.

92. Sumner, J. W., W. L. Nicholson, and R. F. Massung. 1997. PCR amplification and comparison of nucleotide sequences from the *groESL* heat shock operon of *Ehrlichia* species. *J. Clin. Microbiol.* **35:**2087–2092.

93. Sumner, J. W., K. G. Sims, D. C. Jones, and B. E. Anderson. 1993. *Ehrlichia chaffeensis* expresses an immunoreactive protein homologous to the *Escherichia coli* GroEL protein. *Infect. Immun.* **61:**3536–3539.

94. Sumption, K. J., D. J. M. Wright, S. J. Cutler, and B. A. S. Dale. 1995. Human ehrlichiosis in the UK. *Lancet* **346:**1487–1488.

95. Tajima, T., N. Zhi, Q. Lin, Y. Rikihisa, H. W. Horowitz, J. T. Raffalli, G. P. Wormser, and K. E. Hechemy. 2000. Comparison of two recombinant major outer membrane proteins of the human granulocytic ehrlichiosis agent for use in an enzyme-linked immunosorbent assay. *Clin. Diagn. Lab. Immunol.* **7:**652–657.

96. Taylor, M. J., and A. Hoerauf. 1999. *Wolbachia* bacteria of filarial nematodes. *Parasitol. Today* **15:**437–442.

97. Telford, S. R., III, J. E. Dawson, P. Katavolos, C. K. Warner, C. P. Kolbert, and D. H. Persing. 1996. Perpetuation of the agent of human granulocytic ehrlichiosis in a deer tick-rodent cycle. *Proc. Natl. Acad. Sci. USA* **93:**6209–6214.

98. Walker, D. H., and J. S. Dumler. 1996. Emergence of ehrlichioses as human health problems. *Emerg. Infect. Dis.* **2:**18–29.

99. Walker, D. H., and J. S. Dumler. 1997. Human monocytic and granulocytic ehrlichioses. Discovery and diagnosis of emerging tick-borne infections and the critical role of the pathologist. *Arch. Pathol. Lab. Med.* **121:**785–791.

100. Walls, J. J., B. Greig, D. S. Neitzel, and J. S. Dumler. 1997. Natural infection of small mammal species in Minnesota with the agent of human granulocytic ehrlichiosis. *J. Clin. Microbiol.* **35:**853–855.

101. Walls, J. J., M. E. Aguero-Rosenfeld, J. S. Bakken, J. L. Goodman, D. Hossain, R. C. Johnson, and J. S. Dumler. 1999. Inter- and intralaboratory comparison of *Ehrlichia equi* and human granulocytic ehrlichiosis (HGE) agent strains for serodiagnosis of HGE by the immunofluorescent-antibody test. *J. Clin. Microbiol.* **37:**2968–2973.

102. Weiss, E., and J. W. Moulder. 1984. The rickettsias and chlamydias, p. 687–739. *In* N. R. Krieg and J. G. Holt (ed.), *Bergey's Manual of Determinative Bacteriology*, vol. 1. Williams & Wilkins, Baltimore, Md.

103. Weiss, E., J. C. Williams, G. A. Dasch, and Y.-H. Kang. 1989. Energy metabolism of monocytic *Ehrlichia. Proc. Natl. Acad. Sci. USA* **86:**1674–1678.

104. Wong, S. J., G. S. Brady, and J. S. Dumler. 1997. Serological responses to *Ehrlichia equi, Ehrlichia chaffeensis*, and *Borrelia burgdorferi* in patients from New York state. *J. Clin. Microbiol.* **35:**2198–2205.

105. Wong, S. J., and J. A. Thomas. 1998. Cytoplasmic, nuclear, and platelet autoantibodies in human granulocytic ehrlichiosis patients. *J. Clin. Microbiol.* **36:**1953–1959.

106. Wormser, G., D. McKenna, M. Aguero-Rosenfeld, H. Horowitz, J. Munoz, J. Nowakowski, G. Gerina, P. Welch, H. Moorjani, T. Rush, G. Jacquette, A. Stan-

key, R. Falco, M. Rapoport, D. Ackman, J. Talarico, D. White, L. Frielander, R. Gallo, G. Brady, M. Mauer, S. Wong, R. Duncan, L. Kingsley, R. Taylor, G. Birkhead, D. Morse, and J. S. Dumler. 1995. Human granulocytic ehrlichiosis—New York. *Morb. Mortal. Wkly. Rep.* **44:**593–595.

107. **Wormser, G. P., H. W. Horowitz, J. Nowakowski, D. McKenna, J. S. Dumler, S. Varde, I. Schwartz, C. Carbonaro, and M. Aguero-Rosenfeld.** 1997. Positive Lyme disease serology in patients with clinical and laboratory evidence of human granulocytic ehrlichiosis. *Am. J. Clin. Pathol.* **107:**142–147.

108. **Yu, X., P. Brouqui, J. S. Dumler, and D. Raoult.** 1993. Detection of *Ehrlichia chaffeensis* in human tissue by using a species-specific monoclonal antibody. *J. Clin. Microbiol.* **31:**3284–3288.

109. **Yu, X.-J., P. Crocquet-Valdes, L. C. Cullman, and D. H. Walker.** 1996. The recombinant 120-kilodalton protein of *Ehrlichia chaffeensis*, a potential diagnostic tool. *J. Clin. Microbiol.* **34:**2853–2855.

110. **Yu, X.-J., P. Crocquet-Valdes, and D. H. Walker.** 1997. Cloning and sequencing of the gene for a 120-kDa immunodominant protein of *Ehrlichia chaffeensis*. *Gene* **184:**149–154.

111. **Yu, X., J. F. Piesman, J. G. Olson, and D. H. Walker.** 1997. Geographic distribution of different genetic types of *Ehrlichia chaffeensis*. *Am. J. Trop. Med. Hyg.* **56:**679–680.

112. **Zhi, N., N. Ohashi, Y. Rikihisa, H. W. Horowitz, G. P. Wormser, and K. E. Hechemy.** 1998. Cloning and expression of the 44-kilodalton major outer membrane protein gene of the human granulocytic ehrlichiosis agent and application of the recombinant protein to serodiagnosis. *J. Clin. Microbiol.* **36:**1666–1673.

113. **Zhi, N., Y. Rikihisa, H. Y. Kim, G. P. Wormser, and H. W. Horowitz.** 1997. Comparison of major antigenic proteins of six strains of the human granulocytic ehrlichiosis agent by Western immunoblot analysis. *J. Clin. Microbiol.* **35:**2606–2611.

Coxiella

PHILIPPE BROUQUI, THOMAS J. MARRIE, AND DIDIER RAOULT

66

TAXONOMY

Coxiella burnetii has been placed in the subdivision of the class *Proteobacteria*, close to *Rickettsiella grylli*, *Legionella* spp., and *Francisella* spp., on the basis of comparison of the 16S rRNA gene sequences.

DESCRIPTION OF THE GENUS

C. burnetii is a pleomorphic coccobacillus with a gram-negative cell wall (3). It is an obligate intracellular microorganism measuring 0.2 by 0.7 μm. It does not stain with Gram stain but does stain with Giménez stain. It undergoes a developmental cycle in which there are both a large-cell and small-cell variants (41). The small-cell variant attaches to the host cell (usually a macrophage) and is ingested. *C. burnetii* develops within the phagolysosome, where the acidic pH activates its metabolic enzymes. Following maturation to the large-cell variant, sporogenesis begins (41). Spore formation explains why *C. burnetii* is so successful as a pathogen. It can survive in the environment for up to 10 months at 15 to 20°C, for more than 1 month on meat in cold storage, and for more than 40 months in skim milk at room temperature (5). *C. burnetii* was recently shown to survive in free-living amoebae, suggesting a possible alternate mechanism to explain the survival and resistance of the pathogen in the environment (Fig. 1) (33).

C. *burnetii* undergoes phase variation akin to the smooth-to-rough transition of lipopolysaccharides of gram-negative bacteria (67). In nature and in laboratory animals, it exists in the phase I state, in which the organisms react with late-convalescent-phase (45 days) guinea pig sera and only slightly with early-convalescent-phase (21 days) sera (67). Apparently phase II is a deletion mutant of phase I (70), of which the fitness, in vitro, is superior to that of phase I. After numerous passages in cell culture or embryonated eggs, truncation of the lipopolysaccharide occurs, yielding the antigenic form, phase II.

NATURAL HABITATS

C. burnetii, the cause of Q fever, has been identified in arthropods, fish, birds, rodents, marsupials, and livestock (2). Indeed, it naturally infects more than 40 species (including 12 genera) of ticks on five continents (3). However, for unknown reasons, *C. burnetii* transmission to humans via tick bites has seldom been reported and is probably very rare (10). Lice, mites, and parasitic flukes are also infected (44). Bandicoots, rats, rabbits, mice, porcupines, hedgehogs, tortoises, cattle, sheep, goats, dogs, swine, cats, camels, buffaloes, baboons, leopards, hyenas, chickens, ducks, geese, turkeys, pigeons, bats, and shrews have all been infected with this microorganism (30, 44).

The major route of transmission of Q fever to humans is by aerosol following parturition of an infected animal. Infectious particles can stick to wool and dust and can be spread by the wind to distant places. Cases of Q fever may occur miles away from lambing but in the direction that the winds blow (69). Ingestion of milk and milk products is a risk factor for transmission of Q fever (17). Raw milk from cows was considered a risk factor for Q fever in California, and the decrease in the prevalence of Q fever in this state could be partly related to cessation of the practice of drinking raw milk. The consumption of goat cheese made from raw milk was also reported as a risk factor in France (17). More recently, in Canada, an outbreak of Q fever was related to the consumption of pasteurized goat cheese (25). In an experimental animal model, the route of infection (aerosol or intraperitoneal) determined the specific organs that became infected (lung and liver, respectively) (31).

CLINICAL SIGNIFICANCE

The current understanding of the natural history of Q fever is that a nonimmune patient comes into contact with *C. burnetii*, which causes a primary infection that could be asymptomatic or symptomatic (54). The symptomatic primary infection is acute Q fever. The spontaneous evolution of acute infection is usually a complete recovery in the normal host. In immunocompromised hosts, *C. burnetii* can multiply despite an antibody response following primary infection (symptomatic or not). In these cases, because the immune system is unable to control the infection, chronic infection develops. This hypothesis is supported by all available data from humans as well as from animal models (40).

The immune control of Q fever is T-cell dependent but does not lead to *C. burnetii* eradication, and immunosuppression can induce a relapse of infection in apparently cured patients or laboratory animals (61, 62). Therefore, patients with acute Q fever who are immunocompromised

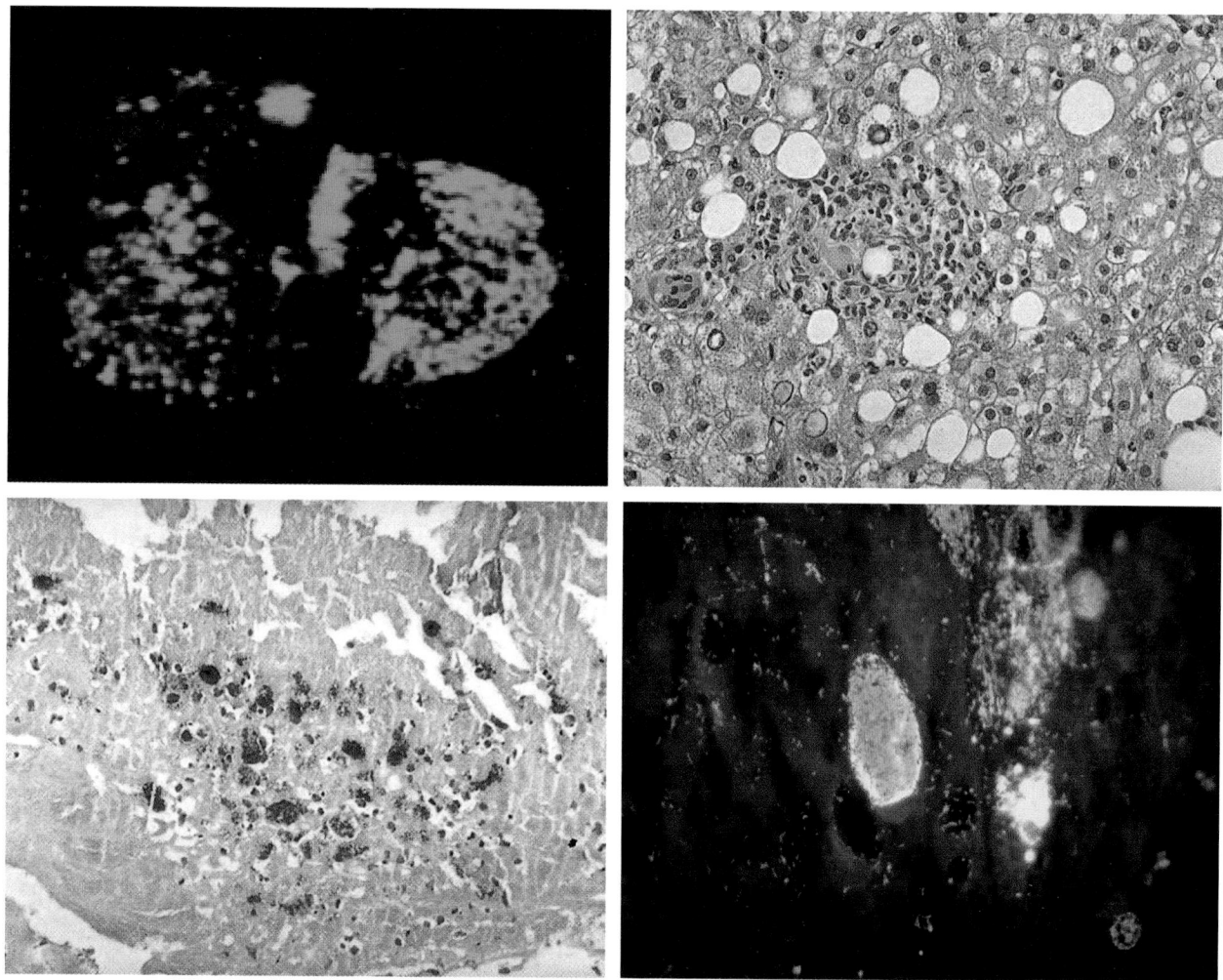

FIGURE 1 (top left)   C. *burnetii* in amoebae. Confocal microscopy of direct fluorescent-antibody stain with anti-C. *burnetii* monoclonal antibodies. Magnification, ×1,000. (Courtesy of B. La Scola, Marseille, France.)

FIGURE 2 (top right)   Hematoxylin and eosin stain of liver biopsy in a patient with acute Q fever, showing a doughnut ring granuloma. Magnification, ×400. (Courtesy of H. Lepidi, Marseille, France.)

FIGURE 3 (bottom left)   Alkaline phosphatase immunohistochemistry on the heart valve from a patient with chronic Q fever endocarditis. C. *burnetii* microorganisms are stained pink within mononuclear cells. Magnification, ×400.

FIGURE 4 (bottom right)   Identification of C. *burnetii* in shell vial culture on day 6 by the use of a specific monoclonal antibody-based direct fluorescent-antibody test. Magnification, ×1,000.

or who have cardiac valve lesions are particularly at risk of developing chronic infection, especially endocarditis (12, 55).

The infection in humans is variable in its clinical expression, severity (varying from asymptomatic to fatal), and natural course. As an acute disease it can manifest as fever, pneumonia, hepatitis, exanthema, myocarditis, pericarditis, meningitis, or encephalitis. In some hosts, acute infection precedes chronic infection; stillbirth or prematurity can result if the patient is pregnant at the time of the infection. Owing to the recruitment of monocytes that may contain C. *burnetii* at sites of vascular injury with inflammation, endocarditis may occur in patients with preexisting valve damage or cancer, and chronic endovascular infection may be the manifestation of chronic Q fever in patients with vascular prostheses or aneurysms (D. Raoult, Editorial, *J. Med. Microbiol.* **44**:77–78, 1996). Following primary infection, 60% of patients will seroconvert without clinical manifestations and only 2% will be hospitalized. A chronic infection develops in fewer than 1% of acutely infected patients and is often associated with a subtle and unique immune defect (40).

Acute Q Fever

The onset is usually abrupt, and patients present with high fever (91%), headaches (51%), myalgias (37%), arthralgias

(29%), and cough (34%) and less frequently with a rash (11%) or a meningeal syndrome (4%). Laboratory investigations show thrombocytopenia (35%), elevated liver enzyme levels (62%), and an elevated erythrocyte sedimentation rate (55%). The chest X ray is abnormal in 27% of patients (55). The clinical presentation varies from country to country in that one of the three major manifestations dominates: isolated fever, hepatitis, or pneumonia. No clear reason for such variations has been identified. Four hypotheses have been proposed: a specific local predominance of a clinical form, strain variability, route of infection, and host specificity.

Clinically isolated fever, without pneumonia or hepatitis, is usually associated with severe headache, and in some patients it persists long enough to meet the criteria for fever of unknown etiology. Pneumonia is the major clinical presentation of Q fever in Nova Scotia (Canada), the Basque country (Spain), and the United Kingdom. Hepatitis is the most common form worldwide including in France and Australia. Usually hepatitis is detected by increased liver enzyme levels; however, a few patients present with jaundice and/or hepatomegaly. Liver biopsy shows inflammatory granulomas, typically organized in the form of a "doughnut"; i.e., the granuloma contains a central lipid vacuole surrounded by a fibrinoid ring (40) (Fig. 2). Neurological manifestations of Q fever, which occur in 1% of large series, include meningitis, meningoencephalitis, and peripheral neuropathy (7). Cardiac involvement occurs in 2% of acutely ill patients. This includes myocarditis, which led to death in two of the eight patients reported to date (20), and pericarditis, which is frequent but nonspecific. C. burnetii has recently been demonstrated to be the most frequently identified cause of pericarditis in Marseille (34), and it is a major cause of pericarditis in Spain and England. Ten percent of persons with Q fever pericarditis develop chronic pericarditis and have recurrences for unidentified reasons.

Chronic fatigue following acute Q fever has been described in Australia and the United Kingdom (1, 46). It was reported that 20% of patients with post-Q fever fatigue syndrome have moderate cytokine dysregulation (46). Q fever in immunocompromised hosts has been reported in patients with cancer (48) as well as in those with human immunodeficiency virus (HIV) infection (53). Twenty-three cases of Q fever during pregnancy have been reported (66). Most of these patients had complications including fetal or newborn death (11 cases) and premature birth (7 cases); only 5 had a normal pregnancy. Half of infected women develop a serological profile of chronic Q fever during pregnancy, and, as in other mammals, C. burnetii can be isolated from milk, placenta, and vaginal discharge. Multiple premature births have been reported in such cases (66), and these patients should probably receive prolonged treatment to eradicate the bacteria because they are subject to relapses during subsequent pregnancies. Patients with a valve lesion, arterial aneurysm, or prosthesis who have an episode of acute Q fever are at very high risk for chronic infection (55). Of acutely infected patients with a preexisting valvulopathy, 38% develop endocarditis within 2 years (12).

Chronic Q Fever

The major clinical form of chronic Q fever is endocarditis. A minimum of 800 cases were reported from 1949 to 2000 (55, 63). In France, Q fever causes 5% of endocarditis cases, with an estimated prevalence of 1 per 10^6 inhabitants per year, which is close to what has been observed in Israel and Switzerland. The clinical presentation of patients with Q fever endocarditis varies according to the length of delay in diagnosis (50). Patients are usually afebrile or have low-grade intermittent fever. Echocardiography is frequently inconclusive and fails to reveal vegetations, so that the diagnosis of endocarditis is easily missed. A clue to the diagnosis is presence of a known valve lesion and unexplained illness (fever, hepatitis, weakness, digital clubbing, weight loss, stroke, or renal insufficiency), an elevated erythrocyte sedimentation rate, increased serum transaminase levels, or thrombocytopenia. In such cases, positive Q fever serology complements the diagnosis made using the modified Duke Criteria (18). Vascular infection is the second most commonly identified manifestation of chronic Q fever. We have diagnosed 25 cases in our laboratory (19, 55), and 6 more were reported from other centers including England, the United States, Switzerland, and Australia (9, 11, 13, 42). Other manifestations of chronic Q fever include osteomyelitis (6), chronic hepatitis in patients with alcoholism (55), pseudotumor of the spleen, inflammatory pseudotumor of the lung, and infection of ventriculoperitoneal drains (35). Recently, a case of vasculitis and pulmonary amyloidoisis (29) followed acute Q fever and resulted in death.

COLLECTION, TRANSPORT, AND STORAGE OF SPECIMENS

Biosafety level 2 practice and facilities are recommended for nonpropagative laboratory procedures, including serological examinations and staining of impression smears. Biosafety level 3 practices and facilities are recommended for activities involving the inoculation, incubation, and harvesting of cell cultures, the necropsy of infected animals, and the manipulation of infected tissues (Centers for Disease Control and Prevention website on biosafety in laboratories when handling C. burnetii: http://www.cdc.gov/od/ohs/biosfty/bmbl4/bmbl4toc.htm). Consequently, although C. burnetii can be isolated from blood and a variety of tissues, this is not feasible in most laboratories. Since the organism can withstand very harsh environmental conditions, it is unlikely that it will die during transport to a suitable laboratory. Blood should be collected in tubes containing EDTA or sodium citrate (heparin interferes with PCR), and the leukocyte layer should be saved for PCR. Solid specimens should be frozen at −80°C until cultured. Most laboratories will depend on serological techniques to diagnose C. burnetii infection. For the diagnosis of acute Q fever, it is best that acute- and convalescent-phase serum samples collected 2 to 4 weeks apart be tested. Serum samples from patients with Q fever present no hazard to laboratory workers when handled using standard biosafety level 2 precautions.

LABORATORY DIAGNOSIS

General approaches to the laboratory diagnosis of C. burnetii infection include direct detection of C. burnetii in tissue, isolation of C. burnetii from blood or from tissue, and serological tests for the detection of antibodies to C. burnetii phase I and phase II antigens.

Direct Detection

C. burnetii can be identified in tissues by a direct immunofluorescence technique. This is of limited utility for the routine diagnosis of *C. burnetii* since, with the exception of heart valve tissue from patients with Q fever endocarditis (4), tissue specimens from patients with acute Q fever are not generally submitted to the laboratory. The main reason for this is that the illness is mild to moderate in severity and death is extremely unusual. However, patients with Q fever endocarditis do have large numbers of *C. burnetii* organisms in the affected valvular tissue. These can be demonstrated by direct immunofluorescence (52) or electron microscopy. Other techniques that can be used to detect *C. burnetii* in tissues include immunoperoxidase immunohistology (4) (Fig. 3) and capture enzyme-linked immunosorbent assays (ELISAs) or enzyme-linked immunofluorescence assays (68). Monoclonal antibodies used in some of these methods are not commercially available and are used predominantly in reference and research laboratories.

PCR has been successfully used to detect DNA in cell cultures and clinical samples (65). Initially, PCR methods used specific hybridization of labeled DNA probes to nucleic acids amplified from clinical samples (22). Several genes have since been used to generate specific primers, including 16S rRNA, 23S rRNA, superoxide dismutase, plasmid-based sequences, and the IS*1111* multicopy insertion sequence (21). The availability of *C. burnetii*-specific primers has allowed the development of a simple and reliable method for the detection of this bacterium, even in paraffin-embedded tissues (64). Furthermore, PCR has proven to be more sensitive than standard culture techniques for retrospective diagnosis from frozen samples and for the follow-up of patients treated for chronic Q fever (65). The amplification of *C. burnetii* DNA from serum samples is less reproducible, and we have failed to reproduce in our laboratory published results from other centers (21). Recently, a TaqMan-based PCR has been used to detect a small amount of *C. burnetii* DNA in bone marrow (24).

Isolation Procedures

Isolation of *C. burnetii* must be done only in a biosafety level 3 containment facility due to its extreme infectivity. This microorganism can be isolated by inoculation of specimens into conventional cell cultures (e.g., Vero cells) (57), embryonated egg yolk sacs (45), or laboratory animals such as mice or guinea pigs (26). The spleen of the inoculated animal is the most useful organ for the recovery of *C. burnetii*. Ground spleen extracts (0.2 to 0.5 ml of a 10% suspension) should be inoculated into embryonated eggs, which die 7 to 9 days later. These methods are used infrequently, but inoculation of animals remains helpful when the organism must be isolated from tissues contaminated with multiple bacteria or in order to obtain phase I *C. burnetii* antigens from phase II cells.

The adaptation of a viral shell vial culture system using human embryonic lung fibroblasts (HEL cells) has improved the isolation of intracellular bacteria, especially *C. burnetii* (36, 56, 57). Plasma and buffy coat from heparinized blood are diluted 1:2 with Eagle's minimal essential medium (EMEM). Tissue specimens are homogenized in sterile phosphate-buffered saline (PBS) and diluted 1:2 in EMEM. Shell vials containing 12-mm-diameter round glass coverslips are seeded with 50,000 HEL cells in 1 ml of EMEM containing 10% fetal calf serum. The cells are incubated for 3 days at 37°C in an atmosphere containing 5% CO_2 until the monolayer is confluent. Then 1 ml of each homogenized specimen is placed into each of three shell vials. A 1-h centrifugation step (700 × g at 23°C) enhances the attachment and penetration of the bacteria into the cells.

The supernatant is removed, and the monolayer is washed twice with PBS. Then 1 ml of EMEM containing 10% fetal calf serum is added to each vial. After an incubation period of 6 days, *C. burnetii* organisms are visualized as short rods by microscopic examination after staining. They are not stained by the Gram stain method but are visible with Giménez stain (24). The presence of *C. burnetii* within the cells is confirmed by an indirect immunofluorescence assay with polyclonal or monoclonal anti-*C. burnetii* antibodies (Fig. 4) (56, 57). Positive cultures are passaged in cells several times to establish the isolated strain.

Serological Tests

The microagglutination test (16, 44), the complement fixation test (14), the indirect immunofluorescent-antibody (IFA) test (14, 43), and ELISA (71) have been used for the serological diagnosis of *C. burnetii* infection.

The IFA test is the serological test of choice for the diagnosis of both acute and chronic Q fever. It is carried out by the procedure of Philip et al. (47) with purified whole-cell antigens at a concentration of 200 μg/ml. Both phase I and phase II cells are used. Each antigen (phase I and phase II cells) is diluted 1:2 with a normal yolk sac (alternatively, serum samples can be diluted in PBS with 3% nonfat powdered milk to avoid nonspecific binding), spotted onto slides, air dried, and fixed in acetone for 15 min at room temperature (approximately 20°C). Each serum sample is diluted in twofold serial dilutions from 1:8 to 1:64 for screening for the presence of antibody. Serum dilutions are added to each antigen spot and incubated in a moist chamber for 1 h at room temperature. Known positive and negative control serum samples are included with each test. Slides are then rinsed three times with PBS before being incubated with a 1:75 dilution of fluorescein isothiocyanate-conjugated antihuman polyvalent (α, γ, or μ chain-specific) immunoglobulin or anti-immunoglobulin G (IgG), anti-IgA, or anti-IgM-specific immunoglobulin for 30 min at 37°C in a moist chamber. The slides are then washed twice in PBS, rinsed in distilled water, and blotted dry. Coverslips are mounted on the slides with glycerol mounting medium. The slides are immediately read on a microscope, with a UV light source, at a magnification of ×400. The end point is the highest dilution showing whole-cell fluorescence. If only screening dilutions are used, the titers of positive samples are then determined to the end point. All samples from a single patient should be run in parallel. The starting serum dilution to be used for testing by the IFA test depends on the level of background antibody in the test population and the antigen preparation. A starting dilution of 1:8 is generally used.

Serum samples from patients with Q fever endocarditis may cross-react with *Bartonella* spp. (32). For patients with a serological diagnosis of *Bartonella* endocarditis, serum samples should also be assayed for *C. burnetii* antibodies. Cross-reaction with other antigens is distinctly unusual. IgM and IgG antibody results can be confounded by the presence of rheumatoid factor; therefore, a rheumatoid factor absorbent is used before determination of IgM and IgG titers (8).

With experimentally infected guinea pigs, ELISA was more sensitive than the IFA test. Antibodies against phase I whole cells were detected by day 9 following infection by ELISA, by day 16 by the IFA tests, and by day 20 by the complement fixation test. The ELISA for the diagnosis of Q fever has not been standardized, rendering comparison of titers from laboratory to laboratory impossible. There are no accepted criteria for the diagnosis of acute versus chronic Q fever by this test.

The complement fixation test is not as sensitive as the IFA test. Serum samples from about 20% of patients with acute Q fever are anticomplementary (37). A prozone phenomenon may be present in serum samples from some patients with chronic Q fever that may result in a false-negative test.

ANTIBIOTIC SUSCEPTIBILITIES

Antibiotic susceptibility testing of *C. burnetii* is difficult since this organism cannot be grown in axenic medium and methods are not standardized; therefore, susceptibility testing should be conducted only in appropriately experienced reference laboratories. Three models of infection have been used: animals, chicken embryos, and cell culture.

Huebner et al. (26) developed a guinea pig model for *C. burnetii* antibiotic susceptibility testing. Although in vivo assays are very important for the testing of antibiotic activity against *C. burnetii* (39), they are very expensive and are not readily available for new antibiotics.

Antibiotic susceptibility in embryonated chicken eggs is performed by injection into the yolk sac just after inoculation of the bacteria. The mean survival time of treated eggs with respect to untreated eggs determines antibiotic efficacy (39). This method is useful for testing the bacteriostatic activities of antibiotics. Thus, Jackson (28) found that terramycin, aureomycin, and chloramphenicol were active against *C. burnetii*. Rifampin, co-trimoxazole, and tetracyclines are bacteriostatic against *C. burnetii*. Penicillin, cephalothin, cycloserine, erythromycin, chloramphenicol, and clindamycin are ineffective. Pefloxacin and ofloxacin demonstrate activity against *C. burnetii* in this model (58).

Raoult et al. developed a shell vial assay with HEL cells for assessment of the bacteriostatic effects of antibiotics against *C. burnetii* (56). Amikacin and amoxicillin were not effective, ceftriaxone and fusidic acid were inconsistently active, while co-trimoxazole, rifampin, doxycycline, tetracycline, minocycline, and clarithromycin (40), as well as sparfloxacin and the quinolones PD 127,391 and PD 131,628 (27), were bacteriostatic. Using the same technique, moxifloxacin demonstrated better activity than ofloxacin and pefloxacin (60) and telithromycin had better activity than erythromycin, with MICs of 1 and 8 μg/ml, respectively (59). Raoult et al. (49), using P388D1 and L929 cells in which multiplication of infected host cells was inhibited with cycloheximide during antibiotic challenges, showed that pefloxacin, rifampin, and doxycycline (49), as well as clarithromycin (40), are bacteriostatic. Hypothesizing that this lack of bactericidal activity was related to antibiotic inactivation by the low pH of the phagolysosomes in which *C. burnetii* is found, Raoult et al. (49) demonstrated that the addition of chloroquine, a lysosomotropic alkalinizing agent, improved the activities of doxycycline and pefloxacin, which then became bactericidal (38). Current recommendation for treatment of chronic Q fever endocarditis is at least 18 months of therapy with doxycycline (100 mg twice daily [b.i.d.]) and chloroquine (200 mg three times daily [t.i.d.]) or at least 3 years of therapy with doxycycline (100 mg b.i.d.) and ofloxacin (200 mg t.i.d.) in patients to whom the first antibiotic regimen cannot be administered (51).

INTERPRETATION AND REPORTING OF RESULTS

The diagnosis of Q fever is based predominantly on serology. Antibodies are usually detectable 2 to 4 weeks after the onset of the infection. The diagnosis of acute Q fever is confirmed by seroconversion (a fourfold or greater increase in antibody levels between acute- and convalescent [10 to 20 days later]-phase serum samples) or the presence of an IgM titer to *C. burnetii* (21).

With chronic Q fever, a single serum sample is diagnostic of both Q fever and chronic disease when high antibody titers are detected against phase I antigen. The complement fixation test lacks sensitivity and should be replaced by microimmunofluorescence, the reference method. This allows testing for antibodies to both phase I and phase II antigens and allows determination of the IgG, IgM, and IgA titers. Phase II titers of IgG and IgM of ≥200 and ≥50, respectively, are diagnostic of acute Q fever. An IgG titer of ≥1,600 against phase I and phase II antigens has a high predictive value for chronic infection (8). In this form of the disease, IgM-specific antibodies are frequently lacking and an increase in IgA antibody levels against both phases is present. To avoid false-negative and false-positive results, IgG should be removed prior to testing for IgM and IgA antibodies (8). A commercial ELISA (PanBio *Coxiella burnetii* immunoglobulin M [IgM] ELISA; QFM-200, Brisbane, Australia) has also been used in the serological diagnosis of acute Q fever, especially for the detection of IgM antibodies (15). Microimmunofluorescence serology is also convenient for the follow-up of patients with chronic infection. In patients with Q fever endocarditis, IgM antibodies, when present at the beginning of the treatment, disappear first, usually within 6 months of treatment. IgA levels decrease next, and this is followed by a decrease in the IgG titer, which never completely disappears (51).

REFERENCES

1. **Ayres, J. G., N. Flint, E. G. Smith, W. S. Tunnicliffe, T. J. Fletcher, K. Hammond, D. Ward, and B. P. Marmion.** 1998. Post-infection fatigue syndrome following Q fever. *Q. J. Med.* **91:**105–123.
2. **Babudieri, B.** 1959. Q fever: a zoonosis. *Adv. Vet. Sci.* **5:**81–182.
3. **Baca, O. G., and D. Paretsky.** 1983. Q fever and *Coxiella burnetii*: a model for host-parasite interactions. *Microbiol. Rev.* **47:**127–149.
4. **Brouqui, P., J. S. Dumler, and D. Raoult.** 1994. Immunohistologic demonstration of *Coxiella burnetii* in the valves of patients with Q fever endocarditis. *Am. J. Med.* **97:**451–458.
5. **Christie, A. B.** 1974. Q fever, p. 876–891. *In* A. B. Christie (ed.), *Infectious Diseases, Epidemiology and Clinical Practice.* Churchill Livingstone, Edinburgh, United Kingdom.
6. **Cottalorda, J., J. L. Jouve, G. Bollini, P. Touzet, A. Poujol, F. Kelberine, and D. Raoult.** 1995. Osteoarticular infection due to *Coxiella burnetii* in children. *J. Pediatr. Orthop. Ser. B* **4:**219–221.
7. **Derrick, E. H.** 1973. The course of infection with *Coxiella burnetii*. *Med. J. Aust.* **1:**1051–1057.
8. **Dupont, H. T., X. Thirion, and D. Raoult.** 1994. Q fever serology: cutoff determination for microimmunofluorescence. *Clin. Diagn. Lab. Immunol.* **1:**189–196.
9. **Duroux-Vouilloz, C., G. Praz, P. Francioli, and O. Peter.** 1998. Q fever with endocarditis: clinical presentation

and serologic follow-up of 21 patients. *Schweiz. Med. Wochenschr.* **128:**521–527. (In German.)

10. Eklund, C. M., R. R. Parker, and D. B. Lackman. 1947. A case of Q fever probably contracted by exposure to ticks in nature. *Public Health Rep.* **62:**1413–1416.

11. Ellis, M. E., C. C. Smith, and M. A. Moffat. 1983. Chronic or fatal Q-fever infection: a review of 16 patients seen in North-East Scotland (1967–80). *Q. J. Med.* **52:** 54–66.

12. Fenollar, F., P. E. Fournier, P. Carrieri, G. Habib, T. Messana, and D. Raoult. 2001. Chronic endocarditis following acute Q fever. *Clin. Infect. Dis.* **33:**312–316.

13. Fergusson, R. J., T. R. Shaw, A. H. Kitchin, M. B. Matthews, J. M. Inglis, and J. F. Peutherer. 1985. Subclinical chronic Q fever. *Q. J. Med.* **57:**669–676.

14. Field, P. R., J. G. Hunt, and A. M. Murphy. 1983. Detection and persistence of specific IgM antibody to *Coxiella burnetii* by enzyme-linked immunosorbent assay: a comparison with immunofluorescence and complement fixation tests. *J. Infect. Dis.* **148:**477–487.

15. Field, P. R., J. L. Mitchell, A. Santiago, D. J. Dickeson, S. W. Chan, D. W. Ho, A. M. Murphy, A. J. Cuzzubbo, and P. L. Devine. 2000. Comparison of a commercial enzyme-linked immunosorbent assay with immunofluorescence and complement fixation tests for detection of *Coxiella burnetii* (Q fever) immunoglobulin M. *J. Clin. Microbiol.* **38:**1645–1647.

16. Fiset, P., R. A. Ormsbee, R. Silberman, M. Peacock, and S. H. Spielman. 1969. A microagglutination technique for detection and measurement of rickettsial antibodies. *Acta Virol.* **13:**60–66.

17. Fishbein, D. B., and D. Raoult. 1992. A cluster of *Coxiella burnetii* infections associated with exposure to vaccinated goats and their unpasteurized dairy products. *Am. J. Trop. Med. Hyg.* **47:**35–40.

18. Fournier, P. E., J. P. Casalta, G. Habib, T. Messana, and D. Raoult. 1996. Modification of the diagnostic criteria proposed by the Duke Endocarditis Service to permit improved diagnosis of Q fever endocarditis. *Am. J. Med.* **100:**629–633.

19. Fournier, P. E., J. P. Casalta, P. Piquet, P. Tournigand, A. Branchereau, and D. Raoult. 1998. *Coxiella burnetii* infection of aneurysms or vascular grafts: report of seven cases and review. *Clin. Infect. Dis.* **26:**116–121.

20. Fournier, P. E., J. Etienne, J. R. Harle, G. Habib, and D. Raoult. 2001. Myocarditis, a rare but severe manifestation of Q fever: report of 8 cases and review of the literature. *Clin. Infect. Dis.* **32:**1440–1447.

21. Fournier, P. E., T. J. Marrie, and D. Raoult. 1998. Diagnosis of Q fever. *J. Clin. Microbiol.* **36:**1823–1834.

22. Frazier, M. E., R. A. Heinzen, L. P. Mallavia, and O. G. Baca. 1992. DNA probes for detecting *Coxiella burnetii* strains. *Acta Virol.* **36:**83–89.

23. Gimenez, D. F. 1964. Staining rickettsiae in yolk sac culture. *Stain Technol.* **30:**135–137.

24. Harris, R. J., P. A. Storm, A. Lloyd, M. Arens, and B. P. Marmion. 2000. Long-term persistence of *Coxiella burnetii* in the host after primary Q fever. *Epidemiol. Infect.* **124:** 543–549.

25. Hatchette, T. F., R. C. Hudson, W. F. Schlech, N. A. Campbell, J. E. Hatchette, S. Ratnam, D. Raoult, C. Donovan, and T. J. Marrie. 2001. Goat-associated Q fever: a new disease in Newfoundland. *Emerg. Infect. Dis.* **7:**413–419.

26. Huebner, R. J., G. A. Hottle, and E. B. Robinson. 1948. Action of streptomycin in experimental infection with Q fever. *Public Health Rep.* **63:**357–362.

27. Jabarit-Aldighieri, N., H. Torres, and D. Raoult. 1992. Susceptibility of *Rickettsia conorii*, *R. rickettsii*, and *Coxiella*

burnetii to PD 127,391, PD 131,628, pefloxacin, ofloxacin, and ciprofloxacin. *Antimicrob. Agents Chemother.* **36:**2529–2532.

28. Jackson, E. B. 1951. Comparative efficacy of several antibiotics on experimental rickettsial infections in embryonated eggs. *Antibiot. Chemother.* **1:**231–241.

29. Kayser, K., M. Wiebel, V. Schulz, and H. J. Gabius. 1995. Necrotizing bronchitis, angiitis, and amyloidosis associated with chronic Q fever. *Respiration* **62:**114–116.

30. Lang, G. H. 1990. Coxiellosis (Q fever) in animals, p. 24–48. *In* T. J. Marrie (ed.), *Q Fever: the Disease*. CRC Press, Inc., Boca Raton, Fla.

31. La Scola, B., H. Lepidi, and D. Raoult. 1997. Pathologic changes during acute Q fever: influence of the route of infection and inoculum size in infected guinea pigs. *Infect. Immun.* **65:**2443–2447.

32. La Scola, B., and D. Raoult. 1996. Serological cross-reactions between *Bartonella quintana*, *Bartonella henselae*, and *Coxiella burnetii*. *J. Clin. Microbiol.* **34:**2270–2274.

33. La Scola, B. L., and D. Raoult. 2001. Survival of *Coxiella burnetii* within free-living amoeba *Acanthamoeba castellanii*. *Clin. Microbiol. Infect.* **7:**75–79.

34. Levy, P. Y., P. Carrieri, and D. Raoult. 1999. *Coxiella burnetii* pericarditis: report of 15 cases and review. *Clin. Infect. Dis.* **29:**393–397.

35. Lohuis, P. J., P. C. Ligtenberg, R. J. Diepersloot, and M. de Graaf. 1994. Q-fever in a patient with a ventriculoperitoneal drain. Case report and short review of the literature. *Neth. J. Med.* **44:**60–64.

36. Marrero, M., and D. Raoult. 1989. Centrifugation-shell vial technique for rapid detection of Mediterranean spotted fever rickettsia in blood culture. *Am. J. Trop. Med. Hyg.* **40:**197–199.

37. Marrie, T. J., and D. Raoult. 1999. *Coxiella*, p. 815–820. *In* P. R. Murray, E. J. Baron, M. A. Pfaller, F. C. Tenover, and R. H. Yolken (ed.), *Manual of Clinical Microbiology*, 7th ed. ASM Press, Washington, D.C.

38. Maurin, M., A. M. Benoliel, P. Bongrand, and D. Raoult. 1992. Phagolysosomal alkalinization and the bactericidal effect of antibiotics: the *Coxiella burnetii* paradigm. *J. Infect. Dis.* **166:**1097–1102.

39. Maurin, M., and D. Raoult. 1993. In vitro susceptibilities of spotted fever group rickettsiae and *Coxiella burnetti* to clarithromycin. *Antimicrob. Agents Chemother.* **37:**2633–2637.

40. Maurin, M., and D. Raoult. 1999. Q fever. *Clin. Microbiol. Rev.* **12:**518–553.

41. McCaul, T. F., and J. C. Williams. 1981. Developmental cycle of *Coxiella burnetii*: structure and morphogenesis of vegetative and sporogenic differentiations. *J. Bacteriol.* **147:**1063–1076.

42. Mejia, A., B. Toursarkissian, R. T. Hagino, J. G. Myers, and M. T. Sykes. 2000. Primary aortoduodenal fistula and Q fever: an underrecognized association? *Ann. Vasc. Surg.* **14:**271–273.

43. Murphy, A. M., and P. R. Field. 1970. The persistence of complement-fixing antibodies to Q-fever (*Coxiella burnetii*) after infection. *Med. J. Aust.* **1:**1148–1150.

44. Ormsbee, R. 1965. Q fever rickettsia, p. 1144–1160. *In* F. L. Horsfall and I. Tamm (ed.), *Viral and Rickettsial Infections of Man*. J. P. Lippincott, Philadelphia, Pa.

45. Ormsbee, R. A. 1952. The growth of *Coxiella burnetii* in embryonated eggs. *J. Bacteriol.* **63:**73–86.

46. Penttila, I. A., R. J. Harris, P. Storm, D. Haynes, D. A. Worswick, and B. P. Marmion. 1998. Cytokine dysregulation in the post-Q-fever fatigue syndrome. *Q. J. Med.* **91:**549–560.

47. Philip, R. N., E. A. Casper, R. A. Ormsbee, M. G. Peacock, and W. Burgdorfer. 1976. Microimmunofluo-

rescence test for the serological study of Rocky Mountain spotted fever and typhus. *J. Clin. Microbiol.* **3:**51–61.

48. **Raoult, D., P. Brouqui, B. Marchou, and J. A. Gastaut.** 1992. Acute and chronic Q fever in patients with cancer. *Clin. Infect. Dis.* **14:**127–130.

49. **Raoult, D., M. Drancourt, and G. Vestris.** 1990. Bactericidal effect of doxycycline associated with lysosomotropic agents on *Coxiella burnetii* in P388D1 cells. *Antimicrob. Agents Chemother.* **34:**1512–1514.

50. **Raoult, D., J. Etienne, P. Massip, S. Iacono, M. A. Prince, P. Beaurain, S. Benichou, J. C. Auvergnat, P. Mathieu, and P. Bachet.** 1987. Q fever endocarditis in the south of France. *J. Infect. Dis.* **155:**570–573.

51. **Raoult, D., P. Houpikian, D. H. Tissot, J. M. Riss, J. Arditi-Djiane, and P. Brouqui.** 1999. Treatment of Q fever endocarditis: comparison of 2 regimens containing doxycycline and ofloxacin or hydroxychloroquine. *Arch. Intern. Med.* **159:**167–173.

52. **Raoult, D., J. C. Laurent, and M. Mutillod.** 1994. Monoclonal antibodies to *Coxiella burnetii* for antigenic detection in cell cultures and in paraffin-embedded tissues. *Am. J. Clin. Pathol.* **101:**318–320.

53. **Raoult, D., P. Y. Levy, H. T. Dupont, C. Chicheportiche, C. Tamalet, J. A. Gastaut, and J. Salducci.** 1993. Q fever and HIV infection. *AIDS* **7:**81–86.

54. **Raoult, D., J. L. Mege, and T. J. Marrie.** Q fever: still a query after all these years. *Emerg. Infect. Dis.,* in press.

55. **Raoult, D., H. Tissot-Dupont, C. Foucault, J. Gouvernet, P. E. Fournier, E. Bernit, A. Stein, M. Nesri, J. R. Harle, and P. J. Weiller.** 2000. Q fever 1985–1998. Clinical and epidemiologic features of 1,383 infections. *Medicine* (Baltimore) **79:**109–123.

56. **Raoult, D., H. Torres, and M. Drancourt.** 1991. Shell-vial assay: evaluation of a new technique for determining antibiotic susceptibility, tested in 13 isolates of *Coxiella burnetii. Antimicrob. Agents Chemother.* **35:**2070–2077.

57. **Raoult, D., G. Vestris, and M. Enea.** 1990. Isolation of 16 strains of *Coxiella burnetii* from patients by using a sensitive centrifugation cell culture system and establishment of the strains in HEL cells. *J. Clin. Microbiol.* **28:**2482–2484.

58. **Raoult, D., M. R. Yeaman, and O. G. Baca.** 1989. Susceptibility of *Coxiella burnetii* to pefloxacin and ofloxacin in ovo and in persistently infected L929 cells. *Antimicrob. Agents Chemother.* **33:**621–623.

59. **Rolain, J. M., M. Maurin, A. Bryskier, and D. Raoult.** 2000. In vitro activities of telithromycin (HMR 3647) against *Rickettsia rickettsii, Rickettsia conorii, Rickettsia africae, Rickettsia typhi, Rickettsia prowazekii, Coxiella burnetii, Bartonella henselae, Bartonella quintana, Bartonella bacilliformis,* and *Ehrlichia chaffeensis. Antimicrob. Agents Chemother.* **44:**1391–1393.

60. **Rolain, J. M., M. Maurin, and D. Raoult.** 2001. Bacteriostatic and bactericidal activities of moxifloxacin against *Coxiella burnetii. Antimicrob. Agents Chemother.* **45:**301–302.

61. **Sidwell, R. W., B. D. Thorpe, and L. P. Gebhardt.** 1964. Studies of latent Q fever infections. I. Effect of whole body X irradiation upon latently infected guinea pig, mice and deer mice. *Am. J. Hyg.* **79:**113–124.

62. **Sidwell, R. W., B. D. Thorpe, and L. P. Gebhardt.** 1964. Studies of latent Q fever infections. II. Effect of multiple cortisone injections. *Am. J. Hyg.* **79:**320–327.

63. **Siegman-Igra, Y., O. Kaufman, A. Keysary, S. Rzotkiewicz, and I. Shalit.** 1997. Q fever endocarditis in Israel and a worldwide review. *Scand. J. Infect. Dis.* **29:**41–49.

64. **Stein, A., and D. Raoult.** 1992. A simple method for amplification of DNA from paraffin-embedded tissues. *Nucleic Acids Res.* **20:**5237–5238.

65. **Stein, A., and D. Raoult.** 1992. Detection of *Coxiella burnetti* by DNA amplification using polymerase chain reaction. *J. Clin. Microbiol.* **30:**2462–2466.

66. **Stein, A., and D. Raoult.** 1998. Q fever during pregnancy: a public health problem in southern France. *Clin. Infect. Dis.* **27:**592–596.

67. **Stoker, M. G. P., and P. Fiset.** 1956. Phase variation of the Nine Mile and other strains of *Rickettsia burnetii. Can. J. Microbiol.* **2:**310–321.

68. **Thiele, D., M. Karo, and H. Krauss.** 1992. Monoclonal antibody based capture ELISA/ELIFA for detection of *Coxiella burnetii* in clinical specimens. *Eur. J. Epidemiol.* **8:**568–574.

69. **Tissot-Dupont, H., S. Torres, M. Nezri, and D. Raoult.** 1999. Hyperendemic focus of Q fever related to sheep and wind. *Am. J. Epidemiol.* **150:**67–74.

70. **Vodkin, M. H., and J. C. Williams.** 1986. Overlapping deletion in two spontaneous phase variants of *Coxiella burnetii. J. Gen. Microbiol.* **132:**2587–2594.

71. **Waag, D., J. Chulay, T. Marrie, M. England, and J. Williams.** 1995. Validation of an enzyme immunoassay for serodiagnosis of acute Q fever. *Eur. J. Clin. Microbiol. Infect. Dis.* **14:**421–427.

ANTIBACTERIAL AGENTS AND SUSCEPTIBILITY TEST METHODS

V

VOLUME EDITOR
JAMES H. JORGENSEN

SECTION EDITORS
MARY JANE FERRARO AND
JOHN D. TURNIDGE

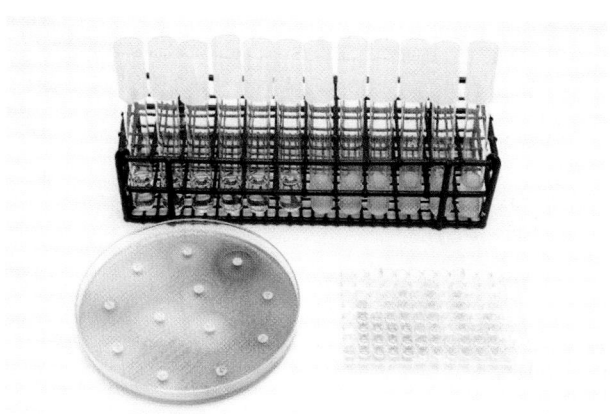

Pseudomonas aeruginosa susceptibility tests performed by disk diffusion, microbroth dilution, and macrobroth dilution.

Antibacterial Agents

JOSEPH D. C. YAO AND ROBERT C. MOELLERING, JR.

67

Antimicrobial chemotherapy has played a vital role in the treatment of human infectious diseases in the 20th century. Since the discovery of penicillin in the 1920s, literally hundreds of antimicrobial agents have been developed or synthesized, and dozens of these are currently available for clinical use. While the broad number and variety of agents available provide a great deal of flexibility for the clinician in the use of these agents, the sheer numbers and continuing development of agents available make it difficult for clinicians to keep up with progress in the field. Similarly, this variety presents significant challenges for the clinical microbiologist, who must decide which agents are appropriate for inclusion in routine and specialized susceptibility testing.

This chapter provides an overview of the antibacterial agents currently marketed in the United States, with major emphasis on their mechanisms of action, spectra of activity, important pharmacologic parameters, and toxicities. Antibiotics that have fallen into disuse or remained investigational are mentioned only briefly.

PENICILLINS

The penicillins (Table 1) are a group of natural and semisynthetic antibiotics containing the chemical nucleus 6-aminopenicillanic acid, which consists of a β-lactam ring fused to a thiazolidine ring (Fig. 1a). The naturally occurring compounds are produced by a number of *Penicillium* spp. The penicillins differ from one another in substitution at position 6, where changes in the side chain may modify the pharmacokinetic and antibacterial properties of the drug.

Mechanism of Action

The major antibacterial action of penicillins is derived from their ability to inhibit a number of bacterial enzymes, namely, penicillin-binding proteins (PBPs), that are essential for peptidoglycan synthesis (291). This ability to inhibit bacterial cell wall enzymes such as the transpeptidases usually confers on the penicillins bactericidal activity against gram-positive bacteria. The bactericidal activity of the penicillins is often related to their ability to trigger membrane-associated autolytic enzymes that destroy the cell wall. Other minor mechanisms of action include inhibition of bacterial endopeptidase and glycosidase, enzymes involved

in bacterial cell growth. There is also recent evidence suggesting that penicillins may inhibit RNA synthesis in some bacteria, causing death without cell lysis, but the significance of these observations remains to be proven (172).

Pharmacology

Oral absorption differs markedly among the penicillins. As a natural congener of penicillin G, penicillin V resists gastric acid inactivation and is better absorbed from the gastrointestinal tract than is penicillin G. Amoxicillin is a semisynthetic analog of ampicillin and has greater gastrointestinal absorption than ampicillin (95 versus 40% absorption). Bacampicillin is an ampicillin ester that is absorbed considerably better from the gastrointestinal tract than is ampicillin or amoxicillin. This ester is inactive until naturally occurring esterases in the intestinal mucosa and serum hydrolyze them to release the parent compound, ampicillin, into the serum. The isoxazolyl penicillins, such as oxacillin, cloxacillin, and dicloxacillin, as well as nafcillin, are acid stable and are also absorbed from the gastrointestinal tract (113), unlike certain other antistaphylococcal penicillins, such as methicillin, which are not acid resistant and cannot be given via the oral route.

Repository forms of penicillin G, available in procaine or benzathine, delay absorption from an intramuscular depot. Procaine penicillin G provides detectable levels for 12 to 24 h, suitable for the treatment of uncomplicated pneumococcal pneumonia and gonorrhea due to fully susceptible organisms. Benzathine penicillin G achieves very low levels in blood for prolonged periods (3 to 4 weeks) and is useful for the therapy of syphilis and for prophylaxis of streptococcal pharyngitis and rheumatic fever.

Penicillins are well distributed to many body compartments, including the lungs, liver, kidneys, muscle, bone, and placenta. Penetration into the eyes, brain, cerebrospinal fluid (CSF), and prostate is poor in the absence of inflammation. These drugs are metabolized to a small degree and are rapidly excreted, essentially unchanged, via the kidneys. With average half-lives of 0.5 to 1.5 h, they are usually administered every 4 to 6 h to maintain effective levels in blood. The renal tubular excretion of penicillins can be blocked by probenecid, thus prolonging their half-lives in serum.

TABLE 1 Penicillins

Natural
  Benzylpenicillin (penicillin G)
  Phenoxymethyl penicillin (penicillin V)

Broad-spectrum
  Aminopenicillins
    Ampicillin
    Amoxicillin
    Bacampicillin
    Pivampicillin
    Carboxypenicillins
    Carbenicillin
    Ticarcillin
  Ureidopenicillins
    Azlocillin
    Mezlocillin
    Piperacillin

Semisynthetic (antistaphylococcal)
  Penicillinase resistant
    Methicillin
    Nafcillin
  Isoxazolyl penicillins
    Cloxacillin
    Dicloxacillin
    Oxacillin
    Flucloxacillin

Penicillin + β-lactamase inhibitor combinations
  Ampicillin-sulbactam (Unasyn)
  Ticarcillin-clavulanate (Timentin)
  Amoxicillin-clavulanate (Augmentin)
  Piperacillin-Tazobactam (Zosyn)

Dosage reduction of most penicillins is necessary only for patients with severe renal insufficiency (creatinine clearance of ≤10 ml/min). Dosages of all penicillins except nafcillin and the isoxazolyl penicillins are adjusted for hemodialysis. Peritoneal dialysis requires dosage reduction of carbenicillin and ticarcillin.

Spectrum of Activity

The penicillins have antibacterial activity against most gram-positive and many gram-negative and anaerobic organisms. Penicillin G is very effective against penicillin-susceptible *Staphylococcus aureus*, *Streptococcus pneumoniae*, *Streptococcus pyogenes*, viridans streptococci, *Streptococcus bovis*, *Neisseria gonorrhoeae*, *Neisseria meningitidis*, *Pasteurella multocida*, anaerobic cocci, *Clostridium* spp., *Fusobacterium* spp., *Prevotella* spp., and *Porphyromonas* spp. However, the occurrence of penicillin-resistant pneumococci has recently been increasing worldwide (147). Penicillin is the drug of choice for syphilis and *Actinomyces* infections. Penicillin V has a spectrum of activity similar to that of penicillin G except that it is less active against *N. gonorrhoeae*. Penicillinase-resistant penicillins, of which methicillin is the prototype, are effective primarily against penicillinase-producing staphylococci (93). The agents are at least 25 times more active than other penicillins against penicillinase-positive *Staphylococcus aureus* and *S. epidermidis*. Although they are also active against *Streptococcus pneumoniae* and *S. pyogenes*, their MICs for these organisms are higher than

those of penicillin G. They are not active against enterococci, members of the family *Enterobacteriaceae*, *Pseudomonas* spp., or members of the *B. fragilis* group.

Ampicillin and amoxicillin have spectra of activity similar to that of penicillin G, but they are more active against enterococci and *Listeria monocytogenes*. Although they are also more active against *Haemophilus influenzae* and *H. parainfluenzae*, up to 25% of *H. influenzae* isolates are resistant, usually because of β-lactamase production. *Salmonella* and *Shigella* spp., including *Salmonella enterica* serovar Typhi, and many strains of *Escherichia coli* and *Proteus mirabilis* are susceptible to these agents. In vivo, ampicillin is more effective against shigellae whereas amoxicillin is more effective against salmonellae. Both of these agents are degraded by β-lactamase and are inactive against many *Enterobacteriaceae* and *Pseudomonas* spp.

The carboxypenicillins and ureidopenicillins have increased activity against gram-negative bacteria that are resistant to ampicillin. Although these drugs are susceptible to staphylococcal penicillinase, they are more stable to hydrolysis by the β-lactamases of the *Enterobacteriaceae* and *Pseudomonas aeruginosa*. Carbenicillin and ticarcillin are relatively active against streptococci as well as against *Haemophilus* spp., *Neisseria* spp., and a variety of anaerobes (100). They inhibit *Enterobacteriaceae* but are inactive against *Klebsiella* spp. Although carboxypenicillins are not particularly active against the enterococci, they may act synergistically with aminoglycosides against these organisms.

The ureidopenicillins have greater in vitro activity against streptococci and enterococci than do the carboxypenicillins, and they inhibit more than 75% of *Klebsiella* spp. (69, 276). They have excellent activity against many *Enterobacteriaceae* and anaerobic bacteria, including members of the *Bacteroides fragilis* group. On a weight basis, their activities in decreasing order of potency against *P. aeruginosa* are as follows: piperacillin, azlocillin > mezlocillin, ticarcillin > carbenicillin (52). These agents also act synergistically with aminoglycosides against *P. aeruginosa*.

Adverse Effects

Common reactions to penicillins include allergic skin rashes, diarrhea, and drug fever. Severe anaphylactic reactions, which can be fatal, may occur in previously sensitized patients rechallenged with penicillins, but, fortunately, such reactions are quite rare. At high doses (usually >30 × 10^6 U/day), penicillin G can cause myoclonic twitching and seizures due to central nervous system toxicity. All of the penicillins may cause interstitial nephritis on an allergic basis, but methicillin is more likely than the other penicillins to cause this complication. Hepatitis has been associated with prolonged use of oxacillin. High-dose carbenicillin can result in sodium overload and hypokalemia. Neutropenia may occur with any of the penicillins. Thrombocytopenia and Coombs-positive hemolytic anemia are rare complications of penicillin therapy. Bleeding tendencies due to interference with platelet function can occur with the use of carboxypenicillins and ureidopenicillins (82). Although pseudomembranous colitis has been associated with all the penicillins, it occurs more frequently with ampicillin than with the others (16).

CEPHALOSPORINS

Cephalosporins are derivatives of the fermentation products of *Cephalosporium acremonium* (also designated *Acre-*

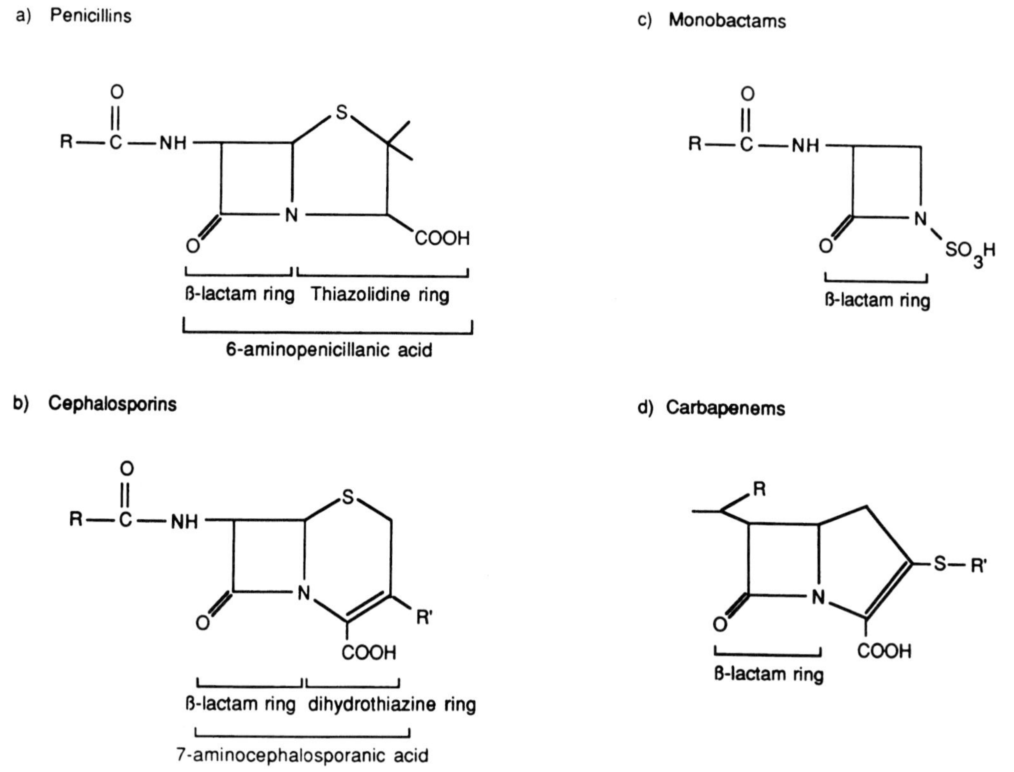

a) Penicillins

c) Monobactams

b) Cephalosporins

d) Carbapenems

FIGURE 1 Chemical structures of β-lactam antibiotics.

monium chrysogenum). They contain a 7-aminocephalosporanic acid nucleus, which consists of a β-lactam ring fused to a dihydrothiazine ring (Fig. 1b). Various substitutions at positions 3 and 7 alter their antibacterial activities and pharmacokinetic properties. Addition of a methoxy group at position 7 of the β-lactam ring results in a new group of compounds called cephamycins, which are highly resistant to a variety of β-lactamases.

Mechanism of Action

Similar to the penicillins, cephalosporins act by binding to PBPs of susceptible organisms, thereby interfering with the synthesis of peptidoglycan of the bacterial cell wall. In addition, these β-lactam agents may produce bactericidal effects by triggering autolytic enzymes in the cell envelope (291).

Pharmacology

Most cephalosporins require parenteral administration, but a growing number are available in oral form. Cephalexin, cephradine, cefadroxil, cefaclor, cefuroxime axetil, cefprozil, loracarbef, cefdinir, cefditoren pivoxil, cefixime, cefpodoxime proxetil, and ceftibuten are given orally and have good gastrointestinal absorption (60 to 90% of the oral dose). Cefuroxime axetil is an acetoxyethyl ester of cefuroxime, and it is deesterified at the intestinal mucosa and absorbed into the bloodstream as cefuroxime. Cefditoren pivoxil and cefpodoxime proxetil are prodrugs that are absorbed and hydrolyzed by esterases in vivo to release the active drugs, cefditoren and cefpodoxime, respectively. Relatively high concentrations of these agents are attained across the placenta and in synovial, pleural, pericardial, and peritoneal fluids. Levels in bile are usually high, especially those of cefoperazone, which is excreted mainly in the bile.

Ceftizoxime, cefotaxime, ceftriaxone, cefoperazone, moxalactam, and cefepime enter the CSF in useful concentrations and are used for the treatment of meningitis. Cefuroxime penetrates inflamed meninges, but levels in CSF are inadequate in providing bactericidal activity against susceptible bacteria.

Cephalothin, cephapirin, and cefotaxime are converted to the desacetyl forms before excretion. All cephalosporins except cefoperazone are excreted primarily by the kidneys, and for these drugs, dosage adjustments are necessary in patients with renal insufficiency (creatinine clearance of <50 ml/min). Like that of the penicillins, the renal excretion of cephalosporins, except for ceftriaxone, is impeded by probenecid. In general, these agents are removed by hemodialysis but not by peritoneal dialysis. Of the cephalosporins, cefonicid and ceftriaxone have the longest elimination half-lives, at 4.5 and 8 h, respectively, permitting once- or twice-daily drug administration in the treatment of serious infections.

Spectrum of Activity

Cephalosporins are classified by a well-accepted but somewhat arbitrary scheme of grouping by generations that is based on general features of their antibacterial activity (Table 2). The first-generation (narrow-spectrum) drugs, exemplified by cephalothin and cefazolin, have good gram-positive activity and relatively modest gram-negative activity. They are active against penicillin-susceptible and -resistant *Staphylococcus aureus* as well as *Streptococcus pneumoniae*, *S. pyogenes*, and other aerobic and anaerobic streptococci. Methicillin-resistant *S. aureus*, *S. epidermidis*, and enterococci are resistant. Some *Enterobacteriaceae*, including many strains of *E. coli*, *Klebsiella* spp., and *Proteus*

TABLE 2 Cephalosporins

Narrow spectrum (first generation)
    Cefadroxil
    Cefazolin
    Cephalexin
    Cephaloridine
    Cephalothin
    Cephapirin
    Cephradine

Expanded spectrum (second generation)
    Cefaclor
    Cefamandole
    Cefonicid
    Ceforanide
    Cefuroxime
    Cefprozil
    Loracarbef

Cephamycins (second generation)
    Cefmetazole
    Cefotetan
    Cefoxitin

Broad spectrum (third generation)
    Cefdinir
    Cefditoren
    Cefixime
    Cefoperazone
    Cefotaxime
    Cefpodoxime
    Ceftazidime
    Ceftibuten
    Ceftizoxime
    Ceftriaxone

Extended spectrum (fourth generation)
    Cefepime
    Cefpirome

mirabilis, are susceptible. *Pseudomonas* spp., including *P. aeruginosa*, many *Proteus* spp., and *Serratia* and *Enterobacter* spp. are resistant. These agents are active against penicillin-susceptible anaerobes except members of the *B. fragilis* group. They have only modest activity against *H. influenzae*.

The second-generation (expanded-spectrum) cephalosporins are stable against certain β-lactamases found in gram-negative bacteria and, as a result, have increased activity against gram-negative organisms. The agents are more active than narrow-spectrum drugs against *E. coli*, *Klebsiella* spp., and *Proteus* spp. Their activity also extends to cover some *Enterobacter* and *Serratia* strains, and they have good activity against *Haemophilus* spp., *Neisseria* spp., and many anaerobes. Cefaclor, cefuroxime, cefamandole, cefonicid, and cefprozil are active against ampicillin-resistant *H. influenzae* and *Moraxella catarrhalis* (266). However, cefamandole exhibits a significant inoculum effect and is not suitable for treating life-threatening infections due to *H. influenzae*. Ceforanide and cefonicid have spectra of antibacterial activities similar to that of cefamandole, but they are less active than cefamandole against gram-positive cocci. Loracarbef belongs to a new class of cephalosporin derivatives known as carbacephems in which the sulfur atom of the dihydrothiazine ring is replaced by a methylene

group to form a tetrahydropyridine ring (51). Since this structural modification of the cephalosporin nucleus is minor, loracarbef is considered a cephalosporin. Its spectrum of antibacterial activity is very similar to those of cefaclor, cefuroxime, and cefprozil. None of the expanded-spectrum agents is active against *Pseudomonas* spp.

Cefoxitin, cefotetan, and cefmetazole belong to a unique group of expanded-spectrum cephalosporins that have marked activity against anaerobes, including members of the *B. fragilis* group (137, 293). Cefotetan is two to four times less active than cefoxitin and cefmetazole against gram-positive cocci, but it is more potent than these two drugs against susceptible *Enterobacteriaceae*. The three drugs are equally active against *H. influenzae*, *M. catarrhalis*, and *N. gonorrhoeae*, including penicillin-resistant strains. While these drugs are comparable in their activities against the *B. fragilis* group, cefoxitin is the most active against *Prevotella* spp., *Porphyromonas* spp., and gram-positive anaerobic cocci. Cefotetan and cefmetazole have the advantage of more prolonged half-lives in serum.

Third-generation (broad-spectrum) cephalosporins are generally less active than the narrow-spectrum agents against gram-positive cocci but are much more active against the *Enterobacteriaceae* and *P. aeruginosa*. Their potent broad spectra of gram-negative activity are due to their stability to β-lactamases and their ability to pass through the outer cell envelopes of gram-negative bacilli (81, 193). There are two subgroups among these agents: those with potent activity against *P. aeruginosa* (ceftazidime and cefoperazone) and those without such activity (ceftizoxime, cefotaxime, and ceftriaxone).

Cefotaxime inhibits more than 90% of strains of *Enterobacteriaceae*, including those resistant to aminoglycosides. Its MICs for 90% of organisms (MIC$_{90}$s) for strains of *E. coli*, *Proteus* spp., and *Klebsiella* spp. tested are <0.5 μg/ml. Its activity against strains of *Serratia marcescens*, *Enterobacter cloacae*, and *Acinetobacter* spp. is variable, and it is inactive against *P. aeruginosa*. It has moderate activity against anaerobes but is inferior to cefoxitin and cefotetan against most of these isolates.

Ceftizoxime and ceftriaxone have spectra of activity similar to that of cefotaxime, with a few exceptions. Ceftriaxone is the most active agent against penicillinase-positive or -negative strains of *N. gonorrhoeae* (85). It is effective as single-dose therapy for infections caused by these organisms (38, 176). Because of its long half-life in serum (the longest of the currently available cephalosporins), ceftriaxone is used frequently in outpatient antibiotic therapy of serious infections, including Lyme disease (177).

Cefoperazone is less active than cefotaxime against many *Enterobacteriaceae* and gram-positive cocci. However, it has activity against *P. aeruginosa*, with an MIC for 50% of organisms (MIC$_{50}$) of ≤16 μg/ml. Its activity against anaerobes is similar to that of cefotaxime (139). Ceftazidime has potent activity against *P. aeruginosa*, with an MIC$_{90}$ of <8 μg/ml (193). It is more active than the ureidopenicillins against these strains. This agent has activity similar to that of cefotaxime against the *Enterobacteriaceae* but is not as active against gram-positive cocci. It has little activity against gram-negative anaerobes.

Cefdinir (48), cefditoren (136, 140), cefixime (12), cefpodoxime (94, 233), and ceftibuten (138, 305) are broad-spectrum oral cephalosporins that are more stable than the narrow- and expanded-spectrum oral cephalosporins against gram-negative bacterial β-lactamases. Compared with the earlier cephalosporins, the newer drugs are equally active against streptococci (MIC$_{90}$s, ≤0.06 μg/ml) but less active against methicillin-susceptible staphylococci (MIC$_{90}$s, 2 μg/ml). With potent activities similar to that of ceftizoxime against many Enterobacteriaceae, H. influenzae, M. catarrhalis, and N. gonorrhoeae (including β-lactamase-producing strains), they are inactive against Pseudomonas, Enterobacter, Serratia, and Morganella spp. and anaerobes. None of the currently available cephalosporins is clinically useful against enterococci.

Cefepime is a so-called fourth-generation (extended-spectrum) cephalosporin approved for clinical use in the United States. Cefepime and cefpirome (formerly HR 810), which is currently undergoing clinical evaluations, have the unique features of reduced affinity for and increased stability to the Bush class I β-lactamases. Therefore, these agents are active against stably derepressed class I β-lactamase mutants of Enterobacteriaceae and P. aeruginosa. In addition, cefepime and cefpirome penetrate well through the gram-negative bacterial outer membrane, due to a quaternary nitrogen substitution that makes them zwitterions (net neutral charge). They are more active in vitro than cefotaxime and ceftriaxone against some Enterobacteriaceae, Proteus, Providencia, Morganella, and Citrobacter (MIC$_{90}$s, ≤0.1 μg/ml) (102, 141, 235). Cefepime has comparable activity to that of ceftazidime against P. aeruginosa with MIC$_{90}$s of ≤4 μg/ml, and it is active against some ceftazidime-resistant strains (219). Against staphylococci (MIC$_{90}$s, ≤2 μg/ml) and streptococci (MIC$_{90}$s, ≤0.12 μg/ml), the activities of this group of drugs are comparable to those of the narrow-spectrum cephalosporins (102, 141). However, they are not active clinically against enterococci or anaerobes.

Adverse Effects

Cephalosporins are generally very well tolerated. The most common side effects are diarrhea and hypersensitivity reactions such as rash, drug fever, and serum sickness. Cross-reactions with these drugs occur in only 3 to 7% of penicillin-allergic patients (143). Other infrequent side effects include pseudomembranous colitis, elevated serum creatinine and transaminase levels, leukopenia, thrombocytopenia, and Coombs-positive hemolytic anemia. These abnormalities are usually mild and reversible. Prolonged use of ceftriaxone has been associated with the formation of gallbladder sludge, which usually resolves after drug therapy is discontinued (238), and, rarely, with cholecystitis.

Disulfiram-like reactions have been described in patients receiving cefamandole, cefotetan, and cefoperazone. This reaction is attributed to the N-methylthiotetrazole side chains of these antibiotics, which are similar to the chemical structure of disulfiram. Hypoprothrombinemia and bleeding tendencies have been observed with these cephalosporins. Causes of the coagulopathy included (i) alteration to healthy gut flora by the antibiotics, thus inhibiting the synthesis of vitamin K and its precursors, and (ii) the N-methythiotetrazole side chain, which inhibits the vitamin K-dependent carboxylase enzyme responsible for converting clotting factors II, VII, IX, and X to their active forms and also prevents regeneration of active vitamin K from its inactive form (236).

OTHER β-LACTAM ANTIBIOTICS

■ Monobactams

Aztreonam is the only monobactam antibiotic currently in clinical use. The monobactams are β-lactams with various side chains affixed to a monocyclic nucleus (Fig. 1c).

Mechanism of Action

Aztreonam binds primarily to PBP 3 of gram-negative aerobes, including P. aeruginosa, thereby disrupting bacterial cell wall synthesis. It is not hydrolyzed by most commonly occurring plasmid- and chromosome-mediated β-lactamases, and it does not induce the production of these enzymes (33).

Pharmacology

Given intravenously, aztreonam is widely distributed to body tissues and fluids. Average serum drug concentrations exceed the MIC$_{90}$s for most Enterobacteriaceae by four- to eightfold for 8 h and are inhibitory to P. aeruginosa for 4 h. It crosses inflamed meninges in sufficient amounts to be potentially therapeutic for meningitis caused by susceptible organisms. Its half-life in serum is about 1.7 h, and it is excreted mainly unchanged by the kidneys. Dosage modification is necessary for patients with renal failure. The drug is removed by both hemodialysis and peritoneal dialysis.

Spectrum of Activity

The antibacterial activity of aztreonam is limited to aerobic gram-negative bacilli, and it inhibits most Enterobacteriaceae, Neisseria spp., and Haemophilus spp., with MIC$_{90}$s of ≤0.5 μg/ml (14, 263). It has significant activity against Enterobacter spp. and Serratia marcescens, with most strains being inhibited at ≤16 μg/ml. However, many Acinetobacter spp., Burkholderia cepacia, and Stenotrophomonas maltophilia are resistant. When combined with aminoglycosides, it shows in vitro synergism against 30 to 60% of aztreonam-susceptible organisms, including P. aeruginosa and aminoglycoside-resistant gram-negative bacilli (32). Bacterial tolerance and inoculum effect are generally not seen with this agent. Aztreonam is not active against gram-positive bacteria or anaerobes.

Adverse Effects

Aztreonam is generally a safe agent, with a toxicity profile similar to those of other β-lactam drugs. Nausea, diarrhea, skin rash, eosinophilia, mild elevation of serum transaminase levels, and transiently elevated serum creatinine level have occurred. It has minimal cross-reactivity with other β-lactams and can be used safely in patients allergic to penicillins or cephalosporins (237). Hematologic abnormalities have not been reported.

■ Carbapenems

Carbapenems are a unique class of β-lactam agents with the widest spectrum of antibacterial activity of the currently available antibiotics. Structurally, they differ from other β-lactams in having a hydroxyethyl side chain in trans configuration at position 6 and lacking a sulfur or oxygen atom in the bicyclic nucleus (Fig. 1d). The unique stereochemistry of the hydroxyethyl side chain confers stability toward β-lactamases. Imipenem (N-formimidoyl thienamycin), a semisynthetic derivative of thienamycin produced by Streptomyces spp., meropenem, and ertapenem are the carbapenems currently available for clinical use (17, 201). Other members of this class currently undergoing preclinical evaluation or clinical trials include biapenem and faropenem.

Mechanism of Action

Carbapenems bind to PBP 1 and PBP 2 of gram-negative and gram-positive bacteria, causing cell elongation and lysis

(252). They are stable toward most plasmid- or chromosome-mediated β-lactamases except those produced by *Stenotrophomonas maltophilia* and some strains of *B. fragilis* (194). Bacterial resistance arises from production of carbapenemases (metallo-β-lactamases) capable of hydrolyzing the carbapenem nucleus and from alteration of the porin channels in the bacterial cell wall, thereby reducing the permeability of the drugs.

Pharmacology

After intravenous administration, the carbapenems are distributed widely in the body but undergo no significant biliary excretion. Imipenem is metabolized and inactivated in the kidneys by a dehydropeptidase I (DHP-I) enzyme found in the brush border of proximal renal tubular cells. To achieve adequate concentrations in serum and urine, a DHP-I inhibitor, cilastatin, was developed; it is combined with imipenem in a 1:1 dosage ratio for clinical use. Cilastatin has no antibacterial activity, nor does it alter the activity of imipenem. It has a renal protective effect by preventing excessive accumulation of potentially toxic imipenem metabolites in the renal tubular cells. Meropenem, ertapenem, faropenem, and biapenem contain a β-methyl group substitution at position C1 of the bicyclic nucleus, resulting in increased stability toward inactivation by human renal DHP-I. These agents do not require concomitant administration of a DHP-I inhibitor.

The pharmacokinetics of imipenem and meropenem are very similar, with elimination half-lives in serum of about 1 h. Peak concentrations of the drugs in serum are about 25 to 35 μg/ml and 55 to 70 μg/ml following 0.5- and 1-g doses, respectively. These drugs penetrate inflamed meninges well, with drug levels of 0.5 to 6 μg/ml in the CSF (53, 201). Ertapenem is highly (>95%) bound to human plasma proteins, with poor penetration into the CSF. Its relatively long plasma half-life of 4 h allows for a once-daily dosing frequency. The peak concentration of 155 μg/ml in serum is reached following a single intravenous dose of 1 g of ertapenem. Dosage adjustment of these carbapenem drugs is necessary for patients with a creatinine clearance of $\leq$30 ml/min. These agents, including cilastin, are effectively removed by hemodialysis.

Spectrum of Activity

In general, all the carbapenems have similar antibacterial potencies with only minor differences. They have excellent in vitro activity against aerobic gram-positive species: staphylococci (penicillin-susceptible and -resistant isolates); viridans streptococci; group A, B, C, and G streptococci; *Bacillus* spp.; and *Listeria monocytogenes*. Imipenem is two- to fourfold more active than meropenem and ertapenem against streptococci and staphylococci, but methicillin-resistant staphylococci are usually resistant to all carbapenems. Although penicillin-resistant pneumococci are associated with elevated carbapenem MICs (MIC$_{90}$s of 0.25 to 2 μg/ml), they remain susceptible to these drugs, with imipenem being the most potent (204). Ertapenem has poor activity against *Enterococcus faecalis*, but these isolates are inhibited by other carbapenems at $\leq$4 μg/ml. However, *E. faecium* isolates are usually resistant.

More than 90% of *Enterobacteriaceae*, including those resistant to other β-lactams and aminoglycosides (199), are susceptible to carbapenems, with the following decreasing order of activity: ertapenem, meropenem > biapenem > imipenem (75, 99, 125, 163, 201). These agents are highly active against clinical isolates of extended-spectrum β-lac-

tamase-producing *K. pneumoniae* and *E. coli*, with MIC$_{90}$s of 0.015 to 0.125 μg/ml (150, 158). Most *Enterobacter* spp., *Citrobacter* spp., and *Serratia* spp. are inhibited by $\leq$2 μg/ml. Although ertapenem is inactive against *Acinetobacter* and *Pseudomonas*, it is 5- to 10-fold more active than other carbapenems against fastidious gram-negative bacteria such as *Haemophilus*, *Moraxella*, *Neisseria*, and *Pasteurella*. Most strains of *P. aeruginosa* are inhibited by other carbapenems at 4 to 8 μg/ml, with meropenem being the most potent agent, including potency against imipenem-resistant strains (99, 125, 157, 214). While they inhibit *Burkholderia cepacia* and *B. stutzeri*, carbapenems are inactive against *S. maltophilia* (65). Emergence of resistant *Pseudomonas* spp. has been observed during therapy with imipenem (302). The drug may show in vitro antagonism when combined with broad-spectrum cephalosporins or extended-spectrum penicillins as a result of its ability to induce class I β-lactamase production (194).

Carbapenems are the most potent β-lactams against anaerobes, with activities comparable to those of clindamycin and metronidazole. The MIC$_{90}$s for anaerobic gram-positive cocci, *Clostridium*, *B. fragilis*, *B. fragilis* group species, *Fusobacterium*, *Porphyromonas*, and *Prevotella* are $\leq$2 μg/ml (107, 163, 214, 295). This class of drugs is also active in vitro against *Actinomyces*, *Nocardia*, and atypical mycobacteria (22, 54, 66, 75, 107).

Adverse Effects

Side effects of carbapenems are similar to those of other β-lactam antibiotics. Nausea, vomiting, and diarrhea occur in up to 5% of patients and are usually associated with parenteral administration of ertapenem and imipenem. Pseudomembranous colitis can occur in patients given carbapenems. Allergic reactions such as drug fever, skin rashes, and urticaria are seen in about 3% of patients. Cross-reactivity with other β-lactam agents is possible but has not been fully studied. Seizures of unclear etiology have occurred in up to 1% of patients receiving ertapenem and imipenem, particularly in the elderly age group and in patients with renal insufficiency or underlying neurologic disorders. Meropenem has not been associated with seizures. Reversible elevation of serum transaminase levels, leukopenia, and thrombocytopenia has been described for carbapenems, but no coagulopathy has been reported.

β-LACTAMASE INHIBITORS

Clavulanic Acid

Clavulanic acid is a naturally occurring, weak antimicrobial agent found initially in cultures of *Streptomyces clavuligerus* (197). It inhibits β-lactamases from staphylococci and many gram-negative bacteria. This agent acts primarily as a "suicide inhibitor" by forming an irreversible acyl enzyme complex with the β-lactamase, leading to loss of activity of the enzyme.

Clavulanic acid acts synergistically with various penicillins and cephalosporins against β-lactamase-producing staphylococci, klebsiellae, *H. influenzae*, *M. catarrhalis*, *N. gonorrhoeae*, *E. coli*, *Proteus* spp., the *B. fragilis* group, *Prevotella* spp., and *Porphyromonas* spp. (8, 100). Plasmid-mediated TEM β-lactamases present in ceftazidime-resistant strains of *K. pneumoniae* and *E. coli* are inactivated by this drug (133, 297). However, the inducible β-lactamases (chromosomal class I) of *Enterobacter*, *Citrobacter*, *Proteus*, *Acinetobacter*, *Serratia*, and *Pseudomonas* spp. are not inhibited by clavulanic acid (148). The combination of clavulanic acid with ampicillin, amoxicillin, or ticarcillin is active in vitro against *Mycobacterium tuberculosis*, which is known to produce β-lactamases (55, 308).

In the United States, clavulanic acid is available for clinical use in a 1:2 or 1:4 combination with oral amoxicillin and in a 1:15 or 1:30 combination with parenteral ticarcillin. The pharmacologic parameters of amoxicillin and ticarcillin are not significantly altered when either drug is combined with clavulanic acid. Amoxicillin-clavulanate is moderately well absorbed from the gastrointestinal tract, with a half-life in serum of about 1 h for each component. One-third of a dose is metabolized, while the remainder is excreted unchanged in the urine. The drug is widely distributed to various body tissues and fluids, but it penetrates uninflamed meninges very poorly.

Adverse reactions are similar to those reported for amoxicillin or ticarcillin used alone. Nausea, vomiting, abdominal cramps, and diarrhea occur in 5 to 10% of patients taking amoxicillin-clavulanate. The incidence of allergic skin reactions is similar to that associated with ampicillin alone.

Sulbactam

Sulbactam is a semisynthetic 6-desaminopenicillin sulfone with weak antibacterial activity (3). It functions as an effective inhibitor of certain plasmid- and chromosome-mediated β-lactamases of *S. aureus*, many *Enterobacteriaceae*, *H. influenzae*, *M. catarrhalis*, *Neisseria* spp., *Legionella* spp., the *B. fragilis* group, *Prevotella* spp., *Porphyromonas* spp., and *Mycobacterium* spp. (98, 182). Sulbactam alone is active against *N. gonorrhoeae*, *N. meningitidis*, some *Acinetobacter* spp., and *Burkholderia cepacia* (134, 183). It acts synergistically with penicillins and cephalosporins against organisms that are otherwise resistant to the β-lactam drugs because of the production of β-lactamases. A combination of sulbactam (8 μg/ml) and ampicillin (16 μg/ml) inhibits most strains of staphylococci, *Klebsiella* spp., *E. coli*, *H. influenzae*, *M. catarrhalis*, *Neisseria* spp., the *B. fragilis* group, *Prevotella* spp., and *Porphyromonas* spp. that are ampicillin resistant (224, 294). Like clavulanic acid, sulbactam does not inhibit the β-lactamases of *Enterobacter*, *Citrobacter*, *Providencia*, indole-positive *Proteus*, *Pseudomonas* spp., or *S. maltophilia*.

For clinical use, sulbactam is combined with ampicillin in a 1:2 ratio as a parenteral preparation. The pharmacologic properties of the drugs are not affected by each other in this combination. Ampicillin-sulbactam penetrates well into body tissues and fluids, including peritoneal and blister fluids. It enters the CSF in the presence of inflamed meninges. Like ampicillin, sulbactam has a half-life in serum of 1 h, and 85% of the drug is excreted unchanged via the kidneys. Since clearances of both sulbactam and ampicillin are affected similarly in patients with impaired renal function, dosage adjustments are similar for the two drugs.

The most common side effects of the ampicillin-sulbactam combination are nausea, diarrhea, and skin rash. Transient eosinophilia and transaminasemia have been reported. Adverse reactions attributed to ampicillin may also occur with the use of ampicillin-sulbactam.

Tazobactam

Tazobactam (formerly YTR 830) is a penicillanic acid sulfone derivative that is structurally related to sulbactam. Like clavulanic acid and sulbactam, tazobactam acts as a suicidal β-lactamase inhibitor (183). Despite having very poor intrinsic antibacterial activity by itself, it is comparable to clavulanate and sulbactam in lowering the MICs by up to 20-fold when combined with various β-lactams against β-lactamase-producing organisms. Tazobactam actively inhibits the β-lactamases of staphylococci, *H. influenzae*, *N. gonorrhoeae*, *E. coli*, the *B. fragilis* group, *Prevotella* spp., and *Porphyromonas* spp. (2, 119, 151). It also has activity against the class I β-lactamases of *Acinetobacter*, *Citrobacter*, *Proteus*, *Providencia*, and *Morganella* spp., but it remains inactive against those of *Enterobacter* spp., *Pseudomonas* spp., *S. maltophilia*, and some *Klebsiella* spp. (148, 151, 183). Of the penicillin–β-lactamase inhibitor combinations, piperacillin-tazobactam is the most active (two- to eightfold lower MICs) against β-lactamase-producing aerobic and anaerobic gram-negative bacilli (78, 151).

Available as a 1:8 ratio dosage combination with piperacillin, tazobactam is administered parenterally. The two drugs do not affect each other's metabolism or pharmacokinetics. High concentrations of both agents are achieved in the intestinal mucosa, lungs, and skin, and the distribution to muscle, fat, prostate, and CSF (in the absence of inflamed meninges) is relatively poor. With a half-life in serum of about 1 h, tazobactam is eliminated mainly via the renal route and is not affected by hepatic failure (248). Major adverse effects of the piperacillin-tazobactam combination are similar to those of piperacillin alone, such as diarrhea, skin rash, and allergic reactions. A mild elevation in serum transaminase levels may be encountered in about 10% of patients.

AMINOGLYCOSIDES AND AMINOCYCLITOLS

Since the first aminoglycoside (aminoglycosidic aminocyclitol), streptomycin, was introduced in 1944, this class of antibiotic has played a vital role in the treatment of serious infections with gram-negative bacteria. Among the unique features of the aminoglycosides is the bactericidal activity against aerobic gram-negative bacilli (including *Pseudomonas* spp.), activity against *M. tuberculosis*, and relatively low incidence of bacterial resistance. The currently available aminoglycosides are derived from *Micromonospora* spp. (gentamicin, sisomicin, and netilmicin) or from *Streptomyces* spp. (streptomycin, neomycin, kanamycin, tobramycin, and paromomycin). The difference in the origin of these compounds accounts for the differences of their suffixes, "micin" versus "mycin." Streptomycin, neomycin, kanamycin, tobramycin, and gentamicin are naturally occurring aminoglycosides, whereas amikacin and netilmicin are semisynthetic derivatives of kanamycin and sisomicin, respectively. Structurally, each of these aminoglycosides contains two or more amino sugars linked by glycosidic bonds to an aminocyclitol ring nucleus.

Spectinomycin is an aminocyclitol antibiotic isolated from *Streptomyces spectabilis*. Although it contains an aminocyclitol nucleus, it is not strictly an aminoglycoside because it does not contain an amino sugar or a glycosidic bond.

Mechanism of Action

Aminoglycosides are bactericidal agents that inhibit bacterial protein synthesis by binding irreversibly to the bacterial 30S ribosomal subunit. The aminoglycoside-bound bacterial ribosomes then become unavailable for translation of mRNA during protein synthesis, thereby leading to cell death (60). The aminoglycosides also cause misreading of the genetic code, with resultant production of nonsense proteins. To reach the intracellular ribosomal binding targets, an aerobic energy-dependent process is necessary to enable successful penetration of the bacterial inner cell membrane by the aminoglycosides. Bacterial uptake of these agents is facilitated by inhibitors of bacterial cell wall synthesis such as β-lactams and vancomycin. This interaction forms the basis of antibacterial synergism between aminoglycosides and β-lactam antibiotics (63, 105).

Spectinomycin acts similarly to the aminoglycosides by binding to the 30S ribosomal subunits and inhibiting protein synthesis. However, it does not cause misreading of the mRNA and is not bactericidal.

Pharmacology

All aminoglycosides have similar pharmacologic properties. Gastrointestinal absorption of these agents is unpredictable and always low. Because of the severe toxicity associated with systemic administration, neomycin is available only for oral and topical use. After intravenous administration, aminoglycosides are freely distributed in the extracellular space but penetrate poorly into the CSF, vitreous fluid of the eye, biliary tract, prostate, and tracheobronchial secretions, even in the presence of inflammation.

In adults with normal renal function, the aminoglycosides have half-lives in serum of about 2 to 3 h. They are primarily excreted, essentially unchanged, via the kidneys. There is considerable variation in the elimination of aminoglycosides among individuals, especially in patients with impaired renal function. Monitoring of serum aminoglycoside levels in these patients is essential for providing adequate therapy and reducing toxicity. With their features of concentration-dependent killing and prolonged postantibiotic effect, aminoglycosides may be administered once daily to achieve maximum bactericidal activity at high concentrations in serum without increased risk of toxicities (18). In renal failure, the drugs accumulate and dosage reductions are necessary. Aminoglycosides are substantially removed by hemodialysis and are removed to a lesser extent by peritoneal dialysis.

Spectrum of Activity

Aminoglycoside antibiotics are active primarily against aerobic gram-negative bacilli and S. aureus. As a group, they are particularly potent against the Enterobacteriaceae, P. aeruginosa, and Acinetobacter spp. Certain differences in antimicrobial spectra among the various aminoglycosides do exist. Kanamycin is limited in its spectrum because of the common resistance of P. aeruginosa and frequent occurrence of plasmid-mediated inactivating enzymes among other gram-negative bacilli (60). It is now used occasionally as a "second-line" drug in combination with other antibiotics for the therapy of mycobacterial infections (283, 284). Similarly, widespread resistance among Enterobacteriaceae has limited the usefulness of streptomycin. As a single agent, streptomycin is used in the therapy of infections due to Francisella tularensis (tularemia) and Yersinia pestis (plague) (169). It is often used in conjunction with tetracycline for the treatment of brucellosis. It has the greatest in vitro activity of the aminoglycosides against M. tuberculosis. It may also be used in combination with penicillin or vancomycin for the treatment of infective endocarditis due to viridans streptococci or enterococci, provided that the organisms do not possess high-level ribosomal or enzymatic resistance to streptomycin (289, 290, 300, 301).

Although gentamicin and tobramycin have very similar antibacterial activity profiles, gentamicin is more active in vitro against Serratia spp. whereas tobramycin is more active against P. aeruginosa (192). However, these minor differences have not been correlated with greater efficacy of one agent over the other. For the most part, gentamicin and tobramycin are susceptible to inactivation by the same modifying enzymes produced by resistant bacteria, except that in contrast to gentamicin, tobramycin can be inactivated by 6-acetyltransferase and 4'-adenyltransferase and has variable susceptibility to 3-acetyltransferase. Netilmicin and amikacin are resistant to many of these aminoglycoside-modifying enzymes and therefore are active against most Enterobacteriaceae that are resistant to gentamicin and tobramycin (186). Netilmicin is intrinsically less active than gentamicin or tobramycin against P. aeruginosa, and most gentamicin-resistant Serratia, Proteus, Providencia, and Pseudomonas isolates are also usually resistant to netilmicin (97). Amikacin is often used as the aminoglycoside of choice when gentamicin and tobramycin resistances are prevalent. In addition, amikacin is active against many Mycobacterium spp. (283, 284). Aminoglycosides are only moderately active against Haemophilus and Neisseria spp. Of the agents active against Bartonella spp., aminoglycosides are the only drugs consistently bactericidal toward this group of organisms (168, 169).

Although active against staphylococci, aminoglycosides are not recommended as single agents for the treatment of staphylococcal infections. Gentamicin is often combined with a penicillin or vancomycin for synergy in the treatment of serious infections due to staphylococci, enterococci, or viridans streptococci (289, 290, 300). The aminoglycosides are not active against anaerobes.

Paromomycin is an aminoglycoside notable for its amebicidal and antihelminthic effects, and it is used clinically for the treatment of intestinal amebiasis and tapeworm infections (175). It has modest antibacterial activity against gram-positive cocci and Enterobacteriaceae, but P. aeruginosa isolates are generally resistant.

Spectinomycin is used primarily for uncomplicated anogenital infections due to N. gonorrhoeae (287), including β-lactamase-producing strains, and gonococci are rarely resistant to this drug (85). It is useful in patients with penicillin allergy. Spectinomycin is ineffective for pharyngeal gonococcal infections, syphilis, or chlamydial infections.

Adverse Effects

Considerable intrinsic toxicity, mainly in the form of nephrotoxicity and auditory or vestibular toxicity, is characteristic of all of the aminoglycosides. The nephrotoxic potential varies among the aminoglycosides, with neomycin being the most toxic and streptomycin the least. This effect is usually reversible when the drug is discontinued. The presence of hypotension, prolonged duration of therapy, preexisting renal insufficiency, and possibly excessive trough serum aminoglycoside concentrations increase the risk of nephrotoxicity.

All aminoglycosides are capable of causing damage to the eighth cranial nerve in humans. Vestibular toxicity is more frequently associated with streptomycin, gentamicin, and tobramycin, whereas auditory toxicity is more typical of kanamycin and amikacin. This frequently irreversible side effect may occur even after discontinuation of the drug and is cumulative with repeated courses of the agent. The ototoxicity is a result of selective destruction of the hair cells in the cochlea. Detectable auditory and vestibular dysfunction has been reported to occur in 3 to 5% of patients receiving gentamicin, tobramycin, or amikacin who underwent audiometric testing and evaluation of vestibular function (83).

Neuromuscular paralysis, which is usually reversible, can occur after rapid intravenous infusion of aminoglycosides. This phenomenon occurs particularly in the setting of myasthenia gravis or concurrent use of succinylcholine during anesthesia. Other minor adverse reactions include local pain and allergic skin rashes. No known serious adverse reactions have been reported for spectinomycin.

QUINOLONES

Quinolones belong to a group of potent antibiotics biochemically related to nalidixic acid, which was developed initially as a urinary "antiseptic." Nalidixic acid and its early analogues, oxolinic acid and cinoxacin, have limited clinical applications as a result of widespread emergence of bacterial resistance. Newer quinolones have been synthesized by modifying the original two-ring quinolone (or naphthyridone) nucleus with different side chain substitutions (6). These new agents, also known as fluoroquinolones, each contain a fluorine atom attached to the nucleus at position 6. Cinoxacin, enoxacin, norfloxacin, lomefloxacin, ciprofloxacin, ofloxacin, levofloxacin, sparfloxacin, trovafloxacin, gatifloxacin, and moxifloxacin are currently available for clinical use in the United States. Temafloxacin and grepafloxacin have been withdrawn from clinical use due to toxicities. Gemifloxacin and sitafloxacin are currently undergoing clinical investigation in the United States.

Mechanism of Action

The primary bacterial target of the quinolones is DNA gyrase, a type II DNA topoisomerase enzyme essential for DNA replication, recombination, and repair (129, 307). Newer fluoroquinolones also inhibit DNA topoisomerase IV. The DNA gyrase A subunit is the main target of quinolones in gram-negative bacteria, whereas topoisomerase IV is the primary target in gram-positive bacteria. Inhibition of these bacterial enzyme targets causes relaxation or decatenation of the supercoiled DNA, leading to termination of chromosomal replication and interference with cell division and gene expression. By inhibiting bacterial DNA synthesis, these agents are bactericidal. However, the antibacterial activity of quinolones is reduced in the presence of low pH, urine, and divalent cations (Mg^{2+} and Ca^{2+}) (307).

Bacterial resistance to quinolones may occur by one or more of the following mechanisms: single-step chromosomal mutations in the structural genes for DNA gyrase and topoisomerase IV, mutations in the regulatory genes governing bacterial outer membrane permeability to the drug, and expression or overexpression of energy-dependent efflux pumps that can actively remove drugs from the bacterial cell (129). Transferable plasmid-mediated resistance to the fluoroquinolones has been reported, but the exact mechanism remains unknown (167).

Pharmacology

Fluoroquinolones are generally well absorbed from the gastrointestinal tract, with the exception of norfloxacin. The oral bioavailability varies from 60 to 95% for the various fluoroquinolones (257, 304). After oral administration, concentrations in serum peak after 1 to 2 h. The presence

of food does not significantly alter the absorption of these drugs. However, coadministration with iron- or zinc-containing multivitamins or with antacids containing aluminum, magnesium, or calcium substantially reduces the gastrointestinal absorption and subsequent peak concentrations of quinolones in serum. The degree of serum protein binding is generally low, ranging from 8% for ofloxacin to 75% for trovafloxacin. The prolonged elimination half-lives of fluoroquinolones, ranging from 3.5 h in ciprofloxacin to 20 h in sparfloxacin, allow for twice- or once-daily dosing (112, 182, 271). Ciprofloxacin, ofloxacin, levofloxacin, trovafloxacin, gatifloxacin, and moxifloxacin are also available for intravenous use. The intravenous formulation of trovafloxacin is prepared as alatrofloxacin mesylate, which is a prodrug of trovafloxacin and is rapidly hydrolyzed in vivo to yield the active drug.

Quinolones have good penetration into the lungs, kidneys, muscle, bone, intestinal wall, and extravascular body fluids. Concentrations in the prostate are about twice those in the serum, and concentrations 25 to 100 times the peak concentrations in serum are achieved in the urine. In the presence of meningeal inflammation, only ofloxacin, levofloxacin, trovafloxacin, gatifloxacin, and moxifloxacin achieve concentrations of >1 μg/ml in the CSF (162, 171). Quinolones penetrate well into phagocytes, such that concentrations within neutrophils and macrophages are as high as 14 times those of concentrations in serum (272). This feature accounts for their excellent in vivo activity against such intracellular pathogens as *Listeria*, *Salmonella*, and *Mycobacterium* spp.

Trovafloxacin and pefloxacin are metabolized mainly by the liver to form glucuronide conjugates, and pefloxacin is converted into norfloxacin in vivo. Ofloxacin exhibits little or no in vivo metabolism, and it is excreted mainly (90%) via the kidneys. The other quinolones are cleared by both hepatic and renal routes in various proportions, with elimination occurring primarily via the kidneys. This renal elimination is blocked by probenecid. Small amounts of these drugs are also excreted in the bile.

Hepatic insufficiency prolongs the elimination half-lives of pefloxacin and trovafloxacin, whereas the clearance of other fluoroquinolones is significantly diminished in the presence of renal failure. All of these drugs are only partially removed by hemodialysis (<15%) and are minimally affected by peritoneal dialysis because of their marked extravascular penetration, as reflected in their very large volumes of distribution.

Spectrum of Activity

Quinolones may be categorized into groups with similar spectra of antibacterial activity (Table 3), analogous to the classification of cephalosporins (6). The narrow-spectrum quinolones are inactive against gram-positive cocci, and their clinical utility is limited by widespread prevalence and rapid emergence of bacterial resistance. Broad-spectrum (second-generation) fluoroquinolones are active against both gram-positive and gram-negative bacteria (182, 267, 279, 307). Increased activity against gram-positive cocci is a major feature of the newer fluoroquinolones (third- and fourth-generation drugs), with potencies two- to eightfold greater than those of broad-spectrum agents (5, 20, 29, 47, 49, 64, 166, 210, 280). MIC$_{90}$s for methicillin-susceptible and -resistant *S. aureus* isolates and coagulase-negative staphylococci are in the range of 0.03 to 1 μg/ml, while methicillin-resistant staphylococci are becoming increasingly resistant to these agents. Although potency against

TABLE 3 Quinolones

Narrow spectrum (first generation)
    Cinoxacin
    Nalidixic acid
    Oxolinic acid

Broad spectrum (second generation)
    Ciprofloxacin
    Enoxacin
    Fleroxacin[a]
    Levofloxacin
    Lomefloxacin
    Norfloxacin
    Ofloxacin
    Pefloxacin[a]
    Rufloxacin[a]

Expanded spectrum (third generation)
    Sparfloxacin[a]
    Tosufloxacin[a]

Extended spectrum (fourth generation)
    Gatifloxacin
    Gemifloxacin[a]
    Moxifloxacin
    Sitafloxacin[a]
    Trovafloxacin

---

[a] Not licensed for clinical use in the United States.

enterococci is lower, gatifloxacin is two- to fourfold and moxifloxacin is four- to eightfold more active than levofloxacin against multidrug-resistant *S. pneumoniae* (MIC$_{90}$s of 0.12 to 1 μg/ml).

In contrast to earlier drugs of this class, many of the expanded- and extended-spectrum quinolones possess potent activity against anaerobes, including members of the *B. fragilis* group and *C. difficile* (44, 73, 200, 250). The relative activities of these newer drugs against all anaerobes, in decreasing order of potency, are as follows: trovafloxacin > moxifloxacin, gatifloxacin, tosufloxacin > sparfloxacin. The more active of these agents inhibit *B. fragilis* group species, *Prevotella*, *Porphyromonas*, *Fusobacterium*, *Clostridium*, and anaerobic gram-positive cocci at concentrations of 0.06 to 2 μg/ml.

The fluoroquinolones possess excellent activity in vivo against *Enterobacteriaceae*, *P. aeruginosa*, *Citrobacter* spp., *Serratia* spp., *Acinetobacter* spp., *H. influenzae*, and gram-negative cocci such as *N. gonorrhoeae*, *N. meningitidis*, and *M. catarrhalis* (20, 23, 24, 47, 49, 64, 166, 277). Enteropathogenic gram-negative bacilli such as *Salmonella*, *Shigella*, *Yersinia enterocolitica*, *Vibrio* spp., *Aeromonas* spp, *Plesiomonas* spp., *Campylobacter jejuni*, and enteroinvasive and enterotoxigenic *E. coli* are all susceptible to the quinolones (77, 307). Clinical studies have shown these drugs to be effective in the prophylaxis and treatment of infectious diarrheas. However, resistance and reduced susceptibility to quinolones have emerged in clinical isolates of *Salmonella*, *Shigella*, and *Campylobacter* spp. (79, 131). *Legionella* spp. are susceptible to these agents; the MICs of most fluoroquinolones for these organisms are 0.12 to 1.0 μg/ml (24, 29, 64, 72). Fluoroquinolones are the first class of oral antibiotics with good activity against *P. aeruginosa*. Ciprofloxacin and trovafloxacin are the most active among these

drugs against *P. aeruginosa*, with MIC$_{90}$s of 0.5 to 1 μg/ml. However, *Burkholderia* spp. and *S. maltophilia* are variably resistant to quinolones (277).

The fluoroquinolones, especially ciprofloxacin, levofloxacin, ofloxacin, and sparfloxacin, are active in vitro against *M. tuberculosis*, *M. fortuitum-chelonae* complex, *M. kansasii*, and *M. xenopi* (61, 267, 311). Their activity against *M. avium* complex is fair to poor. They also exhibit activity against *Chlamydia trachomatis*, *Chlamydophila pneumoniae*, and *Mycoplasma hominis*, with MIC$_{90}$s of 0.1 to 1 μg/ml, but are less potent against *Ureaplasma urealyticum* (77, 144). Ciprofloxacin and pefloxacin inhibit *Rickettsia conorii*, *R. rickettsii*, and *Coxiella burnetii* (221, 222, 310). The broad-spectrum fluoroquinolones also possess potent activity against *Bartonella* spp. (168). Although quinolones possess in vitro activity against *Plasmodium falciparum* at achievable concentrations in serum, they are relatively ineffective when used clinically for the treatment of malaria. *Nocardia* spp. are relatively resistant to the quinolones (22, 66).

No significant inoculum effect has been observed among the bacteria susceptible to quinolones. Combinations of quinolones with β-lactam drugs or aminoglycosides are usually indifferent or additive in their effects against gram-negative and gram-positive bacteria and mycobacteria (307). However, the bactericidal activities of quinolones can be antagonized by rifampin or chloramphenicol.

Adverse Effects

Gastrointestinal symptoms, occurring in up to 10% of patients as nausea, vomiting, abdominal discomfort, and diarrhea, are the most common side effects (7, 156, 253). However, *C. difficile* colitis occurs infrequently with the use of quinolones. Headaches, fatigue, insomnia, dizziness, agitation, and, rarely, seizures can occur. These adverse neurologic effects are usually associated with high dosages in elderly patients or concurrent use of certain nonsteroidal anti-inflammatory drugs.

Allergic reactions are uncommon and often manifest as rash, urticaria, and generalized pruritus. Dose-related photosensitivity occurs most frequently in patients taking fleroxacin, sparfloxacin, and lomefloxacin. Prolongation of the QT interval has also occurred with sparfloxacin and grepafloxacin. Rare laboratory abnormalities occurring during fluoroquinolone therapy include elevations in serum transaminase levels, eosinophilia, leukopenia, and thrombocytopenia. Use of trovafloxacin is limited because it results in rare occurrences of liver dysfunction or failure.

Enoxacin and to a lesser extent ciprofloxacin and pefloxacin increase the levels of theophylline and caffeine in serum as a result of decreased hepatic clearance (7, 216, 298). Other reported drug interactions include augmentation of the anticoagulant effects of warfarin by ciprofloxacin, norfloxacin, and ofloxacin and an increase in serum cyclosporin levels in patients taking ciprofloxacin (216).

Although irreversible cartilage erosions and skeletal abnormalities were observed in studies of quinolone toxicity in animals (7), such effects have not yet been documented clinically. However, quinolones are generally not routinely recommended for use in patients younger than 18 years or in pregnant or nursing mothers. Tendinitis or tendon rupture has occurred with the use of fluoroquinolones.

MACROLIDES

Macrolides have been in use since the early 1950s, with erythromycin being the prototypical antibiotic of this class for over 30 years (288). Their chemical structures consist of a macrocyclic lactone ring attached to two sugar moieties, desosamine and cladinose. They differ from each other in the size (14 to 16 atoms) and substitution pattern of the lactone ring. Erythromycin is a naturally occurring 14-membered macrolide derived from *Streptomyces erythraeus*, and other natural analogs include oleandomycin, spiramycin, and josamycin. Clarithromycin and dirithromycin are 14-membered semisynthetic macrolides, while azithromycin is a 15-membered derivative also known as an azalide, with a nitrogen atom incorporated in its lactone ring. These new macrolides offer significant advantages over erythromycin because of expanded antimicrobial spectra, improved pharmacokinetic parameters, and less frequent adverse effects and drug interactions. Roxithromycin, flurithromycin, and rokitamycin are new macrolides currently available for clinical use in Europe, Asia, and South America (146).

Mechanism of Action

Macrolides are generally bacteriostatic agents that inhibit bacterial RNA-dependent protein synthesis. They may be bactericidal at high drug concentrations and against a low inoculum of bacteria. They bind reversibly to the 23S rRNA of the 50S ribosomal subunits of susceptible organisms, thereby blocking the translocation reaction of polypeptide chain elongation (275). The presence of rRNA methylases is the primary mechanism of macrolide resistance and confers macrolide-lincosamide-streptogramin B (MLS$_B$) coresistance (71). Efflux is also now a common mechanism of resistance in streptococci. Other uncommon mechanisms of resistance to macrolides include the production of macrolide-inactivating enzymes (esterases, phosphorylases, glycosidases) and mutations in 23S rRNA and ribosomal proteins.

Pharmacology

Erythromycin is available in various topical, parenteral (lactobionate and gluceptate), and oral (base stearate, ethylsuccinate, and estolate) preparations. While clarithromycin and dirithromycin are available only in oral forms, azithromycin is formulated for both oral and intravenous administration. When administered orally, erythromycin base is rapidly inactivated by gastric acid whereas the newer macrolides are stable against acid degradation. Intestinal absorption of erythromycin (except for the estolate form) and azithromycin is reduced up to 50% in the presence of food. Peak levels in serum of 2 to 3, 1 to 2, 0.2 to 0.6, and 0.4 μg/ml are reached at 3 h after oral doses of erythromycin (500 mg), clarithromycin (250 mg), dirithromycin (500 mg), and azithromycin (500 mg), respectively. Much higher concentrations of erythromycin are achieved with intravenous infusion. Tissue distributions of macrolides are excellent, with concentrations in various tissues 10- to 100-fold higher than that in serum (299). The high concentrations reached rapidly within neutrophils and macrophages account for their potent activity against some intracellular pathogens (239). They penetrate poorly into the brain and CSF, but they do cross the placenta and are excreted in breast milk.

Erythromycin, clarithromycin, and dirithromycin are metabolized by the liver and excreted primarily in the bile. Azithromycin is excreted largely unchanged in the bile. Clarithromycin exhibits first-pass metabolism, producing a microbiologically active 14-hydroxy derivative that is two to four times more potent than the parent drug against some organisms. Following gastrointestinal absorption, dirithromycin is rapidly converted by nonenzymatic hydrolysis to erythromycylamine, an active derivative with microbiologic activity similar to that of its parent compound. Erythromycin, clarithromycin, 14-hydroxy clarithromycin, azithromycin, and dirithromycin have terminal half-lives in serum of 1.5, 5, 8.5, 41, and 44 h, respectively. Because of its exceptionally high tissue penetration, azithromycin has a half-life in tissue of 2 to 4 days (239). Dosage adjustment of clarithromycin is necessary in patients with moderate to severe renal failure (creatinine clearance of <30 ml/min). Except for clarithromycin, macrolides are removed minimally by hemodialysis or peritoneal dialysis.

Spectrum of Activity

Macrolides are relatively broad-spectrum antibiotics, with activity against gram-positive and some gram-negative bacteria, mycoplasmas, chlamydiae, treponemes, and rickettsiae (122, 239, 299). Erythromycin shows good activity against staphylococci and streptococci, including *S. pneumoniae*, but emergence of resistance among these isolates (especially group A streptococci and *S. pneumoniae*) is a problem in certain parts of the world (42, 147). Erythromycin and dirithromycin exhibit similar in vitro antibacterial activities (19). Clarithromycin is two- to fourfold more active than the other macrolides, and azithromycin is less active than erythromycin against most staphylococci and streptococci (13). These drugs are bactericidal against susceptible strains of streptococci but bacteriostatic against staphylococci and enterococci. Erythromycin-resistant strains display cross-resistance to these drugs, and methicillin-resistant staphylococci and many enterococci are usually resistant to all macrolides. These drugs are also active against *Corynebacterium* spp., *L. monocytogenes*, and *Actinomyces israelii* (13).

The antibacterial activity of macrolides against gram-negative bacilli is influenced by pH, with increasing potency (lower MICs) as the pH rises to 8.5. *H. influenzae* and *M. catarrhalis* are more susceptible to azithromycin (MIC$_{90}$ of 0.5 μg/ml) than to other macrolides (8- to 16-fold higher MIC$_{90}$s) (159, 195, 212). However, additive (and possibly synergistic) activity between clarithromycin and its 14-hydroxy metabolite reduces the MIC of clarithromycin for *H. influenzae* by two- to fourfold (196). Clarithromycin is the most active drug in this class against *Chlamydophila pneumoniae* (MIC$_{90}$ of 0.25 μg/ml) and *Legionella* (MIC$_{90}$ of 0.25 μg/ml) isolates (13). All four macrolides are equally potent against *Bordetella pertussis* and *Mycoplasma pneumoniae*, and erythromycin has long been established as the drug of choice for the therapy of infections due to these pathogens and *Legionella* spp. Macrolides are active against *Campylobacter* spp., *Helicobacter pylori*, *Pasteurella multocida*, *N. meningitidis*, and *Borrelia burgdorferi* (13, 174, 212, 274). Unlike other macrolides, azithromycin is also active in vitro against *E. coli*, *Shigella* spp., *Salmonella* spp., and *Y. enterolitica* (159, 195).

Macrolide antibiotics are effective in vitro against many pathogens that cause sexually transmitted diseases. *N. gonorrheae*, *Haemophilus ducreyi*, *Chlamydia trachomatis*, and *Ureaplasma urealyticum* are all susceptible, but only azithromycin is active against *Mycoplasma hominis* (13, 159). Erythromycin may be used for the treatment of gonorrhea and syphilis in patients who cannot tolerate penicillin G (38, 176), but data on the new macrolides for these indications are limited. Azithromycin is effective as an alternative to tetracyclines for the treatment of genital chlamydial infections (254). As a group, macrolides are among the most potent agents inhibitory toward *Bartonella* spp. (168).

The macrolides have good activity against anaerobic bacteria such as the *B. fragilis* group, *Fusobacterium* spp., *Prevotella* spp., *Porphyromonas* spp., *Propionibacterium acnes*, and anaerobic gram-positive cocci, with MIC_{90}s of 1 to 4 μg/ml (13). Except for dirithromycin, they are active against most *Clostridium* spp., especially *Clostridium perfringens*, with most strains being inhibited at $\leq$1 μg/ml. For this reason, erythromycin is commonly used preoperatively with or without neomycin as oral bowel preparations.

Atypical mycobacteria are more susceptible than M. *tuberculosis* to macrolide antibiotics (159, 196). The MIC_{90}s of clarithromycin and azithromycin for *Mycobacterium avium-intracellulare* complex are in the range of 2 to 4 μg/ml, allowing additive or synergistic killing activity of these organisms within infected macrophages when these drugs are combined with other antimycobacterial drugs (13). Erythromycin is used occasionally to treat infections due to *Mycobacterium scrofulaceum*, M. *kansasii*, and M. *chelonae* (181, 283) and in combination with ampicillin against *Nocardia asteroides* (91).

Spiramycin and the new macrolides offer comparable in vitro activity against *Toxoplasma gondii*, and they are effective in the treatment of toxoplasmosis (175). Although spiramycin has been used to treat cryptosporidiosis, the therapeutic efficacy remains to be proven (58).

Adverse Effects

The incidence of serious side effects related to the use of erythromycin is relatively low. Gastrointestinal irritation, such as abdominal cramps, nausea, vomiting, and diarrhea, is common with oral administration and can occur when the drug is given intravenously. These side effects occur less frequently with dirithromycin, clarithromycin, and azithromycin. Thrombophlebitis is associated with intravenous infusion, but it can be avoided by dilution of the dose in a large volume of fluid and by a slow infusion rate. Hypersensitivity reactions may include skin rash, fever, and eosinophilia. Cholestatic hepatitis occurring in adults has frequently been associated with the estolate form but has also been reported with other forms of erythromycin (259). For this reason, erythromycin estolate is no longer recommended for use in adults.

Reversible hearing loss may occur with use of large doses and very high concentrations of erythromycin in serum ($\geq$4 g/day), usually in elderly patients with renal insufficiency (30, 123). Ototoxicity has also been reported with high doses of clarithromycin and azithromycin used to treat M. *avium-intracellulare* complex infections. Pseudomembranous colitis and superinfection of the gastrointestinal tract or vagina with *Candida* spp. or gram-negative bacilli occur rarely. Concurrent erythromycin therapy increases the levels of theophylline, cyclosporine, and digoxin in serum by interfering with their hepatic metabolism (278). It also increases the anticoagulant effect of warfarin. To date, no clinically significant interactions have been observed between these drugs and dirithromycin, clarithromycin, or azithromycin. However, cardiac arrhythmias have occurred during concurrent use of terfenadine with erythromycin or clarithromycin.

KETOLIDES

Ketolides are semisynthetic derivatives of erythromycin A, having a ketone group instead of an L-cladinose moiety at the 3 position on the erythronolide A ring. This modification of the chemical structure results in increased stability in acid media, noninducibility of MLS_B resistance, and enhanced activity against gram-positive cocci (31). The ketolides currently under clinical development also have a substituted carbamate link between carbon atoms 11 and 12 in the macrolide nucleus. This modification enables them to retain activity against bacteria whose ribosomes have been methylated at position A2058 as a result of acquired methylase genes (31). Various ketolides have been developed and are undergoing preclinical and clinical studies. Telithromycin (formerly HMR 3647) has completed clinical trials in the United States, but as of January 2002 it had not been approved for clinical use by the U.S. Food and Drug Administration. A second ketolide, ABT-773, is currently under development.

Mechanism of Action

Like the macrolide antibiotics, ketolides inhibit the translation function in susceptible organisms at the level of the 50S ribosomal subunit. Specifically, ketolides interact with the bacterial 23S rRNA at domains V and II of the peptidyltransferase site (121). These drugs are also able to inhibit the formation of 30S ribosomal unit. Although ketolides do not induce MLS_B resistance, staphylococci with constitutively expressed MLS_B resistance encoded by *erm* genes are resistant to telithromycin. Active efflux of drug and mutations occurring on 23S rRNA and ribosomal proteins can lead to in vitro resistance to ketolides (31). This class of drugs has a low potential to select for resistance or induce cross-resistance among other MLS_B antimicrobials (62).

Pharmacology

Telithromycin is administered orally as a once-daily dose of 800 mg, with rapid gastrointestinal absorption reaching a mean peak concentration in plasma of 2 μg/ml in 1 to 2 h and steady state in 2 days. A mean trough concentration in plasma of 0.07 μg/ml is attained at 24 h after dosing (191). The oral bioavailability of 57% is unaffected by food ingestion. With about 70% of the drug being protein bound, telithromycin exhibits biphasic elimination from plasma with initial and terminal half-lives of 2 to 3 and 9 to 10 h, respectively. The drug penetrates well into bronchopulmonary, tonsillar, and sinus tissues and middle ear fluid, and it is accumulated by polymorphonuclear neutrophils with an intracellular-to-plasma-concentration ratio of >500 at 24 h. Hepatic metabolism with elimination via feces (~80%) is the main route of excretion, and <15% of the administered dose is eliminated in the urine. Dosage adjustments are not necessary in patients with renal or hepatic impairment (68).

Spectrum of Activity

Ketolides possess a good spectrum of potent activity against respiratory pathogens as well as intracellular bacteria, and telithromycin is designed specifically for the treatment of community-acquired respiratory tract infections. It is more active than macrolides against *S. pneumoniae* isolates, irrespective of penicillin susceptibility, with an MIC_{90} of $\leq$1 μg/ml; and 90% of penicillin-resistant strains are inhibited by telithromycin at 0.25 μg/ml (87, 88). Almost all macrolide-resistant strains of pneumococci are inhibited at

≤0.5 μg/ml, regardless of the underlying mechanism of macrolide resistance. Telithromycin is more active than erythromycin and clarithromycin and as potent as azithromycin against *Haemophilus influenzae* (MIC_{90}s of 2 to 4 μg/ml) and *Moraxella catarrhalis* (MIC_{90}s of 0.06 to 0.125 μg/ml). The activity of telithromycin is unaffected by β-lactamase production in these strains, but the MICs are increased twofold in the presence of 5% CO_2. A significant postantibiotic effect may be observed for up to 9 h with this drug against the major respiratory pathogens (68).

Telithromycin is also active against staphylococci, with MIC_{90}s of 0.125 to 0.25 μg/ml for *S. aureus* and coagulase-negative staphylococci, regardless of the susceptibility of these isolates to oxacillin. However, isolates harboring the constitutive MLS_B mechanism of resistance are resistant to ketolides. Enterococci without underlying resistance to macrolides and clindamycin are susceptible to telithromycin, with MIC_{90}s of 0.125 μg/ml for *Enterococcus faecalis* and *E. faecium*. Higher MIC_{90}s (4 to 8 μg/ml) are observed with erythromycin- or clindamycin-resistant enterococci (240). Telithromycin displays good in vitro activity against beta-hemolytic streptococci and viridans group streptococci, regardless of the susceptibility of these isolates to penicillin G, with all isolates inhibited at ≤0.5 μg/ml. While streptococcal isolates with the *mef*(A) gene-mediated drug efflux mechanism of resistance to erythromycin remain susceptible to telithromycin, the MICs are higher (2 to 16 μg/ml) for the strains with inducible or constitutive *erm* gene-mediated resistance to erythromycin. Other gram-positive cocci, such as *Pediococcus*, *Leuconostoc*, *Stomatococcus*, and *Rhodococcus equi*, are susceptible to telithromycin, with MIC_{90}s of 0.03 to 0.25 μg/ml.

This drug is also very active against gram-positive bacilli, inhibiting *Corynebacterium* (including *C. diphtheriae* and *C. jeikeium*), *Listeria*, *Lactobacillus*, *Actinomyces*, and *Erysipelothrix* spp. at concentrations of ≤0.125 μg/ml (240). Telithromycin is inhibitory (MIC_{90}s of 0.125 to 0.5 μg/ml) to *Peptostreptococcus* spp., *Prevotella* spp., *Porphyromonas* spp., *Bilophila* spp., and *C. perfringens*, but it is not active against other *Clostridium* spp., *Fusobacterium*, *B. fragilis*, and other *B. fragilis* group species (296). This drug has poor activity against other gram-negative bacilli, including the *Enterobacteriaceae*, *Acinetobacter* spp., and *Pseudomonas aeruginosa*.

Intracellular pathogens, such as *Legionella*, *Mycoplasma*, *Chlamydia*, and *Chlamydophila*, are highly susceptible to telithromycin, with drug MIC_{90}s of 0.004 to 0.25 μg/ml (87). *Rickettsia* spp., *Bartonella* spp., *Coxiella burnetii*, and *Francisella tularensis* are also susceptible to this agent. Telithromycin is comparable to the macrolides in its activity against mycobacteria, with MIC_{90}s of 4 μg/ml for *M. chelonei* and *M. avium-intracellulare*, and it is not active against *M. tuberculosis*, *M. bovis*, and other atypical mycobacteria (89).

Adverse Effects

Telithromycin is well tolerated by all patient populations, with gastrointestinal symptoms, such as diarrhea (15%), nausea (9%), vomiting, and dizziness, being the most frequent adverse effects (4). Occurrence of *C. difficile*-associated diarrhea has not been reported in clinical trial studies. Elevation in serum transaminase levels occurs in up to 10% of patients. Since ketolides are substrates and inhibitors of the hepatic cytochrome P-450 CYP3A4 isoenzyme pathway, their potential to lengthen the QT interval is aug-

mented by concomitant administration of other CYP3A4 inhibitors, such as ketoconazole and itraconazole (21).

TETRACYCLINES

Tetracyclines are broad-spectrum bacteriostatic antibiotics with the hydronaphthacene nucleus, which contains four fused rings. The congeners form three groups based on their duration of action. Chlortetracycline, oxytetracycline, and tetracycline are short acting, demeclocycline and methacycline are intermediate acting, and doxycycline and minocycline are long acting.

Mechanism of Action

The tetracyclines act against susceptible microorganisms by inhibiting protein synthesis. They enter bacteria by an energy-dependent process and bind reversibly to the 30S ribosomal subunits of the bacteria (43). This process blocks the access of aminoacyl-tRNA to the RNA-ribosome complex, preventing bacterial polypeptide synthesis. Bacterial resistance to tetracycline occurs as a result of active efflux of the drug from the cell, an altered ribosomal target site that prevents binding of the drug, or production of modifying enzymes that inactivate the drug (251).

Pharmacology

Tetracyclines are incompletely absorbed from the gastrointestinal tract, but their absorption is improved in the fasting state. Ingestion of food, especially dairy products, and other substances such as antacids and iron preparations impairs the absorption of these drugs. Food-mediated interference with absorption is lower with doxycycline and minocycline. These long-acting tetracyclines are more readily absorbed; therefore, lower doses are required. Peak concentrations in serum of 3 to 5 μg/ml are reached in 2 h after standard oral dosages. Intravenous preparations are available, and peak concentrations in serum of 10 to 20 μg/ml are reached in 1 h after intravenous administration. Tetracyclines are usually bacteriostatic at these clinically achievable concentrations in serum.

Tetracyclines are metabolized by the liver and concentrated in the bile. Biliary concentrations of tetracyclines are three- to fivefold higher than the concurrent levels in plasma. These drugs accumulate in the blood of patients with hepatic insufficiency or biliary obstruction. They should be avoided or used cautiously in reduced dosages in patients with impaired liver function.

These antibiotics are excreted primarily in the urine, except for doxycycline, which is excreted 60% as an inactive conjugate via the biliary tract in the feces, with the remaining 40% excreted unchanged in the urine. Renal failure prolongs the half-lives of the tetracyclines except for doxycycline. Therefore, doxycycline is considered the tetracycline of choice for extrarenal infections in the presence of renal failure.

Tissue penetration of these drugs is excellent, but levels in CSF are low even in the presence of meningeal inflammation. Tetracyclines cross the placenta and are incorporated into fetal bone and teeth. They are excreted in high concentrations in human milk. Therefore, tetracyclines are not advised for pregnant or lactating women. Minocycline, the most lipophilic tetracycline at physiologic pH, reaches relatively high concentrations in saliva and tears, making it an ideal antibiotic to eradicate the meningococcal carrier state (120, 126).

Spectrum of Activity

All tetracyclines have similar antimicrobial spectra, with activity against many gram-positive and gram-negative bacteria, mycoplasmas, chlamydiae, rickettsiae, and some protozoa. Many gram-positive aerobic cocci, including *Staphylococcus aureus*, *Streptococcus pyogenes*, and *S. pneumoniae*, are susceptible at concentrations achievable in the serum. However, tetracycline-resistant strains of *S. pneumoniae* are common (147). Although many *E. coli* isolates are susceptible to tetracyclines, pseudomonads and many *Enterobacteriaceae* are resistant. *Shigella* and *Salmonella* spp. are increasingly resistant to these agents (41). Tetracyclines are used mainly for the treatment of acute, uncomplicated urinary tract infections due to *E. coli* (130) and as effective prophylactic therapy for traveler's diarrhea caused by enterotoxigenic *E. coli* (95). With activity against *Burkholderia pseudomallei*, *Brucella* spp., *Vibrio* spp., and *Mycobacterium marinum* (284), they have been used successfully in the treatment of infections due to these bacteria. Their efficacy in the therapy of cholera is diminishing owing to the emergence of resistant *Vibrio cholerae* isolates (309). Minocycline is active against *Nocardia* spp. (66). Many anaerobic bacteria, including members of the *B. fragilis* group and *Actinomyces* spp., are susceptible to tetracyclines (187, 204).

These drugs are useful in the treatment of urethritis and acute pelvic inflammatory diseases caused by *N. gonorrhoeae*, *C. trachomatis*, *U. urealyticum*, and *Mycoplasma hominis*. Emergence of resistance to tetracyclines among *N. gonorrhoeae* strains is increasing (85). The drugs are effective for the treatment of other chlamydial infections (psittacosis, lymphogranuloma venereum, and trachoma) (38, 176). Other infections responsive to tetracyclines include granuloma inguinale, chancroid, relapsing fever, and tularemia.

Tetracyclines are the drugs of choice for treating rickettsial infections (Rocky Mountain spotted fever, endemic and scrub typhus, and Q fever). Many pathogenic spirochetes including *Treponema pallidum* and *Borrelia burgdorferi* are susceptible (38, 176, 177, 188). Protozoans such as *Plasmodium species*, especially *P. falciparum*, and *Entamoeba histolytica* are also inhibited by these drugs (175, 203).

Adverse Effects

Tetracyclines have irritative effects on the upper gastrointestinal tract, producing esophageal ulcerations, nausea, vomiting, and epigastric distress. Alterations in the enteric flora occur with the use of tetracyclines, often resulting in diarrhea, and pseudomembranous colitis can develop after prolonged use. Hypersensitivity reactions are unusual, generally manifesting themselves as urticaria, fixed drug eruptions, morbilliform rashes, and anaphylaxis. Cross-reactivity among tetracyclines is the rule. Photosensitivity reactions consist of an erythematous rash on areas exposed to sunlight and can occur with all analogs, especially demeclocycline (96).

Minocycline has been known to cause dizziness, and benign intracranial hypertension (pseudotumor cerebri) has been described with many of the analogs (285). Tetracyclines can aggravate preexisting renal failure by inhibiting protein synthesis, increasing the azotemia from amino acid metabolism. Tetracyclines cause depression of bone growth, permanent discoloration of the teeth, and enamel hypoplasia when given during tooth and skeletal development

(117). Therefore, these drugs are usually avoided in childhood (<8 years of age) and during pregnancy.

LINCOSAMIDES

The lincosamide antibiotics include lincomycin, which was initially isolated from *Streptomyces lincolnensis*, and clindamycin, which is a chemical modification of lincomycin. The chemical structure of each drug consists of an amino acid linked to an amino sugar. Compared with lincomycin, clindamycin has increased antibacterial activity and improved absorption after oral administration (173). Both drugs are available for parenteral and oral use, but lincomycin is rarely used now in the United States.

Mechanism of Action

Lincosamides bind to the 50S ribosomal subunits of susceptible bacteria and prevent the elongation of peptide chains by interfering with peptidyl transfer, thereby suppressing protein synthesis. The ribosomal binding sites are the same as or closely related to those that bind macrolides, streptogramins, and chloramphenicol (275). Lincosamides can be bactericidal or bacteriostatic, depending on the drug concentration, bacterial species, and inoculum of bacteria.

Pharmacology

About 90% of an oral clindamycin dose is absorbed from the gastrointestinal tract, with no interference from the ingestion of food. A single oral dose of 150 mg yields a peak concentration in serum of 2 to 3 μg/ml in 1 h. Peak levels in serum of 10 to 12 μg/ml are obtained at 1 h after a 600-mg intravenous dose. Therapeutic drug levels in serum are maintained for 6 to 9 h after these dosages (173).

Clindamycin is distributed well in the bones, lungs, pleural fluid, and bile, but it penetrates poorly into CSF, even in patients with meningitis. It readily crosses the placenta and enters fetal tissues. It is actively concentrated in neutrophils and macrophages.

The normal half-life of clindamycin is 2.4 h. Most of the drug is metabolized by the liver and excreted in an inactive form in the urine. Its half-life is prolonged by severe liver dysfunction, necessitating dosage reduction in patients with severe liver disease. Although the drug levels in serum are increased in patients with severe renal failure, dose modification is not essential. The drug is not removed significantly by hemodialysis or peritoneal dialysis.

Spectrum of Activity

Lincosamides have a broad spectrum of activity against the aerobic gram-positive cocci and anaerobes. Clindamycin is more potent than lincomycin against methicillin-susceptible *Staphylococcus* spp., *Streptococcus pneumoniae*, and group A and viridans streptococci (154, 173). The MIC$_{90}$s are in the range of 0.01 to 0.1 μg/ml for these strains. However, resistance to clindamycin has emerged in clinical isolates of these bacteria that are also resistant to erythromycin (42). The prevalence of clindamycin-resistant *S. aureus* may be 15 to 20% in some institutions. Enterococci are uniformly resistant to the lincosamides. All of the *Enterobacteriaceae* are resistant to lincosamides.

Clindamycin is one of the most active antibiotics available against anaerobes, including members of the *B. fragilis* group and *Clostridium perfringens*, with MIC$_{90}$s of ≤2 μg/ml (15, 260). However, clindamycin resistance (which appears to be increasing) is found in 10 to 15% of the *B. fragilis* group, 15 to 20% of *Prevotella* and *Porphyromonas* spp., 10 to

20% of clostridial species, 10% of peptococci, and most *Fusobacterium varium* strains (154, 204, 260). Clindamycin has been used successfully as single-agent therapy for actinomycosis (227), babesiosis (175, 306), and malaria (242). It is also effective in combination with pyrimethamine for toxoplasma encephalitis (57, 226) and in combination with primaquine for *Pneumocystis carinii* pneumonia (268).

Adverse Effects

Clindamycin-associated diarrhea occurs in up to 20% of patients, and use of this drug has been associated with pseudomembranous colitis caused by toxin-producing *C. difficile* (16). This complication is not dose related and may occur after oral or parenteral therapy. Prompt cessation of the antibiotic and initiation of oral vancomycin, metronidazole, or bacitracin therapy is effective in reversing this complication.

Other uncommon side effects include skin rashes, fever, and reversible elevation of serum transaminase levels. Clindamycin can block neuromuscular transmission and may potentiate the action of neuromuscular blocking agents during anesthesia.

GLYCOPEPTIDES AND LIPOPEPTIDES

Vancomycin, a bactericidal antibiotic obtained from *Streptomyces orientales*, is the only glycopeptide marketed for clinical use in the United States. Initially introduced for its efficacy against penicillin-resistant staphylococci, it has become most useful against methicillin-resistant staphylococci and in patients allergic to penicillins or cephalosporins. Teicoplanin (formerly teichomycin A), a new complex glycopeptide chemically related to vancomycin (247), is currently available for clinical use in most countries but not in the United States. Daptomycin (LY 146032) and ramoplanin (MDL 62198) are investigational semisynthetic lipopeptide and lipoglycopeptide antibiotics, respectively, with spectra of activity similar to those of the glycopeptides. Clinical trials of daptomycin are currently in progress for systemic use in humans. Systemic toxicity limits the use of ramoplanin to topical and oral application only.

Mechanism of Action

Glycopeptides inhibit peptidoglycan synthesis in the bacterial cell wall by complexing with the D-alanyl-D-alanine portion of the cell wall precursor (189). Daptomycin also acts by inhibiting bacterial peptidoglycan synthesis, but this is probably secondary to its interference with membrane transport of precursors (1). Resistance to glycopeptides is due to the presence of a complex series of bacterial cytoplasmic enzymes synthesizing abnormal peptidoglycan precursors terminating in D-Ala-D-lactate (instead of D-Ala-D-Ala), thereby markedly lowering the binding affinity with the glycopeptides (76).

Pharmacology

Vancomycin and teicoplanin can be administered orally or parenterally. After oral administration, the drugs are poorly absorbed and high concentrations in stools are achieved, accounting for their efficacy in treating pseudomembranous colitis (86). Peak and trough levels in serum of 20 to 50 and 5 to 15 μg/ml, respectively, are obtained after a 1-g intravenous dose of vancomycin every 12 h in healthy subjects. Similar serum drug concentrations are reached with intravenous teicoplanin, which has the advantage of a longer serum half-life and can be administered once daily. Ther-

apeutic levels of both drugs are achieved in synovial, ascitic, pericardial, and pleural fluids, with variable penetration into the CSF only in the presence of inflamed meninges (118, 178).

Vancomycin and teicoplanin have half-lives in serum of 6 and 45 h, respectively, in patients with healthy renal function, and they are eliminated from the body by glomerular filtration. In patients with severe renal insufficiency, their excretion is prolonged to about 9 days, and they not removed by hemodialysis or peritoneal dialysis.

Intravenous infusion of daptomycin at a dosage of 6 mg/kg results in peak and trough concentrations of 82 and 6 μg/ml, respectively, in serum. About 90% of the drug is bound to plasma protein, with limited metabolism. The elimination half-life is 9 h, and 80% of the drug is excreted via the kidneys, two-thirds as intact drug.

Spectrum of Activity

Glycopeptides and lipopeptides are active mainly against aerobic and anaerobic gram-positive organisms, including methicillin-susceptible and -resistant staphylococci, streptococci, enterococci, *Corynebacterium* spp., *Bacillus* spp., *Listeria monocytogenes*, *Clostridium* spp., and *Actinomyces* spp. The MICs of vancomycin against *Staphylococcus aureus*, *S. epidermidis*, streptococci, and enterococci are typically in the range of 0.25 to 2 μg/ml. The bactericidal activity varies, with MBCs 20-fold higher than MICs for viridans streptococci. These agents are essentially bacteriostatic against enterococci. Teicoplanin (111, 115, 161), ramoplanin (50), and daptomycin (11, 161, 303) are two-to fourfold more active than vancomycin against these gram-positive cocci. Increasing resistance to vancomycin has emerged among clinical isolates of *Enterococcus faecalis* (76, 179), *E. faecium*, and coagulase-negative staphylococci (241). Cross-resistance with teicoplanin is variable in these strains, but most are susceptible to daptomycin and ramoplanin (135, 179), whose MICs are ≤2 μg/ml. Other naturally vancomycin-resistant gram-positive organisms include *Leuconostoc*, *Lactobacillus*, and *Pediococcus* spp., most of which are susceptible to ramoplanin (50, 135, 232).

Vancomycin is useful in the prevention and treatment of endocarditis due to gram-positive bacteria in patients who are allergic to penicillin (56, 300). It is the drug of choice for treating *Corynebacterium jeikeium* infections (104) and may be useful for treating *Chryseobacterium meningosepticum* meningitis (118) and antibiotic-associated *Clostridium difficile* colitis (16, 86).

The glycopeptides and lipopeptides are not active against gram-negative organisms or mycobacteria. They show no cross-resistance with other unrelated antibiotics. They act synergistically with aminoglycosides or rifampin against staphylococci, streptococci, and enterococci (184, 270, 289, 290), and they are bactericidal with aminoglycosides against *Listeria* spp.

Adverse Effects

The most frequent side effects of vancomycin are fever, chills, and phlebitis at the site of infusion. Rapid or bolus infusion of vancomycin causes tingling and flushing of the face, neck, and thorax, known as the red man syndrome, as a result of histamine release by basophils and mast cells (217). This phenomenon is not due to allergic hypersensitivity. Allergic maculopapular or diffuse erythematous rashes can occur in up to 5% of patients (249). Reversible leukopenia or eosinophilia can rarely develop with glycopeptide use.

Hearing loss due to ototoxicity has been described occasionally in patients in whom serum vancomycin concentrations exceed 50 μg/ml, but it is hard to find unequivocal evidence of vancomycin ototoxicity in humans or animals (30). Vancomycin-induced nephrotoxicity has been rare since the recent availability of highly purified vancomycin preparations. However, the risk of nephrotoxicity increases during combination therapy with vancomycin and aminoglycosides.

Teicoplanin is generally well tolerated and does not produce the red man syndrome or nephrotoxicity. It does cause irritation at the site of intravenous infusion, and ototoxicity has been reported (59). Daptomycin has been associated with reversible myopathy in study subjects, but these adverse effects are significantly reduced with lower dosages and once-daily dosing frequency (264).

STREPTOGRAMINS

Streptogramins are natural cyclic peptides produced by *Streptomyces* spp. They are a unique class of antibiotics in which each member of the class is a combination of at least two structurally unrelated components, group A and B streptogramins, acting synergistically against susceptible bacteria (208). Group A streptogramins are polyunsaturated macrolactones consisting of lactam and lactone linkages with an oxazole ring, and the main compounds in this group are pristinamycin II$_A$ and pristinamycin II$_B$. Group B streptogramins are cyclic hexadepsipeptides, with pristinamycin I$_A$ and pristinamycin I$_C$ as the principal compounds. Quinupristin-dalfopristin is the first injectable streptogramin antibiotic combination developed for clinical use in the United States. It is a 30:70 mixture of the semisynthetic streptogramins quinupristin and dalfopristin, which are water-soluble derivatives of pristinamycin I$_A$ and pristinamycin II$_A$, respectively.

Mechanism of Action

The streptogramins exert a synergistic bactericidal effect on susceptible organisms by inhibiting bacterial protein synthesis. They enter bacterial cells via passive diffusion and then bind specifically and irreversibly to the 50S subunits of the 70S bacterial ribosomes. Binding of group A streptogramins to the ribosome induces a conformational change in the ribosome which increases its affinity for group B compounds. Group A streptogramins prevent peptide bond formation during the chain elongation step, while group B components cause release of the incomplete peptide chains from the 50S ribosomal subunit (275).

Acquired bacterial resistance to the streptogramins, which may be chromosomal or plasmid mediated, is due mainly to modification of the drug target by methylation of the bacterial 23S rRNA, resulting in resistance to all macrolides, lincosamides, and group B streptogramins (MLS$_B$ resistance phenotype) but not to group A streptogramins. Active efflux of groups A and B streptogramins and drug inactivation by streptogramin A acetylase and streptogramin B hydrolase have been described.

Pharmacology

Quinupristin-dalfopristin is administered intravenously and has wide distribution into most tissues. Both components are highly protein bound (70 to 90%) and are rapidly cleared from plasma via biliary excretion by hepatic conjugation processes (160). Less than 20% of the administered drug combination is excreted in the urine. Following intra-

venous doses of 7.5 mg/kg, peak concentrations in serum of quinupristin and dalfopristin reach 2.7 and 7.2 μg/ml, respectively, with elimination half-lives of 1 and 0.75 h. The two components penetrate and accumulate in macrophages, and the ratio of peak in vitro cellular to extracellular concentrations is 50:35. The drug combination does not cross the noninflamed blood-brain barrier or placenta to any significant degree. Dosage adjustment is needed for patients with renal insufficiency (creatinine clearance of <30 min/min), and the drug combination is removed in modest amounts by dialysis.

Spectrum of Activity

Streptogramins are active mainly against gram-positive bacteria, with modest activities against selected gram-negative and anaerobic pathogens. Quinupristin-dalfopristin has potent bactericidal activity against methicillin-susceptible and -resistant *Staphylococcus aureus*, coagulase-negative staphylococci, and streptococci, with drug MIC$_{90}$s of ≤1 μg/ml and MBCs within two- to fourfold of the MICs (25, 90). Staphylococci and streptococci, including *Streptococcus pneumoniae*, that are resistant to β-lactam drugs, macrolides, and fluoroquinolones usually remain susceptible to quinupristin-dalfopristin. *E. faecalis* is generally resistant (MIC$_{90}$s of ≤32 μg/ml) to the drug combination, while most *E. faecium* isolates (MIC$_{90}$s of ≤4 μg/ml) are susceptible. Although it is not bactericidal against enterococci, quinupristin-dalfopristin inhibits vancomycin-resistant *E. faecium* (VanA or VanB phenotype), including multidrug-resistant strains, at MIC$_{90}$s of ≤2 μg/ml (160). This drug combination is a major addition to the current therapeutic options for serious multidrug-resistant gram-positive bacterial infections (152, 155, 180, 209). *Neisseria meningitidis*, *N. gonorrhoeae*, *Mycoplasma pneumoniae*, *Chlamydophila pneumoniae*, and *Legionella pneumophila* are all highly susceptible to the drug (MIC$_{90}$s of ≤2 μg/ml). Quinupristin-dalfopristin is also active against *M. catarrhalis* and *H. influenzae*, with drug MIC$_{90}$s of ≤4 μg/ml. *Enterobacteriaceae* and other nonfermenting gram-negative bacilli are resistant.

Among the anaerobes, *Clostridium perfringens* and *C. difficile* are the most susceptible (MIC$_{90}$s of 0.25 μg/ml). Quinupristin-dalfopristin is active against the *Bacteroides fragilis* group (MIC$_{90}$ of 4 μg/ml) as well as other anaerobic bacteria including *Prevotella*, *Porphyromonas*, *Fusobacterium*, *Propionibacterium acnes*, *Lactobacillus*, and peptostreptococci, with drug MIC$_{90}$s of 2 to 4 μg/ml.

Adverse Effects

Phlebitis at the site of intravenous infusion is the major local adverse reaction, and the incidence and severity are dose and concentration related (160, 231). The most common systemic side effects that may lead to discontinuation of therapy are arthralgias and myalgia, both of which are reversible on discontinuation of the combination (180, 220). Elevated levels of serum transaminases and cutaneous reactions such as itching, burning, and erythema of the face, neck, or upper torso also have been reported.

OXAZOLIDINONES

Oxazolidinones are a unique group of synthetic antibiotics originally discovered in the 1970s (93, 165). Two of these drugs, eperezolid and linezolid, were developed for clinical use. Linezolid was eventually chosen for clinical development based on a superior pharmacologic profile.

Mechanism of Action

The oxazolidinones inhibit bacterial protein synthesis by preventing the formation of a functional initiation complex consisting of tRNA^{fMet}, mRNA, and the ribosome (261). Linezolid binds to the ribosome through a primary interaction with the 50S ribosomal subunit, thereby distorting the binding site for tRNA^{fMet} and inhibiting the formation of a functional 70S initiation complex, thus preventing the initiation of translation. In this regard, this class of antibiotics is unique, and there is no cross-resistance with other antibiotics that also inhibit ribosomal protein synthesis. Resistance to linezolid has occurred in clinical isolates of methicillin-resistant *S. aureus* (269) and vancomycin-resistant *E. faecium* (109, 218), as a result of point mutations in bacterial DNA encoding the 23S rRNA.

Pharmacology

Linezolid is available in oral and parenteral forms. Rapid and extensive absorption occurs after oral administration (>95% bioavailability), reaching maximum serum concentrations of 15 to 20 μg/ml within 2 h after an oral dose of 600 mg. The drug is metabolized primarily in the liver, and the elimination half-life is about 5 h. With 30% of the drug being protein bound, it is well distributed in all body tissues, including the CSF. The drug is eliminated via the kidneys, with 30% being excreted unchanged in the urine. No dose adjustment is necessary in patients with renal insufficiency or mild to moderate hepatic impairment, while 20% of a dose is removed by hemodialysis (26).

Spectrum of Activity

As a group, oxazolidinones have varying activity against most gram-positive bacteria and mycobacteria, but the current analogs lack useful activity against most gram-negative bacilli. Linezolid has excellent activity against staphylococci (including methicillin-resistant strains), streptococci, and multidrug-resistant enterococci, with MIC$_{90}$s of 1 to 4 μg/ml (46, 313). The MIC$_{90}$s for penicillin- and cephalosporin-resistant pneumococci are in the range of 0.5 to 2 μg/ml. Although the antibacterial effect of linezolid is generally bacteriostatic, the drug is bactericidal against most strains of pneumococci. Other bacteria that are inhibited by linezolid include *Bacillus cereus*, *Corynebacterium* spp., *Listeria monocytogenes*, *Clostridium* spp., and gram-positive anaerobic cocci. Rapidly growing *Mycobacterium* spp. are also susceptible to linezolid (281). Linezolid is an important therapeutic option for skin and soft tissue infections (258), respiratory tract infections (230), and infections due to methicillin-resistant staphylococci and vancomycin-resistant enterococci (211, 215).

Adverse Effects

The most common drug-related adverse events (≤5% incidence) are diarrhea, headache, and nausea. Prolonged use of linezolid (usually for more than 2 weeks) has led to myelosuppression, including anemia, leukopenia, thrombocytopenia, and pancytopenia, that is reversible upon discontinuation of therapy (114). Although linezolid is a mild inhibitor of monoamine oxidase, there were no reports of clinically significant interactions with adrenergic or serotonergic drugs.

SULFONAMIDES AND TRIMETHOPRIM

Sulfonamides were the first effective systemic antimicrobial agents used in the United States; they were introduced during the 1930s. They are derived from sulfanilamide, which has chemical similarities to p-aminobenzoic acid, a factor essential for bacterial folic acid synthesis. Various substitutions at the sulfonyl radical attached to the benzene ring nucleus enhance the antibacterial activity and also determine the pharmacologic properties of the drug.

Trimethoprim (TMP) is a pyrimidine analog that inhibits the enzyme dihydrofolate reductase, interfering with folic acid metabolism, subsequent pyrimidine synthesis, and one-carbon fragment metabolism in the bacteria. Since TMP and sulfonamides block the bacterial folic acid metabolic pathway at different sites, they potentiate the antibacterial activity of one another and act synergistically against a wide variety of organisms. Such a combination, TMP-sulfamethoxazole (TMP-SMX), also called co-trimoxazole, was introduced clinically in 1968 and has proven to be very effective in the treatment of many infections (229, 234).

Mechanism of Action

Sulfonamides competitively inhibit the bacterial modification of p-aminobenzoic acid into dihydrofolate, whereas TMP inhibits bacterial dihydrofolate reductase. This sequential inhibition of folate metabolism ultimately prevents the synthesis of bacterial DNA (124). Since mammalian cells do not synthesize folic acid, human purine synthesis is not affected significantly by sulfonamides or TMP. The antibacterial effect of these agents may be reduced in patients receiving high doses of folinic acid.

Pharmacology

Sulfonamides are usually administered in the oral and topical forms; the intravenous preparations (sulfadiazine and sulfisoxazole) are rarely used. The sulfonamides vary in their durations of action. Thus, sulfamethizole and sulfisoxazole are short acting, sulfadiazine and SMX are intermediate acting, and sulfadoxine is long acting. Mafenide acetate (Sulfamylon cream) and silver sulfadiazine are applied topically in burn patients and have significant percutaneous absorption. Sulfacetamide is available as an ophthalmic preparation, and various combinations of other sulfonamides are available orally (triple sulfa, or trisulfapyrimidine) or as vaginal creams or suppositories.

The orally administered sulfonamides are absorbed rapidly and completely from the gastrointestinal tract. They are metabolized in the liver by acetylation and glucuronidation and are excreted by the kidneys as free drug and inactive metabolites. Sulfonamides compete for bilirubin-binding sites on plasma albumin and increase the levels of unconjugated bilirubin in blood. For this reason, they should not be given to neonates, in whom increased serum bilirubin levels may cause kernicterus.

Sulfonamides are well distributed throughout the body, with levels in the CSF and synovial, pleural, and peritoneal fluids about 80% of the levels in serum. They readily cross the placenta and enter the fetal circulation. Sulfonamides may be used in patients with renal failure, but the drugs may accumulate during prolonged therapy as a result of reduced renal excretion.

TMP is available only for oral use and is absorbed almost completely from the gastrointestinal tract. After the usual 100-mg dose, peak levels in serum reach 1 μg/ml in 1 to 4 h. This drug is distributed widely in body tissues, including the kidneys, lungs, and prostate, and in body fluids (206). The concentrations in CSF are about 40% of those in serum. Its half-life in serum is about 10 h in healthy subjects and is prolonged in those with renal insufficiency. Up to 80% of a dose is excreted unchanged in the urine by tubular secretion; the remaining fraction is excreted as inactive metabolites by the kidneys or in the bile.

A fixed combination of TMP-SMX in a dose ratio of 1:5 is available for oral and intravenous use. An intravenous dose of 160 mg of TMP with 800 mg of SMX produces average peak levels in serum of 3.4 and 47.3 μg/ml, respectively, in 1 h. Similar peak levels are reached at 2 to 4 h after the same dose is taken orally. Widely distributed in the body, both drugs reach therapeutic levels in the CSF (40% of the levels in serum). Excretion is primarily by the kidneys; dosage reduction is necessary in patients with creatinine clearances of ≤30 ml/min. Both TMP and SMX are removed by hemodialysis and partially by peritoneal dialysis.

Spectrum of Activity

Sulfonamides are inhibitory to a variety of gram-positive and gram-negative bacteria, actinomycetes, chlamydiae, toxoplasmas, and plasmodia. Their in vitro antimicrobial activities are irregular, being strongly influenced by inoculum size and composition of the test media. Susceptibility-testing end points are often difficult to determine because of the presence of hazy growth within zones of inhibition in disk diffusion tests and because of the phenomenon of "trailing" in dilution tests. Sulfadiazine and sulfisoxazole are effective for rheumatic fever prophylaxis, but they are not useful in treating established group A beta-hemolytic streptococcal pharyngitis. These drugs may be used for prophylaxis of close contacts of patients with meningitis due to sulfonamide-susceptible *N. meningitidis*. Sulfisoxazole can be used to treat chlamydial urethritis, and sulfacetamide ophthalmic solution is effective for trachoma and inclusion conjunctivitis.

Sulfadiazine in combination with pyrimethamine has been used successfully to treat toxoplasmosis, and sulfadoxine combined with pyrimethamine (Fansidar) is effective in the prophylaxis and therapy of *Plasmodium falciparum* malaria (175). Sulfonamides are active against *Nocardia asteroides* (66), and they show moderate activity against *Mycobacterium kansasii*, *M. fortuitum*, *M. marinum*, and *M. scrofulaceum* (225). Other uses of sulfonamides include therapy of meliodosis, dermatitis herpetiformis, lymphogranuloma venereum, and chancroid.

Among the gram-negative bacilli, *E. coli* strains were initially susceptible to the sulfonamides, especially at levels achievable in the urine. Therefore, these drugs have been used primarily in the treatment of first-episode acute urinary tract infections due to *E. coli*. However, increasing bacterial resistance has limited their efficacy in recent years. *Serratia marcescens*, *Pseudomonas aeruginosa*, enterococci, and anaerobes are usually resistant to the sulfonamides.

TMP is active in vitro against many gram-positive cocci and most gram-negative bacilli. *P. aeruginosa*, most anaerobes, *Mycoplasma pneumoniae*, *Neisseria* species, *Moraxella catarrhalis*, and mycobacteria are resistant. The MIC varies considerably with the test media used. Like the sulfonamides, TMP is used primarily in the therapy of uncomplicated and recurrent urinary tract infections due to susceptible organisms (130). However, the prevalence of TMP-resistant *Enterobacteriaceae* is increasing (108).

Combinations of TMP with other agents, such as rifampin, polymyxins, and aminoglycosides, have demonstrated in vitro synergistic antibacterial activity against various gram-negative bacilli. TMP combined with dapsone is effective in the treatment of *Pneumocystis carinii* pneumonia in immunocompromised patients.

Many gram-positive cocci, including staphylococci and streptococci, and most gram-negative bacilli, except *P. aeruginosa*, are susceptible to TMP-SMX (34). However, 10 to 50% of strains of *S. pneumoniae* are resistant in many parts of the world (147). The drug combination has variable bactericidal effects on enterococci in vitro, depending on the test media used for susceptibility testing (190). Unlike many bacteria, which can utilize only thymidine for growth, enterococci can use thymidine, thymine, exogenous folinic acid, dihydrofolate, and tetrahydrofolate, resulting in higher drug MICs (25- to 50-fold increase) on media containing these compounds (185). This fact also explains the ineffectiveness of TMP-SMX against enterococci in vivo.

With excellent activity against *Moraxella catarrhalis* and *Haemophilus influenzae*, including β-lactamase-producing strains, TMP-SMX is useful for the therapy of acute otitis media, sinusitis, acute bronchitis, and pneumonia. It has shown excellent results in the prophylaxis and therapy of acute and chronic urinary tract infections (130, 255). It is an effective alternative therapy for uncomplicated urogenital gonorrhea, including cases caused by penicillinase-producing *N. gonorrhoeae* (38, 176). It can also be used for the treatment of chancroid, but resistance to TMP-SMX in *Haemophilus ducreyi* is increasing. The drug combination is also useful in treating infections due to salmonellae, shigellae, enteropathogenic *E. coli*, and *Y. enterocolitica* (188). It has been used successfully for prophylaxis and treatment of traveler's diarrhea (80), but resistance to TMP-SMX in *Shigella* spp. and *E. coli* now severely limits its usefulness in many parts of the world.

Other microorganisms susceptible to TMP-SMX include *Brucella* spp., *Burkholderia pseudomallei*, *B. cepacia*, *Stenotrophomonas maltophilia*, *Mycobacterium kansasii*, *M. marinum*, and *M. scrofulaceum*. *M. tuberculosis* and *M. chelonae* are generally resistant. It is a valuable antibiotic for the treatment of *Nocardia asteroides* infections (282), *B. cepacia* and *S. maltophilia* bacteremia, *Listeria monocytogenes* meningitis, gastroenteritis due to *Isospora belli* and *Cyclospora* spp. (175, 205), and Whipple's disease. In immunocompromised hosts (e.g., those with leukemia or AIDS and organ transplant recipients), TMP-SMX is effective for the prophylaxis and treatment of *Pneumocystis carinii* pneumonia (39, 312).

Adverse Effects

Sulfonamides are known to cause nausea, vomiting, headache, and fever. Hypersensitivity reactions can occur as rashes, vasculitis, erythema nodosum, erythema multiforme, and Stevens-Johnson syndrome (35). Very high doses of less water-soluble sulfonamides such as sulfadiazine may result in crystalluria, with renal tubular deposits of sulfonamide crystals. Bone marrow toxicity with anemia, leukopenia, or thrombocytopenia can occur. Sulfonamides should be avoided in patients with glucose-6-phosphate dehydrogenase deficiency because they can cause hemolytic anemia in such patients. Sulfonamides also potentiate the effects of warfarin, phenytoin, and oral hypoglycemic agents.

In general, TMP is well tolerated. With prolonged use, megaloblastic anemia, neutropenia, and thrombocytopenia can develop, especially in folate-deficient patients. Adverse reactions to TMP-SMX due to either the TMP or, more commonly, the SMX component can occur. Mild gastrointestinal symptoms and allergic skin rashes occur in about 3% of patients (153). Megaloblastic bone marrow changes with leukopenia, thrombocytopenia, or granulocytopenia may develop, usually in patients with preexisting folate deficiency. Nephrotoxicity usually occurs in patients with underlying renal dysfunction. Patients with AIDS have a much higher frequency of adverse reactions (as much as 70%) (110).

POLYPEPTIDES

■ Polymyxins

Polymyxins are a group of related cyclic basic polypeptides originally derived from *Bacillus polymyxa*. They have limited spectra of antimicrobial activity and significant toxicity. Only polymyxins B and E (colistin) are available for therapeutic use in humans.

Mechanism of Action

Acting like detergents or surfactants, members of this group of antibiotics interact with the phospholipids of the bacterial cell membrane, increasing the cell permeability and disrupting osmotic integrity. This process results in leakage of intracellular constituents, leading to cell death. The bactericidal action is reduced in the presence of calcium, which interferes with the attachment of drugs to the cell membrane.

Pharmacology

The polymyxins are usually administered via the parenteral, oral, or topical route. They are not significantly absorbed when given orally or topically, and intramuscular injections can be painful. Peak concentrations in serum of 5 μg/ml are obtained with a total daily dose of intravenous polymyxin B at 2.5 mg (25,000 U)/kg of body weight. Colistin sulfate is given orally for local antibacterial effect in the gut, while colistimethate sodium, a sulfomethyl derivative of colistin, is used for intravenous and intramuscular injections. The half-life of polymyxin B in serum is about 6 to 7 h, and that of colistin is 2 to 4 h. They do not penetrate well into pleural fluid, synovial fluid, or CSF even in the presence of inflammation. Excretion is mostly via the kidneys by glomerular filtration. The levels in serum and the toxicity are increased in patients with renal insufficiency. These drugs are not removed by hemodialysis, but small amounts can be removed by peritoneal dialysis.

Polymyxin is often used topically as 0.1% polymyxin in combination with bacitracin or neomycin for the treatment of skin, mucous membrane, eye, and ear infections. It is poorly absorbed from these surfaces. When the drug is used for irrigation of serous or wound cavities, systemic absorption can be significant enough to produce toxicity.

Spectrum of Activity

Polymyxins are active only against gram-negative bacilli, especially *Pseudomonas* spp. The MIC$_{90}$s for *Pseudomonas* spp., including *P. aeruginosa*, are <8 μg/ml. *Proteus*, *Providencia*, *Serratia*, and *Neisseria* isolates are usually resistant. Emergence of resistance during therapy is rare, and there is no cross-resistance with other antibiotics. Polymyxins B and E have identical antimicrobial spectra and show complete cross-resistance to one another.

The combination of polymyxins with TMP-SMX may be synergistic in the treatment of serious infection due to multiply resistant *Serratia* spp., *P. aeruginosa*, *B. cepacia*, and *S. maltophilia* (65, 228). The polymyxins are usually reserved for serious, life-threatening *Pseudomonas* or gram-negative bacillary infections caused by organisms resistant to all other antibiotics. Aerosolized polymyxins have been used successfully to treat *P. aeruginosa* colonization or respiratory infections in patients with cystic fibrosis or bronchiectasis (84).

Adverse Effects

Neurotoxicity and nephrotoxicity are the two major side effects of polymyxins. Paresthesia with flushing, dizziness, vertigo, ataxia, slurred speech, drowsiness, or mental confusion occurs when levels in serum exceed 1 to 2 μg/ml. Polymyxins also have a curare-like effect that can block neuromuscular transmission. Dose-related renal dysfunction occurs in about 20% of patients receiving appropriate therapeutic dosages. Allergic reactions such as fever and skin rashes are rare, but urticaria and shock after rapid intravenous infusion have occurred.

■ Bacitracin

Originally isolated from *Bacillus licheniformis* (formerly *Bacillus subtilis*), bacitracin is a peptide antibiotic consisting of peptide-linked amino acids. Although it was introduced initially for the systematic treatment of severe staphylococcal infections, it is now restricted mainly to topical use because of its systemic toxicity.

Mechanism of Action

Bacitracin inhibits the dephosphorylation of a lipid pyrophosphate, a step essential for bacterial cell wall synthesis. It also disrupts the bacterial cytoplastic membrane.

Pharmacology

Bacitracin is often used in various topical preparations, such as creams, ointments, antibiotic sprays and powders, and solutions for wound irrigation or bladder instillation. When it is used as a topical antibiotic, no significant amount of bacitracin is absorbed systemically. Large doses used to irrigate serous cavities may be associated with systemic toxicity.

Spectrum of Activity

The drug is active mainly against gram-positive bacteria, especially staphylococci and group A beta-hemolytic streptococci. However, group C and G streptococci are less susceptible, and group B streptococci are resistant (92). *Neisseria* spp. are also susceptible, but gram-negative bacilli are resistant. Bacitracin is often combined with neomycin, polymyxin B, or both in topical preparations to provide broad-spectrum antibacterial coverage. Orally administered bacitracin is effective in treating antibiotic-associated *C. difficile* colitis (70).

Adverse Effects

Systemic administration of bacitracin results in significant nephrotoxicity. Side effects are rare when the drug is given orally or applied topically. The drug is nonirritating to skin and mucous membranes. Allergic skin sensitization is rare.

CHLORAMPHENICOL

Chloramphenicol is a unique antibiotic originally derived from *Streptomyces venezuelae*. It contains a nitrobenzene ring. It is a highly effective broad-spectrum antimicrobial agent with specific indications for use in seriously ill patients. Thiamphenicol is an analog of chloramphenicol with a similar spectrum of antimicrobial activity (198). Only chloramphenicol is available for clinical use in the United States.

Mechanism of Action

The drug is a bacteriostatic agent that inhibits protein synthesis by binding reversibly to the peptidyltransferase component of the 50S ribosomal subunit and preventing the transpeptidation process of peptide chain elongation. At therapeutic concentrations achievable in the serum, it can be bactericidal against common meningeal pathogens such as *S. pneumoniae*, *N. meningitidis*, and *H. influenzae* (162, 198). Bacterial resistance occurs as a result of plasmid-mediated production of chloramphenicol acetyltransferase, which inactivates the drug (244).

Pharmacology

Chloramphenicol is available for topical, oral (as the base or palmitate salt), or parenteral (as the succinate salt) use. It is not absorbed in any significant amount when applied topically, but it is rapidly and completely absorbed from the gastrointestinal tract. After an oral or intravenous dose of 1 g, peak concentrations in serum at 2 h can reach 10 to 15 μg/ml. It diffuses well into many tissues and body fluids, including CSF, where levels are generally 30 to 50% of the concentrations in serum even without meningeal inflammation (245). The antibiotic readily crosses the placental barrier and is present in human milk.

Chloramphenicol is metabolized and inactivated by glucuronidation in the liver, with a half-life of 4 h in adults. The active drug (5 to 10%) and its inactive metabolites are excreted by the kidneys. Careful monitoring of serum chloramphenicol levels, maintaining peak concentrations in serum in the therapeutic range of 10 to 20 μg/ml, is useful for ensuring therapeutic efficacy and reduced toxicity. Patients with hepatic failure have high levels of active drug in serum owing to its prolonged half-life. Dosage modification is not necessary in patients with renal insufficiency, since the metabolites are not as toxic as the active drug. Levels in serum are not affected by hemodialysis or peritoneal dialysis.

Spectrum of Activity

Chloramphenicol is very active against many gram-positive and gram-negative bacteria, chlamydiae, mycoplasmas, and rickettsiae. MIC$_{90}$s for most gram-positive aerobic and anaerobic cocci are ≤12.5 μg/ml (198). However, the drug is often inactive against methicillin-resistant *S. aureus* and *S. epidermidis* and is variably active against enterococci. *N. meningitidis*, *H. influenzae* (ampicillin-resistant and -susceptible strains), and most *Enterobacteriaceae* are susceptible. Its activity against *Serratia* and *Enterobacter* isolates is variable, and *Pseudomonas* spp. are usually resistant. Salmonellae, including *S. enterica* serovar Typhi, are also susceptible, but resistant isolates are being encountered with increasing frequency (41).

Chloramphenicol has excellent activity against anaerobic bacteria, including members of the *B. fragilis* group. Almost all of these isolates are inhibited at concentrations of ≤10 μg/ml (187, 246). It is also active against *Rickettsia* spp. and *Coxiella burnetii*.

Adverse Effects

Bone marrow toxicity is the major complication of chloramphenicol use. This side effect may occur as either dose-related bone marrow suppression or idiosyncratic aplastic anemia. Reversible bone marrow depression with anemia, leukopenia, and thrombocytopenia occurs as a result of a direct pharmacologic effect of the drug on hematopoiesis. High doses (>4 g/day), prolonged therapy, and excessively high levels in serum (>20 μg/ml) predispose patients to develop this type of complication. The second form of bone marrow toxicity is a rare but usually fatal complication that manifests as aplastic anemia. This response is not dose related, and the precise mechanism is unknown. It can occur weeks to months after the use of chloramphenicol, and it can develop after the use of oral, intravenous, or topical preparations.

Gray baby syndrome, characterized by vomiting, abdominal distension, cyanosis, hypothermia, and circulatory collapse, may occur in premature infants and neonates. This toxicity results from the immature hepatic function of neonates, which impairs hepatic inactivation of the drug. Reversible optic neuritis causing decreased visual acuity has been reported in patients receiving prolonged therapy. Chloramphenicol occasionally causes hypersensitivity reactions, including skin rashes, drug fevers, and anaphylaxis. It potentiates the action of warfarin, phenytoin, and oral hypoglycemic agents by competitive inhibition of hepatic microsomal enzymes.

METRONIDAZOLE

Metronidazole is a 5-nitroimidazole derivative that was first introduced in 1959 for the treatment of *Trichomonas vaginalis* infections. It now has an important therapeutic role in the treatment of infections due to anaerobic bacteria and certain protozoan parasites. Tinidazole and ornidazole are other 5-nitroimidazole derivatives, and they are investigational drugs at present in the United States.

Mechanism of Action

Metronidazole owes its bactericidal activity to the nitro group of its chemical structure. After the drug gains entry into the cells of susceptible organisms, the nitro group is reduced by a nitroreductase enzyme in the cytoplasm, generating certain short-lived, highly cytotoxic intermediate compounds or free radicals that disrupt host DNA (74). Resistance to nitroimidazoles may be due to decreased uptake of the drug or to the presence of intracellular enzymes that can scavenge the free-radical intermediates.

Pharmacology

Metronidazole can be administered via the topical, oral, or intravenous route. It is absorbed rapidly and almost completely when given orally. Peak levels in serum of 6 μg/ml are obtained 1 h after an oral dose of 250 mg. Intravenous doses of 7.5 mg/kg result in peak concentrations in serum of 20 to 25 μg/ml. The drug has a half-life in serum of 8 h. Therapeutic levels are achieved in all body tissues and fluids, including abscess cavities and CSF, even in the absence of meningeal inflammation. The drug crosses the placenta and is secreted in breast milk. It is metabolized mainly in the liver, and 60 to 80% is excreted via the kidneys. In patients with impaired hepatic function, plasma clearance of metronidazole is delayed and dosage adjustments are necessary. The pharmacokinetics are minimally affected by renal insufficiency. Metronidazole and its metabolites are removed completely by dialysis.

Spectrum of Activity

Metronidazole exhibits potent activity against almost all anaerobic bacteria, including the B. fragilis group, Fusobacterium, and Clostridium spp. (15). It is one of the few antimicrobial agents with consistent bactericidal activity against members of the B. fragilis group. However, the susceptibility of gram-positive anaerobic cocci is somewhat variable, with $MIC_{90}s$ of 16 $\mu g/ml$ for these organisms. Most strains of the genera Actinomyces and Propionibacterium are resistant. Frequencies of metronidazole-resistant B. fragilis group isolates (MICs of >16 $\mu g/ml$) in the range of 2 to 5% have been reported from various institutions (187, 246). Tinidazole and omidazole are somewhat more potent than metronidazole in their antianaerobe activities. Nitroimidazoles have no activity against aerobic bacteria, including the Enterobacteriaceae.

The drug is effective in the treatment of antibiotic-associated colitis caused by C. difficile (16, 40), with efficacy equivalent to that of oral vancomycin for this indication (265). It is also useful in combination with an aminoglycoside for treating polymicrobial soft tissue infections and mixed aerobic-anaerobic intra-abdominal and pelvic infections.

Metronidazole is active against the protozoa Trichomonas vaginalis, Giardia lamblia, and Entamoeba histolytica. It is the drug of choice for the treatment of trichomoniasis, giardiasis, and intestinal and invasive amebiasis, including amebic liver abscess (103, 175, 262).

Adverse Effects

Metronidazole is generally well tolerated, and adverse side effects are uncommon. It can cause mild gastrointestinal symptoms such as nausea, abdominal cramps, and diarrhea. An unpleasant, metallic taste may be experienced with oral therapy. Metronidazole can potentiate the effect of warfarin and prolong the prothrombin time.

Although metronidazole is carcinogenic in mice and rats, there is no evidence for increased carcinogenicity in humans. Use of this agent in pregnancy, especially during the first trimester and in nursing mothers, however, should be avoided.

RIFAMPIN

Rifampin, also known as rifampicin, is a semisynthetic antibiotic derived from rifamycin B, which belongs to a group of macrocyclic compounds produced by the mold Streptomyces mediterranei. Introduced for clinical use in 1968 as an effective antituberculous drug, this agent has activity against many bacteria. A closely related compound, rifabutin, a derivative of rifamycin S, is another potent antimycobacterial agent, especially against Mycobacterium avium complex (202).

Mechanism of Action

Rifampin exerts its bactericidal effect by forming a stable complex with bacterial DNA-dependent RNA polymerase, preventing the chain initiation process of DNA transcription (292). Mammalian RNA synthesis is not affected, because the mammalian enzyme is much less sensitive to the drug. Rifampin-resistant isolates possess an altered RNA polymerase enzyme, which arises easily from single-step mutations during monotherapy with rifampin.

Pharmacology

The drug is well absorbed after oral administration, reaching peak concentrations in serum of 5 to 10 $\mu g/ml$ in 2 to 4 h following a 600-mg dose. A parenteral preparation is also available. Rifampin is deacetylated in the liver to an active metabolite and excreted in the bile, and it undergoes enterohepatic circulation. The normal half-life in serum varies from 1.5 to 5 h. Dosage adjustments are necessary for patients with severe hepatic dysfunction.

Rifampin is well distributed to almost all body tissues and fluids, reaching concentrations equal to or exceeding that in the serum. Levels in the CSF are highest in the presence of inflamed meninges. It is able to enter phagocytes and kill living intracellular organisms (164), and it crosses the placenta. About 30 to 40% of the drug is excreted in the urine, and it does not accumulate in patients with impaired renal function. Hemodialysis and peritoneal dialysis do not eliminate the drug.

Spectrum of Activity

In addition to its well-known antimycobacterial effects (45), rifampin has a wide spectrum of antimicrobial activity. It is bactericidal against gram-positive cocci such as staphylococci (including methicillin-resistant strains), streptococci, and anaerobic cocci, with drug MICs in the range of 0.01 to 0.5 $\mu g/ml$. It remains an important adjunct in the combination therapy of serious and chronic staphylococcal infections (273). However, it is bacteriostatic against enterococci, with usual MICs of <16 $\mu g/ml$ (184).

Neisseria gonorrhoeae, N. meningitidis, and H. influenzae, including β-lactamase-producing strains, are susceptible to rifampin, which is used frequently in the prophylaxis of meningococcal and H. influenzae type b meningitis (120). MICs for Enterobacteriaceae are ≤12 $\mu g/ml$, while MICs for Serratia marcescens and P. aeruginosa are higher (184). Besides fluoroquinolones, rifampin is one of the most active agents against Legionella pneumophila and other Legionella spp., with MICs of ≤0.03 $\mu g/ml$. Because of its ability to enter phagocytes, rifampin inhibits the growth of Brucella spp. and Coxiella burnetti intracellularly (222), and it is used frequently in the combination therapy of infections due to these organisms. Although chlamydiae are very susceptible to rifampin in vitro, resistance emerges rapidly when rifampin is used alone.

Adverse Effects

Rifampin has many side effects, including gastrointestinal discomfort and hypersensitivity reactions such as drug fever, skin rashes, and eosinophilia. It produces a harmless, orange-red coloration of saliva, tears, urine, and sweat. In up to 20% of patients, an influenza-like syndrome with fever, chills, arthralgias, and myalgias may develop after several months of intermittent therapy (116). This immunologic reaction may be associated with hemolytic anemia, thrombocytopenia, and renal failure. Rifampin-induced hepatitis occurs in <1% of patients and is more frequent during concurrent isoniazid therapy for tuberculosis. The drug is known to antagonize the effect of oral contraceptives and diminish the anticoagulant activity of warfarin.

NITROFURANTOIN

Nitrofurantoin belongs to a class of compounds, the nitrofurans, consisting of a primary nitro group joined to a heterocyclic ring. Its role in human therapeutics is limited to the treatment of urinary tract infections (130).

Mechanism of Action

The precise mechanism of action of nitrofurantoin is unknown. The drug is thought to inhibit various bacterial enzymes and also damage DNA (170).

Pharmacology

The drug is available in microcrystalline (Furadantin) and macrocrystalline (Macrodantin) forms. It is administered orally and is well absorbed from the gastrointestinal tract. Very low levels of the drug are achieved in serum and most body tissues after usual oral doses. With a half-life in serum of about 20 min, two-thirds of the drug is rapidly metabolized and inactivated in various tissues. The remaining one-third is excreted unchanged into the urine. An average dose of nitrofurantoin yields a concentration in urine of 50 to 250 μg/ml in patients with healthy renal function. In alkaline urine, more of the drug is dissociated into the ionized form, with lowered antibacterial activity. Nitrofurantoin accumulates in the sera of patients with creatinine clearances of <60 ml/min. The drug is removed by hemodialysis. The risk of systemic toxicity increases in the presence of severe uremia. It is contraindicated in patients with significant renal impairment and hepatic failure.

Spectrum of Activity

Nitrofurantoin has a broad spectrum of antibacterial activity against gram-positive and gram-negative bacteria, particularly the common urinary tract pathogens. It is active against gram-positive cocci, such as *Staphylococcus aureus*, *S. epidermidis*, *S. saprophyticus*, and *Enterococcus faecalis*, with drug MICs in the range of 4 to 25 μg/ml (127). *Streptococcus pneumoniae*, *S. pyogenes*, *Bacillus subtilis*, and *Corynebacterium* spp. are also susceptible, but they rarely cause urinary tract infections. Over 90% of *E. coli* isolates and many coliform bacteria are susceptible to nitrofurantoin at MICs <32 μg/ml. However, only one-third of *Enterobacter* and *Klebsiella* isolates are susceptible. *Pseudomonas* and most *Proteus* spp. are resistant. Susceptible organisms rarely become resistant to this drug during therapy.

Adverse Effects

Gastrointestinal irritation, with anorexia, nausea, and vomiting, is the most common side effect. Diarrhea and abdominal cramps may occur. Hypersensitivity reactions, such as drug fever, chills, arthralgia, skin rashes, and a lupus-like syndrome, have been observed (128).

Pulmonary reactions are the most common serious side effects associated with nitrofurantoin use. Acute pneumonitis with fever, cough, dyspnea, eosinophilia, and pulmonary infiltrates present on chest X rays can occur after a few days of therapy (128). This immunologically mediated reaction is more common in elderly patients and is rapidly reversible after cessation of therapy. Chronic pulmonary reactions with interstitial pneumonitis leading to irreversible pulmonary fibrosis can occur in patients receiving continuous therapy for 6 months or more.

Peripheral polyneuropathy is a serious side effect, which occurs more often in patients with renal failure. Hemolytic anemia, megaloblastic anemia, and bone marrow suppression with leukopenia can occur. Rare hepatotoxic reactions, such as cholestatic jaundice and chronic active hepatitis, have been reported (243).

FOSFOMYCIN

Fosfomycin, first isolated from cultures of *Streptomyces* spp. in 1969, is a phosphonic acid derivative originally named phosphonomycin (256). In the United States, it is used as single-dose therapy for uncomplicated urinary tract infections due to susceptible organisms (130).

Mechanism of Action

Fosfomycin is bactericidal by inhibiting pyruvyl transferase, a bacterial cytoplasmic enzyme that catalyzes the formation of uridine diphosphate-N-acetylmuramic acid during the first step of peptidoglycan synthesis (142). There is little cross-resistance between fosfomycin and other antibacterial agents, most probably because it differs from other agents in its chemical structure and site of action.

Pharmacology

Originally formulated as sodium and calcium salts for oral and intravenous use, fosfomycin is available in the United States as an oral, water-soluble tromethamine salt. Following oral administration, the compound is rapidly absorbed and converted to the free acid, fosfomycin. With markedly improved oral bioavailability (35 to 40%), fosfomycin has a mean elimination half-life of 5.5 h, and it is primarily excreted unchanged in the urine (207). Following a single oral dose of 3 g, peak concentrations in serum (range, 22 to 32 μg/ml) are achieved within 2 h after administration, with peak concentrations in urine (1,000 to 4,400 μg/ml) occurring within 4 h and remaining high (>128 μg/ml) for 24 to 48 h, sufficient to inhibit most urinary tract pathogens. Peak concentrations in urine are reached later and lowered when the drug is administered with food or antiperistaltic agents. In patients with renal impairment (creatinine clearance of <30 ml/min), peak concentrations of fosfomycin in serum are increased, with decreased urinary elimination and reduced concentrations of the drug in urine.

While the drug is not bound to plasma protein, it is widely distributed in various body fluids and tissues, including the kidneys, prostate, and seminal vesicles, from which it is cleared slowly. Although it crosses the placental barrier, the drug can be used safely during pregnancy if clearly needed.

Spectrum of Activity

Fosfomycin has a broad spectrum of antibacterial activity against most gram-positive and gram-negative bacteria isolated from patients with lower urinary tract infections. *E. coli*, *Serratia*, *Klebsiella*, *Citrobacter*, *Enterobacter* spp., *S. aureus*, and enterococci are generally inhibited by fosfomycin at concentrations of <64 μg/ml (10, 207, 256). Fosfomycin is bactericidal at concentrations that are similar to the MICs, (twofold differences or less). It is more active than TMP and nalidixic acid and similar to norfloxacin and co-trimoxazole in its activity against these organisms (10). At a breakpoint concentration of ≤128 μg/ml, 60, 20, and 80% of isolates of *Pseudomonas* spp., *Morganella morganii*, and *Staphylococcus saprophyticus*, respectively, are susceptible to fosfomycin (213). In multiple-dose use, bacterial resistance to fosfomycin emerges rapidly, and it can be chromosome mediated or, more rarely, plasmid mediated. However, cross-resistance with other antimicrobials has been uncommon (223).

The in vitro activity of fosfomycin is affected by the test medium and conditions (207, 213). Fosfomycin has much greater in vitro activity, and closer correlation with in vivo activity, when the test medium is supplemented with glucose-6-phosphate at 25 μg/ml, which is recommended for susceptibility testing in the agar and broth dilution methods. The disk diffusion testing method utilizes disks containing 200 μg of fosfomycin tromethamine and 50 or 100 μg of glucose-6-phosphate.

Adverse Effects

Mild, self-limiting gastrointestinal disturbances, mainly diarrhea, are the most frequent side effects, occurring in 3 to 5% of patients. Other minor adverse events include headaches, dizziness, rash, and vaginitis.

METHENAMINE

Methenamine is a tertiary amine with properties of a monoacidic base; it is used as a urinary antiseptic. To be activated, it is combined chemically with a poorly metabolized acid and administered as the mandelate (Mandelamine) or hippurate (Hiprex, Urex) salt.

Mechanism of Action

Methenamine has no antibacterial action by itself, but it is converted at acidic pH to ammonia and formaldehyde, which provides the antiseptic action. This hydrolytic process occurs in the urine, and an effective bacteriostatic concentration of formaldehyde is reached at a urine pH of <5.5. Since the serum is at physiologic pH, formaldehyde is not released while methenamine circulates in the body.

Pharmacology

The agent is well absorbed from the gastrointestinal tract and is rapidly excreted in the urine. The elimination half-life is about 4 h. At a urinary pH of 5.0, about 20% of the methenamine excreted in the urine is hydrolyzed to formaldehyde and ammonia. Bactericidal levels of formaldehyde (>20 mg/ml) are generated in the bladder urine at 2 h after oral administration and may be maintained for at least 6 h or until the patient voids (149). The mandelate and hippurate moieties are also rapidly excreted in the urine in active, unchanged forms by glomerular filtration and tubular secretion. The agent is contraindicated in patients with hepatic insufficiency because of the ammonia produced.

Spectrum of Activity

With the liberation of enough formaldehyde into the urine, methenamine is essentially active against all gram-positive and gram-negative bacteria and also against fungi (149). However, it is not effective for treating urinary tract infections due to urea-splitting organisms such as Proteus and Morganella, which can convert urea to ammonium hydroxide, thereby preventing the hydrolysis of methenamine to formaldehyde. Combination with acetohydroxamic acid, a urease inhibitor, has been suggested for treating these infections by Proteus and Morganella. Since bacteria and fungi do not become resistant to formaldehyde, emergence of resistance to methenamine is not a problem.

Methenamine is not useful for acute urinary tract infections. It has been used successfully as prophylactic therapy for recurrent bacteriuria, particularly infections caused by highly resistant gram-negative bacilli or yeasts. It is also effective as prolonged suppressive therapy for chronic bacteriuria in the absence of structural abnormalities of the urinary tract.

Adverse Effects

Methenamine and its acid salts are generally well tolerated. Some patients experience nausea, vomiting, abdominal cramps, and diarrhea. High doses or prolonged administration of the drug can cause urinary tract irritation by the free formaldehyde, resulting in urinary frequency, dysuria, albuminuria, and hematuria. Skin rashes may also occur. To avoid precipitation of urate crystals in the urine, methenamine salts should not be used in patients with gout or hyperuricemia.

MUPIROCIN

Mupirocin, formerly pseudomonic acid A, is a topical antibacterial agent derived from the fermentation products of Pseudomonas fluorescens (101). Structurally, it contains a unique 9-hydroxynonanoic acid moiety. It was developed for the topical treatment of superficial soft tissue infections, particularly those due to staphylococci.

In the United States, mupirocin is available as a 2% ointment or cream (Bactroban). After topical application, <1% of the drug is absorbed systemically, with no detectable levels in the urine or feces. Penetration into the deeper dermal layers of the skin is increased with traumatized skin or use of occlusive dressings. The drug is highly protein bound (95%), and its activity is lowered in the presence of serum. It is most active at moderately acidic pH, with no inoculum effect (286). It is slowly metabolized in the skin to the inactive monic acid.

Mupirocin inhibits isoleucyl-tRNA synthetase, resulting in cessation of bacterial tRNA and protein synthesis (132). It has excellent in vitro activity, primarily against the gram-positive cocci. S. aureus, including methicillin-resistant strains, and coagulase-negative staphylococci are uniformly very susceptible, with drug MIC$_{90}$s of <0.5 μg/ml (36). Emergence of resistant strains of staphylococci can occur with widespread use of mupirocin (27, 28). Most streptococci (including S. pneumoniae, beta-hemolytic streptococci of groups A, B, C, and G, and viridans streptococci) are inhibited by concentrations of ≤1 μg/ml. Resistant bacteria include enterococci, Corynebacterium spp., Erysipelothrix spp., Propionibacterium acnes, gram-positive anaerobes, and most gram-negative bacteria. However, Haemophilus influenzae, Neisseria gonorrhoeae, N. meningitidis, Moraxella catarrhalis, Bordetella pertussis, and Pasteurella multocida are quite susceptible, with drug MICs in the range of 0.02 to 0.025 μg/ml. There is no cross-resistance between mupirocin and other major groups of antibiotics. Clinically, mupirocin is efficacious in the therapy of superficial skin infections, such as impetigo, folliculitis, and burn wound infections, that are caused by staphylococci or streptococci (106). It has been used successfully to eradicate the nasal carriage of S. aureus, including methicillin-resistant strains (37, 67).

No systemic toxic effects have been reported with mupirocin. Local irritation, such as burning, stinging, itch, and rash, which may be due to the polyethylene glycol base in the vehicle ointment, may occur.

APPENDIX
Approximate Concentrations of Antibacterial Agents in Serum

The concentrations of antimicrobial agents listed below are approximations taken from various reports and publications. Several factors can influence the level of antimicrobial agent in individual patients, including inherent differences in the patients themselves, their physical condition, the dosages, and the routes of administration. The values can also be influenced by the assay methods used to obtain them. Therefore, these concentrations should be used only as approximate values, and clinicians should use their knowledge of the patient and the drugs, the recommendations in the U.S. Food and Drug Administration-approved package inserts, and other reputable sources in planning their therapeutic regimens.

Antimicrobial agent	Half-life in serum (h)	Unit dose	Avg peak level in serum (μg/ml)[a]		
			p.o.	i.m.	i.v.[b]
Amikacin	2–2.5	7.5 mg/kg		15–20	20–40
Amoxicillin	1	500 mg	6–8		
Amoxicillin-clavulanate	1.3/1.0	250/125 mg	3.3 (Amox) 1.5 (Clav)		
Ampicillin	1.1	500 mg	2.5–5	8–10	
		1 g			40
Ampicillin-sulbactam	1.1/1.0	3 g			120 (Amp) 60 (Sulb)
		1.5 g			18 (Amp) 13 (Sulb)
Azithromycin	48	500 mg	0.4		3.5
Azlocillin	1	2 g			130
Aztreonam	1.7	1 g		45	90–160
Bacampicillin	1.1	800 mg	13		
Carbenicillin	1.1	1 g		20–30	150
Carbenicillin indanyl sodium	1.1	764 mg	10		
Cefaclor	0.6	500 mg	16		
Cefadroxil	1.5	500 mg	10		
Cefamandole	0.5–1	1 g		20–36	90–140
Cefazolin	1.8	1 g		65	185
Cefepime	2	1 g		30	82
Cefdinir	1.7	300 mg	1.6		
Cefditoren	1.6	200 mg	3.1		
		400 mg	4.4		
Cefixime	3–4	400 mg	3.5		
Cefmetazole	1.5	1 g			70
Cefonicid	4	1 g		98	220
Cefoperazone	2	1 g		65–75	153
Ceforanide	3	1 g		70	125
Cefotaxime	1	1 g		20	40–45
Cefotetan	3–4.5	1 g		50–80	160
Cefoxitin	1	1 g		20–25	55–110
Cefpirome	2	1 g		45	85
Cefpodoxime	2.5	200 mg	2.3		
Cefprozil	1.5	500 mg	10.5		
Ceftazidime	2	1 g		40	70
Ceftibuten	2.5	400 mg	15		
Ceftizoxime	1.5	1 g		39	80–90
Ceftriaxone	6–9	500 mg		40–45	
		1 g			150
Cefuroxime	1.5	750 mg		27	50
Cefuroxime axetil	1.5	500 mg	9		
Cephalexin	0.9	500 mg	18		
Cephalothin	0.6	1 g			30–60
Cephapirin	0.6	1 g			40–70
Cephradine	0.8	500 mg	16		
Chloramphenicol	4	1 g	10–18		10–15
Chlortetracycline	6–9	500 mg	2–4	12	
Cinoxacin	1–1.5	500 mg	15		

(Continued on next page)

Antimicrobial agent	Half-life in serum (h)	Unit dose	Avg peak level in serum (μg/ml)[a]		
			p.o.	i.m.	i.v.[b]
Ciprofloxacin	3.5	400 mg			4.5
		500 mg	3.0		
		750 mg	4.0		
Clarithromycin	5–7	250 mg	1–2		
		500 mg	3–4		
		1,000 mg XL[c]	2–3		
Clinafloxacin	5.2	200 mg	1.5		
Clindamycin	2.5	300 mg	3	6	
		600 mg			10–12
Cloxacillin	0.5	500 mg	10		
Colistimethate sodium	2–4.5	150 mg		5–6	
Daptomycin	9	4 mg/kg			70
		6 mg/kg			82
Demeclocycline	12	300 mg	1–2		
Dicloxacillin	0.5–0.7	500 mg	15		
Dirithromycin	40	500 mg	0.5		
Doxycycline	18–22	100 mg	2.5		4
Enoxacin	4–6	400 mg	3–5		
Ertapenem	4	1 g		70	155
Erythromycin	1.5	500 mg	2–3		
		1 g			10
Fleroxacin	12	400 mg	5		7–8
Fosfomycin	5.7	3 g	25		
		50 mg/kg			275
Fusidic acid	13–19	500 mg	25–30		50
Gatifloxacin	7	400 mg	4		4.5
Gemifloxacin	7–8	800 mg	4		
Gentamicin	2–3	1.5 mg/kg	4–6		4–8
Imipenem	1	500 mg			25–35
Kanamycin	2.2–3	7.5 mg/kg		20–25	
Levofloxacin	6–8	500 mg	5.5		6.5
		750 mg	8.5		12
Lincomycin	5	500 mg	3.5		
		600 mg		10	16–21
Linezolid	5	600 mg	15		15
Lomefloxacin	6.5	400 mg	3		
Loracarbef	1	400 mg	14		
Meropenem	1	500 mg			25–35
Methicillin	0.5	1 g	15		60
Metronidazole	8	500 mg	12		20–25
Mezlocillin	1	1 g			15
		3 g			260
Minocycline	14–16	100 mg	1		
Moxifloxacin	12	400 mg	4.5		4.5
Nafcillin	0.5	500 mg			5–8
		1 g			20–40
Nalidixic acid	1.5	1 g	20–50		
Netilmicin	2.5	2 mg/kg		5–7	6–8
Nitrofurantoin	0.3	100 mg	<2		
Norfloxacin	3.3	400 mg	1.5		
Ofloxacin	5	400 mg	4		
Ornidazole	13	500 mg	10		20
Oxacillin	0.5	500 mg	4–6	14–16	
		1 g			40
Oxytetracycline	9	500 mg	1–2		
Pefloxacin	10	400 mg	3		5.5
Penicillin G	0.5	500 mg	1.5–2.5		
Aqueous		1 × 10^6 U		8–10	10
Benzathine		1.2 × 10^6 U		0.1–0.15	
Procaine		1.2 × 10^6 U		3	

(Continued on next page)

Antimicrobial agent	Half-life in serum (h)	Unit dose	Avg peak level in serum (μg/ml)[a]		
			p.o.	i.m.	i.v.[b]
Penicillin V	0.5	500 mg	3–5		
Piperacillin	1.1	2 g			36
		4 g			240
Piperacillin-tazobactam	1.1/1.0	3.375 g			242 (Pip)
					24 (Tazo)
		4.5 g			298 (Pip)
					34 (Tazo)
Pivampicillin	0.5–1	350 mg	2		
Polymyxin B	6–7	2.5 mg/kg			5
Quinupristin-dalfopristin	1/0.75	7.5 mg/kg			3 (Q)
					7.5 (D)
Rifampin	2–5	600 mg	7–9		10
Sparfloxacin	20	200 mg	1.1		
Spectinomycin	1–2	2 g		100	
Spiramycin	3.8	2 g	3		
Streptomycin	2–3	1 g		25–50	
Sulfadiazine	17	2 g	100–150		
Sulfadoxine	150–200	1 g	50–75		
Sulfamethizole	4–7	2 g	60		
Sulfamethoxazole	10–12	1 g	40		
Sulfisoxazole	5–7	2 g	170		
Teicoplanin	45	200 mg		7	
		400 mg			20–40
Telithromycin	9–10	800 mg	2		
Tetracycline	8	500 mg	4		8
Ticarcillin	1.2	1 g		20–30	
		3 g			190
Ticarcillin-clavulanate	1.2/1.0	3.1 g			330 (Ticar)
					8 (Clav)
Tinidazole	12–14	2 g	40		40
Tobramycin	2–2.8	1.5 mg/kg		4–6	4–8
Trimethoprim	10–12	100 mg	1		
TMP-SMX		160/800 mg	3 (TMP)		9 (TMP)
			46 (SMX)		106 (SMX)
Trovafloxacin (alatrofloxacin i.v.)	11	300 mg			4.5
Vancomycin	6	500 mg			20–40

[a] p.o., oral; i.m., intramuscular; i.v., intravenous.
[b] At 30 min following intravenous infusion.
[c] Extended-release formulation.

REFERENCES

1. **Allen, N. E., J. N. Hobbs, Jr., and W. E. Alborn, Jr.** 1987. Inhibition of peptidoglycan biosynthesis in gram-positive bacteria by LY146032. *Antimicrob. Agents Chemother.* **31:**1093–1099.
2. **Appelbaum, P. C., M. R. Jacobs, S. K. Spangler, and S. Yamabe.** 1986. Comparative activity of β-lactamase inhibitors YTR 830, clavulanate, and sulbactam combined with β-lactams against β-lactamase-producing anaerobes. *Antimicrob. Agents Chemother.* **30:**789–791.
3. **Aswapokee, N., and H. C. Neu.** 1978. A sulfone beta-lactam compound which acts as a beta-lactamase inhibitor. *J. Antibiot.* **31:**1238–1244.
4. **Balfour, J. A., and D. P. Figgitt.** 2001. Telithromycin. *Drugs* **61:**815–829.
5. **Balfour, J. A., and L. R. Wiseman.** 1999. Moxifloxacin. *Drugs* **57:**363–373.
6. **Ball, P.** 2000. Quinolone generations: natural history or natural selection? *J. Antimicrob. Chemother.* **46:**17–24.
7. **Ball, P., L. Mandell, N. Yoshihito, and G. Tillotson.** 1999. Comparative tolerability of the new fluoroquinolone antibacterials. *Drug Saf.* **21:**407–421.
8. **Bansal, M. B., S. K. Chuah, and H. Thadepalli.** 1985. In vitro activity and in vivo evaluation of ticarcillin plus clavulanic acid against aerobic and anaerobic bacteria. *Am. J. Med.* **79**(Suppl. 5B)**:**33–38.
9. **Barradell, L. B., G. L. Plosker, and D. McTavish.** 1993. Clarithromycin: a review of its pharmacological properties and therapeutic use in *Mycobacterium avium-intracellulare* complex infection in patients with acquired immune deficiency syndrome. *Drugs* **46:**289–312.
10. **Barry, A. L., and S. D. Brown.** 1995. Antibacterial spectrum of fosfomycin trometamol. *J. Antimicrob. Chemother.* **35:**228–230.
11. **Barry, A. L., P. C. Fuchs, and S. D. Brown.** 2001. In vitro activities of daptomycin against 2,789 clinical isolates from 11 North American medical centers. *Antimicrob. Agents Chemother.* **45:**1919–1922.
12. **Barry, A. L., and R. N. Jones.** 1987. Cefixime: spectrum of antibacterial activity against 16,016 clinical isolates. *Pediatr. Infect. Dis. J.* **6:**954–957.
13. **Barry, A. L., R. N. Jones, and C. Thornsberry.** 1988. In vitro activities of azithromycin (CP 62,993), clarithromy-

cin (A-56268, TE-031), erythromycin, roxithromycin, and clindamycin. *Antimicrob. Agents Chemother.* **32:**752–754.

14. **Barry, A. L., C. Thornsberry, R. N. Jones, and T. L. Gavan.** 1985. Aztreonam: antibacterial activity, β-lactamase stability, and interpretive standards and quality control guidelines for disk-diffusion susceptibility test. *Rev. Infect. Dis.* **7**(Suppl. 4):S594–S604.

15. **Bartlett, J. G.** 1982. Anti-anaerobic antibacterial agents. *Lancet* **ii:**478–481.

16. **Bartlett, J. G.** 1992. Antibiotic-associated diarrhea. *Clin. Infect. Dis.* **15:**573–579.

17. **Barza, M.** 1985. Imipenem: first of a new class of β-lactam antibiotics. *Ann. Intern. Med.* **103:**552–560.

18. **Bates, R. D., and M. C. Nahata.** 1994. Once-daily administration of aminoglycosides. *Ann. Pharmacother.* **28:**757–766.

19. **Bauernfeind, A.** 1993. In-vitro activity of dirithromycin in comparison with other new and established macrolides. *J. Antimicrob. Chemother.* **31**(Suppl. 3C):39–49.

20. **Bauernfeind, A.** 1997. Comparison of the antibacterial activities of the quinolones BAY 12-8039, gatifloxacin (AM 1155), trovafloxacin, clinafloxacin, levofloxacin and ciprofloxacin. *J. Antimicrob. Chemother.* **40:**639–651. (Erratum: **41:**672, 1998.)

21. **Bearden, D. T., M. M. Neuhauser, and K. W. Garey.** 2001. Telithromycin: an oral ketolide for respiratory infections. *Pharmacotherapy* **21:**1204–1222.

22. **Berkey, P., D. Moore, and K. Rolston.** 1988. In vitro susceptibilities of *Norcardia* species to newer antimicrobial agents. *Antimicrob. Agents Chemother.* **32:**1078–1079.

23. **Beskid, G., and B. L. T. Prosser.** 1993. A multicenter study on the comparative in vitro activity of fleroxacin and three other fluoroquinolones: an interim report from 27 centers. *Am. J. Med.* **94**(Suppl. 3A):2S–8S.

24. **Blondeau, J. M.** 1999. A review of the comparative in-vitro activities of 12 antimicrobial agents, with a focus on five new "respiratory quinolones." *J. Antimicrob. Chemother.* **43**(Suppl. B):1–11.

25. **Bouanchaud, D. H.** 1997. In-vitro and in-vivo antibacterial activity of quinupristin/dalfopristin. *J. Antimicrob. Chemother.* **39**(Suppl. A):15–21.

26. **Bouza, E., and P. Munoz.** 2001. Linezolid: pharmacokinetic characteristics and clinical studies. *Clin. Microbiol. Infect.* **7**(Suppl. 4):75–82.

27. **Boyce, J. M.** 1996. Preventing staphylococcal infections by eradicating nasal carriage of *Staphyloccus aureus*: proceeding with caution. *Infect. Control Hosp. Epidemiol.* **17:**775–779.

28. **Bradley, S. F., M. A. Ramsey, T. M. Morton, and C. A. Kauffman.** 1995. Mupirocin resistance: clinical and molecular epidemiology. *Infect. Control Hosp. Epidemiol.* **16:**354–358.

29. **Brighty, K. E., and T. D. Gootz.** 1997. The chemistry and biological profile of trovafloxacin. *J. Antimicrob. Chemother.* **39**(Suppl. B):1–14.

30. **Brummett, R. E., and K. E. Fox.** 1989. Vancomycin- and erythromycin-induced hearing loss in humans. *Antimicrob. Agents Chemother.* **33:**791–796.

31. **Bryskier, A.** 2000. Ketolides—telithromycin, an example of a new class of antibacterial agents. *Clin. Microbiol. Infect.* **6:**661–669.

32. **Buesing, M. A., and J. H. Jorgensen.** 1984. In vitro activity of aztreonam in combination with newer β-lactams and amikacin against multiply resistant gram-negative bacilli. *Antimicrob. Agents Chemother.* **25:**283–285.

33. **Bush, K., J. S. Freudenberger, and R. B. Sykes.** 1982. Interaction of azthreonam and related monobactams with β-lactamases from gram-negative bacteria. *Antimicrob. Agents Chemother.* **22:**414–420.

34. **Bushby, S. R. M.** 1973. Trimethoprim-sulfamethoxazole: in vitro microbiological aspects. *J. Infect. Dis.* **128**(Suppl.):S442–S462.

35. **Carroll, O. M., P. A. Bryan, and R. J. Robinson.** 1966. Stevens-Johnson syndrome associated with long-acting sulfonamides. *JAMA* **195:**691–693.

36. **Casewell, M. W., and R. L. R. Hill.** 1985. In-vitro activity of mupirocin (pseudomonic acid) against clinical isolates of *Staphylococcus aureus*. *J. Antimicrob. Chemother.* **15:**523–531.

37. **Casewell, M. W., and R. L. R. Hill.** 1986. Elimination of nasal carriage of *Staphylococcus aureus* with mupirocin (pseudomonic acid): a controlled trial. *J. Antimicrob. Chemother.* **17:**365–372.

38. **Centers for Disease Control and Prevention.** 2002. Sexually transmitted diseases treatment guidelines—2002. *Morb. Mortal. Wkly. Rep.* **51**(RR-6):1–78.

39. **Centers for Disease Control and Prevention.** 2002. USPHS/IDSA guidelines for the prevention of opportunistic infections in persons infected with human immunodeficiency virus. *Morb. Mortal. Wkly. Rep.* **51**(RR-8):1–52.

40. **Cherry, R. D., D. Portnoy, M. Jabbari, D. S. Daly, D. G. Kinnear, and C. A. Goresky.** 1982. Metronidazole: an alternate therapy for antibiotic-associated colitis. *Gastroenterology* **82:**849–851.

41. **Cherubin, C. E.** 1981. Antibiotic resistance of *Salmonella* in Europe and the United States. *Rev. Infect. Dis.* **3:**1105–1126.

42. **Cherubin, C. E., and D. B. Azabache.** 1992. While nearly no one was watching: the rise of erythromycin and clindamycin resistance in *Streptococcus pneumoniae* and *Streptococcus pyogenes*. *Antimicrob. Newsl.* **8:**37–44.

43. **Chopra, I., and M. Roberts.** 2001. Tetracycline antibiotics: mode of action, application, molecular biology, and epidemiology of bacterial resistance. *Microbiol. Mol. Biol. Rev.* **65:**232–260.

44. **Chow, A. W., N. Chang, and K. H. Bartlett.** 1985. In vitro susceptibility of *Clostridium difficile* to new β-lactam and quinolone antibiotics. *Antimicrob. Agents Chemother.* **28:**842–844.

45. **Clark, J., and A. Wallace.** 1967. The susceptibility of mycobacteria to rifamide and rifampin. *Tubercle* **48:**144–148.

46. **Clemett, D., and A. Markham.** 2000. Linezolid. *Drugs* **59:**815–827.

47. **Cohen, M. A., M. D. Huband, J. W. Gage, S. L. Yoder, G. E. Roland, and S. J. Gracheck.** 1997. In-vitro activity of clinafloxacin, trovafloxacin, and ciprofloxacin. *J. Antimicrob. Chemother.* **40:**205–211.

48. **Cohen, M. A., E. T. Joannides, G. E. Roland, M. A. Meservey, M. D. Huband, M. A. Shapiro, J. C. Sesnie, and C. L. Heifetz.** 1994. In vitro evaluation of cefdinir (FK482), a new oral cephalosporin with enhanced antistaphylococcal activity and β-lactamase stability. *Diagn. Microbiol. Infect. Dis.* **18:**31–39.

49. **Cohen, M. A., S. L. Yoder, and G. H. Talbot.** 1996. Sparfloxacin worldwide in vitro literature: isolate data available through 1994. *Diagn. Microbiol. Infect. Dis.* **25:**53–64.

50. **Collins, L. A., G. M. Eliopoulos, C. B. Wennersten, M. J. Ferraro, and R. C. Moellering, Jr.** 1993. In vitro activity of ramoplanin against vancomycin-resistant gram-positive organisms. *Antimicrob. Agents Chemother.* **37:**1364–1366.

51. **Cooper, R. D. G.** 1992. The carbacephems: a new beta-lactam antibiotic class. *Am. J. Med.* **92**(Suppl. 6A):2S–6S.

52. **Coppens, L., and J. Klastersky.** 1979. Comparative study of anti-*Pseudomonas* activity of azlocillin, mezlocillin, and ticarcillin. *Antimicrob. Agents Chemother.* **15**:396–399.

53. **Craig, W. A.** 1997. The pharmacology of meropenem, a new carbapenem antibiotic. *Clin. Infect. Dis.* **24**(Suppl. 2):S266–S275.

54. **Cynamon, M. H., and G. S. Palmer.** 1982. In vitro susceptibility of *Mycobacterium fortuitum* to N-formimidoyl thienamycin and several cephamycins. *Antimicrob. Agents Chemother.* **22**:1079–1081.

55. **Cynamon, M. H., and G. S. Palmer.** 1983. In vitro activity of amoxicillin in combination with clavulanic acid against *Mycobacterium tuberculosis.* *Antimicrob. Agents. Chemother.* **24**:429–431.

56. **Dajani, A. S., K. A. Taubert, W. Wilson, A. F. Bolger, A. Bayer, P. Ferrieri, M. H. Gewitz, S. T. Shulman, S. Nouri, J. W. Newburger, C. Hutto, T. J. Pallasch, T. W. Gage, M. E. Levison, G. Peter, and G. Zuccaro, Jr.** 1997. Prevention of bacterial endocarditis: recommendations by the American Heart Association. JAMA **277**:1794–1801.

57. **Dannemann, B., J. A. McCutchan, D. Israelski, D. Antoniskis, C. Leport, B. Luft, J. Nussbaum, N. Clumeck, P. Morlat, J. Chiu, J.-L. Vilde, P. Haseltine, J. Leedom, J. Remington, M. Orellana, D. Feigal, A. Bartok, and the California Collaborative Treatment Group.** 1992. Treatment of toxoplasmic encephalitis in patients with AIDS: a randomized trial comparing pyrimethamine plus clindamycin to pyrimethamine plus sulfadiazine. *Ann. Intern. Med.* **116**:33–43.

58. **Davey, P., J.-C. Pechère, and D. Speller (ed.).** 1988. Spiramycin reassessed. *J. Antimicrob. Chemother.* **22**(Suppl. B):1–210.

59. **Davey, P. G., and A. H. Williams.** 1991. A review of the safety profile of teicoplanin. *J. Antimicrob. Chemother.* **27**(Suppl. B):69–73.

60. **Davies, J. E.** 1983. Resistance to aminoglycosides: mechanisms and frequency. *Rev. Infect. Dis.* **5**(Suppl. 2):S261–S267.

61. **Davies, S., P. D. Sparham, and R. C. Spencer.** 1987. Comparative in-vitro activity of five fluoroquinolones against mycobacteria. *J. Antimicrob. Chemother.* **19**:605–609.

62. **Davies, T. A., B. E. Dewasse, M. R. Jacobs, and P. C. Appelbaum.** 2000. In vitro development of resistance to telithromycin (HMR 3647), four macrolides, clindamycin, and pristinamycin in *Streptococcus pneumoniae.* *Antimicrob. Agents Chemother.* **44**:414–417.

63. **Davis, B. D.** 1982. Bactericidal synergism between β-lactams and aminoglycosides: mechanism and possible therapeutic implications. *Rev. Infect. Dis.* **4**:237–245.

64. **Davis, R., and H. M. Bryson.** 1994. Levofloxacin: a review of its antibacterial activity, pharmacokinetics and therapeutic efficacy. *Drugs* **47**:677–700.

65. **Denton, M., and K. G. Kerr.** 1998. Microbiological and clinical aspects of infection associated with *Stenotrophomonas maltophilia.* *Clin. Microbiol. Rev.* **11**:57–80.

66. **Dewsnup, D. H., and D. N. Wright.** 1984. In vitro susceptibility of *Nocardia asteroides* to 25 antimicrobial agents. *Antimicrob. Agents Chemother.* **25**:165–167.

67. **Doebbeling, B. N., D. L. Breneman, H. C. Neu, R. Aly, B. G. Yangco, H. P. Holley, Jr., R. J. Marsh, M. A. Pfaller, J. E. McGowan, Jr., B. E. Scully, D. R. Reagan, R. P. Wenzel, and the Mupirocin Collaborative Study Group.** 1993. Elimination of *Staphylococcus aureus* nasal carriage in health care workers: analysis of six clinical trials with calcium mupirocin. *Clin. Infect. Dis.* **17**:466–474.

68. **Drusano, G.** 2001. Pharmacodynamic and pharmacokinetic considerations in antimicrobial selection: focus on telithromycin. *Clin. Microbiol. Infect.* **7**(Suppl. 3):24–29.

69. **Drusano, G. L., S. C. Schimpff, and W. L. Hewitt.** 1984. The acylampicillins: mezlocillin, piperacillin, and azlocillin. *Rev. Infect. Dis.* **6**:13–32.

70. **Dudley, M. N., J. C. McLaughlin, G. Carrington, J. Frick, C. H. Nightingale, and R. Quintiliani.** 1986. Oral bacitracin vs vancomycin therapy for *Clostridium difficile*-induced diarrhea: a randomized double-blind trial. *Arch. Intern. Med.* **146**:1101–1104.

71. **Eady, E. A., J. I. Ross, and J. H. Cove.** 1990. Multiple mechanisms of erythromycin resistance. *J. Antimicrob. Chemother.* **26**:461–465.

72. **Edelstein, P. H., E. A. Gaudet, and M. A. C. Edelstein.** 1989. In vitro activity of lomefloxacin (NY-198 or SC 47111), ciprofloxacin, and erythromycin against 100 clinical *Legionella* strains. *Diagn. Microbiol. Infect. Dis.* **12**(Suppl.):93S–95S.

73. **Ednie, L. M., M. R. Jacobs, and P. C. Appelbaum.** 1998. Activities of gatifloxacin compared to those of seven other agents against anaerobic organisms. *Antimicrob. Agents Chemother.* **42**:2459–2462.

74. **Edwards, D. I.** 1993. Nitroimidazole drugs—action and resistance mechanisms. I. Mechanisms of action. *J. Antimicrob. Chemother.* **31**:9–20.

75. **Edwards, J. R.** 1995. Meropenem: a microbiological overview. *J. Antimicrob. Chemother.* **36**(Suppl. A):1–17.

76. **Eliopoulos, G. M.** 1997. Vancomycin-resistant enterococci: mechanism and clinical relevance. *Infect. Dis. Clin. North Am.* **11**:851–865.

77. **Eliopoulos, G. M., and C. T. Eliopoulos.** 1993. Activity in vitro of the quinolones, p. 161–193. *In* D. C. Hooper and J. S. Wolfson (ed.), *Quinolone Antimicrobial Agents,* 2nd ed. American Society for Microbiology, Washington, D.C.

78. **Eliopoulos, G. M., K. Klimm, M. J. Ferraro, G. A. Jacoby, and R. C. Moellering, Jr.** 1989. Comparative in vitro activity of piperacillin combined with the beta-lactamase inhibitor tazobactam (YTR 830). *Diagn. Microbiol. Infect. Dis.* **12**:481–488.

79. **Endtz, H. P., G. J. Ruijs, B. van Klingeren, W. H. Jansen, T. van Reyden, and R. P. Mouton.** 1991. Quinolone resistance in campylobacter isolated from man and poultry following the introduction of fluoroquinolones in veterinary medicine. *J. Antimicrob. Chemother.* **27**:199–208.

80. **Ericsson, C. D., and H. L. DuPont.** 1993. Travelers' diarrhea: approaches to prevention and treatment. *Clin. Infect. Dis.* **16**:616–624.

81. **Fass, R. J.** 1983. Comparative in vitro activities of third-generation cephalosporins. *Arch. Intern. Med.* **143**:1743–1745.

82. **Fass, R. J., E. A. Copelan, J. T. Brandt, M. L. Moeschberger, and J. J. Ashton.** 1987. Platelet-mediated bleeding caused by broad-spectrum penicillins. *J. Infect. Dis.* **155**:1242–1248.

83. **Fee, W. E., Jr.** 1980. Aminoglycoside ototoxicity in the human. *Laryngoscope* **90**(Suppl. 24):1–19.

84. **Feeley, T. W., G. C. DuMoulin, J. Hedley-Whyte, L. S. Bushnell, J. P. Gilbert, and D. S. Feingold.** 1975. Aerosol polymyxin and pneumonia in seriously ill patients. *N. Engl. J. Med.* **293**:471–475.

85. **Fekete, T.** 1993. Antimicrobial susceptibility testing of *Neisseria gonorrhoeae* and implication for epidemiology and therapy. *Clin. Microbiol. Rev.* **6**:22–33.

86. **Fekety, R., J. Silva, B. Buggy, and H. G. Deery.** 1984. Treatment of antibiotic-associated colitis with vancomycin. *J. Antimicrob. Chemother.* **14**(Suppl. D):97–102.

87. **Felmingham, D.** 2001. Microbiological profile of telithromycin, the first ketolide antimicrobial. *Clin. Microbiol. Infect.* **7**(Suppl. 3):2–10.

88. **Felmingham, D., G. Zhanel, and D. Hoban.** 2001. Activity of the ketolide antibacterial telithromycin against typical community-acquired respiratory pathogens. *J. Antimicrob. Chemother.* **48**:33–42.

89. **Fernandez-Roblas, R., J. Esteban, F. Cabria, et al.** 2000. In vitro susceptibilities of rapidly growing mycobacteria to telithromycin (HMR 3647) and seven other antimicrobials. *Antimicrob. Agents Chemother.* **44**:181–182.

90. **Finch, R. G.** 1996. Antibacterial activity of quinupristin/dalfopristin: rationale for clinical use. *Drugs* **51**(Suppl. 1):31–37.

91. **Finland, M., M. C. Bach, C. Garner, and O. Gold.** 1974. Synergistic action of ampicillin and erythromycin against *Nocardia asteroides*: effect of time of incubation. *Antimicrob. Agents Chemother.* **5**:344–353.

92. **Finland, M., C. Garner, C. Wilcox, and L. D. Sabath.** 1976. Susceptibility of beta-hemolytic streptococci to 65 antibacterial agents. *Antimicrob. Agents Chemother.* **9**:11–19.

93. **Ford, C. W., J. C. Hamel, D. Stapert, J. K. Moerman, D. K. Hutchinson, M. R. Barbachyn, and G. E. Zurenko.** 1997. Oxazolidinones: new antibacterial agents. *Trends Microbiol.* **5**:196–200.

94. **Frampton, J. E., R. N. Brogden, H. D. Langtry, and M. M. Buckley.** 1992. Cefpodoxime proxetil: a review of its antibacterial activity, pharmacokinetic properties and therapeutic potential. *Drugs* **44**:889–917.

95. **Freeman, L. D., D. R. Hopper, D. F. Lathen, D. P. Nelson, W. O. Harrison, and D. S. Anderson.** 1983. Brief prophylaxis with doxycycline for the prevention of traveler's diarrhea. *Gastroenterology* **84**:276–280.

96. **Frost, P., G. D. Weinstein, and E. C. Gomez.** 1972. Phototoxic potential of minocycline and doxycycline. *Arch. Dermatol.* **105**:681–683.

97. **Fu, K. P., and H. C. Neu.** 1976. In vitro study of netilmicin compared with other aminoglycosides. *Antimicrob. Agents Chemother.* **10**:526–534.

98. **Fu, K. P., and H. C. Neu.** 1979. Comparative inhibition of β-lactamases by novel β-lactam compounds. *Antimicrob. Agents Chemother.* **15**:171–176.

99. **Fuchs, P. C., A. L. Barry, and S. D. Brown.** 2001. In vitro activities of ertapenem (MK-0826) against clinical bacterial isolates from 11 North American medical centers. *Antimicrob. Agents Chemother.* **45**:1915–1918.

100. **Fuchs, P. C., A. L. Barry, C. Thornsberry, and R. N. Jones.** 1984. In vitro activity of ticarcillin plus clavulanic acid against 632 clinical isolates. *Antimicrob. Agents Chemother.* **25**:392–394.

101. **Fuller, A. T., G. Mellows, M. Woolford, G. T. Banks, K. D. Barrow, and E. B. Chain.** 1971. Pseudomonic acid: an antibiotic produced by *Pseudomonas fluorescens*. *Nature* (London) **234**:416–417.

102. **Fung-Tomc, J. C.** 1997. Fourth-generation cephalosporins. *Clin. Microbiol. Newsl.* **19**:129–136.

103. **Gardner, T. B., and D. R. Hill.** 2001. Treatment of giardiasis. *Clin. Microbiol. Rev.* **14**:114–128.

104. **Geraci, J. E., and W. R. Wilson.** 1981. Vancomycin therapy for infective endocarditis. *Rev. Infect. Dis.* **3**(Suppl.):S250–S258.

105. **Giamarellou, H.** 1986. Aminoglycosides plus β-lactams against gram-negative organisms: evaluation of in vitro synergy and chemical interactions. *Am. J. Med.* **80**(Suppl. 6B):126–137.

106. **Goldfarb, J., D. Crenshaw, J. O'Horo, E. Lemon, and J. L. Blumer.** 1988. Randomized clinical trial of topical mupirocin versus oral erythromycin for impetigo. *Antimicrob. Agents Chemother.* **32**:1780–1783.

107. **Goldstein, E. J. C., D. M. Citron, C. V. Merriam, Y. Warren, and K. L. Tyrrell.** 2000. Comparative in vitro activities of ertapenem (MK-0826) against 1,001 anaerobes isolated from human intra-abdominal infections. *Antimicrob. Agents Chemother.* **44**:2389–2394.

108. **Goldstein, F. W., B. Papadopoulou, and J. F. Acar.** 1986. The changing pattern of trimethoprim resistance in Paris, with a review of worldwide experience. *Rev. Infect. Dis.* **8**:725–737.

109. **Gonzales, R. D., P. C. Schreckenberger, M. B. Graham, S. Kelkar, K. DenBesten, and J. P. Quinn.** 2001. Infections due to vancomycin-resistant *Enterococcus faecium* resistant to linezolid. *Lancet* **357**:1179.

110. **Gordin, F. M., G. L. Simon, C. B. Wofsy, and J. Mills.** 1984. Adverse reactions to trimethoprim-sulfamethoxazole in patients with acquired immunodeficiency syndrome. *Ann. Intern. Med.* **100**:495–499.

111. **Gorzynski, E. A., D. Amsterdam, T. R. Beam, Jr., and C. Rotstein.** 1989. Comparative in vitro activities of teicoplanin, vancomycin, oxacillin, and other antimicrobial agents against bacteremic isolates of gram-positive cocci. *Antimicrob. Agents Chemother.* **33**:2019–2022.

112. **Grasela, D. M.** 2000. Clinical pharmacology of gatifloxacin, a new fluoroquinolone. *Clin. Infect. Dis.* **31**(Suppl. 2):S51–S58.

113. **Gravenkemper, C. F., J. V. Bennett, J. L. Brodie, and W. M. M. Kirby.** 1965. Dicloxacillin: in vitro and pharmacologic comparisons with oxacillin and cloxacillin. *Arch. Intern. Med.* **116**:340–345.

114. **Green, S. L., J. C. Maddox, and E. D. Huttenbach.** 2001. Linezolid and reversible myelosuppression. *JAMA* **285**:1291.

115. **Greenwood, D.** 1988. Microbiological properties of teicoplanin. *J. Antimicrob. Chemother.* **21**(Suppl. A):1–13.

116. **Grosset, J., and S. Leventis.** 1983. Adverse effects of rifampin. *Rev. Infect. Dis.* **5**(Suppl. 3):S440–S446.

117. **Grossman, E. R., A. Walcheck, and H. Freedman.** 1971. Tetracycline and permanent teeth: the relationship between doses and tooth color. *Pediatrics* **47**:567–570.

118. **Gump, D. W.** 1981. Vancomycin for treatment of bacterial meningitis. *Rev. Infect. Dis.* **3**(Suppl.):S289–S292.

119. **Gutmann, L., M. D. Kitzis, S. Yamabe, and J. F. Acar.** 1986. Comparative evaluation of a new β-lactamase inhibitor, YTR 830, combined with different β-lactam antibiotics against bacteria harboring known β-lactamases. *Antimicrob. Agents Chemother.* **29**:955–957.

120. **Guttler, R. B., G. W. Counts, C. K. Avent, and H. N. Beaty.** 1971. Effect of rifampin and minocycline on meningococcal carrier rates. *J. Infect. Dis.* **124**:199–205.

121. **Hansen, L. H., P. Mauvais, and S. Douthwaite.** 1999. The macrolide-ketolide antibiotic binding site is formed by structures in domain II and V of 23S ribosomal RNA. *Mol. Microbiol.* **31**:623–631.

122. **Hardy, D. J., D. M. Hensey, J. M. Beyer, C. Vojtko, E. J. McDonald, and P. B. Fernandes.** 1988. Comparative in vitro activities of new 14-, 15-, and 16-membered macrolides. *Antimicrob. Agents Chemother.* **32**:1710–1719.

123. **Haydon, R. C., J. W. Thelin, and W. E. Davis.** 1984. Erythromycin ototoxicity: analysis and conclusions based on 22 case reports. *Otolaryngol. Head Neck Surg.* **92**:678–684.

124. **Hitchings, G. H.** 1973. Mechanism of action of trimethoprim-sulfamethoxazole. I. *J. Infect. Dis.* **128**(Suppl.): S433–S436.

125. **Hoban, D. J., R. N. Jones, N. Yamane, R. Frei, A. Trilla, and A. C. Pignatari.** 1993. In vitro activity of three carbapenem antibiotics: comparative studies with biapenem (L-627), imipenem, and meropenem against aerobic pathogens isolated worldwide. *Diagn. Microbiol. Infect. Dis.* **17**:299–305.

126. **Hoeprich, P. D., and D. M. Warshauer.** 1974. Entry of four tetracyclines into saliva and tears. *Antimicrob. Agents Chemother.* **5**:330–336.

127. **Hof, H., O. Zak, E. Schweizer, and A. Danzler.** 1984. Antibacterial activities of nitrothiazole derivatives. *J. Antimicrob. Chemother.* **14**:31–39.

128. **Holmberg, L., G. Boman, L. E. Bottiger, B. Eriksson, R. Spross, and A. Wessling.** 1980. Adverse reactions to nitrofurantoin: analysis of 921 reports. *Am. J. Med.* **69**: 733–738.

129. **Hooper, D. C.** 2000. Mechanisms of action and resistance of older and newer fluoroquinolines. *Clin. Infect. Dis.* **31**(Suppl. 2):S24–S28.

130. **Hooton, T. M., and W. E. Stamm.** 1997. Diagnosis and treatment of uncomplicated urinary tract infection. *Infect. Dis. Clin. North Am.* **11**:551–581.

131. **Horiuchi, S., Y. Inagaki, N. Yamamoto, N. Okamura, Y. Imagawa, and R. Nakaya.** 1993. Reduced susceptibilities of *Shigella sonnei* strains isolated from patients with dysentery to fluoroquinolones. *Antimicrob. Agents Chemother.* **37**:2486–2489.

132. **Hughes, J., and G. Mellows.** 1978. Inhibition of isoleucyl-transfer ribonucleic acid synthetase in *Escherichia coli* by pseudomonic acid. *Biochem. J.* **176**:305–318.

133. **Jacoby, G. A.** 1997. Extended-spectrum β-lactamases and other enzymes providing resistance to oxyimino-β-lactams. *Infect. Dis. Clin. North Am.* **11**:875–887.

134. **Jacoby, G. A., and L. Sutton.** 1989. *Pseudomonas cepacia* susceptibility to sulbactam. *Antimicrob. Agents Chemother.* **33**:583–584.

135. **Johnson, A. P., A. H. C. Uttley, N. Woodford, and R. C. George.** 1990. Resistance to vancomycin and teicoplanin: an emerging clinical problem. *Clin. Microbiol. Rev.* **3**:280–291.

136. **Johnson, D. M., D. J. Biedenbach, M. L. Beach, M. A. Pfaller, and R. N. Jones.** 2000. Antimicrobial activity and in vitro susceptibility test development for cefditoren against *Haemophilus influenzae*, *Moraxella catarrhalis*, and *Streptococcus* species. *Diagn. Microbiol. Infect. Dis.* **37**:99–105.

137. **Jones, R. N.** 1989. Review of the in-vitro spectrum and characteristics of cefmetazole (CS-1170). *J. Antimicrob. Chemother.* **23**(Suppl. D):1–12.

138. **Jones, R. N.** 1993. Ceftibuten: a review of antimicrobial activity, spectrum and other microbiologic features. *Pediatr. Infect. Dis. J.* **12**:517–544.

139. **Jones, R. N., and A. L. Barry.** 1983. Cefoperazone: a review of its antimicrobial spectrum, β-lactamase stability, enzyme inhibition, and other in vitro characteristics. *Rev. Infect. Dis.* **5**(Suppl. 1):S108–S126.

140. **Jones, R. N., D. J. Biedenbach, and D. M. Johnson.** 2000. Cefditoren activity against nearly 1000 non-fastidious bacterial isolates and the development of in vitro susceptibility test methods. *Diagn. Microbiol. Infect. Dis.* **37**:143–146.

141. **Jones, R. N., M. A. Pfaller, S. D. Allen, E. H. Gerlach, P. C. Fuchs, and K. E. Aldridge.** 1991. Antimicrobial activity of cefpirome: an update compared to five third-generation cephalosporins against nearly 6,000 recent clinical isolates from five medical centers. *Diagn. Microbiol. Infect. Dis.* **14**:361–364.

142. **Kahan, F. M., J. S. Kahan, P. J. Cassidy, and H. Kropp.** 1974. The mechanism of action of fosfomycin (phosphonomycin). *Ann. N. Y. Acad. Sci.* **235**:364–386.

143. **Kelkar, P. S., and J. T.-C. Li.** 2001. Cephalosporin allergy. *N. Engl. J. Med.* **345**:801–809.

144. **Kenny, G. E., T. M. Hooton, M. C. Roberts, F. D. Cartwright, and J. Hoyt.** 1989. Susceptibilities of genital mycoplasmas to the newer quinolones as determined by the agar dilution method. *Antimicrob. Agents Chemother.* **33**:103–107.

145. **King, A., and I. Phillips.** 2001. The in vitro activity of daptomycin against 514 gram-positive aerobic clinical isolates. *J. Antimicrob. Chemother.* **48**:219–223.

146. **Kirst, H. A., and G. D. Sides.** 1989. New directions for macrolide antibiotics: structural modifications and in vitro activity. *Antimicrob. Agents Chemother.* **33**:1413–1418.

147. **Klugman, K. P.** 1990. Pneumococcal resistance to antibiotics. *Clin. Microbiol. Rev.* **3**:171–196.

148. **Knapp, C. C., J. Sierra-Madero, and J. A. Washington.** 1989. Activity of ticarcillin/clavulanate and piperacillin/tazobactam (YTR 830; CL-298,741) against clinical isolates and against mutants derepressed for class I beta-lactamase. *Diagn. Microbiol. Infect. Dis.* **12**:511–515.

149. **Knight, V., J. W. Draper, E. A. Brady, and C. A. Attmore.** 1952. Methanamine mandelate: antimicrobial activity, absorption and excretion. *Antibiot. Chemother.* **2**:615–635.

150. **Kohler, J., K. L. Dorso, K. Young, G. G. Hammond, H. Rosen, H. Kropp, and L. L. Silver.** 1999. In vitro activities of potent, broad-spectrum carbapenem MK-0826 (L-749,345) against broad-spectrum β-lactamase- and extended-spectrum β-lactamase-producing *Klebsiella pneumoniae* and *Escherichia coli* clinical isolates. *Antimicrob. Agents Chemother.* **43**:1170–1176.

151. **Kuck, N. A., N. V. Jacobus, P. J. Petersen, W. J. Weiss, and R. T. Testa.** 1989. Comparative in vitro and in vivo activities of piperacillin combined with the β-lactamase inhibitors tazobactam, clavulanic acid, and sulbactam. *Antimicrob. Agents Chemother.* **33**:1964–1969.

152. **Lamb, H. M., D. P. Figgitt, and D. Faulds.** 1999. Quinupristin/dalfopristin: a review of its use in the management of serious gram-positive infections. *Drugs* **58**:1061–1097.

153. **Lawson, D. H., and B. J. Paice.** 1982. Adverse reactions to trimethoprim-sulfamethoxazole. *Rev. Infect. Dis.* **4**: 429–433.

154. **Leigh, D. A.** 1981. Antibacterial activity and pharmacokinetics of clindamycin. *J. Antimicrob. Chemother.* **7**(Suppl. A):3–9.

155. **Linden, P. K., R. C. Moellering, C. A. Wood, S. J. Rehm, J. Flaherty, F. Bompart, and G. H. Talbot, for the Synercid Emergency-Use Study Group.** 2001. Treatment of vancomycin-resistant *Enterococcus faecium* infections with quinupristin/dalfopristin. *Clin. Infect. Dis.* **33**:1816–1823.

156. **Lipsky, B. A., and C. A. Baker.** 1999. Fluoroquinolone toxicity profiles: a review focusing on newer agents. *Clin. Infect. Dis.* **28**:352–364.

157. **Livermore, D. M., M. W. Carter, S. Bagel, B. Wide-mann, F. Baquero, E. Loza, H. P. Endtz, N. van Den Braak, C. J. Fernandes, L. Fernandes, N. Frimodt-Moller, L. S. Rasmussen, H. Giamarellou, E. Giamarel-los-Bourboulis, V. Jarlier, J. Nguyen, C. E. Nord, M. J. Struelens, C. Nonhoff, J. Turnidge, J. Bell, R. Zbinden, S. Pfister, L. Mixson, and D. L. Shungu.** 2001. In vitro activities of ertapenem (MK-0826) against recent clinical

bacteria collected in Europe and Australia. 2001. *Antimicrob. Agents Chemother.* **45:**1860–1867.

158. **Livermore, D. M., K. J. Oakton, M. W. Carter, and M. Warner.** 2001. Activity of ertapenem (MK-0826) versus *Enterobacteriaceae* with potent β-lactamases. *Antimicrob. Agents Chemother.* **45:**2831–2837.

159. **Lode, H., K. Borner, P. Koeppe, and T. Schaberg.** 1996. Azithromycin—review of key chemical, pharmacokinetic and microbiological features. *J. Antimicrob. Chemother.* **37**(Suppl. C)**:**1–8.

160. **Low, D. E.** 1995. Quinupristin/dalfopristin: spectrum of activity, pharmacokinetics, and initial clinical experience. *Microb. Drug Resist.* **1:**223–234.

161. **Low, D. E., A. McGeer, and R. Poon.** 1989. Activities of daptomycin and teicoplanin against *Staphylococcus haemolyticus* and *Staphylococcus epidermidis*, including evaluation of susceptibility testing recommendations. *Antimicrob. Agents Chemother.* **33:**585–588.

162. **Lutsar, I., G. H. McCracken, and I. R. Friendland.** 1998. Antibiotic pharmacodynamics in cerebrospinal fluid. *Clin. Infect. Dis.* **27:**1117–1127.

163. **Malanoski, G. J., L. Collins, C. Wennersten, R. C. Moellering, and G. M. Eliopoulos.** 1993. In vitro activity of biapenem against clinical isolates of gram-positive and gram-negative bacteria. *Antimicrob. Agents Chemother.* **37:**2009–2016.

164. **Mandell, G. L.** 1983. The antimicrobial activity of rifampin: emphasis on the relation to phagocytes. *Rev. Infect. Dis.* **5**(Suppl. 3)**:**S463–S467.

165. **Marchese, A., and G. C. Schito.** 2001. The oxazolidinones as a new family of antimicrobial agent. *Clin. Microbiol. Infect.* **7**(Suppl. 4)**:**66–74.

166. **Marco, F., R. N. Jones, D. J. Hoban, A. C. Pignatari, N. Yamane, and R. Frei.** 1994. In-vitro activity of OPC-17116 against more than 6,000 consecutive clinical isolates: a multicentre international study. *J. Antimicrob. Chemother.* **33:**647–654.

167. **Martinez-Martinez, L., A. Pascual, and G. A. Jacoby.** 1998. Quinolone resistance from a transferable plasmid. *Lancet* **351:**797–799.

168. **Maurin, M., S. Gasquet, C. Ducco, and D. Raoult.** 1995. MICs of 28 antibiotic compounds for 14 *Bartonella* (formerly *Rochalimaea*) isolates. *Antimicrob. Agents Chemother.* **39:**2387–2391.

169. **Maurin, M., and D. Raoult.** 2001. Use of aminoglycosides in treatment of infections due to intracellular bacteria. *Antimicrob. Agents Chemother.* **45:**2977–2986.

170. **McCalla, D. R.** 1977. Biological effects of nitrofurans. *J. Antimicrob. Chemother.* **3:**517–520.

171. **McCracken, G. H.** 2000. Pharmacodynamics of gatifloxacin in experimental models of pneumococcal meningitis. *Clin. Infect. Dis.* **31**(Suppl. 2)**:**S45–S50.

172. **McDowell, T. D., and K. E. Reed.** 1989. Mechanism of penicillin killing in the absence of bacterial lysis. *Antimicrob. Agents Chemother.* **33:**1680–1685.

173. **McGehee, R. F., Jr., C. B. Smith, C. Wilcox, and M. Finland.** 1968. Comparative studies of antibacterial activity in vitro and absorption and excretion of lincomycin and clindamycin. *Am. J. Med. Sci.* **256:**279–292.

174. **McNulty, C. A. M., J. Dent, and R. Wise.** 1985. Susceptibility of clinical isolates of *Campylobacter pyloridis* to 11 antimicrobial agents. *Antimicrob. Agents Chemother.* **28:**837–838.

175. **Medical Letter on Drugs and Therapeutics.** 1998. Drugs for parasitic infections. *Med. Lett. Drugs Ther.* **40:**1–12.

176. **Medical Letter on Drugs and Therapeutics.** 1999. Drugs for sexually transmitted diseases. *Med. Lett. Drugs Ther.* **41:**85–90.

177. **Medical Letter on Drugs and Therapeutics.** 2000. Treatment of Lyme disease. *Med. Lett. Drugs Ther.* **42:**37–39.

178. **Moellering, R. C., Jr.** 1984. Pharmacokinetics of vancomycin. *J. Antimicrob. Chemother.* **14**(Suppl. D)**:**43–52.

179. **Moellering, R. C., Jr.** 1991. The enterococcus: a classic example of the impact of antimicrobial resistance on therapeutic options. *J. Antimicrob. Chemother.* **28:**1–12.

180. **Moellering, R. C., Jr., P. K. Linden, J. Reinhardt, E. A. Blumberg, F. Bompart, and G. H. Talbot.** 1999. The efficacy and safety of quinupristin/dalfopristin for the treatment of infections caused by vancomycin-resistant *Enterococcus faecium. J. Antimicrob. Chemother.* **44:**251–261.

181. **Molavi, A., and L. Weinstein.** 1971. In-vitro activity of erythromycin against atypical mycobacteria. *J. Infect. Dis.* **123:**216–219.

182. **Monk, J. P., and D. M. Campoli-Richards.** 1987. Ofloxacin: a review of its antibacterial activity, pharmacokinetic properties and therapeutic use. *Drugs* **33:**346–391.

183. **Moosdeen, F., J. D. Williams, and S. Yamabe.** 1988. Antibacterial characteristics of YTR 830, a sulfone β-lactamase inhibitor, compared with those of clavulanic acid and sulbactam. *Antimicrob. Agents Chemother.* **32:**925–927.

184. **Morris, A. B., R. B. Brown, and M. Sands.** 1993. Use of rifampin in nonstaphylococcal, nonmycobacterial disease. *Antimicrob. Agents Chemother.* **37:**1–7.

185. **Murray, B. E.** 1990. The life and times of the enterococcus. *Clin. Microbiol. Rev.* **3:**46–65.

186. **Muscato, J. J., D. W. Wilbur, J. J. Stout, and R. A. Fahrlender.** 1991. An evaluation of the susceptibility patterns of gram-negative organisms isolated in cancer centres with aminoglycoside usage. *J. Antimicrob. Chemother.* **27**(Suppl. C)**:**1–7.

187. **Musial, C. E., and J. E. Rosenblatt.** 1989. Antimicrobial susceptibilities of anaerobic bacteria isolated at the Mayo Clinic during 1982 through 1987: comparison with results from 1977 through 1981. *Mayo Cin. Proc.* **64:**392–399.

188. **Nadelman, R. B., S. W. Luger, E. Frank, M. Wisniewski, J. J. Collins, and G. P. Wormser.** 1992. Comparison of cefuroxime axetil and doxycycline in the treatment of Lyme disease. *Ann. Intern. Med.* **117:**273–280.

189. **Nagarajan, R.** 1991. Antibacterial activities and modes of action of vancomycin and related glycopeptides. *Antimicrob. Agents Chemother.* **35:**605–609.

190. **Najjar, A., and B. E. Murray.** 1987. Failure to demonstrate a consistent in vitro bactericidal effect of trimethoprim-sulfamethoxazole against enterococci. *Antimicrob. Agents Chemother.* **31:**808–810.

191. **Namour, F., D. H. Wessels, M. H. Pascual, D. Reynolds, E. Sultan, and B. Lenfant.** 2001. Pharmacokinetics of the new ketolide telithromycin (HMR 3647) administered in ascending single and multiple doses. *Antimicrob. Agents Chemother.* **45:**170–175.

192. **Neu, H. C.** 1976. Tobramycin: an overview. *J. Infect. Dis.* **134**(Suppl.)**:**S3–S19.

193. **Neu, H. C.** 1982. The new beta-lactamase-stable cephalosporins. *Ann. Intern. Med.* **97:**408–419.

194. **Neu, H. C.** 1985. Carbapenems: special properties contributing to their activity. *Am. J. Med.* **78**(Suppl 6A)**:**33–40.

195. **Neu, H. C.** 1991. Clinical microbiology of azithromycin. *Am. J. Med.* **91**(Suppl. 3A)**:**12S–18S.

196. **Neu, H. C.** 1991. The development of macrolides: clarithromycin in perspective. *J. Antimicrob. Chemother.* **27**(Suppl. A)**:**1–9.

197. **Neu, H. C., and K. P. Fu.** 1978. Clavulanic acid, a novel inhibitor of beta-lactamases. *Antimicrob. Agents Chemother.* **14:**650–655.

198. **Neu, H. C., and K. P. Fu.** 1980. In vitro activity of chloramphenicol and thiamphenicol analogs. *Antimicrob. Agents Chemother.* **18:**311–316.

199. **Neu, H. C., and P. Lubthavikul.** 1982. Comparative in vitro activity of N-formimidoyl thienamycin against gram-positive and gram-negative aerobic and anaerobic species and its β-lactamase stability. *Antimicrob. Agents Chemother.* **21:**180–187.

200. **Nord, C. E.** 1996. In vitro activity of quinolones and other antimicrobial agents against anaerobic bacteria. *Clin. Infect. Dis.* **23**(Suppl. 1)**:**S15–S18.

201. **Norrby, S. F., K. L. Faulkner, and P. A. Newell.** 1997. Differentiating meropenem and imipenem/cilastatin. *Infect. Dis. Clin. Pract.* **6:**291–303.

202. **O'Brien, R. J., M. A. Lyle, and D. E. Snider, Jr.** 1987. Rifabutin (ansamycin LM 427): a new rifamycin-S derivative for the treatment of mycobacterial diseases. *Rev. Infect. Dis.* **9:**519–530.

203. **Pang, L. W., N. Limsomwong, E. F. Boudreau, and P. Singharaj.** 1987. Doxycycline prophylaxis for falciparum malaria. *Lancet* **i:**1161–1164.

204. **Pankuch, G. A., T. A. Davies, M. R. Jacobs, and P. C. Appelbaum.** 2002. Antipneumococcal activity of ertapenem (MK-0826) compared to those of other agents. *Antimicrob. Agents Chemother.* **46:**42–46.

205. **Pape, J. W., R. I. Verdier, and W. D. Johnson, Jr.** 1989. Treatment and prophylaxis of Isospora belli infection in patients with the acquired immunodeficiency syndrome. *N. Engl. J. Med.* **320:**1044–1047.

206. **Patel, R. B., and P. G. Welling.** 1980. Clinical pharmacokinetics of co-trimoxazole (trimethoprim-sulfamethoxazole). *Clin. Pharmacokinet.* **5:**405–423.

207. **Patel, S. S., J. A. Balfour, and H. M. Bryson.** 1997. Fosfomycin tromethamine. *Drugs* **53:**637–656.

208. **Pechere, J.-C.** 1996. Streptogramins: a unique class of antibiotics. *Drugs* **51**(Suppl. 1)**:**13–19.

209. **Pechere, J.-C.** 1999. Current and future management of infections due to methicillin-resistant staphylococcal infections: the role of quinupristin/dalfopristin. *J. Antimicrob. Chemother.* **44**(Suppl. A)**:**11–18.

210. **Perry, C. M., J. A. Barman Balfour, and H. M. Lamb.** 1999. Gatifloxacin. *Drugs* **58:**683–696.

211. **Perry, C. M., and B. Jarvis.** 2001. Linezolid: a review of its use in the management of serious gram-positive infections. *Drugs* **61:**525–551.

212. **Peters, D. H., H. A. Friedel, and D. McTavish.** 1992. Azithromycin: a review of its antimicrobial activity, pharmacokinetic properties and clinical efficacy. *Drugs* **44:**755–799.

213. **Pfaller, M. A., A. L. Barry, and P. C. Fuchs.** 1993. Evaluation of disk susceptibility testing of fosfomycin tromethamine. *Diagn. Microbiol. Infect. Dis.* **17:**67–70.

214. **Pitkin, D. H., W. Sheikh, and H. L. Nadler.** 1997. Comparative in vitro activity of meropenem versus other extended-spectrum antimicrobials against randomly chosen and selected resistant clinical isolates tested in 26 North American centers. *Clin. Infect. Dis.* **24**(Suppl. 2)**:**S238–S248.

215. **Plouffe, J. F.** 2000. Emerging therapies for serious gram-positive bacterial infections: a focus on linezolid. *Clin. Infect. Dis.* **31**(Suppl. 4)**:**S144–S149.

216. **Polk, R. E.** 1989. Drug-drug interactions with ciprofloxacin and other fluoroquinolones. *Am. J. Med.* **87**(Suppl. 5A)**:**76S–81S.

217. **Polk, R. E., D. P. Healy, L. B. Schwartz, D. T. Rock, M. L. Garson, and K. Roller.** 1988. Vancomycin and the red-man syndrome: pharmacodynamics of histamine release. *J. Infect. Dis.* **157:**502–507.

218. **Prystowsky, J., F. Siddiqui, J. Chosay, D. L. Shinabarger, J. Millichap, L. R. Peterson, and G. A. Noskin.** 2001. Resistance to linezolid: characterization of mutations in rRNA and comparison of their occurrences in vancomycin-resistant enterococci. *Antimicrob. Agents Chemother.* **45:**2154–2156.

219. **Qadri, S. M., B. A. Cunha, Y. Ueno, F. Abumustafa, H. Imambaccus, D. D. Tullo, and P. Domenico.** 1995. Activity of cefepime against nosocomial blood culture isolates. *J. Antimicrob. Chemother.* **36:**531–536.

220. **Raad, I., R. Hachem, H. Hanna, E. Girgawy, K. Rolston, E. Whimbey, R. Husni, and G. Bodey.** 2001. Treatment of vancomycin-resistant enterococcal infections in the immunocompromised host: quinupristin-dalfopristin in combination with minocycline. *Antimicrob. Agents Chemother.* **45:**3202–3204.

221. **Raoult, D., P. Roussellier, V. Galicher, R. Perez, and J. Tamalet.** 1986. In vitro susceptibility of Rickettsia conorii to ciprofloxacin as determined suppressing lethality in chicken embryos and by plaque assay. *Antimicrob. Agents Chemother.* **29:**424–425.

222. **Raoult, D., H. Torres, and M. Drancourt.** 1991. Shell-vial assay evaluation of a new technique for determining antibiotic susceptibility, tested in 13 isolates of Coxiella burnetii. *Antimicrob. Agents Chemother.* **35:**2070–2077.

223. **Reeves, D. S.** 1994. Fosfomycin trometamol. *J. Antimicrob. Chemother.* **34:**853–858.

224. **Retsema, J. A., A. R. English, A. Girard, J. E. Lynch, M. Anderson, L. Brennan, C. Cimochowski, J. Faiella, W. Norcia, and P. Sawyer.** 1986. Sulbactam/ampicillin: in vitro spectrum potency, and activity in models of acute infection. *Rev. Infect. Dis.* **8**(Suppl. 5)**:**S528–S534.

225. **Rodloff, A. C.** 1982. In-vitro susceptibility of nontuberculous mycobacteria to sulphamethoxazole, trimethoprim, and combinations of both. *J. Antimicrob. Chemother.* **9:**195–199.

226. **Rolston, K. V. I., and J. Hoy.** 1987. Role of clindamycin in the treatment of central nervous system toxoplasmosis. *Am. J. Med.* **83:**551–554.

227. **Rose, H. D., and M. W. Rytel.** 1972. Actinomycosis treated with clindamycin. *JAMA* **221:**1052.

228. **Rosenblatt, J. E., and P. R. Stewart.** 1974. Combined activity of sulfamethoxazole, trimethoprim, and polymyxin B against gram-negative bacilli. *Antimicrob. Agents Chemother.* **6:**84–92.

229. **Rubin, R. H., and M. N. Swartz.** 1980. Trimethoprim-sulfamethoxazole. *N. Engl. J. Med.* **303:**426–432.

230. **Rubinstein, E., S. K. Cammarata, T. H. Oliphant, and R. G. Wunderink.** 2001. Linezolid (PNU-100766) versus vancomycin in the treatment of hospitalized patients with nosocomial pneumonia: a randomized, double-blind, multicenter study. *Clin. Infect. Dis.* **32:**402–412.

231. **Rubinstein, E., P. Prokocimer, and G. H. Talbot.** 1999. Safety and tolerability of quinupristin/dalfopristin: administration guidelines. *J. Antimicrob. Chemother.* **44:**37–46.

232. **Ruoff, K. L., D. R. Kuritzkes, J. S. Wolfson, and M. J. Ferraro.** 1988. Vancomycin-resistant gram-positive bacteria isolated from human sources. *J. Clin. Microbiol.* **26:**2064–2068.

233. **Sader, H. S., R. N. Jones, J. A. Washington, P. R. Murray, E. H. Gerlach, S. D. Allen, and M. E. Erwin.** 1993. In vitro activity of cefpodoxime compared with other oral cephalosporins tested against 5,556 recent clinical isolates from five medical centers. *Diagn. Microbiol. Infect. Dis.* **17:**143–150.

234. Salter, A. J. 1982. Trimethoprim-sulfamethoxazole: an assessment of more than 12 years of use. *Rev. Infect. Dis.* **4:**196–236.

235. Sanders, C. C. 1993. Cefepime: the next generation? *Clin. Infect. Dis.* **17:**369–379.

236. Sattler, F. R., M. R. Weitekamp, and J. O. Ballard. 1986. Potential for bleeding with the new beta-lactam antibiotics. *Ann. Intern. Med.* **105:**924–931.

237. Saxon, A., A. Hassner, E. A. Swabb, B. Wheeler, and N. F. Adkinson, Jr. 1984. Lack of cross-reactivity between aztreonam, a monobactam antibiotic, and penicillin in penicillin-allergic subjects. *J. Infect. Dis.* **149:**16–22.

238. Schaad, U. B., J. Wedgwood-Krucko, and H. Tschaeppeler. 1988. Reversible ceftriaxone-associated biliary pseudolithiasis in children. *Lancet* **ii:**1411–1413.

239. Schentag, J. J., and C. H. Ballow. 1991. Tissue-directed pharmacokinetics. *Am. J. Med.* **91**(Suppl. 3A):5S–11S.

240. Schulin, T., C. B. Wennersten, R. C. Moellering, and G. M. Eliopoulos. 1998. In-vitro activity of the new ketolide antibiotic HMR 3647 against Gram-positive bacteria. *J. Antimicrob. Chemother.* **42:**297–301.

241. Schwalbe, R. S., J. T. Stappleton, and P. H. Gilligan. 1987. Emergence of vancomycin resistance in coagulase-negative staphylococci. *N. Engl. J. Med.* **316:**927–931.

242. Seaberg, L. S., A. R. Parquette, I. Y. Gluzman, G. W. Phillips, Jr., T. F. Brodasky, and D. J. Krogstad. 1984. Clindamycin activity against chloroquine-resistant *Plasmodium falciparum. J. Infect. Dis.* **150:**904–911.

243. Sharp, J. R., K. G. Ishak, and H. J. Zimmerman. 1980. Chronic active hepatitis and severe hepatic necrosis associated with nitrofurantoin. *Ann. Intern. Med.* **92:**14–19.

244. Shaw, W. V. 1984. Bacterial resistance to chloramphenicol. *Br. Med. Bull.* **40:**36–41.

245. Smith, A. L. and A. Weber. 1983. Pharmacology of chloramphenicol. *Pediatr. Clin. North Am.* **30:**209–236.

246. Snydman, D. R., L. McDermott, G. J. Cuchural, Jr., D. W. Hecht, P. B. Iannini, L. J. Harrell, S. G. Jenkins, J. P. O'Keefe, C. L. Pierson, J. D. Rihs, V. L. Yu, S. M. Finegold, and S. L. Gorbach. 1996. Analysis of trends in antimicrobial resistance patterns among clinical isolates of *Bacteroides fragilis* group species from 1990 to 1994. *Clin. Infect. Dis.* **23**(Suppl. 1):S54–S65.

247. Somma, S., L. Gastaldo, and A. Corti. 1984. Teicoplanin, a new antibiotic from *Actinoplanes teichomyceticus* nov. sp. *Antimicrob. Agents Chemother.* **26:**917–923.

248. Sörgel, F., and M. Kinzig. 1993. The chemistry, pharmacokinetics and tissue distribution of piperacillin/tazobactam. *J. Antimicrob. Chemother.* **31**(Suppl. A):39–60.

249. Sorrell, T. C., and P. J. Collignon. 1985. A prospective study of adverse reactions associated with vancomycin therapy. *J. Antimicrob. Chemother.* **16:**235–241.

250. Spangler, S. K., M. R. Jacobs, and P. C. Appelbaum. 1996. Susceptibility of anaerobic bacteria to trovafloxacin: comparison with other quinolones and non-quinolone antibiotics. *Infect. Dis. Clin. Pract.* **5**(Suppl. 3):S101–S109.

251. Spear, B. S., N. B. Shoemaker, and A. A. Salyers. 1992. Bacterial resistance to tetracycline: mechanisms, transfer, and clinical significance. *Clin. Microbiol. Rev.* **5:**387–399.

252. Spratt, B. G., V. Jobanputra, and W. Zimmermann. 1977. Binding of thienamycin and clavulanic acid to the penicillin-binding proteins of *Escherichia coli* K-12. *Antimicrob. Agents Chemother.* **12:**406–409.

253. Stahlmann, R., and H. Lode. 1999. Toxicity of quinolones. *Drugs* **58:**37–42.

254. Stamm, W. E. 1991. Azithromycin in the treatment of uncomplicated genital chlamydial infections. *Am. J. Med.* **91**(Suppl. 3A):19S–22S.

255. Stapleton, A., and W. E. Stamm. 1997. Prevention of urinary tract infection. *Infect. Dis. Clin. North Am.* **11:**719–733.

256. Stapley, E. O., D. Hendlin, J. M. Mata, M. Jackson, H. Wallick, S. Hernanadez, S. Mochales, S. A. Currie, and R. M. Miller. 1969. Phosphonomycin. I. Discovery and in vitro biological characterization. *Antimicrob. Agents Chemother.* **9:**284–290.

257. Stein, G. E. 1996. Pharmacokinetics and pharmacodynamics of newer fluoroquinolones. *Clin. Infect. Dis.* **23**(Suppl. 1):S19–S24.

258. Stevens, D. L., L. G. Smith, J. B. Bruss, M. A. McConnell-Martin, S. E. Duvall, W. M. Todd, and B. Hafkin. 2000. Randomized comparison of linezolid (PNU-100766) versus oxacillin-dicloxacillin for treatment of complicated skin and soft tissue infections. *Antimicrob. Agents Chemother.* **44:**3408–3413.

259. Sullivan, D., M. E. Csuka, and B. Blanchard. 1980. Erythromycin ethylsuccinate hepatotoxicity. *JAMA* **243:**1074.

260. Sutter, V. L. 1977. In vitro susceptibility of anaerobes: comparison of clindamycin and other antimicrobial agents. *J. Infect. Dis.* **135**(Suppl.):S7–S12.

261. Swaney, S. M., H. Aoki, M. C. Ganoza, and D. L. Shinabarger. 1998. The oxazolidinone linezolid inhibits initiation of protein synthesis in bacteria. *Antimicrob. Agents Chemother.* **42:**3251–3255.

262. Swedberg, J., J. F. Steiner, F. Deiss, S. Steiner, and D. A. Driggers. 1985. Comparison of single-dose vs one-week course of metronidazole for symptomatic bacterial vaginosis. *JAMA* **254:**1046–1049.

263. Sykes, R. B., and D. P. Bonner. 1985. Aztreonam: first monobactam. *Am. J. Med.* **78**(Suppl. 2A):2–10.

264. Tally, F. P., and M. F. DeBruin. 2000. Development of daptomycin for gram-positive infections. *J. Antimicrob. Chemother.* **46:**523–526.

265. Teasley, D. G., D. N. Gerding, M. M. Olson, L. R. Peterson, R. L. Gebhard, M. J. Schwartz, and J. T. Lee, Jr. 1983. Prospective randomized trial of metronidazole versus vancomycin for *Clostridium difficile*-associated diarrhea and colitis. *Lancet* **ii:**1043–1046.

266. Thornsberry, C. 1992. Review of the in vitro antibacterial activity of cefprozil, a new oral cephalosporin. *Clin. Infect. Dis.* **14**(Suppl. 2):S189–S194.

267. Todd, P. A., and D. Faulds. 1991. Ofloxacin: a reappraisal of its antimicrobial activity, pharmacology and therapeutic use. *Drugs* **42:**825–876.

268. Toma, E., S. Fournier, M. Dumont, P. Bolduc, and H. Deschamps. 1993. Clindamycin/primaquine versus trimethoprim-sulfamethoxazole as primary therapy for *Pneumocystis carinii* pneumonia in AIDS: a randomized, double-blind pilot trial. *Clin. Infect. Dis.* **17:**178–184.

269. Tsiodras, S., H. S. Gold, G. Sakoulas, G. M. Eliopoulos, C. Wennersten, L. Venkataraman, R. C. Moellering, and M. J. Ferraro. 2001. Linezolid resistance in a clinical isolate of *Staphylococcus aureus. Lancet* **358:**207–208.

270. Tuazon, C. U., and H. Miller. 1984. Comparative in vitro activities of teichomycin and vancomycin alone and in combination with rifampin and aminoglycosides against staphylococci and enterococci. *Antimicrob. Agents Chemother.* **25:**411–412.

271. Turnidge, J. 1999. Pharmacokinetics and pharmacodynamics of fluoroquinolones. *Drugs* **58**(Suppl. 2):29–36.

272. **Van der Auwera, P., T. Matsumoto, and M. Husson.** 1988. Intraphagocytic penetration of antibiotics. *J. Antimicrob. Chemother.* **22:**185–192.

273. **Van der Auwera, P., F. Meunier-Carpentier, and J. Kastersky.** 1983. Clinical study of combination therapy with oxacillin and rifampin for staphylococcal infections. *Rev. Infect. Dis.* **5**(Suppl. 3):S515–S522.

274. **Vanhoff, R., B. Gordts, R. Dierickx, H. Coignau, and J. P. Butzler.** 1980. Bacteriostatic and bactericidal activities of 24 antimicrobial agents against *Campylobacter fetus* subsp. *jejuni. Antimicrob. Agents Chemother.* **18:**118–121.

275. **Vannuffel, P., and C. Cocito.** 1996. Mechanism of action of streptogramins and macrolides. *Drugs* **51**(Suppl. 1):20–30.

276. **Verbist, L.** 1979. Comparison of the activities of the new ureidopenicillins, piperacillin, mezlocillin, azlocillin, and Bay k 4999 against gram-negative organisms. *Antimicrob. Agents Chemother.* **16:**115–119.

277. **Visalli, M. A., S. Bajaksouzian, M. R. Jacobs, and P. C. Appelbaum.** 1997. Comparative activity of trovafloxacin, alone and in combination with other agents, against gram-negative nonfermentative rods. *Antimicrob. Agents Chemother.* **41:**1475–1481.

278. **von Rosenstiel, N.-A., and D. Adam.** 1995. Macrolide antibacterials: drug interactions of clinical significance. *Drug Saf.* **13:**105–122.

279. **Wadworth, A. N., and K. L. Goa.** 1991. Lomefloxacin: a review of its antibacterial activity, pharmacokinetic properties and therapeutic use. *Drugs* **42:**1018–1060.

280. **Wagstaff, A. J., and J. A. Balfour.** 1997. Grepafloxacin. *Drugs* **53:**817–824.

281. **Wallace, R. J., Jr., B. A. Brown-Elliott, S. C. Ward, C. J. Crist, L. B. Mann, and R. W. Wilson.** 2001. Activities of linezolid against rapidly growing mycobacteria. *Antimicrob. Agents Chemother.* **45:**764–767.

282. **Wallace, R. J., Jr., E. J. Septimus, T. W. Williams, Jr., R. H. Conklin, T. K. Satterwhite, M. B. Bushby, and D. C. Hollowell.** 1982. Use of trimethoprim-sulfamethoxazole for treatment of infections due to *Norcardia. Rev. Infect. Dis.* **4:**315–325.

283. **Wallace, R. J., Jr., J. M. Swenson, V. A. Silcox, and M. G. Bullen.** 1985. Treatment of non-pulmonary infections due to *Mycobacterium fortuitum* and *Mycobacterium chelonei* on the basis of in vivo susceptibilities. *J. Infect. Dis.* **152:**500–514.

284. **Wallace, R. J., Jr., and K. Wiss.** 1981. Susceptibility of *Mycobacterium marinum* to tetracyclines and aminoglycosides. *Antimicrob. Agents Chemother.* **20:**610–612.

285. **Walters, B. N. J., and S. S. Gubbay.** 1981. Tetracycline and benign intracranial hypertension: report of five cases. *Br. Med. J.* **282:**19–20.

286. **Ward, A., and D. M. Campoli-Richards.** 1986. Mupirocin: a review of its antibacterial activity, pharmacokinetic properties and therapeutic use. *Drugs* **32:**425–444.

287. **Ward, M. E.** 1977. The bactericidal action of spectinomycin on *Neisseria gonorrhoeae. J. Antimicrob. Chemother.* **3:**323–329.

288. **Washington, J. A., II, and W. R. Wilson.** 1985. Erythromycin: a microbial and clinical perspective after 30 years of clinical use. *Mayo Clin. Proc.* **60:**189–203, 271–278.

289. **Watanakunakorn, C., and C. Bakie.** 1973. Synergism of vancomycin-gentamicin and vancomycin-streptomycin against enterococci. *Antimicrob. Agents Chemother.* **4:**120–124.

290. **Watanakunakorn, C., and J. C. Tisone.** 1982. Synergism between vancomycin and gentamicin or tobramycin for methicillin-susceptible and methicillin-resistant *Staphylococcus aureus* strains. *Antimicrob. Agents Chemother.* **22:**903–905.

291. **Waxman, D. J., and J. L. Strominger.** 1983. Penicillin-binding proteins and the mechanism of action of beta-lactam antibiotics. *Annu. Rev. Biochem.* **52:**825–869.

292. **Wehrli, W.** 1983. Rifampin: mechanisms of action and resistance. *Rev. Infect. Dis.* **5**(Suppl. 3):S407–S411.

293. **Wexler, H. M., and S. M. Finegold.** 1988. In vitro activity of cefotetan compared with that of other antimicrobial agents against anaerobic bacteria. *Antimicrob. Agents Chemother.* **32:**601–604.

294. **Wexler, H. M., B. Harris, W. T. Carter, and S. M. Finegold.** 1985. In vitro efficacy of sulbactam combined with ampicillin against anaerobic bacteria. *Antimicrob. Agents Chemother.* **27:**876–878.

295. **Wexler, H. M., D. Molitoris, and S. M. Finegold.** 2000. In vitro activities of MK-826 (L-749,345) against 363 strains of anaerobic bacteria. *Antimicrob. Agents Chemother.* **44:**2222–2224.

296. **Wexler, H. M., E. Molitoris, D. Molitoris, and S. M. Finegold.** 2001. In vitro activity of telithromycin (HMR 3647) against 502 strains of anaerobic bacteria. *J. Antimicrob. Chemother.* **47:**467–469.

297. **Wiedemann, B., C. Kliebe, and M. Kresken.** 1989. The epidemiology of beta-lactamases. *J. Antimicrob. Chemother.* **24**(Suppl. B):1–22.

298. **Wijnands, W. J. A., and T. B. Vree.** 1988. Interaction between the fluoroquinolones and the bronchodilator theophylline. *J. Antimicrob. Chemother.* **22**(Suppl. C):109–114.

299. **Williams, J. D., and A. M. Sefton.** 1993. Comparison of macrolide antibiotics. *J. Antimicrob. Chemother.* **31**(Suppl. C):11–26.

300. **Wilson, W. R., A. W. Karchmer, A. S. Dajani, K. A. Taubert, A. Bayer, D. Kaye, A. L. Bisno, P. Ferrieri, S. T. Shuman, and D. T. Durack.** 1995. Antibiotic treatment of adults with infective endocarditis due to streptococci, enterococci, staphylococci, and HACEK microorganisms. *JAMA* **274:**1706–1713.

301. **Wilson, W. R., R. L. Thompson, C. J. Wilkowske, J. A. Washington II, E. R. Giuliani, and J. E. Geraci.** 1981. Short-term therapy for streptococcal infective endocarditis: combined intramuscular administration of penicillin and streptomycin. *JAMA* **245:**360–363.

302. **Winston, D. J., M. A. McGrattan, and R. W. Busuttil.** 1984. Imipenem therapy of *Pseudomonas aeruginosa* and other serious bacterial infections. *Antimicrob. Agents Chemother.* **26:**673–677.

303. **Wise, R., J. M. Andrews, and J. P. Ashby.** 2001. Activity of daptomycin against gram-positive pathogens: a comparison with other agents and the determination of a tentative breakpoint. *J. Antimicrob. Chemother.* **48:**563–567.

304. **Wise, R., D. Lister, C. A. McNulty, D. Griggs, and J. M. Andrews.** 1986. The comparative pharmacokinetics of five quinolones. *J. Antimicrob. Chemother.* **18**(Suppl. D):71–81.

305. **Wiseman, L. R., and J. A. Balfour.** 1994. Ceftibuten: a review of its antibacterial activity, pharmacokinetic properties and clinical efficacy. *Drugs* **5:**784–808.

306. **Wittner, M., K. S. Rowin, H. B. Tanowitz, J. F. Hobbs, S. Saltzman, B. Wenz, R. Hirsch, E. Chisholm, and G. R. Healy.** 1982. Successful chemotherapy of transfusion babesiosis. *Ann. Intern. Med.* **96:**601–604.

307. **Wolfson, J. S., and D. C. Hooper.** 1989. Fluoroquinolone antimicrobial agents. *Clin. Microbiol. Rev.* **2:**378–424.

308. **Wong, C. S., G. S. Palmer, and M. H. Cynamon.** 1988. In-vitro susceptibility of *Mycobacterium tuberculosis, My-*

cobacterium bovis and *Mycobacterium kansasii* to amoxycillin and ticarcillin in combination with clavulanic acid. *J. Antimicrob. Chemother.* **22:**863–866.

309. **World Health Organization.** 1993. *Guidelines for Cholera Control.* World Health Organization, Geneva, Switzerland.

310. **Yeaman, M. R., L. A. Mitscher, and O. G. Baca.** 1987. In vitro susceptibility of *Coxiella burnetii* to antibiotics, including several quinolones. *Antimicrob. Agents Chemother.* **31:**1079–1084.

311. **Young, L. S., O. G. W. Berlin, and C. B. Inderlied.** 1987. Activity of ciprofloxacin and other fluorinated quinolones against mycobacteria. *Am. J. Med.* **82**(Suppl. 4A)**:**23–26.

312. **Young, L. S., and J. Hindler.** 1987. Use of trimethoprim-sulfamethoxazole singly and in combination with other antibiotics in immunocompromised patients. *Rev. Infect. Dis.* **9**(Suppl. 2)**:**S177–S181.

313. **Zurenko, G. E., B. H. Yagi, R. D. Schaadt, J. W. Allison, J. O. Kilburn, S. E. Glickman, D. K. Hutchinson, M. R. Barbachyn, and S. J. Brickner.** 1996. In vitro activities of U-100592 and U-100766, novel oxazolidone antibacterial agents. *Antimicrob. Agents Chemother.* **40:** 839–845.

Mechanisms of Resistance to Antibacterial Agents*

LOUIS B. RICE, DANIEL SAHM, AND ROBERT A. BONOMO

68

GENERAL CONCEPTS, INOCULUM EFFECTS, AND TOLERANCE

When considering the growing problem of antimicrobial resistance in bacteria, it is worth remembering that resistance is neither a new phenomenon nor unexpected in an environment in which potent antimicrobial agents are used. The diversity of the microbial world and the relatively specific activities of our antimicrobial agents virtually ensure widespread resistance among bacteria. In many cases, this resistance is recognized when an antibiotic is first being tested for development. For example, it is not considered a problem or threat that *Escherichia coli* is resistant to vancomycin. We simply understand that *E. coli* is not within vancomycin's spectrum of activity, and we avoid using vancomycin when *E. coli* infection is known or highly suspected (i.e., it has natural or primary resistance to vancomycin). Conversely, increasing resistance of *E. coli* to ciprofloxacin represents an important problem, since we frequently use the fluoroquinolone class of antimicrobial agents to treat infections in which *E. coli* is likely to be involved. Therefore, when we speak of the problem of resistance, we must recognize that most problems result from expression of resistance by bacteria that are intrinsically susceptible to the antibiotic in question (i.e., acquired resistance).

It is also important to recognize that resistance as a clinical entity is essentially a relative phenomenon, in many ways a problem only indirectly related to the microbiologic techniques often used to detect it. For example, it is possible to incorporate enough ticarcillin into an agar plate to inhibit an ampicillin-resistant *Enterococcus faecium* organism (in many cases this requires about 10,000 µg/ml). Therefore, in one sense, ampicillin-resistant *E. faecium* is "susceptible" to high concentrations of ticarcillin. However, such concentrations cannot be achieved at the site of infection and so ampicillin-resistant *E. faecium* is not considered "susceptible" to ticarcillin. It is the responsibility of the National Committee for Clinical Laboratory Standards (NCCLS), and other standard-setting bodies in different

countries, to make determinations on susceptible, intermediate, and resistant breakpoints for new antimicrobial agents, considering factors such as in vitro susceptibility, pharmacokinetics, and pharmacodynamics. These issues become very important in treating meningitis, where relatively minor increases in the penicillin MIC for *Streptococcus pneumoniae* can foil treatment, but in many cases they are less relevant in the treatment of simple urinary tract infections, given the tendency of many antibiotics to concentrate in the urine.

The "relativity" of resistance is best exemplified by considerations of susceptibility in bacterial strains that exhibit significant inoculum effects, such as those resistant by virtue of producing β-lactamase. β-Lactamase-mediated resistance results from a chemical interaction in which the β-lactamase molecule binds to the β-lactam antibiotic in a manner that ultimately results in the hydrolysis of the critical β-lactam ring structure (Fig. 1). The rapidity and efficiency with which binding and hydrolysis proceed are dependent on the affinity with which the β-lactamase molecule binds the antibiotic and the efficiency of the subsequent hydrolysis. High affinity and rapid hydrolysis mean that the cell wall synthesis machinery (penicillin-binding proteins [PBPs]) can be defended with relatively few β-lactamase molecules compared to the number of β-lactam molecules likely to be present in the vicinity of the PBPs. Low affinity and slow hydrolysis mean that more β-lactamase molecules are necessary for effective resistance but also that resistance can be more easily overcome by adding more antibiotic molecules. Increasing the inoculum of organisms in a solution with a fixed concentration of β-lactam antibiotic has the effect of increasing the number of β-lactamase molecules and can in some instances result in clinically important levels of resistance. A *Klebsiella pneumoniae* strain that produces extended-spectrum β-lactamase TEM-26, for example, may be associated with a standard-inoculum (ca. 10^5 CFU/ml) cefotaxime MIC of 1 µg/ml. However, when the inoculum is increased to 10^7 CFU/ml, the MIC increases to greater than 256 µg/ml (168). This type of resistance is likely to be important when treating a high-inoculum infection such as pneumonia but may be less important when treating a urinary tract infection (142). The existence of inoculum effects has led to the frequent practice of considering all *K. pneumoniae* strains that are resistant to ceftazidime to be resistant to all ceph-

* This chapter contains information presented in chapter 117 by Richard Quintiliani, Jr., Daniel F. Sahm, and Patrice Courvalin in the seventh edition of this Manual.

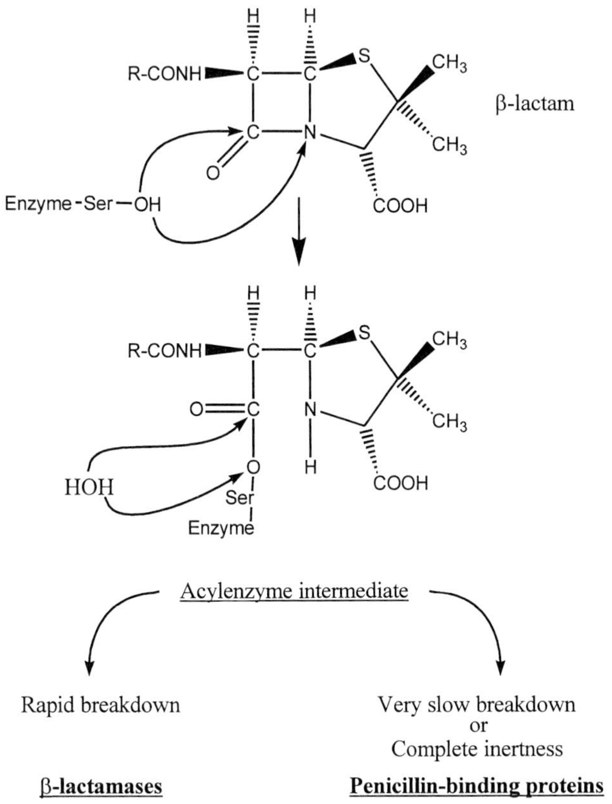

FIGURE 1 Penicillin-interactive, active-site serine pepti-dases and their reactions with β-lactam carbonyl donors. Modified from reference 74 with permission of Annual Reviews (www.annualreviews.org).

alosporins, regardless of the results of in vitro susceptibility tests for other cephalosporins using the standard inoculum.

A second, more amorphous and difficult-to-evaluate concept in considering antimicrobial resistance is that of tolerance, or resistance to killing at antimicrobial concentrations sufficient to inhibit further growth. Tolerance is an unimportant concept for the treatment of most infections, since for therapeutic success it is usually sufficient to inhibit further growth of bacteria (bacteriostatic activity), allowing the patient's immune defenses to kill the growth-inhibited organisms and clean up the debris. In some instances, however, antimicrobial killing of the bacteria (bactericidal activity) is required to yield a high percentage of treatment success. Instances where bactericidal activity is preferred include endocarditis, meningitis, and osteomyelitis, where the immune system has limited access to the infection site. They also include circumstances in which the immune system is severely compromised, such as in patients undergoing high-dose chemotherapy for hematologic malignancies. In these instances, antibiotics that are primarily bacteriostatic, such as the tetracyclines or the macrolides, are considered poor choices for therapy whereas β-lactam antibiotics, which are primarily bactericidal, are preferred. Some bacteria are naturally tolerant to β-lactam antibiotics. Bactericidal activity against the enterococcus, for example, requires two agents, one active against cell wall synthesis and an aminoglycoside (126). Recognition of this bactericidal synergism raised cure rates for enterococcal endocarditis from about 40 to 70% or greater (73, 101,

164). Unfortunately, recent years have seen the proliferation of aminoglycoside-modifying enzymes that negate the synergism and appear to decrease the cure rates for enterococcal endocarditis. Although some level of tolerance to β-lactam antibiotics can be demonstrated for several different bacterial species, the impact on the treatment of clinical infections appears to be less dramatic than with the enterococcus.

Emergence and Spread of Antibiotic Resistance

The emergence of antimicrobial resistance phenotypes is inevitably linked to the clinical (or other) use of the antimicrobial agent against which resistance is directed. One reason for this association is trivial—we do not generally test for resistance to antibiotics that are not in clinical use. The second reason is that nature abhors a vacuum, and so when an effective antibiotic eliminates susceptible members of the flora, resistant varieties soon fill the niche. Once a resistance phenotype has emerged within a previously susceptible species, the rapidity and efficiency with which it spreads are impacted by a host of different factors, including the degree of resistance expressed, the ability of the organism to tolerate the resistance mechanism, linkage to other genes, site of primary colonization, and others. The rapidity and completeness of resistance gene spread are often unpredictable. For example, the staphylococcal β-lactamase gene (conferring resistance to penicillin) was first described shortly after the introduction of penicillin into clinical use and is now almost universally present within staphylococci in the hospital and the community. It was not until the early 1980s that this gene was described in enterococci, and it has never spread widely in this genus. The reverse appears true with the vancomycin resistance genes, which are found widely in E. faecium but have only recently been described in Staphylococcus aureus (39a).

An important cause of the spread of antimicrobial resistance is the failure to adhere to appropriate infection control techniques, both within and outside the hospital. It is well established that strains of methicillin-resistant S. aureus (MRSA) within individual hospitals, and even within entire cities, are often clonally related, as determined by genetic techniques such as pulsed-field gel electrophoresis (170). The spread of these problematic pathogens has been attributed to transmission from patient to patient, presumably by transiently or persistently colonized health care workers (184). The primary site of S. aureus colonization is in the anterior nares. Colonization of the nares facilitates aerosol transmission of the resistant bacteria, particularly during periods of viral upper respiratory infection in the colonized worker. It also facilitates direct transmission, given the frequent contact between hands and nose in many people and frequent poor hand-washing practices by health care workers. The clinical consequences of patient colonization can be significant. Recent studies have shown a direct correlation between patient colonization with an MRSA strain and subsequent infection with the same strain during periods of high risk, such as the postoperative period (99).

Although antibiotic resistance is predominantly a nosocomial problem, resistant bacteria are also spread in the community setting. Sites in which resistant bacteria have been known to spread include day care centers and nursing homes (1, 160). Penicillin-resistant pneumococci have been found to colonize as many as 25% of a day care center's population. Transmission probably reaches its peak in the winter months, when viral upper respiratory infections are prevalent. Prevalence of viral upper respiratory infections works in two ways to increase transmission: (i) it probably increases the inoculum of resistant organisms being spread by those already colonized (see references 99, 170, and 184 for *S. aureus* colonization) and (ii) it makes those who are not colonized more likely to become colonized because of the increased likelihood that they will be receiving antimicrobial therapy. Nursing homes are predisposed to resistance for a variety of reasons, including the debilitated state of much of their population, frequent movement back and forth to tertiary-care hospitals, and frequent use of antimicrobial agents in an effort to ward off hospital admissions.

A final important source for the emergence and spread of antibiotic-resistant bacteria is that of nonhuman niches in which antibiotics are used to excess. It is now well established that antimicrobial use in food animals is associated with both resistance in bacterial species that contaminate food and infect humans, primarily *Salmonella* and *Campylobacter*, or the transfer of resistance determinants to their human counterparts, such as *Enterococcus* (4, 60, 122). Compelling evidence also exists that high rates of ciprofloxacin resistance in *E. coli* can be associated with the use of fluoroquinolones in poultry (56). Finally, the European outbreak of vancomycin-resistant enterococci with the *vanA* determinant was almost certainly fueled by the use of avoparcin (a glycopeptide antibiotic) as a growth promoter in food animals (213). Data are also emerging that the use of antibiotics to promote growth of animals is often expensive and unnecessary, which should prompt all stakeholders in this issue to convene and outline specific instances in which such antimicrobial use will be permitted.

Genetic Bases of Resistance

Acquired antimicrobial resistance results from biochemical processes that are encoded by bacterial genes. A general list of resistance mechanisms is presented in Table 1. To understand the biochemical processes, it is useful to first discuss the genetic underpinnings of resistance and its evolution. Antimicrobial resistance arises by (i) mutation of cellular genes, (ii) acquisition of exogenous resistance genes, or (iii) mutation of acquired genes.

Mutation of Cellular Genes

All antibiotics have targets, which are often (but not always) proteins with important functional responsibilities for cell growth or maintenance. Cellular genes encode these proteins. Interactions between antibiotics and target proteins are often quite specific, and changing a single amino acid, frequently as a result of a single base change in the gene, can sometimes alter these interactions. Perhaps the most familiar example of this type of resistance is resistance to rifampin. Rifampin targets the cellular RNA polymerase (encoded by *rpoB*), and a single point mutation in this gene confers complete resistance (214). This mutation occurs in most bacterial species at a relatively high frequency (ca. 10^{-8}/CFU). Incubating enough cells with inhibitory concentrations of rifampin eliminates susceptible cells and allows the resistant mutants to proliferate. The rifampin in the media is not actually causing resistance but, rather, selecting mutants that occur naturally but which have no selective advantage for survival in the absence of rifampin in the environment. Other examples of mutational resistance include resistance to streptomycin by ribosomal mutation (55), resistance to fluoroquinolones through muta-

tions of cellular topoisomerase (117), and resistance to linezolid by mutations in the rRNA (155).

Resistance mutations may also be found in genes that regulate cellular processes. Perhaps the most completely studied example of regulatory mutation resulting in resistance is the "derepression" of the chromosomal β-lactamase of *Enterobacter* spp. (94). Mutations in a cellular amidase gene (designated *ampD*) result in buildup of a cell wall breakdown product, which has the effect of dramatically increasing the expression of a chromosomal β-lactamase gene (*ampC*). Other examples of regulatory changes include the down-regulation of expression of the porin OMPD2 in *Pseudomonas aeruginosa* associated with resistance to imipenem (111) or the insertion of insertion sequence (IS) elements upstream of a chromosomal carbapenemase conferring imipenem resistance in *Bacteroides fragilis* (147).

Whether mutational resistance is likely to persist depends in some measure on whether the resistance mutation is tolerable to the cell. For example, although decreased expression of OMPD2 appears to be readily achievable for *P. aeruginosa*, the fact that these resistant strains have not spread widely in the 15 years of carbapenem use probably reflects the fact that this porin has functions that are beneficial to the bacterium, favoring reexpression of the porin once the imipenem threat has been dissipated. Similarly, resistance to vancomycin in *S. aureus* has thus far been attributed to marked changes in the composition of the cell wall (186). These changes are unlikely to be favored in an environment free of vancomycin, since *S. aureus* probably "decided" the optimal size and composition of its cell wall a long time ago. The deleterious effects of acquiring resistance are often referred to as fitness cost.

Disadvantageous resistance mutations do not always disappear. Although initial point mutations in the *rpoB* gene that confer rifampin resistance to *Salmonella enterica* serovar Enteritidis appear to decrease the fitness of the organism for survival in vivo, persistence in a live host is frequently associated with compensatory mutations that at least partially restore fitness to the strain while retaining the resistance (rather than mutating back to susceptibility) (23). Similarly, transfer of mutated *pbp5* into *E. faecium* strains is often associated with decreases in the expression of ampicillin resistance, but growth on increased concentrations of ampicillin easily yields colonies that grow well at a higher concentration (167). Similar findings have been reported for *S. aureus* strains transformed with the *mecA* gene encoding methicillin resistance (128). In summary, while mutational resistance often confers a fitness cost, subsequent adaptations frequently make expression of resistance much less costly.

Acquisition of Resistance Genes

If resistance is not achievable through mutation, threatened bacterial species have little choice but to look elsewhere for resistance determinants. They are aided in this effort by the fact that most antimicrobial agents are natural products or derivatives of natural products. Therefore, resistance genes for most antibiotics must exist in the microbial world, either in the species that produce the antibiotic or within species that live in the same ecological niche as the antibiotic producers. The challenge for susceptible human pathogens is to find and acquire these resistance determinants. To assist in this acquisition, bacteria have evolved a range of techniques that promote gene exchange. Perhaps the simplest of these techniques is natural transformation, referring to the ability of some bacterial species to absorb

TABLE 1 Common associations of resistance mechanisms

Antibiotic class	Resistance type	Resistance mechanism	Common example(s)
Aminoglycosides	Decreased uptake	Changes in outer membrane permeability	*P. aeruginosa*
	Enzymatic modification (AMEs)	Phosphotransferase	Wide range of enteric gram-negative bacteria
		Adenyltransferase	Wide range of enteric gram-negative bacteria
		Acetyltransferase	Wide range of enteric gram-negative bacteria
		Bifunctional enzyme	*aac(6′)-aph(2″)* in *S. aureus*, *E. faecium*, and *E. faecalis*
β-Lactams	Altered PBP(s)	PBP2a (additional PBP)	*mecA* in *S. aureus* and coagulase-negative staphylococci
		PBP2x, PBP2b, PBP1a (acquired from other streptococci by transformation	*S. pneumoniae*
		PBP5 (point mutation)	*E. faecium*
	Enzymatic degradation (β-lactamases)	Ambler class A	TEM-1 in *E. coli*, *H. influenzae*, and *N. gonorrhoeae*
			SHV-1 in *K. pneumoniae*
			K-1 (OXY-1) in *K. oxytoca*
			Extended-spectrum β-lactamases (TEM-3+, SHV-2+, and CTX-M types) in *K. pneumoniae* and *E. coli*
			BRO-1 in *M. catarrhalis*
			PC1 in *S. aureus*
			PSE-1 in *P. aeruginosa*
			β-Lactamases of *C. koseri* and *P. vulgaris*
		Ambler class B	L-1 in *S. maltophilia*
			Ccr-A in *B. fragilis*
		Ambler class C	AmpC in *E. cloacae*, *C. freundii*, and similar enzymes in *S. marcescens*, *M. morganii*, *P. stuartii*, and *P. rettgeri*
		Ambler class D	OXA-1 in *E. coli*
Chloramphenicol	Enzymatic degradation	CAT	CAT in *S. pneumoniae*
	Efflux	New membrane transporters	*cmlA* and *flo*-encoded efflux in *E. coli* and *Salmonella* spp.
Glycopeptides	Altered target	Altered peptidoglycan cross-link target (D-Ala–D-Ala to D-Ala–D-Lac or D-Ala–D-Ser) encoded by complex gene cluster	*vanA* and *vanB* gene clusters in *E. faecium* and *E. faecalis*
	Target overproduction	Excess peptidoglycan	Glycopeptide "intermediate" strains of *S. aureus*
Oxazolidinones	Altered target	Mutation leading to reduced binding to active site	G2576U mutation in rRNA in *E. faecium* and *S. aureus*
Macrolides-lincosamides-streptogramins B	Altered target	Ribosomal active-site methylation with reduced binding	*erm*-encoded methylases in *S. aureus*, *S. pneumoniae*, and *S. pyogenes*
Macrolides	Efflux	Mef efflux pump	*mef*-encoded efflux in *S. pneumoniae* and *S. pyogenes*
Streptogramins Streptogramin A	Enzymatic degradation	Acetyltransferases	*vatA*, *vatB*, and *vatC* in *S. aureus*; *vatD*- and *vatE*-encoded enzymes in *E. faecium*

(Continued on next page)

TABLE 1 Common associations of resistance mechanisms *(Continued)*

Antibiotic class	Resistance type	Resistance mechanism	Common example(s)
Quinolones	Altered target	Mutation leading to reduced binding to active site(s) (quinolone-resistance-determining region)	Mutations in *gyrA* in enteric gram-negative bacteria and S. *aureus*
			Mutations in *gyrA* and *parC* in S. *pneumoniae*
	Efflux	New membrane transporters	NorA in S. *aureus*
Rifampin	Altered target	Mutations leading to reduced binding to RNA polymerase	Mutations in *rpoB* in S. *aureus* and M. *tuberculosis*
Tetracyclines	Efflux	New membrane transporters	*tet* genes encoding efflux proteins in gram-positive (mainly group 2) and gram-negative (mainly group 1 [see Table 3]) bacteria
	Altered target	Production of proteins that bind to the ribosome and alter the conformation of the active site (ribosomal protection proteins)	*tet*(M) and *tet*(O) in diverse gram-positive and gram-negative species
Sulfonamides	Altered target	Mutation or recombination of genes encoding DHPS	Found in a wide range of species: E. *coli*, S. *aureus*, S. *pneumoniae*
		Acquisition of new low-affinity DHPS genes	*sul*I and *sul*II in enteric gram-negative bacteria
Trimethoprim	Altered target	Mutations in gene encoding DHFR	S. *aureus*, S. *pneumoniae*, H. *influenzae*
		Acquisition of new low-affinity DHFR genes	*dhfr*I and *dhfr*II encoded, found in a wide range of species
	Overproduction of target	Promoter mutation leading to overproduction of DHFR	E. *coli*

naked DNA molecules from the environment under the appropriate circumstances (79). Once taken up by the susceptible bacterium, these foreign pieces of DNA enter the bacterial chromosome by recombining across regions of sufficient homology. In some cases, functional genes result from this recombination. If the acquired gene encodes a protein that is less susceptible to inhibition than the native protein, a reduction in susceptibility may result. Perhaps the best-studied example of the formation of these "mosaic" genes to confer resistance is penicillin and cephalosporin resistance in *Streptococcus pneumoniae* (79). A variety of mosaic penicillin-binding protein (*pbp*) genes have been described in resistant strains, with the level and degree of resistance determined by the number and nature of gene recombinations.

Most bacteria are incapable of natural transformation, however, and so have developed other mechanisms for acquisition of useful genetic determinants. Perhaps the most commonly employed mechanism for genetic exchange is the transfer of conjugative plasmids (54). These extra-chromosomal replicative DNA forms can encode a large variety of important genes. Some plasmids are relatively narrow in their host range, while others transfer into and replicate within a variety of different species. Transfer fre-

quencies can be very high, as in the F factor of E. *coli* (virtually complete transfer in 1 h) or the pheromone-responsive plasmids found in E. *faecalis* (ca. 10^{-1} transconjugant/recipient CFU in 24 h), or more modest, as observed with the broad-host-range enterococcal plasmids such as pAMB1 (10^{-7} to 10^{-6} transconjugant/recipient CFU in 24 h) (32). Having entered into a new genus on broad-host-range plasmids, resistance determinants can readily transfer onto more frequently transferable plasmids to increase their movement through the new genus. Plasmids may also integrate into the chromosome of the recipient strains, potentially increasing the stability of the genetic information they carry (165).

Bacteria also take advantage of bacterial viruses (bacteriophages) for genetic exchange. These discrete packages deliver to uninfected cells a quantity of DNA approximating the size of their genome (in most cases roughly 40 kb). Designed to incorporate their own genome into the manufactured phage head, they sometimes incorporate bits of chromosomal DNA adjacent to the phage integration site (specialized transduction) and other times incorporate an appropriate-sized plasmid or chromosomal DNA segment unrelated to the integrated phage genome (generalized transduction). Since the staphylococcal β-lactamase gene is frequently identified on nonconjugative plasmids approximately 35 to 40 kb in size and since bacteriophages have been well described in staphylococci for decades, it has been speculated that the high prevalence of β-lactamase production in staphylococci has resulted from bacteriophage-mediated transfer of these plasmids (114). Bacteriophages have also been implicated in the transfer of virulence determinants (62).

Nonreplicative elements known as transposons have also been implicated in the transfer of resistance genes (161). Transposons encode their own ability to transfer between replicons. In some cases, the transposons themselves also encode conjugation functions, which allow them to transfer from bacterial chromosome to bacterial chromosome. The best characterized of these "conjugative transposons" is Tn916, an 18-kb element that was originally described in E. faecalis but that has a very broad host range (162). Tn916 encodes resistance to tetracycline and minocycline through the tet(M) resistance gene. Many different Tn916-like transposons have now been described in enterococci and beyond; some of them, such as Tn1545 from Streptococcus pneumoniae, possess additional resistance genes (conferring resistance to erythromycin and kanamycin)(162). Some investigators have suggested that the conjugation events associated with Tn916-like transposons are akin to cell fusion events, in which portions of the genome distinct from that adjacent to the inserted transposon can exchange via homologous recombination (204). Recently, transposons with structural similarity to Tn916 have been implicated in the transfer of vancomycin resistance between E. faecium strains (38).

Transposons lacking conjugative functions may also transfer between strains. The most common mechanism by which this transfer is presumed to occur is either transient or more permanent integration into transferable plasmids. Among the more common classes of nonconjugative transposons are the Tn3 family elements (including Tn917, conferring erythromycin resistance, and Tn1546, conferring VanA-type vancomycin resistance) (11, 179) and the composite elements formed by mobile IS elements flanking resistance genes (including Tn4001, conferring high-level gentamicin resistance in many gram-positive species) (70).

The precise origin of resistance genes is often difficult to discern, but in some cases it is at least possible to determine that acquired resistance determinants originated in other genera. The VanB-type vancomycin resistance in enterococci, for example, has a guanine-plus-cytosine (G+C) content of nearly 50 mol% (58). The enterococcal genome, in contrast, has an approximately 35 to 38% G+C content. These differences virtually confirm the origin of the VanB determinant in a genus other than Enterococcus. The likely origin appears to be streptomycetes, probably species that manufacture glycopeptide antibiotics, with entry into Enterococcus facilitated by the incorporation of these resistance operons into transposons.

It is worth noting at this point that any concept of the bacterial genome as a fixed entity should be discarded forthwith. Comparison of the genome of E. coli O157:H7 with that of the previously sequenced genome of E. coli K-12 reveals an additional 856 kb of DNA (82). Recent data emanating from a comparative study of 36 S. aureus genomes indicate that 22% of the genome is dispensable, with many of the variable regions constituting presumed pathogenicity islands and regions of antimicrobial resistance (68). Human-pathogenic bacteria have been faced for a considerable time with stiff challenges from the human immune system, as well as from the recent glut of antimicrobial agents. The proliferation of antimicrobial resistance merely represents the logical response of these versatile creatures to this lethal challenge.

Mutation of Acquired Genes

As bacteria have responded to the challenge of antimicrobial agents, so have we responded to the challenge of antibiotic resistance. Our typical response to the appearance of antimicrobial resistance has been a concerted effort to develop novel antimicrobial agents that are active against the resistant strains. The emergence of β-lactamase-mediated resistance to antibiotics is an instructive example of this interplay. Ampicillin was developed as the first penicillin with clinically significant activity against gram-negative bacilli, primarily E. coli. Within a few years of the clinical introduction of ampicillin, strains of E. coli were described that were resistant to this antibiotic by virtue of the production of a plasmid-mediated β-lactamase designated TEM (named after the patient from whom the resistant strain was isolated). S. aureus expressed a similar β-lactamase, prompting a concerted effort on the part of the pharmaceutical industry to develop β-lactam antibiotics resistant to hydrolysis. Among the more successful compounds that were developed were methicillin, with activity against β-lactamase-producing S. aureus; the cephalosporins and carbapenems, with widespread activity against many β-lactamase-producing species; and the β-lactamase inhibitors, which restored the activity of β-lactams susceptible to hydrolysis.

The most successful and widely developed class of β-lactamase-resistant β-lactam antibiotics is the cephalosporins. So many of these agents have been developed for clinical use that they are frequently lumped into "generations" to facilitate remembering their spectra of activity. The "third-generation" or "extended-spectrum" cephalosporins cefotaxime, ceftizoxime, ceftriaxone, and ceftazidime are particularly potent antibiotics that are utterly resistant to hydrolysis by the TEM enzyme. Unfortunately, increasing clinical use of these agents, particularly ceftazidime, was associated with the emergence of resistant gram-negative bacilli, particularly K. pneumoniae (96). Molecular analysis of these resistant strains revealed that the resistance was mediated by β-lactamase and that many of these β-lactamases were derived from the native TEM enzyme through one or more point mutations in the bla_{TEM} gene. The unfortunate realization soon set in that our creative opponents could thwart years and hundreds of millions of dollars in development costs overnight.

Biochemical Mechanisms of Resistance

Modification of the Antibiotic

Many antibiotic-modifying enzymes have been described, including the β-lactamases, the aminoglycoside-modifying enzymes, and chloramphenicol acetyltransferases. Although these enzymes are in many cases acquired, some are intrinsic to certain species. For example, chromosomal β-lactamases are intrinsic to almost all gram-negative bacilli. Expression of these enzymes often occurs only at a very low level, conferring resistance to only very susceptible β-lactams, as with K. pneumoniae resistance to ampicillin through expression of the chromosomal SHV-1 enzyme (166), or to no β-lactams at all, as with E. coli under normal circumstances. In some bacterial genera (notably Enterobacter and Pseudomonas), chromosomal enzymes are under regulatory control, with derangements in these regulatory mechanisms resulting in high-level, broad-spectrum β-lactam resistance (95, 111). In some instances, aminoglycoside-modifying enzymes are intrinsic to bacterial species as well, as with the chromosomal acetyltransferases of *Providencia stuartii* and *Serratia marcescens* (159, 180).

Modifying enzymes in general confer high levels of resistance to the antibiotics against which they have activity. Expression of the TEM-1 β-lactamase by *E. coli*, for example, can increase the ampicillin MIC from 8 to >10,000 μg/ml. Similarly, expression of the bifunctional aminoglycoside resistance enzyme in *E. faecalis* raises the gentamicin MIC from 32–64 to >2,000 μg/ml. As effective as these mechanisms are, however, some antibiotics appear to be immune to inactivating enzymes. Vancomycin has been in clinical use since 1958, yet there are still no examples of vancomycin-modifying enzymes in bacteria.

Modification of the Target Molecule

Since antibiotic interaction with target molecules is generally quite specific, minor alterations of the target molecule can have important effects on antibiotic binding. Numerous examples exist of antibiotic target modification as a mechanism of resistance, including the many erythromycin ribosomal methylases that confer resistance to the macrolide-lincosamide-streptogramin B classes of antibiotics (215). Modifications of PBPs can affect the affinities of these molecules for β-lactam antibiotics, as noted above for *S. pneumoniae*, and especially for ampicillin-resistant *E. faecium* through mutations in PBP5 (79, 167). Modifications of PBPs seem to be a favored mechanism of β-lactam resistance in gram-positive bacteria, whereas β-lactamase production is favored in gram-negative bacilli. Although the reason for this difference is unknown, it is interesting that β-lactamases produced by gram-positive bacteria diffuse into the external medium once produced whereas those produced by gram-negative bacilli are kept within the periplasmic space by the outer membrane. The ability to concentrate β-lactamases enhances their efficacy and may help explain the preference for this mechanism among gram-negative bacilli.

Other important examples of target modifications include the altered cell wall precursors that confer resistance to glycopeptide antibiotics, mutated DNA gyrase and topoisomerase IV conferring resistance to fluoroquinolone antimicrobial agents, ribosomal protection mechanisms conferring resistance to tetracyclines, and RNA polymerase mutations conferring resistance to rifampin. The degree of resistance conferred by target modifications is variable and may be dependent on the ability of the mutated target to perform its normal function. Mutations in PBPs of *S. pneumoniae*, for example, confer a relatively low level of resistance (although one that is significant in the treatment of meningitis) (79), whereas VanA-type vancomycin resistance confers a very high level of resistance to vancomycin in enterococci (12).

Restricted Access to the Target

It is axiomatic that an antibiotic must reach its target in order to be effective. Therefore, when barriers must be crossed by the antibiotic before it can reach its target, strengthening these barriers can be a highly effective mechanism of resistance. All gram-negative bacteria have an outer membrane that must be crossed before the cytoplasmic membrane can be reached. Reductions in the quantities of known or presumed porins (channels for movement of materials across the outer membrane) have been documented as important contributors to resistance to imipenem in *P. aeruginosa*, cefepime in *Enterobacter cloacae*, and cefoxitin or ceftazidime in *K. pneumoniae* (107, 111, 118). In most instances, this restricted entry must be in combination with production of an at least moderately active β-lactamase to confer high-level resistance. Barriers to entry can also exist in the cytoplasmic membrane. Movement of aminoglycosides across the cytoplasmic membrane is an oxygen-dependent process, so that these antibiotics are inactive in anaerobic environments (and hence against strictly anaerobic species) (105).

Efflux Pumps

Among the most active areas of research in antimicrobial resistance is the identification and characterization of pumps that remove one or more antibiotic classes from the bacterial cell. Several classes of pumps have been described in gram-positive and/or gram-negative bacteria. They may be quite selective, or they may have a broad substrate specificity. The majority of these pumps are located in the cytoplasmic membrane and use proton motive force to drive drug efflux. The major families of efflux transporters are (i) the major facilitator superfamily, which includes QacA and NorA/Bmr of gram-positive bacteria and EmrB of *E. coli*; (ii) the small multidrug resistance family, including Smr of *S. aureus* and EmrE of *E. coli*; and (iii) the resistance-nodulation-division family, including AcrAB-TolC of *E. coli* and MexAB-OprM of *P. aeruginosa*. The structure of efflux pumps is shown in Fig. 2. In some instances, combinations of different types of pumps can result in higher levels of resistance than achieved by the activity of a single pump alone (106). Analysis of bacterial genomes has suggested that the number of pumps encoded by many bacterial genomes is considerably greater than was previously realized, suggesting that their contributions to resistance are substantial and have yet to be fully appreciated. Several excellent reviews of pump-mediated resistance have been published (133, 143).

Attribution of resistance to a specific mechanism may be difficult when more than one mechanism is involved. For example, resistance to imipenem in *P. aeruginosa* is contributed to by reduced access (through down-regulation of OmpD) and by production of AmpC β-lactamase (111, 146). Neither mechanism alone is sufficient to yield clinically significant levels of resistance, yet both are required for high levels of resistance to result.

RESISTANCE MECHANISMS FOR DIFFERENT ANTIMICROBIAL CLASSES

Aminoglycoside Resistance

Aminoglycosides (streptomycin, neomycin, gentamicin, tobramycin, paromomycin, amikacin, kanamycin, and netilmicin) are concentration-dependent bactericidal antibiotics that are particularly active against aerobic gram-negative bacilli. The aminoglycosides are a family of molecules containing an aminocyclitol ring (streptidine or 2-deoxystrepamine) and two or more amino sugars linked by glycosidic bonds. As a class, these antibiotics are more effective against *Enterobacteriaceae* than against *Pseudomonas aeruginosa*. Aminoglycosides are not clinically effective against *Shigella* and *Salmonella* spp., although these organisms appear susceptible in vitro. In combination with glycopeptides or β-lactams, they are often used to treat serious

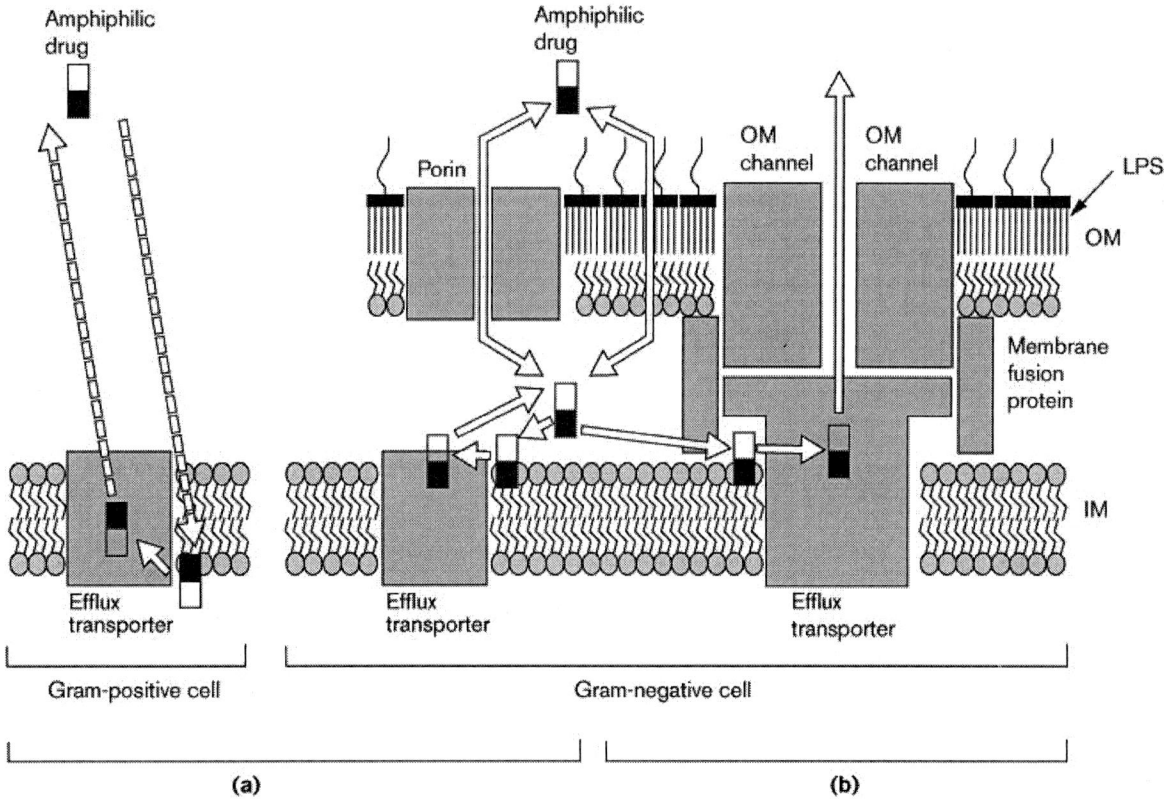

FIGURE 2 Bacterial multidrug pumps exist in one of two configurations. (a) The transporter occurs in the cytoplasmic membrane simply by itself. In gram-positive bacteria (left), drugs enter unhindered and are pumped out to the medium (dashed arrows). In gram-negative bacteria (right), drug molecules that have entered the periplasmic space through porin channels or by directly passing through the lipid bilayer are extruded into the periplasmic space (solid arrows). Drug molecules are shown to first partition into the bilayer of the inner membrane and to then be captured from within the bilayer, but this mechanism may not apply to all transporters. (b) Complex efflux machinery occurs only in gram-negative bacteria. Here the drug molecules are captured and pumped out directly into the medium by an assembly that contains, in addition to the pump, an outer membrane channel and a membrane fusion protein. In both panels, efflux of drug molecules from the cytoplasm may occur but is not shown for simplicity. LPS, lipopolysaccharide; OM, outer membrane; IM, inner membrane. Adapted from reference 133 with permission of Elsevier Science.

infections caused by susceptible gram-positive cocci (as synergistic therapy).

The process of bacterial killing by aminoglycosides is multifactorial. The principal target of aminoglycosides is the 30S subunit of ribosomes (e.g., gentamicin attaches to the highly conserved site A of the *E. coli* 16S rRNA) (125). This binding prevents the elongation of the growing peptide chain by causing misreading or premature termination of peptide synthesis. By interfering with the translation of mRNA, protein production is altered, aberrant proteins are inserted in the cell membrane, cell permeability is increased, more aminoglycosides are taken up into the cell, and cell death ensues.

Resistance to aminoglycosides emerges by one of four mechanisms: (i) alterations in the target site (ribosome) that prevents binding; (ii) loss of cell permeability; (iii) expulsion by efflux pumps; and (iv) enzymatic inactivation by aminoglycoside-modifying enzymes (AMEs). As in the case with β-lactamases, aminoglycoside inactivation by AMEs is the most important in terms of frequency and level

of resistance (15). Furthermore, AMEs can be passed from one bacterium to another via transposons or plasmids (acquired resistance). Numerous reports have also established that these resistance determinants are also encoded on specialized transposable genetic elements called integrons (80, 181, 217).

Resistance Due to Decreased Uptake

Intrinsic resistance most often results from impaired uptake. Chromosomal mutations may also result in resistance, either through a modification of the ribosomal target or through the activation of chromosomal housekeeping genes that modify aminoglycoside molecules. Bacterial cells have multiple copies of the genes that encode rRNA. The presence of mutations in all these genes is extremely rare. Hence, ribosomal mutations are responsible for low-level resistance only.

Intrinsic or acquired resistance secondary to decreased antibiotic uptake confers low-level cross-resistance to all aminoglycosides. Aminoglycosides are highly positively charged compounds that must cross the negatively charged outer membrane (in gram-negative bacteria) and cytoplasmic membrane (in both gram-negative and gram-positive bacteria) before they reach their cytoplasmic ribosomal target. In gram-negative bacteria, the initial step involves cationic binding of aminoglycosides to anionic sites on the outer membrane surface; these sites include lipopolysaccharides, outer membrane proteins, and the polar heads of phospholipids. It has been generally believed that in *E. coli*, aminoglycosides reach the periplasmic space by diffusion through the outer membrane porins, although significant MIC changes due to porin loss have been difficult to demonstrate (176). Studies of *P. aeruginosa* and *E. coli* indicate that uptake across the outer membrane may be due instead to a "self-promoted uptake" mechanism. The cationic aminoglycosides displace divalent cations (e.g., Mg^{2+}) that cross-bridge adjacent lipopolysaccharide molecules, thereby permeabilizing the outer membrane and allowing entry of the antibiotic (98). Consistent with this model, divalent cations have long been known to antagonize the activity of aminoglycosides against gram-negative bacteria (36). However, recent data indicate that, in *P. aeruginosa* at least, a functional efflux pump (MexXY-OprM) is required for cation antagonism of aminoglycoside activity (116). Disruption of the outer membrane may contribute to the bactericidal activity of these drugs since neither inhibition of protein synthesis nor codon misreading alone can adequately account for this activity.

Aminoglycoside-Modifying Enzymes

Aminoglycosides are modified by specific enzymes in the bacterial cell. These enzymes are phosphotransferases (APHs), nucleotidyltransferases or adenyltransferases (ANTs), and acetyltransferases (AACs). AMEs covalently modify specific amino or hydroxyl groups, resulting in aminoglycosides that bind poorly to the target ribosomes. Within each class, there are AMEs with different specific sites of modification.

To understand the site of modification of an AME, one must recall how aminoglycosides are numbered. The streptidine or 2-deoxystreptamine nucleus forms the center for the numbering scheme (from 2-deoxystreptamine are derived all aminoglycosides except streptomycin and spectinomycin). The first sugar moiety at the 4 position has positions numbered with a single prime (1' to 6'); the second sugar moiety at the 6 position has positions numbered with a double prime (1″ to 6″). Hence, AAC(6') acetylates an amino group at the 6' position (via an acetyltransferase) on the amino sugar attached to the 4 position (Fig. 3). Each AME class consists of numerous enzymes that can modify different -OH or -NH₂ groups. These are divided into subclasses. In each subclass, there are different enzyme types that are designated by a Roman numeral, e.g., AAC (3)-I. Isoenzymes are also described and are designated by the lowercase letter a or b and so forth. These isoenzymes are functionally identical and confer identical resistance phenotypes.

Currently, there are seven major phosphotransferases [APH(3'), APH(2″), APH(3″), APH(6), APH(9), APH(4), and APH(7″)], four nucleotidyltransferases [ANT(6), ANT(3″), ANT(4'), and ANT(2″)], and four acetyltransferases [AAC(2'), AAC(6), AAC(1), and AAC(3)]. A bifunctional AME able to acetylate and phosphorylate [AAC(6')-APH(2″)] also exists. This enzyme is found only in *Staphylococcus*, *Enterococcus*, and some streptococci and is responsible for high-level resistance to aminoglycosides (61). The gene *aac(6')-aph(2″)*, which encodes the synthesis of this enzyme,

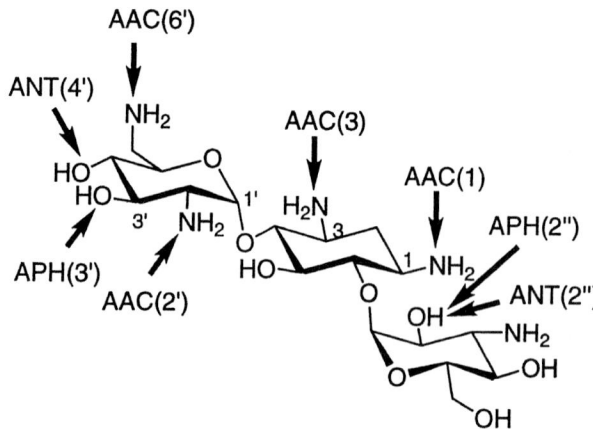

FIGURE 3 Sites of modification on kanamycin B by various aminoglycoside-modifying enzymes. The arrows point to the sites of modification by the specific enzymes, namely, acetyltransferases, phosphotransferases, and nucleotidyltransferases. Reprinted with permission from reference 103.

is present in Tn*4001*-like transposons which are inserted both in plasmids and in the chromosomes of aminoglycoside-resistant isolates. Most methicillin-resistant *Staphylococcus* strains encode this resistance determinant.

Four of these AMEs have been examined by X-ray crystallography (103). These are ANT(4'), AAC(3), AAC(6'), and APH(3') type IIIa. From the overall structure of these AMEs, it is clear that electrostatic interactions (negatively charged binding sites on the enzymes attracted to positively charged groups on the molecule) are critical for binding of aminoglycosides to both the ribosome and the AME.

A large number of AMEs have been described, and the reader is referred to the web site http://www.warn.cas.cz developed by the Schering-Plough group and the Antibiotic Resistance Study Group (15). These enzymes are believed to originate from actinomycetes that synthesize these antibiotics (*Streptomyces* and *Micromonospora* spp.). It is also possible that AMEs originated from enzymes involved in normal cellular respiration (housekeeping functions) (158). In addition to genetic studies, mechanistic investigations have been performed describing how these enzymes inactivate aminoglycosides (14). Suffice it to say, each AME class (ANTs, AACs, APHs) possesses unique mechanisms.

Resistance to β-Lactam Antibiotics

Penicillin-Binding Protein-Mediated Resistance

β-Lactam antibiotics (penicillins, cephalosporins, monobactams, and carbapenems) are the safest and mostly widely used class of antibiotics ever developed. They act by inhibiting the PBPs, the transpeptidases, transglycosylases, and carboxypeptidases that manufacture peptidoglycan. The specific functions of different PBPs have been identified for some bacteria, but the precise ways in which they interact with each other and with cell wall precursors remain largely a mystery. Some are clearly essential for cell viability (generally the high-molecular-weight transpeptidases and transglycosylases), while others appear to be dispensable, with no apparent deleterious effects on cellular structure or function resulting from their absence (most commonly the low-molecular-weight carboxypeptidases). It has long been suspected that some PBPs are redundant and can serve the functions of others. For example, *E. faecium* strains in which all of the PBPs except low-affinity PBP5 are saturated grow normally, implying that PBP5 can perform all of the functions required for cell wall synthesis (218). On the other hand, *E. faecium* strains in which *pbp5* has been deleted grow normally as well, implying that the other PBPs can provide all of these functions (167).

PBPs are all members of a larger family of serine peptidases that also includes most of the β-lactamases. PBPs and β-lactamases interact with β-lactam molecules (which themselves are structural analogues of the peptidyl-D-alanyl-D-alanine termini of peptidoglycan precursors) by catalytically disrupting the β-lactam bond, resulting in a serine ester-linked acylenzyme derivative (Fig. 1). In the case of β-lactamases, a water molecule then hydrolyzes the ester linkage of the acylenzyme intermediate, releasing the irreversibly damaged penicilloyl (or cephalosporyl) moiety and regenerating the active enzyme. PBP–β-lactam acylenzyme derivatives are in general less accommodating to nucleophilic attack by the water molecule, resulting in a persistence of the covalent bond and inactivation of the PBP. The stability of this interaction allows the identification of these proteins by binding to radiolabeled penicillin and is the genesis of their designation as "penicillin-binding proteins." Because β-lactamases serve no definable function in the cell other than to interact with β-lactam molecules, their affinity for the β-lactam and the rapidity with which the reaction proceeds determine their effectiveness and hence the level of resistance. Conversely, since PBPs have a very important alternative function (manufacture of cell wall), the affinity of the interaction between PBPs and the β-lactam is a measure of distraction from their primary functions and thereby often defines the level of susceptibility of the strain.

Inhibition of PBPs interrupts cell wall synthesis, which by itself should inhibit cell growth rather than kill the cell. However, the interaction of β-lactam molecules with PBPs triggers the activity of cell wall-degrading molecules known as autolysins, which rupture the cell, leading to cell death (203). The extent to which these autolytic enzymes are activated correlates in most cases with the cidal activity of a β-lactam against a particular bacterial strain.

Some bacterial species are intrinsically resistant to some β-lactam antibiotics by virtue of decreased PBP affinity. For example, enterococci are resistant to clinically achievable levels of cephalosporin antibiotics because of the presence of low-affinity PBP5. Similar low affinity is demonstrated for the semisynthetic antistaphylococcal penicillins nafcillin and oxacillin, as well as for the antipseudomonal penicillins carbenicillin and ticarcillin. Enterococcal PBP5s are bound with a diminished affinity by ampicillin and the ureidopenicillins mezlocillin and piperacillin, resulting in MICs that are higher than for streptococci but within the achievable concentration range in human serum.

PBP-mediated resistance for normally susceptible bacteria takes several forms, including (i) overproduction of a PBP, (ii) acquisition of a foreign PBP with low affinity, (iii) recombination of a susceptible PBP with more resistant varieties, and (iv) point mutations within PBPs that lower their affinity for the β-lactam antibiotic. PBP-mediated resistance is found predominantly in gram-positive bacteria. However, there are examples of gram-negative bacteria with PBP-mediated resistance, and we will point these out as they come up.

PBP Overexpression

Increased expression of a PBP as a mechanism of conferring resistance is relatively uncommon. Clear examples of settings in which increased quantities of a PBP are associated with resistance include increased levels of methicillin resistance found in *S. aureus* strains that overexpress PBP4 (85) and increased levels of penicillin resistance in *Enterococcus hirae* and *E. faecium* strains that overexpress PBP5 (69, 167). The existence of this mechanism serves as a reminder that, like β-lactamases, susceptibility or resistance depends on the number of β-lactam molecules relative to the number of targets. Increasing the number of target molecules can, under the correct circumstances, result in resistance. Conversely, the effectiveness of imipenem against *E. coli* has been partially attributed to the fact that its primary target is PBP2, which is present in roughly 200 copies, in contrast to PBP3, which is estimated at 2,000 copies. In any case, overproduction of PBPs is a rare mechanism of resistance to β-lactam antibiotics.

Acquisition of Foreign PBPs

Acquisition of a foreign PBP as a mechanism of resistance is best exemplified by the expression of methicillin resistance in *S. aureus* strains by virtue of the expression of PBP2a, a low-affinity PBP not native to *S. aureus* (40). Structural analysis of PBP2a suggests that it possesses both transglycosylase and transpeptidase domains, suggesting that it can perform all of the functions normally assigned to the native *S. aureus* PBPs. PBP2a confers resistance to all β-lactam antibiotics, although it is bound relatively well by ampicillin (41). The fact that virtually all MRSA strains express β-lactamase limits the utility of ampicillin, but in vitro and animal studies suggest that combinations of ampicillin with β-lactamase inhibitors may be effective. To date, there are no clinical data in humans to support using these combinations to treat MRSA infections.

The origin of the *mecA* gene (which encodes PBP2a) is unknown. A *mecA* homologue has been identified in *Staphylococcus sciuri*, a primitive staphylococcal species associated with rodents and primitive mammals (47). The deduced amino acid sequences of the two enzymes exhibited 88% similarity across the entire protein and 91% identity within the transpeptidase domain. *S. sciuri* strains are not methicillin resistant, however, which may be due to the lack of an effective promoter upstream of the gene. *S. sciuri mecA* homologues in which the promoter has spontaneously mutated express higher levels of methicillin resistance in both *S. sciuri* and when cloned on a high-copy-number vector in *S. aureus* (220). Expression of methicillin resistance in *S. aureus* is commonly under regulatory control, either by the product of the upstream *mecI* gene or in *trans* by the homologous *blaI* gene that regulates the expression of β-lactamase (the promoter regions of *mecA* and the *blaZ* β-lactamase genes are similar) (77). The *mecI* and *blaI* repressors are in turn controlled by the *mecR1* and *blaR1* sensors and transducers, although the precise mechanism of this interaction is incompletely understood. The efficiency of induction varies with the mechanism (*blaR1*-*blaI*-mediated induction is faster), leading to complications in detecting the methicillin resistance phenotype. In fact, only a small minority of a resistant population may express high levels of resistance. Several techniques are used in the laboratory to "bring out" the resistance (prolonged incubation, increased salt in the media), and more recently techniques have been developed to bypass phenotypic expression in favor of directly identifying the *mecA* gene or directly detecting the PBP2a protein.

Expression of PBP2a-mediated resistance to β-lactams in *S. aureus* is also influenced by the expression of other genetic loci called *fem* (factors essential for methicillin resistance) or *aux* (auxiliary) genes (20). *fem* and *aux* genes were first identified by transposon mutagenesis of MRSA in an experiment to find insertions that would reduce the expression of resistance. Many *fem* and *aux* factors have now been identified, and all are involved in the formation of the staphylococcal cell wall (40). It appears that even minor perturbations of the normal processes prevent PBP2a from functioning, suggesting that it is a very particular enzyme.

The *mecA* gene is located within a larger (ca. 450 to 60-kb) region of the chromosome known as the *mec* region (92). Although this region is flanked by IS elements, it has not been conclusively demonstrated to be mobile in vitro. In addition, transfer of the *mec* region between staphylococcal strains has never been conclusively documented. The spread of MRSA within institutions is therefore largely due to the transmission of resistant organisms from patient to patient, probably on the hands of transiently colonized health care workers (184). Single strains have spread through entire hospitals and even cities (170).

Resistance Mutations by Recombination with Foreign DNA

Resistance through recombination between native, susceptible PBPs and those of less susceptible species is a phenomenon largely restricted to species that are capable of undergoing natural transformation or of taking up naked DNA from the environment. Prominent among these species are *Streptococcus pneumoniae*, viridans streptococci, *Neisseria gonorrhoeae*, and *Neisseria meningitidis* (79). *S. pneumoniae* contains six PBPs (PBP1a, PBP1b, PBP2a, PBP2b, PBP2x, and PBP3), all of which are subject to recombination with foreign PBPs taken up by transformation. In most cases, resistant *pbp* genes demonstrate mosaic patterns (individual segments of foreign *pbp* genes integrated with the native *pbp* gene) with the foreign DNA in the less penicillin-susceptible viridans streptococci (79). In fact, genetic exchange appears common between these closely related species, with mosaic patterns demonstrable even in PBPs from susceptible *S. mitis* strains (7). Penicillin resistance in *S. pneumoniae* can be established by alterations in PBP2X, PBP2B, and PBP1A, whereas only alterations in PBP2X and PBP1A are required for cephalosporin resistance (17). Penicillin resistance has been detected in *S. pneumoniae* for some time, with cephalosporin resistance emerging more recently, most commonly in strains already resistant to penicillin. However, strains resistant to cephalosporins but susceptible to penicillin have also been reported (189). High-level resistance (≥2 μg/ml) usually implies modification of more than one PBP, sometimes with several mosaic insertions in each one (17).

As with PBP2a-mediated resistance to methicillin *Staphylococcus aureus*, expression of penicillin and cephalosporin resistance in *S. pneumoniae* is dependent on the proper functioning of auxiliary genes. The *fib* locus of *S. pneumoniae* (*fibA* and *fibB*) is analogous to *femA* and *femB* in *S. aureus*. It is involved in the formation of interpeptide bridges, and inactivation of the *fib* locus is associated with a reduction in the number of cross-linked muropeptides and loss of penicillin resistance even in the presence of low-affinity mosaic PBPs (212). The *murM/murN* operon en-

codes enzymes involved in the biosynthesis of branched structured cell wall muropeptides commonly found in penicillin-resistant pneumococci (64). Inactivation of *murM/murN* results in loss of branched chain muropeptides as well as loss of penicillin resistance.

Among gram-negative species, *Neisseria* is well known to be naturally transformable. It is therefore not entirely surprising that strains of both *N. gonorrhoeae* and *N. meningitidis* have been described in which mosaic PBP genes are associated with decreased susceptibility to penicillin (79). Similar to the *S. pneumoniae* picture, the resistant portions of the PBP genes have been acquired from closely related commensal *Neisseria* species that are more resistant to penicillin (193). While penicillin resistance in *N. meningitidis* remains thankfully extremely rare, both β-lactamase-mediated resistance and PBP-mediated resistance to β-lactams in *N. gonorrhoeae* are quite common.

Point Mutations

The final mechanism of PBP-mediated β-lactam resistance results from point mutations within the *pbp* genes that result in lower affinity for the β-lactam in question. This form of mutational resistance is seen most commonly in PBP5 of *E. faecium* strains, raising penicillin MICs from 4–16 to as high as >1,000 μg/ml. High-level penicillin-resistant strains now represent the majority of clinical *E. faecium* isolates in the United States (173). These mutations further reduce the affinity for cephalosporins and other β-lactams with lower affinity for the nonmutated version, an increase in resistance that may have implications for the likelihood that antibiotic use will promote colonization with multiresistant *E. faecium* (52). Most of the mutations occur in the vicinity of one or more of several conserved "boxes" important for β-lactam binding (171). Although it is presumed that multiple mutations lead to higher levels of resistance, a systematic study of the importance of various mutations for the expression of resistance has not been published. In rare instances, point mutations of the *Staphylococcus aureus pbp2* gene have been associated with methicillin resistance, but the importance of this mechanism pales in comparison to expression of PBP2a (78). Among gram-negative species, point mutations of the *ftsI* gene of *Haemophilus influenzae* (encoding the transpeptidase domain of PBP3A and/or PBP3B) have been associated with non-β-lactamase-mediated resistance to ampicillin and cephalosporins in this species (208). Although mutations have also been noted within PBP4 in this species, it is not clear that these have a significant impact on β-lactam susceptibility.

β-Lactamase-Mediated Resistance

PBPs and most β-lactamases are members of a superfamily of active-site serine proteases (74, 120). These enzymes catalytically disrupt the β-lactam (amide) bond to form an acyl enzyme complex (Fig. 1). A conserved serine in the active site (Ser70) acts as the reactive nucleophile in the acylation reaction. In β-lactamases, a critically positioned water molecule then serves as the attacking nucleophile in the deacylation step. Water is important for the efficient hydrolysis of the ester linkage to release the penicilloyl and cephalosporyl moiety. In general, the major difference between PBPs and β-lactamases is in the rate of deacylation. The structure of PBPs does not allow a water molecule ready access. As a result, following β-lactam binding, PBPs undergo slow deacylation compared to β-lactamases, whose rates can be as rapid as 2 to 3,000/s (33).

β-Lactamases are a heterogeneous group of proteins with structural similarities. They are composed of α-helices and a β-pleated sheet (100). The β-pleated sheet is composed of five antiparallel strands. Two schemes are currently used to classify β-lactamases: the Ambler classification scheme and the Bush-Jacoby-Medeiros classification system (6, 34, 35). The Ambler scheme separates β-lactamases into four distinct classes based on similarities in amino acid sequence. Classes A, C, and D are serine β-lactamases, whereas class B enzymes are metallo-β-lactamases that require zinc for activity. The Bush-Jacoby-Medeiros scheme classifies β-lactamases according to functional similarities (substrate and inhibitor profiles). There are four categories and multiple subgroups in the Bush-Jacoby-Medeiros system (Groups 1, 2, 3, and 2a, 2c, 3a, etc.). A comparison of the two classification systems is summarized in Table 2.

β-Lactamases can be chromosome, plasmid, or transposon encoded and produced in a constitutive or inducible manner; they are secreted into the periplasmic space in gram-negative bacteria or into the surrounding medium by their gram-positive counterparts (112). Membrane-associated enzymes have been rarely reported (*Bacillus licheniformis*, *Bacillus cereus*, and *Bacteroides vulgatus*) (120).

Class A β-Lactamases

Sequence comparisons and structural determinations of a number of class A β-lactamases have advanced our knowledge of the catalytic properties of these enzymes. The class A β-lactamases possess four common motifs that create a complex hydrogen-bonding network to fix the β-lactam in the substrate-binding pocket (120). In class A β-lactamases, residues S70-Xaa-Xaa-K73, S130-D131-N132 (SDN loop), and K/R234-T/S235-G236 define the conserved residues critical for β-lactam binding and hydrolysis. In the substrate-binding pocket, the oxyanion hole (as defined by the backbone NH group of Ser70 and Ala237) also serves to attract β-lactams for catalysis (100). The Ω loop (amino acids 160 to 179) is unique in class A β-lactamases. A highly conserved Glu166 that functions as a general base in the catalytic process is located in this loop

(196). Arg164 and Asn179 define the limits, or "neck," of the Ω loop.

Two commonly encountered class A β-lactamases found in members of the *Enterobacteriaceae* are designated TEM-1 and SHV-1. TEM-1 and SHV-1 are primarily penicillinases with little or no activity against cephalosporins. These β-lactamases have received significant attention over the past decade since they are the progenitors of the "extended-spectrum" enzymes now common in many hospitals. Extended-spectrum β-lactamases (ESBLs) are enzymes that have "expanded" or changed their substrate profile because of amino acid mutations, allowing hydrolysis of most cephalosporins (145). Among the TEM and SHV family enzymes, five amino acid residues appear to be most important for conferring the ESBL phenotype: Gly238 and Ala237 (located on the b3 β-pleated sheet), Arg164 and Asp179 (located on the neck of the Ω loop), and Asp104 (located directly across G238 and A237 at the opening of the active-site cavity) (100, 120, 156). These amino acid residues are positioned in the active-site pocket. In particular, the substitution of Gly to Ser, Ala, or Asp at the Ambler position ABL 238 is a common mutation in TEM and SHV ESBLs (www.lahey.org).

The crystal structure of ESBL type β-lactamase TEM-52 has been determined and indicates that important interactions are also formed with residue 243, resulting in a major shift in the b3 β-strand (139). In TEM-52, the hydroxyl of the Gly238Ser substitution forms two new H bonds: one to the Ser243 backbone amide and one to the Ser243 hydroxyl group. This widens the active site and may facilitate the binding of "bulky" oxyimino cephalosporin substrates.

Sites within TEM and SHV that confer resistance to inhibition by β-lactamase inhibitors have also been defined (Met69, Ser130, Arg244, Arg275Leu, and Asn276) (26, 51, 59, 154, 175, 198, 202, 210, 211). In most cases, ESBL mutations render the enzymes more susceptible to inhibition by the mechanism-based inactivators clavulanic acid, sulbactam, and tazobactam, whereas mutations conferring resistance to inhibitors result in reduced activity against cephalosporins. Mutants of TEM β-lactamases are being

TABLE 2 β-Lactamase classification

Bush-Jacoby-Medeiros system	Major subgroups	Ambler system	Main attributes
Group 1 cephalosporinases		C (Cephalosporinases)	Usually chromosomal; resistance to all β-lactams except carbapenems; not inhibited by clavulanate
Group 2 penicillinases (clavulanic acid susceptible)	2a	A (Serine β-lactamases)	Staphylococcal penicillinases
	2b	A	Broad-spectrum: TEM-1, TEM-2, SHV-1
	2be	A	Extended-spectrum: TEM-3–??, SHV-2
	2br	A	Inhibitor resistant TEM (IRT)
	2c	A	Carbenicillin hydrolyzing
	2e	A	Cephalosporinases inhibited by clavulanate
	2f	A	Carbapenemases inhibited by clavulanate
	2d	D (Oxacillin hydrolyzing)	Cloxacillin hydrolyzing (OXA)
Group 3 metallo-β-lactamase	3a	B (Metalloenzymes)	Zinc-dependent carbapenemases
	3b	B	
	3c	B	
Group 4		Not classified	Miscellaneous enzymes, most not yet sequenced

recovered that maintain the ESBL phenotype but also demonstrate inhibitor resistance. These are referred to as complex mutants of TEM (CMT-1 and CMT-2) (63, 187).

Most inhibitor-resistant β-lactamases are variants of the TEM-1 enzyme, with only one description of a clinical isolate expressing SHV resistant to inhibitors (SHV-10) (154). It is possible that the frequency of inhibitor-resistant β-lactamases is underestimated, since many laboratories in the United States do not identify these strains. Piperacillin/tazobactam may be still effective for the treatment of E. coli expressing some inhibitor-resistant TEM β-lactamases (27).

A large number of non-TEM and non-SHV class A ESBLs have been described (29, 30, 136). The most important families include the CTX-M family (Toho-1) and the PER family (PER-1 and PER-2) (137, 163, 207). There are 20 reported CTX-M type β-lactamases (www.lahey.org). These β-lactamases have been found in E. coli, Salmonella enterica serovar Typhimurium, Citrobacter spp., and Enterobacter spp. As a group, they are closest in amino acid identity to chromosomal cephalosporinases of Klebsiella oxytoca β-lactamase (OXY-1) and the chromosomal cephalosporinases of Proteus vulgaris and Citrobacter koseri (C. diversus) (207). They can be divided into three distinct clusters (see www.lahey.org). Unlike most (but not all) TEM- and SHV-derived ESBLs, CTX-M β-lactamases hydrolyze cefotaxime and ceftriaxone better than they do ceftazidime. It appears that CTX-M enzymes are more readily inhibited by tazobactam than they are by clavulanic acid. The first CTX-M-type β-lactamase (MEN-1) was described nearly a decade ago (18). The crystal structure of Toho-1 (a member of the CTX-M family) indicates that the structural flexibility of the active site is important for the ESBL phenotype (91). The crystal structure of PER-1 reveals unique features as well (205).

Other clinically important variants in this class have been described (VEB-1, BES-1, IBI-1, and IBI-2) (29, 30, 148). VEB-1 is the first class A ESBL to be found within an integron. Other β-lactamases found within integrons include IBC-1 and some PSE, OXA, and CARB β-lactamases (29). Although the carbapenems remain quite stable to hydrolysis by most class A β-lactamases, several enzymes of this class are able to hydrolyze the carbapenems (Sme-1, Sme-2, NMC-A, IMI-1, and KPC-1) (149, 221). These enzymes remain rare in North America but are found increasingly in areas of the world in which carbapenems are used in abundance.

Class B β-Lactamases

Unlike the serine-dependent β-lactamases (class A, C, and D β-lactamases), class B β-lactamases are metalloenzymes (157). As such, class B β-lactamases require zinc or another heavy metal for catalysis and their activities are inhibited by chelating agents. With few exceptions (see below), class B β-lactamases confer resistance to a wide range of β-lactam compounds, including cephamycins and carbapenems. Class B β-lactamases are resistant to inactivation by clavulanate, sulbactam, and tazobactam. Aztreonam, a monobactam, is not hydrolyzed and does not act as an inhibitor (157).

Class B β-lactamases can be grouped into three different subclasses; B1, B2, and B3 (71, 157). Subclass B1 contains the metallo-β-lactamase II (BcII) from Bacillus cereus; the CcrA (also named CfiA) β-lactamase from Bacteroides fragilis; the BlaB β-lactamases from Chryseobacterium meningosepticum; the IND-1 β-lactamase from Chryseobacterium indologenes; the IMP β-lactamases found in some clinical isolates of Pseudomonas aeruginosa, Serratia marcescens, Klebsiella pneumoniae, and Acinetobacter baumannii; and the VIM β-lactamases found in some strains of P. aeruginosa. Subclass B2 includes the β-lactamase produced by various species of Aeromonas (CphA, ImiS, and CphA2) and the Sfh-I β-lactamase from Serratia fonticola. Finally, subclass B3 includes the L1 β-lactamases from Stenotrophomonas maltophilia, the GOB β-lactamases from C. meningosepticum, the FEZ-1 β-lactamase from Legionella gormanii, and the THIN-B β-lactamase produced by Janthinobacterium lividum (71).

The atomic structures of a number of class B β-lactamases (Bc-II from B. cereus 569/H/9, CcrA from B. fragilis, L1 from S. maltophilia, and IMP-1 from P. aeruginosa, among others) have been solved (37, 45, 71). Although the genes encoding these β-lactamases show very little primary-structure sequence identity (17–37%), the three-dimensional structures of the known metallo-β-lactamases are similar. The primary structures of Bc-II and CcrA bind two zinc ions in the active site. In contrast, only a single zinc ion is bound by the CphA enzyme from A. hydrophila. L1 from S. maltophilia exists as a tetramer and binds two zinc ions with each subunit (37, 45, 192, 209). The central role of the conserved cysteine in the catalytic mechanism has been reviewed (144).

Because of the metal ion, the catalytic pathway of metallo-β-lactamases does not involve an acyl enzyme intermediate as it does in class A and C β-lactamases (18, 91, 163, 205, 207). The catalytic pathway in class B involves a hydrolytic water molecule (the "bridging" water molecule) that possesses enhanced nucleophilicity due to the proximity to the metal ion. The addition of the hydroxide to the carbonyl carbon of the β-lactam leads to the formation of a transient, noncovalent reaction intermediate.

The majority of metallo-β-lactamases are chromosomally encoded, and their expression may be constitutive or inducible (157). The metallo β-lactamases of B. cereus, S. maltophilia, A. hydrophila, and A. jandaei are inducible. In A. jandaei, regulation of the metallo β-lactamase appears to involve a two-component signal transduction system (3).

Class C β-Lactamases

Ambler Class C (Bush-Jacoby-Medeiros group 1) β-lactamases are produced to a greater or lesser degree by almost all gram-negative bacteria (Salmonella and Klebsiella being the only known exceptions). Chromosomally encoded versions of these enzymes are particularly important in clinical isolates of Citrobacter freundii, Enterobacter aerogenes, E. cloacae, Morganella morganii, Pseudomonas aeruginosa, and Serratia marcescens. Class C β-lactamases hydrolyze cephalosporins (including extended-spectrum cephalosporins) more effectively than they do penicillins.

In comparison to class A enzymes, class C β-lactamases have larger active-site cavities, which may allow them to bind the bulky extended-spectrum cephalosporins (oxyimino-β-lactams) (48, 113). It is claimed that this conformational flexibility and its influence on adjacent structures facilitate the hydrolysis of oxyimino β-lactams by making the acyl-enzyme intermediate more open to attack by water (48, 113). Most class C enzymes are resistant to inhibition by mechanism-based inactivators. The interaction of Class C enzymes with β-lactamase inhibitors is an area of active study (152).

The important structural elements described for class A enzymes are also present in class C β-lactamases. The active-site serine is located near the N terminus of a long helix and is followed on the next helix turn by a lysine (Ser-Xaa-Xaa-Lys). The second element contains an SXN or YXN pattern corresponding to the Ser130-Asp131-Asn132 loop of class A β-lactamases. The opposite side of the active site is marked by (Lys/Arg/His)-(Thr/Ser)-Gly, corresponding to the KTG motif of class A enzymes. The corresponding Glu166 in Class C β-lactamases is not readily apparent, but this role may be filled by the tyrosine in the Tyr-Xaa-Asn motif.

Under normal circumstances in clinically important class C enzyme-producing gram-negative bacilli, β-lactamase production is repressed. The details of the repression are worked out in greatest detail for *Enterobacter* spp. (93, 94). Repression and activation are closely linked to the processes of cell wall synthesis and breakdown. The molecule that serves as both the repressor and the activator of *ampC* transcription is AmpR, a transcriptional regulator of the LysR family. AmpR is present as a repressor by virtue of its interaction with UDP MurNac-pentapeptide, a peptidoglycan precursor molecule. In this form, AmpR is incapable of activating *ampC* and in fact serves as a repressor of *ampR* expression. In the setting of high concentrations of the cell wall breakdown product anhydro-MurNAc-tripeptide (or anhydroMurNac-pentapeptide), however, UDP-MurNAc-pentapeptide is displaced from its site in AmpR, resulting in the conversion of AmpR to an activator of *ampC* transcription.

Increases in *ampC* expression may result from the action of β-lactam antibiotics, some of which cause the release of significant quantities of anhydro-MurNAc-tripeptide and/or pentapeptide from the peptidoglycan. This anhydro-UDP-MurNAc-tripeptide enters the cell through a channel (AmpG) and overwhelms the recycling ability of the cytosolic amidase (AmpD) specific for recycling of muropeptides. Under these circumstances (induction), β-lactamase is produced only as long as the antibiotic is present in the medium.

Constitutive high-level production of AmpC β-lactamase most commonly results from a mutation of the *ampD* gene, reducing the quantity of or eliminating AmpD from the cytoplasm. Under these circumstances, a constant high level of anhydro-MurNAc-tripeptide is present in the cytoplasm, and AmpR serves as a constitutive activator of *ampC* transcription. Constitutive production can also result from deletion of *ampR,* but in this circumstance β-lactamase production generally occurs at a low level.

A recent development has been the discovery of *ampC*-type β-lactamase genes on transferable plasmids. Plasmid-encoded AmpC cephalosporinases are separated into four general groups (163). Group 1 consists of those which originated from the chromosomal AmpC of *C. freundii* (BIL-1, CMY-2, LAT-1, and LAT-2). Members of group 2 are related to the chromosomal cephalosporinase of *E. cloacae* (MIR-1 and ACT-1), members of group 3 are related to the AmpC of *P. aeruginosa* (CMY-1, FOX-1, and MOX-1), and members of group 4 are related to the CMY-1 β-lactamase (CMY-1 cluster). Plasmid-mediated class C β-lactamases have been described in many gram-negative bacteria from all parts of the world. Host strains harboring these enzymes include *K. pneumoniae, E. aerogenes, Salmonella* spp. (serovars Seftenberg and Enteritidis), *E. coli, Proteus mirabilis, Morganella morganii,* and *Klebsiella oxytoca.* The loss of porin proteins in clinical isolates with plasmid-encoded AmpC enzymes may result in resistance to carbapenems (31, 194).

Class D β-Lactamases

The OXA-type (oxacillin-hydrolyzing) β-lactamases have been most commonly found in *Enterobacteriaceae* and in *P. aeruginosa* (131). OXA enzymes confer resistance to penicillins, cloxacillin, oxacillin, and methicillin. They are weakly inhibited by clavulanic acid but are inhibited by sodium chloride (NaCl). Overall, the amino acid identities between class D and class A or class C β-lactamases are only 16%. Their frequent location on mobile genetic elements (plasmids or integrons) facilitates spread (131).

Several OXA β-lactamases (OXA-11 and OXA-14 to OXA-20) are associated with an ESBL phenotype. A comparison of the crystal structure of the OXA-10 β-lactamase with that of the class C enzyme from *Enterobacter cloacae* P99 and of the class A TEM-1 enzyme from *E. coli* shows that the class D and class A enzymes have a common fold (α-helices and β-pleated sheets), although the distribution of secondary-structure elements is different. A remarkable feature is the nearly perfect symmetry of all atoms that constitute the catalytic machinery for acylation (Ser67, Lys70, Ser115, and Lys205 in OXA-10 and Ser70, Lys73, Ser130, and Lys234 in TEM-1). There seems to be an extension of the substrate-binding site (tripeptide strand) in OXA-10. The role of the peptide extension is not known. The "oxyanion hole" is provided by the main chain nitrogen atoms of Ser-67 and Phe-208. There also appears to be a different deacylation mechanism from class A. In class D the same residue (Lys70) is involved in acylation and deacylation (121, 140).

Resistance to Chloramphenicol

Acetyltransferases

Chloramphenicol is a broad-spectrum antimicrobial agent whose use has waned in recent years due to its well-characterized hematologic toxicity and the availability of a wealth of less toxic therapeutic options. The most common mechanism of resistance to chloramphenicol is the elaboration of chloramphenicol acetyltransferases (CATs). A large number of CAT genes have been reported, and these determinants generally confer extremely high levels of resistance to the organisms expressing them. Substantial structural similarities exist between the different CAT variants, although their nucleotide sequences may be quite divergent (130). Chloramphenicol contains two hydroxyl groups that are acetylated in a reaction catalyzed by CAT in which acetyl coenzyme A serves as the acyl donor. Initial acetylation occurs at the C-3 hydroxyl group to give 3-acetoxychloramphenicol (182). Following nonenzymatic rearrangement to 1-acetoxychloramphenicol and reacetylation, the 1,3-diacetoxychloramphenicol product is formed. Neither the mono- nor the diacetoxy derivatives are able to bind to the 50S ribosomal subunit and inhibit prokaryotic peptidyltransferase (182).

In *Staphylococcus aureus,* five structurally similar CATs (A, B, C, D, and that encoded by the prototypic plasmid pC194) have been described (67). The *cat* genes encoding these enzymes are commonly located on small multicopy plasmids, and expression is inducible by a translational attenuation mechanism. *Enterococcus faecalis* and *Streptococcus pneumoniae* also express inducible CAT genes that are similar to the type D gene of *S. aureus.* Two *cat* genes encoding constitutive CAT expression have been described in *Clostridium perfringens. catP* is generally found within transposon Tn*4451,* whereas *catQ* (nearly identical to *catD* of *Clostridium difficile*) is chromosomal.

Three types of CATs (I, II, and III) have been identified in gram-negative bacteria. The widely prevalent type I enzymes are distinguished by their ability to bind and inhibit (without acetylation) the activity of fusidic acid (19). These enzymes are frequently found associated with transposon Tn9 or related elements. Type II CATs are notable for their sensitivity to inhibition by thiol-reactive agents and by their association with *H. influenzae* (129). Most knowledge of the structural features of the CAT enzymes comes from the study of the type III enzyme, for which the tertiary structure is known at high resolution (130). The structural determinants of binding for each substrate are also known for this enzyme.

A second class of chloramphenicol-acetylating enzymes, the xenobiotic acetyltransferases, have been described in the last decade (130). Xenobiotic acetyltransferases are structurally unrelated to classic CATs, and those that have been demonstrated to acetylate chloramphenicol confer only low levels of chloramphenicol resistance even when present at high copy number. Their natural substrate is probably something other than chloramphenicol, explaining their limited ability to acetylate this antibiotic. First described in *Agrobacterium tumefaciens*, they have now been identified in a wide range of species. Included among this class of agents are the virginiamycin acetyltransferases found in *S. aureus* and *E. faecium* (see "Resistance to Macrolides" below). In fact, although they are members of this class, the *vat* genes do not confer resistance to chloramphenicol, nor have they been demonstrated to be able to acetylate chloramphenicol in vitro (130). They are, however, quite adept at acetylating streptogramins.

Decreased Accumulation of Chloramphenicol

As with many other compounds, resistance presumed to be due to barriers to entry in the past has often been discovered to be more commonly due to active efflux. It is now well recognized that chloramphenicol serves as a substrate for many of the MDR efflux pumps that exist in gram-positive and gram-negative bacteria, including those found in *E. coli*, *P. aeruginosa*, *Bacillus subtilis*, and *S. aureus* (133). The first chloramphenicol-specific efflux gene that was described was *cmlA* within the In4 integron of Tn1696 (22). *cmlA* encodes an efflux mechanism that uses chloramphenicol but not florfenicol (a chloramphenicol derivative licensed in 1996 for use in animals in the United States for the treatment of bovine respiratory pathogens) as a substrate. More recently, reports have emerged of gram-negative bacteria that express efflux genes specific for both chloramphenicol and florfenicol (flo_{Pp}, flo_{St}). Perhaps not surprisingly, these resistance genes are being reported with increasing frequency from animal-derived *E. coli* and *Salmonella* isolates (25, 216). In fact, the chloramphenicol resistance expressed by multiresistant *S. enterica* serovar Typhimurium DT104 is most commonly encoded by flo_{St} (25), emphasizing again the potential negative impact of using similar antimicrobial agents in humans and animals.

Resistance to Glycopeptides

Glycopeptide antibiotics (vancomycin and teicoplanin) inhibit cell wall synthesis by binding to the pentapeptide peptidoglycan precursor molecule as it exits the cytoplasmic membrane. This binding prevents the cross-linking (transpeptidation) of peptidoglycan precursors necessary for the formation of normal, stable cell walls. The large size of the glycopeptide molecules also appears to inhibit the other major peptidoglycan linkage reaction (transglycosylation)

by steric hindrance. The specific moiety bound by vancomycin is the terminal D-alanyl-D-alanine of the pentapeptide. The vast majority of bacteria that have been studied have peptidoglycan precursors that are pentapeptides terminating in D-Ala-D-Ala, and therefore are theoretically susceptible to vancomycin. However, the large size of vancomycin exceeds the exclusion limits of the porins in gram-negative outer membranes, so that vancomycin cannot access the target in these species. Hence, vancomycin is active only against bacteria lacking outer membranes, which are predominantly gram positive.

Acquired resistance to vancomycin in gram-positive bacteria comes in three varieties that are largely defined by the species within which they have been described: (i) altered precursor formation in enterococci, (ii) mutational cell wall changes in staphylococci, and (iii) tolerance in pneumococci. The importance of the first type of resistance is characterized more by its prevalence than by the importance of the species as a cause of infection, whereas the other two are defined more by the importance of the species than by their prevalence.

To date, six varieties of enterococcal glycopeptide resistance have been described (VanA through VanE and VanG). Of these, the most clinically important are VanA and VanB (12). VanA and VanB are encoded by similar operons in which three genes (*vanH*, *vanA*, *vanX* or *vanH_B*, *vanB*, and *vanX_B*) are required for the expression of resistance (12). Two other genes (*vanY* and *vanZ* or *vanY_B* and *vanW*) serve to amplify resistance but are not required for its expression (8, 9), and two more genes (*vanS* and *vanR* or *vanS_B* and *vanR_B*) regulate the transcription of the three essential genes (10, 57). The ultimate purpose of these genes is to alter the structure of the pentapeptide precursor from terminating in D-alanyl-D-alanine to terminating in D-alanine-D-lactate, thus reducing the binding affinity of vancomycin to its target roughly 1,000-fold. The sequence of reactions resulting in this structure is outlined in Fig. 4. Since the terminal amino acid is cleaved off of the pentapeptide in the transpeptidation reaction, the final composition of the cell wall is indistinguishable from strains without the resistance determinant. Apparently the PBPs, which facilitate transpeptidation, have no trouble in processing the altered precursors.

VanA enterococci are phenotypically resistant to vancomycin and teicoplanin, whereas VanB strains are resistant to vancomycin but appear susceptible to teicoplanin. This susceptibility results from the fact that teicoplanin does not induce expression of resistance (57). Once the VanB operon is expressed, however, resistance to teicoplanin results. Consequently, teicoplanin has been disappointing as a therapy for infections caused by VanB enterococci, since mutations in the VanB regulatory apparatus resulting in either inducibility by teicoplanin or constitutive expression occur readily during therapy (13, 83, 97).

Both VanA and VanB operons are encoded by transposons. VanA is found exclusively within transposon Tn1546, a 10.4-kb Tn3 family element that is presumed to disseminate between enterococci by integrating into conjugative plasmids (11). The genes of the VanA operon are highly conserved in their sequence when different strains are compared, but the restriction maps of the operons and of Tn1546 often differ markedly among clinical strains (50). These differences result from insertions of a variety of IS elements with or without subsequent deletions of parts of the mobile element, and they have been used by some investigators to establish lineages of strains within defined

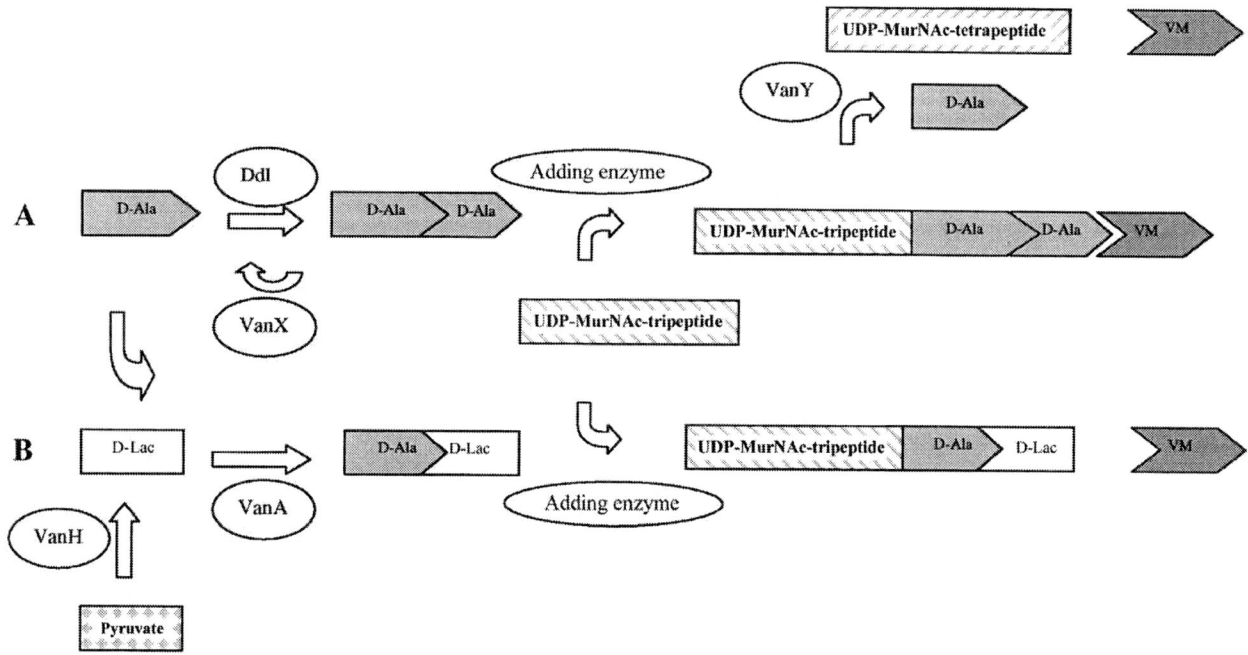

FIGURE 4 Simplified schematic representation of the two pathways for synthesis of peptidoglycan (PG) precursors present in a VanA enterococcus. (A) The upper pathway produces the native PG precursor that is the target for vancomycin. (B) The altered PG precursor produced by the lower pathway binds vancomycin poorly. VanY, encoded by the *vanA* gene cluster, modifies the finished native PG precursor. D-Ala, D-alanine; D-Ala–D-Ala, D-alanyl–D-alanine; D-Ala–D-Lac, D-alanyl–D-lactate; Ddl, D-Ala:D-Ala ligase; D-Lac, D-lactate; UDP-MurNAc, uridine diphosphate-*N*-acetylmuramyl; VM, vancomycin. Reprinted from reference 75 with permission of the University of Chicago Press.

clinical settings. The VanB operon is most commonly encoded on transposons designated Tn*5382* or Tn*1549* (38, 72). These transposons exhibit significant homology to prototype enterococcal conjugative transposon Tn*916* but have yet to be conclusively shown to transpose or to transfer between enterococcal strains by themselves. In contrast to the *vanA* gene, three allelic variants of *vanB* (*vanB1*, *vanB2*, and *vanB3*) have been described. The *vanB2* gene is associated with Tn*5382* (49).

The overwhelming majority of clinical vancomycin-resistant enterococcal (VRE) strains are *E. faecium*, a predilection that remains unexplained (173). In the United States, the vast majority of *E. faecium* strains that are resistant to vancomycin also express high levels of resistance to ampicillin, thereby negating our two most effective and reliable antienterococcal agents. In some strains, this linkage is actually physical, with insertion of Tn*5382* immediately downstream of the *pbp5* gene encoding high-level ampicillin resistance (38). These two determinants transfer between enterococcal chromosomes together by mechanisms that have yet to be determined.

The origin of the vancomycin resistance determinants is obscure, but it is clear by sequence comparisons that they did not develop within the enterococci (see above). Their entry into the enterococcus, markedly delayed considering that vancomycin was introduced into clinical use in 1958, was probably facilitated by the administration of high concentrations of glycopeptides to mammalian gastrointestinal tracts. In Europe, this exposure occurred largely in the gastrointestinal tracts of food animals that were fed the

glycopeptide avoparcin as a growth promoter (213). Evidence is now quite convincing that the animal strains transferred to the European human population through the food chain (191). In the United States, where glycopeptides were never used in animal feeds, the exchange event probably occurred in the gastrointestinal tracts of hospital patients who were given vancomycin orally to treat real or presumed *Clostridium difficile*-associated diarrhea. The U.S. *E. faecium* strains were probably highly adapted to the hospital environment through acquisition of antibiotic resistance and virulence determinants. These differences in origin may explain why VRE infections in European hospitals are quite rare, despite sometimes heavy colonization of the community population, whereas VRE infections in the United States now constitute approximately 25% of all enterococcal infections acquired in the hospital, despite no compelling evidence of colonization in the community at all.

Thankfully, the VanA and VanB operons have remained restricted to *E. faecalis* and *E. faecium*, with few exceptions (151, 153, 195). VanA has been transferred and expressed in *S. aureus* in vitro (135) and has recently been identified in a clinical *S. aureus* isolate (39a).

The VanC operon is intrinsic to the cell wall synthesis machinery of the minor enterococcal species *Enterococcus casseliflavus* (including the biotype formerly classified as *E. flavescens*) and *Enterococcus gallinarum* (104, 132). The peptidoglycan precursor in VanC strains terminates in D-alanine-D-serine, reducing vancomycin affinity about sevenfold and resulting in low levels of resistance. Precursors terminate in D-alanine-D-serine strains of *E. faecalis* with VanE (66), whereas VanD *E. faecium* terminates in D-alanine-D-lactate. The failure to observe dissemination of VanD may be explained in part by the fact that the VanX-equivalent enzyme in *E. faecium* BM4339 appears to be ineffective in an enterococcal background. Resistance was expressed in BM4339 because that strain lacked a functional cellular ligase (*ddl*) gene, eliminating the need for VanX activity to express resistance (39). The *vanG* locus has been described in four *E. faecalis* isolates of Australian origin and possesses some analogous genes to other vancomycin resistance operons, but the biochemical mechanism by which its expression results in resistance remains to be determined (123).

Mutational resistance to glycopeptides in *S. aureus* is a rare clinical entity that most commonly takes the form of reduced susceptibility, rather than frank resistance. These strains, alternatively called VISA (vancomycin-intermediate *S. aureus*) or GISA (glycopeptide-intermediate *S. aureus*), are associated with vancomycin MICs in the 4- to 8-μg/ml range (110). However, within these cultures are smaller populations of cells associated with higher levels of resistance. Animal studies suggest that the level of resistance expressed by GISA strains will reduce the effectiveness of vancomycin therapy (44).

The exact mechanism of glycopeptide resistance in GISA strains remains incompletely understood (28). One consistent finding is a thickened cell wall with increased numbers of unlinked precursors and abnormal septa formation (186). Consistent with this phenotype is the fact that all clinically isolated GISA strains studied have virtually undetectable quantities of PBP4, a low-molecular-weight PBP associated with peptidoglycan cross-linking (65). Restoration of PBP4 on a high-copy-plasmid restores cross-linking and vancomycin susceptibility to these strains. It has been suggested that vancomycin resistance results from the "absorption" of most of the vancomycin by the unlinked precursors (false vancomycin targets) before it can arrive at its true target, the peptidoglycan precursors attached to lipid II as they emerge from the cytoplasmic membrane (88). Further work is required before we understand the details of vancomycin resistance in these rare but troublesome strains.

Glycopeptide resistance has also been reported in coagulase-negative species of staphylococci. In contrast to *S. aureus*, resistance in *S. haemolyticus* has been associated with changes in the composition of the cross-links of the peptidoglycan (21). The mechanism by which this would lead to vancomycin resistance is incompletely understood.

Vancomycin is, in general, a less bactericidal antibiotic than are the β-lactams. Evidence for the importance of this observation can be found in several species. The bacteremia associated with *S. aureus* endocarditis, for example, takes roughly twice as much time to clear with vancomycin treatment than with treatment by the β-lactam oxacillin (108). Recently, reports of vancomycin tolerance in *Streptococcus pneumoniae* have appeared (84). *S. pneumoniae* is the most common cause of bacterial meningitis in most patient populations, and bactericidal therapy is optimal for treatment of this condition. As the prevalence of penicillin and cephalosporin resistance in pneumococci continues to increase around the world, empiric treatment of pneumococcal meningitis with vancomycin is likely to increase. The mechanism of tolerance involves a defect in the autolytic machinery of the cell. However, evidence indicates that the defect may not be the same in each strain, reducing

the likelihood that a rapid genotypic detection method will be feasible. At least one case of presumed recrudescence of meningitis after treatment of a case of vancomycin-tolerant pneumococcal meningitis has been reported (84), but the ultimate importance of these observations remains to be determined.

Resistance to Linezolid

The oxazolidinone antibiotic linezolid inhibits bacterial protein synthesis by interacting with the N-formylmethionyl-tRNA–ribosome–mRNA ternary complex commonly referred to as the initiation complex (185). Linezolid exerts excellent bacteriostatic activity against a wide range of gram-positive pathogens, including methicillin-resistant staphylococci and multiresistant enterococci. Clinical use of this agent has been associated with the emergence of resistant strains, most commonly after prolonged therapy of difficult-to-eradicate bacteria. Resistance has now been described in both *E. faecium* and *S. aureus*, and there are suggestions that the rate of emergence of resistance in *E. faecium* may be significant. Analysis of linezolid-resistant enterococcal laboratory mutants suggests that resistance is associated with a G2576U (*Escherichia coli* numbering scheme) point mutation in the 23S rRNA, although mutations at other positions may also contribute to resistance (155). A G2576U mutation has been described in resistant clinical isolates of *E. faecium* and in the analogous position of the 23S ribosomal subunit of a resistant *S. aureus* isolate (76, 206). Since the 23S subunit genes exist in multiple copies in different bacteria (four in *E. faecalis* and six in *E. faecium*), it has been suggested that more than one copy of the genes must be mutated to confer resistance. No systematic study has yet been done to define the correlation, if any, between the number of mutated genes and the level of phenotypic resistance.

Resistance to Macrolides

Erythromycin (the first macrolide) was initially isolated from *Streptomyces erythraeus*, a soil organism found in the Philippines. There are currently three macrolides in common use: erythromycin, clarithromycin, and azithromycin. Clarithromycin differs from erythromycin only by methylation of the hydroxy group at the C-6 position and azithromycin differs from erythromycin by the addition of a methyl substituted nitrogen atom in the lactone ring. Macrolides inhibit protein synthesis in susceptible organisms by binding reversibly to the peptidyl-tRNA binding region of the 50S ribosomal subunit, inhibiting the translocation of a newly synthesized peptidyl-tRNA molecule from the acceptor site on the ribosome to the peptidyl (donor site). Erythromycin does not bind to mammalian ribosomes. Gram-negative organisms are resistant to erythromycin because entry of erythromycin into the cell is restricted.

Resistance to macrolides occurs by several mechanisms. Among the more important of these mechanisms is methylation of the ribosome, preventing erythromycin binding (215). This methylation is most commonly accomplished by different *erm* (erythromycin ribosomal methylase) genes. Methylated ribosomes confer resistance to macrolides, the related lincosamides (clindamycin), and streptogramin B (MLS$_B$ resistance). Many *erm* genes have been described [*erm*(A) and the related *erm*(TR), *erm*(B) and the related *erm*(AM), *erm*(C), etc.], and resistance is frequently inducible by macrolides but not by clindamycin (iMLS$_B$) (169). In some strains, *erm*-type resistance is expressed constitutively (cMLS_B), resulting in resistance to clindamycin as well.

The second major mechanism of resistance to macrolides is by expression of efflux pumps encoded by *mef* genes (Mef in gram-positive bacteria and Acr-AB-TolC in *H. influenzae* and *E. coli*) (224). The efflux pumps confer resistance to the macrolides but not to clindamycin, hence the phenotypic description of this resistance "M" type. *mef* genes have been studied most extensively in *Streptococcus pneumoniae* [*mef*(E)] and *S. pyogenes* [*mef*(A)], but similar genes have been described in a variety of gram-positive genera. The prevalence of *mef*-mediated resistance versus that mediated by MLS_B-type mechanisms in *S. pneumoniae* varies in different parts of the world. Minor mechanisms of resistance to macrolides include esterases that hydrolyze the antibiotics and point mutations within the genes encoding the 50S ribosomal subunit.

Ketolides belong to a new class of semisynthetic 14-membered-ring macrolides, which differ from erythromycin by having a 3-keto group instead of the neutral sugar L-cladinose. Ketolides bind to an additional site on the bacterial ribosome, increasing their binding affinity relative to other macrolides (53). Telithromycin, a ketolide, is uniformly and highly active against pneumococci (regardless of their susceptibility or resistance to erythromycin and/or penicillin), erythromycin-susceptible *S. pyogenes*, and erythromycin-resistant *S. pyogenes* strains of the M phenotype or iMLS-B or -C phenotype (in which resistance is mediated by a methylase encoded by the *ermTR* gene) (16). Ketolides are less active against erythromycin-resistant *S. pyogenes* strains with the cMLS phenotype or the iMLS-A subtype (where resistance is mediated by a methylase encoded by the *ermAM* gene); these strains range in phenotype from the upper limits of susceptibility to resistant. Methicillin-resistant staphylococci, which commonly express a cMLS_B phenotype, are not susceptible to telithromycin (16).

Quinupristin-dalfopristin is a mixture of semisynthetic streptogramins A and B recently licensed in Europe and the United States. A related streptogramin A and B combination, virginiamycin, has been used for years as a growth promoter in animal feed. Resistance to these mixtures can result from resistance to streptogramin A alone and was first described in staphylococci conferred by genes encoding streptogramin A acetyltransferases [*vat*(A), *vat*(B), and *vat*(C)] or ATP-binding efflux genes [*vga*(A) and *vga*(B)]. The excellent activity of quinupristin-dalfopristin against *E. faecium* makes it an attractive alternative for the treatment of multiresistant *E. faecium* infections, especially since the combination retains good in vitro activity against streptogramin B-resistant strains. Two acetyltransferase-encoding resistance genes have now been described that confer resistance to quinupristin-dalfopristin in *E. faecium*: *vat*(D) [previously *sat*(A)] and *vat*(E) [previously *sat*(G)]. In most cases, these resistance genes are found along with an *erm* resistance gene (190), suggesting that resistance to both streptogramins A and B may be necessary to confer clinically significant levels of resistance to quinupristin-dalfopristin in *E. faecium*. The presence of these resistance genes on transferable plasmids suggests that the potential for their spread within the genus is significant.

Resistance to Quinolones

The fluoroquinolones are among the most widely used antimicrobial agents in both the hospital and community settings. Quinolone antibiotics all act by directly inhibiting

DNA synthesis. Their targets include two type 2 topoisomerases, DNA gyrase and topoisomerase IV. These two enzymes are structurally related in that both exist as tetramers composed of two different subunits (GyrA and GyrB of DNA gyrase; ParC and ParE of topoisomerase IV). DNA gyrase acts to maintain negative supercoiling of DNA, whereas topoisomerase IV separates interlocked daughter DNA strands formed during replication, facilitating segregation into daughter cells. Fluoroquinolones bind to the topoisomerase-DNA complexes and disrupt various cellular processes involving DNA (replication fork, transcription of RNA, DNA helicase) (86, 183, 219). The end result is cellular death by unclear mechanisms.

The affinity of fluoroquinolones for the two targets varies, explaining to some degree the differing potencies of the various agents against different bacterial species. The enzyme for which a particular fluoroquinolone exerts the greatest affinity is referred to as the primary target (5, 24, 141). In general, the primary target of fluoroquinolones in gram-negative bacteria is DNA gyrase whereas in gram-positive bacteria it is topoisomerase IV.

Alterations in Target Enzymes

The most common mechanism of clinically significant levels of fluoroquinolone resistance is through alterations of the topoisomerase enzymes. These alterations are created by spontaneous mutations that occur within the respective genes. In GyrA and ParC, resistance-associated mutations are often localized to a region in the amino terminus of the enzyme that contains the active-site tyrosine that is covalently linked to the broken DNA strand. This 130-bp region of *gyrA* has been referred to as the quinolone resistance-determining region (222). X-ray crystallographic studies of a fragment of the GyrA enzyme suggest that these mutations are clustered in three dimensions, lending support to the hypothesis that the region constitutes a part of the quinolone-binding site (127). Particularly frequent sites for resistance-associated mutations are serine 83 and aspartate 87 of DNA gyrase and serine 79 and aspartate 83 of ParC (146).

Experimental data suggest that point mutations occur singly in roughly 1 in 10^6 to 10^9 cells. The level of resistance conferred by a single point mutation in the primary target enzyme depends on the reduction of enzyme affinity created by the mutation, as well as the affinity of the fluoroquinolone for the secondary target. In this scenario, it is expected that fluoroquinolones exhibiting strong affinity for both target enzymes would be less likely to be associated with the emergence of resistant strains, since the retained activity against the secondary target would be enough to inhibit the bacterium even in the presence of primary target mutation. Fluoroquinolone-species combinations for which single mutations result in significantly higher MICs (such as ciprofloxacin and *S. aureus* or *P. aeruginosa*) would be expected to readily select out resistant mutants in the clinical setting; they have been shown to do so (46).

Most highly resistant strains exhibit more than one mutation in both the GyrA and ParC enzymes, a phenomenon that can be reproduced in the laboratory by serial passage of strains on progressively higher concentrations of fluoroquinolones. It is noteworthy in this context that fluoroquinolone resistance conferred by enzyme mutations is essentially class resistance. In other words, the activity of all fluoroquinolones is impacted by mutations that result in resistance. Therefore, while single point mutations that confer resistance to one fluoroquinolone may not result in

TABLE 3 Examples of bacterial multidrug efflux transporters[a]

Transporter name	Organism	Transporter class	Thought to function with:	Substrates[b]
Gram-positive pumps				
LmrA	*Streptococcus lactis*	ABC		EB, R6G, TPP[+]
QacA	*Staphylococcus aureus*	MFS(14)[c]		EB, QA, chlorhexidine, pentamidine isethionate
LfrA	*Mycobacterium smegmatis*	MFS(14)[c]		EB, AC, QA, FQ
NorA	*Staphylococcus aureus*	MFS(12)[c]		EB, AC, QA, FQ, R6G, TPP[+], puromycin, CP
Bmr	*Bacillus subtilis*	MFS(12)[c]		EB, AC, QA, FQ, R6G, TPP[+], puromycin, CP
Smr	*Staphylococcus aureus*	SMR		EB, CV, QA, methyl viologen, TPP[+]
Gram-negative pumps				
EmrB	*Escherichia coli*	MFS(14)[c]	EmrA, TolC(?)	CCCP, NA, thiolactomycin
AcrB	*Escherichia coli*	RND	AcrA, TolC	EB, AC, Cv, SDS, TX100, bile salts, β-lactams, Nov, Ery, Fus, Tet, CP, mitomycin C, FQ, NA, organic solvents
MexB	*Pseudomonas aeruginosa*	RND	MexA, OprM	β-Lactams, Nov, Ery, Fus, Tet, CP, FQ
MexD	*Pseudomonas aeruginosa*	RND	MexC, OprJ	Fourth-generation cephalosporins, Tet, CP, FQ
MexF	*Pseudomonas aeruginosa*	RND	MexE, OprN	CP, FQ

[a] Adapted from reference 32 with permission of the National Academy of Sciences USA.
[b] Abbreviations: AC, acriflavin; CP, chloramphenicol; CCCP, carbonyl cyanide *m*-chlorophenylhydrazone; CV, crystal violet; EB, ethidium bromide; Ery, erythromycin; FQ, fluoroquinolones; Fus, fusidic acid; NA, nalidixic acid; Nov, novobiocin; QA, quaternary ammonium compounds, including benzalkonium chloride and cetyltrimethylammonium bromide; R6G, rhodamine 6G; SDS, sodium dodecyl sulfate; Tet, tetracyclines; TPP[+], tetrapenylphosphonium; TX100, Triton X-100.
[c] This family consists of proteins with 12 or 14 transmembrane segments.

MICs associated with clinical resistance for another, the MICs of the second fluoroquinolone will inevitably be increased. In the setting of such preexisting mutations, the second fluoroquinolone could then select out an additional mutation that would result in clinically significant levels of resistance. This reasoning has led to the recommendation that the most potent and broadly active fluoroquinolone should always be used first, to prevent the emergence of resistance. The wisdom of this recommendation remains to be tested.

Mutations in GyrB and ParE are far less common than in their companion subunits and tend to cluster in the midportion of the subunit (89). A clear understanding of the impact of these mutations on enzyme structure or function awaits detailed crystallographic studies of enzyme-fluoroquinolone complexes.

Resistance Due to Decreased Intracellular Accumulation

Fluoroquinolones penetrate the outer membrane of gramnegative bacteria through porins, and so the absence of specific porins can impact the level of susceptibility. However, their ability to diffuse through outer and cytoplasmic membranes is sufficient to retain activity against strains solely lacking porins (134). More important in reducing intracellular accumulation of fluoroquinolones is the expression of multidrug resistance pumps (146). Several such pumps have been identified in human-pathogenic bacteria, some of which are listed in Table 3. Efflux pumps in gram-negative bacteria extend from the cytoplasmic membrane through the outer membrane, whereas pumps in

gram-positive bacteria need only traverse the cytoplasmic membrane. These pumps move compounds across the bacterial membranes by proton motive force and are presumed to represent systems by which bacteria rid themselves of toxic materials. Resistance results when the expression of pumps is increased due to mutations within the regulatory genes (225). By themselves, pumps generally confer only a low level of resistance to fluoroquinolones. However, their expression may amplify the level of resistance conferred by point mutations within the topoisomerase genes. By so doing, they may increase the risk that a given fluoroquinolone will select out resistant mutants through single point mutations.

Resistance to Rifampin

Rifampin is particularly active against gram-positive bacteria and mycobacteria. It acts by inhibiting bacterial DNA-dependent RNA polymerase. Point mutations in the chromosomal *rpoB* gene confer resistance to rifampin (214). The frequency with which these point mutations occur precludes the use of rifampin as a single agent for the treatment of bacterial infections.

Resistance to Tetracyclines

The tetracyclines are a group of bacteriostatic antibiotics that act by inhibiting the attachment of aminoacyl-tRNA to the ribosome acceptor site, thereby preventing elongation of the peptide chains of nascent proteins (177). To gain access to the bacterial ribosome, tetracyclines need to enter the cell. In *E. coli* and presumably other gram-negative bacteria, they enter the periplasmic space through outer membrane porins OmpC and OmpF, probably chelated to magnesium ions (177). Once in the periplasmic space, the weakly lipophilic tetracycline molecule dissociates from the magnesium ion and crosses into the cell by diffusing through the lipid bilayer in an energy-dependent process. Once inside the cell, tetracycline-ion complexes bind to the ribosome at a single, high-affinity binding site on the 30S subunit, blocking access of the aminoacyl-tRNA to the ribosome acceptor site. Although the binding of tetracycline to the ribosome is high affinity, it is reversible (42).

Tetracyclines are broad-spectrum and effective antimicrobial agents. Unfortunately, widespread use of tetracyclines to treat clinical infections and for promotion of growth in livestock has been associated with the emergence and dissemination of a variety of resistance determinants. As a consequence, the number of infections for which tetracyclines are considered recommended first-line therapy has been limited for many years (172). The vast majority of tetracycline resistance determinants fall into one of two classes: efflux proteins or ribosomal protection proteins. The designations of the different resistance determinants and their classes are listed in Table 4, extracted from an excellent review of tetracyclines by Chopra and Roberts (43). Initial designations of tetracycline resistance determinants used the prefixes *tet* or *otr*, with letters (A, for example) designating the different determinants. Since the number of resistance determinants now exceeds the number of letters in the alphabet, a system using numbers has been devised (109).

Tetracycline efflux proteins are all membrane associated and are members of the major facilitator superfamily of

TABLE 4 Mechanisms of resistance for characterized *tet* and *otr* genes[a]

Genes[b]
Efflux
tet(A), *tet*(B), *tet*(C), *tet*(D), *tet*(E), *tet*(G), *tet*(H), *tet*(I), *tet*(J), *tet*(Z), *tet*(30)[c] *tet*(31)[c]
tet(K), *tet*(L)
otr(B), *tcr3*[d]
tetP(A)
tet(V)
tet(Y)[e]
Ribosomal protection
tet(M), *tet*(O), *tet*(S), *tet*(W)
tet(Q), *tet*(T)
otr(A), *tetP*(B),[f] *tet*[d]
Enzymatic
tet(X)
Unknown[g]
tet(U), *otr*(C)

[a] Adapted from reference 43.
[b] Grouped according to the scheme in reference 124.
[c] First numbered genes.
[d] These genes have not been given new designations.
[e] Relatedness to groups 1 to 6 is unclear, since the gene has not been studied extensively.
[f] *tetP*(B) is not found alone, and *tetP*(A) and *tetP*(B) are counted as one gene.
[g] *tet*(U) has been sequenced but does not appear to be related to either efflux or ribosomal protection proteins; *otr*(C) has not been sequenced.

proteins. They expel tetracycline from the cell by exchanging a proton for a tetracycline-cation complex. In general, the efflux proteins confer resistance to tetracyclines but tend to spare minocycline (43). The single exception to this rule is the gram-negative Tet(B) protein, which confers resistance to both tetracycline and minocycline. The efflux proteins have been divided into six groups based on amino acid identity. Group 1 consists of Tet efflux proteins that are found primarily in gram-negative species [with the exception of Tet(Z)], whereas group 2 [consisting only of Tet(K) and Tet(L)] is found primarily in gram-positive species. Groups 3 through 6 are small groups consisting of one or two efflux proteins each.

Ribosome protection proteins comprise the other major mechanism of tetracycline resistance. These proteins exhibit homology to elongation factors EF-Tu and EF-G and exhibit ribosome-dependent GTPase activity (174). They act by binding to the ribosome, thereby changing its conformation and inhibiting the binding of tetracycline. Tet(M) and Tet(O) are the best characterized of these proteins. Ribosome protection genes are widespread in bacteria, in many cases as a result of their incorporation into broad-host-range conjugative transposons.

Both efflux proteins and ribosomal protection proteins are regulated in ways such that their expression is increased in the presence of tetracyclines. The gram-negative efflux proteins are regulated by repressors that are divergently transcribed relative to the efflux proteins (87). Binding of the repressor to tetracycline changes the conformation of the repressor so that it can no longer bind to the operator region, resulting in increased transcription of both the efflux protein and the repressor genes. The gram-positive efflux genes are not associated with specific protein repressors, but sequence analysis suggests that these determinants may be regulated by mechanisms similar to translational attenuation (178). Transcription of ribosomal protection genes is augmented by growth in the presence of tetracycline. Sequence analysis of the upstream region suggests that the mechanism of regulation may be transcriptional attenuation (197), but study of this area has been limited.

Intrinsic mechanisms of tetracycline resistance exist in many if not all gram-negative bacteria. Among the best characterized of these systems is the *mar* operon (2). This locus consists of a repressor (MarR) that represses the transcription of *marA*, which encodes a transcriptional activator of a variety of genes. Overexpression of MarA results in decreased expression of OmpF, a porin through which tetracycline enters the periplasmic space, and increased expression of multidrug efflux pump AcrAB, a member of the resistance-nodulation-cell division family of efflux proteins that includes tetracyclines among its substrates. Several similar pump systems have been described in *P. aeruginosa* and other gram-negative bacteria (150). As our knowledge of the genomes of different bacterial species becomes more complete, we will no doubt discover several other pump systems that will affect the levels of susceptibility to tetracyclines and other antibiotics.

The remarkable diversity of species within which tetracycline resistance determinants are found owes much to the inclusion of these resistance genes within broad-host-range transferable genetic elements. These include transferable plasmids in gram-negative species, where *tet* genes may be found included within integrons, and conjugative transposons. Among the best studied of the conjugative transposons is the Tn*916* family, originally described in *E. faecalis* (162). The complete sequence of Tn*916* has been determined and is remarkable for its dearth of restriction enzyme digestion sites [except in the region of the *tet*(M) gene, which appears to be a late arrival to the element] (138). This lack of restriction sites probably facilitates the entry of Tn*916* into a variety of different bacterial species. Transfer of Tn*916*-like elements from enterococci into many other species has been demonstrated in vitro and in animal models, and the remnants of Tn*916*-like sequences in *Neisseria gonorrhoeae* are impressive testimony to its ability to travel widely (162). Transfer of Tn*916*-like elements, which is increased after exposure to tetracycline, has also been suggested to facilitate transfer of unlinked genes, further amplifying the risks associated with overexposure to tetracycline in the environment.

Resistance to Trimethoprim-Sulfamethoxazole

Biosynthesis of several amino acids and purines depends on the availability of tetrahydrofolate (THF). With few exceptions, bacteria are unable to absorb preformed folic acid and hence rely upon their ability to synthesize it. Sulfamethoxazole and trimethoprim are inhibitors of two enzymes (dihydropteroic acid synthase [DHPS] and dihydrofolate reductase [DHFR], respectively) that act sequentially in the manufacture of THF. It is thought that the two inhibitors act synergistically to inhibit folate synthesis, although the mechanism for possible synergism (since sequential blockage of a fully inhibited pathway should not augment resistance) is not clear.

Intrinsic Resistance

Trimethoprim-sulfamethoxazole is a remarkably broad-spectrum antimicrobial agent. Intrinsic resistance is relatively rare and may occur by decreased access to the target enzymes (*P. aeruginosa*) (200), by the presence of low-affinity DHFR enzymes (*Neisseria* spp., *Clostridium* spp., *Brucella* spp., *Bacteroides* spp., *Moraxella catarrhalis*, and *Nocardia* spp.) (201), or by the ability to absorb exogenous folate (*Enterococcus* spp. and *Lactobacillus* spp.) (223) or thymine (*Enterococcus* spp.) (81). The decreased access to the target enzyme in *P. aeruginosa* appears to be associated with both a permeability barrier and active efflux from the cell (102, 119). The percent contribution of each of these mechanisms to resistance remains unclear.

Acquired Resistance to Trimethoprim

Mutational resistance to trimethoprim has been described in several species and involves promoter mutations leading to overproduction of DHFR (in *E. coli*), point mutations within the *dhfr* gene leading to resistance (in *Staphylococcus aureus* and *Streptococcus pneumoniae*), or both mechanisms (in *H. influenzae*) (90). More common is the acquisition of low-affinity *dhfr* genes, of which approximately 20 have been described (90). Expression of the *dhfr*I and variants of *dhfr*II genes, which are most commonly found on plasmids in gram-negative bacteria, increases resistance to levels greatly exceeding clinically achievable concentrations.

Acquired Resistance to Sulfonamides

Point mutations in chromosomal *dhps* genes conferring resistance sulfonamides have been reported in many different species (90). More extensive changes within *dhps* genes resulting in resistance have been reported in *Neisseria meningitidis* and *Streptococcus pyogenes*. In these instances, the extensive changes have suggested the acquisition of at least some parts of the *dhps* genes from other species via transformation and recombination (188, 199). Plasmid-medi-

ated transferable resistance to sulfonamides has been described in gram-negative bacteria for decades (90). In contrast to the diversity in *dhfr* genes, only two acquired low-affinity *dhps* genes (*sulI* and *sulII*) have been described. Genes conferring resistance to sulfonamides are frequently incorporated into multiresistance integrons, which are themselves frequently integrated into transferable plasmids. The transferability of these resistance plasmids and the frequent association with other resistance genes explain in part the widespread nature and persistence of resistance to this antimicrobial combination. One trimethoprim-sulfamethoxazole-resistant *E. coli* strain was recently reported to have spread widely in the United States, causing urinary tract infections in young women in at least two states (115).

REFERENCES

1. **Adcock, P. M., P. Pastor, F. Medley, J. E. Patterson, and T. V. Murphy.** 1998. Methicillin-resistant *Staphylococcus aureus* in two child care centers. *J. Infect. Dis.* **178:**577–580.
2. **Alekshun, M. N., and S. B. Levy.** 1997. Regulation of chromosomally mediated multiple antibiotic resistance: the mar regulon. *Antimicrob. Agents Chemother.* **41:**2067–2075.
3. **Alksne, L. E., and B. A. Rasmussen.** 1997. Expression of the AsbA1, OXA-12, and AsbM1 β-lactamases in *Aeromonas jandaei* AER 14 is coordinated by a two-component regulon. *J. Bacteriol.* **179:**2006–2013.
4. **Allos, B. M.** 2001. *Campylobacter jejuni* infections: update on emerging issues and trends. *Clin. Infect. Dis.* **32:**1201–1206.
5. **Alovero, F. L., X. S. Pan, J. E. Morris, R. H. Manzo, and L. M. Fisher.** 2000. Engineering the specificity of antibacterial fluoroquinolones: benzenesulfonamide modifications at C-7 of ciprofloxacin change its primary target in *Streptococcus pneumoniae* from topoisomerase IV to gyrase. *Antimicrob. Agents Chemother.* **44:**320–325.
6. **Ambler, R. P.** 1980. The structure of β-lactamases. *Philos. Trans. R. Soc. Lond. Ser. B* **289:**321–331.
7. **Amoroso, A., D. Demares, M. Mollerach, G. Gutkind, and J. Coyette.** 2001. All detectable high-molecular-mass penicillin-binding proteins are modified in a high-level beta-lactam-resistant clinical isolate of *Streptococcus mitis*. *Antimicrob. Agents Chemother.* **45:**2075–2081.
8. **Arthur, M., F. Depardieu, C. Molinas, P. Reynolds, and P. Courvalin.** 1995. The vanZ gene of Tn*1546* from *Enterococcus faecium* BM4147 confers resistance to teicoplanin. *Gene* **154:**87–92.
9. **Arthur, M., C. Molinas, and P. Courvalin.** 1992. Sequence of the vanY gene required for production of a vancomycin-inducible D,D-carboxypeptidase in *Enterococcus faecium* BM4147. *Gene* **120:**111–114.
10. **Arthur, M., C. Molinas, and P. Courvalin.** 1992. The VanS-VanR two-component regulatory system controls synthesis of depsipeptide peptidoglycan precursors in *Enterococcus faecium* 4147. *J. Bacteriol.* **174:**2582–2591.
11. **Arthur, M., C. Molinas, F. Depardieu, and P. Courvalin.** 1993. Characterization of Tn*1546*, a Tn*3*-related transposon conferring glycopeptide resistance by synthesis of depsipeptide peptidoglycan precursors in *Enterococcus faecium* BM4147. *J. Bacteriol.* **175:**117–127.
12. **Arthur, M., P. Reynolds, and P. Courvalin.** 1996. Glycopeptide resistance in enterococci. *Trends Microbiol.* **4:**401–407.
13. **Aslangul, E., M. Baptista, B. Fantin, F. Depardieu, M. Arthur, P. Courvalin, and C. Carbon.** 1997. Selection of glycopeptide-resistant mutants of VanB-type *Enterococcus*

faecalis BM4281 in vitro and in experimental endocarditis. *J. Infect. Dis.* **175:**598–605.

14. **Azoulay-Dupuis, E., J. P. Bedos, E. Vallée, D. J. Hardy, R. N. Swanson, and J. J. Pocidalo.** 1991. Antipneumococcal activity of ciprofloxacin, oflaxacin and temafloxacin in an experimental mouse pneumonia model at various stages of disease. *J. Infect. Dis.* **163:**319–324.

15. **Azucena, E., and S. Mobashery.** 2001. Aminoglycoside-modifying enzymes: mechanisms of catalytic processes and inhibition. *Drug Resist. Update* **4:**106–117.

16. **Balfour, J. A., and D. P. Figgitt.** 2001. Telithromycin. *Drugs* **61:**815–829.

17. **Barcus, V. A., K. Ghanekar, M. Yeo, T. J. Coffey, and C. G. Dowson.** 1995. Genetics of high level penicillin resistance in clinical isolates of *Streptococcus pneumoniae.* *FEMS Microbiol. Lett.* **126:**299–303.

18. **Barthelemy, M., J. Peduzzi, H. Bernard, C. Tancrede, and R. Labia.** 1992. Close amino acid sequence relationship between the new plasmid-mediated extended-spectrum beta-lactamase MEN-1 and chromosomally encoded enzymes of *Klebsiella oxytoca. Biochim. Biophys. Acta* **1122:** 15–22.

19. **Bennett, A. D., and W. V. Shaw.** 1983. Resistance to fusidic acid in *Escherichia coli* mediated by the type I variant of chloramphenicol acetyltransferase. A plasmid-encoded mechanism involving antibiotic binding. *Biochem. J.* **215:**29–38.

20. **Berger-Bachi, B., A. Strassle, J. E. Gustafson, and F. H. Kayser.** 1992. Mapping and characterization of multiple chromosomal factors involved in methicillin resistance in *Staphylococcus aureus. Antimicrob. Agents Chemother.* **36:** 1367–1373.

21. **Billot-Klein, D., L. Gutmann, D. Bryant, D. Bell, J. Van Heijenoort, J. Grewal, and D. M. Shlaes.** 1996. Peptidoglycan synthesis and structure in *Staphylococcus haemolyticus* expressing increasing levels of resistance to glycopeptide antibiotics. *J. Bacteriol.* **178:**4696–4703.

22. **Bissonnette, L., S. Champetier, J. P. Buisson, and P. H. Roy.** 1991. Characterization of the nonenzymatic chloramphenicol resistance (cmlA) gene of the In4 integron of Tn*1696*: similarity of the product to transmembrane transport proteins. *J. Bacteriol.* **173:**4493–4502.

23. **Bjorkman, J., I. Nagaev, O. G. Berg, D. Hughes, and D. I. Andersson.** 2000. Effects of environment on compensatory mutations to ameliorate costs of antibiotic resistance. *Science* **287:**1479–1482.

24. **Blanche, F., B. Cameron, F. X. Bernard, L. Maton, B. Manse, L. Ferrero, N. Ratet, C. Lecoq, A. Goniot, D. Bisch, and J. Crouzet.** 1996. Differential behaviors of *Staphylococcus aureus* and *Escherichia coli* type II DNA topoisomerases. *Antimicrob. Agents Chemother.* **40:**2714–2720.

25. **Bolton, L. F., L. C. Kelley, M. D. Lee, P. J. Fedorka-Cray, and J. J. Maurer.** 1999. Detection of multidrug-resistant *Salmonella enterica* serotype Typhimurium DT104 based on a gene which confers cross-resistance to florfenicol and chloramphenicol. *J. Clin. Microbiol.* **37:**1348–1351.

26. **Bonomo, R. A., C. G. Dawes, J. R. Knox, and D. M. Shlaes.** 1995. beta-Lactamase mutations far from the active site influence inhibitor binding. *Biochim. Biophys. Acta* **1247:**121–125.

27. **Bonomo, R. A., S. D. Rudin, and D. M. Shlaes.** 1997. Tazobactam is a potent inhibitor of select class A inhibitor-resistant enzymes. *FEMS Microbiol. Lett.* **48:**59–62.

28. **Boyle-Vavra, S., H. Labischinski, C. C. Ebert, K. Ehlert, and R. S. Daum.** 2001. A spectrum of changes occurs in peptidoglycan composition of glycopeptide-intermediate

29. **Bradford, P. A.** 2001. Extended-spectrum beta-lactamases in the 21st century: characterization, epidemiology, and detection of this important resistance threat. *Clin. Microbiol. Rev.* **14:**933–951.

30. **Bradford, P. A.** 2001. What's new in beta-lactamases? *Curr. Infect. Dis. Rep.* **3:**13–19.

31. **Bradford, P. A., C. Urban, N. Mariano, S. J. Projan, J. J. Rahal, and K. Bush.** 1997. Imipenem resistance in *Klebsiella pneumoniae* is associated with the combination of ACT-1, a plasmid-mediated AmpC beta-lactamase, and the loss of an outer membrane protein. *Antimicrob. Agents Chemother.* **41:**563–569.

32. **Bruand, C., L. Chatelier, S. D. Ehrlich, and L. Janniere.** 1993. A fourth class of theta-replicating plasmids: the pAMβ1 family from Gram-positive bacteria. *Proc. Natl. Acad. Sci. USA* **90:**11668–11672.

33. **Bush, K.** 1988. Beta-lactamase inhibitors from laboratory to clinic. *Clin. Microbiol. Rev.* **1:**109–123.

34. **Bush, K.** 2001. New beta-lactamases in gram-negative bacteria: diversity and impact on the selection of antimicrobial therapy. *Clin. Infect. Dis.* **32:**1085–1089.

35. **Bush, K., G. A. Jacoby, and A. A. Medeiros.** 1995. A functional classification scheme for β-lactamases and its correlation with molecular structure. *Antimicrob. Agents Chemother.* **39:**1211–1233.

36. **Campbell, B. D., and R. J. Kadner.** 1980. Relation of aerobiosis and ionic strength to the uptake of dihydrostreptomycin in *Escherichia coli. Biochim. Biophys. Acta* **593:**1–10.

37. **Carfi, A., S. Pares, E. Duee, M. Galleni, C. Duez, J. M. Frere, and O. Dideberg.** 1995. The 3-D structure of a zinc metallo-β-lactamase from *Bacillus cereus* reveals a new type of protein fold. *EMBO J.* **14:**4914–4921.

38. **Carias, L. L., S. D. Rudin, C. J. Donskey, and L. B. Rice.** 1998. Genetic linkage and cotransfer of a novel, *vanB*-containing transposon (Tn*5382*) and a low-affinity penicillin-binding protein 5 gene in a clinical vancomycin-resistant *Enterococcus faecium* isolate. *J. Bacteriol.* **180:**4426–4434.

39. **Casadewall, B., P. E. Reynolds, and P. Courvalin.** 2001. Regulation of expression of the vanD glycopeptide resistance gene cluster from *Enterococcus faecium* BM4339. *J. Bacteriol.* **183:**3436–3446.

39a.**CDC.** 2002. *Staphylococcus aureus* resistant to vancomycin—United States, 2002. *Morb. Mortal. Wkly. Rep.* **51:** 565–567.

40. **Chambers, H. F.** 1997. Methicillin resistance in staphylococci: molecular and biochemical basis and clinical implications. *Clin. Microbiol. Rev.* **10:**781–791.

41. **Chambers, H. F., M. Sachdeva, and S. Kennedy.** 1990. Binding affinity for penicillin-binding protein 2a correlates with in vivo activity of beta-lactam antibiotics against methicillin-resistant *Staphylococcus aureus. J. Infect. Dis.* **162:**705–710.

42. **Chopra, I., P. M. Hawkey, and M. Hinton.** 1992. Tetracyclines, molecular and clinical aspects. *J. Antimicrob. Chemother.* **29:**245–277.

43. **Chopra, I., and M. Roberts.** 2001. Tetracycline antibiotics: mode of action, applications, molecular biology, and epidemiology of bacterial resistance. *Microbiol. Mol. Biol. Rev.* **65:**232–260.

44. **Climo, M. W., R. L. Patron, and G. L. Archer.** 1999. Combinations of vancomycin and beta-lactams are synergistic against staphylococci with reduced susceptibilities to vancomycin. *Antimicrob. Agents Chemother.* **43:**1747–1753.

45. **Concha, N. O., C. A. Janson, P. Rowling, S. Pearson, C. A. Cheever, B. P. Clarke, C. Lewis, M. Galleni, J. M. Frere, D. J. Payne, J. H. Bateson, and S. S. Abdel-**

Meguid. 2000. Crystal structure of the IMP-1 metallo β-lactamase from *Pseudomonas aeruginosa* and its complex with a mercaptocarboxylate inhibitor: binding determinants of a potent, broad-spectrum inhibitor. *Biochemistry* **39:**4288–4298.

46. **Coronado, V. G., J. R. Edwards, D. H. Culver, and R. P. Gaynes.** 1995. Ciprofloxacin resistance among nosocomial Pseudomonas aeruginosa and Staphylococcus aureus in the United States. National Nosocomial Infections Surveillance (NNIS) System. *Infect. Control Hosp. Epidemiol.* **16:**71–75.

47. **Couto, I., H. de Lencastre, E. Severina, W. Kloos, J. A. Webster, R. J. Hubner, I. S. Sanches, and A. Tomasz.** 1996. Ubiquitous presence of a *mecA* homologue in natural isolates of *Staphylococcus sciuri*. *Microb. Drug Resist.* **2:**377–391.

48. **Crichlow, G. V., A. P. Kuzin, M. Nukaga, K. Mayama, T. Sawai, and J. R. Knox.** 1999. Structure of the extended-spectrum class C β-lactamase of *Enterobacter cloacae* GC1, a natural mutant with a tandem tripeptide insertion. *Biochemistry* **38:**10256–10261.

49. **Dahl, K. H., E. W. Lundblad, T. P. Rokenes, O. Olsvik, and A. Sundsfjord.** 2000. Genetic linkage of the *vanB2* gene cluster to Tn*5382* in vancomycin-resistant enterococci and characterization of two novel insertion sequences. *Microbiology* **146:**1469–1479.

50. **Darini, A. L., M. F. Palepou, and N. Woodford.** 2000. Effects of the movement of insertion sequences on the structure of VanA glycopeptide resistance elements in *Enterococcus faecium*. *Antimicrob. Agents Chemother.* **44:**1362–1364.

51. **Delaire, M., R. Labia, J. P. Samama, and J. M. Masson.** 1992. Site-directed mutagenesis at the active site of *Escherichia coli* TEM-1 beta-lactamase. Suicide inhibitor-resistant mutants reveal the role of arginine 244 and methionine 69 in catalysis. *J. Biol. Chem.* **267:**20600–20606.

52. **Donskey, C. J., J. A. Hanrahan, R. A. Hutton, and L. B. Rice.** 2000. Effect of parenteral antibiotic administration on establishment of colonization with vancomycin-resistant *Enterococcus faecium* in the mouse gastrointestinal tract. *J. Infect. Dis.* **181:**1830–1833.

53. **Douthwaite, S., L. H. Hansen, and P. Mauvais.** 2000. Macrolide-ketolide inhibition of MLS-resistant ribosomes is improved by alternative drug interaction with domain II of 23S rRNA. *Mol. Microbiol.* **36:**183–193.

54. **Dunny, G. M., B. A. B. Leonard, and P. J. Hedberg.** 1995. Pheromone-inducible conjugation in *Enterococcus faecalis*: interbacterial and host-parasite chemical communication. *J. Bacteriol.* **177:**871–876.

55. **Eliopoulos, G. M., B. F. Farber, B. E. Murray, C. Wennersten, and R. Moellering, Jr.** 1984. Ribosomal resistance of clinical enterococcal isolates to streptomycin. *Antimicrob. Agents Chemother.* **25:**398–399.

56. **Ena, J., M. M. Lopez-Perezagua, C. Martinez-Peinado, M. A. Cia-Barrio, and I. Ruiz-Lopez.** 1998. Emergence of ciprofloxacin resistance in *Escherichia coli* isolates after widespread use of fluoroquinolones. *Diagn. Microbiol. Infect. Dis.* **30:**103–107.

57. **Evers, S., and R. Courvalin.** 1996. Regulation of VanB-type vancomycin resistance gene expression by the vanS$_B$-VanR$_B$ two-component regulatory system in *Enterococcus faecalis* V583. *J. Bacteriol.* **178:**1302–1309.

58. **Evers, S., D. F. Sahm, and P. Courvalin.** 1993. The *vanB* gene of vancomycin-resistant *Enterococcus faecalis* V583 is structurally-related to genes encoding D-ala:D-ala ligases and glycopeptide-resistance proteins VanA and VanC. *Gene* **124:**143–144.

59. **Farzaneh, S., E. B. Chaibi, J. Peduzzi, M. Barthelemy, R. Labia, J. Blazquez, and F. Baquero.** 1996. Implication of

Ile-69 and Thr-182 residues in kinetic characteristics of IRT-3 (TEM-32) beta-lactamase. *Antimicrob. Agents Chemother.* **40:**2434–2436.

60. **Ferber, D.** 2000. Antibiotic resistance. Superbugs on the hoof? *Science* **288:**792–794.

61. **Ferretti, J. J., K. S. Gilmore, and P. Courvalin.** 1986. Nucleotide sequence of the gene specifying the bifunctional 6′-aminoglycosideacetyl transferase-2″ aminoglycoside phosphotransferase enzyme in *Streptococcus faecalis* and identification and cloning of the gene regions specifying the two activities. *J. Bacteriol.* **167:**631–638.

62. **Ferretti, J. J., W. M. McShan, D. Ajdic, D. J. Savic, G. Savic, K. Lyon, C. Primeaux, S. Sezate, A. N. Suvorov, S. Kenton, H. S. Lai, S. P. Lin, Y. Qian, H. G. Jia, F. Z. Najar, Q. Ren, H. Zhu, L. Song, J. White, X. Yuan, S. W. Clifton, B. A. Roe, and R. McLaughlin.** 2001. Complete genome sequence of an M1 strain of *Streptococcus pyogenes*. *Proc. Natl. Acad. Sci. USA* **98:**4658–4663.

63. **Fiett, J., A. Palucha, B. Miaczynska, M. Stankiewicz, H. Przondo-Mordarska, W. Hryniewicz, and M. Gniadkowski.** 2000. A novel complex mutant beta-lactamase, TEM-68, identified in a *Klebsiella pneumoniae* isolate from an outbreak of extended-spectrum beta-lactamase-producing klebsiellae. *Antimicrob. Agents Chemother.* **44:**1499–1505.

64. **Filipe, S. R., and A. Tomasz.** 2000. Inhibition of the expression of penicillin resistance in *Streptococcus pneumoniae* by inactivation of cell wall muropeptide branching genes. *Proc. Natl Acad. Sci. USA* **97:**4891–4896.

65. **Finan, J. E., G. L. Archer, M. J. Pucci, and M. W. Climo.** 2001. Role of penicillin-binding protein 4 in expression of vancomycin resistance among clinical isolates of oxacillin-resistant *Staphylococcus aureus*. *Antimicrob. Agents Chemother.* **45:**3070–3075.

66. **Fines, M., B. Perichon, P. Reynolds, D. F. Sahm, and P. Courvalin.** 1999. VanE, a new type of acquired glycopeptide resistance in *Enterococcus faecalis* BM4405. *Antimicrob. Agents Chemother.* **43:**2161–2164.

67. **Fitton, J. E., and W. V. Shaw.** 1979. Comparison of chloramphenicol acetyltransferase variants in staphylococci. Purification, inhibitor studies and N-terminal sequences. *Biochem. J.* **177:**575–582.

68. **Fitzgerald, J. R., D. E. Sturdevant, S. M. Mackie, S. R. Gill, and J. M. Musser.** 2001. Evolutionary genomics of *Staphylococcus aureus*: insights into the origin of methicillin-resistant strains and the toxic shock syndrome epidemic. *Proc. Natl. Acad. Sci. USA* **98:**8821–8826.

69. **Fontana, R., M. Aldegheri, M. Ligozzi, H. Lopez, A. Sucari, and G. Satta.** 1994. Overproduction of a low-affinity penicillin-binding protein and high-level ampicillin resistance in *Enterococcus faecium*. *Antimicrob. Agents Chemother.* **38:**1980–1983.

70. **Galas, D. J., and M. Chandler.** 1989. Bacterial insertion sequences, p. 109–162. *In* D. E. Berg and M. M. Howe (ed.), *Mobile DNA*. American Society for Microbiology, Washington, D.C.

71. **Galleni, M., J. Lamotte-Brasseur, G. M. Rossolini, J. Spencer, O. Dideberg, and J. M. Frere.** 2001. Standard numbering scheme for class B beta-lactamases. *Antimicrob. Agents Chemother.* **45:**660–663.

72. **Garnier, F., S. Taourit, P. Glaser, P. Courvalin, and M. Galimand.** 2000. Characterization of transposon Tn*1549*, conferring VanB-type resistance in *Enterococcus* spp. *Microbiology* **146:**1481–1489.

73. **Geraci, J. E., and W. J. Martin.** 1954. Subacute enterococcal endocarditis: clinical, pathologic and therapeutic considerations in 33 patients. *Circulation* **10:**173–194.

74. **Ghuysen, J. M.** 1991. Serine β-lactamases and penicillin-binding proteins. *Annu. Rev. Microbiol.* **45:**37–67.

75. **Gold, H. S.** 2001. Vancomycin-resistant enterococci: mechanisms and clinical observations. *Clin. Infect. Dis.* **33:**210–219.

76. **Gonzales, R. D., P. C. Schreckenberger, M. B. Graham, S. Kelkar, K. DenBesten, and J. P. Quinn.** 2001. Infections due to vancomycin-resistant *Enterococcus faecium* resistant to linezolid. *Lancet* **357:**1179.

77. **Hackbarth, C. J., and H. F. Chambers.** 1993. *blaI* and *blaR1* regulate β-lactamase and PBP 2a production in methicillin-resistant *Staphylococcus aureus*. *Antimicrob. Agents Chemother.* **37:**1144–1149.

78. **Hackbarth, C. J., T. Kocagoz, S. Kocagoz, and H. F. Chambers.** 1995. Point mutations in *Staphylococcus aureus* PBP 2 gene affect penicillin-binding kinetics and are associated with resistance. *Antimicrob. Agents Chemother.* **39:**103–106.

79. **Hakenbeck, R., and J. Coyette.** 1998. Resistant penicillin-binding proteins. *Cell. Mol. Life Sci.* **54:**332–340.

80. **Hall, R. M.** 1997. Mobile gene cassettes and integrons: moving antibiotic resistance genes in gram-negative bacteria. *Ciba Found. Symp.* **207:**192–202.

81. **Hamilton-Miller, J. M.** 1988. Reversal of activity of trimethoprim against gram-positive cocci by thymidine, thymine and 'folates.' *J. Antimicrob. Chemother.* **22:**35–39.

82. **Hayashi, T., K. Makino, M. Ohnishi, K. Kurokawa, K. Ishii, K. Yokoyama, C. G. Han, E. Ohtsubo, K. Nakayama, T. Murata, M. Tanaka, T. Tobe, T. Iida, T. Takami, T. Honda, C. Sasakawa, N. Ogasawara, T. Yasunaga, S. Kuhara, T. Shiba, M. Hattori, and H. Shinagawa.** 2001. Complete genome sequence of enterohemorrhagic *Escherichia coli* O157:H7 and genomic comparison with a laboratory strain K-12. *DNA Res.* **8:**11–22.

83. **Hayden, M. K., G. M. Trenholm, J. E. Schultz, and D. F. Sahm.** 1993. In vivo development of teicoplanin resistance in a VanB *Enterococcus faecium* isolate. *J. Infect. Dis.* **167:**1224–1227.

84. **Henriques Normark, B., R. Novak, A. Ortqvist, G. Kallenius, E. Tuomanen, and S. Normark.** 2001. Clinical isolates of *Streptococcus pneumoniae* that exhibit tolerance of vancomycin. *Clin. Infect. Dis.* **32:**552–558.

85. **Henze, U. U., and B. Berger-Bachi.** 1995. *Staphylococcus aureus* penicillin-binding protein 4 and intrinsic beta-lactam resistance. *Antimicrob. Agents Chemother.* **39:**2415–2422.

86. **Hiasa, H., D. O. Yousef, and K. J. Marians.** 1996. DNA strand cleavage is required for replication fork arrest by a frozen topoisomerase-quinolone-DNA ternary complex. *J. Biol. Chem.* **271:**26424–26429.

87. **Hillen, W., and C. Berens.** 1994. Mechanisms underlying expression of Tn10 encoded tetracycline resistance. *Annu. Rev. Microbiol.* **48:**345–369.

88. **Hiramatsu, K.** 1998. Vancomycin resistance in staphylococci. *Drug Resist. Updates* **1:**135–150.

89. **Hooper, D. C.** 2001. Emerging mechanisms of fluoroquinolone resistance. *Emerg. Infect. Dis.* **7:**337–341.

90. **Huovinen, P.** 2001. Resistance to trimethoprim-sulfamethoxazole. *Clin. Infect. Dis.* **32:**1608–1614.

91. **Ibuka, A., A. Taguchi, M. Ishiguro, S. Fushinobu, Y. Ishii, S. Kamitori, K. Okuyama, K. Yamaguchi, M. Konno, and H. Matsuzawa.** 1999. Crystal structure of the E166A mutant of extended-spectrum beta-lactamase Toho-1 at 1.8 A resolution. *J. Mol. Biol.* **285:**2079–2087.

92. **Ito, T., Y. Katayama, K. Asada, N. Mori, K. Tsutsumimoto, C. Tiensasitorn, and K. Hiramatsu.** 2001. Structural comparison of three types of staphylococcal cassette chromosome mec integrated in the chromosome in methicillin-resistant *Staphylococcus aureus*. *Antimicrob. Agents Chemother.* **45:**1323–1336.

93. **Jacobs, C.** 1997. Pharmacia Biotech & Science prize. 1997 grand prize winner. Life in the balance: cell walls and antibiotic resistance. *Science* **278:**1731–1732.

94. **Jacobs, C., J.-M. Frere, and S. Normark.** 1997. Cytosolic intermediates for cell wall biosynthesis and degradation control inducible β-lactam resistance in gram-negative bacteria. *Cell* **88:**823–832.

95. **Jacobs, C., B. Joris, M. Jamin, K. Klarsov, J. Van Beeumen, D. Mengin-Lecreulx, J. van Heijenoort, J. T. Park, S. Normark, and J.-M. Frère.** 1995. AmpD, essential for both β-lactamase regulation and cell wall recycling, is a novel cytosolic N-acetylmuramyl-L-alanine amidase. *Mol. Microbiol.* **15:**553–559.

96. **Jacoby, G. A., and A. A. Medeiros.** 1991. More extended-spectrum β-lactamases. *Antimicrob. Agents Chemother.* **35:**1697–1704.

97. **Kaatz, G. W., S. M. Seo, N. J. Dorman, and S. A. Lerner.** 1990. Emergence of teicoplanin resistance during therapy of *Staphylococcus aureus* endocarditis. *J. Infect. Dis.* **162:**103–108.

98. **Kadurugamuwa, J. L., A. J. Clarke, and T. J. Beveridge.** 1993. Surface action of gentamicin on *Pseudomonas aeruginosa*. *J. Bacteriol.* **175:**5798–5805.

99. **Kluytmans, J., A. van Belkum, and H. Verbrugh.** 1997. Nasal carriage of *Staphylococcus aureus*: epidemiology, underlying mechanisms, and associated risks. *Clin. Microbiol. Rev.* **10:**505–520.

100. **Knox, J. R.** 1995. Extended-spectrum and inhibitor-resistant TEM-type beta-lactamases: mutations, specificity, and three-dimensional structure. *Antimicrob. Agents Chemother.* **39:**2593–2601.

101. **Koenig, M. D., and D. Kaye.** 1961. Enterococcal endocarditis: report of nineteen cases with long term follow-up data. *N. Engl. J. Med.* **264:**257–264.

102. **Kohler, T., M. Kok, M. Michea-Hamzehpour, P. Plesiat, N. Gotoh, T. Nishino, L. K. Curty, and J. C. Pechere.** 1996. Multidrug efflux in intrinsic resistance to trimethoprim and sulfamethoxazole in *Pseudomonas aeruginosa*. *Antimicrob. Agents Chemother.* **40:**2288–2290.

103. **Kotra, L. P., J. Haddad, and S. Mobashery.** 2000. Aminoglycosides: perspectives on mechanisms of action and resistance and strategies to counter resistance. *Antimicrob. Agents Chemother.* **44:**3249–3256.

104. **Leclercq, R., S. Dutka-Malen, J. Duval, and P. Courvalin.** 1992. Vancomycin resistance gene *vanC* is specific to *Enterococcus gallinarum*. *Antimicrob. Agents Chemother.* **36:**2005–2008.

105. **Leclercq, R., S. Dutka-Malen, A. Brisson-Noel, C. Molinas, E. Derlot, M. Arthur, J. Duval, and P. Courvalin.** 1992. Resistance of enterococci to aminoglycosides and glycopeptides. *Clin. Infect. Dis.* **15:**495–501.

106. **Lee, A., W. Mao, M. S. Warren, A. Mistry, K. Hoshino, R. Okumura, H. Ishida, and O. Lomovskaya.** 2000. Interplay between efflux pumps may provide either additive or multiplicative effects on drug resistance. *J. Bacteriol.* **182:**3142–3150.

107. **Lee, E. H., M. H. Nicolas, M. D. Kitzis, G. Pialoux, E. Collatz, and L. Gutmann.** 1991. Association of two resistance mechanisms in a clinical isolate of *Enterobacter cloacae* with high-level resistance to imipenem. *Antimicrob. Agents Chemother.* **35:**1093–1098.

108. **Levine, D. P., B. S. Fromm, and B. R. Reddy.** 1991. Slow response to vancomycin or vancomycin plus rifampin in methicillin-resistant *Staphylococcus aureus* endocarditis. *Ann. Intern. Med.* **115:**674–680.

109. **Levy, S. B., L. M. McMurry, T. M. Barbosa, V. Burdett, P. Courvalin, W. Hillen, M. C. Roberts, J. I. Rood, and D. E. Taylor.** 1999. Nomenclature for new

tetracycline resistance determinants. *Antimicrob. Agents Chemother.* **43:**1523–1524.

110. **Linares, J.** 2001. The VISA/GISA problem: therapeutic implications. *Clin. Microbiol. Infect.* **7:**8–15.

111. **Livermore, D. M.** 1992. Interplay of impermeability and chromosomal β-lactamase activity in imipenem-resistant *Pseudomonas aeruginosa. Antimicrob. Agents Chemother.* **36:**2046–2048.

112. **Livermore, D. M.** 1995. β-Lactamases in laboratory and clinical resistance. *Clin. Microbiol. Rev.* **8:**557–584.

113. **Lobkovsky, E., E. M. Billings, P. C. Moews, J. Rahil, R. F. Pratt, and J. R. Knox.** 1994. Crystallographic structure of a phosphonate derivative of the *Enterobacter cloacae* P99 cephalosporinase: mechanistic interpretation of a beta-lactamase transition-state analog. *Biochemistry* **33:**6762–6772.

114. **Lyon, B. R., and R. Skurray.** 1987. Antimicrobial resistance in *Staphylococcus aureus*: genetic basis. *Microbiol. Rev.* **51:**88–134.

115. **Manges, A. R., J. R. Johnson, B. Foxman, T. T. O'Bryan, K. E. Fullerton, and L. W. Riley.** 2001. Widespread distribution of urinary tract infections caused by a multidrug-resistant *Escherichia coli* clonal group. *N. Engl. J. Med.* **345:**1007–1013.

116. **Mao, W., M. S. Warren, A. Lee, A. Mistry, and O. Lomovskaya.** 2001. MexXY-OprM efflux pump is required for antagonism of aminoglycosides by divalent cations in *Pseudomonas aeruginosa. Antimicrob. Agents Chemother.* **45:**2001–2007.

117. **Martinez, J. L., A. Alonso, J. M. Gomez-Gomez, and F. Baquero.** 1998. Quinolone resistance by mutations in chromosomal gyrase genes. Just the tip of the iceberg? *J. Antimicrob. Chemother.* **42:**683–688.

118. **Martinez-Martinez, L., S. Hernandez-Alles, S. Alberti, J. M. Tomas, V. J. Benedi, and G. A. Jacoby.** 1996. In vivo selection of porin-deficient mutants of *Klebsiella pneumoniae* with increased resistance to cefoxitin and expanded-spectrum cephalosporins. *Antimicrob. Agents Chemother.* **40:**342–348.

119. **Maseda, H., H. Yoneyama, and T. Nakae.** 2000. Assignment of the substrate-selective subunits of the MexEF-OprN multidrug efflux pump of *Pseudomonas aeruginosa. Antimicrob. Agents Chemother.* **44:**658–664.

120. **Matagne, A., J. Lamotte-Brasseur, and J. M. Frere.** 1998. Catalytic properties of class A beta-lactamases: efficiency and diversity. *Biochem. J.* **330:**581–598.

121. **Maveyraud, L., D. Golemi, L. P. Kotra, S. Tranier, S. Vakulenko, S. Mobashery, and J. P. Samama.** 2000. Insights into class D beta-lactamases are revealed by the crystal structure of the OXA10 enzyme from *Pseudomonas aeruginosa. Struct. Fold Des.* **8:**1289–1298.

122. **McDonald, L. C., S. Rossiter, C. Mackinson, Y. Y. Wang, S. Johnson, M. Sullivan, R. Sokolow, E. DeBess, L. Gilbert, J. A. Benson, B. Hill, and F. J. Angulo.** 2001. Quinupristin-dalfopristin-resistant *Enterococcus faecium* on chicken and in human stool specimens. *N. Engl. J. Med.* **345:**1155–1160.

123. **McKessar, S. J., A. M. Berry, J. M. Bell, J. D. Turnidge, and J. C. Paton.** 2000. Genetic characterization of *vanG*, a novel vancomycin resistance locus in *Enterococcus faecalis. Antimicrob. Agents Chemother.* **44:**3224–3228.

124. **McMurry, L. M., and S. B. Levy.** 2000. Tetracycline resistance in gram-positive bacteria, p. 660–677. *In* V. A. Fischetti, R. P. Novick, J. J. Ferretti, D. A. Portnoy, and J. I. Rood (ed.), *Gram-Positive Pathogens.* American Society for Microbiology, Washington, D.C.

125. **Mingeot-Leclercq, M. P., Y. Glupczynski, and P. M. Tulkens.** 1999. Aminoglycosides: activity and resistance. *Antimicrob. Agents Chemother.* **43:**727–737.

126. **Moellering, R. C., and A. N. Weinberg.** 1971. Studies on antibiotic synergism against enterococci. II. Effect of various antibiotics on the uptake of 14C-labelled streptomycin by enterococci. *J. Clin. Investig.* **50:**2580–2584.

127. **Morais Cabral, J. H., A. P. Jackson, C. V. Smith, N. Shikotra, A. Maxwell, and R. C. Liddington.** 1997. Crystal structure of the breakage-reunion domain of DNA gyrase. *Nature* **388:**903–906.

128. **Murakami, K., and A. Tomasz.** 1989. Involvement of multiple genetic determinants in high-level methicillin resistance in *Staphylococcus aureus. J. Bacteriol.* **171:**874–879.

129. **Murray, I. A., J. V. Martinez-Suarez, T. J. Close, and W. V. Shaw.** 1990. Nucleotide sequences of genes encoding the type II chloramphenicol acetyltransferases of *Escherichia coli* and *Haemophilus influenzae*, which are sensitive to inhibition by thiol-reactive reagents. *Biochem. J.* **272:**505–510.

130. **Murray, I. A., and W. V. Shaw.** 1997. O-Acetyltransferases for chloramphenicol and other natural products. *Antimicrob. Agents Chemother.* **41:**1–6.

131. **Naas, T., and P. Nordmann.** 1999. OXA-type beta-lactamases. *Curr. Pharm. Des.* **5:**865–879.

132. **Navarro, F., and P. Courvalin.** 1994. Analysis of genes encoding D-alanine-D-alanine ligase-related enzymes in *Enterococcus casseliflavus* and *Enterococcus flavescens. Antimicrob. Agents Chemother.* **38:**1788–1793.

133. **Nikaido, H.** 1998. Multiple antibiotic resistance and efflux. *Curr. Opin. Microbiol.* **1:**516–523.

134. **Nikaido, H., and D. G. Thanassi.** 1993. Penetration of lipophilic agents with multiple protonation sites into bacterial cells: tetracyclines and fluoroquinolones as examples. *Antimicrob. Agents Chemother.* **37:**1393–1399.

135. **Noble, W. C., Z. Virani, and R. G. A. Gee.** 1992. Co-transfer of vancomycin and other resistance genes from *Enterococcus faecalis* NCTC 12201 to *Staphylococcus aureus. FEMS Microbiol. Lett.* **93:**195–198.

136. **Nordmann, P.** 1998. Trends in beta-lactam resistance among *Enterobacteriaceae. Clin. Infect. Dis.* **27**(Suppl. 1): S100–S106.

137. **Nordmann, P., and T. Naas.** 1994. Sequence analysis of PER-1 extended-spectrum β-lactamase from *Pseudomonas aeruginosa* and comparison with class A β-lactamases. *Antimicrob. Agents Chemother.* **38:**104–114.

138. **Oggioni, M. R., C. G. Dowson, J. M. Smith, R. Provvedi, and G. Pozzi.** 1996. The tetracycline resistance gene *tet*(M) exhibits mosaic structure. *Plasmid* **35:**156–163.

139. **Orencia, M. C., J. S. Yoon, J. E. Ness, W. P. Stemmer, and R. C. Stevens.** 2001. Predicting the emergence of antibiotic resistance by directed evolution and structural analysis. *Nat. Struct. Biol.* **8:**238–242.

140. **Paetzel, M., F. Danel, L. de Castro, S. C. Mosimann, M. G. Page, and N. C. Strynadka.** 2000. Crystal structure of the class D beta-lactamase OXA-10. *Nat. Struct. Biol.* **7:**918–925.

141. **Pan, X. S., and L. M. Fisher.** 1999. Streptococcus pneumoniae DNA gyrase and topoisomerase IV: overexpression, purification, and differential inhibition by fluoroquinolones. *Antimicrob. Agents Chemother.* **43:**1129–1136.

142. **Paterson, D. L., W. C. Ko, A. Von Gottberg, J. M. Casellas, L. Mulazimoglu, K. P. Klugman, R. A. Bonomo, L. B. Rice, J. G. McCormack, and V. L. Yu.** 2001. Outcome of cephalosporin treatment for serious infections due to apparently susceptible organisms producing extended-spectrum beta-lactamases: implications

for the clinical microbiology laboratory. *J. Clin. Microbiol.* **39:**2206–2212.

143. **Paulsen, I. T., M. H. Brown, and R. A. Skurray.** 1996. Proton-dependent multidrug efflux systems. *Microbiol. Rev.* **60:**575–608.

144. **Paul-Soto, R., R. Bauer, J. M. Frere, M. Galleni, W. Meyer-Klaucke, H. Nolting, G. M. Rossolini, D. de Seny, M. Hernandez-Valladares, M. Zeppezauer, and H. W. Adolph.** 1999. Mono- and binuclear Zn^{2+}-beta-lactamase. Role of the conserved cysteine in the catalytic mechanism. *J. Biol. Chem.* **274:**13242–13249.

145. **Phillipon, A., R. Labia, and G. A. Jacoby.** 1989. Extended-spectrum β-lactamases. *Antimicrob. Agents Chemother.* **33:**1131–1136.

146. **Piddock, L. J.** 1999. Mechanisms of fluoroquinolone resistance: an update 1994–1998. *Drugs* **58**(Suppl. 2)**:**11–18.

147. **Podglajen, I., J. Breuil, A. Rohaut, C. Monsempes, and E. Collatz.** 2001. Multiple mobile promoter regions for the rare carbapenem resistance gene of *Bacteroides fragilis*. *J. Bacteriol.* **183:**3531–3535.

148. **Poirel, L., T. Naas, M. Guibert, E. B. Chaibi, R. Labia, and P. Nordmann.** 1999. Molecular and biochemical characterization of VEB-1, a novel class A extended-spectrum beta-lactamase encoded by an *Escherichia coli* integron gene. *Antimicrob. Agents Chemother.* **43:**573–581.

149. **Poirel, L., G. F. Weldhagen, T. Naas, C. De Champs, M. G. Dove, and P. Nordmann.** 2001. GES-2, a class A beta-lactamase from *Pseudomonas aeruginosa* with increased hydrolysis of imipenem. *Antimicrob. Agents Chemother.* **45:**2598–2603.

150. **Poole, K., K. Krebes, C. McNally, and S. Neshat.** 1993. Multiple antibiotic resistance in *Pseudomonas aeruginosa*: evidence for involvement of an efflux operon. *J. Bacteriol.* **175:**7363–7372.

151. **Power, E. G. M., Y. H. Abdulla, H. G. Talsania, W. Spice, S. Aathithan, and G. L. French.** 1995. *vanA* genes in vancomycin-resistant clinical isolates of *Oerskovia turbata* and *Arcanobacterium* (*Corynebacterium*) *haemolyticum*. *J. Antimicrob. Chemother.* **36:**595–606.

152. **Powers, R. A., E. Caselli, P. J. Focia, F. Prati, and B. K. Shoichet.** 2001. Structures of ceftazidime and its transition-state analogue in complex with AmpC beta-lactamase: implications for resistance mutations and inhibitor design. *Biochemistry* **40:**9207–9214.

153. **Poyart, C., C. Pierre, G. Quiesne, B. Pron, P. Berche, and P. Trieu-Cuot.** 1997. Emergence of vancomycin resistance in the genus *Streptococcus*: characterization of a *vanB* transferable determinant in *Streptococcus bovis*. *Antimicrob. Agents Chemother.* **41:**24–29.

154. **Prinarakis, E. E., V. Miriagou, E. Tzelepi, M. Gazouli, and L. S. Tzouvelekis.** 1997. Emergence of an inhibitor-resistant beta-lactamase (SHV-10) derived from an SHV-5 variant. *Antimicrob. Agents Chemother.* **41:**838–840.

155. **Prystowsky, J., F. Siddiqui, J. Chosay, D. L. Shinabarger, J. Millichap, L. R. Peterson, and G. A. Noskin.** 2001. Resistance to linezolid: characterization of mutations in rRNA and comparison of their occurrences in vancomycin-resistant enterococci. *Antimicrob. Agents Chemother.* **45:**2154–2156.

156. **Raquet, X., J. Lamotte-Brasseur, E. Fonze, S. Goussard, P. Courvalin, and J. M. Frere.** 1994. TEM beta-lactamase mutants hydrolysing third-generation cephalosporins. A kinetic and molecular modelling analysis. *J. Mol. Biol.* **244:**625–639.

157. **Rasmussen, B. A., and K. Bush.** 1997. Carbapenem-hydrolyzing beta-lactamases. *Antimicrob. Agents Chemother.* **41:**223–232.

158. **Rather, P. N.** 1998. Origins of aminoglycoside modifying enzymes. *Drug Resist. Updates* **1:**285–291.

159. **Rather, P. N., E. Orosz, K. J. Shaw, R. Hare, and G. Miller.** 1993. Characterization and transcriptional regulation of the 2′-N-acetyltransferase gene from *Providencia stuartii*. *J. Bacteriol.* **175:**6492–6498.

160. **Reichler, M. R., A. A. Allphin, R. F. Breiman, J. R. Schreiber, J. E. Arnold, L. K. McDougal, R. R. Facklam, B. Boxerbaum, D. May, R. O. Walton, et al.** 1992. The spread of multiply resistant *Streptococcus pneumoniae* at a day care center in Ohio. *J. Infect. Dis.* **166:**1346–1353.

161. **Rice, L. B.** 2000. Bacterial monopolists: the bundling and dissemination of antimicrobial resistance genes in gram-positive bacteria. *Clin. Infect. Dis.* **31:**762–769.

162. **Rice, L. B.** 1998. Tn916-family conjugative transposons and dissemination of antimicrobial resistance determinants. *Antimicrob. Agents Chemother.* **42:**1871–1877.

163. **Rice, L. B., and R. A. Bonomo.** 2000. beta-Lactamases: which ones are clinically important? *Drug Resist. Update* **3:**178–189.

164. **Rice, L. B., S. B. Calderwood, G. M. Eliopoulos, B. F. Farber, and A. W. Karchmer.** 1991. Enterococcal endocarditis: a comparison of native and prosthetic valve disease. *Rev. Infect. Dis.* **13:**1–7.

165. **Rice, L. B., and L. L. Carias.** 1998. Transfer of Tn5385, a composite, multiresistance element from *Enterococcus faecalis*. *J. Bacteriol.* **180:**714–721.

166. **Rice, L. B., L. L. Carias, A. M. Hujer, M. Bonafede, R. Hutton, C. Hoyen, and R. A. Bonomo.** 2000. High-level expression of chromosomally encoded SHV-1 β-lactamase and an outer membrane protein change confer resistance to ceftazidime and piperacillin-tazobactam in a clinical isolate of *Klebsiella pneumoniae*. *Antimicrob. Agents Chemother.* **44:**362–367.

167. **Rice, L. B., L. L. Carias, R. Hutton-Thomas, F. Sifaoui, L. Gutmann, and S. D. Rudin.** 2001. Penicillin-binding protein 5 and expression of ampicillin resistance in *Enterococcus faecium*. *Antimicrob. Agents Chemother.* **45:**1480–1486.

168. **Rice, L. B., J. D. C. Yao, K. Klimm, G. M. Eliopoulos, and R. C. Moellering, Jr.** 1991. Efficacy of different β-lactams against an extended spectrum β-lactamase-producing *Klebsiella pneumoniae* strain in the rat intra-abdominal abscess model. *Antimicrob. Agents Chemother.* **35:**1243–1244.

169. **Roberts, M. C., J. Sutcliffe, P. Courvalin, L. B. Jensen, J. Rood, and H. Seppala.** 1999. Nomenclature for macrolide and macrolide-lincosamide-streptogramin B resistance determinants. *Antimicrob. Agents Chemother.* **43:**2823–2830.

170. **Roberts, R. B., A. de Lancastre, W. Eisner, E. P. Severina, B. Shopsin, B. N. Kreiswirth, A. Tomasz, and the MRSA Collaborative Study Group.** 1998. Molecular epidemiology of methicillin-resistant *Staphylococcus aureus* in 12 New York hospitals. *J. Infect. Dis.* **178:**164–171.

171. **Rybkine, T., J.-L. Mainardi, W. Sougakoff, E. Collatz, and L. Gutmann.** 1998. Penicillin-binding protein 5 sequence alterations in clinical isolates of *Enterococcus faecium* with different levels of β-lactam resistance. *J. Infect. Dis.* **178:**159–163.

172. **Sabath, L. D.** 1969. Drug resistance of bacteria. *N. Engl. J. Med.* **280:**91–94.

173. **Sahm, D. F., M. K. Marsilio, and G. Piazza.** 1999. Antimicrobial resistance in key bloodstream bacterial

isolates: electronic surveillance with The Surveillance Network Database-USA. *Clin. Infect. Dis.* **29:**259–263.

174. **Sanchez-Pescador, R., J. T. Brown, M. Roberts, and M. S. Urdea.** 1988. Homology of the TetM with translational elongation factors: implications for potential modes of *tet*M-conferred tetracycline resistance. *Nucleic Acids Res.* **16:**1218.

175. **Saves, I., O. Burlet-Schiltz, P. Swaren, F. Lefevre, J. M. Masson, J. C. Prome, and J. P. Samama.** 1995. The asparagine to aspartic acid substitution at position 276 of TEM-35 and TEM-36 is involved in the beta-lactamase resistance to clavulanic acid. *J. Biol. Chem.* **270:**18240–18245.

176. **Sawai, T., R. Hiruma, N. Kawana, M. Kaneko, F. Taniyasu, and A. Inami.** 1982. Outer membrane permeation of beta-lactam antibiotics in *Escherichia coli, Proteus mirabilis*, and *Enterobacter cloacae. Antimicrob. Agents Chemother.* **22:**585–592.

177. **Schnappinger, D., and W. Hillen.** 1996. Tetracyclines: antibiotic action, uptake, and resistance mechanisms. *Arch. Microbiol.* **165:**359–369.

178. **Schwarz, S., M. Cardoso, and H. C. Wegener.** 1992. Nucleotide sequence and phylogeny of the *tet*(L) tetracycline resistance determinant encoded by plasmid pSTE1 from *Staphylococcus hyicus. Antimicrob. Agents Chemother.* **36:**580–588.

179. **Shaw, J. H., and D. B. Clewell.** 1985. Complete nucleotide sequence of macrolide-lincosamide-streptogramin B resistance transposon Tn*917* in *Streptococcus faecalis. J. Bacteriol.* **164:**782–796.

180. **Shaw, K. J., P. Rather, F. Sabatelli, P. Mann, H. Munayyer, R. Mierzwa, G. Petrikkos, R. S. Hare, G. H. Miller, P. Bennett, and P. Downey.** 1992. Characterization of the chromosomal *aac*(6′)-Ic gene from *Serratia marcescens. Antimicrob. Agents Chemother.* **36:**1447–1455.

181. **Shaw, K. J., P. N. Rather, R. S. Hare, and G. H. Miller.** 1993. Molecular genetics of aminoglycoside resistance genes and familial relationships of the aminoglycoside-modifying enzymes. *Microbiol. Rev.* **57:**138–163.

182. **Shaw, W. V.** 1983. Chloramphenicol acetyltransferase: enzymology and molecular biology. *Crit. Rev. Biochem.* **14:**1–46.

183. **Shea, M. E., and H. Hiasa.** 1999. Interactions between DNA helicases and frozen topoisomerase IV-quinolone-DNA ternary complexes. *J. Biol. Chem.* **274:**22747–22754.

184. **Sherertz, R. J., D. R. Reagan, K. D. Hampton, K. L. Robertson, S. A. Streed, H. M. Hoen, R. Thomas, and J. M. Gwaltney, Jr.** 1996. A cloud adult: the *Staphylococcus aureus*-virus interaction revisited. *Ann. Intern. Med.* **124:**539–547.

185. **Shinabarger, D. L., K. R. Marotti, R. W. Murray, A. H. Lin, E. P. Melchior, S. M. Swaney, D. S. Dunyak, W. F. Demyan, and J. M. Buysse.** 1997. Mechanism of action of oxazolidinones: effects of linezolid and eperezolid on translation reactions. *Antimicrob. Agents Chemother.* **41:**2132–2136.

186. **Sieradzki, K., R. B. Roberts, S. W. Haber, and A. Tomasz.** 1999. The development of vancomycin resistance in a patient with methicillin-resistant *Staphylococcus aureus* infection. *N. Engl. J. Med.* **340:**517–523.

187. **Sirot, D., C. Recule, E. B. Chaibi, L. Bret, J. Croize, C. Chanal-Claris, R. Labia, and J. Sirot.** 1997. A complex mutant of TEM-1 beta-lactamase with mutations encountered in both IRT-4 and extended-spectrum TEM-15, produced by an *Escherichia coli* clinical isolate. *Antimicrob. Agents Chemother.* 41:1322–1325.

188. **Skold, O.** 2000. Sulfonamide resistance: mechanisms and trends. *Drug Resist. Update* **3:**155–160.

189. **Smith, A. M., R. F. Botha, H. J. Koornhof, and K. P. Klugman.** 2001. Emergence of a pneumococcal clone with cephalosporin resistance and penicillin susceptibility. *Antimicrob. Agents Chemother.* **45:**2648–2650.

190. **Soltani, M., D. Beighton, J. Philpott-Howard, and N. Woodford.** 2000. Mechanisms of resistance to quinupristin-dalfopristin among isolates of *Enterococcus faecium* from animals, raw meat, and hospital patients in Western Europe. *Antimicrob. Agents Chemother.* **44:**433–436.

191. **Sorensen, T. L., M. Blom, D. L. Monnet, N. Frimodt-Moller, R. L. Poulsen, and F. Espersen.** 2001. Transient intestinal carriage after ingestion of antibiotic-resistant *Enterococcus faecium* from chicken and pork. *N. Engl. J. Med.* **345:**1161–1166.

192. **Spencer, J., A. R. Clarke, and T. R. Walsh.** 2001. Novel mechanism of hydrolysis of therapeutic beta-lactams by *Stenotrophomonas maltophilia* L1 metallo-beta-lactamase. *J. Biol. Chem.* **276:**33638–33644.

193. **Spratt, B. G., Q.-Y. Zhang, D. M. Jones, A. Hutchison, J. A. Brannigan, and C. G. Dowson.** 1989. Recruitment of a penicillin-binding protein gene from *Neisseria flavescens* during the emergence of penicillin resistance in *Neisseria meningitidis. Proc. Natl. Acad. Sci. USA* **86:**8988–8992.

194. **Stapleton, P. D., K. P. Shannon, and G. L. French.** 1999. Carbapenem resistance in *Escherichia coli* associated with plasmid-determined CMY-4 β-lactamase production and loss of an outer membrane protein. *Antimicrob. Agents Chemother.* **43:**1206–1210.

195. **Stinear, T. P., D. C. Olden, P. D. Johnson, J. K. Davies, and M. L. Grayson.** 2001. Enterococcal *vanB* resistance locus in anaerobic bacteria in human faeces. *Lancet* **357:**855–856.

196. **Strynadka, N. C., H. Adachi, S. E. Jensen, K. Johns, A. Sielecki, C. Betzel, K. Sutoh, and M. N. James.** 1992. Molecular structure of the acyl-enzyme intermediate in beta-lactam hydrolysis at 1.7 A resolution. *Nature* **359:**700–705.

197. **Su, Y. A., P. He, and D. B. Clewell.** 1992. Characterization of the *tet*M determinant of Tn*916*: evidence for regulation by transcriptional attenuation. *Antimicrob. Agents Chemother.* **36:**769–778.

198. **Swaren, P., D. Golemi, S. Cabantous, A. Bulychev, L. Maveyraud, S. Mobashery, and J. P. Samama.** 1999. X-ray structure of the Asn276Asp variant of the *Escherichia coli* TEM-1 beta-lactamase: direct observation of electrostatic modulation in resistance to inactivation by clavulanic acid. *Biochemistry* **38:**9570–9576.

199. **Swedberg, G., S. Ringertz, and O. Skold.** 1998. Sulfonamide resistance in *Streptococcus pyogenes* is associated with differences in the amino acid sequence of its chromosomal dihydropteroate synthase. *Antimicrob. Agents Chemother.* **42:**1062–1067.

200. **Then, R. L.** 1982. Mechanisms of resistance to trimethoprim, the sulfonamides, and trimethoprim-sulfamethoxazole. *Rev. Infect. Dis.* **4:**261–269.

201. **Then, R. L., and P. Angehrn.** 1979. Low trimethoprim susceptibility of anaerobic bacteria due to insensitive dihydrofolate reductases. *Antimicrob. Agents Chemother.* **15:**1–6.

202. **Thomson, C. J., and S. G. Amyes.** 1992. TRC-1: emergence of a clavulanic acid-resistant TEM beta-lactamase in a clinical strain. *FEMS Microbiol. Lett.* **70:**113–117.

203. **Tomasz, A.** 1983. Murein hydrolases: enzymes in search of a physiologic function, p. 155–163. *In* R. Hackenbeck, J. Holtje, and H. Labischinski (ed.), *The Target of Penicillin.* Walter de Gruyter, Berlin, Germany.

204. **Torres, O. R., R. Z. Korman, S. A. Zahler, and G. M. Dunny.** 1991. The conjugative transposon Tn*925*: en-

hancement of conjugal transfer by tetracycline in *Enterococcus faecalis* and mobilization of chromosomal genes in both *Bacillus subtilis* and *E. faecalis*. *Mol. Gen. Genet.* **225:**395–400.

205. **Tranier, S., A. T. Bouthors, L. Maveyraud, V. Guillet, W. Sougakoff, and J. P. Samama.** 2000. The high resolution crystal structure for class A beta-lactamase PER-1 reveals the bases for its increase in breadth of activity. *J. Biol. Chem.* **275:**28075–28082.

206. **Tsiodras, S., H. S. Gold, G. Sakoulas, G. M. Eliopoulos, C. Wennersten, L. Venkataraman, R. C. Moellering, Jr., and M. J. Ferraro.** 2001. Linezolid resistance in a clinical isolate of *Staphylococcus aureus*. *Lancet* **358:**207–208.

207. **Tzouvelekis, L. S., E. Tzelepi, P. T. Tassios, and N. J. Legakis.** 2000. CTX-M-type beta-lactamases: an emerging group of extended-spectrum enzymes. *Int. J. Antimicrob. Agents* **14:**137–142.

208. **Ubukata, K., Y. Shibasaki, K. Yamamoto, N. Chiba, K. Hasegawa, Y. Takeuchi, K. Sunakawa, M. Inoue, and M. Konno.** 2001. Association of amino acid substitutions in penicillin-binding protein 3 with beta-lactam resistance in beta-lactamase-negative ampicillin-resistant *Haemophilus influenzae*. *Antimicrob. Agents Chemother.* **45:**1693–1699.

209. **Ullah, J. H., T. R. Walsh, I. A. Taylor, D. C. Emery, C. S. Verma, S. J. Gamblin, and J. Spencer.** 1998. The crystal structure of the L1 metallo-β-lactamase from *Stenotrophomonas maltophilia* at 1.7 A resolution. *J. Mol. Biol.* **284:**125–136.

210. **Vakulenko, S. B., B. Geryk, L. P. Kotra, S. Mobashery, and S. A. Lerner.** 1998. Selection and characterization of beta-lactam–beta-lactamase inactivator-resistant mutants following PCR mutagenesis of the TEM-1 beta-lactamase gene. *Antimicrob. Agents Chemother.* **42:**1542–1548.

211. **Vedel, G., A. Bellaouaj, L. Gilly, R. Labia, A. Phillipon, P. Nevot, and G. Paul.** 1992. Clinical isolates of *Escherichia coli* producing TRI β-lactamases: novel TEM enzymes conferring resistance to β-lactamase inhibitors. *J. Antimicrob. Chemother.* **30:**449–462.

212. **Weber, B., K. Ehlert, A. Diehl, P. Reichmann, H. Labischinski, and R. Hakenbeck.** 2000. The *fib* locus in *Streptococcus pneumoniae* is required for peptidoglycan crosslinking and PBP-mediated beta-lactam resistance. *FEMS Microbiol. Lett.* **188:**81–85.

213. **Wegener, H. C., F. M. Aarestrup, L. B. Jensen, A. M. Hammerum, and F. Bager.** 1999. Use of antimicrobial growth promoters in food animals and *Enterococcus faecium* resistance to therapeutic antimicrobial drugs in Europe. *Emerg. Infect. Dis.* **5:**329–335.

214. **Wehrli, W.** 1983. Rifampin: mechanisms of action and resistance. *Rev. Infect. Dis.* **5**(Suppl. 3)**:**S407–S411.

215. **Weisblum, B.** 1995. Erythromycin resistance by ribosome modification. *Antimicrob. Agents Chemother.* **39:**577–585.

216. **White, D. G., C. Hudson, J. J. Maurer, S. Ayers, S. Zhao, M. D. Lee, L. Bolton, T. Foley, and J. Sherwood.** 2000. Characterization of chloramphenicol and florfenicol resistance in *Escherichia coli* associated with bovine diarrhea. *J. Clin. Microbiol.* **38:**4593–4598.

217. **White, P. A., C. J. McIver, and W. D. Rawlinson.** 2001. Integrons and gene cassettes in the *Enterobacteriaceae*. *Antimicrob. Agents Chemother.* **45:**2658–2661.

218. **Williamson, R., C. LaBouguenec, L. Gutmann, and T. Horaud.** 1985. One or two low affinity penicillin-binding proteins may be responsible for the range of susceptibility of *Enterococcus faecium* to penicillin. *J. Gen. Microbiol.* **131:**1933–1940.

219. **Willmott, C. J., S. E. Critchlow, I. C. Eperon, and A. Maxwell.** 1994. The complex of DNA gyrase and quinolone drugs with DNA forms a barrier to transcription by RNA polymerase. *J. Mol. Biol.* **242:**351–363.

220. **Wu, S. W., H. de Lencastre, and A. Tomasz.** 2001. Recruitment of the *mecA* gene homologue of *Staphylococcus sciuri* into a resistance determinant and expression of the resistant phenotype in *Staphylococcus aureus*. *J. Bacteriol.* **183:**2417–2424.

221. **Yigit, H., A. M. Queenan, G. J. Anderson, A. Domenech-Sanchez, J. W. Biddle, C. D. Steward, S. Alberti, K. Bush, and F. C. Tenover.** 2001. Novel carbapenem-hydrolyzing beta-lactamase, KPC-1, from a carbapenem-resistant strain of *Klebsiella pneumoniae*. *Antimicrob. Agents Chemother.* **45:**1151–1161.

222. **Yoshida, H., M. Bogaki, M. Nakamura, and S. Nakamura.** 1990. Quinolone resistance-determining region in the DNA gyrase *gyrA* gene of *Escherichia coli*. *Antimicrob. Agents Chemother.* **34:**1271–1272.

223. **Zervos, M. J., and D. R. Schaberg.** 1985. Reversal of in vitro susceptibility of enterococci to trimethoprim-sulfamethoxazole by folinic acid. *Antimicrob. Agents Chemother.* **28:**446–448.

224. **Zhong, P., and V. D. Shortridge.** 2000. The role of efflux in macrolide resistance. *Drug Resist. Update* **3:**325–329.

225. **Ziha-Zarifi, I., C. Llanes, T. Kohler, J. C. Pechere, and P. Plesiat.** 1999. In vivo emergence of multidrug-resistant mutants of *Pseudomonas aeruginosa* overexpressing the active efflux system MexA-MexB-OprM. *Antimicrob. Agents Chemother.* **43:**287–291.

Susceptibility Test Methods: General Considerations

JOHN D. TURNIDGE, MARY JANE FERRARO, AND JAMES H. JORGENSEN

69

Determination of the antimicrobial susceptibilities of significant bacterial isolates is one of the principal functions of the clinical microbiology laboratory. From the physician's pragmatic point of view, the results of susceptibility tests are often considered at least as important as the identification of the pathogen involved. This is particularly true in an era of increasing antimicrobial resistance in which treatment options are at times limited to newer, more costly antibacterial agents. As a result, the laboratory must give high priority not only to producing technically accurate data but also to reporting those data to physicians in an easily interpretable manner.

The main objective of susceptibility testing is to predict the outcome of treatment with the antimicrobial agents tested. The implication of the result "susceptible" is that there is a high probability that the patient will respond to treatment with the appropriate dosage of that antimicrobial agent. The result "resistant" implies that treatment with the antimicrobial agent is likely to fail. Most test methods also include an "intermediate" category of susceptibility, which can have several meanings. With agents that can be safely administered at higher doses, this category can imply that higher doses may be required to ensure efficacy or that the agent may prove efficacious if it is normally concentrated in an infected body fluid, e.g., urine. Conversely, for body compartments where drug penetration is restricted even in the presence of inflammation (e.g., cerebrospinal fluid), it suggests that extreme caution should be taken in the use of the agent. It may also represent a "buffer" zone that prevents strains with borderline susceptibility from being incorrectly categorized as resistant.

A further aim of susceptibility testing is to guide the clinician in the selection of the most appropriate agent for a particular clinical problem. In most clinical settings, susceptibility test results are usually obtained 24 to 48 h or more after the patient has been given empirical treatment. The test results may confirm the susceptibility of the organism to the drug initially prescribed or may indicate resistance, in which case alternative therapy will probably be required. The report describing the susceptibility testing results should provide the clinician with alternative agents, to which the organism is susceptible. These alternatives also may be useful if the patient subsequently develops an adverse reaction to the initial antimicrobial agent. There is

a growing emphasis from the professional societies and managed-care organizations to use susceptibility test results to direct therapy toward the most narrow-spectrum, least expensive agent to which the pathogen should respond. This is particularly true for hospitalized patients, in whom the rate of antimicrobial resistance tends to be high, and it is easier to make therapeutic changes for inpatients than for outpatients. This makes the accuracy of susceptibility testing even more critical for effective patient care.

The clinical microbiology laboratory should perform susceptibility testing only with pathogens for which well-standardized methods are available and pathogens whose resistance is known or suspected to be a clinical problem; susceptibility testing should not be performed with normal flora or colonizing organisms. Currently, routine susceptibility testing methods are best standardized for the common aerobic and facultative bacteria and systemic antibacterial agents. For some uncommon or fastidious bacteria and for topical antibacterial agents, simple routine test methods have not been standardized or are not recommended because they are likely to yield inaccurate results. However, testing of such organisms may be performed in reference laboratories by reference MIC methods under special circumstances. With some pathogens (e.g., *Mycobacterium tuberculosis* and invasive yeasts) routine testing is important for patient management, but testing is best performed by specialized laboratories in which test volumes are sufficient to maintain technical proficiency and unusual results are likely to be recognized. Susceptibility methods for certain other pathogens (e.g., mycoplasmas, chlamydiae, campylobacters, helicobacters, legionellae, spirochetes, viruses, protozoa, and helminths) may not be well established at present and are limited to a few specialty laboratories. A number of choices exist in antibacterial susceptibility testing with respect to methodology and selection of agents for routine testing.

SELECTING AN ANTIMICROBIAL SUSCEPTIBILITY TESTING METHOD

Clinical microbiology laboratories can choose from among several conventional or novel methods for performance of routine antibacterial susceptibility testing. These include the broth microdilution, disk diffusion, antibiotic gradient

(15), and automated-instrument methods. In recent years there has been a trend toward the use of commercial broth microdilution and automated-instrument methods instead of the disk diffusion procedure. However, there may be renewed interest in the disk diffusion test because of its inherent flexibility in drug selection and its low cost. The availability of numerous antibacterial agents and the diversity of antibiotic formularies in different institutions have made it difficult for manufacturers of commercial test systems to provide standard test panels that fit everyone's needs. Thus, the inherent flexibility of drug selection that is provided by the disk diffusion test is an undeniable asset of the method. It is also one of the most firmly established and best proven of all susceptibility tests and continues to be updated and refined through frequent (usually annual) NCCLS publications (26). Furthermore, the qualitative interpretive category results of "susceptible," "intermediate," and "resistant" provided by the disk test are readily understood by clinicians. Instrumentation is now available for reading, storing, and interpreting zone diameters and may reduce interobserver reading errors (17, 21).

Advantages of the microdilution or agar gradient diffusion methods include the generation of a quantitative result (i.e., an MIC) rather than a category result, the ability to test accurately some anaerobic or fastidious species that may not be tested by the disk diffusion method (5, 12, 25), and the ancillary benefits of computer systems that accompany many of the microdilution or automated systems (12). Indeed, computerized data management systems are very important in laboratories that may have limited or inflexible laboratory information systems. However, an MIC method should not be chosen on the basis that MICs are routinely more useful to physicians. There is no clear evidence that MICs are more relevant than susceptibility category results to the selection of appropriate antibacterial therapy for most infections (8).

A laboratory may choose to perform rapid, automated antibacterial susceptibility testing in order to generate results faster than can be generated by manual methods. The provision of susceptibility results 1 day sooner than can be provided by conventional methods seems a logical advance in patient care. Two studies have demonstrated both the clinical and economic benefits derived from the use of rapid susceptibility testing and reporting (2, 10). However, rapid susceptibility testing results may not have a substantial impact unless the laboratory uses more aggressive means of communication to make physicians aware of the results (34). This may be because physicians have come to expect antimicrobial susceptibility testing results approximately 48 h after the submission of a specimen or because the results, although generated more rapidly, are still not available soon enough to assist with the initial selection of antimicrobial therapy.

A previously cited shortcoming of rapid susceptibility testing methods was the failure to detect some inducible or subtle resistance mechanisms (11, 16, 32, 33). However, the instruments most notorious for such problems are no longer marketed, and the manufacturers of the remaining instruments have made substantial efforts to correct earlier problems (18, 24, 30, 35) or to extend testing to fastidious organisms (14). It is important to emphasize that accuracy should not be sacrificed in an effort to generate a rapid susceptibility testing result.

SELECTING ANTIBACTERIAL AGENTS FOR ROUTINE TESTING

The laboratory has the responsibility to test and report the antimicrobial agents that are most appropriate for the organism isolated, the site of infection, and the clinical practice setting in which the laboratory functions. The battery of antimicrobial agents routinely tested and reported on by the laboratory will depend on the characteristics of the patients under care in the institution and the likelihood of encountering highly resistant organisms (13). A laboratory serving a tertiary-care medical center which specializes in the care of immunosuppressed patients may need to perform routine tests of agents that are broader in spectrum than those tested by a laboratory that supports a primary-care outpatient practice in which antibiotic-resistant organisms are less commonly encountered.

When a laboratory's routine susceptibility testing batteries are determined, several principles should be followed. First, the antimicrobial agents that are included in the institution's formulary and that are prescribed by physicians on a daily basis should be tested. Second, the species tested strongly influences the choice of antimicrobial agents for testing. NCCLS publishes tables that list the antimicrobial agents appropriate for testing of various groups of aerobic and fastidious bacteria (26). The guidelines indicate the drugs that are most appropriate for testing each organism group and for treatment based on the specimen source (e.g., cerebrospinal fluid, blood, urine, or feces). The lists also include a few agents that may be tested as surrogates for other agents because of the greater ability of a particular agent to detect resistance to closely related drugs (e.g., the use of oxacillin to predict overall β-lactam resistance in staphylococci). This initial list of agents must be tailored to the specific needs of an individual institution through discussions with infectious-disease physicians, pharmacists, and committees concerned with infection control and the institutional formulary (13).

A third important step in defining routine testing batteries is that of ascertaining the availability of specific antimicrobial agents for testing by the laboratory's routine testing methodology. Certain methods (e.g., the disk diffusion, gradient diffusion, or in-house-prepared broth or agar dilution method) allow the greatest flexibility when selecting test batteries. In contrast, some commercial systems may have less flexibility or may involve delays in adding the latest antimicrobial agents approved for clinical use. However, practicality limits the maximum number of drugs that can be tested simultaneously with an isolate by any susceptibility testing method. For example, a maximum of 12 disks can be placed on a 150-mm Mueller-Hinton agar plate and a similar number can ordinarily be accommodated in a microdilution panel if full concentration ranges of each agent are to be included for routine determination of MICs. Some commercial test panels attempt to resolve this problem by testing a larger array of antimicrobial agents, although in a very limited concentration range (perhaps two to four dilutions for each agent).

ESTABLISHING SUSCEPTIBILITY BREAKPOINTS

There is general agreement that the MIC is the most basic laboratory measurement of the activity of an antimicrobial agent against an organism. It is defined as the lowest concentration that will inhibit the growth of a test organism over a defined interval related to the organism's growth rate, most commonly 18 to 24 h. The MIC is the fundamental measurement that forms the basis of most susceptibility testing methods and against which the levels of drug achieved in human body fluids may be compared to determine breakpoints for defining susceptibility.

The conventional technique for measuring the MIC involves exposing the test organism to a series of twofold dilutions of the antimicrobial agent in a suitable culture system, e.g., broth or agar for bacteria. The twofold dilution scheme was originally used because of the convenience of preparing dilutions from a single starting concentration in broth or agar dilution methods. Subsequently, this system proved to be meaningful because an antibiotic's MICs for a single bacterial species in the absence of resistance mechanisms have a statistically normal distribution when plotted on a logarithmic scale. This provides investigators with the opportunity to examine the distributions of MICs for bacterial populations and distinguish abnormal (potentially resistant) from normal (susceptible) strains.

MIC measurements are influenced in vitro by a number of factors including the composition of the medium, the size of the inoculum, the duration of incubation, and the presence of resistant subpopulations of the organism. The in vitro test conditions also do not encompass other factors that can influence in vivo antimicrobial activity. These include sub-MIC effects, postantibiotic effects, protein binding, effects on organism virulence or toxin production, variations in redox potential at sites of infection, and pharmacokinetic changes resulting from different drug levels in blood and at the site of infection over time. Nevertheless, if determined under standardized conditions, MIC measurements provide a fixed reference point for the setting of pharmacodynamic breakpoints with the power to predict efficacy in vivo. Pharmacological breakpoints can be applied directly to routine dilution testing methods that generate MICs, such as the broth microdilution, agar dilution, or gradient methods, and some automated instruments. They also provide reference values for deriving breakpoints for disk diffusion methods.

Breakpoints (or interpretative criteria) are the values that determine the categories of susceptible, intermediate, and resistant. The approach to setting breakpoints varies by organization or regulatory body but, with few exceptions, is based on the agent's MICs. Depending on the approach taken, up to four sources of data can be examined in establishing breakpoints.

(i) MIC distributions. Examination of MIC distributions can indicate the range of MICs for a population of strains that lack any known mechanisms of resistance to the particular drug. These distributions may aid in the recognition of new resistance mechanisms by highlighting strains that fall outside the normal distribution. However, they have limited direct application since the distributions of MICs vary between species, and for some strains for which the MICs are outside the normal population, the MICs may be below clinically derived breakpoints. Such strains may or may not respond to treatment. An example of the latter point is the fact that the penicillin MICs for some β-lactamase-producing organisms or the extended-spectrum cephalosporin MICs of extended-spectrum β-lactamase-producing gram-negative bacilli may be relatively low but do not translate to reliable clinical efficacy. Indeed, knowledge of the presence of specific resistance mechanisms that

inactivate compounds of a particular drug class is very useful in deriving microbiological breakpoints.

(ii) Pharmacokinetics and pharmacodynamics. Pharmacokinetics examines the absorption, distribution, accumulation, and elimination (metabolism and excretion) of a drug in the body over time. These parameters are usually determined in healthy volunteers. A drug's MICs can be compared with the concentration of drug achievable in blood or other body fluids (e.g., cerebrospinal fluid). In the past, breakpoints were chosen so that the MICs for susceptible pathogens would be exceeded by the drug level for most or all of the dosing interval. Newer data that are now considered when establishing breakpoints include pharmacodynamic calculations. Pharmacodynamics is the study of the time course of the action of the drug on the microorganism. For antimicrobial agents, the desired action is pathogen eradication. In vitro pharmacodynamic studies have revealed that agents fall into two classes: those with principally time-dependent antimicrobial action and those with prominent concentration-dependent action. For drugs with time-dependent action, the critical determinant of bacterial killing in vivo is the percentage of time in a dosing interval that the drug concentration is above the MIC ($\%T > $ MIC). For drugs with concentration-dependent action, the important determinant is the area under the concentration-time curve divided by the MIC (AUC/MIC ratio) and/or the peak concentration divided by the MIC (C_{max}/MIC ratio). For β-lactams, macrolides, and glycopeptides, the relevant measure is $\%T > $ MIC, while for aminoglycosides and fluoroquinolones, the AUC/MIC ratio or the C_{max}/MIC ratio is the relevant parameter (9). These values can be used to calculate the maximum MICs or breakpoints that would allow optimum efficacy to be obtained with standard drug dosing schedules.

(iii) Clinical and bacteriological response rates. During clinical trials, the clinical and/or bacteriologic eradication response rates of organisms for which the MICs of new antimicrobial agents have been determined give an indication of the relevance of breakpoints selected by using the MIC distributions and the pharmacokinetic and pharmacodynamic properties of the drug. Response rates of at least 80% may be expected for organisms classified as susceptible, although they can be lower depending on the site and type of infection. While in some countries breakpoints are determined primarily from clinical and bacteriological response rates, NCCLS evaluates clinical and bacteriological response rates in conjunction with population distributions, pharmacokinetics, and pharmacodynamics in establishing the breakpoints in an attempt to provide the best correlation between in vitro test results and clinical outcome (27).

(iv) Zone diameter distributions for disk diffusion methods. Once the MIC breakpoints are selected, disk diffusion breakpoints can be chosen by plotting the zone diameters against the MICs derived from the testing of a large number of strains of various species. A statistical approach that uses the linear regression formula may be used to calculate the appropriate zone diameter intercepts for the predetermined MIC breakpoints. An alternative, pragmatic approach to deriving disk diffusion breakpoints is the use of the error rate-bounded method, in which the zone diameter criteria are selected on the basis of minimization of the disk interpretive errors, especially the very major errors (4, 23) (Fig. 1). Newer statistical techniques are being studied to improve predictive value compared to MICs (7). The newest NCCLS approach focuses on the rate of interpretive errors near the proposed breakpoint versus strains for which the MICs are more than a single log$_2$ dilution from the MIC breakpoints (27). The concept is that errors that occur with isolates whose MICs are very close to the MIC breakpoints are less of a concern than errors with more highly resistant or susceptible strains.

Breakpoints derived by professional groups or regulatory bodies in various countries are often quite similar. However, there can be notable differences in the breakpoints used in different countries for the same agents. The reasons for the differences can be that certain countries use different dosages or administration intervals for some drugs. In addition, some countries are more conservative in assessing the susceptibility to antimicrobial agents and place greater emphasis on the detection of emerging resistance, noted primarily by examination of microorganism population distributions. Technical factors such as the inoculum density, atmosphere of incubation, and test medium can also affect MICs and zone diameters, thereby justifying different interpretive criteria in some countries. These technical differences are summarized in chapter 70. Two non-U.S. methods minimize or avoid the use of an intermediate category of susceptibility, based on the rationale that such results are of little value to the clinician (3, 20). The lack of a "buffer" between susceptible and resistant can result in higher rates of incorrect categorization. It may be safer for a laboratory to employ a method that uses an intermediate category or, if not, to report intermediate results as resistant.

Information on a range of international susceptibility testing methods and/or breakpoints can be downloaded or purchased from the following websites: NCCLS at http://www.nccls.org, the British Society for Antimicrobial Chemotherapy at http://www.bsac.org.uk, the (French) Société Française de Microbiologie at http://www.sfm.assoc.fr, the (German) Deutsches Institut für Normung at http://www.beuth.de, the (Spanish) Sociedad Española de Quimioterapia and Sociedad Española de Enfermedades Infecciosas y Microbiología Clínica at http://www.prous.com/seq/revista/0100/consen2.html, the Swedish Reference Group for Antibiotics at http://www.ltkronoberg.se/ext/raf/RAFENG/Srga.htm, the Danish commercial disk diffusion method at http://www.rosco.dk, and the Australian CDS disk diffusion method at http://www.med.unsw.edu.au/pathology-cds.

FUTURE DIRECTIONS AND NEEDS IN ANTIMICROBIAL SUSCEPTIBILITY TESTING

Antimicrobial resistance is becoming widespread among a variety of clinically significant bacterial species (31, 36). Therefore, the microbiology laboratory plays a key role in the patient management process by providing accurate data on which physicians can base therapy decisions. Susceptibility testing results, however, are also used in surveillance studies and by infection control practitioners to detect and control the spread of antibiotic-resistant organisms (29). Surveillance can be performed at the laboratory, local, regional, national, and international levels through direct interchange of data from laboratory information systems to centralized databases (28). Thus, the accuracy of stored results becomes almost as important as the accuracy of test performance and interpretation.

To meet these challenges and responsibilities, clinical microbiologists must continuously assess and update their susceptibility testing strategies. The first priority is to use accurate and reliable methods, whether they are conventional or perhaps newer molecular methods. Then careful monitoring of test performance with well-characterized control strains that challenge the capability of the testing methods becomes essential. Today, laboratories must use a variety of testing methods, each tailored specifically to a particular species or group of organisms. It is not likely that a single method, whether conventional or commercial, will be optimal for all antimicrobial agents, organisms, and resistance mechanisms. This will require increased education and training for clinical microbiologists in the future. Some assistance may be sought from the computer-based "expert" systems that allow a rapid and accurate view of

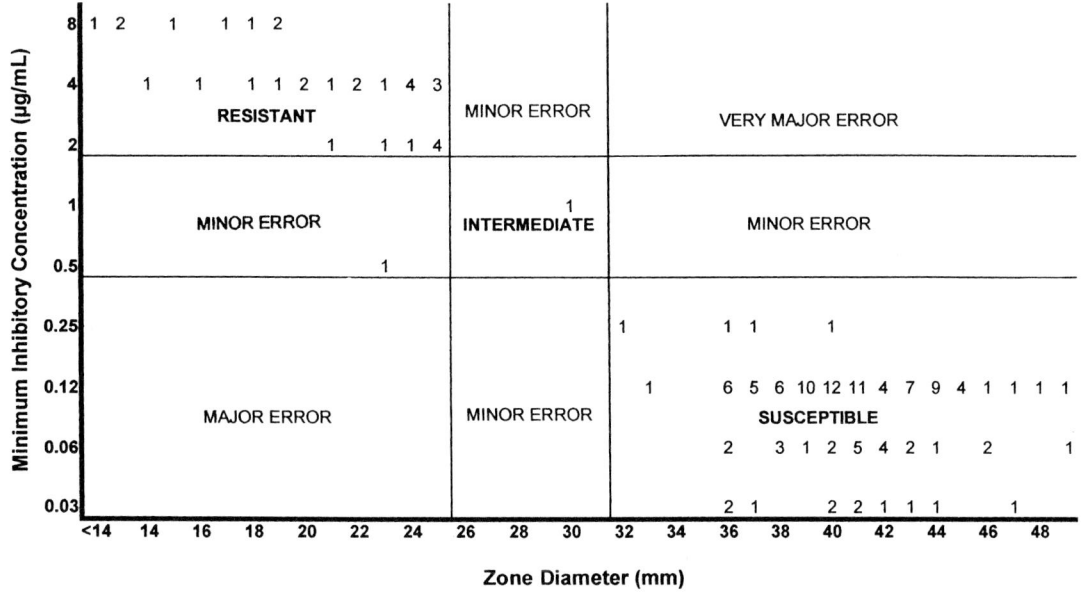

FIGURE 1 Comparison of zone diameters with MICs of a hypothetical antimicrobial agent.

antimicrobial susceptibility profiles and recognition of potential aberrant results or novel resistance mechanisms (6, 30). Rapid progress is also being made on molecular methods that will have practical application in the routine laboratory (1, 19, 22).

More effective means of conveying critical antimicrobial susceptibility testing information to clinicians in a time frame that allows efficient and effective management of patients and in a format that is unambiguous to clinicians in various practice specialties are still needed. Clinical microbiologists should become more proactive in reporting antimicrobial susceptibility results and in cross-linking that information to other databases (e.g., pharmacy prescriptions) to ensure that patients receive the most efficacious cost-effective therapy.

REFERENCES

1. **Allaouchiche, B., H. Jaumain, G. Zambardi, D. Chassard, and J. Freney.** 1999. Clinical impact of rapid oxacillin susceptibility testing using a PCR assay in *Staphylococcus aureus* bacteraemia. *J. Infect.* **39:**198–204.
2. **Barenfanger, J., C. Drake, and G. Kacich.** 1999. Clinical and financial benefits of rapid identification and antimicrobial susceptibility testing. *J. Clin. Microbiol.* **37:**1415–1418.
3. **Bell, S. M.** 1988. Additions and modifications to the range of antibiotics tested by the CDS method of antibiotic sensitivity testing. *Pathology* **20:**303–304.
4. **Brunden, M. N., G. E. Zurenko, and B. Kapik.** 1992. Modification of the error-rate bounded classification scheme for use with two MIC breakpoints. *Diagn. Microbiol. Infect. Dis.* **15:**135–140.
5. **Citron, D. M., M. I. Ostoravi, A. Karlsson, and E. J. C. Goldstein.** 1991. Evaluation of the E test for susceptibility testing of anaerobic bacteria. *J. Clin. Microbiol.* **29:**2197–2203.
6. **Courvalin, P.** 1992. Interpretive reading of antimicrobial susceptibility tests. *ASM News* **58:**368–375.
7. **Craig, B. A.** 2000. Modeling approach to diameter breakpoint determination. *Diagn. Microbiol. Infect. Dis.* **36:**193–202.
8. **Craig, W. A.** 1993. Qualitative susceptibility tests versus quantitative MIC tests. *Diagn. Microbiol. Infect. Dis.* **16:**231–236.
9. **Craig, W. A.** 1998. Pharmacokinetic/pharmacodynamic parameters: rationale for antibacterial dosing of mice and men. *Clin. Infect. Dis.* **26:**1–10.
10. **Doern, G. V., R. Vautour, M. Gaudet, and B. Levy.** 1994. Clinical impact of rapid in vitro antimicrobial susceptibility testing and bacterial identification. *J. Clin. Microbiol.* **32:**1757–1762.
11. **Jett, B., L. Free, and D. F. Sahm.** 1996. Factors influencing the Vitek gram-positive susceptibility system's detection of *vanB*-encoded vancomycin resistance among enterococci. *J. Clin. Microbiol.* **34:**701–706.
12. **Jorgensen, J. H.** 1993. Selection criteria for an antimicrobial susceptibility testing system. *J. Clin. Microbiol.* **31:**2841–2844.
13. **Jorgensen, J. H.** 1993. Selection of antimicrobial agents for routine testing in a clinical microbiology laboratory. *Diagn. Microbiol. Infect. Dis.* **16:**245–249.
14. **Jorgensen, J. H.** 2000. Rapid automated antimicrobial susceptibility testing of *Streptococcus pneumoniae* by use of the bioMerieux VITEK 2. *J. Clin. Microbiol.* **38:**2814–2818.

15. **Jorgensen, J. H., M. J. Ferraro, M. L. McElmeel, J. Spargo, J. M. Swenson, and F. C. Tenover.** 1994. Detection of penicillin and extended-spectrum cephalosporin resistance among *Streptococcus pneumoniae* clinical isolates by use of the E test. *J. Clin. Microbiol.* **32:**159–163.
16. **Katsanis, G. P., J. Spargo, M. J. Ferraro, L. Sutton, and G. A. Jacoby.** 1994. Detection of *Klebsiella pneumoniae* and *Escherichia coli* strains producing extended-spectrum β-lactamases. *J. Clin. Microbiol.* **32:**691–696.
17. **Korgenski, E. K., and J. A. Daly.** 1998. Evaluation of the BIOMIC video reader system for determining interpretive categories of isolates on the basis of disk diffusion susceptibility results. *J. Clin. Microbiol.* **36:**302–304.
18. **Ling, T. K. W., P. C. Tam, Z. K. Liu, and A. F. B. Cheng.** 2001. Evaluation of VITEK 2 rapid identification and susceptibility testing system against gram-negative clinical isolates. *J. Clin. Microbiol.* **39:**2964–2966.
19. **Louie, L., S. O. Matsumura, E. Choi, M. Louie, and A. E. Simor.** 2000. Evaluation of three rapid methods for detection of methicillin resistance in *Staphylococcus aureus. J. Clin. Microbiol.* **38:**2170–2173.
20. **MacGowan, A. P., and R. Wise.** 2001. Establishing MIC breakpoints and the interpretation of in vitro susceptibility tests. *J. Antimicrob. Chemother.* **48**(Suppl. S1):17–28.
21. **Madeiros, A., and J. Crellin.** 2000. Evaluation of the Sirscan automated zone reader in a clinical microbiology laboratory. *J. Clin. Microbiol.* **38:**1688–1693.
22. **Martineau, F., F. J. Picard, L. Grenier, P. H. Roy, M. Ouellette, and M. G. Bergeron for the ESPRIT trial.** 2000. Multiplex PCR assays for the detection of clinically relevant antibiotic resistance genes in staphylococci isolated from patients infected after cardiac surgery. *J. Antimicrob. Chemother.* **46:**527–534.
23. **Metzler, D. M., and R. M. DeHaan.** 1974. Susceptibility tests of anaerobic bacteria: statistical and clinical considerations. *J. Infect. Dis.* **130:**588–594.
24. **Nadler, H. L., C. Dolan, L. Mele, and S. R. Kurtz.** 1985. Accuracy and reproducibility of the AutoMicrobic System Gram-Negative General Susceptibility-Plus card for testing selected challenge organisms. *J. Clin. Microbiol.* **22:**355–360.
25. **NCCLS.** 2001. *Methods for Antimicrobial Susceptibility Testing of Anaerobic Bacteria.* Approved standard M11-A5. NCCLS, Wayne, Pa.
26. **NCCLS.** 2002. *Performance Standards for Antimicrobial Susceptibility Testing.* Twelfth informational supplement. M100-S12. NCCLS, Wayne, Pa.
27. **NCCLS.** 2001. *Development of In Vitro Susceptibility Testing Criteria and Quality Control Parameters.* Approved guideline M23-A2. NCCLS, Wayne, Pa.
28. **Sahm, D. F., J. A. Karlowsky, L. J. Kelly, I. A. Critchley, M. E. Jones, C. Thornsberry, Y. Mauriz, and J. Kahn.** 2001. Need for annual surveillance of antimicrobial resistance in *Streptococcus pneumoniae* in the United States: 2-year longitudinal analysis. *Antimicrob. Agents Chemother.* **45:**1037–1042.
29. **Sahm, D. F., and F. C. Tenover.** 1997. Surveillance for the emergence and dissemination of antimicrobial resistance in bacteria. *Infect. Dis. Clin. N. Am.* **11:**767–785.
30. **Sanders, C. C., M. Peyret, E. S. Moland, S. J. Cavalieri, C. Shubert, K. S. Thomson, J.-M. Boeufgras, and W. E. Sanders, Jr.** 2001. Potential impact of the VITEK 2 System and the Advanced Expert System on the clinical laboratory of a university-based hospital. *J. Clin. Microbiol.* **39:**2379–2385.
31. **Tenover, F. C.** 2001. Development and spread of bacterial resistance to antimicrobial agents. An overview. *Clin. Infect. Dis.* **15**(Suppl.):S108–S115.

32. **Tenover, F. C., J. M. Swenson, C. O'Hara, and S. A. Stocker.** 1995. Ability of commercial and reference antimicrobial susceptibility testing methods to detect vancomycin resistance in enterococci. *J. Clin. Microbiol.* **33:** 1524–1527.
33. **Tenover, F. C., J. Tokars, J. Swenson, S. Paul, K. Splitalny, and W. Jarvis.** 1993. Ability of clinical laboratories to detect antimicrobial-resistant enterococci. *J. Clin. Microbiol.* **31:**1695–1699.
34. **Trenholme, G. M., R. L. Kaplan, P. H. Karahusis, T. Stine, J. Fuhrer, W. Landau, and S. Levin.** 1989. Clinical impact of rapid identification and susceptibility testing of bacterial blood culture isolates. *J. Clin. Microbiol.* **27:** 1342–1345.
35. **Washington, J. A., C. C. Knapp, and C. C. Sanders.** 1988. Accuracy of microdilution and the AutoMicrobic System in detection of β-lactam resistance in gram-negative bacterial mutants with derepressed β-lactamase. *Rev. Infect. Dis.* **10:**824–829.
36. **Williams, R. M.** 2001. Globalization of antimicrobial resistance: epidemiological challenges. *Clin. Infect. Dis.* **15**(Suppl.):S116–S117.

Susceptibility Test Methods: Dilution and Disk Diffusion Methods*

JAMES H. JORGENSEN AND JOHN D. TURNIDGE

70

A number of methods can be used to perform susceptibility tests with antibacterial agents in a clinical laboratory setting or for research purposes, such as assessing the activities of new antimicrobial agents. Susceptibility testing may be performed reliably by either broth or agar dilution or agar diffusion methods. The choice of methodology to be used in individual laboratories may be based on factors such as relative ease of performance, cost, flexibility in selection of drugs for testing, use of automated or semiautomated devices to facilitate testing, and the perceived accuracy of the methodology (40, 42). A misconception may have existed regarding the clinical relevance of determining and routinely reporting MICs versus the interpretive category results (i.e., susceptible, intermediate, or resistant) that are derived by the disk diffusion method. This misconception may be based on the assumption that the dilution test is the inherently more accurate of the two methods. Since there is a direct relationship between the size of the zone of inhibition and the MIC and since MICs and zone diameters for reference strains have similar interlaboratory and intralaboratory reproducibilities, there is little objective evidence that one method is more accurate than the other with the majority of common, rapidly growing bacteria (22, 40). While an MIC may be perceived as more accurate than a result from a disk test, the MIC generated by the standard doubling dilution series may be a concentration somewhere between the concentration inhibiting the organism and the next lowest concentration tested (i.e., usually 1 $\log_2$ dilution lower). For example, an organism may grow in both the presence of an antimicrobial agent at a concentration of 4 μg/ml but does not grow at 8 μg/ml. The actual MIC could be anywhere between 4 and 8 μg/ml. Although we have said that MICs are not inherently more accurate, there are some species with resistance mechanisms that may not be reliably detected by standard disk testing (e.g., vancomycin-intermediate *Staphylococcus aureus*), some species for which the standard disk test is not well calibrated (e.g., *Stenotrophomonas maltophilia* and *Burkholderia cepacia*), some species for which no disk test standards exist (e.g., *Corynebacterium* spp. and *Bacillus* spp.), and some species with mechanisms

of diminished susceptibility for which MICs are needed to guide selection of therapy and appropriate dosing (e.g., penicillin- and cephalosporin-intermediate *Streptococcus pneumoniae*) (22, 35, 43, 44, 53, 54, 68–70).

There may also be the misconception that physicians prefer a quantitative (MIC) result rather than a report of a susceptibility category. To the contrary, few physicians other than those that specialize in infectious diseases have the training or experience to reliably interpret MICs. For that reason, the laboratory is obliged to provide a category interpretation (susceptible, intermediate, or resistant) with each MIC result in order to avoid potential misinterpretation of the data (53). There may be only a limited number of specific clinical indications for determining MICs to assist in patient management. These include primarily testing of isolates from patients with endocarditis or osteomyelitis (22). At this time, the pharmacodynamic principles that relate the importance of the level of antibiotic in serum in relation to the MIC for an organism are useful in determining interpretive breakpoints but are not generally used to optimize therapy for individual patients (23, 31). For research purposes, MICs are useful for evaluating relative degrees of susceptibility of bacteria to various antimicrobial agents and for comparing the rank order of activities of drugs against various species. For clinical laboratory purposes, however, the decision as to whether to perform dilution or disk diffusion testing is usually based on logistical reasons, including ease of performance of a method, its cost, and factors such as selection of a system that can both identify common bacteria and perform susceptibility testing (42). Several commercial systems are now available for performing susceptibility testing; however, a major challenge posed by such systems is the inflexibility of the standard panels of antimicrobial agents that can be tested. The inability to match precisely an institution's antimicrobial agent formulary with drugs readily available in commercial systems has led some laboratories to adopt or retain the highly flexible disk diffusion test for routine use (41).

The selection of antibacterial agents for testing is complicated by the large number of agents available today. Many of these compounds, however, exhibit similar if not identical activities in vitro, so that in some cases, one compound can be tested as a surrogate for one or more closely related compounds. Such extrapolations, which have generally been agreed upon internationally, are listed

---

*This chapter contains information presented in chapter 118 by James H. Jorgensen, John D. Turnidge, and John A. Washington in the seventh edition of this Manual.

in Table 1. Use of these drug surrogates can substantially reduce the number of agents required for testing and in some cases can provide necessary flexibility in adapting commercial test systems for routine use in a variety of institutions. For instance, the susceptibility of a staphylococcus to oxacillin can be extrapolated to indicate the susceptibility of the organism to all currently available penicillinase-stable penicillins, cephalosporins, and carbapenems. It is thus unnecessary to test any of the agents in these chemical classes, with the exception of the beta-lactamase-labile compounds (e.g., penicillin, ampicillin, amoxicillin, and piperacillin) represented by penicillin itself (53, 54). Other extrapolations are possible, especially if there is demonstrated susceptibility to an early member of the chemical class of antimicrobial agent.

It is important that the microbiologist work with the hospital formulary committee to ensure that the antibacterial agents being tested in the laboratory reflect those in the institution's formulary (41). Failure to do so can contribute to antibiotic misuse (57). Guidelines for the selection of antibacterial agents to be tested are routinely published annually by the NCCLS (formerly called the National Committee for Clinical Laboratory Standards) (55) and are summarized in Table 2. While this listing is sometimes regarded rigidly as the standard for selection of those agents to be tested, it should be emphasized that it is a list of agents that should be considered for routine testing only and that many variables go into the decision as to what agents should be tested in any particular setting (41). The NCCLS also cautions that the decision as to which agents should be tested and reported on selectively should be made by the clinical microbiologist in conjunction with the infectious disease practitioner, the pharmacy, and/or the infection control committee (53, 54, 55).

DILUTION METHODS

Dilution susceptibility testing methods are used to determine the minimal concentration, usually in micrograms per milliliter, of antimicrobial agent required to inhibit or kill a microorganism. Procedures for determining antimicrobial inhibitory activity can be carried out by either agar- or broth-based methods. Antimicrobial agents are usually tested at $\log_2$ (twofold) serial dilutions, and the lowest concentration that inhibits the visible growth of an organism is regarded as the MIC. The concentration range used may vary with the drug, the organism being tested, and the site of infection. Ranges should include concentrations that allow determinations of the interpretive categories (i.e., susceptible, intermediate, and resistant) and also the ranges that encompass the expected MICs for quality control reference strains. Other dilution methods include those that test a single or a selected few concentrations of antimicrobial agents (i.e., breakpoint susceptibility testing and single-drug-concentration screens; see below).

Dilution methods offer flexibility in the sense that the standard medium used to test frequently encountered organisms (e.g., staphylococci, enterococci, members of the family *Enterobacteriaceae*, and *Pseudomonas aeruginosa*) may be supplemented or even replaced with another medium to allow accurate testing of various fastidious bacterial species not reliably tested by disk diffusion. Dilution methods are also adaptable to automated systems. In addition, if plates or panels are prepared in-house, the combination of antimicrobial agents to be included is not limited. Any drug available in powder form may be used.

The flexibility of dilution testing is also evident in the reporting formats that may be used. Quantitative results (MICs in micrograms per milliliter) or category results

TABLE 1 Antibacterial susceptibility results that may be extrapolated from other test results

Test drug (result)	Organism(s)	Drugs to which result can be extrapolated
Penicillin G	*Staphylococcus* spp., *Neisseria gonorrhoeae*	Phenoxymethylpenicillin, phenethicillin, ampicillin, amoxicillin, bacampicillin, cyclacillin, hetacillin, carbenicillin, mezlocillin, azlocillin, ticarcillin, piperacillin
Ampicillin	All	Amoxicillin, bacampicillin, cyclacillin, hetacillin
Ampicillin	*Enterococcus* spp.	Penicillin
Oxacillin	*Staphylococcus* spp.	All penicillins including antistaphylococcal penicillins, all cephalosporins, all beta-lactamase inhibitor combinations, all carbapenems, loracarbef
Cephalothin	*Enterobacteriaceae*	Cephapirin, cephradine, cephalexin, cefaclor, and cefadroxil but not other cephalosporins
Erythromycin	Gram-positive cocci	Azithromycin, clarithromycin, dirithromycin, roxithromyxin
Clindamycin	All	Lincomycin
Tetracycline	All (except *Staphylococcus* and *Acinetobacter* spp.)	Doxycycline, minocycline chlortetracycline, demeclocycline, oxytetracycline, methacycline
Sulfisoxazole	All	All sulfonamides
Cephalothin or cefazolin (susceptible)	*Enterobacteriaceae*	Susceptibility to broad-spectrum cephalosporins

TABLE 2 Antimicrobial agents recommended for routine dilution and disk diffusion susceptibility testing[a]

Antimicrobial agent	Group[b] recommended for testing			
	Enterobacteriaceae	Pseudomonas spp. and other non-Enterobacteriaceae	Staphylococci	Enterococci
Penicillins				
Penicillin G			A	A[c,d]
Ampicillin	A			A[c]
Oxacillin[e] or methicillin				A
Ticarcillin[c]	B	A		
Mezlocillin[c]	B	A		
Piperacillin	B	A		
Ampicillin-sulbactam	B			
Amoxicillin-clavulanic acid	B			
Piperacillin-tazobactam	B			
Ticarcillin-clavulanic acid	B	B[f]		
Cephalosporins				
Cephalothin	A[g]			
Cefazolin	A			
Cefamandole	B			
Cefonicid	B			
Cefuroxime	B			
Cefmetazole	B			
Cefoperazone	B	B		
Cefoxitin	B			
Cefotetan	B			
Cefotaxime	B			
Ceftriaxone	B			
Ceftizoxime	B	U		
Ceftazidime	C	A		
Cefepime	B	B		
Other beta-lactams				
Imipenem	B	B		
Meropenem	B	B		
Aztreonam	C	B		
Aminoglycosides[h]				
Gentamicin	A	A	C	C[h]
Netilmicin	C	C		
Tobramycin	C	B		
Amikacin	B	B		
Streptomycin				C[h]
Macrolides				
Azithromycin			B	
Clarithromycin			B	
Erythromycin			B	C
Quinolones				
Ciprofloxacin	B	B	C	U
Gatifloxacin	U		C	
Levofloxacin	B	U	C	U
Lomefloxacin	U	U	U	
Norfloxacin	U	U	U	U
Ofloxacin	U	U	C	
Miscellaneous				
Chloramphenicol	C	C	C	C
Fosfomycin	U			U
Clindamycin			B	
Linezolid			B	B

(Continued on next page)

TABLE 2 *(Continued)*

Antimicrobial agent	Group[b] recommended for testing			
	Enterobacteriaceae	*Pseudomonas* spp. and other non-*Enterobacteriaceae*	Staphylococci	Enterococci
Miscellaneous *(Continued)*				
Mecillinam	U			
Nitrofurantoin	U		U	U
Quinupristin-dalfopristin			C	B
Rifampin			C	C
Sulfisoxazole	U		U	
Tetracycline	C	U[i]	C[i]	U
Trimethoprim-sulfamethoxazole	B	B	B	
Trimethoprim	U		U	
Vancomycin			B	B[d]

[a] Modified from NCCLS standards (53, 54, 55), with permission. Current standards and supplements to them may be obtained from the NCCLS, 940 West Valley Rd., Suite 1400, Wayne, PA 19087-1898.

[b] Group A comprises primary drugs to be tested and reported, group B comprises those to be tested as primary drugs but reported selectively, group C comprises supplemental drugs to be reported selectively, and group U comprises drugs to be tested against urinary isolates only.

[c] Results of tests with penicillin apply to other penicillins (e.g., ampicillin, amoxicillin, carboxypenicillins, and ureidopenicillins) against beta-lactamase-negative enterococci.

[d] Combination therapy consisting of penicillin, ampicillin, or vancomycin and an aminoglycoside is recommended.

[e] Staphylococci resistant to the penicillinase-resistant penicillins should also be considered resistant to penicillins, beta-lactam–beta-lactamase inhibitor combinations, cephalosporins, and carbapenems.

[f] Ticarcillin-clavulanic acid or piperacillin-tazobactam should not be considered a therapeutic alternative for *P. aeruginosa* isolates resistant to carboxy- or ureidopenicillins.

[g] Cephalothin test results may also be used to represent cephapirin, cephradine, cephalexin, cefaclor, cefadroxil, and cefazolin (except against the members of the family *Enterobacteriaceae*). Cefuroxime, cefixime, cefpodoxime, cefprozil, ceftibuten, and loracarbef may be tested separately on a supplemental basis because their activities may be greater than those of cephalothin or cefazolin against the *Enterobacteriaceae*.

[h] For use of aminoglycosides to screen enterococci for synergy resistance, see the sections "Breakpoint Susceptibility Tests" and "Resistance Screens."

[i] Doxycycline or minocycline may be tested on a supplemental basis because of their greater activities against some nonfermentative gram-negative bacilli and staphylococci.

(susceptible, intermediate, or resistant), or both, can be used (53).

DILUTION TESTING: AGAR METHOD

Dilution of Antimicrobial Agents

The solvents and diluents needed to prepare stock solutions of most commonly used antimicrobial agents are presented in the NCCLS document on dilution testing (53).

Preparation, Supplementation, and Storage of Media

Mueller-Hinton agar is the recommended medium for the testing of most commonly encountered aerobic and facultatively anaerobic bacteria (53). The dehydrated agar base is commercially available and should be prepared as described by the manufacturer. Before sterilization, the molten agar is usually distributed into screw-cap tubes in exact aliquots sufficient to dilute the desired antimicrobial concentrations 10-fold. Tubes, one for each drug concentration to be tested, are sterilized by autoclaving at 121°C for 15 min and are allowed to equilibrate to 48 to 50°C in a preheated water bath. Once the tubes are equilibrated, the appropriate volume of antimicrobial agent is added; and the contents of the tubes are mixed by gentle inversion, poured into 100-mm round or square sterile plastic petri plates set on a level surface, and allowed to solidify. For growth controls, plates containing drug-free agar are also prepared. All plates should be poured to a depth of 3 to 4 mm (20 to 25 ml of agar per round plate and 30 ml for square plates), and the pH of each batch should be checked to confirm the acceptable pH range of 7.2 to 7.4 (53).

After sterilization and temperature equilibration of the molten agar, any necessary supplements are aseptically added to the Mueller-Hinton agar. For the testing of streptococci, supplementation with 5% defibrinated sheep or horse blood is recommended (53). However, sheep blood supplementation may antagonize the activities of sulfonamide and trimethoprim against some organisms (12). The presence of blood also affects the results obtained for novobiocin and nafcillin as well as the in vitro activities of cephalosporins against enterococci (16, 61); therefore, blood supplementation should not be used unless necessary for bacterial growth (see chapter 71 for acceptable methods for the testing of fastidious bacterial species). The performance standards of Mueller-Hinton agar have been defined sufficiently such that calcium and magnesium supplementation should not be done (52). The agar should be supplemented with 2% NaCl for the testing of methicillin, nafcillin, or oxacillin against staphylococci (37).

Once prepared, the plates should be sealed in plastic bags and stored at 4 to 8°C. In general, they should be used within 5 days of preparation or as long as the MICs for control strains that are tested routinely are within the acceptable ranges. However, certain agents, e.g., imipenem, cefaclor, and clavulanic acid combinations, are sufficiently labile that plates may not be stored prior to use. Before inoculation, plates that have been stored under refrigeration should be allowed to equilibrate to room temperature, and the agar surface should be dry.

Inoculation Procedures

Variations in inoculum size may substantially affect MIC endpoint determinations; therefore, careful inoculum standardization is required to obtain accurate results. The recommended final inoculum for agar dilution is 10^4 CFU per spot (53). This may be achieved in either of two ways. Four or five colonies are picked from overnight growth on agar-based medium and inoculated into 4 to 5 ml of suitable broth that will support good growth (usually tryptic soy broth). Broths are incubated at 35°C until they are visibly turbid, and then the suspension is diluted until it matches the turbidity of a barium sulfate or equivalent 0.5 McFarland turbidity standard (ca. 10^8 CFU/ml). The standard may be purchased or may be prepared as described in the NCCLS standard (53). The accuracy of the density of the standard should be verified by using a spectrophotometer with a 1-cm light path; for the 0.5 McFarland standard, the absorbance at 625 nm should be 0.08 to 0.10 (53). An alternative inoculum standardization method, one that is preferred by many microbiologists, uses direct suspension of colonies from overnight growth on a nonselective agar medium in broth or saline to a turbidity that matches that of the 0.5 McFarland standard. This approach eliminates the time needed for growing the inoculum in broth (53). In either case, sterile broth or normal saline is used to make a 1:10 dilution of the suspension to give an adjusted concentration of 10^7 CFU/ml (53).

Once the adjusted inoculum is prepared, inoculation of the antimicrobial agent plates should be accomplished within 30 min, since longer delays may lead to changes in inoculum size. By using either a pipette, a calibrated loop, or, more commonly, an inoculum replicating device, 0.001 to 0.002 ml (1 to 2 μl) of the suspension of 10^7 CFU/ml is delivered to the agar surface, resulting in the final desired inoculum of approximately 10^4 CFU per spot. For convenience, use of a replicator is preferred, because a consistent inoculum volume for up to 36 different isolates is simultaneously delivered (66). To use this device, an aliquot of the adjusted inoculum for each isolate is pipetted into the appropriate well of an inoculum seed plate and a multiprong inoculator is used to pick up and gently transfer 0.001 to 0.002 ml from the wells to the agar surfaces. The surface of the agar plates must be dry before inoculation, which should begin with the lowest drug concentration. To check the viability of each test isolate and also as an added check for purity, control plates that do not contain drug are inoculated last. Finally, plates should be clearly marked so that the locations of the different isolates being tested on each plate are known.

Incubation

Inoculated plates are allowed to stand for several minutes until the inocula have been completely absorbed by the medium; then they are inverted and incubated in air at 35°C for 16 to 20 h before being read. To facilitate detection of vancomycin-resistant enterococci and methicillin-resistant or vancomycin-intermediate staphylococci, plates containing vancomycin and either oxacillin or methicillin, respectively, should be incubated for a full 24 h before being read (53). Incubation should not be carried out in the presence of increased levels of CO_2 unless a fastidious organism is being tested (see chapter 71).

Interpretation and Reporting of Results

Before reading and recording of the results obtained with clinical isolates, those obtained with applicable quality control strains tested at the same time should be checked to ensure that their values are within the acceptable ranges (see "Quality Control" below), and the drug-free control plates should be examined for isolate viability and purity.

Endpoints for each antimicrobial agent are best determined by placing the plates on a dark background and examining the plates for the lowest concentration that inhibits visible growth, which is recorded as the MIC. A single colony or a faint haze left by the initial inoculum should not be regarded as growth. If two or more colonies persist at antimicrobial concentrations beyond an otherwise obvious endpoint or if there is no growth at lower concentrations but growth at higher concentrations, the isolate should be subcultured to confirm its purity and the test should be repeated. Substances that may antagonize the antibacterial activities of sulfonamides and trimethoprim may be carried over with the inoculum and cause "trailing," or less definite endpoints (12, 16). Therefore, the MICs of these antimicrobial agents should be interpreted as the endpoint at which 80% or more diminution of growth occurs. Although much less pronounced, trailing endpoints may also occur for some organisms with bacteriostatic agents such as chloramphenicol, the tetracyclines, linezolid, and quinupristin-dalfopristin.

The MIC of each antimicrobial agent is usually recorded in micrograms per milliliter. These quantitative results should be reported with the appropriate corresponding interpretive categories (susceptible, intermediate, or resistant), or the interpretive category may be reported alone. The MIC interpretive standards for these susceptibility categories, as currently recommended by the NCCLS (53), are provided in Table 3. For detailed instructions concerning the use of these criteria and categories, the latest NCCLS standards for dilution testing methods should be consulted (43, 55). Note that the interpretive standards for most of the penicillin-class drugs vary with the organism being tested.

The three interpretive categories are defined as follows. Susceptible indicates that an infection caused by the tested microorganism may be appropriately treated with the usually recommended dose of antibiotic. Intermediate indicates that the isolate may be inhibited by attainable concentrations of certain drugs (e.g., beta-lactams) if higher dosages can be used safely or if the infection involves a body site in which the drug is physiologically concentrated (e.g., the urinary tract). The intermediate category also serves as a buffer zone that prevents slight technical artifacts from causing major interpretive discrepancies. Resistant isolates are not inhibited by the concentration of antimicrobial agent normally achievable with the recommended dose and/or yield results that fall within a range in which specific resistance mechanisms are likely to be present (53).

Advantages and Disadvantages

Dilution testing by the agar method is a well-standardized, reliable susceptibility-testing technique that may be used as a reference for evaluating the accuracies of other testing systems. In addition, the simultaneous testing of a large number of isolates with a few drugs is efficient (such as when new agents are evaluated in the pharmaceutical industry), and microbial contamination or heterogeneity is more readily detected by agar methods than by broth methods. The agar dilution method is considered the reference test method in most of Europe (32), while the broth microdilution method is much more widely used for research and clinical purposes in North America (40). The major disadvantages of the agar method are associated with the time-consuming and labor-intensive tasks of preparing the plates, especially as the number of different antimicrobial

TABLE 3 Interpretive standards for dilution and disk diffusion susceptibility testing[a]

Antimicrobial agent and organism	MIC (μg/ml)			Zone diam (mm)		
	Susceptible	Intermediate	Resistant	Susceptible	Intermediate	Resistant
Penicillins						
Penicillin G						
Staphylococci[b]	≤0.12		≥0.25	≥29		≤28
Enterococci[c]	≤8		≥16	≥15		≤14
Methicillin[d]	≤8		≥16	≥14	10–13	≤9
Oxacillin[d]						
S. aureus	≤2		≥4	≥13	11–12	≤10
Coagulase-negative staphylococci	≤0.25		≥0.5	≥18		≤17
Ampicillin						
Enterobacteriaceae	≤8	16	≥32	≥17	14–16	≤13
Staphylococci	≤0.25		≥0.5	≥29		≤28
Enterococci[c]	≤8		≥16	≥17		≤16
Amoxicillin-clavulanic acid						
Staphylococci	≤4/2		≥8/4	≥20		≤19
Other organisms	≤8/4	16/8	≥32/16	≥18	14–17	≤13
Ampicillin-sulbactam	≤8/4	16/8	≥32/16	≥15	12–14	≤11
Azlocillin	≤64		≥128	≥18		≤17
P. aeruginosa						
Carbenicillin						
P. aeruginosa	≤128	256	≥512	≥17	14–16	≤13
Other gram-negative bacilli	≤16	32	≥64	≥23	20–22	≤19
Mecillinam	≤8	16	≥32	≥15	12–14	≤11
Mezlocillin						
P. aeruginosa	≤64		≥128	≥16		≤15
Other gram-negative bacilli	≤16	32–64	≥128	≥21	18–20	≤17
Piperacillin						
P. aeruginosa	≤64		≥128	≥18		≤17
Other gram-negative bacilli	≤16	32–64	≥128	≥21	18–20	≤17
Piperacillin-tazobactam						
P. aeruginosa	≤64/4		≥128/4	≥18		≤17
Other gram-negative bacilli	≤16/4	32/4–64/4	≥128/4	≥21	18–20	≤17
Staphylococci	≤8/4		≥16/4	≥18		≤17
Ticarcillin						
P. aeruginosa	≤64		≥128	≥15		≤14
Other gram-negative bacilli	≤16	32–64	≥128	≥20	15–19	≤14
Ticarcillin-clavulanic acid						
P. aeruginosa	≤64/2		≥128/2	≥15		≤14
Other gram-negative bacilli	≤16/2	32/2–64/2	≥128/2	≥20	15–19	≤14
Staphylococci	≤8/2		≥16/2	≥23		≤22
Cephalosporins						
Cefaclor	<8	16	≥32	≥18	15–17	≤14
Cefamandole	≤8	16	≥32	≥18	15–17	≤14
Cefazolin	≤8	16	≥32	≥18	15–17	≤14
Cefepime	≤8	16	≥32	≥18	15–17	≤14
Cefetamet	≤4	8	≥16	≥18	15–17	≤14
Cefixime	≤1	2	≥4	≥19	16–18	≤15

(Continued on next page)

TABLE 3 Interpretive standards for dilution and disk diffusion susceptibility testing[a] *(Continued)*

Antimicrobial agent and organism	MIC (µg/ml)			Zone diam (mm)		
	Susceptible	Intermediate	Resistant	Susceptible	Intermediate	Resistant
Cephalosporins *(Continued)*						
Cefmetazole	≤16	32	≥64	≥16	13–15	≤12
Cefonicid	≤8	16	≥32	≥18	15–17	≤14
Cefoperazone	≤16	32	≥64	≥21	16–20	≤15
Cefotaxime	≤8	16–32	≥64	≥23	15–22	≤14
Cefotetan	≤16	32	≥64	≥16	13–15	≤12
Cefoxitin	≤8	16	≥32	≥18	15–17	≤14
Cefpodoxime	≤2	4	≥8	≥21	18–20	≤17
Cefprozil	≤8	16	≥32	≥18	15–17	≤14
Ceftazidime	≤8	16	≥32	≥18	15–17	<14
Ceftibuten	≤8	16	≥32	≥21	18–20	≤17
Ceftizoxime	≤8	16–32	≥64	≥20	15–19	≤14
Ceftriaxone	≤8	16–32	≥64	≥21	14–20	≤13
Cefuroxime axetil	≤4	8–16	≥32	≥23	15–22	≤14
Cefuroxime sodium	≤8	16	≥32	≥18	15–17	≤14
Cephalothin	≤8	16	≥32	≥18	15–17	≤14
Loracarbef	≤8	16	≥32	≥18	15–17	≤14
Moxalactam	≤8	16–32	≥64	≥23	15–22	≤14
Other beta-lactams						
Aztreonam	≤8	16	≥32	≥22	16–21	≤15
Imipenem	≤4	8	≥16	≥16	14–15	≤13
Meropenem	≤4	8	≥16	≥16	14–15	≤13
Aminoglycosides						
Amikacin	≤16	32	≥64	≥17	15–16	≤14
Gentamicin	≤4	8	≥16	≥15	13–14	≤12
Enterococci (high-level resistance)	≤500		>500	≥10	7–9	6
Netilmicin	≤8	16	≥32	≥15	13–14	≤12
Tobramycin	≤4	8	≥16	≥15	13–14	≤12
Streptomycin						
Enterococci (high-level resistance)						
Broth microdilution	≤1,000		>1,000			
Agar based	≤2,000		>2,000	≥10	7–9	6
Glycopeptides						
Teicoplanin	≤8	16	≥32	≥14	11–13	≤10
Vancomycin						
Enterococci	≤4	8–16	≥32	≥17	15–16	≤14
Staphylococci	≤4			≥15	Determine MIC if ≤14	
Macrolides						
Azithromycin	≤2	4	≥8	≥18	14–17	≤13
Clarithromycin	≤2	4	≥8	≥18	14–17	≤13
Dirithromycin	≤2	4	≥8	≥19	16–18	≤15
Erythromycin	≤0.5	1–4	≥8	≥23	14–22	≤13
Quinolones						
Ciprofloxacin	≤1	2	≥4	≥21	16–20	≤15
Enoxacin	≤2	4	≥8	≥18	15–17	≤14

(Continued on next page)

TABLE 3 (Continued)

Antimicrobial agent and organism	MIC (μg/ml)			Zone diam (mm)		
	Susceptible	Intermediate	Resistant	Susceptible	Intermediate	Resistant
Quinolones (Continued)						
Fleroxacin	≤2	4	≥8	≥19	16–18	≤15
Gatifloxacin	≤2	4	≥8	≥18	15–17	≥14
Levofloxacin	≤2	4	≥8	≥17	14–16	≤13
Lomefloxacin	≤2	4	≥8	≥22	19–21	≤18
Nalidixic acid[e]	≤8	16	≥32	≥19	14–18	≤13
Norfloxacin[e]	≤4	8	≥16	≥17	13–16	≤12
Ofloxacin	≤2	4	≥8	≥16	13–15	≥12
Sparfloxacin	≤0.5	1	≥2	≥19	16–18	≥15
Tetracyclines						
Doxycycline	≤4	8	≥16	≥16	13–15	≤12
Minocycline	≤4	8	≥16	≥19	15–18	≤14
Tetracycline	≤4	8	≥16	≥19	15–18	≤14
Other						
Chloramphenicol	≤8	16	≥32	≥18	13–17	≤12
Clindamycin	≤0.5	1–2	≥4	≥21	15–20	≤14
Fosfomycin	≤64	128	≥256	≥16	13–15	≤12
Linezolid						
Enterococci	≤2	4	≥8	≥23	19–22	≤20
Staphylococci	≤2			≥21		
Nitrofurantoin	≤32	64	≥128	≥17	15–16	≤14
Quinupristin-dalfopristin	≤1	2	≥4	≥19	16–18	≤15
Rifampin	≤1	2	≥4	≥20	17–19	≤16
Sulfonamide	≤256		≥512	≥17	13–16	≤12
Trimethoprim[e]	≤8		≥16	≥16	11–15	≤10
Trimethoprim-sulfamethoxazole	≤2/38		≥4/76	≥16	11–15	≤10

[a] Adapted from NCCLS data (53, 54, 55), with permission. The interpretive data are valid only if the methodologies in documents M2-A7 (54) and M7-A5 (53) are followed. NCCLS frequently updates the interpretive tables through new additions of the standards and supplements to them. Users should refer to the most recent additions. The current standards and supplements to them may be obtained from the NCCLS, 940 West Valley Rd., Suite 1400, Wayne, PA 19087-1898.

[b] Penicillin should be used as the class representative for all penicillins (e.g., ampicillin, amoxicillin, mezlocillin, piperacillin, and ticarcillin). Isolates for which MICs are ≤0.03 μg of penicillin per ml generally do not produce a beta-lactamase, whereas those for which MICs are ≥0.25 μg/ml do and should be regarded as resistant to penicillins. Isolates for which penicillin MICs are 0.06 or 0.12 μg/ml should be tested for beta-lactamase.

[c] Therapy for serious enterococcal infections requires high doses of penicillin or ampicillin in combination with an aminoglycoside. Vancomycin may be substituted for the penicillin in instances of penicillin hypersensitivity or of penicillin or ampicillin resistance.

[d] Oxacillin or methicillin may be tested; however, oxacillin is preferred because of its greater stability in vitro. The results from the testing of oxacillin apply also to other penicillinase-resistant penicillins. Oxacillin-resistant staphylococci should be considered resistant to all penicillins, cephalosporins, carbacephems, carbapenems, and beta-lactam–beta-lactamase inhibitor combinations.

[e] For the treatment of urinary tract infections only.

agents to be tested against each isolate increases or if only a few isolates are to be tested.

DILUTION TESTING: BROTH METHODS

The general approaches for broth methods include broth macrodilution, in which the broth volume for each antimicrobial concentration is ≥1.0 ml (usually 2 ml) and is contained in 13- by 100-mm tubes, and broth microdilution, in which antimicrobial dilutions are most often in 0.1-ml volumes contained in wells of microdilution trays.

Broth Macrodilution Methods

Dilution of Antimicrobial Agents

Stock solutions are prepared as discussed in the NCCLS document on dilution testing (53) and are similar to those used for agar dilution tests. As in the agar method, the

actual volumes used for the dilutions would be proportionally increased according to the number of tests being prepared, with a minimum of 1.0 ml needed for each drug concentration. Because addition of the inoculum results in a 1:2 dilution of each concentration, all final drug concentrations must be prepared at twice the actual desired testing concentration (see "Inoculation Procedures" below).

Preparation, Supplementation, and Storage of Media

Cation-adjusted Mueller-Hinton broth (CAMHB) is recommended for the routine testing of commonly encountered nonfastidious organisms (53). Adjustment with the cations Ca^{2+} (20 to 25 mg/liter) and Mg^{2+} (10 to 12.5 mg/liter) is required to ensure acceptable results when aminoglycosides are tested against P. aeruginosa isolates and when tetracycline is tested against other bacteria. However, for convenience and consistency, cation adjustment of Mueller-Hinton broth is now recommended when testing all species and antimicrobial agents (53). Some manufacturers provide Mueller-Hinton broth that already has appropriate concentrations of divalent cations, so the cation content of commercial dehydrated media must be ascertained and care must be taken to supplement the broth with the appropriate cation levels. If adjustment is necessary, it can be accomplished by the addition of suitable volumes of filter-sterilized, chilled CaCl$_2$ stock (3.68 g of CaCl$_2 \cdot$ 2H$_2$O dissolved in 100 ml of deionized water for a concentration of 10 mg of Ca^{2+} per ml) and MgCl$_2$ stock (8.36 g of MgCl$_2 \cdot$ 6H$_2$O in 100 ml of deionized water for a concentration of 10 mg of Mg^{2+} per ml) to the cooled broth (8, 53). Insufficient cation concentrations result in increased aminoglycoside activity (25), while an excess cation content results in decreased aminoglycoside activity against *P. aeruginosa* (7, 25). While the effects of inappropriate calcium and magnesium ion contents are well recognized, other ions, including zinc and manganese, may adversely affect the activities of some drugs, e.g., carbapenems. The NCCLS is developing a consensus standard for manufacturers of Mueller-Hinton broth that attempts to specify all known factors that determine the performance of the medium. Reliable detection of staphylococcal resistance to oxacillin, methicillin, or nafcillin requires that the CAMHB used to test these drugs be supplemented with 2% NaCl (53, 71).

To minimize evaporation and deterioration of antimicrobial agents, tubes should be tightly capped and stored at 4 to 8°C until needed. With most agents, the dilutions should be used within 5 days of preparation or as long as quality control ranges are maintained (see "Quality Control" below). As with agar dilution testing, certain beta-lactam agents are too labile for prolonged storage in final test concentrations.

Inoculation Procedures

The recommended final inoculum is 5 × 10^5 CFU/ml. Isolates are inoculated into a broth that will support good growth (such as tryptic soy broth) and are incubated until they are turbid. The turbidity is adjusted to match that of a 0.5 McFarland standard (approximately 10^8 CFU/ml). Alternatively, four or five colonies from overnight growth on a nonselective agar plate may be directly suspended in broth so that the turbidity matches the turbidity of the McFarland standard (53). This alternative is preferred for the testing of methicillin or oxacillin against staphylococci (53). A portion of the standardized suspension is diluted 1:100 (10^6 CFU/ml) with broth. When 1 ml of this dilution is added to each tube containing 1 ml of the drug diluted in CAMHB, a final inoculum of 5 × 10^5 CFU/ml is achieved. Broth not containing an antimicrobial agent is inoculated as a control for organism viability (growth control). All tubes should be inoculated within 30 min of inoculum preparation, and an aliquot of the inoculum should be plated to check for purity and inoculum density.

Incubation

Tubes are incubated in air at 35°C for 16 to 20 h before the MICs are determined. Incubation should be extended to a full 24 h for the detection of vancomycin-resistant enterococci or methicillin-resistant or vancomycin-intermediate staphylococci (53). Use of increased levels of CO$_2$ is not recommended.

Interpretation and Reporting of Results

Before the MICs for the test strains are read and recorded, the growth controls should be examined for viability, inoculum subcultures should be checked for contamination and appropriate inoculum size, and it should be confirmed that the MICs for the quality control strains are appropriate (see "Quality Control" below). Growth or a lack thereof in the antimicrobial agent-containing tubes is best determined by comparison with the growth control. Generally, growth is indicated by turbidity, a single sedimented button ≥2 mm in diameter, or several buttons with smaller diameters. As with the agar method, trailing endpoints may be seen when trimethoprim or sulfonamides are tested, and the concentration at which 80% or greater diminution of growth compared with that of the growth control occurs should be recorded as the MIC (53). Other interpretation problems include the "skipped tube" phenomenon, in which growth is not observed at one concentration but is observed at lower and higher drug concentrations. Most authorities suggest that when this occurs, the skipped tube should be ignored and the concentration that finally inhibits growth at serially higher concentrations should be recorded as the MIC. If more than one skipped tube occurs or if there is growth in the presence of higher antimicrobial concentrations but not lower ones, the results should not be reported and the test for that drug should be repeated.

The lowest concentration that completely inhibits visible growth of the organism as detected by the unaided eye is recorded as the MIC. The latest NCCLS MIC interpretive standards (55) for the susceptibility categories are provided in Table 3. The definitions of and comments concerning these categories that were given for the agar method also pertain to the broth macrodilution method.

Advantages and Disadvantages

The broth macrodilution method is a well-standardized and reliable reference method that is useful for research purposes or if the testing of the activity of only one drug against a bacterial isolate is needed. However, because of the laborious nature of the procedure and the availability of more convenient dilution systems (i.e., microdilution), this procedure is generally not useful for routine susceptibility testing in most clinical microbiology laboratories.

Broth Microdilution Method

The convenience afforded by the availability of dilution susceptibility testing in microdilution trays has led to the widespread use of broth microdilution methods. The disposable, plastic trays contain a panel of several antimicrobial agents to be tested simultaneously and may be prepared in-house or obtained commercially either frozen or freeze-dried. When commercial systems are used, the manufacturers' recommendations concerning storage, inoculation, incubation, and interpretation should be followed. The primary focus of this section will be the in-house preparation and use of broth microdilution panels. However, most of the principles and practices discussed here are pertinent to the broth microdilution method regardless of the source of the antibiotic panels.

Dilution of Antimicrobial Agents

Antimicrobial stock solutions are prepared as outlined in the NCCLS document on dilution testing (53). The dilution scheme used for agar and broth macrodilution methods is applicable to the antimicrobial dilutions needed for the preparation of broth microdilution panels. A limited number of automated dispensing systems are available and require that at least 10 ml of broth containing each antimicrobial concentration be prepared. From the 10- to 200-ml samples, aliquots of 0.05 or 0.1 ml are simultaneously dispensed to the corresponding wells of each broth microdilution tray with a mechanized dispenser. If 0.05-ml volumes are dispensed, allowances must be made for the 1:2 dilution of the final drug concentration that will occur when the 0.05 ml of inoculum is added (see "Inoculation Procedures" below). When 0.1-ml aliquots are dispensed, the volume of inoculum normally used is sufficiently small ($\leq$0.005 ml) that adjustments in the antimicrobial dilution scheme are not needed. As a general rule, when the inoculum volume is less than 10% of the broth volume in the well, dilution of the antimicrobial concentration by the inoculum does not have to be taken into account (53).

Preparation, Supplementation, and Storage of Media

CAMHB is the recommended medium for broth microdilution testing of nonfastidious organisms and should be prepared as discussed above for the broth macrodilution method. Also, supplementation of the broth with 2% NaCl is required for detection of oxacillin- or methicillin-resistant staphylococci (53). After the antimicrobial dilutions have been dispensed into the plastic trays, they are stacked in groups of 5 to 10, with a tray lid or an empty tray placed on top to minimize contamination and evaporation. Each stack is sealed in a plastic bag and is immediately frozen at $-20°C$ or, preferably, at $-60°C$ or colder. At $-20°C$, preservation is ensured for at least 6 weeks with most drugs, but the shelf life may be extended to months if the trays are stored at -60 to $-70°C$. Exceptions include highly labile compounds such as cefaclor, clavulanic acid, and imipenem, which may not retain their potencies during storage. If thawed, panels must be used or discarded, but not refrozen, since freeze-thaw cycles cause substantial deterioration of beta-lactam antibiotics. For this reason, $-20°C$ household-type freezers with self-defrosting units must not be used.

Inoculation Procedures

As with the macrodilution procedure, the final desired inoculum concentration is 5×10^5 CFU/ml. The isolates may be grown in broth so that the turbidity matches the turbidity of a 0.5 McFarland standard (ca. 1×10^8 to 2×10^8 CFU/ml), or a suspension of that density can be made from colonies grown on a nonselective agar medium following overnight growth (8), which is the method preferred for the detection of methicillin-resistant staphylococci (53). For broth microdilution procedures that require 0.001- to 0.005-ml volumes to inoculate wells containing 0.1 ml of broth, a portion of the suspension with a turbidity matching that of a 0.5 McFarland standard is diluted 1:10 (10^7 CFU/ml) in sterile saline or broth. Multipoint metal or disposable plastic inoculum replicators designed to collect and deliver appropriate volumes are used to transfer the inoculum from the diluted suspension to the wells of the broth microdilution tray, resulting in further dilutions ranging from 1:20 to 1:50, and final inoculum concentrations should be 4×10^5 to 6×10^5 CFU/ml (4×10^4 to 6×10^4 CFU per well). For protocols that use an inoculum volume of 0.05 ml to inoculate 0.05 ml of broth, a 1:100 dilution of a suspension with a turbidity matching that of a 0.5 McFarland standard (ca. 10^6 CFU/ml) is used. When the inoculum is added to the wells, the 1:2 dilution of the inoculum of 1×10^6 CFU/ml results in a final inoculum concentration of 5×10^5 CFU/ml (5×10^4 CFU per well) and also halves the antibiotic concentration in each well. Special care should be taken to confirm the inoculum density on a periodic basis to ensure that the appropriate amount of inoculum is achieved. Moreover, slight deviations from the initial 1:10 dilution described above may be necessary to provide the target inoculum density with some species or organism groups. Insufficient inoculum can be a significant problem with inducible resistance mechanisms of some organisms and may not be recognized as a problem on the basis of the MICs obtained for the very susceptible quality control strains.

Broth microdilution trays should be inoculated within 30 min of inoculum preparation; during preparation, an aliquot should be subcultured to check the purity of the isolates, and colony counts should be set up to check the accuracy of the inoculum concentration. Finally, one well of each panel not containing an antimicrobial agent should be inoculated and used as a growth control, and a second uninoculated well serves as a sterility control.

Incubation

After inoculation, each tray should be covered with plastic tape, sealed in a plastic bag, or tightly fitted with a lid or an empty tray to prevent evaporation during incubation. Trays are incubated in air at 35°C for 16 to 20 h before being read and should not be incubated in stacks of more than four trays for uniform temperature distribution. The incubator should be kept sufficiently humid to avoid evaporation but not so humid that condensation results in contamination problems. A full 24 h of incubation is recommended for the detection of vancomycin-resistant enterococci and methicillin-resistant or vancomycin-intermediate staphylococci (53). Use of increased CO_2 levels during incubation is not recommended.

Interpretation and Reporting of Results

Before the MICs for the clinical isolates are read and recorded, the growth control wells should be examined for organism viability. It is advisable to check inoculum purity by subculture and to verify the inoculum size periodically by quantitative subculture. Also, the appropriateness of the MICs for the quality control strains should be confirmed (see "Quality Control" below). Various viewing devices are available and should be used to facilitate examination of the broth microdilution wells for growth. The simplest and most reliable method may be use of a parabolic magnifying mirror and tray stand that allows clear visual inspection of the undersides of the broth microdilution trays. Growth is best determined by comparison with that in the growth control well and generally is indicated by turbidity throughout the well or by buttons, single or multiple, in the well bottom. The occurrence of trailing endpoints with trimethoprim or sulfonamides should be ignored, and the MIC endpoint should be based on $\geq$80% growth inhibition. Results for drugs for which there is more than one skipped well should not be reported, as with the broth macrodilution test.

The latest NCCLS MIC interpretive criteria (55) for susceptibility categories are given in Table 3. It should be noted that these values are published each year, and only the most recent tables should be used for interpretation of results. The definitions of the interpretive categories and the comments concerning the use of these standards for agar and broth macrodilution methods are also applicable to broth microdilution methods.

Advantages and Disadvantages

The use of broth microdilution trays prepared in-house provides a reliable standardized reference method for susceptibility testing. Inoculation and reading procedures allow relatively convenient simultaneous testing of several antimicrobial agents against individual isolates. Few laboratories have the facilities required for the preparation of broth microdilution trays. However, several sources of commercially prepared antibiotic panels are available. Such products provide trays with wells containing prepared antimicrobial dilutions either frozen or freeze-dried. The former types of trays must be stored frozen in the laboratory, whereas dried panels can be stored at room temperature. Most of these products are accompanied by multipoint inoculating devices or multichannel pipettes. Results of testing may be determined by visual examination or by use of semiautomated or automated instrumentation. However, the versatility of the antimicrobial agent selection available with commercial broth microdilution trays is more limited compared with the selection available by preparing panels in-house.

Breakpoint Susceptibility Tests

Breakpoint susceptibility testing refers to methods by which antimicrobial agents are tested only at the specific concentrations necessary for differentiating between the interpretive categories of susceptible, intermediate, and resistant rather than in the range of five or more doubling-dilution concentrations used to determine MICs. When two drug concentrations adjacent to the breakpoints defining the intermediate and resistant categories are selected, any one of the interpretive categories may be determined. Growth at both concentrations indicates resistance, growth at only the lower concentration signifies an intermediate result, and no growth at either concentration is interpreted as susceptibility.

As for full-range dilution testing, breakpoint methods require the use of appropriately adjusted and supplemented Mueller-Hinton broth or agar. In addition, the standard inoculation, incubation, and interpretation procedures recommended for the full-range dilution methods should be followed.

Considering the limited range of drug concentrations tested, a greater number and variety of antimicrobial agents can be incorporated into a broth microdilution panel set up for breakpoint testing than in panels designed for full-range dilution testing (29). However, convenient quality control procedures to ensure that appropriate concentrations of each antimicrobial agent are present are lacking for the panels used for breakpoint testing. One possible approach is to use one organism for which the modal MIC is equal to or no less than 1 doubling dilution less than the lower or lowest concentration tested and a second organism for which the modal MIC is equal to or no more than 1 doubling dilution greater than the higher or highest concentration tested (53). One of these two quality control organisms should provide on-scale results (53). Despite the theoretical soundness of this approach, routine quality control of panels used for breakpoint testing is more complex and is not readily accomplished in the clinical laboratory.

Resistance Screens

In some circumstances, testing of a single drug concentration may be the most reliable and convenient method for the detection of antimicrobial resistance. The most clinically useful resistance screens are those for staphylococcal resistance to oxacillin (or methicillin) and for resistance of *Enterococcus* spp. to vancomycin or high-level resistance to gentamicin and streptomycin (53). These practical and reliable methods are described in chapter 74.

Gradient Diffusion Method

The E test (AB Biodisk, Solna, Sweden) is a method for quantitative antimicrobial susceptibility testing whereby a preformed antimicrobial gradient from a plastic-coated strip diffuses into an agar medium inoculated with the test organism. In this test, the MIC is read directly from a scale on the top of the strip at the point where the ellipse of organism growth inhibition intercepts the strip. Several strips, each containing a different antimicrobial agent, can be placed radially on the surface of a large round Mueller-Hinton agar plate inoculated with a suspension of a bacterial isolate whose turbidity has been adjusted to match that of a 0.5 McFarland turbidity standard. A number of published evaluations (6, 36, 64) have found good agreement between the MICs obtained by the E test and those obtained by reference dilution methods when staphylococci, enterococci, and gram-negative bacilli with a variety of resistance mechanisms were tested. The E test combines the simplicity and flexibility of the disk diffusion test with the ability to determine the MICs of up to five antimicrobial agents on a single large agar plate. However, E test strips are much more expensive than the paper disks used for diffusion testing, and a simple, mechanized method for simultaneous application of E test strips to the agar plate surface has yet to be devised. The strength of the E test method is its ability to determine an MIC of an infrequently tested drug or to test fastidious or anaerobic bacteria, since the strips may be placed onto various enriched media (see chapters 71 and 72).

QUALITY CONTROL

Quality control recommendations are designed to evaluate the precision and accuracy of test procedures, monitor reagent performance, and evaluate the competencies of the individuals who are conducting the tests.

Reference Strains

A critical element to accomplishing the goals of quality control is the selection and use of reference bacterial strains that are genetically stable and for which the MICs of each antimicrobial agent tested are in the middle of the MIC range (53). That is, the dilutions in a series should encompass at least two concentration increments above and below the previously established MIC for the reference strain. If there are four or fewer dilutions in a series or if nonconsecutive dilutions are tested (i.e., if breakpoint susceptibility testing is performed), quality control for the correct interpretive category rather than an actual MIC or MIC ranges may only be accomplished. *Escherichia coli* ATCC 25922, *P. aeruginosa* ATCC 27853, *Enterococcus faecalis* ATCC 29212, and *S. aureus* ATCC 29213 are the recommended reference strains for both agar and broth dilution methods (53). Beta-lactamase-producing strain *E. coli* ATCC 35218 is recommended only for the testing of penicillin–beta-lactamase inhibitor combinations (53). These organisms may be obtained from the American Type Culture Collection or other reliable commercial sources. For proper storage and subculture procedures, the recommendations of either the NCCLS (53) or the commercial provider should be followed.

MIC Ranges

The acceptable quality control MIC ranges for the various reference strains are given in the NCCLS document on dilution testing (53). Updates of these MIC ranges are published annually (55) and should be readily available in each clinical laboratory. An out-of-control result is defined as an MIC not within the acceptable range. Certain out-of-control results can be directly related to the medium used for testing. High MICs of gentamicin for *P. aeruginosa* ATCC 27853 suggest an inappropriately high cation content or an excessively low pH of the Mueller-Hinton medium, and low MICs indicate an insufficient cation concentration or an elevated pH. Although trimethoprim-sulfamethoxazole is not recommended for the treatment of *E. faecalis* infections, results obtained with strain ATCC 29212 are useful for detecting excessive amounts of substances such as thymidine that interfere with the in vitro activities of antifolate drugs. Trimethoprim-sulfamethoxazole MICs of >0.5/9.5 μg/ml indicate the presence of such interfering substances (53).

Batch and Lot Quality Control

Representative plates, panels, or trays from each new batch prepared in-house or from each new shipment lot obtained from a commercial source should be subjected to quality control and sterility testing. MICs obtained by the testing of reference quality control strains should be within acceptable NCCLS ranges (55). If such accuracy is not achieved, the batch or lot should be rejected or the results obtained with the antimicrobial agent(s) in question should not be reported (see below). Similarly, if selected uninoculated plates or trays fail the sterility check after incubation, the batch or lot should be rejected. In addition to these formal quality control procedures that use reference strains, careful review of susceptibility results obtained during daily testing of clinical isolates is important to identify aberrant or unusual susceptibility patterns possibly indicative of reagent or technical problems.

Quality Control Frequency

In addition to batch and lot testing, quality control tests should be performed daily or at least on every day that the plates or trays are being used to test clinical isolates. When quality control is performed on each day of testing, two consecutive out-of-control MICs or more than two nonconsecutive out-of-control values in 20 consecutive tests indicate problems in the dilution testing procedure that must be identified and solved. However, if accuracy can be sufficiently documented as outlined below, daily testing may be replaced by weekly testing (53, 55).

Each drug-reference strain combination is tested for 30 consecutive testing days to obtain a total of 30 MICs for each combination. If three or fewer MICs per combination are outside the accuracy range, weekly testing may replace daily testing. During weekly testing, a single MIC outside the accuracy range requires that daily testing be performed for 5 consecutive days unless there is an obvious source of error (e.g., contamination, use of an incorrect reference strain, use of an incorrect inoculum density, testing of an

incorrect antimicrobial agent, or use of an incorrect atmosphere of incubation). In such a circumstance, the quality control test needs to be repeated only once. If all five MICs for a problem drug-organism combination are within the accuracy range, weekly testing may be resumed. If one or more of the five MICs for the problem drug-organism combination are outside the accuracy range, daily testing must be initiated and further means to resolve the problem must be pursued. Returning to weekly testing again requires documentation of 30 consecutive days in which three or fewer MICs are outside the accuracy range. If more than three MICs per combination are outside the accuracy range, daily quality control testing must be continued while the problem is being resolved (53, 55).

DISK DIFFUSION TESTING

The disk diffusion method of susceptibility testing allows categorization of most bacterial isolates as susceptible, intermediate, or resistant to a variety of antimicrobial agents. To perform the test, commercially prepared filter paper disks impregnated with a specified single concentration of an antimicrobial agent are applied to the surface of an agar medium that has been inoculated with the test organism. The drug in the disk diffuses through the agar (7). As the distance from the disk increases, the concentration of the antimicrobial agent decreases logarithmically, creating a gradient of drug concentrations in the agar medium surrounding each disk. Concomitant with diffusion of the drug, the bacteria that were inoculated on the surface and that are not inhibited by the concentration of antimicrobial agent continue to multiply until a lawn of growth is visible. In areas where the concentration of drug is inhibitory, no growth occurs, forming a zone of inhibition around each disk.

The disk diffusion procedure has been standardized primarily for the testing of common, rapidly growing bacteria (11, 54). This method should not be used to evaluate the antimicrobial susceptibilities of bacteria that show marked strain-to-strain variability in growth rates, e.g., some glucose-nonfermenting gram-negative bacilli and anaerobic bacteria. The test, however, has been modified to allow reliable testing of certain fastidious bacteria (discussed in chapter 71).

The diameter of the zone of inhibition is influenced by the rate of diffusion of the antimicrobial agent through the agar, which may vary among different drugs depending upon the size of the drug molecule and its hydrophilicity. The zone size, however, is inversely proportional to the MIC, measured as discussed earlier in this chapter. Criteria currently recommended for interpreting zone diameters and MIC results for commonly used antimicrobial agents are listed in Table 3 and are published annually by the NCCLS (54, 55).

Establishing Zone of Inhibition Diameter Interpretive Criteria

The first step in determining interpretive criteria for the disk diffusion test is selection of MIC breakpoints that define susceptibility and resistance categories for each antimicrobial agent. The zone-of-inhibition diameters that correspond to these breakpoints are initially established by testing 300 or more bacterial isolates by both dilution and disk diffusion methods and correlating the zone of inhibition diameters and the MICs of each drug tested (51). The isolates tested should include not only those commonly encountered in clinical laboratories but also those with resistance mechanisms pertinent to the class of antimicrobial agent being tested (15, 51). Organisms evaluated should be those most likely to be tested against the antimicrobial agent in question. The data from these studies are analyzed by preparing a scattergram of values (an example is presented in chapter 69). By convention, each MIC ($\log_2$ scale) is plotted on the y axis, and the corresponding zone of inhibition (arithmetic scale) is plotted on the x axis. Regression analysis can be performed, and a straight regression line showing the best fit is drawn. From this line, an approximate MIC can be inferred from any zone of inhibition diameter. For antimicrobial agents to which isolates are either susceptible or resistant and only infrequently intermediate, regression analysis is not valid. In such cases, the data are plotted as a scattergram, and the interpretive standards are selected to allow optimal separation of the two populations (50, 51). This approach, often called the error-rate-bounded method, may also be used to minimize interpretive errors that can ensue from strict application of the linear regression formula to a data set (50).

Antimicrobial Agent Disks

The amounts of the antimicrobial agents in the disks used for agar diffusion testing are standardized, and in the United States, only a single disk for each drug is recommended (54). The optimal amount of antimicrobial agent per disk is determined early in the development of a new drug by testing disks with several different drug contents that can be evaluated in scattergrams and by the development of regression lines (51). The most desirable concentration of drug per disk is that which produces a zone of inhibition diameter of at least 10 mm for resistant isolates and a zone diameter no larger than 30 mm for susceptible isolates.

Commercially prepared antimicrobial disks usually are supplied in separate containers, each with a desiccant. They must not be used beyond the specified expiration date and should be stored under refrigeration (2 to 8°C) or frozen in a non-frost-free freezer at −20°C or colder until needed. Disks containing a beta-lactam agent should always be stored frozen to ensure that they retain their potency, although a small supply may be stored in the refrigerator for up to 1 week. Unopened disk containers should be removed from the refrigerator or freezer 1 to 2 h before use. This allows the disks to equilibrate to room temperature before the container is opened, thus minimizing the amount of condensation that will occur when warm air comes into contact with the cold disks. A commercially available, mechanical disk-dispensing apparatus can be used and should be fitted with a tight cover, supplied with an adequate desiccant, stored in the refrigerator when not in use, and warmed to room temperature before being opened.

Agar Medium

The recommended medium for disk diffusion testing in the United States is Mueller-Hinton agar (54). This unsupplemented medium has been selected by the NCCLS for several reasons: (i) it demonstrates good batch-to-batch reproducibility for susceptibility testing; (ii) it is low in sulfonamide, trimethoprim, and tetracycline inhibitors; (iii) it supports the growth of most nonfastidious bacterial pathogens; and (iv) years of data and clinical experience regarding its performance have been accrued. Fastidious bacteria, such as *Haemophilus* species, *Neisseria gonorrhoeae*, and streptococci, do not grow satisfactorily on unsupple-

mented Mueller-Hinton agar but can be tested by the disk method with supplemented or modified test media, as discussed in chapter 71.

Plates of Mueller-Hinton agar may be purchased, or the agar may be prepared from a commercially available dehydrated base according to the manufacturer's directions. If the agar is prepared, only formulations that have been tested as described by NCCLS and that have met the acceptance limits recommended by the NCCLS should be used (52). The prepared medium is autoclaved and is immediately placed in a 45 to 50°C water bath. When cool, it is poured into round plastic flat-bottom petri dishes on a level surface to give a uniform depth of about 4 mm (60 to 70 ml of medium for 150-mm plates and 25 to 30 ml of medium for 100-mm plates) and allowed to cool to room temperature. Agar deeper than 4 mm may cause false-positive results for resistance (excessively small zones), whereas agar less than 4 mm deep may be associated with excessively large zones and false-positive results for susceptibility.

Each batch of Mueller-Hinton agar should be checked when the medium is prepared to ensure that the pH is between 7.2 and 7.4 at room temperature, which means that the pH must be measured after the medium has solidified. This can be done by allowing a small amount of agar to solidify around the tip of a pH electrode in a beaker or a cup, by macerating a sufficient amount of agar in neutral distilled water, or by using a properly calibrated surface electrode. A pH outside the range of 7.2 to 7.4 may adversely affect susceptibility test results. If the pH is too low, drugs such as the aminoglycosides, macrolides, and fluoroquinolones will appear to lose potency, whereas others (for example, the penicillins and the tetracyclines) may appear to have excessive activity. The opposite effects are possible if the pH is too high.

Freshly prepared plates may be used on the same day or wrapped in plastic to minimize evaporation and stored in a refrigerator (2 to 8°C). Just before use, if excess moisture is visible on the surface, the plates should be placed in an incubator (35°C) or, with lids ajar, in a laminar-flow hood at room temperature until the moisture evaporates (usually 10 to 30 min). At the time the medium is to be inoculated, no droplets of moisture should be visible on its surface or on the petri dish cover.

Various components of or supplements to Mueller-Hinton medium may affect susceptibility test results; therefore, appropriate quality control procedures (see "Quality Control" below) must be performed and zone diameters must be within acceptable limits. For example, media containing excessive amounts of thymidine or thymine can reverse the inhibitory effects of sulfonamides and trimethoprim, causing zones of growth inhibition to be smaller or less distinct. Organisms may therefore appear to be resistant to these drugs when in fact they are not. Variations in the concentrations of divalent cations, primarily calcium and magnesium, affect the results of aminoglycoside, tetracycline, and colistin tests with *P. aeruginosa* isolates (9, 10). A cation content that is too high reduces zone sizes, whereas a cation content that is too low has the opposite effect. Sheep blood should not be added to Mueller-Hinton medium for the testing of nonfastidious organisms, because the blood can significantly alter the zone diameters for several agents and bacterial species (16).

Inoculation Procedure

To ensure the reproducibility of disk diffusion susceptibility test results, the inoculum must be standardized (11, 54). The inoculum may be prepared by the growth method or by direct suspension from colonies on the agar plate, as described above for dilution testing.

When trimethoprim-sulfamethoxazole is tested by the direct inoculum suspension method, colonies from blood agar medium might carry over enough trimethoprim or sulfonamide antagonists to produce a haze of growth inside the zones of inhibition surrounding susceptible isolates.

The Mueller-Hinton agar plate should be inoculated within 15 min after the inoculum suspension has been adjusted. A sterile cotton swab is dipped into the suspension, rotated several times, and gently pressed on the inside wall of the tube above the fluid level to remove excess inoculum from the swab. The swab is then streaked over the entire surface of the agar plate three times, with the plate rotated approximately 60° each time to ensure even distribution of the inoculum. A final sweep of the swab is made around the agar rim. The lid may be left ajar for 3 to 5 min but for no longer than 15 min to allow any excess surface moisture to be absorbed before the drug-impregnated disks are applied.

Antimicrobial Disks

Within 15 min after the plates are inoculated, selected antimicrobial agent disks are distributed evenly on the surface, with at least 24 mm (center to center) between them. The disks are placed individually with sterile forceps or, more commonly, with a mechanical dispensing apparatus and are then gently pressed down onto the agar surface to provide uniform contact. No more than 12 disks should be placed on one 150-mm plate and no more than 5 disks should be placed on a 100-mm plate to avoid overlapping zones. Some of the antimicrobial agent in the disk diffuses almost immediately; therefore, once a disk contacts the agar surface, the disk should not be moved.

Incubation

No longer than 15 min after disks are applied, the plates are inverted and incubated at 35°C in ambient air. A delay of more than 15 min before incubation permits excess prediffusion of the antimicrobial agents. The interpretive standards for nonfastidious bacteria are based on the results of tests with plates incubated in ambient air, and the zone of inhibition diameters for some drugs, such as the aminoglycosides, macrolides, and tetracyclines, are significantly altered by CO_2; therefore, plates should not be incubated in the presence of increased levels of CO_2. Testing of isolates of some fastidious bacteria, however, requires incubation in 5% CO_2, and the zone diameter criteria for those species have been established on that basis (see chapter 69).

Interpretation and Reporting of Results

Each plate is examined after incubation for 16 to 18 h for all nonfastidious bacterial isolates except staphylococci and enterococci, which must be incubated a full 24 h to allow detection of resistance to oxacillin and vancomycin (54). If plates are inoculated correctly, the inhibition zone diameters are uniformly circular and the lawn of growth is confluent. Growth that consists of individual isolated colonies indicates that the inoculum was too light, and the test must be repeated. The diameters of the zones of complete inhibition, including the diameter of the disk, are measured to

the nearest whole millimeter with calipers or a ruler. With unsupplemented Mueller-Hinton agar, the measuring device is held on the back of the inverted petri dish, which is illuminated with reflected light located a few inches above a black, nonreflecting background.

The zone margin is the area where no obvious growth is visible. When isolates of staphylococci or enterococci are tested, any discernible growth (especially a haze of pinpoint colonies) within the zone of inhibition around the oxacillin disk (for staphylococci) or vancomycin disk (for enterococci) is indicative of resistance. For other bacteria, discrete colonies growing within a clear zone of inhibition may indicate testing of a mixed culture, the colonies of which should be subcultured, reidentified, and retested. However, the presence of colonies within a zone of inhibition may also indicate the selection of high-frequency mutants indicative of eventual resistance to that agent, e.g., *Enterobacter* spp. with penicillins and cephalosporins. With *Proteus* species, if a thin film of swarming growth is visible in an otherwise obvious zone of inhibition, the margin of heavy growth is measured and the film is disregarded. With trimethoprim, the sulfonamides, and combinations of the two agents, antagonists in the medium may allow some minimal growth; therefore, the zone diameter is measured at the obvious margin, and slight growth (20% or less of the lawn of growth) is disregarded.

The zone diameters measured around each disk are interpreted on the basis of guidelines published by the NCCLS, and the organisms are reported as susceptible, intermediate, or resistant to the antimicrobial agents tested (Table 3) (54, 55). The clinical interpretation of the categories of susceptible, intermediate, and resistant has already been provided above under "Dilution Methods." Computer programs that accompany some automated devices that read zone sizes allow the MICs of some antimicrobial agents and for some bacterial isolates to be derived from the linear regression equation (24, 47).

Advantages and Disadvantages

The disk diffusion test has several advantages: (i) it is technically simple to perform and very reproducible, (ii) the reagents are relatively inexpensive, (iii) it does not require any special equipment, (iv) it provides susceptibility category results that are easily understood by clinicians, and (v) it is flexible regarding the selection of antimicrobial agents for testing. The primary limitation of the disk diffusion test is the spectrum of organisms for which it has been standardized. Adequate studies for the development of reliable interpretive standards for disk testing of bacteria not listed in the NCCLS disk diffusion document, including those that may require different media or atmospheres of incubation for adequate growth or that show delayed or variable growth rates, have not been conducted. This includes *S. maltophilia*, *B. cepacia*, *Corynebacterium* spp., *Bacillus* spp., *Aeromonas* spp., and several fastidious gram-positive and gram-negative bacteria not included in this chapter or chapter 71. The disk test is inadequate for the detection of vancomycin-intermediate *S. aureus* (69) and was reported to have difficulties in the past in the detection of some oxacillin-heteroresistant staphylococci (26, 45) and low-level (VanB-type) vancomycin-resistant enterococci (60, 70). A potential disadvantage of disk diffusion susceptibility testing is that it provides a qualitative result, while a quantitative result indicating the degree of susceptibility (MIC) may be desirable in some selected cases, e.g., for the penicillin and cephalosporin susceptibilities of *S.*

pneumoniae and certain viridans group streptococci (see chapter 71).

Quality Control

The goals of a quality control program for disk diffusion tests are to monitor the precision and accuracy of the procedure, the performance of the reagents (medium, disks), and the performance of persons who do the test and read, interpret, and report the results. To best achieve these goals, reference strains are selected for their genetic stability and their usefulness in the disk diffusion test.

Reference Strains

The reference strains recommended for use by the NCCLS to control the disk diffusion procedure when nonfastidious bacteria are tested are *E. coli* ATCC 25922, *P. aeruginosa* ATCC 27853, *S. aureus* ATCC 25923 (not the same strain used for quality control of MIC tests), *E. faecalis* ATCC 29212, and *E. coli* ATCC 35218 (45). *E. coli* ATCC 35218 is recommended only as a control for the testing of beta-lactamase inhibitor combinations containing clavulanic acid, sulbactam, or tazobactam. *E. faecalis* ATCC 29212 can be used to ensure that the levels of inhibitors of trimethoprim or sulfonamides in Mueller-Hinton agar do not exceed acceptable limits and can also be used to control disks containing a high concentration of gentamicin or streptomycin (see chapter 74).

The reference strains listed above should be obtained from a reliable source, and stock cultures should be maintained in such a way that viability is ensured and the opportunity for the selection of resistant variants is minimal (21). The procedures for maintaining and storing working stock cultures are described in the relevant NCCLS standards (51, 53). If an unexplained result indicates that the inherent susceptibility of the strain has been altered, a fresh subculture of that organism should be obtained.

Zone-of-Inhibition Diameter Ranges

The ranges of zone diameters for the reference strains used to monitor the performance of the disk diffusion test are updated frequently and are published annually; therefore, readers should refer to the most recent NCCLS document for this information (55). Generally, the results of 1 in every 20 tests in a series of tests might be out of the accepted limits. If a second result falls outside the stated limits, corrective action must be taken. The action taken and the results of that action must be documented.

Frequency of Testing

Each new batch or lot of Mueller-Hinton agar must be tested with the reference strains listed above before the medium is released for use with clinical specimens, and quality control must be done before a new lot of antimicrobial disks is introduced. Appropriate reference strains also should be tested each day that the disk diffusion test is performed. The frequency of testing, however, may be reduced if satisfactory performance is documented for 30 consecutive days of testing. For each combination of drug and reference strain, no more than 3 of the 30 zone-of-inhibition diameters may be outside the accepted limits published by the NCCLS (54). When this criterion is fulfilled, each reference strain need be tested only once per week and any time a reagent component of the test is changed. However, if a zone-of-inhibition diameter falls outside the acceptable control limits, corrective action must be taken. If the problem appears to be caused by an obvious error such as testing of the wrong disk or the wrong reference strain, contamination of the reference strain, or incubation in the incorrect atmosphere, repeating the test with the appropriate reference strain is acceptable. However, if the cause of the error is not obvious, quality control must be performed daily for a period that will allow discovery of the source of the aberrant result and documentation of how the problem was resolved. This may be accomplished by the same approach described above under "Quality Control" in "Dilution Methods."

ANTIBACTERIAL SUSCEPTIBILITY TESTING METHODS THAT MAY BE USED OUTSIDE THE UNITED STATES

The NCCLS is known for developing laboratory testing standards for use in the United States, including those for antimicrobial susceptibility testing (53, 54). The NCCLS standards are recognized as U.S. national standards by the American National Standards Institute and by federal regulations, including the Clinical Laboratory Improvement Amendments (34), and as standard reference procedures by the U.S. Food and Drug Administration. However, the

TABLE 4 Non-U.S. disk diffusion methods for susceptibility testing

Method (reference)	Country	Society	Agar medium	Comments
BSAC (2)	United Kingdom	BSAC	Iso-Sensitest	
SFM (website)	France	SFM	Mueller-Hinton	Similar to NCCLS
DIN (28)	Germany	DIN	Mueller-Hinton	
SIR (56)	Sweden	SMS[a]	PDM-ASM	
WRG (75)	The Netherlands	WRG	Iso-Sensitest	
Neo-sensitabs (20)	Denmark (also popular in Belgium)		Mueller-Hinton	Uses antimicrobials incorporated into compressed tablets rather than paper disks. Size of tablets results in substantially larger zones than conventional 6-mm disks.
Calibrated dichotomous sensitivity (13, 14)	Australia		Sensitest	Dichotomous (no intermediate category). Disk strengths chosen to give annular radius of inhibition of ~6 mm where possible.

[a] SMS, Swedish Medical Society.

NCCLS procedures are also used by an increasing number of laboratories outside of the United States, including countries in North and South America and in several areas of Europe, Asia, and Australia. However, some countries have committees comprising their own expert microbiologists who establish methods of susceptibility testing for their own countries and interpretive criteria for those tests that may not be the same as those of the NCCLS (18, 32), as described further in chapter 69.

A large number of variations on dilution and diffusion methods are used for routine susceptibility testing outside the United States (Table 4). Many non-U.S. methods are specific to individual countries, having been developed and evolved locally over many years. Like NCCLS methods, there are dilution and diffusion methods. The majority of non-U.S. methods differ from the NCCLS methods in the choice of media, inoculum preparation, and, for diffusion methods, disk content. There is also considerable variation between these methods in terms of the breakpoints and the approaches used to establish the breakpoints (33, 58). Some efforts have been put into harmonizing breakpoints internationally (32, 77, 78), but progress has been slow. European microbiologists, through the European Society of Clinical Microbiology and Infectious Diseases, are moving toward harmonization in their own region and have defined a reference agar dilution MIC method (32). Variations in test methods can cause considerable confusion in laboratories, especially if both NCCLS and non-NCCLS methods are used for different organisms. Thus, it is important to use the breakpoints specified by the methodology, as the tests have been developed and calibrated with those breakpoints. Indeed, the most important message that can be given about the use of these methods is that the method should be followed in all its detail. A considerable amount of time has been spent ensuring the validity of these methods, and deviations can lead to error, unless such deviations have been shown to be comparable to the original method.

Non-NCCLS Breakpoint Methods

Breakpoint methods are essentially broth or agar MIC methods that use a restricted range of antimicrobial concentrations, often only one or two. They are the standard form of susceptibility testing advocated by the Japan Society for Chemotherapy (38, 39) and, as an alternative to disk diffusion testing, by the British Society for Antimicrobial Chemotherapy (BSAC) (1, 17). Both of these societies use techniques for setting breakpoints that differ somewhat from those outlined in chapter 69. BSAC has developed a formula based on the maximum concentration achievable in blood, the level of protein binding, and the elimination half-life of the drug. This is now integrated with other considerations, including pharmacodynamics and clinical outcome data (46). The Japanese Society for Chemotherapy uses both a formula and a comparison with favorable outcome in clinical studies in which the MICs for the pathogens have been determined (5, 62, 63). The Sociedad Española de Quimioterapia has also published breakpoints, which tend to be more conservative, as they are based primarily on MIC distributions (49).

Breakpoint methods may be popular in large laboratories because large numbers of organisms can be tested cost-effectively by using replicators and they provide susceptibility category (i.e., qualitative) endpoints (76). Optical readers are available to facilitate the reading of agar dilution plates (e.g., Mastscanelite [Mast Laboratories, Bootle, United Kingdom]). However, there are considerable diffi-

culties with quality control, including appropriate control strains for which the MICs are near the breakpoints, and the quantification of drug concentrations prior to use (48). In addition, problems with the use of Iso-Sensitest agar (3, 72) and with the incorporation of inhibitors such as p-nitrophenylglycerol (73) or increased agar content (74) to prevent *Proteus* swarming have been reported. In turn, the choice of Mueller-Hinton by the NCCLS has been criticized for not providing luxuriant growth of all organisms (77), suggesting that there is no ideal medium.

International Diffusion Methods

A wide variety of diffusion methods have been developed in different countries over the years. They are quite diverse in their approaches. Almost all have been maintained to a greater or lesser extent because of the widespread popularity of disk testing in general. None appear to offer any major advantage over the modified Kirby-Bauer system (11) advocated by the NCCLS (54). As pointed out above, disk methods are inexpensive and flexible and could become more popular through the use of zone readers and interconnected computers for interpretation of zone diameters (4, 24, 47).

The previously recommended BSAC standard diffusion methods and the comparative and Stokes' methods differed from other diffusion methods in that susceptibility categorization was achieved through comparison with a control strain rather than by reference to a defined set of zone diameters (17). This technique attracted criticism because it was not based upon or derived from correlations with MICs (19) and has now been replaced by a correlated diffusion method (2). For the new BSAC method, Iso-Sensitest agar supplemented for fastidious bacteria with whole defibrinated horse blood with or without β-nicotinamide adenine dinucleotide is recommended. Mueller-Hinton supplemented with 5% sodium chloride is recommended for the detection methicillin or oxacillin resistance in staphylococci. The inoculum is prepared to produce only semiconfluent growth rather than the confluent growth lawn used in the NCCLS method. One important change in the new BSAC method is the elimination of an intermediate category from most organism-antimicrobial combinations (46). The new BSAC methods will be updated at regular intervals with information on new compounds (see the BSAC website [http://www.bsac.org.uk/]).

Since 1980 the Société Française de Microbiologie (SFM) has put considerable effort into standardization of susceptibility testing, and regular updates including breakpoints for new drugs are published frequently (65; Comité de l'Antibiogramme de la Société Française de Microbiologie, Report 2000–2001 [http://www.sfm.asso.fr/Sect4/COMUK.pdf]). Like the NCCLS, SFM has selected Mueller-Hinton medium as the test medium. For diffusion testing, plates can be inoculated by flooding as well as swabbing. In most other aspects this method resembles that of the NCCLS, including the control organisms used and the choice of disk strength. They provide zone diameter breakpoints for drugs available in France and elsewhere that are not approved for clinical use in the United States, e.g., fusidic acid and pristinamycin (65).

The German standards organization, the Deutsches Institut für Normung (DIN), published acceptable methods for diffusion susceptibility testing as early as 1979, with irregular updates published since then (27, 28). It too uses Mueller-Hinton agar but will tolerate the use of other media, provided that the MIC-zone diameter relationships have been determined on that medium. Like the SFM method, the DIN method has much in common with the NCCLS method.

The Swedish SIR or SRGA-M (56, 67) and the Dutch Werkgroep Richtlijnen Gevoeligheidsbepalingen (WRG) (75) methods use still different media. The SIR system is based on the methodology developed by the original International Collaborative Study (30) that was the first to provide a sound theoretical basis to diffusion susceptibility testing. Its recommended medium is either PDM Antibiotic Sensitivity Medium (a Swedish product) or Iso-Sensitest medium. The breakpoints for susceptibility were restructured in 1981 to the more conventional susceptible, intermediate, and resistant categories (67) and were updated in 1997 (59). The MIC breakpoint correlates selected by the SIR system are frequently two- to eightfold lower than those used by other methods. A full summary of the Swedish disk and MIC methodology can be found at the website of the Swedish Reference Group for Antibiotics (http://www.ltkronoberg.se/ext/raf/RAFMETOD/Basmet.htm).

Iso-Sensitest medium is recommended by the WRG system (75), which in other aspects is similar to the NCCLS, SFM, and DIN techniques. Consequently, the zone diameter breakpoints for some drugs are often different, even though they have the same MIC correlates and disk strengths.

A method developed by a commercial firm in Denmark differs technically if not in principle from the other methods. This method uses so-called Neo-sensitabs, which are compressed tablets 9 mm in diameter into which the antibiotic has been incorporated (20). The method and the interpretive zone diameter criteria are updated and published by the manufacturer periodically. Not only are the tablets larger and thicker than conventional 6-mm paper disks but also they usually contain larger amounts of antibiotic, resulting in significantly larger zones of inhibition with most drugs. This has the disadvantage of reducing the number of tablets that can be put on a single plate and still have readable zones. However, the system does have the advantage that the tablets can be stored at room temperature for up to 4 years, obviating the need for storage under refrigeration or freezing. This is an obvious benefit for laboratories in developing countries where reliable refrigeration and power can be a problem.

A diffusion method developed in Australia in 1975 (13, 14) and still widely used in that country has a number of unique features. The calibrated dichotomous sensitivity method uses Sensitest agar and an unusual method for inoculum preparation and is unique in defining just two categories of susceptibility: susceptible and resistant. In order to simplify the reading of test results, each new drug is calibrated against the MIC breakpoint to yield wherever possible a zone diameter of 18 mm. This is achieved by adjusting disk strengths, which in most cases are substantially lower than those used with other methods. The lack of an intermediate category, which increases the risk of serious misclassification (e.g., susceptible instead of resistant), the absence of some common drugs from the range of drugs included in the test, and some unconventional use of surrogate drugs for testing have restricted the widespread adoption of this method. The interpretive criteria are updated regularly and can be found on the website describing the method (http://www.med.unsw.edu.au/pathology-cds).

COMMON SOURCES OF ERROR IN ANTIBACTERIAL SUSCEPTIBILITY TESTING

Potential sources of error in antibacterial susceptibility testing may be categorized as those that relate to the test system and its components, those associated with the test procedure, those peculiar to certain organism and drug combinations, and those that relate to reporting. The most common sources of error encountered in clinical microbiology laboratories are reviewed in the following paragraphs.

Various components of the susceptibility test system may be a source of error. First, the system itself may have limitations regarding the organisms that should be tested. For example, the disk diffusion method should be used only to test rapidly growing bacterial pathogens that have consistent growth rates (those for which interpretive criteria have been developed and published by the NCCLS). Second, the medium used may be a source of error if it fails to conform to the recommended composition and performance. Factors common to both agar-based and broth-based systems are the pH of the medium, which for Mueller-Hinton agar or broth should be between 7.2 and 7.4, and its cation content. The concentration of magnesium and calcium in the broth medium should be that recommended by the NCCLS to ensure reliable results. For the detection of oxacillin-resistant staphylococci, it is essential that the proper amount of sodium chloride be included in the agar or broth used for dilution testing. For agar dilution and disk diffusion, the Mueller-Hinton agar should be 3 to 4 mm deep. Third, the components of the system (antimicrobial disks, agar plates, and trays) must be stored properly, and they should not be used beyond the stated expiration dates.

Steps in the susceptibility test procedure that may be a source of error if they are not performed correctly include inoculum preparation, incubation conditions and duration, endpoint interpretation, and performance of appropriate quality control. The inoculum must be pure, and it must contain an adequate density of bacteria. With rare exceptions, all systems should be incubated in ambient air at 35°C. The incubation time, however, varies. For conventional dilution and disk diffusion systems, incubation for 16 to 20 h and 16 to 18 h, respectively, is recommended except for tests with staphylococci and oxacillin and vancomycin and tests with enterococci and vancomycin, which must be incubated for a full 24 h (53, 54). The endpoints of all susceptibility tests must be measured accurately by following the guidelines published by the NCCLS (53, 54). If endpoints are interpreted by an instrument, the reliability of that instrument must be monitored. Moreover, with all susceptibility test systems, appropriate reference strains must be tested at regular intervals, and any problems that occur must be thoroughly investigated and corrective action must be well documented.

The testing of some bacteria against certain antimicrobial agents may yield misleading results, because these in vitro results do not necessarily correlate with in vivo activity. Examples include narrow- and expanded-spectrum cephalosporins and aminoglycosides tested against fecal isolates of *Salmonella* and *Shigella* spp.; all beta-lactam agents except the penicillinase-resistant penicillins (oxacillin, nafcillin, and methicillin) tested against oxacillin-resistant staphylococci; cephalosporins, aminoglycosides (except concentrations used to detect high-level resistance), clindamycin, and trimethoprim-sulfamethoxazole tested against enterococci; and cephalosporins tested against *Listeria* spp. (53, 54). Therefore, results should not be reported for these combinations of organisms and drugs. Other potential problems associated with reporting are possible transcriptional errors for laboratories that use a manual recording and reporting system and possible errors in the transmission of data for laboratories in which an automated susceptibility test system is interfaced with the laboratory and/or hospital information system.

PROBLEM ORGANISMS AND RESISTANCE MECHANISMS

The dilution and diffusion methods described in this chapter have been developed through careful studies and have been standardized by national professional organizations and diagnostic device manufacturers. Despite this, there are some organisms for which methods have either not yet been standardized (e.g., *Corynebacterium* spp., *Bacillus* spp., *Aeromonas* spp., and *Pasteurella* spp.) or which inexplicably fail to provide reliable results by some of the standard tests (e.g., disk diffusion testing of *S. maltophilia* and *B. cepacia*). Certain other organisms may possess resistance mechanisms that are inducible (VanB-type resistance in some enterococci, the Bush group 1 beta-lactamase in some gram-negative species) or that result in subtle phenotypic expression under standard inoculum and test conditions (oxacillin resistance in some coagulase-negative staphylococci [79], extended-spectrum beta-lactamases [ESBLs] in some members of the family *Enterobacteriaceae* [44]). Reliable detection of these subtle resistance traits may require the use of different or modified test methods that are outlined in chapter 74. The NCCLS has adopted revised MIC and disk diffusion breakpoints for the testing of coagulase-negative staphylococci with oxacillin in an attempt to avoid errors of false susceptibility (53, 54, 68). In contrast, the screening breakpoints for the detection of ESBLs by the use of cefpodoxime have recently been modified by the NCCLS to improve the specificity of that test (55). There is no consensus regarding what level of accuracy is acceptable when selecting a testing method or system for performing antimicrobial susceptibility testing (40). Moreover, it is important to keep in mind that new resistance mechanisms or decreases in susceptibility to important therapeutic agents can arise at any time to challenge our methods of susceptibility testing, e.g., vancomycin-intermediate *S. aureus* (35, 69).

REFERENCES

1. **Andrews, J. M.** 2001. Determination of minimum inhibitory concentrations. *J. Antimicrob. Chemother.* **48**(Suppl. S1):5–16.
2. **Andrews, J. M., for the BSAC Working Party in Susceptibility Testing.** 2001. BSAC standardized disc susceptibility testing method. *J. Antimicrob. Chemother.* **48**(Suppl. S1):43–57.
3. **Andrews, J. M., J. P. Ashby, and R. Wise.** 1990. Problems with Iso-Sensitest agar. *J. Antimicrob. Chemother.* **26**:596–597.
4. **Andrews, J. M., F. J. Boswell, and R. Wise.** 2000. Evaluation of the Oxoid Aura image system for measuring zones of inhibition with the disc diffusion technique. *J. Antimicrob. Chemother.* **46**:535–540.
5. **Arakawa, S., T. Matsui, S. Kamidono, Y. Kawada, H. Kumon, K. Hirai, T. Hirose, T. Matsumoto, K. Yamaguchi, T. Yoshida, K. Watanabe, K. Ueno, A. Saito, and T. Teranishi.** 1998. Derivation of a calculation formula for

6. **Baker, C. N., S. A. Stocker, D. H. Culver, and C. Thornsberry.** 1991. Comparison of the E test to agar dilution, broth microdilution, and agar diffusion susceptibility testing techniques by using a special challenge set of bacteria. *J. Clin. Microbiol.* **29**:533–538.
7. **Barry, A. L.** 1991. Procedures and theoretical considerations for testing antimicrobial agents in agar media, p. 1–16. *In* V. Lorian (ed.), *Antibiotics in Laboratory Medicine,* 3rd ed. The Williams & Wilkins Co., Baltimore, Md.
8. **Barry, A. L., R. E. Badal, and R. W. Hawkinson.** 1983. Influence of inoculum growth phase on microdilution susceptibility tests. *J. Clin. Microbiol.* **18**:645–651.
9. **Barry, A. L., G. H. Miller, C. Thornsberry, R. S. Hare, R. N. Jones, R. R. Lorber, R. Ferraresi, and C. Cramer.** 1987. Influence of cation supplements on activity of netilmicin against *Pseudomonas aeruginosa* in vitro and in vivo. *Antimicrob. Agents Chemother.* **31**:1514–1518.
10. **Barry, A. L., L. B. Reller, G. H. Miller, J. A. Washington, F. D. Schoenknecht, L. R. Peterson, R. S. Hare, and C. Knapp.** 1992. Revision of standards for adjusting the cation content of Mueller-Hinton broth for testing susceptibility of *Pseudomonas aeruginosa* to aminoglycosides. *J. Clin. Microbiol.* **30**:585–589.
11. **Bauer, A. W., W. M. M. Kirby, J. C. Sherris, and M. Turck.** 1966. Antibiotic susceptibility testing by standardized single disk method. *Am. J. Clin. Pathol.* **45**:493–496.
12. **Bauer, A. W., and J. C. Sherris.** 1964. The determination of sulfonamide susceptibility of bacteria. *Chemotherapia* **9**:1–19.
13. **Bell, S. M.** 1975. The CDS method of antibiotic sensitivity testing (calibrated dichotomous sensitivity test). *Pathology* **7**(Suppl.):1–48.
14. **Bell, S. M.** 1988. Additions and modifications to the range of antibiotics tested by the CDS method of antibiotic sensitivity testing. *Pathology* **20**:303–304.
15. **Bradford, P. A., and C. C. Sanders.** 1992. Use of a predictor panel for development of a new disk for diffusion tests with cefoperazone-sulbactam. *Antimicrob. Agents Chemother.* **36**:394–400.
16. **Brenner, V. C., and J. C. Sherris.** 1972. Influence of different media and bloods on the results of diffusion antibiotic susceptibility tests. *Antimicrob. Agents Chemother.* **1**:116–122.
17. **British Society for Antimicrobial Chemotherapy.** 1991. Report of the working party on antibiotic sensitivity testing of the British Society for Antimicrobial Chemotherapy: a guide to sensitivity testing. *J. Antimicrob. Chemother.* **27**(Suppl. D):1–50.
18. **Brown, D. F. J.** 1994. Developments in antimicrobial susceptibility testing. *Rev. Med. Microbiol.* **5**:65–75.
19. **Brown, D. F. J.** 1990. The comparative method for antimicrobial susceptibility testing—time for a change? *J. Antimicrob. Chemother.* **25**:307–312.
20. **Casals, J. B., and N. Pringler.** 1991. *Antibacterial/Antifungal Sensitivity Testing Using Neo-sensitabs®,* 9th ed. Rosco Diagnostica, Taarstrup, Denmark.
21. **Coyle, M. B., M. F. Lampe, C. L. Aitkin, P. Feigl, and J. C. Sherris.** 1976. Reproducibility of control strains for antibiotic susceptibility testing. *Antimicrob. Agents Chemother.* **10**:436–440.
22. **Craig, W. A.** 1993. Qualitative susceptibility tests versus quantitative MIC tests. *Diagn. Microbiol. Infect. Dis.* **16**:231–236.
23. **Craig, W. A.** 1998. Pharmacokinetic/pharmacodynamic parameters for antibacterial dosing of mice and men. *Clin. Infect. Dis.* **26**:1–12.

24. **D'Amato, R. F., L. Hochstein, J. R. Vernaleo, and C. Thornsberry.** 1985. Evaluation of BIOMIC antimicrobial test system. *J. Clin. Microbiol.* **22:**793–798.

25. **D'Amato, R. F., C. Thornsberry, C. N. Baker, and L. A. Kirven.** 1975. Effect of calcium and magnesium ions on the susceptibility of *Pseudomonas* species to tetracycline, gentamicin, polymyxin B, and carbenicillin. *Antimicrob. Agents Chemother.* **7:**596–600.

26. **De Lencastre, H., A. M. Sa Figueiredo, C. Urban, J. Rahal, and A. Tomasz.** 1991. Multiple mechanisms of methicillin resistance and improved methods for detection in clinical isolates of *Staphylococcus aureus. Antimicrob. Agents Chemother.* **35:**632–639.

27. **Deutsches Institut für Normung.** 2000. *Susceptibility Testing of Pathogens to Antimicrobial Agents. Part 3. Agar Diffusion Test.* Publication DIN 58940-3. Beuth Verlag, Berlin, Germany.

28. **Deutsches Institut für Normung.** 2000. *Methods for the Determination of Susceptibility of Pathogens (Except Mycobacteria) to Antimicrobial Agents. Part 4. Evaluation Classes of the Minimum Inhibitory Concentration.* Publication DIN 58940-4. Beuth Verlag, Berlin, Germany.

29. **Doern, G. V.** 1987. Breakpoint susceptibility testing. *Clin. Microbiol. Newsl.* **9:**81–84.

30. **Ericsson, J. M., and J. C. Sherris.** 1971. Antibiotic sensitivity testing. Report of an international collaborative study. *Acta Pathol. Microbiol. Scand. Sect. B Suppl.* **217:**1–90.

31. **Estes, L.** 1998. Review of pharmacokinetics and pharmacodynamics of antimicrobial agents. *Mayo Clin. Proc.* **73:**114–122.

32. **European Committee for Antimicrobial Susceptibility Testing (EUCAST).** 2000. Determination of minimum inhibitory concentration (MICs) of antibacterial agents by agar dilution. EUCAST discussion document. *Clin. Microbiol. Infect.* **6:**509–515.

33. **Ferraro, M. J.** 2001. Should we reevaluate antibiotic breakpoints? *Clin. Infect. Dis.* **33**(Suppl. 3):S227–S229.

34. **Health Care Financing Administration.** 1992. Clinical Laboratory Improvement Amendments of 1988; final rule. *Fed. Regist.* **57:**7137–7186.

35. **Hiramatsu, K., H. Hanaki, T. Ino, K. Yabuta, T. Oguri, and F. C. Tenover.** 1997. Methicillin-resistant *Staphylococcus aureus* clinical strain with reduced vancomycin susceptibility. *J. Antimicrob. Chemother.* **40:**135–146.

36. **Huang, M., P. N. Baker, S. Banerjee, and F. C. Tenover.** 1992. Accuracy of the E test for determining antimicrobial susceptibilities of staphylococci, enterococci, *Campylobacter jejunii,* and gram-negative bacteria resistant to antimicrobial agents. *J. Clin. Microbiol.* **30:**3243–3248.

37. **Huang, M. B., E. T. Gay, C. N. Baker, S. N. Banerjee, and F. C. Tenover.** 1993. Two percent sodium chloride is required for susceptibility testing of staphylococci with oxacillin when using agar-based dilution methods. *J. Clin. Microbiol.* **31:**2683–2688.

38. **Japan Society for Chemotherapy.** 1990. Report of the Committee for Japanese Standards for Antimicrobial Susceptibility Testing for Bacteria. *Chemotherapy* (Tokyo) **38:**102–105. (In Japanese.)

39. **Japan Society for Chemotherapy.** 1993. Report of the Committee for Japanese Standards for Antimicrobial Susceptibility Testing for Bacteria. *Chemotherapy* (Tokyo) **41:**183–189. (In Japanese.)

40. **Jorgensen, J. H.** 1993. Selection criteria for an antimicrobial susceptibility testing system. *J. Clin. Microbiol.* **31:**2841–2844.

41. **Jorgensen, J. H.** 1993. Selection of antimicrobial agents for routine testing in a clinical microbiology laboratory. *Diagn. Microbiol. Infect. Dis.* **16:**245–249.

42. **Jorgensen, J. H., and M. J. Ferraro.** 1998. Antimicrobial susceptibility testing: general principles and contemporary practices. *Clin. Infect. Dis.* **26:**973–980.

43. **Jorgensen, J. H., and M. J. Ferraro.** 2000. Antimicrobial susceptibility testing: special needs for fastidious organisms and difficult-to-detect resistance mechanisms. *Clin. Infect. Dis.* **30:**799–808.

44. **Katsanis, G., J. Spargo, M. J. Ferraro, L. Sutton, and G. A. Jacoby.** 1994. Detection of *Klebsiella pneumoniae* and *Escherichia coli* strains producing extended-spectrum β-lactamases. *J. Clin. Microbiol.* **32:**691–696.

45. **Kiehlbauch, J. A., G. E. Hannett, M. Salfinger, W. Archinal, C. Monserrat, and C. Carlyn.** 2000. Use of the National Committee for Clinical Laboratory Standards guidelines for disk diffusion susceptibility testing in New York State laboratories. *J. Clin. Microbiol.* **38:**3341–3348.

46. **MacGowan, A. P., and R. Wise.** 2001. Establishing MIC breakpoints and the interpretation of in vitro susceptibility tests. *J. Antimicrob. Chemother.* **48**(Suppl. S1):17–28.

47. **Madeiros, A., and J. Crellin.** 2000. Evaluation of the Sirscan automated zone reader in a clinical microbiology laboratory. *J. Clin. Microbiol.* **38:**1688–1693.

48. **McDermott, S. N., and T. F. Hartley.** 1989. New datum handling methods for the quality control of antimicrobial solutions and plates used in the antimicrobial susceptibility test. *J. Clin. Microbiol.* **27:**1814–1825.

49. **Mesa Española de Normalización de la Sensibilidad y Resistancia a los Antimicrobianos (MENSURA).** 2000. Recommendations from MENSURA for selection of antimicrobial agents for susceptibility testing and criteria for the interpretation of antibiograms. *Rev. Esp. Quimio.* **13:**73–86.

50. **Metzler, C., and R. M. DeHaan.** 1974. Susceptibility tests of anaerobic bacteria: statistical and clinical considerations. *J. Infect. Dis.* **130:**588–594.

51. **NCCLS.** 2001. *Development of In Vitro Susceptibility Testing Criteria and Quality Control Parameters.* NCCLS document M23-A2. NCCLS, Wayne, Pa.

52. **NCCLS.** 1996. *Evaluating Production Lots of Dehydrated Mueller-Hinton Agar.* Approved standard M6-A. NCCLS, Wayne, Pa.

53. **NCCLS.** 2000. *Methods for Dilution Antimicrobial Susceptibility Tests for Bacteria That Grow Aerobically.* Approved standard M7-A5. NCCLS, Wayne, Pa.

54. **NCCLS.** 2000. *Performance Standards for Antimicrobial Disk Susceptibility Tests.* Approved standard M2-A7. NCCLS, Wayne, Pa.

55. **NCCLS.** 2002. *Performance Standards for Antimicrobial Susceptibility Testing.* Supplement M100-S12. NCCLS, Wayne, Pa.

56. **Olsson-Liljequist, B., P. Larson, M. Walder, and H. Miorner.** 1997. Antimicrobial susceptibility testing in Sweden. III. Methodology for susceptibility testing. *Scand. J. Infect. Dis.* Suppl. **105:**13–23.

57. **Pestotnik, S. L., R. S. Evans, J. P. Burke, and R. M. Gardner.** 1990. Therapeutic antibiotic monitoring: surveillance using a computerized expert system. *Am. J. Med.* **99:**43–48.

58. **Phillips, I.** 2001. Reevaluation of antibiotic breakpoints. *Clin. Infect. Dis.* **33**(Suppl. 3):S230–S232.

59. **Ringertz, S., B. Olsson-Liljequist, G. Kahlmeter, and G. Kronvall.** 1997. Antimicrobial susceptibility testing in Sweden. II. Species-related zone diameter breakpoints to avoid interpretive errors and guard against unrecognized evolution of resistance. *Scand. J. Infect. Dis.* **105**(Suppl.):8–12.

60. **Rosenberg, J., F. C. Tenover, J. Wong, W. Jarvis, and D. J. Vugia.** 1997. Are clinical laboratories in California

accurately reporting vancomycin-resistant enterococci? *J. Clin. Microbiol.* **35:**2526–2530.

61. **Sahm, D. F., C. N. Baker, R. N. Jones, and C. Thornsberry.** 1984. Influence of growth medium on the in vitro activities of second- and third-generation cephalosporins against *Streptococcus faecalis. J. Clin. Microbiol.* **20:**561–567.

62. **Saito, A.** 1995. Clinical breakpoints for antimicrobial agents in pulmonary infections and sepsis: report of the Committee for Japanese Standards for Antimicrobial Susceptibility Testing of Bacteria. *J. Infect. Chemother.* **1:**83–88.

63. **Saito, A., T. Inamatsu, J. Okada, T. Oguri, H. Kanno, N. Kusano, H. Kumon, K. Yamaguchi, A. Watanabe, and K. Watanabe.** 1999. Clinical breakpoints in pulmonary infections and sepsis: new antimicrobial agents and supplemental information for some agents already released. *J. Infect. Chemother.* **5:**223–226.

64. **Schulz, J. E., and D. F. Sahm.** 1993. Reliability of the E test for detection of ampicillin, vancomycin, and high-level aminoglycoside resistance in *Enterococcus* spp. *J. Clin. Microbiol.* **31:**3336–3339.

65. **Société Française de Microbiologie.** 1996. Report of the Comité de l'Antibiogramme de la Société Française de Microbiologie. 1996. *Clin. Microbiol. Infect. Dis.* **2**(Suppl. 1):S1–S49.

66. **Steers, E., E. L. Foltz, and B. S. Graves.** 1959. An inocula replicating apparatus for routine testing of bacterial susceptibility to antibiotics. *Antibiot. Chemother.* **9:**307–311.

67. **The Swedish Reference Group for Antibiotics.** 1981. A revised system for antibiotic sensitivity testing. *Scand. J. Infect. Dis.* **13:**148–152.

68. **Tenover, F. C., R. N. Jones, J. M. Swenson, B. Zimmer, S. McAllister, and J. H. Jorgensen.** 1999. Methods for improved detection of oxacillin resistance in coagulase-negative staphylococci: results of a multicenter study. *J. Clin. Microbiol.* **37:**4051–4058.

69. **Tenover, F. C., M. V. Lancaster, B. C. Hill, C. D. Steward, S. A. Stocker, G. A. Hancock, C. M. O'Hara, S. K. McAllister, N. C. Clark, and K. Hiramatsu.** 1998. Characterization of staphylococci with reduced suscepti-

bilities to vancomycin and other glycopeptides. *J. Clin. Microbiol.* **36:**1020–1027.

70. **Tenover, F. C., J. M. Swenson, C. M. O'Hara, and S. A. Stocker.** 1995. Ability of commercial and reference antimicrobial susceptibility testing methods to detect vancomycin resistance in enterococci. *J. Clin. Microbiol.* **33:**1524–1527.

71. **Thornsberry, C., and L. K. McDougal.** 1983. Successful use of broth microdilution in susceptibility tests for methicillin-resistant (heteroresistant) staphylococci. *J. Clin. Microbiol.* **18:**1084–1091.

72. **Toohey, M., G. Francis, and N. Stingemore.** 1990. Variation in Iso-sensitest agar affecting β-lactam testing. *Newsl. Antimicrob. Special Interest Group Aust. Soc. Microbiol.* **1**(6):6–8.

73. **Ward, P. B., S. Palladino, J. C. Looker, and P. Feddema.** 1993. *p*-Nitrophenylglycerol in susceptibility testing media alters the MICs of antimicrobials for *Pseudomonas aeruginosa. J. Antimicrob. Chemother.* **31:**489–496.

74. **Ward, P. B., S. Palladino, B. McLaren, R. J. Rathur, and J. C. Looker.** 1993. The effect of increased agar concentration in susceptibility testing media on MICs of antimicrobials for gram-negative bacilli. *J. Antimicrob. Chemother.* **31:**1005–1007.

75. **Werkgroep Richtlijnen Gevoeligheidsbepalingen.** 1981. *Standaardisatie van Gevoeligheidsbepalingen.* Werkgroep Richtlijnen Gevoeligheidsbepalingen, Bilthoven, The Netherlands.

76. **Wheat, P. F.** 1989. The agar-dilution susceptibility technique: past and present. *Clin. Microbiol. Newsl.* **11:**164–166.

77. **Williams, J. D.** 1990. Prospects for standardisation of methods and guidelines for disc susceptibility testing. *Eur. J. Clin. Microbiol. Infect. Dis.* **9:**496–501.

78. **Wise, R., and I. Phillips.** 2000. Towards a common susceptibility testing method? *J. Antimicrob. Chemother.* **45:**919–920.

79. **York, M. K., L. Gibbs, F. Chehab, and G. F. Brooks.** 1996. Comparison of PCR detection of *mecA* with standard susceptibility testing methods to determine methicillin resistance in coagulase-negative staphylococci. *J. Clin. Microbiol.* **34:**249–253.

Susceptibility Test Methods: Fastidious Bacteria

JANET FICK HINDLER AND JANA M. SWENSON

71

Most fastidious bacteria do not grow satisfactorily in standard in vitro susceptibility test systems that use unsupplemented media. For certain fastidious species that are more frequently encountered, such as *Haemophilus influenzae*, *Neisseria gonorrhoeae*, *Streptococcus pneumoniae*, and other *Streptococcus* spp., slight modifications to standard NCCLS disk diffusion and MIC methods have been made to allow reliable testing of these bacteria. The modifications generally involve the use of a test medium with added nutrients and sometimes extended incubation times and/or incubation in an atmosphere with increased levels of CO_2 (Table 1). Specific zone diameter and MIC interpretive criteria have been developed by NCCLS for these bacteria (see examples in Table 2), as have acceptable ranges for recommended quality control (QC) strains. Recently, NCCLS described a standard MIC method for testing *Helicobacter pylori* by an agar dilution procedure (84).

Even though susceptibility test methods for *Moraxella catarrhalis* have not been standardized, testing for *Neisseria meningitidis* and *Listeria monocytogenes* is mentioned in NCCLS documents, although extensive interpretive criteria are not available (86).

NCCLS is currently evaluating methods for testing *Campylobacter* spp.; however, to date, a standard method for testing this genus has not been published. There are no specific recommendations for "other" fastidious bacteria (OFB), such as *Pasteurella*, *Bordetella*, and *Legionella* spp. and various coryneform bacilli. This is in part because (i) infections caused by these bacteria usually respond to drugs of choice, (ii) isolates are infrequently encountered, and (iii) isolates are often difficult to grow or are slow to grow.

In addition to conventional MIC test methods (e.g., agar dilution or broth dilution methods), the E-test MIC determination method has been used to test many types of fastidious bacteria. The E-test approach allows placement of strips on specialized media and the use of various incubation conditions. The limitations of this method include its cost and lack of clearance by the U.S. Food and Drug Administration (FDA) for testing many less commonly encountered fastidious bacteria. Prior to use of the E test for clinical testing in the United States, the FDA clearance status for the particular organism-antimicrobial agent combination should be known. If FDA clearance has not been granted, the results should be interpreted with caution and should be qualified on the patient report.

This chapter summarizes the standard methods recommended by NCCLS for the antimicrobial susceptibility testing of *Streptococcus* spp. (including *S. pneumoniae*), *Haemophilus* spp., *N. gonorrhoeae*, *N. meningitidis*, *L. monocytogenes*, and *H. pylori*. An approach for testing *M. catarrhalis* and *Campylobacter jejuni* is also presented. The incidence of resistance, test methods, and indications for testing and the reporting of results are discussed. Finally, this chapter presents strategies that could be used in the clinical laboratory when requests are made for the testing of a fastidious bacterium for which no standardized susceptibility test method is available.

S. PNEUMONIAE

Incidence of Resistance

Since it was first reported in 1967, penicillin resistance in pneumococci has been steadily increasing worldwide (6, 10). Interpretive criteria for penicillin and *S. pneumoniae* were originally developed for isolates associated with meningitis and are defined by the NCCLS as follows: susceptible, ≤0.06 μg/ml; intermediate, 0.12 to 1 μg/ml; and resistant, ≥2 μg/ml (86). Infections outside of the central nervous system (CNS), such as pulmonary infections, due to strains for which penicillin MICs are in the intermediate range may be treatable with penicillin (44), and recently it has been suggested that penicillin MIC interpretive criteria be revised to reflect this (50). The rates for strains not susceptible to penicillin (including both intermediate and resistant categories) exceed 50% in some parts of the world (16), and in the latest U.S. survey (120), most of the non-penicillin-susceptible strains demonstrated high-level resistance (MICs ≥ 2 μg/ml) rather than intermediate resistance (14 versus 10%). Strains of pneumococci that are susceptible to penicillin generally are susceptible to other β-lactam agents (7); however, as the penicillin MIC increases, the MICs of other β-lactam agents increase also. Pneumococcal strains resistant to cefotaxime or ceftriaxone were not reported until the early 1990s (21, 106). Current rates of resistance to the extended-spectrum cephalosporins vary by location (52), but in a U.S. survey of isolates collected in 1999 to 2000, levels of 14.4% were reported (36). In areas where penicillin resistance is high, the rate of

TABLE 1 Disk diffusion and MIC testing conditions and recommended QC strains for select fastidious bacteria

Organism(s)	Method	Medium[a]	Inoculum source[b]	Incubation atmosphere[c]	Incubation length (h)	Recommended QC strain(s)
S. pneumoniae and Streptococcus spp.	Disk diffusion	MHA + 5% sheep blood	16–18-h growth (from SBA)	5–7% CO_2	20–24	S. pneumoniae ATCC 49619
	Broth microdilution	CAMHB-LHB	16–18-h growth (from SBA)	Ambient air	20–24	S. pneumoniae ATCC 49619
Haemophilus spp.	Disk diffusion	HTM agar	20–24-h growth (from CHOC)	5–7% CO_2	16–18	H. influenzae ATCC 49247, H. influenzae ATCC 49766[d]
	Broth microdilution	HTM broth	20–24-h growth (from CHOC)	Ambient air	20–24	H. influenzae ATCC 49247, H. influenzae ATCC 49766[d]
N. gonorrhoeae	Disk diffusion	GC agar base + supplement	20–24-h growth (from CHOC)	5–7% CO_2	20–24	N. gonorrhoeae ATCC 49226
	Agar dilution	GC agar base + supplement	20–24-h growth (from CHOC)	5–7% CO_2	20–24	N. gonorrhoeae ATCC 49226
N. meningitidis	Broth microdilution	CAMHB-LHB	20–24-h growth (from CHOC)	5–7% CO_2	24	S. pneumoniae ATCC 49619
	Agar dilution	MHA + 5% sheep blood	20–24-h growth (from CHOC)	5–7% CO_2	24	S. pneumoniae ATCC 49619
L. monocytogenes	Broth microdilution	CAMHB-LHB	16–18-h growth (from SBA)	Ambient air	16–20	S. pneumoniae ATCC 49619
H. pylori	Agar dilution	MHA + 5% aged (≥2-wk-old) sheep blood	72-h growth (from SBA)[e]	Microaerobic; produced by gas-generating system for campylobacters	≈72	H. pylori ATCC 43504

[a] HTM, GC agar base, and CAMHB-LHB are defined in the text.
[b] Suspension is in Mueller-Hinton broth or 0.9% NaCl standardized to a 0.5 McFarland standard for disk diffusion. For broth dilution, final organism concentration is 5×10^5 CFU/ml; for agar dilution, final organism concentration is 10^4 CFU/spot. CHOC, chocolate agar; SBA, sheep blood agar.
[c] Incubation temperature, 35°C.
[d] In addition, H. influenzae ATCC 10211 can be used to assess growth-supporting capabilities of HTM. H. influenzae ATCC 49766 is used for QC of select cephalosporins (e.g., cefaclor, cefamandole, and cefuroxime).
[e] Suspension is in 0.9% NaCl standardized to a 2.0 McFarland standard.

resistance to cefotaxime or ceftriaxone would also be expected to be high (54).

Resistance has been described for all classes of antimicrobial agents that are usually considered for treatment of pneumococcal infections, except for the glycopeptides (36, 52, 120). As with penicillin, resistance rates for most of these other classes of antimicrobial agents have risen dramatically. Macrolide resistance in the United States was as high as 25.7% among strains from 33 medical centers in a very recent survey (36). Resistance to macrolides in Asian-Pacific countries is much higher, exceeding 80 to 90% in some areas (16). MICs of erythromycin for pneumococci with macrolide-lincosamide-streptogramin B (MLS)-type resistance (encoded by the ermB gene) are usually ≥64 μg/ml and clindamycin MICs are ≥8 μg/ml, whereas for isolates of the M phenotype (encoded by the mefA gene), erythromycin MICs are in the range of 1 to 32 μg/ml and clindamycin MICs are ≤0.25 μg/ml (36).

Resistance rates for trimethoprim-sulfamethoxazole (TMP-SMX) range from 20 to 36% in the United States (36, 52, 120) and are similar to those outside the United States (52). Resistance rates for fluoroquinolones remain low (59, 100); however, a higher prevalence of resistance to fluoroquinolones has been shown in other countries (27, 51, 119). No resistance to linezolid has been reported to

date (36), and resistance rates for quinupristin-dalfopristin are <1% (36) among S. pneumoniae strains (52, 120).

Reference Test Methods

NCCLS describes both a broth microdilution method and a disk diffusion method for the testing of pneumococci (84–86). Details of these procedures and interpretive criteria are listed in Tables 1 and 2, respectively. The broth microdilution method may be used to test all of the antimicrobial agents recommended by NCCLS for pneumococci. However, with the exception of the oxacillin disk screening test, the disk diffusion method does not work for the β-lactam agents (85, 86, 110). When used to predict susceptibility to penicillin, oxacillin disk diffusion zone diameters of ≥20 mm indicate that the isolate is susceptible to penicillin (86). However, strains with zone diameters of ≤19 mm cannot be readily categorized as resistant, since a strain with an oxacillin zone diameter of ≤19 mm may be penicillin susceptible, intermediate, or resistant (34) when the actual penicillin MIC for the strain is determined. Therefore, if the oxacillin screen test is used without follow-up MIC testing for strains with zones of ≤19 mm, the potential for overstating penicillin resistance is high. NCCLS recommends that for strains isolated from the CNS, the oxacillin screening procedure should not be used and that the labo-

TABLE 2 Interpretive standards for dilution and disk diffusion susceptibility testing of fastidious organisms with antimicrobial agents appropriate for primary testing[a]

Organism and antimicrobial agent	MIC (μg/ml)			Zone diam (mm)		
	Susceptible	Intermediate	Resistant	Resistant	Intermediate	Susceptible
S. pneumoniae						
Cefepime[b]						
Meningitis	≤0.5	1	≥2			
Nonmeningitis	≤1	2	≥4			
Cefotaxime[b]						
Meningitis	≤0.5	1	≥2			
Nonmeningitis	≤1	2	≥4			
Ceftriaxone[b]						
Meningitis	≤0.5	1	≥2			
Nonmeningitis	≤1	2	≥4			
Clindamycin	≤0.25	0.5	≥1	≤15	16–18	≥19
Erythromycin	≤0.25	0.5	≥1	≤15	16–20	≥21
Gatifloxacin	≤1	2	≥4	≤17	18–20	≥21
Levofloxacin	≤2	4	≥8	≤13	14–16	≥17
Meropenem[b]	≤0.25	0.5	≥1			
Moxifloxacin	≤1	2	≥4	≤14	15–17	≥18
Ofloxacin	≤2	4	≥8	≤12	13–15	≥16
Penicillin[c]	≤0.06	0.12–1	≥2			≥20
Sparfloxacin	≤0.5	1	≥2	≤15	16–18	≥19
Tetracycline	≤2	4	≥8	≤18	19–22	≥23
TMP-SMX	≤0.5/9.5	1/19–2/38	≥4/76	≤15	16–18	≥19
Vancomycin[d]	≤1					≤17
Streptococcus spp. other than *S. pneumoniae*						
Ampicillin						
Beta group[d]	≤0.25					≥24
Viridans group[b]	≤0.25	0.5–4	≥8			
Chloramphenicol	≤4	8	≥16	≤17	18–20	≥21
Clindamycin	≤0.25	0.5	≥1	≤15	16–18	≥19
Erythromycin	≤0.25	0.5	≥1	≤15	16–20	≥21
Penicillin						
Beta group[d]	≤0.12					≥24
Viridans group[b]	≤0.12	0.25–2	≥4			
Vancomycin[d]	≤1					≥17
H. influenzae						
Ampicillin	≤1	2	≥4	≤18	19–21	≥22
Ampicillin-sulbactam	≤2/1		≥4/2	≤19		≥20
Cefotaxime[d]	≤2					≥26
Ceftazidime[d]	≤2					≥26
Ceftizoxime[d]	≤2					≥26
Ceftriaxone[d]	≤2					≥26
Cefuroxime sodium (parenteral)	≤4	8	≥16	≤16	17–19	≥20
Chloramphenicol	≤2	4	≥8	≤25	26–28	≥29
Meropenem[d]	≤0.5					≥20
TMP-SMX	≤0.5/9.5	1/19–2/38	≥4/76	≤10	11–15	≥16
N. gonorrhoeae						
Cefixime[d]	≤0.25					≥31
Cefotaxime[d]	≤0.5					≥31
Ceftriaxone[d]	≤0.25					≥35
Ciprofloxacin	≤0.06	0.12–0.5	≥1	≤27	28–40	≥41
Gatifloxacin	≤0.12	0.25	≥0.5	≤33	34–37	≥38
Ofloxacin	≤0.25	0.5–1	≥2	≤24	25–30	≥31
Penicillin	≤0.06	0.12–1	≥2	≤26	27–46	≥47
Tetracycline	≤0.25	0.5–1	≥2	≤30	31–37	≥38

[a] Adapted from NCCLS data (89–91). The interpretive data are valid only if the methodologies in M2-A7 (90) and M7-A5 (89) are followed. NCCLS frequently updates the interpretive tables through new additions of the standards and supplements to them. Users should refer to the most recent additions. The current standards and supplements to them may be obtained from NCCLS, 940 W. Valley Rd., Wayne, PA 19087-1898.

[b] No disk diffusion interpretive criteria defined.

[c] For *S. pneumoniae* penicillin testing, a 1-μg oxacillin disk should be used. If the inhibition zone diameter is ≤19 mm, the MIC of penicillin should be determined.

[d] The absence of resistant strains precludes definition of any result category other than susceptible.

ratory should immediately determine the MICs of penicillin, an extended-spectrum cephalosporin, and vancomycin. Meropenem should also be tested if it is on the institution's formulary (86). MICs would be available without the 24-h delay that a screening test would necessitate if the isolates had oxacillin zones of ≤19 mm.

Along with penicillin, NCCLS recommends primary testing and reporting of erythromycin and TMP-SMX for non-CNS infections. Both drugs can be tested by either the broth microdilution or the disk diffusion method; however, intermittent problems with the pneumococcal QC strain, *S. pneumoniae* ATCC 49619, when TMP-SMX susceptibility was tested by the disk diffusion method have been reported (45).

Commercial Methods for Testing

Several options are available for determining MICs of various antimicrobial agents for pneumococci. The most widely used and evaluated commercial option is the E-test method (AB Biodisk, Solna, Sweden) (56, 63, 64, 70, 74, 105, 112); all drugs recommended by NCCLS for testing against pneumococci except clindamycin have been cleared by the FDA for testing by the E test. The accuracy of the E test has been reported to be >90% for most relevant drugs; however, the number of minor errors with penicillin is relatively high. E-test penicillin MICs are slightly lower than those determined by the reference broth microdilution procedure (56, 63). Since the E test uses incubation in CO_2, the MICs of the macrolides tend to be 1 to 2 dilutions higher than those determined by the broth tests, in which incubation is done in ambient air (97). This is because macrolides are less active at lower pH, which occurs with CO_2 incubation.

Other commercially available FDA-cleared panels or systems specifically designed for testing of pneumococci include Pasco (Difco, Wheatridge, Colo.), MicroScan (Dade MicroScan Inc., West Sacramento, Calif.), Micro-Tech (Aurora, Colo.), Sensititre (Trek Diagnostic Systems, Inc., Westlake, Ohio), and Vitek 2 (bioMerieux, Inc., Hazelwood, Mo.). The Pasco, MicroScan MICroSTREP, and Vitek 2 systems have been evaluated recently and found to produce MICs that are comparable to those determined by the broth microdilution reference method (47, 60, 61, 80).

Strategies for Testing and Reporting of Results

NCCLS has recently revised its recommendations for testing of pneumococci to stipulate that isolates from cerebrospinal fluid (CSF) (rather than isolates from both blood and CSF) be routinely tested by a reliable MIC method to determine susceptibilities to penicillin, cefotaxime or ceftriaxone, meropenem, and vancomycin. Vancomycin may be tested by either the MIC or the disk diffusion method. However, in communities where penicillin resistance is high and resistance to other agents is likely, MIC testing of penicillin, cefotaxime or ceftriaxone, meropenem, vancomycin, and one representative each of the macrolide, fluoroquinolone, and tetracycline classes would be appropriate for testing of strains isolated from blood. Other drugs that might warrant testing if being considered for treatment of infections outside the CNS include cefepime, clindamycin, and rifampin. Infections, such as pneumonia, caused by strains for which the MICs of penicillin are in the intermediate range may be treatable with penicillin or an extended-spectrum cephalosporin if maximal doses are used (44, 50), and it may be appropriate to

include a comment to this effect on the patient report. NCCLS has recently approved a second set of nonmeningitis MIC breakpoints for cefotaxime and ceftriaxone that apply to infections outside the CNS (86). For CSF isolates, only interpretations using the original meningitis breakpoints should be reported; for isolates from infections outside the CNS, both meningitis and nonmeningitis interpretations should be reported (86).

The oxacillin screening procedure should be used only for isolates from patients with non-life-threatening infections, and if the zone diameter is ≤19 mm, at a minimum, the MICs of penicillin and an extended-spectrum cephalosporin should then be determined. Disk diffusion testing is not accurate for the extended-spectrum cephalosporins, and there are no disk diffusion breakpoints for any cephalosporin approved by NCCLS for the testing of pneumococci (86).

STREPTOCOCCI OTHER THAN PNEUMOCOCCI

Incidence of Resistance

Because there are significant differences in susceptibility to β-lactam agents in viridans group versus beta-hemolytic streptococci, there are now separate penicillin, cefotaxime, ceftriaxone, and cefepime interpretive criteria for the two organism groups. As defined by NCCLS (86), the members of the viridans group include strains identified as *Streptococcus mitis*, *S. oralis*, *S. sanguis*, *S. salivarius*, *S. intermedius*, *S. constellatus*, *S. mutans*, and *S. bovis*, as well as the small-colony-forming beta-hemolytic strains with group A, C, F, or G antigen (the *S. anginosus* group, which was previously called *S. milleri*). The beta-hemolytic group includes the large-colony-forming pyogenic strains with group A (*S. pyogenes*), C, or G antigen and strains with group B (*S. agalactiae*) antigen. Although beta-hemolytic streptococci have been uniformly susceptible to penicillin, two reports have described penicillin MICs of 0.25 to 0.5 µg/ml for group B streptococci (13) and group C streptococci (113). The clinical significance of these elevated MICs is not known. Penicillin resistance in viridans group streptococci has been described since the 1970s (20), although the incidence has increased since then. Penicillin resistance rates of >50% for viridans group streptococci are common (2, 35, 115), particularly for *S. mitis* and *S. sanguis*.

Among other classes of agents, resistance has been described for macrolides, lincosamides, tetracyclines, quinupristin-dalfopristin, and fluoroquinolones (1, 35, 115). Single reports of resistance to vancomycin have been noted for *S. bovis* (92) and *S. mitis* (69). The incidence of resistance to most drugs, except for the macrolides, is low; the incidence of resistance to fluoroquinolones is extremely low (28). Resistance to erythromycin is highly variable and is dependent on the degree of erythromycin usage in the community. In Finland, for example, a rate as high as 54% in one city was noted in 1990 for *S. pyogenes* (102). More recently in California, rates varied by county and were reported as high as 32% (124). High-level aminoglycoside resistance has been described for group B and viridans group streptococci (23, 40, 55), the two species for which treatment is likely to include gentamicin or streptomycin.

The MLS-type macrolide resistance in beta-hemolytic streptococci may be either inducible or constitutive (29, 66, 103). If the resistance is inducible, the strains will be resistant to erythromycin (and the other 14- and 15-

membered macrolides) but may appear susceptible to clindamycin unless resistance is induced. A double-disk test using erythromycin and clindamycin that detects inducible resistance in beta-hemolytic streptococci can be performed (81, 103, 124) (see "Reference Test Methods" below). However, the clinical significance of determining inducible resistance to clindamycin when clindamycin is being considered for therapy of a patient infected with an erythromycin-resistant strain is unknown.

Reference Test Methods

Studies by NCCLS to determine interpretive criteria for both MIC and disk diffusion testing have resulted in breakpoints for streptococci that were initially published in 1995. Penicillin and select cephalosporin breakpoints were recently modified as mentioned above. Details for MIC and disk diffusion tests are described in Table 1, and interpretive criteria are listed in Table 2. The disk diffusion test may be used to determine the penicillin susceptibility of beta-hemolytic streptococci; however, the high number of minor errors with penicillin when viridans group streptococci are tested precludes use of the disk diffusion method for that group. Other agents may be tested by either the MIC or the disk method. Aminoglycoside MICs of >1,000 μg/ml for streptococci (121) have been described; however, there are no published methods for screening for high-level aminoglycoside resistance in streptococci.

Susceptibility testing of members of the genera *Abiotrophia* and *Granulicatella* (formerly known as "nutritionally deficient streptococci") can be accomplished by adding 0.001% pyridoxal HCl to the test medium (96). Although penicillin resistance has been described for nutritionally deficient streptococci (96, 114), the results of susceptibility testing may not correlate with treatment outcome (108).

Inducible resistance to clindamycin in beta-hemolytic streptococci can be determined by performing a double-disk test using erythromycin to induce resistance to clindamycin. Mueller-Hinton agar (MHA) supplemented with 5% sheep blood is inoculated as for a disk diffusion test, a 15-μg erythromycin disk and a 2-μg clindamycin disk are placed approximately 12 to 20 mm apart on the agar surface, and the plate is incubated at 35°C overnight; truncation of the clindamycin zone indicates inducible resistance (81, 103). This method, however, has not been thoroughly evaluated and should be considered investigational.

Commercial Test Methods

There have been very few reports of evaluations of commercial susceptibility test systems for streptococci other than pneumococci, although it might be expected that systems capable of testing pneumococci would also perform adequately for other streptococci. The MicroScan panel, MICroSTREP, was recently cleared by the FDA for the testing of these organisms and *S. pneumoniae*. Pasco also has a broth microdilution panel that was recently evaluated and found to perform well (80). The Vitek 2 system can be used for testing of group B streptococci only. The E test has not been extensively evaluated but does appear to be a possible alternative to the reference methods (58; J. Hindler and D. A. Bruckner, *Abstr. 33rd Intersci. Conf. Antimicrob. Agents Chemother.*, abstr. 254, 1993); however, few E-test strips have been cleared by the FDA for diagnostic testing of these organisms in clinical laboratories.

Strategies for Testing and Reporting of Results

Routine testing of beta-hemolytic streptococci is unnecessary since there have been only sporadic reports of penicillin resistance (13, 113). However, if erythromycin is being used to treat infections caused by group A streptococci and treatment failure is suspected, testing might be considered. If clindamycin is being considered for treatment of erythromycin-resistant strains, the determination of inducible clindamycin resistance might also be considered. For viridans group streptococci, penicillin MICs should be determined for strains isolated from blood, especially for patients with infective endocarditis. Disk diffusion is not reliable for the testing of penicillin resistance in viridans group streptococci because it cannot determine the precise levels of penicillin resistance that are needed to guide therapy (121).

H. INFLUENZAE

Incidence of Resistance

Plasmid-mediated β-lactamase-producing *H. influenzae* was first reported in the early 1970s. The incidence of isolates that are ampicillin resistant due to the production of TEM-1 β-lactamase (the most common β-lactamase) continues to be a concern worldwide, with rates ranging from 5% to nearly 40% in various geographic areas (15, 17, 52, 99).

Ampicillin resistance occasionally results from altered penicillin-binding proteins in β-lactamase-negative, ampicillin-resistant (BLNAR) isolates. Blondeau et al. noted that of 566 β-lactamase-negative *H. influenzae* isolates from Canada, 2.7% were resistant and 1.8% showed intermediate susceptibility to ampicillin (17). In contrast, a recent international survey by Sahm et al. did not identify any BLNAR isolates among 2,645 isolates tested (99). Compared with β-lactamase-producing or ampicillin-susceptible *H. influenzae*, BLNAR isolates are less susceptible to amoxicillin-clavulanic acid and to various cephalosporins such as cefaclor, cefuroxime, cefixime, and cefotaxime (12). Recently, Barry et al. studied 143 non-β-lactamase-producing isolates, using four methods; for half of the isolates, the MICs of ampicillin were $\geq$1 μg/ml. In their conclusion, the researchers emphasized the need for a universal definition of BLNAR, along with identification of the optimal method for the testing of such strains and guidelines on interpreting the results before the clinical relevance of such strains can be evaluated (11).

Resistance among *H. influenzae* isolates to broad-spectrum oral cephalosporins (e.g., cefixime and cefpodoxime) is rare, and the overall rate of resistance to expanded-spectrum cephalosporins (e.g., cefuroxime) is 4 to 6%. To date, resistance to extended-spectrum cephalosporins (e.g., ceftriaxone or cefotaxime) has not been reported. The narrower-spectrum, β-lactamase-labile cephalosporins (e.g., cefaclor, loracarbef, and cefprozil) are less active, with resistance rates ranging from 10 to 20% (15, 17, 37, 42, 99).

Resistance to TMP-SMX appears to be increasing, with approximately 10 to 15% resistance among isolates from North America (17, 37). Resistance rates as high as 45% have been reported in Spain (42, 99). Resistance to chloramphenicol, tetracycline, and rifampin is <2% (15, 17, 42), and resistance to fluoroquinolones is very rare (15, 42, 99). Although erythromycin has not been considered a drug of choice for the treatment of infections caused by *H. influenzae*, some of the newer macrolides are more active than erythromycin and may be effective as treatment. Less than 1% of isolates examined in various studies was resistant to azithromycin; however, clarithromycin was less active (15, 42, 99), and 16% of isolates in one study were resistant to this agent (15). The clinical significance of these differences is not known.

Reference Test Methods

β-Lactamase production in *H. influenzae* can easily be detected by the chromogenic cephalosporin, acidometric, or iodometric β-lactamase test method (see chapter 74).

NCCLS has developed standard disk diffusion and MIC methods for the testing of *H. influenzae*, and these methods can also be used to test other *Haemophilus* spp. Specific variables related to each of the methods are listed in Table 1, and interpretive criteria are listed in Table 2. *Haemophilus* test medium (HTM) is recommended and consists of a Mueller-Hinton base, 15 μg of hematin per ml, 15 μg of NAD per ml, and 5 mg of yeast extract per ml. Cation-adjusted Mueller-Hinton broth (CAMHB) is used with the components listed above for the preparation of HTM broth, which also contains 0.2 IU of thymidine phosphorylase per ml (65). Although HTM agar is transparent, some investigators have reported difficulties in measuring zones and poor growth of some strains (49, 79). Broth microdilution tests with HTM generally give clearer endpoints. The problems most often noted with both the disk diffusion and the broth microdilution methods are equivocal endpoints with BLNAR strains with several β-lactams. Because of this, NCCLS recommends that BLNAR strains (which are best detected by tests with ampicillin) be considered resistant to amoxicillin-clavulanic acid, ampicillin-sulbactam, cefalor, cefamandole, cefetamet, cefonicid, cefprozil, cefuroxime, loracarbef, and piperacillin-tazobactam and that the activities of these agents against BLNAR strains not be tested (86).

Commercial Test Methods

Currently, the FDA-cleared broth microdilution panels for testing *Haemophilus* spp. include MicroTech and Sensititre (*H. influenzae* only). The E test has been cleared by the FDA for testing *H. influenzae* with most drugs that would be used for treatment of *Haemophilus* infections (64).

Strategies for Testing and Reporting of Results

β-Lactamase testing detects the most common type of clinically significant resistance in *H. influenzae*. β-Lactamase-positive isolates are ampicillin and amoxicillin resistant. To detect BLNAR strains, an ampicillin disk diffusion or MIC test is required. However, since the incidence of BLNAR is very low, such tests may not be routinely needed, and for practical purposes, a negative β-lactamase test result translates into ampicillin susceptibility. Frequently, the β-lactamase test is the only test routinely performed with clinical isolates. Because of increasing resistance to TMP-SMX, testing should be considered, and NCCLS recommends that this agent be tested and reported routinely (86). Other oral agents that might be considered, such as the oral cephalosporins, newer macrolides, and fluoroquinolones, are predictably active and are often prescribed empirically. Consequently, routine testing of these drugs is generally not useful. However, these and other agents may be tested for surveillance or epidemiological purposes (86).

N. GONORRHOEAE

Incidence of Resistance

During the past two decades, increasing rates of penicillin and tetracycline resistance among *N. gonorrhoeae* isolates have led to the recommendation of ceftriaxone, cefixime, ciprofloxacin, and ofloxacin as the primary agents for uncomplicated gonorrhea instead of penicillin or tetracycline (25, 77, 101). Penicillin resistance is due to the production of a plasmid-associated TEM-1-type β-lactamase (penicillinase-producing *N. gonorrhoeae* [PPNG]) or to mutations in chromosomal genes that result in altered penicillin-binding proteins or diminished outer membrane permeability (chromosomally mediated resistant *N. gonorrhoeae* [CMRNG]). The activities of other β-lactams against PPNG are generally unaltered; however, CMRNG may show decreased susceptibility to other β-lactams (30). Tetracycline resistance in *N. gonorrhoeae* can be plasmid or chromosomally mediated, with plasmid-mediated resistance resulting in a higher level of resistance. The Gonococcal Isolate Surveillance Program (GISP), which tests urethral isolates from male clients visiting sexually transmitted disease clinics throughout the United States, recently demonstrated a decline in the incidence of PPNG from 11.0% in 1991 to 2.1% in 1999. The proportion of isolates with penicillin or tetracycline resistance in 1999 was 28.1%. All 5,180 isolates tested were susceptible to ceftriaxone and cefixime. An elevated ceftriaxone MIC of 0.5 μg/ml was found for only 4 isolates, and for 41 elevated cefixime MICs of 0.5 to 2.0 μg/ml were found (26).

In the 1999 GISP study, 1.0% of the isolates exhibited intermediate susceptibility and 0.4% were resistant to ciprofloxacin (26). However, fluoroquinolone resistance has become widespread throughout Asia. In a recent study of 115 isolates of *N. gonorrhoeae* from female sex workers in the Philippines, the MICs of ciprofloxacin for 49% of isolates were ≥4 μg/ml, and for 63% the MICs were ≥1 μg/ml (5). In Japan in 1997 to 1998, the MICs of ciprofloxacin for 24.4% of 502 *N. gonorrhoeae* isolates from males with urethritis were ≥1 μg/ml (111).

Reference Test Methods

Routine β-lactamase tests readily detect PPNG and can reliably be performed by either the chromogenic cephalosporin, acidimetric, or iodometric method.

NCCLS recommends the use of GC agar base for disk diffusion and agar dilution MIC testing. For both tests, a 1% defined growth supplement must be added; however, in agar dilution tests with imipenem and clavulanate, the growth supplement must be free of cysteine to avoid inhibition of the activities of these two agents (84–86). The agar dilution method is preferred to the broth dilution method for MIC testing because *N. gonorrhoeae* has a tendency to autolyze in liquid media. For other details of testing, see Table 1 and note interpretive criteria in Table 2.

Commercial Test Methods

The only commercial method that has been investigated to any significant extent is the E test, which was reported to produce results comparable to those of conventional reference agar dilution methods (14).

Strategies for Testing and Reporting of Results

Generally, there is no need for routine clinical laboratories to perform antimicrobial susceptibility tests with *N. gonor-*

rhoeae unless there are unusual circumstances. These might include the patient's intolerance to the drugs of choice, treatment failure (assuming that compliance was not an issue), or a disseminated gonococcal infection against which an alternative agent might be preferred. Additionally, if fluoroquinolone resistance is noted in a particular geographic area, testing may be warranted if fluoroquinolones are being prescribed. Some laboratories may perform β-lactamase tests for all isolates if β-lactamase results are requested by the local public health departments for epidemiological purposes. However, many public health departments have eliminated this requirement. Surveillance for established and emerging resistance is generally performed by designated state and local public health agencies.

N. MENINGITIDIS

Incidence of Resistance

Increasing numbers of *N. meningitidis* isolates from the United States and elsewhere that are β-lactamase negative have reduced susceptibility to penicillin (MICs, 0.12 to 1.0 μg/ml), although the frequency of these isolates in different regions varies widely (4, 8, 18, 22, 72, 117, 122). A recent study of 400 isolates obtained in 1998 and 1999 in Spain showed penicillin MICs of 0.12 to 1 μg/ml for 37% of the isolates (117). In contrast, for 3% of 90 *N. meningitidis* isolates from normally sterile sites in 1997 in the United States, the penicillin MICs were 0.12 μg/ml, and for the remaining 87 isolates the penicillin MICs were 0.06 μg/ml (95). The clinical significance of isolates for which penicillin MICs are elevated is uncertain, and penicillin remains the drug of choice for the treatment of meningococcal disease (77, 101). Many infections caused by isolates with reduced susceptibility to penicillin have successfully been treated with high doses of penicillin (109, 122); however, rare reports cited clinical failure (meningitis) when a lower than recommended dose of penicillin was used (116). The broad-spectrum cephalosporins (e.g., ceftriaxone) remain highly active against these isolates (8, 18, 117). In the 1980s, four isolates of β-lactamase-producing *N. meningitidis* were reported (19, 31, 43), and one isolate was reported in 1996 (118); additional isolates have not been noted. Regarding agents used for prophylaxis, resistance to sulfonamides occurs frequently, and resistance to rifampin has been documented on rare occasions (8, 95, 117, 123). There is one report of *N. meningitidis* isolated from CSF from a patient in Australia with decreased susceptibility to ciprofloxacin (MIC, 0.25 μg/ml); however, *N. meningitidis* is typically very susceptible to this agent (MIC, $\leq$0.03 μg/ml) (104).

Strategies for Testing and Reporting of Results

Various broth and agar dilution methods have been used for susceptibility testing of *N. meningitidis*. NCCLS recommends the broth microdilution method using CAMHB with 2 to 5% lysed horse blood (CAMHB-LHB) or the agar dilution method using MHA with 5% sheep blood (both with incubation in 5% CO_2) (86). While incubation in CO_2 is not required, it enhances growth and makes the endpoints easier to read. NCCLS has not yet provided MIC interpretive criteria for *N. meningitidis*. Thus, MICs must be evaluated cautiously. Some provisional MIC breakpoints have been suggested (75, 95).

Although disk diffusion methods (with 2- and 10-IU penicillin disks and 1-μg oxacillin disks) have been exam-

ined for penicillin testing (24), it has been noted that these methods cannot reliably distinguish *N. meningitidis* isolates that are susceptible from those that have decreased penicillin or ampicillin susceptibility (90). Therefore, disk diffusion testing should not be used for these drugs.

Because of the lack of clinical failures with the drugs of choice for the treatment of meningococcal infections, susceptibility testing is probably not warranted in most situations (94, 95). However, if susceptibility testing is required, MIC testing should be performed by one of the two methods suggested by NCCLS, as described above. The E test shows promising results for meningococci and is best used with MHA with 5% sheep blood incubated in CO_2 (75, 89, 90).

M. CATARRHALIS

Incidence of Resistance

More than 90% of M. *catarrhalis* isolates produce β-lactamase (15, 17, 37, 42, 52, 99) and are resistant to amoxicillin, ampicillin, and penicillin. These isolates remain susceptible to amoxicillin-clavulanic acid, which is often prescribed for M. *catarrhalis* infections. Most clinical isolates produce one of two types of chromosomally mediated β-lactamases: BRO-1 or BRO-2 (41, 93). BRO-1-producing strains are 10-fold or more prevalent than BRO-2-producing strains, and ampicillin and penicillin MICs for BRO-1 strains appear to be higher (e.g., $\geq$4.0 μg/ml) than those for BRO-2 strains (e.g., $\leq$0.5 μg/ml) (33, 93). Because of the low MICs for the latter strains, their clinical significance in response to β-lactamase-labile penicillins is questionable. In 1994, a study of isolates from 723 outpatients among 30 medical centers in the United States demonstrated a 6.5% rate of resistance to TMP-SMX (32); however, a similar study in North America in 1997 showed <1% resistance to this agent (37). Hoban et al. reported 2.6% TMP-SMX resistance in Latin America in 1997 to 1999 (52). Resistance to the other drugs recommended for treatment of M. *catarrhalis* infections remains <1% (15, 37, 42, 99).

Strategies for Testing and Reporting of Results

Only the chromogenic cephalosporin method has reliably detected the β-lactamases produced by M. *catarrhalis* (38). Routine β-lactamase testing may not be necessary because of the high incidence of β-lactamase-positive strains. Nevertheless, some advocate reporting of β-lactamase results to highlight the fact that this pathogen is generally unresponsive to some agents (e.g., amoxicillin) commonly prescribed for the treatment of respiratory tract infections. Since M. *catarrhalis* typically responds to the drugs of choice, testing beyond the β-lactamase test is rarely indicated. Current NCCLS protocols do not address antimicrobial susceptibility testing of M. *catarrhalis* other than to suggest that β-lactamase testing be performed (84, 85). Most isolates of M. *catarrhalis* grow satisfactorily in CAMHB and on MHA with ambient air incubation. Despite the lack of standardized test recommendations, Doern and Tubert (38) demonstrated that disk diffusion interpretive criteria for nonfastidious bacteria published by NCCLS in 1984 appear to be satisfactory, at least as they pertain to the susceptible category, for amoxicillin-clavulanic acid, cephalothin, chloramphenicol, erythromycin, tetracycline, and TMP-SMX (82). However, because of the absence of frank resistance to these agents among the 74 clinical isolates of M. *catarrhalis* examined, the investigators were unable to make definitive recommendations pertaining to disk diffusion testing. Disk diffusion and MIC interpretive criteria were defined for ampicillin. These conclusions were made following testing of all isolates by NCCLS reference disk diffusion and MIC methods.

L. MONOCYTOGENES

Incidence of Resistance

L. monocytogenes remains susceptible to the drugs of choice, including ampicillin (or penicillin) and TMP-SMX. In vitro, it is susceptible to other common agents, including chloramphenicol, vancomycin, tetracyclines, and macrolides (73, 76); however, these agents have not proved to be as useful in vivo as the aforementioned agents (53, 57). Although L. monocytogenes may appear susceptible to cephalosporins in vitro, these agents are not effective clinically.

Strategies for Testing and Reporting of Results

Interpretive criteria for ampicillin and penicillin are included in the current NCCLS MIC tables (86). Only criteria for susceptibility (MIC, ≤2.0 μg/ml) are listed because clinical isolates of L. monocytogenes with ampicillin resistance have not been noted. Suggested test parameters include the use of CAMHB-LHB and incubation for 16 to 20 h. L. monocytogenes is not truly fastidious, and testing in Mueller-Hinton broth without the blood supplement has been done satisfactorily (73, 76). It is important to remember that susceptibility to cephalosporins should not be tested or reported for L. monocytogenes, as these results might be misleading (3). This cautionary note is emphasized in NCCLS documents (85) and illustrates why it is inappropriate to indiscriminately report susceptibility results for any agent without knowing if it would be a reasonable therapeutic option. Because cephalosporins are frequently used empirically for the treatment of meningitis, the laboratory should quickly communicate smear or culture findings suspicious for Listeria whenever they occur.

H. PYLORI

Incidence of Resistance

The rates of resistance for H. pylori vary considerably among the agents recommended for therapy (e.g., amoxicillin, clarithromycin, metronidazole, and tetracycline), with resistance to metronidazole being highest. Using the NCCLS reference method, Osato et al. recently reported approximately 35% resistance to metronidazole among 3,193 isolates in the United States (88). In a Korean study that used similar methodologies, 40.6% of 652 isolates were metronidazole resistant (68); however, a study in Japan reported only 12.4% metronidazole resistance among 388 isolates but noted significant differences in various geographic areas (67). Clarithromycin resistance rates were lower, with approximately 11% resistance in the U.S. study and 5.9 and 12.9% resistance observed in the Korean and Japanese studies, respectively. The incidence of resistance to tetracycline and amoxicillin is currently very low (68, 71, 88).

Reference Test Method

NCCLS describes an agar dilution MIC method for the testing of H. pylori. The test medium is MHA supplemented with aged (≥2-week-old) sheep blood. The inoculum is prepared from 72-h-old growth on a blood agar plate to obtain a final concentration of bacteria approximating 10^5 CFU/spot. Incubation is done for 3 days at 35°C in a microaerobic atmosphere produced by a gas-generating system typically used for campylobacters. H. pylori ATCC 43504 has been designated as a QC strain, and currently there are interpretive criteria only for clarithromycin. Other antimicrobial agents that have been studied and for which there are NCCLS QC ranges include amoxicillin, metronidazole, telithromycin (a ketolide), and tetracycline (86). Despite the standardization efforts for the NCCLS method, Osato et al. recently demonstrated discordant results for metronidazole when they tested multiple isolates from different parts of the stomach of individual patients. Incubation of test samples in a microaerobic rather than an anaerobic environment may contribute to the discordance for metronidazole, which is optimally active in an anaerobic environment. Similar problems were not noted for clarithromycin (87).

Commercial Test Methods

Although no commercial methods are FDA cleared for antimicrobial susceptibility testing of H. pylori, several investigators have examined the E test. Osato et al. noted considerably higher rates of resistance to metronidazole among U.S. isolates when comparing E-test and agar dilution results (39 versus 21.6%, respectively). There were no statistical differences for clarithromycin results obtained by the two methods (87, 88). Other investigators noted similar results (78, 91).

Strategies for Testing and Reporting of Results

Because of growth requirements and complex antimicrobial susceptibility testing recommendations, testing of H. pylori is not practical for the routine clinical laboratory. However, because of the significant resistance noted for metronidazole and clarithromycin, testing may be required in select situations, in which case a reliable reference laboratory should be used. Although there are currently no NCCLS interpretive criteria for metronidazole, investigators have used a MIC of >8 μg/ml for resistance (68, 71, 87, 88).

C. JEJUNI

Drugs of Choice for Therapy

Many cases of gastrointestinal disease associated with C. jejuni are self-limiting and do not require antimicrobial therapy. However, in severe cases of gastroenteritis, extraintestinal disease, or disease in patients with underlying conditions, antimicrobial therapy is required (39). The therapy of choice for C. jejuni infections associated with severe gastrointestinal disease is a macrolide (azithromycin, clarithromycin, or erythromycin) or a fluoroquinolone. Alternatives are a tetracycline or gentamicin (77, 101).

Incidence of Resistance

Resistance to macrolides and fluoroquinolones, the drugs of choice for treatment of gastrointestinal infections caused by C. jejuni, is being reported with increasing frequency for human and animal isolates of C. jejuni. Smith et al. examined nearly 5,000 C. jejuni isolates from feces of Minnesota residents and noted an increase in incidence of ciprofloxacin resistance from 1.3% in 1992 to 10.2% in 1998 (107). Of 537 C. jejuni isolates from human fecal specimens obtained during 1997 and 1998 in Spain, 75% were resistant to ciprofloxacin and 3.2% were resistant to erythromycin (98). Resistance among animal isolates, which may subsequently be transmitted to humans, has been associated with the addition of macrolides and fluoroquinolones to animal food as growth-promoting agents (39, 98, 107).

Strategies for Testing and Reporting of Results

There are currently no standard methods for testing of *C. jejuni*. NCCLS is in the process of defining a standard method, and preliminary studies have shown that agar dilution using MHA supplemented with 5% sheep blood and 48-h incubation at 36°C in an atmosphere provided by campylobacter gas-generating systems appears satisfactory. Incubation for 24 h at 42°C is also being evaluated. Disk diffusion methods have been used successfully by some investigators (46, 98), although the NCCLS studies noted that measurement of zones can be very difficult (R. Walker, personal communication). The E test correlated well with agar dilution in a study by Baker et al. when ciprofloxacin, erythromycin, and tetracycline were tested (9), and Hayward had similar success when testing gatifloxacin (48).

Because of the increasing incidence of resistance, testing of individual patient isolates may be warranted in select situations. Submission of isolates to a reference laboratory experienced in testing *C. jejuni* and using an agar dilution method is optimal. Since no standardized method has been described, results generated with any method would have to be qualified as presumptive.

OFB

It is usually unnecessary and inappropriate to perform susceptibility tests with OFB such as *Pasteurella*, *Bordetella*, and *Legionella* spp. and various coryneform bacilli because infections caused by them generally respond to the drugs of choice (101). Many physicians are unaware that susceptibility testing of OFB is complex and that standardized methods and criteria for interpretation of the results are unavailable. Communication of this information will often result in the physician's reconsideration of the request. For serious infections caused by OFB, physicians should be encouraged to seek assistance from an infectious diseases specialist to ensure proper patient management.

On rare occasions, in vitro susceptibility testing of OFB may be required. These occasions might include clinical failure, patient intolerance to the drug(s) of choice, or serious infections against which there are several appropriate drugs that might be prescribed. Additionally, susceptibility testing may aid in species identification (e.g., differentiating *C. jeikeium* from other *Corynebacterium* species). However, because testing is performed by nonstandardized methods, the results must always be interpreted with caution. To guide therapy, reported MIC results can be interpreted by comparing them with the results obtained in various clinical studies documented in the literature. Use of published NCCLS interpretive criteria for nonfastidious bacteria or OFB may result in a misleading report. For example, the typical MIC of penicillin for *Eikenella corrodens* is 1 μg/ml, and penicillin is a drug of choice for the treatment of infections caused by this organism. Use of the penicillin interpretive criteria for staphylococci (with an MIC of $\geq$0.5 indicating resistance) would generate a misleading interpretation of resistance. The impact of unique characteristics of specific organisms (e.g., resistance mechanisms or growth requirements or both) and the types of infections they cause on MIC interpretive criteria can be

appreciated by examining the six different MIC resistance breakpoints for penicillin (e.g., *Staphylococcus*, *Enterococcus*, *S. pneumoniae*, other species of *Streptococcus*, *N. gonorrhoeae*, and *Listeria*) published by NCCLS (86).

The E test has been examined for the testing of a variety of OFB. Many of the data generated have been obtained from comparisons with nonstandardized in vitro test methods, with limited examination of the clinical correlation of the results. Consequently, the results for OFB generated by the E test should also be interpreted with caution in the clinical setting.

A variety of nonstandardized methods of determining the MICs for various OFB have been described in the literature, and they may or may not give comparable results for a given organism. The disk diffusion test should generally not be used because many OFB are slow growing or grow satisfactorily only on an enriched medium. These characteristics can have a significant impact on the diameters of the inhibition zones.

When a nonstandardized method is used, this does not mean that the results are inaccurate; it means that the methods and results have not undergone rigid evaluation to prove that they are meaningful in various clinical settings. In contrast, methods such as those recommended by NCCLS for the testing of *S. pneumoniae*, *Streptococcus* spp., *N. gonorrhoeae*, *H. influenzae*, and *H. pylori* were developed systematically (83) and were subjected to critical review prior to their acceptance as standards (86). Nevertheless, even the standardized methods are not perfect. It is important for laboratory workers to maintain an awareness of the methods available for testing of fastidious bacteria and their strengths and limitations (62). If testing must be performed, it should be done by a laboratory familiar with these limitations.

REFERENCES

1. **Alcaide, F., J. Carratala, J. Liñares, F. Gudiol, and R. Martin.** 1996. In vitro activities of eight macrolide antibiotics and RP-59500 (quinupristin-dalfopristin) against viridans group streptococci isolated from blood of neutropenic cancer patients. *Antimicrob. Agents Chemother.* **40:** 2117–2120.
2. **Alcaide, F., J. Liñares, R. Pallares, J. Carratala, M. A. Benitez, F. Gudiol, and R. Martin.** 1995. In vitro activities of 22 β-lactam antibiotics against penicillin-resistant and penicillin-susceptible viridans group streptococci isolated from blood. *Antimicrob. Agents Chemother.* **39:**2243–2247.
3. **Allerberger, F. J., and M. P. Dierich.** 1992. Listeriosis and cephalosporins. *Clin. Infect. Dis.* **15:**177–178.
4. **Andrews, J. M., and R. Wise.** 2000. In vitro susceptibility of *Neisseria meningitidis*. *J. Antimicrob. Chemother.* **45:**548.
5. **Aplasca De Los Reyes, M. R., V. Pato-Mesola, J. D. Klausner, R. Manalastas, T. Wi, C. U. Tuazon, G. Dallabetta, W. L. Whittington, and K. K. Holmes.** 2001. A randomized trial of ciprofloxacin versus cefixime for treatment of gonorrhea after rapid emergence of gonococcal ciprofloxacin resistance in the Philippines. *Clin. Infect. Dis.* **32:**1313–1318.
6. **Appelbaum, P. C.** 1992. Antimicrobial resistance in *Streptococcus pneumoniae*: an overview. *Clin. Infect. Dis.* **15:**77–83.
7. **Appelbaum, P. C.** 1996. Epidemiology and in vitro susceptibility of drug-resistant *Streptococcus pneumoniae*. *Pediatr. Infect. Dis. J.* **15:**932–934.
8. **Arreaza, L., L. de La Fuente, and J. A. Vazquez.** 2000. Antibiotic susceptibility patterns of *Neisseria meningitidis*

isolates from patients and asymptomatic carriers. *Antimicrob. Agents Chemother.* **44:**1705–1707.

9. **Baker, C. N.** 1992. The E-Test and *Campylobacter jejuni. Diagn. Microbiol. Infect. Dis.* **15:**469–472.

10. **Baquero, F.** 1995. Pneumococcal resistance to beta-lactam antibiotics: a global geographic overview. *Microb. Drug Resist.* **1:**115–120.

11. **Barry, A. L., P. C. Fuchs, and S. D. Brown.** 2001. Identification of beta-lactamase-negative, ampicillin-resistant strains of *Haemophilus influenzae* with four methods and eight media. *Antimicrob. Agents Chemother.* **45:** 1585–1588.

12. **Barry, A. L., P. C. Fuchs, and M. A. Pfaller.** 1993. Susceptibilities of β-lactamase-producing and -nonproducing ampicillin-resistant strains of *Haemophilus influenzae* to ceftibuten, cefaclor, cefuroxime, cefixime, cefotaxime, and amoxicillin/clavulanic acid. *Antimicrob. Agents Chemother.* **37:**14–18.

13. **Betriu, C., M. Gomez, A. Sanchez, A. Cruceyra, J. Romero, and J. J. Picazo.** 1994. Antibiotic resistance and penicillin tolerance in clinical isolates of group B streptococci. *Antimicrob. Agents Chemother.* **38:**2183–2186.

14. **Biedenbach, D. J., and R. N. Jones.** 1996. Comparative assessment of Etest for testing susceptibilities of *Neisseria gonorrhoeae* to penicillin, tetracycline, ceftriaxone, cefotaxime, and ciprofloxacin: investigation using 510(k) review criteria, recommended by the Food and Drug Administration. *J. Clin. Microbiol.* **34:**3214–3217.

15. **Biedenbach, D. J., R. N. Jones, and M. A. Pfaller.** 2001. Activity of BMS284756 against 2,681 recent clinical isolates of *Haemophilus influenzae* and *Moraxella catarrhalis*: report from The SENTRY Antimicrobial Surveillance Program (2000) in Europe, Canada and the United States. *Diagn. Microbiol. Infect. Dis.* **39:**245–250.

16. **Blondeau, J. M., and G. S. Tillotson.** 2001. Antimicrobial susceptibility patterns of respiratory pathogens—a global perspective. *Semin. Respir. Infect.* **15:**195–207.

17. **Blondeau, J. M., D. Vaughan, R. Laskowski, and S. Borsos.** 2001. Susceptibility of Canadian isolates of *Haemophilus influenzae, Moraxella catarrhalis* and *Streptococcus pneumoniae* to oral antimicrobial agents. *Int. J. Antimicrob. Agents* **17:**457–464.

18. **Blondeau, J. M., and Y. Yaschuk.** 1995. In vitro activities of ciprofloxacin, cefotaxime, ceftriaxone, chloramphenicol, and rifampin against fully susceptible and moderately penicillin-resistant *Neisseria meningitidis. Antimicrob. Agents Chemother.* **39:**2577–2579.

19. **Botha, P.** 1988. Penicillin-resistant *Neisseria meningitidis* in southern Africa. *Lancet* **i:**54.

20. **Bourgault, A. M., W. R. Wilson, and J. A. Washington II.** 1979. Antimicrobial susceptibilities of species of viridans streptococci. *J. Infect. Dis.* **140:**316–321.

21. **Bradley, J. S., and J. D. Connor.** 1991. Ceftriaxone failure in meningitis caused by *Streptococcus pneumoniae* with reduced susceptibility to beta-lactam antibiotics. *Pediatr. Infect. Dis. J.* **10:**871–873.

22. **Brown, S., G. Riley, and F. Jamieson.** 2001. *Neisseria meningitidis* with decreased susceptibility to penicillin in Ontario, Canada 1997–2000. *Can. Commun. Dis. Rep.* **27:**73–75.

23. **Buu-Hoi, A., C. Le Bouguenec, and T. Horaud.** 1990. High-level chromosomal gentamicin resistance in *Streptococcus agalactiae* (group B). *Antimicrob. Agents Chemother.* **34:**985–988.

24. **Campos, J., G. Trujillo, T. Seuba, and A. Rodriguez.** 1992. Discriminative criteria for *Neisseria meningitidis* isolates that are moderately susceptible to penicillin and ampicillin. *Antimicrob. Agents Chemother.* **36:**1028–1031.

25. **Centers for Disease Control and Prevention.** 1998. Guidelines for treatment of sexually transmitted diseases. *Morb. Mortal. Wkly Rep.* **47:**1–118.

26. **Centers for Disease Control and Prevention.** 2000. *Sexually Transmitted Diseases Surveillance 1999 Supplement: Gonococcal Isolate Surveillance Project (GISP) Annual Report–1999.* U.S. Department of Health and Human Services, Public Health Service, Atlanta, Ga.

27. **Chen, D. K., A. McGeer, J. C. DeAzavedo, and D. E. Low.** 1999. Decreased susceptibility of *Streptococcus pneumoniae* to fluoroquinolones in Canada. *N. Engl. J. Med.* **343:**233–239.

28. **De Azavedo, J. C. S., L. Trpeski, S. Pong-Porter, S. Matsumura, the Canadian Bacterial Surveillance Network, and D. E. Low.** 1999. In vitro activities of fluoroquinolones against antibiotic-resistant blood culture isolates of viridans group streptococci from across Canada. *Antimicrob. Agents Chemother.* **43:**2299–2301.

29. **De Mouy, D., J. Cavallo, R. LeClercq, R. Fabre, and the Aforcopi-Bio Network.** 2001. Antibiotic susceptibility and mechanisms of erythromycin resistance in clinical isolates of *Streptococcus agalactiae*: French multicenter study. *Antimicrob. Agents Chemother.* **45:**2400–2402.

30. **Dillon, J., and K. H. Yeung.** 1989. β-Lactamase plasmids and chromosomally mediated antibiotic resistance in pathogenic *Neisseria* species. *Clin. Microbiol. Rev.* **2**(Suppl.)**:**S125–S133.

31. **Dillon, J. R., M. Pauze, and K. H. Yeung.** 1983. Spread of penicillinase-producing and transfer plasmids from the gonococcus to *Neisseria meningitidis. Lancet* **i:**779–781.

32. **Doern, G. B., A. B. Brueggemann, G. Pierce, T. Hogan, H. P. Holley, Jr., and A. Rauch.** 1996. Prevalence of antimicrobial resistance among 723 outpatient clinical isolates of *Moraxella catarrhalis* in the United States in 1994 and 1995: results of a 30-center national surveillance study. *Antimicrob. Agents Chemother.* **40:**2884–2886.

33. **Doern, G. V.** 1986. *Branhamella catarrhalis*, an emerging human pathogen. *Diagn. Microbiol. Infect. Dis.* **4:**191–201.

34. **Doern, G. V., A. Brueggemann, and G. Pierce.** 1997. Assessment of the oxacillin disk screening test for determining penicillin resistance in *Streptococcus pneumoniae. Eur. J. Clin. Microbiol. Infect. Dis.* **16:**311–314.

35. **Doern, G. V., M. J. Ferraro, A. Brueggemann, and K. L. Ruoff.** 1996. Emergence of high rates of antimicrobial resistance among viridans group streptococci in the United States. *Antimicrob. Agents Chemother.* **40:**891–894.

36. **Doern, G. V., K. P. Heilmann, H. K. Huyni, P. R. Rhomberg, S. L. Coffman, and A. B. Brueggemann.** 2001. Antimicrobial resistance among clinical isolates of *Streptococcus pneumoniae* in the United States during 1999–2000, including a comparison of resistance rates since 1994–1995. *Antimicrob. Agents Chemother.* **45:**1721–1729.

37. **Doern, G. V., R. N. Jones, M. A. Pfaller, and K. Kugler.** 1999. *Haemophilus influenzae* and *Moraxella catarrhalis* from patients with community-acquired respiratory tract infections: antimicrobial susceptibility patterns from the SENTRY antimicrobial surveillance program (United States and Canada, 1997). *Antimicrob. Agents Chemother.* **43:** 385–389.

38. **Doern, G. V., and T. Tubert.** 1987. Disk diffusion susceptibility testing of *Branhamella catarrhalis* with ampicillin and seven other antimicrobial agents. *Antimicrob. Agents Chemother.* **31:**1519–1523.

39. **Engberg, J., F. M. Aarestrup, D. E. Taylor, P. Gerner-Smidt, and I. Nachamkin.** 2001. Quinolone and macrolide resistance in *Campylobacter jejuni* and *C. coli*: resis-

tance mechanisms and trends in human isolates. *Emerg. Infect. Dis.* **7:**24–34.

40. **Farber, B. F., and Y. Yee.** 1987. High-level aminoglycoside resistance mediated by aminoglycoside-modifying enzymes among viridans streptococci: implications for the therapy of endocarditis. *J. Infect. Dis.* **155:**948–953.

41. **Farmer, T., and C. Reading.** 1982. β-Lactamases of *Branhamella catarrhalis* and their inhibition by clavulanic acid. *Antimicrob. Agents Chemother.* **21:**506–508.

42. **Felmingham, D., and R. N. Gruneberg.** 2000. The Alexander Project 1996–1997: latest susceptibility data from this international study of bacterial pathogens from community-acquired lower respiratory tract infections. *J. Antimicrob. Chemother.* **45:**191–203.

43. **Fontanals, D., V. Pineda, I. Pons, and J. C. Rojo.** 1989. Penicillin-resistant beta-lactamase-producing *Neisseria meningitidis* in Spain. *Eur. J. Clin. Microbiol. Infect. Dis.* **8:**90–91.

44. **Friedland, I. R.** 1995. Comparison of the response to antimicrobial therapy of penicillin-resistant and penicillin-susceptible pneumococcal disease. *Pediatr. Infect. Dis. J.* **14:**885–890.

45. **Fuchs, P. C., A. L. Barry, S. D. Brown, and The Antimicrobial Susceptibility Testing QC Group.** 1997. Interpretive criteria and quality control parameters for testing susceptibilities of *Haemophilus influenzae* and *Streptococcus pneumoniae* to trimethoprim and trimethoprim-sulfamethoxazole. *J. Clin. Microbiol.* **35:**125–131.

46. **Gaudreau, C., and H. Gilbert.** 1997. Comparison of disc diffusion and agar dilution methods for antibiotic susceptibility testing of *Campylobacter jejuni* subsp. *jejuni* and *Campylobacter coli. J. Antimicrob. Chemother.* **39:**707–712.

47. **Guthrie, L., S. Banks, W. Setiawan, and K. B. Waites.** 1999. Comparison of MicroScan MICroSTREP, PASCO, and Sensititre MIC panels for determining antimicrobial susceptibilities of *Streptococcus pneumoniae. Diagn. Microbiol. Infect. Dis.* **33:**267–273.

48. **Hayward, C. L., M. E. Erwin, M. S. Barrett, and R. N. Jones.** 1999. Comparative antimicrobial activity of gatifloxacin tested against *Campylobacter jejuni* including fluoroquinolone-resistant clinical isolates. *Diagn. Microbiol. Infect. Dis.* **34:**99–102.

49. **Heelan, J. S., D. Chesney, and G. Guadagno.** 1992. Investigation of ampicillin-intermediate strains of *Haemophilus influenzae* by using the disk diffusion procedure and current National Committee for Clinical Laboratory Standards guidelines. *J. Clin. Microbiol.* **30:**1674–1677.

50. **Heffelfinger, J. D., S. F. Dowell, J. H. Jorgensen, K. P. Klugman, L. R. Mabry, D. M. Musher, J. F. Plouffe, A. Rakowsky, A. Schuchat, C. G. Whitney, and The Drug-Resistant *Streptococcus pneumoniae* Therapeutic Working Group.** 2000. Management of community-acquired pneumonia in the era of pneumococcal resistance. *Arch. Intern. Med.* **160:**1399–1408.

51. **Ho, P. L., R. W. Yung, D. N. Tsang, T. L. Que, M. Ho, W. H. Seto, T. K. Ng, W. C. Yam, and W. W. Ng.** 2001. Increasing resistance of *Streptococcus pneumoniae* to fluoroquinolones: results of a Hong Kong multicentre study in 2000. *J. Antimicrob. Chemother.* **48:**659–665.

52. **Hoban, D. J., G. V. Doern, A. C. Fluit, M. Roussel-Delvallez, and R. N. Jones.** 2001. Worldwide prevalence of antimicrobial resistance in *Streptococcus pneumoniae, Haemophilus influenzae,* and *Moraxella catarrhalis* in the SENTRY antimicrobial surveillance program, 1997–1999. *Clin. Infect. Dis.* **32:**S81–S93.

53. **Hof, H., T. Nichterlein, and M. Kretschmar.** 1997. Management of listeriosis. *Clin. Microbiol. Rev.* **10:**345–357.

54. **Hofmann, J., M. S. Cetron, M. M. Farley, W. S. Baughman, R. R. Facklam, J. A. Elliott, K. A. Deaver, and**

R. F. Breiman. 1995. The prevalence of drug-resistant *Streptococcus pneumoniae* in Atlanta. *N. Engl. J. Med.* **333:**481–486.

55. **Horodniceanu, T., A. Buu-Hoi, A. Delbos, and G. Bieth.** 1982. High-level aminoglycoside resistance in group A, B, C, D (*Streptococcus bovis*), and viridans streptococci. *Antimicrob. Agents Chemother.* **21:**176–179.

56. **Jacobs, M. R., S. Bajaksouzian, P. C. Appelbaum, and A. Bolmstrom.** 1992. Evaluation of the E test for susceptibility testing of pneumococci. *Diagn. Microbiol. Infect. Dis.* **15:**473–478.

57. **Jones, E. M., and A. P. MacGowan.** 1995. Antimicrobial chemotherapy of human infection due to *Listeria monocytogenes. Eur. J. Clin. Microbiol. Infect. Dis.* **14:**165–175.

58. **Jones, R., D. Johnson, M. Erwin, M. Beach, D. Biedenbach, and M. Pfaller.** 1999. Comparative antimicrobial activity of gatifloxacin tested against *Streptococcus* spp. including quality control guidelines and Etest method validation. *Diagn. Microbiol. Infect. Dis.* **34:**91–98.

59. **Jones, R. N., and M. A. Pfaller.** 2000. In vitro activity of newer fluoroquinolones for respiratory tract infections and emerging patterns of antimicrobial resistance: data from the SENTRY antimicrobial surveillance program. *Clin. Infect. Dis.* **31**(Suppl 2)**:**S16–S23.

60. **Jorgensen, J., M. McElmeel, and S. Crawford.** 1998. Evaluation of the Dade MicroScan MICroSTREP antimicrobial susceptibility testing panel with selected *Streptococcus pneumoniae* challenge strains and recent clinical isolates. *J. Clin. Microbiol.* **36:**788–791.

61. **Jorgensen, J. H., A. L. Barry, M. M. Traczewski, D. F. Sahm, M. L. McElmeel, and S. A. Crawford.** 2000. Rapid automated antimicrobial susceptibility testing of *Streptococcus pneumoniae* by use of the bioMerieux Vitek 2. *J. Clin. Microbiol.* **38:**2814–2818.

62. **Jorgensen, J. H., and M. J. Ferraro.** 2000. Antimicrobial susceptibility testing: special needs for fastidious organisms and difficult-to-detect resistance mechanisms. *Clin. Infect. Dis.* **30:**799–808.

63. **Jorgensen, J. H., M. J. Ferraro, M. L. McElmeel, J. Spargo, J. M. Swenson, and F. C. Tenover.** 1994. Detection of penicillin and extended-spectrum cephalosporin resistance among *Streptococcus pneumoniae* clinical isolates by use of the E Test. *J. Clin. Microbiol.* **32:**159–163.

64. **Jorgensen, J. H., A. W. Howell, and L. A. Maher.** 1991. Quantitative antimicrobial susceptibility testing of *Haemophilus influenzae* and *Streptococcus pneumoniae* by using the E test. *J. Clin. Microbiol.* **29:**109–114.

65. **Jorgensen, J. H., J. S. Redding, L. A. Maher, and A. W. Howell.** 1987. Improved medium for antimicrobial susceptibility testing of *Haemophilus influenzae. J. Clin. Microbiol.* **25:**2105–2113.

66. **Kataja, J., H. Seppala, M. Skurnik, H. Sarkkinen, and P. Huovinen.** 1998. Different erythromycin resistance mechanisms in group C and group G streptococci. *Antimicrob. Agents Chemother.* **42:**1493–1494.

67. **Kato, M., Y. Yamaoka, J. J. Kim, R. Reddy, M. Asaka, K. Kashima, M. S. Osato, F. A. El-Zaatari, D. Y. Graham, and D. H. Kwon.** 2000. Regional differences in metronidazole resistance and increasing clarithromycin resistance among *Helicobacter pylori* isolates from Japan. *Antimicrob. Agents Chemother.* **44:**2214–2216.

68. **Kim, J. J., R. Reddy, M. Lee, J. G. Kim, F. A. El-Zaatari, M. S. Osato, D. Y. Graham, and D. H. Kwon.** 2001. Analysis of metronidazole, clarithromycin and tetracycline resistance of *Helicobacter pylori* isolates from Korea. *J. Antimicrob. Chemother.* **47:**459–461.

69. **Krcmery, V., Jr., S. Spanik, and J. Trupl.** 1996. First report of vancomycin-resistant *Streptococcus mitis* bacteremia in a leukemic patient after prophylaxis with quino-

lones and during treatment with vancomycin. *J. Chemother.* **8:**325–326.

70. **Krisher, K., and A. Linscott.** 1994. Comparison of three commercial MIC systems, E test, fastidious antimicrobial susceptibility panel, and FOX fastidious panel, for confirmation of penicillin and cephalosporin resistance in *Streptococcus pneumoniae. J. Clin. Microbiol.* **32:**2242–2245.

71. **Kusters, J. G., and E. J. Kuipers.** 2001. Antibiotic resistance of *Helicobacter pylori. Symp. Ser. Soc. Appl. Microbiol.* **2001**(30):134S–144S.

72. **Latorre, C., A. Gene, T. Juncosa, C. Munoz, and A. Gonzalez-Cuevas.** 2000. *Neisseria meningitidis:* evolution of penicillin resistance and phenotype in a children's hospital in Barcelona, Spain. *Acta Paediatr.* **89:**661–665.

73. **MacGowan, A. P., H. A. Holt, M. J. Bywater, and D. S. Reeves.** 1990. In vitro antimicrobial susceptibility of *Listeria monocytogenes* isolated in the UK and other *Listeria* species. *Eur. J. Clin. Microbiol. Infect. Dis.* **9:**767–770.

74. **Macias, E. A., E. O. Mason, Jr., H. Y. Ocera, and M. T. LaRocca.** 1994. Comparison of E test with standard broth microdilution for determining antibiotic susceptibilities of penicillin-resistant strains of *Streptococcus pneumoniae. J. Clin. Microbiol.* **32:**430–432.

75. **Marshall, S. A., P. R. Rhomberg, and R. N. Jones.** 1997. Comparative evaluation of Etest for susceptibility testing *Neisseria meningitidis* with eight antimicrobial agents. An investigation using U.S. Food and Drug Administration regulatory criteria. *Diagn. Microbiol. Infect. Dis.* **27:**93–97.

76. **Martinez-Martinez, L., P. Joyanes, A. I. Suarez, and E. J. Perea.** 2001. Activities of gemifloxacin and five other antimicrobial agents against *Listeria monocytogenes* and coryneform bacteria isolated from clinical samples. *Antimicrob. Agents Chemother.* **45:**2390–2392.

77. **Medical Letter.** 2001. The choice of antibacterial drugs, p. 69–78. *In* M. Abramowicz (ed.), *The Medical Letter,* vol. 43. The Medical Letter, New Rochelle, N.Y.

78. **Megraud, F., N. Lehn, T. Lind, E. Bayerdorffer, C. O'Morain, R. Spiller, P. Unge, S. V. van Zanten, M. Wrangstadh, and C. F. Burman.** 1999. Antimicrobial susceptibility testing of *Helicobacter pylori* in a large multicenter trial: the MACH 2 study. *Antimicrob. Agents Chemother.* **43:**2747–2752.

79. **Mendelman, P. M., E. A. Wiley, T. L. Stull, C. Clausen, D. O. Chaffin, and O. Onay.** 1990. Problems with current recommendations for susceptibility testing of *Haemophilus influenzae. Antimicrob. Agents Chemother.* **34:**1480–1484.

80. **Mohammed, J. M., and F. C. Tenover.** 2000. Evaluation of the PASCO Strep Plus broth microdilution antimicrobial susceptibility panels for testing *Streptococcus pneumoniae* and other streptococcal species. *J. Clin. Microbiol.* **38:**1713–1716.

81. **Montanari, M. P., M. Mingoia, E. Giovanetti, and P. E. Varaldo.** 2001. Differentiation of resistance phenotypes among erythromycin-resistant pneumococci. *J. Clin. Microbiol.* **39:**1311–1315.

82. **National Committee for Clinical Laboratory Standards.** 1984. *Performance Standards for Antimicrobial Disk Susceptibility Tests,* 3rd ed. Approved standard M2-A3. National Committee for Clinical Laboratory Standards, Villanova, Pa.

83. **NCCLS.** 2001. *Development of In Vitro Susceptibility Testing Criteria and Quality Control Parameters.* Approved guideline M23-A2. NCCLS, Wayne, Pa.

84. **NCCLS.** 2000. *Methods for Dilution Antimicrobial Susceptibility Tests for Bacteria That Grow Aerobically,* 5th ed. Approved standard M7-A5. NCCLS, Wayne, Pa.

85. **NCCLS.** 2000. *Performance Standards for Antimicrobial Disk Susceptibility Tests,* 7th ed. Approved standard M2-A7. NCCLS, Wayne, Pa.

86. **NCCLS.** 2002. *Performance Standards for Antimicrobial Susceptibility Testing.* Twelfth informational supplement. M100-S12. NCCLS, Wayne, Pa.

87. **Osato, M. S., R. Reddy, S. G. Reddy, R. L. Penland, and D. Y. Graham.** 2001. Comparison of the Etest and the NCCLS-approved agar dilution method to detect metronidazole and clarithromycin resistant *Helicobacter pylori. Int. J. Antimicrob. Agents* **17:**39–44.

88. **Osato, M. S., R. Reddy, S. G. Reddy, R. L. Penland, H. M. Malaty, and D. Y. Graham.** 2001. Pattern of primary resistance of *Helicobacter pylori* to metronidazole or clarithromycin in the United States. *Arch. Intern. Med.* **161:**1217–1220.

89. **Pascual, A., P. Joyanes, L. Martinez-Martinez, A. I. Suarez, and E. J. Perea.** 1996. Comparison of broth microdilution and E-test for susceptibility testing of *Neisseria meningitidis. J. Clin. Microbiol.* **34:**588–591.

90. **Perez-Trallero, E., N. Gomez, and J. M. Garcia-Arenzana.** 1994. Etest as susceptibility test for evaluation of *Neisseria meningitidis* isolates. *J. Clin. Microbiol.* **32:**2341–2342.

91. **Piccolomini, R., G. Di Bonaventura, G. Catamo, F. Carbone, and M. Neri.** 1997. Comparative evaluation of the E test, agar dilution, and broth microdilution for testing susceptibilities of *Helicobacter pylori* strains to 20 antimicrobial agents. *J. Clin. Microbiol.* **35:**1842–1846.

92. **Poyart, C., C. Pierre, G. Quesne, B. Pron, P. Berche, and P. Trieu-Cuot.** 1997. Emergence of vancomycin resistance in the genus *Streptococcus:* characterization of a vanB transferable determinant in *Streptococcus bovis. Antimicrob. Agents Chemother.* **41:**24–29.

93. **Richter, S. S., P. L. Winokur, A. B. Brueggemann, H. K. Huynh, P. R. Rhomberg, E. M. Wingert, and G. V. Doern.** 2000. Molecular characterization of the beta-lactamases from clinical isolates of *Moraxella (Branhamella) catarrhalis* obtained from 24 U.S. medical centers during 1994–1995 and 1997–1998. *Antimicrob. Agents Chemother.* **44:**444–446.

94. **Rosenstein, N. E., B. A. Perkins, D. S. Stephens, T. Popovic, and J. M. Hughes.** 2001. Meningococcal disease. *N. Engl. J. Med.* **344:**1378–1388.

95. **Rosenstein, N. E., S. A. Stocker, T. Popovic, F. C. Tenover, and B. A. Perkins.** 2000. Antimicrobial resistance of *Neisseria meningitidis* in the United States, 1997. The Active Bacterial Core Surveillance (ABCs) Team. *Clin. Infect. Dis.* **30:**212–213.

96. **Ruoff, K.** 1991. Nutritionally variant streptococci. *Clin. Microbiol. Rev.* **4:**184–190.

97. **Sader, H., and L. Del'Alamo.** 2000. Etest compared to broth microdilution: discrepant results when testing macrolides against *Streptococcus pneumoniae* indicate a need for better clinical and serum level/MIC correlation. *Braz. J. Infect. Dis.* **4:**268–270.

98. **Saenz, Y., M. Zarazaga, M. Lantero, M. J. Gastanares, F. Baquero, and C. Torres.** 2000. Antibiotic resistance in *Campylobacter* strains isolated from animals, foods, and humans in Spain in 1997–1998. *Antimicrob. Agents Chemother.* **44:**267–271.

99. **Sahm, D. F., M. E. Jones, M. L. Hickey, D. R. Diakun, S. V. Mani, and C. Thornsberry.** 2000. Resistance surveillance of *Streptococcus pneumoniae, Haemophilus influenzae* and *Moraxella catarrhalis* isolated in Asia and Europe, 1997–1998. *J. Antimicrob. Chemother.* **45:**457–466.

100. **Sahm, D. F., J. A. Karlowsky, L. J. Kelly, I. A. Critchley, M. E. Jones, C. Thornsberry, Y. Mauriz, and J. Kahn.** 2001. Need for annual surveillance of antimicrobial resistance in *Streptococcus pneumoniae* in the United States: 2-year longitudinal analysis. *Antimicrob. Agents Chemother.* **45:**1037–1042.

101. **Sanford, J. P., D. N. Gilbert, R. C. Moellering, Jr., and M. A. Sande.** 2001. *The Sanford Guide to Antimicrobial Therapy,* 2001 ed. Antimicrobial Therapy, Inc., Hyde Park, Vt.

102. **Seppala, A., A. Nissinen, H. Jarvinen, S. Huovinen, T. Henriksson, E. Herva, S. E. Holm, M. Jahkola, M. L. Katila, T. Klaukka, S. Kontiainen, O. Liimatainen, S. Oinonen, L. Passi-Metosomaa, and P. Huovinen.** 1992. Resistance to erythromycin in group A streptococci. *N. Engl. J. Med.* **326:**292–297.

103. **Seppala, H., A. Nissinen, Q. Yu, and P. Huovinen.** 1993. Three different phenotypes of erythromycin-resistant *Streptococcus pyogenes* in Finland. *J. Antimicrob. Chemother.* **32:**885–891.

104. **Shultz, T. R., J. W. Tapsall, P. A. White, and P. J. Newton.** 2000. An invasive isolate of *Neisseria meningitidis* showing decreased susceptibility to quinolones. *Antimicrob. Agents Chemother.* **44:**1116.

105. **Skulnick, M., G. W. Small, P. Lo, M. P. Patel, C. R. Porter, D. E. Low, S. Matsumura, and T. Mazzulli.** 1995. Evaluation of accuracy and reproducibility of E test for susceptibility testing of *Streptococcus pneumoniae* to penicillin, cefotaxime, and ceftriaxone. *J. Clin. Microbiol.* **33:**2334–2337.

106. **Sloas, M. M., F. F. Barrett, P. J. Chesney, B. K. English, B. C. Hill, F. C. Tenover, and R. J. Leggiadro.** 1992. Cephalosporin treatment failure in penicillin- and cephalosporin-resistant *Streptococcus pneumoniae* meningitis. *Pediatr. Infect. Dis. J.* **11:**662–666.

107. **Smith, K. E., J. M. Besser, C. W. Hedberg, F. T. Leano, J. B. Bender, J. H. Wicklund, B. P. Johnson, K. A. Moore, M. T. Osterholm, and the Investigation Team.** 1999. Quinolone-resistant *Campylobacter jejuni* infections in Minnesota, 1992–1998. *N. Engl. J. Med.* **340:**1525–1532.

108. **Stein, D. S., and K. E. Nelson.** 1987. Endocarditis due to nutritionally deficient streptococci: therapeutic dilemma. *Rev. Infect. Dis.* **9:**908–916.

109. **Sutcliffe, E. M., D. M. Jones, S. El-Sheikh, and A. Percival.** 1988. Penicillin-insensitive meningococci in the UK. *Lancet* **i:**657–658.

110. **Swenson, J. M., B. C. Hill, and C. Thornsberry.** 1986. Screening pneumococci for penicillin resistance. *J. Clin. Microbiol.* **24:**749–752.

111. **Tanaka, M., H. Nakayama, M. Haraoka, and T. Saika.** 2000. Antimicrobial resistance of *Neisseria gonorrhoeae* and high prevalence of ciprofloxacin-resistant isolates in Japan, 1993 to 1998. *J. Clin. Microbiol.* **38:**521–525.

112. **Tenover, F. C., C. N. Baker, and J. M. Swenson.** 1996. Evaluation of commercial methods for determining antimicrobial susceptibility of *Streptococcus pneumoniae.* *J. Clin. Microbiol.* **34:**10–14.

113. **Traub, W. H., and B. Leonhard.** 1997. Comparative susceptibility of clinical group A, B, C, F, and G β-hemolytic streptococcal isolates to 24 antimicrobial drugs. *Chemotherapy* **43:**10–20.

114. **Tuohy, M., G. Procop, and J. Washington.** 2000. Antimicrobial susceptibility of *Abiotrophia adiacens* and *Abiotrophia defectiva. Diagn. Microbiol. Infect. Dis.* **38:**189–191.

115. **Tuohy, M., and J. Washington.** 1997. Antimicrobial susceptibility of viridans group streptococci. *Diagn. Microbiol. Infect. Dis.* **29:**277–280.

116. **Turner, P. C., K. W. Southern, N. J. Spencer, and H. Pullen.** 1990. Treatment failure in meningococcal meningitis. *Lancet* **335:**732–733.

117. **Vazquez, J. A., S. Berron, M. J. Gimenez, L. de la Fuente, and L. Aguilar.** 2001. In vitro susceptibility of *Neisseria meningitidis* isolates to gemifloxacin and ten other antimicrobial agents. *Eur. J. Clin. Microbiol. Infect. Dis.* **20:**150–151.

118. **Vazquez, J. A., A. M. Enriquez, L. De la Fuente, S. Berron, and M. Baquero.** 1996. Isolation of a strain of beta-lactamase-producing *Neisseria meningitidis* in Spain. *Eur. J. Clin. Microbiol. Infect. Dis.* **15:**181–182.

119. **Weiss, K., C. Restieri, R. Gautheir, M. Laverdiere, A. McGeer, R. J. Davidson, L. Kilburn, D. J. Bast, J. de Azavedo, and D. E. Low.** 2001. A nosocomial outbreak of fluoroquinolone-resistant *Streptococcus pneumoniae. Clin. Infect. Dis.* **33:**517–522.

120. **Whitney, C. G., M. M. Farley, J. Hadler, L. H. Harrison, C. Lexau, A. Reingold, L. Lefowitz, P. R. Cieslak, M. Cetron, E. R. Zell, J. H. Jorgensen, and A. Schuchat.** 2000. Increasing prevalence of multidrug-resistant *Streptococcus pneumoniae* in the United States. *N. Engl. J. Med.* **343:**1917–1924.

121. **Wilson, W. R., A. W. Karchmer, A. S. Dajani, K. A. Taubert, A. Bayer, D. Kaye, A. L. Bisno, P. Ferrieri, S. T. Shulman, and D. T. Durack.** 1995. Antibiotic treatment of adults with infective endocarditis due to streptococci, enterococci, staphylococci, and HACEK microorganisms. *JAMA* **274:**1706–1713.

122. **Woods, C. R., A. L. Smith, B. L. Wasilauskas, J. Campos, and L. B. Givner.** 1994. Invasive disease caused by *Neisseria meningitidis* relatively resistant to penicillin in North Carolina. *J. Infect. Dis.* **170:**453–456.

123. **Yagupsky, P., S. Ashkenazi, and C. Block.** 1993. Rifampicin-resistant meningococci causing invasive disease and failure of chemoprophylaxis. *Lancet* **341:**1152–1153.

124. **York, M., L. Gibbs, F. Perdreau-Remington, and G. F. Brooks.** 1999. Characterization of antimicrobial resistance in *Streptococcus pyogenes* isolates from the San Francisco Bay area of Northern California. *J. Clin. Microbiol.* **37:**1727–1731.

Susceptibility Test Methods: Anaerobic Bacteria

DIANE M. CITRON AND DAVID W. HECHT

72

The importance of anaerobes as the cause of significant infections, as well as the benefits of specific antimicrobial treatment and prophylaxis against anaerobic bacteria, is well recognized (23, 49). In general, performance of antimicrobial susceptibility testing is viewed as a necessity for effective guidance of antimicrobial therapy. However, when and how susceptibility testing of anaerobes should be performed has been the subject of debate, due in part to several confounding factors and misconceptions (8, 20, 24, 68). For example, specimens obtained from most infections involving anaerobes are polymicrobic, making recovery and identification of individual isolates slow and making determination of antimicrobial susceptibility results unacceptably long to have a consistent impact on individual clinical outcomes. For the clinician, the combination of surgical management and the use of empirical broad-spectrum antimicrobial therapy has limited the correlation of potential antimicrobial resistance with outcome. Such observations have led many laboratories away from the performance of susceptibility testing (33). However, there is substantial evidence that antimicrobial resistance is significant among many anaerobes worldwide and that inappropriate therapy can result in poor clinical responses and increased mortality (48, 55, 56). Recent antimicrobial susceptibility data have also revealed significant differences among individual hospitals on a regional and local basis, suggesting that one medical center's patterns are not applicable to organisms from other institutions (37, 58). Thus, the need for susceptibility testing of anaerobes is considerably more important now than in the past.

At a minimum, individual hospitals should establish patterns of resistance for some anaerobes on a periodic basis, with individual patient isolates being tested as needed to assist in their care. For surveillance purposes, the testing of 75 to 100 isolates representing anaerobes with known resistance, such as members of the *Bacteroides fragilis* group, *Prevotella* spp., *Fusobacterium* spp., *Clostridium* spp., and *Bilophila wadsworthia*, should be considered. Preferably, 30 isolates should be from the *B. fragilis* group and at least 10 of each of the other genera should be tested. The antimicrobial agents to be tested should generally be based on the hospital's formulary, although one agent from each antimicrobial class should be included even if not on the hospital formulary. For individual patient management, susceptibility should be performed when (i) agents are critical for disease management, (ii) long-term therapy is being considered, (iii) anaerobes are isolated from specific body sites, or (iv) a usual regimen fails (Table 1).

This chapter describes currently available methods and their interpretation for susceptibility testing of anaerobes (Table 2). The NCCLS Anaerobe Working Group has established an agar dilution reference method with brucella blood agar as the testing medium (46, 47). This method is not considered generally easy or economical to perform but will serve as the method with which other, more practical methods are compared. At present, alternative testing methods include limited agar dilution, broth microdilution (for the *B. fragilis* group), and the E test. β-Lactamase testing plays a very limited role but can be useful if penicillin therapy is being considered. Broth disk elution and disk diffusion tests are not considered appropriate for anaerobic susceptibility testing since their results do not correlate with the agar dilution reference method (45). The spiral-streak method has not been cleared by the Food and Drug Administration (FDA) for testing of anaerobes, but has been utilized as a research tool (67).

CURRENT PATTERNS OF ANTIBIOTIC RESISTANCE

Susceptibility testing of anaerobes has not been routinely performed at most hospitals (33). As a result, most of the published literature reporting susceptibility of anaerobes is generated by reference laboratories testing a limited number of isolates from one or more medical centers (1, 27, 30, 37, 58). Over the last several years, significant variations in susceptibility results for anaerobes have been reported from different countries, geographic locations within countries, and even hospitals within the same cities (7, 10, 25, 37, 42, 43, 57, 64). Of particular note, the incidence of clindamycin resistance has increased from <10% to >40% for the *B. fragilis* group at some hospitals (37, 58), while resistance to cephalosporins and cephamycins is also rising (37, 58, 59). Some differences in susceptibility results among various reports may be accounted for by the use of different testing methods, lack of uniformity in interpretive breakpoints among countries, and clustering of MICs at the breakpoint for some species with some antimicrobial agent combinations (3, 35). Regardless, it is clear from recent publications that resistance to many classes of antimicrobials among

TABLE 1 Indications for susceptibility testing of anaerobic bacteria

Indication	Examples[a]
Surveillance	
Annual monitoring of isolates at individual medical centers	B. fragilis group, Prevotella spp., Fusobacterium spp., Clostridium spp., B. wadsworthia
Clinical	
Known resistance of a particular species	B. fragilis (clindamycin, cephamycins, piperacillin), Prevotella spp. and Fusobacterium spp. (penicillin, clindamycin)
Failure of a usual therapeutic regimen	Any anaerobe
Pivotal role of antimicrobial agent in clinical outcome	B. fragilis group (osteomyelitis, joint infection)
Need for long-term therapy	B. fragilis group, Prevotella spp. (osteomyelitis, endocarditis, brain abscess, liver abscess, lung abscess)
Infections of specific body sites	Any anaerobe (brain abscess, endocarditis, prosthetic devices or graft, bacteremia)

[a] Examples only, and not intended as inclusive. See the text for specific recommendations.

anaerobes is increasing, and clinicians and laboratories can no longer assume susceptibility of anaerobes to these agents without testing. Further, neither national nor even local data from other institutions are sufficient to predict the susceptibility of anaerobes to antimicrobials at one's own hospital (37, 58). A general outline of current resistance patterns for anaerobic bacteria is provided below.

Gram-Negative Bacilli and Cocci

Bacteroides fragilis Group

Among the 10 members of the B. fragilis group, B. fragilis is generally the most susceptible, although more than 95% of all species are resistant to penicillin and ampicillin. The carboxy- and ureidopenicillins ticarcillin and mezlocillin are somewhat more active than penicillin, but <50% of isolates are susceptible (1, 17). Piperacillin is the most active of the ureidopenicillins against the B. fragilis group, although susceptibility has fallen from approximately 90% to 70% over the last 8 to 10 years (1, 17, 34, 58). The isoxazolyl penicillins, such as oxacillin and nafcillin, are not active against these organisms. The principal mechanism of resistance to penicillins is β-lactamase production (15, 18, 22). Thus, β-lactam–β-lactamase inhibitor combinations, such as ampicillin-sulbactam, amoxicillin-clavulanate, ticarcillin-clavulanate, and piperacillin-tazobactam, are active against nearly all strains of the B. fragilis group, with <2% resistance being cited in most reports (34, 58, 66).

Among the cephalosporins and cephamycins, cefoxitin remains very active against members of the B. fragilis group,

with 80 to 90% of isolates being susceptible. Cefotetan demonstrates activity against B. fragilis similar to that of cefoxitin but is much less active against the other members of the B. fragilis group (1, 2, 16, 17, 65). With the exception of ceftizoxime, broad-spectrum cephalosporins generally have poor activity against most members of the B. fragilis group, inhibiting <50% of isolates (2, 58). Susceptibility to ceftizoxime varies widely among published studies (60 to 90%), probably due to differences in testing methods (3, 11, 50). Narrow-spectrum cephalosporins are not active against members of the B. fragilis group.

A marked decrease in susceptibility to clindamycin among Bacteroides spp. has become widely recognized worldwide, as noted above (37, 58, 62). The clindamycin resistance determinant is frequently located on transferable plasmids and is often linked to transferable tetracycline resistance (62). Among other agents, chloramphenicol, metronidazole, and carbapenems (imipenem and meropenem) are nearly uniformly active against all members of the B. fragilis group in the United States, although imipenem-resistant strains have been reported from Japan (5, 51). Of note, imipenem resistance is mediated by a zinc metalloenzyme that confers resistance to all current β-lactam and β-lactam–β-lactamase inhibitor combination agents and has been reported to be transferable (52). Of additional concern, isolated strains resistant to metronidazole have been reported in France; the resistance is associated with a transferable plasmid (6). Among fluoroquinolone agents, trovafloxacin (a trifluoronaphthyridone) has

TABLE 2 Methods for susceptibility testing of anaerobic bacteria

Method	Medium	Inoculum	Incubation time (h)	Advantages	Disadvantages
Agar dilution[a]	Brucella blood agar	10^5 cells/spot	48	Reference method, multiple isolates tested/antibiotic	Labor-intensive, expensive
Broth microdilution[b]	Supplemented brucella broth	10^6 cells/ml (10^5/well)	48	Economical, commercial panels available, multiple antibiotics/isolate	Limited shelf life of frozen panels
E test	Brucella blood agar	0.5 McFarland, swab plate	24–48	Precise MIC, convenient for individual patient isolates	Expensive for surveillance use

[a] Media are commercially available.
[b] Frozen panels available from PML Microbiologicals, Inc. Lyophilized panels available from Trek Diagnostics.

excellent activity against most members of the *B. fragilis* group; however, it is no longer marketed in most countries, including the United States (36, 38, 46). Other fluoroquinolones such as moxifloxacin and gatifloxacin also exhibit very good but incomplete activity against a broad range of anaerobes (21, 39).

Prevotella and *Porphyromonas*

In general, data on the susceptibility of *Prevotella* and *Porphyromonas* spp. (mostly former *Bacteroides* species) are more limited than those for the *B. fragilis* group. Overall, both genera are more susceptible than the *B. fragilis* group. Currently, about 50% of *Prevotella* spp. are resistant to penicillin and ampicillin due to β-lactamase production, with susceptibility to piperacillin, cefoxitin, cefotetan, and ceftizoxime ranging from 70 to 90% in most published studies (28, 31, 64). Eight percent of *Porphyromonas* spp. strains were reported to produce β-lactamase in a recent survey from Japan (63), as were 10% of strains recovered from serious pelvic infections (D. M. Citron, unpublished data). Susceptibilities of *Porphyromonas* isolates are rarely reported separately in most published literature from the United States, but β-lactamase production is considered rare at present. As with the *B. fragilis* group, both genera are nearly uniformly susceptible to carbapenems, metronidazole, and chloramphenicol.

Other Gram-Negative Bacilli

Penicillin resistance among isolates of the genus *Fusobacterium* has been observed; 19% of isolates in one study were found to be resistant to amoxicillin at 4 μg/ml, with 97% of resistant strains producing β-lactamase (4, 40). In general, >90% of *Fusobacterium* spp. are susceptible to cephalosporins and cephamycins including cefoxitin, cefotetan, and ceftizoxime (40). *Campylobacter rectus* and *C. curvus* (formerly *Wolinella recta* and *W. curva*) vary in their susceptibility to β-lactams but remain very susceptible to chloramphenicol, metronidazole, and clindamycin (41). *Bilophila wadsworthia* is a recently described gram-negative anaerobe from the gastrointestinal tract that frequently produces β-lactamase and therefore is resistant to penicillin and ampicillin. High MIC$_{90}$s are also seen in tests of piperacillin and ceftizoxime, with concentrations clustering near the breakpoints. *B. wadsworthia* is susceptible to clindamycin, cefoxitin, β-lactam–β-lactamase inhibitor combinations, carbapenems, and metronidazole (9). *Campylobacter gracilis* (formerly *Bacteroides gracilis*) was previously considered to be resistant to many β-lactam agents. However, data suggest that when properly identified and tested, this organism is susceptible to most agents tested, including β-lactam–β-lactamase inhibitor combinations, cefoxitin, ceftizoxime, ceftriaxone, and clindamycin (44). Instead, a newly described but more resistant organism, *Sutterella wadsworthensis*, was often isolated from the same samples and identified as *C. gracilis*. *S. wadsworthensis* may demonstrate resistance to clindamycin, ceftizoxime, piperacillin, and/or metronidazole (44).

Gram-Positive Bacilli and Cocci

Non-Spore-Forming Gram-Positive Bacilli

The *Eubacterium* group, *Actinomyces*, *Propionibacterium*, and *Bifidobacterium* are usually susceptible to β-lactam agents including the penicillins, cephalosporins and cephamycins, carbapenems, and β-lactam–β-lactamase inhibitor combinations. *Lactobacillus* spp. are variably susceptible to cephalosporins and may be inhibited effectively only by penicillin (32). New species have recently been added to the *Lactobacillus* genus, and little information on their resistance is available (41). Vancomycin is active against all *Propionibacterium* spp., *Actinomyces* spp., *Eubacterium* spp., and peptostreptococci and some *Lactobacillus* spp., but *L. casei* is usually resistant (12, 29). Most non-spore-forming gram-positive anaerobes are resistant to metronidazole (53).

Spore-Forming Gram-Positive Bacilli

Clostridium perfringens is generally very susceptible to most antianaerobic agents and fluoroquinolones (38). However, nonperfringens *Clostridium* spp. and *C. difficile* have variable susceptibility (28–30, 53). Nonperfringens species may be resistant to clindamycin and β-lactams, while chloramphenicol and metronidazole remain active. *C. difficile* may be resistant to many β-lactams, including cephalosporins, and clindamycin but retains susceptibility to metronidazole and vancomycin, while the vancomycin MICs for *C. innocuum* are 8 to 32 μg/ml (28–30, 53).

Gram-Positive Cocci

At present, only *Peptococcus niger* remains in this genus, and several *Peptostreptococcus* species are being reclassified into other genera (41). In general, these organisms are highly susceptible to all β-lactams, β-lactam–β-lactamase inhibitors, cephalosporins, carbapenems, chloramphenicol, metronidazole, and some fluoroquinolones (38, 53). Some strains may be resistant to clindamycin. Occasionally, microaerophilic streptococci are initially identified as *Peptostreptococcus* spp. and reported to be resistant to metronidazole. The presumptive identification of a metronidazole-resistant *Peptostreptococcus* sp. should prompt further identification of the isolate, since such isolates are rare.

DESCRIPTION OF TEST METHODS

Agar Dilution

Media

The recommended medium is supplemented brucella blood agar, which supports the growth of essentially all anaerobes (47). Brucella base agar is supplemented with hemin (5 μg/ml) and vitamin K$_1$ (1 μg/ml) before being autoclaved, and 5% defibrinated or laked sheep blood is added after the agar has cooled to 48 to 50°C. To prepare hemin stock solution (5 mg/ml), 0.5 g of hemin is dissolved in 10 ml of 1 N NaOH and the solution is brought to 100 ml with distilled water. It is sterilized by autoclaving at 121°C for 15 min. Then 1 ml is added per liter of agar. The stock solution may be stored at 4 to 8°C for 1 month. Vitamin K$_1$ stock solution (10 mg/ml) is prepared by mixing 0.2 ml of vitamin K$_1$ (3-phytylmenadione) with 20 ml of 95% ethanol and added to agar base to achieve a final concentration of 1 μg/ml prior to autoclaving. The stock solution can be stored for up to 6 months at 4°C in a dark bottle. Lysed (laked) sheep blood is prepared by a single cycle of alternate freezing and thawing and does not require clarification by centrifugation. Laked blood may be stored at −20°C for up to 6 months.

The agar is dispensed in 17-ml volumes into test tubes before being autoclaved. After autoclaving, these tubes may be stored at 4 to 8°C for up to 1 month. On the day of the test, the agar is melted by heating and then cooled in a water bath to 48 to 50°C. Laked blood (1 ml) and the antimicrobial dilutions (2 ml) are added, and after the contents are mixed by gently inverting the tubes twice, the plates are poured. After they have solidified, the plates are dried in the incubator by being inverted with the lids ajar for 45 min. The NCCLS recommends that plates not be stored any longer than 7 days in closed containers at 4 to 8°C. However, for research and precise evaluation purposes, storage for no longer than 72 h is recommended. Due to instability, plates containing imipenem or clavulanic acid must be used on the day of preparation.

Inoculum Preparation

The inoculum may be prepared by suspending colonies taken from a 24- to 72-h brucella blood agar plate in brucella broth or other clear broth medium to a density equal to the 0.5 McFarland standard. Alternatively, the initial suspension may be prepared by inoculating five or more colonies into enriched thioglycolate or other broth medium that supports good growth and incubating for 4 to 24 h to obtain adequate turbidity (dilution may be required) (47). Equivalence to a 0.5 McFarland standard can be measured visually or by using a colorimeter or simple photometer device (e.g., from Vitek, Hazelwood, Mo.; Microscan, West Sacramento, Calif.; or Sensititre, Westlake, Ohio). Although photometer measurements are more accurate than visual inspection, use of different broth media can affect photometer readings, requiring the user to verify the inoculum size by performing colony counts.

The organism suspensions are pipetted into the wells of the replicator head (32 to 36 wells) and applied to the plates with a multipronged replicator device that delivers approximately 0.001 ml per spot (10^5 CFU). The drug-free control plates are inoculated first, and then the antimicrobial plates are inoculated, starting with the lowest drug concentration. The plates should be marked to ensure proper orientation.

Contamination by aerobic bacteria during the inoculation procedure can be detected by inoculating drug-free plates and incubating them in an aerobic environment. If thioglycolate or other agar-containing broth medium is used for inoculum preparation, an additional control plate may be inoculated and refrigerated to distinguish inoculum residue that occurs at the time of setting up the MIC tests. Agar dilution plates can be inoculated in an aerobic environment, although the exposure time prior to incubation should be minimized. After the plates are stamped, the inoculation spots should absorb for 10 to 15 min into the medium; then the plates are stacked upside down (to prevent condensation from falling on the spots).

Incubation Conditions

An anaerobic chamber or anaerobic jar equipped with disposable hydrogen-carbon dioxide generators and palladium-coated catalyst pellets or ascorbic acid envelopes is recommended for incubating agar dilution plates. The incubation atmosphere should contain approximately 5% CO_2, and an indicator of anaerobiasis should be included. Incubation is carried out at 35 to 37°C for 44 to 48 h (47).

Interpretation of Results

Since 1993, the NCCLS has defined the end point for agar dilution testing as the concentration at which there is the most marked change from the growth control (45–47). This change is defined as no growth or lighter growth, a haze, multiple tiny colonies, or one to several normal-sized colonies. The technologist should take care to distinguish a

few colonies that may be present as the result of a "splash" from a resistant neighboring isolate from the few colonies that precede full growth of the strain. Plates should be read against a dark background to decrease the appearance of a haze. End points can be difficult to interpret when testing some gram-negative organisms with β-lactams, particularly ceftizoxime and piperacillin. This is especially problematic with many strains of fusobacteria that produce L forms, which appear as transparent hazes in the presence of even very high concentrations of β-lactam agents (40). The current NCCLS document for susceptibility testing of anaerobes now includes a color figure illustrating the end points described above and should be used as an additional guide when using this test method (47). It is important to compare the drug-containing plates to the drug-free control plate when reading the tests, since different species of anaerobic bacteria can have very different-appearing spots, ranging from mucoid-opaque, as with the B. fragilis group, to gray-transparent, as with B. ureolyticus.

MIC results should be interpreted according to criteria recommended by the NCCLS (Table 3) (47). In 1993, an intermediate category was established for anaerobic bacteria (45). For many antimicrobial agents used against anaerobes, a significant percentage of strains have susceptibility test end points that cluster at or near the suggested breakpoints. In a twofold-dilution method, the degree of acceptable variation of end points (usually plus or minus one twofold dilution) does not permit adequate distinction of the qualitative categories. If an intermediate value is determined for any anaerobe, the NCCLS recommends maximum dosages of the antimicrobial agent for therapy. With such dosages, it is believed that organisms with susceptible or intermediate end points are amenable to therapy. This recommendation is predicated upon the presumed surgical intervention that frequently is necessary to treat infections involving these organisms.

TABLE 3 Interpretive categories for MICs for anaerobic bacteria[a]

Antimicrobial agent	MIC (μg/ml)		
	Susceptible	Intermediate	Resistant
Amoxicillin-clavulanic acid	≤4/2	8/4	≥16/8
Ampicillin[b]	≤0.5	1	≥2
Ampicillin-sulbactam	≤8/4	16/8	≥32/16
Cefotetan	≤16	32	≥64
Cefoxitin	≤16	32	≥64
Chloramphenicol	≤8	16	≥32
Clindamycin	≤2	4	≥8
Ertapenem	≤4	8	≥16
Imipenem	≤4	8	≥16
Metronidazole	≤8	16	≥32
Meropenem	≤4	8	≥16
Penicillin[b]	≤0.5	1	≥2
Piperacillin	≤32	64	≥128
Piperacillin-tazobactam	≤32/4	64/4	≥128/4
Tetracycline	≤4	8	≥16
Ticarcillin-clavulanic acid	≤32/2	64/2	≥128/2
Trovafloxacin	≤2	4	≥8

[a] Adapted from reference 47 with permission of the publisher.
[b] Members of the B. fragilis group are presumed to be resistant. Other gram-negative anaerobes may be screened for β-lactamase activity by using a chromogenic cephalosporin test if penicillin therapy is contemplated. Higher levels in blood are achievable; infection with non-β-lactamase-producing organisms, for which the MICs are higher, might be treatable.

Broth Microdilution Test

The broth microdilution procedure has been validated by the NCCLS for testing members of the *B. fragilis* group. The Anaerobe Working Group of the NCCLS is evaluating additional antimicrobial agents and other species for correlation of the broth microdilution method to the reference standard.

Media

Brucella broth supplemented with hemin (5 μg/ml), vitamin K_1, and lysed horse blood is the recommended medium. Microdilution trays may be prepared fresh, frozen after preparation, or purchased commercially as lyophilized or frozen panels. Following the manufacturer's recommendations for storage of commercially prepared panels is recommended, while in-house-prepared trays may be kept at $-70°C$ for up to 6 months if they are stored in sealed plastic bags. Antimicrobial agents should be diluted as specified by the scheme described by the NCCLS (47) and should be prepared in large volumes, 15 to 100 ml, depending on the device used to simultaneously dispense aliquots of 0.1 ml per well into the standard 96-well panels. If the inoculum is to be added via a pipette, the antimicrobial solutions are prepared at twice the desired concentration and dispensed into the wells at 0.05 ml per well; then 0.05 ml of inoculum is added to each well, for a final volume of 0.1 ml. Volumes of less than 0.1 ml are not recommended for testing anaerobes due to loss of liquid by evaporation. Inoculum effects may be exaggerated when smaller volumes are used.

Inoculum Preparation

Inoculum preparation is similar to that in the agar dilution procedure. Organisms may be suspended in a clear broth to equal the turbidity of the 0.5 McFarland standard, or the isolate can be grown for 4 to 24 h in a supplemented thioglycolate or other broth that supports growth of the organism and then diluted to the turbidity of the 0.5 McFarland standard (approximately 1.5×10^8 CFU/ml). The final concentration of organism is 1×10^6 to 2×10^6 CFU/ml (10^5 CFU/well). Depending on the method of tray inoculation, the dilution technique will differ. If 10 μl is added to each well, then the 0.5 McFarland suspension is diluted 1:10. If 50 μl is added, the 0.5 McFarland suspension is diluted 1:50. If a lyophilized tray is used, the 0.5 McFarland suspension is diluted 1:100.

Inoculation Procedure

Frozen trays should be brought to room temperature before the inoculation is performed. Inoculation can be accomplished by using a disposable hand-held 96-prong inoculator, a mechanized dispenser, or a multichannel pipettor within 15 min after inocula are prepared. While the members of the *B. fragilis* group are relatively oxygen tolerant, reducing the trays in an oxygen-free environment prior to inoculation (2 to 4 h) may enhance the growth of certain fastidious anaerobes and reduce the "edge" effect of wells in outer rows being reduced more rapidly than those in inner rows (60). Trays should be reduced prior to inoculation if metronidazole is to be tested, since the antimicrobial activity of metronidazole is dependent on the formation of an active intermediate that requires a reduced atmosphere (60). False resistance can occur with nonfastidious, rapidly growing strains that produce significant growth before metronidazole is reduced to its active form. Control wells should include a well with broth but no drug (growth

control) and an uninoculated well as a sterility check. This well may also be used as a "negative" control for visual comparison with growth in inoculated wells. Alternatively, an uninoculated tray may be incubated as a sterility check, especially if trays are prepared in-house.

It is advisable to perform a colony count and a purity check of the inoculum. This is accomplished by removing 10 μl from the growth control well, diluting it into 10 ml of saline (1:1,000), and spreading 0.1 ml onto the surface of a nonselective blood agar plate for anaerobic incubation. The presence of 100 to 200 colonies indicates an inoculum of 1×10^6 to 2×10^6 CFU/ml. A small amount of material from the growth control well can be inoculated onto a quadrant of a blood agar plate for aerobic incubation to detect aerobic contamination.

Incubation Conditions

Trays are most conveniently incubated in an anaerobic chamber for 40 to 48 h. Alternatively, they can be placed into large anaerobic jars, regular anaerobic jars laid on their side, or anaerobic pouches with the appropriate anaerobic gas generator. No more than four trays should be stacked on top of each other, to ensure uniformity of heating and gas exchange. Trays should not be sealed with sealing tape if set up on the bench, since this will decrease the rate of diffusion of anaerobic gases to the inoculum and may result in poor growth or false resistance to metronidazole.

Interpretation of Results

The plates may be examined using a viewing device, such as a stand with a magnifying mirror. Broth microdilution MIC determinations have criteria similar to those for the agar dilution procedure for reading end points: the concentration at which the most significant reduction in growth is observed is interpreted as the MIC. Similar to that of agar dilution, this decrease in growth may include a tiny, gradually diminishing button of growth, and trailing end points are also observed (47). If the growth in the drug-free growth control well is poor, the test should not be read. At present, breakpoints for broth microdilution are similar to those for agar dilution (47).

E Test

The E test (A-B Biodisk, Solna, Sweden) has been used more frequently for testing anaerobic organisms in recent years, primarily because of its convenience (13, 54). Several studies have determined its utility and indicate that results correlate well with the NCCLS reference approved agar dilution method (13, 54). Rosenblatt and Gustafson (54) have noted that some *Prevotella* and *Bacteroides* strains show very major errors (false susceptibility) with penicillin and ceftriaxone, which are minimized if β-lactamase-positive strains are eliminated from testing. In addition, false resistance to metronidazole among anaerobes has been reported when the E test was used. This phenomenon can be the result of test conditions and medium quality, and it is generally eliminated if test plates are prereduced in an anaerobic chamber overnight before being used (14).

Procedure

The E test consists of plastic strips coated with a gradient of antimicrobial on one side and with an MIC interpretive scale on the other side. The method consists of streaking to confluence (three directions) a 0.5 to 1 McFarland standard of the test organism on a 150-ml-diameter petri dish containing supplemented brucella blood agar. The E-test strips are applied to the surface of the plate in a radial fashion, with the lowest concentration toward the center. If large plates are not available, two strips, one on each half, may be placed on a standard-size plate with the high concentrations of the strips opposite each other. Following 24 to 48 h of anaerobic incubation, an elliptical zone of inhibition is formed. MICs are read at the point of intersection of the ellipse with the interpretive scale of MICs.

Validation for most antimicrobial agents recommended for testing of anaerobes has been confirmed for the E test (54). The complete list of FDA-approved antimicrobials for anaerobe testing is found in the E-test package insert. The E test provides a flexible and simple procedure that is well suited for testing of individual isolates in small laboratories or in laboratories that do not perform batch testing of anaerobe susceptibility. Its main drawback is the relatively high cost of each strip. This can be alleviated somewhat by limiting the number of antimicrobials being tested to a few relevant drugs from the hospital's formulary.

Alternative Test Procedures

Spiral-Streak Method

The spiral-streak method (Spiral Systems Instruments, Bethesda, Md.) also uses a concentration gradient method by distributing an antimicrobial agent radially from the center of an agar plate. Test organisms are placed onto the antimicrobial-containing plate by using radial streaks, and the plates are incubated for 48 h in an anaerobic atmosphere. End points are determined by measuring the length of growth from the center of the plate to the point of inhibition, with data entered into a computer program that determines the concentration of the drug at the end of growth. This method also correlates sufficiently with agar dilution and may be a useful technique for research laboratories; however, it has currently not been cleared for use by the FDA (67).

β-Lactamase Testing

β-lactamase testing of anaerobes can be performed as described by NCCLS (47). Two easily performed methods include a nitrocefin disk assay (Cefinase; BBL, Cockeysville, Md.) and the S1 chromogenic cephalosporin disk (International BioClinical, Inc., Portland, Oreg.). Both tests should be performed as specified by the manufacturers. Hydrolysis of the β-lactam ring by β-lactamases causes a color change on the disks from yellow to red. Most reactions occur within 5 to 10 min, but some β-lactamase-positive *Bacteroides* strains may react more slowly (up to 30 min) (19). When testing *B. wadsworthia*, 1% pyruvate should be added to the testing growth medium for optimal results (61).

β-lactamase testing has limited utility in detecting resistance of anaerobes to certain β-lactam agents. While a chromogenic cephalosporin test is simple and quick, and generally detects β-lactamases produced by species of *Prevotella*, *Porphyromonas*, *Bacteroides*, and other anaerobes, resistance to β-lactam drugs is not always mediated by β-lactamase production (e.g., some strains of *B. distasonis* and *B. fragilis* are resistant owing to alterations of penicillin-binding proteins) (15, 26). Therefore, β-lactamase test results are limited in their clinical application. A positive test does, however, provide clinically relevant information quickly in some situations and can predict resistance to penicillin G and ampicillin.

Quality Control

A quality control program is designed to monitor the accuracy and precision of a susceptibility test procedure, the performance of reagents and equipment, and the performance of persons who conduct the tests. Quality control testing must be performed to demonstrate that any new medium used adequately supports the growth of the test organisms and that antimicrobial agents have not deteriorated during shipping or storage. These tests must be a part of any testing program involving any of the methods described above. Ideally, the quality control strain(s) that most closely resembles the tested organism(s) should be included. The recommended quality control strains are *B. fragilis* ATCC 25285, *B. thetaiotaomicron* ATCC 29741, and *Eubacterium lentum* ATCC 43055. Two quality control strains should be used for each assessment when the agar dilution procedure is used. When an individual strain is being tested by broth microdilution or the E test, one quality control strain should be included. Expected values for quality control strains are published by the NCCLS (47). For some antimicrobial agent-quality control organism combinations, no quality control ranges are recommended due to difficulty in reading the end points.

CONCLUSIONS

Antimicrobial resistance among anaerobes has become a significant problem in recent years, increasing the need for antimicrobial susceptibility testing. Current methods allow accurate surveillance or individual isolate testing by most laboratories. Future studies comparing broth microdilution to the reference agar method will result in better standardization of the more user-friendly method and, possibly, to more widespread commercial availability.

REFERENCES

1. **Aldridge, K. E., D. Ashcraft, K. Cambre, C. L. Pierson, S. G. Jenkins, and J. E. Rosenblatt.** 2001. Multicenter survey of the changing in vitro antimicrobial susceptibilities of clinical isolates of *Bacteroides fragilis* group, *Prevotella*, *Fusobacterium*, *Porphyromonas*, and *Peptostreptococcus* species. *Antimicrob. Agents Chemother.* **45:**1238–1243.
2. **Aldridge, K. E., M. Gelfand, L. D. Reller, L. W. Ayers, C. L. Pierson, R. Schoenknecht, R. L. Tilton, J. Wilkins, A. Henderberg, and D. D. Schiro.** 1994. A five year multicenter study of the susceptibility of the *Bacteroides fragilis* group isolates to cephalosporins, cephamins, penicillins, clindamycin, and metronidazole in the United States. *Diagn. Microbiol. Infect. Dis.* **18:**235–241.
3. **Aldridge, K. E., and D. D. Schiro.** 1994. Major methodology-dependent discordant susceptibility results from *Bacteroides fragilis* group isolates but not other anaerobes. *Diagn. Microbiol. Infect. Dis.* **20:**135–142.
4. **Appelbaum, P. C., S. K. Spangler, and M. R. Jacobs.** 1990. β-Lactamase production and susceptibilities to amoxicillin, amoxicillin-clavulanate, ticarcillin, ticarcillin-clavulanate, cefoxitin, imipenem, and metronidazole of 320 non-*Bacteroides fragilis* isolates and 129 fusobacteria from 28 U.S. centers. *Antimicrob. Agents Chemother.* **34:**1546–1550.
5. **Bandoh, K., K. Ueno, K. Watanabe, and N. Kato.** 1993. Susceptibility patterns and resistance to imipenem in the *Bacteroides fragilis* group species in Japan: a 4-year study. *Clin. Infect. Dis.* **16:**S382–S386.
6. **Bandoh, K., K. Watanabe, Y. Muto, Y. Tanaka, N. Kato, and K. Ueno.** 1992. Conjugal transfer of imipenem resis-

tance in *Bacteroides fragilis*. *J. Antibiot.* (Tokyo) **45:**542–547.

7. **Baquero, F., and M. Reig.** 1992. Resistance of anaerobic bacteria to antimicrobial agents in Spain. *Eur. J. Clin. Microbiol. Infect. Dis.* **11:**1016–1020.

8. **Baron, E. J., D. M. Citron, and H. M. Wexler.** 1990. Anaerobic susceptibility testing-revisited. *J. Clin. Microbiol.* **12:**69–70.

9. **Baron, E. J., G. Ropers, P. Summanen, and R. J. Courcol.** 1997. Bactericidal activity of selected antimicrobial agents against *Bilophila wadsworthia* and *Bacteroides gracilis*. *Clin. Infect. Dis.* **16:**S339–S343.

10. **Bianchini, H., L. B. Fernandez Canigia, C. Bantar, and J. Smayevsky.** 1997. Trends in antimicrobial resistance of the *Bacteroides fragilis* group: a 20-year study at a medical center in Buenos Aires, Argentina. *Clin. Infect. Dis.* **25:**S268–S269.

11. **Borobio, M. V., A. Pascual, M. C. Dominguez, and E. J. Perea.** 1986. Effect of medium, pH, and inoculum size on activity of ceftizoxime and Csh-34343 against anaerobic bacteria. *Antimicrob. Agents Chemother.* **30:**626–627.

12. **Chow, A. W., and N. Cheng.** 1988. In vitro activities of daptomycin (LY146032) and paldimycin (U-70,138F) against anaerobic gram-positive bacteria. *Antimicrob. Agents Chemother.* **32:**788–790.

13. **Citron, D. M., A. Ostavari, A. Karlsson, and E. J. C. Goldstein.** 1991. Evaluation of the epsilometer (E-test) for susceptibility testing of anaerobic bacteria. *J. Clin. Microbiol.* **29:**2197–2203.

14. **Cormican, M. G., M. E. Erwin, and R. N. Jones.** 1996. False resistance to metronidazole by E-test among anaerobic bacteria investigations of contributing test conditions and medium quality. *Diagn. Microbiol. Infect. Dis.* **24:**117–119.

15. **Cuchural, G. J., S. Hurlbut, M. H. Malamy, and F. P. Tally.** 1988. Permeability to β-lactams in *Bacteroides fragilis*. *J. Antimicrob. Chemother.* **22:**785–790.

16. **Cuchural, G. J., F. P. Tally, N. V. Jacobus, K. E. Aldridge, T. J. Cleary, S. M. Finegold, G. B. Hills, P. B. Iannini, J. P. O'Keefe, C. L. Pierson, D. W. Crook, T. A. Russo, and D. W. Hecht.** 1988. Susceptibility of *Bacteroides fragilis* group in the United States: analysis by site of isolation. *Antimicrob. Agents Chemother.* **32:**717–722.

17. **Cuchural, G. J., F. P. Tally, N. V. Jacobus, T. J. Cleary, S. M. Finegold, G. B. Hills, P. B. Iannini, J. P. O'Keefe, and C. L. Pierson.** 1990. Comparative activities of newer beta-lactam agents against members of the *Bacteroides fragilis* group. *Antimicrob. Agents Chemother.* **34:**479–480.

18. **Cuchural, G. J., F. P. Tally, N. V. Jacobus, P. K. Marsh, and J. W. Mayhew.** 1983. Cefoxitin inactivation by *Bacteroides fragilis*. *Antimicrob. Agents Chemother.* **34:**936–940.

19. **Doern, G. V., R. N. Jones, E. H. Gerlach, J. A. Washington, D. J. Biedenbach, A. Brueggemann, M. E. Erwin, C. Knapp, and J. Raymond.** 1995. Multicenter clinical laboratory evaluation of a beta-lactamase disk assay employing a novel chromogenic cephalosporin, S1. *J. Clin. Microbiol.* **33:**1665–1667.

20. **Dougherty, S. H.** 1997. Antimicrobial culture and susceptibility testing has little value for routine management of secondary bacterial peritonitis. *Clin. Infect. Dis.* **25:**S258–S261.

21. **Ednie, L. M., M. R. Jacobs, and P. C. Appelbaum.** 1998. Activities of gatifloxacin compared to those of seven other agents against anaerobic organisms. *Antimicrob. Agents Chemother.* **42:**2459–2462.

22. **Eley, A., and D. Greenwood.** 1986. Beta-lactamases of type culture strains of the *Bacteroides fragilis* group and of strains that hydrolyse cefoxitin, latamoxef and imipenem. *J. Med. Microbiol.* **21:**49–57.

23. **Finegold, S. M.** 1989. Therapy of anaerobic infections, p. 793–818. *In* S. M. Finegold and W. L. George (ed.), *Anaerobic Infections in Humans*. Academic Press, Inc., Orlando, Fla.

24. **Finegold, S. M.** 1997. Perspective on susceptibility testing of anaerobic bacteria. *Clin. Infect. Dis.* **25:**S251–S253.

25. **Fox, A. R., and I. Phillips.** 1987. The antibiotic sensitivity of the *Bacteroides fragilis* group in the United Kingdom. *J. Antimicrob. Chemother.* **20:**477–488.

26. **Georgopapadakou, N. H.** 1993. Penicillin-binding proteins and bacterial resistance to β-lactams. *Antimicrob. Agents Chemother.* **37:**2045–2053.

27. **Goldstein, E. J. C., D. M. Citron, C. V. Merriam, Y. Warren, and K. Tyrrell.** 1999. Activities of telithromycin (HMR 3647, RU 66647) compared to those of erythromycin, azithromycin, clarithromycin, roxithromycin, and other antimicrobial agents against unusual anaerobes. *Antimicrob. Agents Chemother.* **43:**2801–2805.

28. **Goldstein, E. J. C., D. M. Citron, C. V. Merriam, K. Tyrrell, and Y. Warren.** 1999. Activities of gemifloxacin (SB 265805, LB20304) compared to those of other oral antimicrobial agents against unusual anaerobes. *Antimicrob. Agents Chemother.* **43:**2726–2730.

29. **Goldstein, E. J. C., D. M. Citron, C. V. Merriam, Y. Warren, and K. L. Tyrrell.** 2001. Comparative in vitro activities of ertapenem (MK-0826) against 1,001 anaerobes isolated from human intra-abdominal infections. *Antimicrob. Agents Chemother.* **44:**2389–2394.

30. **Goldstein, E. J. C., D. M. Citron, Y. Warren, K. Tyrrell, and C. V. Merriam.** 1999. In vitro activity of gemifloxacin (SB 265805) against anaerobes. *Antimicrob. Agents Chemother.* **43:**2231–2235.

31. **Goldstein, E. J. C., and D. M. Citron.** 1993. Comparative susceptibilities of 173 aerobic and anaerobic bite wound isolates to sparfloxacin, temafloxacin, clarithromycin, and older agents. *Antimicrob. Agents Chemother.* **37:**1150–1153.

32. **Goldstein, E. J. C., D. M. Citron, C. E. Cherubin, and S. L. Hillier.** 1993. Comparative susceptibility of the *Bacteroides fragilis* group species and other anaerobic bacteria to meropenem, imipenem, piperacillin, cefoxitin, ampicillin/sulbactam, clindamycin and metronidazole. *J. Antimicrob. Chemother.* **31:**363–372.

33. **Goldstein, E. J. C., D. M. Citron, R. J. Goldman, M. C. Claros, and S. Hunt-Gerrado.** 1995. United States national hospital survey of anaerobic culture and susceptibility methods, II. *Anaerobe* **1:**309–314.

34. **Hecht, D. W., and L. Lederer.** 1995. Effect of choice of medium on the results of in vitro susceptibility testing of eight antibiotics against the *Bacteroides fragilis* group. *Clin. Infect. Dis.* **20:**S346–S349.

35. **Hecht, D. W., L. Lederer, and J. R. Osmolski.** 1995. Susceptibility results for the *Bacteroides fragilis* group: comparison of the broth microdilution and agar dilution methods. *Clin. Infect. Dis.* **20:**S342–S345.

36. **Hecht, D. W., and J. R. Osmolski.** 1996. Comparison of activities of trovafloxacin (CP-99,219) and five other agents against 585 anaerobes with use of three media. *Clin. Infect. Dis.* **23:**S44–S50.

37. **Hecht, D. W., J. R. Osmolski, and J. P. O'Keefe.** 1993. Variation in the susceptibility of *Bacteroides fragilis* group isolates from six Chicago Hospitals. *Clin. Infect. Dis.* **16:**S357–S360.

38. **Hecht, D. W., and H. M. Wexler.** 1997. In vitro susceptibility of anaerobes to quinolones in the United States. *Clin. Infect. Dis.* **23:**S2–S8.

39. **Hoellman, D. B., L. M. Kelly, M. R. Jacobs, and P. C. Appelbaum.** 2001. Comparative antianaerobic activity of BMS 284756. *Antimicrob. Agents Chemother.* **45:**589–592.

40. **Johnson, C. C.** 1993. Susceptibility of anaerobic bacteria to beta-lactam antibiotics in the United States. *Clin. Infect. Dis.* **16**(Suppl. 4):S371–S376.

41. **Jousimies-Somer, H.** 1997. Recently described clinically important anaerobic bacteria: taxonomic aspects and update. *Clin. Infect. Dis.* **25:**S78–S87.

42. **Labbe, A. C., A. M. Bourgault, J. Vincelette, P. L. Turgeon, and F. Lamothe.** 1999. Trends in antimicrobial resistance among clinical isolates of the *Bacteroides fragilis* group from 1992 to 1997 in Montreal, Canada. *Antimicrob. Agents Chemother.* **43:**2517–2519.

43. **Lubbe, M. M., P. L. Botha, and L. J. Chalkley.** 1999. Comparative activity of eighteen antimicrobial agents against anaerobic bacteria isolated in South Africa. *Eur. J. Clin. Microbiol. Infect. Dis.* **18:**46–54.

44. **Molitoris, E., H. M. Wexler, and S. M. Finegold.** 1997. Sources and antimicrobial susceptibilities of *Campylobacter gracilis* and *Sutterella wadsworthensis*. *Clin. Infect. Dis.* **25:** S264–S265.

45. **National Committee for Clinical Laboratory Standards.** 1993. *Methods for Antimicrobial Susceptibility Testing of Anaerobic Bacteria*, 3rd ed. *Approved Standard M11-A3.* National Committee for Clinical Laboratory Standards, Villanova, Pa.

46. **National Committee for Clinical Laboratory Standards.** 1997. *Methods for Antimicrobial Susceptibility Testing of Anaerobic Bacteria*, 4th ed. *Approved Standard M11-A4.* National Committee for Clinical Laboratory Standards, Wayne, Pa.

47. **National Committee for Clinical Laboratory Standards.** 2001. *Methods for Antimicrobial Susceptibility Testing of Anaerobic Bacteria*, 5th ed. *Approved Standard M11-A5.* National Committee for Clinical Laboratory Standards, Wayne, Pa.

48. **Nguyen, M. H., V. L. Yu, A. J. Morris, L. McDermott, M. W. Wagener, L. Harrell, and D. R. Snydman.** 2001. Antimicrobial resistance and clinical outcome of *Bacteroides* bacteremia: findings of a multicenter prospective observational trial. *Clin. Infect. Dis.* **30:**870–876.

49. **North American Congress on Anaerobic Bacteria and Anaerobic Infections.** 1993. Proceedings of the first North American congress on anaerobic bacteria and anaerobic infections. *Clin. Infect. Dis.* **16:**S159–S411.

50. **O'Keefe, J. P., F. R. Venezio, C. A. DiVincenzo, and K. L. Shatzer.** 1987. Activity of newer beta-lactam agents against clinical isolates of *Bacteroides fragilis* and other *Bacteroides* species. *Antimicrob. Agents Chemother.* **31:** 2002–2004.

51. **Podglajen, I., J. Breuil, and E. Collatz.** 1994. Insertion of a novel DNA sequence, 1S*1186*, upstream of the silent carbapenemase gene *cfiA*, promotes expression of carbapenem resistance in clinical isolates of *Bacteroides fragilis*. *Mol. Microbiol.* **12:**105–114.

52. **Reyssett, G., A. Haggoud, W. Su, and M. Sebald.** 1992. Genetic and molecular analysis of pIP417 and pIP419: *Bacteroides* plasmids encoding 5-nitroimidazole resistance. *Plasmid* **27:**181–190.

53. **Rosenblatt, J.** 1989. Antimicrobic susceptibility of anaerobic bacteria, p. 715–727. *In* S. M. Finegold and W. L. George (ed.), *Anaerobic Infections in Humans.* Academic Press, San Diego, Calif.

54. **Rosenblatt, J. E., and D. R. Gustafson.** 1995. Evaluation of the Etest for susceptibility testing of anaerobic bacteria. *Diagn. Microbiol. Infect. Dis.* **22:**279–284.

55. **Rosenblatt, J. E., and I. Brook.** 1993. Clinical relevance of susceptibility testing of anaerobic bacteria. *Clin. Infect. Dis.* **16:**S446–S448.

56. **Salonen, J. H., E. Eerola, and O. Meurman.** 1998. Clinical significance and outcome of anaerobic bacteremia. *Clin. Infect. Dis.* **26:**1413–1417.

57. **Shore, K. P., S. Pottumarthy, and A. J. Morris.** 1999. Susceptibility of anaerobic bacteria in Auckland: 1991–1996. *N. Z. Med. J.* **112:**424–426.

58. **Snydman, D. R., N. V. Jacobus, L. McDermott, S. Supran, G. J. Cuchural, S. M. Finegold, L. J. Harrell, D. W. Hecht, P. B. Iannini, S. G. Jenkins, C. L. Pierson, J. D. Rihs, and S. L. Gorbach.** 1999. Multicenter study if in vitro susceptibility of the *Bacteroides fragilis* group, 1995 to 1996, with comparison of resistance trends from 1990 to 1996. *Antimicrob. Agents Chemother.* **43:**2417–2422.

59. **Snydman, D. R., L. McDermott, G. J. Cuchural, D. W. Hecht, P. B. Iannini, L. J. Harrell, S. G. Jenkins, J. P. O'Keefe, C. L. Pierson, J. D. Rihs, V. L. Yu, S. M. Finegold, and S. L. Gorbach.** 1996. Analysis of trends in antimicrobial resistance patterns among clinical isolates of *Bacteroides fragilis* group species from 1990 to 1994. *Clin. Infect. Dis.* **23:**S54–S65.

60. **Summanen, P., E. J. Baron, D. M. Citron, C. Strong, H. M. Wexler, and S. M. Finegold.** 1993. *Wadsworth Anaerobic Bacteriology Manual.* Star Publishing Co. Belmont, Calif.

61. **Summanen, P., H. M. Wexler, and S. M. Finegold.** 1992. Antimicrobial susceptibility testing of *Bilophila wadsworthia* by using triphenyltetrazolium chloride to facilitate the endpoint determination. *Antimicrob. Agents Chemother.* **36:**1658–1664.

62. **Tally, F. P., D. R. Snydman, S. L. Gorbach, and M. H. Malamy.** 1979. Plasmid-mediated, transferable resistance to clindamycin and erythromycin in *Bacteroides fragilis*. *J. Infect. Dis.* **139:**83–88.

63. **Tanaka, K., C. Kawamura, K. Fukui, H. Kato, N. Kato, T. Nakamura, K. Watanabe, and K. Ueno.** 1999. Antimicrobial susceptibility and beta-lactamase production of *Prevotella* spp. and *Porphyromonas* spp. *Anaerobe* **5:**461–463.

64. **Tuner, K., and C. E. Nord.** 1992. Antibiotic susceptibility of anaerobic bacteria in Europe. *Clin. Infect. Dis.* **4:**S387–S389.

65. **Wexler, H. M., and S. M. Finegold.** 1988. In vitro activity of cefotetan against anaerobic bacteria compared to other antimicrobial agents. *Antimicrob. Agents Chemother.* **32:** 601–604.

66. **Wexler, H. M., E. Molitoris, and S. M. Finegold.** 1991. Effect of β-lactamase inhibitors on the activities of various β-lactam agents against anaerobic bacteria. *Antimicrob. Agents Chemother.* **25:**1219–1224.

67. **Wexler, H. M., E. Molitoris, P. R. Murray, J. A. Washington, R. J. Zabransky, P. H. Edelstein, and S. M. Finegold.** 1996. Comparison of spiral gradient endpoint and agar dilution methods for susceptibility testing of anaerobic bacteria: a multilaboratory collaborative evaluation. *J. Clin. Microbiol.* **34:**170–174.

68. **Wilson, S. E., and J. Huh.** 1997. In defense of routine antimicrobial susceptibility testing of operative site flora in patients with peritonitis. *Clin. Infect. Dis.* **25:**S254–S257.

Susceptibility Test Methods: Mycobacteria*

CLARK B. INDERLIED AND GABY E. PFYFFER

73

In his review article entitled "The White Plague," M. F. Perutz recounted that Cardinal Richelieu (1585 to 1642), Heinrich Heine (1797 to 1856), Frédéric Chopin (1810 to 1849), Anton Chekhov (1860 to 1904), Franz Kafka (1883 to 1924), George Orwell (1903 to 1950), and Eleanor Roosevelt (1884 to 1962) all had a common fate (126). Each of them died of tuberculosis. For many of these famous cases, it is unknown if the disease was only poorly understood or if management of the disease was simply inadequate or even inappropriate. For some, effective antimicrobial agents for the treatment of tuberculosis had not been discovered or were discovered too late. Streptomycin and p-aminosalicylic acid were not introduced until the late 1940s, and isoniazid, ethambutol, and rifampin were not used to treat tuberculosis until 1952, 1961, and 1968, respectively. Therefore, it is also possible that the more contemporary of these patients were early victims of antimicrobial resistance. In the same article, Professor Perutz related the response of the famous German chemist Gerhard Domagk (1895 to 1964) to Otto Warburg's (1883 to 1970) comment that Domagk "deserved monuments in each valley and every mountain." Domagk, who in 1935 discovered Prontosil (a precursor of sulfanilamide) and 10 years later discovered Conteben (a precursor of isoniazid), replied to Warburg that "no one is interested any longer in diseases that can be cured." Domagk could not have anticipated the extent to which antibiotic resistance would come to complicate the chemotherapy of all infectious diseases, especially tuberculosis. Nevertheless, his words resonate with a particular poignancy for those interested in antimicrobial agents with activity against mycobacteria, in vitro susceptibility testing, and the use of laboratory findings in guiding the treatment of patients with mycobacterial infections.

ANTIMICROBIAL AGENTS

Although a variety of antimicrobial agents are available for the treatment of mycobacterial diseases, not all agents are suitable for treating all types of infections. Furthermore, in the face of antimicrobial resistance, the choice of alternative therapies can be problematic and clinical experience becomes a prevailing factor. For other uncommon mycobacterial infections, the physician is not infrequently faced with a dilemma in choosing a treatment regimen because of a lack of clinical precedence or unclear efficacy. The situation is confounded further by the need to treat mycobacterial infections with a mixture of agents to improve efficacy, to prevent resistance, or to overcome intrinsic resistance. The antimicrobial agents that are used in the treatment of mycobacterial infections are discussed below and in Table 1.

Isoniazid

Isoniazid (isonicotinic acid hydrazide [INH]), a synthetic antimicrobial agent introduced in 1952 for the treatment of tuberculosis, is remarkably specific and potently bactericidal for tubercle bacilli (Fig. 1). INH has comparatively low toxicity and is active against virtually all "wild-type" strains of *Mycobacterium tuberculosis*. While the exact mechanism of action of INH is still not known, its primary effect is on mycolic acid synthesis, as evidenced by the increased fragility of the mycobacterial cell, increased intracellular viscosity, decreased cellular hydrophobicity, and loss of acid fastness (184). Some evidence indicates that INH inhibits a desaturation step in the production of long-chain fatty acids (162) and may also inhibit the elongation of fatty acids and hydroxy lipids (37). In addition, INH appears to interfere with NAD metabolism, energy metabolism, and macromolecular synthesis (41, 185, 186). There is accumulating evidence that INH acts as a prodrug that is "activated" by the catalase-peroxidase encoded by the *kat*G gene (see below) (74, 97, 175), an observation consistent with the well-known correlation between INH resistance and loss of catalase activity.

In 1992, Zhang et al. (194) reported the detection of the *kat*G gene in M. *tuberculosis* and correlated the deletion of this gene with resistance to INH. The *kat*G gene encodes a mycobacterial catalase-peroxidase, and Zhang et al. showed that the transfer of this gene into an INH-resistant strain of M. *smegmatis* conferred susceptibility to INH and that deletion of the gene from clinical isolates of M. *tuberculosis* correlated with INH resistance. In 1994, Banerjee et al. (11) reported that INH and ethionamide resistance in M. *tuberculosis* correlated with

* This chapter contains information presented in chapter 124 by Clark B. Inderlied and Max Salfinger in the seventh edition of this Manual.

TABLE 1 Antimycobacterial agents ranked by clinical utility and candidacy for in vitro susceptibility testing[a]

Mycobacterium species	Antimycobacterial agent			
	Primary or first choice	Secondary or second choice	Tertiary or third choice	Primary resistance likely
M. tuberculosis, M. africanum, M. bovis[b]	INH, RMP, PZA, EMB	SM, ciprofloxacin, ofloxacin, sparfloxacin, rifapentine, ethionamide	Rifabutin, amikacin, levofloxacin, cycloserine, PAS, capreomycin	
M. leprae	Clarithromycin, dapsone, RMP	Ethionamide, prothionamide, minocycline, clofazimine		
M. avium, M. intracellulare	Clarithromycin,[c] azithromycin, EMB	Amikacin, ciprofloxacin, rifabutin	SM, cycloserine, ethionamide	INH, PZA
M. chelonae, M. fortuitum, M. abscessus, M. mucogenicum, M. smegmatis	Amikacin, cefoxitin, ciprofloxacin, clarithromycin, doxycycline or minocycline, sulfonamides	Cefmetazole, imipenem, ofloxacin, tobramycin[d]		INH, PZA, RMP, SM, EMB,[e] clofazimine
M. kansasii	RMP	INH, EMB, clarithromycin	Amikacin, SM, rifabutin, ciprofloxacin, ofloxacin, sulfonamide	PZA
M. scrofulaceum	Lymphadenitis (surgical excision without chemotherapy)	Azithromycin, clarithromycin		INH, PZA
M. marinum	Doxycycline or minocycline, EMB, RMP, sulfonamide	Amikacin, ciprofloxacin, clarithromycin, rifabutin		INH, PZA
M. haemophilum, M. malmoense, M. simiae, M. szulgai, M. xenopi, M. ulcerans	Clarithromycin,[f] EMB,[f] RMP[f]	Amikacin, ciprofloxacin, INH, rifabutin, SM		PZA

[a] First-choice agents are expected to be active against wild-type isolates (i.e., from untreated patients); second- and third-choice agents are less preferable, usually for reasons of toxicity, expense, or unclear efficacy (7). The information in this table was compiled from references 84, 98, 100, and 147, which provide more specific information on the use of these agents for the treatment of various mycobacterial diseases.
[b] M. bovis and M. bovis BCG are considered resistant to PZA (>95%).
[c] Clarithromycin is the class drug for macrolides (azithromycin, clarithromycin, and roxithromycin).
[d] M. chelonae only.
[e] Useful for treating M. smegmatis only.
[f] Proven clinical utility for some but not all species.

a missense mutation in the inhA gene. The inhA gene encodes a protein that has sequence similarity (75% similarity and 40% identity) to the Escherichia coli enzyme EnvM, which may be a component of the mycolic acid biosynthetic pathway. Subsequent studies have

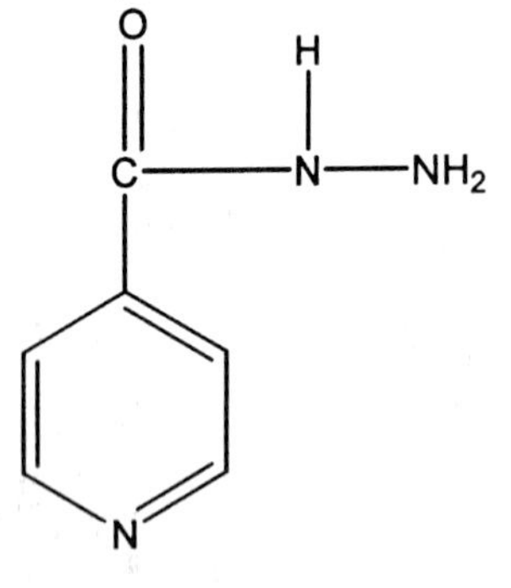

FIGURE 1 Structure of isoniazid.

shown that katG mutations account for 30 to 60% of INH resistance (73, 114) and that inhA mutations confer a low level of INH resistance that may not always be clinically significant (102). Two additional genes have been implicated in INH resistance, the ahpC gene (43, 89, 156, 183, 193) and, quite recently, the kasA gene (103). The ahpC gene encodes an alkyl hydroperoxide reductase subunit, and the kasA gene encodes a putative β-ketoacyl acyl carrier protein synthase. The degree to which mutations in these last genes contribute to INH resistance is not clear, although the role of ahpC appears to be minor. In aggregate, however, mutations in these four genes (katG, inhA, ahpC, and kasA) may account for ~90% of INH resistance (Table 2).

INH is active only against replicating tubercle bacilli; slowly replicating bacilli in the caseous lesions are not readily killed by INH, and dormant bacilli are unlikely to be affected. INH resistance develops rapidly when patients are given monotherapy, and the frequency of INH resistance within a population of tubercle bacilli ranges from 10^{-5} to 10^{-6} (36). Wild-type isolates of M. tuberculosis are inhib-

TABLE 2 Mycobacterial genes with mutations associated with antimicrobial resistance[a]

Antimicrobial agent	Species	Gene	% Resistance[b]	Product	Reference(s)
RMP	M. tuberculosis, M. africanum, M. leprae, M. avium	rpoB	>96	β subunit of RNA polymerase	164, 165, 182
INH	M. tuberculosis	katG		Catalase-peroxidase	73, 116, 164
INH-ethionamide	M. tuberculosis	inhA		envM analog 3-Ketoacyl-acyl carrier protein reductase analog	11
INH	M. tuberculosis, M. leprae	ahpC	90	Subunit of alkyl hydroperoxide reductase	44, 89, 183
INH	M. tuberculosis	kasA		β-Ketoacyl ACP synthase	103
EMB	M. tuberculosis	embB	47–65	Arabinosyltransferase	1, 158
SM	M. tuberculosis, M. smegmatis	rpsL	70	Ribosomal protein S12	52, 90, 117
SM	M. tuberculosis	rrs	70	16S rRNA	52; J. Douglass and L. M. Steyn, Letter, J. Infect. Dis., **167**:1505–1506, 1993
PZA	M. tuberculosis	pncA	72–97	Pyrazinamidase	150, 157
Fluoroquinolone	M. tuberculosis, M. smegmatis	gyrA	75–94	DNA gyrase A subunit	138, 163
Azithromycin-clarithromycin	M. avium, M. intracellulare, M. chelonae, M. abscessus		95	V-domain 23S rRNA	105, 119, 171

[a] Adapted from reference 116.

[b] Estimated percent resistance that can be accounted for by mutations in the respective genes; 90% of the isoniazid resistance can probably be accounted for by mutations in katG, ahpC, inhA, and/or kasA. Percentages are taken in part from reference 2.

ited by INH, with MICs of 0.05 to 0.2 μg/ml (the MICs quoted here are not based on standardized methods and are intended only to convey a sense of the relative potency of certain agents). Other susceptible isolates of slowly growing mycobacteria, such as M. kansasii and M. xenopi, are inhibited by 1 to 5 μg/ml (39). Most other nontuberculous mycobacteria, including the M. avium complex (MAC), M. marinum, M. ulcerans, and all rapidly growing mycobacteria, are resistant to INH. INH is well absorbed when administered orally or intramuscularly; it is distributed throughout the body, and the levels in cerebrospinal fluid (CSF) may equal the levels in plasma in patients with meningeal inflammation or 20% of the levels in plasma in patients without inflammation (3). INH is metabolized in the liver and intestines, primarily by acetylation by an N-acetyltransferase, which can vary significantly from person to person. However, the acetylator phenotype of an individual does not appear to influence either the efficacy of INH or the risk of hepatotoxicity. Adverse drug reactions include infrequent, age-related hepatitis and, less frequently, peripheral neuropathy, hypersensitivity reactions such as fever and rash, and arthralgias.

Rifampin

Rifampin (RMP, rifampicin) is 3,4-(methylpiperazinyl-iminomethylidene)-rifamycin SV; it was introduced in 1968 as a potent antituberculosis agent (Fig. 2). RMP is active against a wide variety of non-acid-fast bacteria and several other slowly growing mycobacteria, notably M. leprae, M. kansasii, M. haemophilum, and M. marinum, but is only variably active against MAC and is inactive against the rapidly growing mycobacteria. RMP inhibits the prokaryotic DNA-dependent RNA polymerase by binding to the β subunit at the presumed catalytic center of the enzyme. The

mammalian RNA polymerase is inhibited by RMP only at significantly higher concentrations than is the prokaryotic enzyme. The RNA polymerase of MAC isolates appears to be susceptible to RMP; therefore, the primary mechanism of intrinsic resistance is most probably impermeability.

Telenti et al. (165) first showed that RMP resistance correlated with changes, primarily amino acid substitutions, within a conserved region of the rpoB gene that encodes the β subunit of the M. tuberculosis RNA polymerase. Subsequent studies showed that >96% of RMP resistance could be attributed to mutations within an 81-bp region of the rpoB gene (116). The molecular basis of RMP resistance in M. leprae is similar to that in M. tuberculosis, and it appears that the same methods can be applied to the detection of RMP resistance in M. leprae (77). Williams et al. (182) developed a rapid PCR-based DNA sequencing method that targets a 305-bp region of the rpoB gene and showed that there was a high degree of sequence similarity (90 to 100%) between the region in M. tuberculosis and the regions in M. leprae, M. avium, and M. africanum. This analysis of 110 RMP-resistant strains of M. tuberculosis identified 16 mutations, 9 of which were identical to those described by Telenti et al. (165) and 7 of which were newly identified mutations. In two strains of RMP-resistant M. avium, missense mutations were detected, but in two other strains, no mutations were detected. This agrees with the observations of Guerrero et al. (59), who showed that mutations in the rpoB gene in M. avium and M. intracellulare are rare and that RMP resistance is most probably a reflection of impermeability to the drug.

RMP is well absorbed from the gastrointestinal tract, and peak concentrations of 5 to 10 μg/ml are reached within 1 to 2 h after an oral dose of 600 mg; concentrations in CSF reach 50% of the levels in plasma in patients with

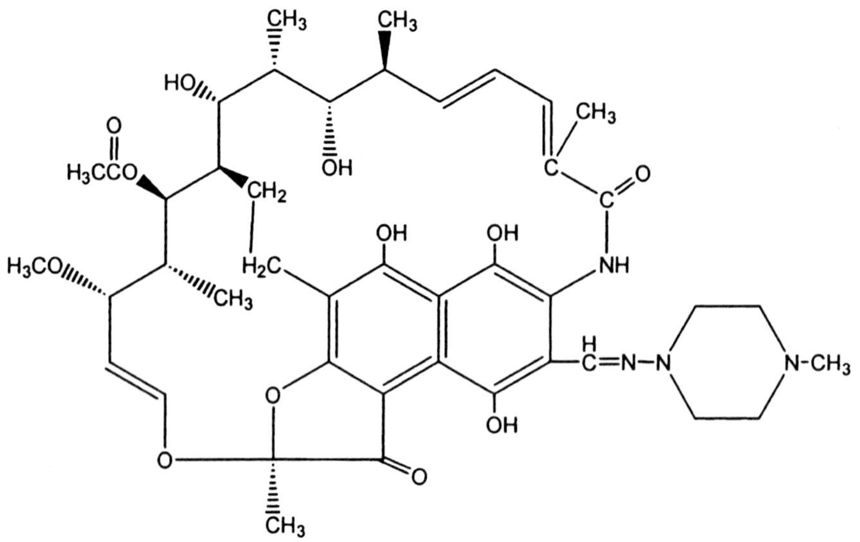

FIGURE 2 Structure of rifampin.

meningeal inflammation. RMP is available in combination with INH as a single capsule (Rifamate) containing 300 mg of RMP and 150 mg of INH and is also available in combination with INH and pyrazinamide as a single capsule (Rifater). RMP concentrations of 0.5 μg/ml are bactericidal for wild-type isolates of M. tuberculosis, and RMP affects intracellular, slowly replicating bacilli in caseous lesions as well as the actively replicating tubercle bacilli in the open pulmonary cavities. Adverse drug reactions include gastrointestinal and hypersensitivity reactions; however, the major effect is hepatotoxicity and a red-orange discoloration of urine, tears, other body fluids, and soft contact lenses. RMP also induces increased hepatic metabolism of a wide variety of other drugs including methadone and birth control pills (3). Of particular concern is the interaction of RMP and, to a somewhat lesser degree, rifabutin with protease inhibitors (saquinavir, ritonavir, and indinavir), which leads to enhanced hepatic metabolism and may result in subtherapeutic levels of the antiviral agents (7).

Pyrazinamide

Pyrazinamide (PZA) is a synthetic derivative (pyrazine analog) of nicotinamide and, in combination with INH, is rapidly bactericidal for replicating forms of M. tuberculosis, with an average MIC of 20 μg/ml (Fig. 3). PZA is inactive against nonreplicating tubercle bacilli and totally inactive against other Mycobacterium species, including M. bovis, MAC, and the rapidly growing mycobacteria. PZA is active

only at acidic pHs; therefore, the pH of the growth medium must be adjusted for accurate measurements of the in vitro activity of the drug. It is most likely that PZA is active only in the acidic milieu of the phagolysosome and, depending on the concentration achieved at the site of the infection, may be bacteriostatic or bactericidal. PZA is hydrolyzed in the liver to the active metabolite pyrazinoic acid, and although the mechanism of action of PZA is unknown, its activity depends on this conversion. M. tuberculosis produces a pyrazinamidase, and most strains of PZA-resistant M. tuberculosis lack this enzyme; however, some PZA-resistant isolates retain pyrazinamidase activity, suggesting that there are other mechanisms of resistance. The lack of pyrazinamidase activity and its correlation with PZA resistance have been associated with mutations in the pncA gene that encodes the enzyme (150, 151, 157). Indeed, it now appears that 72 to 97% of PZA resistance can be attributed to mutations in the pncA gene (Table 2), and one study suggests that this correlation can be used to distinguish between M. tuberculosis and M. bovis (149).

PZA is well absorbed from the gastrointestinal tract and widely distributed throughout the body, with maximum levels in serum of approximately 45 μg/ml 1 to 4 h following an oral dose of 1 g (20 to 25 mg/kg). Hepatotoxicity occurs in a small number of patients; photosensitivity and rash occur rarely. Gout is an important contraindication because of the hyperuricemia associated with PZA therapy. PZA therapy is usually discontinued after the first 2 months of short-course treatment for tuberculosis, whereas INH and RMP treatment is continued for an additional 4 months.

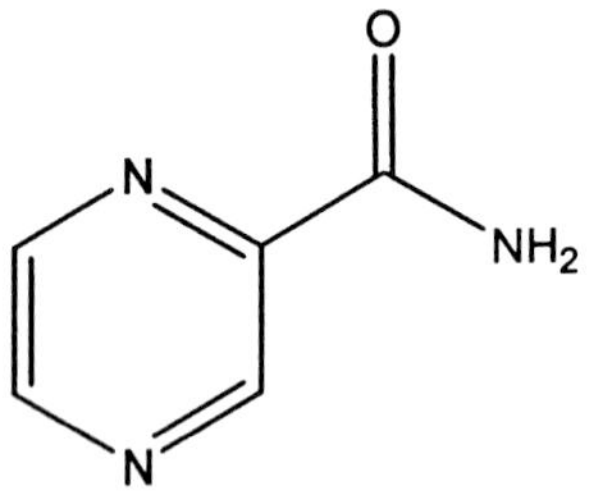

Ethambutol

Ethambutol [dextro-2,2-(ethylenediimino)-di-1-butanol-dihydrochloride (EMB)] is a potent synthetic antituberculosis compound that was introduced in 1961 (Fig. 4). The MICs of EMB tested against wild-type isolates of M. tuberculosis range from 1 to 5 μg/ml, but the activity of the drug against other slowly growing Mycobacterium spp. is much more variable. The primary mechanism of action of EMB is a bacteriostatic inhibition of cell wall synthesis, while evidence points to a specific effect on arabinogalactan syn-

FIGURE 3 Structure of pyrazinamide.

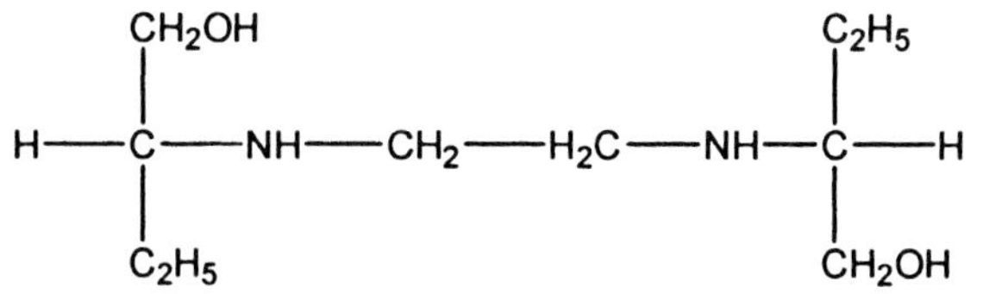

FIGURE 4 Structure of ethambutol.

thesis (161). The frequency of mutation to EMB resistance in *M. tuberculosis* is on the order of 10^{-5}, and there is evidence that EMB resistance in *M. tuberculosis* correlates with a specific mutation (at codon 306) in the *embB* gene, which encodes an arabinosyltransferase (158). Mutations in this codon were associated with MICs of 20 to 40 μg/ml for several EMB-resistant isolates of *M. tuberculosis* (1). Although most MAC isolates are considered intrinsically resistant to EMB, combinations of EMB and other agents, notably quinolones and macrolides, are synergistic (75, 87). It appears that EMB affects the permeability of the MAC cell wall and perhaps increases the intracellular concentration of the other potentially more active drugs (76). Peak concentrations of EMB of 5 μg/ml are achieved in serum 2 to 4 h after a dose of 25 mg/kg. The primary adverse effect associated with EMB is a decrease in visual acuity due to optic neuritis that is related to both the dose and duration of treatment. EMB is not recommended for the treatment of children too young to be monitored for changes in vision unless no other drug is available because of resistance. The effects on vision are generally reversible on discontinuation of drug therapy. A variety of other adverse reactions have been reported, but these are infrequent and sometimes difficult to ascribe to EMB, since they may be due to concurrent therapy with other antituberculosis agents.

Rifabutin and Rifapentine

Rifabutin (ansamycin) is a spiropiperidyl rifamycin with potent in vitro activity against *M. tuberculosis* (71) and MAC (72, 144). Rifapentine is a cyclopentyl rifamycin, which also has potent in vitro activity against *M. tuberculosis*, but its MICs vary somewhat with the test method and medium. Heifets et al. (69) have recently proposed a critical concentration of 0.5 μg/ml to be tested by both the agar proportion method and BACTEC 460TB. The mode of action and mechanism of resistance of rifabutin and rifapentine appear to be identical to those of RMP; however, approximately 30% of RMP-resistant *M. tuberculosis* isolates are susceptible to rifabutin and rifapentine. The latter observation correlates with certain specific mutations in the *rpoB* gene (19). Yang et al. (190) analyzed clinical strains of *M. tuberculosis* for cross-resistance to rifamycins. Alterations at codons 513 and 531 correlate with resistance to RMP, rifabutin, and KRM-1648, a rifamycin derivative. Point mutations at codons 516 and 529, deletion at codon 518, and insertion at codon 514 influence susceptibility to RMP but not to rifabutin or KM-1648, while alteration at codons 515, 521, and 533 did not influence susceptibility to RMP, rifabutin, and KR-1648 (190). These findings were confirmed by analyzing recombinant *M. tuberculosis* clones containing plasmids with specific mutations (180). As with RMP, both rifabutin and rifapentine are metabolized to the corresponding biologically active 25-desacetyl metabolite. Rifabutin decreases the incidence of disseminated MAC disease in human immunodeficiency virus (HIV)-infected

patients when used as a prophylactic agent, and it is approved for that indication (99, 122). The role of rifabutin as a therapeutic agent for MAC disease is unclear, but there may be a significant dose effect (82). In addition to being more active than RMP on a weight basis, rifabutin has a long elimination half-life in humans and concentrates in tissues, notably lung tissues, where the levels are 10-fold higher than in serum. This may account for the reported effectiveness of rifabutin in the therapy of MAC pulmonary infections (50). Rifabutin is absorbed from the gastrointestinal tract and reaches peak levels of 0.5 μg/ml in serum about 4 h after a 300-mg dose. Adverse drug reactions with rifabutin are similar to those observed with RMP, including the above-mentioned important adverse interactions with antiretroviral agents (7, 14). Some unique rifabutin toxicities, including leukopenia, thrombocytopenia, arthralgias, and uveitis when coadministered with clarithromycin, have been described.

Rifapentine was recently approved by the U.S. Food and Drug Administration (FDA) for the treatment of tuberculosis. In a study of 722 patients, 361 received rifapentine plus INH, PZA, and EMB while the remaining patients received RMP in place of rifapentine along with the other drugs (9). In the intensive phase of the study, rifapentine was administered twice a week while RMP was administered daily. In the continuation phase, rifapentine and INH were administered once a week and RMP and INH were administered twice a week. Sputum conversion was somewhat higher in the rifapentine group than in the RMP group: 87 and 81%, respectively. However, relapse was somewhat higher in the rifapentine group than in the RMP group: 10 and 5%, respectively. Rifapentine reaches a peak concentration of 15 μg/ml in serum 5 to 6 h after a 600-mg dose, with a half-life of about 13 h.

Aminoglycosides

The aminoglycosides that are used for the treatment of tuberculosis and other mycobacterial infections include amikacin, kanamycin, and streptomycin (SM). In addition, capreomycin and viomycin, basic peptide antibiotics with a mechanism of action similar to that of the aminoglycosides, are active against *M. tuberculosis* and certain other species of mycobacteria. The other aminoglycosides, gentamicin and tobramycin, are inactive against mycobacteria at the usual concentrations attained in serum (tobramycin is active against *M. chelonae*). Kanamycin is a glycoside of 2-deoxystreptamine, and amikacin is a derivative of kanamycin; thus, there are structural similarities among these antimycobacterial aminoglycosides. The primary mechanism of action of the aminoglycosides is to inhibit the post- to pretranslocation step of protein synthesis by blocking the binding of the aminoacyl-tRNA (e-type binding). Viomycin also blocks aminoacyl-tRNA translocation, and viomycin resistance crosses to capreomycin, suggesting that the mechanism of action is the same. SM MICs for wild-type isolates of *M. tuberculosis* are usually well below the peak concentration of 25 to 50 μg/ml achieved in serum 1 to 2 h after a 1-g intramuscular dose. Amikacin is the most potent of the aminoglycosides, with an average MIC of 1 μg/ml for *M. tuberculosis* and 12.5 μg/ml for *M. chelonae* and *M. abscessus*. There is comparatively little clinical experience with amikacin in the treatment of tuberculosis because the drug is expensive and inconvenient to administer, but amikacin in combination with cefoxitin is standard empirical therapy for serious infections suspected to be caused by rapidly growing mycobacteria. Amikacin also is active against MAC, with about 75% of isolates being susceptible to 30 μg/ml, a MIC which approaches the maximum concentration in serum. In an early uncontrolled trial, amikacin was shown to be the active component of a multiple-drug regimen. Treatment was associated with a positive microbiological and clinical response in HIV-infected patients with disseminated MAC disease (30), but the clinical utility of amikacin for disseminated MAC is uncertain (7). The drug may be useful in an "induction" regimen to clear a bacteremia, and there is laboratory evidence that liposomal amikacin may be more active against tissue infection (127).

The molecular basis of SM resistance (Table 2) in M. tuberculosis was investigated in two studies and shown to result from mutations in the gene that encodes ribosomal protein S12 or from mutations in the 16S rRNA region, which is structurally linked to the S12 protein in the assembled ribosome (52, 117). Finken et al. (52) showed that mutations in the rpsL gene coding for the S12 protein were present in 20 of 38 SM-resistant strains and that there was a mutation in the ssr gene, encoding 16S rRNA, in 9 strains. Nair et al. (117) determined the nucleotide sequence of the rpsL gene and showed that SM resistance, in a small number of isolates, appeared to be a result of point mutations at codon 43 of this gene, a site of SM resistance in E. coli. Meier et al. (105) showed that SM resistance was associated with a single-base (C→T) mutation at position 491 or 512 of the 16S rRNA in two isolates and a single-base (A→G) mutation at position 904 in a third isolate. The latter mutation is equivalent to a mutation in E. coli that correlates with a functional change in the ribosome. Adverse drug reactions associated with aminoglycosides and peptide antibiotics include hearing loss, tinnitus, loss of balance, and renal failure.

Cycloserine

D-Cycloserine (4-amino-3-isooxazolidinone) is an analog of D-alanine that inhibits the synthesis of D-alanyl-D-alanine, an essential component of the mycobacterial cell wall. Cycloserine is active against all mycobacteria as well as several other types of bacteria. The average MICs for M. tuberculosis range from 5 to 20 μg/ml, while peak levels of 20 to 40 μg/ml are achieved in serum 4 h following an oral dose of 250 mg. The drug is widely distributed through the body, including the CSF. There are significant adverse drug reactions associated with cycloserine treatment, notably peripheral neuropathy and central nervous system dysfunction including seizures and psychotic disturbances.

Ethionamide

Ethionamide (2-ethyl-pyridine-4-carbonic acid thioamide) is a derivative of isonicotinic acid and, like INH, blocks mycolic acid synthesis; however, isolates of M. tuberculosis that are resistant to high concentrations of INH are susceptible to ethionamide, suggesting that the site of action may be different from that of INH. However, mutations in the inhA gene have been associated with ethionamide resistance (11). The average MIC for M. tuberculosis is 0.6 to 2.5 μg/ml, and levels of 2 to 20 μg/ml are achieved in serum 3 to 4 h following an oral dose of 0.5 to 1 g. There are significant side effects associated with ethionamide, including gastrointestinal irritation with nausea, vomiting, and cramps, and the presence of neurologic symptoms may require discontinuation of the drug.

Dapsone

Dapsone (diaminodiphenyl sulfone) is a synthetic compound that was first shown to be active against M. leprae in the early 1940s. Dapsone is an antifolate that, like other inhibitors of folic acid synthesis, exerts primarily a bacteriostatic effect and is only weakly bactericidal. Dapsone is administered orally and is well absorbed and distributed throughout the body. Levels in tissue are approximately 2 μg/ml following a 200-mg dose. The drug has a long half-life in serum of 10 to 50 h depending on the individual patient. Adverse drug reactions include gastrointestinal intolerance with nausea, vomiting, anorexia, and methemaglobinemia (common). Hematuria, rash, pruritus, and fever can occur. Traditionally, dapsone is used in combination with RMP and clofazimine for the treatment of leprosy. Acedapsone is a diacetylated form of dapsone with an extraordinarily long half-life of 46 days; as a result, this drug is administered infrequently (e.g., five injections per year), with peak concentrations in tissue occurring 20 to 35 days after administration. Acedapsone is relatively inactive against M. leprae, but in vivo it is deacetylated to the parent compound.

Azithromycin and Clarithromycin

Azithromycin and clarithromycin are important agents in the treatment of all forms of MAC disease, infections caused by rapidly growing mycobacteria, and leprosy. In addition, clarithromycin and azithromycin are effective and approved prophylactic agents for preventing disseminated MAC disease (63, 132). These new macrolides also are useful in the treatment of disease caused by M. marinum, M. haemophilum, and M. kansasii. Indeed, they are viewed as potential cornerstones in the treatment of nontuberculous mycobacterial infections (7). Azithromycin, an azalide (a subclass of macrolides), and clarithromycin are structurally similar to erythromycin and have modifications that improve their acid stability and increase their potency, half-life, achievable concentrations in tissue, and bioavailability without causing toxicity. These macrolides are bacteriostatic agents and inhibit the growth of microorganisms by binding to the 50S subunit of the prokaryotic ribosome, blocking protein synthesis at the peptidyltransferase step. Meier et al. (105) showed that both clarithromycin- and azithromycin-resistant mutants of M. intracellulare have a single-base mutation at adenine-2058 in the 23S rRNA gene (Table 2), a site of mutation or methylation that has been associated with macrolide resistance in other bacteria. This observation was confirmed for M. avium isolates from HIV-infected patients, and MAC resistance breakpoints for clarithromycin and azithromycin were proposed: 32 and 256 μg/ml, respectively (84, 119). The same genetic basis for macrolide resistance was found in M. chelonae and M. abscessus (171).

The in vitro activity of azithromycin against MAC appears to be quite modest, with MICs 32- to 64-fold above the maximum concentration in serum. The remarkable ability of azithromycin to concentrate in tissues most probably accounts for the therapeutic activity of this drug in animal studies and human trials (83, 192; S. L. Koletar, D. J. Williams, and A. Berry, Prog. Abstr. 2nd Int. Conf. Macrolides Azalides Streptogramins, abstr. 292, p. 65, 1994). Azithromycin is rapidly absorbed from the gastrointestinal tract and widely distributed throughout the body. The peak concentrations in serum following a 500-mg dose are 0.4 to 0.6 μg/ml; however, the drug concentrates in tissues to high levels and has a terminal half-life of 68 h. In a small study in humans, the levels of azithromycin in polymorphonuclear neutrophils were nearly 1,000-fold higher than the levels in serum (4, 148).

Clarithromycin inhibits 90% of MAC isolates with MICs of 0.25 to 0.5 μg/ml when measured by a radiometric broth macrodilution method at a neutral to slightly alkaline pH (the activities of all macrolides are strongly influenced by pH). The current recommendation is that clarithromycin be administered at 500 mg twice a day to HIV-infected patients with disseminated MAC disease, but it must be combined with at least one other agent, usually EMB. The peak levels of clarithromycin in serum, 2 to 3 μg/ml, are achieved within 5 to 6 h of a 500-mg dose; the concentrations in tissue are 4 to 5 times greater than the concentrations in serum, and the concentrations in macrophages are 20 to 30 times greater. The elimination half-life is 5 to 7 h following 500 mg twice a day.

A U.S. Public Health Service task force recommended that either azithromycin or clarithromycin be used in combination with a second and perhaps a third agent for the treatment of MAC disease (99). Azithromycin and clarithromycin appear to be equally effective in the treatment of MAC disease, although there is some unconfirmed evidence that clarithromycin is somewhat more potent. Adverse drug reactions, including diarrhea, nausea, abnormal taste, dyspepsia, abdominal pain, and headache, appear to occur with low frequency (less than 3% of patients) for both azithromycin and clarithromycin. Perhaps of particular note, there are many fewer drug interactions with azithromycin than with the other macrolides (5, 14).

Quinolones

Ciprofloxacin, ofloxacin, sparfloxacin, and levofloxacin are fluorinated carboxyquinolones with good in vitro activity against M. tuberculosis and variable activity against MAC and rapidly growing mycobacteria (84). Newer fluoroquinolones such as moxifloxacin and gatifloxacin also are active in vitro against M. tuberculosis. Measurements of the early bactericidal activity of ciprofloxacin in patients with pulmonary tuberculosis suggested that the drug is effective at a high dosage (1,000 mg/day) (155). The mechanism of action of all fluorinated quinolones is inhibition of DNA synthesis as a result of binding to the DNA gyrase (bacterial topoisomerase II). Although this is the presumed mechanism of action in mycobacteria, fewer studies have been performed with mycobacteria than with other microorganisms. Takiff et al. (163) showed that quinolone resistance in M. tuberculosis can be ascribed to mutations in the gyrA and gyrB genes, which encode the DNA gyrase subunits (Table 2).

The MICs of ciprofloxacin against susceptible isolates of M. tuberculosis range from 0.25 to 3 μg/ml. While there are no well verified interpretive standards for testing the activity of ciprofloxacin against mycobacteria, a susceptibility breakpoint of 2 μg/ml for both ciprofloxacin and ofloxacin has been suggested (29) and seems reasonable. Most isolates of M. fortuitum are susceptible to ciprofloxacin, while most isolates of M. chelonae are resistant. The MIC_{90} of ciprofloxacin against MAC is 16 μg/ml, and only 30% of isolates are susceptible to 2 μg/ml (95, 191). Ciprofloxacin is well absorbed from the gastrointestinal tract and is rapidly distributed throughout the body. Maximum concentrations of 2.4 and 4.3 μg/ml are achieved in serum 1 to 2 h after an oral dose of 500 or 750 mg, respectively. The elimination half-life of ciprofloxacin is 4 h in subjects with normal renal function. The MICs of ofloxacin against susceptible isolates

of M. tuberculosis range from 0.5 to 2.5 μg/ml. Maximum ofloxacin concentrations are achieved in serum 1 to 2 h after an oral dose. Following a single 400-mg dose, the concentration of ofloxacin serum is 2.9 μg/ml; after a steady-state dose, it is 4.6 μg/ml. The maximum concentration of levofloxacin in serum is approximately twice that of ofloxacin at the same dosage. The efficacy of ciprofloxacin, ofloxacin, and perhaps the other aforementioned quinolones in the treatment of pulmonary tuberculosis may relate, in part, to the observation that these quinolones concentrate in lung tissue to levels at least four times greater than the concentration in serum (6). A quinolone should be tested as a secondary agent or when resistance to other antituberculous agents is suspected or known (167). Adverse effects with ciprofloxacin and other fluoroquinolones may be less severe than with the other secondary agents (17). However, none of the fluoroquinolone manufacturers indicate that fluoroquinolones can be used to treat tuberculosis, and the use of quinolones in children for any type of infection remains an unresolved question because of lingering concerns about quinolone-associated arthropathy.

p-Aminosalicylic Acid

p-Aminosalicylic acid (PAS) is an antifolate that is active against M. tuberculosis but inactive against most other mycobacteria. There is some evidence that PAS also may affect iron transport in M. tuberculosis and salicylic acid metabolism. The average MIC for susceptible isolates of M. tuberculosis is 1 μg/ml, and peak levels of 7 to 8 μg/ml are achieved in serum 1 to 2 h after a 4-g dose. PAS is incompletely absorbed in the gastrointestinal tract and is associated with significant gastrointestinal side effects; in combination with the need for large dosages (10 to 12 g/day), this leads to frequent problems with adherence.

Clofazimine

Clofazimine [3-(p-chloroanilino)-10-(p-chlorophenyl)-2,10-dihydro-2-isopropyliminophenazine] is a substituted iminophenazine, bright red dye with potent in vitro activity against MAC (its MICs range from 0.1 to 5 μg/ml) but unclear therapeutic efficacy either alone or in combination with other agents. The drug also has potent in vitro activity against M. tuberculosis, but there is little or no information on the in vivo activity. Clofazimine has weak bactericidal activity against M. leprae but is used in combination with RMP and dapsone as a conventional treatment regimen for leprosy. However, it may take up to 50 days of treatment before there is evidence of tissue antimicrobial activity, which may influence the length of time before there is a clinical response in the treatment of M. leprae. Despite its potent in vitro activity, clofazimine appears to offer little in the treatment of disseminated MAC infection (152). Indeed, clofazimine has been associated with higher mortality in two clinical trials (28) compared with trials in which clofazimine was not part of the treatment regimen. Its precise mechanism of action is unknown; however, it is highly lipophilic and binds preferentially to mycobacterial DNA. The absorption of clofazimine following an oral dose is variable and ranges from 45 to 60%. The average concentrations in serum are 0.7 to 1.0 μg/ml following a dose of 100 to 300 mg. The half-life is extraordinarily long (estimated to be 70 days), and the drug tends to be deposited in fatty tissues and cells of the reticuloendothelial system. Adverse drug reactions are limited primarily to a pink or red discoloration of the skin, conjunctiva, cornea, and body fluids and gastrointestinal intolerance including pain, diarrhea, nausea, and vomiting.

Amithiozone

Amithiozone (Thiacetazone, Tibione, or Panthrone) is a thiosemicarbazole that is active against M. *tuberculosis*, with an average MIC for wild-type strains of 1 µg/ml. Resistance develops quickly when monotherapy is given. Peak levels in serum of 1 to 4 µg/ml are achieved 1 to 2 h following an oral dose of 150 mg. Adverse drug reactions include gastrointestinal irritation and bone marrow suppression; hepatotoxicity can occur in patients receiving concomitant INH. Amithiozone in combination with INH has been successfully used for the treatment of tuberculosis in some African countries, where adverse effects are believed to be less severe. However, there is evidence showing an association of Stevens-Johnson syndrome and severe epidermal necrolysis in HIV-infected patients with tuberculosis treated by regimens containing amithiozone (47, 58); and as a result, the World Health Organization recommended that amithiozone not be used to treat HIV-infected patients (124) or patients suspected of being HIV infected. Amithiozone is not available in the United States and is not used in Europe because of the adverse effects.

M. TUBERCULOSIS COMPLEX

Drug Resistance

In the early 1960s, the World Health Organization organized two meetings that led to the description of reliable criteria and techniques for testing mycobacteria for resistance to antituberculosis drugs (25, 26). The critical proportion for resistance on Löwenstein-Jensen slants varied according to the drug, e.g., 1% for INH and RMP and 10% for SM, EMB, PZA, ethionamide, kanamycin, and cycloserine. However, based on the experience of Russel and Middlebrook with 7H10 agar (143), the Centers for Disease Control and Prevention (CDC) recommended Middlebrook 7H10 agar and 1% as the critical proportion for all drugs (94).

Resistance is fundamentally a phenomenon linked to large initial bacterial populations. In lung tuberculosis, the greatest populations are those prevailing in cavities, which can contain 10^7 to 10^9 organisms (Fig. 5), whereas the

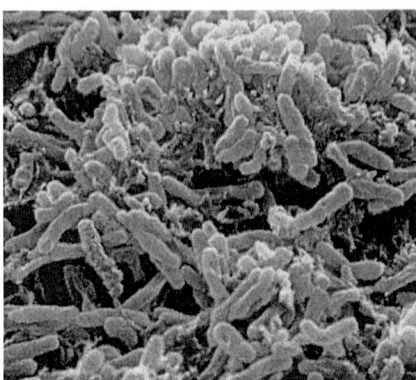

FIGURE 5 Electron micrograph of a population of M. *tuberculosis* bacilli. (Reprinted from D. B. Young, Letter, *Nature* **393:**515–516, 1998, with permission of Eye of Science/Photo Researchers, Inc.).

populations found in hard caseous foci, the most common type of lesion, do not exceed 10^2 to 10^4 organisms (24). The far greater frequency of resistance during the treatment of cavitary tuberculosis was shown as early as 1949 (78, 79). David at CDC (36) demonstrated the probability distribution of drug-resistant mutants and in a fluctuation test showed that M. *tuberculosis* spontaneously mutated to resistance to INH, SM, EMB, and RMP. The average mutation rates for INH, SM, EMB, and RMP were calculated to be 3×10^{-8}, 3×10^{-8}, 1×10^{-7}, and 2×10^{-10} mutation per bacterium per generation, respectively. Thus, the mutation rate for resistance to two drugs is theoretically less than 10^{-15}. Implicit in all the studies of the genetic basis of antimicrobial resistance in M. *tuberculosis* is that the multiple-drug-resistance (MDR) phenotype (minimally defined as simultaneous resistance to INH and RMP) is the result of accumulative mutations rather than the acquisition of an MDR transfer factor (116).

Special-Population Hypothesis

According to the generally accepted theory, resistance appearing during drug treatment is due to the selection and multiplication of the resistant mutants preexisting in the tubercle bacillus population of the host. Inasmuch as the susceptible bacilli are the predominant part of the population, the initial killing involves a greater number of microorganisms and the consequence is a sharp fall in the population of bacilli during the initial period of treatment. The rise due to multiplication of the resistant mutants is revealed later. This "fall-and-rise" phenomenon, as demonstrated in the patient's sputum, was described in the late 1940s (35, 134). In 1979, Mitchison (109) suggested the "special-populations" hypothesis to explain the action of the major antituberculous drugs against the various subpopulations of tubercle bacilli (Fig. 6). The subpopulations include (i) rapidly growing bacilli in the pulmonary lesions, (ii) bacilli that grow in short metabolic spurts and that might be susceptible to RMP but not INH, (iii) bacilli that reside in the acidic environment of the caseous lesions, and (iv) dormant, nonreplicating bacilli. The hypothesis was developed to explain in part the basis of the early bactericidal activity and the later sterilizing activity of antituberculosis agents. Each of the agents of the conventional multiple-drug treatment regimens for tuberculosis is more or less effective in eradicating tubercle bacilli within each of these special populations. Thus, the use of multiple drugs in the treatment of tuberculosis is aimed at both preventing drug resistance and achieving a maximum therapeutic effect. Figure 6 depicts the special-populations hypothesis, as presented by Mitchison in 1992 (110) in his Garrod lecture, altered to include a reference to the observation by Wayne and Sramek (179) that dormant M. *tuberculosis* is susceptible to nitroimidazoles. This study was based on the assumption that dormant tubercle bacilli are in an anaerobic metabolic state and therefore would be susceptible to agents such as metronidazole.

Critical Concentrations

The criteria for defining drug-resistant M. *tuberculosis* were established on an empirical basis, i.e., that there is a certain proportion of drug-resistant mutants above which therapeutic success is less likely to be realized. The procedures used to perform drug susceptibility tests and the criteria for interpreting the results take into account two factors: (i) the critical proportion of drug-resistant mutants and (ii) the critical concentration of the drug in the test medium. On

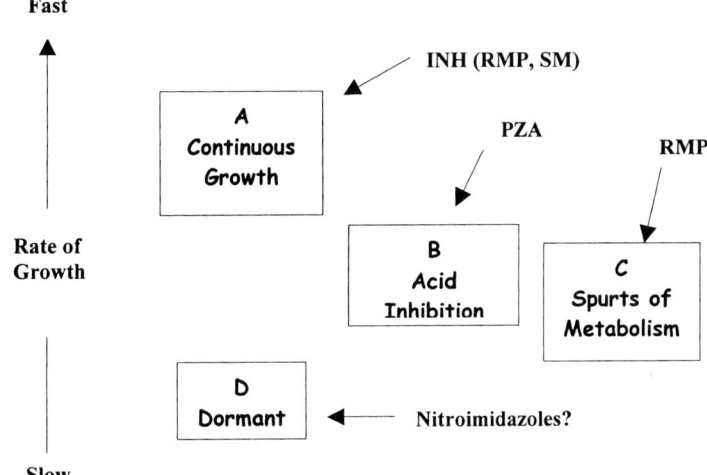

FIGURE 6 Schematic representation of the special-populations hypothesis of Mitchison (110). The model accounts for the action of antimycobacterial agents on different populations of M. tuberculosis bacilli in various sites in the infected host. (A) INH, RMP, and SM are active primarily against bacilli in a continuous state of growth, which are the majority population at the start of treatment. (B) PZA is active only against bacilli within the acidic early caseous lesions that develop within the first 2 months of chemotherapy (110). (C) The comparatively rapid bactericidal activity of RMP is important for the eradication of bacilli that grow for short periods (not long enough to be affected by INH). (D) Some tubercle bacilli may be sequestered in lesions in a metabolically inactive and dormant state; however, there is evidence that these dormant bacilli may actually be in an anaerobic state and susceptible to nitroimidazoles such as metronidazole (179). (Reprinted from reference 110 with permission of Oxford University Press.)

the basis of clinical and bacteriologic studies, the significant proportion of bacilli resistant to an antituberculosis drug, above which a clinical response is unlikely, was generally set at 1%. The critical concentration of a drug is the concentration that inhibits the growth of most cells within the population of a wild-type strain of tubercle bacilli without appreciably affecting the growth of the resistant mutant cells that might be present. In other words, if the proportion of tubercle bacilli that are resistant to the critical concentration of a drug exceeds 1%, it is unlikely that the use of that drug will lead to a therapeutic success. It should be noted that this concentration may not have a direct relationship to the peak level of the drug in serum. The critical concentrations of antituberculosis drugs, in different media, are given in Table 3 (91, 121).

Low versus High Critical Concentrations

On occasion, both the agar proportion and BACTEC 460TB methods may indicate that an M. tuberculosis isolate is resistant to INH, EMB, or SM at the low critical concentration of the drug (Table 3) but susceptible to the same drug at the high concentration. Indeed, it is unclear if testing the low concentration of EMB has any merit, especially since recent evidence indicates that mutations in the embB gene are associated only with resistance at the high concentration (1, 158). Similar studies have not been performed with SM; however, the merit of testing SM at the low concentration must be questioned. If the low concentration of the drug only were tested, the report of "resistant" could potentially mislead a clinician to believe that the drug has no value in the treatment of tuberculosis. Therefore, it is important to test both concentrations of the drugs or, if only the low concentration is tested, to reflex test the higher concentration. The clinician should be alerted that an isolate is resistant to the low concentration but susceptible to the high concentration; therapeutic effect may be achieved with an adjustment in dosage (e.g., INH). The NCCLS recommends that the following comment be appended to the results:

> These results indicate low-level resistance to INH. Some evidence indicates that patients infected with strains exhibiting this level of INH resistance may benefit from continuing therapy with INH. A specialist in the treatment of tuberculosis should be consulted concerning the appropriate therapeutic regimen and dosages (121).

Furthermore, the patient should be closely monitored for the emergence of high-level resistance. A clinician with less experience in the treatment of tuberculosis should seek assistance from a clinician with extensive experience in treating tuberculosis and/or from the local tuberculosis control agency.

Extent of Service

In the United States, mycobacteriology laboratories are classified by the levels or extents of services provided based on criteria proposed by CDC, the American Thoracic Society (ATS), and the College of American Pathologists (CAP). In general, the criteria emphasize the importance of the number of specimens processed, the expertise of the laboratory staff, and the cost-effectiveness of the procedures and protocols (8, 66, 94). The CAP recognizes four levels of service ranging from no mycobacteriologic procedures performed (extent 1) to definitive and comprehensive procedures that may or may not include susceptibility testing

TABLE 3 Critical concentrations of antimycobacterial agents to test against M. *tuberculosis* by radiometric (BACTEC 460TB) or agar proportion methods

Antimicrobial agent	Typical MIC (μg/ml) for susceptible strains	Concn in serum (μg/ml)[c]	Medium and concn (μg/ml)[d]					
			BACTEC 460TB 12B low	BACTEC 460TB 12B high	7H10 low	7H10 high	7H11 low	7H11 high
Primary agents								
INH	0.05–0.2	7	0.1	0.4	0.2	1	0.2	1
RMP	0.5	10	2		1		1	
PZA[a]	20	45	100		NR[f]	NR	NR	
EMB	1–5	2–5	2.5[e]	7.5	5	10	7.5	
Secondary agents								
SM	8	25–50	2[e]	6	2	10	2	10
Capreomycin	1–50	30	1.25[g]		10		10	
Kanamycin	5	14–29	5[g]		5		6	
Cycloserine	5–20	20–40	NR		NR		NR	
Ethionamide	0.6–2.5	2–20	1.25[g]		5		10	
PAS	1	7.5	4[g]		2		8	
Alternative agents								
Rifabutin[b]	0.06–8	0.2–0.5	0.5[g]		0.5/1[g]		0.5[g]	
Rifapentine			0.5[g]		0.5[h]		0.5[h]	
Amikacin	1	16–38	1[g]		4[f]			
Ciprofloxacin	0.25–3	2–4	2[g]					
Ofloxacin	0.5–2.5	3–11	2[g]		2[f]		2	

[a] PZA tested at pH 6 in BACTEC 12B medium.

[b] RMP-susceptible versus RMP-resistant isolates; about 30% of RMP-resistant isolates are rifabutin susceptible.

[c] Concentrations in serum 1 to 4 h after administration of the usual dosage.

[d] Unless otherwise stated, the concentrations shown are from references 70, 119, and 121.

[e] Woodley (187) showed that 2.5 μg of EMB per ml and 2.0 μg of SM per ml tested against susceptible and resistant isolates agreed with the 7H10 proportion method 97 to 99 and 100%, respectively.

[f] NR, no recommendation.

[g] According to reference 128.

[h] According to reference 69.

(extent 4). The ATS recognizes three levels of service (levels I, II, and III); these are roughly equivalent to CAP levels 2, 3, and 4. CAP recommends that susceptibility testing be performed only in an extent 3 or 4 laboratory but that even an extent 4 laboratory might refer isolates to another laboratory with more extensive experience in susceptibility testing of mycobacteria. In general, a CAP extent 4 laboratory should perform susceptibility testing only if the laboratory is capable of identifying the isolate to species and if it regularly performs susceptibility tests on that type of isolate (e.g., at least 10 tests per week). Since certain drugs are tested infrequently (e.g., cycloserine or amikacin), must be prepared from reference powders (e.g., rifabutin or ciprofloxacin), or are problematic (e.g., cycloserine [128]), secondary drug testing should be referred to a laboratory with specific expertise in testing these agents.

When To Perform Susceptibility Tests

Kubica and Dye (94) suggested more than 30 years ago that susceptibility testing of primary drugs be performed at ATS level II laboratories to provide clinically meaningful data in the shortest possible time. Routine testing of all new isolates (from patients not previously treated or not suspected to have primary resistance) was not recommended (10). Given the low incidence of drug resistance in the United States (at that time) and the high probability of successful drug treatment of tuberculosis, it seemed difficult to justify the cost of more frequent testing. While some might argue

that susceptibility testing of initial isolates is not necessary if the incidence of primary drug-resistant tuberculosis is lower than 4%, the arguments for testing are compelling. Testing of initial isolates is consistent with practice in managing nonmycobacterial infections, ensures the most effective treatment for a patient, and contributes to the surveillance database for tuberculosis control. The new edition of the tentative standard on susceptibility testing of mycobacteria and other closely related organisms by NCCLS (121) states that the first isolate of M. *tuberculosis* obtained from each patient should be tested. Susceptibility testing should be repeated if cultures fail to convert to negative after 3 months of therapy or if there is clinical evidence of failure to respond to therapy.

Methods To Test the Susceptibility of *M. tuberculosis*

Methods that are commonly used to test rapidly growing aerobic and facultative anaerobic bacteria are, for a variety of reasons, unsuitable for testing most mycobacterial species. For example, the conventional disk diffusion method is not suitable for testing slowly growing mycobacteria because the drug diffuses throughout the medium before growth of the mycobacteria is significantly affected. The methods generally accepted for determining the antimicrobial susceptibility of mycobacteria are based on the growth of the microorganisms on solid or in liquid medium containing a specified concentration of a single drug. In the past, four growth-based methods have been described: the proportion method, the radiometric or BACTEC 460TB (Becton Dickinson Microbiology Systems, Sparks, Md.) method (a modified proportion method), the absolute-concentration method, and the resistance ratio method. The last two are described elsewhere (70). To date, the agar proportion method and the BACTEC 460TB method are still the most commonly used in the United States and Europe. The technical details of these procedures have been described (61, 70, 84, 153), and only the proportion and BACTEC 460TB methods are discussed further in this chapter, together with the most recent developments in the field of growth-based susceptibility testing based on liquid, nonradiometric medium. These new methods, either manual or fully automated, have been created mainly to overcome the limitations of radiolabeled substrates (in particular, safety and regulatory principles). They include the ESP Culture System II (AccuMed International, Westlake, Ohio) (188), the Mycobacteria Growth Indicator Tube (MGIT; Becton Dickinson) (62, 130), and the MB/BacT ALERT 3D (Bio-Mérieux, Marcy-L'Etoile, France) (133).

Based on the current NCCLS guidelines (121), a rapid susceptibility testing method should be used in conjunction with rapid methods of primary culture and identification to allow the earliest possible detection of resistance. The recommended rapid broth methods for susceptibility testing of M. tuberculosis are commercial systems that have been cleared by the FDA. At present, two such FDA-approved systems are available, i.e., the BACTEC 460TB and the ESP Culture System II. Most importantly, any such rapid method utilized should have been previously demonstrated to generate results that correlate with those obtained with the standardized agar proportion method. Optimally, susceptibility results for M. tuberculosis should be reported within 28 days of receipt of the specimen in the laboratory (18).

Source of Inoculum for Susceptibility Testing

The source of the inoculum for a susceptibility test may be either a smear-positive specimen (direct method) or growth from a primary culture or subculture (indirect method). The direct method is used when antimicrobial resistance is known or suspected. However, the indirect method is considered the standard method for inoculum preparation, and results of the direct method are usually confirmed by subsequent testing by the indirect method. With both the direct and the indirect methods, the inoculum must be a pure culture and careful attention must be given to avoid over- or underinoculation.

For the direct method, the inoculum is either a digested, decontaminated clinical specimen or an untreated, normally sterile body fluid, in which acid-fast bacilli are seen in stained smears. To ensure adequate but not excessive growth in the direct susceptibility test on solid medium, specimens are diluted according to the number of organisms observed in the stained smear of the clinical specimen. A typical dilution scheme is shown in Table 4. Theoretically, this type of inoculum is more representative of the population of the tubercle bacilli in a particular lesion in the host. It is prudent to include an undiluted inoculum, if the smear-positive specimen is from a patient who is receiving antimicrobial therapy, since a significant proportion of the bacilli seen on the smear may be nonviable. The direct susceptibility test has two major advantages. First, results can be reported within 3 weeks from the time of specimen receipt in the laboratory for a majority of smear-positive specimens. Second, the proportion of resistant bacteria

TABLE 4 Guidelines for selection of the dilution of a specimen concentrate prior to inoculation of 7H10 medium for susceptibility testing using the direct method

Dilutions to test[a]	No. of acid-fast bacilli observed with:	
	Carbol fuchsin stain	Fluorochrome stain
Undiluted, 10^{-2}	0	<25
10^{-1}, 10^{-2}	1–10	25–250
10^{-2}, 10^{-3}	>10	>250

[a] Dilutions of concentrated specimen are prepared based on the number of bacilli observed in the initial acid-fast smear. Sterile distilled water is used to prepare the dilutions; the carbol fuchsin stain is examined with the oil immersion objective (1,000×), and the fluorochrome stain is examined with the high-dry objective (450×). If the patient is receiving therapy, not all bacilli observed in the smear may be viable; therefore, the undiluted specimen should be tested as well as the appropriate dilution based on the microscopic criteria given in this table.

better represents the patient's bacterial population. Use of the direct method may be warranted in situations where there is a high prevalence of drug resistance (54). However, cost can become a critical factor when there is a high incidence of smear-positive specimens containing nontuberculous mycobacteria. Also, it is not possible to accurately calibrate the inoculum, which may result in insufficient or excessive growth on drug-free quadrants. In addition, if contaminants grow, results are not interpretable. According to the literature, the total rate of failure for direct susceptibility testing can reach 15% or more, necessitating retesting by the indirect method. The direct method is not recommended for routine use with the BACTEC 460TB or any of the newer, nonradiometric, liquid medium-based procedures at this time, since this application has been the subject of only limited evaluation (96). For the indirect method, the source of the inoculum is a subculture, usually from the primary isolation media. Careful attention should be paid to the selection of colony types so that the final inoculum is representative of all types present to ensure that there is a balance of potentially resistant and susceptible bacilli. The source of inoculum for the liquid medium-based susceptibility testing can be growth on Middlebrook 7H10 or 7H11 agar or an egg-based medium, but growth should take less than 4 weeks from when it was first detected. Turbid growth in a liquid medium (such as Middlebrook 7H9 broth, BACTEC 12B, MGIT, MB/BacT, or ESP Myco) is also acceptable; however, a mixed culture (tubercle bacilli and nontuberculous organisms) can give rise to apparent resistance, especially when the inoculum is derived from a broth culture.

Media Used for Susceptibility Testing

Although a variety of media have been used for drug susceptibility testing of slowly growing mycobacteria, including Middlebrook 7H10 or 7H11 agar and Löwenstein-Jensen media, there is considerable variability in the results. Egg-based media are unsuitable for susceptibility testing, not only because of uncertainty about the potency of the drugs after inspissation but also because phospholipids, proteins, and certain amino acids present in the medium affect some drugs. In an effort to provide uniformity in the testing of mycobacteria, CDC (94) and NCCLS (121) recommend that Middlebrook 7H10 agar supplemented with oleic acid-albumin-dextrose-catalase (OADC) be used as the standard medium for susceptibility testing of slowly growing mycobacteria by the agar-proportion method. A majority of *M. tuberculosis* clinical isolates grow on this medium, and under a dissecting microscope, the transparency of 7H10 agar facilitates the recognition of mixed mycobacterial species or the presence of contaminants. Occasionally, there is insufficient growth of drug-resistant strains of *M. tuberculosis* on 7H10 medium for the test to be valid. With these isolates, 7H11 medium may be substituted for 7H10 agar, but it is necessary to use higher concentrations of some drugs, as shown in Table 3 (64, 84). At present there is no standard formulation for Middlebrook 7H10 agar or OADC (such as there is for Mueller-Hinton medium), and it has been demonstrated that quality control of the medium, especially the OADC supplement, is critical (61).

The medium used for studies with mycobacteria in the BACTEC 460TB instrument is an enriched Middlebrook 7H9 broth containing 4 μCi of [^{14}C]palmitic acid per vial, which is referred to as 7H12 or BACTEC 12B medium. For the newer, nonradiometric systems, the media used are ESP Myco, MGIT, and MB/BacT.

Drugs Used for Susceptibility Testing

Antimicrobial agents for susceptibility testing (reference powders) can be obtained directly from the manufacturer or from commercial sources. In the United States, most antimicrobial agents are also available from U.S. Pharmacopeial Convention, Inc., Reference Standards Order Department, 12601 Twinbrook Parkway, Rockville, MD 20852. The reference powder should be accompanied by information about its assay potency (micrograms per milligram), expiration date, and lot number, as well as the stability and solubility of the agent. Preparations formulated for therapeutic use in humans or animals should not be used. Unopened vials of powders should be stored as specified by the manufacturer, and opened containers should be stored in a desiccator at the recommended temperature. Stock solutions of most agents at 1,000 μg/ml or greater remain stable for at least 6 months at 20°C and for 1 year at 70 to 80°C. Cycloserine solutions at neutral or acidic pH are unstable at room temperature and must be used immediately. If alkalinized with Na$_2$CO$_3$ to a pH of 10, cycloserine stock solutions of 10,000 μg/ml can be stored for 1 week at 5°C or for 1 month at 20°C without loss of activity. Directions provided by the drug manufacturer should be followed in addition to these general recommendations. Paper disks impregnated with standardized amounts of the primary and secondary drugs are available from commercial sources for use in the disk elution modification of the proportion method. Use of these disks obviates errors in weighing and dilution, as well as errors in labeling, since the disks are coded with the drug name and concentration. This technique provides results equivalent to those obtained with solutions prepared from reference powders. Quality control (QC) testing should be performed with each new batch of antimicrobial agent.

Proportion Method

The agar proportion method for susceptibility testing of slowly growing mycobacteria was developed in the early 1960s by G. Canetti (24–26). The method was modified and standardized in the United States and has been considered the standard method of drug testing for *M. tuberculosis* complex in the United States and many European countries for many years. The preferred medium for the proportion test is Middlebrook 7H10 agar. Drugs can either be prepared from reference powders (agar diffusion) or be added as drug-impregnated disks (disk elution) (61). Although reproducibility of results is poor and laboratories are encouraged to use a liquid medium-based assay, PZA can be tested by using the proportion method and a low-pH 7H10 agar; however, 25% of *M. tuberculosis* isolates may fail to grow at pH 5.5 with oleic acid in the medium, and ADC rather than OADC should be used to supplement the medium (23). Heifets and Sanchez (68) have recently developed a new agar medium (pH 6.0) which differs from the conventional Middlebrook 7H10 and 7H11 agar in that animal serum is used instead of OADC.

Inoculum and Incubation

The inoculum can be prepared by the direct or indirect method. When the direct method is used, cultures should be examined weekly for 3 weeks, and even though mature colonies may appear on control media in less than 3 weeks, a report of "susceptible" should not be submitted until week 3. Resistant strains of *M. tuberculosis* complex may be slow to produce visible growth because of metabolic differences compared with susceptible wild-type isolates. If cultures are incubated beyond 3 weeks, degradation of the antimicrobial compound may permit the appearance of colonies of organisms that were susceptible to the initial concentration of the drug. Since the controls are inoculated with a processed specimen, isolated colonies should also be examined for colony morphology and pigmentation differences, as well as for the presence of mixed species of mycobacteria or contaminants. Small colonies of rapid growers, as well as the rough, dry colonies of some MAC strains, are similar in appearance to *M. tuberculosis* colonies on 7H10 agar. Also, rapidly growing mycobacteria may be slow to develop on primary isolation media and rapidly growing mycobacteria will appear as MDR when tested against primary antituberculosis agents. For a test to be valid, the control must show good growth (at least 50 to 150 colonies). Susceptibility testing results must never be reported without a preliminary identification.

When using the indirect method, a sufficient number of colonies must be picked to make a suspension that is equivalent to a McFarland 1 standard or, if there is insufficient growth, a sufficient number should be picked into Dubos Tween-albumin broth and incubated at 35 to 37°C until the turbidity matches a McFarland no. 1 standard. The suspension should not contain clumps of organisms. The actual number of CFU per milliliter is likely to vary from suspension to suspension, so that two dilutions (usually 10^{-2} and 10^{-4}) of the suspension must be used to inoculate two sets of media. If the source of the inoculum is old or if there is scant growth, 10^{-1} and 10^{-3} dilutions should be used or the isolate should be subcultured in broth. QC strains should be tested at dilutions of 10^{-2} and 10^{-3}. Quadrant plates are commonly used for the agar proportion method, and 0.1 ml (about 3 drops from a Pasteur pipette) of each dilution of the inoculum is placed into each quadrant, using one dilution per set of plates. The plates are allowed to dry thoroughly after inoculation, placed in individual CO$_2$-permeable polyethylene bags (clear sandwich bags), and incubated at 35 to 37°C in 5 to 10% CO$_2$ in air. The plates must be protected from light during storage and incubation to prevent the formation of formaldehyde from the medium ingredients. To check strains for purity, blood agar and 7H10 agar plates are inoculated with 1 or 2 drops of the suspension and streaked for isolation.

Reading, Interpreting, and Reporting Results

Purity control plates are examined for contamination after 1 to 2 days; the 7H10 plate should be examined throughout the incubation period, and the blood agar plate should be examined for 1 week. Once the "no-drug" control quadrant of the test isolate or control strain shows at least 50 to 150 colonies, the plates can be read and interpreted. If there are fewer than 50 colonies in the no-drug quadrant by 3 weeks, the test is repeated. Use of the designations 1+ to 4+ to grade the amount of growth is discouraged. The reference agar proportion method employs a percentage calculation to detect resistance or susceptibility. The presence of microcolonies in the drug-containing quadrants should be noted, and the number of colonies observed in each quadrant is reported as a percentage of the number of colonies in the no-drug control quadrant. If the percentage of colonies exceeds 1%, the isolate should be reported as resistant to that drug at the concentration tested. The percentage of resistant colonies can be used as an indicator of therapeutic efficacy and should immediately be reported to the physician, along with the drug concentration and test method.

Quality Control

M. tuberculosis H37Rv (ATCC 27294) is susceptible to all primary and secondary antituberculosis drugs and can be used for QC. Strains of M. tuberculosis that are resistant to INH, RMP, and/or other drugs are available from the American Type Culture Collection; however, these strains are resistant to high concentrations of the respective drugs and are not ideal for QC testing. Also, for safety considerations, it is not advisable to use a single M. tuberculosis strain that is resistant to more than two drugs (121). Aliquots of suspensions of QC strains of M. tuberculosis, adjusted to match a McFarland no. 1 standard in 7H9 broth, can be stored at −70°C for up to 6 months. QC testing should be performed with each new batch of medium or antimicrobial agent, and media should be checked for sterility and shown to support adequate growth. Guthertz et al. (60) demonstrated the importance of controlling for all components of 7H10 agar including lots of Middlebrook 7H10 agar, glycerol, and especially OADC. The issue of which QC results should be available before releasing patient test results was discussed above.

BACTEC 460TB Method

Although one of the new nonradiometric systems has recently been cleared by the FDA for susceptibility testing of M. tuberculosis to primary drugs and other systems are expected to be approved in the near future, the BACTEC 460TB method continues to be important in drug testing. Mycobacteria easily grow in the BACTEC 12B medium containing [^{14}C]palmitic acid. This compound is metabolized, resulting in the production of $^{14}CO_2$; therefore, growth or inhibition of growth in BACTEC 12B medium is measured as changes in the growth-dependent production of CO_2. The instrument quantitatively detects the amount of $^{14}CO_2$ released, expressed in terms of a growth index (GI), and then automatically replaces the headspace with 5 to 10% unlabeled CO_2 in air, thereby maintaining the recommended CO_2 atmosphere. The rate and amount of $^{14}CO_2$ produced are directly proportional to the rate and amount of growth.

The BACTEC 460TB system can be used to test all primary drugs (RMP, INH, PZA, EMB, and SM), as well as the secondary drugs including the newer quinolones and rifamycins (128). The rapid availability of results with the BACTEC 460TB procedure may take precedence over cost considerations. If resistance to a primary drug is suspected, secondary drugs can be tested by the BACTEC 460TB method, provided that the laboratory is qualified. Irrespective of its rapidity, it is prudent to consider the limitations of the BACTEC 460TB method. In some clinical situations, the method might be best considered a screening test, since it does not allow an estimate of the percentage of resistant bacilli and is vulnerable to major errors (false susceptibility or resistance) due to the use of mixed populations of mycobacterial species. Indeed, when an MDR isolate of M. tuberculosis is detected for the first time by the BACTEC 460TB method, the identity of the isolate should be confirmed and the presence of a contaminant or mixed culture should be ruled out before secondary agents are tested. While the importance of promptly reporting an MDR isolate of M. tuberculosis cannot be overstated, the consequences of a false report of multiple resistance must be recognized as well (123). Clinician concerns about discrepancies between susceptibility test results and clinical response or status must be communicated back to the laboratory as part of an effective quality assurance program.

Four of the primary drugs (SM, INH, RMP, and EMB) are available as lyophilized powders in the BACTEC SIRE kit, designed specifically for use with 12B medium and the BACTEC 460TB instrument. Alternatively, stock solutions of these agents can be prepared from reference powders. Lyophilized vials of PZA are also available for the pH 6.0 modified BACTEC PZA test medium. The secondary drugs, including capreomycin, cycloserine, ethionamide, and kanamycin (W. M. Gross and J. E. Hawkins, *Abstr. 86th Annu. Meet. Am. Soc. Microbiol.* 1986, abstr. C-378, p. 391, 1986), as well as newer agents, such as ciprofloxacin, ofloxacin, sparfloxacin, rifapentine, and rifabutin, must be prepared from reference powders. Critical concentrations for most of these drugs have been established, and the results of the radiometric and proportion methods correlate well, except for cycloserine (128).

Inoculum and Incubation

The source of inoculum for susceptibility testing should be fresh growth of actively growing bacilli. If growth from a primary BACTEC 12B vial is used for the inoculum, the daily GI reading should be at least 500 or, even better, between 800 and 900. The higher the GI, the shorter the period until the control vial reaches >30 and the earlier the test results can be interpreted. If the primary vial is past the GI peak or if the vial was kept at room temperature for more than 2 days, a fresh 12B vial should be inoculated. Other types of broth culture (Dubos, Middlebrook 7H9, Septichek AFB, ESP Myco, MGIT, MB/BacT medium) can be used as a source of inoculum; however, it is necessary to ensure that the broth culture is uncontaminated or not mixed. A variety of procedures may be used for mycobacterial purity checks (121). After the inoculum is thoroughly mixed to break up clumps, the turbidity should be adjusted to match a McFarland no. 0.5 standard rather than a McFarland no. 1 standard; a 1:100 dilution of the final inoculum is used as a control. BACTEC diluting fluid or distilled water, but not a broth or other substrate-containing medium, must be used to prepare the dilutions. An undiluted control is used to monitor the growth kinetics of the inoculum and also can serve as a source of inoculum if a test must be repeated.

Also, fresh growth on any solid media may serve as an inoculum source. It is important to harvest several (5 to 10) colonies in order to ensure a representative sample of growth (harvesting from only 2 or 3 single colonies is inadequate), and it is very important to thoroughly homogenize the inoculum in a tube containing 3 to 5 ml of diluting fluid and glass beads. After being vortexed for 1 to 2 min, the tube is left to stand undisturbed for 30 min to allow larger particles to settle, and then the top half of the supernatant is transferred into a new tube. The turbidity is adjusted to match a McFarland no. 0.5 standard, and this suspension is used to inoculate the drug-containing vials. Blood agar and 7H10 plates are inoculated with a few drops of the inoculum suspension to check for purity.

As safety precautions, disposable tuberculin syringes with a permanently attached needle should be used; rubber gloves, respirator, and a gown must be worn; and all steps involving the preparation of inocula and inoculation of vials should be performed in a class II or III biological safety cabinet.

Prior to inoculation, BACTEC 12B vials must be prerun in the BACTEC 460TB instrument to establish a gas phase of 5% CO_2 in air in the headspace of the vial; any vial with an initial GI of 20 must be rejected. Each prerun vial is inoculated with 0.1 ml of the adjusted suspension of the test or QC isolate, and the vials are incubated at $37 \pm 1°C$ (the temperature of incubation is critical) in the dark.

Reading, Interpreting, and Reporting Results

Vials are read on the BACTEC 460TB instrument at intervals of 24 ± 1 h for a minimum of 4 days and until the control vial reaches a GI of 30. For laboratories with limited weekend coverage, an alternative schedule is to inoculate the vials on Friday and first read them on Monday (65). The Monday reading is disregarded, since it reflects 2 days of CO_2 production, and the vials are read daily for at least 3 days (5 days total). Batch testing is discouraged unless the susceptibility test can be started during the same week that the isolate is identified to species, i.e., identified as M. tuberculosis complex. In those situations, to avoid any delay, the isolate should be sent to a reference laboratory that works 7 days a week.

When the GI of the control is 30 after a minimum of 4 days, the difference in GI from one day to the next, designated the ΔGI, should be interpreted as follows:

$$\Delta GI \text{ of control} > \Delta GI \text{ of drug} = \text{Susceptible}$$

$$\Delta GI \text{ of control} < \Delta GI \text{ of drug} = \text{Resistant}$$

If the GI is 500 and remains >500 on the next reading, the isolate should be considered resistant to that drug regardless of the ΔGI (it is necessary to check that the GI of the control was not >30 in less than 3 days to rule out overinoculation). Continued incubation for a few days may allow one to resolve borderline results, but the incubation should not be extended beyond 3 days after the control vial is positive. Susceptibility test results should never be reported without a preliminary or final identification of the isolate as M. tuberculosis complex or M. tuberculosis, especially when the isolate is resistant to a drug(s). Usually, BACTEC 460TB results are straightforward; however, if the ΔGIs are close (within 10%), a preliminary report should be issued as pending and the test should be repeated. In most situations, resistant (especially RMP-resistant) strains should be immediately tested against secondary drugs. Use of the term "borderline," as recommended by the BACTEC manufacturer, is not encouraged, because the definition of this term is unclear and may mislead the clinician into

believing that a drug has no use in the treatment of tuberculosis. Susceptibility test results should be reported without delay. The report should include the test method, the name of the drug, the concentration tested, and the result (susceptible or resistant). It is not possible to report the percent resistance by using the BACTEC 460TB method. Drug resistance should be reported by telephone and/or fax to the requesting physician, the infection control program, and the local tuberculosis control program, and a follow-up hard-copy report should be submitted. It is prudent to confirm the receipt of a fax report in lieu of direct communication with the physician or public health official.

Quality Control

Reference strains with known susceptibility patterns should be tested with each new batch of drug and BACTEC 12B medium. In addition, QC tests should be performed at least once a week in laboratories that perform tests daily or weekly or when a patient isolate is tested if tests are performed less frequently. The H37Rv strain of M. tuberculosis (ATCC 27294), which is susceptible to all standard antituberculosis agents, is commonly used for QC. We recommend that new lots of drugs or media (including new lots of BACTEC 12B medium) be QC tested with the ATCC 27294 strain and at least four concentrations of each drug to be tested. The concentrations tested should define an MIC for the ATCC 27294 strain with concentrations above and below the MIC to detect an out-of-control result. Mutants of H37Rv selected for in vitro resistance to single or multiple drugs are also available; however, these strains are resistant to very high concentrations and are not particularly suitable for QC purposes. In addition, reporting the test results for a patient isolate should not be delayed because of the pending test results for a resistant QC strain. Suspensions of QC strains may be prepared in BACTEC diluting solution and frozen at −70°C in 1-ml test samples for up to 6 months (153). A single tube is thawed for QC testing, and the same procedure as that for clinical isolates is used. At present, there is no published consensus on which QC results should be available before the test results on a patient isolate may be released. However, it seems reasonable that the QC test results for medium components be available and acceptable, as well as the results for the "susceptible" QC strain (e.g., ATCC 27294). The procedure manual should clearly state the corrective action that should be taken when a QC test fails, including the way in which the results for patient isolates should be handled.

Testing PZA

Reliable testing of PZA by the radiometric method is different from testing by the BACTEC 460TB method for the other primary drugs (108), because PZA activity must be measured at pH 5.5 rather than pH 6.8, the usual pH of the growth medium. However, most strains of M. tuberculosis grow poorly at pH 5.5 and some fail to grow altogether (23). As a compromise between testing at the pH for optimum PZA activity and testing at the pH for optimum growth, Salfinger et al. (146) recommended that PZA be tested at pH 5.9 ± 0.1. In addition, to accurately and reliably test PZA, several other adjustments to the standard radiometric method are made. (i) To prepare the inoculum, each isolate must be subcultured in a fresh BACTEC 12B vial supplemented with BACTEC reconstituting fluid, which is an aqueous solution of polyoxyethylene stearate (POES) (154). The isolate is tested daily, and once the GI is 300 to 500, this culture is used for susceptibility testing. Alternatively, a 1:10 dilution of the inoculum (GI = 999 or McFarland no. 0.5) used for testing the other primary drugs is used and the suspension is vigorously homogenized before use. (ii) Either the lyophilized PZA is reconstituted with POES or PZA reference powder is dissolved in POES to achieve a final concentration of 100 μg/ml, the critical concentration for the BACTEC method, which is equivalent to 25 to 50 μg/ml (used in the proportion method) (153). (iii) A special BACTEC 12B medium at pH 6.0 supplemented with POES is used to test PZA. (iv) The PZA-containing vial and the control vial are inoculated with the same suspension; i.e., the inoculum for the control vial should not be diluted. (v) The vials are tested daily until the control vial reaches a GI of 200; if the GI fails to reach 200 within 14 days, the test is uninterpretable. (vi) The isolate is considered susceptible to PZA if the GI of the PZA vial is <10% of the GI of the control vial. If the GIs of the test and control vials are very close, the result is considered borderline and the test must be repeated. (vii) In addition to the use of H37Rv (PZA susceptible) for QC testing, M. bovis BCG (PZA resistant) can be used as a control for PZA resistance. If an isolate tests resistant to PZA, especially if it is resistant to PZA alone, its identity should be confirmed, since M. bovis and M. bovis BCG are PZA resistant whereas the majority of M. tuberculosis isolates are PZA susceptible (M. Salfinger, L. B. Reller, and F. M. Kafader, Abstr. 90th Annu. Meet. Am. Soc. Microbiol. 1990, abstr. U55, p. 150, 1990). This is especially important if the laboratory identifies isolates only to the level of the M. tuberculosis complex. Some M. tuberculosis isolates grow poorly at pH 6.0 (145), and other isolates may be inhibited by the POES supplement (107).

ESP Culture System II
The ESP Culture System II is a fully automated, continuously monitoring system for growth and detection of mycobacteria (188) which allows, in parallel, testing of the susceptibility of M. tuberculosis to major primary drugs (i.e., INH, RMP, EMB, and SM). The ESP II technology is based on detection of pressure changes (gas production or gas consumption due to microbial growth) within the headspace above the broth culture medium in a sealed bottle. The culture medium consists of a Middlebrook 7H9 broth which has been enriched with glycerol and Casitone, and contains a cellulose sponge. Before the medium is inoculated with a test strain, OADC enrichment must be added to a final concentration of 10%.

Inoculum and Incubation
ESP antibiotics are supplied as lyophilate by the manufacturer. Preparation of ESP bottles requires the addition of 1.0 ml of antibiotic solution. The final concentrations in the Myco bottles are as follows: INH, 0.1 μg/ml; RMP, 1.0 μg/ml; EMB, 5.0 μg/ml; and SM, 8.0 μg/ml. INH and EMB can be tested at a higher concentrations (0.4 and 8.0 μg/ml, respectively). For the inoculation of organisms into the ESP Myco bottles, 0.5 ml of a 1:10 dilution from a McFarland no. 1 standard must be added to the drug-containing bottles. The inoculum can be prepared from either solid (e.g., Löwenstein-Jensen) or liquid (e.g., ESP Myco) medium. Cultures are kept in the instrument at 35°C, and growth is automatically monitored.

Reading, Interpreting, and Reporting Results
At the end of the specified incubation period, as determined by the drug-free control bottle for each isolate that

is tested, the isolate is manually determined to be susceptible or resistant to a drug. If the control bottle (without drugs) signals positive, the time to detection is calculated. Drug-containing bottles are monitored for another 3 days after the control bottle turned positive. Results are interpreted according to the following rules: a strain is considered resistant if the time of detection is the same time as or up to 3 days after that for the control bottle; a strain is considered susceptible if no growth occurs in the drug-containing bottle or if the time of detection is more than 3 days after that for the control bottle. The few studies demonstrate good agreement of the ESP Culture System II with the BACTEC 460TB and the agar proportion method and detection times which are very comparable to those obtained by the radiometric method (15, 141).

Quality Control
Each new ESP Myco Susceptibility Kit and/or lots of medium and growth supplement should be tested with strains of M. tuberculosis qualified for QC.

MGIT
In 1995, the MGIT was introduced for the growth and detection of mycobacteria from clinical specimens (62, 130). The MGIT medium consists of a modified Middlebrook 7H9 broth in conjunction with a fluorescence quenching-based oxygen sensor (silicon rubber impregnated with a ruthenium pentahydrate). The fluorescent compound is sensitive to the presence of oxygen dissolved in the medium. The fluorescence of the indicator is quenched in the presence of oxygen, but fluorescence increases as soon as actively respiring microorganisms utilize the dissolved oxygen. Fluorescence is detected using a 365-nm UV transilluminator. Principally, the MGIT system is available as a manual or a fully automated, continuously monitoring system called BACTEC MGIT 960. Apart from using nonradiometric medium, it frees the technician from using syringes. In addition to detecting and monitoring growth, the system can be used for testing of susceptibility to INH, RMP, EMB, PZA, and SM. Fluorescence of the drug-containing tubes is compared with that of the drug-free growth control tube. When using the instrument, the ratio of relative growth between the drug-containing tube and the growth control tube is determined by software algorithms. If the relative growth in the drug tube equals or exceeds that in the growth control tube, the organism is considered resistant to the drug; if the relative growth is less than that in the growth control tube, the organism is considered susceptible.

Four drugs (SIRE, i.e., SM, INH, RMP, and EMB) are designed specifically for use with the MGIT medium and the BACTEC MGIT 960 instrument (MGIT 960 AST set). Stock solutions of these drugs also can be prepared from reference powders. Recently, lyophilized vials of PZA have become available for testing PZA susceptibility based on an adapted protocol utilizing BACTEC MGIT 960 PZA medium at pH 5.9. Similar to the BACTEC 460TB procedure, the BACTEC MGIT 960 employs a two-tier test, with the first tier comprising the four SIRE drugs being tested at drug concentrations equivalent to the critical concentrations of the agar proportion method (i.e., SM, 1.0 μg/ml; INH, 0.1 μg/ml; RMP, 1.0 μg/ml; EMB, 5.0 μg/ml). If there is resistance to INH, EMB, and/or SM, a second test that involves a higher concentration of the drug(s) (SM, 4.0 μg/ml; INH, 0.4 μg/ml; EMB, 7.5 μg/ml) may be used. Although only a few published reports are available for these drugs to date, there is a good correlation between the MGIT and the BACTEC 460TB system or the agar proportion method (13, 142). The same holds true for PZA susceptibility testing (129). The time to results is comparable to that for the radiometric technique. However, ample information regarding second-line drugs is lacking.

Inoculum and Incubation

Inoculum (0.5 ml) for drug susceptibility testing may be prepared from either liquid or solid media. To ensure viability of the colonies, accuracy of results, and reproducibility of dilutions, strict adherence to the guidelines of the manufacturer is imperative. Prior to inoculating the SIRE AST tubes, 0.8 ml of the BACTEC MGIT 960 drug susceptibility testing supplement (OADC) and 100 μl of the drug solution are added to the MGIT. With a liquid source of inoculum, the MGIT must nominally be used no sooner than the day following the instrument's positivity (day 1) and no later than 5 days following the day of the instrument's positivity. If it is older, the isolate must first be subcultured again. With solid media, the isolate can be used no longer than 14 days after the first appearance of colonies on the plate or slant.

If growth from a primary MGIT is taken for susceptibility testing, the suspension can immediately be used for testing. Appropriate dilutions (1:5) have been made for day 3 through 5 positive MGIT 960 tubes prior to inoculation of the drug set to avoid overinoculation. When working with a solid medium source, inoculum preparation includes vortexing with glass beads and two specified settling times to ensure homogeneity of the final cell suspension. The suspension has to be adjusted to a McFarland no. 0.5 equivalent and then diluted 1:5 before inoculation of the MGIT 960 AST set. For the growth control tube, 100 μl of a positive MGIT 960 broth is pipetted into 10 ml of sterile saline to prepare a 1:100 dilution of the growth suspension. From this suspension, 0.5 ml is inoculated into a fresh MGIT without drug. Cultures are kept at 35°C, and growth is automatically monitored.

Reading, Interpreting, and Reporting Results

Drug results are listed automatically on the data report form (S, susceptible; R, resistant; X, invalid result), together with growth units and time to result.

Quality Control

Reference strains with known susceptibility patterns should be tested with each new batch of drug and MGIT medium.

Testing PZA

PZA can reliably be tested by using the novel BACTEC MGIT PZA tube, which contains 7 ml of MGIT broth, modified with a reduced pH (129). Inocula can be prepared either from MGIT medium or from solid medium, such as Löwenstein-Jensen medium. Prior to inoculating the PZA set tubes, 0.8 ml of MGIT PZA supplement and 100 μl of PZA solution (100 μg/ml) are added. MGIT cultures are used no sooner than the day following the instrument's positivity (day 1) and no later than 5 days following the day of positivity. On day 1 and 2 following positivity, the inoculum is used undiluted, while on days 3 to 5, suspensions are diluted 1:5 with sterile saline. Then 0.5 ml is inoculated into the MGIT PZA tubes. The growth control tube is inoculated with 0.5 ml of a 1:10 dilution of the respective suspension. Cultures grown on Löwenstein-Jensen medium are used no later than 14 days after the first

colonies appear on the slant. To ensure homogeneity, a suspension adjusted to a McFarland no. 0.5 equivalent is prepared by using glass beads and then diluted 1:5 prior to inoculation of the MGIT PZA set. All inoculated PZA sets must be loaded into the instrument within 8 h of inoculation. Again, using predefined algorithms, readings are automatically interpreted by the instrument. In contrast to BACTEC 460TB, the PZA "borderline" category no longer exists with this method.

MB/BacT ALERT 3D

The MB/BacT ALERT 3D System (bioMerieux) is another fully automated, nonradiometric system which allows both culture of mycobacteria and susceptibility testing of M. *tuberculosis* (133). With this technology, carbon dioxide is released into the medium by actively metabolizing microorganisms and is detected by a gas-permeable sensor containing an indicator embedded at the bottom of the culture bottles. Color changes are monitored by a reflectometric detection unit, and data are compiled by an internal database management system. Susceptibility testing of M. *tuberculosis* is currently available for INH, RMP, EMB, and SM.

Inoculum and Incubation

Following the instructions of the manufacturer, the MB/BacT process bottles containing a modified Middlebrook 7H9 medium (with casein, bovine serum albumin, and catalase) are supplemented with the following final drug concentrations: INH, 1 μg/ml; RMP, 1 μg/ml; SM, 1 μg/ml; and EMB, 2 μg/ml. Subsequently, bottles are inoculated with 0.5 ml of a suspension of M. *tuberculosis* adjusted to a McFarland no. 2 standard. Two bottles without drugs serve as growth controls, one inoculated with 0.5 ml of the cell suspension adjusted to a McFarland no. 2 standard (control 1) and one with 0.5 ml of the cell suspension (McFarland no. 2 standard) diluted 1:100 (control 2).

Reading, Interpreting, and Reporting Results

At the time that the MB/BacT System recognizes growth in the control 2 bottle, testing is terminated and the growth status of the bottles containing the drugs is determined. An isolate is considered resistant if the drug-containing bottle is positive before or on the same day as the corresponding diluted control bottle (control 2). Susceptibility is defined as the drug-containing bottle remaining negative or becoming positive later than the control 2 bottle. On the basis of preliminary studies, there is excellent agreement of the MB/BacT results with susceptibility data generated by the agar proportion method and BACTEC 460TB (22, 45, 133), in particular for INH and RMP. The manufacturer increased the EMB concentration to 2.5 μg/ml in order to improve the correlation with the results of the agar proportion method (153). The time necessary to determine the susceptibility patterns of M. *tuberculosis* is within what has been observed for the BACTEC 460TB System.

Quality Control

Reference strains with known susceptibility patterns should be tested with each new batch of drug and MB/BacT medium.

M. AVIUM COMPLEX

Clinical Significance

MAC is commonly isolated from a variety of clinical specimens, and isolation of MAC from blood or other sterile sites is almost always clinically significant. However, the isolation of MAC is especially significant in HIV-infected patients with profound CD4 T-cell lymphocytopenia, i.e., ≤75 CD4 T lymphocytes per μl. Although disseminated MAC infection remains a complication in HIV-infected patients, the incidence has significantly decreased due to the introduction of effective prophylaxis and immune system restoration associated with the use of highly active antiretroviral therapy. Also, disseminated MAC disease still occurs in patients who fail to respond to antiretroviral treatment because of resistance, drug intolerance, or lack of compliance. In many of these patients, MAC infection occurs as a relapse of MAC disease rather than as a new infection. MAC is also a cause of chronic pulmonary lung disease and is the leading cause of lung disease due to nontuberculous mycobacteria in the United States. The incidence of MAC lung disease has been steadily increasing in patients with a history of chronic pulmonary disease, including patients with chronic obstructive pulmonary disease and cystic fibrosis. Nevertheless, the detection of MAC in respiratory or gastrointestinal tract specimens can be difficult to interpret, especially in patients who are not clearly at risk for MAC disease. Clinical, histopathologic, and/or radiologic evidence of MAC disease, repeated isolation of MAC, increasing numbers of bacilli in sequential specimens, or the absence of other identifiable causes of signs and symptoms are important factors to consider in assessing the clinical significance of MAC isolates.

Drug Resistance

Most MAC isolates are intrinsically resistant to INH and PZA, and these antimicrobial agents play no role in the treatment of MAC infection (7). The intrinsic antimicrobial resistance was first described as due to the impermeability of the MAC cell envelope (135). However, more recent evidence suggests that INH resistance is due to a lack of a complete antimicrobial effect (12, 104). Cell-free in vitro studies have shown that certain drug targets (e.g., ribosomes, ribosomal subunits, and RNA polymerase) bind the corresponding drugs (e.g., macrolides, aminoglycosides, and rifamycins) and that the target functions are inhibited, yet many of these compounds are ineffective against whole cells. While MAC produces β-lactamase (111), there is otherwise no evidence that MAC actively degrades or inactivates antimicrobial agents.

MAC isolates are variably susceptible to aminoglycosides (amikacin, kanamycin, and SM) and rifamycins (RMP and rifabutin), but these agents should be considered secondary agents, which would be useful in combination with other agents or for salvage therapy. Clarithromycin was approved by the FDA for the treatment of MAC infection, but it must be combined with at least one additional agent, usually EMB (28). Rifabutin, clarithromycin, and azithromycin were approved as prophylactic agents for disseminated MAC infection; however, their mechanism of action as prophylactic agents is unclear.

MAC isolates display at least three colony type variants: a smooth, opaque, and domed type; a smooth, transparent, and flat type; and a rough type. Colony variant types have been associated with certain phenotypic properties, and the smooth, transparent, flat type is generally more virulent and resistant to antimicrobial agents than the opaque type. The conversion between colony types appears to be a phenotypic rather than a genotypic phenomenon and occurs at a high rate. The transparent-to-opaque transition occurs at a rate of approximately 5×10^{-4} per bacterium per generation, while the reverse transition occurs at a rate of approximately 1×10^{-6} per bacterium per generation. The clinical significance of this phenomenon is unknown, and both the transparent and opaque colony types are observed in primary cultures of various clinical specimens. However, the transparent colony type may not be evident unless the specimen is diluted first or streaked for isolation. The occurrence of colony type variants is problematic for susceptibility testing, since there can be a significant difference in susceptibility to agents used to treat MAC infections.

When To Perform Susceptibility Tests

In vitro susceptibility testing of MAC by the methods and interpretive criteria described for M. tuberculosis has little value in guiding antimicrobial therapy. For many antimicrobial agents, there is a lack of a correlation between in vitro susceptibility test results and clinical response. As a result, there are only limited interpretive criteria for defining susceptibility and resistance, principally for the macrolides (azithromycin and clarithromycin). Although wild-type MAC isolates are uniformly susceptible to macrolides, macrolide resistance develops quickly with monotherapy and may eventually develop with combination therapy. An analysis of macrolide-resistant MAC isolates showed that over 95% of clinically significant macrolide resistance in MAC is a consequence of mutations in the V-domain of the 23S rRNA gene (Table 2) (105, 119). Therefore, clinically significant macrolide resistance can be defined as a clarithromycin MIC of ≥32 μg/ml or an azithromycin MIC of ≥256 μg/ml. Predicting in vivo susceptibility is always less reliable; however, a positive clinical and microbiological response is expected if the MICs of clarithromycin and azithromycin are ≤4 and ≤32 μg/ml, respectively.

If a patient has not received macrolide prophylaxis, it is probably unnecessary to perform a susceptibility test on an initial MAC isolate from blood or tissue (7) as a guide to treatment. However, establishing baseline MICs for a MAC isolate may prove invaluable in interpreting susceptibility test results on an isolate from the same patient weeks or months later. Susceptibility testing is also warranted if a patient's history of previous macrolide treatment or prophylaxis is unclear, if a patient relapses, if the infection is intractable, or if the clinical situation is desperate. In the latter regard, testing may assist in deciding how aggressive salvage therapy should be. Indeed, even in the face of macrolide resistance, it may be prudent to continue macrolide treatment because of the disseminated nature of the disease and the lack of serious adverse effects of these drugs.

Test Methods

Broth microdilution and macrodilution and agar dilution methods have been described that measure, in a quantitative manner, the in vitro activity of antimycobacterial agents against MAC. In Europe, an agar dilution method with Mueller-Hinton agar supplemented with OADC is used; however, in the United States, there is consensus that both radiometric broth macrodilution and broth microdilution methods are accurate and reliable. The current recommendations of the NCCLS Subcommittee on Antimycobacterial Susceptibility Testing indicate that susceptibility testing for MAC should be restricted to the newer macrolides (clarithromycin, azithromycin, and roxithromycin) and that test results with clarithromycin can be extended to the other two compounds in this class (121). If other drugs are tested (e.g., EMB, amikacin, and RMP), five concentrations should be tested in increments of 1 $\log_2$

unit. BACTEC 12B medium can be used for macrodilution tests, and either Middlebrook 7H9 or Mueller-Hinton broth supplemented with OADC or OAD can be used for microdilution tests. The issue of pH remains somewhat controversial, and the NCCLS does not make a specific recommendation but states that pH 6.8 and 7.4 are both acceptable, providing that the NCCLS recommended interpretive criteria are followed (Table 5).

Inoculum and Incubation

Currently there are no specific recommendations regarding preparation of the inoculum. The options include the use of "seed" BACTEC vials (subcultures of fresh growth) or the preparation of a suspension of mycobacteria taken directly from an agar plate. However the inoculum is prepared, it is important to avoid the selection of colony type variants during subculture, and only transparent colony types should be tested. The inoculum should be between 10^4 and 10^5 CFU/ml for the radiometric broth macrodilution test and approximately 5×10^5 CFU/ml for the broth microdilution test. The concentration ranges of clarithromycin and azithromycin to test are shown in Table 5.

The period of incubation should not extend beyond 10 days, and the "no-drug" control should not exceed a GI of 999 in less than 4 days in the radiometric test. The end point for the radiometric test is defined by the GI value for the inoculum diluted 1:100, whereas the end point for the broth microdilution assay is visible turbidity. Finally, Tween 80 or other surfactants should not be used to disperse clumps of bacilli because of the potential synergistic effect of the surfactant activity of Tween 80 and antimicrobial agents.

Reporting Results

The activity of all agents should be expressed as an MIC, but interpretive criteria are available only for clarithromycin and azithromycin. The results for other drugs should be reported as MICs without interpretation. Therefore, the testing of agents other than the macrolides should be restricted to situations in which the clinician has extensive experience in the use of these agents in the treatment of MAC disease or for research purposes. However, it is important to recognize that disseminated MAC disease is principally an infection of the blood, macrophages, bone marrow, spleen, and other tissues. Thus, clinical effectiveness is likely to relate to both potent activity and the ability of drugs to accumulate in cells and tissues to levels above the MIC for the infecting microorganism.

Regarding the effect of pH on macrolides (e.g., the MIC_{90} of roxithromycin under mildly alkaline condi-

tions [pH 7.4] drops to approximately 12 $\mu g/ml$) (136), one view is that testing at pH 7.2 to 7.4 is potentially misleading because some MAC isolates grow more slowly (and some fail to grow) at this pH. Thus, MICs measured in this pH range may reflect synergy between a suboptimal pH for growth and inhibitory drug activity (81; S. Beaty, S. Siddiqi, and M. Gnacek, Abstr. 92nd Gen. Meet. Am. Soc. Microbiol. 1992, abstr. U-102, 1992). Also, BACTEC 12B medium is unstable at pH 7.2 to 7.4 because of the poor buffering capacity of the medium at pHs above 7.2. In addition, the intracellular environment of MAC-infected macrophages (i.e., pH 6.0 to 6.5) suggests that macrolides should be tested under the mildly acidic, more clinically relevant conditions. Although MAC can block phagolysosome fusion, the intracellular pH remains in the range of pH 6.0 to 6.5 (125, 137, 160). Blocking phagolysosome fusion prevents a drop to pH 5.0 or lower but does not result in an increase in the intracellular pH to 7.2 to 7.4.

OTHER SLOWLY GROWING MYCOBACTERIA

Nearly 15 years ago, Woods and Washington (189) reviewed the nontuberculous mycobacterioses and concluded that no clear recommendations could be made for treatment of these infections and that the need for susceptibility testing was difficult or impossible to assess. Now, 15 years later, the situation has not appreciably changed. Many mycobacterioses remain quite rare (e.g., those due to M. simiae) or are initially misdiagnosed as tuberculosis, which confuses any analysis of the response to therapy. Nevertheless, for certain species of nontuberculous mycobacteria, there has been an accumulation of information and experience that can be the basis for some recommendations. Susceptibility testing is often helpful with these uncommon species because of the paucity of information about treatment options, and in vitro results provide some rational basis for guiding treatment. Furthermore, baseline information may be useful if there is a microbiologic relapse. However, the vagaries of testing and interpretation of results mandate that the testing be performed in an experienced laboratory and, to better ensure consistency of results, that follow-up testing be performed by the same laboratory.

M. kansasii

Isolates of M. kansasii from patients not previously treated with RMP are predictably susceptible to RMP at 1 $\mu g/ml$, and patients have been successfully treated with RMP, INH, and a third agent, usually EMB (38). However, resis-

TABLE 5 Susceptibility testing of clarithromycin and azithromycin against MAC[a]

Antimicrobial agent	Concn range ($\mu g/ml$) for:		pH	Interpretive criteria			QC (M. avium ATCC 700898)	
	BACTEC	Microtiter		Susceptible ($\mu g/ml$)	Intermediate ($\mu g/ml$)	Resistant ($\mu g/ml$)	Concn range ($\mu g/ml$)	Expected end points ($\mu g/ml$)
Clarithromycin	2–64 or 4, 16, and 64	1–64	6.8	≤16	32	≥64	1, 2, and 4	1–4
Clarithromycin	2–64 or 4, 8, and 32	2–64	7.3–7.4	≤4	8–16	≥32	0.5, 1, and 2	0.5–2
Azithromycin	16–512 or 32, 128, and 512	NR[b]	6.8	≤128	256	≥512	8, 16, and 32	8–32

[a] Data from reference 121.
[b] NR, no recommendation.

tance to RMP can develop during therapy, and a patient's history of RMP therapy may be unknown or unclear. Therefore, susceptibility testing should be performed on initial isolates with RMP at 1 μg/ml by the agar proportion method. There is a good correlation between agar and broth (BACTEC 12B or 7H9 or Mueller-Hinton plus OADC broth microdilution) methods, but unless a laboratory performs a large number of tests on M. kansasii isolates, the agar method is more convenient. Testing of INH and EMB should be discouraged, and reports of resistance to 0.2 or 1 μg of INH per ml or 2 μg of SM per ml should be disregarded (7). The recommendation of the ATS is to treat M. kansasii pulmonary disease with a combination of INH (300 mg), RMP (600 mg), and EMB (25 mg/kg for 2 months and then 15 mg/kg for 18 months), with at least 12 months of negative sputum cultures (7). Alternative agents include rifabutin (for HIV-positive patients treated with protease inhibitors), SM, clarithromycin, amikacin, ciprofloxacin, and trimethoprim-sulfamethoxazole. Tentative testing and interpretive guidelines for these agents are shown in Table 6 (121).

M. marinum

M. marinum is predictably susceptible to RMP and EMB, and alternative agents include clarithromycin, amikacin, tetracycline, doxycycline, minocycline, ciprofloxacin, and trimethoprim-sulfamethoxazole. Routine susceptibility testing of M. marinum isolates should be discouraged. If the infection is intractable or relapses, the methods and interpretive criteria for testing rapidly growing mycobacteria are more likely to provide reliable and clinically useful results. The NCCLS has recommended (i) antimicrobial agents to test, (ii) resistance breakpoints, and (iii) methods (121). Successful treatment may require surgical excision or debridement, and antimicrobial treatment may be necessary only during the perioperative period (7).

M. haemophilum

M. haemophilum is an opportunistic pathogen in immunocompromised patients, and there is some correlation between susceptibility test results and clinical efficacy, although virtually all treatment regimens examined included combinations of agents (159). Wild-type isolates of M. haemophilum appear to be susceptible to quinolones, rifamycins, clarithromycin, and azithromycin and resistant to

TABLE 6 Tentative breakpoint concentrations for antimicrobial agents that might be tested against M. kansasii and selected slowly growing mycobacteria other than tuberculosis[a]

Antimicrobial agent	Resistance breakpoint (μg/ml)
RMP	1–2
Rifabutin	0.5–2
EMB	5
INH	5
SM	10
Clarithromycin	32
Amikacin	10
Ciprofloxacin	2
Trimethoprim-sulfamethoxazole	2/38

[a] Data from reference 121.

PZA and EMB; they are likely to be resistant to INH and SM (16, 159).

M. xenopi, M. szulgai, and M. malmoense

In vitro susceptibility test results for M. xenopi, M. szulgai, and M. malmoense may be helpful because of the paucity of information about the susceptibility patterns of these species. For example, susceptibility testing has been reported to be important to the management of infections caused by M. xenopi (168), but an earlier report indicated that the correlation between susceptibility test results and therapeutic response was inconsistent (189). Pulmonary infections by these three species have been successfully treated with INH, EMB, and RMP, and one report indicated that clarithromycin was effective in the treatment of M. xenopi infections (7). Candidate drugs for testing with these species are the same as for M. kansasii (Table 6). The test method should be either the BACTEC radiometric or agar proportion method; however, there may be advantages to using the BACTEC 460TB method and defining the in vitro susceptibility in terms of an MIC. Extrapolation of the M. tuberculosis "critical concentrations" to these species of mycobacteria may be misleading, since there is some evidence that infections caused by these species can be successfully treated with higher concentrations of INH, SM, and EMB than might be used for M. tuberculosis (7).

M. gordonae

Testing M. gordonae isolates is usually inappropriate because actual disease is quite rare and contamination is common (178). Before testing M. gordonae isolates, one should ask whether the isolate truly is M. gordonae and whether there is convincing evidence that the isolate is playing a role in the disease. Until these questions are answered in the affirmative, susceptibility testing is inappropriate because the results could be misleading and the patient may be misdiagnosed and inadequately treated.

The most prudent approach to the testing of slowly growing mycobacteria other than M. tuberculosis is to restrict it to reference laboratories with extensive experience in working with these species. Interpretation of the susceptibility test results requires good communication between the laboratory and the clinician. Finally, clinicians without experience in the treatment of these mycobacterial infections should consult with their more experienced colleagues.

RAPIDLY GROWING MYCOBACTERIA

Clinical Significance

Rapidly growing mycobacteria are defined as acid-fast bacilli that form visible colonies from a dilute inoculum on a solid medium within 5 to 7 days. It is important to note that this definition does not necessarily apply to the original culture of a patient's specimen. Although there are over 30 species of rapidly growing mycobacteria, disease in humans is restricted to three species: M. fortuitum, M. chelonae, and M. abscessus. These three species are important causes of cutaneous, pulmonary, and nosocomial infection, especially following catheter insertions, augmentation mammaplasty, and cardiac bypass surgery. Disseminated disease is rare and is usually associated with immunodeficiency including that due to corticosteroid therapy, although it is not common in HIV-infected patients (100). M. smegmatis, M. peregri-

num, and *M. mucogenicum* also have been implicated as rare causes of disease in humans (173, 174), and at least two species of rapidly growing mycobacteria are animal pathogens (57). Clinical isolates should be identified to species, and isolates of the *M. fortuitum* group (i.e., *M. fortuitum*, *M. peregrinum*, and *M. fortuitum* third biovariant complex) must be distinguished from the *M. chelonae-M. abscessus* group of rapid growers. Also, the importance of distinguishing rapidly growing from slowly growing mycobacteria isolated from clinical specimens must be emphasized, since conventional antimycobacterial agents (except some aminoglycosides) are ineffective in the treatment of disease caused by rapid growers. Furthermore, this intrinsic resistance to conventional antimycobacterial agents may not be appreciated by clinicians with limited experience in treating these infections. Therefore, it is incumbent on the laboratory to assist in assessing the clinical significance of these isolates and to provide information on appropriate antimicrobial therapy. Isolation of the aforementioned species of rapidly growing mycobacteria from wounds is almost always clinically significant, and susceptibility testing should be performed with antimicrobial agents that have proven therapeutic effectiveness. The isolation of rapidly growing mycobacteria from respiratory specimens is difficult to interpret, but frequently these isolates are not clinically significant. However, the repeated isolation of a rapid grower in pure culture or in predominant numbers from respiratory specimens is consistent with true respiratory tract disease, especially in patients with a history of chronic respiratory disease. In patients with wound infections, debridement and excision of the infected tissue are frequently necessary adjuncts to antimicrobial therapy, although 20% of cases of cutaneous infection are likely to resolve spontaneously without surgical intervention or antimicrobial therapy (172).

Although these mycobacteria are considered rapid growers when subcultured to blood or chocolate agar, primary isolation may take much longer than 5 to 7 days. When rapid growers are the suspected cause of infection based on clinical suspicion, specimens should be inoculated onto Löwenstein-Jensen and/or Middlebrook medium and incubated at both 30 and 37°C to promote their growth, especially for *M. chelonae* and *M. abscessus*. Identification of rapidly growing mycobacteria to species is important because of significant differences in the wild-type susceptibility patterns of the three species most commonly associated with disease in humans.

Methods

Four methods have been described to measure the in vitro susceptibility of rapidly growing mycobacteria: broth microdilution, agar disk elution, disk diffusion, and the E test. Only the broth microdilution method has been approved by the NCCLS (121). A disk diffusion method was described by Hawkins et al. (67), but it has important limitations; notably, there is a lack of verified interpretive criteria, and the disk contents of certain drugs are too low. The E test was evaluated for testing rapid growers and the results were promising (93), but the method has not been widely adopted in clinical laboratories that test these mycobacteria.

Broth Microdilution Method

The broth microdilution method for testing rapidly growing mycobacteria is essentially a modification of the NCCLS standard method for non-acid-fast organisms that grow aerobically (120); it has been described in detail by Brown et al. (21) and is recommended as a laboratory standard (121). This method is most suitable for laboratories that test large numbers of isolates. The antimicrobial agents, concentration range, and interpretive criteria that should be considered for testing rapidly growing mycobacteria by this method are shown in Table 7. Commercially prepared broth microdilution panels can be used if the appropriate drugs are available at the necessary concentrations. Alternatively, broth microdilution panels can be prepared by the method described by Brown et al. (21), which recommends the use of a dispensing device such as the Quick Spense II (Dynatech, Inc., Chantilly, Va.). Once prepared, the plates can be sealed in plastic bags and stored at 70°C for up to 6 months.

TABLE 7 Antimicrobial agents to test against rapidly growing mycobacteria by broth microdilution method[a]

Antimicrobial agent	Concn range (μg/ml)	MIC (μg/ml) for:			QC concn range (μg/ml) for:	
		Susceptible strains	Intermediate strains	Resistant strains	M. peregrinum ATCC 700686[h]	S. aureus ATCC 29213[h]
Amikacin[b]	1–128	≤16	32	≥64	≤1–4	1–4
Cefoxitin[c]	2–256	≤16	32–64	≥128	16–32	1–4
Ciprofloxacin[d]	0.125–16	≤1	2	≥4	≤0.125–0.5	0.125–0.5
Clarithromycin[e]	0.06–64	≤2	4	≥8	≤0.06–0.5	0.125–0.5
Doxycycline[f]	0.25–32	≤1	2–8	≥16	≤0.125–0.5	0.125–0.5
Imipenem	1–64	≤4	8	≥16	2–16	
Sulfamethoxazole	1–64	≤32		≥64	≤1–4	32–128
Tobramycin[g]	1–32	≤4	8	≥16	4–8	0.125–1

[a] Table and footnotes are adapted from reference 121.
[b] Kanamycin may be more active than amikacin against *M. abscessus* and *M. chelonae*. The amikacin MICs of ≥64 μg/ml for *M. abscessus* are unusual and must be confirmed.
[c] Cefoxitin is one dilution higher than the conventional NCCLS-suggested breakpoint; it is the only cephalosporin that should be tested.
[d] Report results only for *M. chelonae*.
[e] Class agent for all newer macrolides. *M. chelonae* and *M. abscessus* should be read at 3 days but not more than 4 days. Trailing across a breakpoint should be interpreted as resistance with *M. fortuitum*.
[f] In general, doxycycline and minocycline are four- to eightfold more active than tetracycline.
[g] Likely to be active against only *M. chelonae*.
[h] Expected range for QC purposes. Potencies of drug preparations also can be tested with *E. coli* ATCC 25922 and *Pseudomonas aeruginosa* ATCC 27853 and compared with expected ranges as described in NCCLS document M7 (120).

Inoculum

Fresh growth is prepared by inoculating a blood agar plate with the test organism and incubating the plate at 30°C for 72 h. The current recommendation is to prepare the inoculum by collecting growth from the blood agar plate with a sterile cotton swab and making a suspension in sterile distilled water that is equivalent to a McFarland no. 0.5 turbidity standard. The final inoculum should be 1×10^5 to 5×10^5 CFU/ml or 1×10^4 to 5×10^4 CFU/100 μl/well of a microtiter plate. The purity of the inoculum should be checked for each isolate, and occasionally the size of the inoculum should be verified by quantitative plate culture, especially if there is a problem with clumping.

Incubation and Reading

The microtiter plates are sealed and incubated for 3 to 5 days at 30°C in air, but they must not be incubated beyond 5 days because of drug instability. If there is not sufficient growth to interpret the results after 5 days of incubation, the test should be repeated. The MIC is defined as the lowest concentration of antimicrobial agent that completely inhibits visible growth. As with other types of bacteria, "trailing" is common when testing the sulfonamides, and the MICs of these agents should be read at approximately 80% inhibition of growth.

Reporting Results

Results are reported as MICs with the interpretive criteria shown in Table 6. Imipenem results should not be reported for M. chelonae and M. abscessus. The NCCLS guidelines should be consulted for further information on testing and reporting results for imipenem (121).

Quality Control

QC strains for monitoring test performance and for verifying the concentration of antimicrobial agents are listed in Table 6. QC tests should be performed on each new batch of test plates once a week or as performed. At present there is very limited interlaboratory proficiency testing available for testing rapidly growing mycobacteria. Therefore, laboratories are encouraged to submit isolates to reference laboratories with extensive experience in testing these mycobacteria for confirmatory tests in lieu of a formal proficiency test program.

Agar Disk Elution Method

The agar disk elution method can be viewed as an adaptation of the disk elution modification of the proportion method for testing M. tuberculosis. The method may be particularly well suited for occasional or infrequent testing of small numbers of isolates. The method has been described in detail elsewhere (20). However, the disk elution method was not included in the most recent NCCLS recommendation (121), most probably because of their recommendation that susceptibility testing of rapidly growing mycobacteria be restricted to laboratories with extensive experience in testing these mycobacteria.

Alternative Susceptibility Testing Methods

In the last decade, drug susceptibility testing of mycobacteria has become a very dynamic field, spawning many new technologies that one day may prove successful in a clinical laboratory. They all comply with the standard set by CDC that susceptibility test results have to be available within 28 days from the time the specimen arrives in the laboratory (18). Some of these techniques are based on improved methods for measuring inhibition of growth, while others are based on molecular assays for both analytes that correlate with growth or direct detection of mutations associated with resistance. Among growth-based strategies is the determination of the MIC of drugs. This procedure, which is labor-intensive, has been greatly facilitated by the E test (AB Biodisk, Solna, Sweden) (86, 176). Although convenient, especially for determining resistance in rapidly growing mycobacteria, use of E-test strips for susceptibility testing of M. tuberculosis remains limited because of the potential hazard arising from the high inoculum needed to inoculate the agar plates (86). Additional methods distinguish viable from nonviable tubercle bacilli by using tetrazolium dye reduction (32, 53, 56, 115) or flow cytometry (112) or use particle-counting immunoassay to quantify mycobacterial antigen (46). Jacobs et al. (85) described a method based on the use of a luciferase reporter mycobacteriophage. The premise was that viable mycobacteria support the infection and multiplication of phages whereas inhibited or killed mycobacteria do not. Therefore, mycobacteria susceptible to INH or RMP supported the phage infection and expressed luciferase. When exposed to INH or RMP, the cells were killed and no light was produced. This assay has recently been modified to allow easy detection of the emitted light with a Polaroid film box (aka the "Bronx box") (140). Cooksey et al. (33) introduced the luciferase gene into M. tuberculosis H37Ra by electroporation of a plasmid containing the luciferase gene linked to the hsp60 promoter. The results of a broth microtiter assay with the luciferase-H37Ra strain were comparable to the results of a conventional broth microdilution assay. Cangelosi et al. (27) described an alternative approach based on the measurement of the precursor rRNA. In this assay, M. tuberculosis nucleic acid is probed with specific pre-16S rRNA stem sequences in the presence or absence of drugs that have a direct or indirect effect on rRNA synthesis. Responses to RMP and ciprofloxacin were detected within 24 and 48 h, respectively. Detectable pre-rRNA was depleted in susceptible cells but remained abundant in resistant cells. The ability of RMP to block the lytic cell cycle of bacteriophage D29 within susceptible M. tuberculosis and hence the production of plaques on a lawn has led to another bacteriophage-based assay for susceptibility testing of M. tuberculosis to a variety of drugs (48, 49).

Mutations in genes that encode targets of antimycobacterial agents (Table 2) can be detected by a variety of methods. A particular focus of such studies has been RMP resistance because of the pivotal role of RMP in the treatment of tuberculosis and other mycobacterial infections, the conserved nature of the genetic basis for resistance (>96% of RMP resistance correlates with mutations in an 81-bp segment of the rpoB gene), and the use of RMP resistance as a surrogate marker of MDR M. tuberculosis. The methods used to detect rpoB mutations include PCR amplification of the target sequence and detection by DNA sequencing (80, 88, 165; V. Sintchenko, P. J. Jelfs, W. K. Chew, and G. L. Gilbert, Letter, J. Antimicrob. Chemother. **44:**294–295, 1999), the line probe assay (34, 42, 101), single-strand conformation polymorphism (51, 166), dideoxy fingerprinting (51), the mismatch RNA-RNA protection assay (118), the heteroduplex generator assay (181), the use of molecular beacons synthesized from modified oligonucleotides (131), and PCR–enzyme-linked immunosorbent assay (55). Similar approaches have been developed for detecting mutations involved in INH (139), EMB and RMP (177), and PZA (40, 113) resistance. Torres et al. (169) have proposed real-time PCR coupled to fluorescence detection for a rapid detection of RMP and INH resistance associated with mutations in M. *tuberculosis*. Most recently, DNA microarray technology described for mycobacterial identification has also been applied to the efficient detection of mutations associated with resistance to TB drugs (106, 128, 170). Undoubtedly, the application of these assays for routine use in the clinical mycobacteriology laboratory is likely to require technical simplification or automation as well as outcome analysis to justify the anticipated increased costs compared with conventional approaches. Indeed, even if these goals are achieved, it is likely that there are many more mutations to be discovered before antimicrobial resistance in M. *tuberculosis* and other mycobacteria can reliably be detected by molecular assays.

NOCARDIA AND OTHER AEROBIC ACTINOMYCETES

Clinical Significance

Nocardia spp. and other aerobic actinomycetes (*Actinomadura*, *Rhodococcus*, *Gordonia*, *Tsukamurella*, and *Streptomyces* spp.) can cause serious disease in healthy hosts, but infections by these microorganisms in immunocompromised hosts can be systemic and life-threatening (31, 92).

Antimicrobial therapy with multiple agents over several months is often necessary to achieve a positive outcome. In vitro susceptibility testing may be of great value in guiding treatment and monitoring for resistance.

Testing Method

The antimicrobial agents that are recommended for primary and secondary in vitro susceptibility testing are listed in Table 8. The broth microdilution method used with rapidly growing mycobacteria can be used to test *Nocardia* and other aerobic actinomycetes. The inoculum should be prepared as a suspension of microorganisms harvested from a blood agar plate that was incubated for 1 to 3 days at 37°C in air. Some species may require extended incubation for up to 5 days in order to have sufficient growth. Presently there are no standard strains available for QC, but standard strains of *Staphylococcus aureus* and *Escherichia coli* can be used for QC of the drug preparations. A previous clinical isolate may be useful as a QC strain for the overall procedure.

Reporting of Results

The MIC interpretive criteria for testing *Nocardia* spp. and other aerobic actinomycetes are shown in Table 8. It should be emphasized that the interpretive criteria, as recommended by the NCCLS in document M24-T2 or the forthcoming M24-A, for amikacin, minocycline, and sulfamethoxazole are different from the criteria for rapidly growing aerobic bacteria recommended by the NCCLS in document M7-A5 (120).

TABLE 8 Antimicrobial agents to test against *Nocardia* and other aerobic actinomycetes[a]

Antimicrobial agent	Concn range (μg/ml)	MIC (μg/ml) for:			QC concn (μg/ml) for[e]:	
		Susceptible strains	Intermediate strains	Resistant strains	*S. aureus* ATCC 29213	*E. coli* ATCC 35218
Primary						
Amikacin[b]	1–16	≤8		≥16	1–4	
Amoxicillin-clavulanic acid	2/1–32/16	≤8/4	16/8	≥32/16	0.12/0.06–0.5/0.25	4/2–16/8
Ceftriaxone	4–64	≤8	16–32	≥64	1–8	
Ciprofloxacin	0.25–4	≤1	2	≥4	0.12–0.5	
Clarithromycin[c]	0.5–8	≤2	4	≥8	0.12–0.5	
Imipenem	1–16	≤4	8	≥16	0.016–0.06	
Linezolid[d]	0.5–8	≤8			1–4	
Minocycline[b]	0.5–8	≤1	2–4	≥8	0.06–0.5	
Sulfamethoxazole[b]	4–64	≤32		≥64	32–128	
or						
Trimethoprim-sulfamethoxazole	0.25/4.75–4/76	≤2/38		≥4/76	≤0.5/9.5	
Tobramycin	1–16	≤4	8	≥16	0.12–1	
Secondary						
Cefepime	2–32	≤8	16	≥32	1–4	
Cefotaxime	4–64	≤8	16–32	≥64	1–4	
Doxycycline	0.5–8	≤1	2–4	≥8	0.12–1	
Gentamicin	1–16	≤4	8	≥16	0.12–1	

[a] Table and footnotes are adapted from reference 121.
[b] The breakpoints for these antimicrobial agents are different from the current NCCLS recommendations.
[c] Used as a class agent for newer macrolides.
[d] Proposed breakpoint. No *Nocardia* isolates with linezolid MICs of >8 μg/ml have been reported.
[e] At present there are no standard quality control strains of *Nocardia* or other aerobic actinomycetes. These standard *S. aureus* and *E. coli* strains should be used for QC of the concentration of antimicrobial agents.

REFERENCES

1. **Alcaide, F., G. E. Pfyffer, and A. Telenti.** 1997. Role of *embB* in natural and acquired resistance to ethambutol in mycobacteria. *Antimicrob. Agents Chemother.* **41:**2270–2273.
2. **Alcaide, F., and A. Telenti.** 1997. Molecular techniques in the diagnosis of drug-resistant tuberculosis. *Ann. Acad. Med. Singapore* **26:**647–650.
3. **Alford, R. H.** 1990. Antimycobacterial agents, p. 350–360. *In* G. L. Mandell, R. G. Douglas, Jr., and J. E. Bennett (ed.), *Principles and Practices of Infectious Diseases.* Churchill Livingstone, Inc., New York, N.Y.
4. **Amsden, G. W.** 1996. Erythromycin, clarithromycin, and azithromycin: are the differences real? *Clin. Ther.* **18:**56–72.
5. **Amsden, G. W.** 1995. Macrolides versus azalides: a drug interaction update. *Ann. Pharm.* **29:**906–917.
6. **Andriole, V. T.** 1990. Quinolones, p. 334–345. *In* G. L. Mandell, R. G. Douglas, Jr., and J. E. Bennett (ed.), *Principles and Practices of Infectious Diseases.* Churchill Livingstone, Inc., New York, N.Y.
7. **Anonymous.** 1997. Diagnosis and treatment of disease caused by nontuberculous mycobacteria. *Am. J. Respir. Crit. Care Med.* **156:**S1–S25.
8. **Anonymous.** 1983. Levels of laboratory services for mycobacterial disease: official statement of the American Thoracic Society. *Am. Rev. Respir. Dis.* **128:**213.
9. **Anonymous.** 1998. *Priftin® (Rifapentine) Prescribing Information.* Hoechst Marion Roussel, Inc., Kansas City, Mo.
10. **Bailey, W. C., J. B. Bass, J. E. Hawkins, G. P. Kubica, and R. J. Wallace.** 1984. Drug susceptibility testing for mycobacteria. *Am. Thorac. Soc. Newsl.* **10:**9–10.
11. **Banerjee, A., E. Dubnau, A. Quemard, V. Balasubramanian, K. S. Um, T. Wilson, D. Collins, G. de Lisle, and W. R. Jacobs, Jr.** 1994. *inhA*, a gene encoding a target for isoniazid and ethionamide in *Mycobacterium tuberculosis. Science* **263:**227–230.
12. **Barry, C. E., III, and K. Mdluli.** 1996. Drug sensitivity and environmental adaptation of mycobacterial cell wall components. *Trends Microbiol.* **4:**275–281.
13. **Bémer, P., F. Palicova, S. Rüsch-Gerdes, S. H. Siddiqi, H. B. Drugeon, and G. E. Pfyffer.** 2002. Multicenter evaluation of fully-automated BACTEC Mycobacteria Growth Indicator Tube 960 System for susceptibility testing of *Mycobacterium tuberculosis. J. Clin. Microbiol.* **40:**150–154.
14. **Benson, C.** 1997. Critical drug interactions with agents used for prophylaxis and treatment of *Mycobacterium avium* infections. *Am. J. Med.* **102:**32–36.
15. **Bergmann, J. S., and G. L. Woods.** 1998. Evaluation of the ESP culture system II for testing susceptibilities of *Mycobacterium tuberculosis* isolates to four primary antituberculous drugs. *J. Clin. Microbiol.* **36:**2940–2943.
16. **Bernard, E. M., F. F. Edwards, T. E. Kiehn, S. T. Brown, and D. Armstrong.** 1993. Activities of antimicrobial agents against clinical isolates of *Mycobacterium haemophilum. Antimicrob. Agents Chemother.* **37:**2323–2326.
17. **Berning, S. E., L. Madsen, M. D. Iseman, and C. A. Peloquin.** 1995. Long-term safety of ofloxacin and ciprofloxacin in the treatment of mycobacterial infections. *Am. J. Respir. Crit. Care Med.* **151:**2006–2009.
18. **Bird, B. R., M. M. Denniston, R. E. Huebner, and R. C. Good.** 1996. Changing practices in mycobacteriology: a follow-up survey of state and territorial public health laboratories. *J. Clin. Microbiol.* **34:**554–559.
19. **Bodmer, T., G. Zurcher, P. Imboden, and A. Telenti.** 1995. Mutation position and type of substitution in the beta-subunit of the RNA polymerase influence in-vitro activity of rifamycins in rifampicin-resistant *Mycobacterium tuberculosis. J. Antimicrob. Chemother.* **35:**345–348.
20. **Brown, B. A., J. M. Swenson, and R. J. Wallace, Jr.** 1992. Agar disk elution test for rapidly growing mycobacteria, p. 5.10.1–5.10.11. *In* H. D. Isenberg (ed.), *Clinical Microbiology Procedures Handbook,* vol. 1. American Society for Microbiology, Washington, D.C.
21. **Brown, B. A., J. M. Swenson, and R. J. Wallace, Jr.** 1992. Broth microdilution test for rapidly growing mycobacteria, p. 5.11.1–5.11.10. *In* H. D. Isenberg (ed.), *Clinical Microbiology Procedures Handbook,* vol. 1. American Society for Microbiology, Washington, D.C.
22. **Brunello, F., and R. Fontana.** 2000. Reliability of the MB/BacT system for testing susceptibility of *Mycobacterium tuberculosis* complex isolates to antituberculous drugs. *J. Clin. Microbiol.* **38:**872–873.
23. **Butler, W. R., and J. O. Kilburn.** 1982. Improved method for testing susceptibility of *Mycobacterium tuberculosis* to pyrazinamide. *J. Clin. Microbiol.* **16:**1106–1109.
24. **Canetti, G.** 1965. Present aspects of bacterial resistance in tuberculosis. *Am. Rev. Respir. Dis.* **92:**687–702.
25. **Canetti, G., W. Fox, A. Khomenko, H. T. Mahler, N. K. Menon, D. A. Mitchison, N. Rist, and N. A. Smelev.** 1969. Advances in techniques of testing mycobacterial drug sensitivity, and the use of sensitivity tests in tuberculosis control programs. *Bull. W. H. O.* **41:**21–43.
26. **Canetti, G., S. Froman, J. Grosset, P. Hauduroy, M. Lagerova, H. T. Mahler, G. Meissner, D. A. Mitchison, and L. Sula.** 1963. Mycobacteria: laboratory methods for testing drug sensitivity and resistance. *Bull. W. H. O.* **29:**565–578.
27. **Cangelosi, G. A., W. H. Brabant, T. B. Britschgi, and C. K. Wallis.** 1996. Detection of rifampin- and ciprofloxacin-resistant *Mycobacterium tuberculosis* by using species-specific assays for precursor rRNA. *Antimicrob. Agents Chemother.* **40:**1790–1795.
28. **Chaisson, R. E., P. Keiser, M. Pierce, W. J. Fessel, J. Ruskin, C. Lahart, C. A. Benson, K. Meek, N. Siepman, and J. C. Craft.** 1997. Clarithromycin and ethambutol with or without clofazimine for the treatment of bacteremic *Mycobacterium avium* complex disease in patients with HIV infection. *AIDS* **11:**311–317.
29. **Chen, C. H., J. F. Shih, P. J. Lindholm-Levy, and L. B. Heifets.** 1989. Minimal inhibitory concentrations of rifabutin, ciprofloxacin, and ofloxacin against *Mycobacterium tuberculosis* isolated before treatment of patients in Taiwan. *Am. Rev. Respir. Dis.* **140:**987–989.
30. **Chiu, J., J. Nussbaum, S. Bozette, J. G. Tilles, L. S. Young, J. Leedom, P. N. R. Heseltine, and J. A. McCutchan.** 1990. Treatment of disseminated *Mycobacterium avium* complex infection in AIDS with amikacin, ethambutol, rifampin, and ciprofloxacin. *Ann. Intern. Med.* **113:**358–361.
31. **Choucino, C., S. A. Goodman, J. P. Greer, R. S. Stein, S. N. Wolff, and J. S. Dummer.** 1996. Nocardial infections in bone marrow transplant recipients. *Clin. Infect. Dis.* **23:**1012–1019.
32. **Collins, L., and S. G. Franzblau.** 1997. Microplate alamar blue assay versus BACTEC 460 system for high-throughput screening of compounds against *Mycobacterium tuberculosis* and *Mycobacterium avium. Antimicrob. Agents Chemother.* **41:**1004–1009.
33. **Cooksey, R. C., J. T. Crawford, W. R. Jacobs, Jr., and T. M. Shinnick.** 1993. A rapid method for screening antimicrobial agents for activities against a strain of *Mycobacterium tuberculosis* expressing firefly luciferase. *Antimicrob. Agents Chemother.* **37:**1348–1352.
34. **Cooksey, R. C., G. P. Morlock, S. Glickman, and J. T. Crawford.** 1997. Evaluation of a line probe assay kit for

characterization of *rpoB* mutations in rifampin-resistant *Mycobacterium tuberculosis* isolates from New York City. *J. Clin. Microbiol.* **35:**1281–1283.

35. **Crofton, J., and D. A. Mitchison.** 1948. Streptomycin resistance in pulmonary tuberculosis. *Br. Med. J.* **2:**1009–1015.

36. **David, H. L.** 1970. Probability distribution of drug-resistant mutants in unselected populations of *Mycobacterium tuberculosis.* *Appl. Microbiol.* **20:**810–814.

37. **Davidson, L. A., and K. Takayama.** 1979. Isoniazid inhibition of the synthesis of monosaturated long-chain fatty acids in *Mycobacterium tuberculosis* H37Ra. *Antimicrob. Agents Chemother.* **16:**104–105.

38. **Davidson, P. D.** 1987. Drug resistance and the selection of therapy for tuberculosis. *Am. Rev. Respir. Dis.* **136:**255–257.

39. **Davidson, P. T.** 1989. The diagnosis and management of disease caused by *M. avium* complex, *M. kansasii,* and other mycobacteria, p. 431–443. *In* D. E. Snider, Jr. (ed.), *Clinics in Chest Medicine,* vol. 10. The W. B. Saunders Co., Philadelphia, Pa.

40. **Davies, A. P., O. J. Billington, T. D. McHugh, D. A. Mitchison, and S. H. Gillespie.** 2000. Comparison of phenotypic and genotypic methods for pyrazinamide susceptibility testing with *Mycobacterium tuberculosis. J Clin. Microbiol.* **38:**3686–3688.

41. **Davis, W. B., and M. M. Weber.** 1977. Specificity of isoniazid on growth inhibition and competition for an oxidized nicotiniamide adenine dinucleotide regulatory site on the electron transport pathway in *Mycobacterium phlei. Antimicrob. Agents Chemother.* **12:**213–218.

42. **De Beenhouwer, H., Z. Lhiang, G. Jannes, W. Mijs, L. Machtelinckx, R. Rossau, H. Traore, and F. Portaels.** 1995. Rapid detection of rifampicin resistance in sputum and biopsy specimens from tuberculosis patients by PCR and line probe assay. *Tubercle Lung Dis.* **76:**425–430.

43. **Deretic, V., W. Philipp, S. Dhandayuthapani, M. H. Mudd, R. Curcic, T. Garbe, B. Heym, L. E. Via, and S. T. Cole.** 1995. *Mycobacterium tuberculosis* is a natural mutant with an inactivated oxidative-stress regulatory gene: implications for sensitivity to isoniazid. *Mol. Microbiol.* **17:**889–900.

44. **Dhandayuthapani, S., M. Mudd, and V. Deretic.** 1997. Interactions of OxyR with the promoter region of the *oxyR* and *ahpC* genes from *Mycobacterium leprae* and *Mycobacterium tuberculosis. J. Bacteriol.* **179:**2401–2409.

45. **Diaz-Infantes, M. S., M. J. Ruiz-Serrano, L. Martinez-Sanchez, A. Ortega, and E. Bouza.** 2000. Evaluation of the MB/BacT Mycobacterium Detection System for susceptibility testing of *Mycobacterium tuberculosis. J. Clin. Microbiol.* **38:**1988–1989.

46. **Drowart, A., C. L. Cambiaso, K. Huygen, E. Serruys, F. Portaels, E. Jann, and J. P. Van Vooren.** 1997. Detection of rifampicin and isoniazid resistances of *Mycobacterium tuberculosis* strains by particle counting immunoassay (PACIA). *Int. J. Tubercle Lung Dis.* **1:**284–288.

47. **Dukes, C. S., J. Sugarman, J. P. Cegielski, G. J. Lallinger, and D. H. Mwakyusa.** 1992. Severe cutaneous hypersensitivity reactions during treatment of tuberculosis in patients with HIV infection in Tanzania. *Trop. Geogr. Med.* **44:**308–311.

48. **Eltringham, I. J., F. A. Drobniewski, J. A. Mangan, P. D. Butcher, and S. M. Wilson.** 1999. Evaluation of reverse transcription-PCR and a bacteriophage-based assay for rapid phenotypic detection of rifampin resistance in clinical isolates of *Mycobacterium tuberculosis. J. Clin. Microbiol.* **37:**3524–3527.

49. **Eltringham, I. J., S. M. Wilson, and F. A. Drobniewski.** 1999. Evaluation of a bacteriophage-based assay (phage amplified biologically assay) as a rapid screen for resistance to isoniazid, ethambutol, streptomycin, pyrazinamide, and ciprofloxacin among clinical isolates of *Mycobacterium tuberculosis. J. Clin. Microbiol.* **37:**3528–3532.

50. **Farr, B. M., and G. L. Mandell.** 1990. Rifamycins, p. 295–303. *In* G. L. Mandell, R. G. Douglas, Jr., and J. E. Bennett (ed.), *Principles and Practices of Infectious Diseases.* Churchill Livingstone, Inc., New York, N.Y.

51. **Felmlee, T. A., Q. Liu, A. C. Whelen, D. Williams, S. S. Sommer, and D. H. Persing.** 1995. Genotypic detection of *Mycobacterium tuberculosis* rifampin resistance: comparison of single-strand conformation polymorphism and dideoxy fingerprinting. *J. Clin. Microbiol.* **33:**1617–1623.

52. **Finken, M., P. Kirschner, A. Meier, A. Wrede, and E. C. Böttger.** 1993. Molecular basis of streptomycin resistance in *Mycobacterium tuberculosis:* alterations of the ribosomal protein S12 gene and point mutations within a functional 16S ribosomal RNA pseudoknot. *Mol. Microbiol.* **9:**1239–1246.

53. **Franzblau, S. G., R. S. Witzig, J. C. McLaughlin, P. Torres, G. Madico, A. Hernandez, M. T. Degnan, M. B. Cook, V. K. Quenzer, R. M. Ferguson, and R. H. Gilman.** 1998. Rapid, low-technology MIC determination with clinical *Mycobacterium tuberculosis* isolates by using the microplate Alamar Blue assay. *J. Clin. Microbiol.* **36:**362–366.

54. **Frieden, T. R., T. Sterling, A. Pablos-Mendez, J. O. Kilburn, G. M. Cauthen, and S. W. Doolery.** 1993. The emergence of drug-resistant tuberculosis in New York City. *N. Engl. J. Med.* **328:**521–526.

55. **Garcia, L., M. Alonso-Sanz, M. J. Rebollo, J. C. Tercero, and F. Chaves.** 2001. Mutations in the *rpoB* gene of rifampin-resistant *Mycobacterium tuberculosis* isolates in Spain and their rapid detection by PCR-enzyme-linked immunosorbent assay. *J. Clin. Microbiol.* **39:**1813–1818.

56. **Gomez-Flores, R., S. Gupta, R. Tamez-Guerra, and R. T. Mehta.** 1995. Determination of MICs for *Mycobacterium avium-M. intracellulare* complex in liquid medium by a colorimetric method. *J. Clin. Microbiol.* **33:**1842–1846.

57. **Good, R. C.** 1985. Opportunistic pathogens in the genus *Mycobacterium. Annu. Rev. Microbiol.* **39:**347–369.

58. **Grosset, J. H.** 1992. Treatment of tuberculosis in HIV infection. *Tubercle Lung Dis.* **73:**378–383.

59. **Guerrero, C., L. Stockman, F. Marchesi, T. Bodmer, G. D. Roberts, and A. Telenti.** 1994. Evaluation of the *rpoB* gene in rifampicin-susceptible and resistant *Mycobacterium avium* and *Mycobacterium intracellulare. J. Antimicrob. Chemother.* **33:**661–663.

60. **Guthertz, L. S., M. E. Griffith, E. G. Ford, J. M. Janda, and T. F. Midura.** 1988. Quality control or individual components used in Middlebrook 7H10 medium for mycobacterial susceptibility testing. *J. Clin. Microbiol.* **26:**2338–2342.

61. **Hacek, D.** 1992. Modified proportion agar dilution test for slowly growing mycobacteria, p. 5.13.1–5.13.15. *In* H. D. Isenberg (ed.), *Clinical Microbiology Procedures Handbook,* vol. 1. American Society for Microbiology, Washington, D.C.

62. **Hanna, B. A., A. Ebrahimzadeh, L. B. Elliott, M. A. Morgan, S. M. Novak, S. Rüsch-Gerdes, M. Acio, D. F. Dunbar, T. M. Holmes, C. H. Rexer, C. Savthyakumar, and A. M. Vannier.** 1999. Multicenter evaluation of the BACTEC MGIT 960 system for recovery of mycobacteria. *J. Clin. Microbiol.* **37:**748–752.

63. **Havlir, D. V., M. P. Dube, F. R. Sattler, D. N. Forthal, C. A. Kemper, M. W. Dunne, D. M. Parenti, J. P. Lavelle, A. White, M. D. Witt, S. A. Bozzette, J. A. McCutchan and the California Collaborative Treatment Group.** 1996. Prophylaxis against disseminated *Mycobac-*

terium avium complex with weekly azithromycin, daily rifabutin, or both. *N. Engl. J. Med.* **335:**392–398.

64. **Hawkins, J. E.** 1984. Drug susceptibility testing, p. 177–193. *In* G. P. Kubica and L. G. Wayne (ed.), *The Mycobacteria: a Sourcebook,* part A. Marcel Dekker, Inc., New York, N.Y.

65. **Hawkins, J. E.** 1986. Non-weekend schedule for BACTEC susceptibility testing of *Mycobacterium tuberculosis. J. Clin. Microbiol.* **23:**934–937.

66. **Hawkins, J. E., R. C. Good, G. P. Kubica, P. R. Gangadharam, H. M. Gruft, and K. D. Stottmeier.** 1983. The levels of service concept in mycobacteriology. *Am. Thorac. Soc. News* **9:**19–25.

67. **Hawkins, J. E., R. J. Wallace, Jr., and B. A. Brown.** 1991. Antibacterial susceptibility tests: mycobacteria, p. 1138–1152. *In* A. Balows, W. J. Hausler, Jr., K. L. Herrmann, H. D. Isenberg, and H. J. Shadomy (ed.), *Manual of Clinical Microbiology,* 5th ed. American Society for Microbiology, Washington, D.C.

68. **Heifets, L., and T. Sanchez.** 2000. New agar medium for testing susceptibility of *Mycobacterium tuberculosis* to pyrazinamide. *J. Clin. Microbiol.* **38:**1498–1501.

69. **Heifets, L., T. Sanchez, J. Vanderkolk, and V. Pham.** 1999. Development of rifapentine susceptibility tests for *Mycobacterium tuberculosis. Antimicrob. Agents Chemother.* **43:**25–28.

70. **Heifets, L. B.** 1991. *Drug Susceptibility in the Chemotherapy of Mycobacterial Infections,* p. 212. CRC Press, Inc. Boca Raton, Fla.

71. **Heifets, L. B., and M. D. Iseman.** 1985. Determination of in vitro susceptibility of mycobacteria to ansamycin. *Am. Rev. Respir. Dis.* **132:**710–711.

72. **Heifets, L. B., M. D. Iseman, P. J. Lindholm-Levy, and W. Kanes.** 1985. Determination of ansamycin MICs for *Mycobacterium avium* complex in liquid medium by radiometric and conventional methods. *Antimicrob. Agents Chemother.* **28:**570–575.

73. **Heym, B., Y. Zhang, S. Poulet, D. Young, and S. T. Cole.** 1993. Characterization of the *katG* gene encoding a catalase-peroxidase required for isoniazid susceptibility of *Mycobacterium tuberculosis. J. Bacteriol.* **175:**4255–4259.

74. **Hillar, A., and P. C. Loewen.** 1995. Comparison of isoniazid oxidation catalyzed by bacterial catalase-peroxidases and horseradish peroxidase. *Arch. Biochem. Biophys.* **323:** 438–446.

75. **Hoffner, S. E., M. Kratz, B. Olsson-Liljequist, S. B. Svenson, and G. Källenius.** 1989. In-vitro synergistic activity between ethambutol and fluorinated quinolones against *Mycobacterium avium* complex. *J. Antimicrob. Chemother.* **24:**317–324.

76. **Hoffner, S. E., S. B. Svenson, and A. E. Beezer.** 1990. Microcalorimetric studies of the initial interaction between antimycobacterial drugs and *Mycobacterium avium. J. Antimicrob. Chemother.* **25:**353–359.

77. **Honore, N., and S. T. Cole.** 1993. Molecular basis of rifampin resistance in *Mycobacterium leprae. Antimicrob. Agents Chemother.* **37:**414–418.

78. **Howard, W. L., F. Maresh, E. E. Mueller, S. A. Yanitelli, and G. F. Woodruff.** 1949. The role of pulmonary cavitation in the development of bacterial resistance to streptomycin. *Am. Rev. Tuberc.* **59:**391–401.

79. **Howlett, H. S., J. B. O'Connor, J. F. Sadusk, J. E. Swift, and F. A. Beardsley.** 1949. Sensitivity of tubercle bacilli to streptomycin: the influence of various factors upon the emergence of resistant strains. *Am. Rev. Tuberc.* **59:**402–414.

80. **Hunt, J. M., G. D. Roberts, L. Stockman, T. A. Felmlee, and D. H. Persing.** 1994. Detection of a genetic locus encoding resistance to rifampin in mycobacterial cultures

and in clinical specimens. *Diagn. Microbiol. Infect. Dis.* **18:**219–227.

81. **Inderlied, C. B.** 1994. Antimycobacterial susceptibility testing: present practices and future trends. *Eur. J. Clin. Micrbiol. Infect. Dis.* **13:**980–993.

82. **Inderlied, C. B., C. A. Kemper, and L. E. M. Bermudez.** 1993. The *Mycobacterium avium* complex. *Clin. Microbiol. Rev.* **6:**266–310.

83. **Inderlied, C. B., P. T. Kolonski, M. Wu, and L. S. Young.** 1989. In vitro and in vivo activity of azithromycin (CP 62,993) against the *Mycobacterium avium* complex. *J. Infect. Dis.* **159:**994–997.

84. **Inderlied, C. B., and K. A. Nash.** 1996. Antimycobacterial agents: in vitro susceptibility testing, spectra of activity, mechanisms of action and resistance, and assays for activity in biologic fluids, p. 127–175. *In* V. Lorian (ed.), *Antibiotics in Laboratory Medicine,* 4th ed. The Williams & Wilkins Co., Baltimore, Md.

85. **Jacobs, W. R., Jr., R. G. Barletta, R. Udani, J. Chan, G. Kalkut, G. Sosne, T. Kieser, G. J. Sarkis, G. F. Hatfull, and B. R. Bloom.** 1993. Rapid assessment of drug susceptibilities of *Mycobacterium tuberculosis* by means of luciferase reporter phages. *Science* **260:**819–822.

86. **Joloba, M. L., S. Bajaksouzian, and M. R. Jacobs.** 2000. Evaluation of Etest for susceptibility testing of *Mycobacterium tuberculosis. J. Clin. Microbiol.* **38:**3834–3836.

87. **Källenius, G., S. G. Svenson, and S. E. Hoffner.** 1989. Ethambutol: a key for *Mycobacterium avium* complex chemotherapy. *Am. Rev. Respir. Dis.* **140:**264.

88. **Kapur, V., L. L. Li, S. Iordanescu, M. R. Hamrick, A. Wanger, B. N. Kreiswirth, and J. M. Musser.** 1994. Characterization by automated DNA sequencing of mutations in the gene (*rpoB*) encoding the RNA polymerase beta subunit in rifampin-resistant *Mycobacterium tuberculosis* strains from New York City and Texas. *J. Clin. Microbiol.* **32:**1095–1098.

89. **Kelley, C. L., D. A. Rouse, and S. L. Morris.** 1997. Analysis of *ahpC* gene mutations in isoniazid-resistant clinical isolates of *Mycobacterium tuberculosis. Antimicrob. Agents Chemother.* **41:**2057–2058.

90. **Kenney, T. J., and G. Churchward.** 1994. Cloning and sequence analysis of the *rpsL* and *rpsG* genes of *Mycobacterium smegmatis* and characterization of mutations causing resistance to streptomycin. *J. Bacteriol.* **176:**6153–6156.

91. **Kent, P. T., and G. P. Kubica.** 1985. *Public Health Mycobacteriology—a Guide for the Level III Laboratory.* U.S. Department of Health and Human Services, Center for Disease Control, Atlanta, Ga.

92. **Kontoyiannis, D. P., K. Ruoff, and D. C. Hooper.** 1998. *Nocardia* bacteremia. Report of 4 cases and review of the literature. *Medicine* **77:**255–267.

93. **Koontz, F.** 1994. E-test for susceptibility testing of rapid growing mycobacteria. *Diagn. Microbiol. Infect. Dis.* **19:** 183–186.

94. **Kubica, G. P., and W. E. Dye.** 1967. *Laboratory Methods for Clinical and Public Health Mycobacteriology.* U.S. Government Printing Office, Washington, D.C.

95. **Leysen, D. C., A. Haemers, and S. R. Pattyn.** 1989. Mycobacteria and the new quinolones. *Antimicrob. Agents Chemother.* **33:**1–5.

96. **Libonati, J. P., C. E. Stager, J. R. Davis, and S. H. Siddiqi.** 1988. Direct antimicrobial drug susceptibility testing of *Mycobacterium tuberculosis* by the radiometric method. *Diagn. Microbiol. Infect. Dis.* **10:**41–48.

97. **Magliozzo, R. S., and J. A. Marcinkeviciene.** 1997. The role of Mn(II)-peroxidase activity of mycobacterial catalase-peroxidase in activation of the antibiotic isoniazid. *J. Biol. Chem.* **272:**8867–8870.

98. **Mandell, G. L., R. G. Douglas, Jr., and J. E. Bennett.** 1992. *Handbook of Antimicrobial Therapy 1992.* Churchill Livingstone, Inc., New York, N.Y.

99. **Masur, H.** 1993. Recommendations on prophylaxis and therapy for disseminated *Mycobacterium avium* complex disease in patients infected with the human-immunodeficiency-virus. *N. Engl. J. Med.* **329:**898–904.

100. **McFarland, E. J., and D. R. Kuritzkes.** 1993. Clinical features and treatment of infection due to *Mycobacterium fortuitum/chelonae* complex, p. 188–202. *In* J. S. Remington and M. N. Swartz (ed.), *Current Clinical Topics in Infectious Diseases*, vol. 13. Blackwell Scientific Publications, Boston, Mass.

101. **McNerney, R., P. Kiepiela, K. S. Bishop, P. M. Nye, and N. G. Stocker.** 2001. Rapid screening of *Mycobacterium tuberculosis* for susceptibility to rifampin and streptomycin. *Int. J. Tuberc. Lung Dis.* **4:**69–75.

102. **Mdluli, K., D. R. Sherman, M. J. Hickey, B. N. Kreiswirth, S. Morris, C. K. Stover, and C. Barry III.** 1996. Biochemical and genetic data suggest that InhA is not the primary target for activated isoniazid in *Mycobacterium tuberculosis. J. Infect. Dis.* **174:**1085–1090.

103. **Mdluli, K., R. A. Slayden, Y. Zhu, S. Ramaswamy, X. Pan, D. Mead, D. D. Crane, J. M. Musser, and C. E. Barry III.** 1998. Inhibition of a *Mycobacterium tuberculosis*-ketoacyl ACP synthase by isoniazid. *Science* **280:**1607–1610.

104. **Mdluli, K., J. Swanson, E. Fischer, R. E. Lee, and C. E. Barry III.** 1998. Mechanisms involved in the intrinsic isoniazid resistance of *Mycobacterium avium. Mol. Microbiol.* **27:**1223–1233.

105. **Meier, A., P. Kirschner, B. Springer, V. A. Steingrube, B. A. Brown, R. J. Wallace, Jr., and E. C. Böttger.** 1994. Identification of mutations in 23S rRNA gene of clarithromycin-resistant *Mycobacterium intracellulare. Antimicrob. Agents Chemother.* **38:**381–384.

106. **Mikhailovich, V. M., S. A. Lapa, D. A. Gryadunov, B. N. Strizhkov, A. Y. Sobolev, O. L. Skotnikova, O. A. I. Rtuganova, A. M. Moroz, V. I. Litvinov, L. K. Shipina, M. A. Vladimirskii, L. N. Chernousova, V. V. Erokhin, and A. D. Mirzabekov.** 2001. Detection of rifampicin-resistant *Mycobacterium tuberculosis* strains by hybridization polymerase chain reaction on a specialized TB-microchip. *Bull. Exp. Biol. Med.* **131:**94–98.

107. **Miller, M. A., L. Thibert, F. Desjardins, S. H. Siddiqi, and A. Dascal.** 1996. Growth inhibition of *Mycobacterium tuberculosis* by polyoxyethylene stearate present in the BACTEC pyrazinamide susceptibility test. *J. Clin. Microbiol.* **34:**84–86.

108. **Miller, M. A., L. Thibert, F. Desjardins, S. H. Siddiqi, and A. Dascal.** 1995. Testing of susceptibility of *Mycobacterium tuberculosis* to pyrazinamide: comparison of Bactec method with pyrazinamidase assay. *J. Clin. Microbiol.* **33:**2468–2470.

109. **Mitchison, D. A.** 1979. Basic mechanisms of chemotherapy. *Chest* **76**(Suppl.):771–781.

110. **Mitchison, D. A.** 1992. The Garrod Lecture. Understanding the chemotherapy of tuberculosis-current problems. *J. Antimicrob. Chemother.* **29:**477–493.

111. **Mizuguchi, Y., M. Ogawa, and T. Udou.** 1985. Morphological changes induced by β-lactam antibiotics in *Mycobacterium avium-intracellulare* complex. *Antimicrob. Agents Chemother.* **27:**541–547.

112. **Moore, A. V., S. M. Kirk, S. M. Callister, G. H. Mazurek, and R. F. Schell.** 1999. Safe determination of susceptibility of *Mycobacterium tuberculosis* to antimycobacterial agents by flow cytometry. *J. Clin. Microbiol.* **37:**479–483.

113. **Morlock, G. P., J. T. Crawford, W. R. Butler, S. E. Brim, D. Sikes, G. H. Mazurek, C. L. Woodley, and R. C. Cooksey.** 2000. Phenotypic characterization of *pncA* mutants of *Mycobacterium tuberculosis. Antimicrob. Agents Chemother.* **44:**2291–2295.

114. **Morris, S., G. H. Bai, P. Suffys, L. Portillo-Gomez, M. Fairchok, and D. Rouse.** 1995. Molecular mechanisms of multiple drug resistance in clinical isolates of *Mycobacterium tuberculosis. J. Infect. Dis.* **171:**954–960.

115. **Mshana, R. N., G. Tadesse, G. Abate, and H. Miorner.** 1998. Use of 3-(4,5-dimethylthiazol-2-yl)-2,5-diphenyl tetrazolium bromide for rapid detection of rifampin-resistant *Mycobacterium tuberculosis. J. Clin. Microbiol.* **36:**1214–1219.

116. **Musser, J. M.** 1995. Antimicrobial agent resistance in mycobacteria: molecular genetic insights. *Clin. Microbiol. Rev.* **8:**496–514.

117. **Nair, J., D. A. Rouse, G. H. Bai, and S. L. Morris.** 1993. The *rpsL* gene and streptomycin resistance in single and multiple drug-resistant strains of *Mycobacterium tuberculosis. Mol. Microbiol.* **10:**521–527.

118. **Nash, K. A., A. Gaytan, and C. B. Inderlied.** 1997. Detection of rifampin resistance in *Mycobacterium tuberculosis* by use of a rapid, simple, and specific RNA/RNA mismatch assay. *J. Infect. Dis.* **176:**533–536.

119. **Nash, K. A., and C. B. Inderlied.** 1995. Genetic basis of macrolide resistance in *Mycobacterium avium* isolated from patients with disseminated disease. *Antimicrob. Agents Chemother.* **39:**2625–2630.

120. **National Committee for Clinical Laboratory Standards.** 2000. *Methods for Dilution Antimicrobial Susceptibility Tests for Bacteria That Grow Aerobically*, 4th ed., vol. M7-A5. NCCLS, Villanova, Pa.

121. **National Committee for Clinical Laboratory Standards.** 2000. *Susceptibility Testing of Mycobacteria. Nocardia and Other Aerobic Actinomycetes; Tentative Standard M24-T2.* NCCLS, Villanova, Pa.

122. **Nightingale, S. D., W. D. Cameron, F. M. Gordin, P. M. Sullam, D. L. Cohn, R. E. Chaisson, L. J. Eron, P. D. Saprti, D. Bihari, D. L. Kaufman, J. J. Stern, D. D. Pearce, W. G. Weinberg, A. LaMarca, and F. P. Siegel.** 1993. Two controlled trials of rifabutin prophylaxis against *Mycobacterium avium* complex infection in AIDS. *N. Engl. J. Med.* **329:**828–833.

123. **Nitta, A. T., P. T. Davidson, M. L. de Koning, and R. J. Kilman.** 1996. Misdiagnosis of multidrug-resistant tuberculosis possibly due to laboratory-related errors. *JAMA* **276:**1980–1983.

124. **Nunn, P., J. Porter, and P. Winstanley.** 1993. Thiacetazone—avoid like poison or use with care. *Trans. R. Soc. Trop. Med. Hyg.* **87:**578–582.

125. **Oh, Y. K., and R. M. Straubinger.** 1996. Intracellular fate of *Mycobacterium avium*: use of dual-label spectrofluorometry to investigate the influence of bacterial viability and opsonization on phagosomal pH and phagosome-lysosome interaction. *Infect. Immun.* **64:**319–325.

126. **Perutz, M. F.** 1994. The white plague. *N. Y. Rev. Books* **XLI:**35–39.

127. **Petersen, E. A., J. B. Grayson, E. M. Hersh, R. T. Dorr, S. M. Chiang, M. Oka, and R. T. Proffitt.** 1996. Liposomal amikacin: improved treatment of *Mycobacterium avium* complex infection in the beige mouse model. *J. Antimicrob. Chemother.* **38:**819–828.

128. **Pfyffer, G. E., D. A. Bonato, A. Ebrahimzadeh, W. Gross, J. Hotaling, J. Kornblum, A. Laszlo, G. Roberts, M. Salfinger, F. Wittwer, and S. Siddiqi.** 1999. Multicenter laboratory validation of susceptibility testing of *Mycobacterium tuberculosis* against classical second-line and newer antimicrobial drugs by using the radiometric

BACTEC 460 technique and the proportion method with solid media. *J. Clin. Microbiol.* **37:**3179–3186.

129. **Pfyffer, G. E., F. Palicova, and S. Rüsch-Gerdes.** 2002. Testing of susceptibility of *Mycobacterium tuberculosis* to pyrazinamide with the nonradiometric BACTEC MGIT 960 system. *J. Clin. Microbiol.* **40:**1670–1674.

130. **Pfyffer, G. E., H. M. Welscher, P. Kissling, C. Cieslak, M. J. Casal, J. Gutierrez, and S. Rüsch-Gerdes.** 1997. Comparison of the Mycobacteria Growth Indicator Tube (MGIT) with radiometric and solid culture for recovery of acid-fast bacilli. *J. Clin. Microbiol.* **35:**364–368.

131. **Piatek, A. S., A. Telenti, M. R. Murray, H. El-Hajj, W. R. Jacobs, Jr., F. R. Kramer, and D. Alland.** 2000. Genotypic analysis of *Mycobacterium tuberculosis* in two distinct populations using molecular beacons: implications for rapid susceptibility testing. *Antimicrob. Agents Chemother.* **44:**103–110.

132. **Pierce, M., S. Crampton, D. Henry, L. Heifets, A. LaMarca, M. Montecalvo, G. P. Wormser, H. Jablonowski, J. Jemsek, M. Cynamon, B. G. Yangco, G. Notario, and J. C. Craft.** 1996. A randomized trial of clarithromycin as prophylaxis against disseminated *Mycobacterium avium* complex infection in patients with advanced acquired immunodeficiency syndrome. *N. Engl. J. Med.* **335:**384–391.

133. **Piersimoni, C., C. Scarparo, A. Callegaro, C. P. Tosi, D. Nista, S. Bornigia, M. Scagnelli, A. Rigon, G. Ruggiero, and A. Goglio.** 2001. Comparison of MB/Bact alert 3D system with radiometric BACTEC system and Lowenstein-Jensen medium for recovery and identification of mycobacteria from clinical specimens: a multicenter study. *J. Clin. Microbiol.* **39:**651–657.

134. **Pyle, M.** 1947. Relative number of resistant tubercle bacilli in sputa of patients before and during treatment with streptomycin. *Proc. Mayo Clin.* **22:**465–473.

135. **Rastogi, N., C. Frehel, A. Ryter, H. Ohayon, M. Lesourd, and H. L. David.** 1981. Multiple drug resistance in *Mycobacterium avium*: is the wall architecture responsible for the exclusion of antimicrobial agents? *Antimicrob. Agents Chemother.* **20:**666–677.

136. **Rastogi, N., K. S. Goh, and A. Bryskier.** 1994. Activities of roxithromycin used alone and in combination with ethambutol, rifampin, amikacin, ofloxacin, and clofazimine against *Mycobacterium avium* complex. *Antimicrob. Agents Chemother.* **38:**1433–1438.

137. **Rathman, M., M. D. Sjaastad, and S. Falkow.** 1996. Acidification of phagosomes containing *Salmonella typhimurium* in murine macrophages. *Infect. Immun.* **64:**2765–2773.

138. **Revel Viravau, V., Q. C. Truong, N. Moreau, V. Jarlier, and W. Sougakoff.** 1996. Sequence analysis, purification, and study of inhibition by 4-quinolones of the DNA gyrase from *Mycobacterium smegmatis*. *Antimicrob. Agents Chemother.* **40:**2054–2061.

139. **Rinder, H., K. Feldmann, E. Tortoli, J. Grosset, M. Casal, E. Richter, M. Rifai, V. Jarlier, M. Vaquero, S. Rüsch-Gerdes, E. Cambau, J. Gutierrez, and T. Loscher.** 1999. Culture-independent prediction of isoniazid resistance in *Mycobacterium tuberculosis* by katG gene analysis directly from sputum samples. *Mol. Diagn.* **4:**145–152.

140. **Riska, P. F., Y. Su, S. Bardarov, L. Freundlich, G. Sarkis, G. Hatfull, C. Carriere, V. Kumar, J. Chan, and W. R. Jacobs, Jr.** 1999. Rapid film-based determination of antibiotic susceptibilities of *Mycobacterium tuberculosis* strains by using a luciferase reporter phage and the Bronx Box. *J. Clin. Microbiol.* **37:**1144–1149.

141. **Ruiz, P., F. J. Zerolo, and M. J. Casal.** 2000. Comparison of susceptibility testing of *Mycobacterium tuberculosis* using the ESP culture system II with that using the BACTEC method. *J. Clin. Microbiol.* **38:**4663–4664.

142. **Rüsch-Gerdes, S., C. Domehl, G. Nardi, M. R. Gismondo, H. M. Welscher, and G. E. Pfyffer.** 1999. Multicenter evaluation of the mycobacteria growth indicator tube for testing susceptibility of *Mycobacterium tuberculosis* to first-line drugs. *J. Clin. Microbiol.* **37:**45–48.

143. **Russel, W. R., and G. Middlebrook.** 1961. *Chemotherapy of Tuberculosis.* Charles C Thomas, Springfield, Ill.

144. **Saito, H., K. Sato, and H. Tomioka.** 1988. Comparative in vitro and in vivo activity of rifabutin and rifampicin against *Mycobacterium avium* complex. *Tubercle* **69:**187–192.

145. **Salfinger, M., and L. B. Heifets.** 1988. Determination of pyrazinamide MICs for *Mycobacterium tuberculosis* at different pHs by the radiometric method. *Antimicrob. Agents Chemother.* **32:**1002–1004.

146. **Salfinger, M., L. B. Reller, B. Demchuk, and Z. T. Johnson.** 1989. Rapid radiometric method for pyrazinamide susceptibility testing of M. *tuberculosis*. *Res. Microbiol.* **140:**301–309.

147. **Sanford, J. P.** 2001. *Guide to Antimicrobial Therapy.* Antimicrobial Therapy, Inc., Dallas, Tex.

148. **Schentag, J. J., and C. H. Ballow.** 1991. Tissue-directed pharmacokinetics. *Am. J. Med.* **91:**5S–11S.

149. **Scorpio, A., D. Collins, D. Whipple, D. Cave, J. Bates, and Y. Zhang.** 1997. Rapid differentiation of bovine and human tubercle bacilli based on a characteristic mutation in the bovine pyrazinamidase gene. *J. Clin. Microbiol.* **35:**106–110.

150. **Scorpio, A., P. Lindholm Levy, L. Heifets, R. Gilman, S. Siddiqi, M. Cynamon, and Y. Zhang.** 1997. Characterization of pncA mutations in pyrazinamide-resistant *Mycobacterium tuberculosis*. *Antimicrob. Agents Chemother.* **41:**540–543.

151. **Scorpio, A., and Y. Zhang.** 1996. Mutations in pncA, a gene encoding pyrazinamidase/nicotinamidase, cause resistance to the antituberculous drug pyrazinamide in tubercle bacillus. *Nat. Med.* **2:**662–667.

152. **Shafran, S. D., J. Singer, D. P. Zarowny, P. Phillips, I. Salit, S. L. Walmsley, I. W. Fong, M. J. Gill, A. R. Rachlis, R. G. Lalonde, M. M. Fanning, C. M. Tsoukas, and the Canadian HIV Trials Network Protocol 010 Study Group.** 1996. A comparison of two regimens for the treatment of *Mycobacterium avium* complex bacteremia in AIDS: rifabutin, ethambutol, and clarithromycin versus rifampin, ethambutol, clofazimine, and ciprofloxacin. *N. Engl. J. Med.* **335:**377–383.

153. **Siddiqi, S. H.** 1992. Radiometric (Bactec) tests for slowly growing mycobacteria, p. 5.14.1–5.14.25. *In* H. D. Isenberg (ed.), *Clinical Microbiology Procedures Handbook*, vol. 1. American Society for Microbiology, Washington, D.C.

154. **Siddiqi, S. H., J. P. Libonati, M. E. Carter, N. M. Hooper, J. F. Baker, C. C. Hwangbo, and L. E. Warfel.** 1988. Enhancement of mycobacterial growth in Middlebrook 7H12 medium by polyoxyethylene stearate. *Curr. Microbiol.* **17:**105–110.

155. **Sirgel, F. A., F. J. Botha, D. P. Parkin, B. W. Van de Wal, R. Schall, P. R. Donald, and D. A. Mitchison.** 1997. The early bactericidal activity of ciprofloxacin in patients with pulmonary tuberculosis. *Am. J. Respir. Crit. Care Med.* **156:**901–905.

156. **Sreevatsan, S., X. Pan, Y. Zhang, V. Deretic, and J. M. Musser.** 1997. Analysis of the oxyR-ahpC region in isoniazid-resistant and -susceptible *Mycobacterium tuberculosis* complex organisms recovered from diseased humans and animals in diverse localities. *Antimicrob. Agents Chemother.* **41:**600–606.

157. Sreevatsan, S., X. Pan, Y. Zhang, B. N. Kreiswirth, and J. M. Musser. 1997. Mutations associated with pyrazinamide resistance in *pncA* of *Mycobacterium tuberculosis* complex organisms. *Antimicrob. Agents Chemother.* **41:** 636–640.

158. Sreevatsan, S., K. E. Stockbauer, X. Pan, B. N. Kreiswirth, S. L. Moghazeh, W. Jacobs, Jr., A. Telenti, and J. M. Musser. 1997. Ethambutol resistance in *Mycobacterium tuberculosis:* critical role of *embB* mutations. *Antimicrob. Agents Chemother.* **41:**1677–1681.

159. Straus, W. L., S. M. Ostroff, D. B. Jernigan, T. E. Kiehn, E. M. Sordillo, D. Armstrong, N. Boone, N. Schneider, J. O. Kilburn, V. A. Silcox, V. LaBombardi, and R. C. Good. 1994. Clinical and epidemiologic characteristics of *Mycobacterium haemophilum,* an emerging pathogen in immunocompromised patients. *Ann. Intern. Med.* **120:**118–125.

160. Sturgill-Koszycki, S., P. H. Schlesinger, P. Chakraborty, P. L. Haddix, H. L. Collins, A. K. Fok, R. D. Allen, S. L. Gluck, J. Heuser, and D. G. Russell. 1994. Lack of acidification in *Mycobacterium* phagosomes produced by exclusion of the vesicular proton-ATPase. *Science* **263:**678–681.

161. Takayama, K., and J. O. Kilburn. 1989. Inhibition of synthesis of arabinogalactan by ethambutol in *Mycobacterium smegmatis. Antimicrob. Agents Chemother.* **33:**1493–1499.

162. Takayama, K., and N. Qureshi. 1984. Structure and synthesis of lipids, p. 315–344. *In* G. P. Kubica and L. G. Wayne (ed.), *The Mycobacteria: a Sourcebook,* part A. Marcel Dekker, Inc., New York, N.Y.

163. Takiff, H. E., L. Salazar, C. Guerrero, W. Philipp, W. M. Huang, B. Kreiswirth, S. T. Cole, W. Jacobs, Jr., and A. Telenti. 1994. Cloning and nucleotide sequence of *Mycobacterium tuberculosis* gyrA and gyrB genes and detection of quinolone resistance mutations. *Antimicrob. Agents Chemother.* **38:**773–780.

164. Telenti, A., N. Honore, C. Bernasconi, J. March, A. Ortega, B. Heym, H. E. Takiff, and S. T. Cole. 1997. Genotypic assessment of isoniazid and rifampin resistance in *Mycobacterium tuberculosis:* a blind study at reference laboratory level. *J. Clin. Microbiol.* **35:**719–723.

165. Telenti, A., P. Imboden, F. Marchesi, D. Lowrie, S. Cole, M. J. Colston, L. Matter, K. Schopfer, and T. Bodmer. 1993. Detection of rifampin-resistance mutations in *Mycobacterium tuberculosis. Lancet* **341:**647–650.

166. Telenti, A., P. Imboden, F. Marchesi, T. Schmidheini, and T. Bodmer. 1993. Direct, automated detection of rifampin-resistant *Mycobacterium tuberculosis* by polymerase chain reaction and single-strand conformation polymorphism analysis. *Antimicrob. Agents Chemother.* **37:** 2054–2058.

167. Tenover, F. C., J. T. Crawford, R. E. Huebner, L. J. Geiter, C. R. Horsburgh, and R. C. Good. 1993. The resurgence of tuberculosis: is your laboratory ready? *J. Clin. Microbiol.* **31:**767–770.

168. Terashima, T., F. Sakamaki, N. Hasegawa, M. Kanazawa, and T. Kawashiro. 1994. Pulmonary infection due to *Mycobacterium xenopi. Intern. Med.* **33:**536–539.

169. Torres, M. J., A. Criado, J. C. Palomares, and J. Aznar. 2000. Use of real-time PCR and fluorimetry for rapid detection of rifampin and isoniazid resistance-associated mutations in *Mycobacterium tuberculosis. J. Clin. Microbiol.* **38:**3194–3199.

170. Troesch, A., H. Nguyen, C. G. Miyada, S. Desvarenne, T. R. Gingeras, P. M. Kaplan, P. Cros, and C. Mabilat. 1999. Mycobacterium species identification and rifampin resistance testing with high-density DNA probe arrays. *J. Clin. Microbiol.* **37:**49–55.

171. Wallace, R., Jr., A. Meier, B. A. Brown, Y. Zhang, P. Sander, G. O. Onyi, and E. C. Böttger. 1996. Genetic basis for clarithromycin resistance among isolates of *Mycobacterium chelonae* and *Mycobacterium abscessus. Antimicrob. Agents Chemother.* **40:**1676–1681.

172. Wallace, R. J., Jr. 1989. The clinical presentation, diagnosis, and therapy of cutaneous and pulmonary infections due to the rapidly growing mycobacteria, M. *fortuitum* and M. *chelonae. Clin. Chest Med.* **10:**419–429.

173. Wallace, R. J., Jr., J. M. Musser, S. I. Hull, V. A. Silcox, L. C. Steele, G. D. Forrester, A. Labidi, and R. K. Selander. 1989. Diversity and sources of rapidly growing mycobacteria associated with infections following cardiac surgery. *J. Infect. Dis.* **159:**708–716.

174. Wallace, R. J., Jr., D. R. Nash, M. Tsukamura, Z. M. Blacklock, and V. A. Silcox. 1988. Human disease due to *Mycobacterium smegmatis. J. Infect. Dis.* **158:**52 59.

175. Wang, J. Y., R. M. Burger, and K. Drlica. 1998. Role of superoxide in catalase-peroxidase-mediated isoniazid action against mycobacteria. *Antimicrob. Agents Chemother.* **42:**709–711.

176. Wanger, A., and K. Mills. 1996. Testing of *Mycobacterium tuberculosis* susceptibility to ethambutol, isoniazid, rifampin, and streptomycin by using Etest. *J. Clin. Microbiol.* **34:**1672–1676.

177. Watterson, S. A., S. M. Wilson, M. D. Yates, and F. A. Drobniewski. 1998. Comparison of three molecular assays for rapid detection of rifampin resistance in *Mycobacterium tuberculosis. J. Clin. Microbiol.* **36:**1969–1973.

178. Wayne, L. G., and H. A. Sramek. 1992. Agents of newly recognized or infrequently encountered mycobacterial diseases. *Clin. Microbiol. Rev.* **5:**1–25.

179. Wayne, L. G., and H. A. Sramek. 1994. Metronidazole is bactericidal to dormant cells of *Mycobacterium tuberculosis. Antimicrob. Agents Chemother.* **38:**2054–2058.

180. Williams, D. L., L. Spring, L. Collins, L. P. Miller, L. B. Heifets, P. R. Gangadharam, and T. P. Gillis. 1998. Contribution of *rpoB* mutations to development of rifamycin cross-resistance in *Mycobacterium tuberculosis. Antimicrob. Agents Chemother.* **42:**1853–1857.

181. Williams, D. L., L. Spring, T. P. Gillis, M. Salfinger, and D. H. Persing. 1998. Evaluation of a polymerase chain reaction-based universal heteroduplex generator assay for direct detection of rifampin susceptibility of *Mycobacterium tuberculosis* from sputum specimens. *Clin. Infect. Dis.* **26:**446–450.

182. Williams, D. L., C. Waguespack, K. Eisenach, J. T. Crawford, F. Portaels, M. Salfinger, C. M. Nolan, C. Abe, V. Sticht-Groh, and T. P. Gillis. 1994. Characterization of rifampin-resistance in pathogenic mycobacteria. *Antimicrob. Agents Chemother.* **38:**2380–2386.

183. Wilson, T. M., and D. M. Collins. 1996. *ahpC,* a gene involved in isoniazid resistance of the *Mycobacterium tuberculosis* complex. *Mol. Microbiol.* **19:**1025–1034.

184. Winder, F. G. 1982. Mode of action of the antimycobacterial agents and associated aspects of the molecular biology of the mycobacteria, p. 353–438. *In* C. Ratledge and J. Stanford (ed.), *The Biology of the Mycobacteria,* vol. 1. *Physiology, Identification and Classification.* Academic Press, Inc., New York, N.Y.

185. Winder, F. G., and P. B. Collins. 1969. The effect of isoniazid on nicotinamide nucleotide concentrations in tubercle bacilli. *Am. Rev. Respir. Dis.* **100:**101–103.

186. Winder, F. G., and P. B. Collins. 1968. The effect of isoniazid on nicotinamide nucleotide levels in *Mycobacterium bovis* strain BCG. *Am. Rev. Respir. Dis.* **97:**719–720.

187. Woodley, C. L. 1986. Evaluation of streptomycin and ethambutol concentrations for susceptibility testing of *Mycobacterium tuberculosis* by radiometric and conventional procedures. *J. Clin. Microbiol.* **23:**385–386.

188. **Woods, G. L., G. Fish, M. Plaunt, and T. Murphy.** 1997. Clinical evaluation of difco ESP culture system II for growth and detection of mycobacteria. *J. Clin. Microbiol.* **35:**121–124.

189. **Woods, G. L., and J. A. Washington, 3rd.** 1987. Mycobacteria other than *Mycobacterium tuberculosis:* review of microbiologic and clinical aspects. *Rev. Infect. Dis.* **9:**275–294.

190. **Yang, B., H. Koga, H. Ohno, K. Ogawa, M. Fukuda, Y. Hirakata, S. Maesaki, K. Tomono, T. Tashiro, and S. Kohno.** 1998. Relationship between antimycobacterial activities of rifampicin, rifabutin and KRM-1648 and *rpoB* mutations of *Mycobacterium tuberculosis. J. Antimicrob. Chemother.* **42:**621–628. (Erratum, **43:**613, 1999.)

191. **Young, L. S., O. G. Berlin, and C. B. Inderlied.** 1987. Activity of ciprofloxacin and other fluorinated quinolones against mycobacteria. *Am. J. Med.* **82:**23–26.

192. **Young, L. S., L. Wiviott, M. Wu, P. Kolonoski, R. Bolan, and C. B. Inderlied.** 1991. Azithromycin for treatment of *Mycobacterium avium-intracellulare* complex infection in patients with AIDS. *Lancet* **338:** 1107–1109.

193. **Zhang, Y., S. Dhandayuthapani, and V. Deretic.** 1996. Molecular basis for the exquisite sensitivity of *Mycobacterium tuberculosis* to isoniazid. *Proc. Natl. Acad. Sci. USA* **93:**13212–13216.

194. **Zhang, Y., B. Heym, B. Allen, D. Young, and S. Cole.** 1992. The catalase-peroxidase gene and isoniazid resistance of *Mycobacterium tuberculosis. Nature* **358:**591–593.

Special Phenotypic Methods for Detecting Antibacterial Resistance*

JANA M. SWENSON, JANET FICK HINDLER, AND JAMES H. JORGENSEN

74

Special phenotypic tests for detecting antibacterial resistance range from the rapid and simple spot β-lactamase test to the more time-consuming and complex minimum bactericidal concentration (MBC) assays. These tests may either supplement or replace traditional testing methods depending on the organism and the assay. This chapter describes tests for detection of high-level aminoglycoside resistance and acquired vancomycin resistance in enterococci, tests for detection of oxacillin resistance in staphylococci, tests for detection of β-lactamases in multiple organisms, and tests for determination of bactericidal activity.

Quality control information is given for all of the tests in each section; however, guidelines for the frequency of quality control testing are not provided, because they have not been determined and may vary depending on laboratory circumstances. A practical approach would be to perform quality control testing each day clinical isolates are tested or less frequently (e.g., weekly) once a laboratory has thoroughly documented that less frequent quality control testing can validate the reliability of the procedures. However, the College of American Pathologists recommends that quality control testing be done daily on β-lactamase tests. Quality control tests should be performed each time new lots of material are put into use.

TESTS TO DETECT RESISTANCE IN ENTEROCOCCI

Systemic enterococcal infections, such as endocarditis, are commonly treated with a cell wall-active agent (either a β-lactam drug or a glycopeptide such as vancomycin) and an aminoglycoside (usually gentamicin or streptomycin). These agents act synergistically to enhance killing (155). However, when an enterococcal strain is resistant to the cell wall-active agent or has high-level resistance (HLR) to the aminoglycoside, there is no synergism and combination therapy will not provide a bactericidal effect (107). Because of this, it is important to detect the presence of resistance

to both the aminoglycoside and the cell wall-active agent individually in order to predict the likelihood of synergy.

Detection of High-Level Resistance to Aminoglycosides

Because aminoglycosides have poor activity against enterococci (MICs range from 8 to 256 μg/ml), they cannot be used as single agents for therapy (54, 107). This intrinsic, moderate-level resistance is due to poor uptake of the aminoglycoside by the cell (107). Acquired aminoglycoside resistance in enterococci is due either to mutations resulting in decreased binding of the agent to the ribosome, as occurs with streptomycin (called ribosomal resistance), or, more commonly, to the acquisition of new genes that encode enzymes that modify aminoglycosides (called acquired resistance). Acquired aminoglycoside resistance usually corresponds to MICs that are significantly above the concentrations normally tested in routine susceptibility tests, e.g., ≥2,000 μg/ml for streptomycin and ≥500 μg/ml for gentamicin, and is designated HLR (107) (see also chapters 30 and 68).

Synergy between an aminoglycoside and a cell wall-active agent can be determined directly by performing complex time-kill studies (83) or can be predicted by using less cumbersome screening tests. Gentamicin and streptomycin are the only two agents that should be tested on a routine basis. All enterococcal isolates that are resistant to gentamicin are considered resistant to tobramycin and amikacin as well. Resistance to streptomycin is mediated by a different resistance mechanism, and, consequently, streptomycin resistance must be determined separately from gentamicin resistance. Isolates of *Enterococcus faecium* are intrinsically resistant to the synergistic actions of amikacin, kanamycin, tobramycin, and netilmicin with cell wall-active agents, irrespective of in vitro testing results for HLR (104). *Enterococcus faecalis* strains that are susceptible to gentamicin may be resistant to kanamycin and amikacin. In vitro tests with amikacin cannot reliably predict HLR to amikacin in *E. faecalis,* but kanamycin could be used to predict HLR to amikacin and kanamycin (143), although optimal methods for testing have not been determined. Recently, the genes for two new enzymes that mediate gentamicin resistance have been described, *aph2″-(Ic)* and *aph2″-(Id)* (22, 178), but neither of the enzymes is detected by the screening methods described below since their pres-

---

* This chapter contains information presented in chapter 121 by Jana M. Swenson, Janet A. Hindler, and Lance R. Peterson in the seventh edition of this Manual.

ence seems to lead to intermediate, not high-level, resistance. Only time-kill or molecular studies will detect the presence of these enzymes. The incidence of strains containing these two novel enzymes is unknown at present.

In 1992, the National Committee for Clinical Laboratory Standards (NCCLS) recognized that confusion existed about methods for detection of HLR to aminoglycosides in enterococci and subsequently published details of agar dilution, broth microdilution, and disk diffusion methods for detecting HLR. These methods are summarized in Table 1 and discussed below.

Agar Dilution Screening Method

Agar plates are prepared with brain heart infusion (BHI) agar supplemented with 500 μg of gentamicin per ml or 2,000 μg of streptomycin per ml (see chapter 70). The plates are inoculated by spotting 10 μl of a suspension that is equivalent to a 0.5 McFarland standard prepared from growth on an 18- to 24-h agar plate, giving a final inoculum of 10^6 CFU per spot. The plates are incubated for a full 24 h in ambient air. The presence of more than one colony or a haze of growth should be read as resistant. For streptomycin, the plates should be reincubated for an additional 24 h if there is no growth at 24 h. Mueller-Hinton agar (MHA), MHA plus 5% sheep blood, or dextrose phosphate agar may be substituted for BHI agar (128), but because growth is better on BHI agar, this is the preferred medium. Commercially prepared agar screen plates are available and have performed well (40, 139, 140). Kanamycin agar screen tests have not been as extensively evaluated and are not standardized, but it has been reported that for determining HLR to both amikacin and kanamycin in *E. faecalis*, kanamycin at 2,000 μg/ml in BHI agar can be used (143).

Broth Microdilution Screening Method

Broth microdilution plates are prepared with single wells containing BHI broth supplemented with 500 μg of gentamicin per ml or 1,000 μg of streptomycin per ml. The final inoculum concentration is that recommended for routine broth microdilution testing, i.e., 5×10^5 CFU/ml. The plates are incubated for 24 h in ambient air. For streptomycin, the plates should be reincubated for an additional 24 h if there is no growth at 24 h. Any growth is interpreted as denoting resistance.

The recommended streptomycin concentration for use in the broth microdilution screen is half that used in the agar dilution screen test. Because this test is often included as part of a routine gram-positive MIC panel, the inoculum is that commonly used in broth microdilution testing (5 × 10^5 CFU/ml). The total number of cells tested in the agar dilution screening procedure (1 × 10^6 CFU/spot) is 20-fold larger than that normally used in the broth microdilution test (5 × 10^4 CFU/0.1-ml well). In order to provide a test that uses a low inoculum and at the same time maximizes the detection of HLR to streptomycin, it was necessary to lower the concentration recommended for testing streptomycin from 2,000 to 1,000 μg/ml in the broth microdilution test. Because of poorer growth and the lower inoculum, Mueller-Hinton broth is inadequate for use in the broth microdilution screen test (159). The performance of other aminoglycosides in this test has not been evaluated.

Disk Diffusion Screening Method

The standard disk diffusion procedure (116) described in chapter 70 (with unsupplemented MHA) is used, except that special high-content disks (gentamicin at 120 μg and streptomycin at 300 μg) are required (144). Zones are measured after 18 to 24 h of incubation in ambient air at 35°C. Isolates with zone diameters of ≥10 mm are categorized as susceptible. The absence of a zone of inhibition corresponds to the presence of HLR. Strains with zone diameters from 7 to 9 mm usually display HLR, but a few are strains for which the MICs are only moderately elevated (159). Therefore, strains giving 7- to 9-mm zones should be tested by either the standard agar or broth microdilution screen method to determine susceptibility or resistance. High-content gentamicin and streptomycin disks are available commercially.

Quality Control

For both gentamicin and streptomycin, *E. faecalis* ATCC 29212 is used as the susceptible control strain and *E. faecalis* ATCC 51299 is used as the resistant control strain (158). Only *E. faecalis* ATCC 29212 is used for control of disk

TABLE 1 Screening methods for detecting vancomycin and high-level aminoglycoside resistance in enterococci

Parameter	Screening procedure			
	Vancomycin agar dilution	Aminoglycoside agar dilution	Aminoglycoside broth microdilution	Aminoglycoside disk diffusion
Medium	BHI agar	BHI agar	BHI broth	MHA
Inoculum	10^5–10^6 CFU/spot	10^6 CFU/spot	5×10^4 CFU/0.1 ml	0.5 McFarland[a]
Incubation (h)	24	24[b]	24[b]	18–24
Drug concn				
Gentamicin	NA[c]	500 μg/ml	500 μg/ml	120 μg/disk
Streptomycin	NA	2,000 μg/ml	1,000 μg/ml	300 μg/disk
Vancomycin	6 μg/ml	NA	NA	NA
End point	>1 colony	>1 colony	Any growth	6 mm = resistant, 7–9 mm = inconclusive,[d] ≥10 mm = susceptible

[a] NCCLS disk diffusion method (116).
[b] If streptomycin is negative at 24 h, reincubate for an additional 24 h.
[c] NA, not applicable.
[d] If the zone is 7 to 9 mm, the test is inconclusive and an agar or broth microdilution test should be performed to confirm susceptibility or resistance.

diffusion tests. The expected quality control limits are 16 to 23 mm for gentamicin (120-µg) disks and 14 to 20 mm for streptomycin (300-µg) disks (118).

Detection of Penicillin and Ampicillin Resistance

Compared to streptococci, for which penicillin MICs are usually ≤0.12 µg/ml, all enterococci are "relatively resistant" to β-lactams, with penicillin MICs usually ≥2 µg/ml (107). Isolates of *E. faecium* are inherently more resistant to penicillin than are isolates of *E. faecalis*; the usual MICs of penicillin for *E. faecium* are 16 to 64 µg/ml, whereas the usual MICs for *E. faecalis* are 2 to 4 µg/ml (44, 104). Ampicillin MICs are generally 1 dilution lower than penicillin MICs (46, 107). This intrinsic relative resistance, as well as higher levels of resistance to penicillin and ampicillin (MICs ≥16 µg/ml), has been associated with changes in penicillin-binding proteins (PBPs), including PBP 5 (39, 46, 107). In addition to changes in PBPs, resistance to β-lactam agents can be mediated by the production of β-lactamase (108), but this is much less common and has been found only in *E. faecalis*.

No screening tests have been described for detection of penicillin and ampicillin resistance. Routine antimicrobial susceptibility tests (see chapter 70) will detect the higher-level resistance due to changes in PBPs, and this will be evident as higher MICs or smaller zones of inhibition. However, routine tests (such as broth microdilution or disk diffusion) will not detect resistance due to β-lactamase in enterococci; an inoculum 100-fold greater than that routinely recommended (e.g., 10^7 CFU/ml) is necessary for resistance to be demonstrated by standard dilution methods (108, 136). The nitrocefin β-lactamase test is recommended for detection of strains that are resistant due to the production of β-lactamase (see "β-Lactamase Tests" below).

As defined by the NCCLS (115), resistance to penicillin and ampicillin corresponds to MICs of ≥16 µg/ml. The NCCLS recommends that results of penicillin susceptibility tests be used to predict susceptibility to ampicillin, amoxicillin, piperacillin, and β-lactam–β-lactamase inhibitor combinations (115, 116). In general, enterococcal strains resistant to penicillin or ampicillin as a result of altered PBPs (MICs, ≥16 µg/ml) should also be considered resistant to imipenem, regardless of the test results (54). β-Lactamase-producing enterococci should be considered resistant to penicillin, ampicillin, and the ureidopenicillins but susceptible to imipenem as well as β-lactam–β-lactamase inhibitor combinations (108).

Torres et al. (177) have recommended that in the absence of aminoglycoside resistance, strains of *E. faecium* for which penicillin MICs were ≤64 µg/ml should be considered potentially susceptible to synergy with an aminoglycoside. In addition, in a recent review, Murray (109) recommended that for strains of *E. faecium* categorized as resistant to both ampicillin and vancomycin, tests to determine the actual MICs might be worthwhile since strains for which ampicillin MICs are 16 to 64 µg/ml may be treatable with ampicillin. Additional clinical studies are needed to clarify the level of ampicillin and penicillin resistance that correlates with the absence of synergy. Currently, most commonly used antimicrobial susceptibility test systems do not include ampicillin concentrations above 16 µg/ml, so that it would be difficult to differentiate borderline resistance (ampicillin MICs, 16 to 32 µg/ml) from higher-level resistance (MICs, ≥64 µg/ml). For a β-lactamase-negative strain, testing of a single concentra-

tion of ampicillin or penicillin at 32 or 64 µg/ml by an agar or broth dilution method with Mueller-Hinton medium and an inoculum normally used for MIC testing (116) could help define the level of resistance. Since ampicillin MICs are generally 1 dilution lower than penicillin MICs (46), it is possible to encounter strains that appear to be susceptible to ampicillin but resistant to penicillin (169). The clinical significance of this finding is unknown. The ampicillin E-test strip covers concentrations from 0.016 to 256 µg/ml and has been shown to reliably detect ampicillin resistance in enterococci (150). This would also likely be true of the penicillin E-test strip.

Detection of Vancomycin Resistance

Definitions of vancomycin resistance in enterococci continue to undergo modifications as more is learned about the genetics and clinical significance of the resistance. As defined by the NCCLS, the MIC interpretive criteria for vancomycin are ≤4 µg/ml for susceptible, 8 to 16 µg/ml for intermediate, and ≥32 µg/ml for resistant. The three most common phenotypes of resistance are (i) high-level vancomycin resistance (MICs, ≥64 µg/ml) with accompanying teicoplanin resistance (MICs, ≥16 µg/ml) (VanA phenotype); (ii) moderate- to high-level vancomycin resistance (MICs, 16 to 512 µg/ml), most commonly without teicoplanin resistance (VanB phenotype); and (iii) intrinsic low-level resistance associated with *Enterococcus gallinarum* and *Enterococcus casseliflavus* (MICs, 2 to 32 µg/ml) (VanC phenotype) (88, 89, 90). Both the VanA and VanB phenotypes are most commonly seen in *E. faecalis* and *E. faecium* but have been found in other species (23). Three additional genotypes have been described recently, *vanD* (122, 128), *vanE* (38), and *vanG* (102). The VanD-type resistance, resulting in HLR to vancomycin (MICs, ≥64 µg/ml) and variable resistance to teicoplanin, has been found only in *E. faecium*. The VanE-type resistance, found in *E. faecalis*, is expressed as intermediate resistance to vancomycin (MICs, 16 µg/ml); the organism remains susceptible to teicoplanin. The VanG phenotype is similar to the VanD phenotype.

Many methods commonly used by clinical laboratories, including the disk diffusion method and the Vitek and MicroScan systems, have had problems detecting low-level vancomycin resistance (both the VanB and VanC types) in enterococci (35, 121, 141, 142, 162, 169, 187). However, most of these systems have shown some improvement in detection (21, 62, 72, 169), and both Vitek and the conventional (but not the Rapid) MicroScan systems are approved for use in the detection of vancomycin resistance in enterococci. In addition, the new Vitek 2 system appears to perform well for detection of vancomycin-resistant enterococci (42, 180). Recommendations for disk diffusion testing of vancomycin (including extending incubation to 24 h and examining zones under transmitted light), published in 1993, have improved the accuracy of the test (112, 160). When the new disk diffusion interpretive criteria for enterococci and vancomycin were proposed, the main problems were with detection of *vanC*-containing strains (160). This continues to be a problem, as reported in more recent studies (35, 85). However, the clinical significance of *vanC*-type resistance is unknown (see below).

Because of the potential failure of some systems to detect the vancomycin resistance expressed by certain enterococcal strains, an agar screening test first described by Willey et al. (187) was studied and adopted by the NCCLS in 1993 (111, 157) (Table 1). The sensitivity and specificity of the agar screen test were very high when it was first evaluated (96 to 99% and 100%, respectively). In recent evaluations, commercially prepared plates also performed well (35, 40, 182). However, there is some confusion among clinical laboratorians about the characterization of susceptibility or resistance for the *vanC*-containing enterococci, *E. gallinarum* and *E. casseliflavus*, because their growth is variable on the agar screen plate. Both of these species intrinsically contain a *vanC* gene, but the MICs of vancomycin for them range from 2 to 32 μg/ml (88). Whether the presence of this gene is associated with therapeutic failures is not known. Since the vancomycin MICs for these strains are often >4 μg/ml, the strains are likely to grow on the agar screen plates, where a higher inoculum and a richer medium may promote growth (40, 139, 157). Most strains of *vanC*-containing enterococci are motile at 30°C; *E. casseliflavus* is typically yellow pigmented. These characteristics have been used to distinguish *vanC*-containing enterococci from other species (12, 40, 41). However, some *E. gallinarum* and *E. casseliflavus* strains may be nonmotile. Because of this, a better test to differentiate them from *E. faecalis* and *E. faecium* is fermentation of 1% methyl-α-D-glucopyranoside (MGP). All *vanC*-containing enterococci acidify MGP, whereas *E. faecium* and *E. faecalis* do not (132) (see also chapter 30).

Agar Dilution Screen

Agar plates are prepared (see chapter 70 for a description of the general procedure for agar plate preparation) with BHI agar supplemented with 6 μg of vancomycin per ml. The plates are inoculated by spotting 1 to 10 μl of a suspension on the agar surface, using growth from an 18- to 24-h agar plate to make a suspension equivalent in turbidity to a 0.5 McFarland standard. The final inoculum is 10^5 to 10^6 CFU per spot. Recently, Jorgensen et al. (77) found that inoculation of the plates with a cotton swab dipped in the 0.5 McFarland suspension was equivalent to using a measured 1- or 10-μl aliquot. After inoculation, the plates are incubated for a full 24 h in ambient air at 35°C. The presence of more than one colony or a haze of growth indicates resistance.

Quality Control

For quality control, *E. faecalis* ATCC 29212 (no growth, i.e., susceptible) and *E. faecalis* ATCC 51299 (growth, i.e., resistant) should be tested (158). Plates made with BHI agars from certain manufacturers may allow light growth of *E. faecalis* ATCC 29212, especially if the higher inoculum (10 μl) is used or the plates are held longer than 24 h.

Reporting Resistance in Enterococci

For any serious enterococcal infection, results of the screen for HLR to gentamicin and streptomycin must be reported in concert with the results of the testing of the cell wall-active agent, because synergy would not be expected if any one of the agents reported is resistant. Helpful suggestions on reporting the results of enterococcal tests are given by Hindler and Sahm (54).

OXACILLIN DISK SCREEN TEST FOR DETECTION OF PENICILLIN RESISTANCE IN PNEUMOCOCCI

A screening test in which a 1-μg oxacillin disk is used to detect penicillin resistance in pneumococci was first de-

scribed following an outbreak caused by *Streptococcus pneumoniae* resistant to multiple antimicrobial agents in South Africa in the 1970s (29, 63, 161). Since then, this test has been used extensively and shown to be highly sensitive but not specific for detection of nonsusceptible pneumococci (30). Strains identified as nonsusceptible by this method may in fact be penicillin susceptible, intermediate, or resistant. Penicillin MIC tests must be performed on any strain that produces a zone diameter of ≤19 mm to determine if it is indeed resistant (30). MIC tests rather than the oxacillin disk screen should be used routinely on strains isolated from cerebrospinal fluid and blood.

DETECTION OF OXACILLIN RESISTANCE IN STAPHYLOCOCCI

Oxacillin-Salt Agar Screening Test

Strains of *Staphylococcus aureus* resistant to both oxacillin and methicillin have most commonly been referred to as methicillin-resistant *S. aureus* (MRSA). However, since methicillin is not readily available in the United States, the resistance is more appropriately referred to as oxacillin resistance (ORSA). NCCLS MIC interpretive criteria for oxacillin and *S. aureus* are ≤2 μg/ml for susceptible and ≥4 μg/ml for resistant (118). At least three different resistance mechanisms contribute to oxacillin resistance in *S. aureus*: (i) production of a supplemental PBP (PBP 2a) encoded by a chromosomal *mecA* gene, (ii) inactivation of the drug by increased production of β-lactamase, and (iii) production of modified intrinsic PBPs (MOD-SA) with altered affinity for the drug (17, 19, 27, 49, 175). From a clinical perspective, it is important to differentiate isolates that have *mecA*-positive resistance, which is the classic type of oxacillin resistance, from the infrequently encountered isolates that have one of the other types of more subtle or borderline resistance, because it may affect therapy. Strains that possess *mecA* (classic resistance) are either heterogeneous or homogeneous in their expression of resistance. With homogeneous expression, virtually all cells express resistance when tested by standard in vitro test methods. However, testing of a heteroresistant isolate results in some cells that appear to be susceptible and others that appear to be resistant. Often only 1 in 10^4 to 1 in 10^8 *mecA*-positive cells in the test population expresses resistance (51, 138, 176). Heterogeneous expression occasionally results in MICs that appear to be borderline, i.e., oxacillin MICs of 2 to 8 μg/ml, and consequently, the isolates may be interpreted as susceptible (MICs, ≤2 μg/ml) (145). Isolates that have classic resistance are usually resistant to other agents such as erythromycin, clindamycin, chloramphenicol, tetracycline, trimethoprim-sulfamethoxazole, older fluoroquinolones, or aminoglycosides. However, some ORSA isolates, such as those recently described in community-onset infections, are not multiply resistant (16). Resistance mediated by β-lactamase or the presence of modified PBPs (MOD-SA) also results in borderline resistance. β-Lactamase-mediated resistance can usually be distinguished from the classic type (*mecA*-positive) of resistance or MOD-SA resistance by the addition of a β-lactamase inhibitor (e.g., clavulanic acid) to the oxacillin MIC test, which lowers the MIC by 2 dilutions or more. Isolates that are resistant by either the β-lactamase or the MOD-SA mechanism usually do not have multiple-drug resistance. The presence of classic resistance in *S. aureus* can be detected simply and reliably by the agar screen test (115) or one of the new rapid methods (see below). Strains with β-lactamase-mediated resistance are unlikely to grow on the agar screen plate; however, MOD-SA strains may grow, depending on the oxacillin MIC for the strains (163).

Although the *mecA* gene has been identified in coagulase-negative staphylococci (49, 176), the agar screen test has not been reliable for detecting oxacillin resistance in this group of bacteria (166) because of the 6-μg/ml oxacillin concentration. For some *mecA*-positive coagulase-negative staphylococci (primarily *Staphylococcus epidermidis*), oxacillin MICs are as low as 0.5 μg/ml (100, 191). Consequently, the NCCLS recently eliminated recommendations for use of the agar screen test for coagulase-negative staphylococci and also modified oxacillin breakpoints to ≤0.25 μg/ml for susceptible and ≥0.5 μg/ml for resistant for coagulase-negative staphylococci (115). However, recent studies found that correlation of these interpretive criteria with the presence or absence of *mecA* is optimum only for *S. epidermidis*, *Staphylococcus haemolyticus*, and, possibly, *Staphylococcus hominis* (45, 61, 95). In other species of coagulase-negative staphylococci that are generally less frequently encountered in clinical specimens, these interpretive criteria are less specific, such that many *mecA*-negative strains test falsely resistant by disk and MIC methods.

Test Method

MHA supplemented with 4% sodium chloride and 6 μg of oxacillin per ml is used for the agar screen method recommended by the NCCLS (115). Plates containing 4% NaCl and 10 μg of methicillin per ml have also been described (174) but are currently not recommended. Because oxacillin is more stable and appears to be superior to other penicillinase-stable penicillins (e.g., methicillin, nafcillin, and the isoxazolyl penicillins cloxacillin, dicloxacillin, and flucloxacillin) in detecting resistance to this group of compounds, it is preferred in the agar screen and other diagnostic tests. Agar screen plates are available from several commercial manufacturers. The procedure for preparing agar dilution plates is outlined in chapter 70.

The optimal methods for inoculation of the agar screen test have recently been clarified (163). Inoculum suspensions are prepared by selecting colonies from overnight growth on a nonselective agar plate. The colonies are transferred to broth (e.g., tryptic soy broth) or saline to produce a suspension that matches the turbidity of a 0.5 McFarland standard. This suspension is used to inoculate the oxacillin agar screen plate by either (i) dipping a cotton swab into the test suspension, expressing the excess liquid from the swab, and inoculating an area 10 to 15 mm in diameter (or streaking the swab onto a quadrant of the agar surface) or (ii) spotting an area 10 to 15 mm in diameter with a 1-μl loop that has been dipped in the suspension (163). Test plates are incubated for a full 24 h at 35°C (no higher) in ambient air and examined for growth of more than one colony, which indicates resistance. Once again, the test is currently not recommended for coagulase-negative staphylococci (115).

Quality Control

S. aureus ATCC 29213 (oxacillin susceptible) and *S. aureus* ATCC 43300 (oxacillin resistant) are the recommended quality control strains.

Other Tests for Detection of Oxacillin Resistance in Staphylococci

Several commercial rapid methods that detect oxacillin resistance in staphylococci have been introduced. They include three latex agglutination tests that detect the presence of PBP 2a, the MRSA-Screen test (Denka-Seikin Co., Ltd., Tokyo, Japan), the PBP 2′ latex agglutination test (Oxoid Limited, Basingstoke, United Kingdom), and the Mastalex test (Mast Diagnostics, Bootle, United Kingdom) (9), as well as a DNA cycling probe assay, Velogene (Alexon-Trend, Inc., Ramsey, Minn.), that detects the presence of the *mecA* gene. All except the Mastalex test have been cleared by the Food and Drug Administration (FDA). The MRSA-Screen test, cleared for use only with *S. aureus*, has been widely evaluated and found to have high sensitivity and specificity for that species (14, 96, 145, 164, 181, 183, 190). Detection of resistance in coagulase-negative staphylococci by the MRSA-Screen test has been less successful, requiring either induction, an increased inoculum, or an increased agglutination time for adequate sensitivity (58, 60, 95, 189). The Oxoid latex agglutination test has been approved by the FDA for testing of both *S. aureus* and coagulase-negative staphylococci, although to date there have been no published evaluations of its performance. Velogene appears to achieve adequate sensitivity and specificity, although it also has not been widely evaluated (2, 96, 163). When confirmation of the presence of the *mecA* gene is required, besides these commercial rapid methods, molecular analysis may also be performed by standard PCR methods (see chapter 75).

Reporting Results

Growth of an *S. aureus* isolate on an oxacillin agar screen plate generally means that the isolate is *mecA* positive. If performed properly, the agar screen method will detect most *mecA*-positive *S. aureus* strains. Occasionally, however, a heteroresistant *mecA*-positive strain is not detected; this may be due in part to a low frequency of resistance expression (14, 135) or to lot-to-lot or manufacturer-to-manufacturer variation in the test medium (53, 55). Testing by broth microdilution may also fail to detect extremely heteroresistant, *mecA*-positive *S. aureus* (145). The oxacillin agar screen test generally does not detect borderline-resistant strains. Although MOD-SA isolates, particularly those associated with MICs of ≥8 μg/ml, may grow on agar screen plates (163), isolates with borderline resistance due to β-lactamase are usually associated with oxacillin MICs of ≤4 μg/ml and do not usually grow on the screen plates. Since both types of borderline-resistant isolates are infrequently encountered in clinical specimens of *S. aureus*, the possibility of their presence minimally affects the utility of the agar screen test.

The NCCLS recommends that oxacillin-resistant staphylococci be reported as resistant to all β-lactam agents, including penicillins, cephems, β-lactam–β-lactamase inhibitor combination agents, and carbapenems. These agents are clinically ineffective against oxacillin-resistant staphylococcal infections, even though they may demonstrate in vitro activity (115, 116). Consequently, an isolate that grows on the oxacillin agar screen plate should be considered resistant to these agents as well as to all penicillinase-stable penicillins. Isolates of *S. aureus* that appear oxacillin resistant by an alternative test method but fail to grow on the agar screen plate are probably borderline resistant and lack *mecA* (84, 106, 135). Much less is known about borderline resistance than about *mecA*-positive resistance since there have been few clinical studies (101); however, in animal-model studies, isolates with β-lactamase-mediated resistance appear to be effectively treated with β-lactam agents (18, 19, 127, 170). If a phenotypically oxacillin-resistant *S. aureus* strain is isolated from a seriously ill patient and is found not to contain the *mecA* gene, the laboratory worker should convey this information to the patient's clinician. The incidence of phenotypically susceptible *mecA*-positive strains of *S. aureus* is not known. However, should phenotypically susceptible strains be isolated from serious infections in patients with a prior history of ORSA infection, confirmation by one of the rapid molecular methods should be considered (145).

DETECTION OF VANCOMYCIN RESISTANCE IN STAPHYLOCOCCI

Strains of staphylococci with reduced susceptibility to vancomycin have been described (15, 56). The MICs for these strains are 4 to 8 μg/ml. The MIC interpretive criteria for vancomycin are currently set at ≤4 μg/ml for susceptible, 8 to 16 μg/ml for intermediate, and ≥32 μg/ml for resistant (118), making these isolates borderline in their resistance to vancomycin. Zone diameters for these strains do not characterize them as being distinct from the normally susceptible population of staphylococci, because all of the isolates tested to date have had zones in the 16- to 19-mm range. The NCCLS recommendations for disk diffusion testing of staphylococci have recently changed, with zones of ≥15 mm denoting susceptibility. No breakpoints for intermediate or resistant are currently set, but it is suggested that strains with zones of <15 mm should be tested by an MIC method (118); however, these new breakpoints will not detect vancomycin-intermediate staphylococci.

A recent study evaluated the performance of commercial susceptibility testing systems for their ability to detect staphylococcal strains with reduced vancomycin susceptibility (167). The performance of the BHI vancomycin agar screen plate that is used to detect vancomycin-resistant enterococci was also evaluated. The vancomycin BHI agar screen plates were inoculated with 10 μl of a 0.5 McFarland suspension of organisms and incubated at 35°C in ambient air for a full 24 h. The vancomycin agar screen plates from four commercial sources (Becton Dickinson Microbiology Systems, Cockeysville, Md.; Hardy Diagnostics, Santa Maria, Calif.; PML Microbiologicals, Wilsonville, Oreg.; and Remel, Lenexa, Kans.) were able to detect eight of eight strains for which the vancomycin MICs were 8 μg/ml (167). In addition, one of three strains for which the vancomycin MIC was 4 μg/ml grew on the selective agar. None of the 24 strains for which the MICs were ≤2 μg/ml grew on the commercial screen plates, making the plates highly sensitive and specific in this limited study. However, in-house-prepared screening agar showed breakthrough growth of susceptible strains, indicating that some lots of BHI may not be suitable for this test. The performance of the commercial susceptibility testing systems evaluated in this study was not as good; however, both the MicroScan (overnight) conventional panels and the E test appeared to perform well when incubated for a full 24 h. The Vitek system (bioMérieux Vitek, Hazelwood, Mo.) tended to report MICs of 4 μg/ml for the isolates for which the MICs by broth microdilution were 8 μg/ml. However, recent software modifications to the Vitek system showed improved performance with these strains (133). For all ORSA isolates

detected, laboratories that use the disk diffusion method to test staphylococci should also consider inoculating a commercial vancomycin agar screen plate in order to identify strains for which the vancomycin MICs are ≥8 μg/ml. The screen plate might also be added to staphylococcal testing protocols that use a commercial test system which has not been shown to reliably detect vancomycin-intermediate *S. aureus*. A recent report by Marlowe et al. (99) provides additional strategies for detecting and confirming the decreased susceptibility of staphylococci to vancomycin.

DETECTION OF ENZYMES MEDIATING RESISTANCE

Detection of antimicrobial agent-modifying enzymes in the clinical laboratory is limited to tests for β-lactamase. Tests for detection of other enzymes, e.g., chloramphenicol acetyltransferase (3, 70), are usually performed only in a research setting. For more detailed information on these and other types of resistance enzymes, refer to chapters 68 and 75.

β-Lactamase Tests

In the clinical laboratory, β-lactamase tests must be used only when they can provide clinically useful information, and the definitions of positive or negative reactions must not be extended beyond their intended meanings. For example, a β-lactamase-positive result for a *Neisseria gonorrhoeae* isolate means that the isolate is resistant to penicillin but does not imply that the isolate is resistant to the extended-spectrum cephalosporin group of β-lactam agents. Similarly, direct β-lactamase tests for members of the family *Enterobacteriaceae* or for *Pseudomonas* spp. (all of which produce a variety of β-lactamases that result in various susceptibilities to β-lactam agents) have little clinical value and should not be used for these species. A list of the organisms for which β-lactamase tests are useful is given in Table 2.

Direct Tests for β-Lactamase Activity

In the direct β-lactamase test, a positive reaction indicates that the isolate is resistant to the β-lactam agents noted in Table 2, but a negative reaction is inconclusive. For example, most ampicillin-resistant *Haemophilus influenzae* isolates produce β-lactamase, which can be detected by direct β-lactamase tests; however, rare strains are ampicillin resistant but β-lactamase negative (7, 31, 37). For the latter, conventional disk diffusion or dilution tests are needed to detect the resistance (see chapter 70). Three direct β-lactamase assays, the acidimetric, iodometric, and chromogenic methods, have been widely used (52, 92). Each method involves testing bacteria grown on nonselective media, and the results are available within 1 to 60 min. The acidimetric and iodometric methods use a colorimetric indicator to detect the presence of penicilloic acid in the reaction vessel following β-lactamase hydrolysis of penicillin. In the acidimetric method, the substrates are citrate-buffered penicillin and a phenol red indicator. A decreasing pH associated with the presence of penicilloic acid results in a color change from red (negative result) to yellow (positive result) (36). The substrates in the iodometric test are phosphate-buffered penicillin plus a starch-iodine complex. Penicilloic acid, if present, reduces the iodine and prevents it from combining with starch, resulting in a colorless reaction (positive); a bluish-purple color corresponds to a negative result (13).

TABLE 2 Bacteria for which β-lactamase tests have been used in the clinical laboratory

Species	Method(s) commonly used	Predicted resistance[a]
Bacteroides spp. and other gram-negative anaerobes, except B. fragilis group	Direct β-lactamase tests[b]	Penicillins[c]
Enterococcus spp.	Direct β-lactamase tests	Penicillins[c]
Haemophilus influenzae	Direct β-lactamase tests	Penicillins[c]
Moraxella catarrhalis	Direct β-lactamase tests (nitrocefin only)	Penicillins[c]
Neisseria gonorrhoeae	Direct β-lactamase tests	Penicillins[c]
Staphylococcus spp.	Direct β-lactamase tests with prior induction	Penicillins[c]
Escherichia coli	NCCLS ESBL screening and confirmation tests	Penicillins, cephems, and aztreonam
Klebsiella pneumoniae and K. oxytoca	NCCLS ESBL screening and confirmation tests	Penicillins, cephems, and aztreonam

[a] A positive result indicates resistance; however, a negative result is inconclusive, since other resistance mechanisms may occur.
[b] Includes chromogenic cephalosporin, acidimetric, and iodometric tests.
[c] A positive result indicates resistance to all penicillinase-labile penicillins, including amoxicillin, ampicillin, azlocillin, carbenicillin, mezlocillin, piperacillin, and ticarcillin.

The chromogenic cephalosporin nitrocefin can be used in a test tube assay (120) but has been incorporated into several filter paper-type disk or strip products that are commercially available and widely used in clinical laboratories. β-Lactamase hydrolysis of the chromogenic cephalosporin molecule causes an electron shift that results in a colored product (120). Although the acidimetric and iodometric methods have varied in performance, perhaps due in part to a lack of experience with these methods, the chromogenic method has been reliable in detecting β-lactamases produced by all of the organisms indicated in Table 2 (74, 119).

The colorimetric β-lactamase tests rely on visualization of a colored product that presumably results from β-lactamase destruction of the substrate β-lactam molecule. However, these tests are not 100% specific, and other substances may yield colored end points. Serum may cause a colored reaction with the nitrocefin test (120), and if reagents are not stored properly, spontaneous degradation of penicillin may produce false-positive acidimetric or iodometric β-lactamase reactions.

While some bacteria (e.g., H. influenzae, N. gonorrhoeae, and enterococci) constitutively produce β-lactamase, others (e.g., staphylococci) may produce detectable amounts of enzyme only after exposure to an inducing agent, which is generally a β-lactam (32). If staphylococci produce a positive β-lactamase result without induction, the results can be reported. However, if no β-lactamase is detected, then the test must be performed on cells that have been exposed to an inducing agent before a negative result is reported. This can be done by testing organisms that have been grown in the presence of subinhibitory concentrations of a β-lactam agent (e.g., 0.25 μg of cefoxitin per ml) in a broth or agar system. Alternatively, growth from around the periphery of the zone surrounding a β-lactam disk (e.g., a 1-μg oxacillin disk) can be tested. A positive result may take longer to develop in staphylococci than in other organisms, and the test should not be considered negative until it has been allowed to react for at least 60 min.

β-Lactamase testing by the chromogenic nitrocefin method with anaerobic gram-negative bacilli other than those from the Bacteroides fragilis group is recommended prior to susceptibility testing (117). Members of the B. fragilis group characteristically produce β-lactamase, and they should be considered penicillin resistant. As with aerobes, resistance to β-lactam drugs is not always mediated by β-lactamase production (e.g., in some strains of Bacteroides distasonis and B. fragilis) (1, 64, 117).

The S. aureus strains recommended by the NCCLS for quality control of routine disk diffusion and dilution tests (115, 116) can be used for quality control of β-lactamase tests. S. aureus ATCC 25923 is β-lactamase negative, whereas S. aureus ATCC 29213 is β-lactamase positive.

Tests for Extended-Spectrum β-Lactamases

The genes generally responsible for β-lactamase-mediated ampicillin resistance in Escherichia coli and Klebsiella spp. can undergo simple point mutations that result in the production of novel β-lactamases that are capable of hydrolyzing extended-spectrum cephalosporins (e.g., cefotaxime, ceftriaxone, ceftizoxime, and ceftazidime) and aztreonam, as well as older β-lactam drugs. These enzymes are referred to as extended-spectrum β-lactamases (ESBLs) (10, 66, 93, 130, 173) and are discussed in chapter 68. At least 100 different types of ESBLs have been noted in several gram-negative species and are associated with a variety of in vitro antimicrobial susceptibility profiles (10, 173).

The in vitro susceptibility results obtained with an isolate that produces ESBLs often defy typical "hierarchy" rules of β-lactam (particularly cephem) activity. Sometimes the more narrow spectrum cephems (particularly the cephamycins, such as cefoxitin or cefotetan) are more active than broad-spectrum agents (20, 105). Several reports suggest that ESBL-producing isolates should be considered resistant to all extended-spectrum penicillins, cephalosporins, and monobactams even if they appear to be susceptible to these agents in vitro (123, 124, 154). The β-lactamase-stable carbapenems (ertapenem, imipenem, meropenem) are active in vitro (4, 65, 73, 131, 152, 153, 188) and appear to be clinically effective against ESBL producers (69, 103, 123, 126). Some ESBL-producing isolates are susceptible to β-lactam–β-lactamase inhibitor combination agents in vitro, but the effectiveness of these agents in vivo is uncertain, particularly if there is a high concentration of organisms at the infection site (67). The genes that code for production of ESBLs are often linked to other resistance genes, so that ESBL-producing isolates are often multiply resistant (e.g., resistant to aminoglycosides and trimethoprim-sulfamethoxazole) (78).

Routine disk diffusion and MIC tests using traditional breakpoints may not always identify isolates that produce ESBLs (68, 71, 78, 105). Thus, the NCCLS has developed new MIC and disk diffusion screening breakpoints for aztreonam, cefotaxime, cefpodoxime, ceftazidime, and ceftriaxone that aid in detecting ESBL-producing *E. coli*, *Klebsiella oxytoca*, and *Klebsiella pneumoniae* isolates (118). ESBL-producing clinical isolates may demonstrate HLR to one or more of the screening drugs (69, 78, 94, 103, 152, 186). Thus, the sensitivity of the screen test increases when more than one screening drug is used (6, 34, 57, 105, 118, 172, 188). Cefpodoxime is most likely to detect isolates producing ESBLs, but this agent lacks specificity, particularly for *E. coli* (43, 105, 171). However, the NCCLS has recently modified the screening breakpoints for cefpodoxime in order to increase the specificity with a minimal effect on the sensitivity (118). Unlike inducible AmpC β-lactamases, ESBLs are inhibited by clavulanic acid, and this property is used to identify ESBLs in the clinical laboratory. These tests are based on enhanced activity when a β-lactam (usually ceftazidime or cefotaxime) is tested with clavulanic acid compared to the activity when the β-lactam is tested alone. The NCCLS describes standard disk diffusion and broth microdilution MIC tests to be used as phenotypic confirmatory tests for the presence of ESBLs in *E. coli*, *K. oxytoca*, and *K. pneumoniae*. For broth microdilution, cefotaxime and ceftazidime are tested with and without 4 μg of clavulanic acid per ml. A decrease in the MIC of ≥3 dilutions for the agents tested in combination with clavulanic acid compared to the values obtained for the agents tested alone indicates the presence of an ESBL. For disk diffusion, the same agents incorporated into disks with and without 10 μg of clavulanic acid are tested. An increase in the zone diameter of ≥5 mm for either of the disks with clavulanic acid indicates the presence of an ESBL. *K. pneumoniae* ATCC 700603 should be included for quality control purposes; accepted ranges are given in the current NCCLS M100-S12 tables (118). Isolates of *E. coli* and *Klebsiella* spp. confirmed to be ESBL producers should be reported as resistant to penicillins (not including β-lactam–β-lactamase inhibitor combinations), cephalosporins (which excludes the cephamycins cefoxitin and cefotetan), and aztreonam (118). For screen-positive strains that do not show a clavulanic acid effect, there are insufficient data to justify modifying reports at present; these isolates should be reported as they test. One of the limitations of the phenotypic confirmatory test is that some ESBL-producing strains may demonstrate a negative confirmatory test result, which may occur as a result of decreased porin production, production of large quantities of ESBL, hyperproduction of a TEM-1 or SHV-1 β-lactamase, production of additional β-lactamases (e.g., AmpC) that are not inhibited by clavulanic acid, or a combination of these (10, 173). Steward et al. (156) showed in a recent study that cefepime with and without clavulanic acid is superior to the current confirmatory test agents (both cefotaxime and ceftazidime with and without clavulanic acid) in detection of ESBLs in some strains that have multiple β-lactam resistance mechanisms. The NCCLS has not addressed the utility of the screening or phenotypic confirmatory tests for detecting ESBLs in members of the family *Enterobacteriaceae* other than *E. coli* and *Klebsiella* spp. In theory, however, they should detect ESBLs in other genera that are normally susceptible to extended-spectrum cephalosporins.

Typically, screening for and confirmation of ESBL production is a two-step process; however, at least one commercial manufacturer has a product that incorporates a confirmatory test on a primary susceptibility test panel (146). The laboratory's ability to detect and report the presence of ESBLs in a timely manner will likely affect the selection of appropriate therapy for patients with infections caused by ESBL-producing strains. Consequently, every laboratory should have a procedure to address detection of ESBLs (87, 124, 131, 154, 168). There is some debate as to the significance of ESBLs in isolates from noninvasive infections, such as uncomplicated urinary tract infections (34, 125). However, regardless of the source, ESBL-producing isolates are important from an infection control perspective.

Tests for Inducible β-Lactamases

Several tests have been described for assessing the ability of *Acinetobacter*, *Citrobacter freundii*, *Enterobacter*, *Morganella*, *Proteus vulgaris*, *Proteus penneri*, *Providencia*, *Pseudomonas aeruginosa*, and *Serratia marcescens* isolates to produce inducible β-lactamases. However, because virtually all isolates of the genera and species mentioned above have the potential to produce inducible β-lactamases, the β-lactamase induction test (8, 24) has limited clinical application. Instead, physicians must maintain an awareness of the organisms that can produce inducible β-lactamases (sometimes with a mutation in gene regulation that causes them to be stably derepressed) and the potential for therapeutic failure if certain β-lactams are used to treat infections caused by these organisms.

DETERMINATION OF BACTERICIDAL ACTIVITIES OF ANTIMICROBIAL AGENTS

Most in vitro susceptibility test methods measure the abilities of antimicrobial agents to inhibit the growth of bacteria. It is also possible to assess the ability of a drug to provide a bactericidal effect on an isolate or group of isolates. This may be useful in managing certain serious infections that have been shown to require bactericidal action for optimal efficacy, for certain patients who are immunosuppressed, and for research purposes to study the pharmacodynamic properties of a new or established antimicrobial agent. The tests most often performed include determination of the MBC, determination of the serum bactericidal titer (SBT), and kinetic time-kill assays. In even the most sophisticated clinical laboratories serving large tertiary-care medical centers, determinations of bactericidal activity probably account for fewer than 1% of all susceptibility tests performed. Thus, these are highly specialized tests performed for very limited indications.

Tests of bactericidal activity have most often been used for selection and monitoring of therapy in patients with infective endocarditis (26, 75, 129, 134, 137, 148, 149, 184), osteomyelitis (75, 110, 129, 134, 185), and, much less commonly, meningitis (129, 137, 147) or in neutropenic cancer patients (79, 82, 151). In most settings, these tests may be favored by certain physicians or specialty groups (e.g., infectious disease specialists) for the management of their patients' very complicated infections but do not represent standard care in all American medical centers. It is important to recognize that the data in support of the use of bactericidal activity determinations for patient management are limited, and early studies were often performed by nonstandardized methods (26, 75, 97, 148, 165). Prior reviews have highlighted the technical problems and lack of expert consensus for interpreting the results of bactericidal activity determinations (97, 98, 134). The perception that the tests are not reproducible may have stifled development of consensus criteria for when and how these tests can best be applied. The lack of standardization of the specific assays has recently been addressed by the NCCLS through publication of standard methods for determining bactericidal activity (113, 114). This section discusses bactericidal testing in a clinical laboratory setting and reflects the consensus standards developed by the NCCLS.

Clinical Use of Bactericidal Testing

For those who favor use of bactericidal tests for management of certain serious infections, a typical sequence is to first determine the MICs and MBCs of a limited number of agents that could be used to treat the patient in order to select the agent with the most favorable (i.e., lowest) MBC relative to the safely achievable levels of the drug. Determination of the MBC provides an opportunity to detect possible tolerance of the patient's isolate to drugs that would normally be considered bactericidal against the species being tested and might result in clinical failure (28, 50, 59, 110, 179). Once one or more drugs has been selected on the basis of the results of MIC and MBC testing and the patient has been started on standard doses of the agent(s), the second step would be to assess the bactericidal activity achieved in the patient by performance of a serum bactericidal test(s). The goal here is to ensure that the dosage regimen provides sufficient bactericidal activity in that patient's blood or, possibly, cerebrospinal fluid. The body fluid (usually serum) is serially diluted and inoculated with the patient's own infecting organism. The SBT test result is expressed as a titer indicating the dilution of serum or body fluid that is bactericidal; in general, a higher titer indicates better activity. If the SBT is deemed to be too low, it may be possible to adjust the dosage regimen, or it may be advisable to select alternative therapy in an effort to avoid a poor therapeutic outcome (134, 184, 185). Performance of the SBT test can also provide an assessment of the effectiveness of drug combinations intended to provide a synergistic effect in order to treat a highly resistant bacterial isolate or an organism not readily killed by single-agent therapy (e.g., *Enterococcus* spp.) (113).

From this description, it should be obvious to the reader that performance of bactericidal tests requires considerable technical proficiency on the part of the laboratory and also a highly informed and experienced clinician to make use of the data. The interpretation of the SBT must take into account knowledge of the key pharmacodynamic property of the antibiotic (i.e., concentration-dependent versus time-dependent killing activity), the location and the seriousness of the infection, the pathogenic potential of the infecting organism, and the potential toxicity and cost of the treatment regimen. Bactericidal testing should not be performed unless there is close communication between the clinical microbiologist and the requesting clinician. Possible pitfalls include selecting potentially more toxic or expensive drugs on the basis of a low MIC or MBC (unless the physician is very knowledgeable about various classes of antimicrobial agents) and raising antibiotic levels to potentially toxic levels in order to achieve a higher or more favorable SBT. Therefore, laboratories should undertake

bactericidal testing only after thorough discussions with their clinician customers.

Determination of the MBC

There are several basic requirements for standardized determination of the MBC. The test may be performed by either the tube broth macrodilution method or the broth microdilution procedure. A detailed description of the methods can be found in the NCCLS document that deals specifically with bactericidal tests (114). In brief, the test usually uses standard cation-adjusted Mueller-Hinton broth (with lysed horse blood supplementation if needed for fastidious organisms) dispensed in 1-ml aliquots in glass tubes (13 by 100 mm) or in 0.1-ml volumes in plastic microdilution trays. A significant component in performance of the MBC test is the inoculum preparation and inoculation procedure. An actively growing (log-phase) inoculum (80) is used (114, 165) rather than an inoculum that is allowed to grow to the stationary phase or fresh colonies simply suspended in broth or saline, as suggested in the standard MIC test (115). Use of a log-phase inoculum is necessary to accurately assess the bactericidal properties of drugs that require actively growing cells to exert a bactericidal effect. In addition, it is important to carefully dispense the standardized inoculum suspension below the meniscus of the broth in each tube or well to prevent splashing that can lead to organisms sticking to the wall of the tube or well above the meniscus rather than being in contact with the drug in the test medium (114). If splashing or aerosolization of the inoculum occurs, viable organisms recovered at the time of the final subculture may represent bacteria that were not sufficiently exposed to the drug during the course of the test and thus would give the erroneous perception that the drug was not bactericidal (80, 114, 165).

After determination of the MIC following incubation at 35°C, quantitative subcultures (usually 0.01 ml) are performed at 24 h (following vortexing or shaking at 20 h) with samples from each tube or well with concentrations at and above the MIC of the drug being tested. The subculture aliquots are streaked across the entire surface of a plate containing a standard growth medium (e.g., sheep blood agar). In order to calculate the degree of killing at each antibiotic concentration, it is necessary that a colony count be performed on the positive control tube or well at the time of initial inoculation of the MIC test. As in the standard MIC procedure, the target inoculum density is 5×10^5 CFU/ml (114, 115). After the subculture plates are incubated for 24 to 48 h, any visible colonies are counted on each subculture plate. The standard definition of the MBC is the reduction of the initial inoculum by ≥99.9% (3 logs) (114). In practice, it is advisable to correct for pipetting error and to account for the Poisson distribution of bacterial cells in a liquid by using statistically derived rejection value tables (114). The tables define the number of colonies that can be tolerated on the basis of the initial inoculum density of each test. If the number of colonies on a particular plate exceeds the rejection value for that test, the antibiotic did not achieve the strict definition of a bactericidal effect at that given concentration of the drug. It is then hoped that the next higher concentration of the drug will have fewer surviving colonies to fulfill the definition of a bactericidal effect. The MBC of an antibiotic should be reported in micrograms per milliliter, in the same manner as the MIC is reported. A given MBC test should be considered invalid if there is evidence of contamination of the inoculum or the subcultured tubes or wells, if there is no growth in the positive control well or tube or if there is growth in the sterility well or tube, or if there are several skipped dilutions in the MIC portion of the test (47, 114).

Assessment of Bactericidal Activity by the Time-Kill Method

Measuring the rate of bactericidal activity by time-kill analysis provides the opportunity to assess the speed with which killing may occur at a given antibiotic concentration. It is a more laborious approach than determination of the MBC and thus may be best reserved for research purposes. It is also possible to assess the activities of drugs in combination in order to recognize synergistic, indifferent, or antagonistic effects of two or more drugs tested together (81, 86, 114). This approach appears to correlate better with in vivo studies of combined drug effects than the alternative checkerboard titration method (5, 11, 25). The details of performance of the time-kill test have been defined in the NCCLS guideline (114). Many of the same critical factors that affect the outcome of the MBC test apply to the performance of time-kill assays, e.g., preparation of an actively growing inoculum and use of quantitative subcultures from antibiotic-containing tubes. The time-kill method requires that multiple samples be removed at various times (e.g., 0, 4, 8, 12, and 24 h) for colony counts, and thus, the volume of medium for each antibiotic concentration tested is usually ≥10 ml contained in a glass

test tube or flask (114). A given antibiotic is often tested at more than one concentration that relates to the previously determined MIC of that agent (e.g., the MIC, two times the MIC, or four times the MIC). When high concentrations (four or more times the MIC) of a drug are tested by the time-kill method, it is necessary to demonstrate that antibiotic carryover has not falsely diminished the number of colonies on subculture plates (114). The results of a time-kill assay are frequently depicted graphically by plotting the colony counts of each antibiotic and concentration tested over time (Fig. 1). A bactericidal effect is again defined as ≥99.9% killing at a specified time (114). When drugs are tested in combination by the time-kill method, synergy is often defined as a ≥2-log decrease in the number of CFU achieved with a drug combination compared to that achieved with the most active drug tested alone (114).

Performance of the Serum Bactericidal Test

The determinations of the serum inhibitory and bactericidal titers are performed in a manner analogous to the MIC and MBC procedures, except that the patient's serum, rather than preweighed and prediluted concentrations of the drug, is used as the source of antibiotic. A guideline that describes the details of the serum bactericidal test has been published by the NCCLS (113). The principal steps in performing the test include (i) obtaining one or more blood samples from the patient at specified intervals, (ii) prepar-

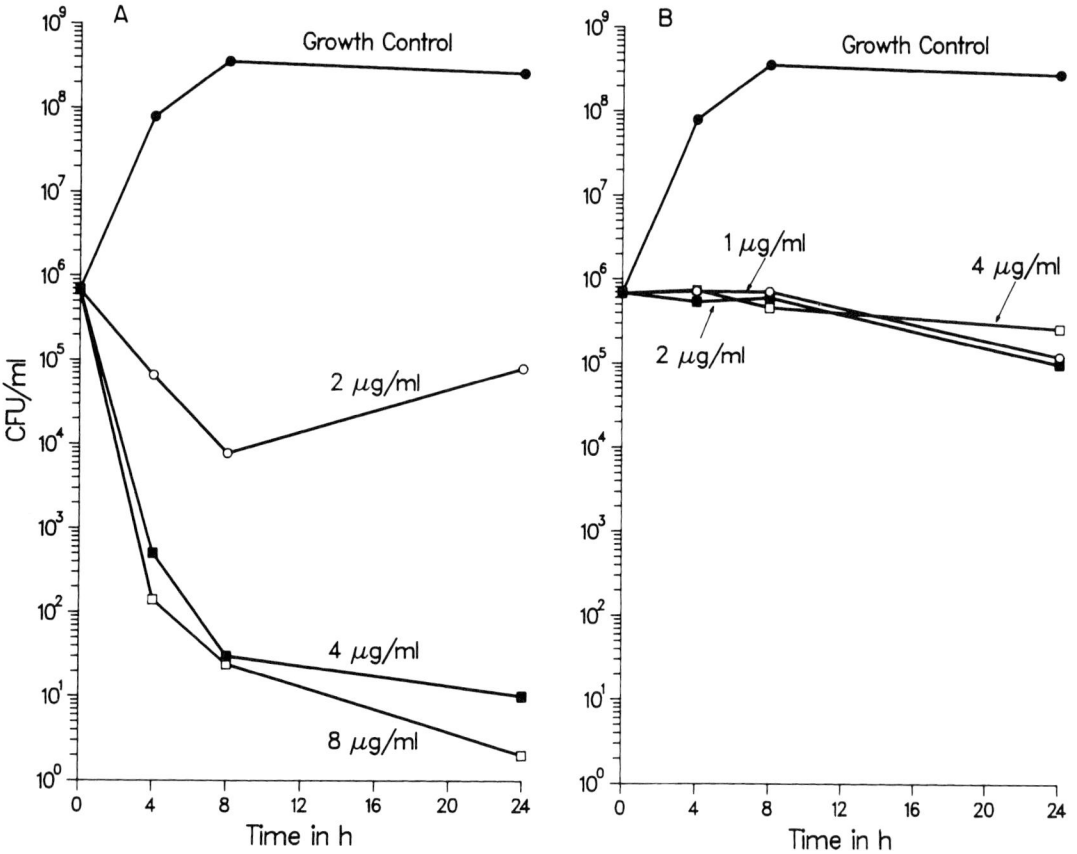

FIGURE 1   Results of time-kill assay of an *E. faecium* isolate. (A) Daptomycin tested at the MIC (2 μg/ml) and at two and four times the MIC, demonstrating a bactericidal effect at two and four times the MIC. (B) Vancomycin tested at the MIC (1 μg/ml) and at two and four times the MIC, without evidence of a bactericidal effect. Reproduced from reference 76 with permission.

ing twofold dilutions of the patient's serum in pooled and pretested human serum in glass tubes or plastic microdilution trays, (iii) inoculating each tube or well with a standardized, actively growing inoculum (as described above for the MBC test) of the patient's own infecting organism in appropriate growth medium (usually cation-adjusted Mueller-Hinton broth), and (iv) incubating for 20 to 24 h (113). Pooled human serum is recommended as the diluent of the patient's serum in each tube or well in order to make protein binding consistent throughout the range of serum dilutions, especially for drugs that are highly protein bound. The pretesting of the pooled human serum includes screening for human immunodeficiency virus type 1 and hepatitis B virus, for antibiotic activity, and for optical clarity (113). In addition, the pooled serum should be heat inactivated immediately prior to use, and the pH should be adjusted to the correct range of 7.2 to 7.4 (113). An alternative to the laborious serum preparation step just described is the creation of a serum ultrafiltrate that precludes the need for a serum diluent (91, 113). The blood samples for testing are usually obtained from the patient shortly after the antibiotic is administered, at the time of the presumed peak level in serum (usually 30 to 60 min after administration), and often immediately prior to administration of the next drug dose (trough level) (113). The end points of the test are indicated by the highest dilution (titer) of the patient's serum sample that prevents visible growth following the incubation period (serum inhibitory titer). Similar to the MBC determination, quantitative subcultures are performed from each dilution of the patient's serum that has prevented visible growth. The SBT is defined as that dilution (titer) that provides a ≥99.9% reduction of the original inoculum of the test based upon the standard rejection value tables (113). Thus, the results of the test are reported as dilutions (the titer) of the patient's serum rather than as a drug concentration (in micrograms per milliliter) as in the MIC and MBC tests.

Interpreting the Results of Bactericidal Determinations

The interpretation of the results of the bactericidal determinations described above has not received the same degree of critical scrutiny or level of consensus standards that has been achieved for interpretation of MIC determina-

tions. However, a few general statements can be made. A favorable MBC would typically be the same as or perhaps 1 to 2 dilutions greater than the MIC of agents that are normally considered bactericidal (e.g., β-lactams, glycopeptides, aminoglycosides, and fluoroquinolones). A principal rationale for performing MBC or kinetic time-kill studies would be to detect an isolate that is not effectively killed by a typically bactericidal drug. This failure to exert a bactericidal effect is often described as tolerance and is defined as an MBC ≥32-fold the MIC of a particular agent (50, 114). Failure to achieve at least a 3-$\log_{10}$ reduction of CFU in the kinetic time-kill assay could likewise signify a tolerant strain (114).

Results of the serum bactericidal test that reflect a high titer of antibacterial activity in the serum suggest that the patient has been dosed adequately, has not experienced abnormal elimination of the antibiotic, and does not have a tolerant bacterial isolate. This perception can be quantified by comparing the peak and trough titers obtained with those that have been shown to correlate with rapid organism eradication in collaborative studies (134, 184, 185). For rapid clearance of bacteremia and optimal time to sterilization of cardiac vegetations, a peak SBT of ≥1:64 and a trough SBT of ≥1:32 should be achieved whenever possible (134, 184). However, lower bactericidal titers do not necessarily signify a poor clinical outcome. In patients with chronic osteomyelitis, limited data have suggested that peak SBTs of ≥1:16 and trough SBTs of ≥1:4 predict clinical cure, while titers as low as 1:2 at the trough have been shown to be satisfactory in acute osteomyelitis (134, 185). Titers of ≥1:8 have generally (80% of cases) been associated with satisfactory outcomes in cancer chemotherapy patients (82).

Limitations of Bactericidal Determinations

As stated earlier, clinical microbiologists and infectious disease specialists are not uniformly convinced of the importance of bactericidal determinations as a routine part of even highly complicated bacterial infections. Part of the controversy over the use of these tests may stem from the fact that the procedures themselves have only recently been standardized to a significant degree. Indeed, there are still several procedural steps in these tests that can be difficult to control (Table 3), not the least of which are the critical

TABLE 3 Technical factors that are critical for reliable determination of MBCs and SBTs and potential pitfalls in those procedure steps

Procedure step	Potential pitfall
Preparation of an actively growing, log-phase inoculum	Use of stationary-phase inoculum will increase the percentage of persisters and potentially result in false tolerance with antibiotics that require rapidly growing cells to exert a bactericidal effect
Delivery of the inoculum aliquot below the meniscus of the broth	Splashing of the inoculum suspension onto the wall of the tube or microdilution well will prevent some cells from contact with the antibiotic and lead to an inaccurate number of colonies upon final subculture
Quantitative subculture of tubes or wells containing drug concentrations at the MIC or higher following incubation	Subculture of too large a volume may cause the problem of antibiotic carryover and persistent inhibition; subculture of an insufficient volume precludes accurate counting of surviving organisms
Determination of ≥99.9% reduction in CFU/ml	Inaccurate pipetting or failure to compensate for a pipetting error or Poisson distribution of bacteria will compromise calculation of the bactericidal end point
Failure to account for protein binding in the SBT test	SBT may be falsely elevated with drugs that are highly protein bound (e.g., >90%)

steps of inoculum preparation and dispensing and the final step of accurately counting the surviving bacteria. Despite full attention to the critical details of these test procedures, confusing results may still occur in the form of the skip tube phenomenon (47) or trailing bactericidal end points due to persisters (114). Persisters are thought to represent a fraction of the bacterial population and occasionally exceed 0.1% of the population due to metabolically inactive cells not effectively eradicated during the test (48). A point of occasional concern is the paradoxical or Eagle effect, in which a bactericidal effect can be demonstrated at a relatively low drug concentration, but cells are found not to be killed at very high drug concentrations relative to the MIC (114). This phenomenon has been attributed to secondary effects of some cell wall-active agents on intracellular processes such as protein synthesis, thereby slowing the growth rate and preventing the drug's principal effect on cell wall synthesis of rapidly growing cells (33). A major contribution of the NCCLS guidelines is the provision of suggested quality control measures, including established MBC ranges for commonly used control organisms (114, 115). Despite these vigorous efforts to standardize these determinations, it is likely that bactericidal tests will continue to be a subject of discussion and be performed at a relatively few institutions for purposes of patient management.

ADDENDUM IN PROOF

In 2002, a single strain of *S. aureus* with high-level resistance to vancomycin (MIC, >128 μg/ml) was isolated from a diabetic patient with peripheral vascular disease and chronic renal failure (Centers for Disease Control and Prevention, *Morb. Mortal. Wkly. Rep.* **51**:565–567, 2002). The isolate was recovered from a dialysis catheter site and a chronic foot ulcer. The vancomycin-resistant *S. aureus* isolate contained the *vanA* gene often found in vancomycin-resistant enterococci in addition to *mecA*. The isolate grew well on the BHI vancomycin screen agar (F. C. Tenover, unpublished observations).

REFERENCES

1. **Aldridge, K. E., D. Ashcraft, K. Cambre, C. L. Pierson, S. G. Jenkins, and J. E. Rosenblatt.** 2001. Multicenter survey of the changing in vitro antimicrobial susceptibilities of clinical isolates of *Bacteroides fragilis* group, *Prevotella, Fusobacterium, Porphyromonas,* and *Peptostreptococcus* species. *Antimicrob. Agents Chemother.* **45**:1238–1243.
2. **Arbique, J., K. Forward, D. Haldane, and R. Davidson.** 2001. Comparison of the Velogene rapid MRSA identification assay, Denka MRSA-Screen assay, and BBL Crystal MRSA ID system for rapid identification of methicillin-resistant *Staphylococcus aureus. Diagn. Microbiol. Infect. Dis.* **40**:5–10.
3. **Azemun, P., T. Stull, M. Roberts, and A. L. Smith.** 1981. Rapid detection of chloramphenicol resistance in *Haemophilus influenzae. Antimicrob. Agents Chemother.* **20**:168–170.
4. **Babini, G. S., and D. M. Livermore.** 2000. Antimicrobial resistance amongst *Klebsiella* spp. collected from intensive care units in Southern and Western Europe in 1997–1998. *J. Antimicrob. Chemother.* **45**:183–189.
5. **Bayer, A. S., and J. O. Morrison.** 1984. Disparity between timed-kill and checkerboard methods for determination of in vitro bactericidal interactions of vancomyin plus rifampin versus methicillin-susceptible and -resistant *Staphylococcus aureus. Antimicrob. Agents Chemother.* **26**:220–223.
6. **Bedenic, B., C. Randegger, A. Boras, and H. Haechler.** 2001. Comparison of five different methods for detection of SHV extended-spectrum β-lactamases. *J. Chemother.* **13**:24–33.
7. **Blondeau, J. M., D. Vaughan, R. Laskowski, and S. Borsos.** 2001. Susceptibility of Canadian isolates of *Haemophilus influenzae, Moraxella catarrhalis* and *Streptococcus pneumoniae* to oral antimicrobial agents. *Int. J. Antimicrob. Agents* **17**:457–464.
8. **Bongaerts, G., and H. Roelofs-Willemse.** 1998. In vitro expression of β-lactam-induced response by clinical gram-negative bacteria with the potential for inducible β-lactamase production. *Scand. J. Infect. Dis.* **30**:579–583.
9. **Brown, D. F., and E. Walpole.** 2001. Evaluation of the Mastalex latex agglutination test for methicillin resistance in *Staphylococcus aureus* grown on different screening media. *J. Antimicrob. Chemother.* **47**:187–189.
10. **Bush, K.** 2001. New β-lactamases in gram-negative bacteria: diversity and impact on the selection of antimicrobial therapy. *Clin. Infect. Dis.* **32**:1085–1089.
11. **Cappelletty, D. M., and M. J. Rybak.** 1996. Comparison of methodologies for synergism testing of drug combinations against resistant strains of *Pseudomonas aeruginosa. Antimicrob. Agents Chemother.* **40**:677–683.
12. **Cartwright, C. P., F. Stock, G. A. Fahle, and V. J. Gill.** 1995. Comparison of pigment production and motility tests with PCR for reliable identification of intrinsically vancomycin-resistant enterococci. *J. Clin. Microbiol.* **33**:1931–1933.
13. **Catlin, B. W.** 1975. Iodometric detection of *Haemophilus influenzae* β-lactamase: rapid presumptive test for ampicillin resistance. *Antimicrob. Agents Chemother.* **7**:265–270.
14. **Cavassini, M., A. Wenger, K. Jaton, D. S. Blanc, and J. Bille.** 1999. Evaluation of MRSA-Screen, a simple anti-PBP 2a slide latex agglutination kit, for rapid detection of methicillin resistance in *Staphylococcus aureus. J. Clin. Microbiol.* **37**:1591–1594.
15. **Centers for Disease Control and Prevention.** 1997. Reduced susceptibility of *Staphylococcus aureus* to vancomycin—Japan, 1996. *Morbid. Mortal. Wkly. Rep.* **46**:765–766.
16. **Centers for Disease Control and Prevention.** 1999. Four pediatric deaths from community-acquired methicillin-resistant *Staphylococcus aureus*—Minnesota and North Dakota, 1997–1999. *Morbid. Mortal. Wkly. Rep.* **48**:707–710.
17. **Chambers, H. F.** 1997. Methicillin resistance in staphylococci: molecular and biochemical basis and clinical implications. *Clin. Microbiol. Rev.* **10**:781–791.
18. **Chambers, H. F., G. Archer, and M. Matsuhashi.** 1989. Low-level methicillin resistance in *Staphylococcus aureus. Antimicrob. Agents Chemother.* **33**:424–428.
19. **Chambers, H. F., and C. J. Hackbarth.** 1992. Methicillin-resistant *Staphylococcus aureus*: genetics and mechanisms of resistance, p. 21–35. *In* M. T. Cafferkey (ed.), *Methicillin-Resistant* Staphylococcus aureus: *Clinical Management and Laboratory Aspects.* Marcel Dekker, Inc., New York, N.Y.
20. **Chanal-Claris, C., D. Sirot, L. Bret, P. Chatron, R. Labia, and J. Sirot.** 1997. Novel extended-spectrum TEM-type β-lactamase from an *Escherichia coli* isolate resistant to ceftazidime and susceptible to cephalothin. *Antimicrob. Agents Chemother.* **41**:715–716.
21. **Chen, Y., S. A. Marshall, P. Winokur, S. Coffman, W. Wllke, P. Murray, C. Spiegel, M. A. Pfaller, G. V. Doern, and R. N. Jones.** 1998. Use of molecular and reference susceptibility testing methods in a multicenter evaluation of MicroScan dried overnight gram-positive MIC panels for detection of vancomycin and high-level

aminoglycoside resistances in enterococci. *J. Clin. Microbiol.* **36:**2996–3001.

22. **Chow, J. W., M. J. Zervos, S. A. Lerner, L. A. Thal, S. Donabedian, D. Jaworski, S. Tsai, K. Shaw, and D. B. Clewell.** 1997. A novel gentamicin resistance gene in *Enterococcus. Antimicrob. Agents Chemother.* **41:**511–514.

23. **Clark, N. C., R. C. Cooksey, B. C. Hill, J. M. Swenson, and F. C. Tenover.** 1993. Characterization of glycopeptide-resistant enterococci from U.S. hospitals. *Antimicrob. Agents Chemother.* **37:**2311–2317.

24. **Cox, V.** 1992. β-Lactamase induction test for gram-negative bacilli, p. 5.7.1–5.7.6. *In* H. D. Isenberg (ed.), *Clinical Microbiology Procedures Handbook.* American Society for Microbiology, Washington, D.C.

25. **D'Alessandri, R. M., D. J. McNeely, and R. M. Kluge.** 1998. Antibiotic synergy and antagonism against clinical isolates of *Klebsiella* species. *Antimicrob. Agents Chemother.* **10:**889–892.

26. **DeGirolami, P. C., and G. Eliopoulos.** 1987. Antimicrobial susceptibility tests and their role in therapeutic drug monitoring. *Clin. Lab. Med.* **7:**499–513.

27. **De Lencastre, H., S. A. Figueiredo, C. Urban, J. Rahal, and A. Tomasz.** 1991. Multiple mechanisms of methicillin resistance and improved methods for detection in clinical isolates of *Staphylococcus aureus. Antimicrob. Agents Chemother.* **35:**632–639.

28. **Denny, A. E., L. R. Peterson, D. N. Gerding, and W. H. Hall.** 1979. Serious staphylococcal infections with strains tolerant to bactericidal antibiotics. *Ann. Intern. Med.* **139:**1026–1031.

29. **Dixon, J. M., A. E. Lipinski, and M. E. Graham.** 1977. Detection and prevalence of pneumococci with increased resistance to penicillin. *Can. Med. Assoc. J.* **117:**1159–1161.

30. **Doern, G. V., A. Brueggemann, and G. Pierce.** 1997. Assessment of the oxacillin disk screening test for determining penicillin resistance in *Streptococcus pneumoniae. Eur. J. Clin. Microbiol. Infect. Dis.* **16:**311–314.

31. **Doern, G. V., A. B. Brueggemann, G. Pierce, H. P. Holley, Jr., and A. Rauch.** 1997. Antibiotic resistance among clinical isolates of *Haemophilus influenzae* in the United States in 1994 and 1995 and detection of β-lactamase-positive strains resistant to amoxicillin-clavulanate: results of a national multicenter surveillance study. *Antimicrob. Agents Chemother.* **41:**292–297.

32. **Dyke, J. W.** 1979. β-Lactamases of *Staphylococcus aureus*, p. 291–310. *In* J. M. Hamilton-Miller (ed.), *β-Lactamases.* Academic Press, Ltd., London, United Kingdom.

33. **Eagle, H., and A. D. Musselman.** 1948. The rate of bacterial action of penicillin in vitro as a function of its concentration and its paradoxically reduced activity at high concentrations against certain organisms. *J. Exp. Med.* **88:**131.

34. **Emery, C. L., and L. A. Weymouth.** 1997. Detection and clinical significance of extended-spectrum β-lactamases in a tertiary-care medical center. *J. Clin. Microbiol.* **35:**2061–2067.

35. **Endtz, H. P., N. Van Den Braak, A. Van Belkum, W. H. Groessens, D. Kreft, A. B. Stroebel, and H. A. Verbrugh.** 1998. Comparison of eight methods to detect vancomycin resistance in enterococci. *J. Clin. Microbiol.* **36:**592–594.

36. **Escamilla, J.** 1976. Susceptibility of *Haemophilus influenzae* to ampicillin as determined by use of a modified, one-minute β-lactamase test. *Antimicrob. Agents Chemother.* **9:**196–198.

37. **Felmingham, D., and R. N. Gruneberg.** 2000. The Alexander Project 1996–1997: latest susceptibility data from this international study of bacterial pathogens from community-acquired lower respiratory tract infections. *J. Antimicrob. Chemother.* **45:**191–203.

38. **Fines, M., B. Perichon, P. Reynolds, D. F. Sahm, and P. Courvalin.** 1999. VanE, a new type of acquired glycopeptide resistance in *Enterococcus facealis* BM4405. *Antimicrob. Agents Chemother.* **43:**2161–2164.

39. **Fontana, R., M. Ligozzi, F. Pittaluga, and G. Satta.** 1996. Intrinsic penicillin resistance in enterococci. *Microb. Drug Resist.* **2:**209–213.

40. **Free, L., and D. Sahm.** 1995. Investigation of the reformulated Remel Synergy Quad plate for detection of high-level aminoglycoside and vancomycin resistance in enterococci. *J. Clin. Microbiol.* **33:**1643–1645.

41. **Freeman, C., A. Robinson, B. Cooper, M. Mazens-Sullivan, R. Quintiliani, Jr., and C. Nightingale.** 1995. In vitro antimicrobial susceptibility of glycopeptide-resistant enterococci. *Diagn. Microbiol. Infect. Dis.* **21:**47–50.

42. **Garcia-Garrote, F., E. Cercenado, and E. Bouza.** 2000. Evaluation of a new system, VITEK 2, for identification and antimicrobial susceptibility testing of enterococci. *J. Clin. Microbiol.* **38:**2108–2111.

43. **Gibb, A. P., and M. Crichton.** 2000. Cefpodoxime screening of *Escherichia coli* and *Klebsiella* spp. by Vitek for detection of organisms producing extended-spectrum β-lactamases. *Diagn. Microbiol. Infect. Dis.* **38:**255–257.

44. **Gordon, S., J. M. Swenson, B. C. Hill, N. E. Pigott, R. R. Facklam, R. C. Cooksey, C. Thornsberry, The Enterococcal Study Group, W. R. Jarvis, and F. C. Tenover.** 1992. Antimicrobial susceptibility patterns of common and unusual species of enterococci causing infections in the United States. *J. Clin. Microbiol.* **30:**2373–2378.

45. **Gradelski, E., L. Valera, L. Aleksunes, D. Bonner, and J. Fung-Tomc.** 2001. Correlation between genotype and phenotype categorization of staphylococci based on methicillin susceptibility and resistance. *J. Clin. Microbiol.* **39:**2961–2963.

46. **Grayson, M. L., G. M. Eliopoulos, C. B. Wennersten, K. L. Ruoff, P. C. De Girolami, M. J. Ferraro, and R. C. Moellering, Jr.** 1991. Increasing resistance to beta-lactam antibiotics among clinical isolates of *Enterococcus faecium*: a 22-year review at one institution. *Antimicrob. Agents Chemother.* **35:**2180–2184.

47. **Gresser-Burns, M. E., C. J. Shanholtzer, L. R. Peterson, and D. N. Gerding.** 1987. Occurrence and reproducibility of the "skip" phenomenon in bactericidal testing of *Staphylococcus aureus. Diagn. Microbiol. Infect. Dis.* **6:**335–342.

48. **Gunnison, J. B., M. A. Fraher, and E. Jawetz.** 1963. Persistence of *Staphylcoccus aureus* in penicillin in vitro. *J. Gen. Microbiol.* **34:**335–349.

49. **Hackbarth, C. J., and H. F. Chambers.** 1989. Methicillin-resistant staphylococci: genetics and mechanisms of resistance. *Antimicrob. Agents Chemother.* **33:**991–994.

50. **Handwerger, S., and A. Tomasz.** 1985. Antibiotic tolerance among clinical isolates of bacteria. *Rev. Infect. Dis.* **7:**368–386.

51. **Hartman, B. J., and A. Tomasz.** 1986. Expression of methicillin resistance in heterogeneous strains of *Staphylococcus aureus. Antimicrob. Agents Chemother.* **29:**85–92.

52. **Hindler, J.** 1997. Antimicrobial susceptibility tests, p. 105–154. *In* H. D. Isenberg (ed.), *Essential Procedures in Clinical Microbiology.* American Society for Microbiology, Washington, D.C.

53. **Hindler, J. A., and C. B. Inderlied.** 1985. Effect of source of Mueller-Hinton agar and resistance frequency on the detection of methicillin-resistant *Staphylococcus aureus. J. Clin. Microbiol.* **21:**205–210.

54. **Hindler, J. A., and D. F. Sahm.** 1992. Controversies and confusion regarding antimicrobial susceptibility testing of enterococci. *Antimicrob. Newsl.* **8:**65–74.

55. **Hindler, J. A., and N. L. Warner.** 1984. Effect of source of Mueller-Hinton agar on detection of oxacillin resistance in *Staphylococcus aureus* using a screening methodology. *J. Clin. Microbiol.* **25:**734–735.

56. **Hiramatsu, K., H. Hanaki, T. Ino, K. Yabuta, T. Oguri, and F. C. Tenover.** 1997. Methicillin-resistant *Staphylococcus aureus* clinical strain with reduced vancomycin susceptibility. *J. Antimicrob. Chemother.* **40:**135–136.

57. **Ho, P. L., D. N. Tsang, T. L. Que, M. Ho, and K. Y. Yuen.** 2000. Comparison of screening methods for detection of extended-spectrum β-lactamases and their prevalence among *Escherichia coli* and *Klebsiella* species in Hong Kong. *APMIS* **108:**237–240.

58. **Horstkotte, M. A., J. K. M. Knobloch, H. Rohde, and D. Mack.** 2001. Rapid detection of methicillin resistance in coagulase-negative staphylococci by a penicillin-binding protein 2a-specific latex agglutination test. *J. Clin. Microbiol.* **39:**3700–3702.

59. **Hunter, T. H.** 1950. Speculations on the mechanism of cure of endocarditis. *JAMA* **144:**527.

60. **Hussain, Z., L. Stoakes, S. Garrow, S. Longo, V. Fitzgerald, and R. Lannigan.** 2000. Rapid detection of *mecA*-positive and *mecA*-negative coagulase-negative staphylococci by an anti-penicillin binding protein 2a slide latex agglutination test. *J. Clin. Microbiol.* **38:**2051–2054.

61. **Hussain, Z., L. Stoakes, V. Massey, D. Diagre, V. Fitzgerald, S. El Sayed, and R. Lannigan.** 2000. Correlation of oxacillin MIC with *mecA* gene carriage in coagulase-negative staphylococci. *J. Clin. Microbiol.* **38:**752–754.

62. **Iwen, P. C., D. M. Kelley, J. Linder, and S. H. Hinrichs.** 1996. Revised approach for identification and detection of ampicillin and vancomycin resistance in *Enterococcus* species by using MicroScan panels. *J. Clin. Microbiol.* **34:**1779–1783.

63. **Jacobs, M. R., H. J. Koornhof, R. M. Robins-Browne, C. M. Stevenson, Z. A. Vermaak, I. Freiman, G. B. Miller, M. A. Witcomb, M. Isaäcson, J. I. Ward, and R. Austrian.** 1978. Emergence of multiply resistant pneumococci. *N. Engl. J. Med.* **299:**735–740.

64. **Jacobs, M. R., S. K. Spangler, and P. C. Appelbaum.** 1992. β-Lactamase production and susceptibility of US and European anaerobic gram-negative bacilli to β-lactams and other agents. *Eur. J. Clin. Microbiol. Infect. Dis.* **11:**1081–1093.

65. **Jacoby, G., P. Han, and J. Tran.** 1997. Comparative in vitro activities of carbapenem L-749,345 and other antimicrobials against multiresistant gram-negative clinical pathogens. *Antimicrob. Agents Chemother.* **41:**1830–1831.

66. **Jacoby, G., A. A. Medeiros, T. F. O'Brien, M. E. Pinto, and J. Jiang.** 1989. Broad-spectrum transmissible β-lactamases. *N. Engl. J. Med.* **319:**723–724.

67. **Jacoby, G. A.** 1998. Epidemiology of extended-spectrum β-lactamases. *Clin. Infect. Dis.* **27:**81–83.

68. **Jacoby, G. A., and P. Han.** 1996. Detection of extended-spectrum β-lactamases in clinical isolates of *Klebsiella pneumoniae* and *Escherichia coli. J. Clin. Microbiol.* **34:**908–911.

69. **Jacoby, G. A., and A. A. Medeiros.** 1991. More extended-spectrum β-lactamases. *Antimicrob. Agents Chemother.* **35:**1697–1704.

70. **Jankins, M.** 1992. Chloramphenicol acetyltransferase test, p. 5.8.1–5.8.7. *In* H. D. Isenberg (ed.), *Clinical Microbiology Procedures Handbook.* American Society for Microbiology, Washington, D.C.

71. **Jarlier, V., M. H. Nicolas, G. Fournier, and A. Philippon.** 1988. Extended broad-spectrum β-lactamases conferring transferable resistance to newer β-lactam agents in Enterobacteriaceae: hospital prevalence and susceptibility patterns. *Rev. Infect. Dis.* **10:**867–878.

72. **Jett, B., L. Free, and D. F. Sahm.** 1996. Factors influencing the Vitek gram-positive susceptibility system's detection of *vanB*-encoded vancomycin resistance among enterococci. *J. Clin. Microbiol.* **34:**701–706.

73. **Jones, R. N.** 2001. Resistance patterns among nosocomial pathogens: trends over the past few years. *Chest* **119:**397S–404S.

74. **Jones, R. N., D. C. Edson, and Microbiology Resource Committee of the College of American Pathologists.** 1991. Antimicrobial susceptibility testing trends and accuracy in the United States. A review of the College of American Pathologists Microbiology Surveys, 1972–1989. *Arch. Pathol. Lab. Med.* **115:**429–436.

75. **Jordan, G. W., and M. M. Kawachi.** 1981. Analysis of serum bactericidal activity in endocarditis, osteomyelitis, and other bacterial infections. *Medicine* **60:**49–61.

76. **Jorgensen, J. H., L. A. Maher, and J. S. Redding.** 1987. In vitro activity of LY146032 (daptomycin) against selected aerobic bacteria. *Eur. J. Clin. Microbiol.* **6:**91–96.

77. **Jorgensen, J. H., M. L. McElmeel, and C. W. Trippy.** 1996. Comparison of inoculation methods for testing enterococci by using vancomycin screening agar. *J. Clin. Microbiol.* **34:**2841–2842.

78. **Katsanis, G. P., J. Spargo, M. J. Ferraro, L. Sutton, and G. A. Jacoby.** 1994. Detection of *Klebsiella pneumoniae* and *Escherichia coli* strains producing extended-spectrum β-lactamases. *J. Clin. Microbiol.* **32:**691–696.

79. **Kiehn, T. E., P. D. Ellner, and D. Budzko.** 1989. Role of the microbiology laboratory in care of the immunosuppressed patient. *Rev. Infect. Dis.* **11**(Suppl. 7):S1706–S1710.

80. **Kim, K. S., and B. F. Anthony.** 1981. Importance of bacterial growth phase in determining minimum bactericidal concentrations of penicillin and methicillin. *Antimicrob. Agents Chemother.* **19:**1075–1077.

81. **King, T. C., D. Schlessinger, and D. J. Krogstad.** 1981. The assessment of antimicrobial combinations. *J. Infect. Dis.* **129:**193.

82. **Klastersky, J., D. Daneau, G. Swings, and D. Weerts.** 1974. Antibacterial activity in serum and urine as a therapeutic guide in bacterial infections. *J. Infect. Dis.* **129:**187–193.

83. **Knapp, C., and J. A. Moody.** 1992. Tests to assess bactericidal activity, p. 5.16.1–5.16.33. *In* H. D. Isenberg (ed.), *Clinical Microbiology Procedures Handbook.* American Society for Microbiology, Washington, D.C.

84. **Knapp, C. C., M. D. Ludwig, J. A. Washington, and H. F. Chambers.** 1996. Evaluation of Vitek GPS-SA card for testing of oxacillin against borderline-susceptible staphylococci that lack *mec. J. Clin. Microbiol.* **34:**1603–1605.

85. **Kohner, P., R. Patel, J. Uhk, K. Garin, M. Hopkins, L. Wegener, and F. Cockerill III.** 1997. Comparison of agar dilution, broth microdilution, E-test, disk diffusion, and automated Vitek methods for testing susceptibilities of *Enterococcus* spp. to vancomycin. *J. Clin. Microbiol.* **35:**3258–3263.

86. **Krogstad, D. J., and R. C. Moellering, Jr.** 1998. Antimicrobial combinations, p. 537–599. *In* V. Lorian (ed.), *Antibiotics in Laboratory Medicine.* The Williams & Wilkins Co., Baltimore, Md.

87. **Lautenbach, E., J. B. Patel, W. B. Bilker, P. H. Edelstein, and N. O. Fishman.** 2001. Extended-spectrum β-lactamase-producing *Escherichia coli* and *Klebsiella pneumoniae*: risk factors for infection and impact of resistance on outcomes. *Clin. Infect. Dis.* **32:**1162–1171.

88. **Leclercq, R., and P. Courvalin.** 1997. Resistance to glycopeptides in enterococci. *Clin. Infect. Dis.* **24:**545–556.

89. **Leclercq, R., S. Dutka-Malen, A. Brisson-Noel, C. Molinas, E. Derlot, M. Arthur, J. Duval, and P. Courvalin.** 1992. Resistance of enterococci to aminoglycosides and glycopeptides. *Clin. Infect. Dis.* **15:**495–501.

90. **Leclercq, R., S. Dutka-Malen, J. Duval, and P. Courvalin.** 1992. Vancomycin resistance gene *vanC* is specific to *Enterococcus gallinarum. Antimicrob. Agents Chemother.* **36:**2005–2008.

91. **Leggett, J. E., S. A. Wolz, and W. A. Craig.** 1989. Use of serum ultrafiltrate in the serum dilution test. *J. Infect. Dis.* **160:**616–623.

92. **Leitch, C.** 1992. β-Lactamase tests, p. 5.3.1–5.3.8. *In* H. D. Isenberg (ed.), *Clinical Microbiology Procedures Handbook.* American Society for Microbiology, Washington, D.C.

93. **Livermore, D. M.** 1995. β-Lactamases in laboratory and clinical resistance. *Clin. Microbiol. Rev.* **8:**557–584.

94. **Livermore, D. M., and M. Yuan.** 1996. Antibiotic resistance and production of extended-spectrum β-lactamases amongst *Klebsiella* spp. from intensive care units in Europe. *J. Antimicrob. Chemother.* **38:**409–424.

95. **Louie, L., A. Majury, J. Goodfellow, M. Louie, and A. E. Simor.** 2001. Evaluation of a latex agglutination test (MRSA-Screen) for detection of oxacillin resistance in coagulase-negative staphylococci. *J. Clin. Microbiol.* **39:**4149–4151.

96. **Louie, L., S. O. Matsumura, E. Choi, M. Louie, and A. E. Simor.** 2000. Evaluation of three rapid methods for detection of methicillin resistance in *Staphylococcus aureus. J. Clin. Microbiol.* **38:**2170–2173.

97. **MacGowan, A., C. McMullin, P. James, K. Bowker, D. Reeves, and L. White.** 1997. External quality assessment of the serum bactericidal test: results of a methodology/interpretation questionnaire. *J. Antimicrob. Chemother.* **39:**277–284.

98. **MacLowry, J. D.** 1989. Perspective. The serum dilution test. *J. Infect. Dis.* **160:**624–626.

99. **Marlowe, E., M. Cohen, J. F. Hindler, K. Ward, and D. A. Bruckner.** 2001. Practical strategies for detecting and confirming vancomycin-intermediate *Staphylococcus aureus*: a tertiary-care hospital laboratory's experience. *J. Clin. Microbiol.* **39:**2637–2639.

100. **Marshall, S. A., W. W. Wilke, M. A. Pfaller, and R. N. Jones.** 1998. *Staphylococcus aureus* and coagulase-negative staphylococci from blood stream infections: frequency of occurrence, antimicrobial susceptibility, and molecular (*mecA*) characterization of oxacillin resistance in the SCOPE program. *Diagn. Microbiol. Infect. Dis.* **30:**205–214.

101. **Massanari, R. M., M. A. Pfaller, D. S. Wakesfield, G. T. Hammons, L. A. McNut, R. F. Woolson, and C. M. Helms.** 1988. Implications of acquired oxacillin resistance in management and control of *Staphylococcus aureus* infections. *J. Infect. Dis.* **158:**701–709.

102. **McKessar, S., A. Berry, J. Bell, J. Turnidge, and J. C. Paton.** 2001. Genetic characterization of *vanG*, a novel vancomycin resistance locus in *Enterococcus faecalis. Antimicrob. Agents Chemother.* **44:**3224–3228.

103. **Meyer, K. S., C. Urban, J. A. Eagan, B. J. Berger, and J. J. Rahal.** 1993. Nosocomial outbreak of *Klebsiella* infection resistant to late-generation cephalosporins. *Ann. Intern. Med.* **119:**353–358.

104. **Moellering, R. C., Jr., O. M. Koraeniowski, M. A. Sande, and C. B. Wennersten.** 1979. Species-specific resistance to antimicrobial synergism in *Streptococcus fae-*

cium and *Streptococcus faecalis. J. Infect. Dis.* **140:**203–208.

105. **Moland, E. S., C. C. Sanders, and K. S. Thomson.** 1998. Can results obtained with commercially available MicroScan microdilution panels serve as an indicator of β-lactamase production among *Escherichia coli* and *Klebsiella* isolates with hidden resistance to expanded-spectrum cephalosporins and aztreonam? *J. Clin. Microbiol.* **36:**2575–2579.

106. **Montanari, M. P., O. Massidda, M. Mingoia, and P. E. Varalco.** 1996. Borderline susceptibility to methicillin in *Staphylococcus aureus*: a new mechanism of resistance? *Microb. Drug Resist.* **2:**257–260.

107. **Murray, B. E.** 1990. The life and times of the enterococcus. *Clin. Microbiol. Rev.* **3:**46–65.

108. **Murray, B. E.** 1992. β-Lactamase-producing enterococci. *Antimicrob. Agents Chemother.* **36:**2355–2359.

109. **Murray, B. E.** 1997. Vancomycin-resistant enterococci. *Am. J. Med.* **102:**284–293.

110. **Musher, D. M., and R. Fletcher.** 1982. Tolerant *Staphylococcus aureus* causing vertebral osteomyelitis. *Ann. Intern. Med.* **93:**796–800.

111. **National Committee for Clinical Laboratory Standards.** 1993. *Methods for Dilution Antimicrobial Susceptibility Tests for Bacteria That Grow Aerobically.* Approved standard M7-A3. National Committee for Clinical Laboratory Standards, Villanova, Pa.

112. **National Committee for Clinical Laboratory Standards.** 1993. *Performance Standards for Antimicrobial Disk Susceptibility Tests.* Approved standard M2-A5. National Committee for Clinical Laboratory Standards, Villanova, Pa.

113. **National Committee for Clinical Laboratory Standards.** 1999. *Methodology for the Serum Bactericidal Test.* Document M21-A. National Committee for Clinical Laboratory Standards, Wayne, Pa.

114. **National Committee for Clinical Laboratory Standards.** 1999. *Methods for Determining Bactericidal Activity of Antimicrobial Agents.* Document M26-A. National Committee for Clinical Laboratory Standards, Wayne, Pa.

115. **NCCLS.** 2000. *Methods for Dilution Antimicrobial Susceptibility Tests for Bacteria That Grow Aerobically; Approved Standard,* 5th ed. NCCLS document M7-A5. NCCLS, Wayne, Pa.

116. **NCCLS.** 2000. *Performance Standards for Antimicrobial Disk Susceptibility Tests; Approved Standard,* 7th ed. NCCLS document M2-A7. NCCLS, Wayne, Pa.

117. **NCCLS.** 2001. *Methods for Antimicrobial Susceptibility Testing of Anaerobic Bacteria; Approved Standard,* 5th ed. NCCLS document M11-A5. NCCLS, Wayne, Pa.

118. **NCCLS.** 2002. *Performance Standards for Antimicrobial Susceptibility Testing; Twelfth Informational Supplement.* NCCLS document M100-S12. NCCLS. Wayne, Pa.

119. **Neumann, M. A., D. F. Sahm, C. Thornsberry, and J. E. McGowan, Jr.** 1991. *Cumitech 6A, New Developments in Antimicrobial Agent Susceptibility Testing: a Practical Guide.* American Society for Microbiology, Washington, D.C.

120. **O'Callaghan, C. H., A. Morris, S. M. Kirby, and A. H. Shingler.** 1972. Novel method for detection of β-lactamases by using a chromogenic cephalosporin substrate. *Antimicrob. Agents Chemother.* **1:**283–288.

121. **Okabe, T., K. Oana, Y. Kawakami, M. Yamaguchi, Y. Takahashi, Y. Okimura, T. Honda, and T. Katsuyama.** 2000. Limitations of Vitek GPS-418 cards in exact detection of vancomycin-resistant enterococci with the *vanB* genotype. *J. Clin. Microbiol.* **38:**2409–2411.

122. **Ostrowsky, B., N. C. Clark, C. Thauvin-Eliopoulos, L. Venkataraman, M. Samore, F. C. Tenover, G. M. Eliopoulos, R. C. Moellering, Jr., and H. S. Gold.** 1999. A

cluster of VanD vancomycin-resistant *Enterococcus fae-cium*: molecular characterization and epidemiology. *J. Infect. Dis.* **180:**1177–1185.

123. **Paterson, D. L.** 2000. Recommendation for treatment of severe infections caused by Enterobacteriaceae producing extended-spectrum β-lactamases (ESBLs). *Clin. Microbiol. Infect.* **6:**460–463.

124. **Paterson, D. L., W. C. Ko, A. Von Gottberg, J. M. Casellas, L. Mulazimoglu, K. P. Klugman, R. A. Bonomo, L. B. Rice, J. G. McCormack, and V. L. Yu.** 2001. Outcome of cephalosporin treatment for serious infections due to apparently susceptible organisms producing extended-spectrum β-lactamases: implications for the clinical microbiology laboratory. *J. Clin. Microbiol.* **39:**2206–2212.

125. **Paterson, D. L., N. Singh, J. D. Rihs, C. Squier, B. L. Rihs, and R. R. Muder.** 2001. Control of an outbreak of infection due to extended-spectrum β-lactamase-producing *Escherichia coli* in a liver transplantation unit. *Clin. Infect. Dis.* **33:**126–128.

126. **Patterson, J. E.** 2000. Extended-spectrum β-lactamases. *Semin. Respir. Infect.* **15:**299–307.

127. **Pefanis, A., C. Thauvin-Eliopoulos, G. Eliopoulos, and R. C. Moellering, Jr.** 1993. Activity of ampicillin-sulbactam and oxacillin in experimental endocarditis caused by β-lactamase-hyperproducing *Staphylococcus aureus*. *Antimicrob. Agents Chemother.* **37:**507–511.

128. **Perichon, B., P. Reynolds, and P. Courvalin.** 1997. VanD-type glycopeptide-resistant *Enterococcus faecium* BM4339. *Antimicrob. Agents Chemother.* **41:**2016–2018.

129. **Peterson, L. R., and C. J. Shanholtzer.** 1992. Tests for bactericidal effects of antimicrobial agents: technical performance and clinical relevance. *Clin. Microbiol. Rev.* **5:**420–432.

130. **Philippon, A., R. Labia, and G. Jacoby.** 1989. Extended-spectrum β-lactamases. *Antimicrob. Agents Chemother.* **33:**1131–1136.

131. **Quinn, J. P.** 1994. Clinical significance of extended-spectrum β-lactamases. *Eur. J. Clin. Microbiol. Infect. Dis.* **13:**39–42.

132. **Ramotar, K., W. Woods, L. Larocque, and B. Toye.** 2000. Comparison of phenotype methods to identify enterococci intrinsically resistant to vancomycin (vanC VRE). *Diagn. Microbiol. Infect. Dis.* **36:**119–124.

133. **Raney, P., P. Williams, J. E. McGowan, Jr., and F. C. Tenover.** 2002. Validation of Vitek version 7.01 software for testing staphylococci against vancomycin. *Diagn. Microbiol. Infect. Dis.* **43:**135–140.

134. **Reller, L. B.** 1986. The serum bactericidal test. *Rev. Infect. Dis.* **8:**803–808.

135. **Resende, C. A., and A. M. Figueiredo.** 1997. Discrimination of methicillin-resistant *Staphylococcus aureus* from borderline-resistant and susceptible isolates by different methods. *J. Med. Microbiol.* **46:**145–149.

136. **Rosenberg, J., F. C. Tenover, J. Wong, W. Jarvis, and D. J. Vugia.** 1997. Are clinical laboratories in California accurately reporting vancomycin-resistant enterococci? *J. Clin. Microbiol.* **35:**2526–2530.

137. **Rosenblatt, J. E.** 1987. Laboratory tests used to guide antimicrobial therapy. *Mayo Clin. Proc.* **62:**799–805.

138. **Sabath, L.** 1977. Chemical and physical factors influencing methicillin resistance of *Staphylococcus aureus* and *Staphylococcus epidermidis*. *J. Antimicrob. Chemother.* **3:**47–51.

139. **Sahm, D. F., S. Boonlayangoor, P. C. Iwen, J. L. Baade, and G. L. Woods.** 1991. Factors influencing determination of high-level aminoglycoside resistance in *Enterococcus faecalis*. *J. Clin. Microbiol.* **29:**1934–1939.

140. **Sahm, D. F., S. Boonlayangoor, and J. E. Schulz.** 1991. Detection of high-level aminoglycoside resistance in enterococci other than *Enterococcus faecalis*. *J. Clin. Microbiol.* **29:**2595–2598.

141. **Sahm, D. F., J. Kissinger, M. S. Gilmore, P. R. Murray, R. Mulder, J. Solliday, and B. Clarke.** 1989. In vitro susceptibility studies of vancomycin-resistant *Enterococcus faecalis*. *Antimicrob. Agents Chemother.* **33:**1588–1591.

142. **Sahm, D. F., and L. Olsen.** 1990. In vitro detection of enterococcal vancomycin resistance. *Antimicrob. Agents Chemother.* **34:**1846–1848.

143. **Sahm, D. F., and C. Torres.** 1988. Effects of medium and inoculum variations on screening for high-level aminoglycoside resistance in *Enterococcus faecalis*. *J. Clin. Microbiol.* **26:**250–256.

144. **Sahm, D. F., and C. Torres.** 1988. High-content aminoglycoside disks for determining aminoglycoside-penicillin synergy against *Enterococcus faecalis*. *J. Clin. Microbiol.* **26:**257–260.

145. **Sakoulas, G., H. S. Gold, L. Venkataraman, P. DeGirolami, G. M. Eliopoulos, and Q. Qian.** 2001. Methicillin-resistant *Staphylococcus aureus*: comparison of susceptibility testing methods and analysis of *mecA*-positive susceptible strains. *J. Clin. Microbiol.* **39:**3946–3951.

146. **Sanders, C. C., A. L. Barry, J. A. Washington, C. Shubert, E. S. Moland, M. M. Traczewski, C. Knapp, and R. Mulder.** 1996. Detection of extended-spectrum β-lactamase-producing members of the family Enterobacteriaceae with Vitek ESBL test. *J. Clin. Microbiol.* **34:**2997–3001.

147. **Scheld, W. M., and M. A. Sande.** 1983. Bactericidal versus bacteriostatic antibiotic therapy of experimental pneumococcal meningitis in rabbits. *J. Clin. Investig.* **71:**411–419.

148. **Schlichter, J. G., and H. MacLean.** 1947. A method for determining the effective therapeutic level in the treatment of subacute bacterial endocarditis with penicillin: a preliminary report. *Am. Heart J.* **34:**209–211.

149. **Schlichter, J. G., H. MacLean, and A. Milzer.** 1949. Effective penicillin therapy in subacute bacterial endocarditis and other chronic infections. *Am. J. Med. Sci.* **217:**600–608.

150. **Schulz, J. E., and D. F. Sahm.** 1993. Reliability of the E test for detection of ampicillin, vancomycin, and high-level aminoglycoside resistance in *Enterococcus* spp. *J. Clin. Microbiol.* **31:**3336–3339.

151. **Scutier, J. P., and J. Klastersky.** 1984. Significance of serum bactericidal activity in gram-negative bacillary bacteremia in patients with and without granulocytopenia. *Am. J. Med.* **76:**429–435.

152. **Shehabi, A. A., A. Mahafzah, I. Baadran, F. A. Qadar, and N. Dajani.** 2000. High incidence of *Klebsiella pneumoniae* clinical isolates resistant to extended-spectrum β-lactam drugs in intensive care units. *Diagn. Microbiol. Infect. Dis.* **36:**53–56.

153. **Sirot, D.** 1995. Extended-spectrum plasmid-mediated β-lactamases. *J. Antimicrob. Chemother.* **36:**19–34.

154. **Siu, L. K., P. L. Lu, P. R. Hsueh, F. M. Lin, S. C. Chang, K. T. Luh, M. Ho, and C. Y. Lee.** 1999. Bacteremia due to extended-spectrum β-lactamase-producing *Escherichia coli* and *Klebsiella pneumoniae* in a pediatric oncology ward: clinical features and identification of different plasmids carrying both SHV-5 and TEM-1 genes. *J. Clin. Microbiol.* **37:**4020–4027.

155. **Standiford, H. D., J. B. deMaine, and W. M. Kirby.** 1970. Antibiotic synergism of enterococci. *Arch. Intern. Med.* **126:**255–259.

156. **Steward, C. D., J. K. Rasheed, S. K. Hubert, J. W. Biddle, P. Raney, G. J. Anderson, P. P. Williams, K. L.**

Brittain, A. Oliver, J. E. McGowan, Jr., and F. C. Tenover. 2001. Characterization of clinical isolates of *Klebsiella pneumoniae* from 19 laboratories using the National Committee for Clinical Laboratory Standards extended-spectrum β-lactamase detection methods. *J. Clin. Microbiol.* **39:**2864–2872.

157. Swenson, J. M., N. Clark, M. J. Ferraro, D. F. Sahm, G. Doern, M. A. Pfaller, L. B. Reller, M. P. Weinstein, R. J. Zabransky, and F. C. Tenover. 1994. Development of a standardized screening method for detection of vancomycin-resistant enterococci. *J. Clin. Microbiol.* **32:**1700–1704.

158. Swenson, J. M., N. C. Clark, D. F. Sahm, M. J. Ferraro, G. Doern, J. Hindler, J. H. Jorgensen, M. A. Pfaller, L. B. Reller, M. P. Weinstein, R. J. Zabransky, and F. C. Tenover. 1995. Molecular characterization and multilaboratory evaluation of *Enterococcus faecalis* ATCC 51299 and quality control of screening tests for vancomycin and high-level aminoglycoside resistance in enterococci. *J. Clin. Microbiol.* **33:**3019–3021.

159. Swenson, J. M., M. J. Ferraro, D. Sahm, N. C. Clark, D. Culver, F. C. Tenover, and The National Committee for Clinical Laboratory Standards Working Group on Enterococci. 1995. Multilaboratory evaluation of screening methods for detection of high-level aminoglycoside resistance in enterococci. *J. Clin. Microbiol.* **33:**3008–3018.

160. Swenson, J. M., M. J. Ferraro, D. F. Sahm, P. Charache, The National Committee for Clinical Laboratory Standards Working Group on Enterococci, and F. C. Tenover. 1992. New vancomycin disk diffusion breakpoints for enterococci. *J. Clin. Microbiol.* **30:**2525–2528.

161. Swenson, J. M., B. C. Hill, and C. Thornsberry. 1986. Screening pneumococci for penicillin resistance. *J. Clin. Microbiol.* **24:**749–752.

162. Swenson, J. M., B. C. Hill, and C. Thornsberry. 1989. Problems with the disk diffusion test for detection of vancomycin resistance in enterococci. *J. Clin. Microbiol.* **27:**2140–2142. (Erratum, **28:**403, 1990.)

163. Swenson, J. M., J. Spargo, F. C. Tenover, and M. J. Ferraro. 2001. Optimal inoculation methods and quality control for the NCCLS oxacillin agar screen test for detection of oxacillin resistance in *Staphylococcus aureus*. *J. Clin. Microbiol.* **39:**3781–3784.

164. Swenson, J. M., P. P. Williams, G. Killgore, C. M. O'Hara, and F. C. Tenover. 2001. Performance of eight methods, including two new rapid methods, for detection of oxacillin resistance in a challenge set of *Staphylococcus aureus* organisms. *J. Clin. Microbiol.* **39:**3785–3788.

165. Taylor, P. C., F. D. Schoenknecht, J. C. Sherris, and E. C. Linner. 1983. Determination of minimum bactericidal concentrations of oxacillin for *Staphylococcus aureus*: influence and significance of technical factors. *Antimicrob. Agents Chemother.* **23:**142–150.

166. Tenover, F. C., R. N. Jones, J. M. Swenson, B. Zimmer, S. McAllister, J. H. Jorgensen, and The NCCLS Staphylococcus Working Group. 1999. Methods for improved detection of oxacillin resistance in coagulase-negative staphylococci: results of a multicenter study. *J. Clin. Microbiol.* **37:**4051–4058.

167. Tenover, F. C., M. V. Lancaster, B. C. Hill, C. D. Steward, S. A. Stocker, G. A. Hancock, C. M. O'Hara, N. C. Clark, and K. Hiramatsu. 1998. Characterization of staphylococci with reduced susceptibility to vancomycin and other glycopeptides. *J. Clin. Microbiol.* **36:**1020–1027.

168. Tenover, F. C., M. J. Mohammed, T. S. Gorton, and Z. F. Dembek. 1999. Detection and reporting of organisms producing extended-spectrum β-lactamases: survey of laboratories in Connecticut. *J. Clin. Microbiol.* **37:**4065–4070.

169. Tenover, F. C., J. M. Swenson, C. M. O'Hara, and S. A. Stocker. 1995. Ability of commercial and reference antimicrobial susceptibility testing methods to detect vancomycin resistance in enterococci. *J. Clin. Microbiol.* **33:**1524–1527.

170. Thauvin-Eliopoulos, E., L. B. Rice, G. M. Eliopoulos, and R. C. Moellering, Jr. 1990. Efficacy of oxacillin and ampicillin-sulbactam combination in experimental endocarditis caused by β-lactamase-hyperproducing *Staphylococcus aureus*. *Antimicrob. Agents Chemother.* **34:**728–732.

171. Thomson, K. S. 2001. Controversies about extended-spectrum and AmpC β-lactamases. *Emerg. Infect. Dis.* **7:**333–336.

172. Thomson, K. S., C. C. Sanders, and E. S. Moland. 1999. Use of microdilution panels with and without β-lactamase inhibitors as a phenotypic test for β-lactamase production among *Escherichia coli*, *Klebsiella* spp., *Enterobacter* spp., *Citrobacter freundii*, and *Serratia marcescens*. *Antimicrob. Agents Chemother.* **43:**1393–1400.

173. Thomson, K. S. and E. Smith Moland. 2000. Version 2000: the new β-lactamases of gram-negative bacteria at the dawn of the new millennium. *Microbes Infect.* **2:**1225–1235.

174. Thornsberry, C., and L. K. McDougal. 1983. Successful use of broth microdilution in susceptibility tests for methicillin-resistant (heteroresistant) staphylococci. *J. Clin. Microbiol.* **18:**1084–1091.

175. Tomasz, A., H. B. Drugeon, H. M. de Lencastre, D. Jabes, L. McDougal, and J. Bille. 1989. New mechanism for methicillin resistance in *Staphylococcus aureus*: clinical isolates that lack the PBP 2a gene and contain modified penicillin-binding proteins with modified penicillin-binding capacity. *Antimicrob. Agents Chemother.* **33:**1869–1874.

176. Tomasz, A., S. Nachman, and H. Leaf. 1991. Stable classes of phenotypic expression in methicillin-resistant clinical isolates of staphylococci. *Antimicrob. Agents Chemother.* **35:**124–129.

177. Torres, C., C. Tenorio, M. Lantero, M. Gastañares, and F. Baquero. 1993. High-level penicillin resistance and penicillin-gentamicin synergy in *Enterococcus faecium*. *Antimicrob. Agents Chemother.* **37:**2427–2431.

178. Tsai, S., M. J. Zervos, D. B. Clewell, S. Donabedian, D. F. Sahm, and J. W. Chow. 1998. A new high-level gentamicin resistance gene, *aph(2")-Id*, in *Enterococcus* spp. *Antimicrob. Agents Chemother.* **42:**1229–1232.

179. Tuomanen, E., D. T. Durack, and A. Tomasz. 1986. Antibiotic tolerance among clinical isolates of bacteria. *Antimicrob. Agents Chemother.* **30:**521–527.

180. van den Braak, N., W. Goessens, A. van Belkum, H. Verbrugh, and H. Endtz. 2001. Accuracy of the VITEK 2 system to detect glycopeptide resistance in enterococci. *J. Clin. Microbiol.* **39:**351–353.

181. van Griethuysen, A., M. Pouw, N. van Leeuwen, M. Heck, P. Willemse, A. Buiting, and J. Kluytmans. 1999. Rapid slide latex agglutination test for detection of methicillin resistance in *Staphylococcus aureus*. *J. Clin. Microbiol.* **37:**2789–2792.

182. Van Horn, K. G., C. A. Gedris, K. M. Rodney, and J. B. Mitchell. 1996. Evaluation of commercial vancomycin agar screen plates for detection of vancomycin-resistant enterococci. *J. Clin. Microbiol.* **34:**2042–2044.

183. van Leeuwen, W. B., C. van Pelt, A. Luijendijk, H. A. Verbrugh, and W. H. F. Goessens. 1999. Rapid detec-

tion of methicillin resistance in *Staphylococcus aureus* isolates by the MRSA-Screen latex agglutination test. *J. Clin. Microbiol.* **37:**3029–3030.

184. **Weinstein, M. P., C. W. Stratton, A. Ackley, H. B. Hawley, P. A. Robinson, B. D. Fisher, D. V. Alcid, D. S. Stevens, and L. B. Reller.** 1985. Multicenter collaborative evaluation of a standardized bactericidal test as a prognostic indicator in infective endocarditis. *Am. J. Med.* **78:**262–269.

185. **Weinstein, M. P., C. W. Stratton, H. B. Hawley, A. Ackley, and L. B. Reller.** 1987. Multicenter collaborative evaluation of a standardized serum bactericidal test as a predictor of therapeutic efficacy in acute and chronic osteomyelitis. *Am. J. Med.* **83:**218–222.

186. **Wiener, J., J. P. Quinn, P. A. Bradford, R. V. Goering, C. Nathan, K. Bush, and R. A. Weinstein.** 1999. Multiple antibiotic-resistant *Klebsiella* and *Escherichia coli* in nursing homes. *JAMA* **281:**517–523.

187. **Willey, B. M., B. N. Kreiswirth, A. E. Simor, G. Williams, S. R. Scriver, A. Phillips, and D. E. Low.** 1992. Detection of vancomycin resistance in *Enterococcus* species. *J. Clin. Microbiol.* **30:**1621–1624.

188. **Winokur, P. L., R. Canton, J. M. Casellas, and N. Legakis.** 2001. Variations in the prevalence of strains expressing an extended-spectrum β-lactamase phenotype and characterization of isolates from Europe, the Americas, and the Western Pacific region. *Clin. Infect. Dis.* **32:**94–103.

189. **Yamazumi, T., I. Furuta, D. Diekema, M. A. Pfaller, and R. N. Jones.** 2001. Comparison of the Vitek gram-positive susceptibility 106 card, the MRSA-Screen latex agglutination test, and *mecA* analysis for detecting oxacillin resistance in a geographically diverse collection of clinical isolates of coagulase-negative staphylococci. *J. Clin. Microbiol.* **39:**3623–3626.

190. **Yamazumi, T., S. A. Marshall, W. W. Wilke, D. J. Diekema, M. A. Pfaller, and R. N. Jones.** 2001. Comparison of the Vitek gram-positive susceptibility 106 card and the MRSA-Screen latex agglutination test for determining oxacillin resistance in clinical bloodstream isolates of *Staphylococcus aureus*. *J. Clin. Microbiol.* **39:**53–56.

191. **York, M. K., L. Gibbs, F. Chelab, and G. F. Brooks.** 1996. Comparison of PCR detection of *mecA* with standard susceptibility testing methods to determine methicillin resistance in coagulase-negative staphylococci. *J. Clin. Microbiol.* **43:**249–253.

Detection and Characterization of Antimicrobial Resistance Genes in Bacteria

J. KAMILE RASHEED AND FRED C. TENOVER

75

Resistance to antimicrobial agents in bacteria is mediated by (i) acquired genes, whose presence in a cell is usually synonymous with a resistance phenotype; (ii) mutations in resident genes that alter a variety of phenotypes, including alteration of target sites and enhanced efflux mechanisms; or (iii) changes in outer membrane proteins (which limit the access of drugs to the cell). A wide variety of DNA probes and PCR assays focused on the detection of acquired resistance genes have been described over the last two decades (32, 202). However, within the last few years, several novel methods of detecting resistance genotypes have evolved. These include real-time PCR assays (e.g., TaqMan [Applied Biosystems, Foster City, Calif.] protocols), ligase chain reaction, cleavase-based assays (including Invader [Third Wave Technology, Inc., Madison, Wis.] assays), and DNA sequence analysis. Methods for correlating increasing antimicrobial resistance with changes in specific outer membrane proteins (such as relating the absence of the OmpC and OmpF porins of *Escherichia coli* via Western blot analysis or the loss of the corresponding *ompC* and *ompF* loci to resistance to cephamycins or extended-spectrum cephalosporins [118, 221]) continue to evolve.

Several genetic assays for detecting resistance genes are now available commercially. These include line probe assays (36, 204) and cycling probe assays (11, 108), the latter of which is Food and Drug Administration cleared for clinical laboratory use. New technology for rapid DNA sequence analysis is making the detection of mutations associated with antibacterial resistance much easier (127, 145). Although we are learning more about the molecular basis of resistance to antifungal and many antiparasitic drugs, molecular tests for detecting such resistance are still in development.

RATIONALE FOR USING GENETIC TESTS TO DETECT RESISTANCE GENES

There are four major reasons to use genetic tests to identify antimicrobial resistance genes or mutations associated with resistance. First, genetic methods are helpful for arbitrating MIC results that are at or near the breakpoint for resistance of bacterial species. For example, isolates of *Staphylococcus aureus* for which the oxacillin MICs are between 2 and 8 μg/ml (borderline resistant) may contain the *mecA* (meth-

icillin) resistance gene determinant or may produce high levels of β-lactamase, which slowly hydrolyzes oxacillin (25, 69). While vancomycin would be the drug of choice for the former cases, penicillinase-stable β-lactams or β-lactam/β-lactamase inhibitor compounds can be used to treat infections caused by β-lactamase-hyperproducing strains (120). A test indicating the absence of *mecA* in an isolate of *S. aureus* suggests that a physician could use an antimicrobial agent other than vancomycin to treat the infection.

Second, genetic methods can be used to detect resistance genes, or mutations that result in resistance, in organisms directly in clinical specimens to guide therapy early in the course of a patient's disease before cultures are positive. For example, PCR assays can detect mutations in the *pbpA* and *pbp2b* loci associated with penicillin resistance in *Streptococcus pneumoniae* (54, 210). Such mutations indicate that the strain has reduced susceptibility to β-lactam agents and may be resistant to multiple drugs.

Third, genetics-based tests are more accurate than resistance phenotypes for monitoring the epidemiologic spread of a particular resistance gene in a hospital or community setting. For example, tracking the spread of the *vanA* vancomycin resistance gene in enterococci by PCR assays has been helpful in documenting the spread of multiresistant enterococci in the United States (29) and Europe (1, 73). Antibiograms cannot differentiate between organisms containing the *vanA* gene and those with derepressed *vanB* genes (60).

Fourth, genetics-based tests can be used as the "gold standard" for resistance when evaluating the accuracy of new susceptibility testing methods that use clinical isolates or stock cultures for which MICs are borderline (46, 188).

GENETIC TESTS FOR RESISTANCE GENES AND DNA SEQUENCING STRATEGIES TO DETECT MUTATIONS ASSOCIATED WITH RESISTANCE

General Guidelines

The ideal genetic test targets nucleic acid sequences within the open reading frame (or coding region) of the resistance gene and avoids sequences outside of the gene that may contain insertion elements or promoter sequences that may be present in susceptible strains or strains with other types of resistance genes. Among the primers that have been described for studying antibacterial resistance are those directed to β-lactamase genes and the genes that encode resistance to aminocyclitols, aminoglycosides, chloramphenicol, glycopeptides, isoniazid, macrolides, mupirocin, quinolones, rifampin, sulfonamides, tetracyclines, and trimethoprim. Examples of PCR primers that target resistance genes or mutations associated with resistance are shown in Table 1. The table is not meant to be exhaustive but, rather, gives an indication of the types of assays that have been described. Appropriate specificity controls (organisms that have a similar resistance pattern but contain resistance genes other than the target gene) should always be included in all reactions using these primers. Examples of DNA probes that can be used to detect resistance genes are described elsewhere (202).

DNA Sequencing

DNA sequence analysis has been particularly helpful for identifying point mutations associated with resistance to fluoroquinolones (46, 74, 88), extended-spectrum β-lactamases (13, 157, 158), and antimycobacterial drugs (127, 192). There are a number of mutations associated with resistance to isoniazid, rifampin, and streptomycin (62, 81, 195). Unfortunately, additional genetic loci associated with resistance must also be involved since only 60% of resistance can be explained by these loci (125). Thus, sequence analysis for predicting resistance in mycobacteria remains a research tool.

AMINOGLYCOSIDE RESISTANCE GENES

The diversity of aminoglycoside resistance genes, which are common in both gram-positive and gram-negative organisms (172), continues to expand with the recognition of additional acetyltransferases, adenylyltransferases, and phosphotransferases. Unfortunately, the lack of consensus sequences among the acetyltransferase and adenylyltransferase genes prohibits the detection of multiple determinants with a single PCR primer set (172), thus making it difficult to use amplification-based tests to predict aminoglycoside resistance, especially in gram-negative organisms. For example, there are at least 13 different variants of the aac(6')-I determinant responsible for resistance to netilmicin, sisomycin, and tobramycin. Some of these determinants also modify amikacin to a degree sufficient to result in resistance (22, 149). Such determinants are found in a wide variety of organisms, including the Enterobacteriaceae (22, 77, 198, 216), Stenotrophomonas maltophilia (100), and enterococci (38, 47). Novel mutations associated with spectinomycin resistance in Neisseria gonorrhoeae and N. meningitidis have also been delineated through sequencing of the rrs 16S rRNA locus (68). Genotypic methods continue to be used to classify new determinants and to aid in epidemiologic studies of antimicrobial resistance (77, 149, 213, 215).

Among the newer aminoglycoside resistance genes reported in gram-positive organisms are those encoding novel phosphotransferases, e.g., aph(2″)-Ib (91) and aph(2″)-Ic (27), which mediate high-level gentamicin resistance in enterococci, and a well-known streptomycin resistance gene of gram-negative bacteria (aadA), which has appeared in Enterococcus faecalis (30). PCR assays can be helpful for identifying strains of gram-positive cocci that carry genes encoding high-level aminoglycoside resistance (95, 188, 213).

DETECTING GENES ASSOCIATED WITH RESISTANCE TO β-LACTAM DRUGS

Oxacillin Resistance in Staphylococci

Detection of oxacillin resistance in staphylococci, which is mediated primarily by the mecA determinant (25), by phenotypic methods continues to be a problem (189), particularly with the coagulase-negative strains (25, 200, 230). A mecA gene probe or PCR assay can differentiate isolates that are borderline resistant to oxacillin due to the production of large quantities of β-lactamase from isolates that are resistant due to the presence of the mecA determinant (120, 126). The rare strains of S. aureus that are resistant to oxacillin by virtue of containing modified penicillin-binding proteins (PBPs) with reduced affinity for oxacillin (the so-called MOD strains) may be misclassified as oxacillin susceptible by the mecA gene test since these strains are truly oxacillin resistant but do not contain the mecA gene (203). Recently, a latex agglutination assay to identify the mecA gene product, i.e., PBP2a or PBP2′, has been introduced for use on isolated colonies of S. aureus (87, 214). In addition, a cycling probe assay that can identify isolates of S. aureus that have mecA is now commercially available (11, 108). These tests provide alternatives to phenotypic tests for the clinical microbiology laboratory, presuming that the caveats of their use are understood. For example, the cycling probe assay has been cleared by the Food and Drug Administration only for use with S. aureus isolates available in pure culture. The test is not cleared for use directly on clinical samples or for use with coagulase-negative staphylococci.

Detection of mecA by PCR in organisms present in blood culture bottles has been reported by Ubukata et al. (211) and Carroll et al. (21). A minimum of 500 CFU of S. aureus was required for detection of mecA, while the number of CFU of coagulase-negative species of staphylococci required to give a positive PCR test was at least 10-fold higher. Detection was accomplished by using a nonradioactive enzyme-linked colorimetric assay. Although detection of mecA carried by a skin contaminant (e.g., a clinically insignificant coagulase-negative staphylococcus) is a potential drawback to this approach, a rapid mecA-negative result could reduce pharmacy costs by alerting the clinician that a semisynthetic penicillin could be used for therapy instead of vancomycin.

Killgore et al. (97) recently reported the use of TaqMan technology in a real-time PCR format to detect the mecA gene in staphylococci. The advantage of the assay is that up to 90 isolates can be screened for mecA in <3 h. The use of branched-DNA technology for detection of mecA has also been reported (99). Thus, rapid screening of multiple isolates of S. aureus, such as may be used in infection control screening for oxacillin-resistant S. aureus, is now feasible.

β-Lactam Resistance in Pneumococci

Resistance to penicillin, extended-spectrum cephalosporins, and other antimicrobial agents in pneumococci has become a global problem (98, 121). Resistance to β-lactams develops when pneumococcal PBPs are remodeled through the acquisition of chromosomal DNA from other pneumo-

TABLE 1 PCR assays for antimicrobial resistance genes

Antimicrobial agent and gene	Primers (5′ → 3′)	Product size	Use	Reference(s)
Aminoglycosides				
aac(6′)-Ia	ATG AAT TAT CAA ATT GTG	558 bp	Detection, probe	149[a]
	TTA CTC TTT GAT TAA ACT			
aac(6′)-Ic	CTA CGA TTA CGT CAA CGG CTG C	130 bp	Detection	77[b]
	TTG CTT CGC CCA CTC CTG CAC C			
aac(3)-Ia	ACC TAC TCC CAA CAT CAG CC	169 bp	Detection	213[c]
	ATA TAG ATC TCA CTA CGC GC			
aac(3)-IV	GTT ACA CCG GAC CTT GGA	675 bp	Detection	75
	AAC GGC ATT GAG CGT CAG			
aph(3′)-VIa	ATA CAG AGA CCA CAT ACA GT	235 bp	Detection	220
	GGA CAA TCA ATA ATA CCA AT			
aad(2″)-Ia	ATG TTA CGC AGC AGG GCA GTC G	188 bp	Detection	215
	CGT CAG ATC AAT ATC ATC GTG C			
aac(6′)-Ie-aph(2″)-Ia	GAG CAA TAA GGG CAT ACC AAA AAT C	485 bp	Detection	91
	CCG TGC ATT TGT CTT AAA AAA CTG G			
aph(2″)-Ib	TAT GGA TCC ATG GTT AAC TTG GAC GCT GAG	920 bp	Detection	91
	ATT AAG CTT CCT GCT AAA ATA TAA ACA TCT CTG CT			
aph(2″)-Ic	TGA CTC AGT TCC CAG AT	880 bp	Probe[d]	27
	AGC ACT GTT CGC ACC AAA			
aph(2″)-Id	GAC CAG GTA GAA AAG GCA ATA GAG CAG	846 bp	Probe[d]	207
	ATA CCA ATC CAT ATA ACC ATA TTC CTT			
aadA	TGA TTT GCT GGT TAC GGT GAC	284 bp	Detection, probe	30
	CGC TAT GTT CTC TTG CTT TTG			
aadE	ACT GGC TTA ATC AAT TTG GG	597 bp	Detection, probe	30
	GCC TTT CCG CCA CCT CAC CG			
Spectinomycin				
rrs (N. meningitidis, N. gonorrhoeae)	CTT ACC TGG TCT TGA CA	373 bp	Sequencing	68
	CGA TTA CTA GCG ATT CC			
β-Lactams				
mecA (staphylococci)	AAA ATC GAT GGT AAA GGT TGG C	533 bp	Detection	126
	AGT TCT GCA GTA CCG GAT TTG C			
mecA (staphylococci)	TGG CTA TCG TGT CAC AAT CG	310 bp	Detection	217
	CTG GAA CTT GTT GAG CAG AG			
bla_SHV	GCC GGG TTA TTC TTA TTT GTC GC	1,017 bp	Sequencing	132
	TCT TTC CGA TGC CGC CGC CAG TCA			
bla_SHV	GGT TAT GCG TTA TAT TCG CC	275 bp	Probe[d]	158[e]
	ATC TTT CGC TCC AGC TGT TC			
bla_TEM	ATG AGT ATT CAA CAT TTC CG	351 bp	Detection, probe	157
	TTA CTG TCA TGC CAT CC			
bla_TEM	ATA AAA TTC TTG AAG ACG AAA	1,079 bp	Oligotyping	112
	GAC AGT TAC CAA TGC TTA ATC A			
bla_CTX-M-2	ATG ATG ACT CAG AGC ATT CG	884 bp	Detection	183
	TTA TTG CAT CAG AAA CCG TG			
bla_CTX-M-9	GTG ACA AAG AGA GTG CAA CGG	857 bp	Detection	165
	ATG ATT CTC GCC GCT GAA GCC			
bla_CTX-M-10	GCT GAT GAG CGC TTT GCG	684 bp	Detection	134
	TTA CAA ACC GTT GGT GAC G			
bla_OXY-1	GCG TAG CGC TGA TTA ACA CG	668 bp	Probe[d]	66
	CCT GCT GCG GCT GGG TAA AA			
bla_PER-1	ATG AAT GTC ATT ATA AAA GC	926 bp	Detection, probe	212
	AAT TTG GGC TTA GGG CAA GAA A			
bla_PER-2	CGC TTC TGC TCT GCT GAT	469 bp	Detection	10
	GGC AGC TTC TTT AAC GCC			
bla_ROB-1	TGT TTG CAA TCG CTG CC	400 bp	Detection	90
	TTA TCG TAC ACT TTC CA			

(Continued on next page)

TABLE 1 *(Continued)*

Antimicrobial agent and gene	Primers (5′ → 3′)	Product size	Use	Reference(s)
bla_{KPC-1}	TGT CAC TGT ATC GCC GTC CTC AGT GCT CTA CAG AAA ACC	1,011 bp	Detection, sequencing	229
bla_{SME-1}	AAC GGC TTC ATT TTT GTT TAG GCT TCC GCA ATA GTT TTA TCA	830 bp	Detection	154
bla_{IMP}	CTA CCG CAG CAG AGT CTT TG AAC CAG TTT TGC CTT ACC AT	587 bp	Detection	169
bla_{VIM}	TCT ACA TGA CCG CGT CTG TC TGT GCT TTG ACA ACG TTC GC	748 bp	Detection	150
$ampC$ (promoter, *E. coli*)	GAT CGT TCT GCC GCT GTG GGG CAG CAA ATG TGG AGC AA	271 bp	Sequencing	20
bla_{OXA-1}	CCA AAG ACG TGG ATG GTT AAA TTC GAC CCC AAG TT	540 bp	Detection	177
bla_{OXA-2}	TTC AAG CCA AAG GCA CGA TAG TCC GAG TTG ACT GCC GGG TTG	703 bp	Detection	183
bla_{OXA-10}	CGT GCT TTG TAA AAG TAG CAG CAT GAT TTT GGT GGG AAT GG	652 bp	Detection	183
$bla_{OXA-10/11}$	TAT CGC GTG TCT TTC GAG TA TTA GCC ACC AAT GAT GCC C	775 bp	Probe[d]	43

Chloramphenicol/florfenicol

$cmlA$	TGT CAT TTA CGG CAT ACT CG ATC AGG CAT CCC ATT CCC AT	456 bp	Detection	75
flo	CAC GTT GAG CCT CTA TAT GG ATG CAG AAG TAG AAC GCG AC	869 bp	Detection	130

Glycopeptide

$vanA$	GCT ATT CAG CTG TAC TC CAG CGG CCA TCA TAC GG	783 bp	Detection	166[f]
$vanA$	GGG AAA ACG ACA ATT GC GTA CAA TGC GGC CGT TA	732 bp	Detection	55
$vanB$	CCC GAA TTT CAA ATG ATT GAA AA CGC CAT CCT CCT GCA AAA	457 bp	Detection, probe	124
$vanB$	CGC CAT ATT CTC CCC GGA TAG AAG CCC TCT GCA TCC AAG CAC	667 bp	Detection	104
$vanB2$	GAG GAT GGG TGC ATC CAG GGA CGT GAA GCC GGG CAG GGT GTT	630 bp	Probe[d]	72
$vanC1$	GAA AGA CAA CAG GAA GAC CGC ATC GCA TCA CAA GCA CCA ATC	796 bp	Detection	29
$vanC2/3$	CGG GGA AGA TGG CAG TAT CGC AGG GAC GGT GAT TTT	484 bp	Detection	93, 167
$vanC3$	GCC TTT ACT TAT TGT TCC GCT TGT TCT TTG ACC TTA	224 bp	Detection	31
$vanD$	TAA GGC GCT TGC ATA TAC CG TGC AGC CAA GTA TCC GGT AA	461 bp	Detection	147
$vanE$	TGT GGT ATC GGA GCT GCA G GTC GAT TCT CGC TAA TCC	513 bp	Detection, probe	61
$vanG$	CGG TTG TGC CGT ACT TGG C GGG TAA AGC CAT AGT CTG GGG C	811 bp	Detection	122

Macrolides, lincosamides, streptogramins

$ermA$	CTT CGA TAG TTT ATT AAT ATT AGT TCT AAA AAG CAT GTA AAA GAA	645 bp	Detection	186
$ermB$	GAA AAG GTA CTC AAC CAA ATA AGT AAC GGT ACT AAA ATT GTT TAC	639 bp	Detection	186
$ermTR$	AGA AGG TTA TAA TGA AAC AGA A GGC ATG ACA TAA ACC TTC AT	212 bp	Detection	160

(Continued on next page)

TABLE 1 PCR assays for antimicrobial resistance genes (*Continued*)

Antimicrobial agent and gene	Primers (5′ → 3′)	Product size	Use	Reference(s)
ermAM	TCA ACC AAA TAA TAA AAC AA	337 bp	Detection	174
	AAT CCT TCT TCA ACA ATC AG			
ermC	ATT TTC TTG TAT TCT TTG TT	349 bp	Detection	174
	TTC CTA AAA ACC AAT CCT AT			
ermF	GCA GAC AGG CGC AAG CAG CAA	606 bp	Detection	162
	ACC ACG TTC CCA TGA GTG GTA TGG			
ermG	AGG GAA AGG TCA TTT TAC TGC	664 bp	Detection	160
	CCC TAC CTA TAA CTA AAC ATT			
mefA	CTA TGA CAG CCT CAA TGC G	1,435 bp	Detection, probe	28
	ACC GAT TCT ATC AGC AAA G			
mefA/mefE	AGT ATC ATT AAT CAC TAG TGC	348 bp	Detection	186
	TTC TTC TGG TAC TAA AAG TGG			
ereA	AGT CGG CGG TTA TTT CAT	746 bp	Detection	174
	TGC TCC CTC ATT TTC ATT TA			
ereB	CGG ATA AAG AAG CAC TAC AC	788 bp	Detection	174
	AAC GAC CTC AGA TAC AGA TG			
mphA	AAC TGT ACG CAC TTG C	837 bp	Detection	186
	GGT ACT CTT CGT TAC C			
msrA/msrB	GTC AAA AAC TGC TAA CAC AAG	343 bp	Detection	174
	AAT AAT ACT GCT AAC GAT AAT			
smp	AAA TTG TTT AAA AAG AAA TC	616 bp	Detection, probe	187
	TTT GAA CCA TAA TAT TCA TC			
vat	CAA TGA CCA TGG ACC TGA TC	615 bp	Detection	5
	AGC ATT TCG ATA TCT CC			
vatB	CCT GAT CCA AAT AGC ATA TAT CC	601 bp	Detection	4
	CTA AAT CAG AGC TAC AAA GTG			
satG (vatE)	CTA TAC CTG ACG CAA ATG C	511 bp	Detection	222
	GGT TCA AAT CTT GGT CCG			
vga	TCT AAT GGT ACA GGA AAG ACA ACG	399 bp	Detection	186
	ATC GTG AGA TAC AAA GAT TAT			
linB	CCT ACC TAT TGT TTG TGG AA	944 bp	Detection	15
	ATA ACG TTA CTC TCC TAT TC			
Mupirocin				
IRS	CCA TGC CTT ACC AGT TGA ATT	1.65 kb	Probe[d]	71
	GGA TCC CCG AGC ACT ATC CGA			
mupA	CCC ATG GCT TAC CAG TTG A	1.65 kb	Detection, probe	156
	CCA TGG AGC ACT ATC CGA A			
mupA	TGA CAA TAG AAA AGG ACA GG	190 bp	Detection	141
	CTC TAA TTC AAC TGG TAA GCC			
ileS-2	GTT TAT CTT CTG ATG CTG AG	237 bp	Detection	133
	CCC CAG TTA CAC CGA TAT AA			
Quinolones				
gyrA (M. tuberculosis)	CAG CTA CAT CGA CTA TGC GA	320 bp	Sequencing	92
	GGG CTT CGG TGT ACC TCA T			
gyrA (A. baumannii)	AAA TCT GCC CGT GTC GTT GGT	343 bp	Sequencing	219
	GCC ATA CCT ACG GCG ATA CC			
gyrA (E. coli)	ACG TAC TAG GCA ATG ACT GG	190 bp	Sequencing	59[g]
	AGA AGT CGC CGT CGA TAG AAC			
gyrA (S. pneumoniae)	TTC TCT ACG GAA TGA ATG	272 bp	Sequencing	88
	GAT ATC ACG AAG CAT TTC CAG			
gyrB (S. pneumoniae)	TTC TCC GAT TTC CTC ATG	458 bp	Sequencing	142
	AGA AGG GTA CGA ATG TGG			
parC (S. pneumoniae)	TGG GTT GAA GCC GGT TCA	361 bp	Sequencing	88
	CAA GAC CGT TGG TTC TTT C			
parE (S. pneumoniae)	CCA ATC TAA GAA TCC TG	357 bp	Sequencing	148
	GCA ATA TAG ACA TGA CC			

(Continued on next page)

TABLE 1 *(Continued)*

Antimicrobial agent and gene	Primers (5′ → 3′)	Product size	Use	Reference(s)
Sulfonamides				
sulA	AGC CAA TCA TGC AAA GAC AG	916 bp	Sequencing	119
	ATT TTC CGC TTC ATC AGC CAG			
sul1	CTT CGA TGA GAG CCG GCG GC	437 bp	Detection	75
	GCA AGG CGG AAA CCC GCG CC			
Dihydropteroate synthase (DHPS) gene (*Pneumocystis carinii*)	TTA CTC CTG ATT CTT TTT TCG ATG GG	259 bp	SSCP[j] assay	110
	GCC TTA ATT GCT TGT TCT GCA ACC			
Tetracycline				
tet(A)	GTA ATT CTG AGC ACT GT	954 bp	Probe[d]	78[h]
	CCT GGA CAA CAT TGC TT			
tet(B)	CAG TGC TGT TGT TGT CAT TAA	528 bp	Detection, sequencing	162
	GCT TGG AAT ACT GAG TGT AA			
tet(E)	GTG ATG ATG GCA CTG GT	1,196 bp	Probe[d]	67[i]
	TGC TGT ACA TCG CTC TT			
tet(M)	GAA CTC GAA CAA GAG GAA AGC	741 bp	Detection	136
	ATG GAA GCC CAG AAA GGA T			
tet(O)	AAC TTA GGC ATT CTG GCT CAC	519 bp	Detection	136
	TCC CAC TGT TCC ATA TCG TCA			
tetA(P)	CAC AGA TTG TAT GGG GAT TAG G	764 bp	Detection, sequencing	109
	CAT TTA TAG AAA GCA CAG TAG C			
tet(Q)	ATT GCG GAA GTG GAG CGG AC	814 bp	Detection	135
	GCC GGA CGG AGG ATT TGA GA			
tet(V)	GAC AAC GGC ATG AAC	405 bp	Detection	50
	GTT CGC GAG CAT GTT C			
tet(W)	GAG AGC CTG CTA TAT GCC AGC	168 bp	Detection	6
	GGG CGT ATC CAC AAT GTT AAC			
Trimethoprim				
dhfrVIII	CTA ACG GCG CTA TCT TCG TGA ACA ACG	300 bp	Detection	185
	TAT GAA TTC TTC CAT GCC ATT CTG CTC GTA G			
dfr1	ACG GAT CCT GGC TGT TGG TTG GAC GC	254 bp	Detection	70
	CGG AAT TCA CCT TCC GGC TCG ATG TC			
dfr9	ATG AAT TCC CGT GGC ATG AAC CAG AAG AT	399 bp	Detection	70
	ATG GAT CCT TCA GTA ATG GTC GGG ACC TC			
dfrA	CCC TGC TAT TAA AGC ACC	262 bp	Detection, sequencing	41
	CAT GAC CAG ATA ACT C			
Ethambutol				
embB (*M. tuberculosis*)	ACG CTG AAA CTG CTG GCG AT	400 bp	SSCP assay	3
	ACA GAC TGG CGT CGC TGA CA			
Pyrazinamide				
pncA (*M. tuberculosis*)	GCT GGT CAT GTT CGC GAT CG	673 bp	Sequencing	182
	CAG GAG CTG CAA ACC AAC TCG			
Rifampin				
rpoB (*M. tuberculosis*)	GGG AGC GGA TGA CCA CCC A	350 bp	Sequencing	92
	GCG GTA CGG CGT TTC GAT GAA C			
rpoB (mycobacteria)	CCA CCC AGG ACG TGG AGG CGA TCA CAC	224 bp	Sequencing	34
	AGT GCG ACG GGT GCA CGT CGC GGA CCT			
Streptomycin				
rpsL (*M. tuberculosis*)	GGC CGA CAA ACA GAA CGT	501 bp	Sequencing	181
	GTT CAC CAA CTG GGT GAC			

(Continued on next page)

TABLE 1 PCR assays for antimicrobial resistance genes (*Continued*)

Antimicrobial agent and gene	Primers (5′ → 3′)	Product size	Use	Reference(s)
rrs (*M. tuberculosis*)	TTG GCC ATG CTC TTG ATG CCC TGC ACA CAG GCC ACA AGG GA	1,140 bp	Sequencing	123
rrs (mycobacteria)	GAT GAC GGC CTT CGG GTT GT TCT AGT CTG CCC GTA TCG CC	238 bp	Sequencing (530 loop)	83
rrs (mycobacteria)	GTA GTC CAC GCC GTA AAC GG AGG CCA CAA GGG AAC GCC TA	238 bp	Sequencing (912–915 domain)	83
Isoniazid				
katG	GAA ACA GCG GCG CTG GAT CGT GTT GTC CCA TTT CGT CGG GG	209 bp	SSCP assay	195
katG	TTT CGG CGC ATG GCC ATG A ACA GCC ACC GAG CAC GAC	894 bp	Sequencing, RFLP[k] analysis	76
inhA	TCG ACG CCG GCG ATG G CCG GTC CGC CGA ACG	905 bp	Sequencing	92
ahpC	ATG CAT TGT CCG CTT TGA TG TTC TAT ACT CAT TGA TT	588 bp	Sequencing	96

[a] This reference also describes primer sets for the detection of *aac(6′)-Ib*, *aac(6′)-Id*, *aac(6′)-If*, *aac(6′)-Ig*, and *aac(6′)-Ih*.

[b] This reference also describes primer sets for the detection of *aac(6′)-Id*, *aac(6′)-Ie*, *aac(6′)-Ig*, *aac(6′)-Ih*, *aac(6′)-Ii*, *aac(6′)-Ij*, *aac(6′)-Il*, and *aac(6′)-IIb*.

[c] This reference also describes primer sets for the detection of *aac(3)-IIa*, *aac(3)-IIIa*, *aac(3)-IVa*, *aad(4′)-Ia*, *aac(6′)/aph(2″)*, and *aph(3′)-IIIa*.

[d] This primer set is used in this study for the synthesis of an intragenic probe, not for direct detection.

[e] This reference also describes primer sets for the detection and sequencing of *bla*$_{SHV}$ and the detection of *bla*$_{TEM}$.

[f] This reference also describes primer sets for the detection of *vanB*, *vanC1*, and *vanC2*.

[g] This reference also describes primer sets for the DNA sequencing of *parC* and *parE* of *E. coli*.

[h] This reference also describes primer sets for the synthesis of probes for *tet*(C), *tet*(D), *tet*(E), *tet*(G), *tet*(H), and *tet*(M).

[i] This reference also describes primer sets for the synthesis of probes for *tet*(A), *tet*(B), *tet*(C), *tet*(D), and *tet*(G).

[j] SSCP, single-strand conformational polymorphism.

[k] RFLP, restriction fragment length polymorphism.

cocci or other streptococcal species (35, 52). Although remodeling is not a random process, it has been difficult to develop PCR primers that can accurately differentiate low-level from high-level penicillin-resistant strains. Using primers to the *pbp2b* gene, Ubukata et al. (210) attempted to resolve this issue. In their assay, the lack of product in the presence of amplification controls suggests that the *pbp2b* gene had been remodeled and therefore mediates resistance. However, such an assay does not reliably indicate which strains could be treated with penicillin instead of an extended-spectrum cephalosporin, as might be desirable for an assay to be used in a clinical laboratory, but it may be used as a screening tool for analyzing large groups of strains for resistance. du Plessis et al. (53) have also attempted to identify penicillin-resistant pneumococci directly in cerebrospinal fluid (CSF) by using PCR primers directed to *pbp2b* sequences.

β-Lactamase Genes in Gram-Negative Organisms

A variety of PCR primer sets have been developed to detect the genes encoding the TEM, SHV, OXA, CTX-M, and AmpC β-lactamases present in gram-negative organisms (Table 1). For example, the *bla*$_{TEM}$ gene has been detected by PCR in many species of *Enterobacteriaceae*, in *Haemophilus* spp., and in *N. gonorrhoeae* (158, 175, 199). While PCR has been used to detect *bla*$_{TEM}$ directly in CSF samples containing *H. influenzae* (199), such assays have not found clinical utility, primarily since extended-spectrum cephalosporins, and not ampicillin, are now used for *H. influenzae* meningitis therapy.

The incidence of nosocomial infections caused by *Klebsiella pneumoniae*, *K. oxytoca* (65, 66, 168, 183), and other *Enterobacteriaceae* that produce extended-spectrum β-lactamases (39, 115) and other enzymes capable of hydrolyzing cefotaxime, ceftriaxone, ceftazidime, and aztreonam is increasing in the United States and around the world (17, 132, 158, 169, 209, 218, 226). Better tools are needed for the rapid recognition and classification of these enzymes (19). Isoelectric focusing is used as a screening test to identify the presence of β-lactamase in clinical isolates, although the test lacks specificity (80, 111, 183). Thus, DNA sequencing has become the "gold standard" for analyzing novel β-lactamase genes (113, 157, 169).

Carbapenemases, including CfiA, IMI-1, IMP-1, KPC-1, Nmc-A, and Sme-1 (128, 159, 169, 229), mediate resistance to imipenem and, in most cases, meropenem. These β-lactamases are present in *Enterobacteriaceae* and *Pseudomonas* species. Phenotypically, it is often difficult to differentiate resistance caused by a carbapenemase from resistance mediated by an AmpC-type enzyme in a strain with decreased permeability to carbapenems due to down regulation of one or more porins (18, 102, 107). Thus, PCR assays involving AmpC and carbapenemase genes can be useful in differentiating the two mechanisms.

CHLORAMPHENICOL RESISTANCE

Genes encoding chloramphenicol acetyltransferases (CAT) are present in both gram-negative and gram-positive organisms and mediate resistance to chloramphenicol (173). DNA probes to the *cat* genes commonly found in gram-negative organisms (*catI*, *catII*, and *catIII*) have been described, but the probes include sequences outside of the open reading frame of the genes and their specificity has not been rigorously ascertained. Probes for the *cat* genes of gram-positive anaerobes, including *Clostridium perfringens* and *C. difficile* (*catP*, *catQ*, and *catD*), are more specific (12, 164, 228). Additional genes that show relatively little DNA sequence homology to those mentioned above are present in staphylococci, streptococci, and aerobic gram-positive bacilli. DNA probes for many of these genes have been described, although their clinical utility has yet to be established. Direct detection of these genes in clinical samples has not been reported, but it may become important as levels of resistance to extended-spectrum β-lactam agents, currently the drugs of choice for treating bacterial meningitis in children, become more pronounced. PCR primers capable of detecting the *cat* genes present in streptococci and enterococci have also been described (205).

RESISTANCE TO VANCOMYCIN AND OTHER GLYCOPEPTIDES

Acquired vancomycin resistance was first noted in enterococci (24, 101) but has subsequently been documented in a variety of other pathogens (143, 151, 152, 184). Resistance is mediated by several different determinants, including *vanA*, *vanB*, *vanC*, *vanD*, *vanE*, and *vanG* (9, 55, 61, 122, 138, 146, 147, 166). PCR has been used to track the epidemiologic spread of *vanA* subtypes in both humans and animals (1, 37, 224). PCR assays also can differentiate among the three unique *vanB* genes, designated *vanB1*, *vanB2*, and *vanB3* (40, 104), and the three *vanC* genes, designated *vanC1*, *vanC2*, and *vanC3* (31). Subtypes of *vanD*, including *vanD1*, *vanD2*, *vanD3*, and *vanD4*, also exist, but differentiation by PCR is difficult (14, 42). PCR has been used to detect *vanA* and *vanB* in enterococci in fecal samples to aid infection control efforts (140, 167). Decreased susceptibility to glycopeptides has been noted in strains of *S. aureus* from Japan, the United States, and elsewhere (23, 82, 197). These strains do not contain the *van* genes recognized in enterococci and other genera (201). Genotypic detection of such strains has yet to be accomplished.

MACROLIDE, LINCOSAMIDE, AND STREPTOGRAMIN RESISTANCE

Several new loci associated with erythromycin resistance have been reported. These include the novel methylase gene *ermTR* originally noted in *Streptococcus pyogenes*, which mediates resistance to macrolides, lincosamides (such as clindamycin), and streptogramins (i.e., the MLS$_B$ resistance phenotype) (44, 94, 160, 170). This resistance phenotype is similar to that of the *ermA*, *ermB*, and *ermC* genes. In contrast, *msrA*, identified primarily in staphylococci, mediates resistance only to macrolides and streptogramins (MS resistance), as does the macrolide efflux gene *mefA* of streptococci (8, 28, 56, 63, 174, 227), which was previously called *mefE* in pneumococci (163). The *mefA* determinant appears to be a common cause of erythromycin resistance in pneumococci in the United States (190). Finally, 23S rRNA mutations and ribosomal protein L4 mutations in pneumococci have also been shown to mediate macrolide resistance (49, 191).

Since most strains of staphylococci that are erythromycin resistant are presumed to be resistant to clindamycin

(which would be correct if they harbored an *erm* gene), *msrA* probes or PCR assays could be used to indicate the presence of *msrA* if clindamycin therapy was to be used (106). Two new phosphotransferases, encoded by *mphA* and *mphB*, have also been shown to mediate resistance to 14-membered ring macrolides in *Escherichia coli* (131, 193).

Because of the introduction of quinupristin-dalfopristin into clinical use, there is increasing interest in mechanisms of streptogramin resistance. These include streptogramin acetyltransferases (*sat* genes), virginiamycin acetyltransferases (*vat* genes), and the efflux pumps encoded by *vgaA* and *vgaB* (16, 178). Mechanisms active against both the streptogramin A and streptogramin B components of quinupristin-dalfopristin are necessary to result in a resistance phenotype. Several of the loci previously classified as *sat* genes have been reclassified as *vat* genes (79, 163, 178, 222, 223). For example, *vatD* is the former *satA*, and *vatE* is the former *satG*. Resistance to the streptogramin B component is mediated by the lactonases VgbA and VgbB, or the *ermB*-encoded methylase. In staphylococci, in particular, many of these genes are clustered.

MUPIROCIN RESISTANCE

Mupirocin is an antistaphylococcal agent that is used to reduce the carriage of staphylococci among infected patients and hospital personnel. A PCR assay has been described that can detect high-level mupirocin resistance (71). However, the practical value of the assay has not been assessed in a clinical laboratory setting.

QUINOLONE RESISTANCE

There are two major mechanisms of quinolone resistance: (i) alteration of the target sites, the organisms' gyrase (*gyrA* and *gyrB*) and topoisomerase (*parC* and *parE*) (59, 84, 192, 194, 206), and (ii) active efflux of the drug out of the cell (48, 59, 144), which limits access of the drug to the target site. Resistance is usually associated with point mutations in the *gyr* or *par* loci. Since DNA probes, in most cases, are not sufficiently sensitive to detect these changes, investigators have used PCR coupled with direct sequencing of the amplification products to identify changes in the nucleotide sequence of the *gyrA*, *gyrB*, *parC*, and *parE* genes (74, 88, 92, 219). The primers, however, appear to be species specific (Table 1).

SULFONAMIDE RESISTANCE

There are two major sulfonamide resistance genes, *sulI* and *sulII*. Both have been cloned and sequenced, and probes have been described for each (155). Neither probe has been used to identify the presence of the gene directly in clinical samples. Interestingly, the *sul* genes are often associated with transposable DNA elements, such as Tn*21* (86, 155), that can shuttle multiple resistance genes from organism to organism. Thus, the *sul* genes can serve as indicators of multiple resistance in gram-negative organisms.

TETRACYCLINE RESISTANCE

Tetracycline resistance is widespread in the bacterial kingdom (105, 180). PCR assays have been developed for the *tet*(A), *tet*(B), *tet*(C), *tet*(D), *tet*(E), *tet*(F), *tet*(H), *tet*(K), *tet*(L), *tet*(M), *tet*(N), *tet*(O), *tet*(Q), *tet*(S), *tet*(U), and *tet*(V) determinants (2, 26, 50, 51, 64, 67, 78, 114, 116,

117, 161, 179, 180, 231). Multiple alleles of several of these determinants exist. For example, S. pneumoniae contains six tet(M) alleles, designated tet(M)1 through tet(M)6, which have been differentiated by restriction analysis of PCR fragments (51). Such epidemiologic studies using genotyping of resistance determinants contribute to our understanding of resistance transfer and evolution. Primers for the tet(M), tet(O), and tet(Q) determinants are useful for detecting tetracycline resistance genes directly in periodontal samples (135, 136), where the presence of resistant organisms may indicate patients who are likely to fail therapy with tetracycline (114). Multiple types of the tet(M) gene also have been recognized through sequence analysis (137).

TRIMETHOPRIM RESISTANCE

The number of genes capable of mediating trimethoprim resistance in bacteria continues to expand (7, 85, 86, 103, 176). DNA probes have proven to be powerful tools for detecting and classifying novel trimethoprim resistance genes (called dhfr) (7, 89, 153). However, because consensus sequences common to all the dhfr genes have not been identified, PCR primers that could simplify the detection of this family of genes have not been developed, although PCR primers for some individual genes have been developed (41, 75, 103, 185). A novel trimethoprim resistance gene, folH, also has been recognized in H. influenzae (45).

DETECTING RESISTANCE IN MYCOBACTERIA

Multidrug-resistant strains of Mycobacterium tuberculosis have been recognized in hospitals in the United States, Southeast Asia, and parts of Europe, where they constitute a major public health problem (57, 58). Consequently, the rapid identification of resistant strains has become a critical issue for the laboratory. PCR assays in conjunction with DNA sequencing have been developed to detect mutations in many loci of the M. tuberculosis genome that are associated with the development of resistance (33, 92, 196, 225). The mechanisms of resistance are described in chapter 73.

GUIDELINES FOR USING GENETIC TESTS

Today, with the exception of commercially prepared cycling probe assays, DNA probes are rarely used to detect resistance genes. Rather, laboratories use PCR assays, which are more accessible and easier to adapt to clinical laboratory use than are DNA probes. The critical issue with PCR assays is the reliability of results. The need for quality control measures, including the use of amplification controls, such as simultaneous amplification of rRNA or rDNA sequences to ensure the availability of amplifiable nucleic acid and absence of inhibitory substances in the reaction, cannot be stressed enough. The temperatures used in PCR assays optimized for use with purified DNA or with DNA from bacterial isolates obtained in pure culture may not be stringent enough to avoid false-positive results when used with clinical samples, such as blood or CSF, where considerably more nonspecific priming can occur (199). It may be necessary to increase the temperatures of the assays, particularly the annealing temperatures, to avoid this problem. The use of control reactions containing no template DNA to identify nonspecific products due to contamination of

Taq polymerase with DNA, such as that caused by cloning-vector DNA, is critical (199, 208).

One should never assume that PCR primers reported in the literature have undergone rigorous testing. Rather, primer sets should be thoroughly tested for specificity, self-complementarity, and dimer formation before use. According to the Clinical Laboratory Improvement Act of 1988, validation of DNA probe and PCR tests by the clinical laboratory in which they are to be used is mandatory before they can be used for analysis of clinical specimens. Methods for validation are published by the NCCLS (129).

Finally, now that cycling probes and PCR assays for detecting and differentiating resistance genes are becoming commercially available, more surveys of resistance mechanisms, such as those described by Eady et al. (56), Kapur et al. (92), Ounissi et al. (139), and Shaw et al. (171), should be undertaken to determine the reservoirs of resistance genes and the way in which resistance genes disseminate in hospitals and community settings. Such studies would also help to determine the frequency with which organisms carry resistance genes that are not expressed. Although still considered experimental, many of the probe and PCR methods for detecting resistance genes described herein are already having a positive effect on guiding therapy early in the course of infection and making the treatment of infectious diseases less empiric.

REFERENCES

1. **Aarestrup, F. M., P. Ahrens, M. Madsen, L. V. Pallesen, R. L. Poulsen, and H. Westh.** 1996. Glycopeptide susceptibility among Danish Enterococcus faecium and Enterococcus faecalis isolates of animal and human origin and PCR identification of genes within the VanA cluster. Antimicrob. Agents Chemother. **40:**1938–1940.

2. **Abraham, L. J., D. I. Berryman, and J. I. Rood.** 1988. Hybridization analysis of the class P tetracycline resistance determinant from the Clostridium perfringens R-plasmid, pCW3. Plasmid **19:**113–120.

3. **Alcaide, F., G. E. Pfyffer, and A. Telenti.** 1997. Role of embB in natural and acquired resistance to ethambutol in mycobacteria. Antimicrob. Agents Chemother. **41:**2270–2273.

4. **Allignet, J., and N. El Solh.** 1995. Diversity among the gram-positive acetyltransferases inactivating streptogramin A and structurally related compounds and characterization of a new staphylococcal determinant, vatB. Antimicrob. Agents Chemother. **39:**2027–2036.

5. **Allignet, J., V. Loncle, C. Simenel, M. Delepierre, and N. El Solh.** 1993. Sequence of a staphylococcal gene, vat, encoding an acetyltransferase inactivating the A-type compounds of virginiamycin-like antibiotics. Gene **130:**91–98.

6. **Aminov, R. I., N. Garrigues-Jeanjean, and R. I. Mackie.** 2001. Molecular ecology of tetracycline resistance: development and validation of primers for detection of tetracycline resistance genes encoding ribosomal protection proteins. Appl. Environ. Microbiol. **67:**22–32.

7. **Amyes, S. G. B., and K. J. Towner.** 1990. Trimethoprim resistance; epidemiology and molecular aspects. J. Med. Microbiol. **31:**1–19.

8. **Arpin, C., H. Daube, F. Tessier, and C. Quentin.** 1999. Presence of mefA and mefE genes in Streptococcus agalactiae. Antimicrob. Agents Chemother. **43:**944–946.

9. **Arthur, M., and R. Quintiliani, Jr.** 2001. Regulation of VanA- and VanB-type glycopeptide resistance in enterococci. Antimicrob. Agents Chemother. **45:**375–381.

10. **Bauernfeind, A., I. Stemplinger, R. Jungwirth, P. Mangold, S. Amann, E. Akalin, Ö. Ang, C. Bal, and**

J. M. Casellas. 1996. Characterization of β-lactamase gene bla$_{PER-2}$, which encodes an extended-spectrum class A β-lactamase. *Antimicrob. Agents Chemother.* **40:**616–620.

11. Bekkaoui, F., J. P. McNevin, C. H. Leung, G. J. Peterson, A. Patel, R. S. Bhatt, and R. N. Bryan. 1999. Rapid detection of the mecA gene in methicillin resistant staphylococci using a colorimetric cycling probe technology. *Diagn. Microbiol. Infect. Dis.* **34:**83–90.

12. Bolivar, F., R. L. Rodriguez, P. J. Greene, M. C. Betlach, H. L. Heyneker, H. W. Boyer, J. H. Crosa, and S. Falkow. 1977. Construction and characterization of new cloning vehicles. II. A multipurpose cloning system. *Gene* **2:**95–113.

13. Bonnet, R., C. Dutour, J. L. M. Sampaio, C. Chanal, D. Sirot, R. Labia, C. De Champs, and J. Sirot. 2001. Novel cefotaximase (CTX-M-16) with increased catalytic efficiency due to substitution Asp-240→Gly. *Antimicrob. Agents Chemother.* **45:**2269–2275.

14. Boyd, D. A., J. Conly, H. Dedier, G. Peters, L. Robertson, E. Slater, and M. R. Mulvey. 2001. Molecular characterization of the vanD gene cluster and a novel insertion element in a vancomycin-resistant enterococcus isolated in Canada. *J. Clin. Microbiol.* **38:**2392–2394.

15. Bozdogan, B., L. Berrezouga, M.-S. Kuo, D. A. Yurek, K. A. Farley, B. J. Stockman, and R. Leclercq. 1999. A new resistance gene, linB, conferring resistance to lincosamides by nucleotidylation in *Enterococcus faecium* HM1025. *Antimicrob. Agents Chemother.* **43:**925–929.

16. Bozdogan, B., and R. Leclercq. 1999. Effects of genes encoding resistance to streptogramins A and B on the activity of quinupristin-dalfopristin against *Enterococcus faecium*. *Antimicrob. Agents Chemother.* **43:**2720–2725.

17. Bradford, P. A. 2001. Extended-spectrum β-lactamases in the 21st century: characterization, epidemiology, and detection of this important resistance threat. *Clin. Microbiol. Rev.* **14:**933–951.

18. Bradford, P. A., C. Urban, N. Mariano, S. J. Projan, J. J. Rahal, and K. Bush. 1997. Imipenem resistance in *Klebsiella pneumoniae* is associated with the combination of ACT-1, a plasmid-mediated AmpC β-lactamase, and the loss of an outer membrane protein. *Antimicrob. Agents Chemother.* **41:**563–569.

19. Bush, K. 2001. New β-lactamases in gram-negative bacteria: diversity and impact on the selection of antimicrobial therapy. *Clin. Infect. Dis.* **32:**1085–1089.

20. Caroff, N., E. Espaze, D. Gautreau, H. Richet, and A. Reynaud. 2000. Analysis of the effects of −42 and −32 ampC promoter mutations in clinical isolates of *Escherichia coli* hyperproducing AmpC. *J. Antimicrob. Chemother.* **45:**783–788.

21. Carroll, K. C., R. B. Leonard, P. L. Newcomb-Gayman, and D. R. Hillyard. 1996. Rapid detection of the staphylococcal mecA gene from BACTEC blood culture bottles by the polymerase chain reaction. *Am. J. Clin. Pathol.* **106:**600–605.

22. Casin, I., F. Bordon, P. Bertin, A. Coutrot, I. Podglajen, R. Brasseur, and E. Collatz. 1998. Aminoglycoside 6′-N-acetyltransferase variants of the Ib type with altered substrate profile in clinical isolates of *Enterobacter cloacae* and *Citrobacter freundii*. *Antimicrob. Agents Chemother.* **42:**209–215.

23. Centers for Disease Control and Prevention. 1997. *Staphylococcus aureus* with reduced susceptibility to vancomycin—United States, 1997. *Morb. Mortal. Wkly. Rep.* **46:**765–766.

24. Cetinkaya, Y., P. Falk, and C. G. Mayhall. 2000. Vancomycin-resistant enterococci. *Clin. Microbiol. Rev.* **13:**686–707.

25. Chambers, H. F. 1988. Methicillin-resistant staphylococci. *Clin. Microbiol. Rev.* **1:**173–186.

26. Charpentier, E., G. Gerbaud, and P. Courvalin. 1993. Characterization of a new class of tetracycline-resistance gene tet(S) in *Listeria monocytogenes* BM4210. *Gene* **131:**27–34.

27. Chow, J. W., M. J. Zervos, S. A. Lerner, L. A. Thal, S. M. Donabedian, D. D. Jaworski, D. Tsai, K. J. Shaw, and D. B. Clewell. 1997. A novel gentamicin resistance gene in *Enterococcus*. *Antimicrob. Agents Chemother.* **41:**511–514.

28. Clancy, J., J. Petitpas, F. Dib-Hajj, W. Yuan, M. Cronan, A. V. Kamath, J. Bergeron, and J. A. Retsema. 1996. Molecular cloning and functional analysis of a novel macrolide-resistance determinant, mefA, from *Streptococcus pyogenes*. *Mol. Microbiol.* **22:**867–879.

29. Clark, N. C., R. C. Cooksey, B. C. Hill, J. M. Swenson, and F. C. Tenover. 1993. Characterization of glycopeptide-resistant enterococci from U.S. hospitals. *Antimicrob. Agents Chemother.* **37:**2311–2317.

30. Clark, N. C., Ø. Olsvik, J. M. Swenson, C. A. Spiegel, and F. C. Tenover. 1999. Detection of a streptomycin/spectinomycin adenylyltransferase gene (aadA) in *Enterococcus faecalis*. *Antimicrob. Agents Chemother.* **43:**157–160.

31. Clark, N. C., L. M. Teixeira, R. R. Facklam, and F. C. Tenover. 1998. Detection and differentiation of vanC-1, vanC-2, and vanC-3 glycopeptide resistance genes in enterococci. *J. Clin. Microbiol.* **36:**2294–2297.

32. Cockerill, F. R., III. 1999. Genetic methods for assessing antimicrobial resistance. *Antimicrob. Agents Chemother.* **43:**199–212.

33. Cockerill, F. R., III, J. R. Uhl, Z. Temesgen, Y. Zhang, L. Stockman, G. D. Roberts, D. L. Williams, and B. C. Kline. 1995. Rapid identification of a point mutation of the *Mycobacterium tuberculosis* catalase-peroxidase (katG) gene associated with isoniazid resistance. *J. Infect. Dis.* **171:**240–245.

34. Cockerill, F. R., III, D. E. Williams, K. D. Eisenach, B. C. Kline, L. K. Miller, L. Stockman, J. Voyles, G. M. Caron, S. K. Bundy, G. D. Roberts, W. R. Wilson, A. C. Whelen, J. M. Hunt, and D. H. Persing. 1996. Prospective evaluation of the utility of molecular techniques for diagnosing nosocomial transmission of multidrug-resistant tuberculosis. *Mayo Clin. Proc.* **71:**221–229.

35. Coffey, T. J., C. G. Dowson, M. Daniels, J. Zhou, C. Martin, B. G. Spratt, and J. M. Musser. 1991. Horizontal transfer of multiple penicillin-binding protein genes, and capsular biosynthetic genes, in natural populations of *Streptococcus pneumoniae*. *Mol. Microbiol.* **5:**2255–2260.

36. Cooksey, R. C., G. P. Morlock, S. Glickman, and J. T. Crawford. 1997. Evaluation of a line probe assay kit for characterization of rpoB mutations in rifampin-resistant *Mycobacterium tuberculosis* isolates from New York City. *J. Clin. Microbiol.* **35:**1281–1283.

37. Coque, T. M., J. F. Tomayko, S. C. Ricke, P. C. Okhyusen, and B. E. Murray. 1996. Vancomycin-resistant enterococci from nosocomial, community, and animal sources in the United States. *Antimicrob. Agents Chemother.* **40:**2605–2609.

38. Costa, Y., M. Galimand, R. Leclercq, J. Duval, and P. Courvalin. 1993. Characterization of the chromosomal aac(6′)-Ii gene specific for *Enterococcus faecium*. *Antimicrob. Agents Chemother.* **37:** 1896–1903.

39. Coudron, P. E., E. S. Moland, and C. C. Sanders. 1997. Occurrence and detection of extended-spectrum β-lactamases in members of the family Enterobacteriaceae at a veterans medical center: seek and you may find. *J. Clin. Microbiol.* **35:**2593–2597.

40. **Dahl, K. H., G. S. Simonsen, Ǿ. Olsvik, and A. Sundsfjord.** 1999. Heterogeneity in the *vanB* gene cluster of genomically diverse clinical strains of vancomycin-resistant enterococci. *Antimicrob. Agents Chemother.* **43:** 1105–1110.

41. **Dale, G. E., H. Langen, M. G. P. Page, R. L. Then, and D. Stüber.** 1995. Cloning and characterization of a novel, plasmid-encoded trimethoprim-resistant dihydrofolate reductase from *Staphylococcus haemolyticus* MUR313. *Antimicrob. Agents Chemother.* **39:**1920–1924.

42. **Dalla Costa, L. M., P. E. Reynolds, H. A. Souza, D. C. Souza, M.-F. I. Palepou, and N. Woodford.** 2000. Characterization of a divergent *vanD*-type resistance element from the first glycopeptide-resistant strain of *Enterococcus faecium* isolated in Brazil. *Antimicrob. Agents Chemother.* **44:**3444–3446.

43. **Danel, F., L. M. C. Hall, D. Gur, and D. M. Livermore.** 1995. OXA-14, another extended-spectrum variant of OXA-10 (PSE-2) β-lactamase from *Pseudomonas aeruginosa. Antimicrob. Agents Chemother.* **39:**1881–1884.

44. **De Azavedo, J. C. S., R. H. Yeung, D. J. Bast, C. L. Duncan, S. B. Borgia, and D. E. Low.** 1999. Prevalence and mechanisms of macrolide resistance in clinical isolates of group A streptococci from Ontario, Canada. *Antimicrob. Agents Chemother.* **43:**2144–2147.

45. **De Groot, R., M. Sluijter, A. De Bruyn, J. Campos, W. H. F. Goessens, A. L. Smith, and P. W. M. Hermans.** 1996. Genetic characterization of trimethoprim resistance in *Haemophilus influenzae. Antimicrob. Agents Chemother.* **40:**2131–2136.

46. **Deguchi, T., M. Yasuda, M. Asano, K. Tada, H. Iwata, H. Komeda, T. Ezaki, I. Saito, and Y. Kawada.** 1995. DNA gyrase mutations in quinolone-resistant clinical isolates of *Neisseria gonorrhoeae. Antimicrob. Agents Chemother.* **39:**561–563.

47. **del Campo, R., C. Tenorio, C. Rubio, J. Castillo, C. Torres, and R. Gómez-Lus.** 2000. Aminoglycoside-modifying enzymes in high-level streptomycin and gentamicin resistant *Enterococcus* spp. in Spain. *Int. J. Antimicrob. Agents* **15:**221–226.

48. **del Mar Tavío, M., J. Vila, J. Ruiz, J. Ruiz, A. M. Martín-Sánchez, and M. T. Jiménez de Anta.** 1999. Mechanisms involved in the development of resistance to fluoroquinolones in *Escherichia coli* isolates. *J. Antimicrob. Chemother.* **44:**735–742.

49. **Depardieu, F., and P. Courvalin.** 2001. Mutation in 23S rRNA responsible for resistance to 16-membered macrolides and streptogramins in *Streptococcus pneumoniae. Antimicrob. Agents Chemother.* **45:**319–323.

50. **De Rossi, E., M. C. J. Blokpoel, R. Cantoni, M. Branzoni, G. Riccardi, D. B. Young, K. A. L. De Smet, and O. Ciferri.** 1998. Molecular cloning and functional analysis of a novel tetracycline resistance determinant, *tet*(V), from *Mycobacterium smegmatis. Antimicrob. Agents Chemother.* **42:**1931–1937.

51. **Doherty, N., K. Trzcinski, P. Pickerill, P. Zawadzki, and C. G. Dowson.** 2000. Genetic diversity of the *tet*(M) gene in tetracycline-resistant clonal lineages of *Streptococcus pneumoniae. Antimicrob. Agents Chemother.* **44:**2979–2984.

52. **Dowson, C. G., A. Hutchison, and B. G. Spratt.** 1989. Extensive re-modelling of the transpeptidase domain of penicillin-binding protein 2B of a penicillin-resistant South African isolate of *Streptococcus pneumoniae. Mol. Microbiol.* **3:**95–102.

53. **du Plessis, M., A. M. Smith, and K. P. Klugman.** 1998. Rapid detection of penicillin-resistant *Streptococcus pneumoniae* in cerebrospinal fluid by a seminested-PCR strategy. *J. Clin. Microbiol.* **36:**453–457.

54. **du Plessis, M., A. M. Smith, and K. P. Klugman.** 1999. Application of *pbp1*A PCR in identification of penicillin-resistant *Streptococcus pneumoniae. J. Clin. Microbiol.* **37:** 628–632.

55. **Dutka-Malen, S., S. Evers, and P. Courvalin.** 1995. Detection of glycopeptide resistance genotypes and identification to the species level of clinically relevant enterococci by PCR. *J. Clin. Microbiol.* **33:**24–27.

56. **Eady, E. A., J. I. Ross, J. L. Tipper, C. E. Walters, J. H. Cove, and W. C. Noble.** 1993. Distribution of genes encoding erythromycin ribosomal methylases and an erythromycin efflux pump in epidemiologically distinct groups of staphylococci. *J. Antimicrob. Chemother.* **31:** 211–217.

57. **Edlin, B. R., J. I. Tokars, M. H. Grieco, J. T. Crawford, J. Williams, E. M. Sordillo, K. R. Ong, J. O. Kilburn, S. W. Dooley, K. G. Castro, W. R. Jarvis, and S. D. Holmberg.** 1992. An outbreak of multidrug-resistant tuberculosis among hospitalized patients with the acquired immunodeficiency syndrome. *N. Engl. J. Med.* **326:**1514–1521.

58. **Espinal, M. A., A. Laszlo, L. Simonsen, F. Boulahbal, S. J. Kim, A. Reniero, S. Hoffner, H. L. Rieder, N. Binkin, C. Dye, R. Williams, and M. C. Raviglione.** 2001. Global trends in resistance to antituberculosis drugs. *N. Engl. J. Med.* **344:**1294–1303.

59. **Everett, M. J., Y. F. Jin, V. Ricci, and L. J. V. Piddock.** 1996. Contributions of individual mechanisms to fluoroquinolone resistance in 36 *Escherichia coli* strains isolated from humans and animals. *Antimicrob. Agents Chemother.* **40:**2380–2386.

60. **Evers, S., D. F. Sahm, and P. Courvalin.** 1993. The *vanB* gene of vancomycin-resistant *Enterococcus faecalis* V583 is structurally related to genes encoding D-Ala:D-Ala ligases and glycopeptide-resistance proteins VanA and VanC. *Gene* **124:**143–144.

61. **Fines, M., B. Perichon, P. Reynolds, D. F. Sahm, and P. Courvalin.** 1999. VanE, a new type of acquired glycopeptide resistance in *Enterococcus faecalis* BM4405. *Antimicrob. Agents Chemother.* **43:**2161–2164.

62. **Finken, M., P. Kirschner, A. Meier, A. Wrede, and E. C. Böttger.** 1993. Molecular basis of streptomycin resistance in *Mycobacterium tuberculosis*: alterations of the ribosomal protein S12 gene and point mutations within a functional 16S ribosomal RNA pseudoknot. *Mol. Microbiol.* **9:**1239–1246.

63. **Fitoussi, F., C. Loukil, I. Gros, O. Clermont, P. Mariani, S. Bonacorsi, I. Le Thomas, D. Deforche, and E. Bingen.** 2001. Mechanisms of macrolide resistance in clinical group B streptococci isolated in France. *Antimicrob. Agents Chemother.* **45:**1889–1891.

64. **Fletcher, H. M., and F. L. Macrina.** 1991. Molecular survey of clindamycin and tetracycline resistance determinants in *Bacteroides* species. *Antimicrob. Agents Chemother.* **35:**2415–2418.

65. **Fournier, B., and P. H. Roy.** 1997. Variability of chromosomally encoded β-lactamases from *Klebsiella oxytoca. Antimicrob. Agents Chemother.* **41:**1641–1648.

66. **Fournier, B., P. H. Roy, P. H. Lagrange, and A. Philippon.** 1996. Chromosomal β-lactamase genes of *Klebsiella oxytoca* are divided into two main groups, bla_{OXY-1} and bla_{OXY-2}. *Antimicrob. Agents Chemother.* **40:**454–459.

67. **Frech, G., and S. Schwarz.** 2000. Molecular analysis of tetracycline resistance in *Salmonella enterica* subsp. *enterica* serovars Typhimurium, Enteritidis, Dublin, Choleraesuis, Hadar and Saintpaul: construction and application of specific gene probes. *J. Appl. Microbiol.* **89:**633–641.

68. **Galimand, M., G. Gerbaud, and P. Courvalin.** 2000. Spectinomycin resistance in *Neisseria* spp. due to muta-

tions in 16S rRNA. *Antimicrob. Agents Chemother.* **44:** 1365–1366.

69. **Geha, D. J., J. R. Uhl, C. A. Gustaferro, and D. H. Persing.** 1994. Multiplex PCR for identification of methicillin-resistant staphylococci in the clinical laboratory. *J. Clin. Microbiol.* **32:**1768–1772.

70. **Gibreel, A., and O. Sköld.** 1998. High-level resistance to trimethoprim in clinical isolates of *Campylobacter jejuni* by acquisition of foreign genes (*dfr1* and *dfr9*) expressing drug-insensitive dihydrofolate reductases. *Antimicrob. Agents Chemother.* **42:**3059–3064.

71. **Gilbart, J., C. R. Perry, and B. Slocombe.** 1993. High-level mupirocin resistance in *Staphylococcus aureus:* evidence for two distinct isoleucyl-tRNA synthetases. *Antimicrob. Agents Chemother.* **37:**32–38.

72. **Gold, H. S., S. Ünal, E. Cercenado, C. Thauvin-Eliopoulos, G. M. Eliopoulos, C. B. Wennersten, and R. C. Moellering, Jr.** 1993. A gene conferring resistance to vancomycin but not teicoplanin in isolates of *Enterococcus faecalis* and *Enterococcus faecium* demonstrates homology with *vanB, vanA,* and *vanC* genes of enterococci. *Antimicrob. Agents Chemother.* **37:**1604–1609.

73. **Gordts, B., H. Van Landuyt, M. Ieven, P. Vandamme, and H. Goossens.** 1995. Vancomycin-resistant enterococci colonizing the intestinal tracts of hospitalized patients. *J. Clin. Microbiol.* **33:**2842–2846.

74. **Griggs, D. J., K. Gensberg, and L. J. V. Piddock.** 1996. Mutations in *gyrA* gene of quinolone-resistant salmonella serotypes isolated from humans and animals. *Antimicrob. Agents Chemother.* **40:**1009–1013.

75. **Guerra, B., S. M. Soto, J. M. Argüelles, and M. C. Mendoza.** 2001. Multidrug resistance is mediated by large plasmids carrying a class 1 integron in the emergent *Salmonella enterica* serotype [4, 5, 12:i:−]. *Antimicrob. Agents Chemother.* **45:**1305–1308.

76. **Haas, W. H., K. Schilke, J. Brand, B. Amthor, K. Weyer, P. B. Fourie, G. Bretzel, V. Sticht-Groh, and H. J. Bremer.** 1997. Molecular analysis of *katG* gene mutations in strains of *Mycobacterium tuberculosis* complex from Africa. *Antimicrob. Agents Chemother.* **41:**1601–1603.

77. **Hannecart-Pokorni, E., F. Depuydt, L. De Wit, E. Van Bossuyt, J. Content, and R. Vanhoof.** 1997. Characterization of the 6′-N-aminoglycoside acetyltransferase gene *aac(6′)-Il* associated with a *sull*-type integron. *Antimicrob. Agents Chemother.* **41:**314–318.

78. **Hansen, L. M., P. C. Blanchard, and D. C. Hirsh.** 1996. Distribution of *tet*(H) among *Pasteurella* isolates from the United States and Canada. *Antimicrob. Agents Chemother.* **40:**1558–1560.

79. **Haroche, J., J. Allignet, S. Aubert, A. E. Van Den Bogaard, and N. El Solh.** 2000. *satG,* conferring resistance to streptogramin A, is widely distributed in *Enterococcus faecium* strains but not in staphylococci. *Antimicrob. Agents Chemother.* **44:**190–191.

80. **Heritage, J., F. H. M'Zali, D. Gascoyne-Binzi, and P. M. Hawkey.** 1999. Evolution and spread of SHV extended-spectrum β-lactamases in gram-negative bacteria. *J. Antimicrob. Chemother.* **44:**309–318.

81. **Heym, B., N. Honoré, C. Truffot-Pernot, A. Banerjee, C. Schurra, W. R. Jacobs, Jr., J. D. van Embden, J. H. Grosset, and S. T. Cole.** 1994. Implications of multidrug resistance for the future of short-course chemotherapy of tuberculosis: a molecular study. *Lancet* **344:**293–298.

82. **Hiramatsu, K., H. Hanaki, T. Ino, K. Yabuta, T. Oguri, and F. C. Tenover.** 1997. Methicillin-resistant *Staphylococcus aureus* clinical strain with reduced vancomycin susceptibility. *J. Antimicrob. Chemother.* **40:**135–136.

83. **Honoré, N., and S. T. Cole.** 1994. Streptomycin resistance in mycobacteria. *Antimicrob. Agents Chemother.* **38:** 238–242.

84. **Hooper, D. C., J. S. Wolfson, E. Y. Ng, and M. N. Swartz.** 1987. Mechanisms of action of and resistance to ciprofloxacin. *Am. J. Med.* **82**(Suppl. 4A):12–20.

85. **Huovinen, P.** 2001. Resistance to trimethoprim-sulfamethoxazole. *Clin. Infect. Dis.* **32:**1608–1614.

86. **Huovinen, P., L. Sundström, G. Swedberg, and O. Sköld.** 1995. Trimethoprim and sulfonamide resistance. *Antimicrob. Agents Chemother.* **39:**279–289.

87. **Hussain, Z., L. Stoakes, S. Garrow, S. Longo, V. Fitzgerald, and R. Lannigan.** 2000. Rapid detection of *mecA*-positive and *mecA*-negative coagulase-negative staphylococci by an anti-penicillin binding protein 2a slide latex agglutination test. *J. Clin. Microbiol.* **38:**2051–2054.

88. **Janoir, C., V. Zeller, M.-D. Kitzis, N. J. Moreau, and L. Gutmann.** 1996. High-level fluoroquinolone resistance in *Streptococcus pneumoniae* requires mutations in *parC* and *gyrA. Antimicrob. Agents Chemother.* **40:**2760–2764.

89. **Jansson, C., A. Franklin, and O. Sköld.** 1992. Spread of a newly found trimethoprim resistance gene, *dhfrIX,* among porcine isolates and human pathogens. *Antimicrob. Agents Chemother.* **36:**2704–2708.

90. **Juteau, J.-M., M. Sirois, A. A. Medeiros, and R. C. Levesque.** 1991. Molecular distribution of ROB-1 β-lactamase in *Actinobacillus pleuropneumoniae. Antimicrob. Agents Chemother.* **35:**1397–1402.

91. **Kao, S. J., I. You, D. B. Clewell, S. M. Donabedian, M. J. Zervos, J. Petrin, K. J. Shaw, and J. W. Chow.** 2000. Detection of the high-level aminoglycoside resistance gene *aph(2″)-Ib* in *Enterococcus faecium. Antimicrob. Agents Chemother.* **44:**2876–2879.

92. **Kapur, V., L.-L. Li, M. R. Hamrick, B. B. Plikaytis, T. M. Shinnick, A. Telenti, W. R. Jacobs, Jr., A. Banerjee, S. Cole, K. Y. Yuen, J. E. Clarridge III, B. N. Kreiswirth, and J. M. Musser.** 1995. Rapid *Mycobacterium* species assignment and unambiguous identification of mutations associated with antimicrobial resistance in *Mycobacterium tuberculosis* by automated DNA sequencing. *Arch. Pathol. Lab. Med.* **119:**131–138.

93. **Kariyama, R., R. Mitsuhata, J. W. Chow, D. B. Clewell, and H. Kumon.** 2000. Simple and reliable multiplex PCR assay for surveillance isolates of vancomycin-resistant enterococci. *J. Clin. Microbiol.* **38:**3092–3095.

94. **Kataja, J., P. Huovinen, M. Skurnik, The Finnish Study Group for Antimicrobial Resistance, and H. Seppälä.** 1999. Erythromycin resistance genes in group A streptococci in Finland. *Antimicrob. Agents Chemother.* **43:**48–52.

95. **Kaufhold, A., A. Podbielski, T. Horaud, and P. Ferrieri.** 1992. Identical genes confer high-level resistance to gentamicin upon *Enterococcus faecalis, Enterococcus faecium,* and *Streptococcus agalactiae. Antimicrob. Agents Chemother.* **36:**1215–1218.

96. **Kelley, C. L., D. A. Rouse, and S. L. Morris.** 1997. Analysis of *ahpC* gene mutations in isoniazid-resistant clinical isolates of *Mycobacterium tuberculosis. Antimicrob. Agents Chemother.* **41:**2057–2058.

97. **Killgore, G. E., B. Holloway, and F. C. Tenover.** 2000. A 5′ nuclease PCR (TaqMan) high-throughput assay for detection of the *mecA* gene in staphylococci. *J. Clin. Microbiol.* **38:**2516–2519.

98. **Klugman, K. P.** 1990. Pneumococcal resistance to antibiotics. *Clin. Microbiol. Rev.* **3:**171–196.

99. **Kolbert, C. P., J. Arruda, P. Varga-Delmore, X. Zheng, M. Lewis, J. Kolberg, and D. H. Persing.** 1998. Branched-DNA assay for detection of the *mecA* gene in oxacillin-resistant and oxacillin-sensitive staphylococci. *J. Clin. Microbiol.* **36:**2640–2644.

100. Lambert, T., M.-C. Ploy, F. Denis, and P. Courvalin. 1999. Characterization of the chromosomal *aac(6′)-Iz* gene of *Stenotrophomonas maltophilia*. Antimicrob. Agents Chemother. **43:**2366–2371.

101. Leclercq, R., E. Derlot, J. Duval, and P. Courvalin. 1988. Plasmid-mediated resistance to vancomycin and teicoplanin in *Enterococcus faecium*. N. Engl. J. Med. **319:**157–161.

102. Lee, E. H., M. H. Nicolas, M. D. Kitzis, G. Pialoux, E. Collatz, and L. Gutmann. 1991. Association of two resistance mechanisms in a clinical isolate of *Enterobacter cloacae* with high-level resistance to imipenem. Antimicrob. Agents Chemother. **35:**1093–1098.

103. Lee, J. C., J. Y. Oh, J. W. Cho, J. C. Park, J. M. Kim, S. Y. Seol, and D. T. Cho. 2001. The prevalence of trimethoprim-resistance-conferring dihydrofolate reductase genes in urinary isolates of *Escherichia coli* in Korea. J. Antimicrob. Chemother. **47:**599–604.

104. Lee, W. G., J. A. Jernigan, J. K. Rasheed, G. J. Anderson, and F. C. Tenover. 2001. Possible horizontal transfer of the *vanB2* gene among genetically diverse strains of vancomycin-resistant *Enterococcus faecium* in a Korean hospital. J. Clin. Microbiol. **39:**1165–1168.

105. Levy, S. B., L. M. McMurry, T. M. Barbosa, V. Burdett, P. Courvalin, W. Hillen, M. C. Roberts, J. I. Rood, and D. E. Taylor. 1999. Nomenclature for new tetracycline resistance determinants. Antimicrob. Agents Chemother. **43:**1523–1524.

106. Lina, G., A. Quaglia, M.-E. Reverdy, R. Leclercq, F. Vandenesch, and J. Etienne. 1999. Distribution of genes encoding resistance to macrolides, lincosamides, and streptogramins among staphylococci. Antimicrob. Agents Chemother. **43:**1062–1066.

107. Livermore, D. M. 1997. Acquired carbapenemases. J. Antimicrob. Chemother. **39:**673–676.

108. Louie, L., S. O. Matsumura, E. Choi, M. Louie, and A. E. Simor. 2000. Evaluation of three rapid methods for detection of methicillin resistance in *Staphylococcus aureus*. J. Clin. Microbiol. **38:**2170–2173.

109. Lyras, D., and J. I. Rood. 1996. Genetic organization and distribution of tetracycline resistance determinants in *Clostridium perfringens*. Antimicrob. Agents Chemother. **40:**2500–2504.

110. Ma, L., and J. A. Kovacs. 2001. Rapid detection of mutations in the human-derived *Pneumocystis carinii* dihydropteroate synthase gene associated with sulfa resistance. Antimicrob. Agents Chemother. **45:**776–780.

111. Mabilat, C., and P. Courvalin. 1990. Development of "oligotyping" for characterization and molecular epidemiology of TEM β-lactamases in members of the family *Enterobacteriaceae*. Antimicrob. Agents Chemother. **34:**2210–2216.

112. Mabilat, C., and S. Goussard. 1993. PCR detection and identification of genes for extended-spectrum β-lactamases, p. 553–559. In D. H. Persing, T. F. Smith, F. C. Tenover, and T. J. White (ed.), *Diagnostic Molecular Microbiology: Principles and Applications*. American Society for Microbiology, Washington, D.C.

113. Mabilat, C., S. Goussard, W. Sougakoff, R. C. Spencer, and P. Courvalin. 1990. Direct sequencing of the amplified structural gene and promoter for the extended-broad-spectrum β-lactamase TEM-9 (RHH-1) of *Klebsiella pneumoniae*. Plasmid **23:**27–34.

114. Manch-Citron, J. N., G. H. Lopez, A. Dey, J. W. Rapley, S. R. MacNeill, and C. M. Cobb. 2000. PCR monitoring for tetracycline resistance genes in subgingival plaque following site-specific periodontal therapy: a preliminary report. J. Clin. Periodontol. **27:**437–446.

115. Mariotte, S., P. Nordmann, and M. H. Nicolas. 1994. Extended-spectrum β-lactamase in *Proteus mirabilis*. J. Antimicrob. Chemother. **33:**925–935.

116. Marshall, B., C. Tachibana, and S. B. Levy. 1983. Frequency of tetracycline resistance determinant classes among lactose-fermenting coliforms. Antimicrob. Agents Chemother. **24:**835–840.

117. Martin, P., P. Trieu-Cuot, and P. Courvalin. 1986. Nucleotide sequence of the *tet*M tetracycline resistance determinant of the streptococcal conjugative shuttle transposon Tn*1545*. Nucleic Acids Res. **14:**7047–7058.

118. Martínez-Martínez, L., M. C. Conejo, A. Pascual, S. Hernández-Allés, S. Ballesta, E. Ramírez De Arellano-Ramos, V. J. Benedí, and E. J. Perea. 2000. Activities of imipenem and cephalosporins against clonally related strains of *Escherichia coli* hyperproducing chromosomal β-lactamase and showing altered porin profiles. Antimicrob. Agents Chemother. **44:**2534–2536.

119. Maskell, J. P., A. M. Sefton, and L. M. C. Hall. 1997. Mechanism of sulfonamide resistance in clinical isolates of *Streptococcus pneumoniae*. Antimicrob. Agents Chemother. **41:**2121–2126.

120. Massanari, R. M., M. A. Pfaller, D. S. Wakefield, G. T. Hammons, L.-A. McNutt, R. F. Woolson, and C. M. Helms. 1988. Implications of acquired oxacillin resistance in the management and control of *Staphylococcus aureus* infections. J. Infect. Dis. **158:**702–709.

121. McDougal, L. K., J. K. Rasheed, J. W. Biddle, and F. C. Tenover. 1995. Identification of multiple clones of extended-spectrum cephalosporin-resistant *Streptococcus pneumoniae* isolates in the United States. Antimicrob. Agents Chemother. **39:**2282–2288.

122. McKessar, S. J., A. M. Berry, J. M. Bell, J. D. Turnidge, and J. C. Paton. 2000. Genetic characterization of *vanG*, a novel vancomycin resistance locus of *Enterococcus faecalis*. Antimicrob. Agents Chemother. **44:**3224–3228.

123. Meier, A., P. Kirschner, F.-C. Bange, U. Vogel, and E. C. Böttger. 1994. Genetic alterations in streptomycin-resistant *Mycobacterium tuberculosis*: mapping of mutations conferring resistance. Antimicrob. Agents Chemother. **38:**228–233.

124. Miele, A., M. Bandera, and B. P. Goldstein. 1995. Use of primers selective for vancomycin resistance genes to determine *van* genotype in enterococci and to study gene organization in VanA isolates. Antimicrob. Agents Chemother. **39:**1772–1778.

125. Morris, S., G. H. Bai, P. Suffys, L. Portillo-Gomez, M. Fairchok, and D. Rouse. 1995. Molecular mechanisms of multiple drug resistance in clinical isolates of *Mycobacterium tuberculosis*. J. Infect. Dis. **171:**954–960.

126. Murakami, K., W. Minamide, K. Wada, E. Nakamura, H. Teraoka, and S. Watanabe. 1991. Identification of methicillin-resistant strains of staphylococci by polymerase chain reaction. J. Clin. Microbiol. **29:**2240–2244.

127. Musser, J. M., V. Kapur, D. L. Williams, B. N. Kreiswirth, D. van Soolingen, and J. D. A. van Embden. 1996. Characterization of the catalase-peroxidase gene (*katG*) and *inhA* locus in isoniazid-resistant and -susceptible strains of *Mycobacterium tuberculosis* by automated DNA sequencing: restricted array of mutations associated with drug resistance. J. Infect. Dis. **173:**196–202.

128. Naas, T., L. Vandel, W. Sougakoff, D. M. Livermore, and P. Nordmann. 1994. Cloning and sequence analysis of the gene for a carbapenem-hydrolyzing class A β-lactamase, Sme-1, from *Serratia marcescens* S6. Antimicrob. Agents Chemother. **38:**1262–1270.

129. **NCCLS.** 1995. *Molecular Diagnostic Methods for Infectious Diseases. Approved Guideline MM3-A*, vol. 15, no. 22. NCCLS, Wayne, Pa.

130. **Ng, L.-K., M. R. Mulvey, I. Martin, G. A. Peters, and W. Johnson.** 1999. Genetic characterization of antimicrobial resistance in Canadian isolates of *Salmonella* serovar Typhimurium DT104. *Antimicrob. Agents Chemother.* **43:**3018–3021.

131. **Noguchi, N., A. Emura, H. Matsuyama, K. O'Hara, M. Sasatsu, and M. Kono.** 1995. Nucleotide sequence and characterization of erythromycin resistance determinant that encodes macrolide 2′-phosphotransferase I in *Escherichia coli. Antimicrob. Agents Chemother.* **39:**2359–2363.

132. **Nüesch-Inderbinen, M. T., H. Hächler, and F. H. Kayser.** 1996. Detection of genes coding for extended-spectrum SHV beta-lactamases in clinical isolates by a molecular genetic method, and comparison with the E Test. *Eur. J. Clin. Microbiol. Infect. Dis.* **15:**398–402.

133. **Nunes, E. L., K. R. dos Santos, P. J. Mondino, M. Bastos, and M. Giambiagi-deMarval.** 1999. Detection of *ileS-2* gene encoding mupirocin resistance in methicillin-resistant *Staphylococcus aureus* by multiplex PCR. *Diagn. Microbiol. Infect. Dis.* **34:**77–81.

134. **Oliver, A., J. C. Pérez-Díaz, T. M. Coque, F. Baquero, and R. Cantón.** 2001. Nucleotide sequence and characterization of a novel cefotaxime-hydrolyzing β-lactamase (CTX-M-10) isolated in Spain. *Antimicrob. Agents Chemother.* **45:**616–620.

135. **Olsvik, B., M. J. Flynn, F. C. Tenover, J. Slots, and I. Olsen.** 1996. Tetracycline resistance in *Prevotella* isolates from periodontally diseased patients is due to the *tet*(Q) gene. *Oral Microbiol. Immunol.* **11:**304–308.

136. **Olsvik, B., I. Olsen, and F. C. Tenover.** 1995. Detection of *tet*(M) and *tet*(O) using the polymerase chain reaction in bacteria isolated from patients with periodontal disease. *Oral Microbiol. Immunol.* **10:**87–92.

137. **Olsvik, B., F. C. Tenover, I. Olsen, and J. K. Rasheed.** 1996. Three subtypes of the *tet*(M) gene identified in bacterial isolates from periodontal pockets. *Oral Microbiol. Immunol.* **11:**299–303.

138. **Ostrowsky, B. E., N. C. Clark, C. Thauvin-Eliopoulos, L. Venkataraman, M. H. Samore, F. C. Tenover, G. M. Eliopoulos, R. C. Moellering, Jr., and H. S. Gold.** 1999. A cluster of VanD vancomycin-resistant *Enterococcus faecium*: molecular characterization and clinical epidemiology. *J. Infect. Dis.* **180:**1177–1185.

139. **Ounissi, H., E. Derlot, C. Carlier, and P. Courvalin.** 1990. Gene homogeneity for aminoglycoside-modifying enzymes in gram-positive cocci. *Antimicrob. Agents Chemother.* **34:**2164–2168.

140. **Padiglione, A. A., E. A. Grabsch, D. Olden, M. Hellard, M. I. Sinclair, C. K. Fairley, and M. L. Grayson.** 2000. Fecal colonization with vancomycin-resistant enterococci in Australia. *Emerg. Infect. Dis.* **6:**534–536.

141. **Palepou, M.-F., A. P. Johnson, B. D. Cookson, H. Beattie, A. Charlett, and N. Woodford.** 1998. Evaluation of disc diffusion and Etest for determining the susceptibility of *Staphylococcus aureus* to mupirocin. *J. Antimicrob. Chemother.* **42:**577–583.

142. **Pan, X.-S., J. Ambler, S. Mehtar, and L. M. Fisher.** 1996. Involvement of topoisomerase IV and DNA gyrase as ciprofloxacin targets in *Streptococcus pneumoniae. Antimicrob. Agents Chemother.* **40:**2321–2326.

143. **Patel, R.** 1999. Enterococcal-type glycopeptide resistance genes in non-enterococcal organisms. *FEMS Microbiol. Lett.* **185:**1–7.

144. **Paulsen, I. T., M. H. Brown, and R. A. Skurray.** 1996. Proton-dependent multidrug efflux systems. *Microbiol. Rev.* **60:**575–608.

145. **Pease, A. C., D. Solas, E. J. Sullivan, M. T. Cronin, C. P. Holmes, and S. P. Fodor.** 1994. Light-generated oligonucleotide arrays for rapid DNA sequence analysis. *Proc. Natl. Acad. Sci. USA* **91:**5022–5026.

146. **Perichon, B., B. Casadewall, P. Reynolds, and P. Courvalin.** 2000. Glycopeptide-resistant *Enterococcus faecium* BM4416 is a VanD-type strain with an impaired D-alanine:D-alanine ligase. *Antimicrob. Agents Chemother.* **44:**1346–1348.

147. **Perichon, B., P. Reynolds, and P. Courvalin.** 1997. VanD-type glycopeptide-resistant *Enterococcus faecium* BM4339. *Antimicrob. Agents Chemother.* **41:**2016–2018.

148. **Perichon, B., J. Tankovic, and P. Courvalin.** 1997. Characterization of a mutation in the *parE* gene that confers fluoroquinolone resistance in *Streptococcus pneumoniae. Antimicrob. Agents Chemother.* **41:**1166–1167.

149. **Ploy, M.-C., H. Giamarellou, P. Bourlioux, P. Courvalin, and T. Lambert.** 1994. Detection of *aac(6′)-I* genes in amikacin-resistant *Acinetobacter* spp. by PCR. *Antimicrob. Agents Chemother.* **38:**2925–2928.

150. **Poirel, L., T. Naas, D. Nicolas, L. Collet, S. Bellais, J.-D. Cavallo, and P. Nordmann.** 2000. Characterization of VIM-2, a carbapenem-hydrolyzing metallo-β-lactamase and its plasmid- and integron-borne gene from a *Pseudomonas aeruginosa* clinical isolate in France. *Antimicrob. Agents Chemother.* **44:**891–897.

151. **Power, E. G. M., Y. H. Abdulla, H. G. Talsania, W. Spice, S. Aathithan, and G. L. French.** 1995. *vanA* genes in vancomycin-resistant clinical isolates of *Oerskovia turbata* and *Arcanobacterium* (*Corynebacterium*) *haemolyticum. J. Antimicrob. Chemother.* **36:**595–606.

152. **Poyart, C., C. Pierre, G. Quesne, B. Pron, P. Berche, and P. Trieu-Cuot.** 1997. Emergence of vancomycin resistance in the genus *Streptococcus*: characterization of a *vanB* transferable determinant in *Streptococcus bovis. Antimicrob. Agents Chemother.* **41:**24–29.

153. **Pulkkinen, L., P. Huovinen, E. Vuorio, and P. Toivanen.** 1984. Characterization of trimethoprim resistance by use of probes specific for transposon Tn7. *Antimicrob. Agents Chemother.* **26:**82–86.

154. **Queenan, A. M., C. Torres-Viera, H. S. Gold, Y. Carmeli, G. M. Eliopoulos, R. C. Moellering, Jr., J. P. Quinn, J. Hindler, A. A. Medeiros, and K. Bush.** 2000. SME-type carbapenem-hydrolyzing class A β-lactamases from geographically diverse *Serratia marcescens* strains. *Antimicrob. Agents Chemother.* **44:**3035–3039.

155. **Rådström, P., G. Swedberg, and O. Sköld.** 1991. Genetic analyses of sulfonamide resistance and its dissemination in gram-negative bacteria illustrate new aspects of R plasmid evolution. *Antimicrob. Agents Chemother.* **35:**1840–1848.

156. **Ramsey, M. A., S. F. Bradley, C. A. Kauffman, and T. M. Morton.** 1996. Identification of chromosomal location of *mupA* gene, encoding low-level mupirocin resistance in staphylococcal isolates. *Antimicrob. Agents Chemother.* **40:**2820–2823.

157. **Rasheed, J. K., G. J. Anderson, H. Yigit, A. M. Queenan, A. Doménech-Sánchez, J. M. Swenson, J. W. Biddle, M. J. Ferraro, G. A. Jacoby, and F. C. Tenover.** 2000. Characterization of the extended-spectrum β-lactamase reference strain. *Klebsiella pneumoniae* K6 (ATCC 700603), which produces the novel enzyme SHV-18. *Antimicrob. Agents Chemother.* **44:**2382–2388.

158. **Rasheed, J. K., C. Jay, B. Metchock, F. Berkowitz, L. Weigel, J. Crellin, C. Steward, B. Hill, A. A. Medeiros, and F. C. Tenover.** 1997. Evolution of extended-spectrum β-lactam resistance (SHV-8) in a strain of *Escherichia coli* during multiple episodes of bacteremia. *Antimicrob. Agents Chemother.* **41:**647–653.

159. **Rasmussen, B. A., K. Bush, D. Keeney, Y. Yang, R. Hare, C. O'Gara, and A. A. Medeiros.** 1996. Characterization of IMI-1 β-lactamase, a class A carbapenem-hydrolyzing enzyme from *Enterobacter cloacae*. *Antimicrob. Agents Chemother.* **40:**2080–2086.

160. **Reig, M., J.-C. Galan, F. Baquero, and J. C. Perez-Diaz.** 2001. Macrolide resistance in *Peptostreptococcus* spp. mediated by *ermTR*: possible source of macrolide-lincosamide-streptogramin B resistance in *Streptococcus pyogenes*. *Antimicrob. Agents Chemother.* **45:**630–632.

161. **Ridenhour, M. B., H. M. Fletcher, J. E. Mortensen, and L. Daneo-Moore.** 1996. A novel tetracycline-resistant determinant, *tet*(U), is encoded on the plasmid pKQ10 in *Enterococcus faecium*. *Plasmid* **35:**71–80.

162. **Roberts, M. C., W. O. Chung, and D. E. Roe.** 1996. Characterization of tetracycline and erythromycin resistance determinants in *Treponema denticola*. *Antimicrob. Agents Chemother.* **40:**1690–1694.

163. **Roberts, M. C., J. Sutcliffe, P. Courvalin, L. B. Jensen, J. Rood, and H. Seppala.** 1999. Nomenclature for macrolide and macrolide-lincosamide-streptogramin B resistance determinants. *Antimicrob. Agents Chemother.* **43:** 2823–2830.

164. **Rood, J. I., S. Jefferson, T. L. Bannam, J. M. Wilkie, P. Mullany, and B. W. Wren.** 1989. Hybridization analysis of three chloramphenicol resistance determinants from *Clostridium perfringens* and *Clostridium difficile*. *Antimicrob. Agents Chemother.* **33:**1569–1574.

165. **Sabaté, M., R. Tarragó, F. Navarro, E. Miró, C. Vergés, J. Barbé, and G. Prats.** 2000. Cloning and sequence of the gene encoding a novel cefotaxime-hydrolyzing β-lactamase (CTX-M-9) from *Escherichia coli* in Spain. *Antimicrob. Agents Chemother.* **44:**1970–1973.

166. **Sahm, D. F., L. Free, and S. Handwerger.** 1995. Inducible and constitutive expression of *vanC-1*-encoded resistance to vancomycin in *Enterococcus gallinarum*. *Antimicrob. Agents Chemother.* **39:**1480–1484.

167. **Satake, S., N. Clark, D. Rimland, F. S. Nolte, and F. C. Tenover.** 1997. Detection of vancomycin-resistant enterococci in fecal samples by PCR. *J. Clin. Microbiol.* **35:**2325–2330.

168. **Saurina, G., J. M. Quale, V. M. Manikal, E. Oydna, and D. Landman.** 2000. Antimicrobial resistance in *Enterobacteriaceae* in Brooklyn, NY: epidemiology and relation to antibiotic usage patterns. *J. Antimicrob. Chemother.* **45:**895–898.

169. **Senda, K., Y. Arakawa, S. Ichiyama, K. Nakashima, H. Ito, S. Ohsuka, K. Shimokata, N. Kato, and M. Ohta.** 1996. PCR detection of metallo-β-lactamase gene (*bla*$_{IMP}$) in gram-negative rods resistant to broad-spectrum β-lactams. *J. Clin. Microbiol.* **34:**2909–2913.

170. **Seppälä, H., M. Skurnik, H. Soini, M. C. Roberts, and P. Huovinen.** 1998. A novel erythromycin resistance methylase gene (*ermTR*) in *Streptococcus pyogenes*. *Antimicrob. Agents Chemother.* **42:**257–262.

171. **Shaw, K. J., R. S. Hare, F. J. Sabatelli, M. Rizzo, C. A. Cramer, L. Naples, S. Kocsi, H. Munayyer, P. Mann, G. H. Miller, L. Verbist, H. Van Landuyt, Y. Glupczynski, M. Catalano, and M. Woloj.** 1991. Correlation between aminoglycoside resistance profiles and DNA hybridization of clinical isolates. *Antimicrob. Agents Chemother.* **35:**2253–2261.

172. **Shaw, K. J., P. N. Rather, R. S. Hare, and G. H. Miller.** 1993. Molecular genetics of aminoglycoside resistance genes and familial relationships of the aminoglycoside-modifying enzymes. *Microbiol. Rev.* **57:**138–163.

173. **Shaw, W. V.** 1983. Chloramphenicol acetyltransferase: enzymology and molecular biology. *Crit Rev. Biochem.* **14:**1–46.

174. **Shortridge, V. D., R. K. Flamm, N. Ramer, J. Beyer, and S. K. Tanaka.** 1996. Novel mechanism of macrolide resistance in *Streptococcus pneumoniae*. *Diagn. Microbiol. Infect. Dis.* **26:**73–78.

175. **Simard, J.-L., and P. H. Roy.** 1993. PCR detection of penicillinase-producing *Neisseria gonorrhoeae*, p. 543–546. *In* D. H. Persing, T. F. Smith, F. C. Tenover, and T. J. White (ed.), *Diagnostic Molecular Microbiology: Principles and Applications*. American Society for Microbiology, Washington, D.C.

176. **Singh, K. V., R. R. Reves, L. K. Pickering, and B. E. Murray.** 1992. Identification by DNA sequence analysis of a new plasmid-encoded trimethoprim resistance gene in fecal *Escherichia coli* isolates from children in day-care centers. *Antimicrob. Agents Chemother.* **36:**1720–1726.

177. **Siu, L. K., J. Y. C. Lo, K. Y. Yuen, P. Y. Chau, M. H. Ng, and P. L. Ho.** 2000. β-Lactamases in *Shigella flexneri* isolates from Hong Kong and Shanghai and a novel OXA-1-like β-lactamase, OXA-30. *Antimicrob. Agents Chemother.* **44:**2034–2038.

178. **Soltani, M., D. Beighton, J. Philpott-Howard, and N. Woodford.** 2000. Mechanisms of resistance to quinupristin-dalfopristin among isolates of *Enterococcus faecium* from animals, raw meat, and hospital patients in Western Europe. *Antimicrob. Agents Chemother.* **44:**433–436.

179. **Sougakoff, W., B. Papadopoulou, P. Nordmann, and P. Courvalin.** 1987. Nucleotide sequence and distribution of gene *tetO* encoding tetracycline resistance in *Campylobacter coli*. *FEMS Microbiol. Lett.* **44:**153–159.

180. **Speer, B. S., N. B. Shoemaker, and A. A. Salyers.** 1992. Bacterial resistance to tetracycline: mechanisms, transfer, and clinical significance. *Clin. Microbiol. Rev.* **5:**387–399.

181. **Sreevatsan, S., X. Pan, K. E. Stockbauer, D. L. Williams, B. N. Kreiswirth, and J. M. Musser.** 1996. Characterization of *rpsL* and *rrs* mutations in streptomycin-resistant *Mycobacterium tuberculosis* isolates from diverse geographic localities. *Antimicrob. Agents Chemother.* **40:** 1024–1026.

182. **Sreevatsan, S., X. Pan, Y. Zhang, B. N. Kreiswirth, and J. M. Musser.** 1997. Mutations associated with pyrazinamide resistance in *pncA* of *Mycobacterium tuberculosis* complex organisms. *Antimicrob. Agents Chemother.* **41:** 636–640.

183. **Steward, C. D., J. K. Rasheed, S. K. Hubert, J. W. Biddle, P. M. Raney, G. J. Anderson, P. P. Williams, K. L. Brittain, A. Oliver, J. E. McGowan, Jr., and F. C. Tenover.** 2001. Characterization of clinical isolates of *Klebsiella pneumoniae* from 19 laboratories using the National Committee for Clinical Laboratory Standards extended-spectrum β-lactamase detection methods. *J. Clin. Microbiol.* **39:**2864–2872.

184. **Stinear, T. P., D. C. Olden, P. D. R. Johnson, J. K. Davies, and M. L. Grayson.** 2001. Enterococcal *vanB* resistance locus in anaerobic bacteria in human faeces. *Lancet* **357:**855–856.

185. **Sundström, L., C. Jansson, K. Bremer, E. Heikkilä, B. Olsson-Liljequist, and O. Sköld.** 1995. A new *dhfrVIII* trimethoprim-resistance gene, flanked by IS*26*, whose product is remote from other dihydrofolate reductases in parsimony analysis. *Gene* **154:**7–14.

186. **Sutcliffe, J., T. Grebe, A. Tait-Kamradt, and L. Wondrack.** 1996. Detection of erythromycin-resistant determinants by PCR. *Antimicrob. Agents Chemother.* **40:** 2562–2566.

187. **Sutcliffe, J., A. Tait-Kamradt, and L. Wondrack.** 1996. *Streptococcus pneumoniae* and *Streptococcus pyogenes* resistant to macrolides but sensitive to clindamycin: a com-

mon resistance pattern mediated by an efflux system. *Antimicrob. Agents Chemother.* **40:**1817–1824.

188. **Swenson, J. M., M. J. Ferraro, D. F. Sahm, N. C. Clark, D. H. Culver, F. C. Tenover, and The National Committee for Clinical Laboratory Standards Study Group on Enterococci.** 1995. Multilaboratory evaluation of screening methods for detection of high-level aminoglycoside resistance in enterococci. *J. Clin. Microbiol.* **33:** 3008–3018.

189. **Swenson, J. M., P. P. Williams, G. Killgore, C. M. O'Hara, and F. C. Tenover.** 2001. Performance of eight methods, including two new rapid methods, for detection of oxacillin resistance in a challenge set of *Staphylococcus aureus* organisms. *J. Clin. Microbiol.* **39:**3785–3788.

190. **Tait-Kamradt, A., J. Clancy, M. Cronan, F. Dib-Hajj, L. Wondrack, W. Yuan, and J. Sutcliffe.** 1997. *mefE* is necessary for the erythromycin-resistant M phenotype in *Streptococcus pneumoniae. Antimicrob. Agents Chemother.* **41:**2251–2255.

191. **Tait-Kamradt, A., J. Davies, M. Cronan, M. R. Jacobs, P. C. Appelbaum, and J. Sutcliffe.** 2000. Mutations in 23S rRNA and ribosomal protein L4 account for resistance in pneumococcal strains selected in vitro by macrolide passage. *Antimicrob. Agents Chemother.* **44:**2118–2125.

192. **Takiff, H. E., L. Salazar, C. Guerrero, W. Philipp, W. M. Huang, B. Kreiswirth, S. T. Cole, W. R. Jacobs, Jr., and A. Telenti.** 1994. Cloning and nucleotide sequence of *Mycobacterium tuberculosis gyrA* and *gyrB* genes and detection of quinolone resistance mutations. *Antimicrob. Agents Chemother.* **38:**773–780.

193. **Taniguchi, K., A. Nakamura, K. Tsurubuchi, A. Ishii, K. O'Hara, and T. Sawai.** 1999. Identification of functional amino acids in the macrolide 2′-phosphotransferase II. *Antimicrob. Agents Chemother.* **43:**2063–2065.

194. **Tankovic, J., B. Perichon, J. Duval, and P. Courvalin.** 1996. Contribution of mutations in *gyrA* and *parC* genes to fluoroquinolone resistance of mutants of *Streptococcus pneumoniae* obtained in vivo and in vitro. *Antimicrob. Agents Chemother.* **40:**2505–2510.

195. **Telenti, A., N. Honoré, C. Bernasconi, J. March, A. Ortega, B. Heym, H. E. Takiff, and S. T. Cole.** 1997. Genotypic assessment of isoniazid and rifampin resistance in *Mycobacterium tuberculosis*: a blind study at reference laboratory level. *J. Clin. Microbiol.* **35:**719–723.

196. **Telenti, A., P. Imboden, F. Marchesi, T. Schmidheini, and T. Bodmer.** 1993. Direct, automated detection of rifampin-resistant *Mycobacterium tuberculosis* by polymerase chain reaction and single-strand conformation polymorphism analysis. *Antimicrob. Agents Chemother.* **37:** 2054–2058.

197. **Tenover, F. C., J. W. Biddle, and M. V. Lancaster.** 2001. Increasing resistance to vancomycin and other glycopeptides in *Staphylococcus aureus. Emerg. Infect. Dis.* **7:**327–332.

198. **Tenover, F. C., D. Filpula, K. L. Phillips, and J. J. Plorde.** 1988. Cloning and sequencing of a gene encoding an aminoglycoside 6′-N-acetyltransferase from an R factor of *Citrobacter diversus. J. Bacteriol.* **170:**471–473.

199. **Tenover, F. C., M. B. Huang, J. K. Rasheed, and D. H. Persing.** 1994. Development of PCR assays to detect ampicillin resistance genes in cerebrospinal fluid samples containing *Haemophilus influenzae. J. Clin. Microbiol.* **32:** 2729–2737.

200. **Tenover, F. C., R. N. Jones, J. M. Swenson, B. Zimmer, S. McAllister, and J. H. Jorgensen for the NCCLS Staphylococcus Working Group.** 1999. Methods for improved detection of oxacillin resistance in coagulase-

negative staphylococci: results of a multicenter study. *J. Clin. Microbiol.* **37:**4051–4058.

201. **Tenover, F. C., M. V. Lancaster, B. C. Hill, C. D. Steward, S. A. Stocker, G. A. Hancock, C. M. O'Hara, N. C. Clark, and K. Hiramatsu.** 1998. Characterization of staphylococci with reduced susceptibilities to vancomycin and other glycopeptides. *J. Clin. Microbiol.* **36:** 1020–1027.

202. **Tenover, F. C., and J. K. Rasheed.** 1999. Genetic methods for detecting antibacterial and antiviral resistance genes, p. 1578–1592. *In* P. R. Murray, E. J. Baron, M. A. Pfaller, F. C. Tenover, and R. H. Yolken (ed.), *Manual of Clinical Microbiology*, 7th ed. American Society for Microbiology, Washington, D.C.

203. **Tomasz, A., H. B. Drugeon, H. M. De Lencastre, D. Jabes, L. McDougal, and J. Bille.** 1989. New mechanism for methicillin resistance in *Staphylococcus aureus*: clinical isolates that lack the PBP 2a gene and contain normal penicillin-binding proteins with modified penicillin-binding capacity. *Antimicrob. Agents Chemother.* **33:** 1869–1874.

204. **Tortoli, E., A. Nanetti, C. Piersimoni, P. Cichero, C. Farina, G. Mucignat, C. Scarparo, L. Bartolini, R. Valentini, D. Nista, G. Gesu, C. P. Tosi, M. Crovatto, and G. Brusarosco.** 2001. Performance assessment of new multiplex probe assay for identification of mycobacteria. *J. Clin. Microbiol.* **39:**1079–1084.

205. **Trieu-Cuot, P., G. De Cespédès, F. Bentorcha, F. Delbos, E. Gaspar, and T. Horaud.** 1993. Study of heterogeneity of chloramphenicol acetyltransferase (CAT) genes in streptococci and enterococci by polymerase chain reaction: characterization of a new CAT determinant. *Antimicrob. Agents Chemother.* **37:**2593–2598.

206. **Truong, Q. C., J.-C. Nguyen Van, D. Shlaes, L. Gutmann, and N. J. Moreau.** 1997. A novel, double mutation in DNA gyrase A of *Escherichia coli* conferring resistance to quinolone antibiotics. *Antimicrob. Agents Chemother.* **41:**85–90.

207. **Tsai, S. F., M. J. Zervos, D. B. Clewell, S. M. Donabedian, D. F. Sahm, and J. W. Chow.** 1998. A new high-level gentamicin resistance gene, *aph(2″)-Id*, in *Enterococcus* spp. *Antimicrob. Agents Chemother.* **42:**1229–1232.

208. **Tyler, K. D., G. Wang, S. D. Tyler, and W. M. Johnson.** 1997. Factors affecting reliability and reproducibility of amplification-based DNA fingerprinting of representative bacterial pathogens. *J. Clin. Microbiol.* **35:**339–346.

209. **Tzouvelekis, L. S., E. Tzelepi, P. T. Tassios, and N. J. Legakis.** 2000. CTX-M-type β-lactamases: an emerging group of extended-spectrum enzymes. *Int. J. Antimicrob. Agents* **14:**137–142.

210. **Ubukata, K., Y. Asahi, A. Yamane, and M. Konno.** 1996. Combinational detection of autolysin and penicillin-binding protein 2B genes of *Streptococcus pneumoniae* by PCR. *J. Clin. Microbiol.* **34:**592–596.

211. **Ubukata, K., S. Nakagami, A. Nitta, A. Yamane, S. Kawakami, M. Sugiura, and M. Konno.** 1992. Rapid detection of the *mecA* gene in methicillin-resistant staphylococci by enzymatic detection of polymerase chain reaction products. *J. Clin. Microbiol.* **30:**1728–1733.

212. **Vahaboglu, H., L. M. C. Hall, L. Mulazimoglu, S. Dodanli, I. Yildirim, and D. M. Livermore.** 1995. Resistance to extended-spectrum cephalosporins, caused by PER-1 β-lactamase, in *Salmonella typhimurium* from Istanbul, Turkey. *J. Med. Microbiol.* **43:**294–299.

213. **Van de Klundert, J. A. M., and J. S. Vliegenthart.** 1993. PCR detection of genes coding for aminoglycoside-modifying enzymes, p. 547–552. *In* D. H. Persing, T. F. Smith,

F. C. Tenover, and T. J. White (ed.), *Diagnostic Molecular Microbiology: Principles and Applications.* American Society for Microbiology, Washington, D.C.

214. **Van Griethuysen, A., M. Pouw, N. Van Leeuwen, M. Heck, P. Willemse, A. Buiting, and J. Kluytmans.** 1999. Rapid slide latex agglutination test for detection of methicillin resistance in *Staphylococcus aureus. J. Clin. Microbiol.* **37:**2789–2792.

215. **Vanhoof, R., J. Content, E. Van Bossuyt, L. Dewit, and E. Hannecart-Pokorni.** 1992. Identification of the *aadB* gene coding for the aminoglycoside-2″-O-nucleotidyltransferase, ANT(2″), by means of the polymerase chain reaction. *J. Antimicrob. Chemother.* **29:**365–374.

216. **Vanhoof, R., H. J. Nyssen, E. Van Bossuyt, E. Hannecart-Pokorni, and the Aminoglycoside Resistance Study Group.** 1999. Aminoglycoside resistance in gram-negative blood isolates from various hospitals in Belgium and the Grand Duchy of Luxembourg. *J. Antimicrob. Chemother.* **44:**483–488.

217. **Vannuffel, P., J. Gigi, H. Ezzedine, B. Vandercam, M. Delmee, G. Wauters, and J.-L. Gala.** 1995. Specific detection of methicillin-resistant *Staphylococcus* species by multiplex PCR. *J. Clin. Microbiol.* **33:**2864–2867.

218. **Vercauteren, E., P. Descheemaeker, M. Ieven, C. C. Sanders, and H. Goossens.** 1997. Comparison of screening methods for detection of extended-spectrum β-lactamases and their prevalence among blood isolates of *Escherichia coli* and *Klebsiella* spp. in a Belgian teaching hospital. *J. Clin. Microbiol.* **35:**2191–2197.

219. **Vila, J., J. Ruiz, P. Goñi, A. Marcos, and T. Jimenez De Anta.** 1995. Mutation in the *gyrA* gene of quinolone-resistant clinical isolates of *Acinetobacter baumannii. Antimicrob. Agents Chemother.* **39:**1201–1203.

220. **Vila, J., J. Ruiz, M. Navia, B. Becerril, I. Garcia, S. Perea, I. Lopez-Hernandez, I. Alamo, F. Ballester, A. M. Planes, J. Martinez-Beltran, and T. J. De Anta.** 1999. Spread of amikacin resistance in *Acinetobacter baumannii* strains isolated in Spain due to an epidemic strain. *J. Clin. Microbiol.* **37:**758–761.

221. **Weber, D. A., C. C. Sanders, J. S. Bakken, and J. P. Quinn.** 1990. A novel chromosomal TEM derivative and alterations in outer membrane proteins together mediate selective ceftazidime resistance in *Escherichia coli. J. Infect. Dis.* **162:**460–465.

222. **Werner, G., B. Hildebrandt, I. Klare, and W. Witte.** 2000. Linkage of determinants for streptogramin A, macrolide-lincosamide-streptogramin B, and chloramphenicol resistance on a conjugative plasmid in *Entero-coccus faecium* and dissemination of this cluster among streptogramin-resistant enterococci. *Int. J. Med. Microbiol.* **290:**543–548.

223. **Werner, G., and W. Witte.** 1999. Characterization of a new enterococcal gene, *satG,* encoding a putative acetyltransferase conferring resistance to streptogramin A compounds. *Antimicrob. Agents Chemother.* **43:**1813–1814.

224. **Willems, R. J. L., J. Top, N. Van den Braak, A. van Belkum, D. J. Mevius, G. Hendriks, M. van Santen-Verheuvel, and J. D. A. van Embden.** 1999. Molecular diversity and evolutionary relationships of Tn*1546*-like elements in enterococci from humans and animals. *Antimicrob. Agents Chemother.* **43:**483–491.

225. **Williams, D. L., C. Waguespack, K. Eisenach, J. T. Crawford, F. Portaels, M. Salfinger, C. M. Nolan, C. Abe, V. Sticht-Groh, and T. P. Gillis.** 1994. Characterization of rifampin resistance in pathogenic mycobacteria. *Antimicrob. Agents Chemother.* **38:**2380–2386.

226. **Winokur, P. L., R. Canton, J. M. Casellas, and N. Legakis.** 2001. Variations in the prevalence of strains expressing an extended-spectrum β-lactamase phenotype and characterization of isolates from Europe, the Americas, and the Western Pacific region. *Clin. Infect. Dis.* **32**(Suppl. 2)**:**S94–S103.

227. **Wondrack, L., M. Massa, B. V. Yang, and J. Sutcliffe.** 1996. Clinical strain of *Staphylococcus aureus* inactivates and causes efflux of macrolides. *Antimicrob. Agents Chemother.* **40:**992–998.

228. **Wren, B. W., P. Mullany, C. Clayton, and S. Tabaqchali.** 1988. Molecular cloning and genetic analysis of a chloramphenicol acetyltransferase determinant from *Clostridium difficile. Antimicrob. Agents Chemother.* **32:**1213–1217.

229. **Yigit, H., A. M. Queenan, G. J. Anderson, A. Domenech-Sanchez, J. W. Biddle, C. D. Steward, S. Alberti, K. Bush, and F. C. Tenover.** 2001. Novel carbapenem-hydrolyzing β-lactamase, KPC-1, from a carbapenem-resistant strain of *Klebsiella pneumoniae. Antimicrob. Agents Chemother.* **45:**1151–1161.

230. **York, M. K., L. Gibbs, F. Chehab, and G. F. Brooks.** 1996. Comparison of PCR detection of *mecA* with standard susceptibility testing methods to determine methicillin resistance in coagulase-negative staphylococci. *J. Clin. Microbiol.* **34:**249–253.

231. **Zhao, J., and T. Aoki.** 1992. Nucleotide sequence analysis of the class G tetracycline resistance determinant from *Vibrio anguillarum. Microbiol. Immunol.* **36:**1051–1060.

Author Index

Subject Index

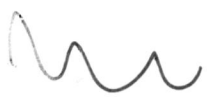